Casarett and Doull's
TOXICOLOGY
The Basic Science of Poisons

What is there that is not poison?
All things are poison and nothing (is)
without poison. Solely the dose
determines that a thing is not a poison.
Paracelsus
(1493–1541)

NOTICE

Medicine is an ever-changing science. As new research and clinical experience broaden our knowledge, changes in treatment and drug therapy are required. The author and the publisher of this work have checked with sources believed to be reliable in their efforts to provide information that is complete and generally in accord with the standards accepted at the time of publication. However, in view of the possibility of human error or changes in medical sciences, neither the author nor the publisher nor any other party who has been involved in the preparation or publication of this work warrants that the information contained herein is in every respect accurate or complete, and they disclaim all responsibility for any errors or omissions or for the results obtained from use of the information contained in this work. Readers are encouraged to confirm the information contained herein with other sources. For example and in particular, readers are advised to check the product information sheet included in the package of each drug they plan to administer to be certain that the information contained in this work is accurate and that changes have not been made in the recommended dose or in the contraindications for administration. This recommendation is of particular importance in connection with new or infrequently used drugs.

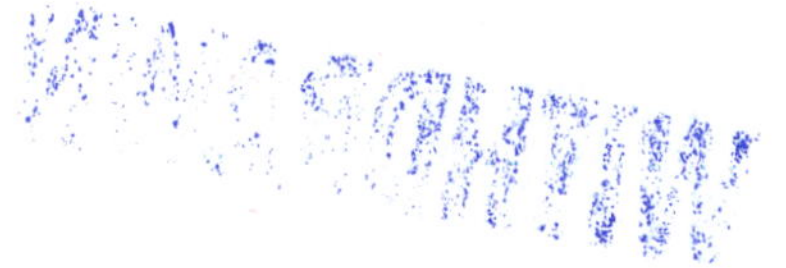

Casarett and Doull's TOXICOLOGY
The Basic Science of Poisons

Sixth Edition

Editor
Curtis D. Klaassen, Ph.D.
Professor of Pharmacology and Toxicology
Department of Pharmacology, Toxicology, and Therapeutics
University of Kansas Medical Center
Kansas City, Kansas

McGraw-Hill
Medical Publishing Division

New York Chicago San Francisco Lisbon London Madrid Mexico City Milan
New Delhi San Juan Seoul Singapore Sydney Toronto

McGraw-Hill
A Division of The McGraw-Hill Companies

CASARETT AND DOULL'S TOXICOLOGY: THE BASIC SCIENCE OF POISONS

1234567890 DOW DOW 0987654321

ISBN 0-07-134721-6

This book was set in Times Roman by TechBooks, Inc.
The editors were Andrea Seils, Susan R. Noujaim, and Lester A. Sheinis.
The production supervisor was Richard C. Ruzycka.
The text designer was Marsha Cohen/Parallelogram.
The cover designer was Janice Bielawa.
The indexer was Barbara Littlewood.
R.R. Donnelley & Sons Company was printer and binder.

This book is printed on acid-free paper.

Library of Congress Cataloging-in-Publication Data is on file for this title at the Library of Congress.

INTERNATIONAL EDITION ISBN 0-07-112453-5

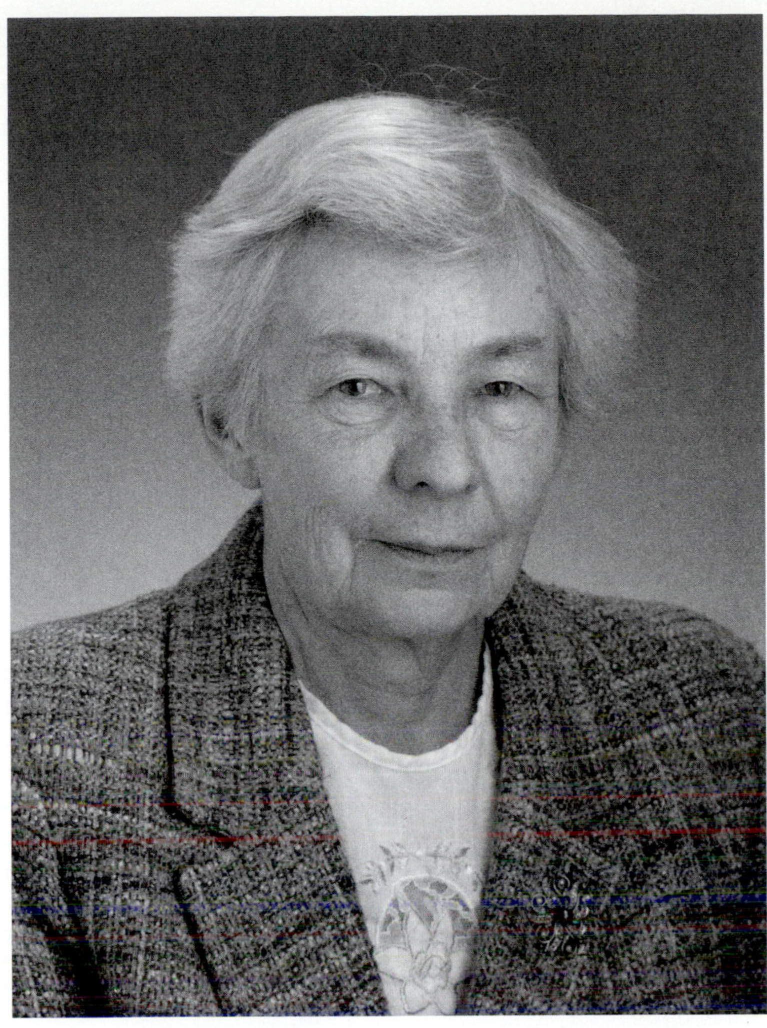

This edition of the textbook is dedicated to the memory of Dr. Mary Amdur, who was a coeditor on editions two through four.

Mary Amdur received her B.S. in Chemistry from the University of Pittsburgh in 1943, and, in just three years, was awarded the Ph.D. in Biochemistry from Cornell. She spent her academic career at the Harvard School of Public Health (1949–1977), Massachusetts Institute of Technology (1977–1989), and the Institute of Environmental Medicine of New York University in Tuxedo Park, New York (1989–1996). She died in February 1998 while flying home from a vacation in Hawaii.

Dr. Amdur was a distinguished toxicologist in the area of air pollution. Her research accomplishments provided seminal contributions to our understanding of the effects of gases and particles on human and animal lungs. She contributed to our knowledge of the adverse effects of sulfuric acid mists and mixtures of gases and particles in the lung. This work had a major role in the establishment of national and international air pollution standards. Her career in toxicology was uniquely distinguished and profound in its impact on public policy and public health.

Dr. Amdur made these accomplishments at a time in which science was strongly male-dominated. Her research career was impaired by a number of barriers, because of this environment (Costa and Gordon, *Toxicol Sci*, 56: 5–7, 2000). In fact, she never was awarded a tenure position at any of the three academic positions where she did her outstanding research.

Dr. Amdur received a number of awards throughout her career. These included the 1974 Donald E. Cummings Memorial Award from the American Industrial Hygiene Association, the 1984 Henry F. Smyth Award from the American Academy of Industrial Hygiene, the 1986 Career Achievement Award from the Inhalation Section of the Society of Toxicology, and the 1989 Herbert E. Stockinger Award from the American Conference of Governmental Industrial Hygienists. In 1997, she became the first woman to receive the Merit Award from the Society of Toxicology.

For those of us who were fortunate to work with Mary Amdur, we will remember not only her scientific accomplishments but also her wit, demeanor, and absolute honesty.

CONTENTS

CONTRIBUTORS

Daniel Acosta, Jr., Ph.D.
Dean and Professor
College of Pharmacy
University of Cincinnati
Cincinnati, Ohio
Chapter 18

Todd A. Anderson, Ph.D.
Assistant Section Leader
The Institute of Environmental and Human Health (TIEHH)
Associate Professor, Department of Environmental Toxicology
Texas Tech
Lubbock, Texas
Chapter 29

Douglas C. Anthony, M.D., Ph.D.
Associate Professor of Pathology
Harvard Medical School
Department of Pathology
Children's Hospital
Boston, Massachusetts
Chapter 16

Robert J. Baker, Ph.D.
Adjunct Professor
The Institute of Environmental and Human Health (TIEHH)
Horn Professor
Department of Biological Sciences
Texas Tech University
Lubbock, Texas
Chapter 29

Catherine M. Bens, M.S.
Senior Research Associate
The Institute of Environmental and Human Health (TIEHH)
Texas Tech
Lubbock, Texas
Chapter 29

John C. Bloom, V.M.D., Ph.D.
Director, Diagnostic and Experimental Medicine
Eli Lilly and Company
Indianapolis, Indiana
Chapter 11

William K. Boyes, Ph.D.
Neurophysiological Toxicology Branch
Neurotoxicology Division
National Health and Environmental Effects Research Laboratory
U.S. Environmental Protection Agency
Research Triangle Park, North Carolina
Chapter 17

John T. Brandt, M.D.
Senior Clinical Research Pathologist
Eli Lilly and Company
Indianapolis, Indiana
Chapter 11

James V. Bruckner, Ph.D.
Professor of Pharmacology and Toxicology
College of Pharmacy
University of Georgia
Athens, Georgia
Chapter 24

George A. Burdock, Ph.D., D.A.B.T.
Burdock and Associates, Inc.
Vero Beach, Florida
Chapter 30

Leigh Ann Burns-Naas, Ph.D.
Senior Toxicology Specialist
Health, Environmental, and Regulatory Affairs
Dow Corning Corporation
Midland, Michigan
Chapter 12

Louis R. Cantilena, Jr., M.D., Ph.D.
Associate Professor of Medicine and Pharmacology
Director, Division of Clinical Pharmacology and Medical Toxicology
Uniformed Services University of the Health Sciences
Bethesda, Maryland
Chapter 32

Charles C. Capen, D.V.M., Ph.D.
Professor and Chairperson
Department of Veterinary Biosciences
Ohio State University
Columbus, Ohio
Chapter 21

James A. Carr, Ph.D.
Adjunct Associate Professor
The Institute of Environmental and Human Health (TIEHH)
Associate Professor, Department of Biological Sciences
Texas Tech University
Lubbock, Texas
Chapter 29

Enrique Chacon, Ph.D.
Vice President of Business Development
Cedra Corporation
Austin, Texas
Chapter 18

Louis A. Chiodo, Ph.D.
Assistant Director
The Institute of Environmental and Human Health (TIEHH)
Professor of Pharmacology
Texas Tech University Health Sciences Center
Lubbock, Texas
Chapter 29

Thomas W. Clarkson, Ph.D.
J. Lowell Orbison Distinguished Alumni Professor
Department of Environmental Medicine
University of Rochester School of Medicine
Rochester, New York
Chapter 23

George P. Cobb III, Ph.D.
Division Leader
The Institute of Environmental and Human Health (TIEHH)
Associate Professor
Department of Environmental Toxicology
Texas Tech
Lubbock, Texas
Chapter 29

David E. Cohen, M.D., M.P.H.
Director of Occupational and Environmental Dermatology
Assistant Professor of Dermatology
New York University School of Medicine
New York, New York
Chapter 19

Daniel L. Costa, Sc.D.
Chief, Pulmonary Toxicology Branch
Experimental Toxicology Division
National Health and Environment Effects Research Laboratory
U.S. Environmental Protection Agency
Research Triangle Park, North Carolina
Chapter 28

Richard L. Dickerson, Ph.D.
Research Scientist, The Institute of Environmental and Human Health (TIEHH)
Associate Professor
Department of Environmental Toxicology
Texas Tech
Lubbock, Texas
Chapter 29

Kenneth R. Dixon, Ph.D.
Section Leader
The Institute of Environmental and Human Health (TIEHH)
Professor
Department of Environmental Toxicology
Texas Tech
Lubbock, Texas
Chapter 29

John Doull, M.D.
Emeritus Professor of Pharmacology and Toxicology
Department of Pharmacology
University of Kansas Medical Center
Kansas City, Kansas
Appendix

Yvonne P. Dragan, Ph.D.
Assistant Professor
Ohio State University
James Cancer Hospital and Solove Research Institute and the Environmental Molecular Science Institute
Columbus, Ohio
Chapter 8

David L. Eaton, Ph.D.
Professor and Associate Dean for Research
School of Public Health and Community Medicine
Department of Environmental Health
University of Washington
Seattle, Washington
Chapter 2

Donald J. Ecobichon, M.D.
Professor
Department of Pharmacology and Toxicology
Queen's University
Kingston, Canada
Chapter 22

Elaine M. Faustman, Ph.D.
Professor
School of Public Health and Community Medicine
Department of Environmental Health
University of Washington
Seattle, Washington
Chapter 4

W. Gary Flamm, Ph.D., F.A.C.T., F.A.T.S.
Flamm Associates
Vero Beach, Florida
Chapter 30

Donald A. Fox, Ph.D.
Professor
College of Optometry
Department of Biochemical and Biophysical Sciences, and Department of Pharmacology and Pharmaceutical Sciences
University of Houston
Houston, Texas
Chapter 17

Lynn T. Frame, Ph.D.
Senior Research Associate
The Institute of Environmental and Human Health (TIEHH)
Texas Tech
Lubbock, Texas
Chapter 29

Michael A. Gallo, Ph.D.
UMDNJ-Robert Wood Johnson Medical School
Piscataway, New Jersey
Chapter 1

Robert A. Goyer, M.D.
Professor Emeritus
University of Western Ontario
London, Ontario, Canada
Chapter 23

Doyle G. Graham, M.D., Ph.D.
Professor and Chair of Pathology
Department of Pathology
Vanderbilt University Medical Center
Nashville, Tennessee
Chapter 16

Zoltán Gregus, M.D., Ph.D., D.Sc.
Professor
Department of Pharmacology and Pharmacotherapy
University of Pécs Medical School
Pécs, Hungary
Chapter 3

Naomi H. Harley, Ph.D.
Research Professor
New York University School of Medicine
Department of Environmental Medicine
New York, New York
Chapter 25

George R. Hoffmann, B.A., M.S., Ph.D.
Anthony and Renee Marlon Professor
Department of Biology
Holy Cross College
Worcester, Massachusetts
Chapter 9

Michael J. Hooper, Ph.D.
Research Scientist
The Institute of Environmental and Human Health (TIEHH)
Associate Professor
Department of Environmental Toxicology
Texas Tech
Lubbock, Texas
Chapter 29

Robert J. Kavlock, Ph.D.
Director, Reproductive Toxicology Division
National Health and Environmental Effects Research Laboratory
United States Environmental Protection Agency
Research Triangle Park, North Carolina
Chapter 10

Ronald J. Kendall, Ph.D.
Director
The Institute of Environmental and Human Health (TIEHH)
Professor and Chair
Department of Environmental Toxicology
Texas Tech
Lubbock, Texas
Chapter 29

Curtis D. Klaassen, Ph.D.
Professor of Pharmacology and Toxicology
Department of Pharmacology, Toxicology, and Therapeutics
University of Kansas Medical Center
Kansas City, Kansas
Chapters 2, 3, 5

Frank N. Kotsonis, Ph.D., D.A.B.T.
Corporate Vice President, Monsanto Company
Worldwide Regulatory Affairs
Skokie, Illinois
Chapter 30

Jerold A. Last, Ph.D.
Professor
Pulmonary/Critical Care Medicine
School of Medicine
University of California, Davis
Davis, California
Chapter 15

Clyde F. Martin, Ph.D.
Special Assistant
The Institute of Environmental and Human Health (TIEHH)
Horn Professor
Department of Mathematics and Statistics
Texas Tech University
Lubbock, Texas
Chapter 29

Scott T. McMurry, Ph.D.
Section Leader
The Institute of Environmental and Human Health (TIEHH)
Assistant Professor
Department of Environmental Toxicology
Texas Tech
Lubbock, Texas
Chapter 29

B. Jean Meade, D.V.M., Ph.D.
Toxicologist
National Institute of Occupational Safety and Health
Morgantown, West Virginia
Chapter 12

Michele A. Medinsky, Ph.D., D.A.B.T.
Toxicology Consultant
Durham, North Carolina
Chapter 7

Russell B. Melchert, Ph.D.
Assistant Professor
Department of Pharmaceutical Sciences
College of Pharmacy
University of Arkansas for Medical Sciences
Little Rock, Arkansas
Chapter 18

Richard A. Merrill, L.L.B., M.A.
Professor of Law
University of Virginia
Charlottesville, Virginia
Chapter 34

Thomas J. Montine, M.D., Ph.D.
Associate Professor of Pathology and Pharmacology
Margaret and George Thorne Professorship in Pathology
Department of Pathology
Vanderbilt University Medical Center
Nashville, Tennessee
Chapter 16

Albert E. Munson, Ph.D.
Director Health Effects Laboratory Division
National Institute of Occupational Safety and Health
Morgantown, West Virginia
Chapter 12

Stata Norton, Ph.D.
Emeritus Professor of Pharmacology and Toxicology
Department of Pharmacology, Toxicology, and Therapeutics
University of Kansas Medical Center
Kansas City, Kansas
Chapter 27

Gilbert S. Omenn, Ph.D., M.D.
Executive Vice President for Medical Affairs
Professor of Internal Medicine, Human Genetics and Public Health
University of Michigan
Ann Arbor, Michigan
Chapter 4

Andrew Parkinson, Ph.D.
CEO
XENOTECH
Kansas City, Kansas
Chapter 6

Reynaldo Patino, Ph.D.
Section Leader
The Institute of Environmental and Human Health (TIEHH)
Associate Professor
Department of Biological Sciences
Texas Tech University
Assistant Unit Leader
Texas Cooperative Fish and Wildlife Research Unit
United States Geological Survey
Lubbock, Texas
Chapter 29

Henry C. Pitot III, M.D., Ph.D.
Professor Emeritus
University of Wisconsin
McArdle Laboratory for Cancer Research and the Center for Environmental Toxicology
Madison, Wisconsin
Chapter 8

Alphonse Poklis, Ph.D.
Professor
Department of Pathology
Medical College of Virginia Campus
Virginia Commonwealth University
Richmond, Virginia
Chapter 31

R. Julian Preston, B.A., M.A., Ph.D.
Director
Environmental Carcinogenesis Division
U.S. Environmental Protection Agency
Research Triangle Park, North Carolina
Chapter 9

Kenneth S. Ramos, Ph.D.
Professor
Department of Physiology and Pharmacology
College of Veterinary Medicine
Texas A&M University
College Station, Texas
Chapter 18

Robert H. Rice, Ph.D.
Professor
University of California/Davis
Department of Environmental Toxicology
Davis, California
Chapter 19

John M. Rogers, Ph.D.
Chief
Developmental Biology Branch
Reproductive Toxicology Division
National Health and Environmental Effects Research Laboratory
United States Environmental Protection Agency
Research Triangle Park, North Carolina
Chapter 10

Karl Rozman, Ph.D.
Professor of Pharmacology and Toxicology
Department of Pharmacology and Toxicology
University of Kansas Medical Center
Kansas City, Kansas
Chapter 5

Findlay E. Russell, M.D., Ph.D.
Department of Pharmacology and Toxicology
College of Pharmacy
University of Arizona
Tucson, Arizona
Department of Neurology
University of Southern California
Los Angeles, California
Department of Neurological Sciences
Loma Linda University
Loma Linda, California
Chapter 26

Rick G. Schnellmann, Ph.D.
Professor and Chair
Pharmaceutical Sciences
Department of Pharmaceutical Sciences
Medical University of South Carolina
Charleston, South Carolina
Chapter 14

Ernest E. Smith, Ph.D.
Research Scientist
The Institute of Environmental and Human Health Center (TIEHH)
Assistant Professor
Department of Environmental Toxicology
Texas Tech
Lubbock, Texas
Chapter 29

Christopher W. Theodorakis, Ph.D.
Assistant Section Leader
The Institute of Environmental and Human Health (TIEHH)
Assistant Professor
Department of Environmental Toxicology
Texas Tech
Lubbock, Texas
Chapter 29

John A. Thomas, Ph.D.
Professor Emeritus
University of Texas Health Science Center–San Antonio
Department of Pharmacology
San Antonio, Texas
Chapter 20

Michael J. Thomas, M.D., Ph.D.
Assistant Professor
University of North Carolina School of Medicine
Division of Endocrinology
Chapel Hill, North Carolina
Chapter 20

Peter S. Thorne, Ph.D.
Professor of Toxicology
Professor of Environmental Engineering (secondary)
University of Iowa College of Public Health
Department of Occupational and Environmental Health
Iowa City, Iowa
Chapter 33

Mary Treinen-Moslen, Ph.D.
William C. Levin Professor of Environmental Toxicology
Toxicology Program
University of Texas Medical Branch
Galveston, Texas
Chapter 13

Jack Valentine, Ph.D.
Research Pharmacokineticist
Research Triangle Institute
Research Triangle Park, North Carolina
Chapter 7

William M. Valentine, D.V.M., Ph.D.
Associate Professor of Pathology
Department of Pathology
Vanderbilt University Medical Center
Nashville, Tennessee
Chapter 16

D. Alan Warren, M.P.H., Ph.D
Toxicologist
Terra, Inc.
Tallahassee, Florida
Chapter 24

Hanspeter R. Witschi, M.D.
Professor of Toxicology
Institute of Toxicology and Environmental Health and Department of Molecular Biosciences
School of Veterinary Medicine
University of California
Davis, California
Chapter 15

PREFACE

The sixth edition of *Casarett and Doull's Toxicology: The Basic Science of Poisons* marks its silver anniversary. The sixth edition, as the previous five, is meant to serve primarily as a text for, or an adjunct to, graduate courses in toxicology. Because the five previous editions have been widely used in courses in environmental health and related areas, an attempt has been made to maintain those characteristics that make it useful to scientists from other disciplines. This edition will again provide information on the many facets of toxicology and especially on the principles, concepts, and modes of thought that are the foundation of the discipline. Mechanisms of toxicity are emphasized. Research toxicologists will find this book an excellent reference source to find updated material in areas of their special or peripheral interests.

The overall framework of the sixth edition is similar to the fifth edition. The seven units are "General Principles of Toxicology" (Unit 1), "Disposition of Toxicants" (Unit 2), "Non-Organ-Directed Toxicity" (carcinogenicity, mutagenicity, and teratogenicity) (Unit 3), "Target Organ Toxicity" (Unit 4), "Toxic Agents" (Unit 5), "Environmental Toxicology" (Unit 6), and "Applications of Toxicology" (Unit 7).

The sixth edition reflects the marked progress made in toxicology the last few years. For example, the importance of apoptosis, cytokines, growth factors, oncogenes, cell cycling, receptors, gene regulation, transcription factors, signaling pathways, transgenic animals, "knock-out" animals, polymorphisms, microarray technology, genomics, proteonomics, etc., in understanding the mechanisms of toxicity are included in this edition. More information on risk assessment is also included. References in this edition include not only traditional journal and review articles, but, for the first time, internet sites.

The editor is grateful to his colleagues in academia, industry, and government who have made useful suggestions for improving this edition, both as a book and as a reference source. The editor is especially thankful to all the contributors, whose combined expertise has made possible a volume of this breadth. I especially recognize John Doull, the original editor of this book, for his continued support.

PREFACE TO THE FIRST EDITION

This volume has been designed primarily as a textbook for, or adjunct to, courses in toxicology. However, it should also be of interest to those not directly involved in toxicologic education. For example, the research scientist in toxicology will find sections containing current reports on the status of circumscribed areas of special interest. Those concerned with community health, agriculture, food technology, pharmacy, veterinary medicine, and related disciplines will discover the contents to be most useful as a source of concepts and modes of thought that are applicable to other types of investigative and applied sciences. For those further removed from the field of toxicology or for those who have not entered a specific field of endeavor, this book attempts to present a selectively representative view of the many facets of the subject.

Toxicology: The Basic Science of Poisons has been organized to facilitate its use by these different types of users. The first section (Unit I) describes the elements of method and approach that identify toxicology. It includes those principles most frequently invoked in a full understanding of toxicologic events, such as dose-response, and is primarily mechanistically oriented. Mechanisms are also stressed in the subsequent sections of the book, particularly when these are well identified and extend across classic forms of chemicals and systems. However, the major focus in the second section (Unit II) is on the systemic site of action of toxins. The intent therein is to provide answers to two questions: What kinds of injury are produced in specific organs or systems by toxic agents? What are the agents that produce these effects?

A more conventional approach to toxicology has been utilized in the third section (Unit III), in which the toxic agents are grouped by chemical or use characteristics. In the final section (Unit IV) an attempt has been made to illustrate the ramifications of toxicology into all areas of the health sciences and even beyond. This unit is intended to provide perspective for the nontoxicologist in the application of the results of toxicologic studies and a better understanding of the activities of those engaged in the various aspects of the discipline of toxicology.

It will be obvious to the reader that the contents of this book represent a compromise between the basic, fundamental, mechanistic approach to toxicology and the desire to give a view of the broad horizons presented by the subject. While it is certain that the editors' selectivity might have been more severe, it is equally certain that it could have been less so, and we hope that the balance struck will prove to be appropriate for both toxicologic training and the scientific interest of our colleague.

L.J.C.
J.D.

Although the philosophy and design of this book evolved over a long period of friendship and mutual respect between the editors, the effort needed to convert ideas into reality was undertaken primarily by Louis J. Casarett. Thus, his death at a time when completion of the manuscript was in sight was particularly tragic. With the help and encouragement of his wife, Margaret G. Casarett, and the other contributors, we have finished Lou's task. This volume is a fitting embodiment of Louis J. Casarett's dedication to toxicology and to toxicologic education.

J.D.

CASARETT AND DOULL'S
TOXICOLOGY
THE BASIC SCIENCE OF POISONS

What is there that is not poison?
All things are poison and nothing (is)
without poison. Solely the dose
determines that a thing is not a poison.
Paracelsus
(1493–1541)

UNIT 1

GENERAL PRINCIPLES OF TOXICOLOGY

CHAPTER 1

HISTORY AND SCOPE OF TOXICOLOGY

Michael A. Gallo

Toxicology has been defined as the study of the adverse effects of xenobiotics and thus is a borrowing science that has evolved from ancient poisoners. Modern toxicology goes beyond the study of the adverse effects of exogenous agents to the study of molecular biology, using toxicants as tools. Historically, toxicology formed the basis of therapeutics and experimental medicine. Toxicology in this century (1900 to the present) continues to develop and expand by assimilating knowledge and techniques from most branches of biology, chemistry, mathematics, and physics. A recent addition to the field of toxicology (1975 to the present) is the application of the discipline to safety evaluation and risk assessment.

The contributions and activities of toxicologists are diverse and widespread. In the biomedical area, toxicologists are concerned with mechanisms of action and exposure to chemical agents as a cause of acute and chronic illness. Toxicologists contribute to physiology and pharmacology by using toxic agents to understand physiological phenomena. They are involved in the recognition, identification, and quantification of hazards resulting from occupational exposure to chemicals and the public health aspects of chemicals in air, water, other parts of the environment, foods, and drugs. Traditionally, toxicologists have been intimately involved in the discovery and development of new drugs and pesticides. Toxicologists also participate in the development of standards and regulations designed to protect human health and the environment from the adverse effects of chemicals. Environmental toxicologists (a relatively new subset of the discipline) have expanded toxicology to study the effects of chemicals in flora and fauna. Molecular toxicologists are studying the mechanisms by which toxicants modulate cell growth and differentiation and cells respond to toxicants at the level of the gene. In all branches of toxicology, scientists explore the mechanisms by which chemicals produce adverse effects in biological systems. Clinical toxicologists develop antidotes and treatment regimes to ameliorate poisonings and xenobiotic injury. Toxicologists carry out some or all of these activities as members of academic, industrial, and governmental organizations. In doing so, they share methodologies for obtaining data about the toxicity of materials and the responsibility for using this information to make reasonable predictions regarding the hazards of the material to people and the environment. These different but complementary activities characterize the discipline of toxicology.

Toxicology, like medicine, is both a science and an art. The science of toxicology is defined as the observational and data-gathering phase, whereas the art of toxicology consists of the utilization of the data to predict outcomes of exposure in human and animal populations. In most cases, these phases are linked because the facts generated by the science of toxicology are used to develop extrapolations and hypotheses to explain the adverse effects of chemical agents in situations where there is little or no information. For example, the observation that the administration of TCDD (2,3,7,8-tetrachlorodibenzo-*p*-dioxin) to female Sprague-Dawley rats induces hepatocellular carcinoma is a fact. However, the conclusion that it will also do so in humans is a prediction or hypothesis. It is important to distinguish facts from predictions. When we fail to distinguish the science from the art, we confuse facts with predictions and argue that they have equal validity, which they clearly do not. In toxicology, as in all sciences, theories have a higher level of certainty than do hypotheses, which in turn are more certain than speculations, opinions, conjectures, and guesses. An insight into modern toxicology and the roles, points of view, and activities of toxicologists can be obtained by examining the historical evolution of the discipline.

HISTORY OF TOXICOLOGY

Antiquity

Toxicology dates back to the earliest humans, who used animal venoms and plant extracts for hunting, warfare, and assassination. The knowledge of these poisons must have predated recorded history. It is safe to assume that prehistoric humans categorized some plants as harmful and others as safe. The same is probably true for the classification of snakes and other animals. The Ebers papyrus (circa 1500 B.C.) contains information pertaining to many recognized poisons, including hemlock (the state poison of the Greeks), aconite (a Chinese arrow poison), opium (used as both a poison and an antidote), and metals such as lead, copper, and antimony. There is also an indication that plants containing substances similar to digitalis and belladonna alkaloids were known. Hippocrates (circa 400 B.C.) added a number of poisons and clinical toxicology principles pertaining to bioavailability in therapy and overdosage, while the Book of Job (circa 400 B.C.) speaks of poison arrows (Job 6:4). In the literature of ancient Greece, there are several references to poisons and their use. Some interpretations of Homer have Odysseus obtaining poisons for his arrows (Homer, circa 600 B.C.). Theophrastus (370–286 B.C.), a student of Aristotle, included numerous references to poisonous plants in *De Historia Plantarum*. Dioscorides, a Greek physician in the court of the Roman emperor Nero, made the first attempt at a classification of poisons, which was accompanied by descriptions and drawings. His classification into plant, animal, and mineral poisons not only remained a standard for 16 centuries but is still a convenient classification (Gunther, 1934). Dioscorides also dabbled in therapy, recognizing the use of emetics in poisoning and the use of caustic agents and cupping glasses in snakebite. Poisoning with plant and animal toxins was quite common. Perhaps the best-known recipient of poison used as a state method of execution was Socrates (470–399 B.C.), whose cup of hemlock extract was apparently estimated to be the proper dose. Expeditious suicide on a voluntary basis also made use of toxicologic knowledge. Demosthenes (385– 322 B.C.), who took poison hidden in his pen, was one of many examples. The mode of suicide calling for one to fall on his sword, although manly and noble, carried little appeal and less significance for the women of the day. Cleopatra's (69–30 B.C.) knowledge of natural primitive toxicology permitted her to use the more genteel method of falling on her asp.

The Romans too made considerable use of poisons in politics. One legend tells of King Mithridates VI of Pontus, whose numerous acute toxicity experiments on unfortunate criminals led to his eventual claim that he had discovered an antidote for every venomous reptile and poisonous substance (Guthrie, 1946). Mithridates was so fearful of poisons that he regularly ingested a mixture of 36 ingredients (Galen reports 54) as protection against assassination. On the occasion of his imminent capture by enemies, his attempts to kill himself with poison failed because of his successful antidote concoction, and he was forced to use a sword held by a servant. From this tale comes the term "mithridatic," referring to an antidotal or protective mixture. The term "theriac" also has become synonymous with "antidote," although the word comes from the poetic treatise *Theriaca* by Nicander of Colophon (204–135 B.C.), which dealt with poisonous animals; his poem "Alexipharmaca" was about antidotes.

Poisonings in Rome reached epidemic proportions during the fourth century B.C. (Livy). It was during this period that a conspiracy of women to remove men from whose death they might profit was uncovered. Similar large-scale poisoning continued until Sulla issued the *Lex Cornelia* (circa 82 B.C.). This appears to be the first law against poisoning, and it later became a regulatory statute directed at careless dispensers of drugs. Nero (A.D. 37–68) used poisons to do away with his stepbrother Brittanicus and employed his slaves as food tasters to differentiate edible mushrooms from their more poisonous kin.

Middle Ages

Come bitter pilot, now at once run on
The dashing rocks thy seasick weary bark!
Here's to my love! O true apothecary!
Thy drugs are quick. Thus with a kiss I die.
Romeo and Juliet, act 5, scene 3

Before the Renaissance, the writings of Maimonides (Moses ben Maimon, A.D. 1135–1204) included a treatise on the treatment of poisonings from insects, snakes, and mad dogs (*Poisons and Their Antidotes*, 1198). Maimonides, like Hippocrates before him, wrote on the subject of bioavailability, noting that milk, butter, and cream could delay intestinal absorption. Malmonides also refuted many of the popular remedies of the day and stated his doubts about others. It is rumored that alchemists of this period (circa A.D. 1200), in search of the universal antidote, learned to distill fermented products and made a 60% ethanol beverage that had many interesting powers.

In the early Renaissance, the Italians, with characteristic pragmatism, brought the art of poisoning to its zenith. The poisoner became an integral part of the political scene. The records of the city councils of Florence, particularly those of the infamous Council of Ten of Venice, contain ample testimony about the political use of poisons. Victims were named, prices set, and contracts recorded; when the deed was accomplished, payment was made.

An infamous figure of the time was a lady named Toffana who peddled specially prepared arsenic-containing cosmetics (*Agua Toffana*). Accompanying the product were appropriate instructions for its use. Toffana was succeeded by an imitator with organizational genius, Hieronyma Spara, who provided a new fillip by directing her activities toward specific marital and monetary objectives. A local club was formed of young, wealthy married women, which soon became a club of eligible young wealthy widows, reminiscent of the matronly conspiracy of Rome centuries earlier. Incidentally, arsenic-containing cosmetics were reported to be responsible for deaths well into the twentieth century (Kallett and Schlink, 1933).

Among the prominent families engaged in poisoning, the Borgias were the most notorious. However, many deaths that were attributed to poisoning are now recognized as having resulted from infectious diseases such as malaria. It appears true, however, that Alexander VI, his son Cesare, and Lucrezia Borgia were quite active. The deft application of poisons to men of stature in the Catholic Church swelled the holdings of the papacy, which was their prime heir.

In this period Catherine de Medici exported her skills from Italy to France, where the prime targets of women were their husbands. However, unlike poisoners of an earlier period, the circle represented by Catherine and epitomized by the notorious Marchioness de Brinvillers depended on developing direct evidence to arrive at the most effective compounds for their purposes. Under the guise of delivering provender to the sick and the poor, Catherine tested toxic concoctions, carefully noting the rapidity of the toxic response (onset of action), the effectiveness of the compound (potency), the degree of response of the parts of the body (specificity, site of action), and the complaints of the victim (clinical signs and symptoms).

The culmination of the practice in France is represented by the commercialization of the service by Catherine Deshayes, who earned the title "La Voisine." Her business was dissolved by her execution. Her trial was one of the most famous of those held by the Chambre Ardente, a special judicial commission established by Louis XIV to try such cases without regard to age, sex, or national origin. La Voisine was convicted of many poisonings, with over 2000 infants among her victims.

Age of Enlightenment

All substances are poisons; there is none which is not a poison. The right dose differentiates a poison from a remedy.

Paracelsus

A significant figure in the history of science and medicine in the late Middle Ages was the renaissance man Philippus Aureolus Theophrastus Bombastus von Hohenheim-Paracelsus (1493–1541). Between the time of Aristotle and the age of Paracelsus, there was little substantial change in the biomedical sciences. In the sixteenth century, the revolt against the authority of the Catholic Church was accompanied by a parallel attack on the godlike authority exercised by the followers of Hippocrates and Galen. Paracelsus personally and professionally embodied the qualities that forced numerous changes in this period. He and his age were pivotal, standing between the philosophy and magic of classical antiquity and the philosophy and science willed to us by figures of the seventeenth and eighteenth centuries. Clearly, one can identify in Paracelsus's approach, point of view, and breadth of interest numerous similarities to the discipline that is now called toxicology.

Paracelsus, a physician-alchemist and the son of a physician, formulated many revolutionary views that remain an integral part of the structure of toxicology, pharmacology, and therapeutics today (Pagel, 1958). He promoted a focus on the "toxicon," the primary toxic agent, as a chemical entity, as opposed to the Grecian concept of the mixture or blend. A view initiated by Paracelsus that became a lasting contribution held as corollaries that (1) experimentation is essential in the examination of responses to chemicals, (2) one should make a distinction between the therapeutic and toxic properties of chemicals, (3) these properties are sometimes but not always indistinguishable except by dose, and (4) one can ascertain a degree of specificity of chemicals and their therapeutic or toxic effects. These principles led Paracelsus to introduce mercury as the drug of choice for the treatment of syphilis, a practice that survived 300 years but led to his famous trial. This viewpoint presaged the "magic bullet" (arsphenamine) of Paul Ehrlich and the introduction of the therapeutic index. Further, in a very real sense, this was the first sound articulation of the dose-response relation, a bulwark of toxicology (Pachter, 1961).

The tradition of the poisoners spread throughout Europe, and their deeds played a major role in the distribution of political power throughout the Middle Ages. Pharmacology as it is known today had its beginnings during the Middle Ages and early Renaissance. Concurrently, the study of the toxicity and the dose-response relationship of therapeutic agents was commencing.

The occupational hazards associated with metalworking were recognized during the fifteenth century. Early publications by Ellenbog (circa 1480) warned of the toxicity of the mercury and lead exposures involved in goldsmithing. Agricola published a short treatise on mining diseases in 1556. However, the major work on the subject, *On the Miners' Sickness and Other Diseases of Miners* (1567), was published by Paracelsus. This treatise addressed the etiology of miners' disease, along with treatment and prevention strategies. Occupational toxicology was further advanced by the work of Bernardino Ramazzini. His classic, published in 1700 and entitled *Discourse on the Diseases of Workers,* set the standard for occupational medicine well into the nineteenth century. Ramazzini's work broadened the field by discussing occupations ranging from miners to midwives and including printers, weavers, and potters.

The developments of the industrial revolution stimulated a rise in many occupational diseases. Percival Pott's (1775) recognition of the role of soot in scrotal cancer among chimney sweeps was the first reported example of polyaromatic hydrocarbon carcinogenicity, a problem that still plagues toxicologists today. These findings led to improved medical practices, particularly in prevention. It should be noted that Paracelsus and Ramazzini also pointed out the toxicity of smoke and soot.

The nineteenth century dawned in a climate of industrial and political revolution. Organic chemistry was in its infancy in 1800, but by 1825 phosgene ($COCl_2$) and mustard gas (bis[B-chloroethyl]sulfide) had been synthesized. These two agents were used in World War I as war gases. By 1880 over 10,000 organic compounds had been synthesized including chloroform, carbon tetrachloride, diethyl ether, and carbonic acid, and petroleum and coal gasification by-products were used in trade (Zapp, 1982). Determination of the toxicologic potential of these newly created chemicals became the underpinning of the science of toxicology as it is practiced today. However, there was little interest during the mid-nineteenth century in hampering industrial development. Hence, the impact of industrial toxicology discoveries was not felt until the passage of worker's insurance laws, first in Germany (1883), then in England (1897), and later in the United States (1910).

Experimental toxicology accompanied the growth of organic chemistry and developed rapidly during the nineteenth century. Magendie (1783–1885), Orfila (1787–1853), and Bernard (1813–1878) carried out truly seminal research in experimental toxicology and laid the groundwork for pharmacology and experimental therapeutics as well as occupational toxicology.

Orfila, a Spanish physician in the French court, was the first toxicologist to use autopsy material and chemical analysis systematically as legal proof of poisoning. His introduction of this detailed type of analysis survives as the underpinning of forensic toxicology (Orfila, 1818). Orfila published the first major work devoted expressly to the toxicity of natural agents (1815). Magendie, a physician and experimental physiologist, studied the mechanisms of action of emetine, strychnine, and "arrow poisons" (Olmsted, 1944). His research into the absorption and distribution of these compounds in the body remains a classic in toxicology and pharmacology. One of Magendie's more famous students, Claude Bernard, continued the study of arrow poisons (Bernard, 1850) but also added works on the mechanism of action of carbon monoxide. Bernard's treatise, *An Introduction to the Study of Experimental Medicine* (translated by Greene in 1949), is a classic in the development of toxicology.

Many German scientists contributed greatly to the growth of toxicology in the late nineteenth and early twentieth centuries. Among the giants of the field are Oswald Schmiedeberg (1838–1921) and Louis Lewin (1850–1929). Schmiedeberg made many contributions to the science of toxicology, not the least of which was the training of approximately 120 students who later populated the most important laboratories of pharmacology and toxicology throughout the world. His research focused on the synthesis of hippuric acid in the liver and the detoxification mechanisms of the liver in several animal species (Schmiedeberg and Koppe, 1869). Lewin, who was educated originally in medicine and the natural sciences, trained in toxicology under Liebreich at the Pharmacological Institute of Berlin (1881). His contributions on the chronic toxicity of narcotics and other alkaloids remain a classic. Lewin also published much of the early work on the toxicity of methanol, glycerol, acrolein, and chloroform (Lewin, 1920, 1929).

MODERN TOXICOLOGY

Toxicology has evolved rapidly during this century. The exponential growth of the discipline can be traced to the World War II era with its marked increase in the production of drugs, pesticides, munitions, synthetic fibers, and industrial chemicals. The history of many sciences represents an orderly transition based on theory, hypothesis testing, and synthesis of new ideas. Toxicology, as a gathering and an applied science, has, by contrast, developed in fits and starts. Toxicology calls on almost all the basic sciences to test its hypotheses. This fact, coupled with the health and occupational regulations that have driven toxicology research since 1900, has made this discipline exceptional in the history of science. The differentiation of toxicology as an art and a science, though arbitrary, permits the presentation of historical highlights along two major lines.

Modern toxicology can be viewed as a continuation of the development of the biological and physical sciences in the late nineteenth and twentieth centuries (Table 1-1). During the second half of the nineteenth century, the world witnessed an explosion in science that produced the beginning of the modern era of medicine, synthetic chemistry, physics, and biology. Toxicology has drawn its strength and diversity from its proclivity to borrowing. With the advent of anesthetics and disinfectants and the advancement of experimental pharmacology in the late 1850s, toxicology as it is currently understood got its start. The introduction of ether, chloroform, and carbonic acid led to several iatrogenic deaths. These unfortunate outcomes spurred research into the causes of the deaths and early experiments on the physiological mechanisms by which these compounds caused both beneficial and adverse effects. By the late nineteenth century the use of organic chemicals was becoming more widespread, and benzene, toluene, and the xylenes went into larger-scale commercial production.

During this period, the use of "patent" medicines was prevalent, and there were several incidents of poisonings from these medicaments. The adverse reactions to patent medicines, coupled with the response to Upton Sinclair's exposé of the meat-packing industry in *The Jungle,* culminated in the passage of the Wiley Bill (1906), the first of many U.S. pure food and drug laws (see Hutt and Hutt, 1984, for regulatory history).

A working hypothesis about the development of toxicology is that the discipline expands in response to legislation, which itself is a response to a real or perceived tragedy. The Wiley bill was the

Table 1-1
Selection of Developments in Toxicology

Development of early advances in analytic methods
Marsh, 1836: development of method for arsenic analysis
Reinsh, 1841: combined method for separation and analysis of As and Hg
Fresenius, 1845, and von Babo, 1847: development of screening method for general poisons
Stas-Otto, 1851: extraction and separation of alkaloids
Mitscherlich, 1855: detection and identification of phosphorus
Early mechanistic studies
F. Magendie, 1809: study of "arrow poisons," mechanism of action of emetine and strychnine
C. Bernard, 1850: carbon monoxide combination with hemoglobin, study of mechanism of action of strychnine, site of action of curare
R. Bohm, ca. 1890: active anthelmintics from fern, action of croton oil catharsis, poisonous mushrooms
Introduction of new toxicants and antidotes
R. A. Peters, L. A. Stocken, and R. H. S. Thompson, 1945: development of British Anti Lewisite (BAL) as a relatively specific antidote for arsenic, toxicity of monofluorocarbon compounds
K. K. Chen, 1934: introduction of modern antidotes (nitrite and thiosulfate) for cyanide toxicity
C. Voegtlin, 1923: mechanism of action of As and other metals on the SH groups
P. Müller, 1944–1946: introduction and study of DDT (dichlorodiphenyltrichloroethane) and related insecticide compounds
G. Schrader, 1952: introduction and study of organophosphorus compounds
R. N. Chopra, 1933: indigenous drugs of India
Miscellaneous toxicologic studies
R. T. Williams: study of detoxication mechanisms and species variation
A. Rothstein: effects of uranium ion on cell membrane transport
R. A. Kehoe: investigation of acute and chronic effects of lead
A. Vorwald: studies of chronic respiratory disease (beryllium)
H. Hardy: community and industrial poisoning (beryllium)
A. Hamilton: introduction of modern industrial toxicology
H. C. Hodge: toxicology of uranium, fluorides; standards of toxicity
A. Hoffman: introduction of lysergic acid and derivatives; psychotomimetics
R. A. Peters: biochemical lesions, lethal synthesis
A. E. Garrod: inborn errors of metabolism
T. T. Litchfield and F. Wilcoxon: simplified dose-response evaluation
C. J. Bliss: method of probits, calculation of dosage-mortality curves

first such reaction in the area of food and drugs, and the worker's compensation laws cited above were a response to occupational toxicities. In addition, the National Safety Council was established in 1911, and the Division of Industrial Hygiene was established by the U.S. Public Health Service in 1914. A corollary to this hypothesis might be that the founding of scientific journals and/or societies is sparked by the development of a new field. The *Journal of Industrial Hygiene* began in 1918. The major chemical manufacturers in the United States (Dow, Union Carbide, and Du Pont) established internal toxicology research laboratories to help guide decisions on worker health and product safety.

During the 1890s and early 1900s, the French scientists Becquerel and the Curies reported the discovery of "radioactivity." This opened up for exploration a very large area in physics, biology, and medicine, but it would not actively affect the science of toxicology for another 40 years. However, another discovery, that of vitamins, or "vital amines," was to lead to the use of the first large-scale bioassays (multiple animal studies) to determine whether these "new" chemicals were beneficial or harmful to laboratory animals. The initial work in this area took place at around the time of World War I in several laboratories, including the laboratory of Philip B. Hawk in Philadelphia. Hawk and a young associate, Bernard L. Oser, were responsible for the development and verification of many early toxicologic assays that are still used in a slightly amended form. Oser's contributions to food and regulatory toxicology were extraordinary. These early bioassays were made possible by a major advance in toxicology: the availability of developed and refined strains of inbred laboratory rodents (Donaldson, 1912).

The 1920s saw many events that began to mold the fledgling field of toxicology. The use of arsenicals for the treatment of diseases such as syphilis (arsenicals had been used in agriculture since the mid-nineteenth century) resulted in acute and chronic toxicity. Prohibition of alcoholic beverages in the United States opened the door for early studies of neurotoxicology, with the discovery that triorthocresyl phosphate (TOCP), methanol, and lead (all products of "bootleg" liquor) are neurotoxicants. TOCP, which is a modern gasoline additive, caused a syndrome that became known as "ginger-jake" walk, a spastic gait resulting from drinking adulterated ginger beer. Mueller's discovery of DDT (dichlorodiphenyltrichloroethane) and several other organohalides, such as hexachlorobenzene and hexachlorocyclohexane, during the late 1920s resulted in wider use of insecticidal agents. Other scientists were hard at work attempting to elucidate the structures and activity of the estrogens and androgens. Work on the steroid hormones led to the use of several assays for the determination of the biological activity of organ extracts and synthetic compounds. Efforts to synthesize steroid-like chemicals were spearheaded by E. C. Dodds and his coworkers, one of whom was Leon Golberg, a young organic chemist. Dodds's work on the bioactivity of the estrogenic compounds resulted in the synthesis of diethylstilbestrol (DES), hexestrol, and other stilbenes and the discovery of the strong estrogenic activity of substituted stilbenes. Golberg's intimate involvement in this work stimulated his interest in biology, leading to degrees in biochemistry and medicine and a career in toxicology in which he oversaw the creation of the laboratories of the British Industrial Biological Research Association (BIBRA) and the Chemical Industry Institute of Toxicology (CIIT). Interestingly, the initial observations that led to the discovery of DES were the findings of feminization of animals treated with the experimental carcinogen 7,12-dimethylbenz[*a*]anthracene (DMBA).

The 1930s saw the world preparing for World War II and a major effort by the pharmaceutical industry in Germany and the United States to manufacture the first mass-produced antibiotics. One of the first journals expressly dedicated to experimental toxicology, *Archiv für Toxikologie,* began publication in Europe in 1930, the same year that Herbert Hoover signed the act that established the National Institutes of Health (NIH) in the United States.

The discovery of sulfanilamide was heralded as a major event in combating bacterial diseases. However, for a drug to be effective, there must be a reasonable delivery system, and sulfanilamide is highly insoluble in an aqueous medium. Therefore, it was originally prepared in ethanol (elixir). However, it was soon discovered that the drug was more soluble in ethylene glycol, which is a dihydroxy rather than a monohydroxy ethane. The drug was sold in glycol solutions but was labeled as an elixir, and several patients died of acute kidney failure resulting from the metabolism of the glycol to oxalic acid and glycolic acid, with the acids, along with the active drug, crystallizing in the kidney tubules. This tragic event led to the passage of the Copeland bill in 1938, the second major bill involving the formation of the U.S. Food and Drug Administration (FDA). The sulfanilamide disaster played a critical role in the further development of toxicology, resulting in work by Eugene Maximillian Geiling in the Pharmacology Department of the University of Chicago that elucidated the mechanism of toxicity of both sulfanilamide and ethylene glycol. Studies of the glycols were simultaneously carried out at the U.S. FDA by a group led by Arnold Lehman. The scientists associated with Lehman and Geiling were to become the leaders of toxicology over the next 40 years. With few exceptions, toxicology in the United States owes its heritage to Geiling's innovativeness and ability to stimulate and direct young scientists and Lehman's vision of the use of experimental toxicology in public health decision making. Because of Geiling's reputation, the U.S. government turned to this group for help in the war effort. There were three main areas in which the Chicago group took part during World War II: the toxicology and pharmacology of organophosphate chemicals, antimalarial drugs, and radionuclides. Each of these areas produced teams of toxicologists who became academic, governmental, and industrial leaders in the field.

It was also during this time that DDT and the phenoxy herbicides were developed for increased food production and, in the case of DDT, control of insect-borne diseases. These efforts between 1940 and 1946 led to an explosion in toxicology. Thus, in line with the hypothesis advanced above, the crisis of World War II caused the next major leap in the development of toxicology.

If one traces the history of the toxicology of metals over the past 45 years, the role of the Chicago group is quite visible. This story commences with the use of uranium for the "bomb" and continues today with research on the role of metals in their interactions with DNA, RNA, and growth factors. Indeed, the Manhattan Project created a fertile environment that resulted in the initiation of quantitative biology, radiotracer technology, and inhalation toxicology. These innovations have revolutionized modern biology, chemistry, therapeutics, and toxicology.

Inhalation toxicology began at the University of Rochester under the direction of Stafford Warren, who headed the Department of Radiology. He developed a program with colleagues such as Harold Hodge (pharmacologist), Herb Stokinger (chemist), Sid Laskin (inhalation toxicologist), and Lou and George Casarett (toxicologists). These young scientists were to go on to become giants in the field. The other sites for the study of radionuclides were Chicago for the "internal" effects of radioactivity and Oak Ridge, Tennessee, for the effects of "external" radiation. The work of the scientists on these teams gave the scientific community data that contributed to the early understanding of macromolecular binding of xenobiotics, cellular mutational events, methods for inhalation toxicology and therapy, and toxicological properties of trace metals, along with a better appreciation of the complexities of the dose-response curve.

Another seminal event in toxicology that occurred during the World War II era was the discovery of organophosphate cholinesterase inhibitors. This class of chemicals, which was discovered by Willy Lange and Gerhard Schrader, was destined to become a driving force in the study of neurophysiology and toxicology for several decades. Again, the scientists in Chicago played major roles in elucidating the mechanisms of action of this new class of compounds. Geiling's group, Kenneth Dubois in particular, were leaders in this area of toxicology and pharmacology. Dubois's students, particularly Sheldon Murphy, continued to be in the forefront of this special area. The importance of the early research on the organophosphates has taken on special meaning in the years since 1960, when these nonbioaccumulating insecticides were destined to replace DDT and other organochlorine insectides.

Early in the twentieth century, it was demonstrated experimentally that quinine has a marked effect on the malaria parasite [it had been known for centuries that chincona bark extract is efficacious for "Jesuit fever" (malaria)]. This discovery led to the development of quinine derivatives for the treatment of the disease and the formulation of the early principles of chemotherapy. The pharmacology department at Chicago was charged with the development of antimalarials for the war effort. The original protocols called for testing of efficacy and toxicity in rodents and perhaps dogs and then the testing of efficacy in human volunteers. One of the investigators charged with generating the data needed to move a candidate drug from animals to humans was Fredrick Coulston. This young parasitologist and his colleagues, working under Geiling, were to evaluate potential drugs in animal models and then establish human clinical trials. It was during these experiments that the use of nonhuman primates came into vogue for toxicology testing. It had been noted by Russian scientists that some antimalarial compounds caused retinopathies in humans but did not apparently have the same adverse effect in rodents and dogs. This finding led the Chicago team to add one more step in the development process: toxicity testing in rhesus monkeys just before efficacy studies in people. This resulted in the prevention of blindness in untold numbers of volunteers and perhaps some of the troops in the field. It also led to the school of thought that nonhuman primates may be one of the better models for humans and the establishment of primate colonies for the study of toxicity. Coulston pioneered this area of toxicology and remains committed to it.

Another area not traditionally thought of as toxicology but one that evolved during the 1940s as an exciting and innovative field is experimental pathology. This branch of experimental biology developed from bioassays of estrogens and early experiments in chemical- and radiation-induced carcinogenesis. It is from these early studies that hypotheses on tumor promotion and cancer progression have evolved.

Toxicologists today owe a great deal to the researchers of chemical carcinogenesis of the 1940s. Much of today's work can be traced to Elizabeth and James Miller at Wisconsin. This husband and wife team started under the mentorship of Professor Rusch, the director of the newly formed McArdle Laboratory for Cancer Research, and Professor Baumann. The seminal research of the Millers led to the discovery of the role of reactive intermediates in carcinogenicity and that of mixed-function oxidases in the endoplasmic reticulum. These findings, which initiated the great works on the cytochrome-P450 family of proteins, were aided by two other major discoveries for which toxicologists (and all other biological scientists) are deeply indebted: paper chromatography in 1944 and the use of radiolabeled dibenzanthracene in 1948. Other major events of note in drug metabolism included the work of Bernard Brodie on the metabolism of methyl orange in 1947. This piece of seminal research led to the examination of blood and urine for chemical and drug metabolites. It became the tool with which one could study the relationship between blood levels and biological action. The classic treatise of R. T. Williams, *Detoxication Mechanisms,* was published in 1947. This text described the many pathways and possible mechanisms of detoxication and opened the field to several new areas of study.

The decade after World War II was not as boisterous as the period from 1935 to 1945. The first major U.S. pesticide act was signed into law in 1947. The significance of the initial Federal Insecticide, Fungicide, and Rodenticide Act was that for the first time in U.S. history a substance that was neither a drug nor a food had to be shown to be safe and efficacious. This decade, which coincided with the Eisenhower years, saw the dispersion of the groups from Chicago, Rochester, and Oak Ridge and the establishment of new centers of research. Adrian Albert's classic *Selective Toxicity* was published in 1951. This treatise, which has appeared in several editions, presented a concise documentation of the principles of the site-specific action of chemicals.

AFTER WORLD WAR II

You too can be a toxicologist in two easy lessons, each of ten years.
Arnold Lehman (circa 1955)

The mid-1950s witnessed the strengthening of the U.S. Food and Drug Administration's commitment to toxicology under the guidance of Arnold Lehman. Lehman's tutelage and influence are still felt today. The adage "You too can be a toxicologist" is as important a summation of toxicology as the often quoted statement of Paracelsus: "The dose makes the poison." The period from 1955 to 1958 produced two major events that would have a long-lasting impact on toxicology as a science and a professional discipline. Lehman, Fitzhugh, and their coworkers formalized the experimental program for the appraisal of food, drug, and cosmetic safety in 1955, updated by the U.S. FDA in 1982, and the Gordon Research Conferences established a conference on toxicology and safety evaluation, with Bernard L. Oser as its initial chairman. These two events led to close relationships among toxicologists from several groups and brought toxicology into a new phase. At about the same time, the U.S. Congress passed and the president of the United States signed the additives amendments to the Food, Drug, and Cosmetic Act. The Delaney clause (1958) of these amendments stated broadly that any chemical found to be carcinogenic in laboratory animals or humans could not be added to the U.S. food supply. The impact of this legislation cannot be overstated. Delaney became a battle cry for many groups and resulted in the inclusion at a new level of biostatisticians and mathematical modelers in the field of toxicology. It fostered the expansion of quantitative methods in toxicology and led to innumerable arguments about the "one-hit" theory of carcinogenesis. Regardless of one's view of Delaney, it has served as an excellent starting point for understanding the complexity of the biological phenomenon of carcinogenicity and the development of risk assessment models. One must remember that at the time of Delaney, the analytic detection level for most chemicals was 20 to 100 ppm (today, parts per quadrillion). Interestingly, the Delaney clause has been invoked only on a few occasions, and it has been stated that Congress added little to the food and drug law with this clause (Hutt and Hutt, 1984).

Shortly after the Delaney amendment and after three successful Gordon Conferences, the first American journal dedicated to toxicology was launched by Coulston, Lehman, and Hayes. *Toxicology and Applied Pharmacology* has been the flagship journal of toxicology ever since. The founding of the Society of Toxicology followed shortly afterward, and this journal became its official publication. The society's founding members were Fredrick Coulston, William Deichmann, Kenneth DuBois, Victor Drill, Harry Hayes, Harold Hodge, Paul Larson. Arnold Lehman, and C. Boyd Shaffer. These researchers deserve a great deal of credit for the growth of toxicology. DuBois and Geiling published their *Textbook of Toxicology* in 1959.

The 1960s were a tumultuous time for society, and toxicology was swept up in the tide. Starting with the tragic thalidomide incident, in which several thousand children were born with serious birth defects, and the publication of Rachel Carson's *Silent Spring* (1962), the field of toxicology developed at a feverish pitch. Attempts to understand the effects of chemicals on the embryo and fetus and on the environment as a whole gained momentum. New legislation was passed, and new journals were founded. The education of toxicologists spread from the deep traditions at Chicago and Rochester to Harvard, Miami, Albany, Iowa, Jefferson, and beyond. Geiling's fledglings spread as Schmiedeberg's had a half century before. Many new fields were influencing and being assimilated into the broad scope of toxicology, including environmental sciences, aquatic and avian biology, cell biology, analytic chemistry, and genetics.

During the 1960s, particularly the latter half of the decade, the analytic tools used in toxicology were developed to a level of sophistication that allowed the detection of chemicals in tissues and other substrates at part per billion concentrations (today parts per quadrillion may be detected). Pioneering work in the development of point mutation assays that were replicable, quick, and inexpensive led to a better understanding of the genetic mechanisms of carcinogenicity (Ames, 1983). The combined work of Ames and the Millers (Elizabeth C. and James A.) at McArdle Laboratory allowed the toxicology community to make major contributions to the understanding of the carcinogenic process.

The low levels of detection of chemicals and the ability to detect point mutations rapidly created several problems and opportunities for toxicologists and risk assessors that stemmed from interpretation of the Delaney amendment. Cellular and molecular toxicology developed as a subdiscipline, and risk assessment became a major product of toxicological investigations.

The establishment of the National Center for Toxicologic Research (NCTR), the expansion of the role of the U.S. FDA, and the establishment of the U.S. Environmental Protection Agency (EPA) and the National Institute of Environmental Health Sciences (NIEHS) were considered clear messages that the government had taken a strong interest in toxicology. Several new journals appeared during the 1960s, and new legislation was written quickly after *Silent Spring* and the thalidomide disaster.

The end of the 1960s witnessed the "discovery" of TCDD as a contaminant in the herbicide Agent Orange (the original discovery of TCDD toxicity was reported in 1957). The research on the toxicity of this compound has produced some very good and some very poor research in the field of toxicology. The discovery of a high-affinity cellular binding protein designated the "Ah" receptor (see Poland and Knutsen, 1982, for a review) at the McArdle Laboratory and work on the genetics of the receptor at NIH (Nebert and Gonzalez, 1987) have revolutionized the field of toxicology. The importance of TCDD to toxicology lies in the fact that it forced researchers, regulators, and the legal community to look at the role of mechanisms of toxic action in a different fashion.

At least one other event precipitated a great deal of legislation during the 1970s: Love Canal. The "discovery" of Love Canal led to major concerns regarding hazardous wastes, chemical dump sites, and disclosure of information about those sites. Soon after Love Canal, the EPA listed several equally contaminated sites in the United States. The agency was given the responsibility to develop risk assessment methodology to determine health risks from exposure to effluents and to attempt to remediate these sites. These combined efforts led to broad-based support for research into the mechanisms of action of individual chemicals and complex mixtures. Love Canal and similar issues created the legislative environment that led to the Toxic Substances Control Act and eventually to the Superfund bill. These omnibus bills were created to cover the toxicology of chemicals from initial synthesis to disposal (cradle to grave).

The expansion of legislation, journals, and new societies involved with toxicology was exponential during the 1970s and 1980s and shows no signs of slowing down. Currently, in the United States there are dozens of professional, governmental, and other scientific organizations with thousands of members and over 120 journals dedicated to toxicology and related disciplines.

In addition, toxicology continues to expand in stature and in the number of programs worldwide. The International Congress of Toxicology is made up of toxicology societies from Europe, South America, Asia, Africa, and Australia and brings together the broadest representation of toxicologists.

The original Gordon Conference series has changed to Mechanisms of Toxicity, and several other conferences related to special areas of toxicology are now in existence. The American Society of Toxicology has formed specialty sections and regional chapters to accommodate the over 5000 scientists involved in toxicology today. Texts and reference books for toxicology students and scientists abound. Toxicology has evolved from a borrowing science to a seminal discipline seeding the growth and development of several related fields of science and science policy.

The history of toxicology has been interesting and varied but never dull. Perhaps as a science that has grown and prospered by borrowing from many disciplines, it has suffered from the absence of a single goal, but its diversification has allowed for the interspersion of ideas and concepts from higher education, industry, and government. As an example of this diversification, one now finds toxicology graduate programs in medical schools, schools of public health, and schools of pharmacy as well as programs in environmental science and engineering and undergraduate programs in toxicology at several institutions. Surprisingly, courses in toxicology are now being offered in several liberal arts undergraduate schools as part of their biology and chemistry curricula. This has resulted in an exciting, innovative, and diversified field that is serving science and the community at large.

Few disciplines can point to both basic sciences and direct applications at the same time. Toxicology—the study of the adverse effects of xenobiotics—may be unique in this regard.

REFERENCES

Albert A: *Selective Toxicity*. London: Methuen, 1951.

Ames BN: Dietary carcinogens and anticarcinogens. *Science* 221:1249–1264, 1983.

Bernard C: Action du curare et de la nicotine sur le systeme nerveux et sur le systme musculaire. *CR Soc Biol* 2:195, 1850.

Bernard C: *Introduction to the Study of Experimental Medicine,* trans. Greene HC, Schuman H. New York: Dover, 1949.

Carson R: *Silent Spring*. Boston: Houghton Mifflin, 1962.

Christison R: *A Treatise on Poisons,* 4th ed. Philadelphia: Barrington & Howell, 1845.

Doll R, Peto R: *The Causes of Cancer,* New York: Oxford University Press, 1981.

Donaldson HH: The history and zoological position of the albino rat. *Natl Acad Sci* 15:365–369, 1912.

DuBois K, Geiling EMK: *Textbook of Toxicology*. New York: Oxford University Press, 1959.

Gunther RT: *The Greek Herbal of Dioscorides*. New York: Oxford University Press, 1934.

Guthrie DA: *A History of Medicine*. Philadelphia: Lippincott, 1946.

Handler P: Some comments on risk assessment, in *The National Research Council in 1979: Current Issues and Studies*. Washington, DC: NAS, 1979.

Hutt PB, Hutt PB II: A history of government regulation of adulteration and misbranding of food. *Food Drug Cosmet J* 39:2–73, 1984.

Kallet A, Schlink FJ: *100,000,000 Guinea Pigs: Dangers in Everyday Foods, Drugs and Cosmetics*. New York: Vanguard, 1933.

Levey M: Medieval arabic toxicology: The book on poisons of Ibn Wahshiya and its relation to early Indian and Greek texts. *Trans Am Philos Soc* 56(7): 1966.

Lewin L: *Die Gifte in der Weltgeschichte: Toxikologische, allgemeinverstandliche Untersuchungen der historischen Quellen*. Berlin: Springer, 1920.

Lewin L: *Gifte und Vergiftungen*. Berlin: Stilke, 1929.

Loomis TA: *Essentials of Toxicology,* 3d ed. Philadelphia: Lea & Febiger, 1978.

Macht DJ: Louis Lewin: Pharmacologist, toxicologist, medical historian. *Ann Med Hist* 3:179–194, 1931.

Meek WJ: *The Gentle Art of Poisoning*. Medico-Historical Papers. Madision: University of Wisconsin, 1954; reprinted from *Phi Beta Pi Quarterly,* May 1928.

Muller P: Uber zusammenhange zwischen Konstitution und insektizider Wirkung. I. *Helv Chim Acta* 29:1560–1580, 1946.

Munter S (ed).: *Treatise on Poisons and Their Antidotes. Vol. II of the Medical Writings of Moses Maimonides*. Philadelphia: Lippincott, 1966.

Nebert D, Gonzalez FJ: P450 genes: Structure, evolution and regulation. *Annu Rev Biochem* 56:945–993, 1987.

Olmsted JMD: *François Magendie: Pioneer in Experimental Physiology and Scientific Medicine in XIX Century France*. New York: Schuman, 1944.

Orfila MJB: *Secours a Donner aux Personnes Empoisonees et Asphyxiees*. Paris: Feugeroy, 1818.

Orfila MJB: *Traite des Poisons Tires des Regnes Mineral, Vegetal et Animal, ou, Toxicologie Generale Consideree sous les Rapports de la Physiologie, de la Pathologie et de la Medecine Legale*. Paris: Crochard, 1814–1815.

Pachter HM: *Paracelsus: Magic into Science*. New York: Collier, 1961.

Pagel W: *Paracelsus: An Introduction to Philosophical Medicine in the Era of the Renaissance*. New York: Karger, 1958.

Paracelsus (Theophrastus ex Hohenheim Eremita): *Von der Besucht*. Dillingen, 1567.

Poland A, Knutson JC: 2,3,7,8-Tetrachlorodibenzo-*p*-dioxin and related halogenated aromatic hydrocarbons, examination of the mechanism of toxicity. *Annu Rev Pharmacol Toxicol* 22:517–554, 1982.

Ramazzini B: *De Morbis Artificum Diatriba*. Modena: Typis Antonii Capponi, 1700.

Robert R: *Lehrbuch der Intoxikationen*. Stuttgart: Enke, 1893.

Schmiedeberg O, Koppe R: *Das Muscarin das giftige Alkaloid des Fliegenpilzes*. Leipzig: Vogel, 1869.

Thompson CJS: *Poisons and Poisoners: With Historical Accounts of Some Famous Mysteries in Ancient and Modern Times*. London: Shaylor, 1931.

U.S. FDA: *Toxicologic Principles for the Safety Assessment of Direct Food Additives and Color Additives Used in Food*. Washington, DC: U.S. Food and Drug Administration, Bureau of Foods, 1982.

Voegtlin C, Dyer HA, Leonard CS: On the mechanism of the action of arsenic upon protoplasm. *Public Health Rep* 38:1882–1912, 1923.

Williams RT: *Detoxication Mechanisms,* 2d ed. New York: Wiley, 1959.

Zapp JA Jr, Doull J: Industrial toxicology: Retrospect and prospect, in Clayton GD, Clayton FE (eds): *Patty's Industrial Hygiene and Toxicology,* 4th ed. New York: Wiley Interscience, 1993, pp 1–23.

SUPPLEMENTAL READING

Adams F (trans.): *The Genuine Works of Hippocrates*. Baltimore: Williams & Wilkins, 1939.

Beeson BB: Orfila—pioneer toxicologist. *Ann Med Hist* 2:68–70, 1930.

Bernard C: Analyse physiologique des proprietes des systemes musculaire et nerveux au moyen du curare. *CR Acad Sci (Paris)* 43:325–329, 1856.

Bryan CP: *The Papyrus Ebers*. London: Geoffrey Bales, 1930.

Clendening L: *Source Book of Medical History*. New York: Dover, 1942.

Gaddum JH: *Pharmacology,* 5th ed. New York: Oxford University Press, 1959.

Garrison FH: *An Introduction to the History of Medicine,* 4th ed. Philadelphia: Saunders, 1929.

Hamilton A: *Exploring the Dangerous Trades*. Boston: Little, Brown, 1943. (Reprinted by Northeastern University Press, Boston, 1985.)

Hays HW: *Society of Toxicology History, 1961–1986*. Washington, DC: Society of Toxicology, 1986.

Holmstedt B, Liljestrand G: *Readings in Pharmacology*. New York: Raven Press, 1981.

CHAPTER 2

PRINCIPLES OF TOXICOLOGY

David L. Eaton and Curtis D. Klaassen

INTRODUCTION TO TOXICOLOGY

Toxicology is the study of the adverse effects of chemicals on living organisms. A *toxicologist* is trained to examine the nature of those effects (including their cellular, biochemical, and molecular mechanisms of action) and assess the probability of their occurrence. Thus, the principles of toxicology are integral to the proper use of science in the process commonly called *risk assessment,* where quantitative estimates are made of the potential effects on human health and environmental significance of various types of chemical exposures (e.g., pesticide residues on food, contaminants in drinking water). The variety of potential adverse effects and the diversity of chemicals in the environment make toxicology a very broad science. Therefore, toxicologists often specialize in one area of toxicology.

Different Areas of Toxicology

The professional activities of toxicologists fall into three main categories: descriptive, mechanistic, and regulatory (Fig. 2-1). Although each has distinctive characteristics, each contributes to the other, and all are vitally important to chemical risk assessment (see Chap. 4).

A *mechanistic toxicologist* is concerned with identifying and understanding the cellular, biochemical, and molecular mechanisms by which chemicals exert toxic effects on living organisms (see Chap. 3 for a detailed discussion of mechanisms of toxicity). The results of mechanistic studies are very important in many areas of applied toxicology. In risk assessment, mechanistic data may be very useful in demonstrating that an adverse outcome (e.g., cancer, birth defects) observed in laboratory animals is directly relevant to humans. For example, the relative toxic potential of organophosphate insecticides in humans, rodents, and insects can be accurately predicted on the basis of an understanding of common mechanisms (inhibition of acetylcholinesterase) and differences in biotransformation for these insecticides among the different species. Similarly, mechanistic data may be very useful in identifying adverse responses in experimental animals that may not be relevant to humans. For example, the propensity of the widely used artificial sweetener saccharin to cause bladder cancer in rats may not be relevant to humans at normal dietary intake rates. This is because mechanistic studies have demonstrated that bladder cancer is induced only under conditions where saccharin is at such a high concentration in the urine that it forms a crystalline precipitate (Cohen, 1999). Dose–response studies suggest that such high concentrations would not be achieved in the human bladder even after extensive dietary consumption.

Mechanistic data also are useful in the design and production of safer alternative chemicals and in rational therapy for chemical poisoning and treatment of disease. For example, the drug thalido-

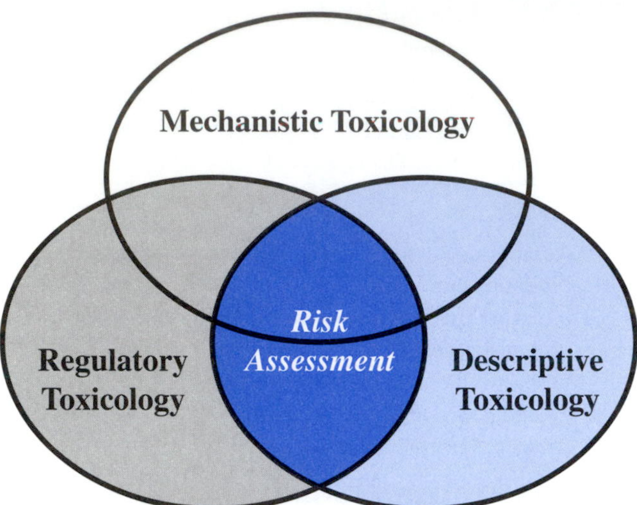

Figure 2-1. Graphical representation of the interconnections between different areas of toxicology.

mide was originally marketed in Europe as a sedative agent for pregnant women. However, it was banned for clinical use in 1962 because of devastating birth defects that occurred if the drug was ingested during a critical period in pregnancy. But mechanistic studies over the past several decades have demonstrated that this drug may have a unique molecular mechanism of action that interferes with the expression of certain genes responsible for blood vessel formation (angiogenesis). With an understanding of this mechanism, thalidomide has been "rediscovered" as a valuable therapeutic agent that may be highly effective in the treatment of certain infectious diseases (e.g., leprosy and AIDS), a variety of inflammatory diseases, and some types of cancer. Obviously, its use in pregnant women is strictly prohibited, but the discovery of this mechanism of action may now allow this drug to be used safely and effectively in the treatment of many other diseases (Lary *et al.,* 1999). In addition to aiding directly in the identification, treatment, and prevention of chemical toxicity, an understanding of the mechanisms of toxic action contributes to the knowledge of basic physiology, pharmacology, cell biology, and biochemistry. For example, studies on the toxicity of fluoroorganic alcohols and acids contributed to the knowledge of basic carbohydrate and lipid metabolism, and knowledge of regulation of ion gradients in nerve axonal membranes has been greatly aided by studies of biological toxins such as tetrodotoxin and synthetic chemicals such as DDT (dichlorodiphenyltrichloroethane). The advent of new technologies in molecular biology and genomics now provide mechanistic toxicologists with the tools to explore exactly how humans may differ from laboratory animals in their response to toxic substances. These same tools are also being utilized to identify individuals who are genetically susceptible to factors in the environment. For example, it is now recognized that a small percentage of the population genetically lacks the ability to detoxify the chemotherapeutic drug, 6-mercaptopurine, used in the treatment of some forms of leukemia. Young children with leukemia who are homozygous for this genetic trait may experience serious toxic effects from a standard therapeutic dose of this drug. Genetic tests are now available that can identify genetically susceptible individuals in advance of treatment (Weinshilboum *et al.,* 1999). This new area of 'toxicogenomics' provides an exciting opportunity in the future for mechanistic toxicologists to identify and protect genetically susceptible individuals from harmful environmental exposures, and to customize drug therapies that enhance efficacy and minimize toxicity, based on their individual genetic makeup.

A *descriptive toxicologist* is concerned directly with toxicity testing, which provides information for safety evaluation and regulatory requirements. The appropriate toxicity tests (as described later in this chapter) in experimental animals are designed to yield information that can be used to evaluate risks posed to humans and the environment by exposure to specific chemicals. The concern may be limited to effects on humans, as in the case of drugs and food additives. Toxicologists in the chemical industry, however, must be concerned not only with the risk posed by a company's chemicals (insecticides, herbicides, solvents, etc.) to humans but also with potential effects on fish, birds, and plants, as well as other factors that might disturb the balance of the ecosystem. Descriptive toxicology studies provide important clues to a chemical's mechanism of action, and thus contribute to the development of mechanistic toxicology through hypothesis generation. Such studies are also a key component of risk assessments that are used by regulatory toxicologists.

A *regulatory toxicologist* has the responsibility for deciding, on the basis of data provided by descriptive and mechanistic toxicologists, whether a drug or another chemical poses a sufficiently low risk to be marketed for a stated purpose. The Food and Drug Administration (FDA) is responsible for allowing drugs, cosmetics, and food additives to be sold in the market according to the Federal Food, Drug and Cosmetic Act (FDCA). The U.S. Environmental Protection Agency (EPA) is responsible for regulating most other chemicals according to the Federal Insecticide, Fungicide and Rodenticide Act (FIFRA), the Toxic Substances Control Act (TSCA), the Resource Conservation and Recovery Act (RCRA), the Safe Drinking Water Act, and the Clean Air Act. The EPA is also responsible for enforcing the Comprehensive Environmental Response, Compensation and Liability Act [CERCLA, later revised as the Superfund Amendments Reauthorization Act (SARA)], more commonly called the Superfund. This regulation provides direction and financial support for the cleanup of waste sites that contain toxic chemicals and may present a risk to human health or the environment. The Occupational Safety and Health Administration (OSHA) of the Department of Labor was established to ensure that safe and healthful conditions exist in the workplace. The Consumer Product Safety Commission is responsible for protecting consumers from hazardous household substances, whereas the Department of Transportation (DOT) ensures that materials shipped in interstate commerce are labeled and packaged in a manner consistent with the degree of hazard they present. Regulatory toxicologists are also involved in the establishment of standards for the amount of chemicals permitted in ambient air, industrial atmospheres, and drinking water, often integrating scientific information from basic descriptive and mechanistic toxicology studies with the principles and approaches used for risk assessment (Chap. 4). Some of the philosophic and legal aspects of regulatory toxicology are discussed in Chap. 34.

In addition to the above categories, there are other specialized areas of toxicology such as forensic, clinical, and environmental toxicology. *Forensic toxicology* is a hybrid of analytic chemistry and fundamental toxicological principles. It is concerned primarily with the medicolegal aspects of the harmful effects of chemicals on humans and animals. The expertise of forensic toxicologists is invoked primarily to aid in establishing the cause of death and determining its circumstances in a postmortem investigation (Chap.

31). *Clinical toxicology* designates an area of professional emphasis in the realm of medical science that is concerned with disease caused by or uniquely associated with toxic substances (see Chap. 32). Generally, clinical toxicologists are physicians who receive specialized training in emergency medicine and poison management. Efforts are directed at treating patients poisoned with drugs or other chemicals and at the development of new techniques to treat those intoxications. *Environmental toxicology* focuses on the impacts of chemical pollutants in the environment on biological organisms. Although toxicologists concerned with the effects of environmental pollutants on human health fit into this definition, it is most commonly associated with studies on the impacts of chemicals on nonhuman organisms such as fish, birds, and terrestrial animals. *Ecotoxicology* is a specialized area within environmental toxicology that focuses more specifically on the impacts of toxic substances on population dynamics in an ecosystem. The transport, fate, and interactions of chemicals in the environment constitute a critical component of both environmental toxicology and ecotoxicology.

Spectrum of Toxic Dose

One could define a *poison* as any agent capable of producing a deleterious response in a biological system, seriously injuring function or producing death. This is not, however, a useful working definition for the very simple reason that virtually every known chemical has the potential to produce injury or death if it is present in a sufficient amount. Paracelsus (1493–1541), a Swiss/German/Austrian physician, scientist, and philosopher, phrased this well when he noted, "What is there that is not poison? All things are poison and nothing [is] without poison. Solely the dose determines that a thing is not a poison."

Among chemicals there is a wide spectrum of doses needed to produce deleterious effects, serious injury, or death. This is demonstrated in Table 2-1, which shows the dosage of chemicals needed to produce death in 50 percent of treated animals (LD_{50}). Some chemicals produce death in microgram doses and are commonly thought of as being extremely poisonous. Other chemicals may be relatively harmless after doses in excess of several grams. It should be noted, however, that measures of acute lethality such as LD_{50} may not accurately reflect the full spectrum of toxicity, or hazard, associated with exposure to a chemical. For example, some chemicals with low acute toxicity may have carcinogenic or teratogenic effects at doses that produce no evidence of acute toxicity.

Table 2-1
Approximate Acute LD_{50}s of Some Representative Chemical Agents

AGENT	LD_{50}, mg/kg*
Ethyl alcohol	10,000
Sodium chloride	4,000
Ferrous sulfate	1,500
Morphine sulfate	900
Phenobarbital sodium	150
Picrotoxin	5
Strychnine sulfate	2
Nicotine	1
d-Tubocurarine	0.5
Hemicholinium-3	0.2
Tetrodotoxin	0.10
Dioxin (TCDD)	0.001
Botulinum toxin	0.00001

*LD_{50} is the dosage (mg/kg body weight) causing death in 50 percent of exposed animals.

CLASSIFICATION OF TOXIC AGENTS

Toxic agents are classified in a variety of ways, depending on the interests and needs of the classifier. In this textbook, for example, toxic agents are discussed in terms of their target organs (liver, kidney, hematopoietic system, etc.), use (pesticide, solvent, food additive, etc.), source (animal and plant toxins), and effects (cancer, mutation, liver injury, etc.). The term *toxin* generally refers to toxic substances that are produced by biological systems such as plants, animals, fungi or bacteria. The term *toxicant* is used in speaking of toxic substances that are produced by or are a by-product of anthropogenic (human-made) activities. Thus, zeralanone, produced by a mold, is a toxin, whereas "dioxin" [2,3,7,8-tetrachlorodibenzo-*p*-dioxin (TCDD)], produced during the combustion of certain chlorinated organic chemicals, is a toxicant. Some toxicants can be produced by both natural and anthropogenic activities. For example, polyaromatic hydrocarbons are produced by the combustion of organic matter, which may occur both through natural processes (e.g., forest fires) and through anthropogenic activities (e.g., combustion of coal for energy production; cigarette smoking). Arsenic, a toxic metalloid, may occur as a natural contaminant of groundwater or may contaminate groundwater secondary to industrial activities. Generally, such toxic substances are referred to as toxicants, rather than toxins, because, although they are naturally produced, they are not produce by biological systems.

Toxic agents also may be classified in terms of their physical state (gas, dust, liquid), their chemical stability or reactivity (explosive, flammable, oxidizer), general chemical structure (aromatic amine, halogenated hydrocarbon, etc.), or poisoning potential (extremely toxic, very toxic, slightly toxic, etc.). Classification of toxic agents on the basis of their biochemical mechanisms of action (e.g., alkylating agent, sulfhydryl inhibitor, methemoglobin producer) is usually more informative than classification by general terms such as irritants and corrosives. But more general classifications such as air pollutants, occupation-related agents, and acute and chronic poisons can provide a useful focus on a specific problem. It is evident from this discussion that no single classification is applicable to the entire spectrum of toxic agents and that combinations of classification systems or a classification based on other factors may be needed to provide the best rating system for a special purpose. Nevertheless, classification systems that take into consideration both the chemical and the biological properties of an agent and the exposure characteristics are most likely to be useful for legislative or control purposes and for toxicology in general.

CHARACTERISTICS OF EXPOSURE

Toxic effects in a biological system are not produced by a chemical agent unless that agent or its metabolic breakdown (biotransformation) products reach appropriate sites in the body at a concentration and for a length of time sufficient to produce a toxic manifestation. Many chemicals are of relatively low toxicity in the "native" form but, when acted on by enzymes in the body, are converted to intermediate forms that interfere with normal cellular biochemistry and physiology. Thus, whether a toxic response occurs is dependent on the chemical and physical properties of the agent, the exposure situation, how the agent is metabolized by the system, and the overall susceptibility of the biological system or subject. Thus, to characterize fully the potential hazard of a specific chemical agent, we need to know not only what type of effect it produces and the dose required to produce that effect but also information about the agent, the exposure, and its disposition by the subject. The major factors that influence toxicity as it relates to the exposure situation for a specific chemical are the route of administration and the duration and frequency of exposure.

Route and Site of Exposure

The major routes (pathways) by which toxic agents gain access to the body are the gastrointestinal tract (ingestion), lungs (inhalation), skin (topical, percutaneous, or dermal), and other parenteral (other than intestinal canal) routes. Toxic agents generally produce the greatest effect and the most rapid response when given directly into the bloodstream (the intravenous route). An approximate descending order of effectiveness for the other routes would be inhalation, intraperitoneal, subcutaneous, intramuscular, intradermal, oral, and dermal. The "vehicle" (the material in which the chemical is dissolved) and other formulation factors can markedly alter absorption after ingestion, inhalation, or topical exposure. In addition, the route of administration can influence the toxicity of agents. For example, an agent that is detoxified in the liver would be expected to be less toxic when given via the portal circulation (oral) than when given via the systemic circulation (inhalation).

Occupational exposure to toxic agents most frequently results from breathing contaminated air (inhalation) and/or direct and prolonged contact of the skin with the substance (dermal exposure), whereas accidental and suicidal poisoning occurs most frequently by oral ingestion. Comparison of the lethal dose of a toxic substance by different routes of exposure often provides useful information about its extent of absorption. In instances when the lethal dose after oral or dermal administration is similar to the lethal dose after intravenous administration, the assumption is that the toxic agent is absorbed readily and rapidly. Conversely, in cases where the lethal dose by the dermal route is several orders of magnitude higher than the oral lethal dose, it is likely that the skin provides an effective barrier to absorption of the agent. Toxic effects by any route of exposure also can be influenced by the concentration of the agent in its vehicle, the total volume of the vehicle and the properties of the vehicle to which the biological system is exposed, and the rate at which exposure occurs. Studies in which the concentration of a chemical in the blood is determined at various times after exposure are often needed to clarify the role of these and other factors in the toxicity of a compound. For more details on the absorption of toxicants, see Chap. 5.

Duration and Frequency of Exposure

Toxicologists usually divide the exposure of experimental animals to chemicals into four categories: acute, subacute, subchronic, and chronic. Acute exposure is defined as exposure to a chemical for less than 24 h, and examples of exposure routes are intraperitoneal, intravenous, and subcutaneous injection; oral intubation; and dermal application. While acute exposure usually refers to a single administration, repeated exposures may be given within a 24-h period for some slightly toxic or practically nontoxic chemicals. Acute exposure by inhalation refers to continuous exposure for less than 24 h, most frequently for 4 h. Repeated exposure is divided into three categories: subacute, subchronic, and chronic. *Subacute exposure* refers to repeated exposure to a chemical for 1 month or less, *subchronic* for 1 to 3 months, and *chronic* for more than 3 months. These three categories of repeated exposure can be by any route, but most often they occur by the oral route, with the chemical added directly to the diet.

In human exposure situations, the frequency and duration of exposure are usually not as clearly defined as in controlled animal studies, but many of the same terms are used to describe general exposure situations. Thus, workplace or environmental exposures may be described as *acute* (occurring from a single incident or episode), *subchronic* (occurring repeatedly over several weeks or months), or *chronic* (occurring repeatedly for many months or years).

For many agents, the toxic effects that follow a single exposure are quite different from those produced by repeated exposure. For example, the primary acute toxic manifestation of benzene is central nervous system (CNS) depression, but repeated exposures can result in bone marrow toxicity and an increased risk for leukemia. Acute exposure to agents that are rapidly absorbed is likely to produce immediate toxic effects but also can produce delayed toxicity that may or may not be similar to the toxic effects of chronic exposure. Conversely, chronic exposure to a toxic agent may produce some immediate (acute) effects after each administration in addition to the long-term, low-level, or chronic effects of the toxic substance. In characterizing the toxicity of a specific chemical, it is evident that information is needed not only for the single-dose (acute) and long-term (chronic) effects but also for exposures of intermediate duration. The other time-related factor that is important in the temporal characterization of repeated exposures is the frequency of exposure. The relationship between elimination rate and frequency of exposure is shown in Fig. 2-2. A chemical that produces severe effects with a single dose may have no effect if the same total dose is given in several intervals. For the chemical depicted by line B in Fig. 2-2, in which the half-life for elimination (time necessary for 50 percent of the chemical to be removed from the bloodstream) is approximately equal to the dosing frequency, a theoretical toxic concentration of 2 U is not reached until the fourth dose, whereas that concentration is reached with only two doses for chemical A, which has an elimination rate much slower than the dosing interval (time between each repeated dose). Conversely, for chemical C, where the elimination rate is much shorter than the dosing interval, a toxic concentration at the site of toxic effect will never be reached regardless of how many doses are administered. Of course, it is possible that residual cell or tissue damage occurs with each dose even though the chemical itself is not accumulating. The important consideration, then, is whether the interval between doses is sufficient to allow for complete repair of tissue damage. It is evident that with any type of repeated exposure, the production of a toxic effect is influenced not only by the frequency of exposure but may, in fact, be totally dependent on the frequency rather than the duration of exposure. Chronic toxic effects may occur, therefore, if the chemical accumulates in the biological system (rate of absorption exceeds the rate of biotransformation and/or excretion), if it produces irreversible toxic effects, or if there is insufficient time for the system to recover from the toxic damage within the exposure frequency interval. For additional discussion of these relationships, consult Chaps. 5 and 7.

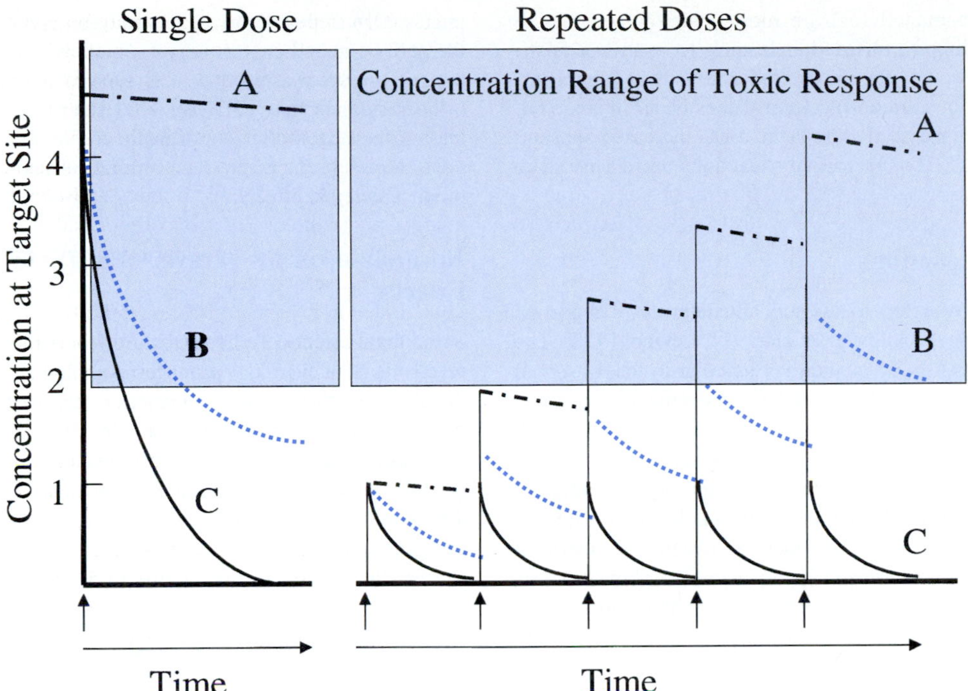

Figure 2-2.** **Diagrammatic view of the relationship between dose and concentration at the target site under different conditions of dose frequency and elimination rate.

Line A. A chemical with very slow elimination (e.g., half-life of 1 year). *Line B.* A chemical with a rate of elimination equal to frequency of dosing (e.g., 1 day). *Line C.* Rate of elimination faster than the dosing frequency (e.g., 5 h). Blue-shaded area is representative of the concentration of chemical at the target site necessary to elicit a toxic response.

SPECTRUM OF UNDESIRED EFFECTS

The spectrum of undesired effects of chemicals is broad. Some effects are deleterious and others are not. In therapeutics, for example, each drug produces a number of effects, but usually only one effect is associated with the primary objective of the therapy; all the other effects are referred to as *undesirable* or *side effects* of that drug for that therapeutic indication. However, some of these side effects may be desired for another therapeutic indication. For example, the "first-generation" antihistamine diphenhydramine (Benadryl) is effective in reducing histamine responses associated with allergies, but it readily enters the brain and causes mild CNS depression (drowsiness, delayed reaction time). With the advent of newer histamine (H_1) receptor antagonists that do not cross the blood-brain barrier and thus do not have this CNS-depressant side effect, the drug is used less commonly today as an antihistamine. However, it is widely used as an "over the counter" sleep remedy in combination with analgesics (e.g., Tylenol PM, Excedrin PM, etc), taking advantage of the CNS-depressant effects. Some side effects of drugs are never desirable and are always deleterious to the well-being of humans. These are referred to as the *adverse, deleterious,* or *toxic* effects of the drug.

Allergic Reactions

Chemical allergy is an immunologically mediated adverse reaction to a chemical resulting from previous sensitization to that chemical or to a structurally similar one. The term *hypersensitivity* is most often used to describe this allergic state, but *allergic reaction* and *sensitization reaction* are also used to describe this situation when preexposure of the chemical is required to produce the toxic effect (see Chap. 12). Once sensitization has occurred, allergic reactions may result from exposure to relatively very low doses of chemicals; therefore population-based dose–response curves for allergic reactions have seldom been obtained. Because of this omission, some people assumed that allergic reactions are not dose-related. Thus, they do not consider the allergic reaction to be a true toxic response. However, for a given allergic individual, allergic reactions are dose-related. For example, it is well known that the allergic response to pollen in sensitized individuals is related to the concentration of pollen in the air. In addition, because the allergic response is an undesirable, adverse, deleterious effect, it obviously is also a toxic response. Sensitization reactions are sometimes very severe and may be fatal.

Most chemicals and their metabolic products are not sufficiently large to be recognized by the immune system as a foreign substance and thus must first combine with an endogenous protein to form an antigen (or immunogen). A molecule that must combine with an endogenous protein to elicit an allergic reaction is called a *hapten.* The hapten-protein complex (antigen) is then capable of eliciting the formation of antibodies, and usually at least 1 or 2 weeks is required for the synthesis of significant amounts of antibodies. Subsequent exposure to the chemical results in an antigen–antibody interaction, which provokes the typical manifestations of allergy. The manifestations of allergy are numerous. They may involve various organ systems and range in severity from minor skin disturbance to fatal anaphylactic shock. The pattern of allergic response differs in various species. In humans, involvement of the skin (e.g., dermatitis, urticaria, and itching) and involvement of the eyes (e.g., conjunctivitis) are most common, whereas in guinea pigs, bronchiolar constriction leading to asphyxia is the most common. However, chemically induced asthma (characterized by bronchiolar constriction) certainly does occur in some humans, and the incidence of allergic asthma has increased substantially in recent years. Hypersensitivity reactions are discussed in more detail in Chap. 12.

Idiosyncratic Reactions

Chemical idiosyncrasy refers to a genetically determined abnormal reactivity to a chemical (Goldstein et al., 1974; Levine, 1978). The response observed is usually qualitatively similar to that observed in all individuals but may take the form of extreme sensitivity to low doses or extreme insensitivity to high doses of the chemical. However, while some people use the term *idiosyncratic* as a catchall to refer to all reactions that occur with low frequency, it should not be used in that manner (Goldstein et al., 1974). A classic example of an idiosyncratic reaction is provided by patients who exhibit prolonged muscular relaxation and apnea (inability to breathe) lasting several hours after a standard dose of succinylcholine. Succinylcholine usually produces skeletal muscle relaxation of only short duration because of its very rapid metabolic degradation by an enzyme that is present normally in the bloodstream called plasma butyrylcholinesterase (also referred to as pseudocholinesterase). Patients exhibiting this idiosyncratic reaction have a genetic polymorphism in the gene for the enzyme butyrylcholinesterase, which is less active in breaking down succinylcholine. Family pedigree and molecular genetic analyses have demonstrated that the presence of low plasma butyrylcholinesterase activity is due to the presence of one or more single nucleotide polymorphisms in this gene (Bartels et al., 1992). Similarly, there is a group of people who are abnormally sensitive to nitrites and certain other chemicals that have in common the ability to oxidize the iron in hemoglobin to produce *methemoglobin,* which is incapable of carrying oxygen to the tissues. The unusual phenotype is inherited as an autosomal recessive trait and is characterized by a deficiency in NADH-cytochrome b5 reductase activity. The genetic basis for this idiosyncratic response has been identified as a single nucleotide change in codon 127, which results in replacement of serine with proline (Kobayashi et al., 1990). The consequence of this genetic deficiency is that these individuals may suffer from a serious lack of oxygen delivery to tissues after exposure to doses of methemoglobin-producing chemicals that would be harmless to individuals with normal NADH-cytochrome b5 reductase activity.

Immediate versus Delayed Toxicity

Immediate toxic effects can be defined as those that occur or develop rapidly after a single administration of a substance, whereas delayed toxic effects are those that occur after the lapse of some time. Carcinogenic effects of chemicals usually have a long latency period, often 20 to 30 years after the initial exposure, before tumors are observed in humans. For example, daughters of mothers who took diethylstilbestrol (DES) during pregnancy have a greatly increased risk of developing vaginal cancer, but not other types of cancer, in young adulthood, some 20 to 30 years after their in utero exposure to DES (Hatch et al., 1998). Also, delayed neurotoxicity is observed after exposure to some organophosphorus insecticides that act by covalent modification of an enzyme referred to as *neuropathy target esterase* (NTE), a neuronal protein with serine esterase activity (Glynn et al., 1999). Binding of certain organophosphates (OP) to this protein initiates degeneration of long axons in the peripheral and central nervous system. The most notorious of the compounds that produce this type of neurotoxic effect is triorthocresylphosphate (TOCP). The effect is not observed until at least several days after exposure to the toxic compound. In contrast, most substances produce immediate toxic effects but do not produce delayed effects.

Reversible versus Irreversible Toxic Effects

Some toxic effects of chemicals are reversible, and others are irreversible. If a chemical produces pathological injury to a tissue, the ability of that tissue to regenerate largely determines whether the effect is reversible or irreversible. Thus, for a tissue such as liver, which has a high ability to regenerate, most injuries are reversible, whereas injury to the CNS is largely irreversible because differentiated cells of the CNS cannot divide and be replaced. Carcinogenic and teratogenic effects of chemicals, once they occur, are usually considered irreversible toxic effects.

Local versus Systemic Toxicity

Another distinction between types of effects is made on the basis of the general site of action. Local effects are those that occur at the site of first contact between the biological system and the toxicant. Such effects are produced by the ingestion of caustic substances or the inhalation of irritant materials. For example, chlorine gas reacts with lung tissue at the site of contact, causing damage and swelling of the tissue, with possibly fatal consequences, even though very little of the chemical is absorbed into the bloodstream. The alternative to local effects is systemic effects. Systemic effects require absorption and distribution of a toxicant from its entry point to a distant site, at which deleterious effects are produced. Most substances except highly reactive materials produce systemic effects. For some materials, both effects can be demonstrated. For example, tetraethyl lead produces effects on skin at the site of absorption and then is transported systemically to produce its typical effects on the CNS and other organs. If the local effect is marked, there may also be indirect systemic effects. For example, kidney damage after a severe acid burn is an indirect systemic effect because the toxicant does not reach the kidney.

Most chemicals that produce systemic toxicity do not cause a similar degree of toxicity in all organs; instead, they usually elicit their major toxicity in only one or two organs. These sites are referred to as the *target organs* of toxicity of a particular chemical. The target organ of toxicity is often not the site of the highest concentration of the chemical. For example, lead is concentrated in bone, but its toxicity is due to its effects in soft tissues, particularly the brain. DDT is concentrated in adipose tissue but produces no known toxic effects in that tissue.

The target organ of toxicity most frequently involved in systemic toxicity is the CNS (brain and spinal cord). Even with many compounds having a prominent effect elsewhere, damage to the CNS can be demonstrated by the use of appropriate and sensitive methods. Next in order of frequency of involvement in systemic toxicity are the circulatory system; the blood and hematopoietic system; visceral organs such as the liver, kidney, and lung; and the skin. Muscle and bone are least often the target tissues for systemic effects. With substances that have a predominantly local effect, the frequency with which tissues react depends largely on the portal of entry (skin, gastrointestinal tract, or respiratory tract).

INTERACTION OF CHEMICALS

Because of the large number of different chemicals an individual may come in contact with at any given time (workplace, drugs, diet, hobbies, etc.), it is necessary, in assessing the spectrum of responses, to consider how different chemicals may interact with each other. Interactions can occur in a variety of ways. Chemical interactions are known to occur by a number of mechanisms, such as alterations in absorption, protein binding, and the biotransformation and excretion of one or both of the interacting toxicants. In addition to these modes of interaction, the response of the organism to combinations of toxicants may be increased or decreased because of toxicologic responses at the site of action.

The effects of two chemicals given simultaneously produce a response that may simply be additive of their individual responses or may be greater or less than that expected by addition of their individual responses. The study of these interactions often leads to a better understanding of the mechanism of toxicity of the chemicals involved. A number of terms have been used to describe pharmacologic and toxicologic interactions. An *additive* effect occurs when the combined effect of two chemicals is equal to the sum of the effects of each agent given alone (example: 2 + 3 = 5). The effect most commonly observed when two chemicals are given together is an additive effect. For example, when two organophosphate insecticides are given together, the cholinesterase inhibition is usually additive. A *synergistic* effect occurs when the combined effects of two chemicals are much greater than the sum of the effects of each agent given alone (example: 2 + 2 = 20). For example, both carbon tetrachloride and ethanol are hepatotoxic compounds, but together they produce much more liver injury than the mathematical sum of their individual effects on liver at a given dose would suggest. *Potentiation* occurs when one substance does not have a toxic effect on a certain organ or system but when added to another chemical makes that chemical much more toxic (example: 0 + 2 = 10). Isopropanol, for example, is not hepatotoxic, but when it is administered in addition to carbon tetrachloride, the hepatotoxicity of carbon tetrachloride is much greater than that when it is given alone. *Antagonism* occurs when two chemicals administered together interfere with each other's actions or one interferes with the action of the other (example: 4 + 6 = 8; 4 + (−4) = 0; 4 + 0 = 1). Antagonistic effects of chemicals are often very desirable in toxicology and are the basis of many antidotes. There are four major types of antagonism: functional, chemical, dispositional, and receptor. *Functional antagonism* occurs when two chemicals counterbalance each other by producing opposite effects on the same physiologic function. Advantage is taken of this principle in that the blood pressure can markedly fall during severe barbiturate intoxication, which can be effectively antagonized by the intravenous administration of a vasopressor agent such as norepinephrine or metaraminol. Similarly, many chemicals, when given at toxic dose levels, produce convulsions, and the convulsions often can be controlled by giving anticonvulsants such as the benzodiazepines (e.g., diazepam). *Chemical antagonism* or *inactivation* is simply a chemical reaction between two compounds that produces a less toxic product. For example, dimercaprol (British antilewisite, or BAL) chelates with metal ions such as arsenic, mercury, and lead and decreases their toxicity. The use of antitoxins in the treatment of various animal toxins is also an example of chemical antagonism. The use of the strongly basic low-molecular-weight protein protamine sulfate to form a stable complex with heparin, which abolishes its anticoagulant activity, is another example. *Dispositional antagonism* occurs when the disposition—that is, the absorption, biotransformation, distribution, or excretion of a chemical—is altered so that the concentration and/or duration of the chemical at the target organ are diminished. Thus, the prevention of absorption of a toxicant by ipecac or charcoal and the increased excretion of a chemical by administration of an osmotic diuretic or alteration of the pH of the urine are examples of dispositional antagonism. If the parent compound is responsible for the toxicity of the chemical (such as the anticoagulant warfarin) and its metabolic breakdown products are less toxic than the parent compound, increasing the compound's metabolism (biotransformation) by administering a drug that increases the activity of the metabolizing enzymes (e.g., a "microsomal enzyme inducer" such as phenobarbital) will decrease its toxicity. However, if the chemical's toxicity is largely due to a metabolic product (as in the case of the organophosphate insecticide parathion), inhibiting its biotransformation by an inhibitor of microsomal enzyme activity (SKF-525A or piperonyl butoxide) will decrease its toxicity. *Receptor antagonism* occurs when two chemicals that bind to the same receptor produce less of an effect when given together than the addition of their separate effects (example: 4 + 6 = 8) or when one chemical antagonizes the effect of the second chemical (example: 0 + 4 = 1). Receptor antagonists are often termed *blockers*. This concept is used to advantage in the clinical treatment of poisoning. For example, the receptor antagonist naloxone is used to treat the respiratory depressive effects of morphine and other morphine-like narcotics by competitive binding to the same receptor. Another example of receptor antagonism is the use of the antiestrogen drug tamoxifen to lower breast cancer risk among women at high risk for this estrogen-related cancer. Tamoxifen competitively block estradiol from binding to its receptor. Treatment of organophosphate insecticide poisoning with atropine is an example not of the antidote competing with the poison for the receptor (cholinesterase) but involves blocking the receptor (cholinergic receptor) for the excess acetylcholine that accumulates by poisoning of the cholinesterase by the organophosphate (see Chap. 22).

TOLERANCE

Tolerance is a state of decreased responsiveness to a toxic effect of a chemical resulting from prior exposure to that chemical or to a structurally related chemical. Two major mechanisms are responsible for tolerance: one is due to a decreased amount of toxicant reaching the site where the toxic effect is produced (*dispositional tolerance*), and the other is due to a reduced responsiveness of a tissue to the chemical. Comparatively less is known about the cellular mechanisms responsible for altering the responsiveness of a tissue to a toxic chemical than is known about dispositional tolerance. Two chemicals known to produce dispositional tolerance are carbon tetrachloride and cadmium. Carbon tetrachloride produces tolerance to itself by decreasing the formation of the reactive metabolite (trichloromethyl radical) that produces liver injury (Chap. 13). The mechanism of cadmium tolerance is explained by induction of metallothionein, a metal-binding protein. Subsequent binding of cadmium to metallothionein rather than to critical macromolecules thus decreases its toxicity.

DOSE RESPONSE

The characteristics of exposure and the spectrum of effects come together in a correlative relationship customarily referred to as the *dose–response relationship*. Whatever response is selected for measurement, the relationship between the degree of response of the biological system and the amount of toxicant administered assumes a form that occurs so consistently as to be considered the most fundamental and pervasive concept in toxicology.

From a practical perspective, there are two types of dose-response relationships: (1) the individual dose–response relationship, which describes the response of an *individual* organism to varying doses of a chemical, often referred to as a "graded" response because the measured effect is continuous over a range of doses, and (2) a quantal dose–response relationship, which characterizes the distribution of responses to different doses in a *population* of individual organisms.

Individual, or Graded, Dose–Response Relationships

Individual dose–response relationships are characterized by a dose-related increase in the severity of the response. The dose relatedness of the response often results from an alteration of a specific biochemical process. For example, Fig. 2-3 shows the dose–response relationship between different dietary doses of the organophosphate insecticide chlorpyrifos and the extent of inhibition of two different enzymes in the brain and liver: acetylcholinesterase and carboxylesterase. In the brain, the degree of inhibition of both enzymes is clearly dose-related and spans a wide range, although the amount of inhibition per unit dose is different for the two enzymes. From the shapes of these two dose–response curves it is evident that, in the brain, cholinesterase is more easily inhibited than carboxylesterase. The toxicologic response that results is directly related to the degree of cholinesterase enzyme inhibition in the brain. Thus, clinical signs and symptoms for chlorpyrifos would follow a dose–response relationship similar to that for brain cholinesterase. However, for many chemicals, more than one effect may result because of multiple different target sites in different tissues. Thus, the observed response to varying doses of a chemical in the whole organism is often complicated by the fact that most toxic substances have multiple sites or mechanisms of toxicity, each with its own "dose–response" relationship and subsequent adverse effect. Note that when these dose–response data are plotted using the base 10 log of the dose on the abscissa (Fig. 2.3*B*), a better "fit" of the data to a straight line occurs. This is typical of many graded as well as quantal dose–response relationships.

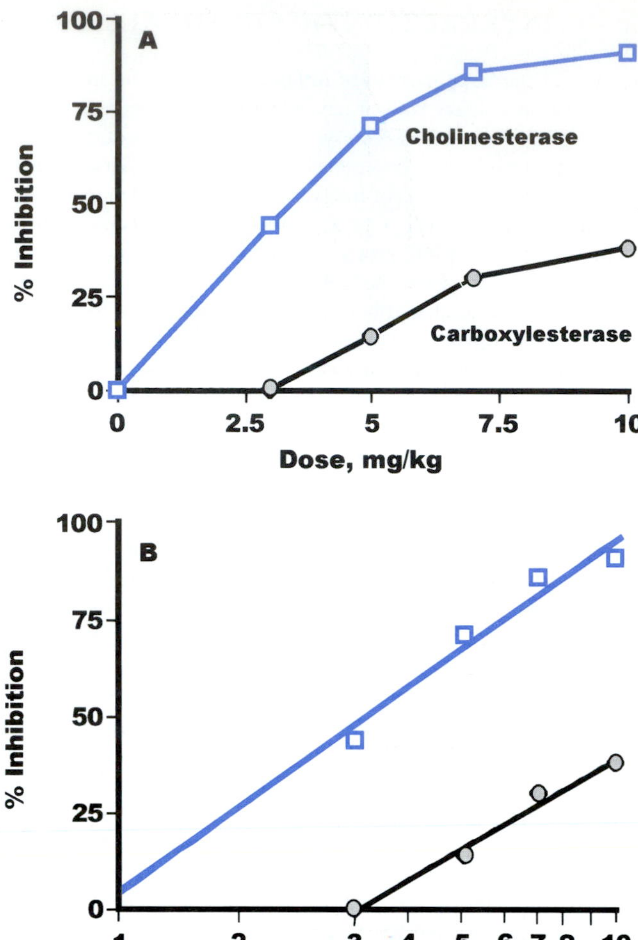

Figure 2-3. Dose–response relationship between different doses of the organophosphate insecticide chlorpyrifos and esterase enzyme inhibition in the brain.

Open circles and blue lines represent acetylcholinesterase activity and closed circles represent carboxylesterase activity in the brains of pregnant female Long-Evans rats given 5 daily doses of chlorpyrifos. *A.* Dose–response curve plotted on an arithmetic scale. *B.* Same data plotted on a semi-log scale. (Data derived from Lassiter et al., Gestational exposure to chloryprifos: Dose response profiles for cholinesterase and carboxylesterase activity. *Toxicol Sci* 52:92–100, 1999, with permission.)

Quantal Dose–Response Relationships

In contrast to the "graded" or continuous-scale dose–response relationship that occurs in individuals, the dose–response relationships in a *population* are by definition quantal—or "all or none"—in nature; that is, at any given dose, an individual in the population is classified as either a "responder" or a "nonresponder." Although these distinctions of "quantal population" and "graded individual" dose–response relationships are useful, the two types of responses are conceptually identical. The ordinate in both cases is simply labeled *the response,* which may be the degree of response in an individual or system or the fraction of a population responding, and the abscissa is the range in administered doses.

In toxicology, the quantal dose response is used extensively. Determination of the median lethal dose (LD_{50}) is usually the first experiment performed with a new chemical. The LD_{50} is the statistically derived single dose of a substance that can be expected to cause death in 50 percent of the animals tested. Typically, groups of animals are dosed at different levels, and the mortality that results in each dose group is recorded. The top panel of Fig. 2-4 shows that quantal dose responses such as lethality exhibit a normal or gaussian distribution. The frequency histogram in this panel also shows the relationship between dose and effect. The bars represent the percentage of animals that died at each dose minus the percentage that died at the immediately lower dose. One can clearly see that only a few animals responded to the lowest dose and the highest dose. Larger numbers of animals responded to doses intermediate between these two extremes, and the maximum frequency of response occurred in the middle portion of the dose range. Thus, we have a bell-shaped curve known as a *normal frequency distribution.* The reason for this normal distribution is that there are differences in susceptibility to chemicals among individ-

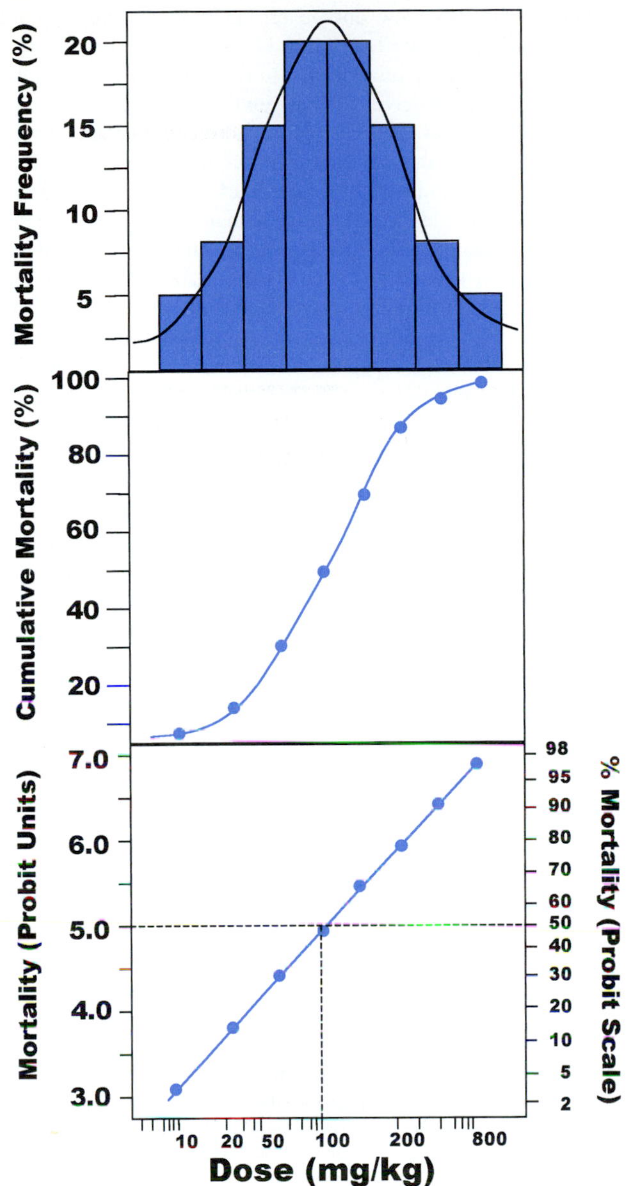

Figure 2-4. Diagram of quantal dose–response relationship.

The abscissa is a log dosage of the chemical. In the top panel the ordinate is mortality frequency, in the middle panel the ordinate is percent mortality, and in the bottom panel the mortality is in probit units (see text).

uals; this is known as biological variation. Animals responding at the left end of the curve are referred to as *hypersusceptible,* and those at the right end of the curve are called *resistant.* If the numbers of individuals responding at each consecutive dose are added together, a cumulative, quantal dose–response relationship is obtained. When a sufficently large number of doses is used with a large number of animals per dose, a sigmoid dose–response curve is observed, as depicted in the middle panel of Fig. 2-4. With the lowest dose (6 mg/kg), 1 percent of the animals die. A normally distributed sigmoid curve such as this one approaches a response of 0 percent as the dose is decreased and approaches 100 percent as the dose is increased; but—theoretically—it never passes through 0 and 100 percent. However, the minimally effective dose of any chemical that evokes a stated all-or-none response is called the *threshold dose* even though it cannot be determined experimentally.

The sigmoid curve has a relatively linear portion between 16 and 84 percent. These values represent the limits of 1 standard deviation (SD) of the mean (and the median) in a population with truly normal or gaussian distribution. However, it is usually not practical to describe the dose–response curve from this type of plot because one does not usually have large enough sample sizes to define the sigmoid curve adequately. In a normally distributed population, the mean ± 1 SD represents 68.3 percent of the population, the mean ± 2 SD represents 95.5 percent of the population, and the mean ± 3 SD equals 99.7 percent of the population. Since quantal dose–response phenomena are usually normally distributed, one can convert the percent response to units of deviation from the mean or normal equivalent deviations (NEDs). Thus, the NED for a 50 percent response is 0; an NED of $+1$ is equated with an 84.1 percent response. Later, it was suggested (Bliss, 1957) that units of NED be converted by the addition of 5 to the value to avoid negative numbers and that these converted units be called *probit units.* The probit (from the contraction of *prob*ability un*it*), then, is an NED plus 5. In this transformation, a 50 percent response becomes a probit of 5, a $+1$ deviation becomes a probit of 6, and a -1 deviation is a probit of 4.

The data given in the top two panels of Fig. 2-4 are replotted in the bottom panel with the mortality plotted in probit units. The data in the middle panel (which was in the form of a sigmoid curve) and the top panel (a bell-shaped curve) form a straight line when transformed into probit units. In essence, what is accomplished in a probit transformation is an adjustment of mortality or other quantal data to an assumed normal population distribution, resulting in a straight line. The LD_{50} is obtained by drawing a horizontal line from the probit unit 5, which is the 50 percent mortality point, to the dose–effect line. At the point of intersection, a vertical line is drawn, and this line intersects the abscissa at the LD_{50} point. It is evident from the line that information with respect to the lethal dose for 90 percent or for 10 percent of the population also may be derived by a similar procedure. Mathematically, it can be demonstrated that the range of values encompassed by the confidence limits is narrowest at the midpoint of the line (LD_{50}) and widest at both extremes (LD_{10} and LD_{90}) of the dose–response curve (dotted lines in Fig. 2-5). In addition to the LD_{50}, the slope of the dose–response curve can also be obtained. Figure 2-5 demonstrates the dose–response curves for the mortality of two compounds. Compound A exhibits a "flat" dose–response curve, showing that a large change in dosage is required before a significant change in response will be observed. However, compound B exhibits a "steep" dose–response curve, where a relatively small change in dosage will cause a large change in response. It is evident that the LD_{50} for both compounds is the same (8 mg/kg). However, the slopes of the dose–response curves are quite different. At one-half of LD_{50} of the compounds (4 mg/kg), less than 1 percent of the animals exposed to compound B would die but 20 percent of the animals given compound A would die.

The *quantal all-or-none response* is not limited to lethality. Similar dose–response curves can be constructed for cancer, liver injury, and other types of toxic responses as well as for beneficial therapeutic responses such as anesthesia or lowering of blood pressure. This is usually performed by measuring a particular parameter (e.g., blood pressure) in a large number of control animals and determining its standard deviation, which is a measure of its vari-

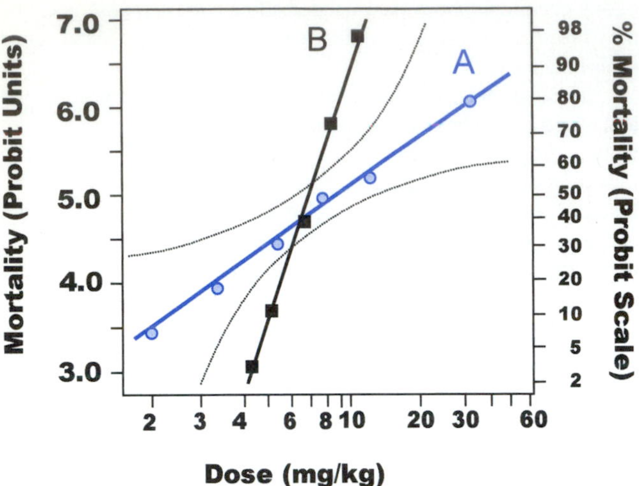

Figure 2-5. Comparison of dose–response relationship for two different chemicals, plotted on a log dose-probit scale.

Note that the slope of the dose–response is steeper for chemical *B* than chemical *A*. Dotted lines represents the confidence limits for chemical *A*.

ability. Because the mean +3 SD represents 99.7 percent of the population, one can assign all animals that lie outside this range after treatment with a chemical as being affected and those lying within this range as not being affected by the chemical. Using a series of doses of the chemical, one thus can construct a quantal dose–response curve similar to that described above for lethality.

In Figs. 2-4 and 2-5 the dosage has been given on a log basis. Although the use of the log of the dosage is empiric, log-dosage plots for normally distributed quantal data provide a more nearly linear representation of the data. It must be remembered, however, that this is not universally the case. Some radiation effects, for example, give a better probit fit when the dose is expressed arithmetically rather than logarithmically. There are other situations in which other functions (e.g., exponentials) of dosage provide a better fit to the data than does the log function. It is also conventional to express the dosage in milligrams per kilogram. It might be argued that expression of dosage on a mole-per-kilogram basis would be better, particularly for making comparisons among a series of compounds. Although such an argument has considerable merit, dosage is usually expressed in milligrams per kilogram.

One might also view dosage on the basis of body weight as being less appropriate than other bases, such as surface area, which is approximately proportional to (body weight)$^{2/3}$. In Table 2-2 selected values are given to compare the differences in dosage by the two alternatives. Given a dose of 100 mg/kg, it can be seen that the dose (milligrams per animal), of course, is proportional to the dose administered by body weight. Surface area is not proportional to weight: While the weight of a human is 3500 times greater than that of a mouse, the surface area of humans is only about 390 times greater than that of mice. Chemicals are usually administered in toxicologic studies as milligrams per kilogram. The same dose given to humans and mice on a weight basis (mg/kg) would be approximately 10 times greater in humans than mice if that dosage were expressed per surface area (mg/cm^2). Cancer chemotherapeutic agents are usually administered on the basis of surface area.

Shape of the Dose–Response Curve

Essential Nutrients The shape of the dose–response relationship has many important implications in toxicity assessment. For example, for substances that are required for normal physiologic function and survival (e.g., vitamins and essential trace elements such as chromium, cobalt, and selenium), the shape of the "graded" dose–response relationship in an individual over the entire dose range is actually U-shaped (Fig. 2-6). That is, at very low doses, there is a high level of adverse effect, which decreases with an increasing dose. This region of the dose–response relationship for essential nutrients is commonly referred to as a *deficiency*. As the dose is increased to a point where the deficiency no longer exists, no adverse response is detected and the organism is in a state of homeostasis. However, as the dose is increased to abnormally high levels, an adverse response (usually qualitatively different from that observed at deficient doses) appears and increases in magnitude with increasing dose, just as with other toxic substances. Thus, it is recognized that high doses of vitamin A can cause liver toxicity and birth defects, high doses of selenium can affect the brain, and high doses of estrogens may increase the risk of breast cancer, even though low doses of all these substances are essential for life.

Hormesis There is considerable evidence to suggest that some nonnutritional toxic substances may also impart beneficial or stimulatory effects at low doses but that, at higher doses, they produce adverse effects. This concept of "hormesis" was first described for

Table 2-2
Comparison of Dosage by Weight and Surface Area

	WEIGHT g	DOSAGE mg/kg	DOSE mg/animal	SURFACE AREA cm^2	DOSAGE mg/cm^2
Mouse	20	100	2	46	0.043
Rat	200	100	20	325	0.061
Guinea pig	400	100	40	565	0.071
Rabbit	1500	100	150	1270	0.118
Cat	2000	100	200	1380	0.145
Monkey	4000	100	400	2980	0.134
Dog	12,000	100	1200	5770	0.207
Human	70,000	100	7000	18,000	0.388

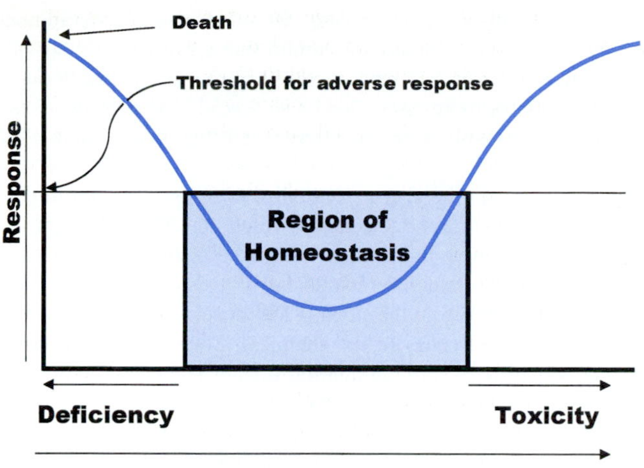

Figure 2-6. Individual dose–response relationship for an essential substance such as a vitamin or trace element.

It is generally recognized that, for most types of toxic responses, a threshold exists such that at doses below the threshold, no toxicity is evident. For essential substances, doses below the minimum daily requirement, as well as those above the threshold for safety, may be associated with toxic effects. The blue-shaded region represents the "region of homeostasis"—the dose range that results in neither deficiency or toxicity.

radiation effects but may also pertain to certain chemical responses (Calabrese and Baldwin, 1999). Thus, in plotting dose versus response over a wide range of doses, the effects of hormesis may also result in a "U-shaped" dose–response curve. In its original development, the concept of hormesis pertained to the ability of substances to stimulate biological systems at low doses but to inhibit them at high doses. The application of the concept of hormesis to whole-animal toxicologic dose–response relationships may also be relevant but requires that the "response" on the ordinate be variant with dose. For example, chronic alcohol consumption is well recognized to increase the risk of esophageal cancer, liver cancer, and cirrhosis of the liver at relatively high doses, and this response is dose-related (curve A, Fig. 2-7). However, there is also substantial clinical and epidemiologic evidence that low to moderate consumption of alcohol reduces the incidence of coronary heart disease and stroke (curve B, Fig. 2-7) (Hanna *et al.,* 1997). Thus, when all responses are plotted on the ordinate, a "U-shaped" dose–response curve is obtained (curve C, Fig. 2-7). U-shaped dose–response relationships have obvious implications for the process of low dose extrapolation in risk assessment.

Another important aspect of the dose–response relationship at low doses is the concept of the threshold. It has long been recognized that acute toxicologic responses are associated with thresholds; that is, there is some dose below which the probability of an individual responding is zero. Obviously, the identification of a threshold depends on the particular response that is measured, the sensitivity of the measurement, and the number of subjects studied. For the individual dose–response relationship, thresholds for most toxic effects certainly exist, although interindividual variability in response and qualitative changes in response pattern with dose make it difficult to establish a true "no effects" threshold for any chemical. The biological basis of thresholds for acute responses is well established and frequently can be demonstrated on the basis of mechanistic information (Aldridge, 1986). The traditional approaches to establishing acceptable levels of exposure to chemicals are inherently different for threshold versus nonthreshold responses. The existence of thresholds for chronic responses is less well defined, especially in the area of chemical carcinogenesis. It is, of course, impossible to scientifically prove the absence of a threshold, as one can never prove a negative. Nevertheless, for the identification of "safe" levels of exposure to a substance, the absence or presence of a threshold is important for practical reasons (Chap. 4). A classic example of the difficulty of establishing thresholds experimentally is provided by the "ED01" study, where over 24,000 mice and 81 different treatment groups were used to determine the shape of the dose–response relationship for the proto-

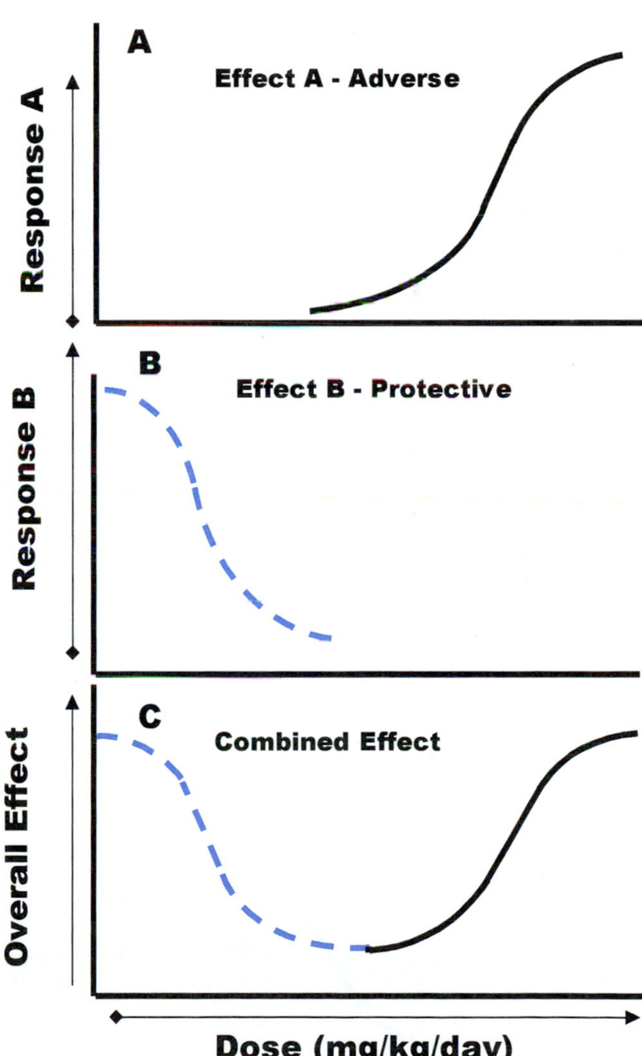

Figure 2-7. Hypothetical dose–response relationship depicting characteristics of hormesis.

Hormetic effects of a substance are hypothesized to occur when relatively low doses result in the stimulation of a beneficial or protective response (*B*), such as induction of enzymatic pathways that protect against oxidative stress. Although low doses provide a potential beneficial effect, a threshold is exceeded as the dose increases and the net effects will be detrimental (*A*), resulting in a typical dose-related increase in toxicity. The complete dose–response curve (*C*) is conceptually similar to the individual dose–response relationship for essential nutrients shown in Fig. 2-6.

typical carcinogen 2-acetylaminofluorene (2-AAF). The study was designed to identify a statistically significant response of 1 percent (0.01 probability). The mice were exposed to 2-AAF at one of seven different doses in the dose range of 30 to 150 ppm (plus 0 dose control) (Littlefield et al., 1979). Eight "sacrifice intervals" were used to determine how quickly tumors developed. The dose–response relationship between 2-AAF exposure and liver and bladder cancer at 24 and 33 months of exposure are shown in Fig. 2-8. Both types of tumors demonstrated increasing incidence with increasing dose, but the shapes of the two curves are dramatically different. For liver tumors, no clear threshold was evident, whereas for bladder tumors, an apparent threshold was evident. However, the apparent threshold, or "no observable adverse effect level" (NOAEL), for bladder cancer was lower at 33 months (45 ppm) than at 24 months (75 ppm). Of course, the ability to detect a low incidence of tumors depends on the number of animals used in the study. Thus, although a threshold (a dose below which no response occurs) appears evident for bladder tumors in Fig. 2-8, one cannot say for certain that tumors would not occur if more animals had been included in the lower-dose groups. (See Chap. 4 for more discussion on statistical issues related to extrapolation of dose–response curves and the determination of NOAELs.)

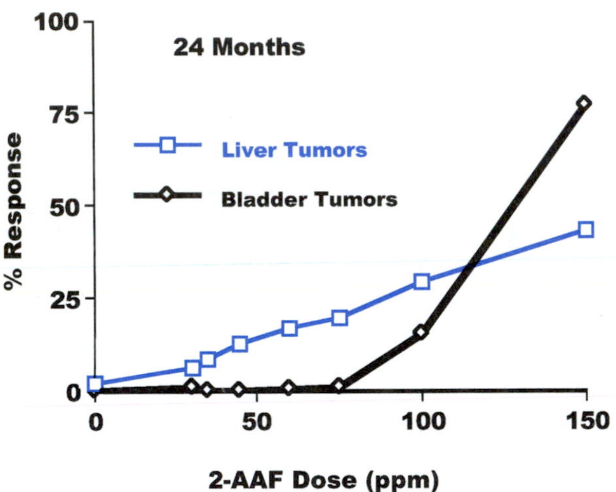

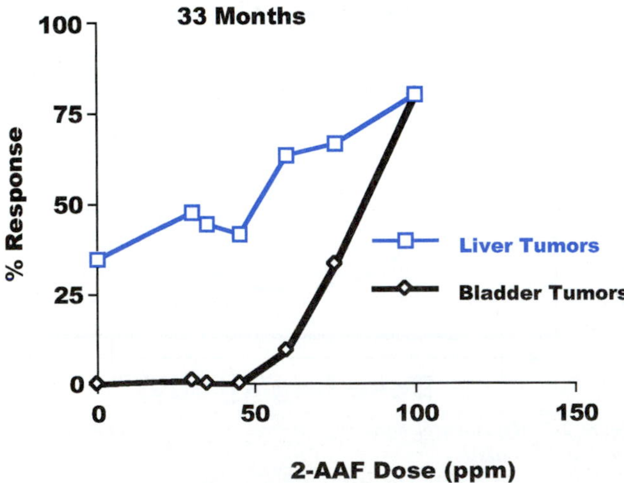

Figure 2-8. Dose–response relationship for carcinogens.

Eight groups of male mice were administered 2-acetylaminofluorine (2-AAF) in the diet from weaning. The percent of animals with liver (*blue line*) or bladder (*black line*) tumors at 24 months (*A*) or 33 months (*B*) are shown. Most of the animals in the high-dose group (150 ppm) did not survive to 33 months; thus, those data are not shown in *B*.

In evaluating the shape of the dose–response relationship in populations, it is realistic to consider inflections in the shape of the dose–response curve rather than absolute thresholds. That is, the slope of the dose–response relationship at high doses may be substantially different from the slope at low doses, usually because of dispositional differences in the chemical. Saturation of biotransformation pathways, protein-binding sites or receptors, and depletion of intracellular cofactors represent some reasons why sharp inflections in the dose–response relationship may occur. For example, the widely used analgesic acetaminophen has a very low rate of liver toxicity at normal therapeutic doses. Even though a toxic metabolite [*N*-acetyl-*p*-benzoquinoneimine (NAPQI)] is produced in the liver at therapeutic doses, it is rapidly detoxified through conjugation with the intracellular antioxidant glutathione. However, at very high doses, the level of intracellular glutathione in the liver is depleted and NAPQI accumulates, causing serious and potentially fatal liver toxicity. This effect is analogous to the rapid change in pH of a buffered solution that occurs when the buffer capacity is exceeded. Some toxic responses, most notably the development of cancer after the administration of genotoxic carcinogens, are often considered to be linear at low doses and thus do not exhibit a threshold. In such circumstances, there is no dose with "zero" risk, although the risk decreases proportionately with a decrease in the dose. The existence or lack of existence of a threshold dose for carcinogens has many regulatory implications and is a point of considerable controversy and research in the field of quantitative risk assessment for chemical carcinogens (Chap. 4).

Assumptions in Deriving the Dose–Response Relationship

A number of assumptions must be considered before dose–response relationships can be used appropriately. The first is that the response is due to the chemical administered. To describe the relationship between a toxic material and an observed effect or response, one must know with reasonable certainty that the relationship is indeed a causal one. For some data, it is not always apparent that the response is a result of chemical exposure. For example, an epidemiologic study might result in the discovery of an "association" between a response (e.g., disease) and one or more variables. Frequently, the data are presented similarly to the presentation of "dose response" in pharmacology and toxicology. Use of the dose response in this context is suspect unless other convincing evidence supports a causal connection between the estimated dose and the measured endpoint (response). Unfortunately, in nearly all retrospective and case-control studies and even in many prospective studies, the dose, duration, frequency, and routes of exposure are seldom quantified, and other potential etiologic factors are frequently present. In its most strict usage, then, the dose–response relationship is based on the knowledge that the effect is a result of a known toxic agent or agents.

A second assumption seems simple and obvious: The magnitude of the response is in fact related to the dose. Perhaps because of its apparent simplicity, this assumption is often a source of misunderstanding. It is really a composite of three other assumptions that recur frequently:

1. There is a molecular target site (or sites) with which the chemical interacts to initiate the response.
2. The production of a response and the degree of response are related to the concentration of the agent at the target site.
3. The concentration at the site is, in turn, related to the dose administered.

The third assumption in using the dose–response relationship is that there exists both a quantifiable method of measuring and a precise means of expressing the toxicity. For any given dose–response relationship, a great variety of criteria or endpoints of toxicity could be used. The ideal criterion would be one closely associated with the molecular events resulting from exposure to the toxicant. It follows from this that a given chemical may have a family of dose–response relationships, one for each toxic endpoint. For example, a chemical that produces cancer through genotoxic effects, liver damage through inhibition of a specific enzyme, and CNS effects via a different mechanism may have three distinct dose–response relationships, one for each endpoint. Early in the assessment of toxicity, little mechanistic information is usually available; thus establishing a dose–response relationship based on the molecular mechanism of action is usually impossible. Indeed, it might not be approachable even for well-known toxicants. In the absence of a mechanistic, molecular ideal criterion of toxicity, one looks to a measure of toxicity that is unequivocal and clearly relevant to the toxic effect. Such measures are often referred to as "effects-related biomarkers." For example, with a new compound chemically related to the class of organophosphate insecticides, one might approach the measurement of toxicity by measuring the inhibition of cholinesterase in blood. In this way, one would be measuring, in a readily accessible system and using a technique that is convenient and reasonably precise, a prominent effect of the chemical and one that is usually pertinent to the mechanism by which toxicity is produced.

The selection of a toxic endpoint for measurement is not always so straightforward. Even the example cited above may be misleading, as an organophosphate may produce a decrease in blood cholinesterase, but this change may not be directly related to its toxicity. As additional data are gathered to suggest a mechanism of toxicity for any substance, other measures of toxicity may be selected. Although many endpoints are quantitative and precise, they are often indirect measures of toxicity. Changes in enzyme levels in blood can be indicative of tissue damage. For example, alanine aminotransferase (ALT) and aspartate aminotransferase (AST) are used to detect liver damage. Use of these enzymes in serum is yet another example of an effects-related biomarker because the change in enzyme activity in the blood is directly related to damage to liver cells. Much of clinical diagnostic medicine relies on effects-related biomarkers, but to be useful the relationship between the biomarker and the disease must be carefully established. Patterns of isozymes and their alteration may provide insight into the organ or system that is the site of toxic effects.

Many direct measures of effects also are not necessarily related to the mechanism by which a substance produces harm to an organism but have the advantage of permitting a causal relation to be drawn between the agent and its action. For example, measurement of the alteration of the tone of smooth or skeletal muscle for substances acting on muscles represents a fundamental approach to toxicological assessment. Similarly, measures of heart rate, blood pressure, and electrical activity of heart muscle, nerve, and brain are examples of the use of physiologic functions as indexes of toxicity. Measurement can also take the form of a still higher level of integration, such as the degree of motor activity or behavioral change.

The measurements used as examples in the preceding discussion all assume prior information about the toxicant, such as its target organ or site of action or a fundamental effect. However, such information is usually available only after toxicologic screening and testing based on other measures of toxicity. With a new substance, the customary starting point in toxicologic evaluation utilizes lethality as an index. Determination of lethality is precise, quantal, and unequivocal and is therefore useful in its own right, if only to suggest the level and magnitude of the potency of a substance. Lethality provides a measure of comparison among many substances whose mechanisms and sites of action may be markedly different. Furthermore, from these studies, clues to the direction of further studies are obtained. This comes about in two important ways. First, simply recording a death is not an adequate means of conducting a lethality study with a new substance. A key element must be a careful, disciplined, detailed observation of the intact animal extending from the time of administration of the toxicant to the death of the animal. From properly conducted observations, immensely informative data can be gathered by a trained toxicologist. Second, a lethality study ordinarily is supported by histologic examination of major tissues and organs for abnormalities. From these observations, one can usually obtain more specific information about the events leading to the lethal effect, the target organs involved, and often a suggestion about the possible mechanism of toxicity at a relatively fundamental level.

Evaluating the Dose–Response Relationship

Comparison of Dose Responses Figure 2-9 illustrates a hypothetical quantal dose–response curve for a desirable effect of a chemical effective dose (ED) such as anesthesia, a toxic dose (TD) effect such as liver injury, and the lethal dose (LD). As depicted in Fig. 2-9, a parallelism is apparent between the (ED) curve and the curve depicting mortality (LD). It is tempting to view the parallel dose–response curves as indicative of identity of mechanism—that is, to conclude that the lethality is a simple extension of the therapeutic effect. While this conclusion may ultimately prove to be correct in any particular case, it is not warranted solely on the basis of the two parallel lines. The same admonition applies to any pair of parallel "effect" curves or any other pair of toxicity or lethality curves.

Therapeutic Index The hypothetical curves in Fig. 2-9 illustrate two other interrelated points: the importance of the selection of the toxic criterion and the interpretation of comparative effect. The concept of the "therapeutic index," which was introduced by Paul Ehrlich in 1913, can be used to illustrate this relationship. Although the therapeutic index is directed toward a comparison of the therapeutically effective dose to the toxic dose of a chemical, it is equally applicable to considerations of comparative toxicity. The *therapeutic index* (TI) in its broadest sense is defined as the ratio of the dose required to produce a toxic effect and the dose needed

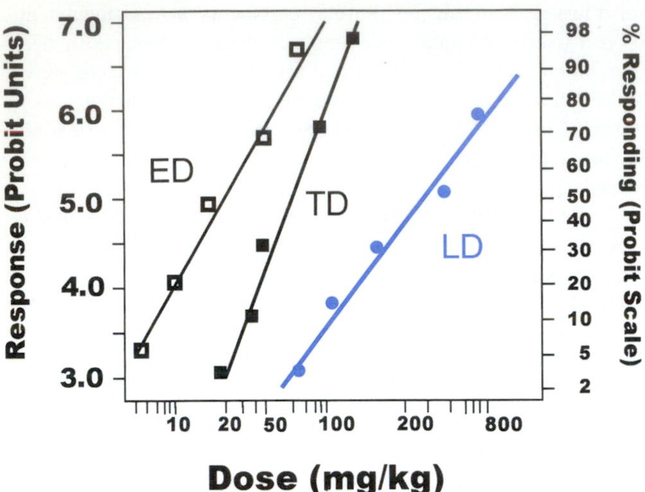

Figure 2-9. Comparison of effective dose (ED), toxic dose (TD), and lethal dose (LD).

The plot is of log dosage versus percentage of population responding in probit units.

to elicit the desired therapeutic response. Similarly, an index of comparative toxicity is obtained by the ratio of doses of two different materials to produce an identical response or the ratio of doses of the same material necessary to yield different toxic effects.

The most commonly used index of effect, whether beneficial or toxic, is the median dose—that is, the dose required to result in a response in 50 percent of a population (or to produce 50 percent of a maximal response). The therapeutic index of a drug is an approximate statement about the relative safety of a drug expressed as the ratio of the lethal or toxic dose to the therapeutic dose:

$$TI = LD_{50}/ED_{50}$$

From Fig. 2-9 one can approximate a therapeutic index by using these median doses. The larger the ratio, the greater the relative safety. The ED_{50} is approximately 20, and the LD_{50} is about 200; thus, the therapeutic index is 10, a number indicative of a relatively safe drug. However, the use of the median effective and median lethal doses is not without disadvantages, because median doses tell nothing about the slopes of the dose–response curves for therapeutic and toxic effects.

Margins of Safety and Exposure One way to overcome this deficiency is to use the ED_{99} for the desired effect and the LD_1 for the undesired effect. These parameters are used in the calculation of the margin of safety:

$$\text{Margin of safety} = LD_1/ED_{99}$$

The quantitative comparisons described above have been used mainly after a single administration of chemicals. However, for chemicals for which there is no beneficial or effective dose and exposures are likely to occur repeatedly, the ratio of LD_1 to ED_{99} has little relevance. Thus, for non drug chemicals, the term *margin of safety* has found use in risk-assessment procedures as an indicator of the magnitude of the difference between an estimated "exposed dose" to a human population and the NOAEL determined in experimental animals.

A measure of the degree of accumulation of a chemical and/or its toxic effects can also be estimated from quantal toxicity data. The *chronicity index* of a chemical is a unitless value obtained by dividing its 1-dose LD_{50} by its 90-dose (90-day) LD_{50}, with both expressed in milligrams per kilogram per day. Theoretically, if no cumulative effect occurs over the doses, the chronicity index will be 1. If a compound were absolutely cumulative, the chronicity index would be 90.

Statistical procedures similar to those used to calculate the LD_{50} can also be used to determine the lethal time 50 (LT_{50}), or the time required for half the animals to die (Litchfield, 1949). The LT_{50} value for a chemical indicates the time course of the toxic effects but does not indicate whether one chemical is more toxic than another.

Frequently, dose–response curves from repeated-dose experimental animal studies (subacute, subchronic, or chronic) are used to estimate the NOAEL, or some other "benchmark" measure of minimal toxic response, such as the dose estimated to produce toxic effects in 10 percent of the population (TD_{10}) (see also Chap. 4). These estimates of minimal toxic dose, derived from quantal dose–response curves, can be used in risk assessment to derive a "margin of exposure" (MOE) index. This index compares the estimated daily exposure, in milligrams per kilogram per day, that might occur under a given set of circumstances to some estimated value from the quantal dose–response relationship (e.g., NOAEL or TD_{10}). Like the MOS, the MOE is often expressed as a ratio of these two values. Thus, for example, if an estimate of human exposure to a pesticide residue yielded a value of 0.001 mg/kg/day, and a TD_{10} of 1 mg/kg/day was determined for that same pesticide, the MOE would be 1000. This value indicates that the estimate of daily exposure under the described set of conditions is 1000 times lower than the estimated daily dose that would cause evident toxicity in 10% of exposed animals. (See Chap. 4 for a more complete discussion of benchmark doses, NOAELs, and MOE.)

Potency versus Efficacy To compare the toxic effects of two or more chemicals, the dose response to the toxic effects of each chemical must be established. One can then compare the potency and maximal efficacy of the two chemicals to produce a toxic effect. These two important terms can be explained by reference to Fig. 2-10, which depicts dose–response curves to four different chemicals for the frequency of a particular toxic effect, such as the production of tumors. Chemical A is said to be more potent than chemical B because of their relative positions along the dosage axis. Potency thus refers to the range of doses over which a chemical produces increasing responses. Thus, A is more potent than B and C is more potent than D. Maximal efficacy reflects the limit of the dose–response relationship on the response axis to a certain chemical. Chemicals A and B have equal maximal efficacy, whereas the maximal efficacy of C is less than that of D.

VARIATION IN TOXIC RESPONSES

Selective Toxicity

Selective toxicity means that a chemical produces injury to one kind of living matter without harming another form of life even though the two may exist in intimate contact (Albert, 1965, 1973). The

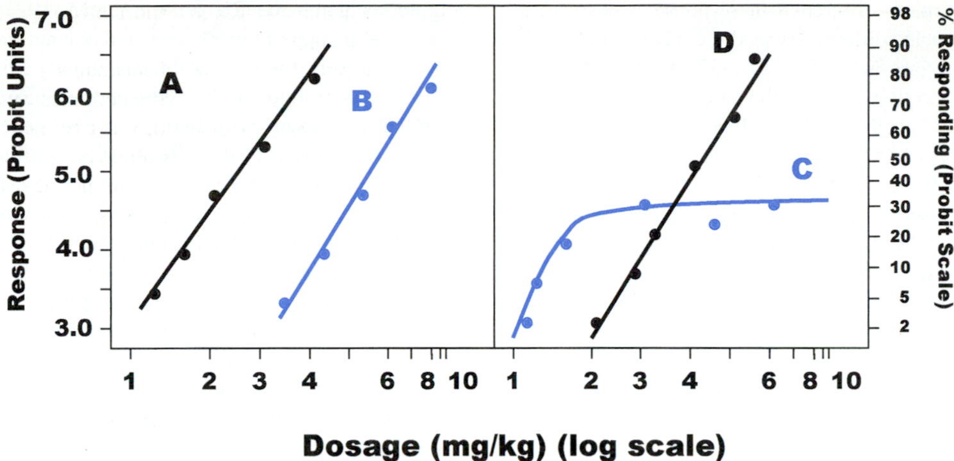

Figure 2-10. Schematic representation of the difference in the dose–response curves for four chemicals (A–D), illustrating the difference between potency and efficacy (see text).

living matter that is injured is termed the *uneconomic form* (or undesirable), and the matter protected is called the *economic form* (or desirable). They may be related to each other as parasite and host or may be two tissues in one organism. This biological diversity interferes with the ability of ecotoxicologists to predict the toxic effects of a chemical in one species (humans) from experiments performed in another species (laboratory animals). However, by taking advantage of the biological diversity, it is possible to develop agents that are lethal for an undesired species and harmless for other species. In agriculture, for example, there are fungi, insects, and even competitive plants that injure the crop, and thus selective pesticides are needed. Similarly, animal husbandry and human medicine require agents, such as antibiotics, that are selectively toxic to the undesirable form but do not produce damage to the desirable form.

Drugs and other chemical agents used for selective toxic purposes are selective for one of two reasons. Either (1) the chemical is equitoxic to both economic and uneconomic cells but is accumulated mainly by uneconomic cells or (2) it reacts fairly specifically with a cytological or a biochemical feature that is absent from or does not play an important role in the economic form (Albert, 1965, 1973). Selectivity resulting from differences in distribution usually is caused by differences in the absorption, biotransformation, or excretion of the toxicant. The selective toxicity of an insecticide spray may be partly due to a larger surface area per unit weight that causes the insect to absorb a proportionally larger dose than does the mammal being sprayed. The effectiveness of radioactive iodine in the treatment of hyperthyroidism (as well as its thyroid carcinogenicity) is due to the selective ability of the thyroid gland to accumulate iodine. A major reason why chemicals are toxic to one but not to another type of tissue is that there are differences in accumulation of the ultimate toxic compound in various tissues. This, in turn, may be due to differences in the ability of various tissues to biotransform the chemical into the ultimate toxic product.

Selective toxicity caused by differences in comparative cytology is exemplified by a comparison of plant and animal cells. Plants differ from animals in many ways—for example, absence of a nervous system, an efficient circulatory system, and muscles as well as the presence of a photosynthetic mechanism and cell walls. The fact that bacteria contain cell walls and humans do not has been utilized in developing selective toxic chemotherapeutic agents, such as penicillin and cephalosporins, that kill bacteria but are relatively nontoxic to mammalian cells.

Selective toxicity also can be a result of a difference in biochemistry in the two types of cells. For example, bacteria do not absorb folic acid but synthesize it from *p*-aminobenzoic acid, glutamic acid, and pteridine, whereas mammals cannot synthesize folic acid but have to absorb it from the diet. Thus, sulfonamide drugs are selectively toxic to bacteria because the sulfonamides, which resemble *p*-aminobenzoic acid in both charge and dimensions, antagonize the incorporation of *p*-aminobenzoic acid into the folic acid molecule—a reaction that humans do not carry out.

Species Differences

Although a basic tenet of toxicology is that "experimental results in animals, when properly qualified, are applicable to humans," it is important to recognize that both quantitative and qualitative differences in response to toxic substances may occur among different species. As discussed above, there are many reasons for selective toxicity among different species. Even among phylogenetically similar species (e.g., rats, mice, guinea pigs, and hamsters), large differences in response may occur. For example, the LD_{50} for the highly toxic dioxin, 2,3,7,8-tetrachlorodibenzo-*p*-dioxin (TCDD), differs by more than 1000-fold between guinea pigs and hamsters. Not only does the lethal dose for TCDD vary widely among species, so do the particular target organs affected. Species differences in response to carcinogenic chemicals represent an important issue in regulatory risk assessment. As discussed in Chap. 4, extrapolation of laboratory animal data to infer human cancer risk is currently a key component of regulatory decision making. The validity of this approach of course depends on the relevance of the experimental animal model to humans. Large differences in carcinogenic response between experimental animal species are not unusual. For example, mice are highly resistant to the hepatocarcinogenic effects of the fungal toxin aflatoxin B_1. Dietary doses as high as 10,000 parts per billion (ppb) failed to produce liver cancer in mice, whereas in rats dietary doses as low as 15 ppb produced a significant increase in liver tumors (Wogan et al., 1974). The mechanistic basis for this dramatic difference in response appears to be entirely related to species differences in the expression of a particular form of glutathione S-transferase (mGSTA3-3) that has unusually high catalytic activity toward the carcinogenic epoxide of aflatoxin (Eaton and Gallagher, 1994). Mice express this enzyme constitutively, whereas rats normally express a closely related form with much less detoxifying activity toward aflatoxin epoxide. Interestingly, rats do possess the gene for a form of glutathione S-transferase with high catalytic activity toward aflatoxin epoxide (rGSTA5-5) that is inducible by certain dietary antioxidants and drugs. Thus, dietary treatment can dramatically change the sensitivity of a species to a carcinogen.

Other examples in which large species differences in response to carcinogens have been observed include the development of renal tumors from 2,3,5-trimethylpentane and *d*-limonene in male rats (Lehman-McKeeman and Caudill, 1992), the production of liver tumors from "peroxisomal proliferators" such as the antilipidemic drug clofibrate and the common solvent trichloroethylene (Roberts, 1999), and the induction of nasal carcinomas in rats after inhalation exposure to formaldehyde (Monticello and Morgan, 1997).

Identifying the mechanistic basis for species differences in response to chemicals is an important part of toxicology because only through a thorough understanding of these differences can the relevance of animal data to human response be verified.

Individual Differences in Response

Even within a species, large interindividual differences in response to a chemical can occur because of subtle genetic differences. Hereditary differences in a single gene that occur in more than 1 percent of the population are referred to as *genetic polymorphism* and may be responsible for idiosyncratic reactions to chemicals, as discussed earlier in this chapter. However, genetic polymorphism may have other important but less dramatic effects than those described for acute idiosyncratic responses (such as that occurring in pseudocholinesterase-deficient individuals after succinylcholine exposure). For example, it is recognized that approximately 50 percent of the Caucasian population has a gene deletion for the enzyme glutathione S-transferase M1. This enzyme has no apparent significant physiologic function, and thus homozygotes for the gene deletion (e.g., those who lack both copies of the normal gene) are functionally and physiologically normal. However, epidemiologic studies have indicated that smokers who are homozygous for the null allele may be at slightly increased risk of developing lung cancer compared with smokers who have one or both copies of the normal gene (Houlston, 1999; Strange and Fryer, 1999). Chapter 6 provides additional examples of genetic differences in biotransformation enzymes that may be important determinants of variability in individual susceptibility to chemical exposures.

Genetic polymorphism in physiologically important genes may also be responsible for interindividual differences in toxic responses. For example, studies in transgenic mice have shown that mice possessing one copy of a mutated *p53* gene (a so-called tumor suppressor gene; see Chap. 8) are much more susceptible to some chemical carcinogens than are mice with two normal copies of the gene (Tennant et al., 1999). In humans, there is evidence that possessing one mutated copy of a tumor suppressor gene greatly increases the risk of developing certain cancers. For example, retinoblastoma is a largely inherited form of cancer that arises because of the presence of two copies of a defective tumor suppressor gene (the Rb gene) (Wiman, 1993). Individuals with one mutated copy of the Rb gene and one normal copy are not destined to acquire the disease (as are those with two copies of the mutated gene), although their chance of acquiring it is much greater than that of persons with two normal Rb genes. This is the case because both copies of the gene must be nonfunctional for the disease to develop. With one mutated copy present genetically, the probability of acquiring a mutation of the second gene (potentially from exposure to environmental mutagens) is much greater than the probability of acquiring independent mutations in both copies of the gene as would be necessary in people with two normal Rb alleles. (See Chap. 8 for additional discussion of tumor suppressor genes.)

As our understanding of the human genome increases, more "susceptibility" genes will be discovered, and it is likely that the etiology of many chronic diseases will be shown to be related to a combination of genetics and environment. Simple blood tests may ultimately be developed that allow an individual to learn whether he or she may be particularly susceptible to specific drugs or environmental pollutants. Although the public health significance of this type of information could be immense, the disclosure of such information raises many important ethical and legal issues that must be addressed before wide use of such tests.

DESCRIPTIVE ANIMAL TOXICITY TESTS

Two main principles underlie all descriptive animal toxicity testing. The first is that the effects produced by a compound in laboratory animals, when properly qualified, are applicable to humans. This premise applies to all of experimental biology and medicine. On the basis of dose per unit of body surface, toxic effects in humans are usually in the same range as those in experimental animals. On a body weight basis, humans are generally more vulnerable than are experimental animals, probably by a factor of about 10. When one has an awareness of these quantitative differences, appropriate safety factors can be applied to calculate relatively safe doses for humans. All known chemical carcinogens in humans, with the possible exception of arsenic, are carcinogenic in some species but not in all laboratory animals. It has become increasingly evident that the converse—that all chemicals carcinogenic in animals are also carcinogenic in humans—is not true (Dybing and Sanner, 1999; Grisham, 1997; Hengstler et al., 1999). However, for regulatory and risk assessment purposes, positive carcinogenicity tests in animals are usually interpreted as indicative of potential human carcinogenicity. If a clear understanding of the mechanism of action of the carcinogen indicates that a positive response in animals is not relevant to humans, a positive animal bioassay may be considered irrelevant for human risk assessment (see Chap. 4). This species variation in carcinogenic response appears to be due in many instances to differences in biotransformation of the procarcinogen to the ultimate carcinogen (see Chap. 6).

The second principle is that exposure of experimental animals to toxic agents in high doses is a necessary and valid method of discovering possible hazards in humans. This principle is based on the quantal dose–response concept that the incidence of an effect in a population is greater as the dose or exposure increases. Practical considerations in the design of experimental model systems require that the number of animals used in toxicology experiments always be small compared with the size of human populations at risk. Obtaining statistically valid results from such small groups of animals requires the use of relatively large doses so that the effect will occur frequently enough to be detected. However, the use of high doses can create problems in interpretation if the response(s) obtained at high doses does not occur at low doses. Thus, for example, it has been shown that bladder tumors observed in rats fed very high doses of saccharin will not occur at the much lower doses of saccharin encountered in the human diet. At the high concentrations fed to rats, saccharin forms an insoluble precipitate in the bladder that subsequently results in chronic irritation of bladder epithelium, enhanced cell proliferation, and ultimately bladder tumors (Cohen, 1998, 1999). In vitro studies have shown that precipitation of saccharin in human urine will not occur at the concentrations that could be obtained from even extraordinary consumption of this artificial sweetener. Examples such as this illustrate the importance of considering the molecular, biochemical, and cellular mechanisms responsible for toxicological responses when extrapolating from high to low dose and across species.

Toxicity tests are not designed to demonstrate that a chemical is safe but to characterize the toxic effects a chemical can produce. There are no set toxicology tests that have to be performed on every chemical intended for commerce. Depending on the eventual use of the chemical, the toxic effects produced by structural analogs of the chemical, as well as the toxic effects produced by the chemical itself, contribute to the determination of the toxicology tests that should be performed. However, the FDA, EPA, and Organization for Economic Cooperation and Development (OECD) have written good laboratory practice (GLP) standards. These guidelines are expected to be followed when toxicity tests are conducted in support of the introduction of a chemical to the market.

The following sections provide an overview of basic toxicity testing procedures in use today. For a detailed description of these tests, the reader is referred to several authoritative texts on this subject (Auletta, 1995; Hayes, 2001; Weathereholtz, 1997).

Acute Lethality

The first toxicity test performed on a new chemical is acute toxicity. The LD_{50} and other acute toxic effects are determined after one or more routes of administration (one route being oral or the intended route of exposure) in one or more species. The species most often used are the mouse and rat, but sometimes the rabbit and dog are employed. Studies are performed in both adult male and female animals. Food is often withheld the night before dosing. The number of animals that die in a 14-day period after a single dosage is tabulated. In addition to mortality and weight, daily examination of test animals should be conducted for signs of intoxication, lethargy, behavioral modifications, morbidity, food consumption, and so on. Acute toxicity tests (1) give a quantitative estimate of acute toxicity (LD_{50}) for comparison with other substances, (2) identify target organs and other clinical manifestations of acute toxicity, (3) establish the reversibility of the toxic response, and (4) provide dose-ranging guidance for other studies.

Determination of the LD_{50} has become a public issue because of increasing concern for the welfare and protection of laboratory animals. The LD_{50} is not a biological constant. Many factors influence toxicity and thus may alter the estimation of the LD_{50} in any particular study. Factors such as animal strain, age and weight, type of feed, caging, pretrial fasting time, method of administration, volume and type of suspension medium, and duration of observation have all been shown to influence adverse responses to toxic substances. These and other factors have been discussed in detail in earlier editions of this textbook (Doull, 1980). Because of this inherent variability in LD_{50} estimates, it is now recognized that for most purposes it is only necessary to characterize the LD_{50} within an order of magnitude range such as 5 to 50 mg/kg, 50 to 500 mg/kg, and so on.

There are several traditional approaches to determining the LD_{50} and its 95 percent confidence limit as well as the slope of the probit line. The reader is referred to the classic works of Litchfield and Wilcoxon (1949), Bliss (1957), and Finney (1971) for a description of the mechanics of these procedures. A computer program in BASIC for determining probit and log-probit or logit correlations has been published (Abou-Setta et al., 1986). These traditional methods for determining LD_{50}s require a relatively large number of animals (40 to 50). Other statistical techniques that require fewer animals, such as the "moving averages" method of Thompson and Weill (Weil, 1952), are available but do not provide confidence limits for the LD_{50} and the slope of the probit line. Finney (1985) has succinctly summarized the advantages and deficiencies of many of the traditional methods. For most circumstances, an adequate estimate of the LD_{50} and an approximation of the 95 percent confidence intervals can be obtained with as few as 6 to 9 animals, using the "up-and-down" method as modified by Bruce (1985). When this method was compared with traditional methods that typically utilize 40 to 50 animals, excellent agreement was obtained for all 10 compounds tested (Bruce, 1987). In mice and rats the LD_{50} is usually determined as described above, but in the larger species only an approximation of the LD_{50} is obtained by increasing the dose in the same animal until serious toxic effects are evident.

If there is a reasonable likelihood of substantial exposure to the material by dermal or inhalation exposure, acute dermal and acute inhalation studies are performed. When animals are exposed acutely to chemicals in the air they breathe or the water they (fish) live in, the dose the animals receive is usually not known. For these situations, the lethal concentration 50 (LC_{50}) is usually determined; that is, the concentration of chemical in the air or water that causes death to 50 percent of the animals. In reporting an LC_{50}, it is imperative that the time of exposure be indicated. The acute dermal toxicity test is usually performed in rabbits. The site of application is shaved. The test substance is kept in contact with the skin for 24 h by wrapping the skin with an impervious plastic material. At the end of the exposure period, the wrapping is removed and the skin is wiped to remove any test substance still remaining. Animals are observed at various intervals for 14 days, and the LD_{50} is calculated. If no toxicity is evident at 2 g/kg, further acute dermal toxicity testing is usually not performed. Acute inhalation studies are performed that are similar to other acute toxicity studies except that the route of exposure is inhalation. Most often, the length of exposure is 4 h.

Although by themselves LD_{50} and LC_{50} values are of limited significance, acute lethality studies are essential for characterizing the toxic effects of chemicals and their hazard to humans. The most meaningful scientific information derived from acute lethality tests comes from clinical observations and postmortem examination of animals rather than from the specific LD_{50} value.

Skin and Eye Irritations

The ability of a chemical to irritate the skin and eye after an acute exposure is usually determined in rabbits. For the dermal irritation test (Draize test), rabbits are prepared by removal of fur on a section of the back by electric clippers. The chemical is applied to the skin (0.5 mL of liquid or 0.5 g of solid) under four covered gauze patches (1 in. square; one intact and two abraded skin sites on each animal) and usually kept in contact for 4 h. The nature of the covering patches depends on whether occlusive, semiocclusive, or nonocclusive tests are desired. For occlusive testing, the test material is covered with an impervious plastic sheet; for semiocclusive tests, a gauze dressing may be used. Occasionally, studies may require that the material be applied to abraded skin. The degree of skin irritation is scored for erythema (redness), eschar (scab) and edema (swelling) formation, and corrosive action. These dermal irritation observations are repeated at various intervals after the covered patch has been removed. To determine the degree of ocular irritation, the chemical is instilled into one eye (0.1 mL of liquid or 100 mg of solid) of each test rabbit. The contralateral eye is used as the control. The eyes of the rabbits are then examined at various times after application.

Controversy over this test has led to the development of alternative in vitro models for evaluating cutaneous and ocular toxicity of substances. The various in vitro methods that have been evaluated for this purpose include epidermal keratinocyte and corneal epithelial cell culture models. These and other in vitro tests have been reviewed recently (Davila et al., 1998).

Sensitization

Information about the potential of a chemical to sensitize skin is needed in addition to irritation testing for all materials that may repeatedly come into contact with the skin. Numerous procedures have been developed to determine the potential of substances to induce a sensitization reaction in humans (delayed hypersensitivity reaction), including the Draize test, the open epicutaneous test, the Buehler test, Freund's complete adjuvant test, the optimization test, the split adjuvant test, and the guinea pig maximization test (Maibach and Patrick, 2001; Rush et al., 1995). Although they differ in regard to route and frequency of duration, they all utilize the guinea pig as the preferred test species. In general, the test chemical is administered to the shaved skin topically, intradermally, or both and may include the use of adjuvant to enhance the sensitivity of the assay. Multiple administrations of the test substance are generally given over a period of 2 to 4 weeks. Depending on the specific protocol, the treated area may be occluded. Some 2 to 3 weeks after the last treatment, the animals are challenged with a nonirritating concentration of the test substance and the development of erythema is evaluated.

Subacute (Repeated-Dose Study)

Subacute toxicity tests are performed to obtain information on the toxicity of a chemical after repeated administration and as an aid to establish doses for subchronic studies. A typical protocol is to give three to four different dosages of the chemicals to the animals by mixing it in their feed. For rats, 10 animals per sex per dose are often used; for dogs, three dosages and 3 to 4 animals per sex are used. Clinical chemistry and histopathology are performed after 14 days of exposure, as described below in the section on subchronic toxicity testing.

Subchronic

The toxicity of a chemical after subchronic exposure is then determined. Subchronic exposure can last for different periods of time, but 90 days is the most common test duration. The principal goals of the subchronic study are to establish a NOAEL and to further identify and characterize the specific organ or organs affected by the test compound after repeated administration. One may also obtain a "lowest observed adverse effect level" (LOAEL) as well as the NOAEL for the species tested. The numbers obtained for NOAEL and LOAEL will depend on how closely the dosages are spaced and the number of animals examined. Determinations of NOAELs and LOAELs have numerous regulatory implications. For example, the EPA utilizes the NOAEL to calculate the *reference dose* (RfD), which may be used to establish regulatory values for "acceptable" pollutant levels (Barnes and Dourson, 1988) (Chap. 4). An alternative to the NOAEL approach referred to as the *benchmark dose* uses all the experimental data to fit one or more dose–response curves (Crump, 1984). These curves are then used to estimate a benchmark dose that is defined as "the statistical lower bound on a dose corresponding to a specified level of risk" (Allen et al., 1994a). Although subchronic studies are frequently the primary or sole source of experimental data to determine both the NOAEL and the benchmark dose, these concepts can be applied to other types of toxicity testing protocols, such as that for chronic toxicity or developmental toxicity (Allen et al., 1994a, 1994b; Faustman et al., 1994) (see also Chap. 4 for a complete discussion of the derivation and use of NOAELs, RfDs, and benchmark doses). If chronic studies have been completed, these data are generally used for NOAEL and LOAEL estimates in preference to data from subchronic studies.

A subchronic study is usually conducted in two species (rat and dog) by the route of intended exposure (usually oral). At least three doses are employed (a high dose that produces toxicity but does not cause more than 10 percent fatalities, a low dose that produces no apparent toxic effects, and an intermediate dose) with 10 to 20 rats and 4 to 6 dogs of each sex per dose. Each animal should be uniquely identified with permanent markings such as ear tags, tattoos, or electronically coded microchip implants. Only healthy animals should be used, and each animal should be housed individually in an adequately controlled environment. Animals should be observed once or twice daily for signs of toxicity, including changes in body weight, diet consumption, changes in fur color or texture, respiratory or cardiovascular distress, motor and behavioral abnormalities, and palpable masses. All premature deaths should be recorded and necropsied as soon as possible. Severely moribund animals should be terminated immediately to preserve tissues and reduce unnecessary suffering. At the end of the 90-day study, all the remaining animals should be terminated and blood and tissues should be collected for further analysis. The gross and microscopic condition of the organs and tissues (about 15 to 20) and the weight of the major organs (about 12) are recorded and evaluated. Hematology and blood chemistry measurements are usually done before, in the middle of, and at the termination of exposure. Hematology measurements usually include hemoglobin concentration, hematocrit, erythrocyte counts, total and differential leukocyte counts, platelet count, clotting time, and prothrombin time. Clinical chemistry determinations commonly made include glucose, calcium, potassium, urea nitrogen, alanine aminotransferase (ALT), serum aspartate aminotransferase (AST), gammaglutamyltranspeptidase (GGT), sorbitol dehydrogenase, lactic dehydrogenase, alkaline phosphatase, creatinine, bilirubin, triglycerides, cholesterol, albumin, globulin, and total protein. Urinalysis is usually performed in the middle of and at the termination of the testing period and often includes determination of specific gravity or osmolarity, pH, proteins, glucose, ketones, bilirubin, and urobilinogen as well as microscopic examination of formed elements. If humans are likely to have significant exposure to the chemical by dermal contact or inhalation, subchronic dermal and/or inhalation experiments may also be required. Subchronic toxicity studies not only characterize the dose–response relationship of a test substance after repeated administration but also provide data for a more reasonable prediction of appropriate doses for chronic exposure studies.

For chemicals that are to be registered as drugs, acute and subchronic studies (and potentially additional special tests if a chemical has unusual toxic effects or therapeutic purposes) must be completed before the company can file an Investigational New Drug (IND) application with the FDA. If the application is approved, clinical trials can commence. At the same time phase I, phase II, and phase III clinical trials are performed, chronic exposure of the animals to the test compound can be carried out in laboratory animals, along with additional specialized tests.

Chronic

Long-term or chronic exposure studies are performed similarly to subchronic studies except that the period of exposure is longer than 3 months. In rodents, chronic exposures are usually for 6 months to 2 years. Chronic studies in nonrodent species are usually for 1 year but may be longer. The length of exposure is somewhat dependent on the intended period of exposure in humans. If the agent is a drug planned to be used for short periods, such as an antimicrobial agent, a chronic exposure of 6 months may be sufficient, whereas if the agent is a food additive with the potential for lifetime exposure in humans, a chronic study up to 2 years in duration is likely to be required.

Chronic toxicity tests are performed to assess the cumulative toxicity of chemicals, but the study design and evaluation often include a consideration of the carcinogenic potential of chemicals so that a separate lifetime feeding study that addresses carcinogenicity does not have to be performed. These studies usually are performed in rats and mice and extend over the average lifetime of the species (18 months to 2 years for mice; 2 to 2.5 years for rats). To ensure that 30 rats per dose survive the 2-year study, 60 rats per group per sex are often started in the study. Both gross and microscopic pathological examinations are made not only on animals that survive the chronic exposure but also on those that die prematurely.

Dose selection is critical in these studies to ensure that premature mortality from chronic toxicity does not limit the number of animals that survive to a normal life expectancy. Most regulatory guidelines require that the highest dose administered be the estimated maximum tolerable dose (MTD). This is generally derived from subchronic studies, but additional longer studies (e.g., 6 months) may be necessary if delayed effects or extensive cumulative toxicity are indicated in the 90-day subchronic study. The MTD has had various definitions (Haseman, 1985). The MTD has been defined by some regulatory agencies as the dose that suppresses body weight gain slightly (i.e., 10 percent) in a 90-day subchronic study (Reno, 1997). However, regulatory agencies may also consider the use of parameters other than weight gain, such as physiological and pharmacokinetic considerations and urinary metabolite profiles, as indicators of an appropriate MTD (Reno, 1997). Generally, one or two additional doses, usually fractions of the MTD (e.g., one-half and one-quarter MTD), and a control group are tested.

The use of the MTD in carcinogenicity has been the subject of controversy. The premise that high doses are necessary for testing the carcinogenic potential of chemicals is derived from the statistical and experimental design limitations of chronic bioassays. Consider that a 0.5 percent increase in cancer incidence in the United States would result in over 1 million additional cancer deaths each year—clearly an unacceptably high risk. However, identifying with statistical confidence a 0.5 percent incidence of cancer in a group of experimental animals would require a minimum of 1000 test animals, and this assumes that no tumors were present in the absence of exposure (zero background incidence).

Figure 2-11 shows the statistical relationship between minimum detectable tumor incidence and the number of test animals per group. This curve shows that in a chronic bioassay with 50 animals per test group, a tumor incidence of about 8 percent could exist even though no animals in the test group had tumors. This example assumes that there are no tumors in the control group. These statistical considerations illustrate why animals are tested at doses higher than those which occur in human exposure. Because it is impractical to use the large number of animals that would be required to test the potential carcinogenicity of a chemical at the doses usually encountered by people, the alternative is to assume that there is a relationship between the administered dose and the tumorigenic response and give animals doses of the chemical that are high enough to produce a measurable tumor response in a reasonable size test group, such as 40 to 50 animals per dose. The limitations of this approach are discussed in Chap. 4.

Recently a new approach for establishing maximum doses for use in chronic animal toxicity testing of drugs has been proposed for substances for which basic human pharmacokinetic data are available (for example, new pharmaceutical agents which have completed phase I clinical trials). For chronic animal studies performed on drugs where single-dose human pharmacokinetic data are available, it has been suggested that a daily dose be used that would provide an area under the curve (AUC) in laboratory ani-

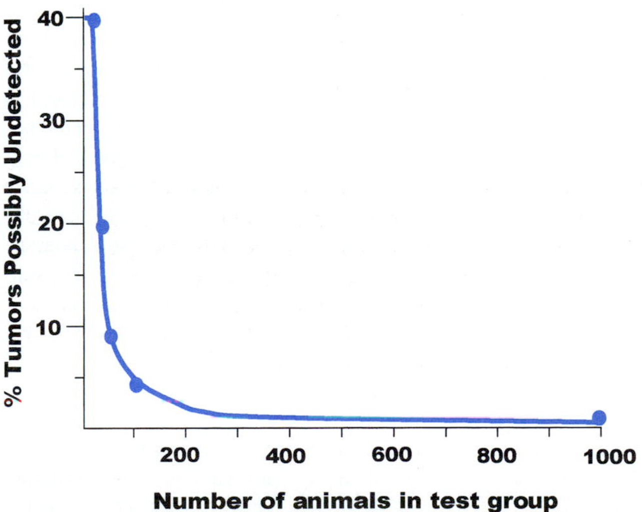

Figure 2-11. Statistical limitations in the power of experimental animal studies to detect tumorigenic effects.

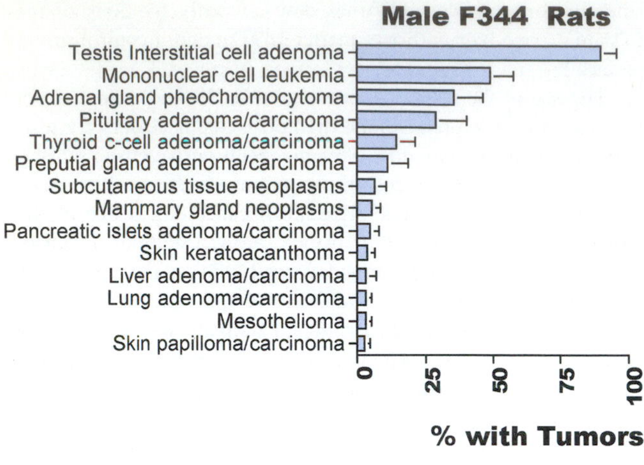

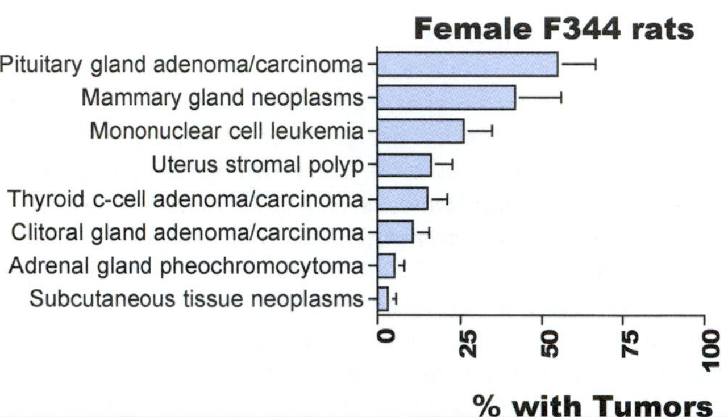

Figure 2-12. Most frequently occurring tumors in untreated control rats from recent NTP 2-year rodent carcinogenicity studies.

The values shown represent the mean ±SD of the percentage of animals developing the specified tumor type at the end of the 2-year study. The values were obtained from 27 different studies involving a combined total of between 1319 and 1353 animals per tumor type.

mals equivalent to 25 times the AUC in humans given the highest (single) daily dose to be used therapeutically. This value would then be used in place of the traditional MTD for chronic bioassays.

Chronic toxicity assays are commonly used to evaluate the potential oncogenicity of test substances (Huff, 1999). Most regulatory guidelines require that both benign and malignant tumors be reported in the evaluation. Statistical increases above the control incidence of tumors (either all tumors or specific tumor types) in the treatment groups are considered indicative of carcinogenic potential of the chemical unless there are qualifying factors that suggest otherwise (lack of a dose response, unusually low incidence of tumors in the control group compared with "historic" controls, etc.). Thus, the conclusion as to whether a given chronic bioassay is positive or negative for carcinogenic potential of the test substance requires careful consideration of background tumor incidence. Properly designed chronic oncogenicity studies require that a concurrent control group matched for variables such as age, diet, housing conditions be used. For some tumor types, the "background" incidence of tumors is surprisingly high. Figure 2-12 shows the background tumor incidence for various tumors in male and female F-344 rats used in 27 National Toxicology Program 2-year rodent carcinogenicity studies. The data shown represent the percent of animals in control (nonexposed) groups that developed the specified tumor type by the end of the 2-year study. These studies involved more than 1300 rats of each sex. Figure 2-13 shows similar data for control (nonexposed) male and female B6C3F1 mice from 30 recent NTP 2-year carcinogenicity studies and includes data from over 1400 mice of each sex. There are several key points that can be derived from these summary data:

1. Tumors, both benign and malignant, are not uncommon events in animals even in the absence of exposure to any known carcinogen.
2. There are numerous different tumor types that develop "spontaneously" in both sexes of both rats and mice, but at different rates.
3. Background tumors that are common in one species may be uncommon in another (for example, testicular interstitial cell adenomas are very common in male rats but rare in male mice; liver adenomas/carcinomas are about 10 times more prevalent in male mice than in male rats).
4. Even within the same species and strain, large gender differences in background tumor incidence are sometimes observed (for example, adrenal gland pheochromocytomas are about seven times more prevalent in male F344 rats than in female F344 rats; lung and liver tumors are twice as prevalent in male B6C3F1 mice as in female B6C3F1 mice).
5. Even when the general protocols, diets, environment, strain and source of animals, and other variables are relatively constant,

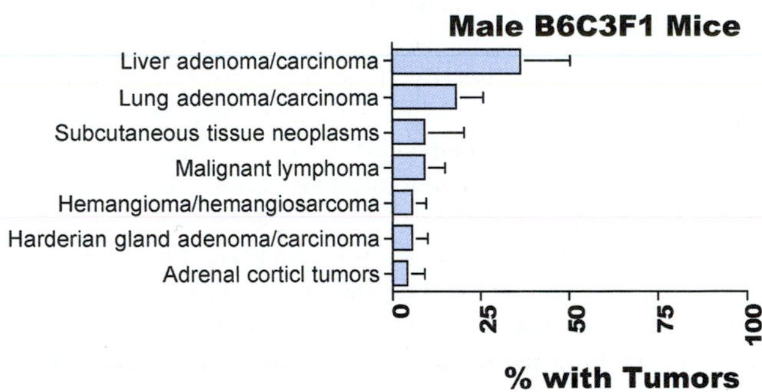

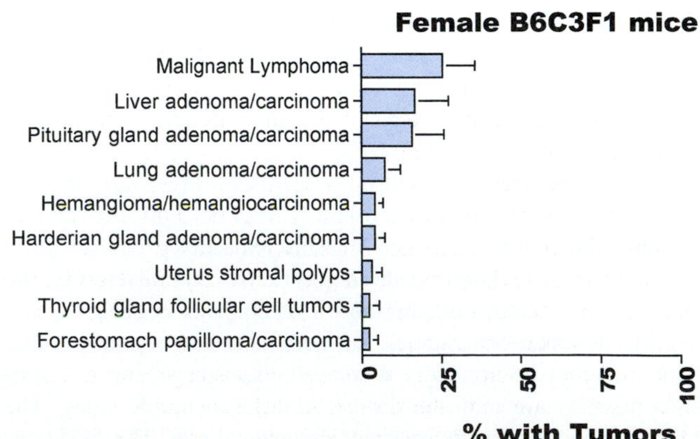

Figure 2-13. Most frequently occurring tumors in untreated control mice from recent NTP 2-year rodent carcinogenicity studies.

The values shown represent the mean ±SD of the percentage of animals developing the specified tumor type at the end of the 2-year study. The values were obtained from 30 different studies involving a total of between 1447 and 1474 animals per tumor type.

background tumor incidence can vary widely, as shown by the relatively large standard deviations for some tumor types in the NTP bioassay program. For example, the range in liver adenoma/carcinoma incidence in 30 different groups of unexposed (control) male B6C3F1 mice went from a low of 10 percent to a high of 68 percent. Pituitary gland adenomas/carcinomas ranged from 12 to 60 percent and 30 to 76 percent in unexposed male and female F344 rats, respectively, and from 0 to 36 percent in unexposed female B6C3F1 mice.

Taken together, these data demonstrate the importance of including concurrent control animals in such studies. In addition, comparisons of the concurrent control results to "historic" controls accumulated over years of study may be important in identifying potentially spurious "false-positive" results. The relatively high variability in background tumor incidence among groups of healthy, highly inbred strains of animals maintained on nutritionally balanced and consistent diets in rather sterile environments highlights the dilemma in interpreting the significance of both positive and negative results in regard to the human population, which is genetically diverse, has tremendous variability in diet, nutritional status, and overall health; and lives in an environment full of potentially carcinogenic substances, both natural and human-made.

Developmental and Reproductive Toxicity

The effects of chemicals on reproduction and development also need to be determined. *Developmental toxicology* is the study of adverse effects on the developing organism occurring anytime during the life span of the organism that may result from exposure to chemical or physical agents before conception (either parent), during prenatal development, or postnatally until the time of puberty. *Teratology* is the study of defects induced during development between conception and birth (see Chap. 10). *Reproductive toxicology* is the study of the occurrence of adverse effects on the male or female reproductive system that may result from exposure to chemical or physical agents (see Chap. 20).

Several types of animal tests are utilized to examine the potential of an agent to alter development and reproduction. Although different countries have often had different testing requirements for reproductive and developmental toxicity, efforts to "harmonize" such testing protocols have resulted in more flexible guidelines for reproductive toxicity testing strategies [see (Christian, 1997) for a summary description of the ICH guidelines]. General fertility and reproductive performance (segment I) tests are usually performed in rats with two or three doses (20 rats per sex per dose) of the test chemical (neither produces maternal toxicity). Males are given the chemical 60 days and females 14 days before mating. The animals are given the chemical throughout gestation and lactation. Typical observations made include the percentage of the females that become pregnant, the number of stillborn and live offspring, and the weight, growth, survival, and general condition of the offspring during the first 3 weeks of life.

The potential of chemicals to disrupt normal embryonic and/or fetal development (teratogenic effects) is also determined in laboratory animals. Current guidelines for these segment II studies call for the use of two species, including one nonrodent species (usually rabbits). Teratogens are most effective when administered during the first trimester, the period of organogenesis. Thus, the animals (usually 12 rabbits and 24 rats or mice per group) are usually exposed to one of three dosages during organogenesis (day 7 to 17 in rodents and days 7 to 19 in rabbits), and the fetuses are removed by cesarean section a day before the estimated time of delivery (gestational days 29 for rabbit, 20 for rat, and 18 for mouse). The uterus is excised and weighed and then examined for the number of live, dead, and resorbed fetuses. Live fetuses are weighed; half of each litter is examined for skeletal abnormalities and the remaining half for soft tissue anomalies.

The perinatal and postnatal toxicities of chemicals also are often examined (segment III). This test is performed by administering the test compound to rats from the 15th day of gestation throughout delivery and lactation and determining its effect on the birthweight, survival, and growth of the offspring during the first 3 weeks of life.

In some instances a multigenerational study may be chosen, often in place of segment III studies, to determine the effects of chemicals on the reproductive system. At least three dosage levels are given to groups of 25 female and 25 male rats shortly after weaning (30 to 40 days of age). These rats are referred to as the F_0 generation. Dosing continues throughout breeding (about 140 days of age), gestation, and lactation. The offspring (F_1 generation) have thus been exposed to the chemical in utero, via lactation, and in the feed thereafter. When the F_1 generation is about 140 days old, about 25 females and 25 males are bred to produce the F_2 generation, and administration of the chemical is continued. The F_2 generation is thus also exposed to the chemical in utero and via lactation. The F_1 and F_2 litters are examined as soon as possible after delivery. The percentage of F_0 and F_1 females that get pregnant, the number of pregnancies that go to full term, the litter size, the number of stillborn, and the number of live births are recorded. Viability counts and pup weights are recorded at birth and at 4, 7, 14, and 21 days of age. The fertility index (percentage of mating resulting in pregnancy), gestation index (percentage of pregnancies resulting in live litters), viability index (percentage of animals that survive 4 days or longer), and lactation index (percentage of animals alive at 4 days that survived the 21-day lactation period) are then calculated. Gross necropsy and histopathology are performed on some of the parents (F_0 and F_1), with the greatest attention being paid to the reproductive organs, and gross necropsy is performed on all weanlings.

The International Commission on Harmonization (ICH) guidelines provide for flexible guidelines that address six "ICH stages" of development: premating and conception (stage A), conception to implantation (stage B), implantation to closure of the hard palate (Stage C), closure of the hard palate to end of pregnancy (stage D), birth and weaning (stage E), and weaning to sexual maturity (stage F). All of these stages are covered in the segment I to segment III studies described above (Christian, 1997).

Numerous short-term tests for teratogenicity have been developed (Faustman, 1988). These tests utilize whole-embryo culture, organ culture, and primary and established cell cultures to examine developmental processes and estimate the potential teratogenic risks of chemicals. Many of these in utero test systems are under evaluation for use in screening new chemicals for teratogenic effects. These systems vary in their ability to identify specific teratogenic events and alterations in cell growth and differentiation. In general, the available assays cannot identify functional or behavioral teratogens (Faustman, 1988).

Mutagenicity

Mutagenesis is the ability of chemicals to cause changes in the genetic material in the nucleus of cells in ways that allow the changes to be transmitted during cell division. Mutations can occur in either of two cell types, with substantially different consequences. Germinal mutations damage DNA in sperm and ova, which can undergo meiotic division and therefore have the potential for transmission of the mutations to future generations. If mutations are present at the time of fertilization in either the egg or the sperm, the resulting combination of genetic material may not be viable, and the death may occur in the early stages of embryonic cell division. Alternatively, the mutation in the genetic material may not affect early embryogenesis but may result in the death of the fetus at a later developmental period, resulting in abortion. Congenital abnormalities may also result from mutations. Somatic mutations refer to mutations in all other cell types and are not heritable but may result in cell death or transmission of a genetic defect to other cells in the same tissue through mitotic division. Because the initiating event of chemical carcinogenesis is thought to be a mutagenic one, mutagenic tests are often used to screen for potential carcinogens.

Numerous in vivo and in vitro procedures have been devised to test chemicals for their ability to cause mutations. Some genetic alterations are visible with the light microscope. In this case, cytogenetic analysis of bone marrow smears is used after the animals have been exposed to the test agent. Because some mutations are incompatible with normal development, the mutagenic potential of a chemical can also be measured by the dominant lethal test. This test is usually performed in rodents. The male is exposed to a single dose of the test compound and then is mated with two untreated females weekly for 8 weeks. The females are killed before term, and the number of live embryos and the number of corpora lutea are determined.

The test for mutagens that has received the widest attention is the *Salmonella*/microsome test developed by Ames and colleagues (Ames et al., 1975). This test uses several mutant strains of *Salmonella typhimurium* that lack the enzyme phosphoribosyl ATP synthetase, which is required for histidine synthesis. These strains are unable to grow in a histidine-deficient medium unless a reverse or back-mutation to the wild type has occurred. Other mutations in these bacteria have been introduced to enhance the sensitivity of the strains to mutagenesis. The two most significant additional mutations enhance penetration of substances into the bacteria and decrease the ability of the bacteria to repair DNA damage. Since many chemicals are not mutagenic or carcinogenic unless they are biotransformed to a toxic product by enzymes in the endoplasmic reticulum (microsomes), rat liver microsomes are usually added to the medium containing the mutant strain and the test chemical. The number of reverse mutations is then quantitated by the number of bacterial colonies that grow in a histidine-deficient medium.

Strains of yeast have recently been developed that detect genetic alterations arising during cell division after exposure to non-genotoxic carcinogens as well as mutations that arise from directly genotoxic carcinogens. This test identifies deletions of genetic material that occur during recombination events in cell division that may result from oxidative damage to DNA, direct mutagenic effects, alterations in fidelity of DNA repair, and/or changes in cell cycle regulation (Galli and Schiestl, 1999). Mutagenicity is discussed in detail in Chap. 9.

Table 2-3
Typical Costs of Descriptive Toxicity Tests

TEST	COST, $
General Acute toxicity	
Acute toxicity (rat; two routes)	6,500
Acute dermal toxicity (rabbit)	3,500
Acute inhalation toxicity (rat)	10,000
Acute dermal irritation (rabbit)	2,000
Acute eye irritation (rabbit)	1,500
Skin sensitization (guinea pig)	5,000
Repeated dose toxicity	
14-day exposure (rat)	45,000
90-day exposure (rat)	110,000
1-year (diet; rat)	250,000
1-year (oral gavage; rat)	300,000
2-year (diet; rat)	685,000
2-year (oral gavage; rat)	860,000
Genetic toxicology tests	
Bacterial reverse mutation (Ames test)	7,000
Mammalian cell forward mutation	25,000
In vitro cytogenetics (CHO cells)	20,000
In vivo micronucleus (mouse)	11,000
In vivo chromosome aberration (rat)	22,500
Dominant lethal (mouse)	85,000
Drosophila sex-linked recessive lethal	55,000
Mammalian bone marrow cytogenetics (in vivo; rat)	22,500
Reproduction	
Segment I (rat)	90,000
Segment II (rat)	63,000
Segment II (rabbit)	72,000
Segment III (rat)	160,000

Other Tests

Most of the tests described above will be included in a "standard" toxicity testing protocol because they are required by the various regulatory agencies. Additional tests also may be required or included in the protocol to provide information relating a special route of exposure (inhalation) or a special effect (behavior). Inhalation toxicity tests in animals usually are carried out in a dynamic (flowing) chamber rather than in static chambers to avoid particulate settling and exhaled gas complications. Such studies usually require special dispersing and analytic methodologies, depending on whether the agent to be tested is a gas, vapor, or aerosol; additional information on methods, concepts, and problems associated with inhalation toxicology is provided in Chaps. 15 and 28. A discussion of behavioral toxicology can be found in Chap. 16. The duration of exposure for both inhalation and behavioral toxicity tests can be acute, subchronic, or chronic, but acute studies are more common with inhalation toxicology and chronic studies are more common with behavioral toxicology. Other special types of animal toxicity tests include immunotoxicology, toxicokinetics (absorption, distribution, biotransformation, and excretion), the development of appropriate antidotes and treatment regimes for poisoning, and the development of analytic techniques to detect residues of chemicals in tissues and other biological materials. The approximate costs of some descriptive toxicity tests are given in Table 2-3.

REFERENCES

Abou-Setta MM, Sorrell RW, Childers CC: A computer program in BASIC for determining probit and log-probit or logit correlation for toxicology and biology. *Bull Environ Contam Toxicol* 36:242–249, 1986.

Albert A: Fundamental aspects of selective toxicity. *Ann NY Acad Sci* 123:5–18, 1965.

Albert A: *Selective Toxicity.* London, Chapman and Hall, 1973.

Aldridge WN: The biological basis and measurement of thresholds. *Annu Rev Pharmacol Toxicol* 26:39–58, 1986.

Allen BC, Kavlock RJ, Kimmel CA, et al: Dose–response assessment for developmental toxicity: II. Comparison of generic benchmark dose estimates with no observed adverse effect levels. *Fundam Appl Toxicol* 23:487–495, 1994a.

Allen BC, Kavlock RJ, Kimmel CA, et al: Dose–response assessment for developmental toxicity: III. Statistical models. *Fundam Appl Toxicol* 23:496–509, 1994b.

Ames BN, McCann J, Yamasaki E: Methods for detecting carcinogens and mutagens with the *Salmonella*/mammalian-microsome mutagenicity test. *Mutat Res* 31:347–364, 1975.

Auletta CS: Acute, Subchronic and chronic toxicology, in Derelanko MJ, Hollinger MA (eds): *CRC Handbook of Toxicology.* Orlando, FL: CRC Press, 1995, pp 51–104.

Barnes DG, Dourson M: Reference dose (RfD): Description and use in health risk assessments. *Regul Toxicol Pharmacol* 8:471–486, 1988.

Bartels CF, James K, La Du BN: DNA mutations associated with the human butyrylcholinesterase J-variant. *Am J Hum Genet* 50:1104–1114, 1992.

Bliss CL: Some principles of bioassay. *Am Sci* 45:449–466, 1957.

Bruce RD: A confirmatory study of the up-and-down method for acute oral toxicity testing. *Fundam Appl Toxicol* 8:97–100, 1987.

Bruce RD: An up-and-down procedure for acute toxicity testing. *Fundam Appl Toxicol* 5:151–157, 1985.

Calabrese EJ, Baldwin LA: Chemical hormesis: its historical foundations as a biological hypothesis. *Toxicol Pathol* 27:195–216, 1999.

Christian M: Reproductive and developmental toxicity studies, in Sipes IG, McQueen CA, Gandolfi AJ (eds.): *Comprehensive Toxicology.* Williams PD, Hottendorf GH (eds): Vol 2. *Toxicological Testing and Evaluation.* New York: Pergamon Press, 1997, pp 145–154.

Cohen SM: Calcium phosphate–containing urinary precipitate in rat urinary bladder carcinogenesis. *IARC Sci Publ* 147:175–189, 1999.

Cohen SM: Cell proliferation and carcinogenesis. *Drug Metab Rev* 30:339–357, 1998.

Crump KS: An improved procedure for low-dose carcinogenic risk assessment from animal data. *J Environ Pathol Toxicol Oncol* 5:339–348, 1984.

Davila JC, Rodriguez RJ, Melchert RB, et al: Predictive value of in vitro model systems in toxicology. *Annu Rev Pharmacol Toxicol* 38:63–96, 1998.

Doull J: Factors influencing toxicity, in Doull J, Klaassen CD, Amdur MO (eds): *Casarett and Doull's Toxicology: The Basic Science of Poisons, 2d ed.* New York: Macmillan, 1980, pp 70–83.

Dybing E, Sanner T: Species differences in chemical carcinogenesis of the thyroid gland, kidney and urinary bladder. *IARC Sci Publ* 147:15–32, 1999.

Eaton DL, Gallagher EP: Mechanisms of aflatoxin carcinogenesis. *Annu Rev Pharmacol Toxicol* 34:135–172, 1994.

Faustman EM: Short-term tests for teratogens. *Mutat Res* 205:355–384, 1988.

Faustman EM, Allen BC, Kavlock RJ, et al.: Dose–response assessment for developmental toxicity: I. Characterization of database and determination of no observed adverse effect levels. *Fundam Appl Toxicol* 23:478–486, 1994.

Finney DJ: The median lethal dose and its estimation. *Arch Toxicol* 56:215–218, 1985.

Finney DJ: *Probit Analysis.* Cambridge, England: Cambridge University Press, 1971.

Galli A, Schiestl RH: Cell division transforms mutagenic lesions into deletion-recombinagenic lesions in yeast cells. *Mutat Res* 429:13–26, 1999.

Glynn P, Read DJ, Lush MJ, et al: Molecular cloning of neuropathy target esterase (NTE). *Chem Biol Interact* 119–120:513–517, 1999.

Goldstein A, Aronow L, Kalman SM: *Principles of Drug Action.* New York: Wiley, 1974.

Grisham JW: Interspecies comparison of liver carcinogenesis: Implications for cancer risk assessment. *Carcinogenesis* 18:59–81, 1997.

Hanna EZ, Chou SP, Grant, BF: The relationship between drinking and heart disease morbidity in the United States: Results from the National Health Interview Survey. *Alcohol Clin Exp Res* 21:111–118, 1997.

Haseman JK: Issues in carcinogenicity testing: Dose selection. *Fundam Appl Toxicol* 5:66–78, 1985.

Hatch EE, Palmer JR, Titus-Ernstoff L, et al: Cancer risk in women exposed to diethylstilbestrol in utero. *JAMA* 280:630–634, 1998.

Hayes, AW, Ed. *Principles and Methods of Toxicology.* 4th Edition. Taylor and Francis, New York, 2001.

Hengstler JG, Van der Burg B, Steinberg P, et al: Interspecies differences in cancer susceptibility and toxicity. *Drug Metab Rev* 31:917–970, 1999.

Houlston RS: Glutathione S-transferase M1 status and lung cancer risk: A meta-analysis. *Cancer Epidemiol Biomarkers Prev* 8:675–682, 1999.

Huff JE: Value, validity, and historical development of carcinogenesis studies for predicting and confirming carcinogenic risk to humans, in Kitchin KT (ed): *Carcinogenicity Testing: Predicting & Interpreting Chemical Effects.* New York: Marcel Dekker, 1999, pp 21–123.

Kobayashi Y, Fukumaki Y, Yubisui T, et al: Serine-proline replacement at residue 127 of NADH-cytochrome b5 reductase causes hereditary methemoglobinemia, generalized type. *Blood* 75:1408–1413, 1990.

Lary, JM, Daniel, KL, Erickson, JD, et al: The return of thalidomide: Can birth defects be prevented? *Drug Saf* 21:161–169, 1999.

Lehman-McKeeman LD, Caudill D: Biochemical basis for mouse resistance to hyaline droplet nephropathy: Lack of relevance of the alpha 2u-globulin protein superfamily in this male rat-specific syndrome. *Toxicol Appl Pharmacol* 112:214–221, 1992.

Levine RR: *Pharmacology: Drug Actions and Reactions.* Boston: Little, Brown, 1978.

Litchfield J, Wilcoxon F: Simplified method of evaluating dose-effect experiments. *J Pharmacol Exp Ther* 96:99–113, 1949.

Litchfield JT: A method for rapid graphic solution of time-percent effective curve. *J Pharmacol Exp Ther* 97:399–408, 1949.

Littlefield NA, Farmer JH, Gaylor DW, et al: Effects of dose and time in a long-term, low-dose carcinogenicity study, in Staffa JA, Mehlman MA (eds): *Innovations in Cancer Risk Assessment (ED01 Study).* Park Forest South, IL: Pathotox Publishers, 1979.

Maibach HI, Patrick E: Dermatotoxicology, in Hayes AW (ed): *Principles and Methods of Toxicology.* New York: Taylor and Francis, 2001, pp 1039–1084.

Monticello TM, Morgan KT: Chemically-induced nasal carcinogenesis and epithelial cell proliferation: A brief review. *Mutat Res* 380:33–41, 1997.

Reno FE: Carcinogenicity studies, in Sipes IG, McQueen CA, Gandolfi AJ (eds.): *Comprehensive Toxicology.* Williams PD, Hottendorf GH (eds): Vol 2. *Toxicological Testing and Evaluation.* New York: Pergamon Press, 1997, pp 121–131.

Roberts RA: Peroxisome proliferators: Mechanisms of adverse effects in rodents and molecular basis for species differences. *Arch Toxicol* 73:413–418, 1999.

Rush RE, Bonnette KL, Douds DA, et al: Dermal irritation and sensitization, in Derelanko MJ, Hollinger MA (eds): *CRC Handobook of Toxicology.* New York: CRC Press, 1995, pp 105–162.

Strange RC, Fryer, AA: The glutathione S-transferases: influence of polymorphism on cancer susceptibility. *IARC Sci Publ* 148:231–249, 1999.

Tennant, RW, Stasiewicz, S, Mennear, J, et al: Genetically altered mouse models for identifying carcinogens. *IARC Sci Publ* 146:123–150, 1999.

Weathereholtz WM: Acute, subchronic and chronic toxicity studies, in Sipes GI, McQueen CA, Gandolfi AJ (eds): *Comprehensive Toxicology.* Williams PD, Hottendorf GH (eds): Vol 2. *Toxicological Testing and Evaluation.* New York: Pergamon Press, 1997, pp 101–120.

Weil C: Tables for convenient calculation of median-effective dose (LD50 or ED50) and instruction in their use. *Biometrics* 8:249–263, 1952.

Weinshilboum RM, Otterness DM, Szumlanski CL: Methylation pharmacogenetics: Catechol O-methyltransferase, thiopurine methyltransferase, and histamine N-methyltransferase. *Annu Rev Pharmacol Toxicol* 39:19–52, 1999.

Wiman KG: The retinoblastoma gene: Role in cell cycle control and cell differentiation. *FASEB J* 7:841–845, 1993.

Wogan GN, Paglialunga S, Newberne, PM: Carcinogenic effects of low dietary levels of aflatoxin B1 in rats. *Food Cosmet Toxicol* 12:681–685, 1974.

CHAPTER 3

MECHANISMS OF TOXICITY

Zoltán Gregus and Curtis D. Klaassen

Depending primarily on the degree and route of exposure, chemicals may adversely affect the function and/or structure of living organisms. The qualitative and quantitative characterization of these harmful or toxic effects is essential for an evaluation of the potential hazard posed by a particular chemical. It is also valuable to understand the mechanisms responsible for the manifestation of toxicity—that is, how a toxicant enters an organism, how it interacts with target molecules, and how the organism deals with the insult.

An understanding of the mechanisms of toxicity is of both practical and theoretical importance. Such information provides a rational basis for interpreting descriptive toxicity data, estimating the probability that a chemical will cause harmful effects, establishing procedures to prevent or antagonize the toxic effects, designing drugs and industrial chemicals that are less hazardous, and developing pesticides that are more selectively toxic for their target organisms. Elucidation of the mechanisms of chemical toxicity has led to a better understanding of fundamental physiologic and biochemical processes ranging from neurotransmission (e.g., curare-type arrow poisons) to deoxyribonucleic acid (DNA) repair (e.g., alkylating agents). Pathologic conditions such as cancer and Parkinson's disease are better understood because of studies on the mechanism of toxicity of chemical carcinogens and 1,2,3,6-tetrahydro-1-methyl-4-phenylpyridine (MPTP), respectively. Continued research on mechanisms of toxicity will undoubtedly continue to provide such insights.

This chapter reviews the cellular mechanisms that contribute to the manifestation of toxicities. Although such mechanisms are dealt with elsewhere in this volume, they are discussed in detail in this chapter in an integrated and comprehensive manner. We provide an overview of the mechanisms of chemical toxicity by relating a series of events that begins with exposure, involves a multitude of interactions between the invading toxicant and the organism, and culminates in a toxic effect. This chapter focuses on mechanisms that have been identified definitively or tentatively in humans or animals.

As a result of the huge number of potential toxicants and the multitude of biological structures and processes that can be impaired, there are a tremendous number of possible toxic effects.

Correspondingly, there are various pathways that may lead to toxicity (Fig. 3-1). A common course is when a toxicant delivered to its target reacts with it, and the resultant cellular dysfunction manisfests itself in toxicity. An example of this route to toxicity is that taken by the puffer fish poison, tetrodotoxin. After ingestion, this poison reaches the voltage-gated Na^+ channels of motoneurons (step 1). Interaction of tetrodotoxin with this target (step 2a) results in blockade of Na^+ channels, inhibition of the activity of motor neurons (step 3), and ultimately skeletal muscle paralysis. No repair mechanisms can prevent the onset of such toxicity.

Sometimes a xenobiotic does not react with a specific target molecule but rather adversely influences the biological (micro) environment, causing molecular, organellar, cellular, or organ dysfunction leading to deleterious effects. For example, 2,4-dinitrophenol, after entering the mitochondrial matrix space (step 1), collapses the outwardly directed proton gradient across the inner membrane by its mere presence there (step 2b), causing mitochondrial dysfunction (step 3), which is manifest in toxic effects such as hyperthemia and seizures. Chemicals that precipitate in renal tubules and block urine formation represent another example for such a course (step 2b).

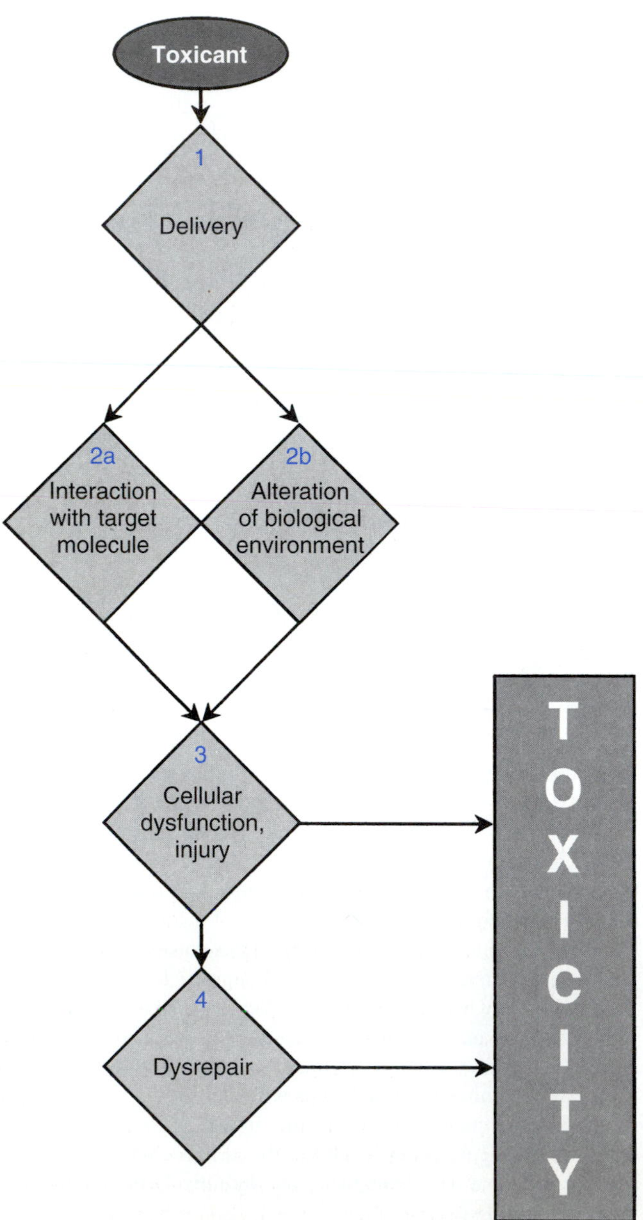

Figure 3-1. Potential stages in the development of toxicity after chemical exposure.

The most complex path to toxicity involves more steps (Fig. 3-1). First, the toxicant is delivered to its target or targets (step 1), after which the ultimate toxicant interacts with endogenous target molecules (step 2a), triggering perturbations in cell function and/or structure (step 3), which initiate repair mechanisms at the molecular, cellular, and/or tissue levels (step 4). When the perturbations induced by the toxicant exceed repair capacity or when repair becomes malfunctional, toxicity occurs. Tissue necrosis, cancer, and fibrosis are examples of chemically induced toxicities whose development follow this four-step course.

STEP 1—DELIVERY: FROM THE SITE OF EXPOSURE TO THE TARGET

Theoretically, the intensity of a toxic effect depends primarily on the concentration and persistence of the ultimate toxicant at its site of action. The ultimate toxicant is the chemical species that reacts with the endogenous target molecule (e.g., receptor, enzyme, DNA, microfilamental protein, lipid) or critically alters the biological (micro)environment, initiating structural and/or functional alterations that result is toxicity. Often the ultimate toxicant is the original chemical to which the organism is exposed (parent compound). In other cases, the ultimate toxicant is a metabolite of the parent compound or a reactive oxygen or nitrogen species (ROS or RNS) generated during the biotransformation of the toxicant. Occasionally, the ultimate toxicant is an endogenous molecule (Table 3-1).

The concentration of the ultimate toxicant at the target molecule depends on the relative effectiveness of the processes that increase or decrease its concentration at the target site (Fig. 3-2). The accumulation of the ultimate toxicant at its target is facilitated by its absorption, distribution to the site of action, reabsorption, and toxication (metabolic activation). Presystemic elimination, distribution away from the site of action, excretion, and detoxication oppose these processes and work against the accumulation of the ultimate toxicant at the target molecule.

Absorption versus Presystemic Elimination

Absorption Absorption is the transfer of a chemical from the site of exposure, usually an external or internal body surface (e.g., skin, mucosa of the alimentary and respiratory tracts), into the systemic circulation. The vast majority of toxicants traverse epithelial barriers and reach the blood capillaries by diffusing through cells. The rate of absorption is related to the concentration of the chemical at the absorbing surface, which depends on the rate of exposure and the dissolution of the chemical. It is also related to the area of the exposed site, the characteristics of the epithelial layer through which absorption takes place (e.g., the thickness of the stratum corneum in the skin), the intensity of the subepithelial microcir-

Table 3-1
Types of Ultimate Toxicants and Their Sources

Parent xenobiotics as ultimate toxicants		
Pb ions		
Tetrodotoxin		
TCDD		
Methylisocyanate		
HCN		
CO		
Xenobiotic metabolites as ultimate toxicants		
Amygdalin	→	HCN
Arsenate	→	Arsenite
Fluoroacetate	→	Fluorocitrate
Ethylene glycol	→	Oxalic acid
Hexane	→	2,5-Hexanedione
Acetaminophen	→	*N*-Acetyl-*p*-benzoquinoneimine
CCl_4	→	$CCl_3OO^{\bullet}$
Benzo[*a*]pyrene (BP)	→	BP-7,8-diol-9,10-epoxide
Benzo[*a*]pyrene (BP)	→	BP-Radical cation
Reactive oxygen or nitrogen species as ultimate toxicants		
Hydrogen peroxide	→	
Diquat, doxorubicin, nitrofurantoin		Hydroxyl radical (HO•)
Cr(V), Fe(II), Mn(II), Ni(II)	→	
Paraquat → $O_2^{\bar{\bullet}}$ + $NO^{\bullet}$		Peroxynitrite ($ONOO^-$)
Endogenous compounds as ultimate toxicants		
Sulfonamides → albumin-bound bilirubin	→	Bilirubin
$CCl_3OO^{\bullet}$ → unsaturated fatty acids	→	Lipid peroxyl radicals
$CCl_3OO^{\bullet}$ → unsaturated fatty acids	→	Lipid alkoxyl radicals
$CCl_3OO^{\bullet}$ → unsaturated fatty acids	→	4-Hydroxynonenal
$HO^{\bullet}$ → proteins	→	Protein carbonyls

culation, and the physicochemical properties of the toxicant. Lipid solubility is usually the most important property influencing absorption. In general, lipid-soluble chemicals are absorbed more readily than are water-soluble substances.

Presystemic Elimination During transfer from the site of exposure to the systemic circulation, toxicants may be eliminated. This is not unusual for chemicals absorbed from the gastrointestinal (GI) tract because they must first pass through the GI mucosal cells, liver, and lung before being distributed to the rest of the body by the systemic circulation. The GI mucosa and the liver may eliminate a significant fraction of a toxicant during its passage through these tissues, decreasing its systemic availability. For example, ethanol is oxidized by alcohol dehydrogenase in the gastric mucosa (Lim et al., 1993), cyclosporine is returned from the enterocyte into the intestinal lumen by P-glycoprotein (an ATP-dependent xenobiotic transporter) and is also hydroxylated by cytochrome P450 (CP3A4) in these cells (Lin et al., 1999), morphine is glucuronidated in the intestinal mucosa and the liver, and manganese is taken up from the portal blood into the liver and excreted into bile. Such processes may prevent a considerable quantity of chemicals from reaching the systemic blood. Thus, presystemic or first-pass elimination reduces the toxic effects of chemicals that reach their target sites by way of the systemic circulation. In contrast, the processes involved in presystemic elimination may contribute to injury of the digestive mucosa, the liver, and the lungs by chemicals such as ethanol, iron salts, α-amanitin, and paraquat because these processes promote their delivery to those sites.

Distribution to and Away from the Target

Toxicants exit the blood during the distribution phase, enter the extracellular space, and may penetrate into cells. Chemicals dissolved in plasma water may diffuse through the capillary endothelium via aqueous intercellular spaces and transcelluar pores called fenestrae and/or across the cell membrane. Lipid-soluble compounds move readily into cells by diffusion. In contrast, highly ionized and hydrophilic xenobiotics (e.g., tubocurarine and aminoglycosides) are largely restricted to the extracellular space unless specialized membrane carrier systems are available to transport them.

During distribution, toxicants reach their site or sites of action, usually a macromolecule on either the surface or the interior of a particular type of cell. Chemicals also may be distributed to the site or sites of toxication, usually an intracellular enzyme, where the ultimate toxicant is formed. Some mechanisms facili-

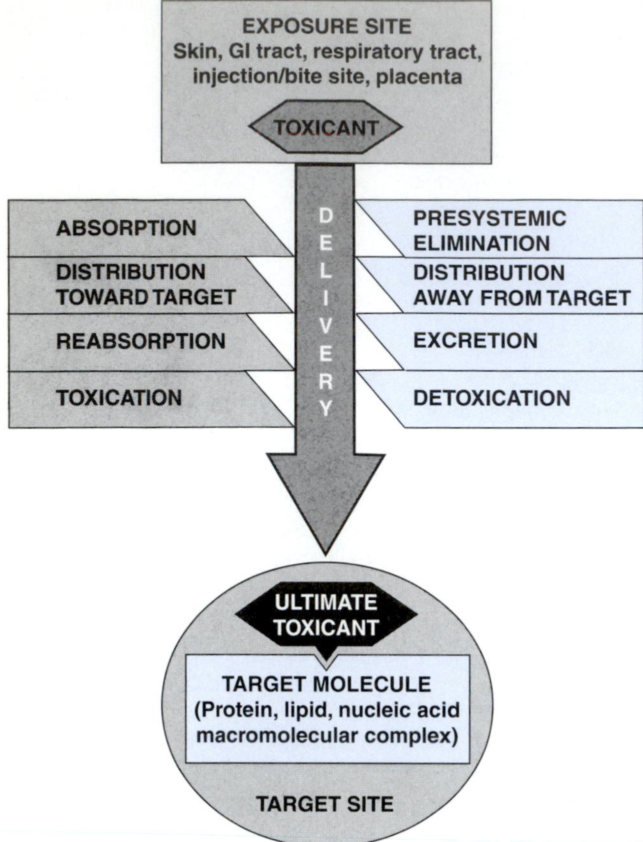

Figure 3-2. The process of toxicant delivery is the first step in the development of toxicity.

Delivery—that is, movement of the toxicant from the site of exposure to the site of its action in an active form—is promoted by the processes listed on the left and opposed by the events indicated on the right.

tate whereas others delay the distribution of toxicants to their targets.

Mechanisms Facilitating Distribution to a Target Distribution of toxicants to specific target sites may be enhanced by (1) the porosity of the capillary endothelium, (2) specialized membrane transport, (3) accumulation in cell organelles, and (4) reversible intracellular binding.

Porosity of the Capillary Endothelium Endothelial cells in the hepatic sinusoids and in the renal peritubular capillaries have larger fenestrae (50 to 150 nm in diameter) that permit passage of even protein-bound xenobiotics. This favors the accumulation of chemicals in the liver and kidneys.

Specialized Transport Across the Plasma Membrane Specialized ion channels and membrane transporters can contribute to the delivery of toxicants to intracellular targets. For example, Na^+,K^+-ATPase promotes intracellular accumulation of thallous ion and voltage-gated Ca^{2+} channels permit the entry of cations such as lead or barium ions into excitable cells. Paraquat enters into pneumocytes, α-amanitin and microcystins enter into hepatocytes (Kröncke et al., 1986), ochratoxin and the cysteine conjugate of mercuric ion enter into renal tubular cells, and an MPTP metabolite (MPP^+) enters into extrapyramidal dopaminergic neurons by means of carrier-mediated uptake. Endocytosis of some toxicant-protein complexes, such as Cd-metallothionein or hydrocarbons bound to the male rat–specific α_{2u}-globulin, by renal proximal tubular cells also can occur. In addition, lipoprotein receptor–mediated endocytosis contributes to entry of lipoprotein-bound toxicants into cells equipped with such transporters. Membrane recycling can internalize catioinic aminoglycosides associated with anionic phopholipides in the brush border membrane of renal tubular cells (Laurent et al., 1990). This process also may contribute to cellular uptake of heavy metal ions. Such uptake mechanisms facilitate the entry of toxicants into specific cells, rendering those cells targets. Thus, carrier-mediated uptake of paraquat by pneumocytes and internalization of aminoglycosides by renal proximal tubular cells expose those cells to toxic concentrations of those chemicals.

Accumulation in Cell Organelles Amphipathic xenobiotics with a protonable amine group and lipophilic character accumulate in lysosomes as well as mitochondria and cause adverse effects there. Lysosomal accumulation occurs by pH trapping, i.e., diffusion of the amine in unprotonated from into the acidic interior of the organelle, where the amine is protonated, preventing its efflux. Binding of the amine to lysosomal phospholipids impairs their degradation and causes phospholipidosis. Mitochondrial accumulation takes place electrophoretically. The amine is protonated in the intermembrane space (to where the mitochondria eject protons). The cation thus formed will then be sucked into the matrix space by the strong negative potential there (−220 mV), where it may impair β-oxidation and oxidative phosphorylation. By such mechanisms, the valued antiarrhytmic drug amiodarone is entrapped in the hepatic lysosomes and mitochondria, causing phospholipidosis (Kodovanti and Mehendale, 1990) and microvesiculas steatosis with other liver lesions (Fromenty and Pessayre, 1997), respectively. The cationic metabolite of MPTP (MPP^+) also electrophoretically accumulates in the mitochondria of dopaminergic neurones, causing mitochondrial dysfunction and cell death.

Reversible Intracellular Binding Binding to the pigment melanin, an intracellular polyanionic aromatic polymer, is a mechanism by which chemicals such as organic and inorganic cations and polycyclic aromatic hydrocarbons can accumulate in melanin-containing cells (Larsson, 1993). The release of melanin-bound toxicants is thought to contribute to the retinal toxicity associated with chlorpromazine and chloroquine, injury to substantia nigra neurons by MPTP and manganese, and the induction of melanoma by polycyclic aromatics.

Mechanisms Opposing Distribution to a Target Distribution of toxicants to specific sites may be hindered by several processes. The processes include (1) binding to plasma proteins, (2) specialized barriers, (3) distribution to storage sites such as adipose tissue, (4) association with intracellular binding proteins, and (5) export from cells.

Binding to Plasma Proteins As long as xenobiotics such as DDT and TCDD are bound to high-molecular-weight proteins or lipoproteins in plasma, they cannot leave the capillaries by diffusion. Even if they exit the bloodstream through fenestrae, they have difficulty permeating cell membranes. Dissociation from proteins is required for most xenobiotics to leave the blood and enter cells. Therefore, strong binding to plasma proteins delays and prolongs the effects and elimination of toxicants.

Specialized Barriers Brain capillaries have very low aqueous porosity because their endothelial cells lack fenestrae and are joined by extremely tight junctions. This blood-brain barrier prevents the access of hydrophilic chemicals to the brain except for those that can be actively transported. Water-soluble toxicants also have restricted access to reproductive cells, which are separated from capillaries by multiple layers to cells. The oocyte is surrounded by the granulosa cells, and the spermatogenic cells are surrounded by Sertoli cells that are tightly joined to form the blood-testis barrier (Chap. 20). Transfer of hydrophilic toxicants across the placenta is also restricted. However, none of these barriers are effective against lipophilic substances.

Distribution to Storage Sites Some chemicals accumulate in tissues (i.e., storage sites) where they do not exert significant effects. For example, highly lipophilic substances such as chlorinated hydrocarbon insecticides concentrate in adipocytes, whereas lead is deposited in bone by substituting for Ca^{2+} in hydroxyapatite. Such storage decreases the availability of these toxicants for their target sites and acts as a temporary protective mechanism. However, insecticides may return to the circulation and be distributed to their target site, the nervous tissue, when there is a rapid lipid loss as a result of fasting. This is thought to contribute to the lethality to pesticide-exposed birds during migration or during the winter months, when food is restricted. The possibility that lead is mobilized from the bone during pregnancy is of concern.

Association with Intracellular Binding Proteins Binding to nontarget intracellular sites also reduces the concentration of toxicants at the target site, at least temporarily. Metallothionein, a cysteine-rich cytoplasmic protein, serves such a function in acute cadmium intoxication (Goering et al., 1995).

Export from Cells Intracellular toxicants may be transported back into the extracellular space. This occurs in brain capillary endothelial cells. These cells contain in their luminal membrane an ATP-dependent membrane transporter known as the multidrug-resistance (mdr) protein, or P-glycoprotein, which extrudes chemicals and contributes to the blood-brain barrier (Schinkel, 1999). Compared to normal mice, mice with disrupted *mdr 1a* gene exhibit 100-fold higher brain levels of and sensitivity to ivermectin, a neurotoxic pesticide and human anthelmintic drug that is one of many P-glycoprotein substrates (Schinkel, 1999). The ooctye is also equipped with the P-glycoprotein that provides protection against chemicals that are substrates for this efflux pump (Elbling et al., 1993).

Excretion versus Reabsorption

Excretion Excretion is the removal of xenobiotics from the blood and their return to the external environment. Excretion is a physical mechanism whereas biotransformation is a chemical mechanism for eliminating the toxicant.

For nonvolatile chemicals, the major excretory structures in the body are the renal glomeruli, which hydrostatically filter small molecules (<60 kDa) through their pores, and the proximal renal tubular cells and hepatocytes, which actively transport chemicals from the blood into the renal tubules and bile canaliculi, respectively. These cells are readily exposed to blood-borne chemicals throught the large endothelial fenestrae; they have membrane transporters that mediate the uptake and luminal extrusion of certain chemicals (Chap. 5). Renal transporters have a preferential affinity for smaller (<300-Da), and hepatic transporters for larger (>400-Da), amphiphilic molecules. A less common "excretory" mechanism consists of diffusion and partition into the excreta on the basis of their lipid content (see below) or acidity. For example, morphine is transferred into milk and amphetamine is transferred into gastric juice by nonionic diffusion. This is facilitated by pH trapping of those organic bases in those fluids, which are acidic relative to plasma (Chap. 5).

The route and speed of excretion depend largely on the physicochemical properties of the toxicant. The major excretory organs—the kidney and the liver—can efficiently remove only highly hydrophilic, usually ionized chemicals such as organic acids and bases. The reasons for this are as follows: (1) In the renal glomeruli, only compounds dissolved in the plasma water can be filtered; (2) transporters in hepatocytes and renal proximal tubular cells are specialized for the secretion of highly hydrophilic organic acids and bases; (3) only hydrophilic chemicals are freely soluble in the aqueous urine and bile; and (4) lipid-soluble compounds are readily reabsorbed by transcellular diffusion.

There are no efficient elimination mechanisms for nonvolatile, highly lipophilic chemicals such as polyhalogenated biphenyls and chlorinated hydrocarbon insecticides. If they are resistant to biotransformation, such chemicals are eliminated very slowly and tend to accumulate in the body upon repeated exposure. Three rather inefficient processes are available for the elimination of such chemicals: (1) excretion by the mammary gland after the chemical is dissolved in the milk lipids; (2) excretion in bile in association with biliary micelles and/or phospholipid vesicles; and (3) intestinal excretion, an incompletely understood transport from the blood into the intestinal lumen. Volatile, nonreactive toxicants such as gases and volatile liquids diffuse from pulmonary capillaries into the alveoli and are exhaled.

Reabsorption Toxicants delivered into the renal tubules may diffuse back across the tubular cells into the peritubular capillaries. This process is facilitated by tubular fluid reabsorption, which increases the intratubular concentration as well as the residence time of the chemical by slowing urine flow. Reabsorption by diffusion is dependent on the lipid solubility of the chemical. For organic acids and bases, diffusion is inversely related to the extent of ionization, because the nonionized molecule is more lipid-soluble. The ionization of weak organic acids such as salicylic acid and phenobarbital and bases such as amphetamine, procainamide, and quinidine is strongly pH-dependent in the physiologic range. Therefore their reabsorption is influenced significantly by the pH of the tubular fluid. Acidification of urine favors the excretion of weak organic bases, while alkalinization favors the elimination of weak organic acids. Carriers for the physiologic oxyanions mediate the reabsorption of some toxic metal oxyanions in the kidney. Chromate and molybdate are reabsorbed by the sulfate transporter, whereas arsenate is reabsorbed by the phosphate transporter.

Toxicants delivered to the GI tract by biliary, gastric, and intestinal excretion and secretion by salivary glands and the exocrine pancreas may be reabsorbed by diffusion across the intestinal mucosa. Because compounds secreted into bile are usually organic acids, their reabsorption is possible only if they are sufficiently lipophilic or are converted to more lipid-soluble forms in the intestinal lumen. For example, glucuronides of toxicants such as diethylstilbestrol and glucuronides of the hydroxylated metabolites of polycyclic aromatic hydrocarbons, chlordecone, and halogenated biphenyls are hydrolyzed by the β-glucuronidase of intestinal microorganisms, and the released aglycones are reabsorbed (Gregus and Klaassen, 1986). Glutathione conjugates of hexachlorobutadiene and trichloroethylene are hydrolyzed by intestinal and pancreatic peptidases, yielding the cysteine conjugates, which are reabsorbed and serve as precursors of additional metabolites with nephrotoxic properties (Dekant et al., 1989).

Toxication versus Detoxication

Toxication A number of xenobiotics (e.g., strong acids and bases, nicotine, aminoglycosides, ethylene oxide, methylisocyanate, heavy-metal ions, HCN, CO) are directly toxic, whereas the toxicity of others is due largely to metabolites. Biotransformation to harmful products is called *toxication* or *metabolic activation.* With some xenobiotics, toxication confers physicochemical properties that adversely alter the microenvironment of biological processes or structures. For example, oxalic acid formed from ethylene glycol may cause acidosis and hypocalcemia as well as obstruction of renal tubules by precipitation as calcium oxalate. Occasionally, chemicals acquire structural features and reactivity by biotransformation that allows for a more efficient interaction with specific receptors or enzymes. For example, the organophosphate insecticide parathion is biotransformed to paraoxon, an active cholinestrase inhibitor; the rodenticide fluoroacetate is converted in the citric acid cycle to fluorocitrate, a false substrate that inhibits aconitase; and fialuridine, an antiviral drug withdrawn because it produced lethal hepatotoxicity in patients, is phosphorylated to the triphosphate, which inhibits DNA polymerase-γ and thus impairs synthesis of mitochondrial DNA (Lewis et al., 1996). Most often, however, toxication renders xenobiotics and occasionally other molecules in the body, such as oxygen and nitric oxide ($^{\bullet}NO$), indiscriminately reactive toward endogenous molecules with susceptible functional groups. This increased reactivity may be due to conversion into (1) electrophiles, (2) free radicals, (3) nucleophiles, or (4) redox-active reactants.

Formation of Electrophiles Electrophiles are molecules containing an electron-deficient atom with a partial or full positive charge that allows it to react by sharing electron pairs with electron-rich atoms in nucleophiles. The formation of electrophiles is involved in the toxication of numerous chemicals (Table 3-2) (Chap. 6). Such reactants are often produced by insertion of an oxygen atom, which withdraws electrons from the atom it is attached to, making that electrophilic. This is the case when aldehydes, ketones, epoxides, arene oxides, sulfoxides, nitroso compounds, phosphonates, and acyl halides are formed (Table 3-2). In other instances, conjugated double bonds are formed, which become polarized by the electron-withdrawing effect of an oxygen, making one of the double-bonded carbons electron-deficient (that is, electrophilic). This occurs when α,β-unsaturated aldehydes and ketones as well as quinones and quinoneimines are produced (Table 3-2). Formation of many of these electrophilic metabolites is catalyzed by cytochrome P450.

Cationic electrophiles are produced as a result of heterolytic bond cleavage. For example, methyl-substituted aromatics such as 7,12-dimethylbenzanthracene and aromatic amines (amides) such as 2-acetylaminofluorene are hydroxylated to form benzylic alcohols and *N*-hydroxy arylamines (amides), respectively (Miller and Surh, 1994). These substances are esterified, typically by sulfotransferases. Heterolytic cleavage of the C—O or N—O bonds of these esters results in a hydrosulfate anion and the concomitant formation of a benzylic carbonium ion or arylnitrenium ion, respectively. The oxidation of metallic mercury to Hg^{2+} and the reduction of CrO_4^{2-} to Cr^{3+} as well as that of AsO_4^{3-} to AsO_3^{2-}/As^{3+} are examples of the formation of electrophilic toxicants from inorganic chemicals.

Formation of Free Radicals A free radical is a molecule or molecular fragment that contains one or more unpaired electrons in its outer orbital. Radicals are formed by (1) accepting an electron or (2) losing an electron or by (3) homolytic fission of a covalent bond.

1. Xenobiotics such as paraquat, doxorubicin, and nitrofurantoin can accept an electron from reductases to give rise to radicals (Fig. 3-3). These radicals typically transfer the extra electron to molecular oxygen, forming a superoxide anion radical ($O_2^{\bar{\bullet}}$) and regenerating the parent xenobiotic, which is ready to gain a new electron (Kappas, 1986). Through this "redox cycling," one electron acceptor xenobiotic molecule can generate many $O_2^{\bar{\bullet}}$ molecules. There are also endogenous sources of $O_2^{\bar{\bullet}}$. This radical is generated in large quantities by NAD(P)H oxidase in activated macrophages and granulocytes during "respiratory burst" and is also produced by the mitochondrial electron transport chain, especially in the "uncoupled" state. The significance of $O_2^{\bar{\bullet}}$ stems to a large extent from the fact that $O_2^{\bar{\bullet}}$ is a starting compound in two toxication pathways (Fig. 3-4); one leading to formation of hydrogen peroxide (HOOH) and then hydroxyl radical ($HO^{\bullet}$), whereas the other produces peroxynitrite ($ONOO^-$) and ultimately nitrogen dioxide ($^{\bullet}NO_2$), and carbonate anion radical ($CO_3^{\bar{\bullet}}$).
2. Nucleophilic xenobiotics such as phenols, hydroquinones, aminophenols, amines, hydrazines, phenothiazines, and thiols are prone to lose an electron and form free radicals in a reaction catalyzed by peroxidases (Aust et al., 1993). Some of these chemicals, such as catechols and hydroquinones, may undergo two sequential one-electron oxidations, producing first semiquinone radicals and then quinones. Quinones are not only reactive electrophiles (Table 3-2) but also electron acceptors with the capacity to initiate redox cycling or oxidation of thiols and NAD(P)H. Polycyclic aromatic hydrocarbons with sufficiently low ionization potential, such as benzo[*a*]pyrene and 7,12-dimethylbenzanthracene, can be converted via one-electron oxidation by peroxidases or cytochrome P450 to radical cations, which may be the ultimate toxicants for these carcinogens (Cavalieri and Rogan, 1992). Like peroxidases, oxyhemoglobin ($Hb\text{-}FeII\text{-}O_2$) can catalyze the oxidation of aminophenols to semiquinone radicals and quinoneimines. This is another example of toxication, because these products, in turn, oxidize ferrohemoglobin (Hb-FeII) to methemoglobin (Hb-FeIII), which cannot carry oxygen.
3. Free radicals also are formed by homolytic bond fission, which can be induced by electron transfer to the molecule (reductive fission). This mechanism is involved in the conversion of CCl_4 to the trichloromethyl free radical ($Cl_3C^{\bullet}$) by an electron transfer from cytochrome P450 or the mitochondrial electron transport chain (reductive dehalogenation) (Recknagel et al., 1989). The $Cl_3C^{\bullet}$ reacts with O_2 to form the even more reactive trichloromethylperoxy radical ($Cl_3COO^{\bullet}$) (Hippeli and Elstner, 1999).

The hydroxyl radical ($HO^{\bullet}$), a free radical of paramount toxicologic significance, also is generated by homolytic fission. Such a process yields large amounts of $HO^{\bullet}$ from water upon ionizing radiation. Reductive homolytic fission of hydrogen peroxide (HOOH) to $HO^{\bullet}$ and HO^- is called the *Fenton reaction* (Fig. 3-4). This is catalyzed by transition metal ions, typically Fe(II) or, Cu(I), Cr(V), Ni(II), or Mn(II), and is a major toxication mechanism for HOOH and its precursor $O_2^{\bar{\bullet}}$ as well as for transition metals. Moreover, the toxicity of chemicals, such as nitrilotriacetic acid, bleomycin, and orellanin (Hippeli and Elstner, 1999), that chelate transition metal ions is also based on Fenton chemistry because chelation in-

Table 3-2
Toxication by Formation of Electrophilic Metabolites

ELECTROPHILIC METABOLITE	PARENT TOXICANT	ENZYMES CATALYZING TOXICATION	TOXIC EFFECT
Nonionic electrophiles			
Aldehydes, ketones			
Acetaldehyde	Ethanol	ADH	Hepatic fibrosis(?)
Zomepirac glucuronide	Zomepirac	GT→isomerization	Immune reaction(?)
2,5-Hexanedione	Hexane	P450	Axonopathy
α,β-Unsaturated aldehydes, ketones			
Acrolein	Allyl alcohol	ADH	Hepatic necrosis
Acrolein	Allyl amine	MAO	Vascular injury
Muconic aldehyde	Benzene	Multiple	Bone marrow injury
4-Hydroxynonenal	Fatty acids	Lipid peroxidation	Cellular injury(?)
Quinones, quinoneimines			
DES-4,4′-quinone	DES	Peroxidases	Carcinogenesis(?)
N-Acetyl-*p*-benzoquinoneimine	Acetaminophen	P450, peroxidases	Hepatic necrosis
Epoxides, arene oxides			
Aflatoxin B_1 8,9-epoxide	Aflatoxin B_1	P450	Carcinogenesis
2-Chlorooxirane	Vinyl chloride	P450	Carcinogenesis
Bromobenzene 3,4-oxide	Bromobenzene	P450	Hepatic necrosis
Benzo[*a*]pyrene 7,8-diol 9,10-oxide	Benzo[*a*]pyrene	P450	Carcinogenesis
Sulfoxides			
Thioacetamide *S*-oxide	Thioacetamide	FMO	Hepatic necrosis
Nitroso compounds			
Nitroso-sulfamethoxazole	Sulfamethoxazole	P450	Immune reaction
Phosphonates			
Paraoxon	Parathion	P450	ChE inhibition
Acyl halides			
Phosgene	Chloroform	P450	Hepatic necrosis
Trifluoroacetyl chloride	Halothane	P450	Immune hepatitis
Thionoacyl halides			
2,3,4,4-Tetrachlorothiobut-3-enoic acid chloride	HCBD	GST→GGT →DP→CβCL	Renal tubular necrosis
Thioketenes			
Chloro-1,2,2-trichlorovinyl-thioketene	HCBD	GST→GGT →DP→CCβL	Renal tubular necrosis
Cationic Electrophiles			
Carbonium ions			
Benzylic carbocation	7,12-DMBA	P450→ST	Carcinogenesis
Carbonium cation	DENA	P450→s.r.	
Nitrenium ions			
Arylnitrenium ion	AAF, DMAB, HAPP	P450→ST	Carcinogenesis
Sulfonium ions			
Episulfonium ion	1,2-dibromoethane	GST	Carcinogenesis
Metal ions			
Mercury(II) ion	Elemental Hg	Catalase	Brain injury
Diaquo-diamino platinate(II)	Cisplatinum	s.r.	Renal tubular necrosis

KEY: AAF = 2-acetylaminofluorene, ADH = alcohol dehydrogenase, CCβL = cysteine conjugate β-lyase; ChE = cholinesterase; DENA = diethylnitrosamine; DMAB = *N,N*-dimethyl-4-aminoazobenzene; 7,12-DMBA = 7,12-dimethylbenzanthracene; DES = diethylstilbestrol; DP = dipeptidase; FMO = flavin-containing monooxygenase; GT = UDP-glucuronosyltransferase; GGT = gamma-glutamyltransferase; GST = glutathione *S*-transferase; HAPP = heterocyclic arylamine pyrolysis products; HCBD = hexachlorobutadiene; P450 = cytochrome P450; ST = sulfotransferase; s.r. = spontaneous rearrangement.

creases the catalytic efficiency of some transition metal ions. The pulmonary toxicity of inhaled mineral particles such as asbestos and silica is caused, at least in part, by the formation of $HO^{\bullet}$ triggered by Fe ions on the particle surface (Vallyathan et al., 1998). Hydrogen peroxide is a direct or indirect by-product of several enzymatic reactions, including monoamine oxidase, xanthine oxidase, and acyl-coenzyme A oxidase. It is produced in large quantities by spontaneous or superoxide dismutase-catalyzed dismutation of $O_2^{\bar{\bullet}}$.

Homolytic cleavage is also thought to be involved in free radical generation from $ONOO^-$ (Squadrito and Pryor, 1998) (Fig. 3-4). The facile reaction of $ONOO^-$ with the ubiquitous

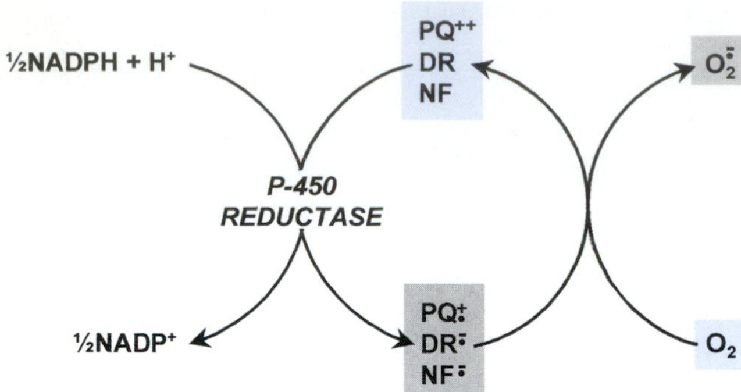

Figure 3-3. Production of superoxide anion radical ($O_2^{\bar{\bullet}}$) by paraquat (PQ^{++}), doxorubicin (DR), and nitrofurantoin (NF).

Note that formation of ($O_2^{\bar{\bullet}}$) is not the final step in the toxication of these xenobiotics, because $O_2^{\bar{\bullet}}$ can yield the much more reactive hydroxyl radical, as depicted in Fig. 3-4.

CO_2 yields nitrosoperoxycarbonate ($ONOOCO_2^-$), which can spontaneously homolyze into two radicals, the oxidant and nitrating agent nitrogen dioxide ($^{\bullet}NO_2$) and the oxidant carbonate anion radical ($CO_3^{\bar{\bullet}}$). Thus, formation of $ONOO^-$ and the latter radicals represent a toxication mechanism for $O_2^{\bar{\bullet}}$ and $^{\bullet}NO$. As $^{\bullet}NO$ is the product of nitric oxide synthase (NOS), this mechanism is especially relevant in and around cells that express NOS consitutively (i.e., neurons and endothelial cells) as well as in and around cells that express the inducible form of NOS in response to cytokines.

Formation of Nucleophiles The formation of nucleophiles is a relatively uncommon mechanism for activating toxicants. Examples include the formation of cyanide from amygdalin, which is catalyzed by bacterial β-glucosidase in the gut; from acrylonitrile after epoxidation and subsequent glutathione conjugation; and from sodium mitroprusside by thiol-induced decomposition. Carbon monoxide is a toxic metabolite of dihalomethanes that undergo oxidative dehalogenation. Hydrogen selenide, a strong nucleophile and reductant, is formed from selenite by reaction with glutathione or other thiols.

Formation of Redox-Active Reactants There are specific mechanisms for the creation of redox-active reactants other than those already mentioned. Examples include the formation of the methemoglobin-producing nitrite from nitrate by bacterial reduction in the intestine or from esters of nitrous or nitric acids in reaction with glutathione. Dapsone hydroxylamine and 5-hydroxyprimaquine, hydroxylated metabolites of the respective drugs, produce methemoglobin by cooxidation (Fletcher et al., 1988). Reductants such as ascorbic acid and reductases such as NADPH-dependent flavoenzymes reduce Cr(VI) to Cr(V) (Shi and Dalai, 1990). Xenobiotic radicals formed in redox cycling (e.g., those depicted in Fig. 3-3) as well as $O_2^{\bar{\bullet}}$ and $^{\bullet}NO$ can reduce Fe(III) bound to ferritin and consequently release it as Fe(II). Cr(V) and Fe(II) thus formed catalyze $HO^{\bullet}$ formation (Fig. 3-4).

In summary, the most reactive metabolites are electron-deficient molecules and molecular fragments such as electrophiles and neutral or cationic free radicals. Although some nucleophiles are reactive (e.g., HCN, CO), many are activated by conversion to electrophiles. Similarly, free radicals with an extra electron cause damage by giving rise to the neutral $HO^{\bullet}$ radical after the formation and subsequent homolytic cleavage of HOOH.

Detoxication Biotransformations that eliminate the ultimate toxicant or prevent its formation are called *detoxications.* In some

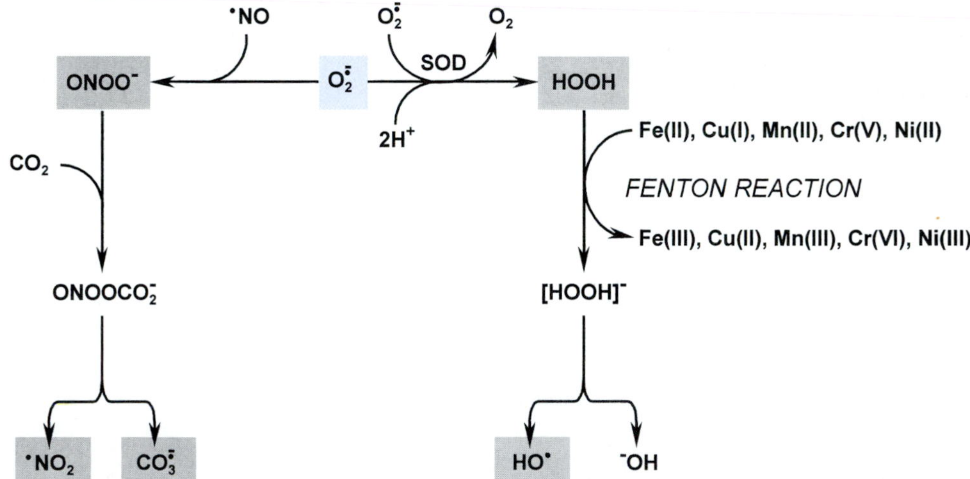

Figure 3-4. Two pathways for toxication of superoxide anion radical ($O_2^{\bar{\bullet}}$) via nonradical products ($ONOO^-$ and HOOH) to radical products ($^{\bullet}NO_2$, $CO_3^{\bar{\bullet}}$ and $HO^{\bullet}$).

In one pathway, conversion of ($O_2^{\bar{\bullet}}$) to HOOH is spontaneous or is catalyzed by superoxide dismutase (SOD). Homolytic cleavage of HOOH to hydroxyl radical and hydroxyl ion is called the Fenton reaction and is catalyzed by the transition metal ions shown. Hydroxyl radical formation is the ultimate toxication for xenobiotics that form $O_2^{\bar{\bullet}}$ (see Fig. 3-3) or for HOOH, the transition metal ions listed, and some chemicals that form complexes with these transiton metal ions. In the other pathway, $O_2^{\bar{\bullet}}$ reacts avidly with nitric oxide ($^{\bullet}NO$), the product of $^{\bullet}NO$ synthase (NOS), forming peroxynitrite ($ONOO^-$). Spontaneous reaction of $ONOO^-$ with carbon dioxide (CO_2) yields nitrosoperoxy carbonate ($ONOOCO_2^-$) that is homolytically cleaved to nitrogen dioxide ($^{\bullet}NO_2$) and carbonate anion radical ($CO_3^{\bar{\bullet}}$). All three radical products indicated in this figure are oxidants, whereas $^{\bullet}NO_2$ is also a nitrating agent.

cases, detoxication may compete with toxication for a chemical. Detoxication can take several pathways, depending on the chemical nature of the toxic substance.

Detoxication of Toxicants with No Functional Groups In general, chemicals without functional groups, such as benzene and toluene, are detoxicated in two phases. Initially, a functional group such as hydroxyl or carboxyl is introduced into the molecule, most often by cytochrome-P450 enzymes. Subsequently, an endogenous acid such as glucuronic acid, sulfuric acid, or an amino acid is added to the functional group by a transferase. With some exceptions, the final products are inactive, highly hydrophilic organic acids that are readily excreted.

Detoxication of Nucleophiles Nucleophiles generally are detoxicated by conjugation at the nucleophilic functional group. Hydroxylated compounds are conjugated by sulfation, glucuronidation, or rarely by methylation, whereas thiols are methylated or glucuronidated and amines and hydrazines are acetylated. These reactions prevent peroxidase-catalyzed conversion of the nucleophiles to free radicals and biotransformation of phenols, aminophenols, catechols, and hydroquinones to electrophilic quinones and quinoneomines. An alternative mechanism for the elimination of thiols and hydrazines is oxidation by flavin-containing monooxygenases (Jakoby and Ziegler, 1990). Some alcohols, such as ethanol, are detoxicated by oxidation to carboxylic acids by alcohol and aldehyde dehydrogenases. A specific detoxication mechanism is the biotransformation of cyanide to thiocyanate by rhodanese.

Detoxication of Electrophiles A general mechanism for the detoxication of electrophilic toxicants is conjugation with the thiol nucleophile glutathione (Ketterer, 1988). This reaction may occur spontaneously or can be facilitated by glutathione *S*-transferases. Metal ions—such as Ag^+, Cd^{2+}, Hg^{2+}, and CH_3Hg^+ ions—readily react with and are detoxicated by glutathione. Specific mechanisms for the detoxication of electrophilic chemicals include epoxide hydrolase-catalyzed biotransformation of epoxides and arene oxides to diols and dihydrodiols, respectively, and carboxylesterase-catalyzed hydrolysis of organophosphate ester pesticides. Others are two-electron reduction of quinones to hydroquinones by DT-diaphorase, reduction of α,β-unsaturated aldehydes to alcohols by alcohol dehydrogenase or oxidation to acids by aldehyde dehydrogenase, and complex formation of thiol-reactive metal ions by metallothionein and the redox-active ferrous iron by ferrin. Covalent binding of electrophiles to proteins can also be regarded as detoxification provided that the protein has no critical function and does not become a neoantigen or otherwise harmful. Carboxylesterases, for example, inactivate organophosphates not only by hydrolysis but also by covalent binding.

Detoxication of Free Radicals Because $O_2^{\bar{\bullet}}$ can be converted into much more reactive compounds (Fig. 3-4), its elimination is an important detoxication mechanism. This is carried out by superoxide dismutases (SOD), high-capacity enzymes located in the cytosol (Cu,Zn-SOD) and the mitochondria (Mn-SOD), which convert $O_2^{\bar{\bullet}}$ to HOOH (Fig. 3-5). Subsequently, HOOH is reduced to water by the selenocysteine-containing glutathione peroxidase in the cytosol or by catalase in the peroxisomes (Fig. 3-5) (Cotgrave et al., 1988).

No enzyme eliminates $HO^\bullet$. While some relatively stable radicals, such as peroxyl radicals, can readily abstract a hydrogen atom from glutathione, α-tocopherol (vitamin E), or ascorbic acid (vitamin C), thus becoming nonradicals, these antioxidants are generally ineffective in detoxifying $HO^\bullet$ (Sies, 1993). This is due to its extremely short half-life (10^{-9} s), which provides little time for the $HO^\bullet$ to reach and react with antioxidants. Therefore the only effective protection against $HO^\bullet$ is to prevent its formation by elimination of its precursor, HOOH, via conversion to water (Fig. 3-5).

$ONOO^-$ (which is not a free radical oxidant) is significantly more stable than $HO^\bullet$ (half-life of about 1 s). Nevertheless, the small biological antioxidant molecules (glutathione, uric acid, ascorbic acid, α-tocopherol) are relatively inefficient in intercepting it because $ONOO^-$ rapidly reacts with CO_2 (Squadrito and Pryor, 1998) to form reactive free radicals (Fig. 3-4). More efficient is the selenocysteine-containing glutathione peroxidase, which can reduce $ONOO^-$ to nitrite (ONO^-) the same way it reduces HOOH to water (Arteel et al., 1999). Selenoprotein P, which contains 10 selenocysteine residues and coats the surface of endothelial cells, also reduces $ONOO^-$ and may serve as a protectant against this oxidant in blood (Arteel et al., 1999; Burk and Hill, 1999). In addition, $ONOO^-$ reacts with oxyhemoglobin, heme-containing peroxidases and albumin, all of which could be important sinks for $ONOO^-$. Furthermore, elimination of the two $ONOO^-$ precursors—i.e., $^\bullet NO$ by reaction with oxyhemoglobin (to yield methemoglobin and nitrate) and $O_2^{\bar{\bullet}}$ by SODs (see above)—is a significant mechanism in preventing $ONOO^-$ buildup (Squadrito and Pryor, 1998).

Peroxidase-generated free radicals are eliminated by electron transfer from glutathione. This results in the oxidation of glutathione, which is reversed by NADPH-dependent glutathione reductase (Fig. 3-6). Thus, glutathione plays an important role in the detoxication of both electrophiles and free radicals.

Detoxication of Protein Toxins Presumably, extra- and intracellular proteases are involved in the inactivation of toxic polypeptides. Several toxins found in venoms, such as α- and β-bungaratoxin, erabutoxin, and phospholipase, contain intramolecular disulfide bonds that are required for their activity. These proteins are inactivated by thioredoxin, an endogenous dithiol protein that reduces the essential disulfide bond (Lozano et al., 1994).

When Detoxication Fails Detoxication may be insufficient for several reasons:

1. Toxicants may overwhelm detoxication processes, leading to exhaustion of the detoxication enzymes, consumption of the cosubtrates, or depletion of cellular antioxidants such as glutathione, ascorbic acid, and α-tocopherol. This results in the accumulation of the ultimate toxicant.
2. Occasionally, a reactive toxicant inactivates a detoxicating enzyme. For example, $ONOO^-$ incapacitates Mn-SOD, which normally would counteract $ONOO^-$ formation (Murphy, 1999) (see Fig. 3-4).

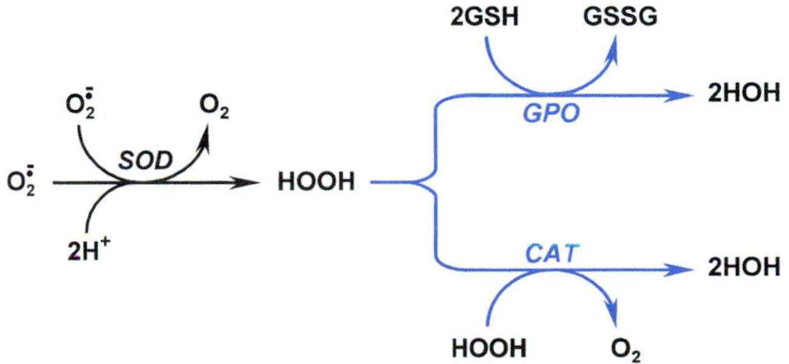

Figure 3-5. Detoxication of superoxide anion radical ($O_2^{\bar{\bullet}}$) by superoxide dismutase (SOD), glutathione peroxidase (GPO), and catalase (CAT).

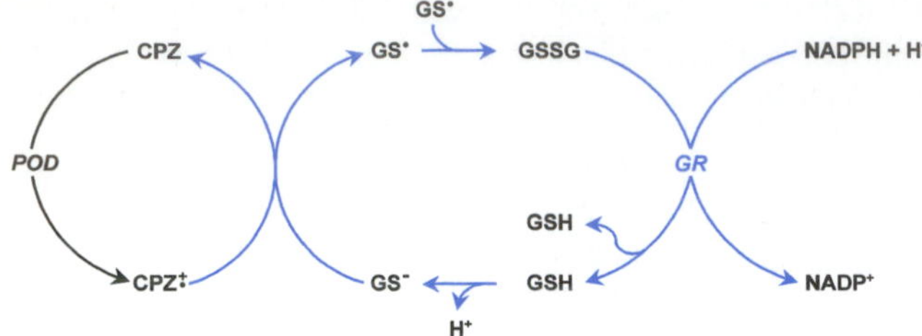

Figure 3-6. Detoxication of peroxidase (POD)–generated free radicals such as chlorpromazine free radical (CPZ⁺•) by glutathione (GSH).

The by-products are glutathione thiyl radical (GS•) and glutathione disulfide (GSSG), from which GSH is regenerated by glutathione reductase (GR).

3. Some conjugation reactions can be reversed. For example, 2-naphthylamine, a bladder carcinogen, is *N*-hydroxylated and glucuronidated in liver, with the glucuronide excreted into urine. While in the bladder, the glucuronide is hydrolyzed, and the released arylhydroxylamine is converted by protonation and dehydration to the reactive electrophilic arylnitrenium ion (Bock and Lilienblum, 1994). Isocyanates and isothiocyanates form labile glutathione conjugates from which they can be released. Thus, methylisocyanate readily forms a glutathione conjugate in the lung after inhalation. From there, the conjugate is distributed to other tissues, where the reactive electrophilic parent compound may be regenerated (Baillie and Kassahun, 1994). Such conjugates are considered transport forms of toxicants.
4. Sometimes detoxication generates potentially harmful byproducts such as the glutathione thiyl radical and glutathione disulfide, which are produced during the detoxication of free radicals (Fig. 3-6). Glutathione disulfide can form mixed disulfides with protein thiols, whereas the thiyl radical (GS•), after reacting with thiolate (GS^-), forms a glutathione disulfide radical anion ($GSSG^{\bullet -}$), which can reduce O_2 to $O_2^{\bullet -}$.

STEP 2—REACTION OF THE ULTIMATE TOXICANT WITH THE TARGET MOLECULE

Toxicity is typically mediated by a reaction of the ultimate toxicant with a target molecule (step 2a in Fig. 3-1). Subsequently, a series of secondary biochemical events occur, leading to dysfunction or injury that is manifest at various levels of biological organization, such as at the target molecule itself, cell organelles, cells, tissues and organs, and even the whole organism. Because interaction of the ultimate toxicant with the target molecule triggers the toxic effect, consideration is given to (1) the attributes of target molecules, (2) the types of reactions between ultimate toxicants and target molecules, and (3) the effects of toxicants on the target molecules (Fig. 3-7). Finally, consideration is given to toxicities that are initiated not by reaction of the ultimate toxicant with target molecules but rather by alteration of the biological (micro)environment in which critical endogenous molecules, cell organelles, cells, and organs operate.

Attributes of Target Molecules

Practically all endogenous compounds are potential targets for toxicants. The identification and characteristics of the target molecules involved in toxicity constitute a major research priority, but a comprehensive inventory of potential target molecules is impossible. Nevertheless, the most prevalent and toxicologically relevant targets are macromolecules such as nucleic acids (especially DNA) and proteins. Among the small molecules, membrane lipids are frequently involved, whereas cofactors such as coenzyme A and pyridoxal rarely are involved.

To be a target, an endogenous molecule must possess the appropriate reactivity and/or steric configuration to allow the ultimate toxicant to enter into covalent or noncovalent reactions. For these reactions to occur, the target molecule must be accessible to a sufficiently high concentration of the ultimate toxicant. Thus, endogenous molecules that are in the vicinity of reactive chemicals or are adjacent to sites where they are formed are frequently targets. The first target for reactive metabolites is often the enzyme responsible for their production or the adjacent intracellular structures. For example, thyroperoxidase, the enzyme responsible for thyroid hormone synthesis, converts some nucleophilic xenobiotics (such as methimazole, amitrole, and resorcinol) into reactive free radical metabolites that inactivate the thyroperoxidase (Engler et al., 1982). This is the basis for the antithyroid as well as the thyroid tumor–inducing effect of these chemicals. Carbon tetrachloride, which is activated by cytochrome P450, destroys this enzyme as well as the neighboring microsomal membranes (Osawa et al., 1995). Several mitochondrial enzymes—including pyruvate dehydrogenase, succinate dehydrogenase, and cytochrome *c* oxidase—are convenient targets for nephrotoxic cysteine conjugates such as dichlorovinyl cysteine, because these conjugates are converted to electrophiles in the same organelle by mitochondrial cysteine conjugate β-lyase (Dekant et al., 1989). Reactive metabolites that are unable to find

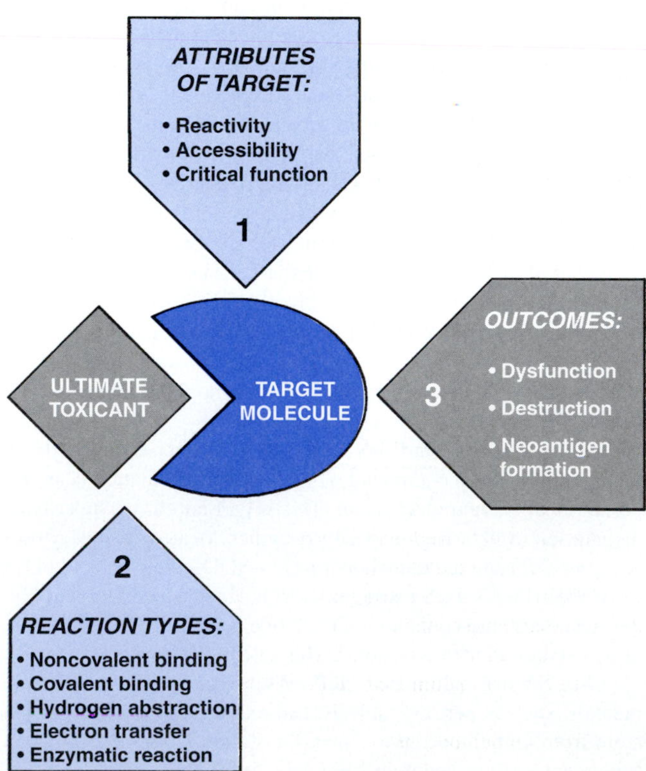

Figure 3-7. Reaction of the ultimate toxicant with the target molecule: the second step in the development of toxicity.

appropriate endogenous molecules in close proximity to their site of formation may diffuse until they encounter such reactants. For example, hard electrophiles such as the arylnitrenium ion metabolite of *N*-methyl-4-aminoazobenzene react readily with hard nucleophilic atoms in nucleic acids, and thus target DNA in the nucleus even though the electrophiles are produced in the cytoplasm.

Not all targets for chemicals contribute to the harmful effects. Thus, while carbon monoxide causes toxicity by binding to ferrohemoglobin, it also associates with the iron in cytochrome P450 with little or no consequence. Covalent binding of toxicants to various intracellular proteins, including enzymes and structural proteins, has been demonstrated, yet it is often uncertain which protein(s) is/are involved in binding that is toxicologically relevant (Cohen et al., 1997; Pumford and Halmes, 1997; Rombach and Hanzlik, 1999). Arylation of some hepatic mitochondrial proteins by acetaminophen might be causally related to the liver injury induced by this drug because the nonhepatotoxic regioisomer of acetaminophen does not readily bind covalently to these proteins (Cohen et al., 1997). In contrast, arylation of a number of hepatic cytoplasmic proteins by acetaminophen is likely to be inconsequential because a nonhepatotoxic regioisomer of this drug also arylates those proteins (Nelson and Pearson, 1990). Covalent binding to proteins without adverse consequences may even represent a form of detoxication by sparing toxicologically relevant targets. This principle is best exemplified by covalent binding of organophosphate insecticides to plasma cholinesterase, which is a significant protective mechanism, as it counteracts phosphorylation of acetylcholinesterase, the target molecule. Thus, to conclusively identify a target molecule as being responsible for toxicity, it should be demonstrated that the ultimate toxicant (1) reacts with the target and adversely affects its function, (2) reaches an effective concentration at the target site, and (3) alters the target in a way that is mechanistically related to the observed toxicity.

Types of Reactions

The ultimate toxicant may bind to the target molecules noncovalently or covalently and may alter it by hydrogen abstraction, electron transfer, or enzymatically.

Noncovalent Binding This type of binding can be due to apolar interactions or the formation of hydrogen and ionic bonds and is typically involved in the interaction of toxicants with targets such as membrane receptors, intracellular receptors, ion channels, and some enzymes. For example, such interactions are responsible for the binding of strychnine to the glycine receptor on motor neurons in the spinal cord, TCDD to the aryl hydrocarbon receptor, saxitoxin to sodium channels, phorbol esters to protein kinase C, and warfarin to vitamin K 2,3-epoxide reductase. Such forces also are responsible for the intercalation of chemicals such as acridine yellow and doxorubicin into the double helix of DNA. These chemicals are toxic because the steric arrangement of their atoms allows them to combine with complementary sites on the endogenous molecule more or less as a key fits into a lock. Noncovalent binding usually is reversible because of the comparatively low bonding energy.

Covalent Binding Being practically irreversible, covalent binding is of great toxicologic importance because it permanently alters endogenous molecules (Boelsterli, 1993). Covalent adduct formation is common with electrophilic toxicants such as nonionic and cationic electrophiles and radical cations. These toxicants react with nucleophilic atoms that are abundant in biological macromolecules, such as proteins and nucleic acids. Electrophilic atoms exhibit some selectivity toward nucleophilic atoms, depending on their charge-to-radius ratio. In general, soft electrophiles prefer to react with soft nucleophiles (low charge-to-radius ratio in both), whereas hard electrophiles react more readily with hard nucleophiles (high charge-to-radius ratio in both). Examples are presented in Table 3-3. Metal ions such as silver and mercury also are classified as soft electrophiles that prefer to react with soft nucleophiles and hard electrophiles such as lithium, calcium, and barium, which react preferentially with hard nucleophiles. Metals falling between these two extremes, such as chromium, zinc, and lead, exhibit universal reactivity with nucleophiles. The reactivity of an electrophile determines which endogenous nucleophiles can react with it and become a target.

Neutral free radicals such as $HO^{\bullet}$, $^{\bullet}NO_2$, and $Cl_3C^{\bullet}$ also can bind covalently to biomolecules. The addition of $Cl_3C^{\bullet}$ to double-bonded carbons in lipids or to lipid radicals yields lipids containing chloromethylated fatty acids. The addition of hydroxyl radicals to DNA bases results in the formation of numerous products, including 8-hydroxypurines, 5-hydroxymethylpyrimidines, and thymine and cytosine glycols (Breen and Murphy, 1995).

Nucleophilic toxicants are in principle reactive toward electrophilic endogenous compounds. Such reactions occur infrequently because electrophiles are rare among biomolecules. Examples include the covalent reactions of amines and hydrazides with the aldehyde pyridoxal, a cosubstrate for decarboxylases. Carbon monoxide, cyanide, hydrogen sulfide, and azide form coordi-

Table 3-3
Examples of Soft and Hard Electrophiles and Nucleophiles

ELECTROPHILES		NUCLEOPHILES
Carbon in polarized double bonds (e.g., quinones, α,β-unsaturated ketones)	Soft ↑	Sulfur in thiols (e.g., cysteinyl residues in proteins and glutathione)
Carbon in epoxides, strained-ring lactones, aryl halides		Sulfur in methionine
Aryl carbonium ions		Nitrogen in primary and secondary amino groups of proteins
Benzylic carbonium ions, nitrenium ions		Nitrogen in amino groups in purine bases in nucleic acids
Alkyl carbonium ions	↓	Oxygen of purines and pyrimidines in nucleic acids
	Hard	Phosphate oxygen in nucleic acids

SOURCE: Based on Coles (1984).

nate covalent bonds with iron in various hemeproteins. Other nucleophiles react with hemoglobin in an electron-transfer reaction (see below).

Hydrogen Abstraction Neutral free radicals, such as those generated in reactions depicted in Fig. 3-4, can readily abstract H atoms from endogenous compounds, converting those compounds into radicals. Abstraction of hydrogen from thiols (R—SH) creates thiyl radicals (R—S•), which are precursors of other thiol oxidation products, such as sulfenic acids (R—SOH) and disulfides (R—S—S—R). Radicals can remove hydrogen from CH_2 groups of free amino acids or from amino acid residues in proteins and convert them to carbonyls. These carbonyls react with amines, forming cross-links with DNA or other proteins. Hydrogen abstraction from deoxyribose in DNA yields the C-4′-radical, the first step to DNA cleavage (Breen and Murphy, 1995). Abstraction of hydrogen from fatty acids produces lipid radicals and initiates lipid peroxidation. As depicted in Fig. 3-8, nitration of tyrosine residues in proteins purportedly involves H abstraction followed by covalent binding between the resultant tyrosyl radical and $^{\bullet}NO_2$ (Squadrito and Pryor, 1998).

Electron Transfer Chemicals can oxidize Fe(II) in hemoglobin to Fe(III), producing methemoglobinemia. Nitrite can oxidize hemoglobin, whereas *N*-hydroxyl arylamines (such as dapsone hydroxylamine), phenolic compounds (such as 5-hydroxy primaquine), and hydrazines (such as phenylhydrazine) are cooxidized with oxyhemoglobin, forming methemoglobin and hydrogen peroxide (Coleman and Jacobus, 1993).

Enzymatic Reactions A few toxins act enzymatically on specific target proteins. For example, ricin induces hydrolytic fragmentation of ribosomes, blocking protein synthesis. Several bacterial toxins catalyze the transfer for ADP-ribose from NAD^+ to specific proteins. For example, diphtheria toxin blocks the function of elongation factor 2 in protein synthesis and cholera toxin activates a G protein through such a mechanism. Snake venoms contain hydrolytic enzymes that destroy biomolecules.

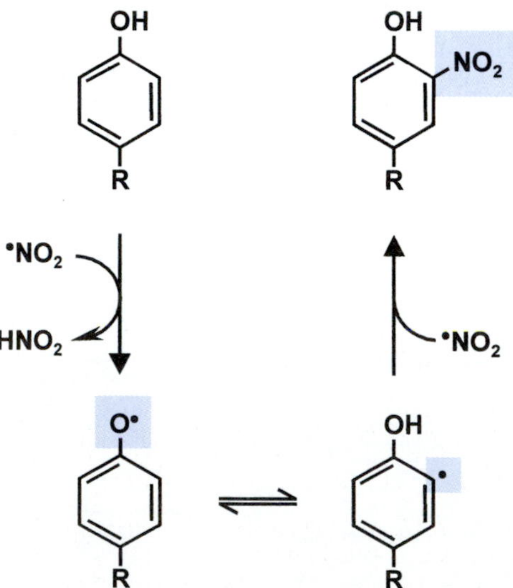

Figure 3-8. Formation of 3-nitrotyrosine residues in proteins by reaction with nitrogen dioxide ($^{\bullet}NO_2$).

($^{\bullet}NO_2$) is the nitrating species generated from $ONOO^-$ (Fig. 3-4). In addition, ($^{\bullet}NO_2$) is a contaminant in cigarette smoke, exhaust of gas engines and stoves, as well as the causative agent of "silo-filler's disease."

In summary, most ultimate toxicants act on endogenous molecules on the basis of their chemical reactivity. Those with more than one type of reactivity may react by different mechanisms with various target molecules. For example, quinones may act as electron acceptors and initiate thiol oxidation or free radical reactions that lead to lipid peroxidation, buy they may also act as soft electrophiles and bind covalently to protein thiols. The lead ion acts as a soft electrophile when it forms coordinate covalent bonds with critical thiol groups in δ-aminolevulinic acid dehydratase, its major target enzyme in heme synthesis (Goering, 1993). However, it behaves like a hard electrophile or an ion when it binds to protein kinase C or blocks calcium channels, substituting for the natural ligand Ca^{2+} at those target sites.

Effects of Toxicants on Target Molecules

Reaction of the ultimate toxicant with endogenous molecules may cause dysfunction or destruction; in the case of proteins, it may render them foreign (i.e., an antigen) to the immune system.

Dysfunction of Target Molecules Some toxicants activate protein target molecules, mimicking endogenous ligands. For example, morphine activates opiate receptors, clofibrate is an agonist on the peroxisome proliferator–activated receptor, and phorbol esters and lead ions stimulate protein kinase C.

More commonly, chemicals inhibit the function of target molecules. Several xenobiotics—such as atropine, curare, and strychnine—block neurotransmitter receptors by attaching to the ligand-binding sites or by interfering with the function of ion channels. Tetrotodoxin and saxitoxin, for example, inhibit opening of the voltage-activated sodium channels in the neuronal membrane, whereas DDT and the pyrethroid insecticides inhibit their closure. Some toxicants block ion transporters, others inhibit mitochondrial electron transport complexes, and many inhibit enzymes. Chemicals that bind to tubulin (e.g., vinblastine, colchicine, paclitaxel, trivalent arsenic) or actin (e.g., cytochalasin B, phalloidin) impair the assembly (polymerization) and/or disassembly (depolymerization) of these cytoskeletal proteins.

Protein function is impaired when conformation or structure is altered by interaction with the toxicant. Many proteins possess critical moities, especially thiol groups, that are essential for catalytic activity or assembly to macromolecular complexes. Proteins that are sensitive to covalent and/or oxidative modification of their thiol groups include the enzymes protein tyrosine phosphatases (Herrlich et al., 1998), glyceraldehyde 3-phosphate dehydrogenase (see Table 3-6), and pyruvate dehydrogenase (see Fig. 3-13), the Ca^{2+} pumps (see Fig. 3-14, Table 3-7), and the transcription factor AP-1, just to name a few. The activity of these and many other proteins is impaired by thiol-reactive chemicals, triggering aberrant signal transduction and/or impaired maintenance of the cell's energy and metabolic homeostasis. Protein tyrosine nitration (see Fig. 3-8) may alter also protein function or may interfere with signaling pathways that involve tyrosine kinases and phosphatases (Arteel et al., 1999).

Toxicants may interfere with the template function of DNA. The covalent binding of chemicals to DNA causes nucleotide mispairing during replication. For example, covalent binding of aflatoxin 8,9-oxide to *N*-7 of guanine results in pairing of the adduct-bearing guanine with adenine rather than cytosine, leading to the formation of an incorrect codon and the insertion of an incorrect amino acid into the protein. Such events are involved in the aflatoxin-induced mutation of the *ras* proto-oncogene and the *p53* tumor suppressor gene (Eaton and Gallagher, 1994). 8-Hydroxyguanine and 8-hydroxyadenine are mutagenic bases produced by $HO^{\bullet}$ that can cause mispairing with themselves as well as with neighboring pyrimidines, producing multiple amino acid substitutions (Breen and Murphy, 1995). Chemicals such as doxorubicin, that intercalate between stacked bases in the double-helical DNA, push adjacent base pairs apart, causing an even greater error in the template function of DNA by shifting the reading frame.

Destruction of Target Molecules In addition to adduct formation, toxicants alter the primary structure of endogenous molecules by means of cross-linking and fragmentation. Bifunctional electrophiles such as 2,5-hexanedione, carbon disulfide, acrolein, 4-hydroxynonenal, and nitrogen mustard alkylating agents cross-link cytoskeletal proteins, DNA, or DNA with proteins. Hydroxyl radicals also can induce cross-linking by converting these macromolecules into either reactive electrophiles (e.g., protein carbonyls), which react with a nucleophilic site in another macromolecule, or radicals, which react with each other. Cross-linking imposes both structural and functional constraints on the linked molecules.

Some target molecules are susceptible to spontaneous degradation after chemical attack. Free radicals such as $Cl_3COO^{\bullet}$ and $HO^{\bullet}$ can initiate peroxidative degradation of lipids by hydrogen abstraction from fatty acids (Recknagel et al., 1989). The lipid radical ($L^{\bullet}$) formed is converted successively to lipid peroxyl radical ($LOO^{\bullet}$) by oxygen fixation, lipid hydroperoxide (LOOH) by hydrogen abstraction, and lipid alkoxyl radical ($LO^{\bullet}$) by the Fe(II)-catalyzed Fenton reaction. Subsequent fragmentation gives rise to hydrocarbons such as ethane and reactive aldehydes such as 4-hydroxynonenal and malondialdehyde (Fig. 3-9). Thus, lipid peroxidation not only destroys lipids in cellular membranes but also generates endogenous toxicants, both free radicals (e.g., $LOO^{\bullet}$, $LO^{\bullet}$) and electrophiles (e.g., 4-hydroxynonenal). These substances can readily react with adjacent molecules, such as membrane proteins, or diffuse to more distant molecules such as DNA.

Apart from hydrolytic degradation by toxins and radiolysis, toxicant-induced fragmentation of proteins is not well documented. There are, however, examples for destruction of the prosthetic group in enzymes. For instance, cytochrome P450 converts allyl isopropyl acetamide into a reactive metabolite, which alkylates the heme moiety of the enzyme. This leads to loss of the altered heme and to porphyria (De Matteis, 1987). Aconitase is attacked by $ONOO^-$ at its $[4Fe\text{-}4S]^{2+}$ cluster, whose one Fe atom is genuinely labile (as is complexed to an inorganic sulfur and not to enzyme-bound cysteines like the others). As a result of the oxidant action of $ONOO^-$, the labile Fe is lost, inactivating the enzyme (Castro et al., 1994) and compromising the citric acid cycle where aconitase functions.

Several forms of DNA fragmentation are caused by toxicants. For instance, attack of DNA bases by $HO^{\bullet}$ can result in the formation of imidazole ring–opened purines or ring–contracted pyrimidines, which block DNA replication. Formation of a bulky adduct at guanine *N*-7 destabilizes the *N*-glycosylic bond, inducing depurination. Depurination results in apurinic sites that are mutagenic. Single-strand breaks typically are caused by hydroxyl radicals via abstraction of H from desoxyribose in DNA yielding the C-4′ radical, followed by $O_2^{\bar{\bullet}}$ addition, Criegee rearrangement, and cleavage of the phosphodiester bond (Breen and Murphy, 1995). Multiple hydroxyl radical attacks on a short length of DNA, which occur after ionizing radiation, cause double-strand breaks that are typically lethal to the affected cell.

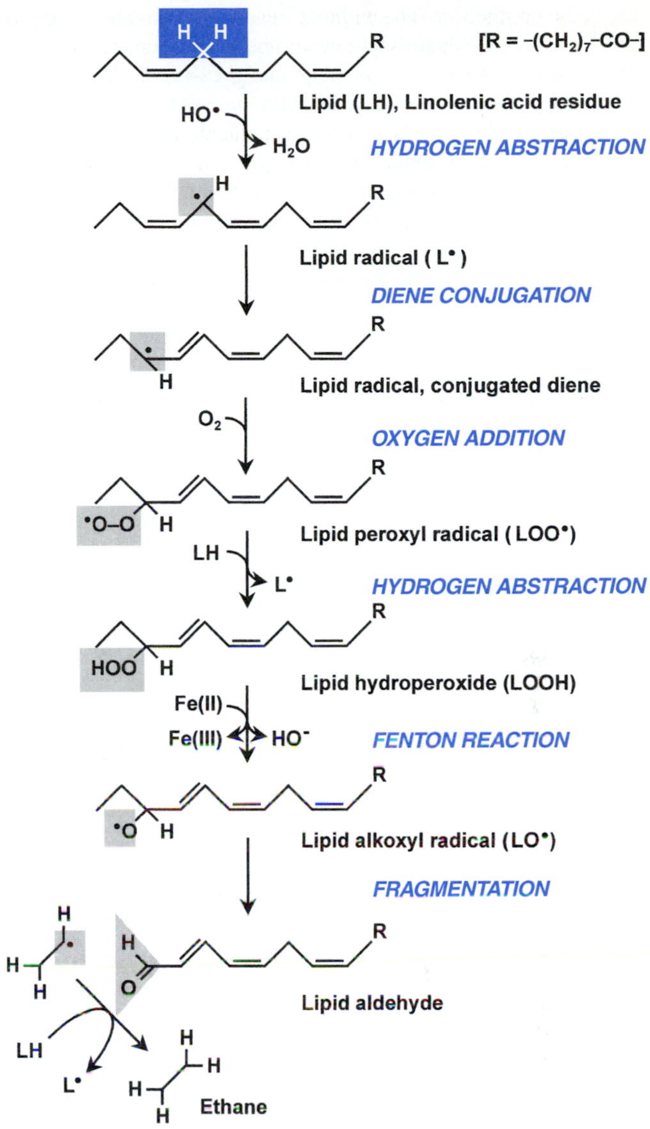

Figure 3-9. Lipid peroxidation initiated by the hydroxyl radical ($HO^{\bullet}$).

Many of the products, such as the radicals and the α,β-unsaturated aldehydes, are reactive, whereas others, such as ethane, are nonreactive but are indicators of lipid peroxidation.

Neoantigen Formation While the covalent binding of xenobiotics or their metabolites is often inconsequential with respect to the function of the immune system, in some individuals these altered proteins evoke an immune response. Some chemicals (e.g., dinitrochlorobenzene, penicillin, nickel) may be sufficiently reactive to bind to proteins spontaneously. Others may obtain reactivity by autooxidation to quinones (e.g., urushiols, the allergens in poison ivy) or by enzymatic biotransformation (Park et al., 1998). For example, cytochrome P450 biotransforms halothane to an electrophile, trifluoroacetyl chloride, which binds as a hapten to various microsomal and cell surface proteins in the liver, inducing antibody production. The immune reaction is thought to be responsible for the hepatitis-like syndrome seen in sensitive patients. Drug-induced lupus and possibly many cases of drug-induced agranulocytosis are mediated by immune reactions triggered by drug-protein adducts. The causative chemicals are typically nucleophiles, such as aromatic amines (e.g., aminopyrine, clozapine, procainamide, and sulfonamides), hydrazines (e.g., hydralazine and isoniazid), and thiols (e.g., propylthiouracil, methimazole, and captopril). These substances can be oxidized by myeloperoxidase discharged from activated granulocytes or by the ROS/RNS such cells produce ($HO^{\bullet}$, $ONOO^{-}$, HOCl, see Fig. 3-22) to reactive metabolites that bind to the surface proteins of these cells, making them antigens (Uetrecht, 1992). Unfortunately, some proteins that bear an adduct can mimic some normal proteins, which thus also can be attacked by the antibodies.

Toxicity Not Initiated by Reaction with Target Molecules

Some xenobiotics do not or do not only interact with a specific endogenous target molecule to induce toxicity but instead alter the biological microenvironment (see step 2b in Fig. 3-1). Included here are (1) chemicals that alter H^+ ion concentrations in the aqueous biophase, such as acids and substances biotransformed to acids, such as methanol and ethylene glycol, as well as protonophoric uncouplers such as 2,4-dinitrophenol and pentachlorophenol, which dissociate their phenolic protons in the mitochondrial matrix, thus dissipating the proton gradient that drives ATP synthesis; (2) solvents and detergents that physicochemically alter the lipid phase of cell membranes and destroy transmembrane solute gradients that are essential to cell functions; and (3) other xenobiotics that cause harm merely by occupying a site or space. For example, some chemicals (e.g., ethylene glycol) form water-insoluble precipitates in the renal tubules. By occupying bilirubin binding sites on albumin, compounds such as the sulfonamides induce bilirubin toxicity (kernicterus) in neonates. Carbon dioxide displaces oxygen in the pulmonary alveolar space and causes asphyxiation.

STEP 3—CELLULAR DYSFUNCTION AND RESULTANT TOXICITIES

The reaction of toxicants with a target molecule may result in impaired cellular function as the third step in the development of toxicity (Fig. 3-1). Each cell in a multicellular organism carries out defined programs. Certain programs determine the destiny of cells—that is, whether they undergo division, differentiation (i.e., express proteins for specialized functions), or apoptosis. Other programs control the ongoing (momentary) activity of differentiated cells, determining whether they secrete more or less of a substance, whether they contract or relax, and whether they transport and metabolize nutrients at higher or lower rates. For regulations of these cellular programs, cells possess signaling networks (such as those shown in Figs. 3-11 and 3-12) that can be activated and inactivated by external signaling molecules. To execute the programs, cells are equipped with synthetic, metabolic, kinetic, transport, and energy-producing system as well as structural elements, organized into macromolecular complexes, cell membranes, and organelles, by which they maintain their own integrity (internal functions) and support the maintenance of other cells (external functions).

As outlined in Fig. 3-10, the nature of the primary cellular dysfunction caused by toxicants, but not necessarily the ultimate outcome, depends on the role of the target molecule affected. If the target molecule is involved in cellular regulation (signaling), dysregulation of gene expression and/or dysregulation of momentary cellular function occurs primarily. However, if the target molecule is involved predominantly in the cell's internal maintenance,

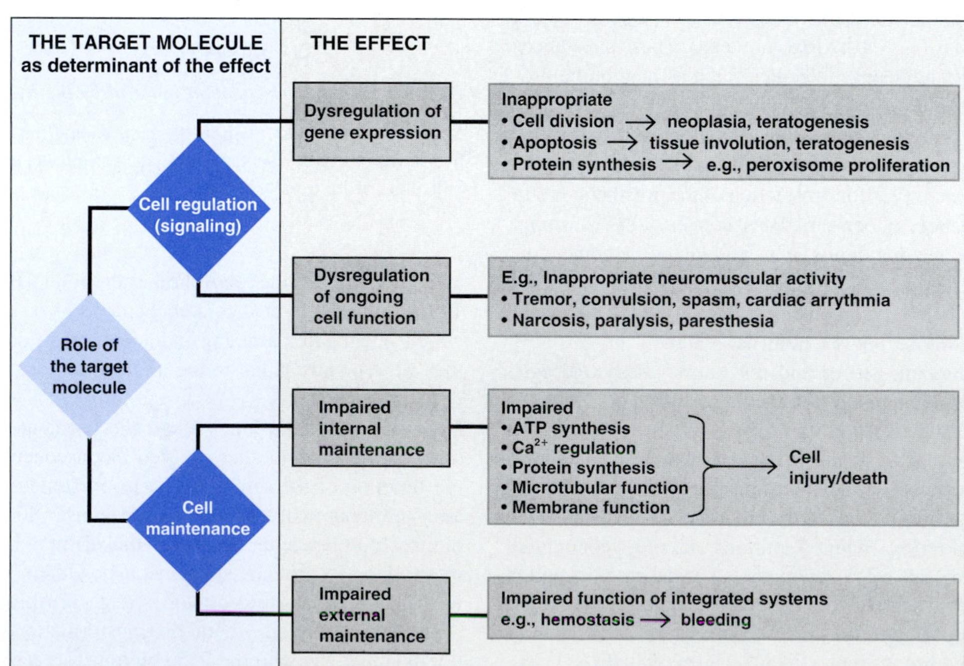

Figure 3-10. The third step in the development of toxicity: alteration of the regulatory or maintenance function of the cell.

the resultant dysfunction can ultimately compromise the survival of the cell. The reaction of a toxicant with targets serving external functions can influence the operation of other cells and integrated organ systems. The following discussion deals with these consequences.

Toxicant-Induced Cellular Dysregulation

Cells are regulated by signaling molecules that activate specific cellular receptors linked to signal transducing networks that transmit the signals to the regulatory regions of genes and/or to functional proteins. Receptor activation may ultimately lead to (1) altered gene expression that increases or decreases the quantity of specific proteins and/or (2) a chemical modification of specific proteins, typically by phosphorylation, that activates or inhibits proteins. Programs controlling the destiny of cells primarily affect gene expression, whereas those regulating the ongoing activities primarily influence the activity of functional proteins; however, one signal often evokes both responses because of branching and interconnection of signaling networks.

Dysregulation of Gene Expression Dysregulation of gene expression may occur at elements that are directly responsible for transcription, at components of the intracellular signal transduction pathway, and at the synthesis, storage, or release of the extracellular signaling molecules.

Dysregulation of Transcription Transcription of genetic information from DNA to mRNA is controlled largely by an interplay between transcription factors (TFs) and the regulatory or promoter region of genes. By binding to nucleotide sequences in this region, activated TFs facilitate the formation of the preinitiation complex, promoting transcription of the adjacent gene. Xenobiotics may interact with the promoter region of the gene, the TFs, or other components of the preinitiation complex. However, altered activation of TFs appears to be the most common modality. Functionally, two types of TFs are known: ligand-activated and signal-activated.

Many natural compounds, such as hormones (e.g., steroids, thyroid hormones) and vitamins (retinoids and vitamin D), influence gene expression by binding to and activating TFs (Table 3-4). Xenobiotics may mimic the natural ligands. For example, fibric acid–type lipid-lowering drugs and phthalate esters substitute for polyunsaturated fatty acids as ligands for the peroxisome proliferator-activated receptor (PPAR) (Poellinger et al., 1992), and Cd^{2+} substitutes for Zn^{2+}, the endogenous ligand of metal-responsive element-binding transcription factor (MTF-1) (Heuchel et al., 1994).

Natural or xenobiotic ligands may cause toxicity mediated by ligand-activated TFs when administered at extreme doses or at critical periods during ontogenesis (Table 3-4). Glucocorticoids induce apoptosis of lymphoid cells. While desirable in the treatment of lymphoid malignancies, this is an unwanted response in many other conditions. TCDD, a ligand of the aryl hydrocarbon receptor (AHR), produces thymic atrophy by causing apoptosis of thymocytes. Estrogens exert mitogenic effects in cells that express estrogen receptors, such as those found in the female reproductive organs, the mammary gland, and the liver. Estrogen-induced proliferation appears to be responsible for tumor formation in these organs during prolonged estrogen exposure (Green, 1992). It has been speculated that environmental xenoestrogens such as DDT, polychlorinated biphenyls, bisphenol A, and atrazine contribute to an increased incidence of breast cancer. Zearalenone, a mycoestrogen feed contaminant, causes vulval prolapse in swine, an example of an estrogen receptor–mediated proliferative lesion. The mitogenic and hepatic tumor-promoting effects of peroxysome proliferators is also receptor-mediated, because it is not observed in PPARα-null mice (Peters et al., 1998). Humans express PPARα at low levels and often in nonfunctional forms and thus, as opposed to rodents, do not exhibit hepatocellular and peroxisomal proliferation. Chemicals that act on ligand-activated TFs, such as glucocorticoids, TCDD, and retinoids, induce fetal malformations that may be regarded as inappropriate gene expression (Armstrong et al., 1992). Candidate target genes are the homeobox genes that determine the body plan during early ontogenesis.

Compounds that act on ligand-activated TFs can also change the pattern of cell differentiation by overexpressing various genes. For example, the PPAR-ligand fibric acid derivatives stimulate genes that encode peroxisomal enzymes and induce proliferation of peroxisomes in rodent liver (Green, 1992).

TCDD, phenobarbital, and pregnenolone 16α-carbonitrile (PCN) activate AHR, the constitutive androstane receptor (CAR), and the pregnane X receptor (PXR), respectively (Table 3-4), thereby exerting their well known cytochrome P450–inducing effects. Genes of other xenobiotic metabolizing enzymes are also activated by these chemicals. For example, TCDD increases the expression of cytochrome-P450 1A1, UDP-glucuronosyltransferase-1, and several subunits of mouse and rat glutathione *S*-transferase because the promoter region of their genes contains a dioxin (or xenobiotic) response element that is recognized by the TCDD-activated Ah receptor complexed with its nuclear translocator protein ARNT. In AHR-null mice, TCDD induces neither these enzymes nor the adverse effects listed in Table 3-4 (Gonzales and Fernandez-Salguero, 1998).

Dysregulation of Signal Transduction Extracellular signaling molecules, such as growth factors, cytokines, hormones, and neurotransmitters, can ultimately activate TFs utilizing cell surface receptors and intracellular signal transducing networks. Figure 3-11 depicts a simplified scheme for such networks and identifies some of the most important signal-activated TFs that control transcriptional activity of genes that influence cell cycle progression and thus determine the fate of cells. Among these TFs are the c-Fos and c-Jun proteins, which bind in dimeric combinations (called AP-1) to the tetradecanoylphorbol acetate (TPA) response element (TRE), for example, in the promoter of cyclin D gene. Another is the c-Myc protein, which, upon dimerizing with Max protein and binding to its cognate nucleotide sequence, transactivates cyclin D and E genes, among others. The cyclins, in turn, accelerate the cell division cycle by activating cyclin-dependent protein kinases (see Figs. 3-21 and 3-24). Mitogenic signaling molecules thus induce cellular proliferation. In contrast, TGF-β induces the expression of cyclin-dependent protein kinase inhibitor proteins (e.g., p27) that mediates its antimitotic effect (Johnson and Walker, 1999) (see Fig. 3-24).

The signal from the cell surface receptors to the TFs is relayed by successive protein-protein interactions and protein phosphorylations. Growth factor receptors (item 6 in Fig. 3-11), exposed on the surface of all cells, are in fact phosphorylating enzymes (i.e., receptor protein tyrosine kinases). Their ligands induce them to phosphorylate themselves, which, in turn, enable these receptors to bind to adapter proteins through which they activate Ras. The active Ras sets in motion the mitogen-activated kinase (MAPK) cascade, involving serial phosphorylations of protein kinases,

Table 3-4
Toxicants Acting on Ligand-Activated Transcription Factors

LIGAND-ACTIVATED TRANSCRIPTION FACTOR	ENDOGENOUS LIGAND	EXOGENOUS LIGAND	EFFECT
Estrogen receptor (ER)	Estradiol	Ethynylestradiol Diethylstilbestrol DDT Zeralenone	Mammary and hepatic carcinogenesis Porcine vulval prolapse
Glucocorticoid receptor (GR)	Cortisol	Dexamethasone	Apoptosis of lymphocytes Teratogenesis (cleft palate)
Retinoic acid receptor (RAR, RXR)	All-*trans*-retinoic acid	13-*cis* retinoic acid	Teratogenesis (craniofacial, cardiac, thymic malformations)
Aryl hydrocarbon receptor (AHR)	Unknown	TCDD PCBs PAHs	Thymic atrophy Wasting syndrome Teratogenesis (cleft palate) Hepatocarcinogenesis in rats Enzyme induction (e.g., ↑ CYP1A1)
Peroxisome proliferator–activated receptor (PPAR)	Fatty acids	Fibrate esters (e.g., clofibrate) Phthalate esters (e.g., DEHP)	Hepatocarcinogenesis in rats Peroxisome proliferation Enzyme induction (e.g., ↑ CYP4A1, ↑ acyl-CoA oxidase)
Constitutive androstane receptor (CAR)	3α,5α-androstenol 3α,5α-androstanol (inhibitors)	Phenobarbital DDT, PCP Chlorpromazine	Enzyme induction (e.g., CYP2B, CYP3A)
Pregnane X receptor (PXR)	Pregnenolone Progesterone	PCN Dexamethasone Spironolactone Cyproterone PCBs Chlordane	Enzyme induction (e.g., ↑ CYP3A)
Metal-responsive element-binding transcription factor (MTF-1)	Zn^{2+}	Cd^{2+}	↑ synthesis of metallothionein

which finally reaches the TFs (Fig. 3-11). Thus, the activity of many signaling elements, ranging from the receptors through the kinases to the transcription factors, is affected by phosphorylation at specific serine, threonine, or tyrosine hydroxyl groups. These signal transducers are typically but not always activated by phosphorylation—that is catalyzed by protein kinases—and are usually inactivated by dephosphorylation, which is carried out by protein phosphatases.

Chemicals may cause aberrant signal transduction in a number of ways, most often by altering protein phosphorylation, occasionally by interfering with the GTPase activity of G proteins (e.g., Ras), by disrupting normal protein-protein interactions or by establishing abnormal ones, or by altering the synthesis or degradation of signaling proteins. Such interventions may ultimately influence cell cycle progression.

Chemically Altered Signal Transduction with Proliferative Effect Xenobiotics that facilitate phosphorylation of signal transducers often promote mitosis and tumor formation. Such are the phorbol esters and fumonisin B that activate protein kinase C (PKC). These chemicals mimic diacylglycerol (DAG), one of the

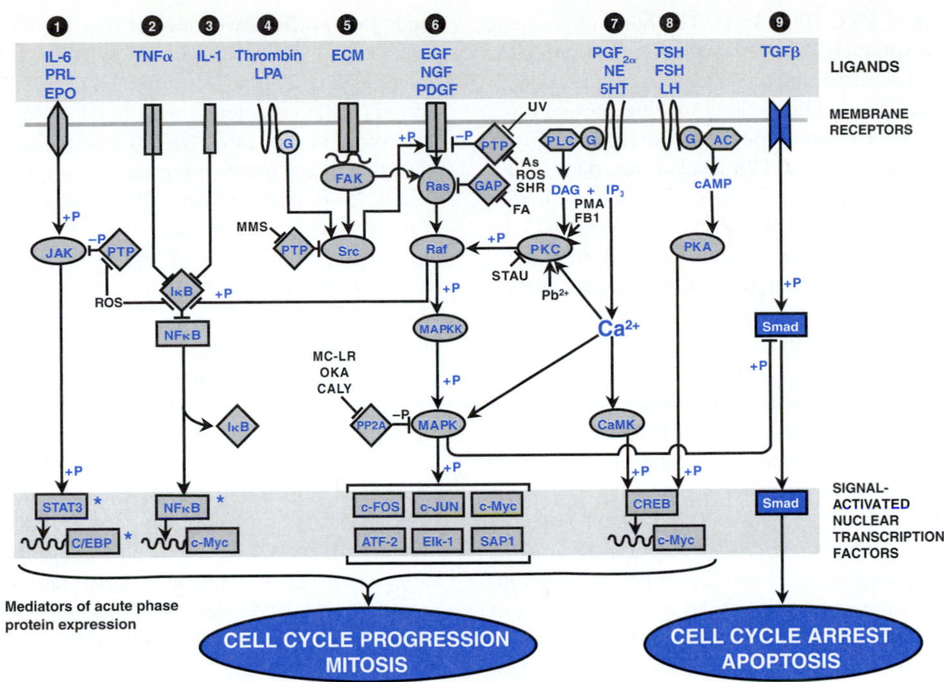

Figure 3-11. Signal transduction pathways from cell membrane receptors to signal-activated nuclear transcription factors that influence transcription of genes involved in cell-cycle regulation.

The symbols of cell membrane receptors are numbered 1–9 and some of their activating ligands are indicated. Circles represent G proteins, oval symbols protein kinases, rectangles transcription factors, wavy lines genes, and diamond symbols inhibitory proteins, such as protein phosphatases (PTP, PP2A), the GTPase-activating protein GAP, and the inhibitory binding protein IκB. Arrowheads indicate stimulation or formation of second messengers (e.g., DAG, IP_3, cAMP, Ca^{2+}), whereas blunt arrows indicate inhibition. Phosphorylation and dephosphorylation are indicated by +P and −P, respectively. Abbreviations for interfering chemicals are printed in black (As = arsenite; CALY = calyculin A; FA = fatty acids; FB1 = fumonisin B; MC-LR = microcystin-LR; OKA = okadaic acid; MMS = methylmethane sulfonate; PMA = phorbol miristate acetate; ROS = reactive oxygen species; SHR = SH-reactive chemicals, such as iodoacetamide; STAU = staurosporin).

In the center of the depicted networks is the pathway activated by growth factors, such as EGF, that acts on a tyrosine kinase receptor (#6) which uses adaptor proteins (Shc, Grb2 and SOS; not shown) to convert the inactive GDP-bound Ras to active GTP-bound form, which in turn activates the MAP-kinase phosphorylation cascade (Raf, MAPKK, MAPK). The phosphorylated MAPK moves into the nucleus and phosphorylates transcription factors thereby enabling them to bind to cognate sequences in the promoter regions of genes to facilitate transcription. There are numerous interconnections between the signal transduction pathways. Some of these connections permit the use of the growth factor receptor (#6)-MAPK "highway" for other receptors (e.g., 4, 5, 7) to send mitogenic signals. For example, receptor (#4) joins in via its G protein β/γ subunits and tyrosine kinase Src; the integrin receptor (#5), whose ligands are constituents of the extracellular matrix (ECM), possibly connects via G-protein Rho (not shown) and focal adhesion kinase (FAK); and the G-protein-coupled receptor (#7) via phospholipase C (PLC)-catalyzed formation of second messengers and activation of protein-kinase C (PKC). The mitogenic stimulus relayed along the growth factor receptor (#6)-MAPK axis can be amplified by, for example, the Raf-catalyzed phosphorylation of IκB, which unleashes NF-κB from this inhibitory protein, and by the MAPK-catalyzed inhibitory phosphorylation of Smad that blocks the cell-cycle arrest signal from the TGF-β receptor (#9). Activation of protein kinases (PKC, CaMK, MAPK) by Ca^{2+} can also trigger mitogenic signaling. Several xenobiotics that are indicated in the figure may dysregulate the signaling network. Some may induce cell proliferation either by activating mitogenic protein kinases (e.g., PKC), or inhibiting inactivating proteins, such as protein phosphatases (PTP, PP2A), GAP or IκB. Others, e.g., inhibitors of PKC, oppose mitosis and facilitate apoptosis.

This scheme is oversimplified and tentative in several details. Virtually all components of the signaling network (e.g., G proteins, PKCs, MAPKs) are present in multiple, functionally different forms whose distribution may be cell specific. The pathways depicted are not equally relevant for all cells. In addition, these pathways regulating gene expression determine not only the fate of cells, but also control certain aspects of the ongoing cellular activity. For example, NF-κB induces synthesis of acute phase proteins.

physiologic activators of PKC (Fig. 3-11). The other physiologic PKC activator Ca^{2+} is mimicked by Pb^{2+}, whose effect on PKCα is concentration-dependent: stimulatory at picomolar concentration, when Pb^{2+} occupies only high-affinity binding sites on PKC, and inhibitory at micromolar concentration, where the low affinity sites are also occupied (Sun et al., 1999). Lead acetate does induce marked hepatocellular proliferation in rats. The activated PKC promotes mitogenic signaling at least in two ways: (1) by phosphorylating Raf, the first protein kinase in the MAPK pathway (Fig. 3-11), and (2) by phosphorylating a protein phosphatase that dephosphorylates the transcription factor c-Jun at specific sites (Thr 231, Ser 234, and Ser 249), thereby permitting its binding to DNA. Protein kinases may also be activated by interacting proteins that had been altered by a xenobiotic. For example, the TCDD-liganded AHR binds to MAPK. This may contribute to the TCDD-induced overexpression of cyclins and cyclin-dependent kinases in guinea pig liver (Ma and Babish, 1999).

Abberant phosphorylation of proteins may result not only from increased phosphorylation by kinases but also from decreased dephosphorylation by phosphatases. Inhibition of phosphatases appears to be the underlying mechanism of the mitogenic effect of various chemicals, oxidative stress, and ultraviolet (UV) irradiation (Herrlich et al., 1999). Protein tyrosine phosphatases and dual-specificity phosphatases (i.e., enzymes that remove phosphate from phosphorylated tyrosine as well as serine and threonine residues) contain a catalytically active cysteine and are susceptible to inactivation by oxidation and covalent reaction with SH-reactive chemicals. Indeed, xenobiotics such as the SH-reactive iodoacetamide, the organometal compound tributyltin, arsenite, and oxidants (e.g., HOOH) cause phosphorylation of the epidermal growth factor (EGF) receptor (item 6 in Fig. 3-11) by interfering with the protein tyrosine phosphatase that would dephosphorylate and thus "silence" this receptor (Herrlich et al., 1999; Chen et al., 1998). Arsenite may also inactivate the dual-specificity phosphatase that dephosphorylates and "silences" certain MAPKs (JNK, p38), whereas methylmethane sulfonate (MMS) appears to inhibit a protein phosphatase that inactivates Src, a protein tyrosine kinase (Herrlich et al., 1999). The thiol oxidizing agent diamide (which increases phosphorylation of MAPKs) and phenolic antioxidants (which form phenoxyl radicals and increase c-Fos and c-Jun expression) (Dalton et al., 1999) may also act by incapacitating protein tyrosine phosphatases. Protein phosphatase 2A (PP2A) is the major soluble ser/thr phosphatase in cells and is likely responsible, at least in part, for reversing the growth factor–induced stimulation of MAPK, thereby keeping the extent and duration of MAPK activity under control (Goldberg, 1999). PP2A also removes an activating phosphate from a mitosis-triggering protein kinase ($p34^{cdc2}$). Several natural toxins are extremely potent inhibitors of PP2A; including the blue-green algae poison microcystin-LG and the dinoflagellate-derived okadaic acid (Toivola and Eriksson, 1999), which are tumor promoters in experimental animals subjected to prolonged low-dose exposure. It is to be noted, however, that acute high-dose exposure to microcystin induces severe liver injury, whereas such exposure to okadaic acid is the underlying cause of the diarrhetic shellfish poisoning. In these conditions, hyperphosphorylation of proteins other than those involved in proliferative signaling (e.g. hepatocellular microfilaments in microcystin poisoning) may be primarily responsible for the pathogenesis.

Apart from phosphatases, there are also inhibitory binding proteins that can keep signaling under control. Such is IκB, which binds to NF-κB, preventing its transfer into the nucleus and its function as a TF. Upon phosphorylation, IκB becomes degraded and NF-κB is set free. Because phosphorylation of IκB can be catalyzed by Raf, a protein kinase in the MAPK cascade (Fig. 3-11), and because the released NF-κB can transactivate the c-Myc gene, NF-κB is an important contributor to proliferative and prolife signaling. In addition, because NF-κB also targets the genes of several cytokines (e.g., TNF-α, IL-1β) and acute phase proteins (e.g., C-reactive protein, α1-acid glycoprotein), and because such cytokines acting on their receptors (items 2 and 3 in Fig. 3-11) also activate NF-κB, this TF plays a leading role also in inflammatory and acute phase reactions (Lee et al., 1998; Waddick and Uckun, 1999). IκB degradation and NF-κB activation can also be induced by oxidative stress, and it appears that peroxides are the reactive oxygen species (ROS) that mediate this effect (Dalson et al., 1999). Activated NF-κB probably contributes to the proliferative and inflammatory response to oxidative stress. NF-κB also protects cells from apoptosis by maintaining c-Myc transcription, which is required for survival (Waddick and Uckun, 1999), and by transactivating the genes of antiapoptotic IAP proteins, which inhibit caspases (Jäättelä, 1999). Another site from which abberant mitogenic signals may originate is the GTP/GDP binding protein Ras, which is active in GTP-bound form but inactive in GDP-bound form. The activity of Ras is normally terminated via stimulation of its own GTPase activity by a GTPase-activating protein (GAP) (Fig. 3-11) that returns Ras into its inactive GDP-bound state. Fatty acids, which may accumulate, for example, in response to phospholipase A activation and exposure to peroxysome proliferators (Rose et al., 1999), inhibit GAP and can delay the turning off of Ras. As discussed in more detail later in the chapter, genotoxic carcinogens may mutate Ras, and if the mutation leads to a loss of its GTPase activity, this would result in a permanent signaling for the MAPK pathway—a condition that contributes to malignant transformation of the affected cell population.

Chemically Altered Signal Transduction with Antiproliferative Effect Downturning of increased proliferative signaling after cell injury may compromise replacement of injured cells. This prediction has been made from a recent study on cultured Hepa 1-6 cells that exhibited the following, seemingly consequential alterations upon exposure to acetaminophen (follow the path in Fig. 3-11): inhibition of Raf $\rightarrow$ diminished degradation of IκB $\rightarrow$ diminished binding of NF-κB to DNA $\rightarrow$ diminished expression of c-Myc mRNA (Boulares et al., 1999). Down-regulation of a normal mitogenic signal is a step away from survival and toward apoptosis. Indeed, staurosporin, an inhibitor of PKC, and gliotoxin, an inhibitor of IκB degradation (Waddick and Uckun, 1999), are potent apoptosis inducers. TGF-β and glucocorticoids increase IκB synthesis and, in turn, decrease NF-κB activation and c-Myc expression (Waddick and Uckun, 1999). These mechanisms may contribute to the apoptotic effect of TGF-β and glucocorticoids, the latter in lymphoid cells.

Dysregulation of Extracellular Signal Production Hormones of the anterior pituitary exert mitogenic effects on endocrine glands in the periphery by acting on cell surface receptors. Pituitary hormone production is under negative feedback control by hormones of the peripheral glands. Perturbation of this circuit adversely affects pituitary hormone secretion and, in turn, the peripheral gland. For example, xenobiotics that inhibit thyroid hormone production (e.g., the herbicide amitrole and the fungicide metabolite ethylenethiourea) or enhance thyroid hormone elimination (e.g., phenobarbital) reduce thyroid hormone levels and increase the secretion of thyroid-stimulating hormone (TSH) because of the reduced feedback inhibition. The increased TSH secretion stimulates cell division in the thyroid gland, which is responsible for the goiters or thyroid tumors caused by such toxicants (Chap. 21). Decreased secretion of pituitary hormone produces the opposite adverse affect, with apoptosis followed by involution of the peripheral target gland. For example, estrogens produce testicular atrophy in males by means of feedback inhibition of gonadotropin secretion. The low sperm count in workers intoxicated with the xenoestrogen chlordecone probably results from such a mechanism.

Dysregulation of Ongoing Cellular Activity Ongoing control of specialized cells is exerted by signaling molecules acting on membrane receptors that transduce the signal by regulating Ca^{2+} entry into the cytoplasm or stimulating the enzymatic formation of intracellular second messengers. The Ca^{2+} or other second messengers ultimately alter the phosphorylation of functional proteins, changing their activity and, in turn, cellular functions almost instantly. Toxicants can adversely affect ongoing cellular activity by disrupting any step in signal coupling.

Dysregulation of Electrically Excitable Cells Many xenobiotics influence cellular activity in excitable cells, such as neurons, skeletal, cardiac, and smooth muscle cells. Cellular functions such as the release of neurotransmitters and muscle contraction are controlled by transmitters and modulators synthesized and released by adjacent neurons. The major mechanisms that control such cells are shown schematically in Fig. 3-12, and chemicals that interfere with these mechanisms are listed in Table 3-5.

Altered regulation of neural and/or muscle activity is the basic mechanism of action of many drugs and is responsible for toxicities associated with drug overdosage, pesticides, and microbial, plant, and animal toxins (Herken and Hucho, 1992). As neu-

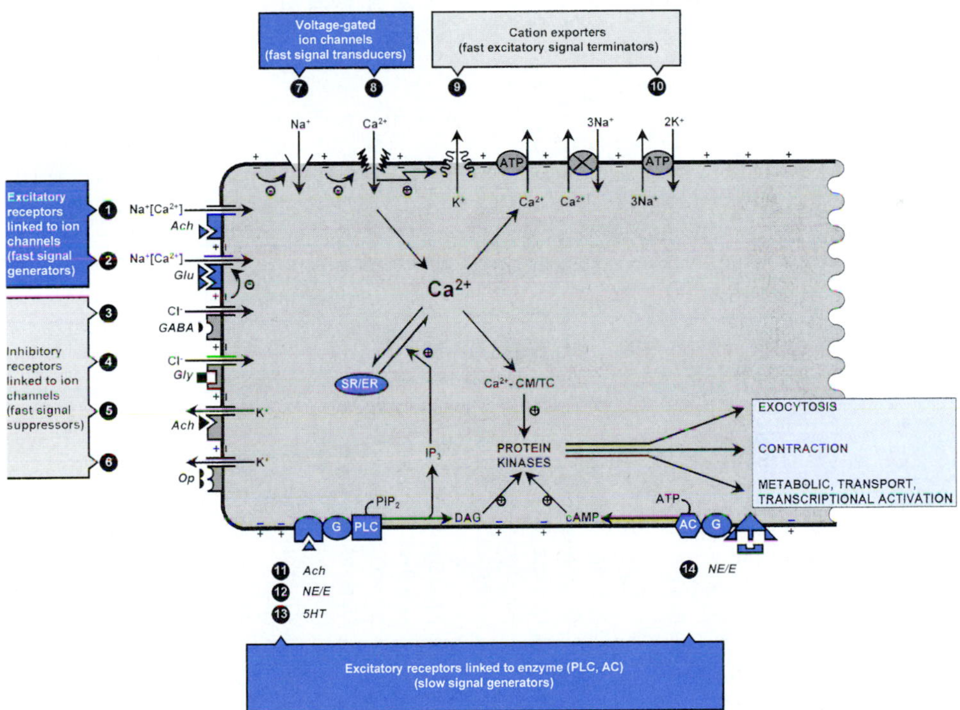

Figure 3-12. Signaling mechanisms for neurotransmitters..

This simplified scheme depicts major cellular signaling mechanisms that are operational in many neurons and muscle and exocrine cells. Chemicals acting on the numbered elements are listed in Table 3-5. Fast signaling is initiated by the opening of ligand-gated Na^+/Ca^{2+} channels (1,2). The resultant cation influx decreases the inside negative potential (i.e., evokes depolarization) and thus triggers the opening of the voltage-gated Na^+ and Ca^{2+} channels (7,8). As a second messenger, the influxed Ca^{2+} activates intracellular Ca^{2+}-binding proteins such as calmodulin (CM) and troponin C (TC), which, in turn, enhance the phosphorylation of specific proteins, causing activation of specific cellular functions. The signal is terminated by channels and transporters (e.g., 9,10) that remove cations from the cells and thus reestablish the inside negative resting potential (i.e., cause repolarization) and restore the resting Ca^{2+} level. Fast signaling can be suppressed by opening the ligand-activated Cl^- or K^+ channels (3-6), which increases the inside negativity (i.e., induces hyperpolarization) and thus counteracts opening of the voltage-gated Na^+ and Ca^{2+} channels (7,8). Signal transduction from other receptors (11–14) is slower because it involves enzymatic generation of second messengers: inositol 1,4,5-trisphosphate (IP_3) and diacylglycerol (DAG) by phospholipase C (PLC) and cyclic AMP (cAMP) by adenylyl cyclase (AC). These messengers influence cellular activities by activating protein kinases directly or by mobilizing Ca^{2+} from the sarcoplasmic or endoplasmic reticulum (SR and ER), as IP_3 does. Ach = acetylcholine; Glu = glutamate; GABA = γ-aminobutyric acid; Gly = glycine; Op = opioid peptides; NE = norepinephrine; E = epinephrine; 5HT = 5-hydroxytryptamine; G = G protein; PIP_2 = phosphatidylinositol 4,5-bisphosphate. Encircled positive and negative signs indicate activation and inhibition, respectively.

Table 3-5

Agents Acting on Signaling Systems for Neurotransmitters and Causing Dysregulation of the Momentary Activity of Electrically Excitable Cells Such as Neurons and Muscle Cells*

Receptor/Channel/Pump		*Agonist/Activator*		*Antagonist/Inhibitor*	
NAME	LOCATION	AGENT	EFFECT	AGENT	EFFECT
1. Acetylcholine nicotinic receptor	Skeletal muscle	Nicotine Anatoxin-a Cytisine *Ind:* ChE inhibitors	Muscle fibrillation, then paralysis	Tubocurarine, lophotoxin α-Bungarotoxin α-Cobrotoxin α-Conotoxin Erabutoxin b *Ind:* botulinum toxin	Muscle paralysis
	Neurons	See above	Neuronal activation	Pb^{2+}, general anesthetics	Neuronal inhibition
2. Glutamate receptor	CNS neurons	*N*-Methyl-*D*-aspartate Kainate, domoate Quinolinate Quisqualate *Ind:* hypoxia, HCN → glutamate release	Neuronal activation → convulsion, neuronal injury ("excitotoxicity")	Phencyclidine Ketamine General anesthetics	Neuronal inhibition → anesthesia Protection against "excitotoxicity"
3. $GABA_A$ receptor	CNS neurons	Muscimol, avermectins sedatives (barbiturates, benzodiazepines) General anaesthetics (halothane) Alcohols (ethanol)	Neuronal inhibition → sedation, general anaesthesia, coma, depression of vital centers	Bicuculline Picrotoxin Pentylenetetrazole Cyclodiene insecticides Lindane *Ind:* isoniazid	Neuronal activation → tremor, convulsion
4. Glycine receptor	CNS neurons, motor neurons	Avermectins (?) General anesthetics	Inhibition of motor neurons → paralysis	Strychnine *Ind:* tetanus toxin	Disinhibition of motor neurons → tetanic convulsion
5. Acetylcholine M_2 muscarinic receptor	Cardiac muscle	*Ind:* ChE inhibitors	Decreased heart rate and contractility	Belladonna alkaloids (e.g., atropine) atropinelike drugs (e.g., TCAD)	Increased heart rate
6. Opioid receptor	CNS neurons, visceral neurons	Morphine and congeners (e.g., heroin, meperidine)	Neuronal inhibition → analgesia, central respiratory depression, constipation, urine retention	Naloxone	Antidotal effects in opiate intoxication

(continued)

7. Voltage-gated Na^+ channel	Neurons, muscle cells, etc.	Aconitine, veratridine Grayanotoxin Batrachotoxin Scorpion toxins Ciguatoxin DDT, pyrethroids	Neuronal activation → convulsion	Tetrodotoxin, saxitoxin μ-Conotoxin Local anaesthetics Phenytoin Quinidine	Neuronal inhibition → paralysis, anesthesia Anticonvulsive action
8. Voltage-gated Ca^+ channel	Neurons, muscle cell, etc.	Maitotoxin (?) Atrotoxin (?) Latrotoxin (?)	Neuronal/muscular activation, cell injury	ω-Conotoxin Pb^2	Neuronal inhibition → paralysis
9. Voltage/Ca^{2+}-activated K^+ Channel	Neurons, muscle cells	Pb^{2+}	Neuronal/muscular inhibition	Ba^{2+} Apamin (bee venom) Dendrotoxin	Neuronal/muscular activation → convulsion/spasm
10. Na^+,K^+-ATPase	Universal			Digitalis glycosides Oleandrin Chlordecone	Increased cardiac contractility, excitability Increased neuronal excitability → tremor
11. Acetylcholine M_3 muscarinic receptor	Smooth muscle, glands	*Ind:* ChE inhibitors	Smooth muscle spasm Salivation, lacrimation	Belladonna alkaloids (e.g., atropine) Atropinelike drugs (e.g., TCAD)	Smooth muscle relaxation → intestinal paralysis, decreased salivation, decreased perspiration
Acetylcholine M_1 muscarinic receptor	CNS neurons	Oxotremorine *Ind:* ChE inhibitors	Neuronal activation → convulsion	See above	
12. Adrenergic alpha$_1$ receptor	Vascular smooth muscle	(Nor)epinephrine *Ind:* cocaine, tyramine amphetamine, TCAD	Vasoconstriction → ischemia, hypertension	Prazosin	Antidotal effects in intoxication with alpha$_1$-receptor agonists
13. 5-HT_2 receptor	Smooth muscle	Ergot alkaloids (ergotamine, ergonovine)	Vasoconstriction → ischemia, hypertension	Ketanserine	Antidotal effects in ergot intoxication
14. Adrenergic beta$_1$ receptor	Cardiac muscle	(Nor)epinephrine *Ind:* cocaine, tyramine amphetamine, TCAD	Increased cardiac contractility and excitability	Atenolol, metoprolol	Antidotal effects in intoxication with beta$_1$-receptor agonists

*Numbering of the signaling elements in this table corresponds to the numbering of their symbols in Fig. 3-12. This tabulation is simplified and incomplete. Virtually all receptors and channels listed occur in multiple forms with different sensitivity to the agents. The reader should consult the pertinent literature for more detailed information. CNS = central nervous system; ChE = cholinesterase; *Ind* = indirectly acting (i.e., by altering neurotransmitter level); TCAD = tricyclic antidepressant.

rons are signal-transducing cells, the influence of chemicals on neurons is seen not only on the neuron affected by the toxicant but also on downstream cells influenced by the primary target. Thus, tetrodotoxin, which blocks voltage-gated Na^+ channels (item 7 in Fig. 3-12) in motor neurons, causes skeletal muscle paralysis. In contrast, cyclodiene insecticides, which block GABA receptors (item 3 in Fig. 3-12) in the central nervous system, induce neuronal excitation and convulsions (Narahashi, 1991).

Perturbation of ongoing cellular activity by chemicals may be due to an alteration in (1) the concentration of neurotransmitters, (2) receptor function, (3) intracellular signal transduction, or (4) the signal-terminating processes.

Alteration in Neurotransmitter Levels Chemicals may alter synaptic levels of neurotransmitters by interfering with their synthesis, storage, release, or removal from the vicinity of the receptor. The convulsive effect of hydrazides is due to their ability to decrease the synthesis of the inhibitory neurotransmitter GABA (Gale, 1992). Reserpine causes its several adverse effects by inhibiting the neuronal storage of norepinephrine, 5-hydroxytryptamine, and dopamine, thereby depleting these transmitters. Skeletal muscle paralysis caused by botulinum toxin is due to inhibition of acetylcholine release from motor neurons and the lacking stimulation of the acethylcholine receptors at the neuromuscular junction (receptor 1 in Fig. 3-12). In contrast, inhibition of acetylcholinesterase by organophosphate or carbamate insecticides or chemical warfare agents (e.g., soman) prevents the hydrolysis of acetylcholine, resulting in massive stimulation of cholinergic receptors (receptors 1, 5, and 10 in Fig. 3-12) and a cholinergic crisis (Table 3-5). Inhibition of the neuronal reuptake of norepinephrine by cocaine or tricyclic antidepressants is responsible for overexcitation of alpha$_1$-adrenergic receptors on vascular smooth muscles, resulting in nasal mucosal ulceration and myocardial infarction in heavy cocaine abusers, whereas overstimulation of beta$_1$-adrenergic receptors contributes to life-threatening arryhthmias. Similar cardiac complications may result from amphetamine abuse, because amphetamine enhances the release of norepinephrine from adrenergic neurons and competitively inhibits neuronal reuptake of this transmitter. A hypertensive crisis can occur with the combined use of tricyclic antidepressants and monoamine oxidase inhibitors, drugs that block different mechanisms of norepinephrine elimination (Hardman et al., 1995).

Toxicant–Neurotransmitter Receptor Interactions Some chemicals interact directly with neurotransmitter receptors, including (1) agonists that associate with the ligand-binding site on the receptor and mimic the natural ligand, (2) antagonists that occupy the ligand-binding site but cannot activate the receptor, (3) activators, and (4) inhibitors that bind to a site on the receptor that is not directly involved in ligand binding. In the absence of other actions, agonists and activators mimic, whereas antagonists and inhibitors block, the physiologic responses characteristic of endogenous ligands. For example, muscimol, a mushroom poison, is an agonist at the inhibitory $GABA_A$ receptor (item 3 in Fig. 3-12), whereas barbiturates, benzodiazepines, general anaesthetics, and alcohols are activators (Narahashi, 1991). Thus, all these agents cause inhibition of central nervous system activity, resulting in sedation, general anesthesia, coma, and ultimately blockade of the medullary respiratory center, depending on the dose administered. There are also similarities in the responses evoked by agonist/activators on excitatory receptors and those elicited by antagonists/inhibitors on inhibitory sites. Thus, glutamate receptor agonists and muscarinic receptor agonists cause neuronal hyperactivity in the brain and ultimately convulsions, as do inhibitors of $GABA_A$ receptor. It is also apparent that chemicals acting as agonists/activators on inhibitory receptors and those acting as antagonists/inhibitors on excitatory receptors may exert similar effects. Moreover, general anesthetic solvents induce general anesthesia not only by activating the inhibitory ligand-gated chloride-ion channels (i.e., $GABA_A$ and glycine receptors; see items 3 and 4, respectively, in Fig. 3-12) but also by inhibiting the excitatory ligand-gated cation channels (i.e., neuronal nicotinic acethylcholine receptor and glutamate receptors; see items 1 and 2, respectively, in Fig. 3-12) (Franks and Lieb, 1998; Perouansky et al., 1998). Because there are multiple types of receptors for each neurotransmitter, these receptors may be affected differentially by toxicants. For example, the neuronal nicotinic acetylcholine receptor is extremely sensitive to inhibition by lead ions, whereas the muscular nicotine receptor subtype is not (Oortgiesen et al., 1993). Other chemicals that produce neurotransmitter receptor–mediated toxicity are listed in Table 3-5.

Some sensory neurons have receptors that are stimulated by chemicals, such as the capsaicin receptor, which is a ligand-gated cation channel (Herken and Hucho, 1992). This receptor mediates the burning sensation of the tongue and reflex stimulation of the lacrimal gland associated with exposure to red pepper and other irritants. Lacrimators in tear gas, which are typically thiol-reactive chemicals, also stimulate these neurons, though their precise mode of action is unclear.

Toxicant–Signal Transducer Interactions Many chemicals alter neuronal and/or muscle activity by acting on signal-transduction processes. Voltage-gated Na^+ channels (item 7 in Fig. 3-12), which transduce and amplify excitatory signals generated by ligand-gated cation channels (receptors 1 and 2 in Fig. 3-12), are activated by a number of toxins derived from plants and animals (Table 3-5) as well as by synthetic chemicals such as DDT, resulting in overexcitation (Narahashi, 1992). In contrast, agents that block voltage-gated Na^+ channels (such as tetrodotoxin and saxitoxin) cause paralysis. The Na^+ channels are also important in signal transduction in sensory neurons; therefore, Na^+-channel activators evoke sensations and reflexes, whereas Na^+-channel inhibitors induce anesthesia. This explains the reflex bradycardia and burning sensation in the mouth that follow the ingestion of monkshood, which contains the Na^+-channel activator aconitine, as well as the use of Na^+-channel inhibitors such as procaine and lidocaine for local anesthesia.

Toxicant–Signal Terminator Interactions The cellular signal generated by cation influx is terminated by removal of the cations through channels or by transporters (Fig. 3-12). Inhibition of cation export may prolong excitation, as occurs with the inhibition of Ca^{2+}-activated K^+ channels (item 9 in Fig. 3-12) by Ba^{2+}, which is accompanied by potentially lethal neuroexcitatory and spasmogenic effects. Glycosides from digitalis and other plants inhibit Na^+,K^+-ATPase (item 10 in Fig. 3-12) and thus increase the intracellular Na^+ concentration, which, in turn, decreases Ca^{2+} export by Ca^{2+}/Na^+ exchange (Fig. 3-12). The resultant rise in the intracellular concentration of Ca^{2+} enhances the contractility and excitability of cardiac muscle. Inhibition of brain Na^+,K^+-ATPase by chlordecone may be responsible for the tremor observed in chlordecone-exposed workers (Desaiah, 1982). Lithium salts, although used therapeutically, have the potential to produce hyperreflexia, tremor, convulsions, diarrhea, and cardiac arrhythmias (Hardman et al., 1995). Lithium also markedly potentiates cholinergically mediated seizures. A possible reason for these toxic effects is inefficient repolarization of neurons and muscle cells in the presence of Li^+. Whereas Li^+ readily enters these cells through Na^+ channels, contributing to the signal-induced depolarization, it is not a substrate for the Na^+,K^+ pump. Therefore, the cells fail to repolarize properly if a fraction of intracellular Na^+ is replaced by Li^+.

Failure of the Na^+,K^+ pump also is believed to contribute to the neuronal damage resulting from hypoxia, hypoglycemia, and cyanide intoxication. Inasmuch as 70 percent of the ATP produced in neurons is used to drive the Na^+,K^+ pump; cessation of ATP synthesis causes a cell to become or remain depolarized. The depolarization-induced release of neurotransmitters such as glutamate from such neurons is thought to be responsible for the hypoxic seizures and further amplification of neuronal injury by the neurotoxic actions of glutamate (Patel et al., 1993).

Dysregulation of the Activity of Other Cells While many signaling mechanisms also operate in nonexcitable cells, disturbance of these processes is usually less consequential. For example, rat liver cells possess $alpha_1$-adrenergic receptors (item 12 in Fig. 3-12) whose activation evokes metabolic changes, such as increased glycogenolysis and glutathione export, through elevation of intracellular Ca^{2+}, which may have toxicologic significance.

Many exocrine secretory cells are controlled by muscarinic acetylcholine receptors (item 11 in Fig. 3-12). Salivation, lacrimation, and bronchial hypersecretion after organophosphate insecticide poisoning are due to stimulation of these receptors. In contrast, blockade of these receptors contributes to the hyperthermia characteristic of atropine poisoning. Kupffer cells, resident macrophages in the liver, secrete inflammatory mediators (see Fig. 3-22) that can harm the neighboring cells. Because Kupffer cells possess glycine receptors, i.e., glycine-gated Cl^- channels (item 4 in Fig. 3-12), the secretory function of these macrophages (e.g., secretion of inflammatory mediators) can be blocked by administration of glycine, which induces hyperpolarization via influx of Cl^-. Such intervention alleviates ethanol-induced liver injury (Yin et al., 1998).

The discovery that some sulfonamides produce hypoglycemia in experimental animals led to the development of oral hypoglycemic agents for diabetic patients. These drugs inhibit K^+ channels in pancreatic beta cells, inducing sequentially depolarization, Ca^{2+} influx through voltage-gated Ca^{2+} channels, and exocytosis of insulin (Hardman et al., 1995). The antihypertensive diazoxide acts in the opposite fashion on K^+ channels and impairs insulin secretion. While this effect is generally undesirable, it is exploited in the treatment of inoperable insulin-secreting pancreatic tumors.

Toxic Alteration of Cellular Maintenance

Numerous toxicants interfere with cellular maintenance functions. In a multicellular organism, cells must maintain their own structural and functional integrity as well as provide supportive functions for other cells. Execution of these functions may be disrupted by chemicals, resulting in a toxic response.

Impairment of Internal Cellular Maintenance: Mechanisms of Toxic Cell Death For survival, all cells must synthesize endogenous molecules; assemble macromolecular complexes, membranes, and cell organelles; maintain the intracellular environment; and produce energy for operation. Agents that disrupt these functions, especially the energy-producing function of mitochondria and protein synthesis controlling function of the genome, jeopardize survival and may cause toxic cell death.

There are three critical biochemical disorders that chemicals inflicting cell death may initiate, namely ATP depletion, sustained rise in intracellular Ca^{2+}, and overproduction of ROS and RNS. In the following discussion, these events and the chemicals that may cause them are individually characterized. Then it is pointed out how their concerted action may induce a bioenergetic catastrophe, culminating in necrosis. Finally, there follows a discussion of the circumstances under which the cell can avoid this disordered decay and how it can execute death by activating catabolic processes that bring about an ordered disassembly and removal of the cell, called apoptosis.

Primary Metabolic Disorders Jeopardizing Cell Survival: ATP Depletion, Ca^{2+} Accumulation, ROS/RNS Generation *Depletion of ATP* ATP plays a central role in cellular maintenance both as a chemical for biosynthesis and as the major source of energy. It is utilized in numerous biosynthetic reactions, activating endogenous compounds by phosphorylation and adenylation, and is incorporated into cofactors as well as nucleic acids. It is required for muscle contraction and polymerization of the cytoskeleton, fueling cellular motility, cell division, vesicular transport, and the maintenance of cell morphology. ATP drives ion transporters such as the Na^+,K^+-ATPase in the plasma membrane, the Ca^{2+}-ATPase in the plasma and the endoplasmic reticulum membranes, and H^+-ATPase in the membrane of lysosomes and neurotransmitter-containing vesicles. These pumps maintain conditions essential for various cell functions. For example, the Na^+ concentration gradient across the plasma membrane generated by the Na^+,K^+ pump drives Na^+-glucose and Na^+-amino acid cotransporters as well as the Na^+/Ca^{2+} antiporter, facilitating the entry of these nutrients and the removal of Ca^{2+}.

Chemical energy is released by hydrolysis of ATP to ADP or AMP. The ADP is rephosphorylated in the mitochondria by ATP synthase (Fig. 3-13). Coupled to oxidation of hydrogen to water, this process is termed *oxidative phosphorylation.* In addition to ATP synthase, oxidative phosphorylation requires the (1) delivery of hydrogen in the form of NADH to the initial electron transport complex; (2) delivery of oxygen to the terminal electron transport complex; (3) delivery of ADP and inorganic phosphate to ATP synthase; (4) flux of electrons along the electron transport chain to O_2, accompanied by ejection of protons from the matrix space across the inner membrane; and (5) return of protons across the inner membrane into the matrix space down an electrochemical gradient to drive ATP synthase (Fig. 3-13).

Several chemicals impede these processes, interfering with mitochondrial ATP synthesis (Commandeur and Vermeuien, 1990; Wallace and Starkow, 2000). These chemicals are divided into five groups (Table 3-6). Substances in class A interfere with the delivery of hydrogen to the electron transport chain. For example, fluoroacetate inhibits the citric acid cycle and the production of reduced cofactors. Class B chemicals such as rotenone and cyanide inhibit the transfer of electrons along the electron transport chain to oxygen. Class C agents interfere with oxygen delivery to the terminal electron transporter, cytochrome oxidase. All chemicals that cause hypoxia ultimately act at this site. Chemicals in class D inhibit the activity of ATP synthase, the key enzyme for oxidative phosphorylation. At this site, the synthesis of ATP may be inhibited in one of four ways: (1) direct inhibition of ATP synthase, (2)

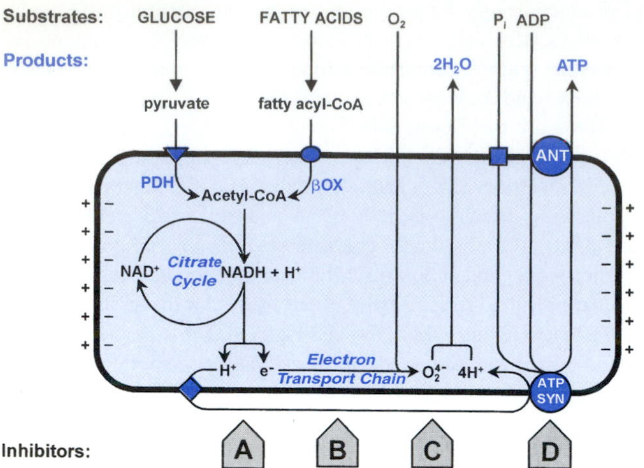

Figure 3-13. ATP synthesis (oxidative phosphorylation) in mitochondria.

Arrows with roman numerals point to the ultimate sites of action of four categories of agents that interfere with oxidative phosphorylation (Table 3-6). For simplicity, this scheme does not indicate the outer mitochondrial membrane and that protons are extruded from the matrix space along the electron transport chain at three sites. βOX = beta-oxidation of fatty acids; e^- = electron; P_i = inorganic phosphate; ANT = adenine nucleotide translocator; ATP SYN = ATP synthase (F_oF_1ATPase).

interference with ADP delivery, (3) interference with inorganic phosphate delivery, and (4) deprivation of ATP synthase from its driving force, the controlled influx of protons into the matrix space. Protonophoric chemicals (uncouplers) such as 2,4-dinitrophenol and pentachlorophenol import protons into the mitochondrial matrix, dissipating the proton gradient that drives the controlled influx of protons into the matrix, which, in turn, drives ATP synthase. Finally, chemicals causing mitochondrial DNA injury, and thereby impairing synthesis of specific proteins encoded by the mitochondrial genome (e.g., subunits of complex I and ATP synthase), are listed in group E. These include the dideoxynucleoside antiviral drugs used against AIDS, such as zidovudine. Table 3-6 lists other chemicals that impair ATP synthesis.

Impairment of oxidative phosphorylation is detrimental to cells because failure of ADP rephosphorylation results in the accumulation of ADP and its breakdown products as well as depletion of ATP. Accordingly, hepatocytes exposed to KCN and iodoacetate exhibit a rapid rise in cytosolic H^+ and Mg^{2+} as a result of the hydrolysis of adenosine di- and triphosphates (existing as Mg salts) and the release of phosphoric acid and Mg^{2+} (Herman et al., 1990). The increased conversion of pyruvate to lactate also may contribute to the acidosis. The lack of ATP compromises the operation of ATP-requiring ion pumps, leading to the loss of ionic and volume-regulatory controls (Buja et al., 1993). Shortly after intracellular acidosis and hypermagnesemia, liver cells exposed to KCN and iodoacetate exhibit a rise in intracellular Na^+, probably as a result of failure of the Na^+ pump, after which plasma membrane blebs appear. The intracellular phosphoric acidosis is beneficial for the cells presumably because the released phosphoric acid forms insoluble calcium phosphate, preventing the rise of cytosolic Ca^{2+}, with its deleterious consequences (see below). In addition, a low pH also directly decreases the activity of phospholipases and inhibits mitochondrial permeability transition (see later). Terminally, the intracellular pH rises, increasing phospholipase activity, and this contributes to irreversible membrane damage (i.e., rupture of the blebs) not only by degrading phospholipids but also by generating endogenous detergents such as lysophospholipids and free fatty acids. The lack of ATP aggravates this condition because the reacylation of lysophospholipids with fatty acids is impaired.

Sustained Rise of Intracellular Ca^{2+} Intracellular Ca^{2+} levels are highly regulated (Fig. 3-14). The 10,000-fold difference between extracellular and cytosolic Ca^{2+} concentration is maintained by the impermeability of the plasma membrane to Ca^{2+} and by transport mechanisms that remove Ca^{2+} from the cytoplasm (Richter and Kass, 1991). Ca^{2+} is actively pumped from the cytosol across the plasma membrane and is sequestered in the endoplasmic reticulum and mitochondria (Fig. 3-14). Because they are equipped with a low-affinity transporter, the mitochondria play a significant role in Ca^{2+} sequestration only when the cytoplasmic levels rise into the micromolar range. Under such conditions, a large amount of Ca^{2+} accumulates in the mitochondria, where it is deposited as calcium phosphate.

Toxicants induce elevation of cytoplasmic Ca^{2+} levels by promoting Ca^{2+} influx into or inhibiting Ca^{2+} efflux from the cytoplasm (Table 3-7). Opening of the ligand- or voltage-gated Ca^{2+} channels or damage to the plasma membrane causes Ca^{2+} to move down its concentration gradient from extracellular fluid to the cytoplasm. Toxicants also may increase cytosolic Ca^{2+} inducing its leakage from the mitochondria or the endoplasmic reticulum. They also may diminish Ca^{2+} efflux through inhibition of Ca^{2+} transporters or depletion of their driving forces. Several chemicals that can cause a sustained rise in cytoplasmic Ca^{2+} levels are listed in Table 3-7. Sustained elevation of intracellular Ca^{2+} is harmful because it can result in (1) depletion of energy reserves, (2) dysfunction of microfilaments, (3) activation of hydrolytic enzymes, and (4) generation of ROS and RNS.

There are at least three mechanisms by which sustained elevations in intracellular Ca^{2+} unfavorably influence the cellular energy balance. First, high cytoplasmic Ca^{2+} levels cause increased mitochondrial Ca^{2+} uptake by the Ca^{2+} "uniporter," which, like ATP synthase, utilizes the inside negative mitochondrial membrane potential ($\Delta\Psi$m) as the driving force. Consequently, mitochondrial Ca^{2+} uptake dissipates $\Delta\Psi$m and inhibits the synthesis of ATP. Moreover, agents that oxidize mitochondrial NADH activate a transporter that extrudes Ca^{2+} from the matrix space (Richter and Kass, 1991). The ensuing continuous Ca^{2+} uptake and export ("Ca^{2+} cycling") by the mitochondria further compromise oxidative phosphorylation. Second, Ca^{2+} may also impair ATP synthesis by causing oxidative injury to the inner membrane by mechanisms described later. Third, a sustained rise in cytoplasmic Ca^{2+} not only impairs ATP synthesis but also increases ATP consumption by the Ca^{2+}-ATPases working to eliminate the excess Ca^{2+}.

A second mechanism by which an uncontrolled rise in cytoplasmic Ca^{2+} causes cell injury is microfilamental dissociation (Nicotera et al., 1992; Leist and Nicotera, 1997). The cellwide network of actin filaments maintains cellular morphology by attachment of the filaments to actin-binding proteins in the plasma membrane. An increase of cytoplasmic Ca^{2+} causes dissociation of actin filaments from α-actinin and fodrin, proteins that promote anchoring of the filament to the plasma membrane. This represents a mechanism leading to plasma membrane blebbing, a condition that predisposes the membrane to rupture.

Table 3-6
Agents Impairing Mitochondrial ATP Synthesis*

A. Inhibitors of hydrogen delivery to the electron transport chain acting on/as
1. Glycolysis (critical in neurons): hypoglycemia; iodoacetate and NO^+ at GAPDH
2. Gluconeogenesis (critical in renal tubular cells): coenzyme A depletors (see below)
3. Fatty acid oxidation (critical in cardiac muscle): hypoglycin, 4-pentenoic acid
4. Pyruvate dehydrogenase: arsenite, DCVC, *p*-benzoquinone
5. Citrate cycle
   (a) Aconitase: fluoroacetate, $ONOO^-$
   (b) Isocitrate dehydrogenase: DCVC
   (c) Succinate dehydrogenase: malonate, DCVC, PCBD-cys, 2-bromohydroquinone, 3-nitropropionic acid, *cis*-crotonalide fungicides
6. Depletors of TPP (inhibit TPP-dependent PDH and α-KGDH): ethanol
7. Depletors of coenzyme A: 4-(dimethylamino)phenol, *p*-benzoquinone
8. Depletors of NADH
   (a) See group A.V.1. in Table 3-7
   (b) Activators of poly(ADP-ribose) polymerase: agents causing DNA damage (e.g., MNNG, hydrogen peroxide, $ONOO^-$)

B. Inhibitors of electron transport acting on/as
1. Inhibitors of electron transport complexes
   (a) NADH–coenzyme Q reductase (complex I): rotenone, amytal, MPP^+, paraquat
   (b) Cycotochrome Q–cytochrome c reductase (complex III): antimycin-A, myxothiazole
   (c) Cytochrome oxidase (complex IV): cyanide, hydrogen sulfide, azide, formate, •NO, phosphine (PH_3)
   (d) Multisite inhibitors: dinitroaniline and diphenylether herbicides, $ONOO^-$
2. Electron acceptors: CCl_4, doxorubicin, menadione, MPP^+

C. Inhibitors of oxygen delivery to the electron transport chain
1. Chemicals causing respiratory paralysis: CNS depressants, convulsants
2. Chemicals causing ischemia: ergot alkaloids, cocaine
3. Chemicals inhibiting oxygenation of Hb: carbon monoxide, methemoglobin-forming chemicals

D. Inhibitors of ADP phosphorylation acting on/as
1. ATP synthase: oligomycin, cyhexatin, DDT, chlordecone
2. Adenine nucleotide translocator: atractyloside, DDT, free fatty acids, lysophospholipids
3. Phosphate transporter: *N*-ethylmaleimide, mersalyl, *p*-benzoquinone
4. Chemicals dissipating the mitochondrial membrane potential (uncouplers)
   (a) Cationophores: pentachlorophenol, dinitrophenol-, benzonitrile-, thiadiazole herbicides, salicylate, cationic amphiphilic drugs (amiodarone, perhexiline), valinomycin, gramicidin, calcimycin (A23187)
   (b) Chemicals permeabilizing the mitochondrial inner membrane: PCBD-cys, chlordecone

E. Chemicals causing mitochondrial DNA damage and impaired transcription of key mitochondrial proteins:
1. Antiviral drugs: zidovudine, zalcitabine, didanosine, fialuridine
2. Ethanol (when chronically consumed)

*The ultimate sites of action of these agents are indicated in Fig. 3-13. DCVC = dichlorovinyl-cysteine; GAPDH = glyceraldehyde 3-phosphate dehydrogenase; α-KGDH = α-ketoglutarate dehydrogenase; MNNG = *N*-methyl-*N*′-nitro-*N*-nitrosoguanidine; MPP^+ = 1-methyl-4-phenylpyridinium; PCBD-cys = pentachlorobutadienyl-cysteine; PDH = pyruvate dehydrogenase; TPP = thyamine pyrophosphate.

A third event whereby high Ca^{2+} levels are deleterious to cells is activation of hydrolytic enzymes that degrade proteins, phospholipids, and nucleic acids (Nicotera et al., 1992; Leist and Nicotera, 1997). Many integral membrane proteins are targets for Ca^{2+}-activated neutral proteases, or calpains (Saido et al., 1994). Calpain-mediated hydrolysis of actin-binding proteins also may cause membrane blebbing. Indiscriminate activation of phospholipases by Ca^{2+} causes membrane breakdown directly and by the generation of detergents. Activation of a Ca^{2+}-Mg^{2+}-dependent endocuclease causes fragmentation of chromatin. Elevated levels of Ca^{2+} can lock topoisomerase II in a form that cleaves but does not religate DNA. In summary, intracellular hypercalcemia activates several process that interfere with the ability of cells to maintain their structural and functional integrity. The relative importance of these processes in vivo requires further definition.

Overproduction of ROS and RNS There are a number of xenobiotics that can directly generate ROS and RNS, such as the redox cyclers (Fig. 3-3) and the transition metals (Fig. 3-4). In ad-

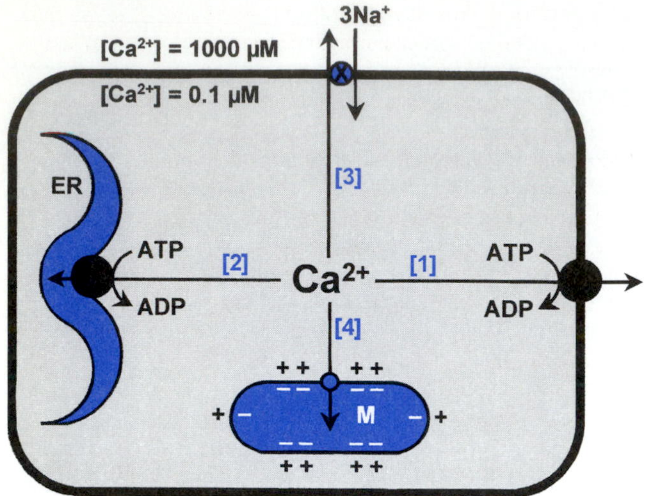

Figure 3-14. Four mechanisms for the elimination of Ca^{2+} from the cytoplasm: Ca^{2+}-ATPase-mediated pumping into (1) the extracellular space as well as (2) the endoplasmic reticulum (ER) and ion-gradient–driven transport into (3) the extracellular space (by the Ca^{2+}/Na^{+} exchanger) as well as (4) the mitochondria (M; by the Ca^{2+} uniporter).

Some chemicals that inhibit these mechanisms are listed in Table 3-7, group B.

dition, overproduction of ROS and RNS can be secondary to the intracellular hypercalcemia, as Ca^{2+} activates enzymes that generate ROS and/or RNS in the following ways:

1. Activation of the dehydrogenases in the citric acid cycle by Ca^{2+} accelerates the hydrogen output from the citrate cycle and, in turn, the flux of electrons along the electron transport chain (see Fig. 3-13). This, together with the suppressed ATP synthase activity (owing to the Ca^{2+}-induced uncoupling), increases the formation of $O_2^{\bar{\bullet}}$ by the mitochondrial electron transport chain.
2. Ca^{2+}-activated proteases proteolytically convert xanthine dehydrogenase into xanthine oxidase, whose byproducts are $O_2^{\bar{\bullet}}$ and HOOH.
3. Neurons and endothelial cells constitutively express NOS that is activated by Ca^{2+}. Given the extremely high reactivity of $^{\bullet}NO$ with $O_2^{\bar{\bullet}}$, co-production of these radicals will inevitably lead to formation of $ONOO^-$, a highly reactive oxidant (Murphy, 1999) (Fig. 3-4). Moreover, $ONOO^-$ can increase its own formation by incapacitating the highly sensitive Mn-SOD, which would eliminate $O_2^{\bar{\bullet}}$, a precursor of $ONOO^-$.

Interplay between the Primary Metabolic Disorders Spells Cellular Disaster The primary derailments in cellular biochemistry discussed above do not remain isolated but interact and amplify each other in a number of ways (Fig. 3-15):

Table 3-7
Agents Causing Sustained Elevation of Cytosolic Ca^{2+}

A. Chemicals inducing Ca^{2+} influx into the cytoplasm
- I. Via ligand-gated channels in neurons:
  1. Glutamate receptor agonists (“excitotoxins”): glutamate, kainate, domoate
  2. “Capsaicin receptor” agonists: capsaicin, resiniferatoxin
- II. Via voltage-gated channels: maitotoxin (?), $HO^{\bullet}$
- III. Via “newly formed pores”: maitotoxin, amphotericin B, chlordecone, methylmercury, alkyltins
- IV. Across disrupted cell membrane:
  1. Detergents: exogenous detergents, lysophospholipids, free fatty acids
  2. Hydrolytic enzymes: phospholipases in snake venoms, endogenous phospholipase A_2
  3. Lipid peroxidants: carbon tetrachloride
  4. Cytoskeletal toxins (by inducing membrane blebbing): cytochalasins, phalloidin
- V. From mitochondria:
  1. Oxidants of intramitochondrial NADH: alloxan, *t*-BHP, NAPBQI, divicine, fatty acid hydroperoxides, menadione, MPP^+
  2. Others: phenylarsine oxide, gliotoxin, $^{\bullet}NO$, $ONOO^-$
- VI. From the endoplasmic reticulum:
  1. IP_3 receptor activators: γ-HCH (lindan), IP_3 formed during “excitotoxicity”
  2. Ryanodine receptor activators: δ-HCH

B. Chemicals inhibiting Ca^{2+} export from the cytoplasm (inhibitors of Ca^{2+}-ATPase in cell membrane and/or endoplasmic reticulum)
- I. Covalent binders: acetaminophen, bromobenzene, CCl_4, chloroform, DCE
- II. Thiol oxidants: cystamine (mixed disulfide formation), diamide, *t*-BHP, menadione, diquat
- III. Others: vanadate, Cd^{2+}
- IV. Chemicals impairing mitochondrial ATP synthesis (see Table 3-6)

KEY: DCE = 1,1-dichloroethylene; *t*-BHP = *t*-butyl hydroperoxide; HCH = hexachlorocyclohexane; MPP^+ = 1-methyl-4-phenylpyridinium; NAPBQI = *N*-acetyl-*p*-benzoquinoneimine.

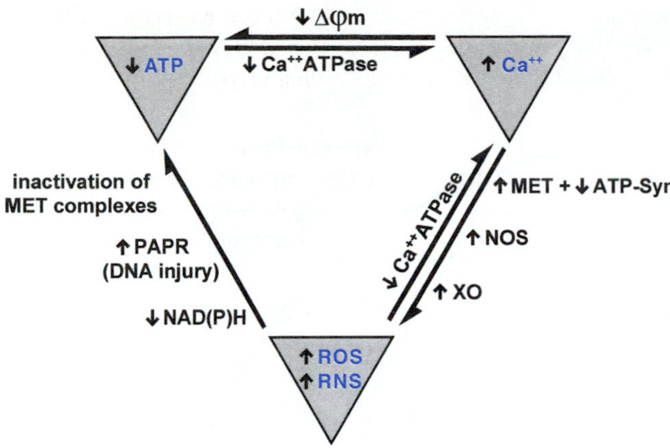

Figure 3-15. Interrelationship between the primary metabolic disorders (ATP depletion, intracellular hypercalcemia, and overproduction of ROS/RNS) that ultimately cause necrosis or apoptosis.

See text for details. ATP-SYN = ATP synthase, MET = mitochondrial electron transport; NOS = nitric oxide synthase; PARP = poly(ADP-ribose) polymerase; ROS = reactive oxygen species; RNS = reactive nitrogen species; XO = xanthine oxidase; $\Delta\Psi m$ = mitochondrial membrane potential.

1. Depletion of cellular ATP reserves deprives the endoplasmic and plasma membrane Ca^{2+} pumps of fuel, causing elevation of Ca^{2+} in the cytoplasm. With the influx of Ca^{2+} into the mitochondria, $\Delta\Psi m$ declines, hindering ATP synthase.
2. As stated above, intracellular hypercalcemia facilitates formation of ROS and RNS, which oxidatively inactivate the thiol-dependent Ca^{2+} pump, which, in turn, aggravates the hypercalcemia.
3. The ROS and RNS can also drain the ATP reserves. •NO is a reversible inhibitor of cytochrome oxidase, NO^+ (nitrosonium cation, a product of •NO) *S*-nitrosylates and thus inactivates glyceraldehyde 3-phosphate dehydrogenase, impairing glycolysis, whereas $ONOO^-$ irreversibly inactivates respiratory chain complexes I, II, III, and aconitase (by reacting with their Fe-S center) (Murphy, 1999). Therefore, •NO and $ONOO^-$ inhibit cellular ATP synthesis.
4. Furthermore, $ONOO^-$ can induce DNA single-strand breaks, which activate poly(ADP-ribose) polymerase (PARP) (Szabó, 1996). As part of the repair strategy, activated PARP transfers multiple ADP-ribose moieties from NAD^+ to nuclear proteins and PARP itself (D'Amours et al., 1999). Consumption of NAD^+ severely compromises ATP synthesis (see Fig. 3-13), whereas resynthesis of NAD^+ consumes ATP. Hence a major consequence of DNA damage by $ONOO^-$ is a cellular energy deficit (Murphy, 1999).

The chain of events and their contribution to the worsening metabolic conditions are somewhat cell-specific. For example, cyanide toxicity in neurons is associated with depolarization and glutamate release (Patel et al., 1993), followed by Ca^{2+} influx through voltage-gated as well as glutamate-gated channels (see items 8 and 12, respectively, in Fig. 3-12). As they express Ca^{2+}-activated NOS, neurons are also prone to generate "nitrosative stress," which affects not only themselves but perhaps more significantly the neighboring astrocytes (Szabó, 1996). In contrast, in cyanide- and iodoacetate-poisoned liver cells, the increase in cytoplasmic Ca^{2+} is not an early event (Herman et al., 1990) and •NO formation is less likely involved. Nevertheless, the interplay of ATP depletion, intracellular hypercalcemia, and overproduction of ROS and RNS, involving multiple vicious cycles (Fig. 3-15), can progressively aggravate the biochemical disorder until it becomes a disaster.

Mitochondrial Permeability Transition (MPT) and the Worst Outcome: Necrosis Mitochrondrial Ca^{2+} uptake, decreased $\Delta\Psi m$, generation of ROS and RNS, depletion of ATP, and consequences of the primary metabolic disorders (e.g., accumulation of inorganic phosphate, free fatty acids, and lysophosphatides) are all considered as causative factors of an abrupt increase in the mitochondrial inner-membrane permeability, termed MPT, believed to be caused by opening of a proteinaceous pore ("megachannel") that spans both mitochondrial membranes (Lemasters et al., 1998; Kroemer et al., 1998). As this pore is permeable to solutes of size $<$1500 Da, its opening permits free influx into the matrix space of protons, causing rapid and complete dissipation of $\Delta\Psi m$ and cessation of ATP synthesis as well as osmotic influx of water, resulting in mitochondrial swelling. Ca^{2+} that had accumulated in the matrix space effluxes through the pore, flooding the cytoplasm. Such mitochondria are not only incapable of synthesizing ATP but even waste the remaining sources because depolarization of the inner membrane forces the ATP synthase to operate in the reverse mode, as an ATPase, hydrolyzing ATP. Then even glycolysis may become compromised by the insufficient ATP supply to the ATP-requiring glycolytic enzymes (hexokinase, phosphofructokinase). A complete bioenergetic catastrophe ensues in the cell if the metabolic disorders evoked by the toxic agent (such as one listed in Tables 3-6 and 3-7) is so extensive that most or all mitochondria in the cell undergo MPT, causing depletion of cellular ATP (see Fig. 3-17). Degradative processes already outlined (e.g., oxidative and hydrolytic degradation of macromolecules and membranes as well as disintegration of intracellular solute and volume homeostasis) will go to completion, causing a complete failure in maintenance of cellular structure and functions and culminating in cell lysis or necrosis.

An Alternative Outcome of MPT: Apoptosis The chemicals that adversely affect the cellular energy metabolism, Ca^{2+} homeostasis and redox state and ultimately cause necrosis, may also induce apoptosis, another form of demise. While the necrotic cell swells and lyses, the apoptotic cell shrinks; its nuclear and cytoplasmic materials condense, and then it breaks into membrane-bound fragments (apoptotic bodies) that are phagocytosed (Wyllie, 1997).

As discussed above, the multiple metabolic defects that a cell suffers in its way to necrosis are causal yet rather random in sequence. In contrast, the routes to apoptosis are ordered, involving cascade-like activation of catabolic processes that finally disassemble the cell. Many details of the apoptotic pathways have been uncovered in recent years, some of which are presented schematically in Fig. 3-16.

It appears that most if not all chemical-induced cell death will involve the mitochondria, and the resulting mitochondrial dysfunction (such as Ca^{2+} accumulation, dissipation of $\Delta\Psi m$, overproduction of ROS/RNS) may ultimately trigger either necrosis or apoptosis, and that MPT is a crucial event in both. Another related event is release into the cytoplasm of cytochrome *c* (cyt *c*), a small hemeprotein that normally resides in the mitochondrial intermembrane space attached to the surface of inner membrane.

The significance of cyt *c* release is twofold (Cai et al., 1998): (1) As cyt *c* is the penultimate link in the mitochondrial electron transport chain, its loss will block ATP synthesis, increase forma-

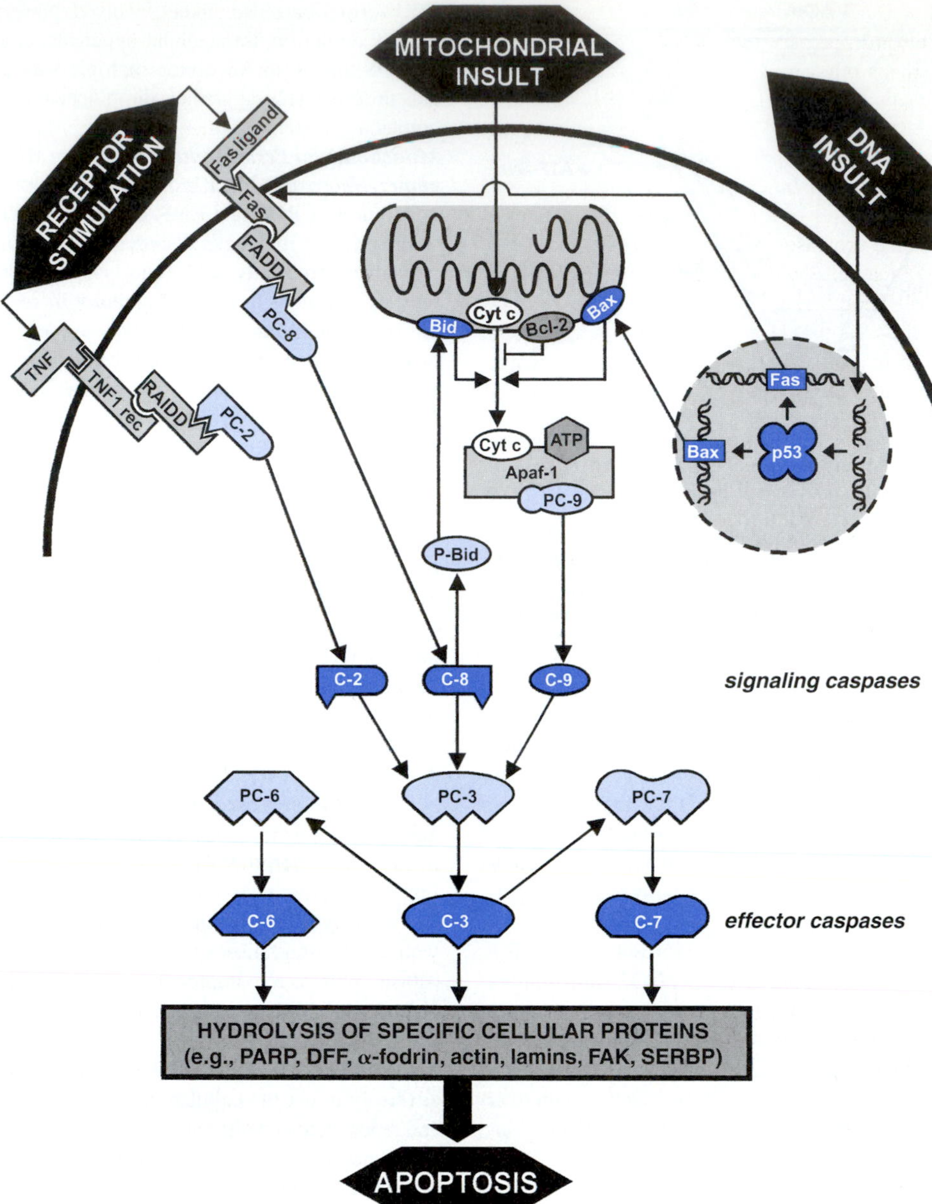

Figure 3-16. Apoptotic pathways initiated by mitochondrial insult, nuclear DNA insult and Fas or TNF receptor-1 stimulation.

The figure is a simplified scheme of three pathways to apoptosis. (1) Mitochondrial insult (see text) ultimately opens the permeability transition pore spanning both mitochondrial membranes and/or causes release of cytochrome c (Cyt c) from the mitochondria. Cyt c release is facilitated by Bax or Bid proteins and opposed by Bcl-2 protein. (2) DNA insult, especially double-strand breaks, activates p53 protein which increases the expression of Bax (that mediates Cyt c release) and the membrane receptor protein Fas. (3) Fas ligand or tumor necrosis factor binds to and activates their respective receptor, Fas and TNF1 receptor. These ligand-bound receptors and the released Cyt c interact with specific adapter proteins (i.e., FADD, RAIDD and Apaf-1) through which they proteolytically activate procaspases (PC) to active caspases (C). The latter in turn cleave and activate other proteins (e.g., the precursor of Bid, P-Bid) and PC-3, a main effector procaspase. The active effector caspase-3 activates other effector procaspases (PC-6, PC-7). Finally, C-3, C-6, and C-7 clip specific cellular proteins, whereby apoptosis occurs. These pathways are not equally relevant in all types of cells and other pathways, such as those employing TGF-β as an extracellular signaling molecule, and ceramide as an intracellular signaling molecule, also exist. DFF = DNA fragmentation factor; FAK = focal adhesion kinase; PARP = poly(ADP-ribose) polymerase; SREBP = sterol regulatory element binding protein.

tion of $O_2^{\bar{\bullet}}$ (instead of O_2^{4-} as shown in Fig. 3-13), and potentially thrust the cell toward necrosis. (2) Simultaneously, the unleashed cyt *c* (and perhaps other proteins set free from the mitochondria) represents a signal or an initial link in the chain of events directing the cell to the apoptotic path (Fig. 3-16). Upon binding, together with ATP, to an adapter protein (Apaf-1), cyt *c* can induce proteolytic cleavage of the Apaf-1-bound latent procaspase-9 to active caspase-9.

Caspases are cysteine proteases (that is, they possess catalytically active cysteine) that clip proteins at specific asparagine residues (Nicholson and Thornberry, 1997). They reside in the cytoplasm in inactive forms, as procaspases, which are proteolytically converted to the active proteases. Some caspases (e.g., 2, 8, and 9) cleave and activate procaspases. Thereby these signaling caspases carry the activation wave to the so-called effector caspases (e.g., 3, 6, and 7), which clip specific cellular proteins, activating or inactivating them. It is the caspase-catalyzed hydrolysis of these specific proteins that accounts directly or indirectly for the morphologic and biochemical alterations in apoptotic cells. For example, proteolytic inactivation of PARP prevents futile DNA repair and wasting of ATP; hydrolytic activation of DNA fragmentation factor induces fragmentation of nuclear DNA; clipping of structural proteins (α-fodrin, actin, lamins) aids in disassembly of the cell; incapacitation of focal adhesion kinase (see Fig. 3-11) permits detachment of the cell from the extracellular matrix; and hydrolytic activation of sterol regulatory element–binding proteins may contribute to accumulation of sterols and externalization of phosphatidylserine in the plasma membrane that identify the apoptotic cell to phagocytes.

The decisive mitochondrial events of cell death, i.e., MPT and release of cyt *c*, are controlled by the Bcl-2 family of proteins, which includes members that facilitate (e.g., Bax, Bad, Bid) and those that inhibit (e.g., Bcl-2, Bcl-XL) these processes. While the death-promoting members probably act directly in the mitochondrial membranes, their death-suppressor counterparts are thought to act predominantly by dimerizing with the death agonists and therefore neutralizing them. Thus, the relative amount of these antagonistic proteins functions as a regulatory switch between cell survival and death (Reed et al., 1998).

The proapoptotic Bax and Bid proteins also represent links whereby death programs initiated extramitochondrically, e.g., by DNA damage in the nucleus or by stimulation of Fas receptors at the cell surface, can engage the mitochondria into the apoptotic process (Green, 1998) (Fig. 3-16). DNA damage (evoked by ionizing and UV radiations, alkylating chemicals, doxorubicin (Adriamycin), and topoisomerase II inhibitors) induces stabilization and activation of p53 protein, a transcription factor, which increases expression of Bax protein (Bates and Vousden, 1998) (see also Fig. 3-25). As discussed further on, DNA damage is potentially mutagenic and carcinogenic, therefore apoptosis of cells with damaged DNA is an important self-defense of the body against oncogenesis. Furthermore, the antitumor drugs targeting the nuclear DNA exert their desirable toxic effects against tumor cells (and also their undesirable cytotoxic effects against rapidly dividing normal cells such as hematopoietic cells and small intestinal mucosal cells) by inducing apoptosis primarily via a p53-dependent mechanism. Stimulation of TNF receptor-1 or Fas can directly activate caspases, nevertheless Fas activation can also engage the mitochondria into the death program via caspase-mediated activation of Bid (Fig. 3-16). The Fas system is involved in cell-mediated cytotoxicity, as cytotoxic T lymphocytes express the Fas ligand that activates Fas in the membrane of potential target cells, such as those of the liver, heart, and the lung. The Fas system also mediates germ cell apoptosis in the testes of rodents exposed to mono-(2-ethylhexyl)phthalate or 2,5-hexanedione, the ultimate toxicant formed from hexane. These chemicals damage the microtubules in the Sertoli cells that normally nurse the germ cells. Unable to support the germ cells, Sertoli cells overexpress the Fas ligand to limit the number of germ cells (which upregulate their Fas receptor) by deleting them via apoptosis (Cohen et al., 1997; Lee et al., 1997).

Thus, apoptosis can be executed via multiple pathways, all involving caspase activation. The route preferred will depend among others on the initial insult (Fig. 3-16) as well as on the type and state of the cell. For example, T lymphocytes lacking the *Bax* gene can still undergo p53-dependent death in response to ionizing radiation, probably by increasing Fas expression (Fig. 3-16), whereas *Bax*-null fibroblasts cannot.

ATP Availability Determines the Form of Cell Death There are several common features in the process of apoptosis and necrosis. First of all, many xenobiotics—such as the hepatotoxin acetaminophen, 1,1-dichloroethylene, thioacetamide, and cadmium as well as the nephrotoxin ochratoxin—can cause both apoptosis and necrosis (Corcoran et al., 1994). Toxicants tend to induce apoptosis at low exposure levels or early after exposure at high levels, whereas they cause necrosis later at high exposure levels. In addition, induction of both forms of cell death by cytotoxic agents may involve similar metabolic disturbances and most importantly MPT (Lemasters et al., 1998; Kroemer et al., 1998; Quian et al., 1999), and blockers of the latter (e.g., cyclosporin A, Bcl-2 overexpression) prevent both apoptosis and necrosis. What determines, then, whether the injured cell undergoes apoptosis or necrosis—which, as emphasized further on, may have a significant impact on the surrounding tissue?

Recent findings suggest that the availability of ATP is critical in determining the form of cell death. In experimental models so different as Ca^{2+}-exposed hepatocytes, Fas-stimulated T lymphocytes, and HOOH-exposed endothelial cells, necrosis occurred instead of apoptosis when cells were depleted of ATP, but apoptosis took place rather than necrosis when ATP depletion was alleviated by providing substrates for ATP generation (Leist et al., 1997; Lemasters et al., 1998; Lelli et al., 1998).

Lemasters et al. (1998) used confocal microscopy to visualize mitochondria in cells exposed to an apoptogenic stimulus and found that MPT does not occur uniformly in all mitochondria. They proposed a model in which the number of mitochondria undergoing MPT (which probably depends on the degree of chemical exposure) determines the severity of cellular ATP depletion and, in turn, the fate of the cell. According to this model (Fig. 3-17), when only a few mitochondria develop MPT, they, and with them the proapoptotic signals (e.g., externalized cyt *c*), are removed by lysosomal autophagy. When MPT involves more mitochondria, the autophagic mechanism becomes overwhelmed and the released cyt *c* initiates caspase activation and apoptosis (Fig. 3-16). When MPT involves virtually all mitochondria, ATP becomes severely depleted for reasons discussed above. Lack of ATP prevents execution of the apoptotic program, which involves ATP-requiring steps, one of which is formation of the complex between Apaf-1, cyt *c*, and pocaspase-9 (Fig. 3-16). Then cytolysis occurs before the caspases come into action.

Induction of Cell Death by Unknown Mechanisms In addition to chemicals that ultimately injure mitochondria by disrupting oxidative phosphorylation and/or control of intracellular Ca^{2+}, there are toxicants that cause cell death by affecting other functions or structures primarily. Included here are (1) chemicals that

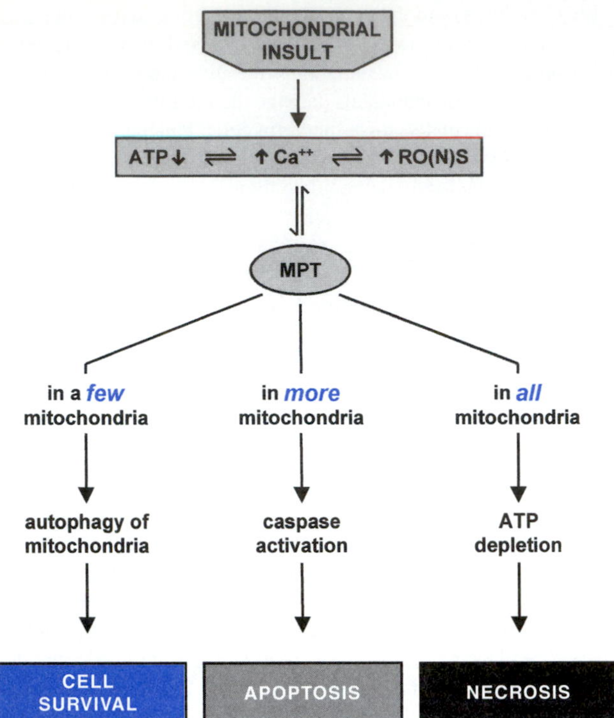

Figure 3-17. "Decision plan" on the fate of injured cell.

See the text for details. MPT = mitochondrial permeability transition; RO(N)S = reactive oxygen or nitrogen species.

directly damage the plasma membrane, such as lipid solvents, detergents, and venom-derived hydrolytic enzymes; (2) xenobiotics that damage the lysosomal membrane, such as aminoglycoside antibiotics and hydrocarbons binding to a_{2u}-globulin; (3) toxins that destroy the cytoskeleton, such as the microfilamental toxins phalloidin and cytochalasins and the microtubular toxins colchicine and 2,5-hexanedione; (4) the protein phosphatase inhibitor hepatotoxin microcystin, which causes hyperphosphorylation of microfilaments and other cellular proteins (Toivola and Eriksson, 1999); and (5) toxins that disrupt protein synthesis, such as α-amanitin and ricin.

The events leading to cell death after exposure to these chemicals are generally unknown. It is likely that cell death caused by these chemicals is ultimately mediated by impairment of oxidative phosphorylation, sustained elevation of intracellular Ca^{2+}, and/or overproduction of ROS/RNS and that it takes the form of necrosis if these processes are abrupt but apoptosis if they are protracted. For example, direct injury of the plasma membrane would lead rapidly to increased intracellular Ca^{2+} levels. Neurofilamental toxins that block axonal transport cause energy depletion in the distal axonal segment. More subtle changes may also underlie the cell death. For example, paclitaxel, an antimicrotubule agent, purportedly causes hyperphosphorylation and inactivation of Bcl-2, which favors opening the MPT pore (Fan, 1999).

Impairment of External Cellular Maintenance Toxicants also may interfere with cells that are specialized to provide support to other cells, tissues, or the whole organism. Chemicals acting on the liver illustrate this type of toxicity. Hepatocytes produce and release into the circulation a number of proteins and nutrients. They remove cholesterol and bilirubin from the circulation, converting them into bile acids and bilirubin glucuronides, respectively, for subsequent excretion into bile. Interruption of these processes may be harmful to the organism, the liver, or both. For example, inhibition of the hepatic synthesis of coagulation factors by coumarins does not harm the liver but may cause death by hemorrhage (Hardman et al., 1995). This is the mechanism of the rodenticidal action of warfarin. In the fasting state, inhibitors of hepatic gluconeogenesis such as hypoglycin may be lethal by limiting the supply of glucose to the brain. Similarly, Reye's syndrome, which is viewed as a hepatic mitochondrial injury caused by a combination of a viral disease (which may induce hepatic NOS) and intake of salicylate (which provokes MPT) (Fromenty and Pessayre, 1997; Lemasters et al., 1998), causes not only hepatocellular injury but also severe metabolic disturbances (hypoglycemia, hyperammonemia) that affect other organs as well. Chemical interference with the β-oxidation of fatty acids or the synthesis, assembly, and secretion of lipoproteins overloads the hepatocytes with lipids, causing hepatic dysfunction (Fromenty and Pessayre, 1997). α-Naphthylisothiocyanate causes separation of the intercellular tight junctions that seal bile canaliculi (Knell et al., 1987), impairing biliary secretion and leading to the retention of bile acids and bilirubin; this adversely affects the liver as well as the entire organism.

STEP 4—REPAIR OR DYSREPAIR

The fourth step in the development of toxicity is inappropriate repair (Fig. 3-1). As noted previously, many toxicants alter macromolecules, which, if not repaired, cause damage at higher levels of the biological hierarchy in the organism. Because repair influences the progression of toxic lesions, mechanisms of repair are categorized in Fig. 3-18 and discussed below in detail.

Molecular Repair

Damaged molecules may be repaired in different ways. Some chemical alterations, such as oxidation of protein thiols and methylation of DNA, are simply reversed. Hydrolytic removal of the molecule's damaged unit or units and insertion of a newly synthesized unit or units often occur with chemically altered DNA and peroxidized lipids. In some instances, the damaged molecule is totally degraded and resynthesized. This process is time-consuming but

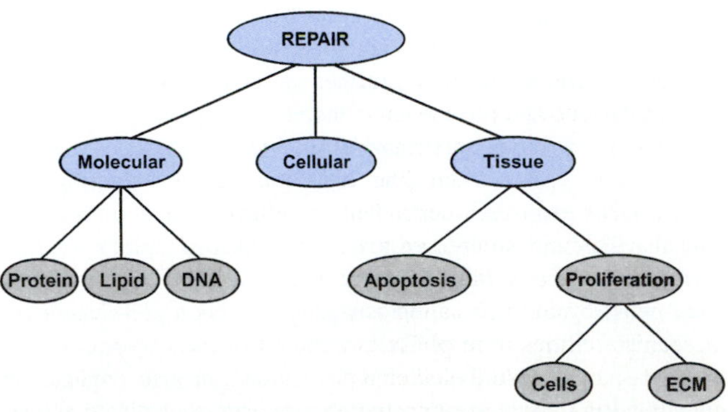

Figure 3-18. Repair mechanisms.

Dysfunction of these mechanisms results in dysrepair, the fourth step in the development of numerous toxic injuries. ECM = extracellular matrix.

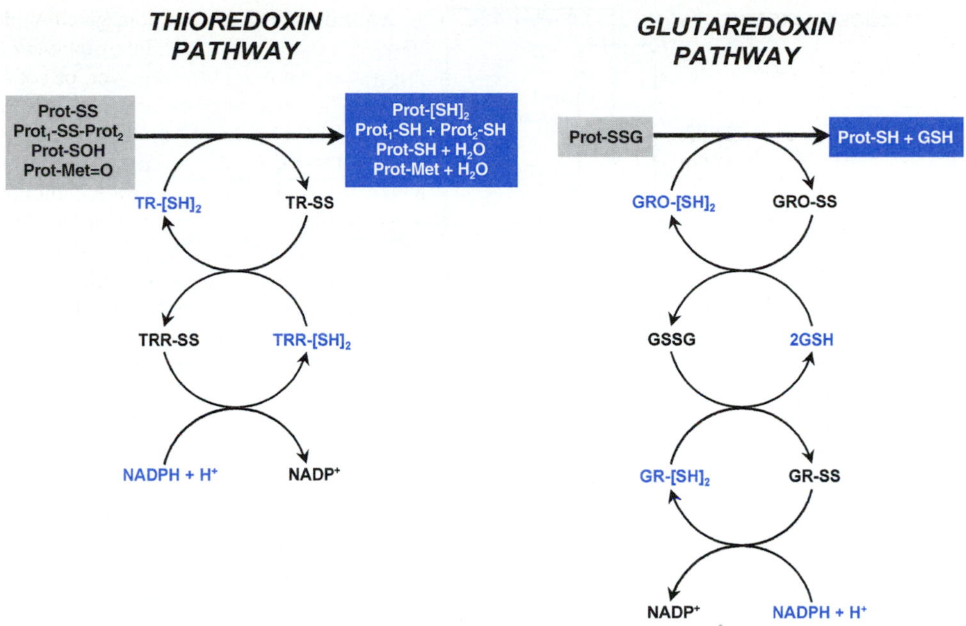

Figure 3-19. Repair of proteins oxidized at their thiol groups.

Protein disulfides (Prot-SS, $Prot_1$-SS-$Prot_2$), protein sulfenic acids (Prot-SOH) and protein methionine sulfoxides (Prot-Met=O) are reduced by thioredoxin (TR-$[SH]_2$) with methionine sulfoxide reductase catalyzing the latter process. Protein-glutathione mixed disulfides (Prot-SSG) are reduced by glutaredoxin (GRO-$[SH]_2$), which is also called thioltransferase. The figure also indicates how TR-$[SH]_2$ and GRO-$[SH]_2$ are regenerated from their disulfides (TR-SS and GRO-SS, respectively). In the mitochondria, TR-SS also can be regenerated by the dithiol dihydrolipoic acid, a component of the pyruvate- and α-ketoglutarate dehydrogenase complexes. GSH = glutathione; GSSG = glutathione disulfide; GR-$[SH]_2$ and GR-SS = glutathione reductase (dithiol and disulfide forms, respectively); TRR-$[SH]_2$ and TRR-SS = thioredoxin reductase (dithiol and disulfide forms, respectively).

unavoidable in cases such as the regeneration of cholinesterases after organophosphate intoxication.

Repair of Proteins Thiol groups are essential for the function of numerous proteins, such as receptors, enzymes, cytoskeletal proteins, and TFs. Oxidation of protein thiols (Prot-SHs) to protein disulfides (Prot-SS, $Prot_1$-SS-$Prot_2$), protein-glutathione mixed disulfides, and protein sulfenic acids (Prot-SOH) as well as oxidation of methionine in proteins to methionine sulfoxide can be reversed by enzymatic reduction (Fernando et al., 1992; Gravina and Mieyal, 1993; Maskovitz et al., 1999) (Fig. 3-19). The endogenous reductants are thioredoxin and glutaredoxin, small, ubiquitous proteins with two redox-active cysteines in their active centers. Because the catalytic thiol groups in these proteins are oxidized, they are recycled by reduction with NADPH generated by glucose-6-phosphate dehydrogenase and 6-phosphogluconate dehydrogenase in the pentose phosphate pathway.

Repair of oxidized hemoglobin (methemoglobin) occurs by means of electron transfer from cytochrome b_5, which is then regenerated by a NADH-dependent cytochrome b_5 reductase (also called methemoglobin reductase). Soluble intracellular proteins are susceptible to denaturation by physical or chemical insults. Molecular chaperones such as the heat-shock proteins are synthesized in large quantities in response to protein denaturation and are important in the refolding of altered proteins (Morimoto, 1993). Damaged proteins can be eliminated also by proteolytic degradation. For example, the immunogenic trifluoroactylated proteins that are formed in the liver during halothane anesthesia are degraded by lysosomal proteases (Cohen et al., 1997). Although the ATP/ubiquitin–dependent proteolytic system is specialized in controlling the level of regulatory proteins (e.g., p53, IκB, cyclins), it can also eliminate damaged or mutated intracellular proteins (Hershko and Ciechanover, 1998). These proteins are first conjugated with ubiquitin, allowing their recognition by proteasomes—large protease complexes in the cytosol that proteolytically degrade them. Removal of damaged and aggregated proteins is especially critical in the eye lens for maintenance of its transparency. Erythrocytes have ATP-independent, nonlysosomal proteolytic enzymes that rapidly and selectively degrade proteins denatured by $HO^{\bullet}$ (Davies, 1987).

Repair of Lipids Peroxidized lipids are repaired by a complex process that operates in concert with a series of reductants as well as with glutathione peroxidase and reductase (Fig. 3-20). Phospholipids containing fatty acid hydroperoxides are preferentially hydrolyzed by phospholipase A2, with the peroxidized fatty acids replaced by normal fatty acids (van Kuijk et al., 1987). Again, NADPH is needed to "repair" the reductants that are oxidized in the process.

Repair of DNA Despite its high reactivity with electrophiles and free radicals, nuclear DNA is remarkably stable, in part because it is packaged in chromatin and because several repair mechanisms are available to correct alterations (Sancar and Sancar, 1988). The mitochondrial DNA, however, lacks histones and efficient repair mechanisms and therefore is more prone to damage.

Direct Repair Certain covalent DNA modifications are directly reversed by enzymes such as DNA photolyase, which cleaves ad-

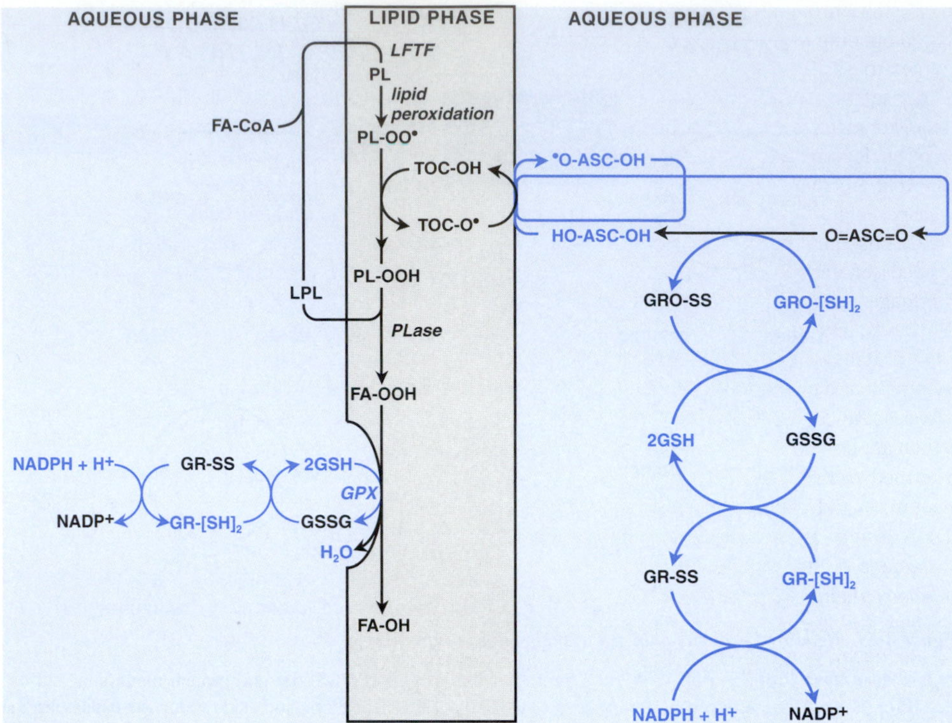

Figure 3-20. Repair of peroxidized lipids.

Phospholipid peroxyl radicals (PL-OO$^\bullet$) formed as a result of lipid peroxidation (Fig. 3-9) may abstract hydrogen from alpha-tocopherol (TOC-OH) and yield phospholipid hydroperoxide (PL-OOH). From the latter, the fatty acid carrying the hydroperoxide group is eliminated via hydrolysis catalyzed by phospholipase (PLase), yielding a fatty acid hydroperoxide (FA-OOH) and a lysophospholipid (LPL). The former is reduced to a hydroxy-fatty acid (FA-OH) by glutathione peroxidase (GPX), utilizing glutathione (GSH), whereas the latter is reacylated to phospholipid (PL) by lysophosphatide fatty acyl-coenzyme A transferase (LFTF), utilizing long-chain fatty acid-coenzyme A (FA-CoA). The figure also indicates regeneration of TOC-OH by ascorbic acid (HO-ASC-OH), regeneration of ascorbic acid from dehydroascorbic acid (O=ASC=O) by glutaredoxin (GRO-[SH]$_2$), and reduction of the oxidized glutaredoxin (GRO-SS) by GSH. Oxidized glutathione (GSSG) is reduced by glutathione reductase (GR-[SH]$_2$), which is regenerated from its oxidized form (GR-SS) by NADPH, the ultimate reductant. Most NADPH is produced during metabolism of glucose via the pentose phosphate shunt. TOC-O$^\bullet$ = tocopheroxyl radical; $^\bullet$O-ASC-OH = ascorbyl radical.

jacent pyrimidines dimerized by UV light. Inasmuch as this chromophore-equipped enzyme uses the energy of visible light to correct damage, its use is restricted to light-exposed cells. Minor adducts, such as methyl groups, attached to the O^6 position of guanine are removed by O^6-alkylguanine-DNA-alkyltransferase (Pegg and Byers, 1992). While repairing the DNA, this alkyltransferase destroys itself, transferring the adduct onto one of its cysteine residues. This results in its inactivation and eventual degradation. Thus, like glutathione, which is depleted during detoxication of electrophiles, O^6-alkylguanine-DNA-alkyltransferase is consumed during the repair of DNA.

Excision Repair Base excision and nucleotide excision are two mechanisms for removing damaged bases from DNA (Chaps. 8 and 9). Lesions that do not cause major distortion of the helix typically are removed by base excision, in which the altered base is recognized by a relatively substrate-specific DNA-glycosylase that hydrolyzes the *N*-glycosidic bond, releasing the modified base and creating an apurinic or apyrimidinic (AP) site in the DNA. For example, 8-hydroxyguanine (8-OH-Gua), a major mutagenic product of oxidative stress, is removed from the DNA by specific 8-OH-Gua DNA glycosylase. The AP site is recognized by the AP endonuclease, which hydrolyzes the phosphodiester bond adjacent to the abasic site. After its removal, the abasic sugar is replaced with the correct nucleotide by a DNA polymerase and is sealed in place by a DNA ligase.

Bulky lesions such as adducts produced by aflatoxins or aminofluorene derivatives and dimers caused by UV radiation are removed by nucleotide-excision repair. An ATP-dependent nuclease recognizes the distorted double helix and excises a number of intact nucleotides on both sides of the lesion together with the one containing the adduct. The excised section of the strand is restored by insertion of nucleotides into the gap by DNA polymerase and ligase, using the complementary strand as a template. This phenomenon, designated "unscheduled DNA synthesis," can be detected by the appearance of altered deoxynucleosides in urine. Excision repair has a remarkably low error rate of less than 1 mistake in 10^9 bases repaired.

Poly(ADP-ribose)polymerase (PARP) appears to be an important contributor in excision repair. Upon base damage or single-strand break, PARP binds to the injured DNA and becomes activated. The active PARP cleaves NAD^+ to use the ADP-ribose moiety of this cofactor for attaching long chains of polymeric ADP-ribose to nuclear proteins, such as histones. Because one ADP-ribose unit contains two negative charges, the poly(ADP-ribosyl)ated proteins accrue negativity and the resultant electrorepulsive force between the negatively charged proteins and DNA causes decondensation of the chromatin structure. It is hypothesized that PARP-mediated opening of the tightly packed chromatin allows the repair enzymes to access the broken DNA and fix it. Thereafter, poly(ADP-ribose) glycohydrolase gains access to the nucleus from its perinuclear localization and reverses the PARP-mediated modification of nuclear proteins (D'Amours et al., 1999). Other features of PARP that are relevant in toxicity—such as destruction of PARP by caspases during apoptosis as well as the significance of NAD^+ (and consequently ATP) wasting by PARP in necrosis—have been discussed earlier in this chapter.

Surveillance for damage by repair systems is not equally vigilant on the two DNA strands, and repair rates are not uniform for all genes (Scicchitano and Hanawalt, 1992). Actively transcribed genes are more rapidly repaired than are nontranscribed genes, and lesions in the transcribed strand that block RNA polymerase are more rapidly repaired than are lesions in the nontranscribed or coding strand. A protein termed *transcription-repair coupling factor* in *Escherichia coli* recognizes and displaces the RNA polymerase that has stalled at a DNA lesion, allowing access by the excision repair enzymes to the damage (Selby and Sancar, 1993).

Recombinational (or Postreplication) Repair Recombinational repair occurs when the excision of a bulky adduct or an intrastrand pyrimidine dimer fails to occur before DNA replication begins (Sancar and Sancar, 1988). At replication, such a lesion prevents DNA polymerase from polymerizing a daughter strand along a sizable stretch of the parent strand that carries the damage. The replication results in two homologous ("sister") yet dissimilar DNA duplexes: one that has a large postreplication gap in its daughter strand and an intact duplex synthesized at the opposite leg of the replication fork. This intact sister duplex is utilized to complete the postreplication gap in the damaged sister duplex. This is accomplished by recombination ("crossover") of the appropriate strands of the two homologous duplexes. After separation, the sister duplex that originally contained the gap carries in its daughter strand a section originating from the parent strand of the intact sister, which in turn carries in its parent strand a section originating from the daughter strand of the damaged sister. This strand recombination explains the phenomenon of "sister chromatid exchange," which is indicative of DNA damage corrected by recombinational repair. This process also repairs double breaks, which can also be repaired by the so-called DNA nonhomologous end-joining system that ligates DNA ends and employs several proteins including DNA-dependent protein kinase. A combination of excision and recombinational repairs occurs in restoration of DNA with interstrand cross-links. The process of recombinational repair at the molecular level has been partially characterized in *E. coli.* Much less is known about this process in eukaryotes.

Cellular Repair: A Strategy in Peripheral Neurons

Repair of damaged cells is not a widely applied strategy in overcoming cellular injuries. In most tissues, injured cells die, with the survivors dividing to replace the lost cells. A notable exception is nerve tissue, because mature neurons have lost their ability to multiply. In peripheral neurons with axonal damage, repair does occur and requires macrophages and Schwann cells. Macrophages remove debris by phagocytosis and produce cytokines and growth factors, which activate Schnwann cells to proliferate and transdifferentiate from myelinating operation mode into a growth-supporting mode. Schwann cells play an indispensable role in promoting axonal regeneration by increasing their synthesis of cell adhesion molecules (e.g., N-CAM), by elaborating extracellular matrix proteins for base membrane construction, and by producing an array of neurotrophic factors (e.g., nerve growth factor, glial–cell line–derived growth factor) and their receptors (Fu and Gordon, 1997). While comigrating with the regrowing axon, Schwann cells physically guide as well as chemically lure the axon to reinnervate the target cell.

In the mammalian central nervous system, axonal regrowth is prevented by growth inhibitory glycoproteins (e.g., NI 35, myelin-associated glycoprotein) and chondroitin sulfate proteoglycans produced by the oligodendrocytes and by the scar produced by astrocytes (Johnson, 1993). Thus, damage to central neurons is irreversible but is compensated for in part by the large number of reserve nerve cells that can take over the functions of lost neurons. For example, in Parkinson's disease, symptoms are not observed until there is at least an 80 percent loss of nigrostriatal neurons.

Tissue Repair

In tissues with cells capable of multiplying, damage is reversed by deletion of the injured cells and regeneration of the tissue by proliferation. The damaged cells are eliminated by apoptosis or necrosis.

Apoptosis: An Active Deletion of Damaged Cells Apoptosis initiated by cell injury can be regarded as tissue repair for two reasons, the first of which is that it may intercept the process leading to necrosis, as discussed earlier (see Fig. 3-17). Necrosis is a more harmful sequala than apoptosis for the tissue in which the injured cell resides. A cell destined for apoptosis shrinks; its nuclear and cytoplasmic materials condense, and then it breaks into membrane-bound fragments (apoptotic bodies) that are phagocytosed (Bursch et al., 1992). During necrosis, cells and intracellular organelles swell and disintegrate with membrane lysis. While apoptosis is orderly, necrosis is a disorderly process that ends with cell debris in the extracellular environment. The constituents of the necrotic cells attract aggressive inflammatory cells, and the ensuing inflammation amplifies cell injury (see further on). With apoptosis, dead cells are removed without inflammation. Second, apoptosis may intercept the process leading to neoplasia by eliminating the cells with potentially mutagenic DNA damage. This function of apoptosis is discussed in more detail in the final section of this chapter.

It must be emphasized, however, that apoptosis of damaged cells has a full value as a tissue repair process only for tissues that are made up of constantly renewing cells (e.g., the bone marrow, the respiratory and gastrointestinal epithelium, and the epidermis of the skin), or of conditionally dividing cells (e.g., hepatic and renal parenchymal cells), because in these tissues the apoptotic cells are readily replaced. The value of apoptosis as a tissue repair strategy is markedly lessened in organs containing nonreplicating and nonreplaceable cells, such as the neurons, cardiac muscle cells, and female germ cells, because deletion of such cells, if extensive, can cause a deficit in the organ's function.

Proliferation: Regeneration of Tissue Tissues are composed of various cells and the extracellular matrix. Tissue elements are anchored to each other by transmembrane proteins. Cadherins allow adjacent cells to adhere to one other, whereas connexins connect neighboring cells internally by association of these proteins into tubular structures (gap junctions). Integrins link cells to the extracellular matrix. Therefore, repair of injured tissues involves not only regeneration of lost cells and the extracellular matrix but also reintegration of the newly formed elements. In parenchymal organs such as liver, kidney, and lung, various types of cells are involved in the process of tissue restoration. Nonparenchymal cells of mesenchymal origin residing in the tissue, such as resident macrophages and endothelial cells, and those migrating to the site of injury, such as blood monocytes, produce factors that stimulate parenchymal cells to divide and stimulate some specialized cells (e.g., the stellate cells in the liver) to synthesize extracellular matrix molecules.

Replacement of Lost Cells by Mitosis Soon after injury, cells adjacent to the damaged area enter the cell division cycle (Fig. 3-21).

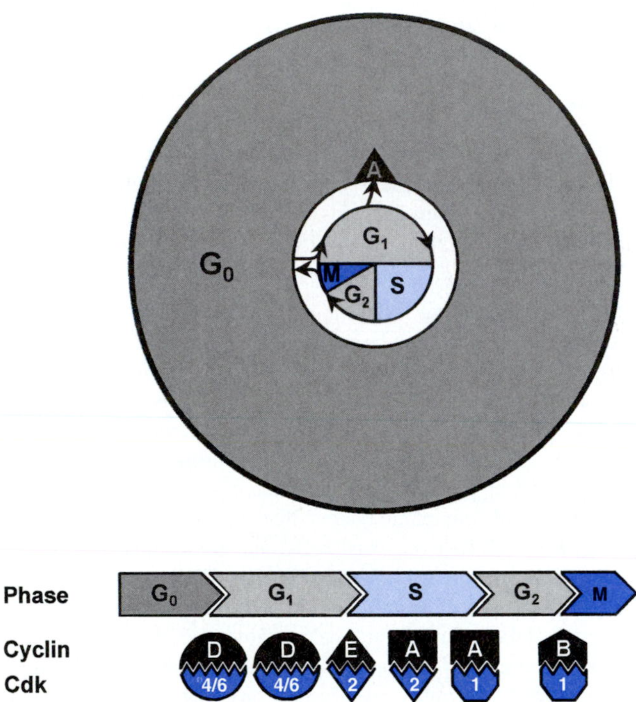

Figure 3-21. The cell division cycle and the participating cyclins and cyclin-dependent protein kinases.

Areas representing phases of the cycle are meant to be proportional to the number of cells in each phase. Normally, most cells are in G_0 phase, a differentiated and quiescent state. After receiving signals to divide, they progress into the G_1 phase of the cell division cycle. G_0/G_1 transition involves activation of immediate early genes so that cells acquire replicative competence. Now increasingly responsive to growth factors, these cells progress to the phase of DNA synthesis (S). If this progression is blocked (e.g., by the accumulated p53 protein), the cells may undergo apoptosis (A). After DNA replication, the cells prepare further for mitosis in the G_2 phase. Mitosis (M) is the shortest phase of the cell cycle (approximately 40 min out of the 40-h-long cycle of hepatocytes) and most likely requires the largest energy expenditure per unit of time. The daughter cells produced may differentiate and enter into the pool of quiescent cells (G_0), substituting for those which had been lost. During the cycle, the levels of various cyclins surge (see figure). These proteins bind to and activate specific cyclin-dependent protein kinases (Cdk, see figure), which, in turn, phosphorylate and thus activate enzymes and other proteins required for DNA replication and cell division (Johnson and Walker, 1999) (see Fig. 3-24). After tissue necrosis, the number of cells entering the cell division cycle markedly increases at areas adjacent to the injury. The proportion of cells that are in S phase in a given period is reflected by the labeling index, whereas the percentage of cells under going mitosis is the mitotic index (see text).

Enhanced DNA synthesis is detected experimentally as an increase in the labeling index, which is the proportion of cells that incorporate administered ^{3}H-thymidine or bromodeoxyuridine into their nuclear DNA during the S phase of the cycle. Also, mitotic cells can be observed microscopically. As early as 2 to 4 h after administration of a low dose of carbon tetrachloride to rats, the mitotic index in the liver increases dramatically, indicating that cells already in the G_2 phase progress rapidly to the M phase. The mitotic activity of the hepatocytes culminates at 36 to 48 h, after a full transit through the cycle, indicating that quiescent cells residing in G_0 enter and progress to mitosis (M). Peak mitosis of nonparenchymal cells occurs later, after activation and replication of parenchymal cells (Burt, 1993). In some tissues, such as intestinal mucosa and bone marrow, stem cells first divide to provide self-renewal and then differentiate to replace more mature cells lost through injury. Stem cells are also located in the liver, in the bile ductules. In toxic liver injury, when hepatocyte replication is impaired, the stem cells proliferate to form the so-called oval cells, which can differentiate into both hepatocytes and biliary epithelial cells (Fausto, 2000). In an ozone-exposed lung, the nonciliated Clara cells and type II pneumocytes undergo mitosis and terminal differentiation to replace, respectively, the damaged ciliated bronchial epithelial cells and type I pneumocytes (Mustafa 1990).

Sequential changes in gene expression occur in the cells that are destined to divide. Early after injury, intracellular signaling turns on, as indicated by activation of protein kinases (e.g., the MAP kinase homolog JNK) as well as transcription factors (e.g., NF-κB, AP-1, C/EBP; see Fig. 3-11), and expression of numerous genes are increased (Fausto, 2000). Among these so-called immediate-early genes are those that code for transcription factors such as c-*fos*, c-*jun* and c-*myc* as well as cytokine-like secreted proteins (Mohn et al., 1991; Zawaski et al., 1993). These primary gene products amplify the initial gene-activation process by stimulating other genes directly or through cell surface receptors and the coupled transducing networks (Fausto and Webber, 1993). A few hours later the so-called delayed-early genes are expressed, such as the Bcl-X_L,which encodes an antiapoptotic protein from the Bcl-2 family (see Fig. 3-16), followed by the genes whose products regulate the cell-division cycle (Fausto, 2000). Not only genes for the cell cycle accelerator proteins (e.g., cyclin D and mdm2; see Fig. 3-24), but also genes whose products decelerate the cell cycle (e.g., p53 and p21; see Fig. 3-24) become temporarily overexpressed, suggesting that this duality keeps tissue regeneration precisely regulated. Thus, genetic expression is reprogrammed so that DNA synthesis and mitosis gain priority over specialized cellular activities. For example, as a result of dedifferentiation, regenerating hepatocytes underexpress cytochrome P450 and hepatic stellate cells cease to accumulate fat and vitamin A.

It has been speculated that the regenerative process is initiated by the release of chemical mediators from damaged cells. The nonparenchymal cells, such as resident macrophages and endothelial cells, are receptive to these chemical signals and produce a host of secondary signaling molecules, cytokines, and growth factors that promote and propagate the regenerative process (Fig. 3-22). The cytokines TNF-α and IL-6 purportedly promote transition of the quiescent cells into cell cycle ("priming"), whereas the growth factors, especially the hepatocyte growth factor (HGF) and transforming growth factor-α (TGF-α), initiate the progression of the "primed" cells in the cycle toward mitosis (Fausto, 2000). Despite its name, neither the formation nor the action of HGF is restricted to the liver. It is produced by resident macrophages and endothelial cells of various organs—including liver, lung, and kidney—

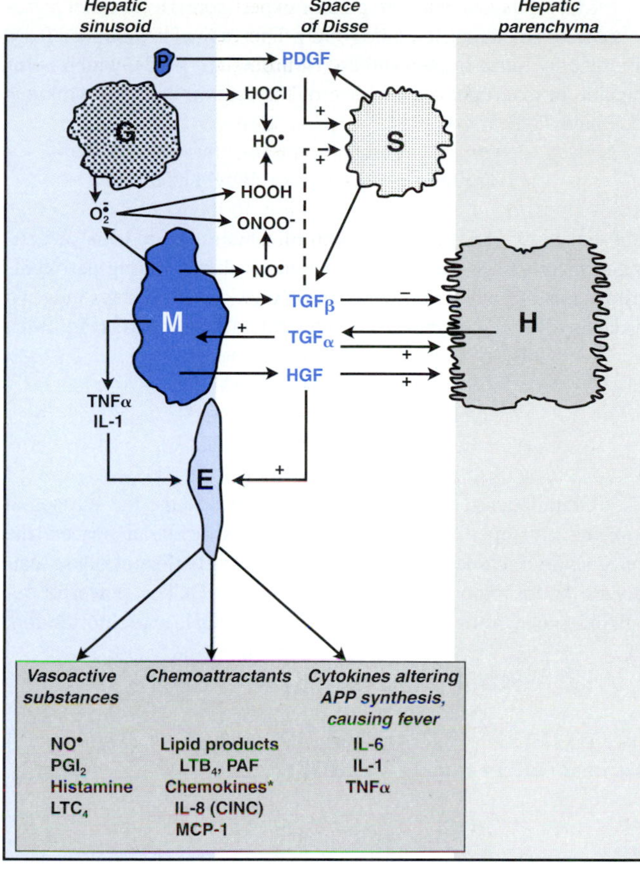

Figure 3-22. Mediators of tissue repair and side reactions to tissue injury in liver: (1) growth factors promoting replacement of cells and the extracellular matrix; (2) mediators of inflammation, acute-phase protein (AAP) synthesis, and fever; and (3) cytotoxic mediators of inflammatory cells.

HGF = hepatocyte growth factor; PDGR = platelet-derived growth factor; TGF-α = transforming growth factor-alpha, TGF-β = transforming growth factor-beta; $NO^{\bullet}$ = nitric oxide; PGI_2 = prostacyclin; LTC_4 = leukotriene C_4; IL = interleukin; LTB_4 = leukotriene B_4; PAF = platelet-activating factor; CINC (the rat homolog of IL-8) = cytokine-induced neutrophil chemoattractant; MCP-1 = monocyte chemotactic protein; TNF = tumor necrosis factor. Cells presented are E = endothelial cells; G = granulocyte; H = hepatocyte; M = macrophage (Kupffer cell); S = stellate cell (also called perisinusoidal, Ito or fat-storing cell). *Rather than the endothelial cells, other stromal cells are the main sources of chemokines (e.g., stellate cells for MCP-1). Solid arrows represent effects of growth factors on cell division, whereas the dashed arrow shows the effect on extracellular matrix formation. Positive and negative signs indicate stimulation and inhibition, respectively. See text for further details.

and in a paracrine manner activates receptors on neighboring parenchymal cells (Fig. 3-22). In rats intoxicated with carbon tetrachloride, the synthesis of HGF in hepatic and renal nonparenchymal cells increases markedly (Noji et al., 1990) and HGF levels in blood rise rapidly (Lindroos et al., 1991). The communication between parenchymal and nonparenchymal cells during tissue repair is mutual. For example, TGF-α, a potent mitogen produced by regenerating hepatocytes, acts both as an autocrine and a paracrine mediator on liver cells as well as on adjacent nonparenchymal cells (Fig. 3-22).

Besides mitosis, cell migration also significantly contributes to restitution of certain tissues. The mucosa of the gastrointestinal tract is an important barrier; therefore replacement of mortally injured epithelial cells is an urgent need. Cells of the residual epithelium rapidly migrate to the site of injury as well as elongate and thin to reestablish the continuity of the surface even before this could be achieved by cell replication. Mucosal repair is dictated not only by growth factors and cytokines operative in tissue repair elsewhere but also by specific factors such as trefoil peptides that are associated with the mucous layer of the gastrointestinal tract and become overexpressed at sites of mucosal injury (Podolsky, 1999).

Replacement of the Extracellular Matrix The extracellular matrix is composed of proteins, glycosaminoglycans, and the glycoprotein and proteoglycan glycoconjugates (Gressner, 1992). In liver, these molecules are synthesized by stellate or fat storing cells located in the space of Disse, between the hepatic sinusoid and the hepatocytes (Fig. 3-22). The stellate cells become activated during liver regeneration, undergoing mitosis and major phenotypic changes. The latter changes include not only increased synthesis and secretion of extracellular matrix constituents but also loss of fat and vitamin A content and expression of actin. Thus, resting stellate cells become transdifferentiated into myofibroblast-like contractile and secretory cells. Activation of stellate cells is mediated chiefly by two growth factors—platelet-derived growth factor (PDGF) and transforming growth factor-β (TGF-β) (Fig. 3-22). Both may be released from platelets (that accumulate and degranulate at sites of injury) and later from the activated stellate cells themselves. The main sources of TGF-β, however, are the neighboring tissue macrophages residing in the hepatic sinusoids (Gressner, 1992). A dramatic increase in TGF-β mRNA levels in Kupffer cells is observed with in situ hybridization after carbon tetrachloride–induced hepatic necrosis (Burt, 1993). Proliferation of stellate cells is induced by the potent mitogen PDGF, whereas TGF-β acts on the stellate cells to stimulate the synthesis of extracellular matrix components, including collagens, fibronectin, tenascin, and proteoglycans. This effect of TGF-β is mediated through activation of JNK (a MAPK homolog) and not through the transcription factor Smad proteins, that relay the signal for the antiproliferative and pro-apoptotic effects of TGF-β (see Fig. 3-11). TGF-β also plays a central role in extracellular matrix formation in other tissues. In the kidney and the lung, for example, TGF-β targets the mesangial cells and the septal fibroblasts, respectively (Border and Ruoslahti, 1992). Remodeling of the extracellular matrix is aided by matrix metalloproteinases, which hydrolyase specific components of the matrix, as well as by tissue inhibitors of matrix metalloproteinases. The former group of these proteins originates from various types of nonparenchymal cells, including inflammatory cells; however, their inhibitors are mainly produced by stellate cells (Arthur et al., 1999).

The way in which tissue regeneration is terminated after repair is unclear, but the gradual dominance of TGF-β, which is a potent antimitogen and apoptogen, over mitogens is a contributing factor in the termination of cell proliferation. Extracellular matrix production may be halted by products of the proliferative response that bind and inactivate TGF-β. The proteoglycan decorin and the positive acute phase protein alpha$_2$-macroglobulin are examples of such products (Gressner, 1992).

Side Reactions to Tissue Injury In addition to mediators that aid in the replacement of lost cells and the extracellular matrix, resident macrophages and endothelial cells activated by cell injury also produce other mediators that induce ancillary reactions with uncertain benefit or harm tissues (Fig. 3-22). Such reactions include inflammation, altered production of acute-phase protein, and generalized reactions such as fever.

Inflammation *Cells and Mediators* Alteration of the microcirculation and accumulation of inflammatory cells are the hallmarks of inflammation. These processes are largely initiated by resident macrophages secreting cytokines such as TNF-α and interleukin-1 (IL-1) in response to tissue damage (Baumann and Gauldie, 1994) (Fig. 3-22). These cytokines, in turn, stimulate neighboring stromal cells, such as the endothelial cells and fibroblasts, to release mediators that induce dilation of the local microvasculature and cause permeabilization of capillaries. Activated endothelial cells also facilitate the egress of circulating leukocytes into the injured tissue by releasing chemoattractants and expressing cell-adhesion molecules, which are cell surface glycoproteins (Jaeschke, 1997). One group of cell-adhesion molecules, called selectins, located on the membrane of endothelial cells, interact with their ligands on the surface of leukocytes, thereby slowing down the flow of these cells and causing them to "roll" on the capillary surface. Subsequently a stronger interaction (adhesion) is established between the endothelial cells and leukocytes with participation of intercellular adhesion molecules (e.g., ICAM-1) expressed on the endothelial cell membrane and integrins expressed on the membrane of leukocytes. This interaction is also essential for the subsequent transendothelial migration of leukocytes. This is facilitated by gradients of chemoattractants that induce expression of leukocyte integrins. Chemoattractants originate from various stromal cells and include chemotactic cytokines (or chemokines), such as the monocyte chemotactic protein-1 (MCP-1) and IL-8 (whose rat homolog is the cytokine-induced neutrophil chemoattractant or CINC), as well as lipid-derived compounds, such as platelet-activating factor (PAF) and leukotriene B_4 (LTB_4). Ultimately all types of cells in the vicinity of injury express ICAM-1, thus promoting leukocyte invasion; the invading leukocytes also synthesize mediators, thus propagating the inflammatory response. Production of most inflammatory mediators is induced by signaling, turned on by TNF-α and IL-1, which results in activation of transcription factors, notably NF-κB and C/EBP (Poli, 1998) (see Fig. 3-11). Genes of many of the proteins mentioned above (e.g., selectins, ICAM-1, MCP-1, IL-8) and below (e.g., inducible nitric oxide synthase, acute phase proteins) as well as the genes of TNF-α and IL-1 themselves contain binding sites for the NF-κB (Lee and Burckart, 1998).

Inflammation Produces Reactive Oxygen and Nitrogen Species Macrophages, as well as leukocytes, recruited to the site of injury undergo a respiratory burst, producing free radicals and enzymes (Weiss and LoBuglio, 1982) (Fig. 3-22). Free radical are produced in the inflamed tissue in three ways, each of which involves a specific enzyme: NAD(P)H oxidase, nitric oxide synthase, or myeloperoxidase.

During the respiratory burst, membrane-bound NAD(P)H oxidase is activated in both macrophages and granulocytes and produces superoxide anion radical ($O_2^{\bar{\bullet}}$) from molecular oxygen:

$$\text{NAD(P)H} + 2O_2 \rightarrow \text{NAD(P)}^+ + H^+ + 2O_2^{\bar{\bullet}}$$

The $O_2^{\bar{\bullet}}$ can give rise to the hydroxyl radical ($HO^\bullet$) in two sequential steps: The first is spontaneous or is catalyzed by superoxide dismutase, and the second, the Fenton reaction, is catalyzed by transition metal ions (see also Fig. 3-4):

$$2O_2^{\bar{\bullet}} + 2H^+ \rightarrow O_2 + \text{HOOH}$$
$$\text{HOOH} + Fe^{2+} \rightarrow Fe^{3+} + HO^- + HO^\bullet$$

Macrophages, but not granulocytes, generate another cytotoxic free radical, nitric oxide ($^\bullet$NO). This radical is produced from arginine by nitric oxide synthase (Wang et al., 1993), which is inducible in macrophages by bacterial endotoxin and the cytokines IL-1 and TNF:

$$\text{L-arginine} + O_2 \rightarrow \text{L-citrulline} + {}^\bullet\text{NO}$$

Subsequently, $O_2^{\bar{\bullet}}$ and $^\bullet$NO, both of which are products of activated macrophages, can react with each other, yielding peroxynitrite anion; upon reaction with carbon dioxide, this decays into two radicals, nitrogen dioxide and carbonate anion radical (Fig. 3-4):

$$O_2^{\bar{\bullet}} + {}^\bullet\text{NO} \rightarrow \text{ONOO}^-$$
$$\text{ONOO}^- + CO_2 \rightarrow \text{ONOOCO}_2^-$$
$$\text{ONOOCO}_2^- \rightarrow {}^\bullet NO_2 + CO_3^{\bar{\bullet}}$$

Granulocytes, but not macrophages, discharge the lysosomal enzyme myeloperoxidase into engulfed extracellular spaces, the phagocytic vacuoles (Wang et al., 1993). Myeloperoxidase catalyzes the formation of hypochlorous acid (HOCl), a powerful oxidizing agent, from hydrogen peroxide (HOOH) and chloride ion:

$$\text{HOOH} + H^+ + Cl^- \rightarrow \text{HOH} + \text{HOCl}$$

Like HOOH, HOCl can form $HO^\bullet$ as a result of electron transfer from Fe^{2+} or from $O_2^{\bar{\bullet}}$ to HOCl:

$$\text{HOCl} + O_2^{\bar{\bullet}} \rightarrow O_2 + Cl^- + HO^\bullet$$

All these reactive chemicals, as well as the discharged lysosomal proteases, are destructive products of inflammatory cells. Although these chemicals exert antimicrobial activity at the site of microbial invasion, at the site of toxic injury they can damage the adjacent healthy tissues and thus contribute to propagation of tissue injury (see "Tissue Necrosis," below). Moreover, in some chemically induced injuries, inflammation plays the leading role. For example, α-naphthyl-isothiocyanate (ANIT), a cholestatic chemical, causes neutrophil- dependent hepatocellular damage. ANIT apparently acts on bile duct epithelial cells, causing them to release chemoattractants for neutrophil cells, which upon invading the liver, injure hepatocytes (Hill et al., 1999). Kupffer cell activation, TNF-α release, and subsequent inflammation are also prominent and causative events in galactosamine-induced liver injury in rats (Stachlewitz et al., 1999).

Altered Protein Synthesis: Acute-Phase Proteins Cytokines released from macrophages and endothelial cells of injured tissues also alter protein synthesis, predominantly in the liver (Baumann and Gauldie, 1994) (Fig. 3-18). Mainly IL-6 but also IL-1 and TNF act on cell surface receptors and increase or decrease the transcriptional activity of genes encoding certain proteins called positive and negative acute-phase proteins, respectively, utilizing primarily the transcription factors NF-κB, C/EBP, and STAT (Poli, 1998; see Fig. 3-12). Many of the hepatic acute-phase proteins, such as C-reactive protein, are secreted into the circulation, and their elevated levels in serum are diagnostic of tissue injury, inflammation, or neoplasm. Increased sedimentation of red blood cells, which is also indicative of these conditions, is due to enrichment of blood plasma with positive acute-phase proteins such as fibrinogen.

Apart from their diagnostic value, positive acute-phase proteins may play roles in minimizing tissue injury and facilitating repair. For example, many of them, such as alpha$_2$-macroglobulin and alpha$_1$-antiprotease, inhibit lysosomal proteases released from the injured cells and recruited leukocytes. Haptoglobin binds hemoglobin in blood, metallothionein complexes metals in the cells, heme oxygenase oxidizes heme to biliverdin, and opsonins facilitate phagocytosis. Thus, these positive acute-phase proteins may be involved in the clearance of substances released upon tissue injury.

Negative acute-phase proteins include some plasma proteins, such as albumin, transthyretin, and transferrin, as well as several forms of cytochrome P450 and glutathione *S*-transferase (Buetler, 1998). Because the latter enzymes play important roles in the toxication and detoxication of xenobiotics, the disposition and toxicity of chemicals may be altered markedly during the acute phase of tissue injury.

Although the acute-phase response is phylogenetically preserved, some of the acute-phase proteins are somewhat species-specific. For example, during the acute phase of tissue injury or inflammation, C-reactive protein and serum amyloid A levels dramatically increase in humans but not in rats, whereas the concentrations of alpha$_1$-acid glycoprotein and alpha$_2$-macroglobulin increase markedly in rats but only moderately in humans.

Generalized Reactions Cytokines released from activated macrophages and endothelial cells at the site of injury also may evoke neurohormonal responses. Thus IL-1, TNF, and IL-6 alter the temperature set point of the hypothalamus, triggering fever. IL-1 possibly also mediates other generalized reactions to tissue injury, such as hypophagia, sleep, and "sickness behavior" (Rothwell, 1991). In addition, IL-1 and IL-6 act on the pituitary to induce the release of ACTH, which in turn stimulates the secretion of cortisol from the adrenals. This represents a negative feedback loop because corticosteroids inhibit cytokine gene expression.

When Repair Fails

Although repair mechanisms operate at molecular, cellular, and tissue levels, for various reasons they often fail to provide protection against injury. First, the fidelity of the repair mechanisms is not absolute, making it possible for some lesions to be overlooked. However, repair fails most typically when the damage overwhelms the repair mechanisms, as when protein thiols are oxidized faster than they can be reduced. In other instances, the capacity of repair may become exhausted when necessary enzymes or cofactors are consumed. For example, alkylation of DNA may lead to consumption of O^6-alkylguanine-DNA-alkyltransferase (Pegg and Byers, 1992), and lipid peroxidation can deplete alpha-tocopherol. Sometimes the toxicant-induced injury adversely affects the repair process itself. Thus, after exposure to necrogenic chemicals, mitosis of surviving cells may be blocked and restoration of the tissue becomes impossible (Soni and Mehendale, 1998). Finally, some types of toxic injuries cannot be repaired effectively, as occurs when xenobiotics are covalently bound to proteins. Thus, toxicity is manifested when repair of the initial injury fails because the repair mechanisms become overwhelmed, exhausted, or impaired or are genuinely inefficient.

It is also possible that repair contributes to toxicity. This may occur in a passive manner, for example, if excessive amounts of NAD^+ are cleaved by PARP when this enzyme assists in repairing broken DNA strands, or when too much NAD(P)H is consumed for the repair of oxidized proteins and endogenous reductants. Either event can compromise oxidative phosphorylation, which is also dependent on the supply of reduced cofactors (see Fig. 3-13), thus causing or aggravating ATP depletion that contributes to cell injury. Excision repair of DNA and reacylation of lipids also contribute to cellular deenergization and injury by consuming significant amounts of ATP. However, repair also may play an active role in toxicity. This is observed after chronic tissue injury, when the repair process goes astray and leads to uncontrolled proliferation instead of tissue remodeling. Such proliferation of cells may yield neoplasia whereas overproduction of extracellular matrix results in fibrosis.

Toxicity Resulting from Dysrepair

Like repair, dysrepair occurs at the molecular, cellular, and tissue levels. Some toxicities involve dysrepair at an isolated level. For example, hypoxemia develops after exposure to methemoglobin-forming chemicals if the amount of methemoglobin produced overwhelms the capacity of methemoglobin reductase. Because this repair enzyme is deficient at early ages, neonates are especially sensitive to chemicals that cause methemoglobinemia. Formation of cataracts purportedly involves inefficiency or impairment of lenticular repair enzyme, such as the endo- and exopeptidases, which normally reduce oxidized crystalline and hydrolyze damaged proteins to their constituent amino acids. Dysrepair also is thought to contribute to the formation of Heinz bodies, which are protein aggregates formed in oxidatively stressed and aged red blood cells. Defective proteolytic degradation of the immunogenic trifluoroacetylated proteins may make halothane-anesthetized patients victims of halothane hepatitis.

Several types of toxicity involve failed and/or derailed repairs at different levels before they become apparent. This is true for the most severe toxic injuries, such as tissue necrosis, fibrosis, and chemical carcinogenesis.

Tissue Necrosis As discussed above, several mechanisms may lead to cell death. Most or all involve molecular damage that is potentially reversible by repair mechanisms. If repair mechanisms operate effectively, they may prevent cell injury or at least retard its progression. For example, prooxidant toxicants cause no lipid fragmentation in microsomal membranes until alpha-tocopherol is depleted in those membranes. Membrane damage ensues when this endogenous antioxidant, which can repair lipids containing peroxyl radical groups (Fig 3-20), becomes unavailable (Scheschonka et al., 1990). This suggests that cell injury progresses toward cell necrosis if molecular repair mechanisms are inefficient or the molecular damage is not readily reversible.

Progression of cell injury to tissue necrosis can be intercepted by two repair mechanisms working in concert: apoptosis and cell proliferation. As discussed above, injured cells can initiate apoptosis, which counteracts the progression of the toxic injury. Apoptosis does this by preventing necrosis of injured cells and the consequent inflammatory response, which may cause injury by releasing cytotoxic mediators. Indeed, the activation of Kupffer cells, the source of such mediators in the liver, by the administration of bacterial lipopolysaccharide (endotoxin) greatly aggravates the hepatotoxicity of galactosamine. In contrast, when the Kupffer cells are selectively eliminated by pretreatment of rats with gadolinium chloride, the necrotic effect of carbon tetrachloride is markedly alleviated (Edwards et, al., 1993). Blockade of Kupffer cell function with glycine (via the inhibitory glycine receptor; see item 4 in Fig. 3-12) also protects the liver from alcohol-induced injury (Yin et al., 1998).

Another important repair process that can halt the propagation of toxic injury is proliferation of cells adjacent to the injured cells. This response is initiated soon after cellular injury. A surge in mitosis in the liver of rats administered a low (nonnecrogenic) dose of carbon tetrachloride is detectable within a few hours. This early cell division is thought to be instrumental in the rapid and complete restoration of the injured tissue and the prevention of necrosis. This hypothesis is corroborated by the finding that in rats pretreated with chlordecone, which blocks the early cell proliferation in response to carbon tetrachloride, a normally nonnecrogenic dose of carbon tetrachloride causes hepatic necrosis (Soni and Mehendale, 1998). The sensitivity of a tissue to injury and the capacity of the tissue for repair are apparently two independent variables, both influencing the final outcome of the effect of injurious chemical—that is, whether tissue restitution ensues with survival or tissue necrosis occurs with death. For example, variations in tissue repair capacity among species and strains of animals appear to be responsible for certain variations in the lethality of hepatotoxicants (Soni and Mehandale, 1998).

It appears that the efficiency of repair is an important determinant of the dose-response relationship for toxicants that cause tissue necrosis. Following chemically induced liver injury, the intensity of tissue repair increases up to a threshold dose, restraining injury, whereupon it is inhibited, allowing unrestrained progression of injury (Soni and Mehendale, 1998). Impaired signaling to mitosis (see Fig. 3-11) caused by high concentrations of acetaminophen may account for lagging repair of the liver damaged by this drug (Boulares et al., 1999), but maintenance of DNA synthesis, mitotic machinery, and energy supply may also be impaired at high-dose chemical exposures. That is, tissue necrosis is caused by a certain dose of a toxicant not only because that dose ensures sufficient concentration of the ultimate toxicant at the target site to initiate injury but also because that quantity of toxicant causes a degree of damage sufficient to compromise repair, allowing for progression of the injury. Experimental observations with hepatotoxicants indicate that apoptosis and cell proliferation are operative with latent tissue injury caused by low (nonnecrogenic) doses of toxicants but are inhibited with severe injury induced by high (necrogenic) doses. For example, 1,1-dichloroethylene, carbon tetrachloride, and thioacetamide all induce apoptosis in the liver at low doses but cause hepatic necrosis after high-dose exposure (Corcoran et al., 1994). Similarly, there is an early mitotic response in the liver to low-dose carbon tetrachloride, but this response is absent after administration of the solvent at necrogenic doses (Soni and Mehendale, 1998). This suggests that tissue necrosis occurs because the injury overwhelms and disables the repair mechanisms, including (1) repair of damaged molecules, (2) elimination of damaged cells by apoptosis, and (3) replacement of lost cells by cell division.

Fibrosis Fibrosis is a pathologic condition characterized by excessive deposition of an extracellular matrix of abnormal composition. Hepatic fibrosis, or cirrhosis, results from chronic consumption of ethanol or intoxication with hepatic necrogens such as carbon tetrachloride and iron. Pulmonary fibrosis is induced by drugs such as bleomycin and amiodarone and prolonged inhalation of oxygen or mineral particles. Doxorubicin may cause cardiac fibrosis, whereas exposure to ionizing radiation induces fibrosis in many organs. Most of these agents generate free radicals and cause chronic cell injury.

Fibrosis is a specific manifestation of dysrepair of the injured tissue. As discussed above, cellular injury initiates a surge in cellular proliferation and extracellular matrix production, which normally ceases when the injured tissue is remodeled. If increased production of extracellular matrix is not halted, fibrosis develops.

The cells that manufacture the extracellular matrix during tissue repair (e.g., stellate cells in liver, fibroblasts-like cells in lungs and skin) are the ones that overproduce the matrix in fibrosis. These cells are controlled and phenotypically altered ("activated") by cytokines and growth factors secreted by nonparenchymal cells, including themselves (see Fig. 3-22). TGF-β appears to be the major mediator of fibrogenesis, although other factors, such as TNF and platelet-derived growth factor, are also involved (Border and Ruoslahti, 1992). Indeed, subcutaneous injection of TGF-β induces local fibrosis, whereas TGF-β antagonists such as anti-TGF-β immunoglobulin and decorin ameliorate experimental fibrogenesis. In several types of experimental fibrosis and in patients with active liver cirrhosis, overexpression of TGF-β in affected tissues has been demonstrated. The increased expression of TGF-β is a common response mediating regeneration of the extracellular matrix after an acute injury. However, while TGF-β production ceases when repair is complete, this does not occur when tissue injury leads to fibrosis. Failure to halt TGF-β overproduction could be caused by continuous injury or a defect in the regulation of TGF-β.

The fibrotic action of TGF-β is due to (1) stimulation of the synthesis of individual matrix components by specific target cells and (2) inhibition of matrix degradation by decreasing the synthesis of matrix metalloproteinases and increasing the level of tissue inhibitors of metalloproteinases (Burt, 1993; Arthur et al., 1999). Interestingly, TGF-β induces transcription of its own gene in target cells, suggesting that the TGF-β produced by these cells can amplify in an autocrine manner the production of the extracellular matrix. This positive feedback may facilitate fibrogenesis (Border and Ruoslahti, 1992).

Fibrosis involves not only excessive accumulation of the extracellular matrix but also changes in its composition. The basement membrane components, such as collagen IV and laminin, as well as the fibrillar type collagens (collagen I and III), which confer rigidity to tissues, increase disproportionately, during fibrogenesis (Gressner, 1992).

Fibrosis is detrimental in a number of ways:

1. The scar compresses and may ultimately obliterate the parenchymal cells and blood vessels.
2. Deposition of basement membrane components between the capillary endothelial cells and the parenchymal cells presents a diffusional barrier which contributes to malnutrition of the tissue cells.
3. An increased amount and rigidity of the extracellular matrix unfavorably affect the elasticity and flexibility of the whole tissue, compromising the mechanical function of organs such as the heart and lungs.
4. Furthermore, the altered extracellular environment is sensed by integrins. Through these transmembrane proteins and the coupled intracellular signal transducing networks (see Fig. 3-11) fibrosis may modulate several aspects of cell behavior, including polarity, motility, and gene expression (Burt, 1993; Raghow, 1994).

Carcinogenesis Chemical carcinogenesis involves insufficient function of various repair mechanisms, including (1) failure of DNA repair, (2) failure of apoptosis, and (3) failure to terminate cell proliferation.

Failure of DNA Repair: Mutation, the Initiating Event in Carcinogenesis. Chemical and physical insults may induce neoplastic transformation of cells by genotoxic and nongenotoxic mechanisms. Chemicals that react with DNA may cause damage such as adduct formation, oxidative alteration, and strand breakage (Fig. 3-23). In most cases, these lesions are repaired or injured cells are eliminated. If neither event occurs, a lesion in the parental DNA strand may induce a heritable alteration, or mutation, in the daughter strand during replication. The mutation may remain silent if it does not alter the protein encoded by the mutant gene or if the mutation causes an amino acid substitution that does not affect the function of the protein. Alternatively, the genetic alteration may be incompatible with cell survival. The most unfortunate scenario for the organism occurs when the altered genes express mutant proteins that reprogram cells for multiplication. When such cells undergo mitosis, their descendants also have a similar propensity for proliferation. Moreover, because enhanced cell division increases the likelihood of mutations, these cells eventually acquire additional mutations that may further increase their growth advantage over their normal counterparts. The final outcome of this process is a nodule, followed by a tumor consisting of transformed, rapidly proliferating cells (Fig. 3-23).

The critical role of DNA repair in preventing carcinogenesis is attested by the human heritable disease xeroderma pigmentosum. Affected individuals exhibit deficient excision repair and a greatly increased incidence of sunlight-induced skin cancers. Cells from these patients are also hypersensitive to DNA-reactive chemicals, including aflatoxin B_1, aromatic amines, polycyclic hydrocarbons, and 4-nitroquinoline-1-oxide (Lehmann and Dean, 1990). Also, mice with ablated PARP gene are extremely sensitive to γ-rays and *N*-methylnitrosourea and show genomic instability, as indicated by increases in the levels of both sister chromatid exchanges and chromatid breaks following DNA damage (D'Amours et al., 1999).

A small set of cellular genes are the targets for genetic alterations that initiate neoplastic transformations. Included are proto-oncogenes and tumor-suppressor genes (Barrett, 1992).

Mutation of Proto-oncogenes Proto-oncogenes are highly conserved genes encoding proteins that stimulate the progression of cells through the cell cycle (Smith et al., 1993). The products of proto-oncogenes include (1) growth factors; (2) growth factor receptors; (3) intracellular signal transducers such as G proteins, protein kinases, cyclins, and cyclin-dependent protein kinases; and (4) nuclear transcription factors. Figure 3-24 depicts several proto-oncogene products that are closely involved in initiating the cell-division cycle. The legend of that figure outlines some important details on the function of these proteins and their interaction with tumor suppressor proteins (to be discussed below). Transient increases in the production or activity of proto-oncogene proteins are required for regulated growth, as during embryogenesis, tissue regeneration, and stimulation of cells by growth factors or hormones. In contrast, permanent activation and/or overexpression of these proteins favors neoplastic transformation. One mechanism whereby genotoxic carcinogens induce neoplastic cell transformation is by producing an activating mutation of a proto-oncogene. Such a mutation is so named because the altered gene (then called an *oncogene*) encodes a permanently active protein that forces the cell into the division cycle. An example of mutational activation of an oncogene protein is that of the Ras proteins.

Ras proteins represent a family of G-proteins with GTP/GDP binding capacity as well as GTPase activity (Anderson et al., 1992).

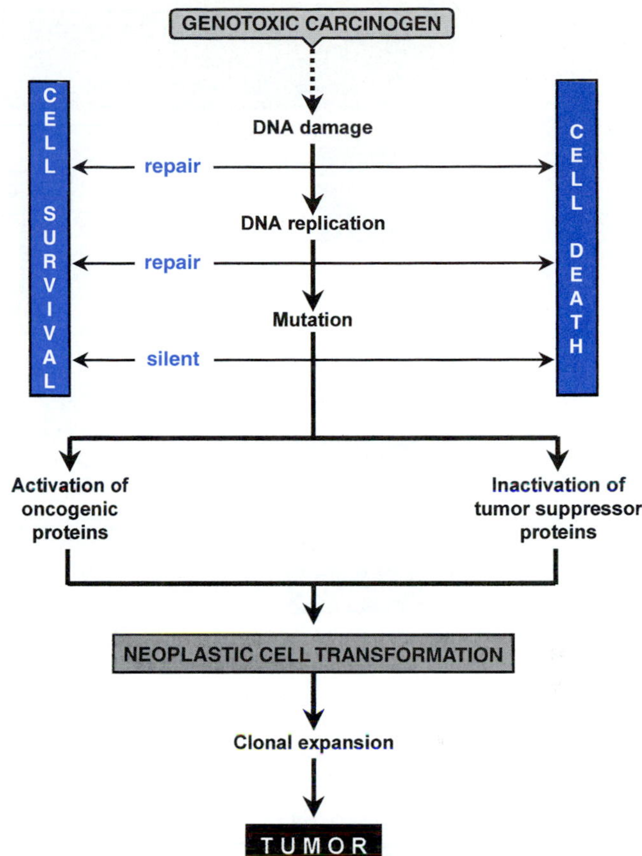

Figure 3-23. The process of carcinogenesis initiated by genotoxic carcinogens (see text for explanation).

They are localized on the inner surface of the plasma membrane and function as crucial mediators in responses initiated by growth factors (see Figs. 3-11 and 3-24). Ras is located downstream from growth factor receptors and nonreceptor protein tyrosine kinases and upstream from mitogen-activated protein kinase (MAPK) cascade whose activation finally upregulates the expression of cyclin D and initiates the mitotic cycle (Fig. 3-24). In this pathway, Ras serves as a molecular switch, being active in the GTP-bound form and inactive in the GDP-bound form. Some mutations of the *ras* gene (e.g., a point mutation in codon 12) dramatically lowers the GTPase activity of the protein. This in turn locks Ras in the permanently active GTP-bound form. Continual rather than signal-dependent activation of Ras can lead eventually to uncontrolled proliferation and transformation. Indeed, microinjection of Ras-neutralizing monoclonal antibodies into cells blocks the mitogenic action of growth factors as well as cell transformation by several oncogenes. Numerous carcinogenic chemicals induce mutations of ras proto-oncogenes that lead to constitutive activation of Ras proteins (Anderson et al., 1992). These include *N*-methyl-*N*-nitrosourea, polycyclic aromatic hydrocarbons, benzidine, aflatoxin B_1, and ionizing radiation. Most of these agents induce point mutations by transversion of G_{35} to T in codon 12.

While mutation-induced constitutive activation of oncogene proteins is a common mechanism in chemical carcinogenesis, overexpression of such proteins also can contribute to neoplastic cell transformation. This may result from (1) sustained transactivation of the promoter region of a proto-oncogene (e.g., the promoter of

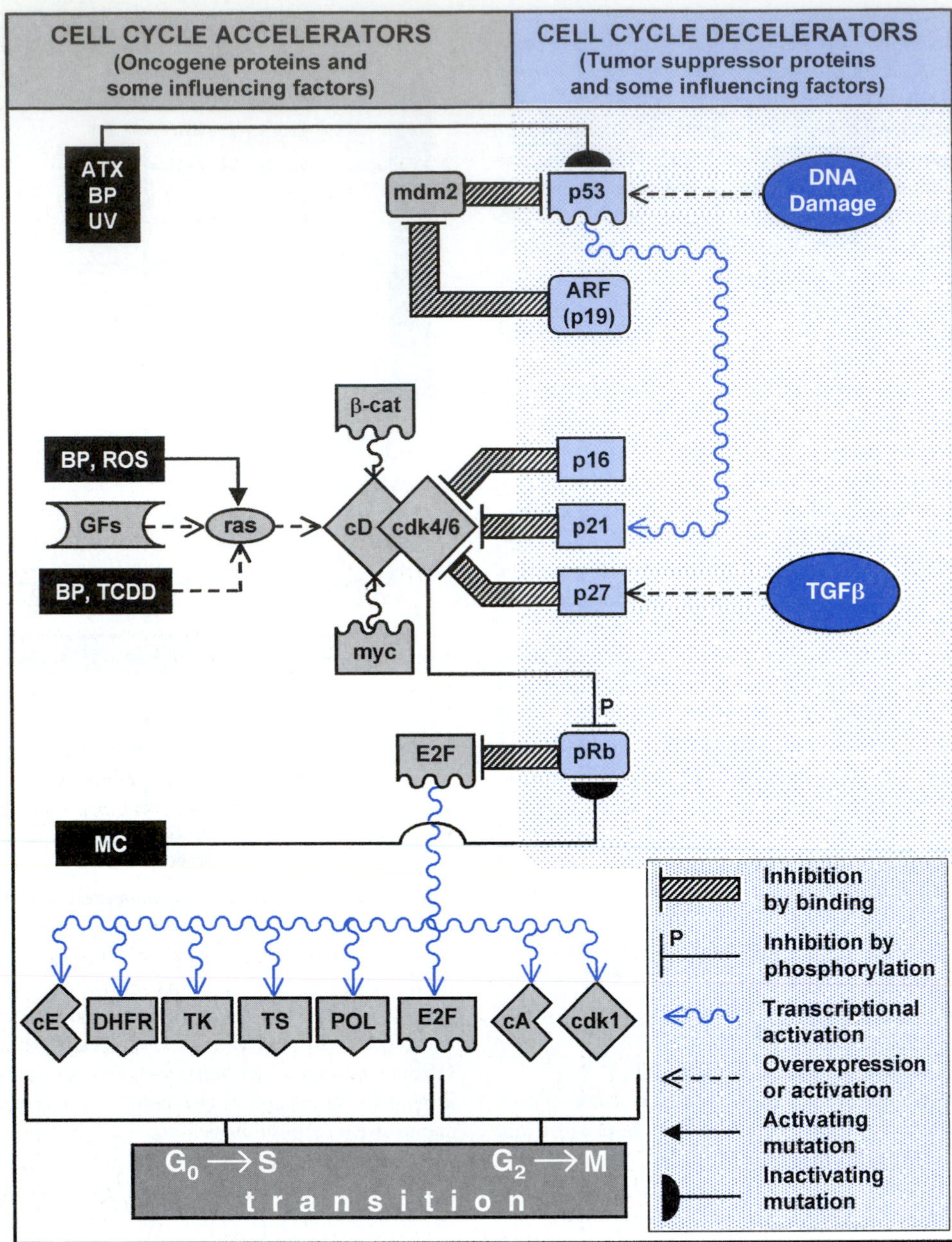

Figure 3-24. Key regulatory proteins controlling the cell division cycle with some signaling pathways and xenobiotics affecting them.

Proteins on the left, represented by gray symbols, accelerate the cell cycle and are oncogenic if permanently active or expressed at high level. In contrast, proteins on the right, represented by blue symbols, decelerate or arrest the cell cycle and thus suppress oncogenesis, unless they are inactivated (e.g., by mutation).

Accumulation of cyclin D (cD) is a crucial event in initating the cell division cycle. cD activates cyclin-dependent protein kinases 4 and 6 (cdk4/6), which in turn phosphorylate the retinoblastoma protein (pRb) causing dissociation of pRb from transcription factor E2F (Johnson and Walker, 1999). Then the unleashed E2F is able to bind to and transactivate genes whose products are essential for DNA synthesis, such as dihydrofolate reductase (DHFR), thymidine kinase (TK), thymidylate synthetase (TS), and DNA polymerase (POL), or are regulatory proteins, such as cyclin E (cE), cyclin A (cA) and cyclin-dependent protein kinase 1 (cdk1), that promote further progression of the cell cycle. Expression of cD is increased, for example, by signals evoked by growth factors (GFs) via ras proteins and by transcription factors, such as myc and β-catenin (β-cat). Some carcinogens, e.g., benzpyrene (BP) and reactive oxygen species (ROS), may cause mutation of the *ras* gene that results in permanently active mutant *ras* protein, but BP as well as TCDD may also induce simple overexpression of normal *ras* protein.

Cell cycle progression is counteracted, for example, by pRb (which inhibits the function of E2F), by cyclin-dependent protein kinase inhibitors (such as p16, p21, and p27), by p53 (that transactivates the *p21* gene), and by ARF (also called p19 that binds to mdm2, thereby neutralizing the antagonistic effect of mdm2 on p53).

ras gene by TCDD- or benzpyrene-ligated Ah receptor; Ramos et al., 1998), (2) an alteration of the regulatory region of proto-oncogenes (e.g., by hypomethylation or translocation) and (3) amplification of the proto-oncogene (Anderson et al., 1992). Gene amplification (i.e., the formation more than one copy) may be initiated by DNA strand breaks, and therefore often observed after exposure to ionizing radiation

Mutation of Tumor-Suppressor Genes Tumor-suppressor genes encode proteins that inhibit the progression of cells in the division cycle. Figure 3-24 depicts such proteins, which include, for example, cyclin-dependent protein kinase inhibitors (e.g., p16, p21, and p27), transcription factors (e.g., p53) that transactivate genes encoding cyclin-dependent protein kinase inhibitors, and proteins (e.g., pRb) that block transcription factors involved in DNA synthesis and cell division. Uncontrolled proliferation can occur when the mutant tumor-suppressor gene encodes a protein that cannot suppress cell division. Inactivating mutations of specific tumor suppressor genes in germ cells are responsible for the inherited predisposition to cancer, as in familial retinoblastoma, Wilms' tumor, familial polyposis, and Li-Fraumeni syndrome (Gennett et al., 1999). Mutations of tumor-suppressor genes in somatic cells contribute to nonhereditary cancers. The best-known tumor suppressor gene involved in both spontaneous and chemically induced carcinogenesis is p53.

The p53 tumor suppressor gene encodes a 53,000-dalton protein with multiple functions (Fig. 3-25). Acting as a transcription factor, the p53 protein (1) transactivates genes whose products arrest the cell cycle (e.g., p21 and gadd 45) or promote apoptosis (e.g., bax and fas receptor) and (2) represses genes that encode antiapoptotic proteins (e.g., bcl-2 and IGF1 receptor) (Asker et al., 1999; Bennett et al., 1999). DNA damage and illegitimate expression of oncogenes (e.g., *c-myc*) stabilizes the p53 protein, causing its accumulation (Fig. 3-25). The accumulated p53 induces cell cycle arrest (permitting DNA repair) or even apoptosis of the affected cells. Thus, p53 eliminates cancer-prone cells from the replicative pool, counteracting neoplastic transformation (Fig. 3-23); therefore it is commonly designated as guardian of the genome.

Indeed, cells that have no p53 are a million times more likely to permit DNA amplification than are cells with a normal level of the suppressor gene. Furthermore, genetically engineered mice with the p53 gene deleted develop cancer by 6 to 9 months of age. These observations attest to the crucial role of the p53 tumor-suppressor gene in preventing carcinogenesis.

Mutations in the p53 gene are found in 50 percent of human tumors and in a variety of induced cancers. The majority are "missense mutations" that change an amino acid and result in a faulty or altered protein (Bennett et al., 1999). The faulty p53 protein forms a complex with endogenous wild-type p53 protein and inactivates it. Thus, the mutant p53 not only is unable to function as a tumor suppressor protein but also prevents tumor suppression by the wild-type p53. Moreover, some observations suggest that the mutant p53 can actively promote cell proliferation, much as an oncogene protein does.

Different carcinogens cause different mutations in the p53 tumor-suppressor gene. An example is the point mutation in codon 249 from AGG to AGT, which changes amino acid 249 in the p53 protein from arginine to serine. This mutation predominates in hepatocellular carcinomas in individuals in regions where food is contaminated with aflatoxin B_1 (Bennett et al., 1999). Because aflatoxin B_1 induces the transversion of G to T in codon 249 of the p53 tumor-suppressor gene in human hepatocytes (Aguilar et al.,

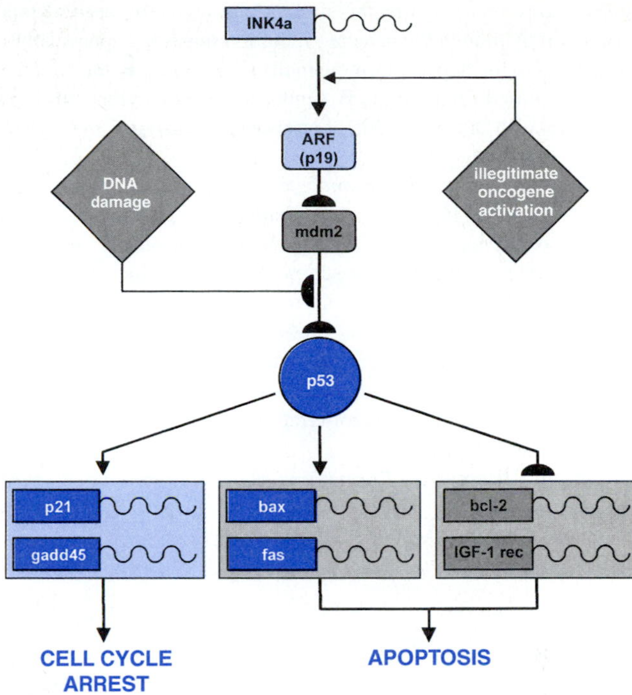

Figure 3-25. The guardian of the genome: p53 tumor suppressor protein—its role and regulation.

The p53 protein is chiefly a gene transcription modulator. For example, it transactivates *p21* (or *waf1*) and *gadd45* genes whose products are inhibitors of cyclin–cyclin-dependent protein kinase complexes and arrest the cell cycle in G_1 and G_2 phases, respectively. p53 also transactivates the genes of pro-apoptotic proteins (e.g., bax and fas; see Fig. 3-16) and transrepresses the genes of anti-apoptotic proteins (e.g., bcl-2 and insulin-like growth factor-1 [IGF-1] receptor), whereby it promotes apoptosis. These (and other) p53-induced pro-apoptotic mechanisms may be cell specific, i.e., all are not necessarily occurring in the same cell at the same time.

The intracellular level and activity of p53 depends primarily on the presence of mdm2 protein, which inactivates p53 and promotes its proteosomal degradation. The influence of mdm2 on p53 may be disrupted by DNA damage (possibly via phosphorylation of p53) and by "illegitimate" oncogene activation. The latter results in overexpression of the ARF (or p19) protein, which in turn, binds to mdm2, releasing p53 from its inactivator mdm2. Both mechanisms thus stabilize p53 protein, thereby greatly increasing its abundance and activity.

By arresting division of cells with potentially mutagenic DNA damage and eliminating such cells, p53 protein counteracts neoplastic development. *p53*-null mice, like *ARF*-null mice, develop tumors with high incidence. Mutational inactivation of the p53 protein is thought to contribute to the carcinogenic effect of aflatoxin B_1, sunlight and cigarette smoke in humans. Overexpression of mdm2 can lead to constitutive inhibition of p53 and thereby promotes oncogenesis even if the *p53* gene is unaltered. See the text for more details.

Signals evoked by DNA damage and TGF-β will ultimately result in accumulation of p53 and p27 proteins, respectively, and deceleration of the cell cycle. In contrast, mutations that disable the tumor suppressor proteins facilitate cell cycle progression and neoplastic conversion and are common in human tumors. Aflatoxin B_1 (ATX), BP and UV light cause such mutations of the *p53* gene (Bennet et al., 1999), whereas *pRb* mutations occur invariably in methylcholanthrene (MC)-induced transplacental lung tumors in mice (Miller, 1999).

1993), it appears likely that this mutation is indeed induced by this mycotoxin. Although the detected mutation in patients presumably contributes to the hepatocarcinogenicity of aflatoxin B_1 in humans, it is not required for aflatoxin B_1–induced hepatocarcinogenesis in rats, as rats do not show this aberration in the transformed liver cells.

Cooperation of Proto-oncogenes and Tumor-Suppressor Genes in Carcinogenesis The accumulation of genetic damage in the form of (1) mutant proto-oncogenes (which encode activated proteins) and (2) mutant tumor-suppressor genes (which encode inactivated proteins) is the main driving force in the transformation of normal cells with controlled proliferative activity to malignant cells with uncontrolled proliferative activity. Because the number of cells in a tissue is regulated by a balance between mitosis and apoptosis, the uncontrolled proliferation results from perturbation of this balance (Fig. 3-26).

Failure of Apoptosis: Promotion of Mutation and Clonal Growth In response to DNA damage caused by UV or gamma irradiation or genotoxic chemicals, the levels of p53 protein in cells increase dramatically (5- to 60-fold) (Levine et al., 1994). As discussed above, the high p53 protein levels block the progression of cells in the G1 phase and allow DNA repair to occur before replication or induce cell death by apoptosis (Fig. 3-25). Consequently, apoptosis eliminates cells with DNA damage, preventing mutation, the initiating event in carcinogenesis.

Preneoplastic cells, or cells with mutations, have much higher apoptotic activity than do normal cells (Bursch et al., 1992). Therefore apoptosis counteracts clonal expansion of the initiated cells and tumor cells. In fact, facilitation of apoptosis can induce tumor regression. This occurs when hormone-dependent tumors are deprived of the hormone that promotes growth and suppresses apoptosis. This is the rationale for the use of tamoxifen, an antiestrogen, and gonadotropin-releasing hormone analogs to combat hormone-dependent tumors of the mammary gland and the prostate gland, respectively (Bursch et al., 1992).

Thus, the inhibition of apoptosis is detrimental because it facilitates both mutations and clonal expansion of preneoplastic cells. Indeed, inhibition of apoptosis plays a role in the pathogenesis of human B-cell lymphomas. In this malignancy, chromosomal

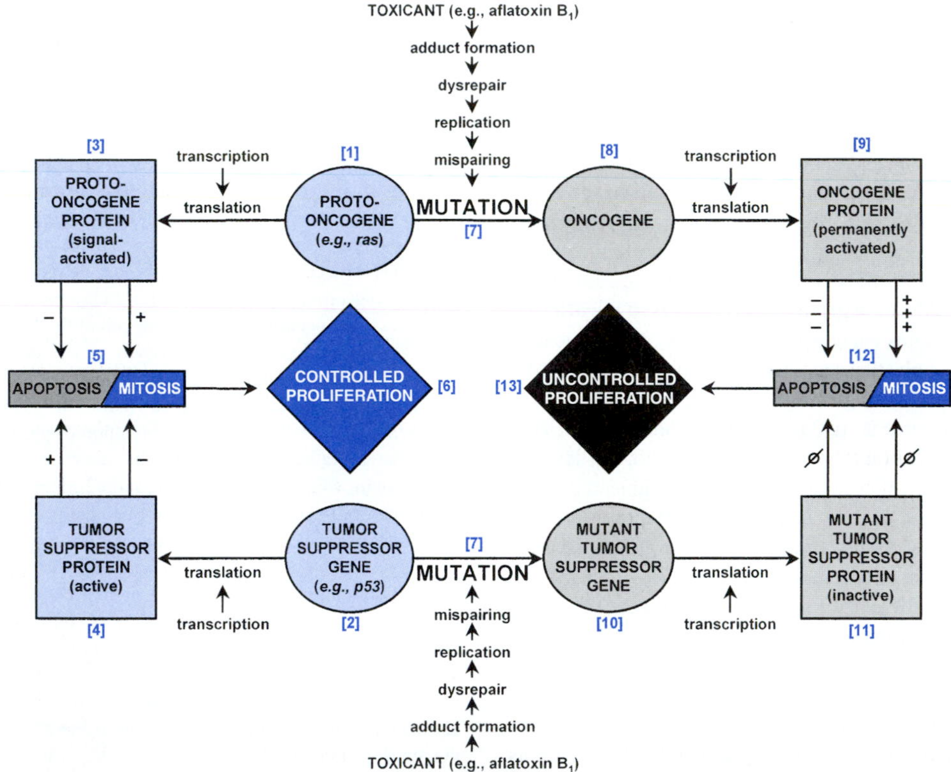

Figure 3-26. A model of cooperation between a proto-oncogene (1) and a tumor suppressor gene (2) before and after mutation.

The model shows that the normal proteins encoded by the cellular proto-oncogenes and the tumor suppressor genes [(3) and (4), respectively] reciprocally influence mitosis and apoptosis (5) and thus ensure controlled cell proliferation (6). However, the balance between the effects of these two types of proteins is offset by a toxicant-induced mutation of their genes (7) if the mutant prot-oncogene (oncogene) (8) encodes a constitutively (i.e., permanently) active oncogene protein (9) and the mutant tumor suppressor gene (10) encodes an inactive tumor suppressor protein (11). Under this condition, the effect of the oncogene protein on mitosis and apoptosis is unopposed (12), resulting in uncontrolled proliferation. Such a scenario may underlie the carcinogenicity of aflatoxin B_1, which can induce mutations in *ras* proto-oncogenes and the *p53* tumor suppressor gene (see text for details). Positive and negative signs represent stimulation and inhibition, respectively; ∅ means "no effect."

translocation brings together the bcl-2 gene and the immunoglobulin heavy-chain locus, resulting in aberrantly increased bcl-2 gene expression. The overexpressed bcl-2 protein, after binding to and inactivating the proapoptotic bax protein (see Fig. 3-16), overrides programmed cell death. Increased levels of bcl-2 are not limited to B-cell lymphoma but are detected in half of the human cancers, and a high bcl-2/bax ratio in a tumor is a marker for poor prognosis (Jäättelä, 1999). Besides bcl-2, other antiapoptotic proteins may also contribute to progression of neoplasia. These include specific heat-shock proteins (Hsp), such as Hsp 70 and 27, as well as a family of "inhibitor of apoptosis proteins" (IAP) that inhibit effector caspases 3 and 7 (see Fig. 3-16). Survivin, a member of the IAP family, is expressed in all cancer cells but not in adult differentiated cells (Jäättelä, 1999).

Inhibition of apoptosis is one mechanism by which phenobarbital, a tumor promoter, promotes clonal expansion of preneoplastic cells. This has been demonstrated in rats given a single dose of *N*-nitrosomorpholine followed by daily treatments with phenobarbital for 12 months to initiate and promote, respectively, neoplastic transformation in liver (Schulte-Hermann et al., 1990). From 6 months onward, phenobarbital did not increase DNA synthesis and cell division in the preneoplastic foci, yet it accelerated foci enlargement. The foci grow because phenobarbital lowers apoptotic activity, allowing the high cell replicative activity to manifest itself. The peroxisome proliferator nafenopin, a nongenotoxic hepatocarcinogen, also suppresses apoptosis in primary rat hepatocyte cultures (Bayly et al., 1994), supporting the hypothesis that this mechanism may play a role in the hepatocarcinogenicity of peroxisome proliferators in rodents.

Failure to Terminate Proliferation: Promotion of Mutation, Proto-Oncogene Expression, and Clonal Growth Enhanced mitotic activity, whether it is induced by oncogenes inside the cell or by external factors such as xenobiotic or endogenous mitogens, promotes carcinogenesis for a number of reasons.

1. First, the enhanced mitotic activity increases the probability of mutations. This is due to activation of the cell-division cycle, which invokes a substantial shortening of the Gl phase. Thus, less time is available for the repair of injured DNA before replication, increasing the chance that the damage will yield a mutation. Although repair still may be feasible after replication, postreplication repair is error-prone. In addition, activation of the cell-division cycle increases the proportion of cells that replicate their DNA at any given time. During replication, the amount of DNA doubles and the DNA becomes unpacked, greatly increasing the effective target size for DNA-reactive mutagenic chemicals.
2. During increased proliferation, proto-oncogenes are overexpressed. These overproduced proto-oncogene proteins may cooperate with oncogene proteins to facilitate the neoplastic transformation of cells. In addition, enhanced mitotic activity indirectly enhances the transcriptional activity of proto-oncogenes and oncogenes by allowing less time for DNA methylation, which occurs in the early postreplication period. Methylation takes place at C_5 of specific cytosine residues in the promoter region of genes and decreases the transcription of genes by inhibiting the interaction of transcription factors with the promoter region. Nonexpressed genes are fully methylated. Hypomethylation of DNA, in contrast, enhances gene expression and may result in overexpression of proto-oncogenes and oncogenes. A "methyl-deficient diet" and ethionine, which deplete *S*-adenosyl-methionine, induce hypomethylation of DNA and cancer, confirming the role of DNA hypomethylation in carcinogenesis (Poirier, 1994).
3. Another mechanism by which proliferation promotes the carcinogenic process is through clonal expansion of the initiated cells to form nodules (foci) and tumors.
4. Finally, cell-to-cell communication through gap junctions and intercellular adhesion through cadherins are temporarily disrupted during proliferation (Yamasaki et al., 1993). Lack of these junctions contributes to the invasiveness of tumor cells. Several tumor promoters, such as phenobarbital, phorbol esters, and peroxisome proliferators, decrease gap junctional intercellular communication. It has been hypothesized that this contributes to neoplastic transformation. It is unclear, however, whether diminished gap junctional communication plays a significant causative role in carcinogenesis or is merely a symptom of cell proliferation.

Nongenotoxic Carcinogens: Promoters of Mitosis and Inhibitors of Apoptosis A number of chemicals cause cancer by altering DNA and inducing a mutation. However, other chemicals do not alter DNA or induce mutations yet induce cancer after chronic administration (Barrett, 1992). These chemicals are designated *nongenotoxic* or *epigenetic carcinogens* and include (1) xenobiotic mitogens (e.g., phenobarbital, phorbol esters, DDT, peroxisomal proliferators, and some other chemicals that promote mitogenic signaling (see Fig. 3-11); (2) endogenous mitogens such as growth factors (e.g., TGF-α) and hormones with mitogenic action on specific cells [e.g., estrogens on mammary gland or liver cells, TSH on the follicular cells of the thyroid gland, and luteinizing hormone (LH) on Leydig cells in testes]; and (3) chemicals that, when given chronically, cause sustained cell injury (such as chloroform and *d*-limonene). Because several of these chemicals promote the development of tumors after neoplastic transformation has been initiated by a genotoxic carcinogen, they are referred to as *tumor promoters*. Despite the initial belief that promoters are unable to induce tumors by themselves, studies suggest that they can do so after prolonged exposure.

Nongenotoxic carcinogens cause cancer by promoting carcinogenesis initiated by genotoxic agents or spontaneous DNA damage (Fig. 3-27). Spontaneous DNA damage, some of which gives rise to mutation, commonly occurs in normal cells (Barrett, 1992). It is estimated that in human cells, 1 out of 10^8 to 10^{10} base pairs suffers spontaneous mutation. Genotoxic carcinogens increase the frequency 10- to 1000-fold. Nongenotoxic carcinogens also increase the frequency of spontaneous mutations through a mitogenic effect and by the mechanisms discussed earlier. In addition, nongenotoxic carcinogens, by inhibiting apoptosis, increase the number of cells with DNA damage and mutations. Both enhanced mitotic activity and decreased apoptotic activity brought about by nongenotoxic carcinogens expand the population of transformed cells, promoting cancer development. In summary, nongenotoxic carcinogens appear to act by enhancing cell division and/or inhibiting apoptosis.

It is easy to recognize that even epigenetic carcinogens of the cytotoxic type act in this manner. As discussed in the section on tissue repair, cell injury evokes the release of mitogenic growth factors such as HGF and TGF-α from tissue macrophages and endothelial cells. Thus, cells in chronically injured tissues are ex-

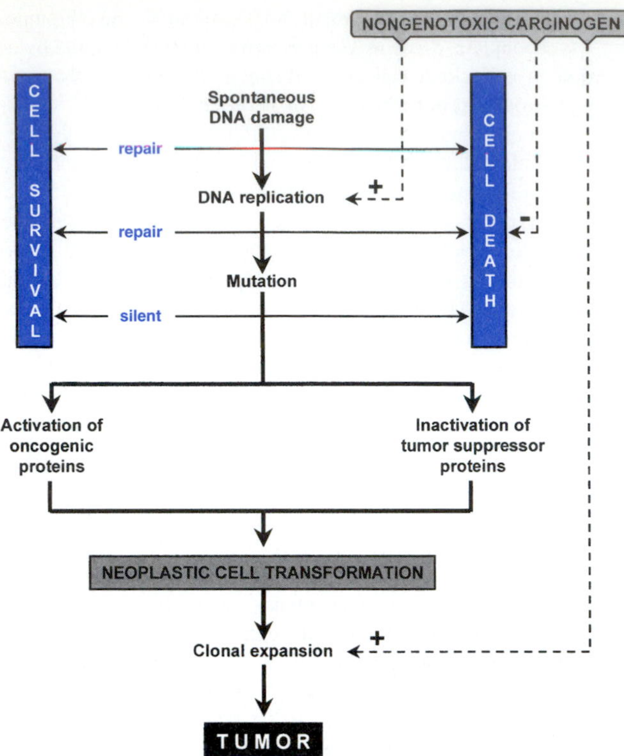

Figure 3-27. The process of carcinogenesis promoted by nongenotoxic carcinogens.

Positive and negative signs represent stimulation and inhibition, respectively. See text for explanation.

posed continuously to endogenous mitogens. Although these growth factors are instrumental in tissue repair after acute cell injury, their continuous presence is potentially harmful because they may ultimately transform the affected cells into neoplastic cells. This view is supported by findings with transgenic mice that overexpress TGF-α. These animals exhibit hepatomegaly at a young age, and 80 percent develop tumors by 12 months (Fausto and Webber, 1993). Mitogenic cytokines secreted by Kupffer cells are apparently involved in hepatocyte proliferation and, possibly, tumor formation induced by peroxysome proliferators in rats (Rose et al., 1999).

It is important to realize that even epigenetic carcinogens can exert a genotoxic effect, although indirectly. For example, chemicals causing chronic cell injury evoke a prolonged inflammatory response, with the free radicals produced by the inflammatory cells causing DNA injury in adjacent cells. Similarly, phorbol esters are not only potent mitogens but also activators of leukocytes, which release DNA-reactive free radicals during their respiratory burst (Weiss and LoBuglio, 1982).

CONCLUSIONS

This overview systematically surveys the mechanisms of the potential events that follow toxicant exposure and contribute to toxicity. This approach is also useful in the search for mechanisms responsible for (1) selective toxicity, that is, differences in the sensitivity to toxicants of various organisms, such as different species and strains of animals, organs, and cells, and (2) alteration of toxicity by exogenous factors such as chemicals and food and physiologic or pathologic conditions such as aging and disease. To identify the mechanisms that underlie selective toxicity or alterations in toxicity, all steps where variations might occur must be considered systematically. Selective or altered toxicity may be due to different or altered (1) exposure; (2) delivery, thus resulting in a different concentration of the ultimate toxicant at the target site; (3) target molecules; (4) biochemical processes triggered by the reaction of the chemical with the target molecules; (5) repair at the molecular, cellular, or tissue level; or (6) mechanisms such as circulatory and thermoregulatory reflexes by which the affected organism can adapt to some of the toxic effects.

In this chapter, a simplified scheme has been used to give an overview of the development of toxicity (Fig. 3-1). In reality, the route to toxicity can be considerably more diverse and complicated. For example, one chemical may yield several ultimate toxicants, one ultimate toxicant may react with several types of target molecules, and reaction with one type of target molecule may have a number of consequences. Thus, the toxicity of one chemical may involve several mechanisms which can interact with and influence each other in an intricate manner.

This chapter has emphasized the significance of the chemistry of a toxicant in governing its delivery to and reaction with the target molecule as well as the importance of the biochemistry, molecular and cell biology, immunology, and physiology of the affected organism in its response to the action of the toxicant. An organism has mechanisms that (1) counteract the delivery of toxicants, such as detoxication; (2) reverse the toxic injury, such as repair mechanisms; and (3) offset some dysfunctions, such as adaptive responses. Thus, toxicity is not an inevitable consequence of toxicant exposure because it may be prevented, reversed, or compensated for by such mechanisms. Toxicity develops if the toxicant exhausts or impairs the protective mechanisms and/or overrides the adaptability of biological systems.

REFERENCES

Aguilar F, Hussain SP, Cerutti P: Aflatoxin Bl induces the transversion of G → T in codon 249 of the p53 tumor suppressor gene in human hepatocytes. *Proc Natl Acad Sci USA* 90:8586–8590, 1993.

Anderson MW, Reynolds SH, You M, Maronpot RM: Role of protooncogene activation in carcinogenesis. *Environ Health Perspect* 98:13–24, 1992.

Armstrong RB, Kim IU, Grippo JF, Levin AA: Retinoids for the future: Investigational approaches for the identification of new compounds. *J Am Acad Dermatol* 27:S38–S42, 1992.

Arteel GE, Briviba K, Sies H: Protection against peroxynitrite. *FEBS Lett* 445:226–230, 1999.

Arthur MJP, Iredale JP, Mann DA: Tissue inhibitors of metalloproteinases: Role in liver fibrosis and alcoholic liver disease. *Alchol Clin Exp Res* 23:940–943, 1999.

Asker C, Wiman KG, Selivanova G: p53-induced apoptosis as a safeguard against cancer. *Biochem Biophys Res Commun* 265:1–6, 1999.

Aust SD, Chignell CF, Bray TM, et al: Free radicals in toxicology. *Toxicol Appl Pharmacol* 120:168–178, 1993.

Baillie TA, Kassahun K: Reversibility in glutathione-conjugate formation. *Adv Pharmacol* 27:163–181, 1994.

Barrett JC: Mechanisms of action of known human carcinogens, in Vainio H, Magee PN, McGregor DB, McMichael AJ (eds): *Mechanisms of Carcinogenesis in Risk Identification.* Lyons, France: International Agency for Research on Cancer, 1992, pp 115–134.

Bates S, Vousden KH: Mechanisms of p53-mediated apoptosis. *Cell Mol Life Sci* 55:28–37, 1999.

Baumann H, Gauldie J: The acute phase response. *Immunol Today* 15:74–80, 1994.

Bayly AC, Roberts RA, Dive C: Suppression of liver cell apoptosis in vitro by the nongenotoxic hepatocarcinogen and peroxisome proliferator nafenopin. *J Cell Biol* 125:197–203, 1994.

Bennett WP, Hussain SP, Vahakangas KH, et al: Molecular epidemiology of human cancer risk: Gene-environment interactions and *p*53 mutation spectrum in human lung cancer. *J Pathol* 187: 8–18, 1999.

Bock KW, Lilienblum W: Roles of uridine diphosphate glucuronosyltransferases in chemical carcinogenesis, in Kauffman FC (ed). *Conjugation-Deconjugation Reactions in Drug Metabolism and Toxicity.* Berlin: Springer-Verlag, 1994, pp 391–428.

Boelsterli UA: Specific targets of covalent drug-protein interactions in hepatocytes and their toxicological significance in drug-induced liver injury. *Drug Metab Rev* 25:395–451, 1993.

Border WA, Ruoslahti E: Transforming growth factor-β in disease: The dark side of tissue repair. *J Clin Invest* 90:1–7, 1992.

Boulares HA, Giardina C, Navarro CL, et al: Modulation of serum growth factor signal transduction in Hepa 1-6 cells by acetaminophen: An inhibition of c-*myc* expression, NF-κB activation, and Raf-1 kinase activity. *Tox Sci* 48:264–274, 1999.

Breen AP, Murphy JA: Reactions of oxyl radicals with DNA. *Free Rad Biol Med* 18:1033–1077, 1995.

Buetler TM: Identification of glutathione S-transferase isozymes and γ-glutamylcysteine synthetase as negative acute-phase proteins in rat liver. *Hepatology* 28:1551–1560, 1998.

Buja LM, Eigenbrodt ML, Eigenbrodt EH: Apoptosis and necrosis: Basic types and mechanisms of cell death. *Arch Pathol Lab Med* 117:1208–1214, 1993.

Burk RF, Hill KE: Orphan selenoproteins. *BioEssays* 21:231–237, 1999.

Bursch W, Oberhammer F, Schulte-Hermann R: Cell death by apoptosis and its protective role against disease. *Trends Pharmacol Sci* 13:245–251, 1992.

Burt AD: C. L. Oakley Lecture (1993): Cellular and molecular aspects of hepatic fibrosis. *J Pathol* 170:105–114, 1993.

Cai J, Yang J, Jones DP: Mitochondrial control of apoptosis: The role of cytochrome *c. Biochim Biophys Acta* 1366:139–149, 1998.

Castro L, Rodriguez M, Radi R: Aconitase is readily inactivated by peroxynitrite, but not by its precursor, nitric oxide. *J Biol Chem* 269:29409–29415, 1994.

Cavalieri EL, Rogan EG: The approach to understanding aromatic hydrocarbon carcinogenesis: The central role of radical cations in metabolic activation. *Pharmacol Ther* 55:183–199, 1992.

Chen W, Martindale L, Holbrook NJ, Liu Y: Tumor promoter arsenite activates extracellular signal-regulated kinase through a signaling pathway mediated by epidermal growth factor receptor and Shc. *Mol Cell Biol* 18:5178–5188, 1998.

Cohen SD, Pumford NR, Khairallah EA, et al: Contemporary issues in toxicology: Selective protein covalent binding and target organ toxicity. *Toxicol Appl Pharmacol* 143:1–2, 1997.

Coleman MD, Jacobus DP: Reduction of dapsone hydroxylamine to dapsone during methaemoglobin formation in human erythrocytes in vitro. *Biochem Pharmacol* 45:1027–1033, 1993.

Coles B: Effects of modifying structure on electrophilic reactions with biological nucleophiles. *Drug Metab Rev* 15:1307–1334, 1984.

Commandeur JNM, Vermeulen NPE: Molecular and biochemical mechanisms of chemically induced nephrotoxicity: A review. *Chem Res Toxicol* 3:171–194, 1990.

Corcoran GB, Fix L, Jones DP, et al: Apoptosis: Molecular control point in toxicity. *Toxicol Appl Pharmacol* 128:169–181, 1994.

Cotgreave IA, Moldeus P, Orrenius S: Host biochemical defense mechanisms against prooxidants. *Annu Rev Pharmacol Toxicol* 28:189–212, 1988.

Cunningham CC, Coleman VVB, Spach PI: The effects of chronic ethanol consumption on hepatic mitochondria energy metabolism. *Alcohol Alcohol* 25:127–136, 1990.

Dalton TP, Shertzer HG, Puga A: Regulation of gene expression by reactive oxygen. *Annu Rev Pharmacol Toxicol* 39:67–101, 1999.

D'Amours D, Desnoyers S, D'Silva I, Poirier GG: Poly(ADP-ribosyl)ation reactions in the regulation of nuclear functions. *Biochem J* 342:249–268, 1999.

Davies KJ: Protein damage and degradation by oxygen radicals: I. General aspects. *J Biol Chem* 262:9895–9901, 1987.

Dekant W, Vamvakas S, Anders MW. Bioactivation of nephrotoxic haloalkenes by glutathione conjugation: Formation of toxic and mutagenic intermediates by cysteine conjugate β-lyase. *Drug Metab Rev* 20:43–83, 1989.

De Matteis F: Drugs as suicide substrates of cytochrome P450, in De Matteis F, Lock EA (eds): *Selectivity and Molecular Mechanisms of Toxicity.* Houndmills, England: Macmillan, 1987, pp 183–210.

Desaiah D: Biochemical mechanisms of chlordecone neurotoxicity: A review. *Neurotoxicology* 3:103–110, 1982.

Eaton DL, Gallagher EP: Mechanisms of aflatoxin carcinogenesis. *Annu Rev Pharmacol Toxicol* 34:135–172, 1994.

Edwards MJ, Keller BJ, Kauffman FC, Thurman RG: The involvement of Kupffer cells in carbon tetrachloride toxicity. *Toxicol Appl Pharmacol* 119:275–279, 1993.

Elbling L, Berger W, Rehberger A, et al: P-Glycoprotein regulates chemosensitivity in early developmental stages of the mouse. *FASEB J* 7:1499–1506, 1993.

Engler H, Taurog A, Nakashima T: Mechanism of inactivation of thyroid peroxidase by thioureylene drugs. *Biochem Pharmacol* 31:3801–3806, 1982.

Fan W: Possible mechanisms of paclitaxel-induced apoptosis. *Biochem Pharmacol* 57:1215–1221, 1991.

Fausto N: Liver regeneration. *J Hepatol* 32:19–31, 2000.

Fausto N, Webber EM: Control of liver growth. *Crit Rev Eukaryot Gene Expr* 3:117–135, 1993.

Fernando MR, Nanri H, Yoshitake S, et al: Thioredoxin regenerates proteins inactivated by oxidative stress in endothelial cells. *Eur J Biochem* 209:917–922, 1992.

Fletcher KA, Barton PF, Kelly JA: Studies on the mechanisms of oxidation in the erythrocyte by metabolites of primaquine. *Biochem Pharmacol* 37:2683–2690, 1988.

Franks NP, Lieb WR: Which molecular targets are most relevant to general anaesthesia? *Toxicol Lett* 100–101:1–8, 1998.

Fromenty B, Pessayre D: Impaired mitochonrial function in microvesicular steatosis. Effects of drugs, ethanol, hormones and cytokines. *J Hepatol* 26:43–53, 1997.

Fu SY, Gordon T: The cellular and molecular basis of peripheral nerve regeneration. *Mol Neurobiol* 14:67–116, 1997.

Gale K: Role of GABA in the genesis of chemoconvulsant seizures. *Toxicol Lett* 64–65:417–428, 1992.

Goering PL: Lead-protein interactions as a basis for lead toxicity. *Neurotoxicology* 14:45–60, 1993.

Goering PL, Waalkes MP, Klaassen CD: Toxicology of cadmium, in Goyer RA, Cherian MG (eds): *Toxicology of Metals: Biochemical Aspects.* Berlin: Springer-Verlag, 1995, pp 189–214.

Goldberg Y: Protein phosphatase 2A: Who shall regulate the regulator? *Biochem Pharmacol* 4:321–328, 1999.

Gonzalez FJ, Fernandez-Salguero P: The aryl hydrocarbon receptor. Studies using the AHR-null mice. *Drug Metab Dispos* 26:1194–1198, 1998.

Gravina SA, Mieyal JJ: Thioltransferase is a specific glutathionyl mixed disulfide oxidoreductase. *Biochemistry* 32:3368–3376, 1993.

Green DR: Apoptotic pathways: The roads to ruin. *Cell* 94:695–698, 1998.

Green S: Nuclear receptors and chemical carcinogenesis. *Trends Pharmacol Sci* 13:251–255, 1992.

Gregus Z, Klaassen CD: Enterohepatic circulation of toxicants, in Rozman K, Hanninien O (eds): *Gastrointestinal Toxicology.* Amsterdam: Elsevier/North Holland, 1986, pp 57–118.

Gressner AM: Hepatic fibrogenesis: The puzzle of interacting cells, fibrogenic cytokines, regulatory loops, and extracellular matrix molecules. *Z Gastroenterol* 30(suppl 1):5–16, 1992.

Hardman JG, Gilman AG, Limbird LL (eds): *Goodman & Gilman's The Pharmacological Basis of Therapeutics,* 9th ed. McGraw-Hill: New York, 1995.

Herken H, Hucho F (eds): *Selective Neurotoxicity.* Berlin: Springer-Verlag, 1992.

Herman B, Gores GJ, Nieminen AL, et al: Calcium and pH in anoxic and toxic injury. *Crit Rev Toxicol* 21:127–148, 1990.

Herrlich P, Rahmsdorf HJ, Bender, K: Signal transduction induced by adverse agents: "Activation by inhibition." The UV response 1997, in Puga A. Wallace KB (eds): *Molecular Biology of the Toxic Response.* Philadelphia: Taylor & Francis, 1999, pp 479–492.

Hershko A, Ciechanover A: The ubiquitin system. *Annu Rev Biochem* 67:425–479, 1998.

Heuchel R, Radtke F, Georgiev O, et al: The transcription factor MTF-1 is essential for basal and heavy metal-induced metallothionein gene expression. *EMBO J* 13:2870–2875, 1994.

Hill DA, Jean PA, Roth RA: Bile duct epithelial cells exposed to alpha-naphthylisothiocyanate produce a factor that causes neutrophil-dependent hepatocellular injury in vitro. *Tox Sci* 47:118–125, 1999.

Hippeli S, Elstner EF: Transition metal ion-catalyzed oxygen activation during pathogenic processes. *FEBS Lett* 443:1–7, 1999.

Jäättelä M: Escaping cell death: Survival proteins in cancer. *Exp Cell Res* 248:30–43, 1999.

Jaeschke H: Cellular adhesion molecules: Regulation and functional significance in the pathogenesis of liver diseases. *Am J Physiol* 273:G602–G611, 1997.

Jakoby WB, Ziegler DM: The enzymes of detoxication. *J Biol Chem* 265:20715–20718, 1990.

Johnson AR: Contact inhibition in the failure of mammalian CNS axonal regeneration. *Bioessays* 15:807–813, 1993.

Johnson DG, Walker CL: Cyclins and cell cycle checkpoints. *Annu Rev Pharmacol Toxicol* 39:295–312, 1999.

Kappus H: Overview of enzyme systems involved in bio-reduction of drugs and in redox cycling. *Biochem Pharmacol* 35:1–6, 1986.

Ketterer B: Protective role of glutathione and glutathione transferases in mutagenesis and carcinogenesis. *Mutat Res* 202:343–361, 1988.

Kodavanti UP, Mehendale HM: Cationic amphiphilic drugs and phospholipid storage disorder. *Pharmacol Rev* 42:327–353, 1990.

Krell H, Metz J, Jaeschke H, et al: Drug-induced intrahepatic cholestasis: Characterization of different pathomechanisms. *Arch Toxicol* 60:124–130, 1987.

Kroemer G, Dallaporta B, Resche-Rigon M: The mitochondrial death/life regulator in apoptosis and necrosis. *Annu Rev Physiol* 60:619–642, 1998.

Kröncke KD, Fricker G, Meier PJ, et al: α-Amanitin uptake into hepatocytes: Identification of hepatic membrane transport systems used by amatoxins. *J Biol Chem* 261:12562–12567, 1986.

Larsson BS: Interaction between chemicals and melanin. *Pigment Cell Res* 6:127–133, 1993.

Laurent G, Kishore BK, Tulkens PM: Aminoglycoside-induced renal phospholipidosis and nephrotoxicity. *Biochem Pharmacol* 40:2383–2392, 1990.

Lee J, Richburg JH, Younkin SC, Boekelheide K: The Fas system is a key regulator of germ cell apoptosis in the testis. *Endocrinology* 138:2081–2088, 1997.

Lee JI, Burckart GJ: Nuclear factor kappa B: important transcription factor and therapeutic target. *J Clin Pharmacol* 38:981–993, 1998.

Lehmann AR, Dean SW: Cancer-prone human disorders with defects in DNA repair, in Cooper CS, Grover PL (eds): *Chemical Carcinogenesis and Mutagenesis II.* Berlin: Springer-Verlag, 1990, pp 71–101.

Leist M, Nicotera P: Calcium and neuronal death. *Rev Physiol Biochem Pharmacol* 132:79–125, 1997.

Leist M, Single B, Castoldi AF, et al: Intracellular adenosine triphosphate (ATP) concentration: a switch in the decision between apoptosis and necrosis. *J Exp Med* 185:1481–1486, 1997.

Lelli JL, Becks LL, Dabrowska MI, Hinshaw DB: ATP converts necrosis to apoptosis in oxidant-injured endothelial cells. *Free Rad Biol Med* 25:694–702, 1998.

Lemasters JJ, Nieminen AL, Qian T, et al: The mitochondrial permeability transition in cell death: A common mechanism in necrosis, apoptosis and autophagy. *Biochim Biophys Acta* 1366:177–196, 1998.

Lewis W, Levine ES, Griniuviene B, et al: Fialuridine and its metabolites inhibit DNA polymerase γ at sites of multiple adjacent analog incorporation, decrease mtDNA abundance, and cause mitochondrial structural defects in cultured hepatoblasts. *Proc Natl Acad Sci* 93:3592–3597, 1996.

Lim RT Jr, Gentry RT, Ito D, et al: First-pass metabolism of ethanol is predominantly gastric. *Alcohol Clin Exp Res* 17:1337–1344, 1993.

Lin JH, Chiba M, Baillie TA: Is the role of the small intestine in first-pass metabolism overemphasized? *Pharmacol Rev* 51:135–137, 1999.

Lindroos PM, Zarnegar R, Michalopoulos GK: Hepatocyte growth factor (hepatopoietin A) rapidly increases in plasma before DNA synthesis and liver regeneration stimulated by partial hepatectomy and carbon tetrachloride administration. *Hepatology* 13:743–750, 1991.

Lozano RM, Yee BC, Buchanan BB: Thioredoxin-linked reductive inactivation of venom neurotoxins. *Arch Biochem Biophys* 309:356–362, 1994.

Ma X, Babish JG: Activation of signal transduction pathways by dioxins. "Activation by inhibition." The UV response 1997. Puga A, Wallace KB (eds): *Molecular Biology of the Toxic Response.* Philadelphia: Taylor & Francis, 1999, pp 493–516.

Meyer M, Schreck R, Baeuerle PA: H_2O_2 and antioxidants have opposite effects on activation of NF-κB and AP-1 in intact cells: AP-1 as secondary antioxidant-responsive factor. *EMBO J* 12:2005–2015, 1993.

Miller JA, Surh Y-J: Sulfonation in chemical carcinogenesis, in Kauffman FC (ed): *Conjugation-Deconjugation Reactions in Drug Metabolism and Toxicity.* Berlin: Springer-Verlag, 1994, pp 429–457.

Miller MS: Tumor suppressor genes in rodent lung carcinogenesis. Mutation of *p*53 does not appear to be an early lesion in lung tumor pathogenesis. *Toxicol Appl Pharmacol* 156:70–77, 1999.

Mohn KL, Laz TM, Hsu JC, et al: The immediate-early growth response in regenerating liver and insulin-stimulated H-35 cells: Comparison with serum-stimulated 3T3 cells and identification of 41 novel immediate-early genes. *Mol Cell Biol* 11:381–390, 1991.

Morimoto RI: Cells in stress: Transcriptional activation of heat shock genes. *Science* 259:1409–1410, 1993.

Moskovitz J, Berlett BS, Poston JM, Stadtman ER: Methionine sulfoxide reductase in antioxidant defense. *Methods Enzymol* 300:239–244, 1999.

Murphy MP: Nitric oxide and cell death. *Biochim Biophys Acta* 1411:401–414, 1999.

Mustafa MG: Biochemical basis of ozone toxicity. *Free Radic Biol Med* 9:245–265, 1990.

Narahashi T: Nerve membrane Na^+ channels as targets of insecticides. *Trends Pharmacol Sci* 13:236–241, 1992.

Narahashi T: Transmitter-activated ion channels as the target of chemical agents, in Kito S et al (eds): *Neuroreceptor Mechanisms in the Brain.* New York: Plenum Press, 1991, pp 61–73.

Nelson SD, Pearson PG: Covalent and noncovalent interactions in acute lethal cell injury caused by chemicals. *Annu Rev Pharmacol Toxicol* 30:169–195, 1990.

Nicholson DW, Thornberry NA: Caspases: Killer proteases. *Trends Biochem Sci* 22:299–306, 1997.

Nicotera P, Bellomo G, Orrenius S: Calcium-mediated mechanisms in chemically induced cell death. *Annu Rev Pharmacol Toxicol* 32:449–470, 1992.

Noji S, Tashiro K, Koyama E, et al: Expression of hepatocyte growth factor gene in endothelial and Kupffer cells of damaged rat livers, as revealed by in situ hybridization. *Biochem Biophys Res Commun* 173:42–47, 1990.

Oortgiesen M, Leinders T, van Kleef RG, Vijverberg HP: Differential neurotoxicological effects of lead on voltage-dependent and receptor-operated ion channels. *Neurotoxicology* 14:87–96, 1993.

Osawa Y, Davila JC, Nakatsuka M, et al: Inhibition of P450 cytochromes by reactive intermediates. *Drug Metab Rev* 27:61–72, 1995.

Park BK, Pirmohamed M, Kitteringham NR: Role of drug disposition in drug hypersensitivity: A chemical, molecular, and clinical perspective. *Chem Res Toxicol* 11:969–988, 1998.

Patel MN, Yim GK, Isom GE: *N*-methyl-*D*-aspartate receptors mediate cyanide-induced cytotoxicity in hippocampal cultures. *Neurotoxicology* 14:35–40, 1993.

Pegg AE, Byers TL: Repair of DNA containing O^6-alkylguanine. *FASEB J* 6:2302–2310, 1992.

Perouansky M, Kirson ED, Yaari Y: Mechanism of action of volatile anesthetics: Effects of halothane on glutamate receptors in vitro. *Toxicol Lett* 100–101:65–69, 1998.

Peters JM, Aoyama T, Cattley RC, et al: Role of peroxisome proliferator-activated receptor α in altered cell cycle regulation in mouse liver. *Carcinogenesis* 19:1989–1994, 1998.

Podolsky DK: Mucosal immunity and inflammation. V. Innate mechanisms of mucosal defense and repair: The best offense is a good defense. *Am J Physiol* 277:G495–G499, 1999.

Poellinger L, Göttlicher M, Gustafsson JA: The dioxin and peroxisome proliferator-activated receptors: Nuclear receptors in search of endogenous ligands. *Trends Pharmacol Sci* 13:241–245, 1992.

Poirier LA: Methyl group deficiency in hepatocarcinogenesis. *Drug Metab Rev* 26:185–199, 1994.

Poli V: The role of C/EBP isoforms in the control of inflammatory and native immunity functions. *J Biol Chem* 273:29279–29282, 1998.

Pryor WA, Squadrito GL: The chemistry of peroxynitrite: A product from the reaction of nitric oxide with superoxide. *Am J Physiol* 268:L699–L722, 1995.

Pumford NR, Halmes NC: Protein targets of xenobiotic reactive intermediates. *Annu Rev Pharmacol Toxicol* 37:91–117, 1997.

Qian T, Herman B, Lemasters JJ: The mitochondrial permeability transition mediates both necrotic and apoptotic death of hepatocytes exposed to Br-A23187. *Toxicol Appl Pharmacol* 154:117–125, 1999.

Raghow R: The role of extracellular matrix in postinflammatory wound healing and fibrosis. *FASEB J* 8:823–831, 1994.

Ramos KS, Zhang Y, Bral CM: Ras activation by benzo[*a*]pyrene, in Puga A, Wallace KB (eds): *Molecular Biology of the Toxic Response.* Philadelphia: Taylor & Francis, 1999, pp 517–530.

Recknagel RO, Glende EA Jr, Dolak JA, Waller RL: Mechanisms of carbon tetrachloride toxicity. *Pharmacol Ther* 43:139–154, 1989.

Reed JC, Jurgensmeier JM, Matsuyama S: Bcl-2 family proteins and mitochondria. *Biochim Biophys Acta* 1366:127–137, 1998.

Richter C, Kass GE: Oxidative stress in mitochondria: Its relationship to cellular Ca^{2+} homeostasis, cell death, proliferation, and differentiation. *Chem Biol Interact* 77:1–23, 1991.

Rombach EM, Hanzlik RP: Detection of adducts of bromobenzene 3,4-oxide with rat liver microsomal protein sulfhydryl groups using specific antibodies. *Chem Res Toxicol* 12:159–163, 1999.

Rose ML, Rusyn I, Bojes HK, et al: Role of Kupffer cells in peroxisome proliferator-induced hepatocyte proliferation. *Drug Metab Rev* 31:87–116, 1999.

Rothwell NJ: Functions and mechanisms of interleukin 1 in the brain. *Trends Pharmacol Sci* 12:430–436, 1991.

Saido TC, Sorimachi H, Suzuki K: Calpain: New perspectives in molecular diversity and physiological-pathological involvement. *FASEB J* 8:814–822, 1994.

Sancar A, Sancar GB: DNA repair enzymes. *Annu Rev Biochem* 57:2967, 1988.

Scheschonka A, Murphy ME, Sies H: Temporal relationships between the loss of vitamin E, protein sulfhydryls and lipid peroxidation in microsomes challenged with different prooxidants. *Chem Biol Interact* 74:233–252, 1990.

Schinkel AH: P-glycoprotein, a gatekeeper in the blood-brain barrier. *Adv Drug Delivery Rev* 36:179–194, 1999.

Schulte-Hermann R, Timmermann-Trosiener I, Barthel G, Bursch W: DNA synthesis, apoptosis, and phenotypic expression as determinants of growth of altered foci in rat liver during phenobarbital promotion. *Cancer Res* 50:5127–5135, 1990.

Scicchitano DA, Hanawalt PC: Intragenomic repair heterogeneity of DNA damage. *Environ Health Perspect* 98:45–51, 1992.

Selby CP, Sancar A: Molecular mechanism of transcription-repair coupling. *Science* 260:53–58, 1993.

Shi X, Dalal NS: NADPH-dependent flavoenzymes catalyze one electron reduction of metal ions and molecular oxygen and generate hydroxyl radicals. *FEBS Lett* 276:189–191,1990.

Sies H: Strategies of antioxidant defense. *Eur J Biochem* 215:213–219, 1993.

Smith MR, Matthews NT, Jones KA, Kung HE: Biological actions of oncogenes. *Pharmacol Ther* 58:211–236, 1993.

Soni MG, Mehendale HM: Role of tissue repair in toxicologic interactions among hepatotoxic organics. *Environ Health Perspect* 106:1307–1317, 1998.

Squadrito GL, Pryor WA: Oxidative chemistry of nitric oxide: The roles of superoxide, peroxynitrite, and carbon dioxide. *Free Rad Biol Med* 25:392–403, 1998.

Stachlewitz RF, Seabra V, Bradford B, et al: Glycine and uridine prevent D-galactosamine hepatoxicity in the rat: Role of the Kupffer cells. *Hepatology* 29:737–145, 1999.

Sun X, Tian X, Tomsig JL, Suszkiw JB: Analysis of differential effects of Pb^{2+} on protein kinase C isozymes. *Toxicol Appl Pharmacol* 156:40–45, 1999.

Szabó C: DNA strand breakage and activation of poly-ADP ribosyltransferase: A cytotoxic pathway triggered by peroxynitrite. *Free Rad Biol Med* 21:855–869, 1996.

Toivola DM, Eriksson JE: Toxins affecting cell signalling and alteration of cytoskeletal structure. *Tox In Vitro* 13:521–530, 1999.

Uetrecht JP: The role of leukocyte-generated reactive metabolites in the pathogenesis of idiosyncratic drug reactions. *Drug Metab Rev* 24:299–366, 1992.

Vallyathan V, Shi X, Castranova V: Reactive oxygen species: Their relation to pneumoconiosis and carcinogenesis. *Environ Health Perspect* 106:1151–1155, 1998.

Van Kuijk FJGM, Sevanian A, Handelman GJ, Dratz EA: A new role for phospholipase A2: Protection of membranes from lipid peroxidation damage. *TIBS* 12:31–34, 1987.

Waddick KG, Uckun FM: Innovative treatment programs against cancer. II. Nuclear factor-κB (NF-κB) as a molecular gartet. *Biochem Pharmacol* 57:9–17, 1999.

Wallace KB, Starkov AA: Mitochondrial targets of drug toxicity. *Annu Rev Pharmacol Toxicol* 40:353–388, 2000.

Wang JF, Komarov P, de Groot H: Luminol chemiluminescence in rat macrophages and granulocytes: The role of NO, O_2/H_2O_2, and HOCl. *Arch Biochem Biophys* 304:189–196, 1993.

Weiss SJ, LoBuglio AF: Phagocyte-generated oxygen metabolites and cellular injury. *Lab Invest* 47:5–18, 1982.

Wyllie AH: Apoptosis: an overview. *Brit Med Bull* 53:451–465, 1997.

Yamasaki H, Krutovskikh V, Mesnil M, et al: Gap junctional intercellular communication and cell proliferation during rat liver carcinogenesis. *Environ Health Perspect* 101(suppl 5):191–197, 1993.

Yin M, Ikejima K, Arteel GE, et al: Glycine accelerates recovery from alcohol-induced liver injury. *J Pharmacol Exp Therap* 286:1014–1019, 1998.

Zawaski K, Gruebele A, Kaplan D, et al: Evidence for enhanced expression of c-*fos*, c-*jun*, and the Ca^{2+}-activated neutral protease in rat liver following carbon tetrachloride administration. *Biochem Biophys Res Commun* 197:585–590, 1993.

CHAPTER 4

RISK ASSESSMENT

Elaine M. Faustman and Gilbert S. Omenn

INTRODUCTION AND HISTORICAL CONTEXT

Toxicologic research and toxicity testing conducted and interpreted by toxicologists constitute the scientific core of an important activity known as risk assessment for chemical exposures. For decades, the American Conference of Governmental Industrial Hygienists (ACGIH) has set threshold limit values for occupational exposures and the U.S. Food and Drug Administration (FDA) has established acceptable daily intakes for pesticide residues and food additives. In 1958, the U.S. Congress instructed the FDA in the Delaney clause to prohibit the addition to the food supply of all substances found to cause cancer in animals or humans. Pragmatically, this policy allowed food sources that had nondetectable levels of these additives to be declared "safe." As advances in analytic chemistry revealed that "nondetects" were not equivalent to "not present," regulatory agencies were forced to develop "tolerance levels" and "acceptable risk levels." Risk assessment methodologies blossomed in the 1970s (Albert, 1994).

Together with the federal regulatory agencies, the White House Office of Science and Technology Policy developed a framework for regulatory decision making (Calkins et al., 1980; ILRG, 1979). The National Research Council then detailed the steps of hazard identification, dose–response assessment, exposure analysis, and characterization of risks (NRC, 1983) in *Risk Assessment in the Federal Government: Managing the Process* (widely known as "The Red Book"). This framework has evolved into the scheme shown in Fig. 4-1, providing a consistent framework for risk assessment across agencies. Figure 4-1 now shows a modified risk framework with bidirectional arrows showing an ideal situation where mechanistic research feeds directly into risk assessments and critical data uncertainty drives research. Initially, attention was focused on cancer risks; in recent years, noncancer endpoints have been examined with similar methods. Continuing advances in toxicology, epidemiology, exposure assessment, biologically based modeling of adverse responses, and modeling of variability and uncertainty have led to improvements in risk assessment. Nevertheless, public policy objectives often require extrapolations that go far beyond the observation of actual effects and reflect different tolerance for risks, generating controversy.

The 1990 Amendments to the U.S. Clean Air Act led to two far-reaching reports triggered by Congressional action to force action on section 112, "Hazardous Air Pollutants." During the previous 20 years only seven substances had been regulated under this section of the law (vinyl chloride, asbestos, benzene, radionuclides, mercury, arsenic, and beryllium), using chemical-by-chemical risk-based analyses, largely because the statute required that the exposure standard provide an "ample margin of safety" below a no-effect level, which was widely agreed to be zero for carcinogens. Congress mandated an entirely new program to control 189 named hazardous air pollutants from point sources with maximum available control technology during the 1990s, to be followed over the next decade with determination of any unacceptable residual risks by methods informed by the mandated reports.

In 1994, the National Academy of Sciences report entitled *Science and Judgment in Risk Assessment* captured in its title the combination of qualitative and quantitative approaches essential to effective assessment of risks (NRC, 1994). This report discusses in detail the challenges and provides approaches for incorporating new scientific findings into the risk assessment process. It also highlights approaches to deal with uncertainty when insufficient scientific information is available. Following up on many of the challenges, the Presidential/Congressional Commission on Risk Assessment and Risk Management (Risk Commission, 1997) formulated a comprehensive framework that is being applied widely. The two crucial concepts are (1) putting each environmental problem or issue into public health and/or ecological context and (2) proactively engaging the relevant stakeholders, often affected or potentially affected community groups, from the very beginning of the six-stage process shown in Fig. 4-2. Particular exposures and potential health effects must be evaluated across sources and exposure pathways and in light of multiple endpoints, not just one chemical, in one environmental medium (air, water, soil, food, products), for one health effect at a time—the general approach up

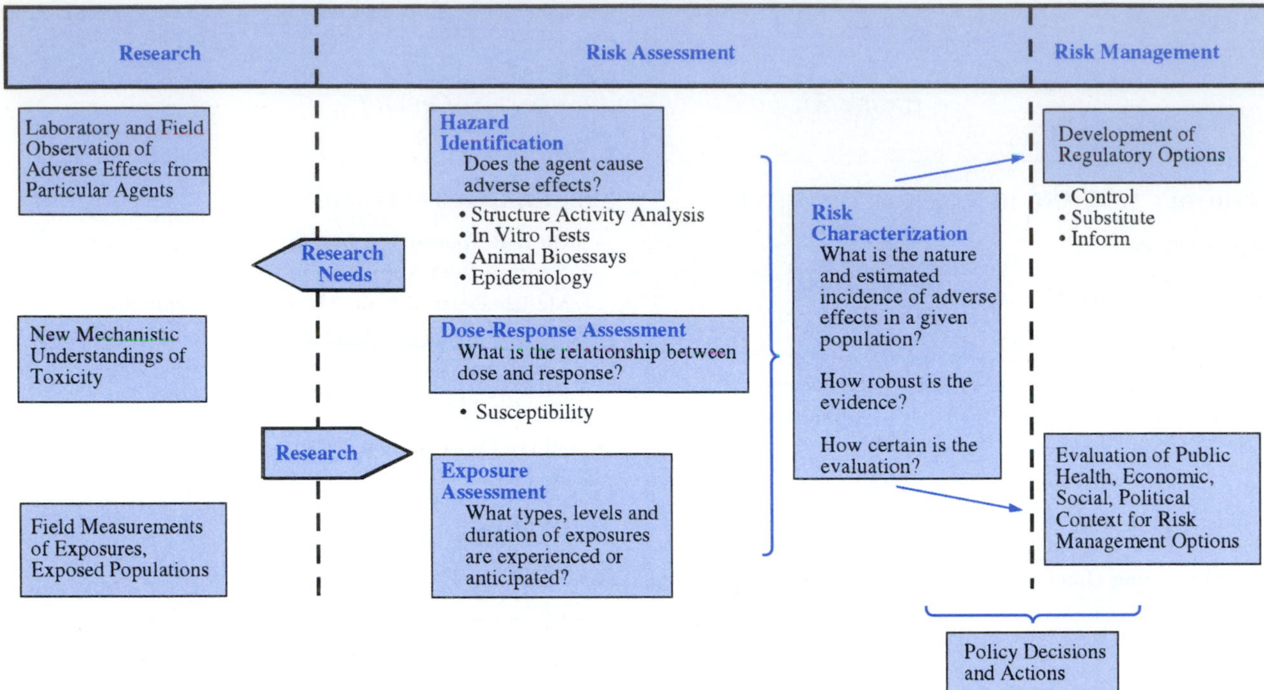

Figure 4-1. Risk assessment/risk management framework.

This framework shows in blue the four key steps of risk assessment: hazard identification, dose-response assessment, exposure assessment, and risk characterization. It shows an interactive, two-way process where research needs from the risk assessment process drive new research, and new research findings modify risk assessment outcomes. (Adapted from NRC, 1983; 1994; Calkins, 1980; Faustman, 1996; Gargas, 1999.)

to the present. A similar framework has been utilized by the Health and Safety Executive Risk Assessment Policy Unit of the United Kingdom (HSE, 2000).

DEFINITIONS

Risk assessment is the systematic scientific characterization of potential adverse health effects resulting from human exposures to hazardous agents or situations (NRC, 1983, 1994; Omenn and Faustman, 2000). *Risk* is defined as the probability of an adverse outcome. The term *hazard* is used in the United States and Canada to refer to intrinsic toxic properties, whereas internationally this term is defined as the probability of an adverse outcome. Risk assessment requires qualitative information about the strength of the evidence and the nature of the outcomes—as well as quantitative assessment of the exposures, host susceptibility factors, and potential magnitude of the risk—and then a description of the uncertainties in the estimates and conclusions. The objectives of risk assessment are outlined in Table 4-1. Analogous approaches are applied to ecologic risks (NRC, 1993a).

The phrase *characterization of risk* may better reflect the combination of qualitative and quantitative analysis. Unfortunately, many toxicologists, public health practitioners, environmentalists, and regulators tend to equate risk assessment with quantitative risk assessment, generating a number (or a number with uncertainty bounds) for an overly precise risk estimate and then ignoring crucial information about the mechanism of effect across species, inconsistent findings across studies, multiple variable health effects, and means of avoiding or reversing the effects of exposures.

Risk management refers to the process by which policy actions are chosen to control hazards identified in the risk assessment/risk characterization stage of the six-stage framework (Fig. 4-2). Risk managers consider scientific evidence and risk estimates—along with statutory, engineering, economic, social, and political factors—in evaluating alternative options and choosing among those options (Risk Commission, 1997). (Chapter 34 discusses approaches to regulatory options.)

Risk communication is the challenging process of making risk assessment and risk management information comprehensible to community groups, lawyers, local elected officials, judges, business people, labor, and environmentalists (Morgan, 1993;

Table 4-1
Objectives of Risk Assessment

1. Balance risks and benefits.
    - Drugs
    - Pesticides
2. Set target levels of risk.
    - Food contaminants
    - Water pollutants
3. Set priorities for program activities.
    - Regulatory agencies
    - Manufacturers
    - Environmental/consumer organizations
4. Estimate residual risks and extent of risk reduction after steps are taken to reduce risks.

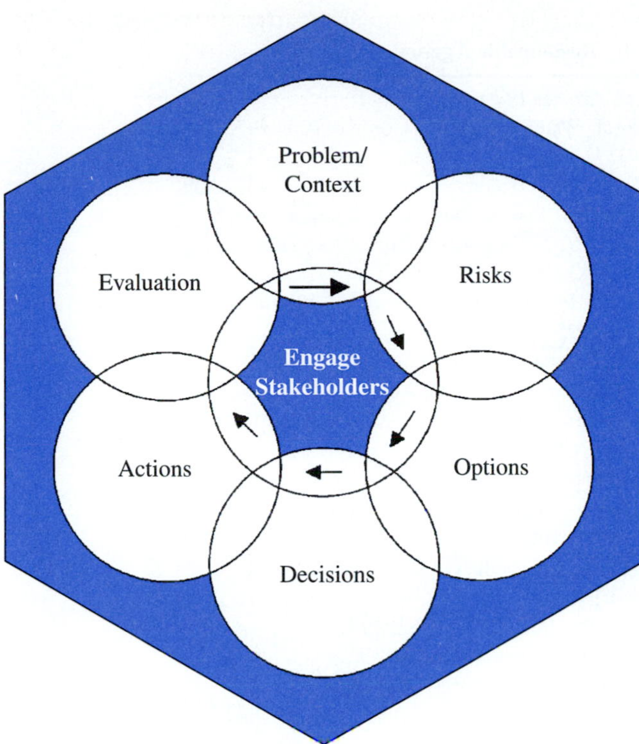

Figure 4-2. Risk management framework for environmental health from the U.S. Commission on Risk Assessment and Risk Management, "Omenn Commission."

The framework comprises six stages: (1) formulating the problem in a broad public health context; (2) analyzing the risks; (3) defining the options; (4) making risk-reduction decisions; (5) implementing those actions; and (6) evaluating the effectiveness of the actions taken. Interactions with stakeholders are critical and thus have been put at the center of the framework. (Omenn 1996; Risk Commission, 1997; Charnley, 1997; Ohanian, 1997.)

Sandman, 1993; NRC, 1996; Fischhoff et al., 1996). A crucial, too-often neglected requirement for communication is listening to the fears, perceptions, priorities, and proposed remedies of these "stakeholders." Often these people have important inputs for various stages of the process, as illustrated in volume 1 of the Risk Commission reports (1997). Sometimes the decision makers and stakeholders simply want to know the "bottom line": is a substance or a situation "safe" or not? Others will be keenly interested in knowing why the risk estimates are uncertain and may be well prepared to challenge underlying assumptions about context and methodology. *Risk perception* is discussed at the end of this chapter.

DECISION MAKING

Risk management decisions are reached under diverse statutes in the United States (Table 4-2).

Some statutes specify reliance on risk alone, while others require a balancing of risks and benefits of the product or activity (Table 4-1). Risk assessments provide a valuable framework for priority setting within regulatory and health agencies, in the chemical development process within companies, and in resource allocation by environmental organizations. Similar statutes and regulatory regimes have been developed in many other countries and through such international organizations as the International Programme for Chemical Safety (IPCS) of the World Health Organization (WHO). Currently, there are significant efforts toward the harmonization of testing protocols and then the assessment of risks and standards.

A major challenge for risk assessment, risk communication, and risk management is to work across disciplines to demonstrate the biological plausibility and clinical significance of the conclusions from epidemiologic, lifetime animal, short-term in vitro and in vivo, and structure-activity studies of chemicals thought to have potential adverse effects. Biomarkers of exposure, effect, or individual susceptibility can link the presence of a chemical in various environmental compartments to specific sites of action in target organs and to host responses (NRC, 1989a, 1989b, 1992a, 1992b). Mechanistic investigations of the actions of specific chemicals can help us penetrate the "black box" approach of simply counting tumors, for example, in exposed animals in routine bioassays. Greater appreciation of the mechanisms and extent of individual variation in susceptibility among humans can improve protection of subgroups of susceptible people and better relate findings in animals to the characterization of risk for humans. Individual behavioral and social risk factors may be critically important both to the risk and the reduction of risk. Finally, public and media attitudes toward local polluters, other responsible parties, and relevant government agencies may lead to what has been labeled "the outrage factor" (Sandman, 1993), greatly influencing the communication process and the choices for risk management.

HAZARD IDENTIFICATION

Assessing Toxicity of Chemicals—Introduction

In many cases, toxicity information for chemicals is limited. For example, the Environmental Protection Agency (EPA) recently evaluated high-production-volume (HPV) chemicals (those produced in excess of 1 million lb/year) to ascertain the availability of chemical hazard data. Their study found that for 43 percent of these HPV chemicals, there were no publicly available studies for any of the basic toxicity endpoints (acute and chronic systemic toxicity, developmental/reproductive toxicity, genotoxicity/mutagenicity, ecotoxicity, and environmental fate). Only 7 percent of the HPV chemicals had a complete set of publicly available studies for these endpoints (EPA, 1998a). International efforts such as the Organization for Economic Development's screening information data set (OECD/SIDS) program are addressing many of these data needs, highlighted by the Environment Defense Fund in the book *Toxic Ignorance* (Roe et al., 1997). Data requirements for specific agents can vary greatly by compound type and applicable regulatory statutes. Table 4-3 shows requirements and 1997 costs for one example class of agents, pesticides (Stevens, 1997; 40 CFR 158.340; EPA, 1998c, 2000b). It also illustrates current international efforts to harmonize these testing guidelines by listing the new harmonized 870 test guidelines (EPA, 2000b). Increasing attention has been focused on this class of chemicals and reviews of available toxicity tests have shown the need for additional developmental neurobehavioral assessments (Makris et al., 1998). In summary, these critical data gaps in evaluating compounds have refocused attention on identifying new approaches that are both informative and cost and time efficient (NRC, 2000).

Table 4-2
Major Toxic Chemical Laws in the United States by Responsible Agency

EPA	Air pollutants	Clean Air Act 1970, 1977, 1990
	Water pollutants	Federal Water Pollution Control Act 1972, 1977
	Drinking water	Safe Drinking Water Act 1974, 1996
	Pesticides	Fungicides, Insecticides, & Rodenticides Act (FIFRA) 1972, Food Quality Protection Act (FQPA) 1996
	Ocean dumping	Marine Protection Research, Sanctuaries Act 1995 Ocean Radioactive Dumping Ban Act 1995
	Toxic chemicals	Toxic Substances Control Act (TSCA) 1976
	Hazardous wastes	Resource Conservation and Recovery Act (RCRA) 1976
	Abandoned hazardous wastes	Superfund (CERCLA) 1980, 1986
CEQ	Environmental impacts	National Environmental Policy Act (NEPA) 1969
OSHA	Workplace	Occupational Safety and Health (OSH) Act 1970
FDA	Foods, drugs, and cosmetics	FDC Acts 1906, 1938, 1962, 1977 FDA Modernization Act 1997
CPSC	Dangerous consumer products	Consumer Product Safety Act 1972
DOT	Transport of hazardous materials	THM Act 1975, 1976, 1978, 1979, 1984, 1990 (×2)

KEY: EPA, Environmental Protection Agency; CEQ, Council for Environmental Quality (now Office of Environmental Policy); OSHA, Occupational Safety and Health Administration; FDA, Food and Drug Administration; CPSC, Consumer Product Safety Commission; DOT, Department of Transportation.

Assessing Toxicity of Chemicals—Methods

Structure/Activity Relationships Given the cost of $1 to $2 million and the 3 to 5 years required for testing a single chemical in a lifetime rodent carcinogenicity bioassay, initial decisions on whether to continue development of a chemical, to submit premanufacturing notice (PMN), or to require additional testing may be based largely on structure/activity relationships (SARs) and limited short-term assays.

An agent's structure, solubility, stability, pH sensitivity, electrophilicity, volatility, and chemical reactivity can be important information for hazard identification. Historically, certain key molecular structures have provided regulators with some of the most readily available information on the basis of which to assess hazard potential. For example, 8 of the first 14 occupational carcinogens were regulated together by the Occupational Safety and Health Administration (OSHA) as belonging to the aromatic amine chemical class. The EPA Office of Toxic Substances relies on structure/activity relationships to meet deadlines to respond to premanufacturing notice for new chemical manufacture under the Toxic Substances Control Act (TSCA). Structural alerts such as *N*-nitroso or aromatic amine groups, amino azo dye structures, or phenanthrene nuclei are clues to prioritize agents for additional evaluation as potential carcinogens. The limited database of known developmental toxicants limits SARs to a few chemical classes, including chemicals with structures related to those of valproic acid, retinoic acid, and glycol ethers (NRC, 2000). For example, a report on developmentally toxic valproic acid derivatives relates their toxicity to activation of peroxisomal proliferation (Lampen et al., 1999).

Structure-activity relationships have been used for assessment of complex mixtures. A prominent application has been EPA's reassessment of risks associated with 2,3,7,8-tetrachlorodibenzo-*p*-dioxin (TCDD) and related chlorinated and brominated dibenzo-*p*-dioxins, dibenzofurans, and planar biphenyls, using toxicity equivalence factors (TEFs), based on induction of the aryl-hydrocarbon (Ah) receptor (EPA, 1994b). The estimated toxicity of environmental mixtures containing these chemicals was calculated as the sum of the product of the concentration of each multiplied by its TEF value. The World Health Organization has organized efforts to reach international consensus on TEFs used for polychlorinated biphenyls (PCBs), polychlorinated dibenzo-*p*-dioxins (PCDDs), and polychlorinated dibenzofurans (PCDFs) for both humans and wildlife (Van den Berg et al., 1998). EPA has issued new nomenclature for TEFs as part of their dioxin reassessment (www.epa.gov/ncea/dioxin.htm). However, it is difficult to predict activity across chemical classes and especially across multiple toxic endpoints using a single biological response. For these TEFs to be valid, all of the endpoints of toxicity must be mediated by the Ah receptor, yet direct measurement of activated Ah receptors in target human tissues is not currently feasible. Compounds within these complex mixtures can compete for the same receptor; thus, TEFs can be overly conservative. Many complex chemical/physical interactions are not easily understood and may be over-simplified. In draft proposals from EPA, cytochrome P450-1A2 (CYP1A2) activity or epidermal growth factor (EGF) receptor concentrations are proposed as activity

Table 4-3
EPA/FIFRA Requirement for Hazard Evaluation of Pesticides

GUIDELINE NO.	REVISED 870 GUIDELINE	TYPE OF TOXICITY STUDY	TEST SYSTEM	OBJECTIVE	APPROXIMATE COST/STUDY (US$)
81-1	1100	Acute oral	Rats	Define toxic dose by ingestion	2000
81-2	1200	Acute dermal	Rabbits	Define toxic dose by absorption through skin	1500
81-3	1300	Acute inhalation	Rats	Define toxic dose by inhalation	5000
81-4	2400	Ocular	Rabbits	Assess eye irritation/injury	1500
81-5	2500	Skin irritation	Rabbits	Assess skin irritation/injury	1000
81-6	2600	Sensitization	Guinea pigs	Assess allergic potential	3000
81-7	6100–6855	Neurotoxicity*†	Hens/rats	Assess nervous system injury	25,000†
84-2	5100–5915	Mutagenicity‡	In vivo/ in vitro	Determine genotoxic potential; screen for carcinogenicity	5,000§
82-1	3050–3465	Range-finding‡ Subacute (28- to 90-day§)	Rats Mice Dogs Rabbits	Determine effects following repeated doses; set dose level for longer studies	70,000 70,000 100,000 75,000
			Rats Mice	Identify target organs; set dose levels for chronic studies	190,000 190,000
83-5 83-2	4200–4300	Carcinogenicity/ Chronic toxicity	Rats Mice	Determine potential to induce tumors; define dose-response relationships (lifetime)	1, 400,000 800,000
83-1			Dogs	Determine long-term toxic effects (1 year)	400,000
83-3 83-4	3550–3800	Reproduction and teratogenicity	Rats Rabbits	Determine potential to cause fetal abnormalities and effects on development, fertility, pregnancy, and development of offspring over at least two generations	505,000
85-1	7485	Toxicokinetics	Rats Mice	Determine and quantitate the metabolic fate of a pesticide	100,000

*Required for organophosphate insecticides only.

†Additional neurotoxicity tests 81-7, 81-8, 82-6, 82-7, and 83-6 have been added to requirements for certain materials and can include tests such as functional observational battery, motor activity, developmental landmarks, and learning and memory assessments (Sette, 1991). Costs listed for this type of study are only those for the initial study, not additional testing.

‡Range-finding studies are not required but provide justification for setting dose levels in required studies. EPA-required studies can include reverse mutation assays in *Salmonella*, forward mutation assays in mammalian cells—e.g., Chinese hamster ovary cells, mouse lymphoma L5178Y (the locus cells)—and in vivo cytogenetics (Dearfield, 1990).

§Indicates per assay cost and represent 1997 estimates using guideline 81 series.

SOURCE: Adapted from Stevens, 1997, and updated with newly revised EPA 870 guideline information (EPA, 2000b). For details on changes in the Health Effects test guidelines reflective of the harmonization of the toxicology guidelines between the Office of Pollution Prevention and Toxics (OPPT) and the Office of Pesticide Programs (OPP) within the EPA and with the Organization for Economic Cooperation and Development (OECD) guidelines, see EPA, 2000b (*http://www.epa.gov/OPPTS_Harmonized/870_Health_Effects_Test_Guidelines*).

surrogates across structurally related dioxin-like compounds for modeling mutation and growth rates.

Computerized SAR methods have given disappointing results in the National Toxicology Program (NTP) 44-chemical rodent carcinogenicity prediction challenge (Ashby and Tennant, 1994; Omenn et al., 1995). Much more focused efforts are those of pharmaceutical companies successfully using three-dimensional (3D) molecular modeling approaches to design ligands (new drugs) that can sterically fit into "receptors of interest." The basis for this strategy is pharmacophore mapping, 3D searching and molecular design, and establishment of 3D quantitative structure– activity relationships (Diener, 1997; Martin, 1993).

In Vitro and Short-Term Tests The next approach for hazard identification comprises in vitro or short-term tests, ranging from bacterial mutation assays performed entirely in vitro to more elaborate short-term tests such as skin-painting studies in mice or altered rat liver–foci assays conducted in vivo. For example, EPA mutagenicity guidelines call for assessment of reverse mutations using the Ames *Salmonella typhimurium* assay; forward mutations using mammalian cells, mouse lymphoma L5178Y, Chinese hamster ovary, or Chinese hamster lung fibroblasts; and in vivo cytogenetics assessment (bone marrow metaphase analysis or micronucleus tests). Chapter 8 discusses uses of these assays for identifying chemical carcinogens and Chap. 9 describes in detail various assays of genetic and mutagenic endpoints. Other assays evaluate developmental toxicity (NRC, 2000; Lewandowski et al., 2000; Brown et al., 1995; Whittaker and Faustman, 1994; Schwetz, 1993; Faustman, 1988), reproductive toxicity (Shelby et al., 1993; Harris et al., 1992; Gray, 1988), neurotoxicity (Costa, 2000; Atterwill et al., 1992), and immunotoxicity (Chap. 12). Less information is available on the extrapolation of these tests results for noncancer risk assessment than for the mutagenicity or carcinogenicity endpoints; however, mechanistic information obtained in these systems has been applied to risk assessment (NRC, 2000; Abbott et al., 1992; EPA, 1994a; Leroux et al., 1996). Overall, progress in developing new in vitro assays has been slow and frustrating.

The Interagency Coordinating Committee on the Validation of Alternative Methods (ICCVAM) of the National Toxicology Program (NTP) has reinvigorated the validation process in the United States as a result of Public Law 103-43 and has put forth recommendations for various short-term/in vitro assays, such as the cell-free corrosivity test, and recommendations for the mouse local lymph node assay for assessing chemical potential to elicit allergic contact dermatitis (NIEHS, 1999). A current review of the frog embryo teratogenicity assay in *Xenopus* (FETAX) by this group is under way.

The validation and application of short-term assays is particularly important to risk assessment because such assays can be designed to provide information about mechanisms of effects; moreover, they are fast and inexpensive compared with lifetime bioassays (McGregor et al., 1999). The NTP rodent carcinogenicity prediction challenge gave promising results for at least the prediction of genotoxic carcinogens; a second round with the next 30 chemicals that entered NTP rodent bioassays has been less successful (Ashby and Tennant, 1994). Validation of in vitro assays, like other kinds of tests, requires determination of their sensitivity (ability to identify true carcinogens), specificity (ability to recognize noncarcinogens as noncarcinogens), and predictive value for the toxic endpoint under evaluation. The societal costs of relying on such tests, with false positives (noncarcinogens classified as carcinogens) and false negatives (true carcinogens not detected) are the subject of a value-of-information model for the testing aspects of risk assessment and risk management (Lave and Omenn, 1986; Omenn and Lave, 1988). (See section below on linking information from hazard identification assessments.)

Current efforts to improve our ability to utilize short-term tests for carcinogenicity prediction include use of multivariate analysis with logistic regression (Kodell et al., 1999) and increased attention to improving the mechanistic basis of short-term testing. Examples of this approach include the several knockout transgenic mouse models proposed for use as shorter-term in vivo assays to identify carcinogens and currently under evaluation by NTP (Nebert and Duffy, 1997; Tennant et al., 1999). A TG.AC transgenic mouse carrying a *V-Ha-ras* gene construct has been shown to develop papillomas and malignant tumors in response to carcinogens and tumor-promoting compounds but is nonresponsive to noncarcinogens. A heterozygous p53 (+/−) mouse with one inactivated allele for p53 gene has been reported to have high sensitivity and specificity. Multiple transgenic assays are under evaluation (Robinson, 1998).

The primary use of short-term tests continues to be for mechanistic evaluations. In that context, results from short-term assays have impacted risk assessments. For example, evidence of nonmutagenicity in both in vitro and in vivo short-term assays continues to play an essential role, allowing regulators to consider nonlinear cancer risk assessment paradigms (EPA, 1999b).

New assay methods from molecular and developmental biology for developmental toxicity risk assessment that acknowledge the highly conserved nature of developmental pathways across species should accelerate use of a broader range of model organisms and assay approaches for noncancer risk assessments (NRC, 2000).

Animal Bioassays The use of animal bioassay data is a key component of the hazard identification process. A basic premise of risk assessment is that chemicals that cause tumors in animals can cause tumors in humans. All human carcinogens that have been adequately tested in animals produce positive results in at least one animal model. Thus, "although this association cannot establish that all agents and mixtures that cause cancer in experimental animals also cause cancer in humans, nevertheless, in the absence of adequate data on humans, it is biologically plausible and prudent to regard agents and mixtures for which there is sufficient evidence of carcinogenicity in experimental animals as if they presented a carcinogenic risk to humans" (IARC, 1994; 2000)—a reflection of the "precautionary principle." In general, the most appropriate rodent bioassays are those that test exposure pathways of most relevance to predicted or known human exposure pathways. Bioassays for reproductive and developmental toxicity and other noncancer endpoints have a similar rationale.

Consistent features in the design of standard cancer bioassays include testing in two species and both sexes, with 50 animals per dose group and near lifetime exposure. Important choices include the strains of rats and mice, the number of doses, and dose levels [typically 90, 50, and 10 to 25 percent of the maximally tolerated dose (MTD)], and the details of the required histopathology (number of organs to be examined, choice of interim sacrifice pathology, etc.). Positive evidence of chemical carcinogenicity can include increases in number of tumors at a particular organ site, induction of rare tumors, earlier induction (shorter latency) of commonly observed tumors, and/or increases in the total number of observed tumors.

However, there are serious problems with the rodent bioassay as a "gold standard" for prediction of human carcinogenicity risk (Risk Commission, 1997; Rodericks et al., 1997; McClain, 1994; Rice et al., 1999; Capen et al., 1999). Tumors may be increased only at the highest dose tested, which is usually at or near a dose that causes systemic toxicity (Ames and Gold, 1990). Second, even without toxicity, the high dose may trigger different events than do low-dose exposures. Table 4-4 presents some mechanistic details about rodent tumor responses that are no longer thought to be directly predictive of cancer risk for humans. Table 4-4 gives examples of both qualitative and quantitative considerations useful for determining relevance of rodent tumor responses for human risk evaluations. An example of qualitative considerations is the male rat kidney tumor observed following exposure to chemicals that bind to a_{2u}-globulin (e.g., unleaded gasoline, 1,4-dichlorobenzene, D-limonene). The a_{2u}-globulin is a male rat-specific low-molecular-weight protein not found in female rats, humans, or other species, including mice and monkeys.

Table 4-4 also illustrates quantitative considerations important for determining human relevance of animal bioassay information. For example, doses of compounds so high as to exceed solubility in the urinary tract outflow lead to tumors of the urinary bladder

Table 4-4
Examples of Mechanistic Considerations for Carcinogens: Explanation for Special Cases of Rodent Bioassay Data Lacking Relevance for Human Risk Evaluation

SYSTEM	TARGET ORGAN	MECHANISM FOR SUSCEPTIBLE SPECIES	SPECIES DIFFERENCES	ILLUSTRATIVE CHEMICAL AGENTS
Urinary tract	Renal tumors in male rats	Chemicals bind to a_{2U}-globulin Accumulation in target kidney cells Increased necrosis Increased regenerative hyperplasia Renal tubular calcification neoplasia	a_{2U}-globulin male rat specific low-molecular weight protein not found in female rats, humans, mice, monkeys	Unleaded gasoline 1,4-Dichlorobenzene D-limonene Isophorons Dimethyl-methylphos-phonate Perchloroethylene Pentachloroethane Hexachloroethane
	Bladder	Reactive hyperplasia from cytotoxic precipitated chemicals	Rodent exposure levels exceed solubility, not relevant for human exposure	Saccharin, melamine, nitrilotriacetic acid, fosetyl-A1
Gastric	Forestomach	Direct oral gavage Local cytotoxicity Hyperplasia	Rodent gavage treatment, exposure conditions not relevant for human exposure	BHA, propionic acid, ethyl acrylate
Endocrine	Thyroid gland tumors	Alteration in thyroid homeostasis Decreased thyroid hormone production Sustained increase in thyroid stimulating hormone (TSH) Thyroid tumors	Lack of thyroid-binding protein in rodents versus humans Decreased $t_{1/2}$ for T_4; increased TSH levels in rodents	Ethylene bisdithio-carbamate, fungicides, amitrol, goitrogens, sulfamethazine
Respiratory	Rat lung	Overwhelming clearance mechanisms	High dose effects seen with rodent models	Various particles, titanium dioxide

SOURCES: Neumann, 1995; Oberdörster, 1995; Omenn, 1995; McClain, 1994; Risk Commission, 1997; Rodericks, 1997.

in male rats following crystal precipitation and local irritation leading to hyperplasia. Such precipitates are known to occur following saccharin or nitriloacetic acid exposure. The decision to exclude saccharin from the NTP list of suspected human carcinogens reaffirms the nonrelevance of such high-dose responses for likely human exposure considerations (Neumann and Olin, 1995; NTP, 2000). A gross overloading of the particle clearance mechanism of rat lungs via directly administered particles, as was seen in titanium dioxide (TDO) exposures, resulted in EPA's delisting TDO as a reportable toxicant for the Clean Air Act Toxic Release Inventory (Oberdörster, 1995; EPA, 1988).

Other rodent responses not likely to be predictive for humans include localized forestomach tumors after gavage. Ethyl acrylate, which produces such tumors, was delisted on the basis of extensive mechanistic studies (NTP, 2000). In general, for risk assessment, it is desirable to use the same route of administration as the likely exposure pathway in humans to avoid such extrapolation issues. Despite the example of forestomach tumors, tumors in unusual sites—like the pituitary gland, the eighth cranial nerve, or the Zymbal gland—should not be dismissed as irrelevant, since organ-organ correlation is often lacking (NRC, 1994).

Rats and mice give concordant positive or negative results in only 70 percent of bioassays, so it is unlikely that rodent/human concordance would be higher (Lave et al., 1988). Haseman and Lockhart (1993) concluded that most target sites in cancer bioassays showed a strong correlation (65 percent) between males and females—especially for forestomach, liver, and thyroid tumors—so they suggested, for efficiency, that bioassays could rely on a combination of male rats and female mice. Even when concordant positive results are observed, there can still be very great differences in potency, as is observed in aflatoxin-induced tumors in rats and mice. In this example, an almost 100,000-fold difference in susceptibility to aflatoxin B_1 (AFB_1)-induced liver tumors is seen between the sensitive rat and trout species versus the more resistant mouse strains. Genetic differences in the expression of cytochrome P450 and glutathione-*S*-transferases explain most of these species differences and suggest that humans may be as sensitive to AFB_1-induced liver tumors as rats (Eaton and Gallagher, 1994).

Critical problems exist in using the hazard identification data from rodent bioassays for quantitative risk assessments. This is because of the limited dose–response data available from these rodent bioassays and nonexistent response information for environmentally relevant exposures. Results thus have traditionally been extrapolated from a dose–response curve in the 10 to 100 percent biologically observable tumor response range down to 10^{-6}

risk estimates (upper confidence limit) or to a benchmark or reference dose-related risk.

Addition of investigations of mechanisms and assessment of multiple noncancer endpoints into the bioassay design represent important enhancements of lifetime bioassays. It is feasible and desirable to tie these bioassays together with mechanistically oriented short-term tests and biomarker and genetic studies in epidemiology (Perera et al., 1991; Perera and Weinstein, 2000). In the example of AFB_1 induced liver tumors, AFB_1-DNA adducts have proved to be an extremely useful biomarker. A highly linear relationship was observed between liver tumor incidence (in rats, mice, and trout) and AFB_1-DNA adduct formation over a dose range of 5 orders of magnitude (Eaton and Gallagher, 1994). Such approaches may allow for an extension of biologically observable phenomena to doses lower than those leading to frank tumor development and help to address the issues of extrapolation over multiple orders of magnitude to predict response at environmentally relevant doses.

Use of Epidemiologic Data in Risk Assessment The most convincing line of evidence for human risk is a well-conducted epidemiologic study in which a positive association between exposure and disease has been observed (NRC, 1983). Epidemiologic studies are essentially opportunistic. Studies begin with known or presumed exposures, comparing exposed versus nonexposed individuals, or with known cases, compared with persons lacking the particular diagnosis. Table 4-5 shows examples of epidemiologic study designs and provides clues on types of outcomes and exposures evaluated. There are important limitations. When the study is exploratory, hypotheses are often weak. Exposure estimates are often crude and retrospective, especially for conditions with long latency before clinical manifestations appear. Generally, there are multiple exposures, especially when a full week or a lifetime is considered. There is always a trade-off between detailed information on relatively few persons and very limited information on large numbers of persons. Contributions from lifestyle factors, such as smoking and diet, are a challenge to sort out. Humans are highly outbred, so the method must consider variation in susceptibility among those who are exposed. The expression of results in terms of odds ratios, relative risks, and confidence intervals may be unfamiliar to nonepidemiologists. Finally, the caveats self-effacing epidemiologists often cite may discourage risk managers and toxicologists!

Nevertheless, human epidemiology studies provide very useful information for hazard identification and sometimes quantitative information for data characterization. Several good illustrations of types of epidemiological studies and their interpretation for toxicological evaluation are given in Checkoway (1994) and Gamble and Battigelli (1991). Three major types of epidemiology study designs are available: cross-sectional studies, cohort studies and case-control studies, as detailed in Table 4-5. Cross sectional studies survey groups of humans to identify risk factors (exposure) and disease but are not useful for establishing cause and effect. Cohort studies evaluate individuals selected on the basis of their exposure to an agent under study. Thus, based on exposure status, these individuals are monitored for development of disease. These prospective studies monitor over time individuals who initially are disease-free to determine the rates at which they develop disease. In case-control studies subjects are selected on the basis of disease status: disease cases and matched cases of disease free individuals. Exposure histories of the two groups are compared to determine key consistent features in their exposure histories. All case-control studies are retrospective studies.

Epidemiologic findings are judged by the following criteria: strength of association, consistency of observations (reproducibility in time and space), specificity (uniqueness in quality or quantity of response), appropriateness of temporal relationship (did the exposure precede responses?), dose–responsiveness, biological plausibility and coherence, verification, and analogy (biological extrapolation) (Hill, 1965). In addition, epidemiologic study designs should be evaluated for their power of detection, appropriateness of outcomes, verification of exposure assessments, completeness of assessing confounding factors, and general applicability of the outcomes to other populations at risk. Power

Table 4-5
Example of Three Types of Epidemiological Study Designs

METHODOLOGICAL ATTRIBUTES	*Type of Study*		
	COHORT	CASE-CONTROL	CROSS-SECTIONAL
Initial classification	Exposure–nonexposure	Disease–nondisease	Either one
Time sequence	Prospective	Retrospective	Present time
Sample composition	Nondiseased individuals	Cases and controls	Survivors
Comparison	Proportion of exposed with disease	Proportion of cases with exposure	Either one
Rates	Incidence	Fractional (%)	Prevalence
Risk index	Relative risk–attributable risk	Relative odds	Prevalence
Advantages	Lack of bias in exposure; yields incidence and risk rates	Inexpensive, small number of subjects, rapid results, suitable for rare diseases, no attrition	Quick results
Disadvantages	Large number of subjects required, long follow-up, attrition, change in time of criteria and methods, costly, inadequate for rare diseases	Incomplete information, biased recall, problem in selecting control and matching, yields only relative risk—cannot establish causation, population of survivors	Cannot establish causation (antecedent consequence); population of survivors; inadequate for rare diseases

SOURCES: Gamble and Battigelli, 1978, 1991.

of detection is calculated using study size, variability, accepted detection limits for endpoints under study, and a specified significance level. (See Healey, 1987, for calculation formulas or computer programs such as EPI-INFO; Dean et al., 1995; or EGRET, 1994, for determination of experimental power of detection.)

Recent advances from the human genome project, increased sophistication and molecular biomarkers, and improved mechanistic bases for epidemiologic hypotheses have allowed epidemiologists to get within the "black box" of statistical associations and move forward our understanding of biological plausibility and clinical relevance. "Molecular epidemiology" is a new focus of human studies where improved molecular biomarkers of exposure, effect, and susceptibility have allowed investigators to more effectively link molecular events in the causative disease pathway. Implications of these improvements for risk assessment are tremendous, as they provide an improved biological basis for extrapolation across the diversity of human populations and allow for improved cross-species comparisons with rodent bioassay information. The biological plausibility of epidemiologic associations will be increased remarkably by the use of biomarkers of exposure, effects, and susceptibility (Perera, et al., 1991; Perera and Weinstein, 2000; Omenn, 2000).

Integrating Qualitative Aspects of Risk Assessment

Qualitative assessment of hazard information should include a consideration of the consistency and concordance of findings. Such assessment should include a determination of the consistency of the toxicologic findings across species and target organs, an evaluation of consistency across duplicate experimental conditions, and the adequacy of the experiments to detect the adverse endpoints of interest.

The National Toxicology Program uses several categories to classify bioassay results, with the category *clear evidence of carcinogenicity* describing bioassays where dose-related increases in malignant or combined malignant and benign neoplasms are seen across all doses, or at least significant increases in two of the four species/sex test groups. NTP's evaluation guidelines specify the additional categories of *some, equivocal, no evidence,* and *inadequate study.*

Qualitative assessment of animal or human evidence is done by many agencies, including the EPA and International Agency for Research on Cancer (IARC). Similar evidence classifications have been used for both the animal and human evidence categories by both agencies. These evidence classifications have included levels of sufficient, limited, inadequate, and no evidence (EPA, 1994a) or *evidence suggesting lack of carcinogenicity* (IARC, 1994; 2000). EPA has also included a specific *no data* category.

These evidence classifications are used for overall weight-of-evidence carcinogenicity classification schemes. Although differing group number or letter categories are used, striking similarities exist between these approaches. EPA's newly proposed changes to their risk assessment guidelines for carcinogenic substances include changes in how likelihood categories are used, with references to categories described as *known, likely,* or *not likely* to be carcinogenic to humans. A category representing a *cannot evaluate* level includes *inadequate data, incomplete or inconclusive data,* and *no data* categories.

In this section we have discussed approaches for evaluating cancer endpoints. Similar weight-of-evidence approaches have been proposed for reproductive risk assessment (refer to *sufficient* and *insufficient evidence* categories in EPA proposed guidelines for reproductive risk in EPA, 1996c). The Institute for Evaluating Health Risks defined an "evaluation process" by which reproductive and developmental toxicity data can be consistently evaluated and integrated to ascertain their relevance for human health risk assessment (Moore et al., 1995). Application of such carefully deliberated approaches for assessing noncancer endpoints should help avoid the tendency to list chemicals as yes or no (positive or negative) without human relevancy information.

For many years there has been an information-sharing process aimed at harmonization of chemical testing regimes and clinical trials methodologies, so that data might be accepted in multiple countries that are members of the Organization for Economic Cooperation and Development (OECD). The United Nations Conference on the Environment in Rio de Janeiro, Brazil, in 1992, established harmonization of risk assessment as one of its goals, with a coordinating role for the International Programme on Chemical Safety. The negotiation in 1994 of the General Agreement on Trade and Tariffs (GATT) and establishment of the World Trade Organization makes harmonization of various aspects of testing, risk assessment, labeling, registration, and standards important elements in trade, not just in regulatory science. Moolenaar (1994) summarized the carcinogen risk assessment methodologies used by various countries as a basis for regulatory actions. He tabulated the risk characterization, carcinogen identification, risk extrapolation, and chemical classification schemes of EPA, U.S. Department of Health and Human Services (DHHS), IARC, ACGIH, Australia, the European Economic Community (EEC), Germany, Netherlands, Norway, and Sweden. The approach of EPA to estimate an upper bound to human risk is unique; all other countries estimate human risk values based on expected incidence of cancer from the exposures under review. The United Kingdom follows a case-by-case approach to risk evaluations for both genotoxic and nongenotoxic carcinogens, with no generic procedures. Denmark, EEC, the United Kingdom (UK), and the Netherlands all divide carcinogens into genotoxic and nongenotoxic agents and use different extrapolation procedures for each. Norway does not extrapolate data to low doses, using instead the TD_{50} to divide category I carcinogens into tertiles by potency. The UK, EEC, and Netherlands all treat nongenotoxic chemical carcinogens as threshold toxicants. A "no observed adverse effect level" (NOAEL) and safety factor are used to set acceptable daily intakes (ADIs). The revised EPA guidelines for cancer risk assessment now propose applying benchmark dose-like methods and consideration of mode-of-action data, which will move the United States toward a more harmonized approach for risk approaches (EPA, 1999).

RISK CHARACTERIZATION

Quantitative considerations in risk assessment include dose—response assessment, exposure assessment, variation in susceptibility, and characterization of uncertainty. For dose–response assessment, varying approaches have been proposed for threshold versus nonthreshold endpoints. Traditionally, threshold approaches have been applied for assessment of noncancer endpoints, and nonthreshold approaches have been used for cancer endpoints. Each approach and its inherent assumptions is discussed below, as are recent efforts to harmonize these approaches.

In general, human exposure data for prediction of human response are quite limited; thus, animal bioassay data have primarily served as the basis for most quantitative risk assessments. However, the risk assessor is normally interested in low environmental exposures of humans, which are well below the experimentally observable range of responses from animal assays. Thus, methods of extrapolation from high dose to low dose and animal risk to human risk are required and make up a major aspect of dose–response assessment.

Dose–Response Assessment

The fundamental basis of the quantitative relationships between exposure to an agent and the incidence of an adverse response is the dose–response assessment. Analysis of dose–response relationships must start with the determination of the critical effects to be quantitatively evaluated. EPA has issued toxicity specific guidelines that are useful in identifying such critical effects (for developmental toxicity, see EPA, 1991b; reproductive toxicity, EPA, 1996c; neurotoxicity, EPA, 1995; cancer, EPA, 1994b, 1996a, 1999). It is usual practice to choose the data sets with adverse effects occurring at the lowest levels of exposure; the "critical" adverse effect is defined as the significant adverse biological effect that occurs at the lowest exposure level (Barnes and Dourson, 1988). Approaches for characterizing threshold dose–response relationships include identification of NOAELs or "lowest observed adverse effect levels" (LOAELs). On the dose–response curve illustrated in Fig. 4-3, the threshold, indicated with a T, represents the dose below which no additional increase in response is observed. The NOAEL is identified as the highest non-statistically significant dose tested; in this example it is point E, at 2 mg/kg body weight. Point F is the LOAEL (2.5 mg/kg body weight), as it is the lowest dose tested with a statistically significant effect.

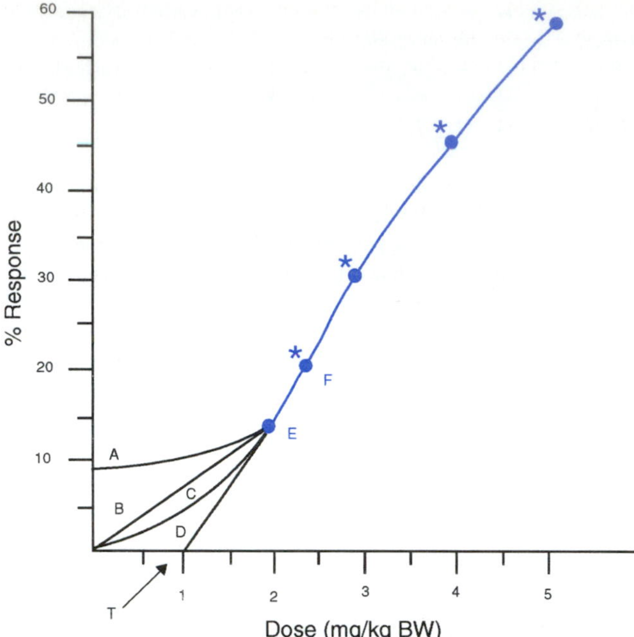

Figure 4-3. Dose–response curve.

This figure is designed to illustrate a typical dose-response curve with "•'s" indicating the biologically determined responses. Statistical significance of these responses is indicated with a * symbol. The threshold dose is shown by T, a dose below which no change in biological response occurs. Point E represents the highest non-statistically significant response point, hence it is the "no observed adverse effect level" (NOAEL) for this example. Point F is the "lowest observed adverse response level" (LOAEL). Curves A to D show possible options for extrapolating the dose-response relationship below the lowest biologically observed data point, E.

In general, animal bioassays are constructed with sufficient numbers of animals to detect low-level biological responses at the 10 percent response range. The risk assessor should always understand the biological significance of the responses being evaluated in order to put such statistical observations in context. *Significance* thus usually refers to both biological and statistical criteria (Faustman et al., 1994) and is dependent upon the number of dose levels tested, the number of animals tested at each dose, and background incidence of the adverse response in the nonexposed control groups. The NOAEL should not be perceived as risk-free, as several reports have shown that the response of NOAELs for continuous endpoints averages 5 percent risk, and NOAELs based on quantal endpoints can be associated with risk of greater than 10 percent (Faustman, et al., 1994, Allen et al., 1994a, 1994b).

As described in Chap. 2, approaches for characterizing dose–response relationships include identification of effect levels such as LD_{50} (dose producing 50 percent lethality), LC_{50} (concentration producing 50 percent lethality), ED_{10} (dose producing 10 percent response), as well as NOAELs (no observed adverse effect levels).

NOAELs have traditionally served as the basis for risk assessment calculations, such as reference doses or acceptable daily intake values. References doses (RfDs) or concentrations (RfCs) are estimates of a daily exposure to an agent that is assumed to be without adverse health impact on the human population. The ADIs are acceptable daily intake values used by WHO for pesticides and food additives to define "the daily intake of chemical, which during an entire lifetime appears to be without appreciable risk on the basis of all known facts at that time" (WHO, 1962) (Dourson et al., 1985). Reference doses (first introduced in Chap. 2) and ADI values typically are calculated from NOAEL values by dividing by uncertainty (UF) and/or modifying factors (MF) (EPA, 1991a; (Dourson and DeRosa, 1991; Dourson and Stara, 1983).

$$\text{RfD} = \text{NOAEL} / (\text{UF} * \text{MF})$$
$$\text{ADI} = \text{NOAEL} / (\text{UF} * \text{MF})$$

In principle, dividing by these factors allows for interspecies (animal-to-human) and intraspecies (human-to-human) variability with default values of 10 each. An additional uncertainty factor can be used to account for experimental inadequacies—for example, to extrapolate from short-exposure-duration studies to a situation more relevant for chronic study or to account for inadequate numbers of animals or other experimental limitations. If only a LOAEL value is available, then an additional 10-fold factor commonly is used to arrive at a value more comparable to a NOAEL. Allen et al. (1994) have shown for developmental toxicity endpoints that application of the 10-fold factor for LOAEL-to-NOAEL conversion is too large. Traditionally, a safety factor of 100 would be used for RfD calculations to extrapolate from a well-conducted animal bioassay (10-fold factor animal to human) and to account for human variability in response (10-fold factor human-to-human variability).

Modifying factors can be used to adjust the uncertainty factors if data on mechanisms, pharmacokinetics, or relevance of the animal response to human risk justify such modification. For example, if there is kinetic information suggesting that rat and human metabolism are very similar for a particular compound, producing the same active target metabolite, then—rather than using a 10-fold uncertainty factor to divide the NOAEL from the animal toxicity study to obtain a human relevant RfD—a factor of 3 for that uncertainty factor might be used. Of particular recent interest is the new extra 10-fold Food Quality and Protection Act (FQPA) factor, added to ensure protection of infants and children (EPA, 1996b). Under this law an additional uncertainty factor is added to ensure protection of children's health; it is currently being used for determining allowable pesticide chemical residues. This factor is designed to take into account potential pre- and postnatal toxicity and to overcome the incompleteness of toxicity and exposure data (FQPA; PL 104-170). Illustrative discussions on how such a legislatively mandated uncertainty factor might be applied are available from EPA (1999) and from Schardein and Scialli (1999) for chlorpyrifos as an example compound.

Recent efforts have focused on using data-derived factors to replace the 10-fold uncertainty factors traditionally used in calculating RfDs and ADIs. Such efforts have included reviewing the human pharmacologic literature from published clinical trials (Silverman et al., 1999) and developing human variability databases for a large range of exposures and clinical conditions (Hattis et al., 1999a, 1999b; Hattis and Silver, 1994). Toward this goal, Renwick has separated the intra-and interspecies uncertainty factors into two components: toxicokinetic (TK) and toxicodynamic (TD) aspects (Renwick, 1991; 1999; Johnson et al., 1997). Figure 4-4 shows these distinctions. A key advantage of this approach is that it provides a structure for incorporating scientific information on specific aspects of the overall toxicologic process into the reference dose calculations; thus, relevant data can replace a portion of the overall "uncertainty" surrounding these extrapolations. Initially Renwick proposed a factor of 4 for the TK and a factor of 2.5 for the TD component for both the interspecies and inter-individual factors (Renwick and Walker, 1993). However, subsequent evaluations have supported the revised WHO (1994) guidance, which retains the 4.0- and 2.5-fold factors for the TK and TD interspecies components but changes both the inter-individual TK and TD factors to 3.2. Such changes highlight the flexibility of this approach to incorporate new conclusions and even compound-specific data (Renwick and Lazarus, 1998).

This overall approach has important implications for how we utilize new toxicologic research. Most efforts to modify the uncertainty factors have focused on more effective use of toxicokinetic information, yet there is also a need to focus on the toxicodynamic aspects of this uncertainty. For example, a Nuclear Regulatory Commission (NRC) report that reviewed how new advances in developmental biology can improve the research relevant for developmental toxicology risk assessment has identified highly conserved cell signaling pathways essential for all development processes across all species (NRC, 2000). Such "dynamic" information is not yet being considered following chemical impacts, but such data on known similarities in comparison of critical pathways across species may be useful in reducing the uncertainty in the TD components of the interspecies portion of the equation. This is one example of how new information may enhance the scientific basis of our approaches for risk assessment.

NOAEL values have also been utilized for risk assessment by evaluating a "margin of exposure" (MOE), where the ratio of the NOAEL determined in animals and expressed as mg/kg/day is compared with the level to which a human may be exposed. For example, human exposures to a specific chemical agent are calculated to be solely via drinking water, and the total daily intake of the compound is 0.04 mg/kg/day. If the NOAEL for neurotoxicity is 100 mg/kg/day, then the MOE would be 2500 for the oral exposure route for neurotoxicity. Such a large value is reassuring to public health officials. Low values of MOE indicate that the human levels of exposure are close to levels for the NOAEL in animals. There is usually no factor included in this calculation for differences in human or animal susceptibility or animal-to-human extrapolation; thus, MOE values of less than 100 have been used by regulatory agencies as flags for requiring further evaluation. A "margin of safety" (MOS) can also be calculated and is frequently utilized in evaluating pharmaceutical agents where an effective therapeutic dose is compared with a dose causing toxicity (see Chap. 2).

The NOAEL approach has been criticized on several points, including that (1) the NOAEL must, by definition, be one of the experimental doses tested; (2) once this is identified, the rest of the

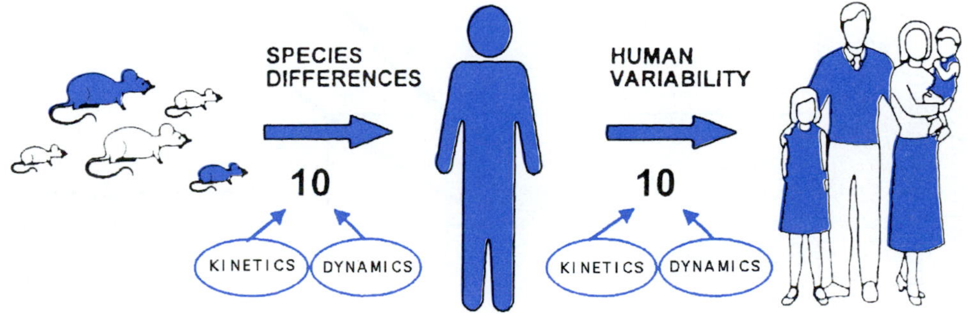

Figure 4-4. Toxicokinetic (TK) and toxicodynamic (TD) considerations inherent in interspecies and inter-individual extrapolations.

Toxicokinetics refers to the processes of absorption, distribution, elimination, and metabolism of a toxicant. *Toxicodynamics* refers to the actions and interactions of the toxicant within the organism and describes processes at organ, tissue, cellular, and molecular levels. This figure shows how uncertainty in extrapolation both across and within species can be considered as being due to two key factors: a kinetic component and a dynamic component. Refer to the text for detailed explanations. (Adapted from Renwick, 1999, 1998.)

dose–response curve is ignored; (3) experiments that test fewer animals result in larger NOAELs and thus larger reference doses, rewarding testing procedures that produce less certain rather than more certain NOAEL values; and (4) the NOAEL approach does not identify the actual responses at the NOAEL and will vary based on experimental design, leading to setting of regulatory limits at varying levels of risk. Because of these limitations, an alternative to the NOAEL approach, the benchmark dose (BMD) method, was first proposed by Crump (1984) and extended by Kimmel and Gaylor (1988). In this approach, the dose response is modeled and the lower confidence bound for a dose at a specified response level [benchmark response (BMR)] is calculated. The BMR is usually specified at 1, 5, or 10 percent. Figure 4-5 shows how a BMD is calculated using a 10 percent benchmark response and a 95 percent lower confidence bound on dose. The BMDx (with x representing the percent benchmark response) is used as an alternative to the NOAEL value for reference dose calculations. Thus, the RfD would be

$$\text{RfD} = \text{BMDx} / \text{UF} * \text{MF}$$

The proposed values to be used for the uncertainty factors and modifying factors for BMDs can range from the same factors as for the NOAEL to lower values due to increased confidence in the response level and increased recognition of experimental variability due to use of a lower confidence bound on dose (Barnes et al., 1995). EPA has developed software for the application of benchmark dose methods (http://www.epa.gov/ncea/bmds.htm) and is developing a technical guidance document to provide guidelines for application of BMDs (EPA, 2000c). These guidelines will address issues of appropriate response levels to be used for various endpoints and how to utilize the LED_x versus ED_x in RfD calculations.

The benchmark dose approach has been applied to study several non-cancer endpoints, including developmental (Allen et al., 1994a, 1994b) and reproductive toxicity (Auton, 1994). The most extensive studies with developmental toxicity have shown that BMD_{05} values were similar to a statistically derived NOAEL for a wide range of developmental toxicity endpoints and that results from using generalized dose–response models were similar to statistical models designed specifically to represent unique features of developmental toxicity testing. A generalized log logistic dose response model offered other advantages in dealing with litter size and intralitter correlations (Allen et al., 1994b).

Advantages of the benchmark dose approach can include (1) the ability to take into account the full dose–response curve, as opposed to focusing on a single test dose as is done in the NOAEL approach; (2) the inclusion of a measure of variability (confidence limit); (3) the use of responses within the experimental range versus extrapolation of responses to low doses not tested experimentally; and (4) the use of a consistent benchmark response level for RfD calculations across studies. Obviously, limitations in the animal bioassays in regard to minimal test doses for evaluation, shallow dose responses, and use of study designs with widely spaced test doses will limit the utility of these assays for any type of quantitative assessments, whether NOAEL- or BMD-based approaches.

Some common environmental exposures—such as those for lead and other criteria air pollutants—are so close to LOAELs that the regulatory agencies use an informal margin-of-safety approach heavily weighted with consideration of technical feasibility (see Risk Commission, 1997).

Nonthreshold Approaches

As Fig. 4-3 shows, numerous dose–response curves can be proposed in the low-dose region of the dose–response curve if a threshold assumption is not made. Because the risk assessor generally needs to extrapolate beyond the region of the dose–response curve for which experimentally observed data are available, the choice of models to generate curves in this region has received lots of attention. For nonthreshold responses, methods for dose–response assessments have also utilized models for extrapolation to de minimus ($10^{-4} - 10^{-6}$) risk levels at very low doses, far below the biologically observed response range and far below the effect levels evaluated for threshold responses. Two general types of dose–response models exist: statistical (or probability distribution models) and mechanistic models (Krewski and Van Ryzin, 1981).

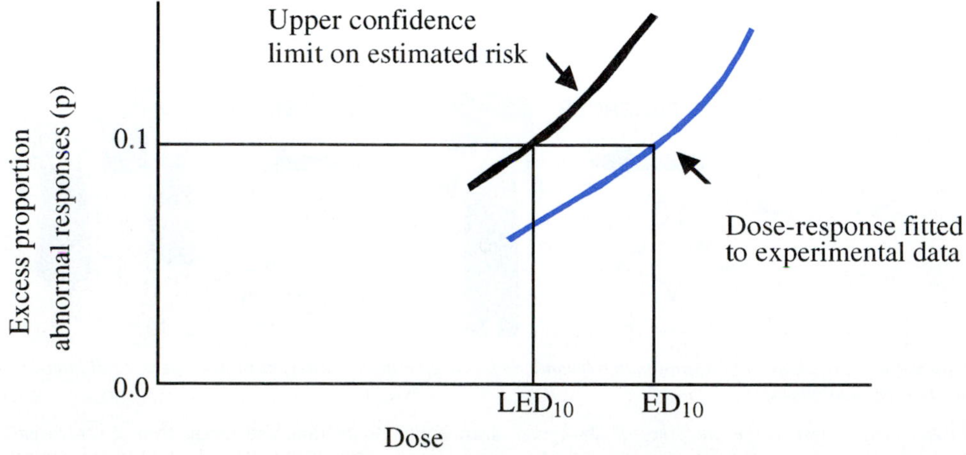

Figure 4-5. Illustration of benchmark dose (BMD) approach.

The LED_{10} is the lower confidence limit of the dose (ED_{10}) associated with a 10 percent incidence of adverse effect. (Based on Kavlock, 1995.)

The distribution models are based on the assumption that each individual has a tolerance level for a test agent and that this response level is a variable following a specific probability distribution function. These responses can be modeled using a cumulative dose–response function. Chapter 2 discusses the common normal distribution pattern (see Fig. 2-3). A log probit model estimates the probability of response at a specified dose (d); thus, $P(d) = \Phi[a + \beta \log d]$, where Φ is the cumulative function for a standard normal distribution of the log tolerances with standard deviations σ and mean μ, a equals μ/σ, and β equals the slope of the probit line $(-1/\sigma)$. The probit curve at low doses usually assumes an S -shape. Chapter 2 discusses determination of the LD_{50} value from such a curve. However, extrapolation of the experimental data from 50 percent response levels to a: "safe", "acceptable," or "de minimus" level of exposure—e.g., one in a million risk above background—illustrates the huge gap between scientific observations and highly protective risk limits (sometimes called *virtually safe doses,* or those corresponding to a 95 percent upper confidence limit on adverse response rates).

The log logistic model was derived from chemical kinetic theory. The probability of response at dose d is defined as $P(d) = [1 - \exp(a + \beta \log d)]^{-1}$. Like the probit model, this model defines sigmoidal curves that are symmetrical around the 50 percent response level; however, the log logistic curves approach the 0 and 100 percent response levels with a more shallow curve shape. The logit and probit curves are indistinguishable in fitting the data in the region of the response curve where experimentally derived data are present (Brown, 1984; Hartung, 1987).

Models Derived from Mechanistic Assumptions

This modeling approach designs a mathematical equation to describe dose–response relationships that are consistent with postulated biological mechanisms of response. These models are based on the idea that a response (toxic effect) in a particular biological unit (animal, human, pup, etc.) is the result of the random occurrence of one or more biological events (stochastic events).

Radiation research has spawned a series of such "hit models" for cancer modeling, where a hit is defined as a critical cellular event that must occur before a toxic effect is produced. These models assume that (1) an infinitely large number of targets exists, for example in the DNA; (2) the organism responds with a toxic response only after a minimum number of targets has been modified; (3) a critical target is altered if a sufficient number of hits occurs; and (4) the probability of a hit in the low dose range of the dose–response curve is proportional to the dose of the toxicant (Brown, 1984).

The simplest mechanistic model is the one-hit (one-stage) linear model in which only one hit or critical cellular interaction is required for a cell to be altered. For example, based on somatic mutation theory, a single mutational change would be sufficient for a cell to become cancerous through a transformational event and dose-independent clonal expansion. The probability statement for these models is $P(d) = 1 - \exp^{(-\lambda d)}$, where λd equals the number of hits occurring during a time period. A single molecule of a genotoxic carcinogen would have a minute but finite chance of causing a mutational event.

As theories of cancer have grown in complexity, so too have these hit-based mechanistic models. Multihit models have been developed that can describe hypothesized single-target multihit events, as well as multitarget, multihit events in carcinogenesis. The probability statements for these models is $P(d) = \int_0^{\lambda d} x^{k-1} \exp(-x)/\Gamma(k)\, dx$, where $\Gamma(k)$ denotes the gamma function with k = critical number of hits for the adverse response. The Weibull model has a dose–response function with characteristics similar to those of the multihit models, where the response equation is $P(d) = 1 - \exp[-\lambda d^k]$. Here again, k = critical number of hits for the toxic cellular response.

Armitage and Doll (1957) developed a multistage model for carcinogenesis that was based on these equations and on the hypothesis that a series of ordered stages was required before a cell could undergo mutation, initiation, transformation, and progression to form a tumor. This relationship was generalized by Crump (1980) by maximizing the likelihood function over polynomials, so that the probability statement is:

$$P(d) = 1 - \exp[-(\lambda_0 + \lambda_1 d^1 + \lambda_2 d^2 + \ldots \lambda_k d^k)]$$

If the true value of λ_1 is replaced with λ_1^* (the upper confidence limit of λ_1), then a linearized multistage model can be derived where the expression is dominated by $(\lambda d^*)d$ at low doses. The slope on this confidence interval, q_1^*, is used by EPA for quantitative cancer assessment. To obtain an upper 95 percent confidence interval on risk, the q_1^* value (risk/Δ dose in mg/kg/day) is multiplied by the amount of exposure (mg/kg/day). Thus, the upper-bound estimate on risk (R) is calculated as:

$$R = q_1^* \,[\text{risk(mg/kg/day)}^{-1}] \times \text{exposure (mg/kg/day)}$$

This relationship has been used to calculate a "virtually safe dose" (VSD), which represents the lower 95 percent confidence limit on a dose that gives an "acceptable level" of risk (e.g., upper confidence limit for 10^{-6} excess risk). The integrated risk information system (IRIS) developed by EPA gives q* values for many environmental carcinogens (EPA, 2000a). Because both the q_1^* and VSD values are calculated using 95 percent confidence intervals, the values are believed to represent conservative, protective estimates. The use of the maximum likelihood estimates (MLE values) from the linearized multistage models has not been accepted due to problems in the stability of MLE estimates at low dose using the linearized multistage (LMS) model.

The EPA has utilized the LMS model to calculate "unit risk estimates" in which the upper confidence limit on increased individual lifetime risk of cancer for a 70-kg human breathing 1 $\mu g/m^3$ of contaminated air or drinking 2 L/day of water containing 1 ppm (1mg/L) is estimated over a 70-year life span. The example given in Fig. 4-7 shows calculation of incremental lifetime cancer risk (ILCR) of skin cancer using soil exposure and q* values for inorganic arsenic.

Toxicologic Enhancements of the Models

Three exemplary areas of research that have improved the models used in risk extrapolation are time to tumor information, physiologically based toxicokinetic modeling, and biologically based dose–response modeling (Albert, 1994). Chapter 7 discusses in detail improvements in our estimation of exposure and offers approaches on how to model "target internal effective dose" in risk assessment rather than just using single-value "external exposure doses." In this chapter we discuss the biologically based dose–response (BBDR) modeling.

BBDR modeling aims to make the generalized mechanistic models discussed in the previous section more clearly reflect specific biological processes. Measured rates are incorporated into the mechanistic equations to replace default or computer-generated values. For example, the Moolgavkar-Venson-Knudson (MVK) model is based on a two-stage model for carcinogenesis, where two mutations are required for carcinogenesis and birth and death rates of cells are modeled through clonal expansion and tumor formation. This model has been applied effectively to human epidemiologic data on retinoblastoma. In animal studies, kidney and liver tumors in the 2-acetylaminofluorene (2-AAF) "mega mouse" study, bladder cancer in saccharin-exposed rats, rat lung tumors following radiation exposure, rat liver tumors following *N*-nitrosomorpholine exposure, respiratory tract tumors following benzo[a]pyrene exposure, and mouse liver tumors following chlordane exposure have been modeled (NRC, 1993a; Cohen and Ellwein, 1990; Moolgavkar and Luebeck, 1990). Additional applications are needed to continue validation of the model (NRC, 1993a). EPA relied on receptor binding theory in its 1994 dioxin risk reassessment (EPA, 1994b) and is currently considering expanded mechanism-based cancer modeling approaches where cytochrome P450 1A2 (CYP1A2) or epidermal growth factor (EGF) receptor concentrations are used as surrogate dose metrics within these two-stage cancer models. Kohn et al. (1993) and Anderson et al. (1993) have used physiologically based toxicokinetics (PBTK) and BBDR information to improve dioxin risk assessment.

Development of biologically based dose–response models for endpoints other than cancer are limited; however, several approaches have been explored in developmental toxicity, utilizing cell cycle kinetics, enzyme activity, litter effects, and cytotoxicity as critical endpoints (Rai and Van Ryzin, 1985; Faustman et al., 1989; Shuey et al., 1994; Leroux et al., 1996, 2000). Of particular interest are approaches that link pregnancy-specific toxicokinetic models with temporally sensitive toxicodynamic models for developmental impacts (Faustman et al., 1999). Unfortunately, there is a lack of specific, quantitative biological information for most toxicants and for most endpoints (NRC, 2000).

In the absence of detailed mechanistic information, EPA has proposed, in their revised cancer guidelines, use of "mode of action" (MOA) information (EPA, 1999). MOA information describes key events and processes leading to molecular and functional effects that would in general explain the overall process of cancer development. In many cases these could be plausible hypothesized MOAs for both cancer and other toxicity endpoints, but the detailed mechanistic nuances might not be fully investigated. EPA has proposed using such MOA information to suggest specific, nondefault approaches for cancer risk assessments and for evaluating toxicity of compounds with common MOAs in cumulative risk assessments (EPA, 1996b, 1998b). For cancer risk assessments, this means using benchmark-like "points of departure" at the ED_{01} or LED_{01} and using a slope from that point that could represent linear or nonlinear options. This would bring quantitative approaches for carcinogens into a similar construct as what is proposed for quantitation of noncancer endpoints. Such approaches are being discussed in EPA's new draft cancer guidelines (EPA, 1999). These build upon guidance developed by the WHO's International Programme on Chemical Safety Harmonization Project (WHO, 2000). Critical to the MOA development is the use of "criteria of causality" considerations, which build on Hill criteria used in epidemiology (Hill, 1965; Faustman et al., 1996; EPA 1999). MOA-based approaches should facilitate incorporation of new scientific information and hence be responsive to the challenges outlined in the 1994 NRC report (NRC, 1994).

One of the key challenges over the next decade for toxicologists doing risk assessments will be interpretation and linking of observations from highly sensitive molecular and genome-based methods with the overall process of toxicity (NRC, 2000; Iyers et al., 1999; Andersen and Barton, 1999; Eisen et al., 1998; Limbird and Taylor, 1998). The basic need for linkage of observations was highlighted in early biomarker work. NRC reports on biomarkers (NRC, 1989a, 1989b, 1992a, 1992b) drew distinctions for biomarkers of effect, exposure, and susceptibility across a continuum of exposure, effect, and disease/toxicity. Biomarkers of early effects, like frank clinical pathology, arise as a function of exposure, response, and time. Early, subtle, and possibly reversible effects can generally be distinguished from irreversible disease states.

Nowhere is the challenge for interpretation of early and highly sensitive responses (biomarkers) made clearer than in the complicated data from gene expression arrays. Because our relatively routine ability to monitor gene responses—up to tens of thousands of them simultaneously—has grown exponentially in the last 5 years, the need for toxicologists to interpret such observations for risk assessment and for the overall process of toxicity has been magnified with equal or greater intensity. Figure 4-6 provides a simplified but illustrative example of multiple biomarker responses with dose or time. For microarray data, each gene response or cluster of genes can have its own pattern of response (peak and overall duration of response). For this to be meaningful for the overall process of toxicity, such responses (e.g., responses B2, B3, and B4) need to be examined in relationship to toxicity. In this example, developmental toxicity could be modeled as response B1 and lethality as B6. In order to describe these responses as relevant for either endpoint of toxicity, the strength, consistency, and coherence of both the temporal and dose relationships would need to be established (Faustman et al., 1999).

Microarray analysis for risk assessment will require much more sophisticated analyses than the cluster analysis techniques currently described in the literature (Eisen et al., 1998). Semiparametric likelihood models and Bayesian inference approaches are promising (Griffith and Brutlage, 2000), as are support vector machine methods (Brown et al., 2000). Because of the vast number of measured responses with gene expression arrays, pattern analysis techniques are being used. However, the extensive databases across chemical classes, pathological conditions, and stages of disease progression that are essential for these analyses are only now being developed through federal funding (NCI Cancer Genome Anatomy Project and NIEHS Environmental Genome Project) and by pharmaceutical agencies and trade organizations. For toxicologists and risk assessors, it will be both exciting and challenging to be faced with interpretation of results from such amazingly sensitive tools (NRC, 2000).

Exposure Assessment

The primary objectives of exposure assessment are to determine source, type, magnitude, and duration of contact with the agent of interest. Obviously, this is a key element of the risk assessment process, as hazard does not occur in the absence of exposure.

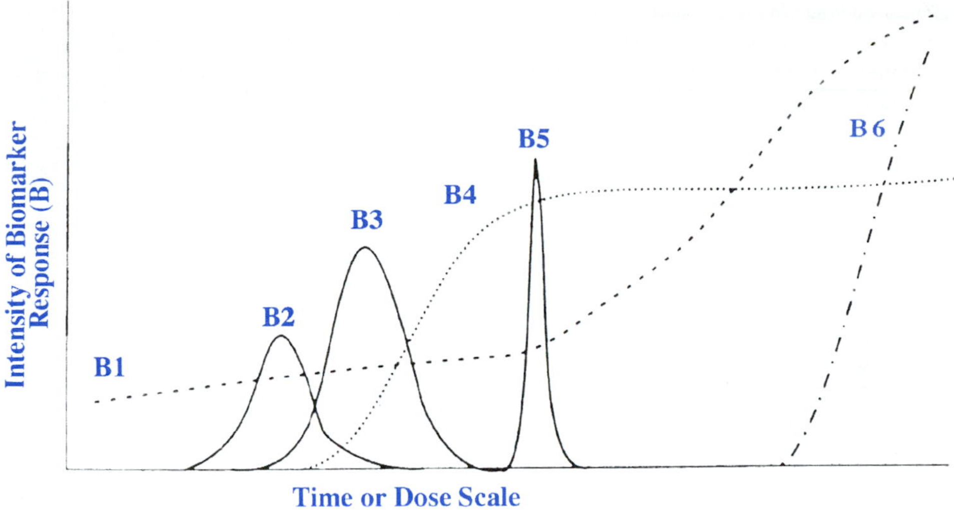

Figure 4-6. Hypothetical biomarker response relationships.

This figure illustrates a variety of dose-related biomarker responses shown as biomarker intensity (B) plotted against dose or time. The text expands upon the potentially complex relationships between biomarkers of early effect versus toxicity that can occur when very sensitive molecular biomarkers are utilized for toxicity assessment. (Adapted from Waterfield and Timbrell, 1999, and Depledge, 1993.)

However, it is also frequently identified as the key area of uncertainty in the overall risk determination. Here, the primary focus is on uses of exposure information in quantitative risk assessment.

Obviously, the primary goal of such calculations is to determine not only the type and amount of total exposure but also to find out specifically how much may be reaching target tissues. A key step in making an exposure assessment is determining what exposure pathways are relevant for the risk scenario under development. The subsequent steps entail quantitation of each pathway identified as a potentially relevant exposure and then summarizing these pathway-specific exposures for calculation of overall exposure. The EPA has published numerous documents which provide guidelines for determining such exposures (EPA, 1992, 1989a). Such calculations can include an estimation of total exposures for a specified population as well as calculation of exposure for highly exposed individuals. The use of a hypothetical maximally exposed individual (MEI) is no longer favored in exposure assessment due to its extremely conservative assumptions at each step of the estimation. However, point estimates of exposure continue to utilize high-end and theoretical upper-bound exposure estimates.

Conceptually such calculations are designed to represent "a plausible estimate" of exposure of individuals in the upper 90th percentile of the exposure distribution. Upper-bound estimations would be "bounding calculations" designed to represent exposures at levels that exceed the exposures experienced by all individuals in the exposure distribution and are calculated by assuming limits for all exposure variables. A calculation for individuals exposed at levels near the middle of the exposure distribution is a central estimate. Figure 4-7 gives example risk calculations using two types of exposure estimation procedures (EPA, 1989a, 1989b, 1992). Part A shows a point estimation method for the calculation of arsenic (As) exposure via a soil ingestion route. In this hypothetical scenario, As exposure is calculated using point estimates, and a lifetime average daily dose (LADD) is calculated as follows:

$$\text{LADD} = \frac{\begin{array}{c}\text{concentration of the}\\ \text{toxicant in the}\\ \text{exposure media}\end{array} \times \begin{array}{c}\text{contact}\\ \text{rate}\end{array} \times \begin{array}{c}\text{contact}\\ \text{fraction}\end{array} \times \begin{array}{c}\text{exposure}\\ \text{duration}\end{array}}{(\text{body weight})\ (\text{lifetime})}$$

Many exposures are now estimated using exposure factors probability distributions rather than single point estimates for the factors within the LADD equation (Finley et al., 1994; Cullen and Frey, 1999). Such approaches can provide a reality check and can be useful for generating more realistic exposure profiles. Part B of Fig. 4-7 shows how this is done using an example arsenic risk scenario with soil As concentration, ingestion rate, exposure duration, frequency, body weight, and bioavailability modeled as distributed variables. Using Monte Carlo simulation techniques, an overall incremental lifetime cancer risk (ILCR) distribution can be generated and a 95th percentile for population risk obtained. The *EPA Exposure Factors Handbook,* which is on-line (http://www.epa.gov/nceawww1/exposure.htm), provides useful information about exposure distributions (EPA, 1989b). This handbook also provides exposure information for specific populations of interest; for example, see Table 4-6 for an example of age-specific exposure information for infants and children for drinking water intake. Exposure data for drinking water, food consumption, soil ingestion, inhalation rates, dermal absorption, product use, and human activity patterns are included on this database.

Additional considerations for exposure assessments include how time and duration of exposures are evaluated in risk assessments. In general, estimates for cancer risk use averages over a lifetime. In a few cases, short-term exposure limits (STELs) are required (for example, ethylene oxide) and characterization of brief but high levels of exposure is required. In these cases exposures are not averaged over the lifetime. With developmental toxicity, a single exposure can be sufficient to produce an adverse developmental effect; thus, daily doses are used, rather than lifetime weighted averages. This is also important due to the time-dependent

A. Ingestion of arsenic from soil-Point Estimation Method

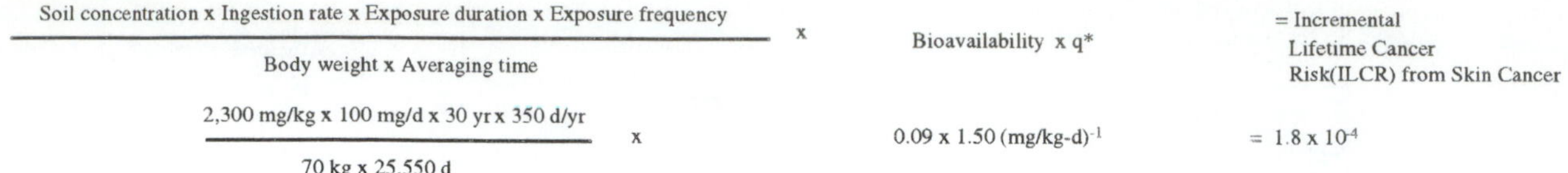

B. Ingestion of arsenic from soil- Probabilistic Methods

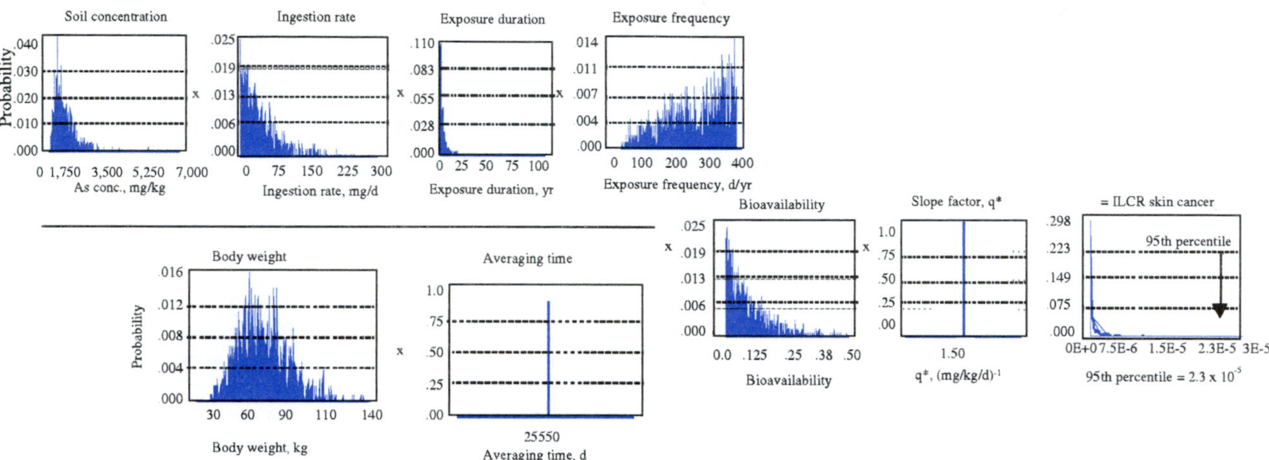

Figure 4-7. Example of risk calculations for incremental lifetime cancer risk (ILCR) of skin cancer due to ingestion of arsenic in soil.

A. Point exposure estimation method for calculation of ILCR. Point estimates for arsenic exposure input parameters are used in this example to calculate the ILCR. This exposure estimate is multiplied by the bioavailability of arsenic in soil to calculate the dose. Multiplication of the dose by the slope factor (q*) yields the lifetime risk. *B.* Probabilistic exposure methods for calculating the incremental lifetime cancer risk (ILCR) from arsenic ingestion. In this example, the soil concentration, ingestion rate, exposure duration and frequency, body weight, and bioavailability are modeled as distributions. Note that q* and averaging time (years) are given as single-point estimations. This method yields a distribution of ILCR, with a 95th percentile upper confidence interval of 2.3×10^{-5}. (From Calabrese, 1989; Davis, 1990; EPA, 1989a, 1989b, 1992, 1999; Israeli, 1992; Brorby, 1993; ATSDR, 1998.)

specificity of many adverse developmental outcomes and invalidation of Haber's law seen with developmental toxicity (Weller et al., 1999; EPA, 1991a).

The Food Quality Protection Act of 1996 has highlighted the need for several additional exposure and risk considerations (EPA, 1996b). These include the need to evaluate total exposures by determining aggregate exposure measures for all exposures to a single substance. Cross-media exposure analyses such as those conducted for lead and mercury are good examples of the value of looking at such total exposures in evaluating human risks. *Cumulative exposures* and *cumulative risk* refer to the total exposure to a group of compounds with similar modes of toxicity. For example, EPA is identifying and categorizing pesticides that act by a common mode of action, and such discussions of cumulative

Table 4-6
Example Exposure Factor Handbook Information: Drinking Water Intake

AGE GROUP	INTAKE (mL/day) MEAN	10th–90th PERCENTILES	INTAKE (mL/kg-day) MEAN	10th–90th PERCENTILES
Infants (<1 year)	302	0–649	43.5	0–101.8
Children (1–10 years)	736	286–1294	35.5	12.5–64.4
Teens (11–19 years)	965	353–1701	18.2	6.5–32.3
Adults (20–64 years)	1366	559–2268	19.9	8.0–33.7
Adults (64+ years)	1459	751–2287	21.8	10.9–34.7
All ages	1193	423–2092	22.6	8.2–39.8

SOURCE: EPA, 1997; Ershow and Cantor, 1989.

exposures to classes of organophosphates with similar modes of toxic action have been used as examples of classes of pesticides for which cumulative exposure and cumulative risk estimates are needed (EPA, 1998b; ILSI, 1999).

Variation in Susceptibility

Toxicology has been slow to recognize the marked variation among humans. Generally, assay results and toxicokinetic modeling utilize means and standard deviations to measure variation, or even standard errors of the mean, to make the range as small as possible. Outliers are seldom investigated. However, in occupational and environmental medicine, physicians are often asked, "Why me, Doc?" when they inform the patient that exposures on the job might explain a clinical problem. The patient insists that he or she is "no less careful than the next person." So it is important to know whether and how this patient might be at higher risk than others. Furthermore, EPA and OSHA are expected under the Clean Air Act and the Occupational Safety and Health Act to promulgate standards that protect the most susceptible subgroups or individuals in the population. By focusing investigators on the most susceptible individuals, there might also be a better chance of recognizing and elucidating underlying mechanisms (Omenn et al., 1990).

Host factors that influence susceptibility to environmental exposures include genetic traits, sex and age, preexisting diseases, behavioral traits (most importantly, smoking), coexisting exposures, medications, vitamins, and protective measures. Genetic studies are of two kinds: (1) investigations of the effects of chemicals and radiation on the genes and chromosomes, which are termed *genetic toxicology* (Chap. 9)—these tests measure evidence and rates of mutations, adduct formation, chromosomal aberrations, sister chromatid exchange, DNA repair and oncogene activation; and (2) ecogenetic studies, identifying inherited variation in susceptibility (predisposition and resistance) to specific exposures, ranging across pharmaceuticals ("pharmacogenetics"), pesticides, inhaled pollutants, foods, food additives, sensory stimuli, allergic and sensitizing agents, and infectious agents. Inherited variation in susceptibility has been demonstrated for all these kinds of external agents. In turn, the ecogenetic variation may affect either the biotransformation systems that activate and detoxify chemicals or the sites of action in target tissues.

Ecogenetics is still in its infancy; development of new methods and specific biomarkers of biotransformation and sites of action of chemicals may permit rapid advances (Nebert, 1999). With the rapid progress on the human genome project, identification of human polymorphisms has greatly expanded. A database of particular interest is the Human DNA Polymorphisms database (http://192.236.17.70:80/genetics), which contains significant information of Human DNA polymorphisms and their analysis. Cytochrome P450 polymorphisms are discussed at http://www.imm.ki.se/CYPalleles.

INFORMATION RESOURCES

The Toxicology Data Network (TOXNET) (http://sis.nlm.nih.gov/sis1/) from the National Library of Medicine provides access to a cluster of databases on toxicology, hazardous chemicals, and related areas including EPA's Integrated Risk Information System (IRIS) (EPA, 2000a), Hazardous Substances Data Bank, the National Cancer Institute's Chemical Carcinogenesis Research Information System, and EPA's Gene-Tox peer-reviewed mutagenicity test database. These information sources vary in the level of assessment included in the database, ranging from just listings of scientific references without comment to extensive peer-reviewed risk assessment information.

The World Health Organization (http://www.who.int) provides chemical-specific information through the International Programme on Chemical Safety (http://www.who.int/pcs/IPCS/index.htm) criteria documents and health and safety documents (WHO, 2000). The International Agency for Research on Cancer (IARC) provides information on specific classes of carcinogens as well as individual agents. The National Institutes for Environmental Health Sciences (NIEHS) National Toxicology Program provides technical reports on the compounds tested as a part of this national program and in its report on carcinogens (ninth report released in year 2000) also provides carcinogen-specific information (http://ehis.niehs.nih.gov/roc/toc9.html).

RISK PERCEPTION AND COMPARATIVE ANALYSES OF RISK

Individuals respond very differently to information about hazardous situations and products, as do communities and whole societies (Fischhoff, 1981, 1993, 1996; Sandman, 1993; NRC, 1996; Risk Commission, 1997; Institute of Medicine, 1999). Understanding these behavioral responses is critical in stimulating constructive risk communication and evaluating potential risk management options. In a classic study, students, League of Women Voters members, active club members, and scientific experts were asked to rank 30 activities or agents in order of their annual contribution to deaths (Slovic et al., 1979). Club members ranked pesticides, spray cans, and nuclear power as safer than did other lay persons. Students ranked contraceptives and food preservatives as riskier and mountain climbing as safer than did others. Experts ranked electric power, surgery, swimming, and x-rays as more risky and nuclear power and police work as less risky than did lay persons. There are also group differences in perceptions of risk from chemicals among toxicologists, correlated with their employment in industry, academia, or government (Neal et al., 1994).

Psychological factors such as dread, perceived uncontrollability, and involuntary exposure interact with factors that represent the extent to which a hazard is familiar, observable, and "essential" for daily living (Lowrance, 1976; Morgan, 1993). Figure 4-8 presents a grid on the parameters controllable/ uncontrollable and observable/not observable for a large number of risky activities; for each of the two paired main factors, highly correlated factors are described in the boxes.

Public demand for government regulations often focuses on involuntary exposures (especially in the food supply, drinking water, and air) and unfamiliar hazards, such as radioactive waste, electromagnetic fields, asbestos insulation, and genetically modified crops and foods. Many people respond very negatively when they perceive that information about hazards or even about new technologies without reported hazards has been withheld by the manufacturers (genetically modified foods) or by government agencies (HIV-contaminated blood transfusions in the 1980s; extent of hazardous chemical or radioactive wastes).

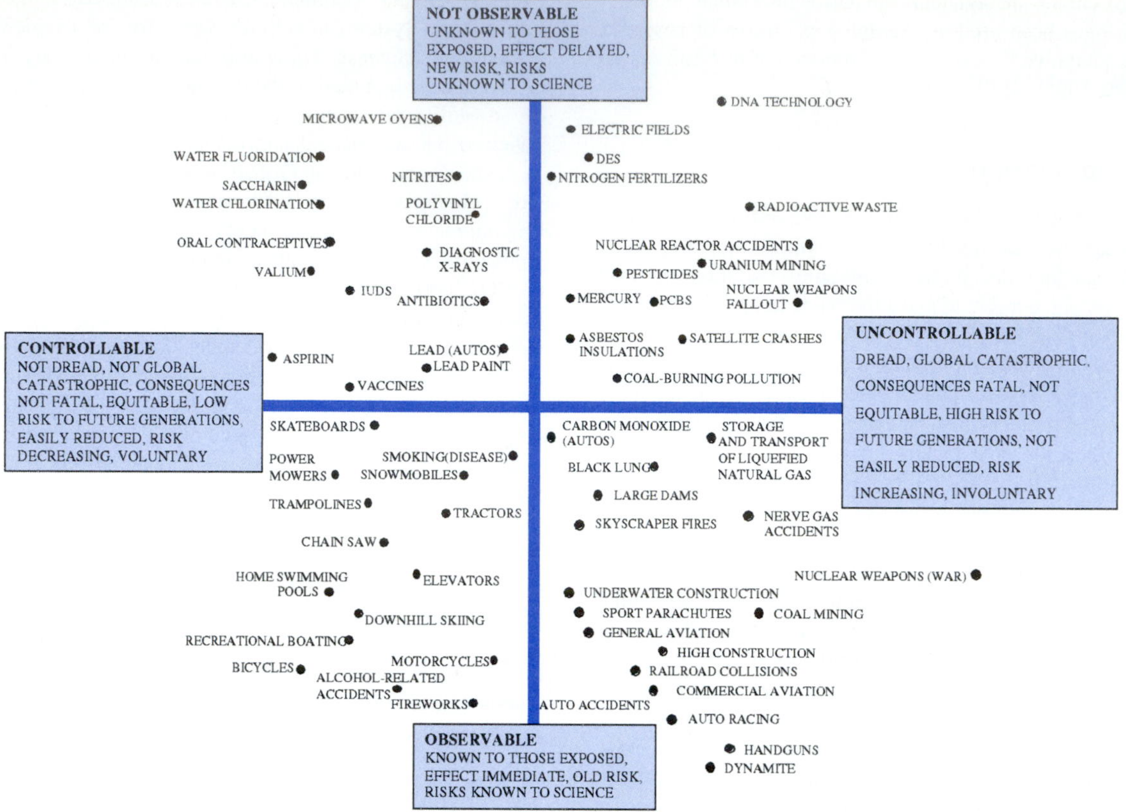

Figure 4-8. Perceptions of risk illustrated using a "risk space" axis diagram.

Risk space has axes that correspond roughly to a hazard's perceived "dreadedness" and to the degree to which it is familiar or observable. Risks in the upper right quadrant of this space are most likely to provoke calls for government regulation. (Morgan, 1993; Slovic, 1988.)

Perceptions of risk led to the addition of an extra safety factor (default value 10) for children in the Food Quality Protection Act of 1996. Engineering-based "as low as reasonably achievable" (ALARA) approaches also reflect the general "precautionary principle," which is strongly favored by those who, justifiably, believe we are far from knowing all risks given the limited toxicity testing (Roe et al., 1997).

A politically controversial matter has been the introduction of organized comparative risk assessment projects. Comparative risk analysis is a planning and decision-influencing tool that ranks various kinds of environmental problems to establish their relative significance and priority for action. Many states have mounted explicit programs. EPA Science Advisory Board reports entitled *Unfinished Business* (EPA, 1987) and *Reducing Risk* (EPA, 1990) were significant priority-setting exercises. This approach is so logical that it may be surprising to learn that comparisons of risks are so controversial. Public health and environmental agency officials routinely practice comparative risk assessment, at least intuitively, in deciding how to allocate their own time, their staff's time, and other resources. They must make judgments about what and how to advise their local communities about potential and definite risks. They must anticipate the question "Compared to what?"

Most people, of course, regularly compare risks of alternative activities—on the job, in recreational pursuits, in interpersonal interactions, and in investments. Since 1993, members of Congress have pressed for the systematic use by federal regulatory agencies of comparisons of similar and dissimilar risks. The aim was to make the benefits and costs of health, safety, and environmental protection more explicit and more comprehensible, with more cost-effective decisions. However, determining how best to conduct comparative risk analyses has proved difficult due to the great variety of health and environmental benefits, the gross uncertainties of dollar estimates of benefits and costs, and the different distributions of benefits and costs across the population. Even more important than these technical challenges was the highly partisan nature of the debate during 1994–1995, as these analytical schemes were linked with strong antiregulatory proposals and characterized by opponents as tactics for avoiding necessary actions.

From the other side of the political spectrum a broad concept called "environmental justice" has emerged, reflecting the ethical guidance that poor, disenfranchised neighborhoods should be protected as much as well-to-do neighborhoods (Rios et al., 1993; Institute of Medicine, 1999). In fact, the poor may need greater protection due to coexisting higher risk factors for poor pregnancy outcomes, impaired growth and development, smoking-related cancers, asthma, lead toxicity, and other health problems. On the other hand, the compelling needs to overcome low rates of prenatal care and childhood immunization, acute lead toxicity from bullets, poor housing, lack of education, and joblessness or low-wage jobs often make hypothetical or long-term relatively low-level estimated risks from chemical pollutant exposures less salient to these communities. One approach to a comprehensive assessment of priorities is the preparation of specific "community risk profiles" (Wernick, 1995).

SUMMARY

The National Research Council and Risk Commission frameworks for risk assessment and risk management provide a consistent databased approach for evaluating risks and taking action to reduce risks. The objectives of risk assessments vary with the issues, risk management needs, and statutory requirements. However, the frameworks are sufficiently flexible to address these various objectives and to accommodate new knowledge while also providing guidance for priority setting in industry, environmental organizations, and government regulatory and public health agencies. Toxicology, epidemiology, exposure assessment, and clinical observations can be linked with biomarkers, cross-species investigations of mechanisms of effects, and systematic approaches to risk assessment, risk communication, and risk management. Advances in toxicology are certain to improve the quality of risk assessments for a broad array of health endpoints as scientific findings substitute data for assumptions and help to describe and model uncertainty more credibly.

REFERENCES

Abbott BD, Harris MW, Birnbaum LS: Comparisons of the effects of TCDD and hydrocortisone on growth factor expression provide insight into their interaction in the embryonic mouse palate. *Teratology* 45:35–53, 1992.

Albert RE: Carcinogen risk assessment in the US Environmental Protection Agency. *Crit Rev Toxicol* 24:75–85, 1994.

Allen BC, Kavlock RJ, Kimmel CA, Faustman EM: Dose response assessments for developmental toxicity: II. Comparison of generic benchmark dose estimates with no observed adverse effect levels. *Fundam Appl Toxicol* 23:487–495, 1994a.

Allen BC, Kavlock RJ, Kimmel CA, Faustman EM: Dose–response assessment for developmental toxicity: III. Statistical models. *Fundam Appl Toxicol* 23:496–509, 1994b.

Ames BN, Gold LS: Too many rodent carcinogens: Mitogenesis increases mutagenesis. *Science* 249:970–971, 1990.

Andersen ME, Barton HA: Biological regulation of receptor-hormone complex c in relation to dose–response assessments of endocrine-active compounds. *Toxicol Sci* 48:38–50, 1999.

Anderson ME, Mills JJ, Gargas ML: Modeling receptor-mediated processes with dioxin: Implications for pharmacokinetics and risk assessment. *Risk Anal* 13:25–36, 1993.

Armitage P, Doll R: A two-stage theory of carcinogenesis in relation to the age distribution of human cancer. *Br J Cancer* 11:161–169, 1957.

Ashby J, Tennant RW: Prediction of rodent carcinogenicity of 44 chemicals: Results. *Mutagenesis* 9:7–15, 1994.

ATSDR: *Toxicological Profile for Arsenic (draft).* Atlanta: U.S. Department of Health and Human Services, 1998; pp 110–113.

Atterwill CK, Johnston H, Thomas SM: Models for the *in vitro* assessment of neurotoxicity in the nervous system in relation to xenobiotic and neurotrophic factor-mediated events. *Neurotoxicology* 13:39–54, 1992.

Auton TR: Calculation of benchmark doses from teratology data. *Regul Toxicol Pharmacol* 19:152–167, 1994.

Barnes DG, Daston GP, Evans JS, et al: Benchmark dose workshop. *Regul Toxicol Pharmacol* 21:296–306, 1995.

Barnes DG, Dourson MJ: Reference dose (RfD): Description and use in health risk assessment. *Regul Toxicol Pharmacol* 8:471–486, 1988.

Brorby G , Finley G: Standard probability density functions for routine use in environmental health risk assessment. In: Society for Risk Analysis annual meeting, Savannah, GA, December, 1993.

Brown CC: High-to low-dose extrapolation in animals, in Rodricks JV, Tardiff RG (eds): *Assessment and Management of Chemical Risks.* Washington, DC: American Chemical Society, 1984, pp 57–79.

Brown MPS, Grundy WN, Lin D, et al: *Proc Natl Acad Sci USA* 97:262–267, 2000.

Brown NA, Spielmann H, Bechter R, et al: Screening chemicals for reproductive toxicity: The current alternatives: The report and recommendations of an ECVAM/ETS workshop (ECVAM Workshop 12). *Alt Lab Anim* 23:868–882, 1995.

Calabrese EJ, Pastides H, Barnes R, et al: How much soil do young children ingest: An epidemiologic study, in Kostecki PT, Calabrese EJ (eds) : *Petroleum Contaminated Soils.* Chelsea, MI: Lewis Publishers, 1989, pp 363–397.

Calkins DR, Dixon RL, Gerber CR, et al: Identification, characterization, and control of potential human carcinogens: A framework for federal decision-making. *J Natl Cancer Inst* 61:169–175, 1980.

Capen CC, Dybing E, Rice JM, Wilbourn JD (eds): *Species Differences in Thyroid Kidney and Urinary Bladder Carcinogenesis* (IARC Scientific Publication No. 147), Lyon, *France:* IARC, 1999.

Charnley G, Omenn GS: A summary of the findings and recommendations of the Commission on Risk Assessment and Risk Management (and accompanying papers prepared for the Commission). *Hum Ecol Risk Assess* 3:701–711, 1997.

Checkoway H: Epidemiology, in Rosenstock L, Cullen M (eds): *Textbook of Clinical Occupational and Environmental Medicine.* Philadelphia: Saunders, 1994, pp 150–168.

Cohen SM, Ellwein LB: Proliferative and genotoxic cellular effects in 2-acetylaminofluorene bladder and liver carcinogenesis: Biological modeling of the EDO1 study. *Toxicol Appl Pharmacol* 104:79–93, 1990.

Costa LG (section ed): Biochemical and molecular neurotoxicology, in Maines MD, Costa LG, Reed DJ, et al (eds): *Current Protocols in Toxicology.* New York: Wiley, 2000.

Crump KS: An improved procedure for low-dose carcinogenic risk assessment from animal data. *J Environ Pathol Toxicol* 5:349–348, 1980.

Crump KS: A new method for determining allowable daily intakes. *Fundam Appl Toxicol* 4:854–871, 1984.

Cullen AC, Frey HC: *Probabilistic Techniques in Exposure Assessment: A Handbook for Dealing with Variability and Uncertainty in Models and Inputs.* New York: Plenum Press, 1999.

Davis S, Waller P, Buschbom R, et al: Quantitative estimates of soil ingestion in normal children between the ages of 2 and 7 years: Population-based estimates using aluminum, silicon, and titanium as soil tracer elements. *Arch Environ Health* 45:112–122, 1990.

Dean AG, Dean JA, Coulombier D, et al: Epi Info, Version 6: A word processing, database, and statistics program for public health on IBM-compatible microcomputers. Atlanta: Centers for Disease Control and Prevention (CDC), 1995.

Dearfield KL: *Pesticide Assessment Guidelines, Subdivision F, Hazard Evaluation, Series 84, Mutagenicity, Addendum 9.* PB91-158394. Washington, DC: National Technical Information Services, 1990.

Depledge MH, Amaral-Mendes JJ, Daniel B, et al: The conceptual basis of the biomarker approach, in Peakall DB, Shugart LR (eds): *Biomarker.* NATO ASI Series. Vol H 68. Berlin: Springer, 1993, p 19.

Diener RM: Safety Assessment of Pharmaceuticals, in Williams P,

Hottendorf G (eds): *Comprehensive Toxicology.* Oxford: Elsevier, 1997, pp 3–16.

Dourson ML, DeRosa CT: The use of uncertainty factors in establishing safe levels of exposure, in Krewski D, Franklin C (eds): *Statistics in Toxicology.* New York: Gordon & Breach, 1991, pp 613–627.

Dourson ML, Hertzberg RC, Hartung R, Blackburn K: Novel methods for the estimation of acceptable daily intake. *Toxicol Ind Health* 1:23–41, 1985.

Dourson ML, Stara JF: Regulatory history and experimental support of uncertainty (safety factors). *Regul Toxicol Pharmacol* 3:224–238, 1983.

Eaton DL, Gallagher EP: Mechanisms of aflatoxin carcinogenesis. *Annu Rev Pharmacol Toxicolo* 34:134–172, 1994.

EGRET, Statistics and Epidemiology Research Corporation (SERC). Seattle: Statistics and Epidemiology Research Corporation, 1994.

Eisen MB, Spellman PT, Brown PO, Botstein D: Cluster analysis and display of genome-wide expression patterns. *Proc Natl Acad Sci USA* 95:14863–14868, 1998.

EPA: *Unfinished Business: A Comparative Assessment of Environmental Problems. Overview Report.* Washington, DC: EPA, 1987.

EPA: Proposed guidelines for assessing female reproductive risk. *Fedl Reg* 53:24834–24847, 1988.

EPA: *Risk assessment guidance for Superfund.* Vol. 1. *Human Health Evaluation Manual,* Part A. Office of Policy Analysis, EPA/540/1-89/002. Washington, DC: Office of Emergency and Remedial Response, 1989.

EPA. *Exposure Factors Handbook.* Final report: EPA. Washington, DC: Office of Health and Environmental Assessment, 1989b (http://www.epa.gov/nceawww1/exposure.htm).

EPA: *Reducing Risk: Setting Priorities and Strategies for Environmental Protection.* Washington, DC: EPA Science Advisory Board, 1990.

EPA: Guidelines for developmental toxicity risk assessment. *Fed Reg* 56:63798–63826, 1991a.

EPA: *Alpha2u-Globulin: Association with Chemically Induced Renal Toxicity and Neoplasia in the Male Rat.* EPA-625/3-91/019F. Washington, DC: EPA, 1991b.

EPA: Guidelines for Exposure Assessment. *Fed Reg* 57:22888–22938, 1992.

EPA: *Guidelines for Carcinogen Risk Assessment* (draft revisions). Washington, DC: Office of Health and Environmental Assessment, Exposure Assessment Group, 1994a.

EPA: *Health Assessment Document for 2,3,7,8-Tetrachlorodibenzo-p-Dioxin (TCDD) and Related Compounds.* Washington, DC: Office of Research and Development, 1994b. [Revisions, September, 2000 *www.epa.gov/ncea/dioxin.htm*].

EPA: *Proposed Guidelines for Neurotoxicity Risk Assessment.* 60:52032–52056. Washington, DC: EPA, 1995.

EPA: Proposed guidelines for ecological risk assessment. *Fed Reg* 61, 1996a.

EPA: *Food Quality Protection Act (FQPA):* Washington, DC: Office of Pesticide Programs, 1996b.

EPA: Guidelines for reproductive toxicity risk assessment. *Fed Reg* 61:56274–56322, 1996c.

EPA: *Aggregate Exposure. Review Document for the Scientific Advisory Panel SAP Public Docket.* Washington, DC: EPA, 1997.

EPA: *Chemical Hazard Availability Study.* Washington, DC: Office of Pollution Prevention and Toxics, 1998a.

EPA: Guidance for identifying pesticides that have a common mechanism of toxicity: Notice of availability and solicitation of public comments. *Fed Reg* 63:42031–42032, 1998b.

EPA: *Health Effects Test Guidelines. OPPTS 870.6300, Developmental Neurotoxicity Study.* Washington, DC: EPA, 1998c.

EPA: *Chlorpyrifos–Report of the FQPA Safety Factor Committee.* HED Doc. No 013296. Washington, DC, 1999a.

EPA: *Guidelines for Carcinogen Risk Assessment, draft.* NCEA-F-0644. Washington, DC: EPA, 1999b.

EPA: *Integrated Risk Information System.* Washington, DC: Office of Research and Development, National Center for Environmental Assessment, 2000a (*http://www.epa.gov/iris/index.html*).

EPA: *Health Effects Test Guidelines: 870 Series Final Guidelines.* Washington, DC: Office of Prevention, Pesticides and Toxic Substances, 2000b. (*http://www.epa.gov/OPPTS_Harmonized/870_Health_Effects_Test_Guidelines*).

EPA: *Benchmark Dose Technical Guidance Document: External Review Draft.* Washington, DC: Risk Assessment Forum, 2000c.

Ershow AG, Cantor KP: *Total Water and Tapwater Intake in The United States:Populations-Based Estimates of Quantities and Sources.* [Bethesda, MD]: Life Sciences Research Office, Federation of American Societies for Experimental Biology, 1989, pp 328–334.

Faustman EM: Short-term test for teratogens. *Mutat Res* 205:355–384, 1988.

Faustman EM, Allen BC, Kavlock RJ, Kimmel CA: Dose–response assessment for developmental toxicity: I. Characterization of data base and determination of no observed adverse effect levels. *Fundaml Appl Toxicol* 23:478–486, 1994.

Faustman EM, Bartell SM: Review of noncancer risk assessment: Applications of benchmark dose methods. *Hum Ecol Risk Assess* 3:893–920, 1997.

Faustman EM, Omenn GS: Risk assessment, in Klaassen CD (ed): *Casarett and Doull's Toxicology,* 5th ed. New York: McGraw-Hill, 1996a, pp 75–88.

Faustman EM, Ponce RA, Seeley MR, Whittaker SG: Experimental approaches to evaluate mechanisms of developmental toxicity, in Hood, R (ed): *Handbook of Developmental Toxicology.* Boca Raton, FL: CRC Press, 1996b, pp 13–41.

Faustman EM, Lewandowski TA, Ponce RA, Bartell SM: Biologically based dose–response models for developmental toxicants: Lessons from methylmercury. *Inhal Toxicol* 11:101–114, 1999.

Faustman EM, Wellington DG, Smith WP, Kimmel CS: Characterization of a developmental toxicity dose response model. *Environ Health Perspect* 79:229–241, 1989.

Finley B, Proctor D, Scott P, et al: Recommended distributions for exposure factors frequently used in health risk assessment. *Risk Anal* 14:533–553, 1994.

Fischhoff B: Cost-benefit analysis: An uncertain guide to public policy. *Ann NY Acad Sci* 363:173–188, 1981.

Fischhoff B, Bostrom A, Quandrel MJ: Risk perception and communication, in Detels R, Holland W, McEwen J, Omenn G (eds): *Oxford Textbook of Public Health.* New York: Oxford University Press, 1996, pp 987–1002.

Fischhoff B, Bostrom A, Quandrel MJ: Risk perception and communication. *Annu Rev Public Health* 14:183–203, 1993.

Gamble JF, Battigelli MC: Epidemiology, in Clayton GD, Clayton FE (eds): *Patty's Industrial Hygiene and Toxicology.* New York: Wiley, 1978, pp 113–127.

Gamble JF, Battigelli MC: Occupational epidemiology: Some guideposts, in Clayton GD, Clayton FE (eds): *Patty's Industrial Hygiene and Toxicology.* New York: Wiley, 1991, pp 35–71.

Gargas ML, Finley BL, Paustenback DJ, Long TF: Environmental health risk assessment: Theory and practice, in Ballantyne B, Marrs T, Syversen T (eds): *General and Applied Toxicology.* New York: Grove's Dictionaries, 1999, pp 1749–1809.

Gray TJB (ed): Application of *In Vitro* Systems in Male Reproductive Toxicology. San Diego, CA: Academic 1988.

Griffith W, Brutlage J: Statistical models for gene expression profiles with phase shift and amplitude scaling. (pending, 2001).

Harris MW, Chapin RE, Lockhart AC, et al: Assessment of a short-term reproductive and developmental toxicity screen. *Fundam Appl Toxicol* 19:186–196, 1992.

Hartung R: Dose–response relationships, in Tardiff R, Rodricks J (eds): *Toxic Substances and Human Risk: Principles of Data Interpretation.* New York: Plenum Press, 1987, pp 29–46.

Haseman JK, Lockhart AM: Correlations between chemically related site-specific carcinogenic effects in long-term studies in rats and mice. *Environ Health Perspect* 101:50–54, 1993.

Hattis D, Banati P, Goble R: Distributions of individual susceptibility among humans for toxic effects: How much protection does the traditional tenfold factor provide for what fraction of which kinds of chemicals and effects? *Ann NY Acad Sci* 895:286–316, 1999a.

Hattis D, Banati P, Goble R, Burmaster DE: Human interindividual variability in parameters related to health risks. *Risk Anal* 19:711–726, 1999b.

Hattis D, Silver K: Human interindividual variability—A major source of uncertainty in assessing risks for noncancer health effects (review). *Risk Anal* 14:421–431, 1994.

Healey GF: Power calculations in toxicology. *ATLA* 15:132–139, 1987.

Hill AB: The environment and disease: Association or causation. *Proc R Soc Med* 58:295–300, 1965.

HSE Health and Safety Executive: *Reducing Risks, Protecting People (discussion document).* Sudbury, Suffolk, UK: HSE Books, 2000.

IARC: *IARC Monographs on the Evaluation of Carcinogenic Risks to Humans.* Vol 60. Lyon, *France:* World Health Organization, 1994.

IARC: *IARC Monographs on the Evaluation of Carcinogenic Risks to Humans.* Vols 1-76. Lyon, *France:* World Health Organization, 2000 (http://www.iarc.fr/index.html).

ILSI: *A Framework for Cumulative Risk Assessment.* Washington, DC: International Life Sciences Institute, 1999.

Institute of Medicine: *Toward Environmental Justice: Research, Education, and Health Policy Needs.* Washington, DC: National Academy Press, 1999.

Israeli M, Nelson CB: Distribution and expected time of residence for United States households. *Risk Anal* 12:65–72, 1992.

Iyer VR, Eisen MB, Ross DT, et al: The transcriptional program in the response of human fibroblasts to serum. *Science* 283:83–87, 1999.

Johnson DE, Wolfgang GHI, Gledin MA, Braeckman RA: Toxicokinetics and toxicodynamics, in Sipes I, McQueen C, Gandolfi A (eds): *Comprehensive Toxicology.* Oxford, UK: Pergamon, Elsevier Sciences, 1997, pp 169–181.

Kavlock RJ, Allen BC, Faustman EM, Kimmel CA: Dose response assessments for developmental toxicity: IV. Benchmark doses for fetal weight changes. *Fundam Appl Toxicol* 26:211–222, 1995.

Kimmel CA, Gaylor DW: Issues in qualitative and quantitative risk analysis for developmental toxicology. *Risk Anal* 8:15–20, 1988.

Kodell RL, Chen JJ, Jackson CD, Gaylor DW: Using short-term tests to predict carcinogenic activity in the long-term bioassay. *Hum Ecol Risk Assess* 5:427–443, 1999.

Kohn MC, Lucier GW, Clark GC, et al: A mechanistic model of effects of dioxin on gene expression in the rat liver. *Toxicol Appl Pharmacol* 120:138–154, 1993.

Krewski D, Van Ryzin J: Dose response models for quantal response toxicity data, in Csorgo M, Dawson D, Rao J, Seleh A (eds): *Statistics and Related Topics.* North-Holland, Amsterdam: , 1981, pp 201–229.

Lampen A, Siehler S, Ellerbeck U, et al: New molecular bioassays for the estimation of the teratogenic potency of valproic acid derivatives in vitro: Activation of the peroxisomal proliferator-activated receptor (PPARdelta). *Toxicol Appl Pharmacol* 160:238–249, 1999.

Lau C, Andersen ME, Crawford-Brown DJ, et al: Evaluation of biologically based dose-response modeling for developmental toxicity: A workshop report. *Regul Toxicol Pharmacol* 31:190–199, 2000.

Lave LB, Ennever F, Rosenkranz HS, Omenn GS: Information value of the rodent bioassay. *Nature* 336:631–633, 1988.

Lave LB, Omenn GS: Cost-effectiveness of short-term tests for carcinogenicity. *Nature* 334:29–34, 1986.

Leroux BG, Leisenring WM, Moolgavkar SH, Faustman EM: A biologically based dose-response model for development. *Risk Anal* 16:449–458, 1996.

Lewandowski TA, Ponce RA, Whittaker SG, Faustman EM: In vitro models for evaluating developmental toxicity, in Gad S (ed): *In Vitro Toxicology.* New York: Taylor & Francis, 2000, pp 139–187.

Limbird LE, Taylor P: Endocrine disruptors signal the need for receptor models and mechanisms to inform policy. *Cell Press* 93:157–163, 1998.

Lowrance WW: *Of Acceptable Risk.* Los Altos, CA: William Kaufmann, 1976.

Makris S, Raffaele K, Sette W, Seed J: *A Retrospective Analysis of Twelve Developmental Neurotoxicity Studies. Draft. Submitted:* Washington, DC: EPA Office of Prevention, Pesticides and Toxic Substances (OPPTS), 1998.

Martin YC: NIDA Research monograph 134, in Rapaka R, Hawks R (eds): *Medications Development: Drug Discovery, Databases, and Computer-Aided Drug Design:* NIH Pub No. 93–3638. Bethesda, MD: National Institutes of Health, 1993, pp 84–102.

McClain RM: Mechanistic considerations in the regulation and classification of chemical carcinogens, in Kotsonis F, Mackey M, Hjelle J (eds): *Nutritional Toxicology.* New York: Raven Press, 1994, pp 278–304.

McGregor DB, Rice JM, Venitt S (eds): *The Use of Short- and Medium-Term Tests for Carcinogens and Data on Genetic Effects in Carcinogenic Hazard Evaluation* (IARC Sci Pub No. 146). Lyon, France: IARC, 1999.

Moolenaar RJ: Carcinogen risk assessment: International comparison. *Regul Toxicol Pharmacol* 20:302–336, 1994.

Moolgavkar SH, Luebeck G: Two-event model for carcinogenesis: Biological, mathematical, and statistical considerations. *Risk Anal* 10:323–341, 1990.

Moore JA, Daston GP, Faustman EM, et al: An evaluative process for assessing human reproductive and developmental toxicity of agents. *Reprod Toxicol* 9:61–95, 1995.

Morgan GM: Risk analysis and management. *Sci Am* 269:32–41, 1993.

Neal N, Malmfors T, Slovic P: Intuitive toxicology: Expert and lay judgments of chemical risks. *Toxicol Pathol* 22:198–201, 1994.

Nebert DW: Pharmacogenetics and pharmacogenomics: Why is this relevant to the clinical geneticist? *Clin Genet* 56:247–258, 1999.

Nebert DW, Duffy JJ: How knockout mouse lines will be used to study the role of drug-metabolizing enzymes and their receptors during reproduction, development, and environmetal toxicity, cancer and oxidative stress. *Biochem Pharmacol* 53:249–254, 1997.

Neumann DA, Olin SS: Urinary bladder carcinogenesis: A working group approach to risk assessment. *Food Chem Toxicol* 33:701–704, 1995.

NIEHS: *Corrositex: An In Vitro Test Method for Assessing Dermal Corrosivity Potential of Chemicals.* 99–4495. Washington, DC: ICCVAM, 1999, pp 33109–33111.

NIEHS: *The Murine Local Lymph Node Assay: A Test Method for Assessing the Allergic Contact Dermatitis Potential of Chemicals/Compounds.* 99–4494. Washington, DC: ICCVAM, 1999, pp 14006–14007.

NRC: *Risk Assessment in the Federal Government: Managing the Process.* Washington, DC: National Academy Press, 1983.

NRC: *Biological markers in pulmonary toxicology.* Washington, DC: National Academy Press, 1989a.

NRC: *Biological Markers in Reproductive Toxicology.* Washington, DC: National Academy Press, 1989b.

NRC: *Biological Markers in Immunotoxicology.* Washington, DC: National Academy Press, 1992a.

NRC: *Environmental Neurotoxicology.* Washington, DC: National Academy Press, 1992b.

NRC Committee on Risk Assessment Methodology: *Issues in Risk Assessment: Use of the Maximum Tolerated Dose in Animal Bioassays for Carcinogenicity.* Washington, DC: National Academy Press, 1993.

NRC: *Science and Judgment in Risk Assessment.* Washington, DC: National Academy Press, 1994.

NRC: *Understanding Risk.* Washington, DC: National Academy Press, 1996.

NRC: *Scientific Frontiers in Developmental Toxicology and Risk Assessment.* Washington, DC: National Research Council, 2000.

NTP: *9th Report on Carcinogens.* Washington, DC: U.S. Department of Human and Health Services, Public Health Service, 2000.

Oberdörster G: Lung particle overload: Implications for occupational exposure to particles. *Regul Toxicol Pharmacol* 21:123–135, 1995.

Ohanian EV, Moore JA, Fowle JR III, et al: Risk characterization: A bridge in informed decision-making. *Fundam Appl Toxicol* 39:81–88, 1997.

Omenn GS: The genomic era: A crucial role for the public health sciences. *Environl Health Perspect* 108:(5):A204–205, 2000.

Omenn GS, Faustman EM: Risk assessment and risk management, in Detels R, Holland W, McEwen J, Omenn G (eds): *Oxford Textbook of Public Health,* 3d ed. New York: Oxford University Press, 1997, pp 969–986. (4th ed. in press.)

Omenn GS, Lave LB: Scientific and cost-effectiveness criteria in selecting batteries of short-term tests. *Mutat Res* 205:41–49, 1988.

Omenn GS, Omiecinski CJ, Eaton DE: Eco-genetics of chemical carcinogens, in Cantor C, Caskey C, Hood L, et al (eds): *Biotechnology and Human Genetic Predisposition to Disease.* New York: Wiley-Liss, 1990, pp 81–93.

Omenn GS, Stuebbe S, Lave L: Predictions of rodent carcinogenicity testing results: Interpretation in light of the Lave-Omenn value-of-information model. *Mol Carcinogen* 14:37–45, 1995.

Perera F, Mayer J, Santella RM, et al: Biologic markers in risk assessment for environmental carcinogens. *Environ Health Perspect* 90:247–254, 1991.

Perera FP, Weinstein IB: Molecular epidemiology: Recent advances and future directions (review). *Carcinogenesis* 21:517–524, 2000.

Rai K, Van Ryzin J: A dose response model for teratological experiments involving quantal responses. *Biometrics* 41:1–10, 1985.

Renwick AG: Safety factors and the establishment of acceptable daily intakes. *Food Addit Contam* 8:135–150, 1991.

Renwick AG: Toxicokinetics, in Ballantyne B, Marrs T, Syversen T (eds): *General and Applied Toxicology.* New York: Grove's Dictionaries, 1999, pp 67–95.

Renwick AG, Lazarus NR: Human variability and noncancer risk assessment-an analysis of the default uncertainty factor. *Regul Toxicol Pharmacol* 27:3–20, 1998.

Renwick AG, Walker R: An analysis of the risk of exceeding the acceptable or tolerable daily intake. *Regul Toxicol Pharmacol* 18:463–480, 1993.

Rice JM, Baan RA, Blettner M, et al: Rodent tumors of urinary bladder, renal cortex, and thyroid gland. IARC Monographs: Evaluations of carcinogenic risk to humans. *Toxicol Sci* 49:166–171, 1999.

Rios R, Poje GV, Detels R: Susceptibility to environmental pollutants among minorities. *Toxicol Industri Health* 9:797–820, 1993.

Risk Commission, the Presidential/Congressional Commission on Risk Assessment and Risk Management, "Omenn Commission": Vol 1: *A Framework for Environmental Health Risk Management.* Vol 2: *Risk Assessment And Risk Management In Regulatory Decision-Making.* Washington DC: Government Printing Office, 1997; www.riskworld.com.

Robinson D: International Life Sciences Institute's role in evaluation of alternative methodology for the assessment of carcinogenic risk. *Toxicol Pathol* 26:474–475, 1998.

Rodericks JV, Rudenko L, Starr TB, Turnbull D: Risk Assessment, in Sipes I, McQueen C, Gandolfi A (eds): *Comprehensive Toxicology.* Oxford, UK: Pergamon, Elsevier Sciences, 1997, pp 315–338.

Roe D, Pease W, Florini K, Silbergeld E: *Toxic Ignorance.* Washington, DC: Environmental Defense Fund, 1997.

Sandman PM: *Responding to Community Outrage: Strategies for Effective Risk Communication.* Fairfax, VA: American Industrial Hygiene Association, 1993.

Schardein JL, Scialli AR: The legislation of toxicologic safety factors: The food quality protection act with chlorpyrifos as a test case. *Reprod Toxicol Rev* 13:1–14, 1999.

Schwetz BA: In vitro approaches in developmental toxicity. *Reprod Toxicol* 7:125–127, 1993.

Sette WF: *Pesticide Assessment Guidelines, Subdivision F, Hazard evaluation, Human and Domestic Animals, Addendum 10,* Neurotoxicity Series 81, 82 and 83, PB91-154617. Washington, DC: National Technical Information Services, 1991.

Shelby MD, Bishop JB, Mason JM, Tindall KR: Fertility, reproduction and genetic disease: Studies on the mutagenic effects of environmental agents on mammalian germ cells. *Environ Health Perspect* 100:283–291, 1993.

Shuey DL, Lau C, Logsdon TR, et al: Biologically based dose-response modeling in developmental toxicology: Biochemical and cellular sequelae of 5-fluorouracil exposure in the developing rat. *Toxicol Appl Pharmacol* 126:129–144, 1994.

Silverman KC, Naumann BD, Holder DJ, et al: Establishing data-derived adjustment factors from published pharmaceutical clinical trial data. *Hum Ecol Risk Assess* 5:1059–1089, 1999.

Slovic P: Risk perception, in Travis C (ed): *Carcinogen Risk Assessment.* New York: Plenum Press, 1988, pp 171–192.

Slovic P, Baruch F, Lichtenstein S: Rating the risks. *Environ* 21:1–20, 36–39, 1979.

Stevens JT: Risk assessment of pesticides, in Williams P, Hottendorf G (eds): *Comprehensive Toxicology.* Oxford, UK: Pergamon, Elsevier Sciences, 1997, pp 17–26.

Tennant RW, Stasiewicz S, Mennear J, et al: Genetically altered mouse models for identifying carcinogens, in McGregor D, Rice J, Venitt S (eds): *The use of Short- and Medium-Term Tests for Carcinogens and Data on Genetic Effects in Carcinogenic Hazard Evaluation.* Lyon, France: IARC Scientific Publications, 146:123–150, 1999.

Van den Berg M, Birnbaum L, Bosveld ATC, et al: Toxic equivalency factors (TEFs) for PCBs, PCDDs, PCDFs for humans and wildlife. *Environ Health Perspect* 106:775–792, 1998.

Waterfield CJ, Timbrell JA: Biomarkers–An overview, in Ballantyne B, Marrs TC, Syversen T (eds): *General and Applied Toxicology.* New York: Grove's Dictionaries, 1999, pp 1841–1854.

Weller E, Long N, Smith A, et al: Dose-rate effects of ethylene oxide exposure on developmental toxicity. *Toxicol Sci* 50:259–270, 1999.

Wernick IK (ed): *Community Risk Profiles: A Tool to Improve Environment and Community Health.* New York: Rockefeller University, 1995.

Whittaker SG, Faustman EM (eds). *In Vitro Assays for Developmental Toxicity.* New York: Raven Press, 1994.

WHO: Principles in governing consumer safety in relation to pesticide residues. *WHO Tech Rep Ser* 240, 1962.

WHO: *Assessing Human Health Risks of Chemicals: Derivation of Guidance Values for Health-Based Exposure Limits.* Geneva: World Health Organization, 1994.

WHO: *International Programme on Chemical Safety (IPCS)/OECD Joint Project on Harmonization of Chemical Hazard: Risk Assessment Terminology. Geneva: WHO,* 2000. (http://www.who.int/pes/rsk_term/term_des.htm).

UNIT 2

DISPOSITION OF TOXICANTS

CHAPTER 5

ABSORPTION, DISTRIBUTION, AND EXCRETION OF TOXICANTS

Karl K. Rozman and Curtis D. Klaassen

INTRODUCTION

As was noted in Chaps. 2 and 3, the toxicity of a substance depends on the dose; that is, the greater the amount of a chemical taken up by an organism, the greater the toxic response. This concept, which is known as *dose response,* requires elaboration, because ultimately it is not the dose but the concentration of a toxicant at the site or sites of action (target organ or tissue) that determines toxicity. It should be noted that the words *toxicant, drug, xenobiotic* (foreign compound), and *chemical* are used interchangeably throughout this chapter, since all chemical entities, whether endogenous or exogenous in origin, can cause toxicity at some dose. The concentration of a chemical at the site of action is proportional to the dose, but the same dose of two or more chemicals may lead to vastly different concentrations in a particular target organ of toxicity. This differential pattern is due to differences in the disposition of chemicals. Disposition may be conceptualized as consisting of absorption, distribution, biotransformation, and excretion. It should be noted, however, that these processes may occur simultaneously. The various factors affecting disposition are depicted in Fig. 5-1. They are discussed in detail in this chapter and Chap. 6. Any or all of these factors may have a minor or major impact on the concentration and thus the toxicity of a chemical in a target organ. For example, (1) if the fraction absorbed or the rate of absorption is low, a chemical may never attain a sufficiently high concentration at a potential site of action to cause toxicity, (2) the distribution of a toxicant may be such that it is concentrated in a tissue other than the target organ, thus decreasing the toxicity, (3) biotransformation of a chemical may result in the formation of less toxic or more toxic metabolites at a fast or slow rate with obvious consequences for the concentration and thus the toxicity at the target site, and (4) the more rapidly a chemical is eliminated from an organism, the lower will be its concentration and hence its toxicity in a target tissue or tissues. Furthermore, all these processes are interrelated and thus influence each other. For example, the rate of excretion of a chemical may depend to a large extent on its distribution and/or biotransformation. If a chemical is distributed to and stored in fat, its elimination is likely to be slow because very low plasma levels preclude rapid renal clearance or other clearances. Some lipid-soluble chemicals are very resistant to biotransformation. Their rate of excretion depends on biotransformation to water-soluble products and/or slow intestinal excretion of the parent compounds. As this brief introduction illustrates, the disposition of xenobiotics is very important in determining the concentration and thus the toxicity of chemicals in organisms.

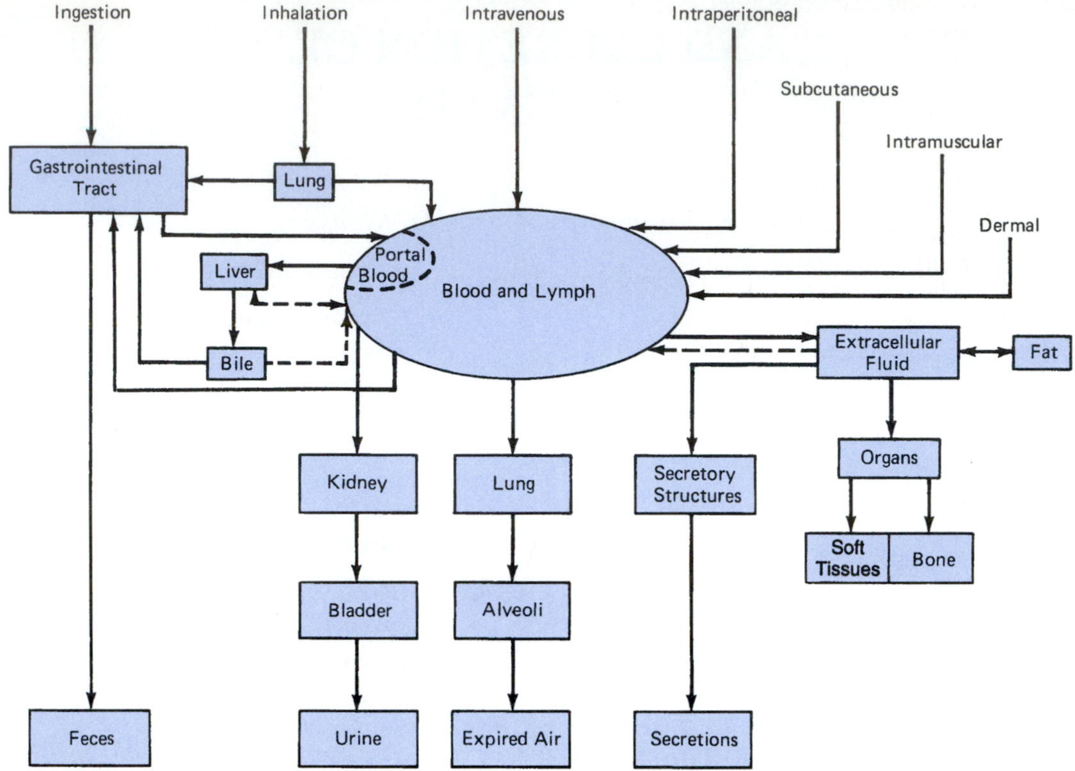

***Figure 5-1.** Routes of absorption, distribution, and excretion of toxicants in the body.*

The quantitation and determination of the time course of absorption, distribution, biotransformation, and excretion of chemicals are referred to as *pharmacokinetics* or *toxicokinetics* (see Chap. 7). Mathematical models are used to describe parts or the whole process of the disposition of a chemical. Calculations based on these models allow a numerical characterization of disposition (half-life, elimination rate constants, tissue profiles, etc.), which is essential for the assessment of the toxicity of a compound. Examination of species differences combined with knowledge of species-specific pathways of handling chemicals often provides the tools that allow toxicologists to predict disposition and its role in the toxicity of a compound for human exposure.

The skin, lungs, and alimentary canal are the main barriers that separate higher organisms from an environment containing a large number of chemicals. Toxicants have to cross one or several of these incomplete barriers to exert their deleterious effects at one site or several sites in the body. Exceptions are caustic and corrosive agents (acids, bases, salts, oxidizers), which act topically. A chemical absorbed into the bloodstream through any of these three barriers is distributed, at least to some extent, throughout the body, including the site where it produces damage. This site is often called the *target organ* or *target tissue.* A chemical may have one or several target organs, and, in turn, several chemicals may have the same target organ or organs. For example, benzene affects the hematopoietic system and carbon tetrachloride injures the liver. Lead and mercury both damage the central nervous system, the kidneys, and the hematopoietic system. It is self-evident that to produce a direct toxic effect in an organ, a chemical must reach that organ. However, indirect toxic responses may be precipitated at distant sites if a toxicant alters regulatory functions. For example, cholestyramine, a nonabsorbable resin, may trap certain acidic vitamins in the intestinal lumen and cause systemic toxicity in the form of various vitamin deficiency syndromes. Several factors other than the concentration influence the susceptibility of organs to toxicants. Therefore, the organ or tissue with the highest concentration of a toxicant is not necessarily the site where toxicity is exerted. For example, chlorinated hydrocarbon insecticides such as dichlorodiphenyltrichloroethane (DDT) attain their highest concentrations in fat depots of the body but produce no known toxic effect in that tissue. A toxicant may also exert its adverse effect directly on the bloodstream, as with arsine gas, which causes hemolysis.

Toxicants are removed from the systemic circulation by biotransformation, excretion, and storage at various sites in the body. The relative contribution of these processes to total elimination depends on the physical and chemical properties of the chemical. The kidney plays a major role in the elimination of most toxicants, but other organs may be of critical importance with some toxic agents. Examples include the elimination of a volatile agent such as carbon monoxide by the lungs and that of lead in the bile. Although the liver is the most active organ in the biotransformation of toxicants, other organs or tissues [enzymes in plasma, kidney, lungs, gastrointestinal (GI) tract, etc.] may also contribute to overall biotransformation. Biotransformation is often a prerequisite for renal excretion, because many toxicants are lipid-soluble and are therefore reabsorbed from the renal tubules after glomerular filtration. After a toxicant is biotransformed, its metabolites may be excreted preferentially into bile, as are the metabolites of DDT, or may be excreted into urine, as are the metabolites of organophosphate insecticides.

In this chapter, the qualitative aspects of absorption, distribution, and excretion are outlined, whereas their quantitative aspects are treated in Chap. 7. The fourth aspect of disposition—the biotransformation of chemicals—is dealt with in Chap. 6. As most toxic agents have to pass several membranes before exerting toxicity, we start with a discussion of some general characteristics of this ubiquitous barrier in the body.

CELL MEMBRANES

Toxicants usually pass through a number of cells, such as the stratified epithelium of the skin, the thin cell layers of the lungs or the gastrointestinal tract, the capillary endothelium, and the cells of the target organ or tissue. The plasma membranes surrounding all these cells are remarkably similar. The thickness of the cell membrane is about 7 to 9 nm. Biochemical, physiologic, and morphologic (electron microscopy) studies have provided strong evidence that membranes consist of a phospholipid bilayer, with polar head groups (phosphatidylcholine, phosphatidylethanolamine) predominating on both the outer and inner surfaces of the membrane and more or less perpendicularly directed fatty acids filling out the inner space. It is also well established that proteins are inserted in the bilayer, and some proteins even cross it, allowing the formation of aqueous pores (Fig. 5-2). Some cell membranes (eukaryotic) have an outer coat or glycocalyx consisting of glycoproteins and glycolipids. The fatty acids of the membrane do not have a rigid crystalline structure but are semifluid at physiologic temperatures. The fluid character of membranes is determined largely by the structure and relative abundance of unsaturated fatty acids. The more unsaturated fatty acids membranes contain, the more fluid-like they are, facilitating more rapid active or passive transport.

A toxicant may pass through a membrane by one of two general processes: (1) passive transport (diffusion according to Fick's law), in which the cell expends no energy, and (2) specialized transport, in which the cell provides energy to translocate the toxicant across its membrane.

Passive Transport

Simple Diffusion Most toxicants cross membranes by simple diffusion. Small hydrophilic molecules (up to a molecular weight of about 600) presumably permeate membranes through aqueous pores (Benz et al., 1980), whereas hydrophobic molecules diffuse across the lipid domain of membranes. The smaller a hydrophilic molecule is, the more readily it traverses membranes by simple diffusion through aqueous pores. Consequently, ethanol is absorbed rapidly from the stomach and intestine and is distributed equally rapidly throughout the body by simple diffusion from blood into all tissues. The majority of toxicants consist of larger organic molecules with differing degrees of lipid solubility. Their rate of transport across membranes correlates with their lipid solubility, which is frequently expressed as octanol/water partition coefficients of the uncharged molecules, or LogP as depicted in Table 5-1. Thus, the amino acids (negative logP) are water-soluble, whereas the environmental contaminants DDT and TCDD are very lipid soluble (high positive logP).

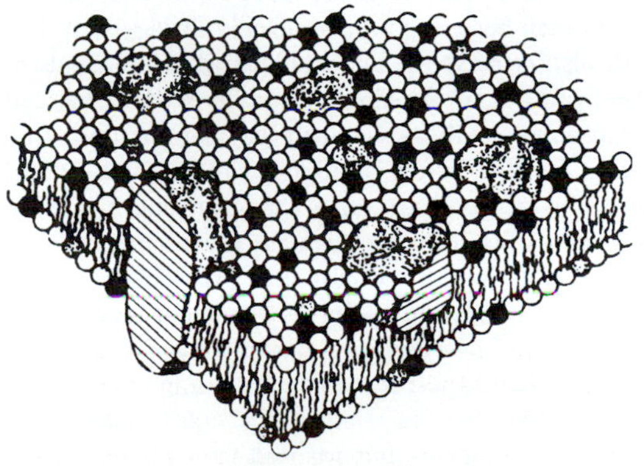

Figure 5-2. Schematic model of a biological membrane.

Table 5-1
Octanol/Water Partition Coefficients (P) of Different Molecules Expressed as LogP

COMPOUND	LogP
Paraquat	Charged molecule
Sulfobromophthalein	Charged molecule
Cephalosporin C	−4.72
Cystine	−4.45
Glycine	−3.21
Glutathione	−3.05
Gluconic acid	−2.89
Cysteine	−2.35
Glucose	−2.21
Edetic acid	−1.93
Ethylene glycol	−1.37
Lead acetate	−0.63
Ouabain	−0.35
P-aminohippuric acid	−0.25
Dimercaprol	0.18
Scopolamine	0.30
Sarin	0.45
Aspirin	1.02
Colchicine	1.19
Atropine	1.32
Benzoic acid	1.88
Benzene	2.14
Salicylic acid	2.19
Digoxin	2.27
Methyl salicylate	2.34
2,4-D	2.73
Warfarin	2.89
Digitoxin	3.05
Parathion	3.47
DDT	6.76
TCDD	7.05

Many chemicals are weak organic acids or bases. In solution, they are ionized according to Arrhenius's theory. The ionized form usually has low lipid solubility and thus does not permeate readily through the lipid domain of a membrane. Some transport of organic anions and cations (depending on their molecular weight) may occur through the aqueous pores, but this is a slow process (except for compounds of very low molecular weight), as the total surface area of aqueous pores is small compared with the total surface area of the lipid domain of a membrane. In general, the nonionized form of weak organic acids and bases is to some extent lipid-soluble, resulting in diffusion across the lipid domain of a membrane. The rate of transport of the nonionized form is proportional to its lipid solubility. The molar ratio of ionized to nonionized molecules of a weak organic acid or base in solution depends on the ionization constant. The ionization constant provides a measure for the weakness of organic acids and bases. The pH at which a weak organic acid or base is 50 percent ionized is called its pK_a or pK_b. Like pH, both pK_a and pK_b are defined as the negative logarithm of the ionization constant of a weak organic acid or base. With the equation $pK_a = 14 - pK_b$, pK_a can also be calculated for weak organic bases. An organic acid with a low pK_a is a relatively strong acid, and one with a high pK_a is a weak acid. The opposite is true for bases. The numerical value of pK_a does not indicate whether a chemical is an organic acid or a base. Knowledge of the chemical structure is required to distinguish between organic acids and bases.

The degree of ionization of a chemical depends on its pK_a and on the pH of the solution. The relationship between pK_a and pH is described by the Henderson-Hasselbalch equations.

$$\text{For acids: } pK_a - \text{pH} = \log \frac{[\text{nonionized}]}{[\text{ionized}]}$$

$$\text{For bases: } pK_a - \text{pH} = \log \frac{[\text{ionized}]}{[\text{nonionized}]}$$

The effect of pH on the degree of ionization of an organic acid (benzoic acid) and an organic base (aniline) is shown in Fig. 5-3. According to the Brönsted-Lowry acid-base theory, an acid is a proton (H^+) donor and a base is a proton acceptor. Thus, the ionized and nonionized forms of an organic acid represent an acid-base pair, with the nonionized moiety being the acid and the ionized moiety being the base. At a low pH, a weak organic acid such as benzoic acid is largely nonionized. At pH 4, exactly 50 percent of benzoic acid is ionized and 50 percent is nonionized, because this is the pK_a of the compound. As the pH increases, more and more protons are neutralized by hydroxyl groups, and benzoic acid continues to dissociate until almost all of it is in the ionized form. For an organic base such as aniline, the obverse is true. At a low pH, when protons are abundant, almost all of aniline is protonated, that is, ionized. This form of aniline is an acid because it can donate protons. As the pH increases, anilinium ions continue to dissociate until almost all the aniline is in the nonionized form, which is the aniline base. As transmembrane passage is largely restricted to the nonionized form, benzoic acid is more readily translocated through a membrane from an acidic environment, whereas more aniline is transferred from an alkaline environment.

Filtration When water flows in bulk across a porous membrane, any solute small enough to pass through the pores flows with it.

pH	Benzoic Acid	% Nonionized	Aniline	% Nonionized
1	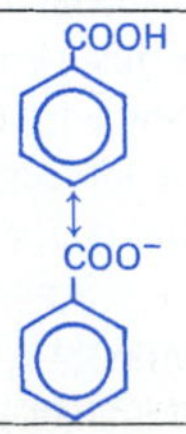 COOH	99.9	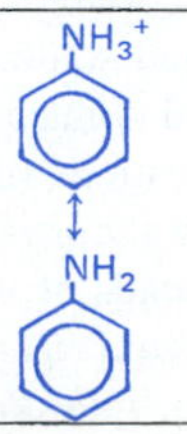 NH_3^+	
2		99		0.1
3		90		1
4		50		10
5	↕	10	↕	50
6	COO^-	1	NH_2	90
7		0.1		99

Figure 5-3. Effect of pH on the ionization of benzoic acid (pK_a 4) and aniline (pK_a = 5).

Passage through these channels is called *filtration,* as it involves bulk flow of water caused by hydrostatic or osmotic force. One of the main differences between various membranes is the size of these channels. In the kidney glomeruli, these pores are relatively large (about 70 nm), allowing molecules smaller than albumin (molecular weight 60,000) to pass through. The channels in most cells are much smaller (<4 nm), permitting substantial passage of molecules with molecular weights of no more than a few hundred (Schanker, 1961, 1962).

Special Transport

There are numerous compounds whose movement across membranes cannot be explained by simple diffusion or filtration. Some compounds are too large to pass through aqueous pores or too insoluble in lipids to diffuse across the lipid domains of membranes. Nevertheless, they are often transported very rapidly across membranes, even against concentration gradients. To explain these phenomena, the existence of specialized transport systems has been postulated. These systems are responsible for the transport across cell membranes of many nutrients, such as sugars and amino and nucleic acids, and also those of some foreign compounds.

Active Transport The following properties characterize an active transport system: (1) chemicals are moved against electrochemical or concentration gradients, (2) the transport system is saturated at high substrate concentrations and thus exhibits a transport maximum (T_m), (3) the transport system is selective for certain structural features of chemicals and has the potential for competitive inhibition between compounds that are transported by the same transporter, and (4) the system requires expenditure of energy, so that metabolic inhibitors block the transport process.

Substances actively transported across cell membranes presumably form a complex with a membrane-bound macromolecular carrier on one side of the membrane. The complex subsequently traverses to the other side of the membrane, where the substance is released. Afterward, the carrier returns to the original surface to repeat the transport cycle.

Significant advances in the understanding of active transport systems for xenobiotics have been made in the last few years. The table below indicates that there are a number of families of xenobiotic transporters. The first family of transporters identified were the multidrug-resistant (mdr) proteins or p-glycoproteins. The gene for this protein was identified in tumor cells resistant to chemotherapeutic anticancer drugs. It was determined that this transporter exudes chemotherapeutic drugs out of the tumor cells, and thus contributes to their resistance. Subsequently, it has been determined that mdr also protects the intact animal from chemicals by exuding chemicals out of intestinal cells, brain endothelial cells, liver cells, and kidney cells as well as protecting the fetus from some chemicals. Another family of proteins are the multi-resistant drug proteins. This family also exudes chemicals out of cells; however, phase II metabolites (glucuronides and glutathione conjugates) appear to be their preferred substrates. The name *organic-anion transporting peptide (oatp) family* is a misnomer because this transporter family transports not only acids, but also bases, and neutral compounds. They appear to be especially important in the hepatic uptake of xenobiotics. In contrast, the organic anion transporter (oat) family is especially important in the renal uptake of anions,

NAME	ABBREVIATION	FUNCTION
Multi-drug–resistant protein or p-glycoprotein	mdr	Decrease GI absorption
		Blood-brain barrier
		Biliary excretion
		Placental barrier
Multi-resistant drug protein	mrp	Urinary excretion
		Biliary excretion
Organic-anion transporting polypeptide	oatp	Hepatic uptake
Organic-anion transporter	oat	Kidney uptake
Organic-cation transporter	oct	Kidney uptake
		Liver uptake
		Placental barrier
Nucleotide transporter	nt	GI absorption
Divalent-metal ion transporter	dmt	GI absorption
Peptide transporter	pept	GI absorption

whereas the organic cation transporter (oct) family is important in both the renal and hepatic uptake of xenobiotics. The nucleotide transporter (nt) family, the divalent-metal ion transporter (dmt), and the peptide transporter (pept) aid in gastrointestinal absorption of nucleotides, metals, and di- and tri-peptides.

Facilitated Diffusion Facilitated diffusion applies to carrier-mediated transport that exhibits the properties of active transport except that the substrate is not moved against an electrochemical or concentration gradient and the transport process does not require the input of energy; that is, metabolic poisons do not interfere with this transport. The transport of glucose from the GI tract across the basolateral membrane of the intestinal epithelium, from plasma into red blood cells, and from blood into the central nervous system (CNS) occurs by facilitated diffusion.

Additional Transport Processes Other forms of specialized transport have been proposed, but their overall importance is not as well established as that of active transport and facilitated diffusion. Phagocytosis and pinocytosis are proposed mechanisms for cell membranes flowing around and engulfing particles. This type of transfer has been shown to be important for the removal of particulate matter from the alveoli by phagocytes and from blood by the reticuloendothelial system of the liver and spleen.

ABSORPTION

The process by which toxicants cross body membranes and enter the bloodstream is referred to as *absorption.* There are no specific systems or pathways for the sole purpose of absorbing toxicants. Xenobiotics penetrate membranes during absorption by the same processes as do biologically essential substances such as oxygen, foodstuffs, and other nutrients. The main sites of absorption are the GI tract, lungs, and skin. However, absorption may also occur from other sites, such as the subcutis, peritoneum, or muscle if a chemical is administered by special routes. Experimentalists and medical professionals often distinguish between parenteral and enteral administration of drugs and other xenobiotics. It is important to know that enteral administration includes all routes pertaining to the alimentary canal (sublingual, oral, and rectal), whereas parenteral administration involves all other routes (intravenous, intraperitoneal, intramuscular, subcutaneous, etc.).

Absorption of Toxicants by the Gastrointestinal Tract

The GI tract is one of the most important sites where toxicants are absorbed. Many environmental toxicants enter the food chain and are absorbed together with food from the GI tract. This site of absorption is of particular interest to toxicologists because suicide attempts frequently involve an overdose of an orally ingested drug. Oral intake is also the most common route by which children are accidentally exposed to poisons.

The GI tract may be viewed as a tube traversing the body. Although it is within the body, its contents can be considered exterior to the body. Therefore, unless a noxious agent has caustic or irritating properties, poisons in the GI tract usually do not produce systemic injury to an individual until they are absorbed.

Absorption of toxicants can take place along the entire GI tract, even in the mouth and rectum. Therefore, drugs such as nitroglycerin are administered sublingually and others are administered rectally, whereas the majority of drugs are given orally. If a toxicant is an organic acid or base, it tends to be absorbed by simple diffusion in the part of the GI tract in which it exists in the most lipid-soluble (nonionized) form. Because gastric juice is acidic and the intestinal contents are nearly neutral, the lipid solubility of weak organic acids or bases can differ markedly in these two areas of the GI tract. One can determine by the Henderson-Hasselbalch equations the fraction of a toxicant that is in the nonionized (lipid-soluble) form and estimate the rate of absorption from the stomach or intestine. According to this equation, a weak organic acid is present mainly in the nonionized (lipid-soluble) form in the stomach and predominantly in the ionized form in the intestine. Therefore, one would expect that weak organic acids are absorbed more readily from the stomach than from the intestine.

In contrast, organic bases (except very weak organic bases) are not in the lipid-soluble form in the stomach but are in that form in the intestine, suggesting that the absorption of such compounds occurs predominantly in the intestine rather than in the stomach. However, the Henderson-Hasselbalch equations have to be interpreted with some qualifications because other factors—such as the mass action law, surface area, and blood flow rate—have to be taken into consideration in examining the absorption of weak organic acids or bases. For example, only 1 percent of benzoic acid is present in the lipid-soluble form in the intestine. Therefore, one might conclude that the intestine has little capacity to absorb this organic acid. However, absorption is a dynamic process. The blood keeps removing benzoic acid from the lamina propria of the intestine, and according to the mass action law, the equilibrium will always be maintained at 1 percent in the nonionized form, providing continuous availability of benzoic acid for absorption. Moreover, absorption by simple diffusion is also proportional to the surface area. Because the small intestine has a very large surface (the villi and microvilli increase the surface area approximately 600-fold), the overall capacity of the intestine for absorption of benzoic acid is quite large. Similar considerations are valid for the absorption of all weak organic acids from the intestine.

The mammalian GI tract has specialized transport systems (carrier-mediated) for the absorption of nutrients and electrolytes (Table 5-2). The absorption of some of these substances is complex and depends on a number of factors. The absorption of iron, for example, depends on the need for iron and takes place in two steps: Iron first enters the mucosal cells and then moves into the blood. The first step is relatively rapid, whereas the second is slow. Consequently, iron accumulates within the mucosal cells as a protein-iron complex termed *ferritin.* When the concentration of iron in blood drops below normal values, some iron is liberated from the mucosal stores of ferritin and transported into the blood. As a consequence, the absorption of more iron from the intestine is triggered to replenish these stores. Calcium is also absorbed by a two-step process: first absorption from the lumen and then exudation into the interstitial fluid. The first step is faster than the second, and therefore intracellular calcium rises in mucosal cells during absorption. Vitamin D is required for both steps of calcium transport.

The GI tract also has at least one active transport system that decreases the absorption of xenobiotics. The multi-drug–resistance transporter (mdr, also termed p-glycoprotein) is localized in enterocytes. When chemicals that are substrates for mdr enter the enterocyte, they are exuded back into the intestinal lumen. Thus, the immunosuppressive drug cyclosporine and the chemotherapeutic anticancer drugs paclitaxel (taxol), colchicine, and vincristine are not readily absorbed from the GI tract for this reason.

Some xenobiotics can be absorbed by the same specialized transport systems. For example, 5-fluorouracil is absorbed by the pyrimidine transport system (Schanker and Jeffrey, 1961), thallium by the system that normally absorbs iron (Leopold et al., 1969), and lead by the calcium transporter (Sobel et al., 1938). Cobalt and manganese compete for the iron transport system (Schade et al., 1970; Thomson et al., 1971a, 1971b). Some dipeptide and oligopeptide transporters have been well characterized and have been shown to play an important role in the active absorption of drugs containing a β-lactam structure (Tsuji et al., 1993; Dantzig et al., 1994). Transepithelial absorption of dipeptides (e.g., glycylsarcosine) and β-lactam antibiotics at low concentrations occurs predominantly by active carrier-mediated mechanisms at both apical and basolateral membranes (Thwaites et al., 1993).

The number of toxicants actively absorbed by the GI tract is low; most enter the body by simple diffusion. Although lipid-

FOR WEAK ACIDS
$pK_a - pH = \log \frac{[\text{nonionized}]}{[\text{ionized}]}$
Benzoic acid $pK_a \approx 4$
Stomach pH ≈ 2 $4 - 2 = \log \frac{[\text{nonionized}]}{[\text{ionized}]}$ $2 = \log \frac{[\text{nonionized}]}{[\text{ionized}]}$ $10^2 = \log \frac{[\text{nonionized}]}{[\text{ionized}]}$ $100 = \log \frac{[\text{nonionized}]}{[\text{ionized}]}$ Ratio favors absorption
Intestine pH ≈ 6 $4 - 6 = \log \frac{[\text{nonionized}]}{[\text{ionized}]}$ $-2 = \log \frac{[\text{nonionized}]}{[\text{ionized}]}$ $10^{-2} = \frac{[\text{nonionized}]}{[\text{ionized}]}$ $\frac{1}{100} = \frac{[\text{nonionized}]}{[\text{ionized}]}$

FOR WEAK BASES
$pK_a - pH = \log \frac{[\text{ionized}]}{[\text{nonionized}]}$
Aniline $pK_a \approx 5$
Stomach pH ≈ 2 $5 - 2 = \log \frac{[\text{ionized}]}{[\text{nonionized}]}$ $3 = \log \frac{[\text{ionized}]}{[\text{nonionized}]}$ $10^3 = \log \frac{[\text{ionized}]}{[\text{nonionized}]}$ $1000 = \log \frac{[\text{ionized}]}{[\text{nonionized}]}$
Intestine pH ≈ 6 $5 - 6 = \log \frac{[\text{ionized}]}{[\text{nonionized}]}$ $-1 = \log \frac{[\text{ionized}]}{[\text{nonionized}]}$ $10^{-1} = \frac{[\text{ionized}]}{[\text{nonionized}]}$ $\frac{1}{10} = \frac{[\text{ionized}]}{[\text{nonionized}]}$ Ratio favors absorption

Table 5-2
Site Distribution of Specialized Transport Systems in the Intestine of Man and Animals

	Location of Absorptive Capacity			
	Small Intestine			
SUBSTRATES	UPPER	MIDDLE	LOWER	COLON
Sugar (glucose, galactose, etc.)	+ +	+ + +	+ +	0
Neutral amino acids	+ +	+ + +	+ +	0
Basic amino acids	+ +	+ +	+ +	?
Gamma globulin (newborn animals)	+	+ +	+ + +	?
Pyrimidines (thymine and uracil)	+	+	?	?
Triglycerides	+ +	+ +	+	?
Fatty acid absorption and conversion to triglyceride	+ + +	+ +	+	0
Bile salts	0	+	+ + +	
Vitamin B_{12}	0	+	+ + +	0
Na^+	+ + +	+ +	+ + +	+ + +
H^+ (and/or HCO_3^- secretion)	0	+	+ +	+ +
Ca^{2+}	+ + +	+ +	+	?
Fe^{2+}	+ + +	+ +	+	?
Cl^-	+ + +	+ +	+	0

SOURCE: Adapted from Wilson TH: *Mechanisms of Absorption.* Saunders, Philadelphia, 1962, pp 40–68.

soluble substances are absorbed by this process more rapidly and extensively than are water-soluble substances, the latter may also be absorbed to some degree. After oral ingestion, about 10 percent of lead, 4 percent of manganese, 1.5 percent of cadmium, and 1 percent of chromium salts are absorbed. If a compound is very toxic, even small amounts of absorbed material produce serious systemic effects. An organic compound that would not be expected to be absorbed on the basis of the pH-partition hypothesis is the fully ionized quaternary ammonium compound pralidoxime chloride (2-PAM; molecular weight 137), yet it is absorbed almost entirely from the GI tract (Levine and Steinberg, 1966). The mechanism by which some lipid-insoluble compounds are absorbed is not entirely clear. It appears that organic ions of low molecular weight (122 to 188) can be transported across the mucosal barrier by paracellular transport, that is, passive penetration through aqueous pores at the tight junctions (Aungst and Shen, 1986), or by active transport as discussed above.

It is interesting to note that even particulate matter can be absorbed by the GI epithelium. Particles of an azo dye, variable in size but averaging several thousand nanometers in diameter, have been shown to be taken up by the duodenum (Barnett, 1959). Emulsions of polystyrene latex particles 22 μm in diameter have been demonstrated to be carried through the cytoplasm of the intestinal epithelium in intact vesicles and discharged into the interstices of the lamina propria, followed by absorption into the lymphatics of the mucosa (Sanders and Ashworth, 1961). Particles appear to enter intestinal cells by pinocytosis, a process that is much more prominent in newborns than in adults (Williams and Beck, 1969). These examples demonstrate some of the principles and the variety of toxicants that can be absorbed at least to some extent by the GI tract.

The resistance or lack of resistance of chemicals to alteration by the acidic pH of the stomach, enzymes of the stomach or intestine, or the intestinal flora is of extreme importance. A toxicant may be hydrolyzed by stomach acid or biotransformed by enzymes of the microflora of the intestine to new compounds with a toxicity greatly different from that of the parent compound. For example, snake venom is much less toxic when administered orally rather than intravenously because it is broken down by digestive enzymes of the GI tract. Ingestion of well water with a high nitrate content produces methemoglobinemia much more frequently in infants than in adults. This is due to the higher pH of the GI tract in newborns, with the consequence of greater abundance of certain bacteria, especially *Escherichia coli,* which convert nitrate to nitrite. Nitrite formed by bacterial action produces methemoglobinemia (Rosenfield and Huston, 1950). Nitrite is also used as a food additive in meats and smoked fish. Some fish, vegetables, and fruit juices contain secondary amines. The acidic environment of the stomach facilitates a chemical reaction between nitrite and secondary amines, leading to the formation of carcinogenic nitrosamines (Chap. 8). Also, the intestinal flora can reduce aromatic nitro groups to aromatic amines that may be goitrogenic or carcinogenic (Thompson et al., 1954). Intestinal bacteria, specifically *Aerobacter aerogenes,* have been shown to degrade DDT to DDE (Mendel and Walton, 1966).

Many factors alter the GI absorption of toxicants. For example, editic acid [ethylenediaminetetraacetic acid (EDTA)] increases the absorption of some toxicants by increasing intestinal permeability. Simple diffusion is proportional not only to surface area and permeability but also to residency time in various segments of the alimentary canal. Therefore, the rate of absorption of a toxicant remaining for longer periods in the intestine increases, whereas that with a shorter residency time decreases. The residency time of a chemical in the intestine depends on intestinal motility. Some agents used as laxatives are known to exert effects on the absorption of xenobiotics by altering intestinal motility (Levine, 1970).

Experiments have shown that the oral toxicity of some chemicals is increased by diluting the dose (Ferguson, 1962; Borowitz et al., 1971). This phenomenon may be explained by more rapid stomach emptying induced by increased dosage volume, which in turn leads to more rapid absorption in the duodenum because of the larger surface area there.

The absorption of a toxicant from the GI tract also depends on the physical properties of a compound, such as lipid solubility, and the dissolution rate. Although it is often generalized that an increase in lipid solubility increases the absorption of chemicals, an extremely lipid-soluble chemical does not dissolve in the GI fluids, and absorption is low (Houston et al., 1974). If the toxicant is a solid and is relatively insoluble in GI fluids, it will have limited contact with the GI mucosa; therefore its rate of absorption will be low. Also, the larger the particle size is, the less will be absorbed, as the dissolution rate is inversely proportional to particle size (Gorringe and Sproston 1964; Bates and Gibaldi, 1970). This explains why metallic mercury is relatively nontoxic when ingested orally and why powdered arsenic is significantly more toxic than its coarse granular form (Schwartze, 1923).

The amount of a chemical entering the systemic circulation after oral administration depends on several factors. First, it depends on the amount absorbed into the GI cells. Further, before a chemical enters the systemic circulation, it can be biotransformed by the GI cells or extracted by the liver and excreted into bile with or without prior biotransformation. The lung can also contribute to the biotransformation or elimination of chemicals before their entrance into the systemic circulation, although its role is less well defined than that of the intestine and liver. This phenomenon of the removal of chemicals before entrance into the systemic circulation is referred to as *presystemic elimination,* or *first-pass effect.*

A number of other factors have been shown to alter absorption. For example, one ion can alter the absorption of another: Cadmium decreases the absorption of zinc and copper, and calcium that of cadmium; zinc decreases the absorption of copper, and magnesium that of fluoride (Pfeiffer, 1977). Milk has been found to increase lead absorption (Kelly and Kostial, 1973), and starvation enhances the absorption of dieldrin (Heath and Vandekar, 1964). The age of animals also appears to affect absorption: Newborn rats absorbed 12 percent of a dose of cadmium, whereas adult rats absorbed only 0.5 percent (Sasser and Jarboe, 1977). While lead and many other heavy metal ions are not absorbed readily from the GI tract, EDTA and other chelators increase the lipid solubility and thus the absorption of complexed ions. Thus, it is important not to give a chelator orally when excess metal is still present in the GI tract after oral ingestion.

The principles of GI absorption may be summarized in the following way. Penetration of amphophilic (having both lipophilic and hydrophilic molecular characteristics) substances across the GI wall occurs according to the basic principles of physicochemistry, with the unstirred water layer representing the rate-determining barrier for the more lipophilic molecules and the epithelial cell membrane representing that for the more hydrophilic compounds. Unlike the skin, which is virtually impenetrable to molecules at the extreme ends of the lipophilicity/hydrophilicity scale, the GI tract can also absorb such compounds. Some extremely hydrophilic compounds are absorbed by active processes, whereas extremely lipophilic compounds [2, 3, 7, 8-tetrachlorodibenzo-*p*-dioxin (TCCD), DDT, polychlorinated biphenyls (PCBs), etc.] ride in on the "coattails" of lipids via the micelles and subsequent biological processes related to lipid metabolism.

In general, gastrointestinal absorption of xenobiotics was thought to be similar between species. The work of Dreyfuss and colleagues illustrates the fallacy of this assumption (Dreyfuss et al., 1978). Absorption of nadolol (calculated from AUC after ip and oral dosing) was essentially complete in the dog, substantially less in humans, and quite limited in the rat (Table 5-3). Urinary and fecal excretion of nadolol support the bioavailability data. However, excretory data further indicate that in addition to the nonabsorbed portion of this compound, biliary and possibly nonbiliary sources also contribute to the fecal excretion of this compound. Calabrese (1984) reported evidence for species differences in the absorption of at least 38 compounds, indicating that nadolol is not an exceptional case.

The rate-limiting barrier in the absorption of most xenobiotics is the unstirred water layer along the intestinal mucosa (Hayton, 1980). The effect of the unstirred water layer as a possible cause of species differences in absorption of xenobiotics has not been investigated. However, Thomson et al. (1983) studied the effect of the unstirred water layer on the absorption of fatty acids and cholesterol. These authors concluded that the thickness of the unstirred water layer may contribute to species differences in the absorption of lipophilic compounds, but other tissue-specific differences must also exist because species differences persisted when the unstirred water layer was diminished as a barrier for hydrophobic compounds by stirring.

Anatomical (allometric) considerations are another likely reason for species differences in intestinal absorption. The relative length of intestinal segments is quite variable (Iatropoulos, 1986), and substantial functional differences exist between such species as ruminants and omnivores (Smith, 1986). Because most xenobiotics are transported across the gastrointestinal mucosa by passive diffusion, and because this transport is surface area– and site-dependent, it can be expected that these factors will be responsi-

Table 5-3
Absorption and Excretion of Radioactivity in Rats, Dogs, and Man after Nadolol Dosages*

SPECIES	DOSE (mg/kg)	ROUTE	PERCENT OF DOSE EXCRETED: URINE	PERCENT OF DOSE EXCRETED: FECES	PERCENT OF DOSE ABSORBED
Rat	20	po	11	84	18
	20	ip	62	31	(100)
Dog	25	po	76	28	102
	25	ip	75	12	(100)
Man	2	po	25	77	34
	2	ip	73	23	(100)

*Modified from Dreyfus et al. (1978).

Table 5-4
pH of the Gastrointestinal Contents of Various Species*

	pH				
SPECIES	STOMACH	JEJUNUM	CECUM	COLON	FECES
Monkey	2.8	6.0	5.0	5.1	5.5
Dog	3.4	6.6	6.4	6.5	6.2
Rat	3.8	6.8	6.8	6.6	6.9
Rabbit	1.9	7.5	6.6	7.2	7.2

*Modified from Smith (1965).

ble for species differences in some instances. Many xenobiotics are weak organic acids or bases. For such compounds, gastrointestinal absorption is dependent on the pH along the gastrointestinal tract. Table 5-4, shows that each segment of the gut reveals considerable species specificity, with differences of up to 2 pH units. This can translate into two orders of magnitude difference in concentration of the undissociated versus dissociated moiety of a weak organic acid or base.

An additional factor that may result in species-dependent absorption of xenobiotics is the gastrointestinal flora. In general, the microflora in animals is remarkably similar, although qualitative and quantitative differences have been reported (Smith, 1965). Notable deviations to this generalization do exist, such as the rabbit and human (Table 5-5). In contrast to other species, the microflora in these two species is very low in the upper gastrointestinal tract. Because absorption of some xenobiotics requires prior bacterial hydrolysis, some species differences may be due to differences in microflora. As an example, cycasin (Rozman and Iatropoulos, 1987) is poorly absorbed by gnotobiotic animals; however, the aglycone of cycasin is readily absorbed. Therefore, species with bacterial β-glucosidase activity in the upper small intestine readily absorb the aglycone (methylazoxymethanol), but species like human, with very low levels of microflora in the upper gastrointestinal tract, may not absorb this compound to any major extent.

Absorption of Toxicants by the Lungs

It is well known that toxic responses to chemicals can result from their absorption after inhalation. The most frequent cause of death from poisoning—carbon monoxide—and probably the most important occupational disease—silicosis—are both due to the absorption or deposition of airborne poisons in the lungs. This site of absorption has been employed in chemical warfare (chlorine and phosgene gas, lewisite, mustard gas) and in the execution of criminals in the gas chamber (hydrogen cyanide).

Toxicants absorbed by the lungs are usually gases (e.g., carbon monoxide, nitrogen dioxide, and sulfur dioxide), vapors of volatile or volatilizable liquids (e.g., benzene and carbon tetrachloride), and aerosols. Because the absorption of inhaled gases and vapor differs from that of aerosols, aerosols are discussed separately below. However, the absorption of gases and vapors is governed by the same principles, and therefore the word *gas* is used to represent both in this section.

Gases and Vapors The absorption of inhaled gases takes place mainly in the lungs. However, before a gas reaches the lungs, it passes through the nose, with its turbinates, which increase the surface area. Because the mucosa of the nose is covered by a film of fluid, gas molecules can be retained by the nose and not reach the lungs if they are very water soluble or react with cell surface components. Therefore, the nose acts as a "scrubber" for water-soluble gases and highly reactive gases, partially protecting the lungs from potentially injurious insults. A case in point is formaldehyde. The drawback of this protective mechanism for the lungs is that a typical nose breather such as a rat develops tumors of the nasal turbinates when chronically exposed to high levels of formaldehyde by inhalation.

Absorption of gases in the lungs differs from intestinal and percutaneous absorption of compounds in that the dissociation of acids and bases and the lipid solubility of molecules are less important factors in pulmonary absorption because diffusion through cell membranes is not rate-limiting in the pulmonary absorption of gases. There are at least three reasons for this. First, ionized molecules are of very low volatility, and consequently their concentration in normal ambient air is insignificant. Second, the epithelial cells lining the alveoli—that is, type I pneumocytes—are very thin and the capillaries are in close contact with the pneumocytes,

Table 5-5
Number of Microbes and their Distribution along the Gastrointestinal Tract of Various Species*

SPECIES	STOMACH	JEJUNUM	COLON	FECES
Monkey	23	24	41	38
Dog	19	20	40	43
Rat	18	23	37	38
Rabbit	4	5	13	13
Man	2	4	10	—

*Modified from Smith (1965) and Hallikainen and Salminen (1986). Expressed as $\log_{10}$ of viable counts.

so that the distance for a chemical to diffuse is very short. Third, chemicals absorbed by the lungs are removed rapidly by the blood, as it takes only about three-fourths of a second for the blood to go through the extensive capillary network in the lungs.

When a gas is inhaled into the lungs, gas molecules diffuse from the alveolar space into the blood and then dissolve. Except for some gases with a special affinity for certain body components (e.g., the binding of carbon monoxide to hemoglobin), the uptake of a gas by a tissue usually involves a simple physical process of dissolving. The end result is that gas molecules partition between the two media: air and blood during the absorptive phase and blood and other tissues during the distributive phase. As the contact of the inspired gas with blood continues in the alveoli, more molecules dissolve in blood until gas molecules in blood are in equilibrium with gas molecules in the alveolar space. At equilibrium, the ratio of the concentration of chemical in the blood and chemical in the gas phase is constant. This solubility ratio is called the *blood-to-gas partition coefficient.* This constant is unique for each gas. Note that only the ratio is constant, not the concentrations, as, according to Henry's law, the amount of gas dissolved in a liquid is proportional to the partial pressure of the gas in the gas phase at any given concentration before or at saturation. Thus, the higher the inhaled concentration of a gas (i.e., the higher the partial pressure), the higher the gas concentration in blood, but the ratio does not change unless saturation has occurred. When equilibrium is reached, the rate of transfer of gas molecules from the alveolar space to blood equals the rate of removal by blood from the alveolar space. For example, chloroform has a high (15) and ethylene a low (0.14) blood/gas phase solubility ratio. For a substance with a low solubility ratio, such as ethylene, only a small percentage of the total gas in the lungs is removed by blood during each circulation because blood is soon saturated with the gas. Therefore, an increase in the respiratory rate or minute volume does not change the transfer of such a gas to blood. In contrast, an increase in the rate of blood flow markedly increases the rate of uptake of a compound with a low solubility ratio because of more rapid removal from the site of equilibrium, that is, the alveolar membranes. It has been calculated that the time to equilibrate between the blood and the gas phase for a relatively insoluble gas is about 8 to 21 min.

Most of a gas with a high solubility ratio, such as chloroform, is transferred to blood during each respiratory cycle so that little if any remains in the alveoli just before the next inhalation. The more soluble a toxic agent is in blood, the more of it will be dissolved in blood by the time equilibrium is reached. Consequently, the time required to equilibrate with blood is very much longer for a gas with a high solubility ratio than for a gas with a low ratio. This has been calculated to take a minimum of 1 h for compounds with a high solubility ratio, although it may take even longer if the gas also has high tissue affinity (i.e., high fat solubility). With these highly soluble gases, the principal factor limiting the rate of absorption is respiration. Because the blood is already removing virtually all of a gas with a high solubility ratio from the lungs, increasing the blood flow rate does not substantially increase the rate of absorption. However, the rate can be accelerated greatly by increasing the rate of respiration, or the minute volume.

Thus, the rate of absorption of gases in the lungs is variable and depends on a toxicant's solubility ratio (concentration in blood/concentration in gas phase before or at saturation) at equilibrium. For gases with a very low solubility ratio, the rate of transfer depends mainly on blood flow through the lungs (perfusion-limited), whereas for gases with a high solubility ratio, it is primarily a function of the rate and depth of respiration (ventilation-limited). Of course, there is a wide spectrum of intermediate behavior between the two extremes, with the median being a blood/gas concentration ratio of about 1.2.

The blood carries the dissolved gas molecules to the rest of the body. In each tissue, the gas molecules are transferred from the blood to the tissue until equilibrium is reached at a tissue concentration dictated by the tissue-to-blood partition coefficient. After releasing part of the gas to tissues, blood returns to the lungs to take up more of the gas. The process continues until a gas reaches equilibrium between blood and each tissue according to the tissue-to-blood partition coefficients characteristic of each tissue. At this time, no net absorption of gas takes place as long as the exposure concentration remains constant, because a steady state has been reached. Of course, if biotransformation and excretion occur, alveolar absorption will continue until a corresponding steady state is established.

Aerosols and Particles The degree of ionization and the lipid solubility of chemicals are very important for oral and percutaneous exposures, whereas water solubility, tissue reactivity, and blood to gas phase partition coefficients are important after exposure to gases and vapors. The important characteristics that affect absorption after exposure to aerosols are the aerosol size and water solubility of a chemical present in the aerosol.

The site of deposition of aerosols depends largely on the size of the particles. This relationship is discussed in detail in Chap. 15. Particles 5 μm or larger usually are deposited in the nasopharyngeal region (Fig. 5-4). Those deposited on the unciliated anterior portion of the nose tend to remain at the site of deposition un-

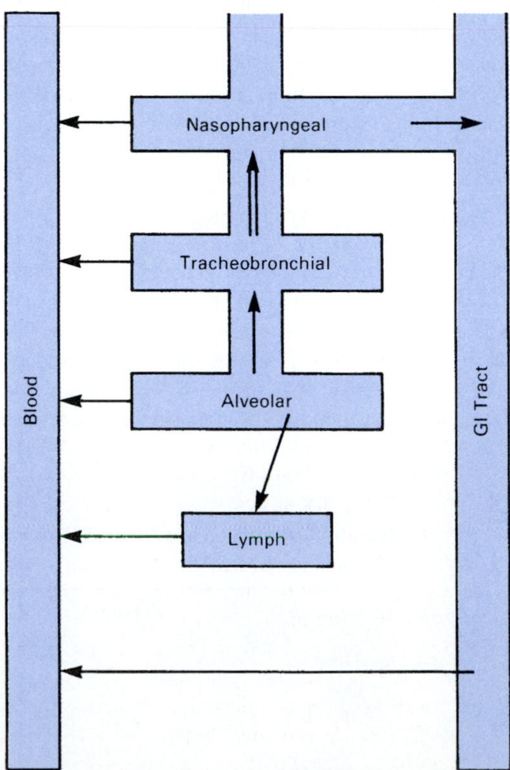

Figure 5-4. Schematic diagram of the absorption and translocation of chemicals by lungs.

til they are removed by nose wiping, blowing, or sneezing. The mucous blanket of the ciliated nasal surface propels insoluble particles by the movement of the cilia. These particles and particles inhaled through the mouth are swallowed within minutes. Soluble particles may dissolve in the mucus and be carried to the pharynx or may be absorbed through the nasal epithelium into blood.

Particles of 2 to 5 μm are deposited mainly in the tracheobronchiolar regions of the lungs, from which they are cleared by retrograde movement of the mucus layer in the ciliated portions of the respiratory tract. The rate of cilia-propelled movement of mucus varies in different parts of the respiratory tract, although in general it is a rapid and efficient transport mechanism. Measurements have shown transport rates between 0.1 and 1 mm per minute, resulting in removal half-lives between 30 and 300 min. Coughing and sneezing greatly increase the movement of mucus and particulate matter toward the mouth. Particles eventually may be swallowed and absorbed from the GI tract.

Particles 1 μm and smaller penetrate to the alveolar sacs of the lungs. They may be absorbed into blood or cleared through the lymphatics after being scavenged by alveolar macrophages.

In addition to gases, liquid aerosols and particles can be absorbed in the alveoli. The mechanisms responsible for the removal or absorption of particulate matter from the alveoli (usually less than 1 μm in diameter) are less clear than those responsible for the removal of particles deposited in the tracheobronchial tree. Removal appears to occur by three major mechanisms. First, particles may be removed from the alveoli by a physical process. It is thought that particles deposited on the fluid layer of the alveoli are aspirated onto the mucociliary escalator of the tracheobronchial region. From there, they are transported to the mouth and may be swallowed, as was mentioned previously. The origin of the thin fluid layer in the alveoli is probably a transudation of lymph and secretions of lipids and other components by the alveolar epithelium. The alveolar fluid flows by an unknown mechanism to the terminal bronchioles. This flow seems to depend on lymph flow, capillary action, the respiratory motion of the alveolar walls, the cohesive nature of the respiratory tract's fluid blanket, and the propelling power of the ciliated bronchioles. Second, particles from the alveoli may be removed by phagocytosis. The principal cells responsible for engulfing alveolar debris are the mononuclear phagocytes, the macrophages. These cells are found in large numbers in normal lungs and contain many phagocytized particles of both exogenous and endogenous origin. They apparently migrate to the distal end of the mucociliary escalator and are cleared and eventually swallowed. Third, removal may occur via the lymphatics. The endothelial cells lining lymphatic capillaries are permeable for very large molecules (molecular weight $>10^6$) and for particles, although the rate of penetration is low above a molecular weight of 10,000 (Renkin, 1968). Nevertheless, the lymphatic system plays a prominent role in collecting high-molecular-weight proteins leaked from cells or blood capillaries and particulate matter from the interstitium and the alveolar spaces. Particulate matter may remain in lymphatic tissue for long periods, and this explains the name "dust store of the lungs."

For the reasons discussed above, the overall removal of particles from the alveoli is relatively inefficient; on the first day only about 20 percent of particles are cleared, and the portion remaining longer than 24 h is cleared very slowly. The rate of clearance by the lungs can be predicted by a compound's solubility in lung fluids. The lower the solubility, the lower the removal rate. Thus, it appears that removal of particles from the lungs is largely due to dissolution and vascular transport. Some particles may remain in the alveoli indefinitely. This may occur when proliferating instead of desquamating alveolar cells ingest dust particles and, in association with a developing network of reticulin fibers, form an alveolar dust plaque or nodule.

Species differences in the absorption of toxicants by the lungs are due to differences in physiology (rate of respiration, blood flow rate, etc.) and to differential exposure conditions (e.g., life span).

Absorption of Toxicants through the Skin

Human skin comes into contact with many toxic agents. Fortunately, the skin is not very permeable and therefore is a relatively good barrier for separating organisms from their environment. However, some chemicals can be absorbed by the skin in sufficient quantities to produce systemic effects. For example, nerve gases such as sarin are readily absorbed by intact skin. Also, carbon tetrachloride can be absorbed through the skin in sufficient quantities to cause liver injury. Various insecticides have caused death in agricultural workers after absorption through intact skin (Chap. 22).

To be absorbed through the skin, a toxicant must pass through the epidermis or the appendages (sweat and sebaceous glands and hair follicles). Sweat glands and hair follicles are scattered in varying densities on the skin. Their total cross-sectional area is probably between 0.1 and 1.0 percent of the total skin surface. Although the entry of small amounts of toxicants through the appendages may be rapid, chemicals are absorbed mainly through the epidermis, which constitutes the major surface area of the skin. Chemicals that are absorbed through the skin have to pass through several cell layers (a total of seven) before entering the small blood and lymph capillaries in the dermis (Fig. 5-5). The rate-determining barrier in the dermal absorption of chemicals is the epidermis. More accurately, it is the stratum corneum (horny layer), the uppermost layer of the epidermis (Dugard, 1983). This is the outer horny layer of the skin, consisting of densely packed keratinized cells that have lost their nuclei and thus are biologically inactive. Passage through the six other cell

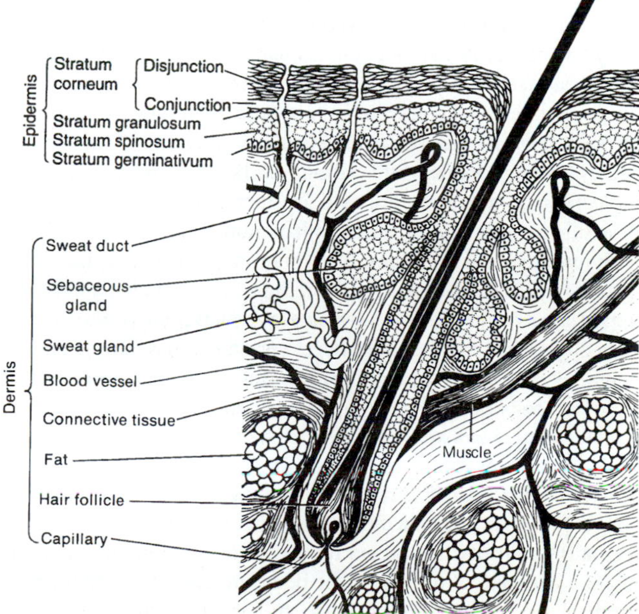

Figure 5-5. Diagram of a cross section of human skin.

layers is much more rapid than is passage through the stratum corneum. Therefore, the most important considerations regarding the dermal absorption of xenobiotics relate to the stratum corneum.

The first phase of percutaneous absorption is diffusion of xenobiotics through the rate-limiting barrier, the stratum corneum. Studies have shown that the stratum corneum is replenished about every 3 to 4 weeks in adults. This complex process includes a gross dehydration and polymerization of intracellular matrix that results in keratin-filled dried cell layers. In the course of keratinization, the cell walls apparently double in thickness owing to the inclusion or deposition of chemically resistant materials. This change in the physical state of the tissue causes a commensurate change in its diffusion barrier property. The transformation is from an aqueous fluid medium that is characterized by liquid state to a dry, keratinous semisolid state with much lower permeability for toxicants by diffusion (permeability by diffusion = diffusivity).

In contrast to the complexity of the GI tract, the skin is a simpler penetration barrier for chemicals because passage through dead cell layers is the rate-determining step. It is clear that all toxicants move across the stratum corneum by passive diffusion. Kinetic measurements suggest that polar and nonpolar toxicants may diffuse through the stratum corneum by different mechanisms. Polar substances appear to diffuse through the outer surface of protein filaments of the hydrated stratum corneum, whereas nonpolar molecules dissolve in and diffuse through the lipid matrix between the protein filaments (Blank and Scheuplein, 1969). The rate of diffusion of nonpolar toxicants is proportional to their lipid solubility and is inversely related to their molecular weight (Marzulli et al., 1965). However, there are limits to the generalization of this theory. The rate of dermal penetration of highly lipophilic chemicals such as TCDD is very limited (Weber et al., 1991). Their solubility in triglycerides is relatively good, but not in phospholipids and other lipids with polar head groups. Because the stratum corneum contains a very low amount of triglycerides (2.8 percent in pigs, 0 percent in humans) and much cholesterol (26.0 percent in pigs, 26.9 percent in humans), some cholesterol esters (4.1 percent in pigs, 10 percent in humans), and various ceramides (44.2 percent in pigs, 41.1 percent in humans), it is not surprising that the absorption of highly lipophilic toxicants through the skin remains quite limited (Wertz and Downing, 1991). Ceramides are moderately lipophilic, as they are amides and/or esters of saturated and unsaturated fatty acids. Thus, the stratum corneum consists of about 75 to 80 percent moderately lipophilic materials. The simple physicochemical fact of *similis similibus solvontur* ("similar dissolves similar") explains the validity of the lipophilicity theory for molecules of moderate lipophilicity that also possess some hydrophilic regions. However, for both extreme ends of the lipophilicity/hydrophilicity spectrum, the stratum corneum represents a nearly impenetrable barrier unless those compounds damage the upper layer of the skin. A slow rate of penetration is possible for such substances via the appendages, provided that they remain in contact with a large skin surface area for prolonged periods.

Human stratum corneum displays significant differences in structure and chemistry from one region of the body to another, and these differences affect the permeability of the skin to chemicals. Skin from the plantar and palmar regions is much different from skin from other areas of the body in that the stratum corneum of the palms and soles is adapted for weight bearing and friction. The stratum corneum of the rest of the body surface is adapted for flexibility and fine sensory discrimination. The permeability of the skin depends on both the diffusivity and the thickness of the stratum corneum. While the stratum corneum is much thicker on the palms and soles (400 to 600 μm in callous areas) than on the arms, back, legs, and abdomen (8 to 15 μm), it has much higher diffusivity per unit thickness. Consequently, toxicants readily cross scrotum skin, since it is extremely thin and has high diffusivity; cross the abdominal skin less rapidly, as it is thicker and exhibits less diffusivity; and cross the sole with the greatest difficulty because the distance to traverse is great even though diffusivity there is highest.

The second phase of percutaneous absorption consists of diffusion of the toxicant through the lower layers of the epidermis (stratum granulosum, spinosum, and germinativum) and the dermis. These cell layers are far inferior to the stratum corneum as diffusion barriers. In contrast to the stratum corneum, they contain a porous, nonselective, aqueous diffusion medium. Toxicants pass through this area by diffusion and enter the systemic circulation through the numerous venous and lymphatic capillaries in the dermis. The rate of diffusion depends on blood flow, interstitial fluid movement, and perhaps other factors, including interactions with dermal constituents.

The absorption of toxicants through the skin varies, depending on the condition of the skin. Because the stratum corneum plays a critical role in determining cutaneous permeability, removal of this layer causes a dramatic increase in the permeability of the epidermis for a variety of large or small molecules, both lipid-soluble and water-soluble (Malkinson, 1964). Agents such as acids, alkalis, and mustard gases that injure the stratum corneum increase its permeability. The most frequently encountered penetration-enhancing damage to the skin results from burns and various skin diseases. Water plays an extremely important role in skin permeability. Under normal conditions, the stratum corneum is partially hydrated, containing about 7 percent water by weight. This amount of water increases the permeability of the stratum corneum approximately tenfold over the permeability that exists when it is completely dry. On additional contact with water, the stratum corneum can increase its weight of tightly bound water up to three- to fivefold, and this results in an additional two- to threefold increase in permeability. Studies of the dermal absorption of toxicants often utilize the method of Draize and associates (1944), wrapping plastic around animals and placing the chemical between the plastic and the skin (occlusive application). This hydrates the stratum corneum and enhances the absorption of some toxicants.

Solvents such as dimethyl sulfoxide (DMSO) also can facilitate the penetration of toxicants through the skin. DMSO increases the permeability of the barrier layer of the skin—that is, the stratum corneum. Little information is available about the mechanism by which DMSO enhances skin permeability. However, it has been suggested that DMSO (1) removes much of the lipid matrix of the stratum corneum, making holes on artificial shunts in the penetration barrier; (2) produces reversible configurational changes in protein structure brought about by the substitution of integral water molecules; and (3) functions as a swelling agent (Allenby et al., 1969; Dugard and Embery, 1969).

Various species have been employed in studying the dermal absorption of toxicants. Considerable species variations have been observed in cutaneous permeability. For many chemicals the skin of rats and rabbits is more permeable, whereas the skin of cats is usually less permeable, while the cutaneous permeability characteristics of guinea pigs, pigs, and monkeys are often similar to those observed in humans (Scala et al., 1968; Coulston and Serrone, 1969; Wester and Maibach, 1977). Species differences in percutaneous absorption account for the differential toxicity of insecticides in insects and humans. For example, the LD_{50} of injected DDT is approximately equal in insects and mammals, but DDT is much less toxic to mammals than to insects when it is applied to the skin. This appears to be due to the fact that DDT is poorly absorbed through the skin of mammals but passes readily through the chitinous exoskeleton of insects. Furthermore, insects have a much greater body surface area relative to weight than do mammals (Winteringham, 1957; Albert, 1965; Hayes, 1965).

Species differences related to dermal absorption of xenobiotics has been appreciated (Calabrese, 1984), perhaps because dermal absorption of endogenous or exogenous compounds may vary by orders of magnitude (Kao et al., 1985). According to Dugard (1983), two factors are important in dermal absorption of chemicals: the appendages (sweat ducts, pilosebaceous ducts) in the early phase of absorption and the stratum corneum in the late and dominating phase of absorption. Both factors are highly species-dependent. Because the stratum corneum is much thicker in humans than in animals, human skin is usually less permeable for xenobiotics than is animal skin. However, the thinner stratum corneum in animals is often compensated for by a relatively thick hair cover, diminishing direct contact of the skin with a xenobiotic. Sweat and pilosebaceous ducts also reveal great species variability. Eccrine sweat glands are located in the pads of the extremities of all mammals. However, the general body surface of man contains 100 to 600/m^2 of coiled tubular sweat glands, whereas rodents and rabbits have none. The number of pilosebaceous ducts in humans and pigs is similar (about 40/cm^2), but rodents may have 100 times more (Calabrese, 1984). Moreover, biotransformations in skin that facilitate absorption also display great species variability (Kao et al., 1985).

Another important potential rate-limiting step in the dermal absorption of chemicals is the cutaneous blood flow. Due to an important thermoregulatory function of the skin in humans as opposed to furred animals, there is a much more extensive vasculature in humans than in most mammals (Calabrese, 1984). This brief discussion illustrates that species differences in the disposition of xenobiotics after dermal exposure may be due to numerous anatomic, physiologic, and biochemical factors.

Absorption of Toxicants after Special Routes of Administration

Toxicants usually enter the bloodstream after absorption through the skin, lungs, or GI tract. However, in studying chemical agents, toxicologists frequently administer them to laboratory animals by special routes. The most common routes are (1) intraperitoneal, (2) subcutaneous, (3) intramuscular, and (4) intravenous. The intravenous route introduces the toxicant directly into the bloodstream, eliminating the process of absorption. Intraperitoneal injection of toxicants into laboratory animals is also a common procedure. It results in rapid absorption of xenobiotics because of the rich blood supply and the relatively large surface area of the peritoneal cavity. In addition, this route of administration circumvents the delay and variability of gastric emptying. Intraperitoneally administered compounds are absorbed primarily through the portal circulation and therefore must pass through the liver before reaching other organs (Lukas et al., 1971). Subcutaneously and intramuscularly administered toxicants are usually absorbed at slower rates but enter directly into the general circulation. The rate of absorption by these two routes can be altered by changing the blood flow to the injection site. For example, epinephrine causes vasoconstriction and will decrease the rate of absorption if it is coinjected intramuscularly with a toxicant. The formulation of a xenobiotic may also affect the rate of absorption; toxicants are absorbed more slowly from suspensions than from solutions.

The toxicity of a chemical may or may not depend on the route of administration. If a toxicant is injected intraperitoneally, most of the chemical enters the liver via the portal circulation before reaching the general circulation. Therefore, an intraperitoneally administered compound may be completely extracted and biotransformed by the liver with subsequent excretion into the bile without gaining access to the systemic circulation. Propranolol (Shand and Rangno, 1972) and lidocaine (Boyes et al., 1970) are two drugs with efficient extraction during the first pass through the liver. Any toxicant displaying the first-pass effect with selective toxicity for an organ other than the liver and GI tract is expected to be much less toxic when administered intraperitoneally than when injected intravenously, intramuscularly, or subcutaneously. For compounds with no appreciable biotransformation in the liver, toxicity ought to be independent of the route of administration if the rates of absorption are equal. This discussion indicates that it is possible to obtain some preliminary information on the biotransformation and excretion of xenobiotics by comparing their toxicity after administration by different routes.

DISTRIBUTION

After entering the blood by absorption or intravenous administration, a toxicant is available for distribution (translocation) throughout the body. Distribution usually occurs rapidly. The rate of distribution to organs or tissues is determined primarily by blood flow and the rate of diffusion out of the capillary bed into the cells of a particular organ or tissue. The final distribution depends largely on the affinity of a xenobiotic for various tissues. In general, the initial phase of distribution is dominated by blood flow, whereas the eventual distribution is determined largely by affinity. The penetration of toxicants into cells occurs by passive diffusion or special transport processes, as was discussed previously. Small water-soluble molecules and ions apparently diffuse through aqueous channels or pores in the cell membrane. Lipid-soluble molecules readily permeate the membrane itself. Very polar molecules and ions of even moderate size (molecular weight of 50 or more) cannot enter cells easily except by special transport mechanisms because they are surrounded by a hydration shell, making their actual size much larger.

Volume of Distribution

Total body water may be divided into three distinct compartments: (1) plasma water, (2) interstitial water, and (3) intracellular water. Extracellular water is made up of plasma water plus interstitial water. The concentration of a toxicant in blood depends largely on its volume of distribution. For example, if 1 g of each of several chemicals were injected directly into the bloodstreams of 70-kg humans, marked differences in their plasma concentrations would be observed depending on the distribution. A high concentration would be observed in the plasma if the chemical were distributed into plasma water only, and a much lower concentration would be reached if it were distributed into a large pool, such as total body water (see below).

The distribution of toxicants is usually complex and cannot be equated with distribution into one of the water compartments

COMPARTMENT	% OF TOTAL	LITERS IN 70-kg HUMAN	PLASMA CONCENTRATION AFTER 1 g OF CHEMICAL
Plasma water	4.5	3	333 mg/liter
Total extracellular water	20	14	71 mg/liter
Total body water	55	38	26 mg/liter
Tissue binding	—	—	0–25 mg/liter

of the body. Binding to and/or dissolution in various storage sites of the body, such as fat, liver, and bone, are usually more important factors in determining the distribution of chemicals.

Some toxicants do not readily cross cell membranes and therefore have restricted distribution, whereas other toxicants rapidly pass through cell membranes and are distributed throughout the body. Some toxicants accumulate in certain parts of the body as a result of protein binding, active transport, or high solubility in fat. The site of accumulation of a toxicant may also be its site of major toxic action, but more often it is not. If a toxicant accumulates at a site other than the target organ or tissue, the accumulation may be viewed as a protective process in that plasma levels and consequently the concentration of a toxicant at the site of action are diminished. In this case, it is assumed that the chemical in the storage depot is toxicologically inactive. However, because any chemical in a storage depot is in equilibrium with the free fraction of toxicant in plasma, it is released into the circulation as the unbound fraction of toxicant is eliminated, for example, by biotransformation.

Storage of Toxicants in Tissues

Since only the free fraction of a chemical is in equilibrium throughout the body, binding to or dissolving in certain body constituents, greatly alters the distribution of a xenobiotic. Toxicants are often concentrated in a specific tissue. Some xenobiotics attain their highest concentrations at the site of toxic action, such as carbon monoxide, which has a very high affinity for hemoglobin, and paraquat, which accumulates in the lungs. Other agents concentrate at sites other than the target organ. For example, lead is stored in bone, but manifestations of lead poisoning appear in soft tissues. The compartment where a toxicant is concentrated can be thought of as a storage depot. Toxicants in these depots are always in equilibrium with the free fraction in plasma. As a chemical is biotransformed or excreted from the body, more is released from the storage site. As a result, the biological half-life of stored compounds can be very long. The following discussion deals with the major storage sites for xenobiotics in the body.

Plasma Proteins as Storage Depot Several plasma proteins bind xenobiotics as well as some physiologic constituents of the body. As depicted in Fig. 5-6, albumin can bind a large number of different compounds. Transferrin, a beta globulin, is important for the transport of iron in the body. The other main metal-binding protein in plasma is ceruloplasmin, which carries most of the copper. The alpha- and beta-lipoproteins are very important in the transport of lipid-soluble compounds such as vitamins, cholesterol, and steroid hormones as well as xenobiotics. The gamma globulins are antibodies that interact specifically with antigens. Compounds possessing basic characteristics often bind to α_1 acid glycoprotein (Wilkinson, 1983).

Many therapeutic agents have been examined with respect to plasma protein binding. The extent of plasma protein binding varies considerably among xenobiotics. Some, such as antipyrine, are not bound; others, such as secobarbital, are bound to about 50 percent; and some, like warfarin, are 99 percent bound. Plasma proteins can bind acidic compounds such as phenylbutazone, basic compounds such as imipramine, and neutral compounds such as digitoxin.

The binding of toxicants to plasma proteins is usually determined by equilibrium dialysis or ultrafiltration. The fraction that passes through the dialysis membrane or appears in the ultrafiltrate is the unbound, or free, fraction. The total concentration is the sum of the bound and free fractions. The bound fraction thus can be determined from the difference between the total and free fractions. The binding of toxicants to plasma proteins can be analyzed through the use of Scatchard plots (Scatchard, 1949). In this analysis, the ratio of bound to free ligand (toxicant) is plotted on the ordinate and the concentration of bound ligand is plotted on the abscissa, depicted in Fig. 5-7. From this analysis, the number of ligand binding sites *(N)* per molecule of protein and the affinity constant of the protein-ligand complex can be determined. The Scatchard plot frequently exhibits nonlinearity, indicating the presence of two or more classes of binding sites with different affinities and capacity characteristics.

Most xenobiotics that are bound to plasma proteins bind to albumin. Albumin is the most abundant protein in plasma and serves as a depot and transport protein for many endogenous and exogenous compounds. Long-chain fatty acids and bilirubin are endogenous ligands with affinity for albumin. There appear to be six

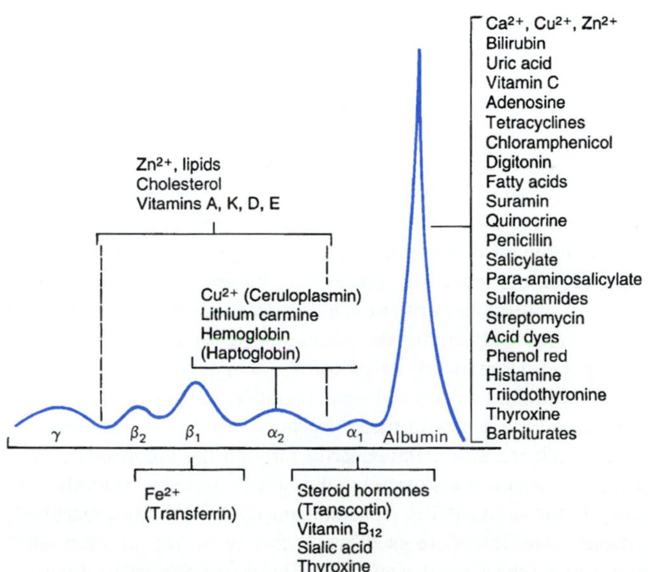

Figure 5-6. Ligand interactions with plasma proteins.

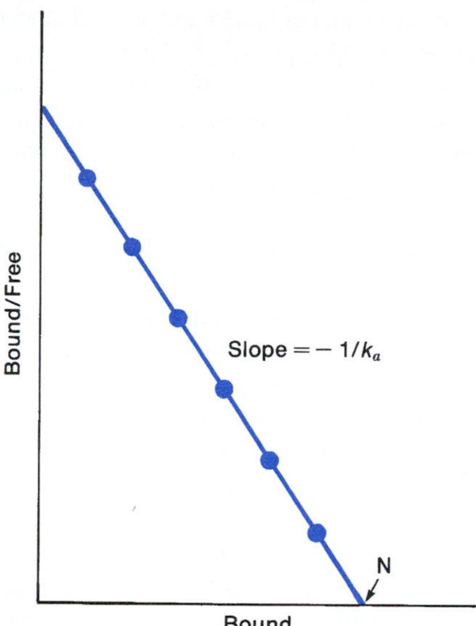

Figure 5-7. Schematic representation of the Scatchard plot for the analysis of the binding of toxicants to proteins.

binding regions on the protein (Kragh-Hansen, 1981). Protein-ligand interactions occur primarily as a result of hydrophobic forces, hydrogen bonding, and Van der Waals forces. Because of their high molecular weight, plasma proteins and the toxicants bound to them cannot cross capillary walls. Consequently, the fraction of toxicant bound to plasma proteins is not immediately available for distribution into the extravascular space or filtration by the kidneys. However, the interaction of a chemical with plasma proteins is a reversible process. As unbound chemical diffuses out of capillaries, bound chemical dissociates from the protein until the free fraction reaches equilibrium between the vascular space and the extravascular space. In turn, diffusion in the extravascular space to sites more distant from the capillaries continues, and the resulting concentration gradient provides the thermodynamic force for continued dissociation of the bound fraction in plasma. Active transport processes are not limited by the binding of chemicals to plasma proteins.

The binding of chemicals to plasma proteins is of special importance to toxicologists because severe toxic reactions can occur if a toxicant is displaced from plasma proteins by another agent, increasing the free fraction of the toxicant in plasma. This will result in an increased equilibrium concentration of the toxicant in the target organ, with the potential for toxicity. For example, if a strongly bound sulfonamide is given concurrently with an antidiabetic drug, the sulfonamide may displace the antidiabetic drug and induce a hypoglycemic coma. Xenobiotics can also compete with and displace endogenous compounds that are bound to plasma proteins. The importance of this phenomenon was demonstrated in a clinical trial comparing the efficacy of tetracycline with that of a penicillin-sulfonamide mixture in the management of bacterial infections in premature infants (Silverman et al., 1956). The penicillin-sulfonamide mixture led to much higher mortality than did the tetracycline, because the sulfonamide displaced a considerable amount of bilirubin from albumin. The bilirubin then diffused into the brain through the not fully developed blood-brain barrier of the newborn, causing a severe form of brain damage termed *kernicterus*.

Most research on the binding of xenobiotics to plasma proteins has been conducted with drugs. However, other chemicals, such as the insecticide dieldrin, also bind avidly to plasma proteins (99 percent). Therefore, it is to be expected that chemical-chemical interactions that alter plasma protein binding occur with many different xenobiotics.

Plasma protein bonding can also give rise to species differences in the disposition of xenobiotics. For example, plasma protein binding of clofibric acid reveals considerable differences between mice, rats, and humans, which roughly correlates with the half-lives of this compound in these species (Table 5-6). Because clofibric acid is primarily eliminated in all three species by glomerular filtration without tubular reabsorption ($pK_a = 3$), differences in the free fraction of this compound in plasma of various species provide part of the explanation for the observed species differences. The other major factor is renal clearance (blood flow–dependent). Additional factors that influence plasma protein binding may also be responsible for species differences, as discussed by Wilkinson (1983). Most important among them are species differences in the concentration of albumin, in binding affinity, and/or in competitive binding of endogenous substances.

Liver and Kidney as Storage Depots The liver and kidney have a high capacity for binding a multitude of chemicals. These two organs probably concentrate more toxicants than do all the other organs combined. Although the mechanisms by which the liver and kidney remove toxicants from the blood have not been established, active transport or binding to tissue components seems to be involved in most cases.

A protein in the cytoplasm of the liver (ligandin) has been identified as having a high affinity for many organic acids. It has been suggested that this protein may be important in the transfer of organic anions from plasma into liver (Levi et al., 1969). This protein also binds azo dye carcinogens and corticosteroids (Litwack et al., 1971). Another protein—metallothionein—has been found to bind cadmium and zinc with high affinities in the kidney and liver. Hepatic uptake of lead illustrates how rapidly liver binds foreign compounds: just 30 min after a single dose, the concentration of lead in liver is 50 times higher than the concentration in plasma (Klaassen and Shoeman, 1974).

Fat as Storage Depot Many organic compounds in the environment are highly lipophilic. This characteristic permits rapid penetration of cell membranes and uptake by tissues. Therefore, it is not surprising that highly lipophilic toxicants are distributed and concentrated in body fat. Such accumulation in adipose tissue has been demonstrated for a number of chemicals, including chlordane, DDT, and polychlorinated and polybrominated biphenyls.

Table 5-6
Plasma Protein Binding and Half-life of Clofibric Acid in the Mouse, Rat, and Man*

SPECIES	PLASMA PROTEIN BINDING (%)	HALF-LIFE (h)
Man	97	21
Rat	75	6
Mouse	45	2

*Modified from Cayen (1980).

Toxicants appear to accumulate in fat by dissolution in neutral fats, which constitute about 50 percent and 20 percent of the body weight of obese individuals and lean athletic individuals, respectively. Thus, large amounts of toxicants with a high lipid/water partition coefficient may be stored in body fat. Storage lowers the concentration of the toxicant in the target organ; therefore, the toxicity of such a compound can be expected to be less severe in an obese person than in a lean individual. However, of more practical concern is the possibility of a sudden increase in the concentration of a chemical in the blood and thus in the target organ of toxicity when rapid mobilization of fat occurs. Several studies have shown that signs of intoxication can be produced by short-term starvation of experimental animals that were previously exposed to persistent organochlorine insecticides.

One frequently overlooked cause of species differences in the distribution of xenobiotics that are stored in fat is the different rate of growth of mammals (Scheufler and Rozman, 1986). As Freeman and colleagues (1988) demonstrated using a physiologically based pharmacokinetic model, tissue and whole body growth contribute more to the distribution and elimination profile of hexachlorobenzene than does excretion.

Bone as Storage Depot Compounds such as fluoride, lead, and strontium may be incorporated and stored in bone matrix. For example, 90 percent of the lead in the body is eventually found in the skeleton.

Skeletal uptake of xenobiotics is essentially a surface chemistry phenomenon, with exchange taking place between the bone surface and the fluid in contact with it. The fluid is the extracellular fluid, and the surface is that of the hydroxyapatite crystals of bone mineral. Many of those crystals are very small, so that the surface is large in proportion to the mass. The extracellular fluid brings the toxicant into contact with the hydration shell of the hydroxyapatite, allowing diffusion through it and penetration of the crystal surface. As a result of similarities in size and charge, F^- may readily displace OH^-, whereas lead or strontium may substitute for calcium in the hydroxyapatite lattice matrix through an exchange-absorption reaction.

Deposition and storage of toxicants in bone may or may not be detrimental. Lead is not toxic to bone, but the chronic effects of fluoride deposition (skeletal fluorosis) and radioactive strontium (osteosarcoma and other neoplasms) are well documented.

Foreign compounds deposited in bone are not sequestered irreversibly by that tissue. Toxicants can be released from the bone by ionic exchange at the crystal surface and dissolution of bone crystals through osteoclastic activity. An increase in osteolytic activity such as that seen after parathyroid hormone administration leads to enhanced mobilization of hydroxyapatite lattice, which can be reflected in an increased plasma concentration of toxicants.

Blood-Brain Barrier

The blood-brain barrier is not an absolute barrier to the passage of toxic agents into the CNS. Instead, it represents a site that is less permeable than are most other areas of the body. Nevertheless, many poisons do not enter the brain in appreciable quantities because of this barrier.

There are four major anatomic and physiologic reasons why some toxicants do not readily enter the CNS. First, the capillary endothelial cells of the CNS are tightly joined, leaving few or no pores between the cells. Second, the brain capillary endothelial cells contain an ATP-dependent transporter, the multi-drug–resistant (mdr) protein that exudes some chemicals back into the blood. Third the capillaries in the CNS are to a large extent surrounded by glial cell processes (astrocytes). Fourth, the protein concentration in the interstitial fluid of the CNS is much lower than that in other body fluids. For small to medium-sized water-soluble molecules, the tighter junctions of the capillary endothelium and the lipid membranes of the glial cell processes represent the major barrier. Lipid-soluble compounds have to traverse not only the membranes of the endothelial cells but also those of glial cell processes. More important, perhaps, the low protein content of the interstitial fluid in the brain greatly limits the movement of water-insoluble compounds by paracellular transport, which is possible in a largely aqueous medium only when such compounds are bound to proteins. These features provide some protection against the distribution of toxicants to the CNS and thus against toxicity.

The effectiveness of the blood-brain barrier varies from one area of the brain to another. For example, the cortex, the lateral nuclei of the hypothalamus, the area postrema, the pineal body, and the posterior lobe of the hypophysis are more permeable than are other areas of the brain. It is not clear whether this is due to the increased blood supply to those areas, a more permeable barrier, or both. In general, the entrance of toxicants into the brain follows the same principle that applies to transfer across other cells in the body. Only the free fraction of a toxicant (i.e., not bound to plasma proteins) equilibrates rapidly with the brain. Lipid solubility plays an important role in determining the rate of entry of a compound into the CNS, as does the degree of ionization, as discussed earlier. In general, increased lipid solubility enhances the rate of penetration of toxicants into the CNS, whereas ionization greatly diminishes it. Pralidoxime (2-PAM), a quaternary nitrogen derivative, does not readily penetrate the brain and is ineffective in reversing the inhibition of brain cholinesterase caused by organophosphate insecticides. It is not clear why some very lipophilic chemicals, such as TCDD, are not readily distributed into the brain, which in fact displays the lowest concentration among all tissues and body fluids (Weber et al., 1993). It is likely, though, that strong binding to plasma proteins or lipoproteins, as well as the composition of the brain (mainly phospholipids), limits the entry of very lipophilic compounds into the brain. Some xenobiotics, although very few, appear to enter the brain by carrier-mediated processes. For example, methylmercury combines with cysteine, forming a structure

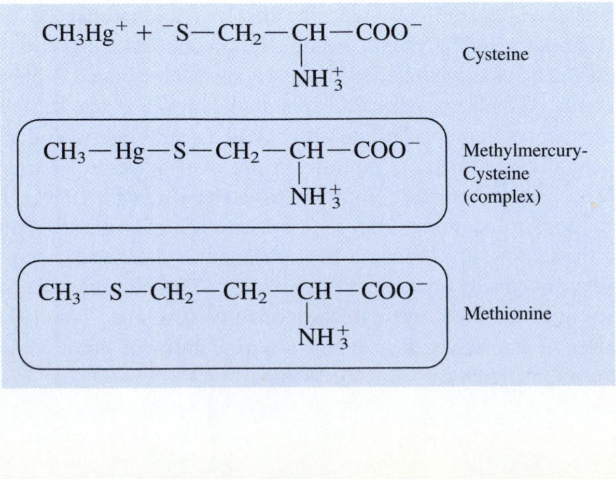

$$CH_3Hg^+ + {}^-S{-}CH_2{-}\underset{\displaystyle NH_3^+}{\underset{|}{CH}}{-}COO^- \quad \text{Cysteine}$$

$$CH_3{-}Hg{-}S{-}CH_2{-}\underset{\displaystyle NH_3^+}{\underset{|}{CH}}{-}COO^- \quad \text{Methylmercury-Cysteine (complex)}$$

$$CH_3{-}S{-}CH_2{-}CH_2{-}\underset{\displaystyle NH_3^+}{\underset{|}{CH}}{-}COO^- \quad \text{Methionine}$$

similar to methionine (see above), and the complex is then accepted by the large neutral amino acid carrier of the capillary endothelial cells (Clarkson, 1987).

Active transport processes decrease the concentration of xenobiotics in the brain. The multidrug resistant protein (mdr) has been demonstrated in endothelial cells in the brain (Schinkel et al., 1994) and is responsible for transporting some chemicals from endothelial cells back into the blood. Ivermectin, an insecticide, has been known to be much more toxic in mdr-null mice (LD50 ≈ 0.4–0.6 mg/kg) than in control mice (50–60 mg/kg). This increased sensitivity to ivermectin in the mdr-null mice is due to 80-fold higher brain ivermectin concentrations.

The blood-brain barrier is not fully developed at birth, and this is one reason why some chemicals are more toxic in newborns than to adults. Morphine, for example, is three to ten times more toxic to newborn than to adult rats because of the higher permeability of the brain of a newborn to morphine (Kupferberg and Way, 1963). Lead produces encephalomyelopathy in newborn rats but not in adults, also apparently because of differences in the stages of development of the blood brain barrier (Pentschew and Garro, 1966).

Passage of Toxicants across the Placenta

For years the term *placental barrier* was associated with the concept that the main function of the placenta is to protect the fetus against the passage of noxious substances from the mother. However, the placenta has many functions: it provides nutrition for the conceptus, exchanges maternal and fetal blood gases, disposes of fetal excretory material, and maintains pregnancy through complex hormonal regulation. Most of the vital nutrients necessary for the development of the fetus are transported by active transport systems. For example, vitamins, amino acids, essential sugars, and ions such as calcium and iron are transported from mother to fetus against a concentration gradient (Young, 1969; Ginsburg, 1971). In contrast, most toxic agents pass the placenta by simple diffusion. The only exceptions are a few antimetabolites that are structurally similar to endogenous purines and pyrimidines, which are the physiologic substrates for active transport from the maternal to the fetal circulation.

Many foreign substances can cross the placenta. In addition to chemicals, viruses (e.g., rubella virus), cellular pathogens (e.g., syphilis spirochetes), globulin antibodies, and erythrocytes (Goldstein et al., 1974) can traverse the placenta. Anatomically, the placental barrier consists of a number of cell layers interposed between the fetal and maternal circulations. The number of layers varies with the species and the state of gestation. Placentas in which the maximum number of cell layers are present (all six layers) are called *epitheliochorial* (Table 5-7). Those in which the maternal epithelium is absent are referred to as *syndesmochorial.* When only the endothelial layer of the maternal tissue remains, the tissue is termed *endotheliochorial;* when even the endothelium is gone, so that the chorionic villi bathe in the maternal blood, the tissue is called *hemochorial.* In some species, some of the fetal layers are absent and are called *hemoendothelial* (Dames, 1968). Within the same species, the placenta may also change its histologic classification during gestation (Amaroso, 1952). For example, at the beginning of gestation, the placenta of a rabbit has six major layers (epitheliochorial), and at the end it has only one (hemoendothelial). One might suspect that a relatively thin placenta such as that of a rat would be more permeable to toxic agents than is the placenta of humans, whereas a thicker placenta such as that of a goat would be less permeable. The exact relationship of the number of layers of the placenta to its permeability has not been investigated. Currently, it is not considered to be of primary importance in determining the distribution of chemicals to the fetus.

The same factors are important determinants of the placental transfer of xenobiotics by passive diffusion (particularly lipid/water solubility), as was discussed above for the passage of molecules across body membranes.

Recently it has been shown that the placenta contains active transport systems that protect the fetus from some xenobiotics. For example, multi-drug–resistant null (mdr null) fetuses are more susceptible to cleft palate produced by a photoisomer of avermectin due to higher concentrations in the mdr null fetuses (Lankas et al., 1998).

The placenta has biotransformation capabilities that may prevent some toxic substances from reaching the fetus (Juchau, 1972). Among the substances that cross the placenta by passive diffusion, more lipid-soluble substances more rapidly attain a maternal-fetal equilibrium. Under steady-state conditions, the concentrations of a toxic compound in the plasma of the mother and fetus are usually the same. The concentration in the various tissues of the fetus depends on the ability of fetal tissue to concentrate a toxicant. For

Table 5-7
Tissues Separating Fetal and Maternal Blood

	MATERNAL TISSUE			FETAL TISSUE			
	Endothelium	*Connective Tissue*	*Epithelium*	*Trophoblast*	*Connective Tissue*	*Endothelium*	*Species*
Epitheliochorial	+	+	+	+	+	+	Pig, horse, donkey
Syndesmochorial	+	+	—	+	+	+	Sheep, goat, cow
Endotheliochorial	+	—	—	+	+	+	Cat, dog
Hemochorial	—	—	—	+	+	+	Human, monkey
Hemoendothelial	—	—	—	—	—	+	Rat, rabbit, guinea pig

SOURCE: Modified from Amaroso EC: Placentation, in Parkes AS (ed): *Marshall's Physiology of Reproduction,* Longmans, Green, London, vol. 2, 1952.

example, the concentration of diphenylhydantoin in the plasma of the fetal goat was about half of that found in the mother. This was due to differences in plasma protein concentration and the binding affinity of diphenylhydantoin to plasma proteins (Shoeman et al., 1972). Also, some organs, such as the liver of the newborn (Klaassen, 1972) and the fetus, do not concentrate some xenobiotics, and therefore lower levels are found in the liver of the fetus. In contrast, higher concentrations of some chemicals, such as lead and dimethylmercury, are encountered in the brain of the fetus because of the fetus's not fully developed blood-brain barrier. Differential body composition between mother and fetus may be another reason for an apparent placental barrier. For example, fetuses have very little fat. Accordingly, and in contrast to the mothers, they do not accumulate highly lipophilic chemicals such as TCDD (Li et al., 1995).

Redistribution of Toxicants

As mentioned earlier, blood flow to and the affinity of an organ or tissue are the most critical factors that affect the distribution of xenobiotics. Chemicals can have an affinity to a binding site (e.g., intracellular protein or bone matrix) or to a cellular constituent (e.g., fat). The initial phase of distribution is determined primarily by blood flow to the various parts of the body. Therefore, a well-perfused organ such as the liver may attain high initial concentrations of a xenobiotic. However, the affinity of less well perfused organs or tissues may be higher for a particular xenobiotic, causing redistribution with time. For example, 2 h after administration, 50 percent of a dose of lead is found in the liver (Klaassen and Shoeman,1974). However, 1 month after dosing, 90 percent of the dose remaining in the body is associated with the crystal lattice of bone. Similarly, 5 min after an intravenous dose of a lipophilic chemical such as TCDD, about 15 percent of the dose is localized in the lungs, but only about 1 percent in adipose tissue. However, 24 h later, only 0.3 percent of the remaining dose is found in the lungs but about 20 percent in adipose tissue (Weber et al., 1993).

EXCRETION

Toxicants are eliminated from the body by several routes. The kidney is perhaps the most important organ for the excretion of xenobiotics, as more chemicals are eliminated from the body by this route than by any other (Chap. 14). Many xenobiotics, though, have to be biotransformed to more water-soluble products before they can be excreted into urine (Chap. 6). The second important route of elimination of many xenobiotics is via feces, and the third, primarily for gases, is via the lungs. Biliary excretion of xenobiotics and/or their metabolites is most often the major source of fecal excretion, but a number of other sources can be significant for some compounds. All body secretions appear to have the ability to excrete chemicals; toxicants have been found in sweat, saliva, tears, and milk (Stowe and Plaa, 1968).

Urinary Excretion

The kidney is a very efficient organ for the elimination of toxicants from the body. Toxic compounds are excreted with urine by the same mechanisms the kidney uses to remove the end products of intermediary metabolism from the body: glomerular filtration, tubular excretion by passive diffusion, and active tubular secretion.

The kidney receives about 25 percent of the cardiac output, about 20 percent of which is filtered at the glomeruli. The glomerular capillaries have large pores (70 nm). Therefore, compounds up to a molecular weight of about 60,000 (proteins smaller than albumin) are filtered at the glomeruli. The degree of plasma protein binding affects the rate of filtration, because protein-xenobiotic complexes are too large to pass through the pores of the glomeruli.

A toxicant filtered at the glomeruli may remain in the tubular lumen and be excreted with urine. Depending on the physicochemical properties of a compound, it may be reabsorbed across the tubular cells of the nephron back into the bloodstream. The principles governing the reabsorption of toxicants across the kidney tubules are the same as those discussed earlier in this chapter for passive diffusion across cell membranes. Thus, toxicants with a high lipid/water partition coefficient are reabsorbed efficiently, whereas polar compounds and ions are excreted with urine. As can be deduced from the Henderson-Hasselbalch equations, bases are excreted (i.e., not reabsorbed) to a greater extent at lower and acids at higher urinary pH values. A practical application of this knowledge is illustrated by the treatment of phenobarbital poisoning with sodium bicarbonate. The percentage of ionization can be increased markedly within physiologically attainable pH ranges for a weak organic acid such as phenobarbital (pK_a 7.2). Consequently, alkalinization of urine by the administration of sodium bicarbonate results in a significant increase in the excretion of phenobarbital (Weiner and Mudge, 1964). Similarly, acceleration of salicylate loss via the kidney can be achieved through the administration of sodium bicarbonate.

Toxic agents can also be excreted from plasma into urine by passive diffusion through the tubule. This process is probably of minor significance because filtration is much faster than excretion by passive diffusion through the tubules, providing a favorable concentration gradient for reabsorption rather than excretion. Exceptions to this generalization may be some organic acids ($pK_a \approx 3$ to 5) and bases ($pK_a \approx 7$ to 9) that would be largely ionized and thus trapped at the pH of urine ($pH \approx 6$). For renal excretion of such compounds, the flow of urine is likely to be important for the maintenance of a concentration gradient, favoring excretion. Thus, diurectics can hasten the elimination of weak organic acids and bases.

Xenobiotics can also be excreted into urine by active secretion. During the last few years a number of transporters have been identified in the kidney. Figure 5-8 illustrates the various families of transporters in the kidney. The organic-anion transporter (oat) family is localized on the basolateral membranes of the proximal tubule. This family is responsible for the renal uptake of organic acids such as *p*-aminohippurate. The organic-cation transporting (oct) family is responsible for the renal uptake of some cations. Once xenobiotics are in the tubular cell, they are exuded into the lumen by multi-drug—resistant protein (mdr) and by multi-resistant drug protein (mrp). In contrast, the organic cation transporter (octn2) and peptide transporter (PEP2) reabsorb chemicals from the tubular lumen.

Some less polar xenobiotics may diffuse into the lumen. In contrast to filtration, protein-bound toxicants are available to active transport. As in all active transport systems, renal secretion of xenobiotics also reveals competition. This fact was put to use

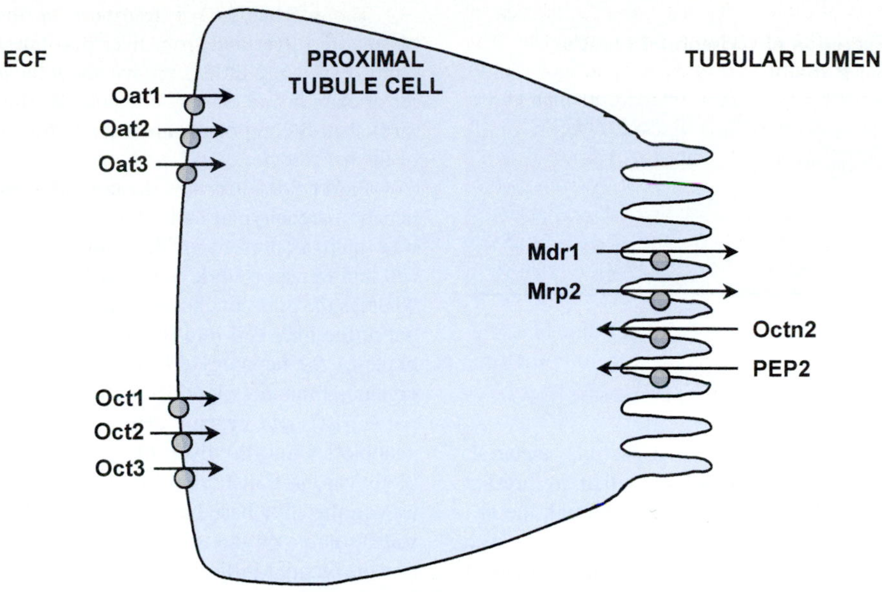

Figure 5-8. Schematic model showing the transport systems in the proximal tubule of the kidney.

The families of transporters are organic anion transporters (oat), organic-cation transporters (oct), multidrug resistant protein (mdr), multiresistant drug protein (mrp), and peptide transporters (PEP). ECF = extracellular fluid.

during World War II, when penicillin was in short supply. Penicillin is actively secreted by the organic acid system of the kidney. To lengthen its half-life and duration of action, another acid was sought to compete with penicillin for renal secretion; probenecid was successfully introduced for this purpose. Uric acid is also secreted actively by renal tubules. It is of clinical relevance that toxicants transported by the organic acid transport system can increase the plasma uric acid concentration and precipitate an attack of gout.

Because many functions of the kidney are incompletely developed at birth, some xenobiotics are eliminated more slowly in newborns than in adults and therefore may be more toxic to newborns. For example, the clearance of penicillin by premature infants is only about 20 percent of that observed in older children (Barnett et al., 1949). It has been demonstrated that the development of this organic acid transport system in newborns can be stimulated by the administration of substances normally excreted by this system (Hirsch and Hook, 1970). Some compounds, such as cephaloridine, are known to be nephrotoxic in adult animals but not in newborns. Because active uptake of cephaloridine by the kidneys is not well developed in newborns, this agent is not concentrated in the tubules and consequently is not nephrotoxic. If the development of active transport in newborns is stimulated, the kidneys take up cephaloridine more readily and nephrotoxicity is observed (Wold et al., 1977). Also, nephrotoxicity can be blocked by probenecid, which competitively inhibits the uptake of cephaloridine into the kidneys (Tune et al., 1977).

The renal proximal tubule reabsorbs small plasma proteins that are filtered at the glomerulus. Thus, if a toxicant binds to those small proteins, it can be carried into the proximal tubule cells and exert toxicity. For example, cadmium bound to metallothionein, a small metal-binding protein, is readily taken up by the kidney, leading to kidney injury (Dorian et al., 1992). Similarly, chemicals such as limonene (present in orange juice) and trimethyl pentane (present in gasoline) bind to α_{2u}-globulin and are taken up by the proximal tubule to produce hyaline droplet nephropathy and eventually renal tumors in male rats (Lehman-McKeeman and Caudill, 1992). Fortunately, α_{2u}-globulin is expressed only by male rats.

Species differences in regard to the urinary excretion of weak organic acids and bases are observed frequently, as the pH of urine varies widely among species. Differences in renal clearance also can occur for compounds filtered at the glomeruli because of differences in plasma protein binding. Interestingly, species variations also can arise as a result of differences in active renal secretion, as has been shown for captopril (Migdalof et al., 1984).

Additional factors affecting the excretion of xenobiotics are exemplified by the disposition of griseofulvin in rats and rabbits (Table 5-8). Rabbits excrete most of a dose of griseofulvin as 6-demethylgriseofulvin in urine. Urinary excretion of this compound is to be expected, because its molecular weight is only 328. Molecules with molecular weight (MW) < 350 tend to be preferentially excreted in urine, whereas those between 350 and 700 are predominately excreted in bile. Because the molecular weight of griseofulvin conjugates is about 500, it is not surprising that rats which biotransform griseofulvin extensively (phase II) excrete much of a dose in bile. This is an example of biotransformation exerting a critical influence on the excretion of a xenobiotic.

Fecal Excretion

Fecal excretion is the other major pathway for the elimination of xenobiotics from the body. Fecal excretion of chemicals is a complex process that is not as well understood as urinary excretion. Several important sources and many more minor sources contribute to the excretion of toxicants via the feces.

Table 5-8
Urinary and Biliary Excretion of Griseofulvin and/or Metabolites in Rats and Rabbits

	*Rats**		*Rabbits**	
	URINE	BILE	URINE	BILE
Total	12	77	78	11
Phase I metabolites	ND†	23	70	3
Phase II metabolites	ND	54	8	8

*Expressed as percent of dose.
†ND, not determined.
SOURCE: Modified from Symchowicz et al. (1967), with permission.

Nonabsorbed Ingesta In addition to indigestible material, varying proportions of nutrients and xenobiotics that are present in food or are ingested voluntarily (drugs) pass through the alimentary canal unabsorbed, contributing to fecal excretion. The physicochemical properties of xenobiotics and the biological characteristics that facilitate absorption were discussed earlier in this chapter. In general, most human-made chemicals are at least to some extent lipophilic and thus are available for absorption. Exceptions include some macromolecules and some essentially completely ionized compounds of higher molecular weight. For example, the absorption of polymers or quaternary ammonium bases is quite limited in the intestine. Consequently, most of a dose of orally administered sucrose polyester, cholestyramine, or paraquat can be found in feces. It is rare for 100 percent of a compound to be absorbed. Therefore, the nonabsorbed portion of xenobiotics contributes to the fecal excretion of most chemicals to some extent.

Biliary Excretion The biliary route of elimination is perhaps the most important contributing source to the fecal excretion of xenobiotics and is even more important for the excretion of their metabolites. The liver is in a very advantageous position for removing toxic agents from blood after absorption from the GI tract, because blood from the GI tract passes through the liver before reaching the general circulation. Thus, the liver can extract compounds from blood and prevent their distribution to other parts of the body. Furthermore, the liver is the main site of biotransformation of toxicants and the metabolites thus formed may be excreted directly into bile. Xenobiotics and/or their metabolites entering the intestine with bile may be excreted with feces: when the physicochemical properties favor reabsorption, an enterohepatic circulation may ensue.

Foreign compounds excreted into bile are often divided into three classes on the basis of ratio of their concentration in bile versus that in plasma. Class A substances have a ratio of nearly 1 and include sodium, potassium, glucose, mercury, thallium, cesium, and cobalt. Class B substances have a ratio of bile to plasma greater than 1 (usually between 10 and 1000). Class B substances include bile acids, bilirubin, sulfobromophthalein, lead, arsenic, manganese, and many other xenobiotics. Class C substances have a ratio below 1 (e.g., inulin, albumin, zinc, iron, gold, and chromium). Compounds rapidly excreted into bile are most likely to be found among class B substances. However, a compound does not have to be highly concentrated in bile for biliary excretion to be of quantitative importance. For example, mercury is not concentrated in bile, yet bile is the main route of excretion for this slowly eliminated substance.

The mechanism of transport of foreign substances from plasma into liver and from liver into bile is not known with certainty. Especially little is known about the mechanism of the transfer of class A and class C compounds. However, it is thought that most class B compounds are actively transported across both sides of the hepatocyte.

Figure 5-9 illustrates the myriad of transporters localized on hepatic parenchymal cells. Sodium-dependent taurocholate peptide (ntcp) is present on the sinusoidal side of the parenchymal cell and transports bile acids such as taurocholate into the liver, whereas the bile salt excretory protein (bsep) transports bile acids out of the liver cell into the bile canaliculi. The sinusoidal membrane of the hepatocyte has a number of transporters including organic-anion polypeptide (oatp) 1 and 2, liver specific transporter (lst), and organic-cation (oct) transporters that transport xenobiotics into the liver. Once inside the hepatocyte, the xenobiotic can be transported into the blood or bile, or often is biotransformed by phase I and II drug metabolizing enzymes to more water-soluble products and then transported into the bile or back into the blood. Multi-drug–resistant protein one (mdr1) and multiresistant drug protein two (mrp2) are responsible for transporting xenobiotics into bile, whereas mrp3 and mrp6 transport xenobiotics back into the blood.

The biliary excretion of two organic acids—sulfobromophthalein (BSP) and indocyanine green (ICG)—has been particularly well examined. The rate of removal of these two dyes has long been used in liver function tests. The test is performed by injecting the dye intravenously and determining its plasma disappearance profile. A lack of proper plasma clearance of BSP or ICG indicates reduced biliary excretion, suggesting liver injury. Bilirubin is also actively transported from plasma into bile. Therefore, jaundice is often observed after a liver injury.

As with renal tubular secretion, toxic agents bound to plasma proteins are fully available for active biliary excretion. The relative importance of biliary excretion depends on the substance and species concerned. It is not known which factors determine whether a chemical will be excreted into bile or into urine. However, low-molecular-weight compounds are poorly excreted into bile while compounds or their conjugates with molecular weights exceeding about 325 can be excreted in appreciable quantities. Glutathione and glucuronide conjugates have a high predilection for excretion into bile. The percentages of a large number of compounds excreted into bile have been tabulated (Klaassen et al., 1981). Marked species variation exists in the biliary excretion of foreign compounds with consequences for the biological half-life of a compound and its toxicity. This species variation in biliary excretion is compound-specific. It is therefore difficult to categorize species into "good" or "poor" biliary excretors. However, in general, rats and mice tend to be better biliary excretors than are other species (Klaassen and Watkins, 1984).

Once a compound is excreted into bile and enters the intestine, it can be reabsorbed or eliminated with feces. Many organic compounds are conjugated before excretion into bile. Such polar metabolites are not sufficiently lipid-soluble to be reabsorbed. However, intestinal microflora may hydrolyze glucuronide and sulfate conjugates, making them sufficiently lipophilic for reabsorption. Reabsorption of a xenobiotic completes an enterohepatic cycle. Repeated enterohepatic cycling may lead to very long half-lives of xenobiotics in the body. Therefore, it is often desirable to interrupt this cycle to hasten the elimination of a toxicant from the body. This principle has been utilized in the treatment of dimethylmercury poisoning; ingestion of a polythiol resin binds the

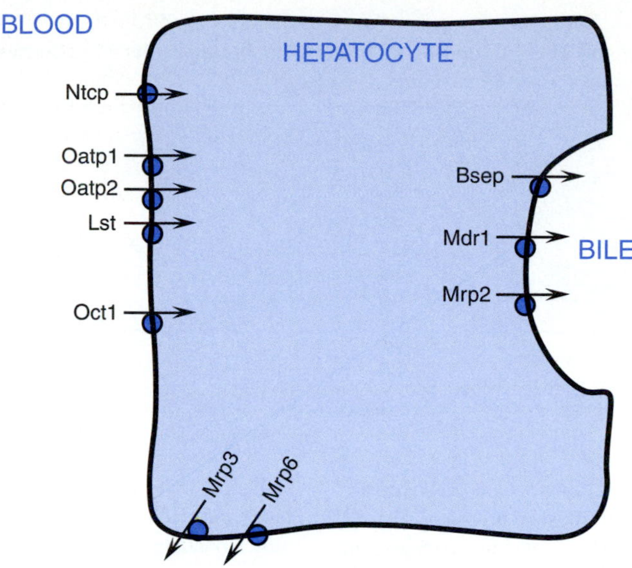

Figure 5-9. Schematic model showing the transport systems in the liver.

ntcp = sodium dependent taurocholate peptide, oatp = organic-anion transporting polypeptide, lst = liver specific transporter, oct = organic-cation transporter, bsep = bile salt excretory protein, mdr = multidrug resistant protein, mrp = multiresistant drug protein.

mercurial and thus prevents its reabsorption (Magos and Clarkson, 1976).

An increase in hepatic excretory function also has been observed after pretreatment with some drugs (Klaassen and Watkins, 1984). For example, it has been demonstrated that phenobarbital increases plasma disappearance by enhancing the biliary excretion of BSP and a number of other compounds. The increase in bile flow caused by phenobarbital appears to be an important factor in increasing the biliary excretion of BSP. However, other factors, such as the induction of some phase II enzymes, also can increase the conjugating capacity of the liver and thus enhance the plasma disappearance and biliary excretion of some compounds. Not all microsomal enzyme inducers increase bile flow and excretion; 3-methylcholanthrene and benzo[a]pyrene are relatively ineffective in this regard.

An increase in biliary excretion can decrease the toxicity of xenobiotics. Phenobarbital treatment of laboratory animals has been shown to enhance the biliary excretion and elimination of methylmercury from the body (Klaassen, 1975; Magos and Clarkson, 1976). Two steroids known to induce microsomal enzymes—spironolactone and pregnenolone-16α-carbonitrile—have also been demonstrated to increase bile production and to enhance biliary excretion of BSP (Zsigmond and Solymoss, 1972). These two steroids have also been shown to decrease the toxicity of several chemicals (Selye, 1970, 1971), including cardiac glycosides (Selye et al, 1969), by increasing their biliary excretion. This in turn decreases the concentration of cardiac glycosides in the heart, their target organ of toxicity (Castle and Lage, 1972, 1973; Klaassen, 1974a).

The hepatic excretory system is not fully developed in newborns, and this is another reason why some compounds are more toxic to newborns than to adults (Klaassen, 1972, 1973a). For example, ouabain is about 40 times more toxic in newborn than in adult rats. This is due to an almost complete inability of the newborn rat liver to remove ouabain from plasma. A decreased excretory function of newborn liver also has been demonstrated for other xenobiotics (Klaassen, 1973b). The development of hepatic excretory function can be promoted in newborns by administering a microsomal enzyme inducer (Klaassen, 1974b).

The toxicity of some compounds can be directly related to their biliary excretion. For example, indomethacin can cause intestinal lesions. The sensitivity of various species to this toxic response is directly related to the amount of indomethacin excreted into bile. The formation of intestinal lesions can be abolished by bile duct ligation (Duggan et al., 1975).

Often the elimination of a compound occurs by different routes in different species, as shown in the case of indomethacin in the dog and the rhesus monkey (Table 5-9). Dogs excrete most of a dose in feces, whereas monkeys excrete the majority of a dose in urine. Both species excrete similarly large quantities of a dose in bile. Because dogs excrete most of a dose in bile as conjugates (MW $>$ 500), it is to be expected that these hydrophilic indomethacin derivatives will not be reabsorbed unless they are hydrolyzed by intestinal bacteria to the reabsorbable parent compound, or to phase I metabolites (which do have good bioavailability). Based on available experimental data, it is not possible to decide with certainty whether or not this is occurring in the dog. It appears that indomethacin undergoes enterohepatic circulation with repeated conjugation in the liver and deconjugation in the small intestine, with a gradual "loss" of conjugates into the large intestine. However, because almost all of fecal excretion consists of indomethacin, it is apparent that the large intestinal flora hydrolyzes the indomethacin conjugates. Limited reabsorption of indomethacin is not surprising (p$K_a \approx 4.5$, colon pH ≈ 8), because more than 99.7 percent of indomethacin is ionized in the large intestine, which has a small surface area (compared to the small intestine). This does not allow for a sufficiently rapid shift in the mass balance to result in substantial reabsorption.

The monkey also reveals extensive enterohepatic recycling of indomethacin (57.7 percent of dose excreted in bile within 2 h). However, most of the biliary excretion consists of parent compound, which is readily reabsorbed in the small intestine, as indi-

Table 5-9
Urinary, Biliary, and Fecal Excretion of Indomethacin and/or Its Metabolites in Dogs and Monkeys after Intravenous Dosage

	Urine		*Bile*		*Feces*	
COMPOUND	DOG	MONKEY	DOG	MONKEY	DOG	MONKEY
Indomethacin	0.6*	10.5	3.8	33.6	68.7	4
Phase I metabolites	4.1	24.2	NI†	NI	2.7	6
Phase II metabolites	3.3	17.9	52.1	8.1	3.1	NI
Total dose excreted	7.9	52.7	55.9	51.7	76.3	10

*Values represent % of dose excreted.
†NI, not identified or very small amounts.
SOURCE: Modified from Hucker et al. (1966) and Yesair et al. (1970), with permission.

cated by the small amount lost into feces (about 10 percent of dose). In contrast to the dog, monkeys excrete most of a dose as phase I metabolites (24.2 percent of dose) and indomethacin (10.5 percent of dose). Because indomethacin has a molecular weight of 358 and phase I metabolites have molecular weights of 220 to 345, these compounds are readily excreted in urine.

Intestinal Excretion It has been shown for a fairly large number of diverse chemicals (e.g., digitoxin, dinitrobenzamide, hexachlorobenzene, ochratoxin A) that their excretion into feces can be explained neither by the unabsorbed portion of an oral dosage nor by excretion into bile (Rozman, 1986). Experiments in bile duct–ligated animals and animals provided with bile fistulas have revealed that the source of many chemicals in feces is a direct transfer from blood into the intestinal contents. This transfer is thought to occur by passive diffusion for most xenobiotics. In some instances, rapid exfoliation of intestinal cells also may contribute to the fecal excretion of some compounds. Intestinal excretion is a relatively slow process. Therefore, it is a major pathway of elimination only for compounds that have low rates of biotransformation and/or low renal or biliary clearance. The rate of intestinal excretion of some lipid-soluble compounds can be substantially enhanced by increasing the lipophilicity of the GI contents—for example, by adding mineral oil to the diet (Rozman, 1986). Active secretion of organic acids and bases also has been demonstrated in the large intestine (Lauterbach, 1977). The importance of active intestinal secretion for fecal elimination has been established only for a few chemicals.

Intestinal Wall and Flora No systematic attempts have been undertaken to assess the role of biotransformation in the intestinal wall in the fecal excretion of xenobiotics. Nevertheless, in recent years evidence has accumulated that mucosal biotransformation and reexcretion into the intestinal lumen occur with many compounds. The significance of these findings for fecal excretion is difficult to judge because further interaction with the intestinal flora may alter these compounds, making them more or less suitable for reabsorption or excretion (Rozman, 1986). More is known about the contribution of the intestinal flora to fecal excretion. It has been estimated that 30 to 42 percent of fecal dry matter originates from bacteria. Chemicals originating from the nonabsorbed portion of an oral dose, the bile, or the intestinal wall are taken up by these microorganism according to the principles of membrane permeability. Therefore, a considerable proportion of fecally excreted xenobiotic is associated with the excreted bacteria. However, chemicals may be profoundly altered by bacteria before excretion with feces, particularly in the large intestine, where intestinal flora are most abundant, and intestinal contents remain for 24 h or longer. It seems that biotransformation by intestinal flora favors reabsorption rather than excretion. Nevertheless, there is evidence that in many instances xenobiotics found in feces derive from bacterial biotransformation. The importance of microbial biotransformation for fecal excretion can be studied by performing experiments in normal versus gnotobiotic animal (animals with no microflora).

Exhalation

Substances that exist predominantly in the gas phase at body temperature are eliminated mainly by the lungs. Because volatile liquids are in equilibrium with their gas phase in the alveoli, they also may be excreted via the lungs. The amount of a liquid eliminated via the lungs is proportional to its vapor pressure. A practical application of this principle is seen in the breath analyzer test for determining the amount of ethanol in the body. Highly volatile liquids such as diethyl ether are excreted almost exclusively by the lungs.

No specialized transport systems have been described for the excretion of toxic substances by the lungs. These substances seem to be eliminated by simple diffusion. Elimination of gases is roughly inversely proportional to the rate of their absorption. Therefore, gases with low solubility in blood, such as ethylene, are rapidly excreted, whereas chloroform, which has a much higher solubility in blood, is eliminated very slowly by the lungs. Trace concentrations of highly lipid-soluble anesthetic gases such as halothane and methoxyflurane may be present in expired air for as long as 2 to 3 weeks after a few hours of anesthesia. Undoubtedly, this prolonged retention is due to deposition in and slow mobilization from adipose tissue of these very lipid-soluble agents. The rate of elimination of a gas with low solubility in blood is perfusion-limited, whereas that of a gas with high solubility in blood is ventilation-limited.

Other Routes of Elimination

Cerebrospinal Fluid A specialized route of removal of toxic agents from a specific organ is represented by the cerebrospinal fluid (CSF). All compounds can leave the CNS with the bulk flow of CSF through the arachnoid villi. In addition, lipid-soluble toxicants also can exit at the site of the blood-brain barrier. It is noteworthy that toxicants also can be removed from the CSF by active transport, similar to the transport systems of the kidneys for the excretion of organic ions.

Milk The secretion of toxic compounds into milk is extremely important because (1) a toxic material may be passed with milk from the mother to the nursing offspring and (2) compounds can be passed from cows to people via dairy products. Toxic agents are excreted into milk by simple diffusion. Because milk is more acidic (pH≈6.5) than plasma, basic compounds may be concentrated in milk, whereas acidic compounds may attain lower concentrations in milk than in plasma (Findlay, 1983; Wilson, 1983). More important, about 3 to 4 percent of milk consists of lipids, and the lipid content of colostrum after parturition is even higher. Lipid-soluble xenoiotics diffuse along with fats from plasma into the mammary gland and are excreted with milk during lactation. Compounds such as DDT and polychlorinated and polybrominated biphenyls, dibenzo-*p*-dioxins, and furans (Van den Berg et al., 1987; Li et al., 1995) are known to occur in milk, and milk can be a major route of their excretion. Species differences in the excretion of xenobiotics with milk are to be expected, as the proportion of milk fat derived from the circulation versus that synthesized de novo in the mammary gland differs widely among species. Metals chemically similar to calcium, such as lead, and chelating agents that form complexes with calcium also can be excreted into milk to a considerable extent.

Sweat and Saliva The excretion of toxic agents in sweat and saliva is quantitatively of minor importance. Again, excretion depends on the diffusion of the nonionized, lipid-soluble form of an agent. Toxic compounds excreted into sweat may produce dermatitis. Substances excreted in saliva enter the mouth, where they are usually swallowed and thus are available for GI absorption.

CONCLUSION

Humans are in continuous contact with toxic agents. Toxicants are in the food we eat, the water we drink, and the air we breathe. Depending on their physical and chemical properties, toxic agents may be absorbed by the GI tract, the lungs, and/or the skin. Fortunately, the body has the ability to biotransform and excrete these compounds into urine, feces, and air. However, when the rate of absorption exceeds the rate of elimination, toxic compounds may accumulate and reach a critical concentration at a certain target site, and toxicity may ensue (Fig. 5-10). Whether a chemical elicits its toxicity depends not only on its inherent potency and site specificity but also on how an organism can handle—that is, dispose of—a particular toxicant. Therefore, knowledge of the disposition of chemicals is of great importance in judging the toxicity of xenobiotics. For example, for a potent CNS suppressant that displays a strong hepatic first-pass effect, oral exposure is of less concern than is exposure by inhalation. Also, two equipotent gases, with the absorption of one being perfusion rate-limited and that of the other being ventilation rate-limited, will exhibit completely different toxicity profiles at a distant site because of differences in the concentrations attained in the target organ.

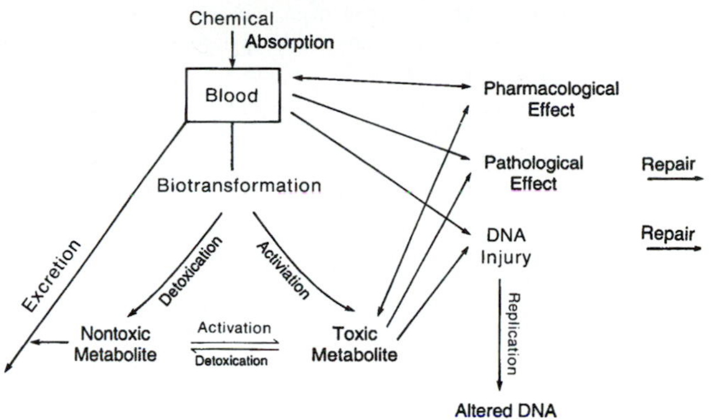

Figure 5-10. Schematic representation of the disposition and toxic effects of chemicals.

Many chemicals have very low inherent toxicity but have to be activated by biotransformation into toxic metabolites; the toxic response then depends on the rate of production of toxic metabolites. Alternatively, a very potent toxicant may be detoxified rapidly by biotransformation. Toxic effects are related to the concentration of the "toxic chemical" at the site of action (in the target organ), whether a chemical is administered or generated by biotransformation in the target tissue or at a distant site. Thus, the toxic response exerted by chemicals is critically influenced by the rates of absorption, distribution, biotransformation, and excretion.

REFERENCES

Albert A: *Selective Toxicity,* 3d ed. London: Methuen, 1965.

Allenby AC, Creasey NH, Edginton JAG, et al: Mechanism of action of accelerants on skin penetration. *Br J Dermatol* 81(suppl 4):4755, 1969.

Amaroso EC: Placentation, in Parks AS (ed): *Marshall's Physiology of Reproduction,* 3d ed. Vol 2. London: Longmans, Green, 1952, pp 127–311.

Aungst B, Shen DD: Gastrointestinal absorption of toxic agents, in Rozman K, Hanninen O (eds): *Gastrointestinal Toxicology.* Amsterdam/New York/Oxford: Elsevier, 1986, pp 29–56.

Barnett HL, McNamara H, Schultz S, Tomposett R: Renal clearances of sodium penicillin G, procaine penicillin G, and inulin in infants and children. *Pediatrics* 3:418–422, 1949.

Barnett RJ: The demonstration with the electron microscope of the end-products of histochemical reactions in relation to the fine structure of cells. *Exp Cell Res* suppl 7:65–89, 1959.

Bates TR, Gibaldi M: Gastrointestinal absorption of drugs, in Swarbrick J (ed): *Current Concepts in the Pharmaceutical Sciences: Biopharmaceutics.* Philadelphia: Lea & Febiger, 1970, pp 57–100.

Benz R, Janko K, Länger P: Pore formation by the matrix protein (porin) to *Escherichia coli* in planar bilayer membranes. *Ann NY Acad Sci* 358:13–24, 1980.

Blank IH, Scheuplein RJ: Transport into and within the skin. *Br J Dermatol* 81(suppl 4):4–10, 1969.

Borowitz JL, Moore PF, Him GKW, Miya TS: Mechanism of enhanced drug effects produced by dilution of the oral dose. *Toxicol Appl Pharmacol* 19:164–168, 1971.

Boyes RN, Adams HJ, Duce BR: Oral absorption and disposition kinetics of lidocaine hydrochloride in dogs. *J Pharmacol Exp Ther* 174:1–8, 1970.

Calabrese EJ: Gastrointestinal and dermal absorption: Interspecies differences. *Drug Metab Rev* 15:1013–1032, 1984.

Castle MC, Lage GL: Effect of pretreatment with spironolactone, phenobarbital or β-diethylaminoethyl diphenylpropylacetate (SKF 525-A) on tritium levels in blood, heart and liver of rats at various times after administration of [^{3}H]digitoxin. *Biochem Pharmacol* 21:1149–1155, 1972.

Castle MC, Lage GL: Enhanced biliary excretion of digitoxin following spironolactone as it relates to the prevention of digitoxin toxicity. *Res Commun Chem Pathol Pharmacol* 5:99–108, 1973.

Cayen MN: Metabolic disposition of antihyperlipidemic agents in man and laboratory animals. *Drug Metab Rev* 11:291–323, 1980.

Clarkson, TW: Metal toxicity in the central nervous system. *Environ Health Perspect* 75:59–64, 1987.

Coulston F, Serrone DM: The comparative approach to the role of nonhuman primates in evaluation of drug toxicity in man: A review. *Ann NY Acad Sci* 162:681–704, 1969.

Dames GS: *Foetal and Neonatal Physiology: A Comparative Study of the Changes at Birth.* Chicago: Year Book, 1968.

Dantzig AH, Duckworth DC, Tabas LB: Transport mechanisms responsible for the absorption of loracarbef, cefixime, and cefuroxime axetil into human intestinal Caco-2 cells. *Biochem Biophys Acta* 1191:7–13, 1994.

Dorian C, Gattone VH II, Klaassen CD: Renal cadmium deposition and injury as a result of accumulation of cadmium-metallothionein (CdMT) by proximal convoluted tubules—A light microscope autoradiographic study with ^{109}CdMT *Toxicol Appl Pharmacol* 114:173–181, 1992.

Dowling RH: Compensatory changes in intestinal absorption. *Br Med Bull* 23:275–278, 1967.

Draize JH, Woodard G, Calvery HO: Methods for the study of irritation and toxicity of substances applied topically to the skin and mucous membranes. *J Pharmacol Exp Ther* 82:377–390, 1944.

Dreyfuss J, Shaw JM, Ross JJ: Absorption of the adrenergic-blocking agent, nadol, by mice, rats, hamsters, rabbits, dogs, monkeys and man: Unusual species differences. *Xenobiotica* 8:503–510, 1978.

Dugard PH: Skin permeability theory in relation to measurements of percutaneous absorption in toxicology, in Marzulli FN, Maibach HI (eds): *Dermatotoxicology,* 2d ed. Washington/New York/London: Hemisphere, 1983, pp 91–116.

Dugard PH, Embery G: The influence of dimethylsulphoxide on the percutaneous migration of potassium butyl [^{35}S]sulphate, potassium methyl [^{35}S]sulphate and sodium [^{35}S]sulphate. *Br J Dermtol* 81(suppl 4):69–74, 1969.

Duggan DE, Hooke KF, Noll RM, Kwan KC: Enterohepatic circulation of indomethacin and its role in intestinal irritation. *Biochem Pharmacol* 24:1749–1754, 1975.

Ferguson HC: Dilution of dose and acute oral toxicity. *Toxicol App Pharmacol* 4:759–762, 1962.

Findlay JWA: The distribution of some commonly used drugs in human breast milk. *Drug Metab Rev* 14:653–686, 1983.

Ginsburg J: Placental drug transfer. *Annu Rev Pharmacol* 11:387–408, 1971.

Goldstein A, Aronow L, Kalman SM (eds): *Principles of Drug Action: The Basis of Pharmacology,* 2d ed. New York: Wiley, 1974.

Gorringe JAL, Sproston EM: The influence of particle size upon the absorption of drugs from the gastrointestinal tract, in Binn TB (ed): *Absorption and Distribution of Drugs.* Baltimore: Williams & Wilkins, 1964, pp 128–139.

Hallikainen A, Salminen S: Foods, food additives and contaminants in gastrointestinal toxicology, in Rozman K, Hänninen O (eds): *Gastrointestinal Toxicology.* Amsterdam/New York/Oxford: Elsevier, 1986, pp 342–362.

Hayton WL: Rate-limiting barriers to intestinal drug absorption: A review. *J Pharmacokin Biopharm* 8:321–334, 1980.

Hayes WJ Jr: Review of the metabolism of chlorinated hydrocarbon insecticides especially in mammals. *Annu Rev Pharmacol* 5:27–52, 1965.

Heath DF, Vandekar M: Toxicity and metabolism of dieldrin in rats. *Br J Ind Med* 21:269–279, 1964.

Hirsch GH, Hook JB: Maturation of renal organic acid transport substrate stimulation by penicillin and *p*-aminohippurate (PAH). *J Pharmacol Exp Ther* 171:103–108, 1970.

Houston JB, Upshall DG, Bridges JW: A re-evaluation of the importance of partition coefficients in the gastrointestinal absorption of nutrients. *J Pharmacol Exp Ther* 189:244–254, 1974.

Hucker HB, Hutt JE, White SD, et al: Studies on the absorption, distribution and excretion of indomethacin in various species. *J Pharmacol Exp Ther* 153:237–249, 1966.

Iatropoulos MJ: Morphology of the gastrointestinal tract, in Rozman K, Hänninen O (eds): *Gastrointestinal Toxicology.* Amsterdam/New York/Oxford: Elsevier, 1986, pp 246–266.

Juchau MR: Mechanisms of drug biotransformation reactions in the placenta. *Fed Proc* 31:48–51, 1972.

Kao J, Patterson FU, Hall J: Skin penetration and metabolism of topically applied chemicals in six mammalian species, including man: An *in vitro* study with benzo(a)pyrene and testosterone. *Toxicol Appl Pharmacol* 81:502–516, 1985.

Kelly D, Kostial K: The effect of milk diet on lead metabolism in rats. *Environ Res* 6:355–360, 1973.

Klaassen CD: Biliary excretion of mercury compounds. *Toxicol Appl Pharmacol* 33:356–365, 1975.

Klaassen CD: Comparison of the toxicity of chemicals in newborn rat to bile duct—ligated and sham-operated rats and mice. *Toxicol Appl Pharmacol* 24:37–44, 1973.

Klaassen CD: Effect of microsomal enzyme inducers on the biliary excretion of cardiac glycosides. *J Pharmacol Exp Ther* 191:201–211, 1974.

Klaassen CD: Hepatic excretory function in the newborn rat. *J Pharmacol Exp Ther* 184:721–728, 1973.

Klaassen CD: Immaturity of the newborn rat's hepatic excretory function for ouabain. *J Pharmacol Exp Ther* 183:520–526, 1972.

Klaassen CD: Stimulation of the development of the hepatic excretory mechanism for ouabain in newborn rats with microsomal enzyme inducers. *J Pharmacol Exp Ther* 191:212–218, 1974.

Klaassen CD, Eaton DL,Cagen SZ: Hepatobiliary disposition of xenobiotics, in Bridges JW, Chasseaud LF (eds): *Progress in Drug Metabolism.* New York: Wiley, 1981, pp 1–75.

Klaassen CD, Shoeman DW: Biliary excretion of lead in rats, rabbits and dogs. *Toxicol Appl Pharmacol* 29:434–446, 1974.

Klaassen CD, Watkins JB: Mechanisms of bile formation, hepatic uptake, and biliary excretion. *Pharmacol Rev* 36:1–67, 1984.

Kragh-Hansen U: Molecular aspects of ligand binding to serum albumin. *Pharmacol Rev* 33:17–53, 1981.

Kupferberg HJ, Way EL: Pharmacologic basis for the increased sensitivity of the newborn rat to morphine. *J Pharmacol Exp Ther* 141:105–112, 1963.

Landas GR, Wise LD, Cartwright ME, et al: Placental p-glycoprotein deficiency enhances susceptibility to chemically induced birth defects in mice. *Reprod Toxicol* 12:457–463, 1998.

Lauterbach F: Intestinal secretion of organic ions and drugs, in Kramer M, Lauterbach F (eds): *Intestinal Permeation.* Amsterdam/Oxford: Excerpta Medica, 1977, pp 173–195.

Lehman-McKeeman LD, Caudill D: α2U-Globulin is the only member of the lipocalin protein superfamily that binds to hyaline droplet inducing agents. *Toxicol Appl Pharmacol* 116:170–176, 1992.

Leopold G, Furukawa E, Forth W, Rummel W: Comparative studies of absorption of heavy metals in vivo and in vitro. *Arch Pharmacol Exp Pathol* 263:275–276, 1969.

Levi AJ, Gatmaitan Z, Arias IM: Two hepatic cytoplasmic protein fractions, Y and Z, and their possible role in the hepatic uptake of bilirubin, sulfobromophthalein, and other anions. *J Clin Invest* 48:2156–2167, 1969.

Levine RR: Factors affecting gastrointestinal absorption of drugs. *Am J Dig Dis* 15:171–188, 1970.

Levine RR, Steinberg GM: Intestinal absorption of pralidoxime and other aldoximes. *Nature* 209:269–271, 1966.

Li X, Weber LWD, Rozman KK: Toxicokinetics of 2,3,7,8-tetrachlorodibenzo-*p*-dioxin (TCDD) in female Sprague-Dawley rats including placental and lactational transfer to fetuses and neonates. *Fundam Appl Toxicol* 27:70–76, 1995.

Litwack G, Ketterer B, Arias IM: Ligandin: A hepatic protein which binds steroids, bilirubin, carcinogens and a number of exogenous organic anions. *Nature* 234:466–467, 1971.

Lukas G, Brindle SD, Greengard P: The route of absorption of intraperitoneally administered compounds. *J Pharmacol Exp Ther* 178: 562–566, 1971.

Magos L, Clarkson TW: The effect of oral doses of a polythiol resin on the excretion of methylmercury in mice treated with cystein, D-penicillamine or phenobarbitone. *Chem Biol Interact* 14:325–335, 1976.

Malkinson FD: Permeability of the stratus corneum, in Montagna W, Lobitz WC Jr (eds): *The Epidermis.* New York: Academic Press, 1964, pp 435–552.

Marzulli FN, Callahan JF, Brown DWC: Chemical structure and skin penetrating capacity of a short series of organic phosphates and phosphoric acid. *J Invest Dermatol* 44:339–344, 1965.

Mendel JL, Walton MS: Conversion of pp-DDT to pp-DDD by intestinal flora of the rat. *Science* 151:1527–1528, 1966.

Migdalof BH, Antonaccio MJ, McKinstry DN, et al: Captopril: Pharmacology, metabolism, and disposition. *Drug Metab Rev* 15: 841–869, 1984.

Pentschew A, Garro F: Lead encephalomyelopathy of the suckling rat and its implication on the porphyrinopathic nervous diseases. *Acta Neuropathol (Berl)* 6:266–278, 1966.

Pfeiffer CJ: Gastroenterologic response to environmental agents-absorption and interactions, in Lee DHK (ed): *Handbook of Physiology. Section 9: Reactions to Environmental Agents.* Bethesda, MD: American Physiological Society, 1977, pp 349–374.

Renkin EM: Capillary permeability, in Mayerson HS (ed): *Lymph and the Lymphatic System.* Springfield, IL: Charles C Thomas, 1968, pp 76–88.

Rosenfield AB, Huston R: Infant methemoglobinemia in Minnesota due to nitrates in well water. *Minn Med* 33:787–796, 1950.

Rozman K: Fecal excretion of toxic substances, in Rozman K, Hänninen O (eds): *Gastrointestinal Toxicology.* Amsterdam/New York/Oxford: Elsevier, 1986, pp 119–145.

Rozman K, Iatropoulos MJ: Gastrointestinal toxicity: Dispositional considerations, in Yacobi A, Skelly JP, Batra VK (eds): *Toxicokinetics in New Drug Development,* New York: American Association of Pharmaceutical Scientist with Pergamon, 1989, pp 199–213.

Sanders E, Ashworth CT: A study of particulate intestinal absorption of hepatocellular uptake: Use of polystyrene latex particles. *Exp Cell Res* 22:137–145, 1961.

Sasser LB, Jarboe GE: Intestinal absorption and retention of cadmium in neonatal rat. *Toxicol Appl Pharmacol* 41:423–431, 1977.

Scala J, McOsker DE, Reller HH: The percutaneous absorption of ionic surfactants. *J Invest Dermatol* 50:371–379, 1968.

Scatchard G: The attraction of proteins for small molecules and ions. *Ann NY Acad Sci* 51:660–672, 1949.

Schade SG, Felsher BF, Glader BE, Conrad ME: Effect of cobalt upon iron absorption. *Proc Soc Exp Biol Med* 134:741–743, 1970.

Schanker LS: Mechanisms of drug absorption and distribution. *Annu Rev Pharmacol* 1:29–44, 1961.

Schanker LS: Passage of drugs across body membranes. *Pharmcol Rev* 74:501–530, 1962.

Schanker LS, Jeffrey J: Active transport of foreign pyrimidines across the intestinal epithelium. *Nature* 190:727–728, 1961.

Scheufler E, Rozman K: Comparative decontamination of hexachlorobenzene exposed rats and rabbits by hexadecane. *J Toxicol Environ Health* 14:353–362, 1984.

Schinkel A, Smith JJM, van Tellingen O, et al: Disruption of the mouse mdr1a p-glycoprotein gene leads to a deficiency in the blood-brain barrier and to increased sensitivity to drugs. *Cell* 47:491–502, 1994.

Schwartze EW: The so-called habituation to arsenic: Variation in the toxicity of arsenious oxide. *J Pharmacol Exp Ther* 20:181–203, 1923.

Selye H: Hormones and resistance. *J Pharm Sci* 60:1–28, 1971.

Selye H, Krajny M, Savoie L: Digitoxin poisoning: Prevention by spironolactone. *Science* 164:842–843, 1969.

Shand DG, Rangno RE: The deposition of propranolol: I. Elimination during oral absorption in man. *Pharmacology* 7:159–168, 1972.

Shoeman DW, Kauffman RE, Azarnoff DL, Boulos BM: Placental transfer of diphenylhydantoin in the goat. *Biochem Pharmacol* 21:1237–1243, 1972.

Silverman WA, Andersen DH, Blanc WA, Crozier DN: A difference in mortality rate and incidence of kernicterus among premature infants allotted to two prophylactic antibacterial regimens. *Pediatrics* 18:614–625, 1956.

Smith GS: Gastrointestinal toxifications and detoxifications in relation to resource management, in Rozman K, Hänninen O (eds): *Gastrointestinal Toxicology,* 3d ed. Amsterdam/New York/Oxford: Elsevier, 1986, pp 223–224.

Smith HW: Observations on the flora of the alimentary tract of animals and factors affecting its composition. *J Pathol Bacteriol* 89:95–107, 1965.

Sobel AE, Gawron O, Kramer B: Influence of vitamin D in experimental lead poisoning. *Proc Soc Exp Biol Med* 38:433–435, 1938.

Stowe CM, Plaa GL: Extrarenal excretion of drugs and chemicals. *Annu Rev Pharmacol* 8:337–356, 1968.

Symchowicz S, Staub MS, Wong KKA: Comparative study of griseofulvin-^{14}C metabolism in the rat and rabbit. *Biochem Pharmacol* 16:2405–2411, 1967.

Thompson RQ, Sturtevant M, Bird OD, Glazko AJ: The effect of metabolites of chloramphenicol (Chloromycetin) on the thyroid of the rat. *Endocrinology* 55:665–681, 1954.

Thomson ABR, Hotke CA, O'Brien BD, Weinstein WM: Intestinal uptake of fatty acids and cholesterol in four animal species and man: Role of unstirred water layer and bile salt micelle. *Comp Biochem Physiol* 75A:221–232, 1983.

Thomson ABR, Olatunbosun D, Valberg LS: Interrelation of intestinal transport system for manganese and iron. *J Lab Clin Med* 78:642–655, 1971a.

Thomson ABR, Valberg LS, Sinclair DG: Competitive nature of the intestinal transport mechanism for cobalt and iron in the rat. *J Clin Invest* 50:2384–2394, 1971b.

Thwaites DT, Brown CD, Hirst BH, Simmons NL: H+-coupled dipeptide (glycylsarcosine) transport across apical and basal borders of human intestinal Caco-2 cell monolayers display distinctive characteristics. *Biochem Biophys Acta* 1151:237–245, 1993.

Tsuji A, Tamai 1, Nakanishi M, et al: Intestinal brush-border transport of the oral cephalosporin antibiotic, cefdinir, mediated by dipeptide and monocarboxylic acid transport systems in rabbits. *J Pharm Pharmacol* 45:996–998, 1993.

Tune BM, Wu KY, Kempson RL: Inhibition of transport and prevention of toxicity of cephaloridine in the kidney: Dose-responsiveness of the rabbit and the guinea pig to probenecid. *J Pharmacol Exp Ther* 202:466–471, 1977.

Van den Berg M, Heeremans C, Veerhoven E, Olie, K: Transfer of polychlorinated dibenzo-*p*-dioxins and dibenzofurans to fetal and neonatal rats. *Fundam Appl Toxicol* 9:635–644, 1987.

Weber LWD, Ernst SW, Stahl BU, Rozman KK: Tissue distribution and toxicokinetics of 2,3,7,8-tetrachloro-dibenzo-*p*-dioxin in rats after intravenous injection. *Fundam Appl Toxicol* 21:523–534, 1993.

Weber LWD, Zesch A, Rozman KK: Penetration, distribution and kinetics of 2,3,7,8-tetrachlorodibenzo-*p*-dioxin in human skin in vitro. *Arch Toxicol* 65:421–428, 1991.

Weiner IM, Mudge GH: Renal tubular mechanisms for excretion of organic acids and bases. *Am J Med* 36:743–762, 1964.

Wertz PhW, Downing DT: Epidermal lipids, in Goldsmith LA (ed): *Physiology, Biochemistry and Molecular Biology of the Skin.* NewYork/Oxford: Oxford University Press, 1991, pp 206–236.

Wester RC, Maibach HI: Percutaneous absorption in man and animal: A perspective, in Drill VA, Lazar P (eds): *Cutaneous Toxicity.* New York: Academic Press, 1977, pp 111–126.

Wilkinson GR: Plasma and tissue binding considerations in drug disposition. *Drug Metab Rev* 14:427–465, 1983.

Williams RM, Beck F: A histochemical study of gut maturation. *J Anat* 105:487–501, 1969.

Wilson JT: Determinants and consequences of drug excretion in breast milk. *Drug Metab Rev* 14:619–652, 1983.

Winteringham FPW: Comparative biochemical aspects of insecticidal action. *Chem Ind* (*Lond*) 1195–1202, 1957.

Wold JS, Joust RR, Owen NV: Nephrotoxicity of cephaloridine in newborn rabbits: Role of the renal anionic transport system. *J Pharmacol Exp Ther* 201:778–785, 1977.

Yesair DW, Callahan M, Remington L, Kensler CJ: Role of the enterohepatic cycle of indomethacin on its metabolism, distribution in tissues and its excretion by rats, dogs, and monkeys. *Biochem Pharmacol* 19:1579–1590, 1970.

Young M: Three topics in placental transport: Amino transport; oxygen transfer; Placental function during labour, in Klopper A, Diczfalusy E (eds): *Foetus and Placenta.* Oxford: Blackwell, 1969, pp 139–189.

Zsigmond G, Solymoss B: Effect of spironolactone, pregnenolone-16 carbonitrile and cortisol on the metabolism and biliary excretion of sulfobromophthalein and phenol-3,6-dibromophthalein disulfonate in rats. *J Pharmacol Exp Ther* 183:499–507, 1972.

CHAPTER 6

BIOTRANSFORMATION OF XENOBIOTICS

Andrew Parkinson

All organisms are exposed constantly and unavoidably to foreign chemicals, or *xenobiotics,* which include both manufactured and natural chemicals such as drugs, industrial chemicals, pesticides, pollutants, pyrolysis products in cooked food, alkaloids, secondary plant metabolites, and toxins produced by molds, plants, and animals. The physical property that enables many xenobiotics to be absorbed through the skin, lungs, or gastrointestinal tract—namely, their lipophilicity—is an obstacle to their elimination, because lipophilic compounds can be readily reabsorbed. Consequently, the elimination of xenobiotics often depends on their conversion to water-soluble chemicals by a process known as *biotransformation,* which is catalyzed by enzymes in the liver and other tissues. An important consequence of biotransformation is that the physical properties of a xenobiotic are generally changed from those favoring absorption (lipophilicity) to those favoring excretion in urine or feces (hydrophilicity). An exception to this general rule is the elimination of volatile compounds by exhalation, in which case biotransformation to nonvolatile, water-soluble chemicals can retard their rate of elimination. Similarly, biotransformation of xenobiotics in the brain and testis (two organs with a barrier to chemical transport) might also be an obstacle to xenobiotic elimination if the metabolites cannot cross the blood-brain or blood-testis barrier.

Without biotransformation, lipophilic xenobiotics would be excreted from the body so slowly that they would eventually overwhelm and kill an organism. This principle is illustrated by comparing the theoretical and observed rates of elimination of barbital and hexobarbital. The theoretical half-life of barbital, which is water-soluble, closely matches the observed elimination half-life of this drug ($t_{1/2}$ 55 to 75 h), which is eliminated largely unchanged. In contrast, the observed elimination half-life of hexobarbital ($t_{1/2}$ 5 to 6 h) is considerably shorter than the theoretical rate of elimination of this highly lipophilic drug ($t_{1/2}$ 2 to 5 months), the difference being that hexobarbital is biotransformed to water-soluble metabolites that are readily excreted.

A change in pharmacokinetic behavior is not the only consequence of xenobiotic biotransformation nor, in some cases, is it the most important outcome. Xenobiotics exert a variety of effects on biological systems. These may be beneficial, in the case of drugs, or deleterious, in the case of poisons. These effects are dependent on the physicochemical properties of the xenobiotic. In many instances, chemical modification of a xenobiotic by biotransformation alters its biological effects. The importance of this principle to pharmacology is that some drugs must undergo biotransformation to exert their pharmacodynamic effect (i.e., it is the metabolite of the drug, and not the drug itself, that exerts the pharmacologic effect). The importance of this principle to toxicology is that many xenobiotics must undergo biotransformation to exert their characteristic toxic or tumorigenic effect (i.e., many chemicals would be considerably less toxic or tumorigenic if they were not converted to reactive metabolites by xenobiotic-biotransforming enzymes). In most cases, however, biotransformation terminates the pharmacologic effects of a drug and lessens the toxicity of xenobiotics. Enzymes catalyzing biotransformation reactions often determine the intensity and duration of action of drugs and play a key role in chemical toxicity and chemical tumorigenesis (Anders, 1985; Jakoby, 1980; Jakoby et al., 1982; Kato et al., 1989).

To a limited extent, the degree to which organisms are exposed to xenobiotics determines their biotransformation capacity. For example, insects that feed on a variety of plants have a greater capacity to biotransform xenobiotics than insects that feed on a limited number of plants; these, in turn, have a greater capacity to biotransform xenobiotics than insects that feed on a single species of plant. Compared with mammals, fish have a low capacity to metabolize xenobiotics, ostensibly because they can eliminate xenobiotics unchanged across their gills. Species differences in the capacity of mammals to biotransform xenobiotics do not simply reflect differences in exposure. However, some chemicals stimulate the synthesis of enzymes involved in xenobiotic biotransformation. This process, known as enzyme induction, is an adaptive and reversible response to xenobiotic exposure. Enzyme induction enables some xenobiotics to accelerate their own biotransformation and elimination (Conney, 1967). The mechanism and consequences of enzyme induction are discussed further on, under "Induction of Cytochrome P450."

GENERAL PRINCIPLES

Basic Properties of Xenobiotic Biotransforming Enzymes

Xenobiotic biotransformation is the principal mechanism for maintaining homeostasis during exposure of organisms to small foreign molecules, such as drugs. In general, xenobiotic biotransformation is accomplished by a limited number of enzymes with broad substrate specificities. The synthesis of some of these enzymes is triggered by the xenobiotic (by the process of enzyme induction), but in most cases the enzymes are expressed constitutively (i.e., they are synthesized in the absence of a discernible external stimulus). The specificity of xenobiotic biotransforming enzymes is so broad that they metabolize a large variety of endogenous chemicals, such as ethanol, acetone, steroid hormones, vitamins A and D, bilirubin, bile acids, fatty acids, and eicosanoids.

Indeed, xenobiotic biotransforming enzymes, or enzymes that are closely related, play an important role in the synthesis of many of these same molecules. For example, several steps in the synthesis of steroid hormones are catalyzed by cytochrome P450 enzymes in steroidogenic tissues. In general, these steroidogenic enzymes play little or no role in the biotransformation of xenobiotics. In the liver, however, other cytochrome P450 enzymes convert steroid hormones to water-soluble metabolites that are excreted in urine or bile, in an analogous manner to the biotransformation and elimination of xenobiotics.

The structure (i.e., amino acid sequence) of a given biotransforming enzyme may differ among individuals, which can give rise to differences in rates of xenobiotic biotransformation. In general, a variant form of a xenobiotic biotransforming enzyme (known as an *allelic variant* or an *allelozyme*) has diminished enzymatic activity compared with that of the wild-type enzyme, although this is not always the case (see "Alcohol Dehydrogenase," below). However, the impact of amino acid substitution(s) on the catalytic activity of a xenobiotic biotransforming enzyme is usually substrate-dependent, such that an allelic variant may interact normally with some substrates (and inhibitors) but abnormally with others. The study of the causes, prevalence, and impact of heritable differences in xenobiotic biotransforming enzymes is known as *pharmacogenetics.*

Biotransformation versus Metabolism

The terms *biotransformation* and *metabolism* are often used synonymously, particularly when applied to drugs. For example, xenobiotic biotransforming enzymes are often called drug-metabolizing enzymes. The term *xenobiotic biotransforming enzymes* is more encompassing, although it conceals the fact that steroids and several other endogenous chemicals are substrates for these enzymes. The term *metabolism* is often used to describe the total fate of a xenobiotic, which includes absorption, distribution, biotransformation, and elimination. However, *metabolism* is commonly used to mean biotransformation, which is understandable from the standpoint that the products of xenobiotic biotransformation are known as *metabolites*. Furthermore, individuals with a genetic enzyme deficiency resulting in impaired xenobiotic biotransformation are described as *poor metabolizers* rather than poor biotransformers. (Individuals with the normal phenotype are called *extensive metabolizers.*)

Stereochemical Aspects of Xenobiotic Biotransformation

Many xenobiotics, especially drugs, contain one or more chiral centers and can therefore exist in two mirror-image forms called stereoisomers or enantiomers. The biotransformation of some chiral xenobiotics occurs stereoselectively—meaning that one enantiomer (stereoisomer) is biotransformed faster than its antipode. For example, the antiepileptic drug Mesantoin, which is a racemic mixture of *R*- and *S*-mephenytoin, is biotransformed stereoselectively in humans, such that the *S*-enantiomer is rapidly hydroxylated (by a cytochrome enzyme called CYP2C19) and eliminated faster than the *R*-enantiomer. The ability of some chiral xenobiotics to inhibit xenobiotic biotransforming enzymes can also occur stereoselectively. For example, quinidine is a potent inhibitor of a human cytochrome P450 enzyme called CYP2D6, on which quinine, its antipode, has relatively little inhibitory effect.

In some cases, achiral molecules (or achiral centers) are converted to a mixture of enantiomeric metabolites, and this conversion may proceed stereoselectively such that one enantiomer is formed preferentially over its antipode. For example, several cytochrome P450 enzymes catalyze the 6-hydroxylation of steroid hormones. Some P450 enzymes (such as CYP2A1) preferentially catalyze the 6α-hydroxylation reaction, whereas other P450 enzymes (such as CYP3A) preferentially catalyze the 6β-hydroxylation reaction (which is a major route of hepatic steroid biotransformation). Ketones can be reduced by carbonyl reductases to a mixture of enantiomeric secondary alcohols, and this often occurs with a high degree of stereoselectivity. For example, pentoxifylline is reduced by carbonyl reductases in blood and liver to a mixture of secondary alcohols, with the major metabolite having an *S*-configuration, as shown in Fig. 6-1. Interestingly, the minor metabolite, a secondary alcohol with the *R*-configuration, has pharmacologic properties distinct from those of its *S*-antipode and its ketone precursor, pentoxifylline. This minor metabolite is known as lisofylline, which is under clinical investigation for the treatment of various diseases.

The reduction of ketones to secondary alcohols is a reversible reaction, and such interconversions can lead to an *inversion of configuration,* in which case a secondary alcohol with, say, an *R*-configuration is oxidized to a ketone (which is achiral); it, in turn, is reduced to a secondary alcohol with an *S*-configuration (i.e., *R*-alcohol → ketone → *S*-alcohol). This interconversion between achiral ketones and enantiomeric secondary alcohols likely explains why the administration of pure *R*-albuterol to human volunteers results in the formation of *S*-albuterol, just as the administration of pure *S*-albuterol leads to the formation of *R*-albuterol (Boulton and Fawcett, 1997).

Phase I and Phase II Biotransformation

The reactions catalyzed by xenobiotic biotransforming enzymes are generally divided into two groups, called phase I and phase II, as shown in Table 6-1 (Williams, 1971). Phase I reactions involve hydrolysis, reduction, and oxidation. These reactions expose or introduce a functional group (–OH, –NH_2, –SH or –COOH), and usually result in only a small increase in hydrophilicity. Phase II biotransformation reactions include glucuronidation, sulfonation (more commonly called sulfation), acetylation, methylation, conjugation with glutathione (mercapturic acid synthesis), and conjugation with amino acids (such as glycine, taurine, and glutamic acid). The cofactors for these reactions (discussed later) react with functional groups that are either present on the xenobiotic or are introduced/exposed during phase I biotransformation. Most phase II biotransformation reactions result in a large increase in xenobiotic hydrophilicity, hence they greatly promote the excretion of foreign chemicals.

Phase II biotransformation of xenobiotics may or may not be preceded by phase I biotransformation. For example, morphine, heroin, and codeine are all converted to morphine-3-glucuronide. In the case of morphine, this metabolite forms by direct conjugation with glucuronic acid. In the other two cases, however, conjugation with glucuronic acid is preceded by phase I biotransformation: hydrolysis (deacetylation) in the case of heroin and *O*-demethylation (involving oxidation by cytochrome P450) in the case of codeine. Similarly, acetaminophen can be glucuronidated and sulfated directly, whereas phenacetin must undergo phase I metabolism (involving *O*-deethylation to acetaminophen) prior to un-

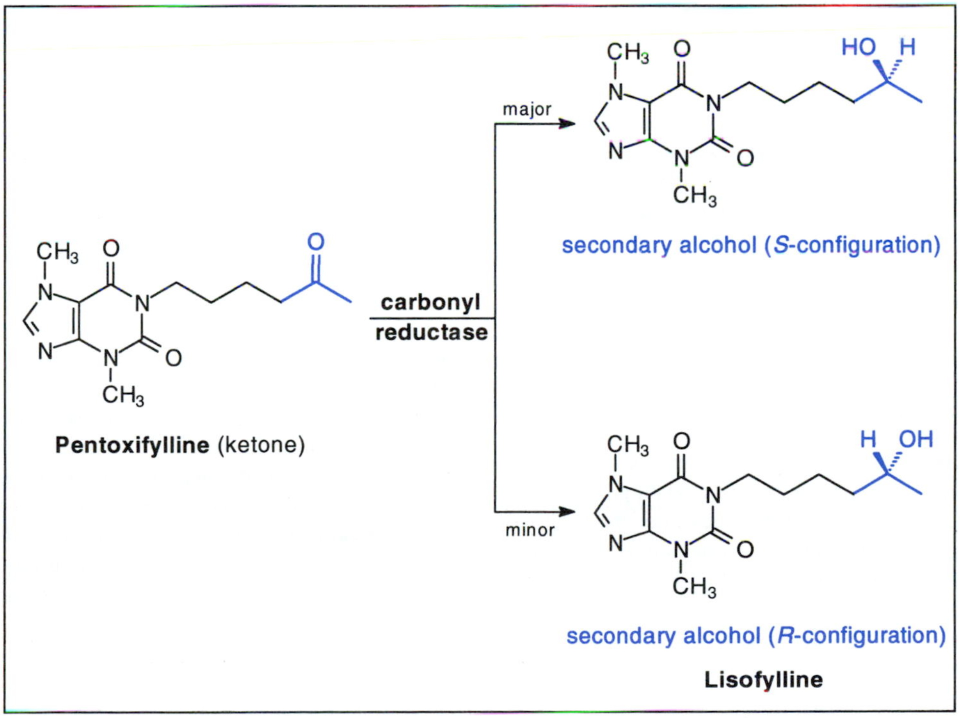

Figure 6-1. Stereochemical aspects of xenobiotic biotransformation: Formation of two enantiomeric metabolites (secondary alcohols) from a single, achiral molecule (a ketone).

Oxidation of a chiral secondary alcohol to an achiral ketone, and subsequent reduction of the ketone to a secondary alcohol of opposite configuration (*e.g., R*-alcohol → ketone → *S*-alcohol) is an example of a process known as *inversion of configuration.*

Table 6-1
General Pathways of Xenobiotic Biotransformation and Their Major Subcellular Location

REACTION	ENZYME	LOCALIZATION
	Phase I	
Hydrolysis	Esterase	Microsomes, cytosol, lysosomes, blood
	Peptidase	Blood, lysosomes
	Epoxide hydrolase	Microsomes, cytosol
Reduction	Azo- and nitro-reduction	Microflora, microsomes, cytosol
	Carbonyl reduction	Cytosol, blood, microsomes
	Disulfide reduction	Cytosol
	Sulfoxide reduction	Cytosol
	Quinone reduction	Cytosol, microsomes
	Reductive dehalogenation	Microsomes
Oxidation	Alcohol dehydrogenase	Cytosol
	Aldehyde dehydrogenase	Mitochondria, cytosol
	Aldehyde oxidase	Cytosol
	Xanthine oxidase	Cytosol
	Monoamine oxidase	Mitochondria
	Diamine oxidase	Cytosol
	Prostaglandin H synthase	Microsomes
	Flavin-monooxygenases	Microsomes
	Cytochrome P450	Microsomes
	Phase II	
	Glucuronide conjugation	Microsomes
	Sulfate conjugation	Cytosol
	Glutathione conjugation	Cytosol, microsomes
	Amino acid conjugation	Mitochondria, microsomes
	Acylation	Mitochondria, cytosol
	Methylation	Cytosol, microsomes, blood

dergoing phase II biotransformation. These examples illustrate how phase I biotransformation is often required for subsequent phase II biotransformation. In general, phase II biotransformation does not precede phase I biotransformation, although there are exceptions to this rule. For example, some sulfated steroids (including some steroid disulfates) are hydroxylated by cytochrome P450.

Nomenclature of Xenobiotic Biotransforming Enzymes

The enzymes involved in xenobiotic biotransformation tend to have broad and overlapping substrate specificities, which precludes the possibility of naming the individual enzymes after the reactions they catalyze (which is how most other enzymes are named). Many of the enzymes involved in xenobiotic biotransformation have been cloned and sequenced; in several cases, arbitrary nomenclature systems have been developed based on the primary amino acid sequence of the individual enzymes.

Distribution of Xenobiotic Biotransforming Enzymes

Xenobiotic biotransforming enzymes are widely distributed throughout the body and are present in several subcellular compartments. In vertebrates, the liver is the richest source of enzymes catalyzing biotransformation reactions. These enzymes are also located in the skin, lung, nasal mucosa, eye, and gastrointestinal tract—which can be rationalized on the basis that these are major routes of exposure to xenobiotics—as well as numerous other tissues, including the kidney, adrenal, pancreas, spleen, heart, brain, testis, ovary, placenta, plasma, erythrocytes, platelets, lymphocytes, and aorta (Gram, 1980; Farrell, 1987; Krishna and Klotz, 1994). Intestinal microflora play an important role in the biotransformation of certain xenobiotics. Within the liver (and most other organs), the enzymes catalyzing xenobiotic biotransformation reactions are located primarily in the endoplasmic reticulum (microsomes) or the soluble fraction of the cytoplasm (cytosol), with lesser amounts in mitochondria, nuclei, and lysosomes (see Table 6-1). Their presence in the endoplasmic reticulum can be rationalized on the basis that those xenobiotics requiring biotransformation for urinary or biliary excretion will likely be lipophilic and, hence, soluble in the lipid bilayer of the endoplasmic reticulum.

By extracting and biotransforming xenobiotics absorbed from the gastrointestinal tract, the liver limits the systemic bioavailability of orally ingested xenobiotics, a process known as *first-pass elimination*. In some cases, xenobiotic biotransformation in the intestine contributes significantly to the first-pass elimination of foreign chemicals. For example, the oxidation of cyclosporine by cytochrome P450 and the conjugation of morphine with glucuronic acid in the small intestine limit the systemic bioavailability of these drugs. Under certain circumstances, oxidation of ethanol to acetaldehyde in the gastric mucosa reduces the systemic bioavailability of alcohol. Some extrahepatic sites contain high levels of xenobiotic biotransforming enzymes, but their small size minimizes their overall contribution to the biotransformation of xenobiotics. For example, certain xenobiotic biotransforming enzymes (such as cytochrome P450 enzymes, flavin monooxygenases, glutathione *S*-transferases, and carboxylesterases) are present in nasal epithelium at levels that rival those found in the liver. The nasal epithelium plays an important role in the biotransformation of inhaled xenobiotics, including odorants, but is quantitatively unimportant in the biotransformation of orally ingested xenobiotics (Brittebo, 1993).

The fact that tissues differ enormously in their capacity to biotransform xenobiotics has important toxicologic implications in terms of tissue-specific chemical injury. Several xenobiotics, such as acetaminophen and carbon tetrachloride, are hepatotoxic due to their activation to reactive metabolites in the liver (Anders, 1985). Cells within an organ also differ in their capacity to biotransform xenobiotics, and this heterogeneity also has toxicologic implications. For example, the cytochrome P450 enzymes that activate acetaminophen and carbon tetrachloride to their reactive metabolites are localized in the centrilobular region of the liver (zone 3), which is why these xenobiotics cause centrilobular necrosis. Species differences in xenobiotic biotransforming enzymes have both toxicologic and pharmacologic consequences, as do factors that influence the activity of xenobiotic biotransforming enzymes (Kato, 1979). For example, the duration of action of hexobarbital (i.e., narcosis) in mice (~10 min), rabbits (~50 min), rats (~100 min), and dogs (~300 min) is inversely related to the rate of hexobarbital biotransformation (i.e., 3-hydroxylation) by liver microsomal cytochrome P450, which follows the rank order mouse > rabbit > rat > dog. The duration of action of hexobarbital in rats can be shortened from ~100 to ~30 min by prior treatment with phenobarbital, which induces cytochrome P450 and thereby increases the rate of hexobarbital 3-hydroxylation. By inducing cytochrome P450, treatment of rats with phenobarbital also increases the hepatotoxic effects of acetaminophen and carbon tetrachloride. Species differences in xenobiotic biotransforming enzymes and factors that affect the pharmacologic or toxicologic effects of xenobiotics are discussed throughout this chapter as each of the major xenobiotic biotransforming enzyme systems is described.

XENOBIOTIC BIOTRANSFORMATION BY PHASE I ENZYMES

Phase I reactions involve hydrolysis, reduction, and oxidation of xenobiotics, as shown in Table 6-1. These reactions expose or introduce a functional group (–OH, $-NH_2$, –SH, or –COOH) and usually result in only a small increase in the hydrophilicity of xenobiotics. The functional groups exposed or introduced during phase I biotransformation are often sites of phase II biotransformation.

Hydrolysis

Carboxylesterases, Pseudocholinesterase, and Paraoxonase Mammals contain a variety of hydrolytic enzymes—namely, carboxylesterases, cholinesterases and organophosphatases—that hydrolyze xenobiotics containing such functional groups as a carboxylic acid ester (procaine), amide (procainamide), thioester (spironolactone), phosphoric acid ester (paraoxon), and acid anhydride [diisopropylfluorophosphate (DFP)], as shown in Fig. 6-2 (Satoh and Hosokawa, 1998). The hydrolysis of carboxylic acid esters, amides, and thioesters is largely catalyzed by carboxylesterases (EC 3.1.1.1), which are located in various tissues and serum, and by two esterases in blood: true acetylcholinesterase (EC 3.1.17), which is located on erythrocyte membranes and is a dimeric enzyme (in contrast to the tetrameric form of the same enzyme found in nervous tissue), and pseudocholinesterase (EC 3.1.1.8), which is also known as butyrylcholinesterase and is located in serum. Phosphoric acid esters are hydrolyzed by paraoxonase, a serum enzyme that is known both as an aryldialkylphosphatase (EC 3.1.8.1) or organophosphatase (for its ability to hydrolyze organophosphates such as paraoxon) and as an arylesterase (for its ability to hydrolyze aromatic carboxylic acid esters such as phenylacetate). Phosphoric acid anhydrides, such as DFP, are hydrolyzed by a related organophosphatase, namely diisopropylfluorophosphatase (EC 3.1.8.2). In the presence of an alcohol, carboxylesterases can catalyze the transesterification of xenobiotics, which accounts for the conversion of cocaine (a methyl ester) to ethylcocaine (the corresponding ethyl ester) (Fig. 6-2). Esterases are not the only enzymes capable of cleaving esters. Aldehyde dehydrogenase has esterase activity. Examples are given later in this chapter (under "Cytochrome P450") in which the cleavage of xenobiotics containing a carboxylic acid ester is catalyzed by cytochrome P450.

Carboxylesterases in serum and tissues and serum cholinesterase collectively determine the duration and site of action of certain drugs. For example, procaine, a carboxylic acid ester, is rapidly hydrolyzed, which is why this drug is used mainly as a local anesthetic. In contrast, procainamide, the amide analog of procaine, is hydrolyzed much more slowly; hence this drug reaches the systematic circulation, where it is useful in the treatment of cardiac arrhythmia. In general, enzymatic hydrolysis of amides occurs more slowly than that of esters, although electronic factors can influence the rate of hydrolysis. The presence of electron-withdrawing substituents weakens an amide bond, making it more susceptible to enzymatic hydrolysis.

In 1953, Aldridge classified esterases based on the nature of their interaction with organophosphates. Esterases that hydrolyze organophosphates are classified as A-esterases; those that are inhibited by organophosphates are classified as B-esterases, whereas those that do not interact with organophosphates are classified as C-esterases. Carboxylesterases and cholinesterase belong to the B-esterase group, which is also known as the family of serine esterase. Organophosphatases such as paraoxonase belong to the A-esterase group.

Although they are not inhibited by organophosphates, A-esterases are inhibited by mercurial compounds that react with free sulfhydryl (–SH) groups, such as *para*-chloromercuribenzoate (PCMB), whereas the opposite is true of B-esterases (i.e., they are inhibited by organophosphates but not by PCMB). Augustinsson (1966) postulated that the major difference between A- and B-esterases is that the former contain a cysteine residue at their active site, whereas the latter contain a serine residue. This hypothesis has been substantiated in the case of B-esterases but not in the case of A-esterases.

Carboxylesterases and cholinesterases are B-esterases with a serine residue at the active site. The mechanism of catalysis by

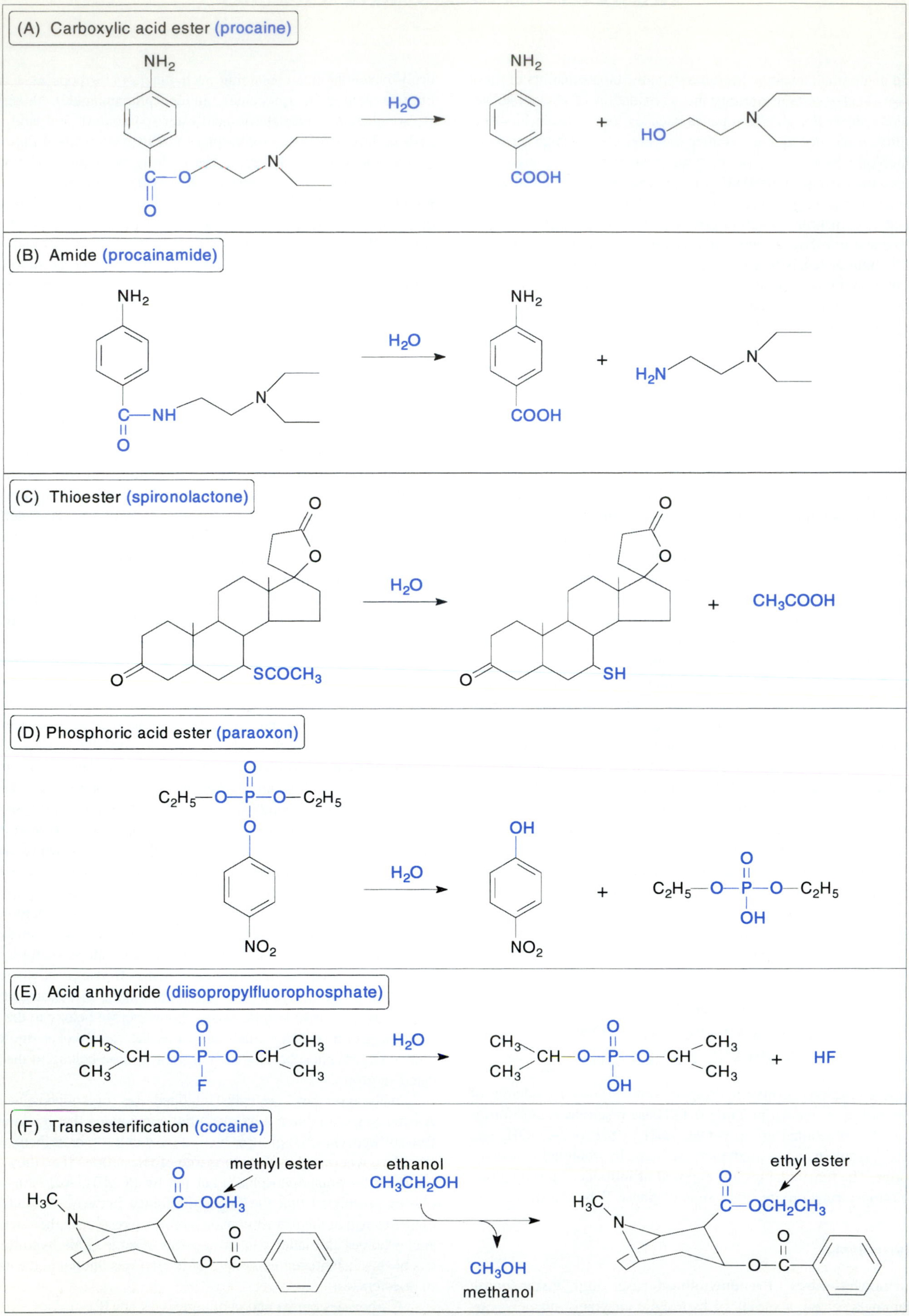

(A) Carboxylic acid ester (procaine)

H_2O

(B) Amide (procainamide)

H_2O

(C) Thioester (spironolactone)

H_2O

$SCOCH_3$ → SH + CH_3COOH

(D) Phosphoric acid ester (paraoxon)

H_2O

(E) Acid anhydride (diisopropylfluorophosphate)

H_2O

+ HF

(F) Transesterification (cocaine)

methyl ester

ethanol

CH_3CH_2OH

CH_3OH

methanol

ethyl ester

Figure 6-2. Examples of reactions catalyzed by carboxylesterases, cholinesterases and organophosphatases.

B-esterases is analogous to the mechanism of catalysis by serine-proteases. In the case of carboxylesterases, for example, it involves charge relay among a catalytic triad comprised of an acidic amino acid residue [glutamate (Glu_{335})], a basic residue [histidine (His_{448})], and a nucleophilic residue [serine (Ser_{203})] (Yan et al., 1994; Satoh and Hosokawa, 1998). Organophosphates bind to the nucleophilic OH-group on the active site serine residue to form a phosphorus-oxygen bond, which is not readily cleaved by water. Therefore, organophosphates bind stoichiometrically to B-esterases and inhibit their enzymatic activity. The mechanism of catalysis of carboxylesterases is discussed in more detail under "Epoxide Hydrolase," below.

Based on the observation that A-esterases are inhibited by PCMB but not by organophosphates, Augustinsson (1966) postulated that organophosphates bind to a nucleophilic SH-group on an active site cysteine residue and form a phosphorus-sulfur bond, which is readily cleaved by water. A strong argument against this postulate is the fact that, when the only potential active site cysteine residue in human paraoxonase (Cys_{283}) is substituted with serine or alanine, there is no loss of catalytic activity (Sorenson et al., 1995). Paraoxonase requires Ca^{2+}, both for stability and catalytic activity, which raises the possibility that the hydrolysis of organophosphates by paraoxonase involves metal-catalyzed hydrolysis, analogous to that proposed for calcium-dependent phospholipase A_2 or zinc-dependent phosphotriesterase activity (Sorenson et al., 1995).

Esterases play an important role in limiting the toxicity of organophosphates. The mechanism of toxicity of organophosphorus pesticides (and carbamate insecticides) involves inhibition of brain acetylcholinesterase, which is a serine-containing esterase that terminates the action of the neurotransmitter, acetylcholine. The symptoms of organophosphate toxicity resemble those caused by excessive stimulation of cholinergic nerves. The covalent interaction between organophosphates and brain acetylcholinesterase is analogous to their binding to the active site serine residue in all B-esterases. As previously mentioned, organophosphates are hydrolyzed by some esterases (the A-esterases, such as paraoxonase) and bind stoichiometrically and, for the most part, irreversibly to carboxylesterases and cholinesterases. Both types of interactions (i.e., hydrolysis and covalent binding) play an important role in the detoxication of these compounds. Numerous studies have shown an inverse relationship between esterase activity and susceptibility to the toxic effect of organophosphates. Factors that decrease esterase activity potentiate the toxic effects of organophosphates, whereas factors that increase carboxylesterase activity have a protective effect. For example, the susceptibility of animals to the toxicity of parathion, malathion, and diisopropylfluorophosphate is inversely related to the level of serum esterase activity. Differences in the susceptibility of several mammalian species to organophosphate toxicity can be abolished by pretreatment with selective esterase inhibitors such as cresylbenzodioxaphosphorin oxide, the active metabolite of tri-*ortho*-tolylphosphate (which is also known as tri-*ortho*-cresylphosphate or TOCP). Esterases are not the only enzymes involved in the detoxication of organophosphorus pesticides. Certain organophosphorus compounds are detoxified by cytochrome P450, flavin monooxygenases, and glutathione *S*-transferases.

Pseudocholinesterase is a tetrameric glycoprotein (Mr 342 kDa) containing four identical subunits, each having one catalytic site. The enzyme hydrolyzes succinylcholine, mivacurium, procaine, chlorpropaine, tetracaine, cocaine, heroin and other drugs. The duration of action of the muscle relaxant succinylcholine is determined by serum pseudocholinesterase. In some individuals (~2 percent of Caucasians), succinylcholine causes prolonged muscular relaxation and apnea, which led to the discovery of an atypical form of pseudocholinesterase ($Asp_{70} \rightarrow Gly_{70}$) (La Du, 1992; Lockridge, 1992). Although this atypical enzyme has markedly diminished activity toward succinylcholine (which is the genetic basis for the exaggerated response to this muscle relaxant in affected individuals), it nevertheless has appreciable activity toward other substrates, such as acetylcholine and benzoylcholine. The normal and atypical pseudocholinesterases are equally sensitive to the inhibitory effect of certain organophosphates, but the atypical enzyme is relatively resistant to the inhibitory effect of dibucaine, a local anesthetic, which forms the basis of a diagnostic test for atypical pseudocholinesterase. The discovery of atypical pseudocholinesterase is of historical interest because it ushered in the new field of pharmacogenetics. Since the initial discovery of atypical pseudocholinesterase in late 1950s, several allelic variants of the enzyme have been identified.

Carboxylesterases are ~60-kDa glycoproteins that are present in a wide variety of tissues, including serum. Most of the carboxylesterase activity in liver is associated with the endoplasmic reticulum, although considerable carboxylesterase activity is present in lysosomes and cytosol. Carboxylesterases generate pharmacologically active metabolites from several ester or amide prodrugs. For example, lovastatin is converted by liver carboxylesterases to the pharmacologically active metabolite, lovastatin β-hydroxyacid, which inhibits HMG-CoA reductase and lowers plasma cholesterol levels. There is some evidence to suggest that therapeutic effect of lovastatin is diminished in individuals with low levels of liver carboxylesterase activity (Tang and Kalow, 1995). Carboxylesterases have also been implicated in the activation of a number of anticancer agents, such as 7-ethyl-10-[4-(1-piperidino)-1-piperidino] carbonyoxycamptothecin (CPT-11), which shows promising activity against a broad range of tumor types, including colorectal and cervical cancer. The anticancer effects of CPT-11 are dependent on its conversion to ethyl camptothecin, which is catalyzed by one or more carboxylesterases. As a result of their ability to hydrolyze prodrugs, carboxylesterases may have clinical applications in the treatment of certain cancers. They might be used, for example, to activate prodrugs in vivo and thereby generate potent anticancer agents in highly selected target sites (e.g., at the surface of tumor cells, or inside the tumor cells themselves). Carboxylesterases might be targeted to tumor sites with hybrid monoclonal antibodies (i.e., bifunctional antibodies that recognize the carboxylesterase and the tumor cell), or the cDNA encoding a carboxylesterase might be targeted to the tumor cells via a viral vector. In the case of CTP-11, this therapeutic strategy would release the anticancer drug, ethyl camptothecin, in the vicinity of the tumor cells, which would reduce the systemic levels and side effects of this otherwise highly toxic drug (Senter et al., 1996).

In addition to xenobiotics, carboxylesterases hydrolyze numerous endogenous compounds, such as palmitoyl-CoA, monoacylglycerol, diacylglycerol, retinyl ester, platelet-activating factor and other esterified lipids. Carboxylesterases can also catalyze the synthesis of fatty acid ethyl esters, which represents a nonoxidative pathway of ethanol metabolism in adipose and certain other tissues. In the case of platelet-activating factor, carboxylesterases catalyze both the deacetylation of PAF and its subsequent esterification with fatty acids to form phosphatidylcholine (Hosokawa and Satoh, 1998).

Certain carboxylesterases also have a physiologic function in anchoring other proteins to the endoplasmic reticulum. For example, the lysosomal enzyme β-glucuronidase is also present in the endoplasmic reticulum, where it is anchored in the lumen by egasyn, a microsomal carboxylesterase. Egasyn binds to β-glucuronidase via its active site serine residue, which effectively abolishes the carboxylesterase activity of egasyn, although there is no corresponding loss of β-glucuronidase activity. The retention of β-glucuronidase in the lumen of the ER is thought to be physiologically significant. Glucuronidation by microsomal UDP-glucuronosyltransferases is a major pathway in the clearance of many endogenous aglycones (such as bilirubin) and xenobiotics (such as drugs). However, hydrolysis of glucuronides by β-glucuronidase complexed with egasyn in the lumen of the endoplasmic reticulum appears to be an important mechanism for recycling endogenous compounds, such as steroid hormones (Dwivedi et al., 1987). The acute-phase response protein, C-response protein, is similarly anchored in the endoplasmic reticulum by egasyn.

A nomenclature system for classifying carboxylesterases has been proposed by Satoh and Hosokawa (1998). The broad substrate specificity of these enzymes precludes the possibility of naming them for the reactions they catalyze, for which reason Satoh and Hosokawa proposed a classification and nomenclature system that is based on a comparison of the amino acid sequences of carboxylesterases (regardless of the species of origin) with the sequence of a human carboxylesterase. Four gene families have been identified (designated CES 1-4) with three subdivisions in the first gene family (namely CES 1A, CES 1B and CES 1C). The first subfamily is further subdivided into three groups (designated CES 1A1, 1A2, and 1A3). Liver microsomes from all mammalian species, including humans, contain at least one carboxylesterase, but the exact number of carboxylesterases expressed in any one tissue or species is not known. Because carboxylesterases are glycoproteins, variations in carbohydrate content can give rise to multiple forms of the same enzyme. Consequently, the large number of carboxylesterases that have been identified by isoelectric focusing and nondenaturing gel electrophoresis probably overestimates the number of genes encoding these enzymes.

Metabolism of xenobiotics by carboxylesterases is not always a detoxication process. Figure 6-3 shows some examples in which carboxylesterases convert xenobiotics to toxic and tumorigenic metabolites.

Peptidases With the advent of recombinant DNA techology, numerous human peptides have been mass-produced for use as drugs, and several recombinant peptide hormones, growth factors, cytokines, soluble receptors, and humanized monoclonal antibodies currently are used therapeutically. To avoid acid-precipitation and proteolytic degradation in the gastrointestinal tract, peptides are administered parenterally. Nevertheless, peptides are hydrolyzed in the blood and tissues by a variety of peptidases, including aminopeptidases and carboxypeptidases, which hydrolyze amino acids at the *N*- and *C*-terminus, respectively, and endopeptidases, which cleave peptides at specific internal sites (trypsin, for example, cleaves peptides on the *C*-terminal side of arginine or lysine residues) (Humphrey and Ringrose, 1986). Peptidases cleave the amide linkage between adjacent amino acids, hence, they function as amidases. As in the case of carboxylesterases, the active site of peptidases contains either a serine or cysteine residue, which initiates a nucleophilic attack on the carbonyl moiety of the amide

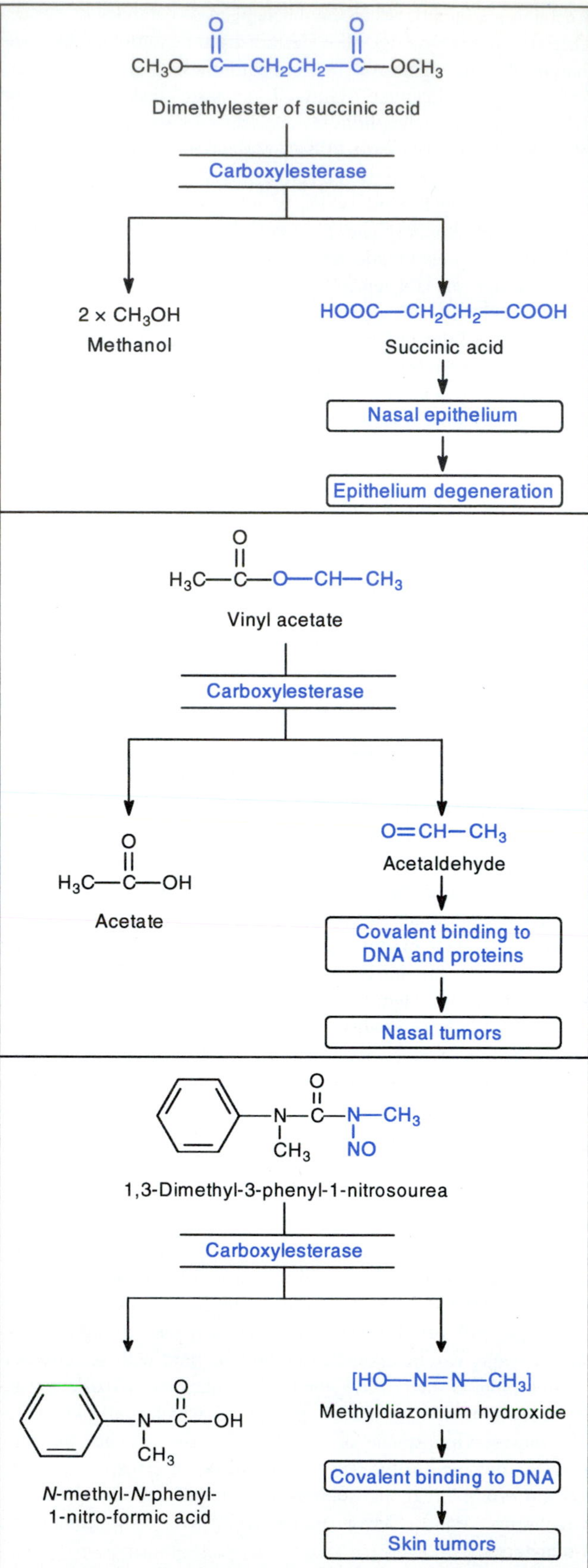

Figure 6-3. Activation of xenobiotics to toxic and tumorigenic metabolites by carboxylesterases.

bond. As previously noted, the mechanism of catalysis by serine proteases, such as chymotrypsin, is similar to that by serine esterases (B-esterases).

Epoxide Hydrolase Epoxide hydrolase catalyzes the *trans*-addition of water to alkene epoxides and arene oxides (oxiranes), which can form during the cytochrome P450-dependent oxidation of aliphatic alkenes and aromatic hydrocarbons, respectively. As shown in Fig. 6-4, the products of this hydrolysis are vicinal diols with a *trans*-configuration (i.e., *trans*-1,2-dihydrodiols); a notable exception being the conversion of leukotriene A_4 (LTA4) to leukotriene B_4 (LTB4), in which case the two hydroxyl groups that result from epoxide hydrolysis appear on nonadjacent carbon atoms. Although the levels vary from one tissue to the next, epoxide hydrolase is present in virtually all tissues, including the liver, testis, ovary, lung, kidney, skin, intestine, colon, spleen, thymus, brain, and heart.

There are five distinct forms of epoxide hydrolase in mammals: microsomal epoxide hydrolase (mEH), soluble epoxide hydrolase (sEH), cholesterol epoxide hydrolase, LTA4 hydrolase, and hepoxilin hydrolase (Beetham et al., 1995). As their names imply, the latter three enzymes appear to hydrolyze endogenous epoxides exclusively and have virtually no capacity to detoxify xenobiotic oxides. LTA4 hydrolase is distinct from the other epoxide hydrolases because it is a bifunctional zinc metalloenzyme that has both epoxide hydrolase and peptidase activity and because the two hydroxyl groups introduced during the conversion of LTA4 to LTB4 are eight carbon atoms apart.

In contrast to the high degree of substrate specificity displayed by the cholesterol, LTA4 and hepoxilin epoxide hydrolases, the microsomal and soluble epoxide hydrolases (mEH and sEH) hydrolyze a wide variety of alkene epoxides and arene oxides. Many epoxides and oxides are intermediary metabolites formed during the cytochrome P450-dependent oxidation of unsaturated aliphatic and aromatic xenobiotics. These electrophilic metabolites might otherwise bind to proteins and nucleic acids and cause cellular toxicity and genetic mutations. Generally, these two forms of epoxide hydrolases and cytochrome P450 enzymes have a similar cellular localization. For example, the distribution of epoxide hydrolase parallels that of cytochrome P450 in liver, lung, and testis. In other words, both enzymes are located in the centrilobular region of the liver (zone 3), in Clara and type II cells in the lung, and in Leydig cells in the testis. The colocalization of epoxide hydrolase and cytochrome P450 presumably ensures the rapid detoxication of alkene epoxides and arene oxides generated during the oxidation metabolism of xenobiotics.

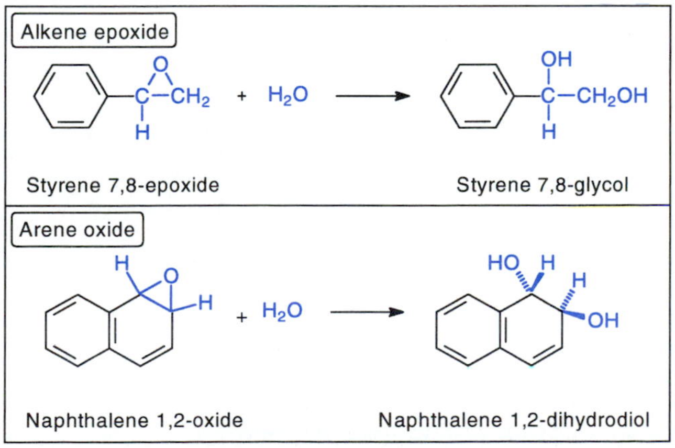

Figure 6-4. Examples of the hydrolyation of an alkene epoxide **(top)** *and an arene oxide* **(bottom)** *by epoxide hydrolase.*

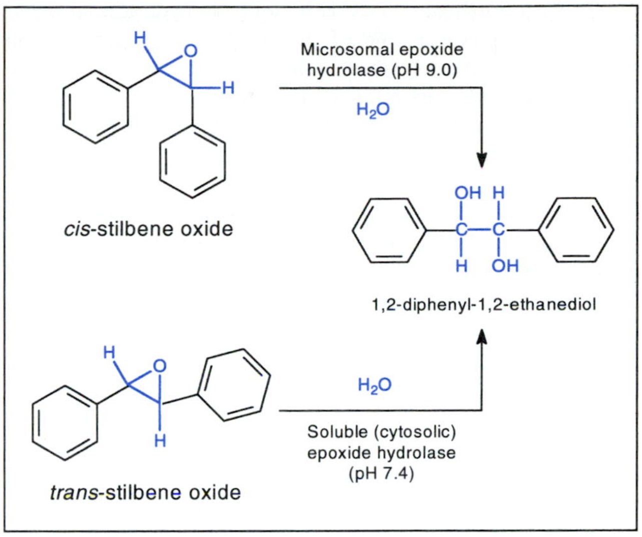

Figure 6-5. Stereoselective hydrolyation of stilbene oxide by microsomal and soluble epoxide hydrolase.

The microsomal and soluble forms of epoxide hydrolase show no evident sequence identity and, not surprisingly, are immunochemically distinct proteins (Beetham et al., 1995). Although both enzymes hydrolyze a broad spectrum of compounds, they exhibit different substrate specificities. For example, mEH rapidly hydrolyzes epoxides on cyclic systems, whereas sEH has little activity toward these compounds. In rat and mouse, these two enzymes can even be distinguished by their stereoselective hydration of stilbene-oxide; mEH preferentially hydrolyzes the *cis*-isomer at pH 9.0, whereas sEH preferentially hydrolyzes the *trans*-isomer at pH 7.4, as shown in Fig. 6-5.

Electrophilic epoxides and arene oxides are constantly produced during the cytochrome P450-dependent oxidation of unsaturated aliphatic and aromatic xenobiotics and are highly reactive to cellular macromolecules such as DNA and protein. Epoxide hydrolases, particularly mEH and sEH, can rapidly convert these potentially toxic metabolites to the corresponding dihydrodiols, which are less reactive and easier to excrete. Thus, epoxide hydrolases are widely considered as a group of detoxication enzymes. In some cases, however, further oxidation of a dihydrodiol can lead to the formation of diol epoxide derivatives that are no longer substrates for epoxide hydrolase because the oxirane ring is protected by bulky substituents that sterically hinder interaction with the enzyme. This point proved to be extremely important in elucidating the mechanism by which polycyclic aromatic hydrocarbons cause tumors in laboratory animals (Conney, 1982). Tumorigenic polycyclic aromatic hydrocarbons, such as benzo[a]pyrene, are converted by cytochrome P450 to a variety of arene oxides that bind covalently to DNA, making them highly mutagenic to bacteria. One of the major arene oxides formed from benzo[a]pyrene, namely the 4,5-oxide, is highly mutagenic to bacteria but weakly mutagenic to mammalian cells. This discrepancy reflects the rapid inactivation of benzo[a]pyrene 4,5-oxide by epoxide hydrolase in mammalian cells. However, one of the arene oxides formed from benzo[a]pyrene, namely benzo[a]pyrene 7,8-dihydrodiol-9,10-oxide, is not a substrate for epoxide hydrolase and is highly mutagenic to mammalian cells and considerably more potent than benzo[a]pyrene as a lung tumorigen in mice.

Benzo[a]pyrene 7,8-dihydrodiol-9,10-oxide is known as a bay-region diolepoxide, and analogous bay-region diolepoxides are now recognized as tumorigenic metabolites of numerous polycyclic aromatic hydrocarbons. A feature common to all bay-region epoxides is their resistance to hydrolyation by epoxide hydrolase, which results from steric hindrance from the nearby dihydrodiol group. As shown in Fig. 6-6, benzo[a]pyrene 7,8-dihydrodiol-9,10-oxide is formed in three steps: Benzo[a]pyrene is converted to the 7,8-oxide, which is converted to the 7,8-dihydrodiol, which is converted to the corresponding 9,10-epoxide. The first and third steps are epoxidation reactions catalyzed by cytochrome P450 or prostaglandin H synthase, but the second step is catalyzed by epoxide hydrolase. Consequently, even though epoxide hydrolase plays a major role in detoxifying several benzo[a]pyrene oxides, such as the 4,5-oxide, it nevertheless plays a role in converting benzo[a]pyrene to its ultimate tumorigenic metabolite, benzo[a]pyrene 7,8-dihydrodiol-9,10-oxide.

Not all epoxides are highly reactive and toxic to the cells that produce them. The major metabolite of carbamazepine is an epoxide, which is so stable that carbamazepine-10,11-epoxide is a major circulating metabolite in patients treated with this antiepileptic drug. (Carbamazepine is converted to a second epoxide, which is less stable and more cytotoxic, as shown under "Cytochrome P450," below.) Vitamin K epoxide is also a nontoxic epoxide, which is formed and consumed during the vitamin K–dependent γ-carboxylation of prothrombin and other clotting factors in the liver. Vitamin K epoxide is not hydrated by epoxide hydrolase but is reduced by vitamin K epoxide reductase. This enzyme is inhibited by warfarin and related coumarin anticoagulants, which interrupt the synthesis of several clotting factors.

Epoxide hydrolase is one of several inducible enzymes in liver microsomes. Induction of epoxide hydrolase is invariably associated with the induction of cytochrome P450, and several cytochrome P450 inducers, such as phenobarbital and *trans*-stilbene oxide, increase the levels of microsomal epoxide hydrolase by up to threefold. In mice, the levels of epoxide hydrolase in liver microsomes can be increased by almost an order of magnitude by antioxidants such as butylated hydroxytoluene (BHT), butylated hydroxyanisole (BHA), and ethoxyquin. Epoxide hydrolase is one of several preneoplastic antigens that are overexpressed in chemically induced foci and nodules that eventually develop into liver tumors. Several alcohols, ketones, and imidazoles stimulate microsomal epoxide hydrolase activity in vitro. Epoxide hydrolase cannot be inhibited by antibodies raised against the purified enzyme, but it

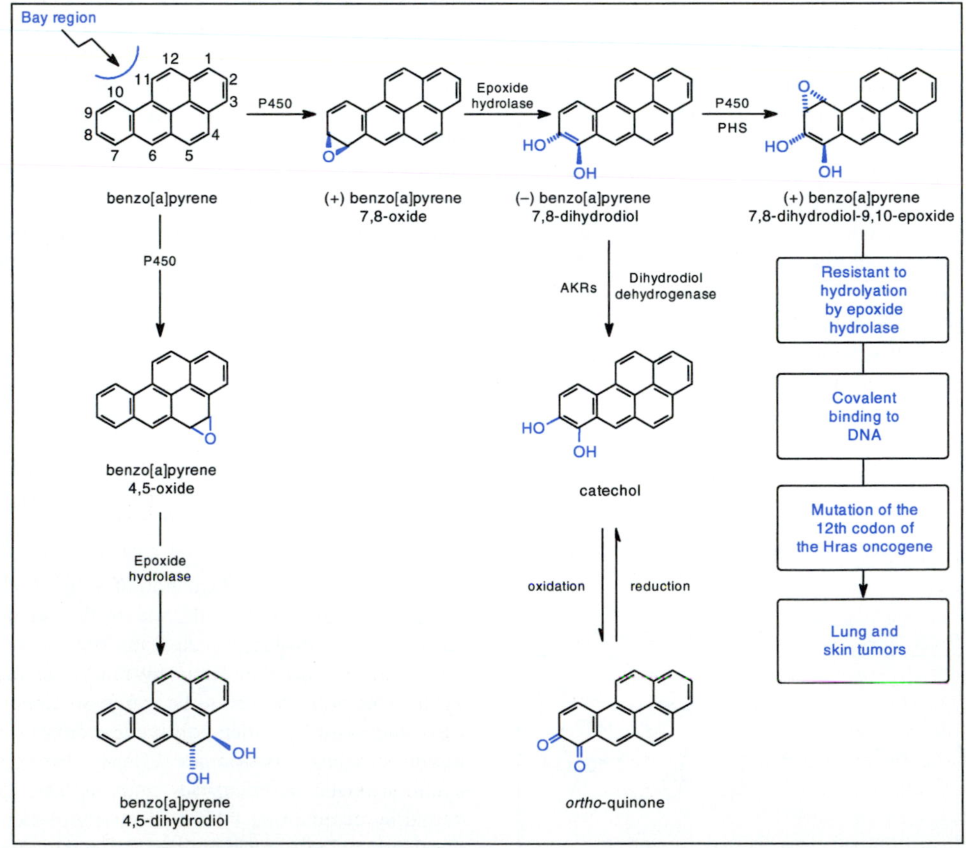

Figure 6-6. Role of epoxide hydrolase in the inactivation of benzo[a]pyrene 4,5-oxide and in the conversion of benzo[a]pyrene to its tumorigenic bay-region diolepoxide.

Also shown is the role of dihydrodiol dehydrogenase, a member of the aldoketo reductase (AKR) superfamily, in the formation of reactive catechol and *ortho*-quinone metabolites of benzo[a]pyrene.

can be inhibited by certain epoxides, such as 1,1,1-trichloropropene oxide and cyclohexene oxide, and certain drugs, such as valpromide (the amide analog of valproic acid) and progabide, a γ-aminobutyric acid (GABA) agonist. These latter two drugs potentiate the neurotoxicity of carbamazepine by inhibiting epoxide hydrolase, leading to increased plasma levels of carbamazepine 10,11-epoxide and presumably the more toxic 2,3-epoxide (Kroetz et al., 1993). Several genetic polymorphisms have been identified in the coding region and the 5′ region (i.e., the regulatory region) of the gene encoding human mEH (Daly, 1999). Two variants involve substitutions at amino acid 113 (Tyr→His) or amino acid 139 (His→Arg), which are encoded by exons 3 and 4, respectively. Although these allelic variant forms of mEH have near normal enzymatic activity (at least 65 percent of normal), they appear to be less stable than the wild-type enzyme. The possibility that these amino acid substitutions might predispose individuals to the adverse effects of antiepileptic drugs has been examined, but no such association was found (Daly, 1999).

The mechanism of catalysis by epoxide hydrolase is similar to that of carboxylesterase, in that the catalytic site comprises three amino acid residues that form a catalytic triad. In mEH, Asp_{226} functions as the nucleophile, His_{431} the base, and both Glu_{376} and Glu_{404} as the acid, as shown in Fig. 6-7. (In sEH, the corresponding residues are Asp_{333}, His_{503}, and Asp_{495}.) The attack of the nucleophile Asp_{226} on the carbon of the oxirane ring initiates enzymatic activity, leading to the formation of an α-hydroxyester-enzyme intermediate, with the negative charge developing on the oxygen atom stabilized by a putative oxyanion hole. The His_{431} residue (which is activated by Glu_{376} and Glu_{404}) activates a water molecule by abstracting a proton (H^+). The activated (nucleophilic) water then attacks the $C\gamma$ atom of Asp_{226}, resulting in the hydrolysis of the ester bond in the acyl-enzyme intermediate, which restores the active enzyme and results in formation of a vicinal diol with a *trans*-configuration (Armstrong, 1999). The second step, namely cleavage of the ester bond in the acyl-enzyme intermediate, resembles the cleavage of the ester or amide bond in substrates for serine esterases and proteases.

Although epoxide hydrolase and carboxylesterase both have a catalytic triad comprising a nucleophilic, basic, and acidic amino acid residue, there are striking differences in their catalytic machinery, which accounts for the fact that carboxylesterases primarily hydrolyze esters and amides whereas epoxide hydrolases primarily hydrolyze epoxides and oxides. In the triad, both enzymes have histidine as the base and either glutamate or aspartate as the acid, but they differ in the type of amino acids for the nucleophile. Even during catalysis, there is a major difference. In carboxylesterases, the same carbonyl carbon atom of the substrate is attacked initially by the nucleophile Ser_{203} to form α-hydroxyester-enzyme ester that is subsequently attacked by the activated water to release the alcohol product. In contrast, two different atoms in epoxide hydrolase are targets of nucleophilic attacks. First the less hindered carbon atom of the oxirane ring is attacked by the nucleophile Asp_{226} to form a covalently bound ester, and next this ester is hydrolyzed by an activated water that attacks the $C\gamma$ atom of the Asp_{226} residue, as illustrated in Fig. 6-7. Therefore, in carboxylesterase, the oxygen introduced into the product is derived from the activated water molecule. In contrast, in epoxide hydrolase, the oxygen introduced into the product is derived from the nucleophile Asp_{226} (Fig. 6-7).

Carboxylesterases and epoxide hydrolases exhibit no primary sequence identity, but they share surprising similarities in the topology of the structure and sequential arrangement of the catalytic triad. Both are members of the α/β-hydrolase fold enzymes, a superfamily of proteins that includes lipases, esterases and haloalkane dehydrogenases (Beetham et al., 1995; Armstrong, 1999). Functionally, proteins in this superfamily all catalyze hydrolytic reactions; structurally, they all contain a similar core segment that comprises eight β-sheets connected by α-helices. They all have a catalytic triad, and the arrangement of the amino acid residues in the triad (i.e., the order of the nucleophile, the acid and the base in the primary sequence) is the mirror image of the arrangement in other hydrolytic enzymes such as trypsin. All three active-site

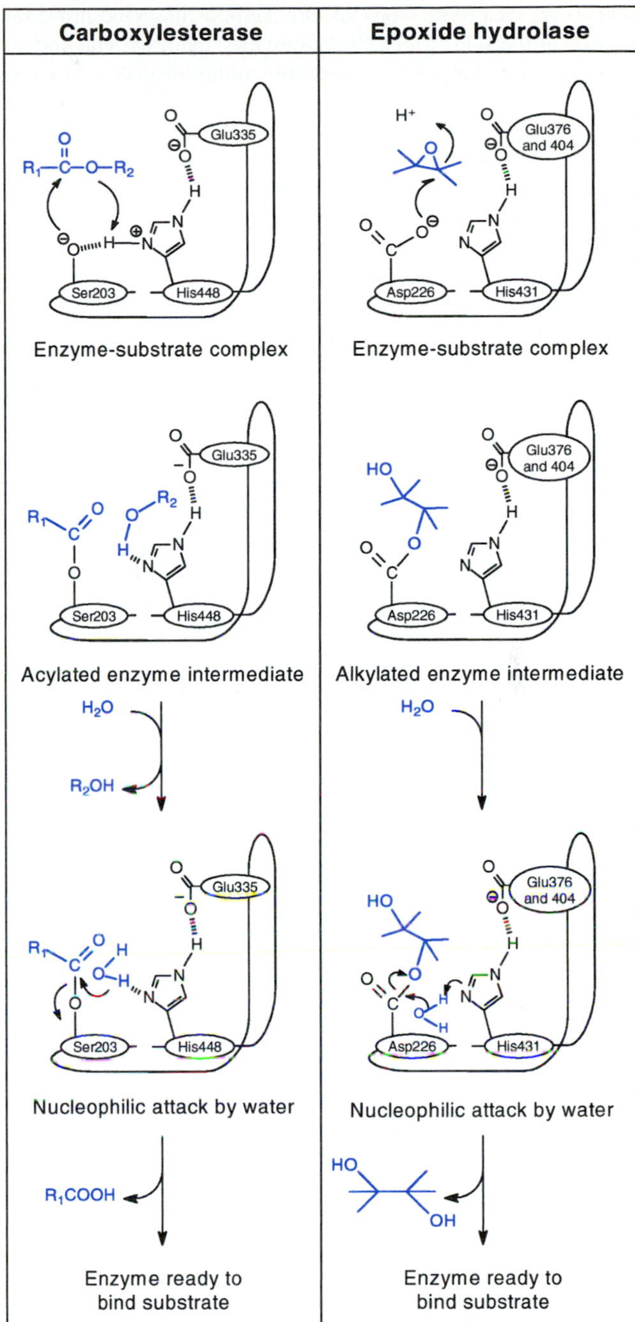

Figure 6-7. Catalytic cycle of microsomal carboxylesterase (left) *and microsomal epoxide hydrolase* (right), *two α/β-hydrolase fold enzymes.*

residues are located on loops that are the best conserved structural features in the fold, which likely provides catalysis with certain flexibility to hydrolyze numerous structurally distinct substrates.

Reduction

Certain metals (e.g., pentavalent arsenic) and xenobiotics containing an aldehyde, ketone, disulfide, sulfoxide, quinone, *N*-oxide, alkene, azo, or nitro group are often reduced in vivo, although it is sometimes difficult to ascertain whether the reaction proceeds enzymatically or nonenzymatically by interaction with reducing agents [such as the reduced forms of glutathione, FAD, FMN and NAD(P)]. Some of these functional groups can be either reduced or oxidized. For example, aldehydes (RCHO) can be reduced to an alcohol (RCH_2OH) or oxidized to a carboxylic acid (RCOOH), whereas sulfoxides (R_1SOR_2) can be reduced to a sulfide (R_1SR_2) or oxidized to a sulfone ($R_1SO_2R_2$). In the case of halogenated hydrocarbons, such as halothane, dehalogenation can proceed by an oxidative or reductive pathway, both of which are catalyzed by the same enzyme (namely cytochrome P450). In some cases, such as azo-reduction, nitro-reduction, and the reduction of some alkenes (e.g., cinnamic acid, $C_6H_5CH{=}CHCOOH$), the reaction is largely catalyzed by intestinal microflora. Many of the reduction reactions described below (including azo-, nitro-, sulfoxide, and *N*-oxide reduction) can be catalyzed by aldehyde oxidase, but this does not appear to be the major enzyme responsible for any of the various reductive pathways of xenobiotic biotransformation.

Azo- and Nitro-Reduction Prontosil and chloramphenicol are examples of drugs that undergo azo- and nitro-reduction, respectively, as shown in Fig. 6-8 (Herwick, 1980). Reduction of prontosil is of historical interest. Treatment of streptococcal and pneumococcal infections with prontosil marked the beginning of specific antibacterial chemotherapy. Subsequently, it was discovered that the active drug was not prontosil but its metabolite, sulfanilamide (*para*-aminobenzene sulfonamide), a product of azo-reduction. During azo-reduction, the nitrogen–nitrogen double bond is sequentially reduced and cleaved to produce two primary amines, a reaction requiring four reducing equivalents. Nitro-reduction requires six reducing equivalents, which are consumed in three sequential reactions, as shown in Fig. 6-8 for the conversion of nitrobenzene to aniline.

Azo- and nitro-reduction are catalyzed by intestinal microflora and by two liver enzymes: cytochrome P450 and NAD(P)H-quinone oxidoreductase (a cytosolic flavoprotein, also known as DT-diaphorase). Under certain circumstances, a third liver enzyme, aldehyde oxidase, may also catalyze azo- and nitro-reduction reactions. The reactions require NAD(P)H and are inhibited by oxygen. The anaerobic environment of the lower gastrointestinal tract is well suited for azo- and nitro-reduction, which is why intestinal microflora contribute significantly to these reactions. Most of the reactions catalyzed by cytochrome P450 involve oxidation of xenobiotics. Azo- and nitro-reduction are examples in which, under conditions of low oxygen tension, cytochrome P450 can catalyze the reduction of xenobiotics.

Nitro-reduction by intestinal microflora is thought to play an important role in the toxicity of several nitroaromatic compounds, including 2,6-dinitrotoluene, which is hepatotumorigenic to male rats. The role of nitro-reduction in the metabolic activation of 2,6-dinitrotoluene is shown in Fig. 6-9 (Long and Rickert, 1982; Mirsalis and Butterworth, 1982). The biotransformation of 2,6-dinitrotoluene begins in the liver, where it is oxidized by cytochrome P450 and conjugated with glucuronic acid. This glucuronide is excreted in bile and undergoes biotransformation by intestinal microflora. One or more of the nitro groups are reduced to amines by nitroreductase, and the glucuronide is hydrolyzed by *β*-glucuronidase. The deconjugated metabolites are absorbed and transported to the liver, where the newly formed amine group is *N*-hydroxylated by cytochrome P450 and conjugated with acetate or sulfate. These conjugates form good leaving groups, which ren-

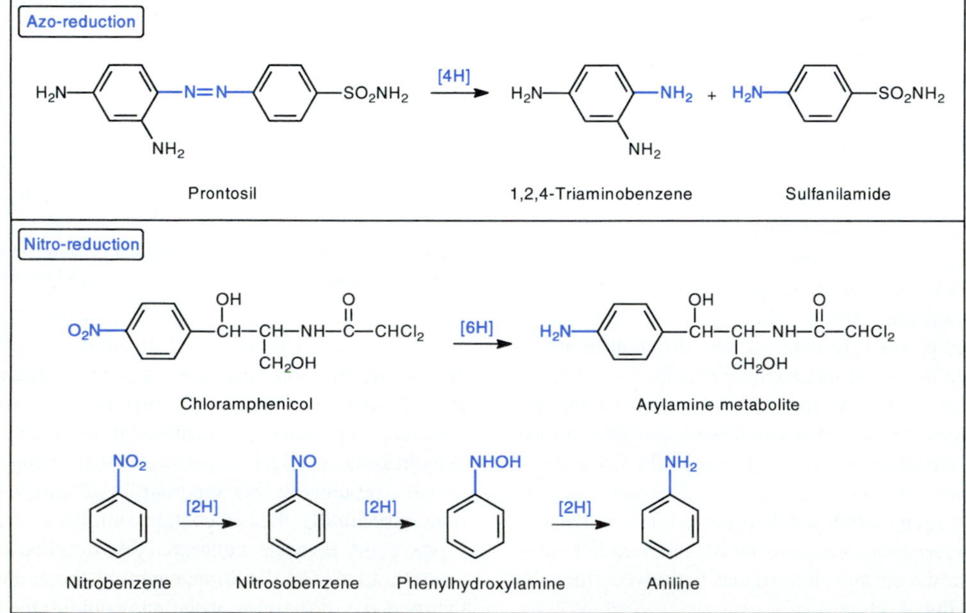

Figure 6-8. Examples of drugs that undergo azo reduction (prontosil) and nitro reduction (chloramphenicol and nitrobenzene).

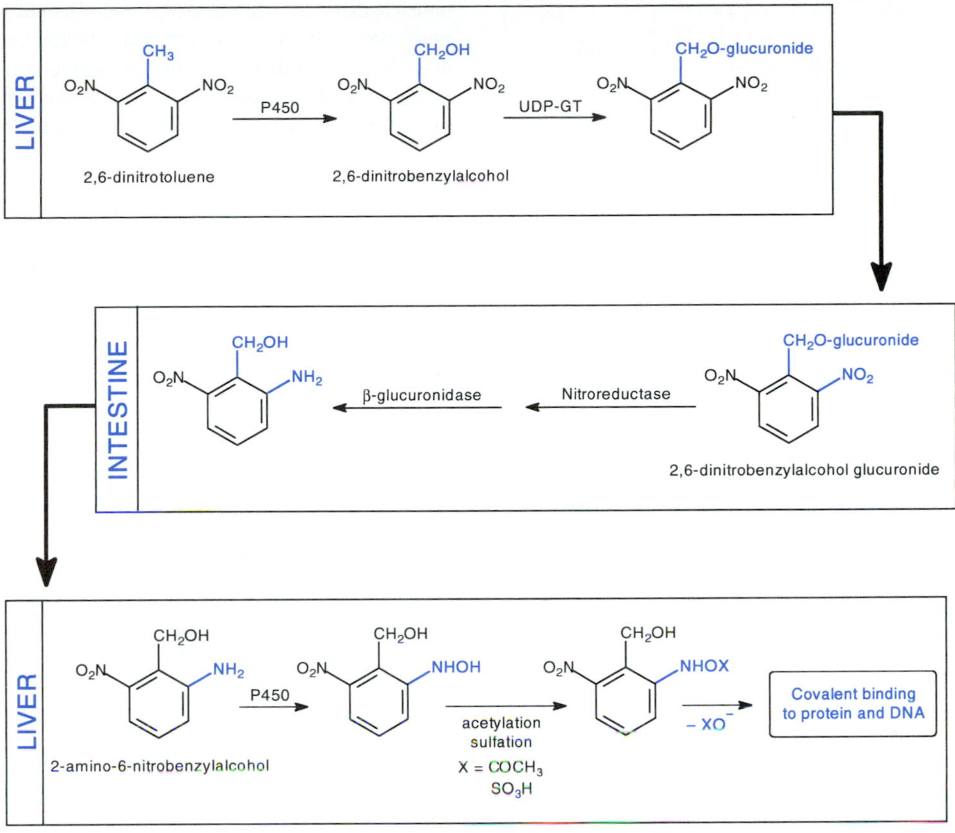

Figure 6-9. Role of nitro reduction by intestinal microflora in the activation of the rat liver tumorigen, 2,6-dinitrotoluene.

der the nitrogen highly susceptible to nucleophilic attack from proteins and DNA; this ostensibly leads to mutations and the formation of liver tumors. The complexity of the metabolic scheme shown in Fig. 6-9 underscores an important principle, namely that the activation of some chemical tumorigens to DNA-reactive metabolites involves several different biotransforming enzymes and may take place in more than one tissue. Consequently, the ability of 2,6-dinitrotoluene to bind to DNA and cause mutations is not revealed in most of the short-term assays for assessing the genotoxic potential of chemical agents. These in vitro assays for genotoxicity do not make allowance for biotransformation by intestinal microflora or, in some cases, the phase II (conjugating) enzymes.

Nitro-reduction by intestinal microflora also plays an important role in the biotransformation of musk xylene (1,3,5-trinitro-2-*t*butyl-4,6-dimethylbenzene). Reduction of one or both of the nitro groups is required for musk xylene to induce (as well as markedly inhibit) liver microsomal cytochrome P450 (namely CYP2B) in rodents (Lehman-McKeeman et al., 1999).

Carbonyl Reduction The reduction of certain aldehydes to primary alcohols and of ketones to secondary alcohols is catalyzed by alcohol dehydrogenase and by a family of carbonyl reductases (Weiner and Flynn, 1989). Carbonyl reductases are monomeric, NADPH-dependent enzymes present in blood and the cytosolic fraction of the liver, kidney, brain, and other tissues. The major circulating metabolite of the antipsychotic drug haloperidol is a secondary alcohol formed by carbonyl reductases in the blood and liver, as shown in Fig. 6-10 (Inaba and Kovacs, 1989). Other xenobiotics that are reduced by carbonyl reductases include pentoxifylline (see Fig. 6-1), acetohexamide, daunorubicin, ethacrynic acid, warfarin, menadione, and 4-nitroacetophenone. The reduction of ketones to secondary alcohols by carbonyl reductases may proceed with a high degree of stereoselectivity, as in the case of pentoxifylline (Fig. 6-1) (Lillibridge et al., 1996). Prostaglandins are possibly physiologic substrates for carbonyl reductases, and they most certainly are substrates for a class of related enzymes known as prostaglandin dehydrogenases (discussed later in this section).

In liver, carbonyl reductase activity is present mainly in the cytosolic fraction, but a different carbonyl reductase is present in the microsomal fraction. These enzymes differ in the degree to which they stereoselectively reduce ketones to secondary alcohols. For example, keto-reduction of pentoxifylline produces two enantiomeric secondary alcohols: one with the *R*-configuration (which is known as lisofylline) and one with the *S*-configuration, as shown in Fig. 6-1. Reduction of pentoxifylline by cytosolic carbonyl reductase results in the stereospecific formation (>95 percent) of the optical antipode of lisofylline, whereas the same reaction catalyzed by microsomal carbonyl reductase produces both lisofylline and its optical antipode in a ratio of about 1 to 5 (Lillibridge et al., 1996).

In rat liver cytosol, the reduction of quinones is primarily catalyzed by DT-diaphorase (see "Quinone Reduction," below), whereas in human liver cytosol, quinone reduction is catalyzed by both DT-diaphorase and carbonyl reductases. Human liver cytosol appears to contain more than one carbonyl reductase. The activity of low- and high-affinity carbonyl reductase activity in human liver cytosol varies about tenfold among individuals (Wong et al., 1993).

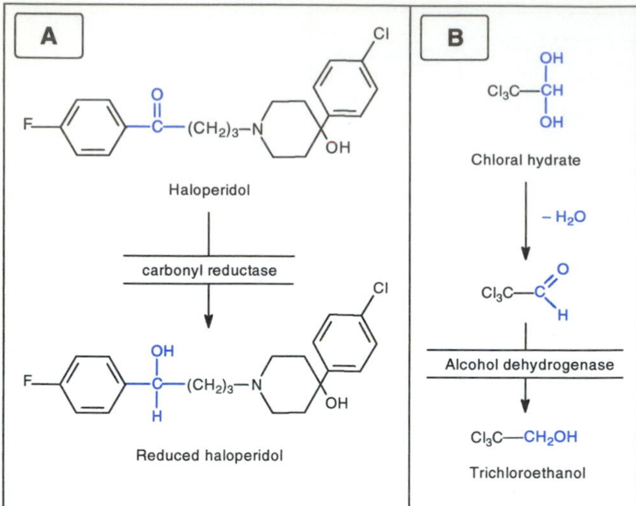

Figure 6-10. Reduction of xenobiotics by carbonyl reductase (A) *and alcohol dehydrogenase* (B).

The number of carbonyl reductases involved in xenobiotic biotransformation is difficult to assess.

Structurally, carbonyl reductases belong to the short-chain dehydrogenase/reductase (SDR) superfamily (which includes certain hydroxysteroid dehydrogenases and prostaglandin dehydrogenases), although certain aldehyde reductases belong to the aldo-keto reductase (AKR) superfamily (which include other hydroxysteroid dehydrogenases and aldose reductases) (Penning, 1997). This latter superfamily of enzymes includes several forms of dihydrodiol dehydrogenase, which are monomeric (~34 kDa), cytosolic NADP(H)-requiring oxidoreductases that oxidize the *trans*-dihydrodiols of various polycyclic aromatic hydrocarbons to the corresponding *ortho*-quinones, which is depicted in Fig. 6-6 (Burczynski and Penning, 2000).

In certain cases, the reduction of aldehydes to alcohols can be catalyzed by alcohol dehydrogenase, as shown in Fig. 6-10 for the conversion of the sedative-hypnotic chloral hydrate to trichloroethanol. Alcohol dehydrogenase typically converts alcohols to aldehydes. In the case of chloral hydrate, the reverse reaction is favored by the presence of the trichloromethyl group, which is a strong electron-withdrawing group.

Disulfide Reduction Some disulfides are reduced and cleaved to their sulfhydryl components, as shown in Fig. 6-11 for the alcohol deterrent disulfiram (Antabuse). As shown in Fig. 6-11, disulfide reduction by glutathione is a three-step process, the last step of which is catalyzed by glutathione reductase. The first steps can be catalyzed by glutathione *S*-transferase, or they can occur nonenzymatically.

Sulfoxide and *N*-Oxide Reduction Thioredoxin-dependent enzymes in liver and kidney cytosol have been reported to reduce sulfoxides, which themselves may be formed by cytochrome P450 or flavin monooxygenases (Anders et al., 1981). It has been suggested that recycling through these counteracting enzyme systems may prolong the half-life of certain xenobiotics. Sulindac is a sulfoxide that undergoes reduction to a sulfide, which is excreted in bile and reabsorbed from the intestine (Ratnayake et al., 1981). This enterohepatic cycling prolongs its duration of action, such that this nonsteroidal anti-inflammatory drug (NSAID) need only be taken twice daily. Diethyldithiocarbamate methyl ester, a metabolite of disulfiram, is oxidized to a sulfine, which is reduced to the parent methyl ester by glutathione. In the latter reaction, two molecules of glutathione (GSH) are oxidized with reduction of the sulfine oxygen to water (Madan et al., 1994), as shown below:

$$R_1R_2C{=}S^+{-}O^- + 2\,GSH \rightarrow R_1R_2C{=}S + GSSG + H_2O$$

Just as sulfoxide reduction can reverse the effect of sulfoxidation, so the reduction of *N*-oxides can reverse the *N*-oxygenation of amines, which is catalyzed by flavin monooxygenases and cytochrome P450. Under reduced oxygen tension, reduction of the *N*-oxides of imipramine, tiaramide, indicine, and *N,N*-dimethylaniline can be catalyzed by mitochondrial and/or microsomal enzymes in the presence of NADH or NADPH (Sugiura and Kato, 1977). The NADPH-dependent reduction of *N*-oxides in liver mi-

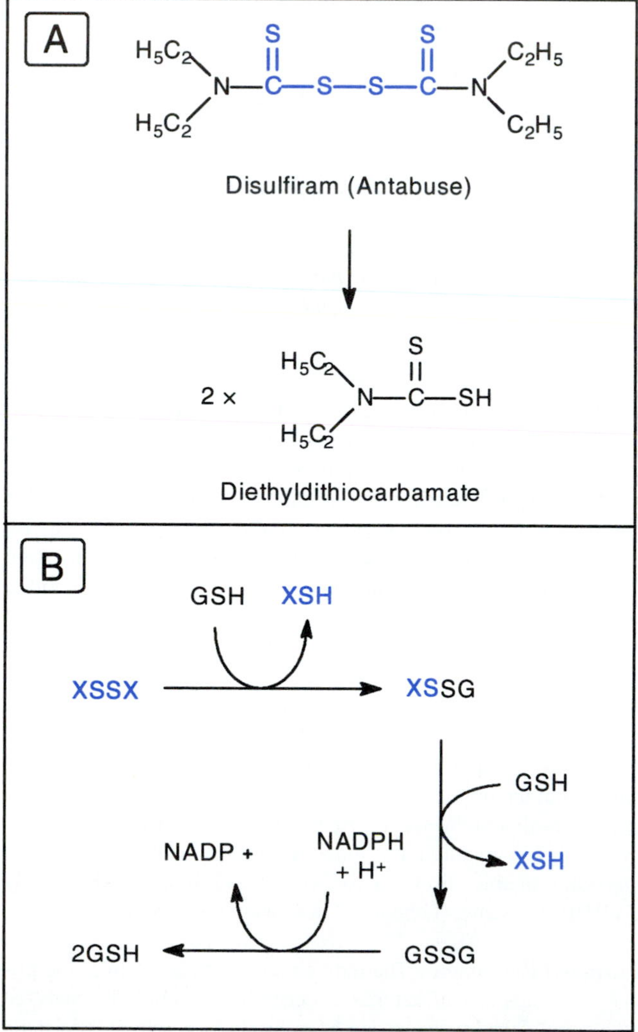

Figure 6-11. Biotransformation of disulfiram by disulfide reduction (A) *and the general mechanism of glutathione-dependent disulfide reduction of xenobiotics* (B).

ABBREVIATIONS: GSH, glutathione; XSSX, xenobiotic disulfide; GSSG, reduced glutathione. The last reaction in *(B)* is catalyzed by glutathione reductase.

crosomes appears to be catalyzed by cytochrome P450 (Sugiura et al., 1976), although in some cases NADPH-cytochrome P450 reductase may play an important role.

As a class, *N*-oxides are not inherently toxic compounds. However, certain aromatic and aliphatic *N*-oxides have been exploited as bioreductive drugs (also known as DNA-affinic drugs) for the treatment of certain cancers and infectious diseases (Wardman et al., 1995). In these cases, *N*-oxides have been used as prodrugs that are converted to cytotoxic or DNA-binding drugs under hypoxic conditions. The fact that *N*-oxides of certain drugs are converted to toxic metabolites under hypoxic conditions is the basis for their selective toxicity to certain solid tumors (namely those that are hypoxic and hence resistant to radiotherapy) and anaerobic bacteria. For example, tirapazamine (SR 4233) is a benzotriazine di-*N*-oxide that is preferentially toxic to hypoxic cells, such as those present in solid tumors, apparently due to its rapid activation by one-electron reduction of the *N*-oxide to an oxidizing nitroxide radical, as shown in Fig. 6-12 (Walton et al., 1992). This reaction is catalyzed by cytochrome P450 and NADPH-cytochrome P450 reductase (Saunders et al., 2000). Two-electron reduction of the di-*N*-oxide, SR 4233, produces a mono-*N*-oxide, SR 4317, which undergoes a second *N*-oxide reduction to SR 4330. Like SR 4233, the antibacterial agent quindoxin is a di-*N*-oxide whose cytotoxicity is dependent on reductive activation, which is favored by anaerobic conditions.

Bioreductive alkylating agents, which include such drugs as mitomycins, anthracyclines, and aziridinylbenzoquinones, represent another class of anticancer agents that require activation by reduction. However, for this class of agents, bioactivation also involves a two-electron reduction reaction, which is largely catalyzed by DT-diaphorase, described in the next section.

Quinone Reduction Quinones can be reduced to hydroquinones by NAD(P)H-quinone oxidoreductase, a cytosolic flavoprotein also known as DT-diaphorase (Ernster, 1987; Riley and Workman, 1992). An example of this reaction is shown in Fig. 6-13. Formation of the relatively stable hydroquinone involves a two-electron reduction of the quinone with stoichiometric oxidation of NAD[P]H *without* oxygen consumption. The two-electron reduction of quinones also can be catalyzed by carbonyl reductase, especially in humans. Although there are exceptions (see below, this section), this pathway of quinone reduction is essentially nontoxic; that is, it is not associated with oxidative stress, unlike the one-electron reduction of quinones by NADPH-cytochrome P450 reductase (Fig. 6-13). In addition to quinones, substrates for DT-diaphorase include a variety of potentially toxic compounds, in-

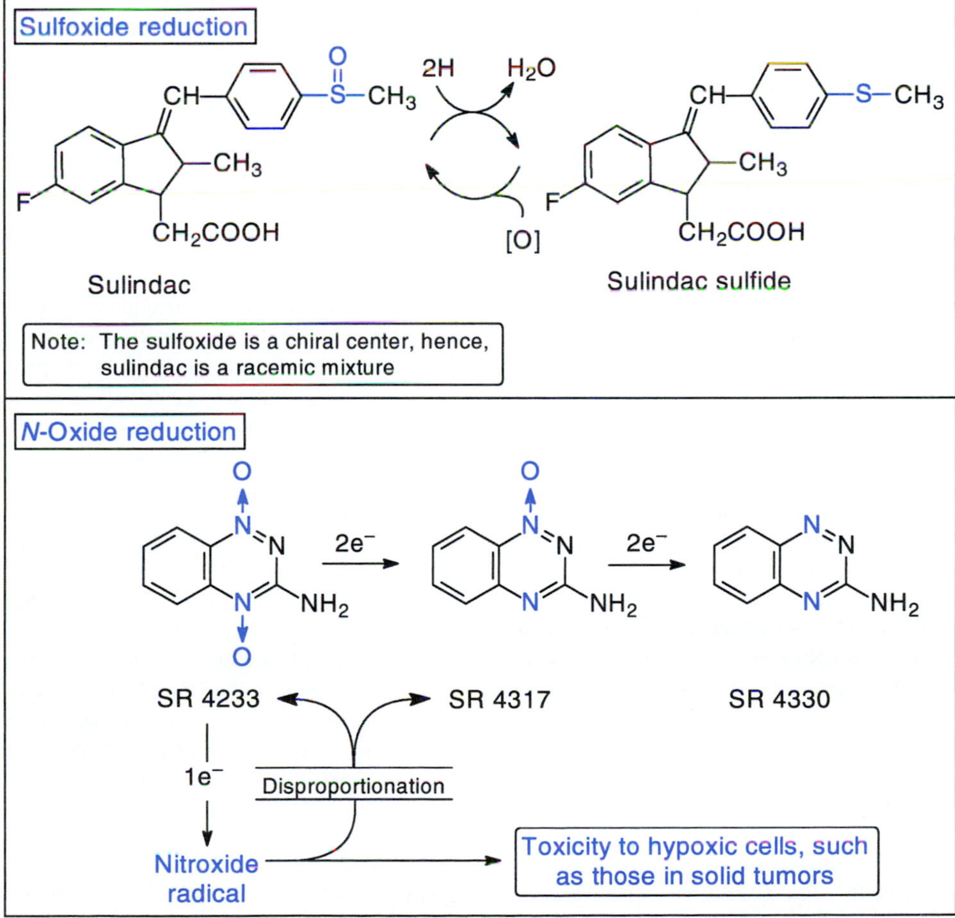

Figure 6-12. Examples of sulfoxide and* N*-oxide reduction.

Note that tirapazamine (3-amino-1,2,4-benzotriazine-1,4-dioxide or SR4233) is a representative of a class of agents that are activated by reduction, which may be clinically useful in the treatment of certain tumors.

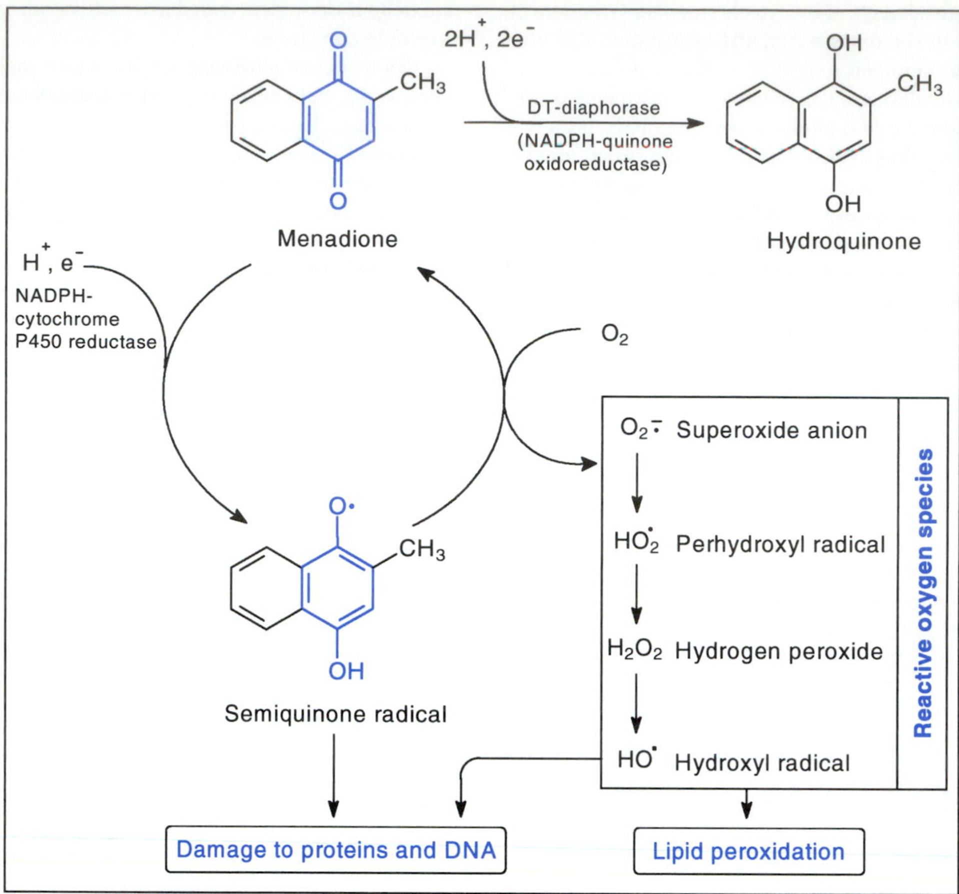

Figure 6-13. ***Two-electron reduction of menadione to a hydroquinone, and production of reactive oxygen species during its one-electron reduction to a semiquinone radical.***

cluding quinone epoxides, quinoneimines, azo dyes, and *C*-nitroso derivatives of arylamines.

The second pathway of quinone reduction is catalyzed by NADPH-cytochrome P450 reductase (a microsomal flavoprotein) and results in the formation of a semiquinone free radical by a one-electron reduction of the quinone. Semiquinones are readily autooxidizable, which leads to nonstoichiometric oxidation of NADPH and oxygen consumption. The oxidative stress associated with autooxidation of a semiquinone free radical, which produces superoxide anion, hydrogen peroxide, and other active oxygen species, can be extremely cytotoxic, as illustrated in Fig. 6-13 for menadione. Oxidative stress appears to be an important component to the mechanism of toxicity of several xenobiotics that either contain a quinone or can be biotransformed to a quinone (Anders, 1985). The production of superoxide anion radicals and oxidative stress are responsible, at least in part, for the cardiotoxic effects of doxorubicin (adriamycin) and daunorubicin (daunomycin), the pulmonary toxicity of paraquat and nitrofurantoin, and the neurotoxic effects of 6-hydroxydopamine. Oxidative stress also plays an important role in the destruction of pancreatic beta cells by alloxan and dialuric acid. Tissues low in superoxide dismutase activity, such as the heart, are especially susceptible to the oxidative stress associated with the redox cycling of quinones. This accounts, at least in part, for the cardiotoxic effects of adriamycin and related anticancer agents.

DT-diaphorase levels are often elevated in tumor cells, which has implications for cancer chemotherapy with agents that are biotransformed by DT-diaphorase (Riley and Workman, 1992). Some cancer chemotherapeutic agents are inactivated by DT-diaphorase, such as SR 4233 (Fig. 6-12), whereas others are activated to cytotoxic metabolites, such as mitomycins, anthracyclines, and aziridinylbenzoquinones. These so-called bioreductive alkylating agents are reduced by DT-diaphorase to generate reactive intermediates that undergo nucleophilic additions with DNA, resulting in single-strand DNA breaks. The reason such drugs are preferentially toxic to tumor cells is that tumor cells, especially those in solid tumors, are hypoxic, and hypoxia induces the synthesis of DT-diaphorase [by a mechanism that involves the activator protein 1 (AP-1) and nuclear factor-κB (NF-κB) response elements in the 5′-promoter region of the DT-diaphorase gene]. Therefore, tumor cells often express high levels of DT-diaphorase, which predisposes them to the toxic effects of mitomycin C and related indolequinones. Interestingly, mitomycin C also up-regulates the expression of DT-diaphorase, which may enable this anticancer drug to stimulate its own metabolic activation in tumor cells (Yao et al., 1997). Induction of DT-diaphorase by mitomycin C, like that by hypoxia, involves transcriptional activation of the AP-1 and NF-κB response elements in the 5′-promoter region of the DT-diaphorase gene. However, whereas activation of the DT-diaphorase AP-1 response element by mitomycin C involves both

Jun and Fos, its activation by hypoxia involves only *jun* family dimers (Yao et al., 1997). Other factors that regulate the expression of DT-diaphorase are described below (this section).

It is now apparent that the structure of the hydroquinones produced by DT-diaphorase determines whether the two-electron reduction of quinones results in xenobiotic detoxication or activation. Hydroquinones formed by two-electron reduction of unsubstituted or methyl-substituted 1,4-naphthoquinones (such as menadione) or the corresponding quinone epoxides are relatively stable to autooxidation, whereas the methoxyl, glutathionyl, and hydroxyl derivatives of these compounds undergo autooxidation with production of semiquinones and reactive oxygen species. The ability of glutathionyl derivatives to undergo redox cycling indicates that conjugation with glutathione does not prevent quinones from serving as substrates for DT-diaphorase. The glutathione conjugates of quinones can also be reduced to hydroquinones by carbonyl reductases, which actually have a binding site for glutathione. In human carbonyl reductase, this binding site is Cys_{227}, which is involved in binding both substrate and glutathione (Tinguely and Wermuth, 1999). Although oxidative stress is an important mechanism by which quinones cause cellular damage (through the intermediacy of semiquinone radicals and the generation of reactive oxygen species), it should be noted that quinones are Michael acceptors, and cellular damage can occur through direct alkylation of critical cellular proteins and/or DNA (reviewed in Bolton et al., 2000).

DT-diaphorase is a dimer of two equal subunits (Mr 27 kDa) each containing FAD. Mouse, rat, and human appear to possess two, three, and four forms of DT-diaphorase, respectively (Riley and Workman, 1992). The human enzymes are encoded by four distinct gene loci (*DIA 1* through *DIA 4*). The fourth gene locus encodes the form of DT-diaphorase known as NADPH-quinone oxidoreductase-1 (NQO_1), which accounts for the majority of DT-diaphorase activity in most human tissues. This enzyme is inducible (see below, this section), and is the ortholog of rat NQO_1. A second, noninducible form of DT-diaphorase, NQO_2, is polymorphically expressed in humans (Jaiswal et al., 1990).

DT-diaphorase is inducible up to tenfold by two classes of agents, which have been categorized as *bifunctional* and *monofunctional* inducers (Prochaska and Talalay, 1992). The bifunctional agents include compounds like β-naphthoflavone, benzo[a]pyrene, 3-methylcholanthrene and 2,3,7,8-tetrachlorodibenzo-*p*-dioxin (TCDD or dioxin), which induce both phase I enzymes (such as the cytochrome P450 enzyme known as CYP1A1) and phase II enzymes (such as glutathione *S*-transferase and uridine diphosphate [UDP]-glucuronosyltransferase). These agents signal through two distinct mechanisms, one involving the XRE (xenobiotic-response element) and one involving the ARE (antioxidant response element), which is also known as the EpRE (electrophilic response element). (Response elements are short sequences of DNA, often located upstream in the 5′-region of a gene, that bind the transcription factors controlling gene expression.) Some enzymes, such as CYP1A1, are largely regulated by the XRE, whereas others, such as glutathione *S*-transferase, are largely regulated by ARE. Some enzymes, such as DT-diaphorase, are regulated by both.

In order to activate the XRE and induce the synthesis of CYP1A1, the so-called bifunctional agents must first bind to a receptor protein called the *Ah* receptor, which is discussed later on under "Induction of Cytochrome P450." Unlike the bifunctional agents, the monofunctional agents do not bind to the *Ah* receptor and, therefore, do not induce CYP1A1. However, like the bifunctional agents, the monofunctional agents can induce the synthesis of those phase II enzymes that are regulated by the ARE (which includes DT-diaphorase).

The monofunctional agents can be subdivided into two chemical classes: those that cause oxidative stress through redox cycling (e.g., the quinone, menadione, and the phenolic antioxidants *tert*-butylhydroquinone and 3,5-di-*tert*-butylcatechol) and those that cause oxidative stress by depleting glutathione (e.g., fumarates, maleates, acrylates, isothiocyanates, and other Michael acceptors that react with glutathione).

As previously mentioned, agents that signal through the XRE do so by binding to the *Ah* receptor. Agents that signal through the ARE do so by an incompletely characterized mechanism. AREs generally contain two AP1/AP1-like elements arranged as inverse or direct repeats with a 3- to 8-base-pair interval and followed by a "GC" box. Several nuclear factors—including Jun, Fos, Fra, and Nrf2 families—bind the ARE and activate transcription of DT-diaphorase and certain phase II enzymes (Favreau and Pickett, 1991; Rushmore et al., 1991; Hayes and Pullford, 1995; Radjendirane and Jaiswal, 1999). The flavonoid β-naphthoflavone, the polycyclic aromatic hydrocarbon benzo[a]pyrene, and the polyhalogenated aromatic hydrocarbon TCDD all induce DT-diaphorase by both mechanisms; the parent compound binds to the *Ah* receptor and is responsible for inducing CYP1A1, as well as DT-diaphorase, via the XRE, whereas electrophilic and/or redox active metabolites of β-naphthoflavone, benzo[a]pyrene, and TCDD are responsible for inducing glutathione *S*-transferase, as well as DT-diaphorase, via the ARE (Radjendirane and Jaiswal, 1999). The situation with benzo[a]pyrene is quite intriguing. This polycyclic aromatic hydrocarbon binds directly to the *Ah* receptor, which binds to the XRE and induces the synthesis of CYP1A1, which in turn converts benzo[a]pyrene to electrophilic metabolites (such as arene oxides and diolepoxides) and redox active metabolites (such as catechols), as shown in Fig. 6-6. These electrophilic and redox active metabolites then induce enzymes that are regulated by the ARE. However, the catechol metabolites of benzo[a]pyrene are further converted by dihydrodiol dehydrogenase to *ortho*-quinones (Fig. 6-6), and are thereby converted back into planar, hydrophobic compounds that are highly effective ligands for the *Ah* receptor (Burczynski and Penning, 2000). This may be toxicologically important, because the *Ah* receptor may translocate *ortho*-quinone metabolites of benzo[a]pyrene into the nucleus, where they might damage DNA (Bolton et al., 2000).

Among the monofunctional agents that apparently induce DT-diaphorase via ARE is sulforaphane, an ingredient of broccoli that may be responsible for the anticarcinogenic effects of this cruciferous vegetable (Zhang et al., 1992). As mentioned above (this section), hypoxia and the anticancer agent mitomycin C are also inducers of DT-diaphorase, which has implications for cancer chemotherapy.

Dihydropyrimidine Dehydrogenase In 1993, fifteen Japanese patients died as a result of an interaction between two oral medications, Sorivudine, a new antiviral drug for herpes zoster, and Tegafur, a prodrug that is converted in the liver to the anticancer agent 5-fluorouracil. The deaths occurred within 40 days of the Japanese government's approval of Sorivudine for clinical use. The mechanism of the lethal interaction between Sorivudine and Tegafur is illustrated in Fig. 6-14 and involves inhibition dihydropyrimidine dehydrogenase, an NADPH-requiring homodimeric protein (Mr ~210 kDa) containing FMN/FAD, and an iron-sulfur cluster in each subunit. The enzyme is located mainly in liver cytosol, where it catalyzes the reduction of 5-fluorouracil and related pyrimidines. Sorivudine is converted in part by gut flora to (*E*)-5-(2-bromovinyl) uracil (BVU), which lacks antiviral activity but is converted by dihydropyrimidine dehydrogenase to a metabolite that binds covalently to the enzyme. The irreversible inactivation (also known as suicidal inactivation) of dihydropyrimidine dehydrogenase by Sorivudine causes a marked inhibition of 5-fluorouracil metabolism, which increases blood levels of 5-fluorouracil to toxic and, in some cases, lethal levels (Ogura et al., 1998; Kanamitsu et al., 2000).

Severe 5-fluorouracil toxicity has also been documented in rare individuals who are genetically deficient in dihydropyrimidine dehydrogenase. The incidence and underlying mechanism of this genetic polymorphism remain to be determined, although its implication is clear: the dosage of 5-fluoroacil should be decreased in individuals devoid of dihydropyrimidine dehydrogenase or substantially lacking in it. Dosage adjustment may also be necessary for heterozygotes (i.e., individuals with a single copy of the active gene) compared with individuals who are homozygous for the wild-type (active) gene (Diasio et al., 1998).

Dehalogenation There are three major mechanisms for removing halogens (F, Cl, Br, and I) from aliphatic xenobiotics (Anders, 1985). The first, known as *reductive dehalogenation,* involves replacement of a halogen with hydrogen, as shown below:

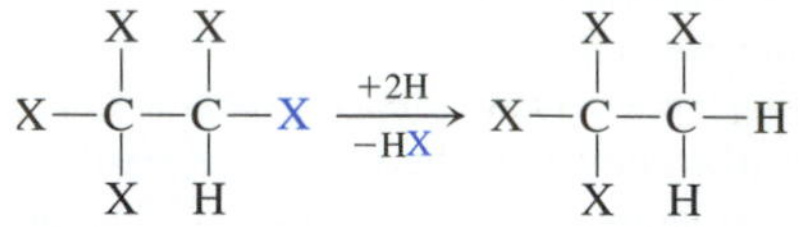

$$\underset{\text{Pentahaloethane}}{X_3C{-}CHX_2} \xrightarrow[-HX]{+2H} \underset{\text{Tetrahaloethane}}{X_3C{-}CH_2X}$$

In the second mechanism, known as *oxidative dehalogenation,* a halogen and hydrogen on the same carbon atom are replaced with oxygen. Depending on the structure of the haloalkane, oxidative dehalogenation leads to the formation of an acylhalide or aldehyde, as shown below:

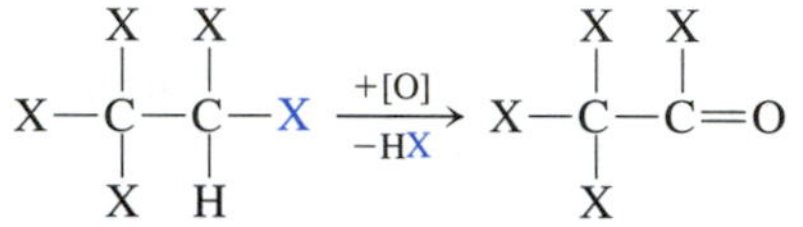

$$\underset{\text{Pentahaloethane}}{X_3C{-}CHX_2} \xrightarrow[-HX]{+[O]} \underset{\text{Tetrahaloacetylhalide}}{X_3C{-}C(X){=}O}$$

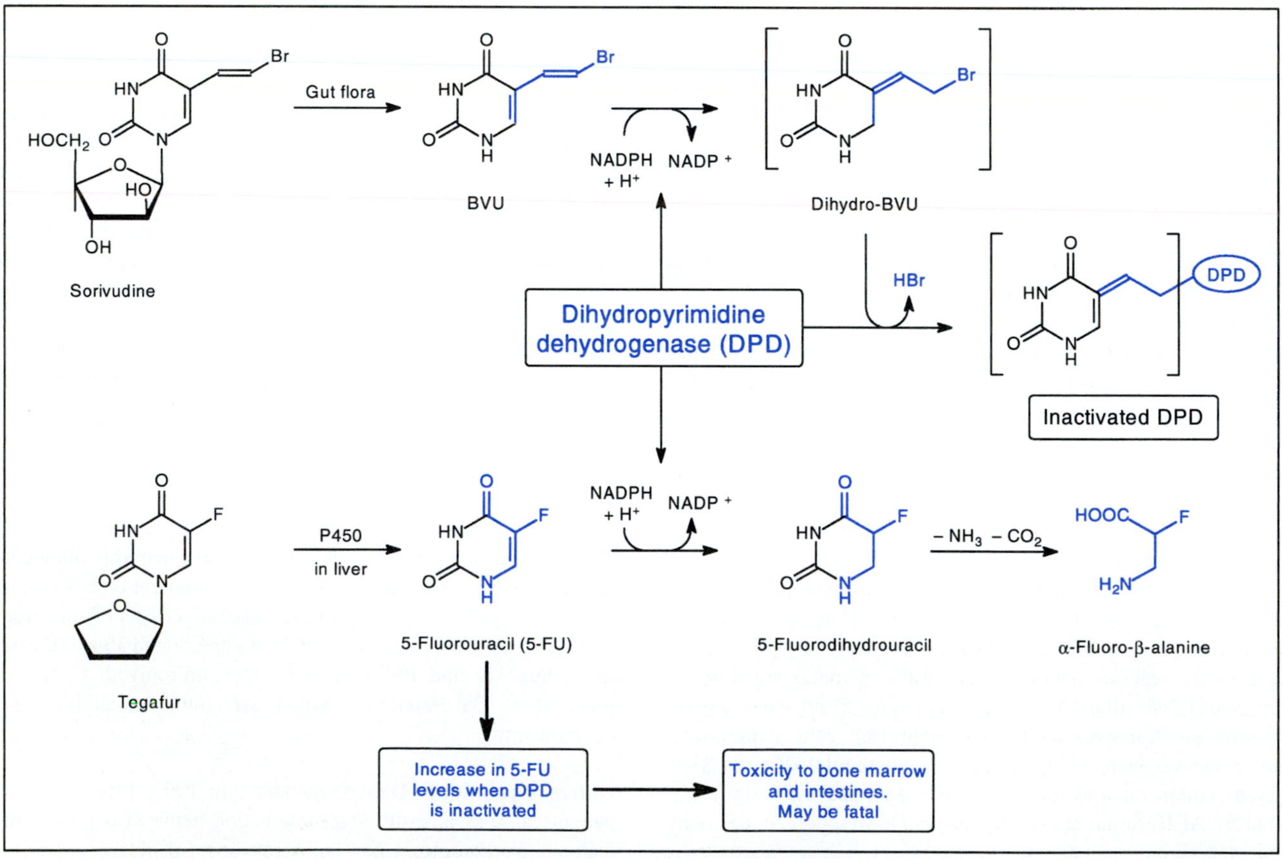

Figure 6-14. Reduction of 5-fluorouracil by dihydropyrimidine dehydrogenase and its inhibition (suicide inactivation) by Sorivudine.

Note: Inhibition of dihydropyrimidine dehydrogenase is the mechanism of fatal interactions between Sorivudine and the 5-fluorouracil prodrug Tegafur.

$$\text{X}{-}\underset{\text{X}}{\overset{\text{X}}{\text{C}}}{-}\underset{\text{H}}{\overset{\text{H}}{\text{C}}}{-}\text{X} \xrightarrow[-\text{HX}]{+[\text{O}]} \text{X}{-}\underset{\text{X}}{\overset{\text{X}}{\text{C}}}{-}\overset{\text{H}}{\text{C}}{=}\text{O}$$

Tetrahaloethane → Trihaloacetaldehyde

A third mechanism of dehalogenation involves the elimination of two halogens on adjacent carbon atoms to form a carbon–carbon double bond, as shown below:

$$\text{X}{-}\underset{\text{X}}{\overset{\text{X}}{\text{C}}}{-}\underset{\text{H}}{\overset{\text{X}}{\text{C}}}{-}\text{X} \xrightarrow[-2\text{HX}]{+2\text{H}} (\text{X})(\text{X})\text{C}{=}\text{C}(\text{X})(\text{H})$$

Pentahaloethane → Trihaloethylene

A variation on this third mechanism is *dehydrohalogenation,* in which a halogen and hydrogen on adjacent carbon atoms are eliminated to form a carbon–carbon double bond.

Reductive and oxidative dehalogenation are both catalyzed by cytochrome P450. (The ability of cytochrome P450 to catalyze both reductive and oxidative reactions is explained later, under "Cytochrome P450.") Dehalogenation reactions leading to double bond formation are catalyzed by cytochrome P450 and glutathione *S*-transferase. These reactions play an important role in the biotransformation and metabolic activation of several halogenated alkanes, as the following examples illustrate.

The hepatotoxicity of carbon tetrachloride (CCl_4) and several related halogenated alkanes is dependent on their biotransformation by reductive dehalogenation. The first step in reductive dehalogenation is a one-electron reduction catalyzed by cytochrome P450, which produces a potentially toxic, carbon-centered radical and inorganic halide. In the case of CCl_4, reductive dechlorination produces a trichloromethyl radical ($\bullet CCl_3$), which initiates lipid peroxidation and produces a variety of other metabolites, as shown in Fig. 6-15. Halothane can also be converted by reductive dehalogenation to a carbon-centered radical, as shown in Fig. 6-16. The mechanism is identical to that described for carbon tetrachloride, although in the case of halothane the radical is generated through loss of bromine, which is a better leaving group than chlorine. Figure 6-16 also shows that halothane can undergo oxidative dehalogenation, which involves oxygen insertion at the C–H bond to generate an unstable halohydrin ($CF_3COHClBr$) that decomposes to a reactive acylhalide (CF_3COCl), which can bind to cellular proteins (particularly to amine groups) or further decompose to trifluoroacetic acid (CF_3COOH).

Both the oxidative and reductive pathways of halothane metabolism generate reactive intermediates capable of binding to proteins and other cellular macromolecules. The relative importance of these two pathways to halothane-induced hepatotoxicity appears to be species-dependent. In rats, halothane-induced hepatotoxicity is promoted by those conditions favoring the reductive dehalogenation of halothane, such as moderate hypoxia (10 to 14% oxygen) plus treatment with the cytochrome P450 inducers phenobarbital and pregnenolone-16α-carbonitrile. In contrast to the situation in rats, halothane-induced hepatotoxicity in guinea pigs is largely the result of oxidative dehalogenation of halothane (Lunam et al., 1989). In guinea pigs, halothane hepatotoxicity is not enhanced by moderate hypoxia and is diminished by the use of deuterated halothane, which impedes the oxidative dehalogenation of halothane because the P450-dependent insertion of oxygen into a carbon–deuterium bond is energetically less favorable (and therefore slower) than inserting oxygen into a carbon–hydrogen bond.

Halothane hepatitis in humans is a rare but severe form of liver necrosis associated with repeated exposure to this volatile anesthetic. In humans as in guinea pigs, halothane hepatotoxicity appears to result from the oxidative dehalogenation of halothane, as shown in Fig. 6-16. Serum samples from patients suffering from halothane hepatitis contain antibodies directed against neoantigens formed by the trifluoroacetylation of proteins. These antibodies have been used to identify which specific proteins in the endoplasmic reticulum are targets for trifluoroacetylation during the oxidative dehalogenation of halothane (Pohl et al., 1989).

The concept that halothane is activated by cytochrome P450 to trifluoroacetylhalide, which binds covalently to proteins and elicits an immune response, has been extended to other volatile anesthetics, such as enflurane, methoxyflurane, and isoflurane. In other words, these halogenated aliphatic hydrocarbons, like halothane, may be converted to acylhalides that form immunogens by bind-

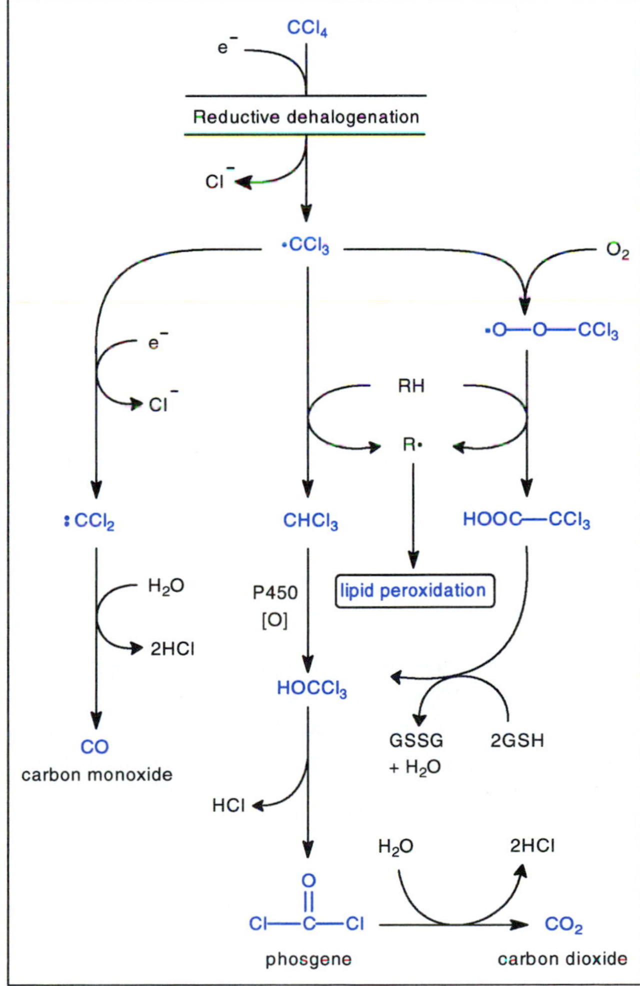

Figure 6-15. Reductive dehalogenation of carbon tetrachloride to a trichloromethyl free radical that initiates lipid peroxidation.

ABBREVIATIONS: RH, unsaturated lipid; R•, lipid dienyl radical; GSH, reduced glutathione; GSSG, oxidized glutathione.

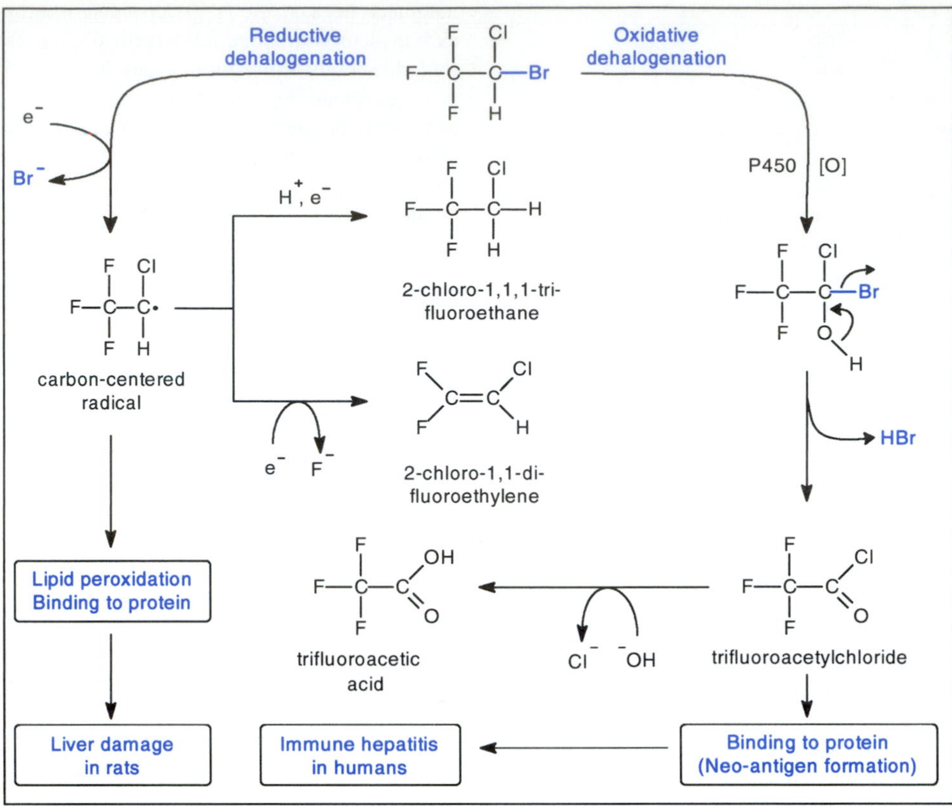

Figure 6-16. Activation of halothane by reductive and oxidative dehalogenation and their role in liver toxicity in rats and humans.

ing covalently to proteins. In addition to accounting for rare instances of enflurane hepatitis, this mechanism of hepatotoxicity can also account for reports of a *cross-sensitization* between enflurane and halothane, in which enflurane causes liver damage in patients previously exposed to halothane.

One of the metabolites generated from the reductive dehalogenation of halothane is 2-chloro-1,1-difluoroethylene (Fig. 6-16). The formation of this metabolite involves the loss of two halogens from adjacent carbon atoms with formation of a carbon–carbon double bond. This type of dehalogenation reaction can also be catalyzed by glutathione *S*-transferases. Glutathione initiates the reaction with a nucleophilic attack either on the electrophilic carbon to which the halogen is attached (mechanism A) or on the halide itself (mechanism B), as shown in Fig. 6-17 for the dehalogenation of 1,2-dihaloethane to ethylene. The insecticide DDT is detoxified by dehydrochlorination to DDE by DDT-dehydrochlorinase, as shown in Fig. 6-18. The activity of this glutathione-dependent reaction correlates well with resistance to DDT in houseflies.

Oxidation

Alcohol, Aldehyde, Ketone Oxidation-Reduction Systems Alcohols, aldehydes, and ketones are oxidized or reduced by a number of enzymes, including alcohol dehydrogenase, aldehyde dehydrogenase, carbonyl reductase, dihydrodiol dehydrogenase, and the molybdenum-containing enzymes, aldehyde oxidase and xanthine dehydrogenase/oxidase. For example, simple alcohols (such as methanol and ethanol) are oxidized to aldehydes (namely formaldehyde and acetaldehyde) by alcohol dehydrogenase. These aldehydes are further oxidized to carboxylic acids (formic acid and acetic acid) by aldehyde dehydrogenase, as shown in Fig. 6-19. NAD^+ is the preferred cofactor for both alcohol and aldehyde dehydrogenase.

Alcohol Dehydrogenase Alcohol dehydrogenase (ADH) is a zinc-containing, cytosolic enzyme present in several tissues including the liver, which has the highest levels, the kidney, the lung, and the gastric mucosa (Agarwal and Goedde, 1992). Human ADH is a dimeric protein consisting of two 40-kDa subunits. The subunits (α, β, γ, π, χ, and sixth subunit known as σ or μ) are encoded by six different gene loci (ADH1 through ADH6). [Although the human ADH subunits α, β, γ, π, and χ are consistently reported to be encoded by genes ADH1 to ADH5, respectively, the sixth subunit (σ or μ) was originally reported to be encoded by gene ADH7. In this review, I have followed the recommendation of Jörnvall and Höög (1995) that the gene encoding the sixth subunit (σ or μ) be designated ADH6.] Updates on ADH nomenclature can be found on the Internet (http://www.gene.ucl.ac.uk./nomenclature/ADH. shtml).

There are three allelic variants of the beta subunit (β_1, β_2, and β_3, which differ by a single amino acid) and two allelic variants of the gamma subunit (γ_1 and γ_2, which differ by two amino acids). Consequently, the human ADH enzymes comprise nine subunits, all of which can combine as homodimers. In addition, the α, β, and γ subunits (and their allelic variants) can form heterodimers with each other (but not with the other subunits, none of which

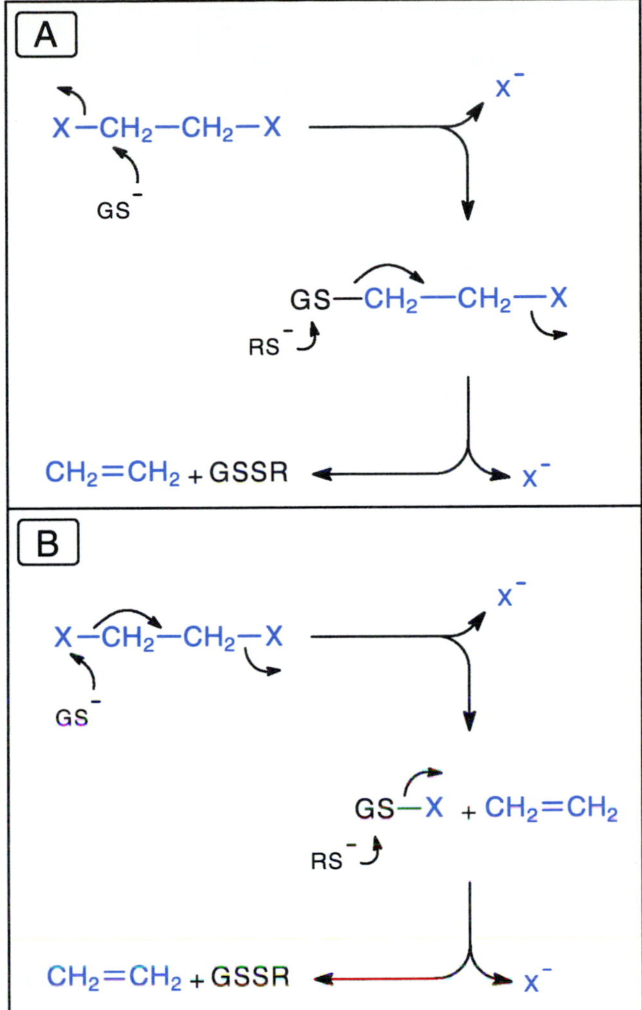

Figure 6-17. Glutathione-dependent dehalogenation of 1,2-dihaloethane to ethylene.

A. Nucleophilic attack on carbon. *B*. Nucleophilic attack on halide.

form heterodimers). The different molecular forms of ADH are divided into four major classes. Class I contains ADH1, ADH2, and ADH3, which can be considered isozymes. ADH1 contains either two alpha subunits or one alpha subunit plus a beta or gamma subunit. ADH2 contains either two beta subunits (which could be β_1, β_2, or β_3) or a beta subunit plus a gamma subunit (which could be γ_1 or γ_2). ADH3 contains two gamma subunits (which could be γ_1 or γ_2). ADH2 enzymes that differ in the type of β subunits are known as allelozymes, as are ADH3 enzymes that differ in the type of γ subunit. Accordingly, ADH2*1 is an allelozyme composed of β_1 units; ADH2*2 is an allelozyme composed of β_2 subunits, and ADH2*3 is an allelozyme composed of β_3 subunits.

Class II contains ADH4, which is made up of two π subunits (named pi because this form of ADH is not inhibited by pyrazole). Class III contains ADH5, which is made up of two χ subunits (for which reason it is also known as chi-ADH). Class IV contains ADH6 (originally named ADH7, as mentioned above), which is made up of two subunits designated σ or μ (Agarwal and Goedde, 1992; Jörnvall and Höög, 1995; Edenberg, 2000).

The class I ADH isozymes (α-ADH, β-ADH, and γ-ADH) are responsible for the oxidation of ethanol and other small aliphatic alcohols, and they are strongly inhibited by pyrazole and its 4-alkyl derivatives (e.g., 4-methylpyrazole). High levels of class I ADH isozymes are expressed in liver and adrenals, with lower levels in kidney, lung, blood vessels [in the case of ADH2 (i.e., β-ADH)] and other tissues, but not brain. Class II ADH (π-ADH) is primarily expressed in liver (with lower levels in stomach), where it preferentially oxidizes larger aliphatic and aromatic alcohols. Class II ADH differs from the class I ADH in that it plays little or no role in ethanol and methanol oxidation, and it is not inhibited by pyrazole. Long-chain alcohols (pentanol and larger) and aromatic alcohols (such as cinnamyl alcohol) are preferred substrates for class III ADH (χ-ADH). Like class II ADH, class III ADH is not inhibited by pyrazole. However, in contrast to class II ADH, which is largely confined to the liver, class III ADH is ubiquitous, being present in virtually all tissues (including brain), where it appears to play an important role in detoxifying formaldehyde. In fact, class III ADH and formaldehyde dehydrogenase are identical enzymes (Koivusalo et al., 1989). Class IV ADH (σ- or μ-ADH) is a low affinity (high K_m), high capacity ADH (high V_{max}), and is the most active of the medium-chain ADHs in oxidizing retinol. It is the major ADH expressed in human stomach and other areas of the gastrointestinal tract (esophagus, gingiva, mouth, and tongue). In contrast the other ADHs, class IV ADH is not expressed in adult human liver. Inasmuch as class IV ADH is expressed in the upper gastrointestinal tract, where chronic alcohol consumption leads to cancer development, there is growing interest in the role of class IV ADH in the conversion of ethanol to acetaldehyde (a suspected upper GI tract carcinogen or cocarcinogen) and in its role in the metabolism of retinol (a vitamin required for epithelial cell growth and differentiation), which might be inhibited by alcohol consumption (Seitz and Oneta, 1998).

The class I isozymes of ADH differ in their capacity to oxidize ethanol. Even the allelozymes, which differ in a single amino acid, differ markedly in the affinity (K_m) and/or capacity (V_{max}) for oxidizing ethanol to acetaldehyde. The homodimer $\beta_2\beta_2$ and heterodimers containing at least one β_2 subunit (i.e., the ADH2*2

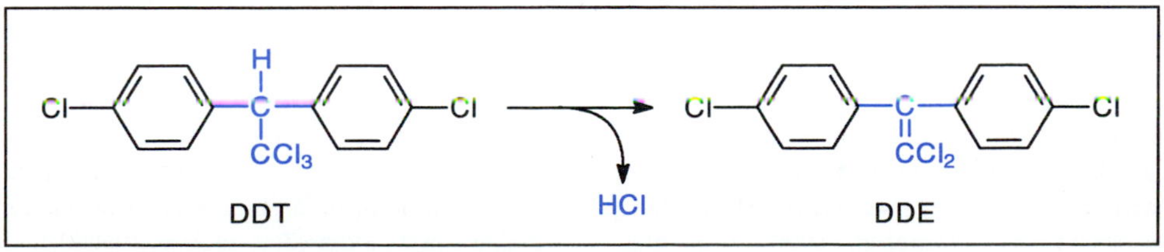

DDT → DDE + HCl

Figure 6-18. Dehydrochlorination of the pesticide DDT to DDE, a glutathione-dependent reaction.

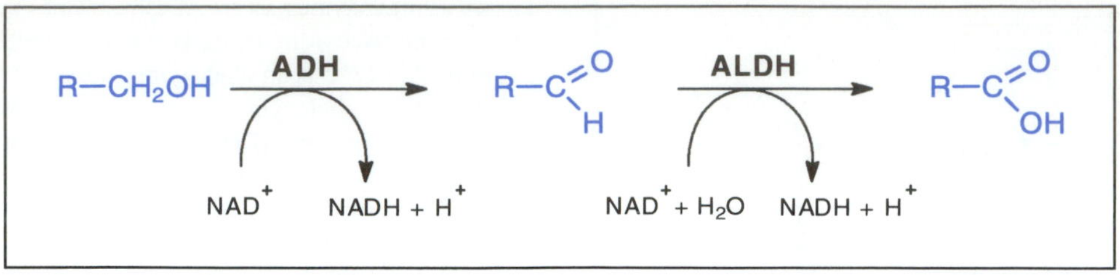

$$R{-}CH_2OH \xrightarrow[NAD^+ \;\rightarrow\; NADH + H^+]{ADH} R{-}C(=O)H \xrightarrow[NAD^+ + H_2O \;\rightarrow\; NADH + H^+]{ALDH} R{-}C(=O)OH$$

Figure 6-19. Oxidation of alcohols to aldehydes and carboxylic acids by alcohol dehydrogenase (ADH) and aldehyde dehydrogenase (ALDH).

allelozymes) are especially active in oxidizing ethanol at physiologic pH. ADH2*2 is known as *atypical* ADH and is responsible for the unusually rapid conversion of ethanol to acetaldehyde in 90 percent of the Pacific Rim Asian population (Japanese, Chinese, Korean). The atypical ADH is expressed to a much lesser degree in Caucasians (<5 percent of Americans, ~8 percent of English, ~12 percent of Germans, and ~20 percent of Swiss), African Americans (<10 percent), Native Americans (0 percent) and Asian Indians (0 percent) (Agarwal and Goedde, 1992). The three ADH2 alleles, ADH2*1 (β_1-ADH), ADH2*2 (β_2-ADH), and ADH2*3 (β_3-ADH), are mainly expressed in Caucasians (up to 95 percent), Pacific Rim Asians (~90 percent) and Africans/African Americans (~24 percent), respectively. These population differences in ADH2 allelozyme expression contribute to ethnic differences in alcohol consumption and toxicity, as discussed in the next section, "Aldehyde Dehydrogenase."

Unlike the allelic variants of ADH2, the allelic variants of ADH3 do not differ markedly in their ability to oxidize ethanol. However, as in the case of the ADH2 allelozymes, the expression of the ADH3 allelozymes also varies from one ethnic group to the next. The two allelozymes of ADH3, namely ADH3*1 (γ_1-ADH) and ADH3*2 (γ_2-ADH) are respectively expressed 50:50 in Caucasians, but 90:10 in Pacific Rim Asians (Li, 2000).

The various class I ADHs in liver oxidize ethanol with a K_m of 50 μM to 4 mM. For comparison, legal intoxication in the United States is defined as a blood alcohol level of 0.1%, which corresponds to 22 mM (Edenberg, 2000). Therefore, during intoxication, the hepatic metabolism of ADH becomes saturated, and the kinetics of ethanol disappearance conform to zero-order kinetics, meaning that a constant amount of ethanol is metabolized per unit time. When the concentration of ethanol falls within the range of K_m, the kinetics of ethanol disappearance conform to a first-order process, meaning that a constant percentage of the remaining ethanol is metabolized per unit time.

Compared with hepatic ADH, gastric ADH has a lower affinity (higher K_m) but higher capacity (larger V_{max}) for oxidizing ethanol, the former being dominated by the class I ADHs, the latter by class IV ADH. Although ethanol is largely biotransformed by hepatic ADH, gastric ADH nevertheless can limit the systemic bioavailability of alcohol. This first-pass elimination of alcohol by gastric ADH can be significant, depending on the manner in which the alcohol is consumed; large doses over a short time produce high ethanol concentrations in the stomach, which compensate for the low affinity (high K_m) of gastric ADH. Young women have lower gastric ADH activity than do men, and gastric ADH activity tends to be lower in alcoholics (Frezza et al., 1990). Some alcoholic women have no detectable gastric ADH, and blood levels of ethanol after oral consumption of alcohol are the same as those that are obtained after intravenous administration. Gastric ADH activity decreases during fasting, which is one reason why alcohol is more intoxicating when it is consumed on an empty stomach. Several commonly used drugs (cimetidine, ranitidine, aspirin) are noncompetitive inhibitors of gastric ADH. Under certain circumstances these drugs increase the systemic availability of alcohol, although the effect is too small to have serious medical, social, or legal consequences (Levitt, 1993). About 30 percent of Asians appear to be genetically deficient in class IV ADH, the main gastric ADH. In addition to biotransforming ethanol and retinol, class IV ADH also detoxifies the dietary carcinogen nitrobenzaldehyde. It has been suggested that a lack of class IV ADH in Japanese subjects may impair their ability to detoxify nitrobenzaldehyde and may possibly be linked to the high rate of gastric cancer observed in the Japanese population (Seitz and Oneta, 1998).

Alcohols can be oxidized to aldehydes by non-ADH enzymes in microsomes and peroxisomes, although these are quantitatively less important than ADH for ethanol oxidation (Lieber, 1999). The microsomal ethanol oxidizing system (formerly known as MEOS) is the cytochrome P450 enzyme CYP2E1. The corresponding peroxisomal enzyme is catalase. The oxidation of ethanol to acetaldehyde by these three enzyme systems is shown in Fig. 6-20.

Aldehyde Dehydrogenase Aldehyde dehydrogenase (ALDH) oxidizes aldehydes to carboxylic acids with NAD^+ as the cofactor. Several ALDH enzymes are involved in the oxidation of xenobiotic aldehydes (Goedde and Agarwal, 1992). The enzymes also have esterase activity (Yoshida et al., 1998). Formaldehyde dehydrogenase, which specifically oxidizes formaldehyde complexed with glutathione, is not a member of the ALDH family but is a class III ADH (Koivusalo et al., 1989). Twelve ALDH genes (known as ALDH1 to 10, SSDH, and MMSDH) have been identified in humans, and a correspondingly large number of ALDH genes appear to be present in other mammalian species. The name, tissue distribution, subcellular location, and major substrate for the 12 human ALDHs are summarized in Table 6-2. The ALDHs differ in their primary amino acid sequences. They may also differ in the quaternary structure. For example, ALDH3 appears to be a dimer of two 85-kDa subunits, whereas ALDH1 and ALDH2 appear to be homotetramers of 54-kDa subunits (Goedde and Agarwal, 1992). In contrast to ALDH1 and ALDH2, which specifically reduce NAD^+, ALDH3 reduces both NAD^+ and $NADP^+$ due to its low affinity for these cofactors.

As shown in Fig. 6-20, ALDH2 is a mitochondrial enzymes that, by virtue of its high affinity, is primarily responsible for oxidizing simple aldehydes, such as acetaldehyde (K_m for acetaldehyde <5 μM at pH 7.4). A genetic polymorphism for ALDH2 has been documented in humans. A high percentage (45 to 53 percent)

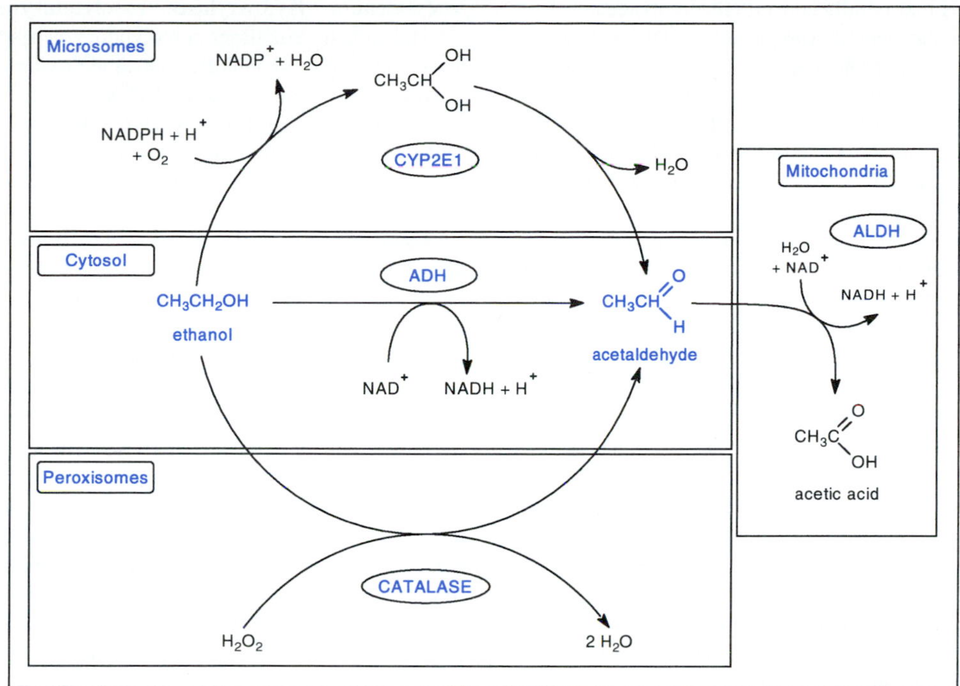

Figure 6-20. Oxidation of ethanol to acetaldehyde by ethanol dehydrogenase (ADH), cytochrome P450 (CYP2E1), and catalase.

Note the oxidation of ethanol to acetic acid involves multiple organelles.

of Japanese, Chinese, Koreans, Taiwanese, and Vietnamese populations are deficient in ALDH2 activity due to a point mutation ($Glu_{487} \rightarrow Lys_{487}$). This inactive allelic variant of ALDH2 is known as ALDH2*2, to distinguish it from the active, wild-type enzyme, ALDH2*1. This same population (i.e., Pacific Rim Asians) also has a high incidence of the atypical form of ADH (i.e., ADH2*2), which means that they rapidly convert ethanol to acetaldehyde but only slowly convert acetaldehyde to acetic acid. (They also have a relatively high prevalence of a deficiency of class IV ADH activity, which impairs gastric metabolism of ethanol.) As a result, many Asian subjects experience a flushing syndrome after consuming alcohol due to a rapid buildup of acetaldehyde, which triggers the dilation of facial blood vessels through the release of catecholamines. Native Americans also experience a flushing syndrome after consuming alcohol, apparently because they express another allelic variant of ALDH2 and/or because acetaldehyde oxidation in blood erythrocytes is impaired in these individuals, possibly due to the expression of a variant form of ALDH1. The functional ge-

Table 6-2
Properties of the Human Aldehyde Dehydrogenases (ALDHs)

ENZYME (ABBREVIATED SYMBOL)	TISSUE	SUBCELLULAR DISTRIBUTION	MAJOR SUBSTRATE
ALDH1	Liver, stomach, etc.	Cytosol	Retinal
ALDH2	Liver, stomach, etc.	Mitochondria	Acetaldehyde
ALDH3	Stomach, lung, etc.	Cytosol	Fatty and aromatic aldehydes
ALDH4	Liver, kidney	Mitochondria	Glutamate, γ-semialdehyde
ALDH5	Testis, liver	Mitochondria	Propionaldehyde
ALDH6	Salivary gland, stomach, kidney	Cytosol	Aliphatic aldehyde, retinal
ALDH7	Kidney, lung	Microsomes	Aliphatic and aromatic aldehydes
ALDH8	Parotid	Microsomes	Unknown
γABHD	Liver, kidney, muscle	Cytosol	Amine aldehyde
FALDH	Liver, heart, muscle	Microsomes	Fatty and aromatic aldehydes
SSDH	Brain, liver, heart	Mitochondria	Succinic semialdehyde
MMSDH	Kidney, liver, heart	Mitochondria	Methylmalonate semialdehyde

KEY: γABHD, 4-aminobutyraldehyde dehydrogenase; FALDH, fatty aldehyde dehydrogenase; SSDH, succinic dehydrogenase; MMSDH, methylmalonate semialdehyde dehydrogenase.

SOURCE: Yoshida et al., 1998.

netic variants of ADH that rapidly convert ethanol to acetaldehyde (i.e., ADH2*2), and the genetic variants of ALDH that slowly detoxify acetaldehyde both protect against heavy drinking and alcoholism. Inhibition of ALDH by disulfiram (Antabuse) causes an accumulation of acetaldehyde in alcoholics. The nauseating effect of acetaldehyde serves to deter continued ethanol consumption (Goedde and Agarwal, 1992). However, it is important to note that a predisposition toward alcoholism is not simply determined by factors that affect the pharmacokinetics of ethanol and its metabolites. Studies in humans and rodents implicate serotonin 1b receptor, dopamine D2 receptor, tryptophan hydroxylase, and neuropeptide Y as candidate targets of genetic susceptibility in the pharmacodynamic actions of ethanol (Li, 2000). Monoamine oxidase may also be a risk modifier for alcoholism, as discussed under "Monoamine Oxidase," further on.

Genetic deficiencies in other ALDHs impair the metabolism of other aldehydes, which is the underlying basis of certain diseases. For example, ALDH4 deficiency disturbs proline metabolism and causes type II hyperprolinemia, symptoms of which include mental retardation and convulsions. A deficiency of ALDH10, which detoxifies fatty aldehydes, disturbs the metabolism of membrane lipids. This is the underlying basis of Sjörgen-Larson syndrome, symptoms of which include ichthyosis, neurologic problems, and oligophrenia (Yoshida et al., 1998).

The toxicologic consequences of an inherited (i.e., genetic) or acquired (e.g., drug-induced) deficiency of ALDH illustrate that aldehydes are more cytotoxic than the corresponding alcohol. This is especially true of allyl alcohol ($CH_2{=}CHCH_2OH$), which is converted by ADH to the highly hepatotoxic aldehyde acrolein ($CH_2{=}CHCHO$). The oxidation of ethanol by ADH and ALDH leads to the formation of acetic acid, which is rapidly oxidized to carbon dioxide and water. However, in certain cases, alcohols are converted to toxic carboxylic acids, as in the case of methanol and ethylene glycol, which are converted via aldehyde intermediates to formic acid and oxalic acid, respectively. Formic and oxalic acids are considerably more toxic than acetic acid. For this reason, methanol and ethylene glycol poisoning are commonly treated with ethanol, which competitively inhibits the oxidation of methanol and ethylene glycol by ADH and ALDH. The potent inhibitor of ADH 4-methylpyrazole (fomepizole) is also used to treat methanol and ethylene glycol poisoning.

The reduction of aldehydes and ketones to primary and secondary alcohols by carbonyl reductases has already been discussed (see "Carbonyl Reduction," above). In contrast to ADH and ALDH, carbonyl reductases typically use NADPH as the source of reducing equivalents. Aldehydes can also be oxidized by aldehyde oxidase and xanthine oxidase, which are discussed below under "Molybdenum Hydroxylases."

Dihydrodiol Dehydrogenase In addition to several hydroxysteroid dehydrogenases and aldose reductases, the aldo-keto reductase (AKR) superfamily includes several forms of dihydrodiol dehydrogenase (Penning, 1997). As previously mentioned in the section on carbonyl reductase, dihydrodiol dehydrogenases are monomeric (~34 kDa), cytosolic, NADP(H)-requiring oxidoreductases that oxidize the *trans*-dihydrodiols of various polycyclic aromatic hydrocarbons to the corresponding *ortho*-quinones, as shown in Fig. 6-6 (Burczynski and Penning, 2000). The conversion of such dihydrodiols to *ortho*-quinones has toxicological implications, which were discussed earlier in the section on "Quinone Reduction."

Molybdenum Hydroxylases (Molybdozymes) Two major molybdenum hydroxylases or molybdozymes participate in the biotransformation of xenobiotics: aldehyde oxidase and xanthine dehydrogenase/xanthine oxidase (XD/XO) (Rettie and Fisher, 1999). Sulfite oxidase is third molybdozyme; it is not described here except to say that sulfite oxidase, as the name implies, oxidizes sulfite, an irritating air pollutant, to sulfate, which is relatively innocuous. All three molybdozymes are flavoprotein enzymes consisting of two identical ~150-kDa subunits, each of which contains FAD, molybdenum, in the form of a pterin molybdenum cofactor $\{[Mo^{VI}(=S)(=O)]^{2+}\}$ and two iron-sulfur (Fe_2S_2) centers (known as FeSI and FeSII). The catalytic cycle involves an interaction between the molybdenum center with a reducing substrate, which results in the reduction of the molybdenum cofactor. After this, reducing equivalents are transferred intramolecularly to the flavin and iron-sulfur centers, with reoxidation occurring via the flavin moiety by molecular oxygen (in the case of aldehyde oxidase and xanthine oxidase) or NAD^+ (in the case of xanthine dehydrogenase). During substrate oxidation, aldehyde oxidase and xanthine oxidase are reduced and then reoxidized by molecular oxygen; hence, they function as true oxidases. The oxygen incorporated into the xenobiotic is derived from water rather than oxygen, which distinguishes the oxidases from oxygenases. The overall reaction is as follows:

$$RH \xrightarrow[-2H^+,-2e^-]{H_2O} ROH$$

Additional details of the catalytic cycle are described below, under "Xanthine Dehydrogenase–Xanthine Oxidase." Xanthine oxidase and aldehyde oxidase catalyze the oxidation of electron-deficient sp^2-hybridized (i.e., double-bonded) carbon atoms found, more often than not, in nitrogen heterocycles, such as purines, pyrimidines, pteridines, and iminium ions. This contrasts with oxidation by cytochrome P450, which generally catalyzes the oxidation of carbon atoms with a high electron density. For this reason, xenobiotics that are good substrates for molybdozymes tend to be poor substrates for cytochrome P450, and vice versa (Rettie and Fisher, 1999). In nitrogen heterocycles, the carbon atom with lowest electron density is adjacent to the nitrogen atom, for which reason xanthine oxidase and aldehyde oxidase tend to hydroxylate the α-carbon atom to form a hydroximine that rapidly tautomerizes to the corresponding α-aminoketone. As the name implies, aldehyde oxidase can convert certain aldehydes to the corresponding carboxylic acid—a property that is also shared by xanthine oxidase, albeit with lower activity. Certain aromatic aldehydes, such as tamoxifen aldehyde and benzaldehyde, are good substrates for aldehyde oxidase and xanthine oxidase, whereas aliphatic aldehydes tend to be poor substrates. Consequently, aldehyde oxidase and xanthine oxidase contribute negligibly to the metabolism of acetaldehyde. Some reactions catalyzed by aldehyde oxidase and xanthine oxidase are shown in Fig. 6-21. Under certain conditions, both enzymes can also catalyze the reduction of xenobiotics containing one or more of the following functional groups: azo, nitro, *N*-oxide, nitrosamine, hydroxamic acid, oxime, sulfoxide, and epoxide. This is discussed further below, in the section entitled "Aldehyde Oxidase."

Xanthine Dehydrogenase–Xanthine Oxidase Xanthine dehydrogenase (XD) and xanthine oxidase (XO) are two forms of the same enzyme that differ in the electron acceptor used in the final step of catalysis. In the case of XD, the final electron acceptor is

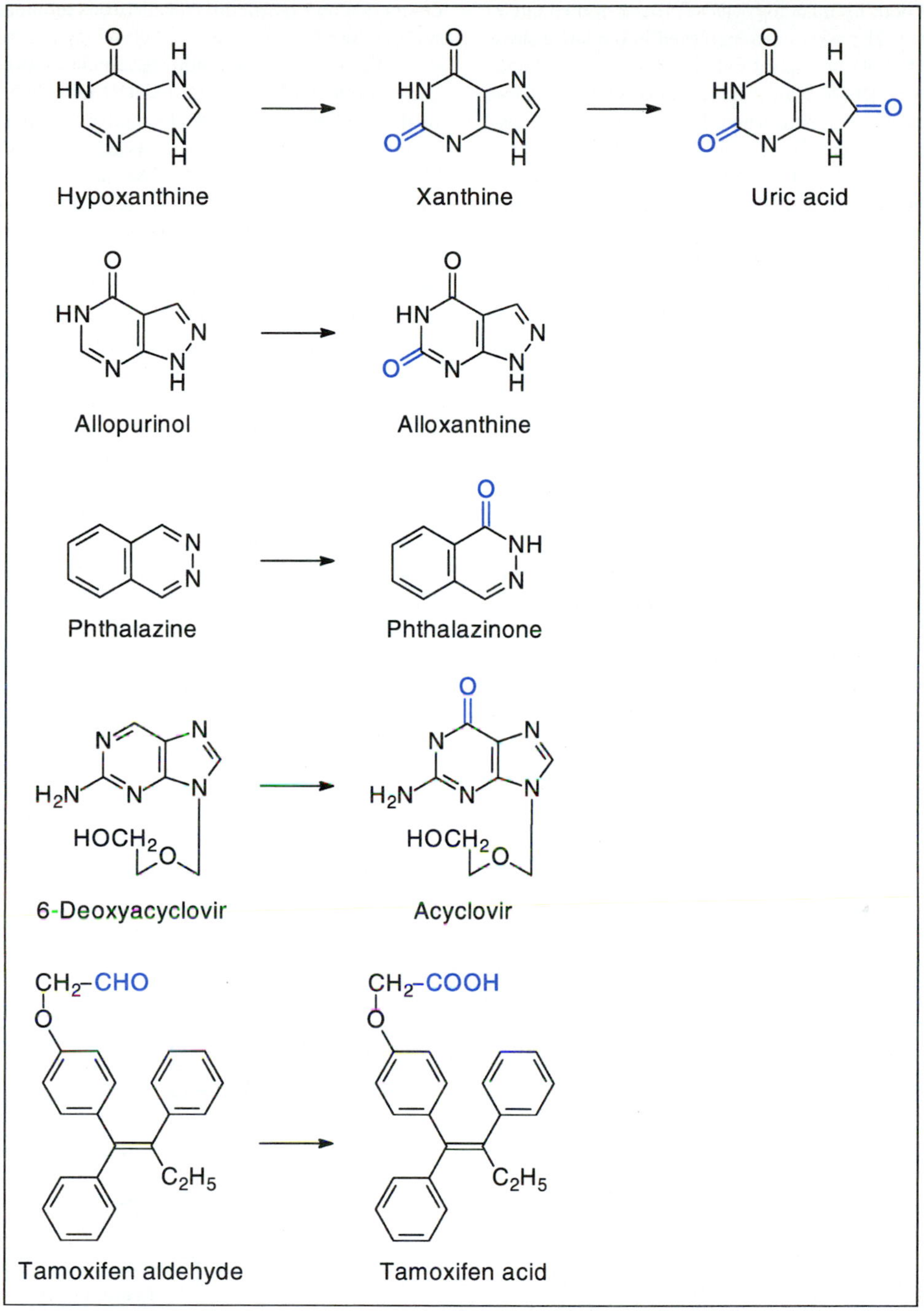

Figure 6-21. Examples of reactions catalyzed by the molybdozymes, xanthine oxidase, and aldehyde oxidase.

NAD^+ (dehydrogenase activity), whereas in the case of XO the final electron acceptor is oxygen (oxidase activity). XD is converted to XO by oxidation of cysteine residues (Cys_{993} and Cys_{1326} of the human enzyme) and/or proteolytic cleavage. The conversion of XD to XO by cysteine oxidation appears to be reversible. Under normal physiologic conditions, XD is the predominant form of the enzyme found in vivo. However, during tissue processing, the dehydrogenase form tends to be converted to the oxidase form, hence, most in vitro studies are conducted with XO or a combination of XO and XD. The induction (up-regulation) of XD and/or the conversion of XD to XO in vivo is thought to play an important role in ischemia-reperfusion injury, lipopolysaccharide (LPS)-mediated tissue injury, and alcohol-induced hepatotoxicity. During ischemia, XO levels increase because hypoxia induces XD/XO gene transcription and because XD is converted to XO. During reperfusion, XO contributes to oxidative stress and lipid peroxidation because the oxidase activity of XO involves the reduction of molecular oxygen, which can lead to the formation of reactive oxygen species of the type shown in Fig. 6-13. Similarly, treatment with LPS, a bacterial endotoxin that triggers an acute inflammatory response, increases XO activity both by inducing XD/XD transcription and by converting XD to XO. The associated increased in oxidative stress has been implicated in LPS-induced cytotoxicity. Ethanol facilitates the conversion of XD to XO, and the conversion of ethanol to acetaldehyde provides a substrate and, hence, a source of electrons for the reduction of oxygen.

Typical reactions catalyzed by XD/XO are shown in Fig. 6-21. XD/XO contributes significantly to the first-pass elimination of several purine derivatives (e.g., 6-mercaptopurine and 2,6-dithiopurine) and limits the therapeutic effects of these cancer chemotherapeutic agents. On the other hand, certain prodrugs are activated by xanthine oxidase. For example, the antiviral prodrugs 6-deoxyacyclovir and 2′-fluoroarabino-dideoxypurine, which are relatively well absorbed after oral dosing, are oxidized by xanthine oxidase to their respective active forms, acyclovir and 2′-fluoroarabino-dideoxyinosine, which are otherwise poorly absorbed (see Fig. 6-21). Furthermore, XD/XO has been implicated in the bioactivation of mitomycin C and related antineoplastic agents, although this bioactivation reaction is also catalyzed by DT-diaphorase (see section entitled "Quinone Reduction," below).

XD/XO catalyzes an important physiologic reaction, namely the sequential oxidation of hypoxanthine to xanthine and uric acid, as shown in Fig. 6-21 (Rajagopalan, 1980). By competing with hypoxanthine and xanthine for oxidation by XD/XO, allopurinol inhibits the formation of uric acid, making allopurinol a useful drug in the treatment of gout (a complication of hyperuricemia). Allopurinol can also be used to evaluate the contribution of XD/XO to xenobiotic biotransformation in vivo. Like allopurinol, hydroxylated coumarin derivatives, such as umbelliferone (7-hydroxycoumarin) and esculetin (7,8-dihydroxycoumarin), are potent inhibitors of XD/XO.

Monomethylated xanthines are preferentially oxidized to the corresponding uric acid derivatives by XD/XO. In contrast, dimethylated and trimethylated xanthines, such as theophylline (1,3-dimethylxanthine) and caffeine (1,3,7-trimethylxanthine), are oxidized to the corresponding uric acid derivatives primarily by cytochrome P450. Through two sequential *N*-demethylation reactions, cytochrome P450 converts caffeine to 1-methylxanthine, which is converted by XD/XO to 1-methyluric acid. The urinary ratio of 1-methylxanthine to 1-methyluric acid provides an in vivo marker of XD/XO activity.

The mechanism of catalysis of xanthine oxidase has been reviewed by Bray et al. (1996). The pteridin molybdenum cofactor $\{[Mo^{VI}(=S)(=O)]^{2+}\}$ contains both a sulfido and oxo ligand. It was once thought that the oxo group was transferred and incorporated into the substrate, such as the C8-position of xanthine. More recent studies suggest that the oxo group does not participate directly in substrate oxidation. Instead, catalysis appears to involve the transient formation of a Mo–C bond between the molybdenum metal center and the C8 position of xanthine, as illustrated in Fig. 6-22. The formation of this Mo-C intermediate is preceded by deprotonation of xanthine (at the C8 position), which reduces the sulfido ligand (Mo=S) to Mo–SH. Deprotonation of xanthine produces a carbanion that reacts with molybdenum to form the Mo–C intermediate, which reacts with water to produce a three-ringed intermediate involving Mo, oxygen and the C8 position of xanthine, which rearranges to yield the hydroxylated substrate (uric acid). The catalytic cycle is completed by the transfer of electrons to

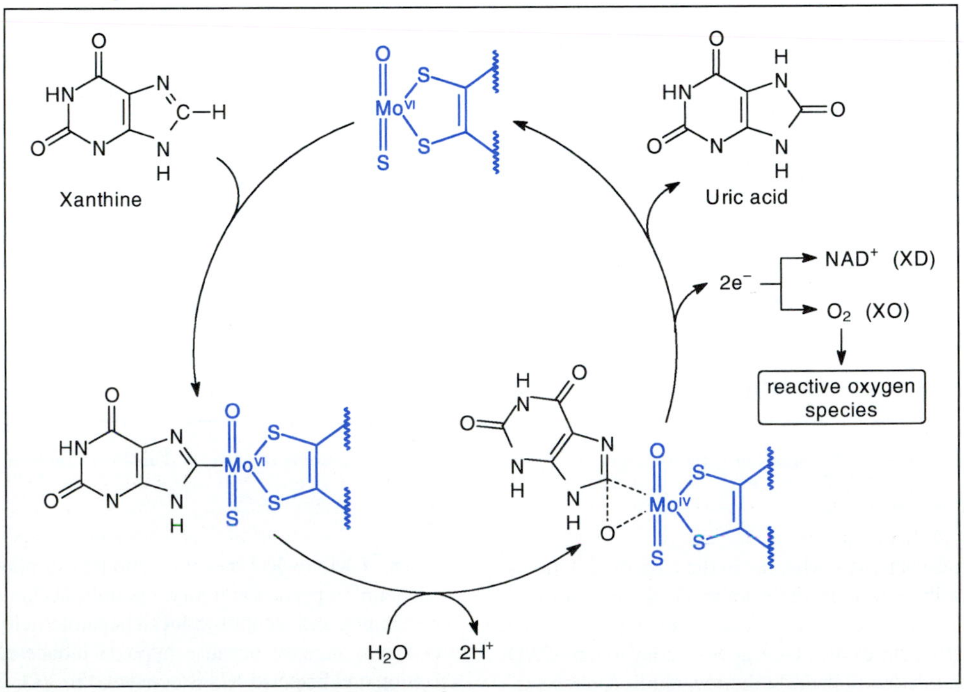

Figure 6-22. Catalytic cycle of xanthine dehydrogenase (XD) and xanthine oxidase (XO).

XD and XO are two forms of the same molybdozyme. During the final step of the catalytic cycle, the enzyme is reoxidized by transferring electrons to NAD^+ (in the case of XD) or oxygen (in the case of XO). The same mechanism of catalysis likely applies to aldehyde oxidase, although there is no dehydrogenase form of this molybdozyme.

NAD^+ (dehydrogenase activity) or oxygen (oxidase activity). A similar mechanism of catalysis likely holds true for aldehyde oxidase.

In humans, XD/XO is a cytosolic enzyme that is widely distributed throughout the body, with the highest levels in heart, brain, liver, skeletal muscle, pancreas, small intestine, colon, and placenta. In humans, XD/XO appears to encoded by a single gene. Although the sequences of two enzymes have been reported in the literature, the first report is now known to describe the sequence of human aldehyde oxidase. A complete deficiency of XD/XO (which may also involve a deficiency of aldehyde oxidase) gives rise to the rare genetic disorder known as xanthinuria.

Aldehyde Oxidase Aldehyde oxidase is the second of two molybdozymes that play an important role in xenobiotic biotransformation, the other being xanthine oxidase (discussed in the preceding section). Whereas xanthine oxidase exists in two forms, a dehydrogenase form (XD) that relays electrons to NAD^+ and an oxidase form (XO) that relays electrons to molecular oxygen, aldehyde oxidase exists only in the oxidase form, apparently because it lacks an NAD^+ binding site (Terao et al., 1998). Another significant difference between these two molybdozymes is that high levels of xanthine oxidase appear to be widely distributed throughout the body, whereas high levels of aldehyde oxidase are found in the liver, with considerably less activity in other tissues, at least in humans. Aside from these differences, many of the features of xanthine oxidase apply to aldehyde oxidase, including subcellular location (cytosol), enzyme structure, and cofactor composition, mechanism of catalysis, preference for oxidizing carbon atoms adjacent to the nitrogen atoms in nitrogen heterocycles, and its preference for oxidizing aromatic aldehydes over aliphatic aldehydes. Furthermore, aldehyde oxidase also transfers electrons to molecular oxygen, which can generate reactive oxygen species and lead to oxidative stress and lipid peroxidation. Therefore, the pathophysiologic features described for xanthine oxidase may similarly apply to aldehyde oxidase, especially in the case of ethanol-induced liver damage.

As shown in Fig. 6-21, aldehyde oxidase can oxidize a number of substituted pyrroles, pyridines, pyrimidines, purines, pteridines, and iminium ions by a mechanism that is presumably similar to that described for xanthine oxidase in the previous section. Aldehyde oxidase can oxidize aldehydes to their corresponding carboxylic acids, but the enzyme shows a marked preference for aromatic aldehydes (e.g., benzaldehyde, tamoxifen aldehyde). Consequently, aldehyde oxidase contributes negligibly to the oxidation of aliphatic aldehydes, such as acetaldehyde. Rodrigues (1994) found that, in a bank of human liver samples, aldehyde oxidase activity toward N^1-methylnicotinamide varied more than 40-fold, whereas activity toward 6-methylpurine varied less than 3-fold. Although this suggests that human liver cytosol contains two or more forms of aldehyde oxidase, subsequent Southern blot analysis has provided evidence for only a single copy of the aldehyde oxidase gene in humans (Terao et al., 1998). On the other hand, two aldehyde oxidase genes have been identified in mice.

A number of physiologically important aldehydes are substrates for aldehyde oxidase, including homovanillyl aldehyde (formed from dopamine), 5-hydroxy-3-indoleacetaldehyde (formed from serotonin), and retinal, which is converted by aldehyde oxidase to retinoic acid, an important regulator of cell growth, differentiation, and morphogenesis. The catabolism of catecholamines by monoamine oxidase produces dihydromandelaldehyde, which is oxidized by aldehyde oxidase to dihydromandelic acid. Therefore, aldehyde oxidase plays an important role in the catabolism of biogenic amines and catecholamines. In humans, the gene for aldehyde oxidase has been mapped to chromosome 2q22-q33, placing it near a genetic marker that cosegregates with the recessive familial form of amyotrophic lateral sclerosis. In mouse brain, aldehyde oxidase is localized in the choroid plexus and motor neurons, which lends further support to the proposal that aldehyde oxidase is a candidate gene for this particular motor neuron disease (Bendotti et al., 1997). Furthermore, combined deficiency of molybdoproteins, which affects aldehyde oxidase and XD/XO, leads to an impairment in the development of the central nervous system and is accompanied by severe neurologic symptoms.

In general, xenobiotics that are good substrates for aldehyde oxidase are poor substrates for cytochrome P450, and vice versa (Rettie and Fisher, 1999). Naphthalene (with no nitrogen atoms) is oxidized by cytochrome P450 but not by aldehyde oxidase, whereas the opposite is true of pteridine (1,3,5,8-tetraazanaphthalene), which contains four nitrogen atoms. The intermediate structure, quinazolone (1,3-diazanaphthalene) is a substrate for both enzymes. This complementarity in substrate specificity reflects the opposing preference of the two enzymes for oxidizing carbon atoms; cytochrome P450 prefers to oxidize carbon atoms with high electron density, whereas aldehyde oxidase (and XD/XO) prefers to oxidize carbon atoms with low electron density. The substrate specificity of aldehyde oxidase differs among mammalian species, with substrate size being the main differentiating factor. The active site of human aldehyde oxidase accommodates much smaller substrates than rabbit or guinea pig aldehyde oxidase. Substituents on a substrate that increase electronegativity tend to enhance V_{max}, whereas substituents that increase lipophilicity tend to increase affinity (decrease K_m). Another interesting species difference is that dogs possess little or no aldehyde oxidase activity. However, aldehyde oxidase in human liver has proven to be rather unstable, which complicates an in vitro assessment of species differences in aldehyde oxidase activity (Rodrigues, 1994; Rettie and Fisher, 1999). A further complication is the observation of species differences in the relative roles of aldehyde oxidase and XD/XO in xenobiotic biotransformation. For example, the 6-oxidation of antiviral deoxyguanine prodrugs is catalyzed exclusively in rats by XD/XO, but by aldehyde oxidase in humans (Rettie and Fisher, 1999).

Aldehyde oxidase is the second of two enzymes involved in the formation of cotinine, a major metabolite of nicotine excreted in the urine of cigarette smokers. The initial step in this reaction is the formation of a double bond (C=N) in the pyrrole ring, which produces nicotine $\Delta^{1',5'}$-iminium ion. Like nicotine, several other drugs are oxidized either sequentially or concomitantly by cytochrome P450 and aldehyde oxidase, including quinidine, azapetine, cyclophosphamide, carbazeran, and prolintane. Other drugs that are oxidized by aldehyde oxidase include bromonidine (an α_2-adrenoceptor agonist), O^6-benzylguanine (a cancer chemotherapeutic agent), quinine (an antimalarial), pyrazinamide (a tuberculostatic agent), methotrexate (an antineoplastic and immunosuppressive agent) and famciclovir (an antiviral prodrug that is converted by aldehyde oxidase to penciclovir). Several pyrimidine derivatives are oxidized by aldehyde oxidase, including 5-ethyl-2(1*H*)-pyrimidone, which is converted by aldehyde oxidase to 5-ethynyluracil. Like Sorivudine, 5-ethynyluracil is a metabolism-dependent (suicide) inactivator of dihydropyrimidine dehydrogenase (see Fig. 6-14).

Menadione, hydralazine, methadone and proadifen are inhibitors of aldehyde oxidase. Menadione is a potent inhibitor of aldehyde oxidase (Ki ~0.1 μM) and can be used together with allopurinol to discriminate between aldehyde oxidase- and xanthine oxidase-catalyzed reactions. Hydralazine has been used to assess the role of aldehyde oxidase in human drug metabolism in vivo. The ability of proadifen to inhibit aldehyde oxidase is noteworthy because this methadone analog, commonly known as SKF 525A, is widely used as a cytochrome P450 inhibitor.

Under certain conditions, aldehyde oxidase and xanthine oxidase can also catalyze the reduction of xenobiotics, including azo-reduction (e.g., 4-dimethylaminoazobenzene), nitro-reduction (e.g., 1-nitropyrene), *N*-oxide reduction (e.g., *S*-(-)-nicotine-1′-*N*-oxide), nitrosamine reduction (e.g., *N*-nitrosodiphenylamine), hydroxamic acid reduction (e.g., *N*-hydroxy-2-acetylaminofluorene), sulfoxide reduction [e.g., sulindac (see Fig. 6-12)] and epoxide reduction [e.g., benzo(9a)pyrene 4,5-oxide]. Oximes (C=NOH) can also be reduced by aldehyde oxidase to the corresponding ketimines (C=NH), which may react nonenzymatically with water to produce the corresponding ketone or aldehyde (C=O) and ammonia. An analogous reaction allows aldehyde oxidase to catalyze the reductive ring-opening of Zonisamide and 1,2-benzisoxazole, which results in formation of an oxo-containing metabolite and ammonia (Sugihara et al., 1996). Xenobiotic reduction by aldehyde oxidase requires anaerobic conditions or the presence of a reducing substrate, such as N^1-methylnicotinamide, 2-hydroxypyrimidine or benzaldehyde. These "cosubstrates" reduce the enzyme, which in turn catalyzes azo-reduction, nitro-reduction, etc., by relaying electrons to xenobiotics (rather than molecular oxygen). These unusual requirements make it difficult to assess the degree to which aldehyde oxidase functions as a reductive enzyme in vivo.

Monoamine Oxidase, Diamine Oxidase, and Polyamine Oxidase Monoamine oxidase (MAO), diamine oxidase (DAO), and polyamine oxidase (PAO) are all involved in the oxidative deamination of primary, secondary, and tertiary amines (Weyler et al., 1992; Benedetti and Dostert, 1994). Substrates for these enzymes include several naturally occurring amines, such as the monoamine serotonin (5-hydroxytryptamine), the diamines putrescine and histamine, and monoacetylated derivatives of the polyamines spermine and spermidine. A number of xenobiotics are substrates for these enzymes, particularly MAO. Oxidative deamination of a primary amine produces ammonia and an aldehyde, whereas oxidative deamination of a secondary amine produces a primary amine and an aldehyde. [The products of the former reaction (i.e., an aldehyde and ammonia) are those produced during the reductive biotransformation of certain oximes by aldehyde oxidase, as described in the preceding section on aldehyde oxidase]. The aldehydes formed by MAO are usually oxidized further by other enzymes to the corresponding carboxylic acids, although in some cases they are reduced to alcohols. Examples of reactions catalyzed by MAO, DAO, and PAO are shown in Fig. 6-23. Monoamine oxidase is located throughout the brain and is present in the liver, kidney, intestine, and blood platelets in the outer membrane of mitochondria. Its substrates include milacemide (Fig. 6-23), a dealkylated metabolite of propranolol (Fig. 6-23), primaquine, haloperidol, doxylamine, β-phenylethylamine, tyramine, catecholamines (dopamine, norepinephrine, epinephrine), tryptophan derivatives (tryptamine, serotonin), and tryptophan analogs known as triptans, which include the antimigraine drugs sumatriptan, zolmitriptan, and rizatriptan.

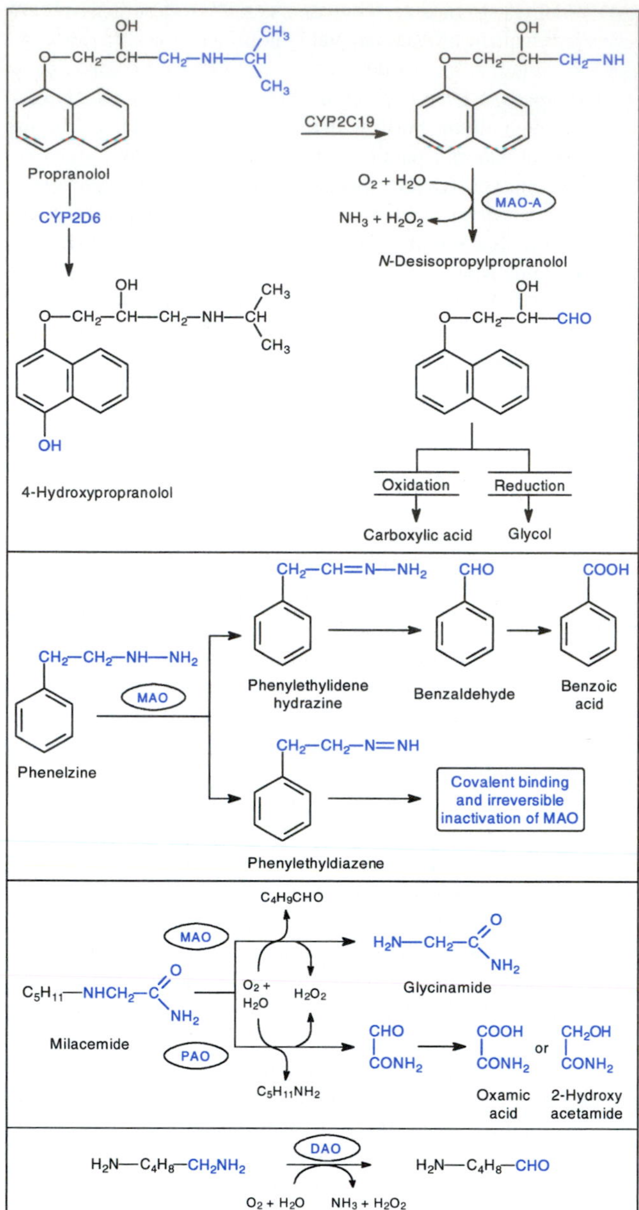

Figure 6-23. Examples of reactions catalyzed by monoamine oxidase (MAO), diamine oxidase (DAO), and polyamine oxidase (PAO).

Note that pheneizine is a metabolism-dependent (mechanism-based) inhibitor of MAO-A and MAO-B.

There are two forms of monoamine oxidase, called MAO-A and MAO-B. MAO-A preferentially oxidizes serotonin (5-hydroxytryptamine), norepinephrine, and the dealkylated metabolite of propranolol. It is preferentially inhibited by clorgyline, whereas MAO-B preferentially oxidizes β-phenylethylamine and benzylamine and is preferentially inhibited by *l*-deprenyl (selegiline). Species differences in the substrate specificity of MAO have been documented. For example, dopamine is oxidized by MAO-B in humans but by MAO-A in rats and by both enzymes in several other mammalian species. Most tissues contain both forms of the enzyme, each encoded by a distinct gene, although some tissues express only one MAO. In humans, for example, only MAO-A is expressed in the placenta, whereas only MAO-B is expressed in blood platelets and lymphocytes. The distribution of MAO in the brain shows little species variation, with the highest concentration of MAO-A in the locus ceruleus and the highest concentration of MAO-B in the raphe nuclei. MAO-A is expressed predominantly in catecholaminergic neurons, whereas MAO-B is expressed largely in serotonergic and histaminergic neurons and glial cells. The distribution of MAO throughout the brain does not always parallel that of its substrates. For example, serotonin is preferentially oxidized by MAO-A, but MAO-A is not found in serotonergic neurons.

MAO-A and -B are encoded by two distinct genes, both localized on the X-chromosome (Xp11.23) and both comprising 15 exons with an identical intron-exon organization, which suggests they are derived from a common ancestral gene (Shih et al., 1999). The amino acid sequence of MAO-A (Mr 59.7 kDa) is 70 percent identical to that of MAO-B (Mr 58.0 kDa). The deletion of both MAO-A and -B gives rise to Norrie disease, an X-linked recessive neurologic disorder characterized by blindness, hearing loss, and mental retardation (Shih et al., 1999). Selective loss of MAO-A (due a point mutation) gives rise to abnormal aggressiveness, whereas alterations in MAO-B have been implicated in Parkinson's disease (discussed later in this section).

The mechanism of catalysis by monoamine oxidase is illustrated below:

$$RCH_2NH_2 + FAD \rightarrow RCH{=}NH + FADH_2$$

$$RCH{=}NH + H_2O \rightarrow RCHO + NH_3$$

$$FADH_2 + O_2 \rightarrow FAD + H_2O_2$$

The substrate is oxidized by the enzyme, which itself is reduced ($FAD \rightarrow FADH_2$). The oxygen incorporated into the substrate is derived from water, not molecular oxygen; hence the enzyme functions as a true oxidase. The catalytic cycle is completed by reoxidation of the reduced enzyme ($FADH_2 \rightarrow FAD$) by oxygen, which generates hydrogen peroxide (which may be a cause of oxidative stress). The initial step in the catalytic cycle appears to be abstraction of hydrogen from the α-carbon adjacent to the nitrogen atom; hence, the oxidative deamination of xenobiotics by MAO is generally blocked by substitution of the α-carbon. For example, amphetamine and other phenylethylamine derivatives carrying a methyl group on the α-carbon atom are not oxidized well by MAO. (Amphetamines can undergo oxidative deamination, but the reaction is catalyzed by cytochrome P450.) The abstraction of hydrogen from the α-carbon adjacent to the nitrogen atom can occur stereospecifically; therefore, only one enantiomer of an α-substituted compound may be oxidized by MAO. For example, whereas MAO-B catalyzes the oxidative deamination of both *R*- and *S*-β-phenylethylamine, only the *R*-enantiomer is a substrate for MAO-A. The oxidative deamination of the dealkylated metabolite of propranolol is catalyzed stereoselectively by MAO-A, although in this case the preferred substrate is the *S*-enantiomer (which has the same absolute configuration as the *R*-enantiomer of β-phenylethylamine) (Benedetti and Dostert, 1994).

Clorgyline and *l*-deprenyl (selegiline) are metabolism-dependent inhibitors (i.e., mechanism-based or suicide inactivators) of MAO-A and MAO-B, respectively. Both enzymes are irreversibly inhibited by phenelzine, a hydrazine that can be oxidized either by abstraction of hydrogen from the α-carbon atom, which leads to oxidative deamination with formation of benzaldehyde and benzoic acid, or by abstraction of hydrogen from the terminal nitrogen atom, which leads to formation of phenylethyldiazene and covalent modification of the enzyme, as shown in Fig. 6-23.

Monoamine oxidase has received considerable attention for its role in the activation of MPTP (1-methyl-4-phenyl-1,2,5,6-tetrahydropyridine) to a neurotoxin that causes symptoms characteristic of Parkinson's disease in humans and monkeys but not rodents (Gerlach et al., 1991). In 1983, Parkinsonism was observed in young individuals who, in attempting to synthesize and use a narcotic drug related to meperidine (demerol), instead synthesized and self-administered MPTP, which causes selective destruction of dopaminergic neurons in the substantia nigra. MPTP crosses the blood–brain barrier, where is it oxidized by MAO in the astrocytes (a type of glial cell) to 1-methyl-4-phenyl-2,3-dihydropyridine ($MPDP^+$), which in turn autooxidizes to the neurotoxic metabolite, 1-methyl-4-phenylpyridine MPP^+, as shown in Fig. 6-24. Because it is transported by the dopamine transporter, MPP^+ concentrates in dopaminergic neurons, where it impairs mitochondrial respiration. The neurotoxic effects of MPTP can be blocked with pargyline (an inhibitor of both MAO-A and MAO-B) and by *l*-deprenyl (a selective inhibitor of MAO-B) but not by clorgyline (a selective inhibitor of MAO-A). This suggests that the activation of MPTP to its neurotoxic metabolite is catalyzed predominantly by MAO-B. This interpretation is consistent with the recent finding that MAO-B knockout mice (i.e., transgenic mice that lack MAO-B) do not sustain damage to the dopaminergic terminals of nigrostriatal neurons after MPTP treatment (Shih et al., 1999).

Genetic and environmental factors both appear to play important roles in the etiology of Parkinson's disease. Apart from MPTP, parkinsongenic neurotoxins to which humans are exposed have not been identified unequivocally, hence, the environmental factors that cause Parkinson's disease remain to be identified. It is interesting that the bipyridyl herbicide paraquat is similar in structure to the toxic metabolite of MPTP, as shown in Fig. 6-24. Some epidemiologic studies have shown a positive correlation between herbicide exposure and the incidence of Parkinsonism in some but not all rural communities. Haloperidol can also be converted to a potentially neurotoxic pyridinium metabolite (Subramanyam et al., 1991).

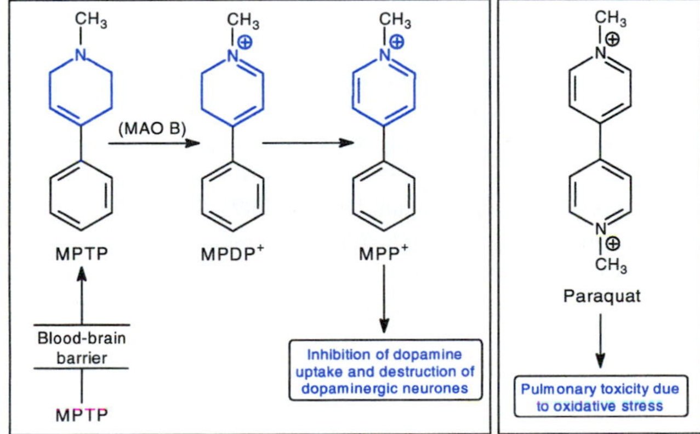

***Figure 6-24.** Activation of MPTP (1-methyl-4-phenyl-1,2,5,6-tetrahydropyridine) to the neurotoxic metabolite, MPP^+(1-methyl-4-phenylpyridine), by monoamine oxidase B.*

The toxic pyridinium metabolite, MPP^+, is structurally similar to the herbicide paraquat. $MPDP^+$, 1-methyl-4-phenyl-2,3-dihydropyridine.

MAO-B may be among the genetic factors that affect susceptibility to Parkinson's disease. MAO-B activity in the human brain increases with aging, perhaps due to a proliferation of glial cells. It has been proposed that increased oxidation of dopamine by MAO-B in the elderly may lead to a loss of dopaminergic neurons in the substantia nigra, which underlies Parkinson's disease. Such damage may be caused by the oxidative stress associated with the oxidative deamination of dopamine by MAO-B. In support of this proposal, it has been found that patients with Parkinson's disease have elevated MAO-B activity in the substantia nigra, and the MAO-B inhibitor *l*-deprenyl (selegiline) delays the progression of symptoms (Sano et al., 1997). Furthermore, there are allelic variants of MAO-B, some of which (such as allele 1 and allele B4) appear to be associated with an increased risk of developing Parkinson's disease (Shih et al., 1999). No such association has been found between Parkinson's disease and MAO-A gene polymorphisms. Recently, cigarette smoking, which carries a number of health risks, has been shown nevertheless to provide some protection against Parkinson's disease (Gorell et al., 1999). Although the mechanism of protection remains to be determined, it is interesting to note that cigarette smokers are known to have decreased levels of MAO-B (and MAO-A) (Shih et al., 1999), the degree of which is proportional to cigarette usage (i.e., it is dose-related) (Whitfield et al., 2000).

MAO-A knockout mice have elevated brain levels of serotonin and a distinct behavioral syndrome, including enhanced aggression in adult males. The enhanced aggressive behavior exhibited by MAO-A knockout mice is consistent with the abnormal aggressive behavior in individuals who lack MAO-A activity due to a point mutation in the MAO-A gene (Shih et al., 1999). Other polymorphisms in the MAO-A gene appear to be risk modifiers for alcoholism among Euro-Americans and Han Chinese (Shih et al., 1999). MAO-B may also be a factor in alcoholism, inasmuch as alcoholics (especially male type 2 alcoholics) tend to have lower MAO activity in platelets, which contain only MAO-B. However, MAO-B activity is not lower in alcoholics when cigarette smoking status is taken into account, which suggests that MAO-B activity tends to be lower in alcoholics because smoking and alcohol and dependence are strongly associated with each other (Whitfield et al., 2000).

Although not present in mitochondria, PAO resembles MAO in its cofactor requirement and basic mechanism of action. Both enzymes use oxygen as an electron acceptor, which results in the production of hydrogen peroxide. The MAO inhibitor pargyline also inhibits PAO. The anticonvulsant milacemide is one of the few xenobiotic substrates for PAO, although it is also a substrate for MAO (Fig. 6-23). By converting milacemide to glycine (via glycinamide), MAO plays an important role in anticonvulsant therapy with milacemide (Benedetti and Dostert, 1994).

Diamine oxidase is a cytosolic, copper-containing pyridoxal phosphate-dependent enzyme present in liver, kidney, intestine, and placenta. Its preferred substrates include histamine and simple alkyl diamines with a chain length of four (putrescine) or five (cadaverine) carbon atoms. Diamines with carbon chains longer than nine are not substrates for DAO, although they can be oxidized by MAO. DAO or a similar enzyme is present in cardiovascular tissue and appears to be responsible for the cardiotoxic effects of allylamine, which is converted by oxidative deamination to acrolein. Although histamine is a substrate for DAO, there is little or no DAO in brain (nor is there a receptor-mediated uptake system for histamine, in contrast to other neurotransmitters). For this reason, the major pathway of histamine metabolism in the brain is by methylation (see "Methylation," below).

Aromatization The conversion of MPTP to MPP^+ (Fig. 6-24) is an example of a reaction involving the introduction of multiple double bonds to achieve some semblance of aromaticity (in this case, formation of a pyridinium ion). Aromatization of xenobiotics is an unusual reaction, but some examples have been documented. A mitochondrial enzyme in guinea pig and rabbit liver can oxidize several cyclohexane derivatives to the corresponding aromatic hydrocarbon, as shown in Fig. 6-25 for the aromatization of cyclohexane carboxylic acid (hexahydrobenzoic acid) to benzoic acid. Mitochondria from rat liver are less active, and those from cat, mouse, dog, monkey, and human are completely inactive. The reaction requires magnesium, coenzyme A, oxygen, and ATP. The first step appears to be the formation of hexahydrobenzoyl-CoA, which is then dehydrogenated to the aromatic product. Glycine stimulates the reaction, probably by removing benzoic acid through conjugation to form hippuric acid (a phase II reaction). The conversion of androgens to estrogens involves aromatization of the A-ring of the steroid nucleus. This reaction is catalyzed by CYP19, one of the cytochrome P450 enzymes involved in steroidogenesis.

Peroxidase-Dependent Cooxidation The oxidative biotransformation of xenobiotics generally requires the reduced pyridine nucleotide cofactors NADPH and NADH. An exception is xenobiotic biotransformation by peroxidases, which couple the reduction of hydrogen peroxide and lipid hydroperoxides to the oxidation of other substrates—a process known as *cooxidation* (Eling et al., 1990). Several different peroxidases catalyze the biotransformation of xenobiotics, and these enzymes occur in a variety of tissues and cell types. For example, kidney medulla, platelets, vascular endothelial cells, the GI tract, brain, lung, and urinary bladder epithelium contain prostaglandin H synthase (PHS); mammary gland epithelium contains lactoperoxidase; and leukocytes contain myeloperoxidase. PHS is one of the most extensively studied peroxidase involved in the xenobiotic biotransformation. This enzyme possesses two catalytic activities: a *cyclooxygenase* that converts arachidonic acid to the cyclic endoperoxide-hydroperoxide PGG_2 (which involves the addition of two molecules of oxygen to each molecule of arachidonic acid) and a *peroxidase* that converts the hydroperoxide to the corresponding alcohol PGH_2 (which can be accompanied by the oxidation of xenobiotics). The conversion of arachidonic acid to PGH_2, which is subsequently converted to a variety of eicosanoids (prostaglandins, thromboxane, and prostacyclin), is shown in Fig. 6-26. PHS and other peroxidases play an important role in the activation of xenobiotics to toxic or tumorigenic metabolites, particularly in extrahepatic tissues that contain low levels of cytochrome P450 (Eling et al., 1990).

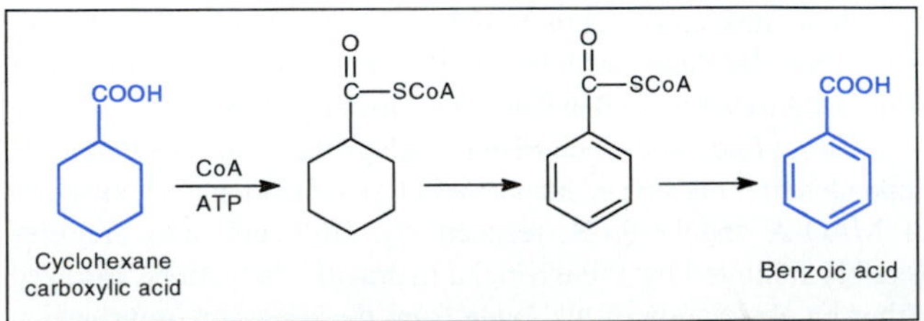

COOH
CoA
ATP
C(=O)—SCoA
C(=O)—SCoA
COOH
Cyclohexane carboxylic acid
Benzoic acid

Figure 6-25. Aromatization of cyclohexane carboxylic acid, a reaction catalyzed by rabbit and guinea pig liver mitochondria.

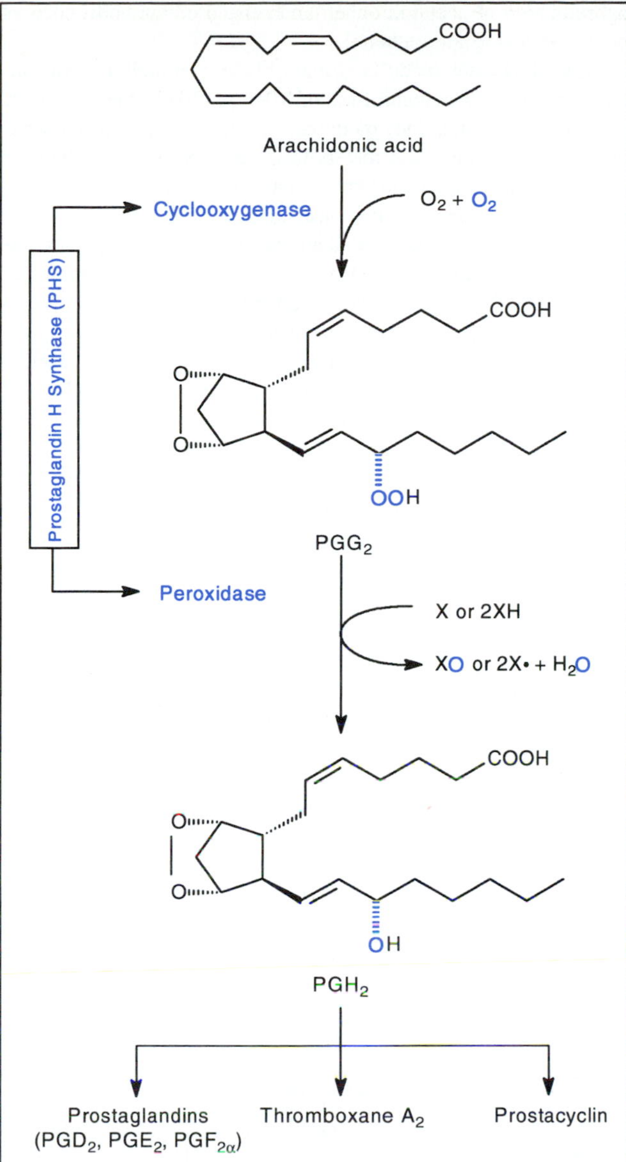

Figure 6-26. Cooxidation of xenobiotics (X) during the conversion of arachidonic acid to PGH_2 by prostaglandin H synthase.

In certain cases, the oxidation of xenobiotics by peroxidases involves direct transfer of the peroxide oxygen to the xenobiotic, as shown in Fig. 6-26 for the conversion of substrate X to product XO. An example of this type of reaction is the PHS-catalyzed epoxidation of benzo[a]pyrene 7,8-dihydrodiol to the corresponding 9,10-epoxide (see Fig. 6-6). Although PHS can catalyze the final step (i.e., 9,10-epoxidation) in the formation of this tumorigenic metabolite of benzo[a]pyrene, it cannot catalyze the initial step (i.e., 7,8-epoxidation), which is catalyzed by cytochrome P450. The 9,10-epoxidation of benzo[a]pyrene 7,8-dihydrodiol can also be catalyzed by 15-lipoxygenase, which is present at high concentrations in human pulmonary epithelial cells, and by peroxyl radicals formed during lipid peroxidation in skin. Cytochrome P450 and peroxyl radicals formed by PHS, lipoxygenase, and/or lipid peroxidation may all play a role in activating benzo[a]pyrene to metabolites that cause lung and skin tumors. These same enzymes can also catalyze the 8,9-epoxidation of aflatoxin B_1, which is one of the most potent hepatotumorigens known. Epoxidation by cytochrome P450 is thought to be primarily responsible for the hepatotumorigenic effects of aflatoxin B_1. However, aflatoxin B_1 also causes neoplasia of rat renal papilla. This tissue has very low levels of cytochrome P450, but contains relatively high levels of PHS, which is suspected, therefore, of mediating the nephrotumorigenic effects of aflatoxin (Fig. 6-27).

The direct transfer of the peroxide oxygen from a hydroperoxide to a xenobiotic is not the only mechanism of xenobiotic oxidation by peroxidases, nor is it the most common. As shown in

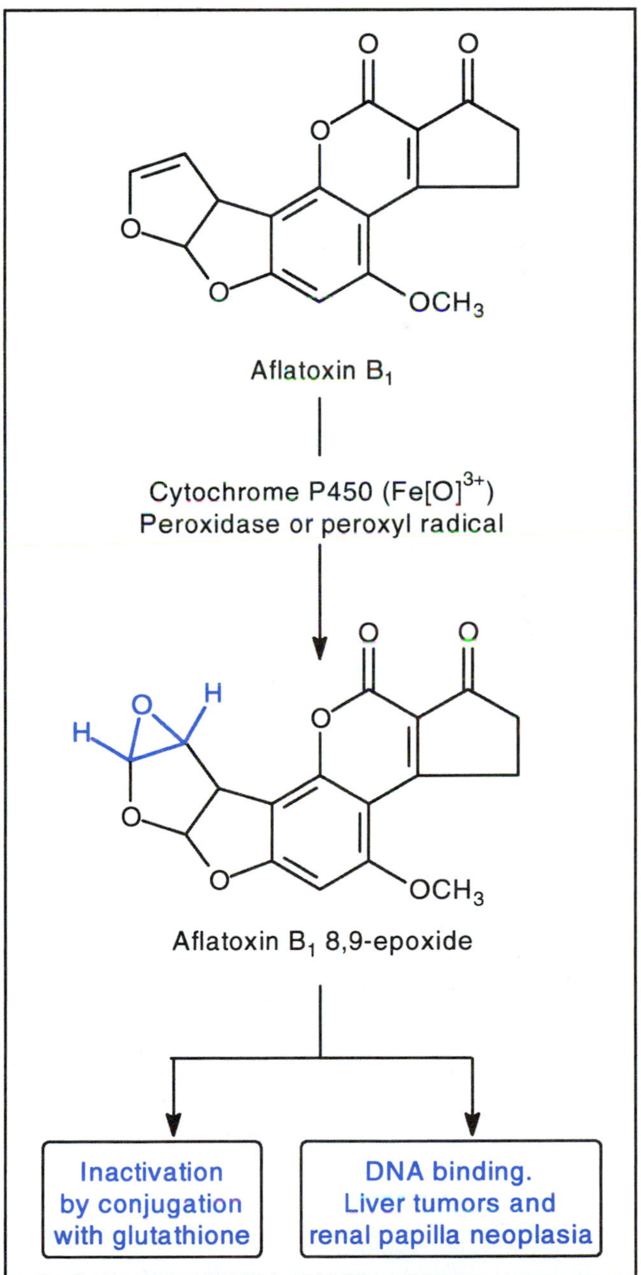

Figure 6-27. Activation of aflatoxin B_1 by cytochrome P450, leading to liver tumor formation, and by peroxidases, leading to renal papilla neoplasia.

Fig. 6-26, xenobiotics that can serve as electron donors, such as amines and phenols, can be oxidized to free radicals during the reduction of a hydroperoxide. In this case, the hydroperoxide is still converted to the corresponding alcohol, but the peroxide oxygen is reduced to water instead of being incorporated into the xenobiotic. For each molecule of hydroperoxide reduced (which is a two-electron process), two molecules of xenobiotic can be oxidized (each by a one-electron process). Important classes of compounds that undergo one-electron oxidation reactions by peroxidase include aromatic amines, phenols, hydroquinones, and polycyclic hydrocarbons. Many of the metabolites produced are reactive electrophiles. For example, polycyclic aromatic hydrocarbons, phenols, and hydroquinones are oxidized to electrophilic quinones. Acetaminophen is similarly converted to a quinoneimine, namely *N*-acetyl-benzoquinoneimine, a cytotoxic electrophile that binds to cellular proteins, as shown in Fig. 6-28. The formation of this toxic metabolite by cytochrome P450 causes centrilobular necrosis of the liver. However, acetaminophen can also damage the kidney medulla, which contains low levels of cytochrome P450 but relatively high levels of PHS; hence, PHS may play a significant role in the nephrotoxicity of acetaminophen. The two-electron oxidation of acetaminophen to *N*-acetyl-benzoquinoneimine by PHS likely involves the formation of a one-electron oxidation product, namely *N*-acetyl-benzosemiquinoneimine radical. Formation of this semiquinoneimine radical by PHS likely contributes to the nephrotoxicity of acetaminophen and related compounds, such as phenacetin and 4-aminophenol.

Like the kidney medulla, urinary bladder epithelium also contains low levels of cytochrome P450 but relatively high levels of PHS. Just as PHS in kidney medulla can activate aflatoxin and acetaminophen to nephrotoxic metabolites, so PHS in urinary bladder epithelium can activate certain aromatic amines—such as benzidine, 4-aminobiphenyl, and 2-aminonaphthalene—to DNA-reactive metabolites that cause bladder cancer in certain species, including humans and dogs. PHS can convert aromatic amines to reactive radicals, which can undergo nitrogen–nitrogen or nitrogen–carbon coupling reactions, or they can undergo a second one-electron oxidation to reactive diimines. Binding of these reactive metabolites to DNA is presumed to be the underlying mechanism by which several aromatic amines cause bladder cancer in humans and dogs. In some cases the one-electron oxidation of an amine leads to *N*-dealkylation. For example, PHS catalyzes the *N*-demethylation of aminopyrine, although in vivo this reaction is mainly catalyzed by cytochrome P450. In contrast to cytochrome P450, PHS does not catalyze the *N*-hydroxylation of aromatic amines.

Many of the aromatic amines known or suspected of causing bladder cancer in humans have been shown to cause bladder tumors in dogs. In rats, however, aromatic amines cause liver tumors by a process that involves *N*-hydroxylation by cytochrome P450,

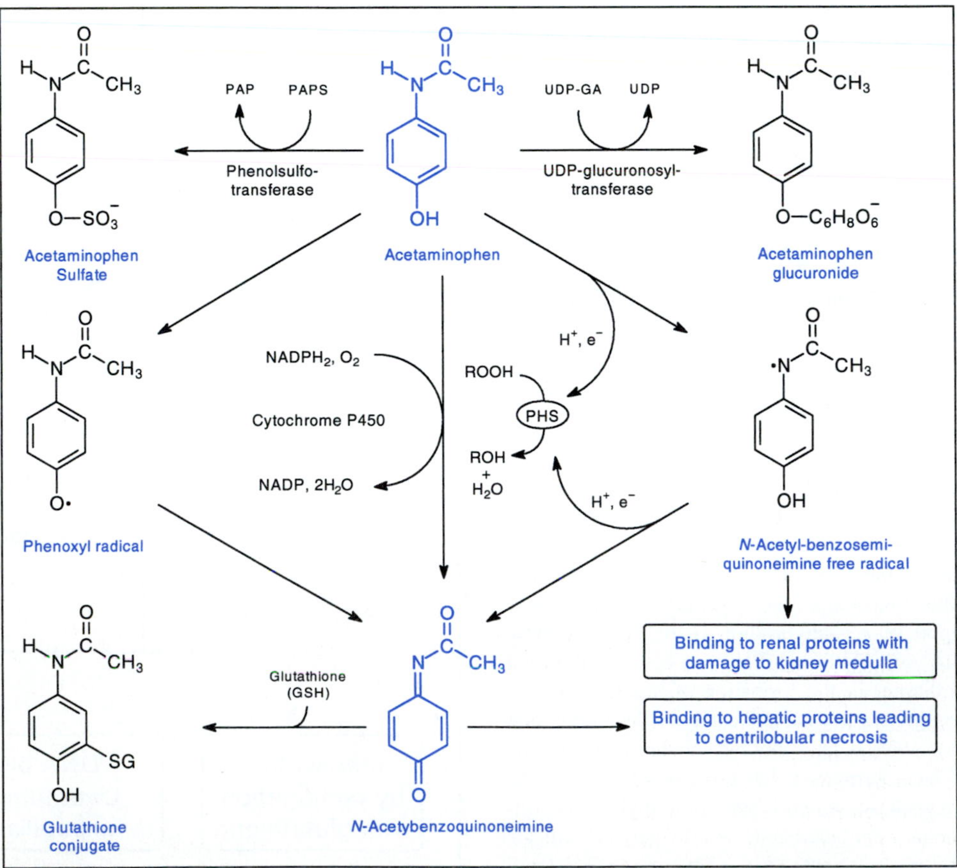

Figure 6-28. Activation of acetaminophen by cytochrome P450, leading to hepatotoxicity, and by prostaglandin H synthase (PHS), leading to nephrotoxicity.

Conjugation with sulfate, glucuronic acid, or glutathione represent detoxication reactions.

followed by conjugation with acetate or sulfate, as shown in Fig. 6-9. This species difference has complicated an assessment of the role of PHS in aromatic amine-induced bladder cancer, because such experiments must be carried out in dogs. However, another class of compounds, the 5-nitrofurans, such as *N*-[4-(5-nitro-2-furyl)-2-thiazole]formamide (FANFT) and its deformylated analog 2-amino-4-(5-nitro-2-furyl)thiazole (ANFT), are substrates for PHS and are potent bladder tumorigens in rats. The tumorigenicity of FANFT is thought to involve deformylation to ANFT, which is oxidized to DNA-reactive metabolites by PHS. The ability of FANFT to cause bladder tumors in rats is blocked by the PHS cyclooxygenase inhibitor aspirin, which suggests that PHS plays an important role in the metabolic activation and tumorigenicity of this nitrofuran. Unexpectedly, combined treatment of rats with FANFT and aspirin causes forestomach tumors, which are not observed when either compound is administered alone. This example underscores the complexity of chemically induced tumor formation. A further complication in interpreting this result is the recent finding that there are two forms of cyclooxygenase: COX-1, which is constitutively expressed in several tissues, and COX-2, which is inducible by growth factors and mediators of inflammation. Increased expression of the latter isozyme has been documented in a number of tumors, including human colorectal, gastric, esophageal, pulmonary, and pancreatic carcinomas (Gupta and DuBois, 1998; Molina et al., 1999). Aspirin and other NSAIDs block the formation of colon cancer in experimental animals, and there is epidemiological evidence that chronic NSAID usage decreases the incidence of colorectal cancer in humans (Gupta and DuBois, 1998). The incidence of intestinal neoplasms in $Apc^{\Delta 716}$ knockout mice is dramatically suppressed by crossing these transgenic animals with COX-2 knockout mice (Oshima et al., 1996). From these few examples it is apparent that cyclooxygenase may play at least two distinct roles in tumor formation—it may convert certain xenobiotics to DNA-reactive metabolites (and thereby *initiate* tumor formation), and it may somehow *promote* subsequent tumor growth, perhaps through formation of growth-promoting eicosanoids.

Many phenolic compounds can serve as reducing substrates for PHS peroxidase. The phenoxyl radicals produced by one-electron oxidation reactions can undergo a variety of reactions, including binding to critical nucleophiles, such as protein and DNA; reduction by antioxidants such as glutathione; and self-coupling. The reactions of phenoxyl radicals are analogous to those of the nitrogen-centered free radicals produced during the one-electron oxidation of aromatic amines by PHS. Peroxidases appear to play an important role in the bone marrow suppression produced by chronic exposure to benzene. Liver cytochrome P450 converts benzene to phenol, which in turn is oxidized to hydroquinone, which can be converted to DNA-reactive metabolites by PHS in bone marrow and by myeloperoxidase in bone marrow leukocytes. The myelosuppressive effect of benzene can be blocked by the PHS inhibitor indomethacin, which suggests an important role for peroxidase-dependent activation in the myelotoxicity of benzene. The formation of phenol and hydroquinone in the liver is also important for myelosuppression by benzene. However, such bone marrow suppression cannot be achieved simply by administering phenol or hydroquinone to mice, although it can be achieved by coadministering hydroquinone with phenol. Phenol stimulates the PHS-dependent activation of hydroquinone. Therefore, bone marrow suppression by benzene involves the cytochrome P450–dependent oxidation of benzene to phenol and hydroquinone in the liver, followed by phenol-enhanced peroxidative oxidation of hydroquinone to reactive intermediates that bind to protein and DNA in the bone marrow (Fig. 6-29). It is noteworthy that the cytochrome P450 enzyme responsible for hydroxylating benzene has been identified as CYP2E1 (see section on cytochrome P450, below). Although CYP2E1was first identified in liver, this same enzyme has been identified in bone marrow, where it can presumably convert benzene to phenol and possibly hydroquinone (Bernauer et al., 2000). The importance of CYP2E1 in the metabolic activation of benzene was recently confirmed by the demonstration that CYP2E1 knockout mice (null mice) are relatively resistant to the myelosuppressive effects of benzene (Gonzalez and Kimura, 1999; Buters et al., 1999).

The ability of phenol to enhance the peroxidative metabolism of hydroquinone is analogous to the interaction between the phenolic antioxidants butylated hydroxytoluene (BHT), and butylated hydroxyanisole (BHA). In mice, the pulmonary toxicity of BHT, which is a relatively poor substrate for PHS, is enhanced by BHA, which is a relatively good substrate for PHS. The mechanism by which BHA enhances the pulmonary toxicity of BHT appears to involve the peroxidase-dependent conversion of BHA to a phenoxyl radical that interacts with BHT, converting it to a phenoxyl radical (by one-electron oxidation) or a quinone methide (by two-electron oxidation), as shown in Fig. 6-30. Formation of the toxic quinone methide of BHT can also be catalyzed by cytochrome P450, which is largely responsible for activating BHT in the absence of BHA.

Several reducing substrates—such as phenylbutazone, retinoic acid, 3-methylindole, sulfite, and bisulfite—are oxidized by PHS to carbon- or sulfur-centered free radicals that can trap oxygen to form a peroxyl radical, as shown in Fig. 6-31 for phenylbutazone. The peroxyl radical can oxidize xenobiotics in a peroxidative manner. For example, the peroxyl radical of phenylbutazone can convert benzo[a]pyrene 7,8-dihydrodiol to the corresponding 9,10-epoxide.

PHS is unique among peroxidases because it can both generate hydroperoxides and catalyze peroxidase-dependent reactions, as shown in Fig. 6-26. Xenobiotic biotransformation by PHS is

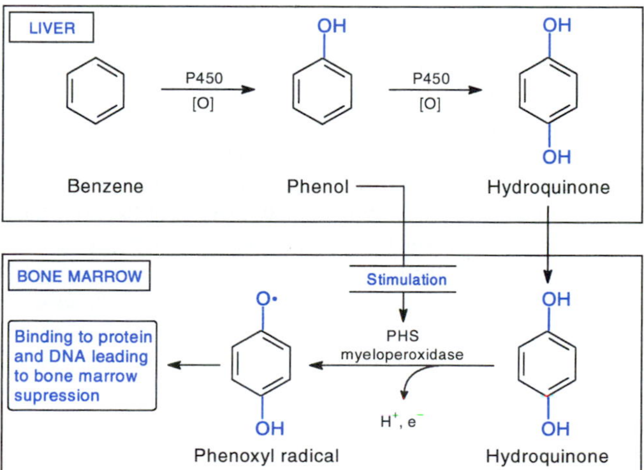

Figure 6-29. Role of cytochrome P450 and peroxidases in the activation of benzene to myelotoxic metabolites.

ABBREVIATION: PHS, prostaglandin H synthase.

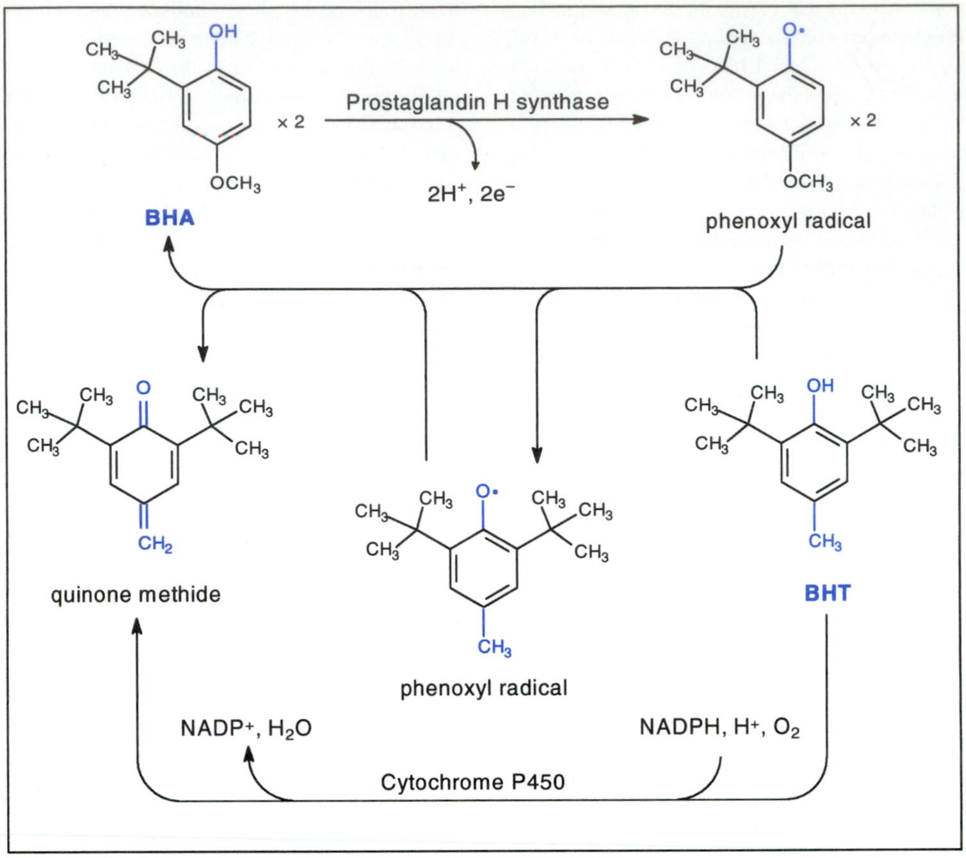

Figure 6-30. Metabolite interaction between the phenolic antioxidants, butylated hydroxytoluene (BHT) and butylated hydroxyanisole (BHA).

Note that activation of BHT to a toxic quinone methide can be catalyzed by cytochrome P450 or, in the presence of BHA, by prostaglandin H synthase.

controlled by the availability of arachidonic acid. The biotransformation of xenobiotics by other peroxidases is controlled by the availability of hydroperoxide substrates. Hydrogen peroxide is a normal product of cellular respiration, and lipid peroxides can form during lipid peroxidation. The levels of these peroxides and their availability for peroxidase reactions depends on the efficiency of hydroperoxide scavenging by glutathione peroxidase and catalase.

Uetrecht and others have implicated myeloperoxidase in the formation of reactive metabolites of drugs that cause agranulocytosis, including clozapine, aminopyrine, vesnarinone, propylthiouracil, dapsone, sulfonamides, procainamide, amodiaquine, and ticlopidine (references to this large body of work can be found in Liu and Uetrecht, 2000). Activation of these drugs involves their oxidation by HOCl, which is the principal oxidant produced by myeloperoxidase (in the presence of hydrogen peroxide and chloride ion) in activated neutrophils and monocytes. In the case of ticlopidine, myeloperoxidase converts the thiophene ring of this antiplatelet drug to a thiophene-*S*-chloride, a reactive metabolite that rearranges to 2-chloroticlopidine (minor) and dehydroticlopidine (major), or reacts with glutathione, as shown in Fig. 6-32. When catalyzed by activated neutrophils, ticlopidine oxidation is inhibited by low concentrations of azide and catalase. When catalyzed by purified myeloperoxidase, ticlopidine oxidation requires hydrogen peroxide and chloride, although all components of this purified system can be replaced with HOCl. It is not known whether drugs that cause agranulocytosis are activated in the bone marrow by neutrophils or their precursors that contain myeloperoxidase or are activated in neutrophils in the general circulation. In the latter case, agranulocytosis would presumably involve an immune response triggered by neoantigens formed in neutrophils by the covalent modification of cellular component by one or more of the reactive metabolites formed by myeloperoxidase.

Flavin Monooxygenases Liver, kidney, and lung contain one or more FAD-containing monooxygenases (FMO) that oxidize the nucleophilic nitrogen, sulfur, and phosphorus heteroatom of a variety of xenobiotics (Ziegler, 1993; Lawton et al., 1994; Cashman, 1995; Rettie and Fisher, 1999; Cashman, 1999). The mammalian FMO gene family comprises five enzymes (designated FMO1 to FMO5) that contain about 550 amino acid residues each and are 50 to 58 percent identical in amino acid sequence across species lines. Each FMO enzyme contains a highly conserved glycine-rich region (residues 4 to 32) that binds 1 mole of FAD (noncovalently) near the active site, which is adjacent to a second highly conserved glycine-rich region (residues 186 to 213) that binds NADPH.

Like cytochrome P450, the FMOs are microsomal enzymes that require NADPH and O_2, and many of the reactions catalyzed by FMO can also be catalyzed by cytochrome P450. Several in vitro techniques have been developed to distinguish reactions catalyzed by FMO from those catalyzed by cytochrome P450. In con-

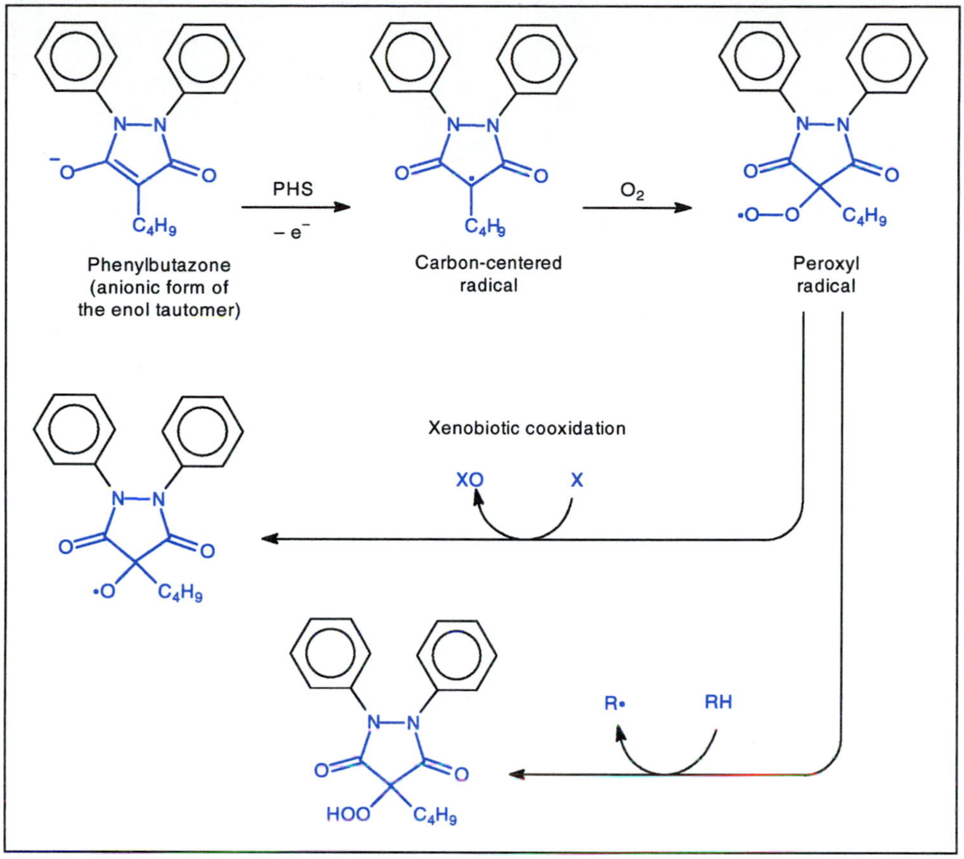

Figure 6-31. Oxidation of phenylbutazone by prostaglandin H synthase (PHS) to a carbon-centered radical and peroxyl radical.

Note that the peroxyl radical can oxidize xenobiotics (X) in a peroxidative manner.

trast to cytochrome P450, FMO is heat-labile and can be inactivated in the absence of NADPH by warming microsomes to 50°C for 1 min. By comparison, cytochrome P450 can be inactivated with nonionic detergent, such as 1% Emulgen 911, which has a minimal effect on FMO activity. The pH optimum for FMO-catalyzed reactions (pH 8 to 10) tends to be higher than that for most (but not all) P450 reactions (pH 7 to 8). Antibodies raised against purified P450 enzymes can be used not only to establish the role of cytochrome P450 in a microsomal reaction but also to identify which particular P450 enzyme catalyzes the reaction. In contrast, antibodies raised against purified FMO do not inhibit the enzyme. The use of chemical inhibitors to ascertain the relative contribution of FMO and cytochrome P450 to microsomal reactions is often complicated by a lack of specificity. For example, cimetidine and SKF 525A, which are well-recognized cytochrome P450 inhibitors, are both substrates for FMO. Conversely, the FMO inhibitor methimazole is known to inhibit several of the P450 enzymes in human liver microsomes (namely CYP2B6, CYP2C9, and CYP3A4). The situation is further complicated by the observation that the various forms of FMO differ in their thermal stability and sensitivity to detergents and other chemical modulators (examples of which are described later in this section).

FMO catalyzes the oxidation of nucleophilic tertiary amines to *N*-oxides, secondary amines to hydroxylamines and nitrones, and primary amines to hydroxylamines and oximes. Amphetamine, benzydamine, chlorpromazine, clozapine, guanethidine, imipramine, methamphetamine, olanzapine, and tamoxifen are examples of nitrogen-containing drugs that are *N*-oxygenated by FMO (and by cytochrome P450 in most cases). FMO also oxidizes several sulfur-containing xenobiotics (such as thiols, thioethers, thiones, and thiocarbamates) and phosphines to *S*- and *P*-oxides, respectively. Cimetidine and sulindac sulfide are examples of sulfur-containing drugs that are converted to sulfoxides by FMO. (Fig. 6-12 shows how sulindac is reduced to sulindac sulfide, only to be oxidized by FMO back to the parent drug in what is often called a futile cycle.) Hydrazines, iodides, selenides, and boron-containing compounds are also substrates for FMO. Examples of FMO-catalyzed reactions are shown in Fig. 6-33*A* and *B*.

In general, the metabolites produced by FMO are the products of a chemical reaction between a xenobiotic and a peracid or peroxide, which is consistent with the mechanism of catalysis of FMO (discussed later in this section). The reactions catalyzed by FMO are generally detoxication reactions, although there are exceptions to this rule, described below (this section). Inasmuch as FMO attacks nucleophilic heteroatoms, it might be assumed that substrates for FMO could be predicted simply from their pKa values (i.e., from a measure of their basicity). Although there is some truth to this—for example, xenobiotics containing an sp^3-hybridized nitrogen atom with a pKa of 5 to 10 are generally good substrates for FMO—predictions of substrate specificity based on

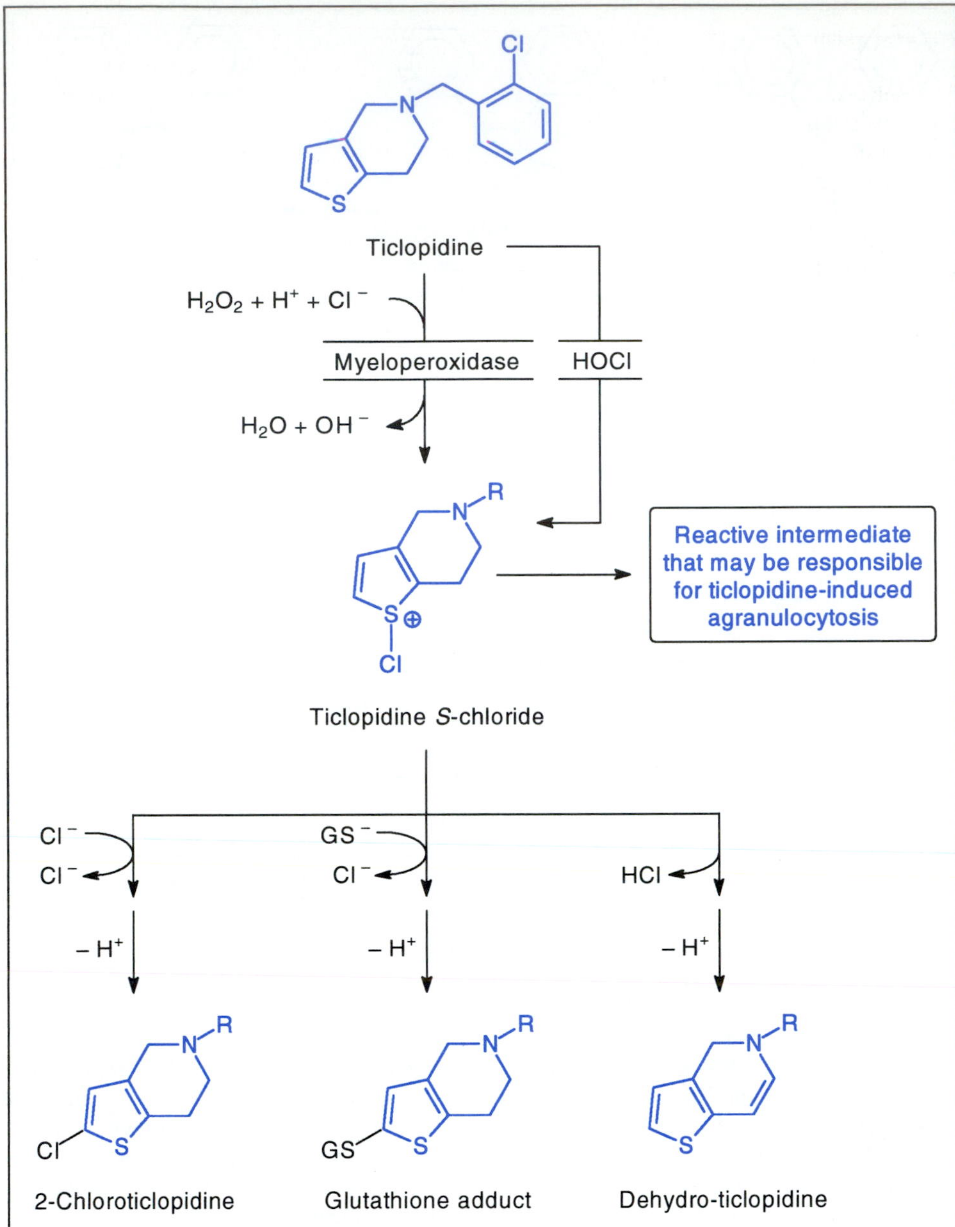

Figure 6-32. Activation of ticlopidine to a reactive thiophene S-chloride by myeloperoxidase.

pKa alone are not very reliable, presumably because steric effects influence access of substrates to the FMO active site (Rettie and Fisher, 1999).

With few exceptions, FMO acts as an electrophilic oxygenating catalyst, which distinguishes it from most other flavoprotein oxidases and monooxygenases (which will be discussed further in the section on cytochrome P450). The mechanism of catalysis by FMO is depicted in Fig. 6-34. After the FAD moiety is reduced to $FADH_2$ by NADPH, the oxidized cofactor, $NADP^+$, remains bound to the enzyme. $FADH_2$ then binds oxygen to produce a peroxide (i.e., the 4a-hydroperoxyflavin of FAD). The peroxide is relatively stable, probably because the active site of FMO comprises nonnucleophilic, lipophilic amino acid residues. During the oxygenation of xenobiotics, the 4a-hydroperoxyflavin is converted to 4a-hydroxyflavin with transfer of the flavin peroxide oxygen to the substrate (depicted as X $\rightarrow$ XO in Fig. 6-34). From this latter step, it is understandable why the metabolites produced by FMO are generally the products of a chemical reaction between a xenobiotic and a peroxide or peracid. The final step in the catalytic cycle involves dehydration of 4a-hydroxyflavin (which restores FAD to its resting, oxidized state) and release of $NADP^+$. This final step is important because it is rate-limiting, and it occurs after substrate oxygenation. Consequently, this step determines the upper limit of the rate of substrate oxidation. Therefore all good substrates for FMO are converted to products at the same maximum rate (i.e., V_{max} is determined by the final step in the catalytic cycle). Binding of $NADP^+$ to FMO during catalysis is important because it prevents the reduction of oxygen to H_2O_2. In the absence of bound

$NADP^+$, FMO would function as an NADPH-oxidase that would consume NADPH and cause oxidative stress through excessive production of H_2O_2.

The oxygenation of substrates by FMO does not lead to inactivation of the enzyme, even though some of the products are strong electrophiles capable of binding covalently to critical and noncritical nucleophiles such as protein and glutathione, respectively. The products of the oxygenation reactions catalyzed by FMO and/or the oxygenation of the same substrates by cytochrome P450 can inactivate cytochrome P450. For example, the FMO-dependent *S*-oxygenation of spironolactone thiol (which is formed by the deacetylation of spironolactone by carboxylesterases, as shown in Fig. 6-2) leads to the formation of an electrophilic sulfenic acid ($R-SH \rightarrow R-SOH$), which inactivates cytochrome P450 and binds covalently to other proteins.

In humans, FMO plays an important role in the biotransformation of several drugs (e.g., benzydamine, cimetidine, clozapine, guanethidine, methimazole, olanzapine, sulindac sulfide, tamoxifen and various dimethylaminoalkyl phenothiazine derivatives such as chlorpromazine and imipramine), xenobiotics (e.g., cocaine, methamphetamine, nicotine, tyramine), and endogenous substrates (e.g., trimethylamine, cysteamine). The major flavin monooxygenase in human liver microsomes, FMO3, is predominantly if not solely responsible for converting (*S*)-nicotine to

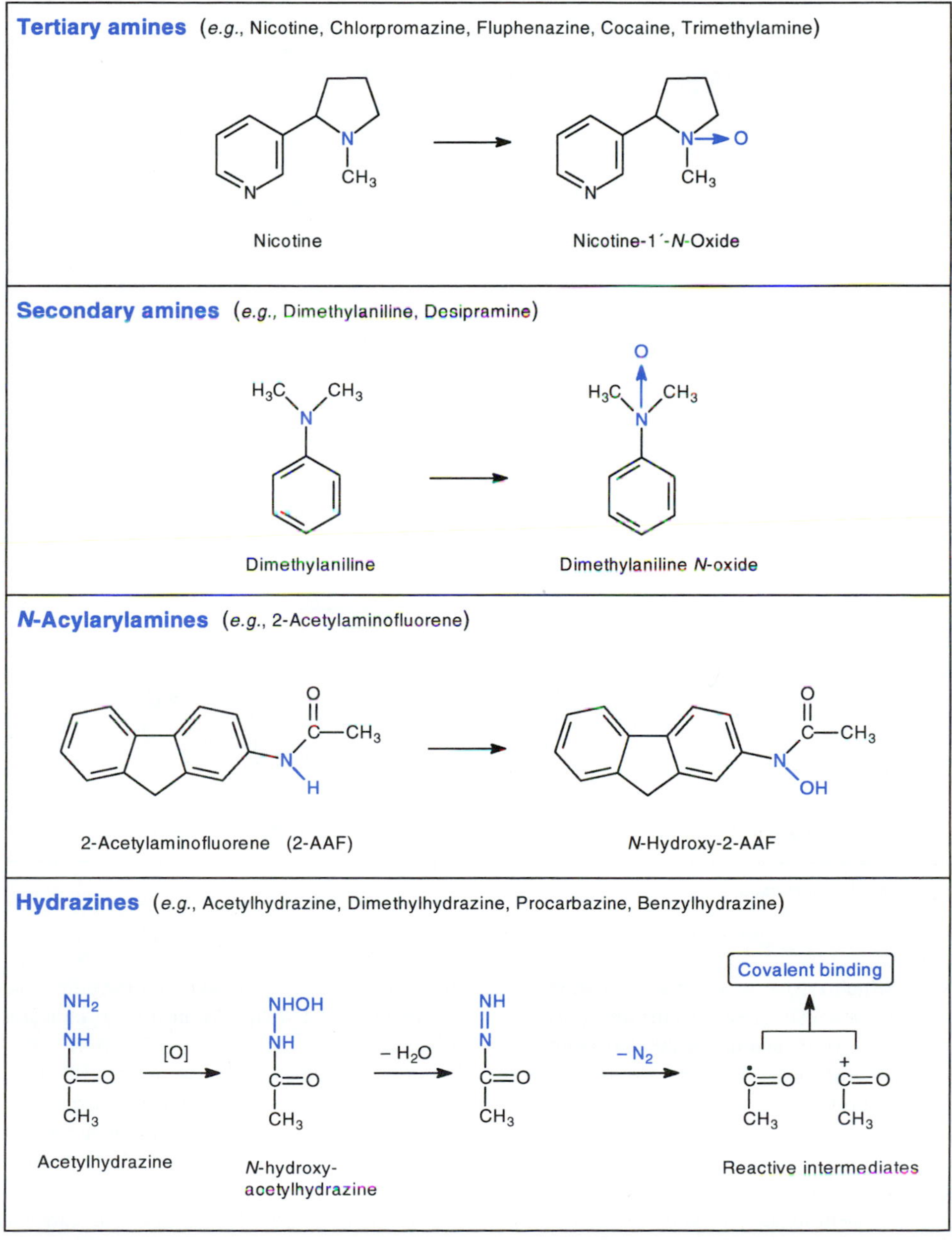

Figure 6-33. **A.** *Examples of reactions catalyzed by flavin monooxygenases (FMO): Nitrogen-containing xenobiotics.* **B.** *Examples of reactions catalyzed by flavin monooxygenases (FMO): Sulfur- and phophorus-containing xenobiotics.*

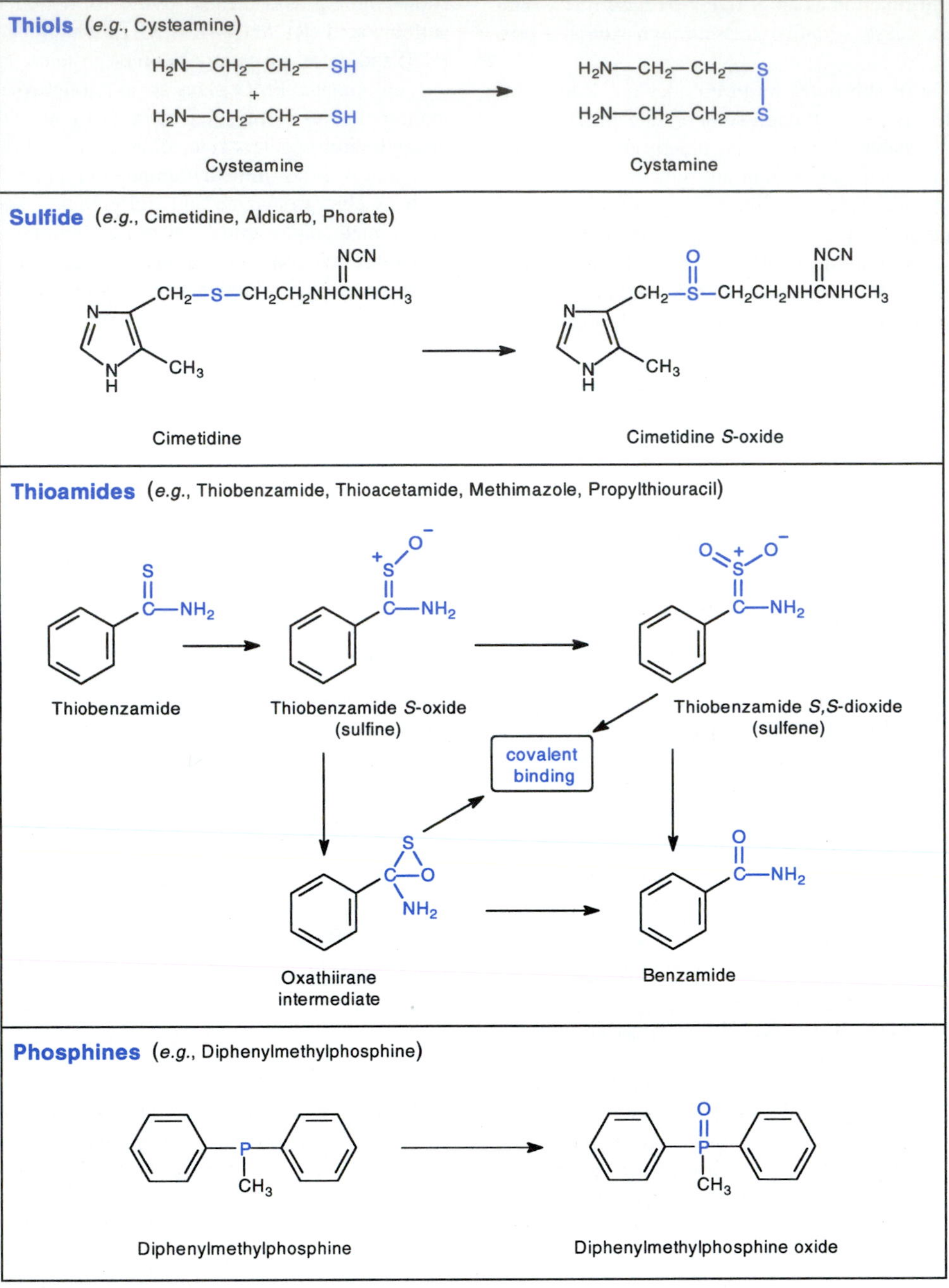

Figure 6-33. (continued)

(*S*)-nicotine *N*-1′-oxide (which is one of the reactions shown in Fig. 6-33*A*). The reaction proceeds stereospecifically; only the *trans* isomer is produced by FMO3, and this is the only isomer of (*S*)-nicotine *N*-1′-oxide excreted in the urine of cigarette smokers or individuals wearing a nicotine patch. Therefore, the urinary excretion of *trans*-(*S*)-nicotine *N*-1′-oxide can be used as an in vivo probe of FMO3 activity in humans. FMO3 is also the principal enzyme involved in the *S*-oxygenation of cimetidine, an H_2 antagonist widely used in the treatment of gastric ulcers and other acid-related disorders (this reaction is shown in Fig. 6-33*B*). Cimetidine is stereoselectively sulfoxidated by FMO3 to an 84:16 mixture of (+) and (−) enantiomers, which closely matches the 75:25 enantiomeric composition of cimetidine *S*-oxide in human urine. Therefore, the urinary excretion of cimetidine *S*-oxide, like that of (*S*)-nicotine *N*-1′-oxide, is an in vivo indicator of FMO3 activity in humans.

Sulindac is a sulfoxide that exists in two stereochemical forms (as do most sulfoxides), and a racemic mixture of *R*- and *S*-sulindac is used therapeutically as a NSAID. As shown in Fig. 6-12, the sulfoxide group in sulindac is reduced to the corresponding sulfide (which is achiral), which is then oxidized back to sulindac (a process often described as futile cycling). In human liver, the sulfoxidation of sulindac sulfide is catalyzed by FMO3 with little or no contribution from cytochrome P450. At low substrate concentrations (30 μM), FMO3 converts sulindac sulfide to *R*- and *S*-sulindac in an 87:13 ratio (Hamman et al., 2000). Consequently,

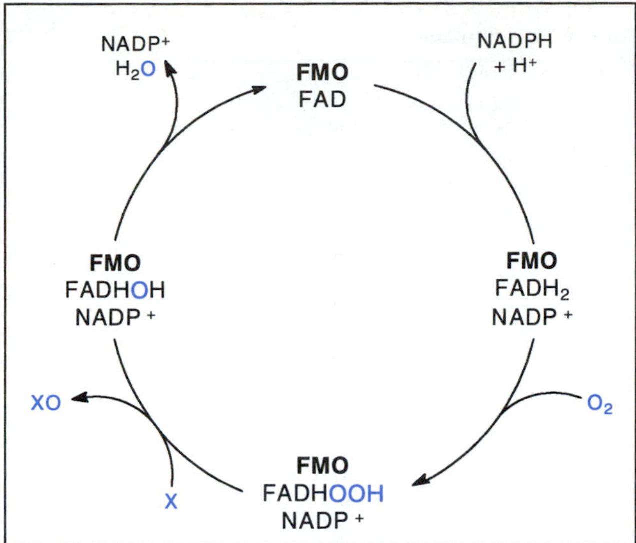

Figure 6-34. Catalytic cycle of flavin monooxygenase (FMO).

X and XO are the xenobiotic substrate and oxygenated product, respectively. The 4a-hydroperoxyflavin and 4a-hydroxyflavin of FAD are depicted as FADHOOH and FADHOH, respectively.

although sulindac is administered as a racemic mixture (i.e., a 1:1 mixture of *R*- and *S*-enantiomers), the reduction of this drug to the corresponding sulfide and its preferential sulfoxidation by FMO3 to *R*-sulindac results in stereoselective enrichment of *R*-sulindac in serum and urine.

In the case of sulindac sulfide, stereoselective sulfoxidation occurs not only with human FMO3 (the major FMO in human liver) but also with porcine FMO1 (the major form expressed in pig liver) and rabbit FMO2 (the major form expressed in rabbit lung) (Hamman et al., 2000). However, this conformity is the exception rather than the rule. For example, in contrast to the stereoselective oxygenation of (*S*)-nicotine and cimetidine by human FMO3 (see above), FMO1 (which is the major FMO expressed in pig, rat, and rabbit liver) converts (*S*)-nicotine to a 1:1 mixture of *cis*- and *trans*-(*S*)-nicotine *N*-1′ -oxide and similarly converts cimetidine to a 1:1 mixture of (+) and (−) cimetidine *S*-oxide, respectively. Therefore, statements concerning the role of FMO in the disposition of xenobiotics in humans may not apply to other species, or vice versa.

Several sulfur-containing xenobiotics are oxygenated by FMO to electrophilic reactive intermediates. Such xenobiotics include various thiols, thioamides, 2-mercaptoimidazoles, thiocarbamates, and thiocarbamides. The electrophilic metabolites of these xenobiotics do not inactivate FMO, but they can covalently modify and inactivate neighboring proteins, including cytochrome P450. Some of these same xenobiotics are substrates for cytochrome P450, and their oxygenation to electrophilic metabolites leads to inactivation of cytochrome P450, a process known variously as metabolism-dependent inhibition, mechanism-based inhibition and suicide inactivation. 2-Mercaptoimidazoles undergo sequential *S*-oxygenation reactions by FMO, first to sulfenic acids and then to sulfinic acids (R–SH → R–SOH → R–SO_2H). These electrophilic metabolites, like the sulfenic acid metabolite produced from spironolactone thiol (see above), bind to critical nucleophiles (such as proteins) or interact with glutathione to form disulfides. The thiocarbamate functionality present in numerous agricultural chemicals is converted by FMO to *S*-oxides (sulfoxides), which can be further oxygenated to sulfones. These reactions involve *S*-oxygenation adjacent to a ketone, which produces strong electrophilic acylating agents, which may be responsible for the toxicity of many thiocarbamate herbicides and fungicides. The hepatotoxicity of thiobenzamide is dependent on *S*-oxidation by FMO and/or cytochrome P450. As shown in Fig. 6-33*B*, the *S*-oxidation of thiobenzamide can lead to the formation of an oxathiirane (a three-membered ring of carbon, sulfur, and oxygen) that can bind covalently to protein (which leads to hepatocellular necrosis) or rearrange to benzamide, a reaction known as *oxidative group transfer*.

Endogenous FMO substrates include cysteamine, which is oxidized to the disulfide, cystamine, and trimethylamine (TMA), which is converted to TMA *N*-oxide (Fig. 6-33*B*). By converting cysteamine to cystamine, FMO may serve to produce a low-molecular-weight disulfide-exchange agent, which may participate in the formation of disulfide bridges during peptide synthesis or the renaturation of proteins. By converting TMA to TMA *N*-oxide, FMO converts a malodorous and volatile dietary product of choline, lecithin, and carnitine catabolism to an inoffensive metabolite. TMA smells of rotting fish, and people who are genetically deficient in FMO3 suffer from trimethylaminuria or *fish-odor syndrome,* which is caused by the excretion of TMA in urine, sweat, and breath (Ayesh and Smith, 1992). The underlying genetic basis of trimethylaminuria is a mutation (Pro_{153} → Leu_{153}) in exon 4 of the FMO3 gene (Dolphin et al., 1997). Although this mutation (and hence trimethylaminuria) occurs only rarely, it is now known to be just one of several mutations that decrease or eliminate FMO3 activity; these other mutations include missense mutations (Met_{66} → Ile_{66}, Met_{82} → Thr_{82}, Arg_{492} → is Trp_{492}) and the nonsense mutation Glu_{305} → X_{305} (Cashman et al., 2000). As might be expected, trimethylaminuria is associated with an impairment of nicotine *N*-oxidation and other pathways of drug biotransformation that are primarily catalyzed by FMO3 (Rettie and Fisher, 1999).

Humans and other mammals express five different flavin monooxygenases (FMO1, FMO2, FMO3, FMO4, and FMO5) in a species- and tissue-specific manner, as shown in Table 6-3 (adapted from Cashman, 1995). For example, the major FMO expressed in human and mouse liver microsomes is FMO3, whereas FMO1 is the major FMO expressed in rat, rabbit, and pig liver. (Although FMO3 is the major FMO in *adult* human liver, the major FMO in *fetal* human liver is FMO1.) In humans, high levels of FMO1 are expressed in the kidney, and low levels of FMO2 are expressed in the lung. However, lung microsomes from other species, particularly rabbit, mouse, and monkey, contain high levels of FMO2. The uncharacteristically low levels of FMO2 in human lung are due to a mutation (a C → T transition at codon 472) in the major human FMO2 allele, which results in the synthesis of a nonfunctional, truncated protein (one lacking the last 64–amino acid residues from the C-terminus) (Dolphin et al., 1998). FMO4 appears to be expressed at low levels in the brain of several mammalian species, where it might terminate the action of several centrally active drugs and other xenobiotics.

The various forms of FMO are distinct gene products with different physical properties and substrate specificities. For example, FMO2 *N*-oxygenates *n*-octylamine, whereas such long aliphatic primary amines are not substrates for FMO1, although they stimulate its activity toward other substrates (in some cases causing a change in stereospecificity). Conversely, short-chain tertiary amines, such as chlorpromazine and imipramine, are sub-

Table 6-3
Putative Tissue Levels of FMO Forms Present in Animals and Humans

	FMO1	FMO2	FMO3	FMO4	FMO5
Liver					
Mouse	Low	NP*	High	?	Low
Rat	High	?*	Low	?	Low
Rabbit	High	NP	Low	?	Low
Human	Very low	Low	High	Very low	Low
Kidney					
Mouse	High	?	High	?	Low
Rat	High	?	High	High	Low
Rabbit	Low	Low	Very low	High	Low
Human	High	Low	?	?	?
Lung					
Mouse	?	High	Very low	NP	Low
Rat	?	?	?	NP	Low
Rabbit	?	Very high	?	NP	NP
Human	?	Low	?	NP	?

* NP, apparently not present. A question mark indicates that no data are available or the presence of an FMO form is in doubt.
SOURCE: Cashman, 1995.

strates for FMO1 but not FMO2. Certain substrates are oxygenated stereospecifically by one FMO enzyme but not another. For example, FMO2 and FMO3 convert (*S*)-nicotine exclusively to *trans*-(*S*)-nicotine *N*-1′-oxide, whereas the *N*-oxides of (*S*)-nicotine produced by FMO1 are a 1:1 mixture of *cis* and *trans* isomers. FMO2 is heat-stable under conditions that completely inactivate FMO1, and FMO2 is resistant to anionic detergents that inactivate FMO1. Low concentrations of bile salts, such as cholate, stimulate FMO activity in rat and mouse liver microsomes but inhibit FMO activity in rabbit and pig liver.

The FMO enzymes expressed in liver microsomes are not under the same regulatory control as cytochrome P450. In rats, the expression of FMO1 is repressed rather than induced by treatment with phenobarbital or 3-methylcholanthrene (although some studies point to of a modest [~3-fold] induction of rat FMO1 by 3-methylcholanthrene). Indole-3-carbinol, which induces the same P450 enzymes as 3-methylcholanthrene, causes a marked decrease in FMO activity in rat liver and intestine. A similar decrease in FMO3 activity occurs in human volunteers following the consumption of large amounts of Brussels sprouts, which contain high levels of indole-3-carbinol and related indoles. The decrease in FMO3 activity may result from direct inhibition of FMO3 by indole-3-carbinol and its derivatives rather than from an actual decrease in enzyme levels (Cashman et al., 1999). The levels of FMO3 and, to a lesser extent, of FMO1 in mouse liver microsomes are sexually differentiated (female > male) due to suppression of expression by testosterone. The opposite is true of FMO1 levels in rat liver microsomes, the expression of which is positively regulated by testosterone and negatively regulated by estradiol. In pregnant rabbits, lung FMO2 is positively regulated by progesterone and/or corticosteroids.

Species differences in the relative expression of FMO and cytochrome P450 appear to determine species differences in the toxicity of the pyrrolizidine alkaloids, senecionine, retrorsine, and monocrotaline. These compounds are detoxified by FMO, which catalyzes the formation of tertiary amine *N*-oxides, but they are activated by cytochrome P450, which oxidizes these alkaloids to pyrroles that generate toxic electrophiles through the loss of substituents on the pyrrolizidine nucleus (details of which appear in the section on cytochrome P450). Rats have a high pyrrole-forming cytochrome P450 activity and a low *N*-oxide forming FMO activity, whereas the opposite is true of guinea pigs. This likely explains why pyrrolizidine alkaloids are highly toxic to rats but not to guinea pigs. Many of the reactions catalyzed by FMO are also catalyzed by cytochrome P450, but differences in the oxidation of pyrrolizidine alkaloids by FMO and cytochrome P450 illustrate that this is not always the case.

Cytochrome P450 Among the phase I biotransforming enzymes, the cytochrome P450 system ranks first in terms of catalytic versatility and the sheer number of xenobiotics it detoxifies or activates to reactive intermediates (Guengerich, 1987; Waterman and Johnson, 1991). The highest concentration of P450 enzymes involved in xenobiotic biotransformation is found in liver endoplasmic reticulum (microsomes), but P450 enzymes are present in virtually all tissues. The liver microsomal P450 enzymes play a very important role in determining the intensity and duration of action of drugs, and they also play a key role in the detoxication of xenobiotics. P450 enzymes in liver and extrahepatic tissues play important roles in the activation of xenobiotics to toxic and/or tumorigenic metabolites. Microsomal and mitochondrial P450 enzymes play key roles in the biosynthesis or catabolism of steroid hormones, bile acids, fat-soluble vitamins, fatty acids, and eicosanoids, which underscores the catalytic versatility of cytochrome P450.

All P450 enzymes are heme-containing proteins. The heme iron in cytochrome P450 is usually in the ferric (Fe^{3+}) state. When reduced to the ferrous (Fe^{2+}) state, cytochrome P450 can bind ligands such as O_2 and carbon monoxide (CO). The complex between ferrous cytochrome P450 and CO absorbs light maximally at 450 nm, from which cytochrome P450 derives its name. The absorbance maximum of the CO complex differs slightly among different P450 enzymes and ranges from 447 to 452 nm. All other hemoproteins that bind CO absorb light maximally at ~420 nm. The unusual absorbance maximum of cytochrome P450 is due to an unusual fifth ligand to the heme (a cysteine-thiolate). The amino acid sequence around the cysteine residue that forms the thiolate bond with the heme moiety is highly conserved in all P450 enzymes (Negishi et al., 1996). When this thiolate bond is disrupted, cytochrome P450 is converted to a catalytically inactive form called cytochrome P420. By competing with oxygen, CO inhibits cytochrome P450. The inhibitory effect of carbon monoxide can be reversed by irradiation with light at 450 nm, which photodissociates the cytochrome P450–CO complex.

These properties of cytochrome P450 are of historical importance. The observation that treatment of rats with certain chemicals, such as 3-methylcholanthrene, causes a shift in the peak absorbance of cytochrome P450 (from 450 to 448 nm) provided some of the earliest evidence for the existence of multiple forms of cytochrome P450 in liver microsomes. The conversion of cytochrome P450 to cytochrome P420 by detergents and phospholipases helped to establish the hemoprotein nature of cytochrome P450. The inhibition of cytochrome P450 by CO and the reversal of this inhibition by photodissociation of the cytochrome P450–CO complex established cytochrome P450 as the microsomal and mitochondrial enzyme involved in drug biotransformation and steroid biosynthesis (Omura, 1999).

The basic reaction catalyzed by cytochrome P450 is monooxygenation in which one atom of oxygen is incorporated into a substrate, designated RH, and the other is reduced to water with reducing equivalents derived from NADPH, as follows:

$$\text{Substrate (RH)} + O_2 + \text{NADPH} + H^+ \rightarrow \text{Product (ROH)} + H_2O + \text{NADP}^+$$

Although cytochrome P450 functions as a monooxygenase, the products are not limited to alcohols and phenols due to rearrangement reactions (Guengerich, 1991). During catalysis, cytochrome P450 binds directly to the substrate and molecular oxygen, but it does not interact directly with NADPH or NADH. The mechanism by which cytochrome P450 receives electrons from NAD(P)H depends on the subcellular localization of cytochrome P450. In the endoplasmic reticulum, which is where most of the P450 enzymes involved in xenobiotic biotransformation are localized, electrons are relayed from NADPH to cytochrome P450 via a flavoprotein called NADPH–cytochrome P450 reductase. Within this flavoprotein, electrons are transferred from NADPH to cytochrome P450 via FMN and FAD. In mitochondria, which house many of the P450 enzymes involved in steroid hormone biosynthesis and vitamin D metabolism, electrons are transferred from NAD(P)H to cytochrome P450 via two proteins; an iron-sulfur protein called ferredoxin and an FMN-containing flavoprotein called ferredoxin reductase (these proteins are also known as adrenodoxin and adrenodoxin reductase). In bacteria such as *Pseudomonas putida,* electron flow is similar to that in mitochondria (NADH → flavoprotein → putidaredoxin → P450).

There are some notable exceptions to the general rule that cytochrome P450 requires a second enzyme (i.e., a flavoprotein) for catalytic activity. One exception applies to two P450 enzymes involved in the conversion of arachidonic acid to eicosanoids, namely thromboxane synthase and prostacyclin synthase. These two P450 enzymes convert the endoperoxide PGH_2 to thromboxane (TXA_2) and prostacyclin (PGI_2) in platelets and the endothelial lining of blood vessels, respectively. In both cases, cytochrome P450 functions as an isomerase and catalyzes a rearrangement of the oxygen atoms introduced into arachidonic acid by cyclooxygenase. The plant cytochrome P450, allene oxide synthase, and certain invertebrate P450 enzymes also catalyze the rearrangement of oxidized chemicals. The second exception are two cytochrome P450 enzymes expressed in the bacterium *Bacillus megaterium,* which are known as BM-1 and BM-3 (or CYP106 and CYP102, respectively). These P450 enzymes are considerably larger than most P450 enzymes because they are linked directly to a flavoprotein. In other words, the P450 moiety and flavoprotein are expressed in a single protein encoded by a single gene. Through recombinant DNA techniques, mammalian P450 enzymes have been linked directly to NADPH–cytochrome P450 reductase and, like the bacterial enzyme, the resultant fusion protein is catalytically active. Most mammalian P450 enzymes are not synthesized as a single enzyme containing both the hemoprotein and flavoprotein moieties, but this arrangement is found in nitric oxide (NO) synthase. In addition to its atypical structure, the P450 enzyme expressed in *B. megaterium,* CYP102, is unusual for another reason: It is inducible by phenobarbital, as are some of the mammalian P450 enzymes (see "Induction of Cytochrome P450," below).

Phospholipids and cytochrome b_5 also play an important role in cytochrome P450 reactions. Cytochrome P450 and NADPH–cytochrome P450 reductase are embedded in the phospholipid bilayer of the endoplasmic reticulum, which facilitates their interaction. When the *C*-terminal region that anchors NADPH–cytochrome P450 reductase in the membrane is cleaved with trypsin, the truncated flavoprotein can no longer support cytochrome P450 reactions, although it is still capable of reducing cytochrome *c* and other soluble electron acceptors. The ability of phospholipids to facilitate the interaction between NADPH–cytochrome P450 reductase and cytochrome P450 does not appear to depend on the nature of the polar head group (serine, choline, inositol, ethanolamine), although certain P450 enzymes (those in the CYP3A subfamily) have a requirement for phospholipids containing unsaturated fatty acids.

Cytochrome b_5 can donate the second of two electrons required by cytochrome P450. Although this would be expected simply to increase the rate of catalysis of cytochrome P450, cytochrome b_5 can also increase the apparent affinity with which certain P450 enzymes bind their substrates; hence, cytochrome b_5 can increase V_{max} and/or decrease the apparent K_m of cytochrome P450 reactions. In both cases, cytochrome b_5 increases V_{max}/K_m, which is a measure of catalytic efficiency and intrinsic clearance. Liver microsomes contain numerous forms of cytochrome P450 but only a single form of NADPH–cytochrome P450 reductase and cytochrome b_5. For each molecule of NADPH–cytochrome P450 reductase in rat liver microsomes, there are 5 to 10 molecules of cytochrome b_5 and 10 to 20 molecules of cytochrome P450. NADPH–cytochrome P450 reductase will reduce electron acceptors other than cytochrome P450, which enables this enzyme to be measured based on its ability to reduce cytochrome-c (which is why NADPH–cytochrome P450 reductase is often called NADPH–cytochrome-c reductase). NADPH–cytochrome P450 reductase can transfer electrons much faster than cytochrome P450 can use them, which more than likely accounts for the low ratio of NADPH–cytochrome P450 reductase to cytochrome P450 in liver microsomes. Low levels of NADPH–cytochrome P450 reductase may also be a safeguard to protect cells from the often deleterious one-electron reduction reactions catalyzed by this flavoprotein (see Fig. 6-13).

The catalytic cycle of cytochrome P450 is shown in Fig. 6-35 (Dawson, 1988; Schlichting et al., 2000). The first part of the cycle involves the activation of oxygen, and the final part involves substrate oxidation, which entails the abstraction of a hydrogen atom or an electron from the substrate followed by oxygen rebound (radical recombination). Following the binding of substrate to the P450 enzyme, the heme iron is reduced from the ferric (Fe^{3+}) to the ferrous (Fe^{2+}) state by the addition of a single electron from NADPH–cytochrome P450 reductase. The reduction of cytochrome P450 is facilitated by substrate binding, possibly because binding of the substrate in the vicinity of the heme moiety converts the heme iron from a low-spin to a high-spin state. Oxygen binds to cytochrome P450 in its ferrous state, and the $Fe^{2+}O_2$ complex is converted to an $Fe^{2+}OOH$ complex by the addition of a proton (H^+) and a second electron, which is derived from NADPH–cytochrome P450 reductase or cytochrome b_5. Introduction of a second proton cleaves the $Fe^{2+}OOH$ complex to produce water and an $(FeO)^{3+}$ complex, which transfers its oxygen atom to the substrate. Release of the oxidized substrate returns cytochrome P450 to its initial state. If the catalytic cycle is interrupted (uncoupled) following introduction of the first electron, oxygen is released as superoxide anion ($O_2^{\bar{\cdot}}$). If the cycle is interrupted after introduction of the second electron, oxygen is released as hydrogen peroxide (H_2O_2). The final oxygenating species, $(FeO)^{3+}$, can be generated directly by the transfer of an oxygen atom from hydrogen peroxide and certain other hydroperoxides, a process known as the peroxide shunt. For this reason certain P450 reactions can be supported by hydroperoxides in the absence of NADPH–cytochrome P450 reductase and NADPH.

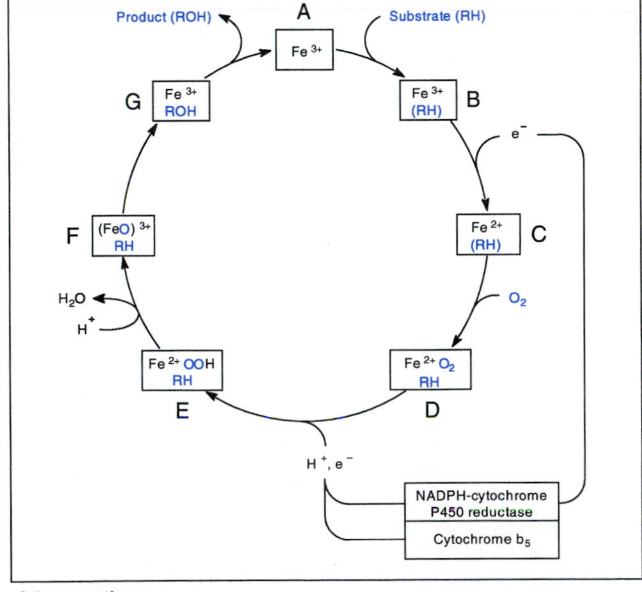

Other reactions

One-electron reduction	**C** (Fe^{2+} RH)	⟶	**A** (Fe^{3+}) + $RH^{\bar{\cdot}}$
Superoxide anion production	**D** (Fe^{2+} O_2 RH)	⟶	**B** (Fe^{3+} RH) + $O_2^{\bar{\cdot}}$
Hydrogen peroxide production	**E** (Fe^{2+}OOH RH) + H^+	⟶	**B** (Fe^{3+}RH) + H_2O_2
Peroxide shunt	**B** (Fe^{3+} RH) + XOOH	⟶	**F** $(FeO)^{3+}$ RH + XOH

Figure 6-35. Catalytic cycle of cytochrome P450.

Cytochrome P450 catalyzes several types of oxidation reactions, including:

1. Hydroxylation of an aliphatic or aromatic carbon
2. Epoxidation of a double bond
3. Heteroatom (*S*-, *N*-, and *I*-) oxygenation and *N*-hydroxylation
4. Heteroatom (*O*-, *S*-, *N*- and *Si*-) dealkylation
5. Oxidative group transfer
6. Cleavage of esters
7. Dehydrogenation

In the first three cases, oxygen from the $(FeO)^{3+}$ complex is incorporated into the substrate, which otherwise remains intact. In the fourth case, oxygenation of the substrate is followed by a rearrangement reaction leading to cleavage of an amine (*N*-dealkylation) or an ether (*O*- and *S*-dealkylation). Oxygen from the $(FeO)^{3+}$ complex is incorporated into the alkyl-leaving group, producing an aldehyde or ketone. In the fifth case, oxygenation of the substrate is followed by a rearrangement reaction leading to loss of a heteroatom (oxidative group transfer). The sixth case, the cleavage of esters, resembles heteroatom dealkylation in that the functional group is cleaved with incorporation of oxygen from the $(FeO)^{3+}$ complex into the leaving group, producing an aldehyde. In the seventh case, two hydrogens are abstracted from the substrate with the formation of a double bond (C=C, C=O, or C=N), with the reduction of oxygen from the $(FeO)^{3+}$ complex to water. It should be noted that this long list of reactions does not encompass all of the reactions catalyzed by cytochrome P450. As noted above (this section), cytochrome P450 can catalyze reductive reactions (such as azo reduction, nitro reduction, and reductive dehalogenation) and isomerization reactions (such as the conversion of PGH_2 to thromboxane and prostacyclin). During the synthesis of steroid hormones, cytochrome P450 catalyzes the cleavage of carbon–carbon bonds, which occurs during the conversion of cholesterol to pregnenolone by side-chain cleavage enzyme (also known as $P450_{scc}$ and CYP11A1) and the aromatization of a substituted cyclohexane, which occurs during the conversion of androgens to estrogens by aromatase (also known as $P450_{aro}$ and CYP19).

Examples of aliphatic and aromatic hydroxylation reactions catalyzed by cytochrome P450 are shown in Figs. 6-36 and 6-37, respectively. The hydroxylation of aromatic hydrocarbons may proceed via an oxirane intermediate (i.e., an arene oxide) that isomerizes to the corresponding phenol. Alternatively aromatic hydroxylation can proceed by a mechanism known as direct insertion. The *ortho*-hydroxylation and *para*-hydroxylation of chlorobenzene proceed via 2,3- and 3,4-epoxidation, whereas *meta*-hydroxylation proceeds by direct insertion, as shown in Fig. 6-38. When aromatic hydroxylation involves direct insertion, hydrogen abstraction (i.e., cleavage of the C–H bond) is the rate-limiting step, so that substitution of hydrogen with deuterium or tritium considerably slows the hydroxylation reaction. This *isotope effect* is less marked when aromatic hydroxylation proceeds via an arene oxide intermediate. Arene oxides are electrophilic and therefore potentially toxic metabolites that are detoxified by such enzymes as epoxide hydrolase (see Fig. 6-6) and glutathione *S*-transferase. Depending on the ring substituents, the rearrangement of arene oxides to the corresponding phenol can lead to an intramolecular migration of a substituent (such as hydrogen or a halogen) from one carbon to the next. This intramolecular migration occurs at the site of oxidation

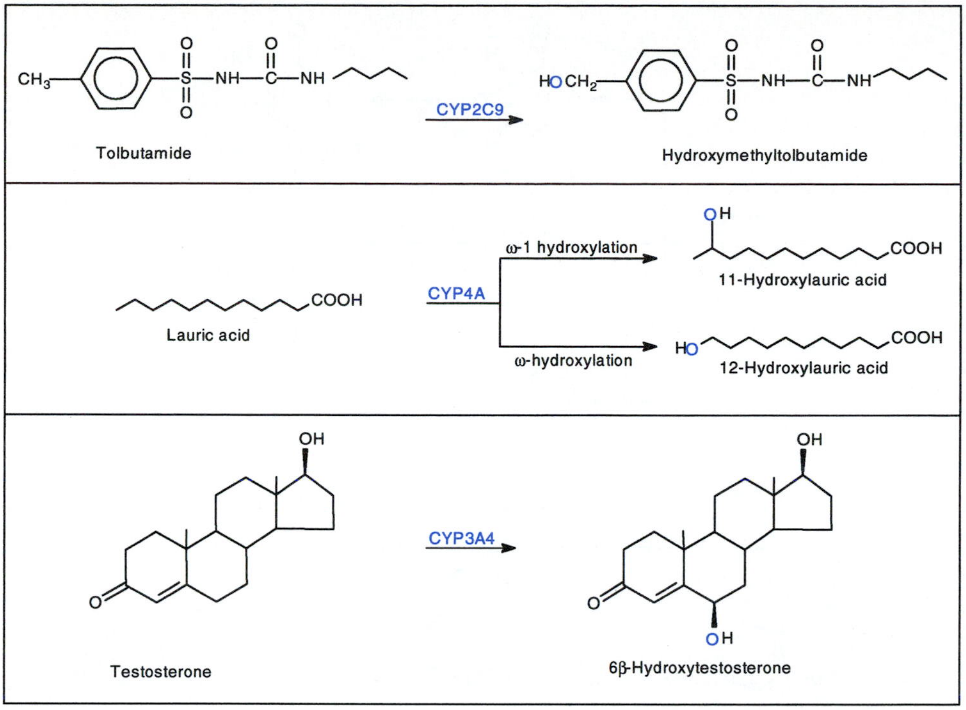

Figure 6-36. Examples of reactions catalyzed by cytochrome P450: Hydroxylation of aliphatic carbon.

and is known as the NIH shift—so named for its discovery at the National Institutes of Health.

Aliphatic hydroxylation involves insertion of oxygen into a C–H bond. As in the case of aromatic hydroxylation by direct insertion, cleavage of the C–H bond by hydrogen abstraction is the rate-limiting step, as shown below:

$$(FeO)^{3+}\ HC{-} \longrightarrow Fe(OH)^{3+}\ {\cdot}C{-} \longrightarrow Fe^{3+}\ HO{-}C{-}$$

In the case of simple, straight-chain hydrocarbons, such as n-hexane, aliphatic hydroxylation occurs at both the terminal methyl groups and the internal methylene groups. In the case of fatty acids and their derivatives (i.e., eicosanoids such as prostaglandins and leukotrienes), aliphatic hydroxylation occurs at the ω-carbon (terminal methyl group) and the ω-carbon (penultimate carbon), as shown for lauric acid in Fig. 6-36. Most P450 enzymes preferentially catalyze the ω-1 hydroxylation of fatty acids and their derivatives, but one group of P450 enzymes (those encoded by the *CYP4A* genes) preferentially catalyzes the ω-hydroxylation of fatty acids, which can be further oxidized to dicarboxylic acids.

Xenobiotics containing a carbon–carbon double bond (i.e., alkenes) can be epoxidated (i.e., converted to an oxirane) in an analogous manner to the oxidation of aromatic compounds to arene oxides. Just as arene oxides can isomerize to phenols, so aliphatic epoxides can isomerize to the corresponding ene-ol, the formation of which may involve an intramolecular migration (NIH shift) of a substituent at the site of oxidation. Like arene oxides, aliphatic epoxides are also potentially toxic metabolites that are inactivated by other xenobiotic-metabolizing enzymes. Oxidation of some aliphatic alkenes and alkynes produces metabolites that are sufficiently reactive to bind covalently to the heme moiety of cytochrome P450, a process variously known as metabolism-dependent inhibition, suicide inactivation, or mechanism-based inhibition. As previously discussed in the section on epoxide hydrolase, not all epoxides are highly reactive electrophiles. Although the 3,4-epoxidation of coumarin produces an hepatotoxic metabolite, the 10,11-epoxidation of carbamazepine produces a stable, relatively nontoxic metabolite (Fig. 6-38).

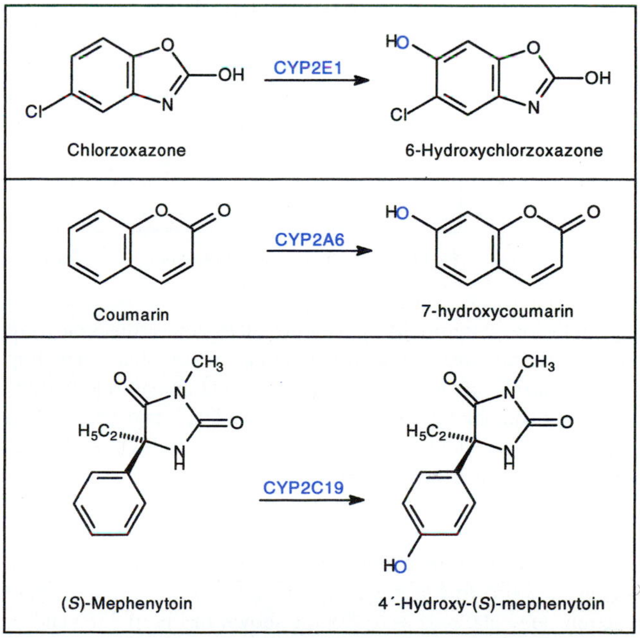

Figure 6-37. Examples of reactions catalyzed by cytochrome P450: Hydroxylation of aromatic carbon.

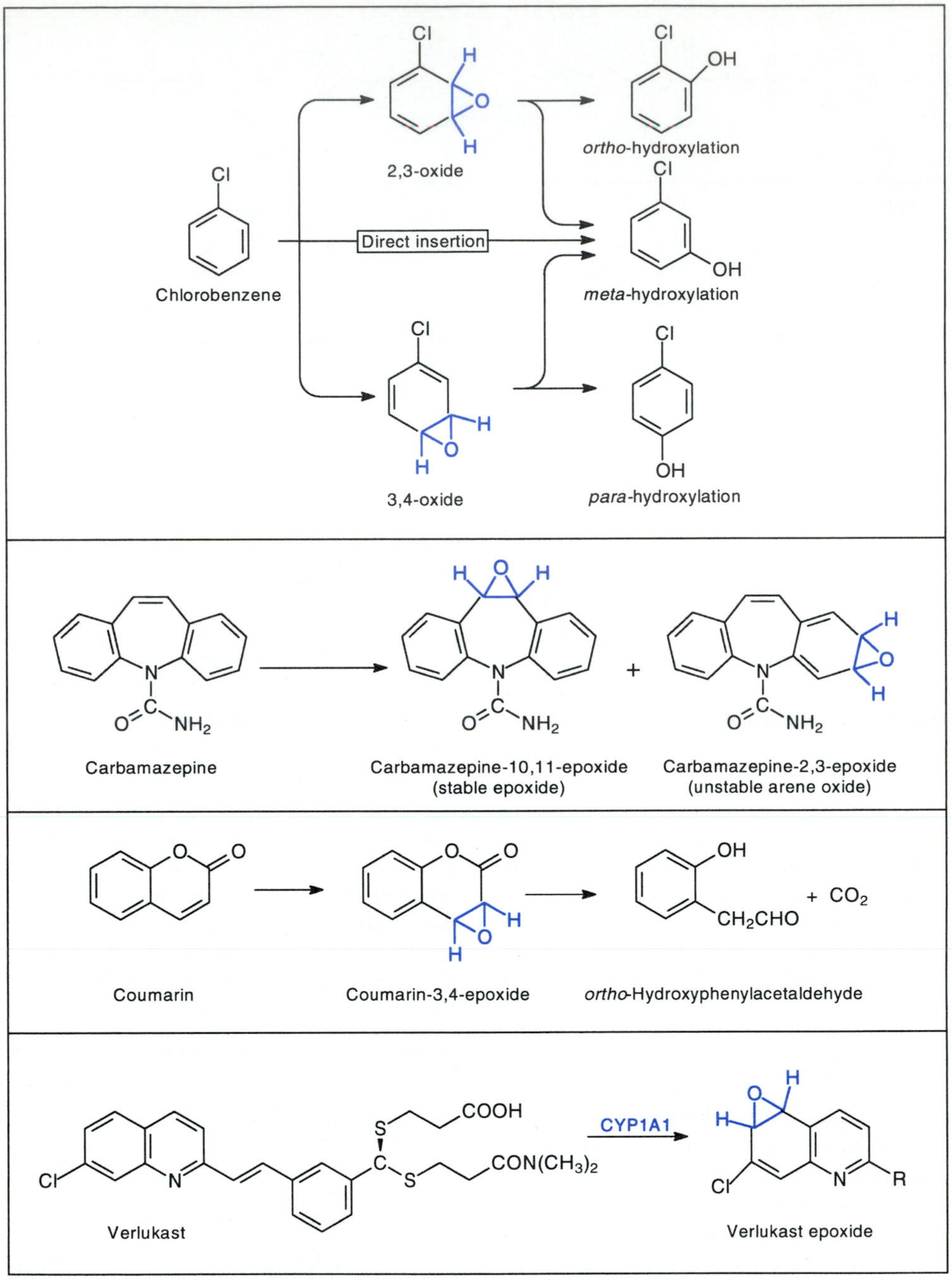

Figure 6-38. Examples of reactions catalyzed by cytochrome P450: Epoxidation.

In the presence of NADPH and O_2, liver microsomes catalyze the oxygenation of several *S*-containing xenobiotics, including chlorpromazine, cimetidine, lansoprazole, and omeprazole. Sulfur-containing xenobiotics can potentially undergo two consecutive sulfoxidation reactions: one that converts the sulfide (S) to the sulfoxide (SO), which occurs during the sulfoxidation of chlorpromazine and cimetidine, and one that converts the sulfoxide (SO) to the sulfone (SO_2), which occurs during the sulfoxidation of omeprazole and lansoprazole, as shown in Fig. 6-39. Albendazole is converted first to a sulfoxide and then to a sulfone. All of these reactions are catalyzed by FMO (as shown in Fig. 6-33*B*) and/or cytochrome P450 (as shown in Fig. 6-39). Both enzymes are efficient catalysts of *S*-oxygenation, and both contribute significantly to the sulfoxidation of various xenobiotics. For example, the sulfoxidation of omeprazole, lansoprazole, chlorpromazine, and phenothiazine by human liver microsomes is primarily catalyzed by a P450 enzyme (namely CYP3A4), whereas the sulfoxidation of cimetidine and sulindac sulfide is primarily catalyzed by a flavin monooxygenase (namely FMO3). In the presence of NADPH and O_2, liver microsomes catalyze the oxygenation of several *N*-containing xenobiotics — including chlorpromazine, doxylamine, oflaxacin, morphine, nicotine, MPTP, methapyrilene, methaqualone, metronidazole, pargyline, pyridine, senecionine, strychnine, trimethylamine, trimipramine, and verapamil—all of which are converted to stable *N*-oxides. Whereas *S*-oxygenation might be catalyzed by both cytochrome P450 and FMO, *N*-oxygenation is more likely to be catalyzed by just one of these enzymes. For example, the conversion of (*S*)-nicotine to *trans-*

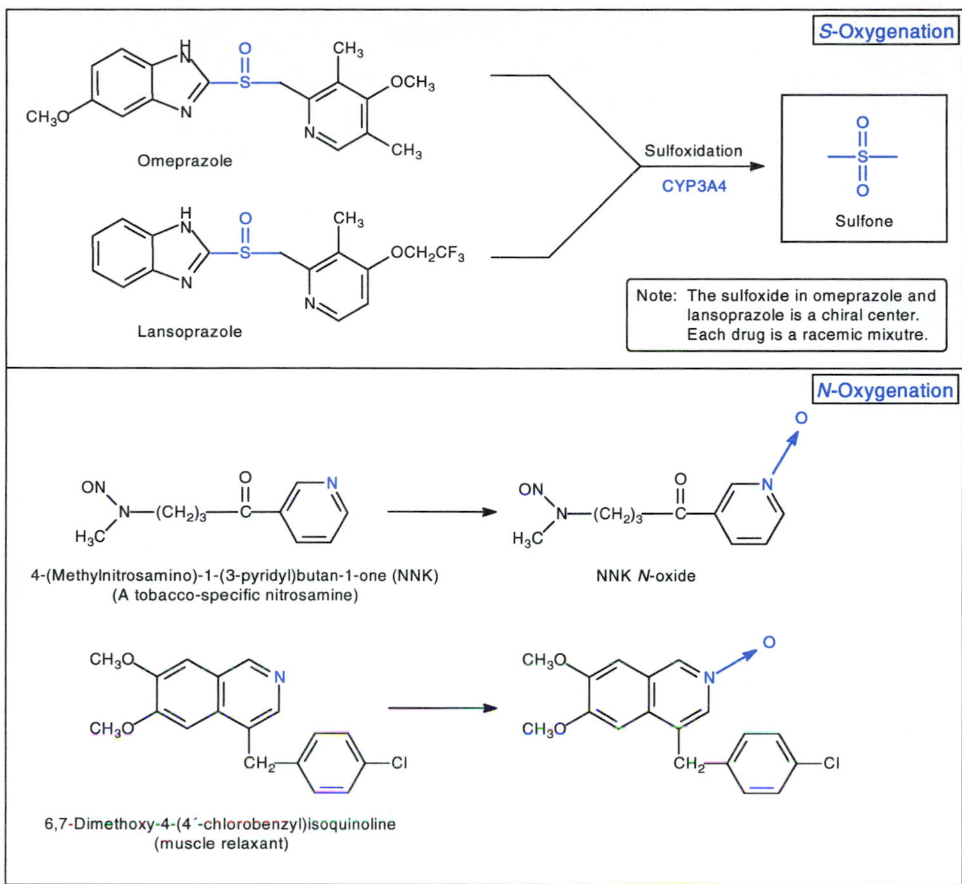

Figure 6-39. Examples of reactions catalyzed by cytochrome P450: Heteroatom oxygenation.

(*S*)-nicotine *N*-1′-oxide by human liver microsomes is catalyzed by FMO3, with little or no contribution from cytochrome P450. Conversely, the conversion of pyridine to its *N*-oxide is primarily catalyzed by cytochrome P450. Both enzymes can participate in the *N*-oxygenation of certain xenobiotics. For example, the *N*-oxygenation of chlorpromazine is catalyzed by FMO3 and, to a lesser extent, by two P450 enzymes (CYP2D6 and CYP1A2). In general, FMO catalyzes the *N*-oxygenation of xenobiotics containing electron-deficient nitrogen atoms, whereas cytochrome P450 catalyzes the *N*-oxygenation of xenobiotics containing electron-rich nitrogen atoms. Therefore, substrates primarily *N*-oxygenated by cytochrome P450 are somewhat limited to pyridine-containing xenobiotics, such as the tobacco-specific nitrosamine NNK and the antihistamine temelastine, and to xenobiotics containing a quinoline or isoquinoline group, such as the muscle relaxant 6,7-dimethoxy-4-(4′-chlorobenzyl)isoquinoline. The initial step in heteroatom oxygenation by cytochrome P450 involves the abstraction of an electron from the heteroatom (*N*, *S* or *I*) by the $(FeO)^{3+}$ complex, as shown below for sulfoxidation.

$$(FeO)^{3+}\ :\overset{|}{\underset{|}{S}} \longrightarrow (FeO)^{2+}\ \overset{+}{\cdot}\overset{|}{\underset{|}{S}} \longrightarrow Fe^{3+}\ O^{-}\!\!-\!\overset{+}{\overset{|}{\underset{|}{S}}}\!-$$

Abstraction of an electron from *N*, *O*, or *S* by the $(FeO)^{3+}$ complex is also the initial step in heteroatom dealkylation, but in this case abstraction of the electron from the heteroatom is quickly followed by abstraction of a proton (H^+) from the α-carbon atom (the carbon atom attached to the heteroatom). Oxygen rebound leads to hydroxylation of the α-carbon, which then rearranges to form the corresponding aldehyde or ketone with cleavage of the α-carbon from the heteroatom, as shown below for the *N*-dealkylation of an *N*-alkylamine:

$$(FeO)^{3+}\ :\overset{|}{\underset{\substack{|\\ CH_2R}}{N}}- \longrightarrow (FeO)^{2+}\ \overset{+}{\cdot}\overset{|}{\underset{\substack{|\\ CH_2R}}{N}}- \longrightarrow$$

$$Fe(OH)^{3+}\ :\overset{|}{\underset{\substack{|\\ \cdot CHR}}{N}}- \longrightarrow Fe^{3+}\ :\overset{|}{\underset{\substack{|\\ HOCHR}}{N}}- \longrightarrow :\overset{|}{\underset{\substack{|\\ H}}{N}}- + O{=}CHR$$

Although the initial steps in heteroatom oxygenation and heteroatom dealkylation are the same (abstraction of an electron from the heteroatom to produce a radical cation), the nature of the radical cation determines whether the xenobiotic will undergo oxygenation or dealkylation. The sulfur radical cations of numerous xenobiotics are sufficiently stable to allow oxygen rebound with the heteroatom itself, which results in *S*-oxygenation. However, this is not generally the case with nitrogen radical cations, which undergo rapid deprotonation at the α-carbon, which in turn results in *N*-dealkylation. In general, therefore, cytochrome P450 catalyzes the *N*-dealkylation, not the *N*-oxygenation, of amines. *N*-Oxygenation by cytochrome P450 can occur if the nitrogen radical cation is stabilized by a nearby electron-donating group (mak-

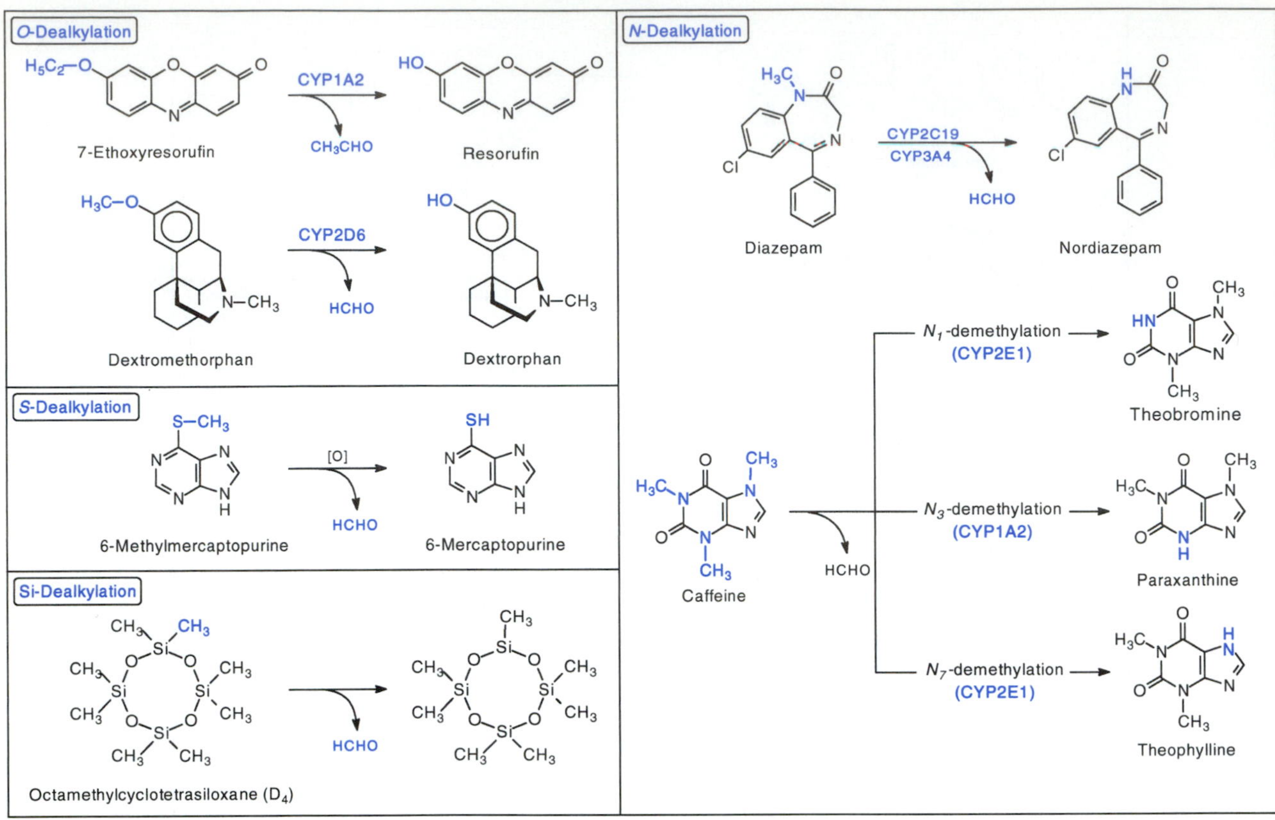

Figure 6-40. Examples of reactions catalyzed by cytochrome P450: Heteroatom dealkylation.

ing the nitrogen electron rich) or if α-protons are either absent (e.g., aromatic amines) or inaccessible (e.g., quinidine). In the case of primary and secondary aromatic amines, *N*-oxygenation by cytochrome P450 usually results in the formation of hydroxylamines, as illustrated in Fig. 6-9. *N*-Hydroxylation of aromatic amines with subsequent conjugation with sulfate or acetate is one mechanism by which tumorigenic aromatic amines, such as 2-acetylaminofluorene, are converted to electrophilic reactive intermediates that bind covalently to DNA (Anders, 1985).

In contrast to cytochrome P450, which oxidizes nitrogen-containing xenobiotics by a radicaloid mechanism involving an initial one-electron oxidation of the heteroatom, the flavin monooxygenases oxidize nitrogen-containing xenobiotics by a heterolytic mechanism involving a two-electron oxidation by the 4a-hydroperoxide of FAD (see Fig. 6-34). These different mechanisms explain why the *N*-oxygenation of xenobiotics by cytochrome P450 generally results in *N*-dealkylation, whereas *N*-oxygenation by the flavin monooxygenases results in *N*-oxide formation. In contrast to cytochrome P450, the flavin monooxygenases do not catalyze *N*-, *O*-, or *S*-dealkylation reactions.

Numerous xenobiotics are *N*-, *O*-, or *S*-dealkylated by cytochrome P450, and some examples of these heteroatom dealkylation reactions are shown in Fig. 6-40. Cytochrome P450 has been shown to catalyze the demethylation of octamethylcyclotetrasiloxane, which is an example of *Si*-demethylation, as shown in Fig. 6-40. The dealkylation of xenobiotics containing an *N*-, *O*-, or *S*-methyl group results in the formation of formaldehyde, which can easily be measured by a simple colorimetric assay to monitor the demethylation of substrates in vitro. The expiration of ^{13}C- or ^{14}C-labeled carbon dioxide following the demethylation of drugs

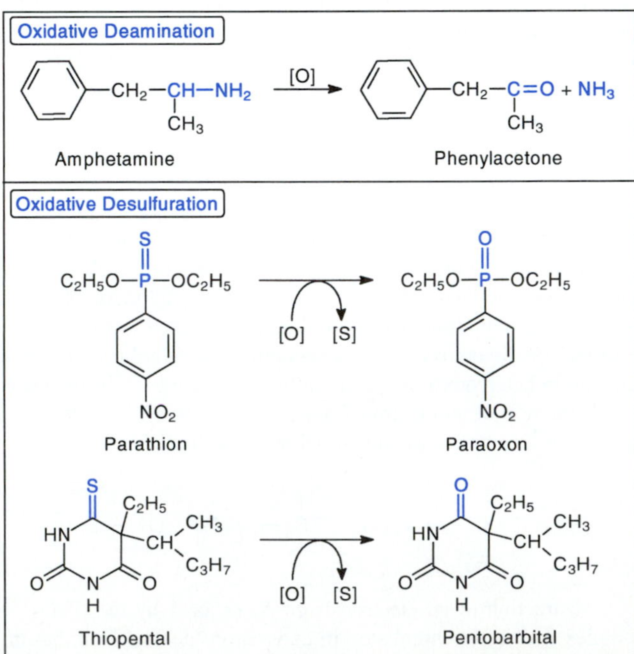

Figure 6-41. Examples of reactions catalyzed by cytochrome P450: Oxidative group transfer.

containing a ^{13}C- or ^{14}C-labeled methyl group has been used to probe cytochrome P450 activity in vivo (Watkins, 1994). The activity of the human P450 enzymes involved in the *N*-demethylation of aminopyrine, erythromycin, and caffeine can be assessed by this technique. Although caffeine has three *N*-methyl groups, all of which can be removed by cytochrome P450, the major pathway in humans involves *N3*-demethylation of caffeine to paraxanthine (see Fig. 6-40).

In addition to *N*-dealkylation, primary amines can also undergo oxidative deamination by cytochrome P450, which is an example of oxidative group transfer. The mechanism is similar to that of *N*-dealkylation: The α-carbon adjacent to the primary amine is hydroxylated, which produces an unstable intermediate that rearranges to eliminate ammonia with the formation of an aldehyde or ketone. The conversion of amphetamine to phenylacetone is an example of oxidative deamination, as shown in Fig. 6-41. Oxidative deamination is also catalyzed by monoamine oxidase (MAO). In the example given above, however, the substrate, amphetamine, contains an α-methyl group which renders it a poor substrate for MAO (as described earlier under *"Monoamine Oxidase, Diamine Oxidase, and Polyamine Oxidase"*).

In addition to oxidative deamination, cytochrome P450 catalyzes two other types of oxidative group transfer, namely oxidative desulfuration and oxidative dehalogenation. In all cases the heteroatom (*N*, *S*, or halogen) is replaced with oxygen. As shown in Fig. 6-42, oxidative desulfuration converts parathion, which has

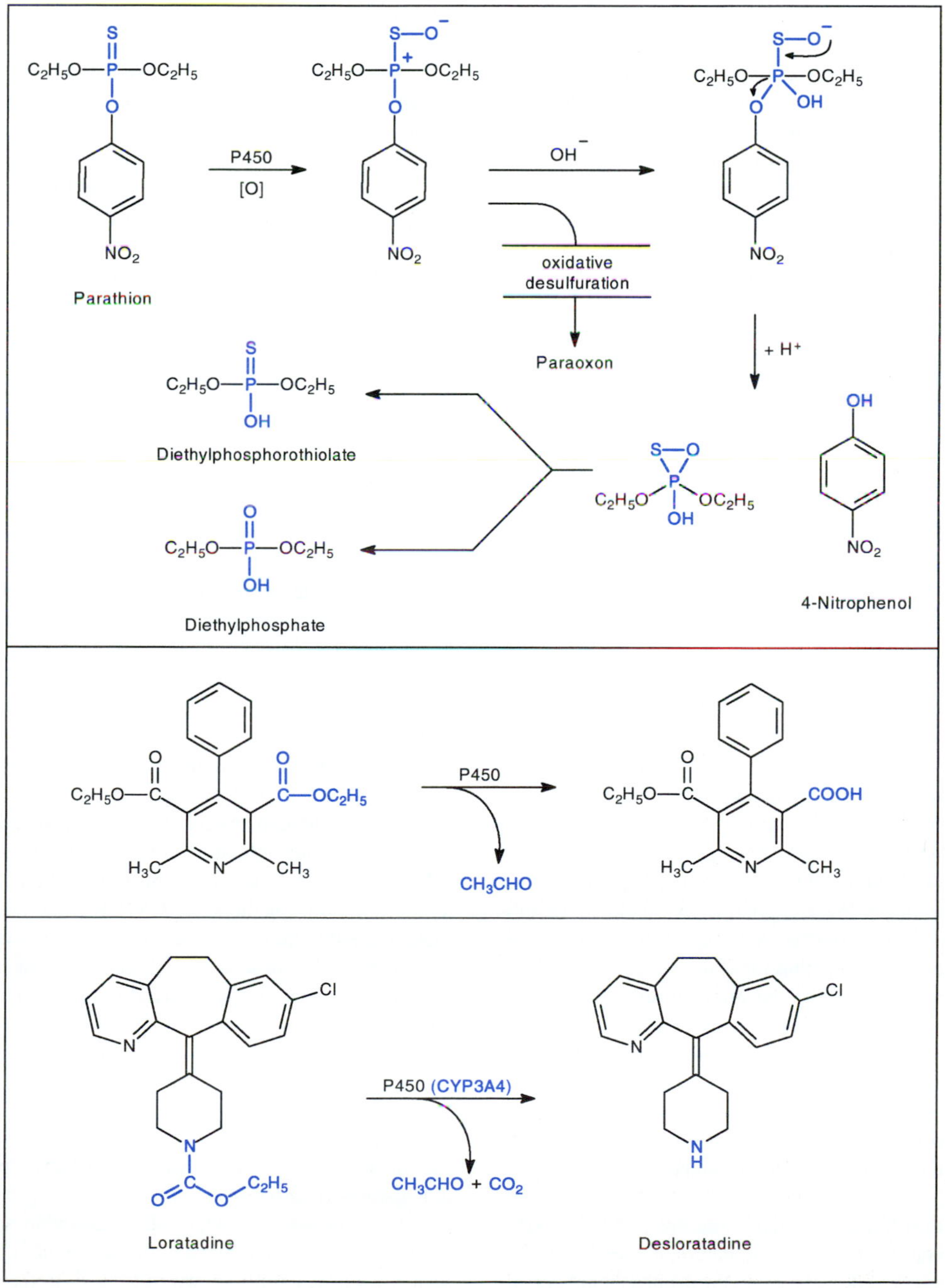

Figure 6-42. Examples of reactions catalyzed by cytochrome P450: Cleavage of esters.

little insecticidal activity, to paraoxon, which is a potent insecticide. The same reaction converts thiopental to pentobarbital. Diethyldithiocarbamate methyl ester, a metabolite of disulfiram, also undergoes oxidative desulfuration. The initial reaction involves *S*-oxidation by cytochrome P450 or FMO to a sulfine ($R_1R_2C{=}S + [O] \rightarrow R_1R_2C \rightarrow S^+{-}O^-$). In the presence of glutathione (GSH) and glutathione *S*-transferase, this sulfine is either converted back to the parent compound ($R_1R_2C{=}S^+{-}O^- + 2\ GSH \rightarrow R_1R_2C{=}S + GSSG + H_2O$) or it undergoes desulfuration ($R_1R_2C{=}S^+{-}O^- + 2\ GSH \rightarrow R_1R_2C{=}O + GSSG + H_2S$) (Madan et al., 1994).

Cytochrome P450 catalyzes both reductive and oxidative dehalogenation reactions (Guengerich, 1991). During oxidative dehalogenation, a halogen and hydrogen from the same carbon atom are replaced with oxygen ($R_1R_2CHX \rightarrow R_1R_2CO$) to produce an aldehyde or acylhalide, as shown in Fig. 6-16 for the conversion of halothane ($CF_3CHClBr$) to trifluoroacetylchloride (CF_3COCl). Oxidative dehalogenation does not involve a direct attack on the carbon–halogen bond, but it involves the formation of an unstable halohydrin by oxidation of the carbon atom bearing the halogen substituent. The carbon–halogen bond is broken during the rearrangement of the unstable halohydrin. When the carbon atom contains a single halogen, the resulting product is an aldehyde, which can be further oxidized to a carboxylic acid or reduced to a primary alcohol. When the carbon atom contains two halogens, the dihalohydrin intermediate rearranges to an acylhalide, which can be converted to the corresponding carboxylic acid (see Fig. 6-16). As discussed previously, aldehydes and, in particular, acylhalides are reactive compounds that can bind covalently to protein and other critical cellular molecules. The immune hepatitis caused by repeated exposure of humans to halothane and related volatile anesthetics is dependent on oxidative dehalogenation by cytochrome P450, with neoantigens produced by the trifluoroacetylation of proteins, as shown in Fig. 6-16.

As shown in Figs. 6-15 and 6-16, cytochrome P450 also can catalyze the reductive dehalogenation of halogenated alkanes and the reduction of certain azo- and nitro-containing xenobiotics (Fig. 6-8). The ability of cytochrome P450 to reduce xenobiotics can be understood from the catalytic cycle shown in Fig. 6-35. Binding of a substrate to cytochrome P450 is followed by a one-electron reduction by NADPH–cytochrome P450 reductase. Under aerobic conditions, reduction of the heme iron to the ferrous state permits binding of oxygen. Anaerobic conditions, in contrast, interrupt the cycle at this point, which allows cytochrome P450 to reduce those substrates capable of accepting an electron. Therefore, cytochrome P450 can catalyze reduction reactions, such as azo-reduction, nitro-reduction, and reductive dehalogenation, particularly under conditions of low oxygen tension. In effect, the substrate rather than molecular oxygen accepts electrons and is reduced. In fact, oxygen acts as an inhibitor of these reactions because it competes with the substrate for the reducing equivalents. The toxicity of many halogenated alkanes is dependent on their biotransformation by reductive dehalogenation. The first step in reductive dehalogenation is a one-electron reduction catalyzed by cytochrome P450, which produces a potentially toxic, carbon-centered radical and inorganic halide. The conversion of CCl_4 to a trichloromethyl radical and other toxic metabolites is shown in Fig. 6-15.

The oxidative desulfuration of parathion involves the production of an intermediate that rearranges to paraoxon (see Fig. 6-41). This same intermediate can decompose to *para*-nitrophenol and diethylphosphorothioic acid, which are the same products formed by the hydrolysis of parathion (Fig. 6-42). In addition to facilitating the hydrolysis of phosphoric acid esters, cytochrome P450 also catalyzes the cleavage of carboxylic acid esters, as shown in Fig. 6-42. Carboxylic acid esters typically are cleaved by carboxylesterases, which results in the formation of an acid and an alcohol ($R_1COOCH_2R_2 + H_2O \rightarrow R_1COOH + R_2CH_2OH$). In contrast, cytochrome P450 converts carboxylic acid esters to an acid plus aldehyde ($R_1COOCH_2\ R_2 + [O] \rightarrow R_1COOH + R_2CHO$), as shown in Fig. 6-42. The deacylation of loratadine is the major route of biotransformation of this nonsedating antihistamine. The reaction is catalyzed predominantly by cytochrome P450 (namely CYP3A4 with a minor contribution from CYP2D6), with little contribution from carboxylesterases.

Cytochrome P450 can also catalyze the dehydrogenation of a number of compounds, including acetaminophen, nifedipine, and related dihydropyridine calcium-channel blockers, sparteine, nicotine, valproic acid, digitoxin, and testosterone, as shown in Fig. 6-43. Dehydrogenation by cytochrome P450 converts acetaminophen to its hepatotoxic metabolite, *N*-acetylbenzoquinoneimine, as shown in Fig. 6-28. Dehydrogenation of digitoxin (dt_3) to 15′-dehydro-dt_3 leads to cleavage of the terminal sugar residue to produce digitoxigenin bisdigitoxoside (dt_2), which can similarly be converted to 9′-dehydro-dt_2, which undergoes digitoxosyl cleavage to digitoxigenin monodigitoxoside (dt_1). In contrast to digitoxin, this latter metabolite is an excellent substrate for glucuronidation. In rats, the P450 enzymes responsible for converting digitoxin to dt_1 (namely the CYP3A enzymes) and the UDP-glucuronosyltransferase responsible for glucuronidating dt_1 are inducible by dexamethasone, pregnenolone-16α-carbonitrile, and spironolactone, all of which protect rats from the toxic effects of digitoxin. The dehydrogenation of nicotine produces nicotine $\Delta^{1',5'}$-iminium ion, which is oxidized by cytosolic aldehyde oxidase to cotinine, a major metabolite of nicotine excreted in the urine of cigarette smokers.

Testosterone is dehydrogenated by cytochrome P450 to two metabolites: 6-dehydrotestosterone, which involves formation of a carbon–carbon double bond, and androstenedione, which involves formation of a carbon–oxygen double bond. The conversion of testosterone to androstenedione is one of several cases where cytochrome P450 converts a primary or secondary alcohol to an aldehyde or ketone, respectively. The reaction can proceed by formation of a *gem*-diol (two hydroxyl groups on the same carbon atom), with subsequent dehydration to a keto group, as shown in Fig. 6-20 for the conversion of ethanol to acetaldehyde. However, *gem*-diols are not obligatory intermediates in the oxidation of alcohols by cytochrome P450, and in fact the conversion of testosterone to androstenedione by CYP2B1 (the major phenobarbital-inducible P450 enzyme in rats) does not involve the intermediacy of a *gem*-diol but proceeds by direct dehydrogenation (Fig. 6-43). In contrast, a *gem*-diol is involved in the formation of androstenedione from *epi*-testosterone (which is identical to testosterone except the hydroxyl group at C17 is in the α-configuration, not the β-configuration). The fact that formation of androstenedione from *epi*-testosterone involves formation of a *gem*-diol, whereas its formation from testosterone does not, makes it difficult to generalize the mechanism by which cytochrome P450 converts alcohols to aldehydes and ketones.

Liver microsomes from all mammalian species contain numerous P450 enzymes, each with the potential to catalyze the various types of reactions shown in Figs. 6-36 through 6-43. In other

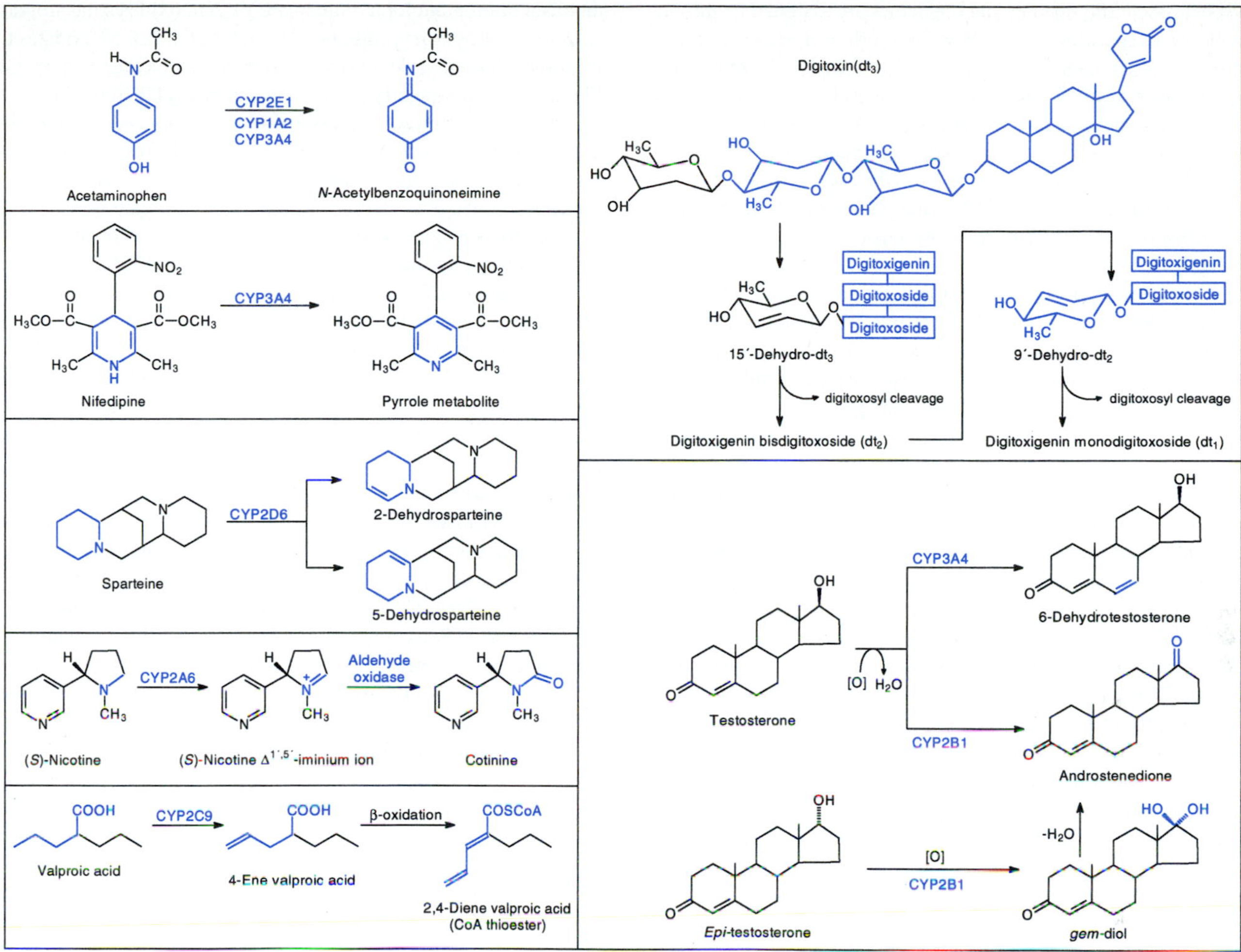

Figure 6-43. Examples of reactions catalyzed by cytochrome P450: Dehydrogenation.

words, all of the P450 enzymes expressed in liver microsomes have the potential to catalyze xenobiotic hydroxylation, epoxidation, dealkylation, oxygenation, dehydrogenation, and so forth. The broad and often overlapping substrate specificity of liver microsomal P450 enzymes precludes the possibility of naming these enzymes for the reactions they catalyze. The amino acid sequence of numerous P450 enzymes has been determined, largely by recombinant DNA techniques, and such sequences now form the basis for classifying and naming P450 enzymes (Gonzalez, 1989; Nelson et al., 1993). In general, P450 enzymes with less than 40 percent amino acid sequence identity are assigned to different gene families (gene families 1, 2, 3, 4, etc.). P450 enzymes that are 40 to 55 percent identical are assigned to different subfamilies (e.g., 2A, 2B, 2C, 2D, 2E, etc.). P450 enzymes that are more than 55 percent identical are classified as members of the same subfamily (e.g., 2A1, 2A2, 2A3, etc.). The liver microsomal P450 enzymes involved in xenobiotic biotransformation belong to three main P450 gene families, namely CYP1, CYP2, and CYP3. Liver microsomes also contain P450 enzymes encoded by the CYP4 gene family, substrates for which include several fatty acids and eicosanoids but relatively few xenobiotics. The liver microsomal P450 enzymes in each of these gene families belong to a single subfamily (i.e., CYP3A and CYP4A), two subfamilies (i.e., CYP1A and CYP1B) or five subfamilies (i.e., CYP2A, CYP2B, CYP2C, CYP2D, and CYP2E). The number of P450 enzymes in each subfamily differs from one species to the next.

Human liver microsomes can contain 15 or more different P450 enzymes (CYP1A1, 1A2, 1B1, 2A6, 2B6, 2C8, 2C9, 2C18, 2C19, 2D6, 2E1, 3A4, 3A5, 3A7, 4A9, and 4A11) that biotransform xenobiotics and/or endogenous substrates (Guengerich, 1994; Wrighton and Stevens, 1992). Other P450 enzymes in human liver microsomes have been described, but they appear to be allelic variants of the aforementioned enzymes rather than distinct gene products. For example, CYP2C10 is an allelic variant of CYP2C9. Unfortunately, a nomenclature system based on structure does not guarantee that structurally related proteins in different species will perform the same function (examples of such functional differences are given later). Some P450 enzymes have the same name in all mammalian species, whereas others are named in a species-specific manner. For example, all mammalian species contain two P450 enzymes belonging to the CYP1A subfamily, and in all cases these are known as CYP1A1 and CYP1A2 because the function and regulation of these enzymes are highly conserved among mammalian species. The same is true of CYP1B1 and CYP2E1. In other words, CYP1A1, CYP1A2, CYP1B1, and CYP2E1 are not species-specific names but rather names given to proteins in all mammalian species. In all other cases, functional or evolutionary relationships are not immediately apparent; hence, the P450 enzymes are named in a species-specific manner and the names are assigned in chronological order regardless of the species of origin. For example, human liver microsomes express CYP2A6, but this is the only functional member of the CYP2A subfamily found in the human liver. The other members of this subfamily (i.e., CYP2A1 to CYP2A5) are the names given to rat and mouse proteins, which were sequenced before the human enzyme. With the exception of CYP1A1, CYP1A2, CYP1B1, and CYP2E1, the names of all of the other P450 enzymes in human liver microsomes refer specifically to human P450 enzymes.

Without exception, the levels and activity of each P450 enzyme have been shown to vary from one individual to the next, due to environmental and/or genetic factors (Meyer, 1994; Shimada et al., 1994). Decreased P450 enzyme activity can result from (1) a genetic mutation that either blocks the synthesis of a P450 enzyme or leads to the synthesis of a catalytically compromised or inactive enzyme, (2) exposure to an environmental factor (such as an infectious disease or a xenobiotic) that suppresses P450 enzyme expression, or (3) exposure to a xenobiotic that inhibits or inactivates a preexisting P450 enzyme. By inhibiting cytochrome P450, one drug can impair the biotransformation of another, which may lead to an exaggerated pharmacologic or toxicologic response to the second drug. In this regard, inhibition of cytochrome P450 mimics the effects of a genetic deficiency in P450 enzyme expression. Increased P450 enzyme activity can result from (1) gene duplication leading to over expression of a P450 enzyme; (2) exposure to environmental factors, such as xenobiotics, that induce the synthesis of cytochrome P450; or (3) stimulation of preexisting enzyme by a xenobiotic.

Although activation of cytochrome P450 has been documented in vitro, it appears to occur in vivo only under special circumstances. Although duplication of functional P450 genes has been documented, induction of cytochrome P450 by xenobiotics is the most common mechanism by which P450 enzyme activity is increased. By inducing cytochrome P450, one drug can stimulate the metabolism of a second drug and thereby decrease or ameliorate its therapeutic effect. A dramatic effect of this type of drug interaction is the induction of ethinylestradiol metabolism by phenobarbital and rifampin, which can ameliorate the contraceptive effect of the former drug and lead to unplanned pregnancy. Allelic variants, which arise by point mutations in the wild-type gene, are another source of interindividual variation in P450 activity. Amino acid substitutions can increase or, more commonly, decrease P450 enzyme activity, although the effect may be substrate-dependent. Examples of genetic factors that influence P450 activity are given later in this section. The environmental factors known to affect P450 levels include medications (e.g., barbiturates, anticonvulsants, rifampin, troglitazone, isoniazid), foods (e.g., cruciferous vegetables, charcoal-broiled beef), social habits (e.g., alcohol consumption, cigarette smoking), and disease status (diabetes, inflammation, viral and bacterial infection, hyperthyroidism, and hypothyroidism). When environmental factors influence P450 enzyme levels, considerable variation may be observed during repeated measures of xenobiotic biotransformation (e.g., drug metabolism) in the same individual. Such variation is not observed when alterations in P450 activity are determined genetically.

Due to their broad substrate specificity, it is possible that two or more P450 enzymes can contribute to the metabolism of a single compound. For example, two P450 enzymes, designated CYP2D6 and CYP2C19, both contribute significantly to the metabolism of propranolol in humans: CYP2D6 oxidizes the aromatic ring to give 4-hydroxypropranolol, whereas CYP2C19 oxidizes the isopropanolamine side chain to give naphthoxylactic acid (see Fig. 6-23). Consequently, changes in either CYP2D6 or CYP2C19 do not markedly affect the disposition of propranolol. Three human P450 enzymes, CYP1A2, CYP2E1, and CYP3A4, can convert the commonly used analgesic, acetaminophen, to its hepatotoxic metabolite, *N*-acetylbenzoquinoneimine (Fig. 6-43). It is also possible for a single P450 enzyme to catalyze two or more metabolic pathways for the same drug. For example, CYP2D6 catalyzes both the *O*-demethylation and 5-hydroxylation (aromatic ring hydroxylation) of methoxyphenamine, and CYP3A4 catalyzes the 3-hydroxylation and *N*-oxygenation of quinidine, the M1-, M17-, and M21-oxidation of cyclosporine, the 1- and 4-hydroxylation of midazolam, the *tert*-butyl-hydroxylation and *N*-dealkylation of terfenadine, and several pathways of testosterone oxidation, including 1β-, 2β-, 6β-, and 15β-hydroxylation and dehydrogenation to 6-dehydrotestosterone (Figs. 6-36 and 6-43).

The pharmacologic or toxic effects of certain drugs are exaggerated in a significant percentage of the population due to a heritable deficiency in a P450 enzyme (Tucker, 1994; Meyer, 1994; Smith et al., 1998). The two major polymorphically expressed P450 enzymes are CYP2D6 and CYP2C19, although allelic variants have been described for nearly all of the human P450 enzymes involved in xenobiotic biotransformation (Smith et al., 1998). Individuals lacking CYP2D6 or CYP2C19 were initially identified as poor metabolizers of debrisoquine and *S*-mephenytoin, respectively. However, because each P450 enzyme has a broad substrate specificity, each genetic defect affects the metabolism of several drugs. The incidence of the poor-metabolizer phenotype varies among different ethnic groups. For example, 5 to 10 percent of Caucasians are poor metabolizers of debrisoquine (an antihypertensive drug metabolized by CYP2D6), whereas less than 1 percent of Japanese subjects are defective in CYP2D6 activity. In contrast, ~20 percent of Japanese subjects are poor metabolizers of *S*-mephenytoin (an anticonvulsant metabolized by CYP2C19), whereas less than 5 percent of Caucasians are so affected. On Vanuatu and some other Pacific islands, as many as 70 percent of the population are CYP2C19 poor metabolizers (Kaneko et al., 1999). Some individuals have been identified as poor metabolizers of tolbutamide and phenytoin, both of which are metabolized by CYP2C9, or as poor metabolizers of coumarin or phenacetin, which are metabolized by CYP2A6 and CYP1A2, respectively. However, the incidence of each of these phenotypes is apparently less than 1 percent of the populations examined to date.

The observation that individuals who are genetically deficient in a particular P450 enzyme are poor metabolizers of one or more drugs illustrates a very important principle—namely that the rate of elimination of drugs can be largely determined by a single P450 enzyme. This observation seems to contradict the fact that P450 enzymes have broad and overlapping substrate specificities. The resolution to this apparent paradox lies in the fact that, although more than one human P450 enzyme can catalyze the biotransformation of a xenobiotic, they may do so with markedly different affinities. Consequently, xenobiotic biotransformation in vivo, where only low substrate concentrations are usually achieved, is often determined by the P450 enzyme with the highest affinity (lowest apparent K_m) for the xenobiotic. For example, the *N*-demethylation of diazepam (shown in Fig. 6-40) and the 5-hydroxylation of omeprazole are both catalyzed by two human

P450 enzymes, namely CYP2C19 and CYP3A4. However, these reactions are catalyzed by CYP3A4 with such low affinity that the *N*-demethylation of diazepam and the 5-hydroxylation of omeprazole in vivo appear to be dominated by CYP2C19 (Kato and Yamazoe, 1994a). When several P450 enzymes catalyze the same reaction, their relative contribution to xenobiotic biotransformation is determined by the kinetic parameter, V_{max}/K_m, which is a measure of in vitro intrinsic clearance at low substrate concentrations (<10 percent of K_m) (Houston, 1994).

Inasmuch as the biotransformation of a xenobiotic in humans is frequently dominated by a single P450 enzyme, considerable attention has been paid to defining the substrate specificity of the P450 enzymes expressed in human liver microsomes (a process commonly referred to as *reaction phenotyping* or *enzyme mapping*). Three in vitro approaches have been developed for reaction phenotyping. Each has its advantages and disadvantages, and a combination of approaches is usually required to identify which human P450 enzyme is responsible for metabolizing a xenobiotic (Wrighton et al., 1993; Rodrigues 1999; Madan et al., 2000). The three approaches to reaction phenotyping are as follows:

1. *Correlation analysis,* which involves measuring the rate of xenobiotic metabolism by several samples of human liver microsomes and correlating reaction rates with the variation in the level or activity of the individual P450 enzymes in the same microsomal samples. This approach is successful because the levels of the P450 enzymes in human liver microsomes vary enormously from sample to sample (up to 100-fold) but vary independently from each other.
2. *Chemical and antibody inhibition,* which involves an evaluation of the effects of known P450 enzyme inhibitors or inhibitory antibodies on the metabolism of a xenobiotic by human liver microsomes. Chemical inhibitors of cytochrome P450, which are discussed later, must be used cautiously because most of them can inhibit more than one P450 enzyme. Some chemical inhibitors are metabolism-dependent (mechanism-based) inhibitors that require biotransformation to a metabolite that inactivates or noncompetitively inhibits cytochrome P450.
3. *Biotransformation by purified or recombinant human P450 enzymes,* which can establish whether a particular P450 enzyme can or cannot biotransform a xenobiotic, but it does not address whether that P450 enzyme contributes substantially to reactions catalyzed by human liver microsomes. The information obtained with purified or recombinant human P450 enzymes can be improved by taking into account large differences in the extent to which the individual P450 enzymes are expressed in human liver microsomes, which is summarized in Table 6-4. Some P450 enzymes, such as CYP1A1 and CYP1B1, are expressed at such low levels in human liver microsomes that they contribute negligibly to the hepatic biotransformation of xenobiotics. Other P450 enzymes are expressed in some but not all livers. For example, CYP3A5 is expressed in ~25 percent of human livers.

These in vitro approaches have been used to characterize the substrate specificity of several of the P450 enzymes expressed in human liver microsomes. Examples of reactions catalyzed by human P450 enzymes are shown in Figs. 6-36 through 6-43, and examples of substrates, inhibitors, and inducers for each P450 enzyme are given in Table 6-5. Additional examples appear in a comprehensive review by Rendic and Di Carlo (1997), and clinically important examples can be found on the Internet at http://www.dml.georgetown.edu/depts/pharmacology/davetab.html (Abernathy and Flockhart, 2000). It should be emphasized that reaction phenotyping in vitro is not always carried out with pharmacologically or toxicologically relevant substrate concentrations. As a result, the P450 enzyme that appears responsible for biotransforming the drug in vitro may not be the P450 enzyme responsible for biotransforming the drug in vivo. This may be particularly true of CYP3A4, which metabolizes several drugs with high capacity but low affinity. The salient features of the major P450 enzymes in human liver microsomes are summarized below (subsequent sections, this chapter).

Table 6-4
Concentration of Individual P450 Enzymes in Human Liver Microsomes

	Specific Content (pmol/mg protein)		
P450 ENZYME	SOURCE (1)	SOURCE (2)	SOURCE (3)
CYP1A2	45	42	15
CYP2A6	68	42	12
CYP2B6	39	1.0	3.0
CYP2C8	64		
CYP2C9	96		
CYP2C18	<2.5		
CYP2C19	19		
CYP2D6	10	5.0	15
CYP2E1	49	22	
CYP3A4	108	98	40
CYP3A5	1.0		
TOTAL	534	344	

SOURCE: Rodrigues, 1999.

CYP1A1/2 All mammalian species apparently possess two inducible CYP1A enzymes, namely CYP1A1 and CYP1A2. Human liver microsomes contain relatively high levels of CYP1A2 but not of CYP1A1, even though this enzyme is readily detectable in the human lung, intestine, skin, lymphocytes, and placenta, particularly from cigarette smokers. In addition to cigarette smoke, inducers of the CYP1A enzymes include charcoal-broiled meat (a source of polycyclic aromatic hydrocarbons), cruciferous vegetables (a source of various indoles), and omeprazole, a proton-pump inhibitor used to suppress gastric acid secretion. In contrast to CYP1A1, CYP1A2 is not expressed in extrahepatic tissues. CYP1A1 and CYP1A2 both catalyze the *O*-dealkylation of 7-methoxyresorufin and 7-ethoxyresorufin (see Fig. 6-40). Reactions preferentially catalyzed by CYP1A1 include the hydroxylation and epoxidation of benzo[a]pyrene (see Fig. 6-6) and the epoxidation of the leukotriene D_4 receptor antagonist, verlukast (Fig. 6-38). CYP1A2 catalyzes the *N*-hydroxylation of aromatic amines, such as 4-aminobiphenyl and 2-aminonaphthalene, which in many cases represents the initial step in the conversion of aromatic amines to tumorigenic metabolites (see Fig. 6-9). CYP1A2 also catalyzes the *O*-dealkylation of phenacetin and the 4-hydroxylation of acetanilide, both of which produce acetaminophen, which can be converted by CYP1A2 and other P450 enzymes

Table 6-5
Examples of Substrates, Inhibitors, and Inducers of the Major Human Liver Microsomal P450 Enzymes Involved in Xenobiotic Biotransformation

	CYP2A6	CYP2B6	CYP2C8	CYP2C9	CYP2C19	CYP2E1
Substrates	Coumarin Butadiene Nicotine	Benzphetamine 7-Benzyloxyresorufin Bupropion Cyclophosphamide 7-Ethoxy-4-trifluoro-methylcoumarin Ifosphamide *S*-Mephenytoin	Arachidonic acid Carbamazepine Paclitaxel (Taxol)	Celecoxib Diclofenac Phenacetin Phenobarbital Phenytoin Piroxicam Tenoxicam Tetrahydrocannabinol Tienilic acid Tolbutamide Torsemide *S*-Warfarin	Citalopram Diazepam Diphenylhydantoin Hexobarbital Imipramine Lansoprazole *S*-Mephenytoin Mephobarbital Omeprazole Pentamidine Phenobarbital Proguanil Propranolol	Acetaminophen Alcohols Aniline Benzene Caffeine Chlorzoxazone Dapsone Enflurane Halogenated alkanes Isoflurane Methylformamide 4-Nitrophenol Nitrosamines Styrene Theophylline
Inhibitors	Diethyldithiocarbamate Letrozole 8-Methoxypsoralen* Pilocarpine Tranylcypromine	9-Ethynylphenathrene Methoxychlor Orphenadrine*	Etoposide Nicardipine Quercetin Tamoxifen *R*-Verapamil	Sulfaphenazole Sulfinpyrazone	Fluconazole Teniposide Tranylcypromine	3-Amino-1,2,4-triazole* Diethyldithiocarbamate Dihydrocapsaicin Dimethyl sulfoxide Disulfiram 4-Methylpyrazole Phenethylisothiocyanate*
Inducers	Barbiturates?	Phenobarbital Phenytoin Rifampin Troglitazone	Not known	Rifampin	Artemisinin? Rifampin	Ethanol Isoniazid

*Metabolism-dependent (mechanism-based) inhibitor.

Table 6-5 (*continued*)

	CYP1A2	CYP2D6			CYP3A4		
Substrates	Acetaminophen Acetanilide Aminopyrine Antipyrine Aromatic amines Caffeine Estradiol Ethoxyresorufin Imipramine Methoxyresorufin Phenacetin Tacrine Theophylline Trimethadone Warfarin	Amiflamine Amitriptyline Aprindine Brofaromine Bufurolol Captopril Chlorpramazine Cinnarizine Citalopram Clonipramine Clozapine Codeine Debrisoquine Deprenyl Desmethylcitalopram Despiramine Dextromethorphan	Dolasetron Encainide Flecainide Fluoxetine Flunarizine Fluphenazine Guanoxan Haloperidol (reduced) Hydrocodone Imipramine Indoramin Methoxyamphetamine Methoxyphenamine Metoprolol Mexiletene Mianserin	Miniaprine Nortriptyline Ondansetron Paroxetine Perhexiline Perphenazine Propafenone Propranolol *N*-Propylajmaline Remoxipride Sparteine Tamoxifen Thioridazine Timolol Tomoxetine Trifluperidol Tropisetron	Acetaminophen Aldrin Alfentanil Amiodarone Aminopyrine Amprenavir Antipyrine Astemizole Benzphetamine Budesonide Carbamazepine Celecoxib Cisapride Cyclophosphamide Cyclosporin Dapsone Delavirdine Digitoxin Diltiazem Diazepam	Erythromycin Ethinylestradiol Etoposide Flutamide Hydroxyarginine Ifosphamide Imipramine Indinavir Lansoprazole Lidocaine Loratadine Losartan Lovastatin Midazolam Nelfinavir Nicardipine Nifedipine Omeprazole Quinidine	Rapamycin Retinoic acid Saquinavir Steroids (e.g., cortisol) Tacrolimus (FK 506) Tamoxifen Taxol Teniposide Terfenadine Tetrahydrocannabinol Theophylline Toremifene Triazolam Trimethadone Troleandomycin Verapamil Warfarin Zatosetron Zonisamide
Inhibitors	Ciprofloxacin Fluvoxamine Furafylline* α-Naphthoflavone	Ajmalicine Celecoxib Chinidin Corynanthine	Fluoxetine Lobelin Propidin	Quinidine Trifluperidol Yohimbine	Amprenavir Clotrimazole Delavirdine Ethinylestradiol* Fluoxetine Gestodene*	Indinavir Itraconazole Ketoconazole Miconazole Nelfinavir Nicardipine	Ritonavir Saquinavir Troleandomycin* Verapamil *Activator:* α-Naphthoflavone
Inducers	Charcoal-broiled beef Cigarette smoke Cruciferous vegetables Omeprazole	None known			Carbamazepine Dexamethasone Glutethimide Nevirapine Phenobarbital	Phenytoin Rifabutin Rifampin Ritonavir? St. John's Wort	Sulfadimidine Sulfinpyrazone Troglitazone Troleandomycin

*Metabolism-dependent (mechanism-based) inhibitor.

to a toxic benzoquinoneimine (Fig. 6-28). The anticholinesterase agent tacrine, which is used in the treatment of Alzheimer's disease, is similarly converted by CYP1A2 to a reactive quinoneimine/quinone methide (Pirmohamed and Park, 1999). As shown in Fig. 6-40, CYP1A2 catalyzes the *N3*-demethylation of caffeine to paraxanthine. By measuring rates of formation of paraxanthine in blood, urine, or saliva or by measuring the exhalation of isotopically labeled CO_2 from ^{13}C- or ^{14}C-labeled caffeine, the *N3*-demethylation of caffeine can be used as an in vivo probe of CYP1A2 activity, which varies enormously from one individual to the next. CYP1A1 and CYP1A2 are both inhibited by α-naphthoflavone. Ellipticine preferentially inhibits CYP1A1, whereas the metabolism-dependent inhibitor furafylline is a specific inhibitor of CYP1A2.

Although CYP1A1 and CYP1A2 are expressed in all mammals, there are species differences in their function and regulation. For example, although CYP1A1 is not expressed in human liver (or in the liver of most other mammalian species), it appears to be constitutively expressed in rhesus monkey and guinea pig liver. Conversely, although CYP1A2 is expressed in human liver (and in most other mammalian species), it does not appear to be constitutively expressed in cynomolgus monkey liver. Polycyclic and polyhalogenated aromatic hydrocarbons appear to induce CYP1A enzymes in all mammalian species. In contrast, omeprazole is an inducer of CYP1A enzymes in humans, but not in mice or rabbits (Diaz et al., 1990). The function of the CYP1A enzymes is fairly well conserved across species, although there are subtle differences. For example, in some species, such as the rat, CYP1A1 is considerably more effective than CYP1A2 as a catalyst of 7-ethoxyresorufin *O*-dealkylation, whereas the opposite is true in other species, such as rabbit. In mice, CYP1A1 and CYP1A2 catalyze the *O*-dealkylation of 7-ethoxyresorufin at comparable rates. In the rat, CYP1A1 preferentially catalyzes the *O*-dealkylation of 7-ethoxyresorufin whereas CYP1A2 preferentially catalyzes the *O*-dealkylation of 7-methoxyresorufin. However, in other species, such as the mouse and the human, CYP1A2 catalyzes the *O*-dealkylation of 7-ethoxyresorufin and 7-methoxyresorufin at about the same rate. There are also species differences in the affinity with which CYP1A2 interacts with xenobiotics. For example, furafylline is a potent, metabolism-dependent inhibitor of human CYP1A2 but a weak inhibitor of rat CYP1A2. Although the levels of CYP1A2 vary enormously from one individual to the next, genetic defects in CYP1A2 are rare (<1 percent).

CYP2A6 Enzymes belonging to the *CYP2A* gene family show marked species differences in catalytic function. For example, the two CYP2A enzymes expressed in rat liver, namely CYP2A1 and CYP2A2, primarily catalyze the 7α- and 15α-hydroxylation of testosterone, respectively. In contrast, the CYP2A enzyme expressed in human liver, namely CYP2A6, catalyzes the 7-hydroxylation of coumarin, as shown in Fig. 6-37. Just as rat CYP2A1 and CYP2A2 have little or no capacity to 7-hydroxylate coumarin, human CYP2A6 has little or no capacity to hydroxylate testosterone. Mouse liver microsomes contain three CYP2A enzymes: a testosterone 7α-hydroxylase (CYP2A1), a testosterone 15α-hydroxylase (CYP2A4), and a coumarin 7-hydroxylase (CYP2A5). Functionally, CYP2A5 can be converted to CYP2A4 by a single amino acid substitution ($Phe_{209} \rightarrow Leu_{209}$). In other words, this single amino substitution converts CYP2A5 from a coumarin 7-hydroxylating to a testosterone 15α-hydroxylating enzyme (Lindberg and Negishi, 1989). The fact that a small change in primary structure can have a dramatic effect on substrate specificity makes it difficult to predict whether orthologous proteins in different species (which are structurally similar but never identical) will catalyze the same reactions.

Differences in CYP2A function have important implications for the adverse effects of coumarin, which is hepatotoxic to rats but not humans. Whereas coumarin is detoxified in humans by conversion to 7-hydroxycoumarin, which is subsequently conjugated with glucuronic acid and excreted, a major pathway of coumarin biotransformation in rats involves formation of the hepatotoxic metabolite, coumarin 3,4-epoxide, as shown in Fig. 6-38. In addition to catalyzing the 7-hydroxylation of coumarin, CYP2A6 converts 1,3-butadiene to butadiene monoxide and nicotine to nicotine $\Delta^{1',5'}$-iminium ion, which is further oxidized by aldehyde oxidase to cotinine, as shown in Fig. 6-43. 8-Methoxypsoralen, a structural analog of coumarin, is a potent, metabolism-dependent inhibitor of CYP2A6. Although the levels of CYP2A6 vary enormously from one individual to the next, genetic defects in this enzyme are rare (<1 percent). Nevertheless, those individuals who lack CYP2A6 appear to have an aversion to cigarette smoking, presumably because they are poor metabolizers of nicotine (Pianezza et al., 1998).

CYP2B6 Enzymes belonging to the CYP2B subfamily have been studied extensively in many species, although only recently was it appreciated that, despite its low levels in human liver, CYP2B6 contributes significantly to the biotransformation of certain xenobiotics (Ekins and Wrighton, 1999). CYP2B6 appears to be the functional gene expressed in human, with CYP2B7 (a splice variant of CYP2B6) unable to encode for a functional enzyme. CYP2B6 catalyzes the *O*-dealkylation of 7-ethoxy-4-trifluromethylcoumarin, the *N*-demethylation of benzphetamine, and the *O*-dealkylation of benzyloxyresorufin; however, these reactions are not selective for CYP2B6. More specific reactions are *S*-mephenytoin *N*-demethylation and the cyclopentyl ring hydroxylation of the phosphodiester inhibitor 3-cyclopentyloxy-*N*-(3,5-dichloro-4-pyridyl)-4-methoxybenzamide (RP 73401). Orphenadrine inhibits CYP2B6, but not selectively. 9-Ethynylphenanthrene has been shown to be a potent metabolism-dependent (mechanism-based) inhibitor of CYP2B6, and appears to be selective. CYP2B6 levels in adult human liver are low, but the enzyme is inducible by rifampin, troglitazone and various anticonvulsant drugs (phenobarbital, phenytoin), which also induce CYP3A4. Phenobarbital (and a host of other xenobiotics) primarily induce the corresponding CYP2B enzymes in other species. For example, CYP2B10, CYP2B1/2, CYP2B11 and CYP2B17 are the major phenobarbital-inducible P450 enzymes in mouse, rat, dog, and cynomolgus monkey, respectively.

CYP2C8 The 6α-hydroxylation of the taxane ring of paclitaxel (which generates a metabolite known as M5, VIII′ and HM3) is a specific marker for CYP2C8 (Rahman et al., 1994). Another pathway of paclitaxel metabolism, aromatic hydroxylation (3′-p-hydroxylaton) to M4 (also known as VII′), is catalyzed by CYP3A enzymes. CYP2C8 catalyzes the 10,11-epoxidation of carbamazepine, although this reaction in human liver microsomes is dominated by CYP3A4/5. The 4-hydroxylation of all-*trans* retinoic acid appears to be catalyzed primarily by CYP2C8, however, members of the CYP3A subfamily may be minor participants as well. CYP2C8 also metabolizes endogenous arachidonic acid to form epoxyeicosatrienoic acids, which are converted by cytosolic epoxide hydrolase dihydroeicosatrienoic acids. It has been speculated that the biologically active eicosanoids may be important in maintaining homeostasis in the liver. The multidrug resistance (MDR) reversing agents *R*-verapamil, tamoxifen, and etoposide (VP-16) inhibit the CYP2C8-dependent metabolism of paclitaxel but also inhibit its metabolism by CYP3A4. Quercetin has been shown to inhibit the CYP2C8-dependent hydroxylation of paclitaxel; however, it may not inhibit CYP2C8 selectively.

CYP2C9 A genetic polymorphism for tolbutamide metabolism was first described in 1978–1979, although its incidence is still unknown (Back and Orme, 1992). Poor metabolizers are defective in CYP2C9, which catalyzes the methyl-hydroxylation of this hypoglycemic agent. Poor metabolizers of tolbutamide are also poor metabolizers of phenytoin, which is consistent with in vitro data suggesting that CYP2C9 catalyzes both the methyl-hydroxylation of tolbutamide and the 4-hydroxylation of phenytoin. The antimalarial naphthoquinone 58C80 is converted to a *t*-butyl hydroxylated metabolite by CYP2C9. CYP2C9 also catalyzes the 7-hydroxylation and, to a lesser extent, the 6-hydroxylation of *S*-warfarin; it also appears to catalyze the 7-hydroxylation of Δ^1-tetrahydrocannabinol. Although CYP2C9 (Arg_{144}, Tyr_{358}, Ile_{359}, Gly_{417}) and its allelic variant CYP2C9 ($Arg_{144} \rightarrow Cys_{144}$) both catalyze the methyl-hydroxylation of tolbutamide (the former being twice as active as the latter), the latter enzyme is virtually devoid of *S*-warfarin 6- and 7-hydroxylase activity (Rettie et al., 1994). This suggests that individuals who express the allelic variant CYP2C9 ($Arg_{144} \rightarrow Cys_{144}$) could be poor metabolizers of warfarin but near normal metabolizers of tolbutamide. CYP2C9 also appears to be responsible for metabolizing several NSAIDs, including the 4′-hydroxylation of diclofenac and the 5′-hydroxylation of piroxicam and tenoxicam. Tienilic acid is also metabolized by CYP2C9, but with potentially deleterious effects. CYP2C9 converts tienilic acid to an electrophilic thiophene sulfoxide, which can react either with water to give 5-hydroxytienilic acid or with a nucleophilic amino acid (Ser_{365}) in CYP2C9 to form a covalent adduct, which inactivates the enzyme (Koenigs et al., 1999). Antibodies directed against the adduct between CYP2C9 and tienilic acid are thought to be responsible for the immunoallergic hepatitis that develops in about 1 out of every 10,000 patients treated with this uricosuric diuretic drug. Sulfaphenazole is a potent inhibitor of CYP2C9, both in vitro and in vivo.

CYP2C18 The functions of CYP2C18 are largely unknown. The mRNA encoding this protein is expressed in all human livers, although the mean value is one-seventh to one-eighth that of the mRNAs encoding CYP2C8 and CYP2C9. The levels of CYP2C18 mRNA vary widely from one liver to the next and vary independently of the mRNAs encoding CYP2C8 and CYP2C9, which tend to be coregulated.

CYP2C19 A genetic polymorphism for the metabolism of *S*-mephenytoin was first described in 1984 (reviewed in Wilkinson et al., 1989). The deficiency affects the 4′-hydroxylation (aromatic ring hydroxylation) of this anticonvulsant drug. The other major pathway of *S*-mephenytoin metabolism, namely *N*-demethylation to *S*-nirvanol, is catalyzed by CYP2B6, so it is not affected. Consequently, poor metabolizers excrete little or no 4′-hydroxymephenytoin in their urine but excrete increased amounts of the *N*-demethylated metabolite, *S*-nirvanol (*S*-phenylethylhydantoin). Interestingly, the P450 enzyme responsible for this genetic polymorphism, namely cytochrome CYP2C19, is highly stereoselective for the *S*-enantiomer of mephenytoin. In contrast to the *S*-enantiomer, the *R*-enantiomer is not converted to 4′-hydroxymephenytoin but is *N*-demethylated to *R*-nirvanol (*R*-phenylethylhydantoin). The formulation of mephenytoin used clinically is mesantoin, which is a racemic mixture of *S*- and *R*-enantiomers. An exaggerated central response has been observed in poor metabolizers administered mephenytoin at doses that were without effect in extensive metabolizers of mephenytoin.

There is considerable interethnic variation in the incidence of the poor-metabolizer phenotype for *S*-mephenytoin. In Caucasians, CYP2C19 is defective in 2 to 5 percent of the population, but it is defective in 12 to 23 percent of Japanese, Chinese, and Korean subjects. On Vanuatu and some other Pacific islands, CYP2C19 is deficient in ~70 percent of the population (Kaneko et al., 1999). Based on clinical observations and/or in vitro analysis, CYP2C19 also appears to metabolize diphenylhydantoin (dilantin), mephobarbital, hexobarbital, propranolol, imipramine, diazepam, omeprazole, and lansoprazole. CYP2C19 also converts proguanil to cycloguanil, its active antimalarial metabolite. Artemisinin, another antimalarial drug, is an effective inducer of CYP2C19 and dramatically induces its own metabolism (Mihara et al., 1999). The monoamine oxidase inhibitor tranylcypromine is a potent but not specific inhibitor of CYP2C19.

CYP2C Enzymes in Other Species The multiplicity, function, and regulation of the CYP2C enzymes vary enormously from one species to the next. For example, whereas the 4′-hydroxylation of *S*-mephenytoin in humans is catalyzed by CYP2C19, this same reaction in rats is catalyzed by a CYP3A enzyme, not a CYP2C enzyme. Conversely, one of the reactions catalyzed by rat CYP2C11, namely the 2α-hydroxylation of testosterone, is not catalyzed by the human CYP2C enzymes (or any of the other P450 enzymes in human liver microsomes).

CYP2D6 In the late 1950s, clinical trials in the United States established that sparteine was as potent as oxytocin for inducing labor at term. However, the duration and intensity of action of sparteine were dramatically increased in ~7 percent of all patients tested. The exaggerated response to sparteine included prolonged (tetanic) uterine contraction and abnormally rapid labor. In some cases, sparteine caused the death of the fetus. The drug was not recommended for clinical use because these side effects were unpredictable and occurred at doses of 100 to 200 mg/kg, which were well tolerated by other patients. The antihypertensive drug debrisoquine was subsequently found to cause a marked and prolonged hypotension in 5 to 10 percent of patients, and a genetic polymorphism for the metabolism of debrisoquine and sparteine was discovered in 1977–1979 (Gonzalez, 1989; Meyer, 1994). Poor metabolizers lack CYP2D6, which catalyzes the 4-hydroxylation of debrisoquine and the Δ^2- and Δ^5-oxidation of sparteine (see Fig. 6-43).

In addition to debrisoquine and sparteine, CYP2D6 biotransforms a large number of drugs, as shown in Table 6-5. Individuals lacking CYP2D6 have an exaggerated response to most but not all of these drugs. For example, even though debrisoquine and propranolol are both biotransformed by CYP2D6, the effects of propranolol are not exaggerated in poor metabolizers of debrisoquine for two reasons. First, 4-hydroxypropranolol is a β-adrenoceptor antagonist, so the 4-hydroxylation of propranolol by CYP2D6 does not terminate the pharmacologic effects of the drug. Second, CYP2D6 is not the only P450 enzyme to biotransform propranolol. As mentioned above, CYP2C19 catalyzes the side-chain oxidation of propranolol to naphthoxylactic acid (see Fig. 6-23). Because CYP2D6 and CYP2C19 both contribute significantly to the biotransformation of propranolol, a deficiency in either one of these enzymes does not markedly alter the pharmacokinetics of this beta blocker. However, in one individual who lacked both enzymes, the total oral clearance of propranolol was markedly reduced (Wilkinson et al., 1989). CYP2D6 catalyzes the *O*-demethylation of codeine to the potent analgesic morphine. Pain control with codeine is reduced in individuals lacking CYP2D6. The biotransformation of substrates for CYP2D6 occurs 5 to 7.5Å from a basic nitrogen, which interacts with an anionic residue (Glu_{301}) in the enzyme's substrate-binding site (Strobl et al., 1993). Quinidine is a potent inhibitor of CYP2D6 because it interacts favorably with the anionic site on CYP2D6, but it cannot be oxidized at sites 5 to 7.5Å from its basic nitrogen atoms. Fluoxetine (and several other selective serotonin-reuptake inhibitors), ajmalicine, and yohimbine are also potent competitive inhibitors of CYP2D6. A poor-metabolizer phenotype can be induced pharmacologically with these potent inhibitors of CYP2D6. Quinine, the levorotatory diasteriomer of quinidine, is not a potent inhibitor of CYP2D6, and neither drug is a potent inhibitor of the CYP2D enzymes expressed in rats. CYP2D6 is one of the few P450 enzymes that efficiently uses the peroxide shunt, so that reactions catalyzed by CYP2D6 can be supported by cumene hydroperoxide.

As shown in Fig. 6-40, CYP2D6 catalyzes the *O*-demethylation of dextromethorphan to dextrorphan, which is glucuronidated and excreted in urine. Dextromethorphan can also be *N*-demethylated, a reaction catalyzed predominantly by CYP3A4 and CYP2B6, but this metabolite is not glucuronidated and excreted in urine. Because the urinary excretion of dextromethorphan is dependent on *O*-demethylation, this over-the-counter antitussive drug can be used to identify individuals lacking CYP2D6, although most poor metabolizers can be identified by DNA analysis (genotyping). There is considerable interethnic variation in the incidence of the poor metabolizer phenotype for debrisoquine/sparteine. In Caucasians, CYP2D6 is defective in 5 to 10 percent of the population, but it is defective in less than 2 percent of African Americans, Africans, Thai, Chinese, and Japanese subjects. Individuals lacking CYP2D6 have an unusually low incidence of some chemically induced neoplastic diseases, such as lung cancer, bladder cancer, hepatocellular carcinoma, and endemic Balkan nephropathy (Idle, 1991; Taningher et al., 1999). It has been hypothesized that CYP2D6 may play a role in the metabolic activation of chemical carcinogens, such as those present in the environment, in the diet, and/or in cigarette smoke. According to this hypothesis, individuals lacking CYP2D6 have a low incidence of cancer because they fail to activate chemical carcinogens. However, CYP2D6 appears to play little or no role in the activation of known chemical carcinogens to DNA-reactive or mutagenic metabolites with the possible exception of the tobacco-smoke specific nitrosamine, 4-(methylnitrosamino)-1-(3-pyridyl)-1-butanone (NNK), which is also activated by other P450 enzymes. Therefore, it remains to be determined whether a deficiency of CYP2D6 is causally or coincidentally related to a low incidence of certain cancers.

CYP2E1 As shown in Fig. 6-20, CYP2E1 was first identified as MEOS, the microsomal ethanol oxidizing system (Lieber, 1999). In addition to ethanol, CYP2E1 catalyzes the biotransformation of a large number halogenated alkanes (Guengerich et al., 1991). CYP2E1 is expressed constitutively in human liver and possibly in extrahepatic tissues, such as the kidney, lung, lymphocytes, and bone marrow, and the enzyme is inducible by ethanol and isoniazid. CYP2E1 catalyzes the *N1*- and *N7*-demethylation of caffeine to theobromine and theophylline, as shown in Fig. 6-40, and it can activate acetaminophen to the hepatotoxic metabolite *N*-acetylbenzoquinoneimine, as shown in Figs. 6-28 and 6-43. The mechanism by which alcohol potentiates the hepatotoxic effects of acetaminophen (Tylenol) is thought to involve increased activation of acetaminophen due to the induction of CYP2E1 and decreased inactivation due to a lowering of glutathione levels. However, the degree to which ethanol consumption increases the risk of acetaminophen-induced hepatotoxicity remains a controversial issue (Prescott, 1999). Induction of CYP2E1 by isoniazid stimulates the dehalogenation of the volatile anesthetics enflurane and isoflurane. In human liver microsomes, CYP2E1 activity can be conveniently measured by the 6-hydroxylation of chlorzoxazone and the hydroxylation of 4-nitrophenol. The 6-hydroxylation of chlorzoxazone can also be catalyzed by CYP1A1, but this enzyme is rarely expressed in human liver. Chlorzoxazone is an FDA-approved muscle relaxant (Paraflex), and the urinary excretion of 6-hydroxychlorzoxazone and the plasma ratio of 6-hydroxychlorzoxazone to chlorzoxazone have been used as noninvasive in vivo probes of CYP2E1. The levels of CYP2E1 are by no means constant among individuals, but they do not exhibit the marked interindividual variation characteristic of other P450 enzymes. CYP2E1 is one of the P450 enzymes that requires cytochrome b_5, which lowers the apparent K_m for several substrates biotransformed by CYP2E1. The function and regulation of CYP2E1 are well conserved among mammalian species.

CYP3A The most abundant P450 enzymes in human liver microsomes belong to the CYP3A gene subfamily, which includes CYP3A4, CYP3A5, and CYP3A7. CYP3A7 is considered a fetal enzyme, whereas the others are considered to be adult forms, although livers from some adults contain CYP3A7 and some fetal livers contain CYP3A5. All human livers appear to contain CYP3A4, although the levels vary enormously (>10-fold) among individuals (Wrighton and Stevens, 1992; Shimada et al., 1994). CYP3A5 is expressed in relatively few livers (10 to 30 percent). One or more of these enzymes is expressed in extrahepatic tissues. For example, CYP3A4 is expressed in the small intestine, whereas CYP3A5 is expressed in 80 percent of all human kidneys.

The CYP3A enzymes biotransform an extraordinary array of xenobiotics and steroids, as shown in Table 6-5 (Thummel and Wilkinson, 1998; Dresser et al., 2000). CYP3A enzymes also catalyze the oxidation of hydroxyarginine to citrulline and nitric oxide. Factors that influence the levels and/or activity of the CYP3A enzymes influence the biotransformation of many of the drugs listed in Table 6-5, and many of these drugs have been shown to inhibit each other's metabolism (Pichard et al., 1990).

In humans, CYP3A enzymes are inducible by numerous drugs, such as rifampin, phenobarbital, phenytoin, and troglitazone (Pichard et al., 1990). Inhibitors of human CYP3A include azole-type antimycotics (e.g., ketoconazole and clotrimazole), macrolide antibiotics (e.g., erythromycin and troleandomycin), HIV protease inhibitors (especially ritonavir), the ethynylprogesterone analog gestodene, and certain flavones or other component(s) present in grapefruit juice (although other flavones, such as α-naphthoflavone, are activators of CYP3A4). Several noninvasive clinical tests of CYP3A activity have been proposed, including the [^{14}C-*N*-methyl]-erythromycin breath test, the plasma clearance of midazolam and nifedipine, and the urinary excretion of 6β-hydroxycortisol (Watkins, 1994). However, for reasons that are not yet understood, there can be marked differences in the results obtained with different tests in the same individuals. Nevertheless, the various noninvasive tests suggest that CYP3A activity varies widely among individuals (>10-fold), but there appear to be no individuals who are completely devoid of CYP3A activity, possibly due to the multiplicity of enzymes in the human CYP3A subfamily.

The function and regulation of the CYP3A enzymes is fairly well conserved among mammalian species, with some notable exceptions. For example, rifampin is an inducer of the CYP3A enzymes in humans and rabbits but not rats or mice, whereas the opposite appears to be true of pregnenolone-16α-carbonitrile (Pichard et al., 1990). In adult rats, the levels of CYP3A2 in males are much greater (>10-fold) than in females, whereas no marked sex difference in CYP3A levels is observed in humans (if anything, the levels of CYP3A enzymes are higher in females than in males).

CYP4A9/11 The CYP4A enzymes in human and other species catalyze the ω- and ω-1 hydroxylation of fatty acids and their derivatives, including prostaglandins, thromboxane, prostacyclin, and leukotrienes. With lauric acid as substrate, the CYP4A enzymes preferentially catalyze the ω-hydroxylation to 12-hydroxylauric acid (see Fig. 6-36), which can be further oxidized to form a dicarboxylic acid. Although CYP4A enzymes also catalyze the ω-1 hydroxylation of lauric acid, other P450 enzymes, including CYP2E1, can contribute significantly to the formation of 11-hydroxylauric acid. The CYP4A enzymes are unusual for ability to preferentially catalyze the ω-hydroxylation of fatty acids over the thermodynamically more favorable reaction leading to ω-1 hydroxylation. Despite their physiologic importance, the CYP4A enzymes appear to play a very limited role in the metabolism of drugs and other xenobiotics.

Activation of Xenobiotics by Cytochrome P450

Biotransformation by cytochrome P450 does not always lead to detoxication, and several examples have been given previously where the toxicity or tumorigenicity of a chemical depends on its activation by cytochrome P450. The role of individual human P450 enzymes in the activation of procarcinogens and protoxicants is summarized in Table 6–6 (adapted from Guengerich and Shimada, 1991). A variety of cytochrome P450–dependent reactions are involved in the activation of the chemicals listed in Table 6-6. The conversion of polycyclic aromatic hydrocarbons to tumor-forming metabolites involves the formation of bay-region diolepoxides, as shown in Fig. 6-6 for the conversion of benzo[a]pyrene to benzo[a]pyrene 7,8-dihydrodiol-9,10, epoxide. Epoxidation generates hepatotoxic metabolites of chlorobenzene and coumarin (Fig. 6-38), and generates an hepatotumorigenic metabolite of aflatoxin B1 (Fig. 6-27).

The initial step in the conversion of aromatic amines to tumor-forming metabolites involves *N*-hydroxylation, as shown for 2-amino-6-nitrobenzylalcohol (Fig. 6-9) and 2-acetylaminofluorene (Fig. 6-33*A*). In the case of acetaminophen, activation to an hepatotoxic metabolite involves dehydrogenation to *N*-acetylbenzoquinoneimine, as shown in Fig. 6-28. A similar reaction converts butylated hydroxytoluene to a toxic quinone methide, as shown in Fig. 6-30. The myelotoxicity of benzene depends on its conversion to phenol and hydroquinone (Fig. 6-29). The toxicity of several organophosphorus insecticides involves oxidative group transfer to the corresponding organophosphate, as shown for the conversion of parathion to paraoxon in Figs. 6-41 and 6-42. The hepatotoxicity of carbon tetrachloride involves reductive dechlorination to a trichloromethyl free radical, which binds to protein and initiates lipid peroxidation, as shown in Fig. 6-15. The hepatotoxicity and nephrotoxicity of chloroform involves oxidative dechlorination to phosgene (Fig. 6-15). Oxidative and reductive dehalo-

Table 6-6
Examples of Xenobiotics Activated by Human P450 Enzymes

CYP1A1
Benzo[a]pyrene and other polycyclic aromatic hydrocarbons
CYP1A2
Acetaminophen
2-Acetylaminofluorene
4-Aminobiphenyl
2-Aminofluorene
2-Naphthylamine
NNK*
Amino acid pyrrolysis products (DiMeQx, MeIQ, MeIQx, Glu P-1, Glu P-2, IQ, PhIP, Trp P-1, Trp P-2)
Tacrine
CYP2A6
N-Nitrosodiethylamine
NNK*
CYP2B6
6-Aminochrysene
Cyclophosphamide
Ifosphamide
CYP2C8, 9, 18, 19
Tienilic acid
Valproic acid
CYP2D6
NNK*
CYP2E1
Acetaminophen
Acrylonitrile
Benzene
Carbon tetrachloride
Chloroform
Dichloromethane
1,2-Dichloropropane
Ethylene dibromide
Ethylene dichloride
Ethyl carbamate
Halothane
N-Nitrosodimethylamine
Styrene
Trichlorothylene
Vinyl chloride
CYP3A4
Acetaminophen
Aflatoxin B_1 and G_1
6-Aminochrysene
Benzo[a]pyrene 7,8-dihydrodiol
Cyclophosphamide
Ifosphamide
1-Nitropyrene
Sterigmatocystin
Senecionine
Tris(2,3-dibromopropyl) phosphate
CYP4A9/11
None known

*NNK, 4-(methylnitrosamino)-1-(3-pyridyl)-1-butanone, a tobacco-specific nitrosamine.

SOURCE: Adapted from Guengerich and Shimada, 1991.

genation both play a role in the activation of halothane, although hepatotoxicity in rats is more dependent on reductive dehalogenation, whereas the immune hepatitis in humans is largely a consequence of oxidative dehalogenation, which leads to the formation of neoantigens (Pohl et al., 1989). Formation of neoantigens (by covalent binding to CYP2C9) is also the mechanism by which the uricosuric diuretic drug tienilic acid causes immune hepatitis (Koenigs et al., 1999).

Some of the chemicals listed in Table 6-6 are activated to toxic or tumorigenic metabolites by mechanisms not mentioned previously. For example, *N*-nitrosodimethylamine, which is representative of a large class of tumorigenic nitrosamines, is activated to an alkylating electrophile by *N*-demethylation, as shown in Fig. 6-44. The activation of ethyl carbamate (urethan) involves two sequential reactions catalyzed by cytochrome P450 (CYP2E1): dehydrogenation to vinyl carbamate followed by epoxidation, as shown in Fig. 6-44. CYP2E1 is one of several P450 enzymes that can catalyze the epoxidation of tetrachloroethylene. The rearrangement of this epoxide to a carbonyl is accompanied by migration of chlorine, which produces the highly reactive metabolite, trichloroacetylchloride, as shown in Fig. 6-44. The toxic pyrrolizidine alkaloids, such as senecionine, are cyclic arylamines that are dehydrogenated by cytochrome P450 (CYP3A4) to the corresponding pyrroles. Pyrroles themselves are nucleophiles, but electrophiles are generated through the loss of substituents on the pyrrolizidine nucleus, as shown in Fig. 6-44 (Mabic et al, 1999).

Cyclophosphamide and ifosphamide are examples of chemicals designed to be activated to toxic electrophiles for the treatment of malignant tumors and other proliferative diseases. These drugs are nitrogen mustards, which have a tendency to undergo intramolecular nucleophilic displacement to form an electrophilic aziridinium species. In the case of cyclophosphamide and ifosphamide, the nitrogen mustard is stabilized by the presence of a phosphoryl oxygen, which delocalizes the lone pair of nitrogen electrons required for intramolecular nucleophilic displacement. For this reason, formation of an electrophilic aziridinium species requires hydroxylation by cytochrome P450, as shown in Fig. 6-44 for cyclophosphamide. Hydroxylation of the carbon atom next to the ring nitrogen leads spontaneously to ring opening and elimination of acrolein. In the resultant phosphoramide mustard, delo-

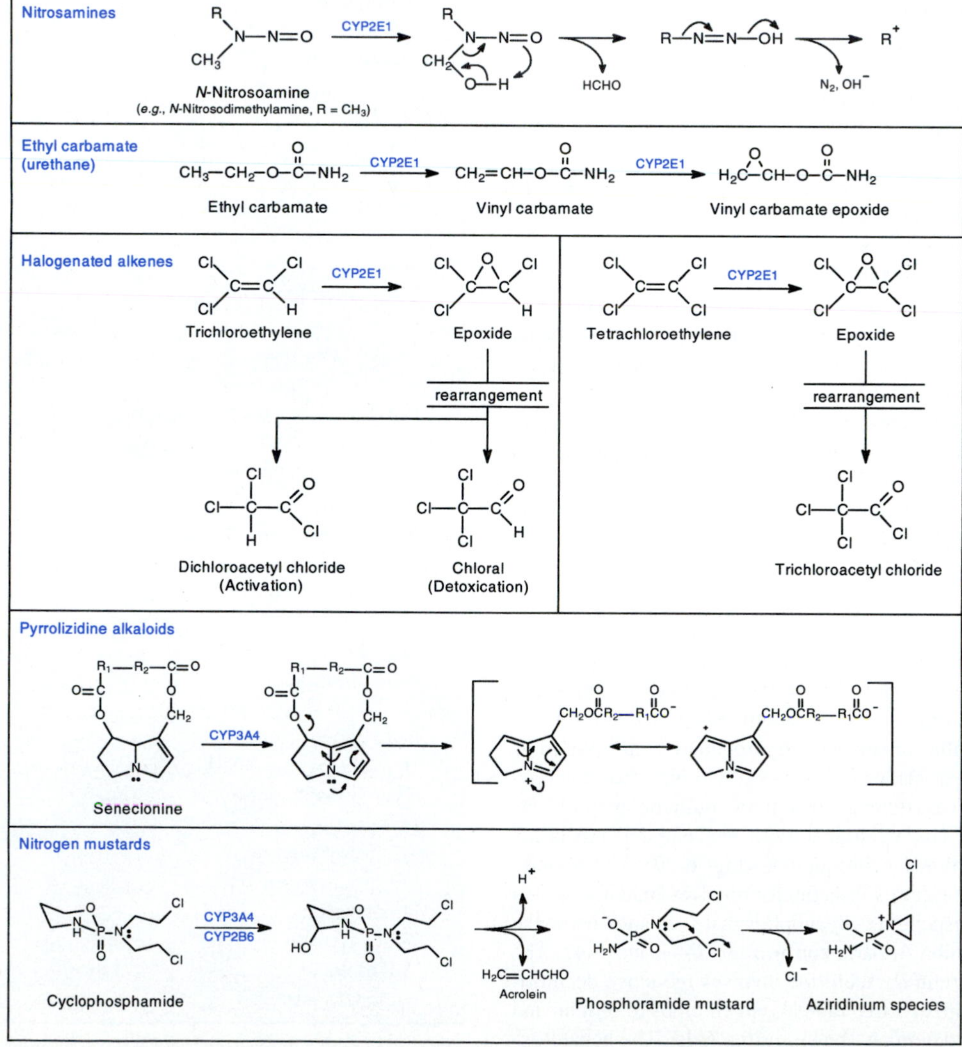

Figure 6-44. Additional mechanisms of cytochrome P450–dependent activation of xenobiotics to reactive (electrophilic) metabolites.

calization of the lone pair of nitrogen electrons to the phosphoryl oxygen is now disfavored by the presence of the lone pair of electrons on the oxygen anion, hence the phosphoramide undergoes an intramolecular nucleophilic elimination to generate an electrophilic aziridinium species. This reaction is catalyzed by CYP3A4 and CYP2B6. Cyclophosphamide is also activated by CYP2B enzymes in rats, one of which (CYP2B12) is expressed in the skin (Friedberg et al., 1992). Activation of cyclophosphamide by P450 enzymes in the skin would generate a cytotoxic metabolite at the base of hair follicles, which may be the reason why hair loss is one of the side effects of cyclophosphamide treatment.

Many of the chemicals listed in Table 6-6 are also detoxified by cytochrome P450 by biotransformation to less toxic metabolites. In some cases, the same P450 enzyme catalyzes both activation and detoxication reactions. For example, CYP3A4 activates aflatoxin B_1 to the hepatotoxic and tumorigenic 8,9-epoxide, but it also detoxifies aflatoxin B_1 by 3-hydroxylation to aflatoxin Q_1. Similarly, CYP3A4 activates senecionine by converting this pyrrolizidine alkaloid to the corresponding pyrrole, but it also detoxifies senecionine through formation of an *N*-oxide (a reaction mainly catalyzed by FMO3). Epoxidation of trichloroethylene by CYP2E1 appears to be both an activation and detoxication pathway, as shown in Fig. 6-44. Rearrangement of trichloroethylene epoxide can be accompanied by migration of chlorine, which produces chloral (trichloroacetaldehyde), or hydrogen, which produces dichloroacetylchloride. Chloral is much less toxic than dichloroacetylchloride, hence, migration of the chlorine during epoxide rearrangement is a detoxication reaction, whereas migration of the hydrogen is an activation reaction. These few examples serve to underscore the complexity of factors that determine the balance between xenobiotic activation and detoxication. Further details of xenobiotic activation are available in recent review articles (Bolton et al., 2000; Mabic et al., 1999; Pirmohamed and Park, 1999; Purohit and Basu, 2000).

P450 Knockout Mice

Several strategies have been developed to explore the role of cytochrome P450 enzymes in the activation of xenobiotics. Cytochrome P450 levels in rodents can be increased by a variety of inducers, which would be expected to enhance xenobiotic toxicity. Alternatively, cytochrome P450 activity can be decreased by various inhibitors, which would be expected to have a protective effect. (Inducers and inhibitors of cytochrome P450 are discussed later in this section.) Various in vitro techniques can be employed, similar to those described earlier in this section for determining the role of human P450 enzymes in drug metabolism. Transgenic mice that lack one or more P450 enzymes, which are commonly referred to as knockout mice or null mice, provide a relatively new strategy to evaluate the role of specific P450 enzymes in xenobiotic activation (Gonzalez and Kimura, 1999; Buters et al., 1999). It should be noted, however, that such transgenic mice often have abnormal phenotypes due to disruption of genes other than the target gene. Moreover, deletion of the same gene can produce markedly different phenotypes, as has been observed in different transgenic mice lacking the *Ah* receptor.

Knockout mice have confirmed the role of several P450 enzymes in the activation of specific xenobiotics. For example, CYP2E1 knockout mice are relatively resistant to the myelotoxic effects of benzene (as previously discussed under "Peroxidase-Dependent Cooxidation"). These same mice are relatively resistant to the toxic effects of chloroform and the lethal effects of acetaminophen. CYP1A2 knockout mice are also relatively more resistant to acetaminophen toxicity, whereas mice lacking both CYP1A2 and CYP2E1 are highly resistant. These results were largely expected based on other evidence implicating CYP2E1 in the activation of benzene, chloroform, and acetaminophen and CYP1A2 in the activation of acetaminophen. However, some results with knockout mice were unexpected. For example, contrary to expectation, CYP1A2 knockout mice were not resistant to hepatotumorigenic effect of 4-aminobiphenyl, even though CYP1A2 was thought to be primarily responsible for catalyzing the initial step in the activation of this carcinogenic amine (i.e., *N*-hydroxylation). On the other hand, the demonstration that CYP1B1 knockout mice are resistant to the toxic and tumorigenic effects of 7,12-dimethylbenzanthracene provides compelling evidence that CYP1B1, which is expressed in numerous extrahepatic tissues, plays a major role in the activation of polycyclic aromatic hydrocarbons to carcinogenic metabolites (Buters et al., 1999).

These studies in knockout mice are relevant to humans because their counterpart can be found in those individuals who lack certain P450 enzymes or other xenobiotic-biotransforming enzymes. Experiments in knockout mice underscore how genetic polymorphisms in the human population are risk modifiers for the development of chemically induced disease.

Inhibition of Cytochrome P450

In addition to predicting the likelihood of some individuals being poor metabolizers due to a genetic deficiency in P450 expression, information on which human P450 enzyme metabolizes a drug can help predict or explain drug interactions (Peck et al., 1993). For example, when administered with azole antifungals (e.g., ketoconazole and itraconazole) or macrolide antibiotics (e.g., erythromycin and troleandomycin), the antihistamine terfenadine (Seldane) can cause torsades de pointes, which in some individuals has apparently led to lethal ventricular arrhythmias (Kivsito et al., 1994). This drug interaction can be rationalized on the basis that terfenadine is normally converted by intestinal and liver CYP3A4 to a tertiary-butyl alcohol, which is further oxidized to a carboxylic acid metabolite. This latter metabolite blocks H1 receptors and does not cross the blood–brain barrier, which is why terfenadine is a nonsedating antihistamine. When formation of the carboxylic acid metabolite is blocked by CYP3A4 inhibitors — such as ketoconazole, itraconazole, erythromycin, or troleandomycin — the plasma levels of the parent drug, terfenadine, become sufficiently elevated to block cardiac potassium channels, which can lead to arrhythmias. In some cases, inhibition of cytochrome P450 is advantageous. For example, ritonavir blocks the CYP3A-dependent metabolism of sequinavir and thereby improves its pharmacokinetic profile. Both these drugs are HIV protease inhibitors, and combined therapy is better than monotherapy in helping to curtail the development of drug-resistant strains of HIV. Ketoconazole and erythromycin inhibit the biotransformation of cyclosporine by intestinal and liver CYP3A4 and consequently increase the bioavailability of cyclosporine and decrease the rate of elimination of this expensive immunosuppressant. However, much higher doses of cyclosporine must be given to patients taking the CYP3A4 inducer rifampin in order to achieve therapeutic levels and immune suppression.

Inhibitory drug interactions generally fall into three categories. The first involves competition between two drugs that are metabolized by the same P450 enzyme. For example, omeprazole and diazepam are both metabolized by CYP2C19. When the two drugs are administered simultaneously, omeprazole decreases the plasma clearance of diazepam and prolongs its plasma half-life. The inhibition of diazepam metabolism by omeprazole is presumed to involve competition for metabolism by CYP2C19 because no such inhibition occurs in individuals who, for genetic reasons, lack this polymorphically expressed P450 enzyme. The second inhibitory drug interaction is also competitive in nature, but the inhibitor is not a substrate for the affected P450 enzyme. The inhibition of dextromethorphan biotransformation by quinidine is a good example of this type of drug interaction. Dextromethorphan is *O*-demethylated by CYP2D6, and the clearance of dextromethorphan is impaired in individuals lacking this polymorphically expressed enzyme. The clearance of dextromethorphan is similarly impaired when this antitussive agent is taken with quinidine, a potent inhibitor of CYP2D6. However, quinidine is not biotransformed by CYP2D6, even though it binds to this enzyme with high affinity ($K_i \sim 100$ nM). Quinidine is actually biotransformed by CYP3A4, and is a weak competitive inhibitor of this enzyme ($K_i > 100\ \mu M$). The COX-2 inhibitor celecoxib (Celebrex) is also a CYP2D6 inhibitor, even though it is metabolized by other P450 enzymes.

The third type of drug interaction results from noncompetitive inhibition of cytochrome P450, and it often involves metabolism-dependent inhibition of cytochrome P450 (also known as mechanism-based or suicide inactivation) (Halpert et al., 1994). The inhibition of terfenadine metabolism by macrolide antibiotics appears to be an example of this type of drug interaction. CYP3A4 converts macrolide antibiotics to a metabolite that binds so tightly (but noncovalently) to the heme moiety of CYP3A4 that it is not released from the enzyme's active site. The noncompetitive inhibition of a P450 enzyme by a metabolism-dependent inhibitor can completely block the metabolism of a drug. As the fatal interactions between macrolide antibiotics and terfenadine indicate, noncompetitive inhibition of cytochrome P450 can have profound consequences. Numerous compounds are activated by cytochrome P450 to metabolites that bind covalently to the heme moiety or surrounding protein. These compounds, known as suicide inactivators, include various halogenated alkanes (CCl_4), halogenated alkenes (vinyl chloride, trichloroethylene), allylic compounds (allylisopropylacetamide and secobarbital), and acetylenic compounds (ethinylestradiol and the ethynylprogesterone, gestodene). Ethinyl derivatives of various P450 substrates have been synthesized as potential selective metabolism-dependent inhibitors of individual P450 enzymes. For example, polycyclic aromatic hydrocarbons are preferred substrates for CYP1A1, and this enzyme can be inactivated by various ethynyl derivatives of naphthalene and pyrene. 9-Ethynylphenanthrene is a metabolism-dependent inhibitor of CYP2B6. Furafylline is a metabolism-dependent inhibitor of CYP1A2, for which the structurally related xanthine, caffeine, is a substrate. Similarly, tienilic acid is metabolism-dependent inhibitor of CYP2C9, whereas 8-methoxypsoralen, which is a derivative of coumarin, is a metabolism-dependent inhibitor of CYP2A6 (Table 6-5).

Induction of Cytochrome P450

In contrast to inhibitors, inducers of cytochrome P450 increase the rate of xenobiotic biotransformation (Conney, 1967, 1982; Batt et al., 1992). Some of the P450 enzymes in human liver microsomes are inducible, as summarized in Table 6-5 (Pichard et al., 1990). Clinically important consequences of P450 enzyme induction include the enhanced biotransformation of cyclosporine, warfarin, and contraceptive steroids by inducers of the CYP3A and CYP2C enzymes and enhanced activation of acetaminophen to its hepatotoxic metabolite *N*-acetylbenzoquinoneimine, by the CYP2E1 inducers ethanol and isoniazid, and possibly by CYP3A enzyme inducers. As an underlying cause of serious adverse effects, P450 induction is generally less important than P450 inhibition, because the latter can cause a rapid and profound increase in blood levels of a drug, which can cause toxic effects and symptoms of drug overdose. In contrast, cytochrome P450 induction lowers blood levels, which compromises the therapeutic goal of drug therapy but does not cause an exaggerated response to the drug. An exception to this rule is the potentiating effect of alcohol and isoniazid on acetaminophen hepatotoxicity, which is in part because of cytochrome P450 induction.

However, even this drug interaction is complicated by the fact that ethanol and isoniazid are inhibitors as well as inducers of CYP2E1 (Zand et al., 1993). Consequently, increased activation of acetaminophen by ethanol and isoniazid is a delayed response, due to the time required for increased synthesis of CYP2E1 and for the inducers to be cleared to the point where they no longer cause an overall inhibition of CYP2E1 activity. CYP3A4 and CYP1A2 are also inducible enzymes capable of activating acetaminophen to a reactive quinoneimine. By inducing CYP3A4, rifampin and barbiturates would be expected to enhance the hepatotoxicity of acetaminophen, and there is some clinical evidence that this does occur. In contrast, induction of CYP1A2 by cigarette smoking or dietary exposure to polycyclic aromatic hydrocarbons (in charcoal-broiled beef) or indole-3-carbinol derivatives (in cruciferous vegetables) has been reported to have no effect on the hepatotoxicity of acetaminophen, even though CYP1A2 induction in rodents potentiates the hepatocellular necrosis caused by acetaminophen.

Induction of cytochrome P450 would be expected to increase the activation of procarcinogens to DNA-reactive metabolites, leading to increased tumor formation. Contrary to expectation, there is little evidence from either human epidemiologic studies or animal experimentation that P450 induction enhances the incidence or multiplicity of tumors caused by known chemical carcinogens. In fact, most evidence points to a protective role of enzyme induction against chemical-induced neoplasia (Parkinson and Hurwitz, 1991). On the other hand, transgenic (knockout) mice lacking the *Ah* receptor were recently shown to be resistant to the carcinogenic effects of benzo[a]pyrene (Shimizu et al., 2000), which suggests that induction of CYP1A1 plays an important role in the carcinogenicity of polycyclic aromatic hydrocarbons (PAH). However, the *Ah* receptor may be critical to PAH carcinogenicity for reasons other than its role in CYP1A1 induction. For example, the *Ah* receptor may transport DNA-reactive metabolites, such as *ortho*-quinones, to the nucleus (see Fig. 6-6; Burczynski and Penning, 2000), or it might regulate the expression of genes that influence tumor promotion, as has been proposed for other receptors that mediate cytochrome P450 induction (discussed later in this section). In this regard it is significant that benzo[a]pyrene is a complete carcinogen (both an initiator and promoter), and that TCDD and other *Ah* receptor ligands are potent tumor promoters.

Cytochrome P450 induction can cause pharmacokinetic tolerance, as in the case of artemisinin [which induces CYP2C19 (Mihara et al., 1999)], in which case larger doses of drug must be administered to achieve therapeutic blood levels due to increased drug biotransformation. In many instances, however, P450 induction does not necessarily enhance the biotransformation of the inducer, in which case the induction is said to be gratuitous. Drugs are also known to induce enzymes that play no role in their biotransformation. For example, omeprazole induces CYP1A2, even though the disposition of this acid-suppressing drug is largely determined by CYP2C19. Some of the most effective inducers of cytochrome P450 are polyhalogenated aromatic hydrocarbons, such as polychlorinated derivatives of dibenzo-*p*-dioxin (PCDDs), dibenzofurans (PCDFs), azobenzenes and azoxybenzenes, biphenyl (PCBs), and naphthalene. In general, highly chlorinated compounds are resistant to biotransformation and cause a prolonged induction of cytochrome P450 and other enzymes. Due to the increased demand for heme, persistent induction of cytochrome P450 can lead to porphyria, a disorder characterized by excessive accumulation of intermediates in the heme biosynthetic pathway. In 1956, widespread consumption of wheat contaminated with the fungicide hexachlorobenzene caused an epidemic of porphyria cutanea tarda in Turkey. Another outbreak occurred in 1964 among workers at a factory in the United States manufacturing 2,4,5-trichlorophenoxyacetic acid (the active ingredient in several herbicides and in the defoliant Agent Orange). The outbreak of porphyria cutanea tarda was caused not by the herbicide itself but by a contaminant, 2,3,7,8-tetrachlorodibenzo-*p*-dioxin, also known as dioxin and TCDD. Drugs that cause P450 induction have not been shown to cause porphyria cutanea tarda under normal circumstances, but phenobarbital, phenytoin, and alcohol are recognized as *precipitating factors* because they cause episodes of porphyria cutanea tarda in individuals with an inherited deficiency in the heme-biosynthetic enzyme uroporphyrinogen decarboxylase.

The mechanism of P450 induction has been studied extensively in rats and other laboratory animals (Gonzalez, 1989; Okey, 1990; Ryan and Levin, 1990; Porter and Coon, 1991). Currently, five classes of P450 enzyme inducers are recognized, which are represented by 3-methylcholanthrene, phenobarbital, pregnenolone-16α-carbonitrile (PCN), clofibric acid, and isoniazid. The first four inducers cause a marked (<10-fold) increase in the rate of transcription of one or more specific P450 enzymes. For each of these four inducers, the *trans*-acting factor that mediates the transcriptional activation of the P450 genes has been identified, as shown in Table 6-7. For the most part, these *trans*-acting factors are ligand-activated receptors that must dimerize with another protein in order to form a DNA-binding protein that can bind to discrete regions of DNA (*cis*-acting factors or response elements) and thereby activate gene transcription (Honkakoski and Negishi, 2000; Waxman, 1999).

Treatment of rats with 3-methylcholanthrene causes a marked (>20-fold) induction of CYP1A1 and CYP1A2. Liver microsomes from untreated rats contain low levels of CYP1A2 and virtually undetectable levels of CYP1A1. In addition to polycyclic aromatic hydrocarbons, such as 3-methylcholanthrene and benzo[a]pyrene, inducers of the CYP1A enzymes include flavones (e.g., β-naphthoflavone), polyhalogenated aromatic hydrocarbons (e.g., TCDD, 3,3′,4,4′,5,5′-hexachlorobiphenyl), acid condensation products of indole-3-carbinol, and certain drugs and food additives (e.g., chlorpromazine, phenothiazine, clotrimazole, ketoconazole, miconazole, isosafrole). Induction of CYP1A1 involves transcriptional activation of the *CYP1A1* gene, which, together with message stabilization, results in an increase in the levels of mRNA and newly synthesized protein.

In the absence of an inducer, transcription of the *CYP1A1* gene is suppressed by a repressor protein, which accounts for the low constitutive levels of CYP1A1 in most species. (Guinea pig and rhesus monkey appear to express CYP1A1 constitutively and hence are exceptions to this general rule). Induction of CYP1A1 involves both derepression and activation of transcription by the *Ah* receptor. Although this cytosolic receptor binds several *a*romatic *h*ydrocarbons, such as 3-methylcholanthrene and benzo[a]pyrene, the ligand with the highest binding affinity is TCDD, which is why the *Ah* receptor is also known as the dioxin receptor (Whitlock, 1993). The *Ah* receptor is normally complexed in a 1:2 ratio with heat-shock protein (hsp90), which dissociate upon binding of ligand to the *Ah* receptor, enabling the receptor to be phosphorylated by tyrosine kinase. The activated *Ah* receptor then enters the nucleus and forms a heterodimer complex with the *Ah*-receptor-nuclear translocator *Arnt*. Inside the nucleus, the *Ah* receptor-*Arnt* complex binds to regulatory sequences [known as *dioxin-responsive elements (DRE)* or *xenobiotic responsive elements (XRE)*] and enhances the transcription of the *CYP1A1* gene and other genes with an XRE or XRE-like sequence in their upstream enhancer region [namely CYP1A2, DT-diaphorase, glutathione *S*-transferase, UDP-glucuronosyltransferase (UGT1A6 and UGT1A7), and aldehyde dehydrogenase]. The XRE is only a small segment of DNA (the consensus sequence is 5′-TXGCGTG-3′, where X is normally T or A), which can be located more than a thousand bases from the initiation site for transcription. The enhancer region of the *CYP1A1* gene contains multiple XREs, which accounts for the marked (<100-fold) increase in CYP1A1 mRNA and protein levels following exposure to ligands for the *Ah* receptor.

Arnt was initially thought to be a cytosolic protein that simply facilitates the translocation of the ligand-bound *Ah* receptor into the nucleus. It is now recognized as an important component of the receptor complex that binds to DNA and activates transcription of genes under the control of the *Ah* receptor. For heterodimer formation, the *Ah* receptor must be bound to ligand and possibly phosphorylated, and *Arnt* must be phosphorylated, ap-

Table 6-7
Receptors Mediating the Induction of P450 Enzymes

P450 ENZYME	RECEPTOR	RECEPTOR LIGAND	CORECEPTOR	CORECEPTOR LIGAND
CYP1A	AhR	TCDD, PAHs, β-NF*	Arnt	None
CYP2B	CARβ	Androstanol,† Phenobarbital?	RXR	9-*cis*-retinoic acid
CYP3A	PXR	PCN, Rifampin	RXR	9-*cis*-retinoic acid
CYP4A	PPARα	Peroxisome proliferators	RXR	9-*cis*-retinoic acid

* TCDD, 2,3,7,8-tetrachlorodibenzo-p-dioxin; PAHs, polycyclic aromatic hydrocarbons; β-NF, β-naphthoflavone.

† Androstanol may represent a physiologic ligand that blocks the constitutive DNA-binding properties of CARβ.

parently by protein kinase C. The *Ah* receptor is often compared with the steroid/thyroid/retinoid family of receptors, which also bind ligands in the cytoplasm and are translocated to the nucleus where they bind to DNA and enhance gene transcription. However, the *Ah* receptor is a novel ligand-activated transcription factor, very distinct from these other receptors. Whereas the steroid/thyroid/retinoid receptors have "zinc-finger" DNA-binding domains and form homodimers, the *Ah* receptor forms a heterodimer with *Arnt;* both of these contain a basic helix-loop-helix (bHLH) domain near their *N*-terminus. The basic region binds DNA and the helix-loop-helix is involved in protein–protein interactions. The XRE recognized by the *Ah* receptor-*Arnt* complex contains a sequence of four base pairs (5′-GCGT-3′) that is part of the recognition motif for other bHLH proteins (Whitlock, 1993).

In mice, the *Ah* receptor is encoded by a single gene, but there are four allelic variants: a low-affinity form known as Ah^{d} (an ~104-kDa protein expressed in strains DBA/2, AKR, and 129) and three high-affinity forms known as Ah^{b-1} (an ~95-kDa protein expressed in C57 mice), Ah^{b-2} (an ~104-kDa protein expressed in BALB/c, C3H, and A mice), and Ah^{b-3} (an ~105-kDa protein expressed in MOLF/Ei mice) (Poland et al., 1994). Mice that express the low-affinity form of the receptor (Ah^{d}) require higher doses (~10 times) of TCDD to induce CYP1A1. Even though they respond to high doses of TCDD, Ah^{d} mice are called *nonresponsive* because it is not possible to administer sufficient amounts of polycyclic aromatic hydrocarbons to cause induction of CYP1A1. Although several genetic alterations give rise to the four allelic variants of the *Ah* receptor, the low-affinity binding of ligands to the Ah^{d} receptor from nonresponsive mice is attributable to a single amino acid substitution ($Ala^{375} \rightarrow Val^{375}$).

In vivo, the Ah^{d} and Ah^{b} genotypes can be distinguished by phenotypic differences in the effects of 3-methylcholanthrene treatment on the duration of action of the muscle relaxant zoxazolamine. Treatment of nonresponsive (Ah^{d}) mice with 3-methylcholanthrene results in no change in zoxazolamine-induced paralysis time. In contrast, such treatment of responsive (Ah^{b}) mice causes an induction of CYP1A1, which accelerates the 6-hydroxylation of zoxazolamine and reduces paralysis time from about 1 h to several minutes.

Some of the genes regulated by the *Ah* receptor contain other responsive elements and their expression is controlled by other transcription factors (Nebert, 1994). To a limited extent, the induction of CYP1A1 by polycyclic aromatic hydrocarbons can also be mediated by another cytosolic receptor known as the 4S-binding protein, which has been identified as the enzyme glycine *N*-methyltransferase. The first intron of the CYP1A1 gene contains a glucocorticoid-responsive element (GRE); hence the induction of CYP1A1 by TCDD can be augmented by glucocorticoids. DT-diaphorase is inducible up to tenfold by two classes of agents: chemicals like 3-methylcholanthrene and TCDD that bind to the *Ah* receptor and chemicals that cause oxidative stress, such as menadione, *tert*-butylhydroquinone, and 3,5-di-*tert*-butylcatechol, which produce reactive oxygen species through redox cycling reactions. These latter effects are mediated by the antioxidant responsive elements (ARE); therefore these enzymes are inducible by so-called *monofunctional* agents that do not induce CYP1A1 (see the section on DT-diaphorase above). The flavonoid β-naphthoflavone, the polycyclic aromatic hydrocarbon benzo[a]pyrene, and the polyhalogenated aromatic hydrocarbon TCDD all induce DT-diaphorase by both mechanisms; the parent compound binds to the *Ah* receptor and is responsible for inducing CYP1A1 as well as DT-diaphorase via the XRE, whereas electrophilic and/or redox active metabolites of β-naphthoflavone, benzo[a]pyrene, and TCDD are responsible for inducing glutathione *S*-transferase as well as DT-diaphorase via the ARE (Radjendirane and Jaiswal, 1999). The ARE core sequence for enzyme induction (5′-**GTGA**CAAA**GC**-3′) is similar to the AP-1 DNA-binding site (5′-TGACTCA-3′), which is regulated by redox status (see the earlier section on quinone reduction).

The enhancer region of *CYP1A2* also contains an XRE (or XRE-like sequences), so inducers of CYP1A1 are also inducers of CYP1A2. However, the induction of CYP1A2 differs from that of CYP1A1 in several respects: it occurs at lower doses of inducer; it often involves stabilization of mRNA or enzyme from degradation, and it requires liver-specific factors. The first of these differences (dose–response) may explain why low-level exposure of humans to CYP1A inducers results in an increase in hepatic levels of CYP1A2 but not CYP1A1. The second of these differences (namely stabilization of mRNA and/or enzyme) apparently explains why compounds that form stable complexes with CYP1A2, such as isosafrole, can induce CYP1A2 even in nonresponsive (Ah^{d}) mice. The third difference (the requirement for hepatic factors) explains why CYP1A2 is not expressed or inducible in extrahepatic tissues, hepatoma-derived cell lines, or isolated hepatocytes cultured under conditions that do not restore liver-specific gene expression. CYP1B1 is also regulated by the *Ah* receptor. In contrast to CYP1A2, CYP1B1 is primarily expressed in extrahepatic tissues, which is also true of human CYP1A1.

Liver microsomes from untreated rats contain low levels of CYP2B2 and extremely low or undetectable levels of CYP2B1, which are structurally related enzymes (97 percent identical) with very similar substrate specificities. Treatment of rats with phenobarbital causes a marked (>20-fold) induction of cytochromes CYP2B1 and CYP2B2. In addition to barbiturates, such as phenobarbital and glutethimide, inducers of the CYP2B enzymes include drugs (e.g., phenytoin, loratadine, doxylamine, griseofulvin, chlorpromazine, phenothiazine, clotrimazole, ketoconazole, miconazole), pesticides (e.g., DDT, chlordane, dieldrin), food additives (e.g., butylated hydroxytoluene and butylated hydroxyanisole), personal care ingredients [e.g., octamethylcyclotetrasiloxane (or D4)] and certain polyhalogenated aromatic hydrocarbons [e.g., 2,2′,4,4′,5,5′-hexachlorobiphenyl and 1,4-bis[2]-(3,5-chloropyridyloxy)benzene or TCPOBOP]. Treatment of rats with phenobarbital also results in a two- to fourfold increase in the levels of CYP2A1, CYP2C6, and CYP3A2, as well as a 50 to 75 percent decrease in the levels of CYP2C11, which is present only in adult male rats. In addition, treatment of rats with phenobarbital generally causes an increase (50 to 300 percent) in the concentration of cytochrome b_5, NADPH-cytochrome P450 (*c*) reductase, epoxide hydrolase, aldehyde dehydrogenase, glutathione *S*-transferase and UDP-glucuronosyltransferase. Indeed treatment of rodents with phenobarbital and related inducers causes hepatocellular hyperplasia and/or hypertrophy, which is accompanied by a proliferation of the endoplasmic reticulum.

The mechanism of induction of CYP2B1 by phenobarbital has not been elucidated in as much detail as the induction of CYP1A1 by TCDD. As in the case of CYP1A1, induction of CYP2B1 involves transcriptional activation of the *CYP2B1* gene, which, together with message stabilization, results in an increase in the levels of mRNA and newly synthesized protein. As shown in Table 6-7,

CYP2B1 induction by phenobarbital appears to be mediated by CAR_β, which must dimerize with another nuclear receptor, the retinoid X receptor (RXR), which is activated by 9-*cis*-retinoic acid. CAR_β is a constitutively activated receptor, meaning it is active as a DNA-binding protein in the absence of a bound ligand. However, androstanol and androstenol have been identified as high affinity CAR_β ligands, although these steroids are not CYP2B1 inducers. It would appear that androstanol and androstenol (or related steroids) bind to CAR_β and *block* its inherent ability to function as a DNA-binding protein. Accordingly, induction by phenobarbital appears to involve the displacement of these androstanes from CAR_β. Once derepressed, CAR_β can dimerize with RXR, enter the nucleus and bind to the phenobarbital-responsive element (PBRE) preceding the CYP2B1 gene and numerous other phenobarbital-responsive genes. The fact that, according to this model, phenobarbital-type inducers need only displace androstanes from CAR_β, which presumably does not require highly specific binding, may help to explain why CYP2B1 inducers lack any discernible structure-activity relationship.

The bacterium *B. megaterium* contains two cytochrome P450 enzymes, known as P450BM-1 and P450BM-3, that are inducible by phenobarbital and other compounds that induce rat CYP2B1 (Liang et al., 1995). The 5′-enhancer regions of these bacterial genes contain a 15-base-pair DNA sequence that, when deleted or mutated, results in P450BM-1 or P450BM-2 expression. A similar 15-base-pair DNA sequence, which is known as the *Barbie box* (after *barbiturate*), is present in the 5′-enhancer region of CYP2B1, CYP2B2, and numerous other mammalian genes that are transcriptionally activated by phenobarbital. All Barbie boxes contain a four base pair sequence (5′-AAAG-3′), making this the likely site of DNA-protein interactions. In the absence of inducer, a repressor protein, Bm3R1, binds to the Barbie box and impedes or prevents transcription of the structural gene. Binding of the inducer to this repressor causes its dissociation from the Barbie box, which results in increased transcription. However, in light of the discoveries surrounding CAR_β, it is now clear that the key feature of the bacterial phenobarbital induction mechanism, namely removal of the repressor protein Bm3R1 from the Barbie box, is not the mechanism of phenobarbital induction in mammals.

Treatment of rodents with PCN causes an induction of CYP3A1 and CYP3A2—two independently regulated CYP3A enzymes with very similar structures (87 percent similar) and substrate specificities. In contrast to CYP3A1, CYP3A2 is present in liver microsomes from untreated rats, although the levels of this enzyme decline markedly after puberty in female rats. Consequently, CYP3A2 is a male-specific protein in mature rats, and it is inducible in mature male but not mature female rats (whereas CYP3A1 is inducible in mature male and female rats). In addition to PCN, inducers of CYP3A enzymes include steroids (e.g., dexamethasone and spironolactone), macrolide antibiotics (e.g., troleandomycin and erythromycin estolate), and azole antifungals (e.g., clotrimazole, ketoconazole, and miconazole). Although it primarily induces the CYP2B enzymes (see above), phenobarbital is also an inducer of CYP3A2.

The induction of CYP3A1, like that of CYP1A1 and CYP2B1, involves transcriptional activation of the structural gene, which, together with message stabilization, results in an increase in the levels of CYP3A1 mRNA and newly synthesized protein. The mechanism of induction of CYP3A1 involves the binding of PCN and related inducers to an orphan receptor known as the pregnane-X receptor (PXR). The ligand-activated PXR dimerizes with RXR (which is activated by 9-*cis*-retinoic acid), and the heterodimer is translocated to the nucleus where it binds to response elements that activate the transcription of CYP3A1 and other PCN-inducible genes. The ligand-binding properties of PXR vary among mammalian species. PCN is a ligand for rodent PXR, whereas rifampin is not. The converse is true of human PXR, which explains why PCN, but not rifampin, is an effective CYP3A inducer in rodents, whereas rifampin, but not PCN, is an effective inducer of human CYP3A4.

In the case of macrolide antibiotics, such as troleandomycin and erythromycin, induction of CYP3A1 involves both transcriptional activation and stabilization of the newly synthesized enzyme against protein degradation. This latter effect involves biotransformation of the macrolide antibiotic to a metabolite that binds tightly to the heme moiety. The induction of CYP3A1 by macrolide antibiotics is often masked by their ability to function as metabolism-dependent inhibitors. The enzyme-inducing effects of clotrimazole, ketoconazole, and miconazole are similarly masked by the ability of these azole antimycotics to bind to and inhibit cytochrome P450 enzymes (including CYP3A1). Substrates and ligands stabilize CYP3A1 by inhibiting its cAMP-dependent-phosphorylation on Ser_{393}, which otherwise denatures the protein and targets it for degradation in the endoplasmic reticulum.

Treatment of male rats with clofibric acid causes a marked induction (up to 40-fold) of CYP4A1, CYP4A2, and CYP4A3, which are three independently regulated CYP4A enzymes with similar substrate specificities (Sundseth and Waxman, 1991). CYP4A1 is expressed in the liver, whereas CYP4A3 is expressed in the liver and kidney. CYP4A2 is expressed in the liver and kidney of male rats, but it is neither expressed nor inducible in female rats. In addition to clofibric acid, inducers of CYP4A enzymes include perfluorodecanoic acid, phthalate ester plasticizers, 2,4-dichlorophenoxyacetic acid (2,4-D), ciprofibrate and other hypolipidemic drugs, aspirin and other NSAIDs, nicotinic acid, dehydroepiandrosterone sulfate, and leukotriene receptor antagonists (MK-0571 and RG 7512). A feature common to all these CYP4A enzyme inducers is their ability to cause proliferation of hepatic peroxisomes.

As in the case of CYP1A1, CYP2B1, and CYP3A1, the induction of CYP4A enzymes by clofibric acid involves transcriptional activation of the structural gene, which results in an increase in the levels of mRNA and newly synthesized protein. The transcription factor that activates the *CYP4A* genes is the peroxisome proliferator-activated receptor (PPARα), a member of the steroid/thyroid/retinoid superfamily of nuclear receptors that regulates transcription of the genes for fatty acyl-CoA oxidase, bifunctional enzyme (enoyl-CoA hydratase/3-hydroxyacyl-CoA dehydrogenase), and fatty acid binding protein (Muerhoff et al., 1992; Demoz et al., 1994). Binding of a peroxisome proliferator to PPARα results in the formation of a heterodimer with RXR, which is activated by 9-*cis*-retinoic acid. The ligand-bound heterodimer of PPARα and RXR binds to a regulatory DNA sequence known as the peroxisome proliferator response element. Three PPREs have been identified in the 5′-enhancer region of the rabbit *CYP4A6* gene. Each of these elements contains a sequence known as DR1, an imperfect repeat of the nuclear receptor binding consensus sequence separated by one nucleotide (PuGGTCA N PuGGTCA). Peroxisome proliferators can bind to PPARα stereoselectively; therefore, the enantiomers of certain drugs differ in their ability to induce CYP4A and cause a proliferation of peroxisomes. Androsterone sulfate and arachidonic acid are physiologic ligands for PPARα.

Treatment of rats with isoniazid causes a two- to fivefold induction of CYP2E1. In sexually mature rats, the levels of liver microsomal CYP2E1 are slightly greater in female than in male rats. In addition to isoniazid, inducers of CYP2E1 include ethanol, acetone, pyrazole, pyridine, ketoconazole, fasting, and uncontrolled diabetes. A common feature of CYP2E1 inducers is their ability to inhibit or be biotransformed by CYP2E1 and/or their ability to increase serum ketone bodies. Like CYP3A1, CYP2E1 is induced both by transcriptional activation of the gene and stabilization of the protein against degradation (Koop and Tierney, 1990). Induction of CYP2E1 can also involve mRNA stabilization and/or increased efficiency of mRNA translation. The mechanism of CYP2E1 induction varies even among closely related inducers. For example, although diabetes and fasting both increase the levels of CYP2E1 mRNA by ~10-fold, the increase with diabetes results from mRNA stabilization, whereas the increase with fasting results from increased gene transcription. Acetone and other substrates stabilize CYP2E1 by blocking its cAMP-dependent-phosphorylation on Ser_{129}, which otherwise causes the denaturation and degradation of this enzyme. The enzyme-inducing effects of ethanol, acetone, pyrazole, pyridine, and isoniazid are often masked in vivo by the binding of these substrates to CYP2E1.

In mature rats, the levels of certain P450 enzymes are sexually differentiated; that is, they are higher in either male or female rats. Male-specific enzymes include CYP2A2, CYP2C11, CYP2C13, CYP3A2, and CYP4A2. The only known female-specific P450 enzyme is CYP2C12, although the levels of several other P450 enzymes are greater in female than male rats, including CYP2A1, CYP2C7, and CYP2E1. These gender-related differences in P450 enzyme expression are due in large part to sex differences in the pattern of secretion of growth hormone, which is pulsatile in male rats and more or less continuous in females (Waxman et al., 1991). Treatment of mature male rats with various xenobiotics perturbs the pattern of growth hormone secretion and causes a partial "feminization" of P450 enzyme expression, which includes decreased expression of CYP2C11. Sex differences in the expression of P450 enzymes occur to a limited extent in mice, but no marked sex differences in P450 expression have been observed in dogs, monkeys, or humans.

Enzymatic assays have been developed to monitor the induction of the aforementioned P450 enzymes. A series of 7-alkoxyresorufin analogs has proven very useful for monitoring the induction of rat and mouse CYP1A and CYP2B enzymes. CYP1A enzymes preferentially catalyze the *O*-dealkylation of 7-methoxyresorufin and 7-ethoxyresorufin, whereas CYP2B enzymes preferentially catalyze the *O*-dealkylation of 7-pentoxyresorufin and 7-benzyloxyresorufin. The effects of treating rats with phenobarbital on the levels of liver CYP2A1, CYP2B1/2, CYP2C11, and CYP3A1/2 can be monitored by changes in specific pathways of testosterone oxidation. For all practical purposes, the rates of testosterone 2α-, 7α-, and 16β-hydroxylation accurately reflect the levels of CYP2C11, CYP2A1, and CYP2B1/2, respectively. The 2β-, 6β-, and 15β-hydroxylation of testosterone collectively reflect the levels of CYP3A1 and/or CYP3A2. Induction of CYP2E1 can be monitored by increases in 4-nitrophenol hydroxylase, aniline 4-hydroxylase, and chlorzoxazone 6-hydroxylase activity, although none of these reactions is specifically catalyzed by CYP2E1. The 12-hydroxylation of lauric acid appears to be catalyzed specifically by CYP4A enzymes. Indeed the ω-hydroxylation of fatty acids and their derivatives (such as eicosanoids) appears to be a physiological function of these enzymes. CYP4A enzymes also catalyze the 11-hydroxylation of lauric acid, but this reaction is also catalyzed by other P450 enzymes, including the CYP2B and CYP2E enzymes. Induction of CYP4A enzymes by clofibric acid increases the ratio 12- to 11-hydroxylauric acid, whereas induction of CYP2B enzymes by phenobarbital or CYP2E1 by isoniazid has the opposite effect.

In addition to measuring certain enzyme activities, changes in the levels of specific P450 enzymes can also be monitored by immunochemical techniques, such as Western immunoblotting. When P450 induction involves increased gene transcription and/or mRNA stabilization, the increase in mRNA levels can be measured by Northern blotting. These techniques are particularly useful for detecting P450 induction by chemicals that bind tightly to the active site of cytochrome P450 enzymes and thus mask their detection by enzymatic assays. Such chemicals include macrolide antibiotics (e.g., erythromycin and troleandomycin), methylenedioxy-containing compounds (e.g., safrole and isosafrole), azole antimycotics (e.g., clotrimazole, ketoconazole, and miconazole) and musk xylene (Lehman-McKeeman et al., 1999).

Numerous phenobarbital-type inducers and peroxisome proliferators are epigenetic tumorigens (Grasso et al., 1991). Rodents treated chronically with these chemicals develop liver and/or thyroid tumors. The liver tumors seem to be a consequence of hepatocellular hyperplasia/hypertrophy and the sustained proliferation of either the endoplasmic reticulum (in the case of CYP2B inducers) or peroxisomes (in the case of CYP4A inducers). The thyroid tumors are the result of UDP-glucuronosyltransferase induction, which accelerates the glucuronidation of thyroid hormones, leading to a compensatory increase in thyroid-stimulating hormone (TSH). Sustained stimulation of the thyroid gland by TSH leads to the development of thyroid follicular tumors. These epigenetic mechanisms of chemical-induced tumor formation do not appear to operate in humans. Prolonged treatment (>35 years) with anticonvulsants, such as phenobarbital or phenytoin, does not increase the incidence of liver or thyroid tumor formation in humans. Prolonged elevation of TSH in humans does not lead to tumor formation but causes goiter, a reversible enlargement of the thyroid gland associated with iodide deficiency and treatment with drugs that block thyroid hormone synthesis. Chemicals that cause peroxisome proliferation in rodents do not do so in humans and other primates, possibly because of low levels of PPARα in primate liver and/or the presence of other transcription factors (such as LXRα and the thyroid hormone receptor) that bind to or near the PPRE consensus site. Gene knockout mice lacking PPARα are refractory to peroxisome proliferation and peroxisome proliferator–induced changes in gene expression (including induction of CYP4A and β-oxidation enzymes). Furthermore, PPARα-null mice are resistant to hepatocarcinogenesis when fed a diet containing WY-14,643, a potent peroxisome proliferator and nongenotoxic carcinogen (Gonzalez et al., 1998).

PHASE II ENZYME REACTIONS

Phase II biotransformation reactions include glucuronidation, sulfonation (more commonly called sulfation), acetylation, methylation, conjugation with glutathione (mercapturic acid synthesis), and conjugation with amino acids (such as glycine, taurine, and glutamic acid) (Paulson et al., 1986). The cofactors for these reactions, which are shown in Fig. 6-45, react with functional groups that are either present on the xenobiotic or are introduced/exposed during phase I biotransformation. With the exception of methylation and acetylation, phase II biotransformation reactions result in a large increase in xenobiotic hydrophilicity, so they greatly promote the excretion of foreign chemicals. Glucuronidation, sulfation, acetylation, and methylation involve reactions with activated or "high-energy" cofactors, whereas conjugation with amino acids or glutathione involves reactions with activated xenobiotics. Most phase II biotransforming enzymes are mainly located in the cytosol; a notable exception is the UDP-glucuronosyltransferases, which are microsomal enzymes (Table 6-1). Phase II reactions generally proceed much faster than phase I reactions, such as those catalyzed by cytochrome P450. Therefore, the rate of elimination of xenobiotics whose excretion depends on biotransformation by cytochrome P450 followed by phase II conjugation is generally determined by the first reaction.

Glucuronidation

Glucuronidation is a major pathway of xenobiotic biotransformation in mammalian species except for members of the cat family (lions, lynxes, civets, and domestic cats) (Miners and Mackenzie, 1992; Mackenzie et al., 1992; Burchell and Coughtrie, 1992; Burchell, 1999; Tukey and Strassburg, 2000). Glucuronidation requires the cofactor uridine diphosphate-glucuronic acid (UDP-glucuronic acid), and the reaction is catalyzed by UDP-glucuronosyltransferases (UGTs), which are located in the endoplasmic reticulum of liver and other tissues, such as the kidney, intestine, skin, brain, spleen, and nasal mucosa (Fig. 6-46). Examples of xenobiotics that are glucuronidated are shown in Fig. 6-47. The site of glucuronidation is generally an electron-rich nucleophilic heteroatom (O, N, or S). Therefore, substrates for glucuronidation contain such functional groups as aliphatic alcohols and phenols (which form *O*-glucuronide ethers), carboxylic acids (which form *O*-glucuronide esters), primary and secondary aromatic and aliphatic amines (which form *N*-glucuronides), and free

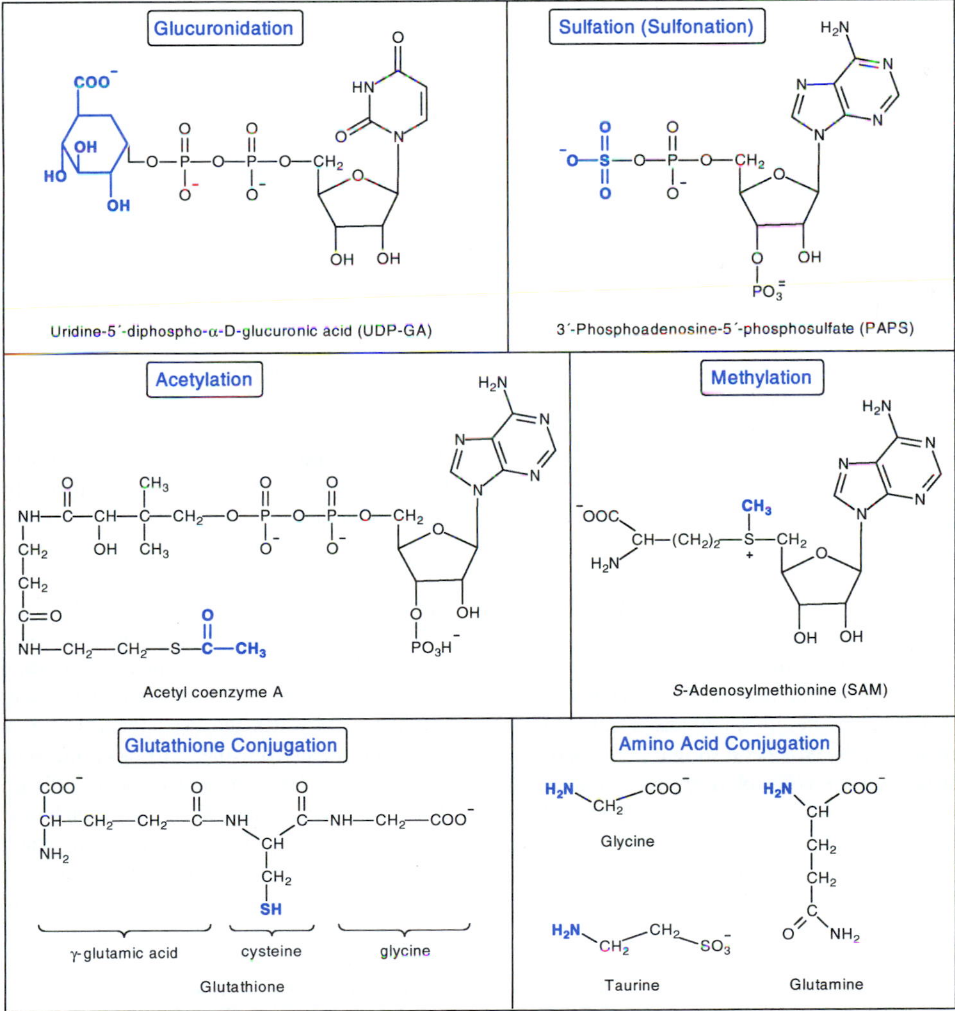

Figure 6-45. Structures of cofactors for phase II biotransformation.

The functional group that reacts with or is transferred to the xenobiotic is shown in blue.

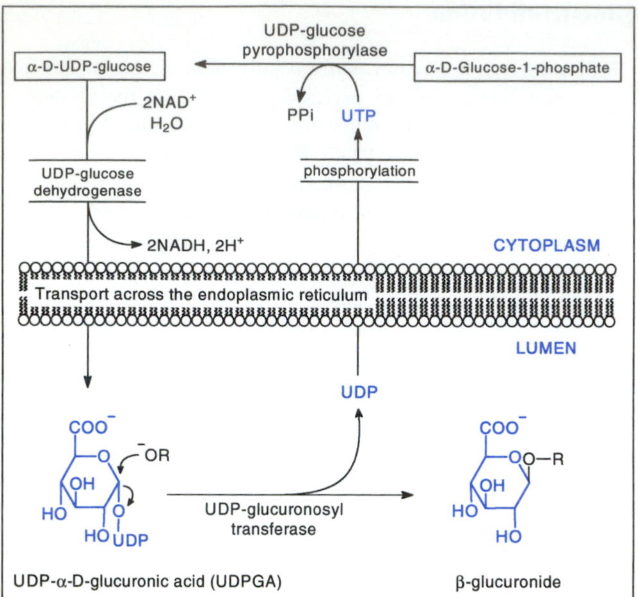

Figure 6-46. Synthesis of UDP-glucuronic acid and inversion of configuration ($\alpha \rightarrow \beta$) during glucuronidation of a phenolic xenobiotic (designated RO^-).

Note that these microsomal enzymes face the lumen of the endoplasmic reticulum.

sulfhydryl groups (which form *S*-glucuronides). In humans and monkeys, more than thirty tertiary amines, including tripelennamine, cyclobenzaprine and imipramine, are substrates for *N*-glucuronidation, which leads to formation of positively charged quaternary glucuronides (Hawes, 1998). Certain xenobiotics—such as phenylbutazone, sulfinpyrazone and feprazone—contain carbon atoms that are sufficiently nucleophilic to form *C*-glucuronides. Coumarin and certain other carbonyl-containing compounds are glucuronidated to form arylenol-glucuronides. In addition to numerous xenobiotics, substrates for glucuronidation include several endogenous compounds, such as bilirubin, steroid hormones, and thyroid hormones. A listing of over 350 UDP-glucuronosyltransferase substrates is available at www.AnnualReview.org (Tukey and Strassburg, 2000).

Glucuronide conjugates of xenobiotics and endogenous compounds are polar, water-soluble conjugates that are eliminated from the body in urine or bile. Whether glucuronides are excreted from the body in bile or urine depends on the size of the aglycone (parent compound or phase I metabolite). In rat, glucuronides are preferentially excreted in urine if the molecular weight of the aglycone is less than 250, whereas glucuronides of larger molecules (aglycones with molecular weight >350) are preferentially excreted in bile. Molecular weight cutoffs for the preferred route of excretion vary among mammalian species. The carboxylic acid moiety of glucuronic acid, which is ionized at physiologic pH, promotes excretion because (1) it increases the aqueous solubility of the xenobiotic and (2) it is recognized by the biliary and renal organic anion transport systems, which enables glucuronides to be secreted into urine and bile. The cofactor for glucuronidation is synthesized from glucose-1-phosphate, and the linkage between glucuronic acid and UDP has an α-configuration, as shown in Fig. 6-46. This configuration protects the cofactor from hydrolysis by β-glucuronidase. However, glucuronides of xenobiotics have a β-configuration. This inversion of configuration occurs because glucuronides are formed by nucleophilic attack by an electron-rich atom (usually O, N, or S) on UDP-glucuronic acid, and this attack occurs on the opposite side of the linkage between glucuronic acid and UDP, as shown in Fig. 6-46. In contrast to the UDP-glucuronic acid cofactor, xenobiotics conjugated with glucuronic acid are substrates for β-glucuronidase. Although present in the lysosomes of some mammalian tissues, considerable β-glucuronidase activity is present in the intestinal microflora. The intestinal enzyme can release the aglycone, which can be reabsorbed and enter a cycle called *enterohepatic circulation,* which delays the elimination of xenobiotics. Nitrogen-glucuronides are more slowly hydrolyzed by β-glucuronidase than *O*- or *S*-glucuronides, whereas *O*-glucuronides tend to be more stable to acid-catalyzed hydrolysis than *N*- or *S*-glucuronides. The potential for glucuronides to be hydrolyzed in the presence of acid or base complicates the analysis of conjugates in urine or feces.

The *C*-terminus of all UDP-glucuronosyltransferases contains a membrane-spanning domain that anchors the enzyme in the endoplasmic reticulum. The enzyme faces the lumen of the endoplasmic reticulum, where it is ideally placed to conjugate lipophilic xenobiotics and their metabolites generated by cytochrome P450 and other microsomal phase I enzymes. The lumenal orientation of UDP-glucuronosyltransferases poses a problem because UDP-glucuronic acid is a water-soluble cofactor synthesized in the cytoplasm. A transporter has been postulated to shuttle this cofactor into the lumen of the endoplasmic reticulum, and it may also shuttle UDP (the byproduct of glucuronidation) back into the cytoplasm for synthesis of UDP-glucuronic acid, as shown in Fig. 6-46. In vitro, the glucuronidation of xenobiotics by liver microsomes can be stimulated by detergents, which disrupt the lipid bilayer of the endoplasmic reticulum and allow UDP-glucuronosyltransferases free access to UDP-glucuronic acid. High concentrations of detergent can inhibit UDP-glucuronosyltransferases, presumably by disrupting their interaction with phospholipids, which are important for catalytic activity.

Radominska-Pandya et al. (1999) have proposed that UDP-glucuronosyltransferases form homo- and heterodimers in the endoplasmic reticulum, which are stabilized by substrate binding (which gains access to the active site by diffusion through the lipid bilayer). According to this model, UDP-glucuronic acid gains access to the active site via a proteinaceous channel formed between the two monomers. After conjugation, the product glucuronide and UDP are expelled into the cytosol by the same channel used for entry of the cofactor, after which the dimer dissociates to allow pairing of the monomers with other UDP-glucuronosyltransferases. This model obviates the need for a transporter to shuttle UDP-glucuronic acid from the cytosol to the lumen of endoplasmic reticulum. It is not known whether such dimerization, if it occurs, alters the substrate specificity of the individual UDP-glucuronosyltransferases, which would have implications for studies designed to determine the substrate specificity of recombinant enzymes, which are invariably expressed individually.

Cofactor availability can limit the rate of glucuronidation of drugs that are administered in high doses and are conjugated extensively, such as aspirin and acetaminophen. In experimental animals, the glucuronidation of xenobiotics can be impaired in vivo by factors that reduce or deplete UDP-glucuronic acid levels, such as diethyl ether, borneol, and galactosamine. The lowering of UDP-glucuronic acid levels by fasting, such as might occur during a se-

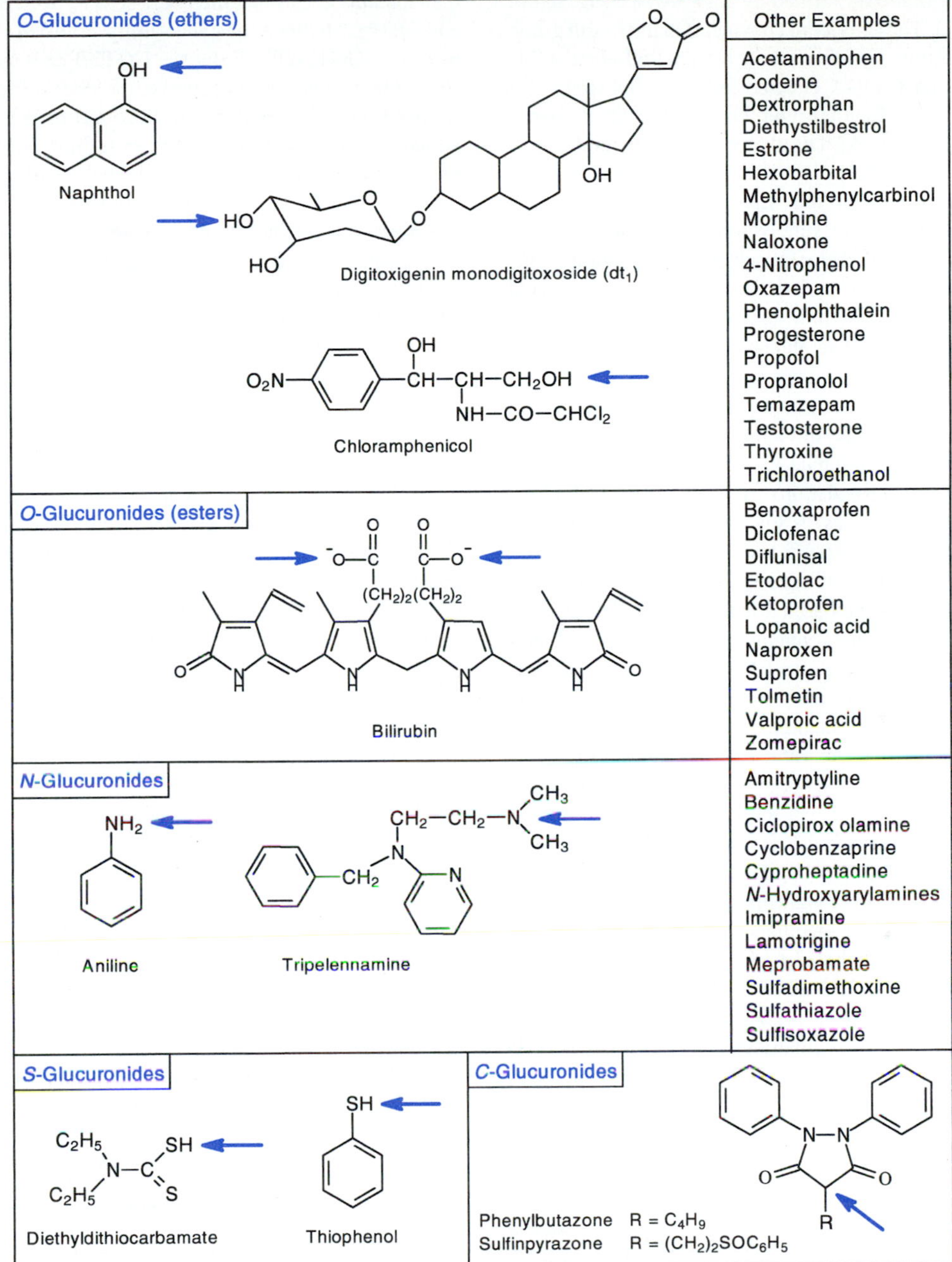

Figure 6-47. Examples of xenobiotics and endogenous substrates that are glucuronidated.

The arrow indicates the site of glucuronidation.

vere toothache, is thought to predispose individuals to the hepatotoxic effects of acetaminophen, although even then hepatotoxicity only occurs with higher-than-recommended doses of this analgesic (Whitcomb and Block, 1994).

The existence of multiple forms of UDP-glucuronosyltransferase was first suggested by the observation that in rats developmental changes in glucuronidation rates were substrate-dependent, and the glucuronidation of xenobiotics could be differentially affected by treatment of rats with chemicals known to induce cytochrome P450. Based on their ontogeny and inducibility, the UDP-glucuronosyltransferase activities in rat liver microsomes were categorized into four groups. The activity of enzyme(s) in the first group peaks 1 to 5 days *before* birth, and it is inducible by 3-methylcholanthrene and other CYP1A enzyme inducers. Substrates for the group 1 enzyme(s) tend to be planar chemicals, such as 1-naphthol, 4-nitrophenol, and 4-methylumbelliferone. The activity of enzyme(s) in the second group peaks ~5 days *after* birth and is inducible by phenobarbital and other CYP2B enzyme inducers. Substrates for the group 2 enzyme(s) tend to be bulky chemicals, such as chloramphenicol, morphine, 4-hydroxybiphenyl, and monoterpenoid alcohols. The activity of enzyme(s) in the third group peaks around the time of puberty (~1 month) and is inducible by PCN and other CYP3A enzyme inducers. Substrates for the group 3 enzyme(s) include digitoxigenin monodigitoxoside

(dt_1), a metabolite of digitoxin formed by CYP3A (see Fig. 6-43), and possibly bilirubin. The activity of enzyme(s) in the fourth group also peak around the time of puberty (~1 month) and is inducible by clofibrate and other CYP4A enzyme inducers. Substrates for the group 4 enzyme(s) include bilirubin but not dt_1, which distinguishes group 3 from group 4 UDP-glucuronosyltransferases.

Although this classification system still has some practical value, it has become evident that the four groups of UDP-glucuronosyltransferases do not simply represent four independently regulated enzymes with different substrate specificities. This realization stems from various studies, including those conducted with Gunn rats, which are hyperbilirubinemic due to a genetic defect in bilirubin conjugation. The glucuronidation defect in Gunn rats is substrate-dependent in a manner that does not match the categorization of UDP-glucuronosyltransferases into the four aforementioned groups. For example, in Gunn rats the glucuronidation of the group 2 substrates, morphine and chloramphenicol, is not impaired, whereas the glucuronidation of 1-naphthol, dt_1 and bilirubin (group 1, 3, and 4 substrates) is low or undetectable. The induction of UDP-glucuronosyltransferase activity by 3-methylcholanthrene, PCN, and clofibric acid is impaired in Gunn rats, whereas the induction by phenobarbital is normal. (Although phenobarbital does not induce the conjugation of bilirubin in Gunn rats, it does so in normal Wistar rats.) Only when the UDP-glucuronosyltransferases were cloned did it become apparent why the genetic defect in Gunn rats affects three of the four groups of UDP-glucuronosyltransferases that are otherwise independently regulated as a function of age and xenobiotic treatment (Owens and Ritter, 1992). It is now apparent that the UDP-glucuronosyltransferases expressed in rat liver microsomes belong to two gene families, UGT1 and UGT2. The former gene family contains at least seven enzymes, all of which belong to the same subfamily designated UGT1A. The individual members of the rat UGT1A subfamily are UGT1A1, 1A2, 1A3, 1A5, 1A6, 1A7, and 1A8. UGT1A4 is not a member of the rat UGT1A subfamily, although additional members may yet be identified. The second UGT gene family in rats is divided into two subfamilies, UGT2A and UGT2B; the former contains a single member (UGT2A1) whereas the second contains at least six members (UGT2B1, 2B2, 2B3, 2B6, 2B8, and 2B12). Members of gene family 2 are all distinct gene products (i.e., UGT2A1 and the six UGT2B enzymes are encoded by seven separate genes). In contrast, members of family 1 are formed from a single gene with multiple copies of the first exon, each of which can be connected in cassette fashion with a common set of exons (exons 2 to 5). This arrangement is illustrated in Fig. 6-48 for the human UGT1 gene locus. In rats, the fourth copy of exon 1 is a pseudogene, hence, there is no UGT1A4 in rats. In humans, the second copy of exon 1 is a pseudogene, hence, there is no UGT1A2 in humans. (The human UGT1A gene locus is discussed later in this section.) The rat UGT1A gene locus is known to contain eight versions of the first exon, which produce seven functional UGT1A enzymes. Additional members of the rat UGT1A subfamily are thought to exist, including one that glucuronidates dt_1, a metabolite of digitoxin (see Fig. 6-43).

A simplified view of the UGT1A gene locus is that the multiple UGT1A enzymes are constructed by linking different substrate binding sites (encoded by multiple copies of exon 1) to a constant portion of the enzyme (encoded by exons 2 to 5). This constant region is involved in cofactor binding and membrane insertion. This method of generating multiple forms of an enzyme from a single gene locus is economical, but it is also the genetic equivalent of putting all of one's eggs in the same basket. Whereas a mutation in any one of the UGT2 enzymes affects a single enzyme, a mutation in the constant region of the UGT1 gene affects all enzymes encoded by this locus. In the Gunn rat, a mutation at codon 415 introduces a premature stop signal, so that all forms of UDP-glucuronosyltransferase encoded by the UGT1 locus are truncated and functionally inactive. The UDP-glucuronosyltransferases known to be encoded by the rat UGT1 locus include the 3-methylcholanthrene-inducible enzyme that conjugates planar molecules like 1-naphthol (UGT1A6 and UGT1A7), the phenobarbital- and clofibric acid-inducible enzyme that conjugates bilirubin (UGT1A1 and, to a lesser extent, UGT1A4), and the PCN-inducible enzyme that conjugates dt_1 (which will be named when the first exon for this enzyme is cloned and localized within the UGT1A gene locus). All of these UGT1 enzymes are defective in Gunn rats.

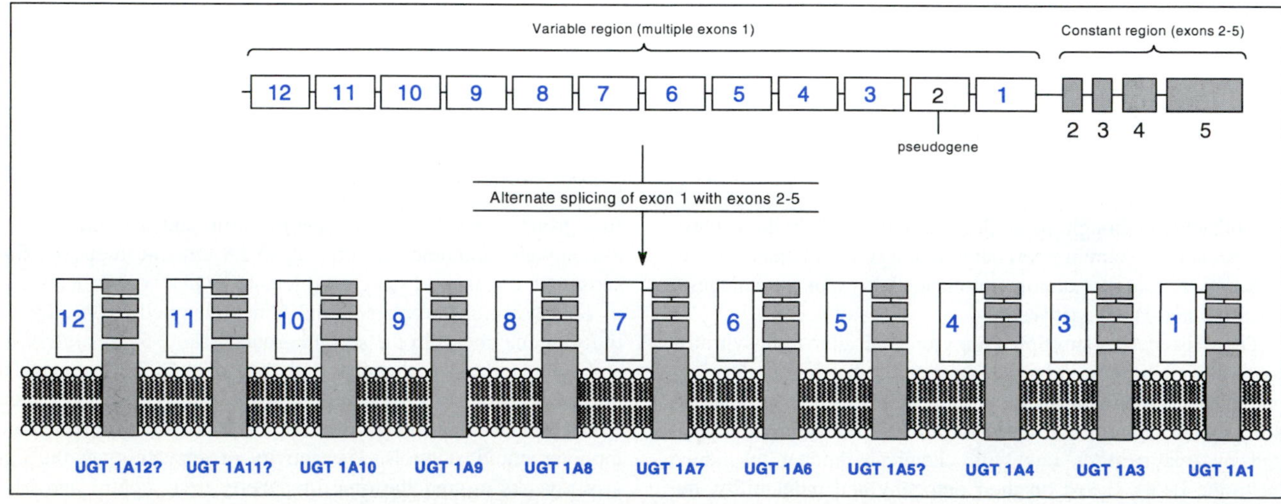

Figure 6-48. Structure of the human UGT 1 locus which encodes multiple forms of UDP-glucuronosyltransferase.

The second family of rat UDP-glucuronosyltransferases, which share less than 50 percent of amino acid sequence identity with the first family, are divided into two subfamilies (UGT2A and UGT2B), and its members are distinct gene products. The single member of the 2A subfamily, UGT2A1, is expressed specifically in olfactory epithelium where it conjugates a wide variety of substrates. The six known members of the rat UGT2B subfamily (UGT2B1, 2, 3, 6, 8, and 12) are expressed in liver and various extrahepatic tissues. Members of the UGT2B subfamily are named in the order they are cloned, regardless of the species of origin (much like the nomenclature system for most of the P450 enzymes). UGT2B enzymes have been cloned from rat (forms 1, 2, 3, 6, 8, and 12), humans (forms 4, 7, 10, 11, 15, and 17), mouse (form 5), and rabbits (forms 13, 14, and 16). A rabbit UDP-glucuronosyltransferase has been classified as UGT2C1; however, UGT2C genes in other mammalians have not been identified. In rats, at least one UGT2B enzyme (UGT2B1) is inducible by phenobarbital. The gene encoding this enzyme is not defective in Gunn rats; therefore, treatment of Gunn rats with phenobarbital induces the glucuronidation of substrates for UGT2B1. However, UGT2B1 does not conjugate bilirubin (a reaction mainly catalyzed by UGT1A1 and/or UGT1A4), which is why phenobarbital cannot induce the conjugation of bilirubin in Gunn rats. UGT2B1 is the main enzyme responsible for catalyzing the 3-*O*-glucuronidation of morphine, which is markedly increased by treatment of rats with phenobarbital. Whereas as Gunn rats are genetically defective in all UGT1A enzymes, LA rats are selectively defective in UGT2B2, which allowed this enzyme to be identified as the principal enzyme responsible for glucuronidating androsterone and triiodothyronine (T_3) in rats (Burchell, 1999). The multiple forms of human UDP-glucuronosyltransferase are also products of either a single UGT1A gene locus (see Fig. 6-48) or multiple UGT2 genes. The human UGT1A locus contains 12 potential copies of the first exon, although only nine transcripts have been identified (UGT1A1, 1A3, 1A4, 1A5, 1A6, 1A7, 1A8, 1A9, and 1A10), all of which are transcribed in vivo into functional enzymes with the possible exception of UGT1A5 (Tukey and Strassburg, 2000). The UGT2 genes expressed in humans include UGT2A1 (which is expressed only in olfactory tissue in an analogous manner to the corresponding rat enzyme), and UGT2B4, 2B7, 2B10, 2B11, 2B15, and 2B17. The tissue distribution and substrate specificity of the human UGT1 and UGT2 enzymes have been reviewed by Tukey and Strassburg (2000). Suffice it to say that these enzymes are expressed in a wide variety of tissues, and some enzymes—including UGT1A7, 1A8, 1A10, 2A1, and 2B17—are expressed only in extrahepatic tissues, which has implications for the common practice of using human liver microsomes to investigate the role of glucuronidation in drug metabolism. Numerous UGT1 and UGT2 enzymes are expressed throughout the gastrointestinal tract, where they contribute significantly to the first-pass elimination of numerous xenobiotics. Several UGT2B enzymes are expressed in steroid-sensitive tissues, such as prostate and mammary gland, where they presumably terminate the effects of steroid hormones.

Probe drugs have been identified for some but not all of the human UDP-glucuronosyltransferases, including UGT1A1 (bilirubin), UGT1A4 (imipramine), UGT1A6 (1-naphthol and possibly acetaminophen), UGT1A8 (propofol), and UGT2B7 (morphine) (Burchell, 1997). The glucuronidation of morphine by UGT2B7 involves conjugation of the phenolic 3-hydroxyl and the alcoholic 6-hydroxyl group in a 7:1 ratio. The 6-*O*-glucuronide is 600 times more potent an analgesic than the parent drug, whereas the 3-*O*-glucuronide is devoid of analgesic activity. UGT2B7 is present in the brain, where it might facilitate the analgesic effect of morphine through formation of the 6-*O*-glucuronide, which presumably does not readily cross the blood-brain barrier and may be retained in the brain longer than morphine (Tukey and Strassburg, 2000).

In humans, Crigler-Najjar syndrome and Gilbert's disease are congenital defects in bilirubin conjugation analogous to that seen in Gunn rats. The major bilirubin-conjugating enzyme in humans is UGT1A1. Genetic polymorphisms in exons 2-5, which affect all enzymes encoded by the UGT1A locus, and polymorphisms in exon 1, which specifically affect UGT1A1, have been identified in patients with Crigler-Najjar syndrome and Gilbert's disease. More than thirty genetic polymorphisms are associated with these diseases (Tukey and Strassburg, 2000). Some polymorphisms are associated with type I Crigler-Najjar syndrome, a severe form of the disease characterized by a complete loss of bilirubin-conjugating activity and marked hyperbilirubinemia, whereas others are associated with the less severe type II Crigler-Najjar syndrome or Gilbert's disease. The milder forms of hyperbilirubinemia respond to phenobarbital, which stimulates bilirubin conjugation presumably by inducing UGT1A1. Type I Crigler-Najjar syndrome is associated with impaired glucuronidation of propofol, 17α-ethinylestradiol and various phenolic substrates for UGT1A enzymes.

There is some evidence for genetic polymorphisms in some of the human UGT2 enzymes. For example, oxazepam is glucuronidated by UGT2B7, which preferentially glucuronidates *S*-oxazepam over its *R*-enantiomer. Ten percent of the population appear to be poor glucuronidators of *S*-oxazepam, which may or may not reflect genetic polymorphisms of the UGT2B7 gene. Such polymorphisms appear to be the underlying cause of alterations in hyodeoxycholate glucuronidation in gastric mucosa (Tukey and Strassburg, 2000). Human UGT1A6 glucuronidates acetaminophen, and the glucuronidation of acetaminophen in humans is enhanced by cigarette smoking and dietary cabbage and brussels sprouts, which suggests that human UGT1A6 is inducible by polycyclic aromatic hydrocarbons and derivatives of indole 3-carbinol (Bock et al., 1994). However, direct evidence for induction of human UGT1A6 is lacking, even though rat UGT1A6 is highly inducible by polycyclic aromatic hydrocarbons and other CYP1A inducers. (It should be noted that the UGT1A enzymes in rat and human are named according to the location of the first exon relative to the shared exons within the UGT1A gene locus. Consequently, the identically named UGT1A enzymes in rats and humans need not necessarily glucuronidate the same substrates nor be under similar regulatory control.) Nevertheless, ligands for the *Ah* receptor, such as those present in cigarette smoke, induce CYP1A2, which would be expected to enhance the hepatotoxicity of acetaminophen. Increased acetaminophen glucuronidation may explain why cigarette smoking does not enhance the hepatotoxicity of acetaminophen. Conversely, decreased glucuronidation may explain why some individuals with Gilbert's syndrome are predisposed to the hepatotoxic effects of acetaminophen (De Morais et al., 1992). Low rates of glucuronidation also predispose humans to the adverse gastrointestinal effects of irinotecan, a derivative of camptothecin (Gupta et al., 1994). Low rates of glucuronidation predispose newborns to jaundice and to the toxic effects of chloramphenicol; the latter was once used prophylactically to prevent opportunistic infections in newborns until it was found to cause severe cyanosis and even death (gray baby syndrome).

Glucuronidation generally detoxifies xenobiotics and potentially toxic endobiotics, such as bilirubin, for which reason glucuronidation is generally considered a beneficial process. However, steroid hormones glucuronidated on the D-ring (but not the A-ring) cause cholestasis, and induction of UDP-glucuronosyltransferase activity has been implicated as an epigenetic mechanism of thyroid tumor formation in rodents (Curran and DeGroot, 1991; McClain, 1989). Inducers of UDP-glucuronosyltransferases cause a decrease in serum thyroid hormone levels, which triggers a compensatory increase in thyroid-stimulating hormone (TSH). During sustained exposure to the enzyme-inducing agent, prolonged stimulation of the thyroid gland by TSH (>6 months) results in the development of thyroid follicular cell neoplasia. Glucuronidation followed by biliary excretion is a major pathway of thyroxine biotransformation in rodents whereas deiodination is the major pathway (up to 85 percent) of thyroxine metabolism in humans. In contrast to the situation in rodents, prolonged stimulation of the thyroid gland by TSH in humans will result in malignant tumors only in exceptional circumstances and possibly only in conjunction with some thyroid abnormality. Therefore, chemicals that cause thyroid tumors in rats or mice by inducing UDP-glucuronosyltransferase activity are unlikely to cause such tumors in humans. In support of this conclusion, extensive epidemiologic data in epileptic patients suggest that phenobarbital and other anticonvulsants do not function as thyroid (or liver) tumor promoters in humans.

In some cases, glucuronidation represents an important event in the toxicity of xenobiotics. For example, the aromatic amines that cause bladder cancer, such as 2-aminonaphthalene and 4-aminobiphenyl, undergo *N*-hydroxylation in the liver followed by *N*-glucuronidation of the resultant *N*-hydroxyaromatic amine. The *N*-glucuronides, which accumulate in the urine of the bladder, are unstable in acidic pH and thus are hydrolyzed to the corresponding unstable, tumorigenic *N*-hydroxyaromatic amine, as shown in Fig. 6-49. A similar mechanism may be involved in colon tumor formation by aromatic amines, although in this case hydrolysis of the *N*-glucuronide is probably catalyzed by β-glucuronidase in intestinal microflora. Some acylglucuronides are reactive intermediates that bind covalently to protein by mechanisms that may or may not result in cleavage of the glucuronic acid moiety, as shown in Fig. 6-49. Several drugs—including the NSAIDs diclofenac, diflunisal, etodolac, ketoprofen, suprofen, and tolmetin—contain a carboxylic acid moiety that is glucuronidated to form a reactive acylglucuronide. Neoantigens formed by binding of acylglucuronides to protein might be the cause of rare cases of NSAID-induced immune hepatitis. Binding of acylglucuronides to protein can involve isomerization reactions that lead to retention of a rearranged glucuronide moiety (Fig. 6-49). Formation of a common neoantigen (i.e., one that contains a rearranged glucuronic acid moiety) might explain the allergic cross-reactivities (cross-sensiti-

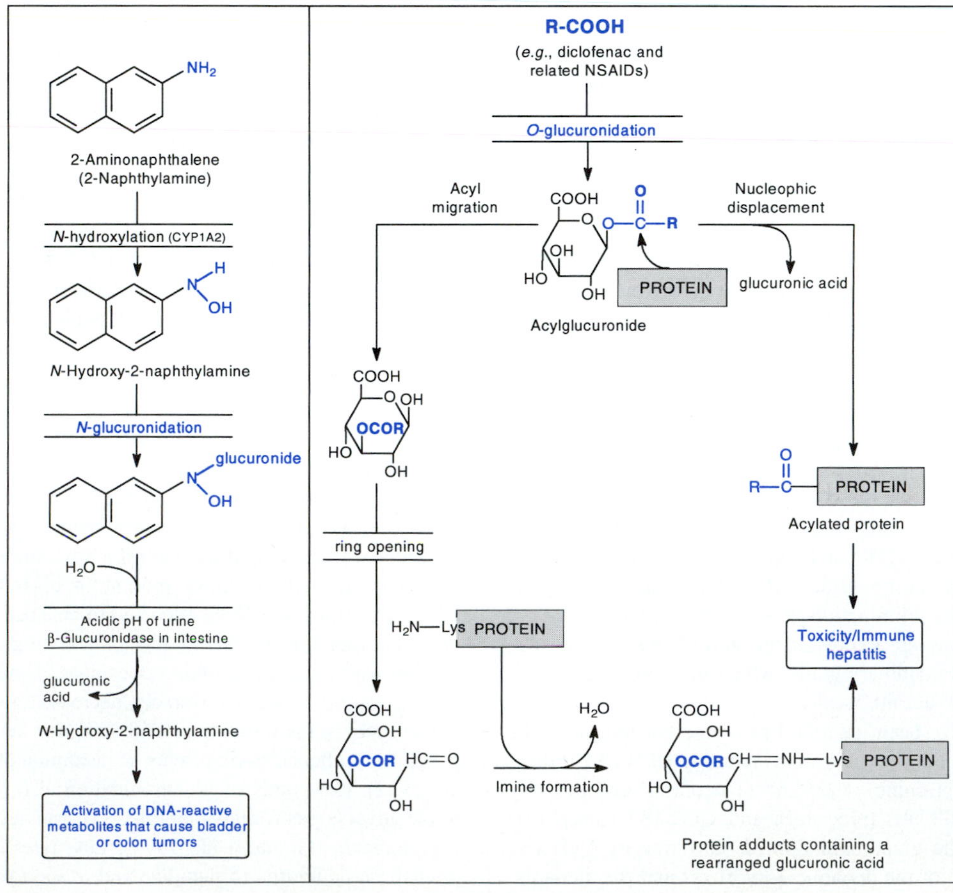

Figure 6-49. Role of glucuronidation in the activation of xenobiotics to toxic metabolites.

zation) observed among different NSAIDs (Spahn-Langguth and Benet, 1992; Kretz-Rommel and Boesterli, 1994).

Sulfation

Many of the xenobiotics and endogenous substrates that undergo *O*-glucuronidation also undergo sulfate conjugation, as illustrated in Fig. 6-28 for acetaminophen (Mulder, 1981; Paulson et al., 1986). Sulfate conjugation generally produces a highly water-soluble sulfuric acid ester. The reaction is catalyzed by sulfotransferases, a large multigene family of soluble (cytosolic) enzymes found primarily in the liver, kidney, intestinal tract, lung, platelets, and brain. The cofactor for the reaction is 3′-phosphoadenosine-5′-phosphosulfate (PAPS), the structure of which is shown in Fig. 6-45. The sulfate conjugation of aliphatic alcohols and phenols, R—OH, proceeds as follows:

$$\mathrm{R{-}OH} + \boxed{\text{phospho-adenosine}}{-}\mathrm{O{-}\overset{O^-}{\underset{O}{P}}{-}O{-}\overset{O}{\underset{O}{S}}{-}O^-} \longrightarrow$$

$$\mathrm{R{-}O{-}\overset{O}{\underset{O}{S}}{-}O^-} + \boxed{\text{phospho-adenosine}}{-}\mathrm{O{-}\overset{O^-}{\underset{O}{P}}{-}O^-} + \mathrm{H^+}$$

Sulfate conjugation involves the transfer of sulfonate not sulfate (i.e., SO_3^- not SO_4^-) from PAPS to the xenobiotic. (The commonly used terms *sulfation* and *sulfate conjugation* are used here, even though *sulfonation* and *sulfonate conjugation* are more appropriate descriptors.) Sulfation is not limited to phenols and aliphatic alcohols (which are often the products of phase I biotransformation), although these represent the largest groups of substrates for sulfotransferases. Certain aromatic amines, such as aniline and 2-aminonaphthalene, can undergo sulfate conjugation to the corresponding sulfamates. The *N*-oxide group in minoxidil and the *N*-hydroxy group in *N*-hydroxy-2-aminonaphthalene and *N*-hydroxy-2-acetylaminofluorene can also be sulfated. In all cases, the conjugation reaction involves nucleophilic attack of oxygen or nitrogen on the electrophilic sulfur atom in PAPS with cleavage of the phosphosulfate bond. Table 6-8 lists some examples of xenobiotics and endogenous compounds that are sulfated without prior biotransformation by phase I enzymes. An even greater number of xenobiotics are sulfated after a hydroxyl group is exposed or introduced during phase I biotransformation.

Carboxylic acids can be conjugated with glucuronic acid but not with sulfate. However, a number of carboxylic acids, such as benzoic acid, naphthoic acid, naphthylacetic acid, salicylic acid, and naproxen, are competitive inhibitors of sulfotransferases (Rao and Duffel, 1991). Pentachlorophenol and 2,6-dichloro-4-nitrophenol are potent sulfotransferase inhibitors because they bind to the enzyme but cannot initiate a nucleophilic attack on PAPS due to the presence of electron-withdrawing substituents in the *ortho*- and *para*-positions on the aromatic ring.

Sulfate conjugates of xenobiotics are excreted mainly in urine. Those excreted in bile may be hydrolyzed by aryl sulfatases present in gut microflora, which contributes to the enterohepatic circulation of certain xenobiotics. Sulfatases are also present in the endoplasmic reticulum and lysosomes, where they primarily hydrolyze sulfates of endogenous compounds presumably in a manner analogous to that described for microsomal β-glucuronidase (Dwivedi et al., 1987) (see comments on egasyn under "Carboxylesterases"). Some sulfate conjugates are substrates for further biotransformation. For example, dehydroepiandrosterone-3-sulfate is 16α-hydroxylated by CYP3A7, the major P450 enzyme expressed in human fetal liver, whereas androstane-3,17-diol-3,17-disulfate is 15β-hydroxylated by CYP2C12, a female-specific P450 enzyme in rats. Sulfation facilitates the deiodination of thyroxine and triiodothyronine and can determine the rate of elimination of thyroid hormones in some species.

Table 6-8
Examples of Xenobiotics and Endogenous Compounds That Undergo Sulfate Conjugation

FUNCTIONAL GROUP	EXAMPLE
Primary alcohol	Chloramphenicol, ethanol, hydroxymethyl polycyclic aromatic hydrocarbons, polyethylene glycols
Secondary alcohol	Bile acids, 2-butanol, cholesterol, dehydroepiandrosterone, doxaminol
Phenol	Acetaminophen, estrone, ethinylestradiol, naphthol, pentachlorophenol, phenol, picenadol, salicylamide, trimetrexate
Catechol	Dopamine, ellagic acid, α-methyl-DOPA
N-oxide	Minoxidil
Aliphatic amine	2-Amino-3,8-dimethylimidazo[4,5,-f]-quinoxaline (MeIQx)* 2-Amino-3-methylinidazo-[4,5-f]-quinoline (IQ)* 2-Cyanoethyl-*N*-hydroxythioacetamide, despramine
Aromatic amine	2-Aminonaphthalene, aniline
Aromatic hydroxylamine	*N*-hydroxy-2-aminonaphthalene
Aromatic hydroxyamide	*N*-hydroxy-2-acetylaminofluorene

*Amino acid pyrolysis products.

The sulfate donor PAPS is synthesized from inorganic sulfate (SO_4^{2-}) and ATP in a two step reaction: The first reaction is catalyzed by ATP sulfurylase, which converts ATP and SO_4^{2-} to adenosine-5′-phosphosulfate (APS) and pyrophosphate. The second reaction is catalyzed by APS kinase, which transfers a phosphate group from ATP to the 3′-position of APS. The major source of sulfate required for the synthesis of PAPS appears to be derived from cysteine through a complex oxidation sequence. Because the concentration of free cysteine is limited, the cellular concentrations of PAPS (~75 μM) are considerably lower than those of UDP-glucuronic acid (~350 μM) and glutathione (~10 mM).

The relatively low concentration of PAPS limits the capacity for xenobiotic sulfation. In general, sulfation is a high-affinity but low-capacity pathway of xenobiotic conjugation, whereas glucuronidation is a low-affinity but high-capacity pathway. Acetaminophen is one of several xenobiotics that are substrates for both sulfotransferases and UDP-glucuronosyltransferases (see Fig. 6-28). The relative amount of sulfate and glucuronide conjugates of acetaminophen is dependent on dose. At low doses, acetaminophen sulfate is the main conjugate formed due to the high affinity of sulfotransferases. As the dose increases, the proportion of acetaminophen conjugated with sulfate decreases, whereas the proportion conjugated with glucuronic acid increases. In some cases, even the absolute amount of xenobiotic conjugated with sulfate can decrease at high doses apparently because of substrate inhibition of sulfotransferase.

Multiple sulfotransferases have been identified in all mammalian species examined. An international workshop approved the abbreviation SULT for sulfotransferase (although ST remains a common abbreviation) and developed a nomenclature system based on amino acid sequences (and, to some extent, function), but the names of the individual forms have not been universally agreed upon. For example, some groups use SULT1A1 to name one of the human phenol sulfotransferases whereas others use it to name the corresponding rat enzyme. The nomenclature system used here is that summarized by Nagata and Yamazoe (2000), which is similar to the nomenclature system developed for cytochrome P450. The sulfotransferases are arranged into gene families that share less than 40 percent amino acid sequence identity. The five gene families identified to date (SULT1–SULT5) are subdivided into subfamilies that are 40 to 65 percent identical. For example, SULT1 is divided into five subfamilies designated SULT1A–SULT1E. Two sulfotransferases that share more than 65 percent similarity are considered individual members of the same subfamily. For example, SULT1A2, SULT1A3, and SULT1A5 are three individual members of the human SULT1A subfamily. The individual sulfotransferases are named in the order they are sequenced without regard to the species of origin. Although five SULT gene families have been identified, these have not been identified in all mammalian species. Furthermore, SULT1 and SULT2 are the only gene families subdivided into subfamilies [five in the case of SULT1 (SULT1A–1E); two in the case of SULT2 (SULT2A and SULT2B)]. Most of the sulfotransferases cloned to date belong to one of two families, SULT1 and SULT2. These two families are functionally different; the SULT1 enzymes catalyze the sulfation of phenols, whereas the SULT2 enzymes catalyze the sulfation of alcohols. A sulfotransferase that catalyzes the sulfonation of amines (to form sulfamates) has been cloned from rabbit, and this enzyme belongs to the SULT3 gene family. The properties of the sulfotransferases encoded by the SULT4 and SULT5 gene families are not known.

Eleven cytosolic sulfotransferases have been cloned from rat, and they belong either to the SULT1 or SULT2 gene families. The individual rat enzymes are SULT1A1, 1B1, 1C1, 1C6, 1C7, 1D2, 1E2, 1E6, 2A1, 2A2, and 2A5 (Nagata and Yamazoe, 2000). The enzymes were previously categorized into five classes based on their catalytic activity. These five functional classes were *arylsulfotransferase,* which sulfates numerous phenolic xenobiotics; *alcohol sulfotransferase,* which sulfates primary and secondary alcohols including nonaromatic hydroxysteroids (for which reason these enzymes are also known as hydroxysteroid sulfotransferases); *estrogen sulfotransferase,* which sulfates estrone and other aromatic hydroxysteroids; *tyrosine ester sulfotransferase,* which sulfates tyrosine methyl ester and 2-cyanoethyl-*N*-hydroxythioacetamide, and *bile salt sulfotransferase,* which sulfates conjugated and unconjugated bile acids. The *arylsulfotransferase* and *estrogen sulfotransferase* are composed largely of SULT1 enzymes, which catalyze the sulfation of phenolic xenobiotics, catechols, and aromatic steroids. The *alcohol sulfotransferase* and *bile salt sulfotransferase* are composed largely of SULT2 enzymes, which catalyze the sulfation of a variety of primary and secondary alcohols, bile acids and hydroxysteroids (such as dehydroepiandrosterone or DHEA). The individual sulfotransferases have broad and overlapping substrate specificities. Consequently, sulfation reactions that are specific for a single sulfotransferase enzyme are the exception rather than the rule.

In rats, sulfotransferase activity varies considerably with the sex and age. In mature rats, phenol sulfotransferase activity (SULT1A activity) is higher in males, whereas alcohol sulfotransferase and bile salt sulfotransferase activities (SULT2 activities) are higher in females. Sex differences in the developmental expression of individual sulfotransferase are the result of a complex interplay between gonadal, thyroidal, and pituitary hormones, which similarly determine sex differences in P450 enzyme expression. However, compared with P450 enzymes, the sulfotransferases are refractory or only marginally responsive to the enzyme-inducing effects of 3-methylcholanthrene and phenobarbital, although one or more individual SULT2 enzymes are inducible by PCN. In general, sulfotransferase activity is low in pigs but high in cats. The high sulfotransferase activity in cats offsets their low capacity to conjugate xenobiotics with glucuronic acid.

Nine genes encoding cytosolic sulfotransferases have been identified in humans, and they belong either to the SULT1 or SULT2 gene families. The individual human enzymes are SULT1A2, 1A3, 1A5, 1B2, 1C2, 1C3, 1E4, 2A3, and 2B1 (Nagata and Yamazoe, 2000). A tenth human sulfotransferase has been identified by the Human Chromosome Project Group. The properties of this sulfotransferase, which is a member of the SULT5 gene family, have yet to be determined. Several of the human SULT genes have multiple initiation sites for transcription, which produces different mRNA transcripts. Consequently, in some cases, different versions of the same human SULT gene have been cloned several times. For example, there are three alternative first exons (exons 1a, 1b, and 1c) in the human SULT1A5 gene (none of which contains a coding region), and five SULT1A5 cDNAs have been cloned from various human tissues, each with a unique 5′-region (Nagata and Yamazoe, 2000).

Human liver cytosol contains two phenol sulfotransferase activities (PST) that can be distinguished by their thermal stability; hence, they are known as TS-PST (*thermally stable*) and TL-PST (*thermally labile*) (Weinshilboum, 1992; Weinshilboum et al., 1997). It is now known that TS-PST actually reflects the activity of two sulfotransferases, namely SULT1A2 and SULT1A3, whereas TL-PST reflects the activity of SULT1A5 (hence, the three members of the SULT1A gene subfamily in human are represented functionally by TS-PST and TL-PST activity). SULT1A2 and SULT1A3 function as homo- and heterodimers, and are co-regulated. Although these two individual sulfotransferases are not catalytically identical, they are sufficiently similar to consider them as the single activity traditionally known as TS-PST.

Because of differences in their substrate specificity, TS-PST and TL-PST are also known as phenol-PST and monoamine-PST, respectively. TL-PST preferentially catalyzes the sulfation of dopamine, epinephrine, and levadopa, whereas TS-PST preferentially catalyzes the sulfation of simple phenols, such as phenol, 4-nitrophenol, minoxidil, and acetaminophen. TS-PST also catalyzes the *N*-sulfation of 2-aminonaphthalene. TS-PST (sensitive) and TL-PST (insensitive) can also be distinguished by differences in their sensitivity to the inhibitory effects of 2,6-dichloro-4-nitrophenol.

The expression of TS-PST in human liver is largely determined by genetic factors, which also determine the corresponding sulfotransferase activity in blood platelets. Inherited variation in platelet TS-PST largely reflects genetic polymorphisms in SULT1A3. An allelic variant of SULT1A3 known as SULT1A3*2 ($Arg_{213} \rightarrow His_{213}$) is associated with low TS-PST activity and decreased thermal stability. This particular genetic polymorphism is common in both Caucasians and Nigerians (with an allele frequency of 0.31 and 0.37, respectively), and is correlated with interindividual variation in the sulfation of acetaminophen. Low TS-PST predisposes individuals to diet-induced migraine headaches, possibly due to impaired sulfation of unidentified phenolic compounds in the diet that cause such headaches.

Human SULT1B2, like the corresponding enzyme in other species, catalyzes the sulfation of thyroid hormones. Genetic polymorphisms in this gene have not been identified, although SULT1B2 levels in human liver cytosol vary widely. SULT1B2 is also expressed in human colon, small intestine and blood leukocytes. Humans have two SULT1C enzymes (SULT1C2 and SULT1C3). Their function has not been determined, although the corresponding rat enzyme (SULT1C1) catalyzes the sulfation of *N*-hydroxy-2-acetylaminofluorene (see Fig. 6-50). High levels of SULT1C2 and 1C3 are expressed in fetal liver and kidney. Hepatic levels decline in adulthood, but significant levels of SULT1C2 and 1C3 are present in adult kidney, stomach and thyroid. Human SULT1E4 has been identified has a high affinity estrogen sulfotransferase. SULT1A3 also catalyzes the sulfation of estrogen, such as 17β-estradiol, but it does so with a much lower affinity than

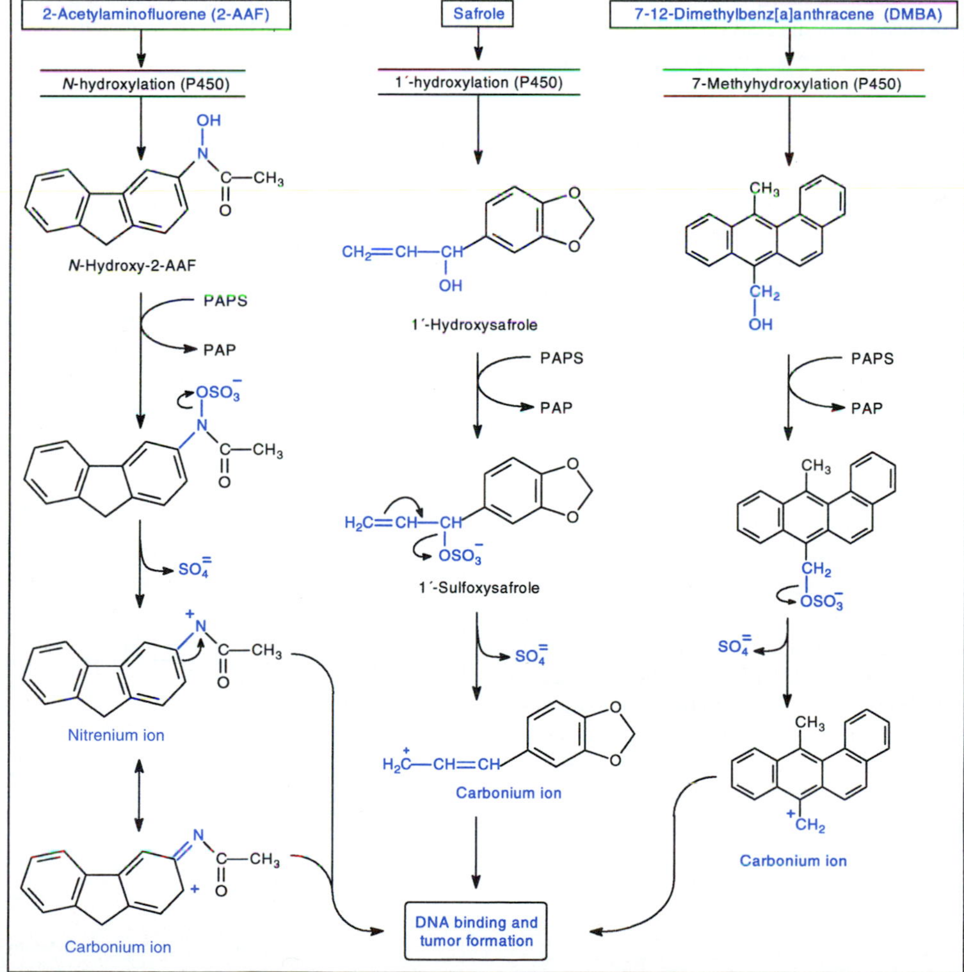

Figure 6-50. Role of sulfation in the generation of tumorigenic metabolites (nitrenium or carbonium ions) of 2-acetylaminofluorene, safrole, and 7,12-dimethylbenz[a]anthracene (DMBA).

does SULT1E4. The sulfation of 17α-ethinylestradiol in human hepatocytes is inducible by rifampin (Li et al., 1999), which raises the possibility that SULT1E4 is an inducible enzyme. In addition to human liver, SULT1E4 is expressed in placenta, breast, and uterine tissue.

SULT2A3 is the human alcohol sulfotransferase long known as DHEA-ST (for its ability to sulfate dehydroepiandrosterone). In addition to DHEA, substrates for SULT2A3 include steroid hormones, bile acids and cholesterol. Furthermore, SULT2A3 converts several procarcinogens to electrophilic metabolites, including hydroxymethyl polycyclic aromatic hydrocarbons, *N*-hydroxy-2-acetylaminofluorene and 1′-hydoxysafrole, as shown in Fig. 6-50. The thermal stability of SULT2A3 is intermediate between that of the two phenol sulfotransferases (TS-PST and TL-PST), and the enzyme is resistant to the inhibitory effects of 2,6-dichloro-4-nitrophenol. SULT2A3 is not expressed in blood platelets, but the activity of this enzyme has been measured in human liver cytosol. SULT2A3 is bimodally distributed, possibly due to a genetic polymorphism, with a high activity group composed of ~25 percent of the population. Several genetic polymorphisms of the SULT2A3 have been identified, but the underlying basis for the high activity group remains to be determined.

Human SULT2B1 is also a DHEA-sulfotransferase. It is expressed in placenta, prostate, and trachea. The SULT2B1 gene can be transcribed from one of two exons, both of which contain coding sequences, hence, two forms of SULT2B1 (known as 2B1a and 2B1b) with different *N*-terminal amino acid sequences can be transcribed by alternate splicing of a single gene. This situation is analogous to the alternative splicing of multiple exons 1 in the UGT1 gene family (see Fig. 6-48).

In general, sulfation is an effective means of decreasing the pharmacologic and toxicologic activity of xenobiotics. There are cases, however, in which sulfation increases the toxicity of foreign chemicals because certain sulfate conjugates are chemically unstable and degrade to form potent electrophilic species. As shown in Fig. 6-50, sulfation plays an important role in the activation of aromatic amines, methyl-substituted polycyclic aromatic hydrocarbons, and safrole to tumorigenic metabolites. To exert its tumorigenic effect in rodents, safrole must be hydroxylated by cytochrome P450 to 1′-hydroxysafrole, which is then sulfated to the electrophilic and tumor-initiating metabolite, 1′-sulfooxysafrole (Boberg et al., 1983). 1′-Hydroxysafrole is a more potent hepatotumorigen than safrole. Two lines of evidence support a major role for sulfation in the hepatotumorigenic effect of 1′-hydroxysafrole. First, the hepatotumorigenic effect of 1′-hydroxysafrole can be inhibited by treating mice with the sulfotransferase inhibitor, pentachlorophenol. Second, the hepatotumorigenic effect of 1′-hydroxysafrole is markedly reduced in brachymorphic mice, which have a diminished capacity to sulfate xenobiotics because of a genetic defect in PAPS synthesis. Brachymorphic mice are undersized because the defect in PAPS synthesis prevents the normal sulfation of glycosaminoglycans and proteoglycans such as heparin and chondroitin, which are important components of cartilage. These particular sulfation reactions are catalyzed by membrane-bound sulfotransferase, which are thought not to play a role in xenobiotic sulfation.

Methylation

Methylation is a common but generally minor pathway of xenobiotic biotransformation. Methylation differs from most other phase II reactions because it generally decreases the water-solubility of xenobiotics and masks functional groups that might otherwise be conjugated by other phase II enzymes. One exception to this rule is the *N*-methylation of pyridine-containing xenobiotics, such as nicotine, which produces quaternary ammonium ions that are water-soluble and readily excreted. Another exception is the *S*-methylation of thioethers to form positively charged sulfonium ions, a reaction catalyzed by thioether methyltransferase (TEMT), which has only been identified in mice (Weinshilboum et al., 1999). The cofactor for methylation is *S*-adenosylmethionine (SAM), the structure of which is shown in Fig. 6-45. The methyl group bound to the sulfonium ion in SAM has the characteristics of a carbonium ion and is transferred to xenobiotics and endogenous substrates by nucleophilic attack from an electron-rich heteroatom (*O*, *N*, or *S*). Consequently, the functional groups involved in methylation reactions are phenols, catechols, aliphatic and aromatic amines, *N*-heterocyclics, and sulfhydryl-containing compounds. The conversion of benzo[a]pyrene to 6-methylbenzo[a]pyrene is a rare example of *C*-methylation. Another reaction that appears to involve *C*-methylation, the conversion of cocaine to ethylcocaine, is actually a transesterification reaction, as shown in Fig. 6-2. Metals can also be methylated. Inorganic mercury and arsenic can both be dimethylated, and inorganic selenium can be trimethylated. The selenium atom in ebselen is methylated following the ring opening of this anti-inflammatory drug. Some examples of xenobiotics and endogenous substrates that undergo *O*-, *N*-, or *S*-methylation are shown in Fig. 6-51. During these

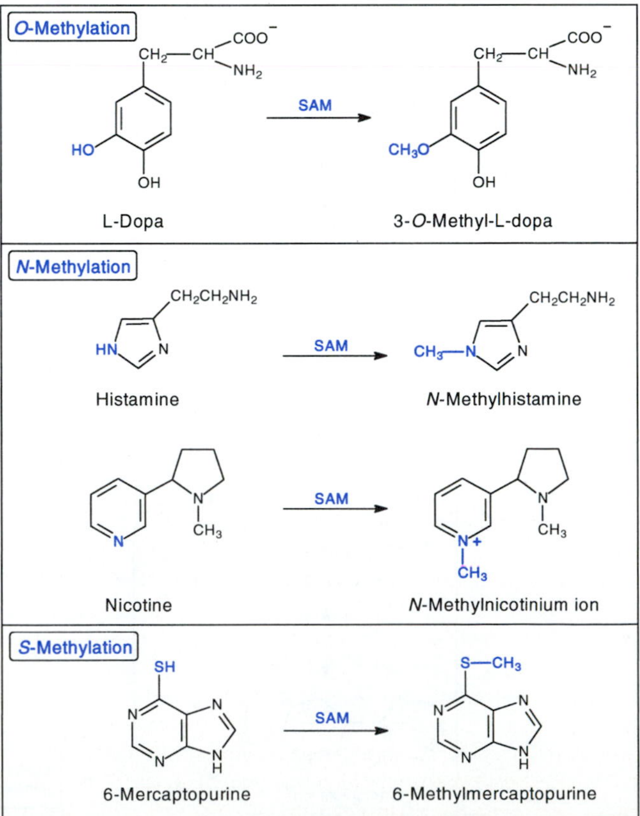

Figure 6-51. Examples of compounds that undergo O-, N-, *or* S-*methylation.*

methylation reactions, SAM is converted to *S*-adenosylhomocysteine.

The *O*-methylation of phenols and catechols is catalyzed by two different enzymes known as phenol *O*-methyltransferase (POMT) and catechol-*O*-methyltransferase (COMT) (Weinshilboum, 1989, 1992b). POMT is a microsomal enzyme that methylates phenols but not catechols, and COMT is both a cytosolic and microsomal enzyme with the converse substrate specificity. COMT plays a greater role in the biotransformation of catechols than POMT plays in the biotransformation of phenols. COMT was originally described as a cytosolic, Mg^{2+}-requiring, monomeric enzyme (Mr 25,000). However, in rats and humans, COMT is encoded by a single gene with two different transcription initiation sites. Transcription at one site produces a cytosolic form of COMT, whereas transcription from the other site produces a membrane-bound form by adding a 50–amino acid segment that targets COMT to the endoplasmic reticulum (Weinshilboum et al., 1999). The cytosolic form of COMT is present in virtually all tissues, including erythrocytes, but the highest concentrations are found in liver and kidney. The membrane-bound form is more highly expressed in brain.

Substrates for COMT include several catecholamine neurotransmitters, such as epinephrine, norepinephrine, and dopamine, and catechol drugs, such as the anti-Parkinson's disease agent L-dopa (3,4-dihydroxyphenylalanine) and the antihypertensive drug methyldopa (α-methyl-3,4-dihydroxyphenylalanine). Catechol estrogens, which are formed by 2- or 4-hydroxylation of the steroid A-ring, are substrates for COMT, as are drugs that are converted to catechols either by two consecutive hydroxylation reactions (as in the case of phenobarbital and diclofenac), by ring opening of a methylenedioxy group (as in the case of stiripentol and 3,4-methylenedioxymethamphetamine), or by hydrolysis of vicinal esters (as in the case of ibopamine). Formation of catechol estrogens, particularly 4-hydroxyestradiol, has been suggested to play an important role in estrogen-induced tumor formation in hamster kidney, rat pituitary, and mouse uterus (Zhu and Liehr, 1993). These tissues contain high levels of epinephrine or dopamine, which inhibit the *O*-methylation of 4-hydroxyestradiol by COMT. Nontarget tissues do not contain high levels of catecholamines, which suggests that 4-hydroxyestradiol induces tumor formation in those tissues that fail to methylate and detoxify this catechol estrogen. These observations in animals are especially intriguing in view of subsequent clinical evidence that low COMT activity appears to be a risk modifier for breast cancer (Weinshilboum et al., 1999).

In humans, COMT is encoded by a single gene with alleles for a low activity form ($COMT^L$) and high activity form ($COMT^H$) (Weinshilboum, 1989, 1992b; Weinshilboum at al., 1999). This polymorphism results from a single G $\rightarrow$ A transition that results in an amino acid substitution (Val $\rightarrow$ Thr) at position 108 in cytosolic COMT and position 158 in microsomal COMT (Weinshilboum et al., 1999). The presence of methionine at position 108 in the cytosolic enzyme not only decreases the catalytic activity of COMT, but it decreases the thermal stability of the enzyme, which has long been used to differentiate $COMT^L$ (thermolabile) from $COMT^H$ (thermostable). In Caucasians, these allelic variants are expressed with equal frequency, so that 25 percent of the population is homozygous for either the low or high activity enzyme, and 50 percent is heterozygous and have intermediate COMT activity. COMT activity is generally higher in Asians and African Americans due to a higher frequency of the $COMT^H$ allele ($\sim$0.75 for Asians and African Americans vs. $\sim$0.5 for Caucasians) (McLeod et al., 1994). The genetically determined levels of COMT in erythrocytes correlates with individual differences in the proportion of L-dopa converted to 3-*O*-methyldopa and the proportion of methyldopa converted to its 3-*O*-methyl metabolite. *O*-Methylation is normally a minor pathway of L-dopa biotransformation, but 3-*O*-methyldopa is the major metabolite when L-dopa is administered with a dopa decarboxylase inhibitor, such as carbidopa or benserazide, which is common clinical practice. High COMT activity, resulting in extensive *O*-methylation of L-dopa to 3-*O*-methyldopa, has been associated with poor therapeutic management of Parkinson's disease and an increased incidence of drug-induced toxicity (dyskinesia). However, there is no evidence that the genetic polymorphism in COMT represents a risk modifier for the development of Parkinson's disease or related disorders, such as schizophrenia (Weinshilboum et al., 1999).

Several *N*-methyltransferases have been described in humans and other mammals, including phenylethanolamine *N*-methyltransferase (PNMT), which catalyzes the *N*-methylation of the neurotransmitter norepinephrine to form epinephrine; histamine *N*-methyltransferase (HNMT), which specifically methylates the imidazole ring of histamine and closely related compounds (Fig. 6-51), and nicotinamide *N*-methyltransferase (NNMT), which methylates compounds containing a pyridine ring, such as nicotinamide and nicotine, or an indole ring, such as tryptophan and serotonin (Weinshilboum, 1989, 1992b; Weinshilboum et al., 1999). PNMT is expressed in the adrenal medulla and in certain regions of the brain, and is not thought to play a significant role in the biotransformation of xenobiotics. However, HNMT and NNMT are expressed in liver, intestine and/or kidney, where they play a role in xenobiotic biotransformation.

Histamine *N*-methyltransferase is a cytosolic enzyme (Mr 33,000). Its activity (which can be measured in erythrocytes) varies sixfold among individuals due to a genetic polymorphism (C $\rightarrow$ T) that results in a point mutation at amino acid residue 105 (Thr $\rightarrow$ Ile). The latter allele (Ile_{105}) is quite common (10 percent frequency) and encodes a variant of HNMT with decreased catalytic activity and thermal stability.

Nicotinamide *N*-methyltransferase activity in human liver, like HNMT activity in erythrocytes, varies considerably from one individual to the next, but it is not known to what extent genetic polymorphisms account for this variation. NNMT is a monomeric, cytosolic enzyme (Mr $\sim$30,000) that appears to a member of a family of methyltransferases that includes PNMT and TEMT (the thioether *S*-methyltransferase present in mouse lung). NNMT catalyzes the *N*-methylation of nicotinamide and structurally related pyridine compounds (including pyridine itself) to form positively charged pyridinium ions. Nicotinic acid (niacin), a commonly used lipid-lowering agent, is converted nicotinamide in vivo, which is then methylated by NNMT (or it is incorporated into nicotinamide adenine dinucleotide, NAD). In contrast to many other methyltransferases, NNMT is not expressed in erythrocytes.

The system that is used to classify human *N*-methyltransferases may not be appropriate for other species. In guinea pigs, for example, nicotine and histamine are both methylated by a common *N*-methyltransferase. Guinea pigs have an unusually high capacity to methylate histamine and xenobiotics. The major route of nicotine biotransformation in the guinea pig is methylation, although *R*-(+)-nicotine is preferentially methylated over its *S*-(−)-enantiomer (Cundy et al., 1985). Guinea pigs also methylate the imidazole ring of cimetidine.

S-Methylation is an important pathway in the biotransformation of sulfhydryl-containing xenobiotics, such as the antihypertensive drug captopril, the antirheumatic agent D-penicillamine, the antineoplastic and immunosuppressive drugs 6-mercaptopurine, 6-thioguanine and azathioprine, metabolites of the alcohol deterrent disulfiram, and the deacetylated metabolite of the antidiuretic, spironolactone. In humans, *S*-methylation is catalyzed by two enzymes, thiopurine methyltransferase (TPMT) and thiol methyltransferase (TMT). A third enzyme, thioether *S*-methyltransferase (TEMT) has been identified in mice (Weinshilboum et al., 1999).

TPMT is a cytoplasmic enzyme that preferentially methylates aromatic and heterocyclic compounds such as the thiopurine drugs 6-mercaptopurine, 6-thioguanine and azathioprine. TMT is a microsomal enzyme that preferentially methylates aliphatic sulfhydryl compounds such as captopril, D-penicillamine, and disulfiram derivatives. Both enzymes are present in erythrocytes at levels that reflect the expression of TPMT and TMT in liver and other tissues. Although TPMT and TMT are independently regulated, their expression in erythrocytes is largely determined by genetic factors. TPMT is encoded by a single gene with alleles for a low activity form ($TPMT^L$) and for a high activity form ($TPMT^H$). The gene frequency of $TPMT^L$ and $TPMT^H$ are 6 and 94 percent, respectively, which produces a trimodal distribution of TPMT activity with low, intermediate and high activity expressed in 0.3, 11.1, and 88.6 percent of the population, respectively. At least eight separate genetic polymorphisms are associated with low TPMT activity. In Caucasians, the allele that is most commonly associated with the $TPMT^L$ phenotype is TPMT*3, which differs from the wild-type enzyme (TPMT*1) at both residue 154 (Ala → Thr) and 240 (Tyr → Cys) (Weinshilboum et al., 1999).

Cancer patients with low TPMT activity are at increased risk for thiopurine-induced myelotoxicity, in contrast to the potential need for higher-than-normal doses to achieve therapeutic levels of thiopurines in patients with TPMT high activity (Weinshilboum, 1989, 1992b). The thiopurine drugs metabolized by TPMT have a relatively narrow therapeutic index, and are used to treat life-threatening illnesses such as acute lymphoblastic leukemia or organ-transplant patients. Phenotyping for the TPMT genetic polymorphism represents one of the first examples in which testing for a genetic variant has entered standard clinical practice (Weinshilboum et al., 1999).

TPMT can be inhibited by benzoic acid derivatives, which also complicates therapy with drugs that metabolized by TPMT. Patients with inflammatory bowel disorders such as Crohn's disease are often treated with thiopurine drugs, which are metabolized by TPMT, and with sulfasalazine or olsalazine, which are potent TPMT inhibitors. The combination of these drugs can lead to thiopurine-induced myelosuppression.

A genetic polymorphism for TMT also has been described, but its pharmacologic and toxicologic significance remain to be determined. The molecular basis for the polymorphism has not been determined, but studies have shown that 98 percent of the fivefold individual variation in erythrocyte TMT activity is due to inheritance, with an allele for high TMT activity having a frequency of 0.12. TMT is relatively specific for aliphatic sulfhydryl compounds such as 2-mercatoethanol, captopril, D-penicillamine and *N*-acetylcysteine. TMT is present in liver microsomes and erythrocyte membranes. TMT is not inhibited by benzoic acid derivatives, but it is inhibited by the cytochrome P450 inhibitor SKF 525A (Weinshilboum et al., 1999). The hydrogen sulfide produced by anaerobic bacteria in the intestinal tract is converted by *S*-methyltransferases to methane thiol and then to dimethylsulfide. Another source of substrates for *S*-methyltransferase are the thioethers of glutathione conjugates. Glutathione conjugates are hydrolyzed to cysteine conjugates, which can either be acetylated to form mercapturic acids or cleaved by beta lyase. This beta lyase pathway converts the cysteine conjugate to pyruvate, ammonia and a sulfhydryl-containing xenobiotic, which is a potential substrate for *S*-methylation.

Acetylation

N-Acetylation is a major route of biotransformation for xenobiotics containing an aromatic amine ($R{-}NH_2$) or a hydrazine group ($R{-}NH{-}NH_2$), which are converted to aromatic amides ($R{-}NH{-}COCH_3$) and hydrazides ($R{-}NH{-}NH{-}COCH_3$), respectively (Evans, 1992). Xenobiotics containing primary aliphatic amines are rarely substrates for *N*-acetylation, a notable exception being cysteine conjugates, which are formed from glutathione conjugates and converted to mercapturic acids by *N*-acetylation in the kidney (see "Glutathione Conjugation," below). Like methylation, *N*-acetylation masks an amine with a nonionizable group, so that many *N*-acetylated metabolites are less water soluble than the parent compound. Nevertheless, *N*-acetylation of certain xenobiotics, such as isoniazid, facilitates their urinary excretion.

The *N*-acetylation of xenobiotics is catalyzed by *N*-acetyltransferases and requires the cofactor acetyl-coenzyme A (acetyl-CoA), the structure of which is shown in Fig. 6-45. The reaction occurs in two sequential steps according to a *ping-pong Bi-Bi* mechanism (Hein, 1988). In the first step, the acetyl group from acetyl-CoA is transferred to an active site cysteine residue within an *N*-acetyltransferase with release of coenzyme A ($E{-}SH + CoA{-}S{-}COCH_3 \rightarrow E{-}S{-}COCH_3 + CoA{-}SH$). In the second step, the acetyl group is transferred from the acylated enzyme to the amino group of the substrate with regeneration of the enzyme. For strongly basic amines, the rate of *N*-acetylation is determined by the first step (acetylation of the enzyme), whereas the rate of *N*-acetylation of weakly basic amines is determined by the second step (transfer of the acetyl group from the acylated enzyme to the acceptor amine). In certain cases (discussed below), *N*-acetyltransferases can catalyze the *O*-acetylation of xenobiotics.

N-Acetyltransferases are cytosolic enzymes found in liver and many other tissues of most mammalian species, with the notable exception of the dog and fox, which are unable to acetylate xenobiotics. In contrast to other xenobiotic-biotransforming enzymes, the number of *N*-acetyltransferases is limited (Vatsis et al., 1995). Humans, rabbits, and hamsters express only two *N*-acetyltransferases, known as NAT1 and NAT2, whereas mice express three distinct forms of the enzymes, namely NAT1, NAT2, and NAT3. *NAT* is the official gene symbol for arylamine *N*-acetyltransferase [EC 2.3.1.5], which reflects the fact that aromatic amines, not aliphatic amines, are the preferred substrates for these enzymes. Individual *N*-acetyltransferases and their allelic variants have been named in the order of their description in the literature, which makes for a somewhat confusing nomenclature system (Vatsis et al., 1995). For example, in humans, the wild-type *NAT1* gene is designated *NAT1*4* (note the use of italics). Although *NAT1*3* is also a human gene (an allelic variant), *NAT1*1* and *NAT1*2* are rabbit genes. Similarly, *NAT2*4* is the human wild-type *NAT2* gene, whereas *NAT2*1* is a chicken gene, *NAT2*2* is a rabbit gene, and *NAT2*3* is a rabbit variant (a deleted gene). The official website for maintaining and updating NAT nomenclature is http://www.louisville.edu/medschool/pharmacology/NAT.html.

In each species examined, NAT1 and NAT2 are closely related proteins (79 to 95 percent identical in amino acid sequence) with an active site cysteine residue (Cys_{68}) in the *N*-terminal region (Grant et al., 1992; Vatsis et al., 1995). Although they are encoded by intronless genes on the same chromosome, NAT1 and NAT2 are independently regulated proteins: NAT1 is expressed in most tissues of the body—including liver, urinary bladder, colon, mammary gland, lung, kidney, small intestine and pineal gland—whereas NAT2 is mainly expressed in liver and intestine. However, most (but not all) of the tissues that express NAT1 also appear to express low levels of NAT2, at least at the level of mRNA (Rychter et al., 1999).

NAT1 and NAT2 also have different but overlapping substrate specificities, although no substrate is exclusively *N*-acetylated by one enzyme or the other. Substrates preferentially *N*-acetylated by human NAT1 include *para*-aminobenzoic acid (PABA), *para*-aminosalicylic acid, sulfamethoxazole, and sulfanilamide, while substrates preferentially *N*-acetylated by human NAT2 include isoniazid, hydralazine, procainamide, dapsone, aminoglutethimide, and sulfamethazine. Some xenobiotics, such as the carcinogenic aromatic amine, 2-aminofluorene, are *N*-acetylated equally well by NAT1 and NAT2.

Several drugs are *N*-acetylated following their biotransformation by phase I enzymes. For example, caffeine is *N3*-demethylated by CYP1A2 to paraxanthine (Fig. 6-40), which is then *N*-demethylated to 1-methylxanthine and *N*-acetylated to 5-acetylamino-6-formylamino-3-methyluracil (AFMU) by NAT2. Other drugs converted to metabolites that are *N*-acetylated by NAT2 include sulfasalazine, nitrazepam, and clonazepam. Examples of drugs that are *N*-acetylated by NAT1 and NAT2 are shown in Fig. 6-52. It should be noted, however, that there are species differences in the substrate specificity of *N*-acetyltransferases. For example, *para*-aminobenzoic acid is preferentially *N*-acetylated by NAT1 in humans and rabbits but by NAT2 in mice and hamsters.

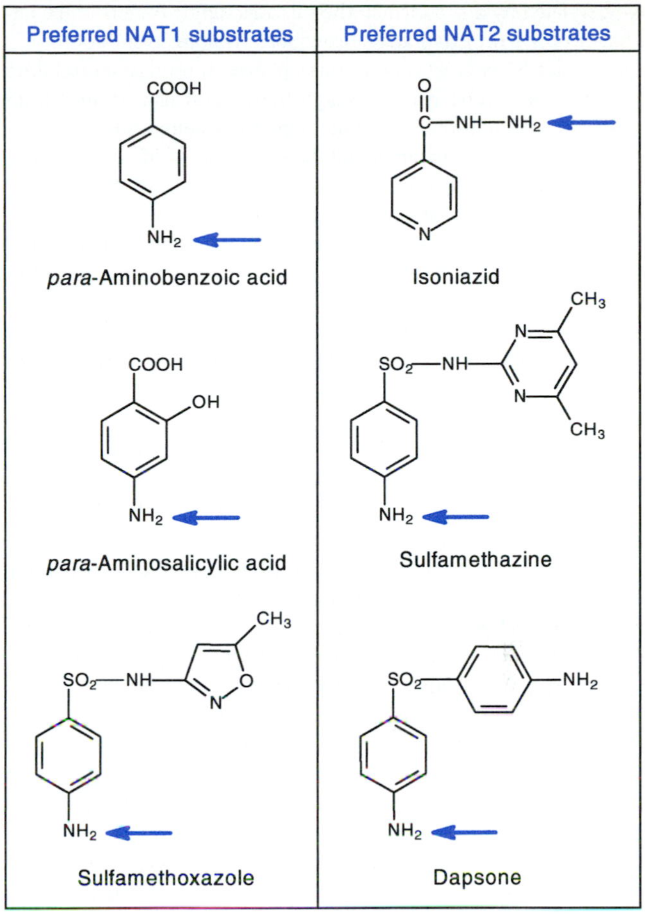

Preferred NAT1 substrates	Preferred NAT2 substrates
para-Aminobenzoic acid	Isoniazid
para-Aminosalicylic acid	Sulfamethazine
Sulfamethoxazole	Dapsone

Figure 6-52. Examples of substrates for the human N*-acetyltransferases, NAT1, and the highly polymorphic NAT2.*

Genetic polymorphisms for *N*-acetylation have been documented in humans, hamsters, rabbits, and mice (Evans, 1992; Grant et al., 1992; Vatsis et al., 1995; Hivonen, 1999; Heim et al., 2000). A series of clinical observations in the 1950s established the existence of *slow* and *fast acetylators* of the antitubercular drug isoniazid. The incidence of the slow acetylator phenotype is high in Middle Eastern populations (e.g., ~70 percent in Egyptians, Saudi Arabians, and Moroccans), intermediate in Caucasian populations (~50 percent in Americans, Australians, and Europeans), and low in Asian populations (e.g., <25 percent of Chinese, Japanese, and Koreans).

The slow acetylator phenotype is caused by various mutations in the *NAT2* gene that either decrease NAT2 activity or enzyme stability (at least 26 allelic variants of human *NAT2* have been documented). For example, a point mutation ($T \rightarrow C$) in nucleotide 341 (which causes the amino acid substitution $Ile_{114} \rightarrow Thr_{114}$) decreases V_{max} for *N*-acetylation without altering the K_m for substrate binding or the stability of the enzyme. This mutation (which is the basis for the *NAT2*5* allele) is the most common cause of the slow acetylator phenotype in Caucasians but is rarely observed in Asians. (Note: There are six known *NAT2*5* alleles, designated *NAT2*5A* through *NAT*5F.* The allele containing just the $Ile_{114} \rightarrow Thr_{114}$ substitution is *NAT2**5D. The others contain this and at least one other nucleotide and/or amino acid substitution.) The *NAT2*7* allele is more prevalent in Asians than Caucasians, and involves a point mutation ($G \rightarrow A$) in nucleotide 857 (which causes the amino acid substitution $Gly_{286} \rightarrow Glu_{286}$), which decreases the stability, rather than the activity, of NAT2. Within the slow NAT2 acetylator phenotype there is considerable variation in rates of xenobiotic *N*-acetylation. This is because different mutations in the *NAT2* gene have different effects on NAT2 activity and/or enzyme stability, and because the *N*-acetylation of "NAT2-substrates" by NAT1 becomes significant in slow acetylators.

NAT1 and NAT2 used to be referred to as *monomorphic* and *polymorphic N*-acetyltransferases because only the latter enzyme was thought to be genetically polymorphic. However, at least 22 allelic variants have now been documented for the human NAT1 gene (almost as many as for the NAT2 gene), although these variants are less prevalent than the NAT2 allelic variants, hence, there is less genetically determined variation in the metabolism of "NAT1 substrates." Nevertheless, there is evidence that phenotypic differences in the *N*-acetylation of *para*-aminosalicylic acid are distributed bimodally, consistent with the existence of low and high activity forms of NAT1. Furthermore, an extremely slow acetylator of *para*-aminosalicylic acid has been identified with mutations in both *NAT1* alleles; one that decreases NAT1 activity and stability and one that encodes a truncated and catalytically inactive form of the enzyme. The incidence and pharmacologic/toxicologic significance of genetic polymorphisms in *NAT1* that produce phenotypically discernible alterations in NAT1 activity remain to be determined.

Genetic polymorphisms in *NAT2* have a number of pharmacologic and toxicologic consequences for drugs that are

N-acetylated by this enzyme. The pharmacologic effects of the antihypertensive drug hydralazine are more pronounced in slow NAT2 acetylators. Slow NAT2 acetylators are predisposed to several drug toxicities, including nerve damage (peripheral neuropathy) from isoniazid and dapsone, systemic lupus erythematosus from hydralazine and procainamide, and the toxic effects of coadministration of the anticonvulsant phenytoin with isoniazid. Slow NAT2 acetylators that are deficient in glucose-6-phosphate dehydrogenase are particularly prone to hemolysis from certain sulfonamides. HIV-infected individuals of the slow acetylator phenotype suffer more often from adverse drug events and, among patients with Stevens-Johnson syndrome, the overwhelming majority are slow acetylators. Fast NAT2 acetylators are predisposed to the myelotoxic effects of amonafide because *N*-acetylation retards the clearance of this antineoplastic drug.

Some epidemiologic studies suggest that rapid NAT2 acetylators are at increased risk for the development of isoniazid-induced liver toxicity, although several other studies contradict these findings and provide convincing evidence that slow NAT2 acetylation is a risk modifier for isoniazid-induced hepatotoxicity. Following its acetylation by NAT2, isoniazid can be hydrolyzed to isonicotinic acid and acetylhydrazine ($CH_3CO-NHNH_2$). This latter metabolite can be *N*-hydroxylated by FMO or cytochrome P450 to a reactive intermediate, as shown in Fig. 6-33*A*. The generation of a reactive metabolite from acetylhydrazine would seem to provide a mechanistic basis for enhanced isoniazid hepatotoxicity in fast acetylators. However, acetylhydrazine can be further acetylated to diacetlyhydrazine ($CH_3CO-NHNH-COCH_3$), and this detoxication reaction is also catalyzed by NAT2. Therefore, acetylhydrazine is both produced and detoxified by NAT2, hence slow acetylation, not fast acetylation, becomes the risk modifier for isoniazid-induced hepatotoxicity, just as it is for isoniazid-induced peripheral neuropathy. Rifampin and alcohol have been reported to enhance the hepatotoxicity of isoniazid. These drug interactions are probably the result of increased *N*-hydroxylation of acetylhydrazine due to cytochrome-P450 induction rather than to an alteration in NAT2 activity.

Isoniazid is an anti-tubercular drug, and its inactivation by NAT2 is interesting from the perspective that several organisms, including *Mycobacterium tuberculosis,* express a NAT2-like enzyme, which has implications for isoniazid-resistance in tuberculosis.

Aromatic amines can be both activated and deactivated by *N*-acetyltransferases (Kato and Yamazoe, 1994b; Hirvonen, 1999; Hein et al., 2000). The *N*-acetyltransferases detoxify aromatic amines by converting them to the corresponding amides because aromatic amides are less likely than aromatic amines to be activated to DNA-reactive metabolites by cytochrome P450, PHS, and UDP-glucuronosyltransferase. However, *N*-acetyltransferases can activate aromatic amines if they are first *N*-hydroxylated by cytochrome P450 because *N*-acetyltransferases can also function as *O*-acetyltransferases and convert *N*-hydroxyaromatic amines (hydroxylamines) to acetoxy esters. As shown in Fig. 6-9, the acetoxy esters of *N*-hydroxyaromatic amines, like the corresponding sulfate esters (Fig. 6-50), can break down to form highly reactive nitrenium and carbonium ions that bind to DNA. *N*-Acetyltransferases catalyze the *O*-acetylation of *N*-hydroxyaromatic amines by two distinct mechanisms. The first reaction, which is exemplified by the conversion of *N*-hydroxyaminofluorene to *N*-acetoxyaminofluorene, requires acetyl-CoA and proceeds by the same mechanism previously described for *N*-acetylation. The second reaction is exemplified by the conversion of 2-acetylaminofluorene to *N*-acetoxyaminofluorene, which does not require acetyl-CoA but involves an intramolecular transfer of the *N*-acetyl group from nitrogen to oxygen. These reactions are shown in Fig. 6-53.

Genetic polymorphisms in *NAT2* have been reported to influence susceptibility to aromatic amine-induced bladder and colon cancer (Evans, 1992; Kadlubar, 1994; Hirvonen, 1999; Hein et al., 2000). Bladder cancer is thought to be caused by bicyclic aromatic amines (benzidine, 2-aminonaphthalene, and 4-aminobiphenyl), whereas colon cancer is thought to be caused by heterocyclic aromatic amines, such as the products of amino acid pyrolysis (e.g., 2-amino-6-methylimidazo[4,5-*b*]pyridine or PhIP, and others listed in Table 6-6). Epidemiologic studies suggest that slow NAT2 acetylators are more likely than fast NAT2 acetylators to develop bladder cancer from cigarette smoking and from occupational exposure to bicyclic aromatic amines. The possibility that slow NAT2 acetylators are at increased risk for aromatic amine-induced cancer is supported by the finding that dogs, which are poor acetylators, are highly prone to aromatic amine-induced bladder cancer. By comparison, fast NAT2 acetylators appear to be at increased risk for colon cancer from heterocyclic aromatic amines.

The influence of acetylator phenotype on susceptibility to aromatic amine-induced cancer can be rationalized on the ability of *N*-acetyltransferases to activate and detoxify aromatic amines and by differences in the substrate specificity and tissues distribution of NAT1 and NAT2 (recall that NAT1 is expressed in virtually all

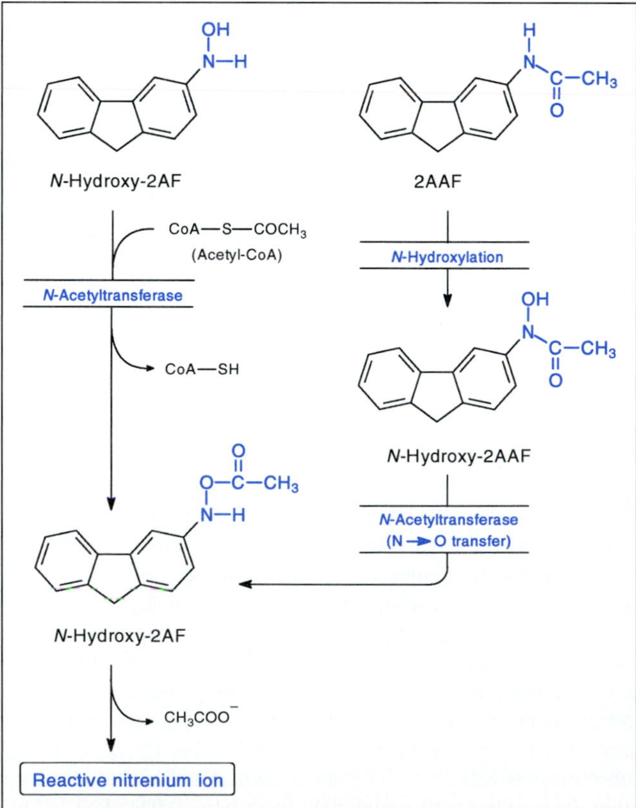

Figure 6-53. Role of N-acetyltransferase in the O-acetylation of N-hydroxy-2-aminofluorene (N-hydroxy-2AF) and the intramolecular rearrangement of N-hydroxy-2-acetylaminofluorene (N-hydroxy-2-AAF).

tissues, whereas NAT2 is expressed mainly in the liver and intestinal tract). Both NAT1 and NAT2 catalyze the *O*-acetylation (activation) of *N*-hydroxy bicyclic aromatic amines, whereas the *O*-acetylation of *N*-hydroxy heterocyclic aromatic amines is preferentially catalyzed by NAT2. Bicyclic aromatic amines can also be *N*-acetylated (detoxified) by NAT1 and NAT2, but heterocyclic aromatic amines are poor substrates for both enzymes. Therefore, the fast acetylator phenotype protects against aromatic amine-induced bladder cancer because NAT2 (as well as NAT1) catalyzes the *N*-acetylation (detoxication) of bicyclic aromatic amines in the liver. In slow acetylators, a greater proportion of the bicyclic aromatic amines are activated through *N*-hydroxylation by CYP1A2. These *N*-hydroxylated aromatic amines can be activated by *O*-acetylation, which can be catalyzed in the bladder itself by NAT1. Recent evidence suggests that a high level of NAT1 in the bladder is a risk modifier for aromatic amine-induced bladder cancer. In addition, the fast acetylator phenotype potentiates the colon cancer-inducing effects of heterocyclic aromatic amines. These aromatic amines are poor substrates for NAT1 and NAT2, so that high levels of NAT2 in the liver do little to prevent their *N*-hydroxylation by CYP1A2. The *N*-hydroxylated metabolites of heterocyclic aromatic amines can be activated by *O*-acetylation, which can be catalyzed in the colon itself by NAT2. The presence of NAT2 (and NAT1) in the colons of fast acetylators probably explains why this phenotype is a risk modifier for the development of colon cancer.

Whether fast acetylators are protected from or predisposed to the cancer-causing effects of aromatic amines depends on the nature of the aromatic amine (bicyclic vs. heterocyclic) and on other important risk modifiers. For example, CYP1A2 plays an important role in the *N*-hydroxylation of both bicyclic and heterocyclic amines, and high CYP1A2 activity has been shown to be a risk modifier for aromatic amine-induced bladder and colon cancer. A single nucleotide polymorphism in intron 1 of CYP1A2 is associated with high inducibility, and this allelic variant is a risk modifier for bladder cancer in smokers or in people who are slow NAT2 acetylators (Brockmöller et al., 1998). It remains to be determined whether the activation of aromatic amines by *N*-glucuronidation and the activation of *N*-hydroxy aromatic amines by sulfation have a similar impact on the incidence of bladder and colon cancer. These and other risk modifiers may explain why some epidemiologic studies, contrary to expectation, have shown that slow NAT2 acetylators are at increased risk for aromatic amine-induced bladder cancer, as was demonstrated recently for benzidine manufacturers in China (Hayes et al., 1993).

The *N*-acetylation of aromatic amines (a detoxication reaction) and the *O*-acetylation of *N*-hydroxy aromatic amines (an activation reaction) can be reversed by a microsomal enzyme called arylacetamide deacetylase (Probst et al., 1994). This enzyme is similar to but distinct from the microsomal carboxylesterases that hydrolyze esters and amides. Whether arylacetamide deacetylase alters the overall balance between detoxication and activation of aromatic amines remains to be determined.

Overall, it would appear that low NAT2 activity increases the risk of bladder, breast, liver, and lung cancers and decreases the risk of colon cancer, whereas low NAT1 activity increases the risk of bladder and colon cancers and decreases the risk of lung cancer (Hirvonen, 1999). The individual risks associated with particular NAT1 and/or NAT2 acetylator genotypes are small, but they increase when considered in conjunction with other susceptibility genes and/or exposure to carcinogenic aromatic and heterocyclic amines. Because of the relatively high frequency of allelic variants of *NAT1* and *NAT2*, the attributable risk of cancer in the population may be high (Hein et al., 2000).

Amino Acid Conjugation

There are two principal pathways by which xenobiotics are conjugated with amino acids, as illustrated in Fig. 6-54. The first involves conjugation of xenobiotics containing a carboxylic acid group with the amino group of amino acids such as glycine, glutamine, and taurine (see Fig. 6-45). This pathway involves activation of the xenobiotic by conjugation with CoA, which produces an acyl-CoA thioether that reacts with the *amino group* of an amino acid to form an amide linkage. The second pathway involves conjugation of xenobiotics containing an aromatic hydroxylamine (*N*-hydroxy aromatic amine) with the *carboxylic acid group* of such amino acids as serine and proline. This pathway involves activation of an amino acid by aminoacyl-tRNA-synthetase, which reacts with an aromatic hydroxylamine to form a reactive *N*-ester (Kato and Yamazoe, 1994b).

The conjugation of benzoic acid with glycine to form hippuric acid was discovered in 1842, making it the first biotransformation reaction discovered (Paulson et al., 1985). The first step in this conjugation reaction involves activation of benzoic acid to an acyl-CoA thioester. This reaction requires ATP and is catalyzed by acyl-CoA synthetase (ATP-dependent acid:CoA ligase). The second step is catalyzed by acyl-CoA:amino acid *N*-acyltransferase, which transfers the acyl moiety of the xenobiotic to the amino group of the acceptor amino acid. The reaction proceeds by a *ping-pong Bi-Bi* mechanism, and involves transfer of the xenobiotic to a cysteine residue in the enzyme with release of coenzyme A, followed by transfer of the xenobiotic to the acceptor amino acid with regeneration of the enzyme. The second step in amino acid conjugation is analogous to amide formation during the acetylation of aromatic amines by *N*-acetyltransferase. Substrates for amino acid conjugation are restricted to certain aliphatic, aromatic, heteroaromatic, cinnamic, and arylacetic acids.

The ability of xenobiotics to undergo amino acid conjugation depends on steric hindrance around the carboxylic acid group, and by substituents on the aromatic ring or aliphatic side chain. In rats, ferrets, and monkeys, the major pathway of phenylacetic acid biotransformation is amino acid conjugation. However, due to steric hindrance, diphenylacetic acid cannot be conjugated with an amino acid, so the major pathway of diphenylacetic acid biotransformation in these same three species is acylglucuronidation. Bile acids are endogenous substrates for glycine and taurine conjugation. However, the activation of bile acids to an acyl-CoA thioester is catalyzed by a microsomal enzyme, cholyl-CoA synthetase, and conjugation with glycine or taurine is catalyzed by a single cytosolic enzyme, bile acid-CoA:amino acid *N*-acyltransferase (Falany et al., 1994). In contrast, the activation of xenobiotics occurs mainly in mitochondria, which appear to contain multiple acyl-CoA synthetases. The second step in the conjugation of xenobiotics with amino acid is catalyzed by cytosolic and/or mitochondrial forms of *N*-acyltransferase. Two different types of *N*-acyltransferases have been purified from mammalian hepatic mitochondria. One prefers benzoyl-CoA as substrate, whereas the other prefers arylacetyl-CoA. Another important difference between the amino acid conjugates of xenobiotics and bile acids is their route of elimination: Bile acids are secreted into bile whereas amino acid conjugates of xenobiotics are eliminated primarily in urine. The addition of an endogenous amino acid to xenobiotics

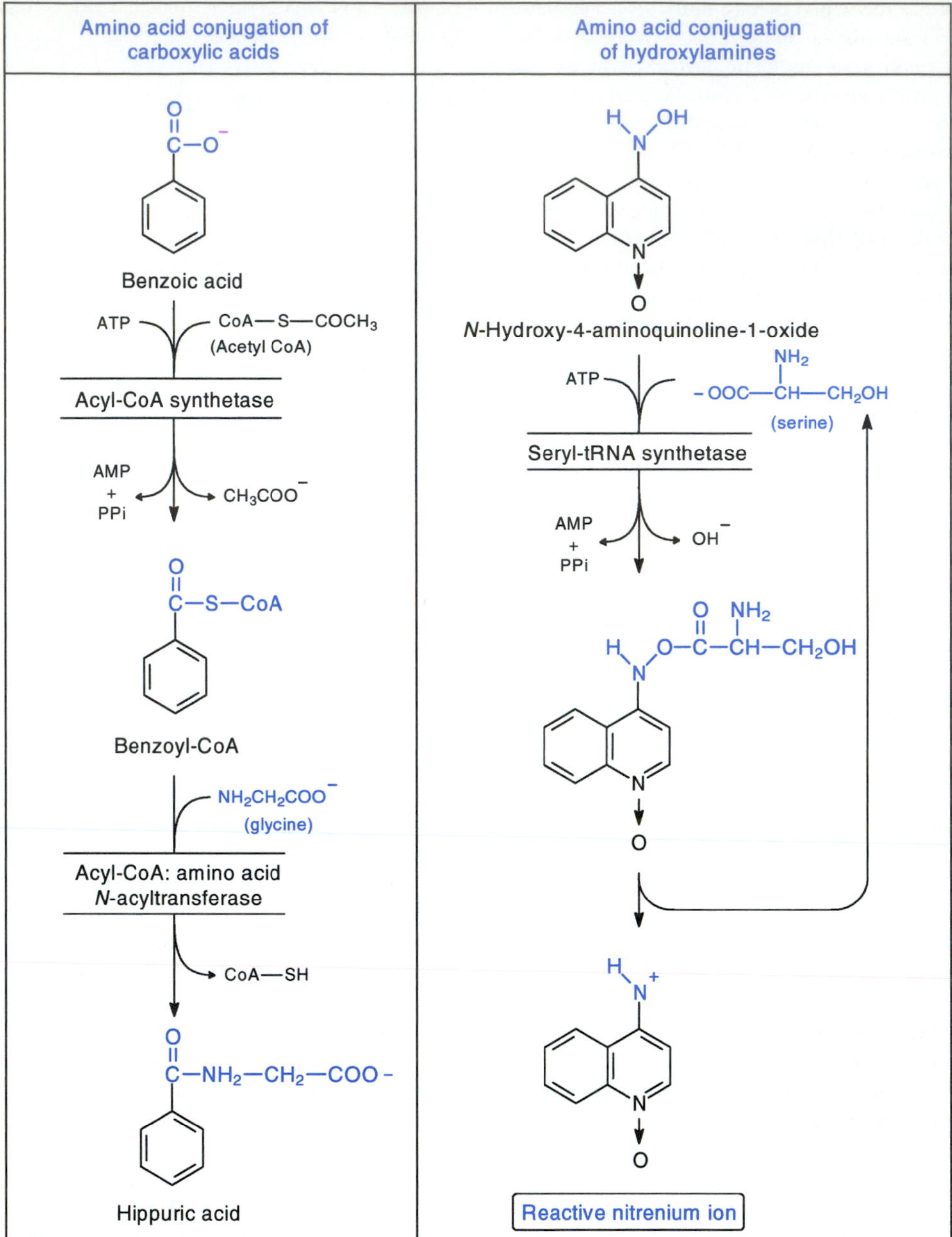

Figure 6-54. Conjugation of xenobiotics with amino acids.

may facilitate this elimination by increasing their ability to interact with the tubular organic anion transport system in the kidney.

In addition to glycine, glutamine, and taurine, acceptor amino acids for xenobiotic conjugation include ornithine, arginine, histidine, serine, aspartic acid, and several dipeptides, such as glycylglycine, glycyltaurine, and glycylvaline. The acceptor amino acid used for conjugation is both species and xenobiotic-dependent. For benzoic, heterocyclic, and cinnamic acids, the acceptor amino acid is glycine, except in birds and reptiles, which use ornithine. Arylacetic acids are also conjugated with glycine except in primates, which use glutamine. In mammals, taurine is generally an alternative acceptor to glycine. Taurine conjugation is well developed in nonmammalian species and carnivores. Whereas most species conjugate bile acids with both glycine and taurine, cats and dogs conjugated bile acids only with taurine. Conjugation of carboxylic acid-containing xenobiotics is an alternative to glucuronidation. Conjugation with amino acids is a detoxication reaction, whereas the glucuronidation of carboxylic acid-containing xenobiotic produces potentially toxic acylglucuronides (see Fig. 6-49). Amino acid conjugation of ibuprofen and related *profens* (2-substituted propionic acid NSAIDs) is significant for two reasons: it limits the formation of potentially toxic acylglucuronides, and it leads to chiral inversion (the interconversion of *R*- and *S*-enantiomers) (Shirley et al., 1994). This latter reaction requires conversion of the profen to its acyl-CoA thioester, which undergoes chiral inversion by 2-arylpropionyl-CoA epimerase (this involves the intermediacy of a symmetrical, conjugated enolate anion). Chiral inversion explains why the *R*- and *S*-enantiomers of several profen NSAIDs have comparable anti-inflammatory effects in vivo, even though the *S*-enantiomers are considerably more potent than their antipodes as inhibitors of cyclooxygenase (the target of NSAID therapy).

In contrast to amino acid conjugation of carboxylic acid-containing xenobiotics, which is a detoxication reaction, amino acid conjugation of *N*-hydroxy aromatic amines (hydroxylamines) is an activation reaction because it produces *N*-esters that can degrade to form electrophilic nitrenium and carbonium ions (Anders, 1985; Kato and Yamazoe, 1994b). Conjugation of hydroxylamines with amino acids is catalyzed by cytosolic aminoacyl-tRNA synthetases and requires ATP (Fig. 6-54). Hydroxylamines activated by aminoacyl-tRNA synthetases include *N*-hydroxy-4-aminoquinoline 1-oxide, which is conjugated with serine, and *N*-hydroxy-Trp-P-2, which is conjugated with proline. [*N*-hydroxy-Trp-P-2 is the *N*-hydroxylated metabolite of Trp-P-2, a pyrolysis product of tryptophan (see Table 6-6)]. It is now apparent that the hydroxylamines formed by the cytochrome P450–dependent *N*-hydroxylation of aromatic amines can potentially be activated by numerous reactions, including *N*-glucuronidation by UDP-glucuronosyltransferase (Fig. 6-49), *O*-acetylation by *N*-acetyltransferase (Fig. 6-9), *O*-sulfation by sulfotransferase (Fig. 6-50), and conjugation with amino acids by seryl- or prolyl-tRNA synthetase (Fig. 6-54).

Glutathione Conjugation

The preceding section described the conjugation of xenobiotics with certain amino acids, including some simple dipeptides, such as glycyltaurine. This section describes the conjugation of xenobiotics with the tripeptide glutathione, which is comprised of glycine, cysteine, and glutamic acid (the latter being linked to cysteine via the γ-carboxyl group, not the usual α-carboxyl group, as shown in Fig. 6-45). Conjugation of xenobiotics with glutathione is fundamentally different from their conjugation with other amino acids and dipeptides (Sies and Ketterer, 1988; Mantle et al., 1987). Substrates for glutathione conjugation include an enormous array of electrophilic xenobiotics, or xenobiotics that can be biotransformed to electrophiles. In contrast to the amides formed by conjugation of xenobiotics to other amino acids, glutathione conjugates are thioethers, which form by nucleophilic attack of glutathione thiolate anion (GS^-) with an electrophilic carbon atom in the xenobiotic. Glutathione can also conjugate xenobiotics containing electrophilic heteroatoms (*O*, *N*, and *S*).

The synthesis of glutathione involves formation of the peptide bond between cysteine and glutamic acid, followed by peptide bond formation with glycine. The first reaction is catalyzed by γ-glutamylcysteine synthetase; the second by glutathione synthetase. At each step, ATP is hydrolyzed to ADP and inorganic phosphate. The first reaction is inhibited by buthionine-*S*-sulfoximine, which can be used in vivo to decrease glutathione levels in experimental animals. The conjugation of xenobiotics with glutathione is catalyzed by a family of glutathione *S*-transferases. These enzymes are present in most tissues, with high concentrations in the liver, intestine, kidney, testis, adrenal, and lung, where they are localized in the cytoplasm (>95 percent) and endoplasmic reticulum (<5 percent).

Substrates for glutathione *S*-transferase share three common features: they are hydrophobic, they contain an electrophilic atom, and they react nonenzymatically with glutathione at some measurable rate. The mechanism by which glutathione *S*-transferase increases the rate of glutathione conjugation involves deprotonation of GSH to GS^- by an active site tyrosinate (Tyr-O^-), which functions as a general base catalyst (Atkins et al., 1993; Dirr et al., 1994). The concentration of glutathione in liver is extremely high (~10 mM); hence, the nonenzymatic conjugation of certain xenobiotics with glutathione can be significant. However, some xenobiotics are conjugated with glutathione stereoselectively, indicating that the reaction is largely catalyzed by glutathione *S*-transferase. Like glutathione, the glutathione *S*-transferases are themselves abundant cellular components, accounting for up to 10 percent of the total cellular protein. These enzymes bind, store, and/or transport a number of compounds that are not substrates for glutathione conjugation. The cytoplasmic protein formerly known as ligandin, which binds heme, bilirubin, steroids, azo-dyes and polycyclic aromatic hydrocarbons, is glutathione *S*-transferase.

As shown in Fig. 6-55, substrates for glutathione conjugation can be divided into two groups: those that are sufficiently electrophilic to be conjugated directly, and those that must first be biotransformed to an electrophilic metabolite prior to conjugation. The second group of substrates for glutathione conjugation includes reactive intermediates produced during phase I or phase II biotransformation, and include oxiranes (arene oxides and alkene epoxides), nitrenium ions, carbonium ions, and free radicals. The conjugation reactions themselves can be divided into two types: *displacement reactions,* in which glutathione displaces an electron-withdrawing group, and *addition reactions,* in which glutathione is added to an activated double bond or strained ring system.

The displacement of an electron-withdrawing group by glutathione typically occurs when the substrate contains halide, sulfate, sulfonate, phosphate, or a nitro group (i.e., good *leaving groups*) attached to an allylic or benzylic carbon atom. Displacement of an electron-withdrawing group from aromatic xenobiotics is decreased by the presence of other substituents that donate electrons to the aromatic ring ($-NH_2$, $-OH$, $-OR$, and $-R$). Conversely, such displacement reactions are increased by the presence of other electron-withdrawing groups ($-F$, $-Cl$, $-Br$, $-I$, $-NO_2$, $-CN$, $-CHO$, and $-COOR$). This explains why 1,2-dichloro-4-nitrobenzene and 1-chloro-2,4-dinitrobenzene, each of which contains three electron-withdrawing groups, are commonly used as substrates for measuring glutathione *S*-transferase activity in vitro. Glutathione *S*-transferase can catalyze the *O*-demethylation of dimethylvinphos and other methylated organophosphorus compounds. The reaction is analogous to the interaction between methyliodide and glutathione, which produces methylglutathione and iodide ion ($GS^- + CH_3I \rightarrow GS{-}CH_3 + I^-$). In this case, iodide is the leaving group. In the case of dimethylvinphos, the entire organophosphate molecule (minus the methyl group) functions as the leaving group.

The addition of glutathione to a carbon–carbon double bond is also facilitated by the presence of a nearby electron-withdrawing group, hence, substrates for this reaction typically contain a double bond attached to $-CN$, $-CHO$, $-COOR$, or $-COR$. The double bond in diethyl maleate is attached to two electron-withdrawing groups and readily undergoes a Michael addition reaction with glutathione, as shown in Fig. 6-55. Diethyl maleate reacts so well with glutathione that it is often used in vivo to decrease glutathione levels in experimental animals. The loop diuretic ethacrynic acid contains an α/β-unsaturated ketone that readily reacts with glutathione and other sulfhydryls by Michael addition. The conversion of acetaminophen to a glutathione conjugate involves addition of glutathione to an activated double bond, which is formed during the cytochrome P450–dependent dehydrogenation of acetaminophen to *N*-acetylbenzoquinoneimine, as shown in Fig. 6-28.

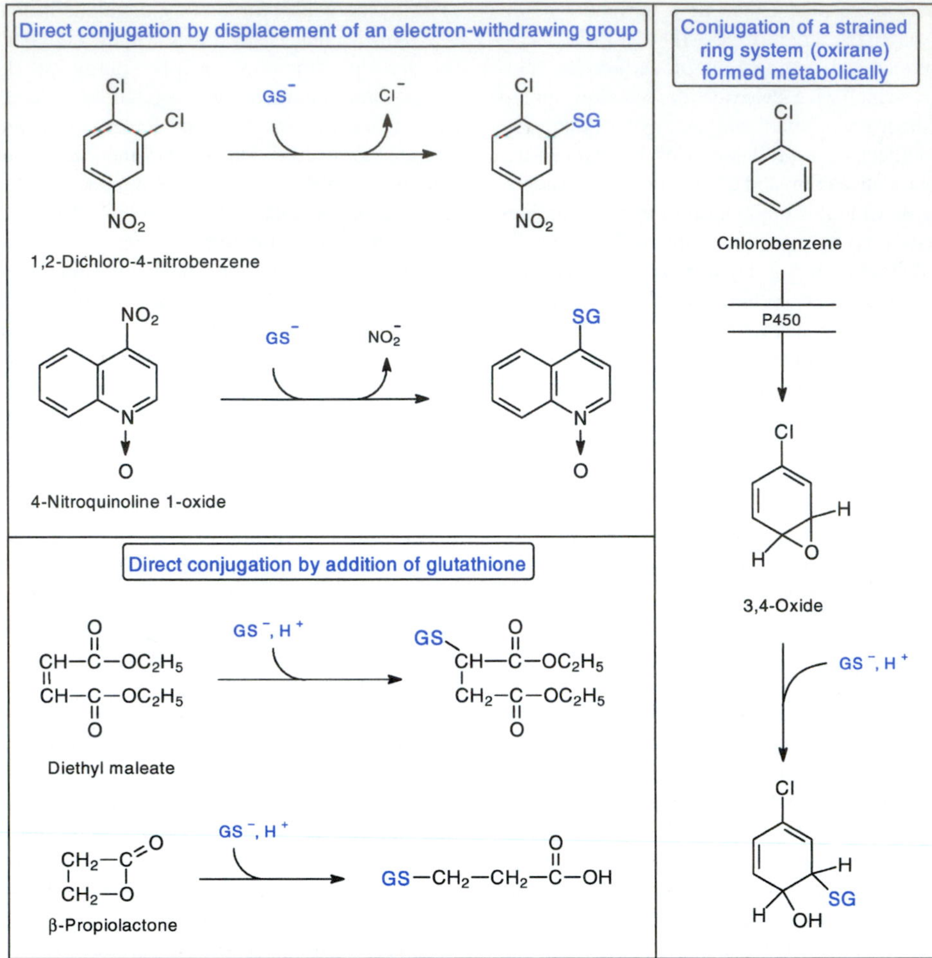

Figure 6-55. Examples of glutathione conjugation of xenobiotics with an electrophilic carbon.

GS^- represents the anionic form of glutathione.

Arene oxides and alkene epoxides, which are often formed by cytochrome P450–dependent oxidation of aromatic hydrocarbons and alkenes, are examples of strained ring systems that open during the addition of glutathione (Fig. 6-55). In many cases, conjugation of arene oxides with glutathione proceeds stereoselectively, as shown in Fig. 6-56 for the 1,2-oxides of naphthalene. The glutathione conjugates of arene oxides may undergo rearrangement reactions, which restore aromaticity and possibly lead to migration of the conjugate to the adjacent carbon atom (through formation of an episulfonium ion), as shown in Fig. 6-56. Conjugation of quinones and quinoneimines with glutathione also restores aromaticity, as shown in Fig. 6-28 for *N*-acetylbenzoquinoneimine, the reactive metabolite of acetaminophen. Compared with glucuronidation and sulfation, conjugation with glutathione is a minor pathway of acetaminophen biotransformation, even though liver contains high levels of both glutathione and glutathione *S*-transferases. The relatively low rate of glutathione conjugation reflects the slow rate of formation of *N*-acetylbenzoquinoneimine, which is catalyzed by cytochrome P450 (Fig. 6-28).

Glutathione can also conjugate xenobiotics with an electrophilic heteroatom (*O*, *N*, and *S*), as shown in Fig. 6-57. In each of the examples shown in Fig. 6-57, the initial conjugate formed between glutathione and the heteroatom is cleaved by a second molecule of glutathione to form oxidized glutathione (GSSG). The initial reactions shown in Fig. 6-57 are catalyzed by glutathione *S*-transferase, whereas the second reaction (which leads to GSSG formation) generally occurs nonenzymatically. Analogous reactions leading to the reduction and cleavage of disulfides have been described previously (see Fig. 6-11). Some of the reactions shown in Fig. 6-57, such as the reduction of hydroperoxides to alcohols, can also be catalyzed by glutathione peroxidase, which is a selenium-dependent enzyme. (For their role in the reduction of hydroperoxides, the glutathione *S*-transferases are sometimes called nonselenium-requiring glutathione peroxidases.) Cleavage of the nitrate esters of nitroglycerin releases nitrite, which can be converted to the potent vasodilator, nitric oxide. The ability of sulfhydryl-generating agents to partially prevent or reverse tolerance to nitroglycerin suggests that glutathione-dependent denitration may play a role in nitroglycerin-induced vasodilation.

Glutathione *S*-transferases catalyze two important isomerization reactions, namely the conversion of the endoperoxide, PGH_2, to the prostaglandins PGD_2 and PGE_2, and the conversion of Δ^5 steroids to Δ^4 steroids, such as the formation of androstenedione from androst-5-ene-3,17-dione. Another physiologic function of glutathione *S*-transferase is the synthesis of leukotriene C_4, which is catalyzed by a microsomal form of the enzyme.

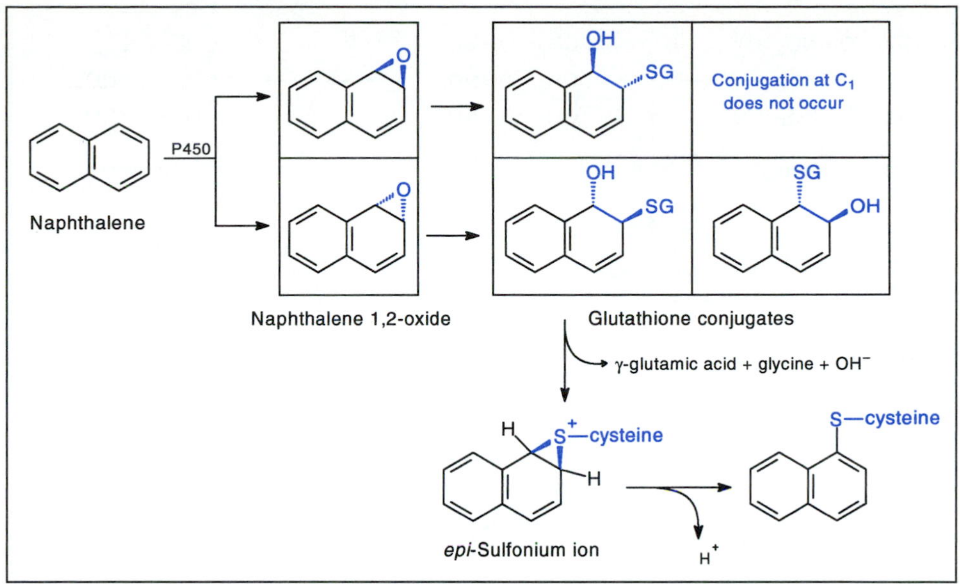

Figure 6-56. Stereoselective conjugation of naphthalene 1,2-oxide and rearrangement of 2-naphthyl to 1-naphthyl conjugates.

Glutathione conjugates formed in the liver can be excreted intact in bile, or they can be converted to mercapturic acids in the kidney and excreted in urine. As shown in Fig. 6-58, the conversion of glutathione conjugates to mercapturic acids involves the sequential cleavage of glutamic acid and glycine from the glutathione moiety, followed by *N*-acetylation of the resulting cysteine conjugate. The first two steps in mercapturic acid synthesis are catalyzed by γ-glutamyltranspeptidase and aminopeptidase M. The glutathione conjugate, leukotriene C_4, is similarly hydrolyzed by γ-glutamyltranspeptidase to form leukotriene D_4, which is hydrolyzed by aminopeptidase M to form leukotriene E_4. Glutathione S-transferases are dimers composed of identical subunits (Mr 23 to 29 kDa), although some forms are heterodimers. Each subunit contains 200 to 240 amino acids and one catalytic site. Numerous subunits have been cloned and sequenced, which forms the basis of a nomenclature system for naming the glutathione *S*-transferases (Mannervick et al., 1992; Hayes and Pulford, 1995; Whalen and Boyer, 1998). Each enzyme is assigned a two-digit number to designate its subunit composition. For example, the homodimers of subunits 1 and 2 are designated 1-1 and 2-2, respectively, whereas the heterodimer is designated 1-2. The soluble glutathione *S*-transferases were initially arranged into four classes designated A, M, P, and T (which refer to alpha, mu, pi, and theta or α, μ, π, and θ). More recently, three additional classes have been identified, namely K (kappa), S (sigma), and Z (zeta) (Hayes and Pulford, 1995; Whalen and Boyer, 1998; Strange et al., 2000). None of these seven gene classes corresponds to the microsomal glutathione *S*-transferase, which appears to have evolved independently. By definition, the subunits in the different classes share less than 40 percent amino acid identity. Generally, the subunits within a class are ~70 percent identical and can form heterodimers, whereas the subunits in different classes are only ~30 percent identical, which appears to prevent dimerization of two subunits from different classes.

Humans express four subunits belonging to the alpha class of glutathione *S*-transferases, designated hGSTA1 to hGSTA4. Rats express at lease five, and possibly as many as eight, GSTA subunits. The first five alpha subunits are known as rGSTA1 to rGSTA5, which are also known as Ya_1, Ya_2, Yc_1, Yk (or Yα), and Yc_2. Rat GSTA1 and GSTA2 are also known as ligandin. Members of the alpha class of glutathione *S*-transferases have basic isoelectric points. They are the major glutathione *S*-transferases in liver and kidney.

Humans express six subunits belonging to the mu class of glutathione *S*-transferases, designated hGSTM1a, –M1b, –M2, –M3, –M4, and –M5. The first two subunits are allelic variants that differ by a single amino acid; hGSTM1a is a "basic variant" with lysine at residue 173, whereas hGSTM1b is an "acidic variant" with asparagine at the corresponding site. Rats express six subunits, designated rGSTM1 to rGSTM6. Rat M1, M2, M3, and M4 are also known as Yb_1, Yb_2, Yb_3, and Yb_4. Members of the mu class of glutathione *S*-transferases have neutral isoelectric points. Human GSTM2 and M3 are expressed in muscle and brain, respectively.

Humans express two subunits belonging to the pi class of glutathione *S*-transferases (hGSTP1a and hGSTP1b), whereas rats express only one subunit (rGSTP1). The two human pi enzymes are allelic variants that differ by a single amino acid (Ile_{105} in hGSTP1a, and Val_{105} in hGSTP1b). However, hGSTP1b is seven times more active that hGST1a in conjugating diol epoxides of polycyclic aromatic hydrocarbons (Strange et al., 2000). Members of the pi class of glutathione *S*-transferases have acidic isoelectric points. They are expressed in the placenta, lung, gut, and other extrahepatic tissues. In rats, GSTP1 is one of several preneoplastic antigens that are overexpressed in chemical-induced tumors.

Humans appear to express two subunits belonging to the theta class of glutathione *S*-transferases (hGSTT1 and hGSTT2), whereas rats appear to express three subunits (rGSTT1 to rGSTT3). A single kappa and single zeta subunit are expressed in humans, but not rats, and are subunits for hGSTK1 and hGSTZ1, respectively. In contrast, a single sigma subunit is expressed in rats, but not humans, and is the subunit for rGSTS1. Alternative names for all glutathione *S*-transferase subunits are summarized in Hayes and Pulford (1995), along with information on their substrate specificity and tissue distribution. The microsomal glutathione *S*-trans-

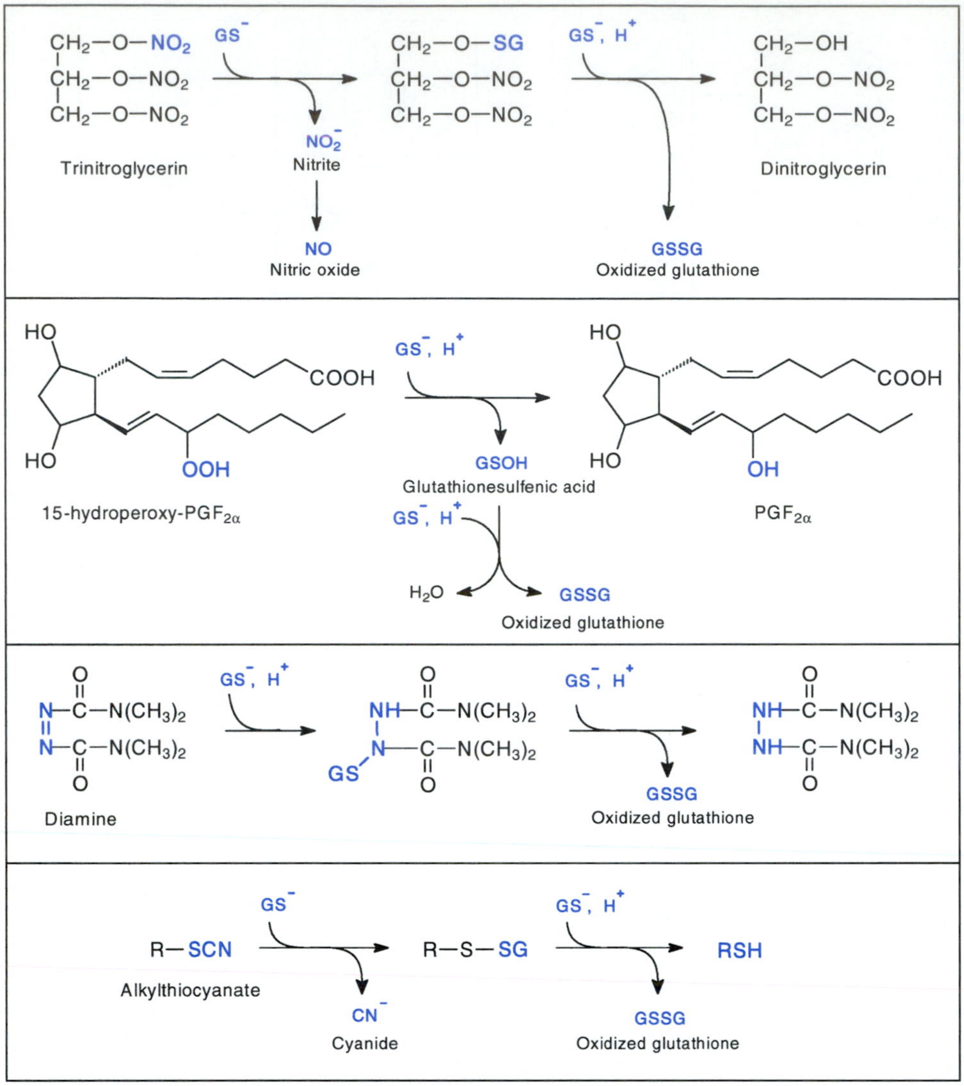

Figure 6-57. Examples of glutathione conjugation of electrophilic heteroatoms.

ferases are distinct from the soluble enzymes. Two microsomal glutathione *S*-transferases have been identified: one is a trimeric enzyme that conjugates xenobiotics with glutathione, the other is a distinct enzyme that conjugates leukotriene A_4 (a lipid epoxide derived of arachidonic acid) with glutathione to form leukotriene C_4. This latter enzyme is known as leukotriene C_4 synthase.

The conjugation of certain xenobiotics with glutathione is catalyzed by all classes of glutathione *S*-transferase. For example, the alpha, mu, and pi classes of human glutathione *S*-transferase all catalyze the conjugation of 1-chloro-2,4-dinitrobenzene. Other reactions are fairly specific for one class of enzymes (Hayes and Pulford, 1995). For example, the alpha glutathione *S*-transferases preferentially isomerize Δ^5 steroids to Δ^4 steroids and reduce linoleate and cumene hydroperoxide to their corresponding alcohols. The mu glutathione *S*-transferases preferentially conjugate certain arene oxides and alkene epoxides, such as styrene-7,8-epoxide. The pi glutathione *S*-transferases preferentially conjugate ethacrynic acid. However, individual members within a class of glutathione *S*-transferases can differ markedly in their substrate specificity. In mice, for example, the alpha glutathione *S*-transferases comprised of Yc subunits (mGSTA3-3) can rapidly conjugate aflatoxin B_1 8,9-epoxide, whereas those comprised of Ya subunits (GSTA1-1) are virtually incapable of catalyzing this reaction (Eaton and Gallagher, 1994).

In rodents, individual members of the alpha and mu class of glutathione *S*-transferases are inducible (generally 2- to 3-fold) by 3-methylcholanthrene, phenobarbital, corticosteroids, oltipraz and various antioxidants (such as ethoxyquin and butylated hydroxyanisole). Several glutathione *S*-transferase substrates (i.e., Michael acceptors) are glutathione *S*-transferase inducers, as are certain nonsubstrates, such as hydrogen peroxide and other reactive oxygen species (Rushmore et al., 1991; Daniel, 1993; Nguyen et al., 1994; Hayes and Pulford, 1995). Induction is usually associated with increased levels of mRNA due to transcriptional activation of the gene encoding a subunit of glutathione *S*-transferase. Not all subunits are induced to the same extent. Treatment of rats with xenobiotics generally increases the hepatic concentration of rGSTA2 and M1 subunits to a greater extent than the rGSTA1 and A3 subunits, which in turn are induced more than rGSTA4 and M2. The rat GSTA5 and P1, which are constitutively expressed at low

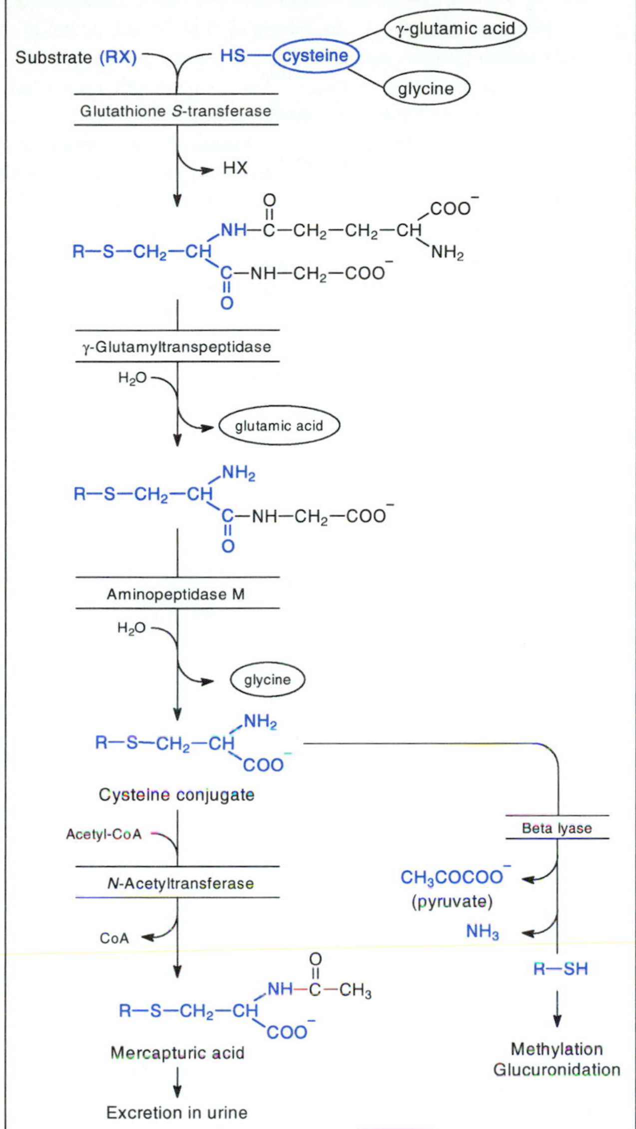

Figure 6-58. Glutathione conjugation and mercapturic acid biosynthesis.

levels in adult rat liver, are dramatically induced by ethoxyquin and coumarin, respectively.

The enhancer regions of the genes encoding some of the rodent glutathione *S*-transferases (such as rGSTA2-2) have been shown to contain a xenobiotic (dioxin)-responsive element (XRE), a putative phenobarbital-responsive element, a glucocorticoid-responsive element (GRE), and an antioxidant responsive element (ARE, which is also known as the electrophile-responsive element, or EpRE). Accordingly, in rodents, certain glutathione *S*-transferase subunits, such as rGSTA1 (Ya_1) and rGSTA1 (Ya_2), are regulated by both *monofunctional* and *bifunctional* agents, as described previously for DT-diaphorase (see "Quinone Reduction" and "Induction of Cytochrome P450," above). Induction of glutathione *S*-transferases by the monofunctional agent sulforaphane is thought to be responsible, at least in part, for the anticancer effects of broccoli (Zhang et al., 1992). It remains to be determined whether factors that regulate the expression of glutathione *S*-transferases in rodents have similar effects in humans, but some differences have been noted. For example, the 5′ promoter region of alpha glutathione *S*-transferase in humans (hGSTA1) lacks the ARE and XRE consensus sequences through which the corresponding rat enzyme is induced. However, such sequences appear to be present in the promoter region of human GSTM4 and GSTP1 genes (Hayes and Pulford, 1995; Whalen and Boyer, 1998). [A functional ARE is also present in the promoter region of human DT-diaphorase (NQO1)]. Therefore, certain subunits of glutathione *S*-transferases are inducible by a variety of mechanisms in rats, and other subunits appear to be inducible by similar mechanisms in humans. Species differences in glutathione *S*-transferase regulation may also stem from differences in xenobiotic biotransformation, especially differences in the formation of electrophiles, Michael acceptors and/or the production of oxidative stress. For example, coumarin is thought be an inducer of GSTP1 in rats because it is converted in rat liver to reactive metabolites, namely coumarin 2,3-epoxide and *ortho*-hydroxyphenylacetaldehyde (see Fig. 6-38). In contrast, the major route of coumarin biotransformation in humans is by 7-hydroxylation, which would not be expected to be associated with glutathione *S*-transferase induction.

Conjugation with glutathione represents an important detoxication reaction because electrophiles are potentially toxic species that can bind to critical nucleophiles, such as proteins and nucleic acids, and cause cellular damage and genetic mutations. All of the enzymes involved in xenobiotic biotransformation have the potential to generate reactive intermediates, most of which are detoxified to some extent by conjugation with glutathione. Glutathione is also a cofactor for glutathione peroxidase, which plays an important role in protecting cells against lipid peroxidation. Resistance to toxic compounds is often associated with an overexpression of glutathione *S*-transferase. Examples include the resistance of insects to DDT (see Fig. 6-18), of corn to atrazine, and of cancer cells to chemotherapeutic agents.

Glutathione *S*-transferase is the major determinant of certain species differences in chemical-induced toxicity. For example, low doses of aflatoxin B_1 cause liver toxicity and tumor formation in rats but not mice, even though rats and mice convert aflatoxin B_1 to the highly reactive 8,9-epoxide at similar rates (this reaction is shown in Fig. 6-27). This species difference arises because mice express high levels of an alpha class glutathione *S*-transferase (mGSTA3-3 or Yc) enabling them to conjugate aflatoxin B_1 8,9-epoxide with glutathione up to fifty times faster than rats (or humans, which are also considered a susceptible species) (Eaton and Gallagher, 1994). Mice become sensitive to the adverse effects of aflatoxin B_1 following treatment with agents that decrease glutathione levels, such as diethyl maleate (which depletes glutathione) or buthionine-*S*-sulfoximine (which inhibits glutathione synthesis). Conversely, treatment of rats with inducers of glutathione *S*-transferase (rGSTA5-5 or Yc_2), such as ethoxyquin, BHA, oltipraz, and phenobarbital, protects them from the hepatotoxic/tumorigenic action of aflatoxin B_1 (Hayes et al., 1994).

The conjugation of aflatoxin B_1 8,9-epoxide with glutathione provides an interesting example of the stereospecificity with which certain glutathione conjugation reactions can occur. Cytochrome P450 converts aflatoxin B_1 to a mixture of *exo*- and *endo*-8,9-epoxides (only a generic 8,9-epoxide is shown in Fig. 6-27; meaning the figure does not indicate whether the oxygen atom is above or below the plane of the ring system). Both enantiomeric epoxides are formed by liver microsomes from mice, rats and humans, but only the *exo*-epoxide binds extensively to DNA (where it binds to the N^7 position of guanine). Mouse alpha-GST (mGSTA3-3) rapidly conjugates the *exo*-epoxide, which accounts for the resistance of this species to aflatoxin-induced hepatotoxicity and tumorigenicity (as described above). Rat and human alpha-glutathione *S*-transferases do not rapidly conjugate either the *exo*- or the *endo*-epoxide (with the exception of the inducible rat glutathione *S*-transferase [A5-5], which is not constitutively expressed in rats to any great extent). However, human mu-GSTs (hGSTM1a-1a and hGSTM2-2) can conjugate aflatoxin B_1 8,9-epoxide, but they preferentially conjugate the relatively innocuous *endo*-isomer (Wang et al., 2000).

Species differences in the detoxication of aflatoxin B_1 8,9-epoxide suggest that individual differences in glutathione *S*-transferase may determine susceptibility to the toxic effects of certain chemicals. In support of this interpretation, a genetic polymorphism for hGSTM1 has been identified, and individuals who are homozygous for the null allele (i.e., those with low glutathione *S*-transferase activity due to complete deletion of the GSTM1 gene) appear to be at increased risk for cigarette smoking–induced lung cancer and bladder cancer (Hayes and Pulford, 1995; Whalen and Boyer, 1998; Strange et al., 2000). Depending on the ethnic group, 22 to 100 percent of the population are homozygous for the GSTM1 null genotype, which results in a complete lack of GSTM1 activity in all tissues. Similarly, theta GST activity is absent from 11 to 58 percent of the population (depending on ethnicity) due to deletion of the GSTT1 gene, which appears to increase susceptibility to development of astrocytoma, meningioma and myelodysplasia. When examined for their individual effect, these null genotypes generally have a small effect on susceptibility, with an odds ratio of 2 or less. However, the odds ratio can increase dramatically when these null glutathione *S*-transferase genotypes are examined in conjunction with other genotypes or with environmental factors (such as exposure to carcinogens). For example, when the GSTM1 null genotype is combined with cigarette smoking and a particular CYP1A1 allele, the odds ratio can increase to 8.9 (in one study) or 21.9 (in another study). Polymorphisms that result in amino substitutions have been reported for most human glutathione *S*-transferase genes; some of which alter glutathione *S*-transferase function. Some of these polymorphisms may also be risk modifiers for certain diseases in an analogous manner to the GSTM1 and GSTT1 null genotypes.

In some cases, conjugation with glutathione enhances the toxicity of a xenobiotic (Monks et al., 1990; Dekant and Vamvakas, 1993). Four mechanisms of glutathione-dependent activation of xenobiotics have been identified, as shown in Fig. 6-59. These mechanisms are (1) formation of glutathione conjugates of haloalkanes, organic thiocyanates, and nitrosoguanides that release a toxic metabolite; (2) formation of glutathione conjugates of vicinal dihaloalkanes that are inherently toxic because they can form electrophilic sulfur mustards; (3) formation of glutathione conjugates of halogenated alkenes that are degraded to toxic metabolites by β-lyase in the kidney; and (4) formation of glutathione conjugates of quinones, quinoneimines, and isothiocyanates that are degraded to toxic metabolites by γ-glutamyltranspeptidase and endopeptidase M in the kidney.

The first mechanism is illustrated by dichloromethane, which is conjugated with glutathione to form chloromethyl-glutathione, which then breaks down to formaldehyde. Both formaldehyde and the glutathione conjugate are reactive metabolites, and either or both may be responsible for dichloromethane-induced tumorigenesis in sensitive species. The rate of conjugation of dichloromethane with glutathione is considerably faster in mice, which are susceptible to dichloromethane-induced tumorigenesis, than in rats or hamsters, which are resistant species.

The second mechanism accounts for the toxicity of dichloroethane and dibromoethane. These vicinal dihaloalkanes are converted to glutathione conjugates that can rearrange to form mutagenic and nephrotoxic episulfonium ions (sulfur half-mustards) (Fig. 6-59). Dichloroethane and dibromoethane can also be oxidized by cytochrome P450 to chloroacetaldehyde and bromoacetaldehyde (by reactions analogous to those shown in Fig. 6-44). Either pathway can potentially account for the toxic and tumorigenic effects of these dihaloalkanes. However, the toxicity and DNA-binding of dihaloalkanes are increased by factors that decrease their oxidation by cytochrome P450 and increase their conjugation with glutathione.

The third mechanism accounts for the nephrotoxicity of several halogenated alkenes. Several halogenated alkenes, such as hexachlorobutadiene, cause damage to the kidney tubules in rats, which leads to carcinoma of the proximal tubules. These nephrotoxic halogenated alkenes are conjugated with glutathione and transported to the kidney for processing to mercapturic acids. The cysteine conjugates, which form by removal of glutamic acid and glycine, are substrates for *N*-acetyltransferase, which completes the synthesis of mercapturic acids, and β-lyase, which removes pyruvate and ammonia from the cysteine conjugate to produce thionylacyl halides and thioketenes. The early damage to renal mitochondria caused by halogenated alkenes is probably because cysteine-conjugate β-lyase is a mitochondrial enzyme.

The fourth mechanism accounts for the nephrotoxicity of bromobenzene, which causes damage to the proximal tubules in rats. Bromobenzene is oxidized by cytochrome P450 in the liver to bromohydroquinone, which is conjugated with glutathione and transported to the kidney (Fig. 6-59). The glutathione conjugate is converted to the cysteine derivative by γ-glutamyltranspeptidase and aminopeptidase M. Substitution of bromohydroquinones with cysteine lowers their redox potential and thereby facilitates their oxidation to toxic quinones. The cysteine conjugates of bromohydroquinone are thought to undergo redox cycling and cause kidney damage through the generation of reactive oxygen species. 4-Aminophenol is thought to cause kidney damage by a similar mechanism, except a benzoquinoneimine is involved in conjugation with glutathione and subsequent damage to proximal tubules of the kidney. Treatment of rats with the glutathione depletor, buthionine-*S*-sulfoximine, protects them against the nephrotoxic effects of 4-aminophenol, which implicates glutathione conjugation in the activation of this compound.

Rhodanese

Rhodanese is a mitochondrial enzyme that converts cyanide to the far less toxic metabolite, thiocyanate. The reaction involves transfer of sulfur from thiosulfate (or another sulfur donor) as follows:

$$\underset{\text{cyanide}}{CN^-} + \underset{\text{thiosulfate}}{S_2O_3^{2-}} \rightarrow \underset{\text{thiocyanate}}{SCN^-} + \underset{\text{sulfite}}{SO_3^{2-}}$$

The sulfite produced by this reaction can be converted to sulfate by the molybdozyme, sulfite oxidase. Cyanide can also be "detoxified" by binding to methemoglobin (the oxidized or ferric form of hemoglobin). 4-Dimethylaminophenol is used to induce methemoglobinemia as an antidote to cyanide poisoning because methemoglobin competes with cytochrome oxidase for the cyanide ion. However, 4-dimethylaminophenol is nephrotoxic to rats, presumably by a mechanism similar to that described above for the

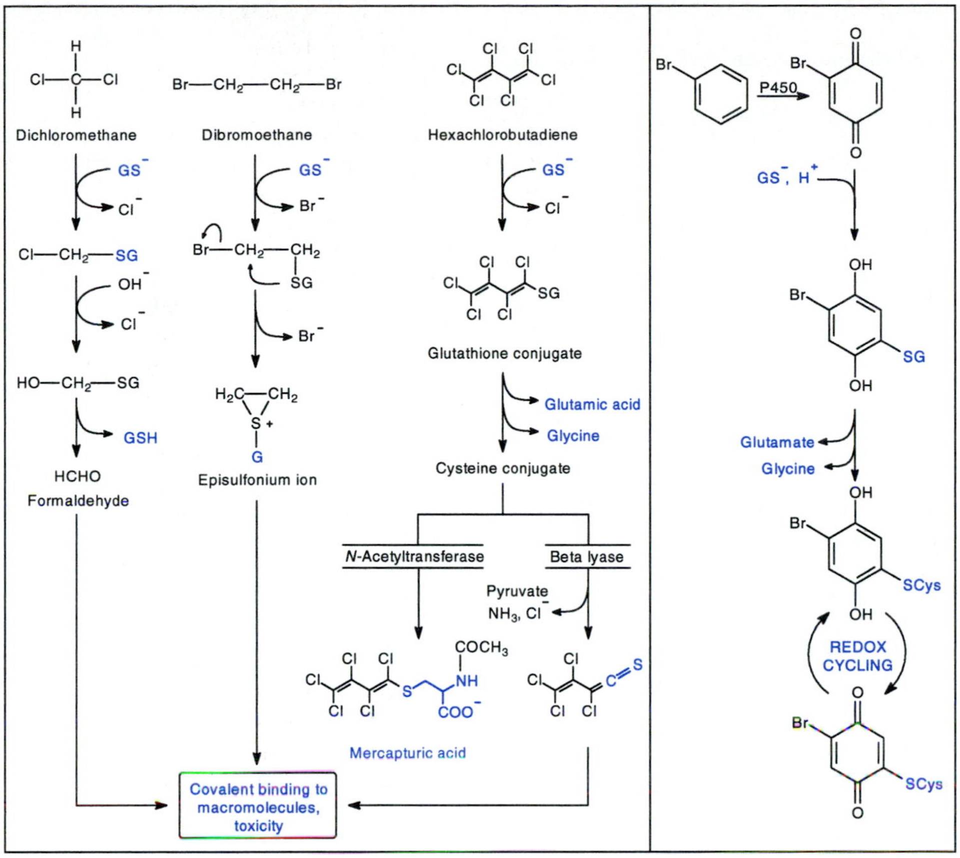

Figure 6-59. Role of glutathione conjugation in the activation of xenobiotics to toxic metabolites.

structural analog, 4-aminophenol (see preceding section and section on "Peroxidase-Dependent Cooxidation").

Phosphorylation—The Dog That Did Not Bark

All phase II conjugation reactions ultimately require ATP, either to activate the xenobiotic for conjugation with glutathione or amino acids or to synthesize high-energy cofactors such as UDP-glucuronic acid and PAPS. The process is inefficient in that several ATP molecules (or their equivalent) are used to synthesize each cofactor molecule. The question arises: Why is ATP not used directly by phase II enzymes? In other words, why are xenobiotics never phosphorylated, which would require less ATP and would achieve the goal of converting xenobiotics to water-soluble conjugates. It is difficult to be certain why this does not occur, but three reasons suggest themselves. First, if xenobiotics could be phosphorylated, high intracellular levels of a xenobiotic might consume so much ATP as to jeopardize cell viability, whereas UDP-glucuronic acid and PAPS can be depleted without killing cells. Second, phosphorylation of endogenous substrates, such as glucose, is a mechanism for trapping endogenous substrates in a cell. This works because the plasmamembrane of all cells is a barrier to the passage of polar compounds by virtue of its hydrophobic properties (lipid bilayer) and its lack of transporters that pump phosphorylated compounds out of the cell. A lipid bilayer is also a physical barrier to other water-soluble conjugates, such as glucuronides and sulfates, but these are transported out of the cell by various transporters. Third, phosphorylation of both small molecules (such as inositol) and proteins (such as membrane-bound receptors and various transcription factors) plays an important role in intracellular and intranuclear signaling. It is possible that some xenobiotics, if they were phosphorylated, might interfere with these regulatory systems and thereby disrupt cellular homeostasis. Whatever the reason, there appears to be strong evolutionary pressure against the conjugation of xenobiotics with phosphoric acid.

REFERENCES

Abernathy DR, Flockhart DA: Molecular basis of cardiovascular drug metabolism: Implications for predicting clinically important drug interactions. *Circulation* 101:1749–1753, 2000.

Agarwal DP, Goedde HW: Pharmacogenetics of alcohol dehydrogenase, in Kalow W (ed): *Pharmacogenetics of Drug Metabolism.* New York: Pergamon Press, 1992, pp 263–280.

Aldridge WN: Serum esterases: Two types of esterases (A and B) hydrolyzing para-nitrophenylacetate, propionate, and a method for their determination. *Biochem J* 53:110–119, 1953.

Anders MW (ed): *Bioactivation of Foreign Compounds.* New York: Academic Press, 1985.

Anders MW, Ratnayake JH, Hanna PE, Fuchs JA: Thioredoxin-dependent sulfoxide reduction by rat renal cytosol. *Drug Metab Dispos* 9:307–310, 1981.

Armstrong RN: Kinetic and chemical mechanism of epoxide hydrolase. *Drug Metab Rev* 31:71–86, 1991.

Atkins WM, Wang RW, Bird AW, et al: The catalytic mechanism of glutathione *S*-transferase (GST): Spectroscopic determination of the pKa of Tyr-9 in rat a1-1 GST. *J Biol Chem* 268:19188–19191, 1993.

Augustinsson KB: Arylesterases. *J. Histochem Cytochem* 12:744–747, 1966.

Ayesh R, Smith RL: Genetic polymorphism of trimethylamine *N*-oxidation, in Kalow W (ed): *Pharmacogenetics of Drug Metabolism*. New York: Pergamon Press, 1992, pp 315–332.

Back DJ, Orme LE: Genetic factors influencing the metabolism of tolbutamide, in Kalow W (ed): *Pharmacogenetics of Drug Metabolism*. New York: Pergamon Press, 1992, pp 737–746.

Batt AM, Siest G, Magdalou J, Galteau M-M: Enzyme induction by drugs and toxins. *Clin Chim Acta* 209:109–121, 1992.

Beetham JK, Grant D, Arand M, et al: Gene evolution of epoxide hydrolases and recommended nomenclature. *DNA Cell Biol* 14:61–71, 1995.

Bell PA, Kasper CB: Expression of rat microsomal epoxide hydrolase in *Escherichia coli*: Identification of a histidyl residue essential for catalysis. *J Biol Chem* 268:14011–14017, 1993.

Benedetti MS, Dostert P: Contribution of amine oxidases to the metabolism of xenobiotics. *Drug Metab Rev* 26:507–535, 1994.

Bendotti C, Prosperini E, Kurosaki M, et al: Selective localization of mouse aldehyde oxidase mRNA in the choroid plexus and motor neurons. *Neuroreport* 8:2343–2349, 1997.

Bernauer U, Vieth B, Ellrich R, et al: CYP2E1 expression in bone marrow and its intra- and interspecies variability: Approaches for a more reliable extrapolation from one species to another in the risk assessment of chemicals. *Arch Toxicol* 73:618–624, 2000.

Boberg EW, Miller EC, Miller JA, et al: Strong evidence from studies with brachymorphic mice and pentachlorophenol that 1′-sulfoöxysafrole is the major ultimate electrophilic and carcinogenic metabolite of 1′-hydroxysafrole in mouse liver. *Cancer Res* 43:5163–5173, 1983.

Bock KW, Schrenk D, Forster A, et al: The influence of environmental and genetic factors on CYP2D6, CYP1A2, and UDP-glucuronosyltransferases in man using sparteine, caffeine, and paracetamol as probes. *Pharmacogenetics* 4:209–218, 1994.

Bolton JL, Trush MA, Penning TM, et al: Role of quinones in toxicology. *Chem Res Toxicol* 13:135–160, 2000.

Boulton DW, Fawcett JP: Pharmacokinetics and pharmacodynamics of single doses of albuterol and its enantiomers in humans. *Clin Pharmacol Ther* 62:138–144, 1997.

Bray RC, Bennet B, Burke JF, et al: Recent studies of xanthine oxidase and related enzymes. *Biochem Soc Trans* 24:99–105, 1996.

Brittebo EB: Metabolism of xenobiotics in the nasal olfactory mucosa: Implications for local toxicity. *Pharmacol Toxicol* 72(suppl III):50–52, 1993.

Brockmöller J, Cascorbi I, Kerb R, et al: Polymorphisms in xenobiotic conjugation and disease predisposition. *Toxicol Lett* 102–103:173–183, 1998.

Burchell B, Coughtrie MWH: UDP-glucuronosyltransferases, in Kalow W (ed): *Pharmacogenetics of Drug Metabolism*. New York: Pergamon Press, 1992, pp 195–225.

Burchell B: Transformation reactions: Glucuronidation, in Woolf TF (ed): *Handbook of Drug Metabolism*. New York: Marcel Dekker, 1999, pp 153–173.

Burczynski ME, Penning TM: Genotoxic polycyclic aromatic hydrocarbon *ortho*-quinones generated by aldo-keto reductases induce CYP1A1 via nuclear translocation of the aryl hydrocarbon receptor. *Cancer Res* 60:908–915, 2000.

Buters JTM, Doehmer J, Gonzalez FJ: Cytochrome P450–null mice. *Drug Metab Rev* 31:437–447, 1999.

Buters JTM, Sakai S, Richter T, et al: Cytochrome P450 CYP1B1 determines susceptibility to 7,12-dimethylbenz[*a*]anthracene–induced lymphomas. *Proc Natl Acad Sci USA* 96:1977–1982, 1999.

Cashman JR: In vitro metabolism: FMO and related oxygenations, in Woolf TF (ed) *Handbook of Drug Metabolism*. New York: Marcel Dekker, 1999, pp 477–505.

Cashman JR: Structural and catalytic properties of the mammalian flavin monooxygenase. *Chem Res Toxicol* 8:165–181, 1995.

Cashman JR, Akerman BR, Forrest SM, Treacy EP: Population-specific polymorphisms of the human *FMO3* gene: Significance for detoxification. *Drug Metab Dispos* 28:169–173, 2000.

Cashman JR, Xiong Y, Lin J, et al: *In vitro* and *in vivo* inhibition of human flavin-containing monooxygenase form 3 (FMO3) in the presence of dietary indoles. *Biochem Pharmacol* 58:1047–1055, 1999.

Conney A: Induction of microsomal enzymes by foreign chemicals and carcinogenesis by polycyclic aromatic hydrocarbons: GHA Clowes Memorial Lecture. *Cancer Res* 42:4875–4917, 1982.

Conney AH: Pharmacological implications of microsomal enzyme induction. *Pharmacol Rev* 19:317–366, 1967.

Cundy KC, Sato M, Crooks PA: Stereospecific in vivo *N*-methylation of nicotine in the guinea pig. *Drug Metab* 13:175–185, 1985.

Curran PG, DeGroot LJ: The effect of hepatic enzyme-inducing drugs on thyroid hormones and the thyroid gland. *Endocrinol Rev* 12:135–150, 1991.

Daly AK: Pharmacogenetics, in Woolf TF (ed): *Handbook of Drug Metabolism.* New York: Marcel Dekker, 1999, pp 175–202.

Daniel V: Glutathione *S*-transferases: Gene structure and regulation of expression. *Crit Rev Biochem Mol Biol* 28:173–207, 1993.

Dawson JH: Probing structure-function relations in heme-containing oxygenases and peroxidases. *Science* 240:433–439, 1988.

Dekant W, Vamvakas S: Glutathione-dependent bioactivation of xenobiotics. *Xenobiotica* 23:873–887, 1993.

Delfino RJ, Smith C, West JG, et al: Breast cancer, passive and active cigarette smoking and N-acetyltransferase 2 genotype. *Pharmacogenetics* 10:461–469, 2000.

DeMorais SMF, Uetrecht JP, Wells PG: Decreased glucuronidation and increased bioactivation of acetaminophen in Gilbert's syndrome. *Gastroenterology* 102:577–586, 1992.

Demoz A, Vaagenes H, Aarsaether N, et al: Coordinate induction of hepatic fatty acyl-CoA oxidase and P4504A1 in rat after activation of the peroxisome proliferator-activated receptor (PPAR) by sulphur-substituted fatty acid analogues. *Xenobiotica* 24:943–956, 1994.

Diasio RB, Beavers TL, Carpenter JT: Familial deficiency of dihydropyrimidine dehydrogenase: Biochemical basis for familial pyrimidinemia and severe 5-fluorouracil–induced toxicity. *J Clin Invest* 81:47–51, 1988.

Diaz D, Fabre I, Daujat M, et al: Omeprazole is an aryl hydrocarbonlike inducer of human hepatic cytochrome P450. *Gastroenterology* 99:737–747, 1990.

Dirr H, Reinemer P, Huber R: X-ray crystal structures of cytosolic glutathione *S*-transferases: Implications for protein architecture, substrate recognition and catalytic function. *Eur J Biochem* 220:645–661, 1994.

Dolphin CT, Beckett DJ, Janmohamed A, et al: The flavin-containing monooxygenase 2 gene (*FMO2*) of humans, but not of other primates, encodes a truncated, nonfunctional protein. *J Biol Chem* 273:30599–30607, 1998.

Dolphin CT, Janmohamed A, Smith RL, et al: A missense mutation, Pro153Leu (C → T), in the gene encoding flavin-containing monooxygenase 3, *FMO3,* underlies fish-odour syndrome. *Nat Genet* 17:491–494, 1997.

Dresser GK, Spence JD, Bailey DG: Pharmacokinetic–pharmacodynamic consequences and clinical relevance of cytochrome P450 3A4 inhibition. *Clin Pharmacokinet* 38(1):41–57, 2000.

Dwivedi C, Downie A, Webb TE. Net glucuronidation in different rat strains: Importance of microsomal β-glucuronidase. *FASEB J* 1:303–307, 1987.

Eaton DL, Gallagher EP: Mechanisms of aflatoxin carcinogenesis. *Annu Rev Pharmacol Toxicol* 34:135–172, 1994.

Edenberg HJ: Regulation of the mammalian alcohol dehydrogenase genes. *Prog Nucl Acid Res Mol Biol* 64:295–341, 2000.

Ekins S, Wrighton SA: The role of CYP2B6 in human xenobiotic metabolism. *Drug Metab Rev* 31(3):719–754, 1999.

Eling TE, Thompson DC, Foureman GL, et al: Prostaglandin H synthase and xenobiotic oxidation. *Annu Rev Pharmacol Toxicol* 30:1–45, 1990.

Ernster L: DT-diaphorase: A historical review. *Chem Scripta* 27A:1–17, 1987.

Evans DAP: *N*-Acetyltransferase, in Kalow W (ed): *Pharmacogenetics of Drug Metabolism*. New York: Pergamon Press, 1992, pp 95–178.

Falany CN, Johnson MR, Barnes S, Diasio RB: Glycine and taurine conjugation of bile acids by a single enzyme: Molecular cloning and expression of human liver bile acid CoA:amino acid *N*-acetyltransferase. *J Biol Chem* 269:19375–19379, 1994.

Farrell GC: Drug metabolism in extrahepatic diseases. *Pharmacol Ther* 35:375–404, 1987.

Favreau LV, Pickett CB: Transcriptional regulation of the rat NAD(P)H: quinone reductase gene. Identification of regulatory elements controlling basal level expression and inducible expression by planar aromatic compounds and phenolic antioxidants. *J Biol Chem* 266:4556–4561, 1991.

Frezza C, DiPadova G, Pozzato M, et al: High blood alcohol levels in women: The role of decreased gastric alcohol dehydrogenase activity and blood ethanol levels. *N Engl J Med* 322:95–99, 1990.

Friedberg T, Grassow MA, Bartlomowiczoesch B, et al: Sequence of a novel CYP2B cDNA coding for a protein which is expressed in a sebaceous gland but not in the liver. *Biochem J* 297:775–783, 1992.

Gerlach M, Riederer P, Przuntek H, Youdim MBH: MPTP mechanisms of neurotoxicity and their implications for Parkinson's disease. *Eur J Pharmacol* 208:273–286, 1991.

Goedde HW, Agarwal DP: Pharmacogenetics of aldehyde dehydrogenase, in Kalow W (ed): *Pharmacogenetics of Drug Metabolism*. New York: Pergamon Press, 1992, pp 281–311.

Gonzalez FJ: The molecular biology of cytochrome P450s. *Pharmacol Rev* 40:243–288, 1989.

Gonzalez FJ, Kimura S: Role of gene knockout mice in understanding the mechanisms of chemical toxicity and carcinogenesis. *Cancer Lett* 143:199–204, 1999.

Gonzalez FJ, Peters JM, Cattley RC: Mechanism of action of the nongenotoxic peroxisome proliferators: Role of the peroxisome proliferator activated receptor α. *J Natl Cancer Inst* 90:1702–1709, 1998.

Gorell JM, Rybicki BA, Johnson CC, Peterson EL: Smoking and Parkinson's disease: A dose–response relationship. *Neurology* 52:115–119, 1999.

Gram TE (ed): *Extrahepatic Metabolism of Drugs and Other Foreign Compounds*. New York: Spectrum, 1980, pp 1–601.

Grant DM, Blum M, Meyers UA: Polymorphisms of *N*-acetyltransferase genes. *Xenobiotica* 22:1073–1081, 1992.

Grasso P, Sharratt M, Cohen AJ: Role of persistent, non-genotoxic tissue damage in rodent cancer and relevance to humans. *Annu Rev Pharmacol Toxicol* 31:253–287, 1991.

Guengerich FP: Catalytic selectivity of human cytochrome P450 enzymes: Relevance to drug metabolism and toxicity. *Toxicol Lett* 70:133–138, 1994.

Guengerich FP: *Mammalian Cytochrome P450*. Boca Raton, FL: CRC Press, 1987.

Guengerich FP: Reactions and significance of cytochrome P450 enzymes. *J Biol Chem* 266:10019–10022, 1991.

Guengerich FP, Kim D-H, Iwasaki M: Role of human cytochrome P450 IIE1 in the oxidation of many low molecular weight cancer suspects. *Chem Res Toxicol* 4:168–179, 1991.

Guengerich FP, Shimada T: Oxidation of toxic and carcinogenic chemicals by human cytochrome P450 enzymes. *Chem Res Toxicol* 4:391–407, 1991.

Gupta E, Lestingi TM, Mick R, et al: Metabolic fate of irinotecan in humans: Correlation of glucuronidation with diarrhea. *Cancer Res* 54:3723–3725, 1994.

Gupta RA, DuBois RN: Aspirin, NSAIDs, and colon cancer prevention. Mechanism? *Gastroenterology* 114:1095–1098, 1999.

Halpert JR, Guengerich FP, Bend JR, Correia MA: Contemporary issues in toxicology: Selective inhibitors of cytochromes P450. *Toxicol Appl Pharmacol* 125:163–175, 1994.

Hamman MA, Haehner-Daniels BD, Wrighton SA, et al: Stereoselective sulfoxidation of sulindac sulfide by flavin-containing monooxygenases. *Biochem Pharmacol* 60:7–17, 2000.

Hawes EM: N^+-Glucuronidation, a common pathway in human metabolism of drugs with a tertiary amine group. *Drug Metab Dispos* 26:830–837, 1998.

Hayes JD, Nguyen T, Judah DJ, et al: Cloning of cDNAs from fetal rat liver encoding glutathione *S*-transferase Yc polypeptides. *J Biol Chem* 269:20707–20717, 1994.

Hayes JD, Pulford DJ: The glutathione-S-transferase supergene family: Regulation of GST and the contribution of the isoenzymes to cancer chemoprotection and drug resistance. *Crit Rev Biochem Mol Biol* 30:445–600, 1995.

Hayes RB, Bi W, Rothman N, et al: *N*-Acetylation phenotype and genotype and risk of bladder cancer in benzidine-exposed workers. *Carcinogenesis* 14:675–678, 1993.

Hein DW, Doll MA, Fretland, AJ et al: Molecular genetics and epidemiology of the *NAT1* and *NAT2* acetylation polymorphisms. *Cancer Epidemiol Biomarkers Prev* 9:29–42, 2000.

Herwick DS: Reductive metabolism of nitrogen-containing functional groups, in Jakoby WB, Bend JR, Caldwell J (eds): *Metabolic Basis of Detoxication*. New York: Academic Press, 1980, pp 151–170.

Hirvonen A: Polymorphic NATs and cancer predisposition, in Ryder W (ed): *Metabolic Polymorphisms and Susceptibility to Cancer.* IARC Sci Pub No 148. Lyon, France: International Agency for Research on Cancer (IARC), 1999, pp 251–270.

Honkakoski P, Negishi M: Regulation of cytochrome P450 (*CYP*) genes by nuclear receptors. *Biochem J* 347:321–337, 2000.

Houston JB: Utility of in vitro drug metabolism data in predicting in vivo metabolic clearance. *Biochem Pharmacol* 47:1469–1479, 1994.

Humphrey MJ, Ringrose PS: Peptides and related drugs: A review of their adsorption, metabolism, and excretion. *Drug Metab Rev* 17:283–310, 1986.

Idle JR: Is environmental carcinogenesis modulated by host polymorphism? *Mutat Res* 247:259–266, 1991.

Inaba T, Kovacs J: Haloperidol reductase in human and guinea pig livers. *Drug Metab Dispos* 17:330–333, 1989.

Jaiswal AK, Burnett P, Adesnik M, McBride OW: Nucleotide and deduced amino acid sequence of a human cDNA (NQO_2) corresponding to a second member of the NAD(P)H: Quinone oxidoreductase gene family: Extensive polymorphism at the NQO_2 gene locus on chromosome 6. *Biochemistry* 29:1899–1906, 1990.

Jakoby WB (ed): *Enzymatic Basis of Detoxication*. Vols 1 and 2. New York: Academic Press, 1980.

Jakoby WB, Bend JR, Caldwell J: *Metabolic Basis of Detoxification: Metabolism of Functional Groups*. New York: Academic Press, 1982, pp 1–375.

Jörnvall H, Höög J-O: Nomenclature of alcohol dehydrogenases. *Alcohol Alcoholism* 30:153–161, 1995.

Kadlubar FF: Biochemical individuality and its implications for drug and carcinogen metabolism: Recent insights from acetyltransferase and cytochrome P4501A2 phenotyping and genotyping in humans. *Drug Metab Rev* 26:37–46, 1994.

Kanamitsu S-I, Ito K, Okuda H, et al: Prediction of in vivo drug–drug interactions based on mechanism-based inhibition from in vitro data: Inhibition of 5-fluorouracil metabolism by (E)-5-(2-bromovinyl)uracil. *Drug Metab Dispos* 28:467–474, 2000.

Kaneko A, Lum JK, Yaviong J, et al: High and variable frequencies of *CYP2C19* mutations: Medical consequences of poor drug metabolism in Vanuatu and other Pacific islands. *Pharmacogenetics* 9:581–590, 1999.

Kato R: Characteristics and differences in the hepatic mixed function oxidases of different species. *Pharmacol Ther* 6:41–98, 1979.

Kato R, Estabrook RW, Cayen MN (eds): *Xenobiotic Metabolism and Disposition*. London: Taylor and Francis, 1989, pp 1–538.

Kato R, Yamazoe Y: The importance of substrate concentration in determining cytochromes P450 therapeutically relevant in vivo. *Pharmacogenetics* 4:359–362, 1994a.

Kato R, Yamazoe Y: Metabolic activation of *N*-hydroxylated metabolites of carcinogenic and mutagenic arylamines and arylamides by esterification. *Drug Metab Rev* 26:413–430, 1994b.

Kivsito KT, Neuvonen PJ, Klotz U: Inhibition of terfenadine metabolism: Pharmacokinetic and pharmacodynamic consequences. *Clin Pharmacokin* 27:1–5, 1994.

Koenigs LL, Peter RM, Hunter AP, et al: Electrospray ionization mass spectrometric analysis of intact cytochrome P450: Identification of tienilic acid adducts to P450 2C9. *Biochemistry* 38:2312–2319, 1999.

Koivusalo M, Baumann M, Uotila L: Evidence for the identity of glutathione-dependent formaldehyde dehydrogenase and class III alcohol dehydrogenase. *FEBS Lett* 257:105–109, 1989.

Koop DR, Tierney DJ: Multiple mechanisms in the regulation of ethanol-inducible cytochrome P450IIE1. *Bioessays* 12:429–435, 1990.

Kretz-Rommel A, Boesterli UA: Mechanism of covalent adduct formation of diclofenac to rat hepatic microsomal proteins: Retention of the glucuronic acid moiety in the adduct. *Drug Metab Dispos* 22:956–961, 1994.

Krishna DR, Klotz U: Extrahepatic metabolism of drugs in humans. *Clin Pharmacokinet* 26:144–160, 1994.

Kroetz DL, Loiseau P, Guyot M, Levy RH: In vivo and in vitro correlation of microsomal epoxide hydrolase inhibition by progabide. *Clin Pharmacol Ther* 54:485–497, 1993.

La Du BN: Human serum paraoxonase/arylesterase, in Kalow W (ed): *Pharmacogenetics of Drug Metabolism*. New York: Pergamon Press, 1992, pp 51–91.

Lawton MP, Cashman JR, Cresteil T, et al: A nomenclature for the mammalian flavin monooxygenase gene family based on amino acid sequence identities. *Arch Biochem Biophys* 308:254–257, 1994.

Lecoeur S, Bonierbale E, Challine D, et al: Specificity of in vitro covalent binding of tienilic acid metabolites to human liver microsomes in relationship to the type of hepatotoxicity: Comparison with two directly hepatotoxic drugs. *Chem Res Toxicol* 7:434–442, 1994.

Lehman-McKeeman LD, Caudill D, Vassallo JD, et al: Effects of musk xylene and musk ketone on rat hepatic cytochrome P450 enzymes. *Toxicol Lett* 111:105–115, 1999.

Levitt MD: Review article: Lack of clinical significance of the interaction between H2-receptor antagonists and ethanol. *Aliment Pharmacol Ther* 7:131–138, 1993.

Li AP, Hartman NR, Lu C, Collins JM, Strong JM: Effects of cytochrome P450 inducers on 17α-ethinylestradiol (EE_2) conjugation by primary human hepatocytes. *Br J Clin Pharmacol* 48:733–742, 1999.

Li T-K: Pharmacogenetics of responses to alcohol and genes that influence alcohol drinking. *J Stud Alcohol* 61:5–12, 2000.

Liang Q, He J-S, Fulco A: The role of barbie box sequences as *cis*-acting elements involved in the barbiturate-mediated induction of cytochromes P450 BM-1 and P450 BM-3 in *Bacillus megaterium*. *J Biol Chem* 270:4438–4450, 1995.

Lieber CS: Microsomal ethanol-oxidizing system (MEOS): The first 30 years (1968–1998)—a review. *Alcoholism Clin Exp Res* 23:991–1007, 1999.

Lillibridge JA, Kalhorn TK, Slattery JT: Metabolism of lisofylline and pentoxifylline in human liver microsomes and cytosol. *Drug Metab Dispos* 24:1174–1179, 1996.

Lindberg R, Negishi M: Alteration of mouse cytochrome P450coh substrate specificity by mutation of a single amino acid residue. *Nature* 336:632–634, 1989.

Liu ZC, Uetrecht JP: Metabolism of ticlopidine by activated neutrophils: Implications for ticlopidine-induced agranulocytosis. *Drug Metab Dispos* 28:726–730, 2000.

Lockridge O: Genetic variants of human serum butyrylcholinesterase influence the metabolism of the muscle relaxant succinylcholine, in Kalow W (ed): *Pharmacogenetics of Drug Metabolism*. New York: Pergamon Press, 1992, pp 15–50.

Long RM, Rickert DE: Metabolism and excretion of 2,6-dinitro-[14C]toluene in vivo and in isolated perfused rat livers. *Drug Metab Dispos* 10:455–458, 1982.

Lunam CA, Hall PM, Cousins MJ: The pathology of halothane hepatotoxicity in a guinea pig model: A comparison with human halothane hepatitis. *Br J Exp Pathol* 70:533–541, 1989.

Mabic S, Castagnoli K, Castagnoli N: Oxidative metabolic bioactivation of xenobiotics, in Woolf TF (ed): *Handbook of Drug Metabolism*. New York: Marcel Dekker, 1999, pp 49–79.

Mackenzie PI, Rodbourne L, Stranks S: Steroid UDP glucuronosyltransferases. *J Steroid Biochem* 43:1099–1105, 1992.

Madan A, Usuki E, Burton LA, et al: In vitro approaches for studying the inhibition of drug-metabolizing enzymes and identifying the drug-metabolizing enzymes responsible for the metabolism of drugs, in Rodrigues AD (ed): New York: Marcel Decker. In press.

Madan A, Williams TD, Faiman MD: Glutathione- and glutathione-*S*-transferase-dependent oxidative desulfuration of the thione xenobiotic diethyldithiocarbamate methyl ester. *Mol Pharmacol* 46:1217–1225, 1994.

Mannervik B, Awasthi YC, Board PG, et al: Nomenclature for human glutathione transferases. *Biochem J* 282:305–308, 1992.

Mantle TJ, Pickett CB, Hayes JD (eds): *Glutathione S-Transferases and Carcinogenesis*. London: Taylor and Francis, 1987, pp 1–267.

McClain RM: The significance of hepatic microsomal enzyme induction and altered thyroid function in rats: Implications for thyroid gland neoplasia. *Toxicol Pathol* 17:294–306, 1989.

McLeod HL, Fang L, Luo X, et al: Ethnic differences in erythrocyte catechol-*O*-methyltransferase activity in black and white Americans. *J Pharmacol Exp Ther* 270:26–29, 1994.

Meyer UA: The molecular basis of genetic polymorphisms of drug metabolism. *J Pharm Pharmacol* 46(suppl 1):409–415, 1994.

Mihara K, Svensson USH, Tybring G, et al: Stereospecific analysis of omeprazole supports artemisinin as a potent inducer of CYP2C19. *Fundam Clin Pharmacol* 13:671–675, 1999.

Miners JO, Mackenzie PI: Drug glucuronidation in humans. *Pharmacol Ther* 51:347–369, 1992.

Mirsalis JC, Butterworth BE: Induction of unscheduled DNA synthesis in rat hepatocytes following in vivo treatment with dinitrotoluene. *Carcinogenesis* 3:241–245, 1982.

Molina MA, Sitja-Arnau M, Lemoine MG, et al: Increased cyclooxygenase-2 expression in human pancreatic carcinomas and cell lines: Growth inhibition by nonsteroidal anti-inflammatory drugs. *Cancer Res* 59:4356–4362, 1999.

Monks TJ, Anders MW, Dekant W, et al: Contemporary issues in toxicology: Glutathione conjugate mediated toxicities. *Toxicol Pharmacol* 106:1–19, 1990.

Muerhoff AS, Griffin KJ, Johnson EF: The peroxisome proliferator-activated receptor mediates the induction of CYP4A6, a cytochrome P450 fatty acid ω-hydroxylase, by clofibric acid. *J Biol Chem* 267:10951–10953, 1992.

Mulder GJ (ed): *Sulfation of Drugs and Related Compounds*. Boca Raton, FL: CRC Press, 1981.

Nagata K, Yamazoe Y: Pharmacogenetics of sulfotransferase. *Annu Rev Pharmacol Toxicol* 40:159–176, 2000.

Nebert D: Drug-metabolizing enzymes in ligand-modulated transcription. *Biochem Pharmacol* 47:25–37, 1994.

Negishi M, Uno T, Darden TA, et al: Structural flexibility and functional versatility of mammalian P450 enzymes. *FASEB J* 10:683–689, 1996.

Nelson DR, Kamataki T, Waxman DJ, et al: The P450 superfamily: Update on new sequences, gene mapping, accession numbers, early trivial names, and nomenclature. *DNA Cell Biol* 12:1–51, 1993.

Nguyen T, Rushmore TH, Pickett CB: Transcriptional regulation of a rat liver glutathione *S*-transferase Ya subunit gene. *J Biol Chem* 269:13656–13663, 1994.

Ogura K, Nishiyama T, Takubo H, et al: Suicidal inactivation of human dihydropyrimidine dehydrogenase by (E)-5-(2-bromovinyl)uracil derived from the antiviral, sorivudine. *Cancer Lett* 122:107–113, 1998.

Okey AB: Enzyme induction in the cytochrome P450 system. *Pharmacol Ther* 45:241–298, 1990.

Omura T: Forty years of cytochrome P450. *Biochem Biophys Res Comm* 266:690–698, 1999.

Oshima M, Dinchuk JE, Kargman SL, et al: Suppression of intestinal polyposis in APC delta716 knockout mice by inhibition of cyclooxygenase-2 (COX-2). *Cell* 87:803–809, 1996.

Owens IS, Ritter JK: The novel bilirubin/phenol UDP-glucuronosyltransferase *UGT1* gene locus: Implications for multiple nonhemolytic familial hyperbilirubinemia phenotypes. *Pharmacogenetics* 2:93–108, 1992.

Parkinson A, Hurwitz A: Omeprazole and the induction of human cytochrome P450: A response to concerns about potential adverse effects. *Gastroenterology* 100:1157–1164, 1991.

Paulson GD, Caldwell J, Hutson DH, Menn JJ (eds): *Xenobiotic Conjugation Chemistry*. Washington, DC: American Chemical Society, 1986, pp 1–358.

Peck CC, Temple R, Collins JM: Understanding consequences of concurrent therapies. *JAMA* 269:1550–1552, 1993.

Penning TM: Molecular endocrinology of hydroxysteroid dehydrogenases. *Endocr Rev* 18:281–305. 1997.

Pianezza ML, Sellers EM, Tyndale RF: Nicotine metabolism defect reduces smoking. *Nature* 393:750, 1998.

Pichard L, Fabre I, Fabre G, et al: Cyclosporin A drug interactions: Screening for inducers and inhibitors of cytochrome P450 (cyclosporin A oxidase) in primary cultures of human hepatocytes and in liver microsomes. *Drug Metab Dispos* 18:595–606, 1990.

Pirmohamed M, Park BK: Metabolic models of cytotoxicity, in Woolf TF (ed): *Handbook of Drug Metabolism*. New York: Marcel Dekker, 1999, pp 443–476.

Pohl LR, Kenna JG, Satoh H, et al: Neoantigens associated with halothane hepatitis. *Drug Metab Rev* 20:203–217, 1989.

Poland A, Palen D, Glover E: Analysis of the four alleles of the murine aryl hydrocarbon receptor. *Mol Pharmacol* 46:915–921, 1994.

Porter TD, Coon MJ: Multiplicity of isoforms, substrates, and catalytic and regulatory mechanisms. *J Biol Chem* 266:13469–13472, 1991.

Prescott LF: Paracetamol, alcohol and the liver. *Br J Clin Pharmacol* 49:291–301, 1999.

Probst MR, Beer M, Beer D, et al: Molecular cloning of a novel esterase involved in the metabolic activation of arylamine carcinogens with high sequence similarity to hormone-sensitive lipase. *J Biol Chem* 269:21650–21656, 1994.

Prochaska HJ, Talalay P: Regulatory mechanisms of monofunctional and bifunctional anticarcinogenic enzyme inducers in murine liver. *Cancer Res* 48:4776–4782, 1992.

Purohit V, Basu AK: Mutagenicity of nitroaromatic compounds. *Chem Res Toxicol* 13:673–692, 2000.

Radjendirane V, Jaiswal AK: Antioxidant response element-mediated 2,3,7,8-tetrachlorodibenzo-*p*-dioxin (TCDD) induction of human NAD(P)H:quinone oxidoreductase 1 gene expression. *Biochem Pharmacol* 58:1649–1655, 1999.

Rahman A, Korzekwa KR, Grogan J, et al: Selective biotransformation of taxol to 6*A*-hydroxytaxol by human cytochrome P450 2C8. *Cancer Res* 54:5543–5546, 1994.

Rajagopalan KV: Xanthine oxidase and aldehyde oxidase, in Jakoby WB (ed): *Enzymatic Basis of Detoxication*. Vol 1. New York: Academic Press, 1980, pp 295–306.

Radominska-Pandya A, Czernik PJ, Little JM, et al: Structural and functional studies of UDP-glucuronosyltransferases. *Drug Metab Rev* 31:817–899, 1999.

Rao SI, Duffel MW: Inhibition of aryl sulfotransferase by carboxylic acids. *Drug Metab Dispos* 19:543–545, 1991.

Ratnayake JH, Hanna PE, Anders MW, Duggan DE: Sulfoxide reduction in vitro reduction of sulindac by rat hepatic cytosolic enzymes. *Drug Metab Dispos* 9:85–87, 1981.

Rendic S, Di Carlo FJ: Human cytochrome P450 enzymes: A status report summarizing their reactions, substrates, inducers and inhibitors. *Drug Metab Rev* 29:413–580, 1997.

Rettie A, Wienkers L, Gonzalez FJ, et al: Impaired (*S*)-warfarin metabolism catalyzed by the R144C allelic variant of CYP2C9. *Pharmacogenetics* 4:39–42, 1994.

Rettie AE, Fisher MB: Transformation enzymes: Oxidative; non-P450, in Woolf TF (ed): *Handbook of Drug Metabolism*. New York: Marcel Dekker, 1999, pp 131–151.

Riley RJ, Workman P: DT-diaphorase and cancer chemotherapy. *Biochem Pharmacol* 43:1657–1669, 1992.

Rodrigues AD: Comparison of levels of aldehyde oxidase with cytochrome P450 activities in human liver in vitro. *Biochem Pharmacol* 48:197–200, 1994.

Rodrigues AD: Intergrated cytochrome P450 reaction phenotyping: Attempting to bridge the gap between cDNA-expressed cytochromes P450 and native human liver microsomes. *Biochem Pharmacol* 57:465–480, 1999.

Rushmore TH, Morton MR, Pickett CB: The antioxidant responsive element: Activation by oxidative stress and identification of the DNA consensus sequence required for functional activity. *J Biol Chem* 266:11632–11639, 1991.

Ryan DE, Levin W: Purification and characterization of hepatic microsomal cytochrome P450. *Pharmacol Ther* 45:153–239, 1990.

Rychter MD, Land SJ, King CM: Histological localization of acetyltransferases in human tissue. *Cancer Lett* 143:99–102, 1999.

Sano M, Ernesto C, Ronald MS, Thomas RG, et al: A controlled trial of selegiline or α-tocopherol, or both as treatment for Alzheimer's disease. *N Engl J Med* 336:1216–1222, 1997.

Satoh T: Role of carboxylesterases in xenobiotic metabolism. *Rev Biochem Toxicol* 8:155–181, 1987.

Satoh T, Hosokawa M: The mammalian carboxylesterases: From molecules to functions. *Annu Rev Pharmacol Toxicol* 38:257–288, 1998.

Saunders MP, Patterson AV, Chinje EC, et al: NADPH: Cytochrome-c (P450) reductase activates tirapazamine (SR4233) to restore hypoxic and oxic cytotoxicity in an aerobic resistant derivative of the A459 lung cancer cell line. *Br J Canc* 82:651–656, 2000.

Schlichting I, Berendzen J, Chu K, et al: The catalytic pathway of cytochrome P450cam at atomic resolution. *Science* 287:1615–1622, 2000.

Seitz HK, Oneta CM: Gastrointestinal alcohol dehydrogenase. *Nutrition Rev* 56:52–60, 1998.

Senter PD, Marquardt H, Thomas BA, et al. The role of rat serum carboxylesterase in the activation of paclitaxel and camptothecin prodrugs. *Cancer Res* 56:1471–1474, 1996.

Shih JC, Chen K, Ridd MJ: Monoamide oxidase: From genes to behavior. *Annu Rev Neurosci* 22:197–217, 1999.

Shimada T, Yamazaki H, Mimura M, et al: Interindividual variations in human liver cytochrome P450 enzymes involved in the oxidation of drugs, carcinogens and toxic chemicals: Studies with liver microsomes of 30 Japanese and 30 Caucasians. *J Pharmacol Exp Ther* 270:414–423, 1994.

Shimizu Y, Nakatsuru Y, Ichinose M, et al: Benzo[a]pyrene carcinogenicity is lost in mice lacking the aryl hydrocarbon receptor. *Proc Nat Acad Sci USA* 97:779–782, 2000.

Shirley MA, Guan X, Kaiser DG, et al: Taurine conjugation of ibuprofen in humans and in rat liver in vitro: Relationship to metabolic chiral inversion. *J Pharmacol Exp Ther* 269:1166–1175, 1994.

Sies H, Ketterer B (eds): *Glutathione Conjugation Mechanisms and Biological Significance*. London: Academic Press, 1988, pp 1–480.

Smith G, Stubbins MJ, Harries LW, Wolf CR: Molecular genetics of the human cytochrome P450 monooxygenase superfamily. *Xenobiotica* 28:1129–1165, 1998.

Sorenson RC, Primo-Parmo SL, Kuo C-L, et al: Reconsideration of the catalytic center and mechanism of mammalian paraoxonase/arylesterase. *Proc Natl Acad Sci USA* 92:7187–7191, 1995.

Spahn-Langguth H, Benet LZ: Acyl glucuronides revisited: Is the glucuronidation process a toxification as well as a detoxification mechanism? *Drug Metab Rev* 24:5–48, 1992.

Strange RC, Jones PW, Fryer AA: Glutathione S-transferase: Genetics and role in toxicology. *Toxicol Lett* 112–113:357–363, 2000.

Strobl GR, von Kruedener S, Stockigt J, et al: Development of a pharmacophore for inhibition of human liver cytochrome P450 2D6: Molecular modeling and inhibition studies. *J Med Chem* 36:1136–1145, 1993.

Subramanyam B, Woolf T, Castagnoli N: Studies on the in vitro conversion of haloperidol to a potentially neurotoxic pyridinium metabolite. *Chem Res Toxicol* 4:123–128, 1991.

Sugihara K, Kitamura S, Tatsumi K: Involvement of mammalian liver cytosols and aldehyde oxidase in reductive metabolism of zonisamide. *Drug Metab Dispos* 24:199–202, 1996.

Sugiura M, Iwasaki K, Kato R: Reduction of tertiary amine *N*-oxides by microsomal cytochrome P450. *Mol Pharmacol* 12:322–334, 1976.

Sugiura M, Kato R: Reduction of tertiary amine *N*-oxides by rat liver mitochondria. *J Pharmacol Exp Ther* 200:25–32, 1977.

Sundseth SS, Waxman DJ: Sex-dependent expression and clofibrate inducibility of cytochrome P450 4A fatty acid ω-hydroxylases. *J Biol Chem* 267:3915–3921, 1992.

Tang B-K, Kalow W: Variable activation of lovastatin by hydrolytic enzymes in human plasma and liver. *Eur J Clin Pharmacol* 47:449–451, 1995.

Taningher M, Malacarne D, Izzotti A, et al: Drug metabolism polymorphisms as modulators of cancer susceptibility. *Mutat Res* 436:227–261, 1999.

Terao M, Kurosaki M, Demontis S, et al: Isolation and characterization of the human aldehyde oxidase gene: Conservation of intron/exon boundaries with xanthine oxidoreductase gene indicates a common origin. *Biochem J* 332:383–393, 1998.

Thummel KE, Wilkinson GR: In vitro and in vivo drug interactions involving human CYP3A. *Annu Rev Pharmaocol Toxicol* 38:389–430, 1998.

Tinguely JN, Wermuth B: Identification of the reactive cysteine residue (Cys227) in human carbonyl reductase. *Eur J Biochem* 260:9–14, 1999.

Tucker GT: Clinical implications of genetic polymorphism in drug metabolism. *J Pharm Pharmacol* 46(suppl 1):417–424, 1994.

Tukey RH, Stassburg CP: Human UDP-glucuronosyltransferases: Metabolism, expression, and disease. *Annu Rev Pharmacol Toxicol* 40:581–616, 2000.

Vatsis KP, Weber WW, Bell DA, et al: Nomenclature for *N*-acetyltransferases. *Pharmacogenetics* 5:1–17, 1995. (Updated in *Pharmacogenetics* 10:291–292, 2000.)

Walton MI, Wolf CR, Workman P: The role of cytochrome P450 and cytochrome P450 reductase in the reductive bioactivation of the novel benzotriazine di-*N*-oxide hypoxic cytotoxin 3-amino-1,2,4-benzotriazine-1,4-dioxide (SR 4233, WIN 59075) by mouse liver. *Biochem Pharmacol* 44:251–259, 1992.

Wang C, Bammler TK, Guo Y, et al: *Mu*-class GSTs are responsible for aflatoxin B_1-8,9-epoxide-conjugating activity in the nonhuman primate *Macaca fascicularis* liver. *Toxicol Sci* 56:26–36, 2000.

Wardman P, Dennis PF, Everett SA, Patel KB, Stratford MR, Tracy M: Radicals from one-electron reduction of nitro compounds, aromatic *N*-oxides and quinones: The kinetic basis for hypoxic-selective, bioreductive drugs. *Biochem Soc Symp* 61:171–194, 1995.

Wardman P, Priyadarsini KI, Dennis MF, et al: Chemical properties which control selectivity and efficacy of aromatic *N*-oxide bioreductive drugs. *Br J Canc (Suppl)* 27:S70–S74, 1996.

Waterman MR, Johnson EF (eds): *Cytochrome P450. Methods in Enzymology*. Vol 206. New York: Academic Press, 1991.

Watkins PB: Noninvasive tests of CYP3A enzymes. *Pharmacogenetics* 4:171–184, 1994.

Waxman DJ: P450 gene induction by structurally diverse xenochemicals: Central role of nuclear receptors CAR, PXR, and PPAR. *Arch Biochem Biophys* 369(1):11–23, 1999.

Waxman DJ, Pampori NA, Ram PA, et al: Interpulse interval in circulating growth hormone patterns regulates sexually dimorphic expression of hepatic cytochrome P450. *Biochemistry* 88:6868–6872, 1991.

Weiner H, Flynn TG (eds): *Enzymology and Molecular Biology of Carbonyl Metabolism 2: Aldehyde Dehydrogenase, Alcohol Dehydrogenase, and Aldo-Keto Reductase*. New York: Liss, 1989.

Weinshilboum R: Methyltransferase pharmacogenetics. *Pharmacol Ther* 43:77–90, 1989.

Weinshilboum R: Sulfotransferase pharmacogenetics, in Kalow W (ed): *Pharmacogenetics of Drug Metabolism*. New York: Pergamon Press, 1992a, pp 227–242.

Weinshilboum RM: Methylation pharmacogenetics: Thiopurine methyltransferase as a model system. *Xenobiotica* 22:1055–1071, 1992b.

Weinshilboum RM, Otterness DM, Atsoy IA, et al: Sulfotransferase molecular biology: cDNAs and genes. *FASEB J* 11:3–14, 1997.

Weinshilboum RM, Otterness DM, Szumlanski CL: Methylation pharmacogenetics: Catechol *O*-methyltransferase, thiopurine methyltransferase, and histamine *N*-methyltransferase. *Annu Rev Pharmacol Toxicol* 39:19–52, 1999.

Weyler W, Hsu YP, Breakefield XO: Biochemistry and genetics of monoamine oxidase, in Kalow W (ed): *Pharmacogenetics of Drug Metabolism*. New York: Pergamon Press, 1992, pp 333–366.

Whalen R, Boyer TD: Human glutathione S-transferases. *Semin Liver Dis* 18:345–358, 1998.

Whitcomb DC, Block GD: Association of acetaminophen hepatotoxicity with fasting and ethanol use. *JAMA* 272:1845–1850, 1994.

Whitfield JB, Pang D, Bucholz KK, et al: Monoamine oxidase: Associations with alcohol dependence, smoking and other measures of psychopathology. *Psychol Med* 20:443–454, 2000.

Whitlock JP: Mechanistic aspects of dioxin action. *Chem Res Toxicol* 6:754–763, 1993.

Wilkinson GR, Guengerich FP, Branch RA: Genetic polymorphism of *S*-mephenytoin hydroxylation. *Pharmacol Ther* 43:53–76, 1989.

Williams RT: *Detoxification Mechanisms*, 2d ed. New York: Wiley, 1971.

Wong JMY, Kalow W, Kadar D, et al: Carbonyl (phenone) reductase in human liver: Inter-individual variability. *Pharmacogenetics* 3:110–115, 1993.

Wrighton SA, Stevens JC: The human hepatic cytochromes P450 involved in drug metabolism. *Crit Rev Toxicol* 22:1–21, 1992.

Wrighton SA, Vandenbranden M, Stevens JC, et al: In vitro methods for assessing human hepatic drug metabolism: Their use in drug development. *Drug Metab Rev* 25:453–484, 1993.

Yan B, Yang D, Brady M, Parkinson A: Rat kidney carboxylesterase: Cloning, sequencing, cellular localization, and relationship to rat liver hydrolase. *J Biol Chem* 269:29688–29696, 1994.

Yao K-S, Hageboutros A, Ford P, O'Dwyer PJ: Involvement of activator protein-1 and nuclear factor-κB transcription factors in the control of the DT-diaphorase expression induced by mitomycin C treatment. *Mol Pharmacol* 51:422–430, 1997.

Yoshida A, Rzhetsky A, Hsu LC, Chang C. Human aldehyde dehydrogenase gene family. *Eur J Biochem* 251:549–557, 1998.

Zand R, Sidney N, Slattery J, et al: Inhibition and induction of cytochrome P4502E1-catalyzed oxidation by isoniazid in humans. *Clin Pharmacol Ther* 54:142–149, 1993.

Zhang Y, Talalay P, Cho C-G, Posner GH: A major inducer of anticarcinogenic protective enzymes from broccoli: Isolation and elucidation of structure. *Proc Natl Acad Sci USA* 89:2399–2403, 1992.

Zhu BT, Liehr JG: Inhibition of the catechol-*O*-methyltransferase-catalyzed *O*-methylation of 2- and 4-hydroxyestradiol by catecholamines: Implications for the mechanism of estrogen-induced carcinogenesis. *Arch Biochem Biophys* 304:248–256, 1993.

Ziegler DM: Recent studies on the structure and function of multisubstrate flavin monooxygenases. *Annu Rev Pharmacol Toxicol* 33:179–199, 1993.

CHAPTER 7

TOXICOKINETICS

Michele A. Medinsky and John L. Valentine

INTRODUCTION

The study of the kinetics of chemicals was originally initiated for drugs and consequently was termed *pharmacokinetics.* However, toxicology is not limited to the study of adverse drug effects but entails an investigation of the deleterious effects of all chemicals. Therefore, the study of the kinetics of xenobiotics is more properly called *toxicokinetics.* Toxicokinetics refers to the modeling and mathematical description of the time course of disposition (absorption, distribution, biotransformation, and excretion) of xenobiotics in the whole organism. The classic way to describe the kinetics of drugs is to represent the body as consisting of one or two compartments even if those compartments have no apparent physiologic or anatomic reality. An alternate approach, physiologically based toxicokinetics, represents the body as a series of mass balance equations that describe each organ or tissue on the basis of physiologic considerations. It should be emphasized that there is no inherent contradiction between the classic and physiologically based approaches. Classic pharmacokinetics, as will be shown, requires certain assumptions that the physiologically based models do not require. Under ideal conditions, physiologic models can predict tissue concentrations, whereas classic models cannot. However, the values of the appropriate parameters are often unknown or inexact, hampering meaningful physiologically based toxicokinetic modeling.

CLASSIC TOXICOKINETICS

Often, it is difficult to obtain relevant biological tissues in order to ascertain a chemical or chemical concentration in the body and then relate that chemical concentration to a toxicologic response. The least invasive and simplest method to gather information on absorption, distribution, metabolism, and elimination of a compound is by sampling blood or plasma over time. If one assumes that the concentration of a compound in blood or plasma is in equilibrium with concentrations in tissues, then changes in plasma chemical concentrations reflect changes in tissue chemical concentrations, and relatively simple pharmacokinetic models can adequately describe the behavior of that chemical in the body. Compartmental pharmacokinetic models consist of a central compartment representing plasma and tissues that rapidly equilibrate with chemical, connected to one or more peripheral compartments that represent tissues that more slowly equilibrate with chemical (Fig. 7-1). Chemical is administered into the central compartment and distributes between central and peripheral compartments. Chemical elimination occurs from the central compartment, which is assumed to contain rapidly perfused tissues capable of eliminating chemical (e.g., kidneys and liver). Advantages of compartmental pharmacokinetic models are that they require no information on tissue physiology or anatomic structure. These models are valuable in predicting the plasma chemical concentrations at different doses, in establishing the time course of chemical in plasma and tissues and the extent of chemical accumulation with multiple doses, and in determining effective dose and dose regimens in toxicity studies (Gibaldi and Perrier, 1982).

One-Compartment Model

The simplest toxicokinetic analysis entails measurement of the plasma concentrations of a xenobiotic at several time points after the administration of a bolus intravenous injection. If the data obtained yield a straight line when they are plotted as the logarithms of plasma concentrations versus time, the kinetics of the xenobiotic can be described with a one-compartment model (Fig. 7-2). Compounds whose toxicokinetics can be described with a one-compartment model rapidly equilibrate, or mix uniformly, between blood and the various tissues relative to the rate of elimination. The one-compartment model depicts the body as a homogeneous unit. This does not mean that the concentration of a compound is the same throughout the body, but it does assume that the changes that

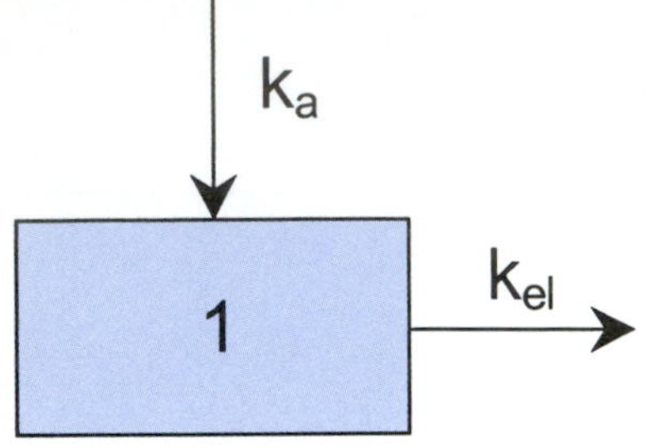

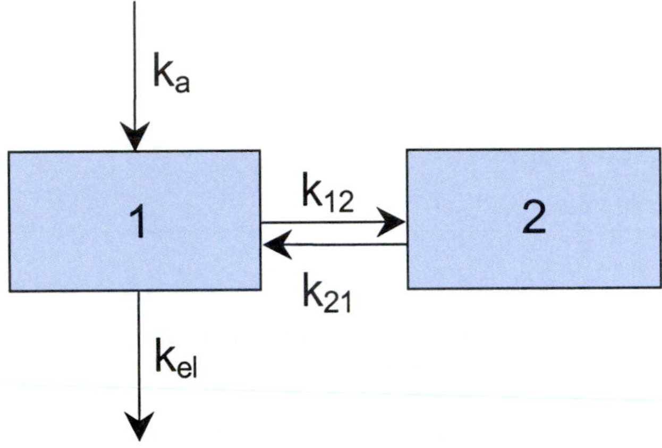

Figure 7-1. ***Compartmental pharmacokinetic models where k_a is the first-order extravascular absorption rate constant into the central compartment (1), k_{el} is the first-order elimination rate constant from the central compartment (1), and k_{12} and k_{21} are the first-order rate constants for distribution of chemical into and out of the peripheral compartment (2) in a two-compartment model.***

occur in the plasma concentration reflect proportional changes in tissue chemical concentrations (Rowland and Tozer, 1980).

In the simplest case, a curve of this type can be described by the expression

$$C = C_0 \times e^{-k_{el} \times t}$$

where C is the blood or plasma chemical concentration over time t, C_0 is the initial blood concentration at time $t = 0$, and k_{el} is the first-order elimination rate constant with dimensions of reciprocal time (e.g., t^{-1}).

Two-Compartment Model

After the rapid intravenous administration of some chemicals, the semilogarithmic plot of plasma concentration versus time does not yield a straight line but a curve that implies more than one dispositional phase. In these instances, the chemical requires a longer time for its concentration in tissues to reach equilibrium with the concentration in plasma, and a multicompartmental analysis of the results is necessary (Fig. 7-2). A multiexponential mathematical equation then best characterizes the elimination of the xenobiotic from the plasma.

Generally, a curve of this type can be resolved into two monoexponential terms (a two-compartment model) and is described by

$$C = A \times e^{-\alpha \times t} + B \times e^{-\beta \times t}$$

where A and B are proportionality constants and α and β are the first-order distribution and elimination rate constants, respectively (Fig. 7-2). During the distribution (α) phase, concentrations of the chemical in the plasma decrease more rapidly than they do in the postdistributional elimination (β) phase. The distribution phase may last for only a few minutes or for hours or days. Whether the distribution phase becomes apparent depends on the time when the first plasma samples are obtained, and on the relative difference in the rates of distribution and elimination. If the rate of distribution is considerably rapid relative to elimination, the timing of blood sampling becomes critical in the ability to distinguish a distribution phase. The equivalent of k_{el} in a one-compartment model is β in a two-compartment model.

Occasionally, the plasma concentration profile of many compounds cannot be described satisfactorily by an equation with two exponential terms—for example, if the chemical has an exceptionally slow distribution into and redistribution out of a deep peripheral compartment or tissue. Sometimes three or four exponential terms are needed to fit a curve to the plot of log C versus time. Such compounds are viewed as displaying characteristics of three- or four-compartment open models. The principles for dealing with such models are the same as those used for the two-compartment open model, but the mathematics are more complex and beyond the scope of this discussion.

Elimination

Elimination includes biotransformation, exhalation, and excretion. The elimination of a chemical from the body whose disposition is described by a one-compartment model usually occurs through a first-order process; that is, the rate of elimination at any time is proportional to the amount of the chemical in the body at that time. First-order reactions occur at chemical concentrations that are not sufficiently high to saturate elimination processes.

The equation for a monoexponential model, $C = C_0 \times e^{-k_{el} \times t}$, can be transformed to a logarithmic equation that has the general form of a straight line, $y = mx + b$:

$$\log C = -(k_{el}/2.303) \times t + \log C_0$$

where log C_0 represents the y-intercept or initial concentration, and $-(k_{el}/2.303)$ represents the slope of the line. The first-order elimination rate constant (k_{el}) can be determined from the slope of the log C versus time plot (*i.e.*, $k_{el} = -2.303 \times slope$). The first-order elimination rate constants k_{el} and β have units of reciprocal time (*e.g.*, $\min^{-1}$ and h^{-1}) and are independent of dose.

Mathematically, the fraction of dose remaining in the body over time (C/C_0) is calculated using the elimination rate constant by rearranging the equation for the monoexponential function and taking the antilog to yield

$$C/C_0 = \text{Anti log } [(-k_{el}/2.303) \times t]$$

Thus, if the elimination rate constant is, for example, 0.3 h^{-1}, the percentage of the dose remaining in the body ($C/C_0 \times 100$) and the percentage of the dose eliminated from the body after 1 h,

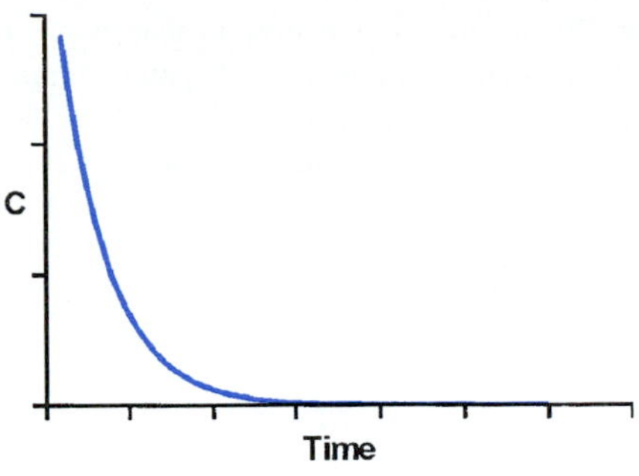

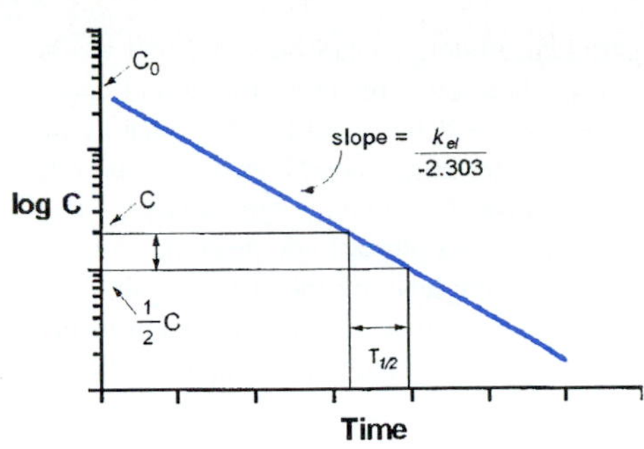

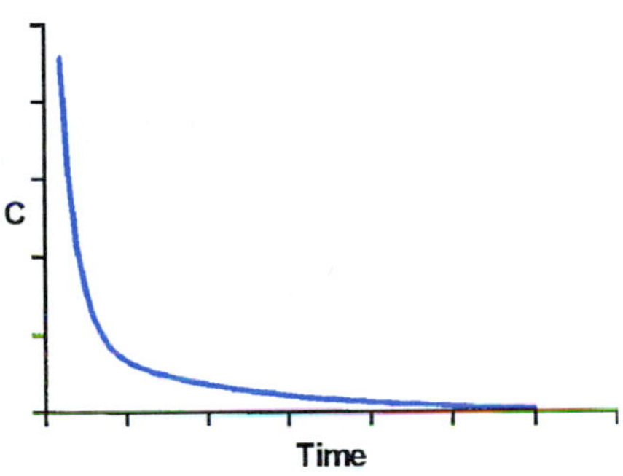

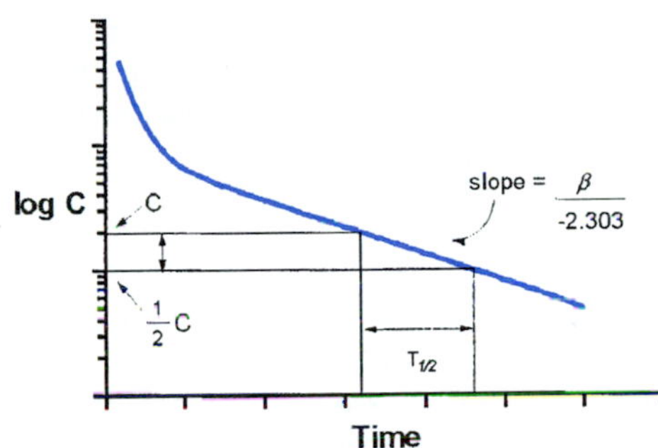

Figure 7-2. Concentration versus time curves of chemicals exhibiting behavior of a one-compartment pharmacokinetic model (top) *and a two-compartment pharmacokinetic model (bottom) on a linear scale* (left) *and a semilogarithmic scale* (right).

Elimination rate constants, k_{el} and β are determined from the slope of the log-linear concentration versus time curve. Half-life ($T_{1/2}$) is the time required for blood or plasma chemical concentration to decrease by one-half. C_0 is the concentration of the chemical at t = 0 determined by extrapolating the log-linear concentration time curve to the Y-axis (t = 0).

i.e., $1 - (C/C_0 \times 100)$, are 74 and 26 percent, respectively, regardless of the dose administered (Table 7-1). The percentage of the total dose eliminated at one hour is said to be independent of dose.

Apparent Volume of Distribution

In a one-compartment model, all chemical is assumed to distribute into plasma and tissues instantaneously. The apparent volume of distribution (V_d) is a proportionality constant that relates the total amount of chemical in the body to the concentration of a xenobiotic in plasma, and is typically described in units of liters or liters per kilogram of body weight (Kato et al., 1987). V_d is the apparent space into which an amount of chemical is distributed in the body to result in a given plasma concentration. For example, envision the body as a tank containing an unknown volume (L) of well mixed water. If a known amount (mg) of dye is placed into the water, the volume of that water can be calculated indirectly by determining the dye concentration (mg/L) that resulted after the dye has equilibrated in the tank simply by dividing the amount of dye added to the tank by the resultant concentration of the dye in water. Synonymously, the apparent volume of distribution of a chemical in the body is determined after intravenous bolus administration, and is mathematically defined as the quotient of the amount of chemical in the body and its plasma concentration. V_d is calculated as

$$V_d = Dose_{iv}/(\beta \times AUC_0^\infty)$$

where $Dose_{iv}$ is the intravenous dose or known amount of chemical in body at time zero; β is the elimination rate constant; and AUC_0^∞ is the area under the chemical concentration versus time curve from time zero to infinity. The product, $\beta \times AUC_0^\infty$, is the concentration of xenobiotic in plasma.

Table 7-1
Elimination of Four Different Doses of a Chemical at 1 Hour After Administration as Described by a One-Compartment Open Model and First-Order Toxicokinetics with a k_{el} of 0.3 h^{-1}

DOSE, mg	CHEMICAL REMAINING, mg	CHEMICAL ELIMINATED, mg	CHEMICAL ELIMINATED, % of dose
10	7.4	2.6	26
30	22	8	26
90	67	23	26
250	185	65	26

For a one-compartment model, V_d can be simplified by the equation $V_d = Dose_{iv}/C_0$, where C_0 is the concentration of chemical in plasma at time zero. C_0 is determined by extrapolating the plasma disappearance curve after intravenous injection to the zero time point (Fig. 7-2). V_d is correctly called the *apparent volume of distribution* because it has no direct physiologic meaning and usually does not refer to a real biological volume. The magnitude of the V_d term is chemical-specific and represents the extent of distribution of chemical out of plasma and into other body tissues (Table 7-2). Thus, for chemicals that readily distribute into extravascular tissues, V_d often exceeds actual body spaces. A chemical with high affinity for tissues will also have a large volume of distribution. In fact, binding to tissues may be so avid that the V_d of a chemical is much larger than the actual body volume. Alternatively, a chemical that predominantly remains in the plasma will have a low V_d that approximates the volume of plasma (Wang et al., 1994). Once the V_d for a chemical is known, it can be used to estimate the amount of chemical remaining in the body at any time if the plasma concentration at that time is also known by the relationship $X_c = V_d \times C_p$, where X_c is the amount of chemical in the body and C_p is the plasma chemical concentration.

Clearance

Chemicals are cleared from the body by various routes, for example, via excretion by the kidneys or intestines, biotransformation by the liver, or exhalation by the lungs. Clearance is an important toxicokinetic concept that describes the rate of chemical elimination from the body (Shargel and Yu, 1993). Clearance is described in terms of volume of fluid containing chemical that is cleared per unit of time. Thus, clearance has the units of flow (milliliters per minute). A clearance of 100 mL/min means that 100 mL of blood or plasma containing xenobiotic is completely cleared in each minute that passes. The overall efficiency of the removal of a chemical from the body can be characterized by clearance. High values of clearance indicate efficient and generally rapid removal, whereas low clearance values indicate slow and less efficient removal of a xenobiotic from the body. *Total body clearance* is defined as the sum of clearances by individual eliminating organs:

$$Cl = Cl_r + Cl_h + Cl_i + \ldots$$

where Cl_r depicts renal, Cl_h hepatic, and Cl_i intestinal clearance. Clearance of xenobiotics from the blood by a particular organ cannot be higher than blood flow to that organ. For example, for a xenobiotic that is eliminated by hepatic biotransformation, hepatic clearance cannot exceed the hepatic blood flow rate even if the maximum rate of metabolism in the liver is more rapid than the rate of hepatic blood flow, because the rate of overall hepatic clearance is limited by the delivery of the xenobiotic to the metabolic enzymes in the liver via the blood. After intravenous, bolus administration, total body clearance is defined as

$$Cl = Dose_{iv}/AUC_0^{\infty}$$

Clearance can also be calculated if the volume of distribution and elimination rate constants are known, and can be defined as $Cl = V_d \times k_{el}$ for a one-compartment model and $Cl = V_d \times \beta$ for a two-compartment model. Clearance is an exceedingly important concept.

Half-Life

Another important and frequently used parameter that characterizes the time course of xenobiotics in an organism is the half-life of elimination ($T_{1/2}$). Half-life is the time required for the blood or plasma chemical concentration to decrease by one-half, and is dependent upon both volume of distribution and clearance. $T_{1/2}$ can be calculated if V_d and Cl are known:

$$T_{1/2} = (0.693 \times V_d)/Cl$$

The above relationship among $T_{1/2}$, V_d and Cl demonstrates that care should be taken in analyses of data when relying upon $T_{1/2}$ as the sole determinant parameter in toxicokinetic studies, since $T_{1/2}$ is influenced by both the volume of distribution for a chemical and the rate by which the chemical is cleared from the blood. For a fixed V_d, $T_{1/2}$ decreases as Cl increases, because chemical is being removed from this fixed volume faster as clearance increases (Fig. 7-3). Conversely, as the V_d increases, $T_{1/2}$ increases for a fixed Cl since the volume of fluid that must be cleared of chemical increases but the rate of clearance does not.

Because of the relationship $T_{1/2} = 0.693 \times k_{el}$, the half-life of a compound can be calculated after k_{el} (or β) has been determined from the slope of the line that designates the elimination phase on the log C versus time plot. The $T_{1/2}$ can also be determined by means of visual inspection of the log C versus time plot, as shown in Fig. 7-2. For compounds eliminated by first-order ki-

Table 7-2
Volume of Distribution (V_d) for Several Chemicals Compared with Volumes of Body Fluid Compartments

CHEMICAL	V_d (L/kg)	BODY COMPARTMENT
Chloroquine	200	
Desmethylimipramine	40	
Tetracycline	1.3	
	0.6	Total body water
Digitoxin	0.5	
	0.27	Extracellular body water
Salicylic acid	0.15	
	0.045	Plasma

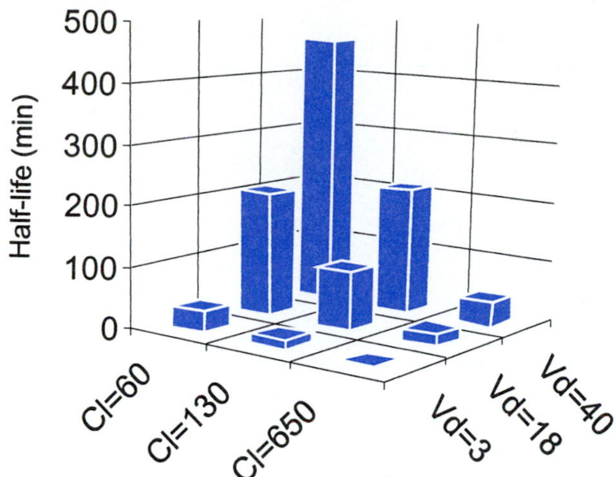

***Figure 7-3. The dependence of* $T_{1/2}$ *on* V_d *and* Cl.**

Renal *Cl* values of 60, 130, and 650 mL/min represent partial reabsorption, glomerular filtration, and tubular secretion, respectively. Values for V_d of 3, 18, and 40 L represent approximate volumes of plasma water, extracellular fluid and total body water, respectively, for an average-sized person.

netics, the time required for the plasma concentration to decrease by one-half is constant. Therefore, xenobiotics eliminated from the body by first-order processes are theoretically never completely eliminated. However, during seven half-lives, 99.2 percent of a chemical is eliminated, and for practical purposes this can be viewed as complete elimination. The half-life of a chemical obeying first-order elimination kinetics is independent of the dose, and does not change with increasing dose.

Saturation Toxicokinetics

As already mentioned, the distribution and elimination of most chemicals occurs by first-order processes. However, as the dose of a compound increases, its volume of distribution or its rate of elimination may change, as shown in Fig. 7-4. This is usually referred to as saturation kinetics. Biotransformation, active transport processes, and protein binding have finite capacities and can be saturated. When the concentration of a chemical in the body is higher than the K_M (chemical concentration at one-half V_{max}, the maximum metabolic capacity), the rate of elimination is no longer proportional to the dose. The transition from first-order to saturation kinetics is important in toxicology because it can lead to prolonged residency time of a compound in the body or increased concentration at the target site of action, which can result in increased toxicity.

Some of the criteria that indicate nonlinear toxicokinetics include the following: (1) The decline in the levels of the chemical in the body is not exponential, (2) AUC_0^∞ is not proportional to the dose, (3) V_d, Cl, k_{el} (or β) *or* $T_{1/2}$ change with increasing dose, (4) the composition of excretory products changes quantitatively or qualitatively with the dose, (5) competitive inhibition by other chemicals that are biotransformed or actively transported by the same enzyme system occurs, and (6) dose-response curves show a nonproportional change in response with an increasing dose, starting at the dose level at which saturation effects become evident.

The elimination of some chemicals from the body is readily saturated. These compounds follow zero-order kinetics. Ethanol is an example of a chemical whose elimination follows zero-order kinetics, with its biotransformation being the rate-limiting step in its elimination (York, 1982). The elimination of ethanol is dependent upon the amount of dose remaining to be eliminated rather than the fraction of dose to be eliminated. As shown in Table 7-3, a constant amount, rather than a constant proportion of ethanol is biotransformed per unit of time regardless of the amount of ethanol present in the body. Important characteristics of zero-order processes are as follows: (1) An arithmetic plot of plasma concentration versus time yields a straight line, (2) the rate or amount of chemical eliminated at any time is constant and is independent of the amount of chemical in the body, and (3) a true $T_{1/2}$ or k_{el} does not exist, but differs depending upon ethanol dose.

By comparison, under first-order elimination kinetics, the elimination rate constant, apparent volume of distribution, clearance and half-life are expected not to change with increasing dose. The important characteristics of first-order elimination are as follows: (1) The rate at which a chemical is eliminated at any time is directly proportional to the amount of that chemical in the body at that time. (2) A semilogarithmic plot of plasma concentration versus time yields a single straight line. (3) The elimination rate constant (k_{el} or β), apparent volume of distribution (V_d), clearance (Cl) and half-life ($T_{1/2}$) are independent of dose. (4) The concentration of the chemical in plasma and other tissues decreases similarly by

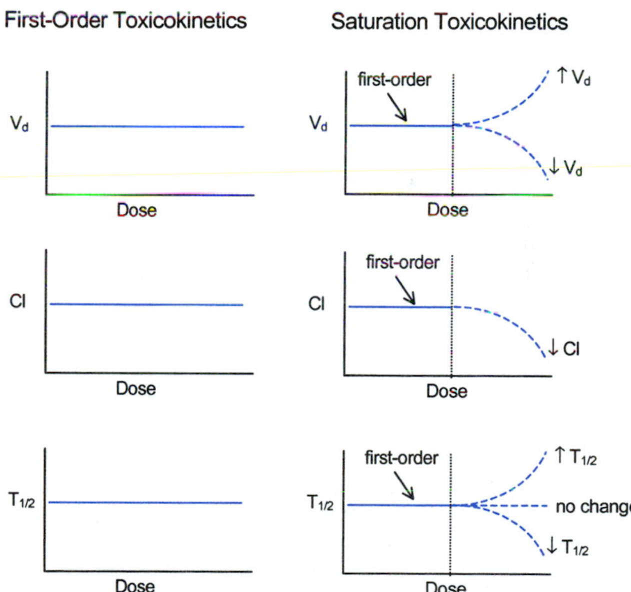

***Figure 7-4.* V_d, Cl *and* $T_{1/2}$ *following first-order toxicokinetics* (left panels) *and changes following saturable toxicokinetics* (right panels).**

Vertical dashed lines represent point of departure from first-order to saturation toxicokinetics. Pharmacokinetic parameters for chemicals that follow first-order toxicokinetics are independent of dose. When protein binding or elimination mechanisms are saturated with increasing dose, pharmacokinetic parameter estimates become dose-dependent. V_d may increase, for example, when plasma protein binding is saturated, allowing more free chemical to distribute into peripheral tissue spaces. Conversely, V_d may decrease with increasing dose if tissue protein binding saturates. Then chemical may redistribute more freely back into plasma. When chemical concentrations exceed the capacity for biotransformation by metabolic enzymes, overall clearance of the chemical decreases. These changes may or may not have effects on $T_{1/2}$ depending upon the magnitude and direction of changes in both V_d and *Cl*.

Table 7-3
Elimination Over Time of a Chemical That Follows Zero-Order Toxicokinetics

TIME, h	ETHANOL REMAINING, mL	ETHANOL ELIMINATED, mL	ETHANOL ELIMINATED, % of that remaining
0	50	0	0
1	40	10	20
2	30	10	25
3	20	10	33
4	10	10	50
5	0	10	100

some constant fraction per unit of time, the elimination rate constant (k_{el} or β).

Bioavailability

For most chemicals in toxicology, exposure occurs by extravascular routes (e.g., inhalation, dermal or oral), and absorption into the systemic circulation is incomplete. The extent of absorption of a xenobiotic can be experimentally determined by comparing the plasma AUC_0^∞ after intravenous and extravascular dosing. The resulting index quantitates the fraction of dosed absorbed systemically and is called *bioavailability* (F). Bioavailability can be determined by using different doses, provided that the compound does not display dose-dependent or saturable kinetics. Pharmacokinetic data following intravenous administration is used as the reference from which to compare extravascular absorption because all chemical is delivered (or 100 percent bioavailable) to the systemic circulation. For example, bioavailability following an oral exposure can be determined as follows:

$$F = (AUC_{po}/Dose_{po}) \times (Dose_{iv}/AUC_{iv})$$

where AUC_{po}, AUC_{iv}, $Dose_{po}$, and $Dose_{iv}$ are the respective area under the plasma concentration versus time curves and doses for oral and intravenous administration. Bioavailabilities for various chemicals range in values between 0 and 1. Complete absorption of chemical is demonstrated when $F = 1$. When $F < 1$, incomplete absorption of chemical is indicated. Bioavailability is an important concept in toxicokinetics. As was discussed earlier, the most critical factor influencing toxicity is not necessarily the dose but rather the concentration of a xenobiotic at the site of action. Xenobiotics are delivered to most organs by the systemic circulation. Therefore, the fraction of a chemical that reaches the systemic circulation is of critical importance in determining toxicity. Several factors can greatly alter this systemic availability, including (1) limited absorption after oral dosing, (2) intestinal first-pass effect, (3) hepatic first-pass effect, and (4) mode of formulation, which affects, for example, dissolution rate or incorporation into micelles (for lipid-soluble compounds).

In summary, for many chemicals, blood or plasma chemical concentration versus time data can be adequately described by a one- or two-compartment, classical pharmacokinetic model when basic assumptions are made (e.g., instantaneous mixing of compartments and first-order kinetics). In some instances, more sophisticated models with increased numbers of compartments will be needed to describe blood or plasma toxicokinetic data; for example if the chemical preferentially distributes into deep peripheral tissues. Modeling and knowledge of toxicokinetic data can be used in deciding on what dose or doses of chemical to use in the planning of toxicology studies (e.g., if specific blood concentrations are desired), in evaluating dose regimens (e.g., intravascular versus extravascular, bolus injection versus infusion or single dosing versus repeated doses), in choosing appropriate sampling times, and in aiding in the evaluation of toxicology data (e.g., what blood or plasma concentrations were achieved to produce a specific response, effects of repeated dosing on accumulation of chemical in the body, etc.).

Computer Software

Several computer software programs are available for compartmental modeling of pharmacokinetic data (e.g., WinNonlin, PKAnalyst, Summit and SAS, among others). Many are menu-driven and operate on Microsoft Windows or Macintosh systems. In general, concentration and time data are entered into a spreadsheet format. The operator then chooses a user-defined model or a specified model from a built-in library to fit curves to concentration versus time data. Convergence of the model occurs through an iterative process to satisfy specific statistical requirements; for example minimizing the sum of square residuals between simulated and observed data. Program outputs include pharmacokinetic parameter estimations and descriptive statistical estimations. A number of software programs also offer graphic output of both test data and model simulations. In summary, a wide variety of options and costs are available that can fit the user's needs.

PHYSIOLOGIC TOXICOKINETICS

The primary difference between *physiologic* compartmental models and *classic* compartmental models lies in the basis underlying the rate constants that describe the transport of chemicals into and out of the compartments (Andersen, 1991). In classic kinetics, the rate constants are defined by the data; thus, these models are often referred to as *data-based.* In physiologic models, the rate constants represent known or hypothesized biological processes, and these models are commonly referred to as *physiologically based.* The concept of incorporating biological realism into the analysis of drug or xenobiotic distribution and elimination is not new. For example, one of the first physiologic models was proposed by Teorell (1937). This model contained all the important determinants in chemical disposition that are considered valid today. Unfortunately, the computational tools required to solve the underlying equations were not available at that time. With advances in computer science, the software and hardware needed to implement physiological models are now well within the reach of toxicologists.

The advantages of physiologically based models compared with classic pharmacokinetics are that (1) these models can provide the time course of distribution of xenobiotics to any organ or tissue, (2) they allow estimation of the effects of changing physiologic parameters on tissue concentrations, (3) the same model can predict the toxicokinetics of chemicals across species by allometric scaling, and (4) complex dosing regimes and saturable processes such as metabolism and binding are easily accommodated (Gargas and Andersen, 1988). The disadvantages are that (1) more information is needed to implement these models compared with classic models, (2) the mathematics can be difficult for many toxicologists to handle, and (3) values for parameters are often ill defined in various species, strains, and disease states. Nevertheless, physiologically based toxicokinetic models are conceptually sound and are potentially useful tools for gaining insight into the kinetics of xenobiotics beyond what classic toxicokinetics can provide.

Basic Model Structure

Physiologic models often look like a number of classic one-compartment models that are linked together. The actual model

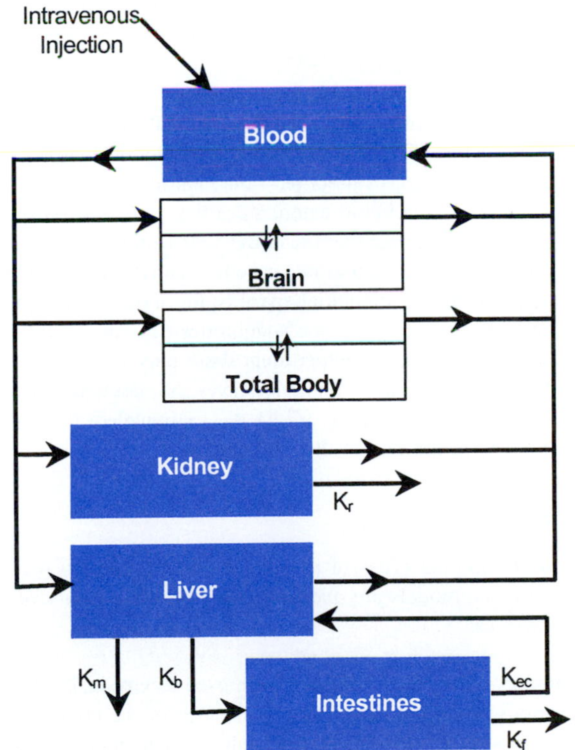

Figure 7-5. Physiologic model for a hypothetical xenobiotic that is soluble in water, has a low vapor pressure (not volatile), and has a relatively large molecular weight* (MW > *100).

This hypothetical chemical is eliminated through metabolism in the liver (K_m), biliary excretion (K_b), renal excretion (K_r) into the urine, and fecal excretion (K_f). The chemical can also undergo enterohepatic circulation (K_{ec}). Perfusion-limited compartments are noted in white and diffusion-limited compartments are noted in blue.

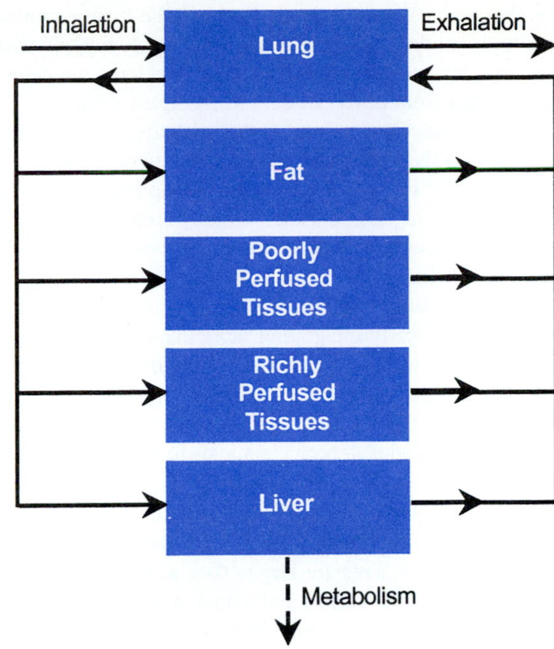

Figure 7-6. Physiological model for a typical volatile organic chemical.

Chemicals for which this model would be appropriate have low molecular weights (MW <100), are soluble in organic solvents, and have significant vapor pressures (volatile). Transport of chemical throughout the body by blood is depicted by the black arrows. Elimination of chemical as depicted by the model includes metabolism (*dashed arrow*) and exhalation (*black arrow*). All compartments are perfusion limited.

structure, or *how* the compartments are linked together, depends on both the chemical and the organism being studied. For example, a physiologic model describing the disposition of a chemical in fish would require a description of the gills (Nichols et al., 1994), whereas a model for the same chemical in mammals would require a lung (Ramsey and Andersen, 1984). Model structures can also vary with the chemicals being studied. For example a model for a nonvolatile, water-soluble chemical, which might be administered by intravenous injection (Fig. 7-5), has a structure different from that of a model for a volatile organic chemical for which inhalation is the likely route of exposure (Fig. 7-6). The route of administration is not the only difference between these two models: For example, the first model has a compartment for the intestines because biliary excretion, fecal elimination, and enterohepatic circulation are presumed important in the disposition of this chemical. The second model has a compartment for fat since fat is an important storage organ for organics. However, the models are not *completely* different. Both contain a liver compartment because the hepatic metabolism of each chemical is an important element of its disposition. It is important to realize that there is no generic physiological model. Models are simplifications of reality and ideally should contain elements believed to be important in describing a chemical's disposition.

In view of the fact that physiologic modeling requires more effort than does classic compartmental modeling, what accounts for the increase in the popularity of the kinetic approach among toxicologists? The answer lies in the potential predictive power of physiologic models. Toxicologists are constantly faced with the issue of extrapolation—from laboratory animals to humans, from high to low doses, from intermittent to continuous exposure, and from single chemicals to mixtures. Because the kinetic constants in physiologic models represent measurable biological or chemical processes, the resultant physiologic models have the potential for extrapolation from observed data to predicted situations.

One of the best illustrations of the predictive power of physiologic models is their ability to extrapolate kinetic behavior from laboratory animals to humans. For example, physiologic models developed for styrene and benzene correctly simulate the concentration of each chemical in the blood of rodents and humans (Ramsey and Andersen, 1984; Travis et al., 1990). *Simulations* are the outcomes or results (such as a chemical's concentration in blood or tissue) of numerically integrating model equations over a simulated time period, using a set of initial conditions (such as intravenous dose) and parameter values (such as organ weights). Both styrene and benzene are volatile organic chemicals; thus, the model structures for the kinetics of both chemicals in rodents and humans is identical to that shown in Fig. 7-6. However, the parameter values for rodents and humans are different. Humans have larger body weights than rodents, and thus weights of organs such as the liver are larger. Because humans are larger, they also breathe more air per unit of time than do rodents, and a human heart pumps a larger volume of blood per unit of time than does that of a rodent, although the rodent's heart beats more times in the same period. The parameters that describe the chemical behavior of styrene and benzene, such as solubility in tissues, are similar in the rodents and human models. This is often the case because the composition of tissues in different species is similar.

For both styrene and benzene there are experimental data for both humans and rodents and the model simulations can be compared with the actual data to see how well the model has performed (Ramsey and Andersen, 1984; Andersen et al., 1984; Travis et al., 1990). The conclusion is that the same model structure is capable of describing the chemicals' kinetics in two different species. Because the parameters underlying the model structure represent measurable biological and chemical determinants, the appropriate values for those parameters can be chosen for each species, forming the basis for successful interspecies extrapolation.

For both styrene and benzene, even though the same model structure is used for both rodents and humans, both the simulated and the observed kinetics of both chemicals differs between rats and humans. The terminal half-life of both organics is longer in the human compared with the rat. This longer half-life for humans is due to the fact that clearance rates for smaller species are faster than those for larger ones. Even though the larger species breathes more air or pumps more blood per unit of time than does the smaller species, blood flows and ventilation rates *per unit of body mass* are greater for the smaller species. The smaller species has more breaths per minute or heartbeats per minute than does the larger one, even though each breath or stroke volume is smaller. These faster flows per unit mass bring more xenobiotic to organs responsible for elimination. Thus, a smaller species can eliminate a xenobiotic faster than a larger one can. Because the parameters in physiologic models represent real, measurable values such as blood flows and ventilation rates, the same model structure can resolve such disparate kinetic behaviors among species.

Compartments

The basic unit of the physiologic model is the lumped compartment, which is often depicted as a box (Fig. 7-7). A *compartment* is a single region of the body with a *uniform* xenobiotic concentration (Rowland, 1984; Rowland, 1985). A compartment may be a particular functional or anatomic portion of an organ, a single blood vessel with surrounding tissue, an entire discrete organ such as the liver or kidney, or a widely distributed tissue type such as fat or skin. Compartments consist of three individual well-mixed phases, or *subcompartments,* that correspond to specific physiologic portions of the organ or tissue. These subcompartments are (1) the *vascular* space through which the compartment is perfused with blood, (2) the *interstitial* space that forms the matrix for the cells, and (3) the *intracellular* space consisting of the cells in the tissue (Gerlowski and Jain, 1983).

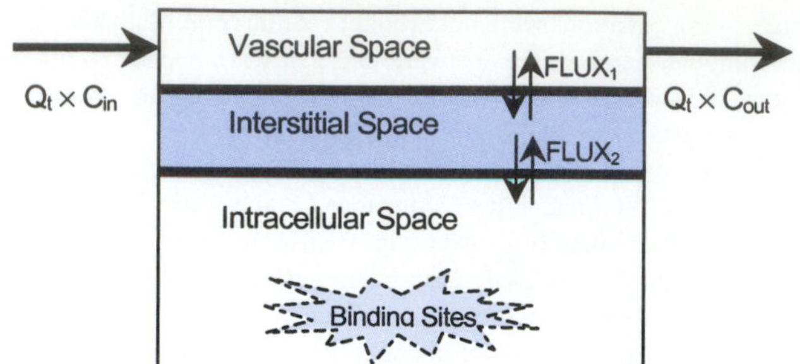

Figure 7-7. Schematic representation of a lumped compartment in a physiologic model.

The blood capillary and cell membranes separating the vascular, interstitial, and intracellular subcompartments are depicted in black. The vascular and interstitial subcompartments are often combined into a single extracellular subcompartment. Q_t is blood flow, C_{in} is chemical concentration into the compartment and C_{out} is chemical concentration out of the compartment.

As shown in Fig. 7-7, the xenobiotic enters the vascular subcompartment at a certain rate in mass per unit of time (e.g., milligrams per hour). The rate of entry is a product of the blood flow rate to the tissue (Q_t, in liters per hour) and the concentration of the xenobiotic in the blood entering the tissue (C_{in}, in milligrams per liter). Within the compartment, the xenobiotic moves from the vascular space to the interstitial space at a certain net rate ($Flux_1$) and moves from the interstitial space to the intracellular space at different net rate ($Flux_2$). Some xenobiotics can bind to cell components; thus, within a compartment there may be both free and bound xenobiotics. The xenobiotic leaves the vascular space at a certain venous concentration (C_{out}). C_{out} is equal to the concentration of the xenobiotic in the vascular space.

Parameters

The most common types of parameters, or information required, in physiologic models are *anatomic, physiologic, thermodynamic,* and *transport.*

Anatomic Anatomic parameters are used to physically describe the various compartments. The *size* of each of the compartments in the physiologic model must be known. The size is generally specified as a volume (milliliters or liters) because a unit density is assumed even though weights are most frequently obtained experimentally. If a compartment contains subcompartments such as those in Fig. 7-7, those volumes also must be known. Volumes of compartments often can be obtained from the literature or from specific toxicokinetic experiments. For example, kidney, liver, brain, and lung can be weighed. Obtaining precise data for volumes of compartments representing widely distributed tissues such as fat or muscle is more difficult. If necessary, these tissues can be removed by dissection and weighed. Among the numerous sources of general information on organ and tissue volumes, Brown et al. (1997) is a good starting point.

Physiologic Physiologic parameters encompass a wide variety of processes in biological systems. The most commonly used physiologic parameters are blood flow, ventilation, and elimination. The blood flow rate (Q_t, in volume per unit time, such as mL/min or L/h) to individual compartments must be known. Additionally, information on the total blood flow rate or *cardiac output* (Q_c) is necessary. If inhalation is the route for exposure to the xenobiotic or is a route of elimination, the alveolar ventilation rate (Q_p) also must be known. Blood flow rates and ventilation rates can be taken from the literature or can be obtained experimentally. Renal clearance rates and parameters to describe rates of biotransformation, or metabolism, are a subset of physiologic parameters and are required if these processes are important in describing the elimination of a xenobiotic. For example, if a xenobiotic is known to be metabolized via a saturable process both V_{max} (the maximum rate of metabolism) and K_M (the concentration of xenobiotic at one-half V_{max}) must be obtained so that elimination of the xenobiotic by metabolism can be described in the model.

Thermodynamic Thermodynamic parameters relate the *total* concentration of a xenobiotic in a tissue (C) to the concentration of *free* xenobiotic in that tissue (C_f). Two important assumptions are that (1) total and free concentrations are in equilibrium with each other and (2) only free xenobiotic can enter and leave the tissue (Lutz et al., 1980). Most often, total concentration is measured experimentally; however, it is the free concentration that is available for binding, metabolism, or removal from the tissue by blood. Various mathematical expressions describe the relationship between these two entities. In the simplest situation, the xenobiotic is a freely diffusible water-soluble chemical that does not bind to any molecules. In this case, the free concentration of the xenobiotic is exactly equal to the total concentration of the xenobiotic: total = free, or $C = C_f$. The affinity of many xenobiotics for tissues of different composition varies. The extent to which a xenobiotic partitions into a tissue is directly dependent on the composition of the tissue and independent of the concentration of the xenobiotic. Thus, the relationship between free and total concentration becomes one of proportionality: total = free × partition coefficient, or $C = C_f \times P$. In this case, P is called a *partition* or *distribution* coefficient. Knowledge of the value of P permits an indirect calculation of the free concentration of xenobiotic or $C_f . C_f = C/P$.

Table 7-4 compares the partition coefficients for a number of toxic volatile organic chemicals. The larger values for the fat/blood partition coefficients compared with those for other tissues suggests that these chemicals distribute into fat to a greater extent than they distribute into other tissues. This has been observed experimentally. Fat and fatty tissue such as bone marrow contain higher concentrations of benzene than do tissues such as liver and blood. Similarly, styrene concentrations in fatty tissue are higher than styrene concentrations in other tissues.

A more complex relationship between the free concentration and the total concentration of a chemical in tissues is also possible. For example, the chemical may bind to saturable binding sites on tissue components. In these cases, nonlinear functions relating the free concentration in the tissue to the total concentration are necessary. Examples in which more complex binding has been used are physiologic models for dioxin and *tertiary*-amyl butyl ether (Andersen et al., 1993; Collins et al., 1999).

Transport The passage of a xenobiotic across a biological membrane is complex and may occur by passive diffusion, carrier-mediated transport, facilitated transport, or a combination of processes (Himmelstein and Lutz, 1979). The simplest of these processes—passive diffusion—is a first-order process described by Fick's law of diffusion. Diffusion of xenobiotics can occur across the blood capillary membrane ($Flux_1$ in Fig. 7-7) or across the cell membrane ($Flux_2$ in Fig. 7-7). *Flux* refers to the rate of transfer of a xenobiotic across a boundary. For simple diffusion, the net flux (milligrams per hour) from one side of a membrane to the other is described as Flux = permeability coefficient × driving force, or

$$Flux = [PA] \times (C_1 - C_2) = [PA] \times C_1 - [PA] \times C_2$$

The permeability coefficient $[PA]$ is often called the *permeability-area cross-product* for the membrane (in units of liters per hour) and is a product of the cell membrane permeability constant (P, in micrometers per hour) for the xenobiotic and the total membrane area (A, in square micrometers). The cell membrane permeability constant takes into account the rate of diffusion of the specific xenobiotic and the thickness of the cell membrane. C_1 and C_2 are the *free* concentrations of xenobiotic on each side of the membrane. For any given xenobiotic, thin membranes, large surface areas, and large concentration differences enhance diffusion.

There are two *limiting conditions* for the transport of a xenobiotic across membranes: *perfusion-limited* and *diffusion-limited.* An understanding of the assumptions underlying the limiting conditions is critical because the assumptions change the way in which the differential equations are written to describe the compartment.

Perfusion-Limited Compartments

A perfusion-limited compartment is also referred to as *blood flow–limited,* or simply *flow-limited.* A flow-limited compartment can be developed if the cell membrane permeability coefficient $[PA]$ for a particular xenobiotic is much greater than the blood flow rate to the tissue (Q_t) or $[PA] >> Q_t$. In this case, the rate of xeno-

Table 7-4
Partition Coefficients for Four Volatile Organic Chemicals

CHEMICAL	BLOOD/AIR	MUSCLE/BLOOD	FAT/BLOOD
Isoprene	3	0.67	24
Benzene	18	0.61	28
Styrene	40	1	50
Methanol	1350	3	11

biotic uptake by tissue subcompartments is limited by the rate at which the blood containing a xenobiotic arrives at the tissue, not by the rate at which the xenobiotic crosses the cell membranes. In most tissues, the rate of entry of a xenobiotic into the interstitial space from the vascular space is not limited by the rate of xenobiotic transport across vascular cell membranes and is therefore perfusion rate limited. In the generalized tissue compartment in Fig. 7-7, this means that transport of the xenobiotic through the loosely knit blood capillary walls of most tissues is rapid compared with delivery of the xenobiotic to the tissue by the blood. As a result, the vascular blood is in equilibrium with the interstitial subcompartment and the two subcompartments are usually lumped together as a single compartment that is often called the *extracellular space.* An important exception to this vascular-interstitial equilibrium relationship is the brain, where the tightly knit blood capillary walls form a barrier between the vascular space and the interstitial space.

As indicated in Fig. 7-7, the cell membrane separates the extracellular compartment from the intracellular compartment. The cell membrane is the most important diffusional barrier in a tissue. Nonetheless, for molecules that are very small (molecular weight <100) or lipophilic, cellular permeability generally does not limit the rate at which a molecule moves across cell membranes. For these molecules, flux across the cell membrane is fast compared with the tissue perfusion rate ($[PA] >> Qt$), and the molecules rapidly distribute through the subcompartments. In this case, the intracellular compartment is in equilibrium with the extracellular compartment, and these tissue subcompartments are usually lumped as a single compartment. This flow-limited tissue compartment is shown in Fig. 7-8. Movement into and out of the entire tissue compartment can be described by a single equation:

$$V_t \times dC/dt = Q_t \times (C_{in} - C_{out})$$

where V_t is the volume of the tissue compartment, C is the concentration of free xenobiotic in the compartment ($V_t \times C$ equals the amount of xenobiotic in the compartment), $V_t \times dC/dt$ is the change in the amount of xenobiotic in the compartment with time expressed as mass per unit of time, Q_t is blood flow to the tissue, C_{in} is xenobiotic concentration entering the compartment, and C_{out} is xenobiotic concentration leaving the compartment. Equations of this type are called mass balance *differential* equations. Differential refers to the term d*x*/dt. Mass balance refers to the requirement that input into one equation must be balanced by outflow from another equation in the physiologic model.

In the perfusion-limited case, C_{out}, or the venous concentration of xenobiotic leaving the tissue, is equal to the free concentration of xenobiotic in the tissue, C_f. As was noted above, C_f (or C_{out}) can be related to the total concentration of xenobiotic in the tissue through a simple linear partition coefficient, $C_{out} = C_f = C/P$. In this case, the differential equation describing the rate of change in the amount of a xenobiotic in a tissue becomes

$$V_t \times dC/dt = Q_t \times (C_{in} - C/P)$$

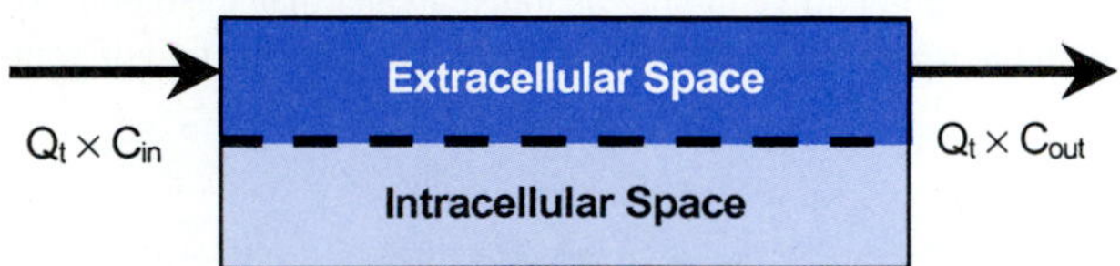

Figure 7-8. Schematic representation of a compartment that is blood-flow–limited.

Rapid exchange between the extracellular space (*blue*) and intracellular space (*light blue*) maintains the equilibrium between them as symbolized by the dashed line. Q_t is blood flow, C_{in} is chemical concentration into the compartment and C_{out} is chemical concentration out of the compartment.

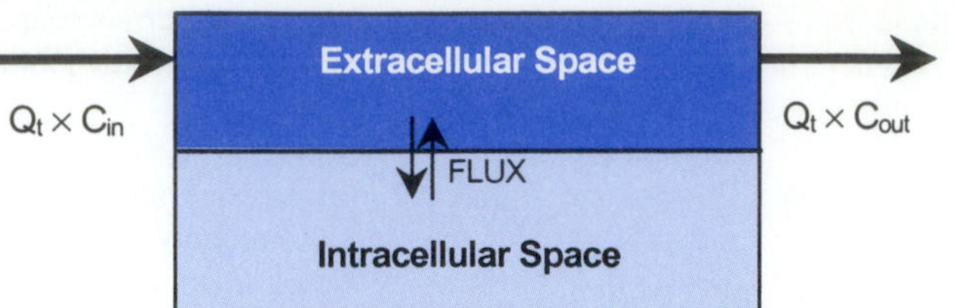

Figure 7-9. Schematic representation of a compartment that is membrane-limited.

Perfusion of blood into and out of the extracellular compartment is depicted by thick arrows. Transmembrane transport (flux) from the extracellular to the intracellular subcompartment is depicted by thin double arrows. Q_t is blood flow, C_{in} is chemical concentration into the compartment and C_{out} is chemical concentration out of the compartment.

The physiologic model shown in Fig. 7-6, which was developed for volatile organic chemicals such as styrene and benzene, is a good example of a model in which all the compartments are described as flow-limited. Distribution of xenobiotic in all the compartments is described by using equations of the type noted above. In a flow-limited compartment, the assumption is that the concentrations of a xenobiotic in all parts of the tissue are in equilibrium. For this reason, the compartments are generally drawn as simple boxes (Fig. 7-6) or boxes with dashed lines that symbolize the equilibrium between the intracellular and extracellular subcompartments (Fig. 7-8). Additionally, with a flow-limited model, estimates of flux are not required to develop the mass balance differential equation for the compartment. Given the information required to estimate flux, this is a simplifying assumption that significantly reduces the number of parameters required in the physiologic model.

Diffusion-Limited Compartments

When uptake into a compartment is governed by cell membrane permeability and total membrane area, the model is said to be *diffusion-limited,* or *membrane-limited.* Diffusion-limited transport occurs when the flux, or the transport of a xenobiotic across cell membranes, is slow compared with blood flow to the tissue. In this case, the permeability-area cross-product $[PA]$ is small compared with blood flow, Q_t, or $PA << Q_t$. The distribution of large polar molecules into tissue cells is likely to be limited by the rate at which the molecules pass through cell membranes. In contrast, entry into the interstitial space of the tissue through the leaky capillaries of the vascular space is usually flow-limited even for large molecules. Figure 7-9 shows the structure of such a compartment. The xenobiotic concentrations in the interstitial and vascular spaces are in equilibrium and make up the extracellular subcompartment where uptake from the incoming blood is flow-limited. The rate of xenobiotic uptake across the cell membrane (into the intracellular space from the extracellular space) is limited by cell membrane permeability and is thus diffusion-limited. Two mass balance differential equations are necessary to describe this compartment:

Extracellular space: $V_{t1} \times dC_1/dt = Q_t \times (C_{in} - C_{out}) - [PA] \times C_1 + [PA] \times C_2$

Intracellular space: $V_{t2} \times dC_2/dt = [PA] \times C_1 - [PA] \times C_2$

Q_t is blood flow, and C is *free* xenobiotic concentration in entering blood (in), exiting blood (out), extracellular space (1), or intracellular space (2). Both equations contain terms for flux, or transfer across the cell membrane, $[PA] \times (C_1 - C_2)$. The physiologic model in Fig. 7-5 is composed of two diffusion-limited compartments each of which contain two subcompartments—extracellular and intracellular space—and several perfusion-limited compartments.

Specialized Compartments

Lung The inclusion of a lung compartment in a physiologic model is an important consideration because inhalation is a common route of exposure to many toxic chemicals. Additionally, the lung compartment serves as an instructive example of the assumptions and simplifications that can be incorporated into physiologic models while maintaining the overall objective of describing processes and compartments in biologically relevant terms. For example, although lung physiology and anatomy are complex, Haggard (1924) developed a simple approximation that sufficiently describes the uptake of many volatile xenobiotics by the lungs. A diagram of this simplified lung compartment is shown in Fig. 7-10. The assumptions inherent in this compartment description are as follows: (1) ventilation is continuous, not cyclic; (2) conducting airways (nasal passages, larynx, trachea, bronchi, and bronchioles) function as inert tubes, carrying the vapor to the pulmonary or gas exchange region; (3) diffusion of vapor across the lung cell and capillary walls is rapid compared with blood flow through the lung; (4) all xenobiotic disappearing from the inspired air appears in the arterial blood (i.e., there is no storage of xenobiotic in the lung tissue and insignificant lung mass); and (5) vapor in the alveolar air and arterial blood within the lung compartment are in rapid equilibrium and are related by P_b, the blood/air partition coefficient (e.g., $C_{alv} = C_{art}/P_b$). P_b is a thermodynamic parameter that quantifies the distribution or partitioning of a xenobiotic into blood compared with air.

In the lung compartment depicted in Fig. 7-10, the rate of inhalation of xenobiotic is controlled by the ventilation rate (Q_p) and the inhaled concentration (C_{inh}). The rate of exhalation of a xenobiotic is a product of the ventilation rate and the xenobiotic concentration in the alveoli (C_{alv}). Xenobiotic also can enter the lung compartment via venous blood returning from the heart, represented by the product of cardiac output (Q_c) and the concentration of xenobiotic in venous blood (C_{ven}). Xenobiotic leaving the lungs via the blood is a function of both cardiac output and the concentration of xenobiotic in arterial blood (C_{art}). Putting these four processes together, a mass balance differential equation can be written for the rate of change in the amount of xenobiotic in the lung compartment (L):

$$dL/dt = Q_p \times (C_{inh} - C_{alv}) + Q_c \times (C_{ven} - C_{art})$$

Because of some of these assumptions, the rate of change in the amount of xenobiotic in the lung compartment becomes equal to zero ($dL/dt = 0$). C_{alv} can be replaced by C_{art}/P_b, and the differential equation can be solved for the arterial blood concentration:

$$C_{art} = (Q_p \times C_{inh} + Q_c \times C_{ven})/(Q_c + Q_p/P_b)$$

This algebraic equation is incorporated into physiologic models for many volatile organics. Because the lung is viewed here as a portal of entry and not as a target organ, the concentration of a xenobiotic delivered to other organs by the blood, or the arterial concentration of that xenobiotic, is of primary interest. The assumptions of continuous ventilation, dead space, rapid equilibration with arterial blood, and no storage of vapor in the lung tissues have worked extremely well with many volatile organics, especially relatively lipophilic chemicals. Indeed, the use of these assumptions simplifies and speeds model calculations and may be entirely adequate for describing the chemical behavior of relatively inert vapors with low water-solubility.

Inspection of the equation for calculating the arterial concentration of the inhaled organic vapor indicates that the term P_b, the xenobiotic-specific blood/air partition coefficient, becomes an important term for simulating the uptake of various volatile organic xenobiotics. As the value for P_b increases, the maximum concentration of the xenobiotic in the blood increases. Additionally, the time to reach the steady-state concentration and the time to clear the xenobiotic also increase with increasing P_b. Fortunately, P_b is readily measured by using in vitro techniques in which a volatile chemical in air is equilibrated with blood in a closed system, such as a sealed vial (Gargas and Andersen, 1988).

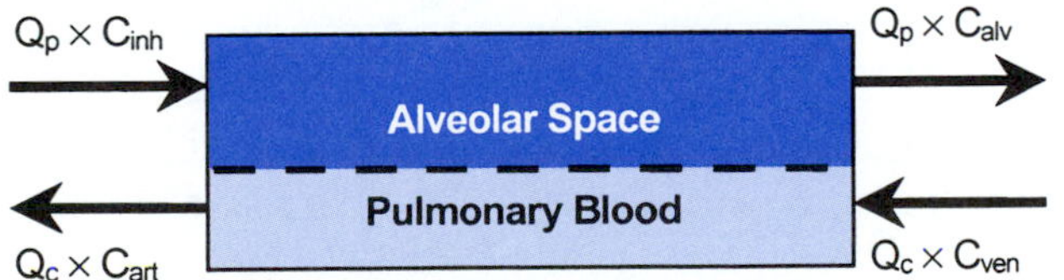

Figure 7-10. Simple model of gas exchange in the alveolar region of the respiratory tract.

Rapid exchange in the lumped lung compartment between the alveolar gas (*blue*) and the pulmonary blood (*light blue*) maintains the equilibrium between them as symbolized by the dashed line. Q_p is alveolar ventilation (L/h); Q_c is cardiac output (L/h); C_{inh} is inhaled vapor concentration (mg/L); C_{art} is concentration of vapor in the arterial blood; C_{ven} is concentration of vapor in the mixed venous blood. The equilibrium relationship between the chemical in the alveolar air (C_{alv}) and the chemical in the arterial blood (C_{art}) is determined by the blood/air partition coefficient P_b, e.g., $C_{alv} = C_{art}/P_b$.

Liver The liver is often represented as a compartment in physiologic models because hepatic biotransformation is an important aspect of the toxicokinetics of many xenobiotics. The effects of multiple factors such as concentration, dose rate, and species on the metabolism of xenobiotics are important in assessing risk. Because the liver is often the major organ for the biotransformation of xenobiotics, the task of metabolism is generally assigned to the liver compartment in physiologic models. A simple compartmental structure for the liver is depicted in Fig. 7-11, where the liver compartment is assumed to be flow-limited. This liver compartment is similar to the general tissue compartment in Fig. 7-8, except that the liver compartment contains an additional process for metabolic elimination. One of the simplest expressions for this process is first-order elimination, which is written

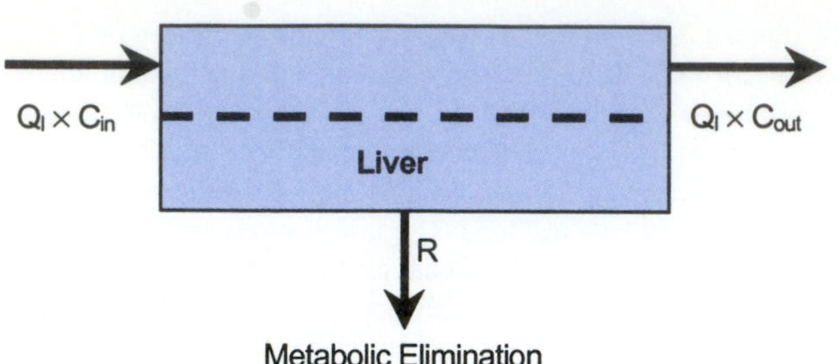

Figure 7-11. Schematic representation of a flow-limited liver compartment in which metabolic elimination occurs.

R, in milligrams per hour, is the rate of metabolism. Q_l is hepatic blood flow, C_{in} is chemical concentration into the liver compartment, and C_{out} is chemical concentration out of the liver compartment.

$$R = C_f \times V_l \times K_f$$

R is the rate of metabolism (milligrams per hour), C_f is the free concentration of xenobiotic in the liver (milligrams per liter), V_l is the liver volume (liters), and K_f is the first-order rate constant for metabolism in units of h^{-1}. A widely used expression for metabolism in physiologic models is the Michaelis-Menten expression for *saturable metabolism* (Andersen, 1981), which employs two parameters, V_{max} and K_M and is written as follows:

$$R = (V_{max} \times C_f)/(K_M + C_f)$$

where V_{max} is the maximum rate of metabolism (in milligrams per hour) and K_M is the Michaelis constant, or xenobiotic concentration at one-half the maximum rate of metabolism (in milligrams per liter). Because many xenobiotics are metabolized by enzymes that display saturable metabolism, the above equation is a key factor in the success of physiologic models for simulation of chemical disposition across a range of doses.

Other, more complex expressions for metabolism also can be incorporated into physiologic models. Bisubstrate second-order reactions, reactions involving the destruction of enzymes, the inhibition of enzymes, or the depletion of cofactors, have been simulated using physiologic models. Metabolism can be also included in other compartments in much the same way as described for the liver.

The usefulness of physiologic models for describing the complex toxicokinetic profiles resulting from saturable metabolism is responsible to a large extent for the popularity of these models. The ability of physiologic models to describe experiments in which metabolism is altered using enzyme inhibitors or genetically modified animals is illustrated in Fig. 7-12. The model used to produce the simulations in this figure accounted for inhalation of xenobiotic, distribution to and uptake by tissues, and various states of metabolism (Jackson et al., 1999). The curves in Fig. 7-12 show that when the maximum metabolic capacity, or V_{max}, is diminished, the uptake of the chemical from the inhalation chamber into the body is reduced.

Blood In a physiologic model, as in a living organism, the tissue compartments are linked together by the blood. Figures 7-5 and 7-6 represent different approaches toward describing the blood in physiologic models. In general, a tissue receives a xenobiotic in the systemic arterial blood. Exceptions are the liver, which receives arterial and portal blood, and the lungs, which receive mixed venous blood. In the body, the venous blood supplies draining from tissue compartments eventually merge in the large blood vessels and heart chambers to form mixed venous blood. In Fig. 7-5, a blood compartment is created in which the input is the sum of the xenobiotic efflux from each compartment ($Q_t \times C_{vt}$). Efflux from the blood compartment is a product of the blood concentration in the compartment and the total cardiac output ($Q_c \times C_{bl}$). The differential equation for the blood compartment in Fig. 7-5 looks like this:

$$dV_{bl} \times C_{bl}/dt = Q_{br} \times C_{vbr} + Q_{tb} \times C_{vtb} + Q_k \times C_{vk} + Q_l \times C_{vl} - Q_c \times C_{bl}$$

where V_{bl} is the volume of the blood compartment; *C* is concentration; *Q* is blood flow; *bl*, *br*, *tb*, *k*, and *l* represent the blood, brain, total body, kidney and liver compartments, respectively; and *vbr*, *vtb*, *vk*, and *vl* represent the venous blood leaving the organs. The venous blood is assumed to contain unbound chemical. Q_c is the total blood flow equal to the sum of the blood flows exiting each organ.

In contrast, the physiologic model in Fig. 7-6 does not have a blood compartment. For simplicity, the blood volumes of the heart and the major blood vessels that are not within organs are assumed to be negligible. The venous concentration of xenobiotic returning to the lungs is simply the weighted average of the xenobiotic concentrations in the venous blood emerging from the tissues:

$$C_v = (Q_l \times C_{vl} + Q_{rp} \times C_{vrp} + Q_{pp} \times C_{vpp} + Q_f \times C_{vf})/Q_c$$

where *C* is concentration; *Q* is blood flow; *v*, *l*, *rp*, *pp*, and *f* represent the venous blood, liver, richly perfused, poorly perfused, and

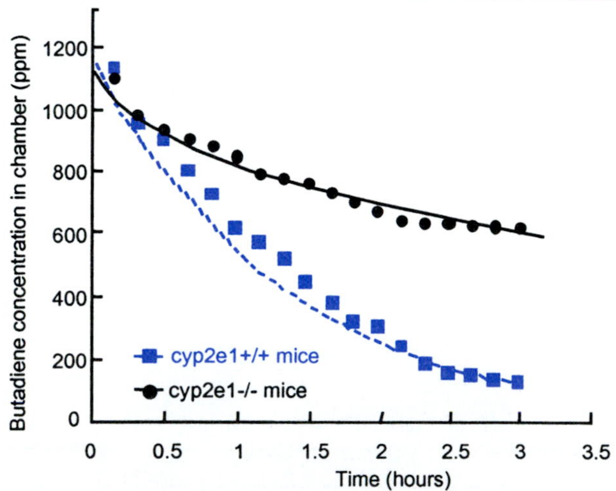

Figure 7-12. Disappearance of butadiene vapor after injection (at t = 0) into a closed chamber containing mice.

The experimental data are the results of measurements of air samples taken from the chamber. The lines are physiologic model simulations of the experiments. After an initial period of equilibration, further decline in the chamber concentration is due to metabolism of butadiene by the mice. The greater the rate of metabolism the faster the decline in the butadiene concentration in the chamber. Mice that do not express the gene for the enzyme CYP2E1 (*black circles*) metabolize less butadiene than mice that do express the gene for CYP2E1 (*blue squares*). [From Jackson et al., 1999, p. 4. Reproduced with permission from CIIT Centers for Health Research.

fat tissue compartments, respectively; and *vl*, *vrp*, *vpp*, and *vf* represent the venous blood leaving the organs. Again the venous blood is assumed to contain unbound chemical. Q_c is the total blood flow equal to the sum of the blood flows exiting each organ.

In the physiologic model in Fig. 7-6, the blood concentration going to the tissue compartments is the arterial concentration (C_{art}) that was calculated above for the lung compartment. The decision to use one formulation as opposed to another to describe blood in a physiologic model depends on the role the blood plays in disposition. If the toxicokinetics after intravenous injection are to be simulated or if binding to or metabolism by blood components is suspected, a separate compartment for the blood that incorporates these additional processes is the best solution. If, as in the case of the volatile organics shown in Fig. 7-6, the blood is simply a conduit to the other compartments, the algebraic solution is acceptable.

CONCLUSION

This chapter provides a basic overview of the simpler elements of physiologic models and the important and often neglected assumptions that underlie model structures. Detailed descriptions of individual models of a wide variety of xenobiotics have been published. Several review articles describing how to construct a model step by step are included in the references. Computer software applications are available for numerically integrating the differential equations that form the models. Investigators have successfully used Advanced Continuous Simulation Language (Pharsight Corp., Palo Alto, CA), Simulation Control Program (Simulation Resources, Inc., Berrien Springs, MI), MATLAB (The MathWorks, Inc., Natick, MA), Microsoft Excel, and SAS software applications to name a few. Choice of software depends on prior experience, familiarity with the computer language used, and cost of the application.

The field of physiologic modeling is rapidly expanding and evolving as toxicologists and pharmacologists develop increasingly more sophisticated applications. Three-dimensional visualizations of xenobiotic transport in fish and vapor transport in the rodent nose, physiologic models of a parent chemical linked in series with one or more active metabolites, models describing biochemical interactions among xenobiotics, and more biologically realistic descriptions of tissues previously viewed as simple lumped compartments are just a few of the most recent applications. Finally, physiologically based *toxicokinetic* models are beginning to be linked to biologically based *toxicodynamic* models to simulate the entire exposure → dose → response paradigm that is basic to the science of toxicology.

REFERENCES

Andersen ME: A physiologically based toxicokinetic description of the metabolism of inhaled gases and vapors: Analysis at steady state. *Toxicol Appl Pharmacol* 60:509–526, 1981.

Andersen ME: Physiological modeling of organic compounds. *Ann Occup Hyg* 35(3):309–321, 1991.

Andersen ME, Gargas ML, Ramsey JC: Inhalation pharmacokinetics: Evaluating systemic extraction, total *in vivo* metabolism, and the time course of enzyme induction for inhaled styrene in rats based on arterial blood:inhaled air concentration ratios. *Toxicol Appl Pharmacol* 73:176–187, 1984.

Andersen ME, Mills JJ, Gargas ML, et al: Modeling receptor-mediated processes with dioxin: Implications for pharmacokinetics and risk assessment. *Risk Anal* 13(1):25–36, 1993.

Brown RP, Delp MD, Lindstedt SL, et al: Physiological parameter values for physiologically based pharmacokinetic models. *Toxicol Ind Health* 13(4):407–484, 1997.

Collins AS, Sumner SCJ, Borghoff SJ, et al: A physiological model for *tert*-amyl alcohol: Hypothesis testing of model structures. *Toxicol Sci* 49:-15–28, 1999.

Gargas ML, Andersen ME: Physiologically based approaches for examining the pharmacokinetics of inhaled vapors, in Gardner DE, Crapo JD, Massaro EJ (eds): *Toxicology of the Lung.* New York: Raven Press, 1988, pp 449–476.

Gerloski LE, Jain RK: Physiologically based pharmacokinetic modeling: Principles and applications. *J Pharm Sci* 72(10):1103–1127, 1983.

Gibaldi M, Perrier D: Pharmacokinetics, 2d ed. New York: Marcel Dekker, 1982.

Haggard HW: The absorption, distribution, and elimination of ethyl ether: II. Analysis of the mechanism of the absorption and elimination of such a gas or vapor as ethyl ether. *J Biol Chem* 49:753–770, 1924.

Himmelstein KJ, Lutz RJ: A review of the applications of physiologically based pharmacokinetic modeling. *J Pharmacokinet Biopharm* 7(2):127–145, 1979.

Jackson TE, Medinsky MA, Butterworth BE, et al: The use of cytochrome P450 2E1 knockout mice to develop a mechanistic understanding of carcinogen biotransformation and toxicity. *CIIT Activ* 19(4):1–9, 1999.

Kato Y, Hirate J, Sakaguchi K, et al: Age-dependent change in warfarin distribution volume in rats: Effect of change in extracellular water volume. *J Pharmacobiodyn* 10:330–335, 1987.

Lutz RJ, Dedrick RL, Zaharko DS: Physiological pharmacokinetics: An *in vivo* approach to membrane transport. *Pharmacol Ther* 11:559–592, 1980.

Nichols J, Rheingans P, Lothenbach D, et al: Three-dimensional visualization of physiologically based kinetic model outputs. *Environ Health Perspect* 102(11):952–956, 1994.

Ramsey JC, Andersen ME: A physiologically based description of the inhalation pharmacokinetics of styrene in rats and humans. *Toxicol Appl Pharmacol* 73:159–175, 1984.

Rowland M: Physiologic pharmacokinetic models and interanimal species scaling. *Pharmacol Ther* 29:49–68, 1985.

Rowland M: Physiologic pharmacokinetic models: Relevance, experience, and future trends. *Drug Metab Rev* 15:55–74, 1984.

Rowland M, Tozer TN: Clinical Pharmacokinetics. Philadelphia: Lea & Febiger, 1980.

Shargel L, Yu ABC: Applied Biopharmaceutics and Pharmacokinetics, 3d ed. Norwalk, CT: Appleton & Lange, 1993.

Teorell T: Kinetics of distribution of substances administered to the body: I. The extravascular modes of administration. *Arch Int Pharmacodyn Ther* 57:205–225, 1937.

Travis CC, Quillen JL, Arms AD. Pharmacokinetics of benzene. *Toxicol Appl Pharmacol* 102:400–420, 1990.

Wang P, Ba ZF, Lu M-C, et al: Measurement of circulating blood volume in vivo after trauma-hemorrhage and hemodilution. *Am J Physiol* 226: R368–R374, 1994.

York JL: Body water content, ethanol pharmacokinetics, and the responsiveness to ethanol in young and old rats. *Dev Pharmacol Ther* 4:106–116, 1982.

UNIT 3

NON-ORGAN-DIRECTED TOXICITY

CHAPTER 8

CHEMICAL CARCINOGENESIS

Henry C. Pitot III and Yvonne P. Dragan

Cancer resulting from exposure to chemicals in the environment, though known for millennia, has taken on new importance in this century. With the advent of advanced technology, new chemical agents enter the environment, although at relatively low levels in most cases, at a prodigious rate. It has been estimated (Korte and Coulston, 1994) that the number of organic chemicals that are continually being brought into the environment (about 300 million tons per year) may include more than 100,000 compounds. Chemical contamination of waste (Landrigan, 1983), the food chain (Foran et al., 1989), and the occupational environment (Anttila et al., 1993) is reportedly substantial. However, other researchers (Ames and Gold, 1990) have noted numerous misconceptions about the relationship of exposure to industrially based environmental chemicals and the incidence of human cancer. Therefore, knowledge about the mechanisms and natural history of cancer development as well as the epidemiology of human cancer is critical to the control and prevention of human neoplastic disease.

HISTORICAL FOUNDATION

The historical foundations for the induction of carcinogenesis by chemicals dates back several thousand years to the description of breast cancer in the Edwin Smith papyrus (Shimkin, 1977). In 1700, Ramazzini described the first example of occupational cancer. He noted the high incidence of breast cancer among nuns, which he attributed to their celibate life. A specific causal relationship between exposure to environmental mixtures and the induction of cancer was reported in 1775 by Percivall Pott, an eminent English physician and surgeon. Pott described the occurrence of cancer of the scrotum in a number of patients with a history of employment as chimney sweeps. With remarkable insight, Pott concluded that the occupation of those men was directly and causally related to their malignant disease. In addition, Pott suggested that the soot to which they were exposed was the causative agent of their condition. While Pott's publication soon led other observers to attribute cancer in various sites to soot exposure, his work had little impact on British public health practice during the succeeding century (Lawley, 1994). Thus, more than a century later, Butlin (1892) reported the relative rarity of scrotal cancer among chimney sweeps on the European continent compared with those in England. This difference was attributed to the relatively low standards of hygiene in Britain and the practice of exposing young "climbing boys" to the combustion products of coal. However, the lesson from Pott's findings has been a long time in the learning. A hundred years after the publication of Pott's monograph, the high incidence of skin cancer among certain German workers was traced to their exposure to coal tar, the chief constituent of the chimney sweeps' soot (Miller, 1978). Even today—more than 200 years after Pott's original scientific report on the association of soot and smoke products with cancer—a large percentage of the world's population is exposed to carcinogenic products that result from the combustion of tobacco and organic fuels.

During the nineteenth century, industrial chemicals, including cutting oils and dyes, were implicated as causative factors in the development of skin and bladder cancer, respectively (Lawley, 1994). Coal tar derivatives became the basis for the dye industry during the middle of the nineteenth century in Europe. Amine-containing aromatics such as 2-naphthylamine and benzidine were discovered and subsequently synthesized and used to yield a variety of chemical species of pigments for coloring a variety of materials. In 1895 Rehn reported the occurrence of bladder cancer in workers in the aniline dye industry. This finding was rapidly supported by other reports (Miller, 1978). Epidemiologic studies incriminated a number of aromatic amines, such as naphthylamines and benzidines, as the inciting agents (Hueper et al., 1938). Today 2-naphthylamine is not used in the U.S. chemical industry and exposure to a variety of other aromatic amines is regulated by law. Thus, the reader may appreciate that the human being was the first experimental animal in which chemical carcinogenesis was studied. Further on, both the development and the data derived from studies of chemical carcinogenesis in animals are considered.

DEFINITIONS

The term *cancer* describes a subset of lesions of the disease neoplasia. *Neoplasia* or the constituent lesion, a *neoplasm,* is defined as a heritably altered, relatively autonomous growth of tissue (Pitot, 1986a). The critical points of this definition are (1) the heritable aspects of neoplasia at the somatic or germ cell level and (2) the relative autonomy of neoplastic cells, reflecting their abnormal regulation of genetic expression, which is inherent in the neoplastic cell or occurs in response to environmental stimuli. Neoplasms may be either *benign* or *malignant*. The critical distinction between these classes is related to the characteristic of successful *metastatic* growth of malignant but not benign neoplasms. *Metastases* are secondary growths of cells from the primary neoplasm. Cancers are malignant neoplasms, whereas the term *tumor* describes space-occupying lesions that may or may not be neoplastic.

The nomenclature of neoplasia depends primarily on whether the neoplasm is benign or malignant and, in the latter case, whether it is derived from epithelial or mesenchymal tissue. For most benign neoplasms, the tissue of origin is followed by the suffix *-oma*: fibroma, lipoma, adenoma, and so on. For malignant neoplasms derived from tissues of mesenchymal origin, the term *sarcoma* is added to the tissue descriptor: fibrosarcoma, osteosarcoma, liposarcoma, and so on. Malignant neoplasms derived from tissues of ectodermal or endodermal (epithelial) origin are termed *carcinomas* with an antecedent tissue descriptor: epidermoid carcinoma (skin), hepatocellular carcinoma, gastric adenocarcinoma, and so on.

In general a *carcinogen* is an agent that causes or induces neoplasia. However, this definition is insufficient by current standards. The following definition may be more appropriate: "A *carcinogen* is an agent whose administration to previously untreated animals leads to a statistically significant increased incidence of neoplasms of one or more histogenetic types as compared with the incidence in appropriate untreated animals" (Pitot, 1986a).

This definition includes the induction of neoplasms that are usually not observed, the earlier induction of neoplasms that usually are observed, and/or the induction of more neoplasms than are usually found. Although it is important to distinguish between agents that induce neoplasms through direct action on the cells that become neoplastic and those which produce neoplasia through indirect actions in the animal as a whole, this is not always possible. Some agents, such as immune suppressants, can increase the incidence of neoplasms in tissues that were previously exposed to carcinogens through indirect effects on the host. When the action of a chemical in causing an increase in neoplasms is known to be indirect—that is, mediated by its effect on cells other than those undergoing carcinogenesis—that agent should not be designated as a carcinogen. Later in this chapter the stages and modifying factors of the process of chemical carcinogenesis are considered, necessitating a further refinement of the term *carcinogen* in relation to the action of specific chemicals in the carcinogenic process.

CARCINOGENESIS BY CHEMICALS

By the turn of this century, studies in humans showed that environmental and possibly internal chemical agents are causative factors in the development of cancer (Shimkin, 1977; Lawley, 1994). However, a systematic study of the mechanisms of chemical carcinogenesis was not possible without defined experimental systems. In 1915, the Japanese pathologists Yamagawa and Ichikawa (1915) described the first production of skin tumors in animals by the application of coal tar to the skin. These investigators repeatedly applied crude coal tar to the ears of rabbits for a number of months, finally producing both benign and later malignant epidermal neoplasms. Later studies demonstrated that the skin of mice is also susceptible to the carcinogenic action of such organic tars. During the next 15 years, extensive attempts were made to determine the nature of the material in the crude tars that caused malignancy. In 1932 Kennaway and associates reported the production of carcinogenic tars by means of pyrolysis of organic compounds consisting only of carbon and hydrogen (Kennaway, 1955).

Organic Chemical Carcinogens

In the early 1930s, several polycyclic aromatic hydrocarbons were isolated from active crude tar fractions. In 1930, the first synthetic carcinogenic polycyclic aromatic hydrocarbon was produced (Miller, 1978). This compound, dibenz-(*a,h*)anthracene (Fig. 8-1), was demonstrated to be a potent carcinogen after repeated painting on the skin of mice. The isolation from coal tar and the synthesis of benzo(*a*)pyrene (3,4-benzpyrene) were achieved in 1932. The structures of several polycyclic aromatic hydrocarbons are shown in Fig. 8-1. Polycyclic hydrocarbons vary in their carcinogenic potencies; for example, the compound dibenz(*a,c*)anthracene has very little carcinogenic activity, while the *a,h* isomer is carcinogenic (Heidelberger, 1970). The more potent polycyclic aromatic hydrocarbon carcinogens are 3-methylcholanthrene and 7,12-dimethylbenz(*a*)anthracene. The carcinogenic dibenzo(*c,q*)carbazole, which has a nitrogen in its central ring, is also considered to be in this class of compounds. Benzo(*e*)pyrene is reportedly inactive in in-

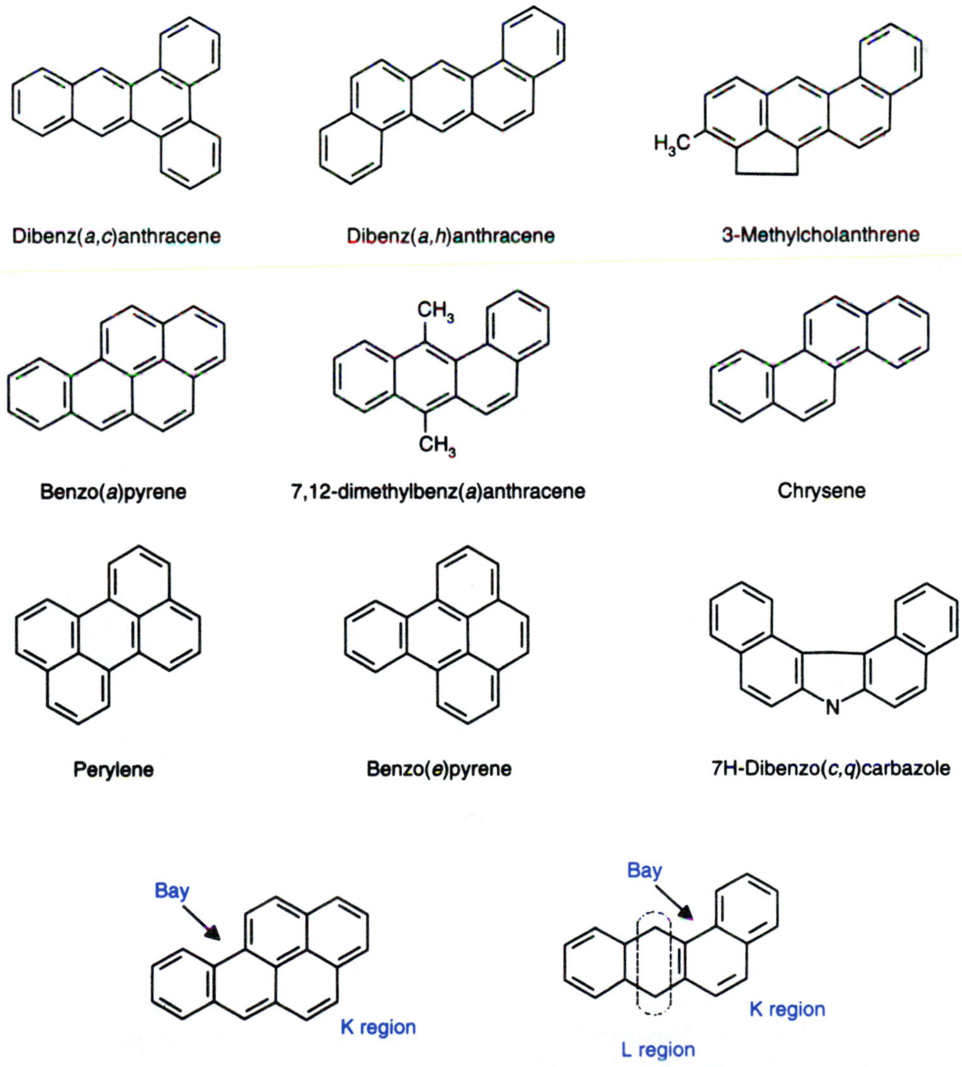

Dibenz(*a,c*)anthracene

Dibenz(*a,h*)anthracene

3-Methylcholanthrene

Benzo(*a*)pyrene

7,12-dimethylbenz(*a*)anthracene

Chrysene

Perylene

Benzo(*e*)pyrene

7H-Dibenzo(*c,q*)carbazole

Bay

K region

Bay

K region

L region

Figure 8-1. Chemical structures of some carcinogenic polycyclic hydrocarbons.

ducing skin cancer in mice but can "initiate" the carcinogenic process. Perylene is inactive as a chemical carcinogen, whereas chrysene may have slight carcinogenic activity.

In 1935, Sasaki and Yoshida opened another field of chemical carcinogenesis by demonstrating that feeding of the azo dye, *o*-aminoazotoluene (3-dimethyl-4-aminoazobenzene) (Fig. 8-2), to rats can result in the development of liver neoplasms. Similarly, Kinosita (1936) demonstrated that the administration of 4-dimethylaminoazobenzene in the diet also causes neoplasms in the liver. A number of analogs of this compound were prepared and tested for carcinogenic potential. Unlike the polycyclic aromatic hydrocarbons, the azo dyes generally did not act at the site of first contact of the compound with the organism but instead at a remote site, the liver.

Another important carcinogen that acts at remote sites is 2-acetylaminofluorene (Fig. 8-2). This chemical induces neoplasms of the mammary gland, ear duct, and liver in rats (Miller et al., 1949) and neoplasms of the bladder in mice (Miller et al., 1964). The aromatic amine 2-naphthylamine and several other aromatic amines are carcinogenic for the urinary bladder in humans (Vainio et al., 1991). The carcinogenic chemical ethyl carbamate is carcinogenic for many tissues in the mouse. Ethyl carbamate was in use in Japan from 1950 to 1975 as a cosolvent for dissolving water-insoluble analgesic drugs (Miller, 1991), but this practice was stopped after 1975. No systematic study of the incidence of cancer in this cohort has been conducted. In addition, certain cytocidal alkylating agents, such as the nitrogen mustards (Fig. 8-2), have been used to treat cancer in humans and are also known to be potent carcinogens in both animals and humans (Vainio et al., 1991). The other three agents depicted on the bottom line of Fig. 8-2 are also alkylating agents that are used industrially. Bis(chloromethyl)ether, a popular intermediate in organic synthetic reactions, has been classified as carcinogenic to humans on the basis of epidemiologic and animal studies (Vainio et al., 1991).

Dimethylnitrosamine is the smallest of the class of dialkylnitrosamines in which the alkyl substituents on the nitrogen linked to the nitroso group may vary widely, including fusion to yield a cyclic aliphatic substituent. Dimethylnitrosamine (Fig. 8-2) is

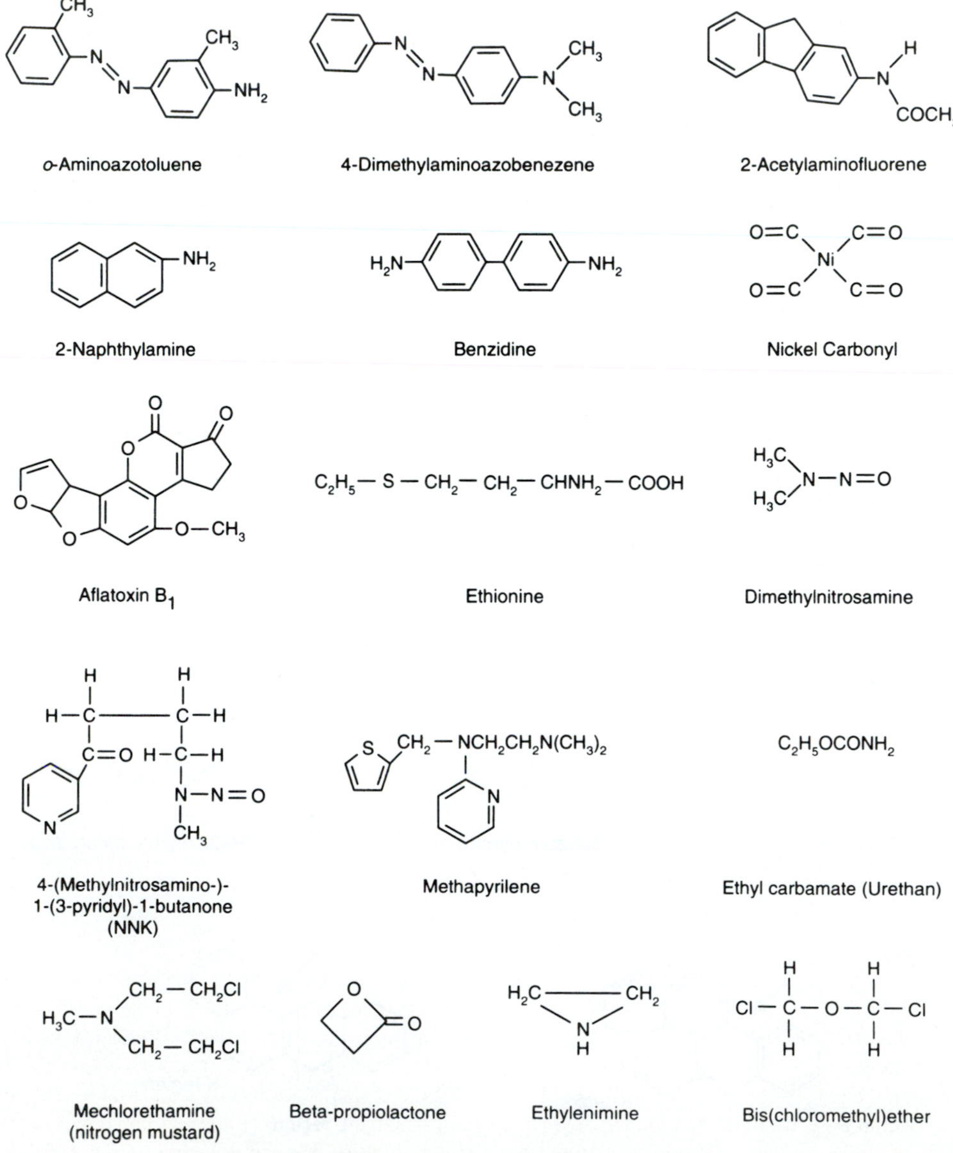

Figure 8-2. Chemical structures of other representative chemical carcinogens.

highly carcinogenic for the liver and kidney in virtually all the mammalian species tested (Schmähl and Habs, 1980). There is substantial epidemiologic evidence for a role of nitroso compounds in the induction of human cancer. The nitrosamine NNK (Fig. 8-2) is produced in tobacco smoke from nicotine, a tobacco alkaloid (Hecht, 1985). This is an extremely potent carcinogen that may play a role in the induction of tobacco-related cancers in humans. Methapyrilene was developed as an antihistamine but is a potent carcinogen in the rat (Mirsalis, 1987). Several investigators (Lijinsky, 1977; Magee and Swann, 1969; Mirvish et al., 1983) have shown that certain dietary components, especially in the presence of high levels of nitrite, may give rise to low levels of nitrosamines or nitrosamides and induce neoplasia of the gastrointestinal tract in experimental animals. The action of bacterial flora in the intestine may enhance the formation of these compounds. There is increasing evidence of an etiologic role for endogenously formed *N*-nitroso compounds in the development of certain human cancers (Bartsch et al., 1990).

Another important environmental and experimental hepatocarcinogenic agent is aflatoxin B_1. This toxic substance is produced by certain strains of the mold *Aspergillus flavus*. Aflatoxin B_1 is one of the most potent hepatocarcinogenic agents known and has produced neoplasms in rodents, fish, birds, and primates (Dragan and Pitot, 1994). This agent is a potential contaminant of many farm products (for example, grain and peanuts) that are stored under warm and humid conditions for some time. Aflatoxin B_1 and related compounds may cause some of the toxic hepatitis and hepatic neoplasia seen in various parts of Africa and the Far East (Wogan, 1992). Other products of molds and fungi are potentially carcinogenic in humans and animals (Schoental, 1985). A number of plants, some of which are edible, also contain chemical carcinogenic agents whose structures have been elucidated (Hirono, 1993).

Ethionine is an antimetabolite of the amino acid methionine. Farber (1963) was the first to show definitively that administration of ethionine in the diet for extended periods can result in the development of liver cancer in rats. This was the first example of direct interference with the metabolism of a normal metabolic constituent, resulting in the development of cancer.

We note here and discuss further later in the chapter that the dose of a chemical carcinogen is very important in relation to its effects just as with any pharmacologic agent. Even though many chemical carcinogens exert their effects by mechanisms somewhat different than many pharmacologic agents, the total administered dose, the rate at which it is given, and a number of other factors in the organism itself each play significant roles in the ultimate carcinogenic response.

Inorganic Chemical Carcinogenesis

In addition to organic compounds such as those illustrated in Figs. 8-1 and 8-2, a number of inorganic elements and their compounds have been shown to be carcinogenic in both animals and humans (Vainio and Wilbourn, 1993). Table 8-1 lists metals that are carcinogenic in some form to humans (part A) and experimental animals (part B) (Sky-Peck, 1986). Many elements and their compounds have not been adequately tested for carcinogenicity in animals, and at this time there is no evidence that such elements exhibit effects in humans on the basis of epidemiologic studies. By contrast, compounds of cadmium, chromium, and nickel have induced malignant neoplasms in humans primarily in industrial and refining situations (Table 8-1, part A) (Magos, 1991). In the case of cadmium, the evidence for carcinogenicity in humans is somewhat limited (Waalkes et al., 1992) because of the variety of confounding factors that occur in situations of human exposure. However, its carcinogenic effect in animals is well documented. By contrast, organonickel compounds, especially nickel carbonyl (Fig. 8-2), are carcinogenic to humans in several tissues, as noted in Table 8-1. Exposures to several metals and their compounds, including lead (Verschaeve et al., 1979) and beryllium (Kuschner, 1981), have been implicated as causes of cancer in humans, but the data are not sufficient to demonstrate such an association unequivocally. In contrast, arsenic and its derivatives present an interesting paradox (Landrigan, 1981) in that there is essentially no experimental evidence to substantiate the carcinogenicity of this element and its compounds in lower animals, whereas the evidence for its carcinogenicity in humans is quite clear (Sky-Peck, 1986).

Film and Fiber Carcinogenesis

A class of chemical carcinogens different from those described thus far is the group of inert plastic and metal films or similar forms that cause sarcomas at the implantation site in some rodents (Brand et al., 1975). The implantation site is usually subcutaneous. Rats and mice are highly susceptible to this form of carcinogenesis, but guinea pigs appear to be resistant (Stinson, 1964). The carcinogenic properties of the implant are to a large extent dependent on its physical characteristics and surface area. Multiple perforations each greater than a certain diameter (for example, 0.4 μm), pulverization, or roughening of the surface of the implant (Ferguson, 1977) markedly reduced the incidence of neoplasms. Plastic sponge implants may also induce sarcomas subcutaneously, and in this instance the yield of tumors is dependent on the thickness of the sponge implant (Roe et al., 1967). The age of the animal at implantation also affects the time that elapses from implantation and tumor development (Paulini et al., 1975).

The chemical nature of the implant is not the critical factor in its ability to transform normal cells to neoplastic cells. Brand and associates (Johnson et al., 1970) studied this phenomenon intensively and demonstrated a variety of kinetic and morphologic characteristics of the process of "foreign-body tumorigenesis" in mice. These investigations have shown that DNA synthesis occurs in the film-attached cell population throughout the preneoplastic phase and that preneoplastic cells may be identified well before neoplasms develop (Thomassen et al., 1978). Brand suggested that such "preneoplastic" cells may be present in normal tissue before implantation and that the implant appears to "create the conditions" required for carcinogenesis of these cells (Brand et al., 1975). Other possible mechanisms for this unique type of carcinogenesis are discussed later in this chapter.

While the epidemiologic evidence that implants of prostheses in humans, such as those used for the repair of hernias and joint replacements, induce the formation of sarcomas is not substantial, there have been a number of isolated reports of neoplasms arising in association with such foreign bodies (Sunderman, 1989). A study in the rat of the carcinogenic potential of a number of materials used in such prostheses demonstrated a small increase in sarcomas in animals with certain metal alloy implants that contained significant amounts of cobalt, chromium, or nickel (Memoli et al., 1986). Of greater significance is the induction of malignant mesothelioma and bronchogenic carcinoma in humans by exposure to asbestos fibers. In this case, the induction of the malignant mesotheliomas

Table 8-1
Carcinogenicity of Metals

A. Metals Causally Associated with Human Cancer

METAL AND SOURCE	MALIGNANCY
Arsenic	
Cu refinery	Pulmonary carcinoma
As pesticides	Lymphoma, leukemia
Chemical plants	Dermal carcinoma
Drinking water (oral)	Hepatic angiosarcoma
Cigarette smoke	
Cadmium	
Cd refinery	Pulmonary carcinoma
Chromium	
Cr refinery	Pulmonary carcinoma
Chrome plating	Gastrointestinal carcinoma
Chromate pigments	
Nickel	
Ni refinery	Pulmonary carcinoma
	Nasolaryngeal carcinoma
	Gastric and renal carcinoma
	Sarcoma (?)

B. Carcinogenicity of Metals in Experimental Animals

METALS	ANIMALS	TUMOR	SITE	ROUTE
Beryllium	Mice, rats, monkeys	Osteosarcoma	Bone	IV, INH
		Carcinoma	Lung	
Cadmium	Mice, rats, chickens	Sarcoma	Injection site	IM, SC, ITS
		Teratoma	Testes	
Cobalt	Rats, rabbits	Sarcoma	Injection site	IM, SC
Chromium	Mice, rats, rabbits	Sarcoma	Injection site	IM, SC, IP,
		Carcinoma	Lung	INH
Iron	Hamsters, mice, rats, rabbits	Sarcoma	Injection site	IM, IP, SC
Nickel	Mice, rats, cats, hamsters, rabbits	Sarcoma	Injection site	IM, ITS, SC
	Guinea pigs, rats	Carcinoma	Lung	INH, IP, IR
		Carcinoma	Kidney	
Lead	Mice, rats	Carcinoma	Kidney	IP, PO, SC
Titanium	Rats	Sarcoma	Injection site	IM
Zinc	Chickens, rats, hamsters	Carcinoma	Testes	ITS
		Teratoma	Testes	

KEY: IV, intravenous; INH, inhalation; IM, intramuscular; SC, subcutaneous; ITS, intratesticular; IP, intraperitoneal; IR, intrarenal; PO, per os.

SOURCE: From Sky-Peck (1986), with permission.

appears to be dependent on the crystal structure rather than the composition of the asbestos both in experimental animals and in humans (Craighead, 1982). In experimental animals, fibers longer than 8 μm and with a diameter less than 1.5 μm induce mesothelioma fairly effectively. Similarly, certain types of asbestos, such as the crocidolite form, are most strongly associated with the occurrence of this neoplasm, whereas exposure to other forms, such as chrysotile, may not be as important a cause of malignant mesothelioma. Thus, in both humans and animals, film and fiber carcinogenesis is largely independent of the chemical nature of the inciting agent.

Hormonal Carcinogenesis

Hormones consist of amines, steroids, and polypeptides. Beatson (1896) was the first to point out that hormones may be causally associated with the development of specific neoplasms. He suggested that a relationship exists between breast cancer and the ovary, the major site of production of female sex hormones.

Hormones play an important physiological role in maintaining the "internal milieu" (Bernard, 1878, 1879). Some cancers may result from abnormal internal production of specific hormones. Alternatively, excessive production or the derangement of the homeostatic mechanisms of an organism may result in neoplastic transformation (Clifton and Sridharan, 1975). Furth (1975) was emphatic in his propositions and demonstrations that disruption of the cybernetic relation between peripheral endocrine glands and the anterior pituitary can result in neoplasia of one of the glands involved (Fig. 8-3). One of the classic examples is the experimental transplantation of normal ovaries into the spleen of castrated rodents (Biskind and Biskind, 1944). This results in a break in the pituitary-gonadal hormone feedback loop. The break occurs because estrogens produced by the ovary are carried by the splenic venous system to the liver. In the liver, the estrogens are metabolized and thus are prevented from entering the general circulation to suppress the pituitary production of gonadotropins. The excessive production of gonadotropins and their constant stimulus of the ovarian fragment in the spleen result ultimately in neoplasia of the ovarian implant.

A similar mechanism is likely to be involved in the production of thyroid neoplasms either by the administration of goitrogens (chemicals that inhibit the synthesis and/or secretion of normal thyroid hormone) or by a marked increase in the circulating levels of thyrotropin secreted by thyrotropin-secreting pituitary neoplasms transplanted into the host. In the former instance, there is a break in the feedback loop and the pituitary gland produces high levels of thyrotropin in the absence of the normal feedback regulation by the thyroid hormone (Furth, 1975). In fact, in humans there is substantial evidence that this may be the mechanism of the development of many thyroid cancers (Williams, 1989). In this case, high levels of circulating thyrotropin result from the unregulated production of this hormone by the transplanted neoplasm (Ueda and Furth, 1967). Thyroidectomy and neonatal gonadectomy result in the development of neoplasms of the pituitary, presumably because of the lack of inhibition by the hormone from the target end organ (Furth, 1975). Chronic administration of pituitary growth hormone also induces a variety of neoplasms in the rat (Moon et al., 1950a, b). Theoretically, then, neoplasms of any of the end organs shown in Fig. 8-3 may be produced by some manipulation that breaks the feedback loop between the pituitary and the target organ.

Some examples of carcinogenesis resulting from the interruption of the cybernetics of hormonal relationships seen in Fig. 8-3 are listed in Table 8-2. In addition to effecting carcinogenesis in the ovary (Biskind and Biskind, 1944), endogenous gonadotropins are involved in the development of adrenocortical and interstitial (Leydig's) cell neoplasms in mice and rats, respectively (Table 8-2). Unleaded gasoline acts like an antiestrogen, thus removing the estrogen protection usually provided against the development of liver neoplasms in the mouse (Standeven et al., 1994) and leading to an increased number of hepatic neoplasms in the female. Phenobarbital acts to decrease serum levels of thyroid hormone (T_3) by stimulating enzymes that metabolize and eliminate the hormone before it can be recycled to the hypothalamus (McClain, 1989). This mechanism is very similar to the effects of goitrogens, which prevent T_3 formation and release from the thyroid. The induction of pituitary adenomas, which themselves produce large amounts of prolactin, is due to an inhibition of the formation of dopamine in the hypothalamus. Dopamine acts like an inhibitor of prolactin synthesis and release by the pituitary. When this inhibition is eliminated by estrogen inhibition of dopamine formation, prolactin-producing pituitary cells replicate at a very high rate. Furthermore, they produce extensive amounts of prolactin, which in turn, in the presence of estrogens, leads to mammary neoplasia (Neumann, 1991).

Figure 8-4 shows some representative structures of hormones, naturally occurring and synthetic, for which there is substantial

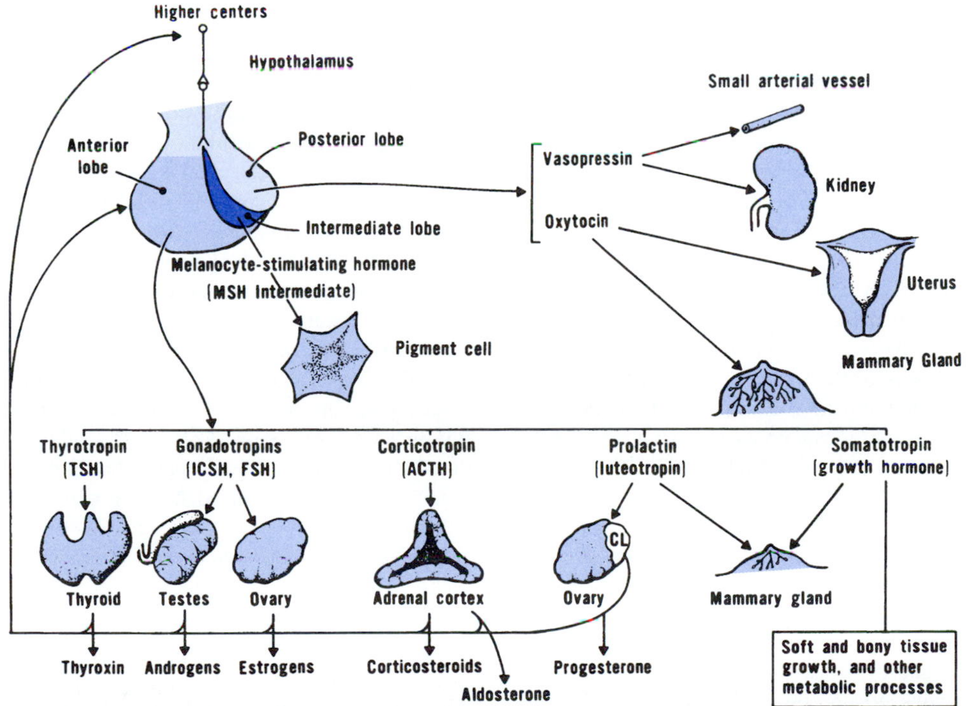

Figure 8-3. Cybernetic relations of the pituitary gland (anterior, intermediate, posterior lobes) with the hypothalamus, other endocrine organs, and tissues of the organism. [After Furth (1975), reproduced with the permission of the author and publisher.]

Table 8-2
Interrupted Cybernetics of Hormonal Carcinogenesis in Rodents

SPECIES/TISSUE	INDUCING AGENT	HORMONAL CARCINOGEN	INTERRUPTED PATHWAY	REFERENCE
Mouse/ovary	Ovary transplant to spleen	Gonadotropin	Estrogen → hypothalamus	Biskind and Biskind, 1944
Rat/thyroid	Goitrogen or thyrotropin-secreting tumor	Thyrotropin	T_3 → hypothalamus	Cf. Furth, 1975
Mouse/adrenal cortex	Ovariectomy	Gonadotropins	Estrogen → hypothalamus	Kawashima et al., 1980
Female mouse/ liver	Unleaded gasoline	Androgens	Estrogen synthesis	Standeven et al., 1994
Rat/thyroid	Phenobarbital	Thyrotropin	T_3 → hypothalamus	McClain, 1989
Rat/pituitary	Estrogens	?	Dopamine → pituitary	Cf. Neumann, 1991
Rat/Leydig cells	Antiantrogens	Gonadotropins	Androgens → hypothalamus	Cf. Neumann, 1991
Rat/mammary gland	Estrogens	Prolactin	Dopamine → pituitary	Cf. Neumann, 1991

evidence of carcinogenicity in lower animals and/or humans. In addition to the structure of growth hormone, two other growth factors expressed in adult tissues—transforming growth factor-α (TGF-α), which is expressed in the small intestine (Barnard et al., 1991), the major salivary glands (Wu et al., 1993), and other tissues (Lee et al., 1993), and insulin-like growth factor-II (IGF-II), which is expressed in the forebrain, uterus, kidney, heart, skeletal muscle, and to a very small degree the liver (Murphy et al., 1987)—may be considered as chemical carcinogens. The carcinogenic action of these two growth factor hormones in vivo has been demonstrated by the use of transgenic mice, among which animals overexpressing TGF-α developed liver neoplasms in dramatic excess of the number seen in controls (Lee et al., 1992), and animals expressing high levels of IGF-II developed excessive numbers of hepatocellular carcinomas and lymphomas (Rogler et al., 1994).

As noted in Table 8-2, neoplasms of the pituitary and the peripheral endocrine organs may be induced by the administration of steroid sex hormones. Although the kidney is not usually considered a peripheral endocrine organ, its cells produce erythropoietin. Synthetic or natural estrogen administration can induce renal cortical carcinomas in male hamsters (Li and Li, 1990), and estradiol induces Leydig cell tumors of the testes in mice (Huseby, 1980). However, a closely related structural analogue, 2-fluoroestradiol, which exhibits significant estrogenic potency, did not induce renal carcinoma in the same sex and species (Liehr, 1983). Recently, the synthetic antiestrogen tamoxifen was found to induce carcinomas of the liver in the rat as well (Williams et al., 1993). Evidence that male hormones by themselves are carcinogenic is not as strong as the data for the carcinogenicity of female hormones. The natural male hormone testosterone does exhibit a weak ability to "transform" hamster embryo cells in culture into a neoplastic phenotype (Lasne et al., 1990). The evidence that synthetic androgens are carcinogenic is somewhat greater, especially in humans. In addition, elevated serum testosterone levels are associated with an increased risk of hepatocellular carcinoma in humans (Yu and Chen, 1993). A number of reports (Mays and Christopherson, 1984; Chandra et al., 1984) have indicated a causative relationship between the administration of synthetic androgens such as oxymetholone (Fig. 8-4*B*) for various clinical conditions and the appearance of hepatocellular neoplasms, predominantly benign.

In addition to apparently direct induction of neoplasia by hormonal stimuli, hormones act in concert with known carcinogenic agents to induce neoplasia. One of the better studied examples of this phenomenon is the induction of mammary adenocarcinomas in rodents. Bittner (1956) demonstrated that three factors are essential for the production of mammary carcinoma in mice: genetic susceptibility, hormonal influence, and a virus transmitted through the milk. The importance of the first two factors has been demonstrated repeatedly in a variety of species, including humans, but incontrovertible evidence for the participation of a virus in mammary carcinogenesis has been obtained only in mice. In the rat, high levels of endogenous prolactin enhance the induction of mammary carcinomas by dimethylbenz(*a*)anthracene (Ip et al., 1980). Chronic treatment with synthetic or natural estrogens alone may induce mammary carcinomas in rodents. Thus, mammary carcinogenesis in rodents is a complicated process that requires several components that may differ from species to species.

Both male and female sex steroid hormones have also been shown to act in concert with known carcinogenic agents to increase the incidence of neoplasia. Various synthetic estrogens administered chronically to animals that had been dosed with a known carcinogen markedly enhanced the development of hepatocellular carcinomas in the rat (Yager and Yager, 1980). Both testosterone and synthetic androgens given with or after chemical carcinogens enhance the induction of adenocarcinomas of the prostate and other accessory sex organs of the male (Hoover et al., 1990). A combi-

Figure 8-4 **A.** ***Structures of polypeptide hormones (hGH, human growth hormone; TGF-α, transforming growth factor alpha; IGF-II, insulin growth factor-II).*** **B.** ***Structures of some naturally occurring (beta-estradiol and testosterone) and synthetic steroid hormones and antihormones.***

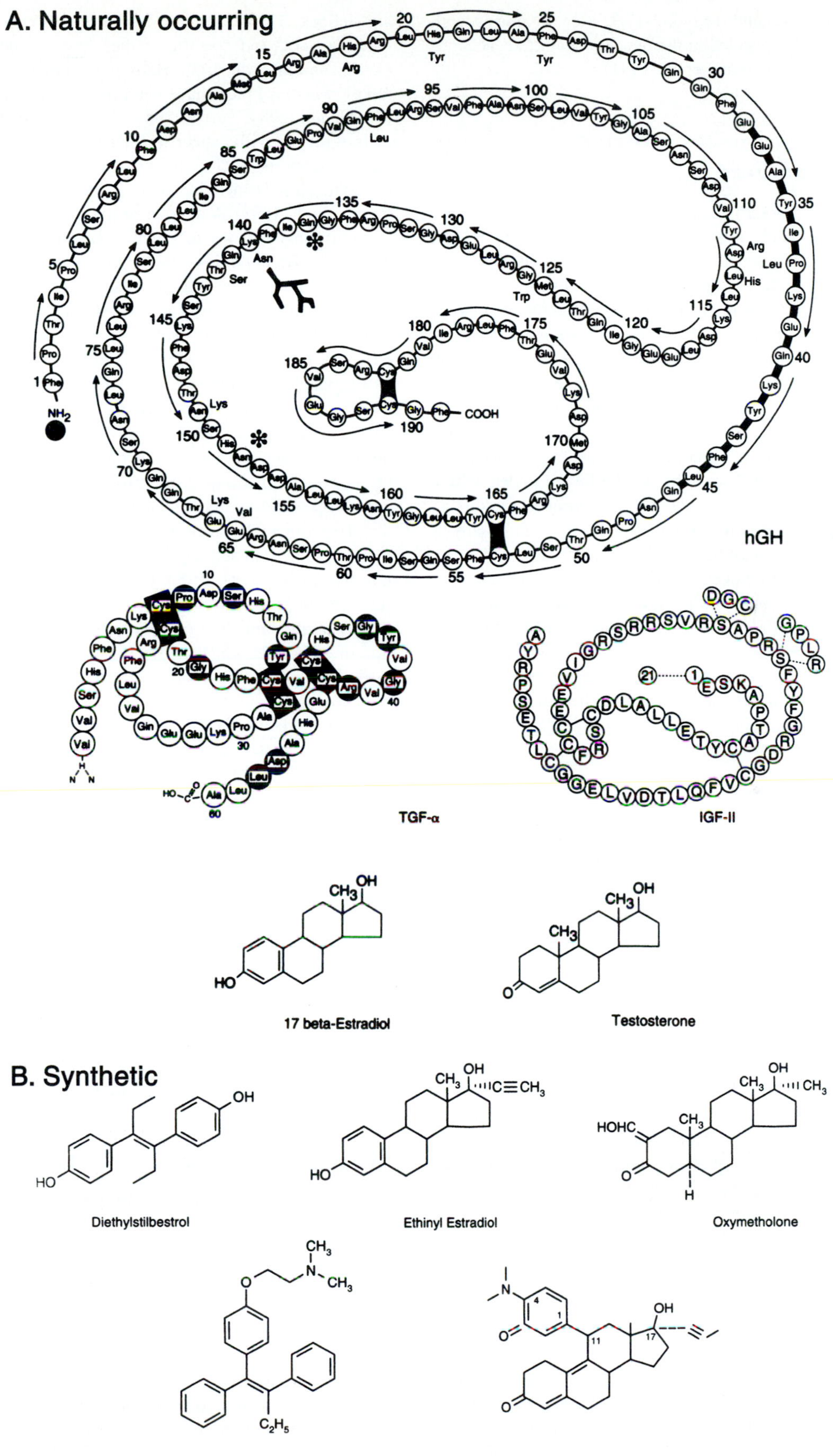
A. Naturally occurring
hGH
TGF-α
IGF-II
17 beta-Estradiol
Testosterone
B. Synthetic
Diethylstilbestrol
Ethinyl Estradiol
Oxymetholone
Tamoxifen
RU 486

nation of testosterone and estradiol-17β after treatment with methylnitrosourea also resulted in the development of adenocarcinomas of the prostate (Bosland et al., 1991).

Chemical Carcinogenesis by Mixtures: Defined and Undefined

While most of this chapter is concerned with the carcinogenic action of specific chemicals, it is relatively unusual for an individual to be exposed to a single carcinogenic agent. Despite this, relatively few detailed studies on mixtures of carcinogenic chemicals have been carried out experimentally. The most common environmental mixtures are those seen in tobacco smoke and other combustion products, including engine exhaust and air pollution (Mauderly, 1993). Interactions between the chemicals in mixtures may be additive, synergistic, or inhibitory (Berger, 1995). In the examples given above, however, the exact chemical nature of components in tobacco smoke or air pollution is not always known and their amounts determined. Thus, one may be forced to deal with a mixture as if it were a single entity or, if the constituents are known, treat the effects of the mixture in an empiric way that usually is related to the most potent component in the mixture.

Studies on the carcinogenic action of defined mixtures of chemicals are usually done with a knowledge of the carcinogenic effect of the chemicals involved. Warshawsky and coworkers (1993) demonstrated that extremely low levels of benzo[*a*]pyrene, which produced no skin tumors on repeated application, resulted in a significant yield of neoplasms when applied in the presence of five noncarcinogenic polycyclic aromatic hydrocarbons. In an earlier study, the administration of two noncarcinogenic aminoazo dyes in the diet of the rat for a year resulted in the appearance of a variety of neoplasms (Neish et al., 1967). More recently, the administration of three to five *N*-nitrosamines resulted in either an additive or synergistic carcinogenic effect of the combinations of the compounds when given at low dose rates (Berger et al., 1987; Lijinsky et al., 1983). In contrast, the administration of a mixture of 40 chemical carcinogens to rats for 2 years at 50 percent of the dose normally used to induce neoplasms in 50 percent of the animals resulted in significant tumor incidences only in the thyroid and liver (Takayama et al., 1989). In a more recent study, ingestion of a mixture of 20 pesticides given at "acceptable daily intake levels" was found to exert no effect on carcinogenesis in rat liver (Ito et al., 1998).

Thus the toxicologic study of complex mixtures not only in the area of carcinogenesis but also as a more general problem in toxicology, is a critical field in human health, as evidenced by disease resulting from a variety of chemical mixtures such as tobacco smoke, diesel exhaust, solvent mixtures, petroleum distillates, and other components of outdoor air pollutants (Feron et al., 1998). As noted above, and as emphasized by others, exposures to chemicals at low, non-toxic doses of the individual constituents may well be of no significant health concern (Cassee et al., 1998). One of the most important chemical mixtures associated with human neoplasia is diet.

Chemical Carcinogenesis by Diet There is substantial evidence in humans to indicate that many dietary components—including excessive caloric intake (Osler, 1987; Lutz and Schlatter, 1992), excessive alcohol intake (IARC, 1987), and a variety of chemical contaminants of the diet including aflatoxin B_1 (Fig. 8-2) (Gorchev and Jelinek, 1985; Lutz and Schlatter, 1992)—are carcinogenic. Other general and specific studies have supported these views (Jensen and Madsen, 1988; Habs and Schmähl, 1980; Miller et al., 1994), whereas others have been more controversial (Willett and MacMahon, 1984; Pariza, 1984). Evidence for the association of dietary factors with cancer incidence in animals is more substantial and supports much of the evidence relating environmental factors to increased cancer incidence in the human (Kritchevsky, 1988; Rogers et al., 1993). A number of the dietary factors implicated in the nutritional etiology of specific human cancers may be seen in Table 8-3 (Trichopoulos, 1989). As noted in the table, the caloric content of diets as well as their individual chemical components are factors in cancer development. Although a relative lack of "antioxidant micronutrients" such as keratinoids, selenium, and the vitamins A, C, and E has been implicated as a factor in the incidence of neoplastic development (Blot et al., 1993; Byers and Perry, 1992), more studies are needed before the effectiveness of these agents in cancer prevention in the human can be established. In addition, food contaminants—either added, occurring endogenously, or as a result of the cooking process—may function as carcinogenic agents in the diet (McGregor, 1998).

Experimental evidence that the lack of available sources of methyl groups can actually induce liver cancer in rats is well documented (Mikol et al., 1983; Ghoshal and Farber, 1984). This observation may be closely related to the earlier studies by Farber (1963) on the induction of liver cancer in rats by the administration of ethionine, which indirectly may cause a lack of available methyl groups in this tissue. Thus, it is apparent that carcinogenesis induced by diet is an extremely complex effect of mixtures of a variety of chemicals. Its importance in human cancer etiology is emphasized further later in this chapter.

MECHANISMS OF CHEMICAL CARCINOGENESIS

Although the discovery that polycyclic hydrocarbons and other chemical compounds can induce cancer in experimental animals gave hope that the complete understanding of the nature of the genesis of neoplasia might be forthcoming, more than 60 years have elapsed since those initial findings, and it appears that we are still a long way from this goal. However, the realization that chemical carcinogens are altered within the living organism by metabolic reactions has brought us much closer to achieving a working understanding of the mechanisms of carcinogenesis.

Metabolism of Chemical Carcinogens in Relation to Carcinogenesis

When it became apparent from the studies of Yoshida and others that chemicals other than polycyclic hydrocarbons were carcinogenic by a variety of metabolic routes, the dilemma of understanding the mechanisms of action of this variety of agents appeared almost insurmountable. It was noted that the excretory metabolites of polycyclic hydrocarbons were hydroxylated derivatives, which usually had little or no carcinogenic activity. Similarly, hydroxylation of the rings of the aromatic amine carcinogens such as 2-acetylaminofluorene (AAF) and 4-dimethyl-aminoazobenzene often resulted in a complete loss of activity. The enzymatic production of these more polar metabolites facilitated the

Table 8-3
Nutritional Etiology of Human Cancer, by Site

CANCER	POSITIVE TOTAL ENERGY BALANCE	LIPIDS	VEGETABLES AND FRUITS	OTHER FIBER, STARCH, CEREALS	PROTEINS	ALCOHOL	β-CAROTENE (VITAMIN A)	VITAMIN C	SALT
Esophagus			−			++	(−)	(−)	(+)
Stomach			−−	(+)			(−)	(−)	+
Large bowel	(+)	+	−	(−)	(+)				
Liver						+			
Pancreas		(+)	(−)						
Gallbladder	(+)								
Lung			(−)				−−		
Bladder									
Kidney	(+)								
Breast*	+	(+)	(−)			(+)	(−)		
Endometrium	+								
Ovary		(+)	(−)						
Prostate	(+)	(+)	(−)						
Cardiovascular	++	++		(−)		−−			+

KEY: ++, +, (+), strong, moderate, and suggestive (but inadequate) evidence, respectively, for a positive (causal) relation;
−−, −, (−), strong, moderate, and suggestive (but inadequate) evidence, respectively, for a negative (protective) relation.
*Height and, for postmenopausal women, obesity are breast cancer risk factors.
SOURCE: Reproduced from Trichopoulos (1989), with permission of the author and publisher.

further metabolism and excretion of the parent compound. The beginning of our present understanding of this dilemma was reported by Elizabeth and James Miller, who first demonstrated that azo dyes became covalently bound to proteins of the liver, but not to proteins of the resulting neoplasms (Miller and Miller, 1947). These initial studies of the Millers led them to suggest that the binding of carcinogens to proteins might lead to the loss or deletion of proteins critical for growth control.

As an extension of this work, Elizabeth Miller (1951) demonstrated the covalent binding of benzo(*a*)pyrene or some of its metabolites to proteins in the skin of mice treated with the hydrocarbon. Later Abell and Heidelberger (1962) described the same phenomenon with another carcinogenic polycyclic hydrocarbon, 3-methylcholanthrene. These findings strongly suggested that a critical step in the induction of cancer by chemicals was the covalent interaction of some form of the chemical with macromolecules. Since the parent compound was incapable of covalent binding directly with macromolecules, the logical conclusion was that the interaction of the chemical with the macromolecule was the result of the metabolic alteration of the parent compound.

Although a number of studies in the 1950s (cf. Weisburger and Weisburger, 1958) demonstrated that ring-hydroxylation was a major pathway in the metabolism of AAF, the Millers and Cramer (Miller et al., 1960) reported that hydroxylation of the nitrogen of the acetylamino group also occurred. They isolated *N*-hydroxy-AAF from the urine of AAF-treated rats and found this metabolite to be more carcinogenic than the parent compound, AAF. Furthermore, *N*-hydroxy-AAF induced neoplasms not observed with the parent compound, such as subcutaneous sarcomas at the site of injection. In animals, such as the guinea pig, that convert little of the AAF to its *N*-hydroxy derivative, cancer of the liver was not produced by feeding the parent compound. These findings strongly supported the suggestion that the parent compound might not be the direct carcinogen; instead, certain metabolic derivatives were active in the induction of neoplasia. These studies paved the way to further investigations of the activation of carcinogens by means of their metabolism (Miller, 1970).

Figure 8-5 depicts a number of metabolic reactions involved in the "activation" of chemicals to the ultimate carcinogenic forms. One may divide such metabolic functions into two general classes (Goldstein and Faletto, 1993). Those involved in phase I metabolism (Fig. 8-5) occur within the endoplasmic reticulum. These reactions involve metabolism by cytochrome P-450 mixed-function oxidases and their reductase as well as the mixed-function amine oxidase. Generally, these metabolic reactions induce biotransformation by converting a substrate to a more polar compound through the introduction of molecular oxygen. Phase II metabolic reactions (Fig. 8-6) are biosynthetic reactions that involve conjugation and occur primarily in the cytosol of the cell. A detailed consideration of xenobiotic metabolism pathways is beyond the scope of this text; the reader is referred to several pertinent reviews (Porter and Coon, 1991; Guengerich, 1992) and Chap. 6 of this book.

As noted in Fig. 8-5, the *N*-hydroxylation of AAF can be followed by esterification of the *N*-hydroxyl group to yield a highly reactive compound capable of nonenzymatic reaction with nucleophilic sites on proteins and nucleic acids. The demonstration of the metabolism of AAF to a highly reactive chemical led the Millers to propose that chemical carcinogens are or can be converted into electrophilic reactants (chemicals with electron-deficient sites). These electrophilic agents exert their carcinogenic effects by covalent interaction with cellular macromolecules (Miller, 1978). Furthermore, the Millers proposed that chemical carcinogens requiring metabolism for their carcinogenic effect be termed procarcinogens, whereas their highly reactive metabolites were termed ultimate carcinogens. Metabolites intermediate between the procarcinogens and ultimate carcinogens were called "proximate" car-

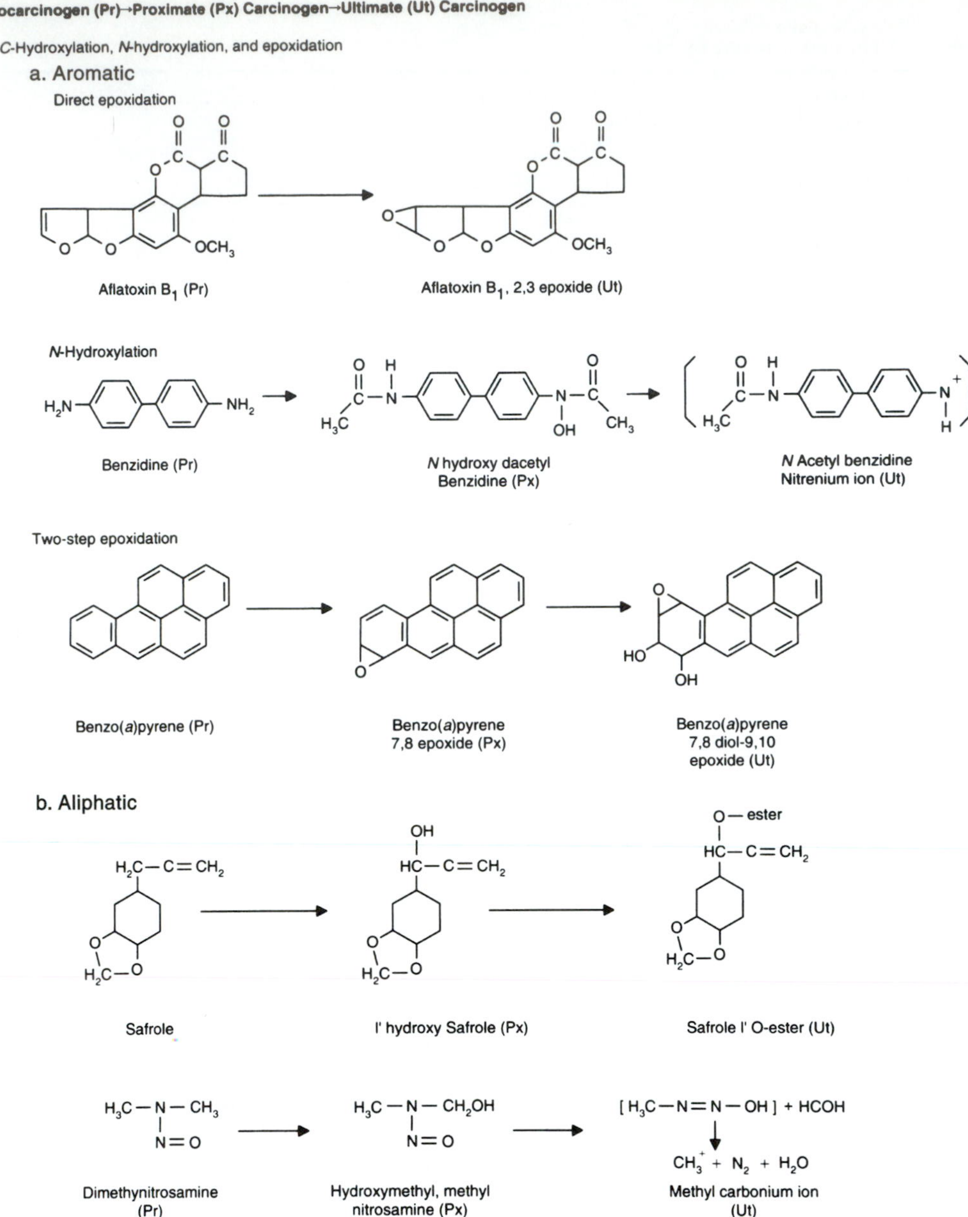

Figure 8-5. ***Structures of representative chemical carcinogens and their metabolic derivatives, the proximate (Px) and ultimate (Ut) carcinogenic forms resulting from the action of phase 1 metabolism of procarcinogens (Pr).***

cinogens. The "ultimate" form of the carcinogen, that is, the form that actually interacts with cellular constituents and probably causes the neoplastic transformation, is the final product shown in the pathways provided in Fig. 8-5. In some instances the structure of the ultimate form of certain carcinogenic chemicals is still not known, while in other cases there may be more than one ultimate carcinogenic metabolite.

After the demonstration by the Millers of the critical significance of electrophilic metabolites in chemical carcinogenesis, the ultimate forms of a number of compounds—specifically of the aromatic amines such as benzidine, naphthylamine, and 4-aminobiphenyl—were described. However, the carcinogenic polycyclic hydrocarbons still posed a problem. Pullman and Pullman (1955) had earlier proposed that the K region (Fig. 8-1) of polycyclic hydrocarbons was important in predicting their carcinogenicity. Boyland (1950) proposed the formation of epoxide intermediates in the metabolism of these chemicals. However, it was not until 1970 that Jerina and associates detected the formation of such an intermediate in a biologic system (Jerina et al., 1970). Other investigations showed that epoxides of polycyclic hydrocarbons could react with nucleic acids and proteins in the absence of any metabolizing system. Surprisingly, K-region epoxides of a number of carcinogenic polycyclic hydrocarbons were weaker carcinogens than the parent hydrocarbons. After this finding, scientific attention shifted to other reactive metabolites of these molecules. Benzo(*a*)pyrene has been used as a model compound in studies of carcinogenic polycyclic hydrocarbons, and some of the metabolic reactions observed in vivo are provided in Figs. 8-5 and 8-6. In

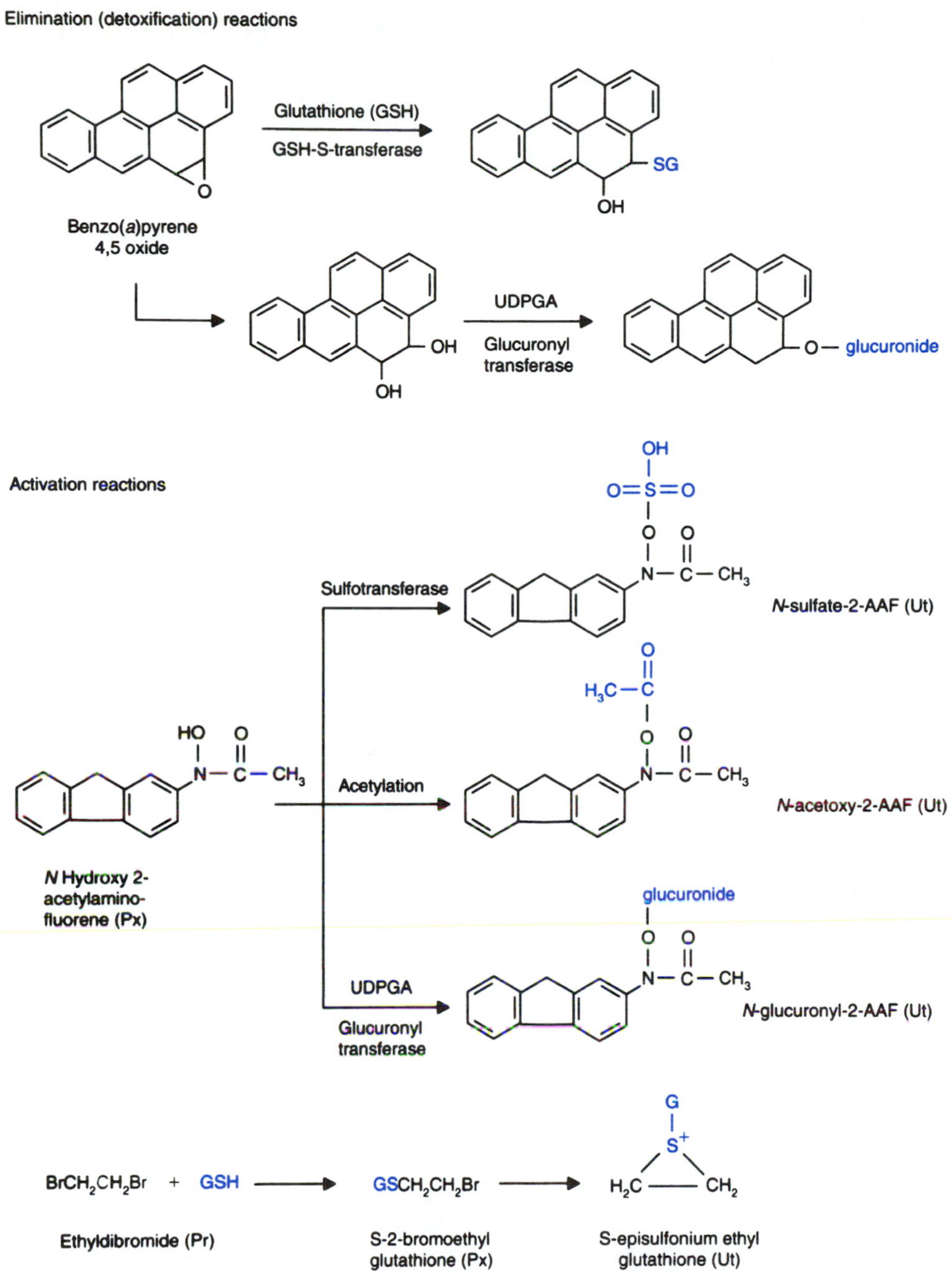

Elimination (detoxification) reactions

Glutathione (GSH)
GSH-S-transferase
SG
OH
Benzo(*a*)pyrene
4,5 oxide
OH
OH
UDPGA
Glucuronyl
transferase
O— glucuronide

Activation reactions

Sulfotransferase
N-sulfate-2-AAF (Ut)
Acetylation
N-acetoxy-2-AAF (Ut)
N Hydroxy 2-
acetylamino-
fluorene (Px)
glucuronide
UDPGA
Glucuronyl
transferase
N-glucuronyl-2-AAF (Ut)

$BrCH_2CH_2Br$ + GSH ⟶ $GSCH_2CH_2Br$ ⟶ H_2C—CH_2 (S^+—G)

Ethyldibromide (Pr)
S-2-bromoethyl
glutathione (Px)
S-episulfonium ethyl
glutathione (Ut)

Figure 8-6. Structures of representative chemical carcinogens and their metabolic derivatives resulting from the action of phase II metabolism of procarcinogens.

1974, Sims and his associates proposed that a diol epoxide of benzo(*a*)pyrene was the ultimate form of this carcinogen (Sims et al., 1974). Subsequent studies by a number of investigators have demonstrated that the structure of this ultimate form is (+)anti-benzo(*a*)pyrene-7,8-dihydrodiol-9,10-epoxide (Yang et al., 1976; also see reviews by: Conney, 1982; Harvey, 1981; Lowe and Silverman, 1984).

One of the ramifications of these findings is the importance of oxidation of the carbons of the "bay region" of potentially carcinogenic polycyclic hydrocarbons. Figure 8-1 indicated the bay regions of benz(*a*)anthracene and benzo(*a*)pyrene. Analogous bay regions may be identified in other polycyclic aromatic hydrocarbons (Fig. 8-1). The bay region is the sterically hindered region formed by the angular benzo ring. Although the bay-region concept has not been tested with all known carcinogenic polycyclic hydrocarbons, it appears to be generally applicable. Several authors (Levin et al., 1978; Conney, 1982) have proposed that epoxidation of the dihydro, angular benzo ring that forms part of a bay region of a polycyclic hydrocarbon may form the ultimate carcinogenic form. In addition, Cavalieri and Rogan (1992) have proposed that radical cations of polycyclic aromatic hydrocarbons formed by oxidation of the parent compound via the cytochrome P-450 pathway are also important intermediates in the formation of ultimate carcinogenic metabolites of these chemicals. Thus, oxidation can result in the metabolic activation of a number of procarcinogens including the PAHs.

Although administration of polypeptide hormones and growth factors can result in neoplasia, these compounds do not possess "ultimate" carcinogenic forms. There is, however, evidence that synthetic steroid hormones, especially estrogens, are metabolized to more reactive intermediates. In the intensively studied estrogen-induced renal neoplasia in hamsters, Zhu and colleagues (1993) have developed substantial evidence that synthetic estrogens are converted to catechol metabolites in significant amounts. These authors have proposed that such metabolites may act as ultimate carcinogenic forms of the synthetic estrogens.

While conjugation with glutathione usually inactivates chemical carcinogens and permits rapid urinary excretion of the conjugate due to water solubility, an exception has recently been described. Both haloalkanes and haloalkenes react with glutathione in a conjugation reaction catalyzed by glutathione *S*-transferase. Halogenated aliphatics may induce neoplasia in several organs, with the kidney as the predominant target site. The glutathione-dependent bioactivation of ethylene dibromide is provided as an example (Fig. 8-6). The proximate carcinogen of ethylene dibromide, glutathione *S*-ethylbromide, spontaneously forms an episulfonium ion as the ultimate carcinogenic form. This highly reactive chemical alkylates DNA at the N^7 position of guanine (Koga et al., 1986). In addition to glutathione conjugates, cysteine *S*-conjugates of several haloalkenes are nephrotoxic and mutagenic (Monks et al., 1990). The actual mechanism of the carcinogenic effect of these two carbon compounds is not clear despite these observations (Monks et al., 1990).

Free Radicals and the Metabolism of Chemical Carcinogens

While phase I and II reactions (see above) catalyze the formation of electrophilic ultimate forms of chemical carcinogens, substantial evidence has accumulated demonstrating a role for free radical reactions in the formation of the ultimate forms of chemical carcinogens (Sun, 1990; Clemens, 1991; Guyton and Kensler, 1993). Free radicals are chemical elements or their compounds that may be positively or negatively charged or neutral but possess a single unpaired electron. In living systems the principal initial source of such free radicals is from the reduction of molecular oxygen by a variety of metabolic pathways including the phase I cytochrome P450 system, mitochondrial oxidation and reduction of oxygen (Kowaltowski and Vercesi, 1999), and enzymes of peroxisomes that produce hydrogen peroxide as a metabolic product (van den Bosch et al., 1992). Several of these forms of "active" oxygen (Fig. 8-7) are also generated during the process of inflammation (Cerutti and Trump, 1991). The superoxide radical may oxidize nitric oxide to the highly reactive peroxynitrite ion which is capable of initiating lipid peroxidation and free radical formation in this species (Hogg and Kalyanaraman, 1999). Most free radicals formed in biological systems are extremely reactive, although a wide range of stabilities are known for a number of different free radical species. While hydrogen peroxide is itself not a free radical, it becomes a source of such on its interaction with transition metals, especially iron, resulting in the formation of the highly reactive hydroxyl free radical, HO· (Fig. 8-7). Although the biological reduction of molecular oxygen is the prime generative pathway for free radical development, free radical intermediates are sometimes formed during the metabolism of chemical carcinogens (Guengerich, 1992), and the metabolic reactions of a number of

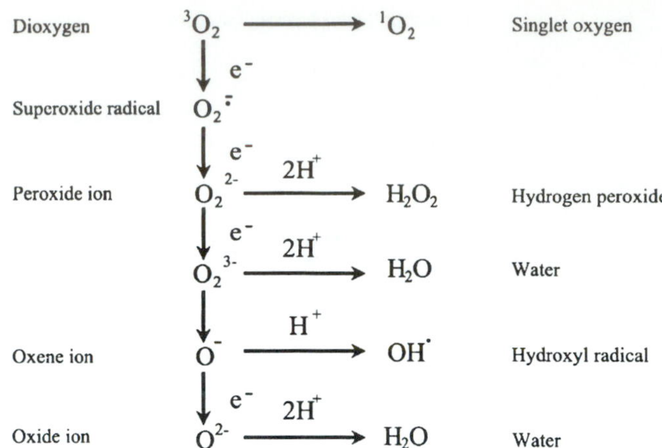

Figure 8-7. Sequential and univalent reduction of molecular oxygen indicating various species produced. [Modified from Martínez-Cayuela (1995), with permission of authors and publishers.]

chemical carcinogens may proceed through free radical intermediates (Floyd, 1981, 1990). Chemical carcinogens—including nitrosamines (Bartsch et al., 1989), nitro compounds (Conaway et al., 1991), and diethylstilbestrol (Wang and Liehr, 1994)—may possess ultimate forms that are free radicals. The formation of free radicals also plays an important role in the carcinogenic effects of ionizing radiation (Biaglow, 1981).

Pathways other than those of the mixed-function oxidase system may also be involved in the bioactivation of chemicals. Marnett (1981) has described the co-oxygenation of polyunsaturated fatty acids, especially arachidonic acid, and polycyclic aromatic hydrocarbons with bioactivation of the hydrocarbon. Such cooxygenation can occur during the synthesis of prostaglandins, a series of autocoids important in normal homeostasis. The prostaglandin H synthetase has two catalytic activities. In the first reaction, the cyclooxygenase activity of prostaglandin H synthetase catalyzes the oxidation of arachidonic acid to the endoperoxidase prostaglandin G_2 (Fig. 8-8). The associated peroxidase activity of prostaglandin H synthase reduces the hydroperoxide prostaglandin G_2 to the alcohol prostaglandin H_2. Many tissues that have a low expression of monooxygenases contain prostaglandin H synthase. In these tissues, compounds can be activated to reactive forms by prostaglandin H synthase, since oxidation by the peroxidase activity often yields a free radical product. The cooxidation of 2-aminofluorene is an example (Fig. 8-8). In the case of benzo(*a*)pyrene 7,8 diol, peroxidase-catalyzed transfer of the free radical from the hydroperoxide to the hydrocarbon results in formation of the ultimate carcinogenic form of benzo(*a*)pyrene, the 7,8 diol 9,10 epoxide. This pathway of metabolic activation of carcinogens, while not ubiquitous, is important in some extrahepatic tissues (Pruess-Schwartz et al., 1989). For example, Wise and colleagues (1984) demonstrated a marked metabolic activation of 2-naphthylamine via the prostaglandin synthase in dog bladder without activation in the liver. Mattammal and associates (1981) have suggested that a number of renal and bladder carcinogens may be activated by this pathway. Several reviews on the role of prostaglandin synthetase in the metabolism of compounds, including their bioactivation in extrahepatic tissues, can be consulted for additional information (Eling et al., 1990; Smith et al., 1991).

In addition to the activation of chemical carcinogens, free radicals may directly react with DNA to produce a variety of struc-

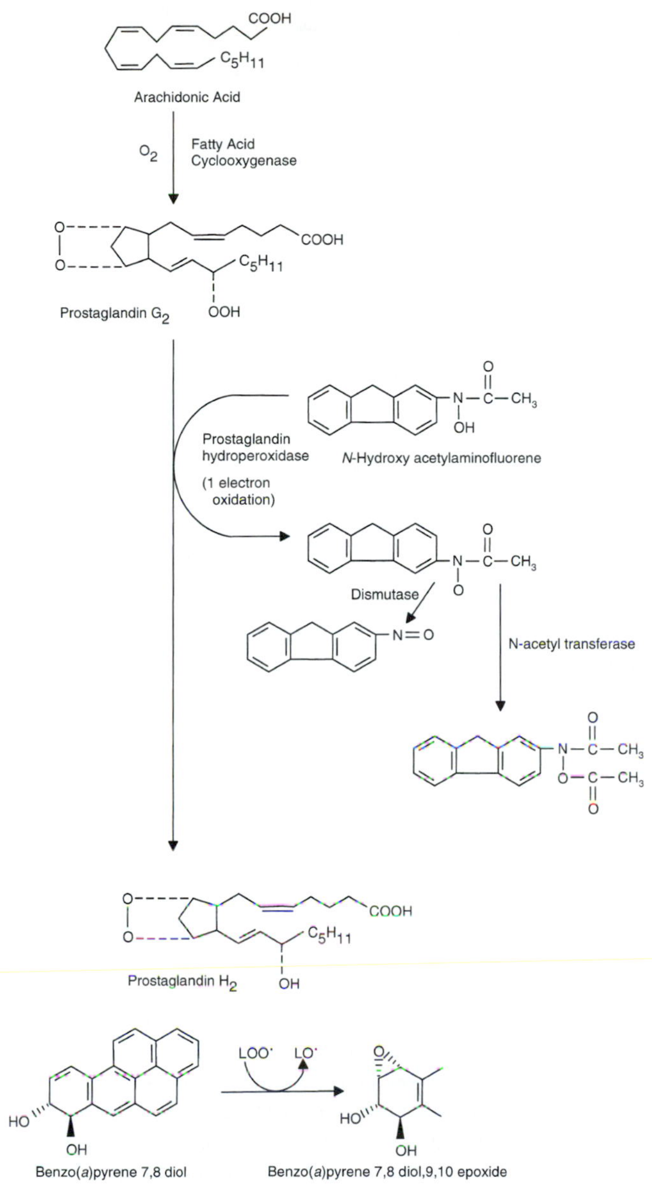

Figure 8-8. The metabolic activation of benzo(a)pyrene 7,8 diol and N-hydroxy 2-acetylaminofluorene during the peroxidation of arachidonic acid.

tural changes in bases. Many of these structures are due to attack by hydroxyl free radicals directly with the DNA base. In a sense such structures are analogous to DNA adducts of carcinogens. The more commonly found of these structures are 8-hydroxy(oxo)guanine and 5-hydroxy-6-hydrothymine. Because of the ubiquitous nature of oxygen free radicals, DNA of all living entities contains a variable number of such structures (Olinski et al., 1998). Under normal circumstances, in mammalian cells there is a quite significant formation of these oxidized DNA bases (see below).

Chemical Structure and Chemical Carcinogenesis

Knowledge of the metabolic activation of chemicals has dramatically advanced our understanding of carcinogenic mechanisms underlying the extreme diversity of chemical structures involved in cancer development. The relationship of chemical structure to carcinogenic activity plays a significant role in the potential identification and mechanism of potential chemical carcinogens. Computerized databases of carcinogenic and noncarcinogenic chemicals have been developed to relate structure to carcinogenic activity in a variety of carcinogens (Enslein et al., 1994; Rosenkranz and Klopman, 1994).

Using the results of rodent bioassays of more than 500 chemicals, Ashby and Paton (1993) studied the influence of chemical structure on both the extent and the target tissue specificity of carcinogenesis for these chemicals. From analysis of the presence of potential electrophilic sites (DNA-reactive), mutagenicity to *Salmonella,* and level of carcinogenicity to rodents, these authors have developed a list of chemical structures that possess a high correlation with the development of neoplasia in rodent tests (Ashby et al., 1989; Tennant and Ashby, 1991). These "structural alerts" signify that a chemical having such structures should be examined closely for carcinogenic potential. These authors have developed a composite model structure indicating the various "structural alerts" that appear to be associated with DNA reactivity or carcinogenicity (Fig. 8-9). The substantial database used to generate these structural alerts indicates the utility of this information for the identification of potential carcinogens and their mechanisms of their action in specific tissues. In addition, investigation of the metabolic activation of such functional groups during the carcinogenic process should provide insight into their role in the induction of cancer.

Mutagenesis and Carcinogenesis

Most chemical carcinogens must be metabolized within the cell before they exert their carcinogenic activity. In this respect, metabolism of some chemicals results in a bioactivation instead of elimination. Thus, metabolic capabilities may underlie how a substance that is not carcinogenic for one species may be carcinogenic for another. This becomes important for carcinogen testing in whole animals for both hazard identification and risk assessment. Such considerations impact directly on the choice of the most sensitive species or the species most similar to humans for these evaluations.

Studies on the induction of liver neoplasms by the food dye *N,N*-dimethyl-4-aminoazobenzene (DAB) provided the first evidence that metabolites of carcinogens could bind to macromolecules. This dye, known as butter yellow, was found to be covalently linked to proteins. Because DAB did not bind to purified protein in vitro and yet could not be extracted from protein after in vivo administration, it was deduced that DAB is metabolized in vivo to a reactive form which covalently binds to cellular macromolecules. The Millers (Miller and Miller, 1947) demonstrated that there was a high degree of correlation between extent of protein binding and carcinogenicity in different species. Because carcinogens are reactive per se or are activated by metabolism to reactive intermediates that bind to cellular components, including DNA, these electrophilic derivatives, which bound to a variety of nucleophilic (electron-dense) moieties in DNA, RNA, and protein, were considered the carcinogenic form of the compounds of interest. Several lines of evidence indicate that DNA is the critical target for carcinogenesis. The first hint that DNA was the target for heritable alterations due to carcinogen administration was from the increased incidence of cancer in genetically prone individuals with defective ability to repair DNA damage (xeroderma pigmentosum; Friedberg, 1992). The second major piece of evidence that DNA was the target of carcinogen action was the observation of carcinogen-induced mutations in specific target genes associated with neoplasia in a multitude of experimental systems. A compar-

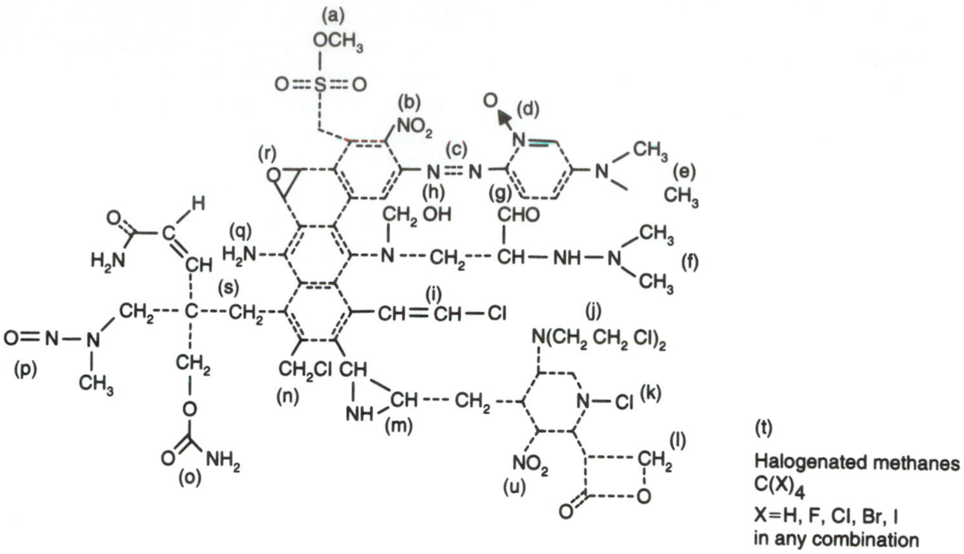

Figure 8-9. The substituents are as follows: (a) alkyl esters of either phosphonic or sulfonic acids; (b) aromatic nitro groups; (c) aromatic azo groups, not per se, but by virtue of their possible reduction to an aromatic amine; (d) aromatic ring,* N*-oxides; (e) aromatic mono and dialkylamino groups; (f) alkyl hydrazines; (g) alkyl aldehydes; (h)* N*-methylol derivatives; (i) monohaloalkenes; (j) a large family of* N *and* S *mustards (β-haloethyl); (k)* N*-chloramines (see below); (l) propiolactones and propiosultones; (m) aromatic and aliphatic aziridinyl derivatives; (n) both aromatic and aliphatic substituted primary alkyl halides; (o) derivatives of urethane (carbamates); (p) alkyl-*N*-nitrosamines; (q) aromatic amines, their* N*-hydroxy derivatives and the derived esters; (r) aliphatic and aromatic epoxides.

The *N*-chloramine substructure (k) has not yet been associated with carcinogenicity, but potent genotoxic activity has been reported for it (discussed in Ashby et al., 1989). Michael-reactive α,β-unsaturated esters, amides, or nitriles form a relatively new class of genotoxin (e.g., acrylamide). However, the structural requirements for genotoxicity have yet to be established, and this structural unit is not shown in the figure. [Adapted from Tennant and Ashby (1991), with permission of the author and publisher.]

ison of DNA adduct formation with biologically effective doses of carcinogens with different potencies demonstrated that the level of DNA damage was relatively similar. Since covalent adducts in DNA could be derived from carcinogenic compounds, the mechanism by which mutations arise and their relationship to carcinogenesis was the next area to be examined in the quest for an understanding of cancer development.

The induction of mutations is due primarily to chemical or physical alterations in the structure of DNA that result in inaccurate replication of that region of the genome. The process of mutagenesis consists of structural DNA alteration, cell proliferation that fixes the DNA damage, and DNA repair that either directly repairs the alkylated base or bases or results in removal of larger segments of the DNA. Electrophilic compounds can interact with the ring nitrogens, exocyclic amino groups, carbonyl oxygens, and the phosphodiester backbone. The reaction of electrophiles with DNA results in alkylation products that are covalent derivatives of the reactive chemical species with DNA. Direct-acting alkylation agents induce preferential binding to highly nucleophilic centers such as the N^7 position of guanine. Less reactive species such as the active form of diethylnitrosamine will also react with the nucleophilic oxygens in DNA. Carcinogenic agents that result in formation of bulky adducts often specifically react with sites in the purine ring. For example, aromatic amines bind to the C^8 position of guanine, while the diol epoxide of polycyclic aromatic hydrocarbons binds to the N^2 and N^6 position of guanine. The position of an adduct in DNA and its chemical and physical properties in that context dictate the types of mutations induced (Essigmann and Wood, 1993). This indicates that different adducts can induce a distinct spectrum of mutations and additionally that any given adduct can result in a multitude of different DNA lesions. Observations on the need for metabolic activation of compounds to their ultimate reactive form were rapidly extended to a number of other compounds, including 2-acetylaminofluorene. In tests of mutagenicity, it was demonstrated that whereas 2-acetylaminofluorene itself is not mutagenic, its sulfate metabolite was highly mutagenic for transforming DNA (Maher et al., 1968). These findings led to the development of mutagenesis assays for the detection of chemical carcinogens from the premise that one could detect carcinogens in highly mutable strains of bacteria given exogenous liver microsomal preparations for in vitro metabolism of the test agent (see below). Cultured mammalian cells have also been developed for evaluation of the mutagenic action of potential carcinogenic agents. Compounds are evaluated in the presence (Michalopoulos et al., 1981) or absence (Li et al., 1991) of metabolic activation systems such as irradiated hepatic feeder layers or hepatic microsomes. The use of these *in vitro* screens of mutagenicity has permitted analysis of the mutational specificity of some carcinogens (Table 8-4). While the data shown in Table 8-4 were derived from bacterial mutagenesis studies, several other systems have also been utilized in attempts to determine mutagenic specificity of various agents (Essigmann and Wood, 1993).

Point mutations, frameshift mutations, chromosomal aberrations, aneuploidy, and polyploidization can be induced by chemi-

Table 8-4
A Comparison of the Mutagenic Spectrum of Aflatoxin B_1 (AFB_1), Benzo[*a*]pyrene Diolepoxide (BPDE), and 2-Acetylaminofluorene (2-AAF)*

MUTATION	AFB_1	BPDE	2-AAF
GC to TA	0.94	0.76	0.88
GC to AT	0.06	0.11	0.06
GC to CG	0.00	0.13	0.06

SOURCE: Modified from Loechler (1989), with permission.

cals with varying degrees of specificity that are, in part, dose–dependent. Mutagenesis can be the result of several different alterations in the physical and chemical nature of DNA. While alkylation of DNA with small alkyl groups or large bulky adducts can result in mutation, other processes may also be involved. Conformation of the DNA has a major impact on the potential mutagenic activity of a compound. This is best demonstrated by the related compounds 2-acetylaminofluorene and 2-aminofluorene, which both form bulky DNA adducts at guanine residues in DNA. The AAF adduct distorts the double helix, while the AF adduct remains outside the helix and does not distort it. The AAF adduct induces frameshift mutations, whereas that of AF induces primarily transversions (Bichara and Fuchs, 1985). Planar agents that can intercalate between the base pairs in DNA can effectively induce frameshift mutations by exacerbating slippage mispairing in repetitive sequences. In addition, agents that lie within the major or minor groove of DNA can perturb nucleosome formation and may alter DNA replication. Some of these agents are potential chemotherapeutic agents. Agents such as irradiation and topoisomerase inhibitors that induce double-strand breaks can also enhance mutagenesis (Eastman and Barry, 1992).

Several mechanisms of mutagenesis exist. The presence of certain alkylation products, such as the O^6 alkyl deoxyguanosine and the O^4 alkyl deoxythymidine, permits a degenerate base pairing able to base pair with the appropriate base as well as an inappropriate base. This can be demonstrated in vitro and in vivo as the induction of transition mutations after treatment with certain alkylating agents (Singer, 1986). Thus, methylating or ethylating agents result in mutations as a result of base mispairing. The active metabolites of numerous compounds, such as PAHs and aromatic amines, can form bulky DNA adducts that block DNA synthesis, resulting in a noncoding lesion. The synthetic machinery employs bypass synthesis to avoid the lethal impact of these unrepaired lesions (Friedberg, 1994). In this condition, the most prevalent base, frequently deoxyadenosine (Shearman and Loeb, 1979), is inserted opposite the offending adducted nucleotide base. Thus, DNA binding and repair, induction of point mutations, and clastogenicity have proven useful as endpoints in the identification of potential carcinogens as well as biomarkers of carcinogen exposure. The role of DNA repair in protection of the genome and in the induction of mutations is an essential component in the mutagenesis process (see below).

Not all chemical carcinogens require intracellular metabolism to become ultimate carcinogens. Examples of direct-acting mutagens include alkylating agents such as β-propiolactone, nitrogen mustard, ethyleneimine, and bis(chloromethyl)ether (Fig. 8-3). Direct-acting carcinogens are typically carcinogenic at multiple sites and in all species examined. A number of the direct-acting alkylating agents, including some used in chemotherapy, are carcinogenic for humans (Vainio et al., 1991).

Macromolecular Adducts Resulting from Reaction with Ultimate Carcinogens

One of the most intriguing problems in chemical carcinogenesis is the chemical characterization of the covalent compounds derived from reactions between the ultimate metabolite of a chemical carcinogen and a macromolecule. The structures of several carcinogens covalently bound to protein and nucleic acids are provided in Fig. 8-10. As noted in the figure, the reaction of the ultimate form of *N*-methyl-4-aminoazobenzene with polypeptides involves a demethylation of methionine and reaction of the electrophilic position ortho to the amino group of the azobenzene with the nucleophilic sulfur of methionine and subsequent loss of the methyl of methionine. The most nucleophilic site in DNA is the N^7 position of guanine, and many carcinogens form covalent adducts at that site. Adducts formed with DNA exhibit stereospecific configurations, as exemplified by the reaction of the epoxide of aflatoxin B_1 with the N^7 position of guanine. The ultimate carcinogenic form of AAF also reacts with guanine at two positions on the DNA base, as shown in the figure. In contrast, ethylene oxide directly alkylates the N^7 position of guanine in DNA (Bolt et al., 1988). An interesting adduction occurs during the metabolism of 2-nitropropane, which results in the formation of 8-aminoguanine possibly from the spontaneous reaction with the highly reactive intermediate (NH_2^+) formed during the metabolism of the nitro group (Sodum et al., 1993). The formation of an additional ring structure in adenine and cytosine occurs with the ultimate form of vinyl chloride and structurally similar carcinogens (Bolt, 1988). For the detailed chemistry of the reactions involved in the formation of such adducts, several reviews are suggested (Miller, 1970, 1978; Weisburger and Williams, 1982; Hathway and Kolar, 1980; and Dipple et al., 1985).

Several carcinogens that adduct DNA by direct methylation, ethylation, or higher alkylations are of considerable experimental and environmental significance. The sites on the individual DNA bases that are alkylated by ethylating and methylating chemicals and the relative proportions of methylated bases present in DNA after reaction with carcinogen-methylating agents are seen in Table 8-5 (Pegg, 1984). The predominant adduct seen with methylating agents such as methylmethane sulfonate is 7-methylguanine. In contrast, ethylation of DNA occurs predominantly in the phosphate backbone. Pegg has argued that the principal carcinogenic adduct is the O^6-alkylguanine. In contrast, Swenberg and associates (1984) reported that O^4-alkylthymine may be a more important adduct for carcinogenesis because this DNA adduct is retained in the DNA for more extended periods than is the O^6-alkylguanine adduct. The importance of the persistence of DNA adducts of ultimate carcinogens are discussed below.

Another common structural change in DNA is the hydroxylation of DNA bases. Such changes have been found in all four of the bases making up DNA (Marnett and Burcham, 1993), but the most commonly analyzed are 5-hydroxymethylthymine (Srinivasan and Glauert, 1990) and 8-hydroxyguanine (Floyd, 1990). These hydroxylated bases have been found in DNA of target organs in animals administered chemical carcinogens but are also present in the DNA of organisms not subjected to any known carcinogenic agent (Marnett and Burcham, 1993). Estimates of a rate of en-

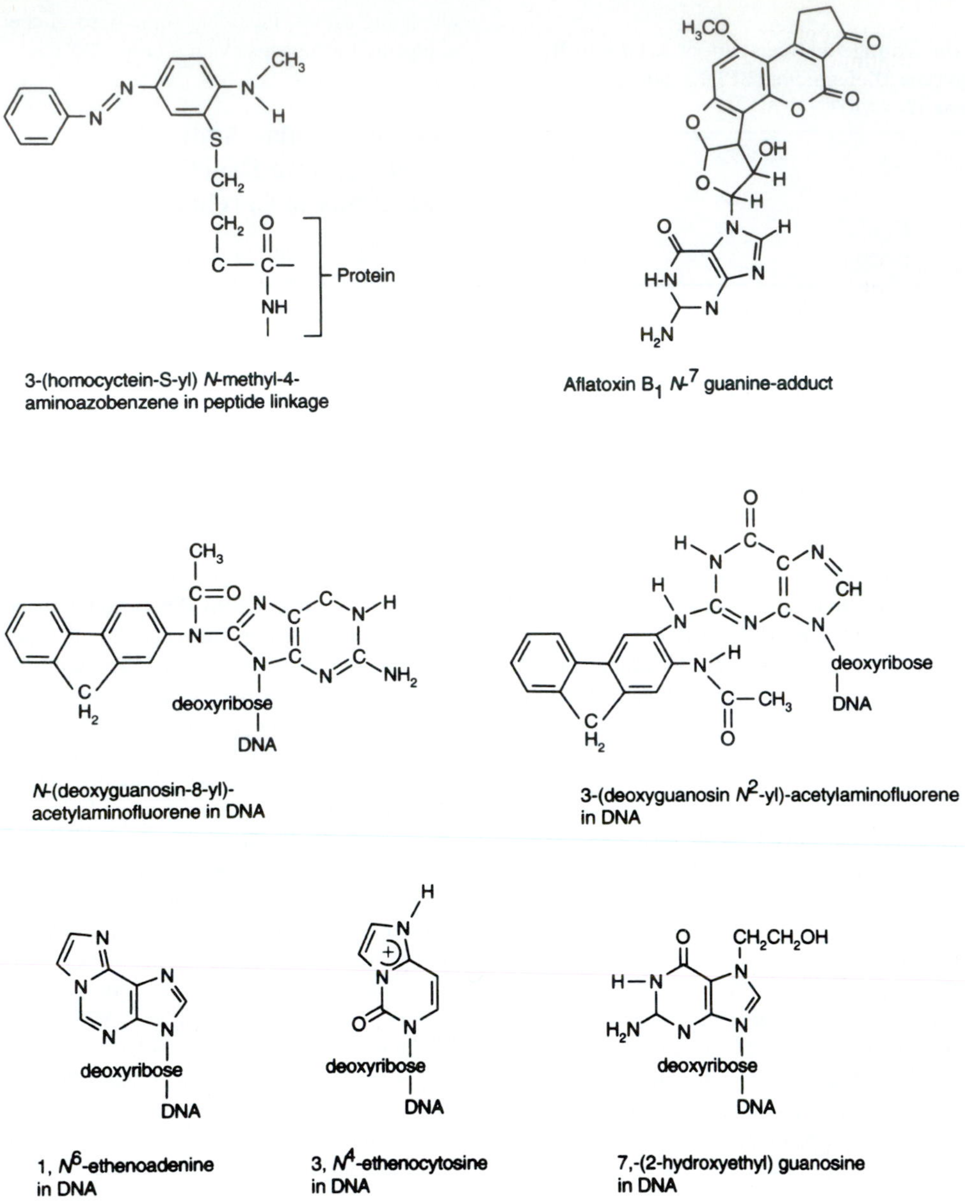

Figure 8-10. Structures of some protein- and nucleic acid-bound forms of certain chemical carcinogens.

The macromolecular linkages are shown schematically. Esters of 2-acetylaminofluorene react predominantly with the 8-position of guanine, whereas the epoxide of aflatoxin B_1 reacts primarily with the N-7 position of guanine. The ethano-adenine and ethano-cytosine adducts result from the reaction of DNA with halogenated acetaldehydes or ultimate forms of vinyl chloride and related structures. 7-(2-Hydroxyethyl)guanosine is a product of the reaction of ethylene oxide with DNA.

dogenous depurination of DNA of 580 bases per hour per cell and DNA strand breaks at a rate of 2300/h per cell have been reported (Shapiro, 1981). These estimates are not incompatible with the presence of oxidative DNA lesions at a level of 10^6 per cell in the young rat and almost twice this in the old rat (Ames et al., 1993). The source of such oxidative damage is presumably from free radical reactions occurring endogenously in the cell that are capable of producing activated oxygen radicals (Floyd, 1990; Ames et al., 1993). Such oxidative reactions, occurring either as a result of an endogenous oxidative phenomenon or from the administration of exogenous chemical and radiation carcinogens, presumably are rapidly repaired by mechanisms discussed below. Thus, endogenous mutations are kept to a minimum.

The best-studied endogenous modification of DNA is the methylation of deoxycytidine residues by the transfer of a methyl group from *S*-adenosylmethionine by DNA methyltransferase (Holliday, 1989; Michalowsky and Jones, 1989). Such methylation results in the heritable expression or repression of specific genes in eukaryotic cells. Genes that are actively transcribed are hypomethylated, whereas those which are hypermethylated tend to be rarely transcribed. When such methylation occurs during development, the expression or repression of specific genes may be "imprinted" by DNA methylation at various stages during development (Barlow, 1993). Chemical carcinogens may inhibit DNA methylation by several mechanisms, including the formation of covalent adducts, single-strand breaks in the DNA alteration in

Table 8-5
Relative Proportions of Methylated Bases Present in DNA after Reaction with Carcinogenic Alkylating Agents

	Percentage of Total Alkylation by	
	DIMETHYLNITROSAMINE *N*-METHYL-*N*-NITROSOUREA 1,2-DIMETHYL-HYDRAZINE	DIETHYLNITROSAMINE *N*-ETHYL-*N*-NITROSOUREA
1-Alkyladenine	0.7	0.3
3-Alkyladenine	8.	4.
7-Alkyladenine	1.5	0.4
3-Alkylguanine	0.8	0.6
7-Alkylguanine	68.	12.
O^6-Alkylguanine	7.5	8.
3-Alkylcytosine	0.5	0.2
O^2-Alkylcytosine	0.1	3.
3-Alkylthymine	0.3	0.8
O^2-Alkylthymine	0.1	7.
O^4-Alkylthymine	0.1–0.7	1–4.
Alkylphosphates	12.	53.

SOURCE: Adapted from Pegg (1984), with permission.

methionine pools, and the direct inactivation of the enzyme, DNA *S*-adenosylmethionine methyltransferase, which is responsible for methylation (Riggs and Jones, 1983). Therefore, the inhibition of DNA methylation by chemical carcinogens may represent a further potential mechanism for carcinogenesis induced by chemicals. Mikol and colleagues (1983) demonstrated the importance of this mechanism in hepatocarcinogenesis; half the animals receiving a diet devoid of methionine and choline for 18 months developed hepatocellular carcinomas and cholangiomas. The methyl-deficient diet induces a drastic hypomethylation of hepatic nuclear DNA (Wilson et al., 1984), which may heritably alter the phenotype of the cell.

Finally, structural changes in DNA of largely unknown character have been reported through the use of ^{32}P-postlabeling (Reddy and Randerath, 1987). In this procedure (Fig. 8-11) DNA is digested to its constituent nucleotides by nucleases and each nucleotide is labeled by using γ^{32}P-labeled ATP and a bacterial kinase, an enzyme that transfers the terminal phosphate of ATP to the available 5′ hydroxyl of the 39 nucleotides to convert all of the nucleotides to a radioactive, biphosphorylated form. Nucleotides of the normal DNA bases are removed by appropriate chromatographic procedures, leaving only those nucleotides that contain structural adducts. Although this technique has been used to demonstrate adduction of DNA by a variety of known chemical carcinogens, it is equally interesting that a number of adducts of unknown structure have been discovered in living cells. Some of these structurally unknown DNA adducts, termed I-compounds (Li and Randerath, 1992), change with dietary modifications, drug administration (Randerath et al., 1992), and species and tissue differences (Li et al., 1990). Li and associates (1995) have presented evidence that at least some of the I-compounds were related to peroxide derivatives of linoleic acid in particular one of the major adducts appears to be derived from 4-hydroxynonenal, a reactive intermediate lipid peroxidation product resulting from free radical reaction with polyunsaturated fatty acids (Chung et al., 1996). I-compounds occur in human fetal tissues (Hansen et al., 1993), increase with age and caloric restriction, but decrease during hepatocarcinogenesis (Randerath et al., 1991). The exact role, if any, of these DNA adducts of unknown structure in the process of carcinogenesis remains a question.

Thus, the role of structural adducts of DNA in carcinogenesis is not a simple one with adduct = mutation = carcinogenesis. Adducts of known carcinogens (Fig. 8-10) may play a significant role in carcinogenesis induced by their procarcinogenic forms, but the function of structurally undefined, endogenously produced adducts such as I-compounds in the carcinogenic process is not so clear. There is not substantial evidence that endogenously formed adducts lead to mutation. Whether a DNA adduct results in the formation is a consequence of its persistence through a period of cell proliferation, which in turn is partially a function of the process of DNA repair.

DNA REPAIR AND CHEMICAL CARCINOGENESIS

Persistence of DNA Adducts and DNA Repair

The extent to which DNA adducts occur after administration of chemical carcinogens depends on the overall metabolism of the chemical agent as well as the chemical reactivity of the ultimate metabolite. Once the adduct is formed, its continued presence in the DNA of the cell depends primarily on the ability of the cellular machinery to repair the structural alteration in the DNA.

It is from such considerations as well as the presumed critical nature of the adduct in the carcinogenic process that a working hypothesis on the relationship between mutagenesis and carcinogenesis has evolved. It has been postulated that the extent of DNA adduct formation and their persistence in the DNA should correlate with the biological effect of the agent (Neumann, 1983). In accordance with this hypothesis, several studies have correlated the persistence of DNA adducts during chemical carcinogenesis with the high incidence of neoplasms in specific tissues (Table 8-6). Among the earliest of these studies was that of Goth and Rajewsky

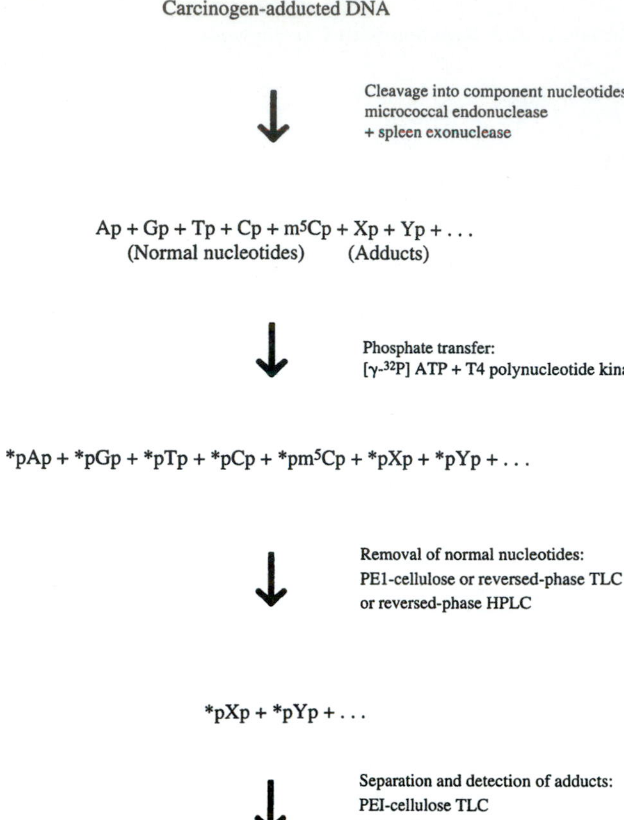

Figure 8-11. The basic features of ^{32}P-postlabeling assay for carcinogen-adducted DNA.

The ^{32}P-assay involves four steps: digestion of DNA, ^{32}P-labeling of the digestion products, removal of ^{32}P-labeled nucleotides not containing adducts, and thin layer chromatography mapping of the [^{32}P] nucleotides with adducts. (Asterisks indicate the position of the ^{32}P-label.) [Modified from Gupta et al. (1982), with permission.]

(1974), who demonstrated the relative persistence of O^6-ethylguanine in DNA of brain but not liver of animals administered ethylnitrosourea at 10 days of age. The rapid loss of the adduct in liver DNA contrasted with the sevenfold slower loss in DNA of the brain. In this study, neoplastic lesions were observed in the brain but not the liver later in life. Swenberg and his associates (1985) demonstrated an analogous situation in the liver, wherein administration of dimethylhydrazine induced a high incidence of neoplasms in hepatic vascular endothelium, but a very low incidence in the hepatocytes. Examination of the analogous adduct O^6-methylguanine demonstrated its rapid removal from the DNA of hepatocytes but much slower removal from the DNA of vascular endothelial cells. Similarly, Kadlubar and his associates (1981) demonstrated that more 2-naphthylamine adducts of guanine persisted in bladder epithelium (urothelium) than in liver after administration of the carcinogen to dogs. The bladder but not the liver is a target for this carcinogen in that species. When the susceptibility to carcinogenesis by diethylnitrosamine was investigated in the same tissue in two different species, significant alkylation and the development of neoplasia were observed in the hamster but not the mouse lung. Thus, the difference in the persistence of DNA adducts plays an important role in target organ and species specificity of select carcinogens.

Although the correlations noted in Table 8-6 support the working hypothesis of the importance of specific adducts during the carcinogenic process, the mere presence of DNA adducts is probably not sufficient for the carcinogenic process to proceed; equally or more important is the persistence of the adducts in the DNA of viable cells. For example, Swenberg and associate (1984) have demonstrated that the O^4-ethylthymine adduct but not the O^6-ethylguanine adduct is stable in liver parenchymal cells after the continuous exposure of rats to diethylnitrosamine. Furthermore, Müller and Rajewsky (1983) found that the O^4-ethylthymine adduct persisted in all organs after the administration of ethylnitrosourea to neonatal or adult rats. By contrast, persistence of DNA adducts of the carcinogenic *trans*-4-aminostilbene does not correlate with tissue susceptibility. While the liver and kidney exhibited the greatest burden and persistence of the adduct and the ear duct glands of Zymbal showed the lowest adduct concentration, it is the latter tissue that is most susceptible to carcinogenesis by this agent (Neumann, 1983). Such differences in susceptibility to carcinogenesis are undoubtedly the result of a number of factors, includ-

Table 8-6
Organ and Species Specificity of Chemical Carcinogenesis in Relation to Persistence of Adducts in DNA

SPECIES	CARCINOGEN	TISSUE	DNA ADDUCT ($t_{1/2}$)	NEOPLASTIC DEVELOPMENT	REFERENCE
Rat (neonates)	ENU*	Liver	O^6EtG (30 h)	±†	(Goth and Rajewsky,
Rat (neonates)	ENU	Brain	O^6EtG (220 h)	+++	1974)
Rat	SDMH	Liver, hepatocytes	O^6MeG (~1.6 days)	±	(Swenberg et al.,
Rat	SDMH	Liver, nonparenchymal cells	O^6MeG (>20 days)	+++	1985)
Dog	2-NA	Liver	N-(dG-8-yl)-2-NA (~2 days)	0	(Kadlubar et al.,
Dog	2-NA	Urothelium	N-(dG-8-yl)-2-NA (>20 days)	+++	1981)
Hamster	DEN	Lung	O^6EtG, (91 h)	+++	(Becker and Shank,
Rat	DEN	Lung	O^6EtG (undetectable)	0	1985)

*ENU, ethylnitrosourea; SDMH, symmetrical dimethylhydrazine; 2-NA, 2-naphthylamine; DEN, diethylnitrosamine; O^6EtG, O^6 ethylguanine; N-(dG-8-yl)-2-NA, N-(deoxyguanosin-8-yl)-2-naphthylamine.

†±, occasional neoplasm; +++, high incidence of neoplasms; 0, no increased incidence of neoplasia above untreated controls.

ing replication of the target cells and repair of the carcinogen-DNA adduct (see below).

Despite exceptions to the working hypothesis, our knowledge of the persistence of covalent adducts of DNA in tissues has been utilized to quantitate the exposure of humans to carcinogenic chemicals and relate the potential risk of neoplastic development to such exposure. The occurrence of adducts of benzo(*a*)pyrene throughout the tissues of exposed animals at unexpectedly similar levels (Stowers and Anderson, 1985) further supports the rationale for the investigation of persistent adducts of DNA and protein as biomarkers of human exposure. Immunologic and highly sensitive chromatographic technologies have been used to demonstrate the presence of adducts of several carcinogenic species (Perera et al., 1991; Shields and Harris, 1991). DNA adducts of carcinogenic PAHs have been demonstrated at relatively high levels in tissues, especially blood cells, of smokers and foundry workers compared with nonexposed individuals (Perera et al., 1991). Huh and coworkers (1989) have demonstrated an increased level of O^4-ethylthymine in the DNA of liver from individuals with no known exposure to ethylating agents, and a statistically significant increased level of ethylation of this base was noted in cancer patients compared with controls. In a more recent study by Hsieh and Hsieh (1993), DNA adducts of aflatoxin B_1 were demonstrated in samples of human placenta and cord blood from patients in Taiwan, an area of high liver cancer incidence. In addition to detection of specific structural DNA adducts, the ^{32}P-postlabeling assay has also been exploited to determine the presence of DNA adducts in human tissues (Beach and Gupta, 1992). As expected, a variety of adducts are found in both normal individuals and those potentially exposed to specific carcinogenic agents. In addition to DNA adducts, specific carcinogens also covalently bind to serum proteins. For example, Bryant and colleagues (1987) showed a five- to sixfold greater level of hemoglobin adducts of 4-aminobiphenyl in smokers than in nonsmokers. While this adduct has a finite lifetime, chronic exposure to cigarette smoke maintains the dramatic increase in the adduct level between these two groups, suggesting a potential use of such determinations in estimating exposure to carcinogenic agents. Thus, the persistence of macromolecular adducts of the ultimate forms of chemical carcinogens may be very important in the carcinogenic mechanism of such agents. However, as noted above, the presence and persistence of DNA adducts is only one factor in the complex process of cancer development.

Mechanisms of DNA Repair

The persistence of DNA adducts is predominantly the result of the failure of DNA repair. The types of structural alterations that may occur in the DNA molecule as a result of interaction with reactive chemical species or directly with radiation are considerable. A number of the more frequently seen structural changes in DNA are schematically represented in Fig. 8-12. The reaction of DNA with reactive chemical species produces adducts on bases, sugars, and the phosphate backbone. In addition, bifunctional reactive chemicals may cause the cross-linking of DNA strands through reaction with two opposing bases. Other structural changes, such as the pyrimidine dimer formation, are specific for ultraviolet radiation, while double-strand DNA breaks are most commonly seen with ionizing radiation (see below). Most of the other lesions depicted in Fig. 8-12 may occur as a result of either chemical or radiation effects on the DNA molecule. To cope with the many structurally distinct types of DNA damage, a variety of mechanisms have evolved to effectively repair each of the types of damage shown in Fig. 8-12. It is estimated that over 100 genes are dedicated to DNA repair, emphasizing the essential nature of the genetic information. A summary of the types of DNA repair most commonly encountered in mammalian systems is given in Table 8-7.

Two types of damage response pathways exist: repair pathways and the tolerance mechanism (Friedberg, 1994). In repair mechanisms the DNA damage is removed, while tolerance mechanisms circumvent the damage without fixing it. Tolerance mechanisms are by definition error-prone. Certain repair mechanisms reverse the DNA damage, for example, removal of adducts from bases and insertion of bases into apurinic/apyrimidinic (AP) sites. An example of direct reversal is provided by the removal of small alkyl groups from the O^6 portion of guanine by alkyltransferases. Alkyltransferases directly transfer the alkyl (methyl or ethyl) group from the DNA base guanine to a cysteine acceptor site in the alkyltransferase protein (Pegg and Byers, 1992). In microorganisms, the intracellular concentration of the alkyltransferase protein is regulated by environmental factors, including the concentration of the alkylating agents. A similar adaptation may occur in certain mammalian tissues in response to DNA-damaging agents and to treatments causing an increase in cell proliferation. In mammalian tissues, the level of the alkyltransferase protein is a major factor in the resistance of some cancer cells to certain chemotherapeutic agents. At least for the alkyltransferase reaction, direct reversal of the premutational lesions restores normal base pairing specificity.

The excisional repair of DNA may involve either the removal of a single altered base having a relatively low-molecular-weight adduct, such as an ethyl or methyl group, and is termed *base excision repair,* or the repair may involve a base with a very large bulky group adducted to it, termed *nucleotide excision repair*. The linkage of two bases seen in the dimerization of pyrimidines by ultraviolet light is also repaired by the latter pathway. This nucleotide excision pathway is represented diagrammatically in Fig. 8-13.

Nucleotide excision repair in multicellular organisms involves a series of reactions noted in the figure. These include recognition of the damage, unwinding of the DNA, 3′ and 5′ sequential dual incisions of the damaged strand, repair synthesis of the eliminated patch, and final ligation. Each of these steps as noted in the figure involves a number of different proteins. In Table 8-8 may be seen a listing of the various proteins occurring in different fractions and their functions in the process of nucleotide excision repair (Petit and Sancar, 1999).

Other studies (cf. Sancar and Tang, 1993; Hanawalt, 1994) have also demonstrated that nucleotide excision repair in many instances occurs simultaneously with gene transcription. In fact, Hanawalt and his associates showed earlier (cf. Bohr et al., 1987) that nucleotide excision repair occurred preferentially in genes which were actively being transcribed. For the final resynthesis of the segment of excised DNA, both the proliferating cell nuclear antigen (PCNA) as well as at least two different DNA polymerases (δ or ε) are needed to complete the repair process together with a ligase (Sancar, 1994).

Since animal cell DNA polymerases are not absolutely faithful in their replication of the template strand, there is the potential for a mutation to occur in the form of one or more mispaired bases during the process outlined above. This possibility is greater in the case of nucleotide excision repair as compared to simple base excision since a much longer base sequence is removed and resynthesized during the nucleotide excision mechanism. The existence and ultimate characterization of a number of the proteins involved

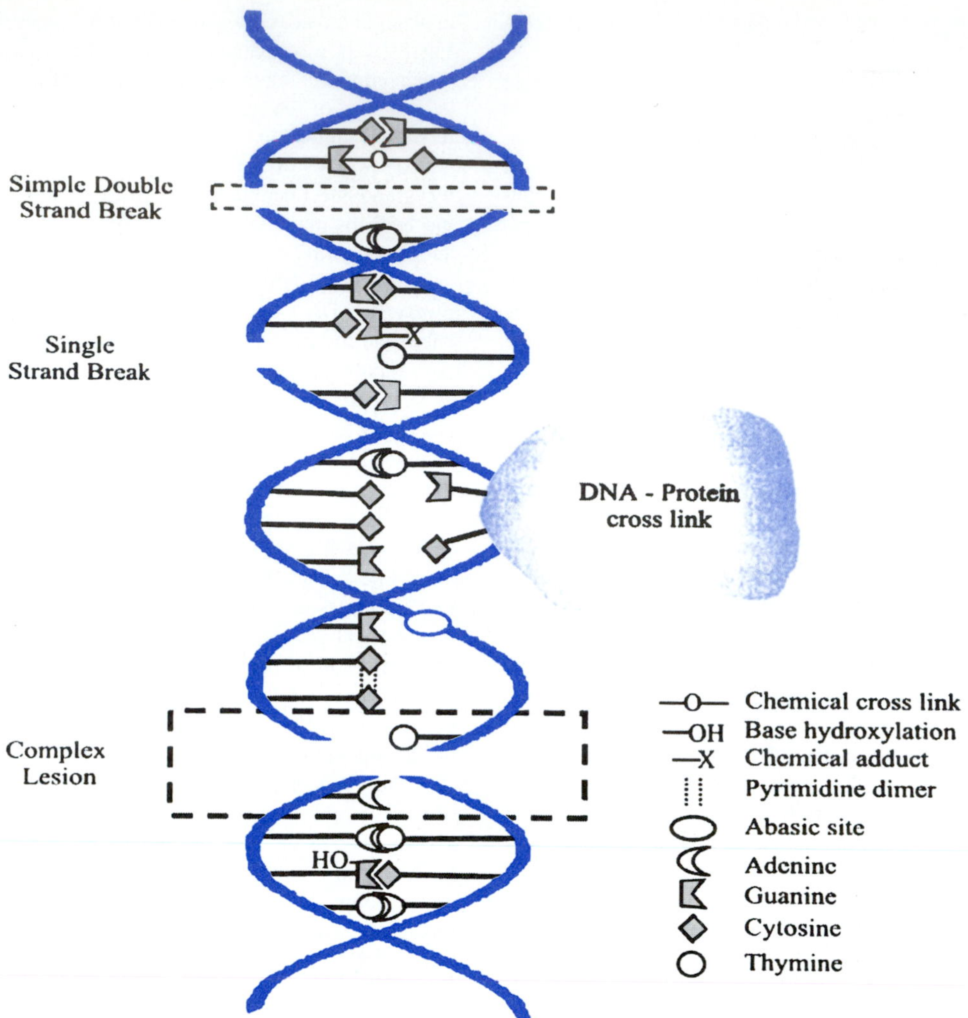

Figure 8-12. Schematic representation of chemical- and radiation-induced lesions in DNA.

Table 8-7
Types of DNA Repair

1. Direct reversal of DNA damage
Alkyltransferases
2. Base excision repair
Glycosylase and AP endonuclease
3. Nucleotide excision repair
T-T, C-C, C-T repair
"Bulky" adduct repair
4. Double-strand-break repair
Homologous recombination (HR)
Nonhomologous DNA end joining (NHEJ)
5. Mismatch repair
Repair of deamination of 5-Me cytosine
Repair of mismatches in DNA due to defective repair, etc.

SOURCE: Modified from Myles and Sancar (1989) and from Lieber (1998), with permission.

in nucleotide excision repair has been the result of human diseases in which defects in this mechanism are known. In particular, the disease, xeroderma pigmentosum, is an autosomal recessive condition in which most patients are highly sensitive to exposure to ultraviolet light. Thus, on chronic exposure to sunlight such individuals have a much greater risk of developing skin cancer than normal individuals. This fact emphasizes the potential importance of altered DNA repair in the development of neoplasia.

While the repair of adducts as indicated above involves several possible pathways, the repair of double DNA strand breaks is more complicated and as a result more prone to error than either the excisional or direct reversal pathways. Single-strand breaks may result from a variety of alterations by chemicals or radiation and, as noted above, during the repair process itself. Double-strand breaks in DNA are largely the result of ionizing radiation or high doses of alkylating carcinogens such as nitrogen mustard or polycyclic hydrocarbons, although even under normal conditions, transient double-strand DNA breaks occur as the result of the normal function of topoisomerases involved in the winding and unwinding of DNA.

In Fig. 8-14 may be noted a schematic diagram of three forms of double-strand DNA repair. Recombinational repair or homologous recombination (HR) is more commonly seen in lower eu-

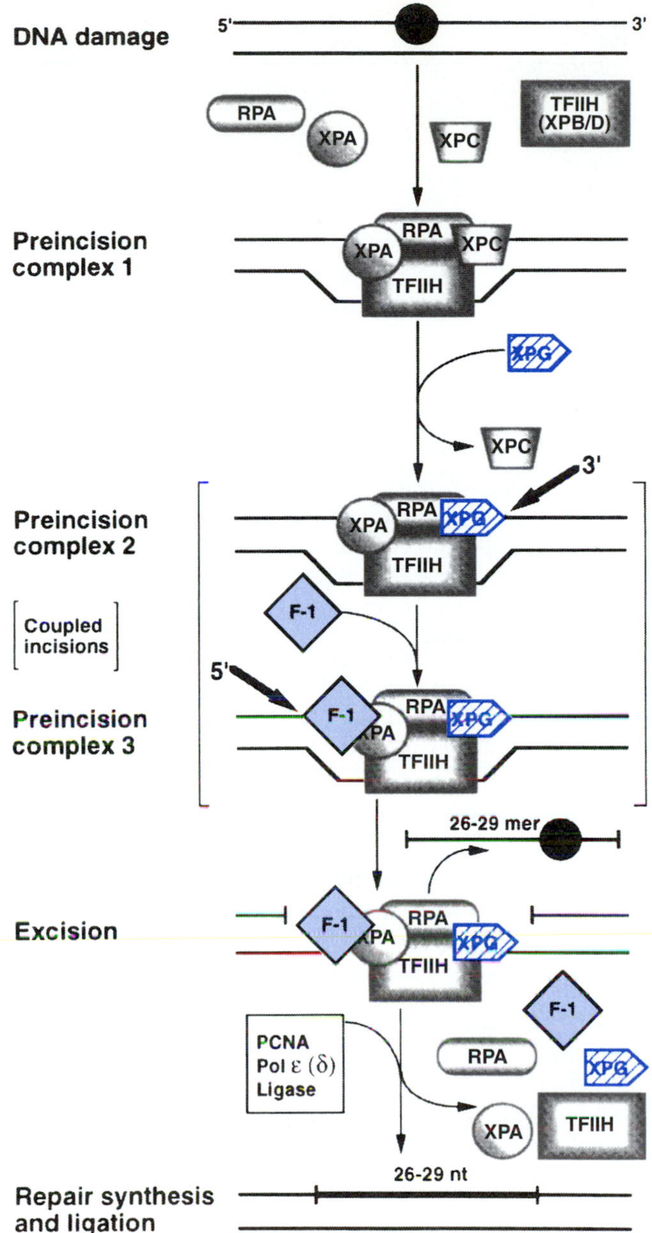

Figure 8-13. Model for transcription-independent nucleotide excision repair of DNA in humans.

1. The damage is first recognized in an ATP-independent step by the short-lived XPA·RPA complex. In a second, ATP-dependent step, the damaged DNA-bound XPA·RPA complex recruits XPC and TFIIH, to form the preincision complex 1 (PIC1). TFIIH possesses both 3′-5′ and 5′-3′ helicase activities, respectively, through its XPB and XPD subunits and unwinds DNA by about 20 base pairs around the damage. 2. XPG binds the PIC1 complex while the molecular matchmaker XPC dissociates, leading to the more stable PIC2 excinuclease complex. 3. PIC2 recruits XPF·ERCC1 (F-1) to form PIC3. XPG makes the 3′ incision and F-1 makes the 5′ incision a fraction of a second later, in a concerted but asynchronous mechanism. 4. The excised damaged fragment is released by the excinuclease complex, leaving in place a post-incision complex whose exact composition is still unclear. The proliferating cell nuclear antigen (PCNA) forms a torus around the DNA molecule associating with DNA polymerase δ and/or ε [Pol ε (δ)] (Tsurimoto, 1998) and a DNA ligase replacing the postincision complex with these repair synthesis proteins. 5. The gap is filled and the repair patch is ligated. [From Petit and Sancar (1999), with permission of authors and publisher.]

karyotes such as yeast while the nonhomologous end joining (NHEJ) pathway of double-strand DNA repair is more commonly seen in higher vertebrates (Van Dyck et al., 1999). The single-strand annealing pathway has not yet been well studied in higher vertebrates. While the exact mechanisms involved in each of these steps are not considered in detail here, the interested reader is referred to more detailed references (Pastink and Lohman, 1999; Lieber, 1998; Featherstone and Jackson, 1999). In general, in the HR and NHEJ pathways, specific proteins interact with the open ends of the DNA, members of the Rad52 group genes in the case of HR (Van Dyck et al., 1999) and the Ku70 and Ku80 proteins in the NHEJ pathway (Featherstone and Jackson, 1999). A DNA-dependent protein kinase (DNA-PKcs) as well as the protein interacting with the DNA ligase (XRCC4) is involved in this mechanism. It should be noted as indicated in the legend to the figure, however, that these mechanisms are quite error-prone and only under the best of circumstances result in a faithful recapitulation of the normal DNA sequence.

Double-strand breaks may occur at sites of single-strand DNA resulting from adduction of bulky molecules, preventing further polymerase action and subsequent endonuclease cleavage and resulting in double-strand breaks and potential chromosomal aberrations (Kaufmann, 1989).

Incorrectly paired nucleotides may occur in DNA as a result of DNA polymerase infidelity, formation and/or repair of apurinic and nucleotide excision sites, double-strand DNA repair, and metabolic modification of specific bases. Mismatch repair can be distinguished from nucleotide excision repair and base excision repair by several characteristics. Nucleotide and base excision repair generally involves the recognition of nucleotides/bases that have been chemically modified or fused to an adjacent nucleotide. In contrast, mismatch repair recognizes normal nucleotides which are either unpaired or paired with a noncomplementary nucleotide (cf. Fishel and Kolodner, 1995). Thus, mismatch repair may become involved in virtually any of the types of DNA repair seen in Table 8-7 with the possible exception of the direct reversal of DNA damage. The various combination of gene products involved in several of the types of mismatch repair are seen in Fig. 8-15. While the nomenclature of the various components varies depending on the phyla—e.g., eukaryotes, yeast, vertebrates—a functional similarity occurs throughout, most faithful in eukaryotes. As noted from the figure, recognition of the mismatch appears to be a major function of the MSH2 (hMSH2 in the human), while MSH3 and MSH6 are involved in the specificity of binding itself (Fishel and Wilson, 1997). Thus, these complexes act as sensors of mismatch as well as other structural changes in the genome (Modrich, 1997; Li et al., 1996; cf. Fishel and Wilson, 1997). As in the case of other types of repair following the recognition and interaction with the mismatch repair proteins, the normal sequence is restored following removal of the mismatch DNA, resynthesis, and ligation (cf. Jiricny, 1998).

As an example of the importance of mismatch DNA repair, the extent of endogenous DNA damage and subsequent repair processes in normal human cells in vivo is seen in Table 8-9. With the possible exception of some single-strand break repair, all the other types of damage are those monitored by the mismatch repair mechanism and repaired under normal conditions. Obviously, a defect in this repair system may result in a dramatic increase in mutational events and in neoplasia.

The critical importance of the fidelity of DNA repair in the maintenance of cellular and organismal homeostasis is apparent

Table 8-8
Proteins Involved in the Nucleotide Excision Repair Process in Humans

FRACTION	PROTEINS	SEQUENCE MOTIF	ACTIVITY OF THE FRACTION	ROLE IN REPAIR
XPA	XPA	Zinc finger	DNA binding	Damage recognition
RPA	p70	Zinc finger	XPA binding	Damage recognition
	p34		DNA binding	
	p11			
TFIIH	XPB	3′-5′ helicase	DNA-dependent ATPase	Formation of preincision complexes PIC 1-2-3
	XPD	5′-3′ helicase	Helicase	Transcription-repair coupling
	p62 (TFB1)		GTF	
	p52			
	p44 (SSL1)	Zinc finger	CAK	
	Cdk7	S/T kinase		
	CycH	Cyclin		
	p34	Zinc finger		
XPC	XPC		DNA binding	Molecular matchmaker
	HHR23B	Ubiquitin		Stabilization of PIC1
XPG	XPG		Nuclease	3′ incision
XPF	XPF		Nuclease	5′ incision
	ERCC1			

KEY: GTF, general transcription factor; CAK, CDK-activating kinase.
SOURCE: Adapted from Petit and Sancar (1999), with permission of authors and publisher.

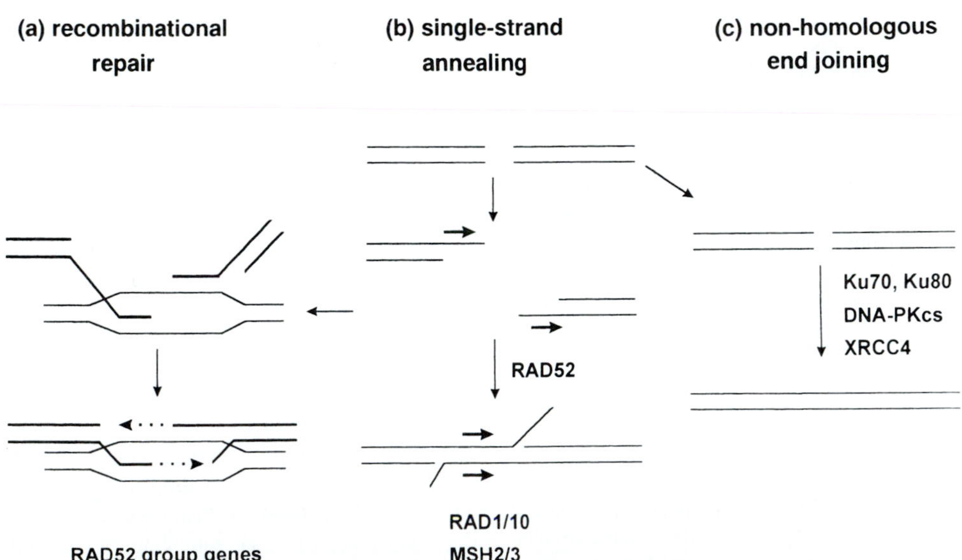

Figure 8-14. Schematic representation of pathways involved in the repair of double-strand breaks in DNA.

(a) The first step in recombinational repair is the formation of 3′ single-stranded tails by exonucleolytic activity followed by invasion of a homologous undamaged donor sequence. Repair synthesis and branch migration lead to the formation of two Holliday junctions, i.e., a single DNA strand linking two double-stranded DNA molecules. Resolution of these intermediate structures results in the formation of two possible crossover and two possible noncrossover products (*not shown*). The fidelity of this repair is dependent on the exact complementation of the unaffected double-strand by the strands undergoing repair. (b) In the single-strand annealing pathway, exposures of regions of homology during resection of the 5′-ends allows formation of joint molecules. Repair of the double-strand break is completed by removal of nonhomologous ends and ligation. As a consequence, a deletion is introduced in the DNA. (c) Nonhomologous end joining is based on religation of the two ends involving a complex of proteins, some of which are indicated in the figure and may involve the deletion and/or insertion of nucleotides. [Adapted from Pastink and Lohman (1999), with permission of authors and publisher.]

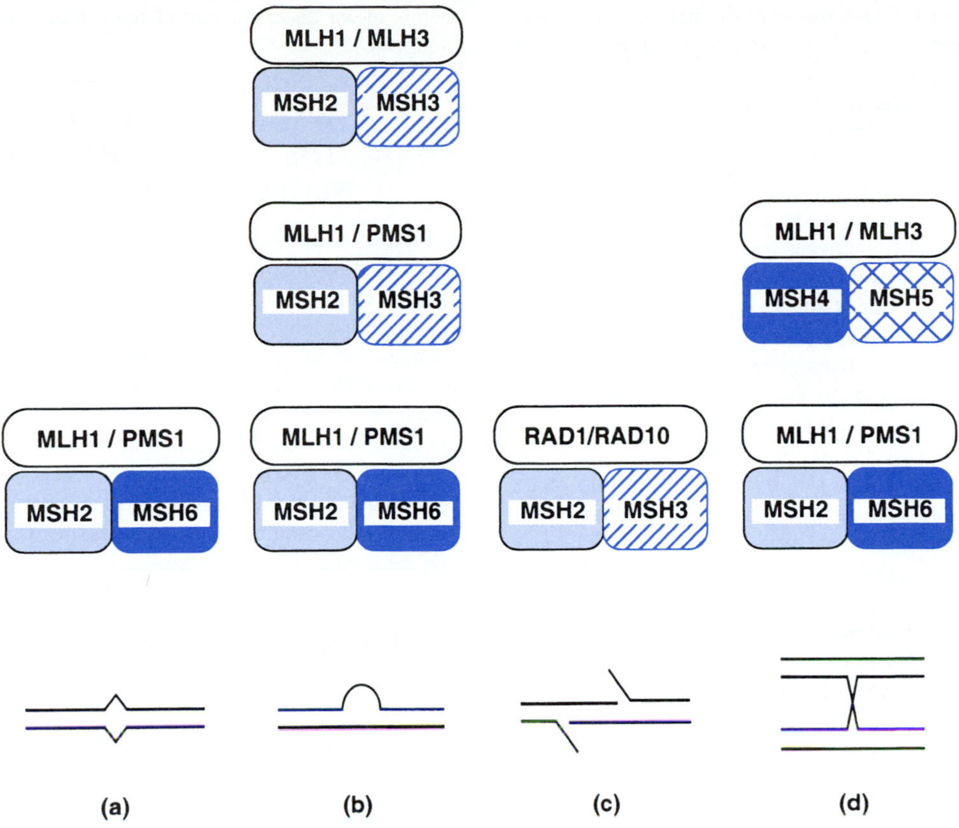

Figure 8-15. Combinational specificities of heterocomplexes of gene products of mismatch repair genes.

(a) Base/base mispairs; (b) insertion/deletion mispairs; (c) 5′ tailed DNA structures generated by single-strand DNA annealing following recombination, e.g. HR; and (d) Holliday junctions. [Adapted from Nakagawa et al. (1999), with permission of authors and publishers.]

from this brief discussion. Because induction of DNA repair processes occurs as a response to genetic damage, the induction can be used as an endpoint for its detection indirectly. In addition, an increase in repair mechanisms above constitutive levels can increase the magnitude of the genotoxic insult. The relative importance of DNA repair in understanding mechanisms of chemical carcinogenesis is most apparent when relating DNA damage and repair to DNA synthesis and cell replication. This is required to exceed the intrinsic capacity of a cell to repair this damage.

DNA Repair, Cell Replication, and Chemical Carcinogenesis

The persistence of DNA adducts in relation to the development of neoplasia in specific tissues (Table 8-6) and differences in the repair of the adducts are critical factors in chemical carcinogenesis. The removal of methyl, ethyl, and similar small alkyl radicals from individual bases is to a great extent dependent on the presence of alkyltransferases (see above). While in some tissues, such as liver,

Table 8-9
Estimates of Endogenous DNA Damage and Repair Processes in Human Cells in Vivo

TYPE OF DAMAGE	ESTIMATED OCCURRENCES OF DAMAGE PER HOUR PER CELL*	MAXIMAL REPAIR RATE, BASE PAIRS PER HOUR PER CELL*
Depurination	1,000	10^4 +
Depyrimidination	55	10^4 +
Cytosine deamination	15	10^4 +
Single-stranded breaks	5,000	2×10^5
N^7-methylguanine	3,500	Not reported
O^6-methylguanine	130	10^4
Oxidation products	120	10^5

*Might be higher or lower by a factor of 2.
SOURCE: Modified from data of the National Academy of Science (1989).

it may be possible to increase the level of such enzymes in response to damage and hormonal or other influences, many tissues do not have an inducible repair mechanisms. Furthermore, some adducts are extremely difficult if not impossible for the cell to repair. An example of such a lesion, the 3-(deoxyguanosine)-N^2-yl-acetylaminofluorene adduct first described by Kriek and his associates (Westra et al., 1976), is depicted in Fig. 8-10. This may in part account for the relatively wide spectrum of neoplasms inducible by this chemical carcinogen.

Of equal importance is the continuous damage to DNA that occurs within cells as a result of ambient mutagens, radiation, and endogenous processes including oxidation, methylation, deamination, and depurination. DNA damage induced by oxidative reactions (oxidative stress) is probably the source of most endogenous DNA damage. Ames et al. (1993) have estimated that the individual reactive "hits" in DNA per cell per day is of the order of 10^5 in the rat and 10^4 in the human as a result of endogenous oxidative reaction. Such reactions can produce alkylation through peroxidative reactions such as those described in Fig. 8-8 or hydroxylation of bases and single-strand breaks (Fig. 8-12). The end product of oxidative damage to DNA can also be interstrand crosslinks and double-strand breaks (Demple and Harrison, 1994) with the potential for subsequent major genetic damage noted below. A more complete listing of the estimates of endogenous DNA damage and repair processes in the human is seen in Table 8-9. The data of this table emphasize the considerable degree and significant variation in types of DNA damage and repair which occurs within each cell of the organism at a molecular level.

Experimental studies in mammalian cells have demonstrated that active oxygen radicals may contribute to clastogenesis directly (Ochi and Kaneko, 1989) and indirectly through the production of lipid peroxides (Emerit et al., 1991). While methods for the repair of some types of oxidative damage including base hydroxylation (Bessho et al., 1993) and single-strand breaks (Satoh and Lindahl, 1994), exist, such repair requires time and may be dependent on many other intracellular factors. Because the formation of a mutation occurs during the synthesis of a new DNA strand by use of the damaged template, cell replication becomes an important factor in the "fixation" of a mutation. The importance of the rate of cell division and DNA synthesis in carcinogenesis has been emphasized by several authors (Ames et al., 1993; Butterworth, 1991; Cohen and Ellwein, 1991). Thus, while many DNA repair mechanisms themselves may not be abnormal in neoplastic cells compared with their normal counterpart, a high rate of cell division will tend to enhance both the spontaneous and induced level of mutation through the chance inability of a cell to repair damage prior to DNA synthesis. An important pathway of DNA repair that is genetically defective in a number of hereditary and spontaneous neoplasms in the human (Umar et al., 1994) is the mismatch repair mechanism that corrects spontaneous and post-replicative base alterations and thus is an important pathway for avoidance of mutation in normal cells. Genetic defects in mismatch repair mechanisms lead to microsatellite DNA and instability with subsequent alteration in the stabilization of the genome itself (Modrich, 1994). Enhanced mitogenesis may also trigger more dramatic genetic alterations including mitotic recombination, gene conversion, and nondisjunction. These genetic changes result in further progressive genetic alterations with a high likelihood of resulting in cancer. The types of mutational events, the numbers of such mutations, and the cellular responses to them thus become important factors in our understanding of the mechanisms of chemical carcinogenesis.

CHEMICAL CARCINOGENS AND THE NATURAL HISTORY OF NEOPLASTIC DEVELOPMENT

A number of chemicals can alter the structure of the genome and/or the expression of genetic information with the subsequent appearance of cancer. However, cancer as a disease usually develops slowly with a long latent period between the first exposure to the chemical carcinogen and the ultimate development of malignant neoplasia. Thus, the process of carcinogenesis (the pathogenesis of neoplasia) involves a variety of biological changes which, to a great extent, reflect the structural and functional alterations in the genome of the affected cell. However, when the biological changes occurring during carcinogenesis are assessed at the molecular level, a better understanding of the mechanisms of cancer development may be generated.

The Pathogenesis of Neoplasia: Biology

Although morphologic changes occurring during the early stages of neoplasia were described during the early decades of this century, it was in the 1940s that a better understanding of the biological changes that occurred following carcinogen exposure was obtained. The first and best-studied model system was that of mouse skin carcinogenesis. The early investigations of Rous and Kidd (1941), Mottram (1944), and Berenblum and Shubik (1947) used the development of benign papillomas as an endpoint for studies of epidermal carcinogenesis in mouse skin induced by polycyclic hydrocarbons. These investigators coined the term "initiation" to designate the initial alteration in individual cells within the tissue resulting from a single subcarcinogenic dose of the chemical carcinogen. In these circumstances, papillomas were obtained only with subsequent chronic, multiple doses of a second agent that by itself was essentially carcinogenic. This latter "stage" was termed *promotion*. Subsequent studies on a mammary adenocarcinoma model in the mouse led to the proposal that processes subsequent to initiation comprised a stage termed *progression* (Foulds, 1954). Foulds's description of this stage emphasized changes characteristic of malignant neoplasia and its evolution to higher degrees of autonomy.

During the last two decades, these investigations have been extended to a variety of tissue systems and to humans (Pitot, 1996). At present the pathogenesis of neoplasia is felt to consist of at least three operationally defined stages beginning with initiation followed by an intermediate stage of promotion, from which evolves the stage of progression. The third stage exhibits many of the characteristics described by Foulds. The biological characteristics of the stages of initiation, promotion, and progression are listed in Table 8-10 (Pitot and Dragan, 1994; Boyd and Barrett, 1990; Harris, 1991). It is in the first and last stage of neoplastic development—initiation and progression—that structural changes in the genome (DNA) can be observed. The structural changes previously discussed are most likely to be involved in the induction of these stages. The intermediate stage of promotion does not appear to involve direct structural changes in the genome of the cell but rather depends on an altered expression of genes.

Table 8-10
Morphologic and Biologic Characteristics of the Stages of Initiation, Promotion, and Progression during Carcinogenesis

INITIATION	PROMOTION	PROGRESSION
Irreversible in viable cells Initiated "stem cell" not morphologically identifiable	Operationally reversible both at the level of gene expression and at the cell level	Irreversible Morphologically discernible alteration in cellular genomic structure resulting from karyotypic instability
Efficiency sensitive to xenobiotic and other chemical factors	Promoted cell population existence dependent on continued administration of the promoting agent	
Spontaneous (endogenous) occurrence of initiated cells	Efficiency sensitive to aging and dietary and hormonal factors Endogenous promoting agents may effect "spontaneous" promotion	Growth of altered cells sensitive to environmental factors during early phase of this stage
Requires cell division for "fixation" Dose-response does not exhibit a readily measurable threshold	Dose-response exhibits measurable threshold and maximal effect	Benign or malignant neoplasms observed in this stage
Relative potency of initiators depends on quantitation of preneoplastic lesions following defined period of promotion	Relative potency of promoters is measured by their effectiveness to cause an expansion of the cell progeny of the initiated population	"Progressor" agents act to advance promoted cells into this stage

Although it may be obvious to the reader, it is important to emphasize that the definition of neoplasia presented at the beginning of the chapter refers only to cells in the stage of progression. Initiated cells almost without exception cannot be identified, and their existence is presumed based on the natural history of neoplastic development. Cells in the stage of promotion are termed *preneoplastic* since their existence is entirely dependent on the continued presence of the promoting agent in the environment. Preneoplasia must be distinguished from premalignant in that the latter terminology also refers to cells in the stage of progression which have not yet expressed their full biologic malignant potential but do have all the characteristics of the stage of progression.

Initiation Until recently the stage of initiation had been characterized and quantitated well after the process of carcinogenesis had begun. As with mutational events (see above), initiation requires one or more rounds of cell division for the "fixation" of the process (Kakunaga, 1975; Columbano et al., 1981). The quantitative parameters of initiation noted in Table 8-10—dose response and relative potency—have been demonstrated in a variety of experimental systems (Pitot et al., 1987; Dragan et al., 1994); however, these parameters may be modulated by alteration of xenobiotic metabolism (Talalay et al., 1988) and by trophic hormones (Liao et al., 1993). The metabolism of initiating agents to nonreactive forms and the high efficiency of DNA repair of the tissue can alter the process of initiation.

One of the characteristics of the stage of initiation is its irreversibility in the sense that the genotype/phenotype of the initiated cell is established at the time of initiation, there is accumulating evidence that not all initiated cells survive over the lifespan of the organism or the period of an experiment. Their demise appears to be due to the normal process of programmed cell death or apoptosis (Wyllie, 1987).

Spontaneous preneoplastic lesions have been described in a number of experimental systems (Maekawa and Mitsumori, 1990; Pretlow, 1994) as well as in the human (Dunham, 1972; Pretlow, 1994; Pretlow et al., 1993). Thus, it would appear that the spontaneous or fortuitous initiation of cells in a variety of tissues is a very common occurrence. If this is true, then the development of neoplasia can be a function solely of the action of agents at the stages of promotion and/or progression.

Promotion As in the stage of initiation, a variety of chemicals have been shown to induce this stage. However, unlike chemicals inducing the stage of initiation, there is no evidence that promoting agents or their metabolites directly interact with DNA or that metabolism is required at all for their effectiveness. In Fig. 8-16 may be seen some representative structures of various promoting agents. Tetradecanoyl phorbol acetate (TPA) is a naturally occurring alicyclic chemical that is the active ingredient of croton oil, a promoting agent used for mouse skin tumor promotion. Saccharin is an effective promoting agent for the bladder, and phenobarbital is an effective promoting agent for hepatocarcinogenesis.

2,3,7,8-Tetrachlorodibenzo-*p*-dioxin (TCDD) is probably the most effective promoting agent known for rat liver carcinogenesis but is also effective in the lung and skin. Estradiol is shown as a representative of endogenous hormones that are effective promoting agents. Both androgens and estrogens, natural and synthetic, are effective promoting agents in their target end organ as well as in liver (Taper, 1978; Sumi et al., 1980; Kemp et al., 1989). Cholic acid enhances preneoplastic and neoplastic lesions in the rat colon (Magnuson et al., 1993), whereas 2,2,4-trimethylpentane and un-

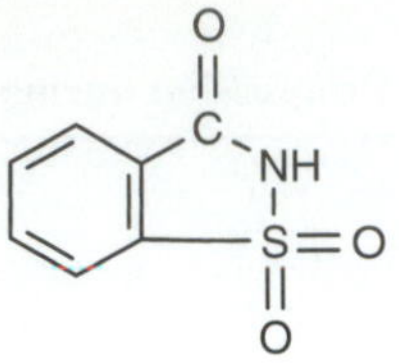

Saccharin

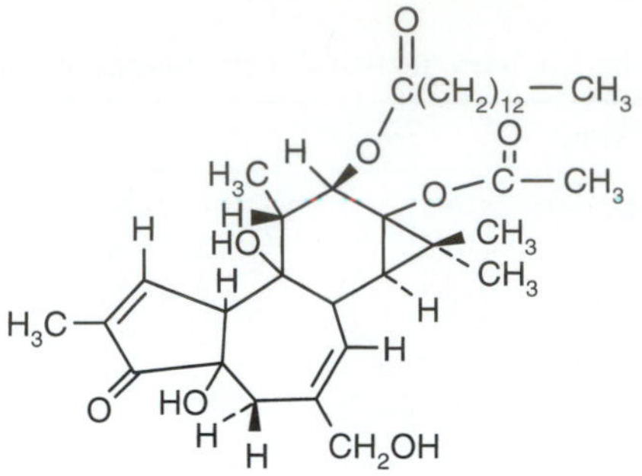

Tetradecanoyl phorbol acetate (TPA)

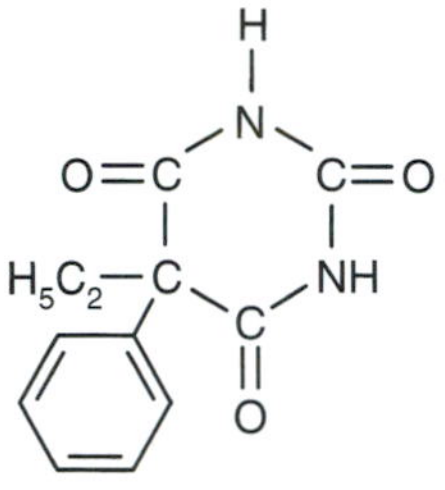

Phenobarbital

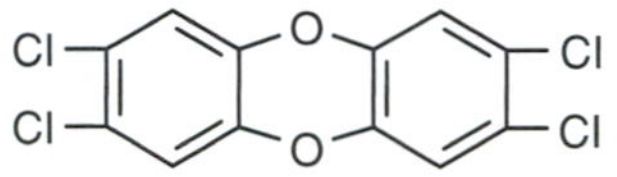

2,3,7,8-Tetrachlorodibenzo-*p*-dioxin

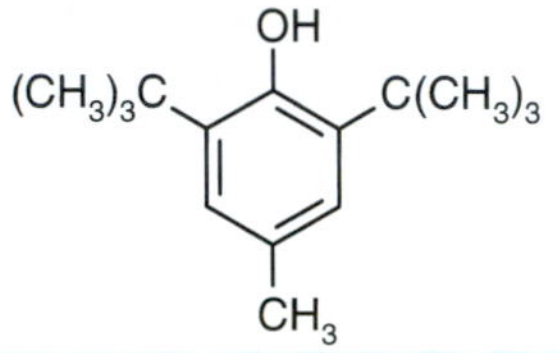

Butylated hydroxytoluene

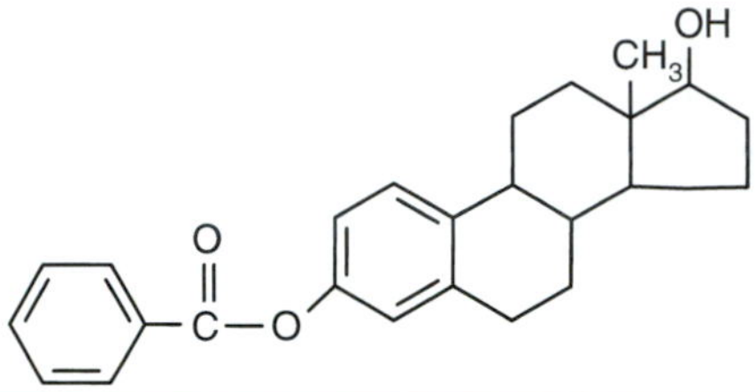

Estradiol benzoate

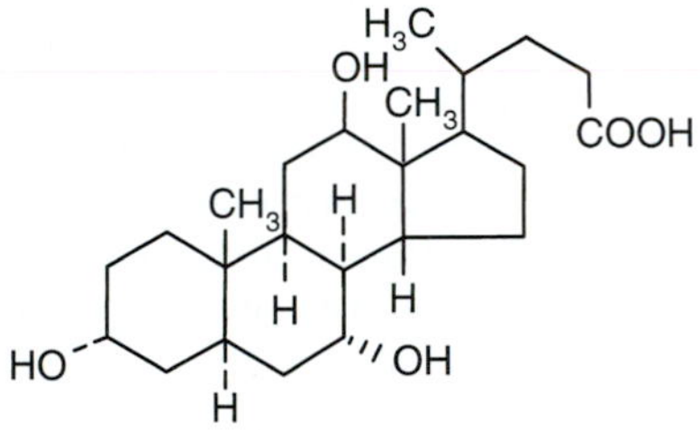

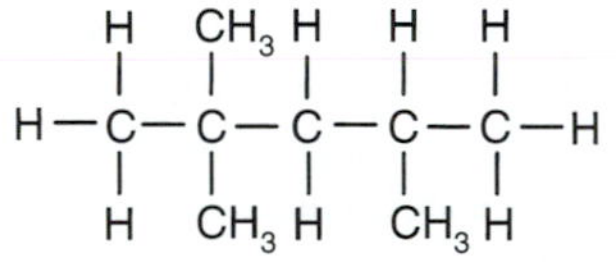

2,2,4-Trimethyl pentane

Cholic acid

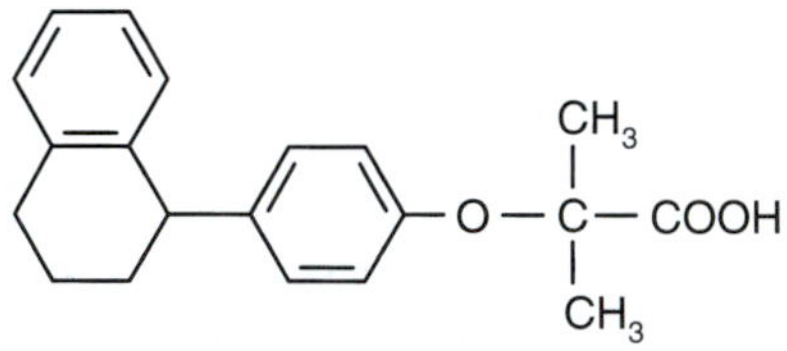

Nafenopin

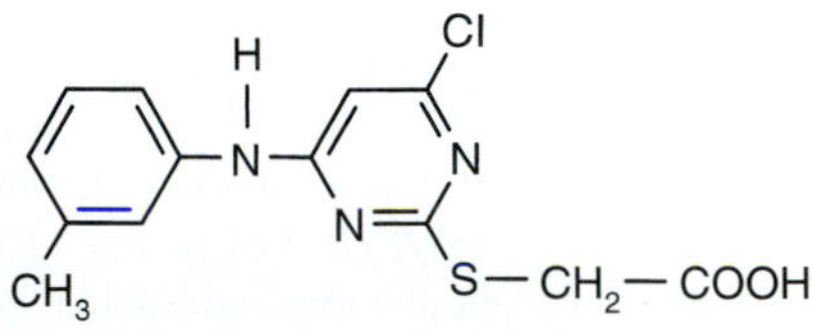

Wy-14,643

Figure 8-16. Structures of representative promoting agents.

leaded gasoline effectively promote renal tubular cell tumors in rats (Short et al., 1989). The final two structures noted—Wy-14,643 and Nafenopin—are two members of the large class of carcinogenic peroxisome proliferators that induce the synthesis of peroxisomes in liver, are effective promoting agents, and on long-term administration at high doses induce hepatic neoplasms (Reddy and Lalwani, 1983). Many other agents including polypeptide hormones (see above), dietary factors including total calories, many other halogenated hydrocarbons, and numerous other chemicals have been found to enhance the development of preneoplastic and neoplastic lesions in one or more systems of carcinogenesis, including the human system.

The distinctive characteristic of promotion as contrasted with initiation or progression is the reversible nature of this stage [Pitot and Dragan, 1995 (Table 8-10)]. Boutwell (1964) first demonstrated that by decreasing the frequency of application of the pro-

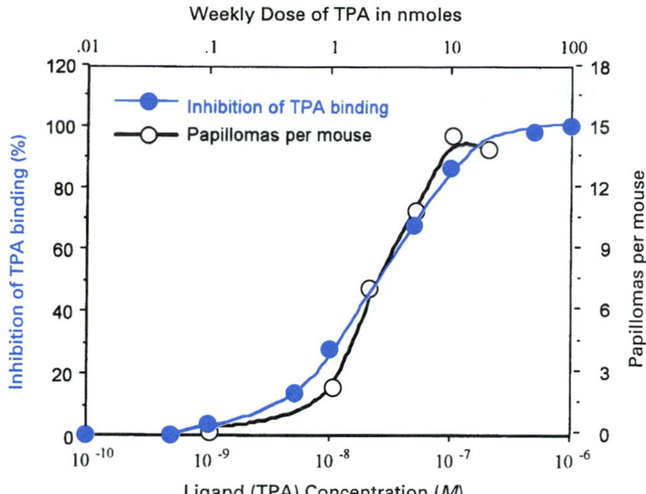

Figure 8-17. Composite showing the specific interaction of the receptor for phorbol esters with its ligand determined as the inhibition of radioactive TPA binding (closed circles).

The tumor response expressed as papillomas per mouse on mice initiated with dimethylbenzanthracene and promoted with various weekly doses of TPA is noted in the open circles [composite graph from data of Ashendel (1985) and from Verma and Boutwell (1980) as published in Pitot (1986a).]

moting agent following initiation in mouse skin there was a lower yield of papillomas in comparison with that obtained by a more frequent application of the promoting agent. Other investigators (Andrews, 1971; Burns et al., 1978) later demonstrated that papillomas developing during promotion in mouse epidermal carcinogenesis regress in large numbers both on removal of the promoting agent and during its continued application. The regression of preneoplastic lesions upon withdrawal of the promoting agents may be due to apoptosis (Schulte-Herrmann et al., 1990). This proposed mechanism is supported by the demonstration that many promoting agents inhibit apoptosis in preneoplastic lesions (Schulte-Herrmann et al., 1993; Wright et al., 1994). Another potential pathway of this operational reversibility is "redifferentiation" or remodeling (Tatematsu et al., 1983). Thus, cells in the stage of promotion are dependent on continued administration of the promoting agent (Hanigan and Pitot, 1985) as implied by the early studies of Furth (1959) on hormonally dependent neoplasia.

Another characteristic of the stage of promotion is its susceptibility to modulation by physiologic factors. The stage of promotion may be modulated by the aging process (Van Duuren et al., 1975) and by dietary and hormonal factors (Sivak, 1979). Glauert and associates (1986) demonstrated that promotion of hepatocarcinogenesis was less effective in rats fed a semisynthetic diet than in those fed a crude, cereal-based diet. The promotion stage of chemically induced rat mammary cancer is also modulated by dietary factors (Cohen et al., 1991) and hormonal (Carter et al., 1988) factors. Many such modulating factors are themselves promoting agents. Several hormones can be carcinogenic. These hormones are effective promoting agents and thus may serve as an exogenous or endogenous source for modulation of cell proliferation during carcinogenesis (Pitot, 1991). Such physiologic agents may be one component of endogenous promotion of initiated cells.

The dose–response relationships of promoting agents exhibit sigmoid-like curves with an observable threshold and maximal effect. Such relationships are depicted in Fig. 8-17, in which the dose–response curve for the binding of the phorbol TPA with its receptor is compared with a dose–response curve for the TPA promotion of dimethylbenzanthracene-initiated papillomas in mouse skin (Ashendel, 1985; Verma and Boutwell, 1980). The threshold effect of promoting agents may be considered a consequence of the reversible nature of their effects at the cellular level (see above). The maximal effect is due to a saturation of ligand binding in the former case and to the promotion of all initiated cells in the latter (Fig. 8-17). Although one may not directly equate the variables in the two processes, the similarity in the shape of the curves is striking (Fig. 8-17). The relative potency of promoting agents may be determined as a function of their ability to induce the clonal growth of initiated cells. Thus, the net rate of growth of preneoplastic lesions can be employed to determine relative potencies for promoting agents (Pitot et al., 1987).

The format of an experimental protocol for the demonstration of initiation and promotion is provided in Fig. 8-18. As noted in the figure, the endpoint of the study, which usually takes from 3 to 6 months, depends on the tissue under investigation, the dose and nature of the initiating and promoting agents utilized, and factors, such as diet and hormonal status, mentioned above. The endpoint analyzed in such studies is properly a preneoplastic lesion (PNL) which develops clonally from initiated cells in the tissue under study. These are altered hepatic foci in the rat or mouse liver (Pitot, 1990), epidermal papillomas for mouse skin (Wigley, 1983), hyperplasia of terminal end buds for rat mammary carcinomas (Purnell, 1980; Russo et al., 1983), and enzyme-altered foci in rat colon carcinogenesis (Pretlow et al., 1993). Administration of the promoting agent for the entire period of the experiment after initiation results in many preneoplastic lesions, whereas alteration of the format of administration of the promoting agent results in the development of very few preneoplastic lesions. This reinforces the fact that the stage of promotion is operationally reversible (Boutwell, 1964) and indicates that a threshold dose effect level may exist.

Progression The transition from early progeny of initiated cells to the biologically malignant cell population constitutes the major part of the natural history of neoplastic development. Foulds recognized the importance of the development of neoplasia beyond the appearance of any initial identifiable lesions (Foulds, 1965).

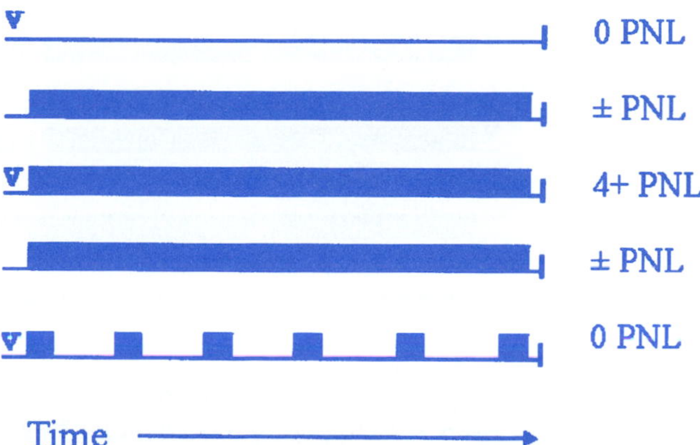

Figure 8-18. General experimental format demonstrating initiation (v) and promotion ▬, for use with carcinogenesis studies in rodent tissues. PN, preneoplastic lesions.

Table 8-11
Putative Progressor Agents in Carcinogenesis

AGENT	INITIATING ACTIVITY	CLASTOGENIC ACTIVITY	CARCINOGENIC ACTIVITY
Arsenic salts	−	+	+
Asbestos fibers	?	+	+
Benzene	−	+	+
Benzoyl peroxide	−	+	±
Hydroxyurea	−	+	±
1,4-Bis[2-(3,5-dichloropyridyloxy)]-benzene	−	+	+
2,5,2′,5′-Tetrachlorobiphenyl	−	+	±

SOURCE: Modified from Pitot and Dragan (1994), with permission.

The characteristics of malignant progression that he observed—growth rate, invasiveness, metastatic frequency, hormonal responsiveness, and morphologic characteristics—vary independently as the disease develops. These characteristics have been ascribed to the karyotypic instability during the irreversible progression stage (Pitot, 1993b). Environmental alterations can influence the stage of progression. For example, exposure to promoting agents can alter gene expression and induce cell proliferation. However, as growth of the neoplasm continues and karyotypic instability evolves, responses to environmental factors may be altered or lost (Noble, 1977; Welch and Tomasovic, 1985). Agents that act only to effect the transition of a cell from the stage of promotion to that of progression may properly be termed *progressor agents*. Some examples are listed in Table 8-11. Such agents presumably have the characteristic of inducing chromosomal aberrations, may not necessarily be capable of initiation, and in some cases may enhance the clastogenesis associated with evolving karyotypic instability. As with the two stages of initiation and promotion, spontaneous progression may also occur. In fact, spontaneous progression would be highly fostered by increased cell replication (Ames et al., 1993).

The experimental demonstration of the stage of progression is somewhat more complex than that of initiation and promotion. In Fig. 8-19 may be seen a general experimental format designed to demonstrate the effect of administration of a progressor agent after a course of initiation and promotion with all of the appropriate controls. However, in this instance the endpoint that is quantitated is the number of neoplastic lesions (NL). In experimental systems, the most effective development of neoplasia involves the continued administration of the promoting agent even after that of the progressor agent. This might be expected because cells early in the stage of progression respond to promoting agents, thus increasing the yield of neoplastic lesions in the experimental system (Table 8-10). As noted, a lower yield, usually still significant, may

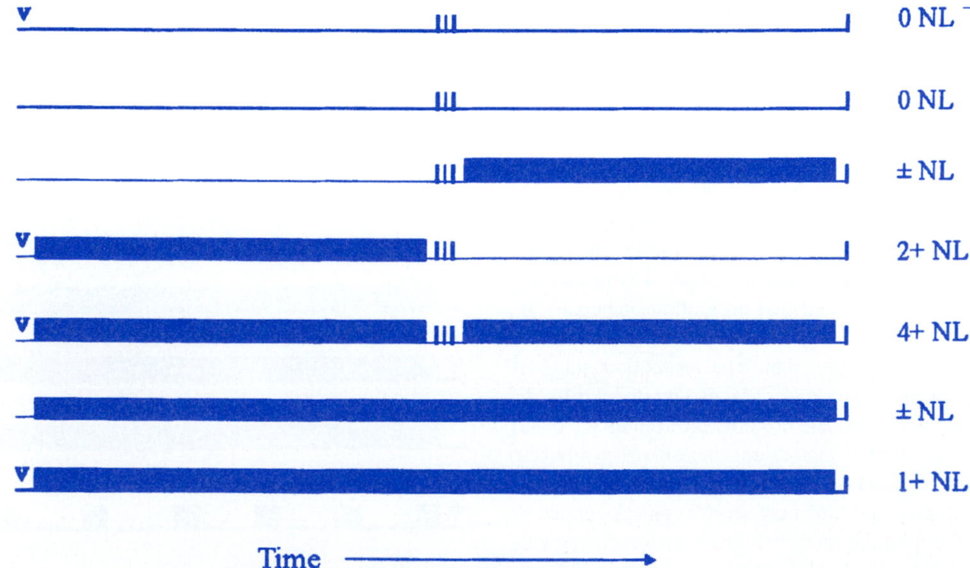

Figure 8-19. General experimental format for demonstration of the stage of progression and the effect of progressor agents in experimental systems.

NL, neoplastic lesions; ±, occasional or infrequent; 1+, few; 2+, some; 4+, many; III, administration of progressor agent as single or several multiple doses; v, initiation; ▬ = promoting agent doses.

be obtained without additional administration of the promoting agent. Because of the duration of the experiment, preneoplastic lesions occur to varying degrees in each of the experimental groups. The difficulty in such studies is the quantitation of the neoplastic lesions which is usually carried out by determining the number and incidence and multiplicity of malignant tumors. However, premalignant lesions already in the stage of progression occur quite commonly (cf. Henson and Albores-Saavedra, 1986), and thus the appropriate endpoint is the quantitation of such lesions. This has been extremely difficult to do, and thus quantitative analyses of the effects of progressor agents remain crude.

Cell and Molecular Mechanisms of the Stages of Carcinogenesis

Although the descriptive and morphologic characteristics of the stages of carcinogenesis are critical to our initial understanding of the pathogenesis of neoplasia, a complete knowledge of the molecular mechanisms of carcinogenesis may be necessary to control the disease through rational therapy, earlier diagnosis, and reasonable methods of prevention. However, our understanding of the molecular mechanisms of carcinogenesis is incomplete. Nonetheless, there has been an exponential explosion of knowledge in this area during the past decade.

Initiation While the morphologic and biological characterization of the stage of initiation has been somewhat limited, mechanistic studies of this stage have been more extensively reported. This is strikingly true in relation to the metabolic activation of chemical carcinogens and the structure of their DNA adducts. As indicated earlier, however, the molecular mechanisms of this stage must conform to the observable biological characteristics of this stage. At least three processes are important in initiation: metabolism, DNA repair, and cell proliferation. Perturbation of any of these pathways have an impact on initiation. While initiated cells are difficult to distinguish morphologically and phenotypically from their normal counterparts, the molecular alterations responsible for initiation may be equally subtle. Table 8-12 lists a number of the molecular mechanistic characteristics of the stages of initiation, promotion, and progression. As already indicated initiating agents or their metabolites are mutagenic to DNA. Thus, carcinogenic agents administered at doses that do not induce neoplasia (incomplete carcinogenesis) are capable of initiating cells in experimental models of multistage carcinogenesis (Boutwell, 1964; Dragan et al., 1994). Furthermore, such subcarcinogenic doses of initiating agents may induce substantial DNA alkylation (Pegg and Perry, 1981; Brambilla et al., 1983; Ward, 1987). The genetic changes necessary to induce the stage of initiation need not be those causing obvious or gross structural chromosomal alterations. Sargent et al. (1989) demonstrated normal karyotypes of cells from altered hepatic foci in the stage of promotion in the rat. A number of investigations have demonstrated specific point mutations in genes which are compatible with those induced in vitro by the adducts resulting from treatment with carcinogenic chemicals (Anderson et al., 1992). The potential genetic targets for initiating agents as well as progressor agents have now been elucidated to some extent. Individual variability, species differences, and organotropism of the stage of initiation are a balance of carcinogen metabolism, cell proliferation, and DNA repair.

Molecular Genetic Targets of DNA-Damaging Carcinogenic Agents Although many genes are affected by the mutagenic action of certain chemical carcinogens, it has long been assumed that mutations in a relatively few specific genes may be most critical to neoplastic transformation. With the discovery and elucidation of the function of viral oncogenes (Bishop, 1985) and their cellular counterparts, proto-oncogenes (Garrett, 1986), the original assumption moved closer to reality. Three different classes of genes have been described that play major roles in the neoplastic process (Table 8-13). Although a variety of other genes involved in DNA repair (Friedburg, 1994; Jass et al., 1994), carcinogen metabolism (Nebert, 1991), and abnormalities in the immune system (Müller, 1990) generate inherited predispositions to the development of neoplasia, it is the products of the proto-oncogenes and cellular oncogenes and the tumor suppressor genes that have been most closely associated with neoplastic transformation (Table 8-13).

Table 8-12
Some Cell and Molecular Mechanisms in Multistage Carcinogenesis

INITIATION	PROMOTION	PROGRESSION
Simple mutations (transitions, transversions, small deletions, etc.) involving the cellular genome.	Reversible enhancement or repression of gene expression mediated via receptors specific for the individual promoting agent.	Complex genetic alterations (chromosomal translocations, deletions, gene amplification, recombination, etc.) resulting from evolving karyotypic instability.
In some species and tissues, point mutations occur in proto-oncogenes and/or potential cellular oncogenes.	Inhibition of apoptosis by promoting agent.	Irreversible changes in gene expression including fetal gene expression, altered MHC gene expression, and ectopic hormone production.
Mutations in genes of signal transduction pathways may result in altered phenotype.	No direct structural alteration in DNA results from action or metabolism of promoting agent.	Selection of neoplastic cells for optimal growth genotype/phenotype in response to the cellular environment and including the evolution of karyotypic instability.

Table 8-13
Characteristics of Proto-oncogenes, Cellular Oncogenes, and Tumor Suppressor Genes

PROTO-ONCOGENES	CELLULAR ONCOGENES	TUMOR SUPPRESSOR GENES
Dominant	Dominant	Recessive
Broad tissue specificity for cancer development	Broad tissue specificity for cancer development	Considerable tissue specificity for cancer development
Germline inheritance rarely involved in cancer development	Germline inheritance rarely involved in cancer development	Germline inheritance frequently involved in cancer development
Analogous to certain viral oncogenes	No known analogs in oncogenic viruses	No known analogs in oncogenic viruses
Somatic mutations activate during all stages of neoplastic development	Somatic mutations activate during all stages of neoplastic development	Germline mutations may initiate, but mutation to neoplasia occurs only during the stage of progression

SOURCE: After Pitot (1993b), with permission.

Table 8-14 shows a listing of a number of functions of proto-oncogenes and cellular oncogenes and tumor suppressor genes, with specific examples and their localization within the cell where known. It is immediately obvious that the oncogenes are involved primarily in cellular growth, signal transduction, and nuclear transcription. Interestingly, similar functions are attributed to known tumor suppressor genes, but in addition at least two of the latter are involved in regulation of the cell cycle. This table is not meant to be all inclusive, and the interested reader is referred to recent reviews and text for a more detailed discussion of these genes and their products (Hunter, 1991; Levine, 1993).

Mutations in proto-oncogenes can result in their activation with subsequent neoplastic transformation similar to that observed following the altered expression of cellular oncogenes. Activation of proto-oncogenes and cellular oncogenes can occur by various means (Table 8-15). Scrutiny of these mechanisms suggests that only point mutations, small insertions and deletions, and possibly altered methylation status are potential events resulting in initiation. The other, more complex alterations in the genome listed would be characteristic of the stage of progression, as will be discussed below.

The activation of proto-oncogenes and cellular oncogenes by specific base mutations, small deletions, and frameshift mutations results from DNA synthesis in the presence of DNA damage including the presence of adducts. Methods for determining such alterations in specimens that consist of only a few hundred or a thou-

Table 8-14
Functions of Representative Oncogenes and Tumor Suppressor Genes

FUNCTIONS OF GENE PRODUCT	GENES	CELL LOCALIZATION
A. Oncogenes		
Growth factors	*sis, fgf*	Extracellular
Receptor/protein tyrosine-kinase	*met, neu*	Extra cell/cell membrane
Protein tyrosine kinase	*src, ret*	Cell membrane/cytoplasmic
Membrane-associated G proteins	*ras, gip-2*	Cell membrane/cytoplasmic
Cytoplasmic protein serine kinases	*raf, pim-1*	Cytoplasmic
Nuclear transcription factors	*myc, fos, jun*	Nuclear
Unknown, undetermined	*bcl-2, crk*	Mitochondrial, cytoplasmic
B. Tumor suppressor genes		
GTPase-activation	NF1	Cell membrane/cytoplasmic
Cell cycle–regulated nuclear transcriptional repressor	RB-1	Nuclear
Cell cycle–regulated nuclear transcription factor	p53	Nuclear
Zinc-finger transcription factor	WT1	Nuclear
Mismatch DNA repair	hMLH1	Nuclear (?)
Zinc-finger transcription factor (?)	BRCA1	Unknown

SOURCES: Part A of the table was extracted from Hunter (1991). Information for part B was obtained from Levine (1993) as well as Papadopoulos et al. (1994) and Bronner et al. (1994), while that for BRCA1 was obtained from Miki et al. (1994) and Futreal et al. (1994).

sand cells have been available only during the last decade (Mies, 1994). The analysis of mutations in specific genes potentially involved in the neoplastic transformation is possible from very small samples by various molecular techniques.

The *ras* genes code for guanosine triphosphatases, which function as molecular switches for signal transduction pathways involved in the control of growth, differentiation, and other cellular functions (Hall, 1994). Table 8-16 lists a number of examples in rodent tissues of specific mutation in two of the *ras* genes, the Ha-*ras* proto-oncogene and the Ki-*ras* cellular oncogene. With the exception of mouse skin, the frequency of such mutations in preneoplastic lesions in experimental animals in the stage of promotion is about 20 to 60 percent. In instances of multistage carcinogenesis in mouse skin, the frequency increases to nearly 100 percent (Bailleul et al., 1989). In general, the mutations noted are those which theoretically could result from DNA-adducts formed by the particular carcinogen. Interestingly, spontaneously occurring neoplasms in mice also exhibit a significant incidence of point mutations in the *ras* proto-oncogenes and cellular oncogenes (Rumsby et al., 1991; Candrian et al., 1991), but neoplasms in corresponding tissues in other species do not necessarily exhibit activating mutations in proto- or cellular oncogenes (Tokusashi et al., 1994; Kakiuchi et al., 1993; Schaeffer et al., 1990). In addition, mutated *ras* genes have been described in normal-appearing mouse skin after dimethylbenz(*a*)anthracene (DMBA) or urethane application (Nelson et al., 1992). By contrast, Cha and associates (1994) recently reported that a very high percentage of untreated rats contained detectable levels of Ha-*ras* mutations in normal mammary tissue. Thus, the mutations seen in neoplasms in untreated animals may result from the selective proliferation of cells containing preexisting mutations.

Thus, while several classes of genes appear appropriate as targets for DNA-damaging carcinogens, the actual role of proto- and cellular oncogene mutations in establishing carcinogenesis is not entirely clear. Among the earliest preneoplastic lesions studied (Table 8-15), less than one-third exhibit mutations in the *ras* gene family, but it is quite possible that other proto- and cellular oncogenes may be targets. Evidence that tumor suppressor genes may be targets for the initiation of early malignant development come largely from studies of genetically inherited neoplasia. In these rare hereditary cancers, one of the alleles of a tumor suppressor gene contains a germline mutation in all cells of the organism (Paraskeva and Williams, 1992; Knudson, 1993).

Promotion Boutwell (1974) was the first to propose that promoting agents may induce their effects through their ability to alter gene expression. During the past decade, our understanding of mechanisms involving the alteration of gene expression by environmental agents has increased exponentially (Morley and Thomas, 1991; Rosenthal, 1994). The regulation of genetic information is mediated through recognition of the environmental effector, hormone, promoting agent, drug, etc., and its specific molecular interaction with either a surface or cytosolic receptor. Several types of receptors exist in cells (Mayer, 1994; Pawson, 1993; Strader et al., 1994) (Fig. 8-20). Plasma membrane receptors may possess a tyrosine protein kinase domain on their intracellular region, while others have multiple transmembrane domains with the intracellular signal transduced through G proteins and cyclic nucleotides (Mayer, 1994). The other general type of receptor mechanism involves a cytosolic receptor that interacts with the ligand (usually lipid-soluble) that has diffused through the plasma membrane. The ligand receptor complex then travels to the nucleus before interacting directly with specific DNA sequences known as response elements.

In both instances is shown in a highly simplified manner the cascade effect of various protein kinases resulting in alterations in transcription as well as cell replication within the nucleus. As shown in the figure, interaction of transmembrane receptors containing a tyrosine protein kinase domain involves initially their dimerization induced by ligand interaction. This activates the protein kinase domain of the receptor causing autophosphorylation. This in turn attracts a cytoplasmic complex, Grb2-Sos to the plasma membrane (Aronheim et al., 1994). Sos is a member of a family of regulatory proteins termed guanine-nucleotide exchange factors (GEFs) (Feig, 1994). Sos association with the G-protein, Ras, stimulates along with other protein interactions the exchange of GDP

Table 8-15
Potential Mechanisms of Oncogene Activation

EVENT	CONSEQUENCE	EXAMPLES
Base mutation in coding sequences	New gene product with altered activity	v-*onc* genes, bladder carcinoma
Deletion in noncoding sequences	Altered regulation of normal gene product	Fibroblast transformation in vitro
Altered promotion for RNA polymerase	Increased transcription of mRNA (normal gene product)	Cell transformation in vitro, lymphoma in chickens
Insertion or substitution with repetitive DNA elements (“transposons”)	Altered regulation of gene product (? normal)	Canine venereal tumor, mouse myeloma
Chromosomal translocation	Altered mRNA, new gene product (?), no altered regulation of gene expression	Burkitt lymphoma in humans, mouse plasmacytoma
Gene amplification	Increased expression of normal gene	Human colon carcinoma, human bladder carcinoma
Hypomethylation of c-*onc* gene	Altered regulation of gene expression (?), normal gene product	Human colon and lung cancer

SOURCE: Adapted from Pitot (1986b), with permission.

Table 8-16
Mutational Activation of *ras* Oncogenes during the Stages of Initiation and Promotion

SPECIES/ TISSUE	CARCINOGEN	LESION	GENE/MUTATION*	FREQUENCY†	REFERENCE
Rat/colon	Azoxymethane	Aberrant crypt foci	K-*ras*/G→A/12	5/16	Shivapurkar et al., 1994
Mouse/liver	Diethylnitros-amine	G6Pase⁻ foci	Ha-*ras*/C→A/61 A→G	12/127	Bauer-Hofmann et al., 1992
Mouse/lung	Urethane	Small adenomas	Ki-*ras*/A→G/61 A→T	32/100	Nuzum et al., 1990
Rat/mammary gland	*N*-methyl-*N*-nitrosourea	Initiated cell clones	H-*ras*/G→A/12	17%	Zhang et al., 1991
Hamster/ pancreas	N-nitroso-*bis* 2-oxopropyl)-amine	Papillary hyperplasia	K-*ras*/G→A/12	12/26	Cerny et al., 1992
Mouse/skin	DMBA/TPA	Papilloma	Ha-*ras*/A→T/61	12/14	Quintanilla et al., 1986

*The numbers in this column refer to the codon position in the cDNA (mRNA) of the gene product.

†The numerator indicates the number of animals exhibiting the mutation; the denominator refers to the total number of animals studied.

with GTP on the Ras α subunit. The GTP-Ras in turn interacts with a cytoplasmic serine-threonine protein kinase, raf, with subsequent activation of its catalytic activity and initiation of a kinase cascade ultimately resulting in the phosphorylation and activation of transcription factors including Jun, Fos, Myc, CREB, and ultimately E2F and Rb, the tumor suppressor gene (Lewis et al., 1998; Janknecht et al., 1995; Roussel, 1998). A number of other transcription factors are also activated by similar pathways involving other pathways such as phospholipase C, phosphatidylinositol kinase, and protein kinase C (Vojtek and Der, 1998; Takuwa and Takuwa, 1996). The rate-limiting step in this process is the mediation of the signal through the G-protein family. The G proteins are targeted to the plasma membrane through lipid moieties, both isoprenoid and fatty acyl, covalently linked to the carboxyl-terminal region of the protein (Yamane and Fung, 1993). In this way the initiation of the signal by the ligand-receptor interaction can be physically related to the rate-limiting G protein activation step. The activation cycle of the G-protein family involves GTP binding to the α subunit of the G protein, such binding being dramatically stimulated by GEF proteins such as Sos. Activation also involves dissociation of the α from the β and γ subunits allowing the α subunit to interact with and activate downstream members of the pathway, a protein kinase, B-raf in the case of the growth factor related pathway or with other membrane molecules such as adenyl cyclase in the case of multiple transmembrane domain receptors (Fig. 8-20). The activated G protein has an extremely short half-life because of the action of RGS (regulator of G-protein signaling) proteins which stimulate GTP hydrolysis to GDP with subsequent reassociation of the G protein in its inactive state (Koelle, 1997).

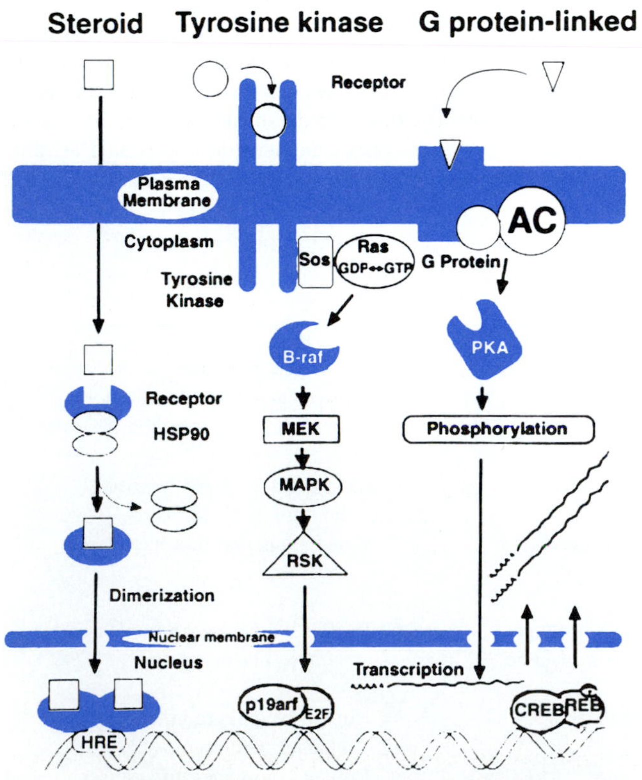

Figure 8-20. Diagram of principal mechanisms of intracellular signal transduction initiated either within the cytosol or at the plasma membrane. [Modified from Mayer (1994), with permission.]

The multiple transmembrane domain receptors (G protein–linked) are in direct association with G proteins and on activation of the receptor by interaction with a ligand may activate a kinase termed a G-protein receptor kinase (GRK) or another effector such as adenyl cyclase (Böhm et al., 1997; Rasenick et al., 1995). In turn, adenyl cyclase produces cyclic AMP, which interacts with the regulatory component of protein kinase A, with a subsequent phosphorylation cascade to the transcription apparatus. In addition to the plasma membrane receptors, gene expression can be regulated through the interaction of cytoplasmic receptors with their ligands as previously discussed. Just as with membrane receptors, the pathways of the cytoplasmic receptors involve multiple interactions with proteins, phosphorylation, and ultimate alteration of transcription through factor interaction with DNA (Weigel, 1996; Pratt and Toft, 1997). In all of these pathways, in addition to alteration of transcription and gene expression, enhancement or inhibition of

Table 8-17
Some Promoter-Receptor Interactions in Target Tissues

PROMOTING AGENT	TARGET TISSUE(S)	RECEPTOR STATUS	TYPE
Tetradecanoylphorbol acetate (TPA)	Skin	Defined (protein kinase C)	Tyrosine kinase/ G protein–linked
2,3,7,8-Tetrachlorodibenzo-*p*-dioxin (TCDD); planar PCBs	Skin, liver	Defined (Ah receptor)	Steroid
Sex steroids (androgens and estrogens)	Liver, mammary tissue, kidney	Defined (estrogen and androgen receptors)	Steroid
Synthetic antioxidants (butylated hydroxytoluene, BHT; butylated hydroxy-anisole, BHA)	Liver, lung, fore-stomach	Postulated	Steroid (?)
Phenobarbital	Liver	Postulated	Unknown
Peroxisome proliferators (WY-14,643, nafenopin, clofibrate)	Liver	Defined [peroxisome proliferator-activated receptor (PPAR)]	Steroid
Polypeptide trophic hormones and growth factors (prolactin, EGF, glucagon)	Liver, skin, mammary gland	Defined or partially characterized	G protein–linked/ tyrosine kinase
Okadaic acid	Skin	Defined (?) (protein phosphatase-2A)	Unknown
Cyclosporine	Liver, lymphoid tissue	Defined (cyclophilin)	Tyrosine kinase/ G protein–linked

SOURCE: Adapted from Pitot and Dragan (1996) with permission of the publisher. Further references may be found in the text. Cyclosporine as a promoter of murine lymphoid neoplasms has been described by Hattori et al. (1988).

cell replication may also be an endpoint which is achieved through transcriptional modulation of the cell cycle.

Many promoting agents exert their effects on gene expression through perturbation of one of the signal transduction pathways, as indicated in Fig. 8-20. One may, in general, classify receptor mechanisms into three broad classes, steroid, tyrosine kinase, and G protein–linked. The majority of the more commonly studied promoting agents exert their actions by mediation of one or more of the receptor pathways indicated in Fig. 8-20. In Table 8-17 are listed some of the best-studied promoting agents known or postulated to be effectors in signal transduction pathways. While protein kinase C (PKC) is not itself one of the three types of receptors noted in Fig. 8-20, it is a mediator of the signal transduction pathways of both the tyrosine kinase and G protein–linked transduction pathways. TPA interacts directly with membrane-bound PKC, displacing the normal activator diacylglycerol and serving to maintain the kinase in its active and soluble form (Ashendel, 1985). The continual activation of this kinase then stimulates further transduction pathways by phosphorylation of specific proteins (Stabel and Parker, 1991). TCDD acts in the steroid pathway via a specific receptor, the Ah receptor, the ligand-receptor complex together with other proteins ultimately altering the transcriptional rate of genes possessing specific regulatory sequences (HRE). In a similar manner, sex steroids, some synthetic antioxidants, and peroxisome proliferators interact with specific soluble receptors and altered gene expression by presumed similar mechanisms to that of TCDD. While in some instances the actual receptor is still not defined, those for polypeptide hormones and growth factors consist of either the tyrosine kinase or G protein–linked types depending on the structure of the polypeptide. The "receptors" for okadaic acid and cyclosporin have been reported to be protein phosphatase 2A and cyclophilin-A respectively (Fujiki and Suganuma, 1993). These proteins, like PKC, are involved in phosphorylation mechanisms of the tyrosine kinase and G protein–linked pathways, although specific sites and mechanisms have not been completely clarified at this time. Thus, the action of promoting agents in altering gene expression may be mediated through specific receptors. This hypothesis provides a reasonable explanation for the tissue specificity demonstrated by many promoting agents. The receptor-ligand concept of promoting agent action is based on the dose–response relationships involving pharmacologic agents. The basic assumptions of such interactions argue that the effect of the agent is directly proportional to the number of receptors occupied by the lig-

Ligand (L) – Receptor (R) Interactions

$$R + L \rightleftharpoons RL\ \text{(complex)}$$

$$K_L = \frac{[R]\cdot[L]}{[RL]}$$

where K_L = the dissociation constant of RL complex

Figure 8-21. Representation of receptor-ligand interaction and dissociation with derivation of the K_L, dissociation constant of the receptor-ligand complex.

and. The intrinsic activity of the chemical and the signal transduction pathways available in the tissue are important factors in the type and degree of response observed.

The Molecular Basis of the Reversibility of the Stage of Tumor Promotion

The theoretical and practical aspects of ligand-receptor interactions have been previously reviewed (cf. Pitot, 1995). Herein we will consider such relationships as they are concerned with the action of tumor promoters. The basic assumption of the ligand-receptor interaction is that the effect of the agent is directly proportional to the number of receptors occupied by that chemical ligand and that a maximum response of the target is obtained only when all receptors are occupied. As seen in Fig. 8-21, a simple bimolecular interaction between the ligand and receptor can be utilized to determine a dissociation constant, K_L of the receptor ligand complex, as noted in the figure. While a variety of mathematical relationships may be derived from this simple equation (cf. Ruffolo, 1992), herein we consider only the dose–response relationship. The dose–response of the receptor-ligand interaction takes the shape of a sigmoidal curve identical to that seen with the inhibition of TPA binding depicted in Fig. 8-17. The figure denotes a threshold response at very low doses and a maximal effect above a specific dose. Theoretically, the linear conversion of the sigmoidal curves such as seen in Fig. 8-17 may indicate effects at even lower doses than those usually studied, but such depends on the association constant of the ligand-receptor complex and the subsequent fate of the complex (Aldridge, 1986). Withdrawal of the ligand reverts the system to its original state. Thus, the regulation of genetic expression that occurs by the ligand-receptor mechanism predicts a threshold and reversible effect unlike that of genotoxic carcinogenic agents, in which an irreversible non-threshold response is assumed on theoretical grounds and can be demonstrated in a variety of instances (Druckrey, 1967; Zeise et al., 1987). Furthermore, at very low doses of some carcinogenic agents, an apparent reversal or "protective" effect of the agent can actually be demonstrated. This phenomenon has been termed *hormesis* (Teeguarden et al., 1998). Regardless of whether this latter effect can be more generalized, it is apparent that both the measured dose response and the receptor mechanisms of tumor promotion imply a no-effect or threshold level for the action of these agents during carcinogenesis. Thus, the stage of tumor promotion, unlike that of initiation and progression, does not involve mutational or structural events in the genome but rather is concerned with the reversible alteration of the expression of genetic information.

The selective induction of proliferation of initiated cell populations was first intimated by the work of Solt and Farber (1976), who used 2-acetylaminofluorene administration as a "selection agent" for the enhancement of proliferation of altered hepatic foci in a modified initiation-promotion protocol. A similar "selection" of certain initiated clones by TPA promotion has also been postulated as occurring during multistage carcinogenesis in mouse skin (cf. DiGiovanni, 1992). Later studies demonstrated that 2-acetylaminofluorene was acting as a promoting agent in this protocol (Saeter et al., 1988). Farber and his colleagues (Roomi et al., 1985) espoused the concept that the lowered xenobiotic metabolism of preneoplastic cell populations gave such cells a competitive advantage in toxic environments such as those provided by the chronic administration of carcinogens. Schulte-Hermann and his associates (1981) have demonstrated that several hepatic promoting agents including phenobarbital, certain steroids, and peroxisome proliferators selectively enhanced the proliferation of cells within preneoplastic lesions in rat liver. A similar effect was reported by Klaunig in preneoplastic and neoplastic hepatic lesions in mice responding to promotion by phenobarbital (Klaunig, 1993). The response of preneoplastic hepatocytes in the rat to partial hepatectomy is also greater than that of normal hepatocytes (Laconi et al., 1994). Preneoplastic hepatocytes in culture exhibit an inherent higher level of replicative DNA synthesis than normal hepatocytes (Xu et al., 1988). Thus, the characteristic of promoting agents at the cell and molecular level to increase cell proliferation of preneoplastic cell populations selectively more than that of their normal counterparts may be the result of altered mechanisms of cell cycle control within the preneoplastic cell.

Cell Cycle Regulation Although the exact mechanism(s) by which promoting agents selectively enhance cell replication in preneoplastic cells is unknown, our understanding of the interaction of ligand-receptor signaling with the cell cycle and its regulation has dramatically increased in recent years. Figure 8-22 diagrams an integration of the cell cycle and apoptosis with the signal transduction pathways (Fig. 8-20). Phosphorylation of the mitogen-activated protein kinase (MAPK) via the signal transduction pathway activates this kinase (Fig. 8-22), which then activates various transcription factors, some of which are noted above in the figure as proto-oncogene products, c-*myc,* c-*jun,* and c-*fos* (Seger and Krebs, 1995). Rb, the retinoblastoma tumor suppressor gene, is made throughout the cell cycle. It becomes highly phosphorylated at the beginning of DNA synthesis (G,1S). This releases a transcription factor, E2F, which is complexed with the highly phosphorylated but not the hypophosphorylated Rb protein. E2F then is available to stimulate the transcription of a variety of genes needed for the transition from G1 and the initiation of DNA synthesis. As we noted above, ligand-receptor interactions can result in the activation of E2F and thus the transcription of genes needed for continuation of the cell cycle. This continuation involves a variety of protein kinases and proteins, known as *cyclins,* which are listed in the figure. Another tumor suppressor gene, the *p53* gene, also plays a role as a transcription factor, preventing continuance of the cell cycle on the occasion of DNA damage (Wu and Levine, 1994). Such a pause allows the cells to repair such damage or, if the damage is excessive, to undergo apoptosis (Fig. 8-22). If the *p53* gene is mutated or absent, such a pause does not occur, and the cell cycle continues replicating despite the presence of damage resulting in mutations and clastogenesis (Lane, 1992; Sander et al., 1993; Dulic et al., 1994). Obviously, the missing mechanistic link is a clear understanding of the selective enhancement of the cell cycle in preneoplastic cells by promoting agents. A variety of possibilities exist, including increased concentrations of receptors or any one or more of the components of the signal transduction pathway, as well as mutations in transcription factors, cyclins, cdks, or other components of the cell cycle. As yet, however, definitive studies to pinpoint such mechanisms have not been performed.

Progression The stage of progression usually develops from cells in the stage of promotion but may develop directly from normal cells, usually as a result of the administration of relatively high, usually cytotoxic doses of complete carcinogenic agents capable of inducing both initiation and progression. In addition, the incorporation into the genome of genetic information such as oncogenic

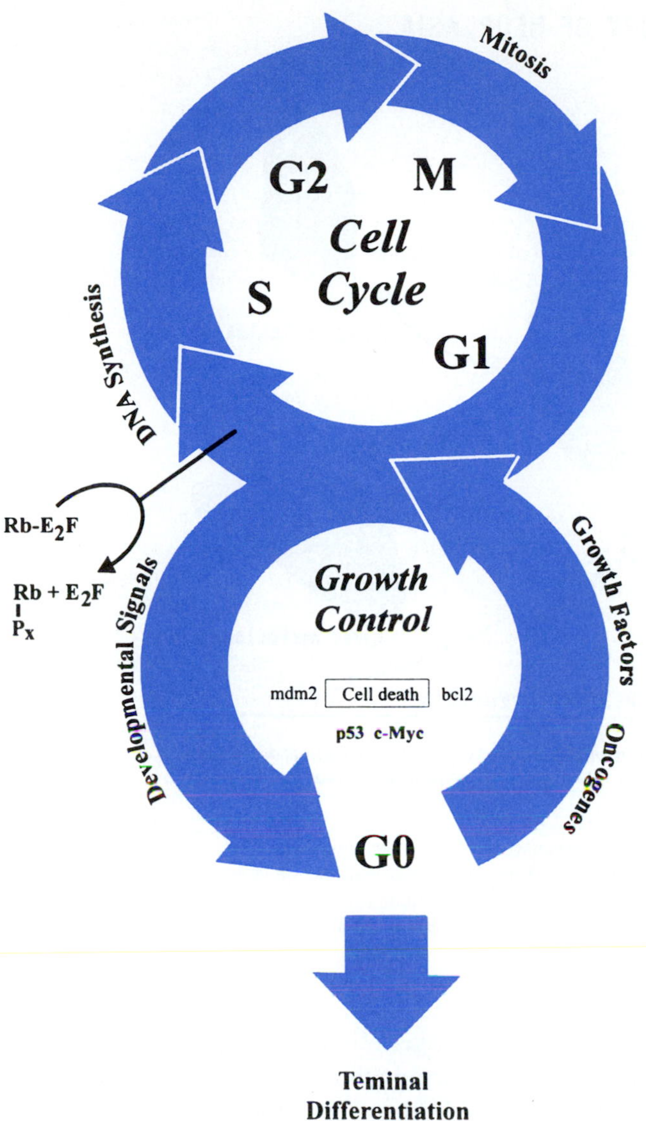

Figure 8-22. Diagram of the cell cycle and its associated cycle to apoptosis or terminal differentiation with potential to return to the active cycle under the influence of growth factors and related components.

Signal transduction may regulate the cell cycle through kinase activation involving the E_2F-Rb interaction or other kinases and related molecules involved in the cell cycle.

viruses, the stable transfection of genetic material, or from spontaneous chromosomal alterations may induce the stage of progression. As noted in Tables 8-10 through 8-12, the major hallmark of the stage of progression is evolving karyotypic instability. It is this molecular characteristic of cells in the stage of progression that potentially leads to multiple "stages" or changes in malignant cells which were first described by Foulds (1954) as "independent characteristics." Foulds noted that cells in the stage of progression might evolve in such a way that the characteristics of invasion, metastatic growth, anaplasia, as well as the rate of growth and responses to hormonal influences changed toward higher and higher degrees of malignancy. Such "independent characteristics" may all be understood as resulting from karyotypic changes that are constantly evolving in cells during the stage of progression. Included in these "characteristics" may be such things as fetal gene expression, the expression of the major histocompatibility complex (MHC) class I and II surface proteins, and the ectopic production of hormones by cells derived from non-hormone-producing tissues as well as several other characteristics of neoplastic cells (Hanahan and Weinberg, 2000). Thus, in some tissues it may be possible to describe multiple "stages" that reflect the evolving karyotypic instability of neoplasms such as in the evolution of colonic (Fearon and Vogelstein, 1992) and other neoplasms (Nowell, 1990). Simultaneous with these changes may be the occurrence of mutated proto- and cellular oncogenes (Liu et al., 1988) and tumor suppressor genes (Yokota and Sugimura, 1993). However, since karyotypic instability is unlikely to lead directly to point mutations in oncogenes and tumor suppressor genes, it is more likely that their appearance reflects the selection of cells better suited to the growth environment of the neoplasm.

The critical molecular characteristic of the stage of progression is karyotypic instability. As pointed out by Harris (1991), the genetic instability of this stage is primarily a reflection of the karyotypic changes seen rather than point mutations or gene amplification. Mechanisms that can lead to karyotypic instability are numerous and include disruption of the mitotic apparatus, alteration in telomere function (Blackburn, 1994), DNA hypomethylation, recombination, gene amplification, and gene transposition (cf. Cheng and Loeb, 1993). The recent demonstration of the role of alterations in mismatch repair genes (see above) in some forms of cancer suggests a potential for both karyotypic and genetic instability. Many neoplasms exhibit one or more of these events, which very likely play a role in the evolution of the carcinogenic process. Numerical and structural genetic changes can occur in populations of cells without adequate repair such as in those with mutant *p53* genes (see above). Histologically distinct neoplasms may exhibit different pathways during their evolution throughout the stage of progression (Heim et al., 1988; Fearon and Vogelstein, 1992).

The Bases for the Stages of Initiation, Promotion, and Progression

In Fig. 8-23 may be seen an artist's conception of the natural history of neoplastic development, beginning with a single initiated cell and resulting in metastatic neoplastic lesions. The bases for the cell and molecular biology of the stages of neoplastic development may be considered in a relatively simple format, as follows:

Initiation results from a simple mutation in one or more cellular genes controlling key regulatory pathways of the cell.

Promotion results from the selective functional enhancement of signal transduction pathways induced in the initiated cell and its progeny by the continuous exposure to the promoting agent.

Progression results from continuing evolution of a basically unstable karyotype.

These seminal characteristics of the three stages of carcinogenesis readily distinguish one from the other and also form a basis for the molecular action of chemicals acting at each of these stages.

Based on a knowledge of the seminal characteristics of each of the stages of carcinogenesis, it is reasonable to classify chemical agents in regard to their primary action during one or more of the stages of carcinogenesis. Table 8-18 presents such a classification. Agents that are capable of initiation and thus are true incomplete carcinogens are unusual, if they exist at all. Although the "pure" initiating activity of certain chemicals in specific tissues has

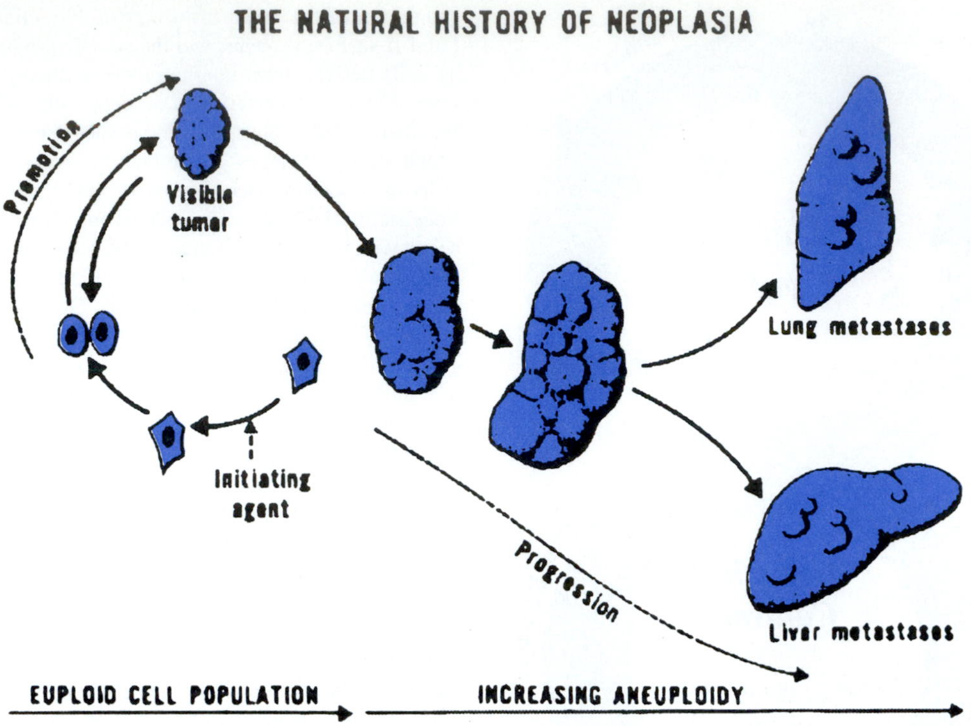

Figure 8-23. The natural history of neoplasia, beginning with the initiated cell after application of an initiating agent (carcinogen), followed by the potentially reversible stage of promotion to a visible tumor, with subsequent progression of this tumor to malignancy.

The relation to karyotype is presented as a generalization on the lower arrows. The reader should again be cautioned that not all neoplastic cells undergo this entire natural history. It is theoretically possible, although this has not yet been definitively shown, that some neoplasms, such as those induced in animals by radiation or high doses of chemical carcinogens, may enter this sequence in the stage of progression, exhibiting aneuploidy, and thus bypass the early euploid cell stages.

been reported (cf. DiGiovanni, 1992), in most instances, at higher doses or in different tissues, such agents can be shown to be carcinogenic, usually acting as complete carcinogens. On the other hand, in distinguishing experimentally between the stages of initiation and promotion, low single doses of complete carcinogens may act to initiate cells, but since they cannot sustain the stage of promotion, they may act de facto as pure initiating agents or incomplete carcinogens. The list of promoting agents and putative promoting agents is, like that of complete carcinogens, growing steadily. Progressor agents in the strict sense of inducing the characteristics noted in Tables 8-10 and 8-12 have not been well characterized. It should be noted, however, that in order to designate a chemical as a complete carcinogen, its ability to induce each of the stages of carcinogenesis is a prerequisite by definition.

Genetic and Nongenetic Mechanisms of Chemical Carcinogenesis in Relation to the Natural History of Cancer Development

Some agents, specifically initiating and progressor agents, possess as a primary aspect of their carcinogenic mechanism the ability to alter the structure of DNA and/or chromosomes. Such "genotoxic" effects have been linked directly to the induction of neoplasia. However, when administered chronically to animals, a number of chemicals induce the development of neoplasia, but there is no evidence of their direct "genotoxic" action on target cells. Considering the effects of chemicals on the development of neoplasia via a multistage process, one may quickly classify such agents as pro-

Table 8-18

Classification of Chemical Carcinogens in Relation to Their Action on One or More Stages of Carcinogenesis

Initiating agent (incomplete carcinogen): a chemical capable only of initiating cells
Promoting agent: a chemical capable of causing the expansion of initiated cell clones
Progressor agent: a chemical capable of converting an initiated cell or a cell in the stage of promotion to a potentially malignant cell
Complete carcinogen: a chemical possessing the capability of inducing cancer from normal cells, usually possessing properties of initiating, promoting, and progressor agents

moting agents acting to expand clones of spontaneously initiated cells. The consequent selective enhancement of cell replication in such initiated cell clones sets the stage for the spontaneous transition of an occasional cell into the stage of progression as discussed above. However, this explanation of "nongenotoxic" carcinogenesis may be oversimplified. Table 8-19 lists a representative sample of chemicals that are nonmutagenic as assessed by induction of mutations in bacteria or mammalian cells, but which, on chronic administration, are carcinogenic in experimental systems. As indicated in the table, a number of these chemicals have been shown to be promoting agents, but some are not. Several of those that are not promoting agents may be classified as putative progressor agents as evidenced by their effectiveness as clastogens in experimental systems (see above). A number of other chemicals (Tennant, 1993) have not been tested for their action at specific stages of carcinogenesis and thus cannot neatly be placed into the classification of Table 8-19.

In addition to the several potential progressor agents such as benzene noted in Table 8-19, other nongenotoxic mechanisms have been proposed to account for carcinogenesis by some of these chemicals (Grasso and Hinton, 1991). One such class are the so-called peroxisome proliferators, so named because on administration they induce an increase in the number and proteins of peroxisomes, primarily in the liver. These compounds now make up a relatively large list of chemicals (Reddy and Lalwani, 1983), which are generally nongenotoxic (Stott, 1988); but many are hepatocarcinogenic and are promoting agents for hepatocarcinogenesis in the rat (Cattley and Popp, 1989). Because of the peroxidative function of many of the enzymes in peroxisomes, Reddy and others (Reddy and Rao, 1989) have proposed that the carcinogenic action of these chemicals may be mediated by an increased oxidative potential for DNA damage in cells treated with such agents. The demonstration of such increased oxidative damage to DNA in livers of peroxisome proliferator–treated rats has been variable (Kasai et al., 1989; Hegi et al., 1990). It should also be remembered that many of the peroxisome proliferators exert their effects through a specific receptor (Issemann and Green, 1990; Motojima, 1993).

Another series of chemical carcinogens that induce renal cell neoplasms in rodents have been found also to induce a dramatic increase in the accumulation of urinary proteins in renal tubular cells. This is observed only in the male rat in which there is an accumulation of the male-specific urinary protein, α_{2u}-globulin, which is correlated with the production of renal neoplasms in male but not female rats. This is found with *d*-limonene (Dietrich and Swenberg, 1991) and unleaded gasoline (Short et al., 1989). Several halogenated hydrocarbons induce α_{2u}-globulin and renal neoplasms in male rats (Konishi and Hiasa, 1994). Compounds that induce α_{2u}-globulin dramatically increase cell proliferation in the kidney as a result of the chronic accumulation of the protein with subsequent cell degeneration. However, this α_{2u}-globulin nephropathy is not itself carcinogenic (Dominick et al., 1991).

Agents that are not mutagenic or genotoxic may induce direct toxicity with sustained tissue damage and subsequent cell proliferation. Both direct DNA toxicity and increased cell proliferation may lead to clastogenesis (Scott et al., 1991) or damage genetic DNA indirectly through oxidative mechanisms. Finally, the cell proliferation resulting from toxicity may selectively induce enhanced replication of an already damaged genome in the initiated cell population. While cell toxicity does not directly induce carcinogenesis, it is capable of enhancing the process. Because many agents that are tested at chronic doses induce at least a mild degree of toxicity, it has been argued that the format of the testing system leads to the induction of neoplasia. Thus, neoplastic development observed with test compound administration may occur as a result of the toxicity and cell proliferation associated with chronic high doses utilized rather than from a direct carcinogenic effect of the agent (Ames and Gold, 1990). Thus, nongenotoxic or nonmutagenic mechanisms of carcinogenesis involve mechanisms

Table 8-19
Some Nonmutagenic Chemical Carcinogens

COMPOUND	SPECIES/TARGET ORGAN	PROMOTING ACTION
Benzene	Rat, mouse/Zymbal gland	−
Butylated hydroxyanisole	Rat, hamster/forestomach	+
Chlorobenzilate	Rat/liver	+
Chloroform	Rat, mouse/liver	+
Clofibrate	Rat/liver	+
Dieldrin	Mouse/liver	+
Diethylhexyl Phthalate	Rat/liver	±
p,p′-Dichlorodiphenyldichloroethylene	Rat/liver	+
1,4 Dioxane	Mouse, rat/liver, Nasal turbinate	NT*
Furfural	Mouse/liver	+
Lindane	Mouse/liver	+
Methapyrilene	Rat/liver	+
Polychlorinated biphenyls	Rat, mouse/liver	+
Reserpine	Mouse/mammary tissue	NT
Saccharin	Rat/bladder	+
2,3,7,8-Tetrachlorodibenzo-p-dioxin	Rat/liver, lung	+
Trichloroethylene	Mouse/liver	+

*NT = not tested.

SOURCE: Modified from Lijinsky (1990) and Tennant (1993), with permission.

as yet uncharacterized. Several types of compounds appear to have primarily a promoting type of effect, including agents that induce P-450s, other mitogenic agents, cytotoxic agents, and many that act through receptor-mediated processes.

CHEMICAL CARCINOGENESIS IN HUMANS

There is substantial evidence that chemical agents can cause cancer in the human. Ramazzini reported in 1700 that breast cancer occurred in a very high incidence in celibate nuns (Wright, 1940). Ramazzini proposed that the development of this neoplasm in this occupational group was the result of their lifestyle, a thesis compatible with present knowledge that endogenous hormone exposure plays a causal role in breast cancer development (Henderson et al., 1982). The initial evidence of an exogenous chemical cause of cancer in the human was related by Hill, who described the association of the use of tobacco snuff with the occurrence of nasal polyps (Hill, 1761). As discussed earlier in this chapter, Pott demonstrated the causal relationship of chimney soot to scrotal cancer in young individuals employed as chimney sweeps. During the last 150 years a number of specific chemicals or chemical mixtures, industrial processes, and lifestyles have been causally related to the increased incidences of a variety of human cancers. The proportion of human cancer caused by a variety of environmental agents is provided in Fig. 8-24 (Doll and Peto, 1981). While this chart is more than two decades old, substantial evidence has accrued in support of these proportional differences. How these proportions were determined and the specific chemicals associated with those segments related to chemical carcinogenesis are the subject of this section.

Epidemiologic and Animal Studies as Bases for the Identification of Chemical Carcinogens in Humans

Epidemiology has been defined as the study of the distribution and determinants of disease (Stewart and Sarfaty, 1978). Epidemiologic methodologies develop their findings from observation rather than controlled experimentation. Animal studies of carcinogenesis provide data from controlled experiments in vivo and in vitro. Because human beings cannot and should not be treated as experimental animals, epidemiologic observations may take a number of forms (Rogan and Brown, 1979; Pitot, 1986a), including the following:

1. *Episodic observations.* Observations of isolated cases of cancer in relation to a specific environmental factor(s) have yielded information in the past as to cause-and-effect relationships. However, deductions from these types of observations must be carefully evaluated in properly designed studies.
2. *Retrospective studies.* Retrospective studies, which are investigations of the histories and habits of groups of individuals who have developed a disease, have been frequent sources of epidemiologic data. An important factor in such investigations is the use of case controls, i.e., individuals not exposed to the variable under study. In many instances, the suitable designation of such controls is the critical component in the study. This type of study is usually the first step in attempting to identify factors that may be causative in the development of human cancer.
3. *Prospective studies.* Prospective investigations involve analyses of the continuing and future development of cancers in individuals with specific social habits, occupational exposures, and so on. Such investigations require large populations, long follow-up periods (usually 10 to 30 years), with a large percentage of both controls and test groups continuing for the duration of the study. Many such investigations are presently under way in the United States and throughout the world.

Epidemiologic studies may be concerned with a single factor or with multiple factors potentially causative of specific human cancers. However, it is rarely possible to identify a single chemical as the sole causative factor in the development of a specific type of human cancer because of the numerous other environmental variables to which the human population or cohort (group under study) is exposed. In addition, environmental factors in the causation of human cancer—including chemical exposure, infection

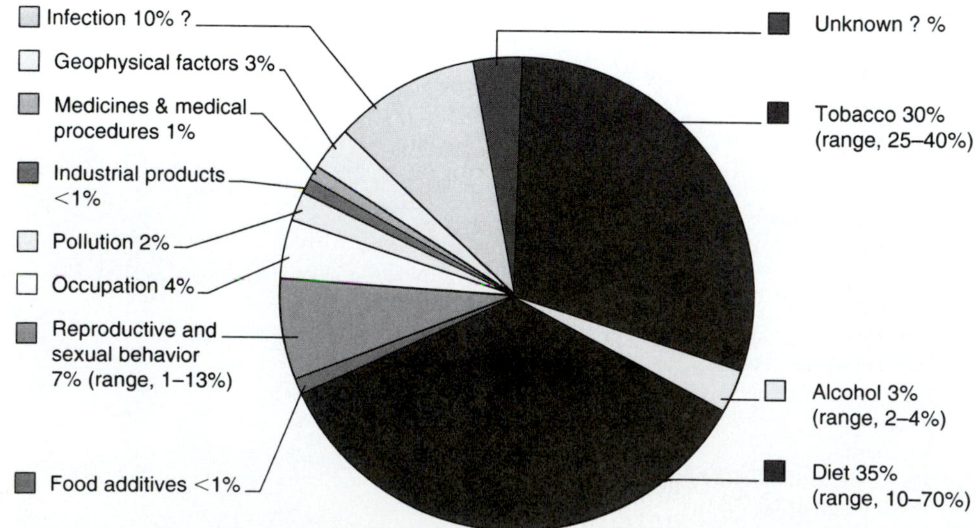

Figure 8-24. Proportions of cancer deaths attributed to various environmental factors [After Doll and Peto (1981), with permission.]

with various parasites, ultraviolet and ionizing radiation, and individual genetic background—may be additive, synergistic, or antagonistic in relation to one another. As a confounding factor, an agent may act at the same or different stages in carcinogenesis.

Epidemiologic studies can identify only factors that are different between two populations and that are sufficiently important in the etiology of the condition under study to play a determining role under the conditions of exposure. Furthermore, on the basis of epidemiologic studies alone, it is usually very difficult to determine whether a specific chemical is or is not carcinogenic to humans. The reasons for this difficulty are the extended periods between first exposure and clinical occurrence of the neoplasm, the high background incidence for many cancers in the general population, the relatively imprecise knowledge of the nature of the exposure in most instances, and other confounding variables. Thus, many negative epidemiologic studies must be considered as inconclusive for indicating the risk factor of relatively weak carcinogens or low doses of carcinogens for the induction of neoplastic disease in the human population (Pitot, 1986a). In view of the fact that epidemiologic studies in themselves are many times insufficient to establish the carcinogenicity of an agent for humans, laboratory studies with laboratory animals in vivo and cells in vitro have been employed to complement or in some cases supplant epidemiologic observations where they exist.

Utilizing both epidemiologic and experimental animal data, several agencies throughout the world have proposed classification of agents based on the evidence for their carcinogenicity in humans. The first scheme that was generally recognized was devised by the International Agency for Research on Cancer (IARC). In the IARC scheme (Table 8-20), the evaluation is based on demonstration of the carcinogenicity of the agent. The terminology that is utilized is as follows (Pitot, 1986a):

1. *Sufficient evidence* of carcinogenicity, which indicates that there is a causal relationship between the agent(s) and human cancer.
2. *Limited evidence* of carcinogenicity, which indicates that a causal interpretation is credible but that alternative explanations, such as chance, bias, or confounding variables, could not be completely excluded.
3. *Inadequate evidence,* which indicates that one of three conditions prevailed: (a) there were few pertinent data; (b) the available studies, while showing evidence of association, did not exclude chance, bias, or confounding variables; (c) studies were available that did not show evidence of carcinogenicity.

For an agent to be classified as carcinogenic to humans (group 1), there must be substantial epidemiologic evidence to support the claim. While epidemiologic studies attempt to examine the human evidence with exposures at biologically relevant doses, such studies are often limited by their expense and the prolonged duration necessary for the detection of clinically relevant malignancy. In addition, numerous confounding variables exist, and the studies usually occur after exposure to a compound (retrospective). In the case of chemicals administered for therapeutic purposes as well as in some industrial exposures, the studies may be well controlled with respect to exposure conditions, but the number of individuals and duration of the exposure are generally limited. Thus, in many investigations with animals, primarily rodents, short-term tests (see below) are used to provide weight to the argument for the potential risk from exposure to the compound. In this instance, the stipulation should be that the endpoint is a qualitative one concerned primarily with hazard identification.

Several other classification schemes exist including that of the Environmental Protection Agency (EPA), the Chemical Manufacturers Association, and the European Community (EC). These classifications agree with respect to classification of compounds that are known human carcinogens but place different emphasis on the results of animal and genotoxicity studies. This is particularly true for single sex or strain-specific effects such as induction of α_2-microglobulin in the rat kidney, peroxisome proliferation in the rodent liver, and thyroid neoplasia in the rodent. Thus, in assessing potential human cancer risk from compound exposure, several factors are considered to provide a greater or lesser concern as to a potential for induction of human cancer from exposure (Table 8-21). Many of these factors are based on the pharmacokinetic and pathologic response similarities of humans and the surrogate test species.

In spite of the limitations of these classifications, an agent cannot be proven to be carcinogenic for the human unless substantial epidemiologic evidence supporting such a claim is available. Despite this restriction, a number of chemical agents, processes, and lifestyles have been shown to be carcinogenic in humans according to the IARC classification.

Table 8-20
IARC Classification of the Evaluation of Carcinogenicity for Human Beings

GROUP	EVIDENCE	EXAMPLES
1. Agent is carcinogenic	Sufficient (human)	Arsenic, aflatoxin, benzene, estrogens, vinyl chloride
2A. Agent is probably carcinogenic	Limited (human) Sufficient (animal)	Benz[*a*]anthracene, DEN, PCBs, styrene oxide
2B. Agent is possibly carcinogenic	Limited (human) or Inadequate (human) Sufficient (animal)	TCDD, styrene, urethane
3. Agent is not classifiable as to carcinogenicity		5-Azacytidine, diazepam
4. Agent is probably not carcinogenic	Inadequate (human) Inadequate (animal)	Caprolactam

Lifestyle Carcinogenesis

Historians have noted that the cancer incidence in the human population appears to go up with the "advancement of civilization." Thus, the more affluent populations tend to have higher general incidences of cancer. A major factor is related to the style of life that the more affluent individual can choose, such lifestyles not always being the most healthy. Chemical factors involved in the development of cancer from lifestyle practices may be related to complex chemical mixtures or, in some instances, related to specific external or internal environmental chemicals. Table 8-22 lists chemical carcinogenic agents associated with lifestyle. Of the agents listed, three—alcoholic beverages, aflatoxins, and dietary intake—are related to the nutritional status of the individual. While aflatoxin has been shown to be a complete carcinogen in experimental animals, the carcinogenic effect of alcoholic beverages and dietary intake is not readily apparent. As noted from the table, elevated risks of several neoplasms in the human result from excessive intake of alcoholic beverages. Since all types of alcoholic beverages are implicated in the variety of studies supporting these claims, ethanol itself and its metabolites appear to be the common components of these beverages that have been implicated as the effective moieties (Blot, 1992). Ethanol is metabolized directly to acetaldehyde, which has been shown to be mutagenic (Garro and Lieber, 1990). There is, however, no evidence that ethanol or alcoholic beverages are complete carcinogens in any system. However, chronic ethanol administration after initiation in rat liver may act to enhance carcinogenesis. In several other organs, ethanol, when given simultaneously with a carcinogenic agent, acts as a cocarcinogen (Seitz and Simanowski, 1988). In support of the promoting action of ethanol in the human, cancer of the oral cavity and pharynx is markedly increased when the individual smokes tobacco as well as abuses alcoholic beverages (Blot, 1992). Furthermore, individuals who are infected with the hepatitis B virus and drink alcoholic beverages excessively are prone to the more rapid appearance of hepatic neoplasms (Ohnishi et al., 1982).

Aflatoxins, especially aflatoxin B_1, which are produced by some strains of a ubiquitous mold *Aspergillus flavus,* are potent hepatocarcinogens in the rodent (Eaton and Groopman, 1994). Epidemiologic studies have demonstrated that in some geographic areas where there has been extensive contamination of foodstuffs by *A. flavus* and its product, aflatoxin, these areas exhibit a high incidence of human liver cancer (Wogan, 1992). Other dietary contaminants—produced directly by organisms such as molds, substances naturally occurring in plants such as the pyrrolizidine alkyloids, and products of the metabolism of dietary components by contaminating molds, which include carcinogenic nitroso compounds (Shixin et al., 1979)—have been demonstrated as carcinogenic in experimental systems. In most of these examples epidemiologic studies are not sufficient to identify them as known human carcinogens (class I in Table 8-20). A number of other known carcinogenic contaminants reportedly also occur in the average diet, and Lutz and Schlatter (1993) have argued that, from risk estimates, one could account for much of the "dietary induced" cancer in the human. Among the contaminants listed are ethanol and a group of carcinogenic heterocyclic amines that are products of the cooking of food; however, Gold and associates (1994) have argued that exposures to any or all of these contaminants in the usual western diet do not pose any significant risk of cancer development to humans.

According to Doll and Peto (1981), the causal relationship between dietary factors and human cancer is quite substantial. To justify this statement, they proposed several mechanisms whereby dietary factors could be causally associated with the induction of human neoplasia, as shown in Table 8-23. We have discussed the first point in relation to aflatoxin and other dietary contaminants that are known carcinogenic agents. With regard to the second point, the exogenous production of heterocyclic amines during cooking leads to their presence in the ingested food (Bogen, 1994). Another potential mechanism is the endogenous formation of carcinogenic agents from dietary constituents as a result of endogenous processes. A principal pathway for the formation of such chemicals is the nitrosation of secondary amines either naturally present in the diet or formed during ingestion, digestion, or metabolism. The source of the nitroso group is from nitrite, most of which is produced endogenously in the human (Leaf et al., 1989). The products of the endogenous nitrosation include nitrosoproline as well as minute amounts of other carcinogens (Bartsch et al., 1990). In addition, a wide variety of other chemicals, most of which may be taken in the diet, are potentially nitrosatable, thus affording the presence of potential carcinogenic nitrosamines (Shephard et al., 1987). While endogenous exposure to such nitroso compounds appears to be fairly ubiquitous, their relevance to the development of human neoplasia is still questionable (Bartsch and Ohshima, 1991). The third point in Table 8-23 involves primarily dietary factors that inhibit the development of cancer. In some instances, as with ethanol (see above), an agent's cocarcinogenic effect when it is given together with a carcinogenic agent is to en-

Table 8-21
Factors Relating to Concern for Potential Human Cancer Induction in Evaluation of Cancer Data

GREAT CONCERN	LESS CONCERN
Human epidemiologic evidence	Negative human epidemiologic data
Genotoxic	Not genotoxic
Multiple species	Single species effect
Tumor site concordance between species	Tumors are species-specific
Multiple tumor sites	No human equivalent to rodent tumor site
Tumors not associated with toxicity	Toxicity associated tumors
Similar metabolism in species	Inconsistent metabolism between species
Induction by multiple routes of exposure	Exposure route not relevant for human
Structural alert	

Table 8-22
Carcinogenic Factors Associated with Lifestyle

CHEMICAL(S), PHYSIOLOGIC CONDITION, OR NATURAL PROCESS	ASSOCIATED NEOPLASM(S)	EVIDENCE FOR CARCINOGENICITY
Alcoholic beverages	Esophagus, liver, oropharynx, and larynx	Sufficient
Aflatoxins	Liver	Sufficient
Betel chewing	Mouth	Sufficient
Dietary intake (fat, protein, calories)	Breast, colon, endometrium, gallbladder	Sufficient
Reproductive history		
1. Late age at 1st pregnancy	Breast	Sufficient
2. Zero or low parity	Ovary	Sufficient
Tobacco smoking	Mouth, pharynx, larynx, lung, esophagus, bladder	Sufficient

SOURCE: Adapted from Pitot (1986a) and Vainio et al. (1991), with permission.

hance the production of neoplasia by a mechanism that enhances the activation of the carcinogenic agent. By contrast, many dietary components have been shown to inhibit the carcinogenic process at the stage of promotion, such as retinoids, while antioxidants such as vitamin E, β-carotene, selenium, etc., may serve to inhibit the metabolic activation of chemical carcinogens by the cytochrome P-450 system or the oxidative changes in DNA that may facilitate spontaneous development of the stage of progression (see above).

The most common mechanism of diet-associated carcinogenesis in the human is through the action of major dietary constituents (fat, carbohydrate, and protein) as promoting agents. Considerable experimental evidence has developed to demonstrate that carbohydrate and lipid are effective promoting agents in the development of several tissue types of neoplasms in different species (Freedman et al., 1990; Wynder et al., 1983).

There is substantial epidemiologic evidence that overnutrition resulting in overweight may increase the incidence of a variety of human cancers (Doll and Peto, 1981). The fact that overnutrition in experimental animals is carcinogenic has been described in numerous publications over several decades (Kritchevsky et al., 1986; Boutwell, 1992). This is most evident when one compares the spontaneous cancer incidence in animals fed a calorically restricted diet with those fed ad libitum. The cancer incidence may differ by four- to sixfold in the two groups. Relatively high levels of dietary fat are associated with increased death rates from cancer of the prostate, colon, and breast in humans (Statland, 1992). However, Willett and associates have argued that, at least for mammary cancer, the fat content of the diet itself does not appear to be the definitive causal agent. Others have argued that the increase in mammary cancer may be related to an increased production of estrogenic and hypophyseal hormones, especially prolactin, as a result of the dietary composition (Henderson et al., 1982).

Endogenous hormone production is also probably related to the phenomenon of the enhanced risk of breast cancer in patients who wait until the fourth decade or more to have their first child. This finding is quite similar to the original observations of Ramazzini on the high incidence of breast cancer in celibate nuns. Doll and Peto (1981) pointed out that cancers of the endometrium, ovary, and breast are significantly less common in women who have borne children early than in women who have had no children. In addition to late first full-term pregnancy, early menarche and late menopause appear to increase the risk of breast cancer in humans (Pike et al., 1983).

Perhaps the most common exogenous cause of human cancer is tobacco smoking and other forms of tobacco abuse. On the basis of their epidemiologic data, Doll and Peto (1981) estimated that 85 to 90 percent of annual lung cancer cases in the United States are a direct result of tobacco use. If we add to this statistic the numbers of cancers of the bladder, gastrointestinal tract, and upper respiratory passages that can be attributed to tobacco smoking, one may conclude that about 30 percent of all cancer deaths in the United States result from this habit. There are substantial data to demonstrate that the complete cessation of tobacco smoking results in a decreasing risk of lung cancer with increasing time after smoking cessation (Reif, 1981). Zatonski and associates (1990) noted that interruption of the smoking habit leads to a significant decrease in laryngeal cancer even when the habit is resumed after the cessation. This finding is very comparable to the intermittent

Table 8-23
Possible Mechanisms of Dietary Carcinogenesis

1. Ingestion of complete carcinogens or initiating or progressor agents	Aflatoxin
2. Exogenous or endogenous production of carcinogens from dietary constituents	Heterocyclic amines *N*-nitrosation
3. Alteration of transport, metabolic activation, or inactivation of carcinogens	Ethanol, vitamins A, E
4. Serve as promoting agents to act on spontaneously initiated cells	Calories, dietary fat

format for promoting agent administration described by Boutwell (1964), which results in little or no tumor promotion even though the final total dose of the promoting agent remains the same. Thus, the stage of tumor promotion occupies the most time and poses the greatest risk in the development of cancer in smokers.

The chewing of tobacco leads to cancer of the mouth. This may also be seen in the Far East, where betel nuts are chewed with or without tobacco in the form of a quid (a packet of betel, tobacco, and other materials). Extracts of the quid have been shown to be carcinogenic in several species (Bhide et al., 1979).

The least is known about the mechanisms of cancer induction by lifestyle factors, but cancers resulting from lifestyle account for two-thirds or more of the chemical induction of this human disease (Fig. 8-24). The stage involved in lifestyle-induced human cancer is primarily that of promotion.

Chemical Carcinogens Associated with Occupations

We have already discussed at least two examples of occupations associated with the development of specific cancers: the report of Ramazzini on the incidence of breast cancer in celibate nuns and that of Pott on the observation of scrotal cancer in men who had been employed as chimney sweeps during their childhood. After these observations, a number of reports of the association of specific cancers with the mining, smelting, dyeing, and lubrication processes and industries were published. It was not until after 1970 that the IARC began intensive studies to establish the carcinogenic risk of chemicals and chemical processes in industry. Table 8-24 lists a number of chemical processes for which there is an established (sufficient) amount of data to implicate these agents as carcinogenic to humans. The same table lists a number of chemicals, some of which are designated as having limited evidence of carcinogenicity in humans (IARC), and for some of which there is established carcinogenic activity only in animals.

The association of occupational exposure to asbestos with the subsequent development of bronchogenic carcinoma and malignant mesothelioma has been well established. The development of bronchogenic carcinoma is seen much more commonly following asbestos exposure than is malignant mesothelioma in those with a history of cigarette smoking. In fact, Muscat and Wynder (1991) found no association between cigarette smoking and mesothelioma incidence in studying patients with the latter disease. Furthermore, Sandén and coworkers (1992), in a study of nearly 4000 shipyard workers exposed to asbestos, found no increased risk of bronchogenic carcinoma 7 to 15 years after exposure to asbestos had ceased. These authors argue that asbestos exposure may act as a promoting agent in relation to the development of bronchogenic carcinoma. In contrast, they argue that the continued risk of mesothelioma years after asbestos exposure indicates its complete carcinogenic action in the development of the latter neoplasm. Other fibrous materials such as fiberglass have been shown to be carcinogenic in the rodent (Stanton et al., 1977), but evidence in the human is not sufficient (Merchant, 1990). Although the mechanism of asbestos induction of cancer is unknown, the type and size of asbestos fibers are significant factors for the carcinogenicity of this material, indicating that a mechanism similar to "plastic film" carcinogenesis is operative (Stanton et al., 1981). In cell culture of Syrian hamster embryo cells, asbestos fibers induce both karyotypic abnormalities and neoplastic transformation (Oshimura et al., 1984). Wood dust carcinogenesis may also be related mechanistically to asbestos carcinogenesis. The induction of cancer by metallic compounds and arsenic has been discussed in this chapter. Aromatic amines used in the chemical and dye industries were known to induce cancer in the human well before the disease was reproduced in experimental animals. In the last century, up to 100 percent of individuals involved in the purification of 2-naphthylamine for use in the dye industry developed bladder cancer (Connolly and White, 1969). Prolonged exposure to benzene has been implicated by several epidemiologic studies in the induction of acute myelogenous leukemia in humans, usually exposed in an occupational setting (Snyder and Kalf, 1994). However, Wallace (1989) has emphasized the ubiquitous nature of benzene exposure to the population in general. Just as with 2-naphthylamine for the demonstration of its animal carcinogenicity in 1938 (Hueper et al., 1938), the induction of leukemia in lower animals by benzene has not yet been reported, although some solid tumors of other organs have been described (Snyder and Kalf, 1994).

There is considerable controversy about several of the agents on the list of suspected human carcinogens to which there is exposure in the workplace. Formaldehyde is a ubiquitous chemical intermediate and is also utilized by several fields in the health sciences. The IARC has labeled the evidence of the carcinogenic potential of formaldehyde in the human as inadequate. However, at relatively high doses, formaldehyde gas is carcinogenic to rodents, but only in the presence of extensive cytotoxicity and cell proliferation (Starr and Gibson, 1985).

Among the most controversial suspected human carcinogenic agents are the phenoxyacetic acids and their contaminating halogenated dioxins. A review by Bond and Rossbacher (1993) indicated no clear evidence of human carcinogenicity of phenoxy herbicides, but a more recent investigation by Hardell and coworkers (1994) that extended earlier investigations argues strongly for a causative relationship with lymphoma. The controversy extends farther because these chemicals are contaminated with polyhalogenated dioxins, specifically TCDD. As noted earlier, this chemical is one of the most potent promoting agents for neoplasia in rodent liver and has an extended half-life of more than 7 years in the human (Pirkle et al., 1989). Fingerhut and colleagues (1991) concluded from a large study of industrial workers that dioxin had induced a small number of soft tissue sarcomas in this cohort. This finding has been disputed by a number of other investigators (Johnson, 1992). The U.S. government has undertaken an extensive study of TCDD as a risk factor in human cancer development.

A less controversial subject is the association of angiosarcoma of the liver with exposure to monomeric vinyl chloride, the basic chemical used in the production of a number of plastics. Although the incidence of this neoplasm even in workers with a history of exposure to vinyl chloride is relatively low (Cooper, 1981), suggesting that the potency of vinyl chloride as a carcinogen is relatively low, the rarity of hepatic angiosarcoma in the general population gives strong support to a causal relationship between exposure to this organic halogen and the induction of hepatic angiosarcoma.

In regard to the general causative relationship between exposure to chemicals in the workplace and the development of human cancer, Doll and Peto (1981) have presented compelling arguments that only about 4 percent of all cancer deaths in the United States could be attributed to occupational circumstances. With strict government regulation of actual and potential industrial health hazards during the last two decades, it is likely that this figure will decrease to even lower levels in the future.

Table 8-24
Exposures to Chemical Carcinogens in the Workplace

AGENT	INDUSTRIES AND TRADES WITH PROVED EXCESS CANCERS AND EXPOSURE	PRIMARY AFFECTED SITE
Established		
Para-aminodiphenyl	Chemical manufacturing	Urinary bladder
Asbestos	Construction, asbestos mining and milling, production of friction products and cement	Pleura, peritoneum, bronchus
Arsenic	Copper mining and smelting	Skin, bronchus, liver
Alkylating agents (mechloro-ethamine hydrochloride and bis[chloromethyl]ether)	Chemical manufacturing	Bronchus
Benzene	Chemical and rubber manufacturing, petroleum refining	Bone marrow
Benzidine, beta-naphthylamine, and derived dyes	Dye and textile production	Urinary bladder
Chromium and chromates	Tanning, pigment making	Nasal sinus, bronchus
Isopropyl alcohol manufacture	Chemical manufacturing	Cancer of paranasal sinuses
Nickel	Nickel refining	Nasal sinus, bronchus
Polynuclear aromatic hydrocarbons (from coke, coal tar, shale, mineral oils, and creosote)	Steel making, roofing, chimney cleaning	Skin, scrotum, bronchus
Vinyl chloride monomer	Chemical manufacturing	Liver
Wood dust	Cabinetmaking, carpentry	Nasal sinus
AGENT	INDUSTRIES AND TRADES	SUSPECTED HUMAN SITES
Suspected		
Acrylonitrile	Chemical and plastics	Lung, colon, prostate
Beryllium	Beryllium processing, aircraft manufacturing, electronics, secondary smelting	Bronchus
Cadmium	Smelting, battery making, welding	Bronchus
Ethylene oxide	Hospitals, production of hospital supplies	Bone marrow
Formaldehyde	Plastic, textile, and chemical production; health care	Nasal sinus, bronchus
Synthetic mineral fibers (e.g., fibrous glass)	Manufacturing, insulation	Bronchus
Phenoxyacetic acid	Farming, herbicide application	Soft tissue sarcoma
Polychlorinated biphenyls	Electrical-equipment production and maintenance	Liver
Organochlorine pesticides (e.g., chlordane, dieldrin)	Pesticide manufacture and application, agriculture	Bone marrow
Silica	Casting, mining, refracting	Bronchus

SOURCE: Modified from Cullen et al. (1990), with permission.

Chemical Carcinogenesis Resulting from Medical Therapy and Diagnosis

In the modern practice of medicine, the original dictum of Hippocrates that a physician should do no harm to a patient has changed as a result of a consideration of the potential benefit to the patient of a specific procedure or therapy in relation to the risk of the procedure or therapy. In general, the risk of intervention to the patient has been unknown or unsuspected, but at a later date the toxic consequences of the therapy have become apparent. A dramatic example of this has been seen with the administration of the synthetic estrogenic compound diethylstilbestrol to pregnant women in order to avert a threatened abortion. While this therapy was originally thought to be beneficial, its risk did not become obvious until many years later. A small percentage of the female offspring of mothers treated with diethylstilbestrol during pregnancy developed clear cell carcinomas of the vagina, usually within a few years after puberty (Herbst, 1981) (Table 8-25). The use of oral contraceptives that contain synthetic steroidal estrogens as the predominant or sole component results in the development of liver cell adenomas (Goldfarb, 1976; Barrows et al., 1988). Regression of a number of adenomas occurred upon withdrawal of the oral contraceptive, suggesting that the effect of these agents is reversible (Steinbrecher et al., 1981). In addition, prolonged use of oral con-

Table 8-25
Carcinogenic Risks of Chemical Agents Associated with Medical Therapy and Diagnosis

CHEMICAL OR DRUG	ASSOCIATED NEOPLASMS	EVIDENCE FOR CARCINOGENICITY
Alkylating agents (cyclophosphamide, melphalan)	Bladder, leukemia	Sufficient
Inorganic arsenicals	Skin, liver	Sufficient
Azathioprine (immunosuppressive drugs)	Lymphoma, reticulum cell sarcoma, skin, Kaposi's sarcoma (?)	Sufficient
Chlornaphazine	Bladder	Sufficient
Chloramphenicol	Leukemia	Limited
Diethylstilbestrol	Vagina (clear cell carcinoma)	Sufficient
Estrogens		
Premenopausal	Liver cell adenoma	Sufficient
Postmenopausal	Endometrium	Limited
Methoxypsoralen with ultraviolet light	Skin	Sufficient
Oxymetholone	Liver	Limited
Phenacetin	Renal pelvis (carcinoma)	Sufficient
Phenytoin (diphenylhydantoin)	Lymphoma, neuroblastoma	Limited
Thorotrast	Liver (angiosarcoma)	Sufficient

traceptives has been associated with increases in the incidence of premenopausal breast cancer in some (White et al., 1994; Olsson et al., 1989; Thomas, 1991) but not all epidemiologic studies (Stanford et al., 1989; Schlesselman et al., 1988). Estrogen therapy has been used successfully to treat a variety of symptoms in postmenopausal women. The administration of estrogens unopposed by progestin is associated with a significantly increased risk of the development of endometrial carcinoma, ranging from 8- to 16-fold (Mack et al., 1976; Henderson et al., 1988). However, when progestogen is given simultaneously with estrogen, no risk of endometrial carcinoma is present, and there is some evidence for protection (Gambrell, 1986). Androgenic steroids, usually in the form of synthetic congeners of testosterone, are associated with hepatocellular carcinomas in humans treated for extended periods for conditions such as aplastic anemia (Hoover and Fraumeni, 1981). Interestingly, recent evidence has suggested that endometrial cancer may be induced by long-term treatment with the antiestrogen tamoxifen (Fisher et al., 1994).

While there are risk-benefit considerations in the use of a number of drugs and hormones in the human, the most striking is the utilization of known carcinogenic agents in the chemotherapy of neoplasia. As noted in Table 8-25, alkylating agents utilized in the treatment of a number of neoplasms are carcinogenic. The development of second neoplasms after chemotherapy and radiation therapy has been most striking in the earlier modalities used to treat Hodgkin's disease. One of the more common secondary neoplasms after treatment with several chemotherapeutic agents is acute myelogenous leukemia, which occurs within the first decade following the curative treatment (Blayney et al., 1987; Swerdlow et al., 1992). Recently, a similar phenomenon has occurred following treatment with a new class of drugs that inhibit DNA topoisomerases, the epipodophyllotoxins (Winick et al., 1993). In a study utilizing combination chemotherapy including epipodophyllotoxins for the treatment of small cell lung cancer, the odds of dying of a secondary or new malignancy were 8 to 1 if the patient survived at least 4 years after therapy (Heyne et al., 1992). In a similar vein, methoxypsoralen, which directly alkylates DNA, has been used in combination with ultraviolet light exposure for the treatment of the autoimmune skin condition psoriasis. Although this treatment is in many ways the treatment of choice, there is distinct evidence that squamous cell carcinoma of the skin is induced by it (Green et al., 1992).

Immunosuppression as a result of genetic abnormalities, therapeutic immunosuppression (as for transplants), and immunosuppression resulting from diseases such as advanced cancer or the acquired immunodeficiency syndrome (AIDS) are associated with increased incidences of a variety of different cancers (Penn, 1989). In these instances, the development of neoplasia is the result of a loss of host resistance to the growth of neoplastic cells, especially those infected with viruses such as the Epstein-Barr virus or one of the herpes simplex viruses (Purtilo and Linder, 1983).

Besides the chemicals listed in Table 8-25, a number of other chemicals that are carcinogenic in lower forms of life are used as drugs in the therapy of a variety of human diseases (Griffith, 1988). Thus, it is clear that some forms of medical therapy and diagnosis pose a carcinogenic risk to humans under certain circumstances. The decision as to which is greater, the benefit to the patient or the risk of producing further pathology, must be made ultimately by the patient in consultation with his or her physician.

THE PREVENTION OF HUMAN CANCER INDUCED BY CHEMICALS

Definitive epidemiologic observations and investigations are the surest way to relate a specific etiologic agent—chemical, physical, or biological—causally with human neoplasms, but epidemiologic studies are still relatively insensitive for identifying causative factors in human cancer. Such studies can identify only factors that are different between two populations and that are sufficiently important to play a determining role under the conditions of exposure. Furthermore, on the basis of epidemiologic studies, it is extremely difficult to determine whether a specific chemical is or is not carcinogenic to humans because of the extended lag period between exposure and clinical occurrence of a neoplasm, the high background incidence of many cancers in the general population, the relatively imprecise knowledge of the nature of the exposure in most instances, and a number of other confounding variables. Only under exceptional circumstances such as the induction of rare and infrequent neoplasms—e.g., vinyl chloride and angiosarcoma (Dannaher et al., 1981)—is it possible to identify an agent as carcinogenic solely on the basis of epidemiologic studies when the incidence of cancer induced by that agent is less than 50 percent more than the occurrence of the resulting cancer in the general human population. Therefore, a "negative" result of an epidemiologic investigation must be considered as inconclusive for determining whether a relatively weak carcinogenic agent has a role in the etiology of human neoplasia. How, then, is it possible to identify actual and potential carcinogenic agents in our environment by methods other than epidemiologic studies? This question has been answered in part by relating the results of additional studies, usually carried out with experimental animals, to the problem of the etiology of human cancer and the risks of environmental agents to populations and/or specific individuals. It is from such studies that government agencies make decisions that ultimately regulate the production and use of, and accordingly the exposures of populations to, agents determined to be actually or potentially carcinogenic for the human.

The ultimate goal of such epidemiologic and basic studies is the prevention of human cancer. There is today sufficient scientific knowledge to allow the prevention of more than 60 percent of human cancers. The failure to achieve such a goal is largely the result of personal and societal decisions well beyond the realm of science. However, since the prevention of disease is by far the most effective and inexpensive mode of health care, it is appropriate that there be a constant and sustained effort to utilize the ever-expanding knowledge of neoplasia to accomplish its control through cancer prevention.

Cancer prevention in humans may in general be grouped into two approaches: active and passive. Table 8-26 depicts an outline of various methods of cancer prevention with an indication of the stage of carcinogenesis toward which the preventive measure is directed. The passive prevention of cancer involves the cessation of smoking, dietary restrictions, and modification of other personal habits such as those of a sexual nature. Active prevention of cancer development is usually accomplished by the administration of an agent to prevent infection by carcinogenic viruses and other organisms or by the intake of chemicals, nutrients, or other factors that may modify or prevent the action of carcinogenic agents. Theoretically, passive cancer prevention or the alteration of one's "carcinogenic" habits can be the most effective and unintrusive method of cancer prevention. However, for many individuals, passive prevention requires external persuasion, such as governmental regulation or peer pressure, to force an alteration of their habits. Obviously, in many instances such methods are doomed to failure. Active cancer prevention, which many consider a form of preventive "therapy," is likely to be the most effective method in this area.

Table 8-26
Modes of the Prevention of Cancer

MODE	STAGE
Passive	
Smoking cessation	Pr, Pg
Dietary restriction	Pr
Moderation of alcohol intake	Pr
Modification of sexual and reproductive habits	I, Pr
Avoidance of excessive ultraviolet exposure	I, Pr
Active	
Dietary modification and supplements	Pr
Vaccination against oncogenic viruses	I, Pr
Application of ultraviolet blocking agents in appropriate situations	I, Pr
Selective screening for certain preneoplastic lesions	I, Pr
Determination of genetic background in relation to neoplastic disease	I, Pr
Administration of antihormones	Pr

KEY: I, initiation; Pr, promotion; Pg, progression.
SOURCE: After Pitot (1993), with permission.

Individuals with hereditary conditions involving alterations in specific oncogenes or tumor suppressor genes constitute a relatively small part of the population. However, genes that may modify the susceptibility of an individual to the development of certain types of neoplasms probably represent significant factors in the development of an important fraction of human cancers (Spitz and Bondy, 1993). In reviewing Table 8-26, one can see that most methods of cancer prevention are linked to action at the stage of promotion. Because this is the reversible stage of neoplastic development, such a finding is not surprising. However, since we still do not know all or even most of the causes of human cancer, the continued identification of agents, especially chemicals, that might induce human cancer is important. While the results of epidemiologic studies, when exhibiting sufficient evidence for a causal relationship, may be considered the "gold standard," such detailed studies, even where feasible, for all the potentially carcinogenic agents existing and entering into our environment would be impossible. Therefore, during the last half century, as knowledge of the mechanisms of carcinogenesis has increased, a significant effort backed by a number of governmental agencies throughout the world was directed toward the development of methods for the identification of potentially carcinogenic agents in the environment by a variety of different systems from bacteria to whole animals. This chapter deals with the identification, characterization, and ultimate estimation of human risk from chemical, biological, and physical agents.

IDENTIFICATION OF POTENTIAL CARCINOGENIC AGENTS

A major factor in determining the carcinogenic potential of an agent is its identification as being carcinogenic. While this statement appears obvious and even redundant, identification of a carcinogen is necessary but not sufficient for determining carcinogenic potential. Still, identification is the starting point, and for this reason it has received the most attention. Generally speaking, the various tests that have been applied to identifying agents with carcinogenic potential may be classified into several general areas. These are seen in Table 8-27. As noted in the table, the time involved in the assay has been arbitrarily separated into short, medium, and long. Short-term assays usually involve days to a few weeks for development of an endpoint; medium-term assays require weeks to some months but much less than a year. Long-term bioassays usually involve $1\frac{1}{2}$ to 2 years of treatment of animals with a test agent. Each of these general categories consists of specific methods. Each of these general categories is considered below in somewhat greater detail.

Short-Term Tests—Mutagenesis Assays

A variety of short-term tests, almost all of which are involved in direct or indirect assays of mutagenicity, both in vivo and in vitro, have now been developed and are used to aid in the identification of potential carcinogens. However, virtually all of these methods are of limited use in directly establishing the estimation of the risk that such chemicals pose for the human population. As noted earlier, a ubiquitous characteristic of neoplastic cells is the presence of a variety of different types of mutations. The fact that many but not all carcinogenic agents are mutagenic or may be metabolized to mutagenic forms further establishes the importance of mutations in the development of the neoplastic process. It is on this basis that short-term tests for mutagenicity were developed to identify potential carcinogenic agents on the basis of their capacity for inducing mutations in DNA in cells in vitro or in vivo.

Table 8-28 lists many of the more commonly used short-term tests for mutagenicity and thus carcinogenic potential. The most widely utilized of these mutagenicity assays was originally developed in *Salmonella typhimurium* by Bruce Ames and associates (Ames et al., 1975). In this assay, bacterial cells that are deficient in DNA repair and lack the ability to grow in the absence of histidine are treated with several dose levels of the test compound, after which reversion to the histidine-positive phenotype is ascertained. Because bacteria differ in their metabolic capabilities compared with mammals, a drug-metabolizing system is added to these assays. Specifically, the 9000 *g* supernatant (S9) that results from centrifuging a liver homogenate prepared from a rat treated with an inducer of multiple P-450s, such as Aroclor 1254, is used in combination with an NADPH regenerating system. The method for performing the *Salmonella* assay (the Ames assay) is depicted in Fig. 8-25. Several different lines of *Salmonella* have been generated to permit the detection of point mutations (TA100, TA1535) and frameshift mutations (TA98, TA1537, TA1538), and the assay is continuously being refined. Typically, five dose levels of the test compound are used in addition to the solvent control. Activation-dependent and activation-independent positive control mutagenic substances are tested concurrently. Certain types of carcinogens are not detected by these bacterial mutagenicity assays, including hormonal carcinogens, metals, agents that have a multiple-target-organ mode of action, and agents with a nongenotoxic mode of action. This bacterial reverse mutation system, when performed in the presence of a mammalian S9 activation system, is, however, a very sensitive screen for the detection of many mutagenic agents.

Table 8-27
General Methods for Identification of Potential Carcinogens

METHODS	TIME FRAME
Short term	
Mutagenesis assays	Several weeks
Transformation in cell culture	1–3 months
Medium term	
Qualitative and quantitative analysis of preneoplasia	2–8 months
Long term	
Chronic bioassay in animals	18–24 months

In addition to the bacterial mutational assay, several in vitro mammalian cell mutation assays exist, including the mouse lymphoma L5178Y (MOLY) assay and the Chinese hamster ovary (CHO) assay. These mammalian mutagenicity assays use either the hypoxanthine-guanine phosphoribosyltransferase (HGPRT) or the thymidine kinase (TK) gene as the endpoint. The basis for these assays is seen in Fig. 8-26. They are similar to the Ames assay in that the phenotypic expression of a mutation in a single-copy gene is compared in treated and untreated cells. These assays are frequently performed in the presence of an exogenous metabolizing source such as an epithelial cell layer that has been irradiated. The mammalian mutation test systems are forward mutation assays in which the heterozygous state of a gene is used as a tool to detect genetic damage that might result in the loss of a phenotype, e.g., growth in the presence of a toxic compound. In CHO cells, the X-linked HPGRT locus is used as the target gene for analysis. This enzyme is important in purine salvage and allows the incorporation of toxic purine analogues such as 6-thioguanine and 8-azaguanine into DNA, resulting in inhibition of cell growth and/or cell death. Alternatively, a mutation in this gene that results in phenotype loss may permit colony formation in the presence of toxic analogs. Assays based on the forward mutation of TK are similar in that colony formation in the presence of a DNA-damaging agent is scored in the presence of a pyrimidine analog. Because these short-term tests are based on the premise that carcinogens damage DNA, their concordance with the chronic bioassay in vivo (see below) is only between 30 and 80 percent. In addition, the results of tests are coincident with each other and tend to detect the same types of carcinogens without providing the battery approach that has been suggested. Among the short-term mutagenicity tests that use mutation as the endpoint, the Ames assay has been the best studied and has been applied to the greatest number of compounds.

Gene Mutation Assays in Vivo Until relatively recently, a measurement of mutational effects in vivo was rather difficult to perform. One of the more popular assays utilized in this area was the dominant lethal assay, in which male mice are exposed to a potential genotoxic stimulus, mated with untreated female mice, and the percentage of pregnancies or number of implants is determined (Lockhart et al., 1992). While the method is relatively easy to perform, relatively few carcinogenic agents have been studied by this method. Similarly, the production of sperm abnormalities in mice by the administration of chemical agents in vivo has not found general use as a short-term mutagenic assay (Wyrobek and Bruce, 1975).

In recent years, with a variety of genetic tools available, genetically engineered cells and animals have been developed that have found use in short-term mutagenesis assays. The four exam-

Table 8-28
Short-Term Tests for Mutagenicity

TEST	ENDPOINT	REFERENCE
Gene mutation assays in vitro		
Prokaryote mutagenesis in vitro (Ames test, etc.)	Back or forward mutations in specific bacterial strains	Maron & Ames, 1983
Mouse lymphoma thymidine kinase (TK)	Mutations in TK	Majeska & Matheson, 1990
Chinese hamster ovary (CHO) and V79 hypoxanthine guanine phosphoribosyltransferase (HGPRT)	Mutations in HGPRT	Li et al., 1987
Gene mutation assays in vivo		
Dominant lethal assay	Death of fertilized egg in mammalian implanted species	Bateman, 1973 Lockhart et al., 1992
Sperm abnormality induction	Microscopically abnormal sperm	Wyrobek & Bruce, 1975
Mutation induction in transgenes in vivo		
$LacZ^-$ mouse	Mutations in $LacZ^-$ gene	Myhr, 1991
LacI mouse	Mutations in LacI gene	cf. Mirsalis et al., 1994
LacI rat	Mutations in LacI gene	de Boer et al., 1996
rpsL mouse	Mutations in rpsL gene	Gondo et al., 1996
Chromosomal alterations in vivo		
Heritable translocation test (mice)	Translocations induced in germ cells	Generoso et al., 1980
Rat bone marrow clastogenesis in vivo	Chromosomal aberrations in bone marrow cells in vivo	Ito et al., 1994
Micronucleus test	Appearance of micronuclei in bone marrow cells in vivo	Tinwell and Ashby, 1994 Heddle et al., 1983
Chromosomal alterations in vitro		
Mitotic recombination, mitotic crossing over, or mitotic gene conversion in yeast	Conversion of heterozygous alleles to homozygous state	Wintersberger & Klein, 1988
Induced chromosomal aberrations in cell lines	Visible alterations in karyotype	Galloway et al., 1985
Sister chromatid exchange	Visible exchange of differentially labeled sister chromatids	Latt, 1981 Murphy et al., 1992
Primary DNA damage		
DNA repair in vivo or in vitro	Unscheduled DNA synthesis and/or DNA strand breaks	Furihata & Matsushima, 1987
Rodent liver: unscheduled DNA synthesis induction	Unscheduled DNA synthesis in rodent liver cells in vivo and/or in vitro	Kennelly, 1995 Steinmetz et al., 1988

ples given in Table 8-28 are those most commonly used for mutational analysis in vivo. The first three involve genetically engineered animals containing transgenes within which are components of the *lac* operon of *Escherichia coli,* a set of coordinately regulated genes involved in lactose metabolism. A schematic representation of the *lac* operon is seen in Fig. 8-27. Some details of the function of the *lac* operon are given in the figure legend. Basically, the *lacI* and *lacZ* genes are the ones utilized in the mutational assays. As noted in the figure, mutations in the *lacI* gene will alter the regulation of expression of the *lacZ* gene, which codes for β-galactosidase activity. Thus, the transgene contains either one or the other of the operons. Mutations in the bacterial transgene are determined by the methods seen in Fig. 8-28. In this technique, DNA is extracted from the tissue of interest, and because of the nature of the transgene, construct may be packaged into a bacterial virus, lambda, which then infects the bacteria, *E. coli,* on a lawn of bacterial growth on a dish as noted in the figure. By selecting appropriate bacterial strains and media, one can isolate mutant phage and analyze the sequence of the *lacI* or *lacZ* gene as appropriate. Thus, one may obtain both the number of mutations per unit DNA from the mouse or, more importantly, the actual sequence changes induced by the mutagenic action of the original agent. The *rpsL* transgene works by a similar mechanism but by a different metabolic pathway (Gondo et al., 1996).

Since several of the transgenic animals are commercially patented, this assay may entail some expense, but is relatively versatile for an in vivo assay for mutagenic identification, and its ability to detect nonmutagenic carcinogens is doubtful. Of interest is the fact that with at least one carcinogenic agent, ethylnitrosourea, the relative sensitivities of mutations induced in the *lacI* transgene and an endogenous gene, *hprt,* were essentially identical (Skopek et al., 1995). Species differences occur with different carcinogens

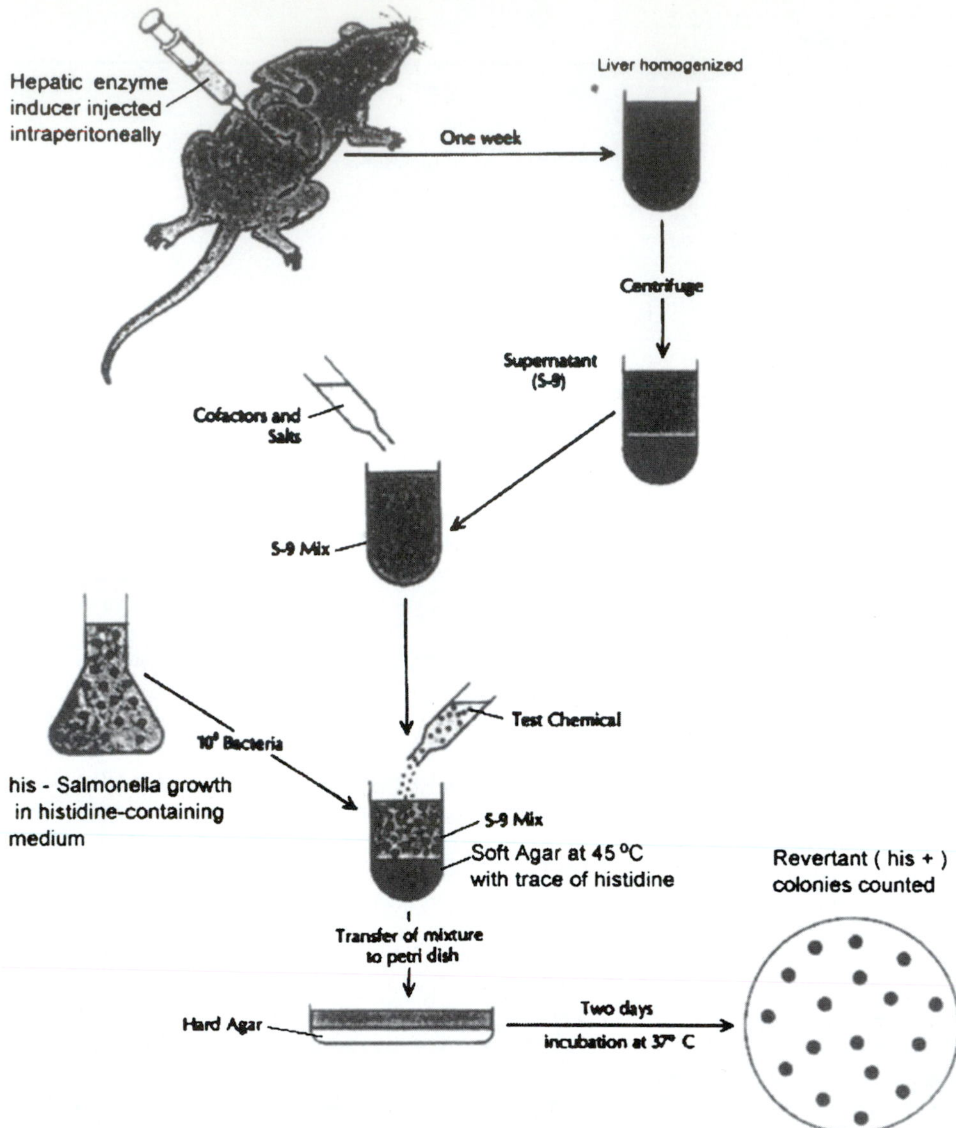

Figure 8-25. Scheme of the Ames test for mutagenesis of chemicals in **Salmonella** *bacterial strains.*

The upper part of the figure outlines the preparation of the S-9 mixture of enzymes and particulates prepared from rodent liver taken from animals previously administered an agent to induce the concentration of such metabolizing enzymes. The *Salmonella,* which require histidine for their growth (his^-), are grown in the presence of histidine, separated from the growth media, and added with the test chemical and S-9 mix as well as soft agar containing a trace of histidine, which allows the cells to undergo one or two divisions (required for mutation fixation). The 5-9 and soft agar mix is transferred to a Petri dish while still warm, incubated for several days, and the colonies that develop in the absence of histidine are counted. [Modified from McCann (1983), with permission of author and publisher.]

in that, for example, aflatoxin B_1 treatment resulted in a much greater number of mutations in the *lacI* rat than in the *lacI* mouse (Dycaico et al., 1996). External ionizing radiation was not very mutagenic in the *lacZ* transgenic mouse (Takahashi et al., 1998), but of interest is the finding that the promoting agent, phenobarbital, enhanced mutation frequency in the livers of *lacZ* transgenic mice treated with diethylnitrosamine (Okada et al., 1997). While a significant number of spontaneous mutations occur in the transgene, as yet this does not appear to be an insurmountable problem (de Boer et al., 1998). Thus, the potential for utilizing such transgenic models for the in vivo assay of mutagenesis is clearly bright. However, their effectiveness in identifying promoting and progressor agents has yet to be validated.

Chromosomal Alterations Chromosomal alterations are extremely common if not ubiquitous in all malignant neoplasms, as was originally suggested by Boveri (1914). Therefore, the induction of chromosomal abnormalities by chemicals in relatively short-term in vivo and in vitro methodologies would logically be considered as an excellent test for carcinogenic potential. Although this has been true in general, the application of various tests for clastogenicity, aneuploidy, and chromatid alterations has not

Mammalian Cell Lines Used for Gene Mutation Studies

Mouse lymphoma L5178Y	TK, HGPRT
CHO	HGPRT
V79 hamster cells	HGPRT

Selection of forward mutations by loss of HPGRT+ phenotype in V79 or chinese hamster ovary cells.

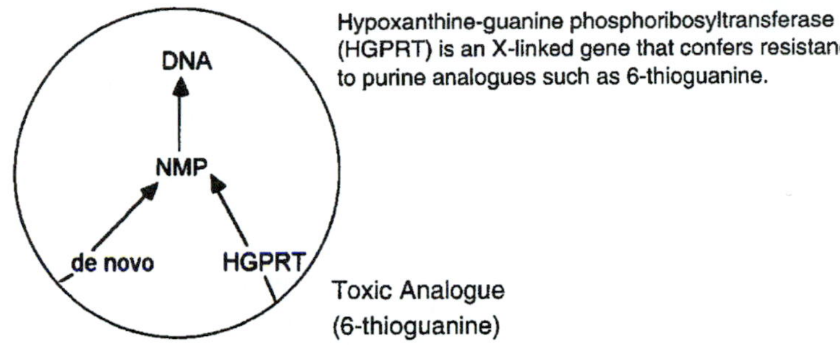

Performed in the presence of an activation system or hepatic feeder layer

Selection of mutagen-induced TK -/- phenotype in TK+/- in mouse lymphoma assay (MOLY) in L5178Y cells. This assay detects forward mutations at the TK locus.

Treat TK (+/-) cells with test compound. Fluoruracil is converted to a toxin, killing the cells. If mutation in TK occurs, FU is not metabolized to a toxin and colonies grow.

DNA

TMP

de novo

TK

Thymidine kinase (TK) confers resistance to pyrimidine analogues. It is a somatic gene.

Toxic analogue (bromodeoxyuridine)

Figure 8-26. Outline of chemically induced mutation in mouse cell lines with thymidine kinase (TK) or hypoxanthine-guanine phosphoribosyltransferase (HGPRT) as the target gene. [Reproduced from Pitot and Dragan (1996), with permission of authors and publisher.]

formed the basis for determining potential carcinogenicity of chemicals. In part, the technology involved is more complicated and expensive than most of the gene mutation assays, and the molecular basis for at least one of the more common tests, that of sister chromatid exchange, is not fully understood. Theoretically, short-term assays for the induction of clastogenicity and related abnormalities would allow the rapid identification of potential progressor agents.

Analysis of chromosomal alterations in vivo was studied in germ cells two decades ago by Generoso et al. (1980) in mice. This procedure, as carried out by these workers, involves the administration of an agent to male mice shortly before breeding and subsequent examination of male offspring for sterility and/or chromosomal abnormalities in both germ and somatic cells. The test is somewhat complex, and thus far only a few very potent mutagenic agents have been found positive in this test. A more commonly employed short-term test for clastogenesis is the micronucleus test, which measures induced clastogenesis in rodent bone marrow in vivo by morphologic evaluation of micronuclei containing chromosome fragments in cell preparations from bone marrow (Heddle et al., 1983). However, this assay also has an occasional false positive, such as vitamin C (Tinwell and Ashby, 1994). With the LEC rat, which exhibits a defect in copper metabolism leading to hepatitis and hepatomas, an increased frequency of chromosome aberrations was seen in the bone marrow after administration of direct-acting alkylating agents that did not need metabolic activation (Ito et al., 1994). However, carcinogenic agents requiring metabolic activation, especially in the liver, induced a lesser amount of chromosomal abnormalities in the bone marrow of these rats than in normal rats.

Studies in vitro of chromosomal alterations have been carried out both in yeast and in cultured mammalian cells. In the former, various genetic end-points are studied, the abnormalities seen being the result of chromosomal alterations (Wintersberger and Klein, 1988). In mammalian cell lines, most of the systems used the same lines as for the gene mutation assays, e.g., Galloway et al. (1985). Relatively few analyses of induced chromosomal alterations have been carried out in normal diploid cells in culture. This test is used much more extensively than most of the other short-term tests involving chromosomal alterations (cf. Ishidate et al., 1988). As might be expected, some discrepancies have arisen between the mutagenic and clastogenic effects of chemicals by these two different systems (cf. Ashby, 1988). Furthermore, chromosomal alterations in these cell lines are sensitive to oxidants (Gille et al.,

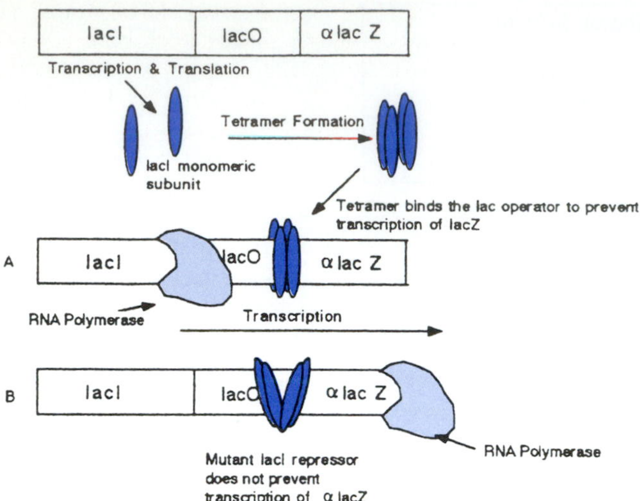

Figure 8-27. Schematic representation of the **lac** *operon in* **E. coli.**

A. The *lacI* gene codes for protein that forms a homotetramer that binds to the *lacO* operator sequence. Binding of the repressor to *lacO* prevents transcription of *lacZ. B.* Transcription of *lacZ* occurs in the presence of the inducing agent, isopropyl-β-thiogalactoside (IPTG). Mutations of the *lacI* may result in partial or complete inactivation of the *lac* repressor, the *lacI* tetrameric protein. Furthermore, mutations in the *lacZ* gene may prevent interaction with the repressor or may be nonfunctional, resulting in no production of the structural gene, *lacZ.* [Reproduced from Provost et al. (1993), with permission of authors and publisher.]

1993; Shamberger et al., 1973; Kirkland et al., 1989), and preferential targets of chemicals in these aneuploid cell lines are chromosomes bearing amplified genes, already indicative of the karyotypic instability of the cell lines being used (Ottagio et al., 1993).

Another short-term test involving changes in chromosomal structure by mechanisms not entirely understood is the technique of "sister chromatid exchange" (SCE). During metaphase, sister chromatids, each of which is a complete copy of the chromosome, are bound together by mechanisms that involve specific proteins (Nasmyth, 1999). SCE reflects an interchange between DNA molecules within different chromatids at homologous loci within a replicating chromosome (Latt, 1981). The detection of SCEs requires methods of differentially labeling sister chromatids. The usual technique is to allow a cell to incorporate a label, usually a halogenated pyrimidine such as bromodeoxyuridine (BrdU), for one replication cycle and then it undergoes a second replication cycle in which the presence of the labeled precursor is actually optional. The procedure has been used in vivo as well as in vitro (DuFrain et al., 1984). In an extensive examination and comparison of the SCE method with cytogenetic changes, the two methods were about 70 percent congruent, again indicating that clastogenesis and SCEs are not identical phenomena (Gebhart, 1981).

Primary DNA Damage The measurement of DNA damage and repair induced by exogenous chemicals, both in vivo and in vitro, has been a relatively common technology used in short-term tests for potential carcinogenicity. The most generally utilized technology involves the analysis of non-replicative DNA synthesis with appropriately labeled precursor nucleotides (cf. Harbach et al., 1991). More sophisticated techniques involve the measurement of DNA strand breakage by eluting DNA fragments from columns to

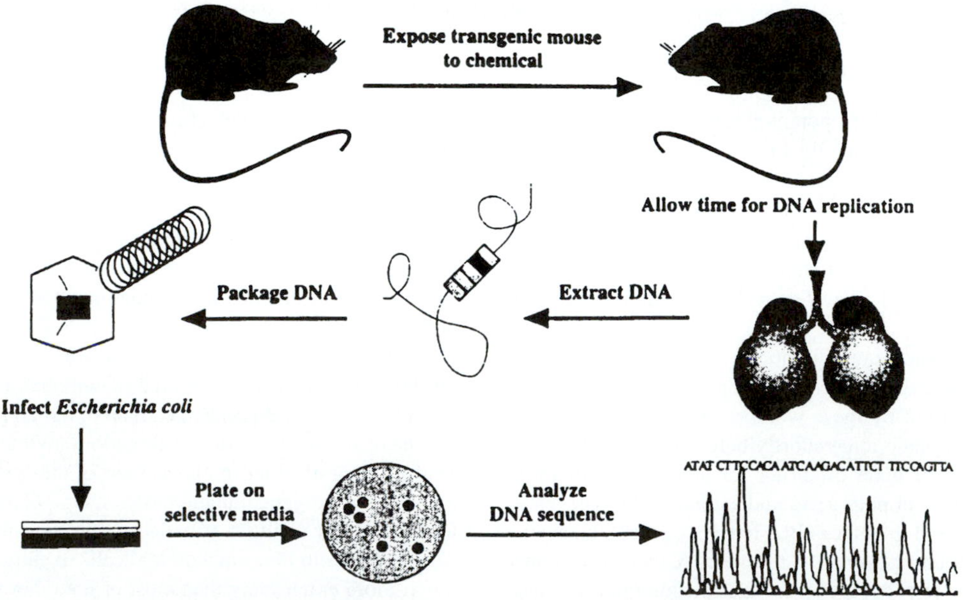

Figure 8-28. Sequence of steps utilized in the determination of the mutagenicity of chemicals in transgenic rodent mutagenicity assays **in vivo.**

The details of the test are briefly discussed in the text or the reader is referred to the original article. [From Recio (1995), reproduced with permission of author and publisher.]

which the DNA is bound with an alkaline solution (Sina et al., 1983; Miyamae et al., 1997). These techniques have been applied to a variety of tissues in cell culture, both primary and cell lines. Primary liver cell cultures have been among the most popular of the tissues utilized (Williams et al., 1989; Strom et al., 1981; Swierenga et al., 1991). While primary hepatocyte cultures have the advantage of an extensive endogenous metabolic apparatus, other workers have attempted to obviate the problem of metabolism of the agent to the active form by administration of the test chemical in vivo, with subsequent explantation of specific organ tissues to culture and measurement of unscheduled DNA synthesis in such cultures (cf. Furihata and Matsushima, 1987). Just as with all of the short-term tests indicated above, the use of DNA repair analysis has limitations, as evidenced by the fact that in an extensive investigation by Williams and his associates (1989) of 167 chemicals testing negative, 44 were carcinogenic. This and the other points raised in this section demonstrate both the usefulness and limitations of short-term tests of mutagenicity and DNA damage for indicating potential carcinogenicity. Regulatory agencies have chosen to approach this problem by requiring a number of different tests to be performed during the study of a particular compound, and these data are taken into account with all of the other information, especially that developed by studies in vivo, as discussed below.

Short-Term Tests—Transformation and Cell Culture

As with other of the short-term tests listed in Table 8-28 and discussed above, determination of the "neoplastic" transformation in cultured cells has also taken the direction of the use of a primary (directly from the animal) culture system in which the cells are diploid and normal in all measurable respects. Another direction is the use of a number of cell lines exhibiting aneuploidy but having reasonably defined cultural characteristics. The techniques for the latter have been somewhat standardized (Dunkel et al., 1991), and an extensive degree of study has been carried out with primary Syrian hamster embryo (SHE) cells in primary culture for predicting the carcinogenic potential of a variety of chemicals (cf. Isfort et al., 1996; Barrett et al., 1984). While these techniques are relatively straightforward, although somewhat more difficult to score in the SHE system, for the most part they suffer from the inability of the cells to metabolize test agents to their ultimate forms. In addition, given the expense required for the establishment and use of tissue culture methodology, this has been a less than popular short-term test for carcinogenic potential.

Chronic Bioassays for Carcinogenicity—Medium- and Long-Term

The ability to induce neoplasia in lower animals has been the basis for our understanding of the pathogenesis of neoplasia. Early studies showing the induction of skin cancer in mice by coal tar derivatives and of liver cancer by organic dyes led to the establishment of model systems in these and other tissues, both for the investigation of cancer development and ultimately for testing of agents for their carcinogenic potential. The administration of chemicals in the diet for extended periods, pioneered in the 1930s by Yoshida and his colleagues (Sasaki and Yoshida, 1935), formed the basis for the establishment of the chronic bioassay of carcinogenicity that is used today. This methodology was espoused by the National Cancer Institute some 30 years after Yoshida's findings (Hadidian et al., 1968), and almost 200 assays of chemicals for their carcinogenic potential by the prolonged feeding to animals was carried out over the next decade (Hottendorf and Pachter, 1985). Parallel to the use of this lifetime model of carcinogenesis in small rodents was the development of various organ-specific model systems, multistage models, and most recently the use of transgenic animals in carcinogen testing. A listing of these animal models is seen in Table 8-29.

Chronic 2-Year Bioassay Today the "gold standard" for determining potential carcinogenic activity of a chemical is through the use of the chronic 2-year bioassay for carcinogenicity in rodents. This assay involves test groups of 50 rats and mice of both sexes and at two or three dose levels of the test agent. The animals should be susceptible but not hypersensitive to the tested effect. In general, two strains are typically used by regulatory agencies in the United States, the B6C3F1 mouse and the F344 rat. The format for the bioassay is seen in Fig. 8-29. Quite simply, animals at about 8 weeks of age are placed on the test agent at the various doses for another 96 weeks of their life span. The test agent may be administered by dietary feeding, by gavage on a regular basis, or by inhalation in rather complex chambers. A variety of pretest analyses are carried out, such as those for acute toxicity, route of administration, and determination of the maximum tolerated dose (MTD). The use of the MTD has been challenged by many, arguing that the toxic effects of high doses of an agent can cause a replicative response in normal cells that could lead to an increase in neoplasia quite secondary to the effects of the agent itself (Cutler et al., 1997; Haseman and Lockhart, 1994). This is supported by the finding of a very high percentage, nearly half in some instances, of agents exhibiting no potential for mutagenicity but inducing neoplasia at the MTD (Gold et al., 1993). Furthermore, these two strains of rodents have a significant spontaneous tumor incidence, as can be noted in Table 8-30.

Because so many research dollars go into carcinogenicity testing and the data resulting from such studies are expected to be useful not only in hazard identification but also in risk estimation, an acceptable scientific protocol with quality assurance must be followed to produce scientifically and statistically valid data. A variety of factors relevant to the acceptable outcome of a carcinogenicity study are considered, including animal husbandry; the identity and purity of the test compound and identification of any

Format for Chronic 2 Year Bioassay for Carcinogenic Potential

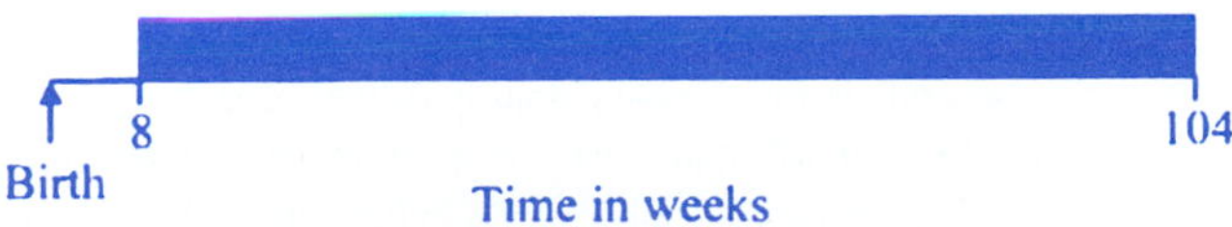

Figure 8-29. Diagram of chronic 2-year bioassay format.

Table 8-29
Animal Models of Neoplastic Development

	ENDPOINT	REFERENCES
Chronic 2-year bioassay	Tumors in all organs	Sontag, 1977
Tissue specific bioassays		
Liver, mouse	Hepatomas	Carmichael et al., 1997
Lung, mouse	Pulmonary adenomas	Shimkin and Stoner, 1975
Brain, rat	Gliomas	Kroh, 1995
Mammary gland, rat/mouse	Adenomas and carcinomas	Dunnick et al., 1995
Medium-term bioassays		
Ito model	Hepatic adenomas and carcinomas	Ito et al., 1989
Newborn mouse	Neoplasms in liver, lung, lymphoid organs	Fujii, 1991
Multistage models of neoplastic development		
Bladder, rat	Papillomas/carcinomas	Hicks, 1980
Colon, rat	Aberrant crypt polyp	Sutherland and Bird, 1994
Epidermis, mouse	Papillomas	DiGiovanni, 1992
Liver, rat	Altered hepatic foci	Pitot et al., 1996
Transgenic mice		
Knockout of *p53* tumor suppressor gene ($p53^{def}$)	Tumors in heterozygous animals having normal phenotype	Donehower, 1996
v-Ha-*ras* with zetaglobin promoter; tandem insertion on chromosome 11 (TG.AC)	Induced transgene expression in skin leads to papilloma development	Spalding et al., 1993

contaminants; the homogeneity, stability, and physical properties of the test compound under various storage conditions; and the solubility, stability, and availability of the test compound in the solvent. In addition, the formulation should be either that which is to be administered to humans or that which permits bioavailability in the test organism. The environment of the rodent is also important, and care should be taken to control for sources of variability in the animals, their diet, and their housing. While the usual comparison in animal studies is the concurrent control, for a number of situations historical controls may be more appropriate (Haseman et al., 1997).

The underlying basis for risk extrapolation from animals to human is that the animal is a good model for human cancer development. In fact, 2-year bioassay models have been used to detect the compounds listed by IARC (Vainio et al., 1991) as known human carcinogens. Also, most known human chemical carcinogens have a carcinogenic potential in animals that supports the results of epidemiologic studies (Vainio et al., 1985). Exceptions include ethanol and arsenic. In addition, it has now become evident that some neoplastic responses to chemicals in animals are unique to the rodent and species as well as the sex involved. These include such responses as thyroid neoplasia (McClain, 1989), the induction of α_{2u}-globulin (Swenberg et al., 1985) resulting in renal neoplasms in male rats, and peroxisome proliferation (Ashby et al., 1994) associated with the induction of hepatic neoplasia in rats. In addition, a significant problem that has arisen in the continued use of the chronic bioassay is the requirement for ad libitum feeding. This results in animals, especially in rats, of extreme weight by the end of the 2 years; many will have died spontaneously prior to the end of the test. Such complications are now being remedied by the use of dietary restriction in the chronic bioassay for the 2-year period. This phenomenon reduces spontaneous cancer incidence and extends lifespan in rodents, and its usefulness in the refinement of the 2-year chronic bioassay is now becoming more appreciated (Keenan et al., 1996; Allaben et al., 1996).

The statistical analysis of results obtained in chronic bioassays has also been difficult when the analysis results in relatively few neoplasms in test animals. As can be seen from Table 8-31, a relatively high percentage of animals must bear tumors before a statistically significant result can be obtained in the face of significant development of spontaneous lesions. Since the latter phenomenon is clearly a problem in these animals (Table 8-30), borderline results become a very difficult problem for regulatory agencies in determining whether or not a compound actually is carcinogenic in the assay or not. An exception to this is when a very unusual histogenetic type of neoplasm not seen spontaneously is found in the test animals at a significant, even very low level (Chu et al., 1981; Basu et al., 1996). The enumeration of all neoplasms versus those in specific tissues also can raise difficulties in interpretation of the bioassay. Despite these criticisms and problems, the chronic 2-year bioassay continues to be the major basis for regulatory action in this country and in many countries throughout the world.

Tissue-Specific Bioassays During the performance of long-term bioassays, it became obvious that certain tissues in specific species exhibited neoplasms more frequently than others when a test agent was administered. From these observations, several tissue-specific bioassays were developed with the objective of a reasonably sensitive assay carried out in a shorter time than the usual chronic 2-year bioassay. The best known of tissue-specific assays is that utilizing the mouse liver. In a recent analysis of chronic bioassays carried out by the National Toxicology Program, Crump et al. reported that 108 of 390 studies indicated a positive carcinogenic response to the test chemical. In 81 of these studies, female mice exhibited significant increases in the incidence of hepatic neoplasms.

Table 8-30
Spontaneous Tumor Incidence (Combined Benign and Malignant) in Selected Sites of the Two Species, B6C3F1 Mice and F344 Rats, Used in the NCI/NTP Bioassay

	B6C3F1 Mice		*F344 Rats*	
SITE	MALE	FEMALE	MALE	FEMALE
Liver				
adenoma	10.3	4.0	3.4	3.0
carcinoma	21.3	4.1	0.8	0.2
Pituitary	0.7	8.3	24.7	47.5
Adrenal	3.8	1.0	19.4	8.0
Thyroid	1.3	2.1	10.7	9.3
Hematopoietic	12.7	27.2	30.1	18.9
Mammary gland	0	1.9	2.5	26.1
Lung	17.1	7.5	2.4	1.2

SOURCE: Adapted from Pitot and Dragan (1996), with permission of publisher.

As noted in Table 8-30, there is a high incidence of spontaneous hepatoma development in mice, more so in the male. This has led to controversy in the interpretation of the significance of the development of mouse hepatomas, especially if they are the only statistically significant increased neoplastic response in the test animals. As a result of this controversy, the interpretation of the significance of the induction of mouse hepatic lesions has been called into question (cf. Dragan et al., 1998; Moch et al., 1996). A further complication of this assay is the fact that in at least one study the majority of the chemicals testing positive exhibited no evidence of an ability to induce DNA damage or mutation (Carmichael et al., 1997).

Another tissue-specific bioassay that was developed by Shimkin and his associates more than two decades ago (Shimkin and Stoner, 1975) is the development of pulmonary adenomas and carcinomas, primarily in strain A mice. The assay was shown to effectively identify a number of relatively potent carcinogenic agents, including a few inorganic carcinogens (Stoner et al., 1976). However, the assay has not been generally accepted as a major component for the determination of carcinogenicity of chemicals, but it has found usefulness in the determination of the molecular mechanisms of pulmonary carcinogenesis in this strain of animals (You et al., 1989; Nuzum et al., 1990). In addition, as noted from Table 8-29, induction of gliomas in the rat brain and of mammary neoplasms in both the rat and the mouse may exhibit potential for tissue-specific bioassays. There have also been attempts to utilize lower vertebrates in the development of tissue-specific bioassays, such as the rainbow trout embryo (Hendricks et al., 1980).

Medium-Term Bioassays While tissue-specific bioassays were directed in part at decreasing the time required for the analysis of carcinogenic potential in vivo, at least two assays have been specifically designated as having reduced the time for the development of an endpoint. The one most intensively used today, primarily in Japan, is the model developed by Dr. Nobuyuki Ito and his colleagues (Ogiso et al., 1990; Shirai, 1997). A diagram of the format for this assay is seen in Fig. 8-30. The entire assay takes only 8 weeks, and the endpoint is nodules and focal lesions in the liver of rats that stain for glutathione *S*-transferase pi (GST-P). The initial "programming" of the liver by administration of a necrogenic

Table 8-31
Percentage of Animals with Tumors (Rx) Administered a Test Agent Required to Obtain Statistical Significance when Compared with Control Animals with Tumors (Co)

PERCENT WITH TUMORS IN CONTROL	*Numbers of Animals* CONTROL	WITH TEST AGENT	PERCENT WITH TUMORS IN Rx
0	50	50	10
	100	50	6
	500	50	4
10	50	50	26
	100	50	22
	500	50	20
20	50	50	38
	100	50	34
	500	50	32
30	50	50	50
	100	50	46
	500	50	44

SOURCE: Adapted from Sontag (1977), with permission.

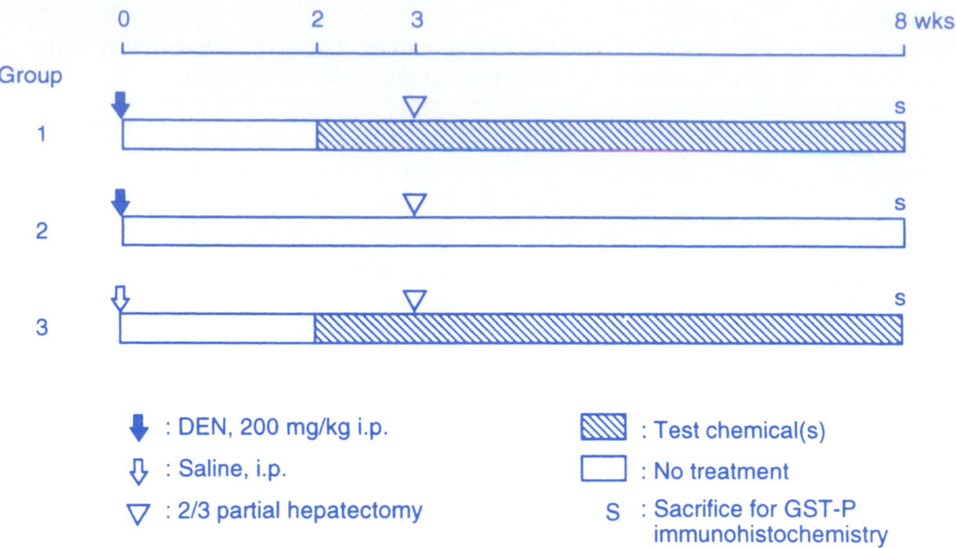

Figure 8-30. The medium-term liver bioassay protocol for identification of potentially carcinogenic agents.

DEN, diethylnitrosamine; GST-P, glutathione *S*-transferase–π. [Reproduced from Shirai (1997), with permission of author and publisher.]

dose of diethylnitrosamine poses some problems in that this dose by itself is carcinogenic, but only after a year or more. Furthermore, this high dose is also clastogenic to rat hepatocytes in vivo (Sargent et al., 1989). However, these authors and their colleagues have demonstrated a significant degree of correlation between long- and medium-term results, indicating the usefulness of this assay as a potential surrogate for the chronic bioassay (Ogiso et al., 1990). More recently these authors have used a slightly modified protocol in which five potent carcinogenic agents are administered for a 4-week period, followed by administration of the test chemical for a subsequent 24- to 32-week period (Ito et al., 1996). Unlike the assay depicted in Fig. 8-29, this more complicated procedure may allow the detection of promoting and progressor agents as well as complete carcinogens in a variety of different tissues. However, outside of Japan these assay procedures have not been generally utilized.

The newborn mouse model of chemical carcinogenesis was initially described by Shubik and his colleagues (Pietra et al., 1959) and later used extensively in studies of mouse hepatocarcinogenesis by Vesselinovitch and his colleagues (1978). More recently, Fujii (1991) has utilized this procedure in the determination of the carcinogenic potential of 45 different chemicals with quite reasonable results. The endpoint of neoplasms in a variety of different tissues, including lung, liver, lymphoid and hematopoietic tissues, is determined within a 1-year period. The assay is relatively inexpensive, utilizing small amounts of the test materials. As yet, however, this assay has not found general usefulness in the determination of carcinogenic potential by regulatory agencies.

Multistage Models of Neoplastic Development

As we have previously noted, the original studies on multistage models of carcinogenesis were developed with the epidermis of the mouse. It was not until some 40 years after those initial experiments that there was some attempt at standardization of the multistage model of carcinogenesis in mouse skin for the analysis of the carcinogenic potential of specific chemicals (Pereira, 1982). The format for such assays was essentially that depicted in Fig. 8-18. Few refinements in the procedure were added with the exception of the use of a genetically susceptible strain of mice, the SENCAR strain, which is now utilized in such tests (Slaga, 1986). This system may also be extended to the potential analysis of progressor agents (Hennings et al., 1993; Warren et al., 1993).

Considerably later than the initial reports of the mouse skin system, Hicks et al. (1975) demonstrated the cocarcinogenic or promoting action of several agents in the development of bladder cancer in the rat. Subsequently, other promoting agents have been demonstrated with this or a related assay, some of which appear to be relatively unique to this tissue for both anatomical and chemical reasons (Cohen and Lawson, 1995; Ito and Fukushima, 1989). At about the same time as the initial report of the multistage bladder model of carcinogenesis, Peraino and associates (1977) reported a multistage model of carcinogenesis in the rat liver. This finding has led to the development of a number of models of multistage carcinogenesis in the rat liver. Solt and Farber (1976) reported a model somewhat analogous to that of Ito and his colleagues, but with an aim directed primarily at studying mechanisms of hepatocarcinogenesis rather than utilizing it as an assay system for potential carcinogens. Shortly thereafter, Pitot et al. (1978) developed a model wherein initiation was performed with a nonnecrogenic dose of the initiating agent, subsequently followed by chronic administration of a promoting agent. The format of these two assay systems are noted in Fig. 8-31. The endpoint of these systems is the quantitative analysis of altered hepatic foci measured by one of several enzymatic markers, the most sensitive being the expression of GSTP (Hendrich et al., 1987). Several studies have investigated the potential for such analyses in the detection of chemical carcinogens (Pereira and Stoner, 1985; Williams, 1989; Oesterle and Deml, 1990). A similar format has been used to study the preneoplastic aberrant crypt foci in the colon of animals administered potential carcinogens (Ghia et al., 1996). However, as yet all such assays utilizing preneoplastic endpoints have not found general usefulness in the identification of potential carcinogenic agents. It

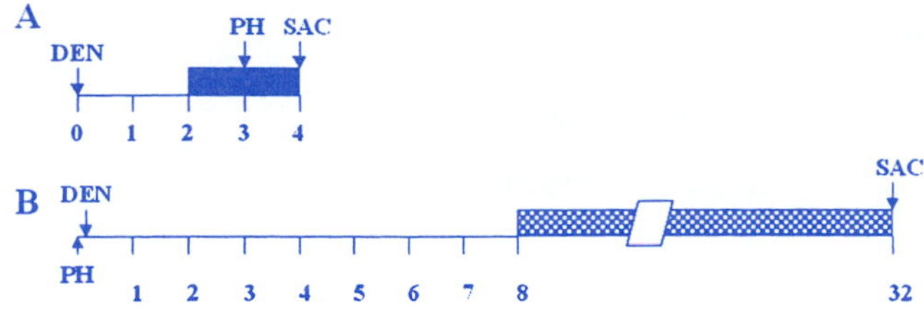

Figure 8-31. Formats of short-term models of multistage hepatocarcinogenesis in the rat.

A. The Solt-Farber model, in which animals are administered a necrogenic dose of diethylnitrosamine followed 2 weeks later by the administration of 0.02% acetylaminofluorene (*shaded bar*) with a 70 percent partial hepatectomy performed after 1 week of AAF feeding and sacrifice 1 week following the surgery. *B.* The Pitot et al. (1978) model, in which a nonnecrogenic dose (10 mg/kg) of DEN is administered 24 h after a partial hepatectomy (PH) and animals are fed a normal diet for 8 weeks, at which time they are placed on a diet containing 0.05 percent phenobarbital for a subsequent 24 weeks and then sacrificed. The endpoint of both models is the quantitation of altered hepatic foci.

is possible that in the future such assays may be useful in distinguishing between agents exerting their carcinogenic effect primarily at one or another of the stages of carcinogenesis.

Transgenic and Knockout Mice as Models of Carcinogenesis

With the advent of the development of transgenic animals as well as gene targeting in mice, recent efforts have been directed towards the development of animal models with specific genetic alterations that make them more susceptible to carcinogenesis by external agents. As noted from Table 8-29, the most popular of these are mice exhibiting one defective allele of the *p53* tumor suppressor gene and a transgenic mouse line (TG·AC) carrying a v-Ha-*ras* oncogene fused to a zeta globin promoter. *p53*-deficient mice develop a high frequency of a variety of spontaneous neoplasms. The incidence of such tumors varies but, in general, all of the homozygous *p53*-defective mice develop neoplasms by 10 months of age, while the heterozygous mice have a 50 percent incidence by 18 months, with over 90 percent incidence by 2 years of age (Donehower, 1996). However, the heterozygous animals did not show an accelerated carcinogenesis of the liver, even when hepatocarcinogens were administered (Dass et al., 1999). In addition to this model system, which mimics the Li-Fraumeni syndrome in humans, a large number of other gene-targeted mutations have been developed in mice but have not yet been utilized as model systems for identifying potential carcinogenic agents (Rosenberg, 1997).

The TG·AC transgenic mouse is one of a large number of potential transgenic mice and rats that might be considered for the study of the development of neoplasia in response to test agents. However, in most cases the expression of the transgene is targeted to a specific tissue, and thus one deals with a tissue-specific development of neoplasia (cf. Goldsworthy et al., 1994). The TG·AC transgenic mouse is very effective in the identification of potential promoting agents for the skin. Administration of the well-known skin-promoting agent, TPA, could induce the development of papillomas after only three to ten applications (Spalding et al., 1993). These investigators also studied several other potential promoting and progressor agents, all of which exhibited a short latency period and high incidence of papilloma induction. Thus, it is apparent that each of these genetic models of carcinogenesis has a role to play in the identification of potential carcinogenic agents. It will require considerable effort to validate each of the models with respect to tissue-specific carcinogenesis by complete carcinogens or by promoting and/or progressor agents (cf. Tennant, 1998).

EVALUATION OF CARCINOGENIC POTENTIAL

The multiple in vivo and in vitro tests described thus far present the experimentalist or the regulator with an extensive amount of data from which to draw conclusions about the carcinogenic potential of the test agent. In addition, epidemiologic studies provide perhaps the most definitive means of estimating the carcinogenic potential to humans from exposure to a specific agent. While such studies, if definitively positive, are the best evidence for carcinogenic potential of an agent to humans, the evidence is usually obtained after an exposure has occurred in a population. In general, epidemiological studies can only detect differences between populations when there is approximately a twofold increase above the background incidence of neoplasia in the control population. Since many more agents than those classified as group 1 by IARC exhibit carcinogenic potential, the in vitro and in vivo tests described earlier have been used as surrogates in attempting to determine carcinogenic potential and risk to the human population. The results of such tests clearly offer qualitative information with respect to the identification of agents exhibiting some potential hazard with respect to one or more aspects of the process of carcinogenesis as we know it today. Major difficulties remain in attempting to extrapolate in a scientific and meaningful way information obtained from in vitro and *in vivo* tests to an estimation of the potential risk of such agents to the human population as inducers of disease, especially neoplasia. As might be expected, a number of problems are involved in the scientific and practical application of information developed from short- and long-term tests to the estimation of human risk.

The Problem of Extrapolation

Since bacterial mutagenicity (Fig. 8-25) is the most widely and extensively utilized test for estimating the qualitative carcinogenic potential of an agent, a number of investigations have been directed toward determining the relationship of bacterial mutagenesis and carcinogenesis of the same chemical, usually in rodents. An early graphical relationship of such a series of tests is seen in Fig. 8-32. Obviously, considerable more efforts have been carried out since the publication of this in 1976 (Sugimura et al., 1976). However, the figure does place in rather definitive terms compounds that exhibit either carcinogenic and/or mutagenic activities. The indicated description of complete carcinogen, promoting agent, initiating agent, etc., is an exercise allowing the further classification of such agents in multistage carcinogenesis. In a far more extensive study, Tennant et al. (1987) related the results of bacterial mutagenicity to carcinogenic potential as determined in the chronic 2-year bioassay and found that the short-term assay detected only about half of the carcinogens as mutagens. These studies and a slightly later one by Ashby (1989) pointed again to the importance of using more than a single short-term assay in attempting to relate DNA structural alterations to potential carcinogenicity. Although the prediction of carcinogenic potential by the bacterial mutagenicity tests

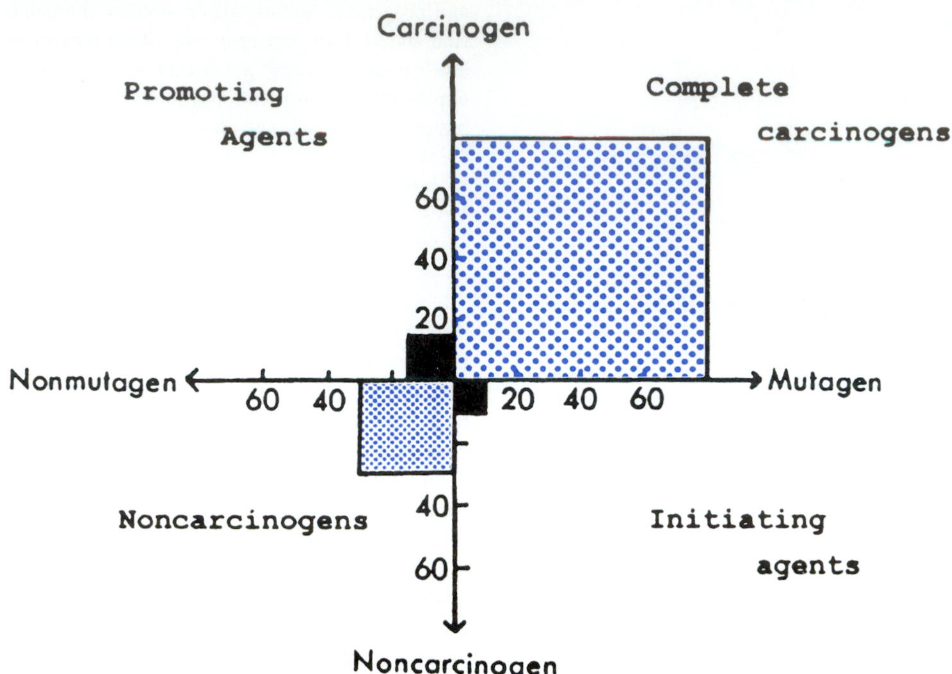

Figure 8-32. Graphic representation of mutagens and nonmutagens in relation to their known carcinogenic potential in animal tests.

The labeling of the quadrants using the classification of Table 8-18 is a further potential extrapolation of these data. [After Sugimura et al. (1976), with permission of authors and publishers.]

together with other short-term tests is in the neighborhood of 60 to 70 percent, it is somewhat surprising that interspecies extrapolation of carcinogenesis in rats and mice is not much greater than this. In an analysis by Gold et al. (1989), chronic bioassays for carcinogenic potential in either mice or rats were only about 70 to 75 percent predictive of carcinogenicity in the other species. In a more recent study (Fung et al., 1993) of 379 chemicals tested by the National Cancer Institute/National Toxicology Program for carcinogenic potential, only slightly more than 50 percent of the chemicals tested exhibited carcinogenicity in at least one organ of one sex of one species. Less than half of these exhibited carcinogenic potential in both species tested, a situation most likely to be indicative of a carcinogenic hazard to humans.

Several other issues are also relevant to cross-species extrapolation, including differences in metabolism of chemical agents between the species. While metabolic schemes are qualitatively similar across species, significant quantitative differences, especially in metabolic rate, partly owing to elimination kinetics, are the rule. Exposure estimation is frequently based on the daily dose administered or on plasma concentration used as a surrogate for concentrations in the tissue. Using plasma concentrations for extrapolation across species assumes that each species responds in the same manner to any given dose of an agent. In the final analysis, it may be that the best basis for cross-species comparison is serum concentration expressed as milligrams per kilogram body weight, since this better predicts tissue concentration-response effects after chronic administration (Allen et al., 1988; Monro, 1992). Thus, it is clear that the problem of extrapolation of both short- and long-term tests to carcinogenic potential in the human is much less than perfect, suggesting an important need for reevaluation and reinterpretation of the tests currently in use. Needless to say, a program to develop better extrapolative endpoints should be a major priority.

The Dose–Response Problem

Another important component in the analysis of assays for carcinogenic potential, both in vivo and in vitro, is that of the dose–response to a particular test agent. The effectiveness of the induction of neoplasia by a chemical agent is dependent on the dose of that agent administered to the test animal. We have already noted the importance of dose–response curves for the stages of initiation and promotion. The differences in the shapes of the curves for these two processes are of considerable significance in assessing carcinogenic potential and risk.

Other factors may also influence a dose–response curve, such as the toxicity of the agent, the bioavailability of the agent, and the metabolic or pharmacokinetic characteristics of the agent within the living organism. A classic dose–response of a complete carcinogen and some of its ramifications are seen in Fig. 8-33 (Druckrey et al., 1963). In this figure, curve 1 shows the relationship between the daily dose administered and the median total dose of animals developing carcinoma. Thus, the left ordinate indicates the sum of all doses administered up to a 50 percent tumor incidence, thus relating the total dose to the tumor incidence. In this way the straight line relationship, if extrapolated, would proceed through the origin. Curve 2 relates the daily dose of carcinogen to the median induction time of the appearance of the first neoplasm. While extrapolation of curve 1 through the origin indicates that there is no dose at which some incidence of neoplasms is not apparent, it should be noted that if the daily dose is less than 0.1 mg/kg, no experimental data points are available. Furthermore, extrapolation of curve 2 to this low-dose region indicates that at doses lower than 0.1 mg/kg, the rats used in this experiment and whose lifetime is approximately 1000 days will not live sufficiently long for carcinomas to appear. In the assay depicted in Fig. 8-33, the

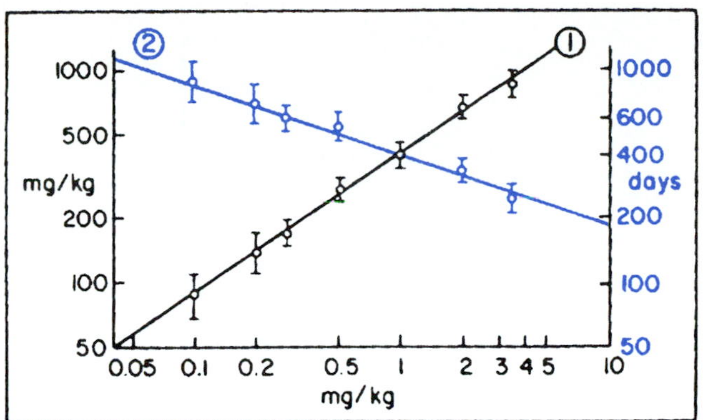

Figure 8-33. Dose–response relation seen in the chronic feeding of 4-dimethylaminostilbene to rats.

1. Relation between the daily dose and the median total dose for animals that developed carcinoma. 2. Relation between daily dose and median induction time. The abscissa shows the daily dose; the ordinate on the left is the total dose administered, and on the right is the time from the beginning of the experiment. All scales are logarithmic. [Modified from Druckrey et al. (1963), with permission.]

animals were administered a carcinogenic agent at a constant rate in the diet. Littlefield and Gaylor (1985) noted that with another complete carcinogen, 2-acetylaminofluorene, both the dose rate and the total dose administered are important in the final analysis. These workers demonstrated that when the total doses of this test agent were similar, the higher dose rates with shorter time periods induced a higher prevalence of neoplasms.

The use of the MTD has been criticized because of the toxicity it induces, paralleled by an increase in cell proliferation in a number of susceptible organs (Ames and Gold, 1990). At the other end of the dose–response curve the problem of the presence or absence of a threshold (no-effect level) of a carcinogenic agent is still hotly debated. We have already noted that, on theoretical grounds, agents capable of damaging DNA might not be expected to exhibit a threshold, whereas those exerting their effects through complicated receptor-mediated pathways, as with promoting agents, would be expected to exhibit a threshold of their effects (Aldridge, 1986). In addition, carcinogenic agents, whether DNA damaging or not, may exhibit a lower than control effect at very low doses (Kitchin et al., 1994; Teeguarden et al., 1998). Despite these observations, as well as the data depicted in Fig. 8-33 and our knowledge of the mechanism of action of promoting agents, regulatory agencies have not seen fit in general to alter the philosophy that carcinogenic agents do not have threshold dose levels. As we shall see, this philosophy has permeated much of the regulatory action taken to date with respect to agents shown to be carcinogenic in any form of life.

In most epidemiologic studies it has not been possible to determine the doses of the agents to which humans have been exposed, and only occasional, rather crude retrospective dose–response curves are available. However, a summary was made by the Meselson Committee (1975) of dose levels of several known human carcinogens that appear to be carcinogenic for certain human populations. These estimated levels were compared with levels of these agents known to produce neoplasms in animals (Table 8-32). They show that the cumulative doses required per unit of body weight for tumor induction in the human and in experimental animals are of the same order of magnitude for four of the six agents. However, a more detailed comparison would require a correction for the short observation time in many of the studies on humans (as in the case of diethylstilbestrol and vinyl

Table 8-32
Approximate Total Doses for Tumor Induction in Humans and Experimental Animals

	Human		*Animal*	
AGENT	DOSE AND ORGAN	INCIDENCE (%)	DOSE, SPECIES, AND ORGAN	INCIDENCE* (%)
Benzidine	50–200 mg/kg† (bladder)‡	22–50	10,000 mg/kg† (mouse liver)‡	67
			50–100 mg/kg (rat mammary gland)	50–80 (2)*
Chlornaphazine	2000 mg/kg (bladder)	16.0	75–4800 mg/kg (mouse lung)	40–100 (38)
Diethylstilbestrol	0.5–300 mg/kg (vaginal and cervical adenocarcinoma)	0.2	2–13 mg/kg (male mouse mammary gland)	4–27
			400 mg/kg (newborn female mouse cervix and vagina)	33
Aflatoxin B_1	0.1 mg/kg (liver)	0.5	1.25–6.0 mg/kg (mouse liver)	23–100 (3)
			0.3–1.5 mg/kg (rat liver)	19–100
Vinyl chloride	70,000 mg/kg (liver)	0.2	30,000 mg/kg (mouse lung and mammary gland)	25, lung 13, mammary
			40,000 mg/kg (rat kidney and liver)	9, kidney 6, liver
Cigarette smoke	From 1000 cigarettes/kg (lung)	2.5	From 400 cigarettes/kg (mouse lung)	4.9 (1.3)
			From 6000 cigarettes/kg (hamster larynx)	6

*Tumor incidence in control groups of animals, given in parentheses. When not designated, control incidence was 0 or not stated.

†The average dose of the group(s).

‡The organ affected and species (for the animals) are noted in parentheses.

SOURCE: Meselson Committee (1975).

Table 8-33
Some Methods for the Measurement of the Potency of Carcinogens

RELATIONSHIP	DESCRIPTION	REFERENCE
Absolute		
Carcinogenic (Iball) index = $\frac{\text{\% of tumors (animals with)}}{\text{Average latent period in days}}$	The percentage number of tumor-bearing animals was calculated from the total number of animals used in the particular assay or from the total number of animals surviving at the time the first tumor became manifest (Hueper, 1963).	Iball, 1939
$K = \frac{\ln 2}{D_{1/2}}$	$D_{1/2}$ is the total animal dose which gives a 50% incidence of cancer after a 2-year exposure. K is defined as potency.	Meselson and Russell, 1977
$R = -\ln(1 - p) = \alpha + \beta d$	R = potency where p is the probability of developing cancer at dose d, and α and β are derived constants.	Crouch and Wilson, 1979
$TD_{50} = \log(2)/b$	The TD_{50} (carcinogenic potency) of a chemical is defined as the dose rate (mg/kg body weight/day, b) which, if administered chronically for a standard period, would halve the probability of an animal remaining without any neoplasia (Bernstein, 1985).	Peto et al., 1984
Relative		
Relative potency = $\frac{\text{Dose of a reference compound needed to produce a specific effect in a particular bioassay (reference dose)}}{\text{Dose of a test compound needed to produce the same magnitude of the same effect in the same bioassay (test dose)}}$	The relative potency of a given agent is defined as the ratio of the dose of that chemical required to induce carcinogenesis in a particular bioassay, relative to the dose of another (reference) agent required to produce the same outcome in the same type of bioassay.	Glass et al., 1991
Multistage		
Initiation Index = #AHF/liver/mmole/kg body weight	Index based on administration of a single dose of initiating agent in mmole/kg body weight.	Pitot et al., 1987
Promotion Index = $V_f/V_c \times \text{mmol}^{-1} \times \text{weeks}^{-1}$	V_f is the total volume fraction (%) occupied by AHF in the livers of rats treated with the test agent, and V_c is the total volume of AHF in control animals, which have only been initiated. The dose rate of administration of the promoting agent is expressed as millimoles/week.	Pitot et al., 1987

chloride), since many cancers in humans do not appear for 20 to 30 years after exposure. In addition, both vinyl chloride and diethylstilbestrol cause a very rare neoplasm in humans that is not usually seen in experimental animals. Thus, the effective doses of several agents known to be carcinogenic for humans and rodents are not markedly dissimilar in the two species. If this conclusion can be extended to other chemical carcinogens in the human environment, then both the qualitative and quantitative extrapolations of such findings in the animal to the human situation have some degree of validity.

The Problem of the Potency of Carcinogenic Agents

It should be apparent to the student by now that not all carcinogenic agents are equally effective in inducing neoplasia, i.e., they exhibit differing carcinogenic potencies. The potency of an agent to induce neoplasia has been simply defined as the slope of the dose–response curve for induction of neoplasms (Choy, 1996). However, such a definition has generally not been the basis for estimates of carcinogenic potency based on data from chronic bioassays with continuous administration of the agent. In Table 8-33 may be seen a listing of some methods for the measurement of the potency of carcinogens, beginning with the early study by Iball (1939) resulting in the Iball Index, which was used for a number of years thereafter. The relationship of Meselson and Russell (1977) may also be derived from the results of bacterial mutagenesis assays. The potency relationship developed by Crouch and Wilson (1979) is dependent on a linear, no-threshold extrapolation of the animal bioassay result, giving the slope as β in the equation seen in the table (Barr, 1985). The TD_{50} has been extensively used, and values were recently compiled by Gold and Zeiger (1997) for a large number of chemicals. The range of carcinogenic potencies developed from such a relationship may be seen in Fig. 8-34. Tennant and his associates (Dybing et al., 1997) have modified the TD_{50} potency relationship, using a different fraction of animals that develop neoplasms. The T_{25} is defined by these workers as the chronic dose rate in mg/kg body weight/day that will give 25 percent of the animals neoplasms at a specific tissue site, after correction for spontaneous incidence, within the standard lifetime of the test species. As expected, since the relationship is basically the same as that noted in Table 8-33 except for only half the percentage, the T_{25} values are usually roughly one-half those of the TD_{50} values. Pepelko (1991) has pointed out one of the difficulties of these absolute potency measurements in that differences in solubility, bioavailability, and some other pharmacokinetic parameters do cause considerable variability in some of the potency values reported.

While the four relationships noted in the table under "absolute" do analyze carcinogenic potency of a chemical from the data on the bioassay of that chemical alone, Glass and associates (1991) did propose a relative potency relationship that has some degree of flexibility and may have some application in risk assessment different from the absolute analyses. Pitot et al. (1987) have attempted to determine indices relating the stages of initiation and promotion to the potency of the agents inducing such stages. In the case of the initiation index, which is relatively straightforward, the values obtained are absolute. In the case of the promoting index, the value is always given in relation to the nontreated control, which does develop focal lesions

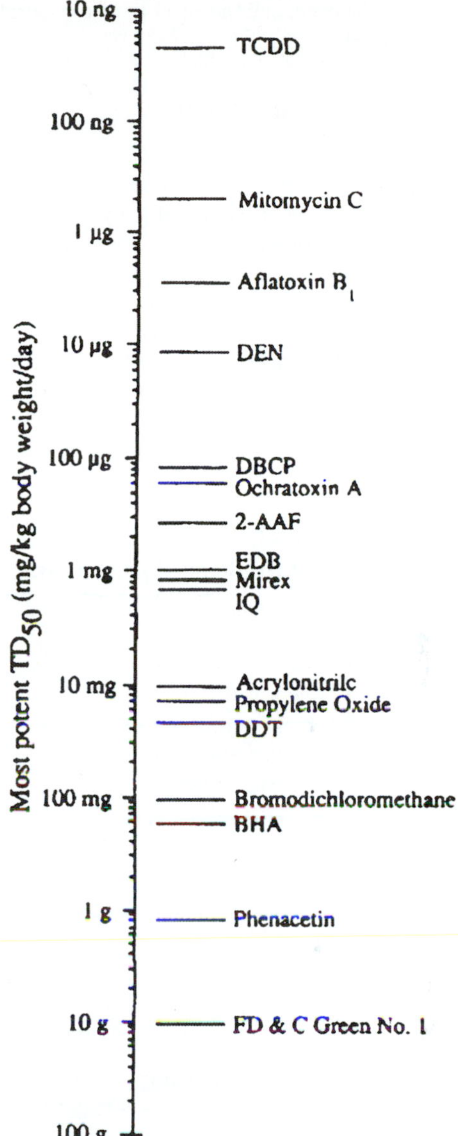

Figure 8-34. *Range of carcinogenic potency as determined by the* TD_{50} *potency relationship of Peto et al. (1984).*

[Adapted from Gold et al. (1998), with permission of authors and publisher.]

from endogenous promotion of spontaneously initiated hepatocytes. However, these measures of initiating and promoting potencies have been applied only to multistage hepatocarcinogenesis in the rat. However, it is quite feasible to extend such analyses to multistage carcinogenesis in a number of other solid organs where the immediate results of initiation can be quantitated and the relative growth of lesions from the initiated cell population can be determined with some degree of accuracy (Pitot et al., 1987).

RELATION (EXTRAPOLATION) OF BIOASSAY DATA TO HUMAN RISK

Campbell (1980) suggested the thesis that the risk (R) of some agent or event can be estimated as a function of the product of the probability (P) of the event and the severity of the harmfulness of the event or agent (H):

$$R = P \times H$$

From the simplest viewpoint, the risk taker may accept harm of greater severity (high value of H) only if the probability of occurrence (P) is very low. Conversely, events that are only modestly harmful (low value of H) may be acceptable at higher levels of frequency or probability. From this argument, safety may be taken as a measure of acceptability of some degree of risk.

Table 8-34, taken from the work of Oser (1978) and Upton (1980), lists the risk of death classified in relation to specific activities. From this table, all of the activities listed exhibit some degree of risk or probability (P) of death or harm (H). The important point to note is that the probability of risk per million persons per year ranges from 0.1 for lightning striking to 20,000 in the case of motorcycling. A careful person presumably compares the risks of any event to his or her health with the benefits that will potentially accrue before making a decision. Relatively few people may actually do this, and even when they do, precisely what index is chosen as the indicator of relative safety is a function of the value judgment of each individual.

As to the risk of cancer, the harm (H) is considered by most laypersons to be extremely great. In view of this concern by the public, the U.S. government through its regulatory agencies, such as the Environmental Protection Agency (EPA), the Food and Drug Administration (FDA), and others, has assumed a major role in practical considerations of human risk from environmental agents. Two theorems are the basis for the estimations of human risk from carcinogenic agents in the environment.

Table 8-34
Risk of Death, by Type of Activity

ACTIVITY	RISK OF DEATH PER MILLION PERSONS PER YEAR
Travel	
Motorcycling	20,000
Pedestrian	40
Automobile	20–30
Airplane	9
Sports	
Car racing	1,200
Rock climbing	1,000
Canoeing	400
Skiing	170
Power boating	30
Swimming (recreational)	19–30
Bicycling	10
Eating and drinking	
Alcohol—one bottle of wine/day	75
Alcohol—one bottle of beer/day	20
Low-level radiation	
Coal mining (black lung disease, 1969)	8,000
Nuclear plant worker (0.8 rem/year, average) (radiation-induced cancer)	80
Airline pilot (0.3 rem/year, average) (radiation-induced cancer)	30
Grand Central Station (40 h/week, 0.12 rem/year)	12
Jet air travel, general population (0.47 mrem/year) (radiation-induced cancer)	0.047
Miscellaneous	
Smoking 20 cigarettes/day	2,000–5,000
Pregnancy	230
Abortion after 14 weeks	70
Contraceptive pills	20
Home accidents	12
Vaccination against smallpox	3
Earthquakes (California)	1.7
Hurricanes	0.4
Lightning	0.1

SOURCE: After Oser (1978) and Upton (1980), with permission.

1. A threshold (no-effect) level for a carcinogenic agent cannot be determined with any degree of accuracy.
2. All carcinogenic agents produce their effects in an irreversible manner, so that the actions of small amounts of carcinogenic agents in our environment are additive—producing a "carcinogenic burden" for the average individual during his or her lifetime.

These bases may be considered as default assumptions that are utilized if there is not sufficient evidence to alter these assumptions. Recent guidelines by the EPA have indicated that at least one regulatory agency is beginning to consider and even include in their final disposition of the regulation of a chemical data that may alter these default assumptions (Page et al., 1997). Since we have already noted the presence of thresholds of promoting agents as well as their reversibility, such data may become useful in consideration of regulation of chemicals in the future. However, the gold standard chronic 2-year bioassay that is utilized as the mainstay in regulation of both industrial and pharmaceutical chemicals does not distinguish between initiating, promoting, and progressor agents; it will require substantial additional studies to give cause to alter the default assumptions. As noted above, scientific risk estimation should be carried out with the full knowledge of the action of the carcinogenic agent as a complete carcinogen, or as having a major action at one or more of the stages of carcinogenesis.

The extrapolation of bioassay data to human risk estimation is one of the most difficult problems that has faced society and will face us for years to come as numerous new chemicals enter the environment. In attempting to predict the behavior of a chemical in the human from data obtained from bioassays, a number of factors should be considered in extrapolation of bioassay data to human risk (Kraybill, 1978). These include:

- Reproducibility of experimental data
- Tumor incidence in experimental animals on a dose–dependent basis
- Relative approximation of experimental dose to that of human exposure
- Acceptable design and statistical evaluation of bioassay
- Consensus on interpretation of histopathologic changes
- Availability of biochemical, metabolic, and pharmacokinetic data to be considered in final decision making

Not included in these factors proposed more than two decades ago is a knowledge of the action of the agent as an initiating, promoting, or progressor agent. Unfortunately, not all of these factors are taken into account when regulatory decisions are made at the governmental level concerning specific compounds in our environment. Newer requirements for more extensive studies of compounds that would satisfy these factors are a goal to be achieved but as yet not attained.

Another consideration in determination of human risk is whether or not the estimation is qualitative or quantitative. Qualitative risk estimation is much easier to develop based on qualitative analyses of the variety of bioassay procedures utilized. IARC as well as regulatory agencies throughout the world take very seriously the qualitative finding of induction of neoplasia in one or two species of animals as a qualitative indication of risk of carcinogenicity to the human. However, quantitative risk analysis is much more difficult. In fact, a number of epidemiologists have refused to make such quantitative relationships on the basis of animal data and would only use data in the human to carry out such estimates. Still, as we have seen from the utilization of various "safe" doses of carcinogenic agents and a variety of other factors, quantitative risk assessment has been and is being applied to human risk situations of specific chemicals and mixtures. Paramount in such considerations are the use of mathematical models in which, making a variety of assumptions, one may develop quantitative risk estimates for the human. We will consider some of these models below.

STATISTICAL ESTIMATES OF HUMAN RISK FROM BIOASSAY DATA BY USING MATHEMATICAL MODELS

The statistical analyses of whole-animal bioassay data have employed over the years a number of mathematical models in an attempt to relate experimental data to the human situation, especially for the purposes of quantitating human risk inso far as is possible. As Gaylor and Shapiro (1979) have pointed out, "There is no choice but to extrapolate." This means, in essence, that because of the insensitivity of epidemiologic studies and the number and quantity of actual and potential carcinogens in our environment, one must make every attempt possible to relate data from bioassay studies to the human condition, especially the potential risk to the public. Most of these mathematical models have as a basic tenet the assumption that carcinogenic agents lack a threshold, act irreversibly, and have effects that are additive. Equations for some of the more commonly used models are given in Table 8-35. None of these

Table 8-35
Mathematical Models Used in the Extrapolation of the Risk of Carcinogenic Agents to the Human

	EQUATION FOR THE PROBABILITY (P) OF TUMOR INDUCTION AT DOSE d
One-hit (linear) model	$P(d) = 1 - e^{(-\lambda d)}$
Multihit (k-hit) model	$P(d) = 1 - \sum_{i=0}^{k-1} (\lambda d)^i e^{-\lambda d}/i!$
Multistage model	$P(d) = 1 - \exp[-(\alpha_1 + \beta_1 d) \ldots (\lambda_k + \beta_k d)]$
Extreme value model	$P(d) = 1 - \exp[-\exp(\alpha + \beta \log_{10} d)]$
Log-probit model	$P(d) = \Phi\ (\alpha + \beta \log_{10} d)$

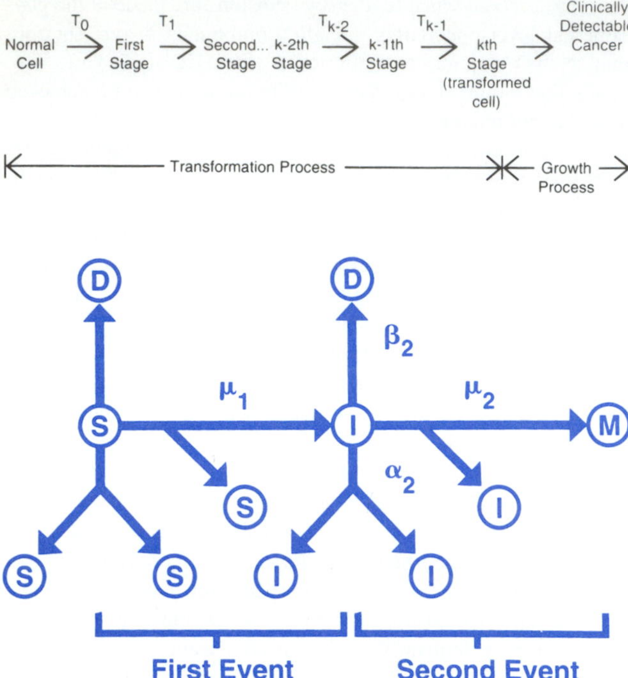

Figure 8-35. The Armitage and Doll (upper) and MKV (lower) models of multistage carcinogenesis.

In the former, the number of stages is unspecified (T_k), and the transition between them is irreversible. In the MKV model, the fates of stem cells (S) and intermediate (I) cells are death (D) or proliferation. Rarely, I cells undergo (M_2 to malignancy (M). The rates of replication (α_2) and apoptosis (β_2) for I cells are indicated, and similar rates for S cells are implied. μ_1 and μ_2 are the rates of the first genetic event (initiation) and the second genetic event (progression). [Adapted from Pitot and Dragan (1996), with permission of publishers.]

models can prove or disprove the existence of a threshold of response, and none can be completely verified on the basis of biological argument; however, the models have been useful in data evaluation and are presently being used by some federal agencies in extrapolating experimental data to the human risk situation. One of the most commonly used techniques is the log-probit model. In the earlier use of this model, the procedure was to regard every agent as carcinogenic. On this assumption, one must determine some "safe" dosage level at which the risk calculated would not exceed some very small level such as 1 in 100 million or 10^{-8}.

The linear multistage model, first proposed by Armitage and Doll (1954), incorporates the idea of multiple steps into a statistical approach for risk analysis. This multistage model (Fig. 8-35) incorporates one aspect of the pathogenesis of neoplastic development, that of multiple stages, but cell cycle–dependent processes, the dynamics of cell kinetics, birth rate, and death rate are not considered. Furthermore, the transition from one stage to the next is considered irreversible. Despite these deficiencies, the linearized multistage model is one of the most commonly utilized models at the present time. At a low dose the multistage model is used to fit the observed tumor incidence data to a polynomial of the dose as noted in Table 8-35. The linear multistage model is not appropriate for estimating low-dose carcinogenic potency for many chemicals. In most cases, the dose response of high doses of testing differs substantially from the considerably lower doses for exposure. Pharmacokinetic and pharmacodynamic models provide information that can help bridge the gap between the high dose and low dose scenarios (Anderson, 1989). A second problem is associated with extrapolation of lifetime exposure of animals to the MTD of a compound to the less than lifetime exposure common for humans. This problem has been addressed by the EPA through the use of the Weibull model (Hanes and Wedel, 1985), which assumes that risk is greater when encountered at a younger age, and, once exposure occurs, risk continues to accrue despite the cessation of exposure. However, observations in humans and experimental animals have demonstrated that in many cases risk decreases after exposure ceases, as would be true if the agent were a promoting agent.

More recently, biomathematical modeling of cancer risk assessment has been used in an attempt to relate such models more closely to the biological characteristics of the pathogenesis of neoplasia. The best known of these biologically based models is that described originally by Moolgavkar, Venzon, and Knudson, termed the MVK model (Moolgavkar, 1986). This model, which is depicted in Fig. 8-35, reproduces quite well the multistage characteristics of neoplastic development with μ_1, the rate at which normal cells are converted to "intermediate" cells (initiated cells), and μ_2, the rate at which intermediate cells are converted to neoplastic (N) cells. These rates model the rates of initiation and progression in multistage carcinogenesis, while the stage of promotion represents the expansion of the intermediate cell population, which is a function of α_2, the rate of division of "intermediate cells," and β_2, the rate of differentiation and/or death of intermediate cells. Other factors in the model that are also true in biology are the rate of replication and cell death of normal or stem cells. While this model originally was developed to explain certain epidemiologic characteristics of breast cancer incidence and mortality in humans (Moolgavkar, 1986), it has found potential application in a variety of multistage models including that of rat liver (Luebeck et al., 1991). Application of the model to risk assessment problems has not found wide use, but this may change in the next few years (Anderson et al., 1992). In addition, integration of biological data, including pharmacokinetic and pharmacodynamic parameters, should aid in the development of a more biologically based risk assessment model.

REGULATION OF CARCINOGENIC RISK AT THE FEDERAL LEVEL

At least four federal agencies have as their primary responsibility the regulation of risk. These agencies include the Consumer Products Safety Commission (CPSC), the EPA, the FDA, and the Occupational Safety and Health Administration (OSHA). At least two types of regulations affect risk analysis; these include regulations similar to the Clean Water Act, which imposes technology-based standards that are dictated by the best available technology, and the Clean Air Act, which imposes health- or risk-based standards to protect human health by providing an ample margin of safety. A number of laws have been passed that control exposure to carcinogens in food, drugs, and the environment (Table 8-36). Perhaps the most controversial is the Food, Drug, and Cosmetic Act of 1938, including the 1958 amendment known as the Delaney amendment. The Delaney amendment was passed to curtail any possible use of additives in food and drugs that had been demonstrated to induce cancer in humans or animals. This law ignores the presence of endogenous or endogenously produced compounds

Table 8-36
Selected Federal Laws for Regulation of Toxic and Carcinogenic Agents

NAME OF ACT AND YEAR PASSED AND AMENDED	AREA OF CONCERN
Food Drug and Cosmetic Act (FDC): 1906, 1938, amended 1958 (Delaney), 1960, 1962, 1968, 1976, 1980, 1984, 1986, 1987, 1990, 1992	Food, drugs, cosmetics, food additives, color additives, new drugs, animal feed additives, medical devices.
Federal Insecticide, Fungicide, and Rodenticide Act (FIFRA): 1948, amended 1972, 1975, 1976	Pesticides
Clean Air Act: 1970, amended 1974, 1977, 1978, 1980, 1981, 1982, 1983, 1990	Air pollutants
Clean Water Act: 1972, amended 1977–1983, 1987, 1988, 1990, 1992; originally the Federal Water Control Act	Water pollutants
Occupational Safety and Health Act (OSHA): 1970, amended 1974, 1978, 1979, 1982, 1990, 1992	Workplace exposure to toxicants
Toxic Substances Control Act (TOSCA): 1976, amended 1981, 1983, 1984, 1986, 1988, 1990, 1992	Hazardous chemicals not covered elsewhere, including premarket review

SOURCE: Adapted from Office of Science and Technology Policy (1986).

that have carcinogenic action. For example, nitrites are effective bacteriocidal agents when used at low levels as food additives, but nitrites are produced extensively in vivo during normal metabolism of nitrogenous compounds, especially when nitrates are present in the diet (Rogers, 1982). High doses of nitrites given with secondary amines result in the formation of nitrosamines, which are carcinogenic in rodents (Rogers, 1982). Thus, a number of difficulties are encountered when food and additives are regulated with strict adherence to the Delaney amendment.

Besides science, a major driving force in legislative actions concerning the regulation of carcinogenic or potentially carcinogenic chemicals in the environment is the benefit obtained from such regulation. The saccharin-cyclamate debates were an interesting example of this (Kraybill, 1976). Saccharin is carcinogenic at a very high dose in rat uroepithelium (Anderson et al., 1988). After considerable debate, the U.S. Congress passed a law permitting the use of this "carcinogenic" compound as an artificial sweetener because of its low cost and benefit to a variety of individuals, especially diabetics. Recently, the courts rejected the use of two food colorings in drugs and cosmetics on the basis of an interpretation of the Delaney amendment as prohibitive of the use of additives even when only minimal risk can be demonstrated. The EPA faces a difficult situation in the regulation of pesticides when it attempts to balance the requirement of the Federal Insecticide, Fungicide, and Rodenticide Act (FIFRA), which requires a balance of risk and benefit in the application of pesticides to raw agricultural products, and the zero tolerance for carcinogens in processed foodstuffs mandated by the Delaney amendment. OSHA is responsible for regulating workers' exposure to potential toxins, including carcinogens. The statutes require that feasibility be considered in concert with lack of effect on workers' health. In the case of *Industrial Union Department v American Petroleum Institute,* the Supreme Court found that the allowable levels of a compound (i.e., benzene) could be established only if a significant risk from exposure could be demonstrated and that this risk could be lessened by a change in practice. In the final analysis, a significant proportion of risk to the average citizen is based on the perception of risk.

International Aspects of Environmental Regulation

Other countries have both preceded and followed legal actions in the United States in regulating noxious and carcinogenic agents that can and do occur in the human environment. The United Kingdom passed a Clean Air Act some three decades ago, well before such legislation appeared in the United States (cf. Hall, 1976). This same nation passed legislation regulating pollution in natural waters within the country at about the same time as similar legislation was enacted in the United States. The European Common Market has also advanced several programs in the area of environmental pollution, especially as related to air and water environments. More generally, they have established an environmental program that concerns itself with the impact of factors involving alterations in the environment, waste disposal, and educational programs (cf. Johnson, 1976). Other countries throughout the world have recognized the importance of controlling potentially damaging agents and have acted accordingly.

RISK-BENEFIT CONSIDERATIONS IN THE REGULATION OF ACTUAL AND POTENTIAL CARCINOGENIC ENVIRONMENTAL HAZARDS

We have briefly reviewed the methods for determining the actual and potential carcinogenic agents in our environment, methods for the estimation of risk to the human population of such agents, and the governmental approach to the regulation of such agents in our environment. An equally important consideration includes somewhat undefined concepts such as benefit-risk analysis, cost-

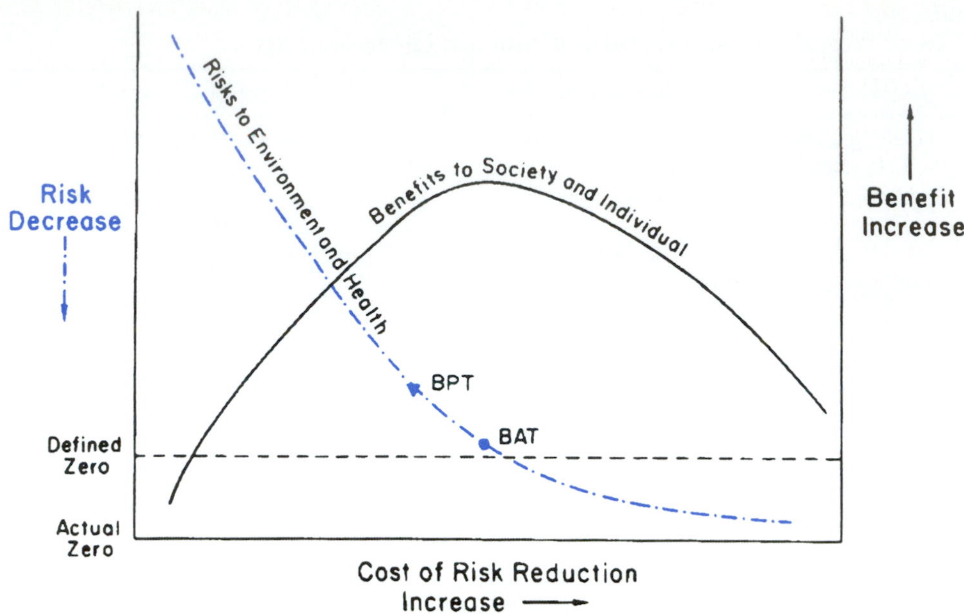

Figure 8-36. Risk-cost-benefit relation emphasizing the impact of cost control on all risks and demonstrating the loss of benefit beyond a certain cost of risk reduction.

BPT, best practicable technology; BAT, best available technology. [Modified from Blair and Hoerger (1979), with permission.]

effectiveness, and risk-cost analysis in the regulation of hazardous agents in our environment. These concepts are concerned with such traditional regulatory terms as "safe," "lowest feasible," and "best practicable technology."

Some of the regulatory legislation leaves no latitude for considerations of benefit versus risk. This is the case with the Delaney amendment, a simplistic legal statement that can create major problems when the regulatory agencies are faced with obeying the law. Problems also arose with respect to nitrite, since the benefits of removing nitrites as preservatives in packaged meats were balanced against the risk of bacterial contamination, especially by *Clostridium botulinum,* in nonpreserved packaged products. Federal regulatory agencies decided that these data were insufficient to ban nitrites under the Delaney clause, and thus nitrite continues to be widely used as a preservative, although at lower levels.

Attempts have been made to quantitate and characterize risks versus benefits. One way is to consider risks to the environment and to health as opposed to risks to society and to general aspects of health. It is evident that reduction in risk from direct exposure to an environmental factor will, at some level of additional cost of control, create new risks to society in terms of increased costs of products, availability of services, personal freedoms, employment, and so on. This relation is shown in Fig. 8-36. In controlling risks to the environment and to health there is a point beyond which the benefits to society and the individual begin to decrease because of the cost, both financial and otherwise, incurred in reducing risk toward actual zero. As was implied previously, there are very rare instances in which actual zero risk is obtained in any circumstance. The points for best practicable technology (BPT) and for best available technology (BAT) are seen on the risk curve. Clearly BPT in risk reduction is less costly than BAT.

More extensive risk-benefit analyses have been published, such as those of Moll and Tihansky (1977), in which dollar values have been estimated for each life that could potentially be saved by eliminating a specific agent from the environment. They also point out that the risks of specific agents in industrial situations may be far greater than those to society as a whole. An example is asbestos, which, though clearly hazardous to some industrial workers, causes little or no hazard at the levels of exposure of the population in general. In this respect, Samuels (1979) has pointed to the potential fallacy in many benefit-risk determinations unless one takes into consideration the concept of *necessary risk,* especially as related to occupational and industrial hazards. This concept stresses the importance of making every effort to eliminate hazardous agents in our environment that are important to society by replacing them with equally useful but less hazardous or nonhazardous components. If this cannot be done and a necessary risk is present, this consideration must be balanced against the benefits.

REFERENCES

Abell CW, Heidelberger C: Interaction of carcinogenic hydrocarbons with tissues: VIII. Binding of tritium-labeled hydrocarbons to the soluble proteins of mouse skin. *Cancer Res* 22:931–946, 1962.

Aldridge WN: The biological basis and measurement of thresholds. *Annu Rev Pharmacol Toxicol* 26:39–58, 1986.

Allaben WT, Turturro A, Leakey JEA, et al: FDA points-to-consider documents: The need for dietary control for the reduction of experimental variability within animal assays and the use of dietary restriction to achieve dietary control. *Toxicol Pathol* 24:776–781, 1996.

Allen B, Crump K, Shipp A: Correlation between carcinogenic potency of chemicals in animals and humans. *Risk Anal* 8:531–561, 1988.

Ames BN, Gold LS: Chemical carcinogenesis: Too many rodent carcinogens. *Proc Natl Acad Sci USA* 87:7772–7776, 1990.

Ames BN, Gold LS: Misconceptions on pollution and the causes of cancer. *Angew Chem Int Ed Engl* 29:1197–1208, 1990.

Ames BN, McCann J, Yamasaki E: Methods for detecting carcinogens and mutagens with the *Salmonella*/mammalian-microsome mutagenicity test. *Mutat Res* 31:347–364, 1975.

Ames BN, Shigenaga MK, Gold LS: DNA lesions, inducible DNA repair, and cell division: Three key factors in mutagenesis and carcinogenesis. *Environ Health Perspect* 93:35–44, 1993.

Anderson ME: Tissue dosimetry, physiologically based pharmacokinetic modeling, and cancer risk assessment. *Cell Biol Toxicol,* 5:405–415, 1989.

Anderson ME, Krishnan K, Conolly RB, McClellan RO: Mechanistic toxicology research and biologically based modeling: partners for improving quantitative risk assessments. *Chem Indust Inst Toxicol* 12:1–7, 1992.

Anderson MW, Reynolds SH, You M, Maronpot RM: Role of proto-oncogene activation in carcinogenesis. *Environ Health Perspect* 98:13–24, 1992.

Anderson R, Lefever F, Maurer J: Comparison of the responses of male rats to dietary sodium saccharin exposure initiated during nursing with responses to exposure initiated to weaning. *Food Che Toxicol* 26:899–907, 1988.

Andrews EJ: Evidence of the nonimmune regression of chemically induced papillomas in mouse skin. *J Natl Cancer Inst* 47:653–665, 1971.

Anttila A, Sallmén M, Hemminki K: Carcinogenic chemicals in the occupational environment. *Pharmacol Toxicol* 72:69–76, 1993.

Armitage P, Doll R: The age distribution of cancer and a multi-stage theory of carcinogenesis. *Br J Cancer* 8:1–12, 1954.

Aronheim A, Engelberg D, Li N, et al: Membrane targeting of the nucleotide exchange factor Sos is sufficient for activating the Ras signaling pathway. *Cell* 78:949–961, 1994.

Ashby J: An opinion on the significance of the 19 non-clastogenic gene-mutagens reported by Tennant et al (1987). *Mutagenesis* 3:463–465, 1988.

Ashby J: Origins of current uncertainties in carcinogen/mutagen screening. *Environ Mol Mutagen* 16:51–59, 1989.

Ashby J, Brady A, Elcombe CR, et al: Mechanistically-based human hazard assessment of peroxisome proliferator-induced hepatocarcinogenesis *Human Exp Toxicol* 13:S1–S117, 1994.

Ashby J, Paton D: The influence of chemical structure on the extent and sites of carcinogenesis for 522 rodent carcinogens and 55 different human carcinogen exposures. *Mutat Res* 286:3–74, 1993.

Ashby J, Tennant RW, Zeiger E, Stasiewicz S: Classification according to chemical structure, mutagenicity to *Salmonella* and level of carcinogenicity of a further 42 chemicals tested for carcinogenicity by the U.S. National Toxicology Program. *Mutat Res* 223:73–103, 1989.

Ashendel CL: The phorbol ester receptor: A phospholipid-regulated protein kinase. *Biochim Biophys Acta* 822:219–242, 1985.

Bailleul B, Brown K, Ramsden M, et al: Chemical induction of oncogene mutations and growth factor activity in mouse skin carcinogenesis. *Environ Health Perspect,* 81:23–27, 1989.

Barlow DP: Methylation and imprinting: From host defense to gene regulation? *Science* 260:309–310, 1993.

Barnard JA, Polk WH, Moses HL, Coffey RJ: Production of transforming growth factor-α by normal rat small intestine. *Am J Physiol,* 261:C994–C1000, 1991.

Barr JT: The calculation and use of carcinogenic potency: A review. *Regul Toxicol Pharmacol* 5:432–459, 1985.

Barrett JC, Hesterberg TW, Thomassen DG: Use of cell transformation systems for carcinogenicity testing and mechanistic studies of carcinogenesis. *Pharmacol Rev* 36:53S–70S, 1984.

Barrows GH, Mays ET, Christopherson WM: Steroid related neoplasia in human liver, in Miller RW et al (eds): *Unusual Occurrences as Clues to Cancer Etiology.* Tokyo: Japan Science Society Press/Taylor & Francis, 1988, pp 47–59.

Bartsch H, Hietanen E, Malaveille C.: Carcinogenic nitrosamines: Free radical aspects of their action. *Free Radic Biol Med* 7:637–644, 1989.

Bartsch H, Ohshima H: Endogenous *N*-nitroso compounds: How relevant are they to human cancer? in Rhoads JE, Fortner J (eds): *General Motors Cancer Research Foundation.* Philadelphia: Lippincott, 1989, pp 304–317.

Bartsch H, Ohshima H, Shuker DEG, et al: Exposure of humans to endogenous *N*-nitroso compounds: Implications in cancer etiology. *Mutat Res* 238:255–267, 1990.

Basu AP, Gaylor DW, Chen JJ: Estimating the probability of occurrence of tumor for a rare cancer with zero occurrence in a sample *Regul Toxicol Pharmacol* 23:139–144, 1996.

Bateman AJ: The dominant lethal assay in the mouse, in *Agents and Actions.* Vol 3, No 2. Basel: Birkhäuser Verlag, 1973, pp 73–76.

Bauer-Hofmann R, Klimek F, Buchmann A, et al: Role of mutations at codon 61 of the c-Ha-*ras* gene during diethylnitrosamine-induced hepatocarcinogenesis in C3H/He mice. *Mol Carcinog* 6:60–67, 1992.

Beach AC, Gupta RC: Human biomonitoring and the ^{32}P-postlabeling assay. *Carcinogenesis* 13:1053–1074, 1992.

Beatson GT: On the treatment of inoperable cases of carcinoma of the mamma: Suggestions for a new method of treatment, with illustrative cases. *Lancet* 2:104–107, 1896.

Becker RA, Shank RC: Kinetics of formation and persistence of ethylguanines in DNA of rats and hamsters treated with diethylnitrosamine. *Cancer Res* 45:2076–2084, 1985.

Berenblum I, Shubik P: A new quantitative approach to the study of stages of chemical carcinogenesis in the mouse's skin. *Br J Cancer* 1:383, 1947.

Berger MR: Synergism and antagonism between chemical carcinogens in Arcos JC, Argus MF, Woo YT (eds): *Chemical Induction of Cancer.* Basel: Birkhäuser, 1995, pp 23–49.

Berger MR, Schmähl D, Zerban H: Combination experiments with very low doses of three genotoxic *N*-nitrosamines with similar organotropic carcinogenicity in rats. *Carcinogenesis* 8:1635–1643, 1987.

Bernard C: Leçons sur les phénomènes de la vie. Paris: Baillière, 1878, 1879.

Bessho T, Roy R, Yamamoto K, et al: Repair of 8-hydroxyguanine in DNA by mammalian *N*-methylpurine-DNA glycosylase. *Proc Natl Acad Sci, USA* 90:8901–8904, 1993.

Bhide SV, Shivapurkar NM, Gothoskar SV, Ranadive KJ: Carcinogenicity of betal quid ingredients: Feeding mice with aqueous extract and the polyphenol fraction of betel nut. *Br J Cancer* 40:922–926, 1979.

Biaglow JE: The effects of ionizing radiation on mammalian cells. *J Chem Educ,* 58:144–156, 1981.

Bichara M, Fuchs RPP: DNA binding and mutation spectra of the carcinogen *N*-2-aminofluorene in *Escherichia coli:* A correlation between the conformation of the premutagenic lesion and the mutation specificity. *J Mol Biol* 183:341–351, 1985.

Bishop JM: Viral oncogenes. *Cell* 42:23–38, 1985.

Biskind MS, Biskind GR: Development of tumors in the rat ovary after transplantation into the spleen. *Proc Soc Exp Biol Med* 55:176–179, 1944.

Bittner JJ: Mammary cancer in C3H mice of different sublines and their hybrids. *J Natl Cancer Inst* 16:1263–1286, 1956.

Blackburn EH: Telomeres: No end in sight. *Cell* 77:621–623, 1994.

Blair EH, Hoerger FD: Risk/benefit analysis as viewed by the chemical industry. Ann NY Acad Sci 329:253–262, 1979.

Blayney DW, Longo DL, Young RC, et al: Decreasing risk of leukemia with prolonged follow-up after chemotherapy and radiotherapy for Hodgkin's disease. *N Engl J Med* 316:710–714, 1987.

Blot WJ: Alcohol and cancer. *Cancer Res* 52:2119s–2123s, 1992.

Blot WJ, Li JY, Taylor PR, et al: Nutrition intervention trials in Linxian, China: Supplementation with specific vitamin/mineral combinations, cancer incidence, and disease-specific mortality in the general population. *J Natl Cancer Inst* 85:1483–1492, 1993.

Bogen KT: Cancer potencies of heterocyclic amines found in cooked foods. *Food Chem Toxicol* 32:505–515, 1994.

Böhm SK, Grady EF, Bunnett NW: Regulatory mechanisms that modulate signalling by G-protein-coupled receptors. *Biochem J* 322:1–18, 1997.

Bohr VA, Phillips DH, Hanawalt PC: Heterogeneous DNA damage and repair in the mammalian genome. Cancer Res 47:6426–6436, 1987.

Bolt HM: Roles of etheno-DNA adducts in tumorigenicity of olefins. *CRC Crit Rev Toxicol* 18:299–309, 1988.

Bolt HM, Peter H, Föst U: Analysis of macromolecular ethylene oxide adducts. *Int Arch Occup Environ Health* 60:141–144, 1988.

Bond GG, Rossbacher R: A review of potential human carcinogenicity of the chlorophenoxy herbicides MCPA, MCPP, and 2,4-DP. *Br J Indust Med* 50:340–348, 1993.

Bosland MC, Dreef-Van Der Meulen HC, Sukumar S, et al: Multistage prostate carcinogenesis: The role of hormones. *Int Symp Princess Takamatsu Cancer Res Fund* 22:109–123, 1991.

Boutwell RK: Caloric intake, dietary fat level, and experimental carcinogenesis, in Jacobs MN (ed): *Exercise, Calories, Fat, and Cancer*. New York: Plenum Press, 1992.

Boutwell RK: Function and mechanism of promoters of carcinogenesis. *CRC Crit Rev Toxicol,* 2:419–443, 1974.

Boutwell RK: Some biological aspects of skin carcinogenesis. *Progr Exp Tumor Res* 4:207–250, 1964.

Boveri T: Zur Frage der Enstebung maligner Tumorgen. Jena: Fischer, 1914.

Boyd JA, Barrett JC: Genetic and cellular basis of multistep carcinogenesis. *Pharmacol Ther* 46:469–486, 1990.

Boyland E: The biological significance of metabolism of polycyclic compounds. *Biochem Soc Symp* 5:40–54, 1950.

Brambilla G, Carlo P, Finollo R, et al: Viscometric detection of liver DNA fragmentation in rats treated with minimal doses of chemical carcinogens. *Cancer Re* 43:202–209, 1983.

Brand KG, Buoen LC, Johnson KH, Brand I: Etiological factors, stages, and the role of the foreign body in foreign body tumorigenesis: A review. *Cancer Res* 35:279–286, 1975.

Bronner CE, Baker SM, Morrison PT, et al: Mutation in the DNA mismatch repair gene homologue *hMLH 1* is associated with hereditary non-polyposis colon cancer. *Nature* 368:258–261, 1994.

Bryant MS, Skipper PL, Tannenbaum SR, MacLure M: Hemoglobin adducts of 4-aminobiphenyl in smokers and nonsmokers. *Cancer Res* 47:602–608, 1987.

Burns FJ, Vanderlaan M, Snyder E, Albert RE: Induction and progression kinetics of mouse skin papillomas, in Slaga TJ, Sivak A, Boutwell RK (eds): *Carcinogenesis.* Vol 2. *Mechanism of Tumor Promotion and Cocarcinogenesis*. New York: Raven Press, 1978, pp 91–96.

Butlin HJ: Three lectures on cancer of the scrotum in chimney-sweeps and others: I. Secondary cancer without primary cancer: II. Why foreign sweeps do not suffer from scrotal cancer. III. Tar and paraffin cancer. *Br Med J* 1:1341–1346, 1892; 2:1–6, 66–71, 1892.

Butterworth BE: Chemically induced cell proliferation as a predictive assay for potential carcinogenicity, in *Chemically Induced Cell Proliferation: Implications for Risk Assessment*. New York: Wiley-Liss, 1991, pp 457–467.

Byers T, Perry G: Dietary carotenes, vitamin C, and vitamin E as protective antioxidants in human cancers. *Annu Rev Nutr* 12:139–159, 1992.

Campbell TC: Chemical carcinogens and human risk assessment. *Fed Proc* 39:2467–2484, 1980.

Candrian U, You M, Goodrow T, et al: Activation of protooncogenes in spontaneously occurring non-liver tumors from C57BL/6 × C3H F_1 mice. *Cancer Res* 51:1148–1153, 1991.

Carmichael NG, Enzmann H, Pate I, Waechter F: The significance of mouse liver tumor formation for carcinogenic risk assessment: Results and conclusions from a survey of ten years of testing by the agrochemical industry. *Environ Health Perspect* 105:1196–1203, 1997.

Carter JH, Carter HW, Meade J: Adrenal regulation of mammary tumorigenesis in female Sprague-Dawley rats: Incidence, latency, and yield of mammary tumors. *Cancer Res* 48:3801–3807, 1988.

Cassee FR, Groten JP, van Bladeren PJ, Feron VJ: Toxicological evaluation and risk assessment of chemical mixtures. *Crit Rev Toxicol* 28:73–101, 1998.

Cattley RC, Popp JA: Differences between the promoting activities of the peroxisome proliferator WY-14,643 and phenobarbital in rat liver. *Cancer Res* 49:3246–3251, 1989.

Cavalieri EL, Rogan EG: The approach to understanding aromatic hydrocarbon carcinogenesis: The central role of radical cations in metabolic activation. *Pharmacol Ther* 55:183–199, 1992.

Cerny WL, Mangold KA, Scarpelli DG: K-*ras* mutation is an early event in pancreatic duct carcinogenesis in the Syrian golden hamster. *Cancer Res* 52:4507–4513, 1992.

Cerutti PA, Trump BF: Inflammation and oxidative stress in carcinogenesis. *Cancer Cells* 3:1–6, 1991.

Cha RS, Thilly WG, Zarbl H: *N*-Nitroso-*N*-methylurea-induced rat mammary tumors arise from cells with preexisting oncogenic *Hras1* gene mutations. *Proc Natl Acad Sci USA,* 91:3749–3753, 1994.

Chandra RS, Kapur SP, Kelleher J, et al: Benign hepatocellular tumors in the young. *Arch Pathol Lab Med* 108:168–171, 1984.

Cheng KC, Loeb LA: Genomic instability and tumor progression: Mechanistic considerations. *Adv Cancer Res* 60:121–156, 1993.

Choy WN: Principles of genetic toxicology, in Fan AM, Chang LW (eds): *Toxicology and Risk Assessment: Principles, Methods, and Applications.* New York: Marcel Dekker, 1996, pp 25–36.

Chu KC, Cueto C Jr, Ward JM: Factors in the evaluation of 200 National Cancer Institute carcinogen bioassays. *J Toxicol Environ Health* 8:251–280, 1981.

Chung FL, Chen HJC, Nath RG: Lipid peroxidation as a potential endogenous source for the formation of exocyclic DNA adducts. *Carcinogenesis* 17:2105–2111, 1996.

Clemens MR: Free radicals in chemical carcinogenesis. *Klin Wochenschr* 69:1123–1134, 1991.

Clifton KH, Sridharan BN: Endocrine factors and tumor growth, in Becker FF (ed): *Cancer—A Comprehensive Treatise,* Vol 3. New York: Plenum Press, 1975, pp 249–285.

Cohen LA, Kendall ME, Zang E, et al: Modulation of *N*-nitrosomethylurea-induced mammary tumor promotion by dietary fiber and fat. *J Natl Cancer Inst* 83:496–501, 1991.

Cohen SM, Ellwein LB: Genetic errors, cell proliferation, and carcinogenesis. *Cancer Res* 51:6493–6505, 1991.

Cohen SM, Lawson TA: Rodent bladder tumors do not always predict for humans. *Cancer Lett* 93:9–16, 1995.

Columbano A, Rajalakshmi S, Sarma DSR: Requirement of cell proliferation for the initiation of liver carcinogenesis as assayed by three different procedures. *Cancer Res* 41:2079–2083, 1981.

Conaway CC, Nie G, Hussain NS, Fiala ES: Comparison of oxidative damage to rat liver DNA and RNA by primary nitroalkanes, secondary nitroalkanes, cyclopentanone oxime, and related compounds. *Cancer Res* 51:3143–3147, 1991.

Conney AH: Induction of microsomal enzymes by foreign chemicals and carcinogenesis by polycyclic aromatic hydrocarbons: GHA Clowes Memorial Lecture. *Cancer Res* 42:4875–4917, 1982.

Connolly JG, White EP: Malignant cells in the urine of men exposed to beta-naphthylamine. *Can Med Assoc J* 100:879–882, 1969.

Cooper WC: Epidemiologic study of vinyl chloride workers: Mortality through December 31, 1972. *Environ Health Perspect* 41:101–106, 1981.

Craighead JE: Asbestos-associated diseases. *Arch Pathol Lab Med* 106:542–597, 1982.

Crouch E, Wilson R: Interspecies comparison of carcinogenic potency. *J Toxicol Environ Health* 5:1095–1118, 1979.

Cullen MR, Cherniack MG, Rosenstock L: Occupational medicine. *N Engl J Med* 322:675–682, 1990.

Cutler NR, Sramek JJ, Greenblatt DJ, et al: Defining the maximum tolerated dose: Investigator, academic, industry and regulatory perspectives. *J Clin Pharmacol* 37:767–783, 1997.

Dannaher CL, Tamburro CH, Yam LT: Occupational carcinogenesis: The Louisville experience with vinyl chloride-associated hepatic angiosarcoma. *Am J Med* 70:279–287, 1981.

Dass, SB, Bucci TJ Heflich RH, Casciano DA: Evaluation of the transgenic $p53^{+/-}$ mouse for detecting genotoxic liver carcinogens in a short-term bioassay. *Cancer Lett* 143:81–85, 1999.

de Boer JG, Erfle H, Holcroft J, et al: Spontaneous mutants recovered from liver and germ cell tissue of low copy number *lac*I transgenic rats. *Mutat Res* 352:73–78, 1996.

de Boer JG, Provost S, Gorelick N, et al: Spontaneous mutation in *lacI* transgenic mice: A comparison of tissues. *Mutagenesis* 13:109–114, 1998.

Demple B, Harrison L: Repair of oxidative damage to DNA: Enzymology and biology. *Annu Rev Biochem* 63:915–948, 1994.

Dietrich DR, Swenberg JA: The presence of α_{2u}-globulin is necessary for d-Limonene promotion of male rat kidney tumors. *Cancer Res* 51:3512–3521, 1991.

DiGiovanni J: Multistage carcinogenesis in mouse skin. *Pharmacol Ther* 54:63–128, 1992.

Dipple A, Michejda CJ, Weisburger EK: Metabolism of chemical carcinogens. *Pharm Ther* 27:265–296, 1985.

Doll R, Peto R: *The Causes of Cancer.* New York: Oxford University Press, 1981.

Dominick MA, Robertson DG, Bleavins MR, et al: α_{2u}-Globulin nephropathy without nephrocarcinogenesis in male Wistar rats administered 1-(aminomethyl)cyclohexaneacetic acid. *Toxicol Appl Pharmacol* 111:375–387, 1991.

Donehower LA: The p53-deficient mouse: A model for basic and applied cancer studies. *Semin Cancer Biol* 7:269–278, 1996.

Dragan Y, Klaunig J, Maronpot R, Goldsworthy T: Mechanisms of susceptibility to mouse liver carcinogenesis. *Toxicol Sci* 41:3–7, 1998.

Dragan YP, Hully JR, Nakamura J, et al: Biochemical events during initiation of rat hepatocarcinogenesis. *Carcinogenesis* 15:1451–1458, 1994.

Dragan YP, Pitot HC: Aflatoxin carcinogenesis in the context of the multistage nature of cancer, in *The Toxicology of Aflatoxins: Human Health, Veterinary, and Agricultural Significance.* New York: Academic Press, 1994, pp 179–206.

Druckrey H: Quantitative aspects in chemical carcinogenesis, in Truhant R, (ed): *Potential Carcinogenic Hazards from Drugs. Evaluation of Risks.* UICC Monograph Series. Vol 7. Berlin: Springer-Verlag, 1967, pp 60–77.

Druckrey H, Schmähl D, Dischler W: Dosis-Wirkungs-Beziehungen bei der Krebserzeugung durch 4-Dimethylamino-stilben bei Ratten. *Z Krebsforsch* 65:272–288, 1963.

DuFrain RJ, McFee AF, Linkous S, et al: In vivo SCE analysis using bromodeoxyuridine, iododeoxyuridine, and chlorodeoxyuridine. *Mutat Res* 139:57–60, 1984.

Dulic V, Kaufmann WK, Wilson SJ, et al: p53-Dependent inhibition of cyclin-dependent kinase activities in human fibroblasts during radiation-induced G1 arrest. *Cell* 76:1013–1023, 1994.

Dunham LJ: Cancer in man at site of prior benign lesion of skin or mucous membrane: A review. *Cancer Res* 32:1359–1374, 1972.

Dunkel VC, Rogers C, Swierenga SHH, et al: Recommended protocols based on a survey of current practice in genotoxicity testing laboratories: III. Cell transformation in C3H/10T1/2 mouse embryo cell, BALB/c 3T3 mouse fibroblast and Syrian hamster embryo cell cultures. *Mutat Res* 246:285–300, 1991.

Dunnick JK, Elwell MR, Huff J, Barrett JC: Chemically induced mammary gland cancer in the National Toxicology Program's carcinogenesis bioassay. *Carcinogenesis* 16:173–179, 1995.

Dybing E, Sanner T, Roelfzema H, et al: T25: A simplified carcinogenic potency index: Description of the system and study of correlations between carcinogenic potency and species/site specificity and mutagenicity. *Pharmacol Toxicol* 80:272–279, 1997.

Dycaico MJ, Stuart GR, Tobal GM, et al: Species-specific differences in hepatic mutant frequency and mutational spectrum among lambda/*lacI* transgenic rats and mice following exposure to aflatoxin B_1. *Carcinogenesis* 17:2347–2356, 1996.

Eastman A, Barry MA: The origins of DNA breaks: A consequence of DNA damage, DNA repair, or apoptosis? *Cancer Invest* 10:229–240, 1992.

Eaton DL, Groopman JD, eds: *The Toxicology of Aflatoxins—Human Health, Veterinary, and Agricultural Significance.* San Diego, CA: Academic Press, 1994.

Eling TE, Thompson DC, Foureman GL, et al: Prostaglandin H synthase and xenobiotic oxidation. *Annu Rev Pharmacol Toxicol* 30:1–45, 1990.

Emerit I, Khan SH, Esterbauer H: Hydroxynonenal, a component of clastogenic factors? *Free Radic Biol Med* 10:371–377, 1991.

Enslein K, Gombar VK, Blake B: Use of SAR in computer-assisted prediction of carcinogenicity and mutagenicity of chemicals by the *TOPKAT* program. *Mutat Res* 305:47–61, 1994.

Essigmann JM, Wood ML: The relationship between the chemical structures and mutagenic specificities of the DNA lesions formed by chemical and physical mutagens. *Toxicol Lett* 67:29–39, 1993.

Farber E: Ethionine carcinogenesis. *Adv Cancer Res* 7:383–474, 1963.

Fearon ER, Vogelstein B: A genetic model for colorectal tumorigenesis. *Cell* 61:759–761, 1992.

Featherstone C, Jackson SP: Ku, a DNA repair protein with multiple cellular functions? Mutat Res 434:3–15, 1999.

Feig LA: Guanine-nucleotide exchange factors: A family of positive regulators of Ras and related GTPases. *Curr Opin Cell Biol* 6:204–211, 1994.

Ferguson DJ: Cellular attachment to implanted foreign bodies in relation to tumorigenesis. *Cancer Res* 37:4367–4371, 1977.

Feron VJ, Cassee FR, Groten JP: Toxicology of chemical mixtures: international perspective. *Environ Health Perspect* 106:1281–1289, 1998.

Fingerhut MA, Halperin WE, Marlow DA, et al: Cancer mortality in workers exposed to 2,3,7,8-tetrachlorodibenzo-*p*-dioxin. *N Engl J Med* 324:212–218, 1991.

Fischer B, Constantino JP, Redmond CK, et al: Endometrial cancer in tamoxifen-treated breast cancer patients: Findings from the National Surgical Adjuvant Breast and Bowel Project (NSABP) B-14. *J Natl Cancer Inst* 86:527–537, 1994.

Fishel R, Kolodner RD: Identification of mismatch repair genes and their role in the development of cancer. *Curr Opin Genet Dev* 5:382–395, 1995.

Fishel R, Wilson T: MutS homologs in mammalian cells. *Curr Opin Genet Dev* 7:105–113, 1997.

Floyd RA: Free-radical events in chemical and biochemical reactions involving carcinogenic arylamines. *Radiat Res* 86:243–263, 1981.

Floyd RA: Role of oxygen free radicals in carcinogenesis and brain ischemia. *FASEB J* 4:2587–2597, 1990.

Foran JA, Cox M, Croxton D: Sport fish consumption advisories and projected cancer risks in the Great Lakes basin. *Am J Public Health* 79:322–325, 1989.

Foulds L: Multiple etiologic factors in neoplastic development. *Cancer Res* 25:1339–1347, 1965.

Foulds L: The experimental study of tumor progression: A review. *Cancer Res* 14:327–339, 1954.

Freedman LS, Clifford C, Messina M: Analysis of dietary fat, calories, body weight, and the development of mammary tumors in rats and mice: A review. *Cancer Res* 50:5710–5719, 1990.

Friedberg EC: DNA repair: Looking back and peering forward. *Bioessays* 16:645–649, 1994.

Friedberg EC: Xeroderma pigmentosum, Cockayne's syndrome, helicases, and DNA repair: What's the relationship? *Cell* 71:887–889, 1992.

Fry RJM, Ley RD, Grube D, Staffeldt E: Studies on the multistage nature of radiation carcinogenesis, in Hecker E, Fusenig NE, Kunz W, et al (eds): *Carcinogenesis—A Comprehensive Survey.* Vol 7. *Cocarcinogenesis and Biological Effects of Tumor Promoters.* New York: Raven Press, 1982, pp 155–165.

Fujii K: Evaluation of the newborn mouse model for chemical tumorigenesis. *Carcinogenesis* 12:1409–1415, 1991.

Fujiki H, Suganuma M: Tumor promotion by inhibitors of protein phosphatases 1 and 2A: The okadaic acid class of compounds. *Adv Cancer Res* 61:143–194, 1993.

Fung VA, Huff J, Weisburger EK, Hoel DG: Predictive strategies for selecting 379 NCI/NTP chemicals evaluated for carcinogenic potential: Scientific and public health impact. *Fundam Appl Toxicol* 20:413–436, 1993.

Furihata C, Matsushima T: Use of in vivo/in vitro unscheduled DNA synthesis for identification of organ-specific carcinogens. *CRC Crit Rev Toxicol* 17:245–277, 1987.

Furth J: A meeting of ways in cancer research: Thoughts on the evolution and nature of neoplasms. *Cancer Res* 19:241–256, 1959.

Furth J: Hormones as etiological agents in neoplasia, in Becker FF (ed): *Cancer—A Comprehensive Treatise*. Vol 1. New York: Plenum Press, 1975, pp 75–120.

Futreal PA, Liu Q, Shattuck-Eidens D, et al: *BRCA1* mutations in primary breast and ovarian carcinomas. *Science* 266:120–122, 1994.

Galloway SM, Bloom AD, Resnick M, et al: Development of a standard protocol for in vitro cytogenesis testing with Chinese hamster ovary cells: Comparison of results for 22 compounds in two laboratories. *Environ Mutagen 7:*1–51, 1985.

Gambrell RD Jr: Cancer and the use of estrogens. *Int J Fertil* 31:112–122, 1986.

Garrett CT: Oncogenes. *Clin Chim Acta* 156:1–40, 1986.

Garro AJ, Lieber CS: Alcohol and cancer. *Annu Rev Pharmacol Toxicol* 30:219–249, 1990.

Gaylor DW, Shapiro RE: Extrapolation and risk estimation for carcinogenesis. *Adv Med Toxicol* 1:65–87, 1979.

Gebhart E: Sister chromatid exchange (SCE) and structural chromosome aberration in mutagenicity testing. *Hum Genet* 58:235–254, 1981.

Generoso WM, Bishop JB, Gosslee DG, et al: Heritable translocation test in mice. *Mutat Res* 76:191–215, 1980.

Ghia M, Mattioli F, Mereto E: A possible medium-term assay for detecting the effects of liver and colon carcinogens in rats. *Cancer Lett* 105:71–75, 1996.

Ghoshal AK, Farber E: The induction of liver cancer by dietary deficiency of choline and methionine without added carcinogens. *Carcinogenesis* 5:1367–1370, 1984.

Gille JJP, van Berkel CGM, Joenje H: Mechanism of hyperoxia-induced chromosomal breakage in Chinese hamster cells. *Environ Mol Mutagen* 22:264–270, 1993.

Glass LR, Easterly CE, Jones TD, Walsh PJ: Ranking of carcinogenic potency using a relative potency approach. *Arch Environ Contam Toxicol* 21:169–176, 1991.

Glauert HP, Schwarz M, Pitot HC: The phenotypic stability of altered hepatic foci: Effect of the short-term withdrawal of phenobarbital and of the long-term feeding of purified diets after the withdrawal of phenobarbital. *Carcinogenesis* 7:117–121, 1986.

Gold LS, Bernstein L, Magaw R, Slone TH: Interspecies extrapolation in carcinogenesis: Prediction between rats and mice *Environ Health Perspect* 81:211–219, 1989.

Gold LS, Manley NB, Slone TH, Garfinkel, GB, et al: The fifth plot of the carcinogenic potency database: Results of animal bioassays published in the general literature through 1988 and by the National Toxicology Program through 1989. *Environ Health Perspect* 100:65–135, 1993.

Gold LS, Slone TH, Ames BN: What do animal cancer tests tell us about human cancer risk? Overview of analyses of the carcinogenic potency database. *Drug Metab Rev* 30:359–404, 1998.

Gold LS, Slone TH, Manley NB, Ames BN: Heterocyclic amines formed by cooking food: Comparison of bioassay results with other chemicals in the Carcinogenic Potency Database. *Cancer Lett* 83:21–29, 1994.

Gold LS, Zeiger E (eds): *Handbook of Carcinogenic Potency and Genotoxicity Databases.* Boca Raton, FL: CRC Press, 1997.

Goldfarb S: Sex hormones and hepatic neoplasia. *Cancer Res* 36:2584–2588, 1976.

Goldstein JA, Faletto MB: Advances in mechanisms of activation and deactivation of environmental chemicals. *Environ Health Perspect* 100:169–176, 1993.

Goldsworthy TL, Recio L, Brown K, et al: Transgenic animals in toxicology. *Fundam Appl Toxicol* 22:8–19, 1994.

Gondo Y, Shioyama Y, Nakao K, Katsuki M: A novel positive detection system of in vivo mutations in *rpsL (strA)* transgenic mice. *Mutat Res* 360:1–14, 1996.

Gorchev HG, Jelinek CF: A review of the dietary intakes of chemical contaminants. *Bull WHO* 63:945–962, 1985.

Goth R, Rajewsky MF: Persistence of O^6-ethylguanine in rat-brain DNA: Correlation with nervous system-specific carcinogenesis by ethylnitrosourea. *Proc Natl Acad Sci USA* 71:639–643, 1974.

Grasso P, Hinton RH: Evidence for and possible mechanisms of nongenotoxic carcinogenesis in rodent liver. *Mutat Res* 248:271–290, 1991.

Green C, Diffey BL, Hawk JLM: Ultraviolet radiation in the treatment of skin disease. *Phys Med Biol* 37:1–20, 1992.

Griffith RW: Carcinogenic potential of marketed drugs. *J Clin Res Drug Dev* 2:141–144, 1988.

Guengerich FP: Metabolic activation of carcinogens. *Pharm Ther* 54:17–61, 1992.

Gupta RC, Reddy MV, Randerath K: ^{32}P-postlabeling analysis of nonradioactive aromatic carcinogen-DNA adducts. *Carcinogenesis* 3:1081–1092, 1982.

Guyton KZ, Kensler TW: Oxidative mechanisms in carcinogenesis. *Br Med Bull* 49:523–544, 1993.

Habs M, Schmähl D: Diet and cancer. *J Cancer Res Clin Oncol* 96:1–10, 1980.

Hadidian Z, Fredrickson TN, Weisburger EK, et al: Tests for chemical carcinogens. Report on the activity of derivatives of aromatic amines, nitrosamines, quinolines, nitroalkanes, amides, epoxides, aziridines, and purine antimetabolites. *J Natl Cancer Inst* 41:985–1036, 1968.

Hall A: A biochemical function for ras at last. *Science* 264:1413–1414, 1994.

Hall TW: Environmental regulation: An international view. I. Britain. *Chem Soc Rev* 5:431–440, 1976.

Hanahan D, Weinberg RA: The hallmarks of cancer. *Cell* 100:57–70, 2000.

Hanawalt PC: Transcription-coupled repair and human disease. *Science* 266:1957–1958, 1994.

Hanes B, Wedel T: A selected review of risk models: One hit, multihit, multistage, probit, Weibull, and pharmacokinetic. *J Am Coll Toxicol* 4:271–278, 1985.

Hanigan MH, Pitot HC: Growth of carcinogen-altered rat hepatocytes in the liver of syngeneic recipients promoted with phenobarbital. *Cancer Res* 45:6063–6070, 1985.

Hansen C, Asmussen I, Autrup H: Detection of carcinogen-DNA adducts in human fetal tissues by the ^{32}P-postlabeling procedure. *Environ Health Perspect* 99:229–231, 1993.

Harbach PR, Rostami HJ, Aaron CS, et al: Evaluation of four methods for scoring cytoplasmic grains in the in vitro unscheduled DNA synthesis (UDS) assay. *Mutat Res* 252:139–148, 1991.

Hardell L, Eriksson M, Degerman A: Exposure to phenoxyacetic acids, chlorophenols, or organic solvents in relation to histopathology, stage, and anatomical localization of non-Hodgkin's lymphoma. *Cancer Res* 54:2386–2389, 1994.

Harris CC: Chemical and physical carcinogenesis: Advances and perspectives for the 1990s. *Cancer Res* 51:5023s–5044s, 1991.

Harvey RG: Activated metabolites of carcinogenic hydrocarbons. *Acc Chem Res* 14:218–226, 1981.

Haseman JK, Boorman GA, Huff J: Value of historical control data and other issues related to the evaluation of long-term rodent carcinogenicity studies. *Toxicol Pathol* 25:524–527, 1997.

Haseman JK, Lockhart A: The relationship between use of the maximum tolerated dose and study sensitivity for detecting rodent carcinogenicity. *Fundam Appl Toxicol* 22:382–391, 1994.

Hathway DE, Kolar GF: Mechanisms of reaction between ultimate chemical carcinogens and nucleic acid. *Chem Soc Rev* 9:241–253, 1980.

Hattori A, Kunz HW, Gill TJ III, et al: Diversity of the promoting action of cyclosporine on the induction of murine lymphoid tumors. *Carcinogenesis* 9:1091–1094, 1988.

Hecht SS: Chemical carcinogenesis: An overview. *Clin Physiol Biochem* 3:89–97, 1985.

Heddle JA, Hite M, Kirkhart B, et al: The induction of micronuclei as a measure of genotoxicity. A report of the U.S. Environmental Protection Agency Gene-Tox Program. *Mutat Res* 123:61–118, 1983.

Hegi ME, Ulrich D, Sagelsdorff P, Richter C, Lutz WK: No measurable increase in thymidine glycol or 8-hydroxydeoxyguanosine in liver DNA of rats treated with nafenopin or choline-devoid low-methionine diet. *Mutat Res* 238:325–329, 1990.

Heidelberger C: Chemical carcinogenesis, chemotherapy: Cancer's continuing core challenges. GHA Clowes Memorial Lecture. *Cancer Res* 30:1549–1569, 1970.

Heim S, Mandahl N, Mitelman F: Genetic convergence and divergence in tumor progression. *Cancer Res* 48:5911–5916, 1988.

Henderson BE, Ross R, Bernstein L: Estrogens as a cause of human cancer: The Richard and Hinda Rosenthal Foundation Award Lecture. *Cancer Res* 48:246–253, 1988.

Henderson BE, Ross RK, Pike MC, Casagrande JT: Endogenous hormones as a major factor in human cancer. *Cancer Res* 42:3232–3239, 1982.

Hendrich S, Campbell HA, Pitot HC: Quantitative stereological evaluation of four histochemical markers of altered foci in multistage hepatocarcinogenesis in the rat. *Carcinogenesis* 8:1245–1250, 1987.

Hendricks JD, Wales JH, Sinnhuber RO, et al: Rainbow trout (*Salmo gairdneri*) embryos: A sensitive animal model for experimental carcinogenesis. *Fed Proc* 39:3222–3229, 1980.

Hennings H, Glick AB, Greenhalgh DA, et al: Critical aspects of initiation, promotion, and progression in multistage epidermal carcinogenesis. *Proc Soc Exp Biol Med* 202:1–18, 1993.

Henson DE, Albores-Saavedra J: *The Pathology of Incipient Neoplasia.* Philadelphia: Saunders, 1986.

Herbst AL: Clear cell adenocarcinoma and the current status of DES-exposed females. *Cancer* 48:484–488, 1981.

Heyne KH, Lippman SM, Lee JJ, et al: The incidence of second primary tumors in long-term survivors of small-cell lung cancer. *J Clin Oncol* 10:1519–1524, 1992.

Hicks RM: Multistage carcinogenesis in the urinary bladder. *Br Med Bull* 36:39–46, 1980.

Hicks RM, Wakefield J St J, Chowaniec J: Evaluation of a new model to detect bladder carcinogens or co-carcinogens, results obtained with saccharin, cyclamate and cyclophosphamide. *Chem Biol Interact* 11:225–233, 1975.

Hill J: *Cautions Against the Immoderate Use of Snuff,* 2d ed. London, 1761.

Hirono I: Edible plants containing naturally occurring carcinogens in Japan. *Jpn J Cancer Res* 84:997–1006, 1993.

Hogg N, Kalyanaraman B: Nitric oxide and lipid peroxidation. *Biochim Biophys Acta* 1411:378–384, 1999.

Holliday R: A different kind of inheritance. *Sci Am* 260:60–73, 1989.

Hoover DM, Best KL, McKenney BK, et al: Experimental induction of neoplasia in the accessory sex organs of male Lobund-Wistar rats. *Cancer Res* 50:142–146, 1990.

Hoover R, Fraumeni JF Jr: Drug-induced cancer. *Cancer* 47:1071–1080, 1981.

Hottendorf GH, Pachter IJ: Review and evaluation of the NCI/NTP carcinogenesis bioassays. *Toxicol Pathol* 13:141–146, 1985.

Hsieh LL, Hsieh T: Detection of aflatoxin B1-DNA adducts in human placenta and cord blood. *Cancer Res* 53:1278–1280, 1993.

Hueper WC, Wiley FH, Wolfe HD: Experimental production of bladder tumors in dogs by administration of beta-naphthylamine. *J Ind Hyg Toxicol* 20:46–84, 1938.

Huh NH, Satoh MS, Shiga J, et al: Immunoanalytical detection of O^4-ethylthymine in liver DNA of individuals with or without malignant tumors. *Cancer Res* 49:93–97, 1989.

Hunter T: Cooperation between oncogenes. *Cell* 64:249–270, 1991.

Huseby RA: Demonstration of a direct carcinogenic effect of estradiol on Leydig cells of the mouse. *Cancer Res* 40:1006–1013, 1980.

IARC Monographs on the Evaluation of Carcinogenic Risks to Humans: Alcohol Drinking. International Agency for Research on Cancer, Lyons, France, 44:101–105, 1987.

Iball J: The relative potency of carcinogenic compounds. *Am J Cancer* 35:188–190, 1939.

Ip C, Yip P, Bernardis LL: Role of prolactin in the promotion of dimethylbenz[*a*]anthracene-induced mammary tumors by dietary fat. *Cancer Res* 40:374–378, 1980.

Isfort RJ, Kerckaert GA, LeBoeuf RA: Comparison of the standard and reduced pH Syrian hamster embryo (SHE) cell in vitro transformation assays in predicting the carcinogenic potential of chemicals. *Mutat Res* 356:11–63, 1996.

Ishidate M Jr, Harnois MC, Sofuni T: A comparative analysis of data on the clastogenicity of 951 chemical substances tested in mammalian cell cultures. *Mutat Res* 195:151–213, 1988.

Issemann I, Green S: Activation of a member of the steroid hormone receptor superfamily by peroxisome proliferators. *Nature* 347:645–650, 1990.

Ito Y, Fujie K, Matsuda S, et al: Long-Evans A and C rat strains susceptible to clastogenic effects of chemicals in the bone marrow cells. *Jpn J Cancer Res* 85:26–31, 1994.

Ito N, Fukushima S: Promotion of urinary bladder carcinogenesis in experimental animals. *Exp Pathol* 36:1–15, 1989.

Ito N, Hasegawa R, Imaida K, et al: Effects of ingestion of 20 pesticides in combination at acceptable daily intake levels on rat liver carcinogenesis. *Food Chem Toxicol* 33:159–163, 1995.

Ito N, Hasegawa R, Imaida K, et al: Medium-term liver and multi-organ carcinogenesis bioassays for carcinogens and chemopreventive agents. *Exp Toxic Pathol* 48:113–119, 1996.

Ito N, Imaida K, Hasegawa R, Tsuda H: Rapid bioassay methods for carcinogens and modifiers of hepatocarcinogenesis. *CRC Crit Rev Toxicol* 19:385–415, 1989.

Ito N, Imaida K, Hirose M, Shirai T: Medium-term bioassays for carcinogenicity of chemical mixtures. *Environ Health Perspect* 106:1331–1336, 1998.

Janknecht R, Cahill MA, Nordheim A: Signal integration at the c-*fos* promoter. *Carcinogenesis* 16:443–450, 1995.

Jass JR, Stewart SM, Stewart J, Lane MR: Hereditary non-polyposis colorectal cancer—Morphologies, genes and mutations. *Mutat Res* 310:125–133, 1994.

Jensen H, Madsen JL: Diet and cancer. *Acta Med Scand* 223:293–304, 1988.

Jerina DM, Daly JW, Witkop B, et al: 1,2-Naphthalene oxide as an intermediate in the microsomal hydroxylation of naphthalene. *Biochemistry* 9:147–156, 1970.

Jiricny J: Replication errors: cha(lle)nging the genome. *EMBO J* 17:6427–6436, 1998.

Johnson ES: Human exposure to 2,3,7,8-TCDD and risk of cancer. *Crit Rev Toxicol* 21:451–462, 1992.

Johnson KH, Buoen LC, Brand I, Brand KG: Polymer tumorigenesis: Clonal determination of histopathological characteristics during early preneoplasia, relationships to karyotype, mouse strain, and sex. *J Natl Cancer Inst* 44:785–793, 1970.

Johnson SP: Environmental regulation: An international view. II. European economic community. *Chem Soc Rev* 5:441–451, 1976.

Kadlubar FF, Anson JF, Dooley KL, Beland FA: Formation of urothelial and hepatic DNA adducts from the carcinogen 2-naphthylamine. *Carcinogenesis* 2:467–470, 1981.

Kakiuchi H, Ushijima T, Ochiai M, et al: Rare frequency of activation of the Ki-*ras* gene in rat colon tumors induced by heterocyclic amines:

Possible alternative mechanisms of human colon carcinogenesis. *Mol Carcinogen* 8:44–48, 1993.

Kakunaga T: The role of cell division in the malignant transformation of mouse cells treated with 3-methylcholanthrene. *Cancer Res* 35:1637–1642, 1975.

Kasai H, Okada Y, Nishimura S, et al: Formation of 8-hydroxydeoxyguanosine in liver DNA of rats following long-term exposure to a peroxisome proliferator. *Cancer Res* 49:2603–2605, 1989.

Kaufmann WK: Pathways of human cell post-replication repair. *Carcinogenesis* 10:1–11, 1989.

Kawashima S, Wakabayashi K, Nishizuka Y: Low incidence of nodular hyperplasia of the adrenal cortex after ovariectomy in neonatally estrogenized mice than in the controls. *Proc Japan Acad* 56:350–354, 1980.

Keenan KP, Laroque P, Ballam G, et al: The effects of diet, *ad libitum* overfeeding, and moderate dietary restriction on the rodent bioassay: The uncontrolled variable in safety assessment. *Toxicol Pathol* 24:757–768, 1996.

Kemp CJ, Leary CN, Drinkwater NR: Promotion of murine hepatocarcinogenesis by testosterone is androgen receptor-dependent but not cell autonomous. *Proc Natl Acad Sci USA* 86:7505–7509, 1989.

Kennaway E: The identification of a carcinogenic compound in coal-tar. *Br Med J* 2:749–752, 1955.

Kennelly JC: Design and interpretation of rat liver UDS assays. *Mutagenesis* 10:215–221, 1995.

Kinosita R: Researches on the cancerogenesis of the various chemical substances. *Gann* 30:423–426, 1936.

Kirkland DJ, Marshall RR, McEnaney S, et al: Aroclor-1254-induced rat-liver S9 causes chromosomal aberrations in CHO cells but not human lymphocytes: A role of active oxygen? *Mutat Res* 214:115–122, 1989.

Kitchin KT, Brown JL, Setzer R: Dose-response relationship in multistage carcinogenesis: promoters. *Environ Health Perspect Suppl* 1:255–264, 1994.

Klaunig JE: Selection induction of DNA synthesis in mouse preneoplastic and neoplastic hepatic lesions after exposure to phenobarbital. *Environ Health Perspect* 101:235–240, 1993.

Knudson AG: Antioncogenes and human cancer. *Proc Natl Acad Sci USA* 90:10914–10921, 1993.

Koelle MR: A new family of G-protein regulators—the RGS proteins. *Curr Opin Cell Biol* 9:143–147, 1997.

Koga N, Inskeep PB, Harris TM, Guengerich FP: *S*-[2-N^7-Guanyl)-ethyl] glutathione, the major DNA adduct formed from 1,2-dibromoethane. *Biochemistry* 25:2192–2198, 1986.

Konishi N, Hiasa Y: Renal carcinogenesis, in Waalkes MP, Ward JM (eds): *Carcinogenesis* New York: Raven Press, 1994, pp 123–159.

Korte F, Coulston F: Some consideration of the impact of energy and chemicals on the environment. *Regul Toxicol Pharmacol* 19:219–227, 1994.

Kowaltowski AJ, Vercesi AE: Mitochondrial damage induced by conditions of oxidative stress. *Free Radic Biol Med* 26:463–471, 1999.

Kraybill H: Food chemicals and food additives, in Newberne P (ed): *Trace Substances and Health: A Handbook.* Part I. New York: Marcel-Dekker, 1976, pp 245–318.

Kraybill HF: Proper perspectives in extrapolation of experimental carcinogenesis data to humans. *Food Technol* 32:62–64, 1978.

Kritchevsky D: Dietary effects in experimental carcinogenesis: Animal models, in Beynen AC, West CE (eds): *Use of Animal Models for Research in Human Nutrition Comparative Animal Nutrition.* Vol 6. Basel: Karger, 1988, pp 174–185.

Kritchevsky D, Weber MM, Buck CL, Klurfeld DM: Calories, fat and cancer. *Lipids* 21:272–274, 1986.

Kroh H: Chemical neuroncogenesis of the central nervous system. *J Neuropathol Exp Neurol Suppl* 54:48S–49S, 1995.

Kuschner M: The carcinogenicity of beryllium. *Environ Health Persp* 40:101–105, 1981.

Laconi E, Vasudevan S, Rao PM, et al: An earlier proliferative response of hepatocytes in γ-glutamyl transferase positive foci to partial hepatectomy. *Cancer Lett* 81:229–235, 1994.

Landrigan PJ: Arsenic—State of the art. *Am J Ind Med* 2:5–14 1981.

Landrigan PJ: Epidemiologic approaches to persons with exposures to waste chemicals. *Environ Health Perspect* 48:93–97, 1983.

Lane DP: p53, guardian of the genome. *Cancer* 358:15–16, 1992.

Lasne C, Lu YP, Orfila L, et al: Study of various transforming effects of the anabolic agents trenbolone and testosterone on Syrian hamster embryo cells. *Carcinogenesis* 11:541–547, 1990.

Latt SA: Sister chromatid exchange formation. *Annu Rev Genet* 15:11–55, 1981.

Lawley, PD: Historical origins of current concepts of carcinogenesis. *Adv Cancer Res* 65:17–111, 1994.

Leaf CD, Wishnok JS, Tannenbaum SR: Mechanisms of endogenous nitrosation. *Cancer Surv* 8:323–334, 1989.

Lee DC, Luetteke NC, Qiu TH, et al: Transforming growth factor-alpha. Its expression, regulation, and role in transformation, in Tsang RC, Lemons JA, Balistren WF (eds): *Growth Factors in Perinatal Development.* New York: Raven Press, 1993, pp 21–38.

Lee GH, Merlino G, Fasuto N: Development of liver tumors in transforming growth factor α transgenic mice. *Cancer Res* 52:5162–5170, 1992.

Levin W, Thakker DR, Wood AW, et al: Evidence that benzo[*a*]anthracene 3,4-diol-1,2-epoxide is an ultimate carcinogen on mouse skin. *Cancer Res* 38:1705–1710, 1978.

Levine AJ: The tumor suppressor genes. *Annu Rev Biochem,* 62:623–651, 1993.

Lewis TS, Shapiro PS, Ahn NG: Signal transduction through MAP kinase cascades. *Adv Cancer Res* 74:49–139, 1998.

Li AP, Aaron CS, Auletta AE, et al: An evaluation of the roles of mammalian cell mutation assays in the testing of chemical genotoxicity. *Regul Toxicol Pharmacol* 14:24–40, 1991.

Li AP, Carver JH, Choy WN, et al: A guide for the performance of the Chinese hamster ovary cell/hypoxanthine guanine phosphoribosyl transferase gene mutation assay. *Mutat Res* 189:135–141, 1987.

Li D, Randerath K: Modulation of DNA modification (I-compound) levels in rat liver and kidney by dietary carbohydrate, protein, fat, vitamin, and mineral content. *Mutat Res* 275:47–56, 1992.

Li D, Wang M, Liehr JG, Randerath K: DNA adducts induced by lipids and lipid peroxidation products: Possible relationships to I-compounds. *Mutat Res* 344:117–126, 1995.

Li D, Xu D, Randerath K: Species and tissue specificities of I-compounds as contrasted with carcinogen adducts in liver, kidney and skin DNA of Sprague-Dawley rats, ICR mice and Syrian hamsters. *Carcinogenesis* 11:2227–2232, 1990.

Li GM, Wang H, Romano LJ: Human MutSα specifically binds to DNA containing aminofluorene and acetylaminofluorene adducts. *J Biol Chem* 271:24084–24088, 1996.

Li JJ, Li SA: Estrogen carcinogenesis in hamster tissues: A critical review. *Endocr Rev* 11:524–531, 1990.

Liao D, Porsch-Hällström I, Gustafsson JA, Blanck A: Sex differences at the initiation stage of rat liver carcinogenesis—Influence of growth hormone. *Carcinogenesis* 14:2045–2049, 1993.

Lieber MR: Pathological and physiological double-strand breaks. *Am J Pathol* 153:1323–1332, 1998.

Liehr JG: 2-Fluoroestradiol. Separation of estrogenicity from carcinogenicity. *Mol Pharmacol* 23:278–281, 1983.

Lijinsky W: Nitrosamines and nitrosamides in the etiology of gastrointestinal cancer. *Cancer* 40:2446–2449, 1977.

Lijinsky W: Non-genotoxic environmental carcinogens. *J Environ Sci Health* C8(1):45–87, 1990.

Lijinsky W, Reuber MD, Riggs C: Carcinogenesis by combinations of *N*-nitroso compounds in rats. *Food Chem Toxicol* 21:601–605, 1983.

Littlefield NA, Gaylor DW: Influence of total dose and dose rate in carcinogenicity studies. *J Toxicol Environ Health* 15:545–560, 1985.

Liu E, Dollbaum C, Scott G, et al: Molecular lesions involved in the progression of a human breast cancer. *Oncogene* 3:323–327, 1988.

Lockhart AMC, Piegorsch WW, Bishop JB: Assessing overdispersion and dose-response in the male dominant lethal assay. *Mutat Res* 272:35–58, 1992.

Loechler EL: Adduct-induced base-shifts: A mechanism by which the adducts of bulky carcinogens might induce mutations. *Biopolymers* 28:909–927, 1989.

Lowe JP, Silverman BD: Predicting carcinogenicity of polycyclic aromatic hydrocarbons. *Chem Res* 17:332–338, 1984.

Luebeck E, Moolgavkar S, Buchman A, Schwarz M: Effects of polychlorinated biphenyls in rat liver: Quantitative analysis of enzyme-altered foci. *Toxicol Appl Pharmacol* 111:469–484, 1991.

Lutz WK, Schlatter J: Chemical carcinogens and overnutrition in diet-related cancer. *Carcinogenesis* 13:2211–2216, 1992.

Lutz WK, Schlatter J: The relative importance of mutagens and carcinogens in the diet. *Pharmacol Toxicol* 72:s104–s107, 1993.

Mack TM, Pike MC, Henderson BE, et al: Estrogens and endometrial cancer in a retirement community. *N Engl J Med* 294:1262–1267, 1976.

Maekawa A, Mitsumori K: Spontaneous occurrence and chemical induction of neurogenic tumors in rats influence of host factors and specificity of chemical structure. *Crit Rev Toxicol* 20:287–310, 1990.

Magee PN, Swann PF: Nitroso compounds. *Br Med Bull* 25:240–244, 1969.

Magnuson BA, Carr I, Bird RP: Ability of aberrant crypt foci characteristics to predict colonic tumor incidence in rats fed cholic acid. *Cancer Res* 53:4499–4504, 1993.

Magos L: Epidemiological and experimental aspects of metal carcinogenesis: Physicochemical properties, kinetics, and the active species. *Environ Health Perspect* 95:157–189, 1991.

Maher VM, Miller EC, Miller JA, Szybalski W: Mutations and decreases in density of transforming DNA produced by derivatives of the carcinogens 2-acetylaminofluorene and *N*-methyl-4-aminoazobenzene. *Mol Pharmacol* 4:411–426, 1968.

Majeska JB, Matheson DW: Development of an optimal S9 activation mixture for the L5178 TK± mouse lymphoma mutation assay. *Environ Mol Mutagen* 16:311–319, 1990.

Marnett LJ: Polycyclic aromatic hydrocarbon oxidation during prostaglandin biosynthesis. *Life Sci* 29:531–546, 1981.

Marnett LJ, Burcham PC: Endogenous DNA adducts: Potential and paradox. *Chem Res Toxicol* 6:771–785, 1993.

Maron DM, Ames BN: Revised methods for the *Salmonella* mutagenicity test. *Mutat Res* 113:173–215, 1983.

Martínez-Cayuela M: Oxygen free radicals and human disease. *Biochimie* 77:147–161, 1995.

Mattammal MB, Zenser TV, Davis BB: Prostaglandin hydroperoxidase-mediated 2-amino-4-(5-nitro-furyl)[^{14}C]thiazole metabolism and nucleic acid binding. *Cancer Res* 41:4961–4966, 1981.

Mauderly JL: Toxicological approaches to complex mixtures. *Environ Health Perspect* 101:155–165, 1993.

Mayer EA: Signal transduction and intercellular communication, in Walsh JH, Dockray GJ (eds): *Gut Peptides: Biochemistry and Physiology.* New York: Raven Press, 1994, pp 33–73.

Mays ET, Christopherson W: Hepatic tumors induced by sex steroids. *Semin Liver Dis* 4:147–157, 1984.

McCann J: In vitro testing for cancer-causing chemicals. Hosp Pract 73–85, 1983.

McClain RM: The significance of hepatic microsomal enzyme induction and altered thyroid function in rats: Implications for thyroid gland neoplasia. *Toxicol Pathol* 17:294–306, 1989.

McGregor D: Diets, food components and human cancer. *Biotherapy* 11:189–200, 1998.

Memoli VA, Urban RM, Alroy J, Galante JO: Malignant neoplasms associated with orthopedic implant materials in rats. *J Orthop Res* 4:346–355, 1986.

Merchant JA: Human epidemiology: A review of fiber type and characteristics in the development of malignant and nonmalignant disease. *Environ Health Perspect* 88:287–293, 1990.

Meselson M, Russell K: Carcinogenic and mutagenic potency, in Hiatt HH, Watson JD, Weinsten JA (eds): *Origins of Human Cancer.* Book C. *Cold Spring Harbor Conferences on Cell Proliferation*. Cold Spring Harbor, NY: Cold Spring Harbor Laboratory, 1977.

Meselson MS, Chairman: *Pest Control: An Assessment of Present and Alternative Technologies.* Vol 1. *Contemporary Pest Control Practices and Prospects: The Report of the Executive Committee.* Washington, DC: National Academy of Sciences, 1975.

Michalopoulos, G, Strom SC, Kligerman AD, et al: Mutagenesis induced by procarcinogens at the hypoxanthine-guanine phosphoribosyl transferase locus of human fibroblasts cocultured with rat hepatocytes. *Cancer Res* 41:1873–1878, 1981.

Michalowsky LA, Jones PA: DNA methylation and differentiation. *Environ Health Perspect* 80:189–197, 1989.

Mies C: Molecular biological analysis of paraffin-embedded tissues. *Hum Pathol* 25:555–560, 1994.

Miki Y, Swensen J, Shattuck-Eidens D, et al: A strong candidate for the breast and ovarian cancer susceptibility gene *BRCA1*. *Science* 266:66–71, 1994.

Mikol YB, Hoover KL, Creasia D, Poirier L: Hepatocarcinogenesis in rats fed methyl-deficient, amino acid-defined diets. *Carcinogenesis* 4:1619–1629, 1983.

Miller AB, Berrino F, Hill M, et al: Diet in the aetiology of cancer: a review. *Eur J Cancer* 30A:207–220, 1994.

Miller EC: Some current perspectives on chemical carcinogenesis in humans and experimental animals: Presidential address. *Cancer Res* 38:1479–1496, 1978.

Miller EC: Studies on the formation of protein-bound derivatives of 3,4-benzopyrene in the epidermal fraction of mouse skin. *Cancer Res* 11:100–108, 1951.

Miller EC, Miller J, Enomoto M: The comparative carcinogenicities of 2-acetylaminofluorene and its *N*-hydroxy metabolite in mice, hamsters, and guinea pigs. *Cancer Res* 24:2018–2026, 1964.

Miller EC, Miller JA: The presence and significance of bound aminoazo dyes in the livers of rats fed p-dimethylaminoazobenzene. *Cancer Res* 7:468–480, 1947.

Miller EC, Miller JA, Sandin RB, Brown RK: The carcinogenic activities of certain analogues of 2-acetylaminofluorene in the rat. *Cancer Res* 9:504–509, 1949.

Miller JA: Carcinogenesis by chemicals: An overview-GHA. Clowes Memorial Lecture. *Cancer Res* 30:559–576, 1970.

Miller JA: The need for epidemiological studies of the medical exposures of Japanese patients to the carcinogen ethyl carbamate (urethane) from 1950 to 1975. *Jpn J Cancer Res* 82:1323–1324, 1991.

Miller JA, Cramer JW, Miller EC: The *N*- and ring-hydroxylation of 2-acetylaminofluorene during carcinogenesis in the rat. *Cancer Res* 20:950–962, 1960.

Mirsalis JC: Genotoxicity, toxicity, and carcinogenicity of the antihistamine methapyrilene. *Mutat Res* 185:309–317, 1987.

Mirsalis JC, Monforte JA, Winegar RA: Transgenic animal models for measuring mutations *in vivo*. *Crit Rev Toxicol* 24:255–280, 1994.

Mirvish SS, Salmasi S, Cohen SM, et al: Liver and forestomach tumors and other forestomach lesions in rats treated with morpholine and sodium nitrite, with and without sodium ascorbate. *J Natl Cancer Inst,* 71:81–85, 1983.

Miyamae Y, Iwasaki, K, Kinae, N, et al: Detection of DNA lesions induced by chemical mutagens using the single-cell gel electrophoresis (Comet) assay. 2. Relationship between DNA migration and alkaline condition. *Mutat Res* 393:107–113, 1997.

Moch RW, Dua PN, Hines FA: Problems in consideration of rodent hepatocarcinogenesis for regulatory purposes. *Toxicol Pathol* 24:138–146, 1996.

Modrich P: Mismatch repair, genetic stability, and cancer. *Science* 266:1959–1960, 1994.

Modrich P: Strand-specific mismatch repair in mammalian cells. *J Biol Chem* 272:24727–24730, 1997.

Moll KD, Tihansky DP: Risk-benefit analysis for industrial and social needs. *Am Ind Hyg Assoc J* 38:153–161, 1977.

Monks TJ, Anders MW, Dekant W, et al: Contemporary issues in toxicology. Glutathione conjugate mediated toxicities. *Toxicol Appl Pharmacol* 106:1–19, 1990.

Monro A: What is an appropriate measure of exposure when testing drugs for carcinogenicity in rodents. *Toxicol Appl Pharmacol* 112:171–181, 1992.

Moolgavkar SH: Carcinogenesis modeling: from molecular biology to epidemiology. *Annu Rev Public Health* 7:151–169, 1986.

Moon HD, Simpson ME, Li CH Evans HM: Neoplasms in rats treated with pituitary growth hormone. I. Pulmonary and lymphatic tissues. *Cancer Res* 10:297, 1950a.

Moon HD, Simpson ME, Li CH, Evans HM: Neoplasms in rats treated with pituitary growth hormone. III. Reproductive organs. *Cancer Res* 10:549, 1950b.

Morley SJ, Thomas G: Intracellular messengers and the control of protein synthesis. *Pharmacol Ther* 50:291–319, 1991.

Motojima K: Peroxisome proliferator-activated receptor (PPAR): Structure, mechanisms of activation and diverse functions. *Cell Struct Funct* 18:267–277, 1993.

Mottram JC: A developing factor in experimental blastogenesis. *J Pathol Bacteriol* 56:181–187, 1944.

Müller H: Recessively inherited deficiencies predisposing to cancer. *Anticancer Res* 10:513–518, 1990.

Müller R, Rajewsky MF: Enzymatic removal of O^6-ethylguanine versus stability of O^4-ethylthymine in the DNA of rat tissues exposed to the carcinogen ethylnitrosourea: Possible interference of guanine-O^6 alkylation with 5-cytosine methylation in the DNA of replicating target cells. *Z Naturforsch* 38:1023–1029, 1983.

Murphy LJ, Bell GI, Friesen HG: Tissue distribution of insulin-like growth factor I and II messenger ribonucleic acid in the adult rat. *Endocrinology* 120:1279–1282, 1987.

Murphy SA, Tice RR, Smith MG, Margolin BH: Contributions to the design and statistical analysis of in vivo SCE experiments. *Mutat Res* 271:39–48, 1992.

Muscat JE, Wynder EL: Cigarette smoking, asbestos exposure, and malignant mesothelioma. *Cancer Res* 51:2263–2267, 1991.

Myhr BC: Validation studies with Muta Mouse: A transgenic mouse model for detecting mutations in vivo. *Environ Mol Mutag* 18:308–315, 1991.

Myles GM, Sancar A: DNA repair. *Chem Res Toxicol* 2:197–226, 1989.

Nakagawa T, Datta A, Kolodner RD: Multiple functions of MutS- and MutL-related heterocomplexes. *Proc Natl Acad Sci USA* 96:14186–14188, 1999.

Nasmyth K: Separating sister chromatids *Trends Biochem Sci* 24:98–104, 1999.

National Academy of Science: Biological significance of DNA adducts and protein adducts, in *Drinking Water and Health.* Vol 9. Washington DC: National Academy Press, 1989, pp 6–37.

Nebert DW: Role of genetics and drug metabolism in human cancer risk. *Mutat Res* 247:267–281, 1991.

Neish WJP, Parry EW, Ghadially FN: Tumour induction in the rat by a mixture of two non-carcinogenic aminoazo dyes. *Oncology* 21:229–240, 1967.

Nelson MA, Futscher BW, Kinsella T, et al: Detection of mutant Ha-*ras* genes in chemically initiated mouse skin epidermis before the development of benign tumors. *Proc Natl Acad Sci USA* 89:6398–6402, 1992.

Neumann F: Early indicators for carcinogenesis in sex-hormone-sensitive organs. *Mutat Res* 248:341–356, 1991.

Neumann HG: Role of extent and persistence of DNA modifications in chemical carcinogenesis by aromatic amines. *Recent Results Cancer Res* 84:77–89, 1983.

Noble RL: Hormonal control of growth and progression in tumors of Nb rats and a theory of action. *Cancer Res* 37:82–94, 1977.

Nowell PC: Cytogenetics of tumor progression. *Cancer* 65:2172–2177, 1990.

Nuzum EO, Malkinson AM, Beer DG: Specific Ki-*ras* codon 61 mutations may determine the development of urethan-induced mouse lung adenomas or adenocarcinomas. *Mol Carcinog* 3:287–295, 1990.

Ochi T, Kaneko M: Active oxygen contributes to the major part of chromosomal aberrations in V79 Chinese hamster cells exposed to *N*-hydroxy-2-naphthylamine. *Free Radic Res Commun* 5:351–358, 1989.

Oesterle D, Deml E: Detection of chemical carcinogens by means of the "rat liver foci bioassay." *Exp Pathol* 39:197–206, 1990.

Office of Science and Technology Policy: Chemical carcinogens: A review of the science and its associated principles. U.S. Interagency Staff Group on Carcinogens. *Environ Health Perspect* 67:201–282, 1986.

Ogiso T, Tatematsu M, Tamano S, et al: Correlation between medium-term liver bioassay system data and results of long-term testing in rats. *Carcinogenesis* 11:561–566, 1990.

Ohnishi K, Iida S, Iwama S, et al: The effect of chronic habitual alcohol intake on the development of liver cirrhosis and hepatocellular carcinoma: Relation to hepatitis B surface antigen carriers. *Cancer* 49:672–677, 1982.

Okada N, Honda A, Kawabata M, Yajima N: Sodium phenobarbital-enhanced mutation frequency in the liver DNA of *lacZ* transgenic mice treated with diethylnitrosamine. *Mutagenesis* 12:179–184, 1997.

Olinski R, Jaruga P, Zastawny TH: Oxidative DNA base modifications as factors in carcinogenesis. *Acta Biochim Polonica* 45:561–572, 1998.

Olsson H, Möller TR, Ranstam J: Early oral contraceptive use and breast cancer among premenopausal women: Final report from a study in southern Sweden. *J Natl Cancer Inst* 81:1000–1004, 1989.

Oser BL Benefit/risk: Whose? What? How much? *Food Technol* 32:55–58, 1978.

Oshimura M, Hesterberg TW, Tsutsui T, Barrett JC: Correlation of asbestos-induced cytogenetic effects with cell transformation of Syrian hamster embryo cells in culture. *Cancer Res* 44:5017–5022, 1984.

Osler M: Obesity and cancer. *Dan Med Bull* 34:267–274, 1987.

Ottagio L, Bonatti S, Cavalieri Z, Abbondandolo A: Chromosomes bearing amplified genes are a preferential target of chemicals inducing chromosome breakage and aneuploidy. *Mutat Res* 301:149–155, 1993.

Page NP, Singh DV, Farland W, et al: Implementation of EPA revised cancer assessment guidelines: Incorporation of mechanistic and pharmacokinetic data. *Fundam Appl Toxicol* 37:16–36, 1997.

Papadopoulos N, Nicolaides N, Wei Y, et al: Mutation of a mutL homolog in hereditary colon cancer. *Science* 263:1559–1560, 1994.

Paraskeva C, Williams AC: Promotability and tissue specificity of hereditary cancer genes: Do hereditary cancer patients have a reduced requirement for tumor promotion because all their somatic cells are heterozygous at the predisposing locus? *Mol Carcinog* 5:4–8, 1992.

Pariza MW: A perspective on diet, nutrition, and cancer. *JAMA* 251:1455–1458, 1984.

Pastink A, Lohman PHM: Repair and consequences of double-strand breaks in DNA. *Mutat Res* 428:141–156, 1999.

Paulini K, Beneke G, Körner B, Enders R: The relationship between the latent period and animal age in the development of foreign body sarcomas. *Beitr Pathol* 154:161–169, 1975.

Pawson T: Signal transduction–A conserved pathway from the membrane to the nucleus. *Dev Genet* 14:333–338, 1993.

Pegg AE: Methylation of the O^6 position of guanine in DNA is the most likely initiating event in carcinogenesis by methylating agents. *Cancer Invest* 2:223–231, 1984.

Pegg AE, Byers TL: Repair of DNA containing O^6-alkylguanine. *FASEB J* 6:2302–2310, 1992.

Pegg AE, Perry W: Alkylation of nucleic acids and metabolism of small doses of dimethylnitrosamine in the rat. *Cancer Res* 41:3128–3132, 1981.

Penn I: Why do immunosuppressed patients develop cancer? *Crit Rev Oncog* 1:27–52, 1989.

Pepelko WE: Effect of exposure route on potency of carcinogens. *Reg Toxicol Pharmacol* 13:3–17, 1991.

Peraino C, Fry RJM, Staffeldt E: Effects of varying the onset and duration of exposure to phenobarbital on its enhancement of 2-acetylaminofluorene-induced hepatic tumorigenesis. *Cancer Res* 37:3623–3627, 1977.

Pereira MA: Mouse skin bioassay for chemical carcinogens. *J Am Coll Toxicol* 1:47–74, 1982.

Pereira MA, Stoner GD: Comparison of rat liver foci assay and strain A mouse lung tumor assay to detect carcinogens: a review. *Fundam Appl Toxicol* 5:688–699, 1985.

Perera F, Mayer J, Santella RM, et al: Biologic markers in risk assessment for environmental carcinogens. *Environ Health Perspect* 90:247–254, 1991.

Petit C, Sancar A: Nucleotide excision repair: From *E. coli* to man. *Biochimie* 81:15–25, 1999.

Peto R, Pike MC, Bernstein L, et al: The TD_{50}: A proposed general convention for the numerical description of the carcinogenic potency of chemicals in chronic-exposure animal experiments. *Environ Health Perspect* 58:1–8, 1984.

Pietra G, Spencer K, Shubik P: Response of newly born mice to a chemical carcinogen. *Nature* 183:1689, 1959.

Pike MC, Krailo MD, Henderson BE, et al: "Hormonal" risk factors, "breast tissue age" and the age-incidence of breast cancer. *Nature* 303:767–770, 1983.

Pirkle JL, Wolfe WH, Patterson DG: Estimates of the half-life of 2,3,7,8-tetrachlorodibenzo-*p*-dioxin in Vietnam veterans of operation ranch hand. *J Toxicol Environ Health* 27:165–171, 1989.

Pitot HC: Altered hepatic foci: Their role in murine hepatocarcinogenesis. *Annu Rev Pharmacol Toxicol* 30:465–500, 1990.

Pitot HC: Endogenous carcinogenesis: the role of tumor promotion. *Proc Soc Exp Biol Med* 198:661–666, 1991.

Pitot HC: *Fundamentals of Oncology,* 3d ed. New York: Marcel Dekker, 1986a.

Pitot HC: Multistage carcinogenesis—Genetic and epigenetic mechanisms in relation to cancer prevention. *Cancer Detect Prev* 17:567–573, 1993.

Pitot HC: Oncogenes and human neoplasia. *Clin Lab Med* 6:167–179, 1986b.

Pitot HC: Stages in neoplastic development, in Schottenfeld D, Fraumeni JF (eds): *Cancer Epidemiology and Prevention*, 2d ed. Oxford, England: Oxford University Press, 1996, pp 65–79.

Pitot HC: The molecular biology of carcinogenesis. *Cancer* 72:962–970, 1993b.

Pitot HC: The role of receptors in multistage carcinogenesis. *Mutat Res* 333:3–14, 1995.

Pitot HC, Barsness L, Goldsworthy T, Kitagawa T: Biochemical characterization of stages of hepatocarcinogenesis after a single dose of diethylnitrosamine. *Nature* 271:456–458, 1978.

Pitot HC, Dragan YP: Chemical carcinogenesis, in Klaasen CD (ed): *Casarett and Doull's Toxicology—The Basic Science of Poisons,* 5th ed. New York: McGraw-Hill, 1996, pp 201–267.

Pitot HC, Dragan YP: Chemical induction of hepatic neoplasia, in Arias IM, Boyer JL, Fausto N, et al (eds): *The Liver: Biology and Pathobiology,* 3d ed. New York: Raven Press, 1994.

Pitot HC, Dragan YP: The instability of tumor promotion in relation to human cancer risk. In McClain M, Slaga TJ, LeBoeuf R, Pitot HC (eds): *Growth Factors and Tumor Promotion: Implications for Risk Assessment, Progress in Clinical and Biological Research.* Vol 391. New York: Wiley, 1995, pp 21–38.

Pitot HC, Dragan YP, Teeguarden J, et al: Quantitation of multistage carcinogenesis in rat liver. *Toxicol Pathol* 24:119–128, 1996.

Pitot HC: The dynamics of carcinogenesis: Implications for human risk. *CIIT Act* 13:1–6, 1993a.

Pitot HC, Goldsworthy TL, Moran S, et al: A method to quantitate the relative initiating and promoting potencies of hepatocarcinogenic agents in their dose-response relationship to altered hepatic foci. *Carcinogenesis* 8:1491–1499, 1987.

Porter TD, Coon MJ: Cytochrome P-450: Multiplicity of isoforms, substrates, and catalytic and regulatory mechanisms. *J Biol Chem* 266:13469–13472, 1991.

Pratt WB, Toft DO: Steroid receptor interactions with heat shock protein and immunophilin chaperones. *Endocr Rev* 18:306–360, 1997.

Pretlow TP: Alterations associated with early neoplasia in the colon, in Pretlow TG, Pretlow TP (eds): *Biochemical and Molecular Aspects of Selected Cancers.* Vol 2. San Diego, CA: Academic Press, 1994, pp 93–114.

Pretlow TP, O'Riordan MA, Spancake KM, Pretlow TG: Two types of putative preneoplastic lesions identified by hexosaminidase activity in whole-mounts of colons from F344 rats treated with carcinogen. *Am J Pathol* 142:1695–1700, 1993.

Provost GS, Kretz PL, Hamner RT, et al: Transgenic systems for in vivo mutation analysis. *Mutat Res* 288:133–149, 1993.

Pruess-Schwartz D, Nimesheim A, Marnett LJ: Peroxyl radical- and cytochrome P-450-dependent metabolic activation of (+)-7,8-dihydroxy-7,8-dihydrobenzo(*a*)pyrene in mouse skin *in vitro* and *in vivo. Cancer Res* 49:1732–1737, 1989.

Pullman A, Pullman B: Electronic structure and carcinogenic activity of aromatic molecules. New developments. *Adv Cancer Res* 3:117–169, 1955.

Purnell DM: The relationship of terminal duct hyperplasia to mammary carcinoma in 7,12-dimethylbenzo(α)anthracene-treated LEW/Mai rats. *Am J Pathol* 98:311–324, 1980.

Purtilo DT, Linder J: Oncological consequences of impaired immune surveillance against ubiquitous viruses. *J Clin Immunol* 3:197–206, 1983.

Quintanilla M, Brown K, Ramsden M, Balmain A: Carcinogen-specific mutation and amplification of Ha-*ras* during mouse skin carcinogenesis. *Nature* 322:78–80, 1986.

Randerath E, Hart RW, Turturro A, et al: Effects of aging caloric restriction on I-compounds in liver, kidney and white blood cell DNA of male Brown-Norway rats. *Mech Ageing Dev* 58:279–296, 1991.

Randerath K, van Golen KL, Dragan YP, Pitot HC: Effects of phenobarbital on I-compounds in liver DNA as a function of age in male rats fed two different diets. *Carcinogenesis* 13:125–130, 1992

Rasenick MM, Caron MG, Dolphin AC, et al: Receptor-G protein-effector coupling: Coding and regulation of the signal transduction process, in Cuello AC, Collier B (eds): *Pharmacological Sciences: Perspectives for Research and Therapy in the Late 1990s.* Basel: Birkhäuser Verlag, 1995, pp 91–102.

Recio L: Transgenic animal models and their application in mechanistically based toxicology research. *Chem Ind Inst Toxicol* 15:1–7, 1995.

Reddy JK, Lalwani ND: Carcinogenesis by hepatic peroxisome proliferators: Evaluation of the risk of hypolipidemic drugs and industrial plasticizers to humans. *CRC Crit Rev Toxicol* 12:1–58, 1983.

Reddy JK, Rao MS: Oxidative DNA damage caused by persistent peroxisome proliferation: Its role in hepatocarcinogenesis. *Mutat Res* 214:63–68, 1989.

Reddy MV, Randerath K: ^{32}P-Postlabeling assay for carcinogen-DNA adducts: Nuclease P_1-mediated enhancement of its sensitivity and applications. *Environ Health Perspect* 76:41–47, 1987.

Reif AE: Effect of cigarette smoking on susceptibility to lung cancer. *Oncology* 38:76–85, 1981.

Riggs AD, Jones PA: 5-Methylcytosine, gene regulation, and cancer. *Adv Cancer Res* 40:1–30, 1983.

Roe FJC, Dukes CE, Mitchley BCV: Sarcomas at the site of implantation of a polyvinyl plastic sponge: Incidence reduced by use of thin implants. *Biochem Pharmacol* 16:647–650, 1967.

Rogan WJ, Brown SM: Some fundamental aspects of epidemiology: A guide for laboratory scientists. *Fed Proc* 38:1875–1879, 1979.

Rogers A: Nitrosamines, in Newberne P (ed): *Trace Substances and Health: A Handbook.* Part 2. New York: Marcel Dekker,1982, pp 47–80.

Rogers AE, Zeisel SH, Groopman J: Diet and carcinogenesis. *Carcinogenesis* 14:2205–2217, 1993.

Rogler CE, Yang D, Rossetti L, et al: Altered body composition and increased frequency of diverse malignancies in insulin-like growth factor-II transgenic mice. *J Biol Chem* 269:13779–13784, 1994.

Roomi MW, Ho R K, Sarma DSR, Farber E: A common biochemical pattern in preneoplastic hepatocyte nodules generated in four different models in the rat. *Cancer Res* 45:564–571, 1985.

Rosenberg MP, Gene knockout and transgenic technologies in risk assessment: The next generation. *Mol Carcinog* 20:262–274, 1997.

Rosenkranz HS, Klopman G: Structural implications of the ICPEMC method for quantifying genotoxicity data. *Mutat Res* 305:99–116, 1994.

Rosenthal N: Molecular medicine. Regulation of gene expression. *N Engl J Med* 331:931–933, 1994.

Rous P, Kidd JG: Conditional neoplasms and sub-threshold neoplastic states: A study of the tar tumors of rabbits. *J Exp Med* 73:369–390, 1941.

Roussel MF: Key effectors of signal transduction and G1 progression. *Adv Cancer Res* 74:1–24, 1998.

Ruffolo RR Jr: Fundamentals of receptor theory: Basics for shock research. *Circ Shock* 37:176–184, 1992.

Rumsby PC, Barrass NC, Phillimore HE, Evans JG: Analysis of the Ha-*ras* oncogene in C3H/He mouse liver tumors derived spontaneously or induced with diethylnitrosamine or phenobarbitone. *Carcinogenesis* 12:2331–2336, 1991.

Russo J, Tait L, Russo IH: Susceptibility of the mammary gland to carcinogenesis: III. The cell of origin of rat mammary carcinoma. *Am J Pathol* 113:50–66, 1983.

Saeter G, Schwarze PE, Nesland JM, Seglen PO: 2-Acetylaminofluorene promotion of liver carcinogenesis by a non-cytotoxic mechanism. *Carcinogenesis* 9:581–587, 1988.

Samuels SW: The fallacies of risk/benefit analysis. *Ann NY Acad Sci* 329:267–273, 1979.

Sancar A: Mechanisms of DNA excision repair. *Science* 266:1954–1956, 1994.

Sancar A., Tang MS: Nucleotide excision repair. *Photochem Photobiol* 57:905–921, 1993.

Sandén A, Järvholm B, Larsson S, Thiringer G: The risk of lung cancer and mesothelioma after cessation of asbestos exposure: A prospective cohort study of shipyard workers. *Eur Respir J* 5:281–285, 1992.

Sander CA, Yano T, Clark HM, et al: p53 Mutation is associated with progression in follicular lymphomas. *Blood* 82:1994–2004, 1993.

Sargent L, Xu Yh, Sattler GL, et al: Ploidy and karyotype of hepatocytes isolated from enzyme-altered foci in two different protocols of multistage hepatocarcinogenesis in the rat. *Carcinogenesis* 10:387–391, 1989.

Sasaki T, Yoshida T: Experimentelle Erzeugung des Lebercarcinoms durch Fütterung mit o-Amidoazotoluol. *Virchows Arch Abt A Pathol Anat* 295:175–200, 1935.

Satoh MS, Lindahl T: Enzymatic repair of oxidative DNA damage. *Cancer Res* 54:1899s–1901s, 1994.

Schaeffer BK, Zurlo J, Longnecker DS: Activation of c-Ki-*ras* not detectable in adenomas or adenocarcinomas arising in rat pancreas. *Mol Carcinog* 3:165–170, 1990.

Schlesselman JJ, Stadel BV, Murray P, Shenghan L: Breast cancer in relation to early use of oral contraceptives. *JAMA* 259:1828–1833, 1988.

Schmähl D, Habs M: Carcinogenicity of *N*-nitroso compounds. Species and route differences in regard to organotropism. *Oncology* 37:237–242, 1980.

Schoental R: Trichothecenes, zearalenone, and other carcinogenic metabolites of *Fusarium* and related microfungi. *Adv Cancer Res* 45:217–274, 1985.

Schulte-Hermann R, Bursch W, Kraupp-Grasl B, et al: Cell proliferation and apoptosis in normal liver and preneoplastic foci. *Environ Health Perspect* 101:87–90, 1993.

Schulte-Hermann R, Ohde G, Schuppler J, Timmermann-Trosiener I: Enhanced proliferation of putative preneoplastic cells in rat liver following treatment with the tumor promoters phenobarbital, hexachlorocyclohexane, steroid compounds, and nafenopin. *Cancer Res* 41:2556–2562, 1981.

Schulte-Hermann R. Timmermann-Trosiener I. Barthel G. Bursch W: DNA synthesis, apoptosis, and phenotypic expression as determinants of growth of altered foci in rat liver during phenobarbital promotion. *Cancer Res* 50:5127–5135, 1990.

Scott D, Galloway SM, Marshall RR, et al: Genotoxicity under extreme culture conditions. *Mutat Res* 257:147–204, 1991.

Seger R, Krebs EG: The MAPK signaling cascade. *FASEB J* 9:726–735, 1995.

Seitz HK, Simanowski UA: Alcohol and carcinogenesis. *Annu Rev Nutr* 8:99–119, 1988.

Shamberger RJ, Baughman FF, Kalchert SL, et al: Carcinogen-induced chromosome breakage decreased by antioxidants. *Proc Natl Acad Sci* USA 70:1461–1463, 1973.

Shapiro R: Damage to DNA caused by hydrolysis, in Seeberg E, Kleppe K (eds): *Chromosome Damage and Repair*. New York: Plenum Press, 1981, pp 3–18.

Shearman CW, Loeb LA: Effects of dupurination on the fidelity of DNA synthesis. *J Mol Biol* 128:197–218, 1979.

Shephard SE, Schlatter Ch, Lutz WK: Assessment of the risk of formation of carcinogenic *N*-nitroso compounds from dietary precursors in the stomach. *Fundam Chem Toxicol* 25:91–108, 1987.

Shields PG, Harris CC: Molecular epidemiology and the genetics of environmental cancer. *JAMA* 266:681–687, 1991.

Shimkin MB: *Contrary to Nature*. Washington, DC: U.S. Department of Health, Education, and Welfare, Public Health Service, National Institutes of Health, 1977.

Shimkin MB, Stoner GD: Lung tumors in mice: Application to carcinogenesis bioassay. *Adv Cancer Res* 21:1–58, 1975.

Shirai T: A medium-term rat liver bioassay as a rapid in vivo test for carcinogenic potential: A historical review of model development and summary of results from 291 tests. *Toxicol Pathol* 25:453–460, 1997.

Shivapurkar N, Tang Z, Ferreira A, et al: Sequential analysis of K-*ras* mutations in aberrant crypt foci and colonic tumors induced by azoxymethane in Fischer-344 rats on high-risk diet. *Carcinogenesis* 15:775–778, 1994.

Shixin L, Mingxin L, Chuan J, et al: An *N*-nitroso compound, *N*-3-methylbutyl-*N*-1-methylacetonylnitrosamine, in cornbread inoculated with fungi. *Sci Sin* 22:601, 1979.

Short BG, Steinhagen WH, Swenberg JA: Promoting effects of unleaded gasoline and 2,2,4-trimethylpentane on the development of atypical cell foci and renal tubular cell tumors in rats exposed to *N*-ethyl-*N*-hydroxyethylnitrosamine. *Cancer Res* 49:6369–6378, 1989.

Sims P, Grover PL, Swaisland A, et al: Metabolic activation of benzo[*a*]pyrene proceeds by a diol-epoxide. *Nature* 252:326–328, 1974.

Sina JF, Bean CL, Dysart GR, et al: Evaluation of the alkaline elution/rat hepatocyte assay as a predictor of carcinogenic/mutagenic potential. *Mutat Res* 113:357–391, 1983.

Singer B: *O*-Alkyl pyrimidines in mutagenesis and carcinogenesis: Occurrence and significance. *Cancer Res* 46:4879–4885, 1986.

Sivak A: Cocarcinogenesis. *Biochim Biophys Acta* 560:67–89, 1979.

Skopek TR, Kort KL, Marino DR: Relative sensitivity of the endogenous *hprt* gene and *lacI* transgene in ENU-treated Big Blue B6C3F1 mice. *Environ Mol Mutagen* 26:9–15, 1995.

Sky-Peck HH: Trace metals and neoplasia. *Clin Physiol Biochem* 4:99–111, 1986.

Slaga TJ: SENCAR mouse skin tumorigenesis model versus other strains and stocks of mice. *Environ Health Perspect* 68:27–32, 1986.

Smith BJ, Curtis JF, Eling TE: Bioactivation of xenobiotics by prostaglandin H synthase. *Chem Biol Interact* 79:245–264, 1991.

Snyder R, Kalf GF: A perspective on benzene leukemogenesis. *Crit Rev Toxicol* 24:177–209, 1994.

Sodum RS, Nie G, Fiala ES: 8-Aminoguanine: A base modification produced in rat liver nucleic acids by the hepatocarcinogen 2-nitropropane. *Chem Res Toxicol* 6:269–276, 1993.

Solt D, Farber E: New principle for the analysis of chemical carcinogenesis. *Nature* 263:701–703, 1976.

Sontag JM: Aspects in carcinogen bioassay, in Hiatt H, Watson J, Winsten J (eds): *Origins of Human Cancer.* Cold Spring Harbor, NY: Cold Spring Harbor Laboratory, 1977.

Spalding JW, Momma J, Elwell MR, Tennant RW: Chemically induced skin carcinogenesis in a transgenic mouse line (TG·AC) carrying a v-Ha-*ras* gene. *Carcinogenesis* 14:1335–1341, 1993.

Spitz MR, Bondy ML: Genetic susceptibility to cancer. *Cancer* 72:991–995, 1993.

Srinivasan S, Glauert HP: Formation of 5-hydroxymethyl-2′-deoxyuridine in hepatic DNA of rats treated with γ-irradiation, diethylnitrosamine, 2-acetylaminofluorene or the peroxisome proliferator ciprofibrate. *Carcinogenesis* 11:2021–2024, 1990.

Stabel S, Parker PJ: Protein kinase C. *Pharm Ther* 51:71–95, 1991.

Standeven AM, Wolf DC, Goldsworthy TL: Investigation of antiestrogenicity as a mechanism of female mouse liver tumor induction by unleaded gasoline. *Chem Ind Inst Toxicol* 14:1–5, 1994.

Stanford JL, Brinton LA, Hoover RN: Oral contraceptives and breast cancer: Results from an expanded case-control study. *Br J Cancer* 60:375–381, 1989.

Stanton MF, Layard M, Tegeris A, et al: Carcinogenicity of fibrous glass: Pleural response in the rat in relation to fiber dimension. *J Natl Cancer Inst* 58:387–603, 1977.

Stanton MF, Layard M, Tegeris A, et al: Relation of particle dimension to carcinogenicity in amphibole asbestoses and other fibrous minerals. *J Natl Cancer Inst* 67:965–975, 1981.

Starr TB, Gibson JE: The mechanistic toxicology of formaldehyde and its implications for quantitative risk estimation. *Annu Rev Pharmacol Toxicol* 25:745–767 1985.

Statland BE: Nutrition and cancer. *Clin Chem* 38:1587–1594, 1992.

Steinbrecher UP, Lisbona R, Huang SN, Mishkin S: Complete regression of hepatocellular adenoma after withdrawal of oral contraceptives. *Dig Dis Sci* 26:1045–1050, 1981.

Steinmetz KL, Green CE, Bakke JP, et al: Induction of unscheduled DNA synthesis in primary cultures of rat, mouse, hamster, monkey, and human hepatocytes. *Mutat Res* 206:91–102, 1988.

Stewart BW, Sarfaty GA: Environmental chemical carcinogenesis. *Med J Aust* 1:92–95, 1978.

Stinson NE: The tissue reaction induced in rats and guinea-pigs by polymethylmethacrylate (acrylic) and stainless steel (18/8/Mo). *Br J Exp Pathol* 45:21–29, 1964.

Stoner GD, Shimkin MB, Troxell MC, et al: Test for carcinogenicity of metallic compounds by the pulmonary tumor response in strain A mice. *Cancer Res* 36:1744–1747, 1976.

Stott WT: Chemically induced proliferation of peroxisomes: Implications for risk assessment. *Regul Toxicol Pharmacol* 8:125–159, 1988.

Stowers SJ, Anderson MW: Formation and persistence of benzo(*a*)pyrene metabolite-DNA adducts. *Environ Health Perspect* 62:31–39, 1985.

Strader CD, Fong TM, Tota MR, et al: Structure and function of G protein-coupled receptors. *Annu Rev Biochem* 63:101–132, 1994.

Strom S, Kligerman AD, Michalopoulos G: Comparisons of the effects of chemical carcinogens in mixed cultures of rat hepatocytes and human fibroblasts. *Carcinogenesis* 2:709–715, 1981.

Sugimura T, Sato S, Nagao M, et al: Overlapping of carcinogens and mutagens, in Magee PN et al (eds): *Fundamentals in Cancer Prevention.* Baltimore: University Park Press, 1976, pp 191–215.

Sumi C, Yokoro K, Kajitani T, Ito A: Synergism of diethylstilbestrol and other carcinogens in concurrent development of hepatic, mammary, and pituitary tumors in castrated male rats. *J Natl Cancer Inst* 65:169–175, 1980.

Sun Y: Free radicals, antioxidant enzymes, and carcinogenesis. *Free Radic Biol Med* 8:583–599, 1990.

Sunderman FW Jr: Carcinogenicity of metal alloys in orthopedic prostheses: Clinical and experimental studies. *Fund Appl Toxicol* 13:205–216, 1989.

Sutherland LAM, Bird RP: The effect of chenodeoxycholic acid on the development of aberrant crypt foci in the rat colon. *Cancer Lett* 76:101–107, 1994.

Swenberg JA, Dyroff MC, Bedell MA, et al: O^4-Ethyldeoxythymidine, but not O^6-ethyldeoxyguanosine, accumulates in hepatocyte DNA of rats exposed continuously to diethylnitrosamine. *Proc Natl Acad Sci USA* 81:1692–1695, 1984.

Swenberg JA, Richardson FC, Boucheron JA, Dyroff MC: Relationships between DNA adduct formation and carcinogenesis. *Environ Health Perspect* 62:177–183, 1985.

Swerdlow AJ, Douglas AJ, Hudson G, et al: Risk of second primary cancers after Hodgkin's disease by type of treatment: Analysis of 2846 patients in the British National Lymphoma Investigation. *Br Med J* 304:1137–1143, 1992.

Swierenga SHH, Bradlaw JA, Brillinger RL, et al: Recommended protocols based on a survey of current practice in genotoxicity testing laboratories: I. Unscheduled DNA synthesis assay in rat hepatocyte cultures. *Mutat Res* 246:235–253, 1991.

Takahashi S, Kubota Y, Sato H: Mutant frequencies in *lacZ* transgenic mice following the internal irradiation from ^{89}Sr or the external γ-ray irradiation. *J Radiat Res* 39:53–60, 1998.

Takayama S, Hasegawa H, Ohgaki H: Combination effects of forty carcinogens administered at low doses to male rats. *Jpn J Cancer Res* 80:732–736, 1989.

Takuwa N, Takuwa Y: Signal transduction of cell-cycle regulation: Its temporo-spacial architecture. *Jpn J Physiol* 46:431–449, 1996.

Talalay P, De Long MJ, Prochaska HJ: Identification of a common chemical signal regulating the induction of enzymes that protect against chemical carcinogenesis. *Proc Natl Acad Sci USA* 85:8261–8265, 1988.

Taper HS: The effect of estradiol-17-phenylpropionate and estradiol benzoate on *N*-nitrosomorpholine-induced liver carcinogenesis in ovariectomized female rats. *Cancer* 42:462–467, 1978.

Tatematsu M, Nagamine Y, Farber E: Redifferentiation as a basis for remodeling of carcinogen-induced hepatocyte nodules to normal appearing liver. *Cancer Res* 43:5049–5058, 1983.

Teeguarden JG, Dragan YP, Pitot HC Implications of hormesis on the bioassay and hazard assessment of chemical carcinogens. *Hum Exp Toxicol* 17:254–258, 1998.

Tennant RW: Evaluation and validation issues in the development of transgenic mouse carcinogenicity bioassays. *Environ Health Perspect* 106:473–476, 1998.

Tennant RW: A perspective on nonmutagenic mechanisms in carcinogenesis. *Environ Health Perspect Suppl* 101:231–236, 1993.

Tennant RW, Ashby J: Classification according to chemical structure, mutagenicity to *Salmonella* and level of carcinogenicity of a further 39 chemicals tested for carcinogenicity by the U.S. National Toxicology Program. *Mutat Res* 257:209–227, 1991.

Tennant RW, Spalding JW, Stasiewicz S, et al: Comparative evaluation of genetic toxicity patterns of carcinogens and noncarcinogens: Strategies for predictive use of short-term assays. *Environ Health Perspect* 75:87–95, 1987.

Thomas DB: Oral contraceptives and breast cancer: Review of the epidemiologic literature. *Contraception* 43:597–642, 1991.

Thomassen MJ, Buoen LC, Brand I, Brand KG: Foreign-body tumorigenesis in mice: DNA synthesis in surface-attached cells during preneoplasia. *J Natl Cancer Inst* 61:359–363, 1978.

Tinwell H, Ashby J: Comparative activity of human carcinogens and NTP rodent carcinogens in the mouse bone marrow micronucleus assay: An integrative approach to genetic toxicity data assessment. *Environ Health Perspect* 102:758–762, 1994.

Tokusashi Y Fukuda I, Ogawa, K: Absence of *p53* mutations and various frequencies of Ki-*ras* exon 1 mutations in rat hepatic tumors induced by different carcinogens. *Mol Carcinogen* 10:45–51, 1994.

Trichopoulos D: Epidemiology of diet and cancer, in Rhoads JE, Fortner J (eds): *Accomplishments in Cancer Research.* Philadelphia: Lippincott, 1989, pp 318–324.

Tsurimoto T: PCNA, a multifunctional ring on DNA. *Biochim Biophys Acta* 1443:23–39, 1998.

Ueda G, Furth J: Sacromatoid transformation of transplanted thyroid carcinoma. *Arch Pathol* 83:3, 1967.

Umar A, Boyer JC, Thomas DC, et al: Defective mismatch repair in extracts of colorectal and endometrial cancer cell lines exhibiting microsatellite instability. *J Biol Chem* 269:14367–14370, 1994.

Upton AC: Radiation injury: Past, present and future, in Hill RB, Terzian JA (eds): *Topics in Environmental Pathology: Elements of a Curriculum for Students of Medicine*. Assoc. Univ. Res. Education Pathol., Bethesda, MD, 1980.

Vainio H, Coleman M, Wilbourn J: Carcinogenicity evaluations and ongoing studies: The IARC databases. *Environ Health Perspect* 96:5–9, 1991.

Vainio H, Hemminki K, Wilbourn J: Data on the carcinogenicity of chemicals in the IARC Monographs programme. *Carcinogenesis* 6:1653–1665, 1985.

Vainio H, Wilbourn J: Cancer etiology: Agents causally associated with human cancer. *Pharmacol Toxicol* 72:4–11, 1993.

van den Bosch H, Schutgens RBH, Wanders RJA, Tager JM: Biochemistry of peroxisomes. *Annu Rev Biochem* 61:157–197, 1992.

Van Duuren BL, Sivak A, Katz C, et al: The effect of aging and interval between primary and secondary treatment in two-stage carcinogenesis on mouse skin. *Cancer Res* 35:502–505, 1975.

Van Dyck E, Stasiak AZ, Stasiak A, West SC: Binding of double-strand breaks in DNA by human Rad52 protein. *Nature* 398:728–731, 1999.

Verma AK, Boutwell RK: Effects of dose and duration of treatment with the tumor-promoting agent, 12-O-tetradecanoylphorbol-13-acetate on mouse skin carcinogenesis. *Carcinogenesis* 1:271–276, 1980.

Verschaeve L, Driesen M, Kirsch-Volders M, et al: Chromosome distribution studies after inorganic lead exposure. *Hum Genet* 49:147–158 1979.

Vesselinovitch SD, Mihailovich N, Rao KVN: Morphology and metastatic nature of induced hepatic nodular lesions in C57BL × C3H F_1 mice. *Cancer Res* 38:2003–2010, 1978.

Vojtek AB, Der CJ: Increasing complexity of the Ras signaling pathway. *J Biol Chem* 273:19925–19928, 1998.

Waalkes MP, Coogan TP, Barter RA: Toxicological principles of metal carcinogenesis with special emphasis on cadmium. *Crit Rev Toxicol* 22:175–201, 1992.

Wallace LA: The exposure of the general population to benzene. *Cell Biol Toxicol* 5:297–314, 1989.

Wang MY, Liehr JG: Identification of fatty acid hydroperoxide cofactors in the cytochrome P450-mediated oxidation of estrogens to quinone metabolites. *J Biol Chem* 269:284–291, 1994.

Ward EJ: Persistent and heritable structural damage induced in heterochromatic DNA from rat liver by *N*-nitrosodimethylamine. *Biochemistry* 26:1709–1717, 1987.

Warren BS, Naylor MF, Winberg LD, et al: Induction and inhibition of tumor progression. *Proc Soc Exp Biol Med* 202:9–15, 1993.

Warshawsky D, Barkley W, Bingham E: Factors affecting carcinogenic potential of mixtures. *Fund Appl Toxicol* 20:376–382, 1993.

Weigel NL: Steroid hormone receptors and their regulation by phosphorylation. *Biochem J* 319:657–667, 1996.

Weisburger EK, Weisburger JH: Chemistry, carcinogenicity and metabolism of 2-fluorenamine and related compounds. *Adv Cancer Res* 5:331–431, 1958.

Weisburger JH, Williams GH: Metabolism of chemical carcinogens, in Becker FF (ed): *Cancer: A Comprehensive Treatise.* Vol 1. New York: Plenum Press, 1982, pp 241–333.

Welch DR, Tomasovic SP: Implications of tumor progression on clinical oncology. *Clin Exp Metast* 3:151–188, 1985.

Westra JG, Kriek E, Hittenhausen H: Identification of the persistently bound form of the carcinogen *N*-acetyl-2-aminofluorene to rat liver DNA in vivo. *Chem Biol Interact* 15:149–164, 1976.

White E, Malone KE, Weiss NS, Daling JR: Breast cancer among young U.S. women in relation to oral contraceptive use. *J Natl Cancer Inst* 86:505–514, 1994.

Wigley CB: Experimental approaches to the analysis of precancer. *Cancer Surv* 2:495–515, 1983.

Willett WC, MacMahon B: Diet and cancer—An overview. *N Engl J Med* 310:633–638, 697–701, 1984.

Williams ED: TSH and thyroid cancer, in Pfeiffer EF, Reaven GM (eds): *Hormone and Metabolic Research.* Suppl Series. Vol 23. New York: Theime, 1989, pp 72–75 .

Williams GM: The significance of chemically induced hepatocellular altered foci in rat liver and application to carcinogen detection. *Toxicol Pathol* 17:663–674, 1989.

Williams GM, Iatropoulos MJ, Djordjevic MV, Kaltenberg OP: The triphenylethylene drug tamoxifen is a strong liver carcinogen in the rat. *Carcinogenesis* 14:315–317, 1993.

Williams GM, Mori H, McQueen CA: Structure-activity relationships in the rat hepatocyte DNA-repair test for 300 chemicals. *Mutat Res* 221:263–286, 1989.

Wilson MJ, Shivapurkar N, Poirier LA: Hypomethylation of hepatic nuclear DNA in rats fed with a carcinogenic methyl-deficient diet. *Biochem J* 218:987–990, 1984.

Winick NJ, McKenna RW, Shuster JJ, et al: Secondary acute myeloid leukemia in children with acute lymphoblastic leukemia treated with etoposide. *J Clin Oncol* 11:209–217, 1993.

Wintersberger U, Klein F: Yeast-mating-type switching: A model system for the study of genome rearrangements induced by carcinogens. *Ann NY Acad Sci* 534:513–520, 1988.

Wise RW, Zenser TV, Kadlubar FF, Davis BB: Metabolic activation of carcinogenic aromatic amines by dog bladder and kidney prostaglandin H synthase. *Cancer Res* 44:1893–1897, 1984.

Wogan GN: Aflatoxins as risk factors for hepatocellular carcinoma in humans. *Cancer Res* 52:2114s–2118s, 1992.

Wright SC, Zhong J, Larrick J: Inhibition of apoptosis as a mechanism of tumor promotion. *FASEB J* 8:654–660, 1994.

Wright WC: *De Morbis Artificum* by Bernardino Ramazzini. The Latin Text of 1713. Chicago: University of Chicago Press, 1940, p 191.

Wu HH, Kawamata H, Wang DD, Oyasu R: Immunohistochemical localization of transforming growth factor α in the major salivary glands of male and female rats. *Histochem J* 25:613–618, 1993.

Wu X, Levine AJ: p53 and E2F-1 cooperate to mediate apoptosis. *Proc Natl Acad Sci USA* 91:3602–3606, 1994.

Wyllie AH: Apoptosis: Cell death in tissue regulation. *J Pathol* 153:313–316, 1987.

Wynder EL, Weisburger JH, Horn C: On the importance and relevance of tumour promotion systems in the development of nutritionally linked cancers. *Cancer Surv* 2:557–576, 1983.

Wyrobek AJ, Bruce WR: Chemical induction of sperm abnormalities in mice. *Proc Natl Acad Sci USA* 72:4425–4429, 1975.

Xu YH, Sattler GL, Pitot HC: A method for the comparative study of replicative DNA synthesis in GGT-positive and GGT-negative hepatocytes in primary culture isolated from carcinogen-treated rats. *In Vitro Cell Dev Biol* 24:995–1000, 1998.

Yager JD, Yager R: Oral contraceptive steroids as promoters of hepatocarcinogenesis in female Sprague-Dawley rats. *Cancer Res* 40:3680–3685, 1980.

Yamagawa K, Ichikawa K: Experimentelle Studie über die Pathogenese der Epithelialgeschwülste. *Mitteilungen Med Fakultät Kaiserl Univ Tokyo* 15:295–344, 1915.

Yamane HK, Fung BKK: Covalent modifications of G-proteins. *Annu Rev Pharmacol Toxicol* 32:201–241, 1993.

Yang SK, McCourt DW, Roller PP, Gelboin HV: Enzymatic conversion of benzo[*a*]pyrene leading predominantly to the diol-epoxide *r*-7,*t*-8-dihydroxy-*t*-9,10-oxy-7,8,9,10-tetrahydrobenzo[*a*]pyrene through a single enantiomer of *r*-7, *t*-8-dihydroxy-7,8-dihydrobenzo[*a*]pyrene. *Proc Natl Acad Sci USA* 73:2594–2598, 1976.

Yokota J, Sugimura T: Multiple steps in carcinogenesis involving alterations of multiple tumor suppressor genes. *FASEB J* 7:920–925, 1993.

You M, Candrian U, Maronpot RR, et al: Activation of the Ki-*ras* protooncogene in spontaneously occurring and chemically induced lung tumors of the strain A mouse. *Proc Natl Acad Sci USA* 86:3070–3074, 1989.

Yu MW, Chen CJ: Elevated serum testosterone levels and risk of hepatocellular carcinoma. *Cancer Res* 53:790–794, 1993.

Zatonski W, Becher H, Lissowska J: Smoking cessation: Intermediate nonsmoking periods and reduction of laryngeal cancer risk. *J Natl Cancer Inst* 82:1427–1428, 1990.

Zeise L, Wilson R, Crouch E: Dose response relationships for carcinogens: A review. *Environ Health Perspect* 73:259–308, 1987.

Zhang R, Haag JD, Gould MN: Quantitating the frequency of initiation and cH-ras mutation in *in situ N*-methyl-*N*-nitrosourea-exposed rat mammary gland. *Cell Growth Diff* 2:1–6, 1991.

Zhu BT, Roy D, Liehr JG: The carcinogenic activity of ethinyl estrogens is determined by both their hormonal characteristics and their conversion to catechol metabolites. *Endocrinology* 132:577–583, 1993.

CHAPTER 9

GENETIC TOXICOLOGY

R. Julian Preston and George R. Hoffmann

WHAT IS GENETIC TOXICOLOGY?

Genetic toxicology is a branch of the field of toxicology that assesses the effects of chemical and physical agents on the hereditary material (DNA) and on the genetic processes of living cells. Such effects can be assessed directly by measuring the interaction of agents with DNA or more indirectly through the assessment of DNA repair or the production of gene mutations or chromosome alterations. Given the risk assessment framework of this chapter, it is important at the outset to distinguish between genotoxicity and mutagenicity. Genotoxicity covers a broader spectrum of endpoints than mutagenicity. For example, unscheduled DNA synthesis, sister chromatid exchanges, and DNA strand breaks are measures of genotoxicity, not mutagenicity, because they are not themselves transmissible events from cell to cell or generation to generation.

This chapter discusses the history of the development of the field of genetic toxicology, the use of genetic toxicologic data in cancer and genetic risk assessment, the mechanisms underlying genetic toxicology assays, the assays that can be used for detecting genotoxic endpoints, the use of the same assays for better understanding mechanisms of mutagenesis, and new methods for the assessment of genetic alterations. The field is evolving rapidly, and the present snapshot will set the stage for considering this evolution.

HISTORY OF GENETIC TOXICOLOGY

The field of genetic toxicology can be considered to have its roots in the pioneering work of H.J. Muller (1927), who showed that x-rays could induce phenotypically described mutations in the fruit fly, *Drosophila.* In his studies he showed not only that radiation exposures could increase the overall frequencies of mutations but also that the types of mutations induced were exactly the same in effect, or phenotype, as those observed in the absence of radiation exposure. Thus, the induced mutagenic responses must be assessed in relation to background mutations. As a conclusion to this study of radiation-induced mutations, Muller predicted the utility of mutagenesis for gene mapping and for parallel mutagenic responses in germ cells.

Karl Sax (1938) built upon Muller's original studies of radiation-induced mutagenicity by showing that x-rays could also induce structural alterations to chromosomes in *Tradescantia* pollen grains. Sax and his colleagues, notably in the absence of a knowledge of DNA structure and chromosomal organization, showed that at least two critical lesions in a nuclear target are required for the production of an exchange within (intrachromosome) or between (interchromosome) chromosomes. We know now that the lesions identified by Sax are DNA double-strand breaks (dsb), base damages (bd), or multiply damaged sites (mds) (reviewed by Ward, 1988). In addition, Sax and colleagues (Sax, 1939; Sax and Luippold, 1952) showed that the yield of chromosome aberrations was reduced if the total dose of x-rays was delivered over extended periods of time or split into two fractions separated by several hours. These observations led to the concept of restitution of radiation-induced damage, which was later recognized as involving specific DNA repair processes (see below).

Consideration of the genetic effects of exogenous agents on cells was expanded to include chemicals in 1946, when Charlotte Auerbach and colleagues reported that nitrogen mustards could induce mutations in *Drosophila* and that these mutations were phenotypically similar to those induced by x-rays (Auerbach and Robson, 1946). Thus, the field of chemical mutagenesis was initiated to run in parallel with studies of radiation mutagenesis. These original studies of Auerbach (actually conducted in 1941) are placed in a historical and biological perspective by the delightful review of Geoffrey Beale (1993).

While the scientific value of the analysis of mutations in *Drosophila* was clear, there was an impression that the practical application to human populations was too wide a step. Thus, a research effort of great magnitude was initiated to attempt to assess radiation-induced mutations in mice. This effort resulted in the publication by William Russell (1951) of data on x-ray–induced mutations using a mouse specific-locus mutation assay. These data clearly showed that the type of results obtained with *Drosophila* could be replicated in a mammalian system. The mouse tester strain developed for the specific-locus assay has recessive mutations at seven loci coding for visible mutations, such as coat color, eye color, and ear shape. This homozygous recessive tester strain can be used for identifying recessive mutations induced in wild-type genes at the same loci in other mice. It was noteworthy that the mutation rate for x-ray-induced mutations in germ cells was similar in mouse and *Drosophila.* Subsequent studies by Lee Russell (Russell et al., 1981) showed that chemicals could induce mutations at the same seven loci.

Over the next 20 years, genetic toxicologists investigated the induction of mutations and chromosomal alterations in somatic and germ cells largely following exposures to radiations. The ability to grow cells in vitro, either as primary cultures or as transformed cell lines, enhanced these quantitative studies. The in vitro culture of human lymphocytes, stimulated to reenter the cell cycle by phytohemagglutinin, greatly expanded the information on the assessment of chromosomal alterations in human cells [an excellent review by Hsu (1979) is recommended]. It also became feasible to use cytogenetic alterations in human lymphocytes as a biodosimeter for assessing human exposures to ionizing radiations (Bender and Gooch, 1962).

Two events during the 1970s served to expand the utility of mutagenicity data into the realm of risk assessment. The Millers and their colleagues (Miller and Miller, 1977) showed that chemical carcinogens could react to form stable, covalent derivatives with DNA, RNA, and proteins both in vitro and in vivo. In addition, they reported that these derivatives could require the metabolism of the parent chemical to form reactive metabolites. This metabolism is required for some chemicals to become carcinogens. Metabolic capability is endogenous in vivo, but most cell lines in vitro have lost this capacity. To overcome this for in vitro mutagenicity studies, Heinrich Malling and colleagues developed an exogenous metabolizing system based upon a rodent liver homogenate (S9) (Malling and Frantz, 1973). While this exogenous metabolism system has had utility, it does have drawbacks related to species and tissue specificity. The development of transgenic cell lines containing inducible P450 genes has overcome this drawback to some extent (Crespi and Miller, 1999).

The second development in the 1970s that changed the field of genetic toxicology was the development by Bruce Ames and colleagues (Ames et al., 1975) of a simple, inexpensive mutation assay with the bacterium *Salmonella typhimurium.* This assay can be used to detect chemically induced reverse mutations at the histidine loci and can incorporate the exogenous metabolizing S9 system described above. The Ames assay, as it is generally called, has been expanded and modified to enhance its specificity as discussed below (under "Gene Mutations in Prokaryotes"). The assay has been used extensively, especially for hazard identification, as part of the cancer risk-assessment process. This use was based on the assumption that carcinogens were mutagens, given that cancer required mutation induction. This latter dogma proved to be somewhat inhibitory, in some ways, to the field of genetic toxicology because it provided a framework that was too rigid. Nonetheless, over the decade of the mid-1970s to mid-1980s somewhere on the order of 200 short-term assays were developed for screening potentially carcinogenic chemicals. The screens included mutagenicity, DNA damage, DNA repair, and cell killing or other genotoxic activities. Several international collaborative studies were organized to establish the sensitivity and specificity of a select group of assays as well as to assess interlaboratory variation (IPCS, 1988). In summary, most assays were able to detect carcinogens or noncarcinogens with an efficiency of about 70 percent as compared with the outcome of cancer bioassays. There are a number of possible reasons for the imperfect correspondence, the most likely being that there is a group of chemical carcinogens that do not induce cancer by a direct mutagenic action. The latter point was addressed to some extent by Tennant et al. (1987), who compared the effectiveness of a small standard battery of well-characterized short-term assays to identify carcinogens. Again, this battery predicted about 70 percent of known carcinogens. Subsequently, the lack of a tight correlation between carcinogenicity and mutagenicity (and the converse, noncarcinogenicity and nonmutagenicity) was found to be due to the fact that some chemicals were not directly mutagenic but instead induced the damage necessary for tumor development indirectly by, for example, clonally expanding preexisting mutant cells (i.e., tumor promotion). This class of chemicals has been given the rather unfortunate name of *nongenotoxic* to contrast them with genotoxic ones; the classification as *not directly mutagenic* is more appropriate. In the past 10 years or so, emphasis has been placed on identifying mechanisms whereby nondirectly mutagenic chemicals can be involved in tumor production.

Those identified include cytotoxicity with regenerative cell proliferation, mitogenicity, receptor-mediated processes, changes in methylation status, and alterations in cell–cell communication.

In the past 10 years or so, the field of genetic toxicology has moved away from the short-term assay approach for assessing carcinogenicity to a much more mechanistic approach, fueled to quite an extent by the advances in molecular biology. The ability to manipulate and characterize DNA, RNA, and proteins and to understand basic cellular processes and how they can be perturbed has advanced enormously over this period. Knowing how to take advantage of these technical developments is paramount. This chapter addresses current genetic toxicology: the assays for qualitative and quantitative assessment of cellular changes induced by chemical and physical agents, the underlying molecular mechanisms for these changes, and how such information can be incorporated in cancer and genetic risk assessments. In addition, the way forward for the field is addressed in the form of an epilogue. Thus, the preceding historical overview sets the stage for the rest of the chapter.

HEALTH IMPACT OF GENETIC ALTERATIONS

The importance of mutations and chromosomal alterations for human health is evident from their roles in genetic disorders and cancer. Therefore, mutations in both germ cells and somatic cells must be considered here.

Somatic Cells

An association between mutation and cancer has long been evident on indirect grounds, such as a correlation between the mutagenicity and carcinogenicity of chemicals, especially in biological systems that have the requisite metabolic activation capabilities. Moreover, human chromosome instability syndromes and DNA repair deficiencies are associated with increased cancer risk (Friedberg, 1985). Cancer cytogenetics has greatly strengthened the association in that specific chromosomal alterations, including deletions, translocations, and inversions, have been implicated in many human leukemias and lymphomas as well as in some solid tumors (Rabbitts, 1994).

Critical evidence that mutation plays a central role in cancer has come from molecular studies of oncogenes and tumor suppressor genes. Oncogenes are genes that stimulate the transformation of normal cells into cancer cells (Bishop, 1991). They originate when genes called proto-oncogenes, involved in normal cellular growth and development, are genetically altered. Normal regulation of cellular proliferation requires a balance between factors that promote growth and those that restrict it. Mutational alteration of proto-oncogenes can lead to overexpression of their growth-stimulating activity, whereas mutations that inactivate tumor suppressor genes, which normally restrain cellular proliferation, free cells from their inhibitory influence (Hanahan and Weinberg, 2000).

The action of oncogenes is genetically dominant in that a single active oncogene is expressed even though its normal allele is present in the same cell. Proto-oncogenes can be converted into active oncogenes by point mutations or chromosomal alterations. Base-pair substitutions in *ras* proto-oncogenes are found in many human tumors (Bishop, 1991; Barrett, 1993). Among chromosomal alterations that activate proto-oncogenes, translocations are especially prevalent (Rabbitts, 1994). For example, Burkitt's lymphoma involves a translocation between the long arm of chromosome 8, which is the site of the *c-MYC* oncogene, and chromosome 14 (about 90 percent of cases), 22, or 2. A translocation can activate a proto-oncogene by moving it to a new chromosomal location, typically the site of a T-cell receptor or immunoglobulin gene, where its expression is enhanced. This mechanism applies to Burkitt's lymphoma and various other hematopoietic cancers. Alternatively, the translocation may join two genes, resulting in a protein fusion that contributes to cancer development. Fusions have been implicated in other hematopoietic cancers and some solid tumors (Rabbitts, 1994). Like translocations, other chromosomal alterations can activate proto-oncogenes, and genetic amplification of oncogenes can magnify their expression (Bishop, 1991).

Mutational inactivation or deletion of tumor suppressor genes has been implicated in many cancers. Unlike oncogenes, the cancer-causing alleles that arise from tumor suppressor genes are typically recessive in that they are not expressed when they are heterozygous (Evans and Prosser, 1992). However, several genetic mechanisms, including mutation, deletion, chromosome loss, and mitotic recombination, can inactivate or eliminate the normal dominant allele, leading to the expression of the recessive cancer gene in a formerly heterozygous cell (Cavenee et al., 1983). The inactivation of tumor suppressor genes has been associated with various cancers, including those of the eye, kidney, colon, brain, breast, lung, and bladder (Fearon and Vogelstein, 1990; Marshall, 1991). Gene mutations in a tumor suppressor gene on, chromosome 17 called *P53* occur in many different human cancers, and molecular characterization of *P53* mutations has linked specific human cancers to mutagen exposures (Harris, 1993; Aguilar et al., 1994).

In the simplest model for the action of tumor suppressor genes, two events are required for the development of the cancer, because both normal alleles must be inactivated or lost (Knudson, 1997). In sporadic forms of the cancer (i.e., no family history), the two genetic events occur independently, but in familial forms (e.g., familial retinoblastoma), the first mutation is inherited, leaving the need for only a single additional event for expression. The strong predisposition to cancer in the inherited disease stems from the high likelihood that a loss of heterozygosity will occur by mutation, recombination, or aneuploidy in at least one or a few cells in the development of the affected organ. The simple model involving two events and a single pair of alleles cannot explain all observations concerning tumor suppressor genes, because many cancers involve more than one tumor suppressor gene. For example, the childhood kidney tumor called Wilms' tumor can be caused by damage in at least three different genes (Marshall, 1991), and colorectal carcinomas are often found to have lost not only the wild-type *P53* tumor suppressor gene but also other tumor suppressor genes (Fearon and Vogelstein, 1990; Stoler et al., 1999). Moreover, a single mutation in a tumor suppressor gene, even though not fully expressed, may contribute to carcinogenesis. For example, a single *P53* mutation in a developing colorectal tumor may confer a growth advantage that contributes to the development of the disease (Venkatachalam et al., 1998). Subsequent loss of heterozygosity will increase the growth advantage as the tumor progresses from benign to malignant (Fearon and Vogelstein, 1990).

Many cancers involve both activation of oncogenes and inactivation of tumor suppressor genes (Bishop, 1991; Fearon and Vogelstein, 1990). The observation of multiple genetic changes supports the view that cancer results from an accumulation of genetic alterations and that carcinogenesis is a multistep process (Stoler et al., 1999; Kinzler et al., 1996; Hahn et al., 1999). At least three stages can be recognized in carcinogenesis: initiation, promotion, and progression (Barrett, 1993). *Initiation* involves the induction of a genetic alteration, such as the mutational activation of a *ras* proto-oncogene by a mutagen. It is an irreversible step that starts the process toward cancer. *Promotion* involves cellular proliferation in an initiated cell population. Promotion can lead to the development of benign tumors such as papillomas. Agents called promoters stimulate this process. Promoters may be mutagenic but are not necessarily so. *Progression* involves the continuation of cell proliferation and the accumulation of additional irreversible genetic changes; it is marked by increasing genetic instability and malignancy. More recent studies are beginning to change this view, leading to the concept of acquired capabilities (Hanahan and Weinberg, 2000).

Gene mutations, chromosome aberrations, and aneuploidy are all implicated in the development of cancer. Mutagens and clastogens contribute to carcinogenesis as initiators. Their role does not have to be restricted to initiation, however, in that mutagens, clastogens, and aneugens may contribute to the multiple genetic alterations that characterize progression or development of acquired capabilities. Other agents that contribute to carcinogenesis, such as promoters, need not be mutagens. However, the role of mutations is critical, and analyzing mutations and mutagenic effects is essential for understanding and predicting chemical carcinogenesis.

Germ Cells

The relevance of gene mutations to health is evident from the many disorders that are inherited as simple Mendelian characteristics (Mohrenweiser, 1991). About 1.3 percent of newborns suffer from autosomal dominant (1 percent), autosomal recessive (0.25 percent), or sex-linked (0.05 percent) genetic diseases (National Research Council, 1990; Sankaranarayanan, 1998). Molecular analysis of the mutations responsible for Mendelian diseases has revealed that almost half these mutations are base-pair substitutions; of the remainder, most are small deletions (Sankaranarayanan, 1998).

Many genetic disorders (e.g., cystic fibrosis, phenylketonuria, Tay-Sachs disease) are caused by the expression of recessive mutations. These mutations are mainly inherited from previous generations and are expressed when an individual inherits the mutant gene from both parents. New mutations make a larger contribution to the incidence of dominant diseases than to that of recessive diseases because only a single dominant mutation is required for expression. Thus, new dominant mutations are expressed in the first generation. If a dominant disorder is severe, its transmission between generations is unlikely because of reduced fitness. For dominants with a mild effect, reduced penetrance, or a late age of onset, however, the contribution from previous generations is apt to be greater than that from new mutations. Estimating the proportion of all Mendelian genetic disease that can be ascribed to new mutations is not straightforward; a rough estimate is 20 percent (Wyrobek, 1993; Shelby, 1994).

Besides causing diseases that exhibit Mendelian inheritance, gene mutations undoubtedly contribute to human disease through the genetic component of disorders with a complex etiology. Some 3 percent (National Research Council, 1990) or 5 to 6 percent (Sankaranarayanan, 1998) of infants are affected by congenital abnormalities; if one includes multifactorial disorders that often have a late onset, such as heart disease, hypertension, and diabetes, the proportion of the population affected increases to more than 60 percent (National Research Council, 1990; Sankaranarayanan, 1998). Such frequencies are necessarily approximate because of differences among surveys in the reporting and classification of disorders. A higher prevalence would be found if less severe disorders were included in the tabulation. Nevertheless, such estimates provide a sense of the large impact of genetic disease.

Refined cytogenetic methods have led to the discovery of minor variations in chromosome structure that have no apparent effect. Nevertheless, other chromosome aberrations cause fetal death or serious abnormalities. Aneuploidy (gain or loss of one or more chromosomes) also contributes to fetal deaths and causes disorders such as Down's syndrome. About 4 infants per 1000 have syndromes associated with chromosomal abnormalities, including translocations and aneuploidy. The majority of these syndromes (about 85 percent) result from trisomies (National Research Council, 1990). Much of the effect of chromosomal abnormalities occurs prenatally. It has been estimated that 5 percent of all recognized pregnancies involve chromosomal abnormalities, as do about 6 percent of infant deaths and 30 percent of all spontaneous embryonic and fetal deaths (Mohrenweiser, 1991). Among the abnormalities, aneuploidy is the most common, followed by polyploidy. Structural aberrations constitute about 5 percent of the total. Unlike gene mutations, many of which are inherited from the previous generation, about 85 percent of the chromosomal anomalies detected in newborns arise de novo in the germ cells of the parents (Mohrenweiser, 1991). The frequency of aneuploidy assessed directly in human sperm initially by standard karyotyping and more recently by fluorescence in situ hybridization (FISH) is 3 to 4 percent; about 0.4 percent are sex chromosome aneuploidies (Martin et al., 1991; Martin et al., 1996). The frequency of aneuploidy in human oocytes is about 18 percent (Martin et al., 1991).

CANCER AND GENETIC RISK ASSESSMENTS

Cancer Risk Assessment

The formalized process for conducting a cancer risk assessment has many variations based upon national requirements and regulations. A summary of some of the different approaches can be found in Moolenaar (1994). There are ongoing attempts, for example, by the International Program on Chemical Safety (IPCS), to develop a harmonized approach to cancer (and genetic) risk assessments. However, no unified approach is currently available. Thus, for the purpose of this chapter, the formalized approach developed by the U.S. Environmental Protection Agency (EPA) based upon the paradigm presented by the National Research Council (National Research Council, 1983) is described here for depicting the use of genetic toxicology in the risk assessment process.

Genetic toxicology data have been used until recently solely for hazard identification. Namely, if a chemical is directly mutagenic, then tumors are produced by this chemical via direct mutagenicity. This has led, in turn, to the use of the default linear extrapolation from the rodent bioassay tumor data to exposure levels consistent with human environmental or occupational exposures (EPA, 1986). The assessment of risk requires the application of a series of default options—for example, from laboratory animals to humans, from large to small exposures, from intermittent to chronic lifetime exposures, and from route to route of exposure. Default options are "generic approaches, based on general scientific knowledge and policy judgement that are applied to various elements of the risk assessment process when specific scientific information is not available" (National Research Council, 1994). The default options have been in some ways the Achilles' heel of the cancer risk-assessment process, since they have a very significant impact on low exposure risk but are based on an uncertain data base. This concern led the EPA (1996) to develop a very different approach, described in the *Proposed Guidelines for Carcinogen Risk Assessment.* In these proposed guidelines, the emphasis is on using mechanistic data, when available, to inform the risk assessment process, particularly for dose–response assessment. The goal is to develop biologically based dose–response models for estimating cancer risk at low environmental exposures. This does, in general, bring the EPA approach into some harmony with those in other countries (Moolenaar, 1994), where a more narrative approach to risk assessment is preferred to a strictly quantitative one. The outcome of a more mechanistically based cancer risk-assessment process is that there is a greater impetus to developing a database for mechanisms in addition to the yes/no interpretation of genotoxicity assays. The same group of genotoxicity assays can be used for the collection of both types of information. The advent of molecular biology techniques has certainly aided in the pursuit of mechanisms of mutagenicity and carcinogenicity. It is anticipated that the cancer risk-assessment process will evolve as new types of data are obtained.

In this regard, some of the issues that remain to be more firmly elucidated are (1) the relative sensitivities of different species (particularly rodent and human) to the induction of organ-specific mutations and tumors by chemicals and radiation; (2) the shape of the dose response for genetic alterations and tumors at low (environmental) exposure levels, especially for genotoxic chemicals; and (3) the relative sensitivity of susceptible subpopulations of all types. A better understanding of these major issues will greatly reduce the uncertainty in cancer risk assessments by, in part, replacing default options with biological data.

Genetic Risk Assessment

The approach for conducting a genetic risk assessment is less well defined than that for cancer risk. In fact, only a handful of genetic risk assessments have been conducted. An in-depth discussion of the topic can be found in the book *Methods for Genetic Risk Assessment* (Brusick, 1994). The reader is also referred to the genetic risk for ethylene oxide developed by the EPA (Rhomberg et al., 1990) and the discussion of this and a recalculation presented by Preston et al. (1995). These two articles serve to highlight the difficulties with and uncertainties in genetic risk assessments.

The general approach is to use rodent germ cell and somatic cell data for induced genetic alterations and human data for induced genetic alterations in somatic cells (when available) to estimate the frequency of genetic alterations in human germ cells. This is the "parallelogram approach" (Fig. 9-1) first used by Brewen and Preston (1974) for x-irradiation and subsequently more fully developed for chemical exposures by Sobels (1982). The aim of this approach is to develop two sensitivity factors: (1) somatic to germ cell in the rodent and (2) rodent to human using somatic cells. These factors can then be used to estimate genetic alterations in human germ cells. Of course, for a complete estimate of genetic risk, it is necessary to obtain an estimate of the frequency of genetic alterations transmitted to the offspring. In addition, separate genetic risk assessments need to be conducted for males and females, given the considerable difference in germ cell development and observed and predicted sensitivity differences.

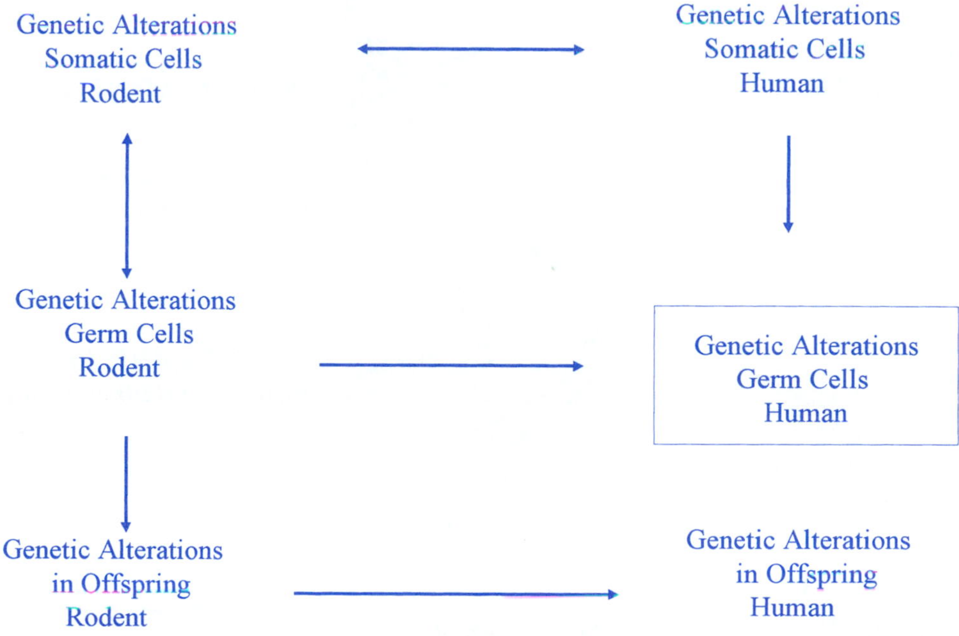

Figure 9-1. Parallelogram approach for genetic risk assessment.

Data obtained for genetic alterations in rodent somatic and germ cells and human somatic cells are used to estimate the frequency of the same genetic alterations in human germ cells. The final step is to estimate the frequency of these genetic alterations that are transmitted to offspring.

MECHANISMS OF INDUCTION OF GENETIC ALTERATIONS

DNA Damage

The types of DNA damage produced by ionizing radiations, nonionizing radiations, and chemicals are many and varied, ranging from single- and double-strand breaks in the DNA backbone to cross-links between DNA bases and between DNA bases and proteins and chemical addition to the DNA bases (adducts) (Fig. 9-2). The aim of this section is to introduce the topic of DNA damage because such damage is the substrate for the formation of genetic alterations and genotoxicity in general. However, much greater detail can be found in recent reviews that are referenced at the appropriate places.

Ionizing Radiations Ionizing radiations such as x-rays, gamma rays, and alpha particles produce DNA single- and double-strand breaks and a broad range of base damages (Ward, 1994; Wallace, 1994; Goodhead, 1994). The relative proportions of these different classes of DNA damage vary with type of radiation. For example, single-strand breaks and base damages predominate with

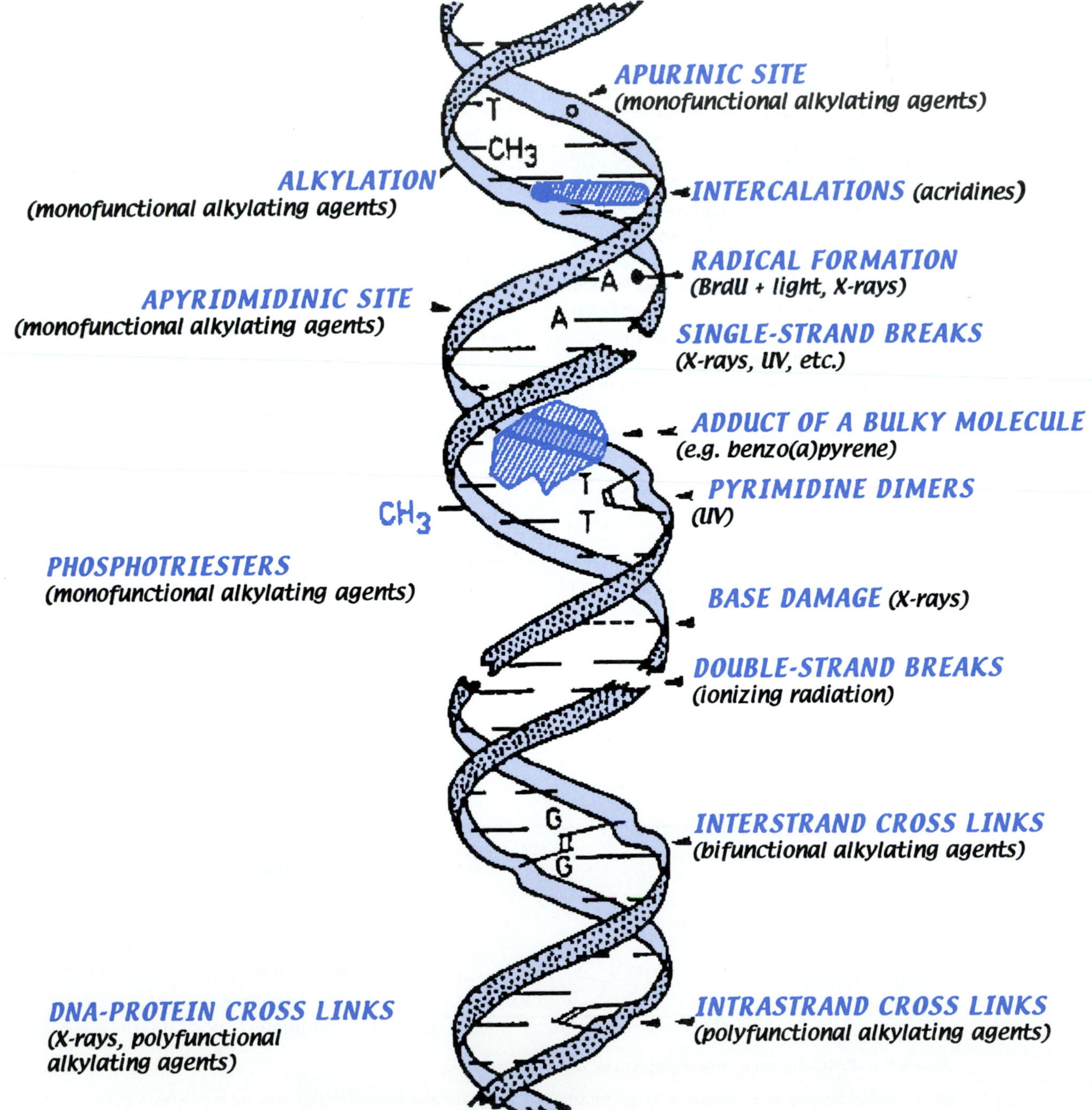

Figure 9-2. Spectrum of DNA damage induced by physical and chemical agents.

x-rays, for which ionization density is sparse, whereas the frequencies of single- and double-strand breaks are more similar with alpha particles, for which ionization density is dense. The frequencies of individual base damages have been assessed using monoclonal antibodies, for example (Le et al., 1998), but only a very few of the total spectrum have so far been studied.

Ultraviolet Light Ultraviolet light (a nonionizing radiation) induces two predominant lesions, cyclobutane pyrimidine dimers and 6,4-photoproducts. These lesions have been studied extensively because they can both be quantitated by chemical and immunological methods (Friedberg et al., 1995).

In part because of this feature, the repair of cyclobutane dimers and 6,4-photoproducts has been extremely well characterized, as discussed below.

Chemicals Chemicals can produce base alterations either directly as adducts or indirectly by intercalation of a chemical between the base pairs (e.g., 9-aminoacridine) (see Heflich, 1991, for a review). Many electrophilic chemicals react with DNA, forming covalent addition products (adducts). The DNA base involved and the positions on DNA bases can be specific for a given chemical. Such specificity of DNA damage can result in a spectrum of mutations that is chemical specific, i.e., a fingerprint of sorts (Dogliotti et al., 1998). Some alkylated bases can mispair, causing mutations when DNA is replicated. Alkylated bases can also lead to secondary alterations in DNA. For example, the alkyl group of an N7-alkylguanine adduct, which is a major adduct formed by many alkylating agents, labilizes the bond that connects the base to deoxyribose, thereby stimulating base loss. Base loss from DNA leaves an apurinic or apyrimidinic site, commonly called an AP site. The insertion of incorrect bases into AP sites causes mutations (Laval et al., 1990).

Bulky DNA adducts formed, for example, by metabolites of benzo(a)pyrene or N-2-acetylaminofluorene are recognized by the cell in a similar way to UV damages and are repaired similarly (see below). Such adducts can also hinder polymerases and cause mutation as a consequence of errors that they trigger in replication.

Endogenous Agents Endogenous agents are responsible for several hundred DNA damages per cell per day (Lindahl, 2000). The majority of these damages are altered DNA bases (e.g., 8-oxoguanine and thymine glycol) and AP sites. The cellular processes that can lead to a DNA damage are oxygen consumption that results in the formation of reactive active oxygen species (e.g., superoxide $^{\cdot}0_2$, hydroxyl free radicals $^{\cdot}$OH, and hydrogen peroxide) and deamination of cytosines and S-methylcytosines leading to uracils and thymines, respectively. The process of DNA replication itself is error-prone, and an incorrect base can be added by the polymerase. The frequencies of these endogenously produced DNA damages can be increased by exogenous (genotoxic) agents.

DNA Repair

The cell is faced with the problem of how to cope with the quite extensive DNA damage that it sustains. In a general sense, two processes are present to achieve this. If the damage is extensive, the cell can undergo apoptosis (programmed cell death), effectively releasing it from becoming a mutant cell (Evan and Littlewood, 1998). If the damage is less severe, cells have developed a range of repair processes that are part of a generalized cellular DNA damage response network that returns the DNA to its undamaged state (error-free repair) or to an improved but still altered state (error-prone repair). The basic principles underlying most repair processes are damage recognition, removal of damage (except for strand breaks or cleavage of pyrimidine dimers), repair DNA synthesis, and ligation. In order to achieve this for different types of DNA lesions, cells have modified the protein complexes used for other housekeeping processes (e.g., transcription, replication, and recombination). The present chapter presents a brief outline of the major classes of DNA repair; much greater detail can be found in the reviews provided for each section and a general review by Van Houten and Albertini (1995).

Base Excision Repair The major pathways by which DNA base damages are repaired involve a glycosylase that removes the damaged base, causing the production of an apurinic or apyrimidinic site that can be filled by the appropriate base or processed further (McCullough et al., 1999; Demple and Harrison, 1994; Seeberg et al., 1995; Wood, 1996). The resulting gap from this further processing can be filled by a DNA polymerase, followed by ligation to the parental DNA. The size of the gap is dependent upon the particular polymerase involved in the repair (i.e., polymerase β for short patches; polymerase δ or ϵ for longer patches). Oxidative damages, either background or induced, are important substrates for base excision repair (Lindahl, 2000).

Nucleotide Excision Repair The nucleotide excision repair (NER) system provides the cell's ability to remove bulky lesions from DNA. In the past decade, the NER process has been studied extensively, and a complete characterization of the genes and proteins involved has been obtained (Aboussekhra et al., 1995; Sancar, 1995; Lehmann, 1995; Benhamou and Sarasin, 2000). NER uses about 30 proteins to remove a damage-containing oligonucleotide from DNA. The basic steps are damage recognition, incision, excision, repair synthesis, and ligation. The characterization of these steps has been enhanced by the use of rodent mutant cell lines and cells from individuals with the UV-sensitivity, skin cancer–prone syndrome xeroderma pigmentosum (XP, for which there are at least seven distinct genetic complementation groups). Of particular interest is the link between NER and transcription, for which the DNA damage in actively transcribing genes, and specifically the transcribed strand, is preferentially and thus more rapidly repaired than the DNA damage in the rest of the genome (Lomnel et al., 1995). Thus, the cell protects the integrity of the transcription process. This link between transcription and repair appears to be provided by two factors: (1) when a bulky lesion is located on the transcribed strand of an active gene, RNA polymerase II is blocked, thus providing a signal for recruiting the NER complex, and (2) a major component of the NER complex is the TFII H basal transcription factor. The involvement of TFII H in repair also provides some specificity to the incisions in the DNA required to remove the damaged nucleotide. An incision on the 3′ side of the damage is made first by the XPG protein followed by one on the 5′ side by the XPF-ERRC1 complex. The lesion is removed in the 27-30 nucleotide segment formed by the two incisions. The gap is filled by polymerase δ or ϵ in the presence of replication factor C and proliferating cell nuclear antigen (PCNA). Ligation by DNA ligase I completes the process. This NER process has been reconstituted in vitro, allowing for complete characterization, kinetic studies, and estimates of fidelity (Aboussekhra et al., 1995).

Double-Strand Break Repair Cell survival is seriously compromised by the presence of broken chromosomes. Unrepaired double-strand breaks trigger one or more DNA damage response systems to either check cell-cycle progression or induce apoptosis. In order to reduce the probability of persistent DNA double-strand breaks, cells have developed an array of specific repair pathways. These pathways are largely similar across a broad range of species from yeast to humans, although the most frequently used one is different among species. There are two general pathways for repair of DNA double-strand breaks: homologous recombination and nonhomologous end-joining. These two can be considered as being in competition for the double-strand break substrate (Haber, 2000).

Homologous Recombination Eukaryotes undergo homologous recombination as part of their normal activities both in germ cells (meiotic recombination) and somatic cells (mitotic recombination). The repair of double-strand breaks (and single-strand gaps) basically uses the same process and complex of proteins, although some different protein–protein interactions are involved (Shinohara and Ogawa, 1995). In eukaryotes, the process has been characterized most extensively for yeast, but evidence is accumulating that a very similar process occurs in mammalian cells, including human (Johnson et al., 1999). The basic steps in double-strand break repair are as follows. The initial step is the production of a 3′-ended single-stranded tail by exonucleases or helicase activity. Through a process of strand invasion, whereby the single-stranded tail invades an undamaged homologous DNA molecule, together with DNA synthesis, a so-called Holliday junction DNA complex is formed. By cleavage of this junction, two DNA molecules are produced (with or without a structural crossover), neither of which now contain a strand break. Additional models have been proposed but probably play a minor role in mammalian cells (Haber, 2000). A detailed description of the specific enzymes known to be involved can be found in Shinohara and Ogawa (1995).

Nonhomologous End-Joining (NHEJ) The characterization of NHEJ in mammalian cells was greatly enhanced by the observation that mammalian cell lines that are hypersensitive to ionizing radiation are also defective in the V(D)J recombination process, which is the means by which the huge range of an antibody's antigen-binding sites and T-cell receptor proteins are generated during mammalian lymphoid cell development. V(D)J recombination requires the production of double-strand breaks, recombination of DNA pieces, and subsequent religation. A major component of the NHEJ repair complex is a DNA-dependent protein kinase (DNA-PK). This protein, a serine/threonine kinase, consists of a catalytic subunit (DNA-PK_{cs}) and a DNA-end-binding protein consisting of KU70 and KU80 subunits. The specific role of DNA-PK in the repair of double-strand breaks is unclear in mammalian cells; a detailed discussion of what is known and some possible models of NHEJ is presented in the review by Critchlow and Jackson (1998). Perhaps the most viable role of DNA-PK is to align the broken DNA ends to facilitate their ligation. In addition, DNA-PK might serve as a signal molecule for recruiting other repair proteins known to be involved in yeast and to some extent in mammalian cells. The final ligation step is performed by DNA ligase IV in human cells.

Mismatch Repair The study of DNA mismatch repair systems has received considerable attention over the past few years, in part because an association has been demonstrated between genetic defects in mismatch repair genes and the genomic instability associated with cancer susceptibility syndromes and sporadic cancers. In general, DNA mismatch repair systems operate to repair mismatched bases formed during DNA replication, genetic recombination, and as a result of DNA damage induced by chemical and physical agents. Detailed reviews can be found in Kolodner (1995), Jiricny (1998), and Modrich and Lahue (1996).

The principal steps in all cells from prokaryotes to human are damage recognition by a specific protein that binds to the mismatch, stabilizing of the binding by the addition of one or more proteins, cutting the DNA at a distance from the mismatch, excision past the mismatch, resynthesis, and ligation. In some prokaryotes, the cutting of the DNA (for DNA replication mismatches) is directed to the strand that contains the incorrect base by using the fact that recently replicated DNA is unmethylated at *N*6-methyladenine at a GATC sequence. The question of whether or not strand-specific mismatch repair occurs in mammalian cells has not been resolved, although some evidence does point to its occurrence (Modrich, 1997). Strand-specificity for DNA mismatches resulting from induced DNA damage has not been identified.

***0^6*-Methylguanine-DNA Methyltransferase Repair** The main role for *0^6*-methylguanine-DNA methyltransferase (MGMT) is to protect cells against the toxic effects of simple alkylating agents. The methyl group is transferred from *0^6*-methylguanine in DNA to a cysteine residue in MGMT. The adducted base is reverted to a normal one by the enzyme, which is itself inactivated by the reaction. Details of the MGMT enzyme properties and the gene isolation and characterization can be found in Tano et al. (1990) and Grombacher et al. (1996).

The probability that induced DNA damage can be converted into a genetic alteration is influenced by the particular repair pathway(s) recruited, the rate of repair of the damage and the fidelity and completeness of the repair. The mechanisms of induction of gene mutations and chromosome alterations discussed in the following sections build upon the assessment of probability of repair versus misrepair versus nonrepair that can be derived from a knowledge of the mechanism of action of the different DNA repair mechanisms. The preceding sections, together with the references provided, should assist in this assessment.

Formation of Gene Mutations

Somatic Cells Gene mutations are considered to be small DNA-sequence changes confined to a single gene; larger genomic changes are considered below, under "Formation of Chromosomal Alterations." The classes of gene mutations are broadly based substitutions and small additions or deletions. More detailed classifications can be found in the review by Ripley (1991). Base substitutions are the replacement of the correct nucleotide by an incorrect one; they can be further subdivided as transitions where the change is purine for purine or pyrimidine for pyrimidine; and transversions where the change is purine for pyrimidine and vice versa. Frameshift mutations are strictly the addition or deletion of one or a few base pairs (not in multiples of three) in protein coding regions. The definition is more generally extended to include such additions and deletions in any DNA region. For the discussion of the mechanism of induction of gene mutations and chromosomal alterations, it is necessary to distinguish chemicals by their general mode of action. Chemicals that can produce genetic alterations with similar effectiveness in all stages of the cell cycle are called radiomimetic, since they act like radiation in this regard. Chemicals that produce genetic alterations far more effectively in the S phase are described as nonradiomimetic. The great majority of chemicals are nonradiomimetic; the radiomimetic group includes bleomycin, streptonigrin, neocarzinostatin and 8-ethyoxycaffeine.

Gene mutations can arise in the absence of specific exogenous exposures to radiations and chemicals. The great majority of so-called spontaneous (background) mutations arise from *replication* of an altered template. These DNA alterations are either the result of oxidative damage or are produced from the deamination of 5-methyl cytosine to thymine at CpG sites resulting in G:C $\rightarrow$ A:T transitions. Mutations induced by ionizing radiations tend to be deletions ranging in size from a few bases to multilocus events (Thacker, 1992). The rapid rate of repair of the majority of radiation-induced DNA damages greatly reduces the probability of DNA lesions being present at the time of DNA replication. Thus, mutations induced by ionizing radiations are generally the result of errors of *DNA repair* (Preston, 1992). The low frequency of gene mutations are produced from any unrepaired DNA base damage present during DNA replication.

Gene mutations produced by a majority of chemicals and nonionizing radiations are base substitutions, frameshifts and small deletions. Of these mutations, a very high proportion are produced by errors of DNA *replication* on a damaged template. Thus, the probability of a DNA adduct, for example, being converted into a mutation is determined by the amount of induced DNA adducts that remain in the DNA at the time that it is replicated. Thus, relative mutation frequency will be the outcome of the race between repair and replication, i.e., the more repair that takes place prior to replication the lower the mutation frequency for a given amount of induced DNA damage. Significant regulators of the race are cell cycle checkpoint genes (e.g., *P53*) since, if the cell is checked from entering the S phase at a G_1/S checkpoint, then more repair can take place prior to the cell starting to replicate its DNA (Mercer, 1998).

The proportion of chemically-induced gene mutations that result from DNA repair errors is low, given that the DNA repair processes involved are error-free, and that, as a generalization, repair of chemically-induced DNA damage is slower than for ionizing radiation damage, leading to the balance tipping towards replication prior to repair, especially for cells in the S phase at the time of exposure.

Germ Cells The mechanism of production of gene mutations in germ cells is basically the same as in somatic cells. Ionizing radiations produce mainly deletions via errors of DNA repair; the majority of chemicals induce base substitutions, frameshifts and small deletions by errors of DNA replication (Favor, 1999).

An important consideration for assessing gene mutations induced by chemicals in germ cells is the relationship between exposure and the timing of DNA replication. Figure 9-3 depicts the stages in oogenesis and spermatogenesis when DNA replicates. A few features are worthy of note. The spermatogonial stem cell in humans and rodents has a long cell cycle time, 8 days or longer, with only a small fraction being occupied by the S phase. Thus, the probability of DNA repair taking place prior to DNA replication is high, for both acute and chronic treatments. However, for considerations of genetic risk, it is the spermatogonial stem cell that is the major contributor since it is present, in general, throughout the reproductive lifetime of an individual. Each time a sper-

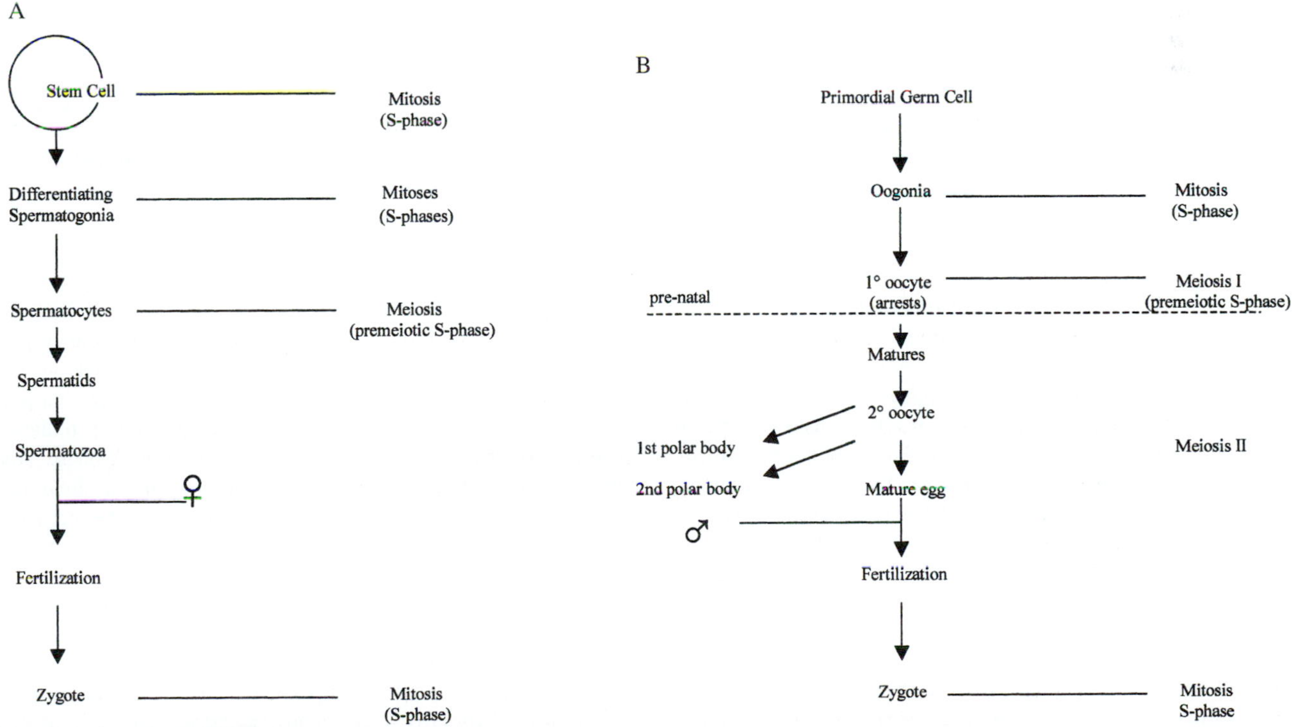

Figure 9-3. The stages of spermatogenesis (A) and oogenesis (B) indicating the periods of cell division and DNA replication (S phase).

matogonial stem cell divides it produces a differentiating spermatogonium and a stem cell. Thus, the stem cell can accumulate genetic damage from chronic exposures. Differentiating spermatogonia, as far as the induction of gene mutation is concerned, are the same as mitotically dividing somatic cells.

The next S phase after gametogenesis occurs in the zygote, formed following fertilization. This fact needs to be balanced by the lack of DNA repair in late spermatids and sperm. Thus, DNA damage induced in these stages will remain until the zygote. Postmeiotic germ cells are particularly sensitive to mutation induction by nonradiomimetic chemicals, especially following acute exposures. The fairly short duration of this stage (approximately 21 days in the mouse) means that their contribution to genetic risk following chronic exposures is quite small.

For oogenesis (Fig. 9-3) similar observations on gene mutation induction and timing of S phase can be made. In this case the primary oocyte arrests prior to birth, and there is no further S phase until the zygote. For this reason the oocyte is resistant to the induction of gene mutations by nonradiomimetic chemicals but not to radiation, for which DNA repair is the mode of formation of mutations, and DNA repair occurs in oocytes (Brewen and Preston, 1982).

These mechanistic aspects of the production of gene mutations (and chromosome alterations described in the following two sections) by chemicals and radiations in somatic and germ cells are most important in considerations of the design of genetic toxicology assays, the interpretation of the data generated, and the incorporation of the data into cancer and genetic risk assessments.

Formation of Chromosomal Alterations

Somatic Cells ***Structural Chromosome Aberrations*** There are components of the formation of chromosome aberrations, sister chromatid exchanges (the apparently reciprocal exchange between the sister chromatids of a single chromosome) and gene mutations that are common. In particular, damaged DNA serves as the substrate leading to all these events. However, chromosome aberrations induced by ionizing radiations are generally formed by errors of DNA repair, whereas those produced by nonradiomimetic chemicals are generally formed by errors of DNA replication on a damaged DNA template.

The DNA repair errors that lead to the formation of chromosome aberrations following ionizing radiation (and radiomimetic chemical) exposure arise from misligation of double-strand breaks or interaction of coincidentally repairing regions during nucleotide excision repair of damaged bases. The details of the DNA damage types and their repair are described above. Thus, the overall kinetics and fidelity of DNA repair influence the sensitivity of cells to the induction of chromosomal aberrations produced by misrepair. The broad outcomes of misrepair are that incorrect rejoining of chromosomal pieces during repair leads to chromosomal exchanges within (e.g., inversions and interstitial deletions) and between (e.g., dicentrics and reciprocal translocations) chromosomes. In fact, using fluorescence in situ hybridization, it can be shown that very complex rearrangements take place (Anderson et al., 2000). Failure to rejoin double-strand breaks or to complete repair of other types of DNA damage leads to terminal deletions.

Acentric fragments arise from interstitial deletions, terminal deletions, and the formation of dicentric chromosomes and rings. The failure to incorporate an acentric fragment into a daughter nucleus at anaphase/telophase, or the failure of a whole chromosome to segregate at anaphase to the cellular poles, can result in the formation of a micronucleus that resides in the cytoplasm.

Errors of DNA replication on a damaged template can lead to a variety of chromosomal alterations. The majority of these involve deletion or exchanges of individual chromatids (chromatid-type aberrations). Thus, nonradiomimetic chemicals induce only chromatid-type aberrations, whereas radiations and radiomimetic chemicals induce chromatid-type aberrations in the S and G_2 phases of the cell cycle, but chromosome-type aberrations affecting both chromatids in G_1. The reason for this latter observation is that the G_1 chromosome behaves as a single DNA molecule and aberrations formed in it will be replicated in the S phase to involve both chromatids. This distinction is important for considerations of outcome of the aberrations and probability of an effect on cells, since for chromatid-type aberrations, one chromatid remains intact and genetically unaltered (Preston et al., 1995).

Numerical Chromosome Changes Numerical changes (e.g., monosomics, trisomics, and ploidy changes) can arise from errors in chromosomal segregation. The complexity of the control and the mechanics of the mitotic process means that alteration of various cellular components can result in failure to segregate the sister chromatids to separate daughter cells or in failure to segregate a chromosome to either pole (Bickel and Orr-Weaver, 1996; Preston, 1996). The mechanisms underlying chromosomal loss are pertinent to those involved in the formation of micronuclei.

A limited set of chemicals has been demonstrated to cause aneuploidy through interaction with components of chromosome movement (Preston, 1996; Aardema et al., 1998). These include benomyl, griseofulvin, nocodazole, colchicine, colecemid, vinblastine, and paclitaxel. These chemicals affect tubulin polymerization or spindle microtubule stability. To date, other mechanisms of aneuploidy induction by chemicals have not been firmly identified.

Sister Chromatid Exchange Sister chromatid exchanges (SCE) are produced during the S phase and are presumed to be a consequence of errors in the replication process, perhaps at the sites of stalled replication complexes (Painter, 1980; Heartlein et al., 1983; Preston, 1991). It is, in fact, this mode of action that makes assays for SCE less than ideal for detecting effects due directly to a chemical exposure. The creation of intracellular conditions that slow the progress of DNA replication, for example, could lead to the formation of SCE.

Germ Cells The formation of chromosomal alterations in germ cells is basically the same as that for somatic cells, namely via misrepair for ionizing radiations and radiomimetic chemicals for treatments in G_1 and G_2, and by errors of replication for all radiations and chemicals for DNA damage present during the S phase. Also, the restrictions on the timing of formation of chromosomal alterations induced by nonradiomimetic chemicals in germ cells is as described above for gene mutations, namely at the specific stages where DNA synthesis occurs, as depicted in Fig. 9-3.

The types of aberrations formed in germ cells are the same as those formed in somatic cells (e.g., deletions, inversions, translocations), although their appearance in diplotene/diakinesis of meiosis I, where analysis is frequently conducted, is rather different because of the homologous chromosome pairing that takes place in meiotic cells (see the review by Leonard, 1973). The specific segregation of chromosomes during meiosis influences the probability of recovery of an aberration, particularly a reciprocal translocation, in the offspring of a treated parent. This is discussed in detail in Preston et al. (1991).

ASSAYS FOR DETECTING GENETIC ALTERATIONS

Introduction to Assay Design

Genetic toxicology assays are used to identify germ cell mutagens, somatic cell mutagens, and potential carcinogens. They detect diverse kinds of genetic alterations that are relevant for human health, including gene mutations, chromosome aberrations, and aneuploidy. Over the last three decades, hundreds of chemicals have been evaluated for genotoxic effects. Genetic toxicology assays serve two interrelated but distinct purposes in the toxicologic evaluation of chemicals: (1) identifying mutagens for purposes of hazard identification, and (2) characterizing dose–response relationships and mutagenic mechanisms, both of which contribute to an understanding of genetic and carcinogenic risks.

A common experience in surveying the mutagenicity literature is encountering a bewildering array of assays in viruses, bacteria, fungi, cultured mammalian cells, plants, insects, and mammals. More than 200 assays for mutagens have been proposed, and useful information has been obtained from many of them. Fortunately, however, most genetic toxicology testing and evaluation relies on relatively few assays.

Table 9-1 lists key assays that have a prominent place in genetic toxicology and for regulatory considerations. Table 9-2 is a more comprehensive list that provides literature citations to many of the assays that one might encounter in the genetic toxicology literature. Even this extensive table is not exhaustive, in that it emphasizes methods of applied genetic toxicology and not those whose use has been restricted largely to studies of mutational mechanisms. The commonly used assays have relied on phenotypic effects as indicators of gene mutations or small deletions and on cytologic methods for observing gross chromosomal damage. Detailed information on assay design, testing data, controls, sample sizes, and other factors in effective testing is found in the references cited.

Some assays for gene mutations detect forward mutations whereas others detect reversion. Forward mutations are genetic alterations in a wild-type gene and are detected by a change in phenotype caused by the alteration or loss of gene function. In contrast, a back mutation or reversion is a mutation that restores gene function in a mutant and thereby brings about a return to the wild-type phenotype. In principle, forward-mutation assays should respond to a broad spectrum of mutagens because any mutation that interferes with gene expression should confer the detectable phenotype. In contrast, a reversion assay might be expected to have a more restricted mutational response because only mutations that correct or compensate for the specific mutation in a particular mutant will be detected. In fact, some reversion assays respond to a broader spectrum of mutational changes than one might expect because mutations at a site other than that of the original mutation (i.e., a suppressor mutation) can sometimes confer the detected phenotype. Both forward mutation assays and reversion assays are used extensively in genetic toxicology.

The simplest gene mutation assays rely on selection techniques to detect mutations. A selection technique is a means of imposing experimental conditions under which only cells or organisms that have undergone mutation can grow. Selection techniques greatly facilitate the identification of rare cells that have experienced mutation among the many cells that have not. Forward mu-

Table 9-1
Principal Assays in Genetic Toxicology

I. Pivotal assays
  A. A well-characterized assay for gene mutations
    The *Salmonella*/mammalian microsome assay (Ames test)
  B. A mammalian assay for chromosome damage in vivo
    Metaphase analysis or micronucleus assay in rodent bone marrow
II. Other assays offering an extensive database or unique genetic endpoint
  A. Assays for gene mutations
    E. coli WP2 tryptophan reversion assay
    TK or HPRT forward mutation assays in cultured mammalian cells
    Drosophila sex-linked recessive lethal assay
  B. Cytogenetic analysis in cultured Chinese hamster or human cells
    Assays for chromosome aberrations and micronuclei
    Assays for aneuploidy
  C. Other indicators of genetic damage
    Mammalian DNA damage and repair assays
    Mitotic recombination assays in yeast and *Drosophila*
  D. Mammalian germ-cell assays
    Mouse-specific locus tests
    Assays for skeletal or cataract mutations in mice
    Cytogenetic analysis and heritable translocation assays
    DNA damage and repair in rodent germ cells
    Dominant lethal assay

Table 9-2
Overview of Genetic Toxicology Assays

ASSAYS	SELECTED LITERATURE CITATIONS
I. DNA damage and repair assays	
A. Direct detection of DNA damage	
Alkaline elution assays for DNA strand breakage	Elia et al., 1994
Comet assay for DNA strand breakage	Fairbairn et al., 1995; Tice et al., 2000
Assays for chemical adducts in DNA	Chang et al., 1994; Kriek et al., 1998; Phillips et al., 2000
B. Bacterial assays for DNA damage	
Differential killing of repair-deficient and wild-type strains	Hamasaki et al., 1992
Induction of the SOS system by DNA damage in *E. coli*	Quillardet and Hofnung, 1993
C. Assays for repairable DNA damage in mammalian cells	
Unscheduled DNA synthesis (UDS) in rat hepatocytes	Madle et al., 1994
UDS in rodent hepatocytes in vivo	Madle et al., 1994
II. Prokaryote gene mutation assays	
A. Bacterial reverse mutation assays	
Salmonella/mammalian microsome assay (Ames test)	Kirkland et al., 1990; Maron and Ames, 1983
E. coli WP2 tryptophan reversion assay	Kirkland et al., 1990; Gatehouse et al., 1994
Salmonella-specific base-pair substitution assay (Ames-II assay)	Gee et al., 1994; Gee et al., 1998
E. coli lacZ–specific reversion assay	Cupples and Miller, 1989; Cupples et al., 1990
B. Bacterial forward mutation assays	
E. coli lacI assay	Calos and Miller, 1981; Halliday and Glickman, 1991
Arabinose resistance in *Salmonella*	Jurado et al., 1994
III. Assays in nonmammalian eukaryotes	
A. Fungal assays for gene mutations	
Reversion of auxotrophs in Neurospora or yeast	Zimmermann et al., 1984
Forward mutations and deletions in red adenine mutants	Zimmermann et al., 1984
B. Fungal assays for aneuploidy	
Genetic detection of mitotic chromosome loss and gain in yeast	Aardema et al., 1998; Zimmermann et al., 1984; Parry, 1993
Meiotic nondisjunction in yeast or Neurospora	Zimmermann et al., 1984
C. Fungal assays for induced recombination	
Mitotic crossing over and gene conversion assays in yeast	Zimmermann, 1992
D. Plant assays	
Gene mutations affecting chlorophyll in seedlings or waxy in pollen	Grant, 1994
Tradescantia stamen hair-color mutations	Grant, 1994
Chromosome aberrations or micronuclei in mitotic or meiotic cells	Grant, 1994
Aneuploidy detected by pigmentation or cytogenetics	Aardema et al., 1998; Grant, 1994; Parry, 1993
E. Drosophila assays	
Sex-linked recessive lethal test in germ cells	Mason et al., 1987
Heritable translocation assays	Mason et al., 1987
Sex chromosome loss tests for aneuploidy	Aardema et al.; Osgood and Cyr, 1998
Induction of mitotic recombination in eyes or wings	Vogel et al., 1999
IV. Mammalian gene mutation assays	
A. In vitro assays for forward mutations	
TK mutations in mouse lymphoma or human cells	Kirkland et al., 1990; Moore et al., 2000
HPRT mutations in Chinese hamster or human cells	DeMarini et al., 1989
XPRT mutations in Chinese hamster AS52 cells	DeMarini et al., 1989
B. In vivo assays for gene mutations in somatic cells	
Mouse spot test (somatic cell specific locus test)	Styles and Penman, 1985
HPRT mutations (6-thioguanine-resistance) in rodent lymphocytes	Cariello and Skopek, 1993
C. Transgenic assays	
Gene mutations in the bacterial lacI gene in mice and rats	Mirsalis et al., 1994; Vijg and van Steeg, 1998
Gene mutations in the bacterial lacZ gene in mice	Mirsalis et al., 1994; Vijg and van Steeg, 1998
Gene mutations in the phage cII gene in lacI or lacZ transgenic mice	Swiger et al., 1999
V. Mammalian cytogenetic assays	

(*continued*)

Table 9-2
Overview of Genetic Toxicology Assays (*continued*)

ASSAYS	SELECTED LITERATURE CITATIONS
A. Chromosome aberrations	
Metaphase analysis in cultured Chinese hamster or human cells	Kirkland et al., 1990; Ishidate et al., 1988; Galloway et al., 1994
Metaphase analysis of rodent bone marrow or lymphocytes in vivo	Kirkland et al., 1990; Preston et al., 1981; Tice et al., 1994
B. Micronuclei	
Cytokinesis-block micronucleus assay in human lymphocytes	Fenech, 1993; Fenech, 1997
Micronucleus assay in mammalian cell lines	Miller et al., 1998; Kirsch-Volders et al., 2000
In vivo micronucleus assay in erythrocytes	Heddle et al., 1991; Hayashi et al., 1994; Hayashi et al., 2000
C. Sister chromatid exchange	
SCE in human cells or Chinese hamster cells	Tucker et al., 1993
SCE in rodent tissues, especially bone marrow	Tucker et al., 1993
D. Aneuploidy in mitotic cells	
Mitotic disturbance seen by staining spindles and chromosomes	Parry, 1998
Hyperploidy detected by chromosome counting	Aardema et al., 1998; Galloway and Ivett, 1986
Chromosome gain or loss in cells with intact cytoplasm	Natarajan, 1993
Micronucleus assay with centromere labeling	Aardema et al., 1998; Natarajan, 1993; Lynch and Parry, 1993
Hyperploid cells in vivo in mouse bone marrow	Aardema et al., 1998; Zimmermann et al., 1984
Mouse bone marrow micronucleus assay with centromere labeling	Aardema et al., 1998; Heddle et al., 1991; Adler et al., 1994
VI. Germ cell mutagenesis	
A. Measurement of DNA damage	
Molecular dosimetry based on mutagen adducts	Russell and Shelby, 1985
UDS in rodent germ cells	Bentley et al., 1994
Alkaline elution assays for DNA strand breaks in rodent testes	Bentley et al., 1994
B. Gene mutations	
Mouse-specific locus test for gene mutations and deletions	Kirkland et al., 1990; Ehling, 1991; Russell and Russell, 1992
Mouse electrophoretic specific locus test	Lewis, 1991
Dominant mutations causing mouse skeletal defects or cataracts	Ehling, 1991
C. Chromosomal aberrations	
Cytogenetic analysis in oocytes, spermatogonia, or spermatocytes	Kirkland et al., 1990; Tease, 1992
Micronuclei in mouse spermatids	Hayashi et al., 2000; Lähdetie et al., 1994
Mouse heritable translocation test	Russell and Shelby, 1985
D. Dominant lethal mutations	
Mouse or rat dominant lethal assay	Adler et al., 1994
E. Aneuploidy	
Cytogenetic analysis for aneuploidy arising by nondisjunction	Aardema et al., 1998; Adler, 1993; Allen et al., 1986
Sex chromosome loss test for nondisjunction or breakage	Russell and Shelby, 1985; Adler, 1993
Micronucleus assay in spermatids with centromere labeling	Aardema et al., 1998

tations and reversions can both be detected by selection techniques in microorganisms and cultured mammalian cells. Because of their speed, low cost, and ease of detecting events that occur at low frequency (i.e., mutation), assays in microorganisms and cell cultures have figured prominently in genetic toxicology.

Studying mutagenesis in intact animals requires assays of more complex design than the simple selection methods used in microorganisms and cultured cells. Genetic toxicology assays therefore range from inexpensive short-term tests that can be performed in a few days to complicated assays for mutations in mammalian germ cells. Even in complex multicellular organisms, however, there has been an emphasis on designing assays that detect mutations with great efficiency. Nevertheless, there remains a gradation in which an increase in relevance for human risk entails more elaborate and costly tests. The most expensive mammalian tests are typically reserved for agents of special importance in basic research or risk assessment, whereas the simpler assays can be applied more broadly.

Because of their reliance on cytologic rather than genetic methods, cytogenetic assays differ in design from typical gene mutation assays. The goal in cytogenetic assays is to apply methodology that permits the unequivocal visual recognition of cells that have experienced genetic damage. The alterations measured include chromosome aberrations, micronuclei, SCE and changes in chromosome numbers. Cytogenetic assays are listed in Tables 9-1 and 9-2 and discussed later in this chapter.

In all mutagenicity testing, one must be aware of possible sources of error. Factors to consider in the application of mutagenicity assays are the choice of suitable organisms and growth conditions, appropriate monitoring of genotypes and phenotypes, effective experimental design and treatment conditions, inclusion of proper positive and negative controls, and sound methods of data analysis (Kirkland et al., 1990).

Many compounds that are not themselves mutagenic or carcinogenic can be activated into mutagens and carcinogens by mammalian metabolism. Such compounds are called promutagens and procarcinogens. Because microorganisms and mammalian cell cultures lack many of the metabolic capabilities of intact mammals, provision must be made for metabolic activation in order to detect promutagens in many genetic assays. The most common means of doing so is to include an in vitro metabolic activation system derived from a mammalian tissue homogenate in the microbial or cell culture assay. For example, the promutagens dimethylnitrosamine and benzo[a]pyrene are not themselves mutagenic in bacteria, but they are mutagenic in bacterial assays if the bacteria are treated with the promutagen in the presence of a homogenate from mammalian liver.

The most widely used metabolic activation system in microbial and cell culture assays is a postmitochondrial supernatant from a rat liver homogenate, along with appropriate buffers and cofactors (Kirkland et al., 1990; Maron and Ames, 1983). The standard liver metabolic activation system is called an S9 mixture, designating a supernatant from centrifugation at $9000 \times g$. Most of the short-term assays in Table 9-2 require exogenous metabolic activation to detect promutagens. Exceptions are those in intact mammals and a few simpler assays, such as the detection of unscheduled DNA synthesis (UDS) in cultured hepatocytes (Madle et al., 1994), that have a high level of endogenous cytochrome P450 metabolism.

Rat liver S9 should be thought of as providing a broad assemblage of metabolic reactions, but not necessarily the same as those of hepatic metabolism in an intact rat. Alternative metabolic activation systems based on homogenates from other species or organs have found some use, but such variations may similarly differ from the species or organs of their origin. Therefore, alternative metabolic activation systems tend to be more useful if chosen for mechanistic reasons rather than simply testing another species or organ. For example, metabolism by intact hepatocytes (Langenbach and Oglesby, 1983) can preserve elements of cellular compartmentalization of reactions altered in tissue homogenation. Likewise, a system that includes a reductive reaction not encompassed by standard S9 is required for detecting the mutagenicity of some azo dyes and nitro compounds (Dellarco and Prival, 1989). Despite their usefulness, in vitro metabolic activation systems, however well refined, cannot mimic mammalian metabolism perfectly. There are differences among tissues in reactions that activate or inactivate foreign compounds, and organisms of the normal flora of the gut can contribute to metabolism in intact mammals. Agents that induce enzyme systems or otherwise alter the physiologic state can also modify the metabolism of toxicants, and the balance between activation and detoxication reactions in vitro may differ from that in vivo.

An interesting development with respect to metabolic activation is the expression of human enzymes in microorganisms or cell cultures. The incorporation of human genes into Salmonella tester strains derived from the Ames assay permits the activation of promutagens (e.g., 2-aminoanthracene or 2-aminofluorene) by human cytochrome P4501A2 without an S9 mixture (Josephy et al., 1995). Mammalian cell lines have also been genetically engineered to express human enzymes of metabolic activation (Sawada and Kamataki, 1998). Many cell lines stably expressing a single form of P450 have been established. Mutagenesis can be measured through such endpoints as *HPRT* mutations and cytogenetic alterations, and the cells are well suited to analyzing the contribution of different enzymes to the activation of promutagens. Cell lines that express various combinations of phase I and phase II enzymes are being developed (Sawada and Kamataki, 1998).

DNA Damage and Repair Assays

Some assays measure DNA damage itself rather than mutational consequences of DNA damage. They may do so directly, through such indicators as chemical adducts or strand breaks in DNA, or indirectly, through measurement of biological repair processes. Adducts in DNA can be detected by ^{32}P-postlabeling, immunologic methods using antibodies against specific adducts, or fluorometric methods in the case of such fluorescent compounds as polynuclear aromatic hydrocarbons and aflatoxin (Chang et al., 1994; Kriek et al., 1998; Phillips et al., 2000). The ^{32}P-postlabeling technique is highly sensitive and applicable to diverse mutagens. The measurement of adducts is useful in human monitoring and molecular dosimetry in that DNA adducts have been quantified after human exposure to various chemicals (Chang et al., 1994; Kriek et al., 1998; Phillips et al., 2000). DNA strand breakage can be measured by alkaline elution and electrophoretic methods (Elia et al., 1994). The applicability of DNA damage assays to rodent testes (Bentley et al., 1994) makes these methods helpful in interpreting risks to germ cells.

A rapid method of measuring DNA damage that has grown in importance over the last decade is the single-cell gel electrophoresis assay, also called the comet assay (Fairbairn et al., 1995; Tice et al., 2000). In this assay cells are incorporated into agarose on slides, lysed so as to liberate their DNA, and subjected to electrophoresis. The DNA is stained with a fluorescent dye for observation and image analysis. Because broken DNA fragments migrate more quickly than larger pieces of DNA, a blur of fragments (a "comet") is observed when the DNA is extensively damaged. The extent of DNA damage can be estimated from the length and other attributes of the comet tail. Variations in the procedure permit the assay's use for the general detection of DNA strand breakage under alkaline conditions (Fairbairn et al., 1995; Tice et al., 2000) or the preferential detection of double-strand breaks under neutral conditions (Fairbairn et al., 1995). Although the comet assay is relatively new and needs further study before its ultimate utility is clear, it appears to be a rapid and sensitive indicator of DNA damage with broad applicability. Though it has most commonly been used with human lymphocytes (Fairbairn et al., 1995) and other mammalian cells (Tice et al., 2000), it can be adapted to diverse species, including plants, worms, mollusks, fish, and amphibians (Cotelle and Férard, 1999). This adaptability suggests that it will find diverse uses in environmental genetic toxicology.

The occurrence of DNA repair can serve as a readily measured indicator of DNA damage. Repair assays have been developed in microorganisms, cultured mammalian cells, and intact mammals (Table 9-2), and some of these assays remain in use. Greater toxicity of a chemical in DNA repair–deficient strains than in their repair-proficient counterparts has served as an indicator of DNA damage in bacteria (e.g., *polA*$^-$ and *polA*$^+$ in *Escherichia coli* or *rec*$^-$ and *rec*$^+$ in *Bacillus subtilis*) (Hamasaki et al., 1992). The induction of bacterial SOS functions, indicated by phage induction or by colorimetry in the SOS chromotest, can similarly serve as a general indicator of genetic damage (Quillardet and Hofnung, 1993). The most common repair assay in mammalian cells is an assay for UDS, which is a measure of excision repair. The occurrence of UDS indicates that the DNA had been damaged (Madle et al., 1994). However, it is to be stressed that the absence of UDS does not denote an absence of DNA damage, because of low sensitivity of the assay and the occurrence of classes of damage that are not actively excised. Though bacterial repair assays have declined in usage over the years, UDS assays continue to be used because of their applicability to cultured hepatocytes with endogenous cytochrome P450 enzyme activities and to tissues of intact animals, including hepatocytes (Madle et al., 1994) and germinal tissue (Bentley et al., 1994).

Gene Mutations in Prokaryotes

The most common means of detecting mutations in microorganisms is selecting for reversion in strains that have a specific nutritional requirement differing from wild-type members of the species; such strains are called auxotrophs. For example, the widely used assay developed by Bruce Ames and his colleagues is based on measuring reversion in a series of histidine auxotrophs in *Salmonella typhimurium.* In the Ames assay one measures the frequency of histidine-independent bacteria that arise in a histidine-requiring strain in the presence or absence of the chemical being tested. Auxotrophic (nutrient deficient) bacteria are treated with the chemical of interest by one of several procedures (e.g., a plate-incorporation assay or a preincubation test) and plated on medium that is deficient in histidine (Kirkland et al., 1990; Maron and Ames, 1983). The assay is conducted using several genetically different strains so that reversion by base-pair substitutions and frameshift mutations in several DNA sequence contexts can be detected and distinguished. Besides the histidine alleles that provide the target for measuring mutagenesis, the Ames tester strains contain other genes and plasmids that enhance the assay. The principal strains of the Ames test and their characteristics are summarized in Table 9-3. Since *S. typhimurium* does not have a capacity for metabolism of promutagens comparable to mammalian tissues, the assay is generally performed in the presence and absence of a rat liver S9 metabolic activation system. Hence, the Ames assay is also commonly called the *Salmonella*/microsome assay.

Though simplicity is a great merit of microbial assays, it can also be deceptive. Even assays that are simple in design and application can be performed incorrectly. For example, in the Ames assay one may see very small colonies in the Petri dishes at highly toxic doses (Kirkland et al., 1990; Maron and Ames, 1983). Counting such colonies as revertants would be an error because they may actually be nonrevertant survivors that grew on the low concentration of histidine in the plates. Were there millions of survivors, the amount of histidine would have been insufficient to allow any of them (except real revertants) to form colonies. This artifact is easily avoided by checking that there is a faint lawn of bacterial growth in the plates; one can also confirm that colonies are revertants by streaking them on medium without histidine to be sure that they grow in its absence. Such pitfalls exist in all mutagenicity tests. Anyone performing mutagenicity tests must, therefore, have detailed familiarity with the laboratory application and literature of the assay and be observant about the responsiveness of the assay.

Though most frequently used as a testing assay, the *Salmonella*/microsome system also provides information on molecular mechanisms of mutagenesis. The primary reversion mechanisms, summarized in Table 9-3, were initially determined by genetic and biochemical means (Maron and Ames, 1983). An ingenious method called allele-specific colony hybridization has greatly facilitated the molecular analysis of revertants in the Ames assay (Koch et al., 1994), and many spontaneous and induced revertants have been cloned or amplified by polymerase chain reaction (PCR) and sequenced (Levine et al., 1994; DeMarini, 2000).

The development of *Salmonella* strains that revert only by a single class of point mutation has made the identification of specific base-pair substitutions more straightforward. These strains (TA7001-TA7006) each revert from *his*$^-$ to *his*$^+$ by a single kind of mutation (e.g., G:C to T:A), and collectively they permit the specific detection of all six possible base pair substitutions (Gee et al., 1994; Gee et al., 1998). Specific reversion assays are also available in *E. coli.* A versatile system based on reversion of *lacZ* mutations in *E. coli* permits the specific detection of all six possible base-pair substitutions (Cupples and Miller, 1989) and frameshift mutations in which one or two bases have been added or deleted in various sequence contexts (Cupples et al., 1990). The broader understanding of mutational mechanisms that comes from refined genetic assays and molecular analysis of mutations can contribute to the interpretation of mutational hazards.

Though information from the Ames assay has become a standard in genetic toxicology testing, equivalent information can be obtained from other bacterial assays. Like the Ames assay, the WP2 tryptophan reversion assay in *E. coli* (Kirkland et al., 1990; Gatehouse et al., 1994) incorporates genetic features that enhance assay sensitivity, can accommodate S9 metabolic activation, and performs well in many laboratories. Mutations are detected by selecting for reversion from *trp*$^-$ to *trp*$^+$.

Bacterial forward mutation assays, such as a selection for arabinose resistance in *Salmonella* (Jurado et al., 1994), are also used in research and testing, though less extensively than the reversion assays. A versatile forward mutation assay that has contributed greatly to an understanding of mutagenic mechanisms is the *lacI* system in *E. coli* (Calos and Miller, 1981; Halliday and Glickman, 1991). Mutations in the *lacI* gene, which encodes the repressor of the lactose operon, are easily identified by phenotype, cloned or amplified by the polymerase chain reaction, and sequenced. The *lacI* gene is widely used as a target for mutagenesis in *E. coli* and in transgenic mice, and more than 30,000 *lacI* mutants have been sequenced (Mirsalis et al., 1994).

Gene Mutations in Nonmammalian Eukaryotes

Many early studies of mutagenesis used yeasts, mycelial fungi, plants, and insects as experimental organisms. Though well-characterized genetic systems permit the detection of a diverse array

Table 9-3
The Ames Assay: Tester Strains and Their Characteristics

I. Standard Tester Strains of Salmonella typhimurium

STRAIN	TARGET ALLELE	CHROMOSOMAL GENOTYPE	PLASMIDS
TA1535	*hisG46*	*hisG46 rfa ΔuvrB*	None
TA100	*hisG46*	*hisG46 rfa ΔuvrB*	pKM101 (*mucAB* Ap^r)
TA1538	*hisD3052*	*hisD3052 rfa ΔuvrB*	None
TA98	*hisD3052*	*hisD3052 rfa ΔuvrB*	pKM101 (*mucAB* Ap^r)
TA1537	*hisC3076*	*hisC3076 rfa ΔuvrB*	None
TA97	*hisD6610*	*hisD6610 hisO1242 rfa ΔuvrB*	pKM101 (*mucAB* Ap^r)
TA102	*hisG428*	*hisD(G)8476 rfa*	pKM101 (*mucAB* Ap^r) and pAQ1 (*hisG428* Tc^r)

II. Genetic Characteristics of the Ames Tester Strains

CHARACTERISTIC	RATIONALE FOR INCLUSION IN THE TESTER STRAIN
rfa	Alters the lipopolysaccharide wall, conferring greater permeability to mutagens.
ΔuvrB	Deletes the excision repair system, increasing sensitivity to many mutagens.
mucAB	Enhances sensitivity to some mutagens whose activity depends on the SOS system.
Ap^r	Permits selection for the presence of pKM101 by ampicillin-resistance.
hisO1242	Affects regulation of histidine genes, enhancing revertibility of *hisD6610* in TA97.
hisD(G)8476	Eliminates the chromosomal *hisG* gene in TA102, making the bacteria histidine auxotrophs in which reversion of *hisG428* on pAQ1 can be measured.
Tc^r	Permits selection for the presence of pAQ1 in TA102 by tetracycline resistance.

III. Mechanisms of Reversion Detected by the Ames Tester Strains

STRAIN	PRIMARY TARGET	SIZE (bp) OF FULL TARGET	PRIMARY MUTATIONS
TA1535, TA100	CC GG	15	GC → TA GC → AT TA → GC
TA1538, TA98	CGCGCGCG GCGCGCGC	76	ΔGC or ΔCG Complex frameshifts
TA104	TAA ATT	12	GC → TA GC → AT AT → TA AT → CG AT → GC
TA1537	CCCCC GGGGG	20	ΔG or ΔC

of genetic alterations in these organisms (Table 9-2), assays in nonmammalian eukaryotes have been largely supplanted in genetic toxicology by bacterial and mammalian systems. Exceptions are to be found where the nonmammalian eukaryotes permit the study of genetic endpoints that are not readily analyzed in mammals or where the organism has special attributes that fit a particular application.

The fruit fly, *Drosophila*, has long occupied a prominent place in genetic research. In fact, the first unequivocal evidence of chemical mutagenesis was obtained in Scotland in 1941 when Charlotte Auerbach and J.M. Robson demonstrated that mustard gas is mutagenic in *Drosophila. Drosophila* continues to be used in modern mutation research (Potter and Turenchalk, 2000) but its role in genetic toxicology is now more limited. The *Drosophila* assay of greatest historical importance is the sex-linked recessive lethal (SLRL) test. A strength of the SLRL test is that it permits the detection of recessive lethal mutations at 600 to 800 different loci on the X chromosome by screening for the presence or absence of wild-type males in the offspring of specifically designed crosses (Mason et al., 1987). The genetic alterations include gene mutations and small deletions. The spontaneous frequency of SLRLs is about 0.2 percent, and a significant increase over this frequency in the lineages derived from treated males indicates mutagenesis. Though it requires screening large numbers of fruit fly vials, the SLRL test yields information about mutagenesis in germ cells, which is lacking in all microbial and cell culture systems. However, means of exposure, measurement of doses, metabolism, and gametogenesis in *Drosophila* differ from those in mammalian toxicology, therefore potentially limiting their relevance to human genetic risk. *Drosophila* assays are also available for studying the induction of chromosome abnormalities in germ cells, specifically heritable translocations (Mason et al., 1987) and sex-chromosome loss (Osgood and Cyr, 1998).

Genetic and cytogenetic assays in plants (Grant, 1994) also occupy a more restricted niche in modern genetic toxicology than they did years ago. However, plant assays continue to find use in special applications, such as in situ monitoring for mutagens (Lewtas, 1991) and exploration of the metabolism of promutagens by agricultural plants. In in situ monitoring, one looks for evidence of mutagenic effects in organisms that are grown in the environment of interest. Natural populations of organisms can also be examined for evidence of genetic damage. For example, frequencies of chlorophyll mutations in red mangroves have been correlated with concentrations of polycyclic hydrocarbons in the sediments in which they were growing (Klekowski et al., 1994). While studies of natural populations are of obvious interest, they require utmost precaution when characterizing the environments and defining appropriate control populations.

Assays in nonmammalian eukaryotes continue to be important in the study of induced recombination. Recombinagenic effects in yeast have long been used as a general indicator of genetic damage (Zimmermann et al., 1984), and interest in the induction of recombination has increased as recombinational events have been implicated in the etiology of cancer (Sengstag, 1994). The best characterized assays for recombinagens are those that detect mitotic crossing over and mitotic gene conversion in the yeast *Saccharomyces cerevisiae* (Zimmermann, 1992; Howlett and Schiestl, 2000). Hundreds of chemicals have been tested for recombinagenic effects in straightforward yeast assays. In yeast strain D7, for example, mitotic crossing over involving the *ade2* locus is detected on the basis of pink and red colony color, and mitotic gene conversion at the *trp5* locus is detected by selection for growth without tryptophan. Strategies have also been devised to detect recombinagenic effects in mycelial fungi, cultured mammalian cells, plants, and mice (Hoffmann, 1994), and at least 350 chemicals have been evaluated in *Drosophila* somatic cell assays in which recombinagenic effects are detected by examining wings or eyes for regions in which recessive alleles are expressed in heterozygotes (Vogel et al., 1999).

Gene Mutations in Mammals

Gene Mutations in Vitro Mutagenicity assays in cultured mammalian cells have some of the same advantages as microbial assays with respect to speed and cost, and they follow quite similar approaches. The most widely used assays for gene mutations in mammalian cells detect forward mutations that confer resistance to a toxic chemical (DeMarini et al., 1989). For example, mutations in the gene encoding hypoxanthine-guanine phosphoribosyltransferase (HPRT enzyme; *HPRT* gene) confer resistance to the purine analog 6-thioguanine (Walker et al., 1999), and thymidine kinase mutations (TK enzyme; *TK* gene) confer resistance to the pyrimidine analog trifluorothymidine (Moore et al., 2000). *HPRT* and *TK* mutations may therefore be detected in cultured cells by attempting to grow cells in the presence of purine analogs and pyrimidine analogues, respectively. For historical reasons, *HPRT* assays have most commonly been conducted in Chinese hamster or human cells and *TK* assays in mouse lymphoma cells or human cells. Although forward-mutation assays typically respond to diverse mechanisms of mutagenesis, there are exceptions. For example, resistance to ouabain results from a specific alteration in the target gene, and alterations that eliminate the gene function are lethal (DeMarini et al., 1989); therefore, ouabain resistance is not useful for general mutagenicity testing.

Gene Mutations in Vivo In vivo assays involve treating intact animals and analyzing genetic effects in appropriate tissues. The choice of suitable doses, treatment procedures, controls, and sample sizes is critical in the conduct of in vivo tests. Mutations may be detected either in somatic cells or in germ cells. Germ cell mutagenesis is of special interest with respect to risk for future generations and is discussed later in the chapter.

The mouse spot test is a traditional genetic assay for gene mutations in somatic cells (Styles and Penman, 1985). Visible spots of altered phenotype in mice heterozygous for coat color genes indicate mutations in the progenitor cells of the altered regions. The spot test is less used today than other somatic cell assays or than its germ cell counterpart, the mouse specific-locus test. Cells from intact animals that are amenable to positive selection for mutants form the basis for efficient in vivo mutation detection in assays analogous to those used in mammalian cell cultures. Lymphocytes with mutations in the *HPRT* gene are readily detected by selection for resistance to 6-thioguanine. The *HPRT* assay in mice, rats, and monkeys (Walker et al., 1999; Casciano et al., 1999) is of special interest because it permits comparisons to the measurement of *HPRT* mutations in humans, an important assay in human mutational monitoring (Cole and Skopek, 1994; Albertini and Hayes, 1997).

Besides determining whether agents are mutagenic, mutation assays provide information on mechanisms of mutagenesis that contribute to an understanding of mutational hazards. Base substitutions and large deletions, which may be indistinguishable on the basis of phenotype, can be differentiated through the use of probes for the target gene and Southern blotting, in that base substitutions are too subtle to be detectable on the blots, whereas gross structural alterations are visible (Cole and Skopek, 1994; Albertini and Hayes, 1997). Molecular analysis has been used to determine proportions of mutations ascribable to deletions and other structural alterations in several assays, including the specific-locus test for germ cell mutations in mice (Favor, 1999) and the human *HPRT* assay (Cole and Skopek, 1994). Gene mutations have been characterized at the molecular level by DNA sequence analysis both in transgenic rodents (Mirsalis et al., 1994) and in endogenous mammalian genes (Cariello and Skopek, 1993). Many *HPRT* mutations from human cells in vitro and in vivo have been analyzed at the molecular level and classified with respect to base-pair substitutions, frameshifts, small deletions, large deletions, and other alterations (Cole and Skopek, 1994).

Transgenic Assays Transgenic animals are products of DNA technology in which the animal contains foreign DNA sequences that have been added to the genome and are transmitted through the germ line. The foreign DNA is therefore represented in all the somatic cells of the animal. Mutagenicity assays in transgenic animals show promise of combining in vivo metabolic activation and pharmacodynamics with simple microbial detection systems, permitting refined analyses of mutations induced in diverse mammalian tissues (Mirsalis et al., 1994; Heddle et al., 2000).

The transgenic animals that have figured most heavily in genetic toxicology are mice that carry *lac* genes from *E. coli.* The bacterial genes were introduced into mice by injecting a vector carrying the genes into zygotes, described in Mirsalis et al. (1994). The strains are commonly referred to by their commercial names—the "Big Blue Mouse" and "MutaMouse." The former uses *lacI* as a target for mutagenesis, and the latter uses *lacZ.* After mutagenic treatment of the transgenic animals, the *lac* genes are recovered from the animal, packaged in phage λ, and transferred to *E. coli* for mutational analysis. Mutant plaques are identified on the basis of phenotype, and mutant frequencies can be calculated for different tissues of the treated animals (Mirsalis et al., 1994). The *cII* locus may be used as a second target gene in both the *lacZ* and *lacI* assays (Swiger et al., 1999). Its use offers technical advantages as a small, easily sequenced target in which independent mutations may be detected readily by positive selection, and it permits interesting comparisons both within and between assays (Swiger et al., 1999). Other transgenic assays are under development and offer the prospect of expanding the versatility of transgenic assays. The *gpt* delta mouse, for example, offers the prospect of detecting large deletions that are induced by many mutagens and clastogens but not readily detected in the *lacI* and *lacZ* transgenic systems (Okada et al., 1999).

Various mutagens, including alkylating agents, nitrosamines, procarbazine, cyclophosphamide, and polycyclic aromatic hydrocarbons have been studied in transgenic mouse assays, and mutant frequencies have been analyzed in such diverse tissues as liver, skin, spleen, kidney, bladder, small intestine, bone marrow, and testis (Morrison and Ashby, 1994). Tissue-specific mutant frequencies can be compared to the distribution of adducts among tissues and to the site-specificity of carcinogenesis (Mirsalis et al., 1994). An important issue that remains to be unequivocally resolved is the extent to which transgenes resemble endogenous genes. Though their mutational responses tend to be comparable (Swiger et al., 1999), some differences have been noted (Burkhart and Malling, 1993; Vijg and van Steeg, 1998), and questions have been raised about the relevance of mutations that might be recovered from dying or dead animal tissues (Burkhart and Malling, 1994). Therefore, transgenic animals offer promising models for the study of chemical mutagenesis, but they must be further characterized before their ultimate place in hazard assessment is clear.

Mammalian Cytogenetic Assays

Chromosome Aberrations Genetic assays as generally conducted (i.e., in the absence of DNA sequencing) are indirect, in that one observes a phenotype and reaches conclusions about genes. In contrast, cytogenetic assays use microscopy for direct observation of the effect of interest. In conventional cytogenetics, metaphase analysis is used to detect chromosomal anomalies, especially unstable chromosome and chromatid aberrations. A key factor in the design of cytogenetic assays is obtaining appropriate cell populations for treatment and analysis (Kirkland et al., 1990; Preston et al., 1981; Ishidate et al., 1988; Galloway et al., 1994). Cells with a stable, well-defined karyotype, short generation time, low chromosome number, and large chromosomes are ideal for cytogenetic analysis. For this reason, Chinese hamster cells have been used widely in cytogenetic testing. Other cells are also suitable, and human cells, especially peripheral lymphocytes, have been used extensively. Cells should be treated during a sensitive period of the cell cycle (typically S), and aberrations should be analyzed at the first mitotic division after treatment so that the sensitivity of the assay is not reduced by unstable aberrations being lost during cell division. Examples of chromosome aberrations are shown in Fig. 9-4.

Cytogenetic assays require careful attention to growth conditions, controls, doses, treatment conditions, and time intervals between treatment and the sampling of cells for analysis (Kirkland et al., 1990). Data collection is a critical step in cytogenetic analysis. It is essential that sufficient cells be analyzed because a negative result in a small sample is equivocal. Results should be recorded for specific classes of aberrations, not just as an overall index of aberrations per cell. The need for detailed data is all the more important because of nonuniformity in the classification of aberrations and disagreement on whether small achromatic (i.e., unstained) gaps in chromosomes are true chromosomal aberrations. Gaps should be quantified but not pooled with other aberrations.

In interpreting results on the induction of chromosome aberrations in cell cultures, one must be alert to the possibility of artifacts associated with extreme assay conditions because aberrations induced under such circumstances may not be a reflection of a chemical-specific genotoxicity (Scott et al., 1991; Galloway, 2000). Questionable positive results have been found at highly cytotoxic doses (Galloway, 2000), high osmolality, and pH extremes (Scott et al., 1991). The possibility that metabolic activation systems may be genotoxic also warrants scrutiny (Scott et al., 1991). While excessively high doses may lead to artifactual positive responses, the failure to test to sufficiently high doses also undermines the utility of a test; therefore, testing should be extended to a dose at which some cytotoxicity is observed, such as a reduction in the mitotic index (the proportion of cells in division), or to an arbitrary limit of about 10 mM if the chemical is nontoxic (Kirkland et al., 1990).

In vivo assays for chromosome aberrations involve treating intact animals and later collecting cells for cytogenetic analysis (Kirkland et al., 1990; Preston et al., 1981; Tice et al., 1994). The main advantage of in vivo assays is that they include mammalian metabolism, DNA repair, and pharmacodynamics. The target is a tissue from which large numbers of dividing cells are easily prepared for analysis, so bone marrow from rats, mice, or Chinese hamsters is most commonly used. An exception is the analysis of interphase cells by FISH, described below. Lymphocytes are another suitable target when stimulated to divide with a mitogen such as phytohemagglutinin. In any case, effective testing requires dosages and routes of administration that ensure adequate exposure of the target cells, proper intervals between treatment and collecting cells, and sufficient numbers of animals and cells analyzed (Kirkland et al., 1990).

FISH is a recent development in cytogenetic analysis; in this procedure, a nucleic acid probe is hybridized to complementary sequences in chromosomal DNA. The probe is labeled with a fluorescent dye so that the chromosomal location to which it binds is visible by fluorescence microscopy. Composite probes have been developed from sequences unique to specific human chromosomes, giving a uniform fluorescent label over the entire chromosome. Slides prepared for standard metaphase analysis are suitable for

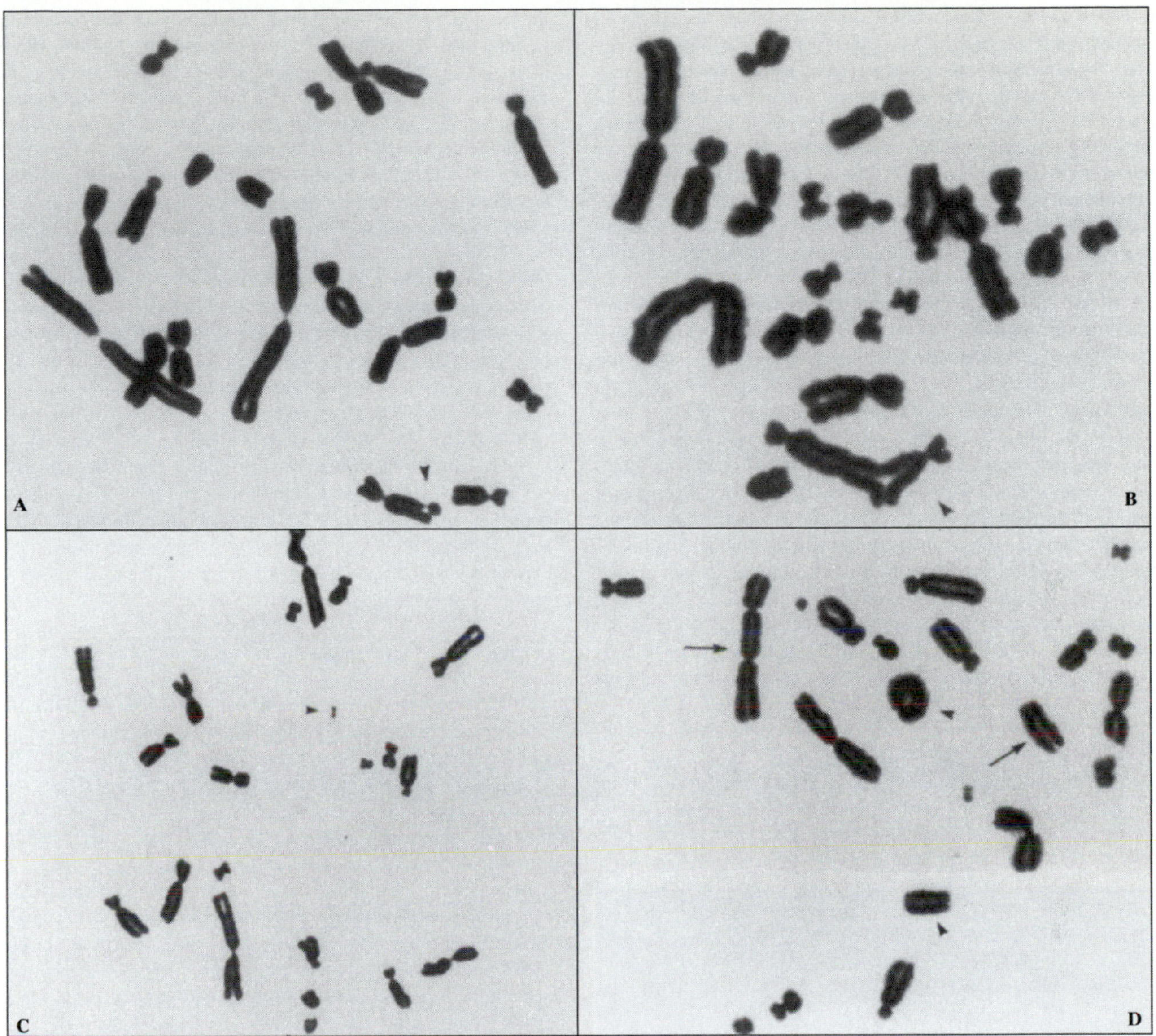

Figure 9-4. Chromosome aberrations induced by x-rays in Chinese hamster ovary (CHO) cells.

A. A chromatid deletion (➤). *B.* A chromatid exchange called a triradial (➤). *C.* A small interstitial deletion (➤) that resulted from chromosome breakage. *D.* A metaphase with more than one aberration: a centric ring plus an acentric fragment (➤) and a dicentric chromosome plus an acentric fragment (→).

FISH after they have undergone a simple denaturation procedure. The use of whole-chromosome probes is commonly called "chromosome painting."

Chromosome painting facilitates cytogenetic analysis, because aberrations are easily detected by the number of fluorescent regions in a painted metaphase. For example, if chromosome 4 were painted with a probe while the other chromosomes were counterstained in a different color, one would see only the two homologs of chromosome 4 in the color of the probe in a normal cell. However, if there were a translocation or a dicentric chromosome and fragment involving chromosome 4, one would see three areas of fluorescence—one normal chromosome 4 and the two pieces involved in the chromosome rearrangement. Aberrations are detected only in the painted portion of the genome, but this disadvantage may be offset by painting a few chromosomes simultaneously with probes of different colors (Tucker et al., 1993). FISH reduces the time and technical skill required to detect chromosome aberrations, and it permits the scoring of stable aberrations, such as translocations and insertions, that are not readily detected in traditional metaphase analysis of unbanded chromosomes. Additionally, some chromosome analysis can be conducted using FISH in interphase cells. Though not routinely used in genotoxicity testing, FISH is a valuable research tool for studying clastogens and is having a substantial impact in monitoring human populations for chromosomal damage.

Micronuclei Metaphase analysis is time-consuming and requires considerable skill, so there is interest in the development of simpler cytogenetic assays, of which micronucleus assays have become increasingly important. Micronuclei are chromatin-containing bodies that represent chromosomal fragments or sometimes whole chromosomes that were not incorporated into a daughter nucleus at mitosis. Since micronuclei usually represent acentric chromosomal fragments, they are most commonly used as simple indicators of chromosomal damage. However, the ability to detect micronuclei containing whole chromosomes has led to their use for detecting aneuploidy as well. Micronucleus assays may be conducted in primary cultures of human lymphocytes (Fenech, 1993; Fenech, 1997), mammalian cell lines (Miller et al., 1998; Kirsch-Volders et al., 2000), or in mammals in vivo (Heddle et al., 1991; Hayashi et al., 1994; Hayashi et al., 2000).

Micronucleus assays in lymphocytes have been greatly improved by the cytokinesis-block technique in which cell division is inhibited with cytochalasin B, resulting in binucleate and multinucleate cells (Fenech, 1993; Fenech, 1997; Kirsch-Volders et al., 2000). In the cytokinesis-block assay in human lymphocytes, nondividing (G_0) cells are treated with ionizing radiation or a radiomimetic chemical and then stimulated to divide with the mitogen phytohemagglutinin. Alternatively, the lymphocytes may be exposed to the mitogen first, so that the subsequent mutagenic treatment with radiations, or radiomimetic and nonradiomimetic chemicals, includes the S period of the cell cycle. In either case, cytochalasin B is added for the last part of the culture period, and micronuclei are counted only in binucleate cells so as to ensure that the cells have undergone a single nuclear division that is essential for micronucleus development. The assay thereby avoids confusion owing to differences in cellular proliferation kinetics. Micronuclei in a binucleate human lymphocyte are shown in - Fig. 9-5.

The in vivo micronucleus assay is most often performed by counting micronuclei in immature (polychromatic) erythrocytes in the bone marrow of treated mice, but it may also be based on peripheral blood (Heddle et al., 1991; Hayashi et al., 1994; Hayashi et al., 2000). Micronuclei remain in the cell when the nucleus is extruded in the maturation of erythroblasts. In vivo micronucleus assays are increasingly used in genotoxicity testing as a substitute for bone marrow metaphase chromosome analysis. Micronucleus assays in mammalian tissues other than bone marrow and blood are useful for mechanistic studies and research but are less often applied to genotoxicity testing (Hayashi et al., 2000).

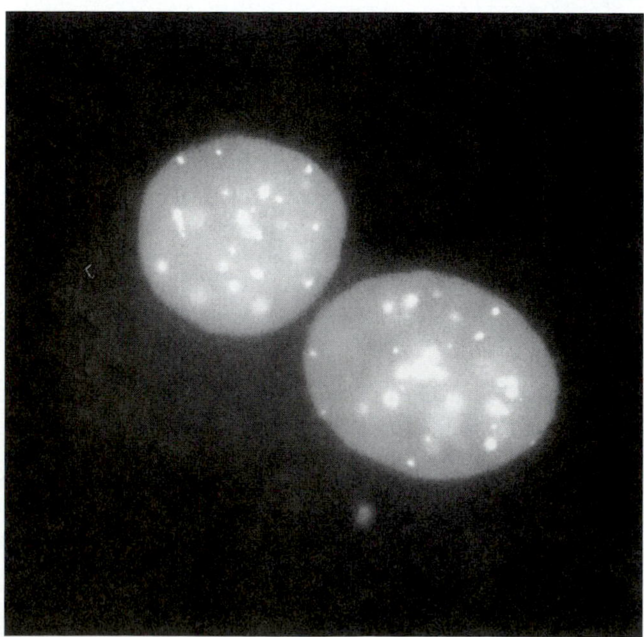

Figure 9-5. Micronucleus in a human lymphocyte.

The cytochalasin B method was used to inhibit cytokinesis that resulted in a binucleate nucleus. The micronucleus resulted from failure of an acentric chromosome fragment or a whole chromosome being included in a daughter nucleus following cell division. (Kindly provided by James Allen, Jill Barnes, and Barbara Collins.)

Sister Chromatid Exchange SCE, in which apparently reciprocal segments have been exchanged between the two chromatids of a chromosome, is visible cytologically through differential staining of chromatids. Figure 9-6 shows SCE in human cells. Many mutagens induce SCE in cultured cells and in mammals in vivo (Tucker et al., 1993). Despite the convenience and responsiveness of SCE assays, data on SCE are less informative than data on chromosome aberrations. There is uncertainty about the underlying mechanisms by which SCEs are formed and how DNA damage or perturbations of DNA synthesis stimulate their formation. SCE assays are therefore best regarded as general indicators of mutagen exposure, analogous to DNA damage and repair assays, rather than measures of a mutagenic effect.

Aneuploidy Although assays for aneuploidy are not yet as refined as those for gene mutations and chromosome aberrations, they are being developed (Aardema et al., 1998). Some of the methods are restricted to specific targets, such as the mitotic spindle in an assay for effects on the polymerization of tubulin in vitro (Parry, 1993). Most, however, measure aneuploidy itself and should therefore encompass all relevant cellular targets. Assays include chromosome counting (Aardema et al., 1998), the detection of micronuclei that contain kinetochores (Aardema et al., 1998; Natarajan, 1993), and the observation of abnormal spindles or spindle-chromosome associations in cells in which spindles and chromosomes have been differentially stained (Parry, 1998). Recently, FISH-based assays have been developed for the assessment of aneuploidy in interphase somatic cells (Rupa et al., 1997) and in sperm (Baumgarthner et al., 1999).

A complication in chromosome counting is that a metaphase may lack chromosomes because they were lost during cell preparation for analysis, rather than having been absent from the living cell. To avoid this artifact, cytogeneticists generally use extra chromosomes (i.e., hyperploidy) rather than missing chromosomes (i.e., hypoploidy) as an indicator of aneuploidy in chromosome preparations from mammalian cell cultures (Aardema et al., 1998; Galloway and Ivett, 1986) or mouse bone marrow (Adler, 1993). A promising means of circumventing this difficulty is growing and treating cells on a glass surface and then making chromosome preparations in situ, rather than dropping cells onto slides from a cell suspension. By counting chromosomes in intact cells, one can collect data for both hyperploidy and hypoploidy (Natarajan, 1993). It has been suggested that counting polyploid cells, which is technically straightforward, may be an efficient way to detect aneugens (Aardema et al., 1998), but there remains some disagreement on the point (Parry, 1998).

Micronucleus assays can detect aneugens as well as clastogens. Micronuclei that contain whole chromosomes are not readily distinguished from those containing chromosome fragments in typically stained preparations, though chromosome-containing ones tend to be somewhat larger (Natarajan, 1993). However, the

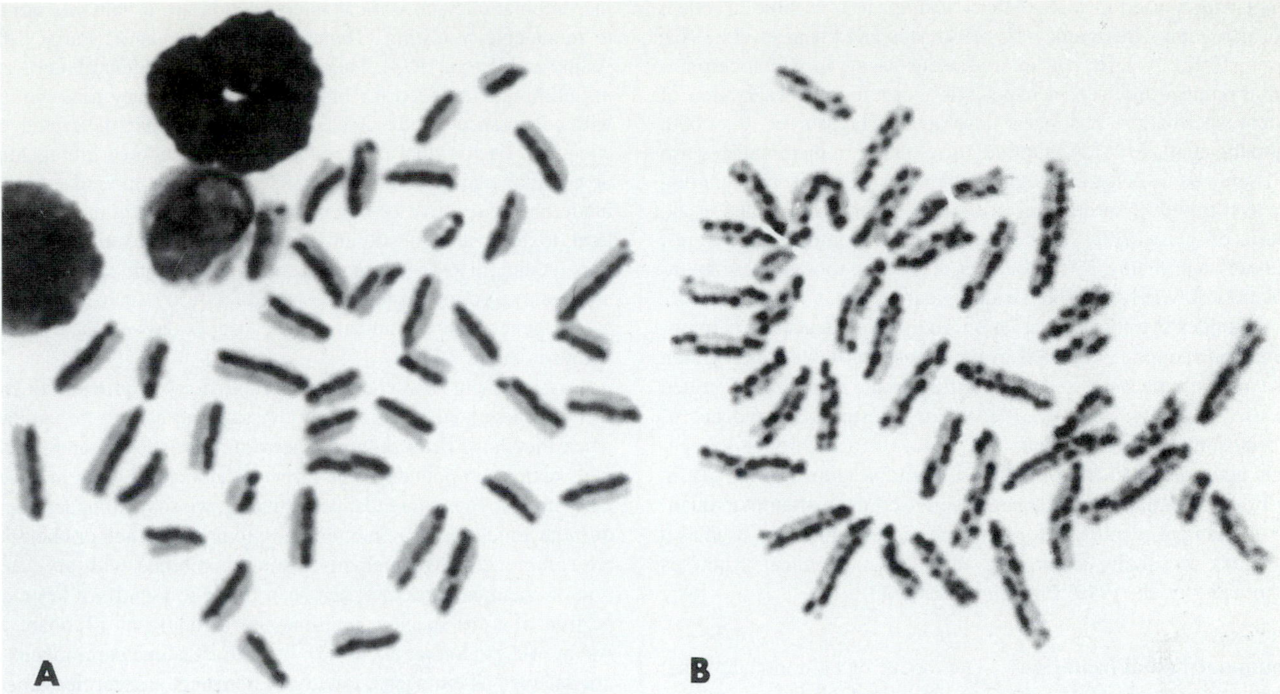

Figure 9-6. Sister chromatid exchanges (SCE) in human lymphocytes.

A. SCE in untreated cell. *B.* SCE in cell exposed to ethyl carbamate. The treatment results in a very large increase in the number of SCE. (Kindly provided by James Allen and Barbara Collins.)

presence of the spindle attachment region of a chromosome (kinetochore) in a micronucleus can indicate that it contains a whole chromosome. Aneuploidy may therefore be detected by means of antikinetochore antibodies with a fluorescent label or FISH with a probe for centromere-specific DNA (Natarajan, 1993; Lynch and Parry, 1993). Micronuclei containing kinetochores or centromeric DNA may be detected both in cell culture assays (Aardema et al., 1998; Lynch and Parry, 1993) and mouse bone marrow in vivo (Heddle et al., 1991; Adler, 1993). Frequencies of micronuclei ascribable to aneuploidy and to clastogenic effects may therefore be determined concurrently by tabulating micronuclei with and without kinetochores.

Germ Cell Mutagenesis

Gene Mutations Germ cell mutagenesis is of special interest as an indicator of genetic damage that enters the gene pool and is transmitted through generations. Mammalian germ cell assays provide the best basis for assessing risks to human germ cells and therefore hold a central place in genetic toxicology despite their relative complexity and expense. The design of the test must compensate for the fact that mutation occurs at low frequency, and even the simplest animal systems face a problem of there being a sufficiently large sample size. One can easily screen millions of bacteria or cultured cells by selection techniques, but screening large numbers of mice poses practical limitations. Therefore, germ cell studies must offer a straightforward, unequivocal identification of mutants with minimal labor.

The mouse specific-locus test detects recessive mutations that produce easily analyzed, visible phenotypes (coat pigmentation and ear size) conferred by seven genes (Favor, 1999; Russell and Shelby, 1985; Ehling, 1991; Russell and Russell, 1992). Mutants may be classified as having point mutations or chromosomal alterations on the basis of genetic and molecular analysis (Favor, 1999). The assay has been important in assessing genetic risks of ionizing radiation and has been used to study various chemical mutagens. Other gene mutation assays in mouse germ cells detect, for example, recessive mutations that cause electrophoretic changes in proteins (Lewis, 1991) and dominant mutations that cause skeletal abnormalities or cataracts (Ehling, 1991).

Mammalian assays permit the measurement of mutagenesis at different germ cell stages (Favor, 1999). Late stages of spermatogenesis are often found to be sensitive to mutagenesis, but spermatocytes, spermatids, and spermatozoa are transitory. Mutagenesis in stem cell spermatogonia and resting oocytes is of special interest in genetic risk assessment because of the persistence of these stages throughout reproductive life (discussed above, with mechanisms of induction of mutations and chromosome alterations in germ cells). Chemical mutagens show specificity with respect to germ cell stages. For example, ethylnitrosourea and chlorambucil are both potent mutagens in the mouse specific-locus test, but the former induces primarily point mutations in spermatogonia, whereas the latter mostly induces deletions in spermatids (Russell and Russell, 1992). The ratio of deletions to point mutations is not only a function of the nature of the mutagen but depends on germ-cell stage, as some mutagens induce higher proportions of gross alterations in late stages of spermatogenesis than in spermatogonia (Favor, 1999; Lewis, 1991).

Chromosomal Alterations Knowledge of the induction of chromosome aberrations in germ cells is important for assessing risks to future generations. Although metaphase analysis of germ cells is not widely used in mutagenicity testing, it is feasible in rodent spermatogonia, spermatocytes, or oocytes (Kirkland et al., 1990; Tease, 1992). A germ cell micronucleus assay, in which chromosomal damage induced in meiosis is measured by observation of rodent spermatids, has been developed (Hayashi et al., 2000; Lähdetie et al., 1994). Aneuploidy originating in mammalian germ cells may be detected cytologically through chromosome counting for hyperploidy (Aardema et al., 1998; Adler, 1993; Allen et al., 1986) or genetically in the mouse sex-chromosome loss test (Russell and Shelby, 1985; Allen et al., 1986), though these methods are not widely used in toxicological testing.

Besides cytologic observation, indirect evidence for chromosome aberrations is obtained in the mouse heritable translocation assay, which measures reduced fertility in the offspring of treated males (Russell and Shelby, 1985). This presumptive evidence of chromosomal rearrangements can be confirmed through cytogenetic analysis. Data from the mouse heritable translocation test in postmeiotic male germ cells have been used in an attempt to quantify human germ cell risk for ethylene oxide, a mutagen used as a fumigant, sterilizing agent, and reactant in chemical syntheses (Rhomberg et al., 1990; Preston et al., 1995).

Dominant Lethal Mutations The mouse or rat dominant lethal assay (Adler et al., 1994) offers an extensive data base on the induction of genetic damage in mammalian germ cells. In the most commonly used version of the assay, males are treated on an acute or subchronic basis with the agent of interest and then mated with virgin females at appropriate intervals. The females are killed and necropsied during pregnancy so that embryonic mortality may be characterized and quantified. Most dominant lethal mutations, manifested as intrauterine deaths, are thought to arise from chromosomal anomalies.

Development of Testing Strategies

Concern about adverse effects of mutation on human health, principally carcinogenesis and the induction of transmissible damage in germ cells, has provided the impetus to identify environmental mutagens. Priorities must be set for testing, because it is not feasible to conduct multiple tests of all chemicals to which people are exposed. Such factors as production volumes, intended uses, the extent of human exposure, environmental distribution, and effects that may be anticipated on the basis of chemical structure or previous testing must be considered in order to ensure that compounds with the greatest potential for adverse effects receive the most comprehensive study. The most obvious use of genetic toxicology assays is screening chemicals to detect mutagens, but they are also used to obtain information on mutagenic mechanisms and dose responses that contribute to an evaluation of hazards. Besides testing pure chemicals, environmental samples are tested (DeMarini, 1991; DeMarini, 1998) because many mutagens exist in complex mixtures.

The first indication that a chemical is a mutagen often lies in chemical structure. Potential electrophilic sites in a molecule serve as an alert to possible mutagenicity and carcinogenicity, because such sites confer reactivity with nucleophilic sites in DNA (Tennant and Ashby, 1991). Attempts to formalize the structural prediction through automated computer programs have not yet led to an ability to make exact predictions of mutagenicity and carcinogenicity of new chemicals (Parry, 1994; Richard, 1998), but structural alerts in combination with critical interpretation are a valuable adjunct to mutagenicity testing (Tennant and Ashby, 1991; Parry, 1994; Ashby and Paton, 1993). Though informative, structural alerts cannot eliminate the need for biological data, and they must be used with cognizance of other factors that can influence the effects of a chemical. Factors that may reduce the likelihood of mutagenicity or carcinogenicity of a structurally alerting compound are steric hindrance of reactive or potentially reactive substituents, metabolism, toxicity, and substituents that enhance the chemical's excretion (Ashby, 1994). Moreover, some agents that lack structural alerts may stimulate mutagenesis indirectly by such mechanisms as the generation of radicals that cause oxidative DNA damage (Clayson et al., 1994).

Assessment of a chemical's genotoxicity requires data from well-characterized genetic assays. Assays are said to be validated when they have been shown to perform reproducibly and reliably with many compounds from diverse chemical classes in several laboratories. To explore test performance, we shall consider the use of mutagenicity assays in attempting to predict whether chemicals are carcinogens. Mutagenicity testing, combined with an evaluation of chemical structure, has been found to identify a large proportion of trans-species, multiple-site carcinogens (Tennant and Ashby, 1991; Gold et al., 1993). In contrast, some carcinogens are not detected as mutagens. Putatively nongenotoxic carcinogens often give responses that are more specific with respect to species, sites, and conditions (Ashby and Paton, 1993; Gold et al., 1993). In predicting carcinogenicity, one should consider both the sensitivity and the specificity of an assay. Sensitivity refers to the proportion of carcinogens that are positive in the assay, whereas specificity is the proportion of noncarcinogens that are negative (Tennant et al., 1987; McGregor et al., 1999). Sensitivity and specificity both contribute to the predictive reliability of an assay. The commonly held view that deficiencies in the sensitivity or specificity of individual assays may be circumvented by using assays in complementary combinations called tiers or batteries has fallen into disfavor because, rather than offsetting each other's strengths and weaknesses, genetic toxicology assays are often consistent with one another (Tennant et al., 1987; Ashby and Tennant, 1991; Kim and Margolin, 1999).

Rather than trying to assemble batteries of complementary assays, it is prudent to emphasize mechanistic considerations in choosing assays. Such an approach makes a sensitive assay for gene mutations (e.g., the Ames assay) and an assay for clastogenic effects in mammals pivotal in the evaluation of genotoxicity, and this is the basis for our highlighting these assays in Table 9-1. The Ames assay has performed reliably with hundreds of compounds in laboratories throughout the world. Other bacterial assays and mammalian cell assays also provide useful information on gene mutations. Beyond gene mutations, one should evaluate damage at the chromosomal level with a mammalian in vitro or in vivo cytogenetic assay. Cytogenetic assays in rodents are especially useful for this purpose because they combine a well-validated genetic assay with mammalian pharmacodynamics and metabolism. The other assays in Table 9-1 offer an extensive data base on chemical mutagenesis (*Drosophila* SLRL), a unique genetic endpoint (i.e., aneuploidy; mitotic recombination), applicability to diverse organisms and tissues (i.e., DNA damage assays, such as the comet assay), or special importance in the assessment of genetic risk (i.e., germ cell assays). The more extensive listing of assays in Table 9-2 provides references that can be helpful in interpreting genetic toxicology data in the scientific literature.

HUMAN POPULATION MONITORING

For cancer risk assessment considerations, the human data utilized most frequently, absent epidemiologic data, are those collected from genotoxicity assessment in human populations. The studies conducted most frequently are for chromosome aberrations, micronuclei, and sister chromatid exchanges (SCE) in peripheral lymphocytes. Cytogenetic alterations have also been assessed in a small number of bone marrow samples. Mutations at the *HPRT* locus have been assessed in peripheral lymphocytes, and glycophorin A variants have been studied in red blood cells.

An important component of any population monitoring study is the selection of the study groups, namely, those individuals who are potentially exposed and the unexposed controls. The size of each study group should be sufficiently large to avoid any confounder having undue influence. Certain characteristics should be matched among exposed and unexposed groups. These include age, sex, smoking status, and general dietary features. Certain characteristics are exclusionary, namely, current or recent medication, radiation exposure, and certain illnesses. It is possible to develop a lengthy list of additional possible confounders of response that would make the selection of suitable study groups very difficult indeed. Study groups of 20 or more individuals can be used as a reasonable substitute for exact matching because confounders will be less influential on chromosome alteration or mutation frequency in larger groups, as mentioned above (discussed in Au et al., 1998). In some instances, it might be informative to compare exposed groups with a historical control, as well as to a concurrent control.

The magnitude of different known confounders varies quite considerably among studies, based in part on the size of the study populations. Some general indication of the magnitude of the effects of age and smoking status on the frequencies of chromosome aberrations and SCE is presented to illustrate the importance of accounting for confounders in the design of a population monitoring study. The comparisons presented are for large studies only. For chromosome aberrations, the frequency of aberrations has been reported in one large study to be about 50 percent higher in smokers (1.5 aberrations per 100 cells in smokers versus 1.0 per 100 cells in the nonsmokers) (Galloway et al., 1986) and in another no difference between smokers and nonsmokers (Bender et al., 1988). The complete data set has been reviewed recently by Au et al. (1998). In general, the frequency of SCE is increased by about one SCE per cell in smokers compared with nonsmokers (Bender et al., 1988; Barale et al., 1998). The study by Barale et al. (1998) also reported a dose response association between SCE frequency and smoking level. The frequency of aberrations, particularly chromosome-type exchanges, has been shown to increase with age of subject. Galloway et al. (1986) reported an increase from 0.8 per 100 cells at about 25 years of age to about 1.5 at 60. Bender et al. (1988) reported an increase with age only for chromosome-type dicentric aberrations, but the increase over a broad age range was small and just statistically significant. Ramsey et al. (1995), using chromosome painting techniques reported that individuals 50 years and older had frequencies of stable aberrations, dicentrics, and acentric fragments that were 10.6-fold, 3.3-fold, and 2.9-fold, respectively, greater than the frequency in cord bloods. Bender et al. (1998) did not find an increase in SCE frequency with the increasing age of the subject. The differences among the results from these large control studies emphasize the difficulty of adequately accounting for confounders (age and smoking presented here) when only a small control group is used, as is frequently the case.

Similar sources of variation have been identified for the monitoring of individuals for *HPRT* mutations. The data are reviewed in detail by Albertini and Hayes (1997). There is less information on sources of variation of glycophorin A variants although quite considerable interindividual variation exists (reviewed in Cole and Skopek, 1994).

For cytogenetic assays (chromosome aberrations, sister chromatid exchanges, and micronuclei) the alterations are produced as a consequence of errors of DNA replication, as discussed in previous sections. From the nature of the alterations, assessed in traditional cytogenetic assays, in which nontransmissible alterations are analyzed, it can be established that these alterations were produced at the first in vitro S phase. Irrespective of the duration of exposure, the frequency of cytogenetic alterations will be proportional to that fraction of the DNA damage that remains at the time of in vitro DNA replication. All the DNA damage induced by potent clastogens that results in chromosome alterations is repaired within a relatively short time after exposure for G_0 human lymphocytes. Thus, for chronic exposures the lymphocyte cytogenetic assay as typically conducted is insensitive.

It is now possible to analyze reciprocal translocations using FISH methods (reviewed in Tucker et al., 1997), and because this aberration type is transmissible from cell generation to generation, its frequency can be representative of an accumulation over time of exposure. The importance of this is that stable chromosome aberrations observed in peripheral lymphocytes exposed in vivo, but assessed following in vitro culture, are produced in vivo in hematopoietic stem cells or other precursor cells of the peripheral lymphocytes pool. To date, population cytogenetic monitoring studies involving the analysis of reciprocal translocations in chemically exposed individuals or radiation-exposed individuals have been conducted quite rarely (Smith et al., 1998; Lucas et al., 1992). To date, the overall sensitivity of the FISH analysis of reciprocal translocations for assessing effects of chronic, low level of exposure to chemical clastogens has not been established. However, a cautionary note is provided by the recent study by Director et al. (1998), who showed that there was no increase in reciprocal translocations assessed by FISH following exposure to cyclophosphamide (0, 32, 64, or 96 ppm) or urethane (0, 5000, 10,000, or 15,000 ppm) for up to 12 weeks. In contrast, recent data from the present author's laboratory (Preston et al., unpublished) have shown that exposure of male mice to ethylene oxide at concentrations of 0, 25, 50, 100, 200 ppm for 6, 12, 24, or 48 weeks resulted in a time and concentration-dependent increase in reciprocal translocations assessed by FISH.

Another factor that certainly affects the utility of population monitoring data on reciprocal translocations using FISH is that the frequency of reciprocal translocations increases significantly with increasing age (Ramsey et al., 1995), but to a lesser extent for nontransmissible aberrations (Bender et al., 1988). Ramsey et al. (1995) provided data on the influence of other confounders on the frequency of reciprocal translocations in human groups. These confounders include smoking, consumption of diet drinks and/or diet sweeteners, exposure to asbestos or coal products, and having a previous major illness. This reemphasizes the point that the selection of study groups and accounting for confounders is essential for a human population cytogenetic monitoring study to be of utility.

Thus, very few of the published studies of cytogenetic population monitoring for individuals have analyzed the appropriate endpoint for detecting the genetic effects of long-term exposure to chemicals. It is quite surprising that positive responses have been reported for increases in unstable, chromatid aberrations because these are nontransmissible, and as noted above are induced at the first in vitro S phase.

The *HPRT* mutation assay can assess the frequency of induced mutations in stem cells or other procursor cells, since a proportion of the mutations are induced as nonlethal events. The transmissible proportion will be greater for agents that do not induce large deletions; this will include the majority of nonradiomimetic chemicals. Induction of mutations in lymphocyte precursor cells will lead to clonal expansion of the mutation in the peripheral pool. However, assessment of the T-cell antigen receptor status of the mutant clones permits a correction for clonal expansion. The population of cells derived from any particular stem cell has a unique antigen receptor status (Albertini and Hayes, 1997). The GPA assay can similarly be used for the assessment of chronic exposures or for estimating exposures at some long time after exposure (Albertini and Hayes, 1997). The predictive value of the assay for adverse health outcome appears to be limited, but it can provide an estimate of exposure.

The potential for cytogenetic endpoints being predictive of relative cancer risk has been addressed in recent reports from the European Study Group on Cytogenetic Biomarkers and Health (Hagmar et al., 1998a; Hagmar et al., 1998b). A study group selected for cytogenetic studies consisted of individuals with reported occupational exposure and unexposed controls. The association between cancer and the frequency of unstable chromosome aberrations in the study groups was not based on exposure status, but rather on the relative frequency of chromosome aberrations, namely, low (1 to 33 percentiles), medium (34 to 66 percentiles), and high (67 to 100 percentiles). In general, the higher the relative frequency of unstable aberrations, the greater the risk of cancer death for all tumors combined. The authors make it clear that there is insufficient information on exposure for it to be used as a predictor of cancer development. In fact, the data indicate that individuals with higher frequencies of chromosome aberrations for whatever reason (genetic or environmental) are *as a group* at greater risk of dying from cancer. This is very different from concluding that exposures to mutagens that result in a higher frequency of chromosome aberrations in peripheral lymphocytes leads to an increased risk of cancer, especially for specific tumor types. The relevance of exposure to mutagenic chemicals in these studies by Hagmar et al. (1998a; 1998b) is uncertain because there was no association between increased SCE frequencies and increased cancer mortality.

This latter concern was addressed by the same group (Bonassi et al., 2000) in a more recent study. The study again showed that there was a significantly increased risk for subjects with a high level of chromosome aberrations compared to those with a low level in both a Nordic and Italian cohort. Of particular relevance to risk assessment, the relationships were not affected by the inclusion of occupational exposure level or smoking. The risk for high versus low levels of chromosome aberrations was similar in individuals heavily exposed to carcinogens and in those who had never, to their knowledge, been exposed to any specific environmental carcinogen. These data highlight the need to use caution when considering the relevance of chromosome aberration data in cancer risk assessment.

NEW APPROACHES FOR GENETIC TOXICOLOGY

In the past 15 years, the field of genetic toxicology has moved into the molecular era. The potential for advances in our understanding of basic cellular processes and how they can be perturbed is enormous. The ability to manipulate and characterize DNA, RNA, and proteins has been at the root of this advance in knowledge. However, the development of sophisticated molecular biology does not in itself imply a corresponding advance in the utility of genetic toxicology and its application to risk assessment. Knowing the types of studies to conduct and knowing how to interpret the data remain as fundamental as always. Measuring finer and finer detail can perhaps complicate the utility of the various mutagenicity assays. There is a need for genetic toxicology to avoid the temptation to use more and more sophisticated techniques to address the same questions and in the end make the same mistakes as have been made previously. How successful we are in designing informative studies perhaps cannot be judged at this time. However, the following examples of recent approaches to obtaining data for enhancing our ability to use noncancer (genotoxicity) data in a mechanistically based cancer (and genetic) risk assessment process provide some encouragement. Several recent developments (e.g., the use of transgenic animals, the comet assay for assessing DNA damages) have already been described in the appropriate assay section above since they are currently in general use.

Advances in Cytogenetics

Until quite recently, the analysis of chromosome alterations relied on conventional chromosome staining with DNA stains such as Giemsa or on the process of chromosome banding. Both approaches require considerable expenditure of time and a rather high level of expertise. However, chromosome banding does allow for the assessment of transmissible aberrations such as reciprocal translocations and inversions with a fairly high degree of accuracy. Knowing the induction frequency of such aberrations is very important, given that they are not lethal to the cell and constitute by far the major class observed in inherited genetic defects and a significant fraction of the alterations observed in tumors. In addition, since stable aberrations are transmissible from parent to daughter cell, they represent effects of chronic exposures. The more readily analyzed but cell lethal, nontransmissible aberrations such as dicentrics and deletions reflect only recent exposures and then only when analyzed at the first division after exposure. (For a more detailed explanation, see Preston, 1998.)

The relative ease with which specific chromosomes, specific genes, and chromosome alterations can be detected has been radically enhanced by the development of FISH (Trask et al., 1993). In principle, the technique relies on amplification of DNA from particular genomic regions such as whole chromosomes or gene regions and the hybridization of these amplified DNAs to metaphase chromosome preparations or interphase nuclei. Regions of hybridization can be determined by the use of fluorescent antibodies that detect modified DNA bases incorporated during amplification or by incorporating fluorescent bases during amplification. The fluorescently labeled, hybridized regions are detected by fluorescence microscopy, and the signal can be increased in strength by computer-enhanced processes. The level of sophistication has increased so much that all 24 different human chromosomes (22 autosomes, X and Y) can be individually detected

(Macville et al., 1997), as can all mouse chromosomes (Liyanage et al., 1996). Alterations in tumors can also be detected on a whole-genome basis (Coleman et al., 1997; Veldman et al., 1997).

There is an extensive literature on the use of FISH for karyotyping tumors and in gene mapping but less on its utility for genetic toxicology studies, especially the assessment of stable chromosome aberrations at long periods after exposure or after long-term exposures. Three particular studies do, however, serve to exemplify the use of FISH in genetic toxicology.

Lucas et al. (1992) demonstrated that stable chromosomal aberrations could be detected in individuals decades after exposure to atomic bombs in Japan. How these frequencies relate to frequencies at the time of exposure is not known with any certainty, given the fact that induced frequencies were not measured since appropriate techniques were not available at that time.

A recent study by Tucker et al. (1997) provided some assessment of the utility of FISH for the analysis of radiation-induced, stable chromosome alterations at various times after exposure. The frequency of reciprocal translocations induced by gamma rays in rat peripheral lymphocytes decreased with time after exposure, reaching a plateau of four days that was 55 to 65 percent of the induced frequency and with a dose dependency. This result suggests that reciprocal translocations fall into two classes, stable and unstable (cell-lethal). Additional work is required to clarify this conclusion and to extend the studies to effects of chemicals.

FISH methods have also allowed for an accurate and sensitive assessment of chromosomal alterations present in tumors. The particular advance that makes this assessment feasible is known as comparative genomic hybridization (CGH) (Kallioniemi et al., 1992). CGH results in the ability to identify the role of chromosomal structural and numerical alterations in tumor development. The genomic instability present in all tumor types appears to have a specific genetic basis, as shown elegantly for colon cancer by Vogelstein and colleagues (Cahill et al., 1998). For CGH, tumor and control DNAs are differentially labeled with fluorescence probes and cohybridized to normal metaphase chromosome preparations. The ratio of the fluorescence intensities of hybridized tumor and control DNA indicates regions of normal genomic content as well as those regions that are over- or underrepresented in tumors. The CGH method is being adapted for automated screening approaches using biochips (Solinas-Tolado et al., 1997). Assessing genetic alterations such as specific gene deletions in single metastatic tumor cells is feasible with a slightly different approach (Pack et al., 1997).

The types of FISH approaches described here undoubtedly indicate the direction in which cytogenetic analysis will proceed. The types of data collected will affect our understanding of how tumors develop. Data on the dose-response characteristics for a specific chromosomal alteration as a proximate marker of cancer can enhance the cancer risk assessment process by describing effects of low exposures that are below those for which tumor incidence can be reliably assessed. Cytogenetic data of the types described above can also improve extrapolation from data generated with laboratory animals to humans.

Molecular Analysis of Mutations and Gene Expression

With the advent of molecular biology techniques, the exact basis of a mutation at the level of the DNA sequence can be established. In many cases, the genetic basis of human disease can be determined even though human genes have long DNA sequences and a complex genomic arrangement. Molecular biology techniques have also enabled a distinction to be made between background mutations and those induced by specific agents. The latter observations are addressed by analyzing the mutational spectra in target genes in laboratory animals and in humans (DeMarini, 2000). For reasons of inherent sensitivity of available methods, the genes analyzed for mutations are ones for which mutated forms can be selected. The confounding factor of many normal cells, which far outnumber a few mutant cells in an exposed cellular population, can be removed. Methods to overcome this drawback are currently being developed, and particular methods such as ligation-mediated polymerase chain reaction (PCR) are close to the required sensitivity level (Albertini and Hayes, 1998).

A giant step forward in the ability to detect and characterize mutations at both the DNA and RNA level has been provided by the development of chip technology (Southern, 1996) and array-based assay systems (Woldicka et al., 1997). With hybridization of test DNAs to oligonucleotide arrays, specific genetic alterations or their cellular consequences can be determined rapidly and automatically. Cost remains a limiting factor, but the potential for assessing specific cellular changes following chemical exposure is enormous.

Until recently, alterations in gene expression following specific exposures or for specific genotypes were analyzed gene by gene. Such an approach makes it difficult to assess changes in gene expression that occur in a concerted fashion. Recent advances using cDNA microarray technologies have allowed the measurement of changes in expression of hundreds or even thousands of genes at one time (Harrington et al., 2000). The level of expression at the mRNA level is measured by amount of hybridization of isolated cDNA's to oligonucleotide fragments from known genes or expressed sequence tags (EST) on a specifically laid out grid. Although this technique holds great promise for establishing a cell's response to exposure to chemical or physical agents in the context of normal cellular patterns of gene expression, it remains to be established how to analyze the vast amounts of data that can and are being obtained and what magnitude of change in gene expression constitutes an adverse effect as far as cellular phenotype is concerned. Extrapolating the responses to organs and whole animals represents a challenge still to be addressed.

CONCLUSIONS

The field of genetic toxicology has had an overall life of about seventy years and has undergone several rebirths during this period. Genetic toxicology began as a basic research field with demonstrations that ionizing radiations and chemicals could induce mutations and chromosome alterations in plant, insect, and mammalian cells. The development of a broad range of short-term assays for genetic toxicology served to identify many mutagens and address the relationship between mutagens and cancer-causing agents, or carcinogens. The inevitable failure of the assays to be completely predictive resulted in the identification of nongenotoxic carcinogens. In 1980, genetic toxicology moved toward gaining a better understanding of the mutagenic mechanisms underlying carcinogenicity and heritable effects. With this improved understanding, genetic toxicology studies began to turn away from hazard identification alone and move toward quantitative risk assessment. Major advances in our knowledge of mechanisms of cancer formation have been fueled by truly amazing progress in molecular biology. Genetic toxicology has begun to take advantage of the knowledge that cancer is a genetic disease with multiple steps, many of which require a mutation. The identification of chromosome alterations involved in tumor formation has been facilitated greatly by the use of FISH. The ability to distinguish between background and induced mutations can in some cases be achieved by mutation analysis at the level of DNA sequence. Key cellular processes related to mutagenesis have been identified, including multiple pathways of DNA repair, cell cycle controls, and the role of checkpoints in ensuring that the cell cycle does not proceed until the DNA and specific cellular structures are checked for fidelity. These observations have enhanced our knowledge of the importance of genotype in susceptibility to cancer. Recent developments in genetic toxicology have greatly improved our understanding of basic cellular processes and alterations that can affect the integrity of the genetic material and its functions. The ability to detect and analyze mutations in mammalian germ cells continues to improve and can contribute to a better appreciation for the long-term consequences of mutagenesis in human populations. Improvements in the qualitative assessment of mutation in somatic cells and germ cells have been paralleled by advances in the ability to assess genetic alterations quantitatively, especially in ways that enhance the cancer and genetic risk assessment process.

ACKNOWLEDGMENTS

We would like to recognize the outstanding secretarial support provided by Carolyn P. Fowler in the preparation of this chapter. The authors also thank Drs. David DeMarini, James Allen, and Les Recio for their valuable comments as part of the review of the chapter.

This document has been reviewed in accordance with the U.S. Environmental Protection Agency policy and approved for publication. Mention of trade names or commercial products does not constitute endorsement or recommendation for use.

REFERENCES

Aardema MJ, Albertini S, Arni P, et al: Aneuploidy: A report of an ECETOC task force. *Mutat Res* 410:3–79, 1998.

Aboussekhra A, Biggerstaff M, Shivji MK, et al: Mammalian DNA nucleotide excision repair reconstituted with purified protein components. *Cell* 80:859–868, 1995.

Adler I-D: Synopsis of the in vivo results obtained with the 10 known or suspected aneugens tested in the CEC collaborative study. *Mutat Res* 287:131–137, 1993.

Adler I-D, Shelby MD, Bootman J, et al: Summary report of the working group on mammalian germ cell tests. *Mutat Res* 312:313–318, 1994.

Aguilar F, Harris CC, Sun T, et al: Geographic variation of p53 mutational profile in nonmalignant human liver. *Science* 264:1317–1319, 1994.

Albertini RJ, Hayes RB: Somatic cell mutations in cancer epidemiology. *IARC Sci Pub* 142:159–184, 1997.

Allen JW, Liang JC, Carrano AV, Preston RJ: Review of literature on chemical-induced aneuploidy in mammalian germ cells. *Mutat Res* 167:123–137, 1986.

Ames BN, McCann J, Yamasaki E: Methods for detecting carcinogens and mutagens with the Salmonella/mammalian-microsome mutagenicity test. *Mutat Res* 31:347–364, 1975.

Anderson RM, Marsden SJ, Wright EG, et al: Complex chromosome aberrations in peripheral blood lymphocytes as a potential biomarker of exposure to high-LET alpha-particles. *Int J Radiat Biol* 76:31–42, 2000.

Ashby J: Two million rodent carcinogens? The role of SAR and QSAR in their detection. *Mutat Res* 305:3–12, 1994.

Ashby J, Paton D: The influence of chemical structure on the extent and sites of carcinogenesis for 522 rodent carcinogens and 55 different human carcinogen exposures. *Mutat Res* 286:3–74, 1993.

Ashby J, Tennant RW: Definitive relationships among chemical structure, carcinogenicity and mutagenicity for 301 chemicals tested by the U.S. NTP. *Mutat Res* 257:229–306, 1991.

Au WW, Gajas-Salazar N, Salama S: Factors contributing to discrepancies in population monitoring studies. *Mutat Res* 400:467–478, 1998.

Auerbach C, Robson JM: Chemical production of mutations. *Nature* 157:302, 1946.

Barale R, Chelotti L, Davini T, et al: Sister chromatid exchange and micronucleus frequency in human lymphocytes of 1,650 subjects in an Italian population: II. Contribution of sex, age, and lifestyle. *Environ Mol Mutagen* 31:228–242, 1998.

Barrett JC: Mechanisms of multistep carcinogenesis and carcinogen risk assessment. *Environ Health Prospect* 100:9–20, 1993.

Baumgarthner A, Van Hummelen P, Lowe XR, et al: Numerical and structural chromosomal abnormalities detected in human sperm with a combination of multicolor FISH assays. *Environ Mol Mutagen* 33:49–58, 1999.

Beale G: The discovery of mustard gas mutagenesis by Auerbach and Robson in 1941. *Genetics* 134:393–399, 1993.

Bender MA, Gooch PC: Persistent chromosome aberrations in irradiated human subjects. *Radiat Res* 16:44–53, 1962.

Bender MA, Preston RJ, Leonard RC, et al: Chromosomal aberration and sister-chromatid exchange frequencies in peripheral blood lymphocytes of a large human population sample. *Mutat Res* 204:421–433, 1988.

Bender MA, Preston RJ, Leonard RC, et al: Chromosomal aberration and sister-chromatid exchange frequencies in peripheral blood lymphocytes of a large human population sample. II. Extension of age range. *Mutat Res* 212:149–154, 1988.

Benhamou S, Sarasin A: Variability in nucleotide excision repair and cancer risk: A review. *Mutat Res* 462:149–158, 2000.

Bentley KS, Sarrif AM, Cimino MC, Auletta AE: Assessing the risk of heritable gene mutation in mammals: *Drosophila* sex-linked recessive lethal test and tests measuring DNA damage and repair in mammalian germ cells. *Environ Mol Mutagen* 23:3–11, 1994.

Bickel SE, Orr-Weaver TL: Holding chromatids together to ensure they go their separate ways. *Bioessays* 18:293–300, 1996.

Bishop JM: Molecular themes in oncogenesis. *Cell* 64:235–248, 1991.

Bonassi S, Hagmar L, Strömberg U, et al: Chromosomal aberrations in lymphocytes predict human cancer independently of exposure to carcinogens. *Cancer Res* 60:1619–1625, 2000.

Brewen JG, Preston RJ: Cytogenetic analysis of mammalian oocytes in mutagenicity studies, in Hsu TC (ed): *Cytogenetic Assays of Environmental Mutagens.* Totowa, NJ: Allanheld, Osmun, 1982, pp 277–287.

Brewen JG, Preston RJ: Cytogenetic effects of environmental mutagens in mammalian cells and the extrapolation to man. *Mutat Res* 26:297–305, 1974.

Brusick JD (ed): *Methods for Genetic Risk Assessment.* Boca Raton, FL: CRC Press, 1994.

Burkhart JG, Malling HV: Mutagenesis and transgenic systems: Perspective from the mutagen, N-ethyl-N-nitrosourea. *Environ Mol Mutagen* 22:1–6, 1993.

Burkhart JG, Malling HV: Mutations among the living and the undead. *Mutat Res* 304:315–320, 1994.

Cahill DP, Lengauer C, Yu J, et al: Mutations of mitotic checkpoint genes in human cancers. *Nature* 392:300–303, 1998.

Calos MP, Miller JH: Genetic and sequence analysis of frameshift mutations induced by ICR-191. *J Mol Biol* 153:39–66, 1981.

Cariello NF, Skopek TR: Analysis of mutations occurring at the human *hprt* locus. *J Mol Biol* 231:41–57, 1993.

Casciano DA, Aidoo A, Chen T, et al: *Hprt* mutant frequency and molecular analysis of *Hprt* mutations in rats treated with mutagenic carcinogens. *Mutat Res* 431:389–395, 1999.

Cavenee WK, Dryja TP, Phillips RA, et al: Expression of recessive alleles by chromosomal mechanisms in retinoblastoma. *Nature* 305:779–784, 1983.

Chang LW, Hsia SMT, Chan P-C, Hsieh L-L: Macromolecular adducts: Biomarkers for toxicity and carcinogenesis. *Annu Rev Pharmacol Toxicol* 34:41–67, 1994.

Clayson DB, Mehta R, Iverson F: Oxidative DNA damage—The effects of certain genotoxic and operationally non-genotoxic carcinogens. *Mutat Res* 317:25–42, 1994.

Cole J, Skopek TR: Somatic mutant frequency, mutation rates and mutational spectra in the human population in vivo. *Mutat Res* 304:33–105, 1994.

Coleman AE, Schrock E, Weaver Z, et al: Previously hidden chromosome aberrations in t(12;15)-positive BALB/c plasmacytomas uncovered by multicolor spectral karyotyping. *Cancer Res* 57:4585–4592, 1997.

Cotelle S, Férard JF: Comet assay in genetic ecotoxicology. *Environ Mol Mutagen* 34:246–255, 1999.

Crespi CL, Miller VP: The use of heterologously expressed drug metabolizing enzymes—state of the art and prospects for the future. *Pharmacol Ther* 84:121–131, 1999.

Critchlow SE, Jackson SP: DNA end-joining from yeast to man. *Trends Biochem Sci* 23:394–398, 1998.

Cupples CG, Cabrera M, Cruz C, Miller JH: A set of *lacZ* mutations in *Escherichia coli* that allow rapid detection of specific frameshift mutations. *Genetics* 125:275–280, 1990.

Cupples CG, Miller JH: A set of *lacZ* mutations in *Escherichia coli* that allow rapid detection of each of the six base substitutions. *Proc Natl Acad Sci USA* 86:5345–5349, 1989.

Dellarco VL, Prival MJ: Mutagenicity of nitro compounds in *Salmonella typhimurium* in the presence of flavin mononucleotide in a preincubation assay. *Environ Mol Mutagen* 13:116–127, 1989.

DeMarini DM: Environmental mutagens/complex mixtures, in Li AP, Heflich RH (eds): *Genetic Toxicology: A Treatise.* Boca Raton, FL: CRC Press, 1991, pp 285–302.

DeMarini DM: Influence of DNA repair on mutation spectra in *Salmonella. Mutat Res* 450:5–17, 2000.

DeMarini DM: Mutation spectra of complex mixtures. *Mutat Res* 411:11–18, 1998.

DeMarini DM, Brockman HE, de Serres FJ, et al: Specific-locus mutations induced in eukaryotes (especially mammalian cells) by radiation and chemicals: A perspective. *Mutat Res* 220:11–29, 1989.

Demple B, Harrison L: Repair of oxidative damage to DNA: Enzymology and biology. *Annu Rev Biochem* 63:915–948, 1994.

Director AE, Tucker JD, Ramsey MJ, Nath J: Chronic ingestion of clastogens by mice and the frequency of chromosome aberrations. *Environ Mol Mutagen* 32:139–147, 1998.

Dogliotti E, Hainant P, Hernandez T, et al: Mutation spectra resulting from carcinogenic exposures: From model systems to cancer-related genes. *Recent Results Cancer Res* 154:97–124, 1998.

Ehling UH: Genetic risk assessment. *Annu Rev Genet* 25:255–280, 1991.

Elia MC, Storer R, McKelvey TW, et al: Rapid DNA degradation in primary rat hepatocytes treated with diverse cytotoxic chemicals: Analysis by pulsed field gel electrophoresis and implications for alkaline elution assays. *Environ Mol Mutagen* 24:181–191, 1994.

EPA (U.S. Environmental Protection Agency): *Guidelines for Carcinogen Risk Assessment. Fed Reg* 51:33992–34003, 1986.

EPA (U.S. Environmental Protection Agency): *Proposed Guidelines for Carcinogen Risk Assessment.* EPA/600P/P-92/003c. Office of Research and Development. Washington, DC: U.S. Environmental Protection Agency, 1996.

Evan G, Littlewood T: A matter of life and cell death. *Science* 281:1317–1322, 1998.

Evans HJ, Prosser J: Tumor-suppressor genes: Cardinal factors in inherited predisposition to human cancers. *Environ Health Perspect* 98:25–37, 1992.

Fairbairn DW, Olive PL, O'Neill KL: The comet assay: A comprehensive review. *Mutat Res* 339:37–59, 1995.

Favor J: Mechanisms of mutation induction in germ cells of the mouse as assessed by the specific-locus test. *Mutat Res* 428:227–236, 1999.

Fearon ER, Vogelstein B: A genetic model for colorectal tumorigenesis. *Cell* 61:759–767, 1990.

Fenech M: The cytokinesis-block micronucleus technique: A detailed description of the method and its application to genotoxicity studies in human populations. *Mutat Res* 285:35–44, 1993.

Fenech M: The advantages and disadvantages of the cytokinesis-block micronucleus method. *Mutat Res* 392:11–18, 1997.

Friedberg EC: *DNA Repair.* New York: Freeman, 1985.

Friedberg EC, Walker GC, Siede W: *DNA Repair and Mutagenesis.* Washington, DC: ASM Press, 1995.

Galloway SM: Cytotoxicity and chromosome aberrations in vitro: Experience in industry and the case for an upper limit on toxicity in the aberration assay. *Environ Mol Mutagen* 35:191–201, 2000.

Galloway SM, Aardema MJ, Ishidate M Jr, et al: Report from working group on in vitro tests for chromosomal aberrations. *Mutat Res* 312:241–261, 1994.

Galloway SM, Berry PK, Nichols WW, et al: Chromosome aberrations in individuals occupationally exposed to ethylene oxide, and in a large control population. *Mutat Res* 170:55–74, 1986.

Galloway SM, Ivett JL: Chemically induced aneuploidy in mammalian cells in culture. *Mutat Res* 167:89–105, 1986.

Gatehouse D, Haworth S, Cebula T, et al: Recommendations for the performance of bacterial mutation assays. *Mutat Res* 312:217–233, 1994.

Gee P, Maron DM, Ames BN: Detection and classification of mutagens: A set of base-specific *Salmonella* tester strains. *Proc Natl Acad Sci USA* 91:11606–11610, 1994.

Gee P, Sommers CH, Melick AS, et al: Comparison of responses of base-specific *Salmonella* tester strains with the traditional strains for identifying mutagens: The results of a validation study. *Mutat Res* 412:115–130, 1998.

Gold LS, Slone TH, Stern BR, Bernstein L: Comparison of target organs of carcinogenicity for mutagenic and non-mutagenic chemicals. *Mutat Res* 286:75–100, 1993.

Goodhead DT: Initial events in the cellular effects of ionizing radiations: Clustered damage in DNA. *Int J Radiat Biol* 65:7–17, 1994.

Grant WF: The present status of higher plant bioassays for the detection of environmental mutagens. *Mutat Res* 310:175–185, 1994.

Grombacher T, Mitra S, Kaina B: Induction of the alkyltransferase (MGMT) gene by DNA damaging agents and the glucocorticoid dexamethasone and comparison with the response of base excision repair. *Carcinogenesis* 17:2329–2336, 1996.

Haber JE: Partners and pathways: Repairing a double-strand break. *Trends Genet* 16:259–264, 2000.

Hagmar L, Bonassi S, Strömberg U, et al: Cancer predictive value of cytogenetic markers used in occupational health surveillance programs: A report from an ongoing study by the European Study Group on Cytogenetic Biomarkers and Health. *Mutat Res* 405:171–178, 1998a.

Hagmar L, Bonassi S, Strömberg U, et al: Chromosomal aberrations in lymphocytes predict human cancer: A report from the European Study Group on Cytogenetic Biomarkers and Health (ESCH). *Cancer Res* 58:4117–4121, 1998b.

Hahn WC, Counter CM, Lundberg AS, et al: Creation of human tumor cells with defined genetic elements. *Nature* 400:464–468, 1999.

Halliday JA, Glickman BW: Mechanisms of spontaneous mutation in DNA repair-proficient *Escherichia coli. Mutat Res* 250:55–71, 1991.

Hamasaki T, Sato T, Nagase H, Kito H: The genotoxicity of organotin compounds in SOS chromotest and rec-assay. *Mutat Res* 280:195–203, 1992.

Hanahan D, Weinberg RA: The hallmarks of cancer. *Cell* 100:57–70, 2000.

Harrington CA, Rosenow C, Retief J: Monitoring gene expression using DNA microarrays. *Curr Opin Microbiol* 3:285–291, 2000.

Harris CC: P53: At the crossroads of molecular carcinogenesis and risk assessment. *Science* 262:1980–1981, 1993.

Hayashi M, MacGregor JT, Gatehouse DG, et al: In vivo rodent erythrocyte micronucleus assay: II. Some aspects of protocol design including repeated treatments, integration with toxicity testing, and automated scoring. *Environ Mol Mutagen* 35:234–252, 2000.

Hayashi M, Tice RR, MacGregor JT, et al: In vivo rodent erythrocyte micronucleus assay. *Mutat Res* 312:293–304, 1994.

Heartlein MW, O'Neill JP, Preston RJ: SCE induction is proportional to substitution in DNA for thymidine by CldU. *Mutat Res* 107:103–109, 1983.

Heddle JA, Cimino MC, Hayashi M, et al: Micronuclei as an index of cytogenetic damage: Past, present, and future. *Environ Mol Mutagen* 18:277–291, 1991.

Heddle JA, Dean S, Nohmi T, et al: In vivo transgenic mutation assays. *Environ Mol Mutagen* 35:253–259, 2000.

Heflich RH: Chemical mutagens, in Li AP, Heflich RH (eds): *Genetic Toxicology: A Treatise.* Boca Raton, FL: CRC Press, 1991, pp 143–202.

Hoffmann GR: Induction of genetic recombination: Consequences and model systems. *Environ Mol Mutagen* 23 (suppl 24):59–66, 1994.

Howlett NG, Schiestl RH: Simultaneous measurement of the frequencies of intrachromosomal recombination and chromosome gain using the yeast DEL assay. *Mutat Res* 454:53–62, 2000.

Hsu TC: *Human and Mammalian Cytogenetics: An Historical Perspective.* New York: Springer-Verlag, 1979.

International Program on Chemical Safety: *Evaluation of Short-Term Tests for Carcinogens, Volumes I and II.* Ashby J, de Serres FJ, Shelby MD, et al. (eds): Cambridge, England: Cambridge University Press, 1988.

Ishidate M Jr, Harnois MC, Sofuni T: A comparative analysis of data on the clastogenicity of 951 chemical substances tested in mammalian cell cultures. *Mutat Res* 195:151–213, 1988.

Jiricny J: Eukaryotic mismatch repair: An update. *Mutat Res* 409:107–121, 1998.

Johnson RD, Liu N, Jasin M: Mammalian XRCC2 promotes the repair of DNA double-strand breaks by homologous recombination. *Nature* 401:397–399, 1999.

Josephy PD, DeBruin LS, Lord HL, et al: Bioactivation of aromatic amines by recombinant human cytochrome P4501A2 expressed in Ames tester strain bacteria: A substitute for activation by mammalian tissue preparations. *Cancer Res* 55:799–802, 1995.

Jurado J, Alejandre-Durán E, Pueyo C: Mutagenicity testing in *Salmonella typhimurium* strains possessing both the His reversion and Ara forward mutation systems and different levels of classical nitroreductase or o-acetyltransferase activities. *Environ Mol Mutagen* 23:286–293, 1994.

Kallioniemi A, Kallioniemi O-P, Sudar D, et al: Comparative genomic hybridization for molecular cytogenetic analysis of solid tumors. *Science* 258:818–821, 1992.

Kim BS, Margolin BH: Prediction of rodent carcinogenicity utilizing a battery of in vitro and in vivo genotoxicity tests. *Environ Mol Mutagen* 34:297–304, 1999.

Kinzler KW, Vogelstein B: Lessons from hereditary colorectal cancer. *Cell* 87:159–170, 1996.

Kirkland DJ, Gatehouse DG, Scott D, et al (eds): *Basic Mutagenicity Tests: UKEMS Recommended Procedures.* New York: Cambridge University Press, 1990.

Kirsch-Volders M, Sofuni T, Aardema M, et al: Report from the in vitro micronucleus assay working group. *Environ Mol Mutagen* 35:167–172, 2000.

Klekowski EJ Jr, Corredor JE, Morell JM, Del Castillo CA: Petroleum pollution and mutation in mangroves. *Marine Pollution Bull* 28:166–169, 1994.

Knudson AG: Hereditary predisposition to cancer. *Ann NY Acad Sci* 833: 58–67, 1997.

Koch WH, Henrikson EN, Kupchella E, Cebula TA: *Salmonella typhimurium* strain TA100 differentiates several classes of carcinogens and mutagens by base substitution specificity. *Carcinogenesis* 15:79–88, 1994.

Kolodner RD: Mismatch repair: Mechanisms and relationship to cancer susceptibility. *Trends Biochem Sci* 20:397–401, 1995.

Kriek E, Rojas M, Alexandrov K, Bartsch H: Polycyclic aromatic hydrocarbon-DNA adducts in humans: Relevance as biomarkers for exposure and cancer risk. *Mutat Res* 400:215–231, 1998.

Lähdetie J, Keiski A, Suutari A, Toppari J: Etoposide (VP-16) is a potent inducer of micronuclei in male rat meiosis: Spermatid micronucleus test and DNA flow cytometry after etoposide treatment. *Environ Mol Mutagen* 24:192–202, 1994.

Langenbach R, Oglesby L: The use of intact cellular activation systems in genetic toxicology assays, in de Serres FJ (ed): *Chemical Mutagens: Principles and Methods for Their Detection.* Vol 8. New York: Plenum Press, 1983, pp 55–93.

Laval J, Boiteux S, O'Connor TR: Physiological properties and repair of apurinic/apyrimidinic sites and imidazole ring-opened guanines in DNA. *Mutat Res* 233:73–79, 1990.

Le XC, Xing JZ, Lee J, et al: Inducible repair of thymine glycol detected by an ultrasensitive assay for DNA damage. *Science* 280:1066–1069, 1998.

Lehmann AR: Nucleotide excision repair and the link with transcription. *Trends Biochem Sci* 20:402–405, 1995.

Léonard A: Observations on meiotic chromosomes of the male mouse as a test of the potential mutagenicity of chemicals in mammals, in Hollaender A (ed): *Chemical Mutagens: Principles and Methods for Their Detection.* Vol 3. New York: Plenum Press, 1973, p 21.

Levine JG, Schaaper RM, DeMarini DM: Complex frameshift mutations mediated by plasmid pKM101: Mutational mechanisms deduced from 4-aminobiphenyl-induced mutation spectra in *Salmonella. Genetics* 136:731–746, 1994.

Lewis SE: The biochemical specific-locus test and a new multiple-endpoint mutation detection system: Considerations for genetic risk assessment. *Environ Mol Mutagen* 18:303–306, 1991.

Lewtas J: Environmental monitoring using genetic bioassays, in Li AP, Heflich RH (eds): *Genetic Toxicology: A Treatise.* Boca Raton, FL: CRC Press, 1991, pp 359–374.

Lindahl T: Suppression of spontaneous mutagenesis in human cells by DNA base excision-repair. *Mutat Res* 462:129–135, 2000.

Liyanage M, Coleman A, duManoir S, et al: Multicolour spectral karyotyping of mouse chromosomes. *Nat Genet* 14:312–315, 1996.

Lomnel L, Carswell-Crumpton C, Hanawalt PC: Preferential repair of the transcribed DNA strand in the dihydrofolate reductase gene throughout the cell cycle in UV-irradiated human cells. *Mutat Res* 366:181–192, 1995.

Lucas JN, Awa A, Straume T, et al: Rapid translocation analysis in humans decades after exposure to ionizing radiation. *Int J Radiat Biol* 62:53–63, 1992.

Lynch AM, Parry JM: The cytochalasin-B micronucleus/kinetochore assay in vitro: Studies with 10 suspected aneugens. *Mutat Res* 287:71–86, 1993.

Macville M, Veldman T, Padilla-Nash H, et al: Spectral karyotyping, a 24-colour FISH technique for the identification of chromosomal rearrangements. *Histochem Cell Biol* 108:299–305, 1997.

Madle S, Dean SW, Andrae U, et al: Recommendations for the performance of UDS tests in vitro and in vivo. *Mutat Res* 312:263–285, 1994.

Malling HV, Frantz CN: In vitro versus in vivo metabolic activation of mutagens. *Environ Health Prospect* 6:71–82, 1973.

Maron DM, Ames BN: Revised methods for the *Salmonella* mutagenicity test. *Mutat Res* 113:173–215, 1983.

Marshall CJ: Tumor suppressor genes. *Cell* 64:313–326, 1991.

Martin RH, Ko E, Rademaker A: Distribution of aneuploidy in human gametes: Comparison between human sperm and oocytes. *Am J Med Genet* 39:321–331, 1991.

Martin RH, Spriggs E, Rademaker AW: Multicolor fluorescence *in situ* hybridization analysis of aneuploidy and diploidy frequencies in 225, 846 sperm from 10 normal men. *Biol Reprod* 54:394–398, 1996.

Mason JM, Aaron CS, Lee WR, et al: A guide for performing germ cell mutagenesis assays using *Drosophila melanogaster. Mutat Res* 189: 93–102, 1987.

McCullough AK, Dodson ML, Lloyd RS: Initiation of base excision repair: Glycosylase mechanisms and structures. *Annu Rev Biochem* 68:255–285, 1999.

McGregor DB, Rice JM, Venitt S (eds): *The Use of Short- and Medium-term Tests for Carcinogens and Data on Genetic Effects in Carcinogenic Hazard Evaluation.* IARC Sci Pub No. 146 Lyon, France: IARC, 1999.

Mercer WE: Checking on the cell cycle. *J Cell Biochem Suppl* 30–31:50–54, 1998.

Miller B, Pötter-Locher F, Seelbach A, et al: Evaluation of the in vitro micronucleus test as an alternative to the in vitro chromosomal aberration assay: Position of the GUM working group on the in vitro micronucleus test. *Mutat Res* 410:81–116, 1998.

Miller JA, Miller EC: Ultimate chemical carcinogens as reactive mutagenic electrophiles, in Hiatt HH, Watson JD, Winsten JA (eds): *Origins of Human Cancer.* Cold Spring Harbor, NY: Cold Spring Harbor Laboratory Press, 1977, pp 605–628.

Mirsalis JC, Monforte JA, Winegar RA: Transgenic animal models for measuring mutations *in vivo. Crit Rev Toxicol* 24:255–280, 1994.

Modrich P: Strand-specific mismatch repair in mammalian cells. *J Biol Chem* 272:24727–24730, 1997.

Modrich P, Lahue R: Mismatch repair in replication fidelity, genetic recombination, and cancer biology. *Annu Rev Biochem* 65:101–133, 1996.

Mohrenweiser HW: Germinal mutation and human genetic disease, in Li AP, Heflich RH (eds): *Genetic Toxicology: A Treatise.* Boca Raton, FL: CRC Press, 1991, pp 67–92.

Moolenaar RJ: Carcinogen risk assessment: International comparison. *Reg Tox Pharmacol* 20:302–336, 1994.

Moore MM, Honma M, Clements J, et al: Mouse lymphoma thymidine kinase locus gene mutation assay: International workshop on genotoxicity test procedures workgroup report. *Environ Mol Mutagen* 35:185–190, 2000.

Morrison V, Ashby J: A preliminary evaluation of the performance of the Muta™ Mouse (*lacZ*) and Big Blue™ (*lacI*) transgenic mouse mutation assays. *Mutagenesis* 9:367–375, 1994.

Muller HJ: Artificial transmutation of the gene. *Science* 66:84–87, 1927.

Natarajan AT: An overview of the results of testing of known or suspected aneugens using mammalian cells in vitro. *Mutat Res* 287:113–118, 1993.

NRC (National Research Council): *Risk Assessment in the Federal Government: Managing the Process.* Washington, DC: National Academy Press, 1983.

NRC (National Research Council) Committee on the Biological Effects of Ionizing Radiations: *Health Effects of Exposure to Low Levels of Ionizing Radiation: BEIR V.* Washington, DC: National Academy Press, 1990.

NRC (National Research Council): *Science and Judgment in Risk Assessment,* Washington, DC: National Academy Press, 1994.

Okada N, Masumura K, Nohmi T, Yajima N: Efficient detection of deletions induced by a single treatment of mitomycin C in transgenic mouse *gpt* delta using the Spi(-) selection. *Environ Mol Mutagen* 34: 106–111, 1999.

Osgood CJ, Cyr K: Induction by nitriles of sex chromosome aneuploidy: Tests of mechanism. *Mutat Res* 403:149–157, 1998.

Pack S, Vortmeyer AO, Pak E, et al: Detection of gene deletion in single metastatic tumor cells in lymph node tissue by fluorescent in-situ hybridization. *Lancet* 350:264–265, 1997.

Painter RB: A replication model for sister-chromatid exchange. *Mutat Res* 70:337–341, 1980.

Parry JM: An evaluation of the use of in vitro tubulin polymerisation, fungal and wheat assays to detect the activity of potential chemical aneugens. *Mutat Res* 287:23–28, 1993.

Parry JM: Detecting chemical aneugens: A commentary to 'Aneuploidy: A report of an ECETOC task force.' *Mutat Res* 410:117–120, 1998.

Parry JM: Detecting and predicting the activity of rodent carcinogens. *Mutagenesis* 9:3–5, 1994.

Phillips DH, Farmer PB, Beland FA, et al: Methods of DNA adduct determination and their application to testing compounds for genotoxicity. *Environ Mol Mutagen* 35:222–233, 2000.

Potter CJ, Turenchalk GS, Xu T: *Drosophila* in cancer research. *Trends Genet* 16:33–39, 2000.

Preston RJ: A consideration of the mechanisms of induction of mutations in mammalian cells by low doses and dose rates of ionizing radiation. *Adv Radiat Biol* 16:125–135, 1992.

Preston, RJ: Aneuploidy in germ cells: Disruption of chromosome mover components. *Environ Mol Mutagen* 28:176–181, 1996.

Preston RJ: Chromosomal changes, in McGregor DB, Rice JM, Venitt S (eds): *The Use of Short- and Medium-Term Tests for Carcinogens and Data on Genetic Effects in Carcinogenic Hazard Evaluation.* IARC Sci Pub 146. Lyon, France: IARC, 1999, pp 395–408.

Preston, RJ: Mechanisms of induction of chromosomal alterations and sister chromatid exchanges, in Li AP, Heflich RF (eds): *Genetic Toxicology: A Treatise.* Boca Raton, FL: CRC Press, 1991, pp 41–66.

Preston RJ, Au W, Bender MA, et al: Mammalian in vivo and in vitro cytogenetic assays: A report of the U.S. EPA's Gene-Tox Program. *Mutat Res* 87:143–188, 1981.

Preston RJ, Fennell TR, Leber AP, et al: Reconsideration of the genetic risk assessment for ethylene oxide exposures. *Environ Mol Mutagen* 26:189–202, 1995.

Quillardet P, Hofnung M: The SOS chromotest: A review. *Mutat Res* 297:235–279, 1993.

Rabbitts TH: Chromosomal translocations in human cancer. *Nature* 372: 143–149, 1994.

Ramsey MJ, Moore DH, Briner JF, et al: The effects of age and lifestyle factors on the accumulation of cytogenetic damage as measured by chromosome painting. *Mutat Res* 338:95–106, 1995.

Rhomberg L, Dellarco VL, Siegel-Scott C, et al: Quantitative estimation of the genetic risk associated with the induction of heritable translocations at low-dose exposure: Ethylene oxide as an example. *Environ Mol Mutagen* 16:104–125, 1990.

Richard AM: Structure-based methods for predicting mutagenicity and carcinogenicity: Are we there yet? *Mutat Res* 400:493–507, 1998.

Ripley LS: Mechanisms of gene mutations, in Li AP, Heflich RH (eds): *Genetic Toxicology: A Treatise.* Boca Raton, FL: CRC Press, 1991, pp 13–40.

Rupa DS, Schuler M, Eastmond DA: Detection of hyperdiploidy and breakage affecting the 1cen-1q12 region of cultured interphase human lymphocytes treated with various genotoxic agents. *Environ Mol Mutagen* 29:161–167, 1997.

Russell LB, Russell WL: Frequency and nature of specific-locus mutations induced in female mice by radiations and chemicals: A review. *Mutat Res* 296:107–127, 1992.

Russell LB, Selby PB, Von Halle E, et al: The mouse specific-locus test with agents other than radiations: Interpretation of data and recommendations for future work. *Mutat Res* 86:329–354, 1981.

Russell LB, Shelby MD: Tests for heritable genetic damage and for evidence of gonadal exposure in mammals. *Mutat Res* 154:69–84, 1985.

Russell WL: X-ray-induced mutations in mice. *Cold Spring Harb Symp Quant Biol* 16:327–336, 1951.

Sancar A: Excision repair in mammalian cells. *J. Biol Chem* 27: 15915–15918, 1995.

Sankaranarayanan K: Ionizing radiation and genetic risks: IX. Estimates of the frequencies of mendelian diseases and spontaneous mutation rates in human populations: A 1998 perspective. *Mutat Res* 411: 129–178, 1998.

Sawada M, Kamataki T: Genetically engineered cells stably expressing cytochrome P450 and their application to mutagen assays. *Mutat Res* 411:19–43, 1998.

Sax K: Induction by X-rays of chromosome aberrations in *Tradescantia* microspores. *Genetics* 23:494–516, 1938.

Sax K: The time factor in X-ray production of chromosome aberrations. *Proc Natl Acad Sci USA* 25:225–233, 1939.

Sax K, Luippold H: The effects of fractional x-ray dosage on the frequency of chromosome aberrations. *Heredity* 6:127–131, 1952.

Scott D, Galloway SM, Marshall RR, et al: Genotoxicity under extreme culture conditions. *Mutat Res* 257:147–204, 1991.

Seeberg E, Eide L, Bjoras M: The base excision repair pathway. *Trends Biochem Sci* 20:391–397, 1995.

Sengstag C: The role of mitotic recombination in carcinogenesis. *Crit Rev Toxicol* 24:323–353, 1994.

Shelby MD: Human germ cell mutagens. *Environ Mol Mutagen* 23 (suppl 24):30–34, 1994.

Shinohara A, Ogawa T: Homologous recombination and the roles of double-strand breaks. *Trends Biochem Sci* 20:387–391, 1995.

Smith MT, Zhang L, Wang Y, et al: Increased translocations and aneusomy in chromosomes 8 and 21 among workers exposed to benzene. *Cancer Res* 58:2176–2181, 1998.

Sobels FH: The parallelogram: An indirect approach for the assessment of genetic risks from chemical mutagens, in Bora KC, Douglas GR, Nestman ER (eds): *Progress in Mutation Research* 3:323–327, 1982.

Solinas-Toldo S, Lampel S, Stilgenbauer S, et al: Matrix-based comparative genomic hybridization: Biochips to screen for genomic imbalances. *Genes Chromosomes Cancer* 20:399–407, 1997.

Southern EM: DNA chips: Analyzing sequence by hybridization to oligonucleotides on a large scale. *Trends Genet* 12:110–115, 1996.

Stoler DL, Chen N, Basik M, et al: The onset and extent of genomic instability in sporadic colorectal tumor progression. *Proc Natl Acad Sci USA* 96:15121–15126, 1999.

Styles JA, Penman MG: The mouse spot test: Evaluation of its performance in identifying chemical mutagens and carcinogens. *Mutat Res* 154:183–204, 1985.

Swiger RR, Cosentino L, Shima N, et al: The *cII* locus in the Muta Mouse system. *Environ Mol Mutagen* 34:201–207, 1999.

Tano K, Shiota S, Collier J, et al: Isolation and structural characterization of a cDNA clone encoding the human DNA repair protein for 0^6-alkylguanine. *Proc Natl Acad Sci USA* 87:686–690, 1990.

Tease C: Radiation- and chemically-induced chromosome aberrations in mouse oocytes: A comparison with effects in males. *Mutat Res* 296:135–142, 1992.

Tennant RW, Ashby J: Classification according to chemical structure, mutagenicity to Salmonella and level of carcinogenicity of a further 39 chemicals tested for carcinogenicity by the U.S. National Toxicology Program. *Mutat Res* 257:209–227, 1991.

Tennant RW, Margolin BH, Shelby MD, et al: Prediction of chemical carcinogenicity in rodents from in vitro genetic toxicity assays. *Science* 236:933–941, 1987.

Thacker J: Radiation-induced mutation in mammalian cells at low doses and dose rates. *Adv Radiat Biol* 16:77–124, 1992.

Tice RR, Agurell E, Anderson D, et al: Single cell gel/comet assay: Guidelines for in vitro and in vivo genetic toxicology testing. *Environ Mol Mutagen* 35:206–221, 2000.

Tice RR, Hayashi M, MacGregor JT, et al: Report from the working group on the in vivo mammalian bone marrow chromosomal aberration test. *Mutat Res* 312:305–312, 1994.

Trask BJ, Allen S, Massa H, et al: Studies of metaphase and interphase chromosomes using fluorescence in situ hybridizaiton. *Cold Spring Harb Symp Quant Biol* 58:767–775, 1993.

Tucker JD, Auletta A, Cimino M, et al: Sister-chromatid exchange: Second report of the Gene-Tox program. *Mutat Res* 297:101–180, 1993.

Tucker JD, Breneman JW, Briner JF, et al: Persistence of radiation-induced translocations in rat peripheral blood determined by chromosome painting. *Environ Mol Mutagen* 30:264–272, 1997.

Tucker JD, Ramsey MJ, Lee DA, Minkler JL: Validation of chromosome painting as a biodosimeter in human peripheral lymphocytes following acute exposure to ionizing radiation in vitro. *Int J Radiat Biol* 64:27–37, 1993.

Van Houten B, Albertini R: DNA damage and repair, in Craighead JE (ed): *Pathology of Environmental and Occupational Disease.* St. Louis: Mosby-Year Book, 1995, pp 311–327.

Veldman T, Vignon C, Schrock E, et al: Hidden chromosome abnormalities in haematological malignancies detected by multicolour spectral karyotyping. *Nat Genet* 15:406–410, 1997.

Venkatachalam S, Shi YP, Jones SN, et al: Retention of wild-type p53 in tumors from p53 heterozygous mice: Reduction of p53 dosage can promote cancer formation. *EMBO J* 17:4657–4667, 1998.

Vijg J, van Steeg H: Transgenic assays for mutations and cancer: Current status and future perspectives. *Mutat Res* 400:337–354, 1998.

Vogel EW, Graf U, Frei HJ, Nivara MM: The results of assays in *Drosophila* as indicators of exposure to carcinogens. *IARC Sci Publ* 146:427–470, 1999.

Walker VE, Jones IM, Crippen TL, et al: Relationships between exposure, cell loss and proliferation, and manifestation of *Hprt* mutant T cells following treatment of preweanling, weanling, and adult male mice with N-ethyl-N-nitrosourea. *Mutat Res* 431:371–388, 1999.

Wallace SS: DNA damages processed by base excision repair: Biological consequences. *Int J Radiat Biol* 66:579–589, 1994.

Ward JF: DNA damage produced by ionizing radiation in mammalian cells: Identities, mechanisms of formation, and reparability. *Prog Nucl Acid Res Mol Biol* 35:95–125, 1988.

Ward JF: The complexity of DNA damage: Relevance to biological consequences. *Int J Radiat Biol* 66:427–432, 1994.

Wodicka L, Dong H, Mittmann M, et al: Genome-wide expression monitoring in *Saccharomyces cerevisiae. Nature Biotech* 15:1359–1367, 1997.

Wood RD: DNA repair in eukaryotes. *Annu Rev Biochem* 65:135–167, 1996.

Wyrobek AJ: Methods and concepts in detecting abnormal reproductive outcomes of paternal origin. *Reprod Toxicol* 7:3–16, 1993.

Zimmermann FK: Tests for recombinagens in fungi. *Mutat Res* 284: 147–158, 1992.

Zimmermann FK, von Borstel RC, von Halle ES, et al: Testing of chemicals for genetic activity with *Saccharomyces cerevisiae:* A report of the U.S. Environmental Protection Agency Gene-Tox Program. *Mutat Res* 133:199–244, 1984.

CHAPTER 10

DEVELOPMENTAL TOXICOLOGY

John M. Rogers and Robert J. Kavlock

HISTORY

Developmental toxicology encompasses the study of pharmacokinetics, mechanisms, pathogenesis, and outcome following exposure to agents or conditions leading to abnormal development. Manifestations of developmental toxicity include structural malformations, growth retardation, functional impairment, and/or death of the organism. Developmental toxicology so defined is a relatively new science, but teratology, or the study of structural birth defects, as a descriptive science precedes written language. For example, a marble sculpture from southern Turkey, dating back to 6500 B.C., depicts conjoined twins (Warkany, 1983), and Egyptian wall paintings of human conditions such as cleft palate and achondroplasia have been dated as early as 5000 years ago. It is believed that mythologic figures such as the cyclops and sirens took their origin in the birth of severely malformed infants (Thompson, 1930; Warkany, 1977). The Babylonians, Greeks, and Romans believed that abnormal infants were reflections of stellar events and as such were considered to be portents of the future. Indeed, the Latin word *monstrum,* from *monstrare* (to show) or *monere* (to warn), is derived from this perceived ability of malformed infants to foretell the future. In turn, derivation of the word *teratology* is from the Greek word for monster, *teras.*

Hippocrates and Aristotle considered that abnormal development could originate in physical causes such as uterine trauma or pressure, but Aristotle also shared a widespread belief that maternal impressions and emotions could influence the development of the child. He advised pregnant women to gaze at beautiful statuary to increase their child's beauty. Though this theory may sound fanciful, it is present in diverse cultures throughout recorded history; indeed, we now know that maternal stress can be deleterious to the developing conceptus (Chernoff et al., 1989).

Another belief, the hybrid theory, held that interbreeding between humans and animals was a cause of congenital malformations (Ballantyne, 1904). Again, such hybrid creatures abound in mythology, including centaurs, minotaurs, and satyrs. Into the seventeenth century, cohabitation of humans with demons and witches was blamed for the production of birth defects. Birth defects were also viewed to represent God's retribution on the parents of the malformed infant and on society.

In 1649, the French surgeon Ambrois Paré expounded the theory of Aristotle and Hippocrates by writing that birth defects could result from narrowness of the uterus, faulty posture of the pregnant woman, or physical trauma, such as a fall. Amputations were thought to result from amniotic bands, adhesions, or twisting of the umbilical cord. This conjecture has proven to be true. With the blossoming of the biological sciences in the sixteenth and seventeenth centuries, theories of the causation of birth defects with basis in scientific fact began to emerge. In 1651, William Harvey put forth the theory of developmental arrest, which stated that malformations resulted from incomplete development of an organ or structure. One example given by Harvey was harelip in humans, a condition that represents a normal early developmental stage. Much later, the theory of developmental arrest was solidified by the experiments of Stockard (1921) using eggs of the minnow, *Fundulus heteroclitus*. By manipulating the chemical constituents and temperature of the growth medium, he produced malformations in the embryos, the nature of which depended on the stage of the insult. He concluded that developmental arrest explained all malformations except those of hereditary origin (Barrow, 1971).

With the advent of the germplasm theory elucidated by Weissmann in the 1880s and the rediscovery of Mendel's laws in 1900, genetics as the basis for some birth defects was accepted. In 1894, Bateson published his treatise on the study of variations in animals as a tool for understanding evolution, inferring that inheritance of such variations could be a basis for speciation (Bateson, 1894). His study contains detailed descriptions and illustrations of such human birth defects as polydactyly and syndactyly, supernumerary cervical and thoracic ribs, duplicated appendages, and horseshoe (fused) kidneys. In this volume, Bateson coined the term *homeosis* to denote morphologic alterations in which one structure has taken on the likeness of another. Study of such alterations in mutants of the fruit fly *Drosophila* and, more recently, the mouse have served as the basis for much of the recent knowledge of the genetic control of development. *Homeobox genes* are found throughout the animal and plant kingdoms and direct embryonic pattern formation (Graham et al., 1989). Acceptance of a genetic basis of birth defects was furthered with studies of human inborn errors of metabolism in the first decade of the twentieth century.

Modern experimental teratology began in the early nineteenth century with the work of Etienne Geoffrey Saint-Hilaire. Saint-Hilaire produced malformed chick embryos by subjecting eggs to various environmental conditions including physical trauma (jarring, inversion, pricking) and toxic exposures. In the latter part of the nineteenth century, Camille Dareste experimented extensively with chick embryos, producing a wide variety of malformations by administering noxious stimuli, physical trauma, or heat shock at various times after fertilization. He found that timing was more important than the nature of the insult in determining the type of malformation produced. Among the malformations described and beautifully illustrated by Dareste (1877, 1891) were the neural tube defects anencephaly and spina bifida, cyclopia, heart defects, situs inversus, and conjoined twins. Many of the great embryologists of the nineteenth and twentieth centuries, including Loeb, Morgan, Driesch, Wilson, Spemann and Hertwig, performed teratological manipulations using various physical and chemical probes to deduce principles of normal development.

In the early twentieth century, a variety of environmental conditions (temperature, microbial toxins, drugs) were found to perturb development in avian, reptilian, fish, and amphibian species. However, despite the already rich literature of nonmammalian teratologic experiments, mammalian embryos were thought to be resistant to induction of malformations and to be either killed outright or protected by the maternal system from adverse environmental conditions. The first reports of induced birth defects in mammalian species were published in the 1930s and were the result of experimental maternal nutritional deficiencies. Hale (1935) produced malformations including anophthalmia and cleft palate in offspring of sows fed a diet deficient in vitamin A. Beginning in 1940, Josef Warkany and coworkers began a series of experiments in which they demonstrated that maternal dietary deficiencies and other environmental factors could affect intrauterine development in rats (Warkany and Nelson, 1940; Warkany, 1945; Warkany and Schraffenberger, 1944; Wilson et al., 1953). These experiments were followed by many other studies in which chemical and physical agents—e.g., nitrogen mustard, trypan blue, hormones, antimetabolites, alkylating agents, hypoxia, and x-rays, to name a few—were clearly shown to cause malformations in mammalian species (Warkany, 1965).

The first human epidemic of malformations induced by an environmental agent was reported by Gregg (1941), who linked an epidemic of rubella virus infection in Austria to an elevation in the incidence of eye, heart, and ear defects as well as to mental retardation. Heart and eye defects predominated with infection in the first or second months of pregnancy, whereas hearing and speech defects and mental retardation were most commonly associated with infection in the third month. Later, the risk of congenital anomalies associated with rubella infection in the first four weeks of pregnancy was estimated to be 61 percent; in weeks five to eight, 26 percent; and in weeks nine to twelve, 8 percent (Sever, 1967). It has been estimated that in the United States alone approximately 20,000 children have been impaired as a consequence of prenatal rubella infections (Cooper and Krugman, 1966).

Although embryos of mammals, including humans, were found to be susceptible to common external influences such as nutritional deficiencies and intrauterine infections, the impact of these findings was not great at the time (Wilson, 1973). That changed, however, in 1961, when the association between thalidomide ingestion by pregnant women and the birth of severely malformed infants was established (see "Scope of the Problem," below).

SCOPE OF PROBLEM—THE HUMAN EXPERIENCE

Successful pregnancy outcome in the general population occurs at a surprisingly low frequency. Estimates of adverse outcomes include postimplantation pregnancy loss, 31 percent; major birth defects, 2 to 3 percent at birth and increasing to 6 to 7 percent at 1 year as more manifestations are diagnosed; minor birth defects, 14 percent; low birth weight, 7 percent; infant mortality (prior to 1 year of age), 1.4 percent; and abnormal neurologic function, 16 to 17 percent (Schardein, 1993). Thus, less than half of all human conceptions result in the birth of a completely normal, healthy infant. Reasons for the adverse outcomes are largely unknown. Brent and Beckman (1990) attributed 15 to 25 percent of human birth defects to genetic causes, 4 percent to maternal conditions, 3 percent to maternal infections, 1 to 2 percent to deformations (e.g., mechanical problems such as umbilical cord limb amputations), <1 percent to chemicals and other environmental influences, and 65 percent to unknown etiologies. These estimates are not dramatically different from those suggested by Wilson (1977). Regardless of the etiology, the sum total represents a significant health burden in light of the 2 million annual births in the United States.

It has been estimated that more that 4100 chemicals have been tested for teratogenicity, with approximately 66 percent shown to be nonteratogenic, 7 percent teratogenic in more than one species, 18 percent teratogenic in most species tested and 9 percent producing equivocal experimental results (Schardein, 2000). In contrast, only about 35 to 40 chemicals, chemical classes, or conditions (Table 10-1) have been documented to alter prenatal development in humans (Schardein and Keller, 1989; Shepard, 1998). Review of several human developmental toxicants provides both a historical view of the field of developmental toxicology and an illustration of some of key principles presented below.

Thalidomide

In 1960, a large increase in newborns with rare limb malformations was recorded in West Germany. The affected individuals had amelia (absence of the limbs) or various degrees of phocomelia (reduction of the long bones of the limbs), usually affecting the arms more than the legs and usually involving both left and right sides, although to differing degrees. Congenital heart disease; ocular, intestinal, and renal anomalies; and malformations of the external and inner ears were also involved. However, the limb defects were characteristic. Limb reduction anomalies of this nature are exceedingly rare. At the university clinic in Hamburg, for example, no cases of phocomelia were reported between 1940 and 1959. In 1959 there was a single case; in 1960, there were 30 cases; and in 1961, a total of 154 cases (Taussig, 1962). The unusual nature of the malformations was key in unraveling the epidemic. In 1961, Lenz and McBride, working independently in Germany and Australia, identified the sedative thalidomide as the causative agent (McBride, 1961; Lenz, 1961, 1963). Thalidomide had been introduced in 1956 by Chemie Grunenthal as a sedative/hypnotic and was used throughout much of the world as a sleep aid and to ameliorate nausea and vomiting in pregnancy. It had no apparent toxicity or addictive properties in humans or adult animals at therapeutic exposure levels. The drug was widely prescribed at an oral dose of 50 to 200 mg/day. There were a few reports of peripheral neuritis attributable to thalidomide, but only in patients with long-term use for up to 18 months (Fullerton and Kermer, 1961). Following the association with birth defects, thalidomide was withdrawn from the market by Grunenthal in November 1961 and case

Table 10-1
Human Developmental Toxicants

Radiation	**Drugs/Chemicals**
Therapeutic	Androgenic chemicals
Radioiodine	Angiotensin converting enzyme inhibitors
Atomic fallout	Captopril, enalapril
	Antibiotics
	Tetracylines
	Anticancer drugs
	Aminopterin, methylaminopterin, cyclophosphamide, busulfan
	Anticonvulsants
	Diphenylhydantoin, trimethadione, valproic Acid
Infections	
Rubella virus	Antithyroid drugs
Cytomegalovirus (CMV)	Methimazole
Herpes simplex virus I and II	Chelators
Toxoplasmosis	Penicillamine
Venezuelan equine encephalitis virus	Chlorobiphenyls
Syphilis	Cigarette smoke
Parvovirus B-19 (erythema infectiosum)	Cocaine
Varicella virus	Coumarin anticoagulants (warfarin)
	Ethanol
	Ethylene oxide
	Fluconazole, high dosage
Maternal Trauma and Metabolic Imbalances	Diethylstilbestrol
Alcoholism	Iodides
Amniocentesis, early	Lithium
Chorionic villus sampling (before day 60)	Metals
	Mercury (organic), lead
Cretinism, endemic	Methylene blue via intraamniotic injection
Diabetes	Misoprostol
Folic acid deficiency	Retinoids
Hyperthermia	13-*cis*-retinoic acid, Etretinate
Phenylketonuria	Thalidomide
Rheumatic disease and congenital heart block	Toluene abuse
Sjögren's syndrome	
Virilizing tumors	

SOURCE: Adapted from Shepard (1998), with permission.

reports ended in mid-1962 as exposed pregnancies were completed. All told, an estimated 5850 malformed infants were born worldwide (Lenz, 1988). Quantitative estimates of malformation risks from exposure have been difficult to compile but are believed to be in the range of one in two to one in ten (Newman, 1985). Due to concerns regarding the severity of the peripheral neuritis and subsequent questions with regard to safety in pregnancy, thalidomide did not receive marketing approval by the U.S. Food and Drug Administration (FDA) prior to its removal from the world market following the epidemic.

As a result of this catastrophe, regulatory agencies in many countries began developing animal testing requirements, separate from chronic toxicity studies, for evaluating the effects of drugs on pregnancy outcomes (Stirling et al., 1997). In the United States, the discussions ultimately led to the development of the Segment I, II, and III testing protocols (Kelsey, 1988). Details and evolution of safety testing requirements for assessment of pregnancy outcomes are found later in this chapter.

It is both ironic and telling that the chemical largely responsible for the advent of modern regulation of potential developmental toxicants presents a very complex pattern of effects in various animal species. It has been tested for prenatal toxicity in at least 19 laboratory species. Malformations and increased resorptions have been observed in some studies in rats, while generally no effects were reported in studies with hamsters or most mouse strains. Effects similar to those observed in humans have been reported for several rabbit strains and in eight of nine primate species. The potency of thalidomide ranges from approximately 1 to 100 mg/kg among sensitive species. In this ranking the human sensitivity was estimated to be 1 mg/kg (Schardein, 1993).

Studies of the relationship between periods of drug use and type of malformation induced established that thalidomide was teratogenic between 20 and 36 days after fertilization (Lenz and Knapp, 1962). Because of its short half-life, teratogenic potency, and good records/recall of drug use, fairly concise timetables of susceptibility can be constructed (Lenz and Knapp, 1962; Nowack, 1965; Neubert and Neubert, 1997; Miller and Stromland, 1999). During the susceptible period of 20 to 36 days postfertilization, anotia (missing ear) was the defect induced earliest, followed by thumb, upper extremity, lower extremity, and triphalangeal thumb (Miller and Stromland, 1999).

Research to understand the species and strain differences in response to thalidomide has met with limited success. Extensive structure-activity studies involving analogs of thalidomide found strict structural requirements (e.g., an intact phthalimide or phthalimidine group) but shed little light on potential mechanisms (Jonsson, 1972; Schumacher, 1975; Helm, 1981). Stephens (1988) reviewed 24 proposed mechanisms, including biochemical alterations involving vitamin B, glutamic acid, acylation, nucleic acids, and oxidative phosphorylation; cellular mechanisms including cell death and cell-cell interactions; and tissue level mechanisms including inhibition of nerve and blood vessel outgrowth. None was considered sufficient by that reviewer. More recent hypotheses concerning the mechanism of thalidomide teratogenesis include effects on angiogenesis (D'Amato et al., 1994; Joussen et al., 1999; Sauer et al., 2000), integrin regulation (Neubert et al., 1996), oxidative DNA damage (Parman et al., 1999), TNF-α inhibition (Argiles et al., 1998), growth factor antagonism (Stephens et al., 1998; Stephens and Fillmore, 2000), and effects on glutathione and redox status (Hansen et al., 1999).

Research on alterations in immune function and angiogenesis has opened the possibility of expanded use of thalidomide in diseases including HIV infection, arthritis, myeloma, diabetic retinopathy, and macular degeneration (Adler, 1994; Calabrese and Fleischer, 2000). Thalidomide has recently been approved by the FDA for oral ulcers associated with AIDS and for erythema nodosum leprosum, an inflammatory complication of Hansen's disease (leprosy). An unprecedented level of safeguards, embodied in the STEPS program (System of Thalidomide Education and Prescribing Safety), surrounds thalidomide use to prevent accidental exposure during pregnancy, including required registration of all prescribers, pharmacies, and patients, required use of contraception, and periodic pregnancy testing for patients of childbearing ability (Lary et al., 1999).

Diethylstilbestrol

Diethylstilbestrol (DES) is a synthetic nonsteroidal estrogen widely used from the 1940s to the 1970s in the United States to prevent threatened miscarriage by stimulating synthesis of estrogen and progesterone in the placenta. Between 1966 and 1969, seven young women between the ages of 15 and 22 were seen at Massachusetts General Hospital with clear cell adenocarcinoma of the vagina. This tumor had never before been seen in patients younger than 30. An epidemiologic case-control study subsequently found an association with first-trimester DES exposure (reviewed in Poskranzer and Herbst, 1977). The Registry of Clear Cell Adenocarcinoma of the Genital Tract of Young Females was established in 1971 to track affected offspring. Maternal use of DES prior to the 18th week of gestation appeared to be necessary for induction of the genital tract anomalies in offspring. The incidence of genital tract tumors peaked at age 19 and declined through age 22, with absolute risk of clear cell adenocarcinoma of the vagina and cervix estimated to be 0.14 to 1.4 per 1000 exposed pregnancies (Herbst et al. 1977). However, the overall incidence of noncancerous alterations in the vagina and cervix was estimated to be as high as 75 percent (Poskranzer and Herbst, 1977). In male offspring of exposed pregnancies, a high incidence of epididymal cysts, hypotrophic testes, and capsular induration along with low ejaculated semen volume and poor semen quality were observed (Bibbo et al., 1977). The realization of the latent and devastating manifestations of prenatal DES exposure has broadened our concept of the magnitude and scope of potential adverse outcomes of intrauterine exposures and foreshadowed today's interest in "endocrine disruptors" (Colburn et al., 1993).

Ethanol

The developmental toxicity of ethanol has been a recurrent concern throughout history and can be traced to biblical times (e.g., Judges 13:3-4), yet only since the description of the Fetal Alcohol Syndrome (FAS) by Jones and Smith in the early 1970s (Jones and Smith, 1973; Jones et al., 1973) has a clear recognition and acceptance of alcohol's developmental toxicity occurred. Since that time, there have been hundreds of clinical, epidemiologic, and experimental studies of the effects of ethanol exposure during gestation.

The FAS comprises craniofacial dysmorphism, intrauterine and postnatal growth retardation, retarded psychomotor and intellectual development, and other nonspecific major and minor abnormalities (Abel, 1982). The average IQ of FAS children has been reported to be 68 (Streissguth et al., 1991a) and changes little over time (Streissguth et al., 1991b). Full-blown FAS has been observed only in children born to alcoholic mothers, and among alcoholics the incidence of FAS has been estimated at 25 per 1000 (Abel, 1984). Numerous methodologic difficulties are involved in attempting to estimate the level of maternal ethanol consumption associated with FAS, but estimates of a minimum of 3 to 4 oz of alcohol per day have been made (Clarren et al., 1987; Ernhart et al., 1987).

In utero exposure to lower levels of ethanol has been associated with a wide range of effects, including isolated components of FAS and milder forms of neurologic and behavioral disorders. These more subtle expressions of the toxicity of prenatal ethanol exposure have been termed Fetal Alcohol Effects (FAE) (Clarren, 1982). Alcohol consumption can affect birth weight in a dose-related fashion even if the mother is not alcoholic. Little (1977) studied prospectively 800 women to evaluate the effects of drinking on birth weight. After adjusting for smoking, gestational age, maternal height, age, parity, and sex of the child, it was found that for each ounce of absolute ethanol consumed per day during late pregnancy there was a 160-g decrease in birth weight. Effects of maternal alcohol consumption during pregnancy on attention, short-term memory, and performance on standardized tests have been noted in a longitudinal prospective study of 462 children (Streissguth et al., 1994a,b). Alcohol intake was related to these effects, the number of drinks per drinking occasion being the strongest predictor.

One animal model of FAS in which pathogenesis of the craniofacial effects has been extensively studied involves intraperitoneal injection of ethanol to pregnant C57Bl/6J mice in early pregnancy when embryos are undergoing gastrulation (Sulik et al., 1981; Sulik and Johnston, 1983). Following such exposures, term fetuses exhibit many of the features of FAS, including microcephaly, microphthalmia, short palpebral fissures, deficiencies of the philtral region, and a long upper lip. The specific set of craniofacial malformations produced in offspring depends on the time of exposure. The mechanisms by which ethanol exerts its teratogenic effects are not understood but probably involve a complex combination of maternal factors and biochemical/cellular effects in the embryo (Rogers and Daston, 1997). Excess cell death in sensitive cell populations appears to be a common finding (Kotch and Sulik, 1992).

Tobacco Smoke

Prenatal and early postnatal exposure to tobacco smoke or its constituents may well represent the leading cause of environmentally induced developmental disease and morbidity today. Approximately 25 percent of women in the United States continue to smoke during pregnancy, despite public health programs aimed at curbing this behavior. Because of the high number of pregnant smokers and the relative accuracy of assessing smoking during pregnancy, results of epidemiologic studies provide a well-characterized picture of the consequences of developmental tobacco smoke exposure. These include spontaneous abortions; perinatal deaths; increased risk of sudden infant death syndrome (SIDS); increased risk of learning, behavioral, and attention disorders; and lower birth weight (Slotkin, 1998; Fried et al., 1998; Tuthill et al., 1999; Haug et al., 2000). One component of tobacco smoke, nicotine, is a known neuroteratogen in experimental animals and can by itself produce many of the adverse developmental outcomes associated with tobacco smoke (Slotkin, 1998). Perinatal exposure to tobacco smoke can also affect branching morphogenesis and maturation of the lung, leading to altered physiologic function (Pinkerton and Joad, 2000; Gilliland et al., 2000). Dempsey and coworkers (2000) found that hypertonia among cocaine-exposed infants was associated not with maternal cocaine usage (as determined by fetal meconium analyses for the cocaine metabolite benzoylecgonine) but rather with maternal urine cotinine levels (a nicotine metabolite). It is important to keep in mind that environmental (passive) tobacco smoke also represents a significant risk to the pregnant nonsmoker (e.g., Windham et al., 2000), as inhaled doses in some situations are similar to those for light smokers.

Cocaine

Cocaine, a plant alkaloid derived from coca, is a local anesthetic with vasoconstrictor properties. During the 1980s, as more potent forms became widely available, cocaine abuse became an epidemic health problem. It has been estimated that up to 45 percent of pregnancies at an urban teaching hospital and 6 percent in a suburban hospital had recent cocaine exposure. Effects on the fetus are complicated and controversial and demonstrate the difficulty of monitoring the human population for adverse reproductive outcomes (reviewed in Scanlon, 1991; Volfe, 1993). Accurate exposure ascertainment is difficult, as many confounding factors—including socioeconomic status and concurrent use of cigarettes, alcohol, and other drugs of abuse—may be involved. In addition, reported effects on the fetus and infant (neurologic and behavioral changes) are difficult to identify and quantify. Nevertheless, a plethora of adverse effects appear to be reliably associated with cocaine exposure in humans, including abruptio placentae; premature labor and delivery; microcephaly; altered prosencephalic development; decreased birth weight; a neonatal neurologic syndrome of abnormal sleep, tremor, poor feeding, irritability, and occasional seizures; and SIDS. Congenital malformations of the genitourinary tract have also been reported (Lutiger et al., 1991), and kidney and bladder function is diminished in fetuses of pregnant women using cocaine (Mitra, 1999). Moreover, fetal cocaine exposure has been associated with impaired neonatal auditory processing (Potter et al., 2000). Fetal cocaine exposure was estimated by chemical analysis of fetal meconium, which can provide a measure of developmental exposure to xenobiotic agents ranging from food additives to over-the-counter medications to drugs of abuse (Ostrea et al., 1998).

Retinoids

The ability of excess vitamin A (retinol) to induce malformations has been known for at least forty years (Cohlan, 1954). Effects on the developing embryo include malformations of the face, limbs, heart, central nervous system, and skeleton. Similar malformations were later shown to be induced by retinoic acid administration in the mouse (Kochhar, 1967) and hamster (Shenefelt, 1972). Since those observations, knowledge relating to the effects of retinol, retinoic acid, and structurally related chemicals that bind to and activate specific nuclear receptors that then regulate a variety of transcriptional events has been expanding rapidly (Chambon, 1994;

Lohnes et al., 1994; Mendelsohn et al., 1994; Collins and Mao, 1999; Arafa et al., 2000). The RXR-alpha receptor appears to play an important role in cleft palate induced by retinoic acid (Nugent et al., 1999). The teratogenic effects of vitamin A and retinoids have been reviewed (Nau et al., 1994; Collins and Mao, 1999). Recently, a link between retinoids and schizophrenia has been proposed, supported by three lines of evidence (Goodman, 1998). First, congenital anomalies similar to those caused by retinoid dysfunction are found in schizophrenics and their relatives; second, genetic loci that are putatively involved in schizophrenia are also the loci of genes in the retinoid cascade; and third, transcriptional activation of candidate schizophrenia genes as well as that of the dopamine D2 receptor is regulated by retinoic acid.

Beginning in 1982, one retinoid, 13-*cis*-retinoic acid (isotretinoin or Accutane), was marketed as an effective treatment of recalcitrant cystic acne. Despite clear warnings against use in pregnancy on the label of this prescription drug (FDA pregnancy category X), an extensive physician and patient education program, and restrictive requirements for prescription to women of child-bearing potential, infants with pathognomonic malformations involving the ears, heart, brain, and thymus began to be reported as early as 1983 (Rosa, 1983; Lammer et al., 1985). Among 115 exposed pregnancies not electively terminated, 18 percent ended in spontaneous abortion and 28 percent of the live-born infants had at least one major malformation (Dai et al., 1992). In another prospective study, there was nearly a doubling of the risk for premature delivery after first-trimester exposure, and about 50 percent of the exposed children had full-scale IQ scores below 85 at age 5 (Lammer, 1992).

Valproic Acid

Valproic acid, or 2-propylpentanoic acid, is an anticonvulsant first marketed in Europe in 1967 and in the United States in 1978. In 1982, Elizabeth Robert reported that of 146 cases of spina bifida aperta contained in a birth defects surveillance system in Lyon, France, nine of the mothers had taken valproate during the first trimester. The odds ratio for this finding in a case-control study was 20.6, and the estimated risk of a valproate-exposed woman having a child with spina bifida was 1.2 percent, a risk similar to that for women with a previous child with a neural tube defect (Centers for Disease Control, 1982). The report was quickly confirmed in other areas of the world through the efforts of the International Clearinghouse of Birth Defect Registries (Centers for Disease Control, 1983). Because of the relatively low risk, the fact that epileptic women are already at elevated risk for birth defects, and that the majority of pregnant epileptics are on drug therapy (including several known teratogens), it was fortunate that several events came together that allowed the determination of valproate as a human teratogen. These included the active birth defects registry, an interest by Robert in the genetics of spina bifida, a question on epilepsy and anticonvulsant use in Robert's survey, and the prevalence of valproate monotherapy for epilepsy in that region (Lammer et al., 1987). While these findings spurred a great deal of research on the effects of valproate in multiple species, including interesting results on the effects of enantiomers of valproate analogs, the mechanism of action, as for most developmental toxicants, remains elusive (Nau et al., 1991; Ehlers et al., 1992; Hauck and Nau, 1992). Use of inbred mouse strains differing in their sensitivity to valproate-induced teratogenesis has revealed several candidate genes conferring sensitivity in that species (Finnell et al., 1997; Craig et al., 2000; Bennett et al., 2000; Faiella et al., 2000).

PRINCIPLES OF DEVELOPMENTAL TOXICOLOGY

Principles of teratology were put forth by Jim Wilson in 1959 and in his watershed monograph *Environment and Birth Defects* (Wilson, 1973) (Table 10-2). Although much progress has been made in the ensuing decades, these basic principles have withstood the test of time and remain basic to developmental toxicology.

Critical Periods of Susceptibility and Endpoints of Toxicity

Basic familiarity with principles of normal development is prerequisite to understanding abnormal development. Development is characterized by change: change in size, changes in biochemistry and physiology, changes in form and functionality. These changes are orchestrated by a cascade of factors regulating gene transcription, the first of which are maternally inherited and present in the egg prior to fertilization. In turn, these factors activate regulatory genes in the embryonic genome, and sequential gene activation continues throughout development. Intercellular and intracellular signaling pathways essential for normal development have been elucidated and rely on transcriptional, translational, and posttranslational controls (e.g., phosphorylation).

Because of the rapid changes occurring during development, the nature of the embryo/fetus as a target for toxicity is also changing. While the basic tenets of toxicology discussed elsewhere in this text also apply during development, the principle of critical

Table 10-2
Wilson's General Principles of Teratology

I. Susceptibility to teratogenesis depends on the genotype of the conceptus and the manner in which this interacts with adverse environmental factors.
II. Susceptibility to teratogenesis varies with the developmental stage at the time of exposure to an adverse influence.
III. Teratogenic agents act in specific ways (mechanisms) on developing cells and tissues to initiate sequences of abnormal developmental events (pathogenesis).
IV. The access of adverse influences to developing tissues depends on the nature of the influence (agent).
V. The four manifestations of deviant development are death, malformation, growth retardation, and functional deficit.
VI. Manifestations of deviant development increase in frequency and degree as dosage increases, from the no effect to the totally lethal level.

SOURCE: From Wilson (1959, 1973), with permission.

periods of sensitivity based on developmental stage of the conceptus is a primary and somewhat unique consideration. In this section we discuss normal developmental stages in the context of their known and potential susceptibility to toxicants. It should be made clear, however, that development is a continuum. Therefore, these stages are used for descriptive purposes and do not necessarily represent discrete developmental events. Timing of some key developmental events in humans and experimental animal species is presented in Table 10-3.

As a logical starting point, *gametogenesis* is the process of forming the haploid germ cells, the egg and sperm. These gametes fuse in the process of *fertilization* to form the diploid *zygote,* or one-celled embryo. Gametogenesis and fertilization are vulnerable to toxicants, but this is the topic of another chapter in this text. It is now known that the maternal and paternal genomes are not equivalent in their contributions to the zygotic genome. The process of *imprinting* occurs during gametogenesis, conferring to certain allelic genes a differential expressivity depending on whether they are of maternal or paternal origin (Latham, 1999). Because imprinting involves cytosine methylation and changes in chromatin conformation, this process may be susceptible to toxicants that affect these targets (Murphy and Jirtle, 2000). Although a plausible target for toxicity, imprinting is not well understood and at present there are no documented examples of toxicant effects on this process. Toxic effects on imprinting could conceivably play a role in paternally mediated developmental toxicity, a topic that is not discussed here but which has received increased attention in the recent literature (Olshan and Mattison, 1995).

Exposure to toxicants during a brief period (~6 h) immediately following fertilization has been demonstrated to result in malformed fetuses for a number of chemicals including ethylene oxide (Generoso et al., 1987), ethylmethane sulfonate, ethylnitrosourea, and triethylene melamine (Generoso et al., 1988). The mechanisms underlying these unexpected findings have not been elucidated but probably do not involve point mutations.

Following fertilization, the embryo moves down the fallopian tube and implants in the wall of the uterus. The *preimplantation* period comprises mainly an increase in cell number through a rapid series of cell divisions with little growth in size (*cleavage* of the zygote) and cavitation of the embryo to form a fluid-filled blastocoele. This stage, termed the *blastocyst,* consisting of about a thousand cells, may contain as few as three cells destined to give rise to the embryo proper (Markert and Petters, 1978), and these cells are within a region called the *inner cell mass.* The remainder of the blastocyst cells give rise to extraembryonic membranes and support structures (e.g., trophoblast and placenta). However, the fates of the cells in the early embryo are not completely determined at this stage. The relatively undifferentiated preimplantation embryo has great restorative (regulative) growth potential (Snow and Tam, 1979). Experiments of Moore et al. (1968) demonstrated that single cells from eight-celled rabbit embryos are capable of producing normal offspring.

Toxicity during preimplantation is generally thought to result in no or slight effect on growth (because of regulative growth) or in death (through overwhelming damage or failure to implant). Preimplantation exposure to DDT, nicotine, or methylmethane sulfonate results in body and/or brain weight deficits and embryo lethality, but not malformations (Fabro, 1973; Fabro et al., 1984). However, there are also examples of toxicant exposure during the preimplantation period leading to fetal malformations. Treatment of pregnant mice with methylnitrosourea on days 2.5, 3.5, and 4.5 of gestation resulted in neural tube defects and cleft palate (Takeuchi, 1984). Cyproterone acetate and medroxyprogesterone acetate are capable of producing malformations when administered on day 2 of gestation (Eibs et al., 1982). Rutledge and coworkers (Rutledge et al., 1994) produced hind-limb and lower body duplications by treating pregnant mice with all-*trans* retinoic acid on gestation day 4.5 to 5.5, at which time the embryos are at the late blastocyst and proamniotic stages. This finding suggests that patterning of the limbs and lower body may begin prior to gastrula-

Table 10-3
Timing of Key Developmental Events in Some Mammalian Species

	RAT	RABBIT	MONKEY	HUMAN
Blastocyst formation	3–5	2.6–6	4–9	4–6
Implantation	5–6	6	9	6–7
Organogenesis	6–17	6–18	20–45	21–56
Primitive streak	9	6.5	18–20	16–18
Neural plate	9.5	—	19–21	18–20
First somite	10	—	—	20–21
First branchial arch	10	—	—	20
First heartbeat	10.2	—	—	22
10 Somites	10–11	9	23–24	25–26
Upper limb buds	10.5	10.5	25–26	29–30
Lower limb buds	11.2	11	26–27	31–32
Testes differentiation	14.5	20	—	43
Heart septation	15.5	—	—	46–47
Palate closure	16–17	19–20	45–47	56–58
Urethral groove closed in male	—	—	—	90
Length of gestation	21–22	31–34	166	267

*Developmental ages are days of gestation.

SOURCE: Adapted from Shepard (1992, 1998), with permission.

tion. Because of the rapid mitoses occurring during the preimplantation period, chemicals affecting DNA synthesis or integrity or those affecting microtubule assembly would be expected to be particularly toxic if given access to the embryo.

Following implantation the embryo undergoes *gastrulation.* Gastrulation is the process of formation of the three primary germ layers—the *ectoderm, mesoderm,* and *endoderm.* During gastrulation, cells migrate through a structure called the *primitive streak,* and their movements set up basic morphogenetic fields in the embryo (Smith et al., 1994). As it is a prelude to organogenesis, the period of gastrulation is quite susceptible to teratogenesis. A number of toxicants administered during gastrulation produce malformations of the eye, brain and face. These malformations are indicative of damage to the anterior neural plate, one of the regions defined by the cellular movements of gastrulation.

The formation of the neural plate in the ectoderm marks the onset of *organogenesis,* during which the rudiments of most bodily structures are established. This is a period of heightened susceptibility to malformations and extends from approximately the third to the eighth weeks of gestation in humans. Within this short period, the embryo undergoes rapid and dramatic changes. At 3 weeks of gestation, the human conceptus is in most ways indistinguishable from other mammalian and indeed other vertebrate embryos, consisting of only a few cell types in a trilaminar arrangement. By 8 weeks, the conceptus, which can now be termed a fetus, has a form clearly recognizable as human. The rapid changes of organogenesis require cell proliferation, cell migration, cell-cell interactions, and morphogenetic tissue remodeling. These processes are exemplified by the *neural crest* cells. These cells originate at the border of the *neural plate* and migrate to form a wide variety of structures throughout the embryo. Neural crest cells derived from segments of the hindbrain (*rhombomeres*) migrate to form bone and connective tissues in the head (Krumlauf, 1993; Vaglia and Hall, 1999).

Within organogenesis, there are periods of peak susceptibility for each forming structure. This is nicely illustrated by the work of Shenefelt (1972), who studied the developmental toxicity of carefully timed exposures to retinoic acid in the hamster. The incidence of some of the defects seen after retinoic acid administration at different times in development are shown in Fig. 10-1. The peak incidence of each malformation coincides with the timing of key developmental events in the affected structure. Thus, the specification of developmental fields for the eyes is established quite early, and microphthalmia has an early critical period. Establishment of rudiments of the long bones of the limbs occurs later, as does susceptibility to shortened limbs. The palate has two separate peaks of susceptibility, the first corresponding to the early establishment of the palatal folds and the second to the later events leading to palatal closure. Notice also that the total incidence of malformations is lower prior to organogenesis but increases to 100 percent by gestation day $7^3/_4$. The processes underlying the development of normal structures are poorly understood but involve a number of key events. A given toxicant may affect one or several developmental events, so the pattern of sensitivity of a structure can change depending on the nature of the toxic insult. Cleft palate is induced in mouse fetuses following maternal exposure to methanol as early as day 5 of gestation, with a peak sensitivity at day 7 and little or no sensitivity after day 9 (Rogers et al., 1994). In contrast, the typical peak critical period for induction of cleft palate for most agents is between gestation days 11 and 13. In a large series of experiments in NMRI mice, Neubert's group found

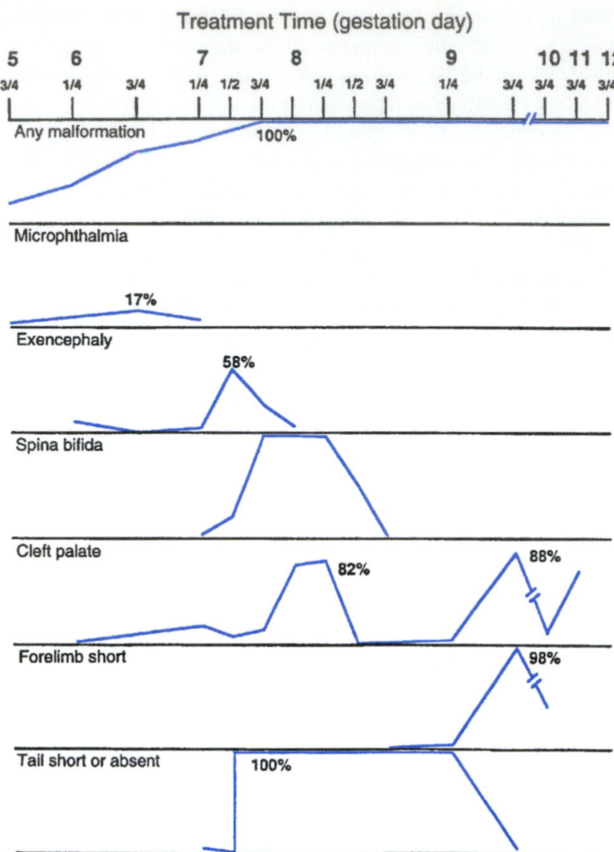

Figure 10-1. Critical periods of sensitivity for induction of various defects by retinoic acid in the hamster.

Incidence of defects are estimates for the embryo/fetal LD_{50} maternal dosage. Note in the top panel that fewer malformations are induced on days 5 to 6, prior to organogenesis, indicating that during this period embryos for the most part either die or recover. Likelihood of malformation increases rapidly during gastrulation and reaches 100 percent during organogenesis. Peak incidence for each defect are enumerated and reflect timing of critical events in the development of each structure. [Modified from Shenefelt (1972), with permission.]

that the day of peak sensitivity to the induction of cleft palate was day 11 for TCDD, day 12 for 2,4,5-trichlorophenoxyacetic acid, and day 13 for dexamethasone (Neubert et al., 1973). Detection of unexpected critical periods like that for induction of cleft palate by methanol may provide clues to normal developmental processes not presently understood.

The end of organogenesis marks the beginning of the *fetal period* (from days 56 to 58 to birth in humans), characterized primarily by tissue differentiation, growth, and physiologic maturation. This is not to say that formation of the organs is complete but that almost all organs are present and grossly recognizable. Further development of organs proceeds during the fetal period to attain requisite functionality prior to birth, including fine structural morphogenesis (e.g., neural outgrowth and synaptogenesis, branching morphogenesis of the bronchial tree and renal cortical tubules) as well as biochemical maturation (e.g., induction of tissue-specific enzymes and structural proteins). One of the latest organogenetic events is closure of the urethral groove in the male, which occurs at about gestation day 90. Failure of this event produces hypospadias, a ventral clefting of the penis.

Exposure during the fetal period is most likely to result in effects on growth and functional maturation. Functional anomalies of the central nervous system and reproductive organs—including behavioral, mental, and motor deficits as well as decreases in fertility—are among the possible adverse outcomes. These manifestations are not apparent prenatally and require careful postnatal observation and testing of offspring. Such postnatal functional manifestations can be sensitive indicators of in utero toxicity, and reviews of postnatal functional deficits of the central nervous system (Rodier et al., 1994), immune system (Holladay and Luster, 1994) and heart, lung, and kidneys (Lau and Kavlock, 1994) are available. Major structural alterations can occur during the fetal period, but these generally result from *deformations* (disruption of previously normal structures) rather than malformations. The extremities may be affected by amniotic bands, wrapping of the umbilical cord, or vascular disruptions, leading to loss of distal structures.

There is a paucity of data concerning the long-term effects of toxic exposure during the fetal period. Some effects could require years to become apparent (such as those noted for DES in above), and others may even result in the onset of senescence and/or organ failure late in life. In rats, prenatal exposure to high dosages of ethanol during the second half of pregnancy shortens life span of the offspring, by about 20 weeks in females and 2.5 to 7 weeks in males (Abel et al., 1987).

Dose–Response Patterns and the Threshold Concept

The major effects of prenatal exposure, observed at the time of birth in developmental toxicity studies, are embryo lethality, malformations, and growth retardation. The relationship between these effects is complex and varies with the type of agent, the time of exposure, and the dose. For some agents these endpoints may represent a continuum of increasing toxicity, with low dosages producing growth retardation and increasing dosages producing malformations and then lethality. Malformations and/or death can occur in the absence of any effect on intrauterine growth, but this is unusual. Likewise, growth retardation and embryo lethality can occur without malformations. Agents producing the latter pattern of response would be considered embryotoxic or embryolethal but not teratogenic (unless it were subsequently established that death was due to a structural malformation).

Another key element of the dose–response relationship is the shape of the dose–response curve at low exposure levels. Because of the high restorative growth potential of the mammalian embryo, cellular homeostatic mechanisms, and maternal metabolic defenses, mammalian developmental toxicity has generally been considered a threshold phenomenon. Assumption of a threshold means that there is a maternal dosage below which an adverse response is not elicited. Daston (1993) summarized two approaches for establishing the existence of a threshold. The first, exemplified by a large teratology study on 2,4,5-T (Nelson and Holson, 1978), suggests that no study is capable of evaluating the dose–response at low response rates (e.g., 805 litters per dose would be necessary to detect the relatively high rate of a 5 percent increase in resorptions). The second approach is to determine whether a threshold exists for the mechanism responsible for the observed effect. While relatively few mechanisms are known, it is clear that cellular and embryonic repair mechanisms and dose-dependent kinetics both support the plausibility of a mechanistic threshold. Lack of a threshold implies that exposure to any amount of a toxic chemical, even one molecule, has the potential to cause developmental toxicity. One mechanism of abnormal development for which this might be the case is gene mutation. A point mutation in a critical gene could theoretically be induced by a single hit or single molecule, leading to a deleterious change in a gene product and consequent abnormal development. This, of course, carries the large assumption that the molecule could traverse the maternal system and the placenta and enter a critical progenitor cell in the embryo. An effect on a single cell might result in abnormal development at the zygote (one-cell) stage, the blastocyst stage (when only a few cells in the inner cell mass are embryo progenitors), or during organogenesis, when organ rudiments may consist of only a few cells.

An apparent threshold for developmental toxicity based at least in part on cellular homeostatic mechanisms is demonstrated in studies of biological mechanisms underlying the developmental dose–response for 5-fluorouracil (Shuey et al, 1994; see also "Safety Assessment," further on). This agent inhibits the enzyme thymidylate synthetase (TS), thus interfering with DNA synthesis and cell proliferation. Significant embryonal TS inhibition can be measured at maternal dosages an order of magnitude below those required to produce malformations and about fivefold below those affecting fetal growth (Figure 10-2). The lack of developmental toxicity despite significant TS inhibition probably reflects ability of the embryo to compensate for imbalances in cellular nucleotide pool sizes.

In the context of human health risk assessment, it is also important to consider the distinction between individual thresholds and population thresholds. There is wide variability in the human population, and a threshold for a population is defined by the threshold of the most sensitive individual in the population (Gaylor et al., 1988). Indeed, even though the biological target of a devel-

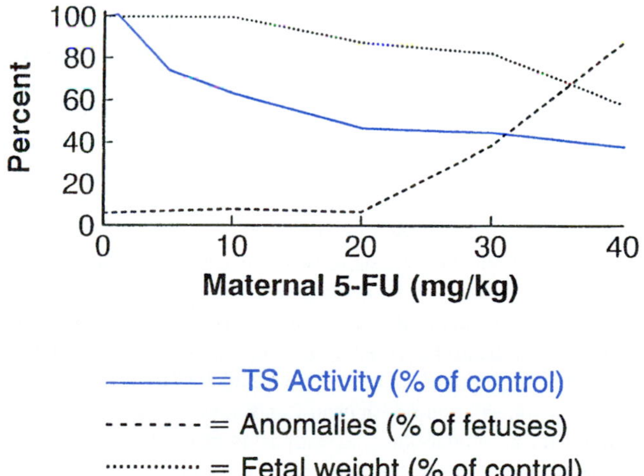

Figure 10-2. Relationship between inhibition of embryonal thymidylate synthetase (TS) and adverse fetal outcome following maternal 5-fluorouracil (5-FU) administration on gestation day 14 in the rat.

5-FU inhibits embryonal TS activity at low dosages, with most of the inhibition occurring below 20 mg/kg. Fetal weight is affected at 20 mg/kg and above, while incidence of anomalies increases only at 30 mg/kg and above. Anomalies include edema, skull dysmorphology, orbital hemorrhage, wavy ribs, cleft palate, brachygnathia and hindlimb defects. [Based on Shuey et al. (1994) and Lau et al. (1992) and unpublished observations.]

opmental toxicant may be thresholded, background factors such as health status or concomitant exposures may render an individual at or even beyond the threshold for failure of that biological process. Any further toxic impact on that process, even one molecule, would theoretically increase risk.

MECHANISMS AND PATHOGENESIS OF DEVELOPMENTAL TOXICITY

The term *mechanisms* is used here to refer to cellular-level events that initiate the process leading to abnormal development. *Pathogenesis* comprises the cell-, tissue-, and organ-level sequelae that are ultimately manifest in abnormality. Mechanisms of teratogenesis listed by Wilson (1977) include mutations, chromosomal breaks, altered mitosis, altered nucleic acid integrity or function, diminished supplies of precursors or substrates, decreased energy supplies, altered membrane characteristics, osmolar imbalance, and enzyme inhibition. While these cellular insults are not unique to development, they may relatively quickly trigger unique pathogenetic responses in the embryo, such as reduced cell proliferation, cell death, altered cell-cell interactions, reduced biosynthesis, inhibition of morphogenetic movements, or mechanical disruption of developing structures.

Experimental studies of cyclophosphamide (CP), a teratogenic chemotherapeutic agent, provide an example of current approaches to understanding teratogenic mechanisms and pathogenesis. Much of this and other mechanistic work was made possible by the advent of whole rodent embryo culture techniques, which involve removing rodent embryos from the uterus at the beginning of organogenesis and growing them in serum-containing culture media (New, 1978; Sadler and Warner, 1984). Embryos will grow normally for about 48 h, completing most of organogenesis. The ability to grow embryos in isolation allows direct exposure, manipulation, and observation of the organogenesis-stage embryo.

Using the embryo culture system, Fantel et al. (1979) and Sanyal et al. (1979) showed that hepatic S9 fractions and cofactors were needed to elicit abnormal development by CP, demonstrating that it must be metabolically activated to be teratogenic. Activation of CP was inhibited by metyrapone or carbon monoxide, indicating involvement of P450 monooxygenases. Of the CP metabolites (Fig. 10-3), 4-hydroxycyclophosphamide (4OHCP) and aldophosphamide (AP) are unstable. A stable derivative of 4OHCP, 4-hydroperoxy-cyclophosphamide (4OOHCP) was tested in vivo (Hales, 1982) and in whole embryo culture (Mirkes, 1987). In the latter study, the morphology of the treated embryos was indistinguishable from that of embryos cultured with CP and an activating system. Spontaneous conversion of 4OOHCP to 4OHCP and then to phosphoramide mustard and acrolein occurs rapidly, and these further metabolites, as well as 4-ketocyclophosphamide (4-ketoCP) and carboxyphosphamide (CaP), have also been studied for their teratogenicity. It appears that 4OHCP is not teratogenic (Hales, 1983) and toxicity elicited by 4-ketoCP is dissimilar to that of activated CP (Mirkes et al., 1981). Subsequent work centered on the two remaining metabolites, PM and AC. Mirkes et al. (1981) demonstrated that the effects of PM on cultured rat embryos were indistinguishable from those of activated CP. Hales (1982) administered CP, PM, or AC to gestation day 13 rat embryos by intraamniotic injection. CP and AC caused hydrocephaly, open eyes, cleft palate, micrognathia, omphalocele and tail and limb defects, while PM produced only hydrocephaly and tail and limb defects. Thus, both PM and AC appear to be teratogenic metabolites of CP.

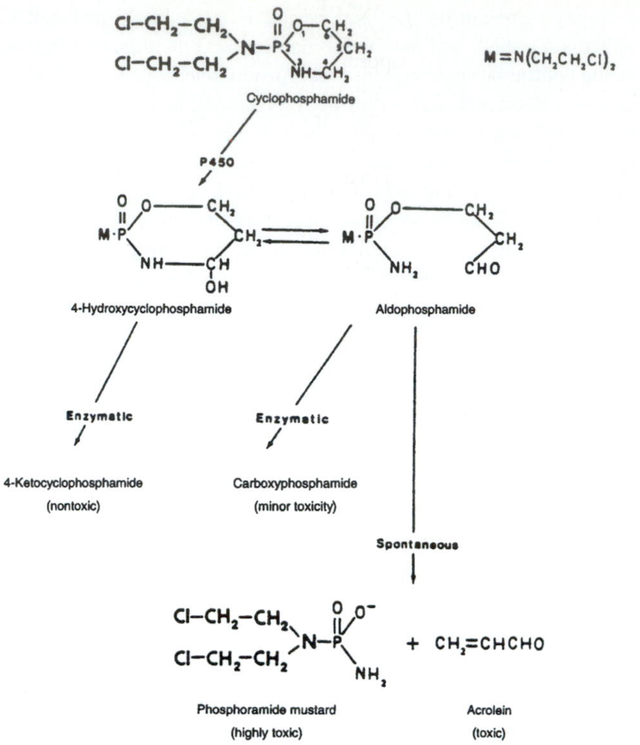

Figure 10-3. Metabolic pathway for cyclophosphamide. [From Mirkes (1985b), with permission.]

What are the cell and molecular targets of activated CP, and what is the nature of the interaction? Experiments with (^{3}H)CP show that approximately 87 percent of bound radioactivity is associated with protein, 5 percent with DNA, and 8 percent with RNA (Mirkes, 1985a). Using alkaline elution, it was demonstrated that CP and PM produce single-strand DNA breaks and DNA-DNA and DNA-protein cross-linking. To determine whether DNA cross-linking is essential for teratogenicity, a monofunctional derivative of PM, capable of producing single-strand breaks but not cross-links in DNA, was tested. Although higher concentrations were needed, this derivative produced the same spectrum of effects as PM (Mirkes et al., 1985). Later, Little and Mirkes (1990) showed that 4-hydroperoxydechlorocyclophosphamide, a CP analog that yields AC and a nonalkylating derivative of PM, did not produce DNA damage when embryos were exposed in serum-containing medium. Using radiolabeled CP, they further found that AC preferentially binds to protein and shows high incorporation into the yolk sac, while PM binds preferentially to DNA. Hales (1989) showed that PM and AC have strikingly different effects on limb buds in culture. These results indicate that PM and AC have different targets in the embryo and that PM is responsible for CP-induced DNA damage.

How do chemical insults at the cell and molecular level translate to a birth defect? To illustrate pathogenesis, we will consider inhibition of cell cycle perturbations and cell death, and continue with our example of cyclophosphamide. Cell death plays a critical role in normal morphogenesis. The term *programmed cell death* (pcd) refers to a specific type of cell death, *apoptosis,* under genetic control in the embryo (Lavin and Watters, 1993). Apoptosis is necessary for sculpting the digits from the hand plate, for instance, and for assuring appropriate functional connectivity between the central nervous system and distal structures. Cell proliferation is obviously essential for development. Cells within the primitive streak of the gastrula-stage rat embryo have the shortest known cell cycle time of any mammalian cell, 3 to 3.5 h (MacAuley et al., 1993). Cell proliferation rates change both spatially and temporally during ontogenesis, as can be demonstrated by examining the proportion of cells in S phase over time in different tissues during mid- to late gestation (Fig. 10-4). There is a delicate balance between cell proliferation, cell differentiation, and apoptosis in the embryo, and one molecular mechanism discussed above (DNA damage) might lead to the cell cycle perturbations and cell death induced by CP in specific cell populations.

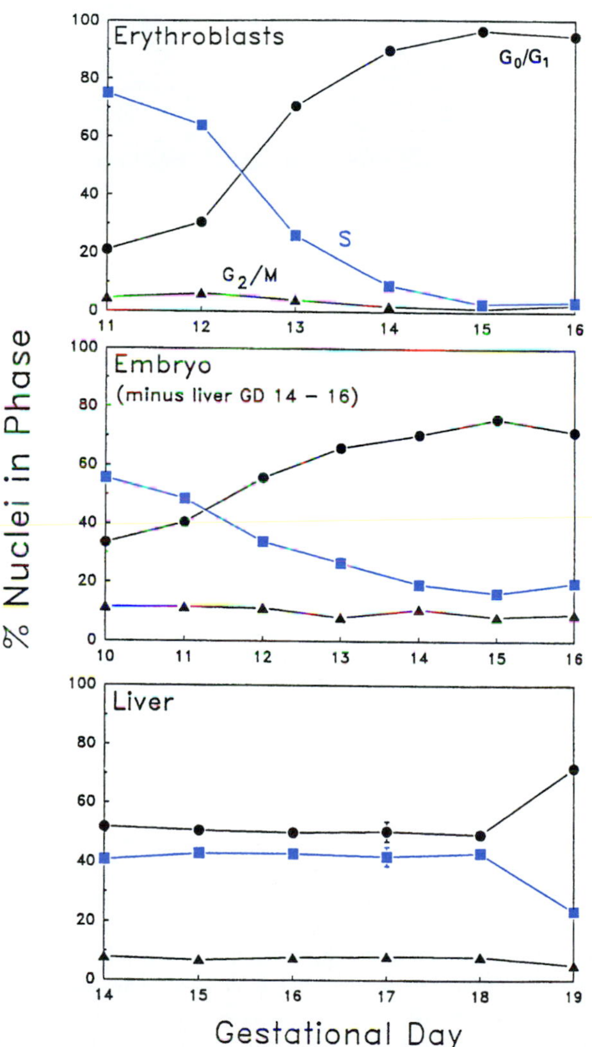

Figure 10-4. Normal developmental changes in cell cycle distributions in erythroblasts, embryo (minus the liver after GD 13), and fetal liver.

Percentages of cells in: ● G_0/G_1; ■ S; and ▲ G_2/M are shown for rat embryos between gestation days 10 and 19 (note changing x-axis range).

The proportion of cells in S phase generally reflects proliferation rate, which decreases with developmental stage in the embryo and erythroblasts. The percentage of S-phase cells in the fetal liver remains fairly high and constant until near term, when a growth spurt occurs. [From Elstein et al. (1993), with permission.]

Maternal cyclophosphamide treatment on gestation day 10 in the rat causes an S-phase cell cycle block as well as widespread cell death in the embryo (Fig. 10-5). In agreement with the S-phase cell cycle block, cell death is observed in areas of rapid cell proliferation (Chernoff et al., 1989; Francis et al., 1990). Similar blockage of the embryonal cell cycle and cell death were observed using activated CP in whole embryo culture (Little and Mirkes, 1992). The embryonal neuroepithelium is quite sensitive to CP-induced cell death, while the heart is resistant. Differences in cell cycle length may, in part, underlie this differential sensitivity. The neuroepithelium of the day 10 rat embryo has a cell cycle time of approximately 9.5 h, while the cell cycle length in the heart was estimated to be 13.4 h. This difference is due to a longer G_0/G_1 phase in the heart cells compared to the neuroepithelium (Mirkes et al, 1989). Damage to DNA by PM occurs predominately in S phase (Little and Mirkes, 1992), which constitutes a relatively greater proportion of the cell cycle in the heart than in the neuroepithelium.

Damage to DNA can inhibit cell cycle progression at the G_1-S transition, through the S phase, and at the G_2-M transition. If DNA damage is repaired, the cell cycle can return to normal, but if damage is too extensive or cell cycle arrest too long, apoptosis may be triggered. The relationship between DNA damage and repair, cell cycle progression, and apoptosis is depicted in Fig. 10-6. An increasing number of genes are being identified that play a role in apoptosis (White, 1993). The p53 gene, which may function as a tumor suppressor, can promote apoptosis or growth arrest. Apoptosis occurring during normal development does not require this gene, as p53-deficient embryos develop normally. However, p53 may be critical for induction of growth arrest or apoptosis in response to DNA damage. The incidence of benzo[a]pyrene-induced fetal resorptions and postpartum death were increased 3-fold and over 10-fold, respectively, in offspring of heterozygous p53-deficient (p/+) pregnant mice compared to normal homozygous (+ / +) controls (Harrison et al., 1994). Growth factors and some cytokines (IL-3, IL-6) can prevent p53-dependent apoptosis. Expression of c-myc produces continued DNA synthesis, which may precipitate apoptosis in the face of DNA damage. Bcl-2 functions as a repressor of apoptosis and functions in conjunction with Bax, a homolog that dimerizes with itself or with Bcl-2. Bax homodimers favor cell death while Bcl-2/Bax heterodimers inhibit cell death (Oltvai and Korsmeyer, 1994).

From the multiple checkpoints and factors present to regulate the cell cycle and apoptosis, it is clear that different cell populations may respond differently to a similar stimulus, in part because cellular predisposition to apoptosis can vary. In regard to the induction of cell death in the neuroepithelium but not the heart by CP, it may be relevant that a portion of the cells from the neuroepithelium undergoes apoptosis normally during this stage of development, indicating competence to respond to an appropriate signal. Conversely, although diverse environmental agents including ethanol, 13-*cis* retinoic acid, ionizing radiation, and hyperthermia are able to induce characteristic patterns of cell death in the embryo (Sulik, et al., 1988), none of them effect cell death in the heart. Recently, Mirkes and Little (1998) have shown that treatment of postimplantation mouse embryos with hyperthermia, cyclophosphamide or sodium arsenate induced DNA fragmentation, activation of caspase-3, and cleavage of poly (ADP-ribose) polymerase (PARP) along with apoptosis in some embryonal tissues,

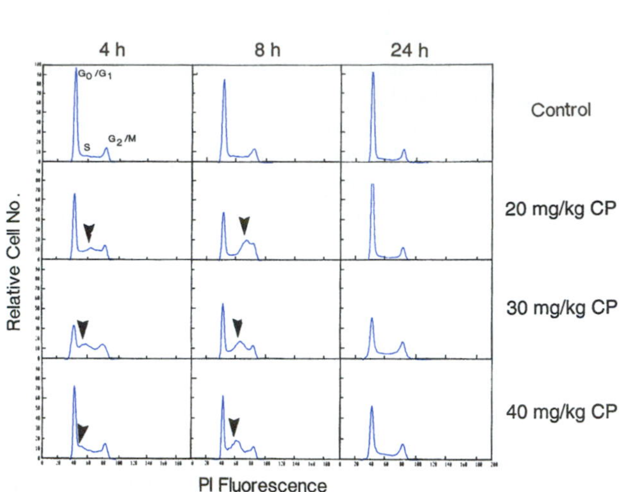

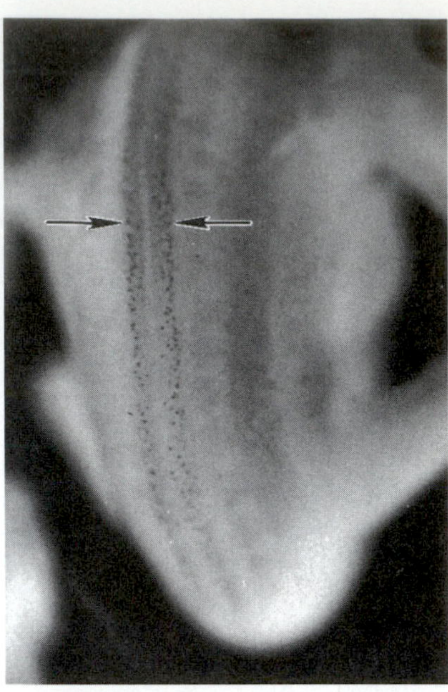

Figure 10-5. Maternal cyclophosphamide (CP) administration on gestation day 10 in CD-1 mice produces perturbations of the embryonal cell cycle and cell death in areas of rapid proliferation.

Left: Cells are inhibited from progressing through the S (DNA synthetic) phase of the cell cycle, indicated by the abnormal population of cells (*arrowheads*) accumulating at progressively earlier stages of S phase 4 and 8 h after increasing maternal CP dosages. The upper panels show the normal GD 10-11 distributions, with the G_0/G_1, S, and G_2/M peaks identified in the upper left panel. By 24 h postdosing, cell cycle distributions have returned to normal at 20 mg/kg, but remain abnormal at higher dosages. *Right:* Nile blue sulfate staining of a mouse embryo 24 h after maternal CP dosing shows cell death (*stippling along either side of the midline, arrows*) in the neural tube, one of the most sensitive target sites for CP. [Adapted from Chernoff et al. (1989), with permission.]

but none of these events occurred in the heart. Subsequently, these investigators demonstrated that these agents can induce changes in embryonal mitochondria resulting in release of cytochrome *c* and activation of caspase-9, the upstream activator of caspase-3. In agreement with the observed lack of apoptosis in the heart, this tissue was also refractory to teratogen-induced cytochrome *c* release from mitochondria (Mirkes and Little, 2000).

In addition to affecting proliferation and cell viability, molecular and cellular insults can affect essential processes such as cell migration, cell-cell interactions, differentiation, morphogenesis, and energy metabolism. Although the embryo has compensatory mechanisms to offset such effects, production of a normal or malformed offspring will depend on the balance between damage and repair at each step in the pathogenetic pathway.

Advances in the Molecular Basis of Dysmorphogenesis

Our still fragmentary understanding of normal development, combined with the small size and inaccessibility of the mammalian embryo, have made the elucidation of mechanisms of abnormal development a daunting task. Now, rapid advances in molecular biology and related technologies are bringing new understanding of mechanisms of normal and abnormal development. Targeted gene disruption by homologous recombination (gene "knockout") has been used to study the function of members of the retinoic acid receptor (RAR) family of nuclear ligand-inducible transcription factors. Chambon and colleagues have produced mice lacking several of these receptors either singly or as double knockouts. Single-receptor isoform mutants were often unaffected, suggesting functional redundancy. Double mutants were invariably nonviable and presented widespread malformations of the skeleton and viscera (Lohnes et al., 1994; Mendelsohn et al., 1994). The compound RARγ-RARβ null mouse exhibits syndactyly, indicating that retinoic acid plays a role in interdigital cell death (Dupe et al., 1999).

The use of synthetic antisense oligonucleotides allows temporal and spatial restriction of gene ablation. In this technique, 15-25-mer oligonucleotides are synthesized that are complimentary to the mRNA to be disrupted (Helene et al., 1990). These probes can enter embryonal cells, and hybridization with cellular mRNA causes disruption of native message. In this way, gene function can be turned off at specific times. Added advantages of the antisense approach are the ability to ablate multiple gene family members (by making the antisense probes to regions of sequence homology) and the much shorter-time frame for the experiments (Sadler and Hunter, 1994). The proto-oncogenes Wnt-1 and Wnt-3a have been implicated in the development of the midbrain and hindbrain. Augustine et al. (1993) attenuated Wnt-1 expression using antisense oligonucleotide inhibition in mouse embryos developing in culture. Exposure during neurulation produced mid- and hindbrain malformations similar to those seen in Wnt-1 null mutant mice, as well as cardiac anomalies not observed in Wnt-1 knockouts created by homologous recombination. Antisense attenuation of Wnt-3a

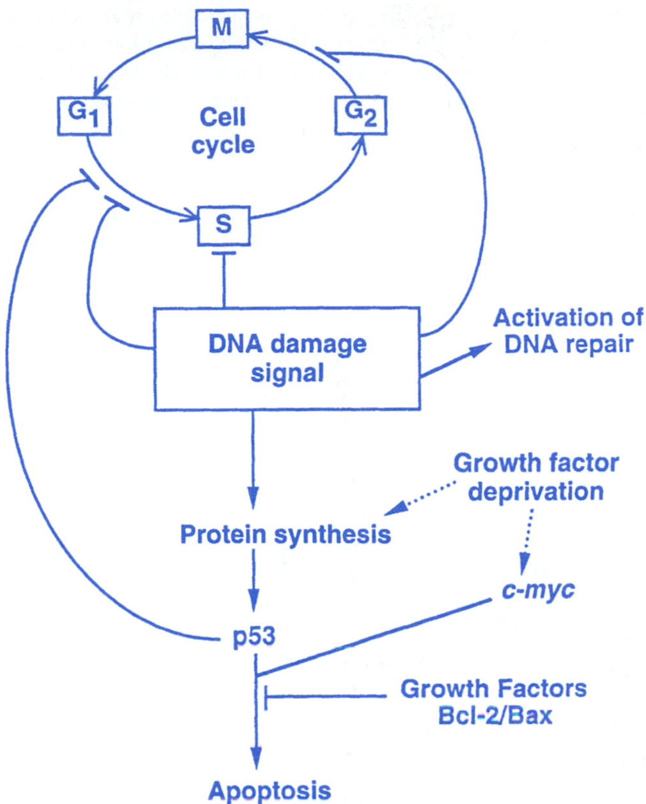

Figure 10-6. Relationships between DNA damage and the induction of cell cycle arrest or apoptosis.

DNA damage can signal inhibition of the cell cycle between G_1 and S, in S phase or between G_2 and mitosis. The signal(s) can also activate DNA repair mechanisms and synthesis of proteins, including p53, that can initiate apoptosis. Growth factors and products of the proto-oncogene *c-myc* and the Bcl-2/Bax gene family, as well as differentiation state and cell cycle phase, are important determinants of the ultimate outcome of embryonal DNA damage.

caused anomalies of the forebrain, midbrain, and spinal cord. Simultaneously attenuating both Wnt-1 and Wnt-3a targeted all brain regions and worsened the effect on the spinal cord, suggesting that these genes may serve a complementary function in the development of the central nervous system.

Gain of gene function can also be studied by engineering genetic constructs with an inducible promoter attached to the gene of interest. Ectopic gene expression can be made ubiquitous or site-specific depending on the choice of promoter to drive expression. Ectopic expression of the Hoxa-7 gene induced in mouse embryos by attaching it to the chicken β-actin promoter resulted in a phenotype exhibiting multiple craniofacial and cervical vertebral malformations (Balling et al., 1989; Kessel et al., 1990). Transient overexpression of specific genes can be accomplished by adding extra copies using adenoviral transduction. In proof-of-concept, Hartig and Hunter (1998) injected the adenoviral vector containing either the bacterial beta-galactosidase or green fluorescent protein reporter gene under the control of the human cytomegalovirus early gene promoter into the intraamniotic space of neurulation-stage mouse embryos and achieved intense gene expression in the neuroepithelium.

Reporter transgenes contain a gene with a readily detectable product fused downstream of a selected regulatory region. The *Escherichia coli lacZ* (β-galactosidase) gene is commonly used for this purpose. Cell lineage studies can be carried out by fusing *lacZ* to a constitutive regulatory sequence and introducing the construct into a somatic cell early in ontogenesis. The reporter gene will then be expressed in and mark all progeny of the transfected cell. This method has been used to study postimplantation development in the mouse embryo (Sanes et al., 1986), although intracellular injection of fluorescent dyes has also proven highly reliable for cell lineage studies (e.g., Smith et al., 1994). The pattern of expression of a particular gene of interest can be discriminated by fusing upstream regulatory elements of the gene to *lacZ,* which will then be transcribed under control of those upstream elements (Zakany et al., 1990).

Retinoic acid (RA) can activate hox genes in vitro, and the 3' hox genes have multiple RA response elements (RAREs). Evidence that RA-induced malformations in mouse embryos are related to changes in hox expression was first provided by staining of hox-*lacZ* transgenic embryos (Marshall, 1992). Within a few hours of RA treatment, hoxb-1 expression extends anteriorly, suggesting that hox genes could be direct targets of RA induction. Regions of altered hox expression could be manifest as abnormal cell fate and morphogenesis (Marshall, 1996; Collins and Mao, 1999). One of the best examples of hox-mediated retinoid teratogenicity is the effect on the developing hindbrain. Identity of the hindbrain segments (rhombomeres) is in part conferred by anterior expression boundaries of specific hox genes, and these boundaries are altered in distinct ways by retinoid treatment. Alterations in expression boundaries for the genes correlate with phenotypic changes seen in the hindbrain at later developmental stages, including transformation of rhombomeres to a phenotype usually associated with a more caudal rhombomere.

PHARMACOKINETICS AND METABOLISM IN PREGNANCY

The manner in which chemicals are absorbed during pregnancy and the extent to and form in which they reach the conceptus are important determinants of whether the agent can impact development. The maternal, placental, and embryonic compartments comprise independent yet interacting systems that undergo profound changes throughout the course of pregnancy. Changes in maternal physiology during pregnancy involve hepatic metabolism, the gastrointestinal tract, cardiovascular system, excretory system, and the respiratory system (Hytten, 1984; Krauer, 1987; Mattison et al., 1991). While these physiologic changes are necessary to support the growing needs of the conceptus in terms of energy supply and waste elimination, the alterations can have significant impact on the uptake, distribution, metabolism, and elimination of xenobiotics. For example, decreases in intestinal motility and increases in gastric emptying time result in longer retention time of ingested chemicals in the upper gastrointestinal tract. Cardiac output increases by 50 percent during the first trimester in humans and remains elevated throughout pregnancy, while blood volume increases and plasma proteins and peripheral vascular resistance decrease. The relative increase in blood volume over red cell volume leads to borderline anemia and a generalized edema with a 70 percent elevation of extracellular space. Thus, the volume of distribution of a chemical and the amount bound by plasma proteins may change considerably during pregnancy. Renal blood flow and glomerular filtration are also increased in many species during pregnancy. Increases in tidal volume, minute ventilation, and minute O_2 uptake can result in increased pulmonary distribution of gases and decreases in time to reach alveolar steady state.

In addition to changes in maternal physiology, limited available evidence suggests that relative rates of drug metabolizing enzymes also change during pregnancy (Juchau, 1981; Juchau and Faustman-Watts, 1983). Decreased hepatic monooxygenase activity has been observed during pregnancy in rats and has been attributed to decreased enzyme levels and to competitive inhibition by circulating steroids (Neims, 1976). Another factor that contributes to lower monooxygenase activity is that pregnant rats appear to be less responsive to induction of hepatic monooxygenases by phenobarbital (but not 3-methylcholanthrene) than are nonpregnant females (Guenther and Mannering, 1977). Despite the absence of a comprehensive literature on this subject, there appears to be an overall decrease in hepatic xenobiotic biotransformation during pregnancy. Clearly, maternal handling of a chemical bears considerable weight in determining the extent of embryotoxicity. In one of the few studies of its type, a linear combination of the 45-min and the 24-h maternal blood concentrations was able to predict the litter response rate for pregnant rats dosed with 500 mg/kg sodium salicylate on gestation day 11 (Kimmel and Young, 1983). These two kinetic parameters probably reflect the influence of the peak drug concentration as well as the cumulative area under the concentration-time curve in inducing developmental disturbances.

The placenta plays a central role in influencing embryonic exposure by helping to regulate blood flow, by offering a transport barrier, and by metabolizing chemicals (Slikker and Miller, 1994). Functionally, the placenta acts as a lipid membrane that permits bidirectional transfer of substances between maternal and fetal compartments. The transfer depends on three major elements: the type of placentation, the physicochemical properties of the chemical, and rates of placental metabolism. Although there are marked species differences in types of placentas, orientation of blood vessels, and numbers of exchanging layers, these do not seem to play a dominant role in placental transfer of most chemicals. It is important to note that virtually any substance present in the maternal plasma will be transported to some extent by the placenta. The passage of most drugs across the placenta seems to occur by simple passive diffusion, the rate of which is proportional to the diffusion constant of the drug, the concentration gradient across the maternal and embryonic plasma, the area of exchange, and the inverse of the membrane thickness (Nau, 1992). Important modifying factors to the rate and extent of transfer include lipid solubility, molecular weight, protein binding, the type of transfer (passive diffusion, facilitated or active transport), the degree of ionization, and placental metabolism. Weak acids appear to be rapidly transferred across the placenta, due in part to the pH gradient between the maternal and embryonic plasma which can trap ionized forms of the drug in the slightly more acidic embryonic compartment (Nau and Scott, 1986). Blood flow probably constitutes the major rate-limiting step for more lipid-soluble compounds.

Quantitating the form, amount, and timing of chemical delivery to the embryonic compartment relative to concurrent developmental processes is an important component of understanding mechanisms of embryotoxicity and species differences in embryonic sensitivity (Nau, 1986). The small size of the conceptus during organogenesis and the fact that the embryo is changing at a rapid rate during this period makes assessment of toxicokinetics difficult. Nevertheless, there has been considerable progress in this area (Nau and Scott, 1987; Clark, 1993). Increasingly sensitive analytical methods are now providing evidence to challenge the historical view, particularly for cytochrome P450–dependent monooxygenases, that the early embryo has low metabolic capabilities (Juchau et al., 1992). Using an embryo culture system, Juchau and coworkers demonstrated that the rat conceptus was able to generate sufficient amounts of metabolites of the proteratogen 2-acetylaminofluorene (2-AAF) to induce dysmorphogenesis, and that the proximate toxicant, the 7-hydroxy metabolite, was different from the metabolite responsible for 2-AAF mutagenesis and carcinogenesis. Prior exposure of the dams to 3-methylcholanthrene increased the sensitivity of the cultured embryos to 2-AAF, thus demonstrating the inducibility of at least some cytochromes in the conceptus. These investigators later showed that embryos could further metabolize the 7-hydroxy metabolite to an even more toxic catechol. No previous induction was necessary for this activation step, demonstrating the presence of constitutive metabolizing enzymes in the embryo. Although the rates of metabolism for these activation steps may be low relative to the maternal liver, they occur close to the target site of the embryo or even within it and thus are significant in terms of inducing embryotoxicity.

The advent of physiologically based pharmacokinetic models has provided the framework to integrate what is known about physiologic changes during pregnancy, both within and between species, with aspects of drug metabolism and embryonic development into a quantitative description of the events. Gabrielson and coworkers (Gabrielson and Paalkow, 1983; Gabrielson and Larsson, 1990) were among the first investigators to develop physiologically based models of pregnancy, and others (Fisher et al., 1989; O'Flaherty et al., 1992; Clark et al., 1993; Luecke et al., 1994, 1997; Young, 1998) have added to their comprehensiveness. The pregnancy model of O'Flaherty and coworkers describes the entire period of gestation, and consists of the uterus, mammary tissue, maternal fat, kidney, liver, other well-perfused maternal tissues, embryo/fetal tissues and yolk sac, and chorioallantoic placentas. It takes into account the growth of various compartments during pregnancy (including the embryo itself), as well as changes in blood flow and the stage-dependent pH gradients between maternal and embryonic plasma. Transfer across the placenta in the model is diffusion limited. The utility of the model was evaluated using 5,5′-dimethyloxazolidine-2,4-dione (DMO), a weak acid that is not appreciably bound to plasma proteins and is eliminated by excretion in the urine. The model demonstrated that the whole body disposition of DMO, including distribution to the embryo, can be accounted for solely on the basis of its pK_a and of the pH and volumes of body fluid spaces. Differences between the disposition of DMO by the pregnant mouse and rat are consistent simply with differences in fluid pH.

The solvent 2-methoxyethanol is embryotoxic and teratogenic in all species tested to date. The proximate teratogen appears to be the metabolite 2-methoxyacetic acid (2-MAA). A physiologically based pharmacokinetic model has been developed for the pregnant mouse (Terry et al., 1995). Pharmacokinetics and tissue partition coefficients for 2-MAA were determined at different stages of embryonal development, and various models were tested based on the alternative hypotheses involving (1) blood-flow limited delivery of 2-MAA to model compartments, (2) pH trapping of ionized 2-MAA within compartments, (3) active transport of 2-MAA into compartments, and (4) reversible binding of 2-MAA within compartments. While the blood-flow limited model best predicted gestation day 8 dosimetry, the active transport models better described dosimetry on gestation days 11 and 13. Using published data on biotransformation of 2-methoxyethanol to ethylene glycol and 2-MAA in rats, Hays et al. (2000) have adapted the pregnant mouse PBPK model to the pregnant rat and successfully predicted tissue levels of 2-MAA following oral or intravenous administration of 2-methoxyethanol. The next step was to extrapolate this model to the inhalation route of exposure, and to model both rats and humans (Gargas et al., 2000). The extrapolation of the model enabled predictions of the exposures needed for pregnant women to reach blood concentrations (Cmax or AUC) equivalent to those in pregnant rats exposed to the no observed adverse effect level (NOAEL) or LOAEL for developmental toxicity. The body of work on PBPK modeling of 2-methoxyethanol is exemplary of the power of these techniques for extrapolating across dose, developmental stage, route, and species.

Maternal metabolism of xenobiotics is an important and variable determinant of developmental toxicity. As for other health endpoints, the developing field of pharmacogenomics offers hope for increasing our ability to predict susceptible subpopulations based on empirical relationships between maternal genotype and fetal phenotype. These relationships will hopefully guide further work to elucidate mechanisms of toxicant-induced abnormal development.

RELATIONSHIPS BETWEEN MATERNAL AND DEVELOPMENTAL TOXICITY

Although all developmental toxicity must ultimately result from an insult to the conceptus at the cellular level, the insult may occur through a direct effect on the embryo/fetus, indirectly through toxicity of the agent to the mother and/or the placenta, or a combination of direct and indirect effects. Maternal conditions capable of adversely affecting the developing organism include decreased uterine blood flow, maternal anemia, altered nutritional status, toxemia, altered organ function, autoimmune states, diabetes, electrolyte or acid-base disturbances, decreased milk quantity or quality, and abnormal behavior (Chernoff et al., 1989; Daston, 1994). Induction or exacerbation of such maternal conditions by toxic agents and the degree to which they manifest in abnormal development are dependent on maternal genetic background, age, parity, size, nutrition, disease, stress, and other health parameters and exposures (DeSesso, 1987; Chernoff, et al., 1989). These relationships are depicted in Fig. 10-7. In this section we will discuss maternal conditions known to adversely affect the conceptus, as well as examples of xenobiotics whose developmental toxicity results completely or in large part from maternal or placental toxicity.

The distinction between direct and indirect developmental toxicity is important for interpreting safety assessment tests in pregnant animals, as the highest dosage level in these experiments is chosen based on its ability to produce some maternal toxicity (e.g., decreased food or water intake, weight loss, clinical signs). However, maternal toxicity defined only by such manifestations gives little insight to the toxic actions of a xenobiotic. When developmental toxicity is observed only in the presence of maternal toxicity, the developmental effects may be indirect; however, understanding of the physiologic changes underlying the observed maternal toxicity and elucidation of the association with developmental effects is needed before one can begin to address the relevance of the observations to human safety assessment. Many known human developmental toxicants, including ethanol and cocaine, adversely affect the embryo/fetus predominately at maternally toxic levels, and part of their developmental toxicity may be ascribed to secondary effects of maternal physiological disturbances. For example, the nutritional status of alcoholics is generally inadequate, and effects on the conceptus may be exacerbated by effects of alcohol on placental transfer of nutrients. Effects of chronic alcohol abuse on maternal folate and zinc metabolism may be particularly important in the induction of fetal alcohol syndrome (Dreosti, 1994).

Maternal Factors Affecting Development

Genetics The genetic makeup of the pregnant female has been well documented as a determinant of developmental outcome in both humans and animals. The incidence of cleft lip and/or palate [CL(P)], which occurs more frequently in whites than in blacks, has been investigated in offspring of interracial couples in the United States (Khoury et al., 1983). Offspring of white mothers had a higher incidence of CL(P) than offspring of black mothers after correcting for paternal race, while offspring of white fathers did not have a higher incidence of CL(P) than offspring of black fathers after correcting for maternal race.

Among experimental animals, the "A" family of inbred mice has a high spontaneous occurrence of cleft lip and palate (Kalter, 1979). Two related mouse strains, A/J and CL/Fr, produce spontaneous CL(P) at 8 to 10 percent and 18 to 26 percent frequencies, respectively. The incidence of CL(P) in offspring depends on the genotype of the mother rather than that of the embryo (Juriloff and Fraser, 1980). The response to vitamin A of murine embryos heterozygous for the curly-tail mutation depends on the genotype of the mother (Seller et al., 1983). The teratogenicity of phenytoin has been compared in several inbred strains of mice. The susceptibility of offspring of crosses between susceptible A/J mice and resistant C57BL/6J mice was determined by the maternal, but not the embryonic genome (Hansen and Hodes, 1983). New genomic approaches have begun to identify genes associated with differential susceptibility of mouse strains to valproic acid (Finnell et al., 1997; Craig et al., 2000; Bennett et al., 2000; Faiella et al., 2000).

Disease Chronic hypertension is a risk factor for the development of preeclampsia, eclampsia, and toxemia of pregnancy, and hypertension is a leading cause of pregnancy-associated maternal deaths. Uncontrolled maternal diabetes mellitus is a significant cause of prenatal morbidity. Certain maternal infections can adversely effect the conceptus (e.g., rubella virus, discussed earlier), either through indirect disease-related maternal alterations or direct transplacental infection. Cytomegalovirus infection is associated with fetal death, microcephaly, mental retardation, blindness, and deafness (MacDonald and Tobin, 1978) and maternal infection with *Toxoplasma gondii* is known to induce hydrocephaly and chorioretinitis in infants (Alford et al., 1974).

One factor common to many disease states is hyperthermia. Hyperthermia is a potent experimental animal teratogen (Edwards, 1986), and there is a body of evidence associating maternal febrile illness during the first trimester of pregnancy with birth defects in

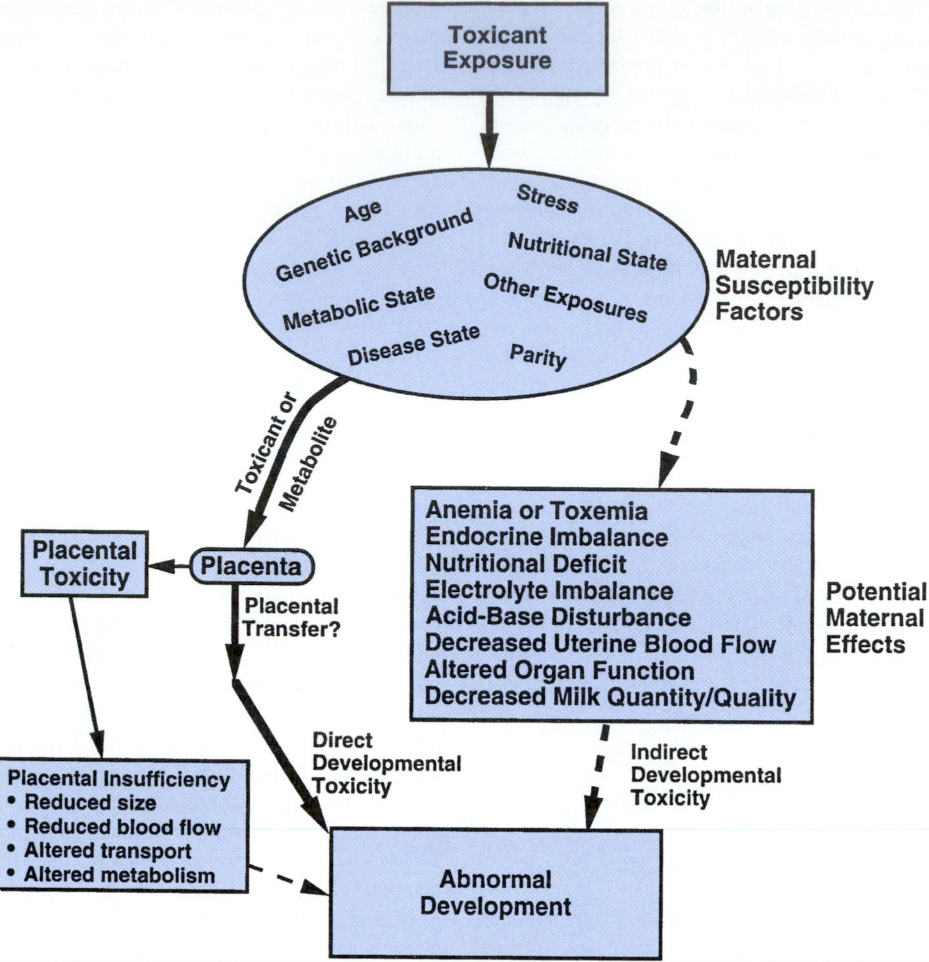

Figure 10- 7. Interrelationships between maternal susceptibility factors, metabolism, induction of maternal physiologic or functional alterations, placental transfer and toxicity, and developmental toxicity.

A developmental toxicant can cause abnormal development through any one or a combination of these pathways. Maternal susceptibility factors determine the predisposition of the mother to respond to a toxic insult, and the maternal effects listed can adversely affect the developing conceptus. Most chemicals traverse the placenta in some form, and the placenta can also be a target for toxicity. In most cases, developmental toxicity is probably mediated through a combination of these pathways.

humans, most notably malformations of the central nervous system (Warkany, 1986; Milunsky, et al., 1992).

Nutrition A wide spectrum of dietary insufficiencies ranging from protein-calorie malnutrition to deficiencies of vitamins, trace elements and/or enzyme cofactors is known to adversely affect pregnancy (Keen et al., 1993). Among the most significant findings related to human nutrition and pregnancy outcome in recent years are results of studies in which pregnant women at risk for having infants with neural tube defects (NTDs) were supplemented with folate (Wald, 1993). The largest and most convincing study is the Medical Research Council (MRC) Vitamin Study, in which supplementation with 4 mg of folic acid reduced NTD recurrence by over 70 percent (MRC, 1991; Bendich, 1993). Results of these studies have prompted the U.S. Centers for Disease Control and Prevention to recommend folate supplementation for women of childbearing age and folate supplementation of some foodstuffs.

Stress Diverse forms of maternal toxicity may have in common the induction of a physiologic stress response. Understanding potential effects of maternal stress on development may help interpret developmental toxicity observed in experimental animals at maternally toxic dosages. Various forms of physical stress have been applied to pregnant animals in attempts to isolate the developmental effects of stress. Subjecting pregnant rats or mice to noise stress throughout gestation can produce developmental toxicity (Kimmel et al., 1976; Nawrot et al., 1980, 1981). Restraint stress produces increased fetal death in rats (Euker and Riegle, 1973) and cleft palate (Barlow et al., 1975), fused and supernumerary ribs, and encephaloceles in mice (Beyer and Chernoff, 1986).

Objective data on effects of stress in humans are difficult to obtain. Nevertheless, studies investigating the relationship of maternal stress and pregnancy outcome have indicated a positive correlation between stress and adverse developmental effects, including low birth weight and congenital malformations (Stott, 1973; Gorsuch and Key, 1974).

Placental Toxicity The placenta is the interface between the mother and the conceptus, providing attachment, nutrition, gas exchange, and waste removal. The placenta also produces hormones critical to the maintenance of pregnancy, and it can metabolize and/or store xenobiotics. Placental toxicity may compromise these functions and produce or contribute to untoward effects on the conceptus. Slikker and Miller (1994) list 46 toxicants known to be toxic to the yolk sac or chorioallantoic placenta, including metals such as cadmium (Cd), arsenic or mercury, cigarette smoke, ethanol, cocaine, endotoxin and sodium salicylate (Daston, 1994; Slikker and Miller, 1994). Cd is among the best studied of these, and it appears that the developmental toxicity of Cd during mid- to late gestation involves both placental toxicity (necrosis, reduced blood flow) and inhibition of nutrient transport across the placenta. Maternal injection of Cd during late gestation results in fetal death in rats, despite little cadmium entering the fetus (Parizek, 1964; Levin and Miller, 1980). Fetal death occurs concomitant with reduced uteroplacental blood flow within 10 h (Levin and Miller, 1980). The authors' conclusion that fetal death was caused by placental toxicity was supported by experiments in which fetuses were directly injected with Cd. Despite fetal Cd burdens almost tenfold higher than those following maternal administration, only a slight increase in fetal death was observed.

Cd is a transition metal similar in its physicochemical properties to the essential metal zinc (Zn). Cadmium interferes with Zn transfer across the placenta (Ahokas et al., 1981; Sorell and Graziano, 1990), possibly via metallothionein (MT), a metal-binding protein induced in the placenta by Cd. Because of its high affinity for Zn, MT may sequester Zn in the placenta, impeding transfer to the conceptus (induction of maternal hepatic MT by Cd or other agents can also induce fetal Zn deficiency, as discussed below). Cadmium inhibits Zn uptake by human placental microvesicles (Page et al., 1992) suggesting that Cd may also compete directly with Zn for membrane transport. Cadmium may also competitively inhibit other Zn-dependent processes in the placenta. Coadministration of Zn ameliorates the developmental toxicity of administered Cd, further indicating that interference of Cd with Zn metabolism is a key to its developmental toxicity (Ferm and Carpenter, 1967, 1968; Daston, 1982).

Maternal Toxicity A retrospective analysis of relationships between maternal toxicity and specific types of prenatal effects found species-specific associations between maternal toxicity and specific adverse developmental effects. Yet, among rat, rabbit, and hamster studies, 22 percent failed to show any developmental toxicity in the presence of significant maternal toxicity (Khera, 1984, 1985). The approach of tabulating literature data suffers from possible bias in the types of studies published (e.g., negative results may not be published), incomplete reporting of maternal and developmental effects, and lack of standard criteria for the evaluation of maternal and developmental toxicity. In a study designed to test the potential of maternal toxicity to affect development, Kavlock et al. (1985) acutely administered 10 structurally unrelated compounds to pregnant mice at maternotoxic dosages. Developmental effects were agent-specific, ranging from complete resorption to lack of effect. An exception was an increased incidence of supernumerary ribs (ribs on the first lumbar vertebra), which occurred with 7 of the 10 compounds. Chernoff et al. (1990) dosed pregnant rats for 10 days with a series of compounds chosen because they exhibited little or no developmental toxicity in previous studies. When these compounds were administered at high dosages producing maternal toxicity (weight loss or lethality), a variety of adverse developmental outcomes was noted, including increased intrauterine death (two compounds), decreased fetal weight (two compounds), supernumerary ribs (two compounds), and enlarged renal pelves (two compounds). In addition, two of the compounds produced no developmental toxicity despite substantial maternal toxicity. These diverse developmental responses led the authors to conclude that maternal toxicity defined by weight loss or mortality is not associated with any consistent syndrome of developmental effects in the rat.

There have been a number of studies directly relating specific forms of maternal toxicity to developmental toxicity, including those in which the test chemical causes maternal effects that exacerbate the agent's developmental toxicity, as well as instances in which developmental toxicity is thought to be the direct result of adverse maternal effects. However, clear delineation of the relative role(s) of indirect maternal and direct embryo/fetal toxicity is difficult.

Acetazolamide inhibits carbonic anhydrase and is teratogenic in mice (Hirsch and Scott, 1983). Although maternal weight loss is not correlated with malformation frequency, maternal hypercapnia potentiates the teratogenicity of acetazolamide. In C57Bl/6J mice, maternal hypercapnia alone results in right forelimb ectrodactyly, the characteristic malformation induced by acetazolamide. Correction of maternal acidosis failed to reduce developmental toxicity, suggesting that the primary teratogenic factor was elevated maternal plasma CO_2 tension (Weaver and Scott, 1984a,b).

Diflunisal, an analgesic and anti-inflammatory drug, causes axial skeletal defects in rabbits. Developmentally toxic dosages resulted in severe maternal anemia (hematocrit = 20–24 percent vs. 37 percent in controls) and depletion of erythrocyte ATP levels (Clark et al., 1984). Teratogenicity, anemia, and ATP depletion were unique to the rabbit among the species studied. A single dose of diflunisal on day 5 of gestation produced a maternal anemia that lasted through day 15. Concentration of the drug in the embryo was less than 5 percent of the peak maternal blood level, and diflunisal was cleared from maternal blood before day 9, the critical day for induction of similar axial skeletal defects by hypoxia. Thus, the teratogenicity of diflunisal in the rabbit was probably due to hypoxia resulting from maternal anemia.

Phenytoin, an anticonvulsant, can affect maternal folate metabolism in experimental animals, and these alterations may play a role in the teratogenicity of this drug (Hansen and Billings, 1985). Further, maternal heart rates were monitored on gestation day 10 after administration to susceptible A/J mice and resistant C57Bl/6J mice (Watkinson and Millikovsky, 1983). Heart rates were depressed by phenytoin in a dose-related manner in the A/J mice but not in C57Bl/6J mice. A mechanism of teratogenesis was proposed relating depressed maternal heart rate and embryonic hypoxia. Supporting studies have demonstrated that hyperoxia reduces the teratogenicity of phenytoin in mice (Millicovsky and Johnston, 1981). Reduced uterine blood flow, has been proposed as a mechanism of teratogenicity caused by hydroxyurea, which produces elevated systolic blood pressure, altered heart rate, decreased cardiac output, severely decreased uterine blood flow, and increased vascular resistance in pregnant rabbits (Millicovsky et al., 1981). Embryos exhibited craniofacial and pericardial hemorrhages immediately after treatment (Millicovsky and DeSesso, 1980a), and identical embryopathies were achieved by clamping the uterine ves-

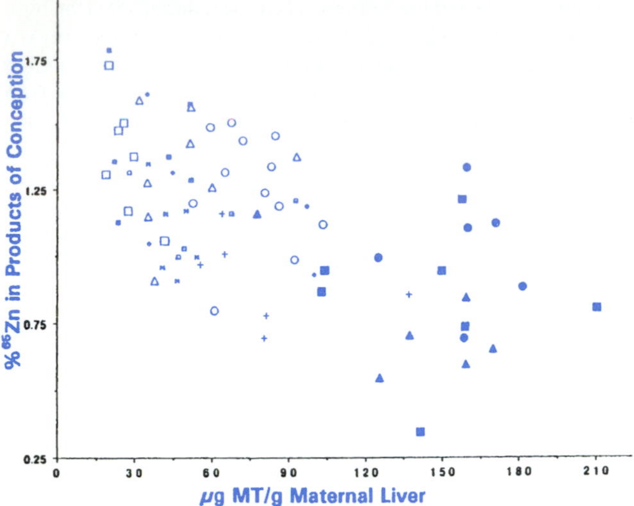

Figure 10-8. Transfer of ^{65}Zn to the products of conception as a function of maternal hepatic metallothionein (MT) concentration.

Pregnant rats were dosed on gestation day 11 with: ● α-hederin; □ dimethylsulfoxide; □ ethanol; ▴ urethane; +melphalan; ♦ acidified alcohol; or □ styrene, or were ○ food-deprived or ▵ food-restricted. □: Saline control. Eight hours after dosing, dams were orally gavaged with a diet slurry containing ^{65}Zn. The amount of ^{65}Zn transferred to the conceptuses was inversely correlated with the degree of treatment-related maternal hepatic MT induction. [Adapted from Taubeneck et al. (1994) with permission.]

sels of pregnant rabbits for 10 minutes (Millicovsky and DeSesso, 1980b).

Metallothionein synthesis is inducible by a wide variety of chemical and physical agents including metals, alcohols, urethane, endotoxin, alkylating agents, hyper- or hypothermia, and ionizing radiation (Daston, 1994). MT synthesis is also induced by endogenous mediators such as glucocorticoids and certain of the cytokines (Klaassen and Lehman-McKeeman, 1989). A mechanism common to the developmental toxicity of these diverse agents may be Zn deficiency of the conceptus secondary to induction of maternal MT. Induction of MT synthesis can produce hepatic MT concentrations over an order of magnitude higher than normal, leading to substantial sequestration of circulating Zn in maternal liver, lowered plasma Zn concentrations, and reduced Zn availability to the conceptus. Embryofetal zinc deficiency secondary to maternal hepatic MT induction has been demonstrated for diverse chemicals including valproic acid (Keen et al., 1989), 6-mercaptopurine (Amemiya et al., 1986, 1989), urethane (Daston et al., 1991), ethanol, and α-hederin (Taubeneck et al., 1994). In a study combining data for many of these compounds, Taubeneck and coworkers (1994) found a strong positive relationship between maternal hepatic MT induction and maternal hepatic ^{65}Zn retention, and a negative relationship between maternal MT induction and ^{65}Zn distribution to the litter (Fig. 10-8).

DEVELOPMENTAL TOXICITY OF ENDOCRINE-DISRUPTING CHEMICALS

One of the most pressing environmental issues facing developmental and reproductive toxicology in recent years has been the growing concern that exposure to chemicals that can interact with the endocrine system may pose a serious health hazard (Toppari, et al., 1996; Kavlock et al 1996; National Research Council, 1999). An "endocrine disruptor" has been broadly defined as "an exogenous agent that interferes with the production, release, transport, metabolism, binding, action, or elimination of natural hormones responsible for the maintenance of homeostasis and the regulation of developmental processes" (Kavlock et al., 1996). Due to the critical role of hormones in directing differentiation in many tissues, the developing organism is particularly vulnerable to fluctuations in the timing or intensity of exposure to chemicals with hormonal (or antihormonal) activity. Chemicals from a wide variety of chemical classes (e.g., pesticides, herbicides, fungicides, plasticizers, surfactants, organometals, halogenated polyaromatic hydrocarbons, phytoestrogens) have been shown to induce developmental toxicity via at least four modes of action involving the endocrine system: (1) by serving as steroid receptors ligands; (2) by modifying steroid hormone metabolizing enzymes; (3) by perturbing hypothalamic-pituitary release of trophic hormones; and (4) by as yet uncharacterized proximate modes of action. Interactions with the functions of estrogens, androgens, and thyroid hormones have been the most studied.

Laboratory Animal Evidence

Chemicals with estrogenic activity are a well-described class of developmental toxicants based on standard criteria of causing specific malformations during critical developmental periods of relatively short duration (Schardein, 2000). Estrogens induce pleiotropic effects, acting on many types of cells with estrogen receptors, and can display cell and organ-specific agonist and antagonist actions. The pattern of outcomes is generally similar across different estrogens, although not all possible outcomes have been described for each. Diethylstilbestrol (DES) provides one of the most well characterized examples of the effects of an estrogen on development. Manifestations of DES exposure include malformations and adverse functional alterations of the male and female reproductive tract and brain. In the CD-1 mouse, effective exposures are in the range of 0.01 to 100 µg/kg on GD 9-16 (Newbold, 1995). At the higher end of the exposure range (10 to 100 µg/kg), total sterility of female offspring is noted, due in part to structural abnormalities of the oviduct, uterus, cervix, and vagina and to depletion and abnormalities of ovarian follicles. In adulthood, male offspring show hypospadias, while females exhibit excessive vaginal keratinization and epidermoid tumors of the vagina. Vaginal adenocarcinoma is seen at dosages as low as 2.5 µg/kg. Benign uterine tumors (leiomyomas) are seen as low as 0.1 µg/kg. In male offspring, sterility is observed at high doses, the result of retained rete testes and Mullerian duct remnants, abnormal sperm morphology and motility, lesions in the reproductive tract (including cryptorchidism and rete testis adenocarcinoma), abnormal reproductive tract secretions, and inflammation (Newbold, 1995). Other estrogenic (or anti-estrogenic) developmental toxicants include estradiol (Biegel et al., 1998, Cook et al., 1998), ethynyl estradiol, antiestrogenic drugs such as tamoxifen and clomiphene citrate (Branham et al., 1988), and pesticides and industrial chemicals such as methoxychlor (Gray et al., 1989), *o,p'*-DDT (Heinrichs et al., 1971), kepone (Gellert, 1978; Guzelian, 1982), Zdioxins (Mably et al., 1992, Gray et al., 1997a, b), bisphenol A (Nagel et al., 1997), and phytoestrogens such as genistein and coumestrol (Medlock et al., 1995). Female offspring are generally more sensitive than males and altered pubertal development, reduced fertility, and reproductive tract anomalies are common findings.

While most of the studies on estrogens have indicated traditional dose–response patterns of effect, with severity and incidence increasing with dose, vom Saal and coworkers (vom Saal et al., 1997; Nagel et al., 1997) have reported that unusual dose–response patterns may occur for endocrine effects on some endpoints. In their studies, a 50 percent elevation in fetal serum estradiol concentration resulting from implantation of estradiol–containing Silastic capsules on days 13 to 19 of gestation in mice caused a 30 percent increase in adult prostate weight, whereas higher maternal serum concentrations were associated with decreased adult prostate weight. A similar pattern was observed for DES given on days 11 to 17 of gestation, as increased adult prostate weights were seen between 0.02 and 20 ng/kg/day, whereas 200 ng/kg/day resulted in smaller prostates. Bisphenol A (2 or 20 μg/kg/day on gestation days 11 to 17) also increased adult prostate weight in these mice. These examples indicate an inverted U-shaped dose–response curve for this endpoint, and bring into question the design of hazard identification studies in the risk assessment of endocrine-mediated developmental responses. However, the issue is controversial, as other researchers using similar testing paradigms have not seen this pattern (e.g., Cagen et al., 1999).

Antiandrogens represent another major class of endocrine disrupting chemicals. Principal manifestations of developmental exposure to an antiandrogen are generally restricted to males, and include hypospadias, retained nipples, reduced testes and accessory sex gland weights, and decreased sperm production. Examples of chemicals known to affect development via an antiandrogenic mechanism include pharmaceuticals such as the androgen receptor antagonist flutamide (Imperato-McGinley et al., 1992) and the 5α-reductase inhibitor finasteride (Clark et al., 1990), and environmentally relevant compounds such as the fungicide vinclozolin (Gray et al., 1994) and the DDT metabolite *p,p′*-DDE (Kelce et al., 1995; You et al., 1998) which are both androgen receptor antagonists. Recently, a phthalate ester (dibutylphthalate) has been shown to induce an antiandrogen phenotype in developing rats, but the effect does not appear to be mediated by direct interaction with the androgen receptor (Mylchreest et al., 1998, 1999). Hypothyroidism causes growth retardation, cognitive deficits, delayed eye opening, hyperactivity, and auditory defects in rodents. The most commonly used chemical to induce these outcomes is propylthiouracil. Polychlorinated biphenyls (PCBs) may act at several sites to lower thyroid hormone levels during development, and cause body weight and auditory deficits (Goldey et al., 1995; Goldey and Crofton, 1998). PCBs also cause learning deficits and alter locomotor activity patterns in rodents (Eriksson et al., 1991; Schantz et al., 1995) and monkeys (Bowman, 1982; Schantz et al., 1991). Some effects, such as deficits in spatial learning ability, closely resemble those seen following neonatal hypothyroidism (Porterfield, 1994). Interestingly, hypothyroidism induced by neonatal treatment of rats with Arochlor 1254 also increases testis weight and sperm production by prolonging the period in which Sertoli cell proliferation is possible (Cooke, Zhao, and Hansen, 1996).

Human Evidence

Despite the biological plausibility of effects demonstrated in numerous laboratory studies, it is not clear whether human health is being adversely impacted from exposures to endocrine disruptors present in the environment. In part this is due to the extraordinary difficulty in demonstrating cause-and-effect relationships in epidemiologic studies where the signals may be weak, the effects evident only long after an exposure, and the endpoints sensitive to a number of other factors. Reports in humans which are or may be relevant to developmental toxicity from endocrine disruption are of two types: (1) Observations of adverse effects on reproductive system development and function following exposure to chemicals with known endocrine activities that are present in medicines, contaminated food, or the workplace. These have tended to involve relatively higher exposure to chemicals with known endocrine effects. (2) Epidemiologic evidence of increasing trends in reproductive and developmental adverse outcomes that have an endocrine basis. With the exception of the classic case of DES (Herbst and Bern, 1981), evidence is either lacking to support a definitive link to an exposure, or appears to be variable across study populations as to whether the responses are observed at all. For example, secular trends have been reported for cryptorchidism (Toppari et al., 1996); hypospadias (Toppari et al., 1996; Pauluzzi et al., 1997; Pauluzzi, 1999); semen quality (Carlsen et al., 1992; Skakkebaek and Keiding, 1994; Olsen et al., 1995; Swan et al., 1997; Auger et al., 1995; de Mouzon et al., 1996; Irvine et al., 1996; Vierula et al., 1996; Bujan et al., 1996; Fisch and Goluboff, 1996), and testicular cancer (Toppari et al., 1996), but due to the lack of exposure assessment, such studies provide limited evidence of a cause and effect relationship.

The most convincing evidence for effects of endocrine-disrupting chemicals in humans comes from reports of neurobehavioral changes and learning deficits in children exposed to PCBs in utero or lactationally, either through their mothers' consumption of PCB-contaminated fish (Jacobson et al., 1990; Jacobson and Jacobson, 1996) or through exposure to background levels of PCBs in the United States (Rogan and Gladen, 1991) or the Netherlands (Koopman-Esseboom et al., 1996). In addition, there have been two occurrences of high level exposure to contaminated rice oil (in Japan in 1968 and in Taiwan in 1979) in which alterations in development of ectodermal tissues and delays in neurological development were seen (Hsu et al., 1985, Yu et al., 1991; Guo et al., 1994; Schecter et al., 1994). In these cases, there was co-exposure to polychlorinated dibenzofurans as well as PCBs. The precise mode of action of the developmental neurotoxicity of PCBs is, however, not yet understood.

Impact on Screening and Testing Programs

The findings of altered reproductive development following early life stage exposures to endocrine disrupting chemicals helped prompt revision of traditional safety evaluation tests such as those recently issued by the EPA (US EPA, 1997). These now include assessments of female estrous cyclicity, sperm parameters (total number, percent progressively motile and sperm morphology in both the parental and F1 generations), the age at puberty in the F1s (vaginal opening in the female, preputial separation in the males); an expanded list of organs for either pathology, gravimetric analysis, and/or histopathology to identify and characterize effects at the target organ; as well as some triggered endpoints including anogenital distance in the F2s and primordial follicular counts in the parental and F1 generations. For the new prenatal developmental toxicity test guidelines, one important modification aimed at improved detection of endocrine disruptors was the expansion of the period of dosing from the end of organogenesis (i.e., palatal closure) to the end of pregnancy in order to include the developmental period of urogenital differentiation.

Over the past several years, two environmental laws enacted by the U.S. Congress specifically require the testing of pesticides and other chemicals found in or on food or in drinking water sources be tested for their potential to cause "estrogenic or other endocrine effects in humans." The Food Quality Protection Act of 1996 (FQPA) and the Safe Drinking Water Act Amendments of 1996 (SDWA) require the EPA to, within 2 years of enactment, develop a screening program using appropriate, valid test systems to determine whether substances may have estrogenic or other endocrine effects in humans. The screening program must undergo a public comment period and peer review and be implemented within 3 years. The laws require that the manufacturers, registrants, or importers conduct the testing of the pesticides and other substances according to the program the EPA develops. An external advisory to EPA, the Endocrine Disruptor Screening and Testing Advisory Committee (EDSTAC), has recommended a battery of assays both for screening and testing potential EDCs that will be used to address the mandates of the FQPA and SDWA (US EPA, 1998). The assays are intended to detect potential interaction with both the sex steroids (estrogen and testosterone) and with thyroid hormone function, and include assessment of both potential human health effects and effects in wildlife. To help prioritize chemicals for screening and testing, the EDSTAC recommended a high through put screening (HTPS) cell-based, receptor-mediated gene transcription assay for chemicals that act either as agonists or antagonists for the estrogen, androgen, or thyroid receptor. It has been estimated that perhaps 15,000 chemicals would be evaluated in the HTPS. The EDSTAC recommendation for the "tier 1" screening (T1S) battery includes three in vitro assays and five in vivo assays. The in vitro assays in T1S include an estrogen receptor binding or transcriptional activation assay; an androgen receptor binding or transcriptional activation assay; and a steroidogenesis assay using minced testis. The five in vivo screens recommended include the rodent 3-day uterotrophic assay; a rodent 20-day pubertal female assay for effects on thyroid function; a male rodent 5-7 day Hershberger assay; a frog metamorphosis assay for thyroid effects; and a fish partial life cycle test. It is estimated that perhaps as many as 1500 chemicals would enter the T1S, and positive chemicals would move into a second level (T2T) where more defined toxicological responses would be characterized. Protocols for these assays are currently being developed, and they should be in use within the 5 year time frame set forth in the legislation.

MODERN SAFETY ASSESSMENT

Experience with chemicals that have the potential to induce developmental toxicity indicates that both laboratory animal testing and surveillance of the human population (i.e., epidemiologic studies) are necessary to provide adequate public health protection. Laboratory animal investigations are guided both by regulatory requirements for drug or chemical marketing as well as by the basic desire to understand mechanisms of toxicity.

Regulatory Guidelines for in Vivo Testing

Prior to the thalidomide tragedy, safety evaluations for reproductive effects were limited in both the types of chemicals evaluated and the sophistication of the endpoints. Subsequently, the FDA issued more extensive testing protocols (termed Segments I, II, and III) for application to a broader range of agents (US FDA, 1966). These testing protocols, with minor variations, were adopted by a variety of regulatory agencies around the world and remained similar for nearly thirty years. Several factors including the historical experience of testing thousands of chemicals, increased knowledge of basic reproductive processes, the ever-increasing cost of testing, the acknowledged redundancy and overlap of required protocols, a growing divergence in study design requirements of various countries, and the expanding international presence of the pharmaceutical industry have succeeded in producing new and streamlined testing protocols that have been accepted internationally (US FDA, 1994). These guidelines, the result of the International Conference of Harmonization of Technical Requirements for Registration of Pharmaceuticals for Human Use (ICH), specifically include considerable flexibility in implementation depending on the particular circumstances of the agent under evaluation. Rather than specify study and technical details, they rely on the investigator to meet the primary goal of detecting and bringing to light any indication of toxicity to reproduction. Palmer (1993) has provided an overview of issues relevant to implementing the ICH guideline. Key elements of the FDA Segment I, II and III studies, the ICH protocols, and the OECD equivalent of the FDA Segment II test are provided in Table 10-4. In each protocol, guidance is provided on species/strain selection, route of administration, number and spacing of dosage levels, exposure duration, experimental sample size, observational techniques, statistical analysis, and reporting requirements. Details are available in the original publications as well as in several reviews (e.g., Manson, 1994; Claudio et al., 1999). Variation of these protocols also exist that include extensions of exposure to early or later time points in development and extensions of observations to postnatal ages with more sophisticated endpoints. For example, the EPA has developed a Developmental Neurotoxicity Protocol for the rat that includes exposure from gestation day 6 though lactation day 10, and observation of postnatal growth, developmental landmarks of puberty (balanopreputial separation, vaginal opening), motor activity, auditory startle, learning and memory, and neuropathology at various ages through postnatal day 60 (US EPA, 1998).

The general goal of these regulatory studies is to identify the NOAEL, which is the highest dosage level that does not produce a significant increase in adverse effects in the offspring. These NOAELs are then used in the risk assessment process (see below) to assess the likelihood of effects in humans given certain exposure conditions.

Multigeneration Tests

Information pertaining to developmental toxicity can also be obtained from studies in which animals are exposed to the test substance continuously over one or more generations. For additional information on this approach, see Chap. 20.

Children's Health and the Food Quality Protection Act

In 1993, the National Academy of Sciences published a report entitled "Pesticides in the Diets of Infants and Children," which brought to light the fact that infants and children differ both qual-

Table 10-4

Summary of in Vivo Regulatory Protocol Guidelines for Evaluation of Developmental Toxicity

STUDY	EXPOSURE	ENDPOINTS COVERED	COMMENTS
***Segment I*:** Fertility and general reproduction study	Males: 10 weeks prior to mating Females: 2 weeks prior to mating	Gamete development, fertility, pre- and post implantation viability, parturition, lactation	Assesses reproductive capabilities of male and female following exposure over one complete spermatogenic cycle or several estrous cycles.
***Segment II*:** Teratogenicity test	Implantation (or mating) through end of organogenesis (or term)	Viability and morphology (external, visceral, and skeletal) of conceptuses just prior to birth	Shorter exposure to prevent maternal metabolic adaptation and to provide high exposure to the embryo during gastrulation and organogenesis. Earlier dosing option for bioaccumulative agents or those impacting maternal nutrition. Later dosing option covers male reproductive tract development and fetal growth and maturation.
***Segment III*:** Perinatal study	Last trimester of pregnancy through lactation	Postnatal survival, growth and external morphology	Intended to observe effects on development of major organ functional competence during the perinatal period, and thus may be relatively more sensitive to adverse effects at this time.
***ICH 4.1.1*:** Fertility protocol	Males: 4 weeks prior to mating Females: 2 weeks prior to mating	Males: Reproductive organ weights and histology, sperm counts and motility Females: Viability of conceptuses at mid-pregnancy or later	Improved assessment of male reproductive endpoints; shorter treatment duration than Segment I.
***ICH 4.1.2*:** Effects on prenatal and postnatal development, including maternal function	Implantation through end of lactation	Relative toxicity to pregnant versus non-pregnant female; postnatal viability, growth, development and functional deficits (including behavior, maturation, and reproduction)	Similar to Segment I study.
***ICH 4.1.3*:** Effects on embryo/fetal development	Implantation through end of organogenesis	Viability and morphology (external, visceral, and skeletal) of fetuses just prior to birth.	Similar to Segment II study. Usually conducted in two species (rodent and nonrodent).
OECD 414 Prenatal developmental toxicity study	Implantation (or mating) through day prior to cesarean section	Viability and morphology (external, visceral, and skeletal) of fetuses just prior to birth.	Similar to Segment II study. Usually conducted in two species (rodent and nonrodent).

itatively and quantitatively from adults in their exposure to pesticide residues in food because of different dietary composition and intake patterns and different activities (NRC, 1993). This report, along with the report from the International Life Sciences Institute entitled "Similarities and Differences between Children and Adults" (Guzelian et al., 1992) provided background and impetus for passage of the Food Quality Protection Act (FQPA) of 1996. The FQPA incorporates an additional tenfold safety factor for children, cumulative effects of toxicants acting through a common mode of action, aggregate exposure (i.e., same toxicant from different sources), and endocrine disruption (see above). The inclusion (at the discretion of the EPA) of the tenfold factor for calculating allowable intakes for children affects most strongly the pesticide industry, whose products appear as residues in food. The application of this safety factor is controversial, in part because its opponents claim that developmental susceptibility is already considered in other tests, such as the Segment II test for prenatal toxicity, the two-generation test, and the developmental neurotoxicity test. On the other hand, proponents applaud the measure and point to the numerous factors that may increase the exposure of infants and children to environmental toxicants and their susceptibility to harm from these exposures. Children have different diets than adults and also have activity patterns that change their exposure profile compared to adults, such as crawling on the floor or ground, putting their hands and foreign objects in their mouths, and raising dust and dirt during play. Even the level of their activity (i.e., closer to the ground) can affect their exposure to some toxicants. In addition to exposure differences, children are growing and developing, which makes them more susceptible to some types of insults. Effects of early childhood exposure, including neurobehavioral effects and cancer, may not be apparent until later in life. Debate continues over the approach to be used in risk assessment in consideration of infants and children.

Alternative Testing Strategies

A variety of alternative test systems have been proposed to refine, reduce, or replace reliance on the standard regulatory mammalian tests for assessing prenatal toxicity (Table 10-5). These can be grouped into assays based on cell cultures, cultures of embryos in vitro (including submammalian species), and short term in vivo tests. Some effort has been made to qualitatively and quantitatively compile results across both the standard and the alternative tests (Faustman, 1988; Kavlock, et al., 1991). Daston (1996) has discussed the theoretical and empirical underpinnings supporting the use of a number of these systems. Yet, validation of these alternative tests continues to be a major and as yet unresolved issue (Neubert, 1989; Welsch, 1990). Much of the early validation work used a selection of chemicals proposed by Smith et al. (1983) which has been criticized as being biased toward direct acting cytotoxicants and for not factoring in potential confounding of fetal effects by maternal toxicity (Johnson, 1985; Brown 1987). Lacking an accepted standard, assessing the significance of the sensitivity and specificity of results from the tests has been problematic. While it was initially hoped that the alternative approaches would become generally applicable to all chemicals, and help prioritize full scale testing, this has not been accomplished. Indeed, given the complexity of embryogenesis and the multiple mechanisms and target site of potential teratogens, it was perhaps unrealistic to have expected a single test, or even a small battery, to accurately prescreen the activity of chemicals in general. To date, their primary success has come from evaluating the relative potency of series of congeners when the prototype chemical has demonstrated appropriate concordance with the in vivo result (Kavlock, 1993). Over the past several years, a validation study of three in vitro embryotoxicity assays, the rat embryo limb bud micromass assay, the mouse embryonic stem cell test, and the rat embryo culture test, has been carried out (Genschow et al., 2000). This study involves interlaboratory blind trials to validate these assays, and the approach involves the development of "prediction models" which mathematically combine assay endpoints to determine which combination and formulation are most predictive of mammalian in vivo results.

An exception to the poor acceptance of alternate tests for prescreening for developmental toxicity is the in vivo test developed by Chernoff and Kavlock (1982). In this test, pregnant females are exposed during the period of major organogenesis to a limited number of dosage levels near those inducing maternal toxicity, and offspring are evaluated over a brief neonatal period for external malformations, growth, and viability. It has proven reliable over a large number of chemical agents and classes (Hardin et al., 1987), and a regulatory testing guideline has been developed (US EPA, 1985).

Epidemiology

Reproductive epidemiology is the study of the possible statistical associations between specific exposures of the father or pregnant woman and her conceptus and the outcome of pregnancy. In rare situations, such as rubella, thalidomide, and isotretinoin, where a relatively high risk exists and the outcome is a rare event, formal studies may not be needed to identify causes of abnormal birth outcomes. The plausibility of linking a particular exposure with a series of case reports increases with the rarity of the defect, the rarity of the exposure in the population, a small source population, a short time span for study, and biological plausibility for the association (Khoury et al., 1991). In other situations, such as occurred with ethanol and valproic acid, associations are sought through either a case-control or a cohort approach. Both approaches require accurate ascertainment of abnormal outcomes and exposures, and a large enough effect and study population to detect an elevated risk. Therein lies one of the difficulties for epidemiologists studying abnormal reproductive outcomes. For example, it has been estimated that the monitoring of more than 1 million births would have been necessary to detect a statistically significant increase in the frequency of spina bifida following the introduction of valproic acid in the United States, where the frequency of exposure was less than 1 in 1000 pregnancies and the risk was only a doubling over the background incidence (Khoury et al., 1987). Another challenge to epidemiologists is the high percentage of human pregnancy wastage, perhaps as much as 31 percent in the peri-implantation period (Wilcox et al., 1988) and an additional 15 percent that are clinically recognized. Therefore, pregnancy failures related to a particular exposure may go undetected in the general population. Furthermore, with the availability of prenatal diagnostic procedures, additional pregnancies of malformed embryos (particularly neural tube defects) are electively aborted. Thus, the incidence of abnormal outcomes at birth may not reflect the true rate of abnormalities, and the term prevalence, rather than incidence, is preferred when the denominator is the number of live births rather than total pregnancies. Other issues particularly relevant to reproductive epidemiology include homogeneity, recording proficiency and confounding. Homogeneity refers to the fact that a particular

Table 10-5
Brief Survey of Alternative Test Methodologies for Developmental Toxicity

ASSAY	BRIEF DESCRIPTION AND ENDPOINTS EVALUATED	CONCORDANCE*	REFERENCE(S)
Mouse ovarian tumor	Labelled mouse ovarian tumor cells added to culture dishes with concanavalin A coated disks for 20 min. Endpoint is inhibition of attachment of cells to disks.	Sensitivity: 19/31; 19/30 Specificity: 7/13; 5/13	Steele et al., 1988 (results from two labs)
Human embryonic palatal mesenchyme	Human embryonic palatal mesenchyme cell line grown in attached culture. Cell number assessed after 3 days.	Sensitivity: 21/31; 21/30 Specificity: 7/13; 5/13	Steele et al., 1988 (results from two labs)
Micromass culture	Midbrain and limb bud cells dissociated from rat embryos and grown in micromass culture for 5 days. Cell proliferation and biochemical markers of differentiation assessed.	Sensitivity: 25/27; 20/33; 11/15 Specificity: 17/19; 18/18; 8/10 Accuracy: 81%	Flint and Orton, 1984 Renault et al., 1989 Uphill et al., 1990 Genschow et al., 2000
Mouse embryonic stem cell (EST) test	(1) Mouse ESTs in 96-well plates assessed for differentiation and cytotoxicity after 7 days. (2) Mouse ESTs and 3T3 cells in 96-well plates assessed for viability after 3 and 5 days. ESTs grown for 3 days in hanging drops form embryoid bodies which are plated and examined after 10 days for differentiation into cardiocytes.	a) Sensitivity: 11/15 Specificity: 7/10 b) Accuracy:79%	(1) Newall and Beedles, 1996 (2) Scholz et al., 1999 Genschow et al., 2000
Chick embryo neural retina cell culture	Neural retinas of day 6.5 chick embryos dissociated and grown in rotating suspension culture for 7 days. Endpoints include cellular aggregation, growth, differentiation, and biochemical markers.	Sensitivity: 36/41 Specificity: 14/17	Daston et al., 1991 Daston et al., 1995a (concordances combined)
Drosophila	Fly larvae grown from egg disposition through hatching of adults. Adult flies examined for specific structural defects (bent bristles and notched wing).	Sensitivity: 10/13 Specificity: 4/5	Lynch et al., 1991
Hydra	*Hydra attenuata* cells are aggregated to form an "artificial embryo" and allowed to regenerate. Dose response compared to that for adult *Hydra* toxicity.	Sensitivity: n/a Specificity: n/a	Johnson and Gabel, 1982
FETAX	Mid-blastula stage *Xenopus* embryos exposed for 96 h and evaluated for viability, growth, morphology.	Sensitivity: n/a Specificity: n/a	Bantle, 1995 Fort et al., 2000
Rodent whole embryo culture	Postimplantation rodent embryos grown in vitro for up to two days and evaluated for growth and development. 3T3 cytotoxicity assay added by Genschow et al. (2000).	Accuracy: 84% (rat embryo culture with 3T3 cyto-toxicity assay)	Webster et al., 1997 Genschow et al., 2000
Chernoff/Kavlock assay	Pregnant mice or rats exposed during organogenesis and allowed to deliver. Postnatal growth, viability and gross morphology of litters assessed.	Sensitivity: 49/58 Specificity: 28/34	Hardin et al., 1987

*Authors interpretation. Sensitivity: correct identification of "positive" chemicals. Specificity: correct identification of "negative" compounds. Accuracy: correct classification of test agents as non-, weakly, or strongly teratogenic. Accuracy values are from Genschow et al. (2000).

outcome may be described differently by various recording units and that, even given a specific outcome, there can be multiple pathogenetic origins (e.g., cleft palate could arise by a variety of mechanisms). Recording difficulties relate to inconsistencies of definitions and nomenclature, and to difficulties in ascertaining or recalling outcomes as well as exposures. For example, birth weights are usually accurately determined and recalled, but spontaneous abortions and certain malformations may not be. Last, confounding by factors such as maternal age and parity, dietary factors, diseases and drug usage, and social characteristics must be accounted for in order to control for variables that affect both exposure and outcome (Khoury et al., 1992).

Epidemiologic studies of abnormal reproductive outcomes are usually undertaken with three objectives in mind: the first is scientific research into the causes of abnormal birth outcomes and usually involves analysis of case reports or clusters; a second aim is prevention and is targeted at broader surveillance of trends by birth defect registries around the world; and the last objective is informing the public and providing assurance. In this regard, it is informative to consider the review by Schardein (1993) of the method and year by which humans teratogens were detected. For 23 of 28 chemicals (including nine cancer therapeutics, androgenic hormones, antithyroid drugs, aminoglycoside antibiotics, coumarin anticoagulants, diethylstilbestrol, methylmercury, hydantoins, primidone, penicillamine, lithium, vitamin A, and retinoic acid), case reports presented the first evidence in humans. For two of these (diethylstilbestrol and lithium), the case reports were soon followed by registries that provided confirmation, while for two others (methyl mercury and hydantoins) follow-up epidemiology studies added support. For only four chemicals, alcohol, PCBs, carbamazepine, and cocaine, did an analytical epidemiological study provide the first human evidence. Evidence for one chemical, valproic acid, was first obtained by analysis of a birth defect registry. For the 28 chemicals in that review, human evidence of developmental toxicity preceded published animal evidence in eleven instances. Cohort studies, with their prospective exposure assessment and ability to monitor both adverse and beneficial outcomes, may be the most methodologically robust approach to identifying human developmental toxicants. The lack of cohort studies demonstrating risk for pregnancy may be in part due to the difficulty in making such associations, but may also reflect the fact that use in pregnancy is not associated with increased risk for the majority of drugs (Irl and Hasford, 2000).

As the human genome project comes to completion, we will have found most of the 100,000 or so human genes (Collins, 1998), and tests for over 700 genes are already available (Pagon, 1998). With ongoing genetic research, information on differential genetic susceptibility to birth defects will be accruing (Khoury, 2000). This new knowledge promises to elucidate links between genetics and disease susceptibility at a pace not possible previously. Understanding the genetic basis of susceptibility to environmentally induced birth defects will not only allow more inclusive risk assessments but should also lead to a better understanding of the mechanisms of action of developmental toxicants.

Concordance of Data

There have been several extensive reviews of the similarity of responses of laboratory animals and humans for developmental toxicants. In general, these studies support the assumption that results from laboratory tests are predictive of potential human effects. Concordance is strongest when there are positive data from more than one test species, although even in this case the results are not applicable to extrapolating specific types of effects across species. The predictiveness of animal data for presumed negative human developmental toxicants is less than that for positive agents, a finding probably related to the problems associated with ascertaining a negative response in humans as well as issues of inappropriate design or interpretation of animal studies. In a quantitative sense, the few comparisons that have been made suggest that humans tend to be more sensitive to developmental toxicants than is the most sensitive test species. While concordance among species for agents reported as positive is high, often special steps must be taken retrospectively to produce an animal model that reflects the nature of outcome in humans (e.g., valproic acid (Ehlers et al., 1992)).

Frankos (1985) reviewed data for 38 compounds having demonstrated or suspect activity in humans; all except tobramycin, which caused otologic defects, were positive in at least one and 76 percent were positive in more than one test species. Predictiveness was highest in the mouse (85 percent) and rat (80 percent), with lower rates for rabbits (60 percent) and hamsters (40 percent). Frankos identified 165 chemicals with no evidence of human effects; only 29 percent were negative in all species tested while 51 percent were negative in more than one species. Schardein and Keller (1989) examined concordance by species and developmental manifestation for 51 potential human developmental toxicants that had adequate animal data (three human developmental toxicants did not). Thalidomide received the widest testing, with data from 19 species; 53 percent had data from 3 species, while 18 percent had data from four or five species. Across all chemicals, the most common findings in humans, rabbits, and monkeys were spontaneous abortion and fetal/neonatal death followed by malformations and then growth retardation. In the rat, prenatal death, growth retardation, and then malformations was the typical pattern. The concordance of results is presented in Table 10-6. All species showed at least one positive response for 64 percent of the human developmental toxicants and, with only a single exception, all of the potential human developmental toxicants showed a positive response in at least one species. Overall, the match to the human, regardless of the nature of the developmental response, was rat, 98 percent; mouse, 91 percent; hamster, 85 percent; monkey, 82 percent; and rabbit, 77 percent. Jelovsek et al. (1989) reviewed the predictiveness of animal data for 84 negative human developmental toxicants, 33 with unknown activity, 26 considered suspicious and 32 considered positive. Variables considered included the response of each species, the number of positive and negative species, percent positive and negative species, and mutagenicity and carcinogenicity. The compounds were correctly classified 63–91 percent of the time based on animal data, depending upon how the suspect and unknown human toxicants were considered. The various models had a sensitivity of 62–75 percent, a positive predictive value of 75–100 percent, and a negative predictive value of 64 to 91 percent.

In addition to qualitative comparisons among species, several attempts at quantitative comparisons of potencies have been developed, although these have been based upon administered dosage and have not attempted to factor in pharmacokinetic differences. Schardein and Keller (1989) estimated the human and animal "threshold" dosages for 21 chemicals. In only two cases, aminopterin and carbon disulfide, were developmental effects seen at lower dosages in animal studies than were believed to cause effects in humans. For the other chemicals, ratios of the "threshold"

Table 10-6
Predictiveness of Animal Data for 51 Potential Human Developmental Toxicants

		MOUSE	RAT	MONKEY	RABBIT	HAMSTER
Potential human developmental toxicants tested (%)		86	96	33	61	26
Concordance by class	G[1]	61	57	65	39	39
	D	75	71	53	52	54
	M	71	67	65	65	62
	All	91	98	82	77	85
False positives	G	25	33	6	19	8
	D	11	16	18	10	0
	M	14	12	6	7	15
False negatives	G	10	14	29	39	54
	D	14	12	29	39	46
	M	11	25	29	29	23

KEY: G, growth retardation; D, death of conceptus; M, malformation; All, either growth, death, or malformations.
SOURCE: Adapted from Schardein and Keller (1989), with permission.

dosages in the most sensitive animals to those in humans ranged from 1.2 to 200. Newman et al. (1993) looked at the data for four well-characterized human developmental toxicants: valproic acid, isotretinoin, thalidomide, and methotrexate. The monkey was the most sensitive test species for the first three chemicals, while the rabbit was the most sensitive to methotrexate. Base upon the NOAEL of the most sensitive test species, human embryos were 0.9 to approximately 10 times more sensitive.

Elements of Risk Assessment

The extrapolation of animal test data for developmental toxicity follows two basic directions, one for drugs where exposure is voluntary and usually to high dosages, the other for environmental agents where exposure is generally involuntary and to low levels. For drugs, a use-in-pregnancy rating is utilized (US FDA, 1979). In this system the letters A, B, C, D, and X are used to classify the evidence that a chemical poses a risk to the human conceptus. For example, drugs are placed in category A if adequate, well-controlled studies in pregnant humans have failed to demonstrate a risk, and in category X (contraindicated for pregnancy) if studies in animals or humans, or investigational or postmarketing reports have shown fetal risk which clearly outweighs any possible benefit to the patient. The default category is C (risks cannot be rule out), assigned when there is a lack of human studies and animal studies are either lacking or are positive for fetal risk, but the benefits may justify the potential risk. Categories B and D represent areas of relatively lesser, or greater concern for risk, respectively. Manson (1993) reviewed the 1992 Physicians' Desk Reference and found 7 percent of the 1033 drugs belonged to category X, 66 percent to category C, and only 0.7 percent to category A. The FDA categorization procedure has been criticized (Teratology Society, 1994) as being too reliant on risk/benefit comparisons, especially given that the magnitude of risk is often unknown, or the benefits are not an issue (e.g., after the drug in question has been taken during early pregnancy and the question is then directed to the management of the exposed pregnancy). The FDA system has also been criticized for demanding an unrealistically high quality of data for assignment to category A (negative controlled studies in pregnant women) and overuse of category C, interpreted as "risks cannot be ruled out" (Sannerstedt et al., 1996). This is an important issue, because presently the perception of teratogenic risk is strong among both patients and prescribers even for safe drugs (Pole et al., 2000).

For environmental agents, the purpose of the risk assessment process for noncancer endpoints such as developmental toxicity is generally to define the dose, route, timing, and duration of exposure which induces effects at the lowest level in the most relevant laboratory animal model (US EPA, 1991). The exposure associated with this "critical effect" is then subjected to a variety of safety or uncertainty factors in order to derive an exposure level for humans that is presumed to be relatively safe (see Chap. 4, "Risk Assessment"). The principal uncertainty factors include one for interspecies extrapolation and one for variability in the human population. The default value for each of these factors is 10. In the absence of firm evidence upon which to base decisions on whether or not to extrapolate animal test data, certain default assumptions are generally made. They include (1) an agent that produces an adverse developmental effect in experimental animals will potentially pose a hazard to humans following sufficient exposure during development; (2) all four manifestations of developmental toxicity (death, structural abnormalities, growth alterations, and functional deficits) are of concern; (3) the specific types of developmental effects seen in animal studies are not necessarily the same as those that may be produced in humans; (4) the most appropriate species is used to estimate human risk when data are available (in the absence of such data, the most sensitive species is appropriate); and (5) in general, a threshold is assumed for the dose–response curve for agents that produce developmental toxicity.

One of the more troubling and subjective aspects of risk assessment for developmental toxicants is distinguishing between adverse effects (defined as an unwanted effect determined to be detrimental to health) and lesser effects, which while different than those observed in control groups, are not considered significant to human health. Considerations relevant to this issue can be categorized into two areas: (1) the observance of the finding and related events in the same or associated experiments; and (2) the understanding of the biology of the effect. The interpretation of reduced fetal growth in developmental toxicity studies illustrates most of the issues. While we have accepted definitions of low birth weight in humans and understand how intrauterine growth retardation translates to an elevated risk of infant mortality and mental retardation, we do not have similar knowledge for fetal weight in rodents, and we seldom even know if reduced fetal weight recorded in prenatal toxicity studies persists beyond birth. Further complicating matters, recent epidemiological evidence suggests that birth weight in humans is a predictor of adult-onset diseases including hypertension, cardiovascular disease, and diabetes (Rich-Edwards, et al., 1999; Osmond and Barker, 2000). Exposure to famine prenatally is also predictive of obesity at 50 years of age in women (Ravelli et al., 1999) and obstructive airway disease in adulthood (Lopuhaa et al., 2000). Animal models of the long-term latent effects of prenatal conditions and toxic exposures have not been developed.

New Approaches

The Benchmark-Dose Approach The use of safety or uncertainty factors applied to an experimentally derived NOAEL to arrive at a presumed safe level of human exposure is predicated on the risk assessment assumption that a threshold for developmental toxicity exists (see "Principles of Developmental Toxicology," above). A threshold should not be confused with the NOAEL, as the NOAEL is dependent entirely on the power of the study and, as will be seen later, is associated with risks perhaps on the order of 5 percent over the control incidence in typical studies. Also, the value obtained by the application of uncertainty factors to the NOAEL should not be confused with a threshold, as this exposure is only assumed to be without appreciable added risk.

The use of the NOAEL in the risk assessment process has been criticized for several reasons. For example, since it is dependent on statistical power to detect pair-wise differences between a treated and a control group, the use of larger sample sizes and more dose groups (which might better characterize the dose–response relationship) can only yield lower NOAELs, and thus better experimental designs are actually penalized by this approach. In addition, the NOAEL is limited to an experimental dose level, and an experiment might need to be repeated to develop a NOAEL for risk assessment. A final point relates to the fact that, given varying experimental designs and variability of control values, NOAELs actually represent different levels of risk across studies.

Crump (1984) proposed using a mathematical model to estimate the lower confidence bounds on a predetermined level of risk [the "benchmark dose" (BMD)]) as a means of avoiding many of the disadvantages of the NOAEL. The application of this approach to a large compilation of Segment II type data sets (Faustman et al.,

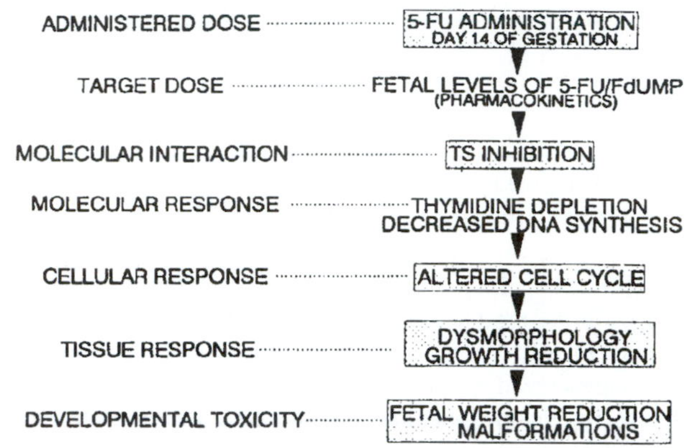

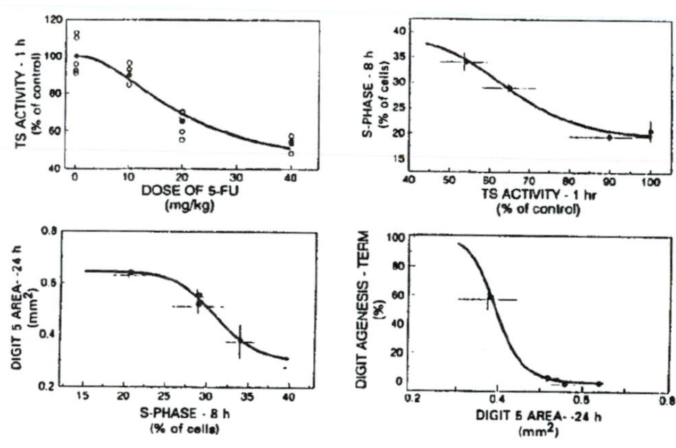

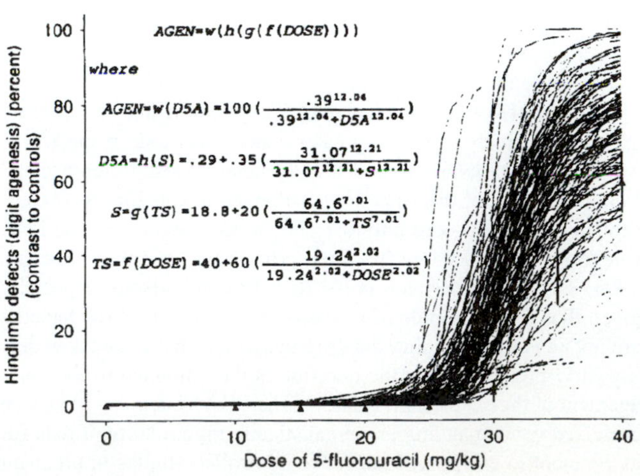

Figure 10-9. Biologically based dose response modeling of the developmental toxicity of 5-fluorouracil (5-FU) following maternal administration on gestation day 14.

Top: Proposed model for the developmental toxicity of 5-FU based on thymidylate synthetase (TS) inhibition, decreased DNA synthesis, cell cycle alterations, and growth deficits and hind-limb dysmorphogenesis. Shaded events were measured experimentally.

Middle: Relationships between successive endpoints are shown in these four panels (hind-limb bud TS activity versus 5-FU dose, S-phase accumulation versus TS activity, limb digit 5 area at 24 h postdose versus proportion of cells in S phase, and digit agenesis at term versus limb digit 5 area at 24 h). Data were fitted with Hill equations.

Bottom: Model for induction of hind-limb defects induced by 5-FU, generated by integration of the individual Hill equations describing the relationships between successive model endpoints as presented in the middle panels. These individual equations are listed here, and the curves were generated by Monte Carlo simulation to estimate variability around the predicted relationship. The simulation results indicate that variability in the intermediate endpoints can account for differences between the predicted and actual dose response. AGEN: digit agenesis at term; D5A: digit 5 area; S: percent of cells in S phase. [Adapted from Shuey et al. (1994), with permission.]

1994; Allen, et al., 1994a,b; Kavlock, 1995) demonstrated that a variety of mathematical models, including those that incorporate developmental-specific features such as litter size and intra-litter correlations, can be readily applied to standard test results. On average, benchmark doses based on a 5 percent added risk of effect calculated on quantal endpoints (e.g., whether an implant was affected or not) were approximately equivalent to traditionally determined NOAELs. When the litter was used as the unit of response (did it contain at least one affected implant?), benchmarks calculated for a 10 percent added risk were most similar to the correspondingly determined NOAEL. Discrepancies between the benchmark dose and the NOAEL were most pronounced when one or more of the following conditions were present: a shallow dose–response, small sample sizes, wide spacing of experimental dosage levels, or more than the typical number of dose levels. These features tend to make determination of the NOAEL more problematic (usually higher) and the confidence limits around the maximum likelihood estimate broader (resulting in lower BMDs).

Biologically Based Dose–Response Modeling The introduction of statistical dose–response models for noncancer endpoints is the first step in developing quantitative, mechanistic models that will help reduce the major uncertainties of high-to-low dose and species-to-species extrapolation of experimental data. These biologically based dose–response models integrate pharmacokinetic information on target tissue dosimetry with molecular/biochemical responses, cellular/tissue responses, and developmental toxicity (O'Flaherty, 1997; Lau and Setzer, 2000). Gaylor and Razzaghi (1992) proposed a model which related induction of cleft palate to fetal growth inhibition, and Gaylor and Chen (1993) proposed a model relating fetal weight and the probability of fetal abnormality. Shuey et al. (1994) presented a model using the cancer chemotherapeutic 5-fluorouracil (Fig. 10-9). They postulated that the developmental toxicity observed in the term fetus was due to an active metabolite (FdUMP) inhibiting the enzyme thymidylate synthetase, with subsequent depletion of thymidine, decreased DNA synthetic rates, reduced cell proliferation, and, ultimately, reduce tissue growth and differentiation. Each step in the process was determined experimentally and the relationships were described by Hill equations. The individual equations were then linked in an integrated model to describe the entire relationship between administered dose and the incidence of hind limb defects. While this is still an empirically based model, the process clearly demonstrated the utility of the approach in understanding the relative importance of various pathways of abnormal development in the ultimate manifestation and in providing a basis for models which could incorporate species-specific response parameters. Leroux and coworkers (1996) took a more theoretical approach, using a cell kinetic model in which a progenitor cell would either divide, differentiate, or die, each event proceeding at a certain rate. These authors constructed a stochastic model based on the premise that a malformation occurs when the number of differentiated cells is less than a critical number for a given stage of development. Ultimately, BBDR models will need to be generalizable across dose, route of exposure, species, and perhaps even chemicals of similar mechanistic classes.

PATHWAYS TO THE FUTURE

Since the last edition of this text, The National Research Council has assembled a committee to assess the state of the science in the area of mechanisms of normal and abnormal development and to explore opportunities to bring new knowledge and approaches to bear on developmental toxicology and risk assessment. In 2000, the committee released its report, "Scientific Frontiers in Developmental Toxicology and Risk Assessment" (NRC, 2000). The report presents a number of exciting findings and ideas, and should serve as a framework to help advance the field of developmental toxicology in the next decade.

The NRC committee reports that major discoveries have been made about mechanisms of normal development, that these mech-

Table 10-7
The 17 Intercellular Signaling Pathways Used in Development by Most Metazoans

PERIOD DURING DEVELOPMENT	SIGNALING PATHWAY
Before organogenesis; later for growth and tissue renewal	1. Wingless-Int pathway 2. Transforming growth factor β pathway 3. Hedgehog pathway 4. Receptor tyrosine kinase pathway 5. Notch-Delta pathway 6. Cytokine pathway (STAT pathway)
Organogenesis and cytodifferentiation; later for growth and tissue renewal	7. Interleukin-1-toll nuclear factor-kappa B pathway 8. Nuclear hormone receptor pathway 9. Apoptosis pathway 10. Receptor phosphotyrosine phosphatase pathway
Larval and adult physiology	11. Receptor guanylate cyclase pathway 12. Nitric oxide receptor pathway 13. G-protein coupled receptor (large G proteins) pathway 14. Integrin pathway 15. Cadherin pathway 16. Gap junction pathway 17. Ligand-gated cation channel pathway

SOURCE: Modified from NRC (2000).

anisms are conserved in diverse animals, many of which have been used extensively in developmental biology and genetics, including the fruit fly, roundworm, zebrafish, frog, chick and mouse. Seventeen conserved intercellular signaling pathways are described which are used repeatedly at different times and locations during development of these and other animal species, as well as in humans (Table 10-7). The conserved nature of these key pathways provides a strong scientific rationale for using these animal models to advantage for developmental toxicology. Not only are these organisms advantageous for developmental toxicity studies due to their well-known genetics and embryology and their rapid generation time, but they are also amenable to genetic manipulation to enhance the sensitivity of specific developmental pathways or to incorporate human genes, such as those of drug metabolizing enzymes, to answer questions of interspecies extrapolation.

The Hedgehog signaling pathway serves as an example of the exciting linkages being made between embryology, genetics, and toxicology. This pathway, first discovered in *Drosophila,* is also present in vertebrates and is important in the development of a number of organs including the central nervous system, the limbs and the face. Ligands for the hedgehog family receptors require proteolytic cleavage and addition of cholesterol for activation, and this pathway is exemplified by the Sonic Hedgehog (SHH) pathway in Fig. 10-10. The receptor for the SHH ligand, called *patched (ptc),* is associated with and normally represses function of the membrane protein *smoothened (smo).* Binding of SHH to *ptc* derepresses function of *smo,* leading to activation of specific transcription factors and transcription of target genes. Mutations of the SHH gene lead to holoprosencephaly (a malformation involving the forebrain and associated structures) in mice and humans. Toxicologically, cyclopamine and jervine, plant alkaloids that bind to *ptc,* can induce holoprosencephaly in animals. Further, covalent binding of cholesterol is required for SHH activity, and cholesterol synthesis inhibitors have also been shown to cause holoprosencephaly. Understanding of the biochemistry and function of this signaling pathway in normal development elucidates the mechanisms of toxicity leading to holoprosencephaly. Conversely, use of

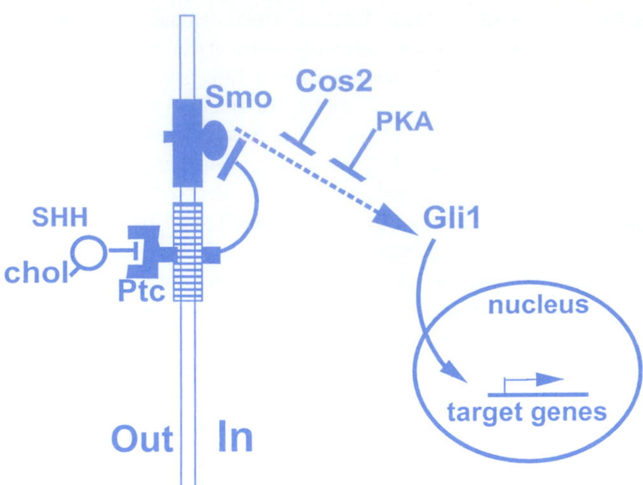

Figure 10-10. Diagram showing the transduction of the Sonic Hedgehog (SHH) signal through the patched (ptc) and smoothened (smo) receptor complex.

The SHH protein requires proteolytic cleavage and covalent binding to cholesterol (chol) prior to binding to ptc. Binding to ptc derepresses smo, which activates a signal cascade of transcription factor (gli) activation and target-gene transcription.

such specific toxicants as pharmacological probes allows confirmation of the role of this pathway in brain development.

Other avenues of increased understanding and progress enumerated in the NRC report include increased understanding of human genetic polymorphisms and their contribution to susceptibility to birth defects, use of sensitized animal models for high to low dose extrapolation, use of stress/checkpoint pathways as indicators of developmental toxicity, implementation of bioinformatic systems to improve data archival and retrieval, and increased multidisciplinary education and research on the causes of birth defects. Hopefully, there will be much to report on the progress of these efforts by the next addition of this text.

REFERENCES

Abel EL: Factors affecting the outcome of maternal alcohol exposure: I. Parity. *Neurobehav Toxicol Teratol* 3:49–51, 1984.

Abel EL: Consumption of alcohol during pregnancy: A review of effects on growth and development of offspring. *Hum Biol* 54:421–453, 1982.

Abel EL, Church MW, Dintcheff BA: Prenatal alcohol exposure shortens life span in rats. *Teratology* 36:217–220, 1987.

Adler T: The return of thalidomide. *Science News* 146:424–425, 1994.

Ahokas RA, Dilts PV Jr, LaHaye EB: Cadmium-induced fetal growth retardation: Protective effect of excess dietary zinc. *Am J Obstet Gynecol* 136:216–221, 1980.

Alford CA, Stagno S, Reynolds DW: Perinatal infections caused by viruses, *Toxoplasma,* and *Treponema pallidum,* in Aldjem S, Brown AK (eds): *Clinical Perinatology.* St. Louis: Mosby, 1974, p 31.

Allen BC, Kavlock RJ, Kimmel CA, Faustman EM: Dose response assessment for developmental toxicity: II. Comparison of generic benchmark dose models with No Observed Adverse Effect Levels. *Fundam Appl Toxicol* 23:487–495, 1994a.

Allen BC, Kavlock RJ, Kimmel CA, Faustman EM: Dose response assessment for developmental toxicity: III. Statistical models. *Fundam Appl Toxicol* 23:496–509, 1994b.

Amemiya K, Hurley LS, Keen CL: Effect of the anticarcinogenic drug 6-mercaptopurine on mineral metabolism in the mouse. *Toxicol Lett* 25:55–62, 1985.

Amemiya K, Hurley LS, Keen CL: Effect of 6-mercaptopurine on 65Zn distribution in the pregnant rat. *Teratology* 39:387–393, 1989.

Arafa HM, Elmazar MM, Hamada FM, et al: Selective agonists of retinoic acid receptors: Comparative toxicokinetics and embryonic exposure. *Arch Toxicol* 73:547–556, 2000.

Argiles JM, Carbo N, Lopez-Soriano FJ: Was tumour necrosis factor-alpha responsible for the fetal malformations associated with thalidomide in the early 1960's? *Med Hypotheses* 50:313–318, 1998.

Auger J, Kunstmann JM, Czyglik F, Jouannet P: Decline in semen quality among fertile men in Paris during the past 20 years. *N Engl J Med* 332:281–285, 1995.

Augustine K, Liu ET, Sadler TW: Antisense attenuation of Wnt-1 and Wnt-3a expression in whole embryo culture reveals roles for these genes in craniofacial, spinal cord, and cardiac morphogenesis. *Dev Genet* 14:500–520, 1993.

Ballantyne JW: *Manual of Antenatal Pathology and Hygiene: The Embryo.* Edinburgh: Green and Sons, 1904.

Balling R, Mutter G, Gruss P, Kessel M: Craniofacial abnormalities induced by ectopic expression of the homeobox gene Hox-1.1 in transgenic mice. *Cell* 58:337–347, 1989.

Bantle JA: FETAX: A developmental toxicity assay using frog embryos, in Rand G (ed): *Fundamentals of Aquatic Toxicology: Effects, Environmental Fate, Risk Assessment,* 2d ed. Washington, DC: Taylor and Francis, 1995, pp 207–230.

Barlow SM, McElhatton PR, Sullivan FM: The relation between maternal restraint and food deprivation, plasma corticosterone, and cleft palate in the offspring of mice. *Teratology* 12:97–103, 1975.

Barrow MV: A brief history of teratology to the early 20th century. *Teratology* 4:119–130, 1971.

Bateson W: *Materials for the Study of Variation Treated with Especial Regard to Discontinuity in the Origin of Species.* London: Macmillan, 1894.

Bennett GD, Wlodarczyk B, Calvin JA, et al: Valproic acid-induced alterations in growth and neurotrophic factor. *Reprod Toxicol* 14:1–11, 2000.

Beyer PE, Chernoff N: The induction of supernumerary ribs in rodents: Role of maternal stress. *Teratogenesis Carcinog Mutagen* 6:419–429, 1986.

Bibbo M, Gill W, Azizi F, et al: Follow-up study of male and female offspring of DES-exposed mothers. *Obstet Gynecol* 49:1–8, 1977.

Biegel LB et al: 90-day feeding and one-generation study reproduction study in Crl:CR BR rat with 17β-estradiol. *Toxicol Sci* 44:116–142, 1998.

Bowman RE: Behavioral sequelae of toxicant exposure during neurobehavioral development, in Hunt VR, Smith MK, Worth D (eds): *Banbury Report 11: Environmental Factors in Human Growth and Development.* Cold Spring Harbor, NY: Cold Spring Harbor Laboratory Press, 1982, pp 283–294.

Branham WS, Zehr DR, Chen JJ, Sheehan DM: Uterine abnormalities in rats exposed neonatally to diethylstilbestrol, ethynylestradiol, or clomiphene citrate. *Toxicology* 51:201–212, 1998.

Brent RL, Beckman DA: Environmental teratogens. *Bull NY Acad Med* 66:123–163, 1990.

Brown N: Teratogenicity testing in vitro: Status of validation studies. *Arch Toxicol Suppl* 11:105–114, 1987.

Bujan L, Mansat A, Pontonnier F, Mieusset R: Time series analysis of sperm concentration in fertile men in Toulouse, France between 1977 and 1992. *Br Med J* 312:471–472, 1996.

Cagen SZ, Waechter JM, Dimond SS, et al: Normal reproductive organ development in CF-1 mice following prenatal exposure to Bisphenol A. *Toxicol Sci* 50:36–44, 1999.

Calabrese L, Fleischer AB: Thalidomide: Current and potential clinical applications. *Am J Med* 108:487–495, 2000.

Capecchi MR: Altering the genome by homologous recombination. *Science* 244:1288–1292, 1989.

Carlsen E, Giwercman A, Keiding N, Skakkebaek NE: Evidence for decreasing quality of semen during past 50 years. *Br Med J* 305:609–613, 1992.

Centers for Disease Control: *MMWR* 32(33):438–439, 1983.

Centers for Disease Control: *MMWR* 31(42):565–566, 1982.

Chambon P: The retinoid signaling pathway: molecular and genetic analyses. *Semin Cell Biol* 5:115–125, 1994.

Chernoff N, Kavlock RJ: An in vivo teratology screen utilizing pregnant mice. *J Environ Toxicol Health* 10:541–550, 1982.

Chernoff N, Rogers JM, Alles AJ, et al: Cell cycle alterations and cell death in cyclophosphamide teratogenesis. *Teratogenesis Carcinog Mutagen* 9:199–209, 1989.

Chernoff N, Setzer RW, Miller DM, et al: Effects of chemically-induced maternal toxicity on prenatal development in the rat. *Teratology* 42:651–658, 1990.

Clark DO: Pharmacokinetic studies in developmental toxicology: Practical considerations and approaches. *Toxicol Meth* 3:223–251, 1993.

Clark DO, Elswick BA, Welsch F, Conolly R: Pharmacokinetics of 2-methoxyethanol and 2-methoxyacetic acid in the pregnant mouse: A physiologically based mathematical model. *Toxicol Appl Pharmacol* 121:239–252, 1993.

Clark RL, Antonello JM, Grosman SJ, et al: External genitalia abnormalities in male rats exposed in utero to finasteride, a 5α-reductase inhibitor. *Teratology* 42:91–100, 1990.

Clark RL, Robertson RT, Minsker DH, et al: Diflunisal-induced maternal anemia as a cause of teratogenicity in rabbits. *Teratology* 30:319–332, 1984.

Clarren SK: The diagnosis and treatment of fetal alcohol syndrome. *Comprehensive Therapy* 8:41–46, 1982.

Clarren SK, Sampson PD, Larsen J, et al: Facial effects of fetal alcohol exposure: Assessment by photographs and morphometric analysis. *Am J Med Genet* 26:651–666, 1987.

Claudio L, Bearer CF, Wallinga D: Assessment of the US Environmental Protection Agency methods for identification of hazards to developing organisms: Part II. The developmental toxicity testing guideline. *Am J Ind Med* 35:554–563, 1999.

Cohlan SQ: Congenital anomalies in the rat produced by excessive intake of vitamin A during pregnancy. *Pediatrics* 13:556–567, 1954.

Colburn T, vom Saal FS, Soto AM: Developmental effects of endocrine-disrupting chemicals in wildlife and humans. *Environ Health Perspect* 378–384, 1993.

Collins FS, Patrinos A, Jordan E, et al: New goals for the US Human Genome Project: 1998–2003. *Science* 282:682–689, 1998.

Collins MD, Mao GE: Teratology of retinoids. *Annu Rev Pharmacol Toxicol* 39:399–430, 1999.

Cook JC, Johnson L, O'Connor JC, et al: Effects of dietary 17β-estradiol exposure on serum hormone concentrations and testicular parameters in male Crl:CD BR rats. *Toxicol Sci* 44:155–168, 1998.

Cooke PS, Zhao YD, Hansen L: Neonatal polychlorinated biphenyl treatment increases adult testis size and sperm production in the rat. *Toxicol Appl Pharmacol* 136:112–117, 1996.

Cooper LZ, Krugman S: Diagnosis and management: Congeneital rubella. *Pediatrics* 37:335–342, 1966.

Craig JC, Bennett GD, Miranda RC, et al: Ribonucleotide reductase subunit R1: A gene conferring sensitivity to valproic acid-induced neural tube defects in mice. *Teratology* 61:305–313, 2000.

Crump K: A new method for determining allowable daily intakes. *Fundam Appl Toxicol* 4:854–871, 1984.

Dai WS, LaBraico JM, Stern RS: Epidemiology of isotretinoin exposure during pregnancy. *J Am Acad Dermatol* 26:599–606, 1992.

D'Amato RJ, Loughman MS, Flynn E, Folkman J: Thalidomide is an inhibitor of angiogenesis. *Proc Natl Acad Sci* 91:4082–4085, 1994.

Dareste C: *Récherches sur la production artificielle des monstruositiés, ou essais de tératogénie expérimentale,* 2d ed. Paris: Reinwald, 1891.

Dareste C: *Récherches sur la production artificielle des monstruositiés, ou essais de tératogénie expérimentale.* Paris: Reinwald, 1877.

Daston GP: The theoretical and empirical case for in vitro developmental toxicity screens, and potential applications. *Teratology* 53:339–344, 1996.

Daston GP: Relationships between maternal and developmental toxicity, in Kimmel CA, Buelke-Sam J (eds): *Developmental Toxicology,* 2d ed. New York: Raven Press, pp 189–212, 1994.

Daston GP: Do thresholds exist for developmental toxicants? A review of the theoretical and experimental evidence, in Kalter H (ed): *Issues and Review in Teratology.* New York: Plenum Press, 1993, pp 169–197.

Daston GP: Fetal zinc deficiency as a mechanism for cadmium-induced toxicity to the developing rat lung and pulmonary surfactant. *Toxicology* 24:55–63, 1982.

Daston GP, Baines D, Elmore E, et al: Evaluation of chick embryo neural retina cell culture as a screen for developmental toxicants. *Fundam Appl Toxicol* 26:203–210, 1995.

Daston GP, Baines D, Yonker JE: Chick embryo neural retinal cell culture as a screen for developmental toxicity. *Toxicol Appl Pharmacol* 109:352–366, 1991.

de Mouzon J, Thonneau P, Spira A, Multigner L: Semen quality has declined among men born in France since 1950. *Br Med J* 313:43, 1996.

Dempsey DA, Hajnal BL, Partridge JC, et al: Tone abnormalities are associated with maternal cigarette smoking during pregnancy in in utero cocaine-exposed infants. *Pediatrics* 106:79–85, 2000.

DeSesso JM: Maternal factors in developmental toxicity. *Teratogenesis Carcinog Mutagen* 7:225–240, 1987.

Dreosti IE: Nutritional factors underlying the expression of the fetal alcohol syndrome. *Ann NY Acad Sci* 678:193–204, 1993.

Dupe V, Ghyselinck NB, Thomazy V, et al: Essential roles of retinoic acid signaling in interdigital apoptosis and control of BMP-7 expression in mouse autopods. *Dev Biol* 208:30–43, 1999.

Edwards MJ: Hyperthermia as a teratogen: A review of experimental studies and their clinical significance. *Teratog Carcinog Mutag* 6:563–582, 1986.

Ehlers K, Sturje H, Merker H-J, Nau H: Spina bifida aperta induced by valproic acid and by all-*trans*-retinoic acid in the mouse: Distinct differences in morphology and periods of sensitivity. *Teratology* 46:117–130, 1992.

Eibs HG, Speilman H, Hagele M: Teratogenic effects of cyproterone acetate and medroxyprogesterone treatment during the pre- and postimplantation period of mouse embryos. *Teratology* 25:27–36, 1982.

Elstein KH, Zucker RM, Andrews JE, et al: Effects of developmental stage and tissue type on embryo/fetal DNA distributions and 5-fluorouracil-induced cell-cycle perturbations. *Teratology* 48:355–363, 1993.

Eriksson P, Lundkvist U, Fredricksson A: Neonatal exposure to 3,4,3′,4′-tetrachlorobiphenyl: Changes in spontaneous behavior and cholinergic muscarinic receptors in the adult mouse. *Toxicology* 69:27–34, 1991.

Ernhart CB, Sokol RJ, Martier S, et al: Alcohol teratogenicity in the human: A detailed assessment of specificity, critical period and threshold. *Am J Obstet Gynecol* 156:33–39, 1987.

Euker JS, Riegle GD: Effect of stress on pregnancy in the rat. *J Reprod Fertil* 34:343–346, 1973.

Fabro S: Passage of drugs and other chemicals into the uterine fluids and preimplantation blastocyst, in Boreus L (ed): *Fetal Pharmacology.* New York: Raven Press, 1973, pp 443–461.

Fabro S, McLachlan JA, Dames NM: Chemical exposure of embryos during the preimplantation stages of pregnancy: Mortality rate and intrauterine development. *Am J Obstet Gynecol* 148:929–938, 1984.

Faiella A, Wernig M, Consalez GG, et al: A mouse model for valproate teratogenicity: Parental effects, homeotic transformations, and altered HOX expression. *Hum Mol Genet* 9:227–236, 2000.

Fantel AG, Greenaway JC, Juchau MR, Shepard TH: Teratogenic bioactivation of cyclophosphamide in vitro. *Life Sci* 25:67–72, 1979.

Faustman EM: Short-term tests for teratogens. *Mutat Res* 205:355–384, 1988.

Faustman EM, Allen BC, Kavlock RJ, Kimmel CA: Dose response assessment for developmental toxicity: I. Characterization of database and determination of No Observed Adverse Effect Levels. *Fundam Appl Toxicol* 23:478–486, 1994.

Ferm VH, Carpenter SJ: Teratogenic effect of cadmium and its inhibition by zinc. *Nature* 216:1123, 1967.

Finnell RH, Wlodarczyk BC, Craig JC, et al: Strain-dependent alterations in the expression of folate pathway genes following teratogenic exposure to valproic acid in a mouse model. *Am J Med Genet* 70:303–311, 1997.

Fisch H, Goluboff ET: Geographic variation in sperm counts: A potential cause of bias in studies of semen quality. *Fertil Steril* 65:1044–1046, 1996.

Fisher JW, Whitaker TA, Taylor DH, et al: Physiologically based pharmocokinetic modeling of the pregnant rat: A multiroute exposure model for trichloroethylene and its metabolite, trichloroacetic acid. *Toxicol Appl Pharmacol* 99:395–414, 1989.

Flint OP, Orton TC: An in vitro assay for teratogens with culture of rat embryo midbrain and limb bud cells. *Toxicol Appl Pharmacol* 76:383–395, 1984.

Fort DJ, Stover EL, Farmer DR, Lemen JK: Assessing the predictive validity of frog embryo teratogenesis assay—*Xenopus* (FETAX). *Teratogenesis Carcinog Mutagen* 20:87–98, 2000.

Francis BM, Rogers JM, Sulik KK, et al: Cyclophosphamide teratogenesis: Evidence for compensatory responses to induced cellular toxicity. *Teratology* 42:473–482, 1990.

Frankos VH: FDA perspectives on the use of teratology data for human risk assessment. *Fundam Appl Toxicol* 5:615–622, 1985.

Fried PA, Watkinson B, Gray R: Differential effects on cognitive functioning in 9- to 12-year olds prenatally exposed to cigarettes and marihuana. *Neurotoxicol Teratol* 20:293–306, 1998.

Fullerton PM, Kermer M: Neuropathy after intake of thalidomide. *Br Med J* 2:855–858, 1961.

Gabrielson JL, Larson KS: Proposals for improving risk assessment in reproductive toxicology. *Pharmacol Toxicol* 66:10–17, 1990.

Gabrielson JL, Paalkow LK: A physiological pharmacokinetic model for morphine disposition in the pregnant rat. *J Pharmacokinet Biopharm* 11:147–163, 1983.

Gargas ML, Tyler TR, Sweeney LM, et al: A toxicokinetic study of inhaled ethylene glycol monomethyl ether (2-ME) and validation of a physiologically based pharmacokinetic model for the pregnant rat and human. *Toxicol Appl Pharmacol* 165:53–62, 2000.

Gaylor DW, Chen JJ: Dose response models for developmental malformations. *Teratology* 47:291–297, 1993.

Gaylor DW, Razzaghi M: Process of building biologically based dose response models for developmental defects. *Teratology* 46:573–581, 1992.

Gaylor DW, Sheehan DM, Young JF, Mattison DR: The threshold dose question in teratogenesis. *Teratology* 38:389–391, 1988.

Gellert RJ: Kepone, mirex, dieldrin and aldrin: Estrogenic activity and the induction of persistent vaginal estrus and anovulation in rats following prenatal treatment. *Environ Res* 16:131–138, 1979.

Generoso WM, Rutledge JC, Cain KT, et al: Mutagen-induced fetal anomalies and death following treatment of females within hours after mating. *Mutat Res* 199:175–181, 1988.

Generoso WM, Rutledge JC, Cain KT, et al: Exposure of female mice to ethylene oxide within hours after mating leads to fetal malformations and death. *Mutat Res* 176:269–274, 1987.

Genschow E, Scholz G, Brown N, et al: Development of prediction models for three in vitro embryotoxicity tests in an ECVAM validation study. *In Vitro Mol Toxicol* 13:51–65, 2000.

Gilliland FD, Berhane K, McConnell R, et al: Maternal smoking during pregnancy, environmental tobacco smoke exposure and childhood lung function. *Thorax* 55:271–276, 2000.

Goldey ES, Crofton KM: Thyroxine replacement attentuates hypothyroxinemia, hearing loss and motor deficits following developmental exposure to Arochlor 1254 in rats. *Toxicol Sci* 45:94–105, 1998.

Goldey ES, Kehn LS, Lau C, et al: Developmental exposure to polychlorinated biphenyls (Arochlor 1254) reduces circulating thyroid hormone concentrations and causes hearing deficits in rats. *Toxicol Appl Pharmacol* 135:77–88, 1995.

Goodman AB: Three independent lines of evidence suggest retinoids as causal to schizophrenia. *Proc Natl Acad Sci USA* 95:7240–7244, 1998.

Gorsuch RL, Key MK: Abnormalities of pregnancy as a function of anxiety and life stress. *Psychosom Med* 36:352–362, 1974.

Graham A, Papoalopulu N, Krumlauf R: The murine and *Drosophila* homeobox gene complexes have common features of organization and expression. *Cell* 57:367–378, 1989.

Gray LE, Ostby J, Kelce WR: A dose–response analysis of the reproductive effects of a single gestational dose of 2,3,7,8-tetrachloro-p-dioxin (TCDD) in male Long Evans Hooded rat offspring. *Toxicol Appl Pharmacol* 146:11–20, 1997a.

Gray LE, Ostby J, Ferrell J,et al: A dose–response analysis of methoxychlor-induced alterations of reproductive development and function in the rat. *Fundam Appl Toxicol* 12:92–108, 1989.

Gray LE, Ostby JS, Kelce WR: Developmental effects of an environmental anti-androgen: The fungicide vinclozolin alters sex differentiation of the male rat. *Toxicol Appl Pharmacol* 129:46–52, 1994.

Gray LE, Wold C, Mann P, Ostby JS: In utero exposure to low doses of 2,3,7,8-tetrachloro-p-dioxin (TCDD) alters reproductive development of female Long Evans Hooded rat offspring. *Toxicol Appl Pharmacol* 146:237–244, 1997b.

Gregg NM: Congenital cataract following German measles in the mother. *Trans Ophthalmol Soc Aust* 3:35–40, 1941.

Guenther TM, Mannering GT: Induction of hepatic monooxygenase systems of pregnant rats with phenobarbital and 3-methylcholanthrene. *Biochem Pharmacol* 26:577–584, 1977.

Guo YL, Lin CJ, Yao WJ, Ryan JJ, Hsu CC: Musculoskeletal changes in children prenatally exposed to polychlorinated biphenyls and related compounds (Yu-Cheng children). *J Toxicol Environ Health* 41:83–93, 1994.

Guzelian PS: Comparative toxicology of chlordecone (kepone) in humans and experimental animals. *Annu Rev Pharmacol Toxicol* 22:89–113, 1982.

Guzelian PS, Henry CJ, Olin SS (eds): *Similarities and Differences Between Children & Adults: Implications for Risk Assessment.* Washington, DC: ILSI Press, 1992.

Hale F: Pigs born without eyeballs. *J Hered* 27:105–106, 1935.

Hales B: Comparison of the mutagenicity of cyclophosphamide and its active metabolites, 4-hydroxycyclophosphamide, phosphoramide mustard and acrolein. *Cancer Res* 42:3018–3021, 1982.

Hales B: Relative mutagenicity and teratogenicity of cyclophosphamide and two of its structural analogs. *Biochem Pharmacol* 32:3791–3795, 1983.

Hales BF: Effects of phosphoramide mustard and acrolein, cytotoxic metabolites of cyclophosphamide, on mouse limb development in vitro. *Teratology* 40:11–20, 1989.

Hansen DK, Billings RE: Phenytoin teratogenicity and effects on embryonic and maternal folate metabolism. *Teratology* 31:363–371, 1985.

Hansen DK, Hodes ME: Comparative teratogenicity of phenytoin among several inbred strains of mice. *Teratology* 28:175–179, 1983.

Hansen JM, Carney EW, Harris C: Differential alteration by thalidomide of the glutathione content of rat vs rabbit conceptuses in vitro. *Reprod Toxicol* 13:547–554, 1999.

Hardin BD, Becker RJ, Kavlock RJ, et al: Overview and summary: Workshop on the Chernoff/Kavlock preliminary developmental toxicity test. *Teratogenesis Carcinog Mutagen* 7:119–127, 1987.

Harrison ML, Nicol CJ, Wells PJ: Tumor supressor genes and chemical teratogenesis: Benzo[a]pyrene embryopathy and cytochromes p-450 activities in p53-deficient transgenic mice. *Toxicologist* 14:246, 1994.

Hartig PC, Hunter ES III: Gene delivery to the neurulating embryo during culture. *Teratology* 58:103–112, 1998.

Hauck R-S, Nau H: The enantiomers of the valproic acid analogue 2-*n*-propylpentyoic acid (4-yn-VPA): Asymmetric synthesis and highly stereoselective teratogenicity in mice. *Pharm Res* 9:850–854, 1992.

Haug K, Irgens LM, Skjaerven R, et al: Maternal smoking and birthweight: Effect modification of period, maternal age and paternal smoking. *Acta Obstet Gynecol Scand* 79:485–489, 2000.

Hays SM, Elswick BA, Blumenthal GM, et al: Development of a physiologically based pharmacokinetic model of 2-methoxyethanol and 2-methoxyacetic acid disposition in pregnant rats. *Toxicol Appl Pharmacol* 163:67–74, 2000.

Heinrichs WL, Gellert RJ, Bakke JL, Lawrence NL: DDT administered to neonatal rats induces persistent estrus syndrome. *Science* 173:642–643, 1971.

Helene C, Toulme JJ: Specific regulation of gene expression by antisense, sense and antigene nucleic acids. *Biochim Biophys Acta* 1049:99–125, 1990.

Helm FC, Frankus E, Friderichs E, et al: Comparative teratological investigation of compounds structurally related to thalidomide. *Arnz Forsch Drug Res* 31:941–949, 1981.

Herbst AL, Bern HA: *Developmental Effects of Diethylstibestrol in Pregnancy.* New York: Thieme-Stratton, 1981.

Herbst AL, Cole P, Colton T, et al: Age-incidence and risk of diethylstilbestrol-related clear cell adenocarcinoma of the vagina and cervix. *Am J Obstet Gynecol* 128:43–50, 1977.

Hirsch KS, Scott WJ Jr: Searching for the mechanism of acetazolamide teratogenesis, in Kalter H (ed): *Issues and Reviews in Teratology.* Vol 1. New York: Plenum Press, 1983, pp 309–347.

Holladay SD, Luster MI: Developmental immunotoxicology, in Kimmel CA, Buelke-Sam J (eds): *Developmental Toxicology,* 2d ed. New York: Raven Press, 1994, pp 93–117.

Hsu S-T, Ma C-I, Hsu SK, et al: Discovery and epidemiology of PCB poisoning in Taiwan: A four-year followup. *Environ Health Perspect* 59:5–10, 1985.

Hytten FE: Physiologic changes in the mother related to drug handling, in Krauer B, Hytten F, del Pozo E (eds): *Drugs and Pregnancy.* New York: Academic Press, 1984, pp 7–17.

Imperato-McGinley J, Sanchez R, Spencer JR, Yee B, Vaughan ED: Comparison of the effects of the 5α-reductase inhibitor finasteride and the antiandrogen flutamide on prostate and genital differentiation: Dose–response studies. *Endocrinology* 131:1149–1156, 1992.

Irl C, Hasford J: Assessing the safety of drugs in pregnancy: The role of prospective cohort studies. *Drug Saf* 22:169–77, 2000.

Irvine S, Cawood E, Richardson D, et al: Evidence of deteriorating semen quality in the United Kingdom: Birth cohort study in 577 men in Scotland over 11 years. *Br Med J* 312:467–471, 1996.

Jacobson J, Jacobson S: Intellectual impairment in children exposed to polychlorinated biphenyls in utero. *N Engl J Med* 335:783–789, 1996.

Jacobson J, Jacobson S, Humphrey H: Effects of exposure to PCBs and related compounds on growth and activity in children. *Neurotoxicol Teratol* 12:319–326, 1990.

Jelovsek FR, Mattison DR Chen JJ: Prediction of risk for human developmental toxicity: How important are animal studies for hazard identification? *Obstet Gynecol* 74:624–636, 1989.

Johnson EM: A review of advances in prescreening for teratogenic hazards, in *Progress in Drug Research.* Vol 29. Basel: Birkhauser, 1985, pp 121–154.

Johnson EM, Gabel BEG: Application of the hydra assay for rapid detection of developmental hazards. *J Am Coll Toxicol* 1:57–71, 1982.

Jones KL, Smith DW: Recognition of the fetal alcohol syndrome in early infancy. *Lancet* 2:999–1001, 1973.

Jones KL, Smith DW, Ulleland CN, Streissguth AP: Pattern of malformation in offspring of chronic alcoholic mothers. *Lancet* 1:1267–1271, 1973.

Jonsson NA: Chemical structure and teratogenic properties. *Acta Pharm Suecia* 9:521–542, 1972.

Joussen AM, Germann T, Kirchhof B: Effect of thalidomide and structurally related compounds on cornela angiogenesis is comparable to their teratological potency. *Graefes Arch Clin Exp Ophthalmol* 237:952–961, 1999.

Juchau MR: Enzymatic bioactivation and inactivation of chemical teratogens and transplacental carcinogens/mutagens, in Juchau MR (ed): *The Biochemical Basis of Chemical Teratogenesis.* New York: Elsevier/ North Holland, 1981, pp 63–94.

Juchau MR Faustman-Watts EM: Pharmacokinetic considerations in the maternal-placental unit. *Clin Obstet Gynecol* 26:379–390, 1983.

Juchau MR, Lee QP; Fantel AG: Xenobiotic biotransformation/bioactivation in organogenesis-stage conceptual tissues: Implications for embryotoxicity and teratogenesis. *Drug Metab Rev* 24:195–238, 1992.

Juriloff DM, Fraser FC: Genetic maternal effects on cleft lip frequency in A/J and CL/Fr mice. *Teratology* 21:167–175, 1980.

Kalter H: The history of the A family of mice and the biology of its congenital malformations. *Teratology* 20:213–232, 1979.

Kavlock RJ: Structure-activity approaches in the screening of environmental agents for developmental toxicity. *Reprod Toxicol* 7:113–116, 1993.

Kavlock RJ, Allen BC, Faustman EM, Kimmel CA: Dose response assessment for developmental toxicity: IV. Benchmark doses for fetal weight changes. *Fundam Appl Toxicol* 26:211–222, 1995.

Kavlock RJ, Chernoff N, Rogers EH: The effect of acute maternal toxicity on fetal development in the mouse. *Teratogenesis Carcinog Mutagen* 5:3–13, 1985.

Kavlock RJ, Daston GP, DeRosa D, et al: Research needs for the risk assessment of health and environmental effects of endocrine disruptors: A report of the US EPA-sponsored workshop. *Environ Health Perspect* 104(suppl 4):715–740, 1996.

Kavlock RJ, Greene JA, Kimmel GL, et al: Activity profiles of developmental toxicity: Design considerations and pilot implementation. *Teratology* 43:159–185, 1991.

Keen CL, Bendich A, Willhite, CC (eds): Maternal nutrition and pregnancy outcome. *Ann NY Acad Sci* 678:1–372, 1993.

Keen CL, Peters JM, Hurley LS: The effect of valproic acid on ^{65}Zn distribution in the pregnant rat. *J Nutr* 119:607–611, 1989.

Kelce WR, Stone CR, Laws SC, et al: Persistent DDT metabolite p,p′-DDE is a potent androgen receptor antagonist. *Nature* 375:581–585, 1995.

Kelsey FO: Thalidomide update: Regulatory aspects. *Teratology* 38:221–226, 1988.

Kessel M, Balling R, Gruss P: Variations of cervical vertebrae after expression of a Hox-1.1 transgene in mice. *Cell* 61:301–308, 1990.

Khera KS: Maternal toxicity: A possible etiological factor in embryo/fetal deaths and fetal malformations of rodent-rabbit species. *Teratology* 31:129–153, 1985.

Khera KS: Maternal toxicity—A possible factor in fetal malformations in mice. *Teratology* 29:411–416, 1984.

Khoury MJ: Genetic susceptibility to birth defects in humans: From gene discovery to public health action. *Teratology* 61:17–20, 2000.

Khoury MJ, Erickson JD, James LM: Maternal factors in cleft lip with or without palate: Evidence from interracial crosses in the United States. *Teratology* 27:351–357, 1983.

Khoury MJ, Holtzman NA: On the ability of birth defects monitoring systems to detect new teratogens. *Am J Epidemiol* 126:136–143, 1987.

Khoury MJ, James LM; Flanders D, Erickson JD: Interpretation of recurring weak associations obtained from epidemiologic studies of suspected human teratogens. *Teratology* 46:69–77, 1992.

Khoury MJ, James LM, Lynberg MC: Quantitative analysis of associations between birth defects and suspected human teratogens. *Am J Med Genet* 40:500–505, 1991.

Kimmel CA, Cook RO, Staples RE: Teratogenic potential of noise in rats and mice. *Toxicol Appl Pharmacol* 36:239–245, 1976.

Kimmel CA, Young JF: Correlating pharmacokinetics and teratogenic endpoints. *Fundam Appl Toxicol* 3:250–255, 1983.

Klaassen CD, Lehman-McKeeman LD: Induction of metallothionein. *J Amer Coll Toxicol* 8:1315–1321, 1989.

Kochhar DM: Teratogenic activity of retinoic acid. *Acta Pathol Microbiol Scand* 70:398–404, 1967.

Koopman-Esseboom C, Weisglas-Kuperus N, de Ridder MAJ, et al: Effects of polychlorinated biphenyl/dioxin exposure and feeding type on infants mental and psychomotor development. *Pediatrics* 97:700–706, 1996.

Kotch LE, Sulik KK: Experimental fetal alcohol syndrome: proposed pathogenic basis for a variety of associated facial and brain anomalies. *Am J Med Genet* 44:168–176, 1992.

Krauer B: Physiological changes and drug disposition during pregnancy, in Nau H, Scott WJ (eds): *Pharmacokinetics in Teratogenesis.* Vol 1. Boca Raton, FL: CRC Press, 1987, pp 3–12.

Krumlauf R: *Hox* genes and pattern formation in the branchial region of the vertebrate head. *Trends Genet* 9:106–112, 1993.

Lammer EJ: Retinoids: Interspecies comparisons and clinical results, in Sundwall A, Danielsson BR, Hagberg O, et al (eds): *Developmental Toxicology—Preclinical and Clinical Data in Retrospect.* Stockholm: Tryckgruppen, 1992, pp 105–109.

Lammer EJ, Chen DT, Hoar RM, et al: Retinoic acid induced embryopathy. *N Engl J Med* 313:837–841, 1985.

Lammer EJ, Sever LE, Oakley GP Jr: Teratogen update: Valproic acid. *Teratology* 35:465–473, 1987.

Lary JM, Daniel KL, Erickson JD, et al: The return of thalidomide: Can birth defects be prevented? *Drug Saf* 21:161–169, 1999.

Latham KE: Epigenetic modification and imprinting of the mammalian genome during development. *Curr Top Dev Biol* 43:1–49, 1999.

Lau C, Kavlock RJ: Functional toxicity in the developing heart, lung and kidney, in Kimmel CA, Buelke-Sam J (eds): *Developmental Toxicology,* 2d ed. New York: Raven Press, 1994, pp 119–188.

Lau C, Setzer RW: Biologically based risk assessment models for developmental toxicity, in Tuan RS, Lo CW (eds): *Developmental Biology Protocols.* Vol II. Totowa, NJ: Humana Press, 2000, pp 271–281.

Lavin M, Watters D (eds): *Programmed Cell Death: The Cellular and Molecular Biology of Apoptosis.* Chur, Switzerland: Harwood Academic Publishers, 1993.

Lenz W: A short history of thalidomide embryopathy. *Teratology* 38:203–215, 1988.

Lenz W: Das thalidomid-syndrom. *Fortschr Med* 81:148–153, 1963.

Lenz W: Kindliche Missbildungen nach Medikament-Einnahme während der Gravidität? *Dtsch Med Wochenschr* 86:2555–2556, 1961.

Lenz W, Knapp K: Die thalidomide-embryopathie. *Dtsch Med Wochenschr* 87:1232–1242, 1962.

Leroux BG, Leisenring WM, Moolgavkar SH, Faustman EM: A biologically-based dose–response model for developmental toxicology. *Risk Anal* 16:449–458, 1996.

Levin AA, Miller RK: Fetal toxicity of cadmium in the rat: Maternal vs. fetal injections. *Teratology* 22:1–5, 1980.

Little SA, Mirkes PE: Effects of 4-hydroperoxycyclophosphamide (4-OOH-CP) and 4-hydroperoxydichlorocyclophosphamide (4-OOH-deClCP) on the cell cycle of postimplantation rat embryos. *Teratology* 45:163–173, 1992.

Little SA, Mirkes PE: Relationship of DNA damage and embryotoxicity induced by 4-hydroperoxydichlorocyclophosphamide in postimplantation rat embryos. *Teratology* 41:223–231, 1990.

Little RE: Moderate alcohol use during pregnancy and decreased infant birth weight. *Am J Public Health* 67:1154–1156, 1977.

Lohnes D, Mark M, Mendelsohn C, et al: Function of the retinoic acid receptors (RARs) during development: I. Craniofacial and skeletal abnormalities in RAR double mutants. *Development* 120:2723–2748, 1994.

Lopuhaa CE, Roseboom TJ, Osmond C, et al: Atopy, lung function, and obstructive airways disease after prenatal exposure to famine. *Thorax* 55:555–561, 2000.

Luecke RH, Wosilait WD, Pearce BA, Young JF: A physiologically based pharmacokinetic computer model for human pregnancy. *Teratology* 49:90–103, 1994.

Luecke RH, Wosilait WD, Young JF: Mathematical analysis for teratogenic sensitivity. *Teratology* 55:373–380, 1997.

Lutiger B, Graham K, Einarson TR, Koren G: Relationship between gestational cocaine use and pregnancy outcome: A meta-analysis. *Teratology* 44:405–414, 1991.

Lynch DW, Schuler RL, Hood RD, Davis DG: Evaluation of *Drosophila* for screening developmental toxicants: Test results with eighteen chemicals and presentation of new *Drosophila* bioassay. *Teratogenesis Carcinog Mutagen* 11:147–173, 1991.

Mably TA, Bjerke DL, Moore RW, et al: In utero and lactational exposure of male rats to 2,3,7,8-tetrachlorodibenzo-p-dioxin. 3. Effects on spermatogenesis and reproductive capability. *Toxicol Appl Pharmacol* 114:118–126, 1992.

MacAuley AM, Werb Z, Mirkes PE: Characterization of the unusually rapid cell cycles during rat gastrulation. *Development* 117:873–883, 1993.

MacDonald H, Tobin JOH: Congenital cytomegalovirus infection: A collaborative study on epidemiological, clinical and laboratory findings. *Dev Med Child Neurol* 20:271–282, 1978.

MacNeish JD, Scott WJ, Potter SS: Legless, a novel mutation found in PHT1-1 transgenic mice. *Science* 241:837–839, 1988.

Manson JM: Testing of pharmaceutical agents for reproductive toxicity, in Kimmel CA, Buelke-Sam J (eds): *Developmental Toxicology,* 2d ed. New York: Raven Press, 1994, pp 379–402.

Markert CL, Petters RM: Manufactured hexaparental mice show that adults are derived from three embryonic cells. *Science* 202:56–58, 1978.

Marshall H, Morrison A, Studer M, et al: Retinoids and hox genes. *FASEB J* 10:969–978, 1996.

Marshall H, Nonchev S, Sham MH, et al: Retinoic acid alters hindbrain Hox code and induces transformation of rhombomeres 2/3 into a 4/5 identity. *Nature* 360:737–741, 1992.

Mattison DR, Blann E, Malek A: Physiological alterations during pregnancy: Impact on toxicokinetics. *Fundam Appl Toxicol* 16:215–218, 1991.

McBride WG: Thalidomide and congenital anomalies. *Lancet* 2 :1358, 1961.

Medlock KL, Branham WS, Sheehan DM: Effects of coumestrol and equol on the developing reproductive tract of the rat. *Proc Soc Exp Biol Med* 208:67–71, 1995.

Mendelsohn C, Lohnes D, Décimo D, et al: Function of the retinoic acid receptors (RARs) during development: II. Multiple abnormalities at various stages of organogenesis in RAR double mutants. *Development* 120:2749–2771, 1994.

Miller MT, Stromland K: Teratogen update: thalidomide: A review with a focus on ocular findings and new potential uses. *Teratology* 60:306–321, 1999.

Millicovsky G, DeSesso JM: Cardiovascular alterations in rabbit embryos in situ after a teratogenic dose of hydroxyurea: An in vivo microscopic study. *Teratology,* 22:115–124, 1980.

Millicovsky G, DeSesso JM: Differential embryonic cardiovascular responses to acute maternal uterine ischemia: An in vivo microscopic study of rabbit embryos with either intact or clamped umbilical cords. *Teratology* 22:335–343, 1980.

Millicovsky G, DeSesso JM, Kleinman LI Clark KE: Effects of hydroxyurea on hemodynamics of pregnant rabbits: A maternally mediated mechanism of embryotoxicity. *Am J Obstet Gynecol* 140:747–752, 1981.

Millicovsky G, Johnston MC: Maternal hyperoxia greatly reduces the incidence of phenytoin-induced cleft lip and palate in A/J mice. *Science* 212:671–672, 1981.

Milunsky A, Ulcickas M, Rothman KJ, et al: Maternal heat exposure and neural tube defects. *JAMA* 268:882–885, 1992.

Mirkes PE: Molecular and metabolic aspects of cyclophosphamide teratogenesis, in Welsch F (ed): *Approaches to Elucidate Mechanisms in Teratogenesis.* Washington, DC: Hemisphere, 1987, pp 123–147.

Mirkes PE: Simultaneous banding of rat embryo DNA, RNA and protein in cesium trifluoroacetate gradients. *Anal Biochem* 148:376–383, 1985a.

Mirkes PE: Cyclophosphamide teratogenesis: A review. *Teratogenicity Carcinog Mutagen* 5:75–88, 1985b.

Mirkes PE, Fantel AG, Greenaway JC, Shepard TH: Teratogenicity of cyclophosphamide metabolites: Phosphoramide mustard, acrolein, and 4-ketocyclophosphamide on rat embryos cultured in vitro. *Toxicol Appl Pharmacol* 58:322–330, 1981.

Mirkes PE, Greenaway JC, Hilton J, Brundrett R: Morphological and biochemical aspects of monofunctional phosphoramide mustard teratogenicity in rat embryos cultured in vitro. *Teratology* 32:241–249, 1985.

Mirkes PE, Little SA: Cytochrome c release from mitochondria of early postimplantation murine embryos exposed to 4-hydroperoxycyclophosphamide, heat shock, and staurosporine. *Toxicol Appl Pharmacol* 62:197–206, 2000.

Mirkes PE, Little SA: Teratogen-induced cell death in postimplantation mouse embryos: Differential tissue sensitivity and hallmarks of apoptosis. *Cell Death Differ* 5:592–600, 1998.

Mirkes PE, Ricks JL, Pascoe-Mason JM: Cell cycle analysis in the cardiac and neuroepithelial tissues of day 10 rat embryos and the effects of phosphoramide mustard, the major teratogenic metabolite of cyclophosphamide. *Teratology* 39:115–120, 1989.

Mitra SC: Effects of cocaine on fetal kidney and bladder function. *J Maternal Fetal Med* 8:262–269, 1999.

Moore NW, Adams CE, Rowson LEA: Developmental potential of single blastomeres of the rabbit egg. *J Reprod Fertil* 17:527–531,

MRC Vitamin Study Research Group [prepared by Wald N with assistance from Sneddon J, Frost C, Stone R]: Prevention of neural tube defects: Results of the MRC vitamin study. *Lancet* 338:132–137, 1991.

Murphy SK, Jirtle RL: Imprinted genes as potential genetic and epigenetic toxicologic targets. *Environ Health Perspect* 108(suppl 1):5–11, 2000.

Mylchreest E, Cattley RC, Foster PM: Male reproductive tract malformations in rats following gestational and lactational exposure to di(n-butyl)phthalate: An anti-androgenic mechanism? *Toxicol Sci* 43:67–60, 1998.

Mylchreest E, Sar M, Cattley RC, Foster PM: Disruption of androgen-regulated male reproductive development by di(*n*-butyl)phthalate during late gestation in rats is different from flutamide. *Toxicol Appl Pharmacol* 156:81–95, 1999.

Nagel SC, vom Saal FS, Thayer KA, et al: Relative binding affinity–serum modified access (RBA–SMA) assay predicts the relative in vivo bioactivity of the xenoestrogens bisphenol A and octylphenol. *Environ Health Perspect* 105:70–76, 1997.

National Research Council: *Hormonally Active Agents in the Environment.* Washington, DC: National Academy Press, 1999.

National Research Council: *Pesticides in the Diets of Infants and Children.* Washington, DC: National Academy Press, 1993.

National Research Council: *Scientific Fromtiers in Developmental Toxicology and Risk Assessment.* Washington, DC: National Academy Press, 2000.

Nau H: Physicochemical and structural properties regulating placenta drug transfer, in Polin RA, Fox WW (eds): *Fetal and Neonatal Physiology.* Vol 1. Philadelphia: Saunders, 1992, pp 130–149.

Nau H: Species differences in pharmacokinetics and drug teratogenesis. *Environ Health Perspect* 70:113–129, 1986.

Nau H, Chahoud I, Dencker L, et al: Teratogenicity of vitamin A and retinoids, in Blomhoff R (ed): *Vitamin A in Health and Disease.* New York: Marcel Dekker, 1994, pp 615–664.

Nau H, Hauck R-S, Ehlers K: Valproic acid induced neural tube defects in mouse and human: Aspects of chirality, alternative drug development, pharmacokinetics and possible mechanisms. *Pharmacol Toxicol* 69:310–321, 1991.

Nau H, Scott WJ: *Pharmacokinetics in Teratogenesis.* Vols I and II. Boca Raton, FL: CRC Press, 1987.

Nau H, Scott WJ: Weak acids may act as teratogens by accumulating in the basic milieu of the early mammalian embryo. *Nature* 323: 276–278, 1986.

Nawrot PS, Cook RO, Hamm CW: Embryotoxicity of broadband high-frequency noise in the CD-1 mouse. *J Toxicol Environ Health* 8:151–157, 1981.

Nawrot PS, Cook RO, Staples RE: Embryotoxicity of various noise stimuli in the mouse. *Teratology* 22:279–289, 1980.

Neims AH, Warner M, Loughnan PM, Aranda JV: Developmental aspects of the hepatic cytochrome P_{450} monooxygenase system. *Annu Rev Pharmacol Toxicol* 16:427–444, 1976.

Nelson CJ, Holson JF: Statistical analysis of teratologic data: Problems and recent advances. *J Environ Pathol Toxicol* 2:187–199, 1978.

Neubert D: In-vitro techniques for assessing teratogenic potential, in Dayan AD, Paine AJ (eds): *Advances in Applied Toxicology.* London: Taylor and Francis,1989, pp 191–211.

Neubert D, Zens P, Rothenwallner A, Merker H-J: A survey of the embryotoxic effects of TCDD in mammalian species. *Environ Health Perspect* 5:63–79, 1973.

Neubert R, Hinz N, Thiel R, Neubert D: Down-regulation of adhesion receptors on cells of primate embryos as a probable mechanism of the teratogenic action of thalidomide. *Life Sci* 58:295–316, 1996.

Neubert R, Neubert D: Peculiarities and possible mode of actions of thalidomide, in Kavlock RJ, Daston GP (eds): *Drug Toxicity in Embryonic Development, II.* Berlin Heidelberg: Springer-Verlag, 1997, pp 41–119.

Neubert R, Nogueira AC, Neubert D: Thalidomide derivatives and the immune system: I. Changes in the pattern of integrin receptors and other surface markers on T lymphocyte subpopulations of marmoset blood. *Arch Toxicol* 67:1–17, 1993.

New DAT: Whole embryo culture and the study of mammalian embryos during organogenesis. *Biol Rev* 5:81–94, 1978.

Newall DR, Beedles KE: The stem cell test: An in vitro assay for teratogenic potential. Results of a blind trial with 25 compounds. *Toxicol in Vitro* 10:229–240, 1996.

Newbold RR: Cellular and molecular effects of developmental exposure to diethylstilbestrol: Implications for other environmental estrogens. *Environ Health Perspect* 103(suppl. 7):83–87, 1995.

Newman CGH: Teratogen update: Clinical aspects of thalidomide embryopathy—A continuing preoccupation. *Teratology* 32:133–144, 1985.

Newman LM, Johnson EM, Staples RE: Assessment of the effectiveness of animal developmental toxicity testing for human safety. *Reprod Toxicol* 7:359–390, 1993.

Nugent P, Sucov HM, Pisano MM, Greene RM: The role of RXR-alpha in retinoic acid–induced cleft palate as assessed with the RXR-alpha knockout mouse. *Int J Dev Biol* 43:567–570, 1999.

O'Flaherty EJ: Pharmacokinetics, pharmacodynamics, and prediction of developmental abnormalities. *Reprod Toxicol* 11:413–416, 1997.

O'Flaherty EJ, Scott WJ, Shreiner C, Beliles RP: A physiologically based kinetic model of rat and mouse gestation: Disposition of a weak acid. *Toxicol Appl Pharmacol* 112:245–256, 1992.

Olsen GW, Bodner KM, Ramlow JM, Ross CE, Lipshultz LI: Have sperm counts been reduced 50 percent in 50 years? A statistical model revisited. *Fertility and Sterility* 63:887–893 1995.

Olshan A, Mattison D (eds): *Male-Mediated Developmental Toxicity.* New York: Plenum Press, 1995.

Oltvai ZN, Korsmeyer SJ: Checkpoints of dueling dimers foil death wishes. *Cell* 79:189–192, 1994.

Osmond C, Barker DJ: Fetal, infant, and childhood growth are predictors of coronary heart disease, diabetes, and hypertension in adult men and women. *Environ Health Perspect* 108(suppl 3):545–553, 2000.

Osmond C, Barker DJP, Winter PD: Early growth and death from cardiovascular disease in women. *Br Med J* 307:1519–1524, 1993.

Ostrea EM Jr, Matias O, Keane C, Mac E, Utarnachitt R, Ostrea A, Mazhar M: Spectrum of gestational exposure to illicit drugs and other xenobiotic agents in newborn infants meconium analysis. *J Pediatr* 133:513–515, 1998.

Page K, Abramovich D, Aggett P et al: Uptake of zinc by the human placenta microvillus border membranes and characterization of the effects of cadmium on the process. *Placenta* 13:151–162, 1992.

Pagon RA, Covington M, Tarczy-Hornoch P: Helix: A directory of medical genetics laboratories. *http://www.genetests.org,* 1998.

Palmer AK: Implementing the ICH guideline for reproductive toxicity, in *Current Issues in Drug Development.* II., Huntingdon Research Centre, 1993, pp 1–21.

Parizek J: Vascular changes at sites of estrogen biosynthesis produced by parenteral injection of cadmium salts: The destruction of the placenta by cadmium salts. *J Reprod Fertil* 7:263–265, 1964.

Parman T, Wiley MJ, Wells PG: Free radical-mediated oxidative DNA damage in the mechanism of thalidomide teratogenicity. *Nat Med* 5:582–585, 1999.

Paulozzi LJ: International trends in rates of hypospadias and cryptorchidism. *Environ Health Perspect* 107:297–302, 1999.

Paulozzi LJ, Erickson JD, Jackson RJ: Hypospadias trends in two American surveillance systems. *Pediatrics* 100:831–834, 1997.

Pinkerton KE, Joad JP: The mammalian respiratory system and critical windows of exposure for children's health. *Environ Health Perspect* 108(suppl 3):457–462, 2000.

Pole M, Einarson A, Pairaudeau N, et al: Drug labeling and risk perceptions of teratogenicity: A survey of pregnant Canadian women and their health professionals. *J Clin Pharmacol* 40:573–577, 2000.

Porterfield SP: Vulnerability of the developing brain to thyroid abnormalities: Environmental insults to the thyroid system. *Environ Health Perspect* 102(suppl 2):125–130, 1994.

Poskanzer D, Herbst AL: Epidemiology of vaginal adenosis and adenocarcinoma associated with exposure to stilbestrol in utero. *Cancer* 39:1892–1895, 1977.

Potter SM, Zelazo PR, Stack DM, Papageorgiou AN: Adverse effects of fetal cocaine exposure on neonatal auditory information processing. *Pediatrics* 105:E40, 2000.

Ravelli AC, van Der Meulen JH, Osmond C, et al: Obesity at the age of 50 y in men and women exposed to famine prenatally. *Am J Clin Nutr* 70:811–816, 1999.

Renault J-Y, Melcion C, Cordier A: Limb bud cell culture for in vitro teratogen screening: Validation of an improved assessment method using 51 compounds. *Teratogenicity Carcinog Mutagen* 9:83–96, 1989.

Rich-Edwards JW, Colditz GA, Stampfer MJ, et al: Birthweight and the risk of type 2 diabetes in adult women. *Ann Intern Med* 130:278–284, 1999.

Rodier PM, Cohen IR, Buelke-Sam J: Developmental neurotoxicology: Neuroendocrine manifestations of CNS insult, in Kimmel CA, Buelke-Sam J (eds): *Developmental Toxicology,* 2d ed. New York: Raven Press, 1994, pp 65–92.

Rogan WJ, Gladen BC: PCBs, DDE and child development at 18 and 24 months. *Am J Epidemiol* 1:407–413, 1991.

Rogers JM, Daston GP: Alcohols: Ethanol and methanol, in Kavlock RJ, Daston GP (eds): *Drug Toxicity in Embryonic Development II.* Berlin Heidelberg: Springer-Verlag, 1997, pp 333–405.

Rogers JM, Mole ML: Critical periods of sensitivity to the developmental toxicity of inhaled methanol in the CD-1 mouse. *Teratology* 55: 364–372, 1997.

Rogers JM, Mole ML, Chernoff N, et al: The developmental toxicity of inhaled methanol in the CD-1 mouse, with quantitative dose–response modeling for estimation of benchmark doses. *Teratology* 47:175–188, 1993.

Rosa FW: Teratogenicity of isotretinoin. *Lancet* 2:513, 1983.

Rutledge JC, Shourbaji AG, Hughes LA, et al: Limb and lower-body duplications induced by retinoic acid in mice. *Proc Natl Acad Sci USA* 91:5436–40, 1994.

Sadler TW, Hunter ES: Principles of abnormal development: Past, present and future, in Kimmel CA, Buelke-Sam J (eds): *Developmental Toxicology,* 2d ed. New York: Raven Press, 1994, pp. 53–63.

Sadler TW, Warner CW: Use of whole embryo culture for evaluating toxicity and teratogenicity. *Pharmacol Rev* 36:145S–150S, 1984.

Sanes JR, Rubenstein LR, Nicolas JF: Use of a recombinant retrovirus to study postimplantation cell lineage in mouse embryos. *EMBO J* 5:3133–3142, 1986.

Sannerstedt R, Lundborg P, Danielsson BR, et al: Drugs during pregnancy: An issue of risk classification and information to prescribers. *Drug Saf* 14:69–77, 1996.

Sanyal MK, Kitchin KT, Dixon RL: Anomalous development of rat embryos cultured in vitro with cyclophosphamide and microsomes. *Pharmacologist* 21:A231, 1979.

Sauer H, Gunther J, Hescheler J, Wartenberg M: Thalidomide inhibits angiogenesis in embryoid bodies by the generation of hydroxyl radicals. *Am J Pathol* 56:151–158, 2000.

Scanlon JW: The neuroteratology of cocaine: Background, theory, and clinical implications. *Reprod Toxicol* 5:89–98, 1991.

Schantz SL, Levin ED, Bowman RE: Long-term neurobehavioral effects of perinatal PCB exposure in monkeys. *J Environ Toxicol Chem* 10:747–756, 1991.

Schantz SL, Moshtaghian J, Ness DK: Spatial learning deficits in adult rats exposed to ortho-substituted PCB congeners during gestation and lactation. *Fundam Appl Toxicol* 26:117–126, 1995.

Schardein JL: *Chemically Induced Birth Defects,* 3d ed. New York: Marcel Dekker, 2000.

Schardein JL: *Chemically Induced Birth Defects,* 2d ed. New York: Marcel Dekker, 1993.

Schardein JL, Keller KA: Potential human developmental toxicants and the role of animal testing in their identification and characterization. *CRC Crit Rev Toxicol* 19:251–339, 1989.

Schecter A, Ryan JJ, Masuda Y, et al: Chlorinated and brominated dioxins and dibenzofurans in human tissue following exposure. *Environ Health Perspect* 102(suppl 1):135–147, 1994.

Scholz G, Pohl I, Genschow E, et al: Embryotoxicity screening using embryonic stem cells in vitro: Correlation to in vivo teratogenicity. *Cells Tissues Organs* 165:203–211, 1999.

Schumacher HJ: Chemical structure and teratogenic properties, in Shepard T, Miller R, Marois M (eds): *Methods for Detection of Environmental Agents That Produce Congenital Defects.* New York: American Elsevier, 1975, pp 65–77.

Seller MJ, Perkins KJ, Adinolfi M: Differential response of heterozygous curly-tail mouse embryos to vitamin A teratogenesis depending on maternal genotype. *Teratology* 28:123, 1983.

Sever JL: Rubella as a teratogen. *Adv Teratol* 2:127–138, 1967.

Shenefelt RE: Morphogenesis of malformations in hamsters caused by retinoic acid: Relation to dose and stage of treatment. *Teratology* 5: 103–118, 1972.

Shepard TH: *Catalog of Teratogenic Agents,* 7th ed. Baltimore: The Johns Hopkins University Press, 1992.

Shepard TH: *Catalog of Teratogenic Agents,* 9th ed. Baltimore: The Johns Hopkins University Press, 1998.

Shuey DL, Lau C, Logsdon TR, et al: Biologically based dose–response modeling in developmental toxicology: Biochemical and cellular sequelae of 5-fluorouracil exposure in the developing rat. *Toxicol Appl Pharmacol* 126:129–144, 1994.

Skakkebaek NE, Keiding N: Changes in semen and the testis. *Br Med J* 309:1316–1317, 1994.

Slikker W, Miller RK: Placental metabolism and transfer: Role in developmental toxicology, in Kimmel CA, Buelke-Sam J (eds): *Developmental Toxicology,* 2d ed. New York: Raven Press, 1994, pp 245–283.

Slotkin TA: Fetal nicotine or cocaine exposure: Which one is worse? *J Pharmacol Exp Ther* 285:931–945, 1998.

Smith JL, Gesteland KM, Schoenwolf GC: Prospective fate map of the mouse primitive streak at 7.5 days of gestation. *Dev Dynam* 201:279–289, 1994.

Smith MK, Kimmel GL, Kochhar DM, et al: A selection of candidate compounds for in vitro teratogenesis test validation. *Teratogenicity Carcinog Mutagen* 3:461–480, 1983.

Snow MHL, Tam PPL: Is compensatory growth a complicating factor in mouse teratology? *Nature* 279:555–557.

Sorrell TL, Graziano JH: Effect of oral cadmium exposure during pregnancy on maternal and fetal zinc metabolism in the rat. *Toxicol Appl Pharmacol* 102:537–545, 1990.

Stephens TD: Proposed mechanisms of action in thalidomide embryopathy. *Teratology* 38:229–239, 1988.

Stephens TD, Bunde CJW, Torres RD, et al: Thalidomide inhibits limb development throught its antagonism of IFG-I + FGF-2 + heparin (abstr). *Teratology* 57:112, 1998.

Stephens TD, Fillmore BJ: Hypothesis: thalidomide embryopathy: Proposed mechanism of action. *Teratology* 61:189–195, 2000.

Stirling DI, Sherman M, Strauss S: Thalidomide: A surprising recovery. *J Am Pharmacol Assoc* NS37:307–313, 1997.

Stockard CR: Developmental rate and structural expression: An experimental study of twins, "double monsters," and single deformities, and the interaction among embryonic organs during their origin and development. *Am J Anat* 28:115–277, 1921.

Stott DH: Follow-up study from birth of the effects of prenatal stress. *Dev Med Child Neurol* 15:770–787, 1973.

Streissguth AP, Aase JM, Clarren SK, et al: Fetal alcohol syndrome in adolescents and adults. *JAMA* 265:1961–1967, 1991a.

Streissguth AP, Barr HM, Olson HC, et al: Drinking during pregnancy decreases word attack and arithmetic scores on standardized tests: adolescent data from a population-based prospective study. *Alcohol Clin Exp Res* 18:248–254, 1994a.

Streissguth AP, Randels SP, Smith DF: A test-retest study of intelligence in patients with fetal alcohol syndrome: implications for care. *J Am Acad Child Adolesc Psychiatry* 30:584–587, 1991b.

Streissguth AP, Sampson PD, Olson HC, et al: Maternal drinking during pregnancy: Attention and short-term memory in 14-year-old offspring: A longitudinal prospective study. *Alcohol Clin Exp Res* 18:202–218, 1994b.

Sulik KK, Cook CS, Webster WS: Teratogens and craniofacial malformations: Relationships to cell death. *Development* 103(suppl):213–231, 1988.

Sulik KK, Johnston MC: Sequence of developmental alterations following acute ethanol exposure in mice: Craniofacial features of the fetal alcohol syndrome. *Am J Anat* 166:257–269, 1983.

Sulik KK, Johnston MC, Webb MA: Fetal alcohol syndrome: Embryogenesis in a mouse model. *Science* 214:936–938, 1981.

Swann SH, Elkin EP, Fenster L: Have sperm counts declined? A reanalysis of global trend data. *Environ Health Perspect* 105:1228–1232, 1997.

Takeuchi IK: Teratogenic effects of methylnitrosourea on pregnant mice before implantation. *Experientia* 40:879–881, 1984.

Taubeneck MW, Daston GP, Rogers JM, Keen CL: Altered maternal zinc metabolism following exposure to diverse developmental toxicants. *Reprod Toxicol* 8:25–40, 1994.

Taussig HB: A study of the German outbreak of phocomelia: The thalidomide syndrome. *JAMA* 180:1106, 1962.

Teratology Society: FDA classification system of drugs for teratogenic risk. *Teratology* 49:446–447, 1994.

Terry KK, Elswick BA, Welsch F, Connolly RB: Development of a physiologically based pharmacokinetic model describing 2-methoxyacetic acid disposition in the pregnant mouse. *Toxicol Appl Pharmacol* 132:103–114, 1995.

Thompson CJS: *Mystery and Lore of Monsters.* London: Williams and Norgate, 1930.

Toppari J, Larsen JC, Christiansen P, et al: Male reproductive health and environmental xenoestrogens. *Environ Health Perspect* 104(suppl 4):741–776, 1996.

Tuthill DP, Stewart JH, Coles EC, et al: Maternal cigarette smoking and pregnancy outcome. *Paediatr Perinatol Epidemiol* 13:245–253, 1999.

U.S. EPA: Endocrine Screening Program: Statement of Policy. *Fed Reg* 63(248):71542–71568, 1998.

U.S. EPA: Guidelines for Developmental Toxicity Risk Assessment; Notice. *Fed Reg* 56:63798–63826, 1991.

U.S. Environmental Protection Agency: Health Effects Test Guidelines. OPPTS 870.3700. Prenatal Developmental Toxicity Study. EPA 712-C-98-207, 1998.

U.S. EPA: *Pesticide Assessment Guidelines, subdivision F, Hazard Evaluation: human and domestic animals, addendum 10: neurotoxicity.* Series 81, 82, and 83. EPA 540/09-91-123 PB 91-154617, 1991.

U.S. EPA: *Special Report on Environmental Endocrine Disruption: An Effects Assessment and Analysis.* US Environmental Protection Agency, EPA/630/R-012., Washington, DC: US EPA, February, 1997.

U.S. EPA: Toxic Substance Control Act Testing Guidelines. Final Rules: Preliminary developmental toxicity screen. *Fed Reg* 50:39428–39429, 1985.

U.S. FDA: *Guidelines for Reproduction Studies for Safety Evaluation of Drugs for Human Use.* Rockville, MD: US FDA, 1966.

U.S. FDA: International Conference on Harmonization; Guideline on Detection of Toxicity to Reproduction for Medicinal Products; Availability; Notice. *Fed Reg* 59:48746–48752, 1994.

U.S. FDA: Labeling and prescription drug advertising: Content and format for labeling for human prescription drugs. *Fed Reg* 44:37434–37467, 1979.

Uphill PF, Wilkins SR, Allen JA: In vitro micromass teratogen test: Results from a blind trial of 25 compounds. *Toxicol in Vitro* 4:623–626, 1990

Vaglia JL, Hall BK: Regulation of neural crest cell populations: Occurrence, distribution and underlying mechanisms. *Int J Dev Biol* 43: 95–110, 1999.

Vierula M, Niemi M, Keiski A, et al: High and unchanged sperm counts of Finnish men. *Int J Androl* 19:11–17, 1996.

Volfe JJ: Effects of cocaine on the fetus. *N Engl J Med* 327:399–407, 1992.

vom Saal FS, Timms BG, Montano MM, et al: Prostate enlargement in mice due to fetal exposure to low doses of estradiol or diethylstilbestrol and opposite effects at high doses. *Proc Natl Acad Sci USA* 94:2056–2061, 1997.

Wald N: Folic acid and the prevention of neural tube defects, in Keen CL, Bendich A, Willhite CC (eds): Maternal Nutrition and Pregnancy Outcome. *Ann NY Acad Sci* 678:112–129, 1993.

Warkany J: Development of experimental mammalian teratology, in Wilson JG, Warkany J (eds): *Teratology: Principles and Techniques.* Chicago: University of Chicago Press, 1965, pp 1–11.

Warkany J: History of teratology, in *Handbook of Teratology.* Vol 1. New York: Plenum Press,1977, pp 3–45.

Warkany J: Manifestations of prenatal nutritional deficiency. *Vit Horm* 3: 73–103, 1945.

Warkany J: Teratogen update: Hyperthermia. *Teratology* 33:365–371, 1986.

Warkany J: Teratology: Spectrum of a science, in Kalter H (ed): *Issues and Reviews in Teratology.* Vol 1. New York: Plenum Press, 1983, pp 19–31.

Warkany J, Nelson RC: Appearance of skeletal abnormalities in the offspring of rats reared on a deficient diet. *Science* 92:383–384, 1940.

Warkany J, Schraffenberger E: Congenital malformations induced in rats by roentgen rays. *Am J Roentgenol Radium Ther* 57:455–463, 1944.

Watkinson WP, Millicovsky G: Effects of phenytoin on maternal heart rate in A/J mice: Possible role in teratogenesis. *Teratology* 28:1–8, 1983.

Weaver TE, Scott WJ Jr: Acetazolamide teratogenesis: Association of maternal respiratory acidosis and ectrodactyly in C57BL/6J mice. *Teratology* 30:187–193, 1984a.

Weaver TE, Scott WJ Jr: Acetazolamide teratogenesis: Interactions of maternal metabolic and respiratory acidosis in the induction of ectrodactyly in C57BL/6J mice. *Teratology* 30:195–202, 1984b.

Webster WS, Brown-Woodman PD, Ritchie HE: A review of the contribution of whole embryo culture to the determination of hazard and risk in teratogenicity testing. *Int J Dev Biol* 41:329–335, 1997.

Welsch F: Short term methods of assessing developmental toxicity hazard, in Kalter H (ed): *Issues and Review in Teratology.* Vol 5. New York: Plenum Press, 1990, pp 115–153.

White E: Death defying acts: A meeting review on apoptosis. *Genes Dev* 7:2277–2284, 1993.

Wilcox AJ, Weinberg CR, O'Connor JF, et al: Incidence of early loss of pregnancy. *N Engl J Med* 319:189–194, 1988.

Wilson JG: *Environment and Birth Defects.* New York: Academic Press, 1973.

Wilson JG: Embryotoxicity of drugs in man, in Wilson JG, Fraser FC (eds): *Handbook of Teratology.* New York: Plenum Press, 1977, p. 309–355.

Wilson JG, Roth CB, Warkany J: An analysis of the syndrome of malformations induced by maternal vitamin A deficiency: Effects of restoration of vitamin A at various times during gestation. *Am J Anat* 92:189–217, 1953.

Windham GC, Hopkins B, Fenster L, Swan SH: Prenatal active or passive tobacco smoke exposure and the risk of preterm delivery or low birth weight. *Epidemiology* 11:427–433, 2000.

You L, Casanova M, Archibeque-Engel S, et al: Impaired male sexual development in perinatal Sprague-Dawley and Long-Evans Hooded rats exposed in utero and lactationally to pp′-DDE. *Toxicol Sci* 45: 162–173, 1998.

Young JF: Physiologically-based pharmacokinetic model for pregnancy as a tool for investigation of developmental mechanisms. *Comput Biol Med* 28:359–364, 1998.

Yu M-L, Hsu C-C, Gladen B, Rogan WJ: In utero PCB/PCDF exposure: Relation of developmental delay to dysmorphology and dose. *Neurotoxicol Teratol* 13:195–202, 1991.

Zakany J, Tuggle CK, Nguyen-Huu CM: The use of *lacZ* gene fusions in the studies of mammalian development: Developmental regulation of mammalian homeobox genes in the CNS. *J Physiol Paris* 84:21–26, 1990.

UNIT 4

TARGET ORGAN TOXICITY

CHAPTER 11

TOXIC RESPONSES OF THE BLOOD

John C. Bloom and John T. Brandt

BLOOD AS A TARGET ORGAN

Hematotoxicology is the study of adverse effects of drugs, nontherapeutic chemicals and other agents in our environment on blood and blood-forming tissues (Bloom, 1997). This subspecialty draws on the discipline of hematology and the principles of toxicology. Scientific understanding of the former began with the contributions of Leeuwenhoek and others in the seventeenth century, with the microscopic examination of blood (Wintrobe, 1985). Hematology was later recognized as an applied laboratory science but limited to quatitation of formed elements of the blood and the study of their morphology, along with that of bone marrow, spleen, and lymphoid tissues. It is now a diverse medical specialty, which—perhaps more than any other discipline—has made tremendous contributions to molecular medicine (Kaushansky, 2000).

The vital functions that blood cells perform, together with the susceptibility of this highly proliferative tissue to intoxication, makes the hematopoietic system unique as a target organ. Accordingly, it ranks with liver and kidney as one of the most important considerations in the risk assessment of individual patient populations exposed to potential toxicants in the environment, workplace, and medicine cabinet.

The delivery of oxygen to tissues throughout the body, maintaining vascular integrity and providing the many affector and effector immune functions necessary for host defense, requires a prodigious proliferative and regenerative capacity. The various blood cells (erythrocytes, granulocytes, and platelets) are each produced at a rate of approximately 1 to 3 million per second in a healthy adult and up to several times that rate in conditions where demand for these cells is high, as in hemolytic anemia or suppurative inflammation (Testa and Molineux, 1993). As with intestinal mucosa and gonads, this characteristic makes hematopoietic tissue a particularly sensitive target for cytoreductive or antimitotic agents, such as those used to treat cancer, infection, and immune-mediated disorders. This tissue is also susceptible to secondary effects of toxic agents that affect the supply of nutrients, such as iron; the clearance of toxins and metabolites, such as urea; or the production of vital growth factors, such as erythropoietin.

The consequences of direct or indirect damage to blood cells and their precursors are predictable and potentially life-threatening. They include hypoxia, hemorrhage, and infection. These effects may be subclinical and slowly progressive or acute and fulminant, with dramatic clinical presentations. Hematotoxicity is usually assessed in the context of risk versus benefit. It may be used to define dosage in treatment modalities in which these effects are limiting, such as those employing certain anticancer, antiviral, and antithrombotic agents.

Hematotoxicity is generally regarded as unacceptable, however, in treatments for less serious illnesses, such as mild hypertension or arthritis or following exposure to contaminated foods or environmental contaminants. Risk-versus-benefit decisions involving hematotoxicity may be controversial, especially when the incidence of these effects is very low. Whether the effect is linked to the pharmacologic action of the agent, as with cytoreductive or thrombolytic agents, or unrelated to its intended action, the right balance between risk and benefit is not always clear.

Hematotoxicity may be regarded as *primary,* where one or more blood components are directly affected, or *secondary,* where the toxic effect is a consequence of other tissue injury or systemic disturbances. Primary toxicity is regarded as among the more common serious effects of xenobiotics, particularly drugs (Magee and Beeley, 1991). Secondary toxicity is exceedingly common, due to the propensity of blood cells to reflect a wide range of local and systemic effects of toxicants on other tissues. These secondary effects on hematopoietic tissue are often more reactive or compensatory than toxic and provide the toxicologist with an important and accessible tool for monitoring and characterizing toxic responses.

HEMATOPOIESIS

The production of blood cells, or hematopoiesis, is a highly regulated sequence of events by which blood cell precursors proliferate and differentiate to meet the relentless needs of oxygen transport, host defense and repair, hemostasis, and other vital functions described previously. The bone marrow is the principal site of hematopoiesis. The spleen has little function in blood cell production in the healthy human but plays a critical role in the clearance of defective or senescent cells, as well in host defense. In the human fetus, hematopoiesis can be found in the liver, spleen, bone marrow, thymus and lymph nodes. The bone marrow is the dominant hematopoietic organ in the latter half of gestation and the only blood cell producing organ at birth (Moore, 1975). All marrow is active, or "red marrow," at birth (Hudson, 1965). During early childhood, hematopoiesis recedes in long bones and, in adults, is confined to the axial skeleton and proximal humerus and femur (Custer and Ahlfeldt, 1932). The marrow in the distal long bones becomes "yellow" or fatty. When demand for blood cell production is great, as with certain disease states, fatty marrow can be reactivated as sites of hematopoiesis (Fig. 11-1). This can be useful in toxicology studies as a marker of sustained hematopoietic stress, as exemplified in studies on the hematopathology of cephalosporin toxicity in the dog (Bloom et al., 1987). Under extreme conditions, embryonic patterns of hematopoiesis may reappear as *extramedullary hematopoiesis* (Young and Weiss, 1997).

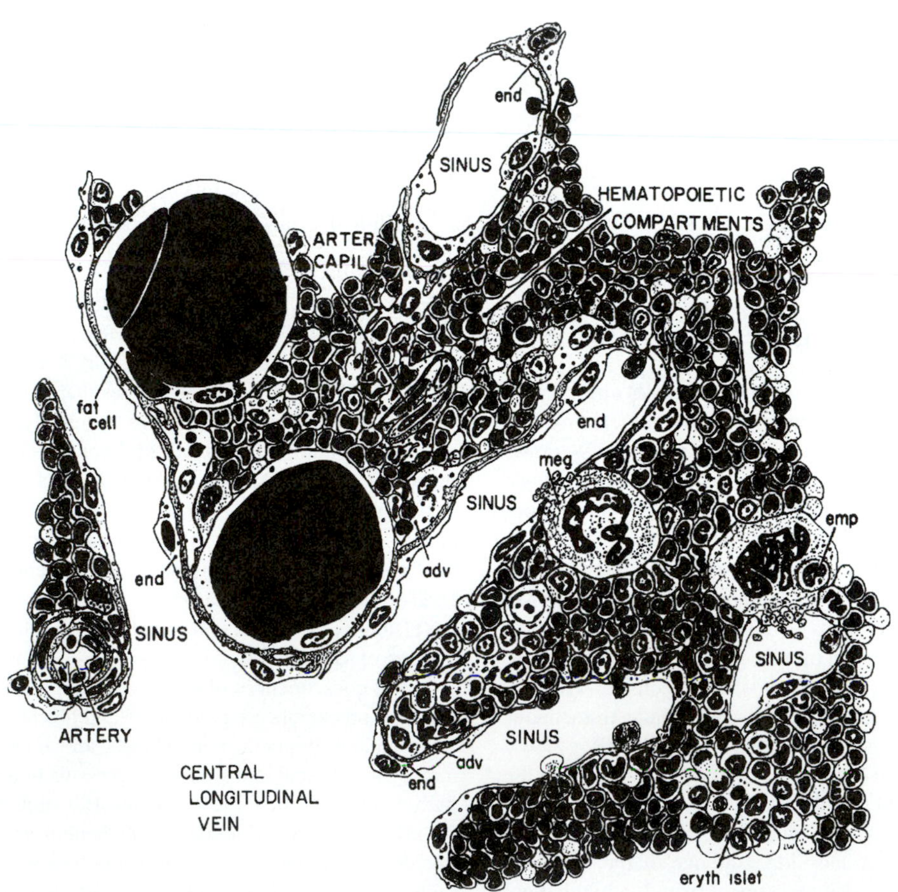

Figure 11-1

Bone marrow schema. Several venous sinuses (SINUS), cut longitudinally, drain into the central longitudinal vein, cut in cross section. A branch of the nutrient artery (ARTERY) and an arterial capillary (ARTER CAPIL) are present. The circulation in the bone marrow, as in the other tissues of the body save the spleen, is "closed"; that is, there is endothelial continuity from artery into vein. Veins in bone marrow have in common with veins elsewhere the primary function of returning blood to the heart. Marrow veins, in addition, possess the distinc-

While the central function of bone marrow is hematopoiesis and lymphopoiesis, bone marrow is also one of the sites of the mononuclear phagocyte system (MPS), contributing monocytes that differentiate into a variety of MPS cells located in liver (Kupffer cells), spleen (littoral cells), lymph nodes, and other tissues. Conventional histologic and cytologic sampling of bone marrow reveals a very limited picture of an exceedingly complex tissue containing erythroid, granulocytic, megakaryocytic, MPS, and lymphoid precursors in varied stages of maturation; stromal cells; and vasculature all encased by bone (Fig. 11-1). Routine examinations of such specimens in our pathology and toxicology laboratories cannot possibly reveal the sophisticated interactions that mediate lineage commitment, proliferation, differentiation, acquisition of functional characteristics, and trafficking that results in the delivery of mature cells to the circulation, as required in sickness and in health. This exquisite and homeostatic regulation of blood cell production involves a complex interplay of developing cells with stromal cells, extracellular matrix components, and cytokines that make up the *hematopoietic inductive microenvironment,* or HIM (Young and Weiss, 1997). Our understanding of how the array of hematopoietic growth factors interact within the HIM is growing rapidly (Kaushansky, 2000). This knowledge, through DNA recombinant technology, continues to yield sophisticated tools and promising therapies that present new pharmacologic and toxicologic challenges.

tive function of receiving blood cells produced and stored in the marrow and carrying them to thymus or spleen, or into the general circulation, for further maturation, widespread distribution and function. The hematopoietic compartments of the bone marrow consist of hematopoietic cells in varying stages of differentiation supported by a fibroblastic stroma. They lie between the most proximal veins, termed venous sinuses or vascular sinuses. When hematopoiesis is rather quiet and few nascent blood cells cross the wall of vascular sinuses, moving from hematopoietic compartments into the sinus lumen, the wall of the sinus tends to be trilaminar, consisting of endothelium (end), wispy basement membrane (in stipple), and adventitial reticular cells (adv) that form an incomplete outermost layer and branch out into the hematopoietic compartment, forming a scaffolding enclosing and supporting the hematopoietic cells. Thus, adventitial reticular cells are both vascular, as the outermost wall of the vascular sinus, and stromal, branching into the perivascular hematopoietic space, holding the vascular sinus in place and supporting hematopoietic cells. Where hematopoietic cell traffic across the wall of the venous sinus is heightened, the adventitial cell cover is retracted and a larger expanse of endothelium, covered only by wisps of basement membrane, is exposed to the hematopoietic cells, facilitating their transmural cell passage. Where transmural cell passage is greatly reduced, adventitial cells accumulate fat and become rounded and bulky, now termed adipocytes, impeding hematopoietic cell passage, and occupying space in the hematopoietic compartment which, when they transform again to adventitial cells flattened upon veins, they yield to hematopoiesis. These fibroblastic stromal cells in the marrow of central bones can modulate readily to and from adventitial cell and adipocyte and retain their granulocyte inductive capacities in either form. In the distal limb and tail bones, where there is little hematopoiesis, they assume the adipocyte form in such large numbers that the marrow is grossly yellow. These adipocytes lose fat only in marked hematopoietic stress, as in spherocytic and other severe anemias where this marrow becomes hematopoietic and grossly red. In such stress, moreover, barrier cells may augment or replace adventitial reticular cells and even endothelial cells. Thus, adventitial cells/adipocytes, by their disposition and bulk, mechanically regulate hematopoiesis and blood cell delivery. In addition, they do so in a subtle manner, through paracrine secretion of several small-protein regulatory factors termed cytokines, which include interleukins. [Reprinted from Young and Weiss (1997) with permission from the authors and Elsevier Science.]

TOXICOLOGY OF THE ERYTHRON

The Erythrocyte

Erythrocytes (red blood cells, or RBCs) make up 40 to 45 percent of the circulating blood volume and serve as the principal vehicle of transportation of oxygen from the lungs to the peripheral tissues. In addition, erythrocytes are involved in the transport of carbon dioxide from tissues to the lung and in the maintenance of a constant pH in blood despite the ever changing concentration of carbon dioxide (Hsia, 1998). Erythrocytes help modulate the inflammatory response through clearance of immune complexes containing complement components and through interaction with nitric oxide, a potent vasodilator (Hebert, 1991). An area of developing interest is the role of erythrocytes as a carrier and/or reservoir for drugs and toxins (Schrijvers et al., 1999). The effect of xenobiotics on erythrocytes has been extensively evaluated, both because of the ready access to the tissue and the frequency with which xenobiotics cause changes in this critical tissue.

Xenobiotics may affect the production, function and/or survival of erythrocytes. These effects are most frequently manifest as a change in the circulating red cell mass, usually resulting in a decrease (anemia). Occasionally, agents that affect the oxygen affinity of hemoglobin lead to an increase in the red cell mass (erythrocytosis), but this is distinctly less common. Shifts in plasma volume can alter the relative concentration of erythrocytes (and hemoglobin concentration) and can be easily confused with true anemia or erythrocytosis.

There are two general mechanisms that lead to true anemia—either decreased production or increased destruction of erythrocytes. Both mechanisms may be operative in some disorders, or a combination may arise due to the imposition of a second disorder on a compensated underlying problem. For example, patients with compensated congenital hemolytic anemias are very susceptible to additional insults, such as parvovirus infection, that may precipitate an acute drop in a previously stable red cell mass.

Evaluation of a peripheral blood sample can provide evidence for the underlying mechanism of anemia (Lee, 1999a). The usual parameters of a complete blood count (CBC)—including the red blood cell (RBC) count, hemoglobin concentration (Hbg) and hematocrit (also referred to as packed cell volume, or PCV)—can establish the presence of anemia. Two additional parameters that are helpful in classifying an anemia are the mean corpuscular volume (MCV) and the reticulocyte count. Increased destruction is usually accompanied by an increase in reticulocytes (young erythrocytes containing residual RNA), which are easily enumerated using appropriate stains. Two related processes contribute to the increased number of reticulocytes in humans. First, increased destruction is accompanied by a compensatory increase in bone marrow production, with an increase in the number of cells being released from the marrow into the circulation. Second, during compensatory erythroid hyperplasia, the marrow releases reticulocytes earlier in their life span and thus the reticulocytes persist for a longer period in the peripheral blood. Other readily performed parameters helpful in the evaluation of the human erythron include: erythrocyte morphology (e.g., megaloblastic changes, erythrocyte fragmentation, sickled RBCs); serum concentration of haptoglobin, lactic dehydrogenase (LD), free hemoglobin, vitamin B_{12}, fo-

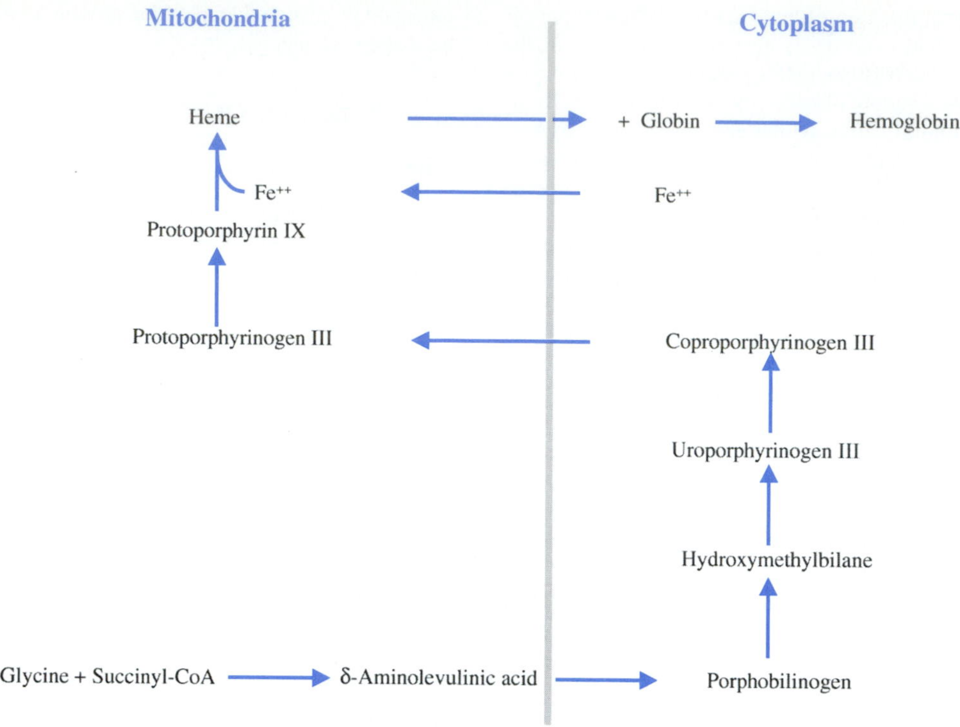

Figure 11-2

The synthesis of heme involves a series of reactions that occur in the cytoplasm and mitochondria of erythroblasts. The initial step in the pathway is the mitochondria synthesis of δ-aminolevulinic acid, a step that is commonly affected by xenobiotics, including lead. Ferrochelatase catalyzes the incorporation of ferrous iron into the tetrapyrrole protoporphyrin IX. Inhibition of the synthetic pathway leading to protoporphyrin IX, as occurs in the sideroblastic anemias, can cause an imbalance between iron concentration and ferrochelatase activity, resulting in iron deposition within mitochondria. Mitochondrial accumulation of iron is the hallmark lesion of the sideroblastic anemias.

late, iron, and ferritin; direct and indirect red cell antiglobulin tests; and bone marrow morphology (Lee, 1999a).

Alterations in Red Cell Production

Erythrocyte production is a continuous process that is dependent on frequent cell division and a high rate of hemoglobin synthesis. Adult hemoglobin (hemoglobin A), the major constituent of the erythrocyte cytoplasm, is a tetramer composed of two α- and two β-globin chains, each with a heme residue located in a stereospecific pocket of the globin chain. Synthesis of hemoglobin is dependent on coordinated production of globin chains and heme moieties. Abnormalities that lead to decreased hemoglobin synthesis are relatively common (e.g., iron deficiency) and are often associated with a decrease in the MCV and hypochromasia (increased central pallor of RBCs on stained blood films due to the low hemoglobin concentration).

An imbalance between α- and β-chain production is the basis of congenital thalassemia syndromes and results in decreased hemoglobin production and microcytosis (Weatherall, 1997). Xenobiotics can affect globin-chain synthesis and alter the composition of hemoglobin within erythrocytes. This is perhaps best demonstrated by hydroxyurea, which has been found to increase the synthesis of γ globin chains. The γ globin chains are a normal constituent of hemoglobin during fetal development, replacing the β chains in the hemoglobin tetramer (hemoglobin F, $\alpha_2\gamma_2$). Hemoglobin F has a higher affinity for oxygen than hemoglobin A and can protect against crystallization (sickling) of deoxyhemoglobin S in sickle cell disease (Steinberg, 1999).

Synthesis of heme requires incorporation of iron into a porphyrin ring (Fig. 11-2) (Ponka, 1997; Dessypris, 1999). Iron deficiency is usually the result of dietary deficiency or increased blood loss. Any drug that contributes to blood loss, such as nonsteroidal anti-inflammatory agents, with their increased risk of gastrointestinal ulceration and bleeding, may potentiate the risk of developing *iron deficiency anemia.* Defects in the synthesis of porphyrin ring of heme can lead to *sideroblastic anemia,* with its characteristic accumulation of iron in bone marrow erythroblasts. The accumulated iron precipitates within mitochondria, causing the intracellular injury and the characteristic staining pattern of ringed sideroblasts evident on iron stains such as Prussian blue. A number of xenobiotics (Table 11-1) can interfere with one or more of the steps in erythroblast heme synthesis and result in sideroblastic

Table 11-1
Xenobiotics Associated with Sideroblastic Anemia

Ethanol	Chloramphenicol
Isoniazid	Cooper chelation/deficiency
Pyrazinamide	Zinc intoxication
Cycloserine	Lead intoxication

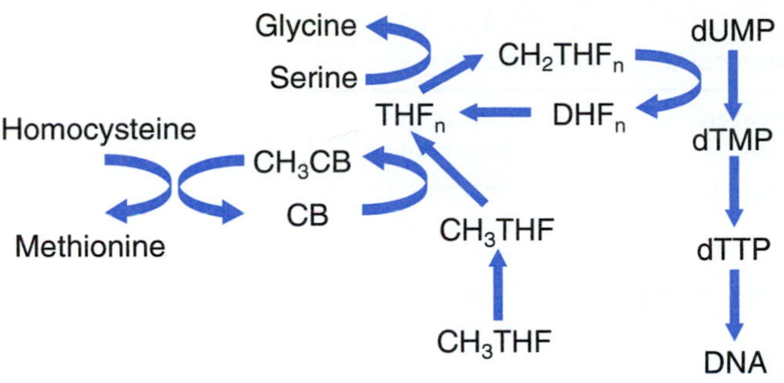

Figure 11-3

Both tetrahydrofolate (THF) and cobalamin (CB, or vitamin B_{12}) are necessary for the synthesis of thymidine (dTMP) for incorporation into DNA. Folate enters the cell as a monoglutamate (CH_3THF) but is transformed to a polyglutamate within the cell, a step that helps prevent leakage of folate back across the cell membrane. However, CH_3THF cannot be conjugated with glutamate. CB is necessary for demethylation of the folate, allowing formation of conjugated (polyglutamate) folate (THF_n). In the absence of CB, folate levels within the cell drop, causing a functional deficiency of folate and impairing synthesis of thymidine.

anemia (Fiske et al., 1994; May and Fitzsimons, 1994; Bottomley, 1999).

All of the hematopoietic elements of the marrow are dependent on continuous proliferation to replace the circulating cells. This requires active DNA synthesis and frequent mitoses. Folate and vitamin B_{12} are necessary to maintain synthesis of thymidine for incorporation into DNA (Fig. 11-3). Deficiency of folate and/or vitamin B_{12} results in *megaloblastic anemia,* with its characteristic morphologic and biochemical changes (Table 11-2), which commonly affect erythroid, myeloid, and megakaryocytic lineages. A number of xenobiotics may contribute to a deficiency of vitamin B_{12} and/or folate (Table 11-3), leading to megaloblastic anemia (Tapp and Savarirayan, 1997; Lee, 1999b; Lee, 1999c).

Many of the antiproliferative agents used in the treatment of malignancy predictably inhibit hematopoiesis, including erythropoiesis. The resulting bone marrow toxicity may be dose-limiting, as previously discussed. The development of recombinant forms of some of the cytokines that regulate hematopoiesis has helped shorten the duration of suppression, and new agents are being developed that may help protect against the marrow toxicity of these agents (Capizzi, 1999).

Table 11-3
Xenobiotics Associated with Megaloblastic Anemia

B_{12} DEFICIENCY	FOLATE DEFICIENCY
Paraminosalicylic acid	Phenytoin
Colchicine	Primidone
Neomycin	Carbamazepine
Ethanol	Phenobarbital
Omeprazole	Sulfasalazine
Hemodialysis	Cholestyramine
Zidovudine	Triamterine
Fish tapeworm	Malabsorption syndromes
	Antimetabolites

Drug-induced *aplastic anemia* may represent either a predictable or idiosyncratic reaction to a xenobiotic. This life-threatening disorder is characterized by peripheral blood pancytopenia, reticulocytopenia, and bone marrow hypoplasia (Young and Maciejewski, 1997; Young, 1999). Agents such as benzene and radiation have a *predictable* effect on hematopoietic progenitors, and the resulting aplastic anemia corresponds to the magnitude of the exposure to these agents. In contrast, idiosyncratic aplastic anemia does not appear to be related to the dose of the agent initiating the process. A long list of agents has been associated with the development of aplastic anemia (Table 11-4), many of which have been reported in only a few patients. The mechanism(s) of aplasia in affected patients is(are) still unknown. Immune mechanisms have long been thought to contribute to the development of the idiosyncratic form of drug-induced aplastic anemia. However, it has been difficult to obtain definitive evidence for humoral and/or cellular mechanisms of marrow suppression (Young, 2000).

Pure red cell aplasia is a syndrome in which the decrease in marrow production is limited to the erythroid lineage. Pure red cell aplasia is an uncommon disorder that may be seen in a variety of clinical settings. A number of drugs have been implicated in the development of red cell aplasia, but many of these represent single case reports (Thompson and Gales, 1996; Marseglia and Locatelli, 1998; Misra et al., 1998; Blanche et al., 1999). As pure red cell aplasia also occurs sporadically, the linkage between drug

Table 11-2
Laboratory Features of Megaloblastic Anemia

MORPHOLOGY	BIOCHEMISTRY
Peripheral blood	Peripheral blood
Pancytopenia	Decreased B_{12} and/or folate
Macrocytosis (↑MCV)	Increased LD
Oval macrocytes	Antiparietal cell antibodies
Hypersegmented neutrophils	Antibody to intrinsic factor
Variation in RBC shape	Increased serum iron
Bone marrow	Hypokalemia
Erythroid hyperplasia	
Megaloblastic anemia	
Giant band neutrophils	
Giant metamyelocytes	

Table 11-4
Drugs and Chemicals Associated with the Development of Aplastic Anemia

Chloramphenicol	Organic arsenicals	Quinacrine
Methylphenylethylhydantoin	Trimethadione	Phenylbutazone
Gold	Streptomycin	Benzene
Penicillin	Allopurinol	Tetracycline
Methicillin	Sulfonamides	Chlortetracycline
Sulfisoxazole	Sulfamethoxypyridazine	Amphotericin B
Mefloquine	Ethosuximide	Felbamate
Carbimazole	Methylmercaptoimidazole	Potassium perchlorate
Propylthiouracil	Tolbutamide	Pyrimethamine
Chlorpropamide	Carbutamide	Tripelennamine
Indomethacin	Carbamazepine	Diclofenac
Meprobamate	Chlorpromazine	Chlordiazepoxide
Mepazine	Chlorphenothane	Parathion
Thiocyanate	Methazolamide	Dinitrophenol
Bismuth	Mercury	Chlordane
Carbon tetrachloride	Cimetidine	Metolazone
Azidothymidine	Ticlopidine	Isoniazid
Trifluoperazine	D-penicillamine	

exposure and pathogenesis of the aplasia remains speculative for some agents. The drugs most clearly implicated in this idiosyncratic reaction, and for which there are multiple case reports, include isoniazid, phenytoin, and azathioprine. The mechanism of drug-induced pure red cell aplasia is unknown, but some evidence suggests that it may be immune-mediated. It has been suggested that genetic variation may play a role in the susceptibility to the development of pure red cell aplasia (Marseglia and Locatelli, 1998). Patients with drug-induced red cell aplasia should not be reexposed to the purported offending agent.

Alterations in the Respiratory Function of Hemoglobin

Hemoglobin is necessary for effective transport of oxygen and carbon dioxide between the lungs and tissues. The respiratory function of hemoglobin has been studied in detail, revealing an intricately balanced system for the transport of oxygen from the lungs to the tissues (Hsia, 1998). Electrostatic charges hold the globin chains of deoxyhemoglobin in a "tense" (T) conformation characterized by a relatively low affinity for oxygen. Binding of oxygen alters this conformation to a "relaxed" (R) conformation that is associated with a 500-fold increase in oxygen affinity. Thus the individual globin units show cooperativity in the binding of oxygen, resulting in the familiar sigmoid shape to the oxygen dissociation curve (Fig. 11-4). The ability of hemoglobin to safely and efficiently transport oxygen is dependent on both intrinsic (homotropic) and extrinsic (heterotropic) factors that affect the performance of this system.

Homotropic Effects Perhaps one of the most important homotropic properties of oxyhemoglobin is the slow but consistent oxidation of heme iron to the ferric state to form methemoglobin. Methemoglobin is not capable of binding and transporting oxygen. In addition, the presence of methemoglobin in a hemoglobin tetramer has allosteric effects that increase the affinity of oxyhemoglobin for oxygen, resulting in a leftward shift of the oxygen dissociation curve (Fig. 11-4). The combination of decreased oxygen content and increased affinity may significantly impair delivery of oxygen to tissues when the concentration of methemoglobin rises beyond critical levels (Hsia, 1998, Ranney and Sharma, 1995).

Not surprisingly, the normal erythrocyte has metabolic mechanisms for reducing heme iron back to the ferrous state; these mechanisms are normally capable of maintaining the concentration of methemoglobin at less than 1% of the total hemoglobin (Coleman and Coleman, 1996). The predominant pathway is cytochrome b_5 methemoglobin reductase, which is dependent on reduced nicotine adenine dinucleotide (NADH) and is also known as NADH-diaphorase. An alternate pathway involves a reduced nicotine adenine dinucleotide phosphate (NADPH) diaphorase that reduces a flavin that in turn reduces methemoglobin. This pathway usually accounts for less than 5 percent of the reduction of methemoglobin, but its activity can be greatly enhanced by methylene blue, which is reduced to leukomethylene blue by NADPH-diaphorase. Leukomethylene blue then reduces methemoglobin to deoxyhemoglobin.

A failure of these control mechanisms leads to increased levels of methemoglobin, or *methemoglobinemia.* The most common cause of methemoglobinemia is exposure to an oxidizing xenobiotic that overwhelms the NADH-diaphorase system. A large number of chemicals and therapeutic agents may cause methemoglobinemia (Table 11-5) (Coleman and Coleman, 1996; Khan and Kruse, 1999; Lukens, 1999; Nguyen et al., 2000). These agents may be divided into direct oxidizers, which are capable of inducing methemoglobin formation when added to erythrocytes in vitro or in vivo, and indirect oxidizers, which do not induce methemoglobin formation when exposed to erythrocytes in vitro but do so after metabolic modification in vivo. Nitrites appear to be able to interact directly with heme to facilitate oxidation of heme iron, but the precise mechanism that leads to methemoglobin formation is unknown for many of the other substances listed in Table 11-5.

The development of methemoglobinemia may be slow and insidious or abrupt in onset, as with the use of some topical anes-

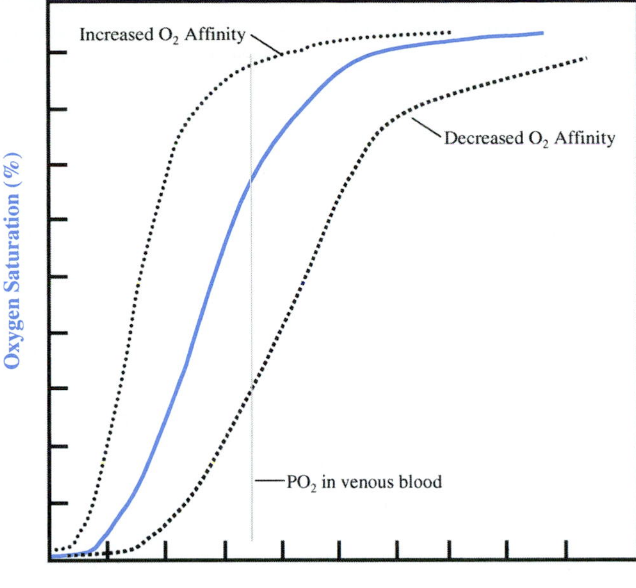

Figure 11-4

The normal oxygen dissociation curve *(solid line)* has a sigmoid shape due to the cooperative interaction between the four globin chains in the hemoglobin molecule. Fully deoxygenated hemoglobin has a relatively low affinity for oxygen. Interaction of oxygen with one heme-iron moiety induces a conformational change in that globin chain. Through surface interactions, that conformational change affects the other globin chains, causing a conformational change in all of the globin chains that increases their affinity for oxygen. Homotropic and heterotropic parameters also affect the affinity of hemoglobin for oxygen. An increase in oxygen affinity results in a shift to the left in the oxygen-dissociation curve. Such a shift may decrease oxygen delivery to the tissues. A decrease in oxygen affinity results in a shift to the right in the oxygen dissociation curve, facilitating oxygen delivery to the tissues.

thetics (Khan and Kruse, 1999; Nguyen et al., 2000). Most patients tolerate low levels (<10%) of methemoglobin without clinical symptoms. Cyanosis is often evident when the methemoglobin concentration exceeds 5 to 10%. Levels above 20% are generally clinically significant and some patients may begin to manifest symptoms related to tissue hypoxemia at methemoglobin levels between 10 and 20%. The severity of clinical manifestations increases as the concentration rises above 20 to 30%, with methemoglobin levels above 70% usually being fatal. Administration of methylene blue is effective in rapidly reversing methemoglobinemia through activation of the NADPH diaphorase pathway. The effect of methylene blue is dependent on an adequate supply of NADPH. Consequently, methylene blue is not effective in patients with glucose-6-phosphate dehydrogenase (G-6-PD) deficiency because of the decreased capacity to form NADPH (Coleman and Coleman, 1996).

Heterotropic Effects There are three major heterotropic effectors of hemoglobin function: pH, erythrocyte 2,3-bisphosphoglycerate (2,3-BPG, formerly designated 2,3-diphosphoglycerate) concentration, and temperature (Ranney and Sharma, 1995; Hsia, 1998). A decrease in pH (e.g., lactic acid, carbon dioxide) lowers the affinity of hemoglobin for oxygen; that is, it causes a right-shift in the oxygen dissociation curve, facilitating the delivery of oxygen to tissues (Fig. 11-4). As bicarbonate and carbon dioxide equilibrate in the lung, the hydrogen ion concentration decreases, increasing the affinity of hemoglobin for oxygen and facilitating oxygen uptake. Thus the buffering capacity of hemoglobin also serves to improve oxygen uptake and delivery.

The binding site for 2,3-BPG is located in a pocket formed by the two β chains of a hemoglobin tetramer. Binding of 2,3-BPG to deoxyhemoglobin results in stabilization of the "T" conformation, with reduced oxygen affinity (a shift to the right of the oxygen dissociation curve). The conformational change induced by binding of oxygen alters the binding site for 2,3-BPG and results in release of 2,3-BPG from hemoglobin. This facilitates uptake of more oxygen for delivery to tissues. The concentration of 2,3-BPG increases whenever there is tissue hypoxemia but may decrease in the presence of acidosis or hypophosphatemia. Thus hypophosphatemia may result in a left shift of the oxygen dissociation curve.

Clofibric acid and bezafibrate are capable of lowering the oxygen affinity of hemoglobin, analogous to 2,3-BPG, without damage to the erythrocyte or hemoglobin (Poyart et al., 1994). However, the association constant of bezafibrate for hemoglobin is too low for there to be a practical effect in vivo. Work continues on bezafibrate derivatives that may lower oxygen affinity and enhance tissue oxygenation. In contrast, some aromatic benzaldehydes have been shown to increase the oxygen affinity and shift the dissociation curve to the left. It was thought that these compounds may be useful in preventing the sickling of deoxyhemoglobin S in patients with sickle cell disease. However, these and other agents evaluated for their effect on hemoglobin oxygen affinity have not progressed into clinical usage (Poyart et al., 1994; Papassotirion et al., 1998).

The oxygen affinity of hemoglobin decreases as the body temperature increases (Hsia, 1998). This facilitates delivery of oxygen to tissues during periods of extreme exercise and febrile illnesses associated with increased temperature. Correspondingly, oxygen affinity increases during hypothermia, which may lead to decreased oxygen delivery under these conditions. This must be taken into consideration during surgical procedures during which there is induction of deep hypothermia.

Table 11-5
Xenobiotics Associated with Methemoglobinemia

THERAPEUTIC AGENTS	ENVIRONMENTAL AGENTS
Benzocaine	Nitrites
Lidocaine	Nitrates
Prilocaine	Nitrobenzenes
Dapsone	Aniline dyes
Amyl nitrate	Butyl nitrite
Isobutyl nitrite	Potassium chlorate
Nitroglycerine	Gasoline additives
Primaquine	Aminobenzenes
Sulfonamide	Nitrotoluenes
Phenacetin	Trinitrotoluene
Nitric oxide	Nitroethane
Phenazopyridine	
Metoclopramide	
Flutamide	
Silver nitrate	
Quinones	
Methylene blue	

The respiratory function of hemoglobin may also be impaired by blocking of the ligand binding site by the interaction with other substances, most notably carbon monoxide (Hsia, 1998). Carbon monoxide has a relatively low rate of association with deoxyhemoglobin but shows high affinity once bound. The affinity is about 200 times that of oxygen, and thus persistent exposure to a carbon monoxide concentration of 0.1% may lead to 50% saturation of hemoglobin. Binding of carbon monoxide also results in stabilization of the hemoglobin molecule in the high-affinity "R" conformation. Consequently, the oxygen dissociation curve is shifted to the left, further compromising oxygen delivery to the tissues. Carbon monoxide is produced at low levels by the body and equilibrates across the pulmonary capillary/alveolar bed. The major sources of significant exposure to carbon monoxide are smoking and burning of fossil fuels (including automobiles). Heavy smoking during pregnancy can result in significant levels of carboxyhemoglobin in fetal blood and diminished oxygenation of fetal tissues.

Methemoglobin can combine reversibly with a variety of chemical substances, including cyanide, sulfides, peroxides, fluorides, and azides (Coleman and Coleman, 1996; Lukens, 1999). The affinity of methemoglobin for cyanide is utilized in two settings. First, nitrites are administered in cyanide poisoning to form methemoglobin, which then binds free cyanide, sparing other critical cellular respiratory enzymes. Second, formation of cyanmethemoglobin by reaction of hemoglobin with potassium ferricyanide is a standard method for measurement of hemoglobin concentration.

Nitric oxide, an important vasodilator that modulates vascular tone, binds avidly to heme iron. An additional function of erythrocytes is related to this interaction, which can influence the availability of nitric oxide in parts of the circulation (Everse and Hsia, 1997; Hsia, 1998). Solutions of hemoglobin have been evaluated as a potential replacement for red blood cell transfusions. However, these trials have been halted due to the toxicity associated with administration of hemoglobin solutions. Vascular instability is one of the complications associated with infusion of hemoglobin solutions and is thought to be related to the scavenging of essential nitric oxide by the administered hemoglobin (Hess et al., 1993; Everse and Hsia, 1997).

Alterations in Erythrocyte Survival

The normal survival of erythrocytes in the circulation is about 120 days (Dessypris, 1999). During this period the erythrocytes are exposed to a variety of oxidative injuries and must negotiate the tortuous passages of the microcirculation and the spleen. This requires a deformable cell membrane and energy to maintain the sodium-potassium gradients and repair mechanisms. Very little protein synthesis occurs during this time, as erythrocytes are anucleate when they enter the circulation and residual mRNA is rapidly lost over the first 1 to 2 days in the circulation. Consequently, senescence occurs over time until the aged erythrocytes are removed by the spleen, where the iron is recovered for reutilization in heme synthesis. Any insult that increases oxidative injury, decreases metabolism, or alters the membrane may cause a decrease in erythrocyte concentration and a corresponding anemia.

Anemia due to increased red cell destruction (hemolytic anemia) is usually characterized by reticulocytosis in the peripheral blood and erythroid hyperplasia of the bone marrow (Lee, 1999a). As reticulocytes tend to be somewhat larger than older erythrocytes, there may be a mild increase in the MCV. The presence of increased numbers of reticulocytes is often evident on the peripheral blood film in the form of polychromatophilic erythrocytes. The residual RNA present in these cells gives the cytoplasm a blue-gray cast on Wright-stained blood films. Depending on where erythrocyte destruction occurs, the concentration of haptoglobin may be decreased, serum LD may be increased, and serum free hemoglobin may be increased. The acquired hemolytic anemias are often divided into immune-mediated and non-immune mediated types.

Nonimmune Hemolytic Anemia

Microangiopathic Anemias Intravascular fragmentation of erythrocytes gives rise to the *microangiopathic hemolytic anemias* (Tabbara, 1992; Ruggenenti and Remuzzi, 1998). The hallmark of this process is the presence of schistocytes (fragmented RBCs) in the peripheral blood. These abnormal cellular fragments are usually promptly cleared from the circulation by the spleen. Thus their presence in peripheral blood samples indicates either an increased rate of formation or abnormal clearance function of the spleen. The formation of fibrin strands in the microcirculation is a common mechanism for RBC fragmentation. This may occur in the setting of disseminated intravascular coagulation, sepsis, the hemolytic-uremic syndrome, and thrombotic thrombocytopenic purpura. The erythrocytes are essentially sliced into fragments by the fibrin strands that extend across the vascular lumen and impede the flow of erythrocytes through the vasculature. Excessive fragmentation can also be seen in the presence of abnormal vasculature, as occurs with damaged cardiac valves, arteriovenous malformations, vasculitis, and widely metastatic carcinoma (Nesher et al., 1994; Rytting et al., 1996; Gordon and Kwaan, 1999). The high shear associated with malignant hypertension may also lead to RBC fragmentation.

Other Mechanical Injuries March hemoglobinuria is an episodic disorder characterized by destruction of RBCs during vigorous exercise or marching (Sagov, 1970; Abarbanel et al., 1990). The erythrocytes appear to be destroyed by mechanical trauma in the feet. Sufficient hemoglobin may be released to cause hemoglobinuria. The disorder should be distinguished from other causes of intermittent hemoglobinuria such as paroxysmal nocturnal hemoglobinuria. The introduction of improved footgear for athletes and soldiers has significantly decreased the incidence of this problem.

Major thermal burns are also associated with a hemolytic process. The erythrocyte membrane becomes unstable as the temperature increases. With major burns there can be significant heat-dependent lysis of erythrocytes. Small RBC fragments break off, with resealing of the cell membrane. These cell fragments usually assume a spherical shape and are not as deformable as normal erythrocytes. Consequently, these abnormal cell fragments are removed in the spleen, leading to an anemia. The burden of RBC fragments may impair the phagocytic function of the spleen, contributing to the increased susceptibility to endotoxic shock following major burns (Schneiderkraut and Loeggering, 1984; Hatherill et al., 1986)

Infectious Diseases A wide variety of infectious diseases may be associated with significant hemolysis, either by direct effect on the erythrocyte or development of an immune-mediated hemolytic process (Berkowitz, 1991; Lee, 1999d). The most common agents that directly cause hemolysis include malaria, babesiosis, clostridial infections, and bartonellosis. Erythrocytes are parasitized in malaria and babesiosis, leading to their destruction.

Clostridial infections are associated with release of hemolytic toxins that enter the circulation and lyse erythrocytes. The hemolysis can be severe with significant hemoglobinuria, even with apparently localized infections. *Bartonella bacilliformis* is thought to adhere to the erythrocyte, leading to rapid removal from the circulation. The hemolysis can be severe and the mortality rate in this disorder (Oroya fever) is high.

Oxidative Hemolysis Molecular oxygen is a reactive and potentially toxic chemical species; consequently the normal respiratory function of erythrocytes generates oxidative stress on a continuous basis. The major mechanisms that protect against oxidative injury in erythrocytes include NADH-diaphorase, superoxide dismutase, catalase, and the glutathione pathway (Coleman and Coleman, 1996; Everse and Hsia, 1997). As indicated previously, a small amount of methemoglobin is continuously formed during the process of loading and unloading of oxygen from hemoglobin. Formation of methemoglobin is associated with formation of superoxide free radicals, which must be detoxified to prevent oxidative injury to hemoglobin and other critical erythrocyte components. Under physiologic conditions, superoxide dismutase converts superoxide into hydrogen peroxide, which is then metabolized by catalase and glutathione peroxidase (Fig. 11-5).

A number of xenobiotics, particularly compounds containing aromatic amines, are capable of inducing oxidative injury in erythrocytes (Table 11-6) (Yoo and Lessin, 1992; Jollow et al., 1995; Everse and Hsia, 1997; Nohl and Stolze, 1998). These agents appear to potentiate the normal redox reactions and are capable of overwhelming the usual protective mechanisms. The interaction between these xenobiotics and hemoglobin leads to the formation of free radicals that denature critical proteins, including hemoglobin, thiol-dependent enzymes, and components of the erythrocyte membrane. In the presence of hydrogen peroxide and xenobiotics such as hydroxylamine, hydroxamic acid, and phenolic compounds, a reactive ferryl (Fe^{+4}) hemoglobin intermediate may be formed according to the following reaction:

$$H_2O_2 + \text{Hgb–}Fe^{3+} \rightarrow H_2O + \text{Hgb}(\bullet+)\text{–}Fe^{4+}\text{–}O^-$$

In this intermediate, referred to as compound 1, tyrosine may donate the extra electron, turning it into a reactive free radical. Compound 1 may undergo further reaction with organic compounds (AH_2 in equations below) to yield additional free radicals according to the following reactions:

$$\text{Hgb}(\bullet+)\text{–}Fe^{4+}\text{–}O^- + AH_2 \rightarrow \text{Hgb–}Fe^{4+}\text{–}O^- + AH\bullet + H^+$$

$$\text{Hgb–}Fe^{4+}\text{–}O^- + AH_2 + H^+ \rightarrow \text{Hgb–}Fe^{3+} + AH\bullet + H_2O$$

Hemoglobin contains exposed free cysteines (β93) that are critical for the structural integrity of the molecule. Oxidation of these groups can denature hemoglobin and decrease its solubility. The oxidized, denatured hemoglobin species comprise what has been designated sulfhemoglobin. The denatured hemoglobin can form aggregates that bind to the cell membrane to form inclusions called *Heinz bodies,* a hallmark of oxidative injury to erythrocytes (Jandl, 1987). Heinz bodies can be visualized by use of phase-contrast microscopy or supravital stains such as crystal violet. These membrane-associated inclusions impair the deformability of the erythrocyte membrane and thus impede movement of erythrocytes through the microcirculation and the spleen. Heinz bodies are effectively removed from the erythrocyte by the spleen, so they are not often observed in peripheral blood samples from patients despite ongoing oxidative injury. However, the culling of Heinz bodies can alter the morphology of the affected cells, giving rise to what are called "bite" cells and "blister" cells, which may provide an important clue as to the ongoing process (Yoo and Lessin, 1992). These cells look as though a portion of the cytoplasm had been cut away. Heinz body formation can be induced by in vitro exposure to oxidizing agents and patients with oxidative hemolysis often show increased in vitro formation of Heinz bodies.

Oxidative denaturation of the globin chain decreases its affinity for the heme group, which may dissociate from the globin chain during oxidative injury. The ferric iron in the heme ring may react with chloride to form a complex called hemin. Hemin is hy-

Table 11-6
Xenobiotics Associated with Oxidative Injury

Acetanilide	Phenylhydrazine
Naphthalene	Nitrobenzene
Nitrofurantoin	Phenacetin
Sulfamethoxypyridazine	Phenol
Aminosalicylic acid	Hydroxylamine
Sodium sulfoxone	Methylene blue
Dapsone	Toluidine blue
Phenazopyridine	Furazolidone
Primaquine	Nalidixic acid
Chlorates	Sulfanilamide
Sulfasalazine	

$$\text{HgbFe}^{++}O_2 \rightleftarrows \text{HgbFe}^{++} + O_2 \quad (1)$$

$$\text{HgbFe}^{++}O_2 \rightleftarrows \text{HgbFe}^{+++} + O_2^- \quad (2)$$

$$2O_2^- + 2H^+ \xrightarrow[\text{Dismutase}]{\text{Superoxide}} O_2 + H_2O_2 \quad (3)$$

$$2\,H_2O_2 \xrightarrow{\text{Catalase}} H_2O + O_2 \quad (4)$$

$$H_2O_2 + \text{GSH} \xrightarrow[\text{Peroxidase}]{\text{Glutathione}} \text{GSSH} + H_2O \quad (5)$$

$$O_2^- + \text{GSH} \xrightarrow[\text{Peroxidase}]{\text{Glutathione}} \text{GSSH} + H_2O \quad (6)$$

Figure 11-5

Oxygen normally exchanges with the ferrous iron of deoxyhemoglobin [Eq. (1)]. Oxygen can "capture" one of the iron electrons, resulting in the generation of methemoglobin (HgbFe^{3+}) and superoxide (O_2^-) [Eq. (2)]. Superoxide must be detoxified or it can lead to oxidative injury within the cell. The pathways involved include superoxide dismutase [Eq. (3)], catalase [Eq. (4)], and glutathione peroxidase [Eqs. (5 and 6)]. A supply of reduced glutathione (GSH) is necessary to prevent excessive oxidative injury.

drophobic and intercalates into the erythrocyte membrane from which it is removed by interaction with albumin. However, if the rate of hemin formation exceeds the rate of removal by albumin, hemin accumulates in the membrane, where it can cause rapid lysis of the erythrocyte (Everse and Hsia, 1997).

The generation of free radicals may also lead to peroxidation of membrane lipids (Jandl, 1987). This may affect the deformability of the erythrocyte and the permeability of the membrane to potassium. The alteration of the Na^+/K^+ gradient is independent of injury to the Na^+/K^+ pump and is potentially lethal to the affected erythrocyte. Oxidative injury also impairs the metabolic machinery of the erythrocyte, resulting in a decrease in the concentration of ATP (Tavazzi et al., 2000). Damage to the membrane can also permit leakage of denatured hemoglobin from the cell. Such free denatured hemoglobin can be toxic on its own. Free hemoglobin may irreversibly bind nitric oxide, resulting in vasoconstriction. Released hemoglobin may form nephrotoxic hemoglobin dimers, leading to kidney damage (Everse and Hsia, 1997).

Oxidative injury thus results in a number of changes that decrease the viability of erythrocytes. Protection against many of the free radical-induced modifications is mediated by reduced glutathione. Formation of reduced glutathione is dependent on NADPH and the hexose monophosphate shunt (Fig. 11-6). Significant oxidative injury usually occurs when the concentration of the xenobiotic is high enough (either due to high exposure or decreased metabolism of the xenobiotic) to overcome the normal protective mechanisms, or, more commonly, when there is an underlying defect in the protective mechanisms.

The most common enzyme defect associated with oxidative hemolysis is glucose-6-phosphate dehydrogenase (G-6-PD) deficiency, a relatively common sex-linked disorder characterized by alterations in the primary structure of G-6-PD that diminish its functional activity (Beutler, 1996; Weatherall, 1997). It is often clinically asymptomatic until the erythrocytes are exposed to oxidative stress. The stress may come from the host response to infection or exposure to xenobiotics. The level of G-6-PD normally decreases as the erythrocytes age. In the African type of G-6-PD deficiency, the enzyme is less stable than normal; thus the loss of activity is accelerated compared to normals. In the Mediterranean type of G-6-PD deficiency, the rate of loss of enzyme activity is even higher. Consequently, the older erythrocytes with the lowest levels of G-6-PD are most susceptible to hemolysis, with the degree of hemolysis affected by the residual amount of enzyme activity as well as the magnitude of the oxidative injury.

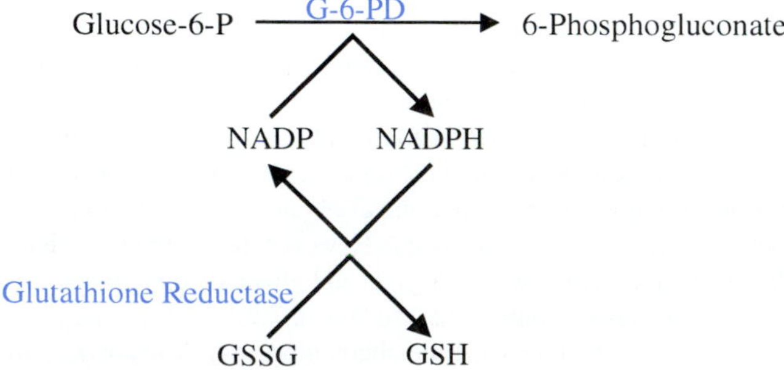

Figure 11-6

The hexose monophosphate shunt in the erythrocyte is critical for generation of NADPH, which helps maintain an intracellular supply of reduced glutathione (GSH). With a deficiency of glucose-6-phosphate dehydrogenase (G-6-PD), the rate-limiting step in this pathway, the cellular levels of GSH are reduced. Such cells show increased susceptibility to oxidative injury. Acute exposure of such cells to an oxidizing agent can result in rapid hemolysis.

Erythrocyte reduced glutathione is rapidly depleted upon exposure to an oxidizing agent in patients with G-6-PD deficiency. This leads to the series of oxidative injuries described above with the development of intra- and extravascular hemolysis. Oxidative hemolysis is usually reversible if the process is promptly recognized and the offending agent is removed. Occasionally the hemolysis may be sufficiently severe to result in death or serious morbidity (e.g., renal failure).

Nonoxidative Chemical-Induced Hemolysis Exposure to some xenobiotics is associated with hemolysis without significant oxidative injury (Lee, 1999d). Arsenic hydride is a gas that is formed during several industrial processes. Inhalation of the gas can result in severe hemolysis, with anemia, jaundice, and hemoglobinuria. The mechanism of hemolysis in arsine toxicity is not understood. Lead poisoning is associated with defects in heme synthesis and a shortening of erythrocyte survival. The cause of the hemolysis is uncertain, but lead can cause membrane damage and interfere with the Na^+/K^+ pump. These effects may cause premature removal of erythrocytes from the circulation. Excess copper has been associated with hemolytic anemia. The pathogenesis may relate to inhibitory effects on the hexose monophosphate shunt and the Embden-Meyerhof pathway. Ingestion of excess chromium may result in a hemolytic anemia and thrombocytopenia, although the mechanism is not known (Cerulli et al., 1998). Significant hemolysis may also occur with biologic toxins found in insect and snake venoms (Gibly et al., 1998; Lee, 1999d).

Immune Hemolytic Anemia Immunologic destruction of erythrocytes is mediated by the interaction of IgG or IgM antibodies with antigens expressed on the surface of the erythrocyte (Parker and Foerster, 1999). In the case of autoimmune hemolytic anemia the antigens are intrinsic components of the patient's own erythrocytes. A large number of drugs have been associated with enhanced binding of immunoglobulin to the erythrocyte surface and shortened RBC survival.

A number of mechanisms have been implicated in xenobiotic-mediated antibody binding to erythrocytes (Parker and Foerster, 1999). Some drugs, of which penicillin is a prototype, appear to bind to the surface of the cell, with the "foreign" drug acting as a *hapten* and eliciting an immune response. The antibodies that arise in this type of response only bind to drug-coated erythrocytes. Other drugs, of which quinidine is a prototype, bind to components of the erythrocyte surface and induce a conformational change in one or more components of the membrane. This type of interaction can give rise to a confusing array of antibody specificities. Some of the antibodies recognize only the *drug-membrane component* complex; others are specific for the membrane component, but only when drug is present; while still others may recognize the membrane component in the presence or absence of the drug. A third mechanism, for which α-methyldopa is a prototype, results in production of a *drug-induced autoantibody* that cannot be distinguished from the antibodies arising in idiopathic autoimmune hemolytic anemia. The mechanism for induction of this group of antibodies is not understood. A variant of this type of response is the augmentation of autoimmune hemolytic anemia that may occur during therapy of some lymphoproliferative disorders. Autoimmune phenomena, including autoimmune hemolytic anemia, are known to occur in lymphoproliferative disorders such as chronic lymphocytic leukemia. Treatment of these disorders with some agents has been associated with worsening of the hemolytic anemia (Gonzalez et al., 1998). It has been hypothesized that therapy further disrupts regulation of the autoimmune phenomenon, allowing increased antibody production.

Some xenobiotics are associated with *nonspecific deposition of proteins* on erythrocytes. This was first associated with cephalosporins but has also been seen with other agents, including cisplatin and the beta-lactamase inhibitors sulbactam and clavulanate (Garritty and Arndt, 1998). Immunoglobulin and complement proteins may be among the proteins deposited on the erythrocyte surface. These proteins may cause a positive direct antiglobulin test, suggesting a drug-induced antibody response. However, there is no evidence of a drug-dependent antibody in the patient's serum, and drug-treated erythrocytes may bind antibody from normal non-drug exposed serum. This form of antibody deposition is generally not associated with hemolysis, although the possibility of hemolysis related to this type of reaction has been raised (Garratty and Arndt, 1998).

The interaction of immunoglobulins with erythrocytes leads to hemolysis through one of two pathways (Parker and Foerster, 1999). The first involves activation of complement with formation of the membrane attack complex (C5b-9); this is the pathway responsible for immune-mediated *intravascular hemolysis.* The second is phagocytosis of erythrocytes that have been opsonized by IgG and/or complement components; this is the pathway responsible for immune-mediated *extravascular hemolysis.* Extravascular hemolysis is the more common of these two mechanisms. This is due in part to the orchestration of factors necessary to achieve lytic activation of complement on erythrocytes.

Lytic activation of complement depends on the isotype of the antibody, the titer of the antibody, the antigen density on the surface of the erythrocyte, and the integrity of erythrocyte defense mechanisms against complement activation. IgM antibodies are more efficient activators of complement than IgG antibodies due to their polyvalent composition. Indeed, complement-mediated lysis is the major mechanism for IgM-mediated hemolysis, as phagocytes do not have specific receptors for the Fc portion of IgM to mediate ingestion of IgM opsonized erythrocytes. High-titer antibodies and a high density of antigens are required to initiate sufficient complement activation to overcome the natural erythrocyte defense mechanisms. Two important regulators of complement activation that are present on erythrocytes are decay accelerating factor (CD55) and membrane inhibitor of reactive lysis (CD59). The importance of these regulators is evident in the enhanced hemolysis that occurs in when these proteins are missing, as in *paroxysmal nocturnal hemoglobinuria* (Nishimura et al., 1999).

Non-lytic activation of complement and binding of IgG results in opsonization of the erythrocyte. Such opsonized erythrocytes are removed by the phagocytic system, particularly in the spleen. The rate of phagocytosis is affected by the concentration of opsonins on the surface and by the presence of both complement components and IgG. Consequently, the higher the concentration of IgG on the surface of the erythrocyte, the greater the rate of phagocytosis.

The clinical phenotype of drug-induced hemolytic anemia is quite variable, due to the complexity of the interactions involved. In some patients with a high-titer antibody, exposure to the offending drug may lead to rapid intravascular hemolysis, with the potential for serious morbidity or even mortality. In other patients, erythrocyte survival is modestly reduced and reasonably well compensated for by erythroid hyperplasia in the bone marrow. In some cases, patients may have evidence of erythrocyte-associated IgG without any detectable effect on erythrocyte survival.

Drug-induced intravascular hemolysis is often a dramatic clinical event and may be associated with fever, chills, back pain, hypotension, a rapid fall in hemoglobin concentration, a decrease in serum haptoglobin, a marked increase in serum LD, and hemoglobinuria (Tabarra, 1992). The clinical picture of extravascular hemolysis depends on the rate of hemolysis but is usually less dramatic. Often there is evidence of reticulocytosis, polychromasia, spherocytosis, a moderate increase in serum LD, and an increase in serum bilirubin. Serologic studies usually show evidence of IgG and/or complement on the surface of erythrocytes, although it may be difficult to document that antibody binding is drug-dependent. The mainstay of therapy in patients with drug-induced hemolytic anemia is removal of the offending agent and avoidance of reexposure.

TOXICOLOGY OF THE LEUKON

Components of Blood Leukocytes

The leukon consists of leukocytes, or white blood cells. They include granulocytes, which may be subdivided into neutrophils, eosinophils and basophils; monocytes; and lymphocytes. Granulocytes and monocytes are nucleated ameboid cells that are phagocytic. They play a central role in the inflammatory response and host defense. Unlike the RBC, which resides exclusively within blood, granulocytes and monocytes merely pass through the blood on their way to the extravascular tissues, where they reside in large numbers.

Granulocytes are defined by the characteristics of their cytoplasmic granules as they appear on a blood smear stained with a polychromatic (Romanovsky) stain. Neutrophils, the largest component of blood leukocytes, are highly specialized in the mediation of inflammation and the ingestion and destruction of pathogenic microorganisms. The turnover of the neutrophil is enormous and increases dramatically in times of inflammation and infection, elevating the number of these cells released from the bone marrow. Eosinophils and basophils modulate inflammation through the release of various mediators and play an important role in other homeostatic functions. All these are influenced by humoral immunity, as discussed in greater detail in Chap. 12.

In the world of clinical and experimental toxicology, the neutrophil is the focus of concern when evaluating granulocytes as possible targets for drug and nontherapeutic chemical effects. Eosinophils and basophils are far more difficult to study, with changes in these populations most frequently associated with reactions to other target organ or systemic toxicity. Examples include the eosinophilia observed with the toxic oil syndrome that resulted from exposure to rapeseed oil denaturated in aniline utilized in northwestern Spain (Kilbourne et al., 1991); and the eosinophilia-myalgia syndrome associated with L-tryptophan preparations contaminated with 1, 1-ethylidene-bis [tryptophan] (Varga et al., 1992).

Evaluation of Granulocytes

The most informative test to assess the neutrophil compartment is the blood neutrophil count. Accurate interpretation requires an understanding of neutrophil kinetics and the response of this tissue to physiologic and pathologic changes. In the blood, neutrophils are distributed between *circulating* and *marginated* pools, which are of equal size in man and in constant equilibrium (Athens et al., 1961; Athens et al., 1961). A blood neutrophil count assesses only the circulating pool, which remains remarkably constant (1800 to 7500 μL^{-1}) in a healthy adult human (Williams et al., 1995), considering that the number of neutrophils that pass through the blood to the tissues is estimated to be 62 to 400 $\times 10^7$ cells/kg/day (Dancey, 1976). Mature (segmented) and a few immature (band) neutrophils can be identified on blood films stained with Wright or Giemsa stain. During inflammation, a "shift to the left" may occur, which refers to an increased number of immature (nonsegmented) granulocytes in the peripheral blood, which may include bands, metamyelocytes, and occasionally myelocytes (Cannistra and Griffin, 1988). During such times, neutrophils may also show "toxic" granulation, Döhle bodies, and cytoplasmic vacuoles (Bainton, 1995). These morphologic changes may be prominent in sepsis or as a result of drug or chemical intoxication.

Neutrophil kinetics and response to disease will vary substantially among animal species. Thus, a thorough understanding of these features in any animal model used in investigative toxicology is required before informed interpretations can be made. In the human, clinically significant neutropenia occurs when the blood neutrophil count is less than 1000 μL^{-1}, but serious recurrent infections do not usually occur until counts fall below 500 μL^{-1} (Williams et al., 1995). In order to fully characterize such changes or understand the pathogenesis of the abnormality, bone marrow must be examined using marrow aspirates and biopsies. These provide information on rates of production, bone marrow reserves, abnormalities in cell distribution and occasionally specific clues as to etiology. In vitro stem cell assays may be used to assess the granulocyte progenitor cell compartment, which may include granulocyte-monocyte colony-forming cells (CFU-GM) performed in a semisolid medium, such as agar or methylcellulose, that contains appropriate growth factors. Normal human marrow specimens contain approximately 50 to 1000 CFU-GM per 10^6 nucleated cells cultured (Liesveld and Lichtman, 1997). Marrow neutrophil reserves can be assessed in vitro after administration of granulocyte colony stimulating factor, or G-CSF (Demirer and Bensinger, 1995), which stimulates increased production and release on neutrophil precursors. Glucocorticoids (Peters et al., 1972) and epinephrine (Babior and Golde, 1995) may also be used for this purpose but are rarely used in a clinical setting. The degree of proliferation in the granulocyte compartment can also be assessed using ^{3}H-thymidine suicide assays or DNA binding dyes with fluorescence-activated cell sorting analyses (Keng, 1986). Assessment of neutrophil function—including adhesion to endothelium, locomotion, chemotaxis, phagocytosis, and metabolic pathways critical to microbe killing—is discussed in Chap. 12.

Toxic Effects on Granulocytes

Effects on Proliferation As with other hematopoietic tissue, the high rate of proliferation of neutrophils makes their progenitor and precursor granulocyte pool particularly susceptible to inhibitors of mitosis. Such effects by cytotoxic drugs are generally nonspecific, as they similarly affect cells of the dermis, gastrointestinal tract, and other rapidly dividing tissues. Agents that affect both neutrophils and monocytes pose a greater risk for toxic sequelae, such as infection (Dale, 1995). Such effects tend to be dose-related, with mononuclear phagocyte recovery preceding neutrophil recovery (Arneborn and Palmblad, 1982).

Various cytoreductive agents, such as the antimetabolites methotrexate and cytosine arabinoside, may inhibit DNA synthesis (i.e., the S phase of the mitotic cycle), or the G2 period, where RNA and protein synthesis proceed prior to the mitotic, or M phase, as is the case with daunorubicin (Minderman et al., 1994). Alkylating agents like cyclophosphamide, cisplatin, and the nitrosureas are toxic to resting and actively dividing cells, where maximum effects are usually seen 7 to 14 days after exposure. Cytokines may enhance these effects, perhaps through driving cells into S phase (Smith et al., 1994). Lindane, an insecticide used to treat seeds and soil, has been associated with leukopenia (Parent-Massin et al., 1994). It is cytotoxic for human CFU-GMs at concentrations observed in blood and adipose tissue from exposed human subjects. An example of agents affecting mature cells is methylmethacrylate monomer, which is used in orthopedic surgical procedures and is cytotoxic to both neutrophils and monocytes at clinically relevant concentrations (Dahl et al., 1994).

Effects on Function While there are a variety of disorders associated with defects in the parameters of neutrophil function discussed above, demonstrable in vivo effects associated with drugs and toxins are surprisingly few (Smolen and Boxer, 1995). Examples include ethanol and glucocorticoids, which impair phagocytosis and microbe ingestion in vitro and in vivo (Brayton et al., 1970). Iohexol and ioxaglate, components of radiographic contrast media, have also been reported to inhibit phagocytosis (Lillevang et al., 1994). Superoxide production, required for microbial killing and chemotaxis, has been reported to be reduced in patients using parenteral heroin as well as in former opiate abusers on long-term methadone maintenance (Mazzone et al., 1994). Chemotaxis is also impaired following treatment with zinc salts in antiacne preparations (Dreno et al., 1992).

Idiosyncratic Toxic Neutropenia Of greater concern are agents that unexpectedly damage neutrophils and granulocyte precursors—particularly to the extent of inducing *agranulocytosis,* which is characterized by a profound depletion in blood neutrophils to less than 500 μL^{-1} (Pisciotta, 1997). Such injury occurs in specifically conditioned individuals, and is therefore termed "idiosyncratic." Mechanisms of idiosyncratic damage often do not relate to pharmacologic properties of the parent drug, which makes managing this risk a particular challenge to hematologists and toxicologists. Preclinical toxicology is rarely predictive of these effects, which are generally detected and characterized following exposure of a large population to the agent (Szarfman et al., 1997).

Idiosyncratic xenobiotic-induced agranulocytosis may involve a sudden depletion of circulating neutrophils concommitant with exposure, which may persist as long as the agent or its metabolites persist in the circulation. Hematopoietic function is usually restored when the agent is detoxified or excreted. Suppression of granulopoiesis, however, is more prevalent than peripheral lysis of neutrophils and is asymptomatic unless sepsis supervenes (Pisciotta, 1997). The onset of leukopenia in the former is more gradual but may be precipitous if lysis of circulating neutrophils also occurs. The pattern of the disease varies with the stage of granulopoiesis affected, which has been well defined for several agents that cause bone marrow toxicity (Table 11-7). Toxicants affecting uncommitted stem cells induce total marrow failure, as seen in aplastic anemia, which generally carries a worse prognosis than agents affect-

Table 11-7
Stages of Granulocytopoiesis: Site of Xenobiotic-Induced Cellular Damage

STAGE OF DEVELOPMENT	DISEASE	OFFENDING DRUGS
Uncommitted (totipotential) stem cell	Aplastic anemia	Chloramphenicol
CFU-S		Gold salts
		Phenylbutazone
		Phenytoin
		Mephenytoin
		Carbamazepine
Committed stem cell	Aplastic anemia	Carbamazepine
	Agranulocytosis	Chlorpromazine
CFU-G		Carbamazepine
		Clozapine
CFU-E	Pure red cell aplasia	
BFU-E		Phenytoin
Morphologically recognizable precursors	Hypoplastic marrow	Most cancer chemotherapy agents
Dividing pool	Hypoplastic marrow	Chloramphenicol
Promyelocyte		Alcohol
Myelocyte		
Nondividing pool	Agranulocytosis	Clozapine
Metamyelocytes, bands		Phenothiazines, etc.
PMNs		
Peripheral blood lysis	Agranulocytosis	Clozapine, etc.
PMNs		Aminopyrine
Tissue pool		

SOURCE: Modified from Pisciotta, 1997, with permission from Elsevier Science.

ing more differentiated precursors (e.g., CFU-G). It is thought that, in the latter case, surviving uncommitted stem cells eventually produce recovery, provided that the risk of infection is successfully managed during the leukopenic episodes (Pisciotta, 1997).

Mechanisms of Toxic Neutropenia Toxic neutropenia may be classified according to mechanism as *immune-mediated* or *non–immune-mediated.* In immune-mediated neutropenia, antigen-antibody reactions lead to destruction of peripheral neutrophils, granulocyte precursors, or both. As with RBCs, an immunogenic xenobiotic can act as a hapten, where the agent must be physically present to cause cell damage, alternatively, may induce immunogenic cells to produce antineutrophil antibodies that do not require the drug to be present. Xenobiotic-induced immune-mediated damage may also be cell-mediated (Pisciotta, 1997).

Detection of xenobiotic induced neutrophil antibodies is considerably more difficult than those of RBCs or platelets. Several assays have been used, which can be grouped into four categories: those measuring endpoints of leukoagglutination, cytotoxic inhibition of neutrophil function, or immunoglobulin binding and those using cell-mediated mechanisms. Among the specific challenges these assays pose are the tendency of neutrophils to stick to each other in vitro, attract immunoglobulin nonspecifically to their surface, and reflect membrane damage through indirect and semiquantitative changes (Pisciotta, 1997). The reader is referred elsewhere for a more detailed discussion of assays for immune-mediated neutrophil damage (Minchinton and Waters, 1984; Hagen et al., 1993).

Non–immune-mediated toxic neutropenia often shows a genetic predisposition (Pisciotta, 1973). Direct damage may cause inhibition of granulopoiesis or neutrophil function. It may entail failure to detoxify or excrete a xenobiotic or its metabolites, which subsequently build up to toxic proportions (Gerson et al., 1983; Gerson and Melzer, 1992; Uetrecht, 1990). Some studies suggest that a buildup of toxic oxidants generated by leukocytes can result in neutrophil damage, as with the reactive intermediates derived from the interaction between clozapine, an atypical antipsychotic, and neutrophils. The resulting superoxide and hypochlorous acid production by the myeloperoxidase system are thought to contribute to clozapine-induced neutropenia (Uetrecht, 1992).

While many drugs and nontherapeutic agents have been associated with neutropenia (Young, 1994; Watts, 1999), the mechanism of this effect has been established in relatively few of these toxicants. Examples of agents associated with immune and non-immune neutropenia/agranulocytosis are listed in Table 11-8.

LEUKEMOGENESIS AS A TOXIC RESPONSE

Human Leukemias

Leukemias are proliferative disorders of hematopoietic tissue that are monoclonal in origin and thus originate from individual bone marrow cells. Historically they have been classified as myeloid or lymphoid, referring to the major lineages for erythrocytes/granulocytes/thrombocytes or lymphocytes, respectively. Because the degree of leukemic cell differentiation has also loosely correlated with the rate of disease progression, poorly differentiated phenotypes have been designated as "acute," whereas well-differentiated ones are referred to as "chronic" leukemias. The classification of

Table 11-8
Examples of Toxicants That Cause Immune and Non-immune Idiopathic Neutropenia

DRUGS ASSOCIATED WITH WBC ANTIBODIES	DRUGS NOT ASSOCIATED WITH WBC ANTIBODIES
Aminopyrine	INH
Propylthiouracil	Rifampicin
Ampicillin	Ethambutol
Metiamide	Allopurinol
Dicloxacillin	Phenothiazines/CPZ
Phenytoin	Flurazepam
Aprindine	HCTZ
Azulfidine	
Chlorpropamide	
CPZ/Phenothiazines	
Procainamide	
Nafcillin	
Tolbutamide	
Lidocaine	
Methimazole	
Levamisole	
Gold	
Quinidine	
Clozapine	

SOURCE: Modified from Pisciotta, 1997, with permission from Elsevier Science.

human leukemias proposed by the French-American-British (FAB) Cooperative Group has become convention, based on the above and other morphologic features (Bennett et al., 1985; Levine and Bloomfield, 1992; Bennett et al., 1982). It provides the diagnostic framework for classifying chronic lymphocytic leukemia (CLL), chronic myelogenous leukemia (CML), acute lymphoblastic leukemia (ALL), acute myelogenous leukemia (AML), and the myelodysplastic syndromes (MDS), along with various subtypes of these disorders. These early correlations imply that the biology and clinical features of these proliferative disorders relate to the stage of differentiation of the target cell, which is now being linked to individual gene alterations, as well as epigenetic factors such as cytokine stimulation. Evidence for these mechanisms is rapidly emerging and supports the notion that leukemogenesis is a multievent progression (Vogelstein et al., 1988; Williams and Whittaker, 1990; Varmua and Weinberg, 1993; Pedersen-Bjergaard et al., 1995). These studies suggest that factors involved in the regulation of hematopoiesis also influence neoplastic transformation. Such factors include cellular growth factors (cytokines), protooncogenes and other growth-promoting genes, as well as additional factors that govern survival, proliferation, and differentiation.

Mechanisms of Toxic Leukemogenesis

The understanding that certain chemicals and radiation can dysregulate hematopoiesis, resulting in leukemogenesis, is a relatively recent one. While suggested by Hunter as early as 1939, following his observations on benzene exposure and AML (Hunter, 1939), it was not until the introduction of radiation and chemotherapy as treatments for neoplasia that these agents became associated with blood dyscrasias that included (or led to) AML (Casciato and Scott, 1979; Foucar et al., 1979; Andersen et al., 1981). The notion emerged that myelotoxic agents, under certain circumstances, can be leukemogenic.

Curiously, AML is the dominant leukemia associated with drug or chemical exposure, followed by MDS (Casciato and Scott, 1979; Andersen et al., 1981; Irons, 1997). The evidence that this represents a continuum of one toxic response is compelling (Irons, 1997). This has also been linked to cytogenetic abnormalities, particularly the loss of all or part of chromosomes 5 and 7. Remarkably, the frequency of these deletions in patients who develop MDS and/or AML after treatment with alkylating or other antineoplastic agents ranges from 67 to 95 percent, depending on the study (Rowley et al., 1981; LeBeau, 1986; Pedersen-Bjergaard, 1984; Johansson et al., 1987; Bitter et al., 1987). Some of these same changes have been observed in AML patients occupationally exposed to benzene (Bitter et al., 1987; Mitelman et al., 1978; Mitelman et al., 1981; Golomb et al., 1982; Fagioli et al., 1992; Cuneo et al., 1992), who also show aneuploidy with a high frequency of involvement of chromosome 7 (Irons, 1997). The relatively low frequency of deletions in chromosomes 5 and 7 in de novo as compared with secondary AML suggests that these cytogenetic markers can be useful in discriminating between toxic exposures and other etiologies of this leukemia (Irons, 1997). These observations, together with the understandings on the pathogenesis of leukemia previously discussed, led Irons to propose a model for the evolution of toxic, or secondary, leukemogenesis, which is illustrated in Fig. 11-7 (Irons, 1997).

Other forms of leukemia—including CML, CLL, ALL, and multiple myeloma—have shown weak correlations with occupational exposure or treatment with alkylating agents (Irons, 1997). The latter has been repeatedly associated with exposure to benzene, although a causal relationship has yet to be demonstrated (Bergsagel et al., 1999).

Leukemogenic Agents

Most *alkylating agents* used in cancer chemotherapy can cause MDS and/or AML, including cyclophosphamide, melphalan, busulfan, chlorambucil, and nitrosurea compounds such as carmustine, or BCNU (Casciato and Scott, 1979; Greene et al, 1986). Other oncolytic agents implicated include azathioprine, procarbazine, doxorubicin, and bleomycin (Carver et al., 1979; Valagussa et al., 1979; Vismans et al., 1980). The risk these agents pose varies considerably with the therapeutic regimen. The incidence of MDS/AML in patients treated with alkylating agents has been reported to be 0.6 to 17 percent, with an average of 100-fold relative risk. Moreover, treatment-related MDS is associated with a substantially higher rate of transformation to AML than is primary or spontaneous MDS (Bitter et al., 1987; Kantarjian et al., 1986).

Of the *aromatic hydrocarbons,* only benzene has been proven to be leukemogenic. Substituted aromatic hydrocarbons have long been suspected to be causative, due to the fact that preparations of xylene and toluene in the past contained as much as 20% benzene (Browning, 1965). There is no clinical or experimental evidence that substituted benzenes cause leukemia (Irons, 1997).

Treatment with *topoisomerase II inhibitors,* particularly the epipodophyllotoxins etoposide and teniposide, can induce AML, the clinical course of which has the following distinguishing characteristics: (1) the absence of a preleukemic phase, (2) a short latency period, (3) frequent involvement of an M4/5 subtype, and (4) balanced chromosome aberrations involving chromosomes 11q23

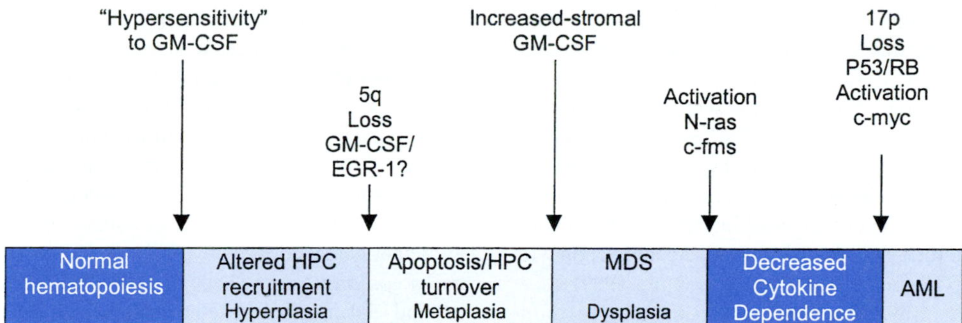

Figure 11-7

Hypothetical model for the evolution of s-AML involving 5q-. Schematic representation of one model for tumor progression consistent with frequently observed events in the development of AML secondary to drug or chemical exposure. Altered myeloid progenitor cell proliferation leads to increased division in the target cell population, which results in clonal loss of heterozygosity due to nondysjunction (e.g., 5q-). The resulting haploinsufficiency of a gene, such as GM-CSF, results in increased cell turnover, abnormal maturation, and ineffective hematopoiesis (i.e., MDS) in the abnormal clone. This is subsequently followed by activation of additional proto-oncogenes that result in progressive growth and survival independence in successive subclones and the development of overt AML. [Adapted from Irons (1997), with permission from Elsevier Science.]

and 21q22 (Murphy, 1993). Similar cytogenetic features have been observed following treatment with doxorubicin or dactinomycin (intercalating topoisomerase II inhibitors) in conjunction with alkylating agents and irradiation (Sandoval et al., 1993).

Exposure to *high-dose γ- or x-ray radiation* has long been associated with ALL, AML, and CML, as demonstrated in survivors of the atom bombings of Nagasaki and Hiroshima (Cartwright, 1992; Shimizu et al., 1989). Less clear is the association of these diseases with low-dose radiation secondary to fallout or diagnostic radiographs (Cartwright, 1992).

Other *controversial agents* include 1, 3-butadiene, nonionizing radiation (electromagnetic, microwave, infrared, visible, and the high end of the ultraviolet spectrum), and cigarette smoking, for which published studies on the relationship to leukemia incidence is confusing, contradictory, or difficult to interpret based on dose response (Irons, 1997).

TOXICOLOGY OF PLATELETS AND HEMOSTASIS

Hemostasis is a multicomponent system responsible for preventing the loss of blood from sites of vascular injury and maintaining circulating blood in a fluid state. Loss of blood is prevented by formation of stable hemostatic plugs mediated by the procoagulant arm of hemostasis. This procoagulant response is normally limited to sites of vascular injury by the multicomponent regulatory arm of hemostasis. The dynamically modulated balance between procoagulant and regulatory pathways permits a rapid, localized response to injury. The major constituents of the hemostatic system include circulating platelets, a variety of plasma proteins, and vascular endothelial cells. Alterations in these components or systemic activation of this system can lead to the clinical manifestations of deranged hemostasis, including excessive bleeding and thrombosis. The hemostatic system is a frequent target of therapeutic intervention as well as inadvertent expression of the toxic effect of a variety of xenobiotics. This section briefly reviews the inadvertent effects of xenobiotics on hemostasis and the toxic effects of agents used to manipulate the hemostatic system.

Toxic Effects on Platelets

The Thrombocyte Platelets are essential for formation of a stable hemostatic plug in response to vascular injury. Platelets initially adhere to the damaged wall through binding of von Willebrand factor (vWF) with the platelet glycoprotein Ib/IX/V (GP Ib/IX/V) receptor complex (Sadler, 1998; Andrews et al., 1999). Ligand binding to GP Ib/IX/V or interaction of other platelet agonists (e.g., thrombin, collagen, ADP, thromboxane A_2) with their specific receptors initiates biochemical response pathways that lead to shape change, platelet contraction, platelet secretion of granule contents, activation of the GP IIb/IIIa receptor and externalization of phosphatidylserine (Solum, 1999; Ware and Coller, 1999). Activation of the GP IIb/IIIa receptor permits fibrinogen and other multivalent adhesive molecules to form crosslinks between nearby platelets, resulting in platelet aggregation (Plow, 1999). Xenobiotics may interfere with the platelet response by causing thrombocytopenia or interfering with platelet function; some agents are capable of affecting both platelet number and function.

Thrombocytopenia Like anemia, thrombocytopenia may be due to decreased production or increased destruction. Thrombocytopenia is a common side effect of intensive chemotherapy, due to the predictable effect of antiproliferative agents on hematopoietic precursors, including those of the megakaryocytic lineage. Thrombocytopenia is a clinically significant component of idiosyncratic xenobiotic-induced aplastic anemia. Indeed, the initial manifestation of aplastic anemia may be mucocutaneous bleeding secondary to thrombocytopenia. A few agents—including thiazide diuretics, diethylstilbestrol, recombinant GM-CSF, and procarbazine—have been associated with isolated suppression of thrombopoiesis. The mechanisms by which this occurs are not known (George, 1999).

Exposure to xenobiotics may cause increased immune-mediated platelet destruction through any one of several mechanisms (Table 11-9) (Aster, 1999). Some drugs function as haptens, binding to platelet membrane components and eliciting an immune response that is specific for the hapten. The responding antibody then binds to the hapten on the platelet surface, leading to removal of the antibody-coated platelet from the circulation. This type of antibody interaction can often be blocked in vitro by excess soluble drug that binds to the antibody and prevents its interaction with the platelet surface (George et al., 1998; Rizvi et al., 1999).

A second mechanism of immune thrombocytopenia is initiated by xenobiotic-induced exposure of a neoepitope on a platelet membrane glycoprotein. This elicits an antibody response, with the responding antibody binding to this altered platelet antigen in the presence of drug, resulting in removal of the platelet from the circulation by the mononuclear phagocytic system. The epitope specificity can be quite selective, as there is often little or no cross-reactivity between drugs having a very similar structure (e.g., quinine and quinidine). This type of interaction is not inhibited in vitro by excess soluble drug, as the antibody target is a platelet-dependent epitope. Quinidine is a prototype of this type of mechanism and can induce antibodies directed at GP Ib/IX/V, GP IIb/IIIa and/or platelet endothelial cell adhesion molecule-1 (PECAM-1) (George et al., 1998; Aster, 1999; Rizvi et al., 1999).

The diagnosis of drug-dependent antiplatelet antibodies can be quite difficult. A number of assays have been described for measurement of platelet-associated immunoglobulin, but the sensitivity and specificity of these assays have not been established. Therefore, these assays are not used in routine clinical practice. Consequently, the diagnosis is usually established by observing the resolution of thrombocytopenia following discontinuation of the offending drug. In most cases, the platelet count returns to normal within 5 to 10 days of drug discontinuation. Although a large number of agents have been implicated in the development of immune thrombocytopenia, the supporting evidence in many cases is weak (George et al., 1998; Rizvi et al., 1999).

Thrombocytopenia is an uncommon but serious complication of inhibitors of GP IIb/IIIa such as abciximab (Nurden et al., 1999; Tcheng, 2000). The mechanism appears to be related to exposure of epitopes on GP IIb/IIIa that react with naturally occurring antibodies. Because the reaction is dependent on antibodies formed prior to exposure to drug, it may occur shortly after the first exposure to the drug. This mechanism appears to be similar to the mechanism underlying EDTA-dependent platelet clumping and satellitosis resulting in pseudothrombocytopenia. In the latter situation, anticoagulation with EDTA results in chelation of calcium and a conformational change in GP IIb/IIIa that allows antibody to bind and mediate platelet clumping or binding to neutrophils (platelet satellitosis). Ligand binding is known to alter the conformation of GP IIb/IIIa. The GP IIb/IIIa inhibitors bind at the ligand binding site and also cause a conformational change in GP IIb/IIIa, permitting naturally occurring antibodies to bind to and initiate clearance of platelets by the mononuclear phagocytic system. Thus, exposure of epitopes that react with naturally occurring antibodies represents a third mechanism of immune-mediated platelet destruction.

Heparin-induced thrombocytopenia (HIT) represents a fourth mechanism of immune-mediated platelet destruction. This disorder is due to the development of antibodies that react with a multimolecular complex formed by the interaction between heparin and a protein, usually platelet factor 4 (PF 4) (Amiral and Meyer, 1998; Warkentin et al., 1998; Visentin, 1999; Warkentin, 1999). When the relative concentration of heparin to PF 4 is appropriate, formation of this complex is associated with exposure of a neoepitope on PF 4 (or another target protein) and development of an IgG response to the neoepitope. The IgG then binds to the PF 4-heparin complex to form an immune complex that binds to the platelet Fc receptor, FcγRIIa. Clustering of platelet FcγRIIa by the immune complex activates biochemical signaling pathways mediated by the cytoplasmic domain of FcγRIIa. This results in platelet activation

Table 11-9
Mechanism of Immune-Mediated Thrombocytopenia

MECHANISM	PROTOTYPIC AGENT	ANTIGEN/ EPITOPE	PLATELET EFFECT	CLINICAL EFFECT
Hapten-directed antibody	Penicillin	Drug	Opsonization ↑ Clearance	Bleeding
Acquired antibody to drug-induced epitope	Quinidine	Drug-GP Ib/IX/V Drug-GP IIb/IIIa	Opsonization ↑ Clearance +/− ↓ Function	Bleeding
Natural antibody to drug-induced epitope	Abciximab	GP IIb/IIIa	Opsonization ↑ Clearance	Bleeding
Immune complex	Heparin	PF 4–heparin complex	Platelet activation Platelet aggregation ↑ Clearance	Thrombosis
Thrombotic thrombocytopenic purpura (TTP)	Ticlopidine	VWF-cleaving protease	Platelet activation Platelet aggregation ↑ Clearance	Microvascular thrombosis Microangiopathic hemolytic anemia
Hemolytic-uremic syndrome	Mitomycin	Unknown	Platelet activation Platelet aggregation ↑ Clearance	Microvascular thrombosis Microangiopathic hemolytic anemia Renal failure

and aggregation. During the process of platelet activation, platelet microparticles that promote thrombin generation are released. Consequently, HIT is associated with both thrombocytopenia and an increased risk of arterial and venous thrombosis. Other drug-antibody complexes (e.g., streptokinase-IgG) may trigger platelet activation and thrombocytopenia through a similar mechanism (Deckmyn et al., 1998; McRedmond et al., 2000).

Thrombotic thrombocytopenic purpura (TTP) is a syndrome characterized by the sudden onset of thrombocytopenia, a microangiopathic hemolytic anemia, and multisystem organ failure, which often includes neurologic dysfunction. The syndrome tends to occur following an infectious disease but may also occur following administration of some pharmacologic agents. The pathogenesis of TTP appears to be related to the ability of unusually large vWF multimers to activate platelets, even in the absence of significant vascular damage. Although these large multimers are normally secreted into blood by endothelial cells, they are normally processed into smaller multimers by a protease present in plasma. Acquired TTP is associated with the development of an antibody that inhibits this protease, permitting the very large vWF multimers to persist in the circulation (Furlan et al., 1998; Tsai and Lian, 1998). Consequently, these multimers bind to platelet GP Ib/IX/V and induce platelet activation and aggregation. The organ failure and hemolysis in TTP is due to the formation of platelet-rich microthrombi throughout the circulation. The development of TTP or TTP-like syndromes has been associated with drugs such as ticlopidine, clopidogrel, cocaine, mitomycin, and cyclosporine (Durand and Lefevre, 1991; Bennett et al., 1998; Bennett et al., 1999; Steinhubl et al., 1999; Volcy et al., 2000).

The hemolytic uremic syndrome (HUS) is a disorder characterized by clinical features similar to those of TTP, with microangiopathic hemolytic anemia, thrombocytopenia, and renal failure (Ruggenenti and Remuzzi, 1998; van de Kar and Monnens, 1998). Neurologic complications tend to be less severe, while renal failure often dominates the clinical picture. Sporadic cases of HUS have been linked to infection with verocytotoxin-producing *Escherichia coli,* but they may also occur during therapy with some drugs, including mitomycin. In contrast to TTP, the vWF-cleaving protease is normal in patients with HUS (Furlan et al., 1998). In the past it was difficult to distinguish between TTP and HUS, but it is now clear that these two syndromes represent distinct disorders. The pathogenesis of the thrombocytopenia and microangiopathic changes in HUS is still uncertain, but there is experimental evidence suggesting that it is related to endothelial cell injury, with subsequent platelet activation and thrombus formation.

Desmopressin, a vasopressin analog, is an example of nonimmune-mediated increased platelet destruction. Desmopressin induces a two- to fivefold increase in the plasma concentration of vWF and factor VIII. It is commonly used in the treatment of patients with von Willebrand's disease and other mild bleeding syndromes. Desmopressin has been associated with the development or accentuation of thrombocytopenia in some patients with type 2B von Willebrand disease. The thrombocytopenia in such cases is related to the release of an abnormal vWF from endothelial cells. The abnormal vWF has enhanced affinity for GP Ib/IX/V and the interaction of the vWF with its receptor leads to platelet clearance from the circulation (Mannucci, 1998).

Toxic Effects on Platelet Function Platelet function is dependent on the coordinated interaction of a number of biochemical response pathways. A variety of drugs and foods have been found to inhibit platelet function, either in vivo or in vitro (George and Shattil, 1991; Schafer, 1995; Baker and Hankey, 1999; Quinn and Fitzgerald, 1999). Major drug groups that affect platelet function include nonsteroidal anti-inflammatory agents, β-lactam-containing antibiotics, cardiovascular drugs, particularly beta blockers, psychotropic drugs, anesthetics, antihistamines, and some chemotherapeutic agents. The effect of these agents can vary between individuals, perhaps due to subclinical variations in underlying platelet function. For example, about 5 percent of the population appears to be significantly more sensitive to the platelet inhibitor action of aspirin than the remainder of the population. In addition, exposure to medications having a modest antiplatelet effect may unmask an unrecognized subclinical intrinsic platelet function disorder. Therefore it is important to fully evaluate the onset of mucocutaneous bleeding when it occurs in patients exposed to agents that might affect platelet function.

Xenobiotics may interfere with platelet function through a variety of mechanisms. Some drugs inhibit the phospholipase A_2/cyclooxygenase pathway and synthesis of thromboxane A_2 (e.g., nonsteroidal anti-inflammatory agents). Other agents appear to interfere with the interaction between platelet agonists and their receptors (e.g., antibiotics, ticlopidine, clopidogrel). As the platelet response is dependent on rapid increase in cytoplasmic calcium, any agent that interferes with translocation of calcium may inhibit platelet function (e.g., calcium channel blockers). Occasionally, drug-induced antibodies will bind to a critical platelet receptor and inhibit its function. The functional defect induced by such antibodies may potentiate the bleeding risk associated with the xenobiotic-induced thrombocytopenia. In some cases, the mechanism of inhibition is not known.

The effect of xenobiotics on platelet function can be studied following in vitro exposure of platelets to the agent of interest. However, evaluation following in vivo exposure is preferred, as metabolites of the parent compound may contain the platelet inhibitory activity. The most common method of assessing platelet function is turbidometric platelet aggregation using platelet-rich plasma, but alternate techniques are available, including the PFA 100 analyzer, flow cytometry, and whole-blood impedance aggregometry (Schmitz et al., 1998; Harrison et al., 1999; Michelson and Furman, 1999).

Toxic Effects on Fibrin Clot Formation

Coagulation Fibrin clot formation is the result of sequential activation of a series of serine proteases that culminates in the formation of thrombin (Mann, 1999). Thrombin is a multifunctional enzyme that converts fibrinogen to fibrin; activates factors V, VIII, XI, XIII, protein C, and platelets; and interacts with a variety of cells (e.g., leukocytes and endothelial cells), activating cellular signaling pathways. The coagulation cascade is initiated when blood is exposed to tissue factor, a membrane protein not normally found in circulating blood but present in most extravascular tissues. The reactions of the coagulation cascade require a negatively charged phospholipid surface for interaction of the enzymes with their substrates. This surface is usually provided by the activated platelet after translocation of phosphatidylserine to the external membrane leaflet. The requirement for phospholipid helps to localize thrombin formation to sites of vascular damage where platelets are being activated.

The most common toxic effects of xenobiotics on fibrin clot formation are related to a decreased level of one or more of the critical proteins necessary for this process. The decrease in clotting factor activity may be due to decreased synthesis of the protein(s) or increased clearance from the circulation. Decreased synthesis is most often a reflection of hepatocellular damage or interference with vitamin K metabolism, as discussed below, whereas increased clearance is usually associated with the development of an antibody to a specific coagulation factor.

Decreased Synthesis of Coagulation Proteins The majority of proteins involved in the coagulation cascade are synthesized in the liver. Therefore, any agent that impairs liver function may cause a decrease in production of coagulation factors. The common tests of the coagulation cascade, the prothrombin time (PT) and activated partial thromboplastin time (aPTT), may be used to screen for liver dysfunction and a decrease in clotting factors. These assays are often performed as part of the safety evaluation of a new chemical entity. The half-life of clotting factors in the circulation varies significantly, with factor VII having the shortest half-life. Therefore, with acute toxicity (e.g., acetaminophen overdose), the effect on blood coagulation may be first seen as a decrease in the level of factor VII. Such a decrease would lead to prolongation of the PT with a normal aPTT. With a more chronic process, either the PT or aPTT or both may be affected.

Factors II, VII, IX, and X are dependent on vitamin K for their complete synthesis (Nelsestuen et al., 2000). Anything that interferes with vitamin K metabolism may lead to a deficiency of these factors and a bleeding tendency. This may occur with agents that interfere with absorption of vitamin K from the intestine or with agents that interfere with the reduction of vitamin K epoxide (Table 11-10). The combination of antibiotic therapy and limited oral intake is a common cause of acquired deficiency of vitamin K-dependent proteins among hospitalized patients (Chakraverty et al., 1996). The "super rodenticides" are another cause of acquired vitamin K deficiency (Chua and Friedenberg, 1998; Berry et al., 2000). These agents have a very prolonged half-life in vivo; thus the coagulation defect may persist for weeks or months following exposure. Rodenticide exposure may occur accidentally, as part of a Munchausen syndrome, in association with a suicide attempt, or as part of a homicide attempt. At times it may be important to distinguish between a true vitamin K deficiency and interference with the reduction of vitamin K epoxide. This is most readily accomplished by measuring the level of vitamin K and vitamin K epoxide in serum or plasma. In the case of vitamin K deficiency, vitamin K and vitamin K epoxide are both decreased; whereas in the case of inhibition of vitamin K reduction, vitamin K epoxide is significantly increased. Specific rodenticides may be measured using HPLC techniques, but it is important to specify which active agent (e.g., brodifacoum) should be measured, as the assays may not show cross-reactivity between agents.

Increased Clearance of Coagulation Factors Idiosyncratic reactions to xenobiotics include the formation of antibodies that react with coagulation proteins. These antibodies bind to the coagulation factor, forming an immune complex that is rapidly cleared from the circulation and resulting in deficiency of the factor. The antibody is often reversible over time if the initiating agent is withdrawn. However, during the acute phase, these patients may have life-threatening bleeding. The factors that are most often affected include factor VIII, factor V, factor XIII, vWF, prothrombin, and thrombin (Table 11-11) (Muntean et al., 1997; Sallah, 1997; Tefferi and Nichols, 1997; Bossi et al., 1998; Knobl and Lechner, 1998; van Genderen and Michiels, 1998; Pruthi and Nichols, 1999). In addition to causing increased clearance from the circulation, these antibodies often inhibit the function of the coagulation factor. This allows analysis of the antibody through evaluation of its interaction with a normal coagulation factor in vitro.

Lupus anticoagulants are antibodies that interfere with in vitro phospholipid-dependent coagulation reactions (Roubey, 1999). Although it was once hypothesized that these antibodies were directed against phospholipid, it is now evident that lupus anticoagulants are directed against phospholipid binding proteins, including prothrombin and β_2-glycoprotein 1. These antibodies usually do not cause a deficiency of any specific coagulation factor. However, in vivo, these antibodies can potentiate procoagulant mechanisms and interfere with the protein C system. Consequently, these antibodies have been associated with an increased risk of thrombosis (Roubey, 1998). The development of lupus anticoagulants has been seen in association with a variety of medications (Table 11-12) (Triplett and Brandt, 1988; List and Doll, 1989; Vargas-Alarcon et al., 1997).

Table 11-10
Conditions Associated with Abnormal Synthesis of Vitamin K–Dependent Coagulation Factors

Warfarin and analogues	Intravenous α-tocopherol
Rodenticides (e.g., brodifacoum)	Dietary deficiency
Broad-spectrum antibiotics	Cholestyramine resin
N-methyl-thiotetrazole cephalosporins	Malabsorption syndromes

Table 11-11
Relationship between Xenobiotics and the Development of Specific Coagulation Factor Inhibitors

COAGULATION FACTOR	XENOBIOTIC
Thrombin	Topical bovine thrombin
	Fibrin glue
Factor V	Streptomycin
	Penicillin
	Gentamicin
	Cephalosporins
	Topical bovine thrombin
Factor VIII	Penicillin
	Ampicillin
	Chloramphenicol
	Phenytoin
	Methyldopa
	Nitrofurazone
	Phenylbutazone
Factor XIII	Isoniazid
	Procainamide
	Penicillin
	Phenytoin
	Practolol
Von Willebrand Factor	Ciprofloxacin
	Hydroxyethyl starch
	Valproic acid
	Griseofulvin
	Tetracycline
	Pesticides

Table 11-12
Xenobiotics Associated with the Development of Lupus Anticoagulants

Chlorpromazine	Antibiotics
Procainamide	Phenytoin
Hydralazine	Viral infections
Quinidine	

Toxicology of Agents Used to Modulate Hemostasis

Patients with bleeding or thrombotic problems are commonly encountered in clinical practice. A variety of agents are available to treat such patients, ranging from recombinant hemostatic proteins to chemical entities that modulate the activity of the coagulation system. The major toxicologic reactions to plasma-derived products are infectious diseases (e.g., hepatitis C) and allergic reactions, which can be severe. The use of some products, such as activated concentrates of vitamin K-dependent proteins (e.g., Autoplex and FEIBA), has been associated with the development of disseminated intravascular coagulation and/or thrombosis in some patients (Mannucci, 1998).

Oral Anticoagulants Oral anticoagulants (warfarin) interfere with vitamin K metabolism by preventing the reduction of vitamin K epoxide, resulting in a functional deficiency of reduced vitamin K (Freedman, 1992; Hirsh et al., 1998). These agents are widely used for prophylaxis and therapy of venous and arterial thrombosis. The therapeutic window for oral anticoagulants is relatively narrow, and there is considerable interindividual variation in the response to a given dose. The consequence of insufficient anticoagulant effect is an increased risk of thromboembolism, while the consequence of excessive anticoagulation is an increased risk of bleeding. A number of factors affect the individual response to oral anticoagulants. For these reasons, therapy with these agents must be routinely monitored to maximize both safety and efficacy. This is routinely performed with the PT, with results expressed in terms of the international normalized ratio (INR). The INR represents the PT ratio that would have been obtained had an international standard PT reagent been used to perform the PT (Hirsh et al., 1998).

Oral anticoagulants are readily absorbed from the gastrointestinal tract and bind avidly to albumin in the circulation. Warfarin and the related coumarin derivatives consist of racemic mixtures of *R*- and *S*-enantiomers. The two enantiomers differ in terms of their potency and metabolism, with the *S*-enantiomer of warfarin being more potent and having a shorter half-life than the *R*-enantiomer. The *S*-enantiomer is metabolized primarily by the cytochrome P450 isoenzyme CYP2C9 while the *R*-enantiomer is metabolized primarily by CYP1A2 and CYP3A4 (Kaminsky and Zhang, 1997). Genetic polymorphisms of CYP2C9 have been described that influence the activity of this enzyme. A $C_{472} \rightarrow T$ base substitution in the gene results in an Arg → Cys substitution at amino acid 144, while an $A_{1061} \rightarrow T$ results in an Ile → Leu substitution at amino acid 359. Three distinct alleles involving these polymorphisms have been identified in clinical studies (Furuya et al., 1995; Bhasker et al., 1997; Miners and Birkett, 1998; Steward et al., 1998; Aithal et al., 1999). The Arg144/Ile359 allele (CYP2C9*1) represents the wild type, with a frequency in the Caucasian population of about 0.79 to 0.86. The Cys144/Ile359 allele (CYP2C9*2) has a frequency of about 0.08 to 0.12 and the Arg144/Leu359 allele (CYP2C9*3) has a frequency of about 0.03 to 0.09. Patients who are heterozygous for CYP2C9*2 or CYP2C9*3 require significantly less warfarin for maintenance in the therapeutic range than patients who are homozygous for CYP2C9*1. In addition, the heterozygotes for Cys144 or Leu359 have a higher frequency of overdosage during the initiation of therapy and a higher rate of bleeding during the first several weeks of therapy. A patient homozygous for CYP2C9*3 was found to be exceedingly sensitive to the effect of warfarin, requiring less than 0.5 mg/day for effective therapy, about one-tenth the amount of drug required for the average patient (Steward et al., 1998).

Genetic variation in the vitamin K-dependent proteins may also affect the response to warfarin. Mutation of Ala-10 in the propeptide of factor IX has been associated with a marked decrease in factor IX and recurrent bleeding during oral anticoagulant therapy (Quenzel et al., 1997; Oldenburg et al, 1998). Ala-10 is a highly conserved amino acid in the region of the molecule that serves as a recognition site for the vitamin K-dependent carboxylase. Recombinant factor IX variants with Glu replacing Ala-10 have been constructed; these variants were found to be resistant to carboxylation in vitro. The factor IX levels are normal in the absence of oral anticoagulants in the patients with the mutation, but they are severely depressed when the PT is in the therapeutic range during oral anticoagulant therapy. This is because the PT is insensitive to the concentration of factor IX. Despite the PT being in the "therapeutic range" these patients are at increased risk of bleeding.

A number of xenobiotics, including foods, have been found to affect the response to oral anticoagulants (Freedman and Olatidoye, 1994; Wells et al., 1994; Harder and Thurmann, 1996; Takahashi et al., 1999). Perhaps the most common mechanism for interference with oral anticoagulants is mediated by inhibition of CYP2C9. The half-life of the *S*-enantiomer is significantly prolonged by such agents, leading to overdosage at what would ordinarily be a therapeutic dose. Other mechanisms of interference include induction of CYP2C9, which tends to diminish the effect of warfarin by shortening its half-life; interference with absorption of warfarin from the gastrointestinal tract; displacement of warfarin from albumin in plasma, which temporarily increases the bioavailability of warfarin until equilibrium is reestablished; diminished vitamin K availability, either due to dietary deficiency or interference with the absorption of this lipid-soluble vitamin; and inhibition of the reduction of vitamin K epoxide, which potentiates the effect of oral anticoagulants.

Just as other drugs interfere with the action of oral anticoagulants, administration of oral anticoagulants may affect the activity of other medications, particularly those that are metabolized by CYP2C9. Dicumarol administration prolongs the half-life of chlorpropamide and phenytoin, resulting in hypoglycemia in the case of chlorpropamide and an increased plasma drug concentration in the case of phenytoin. Bis-hydroxycoumarin, but not warfarin, potentiates the activity of tolbutamide, resulting in enhanced hypoglycemia (Harder and Thurmann, 1996).

Oral anticoagulants have been associated with the development of warfarin-induced skin necrosis (Sallah et al., 1997; Esmon et al., 1999). This disorder is due to the development of extensive microvascular thrombosis in the affected skin. This uncommon toxic effect is believed to be due to a rapid drop in protein C following administration of the drug, resulting in impaired protein C function. As protein C has a much shorter half-life than prothrombin and factor X, the level of protein C drops more rapidly than that of these other coagulation factors once oral anticoagulant therapy is initiated. This effect is proportional to the dose of warfarin used to initiate therapy, with a more marked drop occurring at higher doses (Harrison et al., 1997). Thus the risk of developing warfarin-induced skin necrosis increases with the dose of warfarin used to initiate therapy, particularly when the initial dose exceeds 10 mg per day. Native prothrombin can interfere with the function of the protein C system in a concentration-dependent manner. During the early phases of anticoagulation, the ratio of prothrombin to protein C rises due to the differences in their half-lives. This causes further impairment of protein C function and may contribute to warfarin-induced skin necrosis (Esmon et al., 1999; Smirnov et al., 1999). Patients who are deficient in protein C or protein S at the start of therapy (e.g., congenital deficiency) are at a higher risk of developing this complication. In addition, the affected patients often have an underlying acute illness associated with ongoing activation of the procoagulant pathways.

Vitamin K is necessary for the synthesis of proteins other than the coagulation-related factors, including osteocalcin, a major component of bone. Perhaps because of this, long-term administration of warfarin has been associated with bone demineralization (Philip et al., 1995). This effect can be important in patients with borderline bone density. Administration of warfarin during pregnancy, particularly the first 12 weeks of pregnancy, is associated with congenital anomalies in 25 to 30 percent of exposed infants (Ginsberg and Hirsh, 1998). Many of the anomalies are related to abnormal bone formation. It is thought that warfarin may interfere with synthesis of proteins critical for normal structural development.

Heparin Heparin is a widely used anticoagulant for both prophylaxis and therapy of acute venous thromboembolism (Hirsh et al., 1998). In many hospitals, the majority of patients are exposed to this potent anticoagulant at some point during their hospitalization. The major complication associated with heparin therapy is bleeding, a direct manifestation of its anticoagulant activity. The risk of bleeding is related to the intensity of therapy, the patient's body mass and underlying condition, and the presence of other hemostatic defects (e.g., thrombocytopenia). The APTT is commonly used to monitor therapy with unfractionated heparin, but there are significant problems with standardization of this assay for monitoring purposes. An alternative to the APTT is determination of heparin concentration in plasma, using a functional assay based on the inhibition of thrombin or factor Xa (Olson et al., 1998).

As discussed in the section on platelets, heparin administration is also associated with the development of HIT. For unknown reasons, this complication occurs more frequently with heparin derived from bovine sources than with that derived from porcine sources. The incidence of HIT is also significantly higher in patients receiving unfractionated heparin than it is in patients receiving low-molecular-weight heparin (Warkentin et al., 1995).

Long term administration of heparin is associated with an increased risk of clinically significant osteoporosis (Ginsberg et al., 1990; Levine and Anderson, 1990). The mechanism underlying the development of osteoporosis in these patients is not known. Patients may suffer from spontaneous vertebral fractures and demineralization of long bones of the arms and legs. The risk of osteoporosis may be less with low-molecular-weight heparin as compared to unfractionated heparin.

Heparin administration may also cause a transient rise in serum transaminases (Dukes et al., 1984; Schwartz et al., 1985; Monreal et al., 1989; Guevara et al., 1993). The changes may suggest significant liver dysfunction. However, the rise is rapidly reversible upon discontinuation of heparin and may reverse even before heparin is discontinued. The elevation of serum transaminases has not been associated with chronic liver dysfunction. The mechanism of heparin-induced increase in transaminases is not known.

Fibrinolytic Agents Fibrinolytic agents are used in the treatment of acute thromboembolic disease with the goal of dissolving the pathogenic thrombus (Curzen et al., 1998; Collen, 1999). Each of these drugs works by converting plasminogen, an inactive zymogen, to plasmin, an active proteolytic enzyme. Plasmin is normally tightly regulated and is not freely present in the circulation. However, administration of fibrinolytic agents regularly results in the generation of free plasmin leading to systemic fibrin(ogen)olysis. The toxicology of the fibrinolytic agents can be divided into toxic effects of systemic plasmin activation and toxic effects of the activators themselves.

Systemic fibrinolysis is associated with the development of a complex coagulopathy characterized by a decrease in fibrinogen, factor V, factor VIII, α_2-antiplasmin; an increase in circulating fibrin split products; degradation of platelet GP Ib/IX/V and IIb/IIIa; degradation of endothelial cell glycoproteins; degradation of fibronectin and thrombospondin; and prolongation of the PT, APTT, and thrombin time. All of these effects potentiate the risk of bleeding. Anatomic locations that are frequently involved in bleeding complications include the cerebral circulation and sites of recent vascular access. As systemic plasmin can lyse physiologic as well as pathologic thrombi, reactivation of bleeding from sites of vascular access is not uncommon. Platelet inhibitors and heparin are commonly used in conjunction with fibrinolytic therapy to prevent recurrent thrombosis. As one might expect, the use of anticoagulants in the setting of systemic fibrinolysis may also contribute to the risk of bleeding.

Another complication associated with fibrinolysis is recurrent thrombosis at the site of pathologic thrombosis. While rethrombosis may be related to underlying damage to the vascular wall, there is some evidence that fibrinolytic therapy may contribute to this process. For example, plasmin, in appropriate concentrations can actually induce platelet activation (McRedmond et al., 2000). This process may be mediated by plasmin or streptokinase/plasminogen cleavage of the platelet thrombin receptor (protease activated receptor-1). Cleavage of the receptor is associated with activation of the platelet biochemical signaling pathways. There is sufficient "cross-talk" between the fibrinolytic system and the contact system of coagulation that one could also anticipate increased thrombin generation occurring as a result of fibrinolytic therapy (Schmaier et al., 1999).

Streptokinase is a protein derived from group C β-hemolytic streptococci and is antigenic in humans. Antibody formation to streptokinase occurs commonly in association with streptococcal infections as well as exposure to streptokinase. Acute allergic reactions may occur in 1 to 5 percent of patients exposed to streptokinase, and these allergic reactions may consist of minor symptoms such as hives and fever as well as major, life-threatening anaphylactic reactions. In addition, delayed hypersensitivity reactions associated with severe morbidity may occur (Siebert et al., 1992; Curzen et al., 1998). Allergic reactions also occur with other fibrinolytic agents containing streptokinase (e.g., anisoylated plasminogen-streptokinase complex) or streptokinase-derived peptides. The immune complex formed by IgG and streptokinase is capable of binding to and clustering platelet FcγRIIa, initiating platelet activation and aggregation (McRedmond et al., 2000).

Urokinase and recombinant plasma transminogen activator (t-PA) are generally not associated with allergic reactions. However, work is progressing on a number of genetically engineered forms of t-PA. Whether or not such mutant forms of t-PA are immunogenetic has not been firmly established.

Inhibitors of Fibrinolysis Inhibitors of fibrinolysis are commonly used to control bleeding in patients with congenital abnormalities of hemostasis, such as von Willebrand disease. Tranexamic acid and ε-aminocaproic acid are small molecules that block the binding of plasminogen and plasmin to fibrin and other substrate proteins through interaction with lysine binding sites on plasmin(ogen). They are relatively well tolerated. However, there is some evidence that administration of these agents may increase the risk of thrombosis due to the inhibition of the fibrinolytic system (Mannucci, 1998). In a single case, intravenous infusion of ε-aminocaproic in a patient with chronic renal failure was associated with acute hyperkalemia (Perazella and Biswas, 1999).

Aprotinin is a naturally occurring polypeptide inhibitor of serine proteases. It is usually derived from bovine material and consequently is immunogenic when administered to humans. Aprotinin is given by intravenous infusion, as it is inactive when given orally. Allergic reactions in response to aprotinin have been reported, ranging from minor cutaneous manifestations to anaphylactic reactions (Peters and Noble, 1999).

RISK ASSESSMENT

Assessing the risk that exposure to new drugs, chemical products, and other agents pose to humans—in terms of significant toxic effects on hematopoiesis and the functional integrity of blood cells and hemostatic mechanisms—can be logistically and intellectually challenging. This is due in part to the complexity of hematopoiesis and the range of important tasks that these components perform, as previously discussed. A central issue in drug and nontherapeutic chemical development is the *predictive value* of preclinical toxicology data and the expansive but inevitably limited preregistration clinical database for the occurrence of significant hematotoxicity upon broad exposure to human populations. Appropriately, this area of well-resourced applied toxicology is highly regulated yet provides unique and exciting opportunities for sophisticated, well-controlled research (Bloom, 1993).

Preclinical Risk Assessment

Animal Models and Hematologic Monitoring Most preclinical studies that assess the potential for candidate drugs or nontherapeutic chemicals to induce hematotoxicity in humans are performed in industry as part of the routine safety evaluation of these molecules. These studies are largely prescribed by government regulatory bodies of the various countries and regions, including the United States, the European Union, and Japan (Hall, 1992, 1997). The issues relating to the assessment of blood as a target organ that confront the industrial toxicologist are largely similar to those of other target organs and include the selection of the appropriate animal model, how to best monitor for hematotoxicity, and the appreciation of species differences in responding to hematotoxic insults.

Selection of a species that is practical to study and predictive for hematotoxicity in humans is always a challenge. While this is driven in part by regulatory requirements (Hall, 1992), the selection is influenced by other considerations, including having a pharmacokinetic profile comparable to that of man; prior information on sensitivity of a particular species to a class of compounds; the ability to fully characterize effects on peripheral blood and bone marrow; and practical considerations, such as logistics and economics (Bloom, 1993). These become of particular importance in choosing a model to fully characterize the toxicity of an agent known to have an hematotoxic potential.

Of the commonly used animal species, rats and mice offer the advantage of their small size, which favorably impacts test compound requirements and number of subjects that can be economically housed and tested. Both have been well characterized hematologically (Jain, 1986; Smith, 1995; Valli and McGrath, 1997). Blood volume limitations, however, often prohibit the frequent, or serial, evaluation of blood and bone marrow required to characterize the progression of an hematotoxic effect. While this can be addressed in part through serial sacrifices, the inability to fully characterize individual animals poses a significant disadvantage.

Serial blood and bone marrow sampling is practical in larger species, such as the dog and monkey. These models offer the additional advantage of being hematologically more similar to humans as regards hematopoiesis and blood cell kinetics, which in the monkey extends to immunohematologic features (Ladiges, 1990; Shifrine et al., 1980). The latter species, however, presents more interanimal hematologic variability, particularly in wild-caught primates, due to temperament, vascular access, and other influences such as nutritional status and infection.

Tests used to assess blood and bone marrow in preclinical toxicology studies will vary with the phase or objective of the evaluation (acute, subacute, chronic), the intended use of the agent, and what is understood or suspected regarding the toxicologic profile of the xenobiotic. Ideally, the studies in aggregate should provide information on the effects of single- and multiple-dose exposure on erythrocyte parameters (RBC, Hbg, PCV, MCV, MCHC), leukocyte parameters (WBC and absolute differential counts), thrombocyte counts, screening coagulation tests (PT, aPTT), peripheral blood cell morphology, and bone marrow cytologic and histologic examinations (Bloom, 1993; Weingand et al., 1996). Additional tests should be employed in a problem-driven fashion, as required to better characterize findings from the aforementioned screening efforts or to more fully explore a class-specific effect or other hematotoxicologic potential of concern (Bloom, 1993). Examples of these tests are listed in Table 11-13. While much progress has been made in validating many of the more specialized assays in our principal animal models, additional validation that addresses laboratory- and species-specific preanalytic and analytic variables is often required.

Because hematologic features and response to disease can vary substantially among animal species, it is essential that the toxicologist fully understands the hematology of the animal model used for preclinical risk assessment. While complete and accurate reference data are helpful, they do not provide information on pathophysiology that may be species-specific and required to accurately interpret the preclinical data. Examples of these features include the relative influence of preanalytic variables (blood collection technique, nutritional status, sample stability), response to blood loss or hemolysis, stress effects on the leukogram, susceptibility to secondary effects associated with other target organ toxi-

Table 11-13
Examples of Problem-Driven Tests Used to Characterize Hematologic Observations in Preclinical Toxicology

Reticulocyte count
Heinz body preparation
Cell-associated antibody assays (erythrocyte, platelet, neutrophil)
Erythrocyte osmotic fragility test
Erythrokinetic/ferrokinetic analyses
Cytochemical/histochemical staining
Electron microscopy
In vitro hematopoietic clonogenic assays
Platelet aggregation
Plasma fibrinogen concentration
Clotting factor assays
Thrombin time
Bleeding time

city, etc. It is beyond the scope of this chapter to fully discuss the comparative hematology of laboratory animals, which is provided in several excellent reviews (Jain, 1986; Valli and McGrath, 1997; Smith, 1995).

Applications of in Vitro Bone Marrow Assays As with other target-organ risk assessment, in vitro methods for assessing potential hematotoxicity are attractive in that they are faster and less expensive than in vivo studies while providing data that often suggest or clarify the mechanism of a toxic effect. Drug- or chemical-induced bone marrow suppression can result from effects on specific hematopoietic stem cells or on the hematopoietic microenvironment. These effects can be distinguished and confirmed using short-term clonogenic assays and long-term functional assays, respectively (Deldar, 1994; Williams, 1988; Naughton et al., 1992). The former include burst-forming-unit erythroid (BFU-E), colony-forming-unit erythroid (CFU-E), colony-forming-unit granulocyte/monocyte (CFU-GM), colony-forming-unit megakaryocyte (CFU-MK), and colony-forming-unit granulocyte, erythroid, megakaryocyte, monocyte (CFU-GEMM), which have been developed for several laboratory animal species (Deldar and Parchment, 1997). It is therefore possible to examine effects on the myeloid, erythroid and megakaryocytic lineages in a fashion where concentrations of the agent are tightly controlled as is duration of exposure to it.

In vitro clonogenic assays are best used in a preclinical setting in combination with in vivo testing. Used in this way, the predictive value of these assays is enhanced. This has been particularly true for anticancer and antiviral drugs, where the in vitro component of risk assessment has been used for therapeutic index-based screening to identify less myelosuppressive analogs, structure-toxicity relationships, and new-drug lead candidates (Deldar and Stevens, 1993; Parchment et al., 1993). Other advantages of the in vitro hematopoietic stem cell assays include the opportunities they provide to test combinations of agents as well as their metabolites and effects of serum and other cell components, such as lymphocytes (Deldar and Parchment, 1997). Perhaps most important is the ability to test human hematopoietic cells directly in a preclinical setting, thus obviating extrapolation considerations. Concern for possible metabolic activation can be addressed by culturing the target cells in question with metabolizing systems in a cell-free extract (s9), with isolated hepatocytes, or with other CYP450-expressing cell types (Frazier, 1992).

Perhaps the most interesting use of these in vitro clonogenic assays in risk assessment has been their role in making practical interspecies comparisons regarding sensitivity to a particular agent or group of drugs or chemicals. Comparisons to the sensitivity of human cells can be made that have implications for the relative predictive value of various animal models for hematotoxicity in humans. Examples include the resistance of murine CFU-GM to the anticancer drug topotecan relative to that of the canine and human cells (Deldar, 1993). This is consistent with the early observations of Marsh, that the dog is a particularly predictive model for the myelosuppression associated with anticancer drugs in humans (Marsh, 1985). Thus, while some agents show comparable suppressive activity across species lines (doxorubicin, pyrazoloacridine, hepsulfan, cyclopentenyl cytosine), others, such as camptothecins, carboxyamidotriazole and fostriecin, show differences of as much as three log concentrations (Reagan et al., 1993; Horikoshi and Murphy, 1982; Du et al., 1991). A more detailed discussion on the application of in vitro hematopoietic clonogenic assays for preclinical screening and mechanistic studies is provided by Deldar and Parchment (1997).

While this discussion has focused on in vitro hematopoietic clonogenic assays in the context of risk assessment, these assays have also proven to be extraordinarily useful tools for investigating mechanisms of toxic cytopenia in humans (Deldar, 1994). Parchment and Murphy review the application of these to four categories of hematologic toxicity observed clinically: (1) the reversible cytopenia following acute exposure to a cytotoxic or cytostatic agent; (2) the permanent loss in the production of a mature blood cell type(s); (3) cytosis, or the dramatic increase in blood cell counts following single or repeated toxicant exposure; and (4) the progressive loss or one or more blood cell lineages during chronic exposure to a toxicant (Parchment and Murphy, 1997). In all these circumstances, in vitro and ex vivo hematopoietic clonogenic assays have proven useful in understanding the mechanism(s) of these toxic effects and formulating strategies for risk management and treatment.

Clinical Trials and Risk Assessment

As with preclinical risk assessment, most of the clinical research on hematotoxicity is driven by regulatory requirements and supported by the drug, cosmetic, and chemical industries. The challenges and opportunities this presents are similar to those in preclinical development with the following differences. Most clinical studies involve actual patients with the targeted disease, in contrast to the inbred, healthy, well-defined animals employed in preclinical studies. This presents additional variables and challenges to manage. Second, the scale of clinical trials, the volume of data produced, and the resources required exceed by orders of magnitude those of preclinical studies. Third, many clinical trials involve research cooperative groups that represent a network of clinical scientists from academic medical centers, such as the Eastern Cooperative Oncology Group (ECOG), the AIDS Clinical Trial Group (ACTG), Thrombolysis in Myocardial Infarction (TIMI), and others. Most of the information on drug- or chemical-induced hematotoxicity in humans is collected through this industry-sponsored and highly regulated clinical research.

Table 11-14
WHO Grading Criteria for Subacute and Acute Hematotoxicity

HEMATOLOGICAL PARAMETERS (ADULTS)	GRADE 0	GRADE 1	GRADE 2	GRADE 3	GRADE 4
Hemoglobin (g dL^{-1})	11.0	9.5–10.5	8.0–9.4	6.5–7.9	6.5
(nmol/L)	(6.8)	(6.5–6.7)	(4.95–5.8)	(4.0–4.9)	(4.0)
Leukocytes (1000 μL^{-1})	4.0	3.0–3.9	2.0–2.9	2.0–1.9	1.0
Granulocytes (1000 μL^{-1})	2.0	1.5–1.9	1.0–1.4	0.5–0.9	0.5
Platelets (1000 μL^{-1})	100	75–99	50–74	25–49	<25
Hemorrhage, blood loss	None	Petechiae	Mild	Gross	Debilitating

SOURCE: WHO, 1979.

It is well understood that the ways in which drugs and nontherapeutic chemicals affect the hematopoietic system are influenced by both the nature of the agent and the response of the subject or target population. As discussed previously, many agents are known to induce dose-dependent hematotoxicity in a fashion that is highly predictable. Others cause toxicity in a small number of susceptible individuals, and these often include agents not otherwise hematotoxic in most individuals (Patton and Duffull, 1994). As previously discussed these *idiosyncratic reactions* present the biggest challenge as regards detection and characterization before human patients or populations are broadly exposed. They include aplastic anemia, thrombocytopenia, hemolysis and leukopenia, which may be immune-mediated (Salama and Muller-Eckhardt, 1992) or related to other mechanisms, such the generation of a toxic metabolite (Gerson et al., 1983), as previously discussed.

The chemical structure can be a risk factor if it is similar to that of other known toxicants. Patient or population-related risk factors include pharmacogenetic variations in drug metabolism and detoxification that lead to reduced clearance of the agent or production of novel intermediate metabolites (Gerson et al., 1993; Cunningham et al., 1974; Mason and Fisher, 1992), histocompatibility antigens (Frickhofen et al., 1990), interaction with drugs or other agents (West et al., 1988), increased sensitivity of hematopoietic precursors to damage (Vincent, 1986), preexisting disease of the bone marrow, and metabolic defects that predispose to oxidative or other stresses associated with the agent (Stern, 1989).

In drug development, the clinical evaluation of candidate molecules is usually performed in three phases: *Phase I* examines the effect of single and multiple increasing doses in small numbers of normal and/or patient volunteers. Pharmacokinetic properties are usually addressed, as well as the routes of excretion and metabolism; and the assessment of active and inactive metabolites. The emphasis is usually on safety assessment. *Phase II* includes controlled studies in the target patient population that examine both safety and efficacy. They explore dose response and usually provide the first indication of benefit versus risk. *Phase III* entails larger studies designed to confirm efficacy in an expanded patient population and evaluate less frequent adverse effects, such as the aforementioned idiosyncratic blood dyscrasias.

Development of demonstrably hematotoxic drugs is usually stopped in phase I or II unless the indications include life-threatening conditions, where toxicity is acceptable (e.g., anticancer drugs). Thus, drugs tested in phase III generally show an acceptable safety profile in most subjects at the doses used. Even phase III studies, however, are not usually powered to detect the low incidence of idiosyncratic hematotoxicity previously discussed (Levine and Szarfman, 1996). In order to detect one adverse event affecting 1 percent of an exposed patient population at a 95 percent confidence level, a trial must include approximately 300 subjects (O'Neill, 1988). Most clinical databases supporting new drug applications cannot be used to rule out events that occur below 1 per 500 exposures (Szarfman et al., 1997). Thus, rare, delayed or cumulative toxicity is often missed in preregistration clinical trials.

Detection of low-incidence hematotoxicity is usually achieved through postmarketing surveillance, such as the Med Watch program introduced by the FDA in 1993 (Szarfman et al., 1997). Other countries that practice comprehensive postmarketing surveillance include Canada, the United Kingdom, Sweden, Germany, France, Australia, and New Zealand. Adverse event data, including serious hematotoxicity, are provided to the WHO; this information is compiled by a computer-based recording system employing WHO terminology and system and organ classifications for adverse reactions (Edwards, 1990). Examples of iatrogenic blood dyscrasias detected through postmarketing surveillance include the hemolysis and thrombocytopenia associated with the antibiotic temafloxacin; the aplastic anemia linked to the antiepileptic felbamate; the hemolysis caused by the antidepressant nomifensine; and the agranulocytosis associated with the antiarrhythmic aprindine (Szarfman et al., 1997).

The WHO has also established criteria for grading hematotoxicity (WHO, 1997), which is summarized in Table 11-14. These have been particularly useful in establishing and communicating treatment strategies and guidelines for agents known to suppress hematopoiesis (cytoreductive oncolytic, immunosuppressive, and antiviral agents, etc.) and for which this limiting toxicity is used to establish maximum tolerated doses for individual patients.

Greater risk is acceptable with these agents due to the life-threatening conditions they are used to treat. Similar risk–benefit decisions are also made regarding the use of agents that cause blood dyscrasias in an idiosyncratic fashion, as previously discussed. Some are used to treat nonmalignant or life-threatening conditions, the risk of which is managed through rigorous laboratory monitoring. Examples include felbamate and ticlopidine, as discussed above, and the antischizophrenic drug clozapine, associated with agranulocytosis (Alvir et al., 1993). Postmarketing surveillance plays a critical role in measuring the effectiveness of such monitoring.

REFERENCES

Abarbanel J, Benet AE, Lask D, et al: Sports hematuria. *J Urol* 143:887–890, 1990.

Aithal GP, Day CP, Kesteven PJ, et al: Association of polymorphisms in the cytochrome P450 CYP2C9 with warfarin dose requirement and risk of bleeding complications. *Lancet* 353:717–719, 1999.

Alvir JM, Lieberman JA, Safferman AZ, et al: Colzapine-induced agranulocytosis. Incidence and risk factors in the United States. *N Engl J Med* 329:162–167, 1993.

Amiral J, Meyer D: Heparin-induced thrombocytopenia: Diagnostic tests and biological mechanisms. *Baillieres Clin Haematol* 11:447–460, 1998.

Andersen RL, Bagby, Jr GC, Richert-Boe K, et al: Therapy-related preleukemic syndrome. *Cancer* 47:1867–1871, 1981.

Andrews RK, Shen Y, Gardiner EE, et al: The glycoprotein Ib-IX-V complex in platelet adhesion and signaling. *Thromb Haemost* 82:357–364, 1999.

Arneborn P, Palmblad J: Drug-induced neutropenia—A survey for Stockholm 1973–1978. *Acta Med Scand* 212:289–292, 1982.

Aster RH: Drug-induced immune thrombocytopenia: An overview of pathogenesis. *Semin Hematol* 36:2–6, 1999.

Athens JW, Raab SO, Haab OP, et al: Leukokinetic studies: III. The distribution of granulocytes in the blood of normal subjects. *J Clin Invest* 40:159–164, 1961.

Athens JW, Raab SO, Haab OP, et al: Leukokinetic studies. IV. The total circulating and marginal granulocyte pools and the granulocyte turnover rate in normal subjects. *J Clin Invest* 40:989–995, 1961.

Babior BM, Golde DW: Production, distribution and fate of neutrophils, in Beutler E, Lichtman MA, Coller BS, Kipps TJ (eds): *Williams Hematology,* 5th ed. New York: McGraw-Hill, 1995, pp 773–779.

Bainton DF: Morphology of neutrophils, eosinophils and basophils, in Beutler E, Lichtman MA, Coller BS, Kipps TJ (eds): *Williams Hematology,* 5th ed. New York: McGraw-Hill, 1995, pp 753–779.

Baker RI, Hankey GJ: Antiplatelet drugs. *Med J Aust* 170:379–382, 1999.

Bennett CL, Davidson CJ, Raisch DW, et al: Thrombotic thrombocytopenic purpura associated with ticlopidine in the setting of coronary artery stents and stroke prevention. *Arch Intern Med* 159:2524–2528, 1999.

Bennett CL, Weinberg PD, Rozenberg-Ben-Dror K, et al: Thrombotic thrombocytopenic purpura associated with ticlopidine. A review of 60 cases. *Ann Intern Med* 128:541–544, 1998.

Bennett JM, Catovsky D, Daniel MT, et al: Proposals for the classification of the myelodysplastic syndromes. *Br J Haematol* 51:189–199, 1982.

Bennett JM, Catovsky D, Daniel MT, et al: Proposed revised criteria for the classification of acute myeloid leukemia. A report on the French-American-British Cooperative Group. *Ann Intern Med* 103:620–625, 1985.

Bergsagel DE, Wong O, Bergsagel PL, et al: Benzene and multiple myeloma: Appraisal of the scientific evidence. *Blood* 94:1174–1182, 1999.

Berkowitz FE: Hemolysis and infection: Categories and mechanisms of their interrelationship. *Rev Infect Dis* 13:1151–1162, 1991.

Berry RG, Morrison JA, Watts JW, et al: Surreptitious superwarfarin ingestion with brodifacoum. *South Med J* 93:74–75, 2000.

Beutler E: G6PD: Population genetics and clinical manifestations. *Blood Rev* 10:45–52, 1996.

Bhasker CR, Miners JO, Coulter S, et al: Allelic and functional variability of cytochrome P4502C9. *Pharmacogenetics* 7:51–58, 1997.

Bitter MA, LeBeau MM, Rowley JD, et al: Associations between morphology, karyotype and clinical features in myeloid leukemia. *Hum Pathol* 18:211–225, 1987.

Blanche P, Silberman B, Barreto L, et al: Reversible zidovudine-induced pure red cell aplasia. *AIDS* 13:1586–1587, 1999.

Bloom JC: Introduction to hematotoxicology, in Sipes IG, McQueen CA, Gandolfi AJ (eds): *Comprehensive Toxicology.* Vol. 4. Oxford: Pergamon Press, 1997, pp 1–10.

Bloom JC: Principles of hematotoxicology: Laboratory assessment and interpretation of data. *Toxicol Pathol* 21:130–134, 1993.

Bloom JC, Lewis HB, Sellers TS, et al: The hematopathology of cefonicid- and cefazedone-induced blood dyscrasias in the dog. *Toxicol Appl Pharmacol* 90:143–155, 1987.

Bossi P, Cabane J, Ninet J, et al: Acquired hemophilia due to factor VIII inhibitors in 34 patients. *Am J Med* 105:400–408, 1998.

Bottomly SS: Sideroblastic anemia, in Lee CR, Foerster J, Lukens J, Paraskevas P, Greer JP, Rodgers GM (eds): *Wintrobe's Clinical Hematology,* 10th ed. Philadelphia: Lippincott Williams & Wilkins, 1999, pp 1022–1045.

Brayton RG, Stokes PE, Schwartz MS, et al: Effect of alcohol and various diseases on leukocyte mobilization, phagocytosis and intracellular bacterial killing. *N Engl J Med* 282:123–128, 1970.

Browning E: *Toxicity and Metabolism of Industrial Solvents,* 256th ed. London: Elsevier, 1965, p 3.

Cannistra SA, Griffin JD: Regulation of the production and function of granulocytes and monocytes. *Semin Hematol* 25:173–188, 1988.

Capizzi RL: The preclinical basis for broad-spectrum selective cytoprotection of normal tissues from cytotoxic therapies by amifostine. *Semin Oncol* 26:3–21, 1999.

Cartwright RA: Leukaemia epidemiology and radiation risks. *Blood Rev* 6:10–14, 1992.

Carver JH, Hatch FT, Branscomb EW: Estimating maximum limits to mutagenic potency from cytotoxic potency. *Nature* 279:154–156, 1979.

Casciato DA, Scott JL: Acute leukemia following prolonged cytotoxic agent therapy. *Medicine* (Baltimore) 58(1):32–47, 1979.

Cerulli J, Grabe DW, Gauthier I, et al: Chromium picolinate toxicity. *Ann Pharmacother* 32:428–431, 1998.

Chakraverty R, Davidson S, Peggs K, et al: The incidence and cause of coagulopathies in an intensive care population. *Br J Haematol* 93:460–463, 1996.

Chua JD, Friedenberg WR: Superwarfarin poisoning. *Arch Intern Med* 158:1929–1932, 1998.

Coleman MD, Coleman NA: Drug-induced methaemoglobinaemia: Treatment issues. *Drug Saf* 14:394–405, 1996.

Collen D: The plasminogen (fibrinolytic) system. *Thromb Haemost* 82:259–270, 1999.

Cuneo A, Fagioli F, Pazzi I, et al: Morphologic, immunologic and cytogenic studies in acute myeloid leukemia following occupational exposure to pesticides and organic solvents. *Leuk Res* 16:789–796, 1992.

Cunningham JL, Leyland MJ, Delmore IW, et al: Acetanilide oxidation in phenylbutazone-associated hypoplastic anemia. *Br Med J* 3:313–317, 1974.

Curzen N, Haque R, Timmis A: Applications of thrombolytic therapy. *Intens Care Med* 24:756–768, 1998.

Custer RP, Ahlfeldt FE: Studies on the structure and function of bone marrow. *J Lab Clin Med* 17:960–962, 1932.

Dahl OE, Garvik LJ, Lyberg T: Toxic effects of methylmethacrylate monomer on leukocytes and endothelial cells *in vitro. Acta Orthopaed Scand* 65:147–153, 1994.

Dale DC: Neutropenia, in Beutler E, Lichtman MA, Coller BS, Kipps TJ (eds): *Williams Hematology* 5th ed. New York: McGraw-Hill, 1995, pp 815–824.

Dancey JT, Deubelbeiss KA, Harker LA, et al: Neutrophil kinetics in man. *J Clin Invest* 58: 705–715, 1976.

Deckmyn H, Vanhoorelbeke K, Peerlinck K: Inhibitory and activating human antiplatelet antibodies. *Baillieres Clin Haematol* 11:343–359, 1998.

Deldar A: Drug-induced blood disorders: Review of pathogenetic mechanisms and utilization of bone marrow cell culture technology as an investigative approach. *Curr Topics Vet Res* 1:83–101, 1994.

Deldar A, Parchment RE: Preclinical risk assessment for hematotoxicity: Animal models and *in vitro* systems, in Sipes IG, McQueen CA, Gandolfi AJ (eds): *Comprehensive Toxicology.* Vol 4. Oxford, England: Pergamon Press, 1997, pp 321–333.

Deldar A, Stevens CE: Development and application of *in vitro* models of hematopoiesis to drug development. *Toxicol Pathol* 21:231–240, 1993.

Demirer T, Bensinger WI: Optimization of peripheral blood stem cell collection. *Curr Opin Hematol* 3:219–226, 1995.

Dessypris EN: Erythropoiesis, in Lee CR, Foerster J, Lukens J, Paraskevas P, Greer JP, Rodgers GM (eds): *Wintrobe's Clinical Hematology,* 10th ed. Philadelphia: Lippincott Williams & Wilkins, 1999, pp 169–192.

Dreno B, Trossaert M, Boiteau HL, et al: Zinc salts effects on granulocyte zinc concentrations and chemotaxis in acne patients. *Acta Derm Venereol* 72:250–252, 1992.

Du DL, Volpe DA, Grieshaber CK, et al: Comparative toxicity of fostriecin, hepsulfam and pyrazine diazohydroxide to human and murine hematopoietic progenitor cells *in vitro. Invest New Drugs* 9:149–157, 1991.

Dukes GE Jr, Sanders SW, Russo J Jr, et al: Transaminase elevations in patients receiving bovine or porcine heparin. *Ann Intern Med* 100:646–650, 1984.

Durand JM, Lefevre P: Mitomycin-induced thrombotic thrombocytopenic purpura: Possible successful treatment with vincristine and cyclophosphamide. *Haematologica* 76:421–423, 1991.

Edwards IR, Lidquist M, Wholm BE, et al: Quality criteria for early signals of possible adverse drug reactions. *Lancet* 336:156–158, 1990.

Esmon CT, Gu JM, Xu J, et al: Regulation and functions of the protein C anticoagulant pathway. *Haematologica* 84:363–368, 1999.

Everse J, Hsia N: The toxicities of native and modified hemoglobins. *Free Radic Biol Med* 22:1075–1099, 1997.

Fagioli F, Cuneo A, Piva N, et al: Distinct cytogenetic and clinicopathologic features in acute myeloid leukemia after occupational exposure to pesticides and other organic solvents. *Cancer* 70:77–85, 1992.

Fiske DN, McCoy HE III, Kitchens CS: Zinc-induced sideroblastic anemia: Report of a case, review of the literature, and description of the hematologic syndrome. *Am J Hematol* 46:147–150, 1994.

Foucar K, McKenna RW, Bloomfield CD, et al: Therapy-related leukemia: A panmyelosis. *Cancer* 43:1285–1294, 1979.

Frazier JM: *In vitro* toxicity testing: Applications to safety evaluation, in Frazier JM (ed): *In Vitro Toxicity Testing Applications to Safety Evaluation.* New York: Marcel Dekker, 1992, pp 5–7.

Freedman MD: Oral anticoagulants: Pharmacodynamics, clinical indications and adverse effects. *J Clin Pharmacol* 32:196–209, 1992.

Freedman MD, Olatidoye AG: Clinically significant drug interactions with the oral anticoagulants. *Drug Saf* 10:381–394, 1994.

Frickhofen N, Liu JM, Young NS: Etiologic mechanisms of hematopoietic failure. *Am J Pediatr Hematol Oncol* 12:385–395, 1990.

Furlan M, Robles R, Galbusera M, et al: von Willebrand factor-cleaving protease in thrombotic thrombocytopenic purpura and the hemolytic-uremic syndrome. *N Engl J Med* 339:1578–1584, 1998.

Furuya H, Fernandez-Salguero P, Gregory W, et al: Genetic polymorphism of CYP2C9 and its effect on warfarin maintenance dose requirement in patients undergoing anticoagulation therapy. *Pharmacogenetics* 5:389–392, 1995.

Garratty G, Arndt PA: Positive direct antiglobulin tests and haemolytic anaemia following therapy with beta-lactamase inhibitor containing drugs may be associated with nonimmunologic adsorption of protein onto red blood cells. *Br J Haematol* 100:777–783, 1998.

Gerson SL, Melzer H: Mechanisms of clozapine-induced agranulocytosis. *Drug Saf* 7:17–25, 1992.

Gerson WT, Fine D, Spielberg SP, et al: Anticonvulsant-induced aplastic anemia: Increased susceptibility to toxic drug metabolites *in vitro. Blood* 61:889–893, 1983.

George JN: Thrombocytopenia due to diminished or defective platelet production, in Beutler E, Lichtman MA, Coller BS, Kipps TJ (eds): *Williams Hematology,* 5th ed. New York: McGraw-Hill, 1995, pp 1281–1289.

George JN, Raskob GE, Shah SR, et al: Drug-induced thrombocytopenia: A systematic review of published case reports. *Ann Intern Med* 129:886–890, 1998.

George JN, Shattil SJ: The clinical importance of acquired abnormalities of platelet function. *N Engl J Med* 324:27–39, 1991.

Gibly RL, Walter FG, Nowlin SW, et al: Intravascular hemolysis associated with North American crotalid envenomation. *J Toxicol Clin Toxicol* 36:337–343, 1998.

Ginsberg JS, Hirsh J: Use of antithrombotic agents during pregnancy. *Chest* 114:524S–530S, 1998.

Ginsberg JS, Kowalchuk G, Hirsh J, et al: Heparin effect on bone density. *Thromb Haemost* 64:286–289, 1990.

Golomb HM, Alimena G, Rowley JD, et al: Correlation of occupation and karyotype in adults with acute nonlymphocytic leukemia. *Blood* 60:404–411, 1982.

Gonzalez H, Leblond V, Azar N, et al: Severe autoimmune hemolytic anemia in eight patients treated with fludarabine. *Hematol Cell Ther* 40:113–118, 1998.

Gordon LI, Kwaan HC: Thrombotic microangiopathy manifesting as thrombotic thrombocytopenic purpura/hemolytic uremic syndrome in the cancer patient. *Semin Thromb Hemost* 25:217–221, 1999.

Greene MH, Harris EL, Gershenson DM, et al: Melphalan may be a more potent leukemogen than cyclophosphamide. *Ann Intern Med* 105:360–367, 1986.

Guevara A, Labarca J, Gonzalez-Martin G: Heparin-induced transaminase elevations: A prospective study. *Int J Clin Pharmacol Ther Toxicol* 31:137–141, 1993.

Hagen EC, Ballieux BE, van Es LA, et al: Antineutrophil cytoplasmic autoantibodies: A review of the antigens involved, the assays, and the clinical and possible pathogenic consequences. *Blood* 81:1996–2002, 1993.

Hall RL: Clinical pathology for preclinical safety assessment: Current global guidelines. *Toxicol Pathol* 20:472–476, 1992.

Hall RL: Evaluation and interpretation of hematologic data in preclinical toxicology, in Sipes IG, McQueen CA, Gandolfi AJ (eds): *Comprehensive Toxicology.* Vol 4. Oxford: Pergamon Press, 1997, pp 321–333.

Harder S, Thurmann P: Clinically important drug interactions with anticoagulants. An update. *Clin Pharmacokinet* 30:416–444, 1996.

Harrison L, Johnston M, Massicotte MP, et al: Comparison of 5-mg and 10-mg loading doses in initiation of warfarin therapy. *Ann Intern Med* 126:133–136, 1997.

Harrison P, Robinson MS, Mackie IJ, et al: Performance of the platelet function analyser PFA-100 in testing abnormalities of primary haemostasis. *Blood Coagul Fibrinolysis* 10:25–31, 1999.

Hatherill JR, Till GO, Bruner LH, et al: Thermal injury, intravascular hemolysis, and toxic oxygen products. *J Clin Invest* 78:629–636, 1986.

Hebert LA: The clearance of immune complexes from the circulation of man and other primates. *Am J Kidney Dis* 17:352–361, 1991.

Hess JR, MacDonald VW, Brinkley WW: Systemic and pulmonary hypertension after resuscitation with cell-free hemoglobin. *J Appl Physiol* 74:1769–1778, 1993.

Hirsh J, Dalen JE, Anderson DR, et al: Oral anticoagulants: Mechanism of action, clinical effectiveness, and optimal therapeutic range. *Chest* 114:445S–469S, 1998.

Hirsh J, Warkentin TE, Raschke R, et al: Heparin and low-molecular-weight heparin: Mechanisms of action, pharmacokinetics, dosing considerations, monitoring, efficacy, and safety. *Chest* 114:489S–510S, 1998.

Horikoshi A, Murphy, Jr. MJ: Comparative effects of chemotherapeutic drugs on human and murine hematopoietic progenitors *in vitro. Chemotherapy* 28:480–501, 1982.

Hsia CC: Respiratory function of hemoglobin. *N Engl J Med* 338:239–247, 1998.

Hudson G: Bone marrow volume in the human foetus and newborn. *Br J Haematol* 11:446–452, 1965.

Hunter FT: Chronic exposure of benzene. II. The clinical effects. *J Ind Hyg Toxicol* 21:331, 1939.

Irons RD: Leukemogenesis as a toxic response, in Sipes IG, McQueen CA, Gandolfi AJ (eds): *Comprehensive Toxicology.* Vol 4. Oxford: Pergamon Press, 1997, pp 175–199.

Jain NC: *Schalm's Veterinary Hematology,* 4th ed. Philadelphia: Lea & Febiger, 1986.

Jandl JH: *Blood: Textbook of Hematology.* Boston: Little Brown, 1987, pp 335–349.

Johannsson B, Mertens F, Heim S, et al: Cytogenetics of secondary myelodysplasia (sMDS) and acute nonlymphocytic leukemia (sAMLL). *Eur J Haematol* 47:17–27, 1987.

Jollow DJ, Bradshaw TP, McMillan DC: Dapsone-induced hemolytic anemia. *Drug Metab Rev* 27:107–124, 1995.

Kaminsky LS, Zhang ZY: Human P450 metabolism of warfarin. *Pharmacol Ther* 73:67–74, 1997.

Kantarjian HM, Keating MJ, Walters RS, et al: Therapy-related leukemia and myelodysplastic syndrome: Clinical, cytogenetic and prognostic features. *J Clin Oncol* 14(12):1748–1757, 1986.

Kaushansky K: Blood: New designs for a new millennium. *Blood* 95:1–6, 2000.

Keng PC: Use of flow cytometry in the measurement of cell mitotic cycle. *Int J Cell Cloning* 4:295–311, 1986.

Khan NA, Kruse JA: Methemoglobinemia induced by topical anesthesia: A case report and review. *Am J Med Sci* 318:415–418, 1999.

Kilbourne EM, Posada de la Paz M, Abaitua Borda I, et al: Toxic oil syndrome: A current clinical and epidemiologic summary, including comparisons with eosinophilia-myalgia syndrome. *J Am Coll Cardiol* 18:711–717, 1991.

Knobl P, Lechner K: Acquired factor V inhibitors. *Baillieres Clin Haematol* 11:305–318, 1998.

Ladiges WC, Storb R, Thomas ED: Canine models of bone marrow transplantation. *Lab Anim Sci* 40:11–15, 1990.

LeBeau MM, Albain KS, Larson RA, et al: Clinical and cytogenetic correlations in 63 patients with therapy-related myelodysplastic syndromes and acute nonlymphocytic leukemia: Further evidence for characteristic abnormalities of chromosomes no. 5 and 7. *J Clin Oncol* 4(3):325–345, 1986.

Lee GR: Acquired hemolytic anemia resulting from direct effects of infectious, chemical or physical agents, in Lee CR, Foerster J, Lukens J, Paraskevas P, Greer JP, Rodgers GM (eds): *Wintrobe's Clinical Hematology,* 10th ed. Philadelphia: Lippincott Williams & Wilkins, 1999, pp 1289–1304.

Lee GR: Anemia: A diagnostic strategy, in Lee CR, Foerster J, Lukens J, Paraskevas P, Greer JP, Rodgers GM (eds): *Wintrobe's Clinical Hematology,* 10th ed. Philadelphia: Lippincott Williams & Wilkins, 1999, pp 908–940.

Lee GR: Folate deficiency: Causes and management, in Lee CR, Foerster J, Lukens J, Paraskevas P, Greer JP, Rodgers GM (eds): *Wintrobe's Clinical Hematology,* 10th ed. Philadelphia: Lippincott Williams & Wilkins, 1999, pp 965–972.

Lee GR: Pernicious anemia and other causes of vitamin B12 (cobalamin) deficiency, in Lee CR, Foerster J, Lukens J, Paraskevas P, Greer JP, Rodgers GM (eds): *Wintrobe's Clinical Hematology,* 10th ed. Philadelphia: Lippincott Williams & Wilkins, 1999, pp 941–964.

Levine EG, Bloomfield CD: Leukemias and myelodysplastic syndromes secondary to drug, radiation and environmental exposure. *Semin Oncol* 19(1):47–84, 1992.

Levine JG, Szarfman A: Standardized data structures and visualization tools: A way to accelerate the regulatory review of the integrated summary of safety of new drug applications. *Biopharm Rep* 4: 1996.

Levine MN, Anderson DR: Side-effects of antithrombotic therapy. *Baillieres Clin Haematol* 3:815–829, 1990.

Liesveld JL, Lichtman MA: Evaluation of granulocytes and mononuclear phagocytes, in Sipes IG, McQueen CA, Gandolfi AJ (eds): *Comprehensive Toxicology.* Vol 4. Oxford: Pergamon Press, 1997, pp 123–144.

Lillevang ST, Albertsen M, Rasmessen F, et al: Effect of radiographic contrast media on granulocyte phagocytosis of *Escherichia coli* in a whole blood flow cytometric assay. *Invest Radiol* 29:68–71, 1994.

List AF, Doll DC: Thrombosis associated with procainamide-induced lupus anticoagulant. *Acta Haematol* 82:50–52, 1989.

Lukens JN: Methemoglobinemia and other disorders accompanied by cyanosis, in Lee CR, Foerster J, Lukens J, et al. (eds): *Wintrobe's Clinical Hematology,* 10th ed. Philadelphia: Lippincott Williams & Wilkins, 1999, pp 1046–1055.

Magee P, Beeley L: Drug-induced blood dyscrasias (1). *Pharm J* 246:150–151, 1991.

Mann KG: Biochemistry and physiology of blood coagulation. *Thromb Haemost* 82:165–174, 1999.

Mannucci PM: Hemostatic drugs. *N Engl J Med* 339:245–253, 1998.

Marseglia GL, Locatelli F: Isoniazid-induced pure red cell aplasia in two siblings. *J Pediatr* 132:898–900, 1998.

Marsh JC: Correlation of hematologic toxicity of antineoplastic agents with their effects on bone marrow stem cells: Interspecies studies using an *in vitro* assay. *Exp Hematol* 13(16):16–22, 1985.

Mason RP, Fisher V: Possible role of free radical formation in drug-induced agranulocytosis. *Drug Saf* 7:45–50, 1992.

Mazzone A, Mazzucchelli I, Fossati G, et al: Granulocyte defects and opioid receptors in chronic exposure to heroin or methadone in humans. *Int J Immunopharmacol* 16:959–967, 1994.

McRedmond JP, Harriott P, Walker B, et al: Streptokinase-induced platelet activation involves antistreptokinase antibodies and cleavage of protease-activated receptor-1. *Blood* 95:1301–1308, 2000.

Michelson AD, Furman MI: Laboratory markers of platelet activation and their clinical significance. *Curr Opin Hematol* 6:342–348, 1999.

Minchinton RM, Waters AH: The occurrence and significance of neutrophil antibodies. *Br J Haematol* 56:521–528, 1984.

Minderman H, Linssen P, van der Lely N: Toxicity of idarubicin and doxorubicin towards normal and leukemic human bone marrow progenitors in relation to their proliferative state. *Leukemia* 8:382–387, 1994.

Miners JO, Birkett DJ: Cytochrome P4502C9: An enzyme of major importance in human drug metabolism. *Br J Clin Pharmacol* 45:525–538, 1998.

Misra S, Moore TB, Ament ME, et al: Red cell aplasia in children on tacrolimus after liver transplantation. *Transplantation* 65:575–577, 1998.

Mitelman F, Brandt L, Nilsson PG: Relation among occupational exposure to potential mutagenic/carcinogenic agents, clinical findings and bone marrow chromosomes in acute nonlymphocytic leukemia. *Blood* 52:1229–1237, 1978.

Mitelman F, Nilsson PG, Brandt L, et al: Chromosome pattern, occupation and clinical features in patients with acute nonlymphocytic leukemia. *Cancer Genet Cytogenet* 4:197–214, 1981.

Monreal M, Lafoz E, Salvador R, et al: Adverse effects of three different forms of heparin therapy: Thrombocytopenia, increased transaminases, and hyperkalaemia. *Eur J Clin Pharmacol* 37:415–418, 1989.

Moore MAS: Embryologic and phylogenetic development of the haematopoietic system. *Adv Biosci* 16:87–103, 1975.

Muntean W, Zenz W, Edlinger G, et al: Severe bleeding due to factor V inhibitor after repeated operations using fibrin sealant containing bovine thrombin. *Thromb Haemost* 77:1223, 1997.

Murphy SB: Secondary acute myeloid leukemia following treatment with epipodophyllotoxins. *J Clin Oncol* 11:199–201, 1993.

Naughton BA, Sibanda B, Azar L, et al: Differential effects of drugs upon hematopoiesis can be assessed in long-term bone marrow cultures established on nylon screens. *Pro Soc Exp Biol Med* 199:481–490, 1992.

Nelsestuen GL, Shah AM, Harvey SB: Vitamin K-dependent proteins. *Vitam Horm* 58:355–389, 2000.

Nesher G, Hanna VE, Moore TL, et al: Thrombotic microangiographic hemolytic anemia in systemic lupus erythematosus. *Semin Arthritis Rheum* 24:165–172, 1994.

Nishimura J, Murakami Y, Kinoshita T: Paroxysmal nocturnal hemoglobinuria: An acquired genetic disease. *Am J Hematol* 62:175–182, 1999.

Nohl H, Stolze K: The effects of xenobiotics on erythrocytes. *Gen Pharmacol* 31:343–347, 1998.

Nurden AT, Poujol C, Durrieu-Jais C, et al: Platelet glycoprotein IIb/IIIa inhibitors: Basic and clinical aspects. *Arterioscler Thromb Vasc Biol* 19:2835–2840, 1999.

Oldenburg J, Quenzel EM, Harbrecht U, et al: Missense mutations at ALA-10 in the factor IX propeptide: An insignificant variant in normal life but a decisive cause of bleeding during oral anticoagulant therapy. *Br J Haematol* 98:240–244, 1997.

Olson JD, Arkin CF, Brandt JT, et al: College of American Pathologists Conference XXXI on laboratory monitoring of anticoagulant therapy: Laboratory monitoring of unfractionated heparin therapy. *Arch Pathol Lab Med* 122:782–798, 1998.

O'Neill R: Assessment of safety, in Peace KE (ed.): *Biopharmaceutical Statistics for Drug Development.* New York: Marcel Dekker, 1988.

Papassotiriou I, Kister J, Griffon N, et al: Modulating the oxygen affinity of human fetal haemoglobin with synthetic allosteric modulators. *Br J Haematol* 102:1165–1171, 1998.

Parchment RE, Huang M, Erickson-Miller CK: Roles for *in vitro* myelotoxicity tests in preclinical drug development and clinical trial planning. *Toxicol Pathol* 21:241–250, 1993.

Parchment RE, Murphy MJ: Human hematopoietic stem cells: Laboratory assessment and response to toxic injury, in Sipes IG, McQueen CA, Gandolfi AJ (eds.): *Comprehensive Toxicology.* Vol 4. Oxford, England: Pergamon Press, 1997, pp 303–320.

Parent-Massin D, Thouvenot D, Rio B, et al: Lindane haematotoxicity confirmed by *in vitro* tests on human and rat progenitors. *Human Exp Toxicol* 13:103–106, 1994.

Parker CJ, Foerster J: Mechanisms of immune destruction of erythrocytes, in Lee CR, Foerster J, Lukens J, Paraskevas P, Greer JP, Rodgers GM (eds): *Wintrobe's Clinical Hematology,* 10th ed. Philadelphia: Lippincott Williams & Wilkins, 1999, pp 1191–1209.

Patton WN, Duffull SF: Idiosyncratic drug-induced hematological abnormalities: Incidence, pathogenesis, management and avoidance. *Drug Saf* 11:445–462, 1994.

Pedersen-Bjergaard J, Pedersen M, Roulston D, et al: Different genetic pathways in leukemogenesis for patients presenting with therapy-related myelodysplasia acute myeloid leukemia. *Blood* 86:3542–3552, 1995.

Pedersen-Bjergaard J, Philip P, Pedersen NT, et al: Acute nonlymphocytic leukemia, preleukemia, and acute myeloproliferative syndrome secondary to treatment of other malignant diseases. II. Bone marrow cytology, cytogenetica, results of HLA typing, response to antileukemic chemotherapy, and survival in a total series of 55 patients. *Cancer* 54:452–462, 1984.

Perazella MA, Biswas P: Acute hyperkalemia associated with intravenous epsilon-aminocaproic acid therapy. *Am J Kidney Dis* 33:782–785, 1999.

Peters DC, Noble S: Aprotinin: An update of its pharmacology and therapeutic use in open heart surgery and coronary artery bypass surgery. *Drugs* 57:233–260, 1999.

Peters WP, Holland JF, Senn H, et al: Corticosteroid administration and localized leukocyte mobilization in marrow. *N Engl J Med* 286:342–345, 1972.

Philip WJ, Martin JC, Richardson JM, et al: Decreased axial and peripheral bone density in patients taking long-term warfarin. *QJM* 88:635–640, 1995.

Pisciotta AV: Immune and toxic mechanisms in drug-induced agranulocytosis. *Semin Hematol* 10:279–310, 1973.

Pisciotta AV: Response of granulocytes to toxic injury, in Sipes IG, McQueen CA, Gandolfi AJ (eds): *Comprehensive Toxicology. Vol 4.* Oxford, England: Pergamon Press, 1997, pp 123–144.

Plow EF, Byzova T: The biology of glycoprotein IIb-IIIa. *Coron Artery Dis* 10:547–551, 1999.

Ponka P: Tissue-specific regulation of iron metabolism and heme synthesis: Distinct control mechanisms in erythroid cells. *Blood* 89:1–25, 1997.

Poyart C, Marden MC, Kister J: Bezafibrate derivatives as potent effectors of hemoglobin. *Methods Enzymol* 232:496–513, 1994.

Pruthi RK, Nichols WL: Autoimmune factor VIII inhibitors. *Curr Opin Hematol* 6:314–322, 1999.

Quenzel EM, Hertfelder HJ, Oldenburg J: Severe bleeding in two patients due to increased sensitivity of factor IX activity to phenprocoumon therapy. *Ann Hematol* 74:265–268, 1997.

Quinn MJ, Fitzgerald DJ: Ticlopidine and clopidogrel. *Circulation* 100:1667–1672, 1999.

Ranney HM, Sharma V: Structure and function of hemoglobin, in Beutler E, Lichtman MA, Coller BS, Kipps TJ (eds): *Williams Hematology,* 5th ed. New York: McGraw-Hill, 1995, pp 417–425.

Reagan WJ, Handy V, McKamey A, et al: Effects of doxorubicin on the canine erythroid and myeloid progenitor cells and bone marrow microenvironment. *Comp Haematol* 3:96–101, 1993.

Rizvi MA, Shah SR, Raskob GE, et al: Drug-induced thrombocytopenia. *Curr Opin Hematol* 6:349–353, 1999.

Roubey RA: Immunology of the antiphospholipid syndrome: Antibodies, antigens, and autoimmune response. *Thromb Haemost* 82:656–661, 1999.

Roubey RA: Mechanisms of autoantibody-mediated thrombosis. *Lupus* 7:S114–S119, 1998.

Rowley JD, Golomb HM, Vardiman JW: Nonrandom chromosome abnormalities in acute leukemia and dysmyelopoietic syndromes in patients with previously treated malignant disease. *Blood* 58:759–767, 1981.

Ruggenenti P, Remuzzi G: Pathophysiology and management of thrombotic microangiopathies. *J Nephrol* 11:300–310, 1998.

Rytting M, Worth L, Jaffe N: Hemolytic disorders associated with cancer. *Hematol Oncol Clin North Am* 10:365–376, 1996.

Sadler JE: Biochemistry and genetics of von Willebrand factor. *Annu Rev Biochem* 67:395–424, 1998.

Sagov SE: March hemoglobinuria treated with rubber insoles: Two case reports. *J Am Coll Health Assoc* 19:146, 1970.

Salama A, Muller-Echkardt C: Immune-mediated blood cell dyscrasia related to drugs. *Semin Hematol* 29:54–63, 1992.

Sallah S: Inhibitors to clotting factors. *Ann Hematol* 75:1–7, 1997.

Sallah S, Thomas DP, Roberts HR: Warfarin and heparin-induced skin necrosis and the purple toe syndrome: Infrequent complications of anticoagulant treatment. *Thromb Haemost* 78:785–790, 1997.

Sandoval C, Rui CH, Bowman LC, et al: Secondary acute myeloid leukemia in children previously treated with alkylating agents, intercalating topoisomerase II inhibitors and irradiation. *J Clin Oncol* 11:1039–1045, 1993.

Schafer AI: Effects of nonsteroidal antiinflammatory drugs on platelet function and systemic hemostasis. *J Clin Pharmacol* 35:209–219, 1995.

Schmaier AH, Rojkjaer R, Shariat-Madar Z: Activation of the plasma kallikrein/kinin system on cells: A revised hypothesis. *Thromb Haemost* 82:226–233, 1999.

Schmitz G, Rothe G, Ruf A, et al: European Working Group on Clinical Cell Analysis: Consensus protocol for the flow cytometric characterisation of platelet function. *Thromb Haemost* 79:885–896, 1998.

Schneidkraut MJ, Loegering DJ: Effect of extravascular hemolysis on the RES depression following thermal injury. *Exp Mol Pathol* 40:271–279, 1984.

Schrijvers D, Highley M, De Bruyn E, et al: Role of red blood cells in pharmacokinetics of chemotherapeutic agents. *Anticancer Drugs* 10:147–153, 1999.

Schwartz KA, Royer G, Kaufman DB, et al: Complications of heparin administration in normal individuals. *Am J Hematol* 19:355–363, 1985.

Shifrine M, Wilson FD: *The Canine as a Biomedical Research Model: Im-*

munological, Hematological and Oncological Aspects. Springfield, IL: Technical Information Center, US Department of Commerce, 1980.

Shimizu Y, Kato H, Schull WJ, et al: Studies of the mortality of A-bomb survivors. 9. Mortality, 1950–1985: Part 1. Comparision of risk coefficients for site-specific cancer mortality based on the DS86 and T65DR shielded kerma and organ doses. *Radiat Res* 118:502–524, 1989.

Siebert WJ, Ayres RW, Bulling MT, et al: Streptokinase morbidity—More common than previously recognized. *Aust N Z J Med* 22:129–133, 1992.

Smirnov MD, Safa O, Esmon NL, et al: Inhibition of activated protein C anticoagulant activity by prothrombin. *Blood* 94:3839–3846, 1999.

Smith JE: Comparative hematology, in Beutler E, Lichtman MA, Coller BS, Kipps TJ (eds): *Williams Hematology*, 5th ed. New York: McGraw-Hill, 1995, pp 77–85.

Smith MA, Smith JG, Provan AB, et al: The effect of rh-cytokines on the sensitivity of normal human CPU-GM progenitors to Ara C and on the S-phase activity of light density human bone marrow cells. *Leuk Res* 18:105–110, 1994.

Smolen JE, Boxer LA: Functions of neutrophils, in Beutler E, Lichtman BS, Coller BS, Kipps TJ (eds): *Williams Hematology*, 5th ed. New York: McGraw-Hill, 1995, pp 779–798.

Solum NO: Procoagulant expression in platelets and defects leading to clinical disorders. *Arterioscler Thromb Vasc Biol* 19:2841–2846, 1999.

Steinberg MH: Management of sickle cell disease. *N Engl J Med* 340:1021–1030, 1999.

Steinhubl SR, Tan WA, Foody JM, et al: Incidence and clinical course of thrombotic thrombocytopenic purpura due to ticlopidine following coronary stenting. EPISTENT Investigators. Evaluation of Platelet IIb/IIIa Inhibitor for Stenting. *JAMA* 281:806–810, 1999.

Stern A: Drug-induced oxidative denaturation in red blood cells. *Hematology* 26:301–306, 1989.

Steward DJ, Haining RL, Henne KR, et al: Genetic association between sensitivity to warfarin and expression of CYP2C9*3. *Pharmacogenetics* 7:361–367, 1997.

Szarfman A, Talarico L, Levine JG: Analysis and risk assessment of hematological data from clinical trials, in Sipes IG, McQueen CA, Gandolfi A (eds): *Comprehensive Toxicology*. Vol 4. Oxford, England: Pergamon Press, 1997, pp 363–379.

Tabbara IA: Hemolytic anemias. Diagnosis and management. *Med Clin North Am* 76:649–668, 1992.

Takahashi H, Sato T, Shimoyama Y, et al: Potentiation of anticoagulant effect of warfarin caused by enantioselective metabolic inhibition by the uricosuric agent benzbromarone. *Clin Pharmacol Ther* 66:569–581, 1999.

Tapp H, Savarirayan R: Megaloblastic anaemia and pancytopenia secondary to prophylactic cotrimoxazole therapy. *J Paediatr Child Health* 33:166–167, 1997.

Tavazzi B, Di Pierro D, Amorini AM, et al: Energy metabolism and lipid peroxidation of human erythrocytes as a function of increased oxidative stress. *Eur J Biochem* 267:684–689, 2000.

Tcheng JE: Clinical challenges of platelet glycoprotein IIb/IIIa receptor inhibitor therapy: Bleeding, reversal, thrombocytopenia, and retreatment. *Am Heart J* 139:S38–S45, 2000.

Tefferi A, Nichols WL: Acquired von Willebrand disease: Concise review of occurrence, diagnosis, pathogenesis, and treatment. *Am J Med* 103:536–540, 1997.

Testa NG, Molineux G: *Haemopoiesis: A Practical Approach*. Oxford, England: IRL Press/Oxford University Press, 1993.

Thompson DF, Gales MA: Drug-induced pure red cell aplasia. *Pharmacotherapy* 16:1002–1008, 1996.

Triplett DA, Brandt JT: Lupus anticoagulants: Misnomer, paradox, riddle, epiphenomenon. *Hematol Pathol* 2:121–143, 1988.

Tsai HM, Lian EC: Antibodies to von Willebrand factor-cleaving protease in acute thrombotic thrombocytopenic purpura. *N Engl J Med* 339:1585–1594, 1998.

Uetrecht JP: Drug metabolism by leukocytes and its role in drug-induced lupus and other idiosyncratic drug reactions. *Crit Rev Toxicol* 20:213–235, 1990.

Uetrecht JP: Metabolism of clozapine by neutrophils: Possible implications for clozapine-induced agranulocytosis. *Drug Saf* 7:51–56, 1992.

Valagussa P, Kenda R, Fossati F, et al: Incidence of 2d malignancies in Hodgkin's-Disease (HD) after various forms of treatment (abstr). *Proc Am Soc Clin Oncol* 20:360, 1979.

Valli VE, McGrath JP: Comparative leukocyte biology and toxicology, in Sipes IG, McQueen CA, Gandolfi AJ (eds): *Comprehensive Toxicology*. Vol 4. Oxford, England: Pergamon Press, 1997, pp 201–215.

van de Kar NC, Monnens LA: The haemolytic-uraemic syndrome in childhood. *Baillieres Clin Haematol* 11:497–507, 1998.

van Genderen PJ, Michiels JJ: Acquired von Willebrand disease. *Baillieres Clin Haematol* 11:319–330, 1998.

Varga J, Vitto J, Jiminez SA: The cause and pathogenesis of the eosinophilia-myalgia syndrome. *Ann Intern Med* 116:140–147, 1992.

Vargas-Alarcon G, Yamamoto-Furusho JK, Zuniga J, et al: HLA-DR7 in association with chlorpromazine-induced lupus anticoagulant (LA). *J Autoimmun* 10:579–583, 1997.

Varmus H, Weinberg RA: *Genes and the Biology of Cancer*. New York: Scientific American Library, 1993.

Visentin GP: Heparin-induced thrombocytopenia: Molecular pathogenesis. *Thromb Haemost* 82:448–456, 1999.

Vismans JJ, Briet E, Meijer K, et al: Azathioprine and subacute myelomonocytic leukemia. *Acta Med Scand* 207:315–319, 1980.

Vincent PC: Drug-induced aplastic anemia and agranulocytosis: Incidence and mechanism. *Drugs* 31:52–63, 1986.

Vogelstein B, Fearon ER, Hamilton SR, et al: Genetic alterations during colorectal-tumor development. *N Engl J Med* 319:525–532, 1988.

Volcy J, Nzerue CM, Oderinde A, et al: Cocaine-induced acute renal failure, hemolysis, and thrombocytopenia mimicking thrombotic thrombocytopenic purpura. *Am J Kidney Dis* 35:E3, 2000.

Ware JA, Coller BS: Platelet morphology, biochemistry and function, in Beutler E, Lichtman MA, Coller BS, Kipps TJ (eds): *Williams Hematology*, 5th ed. New York: McGraw-Hill, 1995, pp 1161–1201.

Warkentin TE: Heparin-induced thrombocytopenia: A clinicopathologic syndrome. *Thromb Haemost* 82:439–447, 1999.

Warkentin TE, Chong BH, Greinacher A: Heparin-induced thrombocytopenia: Towards consensus. *Thromb Haemost* 79:1–7, 1998.

Warkentin TE, Levine MN, Hirsh J, et al: Heparin-induced thrombocytopenia in patients treated with low-molecular-weight heparin or unfractionated heparin. *N Engl J Med* 332:1330–1335, 1995.

Watts RG: Neutropenia, in Lee GR, Foerster J, Lukens J, Paraskevas F, Greer JP, Rodgers GM (eds): *Wintrobe's Clinical Hematology*. Vol 2. Philadelphia: Lippincott Williams & Wilkins, 1999, pp 1862–1888.

Weatherall DJ: The thalassaemias. *Br Med J* 314:1675–1678, 1997.

Weingand K, Brown G, Hall R, et al: Harmonization of animal clinical pathology testing in toxicity safety studies. *Fundam Appl Toxicol* 29:198–201, 1996.

Wells PS, Holbrook AM, Crowther NR, et al: Interactions of warfarin with drugs and food. *Ann Intern Med* 121:676–683, 1994.

West BC, DeVault, Jr. GA, Clement JC, et al: Aplastic anemia associated with parenteral chloramphenicol: Review of 10 cases, including the second case of possible increased risk with cimetidine. *Rev Infect Dis* 10:1048–1051, 1988.

WHO: World Health Organization handbook for reporting results of cancer treatments. Offset Publication No. 48. Geneva: WHO, 1979.

William CL, Whittaker MH: The molecular biology of acute myeloid leukemia. Proto-oncogene expression and function in normal and neoplastic myeloid cells. *Clin Lab Med* 10:769–796, 1990.

Williams LH, Udupa KB, Lipschitz DA: Long-term bone marrow culture as a model for host toxicity: The effect of methotrexate on hematopoiesis and adherent layer function. *Exp Hematol* 16:80–87, 1988.

Williams WJ, Morris MW, Nelson DA: Examination of blood, in Beutler

E, Lichtman MA, Coller BS, Kipps TJ (eds): *Williams Hematology,* 5th ed. New York: McGraw-Hill, 1995, pp 8–15.

Wintrobe MM: *Hematology, The Blossoming of Science: A Story of Inspiration and Effort.* New York: Lea & Febiger, 1985.

Yoo D, Lessin LS: Drug-associated "bite cell" hemolytic anemia. *Am J Med* 92:243–248, 1992.

Young KM, Weiss L: Hematopoiesis: Structure-function relationships in bone marrow and spleen, in Sipes IG, McQueen AC, Gandolfi AJ (eds): *Comprehensive Toxicology*. Vol 4. Oxford, England: Pergamon Press, 1997, pp 11–34.

Young NS: Acquired aplastic anemia. *JAMA* 282:271–278, 1999.

Young NS: Agranulocytosis. *JAMA* 271:935–938, 1994.

Young NS: Hematopoietic cell destruction by immune mechanisms in acquired aplastic anemia. *Semin Hematol* 37:3–14, 2000.

Young NS, Maciejewski J: The pathophysiology of acquired aplastic anemia. *N Engl J Med* 336:1365–1372, 1997.

CHAPTER 12

TOXIC RESPONSES OF THE IMMUNE SYSTEM

Leigh Ann Burns-Naas, B. Jean Meade, and Albert E. Munson

Immunity, by definition, is a homeostatic condition in which the body maintains protection from infectious disease. It is a series of delicately balanced, complex, multicellular, and physiologic mechanisms that allow an individual to distinguish foreign material from "self" and to neutralize and/or eliminate the foreign matter. It is characterized by a virtually infinite repertoire of specificities, highly specialized effectors, complex regulatory mechanisms, and an ability to travel throughout the body. The immune system provides the means to initiate rapid and highly specific responses against a myriad of potentially pathogenic organisms. Indeed, the conditions of genetically determined immunodeficiency and of acquired immunodeficiency syndrome (AIDS) graphically highlight the importance of the immune system in the host's defense against microbial infection. In addition, evidence is rapidly building that the immune system plays a role in tumor identification and rejection (immune surveillance).

In light of the central role that the immune system plays in the maintenance of the health of the individual, the interaction of xenobiotics (pharmacologic agents, environmental contaminants, and other chemicals) with the various components of the immune system has become an area of profound interest. Indeed, in some instances, the immune system has been shown to be compromised (decreased lymphoid cellularity, alterations in lymphocyte subpopulations, decreased host resistance, altered specific immune function responses) in the absence of observed toxicity in other organ systems. Decreased immunocompetence (immunosuppression) may result in repeated, more severe, or prolonged infections as well as the development of cancer. Immunoenhancement may lead to immune-mediated diseases such as hypersensitivity responses or autoimmune disease (Fig. 12-1). Because of the potentially profound effects resulting from disruption of the delicately balanced immune system, there is a need to understand the cellular, biochemical, and molecular mechanisms of xenobiotic-induced immunomodulation. With the availability of sensitive, reproducible, and predictive tests, it is now apparent that the inclusion of immunotoxicity testing may represent a significant adjunct to routine

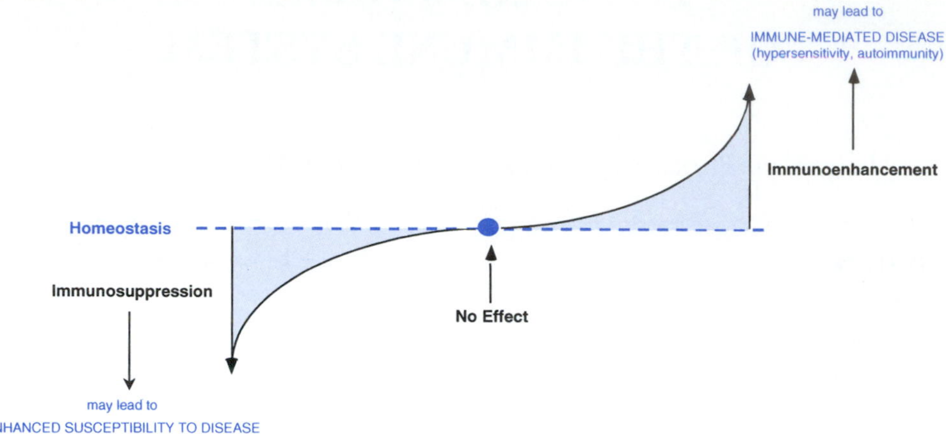

Figure 12-1. Potential consequences of immunomodulation.

safety evaluations for therapeutic agents, biological agents, and chemicals now in development.

This chapter provides (1) an overview of basic concepts in immunology (structure, components, and functions), which are important to the understanding of the impact xenobiotics may have on the exposed individual; (2) a summary of selected current methods utilized to assess immune function; and (3) a brief review of current information on the immunomodulation (immunosuppression, hypersensitivity, and autoimmunity) induced by a variety of xenobiotics. This chapter is not meant to be an immunology textbook nor an exhaustive review of the mechanisms of immunotoxicity of a myriad of xenobiotics. For detailed information on immunology, the reader is referred to two texts, the first edited by Paul (1999), the second edited by Roitt and colleagues (1993). For a more comprehensive review of immunotoxicology, the reader is referred to texts edited by Dean and colleagues (1994), Smialowicz and Holsapple (1996), and Lawrence (1997).

THE IMMUNE SYSTEM

Unlike most organ systems, the immune system has the unique quality of not being confined to a single site within the body. It comprises numerous lymphoid organs (Table 12-1) and numerous different cellular populations with a variety of functions. The bone marrow and the thymus contain microenvironments capable of supporting the production of mature T and B lymphocytes and myeloid cells, such as macrophages and polymorphonuclear cells from nonfunctional precursors (stem cells), and are thus referred to as primary lymphoid organs. With regard to T and B cells, key events that occur in both primary and secondary organs are (1) acquisition of the ability to recirculate and become localized in appropriate places in the periphery (homing capacity), (2) the ability to recognize antigen (rearrangement of the T-cell receptor and the B-cell antigen receptor germline genes), and (3) the ability to interact with accessory cells (through the expression of various cell surface molecules and the development of biochemical signaling pathways) to allow differentiation into both effector and memory cell populations.

The bone marrow is the site of origin of the pluripotent stem cell, a self-renewing cell from which all other hematopoietic cells are derived (Figs. 12-2 and 12-6). During gestation, this cell is found in the embryonic yolk sac and fetal liver; subsequently, it migrates to the bone marrow. Within the bone marrow, the cells of the immune system developmentally "commit" to either the lymphoid or myeloid lineages. Cells of the lymphoid lineage make a further commitment to become either T cells or B cells. Because of their critical role in initiation and regulation of immune responses, T cell precursors are programmed to leave the bone marrow and migrate to the thymus, where they undergo "thymic education" for recognition of self and nonself. This is discussed in more detail under "Cellular Components" in the section below titled "Acquired (Adaptive) Immunity."

Mature naive or virgin lymphocytes (those T and B cells that have never undergone antigenic stimulation) are first brought into contact with exogenously derived antigens within the highly organized microenvironment of the spleen and lymph nodes, otherwise known as the secondary lymphoid organs. These organs can be thought of as biological sieves. The spleen serves as a filter for the blood, removing both foreign antigens and any circulating dead cells and cellular debris. The lymph nodes are part of a network of lymphatic veins that filter antigens from the fluid surrounding the tissues of the body. Key events that occur within the secondary lymphoid organs are (1) specific antigen recognition in the context of the major histocompatibility complex (MHC) class II, (2) clonal expansion (proliferation) of antigen-specific cells, and (3)

Table 12-1
Organization of the Immune System: Lymphoid Tissue

CLASSIFICATION	LYMPHOID ORGANS
Primary	Bone marrow
	Thymus
Secondary	Spleen
	Lymph nodes
Tertiary	Skin-associated lymphoid tissue (SALT)
	Mucosal lamina propria (MALT)
	Gut-associated lymphoid tissue (GALT)
	Bronchial-associated lymphoid tissue (BALT)
	Cells lining the genitourinary tract

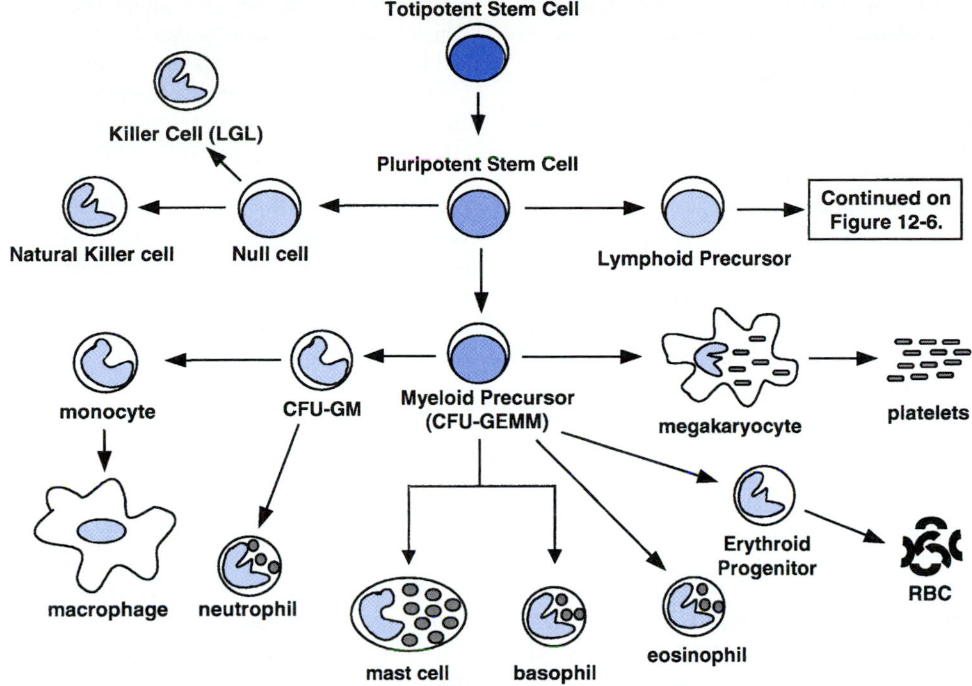

Figure 12-2. Development of the cellular components of the immune system.

differentiation of antigen-stimulated lymphocytes into effector and memory cells.

Lymphoid tissues associated with the skin (skin-associated lymphoid tissue, or SALT) and mucosal lamina propria (mucosa-associated lymphoid tissue, or MALT) can be classified as tertiary lymphoid tissues. Tertiary lymphoid tissues are primarily effector sites where memory and effector cells exert immunologic and immunoregulatory functions. Although in a broad interpretation this would include essentially all tissues of the body, tertiary lymphoid tissues are associated primarily with the surfaces lining the intestines (gut-associated lymphoid tissue, or GALT), respiratory tract (bronchial-associated lymphoid tissue, or BALT), and the genitourinary tract, since these tissues have access directly to the external environment. For extensive reviews of respiratory, mucosal, and dermal immunology and immunotoxicology, the reader is referred to chapters in Smialowicz and Holsapple (1996) and in Lawrence (1997).

Innate Immunity

General Considerations Mammalian immunity can be classified into two functional divisions: innate immunity and acquired (adaptive) immunity (Table 12-2). Innate immunity acts as a first line of defense against infectious agents, eliminating most potential

Table 12-2
Innate verses Acquired Immunity

CHARACTERISTIC	INNATE IMMUNITY	ACQUIRED IMMUNITY
Cells involved	Polymorphonuclear cells (PMN) Monocyte/macrophage NK cells	T cells B cells Macrophages NK cells
Primary soluble mediators	Complement Lysozyme Acute phase proteins Interferon-α/β Other cytokines	Antibody Cytokines
Specificity of response	None	Yes (very high specificity)
Response enhanced by repeated antigen challenge	No	Yes

pathogens before significant infection occurs. It is characterized by being *nonspecific* and includes physical and biochemical barriers both inside and outside of the body as well as immune cells designed for specific responses. Unlike acquired immunity, there is no immunologic memory associated with innate immunity. Therefore, in a normal healthy adult, the magnitude of the immune response to a foreign organism is the same for a secondary or tertiary challenge as it is for the primary exposure.

Externally, the skin provides an effective barrier, as most organisms cannot penetrate intact skin. Most infectious agents enter the body through the respiratory system, gut, or genitourinary tract. Innate defenses present to combat infection from pathogens entering through the respiratory system include mucus secreted along the nasopharynx, the presence of lysozyme in most secretions, and cilia lining the trachea and main bronchi. In addition, reflexes such as coughing, sneezing, and elevation in body temperature are also a part of innate immunity. Pathogens that enter the body via the digestive tract are met with severe changes in pH (acid) within the stomach and a host of microorganisms living in the intestines.

Cellular Components: NK, PMN, Macrophage Two general types of cells are involved in nonspecific (innate) host resistance: natural killer (NK) cells and professional phagocytes (Table 12-3). Like other immune cells, NK cells are derived from the bone marrow stem cell. It is not yet clear exactly how the NK lineage progresses; however, NK cells do possess several surface markers which have been used to define T cells, suggesting that the NK cell is a derivative of a lymphoid precursor cell. The vast majority of NK cells express CD16 (Fc receptor for IgG) on their surface. Although apparently derived from a similar lineage as the T cell, NK cells do not express cell surface CD3 (T cell receptor-associated protein complex) or either chain of the T-cell receptor (TCR). NK cells are located primarily in the spleen, blood, and peritoneal exudate, although they are occasionally found in lymph node tissue as well. For their part in innate immunity, NK cells can recognize virally infected and malignant changes on the surface of cells as well as the Fc portion of IgG on an antibody-coated target cell. The latter recognition is utilized in cell-mediated immunity. Using surface receptors, the NK cell binds and undergoes cytoplasmic reorientation so that cytolytic granules (perforins and enzymatic proteins) are localized near the target cell. These granules are then expelled onto the surface of the target cell. The result of this process is the induction of apoptosis (DNA fragmentation, membrane blebbing, and cellular disintegration) of the target cell.

Phagocytic cells include polymorphonuclear cells (PMN; neutrophil) and the monocyte/macrophage. The precursors of the macrophage and PMN develop from pluripotent stem cells that have become committed to the myeloid lineage (Fig. 12-2). Evidence exists that there are bipotentiating reactive precursors for PMN and macrophage and that differentiation into one or the other

Table 12-3
Characteristics of Selected Immune Cells

PROPERTIES	MONOCYTE/ MACROPHAGE	T CELLS	B CELLS	NK CELLS
Phagocytosis	Yes	No	No	No
Adherence	Yes	No	No	No
Surface receptors:				
Antigen receptors	No	Yes	Yes	No
Complement	Yes	No	Yes	Yes
Fc region of Ig	Yes	Some	Yes	Yes
Surface markers	CD64 CD11b	CD4 CD8 CD3 Thy-1(mouse)	Ig	CD16 Asialo-GM1 (mouse) CD11b
Proliferation in response to:				
Allogeneic cells (MLR)	No	Yes	No	No
Lipopolysaccharide (LPS)	No	No	Yes	No
Phytohemagglutinin (PHA)	No	Yes	No	No
Concanavalin A (Con A)	No	Yes	No	No
Anti-Ig + IL-4	No	No	Yes	No
Anti-CD3 + IL-2	No	Yes	No	No
Effector functions:				
Antibody production	No	No	Yes	No
Cytokine production	Yes	Yes	Yes	Yes
Bactericidal activity	Yes	No	No	No
Tumor cell cytotoxicity	Yes	Yes	No	Yes
Immunologic memory	No	Yes	Yes	No

SOURCE: Modified from Dean JH, Murray MJ: Toxic responses of the immune system, in Amdur MO, Doull J, Klaassen CD (eds): *Casarett and Doull's Toxicology: The Basic Science of Poisons,* 4th ed. New York: Pergammon Press, 1991, p 286.

is dependent upon the interaction with specific colony-stimulating factors (CSFs) such as macrophage-CSF (M-CSF), granulocyte-CSF (G-CSF), granulocyte-macrophage-CSF (GM-CSF), interleukin-3 (IL-3), and others (Unanue, 1993). Within the bone marrow, both cell types undergo several rounds of replication before entering the bloodstream where they circulate for about 10 h and then enter the tissues where they perform effector functions for about 1 to 2 days. PMNs are capable of passing through the cell membrane of the blood vessels and thereby represent a primary line of defense against infectious agents. They are excellent phagocytic cells and can eliminate most microorganisms. Their phagocytic activity is greatly enhanced by the presence of complement and antibody deposited on the surface of the foreign target. They are also important in the induction of an inflammatory response.

Macrophages are terminally differentiated monocytes. Upon exiting the bone marrow, monocytes circulate within the bloodstream for about 1 day. At that time, they begin to distribute to the various tissues where they can then differentiate into macrophages. Macrophages can be found in all tissues, most notably in the liver, lung, spleen, kidney, and brain. Within different tissues, macrophages have distinct properties and vary in extent of surface receptors, oxidative metabolism, and expression of MHC class II. This is likely due to the factors present within the microenvironment in which the monocyte differentiates. The liver macrophages, or Kupffer cells, are primarily responsible for particulate and microbial clearance from the blood. They express high levels of MHC class II, are actively phagocytic, and release several soluble mediators. Thus, they are the primary cells responsible for the acute phase response. Alveolar macrophages remove foreign particulate matter from the alveolar space. They are self-renewing and have a particularly long lifespan. These cells can be harvested by broncheoalveolar lavage and actively secrete proteases and bactericidal enzymes such as lysozyme. Splenic macrophages also phagocytose particulate material and polysaccharides from the blood and tissue. However, unlike other tissue macrophages, they are more diverse within the tissue and their level of expression of MHC class II and their stage of differentiation appears to be dependent upon where within the splenic architecture the macrophages are located. Mononuclear phagocytes within the central nervous system (CNS) are known as microglia and are responsible for antigen presentation in immunologic diseases of the CNS. Microglia have a very slow turnover time, and thus recruitment of monocytes to areas of inflammation within the CNS is also slow.

Should PMNs be unable to contain an infection, macrophages are then recruited to the site of infection. Although macrophages are phagocytic by nature, their bactericidal activity can be augmented by lymphokines produced by T cells that recognize a specific microbial antigen. Macrophages are unique cells within the immune system because they play roles in both the innate arm of immunity (as phagocytic cells) and the acquired arm (as antigen-presenting cells). They adhere well to glass or plastic, are recruited to sites of inflammation by chemotactic factors, can be activated by cytokines to become more effective killers, and can produce cytokines, such as IL (interleukin)-1, IL-6, and TNF (tumor necrosis factor), that act in a paracrine and autocrine fashion. Macrophages also play critical roles as scavengers in the daily turnover of senescent tissues such as red cell nuclei from maturing red cells, PMNs, and plasma cells. The importance of phagocytic cells to the organism can be seen in individuals with spontaneous or induced reduction in the numbers or activity of these cells. This condition is associated with repeated and sometimes fatal bacterial and fungal infections.

Soluble Factors: Acute-Phase Proteins and Complement In addition to the cellular components of innate immunity, there are several soluble components (Table 12-2). These are the acute-phase response and the complement cascade. Upon infection, macrophages (Kupffer cells, in particular) become activated and secrete a variety of cytokines, which are carried by the bloodstream to distant sites. This global response to foreign agents is termed the *acute-phase response* and consists of fever and large shifts in the types of serum proteins synthesized by hepatocytes, such as serum amyloid A, serum amyloid P, and C-reactive protein. These proteins increase rapidly to concentrations up to 100 times the normal concentration and stay elevated through the course of infection. These proteins can bind to bacteria and facilitate the binding of complement and the subsequent uptake of the bacteria by phagocytic cells. This process of protein coating to enhance phagocytosis is termed *opsonization.*

The complement system is a series of about 30 serum proteins whose primary functions are the modification of membranes of infectious agents and the promotion of an inflammatory response. The components of the complement cascade interact with each other and with other elements of both the innate and acquired arms of immunity. Complement activation occurs with each component sequentially, acting on others in a manner similar to the blood clotting cascade (Fig. 12-3). Early components of the cascade are often modified serine proteases, which activate the system but have limited substrate specificity. Several components are capable of binding to microbial membranes and serve as ligands for complement receptors associated with the membrane. The final components, which are related structurally, are also membrane-binding proteins that can enter into the membrane and disrupt membrane integrity (membrane attack complex). And finally, there are several regulatory complement proteins designed to protect the host from inadvertent damage.

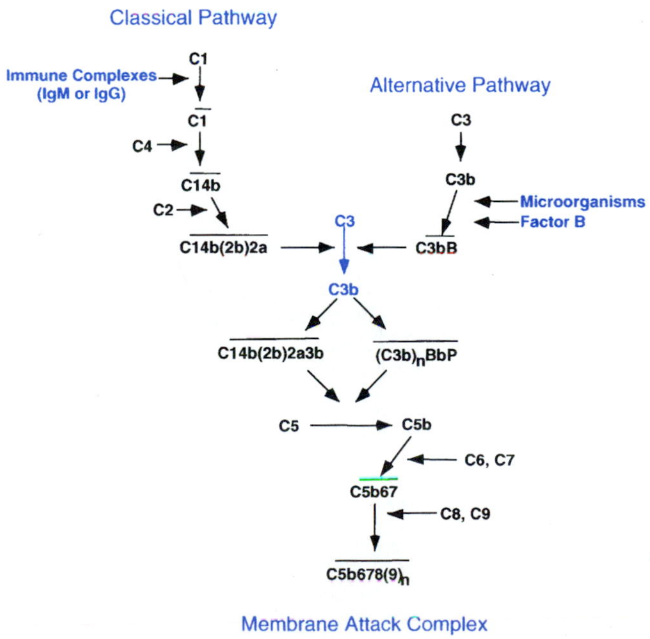

Figure 12-3. The complement cascade.

Two pathways have been identified in the complement cascade. The classic pathway is involved when antibody binds to the microorganism. Because specific antibody defines the target, this is a mechanism by which complement aids effectors of the acquired side of immunity. The second, or alternative pathway, is used to assist the innate arm of immunity. For this cascade, it is not necessary for the host to have prior contact with the pathogen, since several microbial proteins can alone initiate this pathway. Whatever the mechanism of activation, the results are the same. The complement-coated material is targeted for elimination by interaction with complement receptors on the surface of circulating immune cells.

Acquired (Adaptive) Immunity

General Considerations If the primary defenses against infection (innate immunity) are breached, the acquired arm of the immune system is activated and produces a specific immune response to each infectious agent, which usually eliminates the infection. This branch of immunity is also capable of remembering the pathogen and can protect the host from future infection by the same agent. Therefore, the two key features which distinguish acquired immunity are *specificity* and *memory*. This means that in a normal healthy adult, the speed and magnitude of the immune response to a foreign organism is greater for a secondary challenge than it is for the primary challenge (Table 12-2). This is the principle exploited in vaccination.

Acquired immunity may be further subdivided into cell-mediated immunity (CMI) and humoral immunity. CMI, in its broadest sense, includes all immunologic activity in which antibody plays a minimal role. Humoral immunity is directly dependent upon the production of antigen-specific antibody by B cells and involves the coordinated interaction of antigen-presenting cells, T cells, and B cells. A more detailed discussion of both CMI and humoral immunity appears later.

Essential to the development of specific immunity is the recognition of antigen and the generation of an antibody that can bind to it. An antigen (sometimes referred to as an immunogen or allergen) is defined functionally as a substance that can elicit the production of a specific antibody and can be specifically bound by that antibody. Antigens are usually (but not absolutely) biological molecules that can be cleaved and rearranged for presentation. They may be either proteins, carbohydrates (often bacterial), lipids, nucleic acids, or human-engineered substances, and they must be foreign (nonself) or occult (hidden, sequestered). Generally, antigens are about 10 kDa or larger in size. Smaller antigens are termed *haptens* and must be conjugated with carrier molecules (larger antigens) in order to elicit a specific response. However, once a response is made, the hapten can interact with the specific antibody in the absence of the carrier.

Antibodies are produced by B cells and are also defined functionally by the antigen with which they react (i.e., anti-sheep red blood cell IgM, or anti-sRBC IgM). Because the immune system generates antibody to thousands of antigens with which the host may or may not ever come into contact, general antibody of unknown specificity is referred to as *immunoglobulin* (e.g., serum immunoglobulin or serum IgM) until it can be defined by its specific antigen (e.g., anti-sRBC IgM). A simple way to view this point is that an antibody is an immunoglobulin, but immunoglobulin is not necessarily antibody. There are five types of immunoglobulin that are related structurally (Table 12-4): IgM, IgG (and subsets), IgE, IgD, and IgA. All immunoglobulins are made up of heavy and light chains and of constant and variable regions. It is the variable regions that determine antibody specificity (Fig. 12-4). It is the variable region that interacts with antigen, while the Fc region mediates effector functions such as complement fixation (IgM and some IgG subclasses) and phagocyte binding (via Fc receptors). Antibodies subserve several functions in acquired immunity: (1) opsonization (coating of a pathogen with antibody to enhance Fc receptor-mediated endocytosis by phagocytic cells); (2) initiation of the classic pathway of complement-mediated lysis; (3) neutraliza-

Table 12-4
Properties of Immunoglobulin Classes and Subclasses

CLASS	MEAN SERUM CONCENTRATION, mg/mL	HUMAN HALF-LIFE DAYS	BIOLOGICAL PROPERTIES
IgG			Complement fixation (selected subclasses) Crosses placenta Heterocytotropic antibody
Subclasses			
IgG_1	9	21	
IgG_2	3	20	
IgG_3	1	7	
IgG_4	1	21	
IgA	3	6	Secretory antibody
IgM	1.5	10	Complement fixation Efficient agglutination
IgD	0.03	3	Possible role in antigen-triggered lymphocyte differentiation
IgE	0.0001	2	Allergic responses (mast cell degranulation)

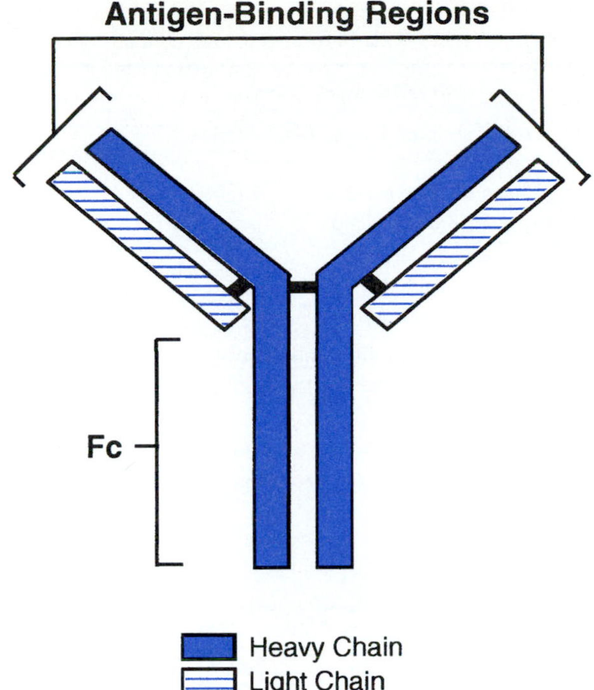

Figure 12-4. Immunoglobulin structure.

tion of viral infection by binding to viral particles and preventing further infection; and (4) enhancement of the specificity of effectors of CMI by binding to specific antigens on target cells, which are then recognized and eliminated by effector cells such as NK or cytotoxic T lymphocytes (CTL).

During an immune response, the cells of the immune system must be able to communicate to coordinate all the activities that occur during the recognition and elimination of foreign antigens. Connecting all the cells of the immune system with each other as well as with other non-immune cell types within the body is a vast network of soluble mediators: the cytokines. Nearly all immune cells secrete cytokines, which may have local or systemic effects. Table 12-5 provides a brief summary of the sources and functions of cytokines of interest in the immune system. Although it would appear that many cytokines have related functions, these functions are not often identical, and a single cytokine may have multiple effects on a variety of cell types. Since cytokines work to tightly regulate immune responses, some induce synthesis of other cytokines and inflammatory mediators, while others inhibit this process. Although the actual number of cytokines (lymphokines, monokines, chemokines, etc.) may not be altogether that large, the complexity of the network is magnified severalfold by the multitude of biological actions of each cytokine and the diversity of cells secreting each mediator.

Cellular Components: APCs, T Cells, B Cells In order to elicit a specific immune response to a particular antigen, that antigen must be taken up and processed by accessory cells for presentation to lymphocytes. Accessory cells that perform this function are termed antigen-presenting cells (APCs) and include the macrophage, follicular dendritic cell (FDC), Langerhans dendritic cell, and B cells. A description of the macrophage is found in the section above titled "Cellular Components of Innate Immunity"; however, the macrophage also plays a critical role as an APC in acquired immunity. Unique among the APCs is the FDC. Unlike hematopoietic cells, the FDC is not derived from the bone marrow stem cell. It is found in secondary lymphoid organs and binds antigen-antibody complexes, but it does not internalize and process the antigen. Instead, the primary function of the FDC is in the persistence of antigen within the secondary lymphoid tissues and the presentation of antigen to B cells. This is believed to be critical for the maintenance of memory for B cells and the induction of high-affinity B cell clones. Although thought of more for its ability to produce immunoglobulin, the B cell can also serve as an APC, and in low antigen concentrations this cell is equally as competent as the macrophage in serving this function. The Langerhans dendritic cell is also a bone marrow–derived cell, but its lineage is distinct from that of the macrophage. It is found primarily in the epidermis, mucosal epithelium, and lymphoid tissues. The Langerhans dendritic cell can migrate into the lymphatic system, where it serves as an APC in the lymph nodes. This cell plays a primary role in contact sensitization.

The interaction of APCs and lymphocytes is critical for the development of an immune response. With the exception of the FDC, APCs internalize the antigen either by phagocytosis, pinocytosis, or receptor-mediated endocytosis (via antigen, Fc, or complement receptors). Following internalization, antigen is processed (intracellular denaturation and catabolism) through several cytoplasmic compartments, and a piece of the antigen (peptide fragments about 20 amino acids in length) becomes physically associated with major histocompatibility complex (MHC) class II (Fig. 12-5). This MHC class II-peptide complex is then transported to the surface of the cell and can interact in a specific manner with lymphocytes. For most APCs, an immunogenic determinant is expressed on the surface of the APC within an hour after internalization, although this is slightly longer for B cells (3 to 4 h). In addition to processing and presentation, pieces of processed antigen may be expelled into the extracellular space. These pieces of processed antigen can then bind in the peptide groove of empty MHC class II on the surface of other APCs for the presentation of that peptide fragment to lymphocytes.

Not only are B lymphocytes capable of serving as APCs, but they are also the effector cells of humoral immunity, producing a number of isotypes of immunoglobulin (Ig) with varying specificities and affinities. Like other immune cells, the B cell develops in the bone marrow from the pluripotent stem cell and becomes committed to the B-cell lineage when the cell begins to rearrange its Ig genes (Fig. 12-6). If, after several attempts, the cell is un-

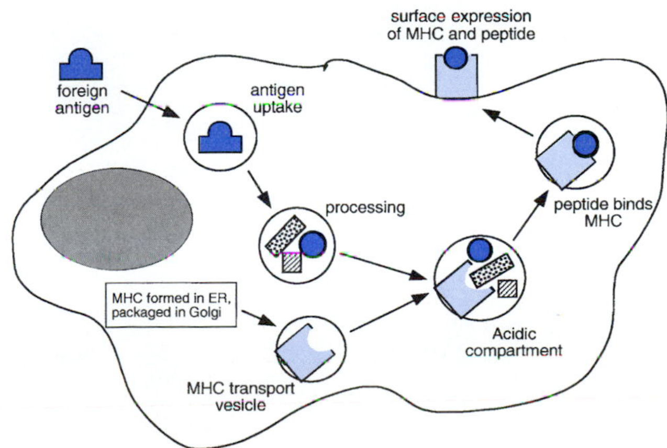

Figure 12-5. General schematic of antigen processing and presentation.

Table 12-5
Cytokines: Sources and Functions in Immune Regulation

CYTOKINE	SOURCE	PHYSIOLOGIC ACTIONS
IL-1	Macrophages B cells Several nonimmune cells	Activation and proliferation of T cells (Th2>Th1) Proinflammatory Induces fever and acute-phase proteins Induces synthesis of IL-8 and TNF-α
IL-2	T cells	Primary T-cell growth factor Growth factor for B cells and NK cells Enhances lymphokine production
IL-3	T cells Mast cells	Stimulates the proliferation and differentiation of stromal cells, progenitors of the macrophage, granulocyte, and erythroid lineages
IL-4	T cells Mast cells Stromal cells Basophils CD4$^+$/NK1.1$^+$ cells	Proliferation of activated T (Th2>Th1) and B cells B-cell differentiation and isotype switching may inhibit some macrophage functions Antagonizes IFN-γ Inhibits IL-8 production
IL-5	T cells Mast cells	Proliferation and differentiation of eosinophils Promotes B-cell isotype switching Synergizes with IL-4 to induce secretion of IgE
IL-6	Macrophages Activated T cells B cells Fibroblasts Keratinocytes Endothelial cells Hepatocytes	Enhances B-cell differentiation and immunoglobulin secretion Induction of acute phase proteins by liver Proinflammatory Proliferation of T cells and increased IL-2 receptor expression Synergizes with IL-4 to induce secretion of IgE
IL-7	Stromal cells Epithelial cells	Proliferation of thymocytes (CD4$^-$/CD8$^-$) Proliferation of pro- and pre-B cells (mice) T-cell growth
IL-8	Macrophages Platelets Fibroblasts NK cells Keratinocytes Hepatocytes Endothelial cells	Activation and chemotaxis of monocytes, neutrophils, basophils and T cells Proinflammatory
IL-9	Th cells	T-cell growth factor (primarily CD4$^+$ cells) Enhances mast-cell activity Stimulates growth of early erythroid progenitors
IL-10	T cells Macrophages B cells	Inhibits macrophage cytolytic activity and macrophage activation of T cells General inhibitor of cytokine synthesis by Th1 cells (in presence of APCs) Enhances CD8$^+$ T cell cytolytic activity Enhances proliferation of activated B cells Mast-cell growth Anti-inflammatory Inhibits endotoxin shock
IL-11	Fibroblasts Stromal cells	Megakaryocyte growth factor Enhances T cell–dependent B-cell immunoglobulin synthesis Enhances IL-6–induced plasma cell differentiation Stimulates platelets, neutrophils, and erythrocytes Induces acute-phase proteins

(continued)

Table 12-5
Cytokines: Sources and Functions in Immune Regulation *(continued)*

CYTOKINE	SOURCE	PHYSIOLOGIC ACTIONS
IL-12	Macrophages B cells	Proliferation and cytolytic action of NK cells Activation, proliferation, and cytolytic action of CTL Stimulates production of IFN-γ Proliferation of activated T cells Decreases IgG1 and IgE primary response
IL-13	T cells	Stimulates class II expression on APC Enhances antigen processing by APC Enhances B-cell differentiation and isotype switching Anti-inflammatory (inhibits synthesis of proinflammatory cytokines) Inhibits antibody-dependent cellular cytotoxicity (ADCC)
IL-14	T cells Some malignant B cells	Enhances B-cell proliferation Inhibition of immunoglobulin secretion Selective expansion of some B-cell subpopulations
IL-15	Activated monocytes Macrophages Several nonimmune cells	NK-cell activation T-cell proliferation Mast-cell growth
IL-16	T cells Mast cells Eosinophils	Chemoattractant for T cells, eosinophils, and monocytes Promotes $CD4^+$ T-cell adhesion Increases expression of IL-2 receptor Promotes synthesis of IL3, GM-CSF, and IFN-γ Proinflammatory May exacerbate allergic reactions
IL-17	$CD4^+$ memory T cells	Induced production of IL-6, IL-8, G-CSF, and PGE_2 Enhances proliferation of activated T cells Inducer of stromal cell–derived proinflammatory cytokines Inducer of stromal cell–derived hematopoietic cytokines
IL-18	Hepatocytes	Synergizes with IL-12 to enhance the activity of Th1 cells Enhances production of IFN-γ
Interferon-α/β (IFN-α/β) (Type 1 IFN)	Leukocytes Epithelial cells Fibroblasts	Induction of class I expression Antiviral activity Stimulation of NK cells
Interferon-γ (IFN-γ)	T cells NK cells Epithelial cells Fibroblasts	Induction of class I and II Activates macrophages (as APC and cytolytic cells) Improves CTL recognition of virally infected cells
Tumor necrosis factor (TNF-α) and lymphotoxin (TNF-β)	Macrophages Lymphocytes Mast cells	Induces inflammatory cytokines Increases vascular permeability Activates macrophages and neutrophils Tumor necrosis (direct action) Primary mediator of septic shock Interferes with lipid metabolism (result is cachexia) Induction of acute phase proteins
Transforming growth factor-β (TGF-β)	Macrophages Megakaryocytes Chondrocytes	Enhances monocyte/macrophage chemotaxis Enhances wound healing: angiogenesis, fibroblast proliferation, deposition of extracellular matrix Inhibits T- and B-cell proliferation Inhibits macrophage cytokine synthesis Inhibits antibody secretion Primary inducer of isotype switch to IgA
GM-CSF	T cells Macrophages Endothelial cells Fibroblasts	Stimulates growth and differentiation of monocytes and granulocytes

(continued)

Table 12-5
Cytokines: Sources and Functions in Immune Regulation *(continued)*

CYTOKINE	SOURCE	PHYSIOLOGIC ACTIONS
Migration inhibitory factor (MIF)	T cells Anterior pituitary cells Monocytes	Inhibits macrophage migration Proinflammatory (induces TNF-α production by macrophages) Appears to play a role in delayed hypersensitivity responses May be a counterregulator of glucocorticoid activity
Erythropoietin (EPO)	Endothelial cells Fibroblasts	Stimulates maturation of erythrocyte precursors

SOURCE: Information on selected cytokines taken from Ruddle (1992), Quesniaux (1992), Paul and Seder (1994), Zurawski and de Vries (1994), Lawrence (1997), and Paul (1999).

successful at rearranging its Ig genes, it dies. Following Ig rearrangement, these cells express heavy chains in their cytoplasm and are termed pre-B cells. Expression of surface IgM and IgD indicates a mature B cell. Mature B cells are found in the lymph nodes, spleen, and peripheral blood. Upon antigen binding to surface Ig, the mature B cell becomes activated and, after proliferation, undergoes differentiation into either a memory B cell or an antibody-forming cell (AFC; plasma cell), actively secreting antigen-specific antibody. A broad description of several B-cell characteristics can be found in Table 12-3.

At a specified time following their commitment to the T-cell lineage, pre-T cells migrate from the bone marrow to the thymus where, in a manner analogous to their B-cell cousins, they begin to rearrange their TCRs (Fig. 12-6). This receptor consists of two chains (α and β, or γ and δ) and is critical for the recognition of MHC + peptide on APCs. At this time, the T cells begin to express the surface marker CD8. CD8 (and CD4) are coreceptors expressed by T cells and are involved in the interaction of the T cell with the APC. T cells bearing the γ/δ TCR subsequently lose expression of CD8 and proceed to the periphery. T cells with the α/βTCR gain surface expression of both the TCR and CD4 and are termed *immature double-positive cells* ($CD4^+/CD8^+$). These immature cells then undergo positive selection to eliminate cells that cannot interact with MHC. Following this interaction, TCR expression increases. Any of these T cells that interact with MHC + self peptide are then eliminated (negative selection). The double-positive cells then undergo another selection process whereby they lose expression of either CD4 or CD8 and then proceed to the periphery as mature single-positive cells ($CD4^+$ or $CD8^+$) with a high level of TCR expression. This rigorous selection process produces T cells that can recognize MHC + foreign peptides and eliminates autoreactive T cells. Generally, T cells that express CD8 mediate cell killing (CTL) or suppressor activity (T suppressor cells). Lymphocytes that participate in delayed hypersensitivity reaction (DHR) or that provide "B-cell help" in humoral responses (helper T cells; Th1 and Th2) express CD4 on their surface. A broad description of several T-cell characteristics can be found in Table 12-3.

Humoral and Cell-Mediated Immunity

The activation of antigen-specific T cells begins with the interaction of the T-cell receptor with MHC class II + peptide. This interaction is strengthened by the presence of co-receptors such as CD4, LFA-3, CD2, LFA-1, and ICAM-1 and involves the bilateral exchange of information, triggering a cascade of biochemical events that ultimately leads to the activation of not only the T cell but the APC as well. Although the macrophage or dendritic cell is traditionally thought of as the APC involved in humoral responses, B cells can also subserve this function. In fact, many believe that, in low antigen concentrations, the B cell serves as the primary APC because of the presence of the high-affinity Ig receptor on the surface of the B cell.

Upon activation and in the presence of IL-1 secreted by the APC, T cells begin to express high-affinity receptors for the major T-cell growth factor, IL-2. In addition, T cells begin to produce IL-2, which can act in an autocrine fashion (on IL-2 receptors on the same T cell) or paracrine fashion (IL-2 receptors on other T cells or on B cells). As T cells begin to undergo clonal expansion (proliferation), they secrete numerous lymphokines (cytokines secreted from lymphocytes; Table 12-5) which can influence (1) the strength of an immune response, (2) the down-regulation of the immune response, (3) the isotype of antibody secreted by the AFC, (4) the activation of cells involved in cell-mediated immunity, and (5) the modulation of activities of numerous immune and nonimmune cells. The next step in the generation of the humoral response is the interaction of activated T cells with B cells. This may be a direct interaction of the T cell with B cell (antigen-specific) or may simply involve the production of lymphokines (such as IL-2, IL-4, IL-6, and TNF-α and TNF-β), which lead to B-cell growth and differentiation into AFCs or memory B cells. A general diagram of the cellular interactions involved in the humoral immune response is given in Fig. 12-7. The production of antigen-specific IgM requires 3 to 5 days after the primary (initial) exposure to antigen (Fig. 12-8). Upon secondary antigen challenge, the B cells undergo isotype switching, producing primarily IgG antibody, which is of higher affinity. In addition, there is a higher serum antibody titer associated with a secondary antibody response.

Cell-mediated immunity (CMI), in its broadest sense, includes all immunologic activity in which antibody plays a minimal role. However, for purposes of discussion here, CMI is more specifically defined as the T-cell–mediated response such as DHR or CTL activity, antibody-dependent cellular cytotoxicity (ADCC) mediated by NK cells, and soluble factor–mediated macrophage cytotoxic responses. Whether an antigen will elicit a primarily cell-mediated or humoral response (or a combination of both) is dependent upon numerous factors. However, it should be noted that there is often an interplay between these two branches of acquired

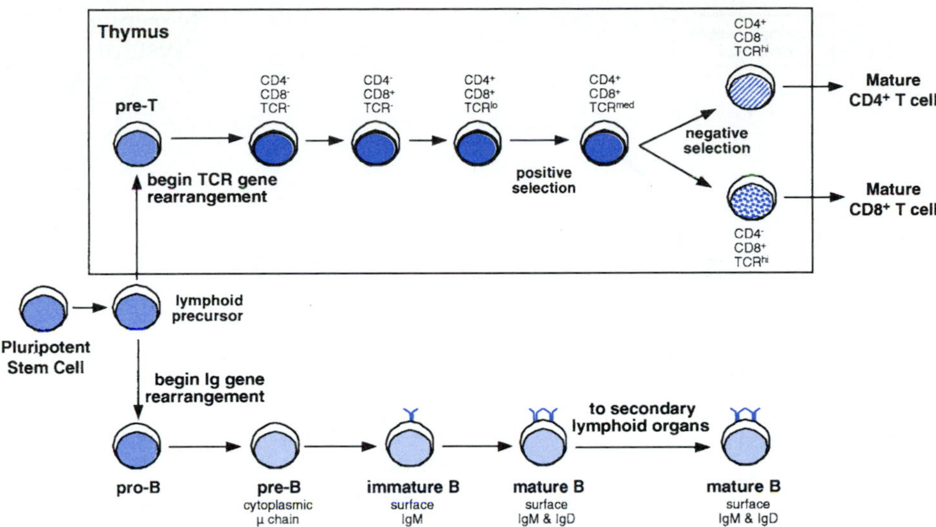

Figure 12-6. Development and differentiation of T and B cells.

immunity. Cells are involved in the initiation of antibody responses and antibody is often an essential player in cell-mediated responses.

There are two general forms of cell-mediated immunity, referred to as delayed-type hypersensitivity and cell-mediated cytotoxicity. Delayed-type hypersensitivity is presented later in this chapter in the section titled "Immune-Mediated Disease." Cell-mediated cytotoxicity responses may occur in numerous ways: (1) MHC class I-dependent recognition of specific antigens (such as viral particles) by CTL, (2) the indirect antigen-specific recognition by the binding of antibody-coated target cells to NK cells via Fc receptors on the latter, and (3) receptor-mediated recognition of complement-coated foreign targets by macrophage. Let us consider the first two together, since their mechanisms of cytotoxicity are similar.

In cell-mediated cytotoxicity, the effector cell (CTL or NK) binds in a specific manner to the target cell (Fig. 12-9). The majority of CTLs express CD8 and recognize either foreign MHC class I on the surface of allogeneic cells, or antigen in association with self MHC class I (e.g., viral particles). In acquired immunity, NK recognition of target cells may be considered antigen-specific because the mechanism of recognition involves the binding of the Fc portion of antigen-specific antibody coating a target cell to the NK via its Fc receptors. Once the CTL or NK cells interact with the target cell, the effector cell undergoes cytoplasmic reorientation so that cytolytic granules are oriented along the side of the effector, which is bound to the target. The effector cell then releases the contents of these granules onto the target cell. The target cell may be damaged by the perforins or enzymatic contents of the cy-

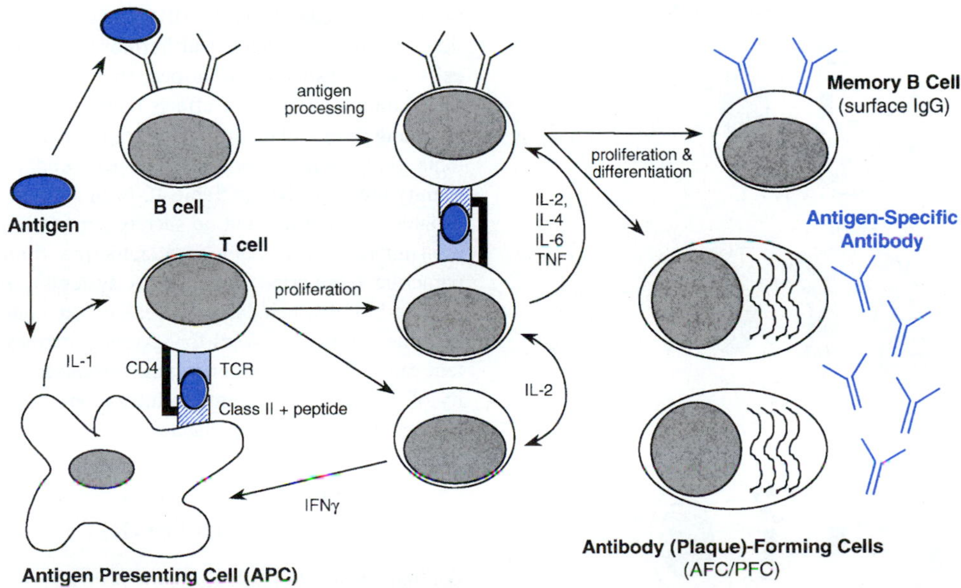

Figure 12-7. Cellular interactions in the antibody response.

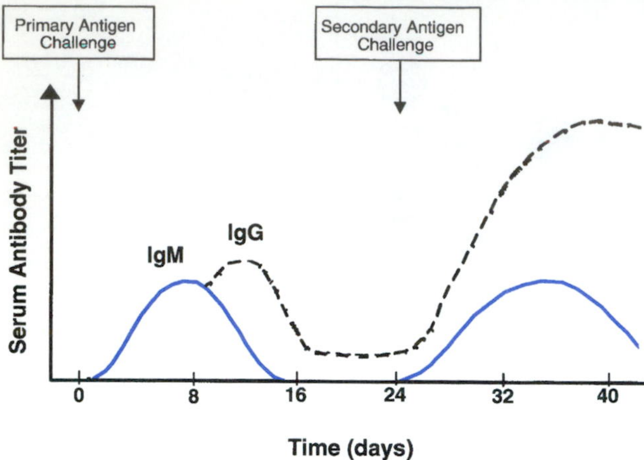

Figure 12-8. Kinetics of the antibody response.

tolytic granules. In addition, the target is induced to undergo programmed cell death (apoptosis). Once it has degranulated, the effector cell can release the dying target and move on to kill other target cells.

Macrophages are the most promiscuous of the immune cells in that they play roles in both innate and acquired (both humoral and cell-mediated) immunity. Their role in cell-mediated cytotoxicity involves activation by T-cell–derived lymphokines (such as interferon-gamma, or IFN-γ) and subsequent recognition of complement-coated target cells via complement receptors present on

1. Identification and engagement of target by effector.

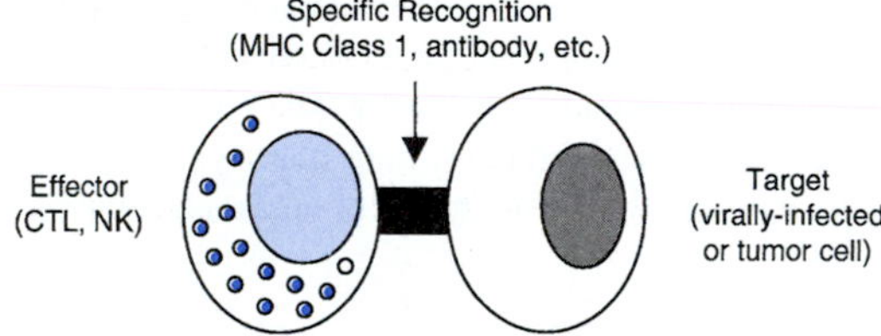

2. Strengthening of interaction and cytoplasmic re-orientation of effector.

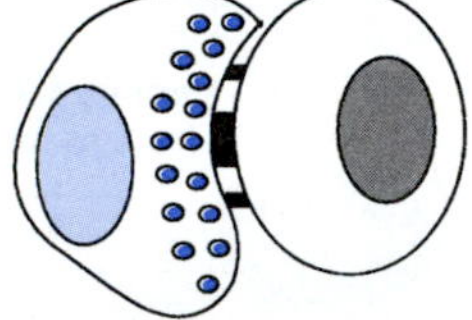

3. Degranulation of effector onto target.

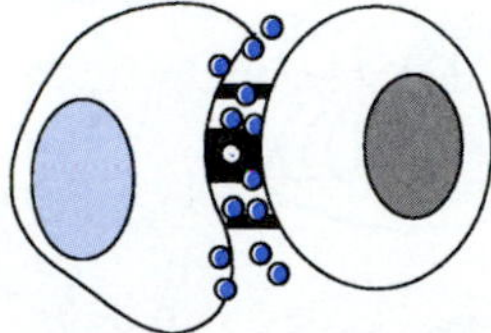

4. Disengagement of effector and death of target.

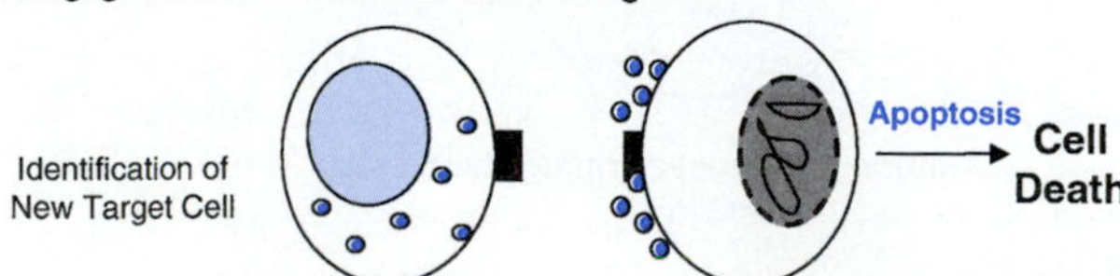

Figure 12-9. Cell-mediated cytotoxicity.

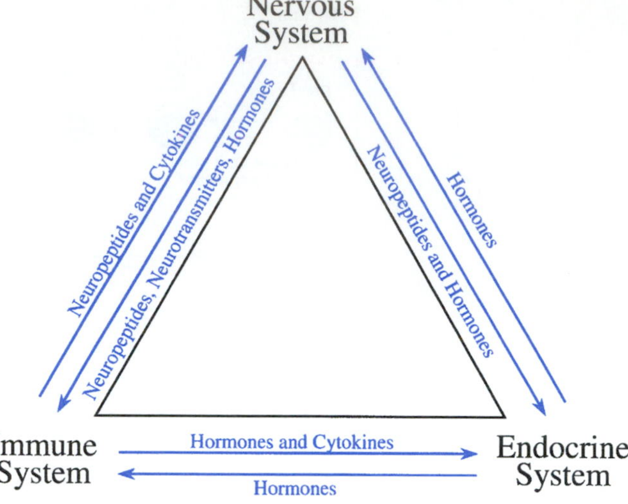

Figure 12-10. Triad of regulatory influence.

the surface of the macrophage. The result is enhanced phagocytic ability and the synthesis and release of hydrogen peroxide, nitric oxide, proteases, and TNF, all of which serve obvious cytolytic functions.

Neuroendocrine Immunology

There is overwhelming evidence that cytokines, neuropeptides, neurotransmitters, and hormones—as well as their receptors—are an integral and interregulated part of the central nervous system, the endocrine system, and the immune system. This blossoming area of immunology has been extensively reviewed elsewhere (Sanders, 1997; Weigent and Blalock, 1995), as has its new place in immunotoxicology (Fuchs and Sanders, 1994). Previous assumptions that the proteins secreted from these regulatory systems (nervous and endocrine) exerted unidirectional actions on the immune system have been shown to be erroneous, as the triad of influence these three systems exert over one another is bidirectional on all three sides (Fig. 12-10). Because receptors for neuropeptides, neurotransmitters, and hormones are present on lymphoid cells, it is reasonable to suspect that some chemicals may exert their immunomodulatory effects indirectly on the immune system by acting to modulate the activity of the nervous or endocrine systems. Some selected outcomes of neuroendocrine actions on immunity are described in Table 12-6. In addition, immune cells are capable of secreting and do secrete peptide hormones and neurotransmitters, which can have autocrine (immune system) and paracrine (endocrine and nervous systems) effects. Because the triad is bidirectional (and the cells of the endocrine and nervous systems possess receptors for several cytokines), the immune system can influence neuroendocrine responses. Due to the complexity of this subject, immune influence on neuroendocrine function is not considered in this chapter.

ASSESSMENT OF IMMUNOLOGIC INTEGRITY

For many years, toxicologists have been aware that xenobiotics can have significant effects on the immune system. However, it has only been in recent years that the subdiscipline of immunotoxi-

Table 12-6
Reported Influences of Neuroendocrine Factors on Immunity*

	CYTOKINE PRODUCTION	NK ACTIVITY	MACROPHAGE ACTIVITY	T CELL ACTIVITY	HUMORAL IMMUNITY
ACTH	↓	↓	↓	↓	↓
Prolactin	↑	?	↑	↑	↑
Growth Hormone	↑	↑	↑	↑	↑
α Endorphins	↑	↑	↑	↓	↓
β Endorphins	↑	↑	↑	↓	↑
Enkephalins	↑	↑	?	?	↓
Substance P	?	↑	↑	↑	↑
hCG	?	↓	?	↓	?
Chemical sympathectomy	↑	?	?	↑ ↓	↑
Norepinephrine	?	?	?	↓	↑ ↓
Epinephrine	?	?	?	↓	↑ ↓

*Data from Madden et al. (1995); Blalock (1989); Weigent and Blalock (1995); Sanders (1997); and Lawrence and Kim (2000).

KEY: ACTH, adrenocorticotropin; hCG, human chorionic gonadotropin; ↑, generally enhanced responses; ↓, generally decreased responses; ↑ ↓, both enhanced and suppressed responses have been reported and may depend on receptor types or subclass of chemical or time of exposure relative to antigen challenge; ?, generally unknown or not reported in the references utilized.

cology has come into its own, with a battery of tests to evaluate immunocompetence. Among the unique features of the immune system is the ability of immune cells to be removed from the body and to function in vitro. This unique quality offers the toxicologist an opportunity to comprehensively evaluate the actions of xenobiotics on the immune system by providing an excellent system for dissecting the cellular, biochemical, and molecular mechanisms of action of multitudes of xenobiotics. While standard toxicologic endpoints such as organ weights, cellularity, and enumeration of cell subpopulations are important components in assessing immune injury, by far the most sensitive indicators of immunotoxicity are the tests that challenge the various immune cells to respond functionally to exogenous stimuli (reviewed in White, 1992). This section focuses on selected in vivo and in vitro tests currently used for evaluating immunotoxicity.

Methods to Assess Immunocompetence

General Assessment Central to any series of studies evaluating immunocompetence is the inclusion of standard toxicologic studies, because any immunologic findings should be interpreted in conjunction with effects observed on other target organs. Standard toxicologic studies that are usually evaluated include body and selected organ weights, general observations of overall animal health, selected serum chemistries, hematologic parameters, and status of the bone marrow (ability to generate specific colony-forming units). In addition, histopathology of lymphoid organs—such as the spleen, thymus, and lymph nodes—may provide insight into potential immunotoxicants. Because of the unique nature of the immune system, there are several experimental approaches that may be taken to assess immunotoxicity and to evaluate the mechanisms of action of xenobiotics. These are depicted in Fig. 12-11 and vary with respect to in vivo or in vitro exposure, immunologic challenge, or immunologic evaluation (immune assay). As an example, the plaque-forming cell assay [Fig. 12-11 (2)] is an ex vivo assay where xenobiotic exposure and antigen challenge occur in vivo and the immune response is evaluated in vitro. In contrast [as depicted in Fig. 12-11 (4)], splenocytes can be removed from a naive animal, exposed to xenobiotic and antigen in vitro, and evaluated in vitro. An example of this would be the in vitro–generated PFC response (Mishell-Dutton assay; Mishell and Dutton, 1967).

Using fluorescently labeled monoclonal antibodies to cell surface markers (Table 12-3) in conjunction with a flow cytometer, it is now possible to accurately enumerate lymphocyte subsets. Antibodies are available to the T-cell surface markers CD4, CD8, and CD3 (among others). Dual colored fluorochromes allow cells to be stained for two markers simultaneously. In this manner, the number of $CD4^+$ and $CD8^+$ cells can be determined simultaneously on a single sample of cells. In the thymus, this dual staining also helps determine the number of $CD4^+/CD8^+$ (double positive) and $CD4^-/CD8^-$ (double negative) cells residing in this organ (Fig. 12-12). This gives the researcher insight into which specific T-cell subsets are targeted and whether the xenobiotic may affect T-cell maturation. Antibodies available to surface immunoglobulin (Ig) and to B220 (the CD45 phosphatase on B cells) help determine the numbers of B cells. Surface markers can reveal significant alterations in lymphocyte subpopulations, and in many instances this is indicative of alterations in immunologic integrity. Indeed, an indicator of AIDS is the changes observed in $CD4^+$ T-cell numbers. Luster and coworkers (1992) have reported that, in conjunction with two or three functional tests, the enumeration of lymphocyte subsets can greatly enhance the detection of immunotoxic chemicals. However, it is important to keep in mind that although surface marker analysis can indicate shifts in lymphocyte populations, functional analysis of the immune system offers greater sensitivity for the detection of immunotoxicity.

Flow cytometry can be useful in immunotoxicology as a tool to assess mechanism of action beyond evaluation of surface markers. These include evaluation of the effects of chemicals in the cell cycle, intracellular free calcium, cellular viability assessment, induction of apoptosis, evaluation of p53, DNA strand breaks (TUNEL assay), membrane potential, intracellular pH, oxidative stress, and membrane lipophilicity (reviewed in Burchiel et al., 1997 and 1999). Flow cytometry has applications in cell sorting and high throughput screening, and there is interest in the utility of this tool in the refinement of certain cellular immune and hypersensitivity assays. A key to acceptance of flow cytometric

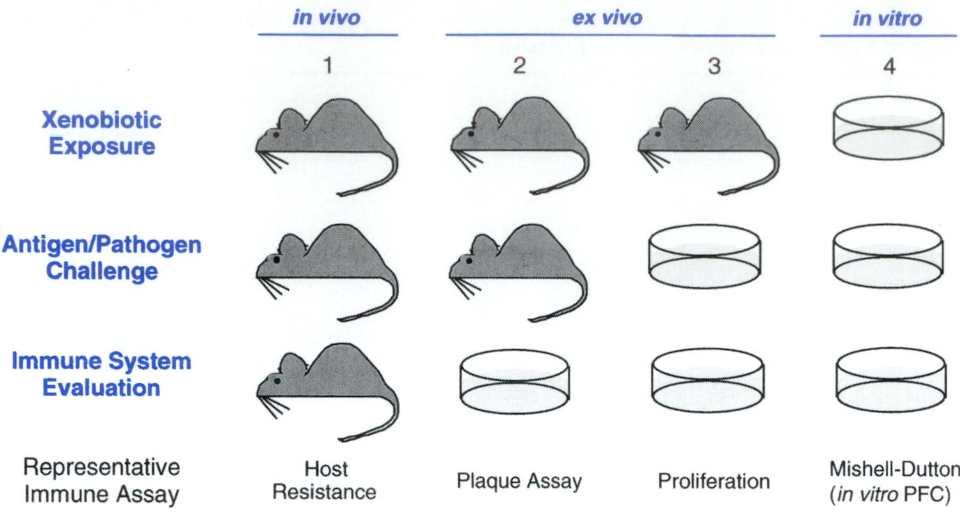

Figure 12-11. Approaches to assessing the immunotoxicity of xenobiotics.

methods for immunotoxicity assessment is assay validation. This concept is supported by one of the conclusions of a workshop focusing on the application of flow cytometry in immunotoxicity assessments. The workshop concluded that while immunophenotyping certainly has a place in the field of immunotoxicology (e.g., used in conjunction with functional tests to identify immunotoxic chemicals; as a method to assess mechanism of action), more research is needed in both the human and the animal before immunophenotyping alone is sufficiently validated for use in predicting chemical-induced effects on human health (ILSI, 1999).

Functional Assessment ***Innate Immunity*** As described earlier, innate immunity encompasses all those immunologic responses that do not require prior exposure to an antigen and that are nonspecific in nature. These responses include recognition of tumor cells by NK cells, phagocytosis of pathogens by

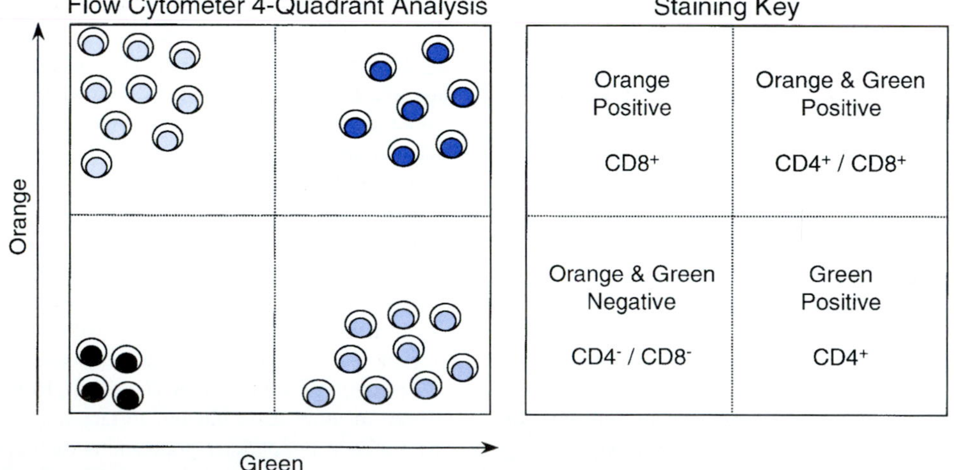

Figure 12-12. Flow cytometry.

In this example, cells from the thymus are stained simultaneously with a fluorescent PE-conjugated (orange) antibody to CD8 and a fluorescent FITC-conjugated (green) antibody. When analyzed on a flow cytometer, the instrument is requested to display a four-quadrant analysis (*left*). Increasing fluorescent intensity (brightness) is indicated by the arrows on each axis. The key to this analysis is displayed on the right. Cells which possess only CD8 fluoresce orange ($CD8^+$) and are displayed in the upper left quadrant (*light blue*). Cells that possess only CD4 fluoresce green ($CD4^+$) and are displayed in the lower right quadrant (*medium blue*). Cells that possess both CD8 and CD4 fluoresce both orange and green ($CD4^+/CD8^+$; double positives) and are displayed in the upper right *quadrant* (*dark blue*). Cells that do not possess either CD8 or CD4 do not fluoresce ($CD4^-/CD8^-$; double negatives) and are displayed in the lower left quadrant (*black*). The instrument can then be requested to determine the percentage of cells in each quadrant. In a typical mouse thymus, there are approximately 8 to 13 percent $CD4^+$, 2 to 5 percent $CD8^+$, 80- to 85 percent $CD4^+/CD8^+$, and 2 to 5 percent $CD4^-/CD8^-$ cells.

macrophages, and the lytic activity of the components of the complement cascade.

To evaluate phagocytic activity, macrophages are harvested from the peritoneal cavity [peritoneal exudate (PE) cells] and are allowed to adhere in 24-well tissue culture plates. The cells are then incubated with chromated chicken red blood cells (^{51}Cr-cRBCs). Following incubation, the supernatant, containing ^{51}Cr-cRBCs that have not been bound by macrophages, is removed. The cRBCs which are bound to the macrophages, but which have not been phagocytized, are removed by a brief incubation with ammonium chloride. Finally, macrophages are lysed with NaOH and radioactivity in the lysate is counted to determine the amount of phagocytosis that occurred. A set of control wells is needed to determine DNA content for each set of wells. Data are presented as a specific activity for adherence and phagocytosis (adhered or phagocytized cpm/DNA content) since xenobiotics altering adherence will have a significant effect on the results.

Another method to evaluate phagocytosis, but which does not require radioactivity, begins similarly to the ^{51}Cr-cRBC assay. Peritoneal macrophages are allowed to adhere to each chamber of a tissue culture slide. After adherence, macrophages are washed and incubated with latex covaspheres. At the end of incubation, cells are fixed in methanol and stained in methylene chloride. Macrophages containing five covaspheres or more are counted as positive and data are expressed as a percentage of phagocytosis (the ratio of macrophages with $\geq$5 covaspheres to total macrophages counted).

The previous macrophage assays are conducted in vitro after chemical exposure either in vivo or in vitro. If an in vivo assay of the ability of tissue macrophages to phagocytose a foreign antigen is required, the functional activity of the reticuloendothelial system can be evaluated. Intravenously injected radiolabeled sheep red blood cells (^{51}Cr-sRBCs) are removed by the tissue macrophage from the circulation and sequestered for degradation in organs such as the liver, spleen, lymph nodes, lung, and thymus. Clearance of the ^{51}Cr-sRBCs is monitored by sampling of the peripheral blood. When steady state has been attained, animals are euthanized and organs are removed and counted in a gamma counter to assess uptake of the ^{51}Cr-sRBCs.

Evaluation of the ability of NK cells to lyse tumor cells is achieved using the YAC-1 cell line as a tumor target for an in vitro cytotoxicity assay. YAC-1 cells are radiolabeled with ^{51}Cr and incubated (in 96-well microtiter plates) in specific effector-to-target ratios with splenocytes from xenobiotic-exposed and nonexposed animals. During an incubation step, splenic NK cells (effectors) lyse the ^{51}Cr-YAC-1 cells, releasing ^{51}Cr into the supernatant. At the end of the incubation, plates are centrifuged and the supernatant is removed and counted on a gamma counter. After correcting for spontaneous release (which should be $<$10 percent), specific release of ^{51}Cr is calculated for each effector-to-target ratio and compared to the specific release from control animals.

Acquired Immunity—Humoral The plaque-(antibody)forming cell (PFC or AFC) assay is a sensitive indicator of immunologic integrity for several reasons. It is a test of the ability of the host to mount an antibody response to a specific antigen. When the particulate T-dependent antigen (an antigen that requires T cells to help B cells make antibody) sheep erythrocytes (sRBCs) is used, this response requires the coordinated interaction of several different immune cells: macrophages, T cells, and B cells. Therefore, an effect on any of these cells (e.g., antigen processing and presentation, cytokine production, proliferation, or differentiation) can have a profound impact on the ability of B cells to produce antigen-specific antibody. Other antigens, termed T cell-independent antigens, such as DNP-Ficoll or TNP-LPS (lipopolysaccharide), can be used that bypass the requirement for T cells in eliciting antibody production by B cells.

A standard PFC assay involves immunizing control and xenobiotic-exposed mice either intravenously or intraperitoneally with the sRBC. The antigen is taken up in the spleen and an antibody response occurs. Four days after immunization, spleens are removed and splenocytes are mixed with sRBC, complement, and agar. This mixture is plated onto petri dishes and covered with a cover slip. After the agar hardens the plates are incubated for 3 h at 37°C. During this time, B cells secrete anti-sRBC IgM antibody. When the IgM and complement coat the surrounding sRBCs, areas of hemolysis (plaques) appear which can be enumerated (Fig. 12-13). At the center of each plaque is a single B cell (antibody- or plaque-forming cell; AFC or PFC). Data are usually presented as IgM PFC (or AFC) per million splenocytes. IgG PFC can also be enumerated by slight modifications of this same assay. This isotype switching (from IgM to IgG) is important in secondary responses in which memory B cells respond more quickly to an antigen.

More recently, it has become evident that the PFC assay can be evaluated in vivo using serum from peripheral blood of immunized mice and an enzyme-linked immunosorbent assay (ELISA; Fig. 12-14). Although the optimal response is delayed by 1 to 2 days (compared to the PFC assay), this assay takes into account antigen-specific antibody secreted by B cells in the spleen as well as B cells residing in the bone marrow. Like the PFC assay, mice (or other experimental animals) are immunized with sRBCs and 6 days later peripheral blood is collected. Serum from each sample is serially diluted and incubated in microtiter plates that have been coated with sRBC membranes. The membranes serve as the antigen to which sRBC-specific IgM or IgG will bind. After incubation of the test sera and a wash step, an enzyme-conjugated monoclonal antibody (the secondary antibody) against IgM (or IgG) is added. This antibody recognizes the IgM (or IgG) and binds specifically to that antibody. After incubation and a wash step, the enzyme substrate (chromogen) is added. When the substrate comes into contact with the enzyme on the secondary antibody, a color change occurs which can be detected by measuring absorbance with a plate reader. Since this is a kinetic assay (color develops over time and is dependent upon concentration of anti-sRBC antibody in the test sera), it is important to establish control concentration–response curves so that data can be evaluated in the linear range of the curve. Data are usually expressed in arbitrary optical density (OD) units. Advantages of the ELISA over the PFC assay are the ability to conduct in vivo analyses and to attain a greater degree of flexibility, since serum samples can be stored frozen for analysis at a later date.

One final assay measures the ability of B cells to undergo blastogenesis and proliferation, which are critical steps in the generation of an antibody response. This is achieved in microtiter plates by stimulating splenocytes with a monoclonal antibody to surface Ig (anti-Ig) in the presence of IL-4, or with the B-cell mitogen LPS. Proliferation is evaluated 2 to 3 days after stimulation by measuring uptake of ^{3}H-thymidine into the DNA of the cultured cells. Data are usually expressed as mean counts per minute for each treatment group. These studies are usu-

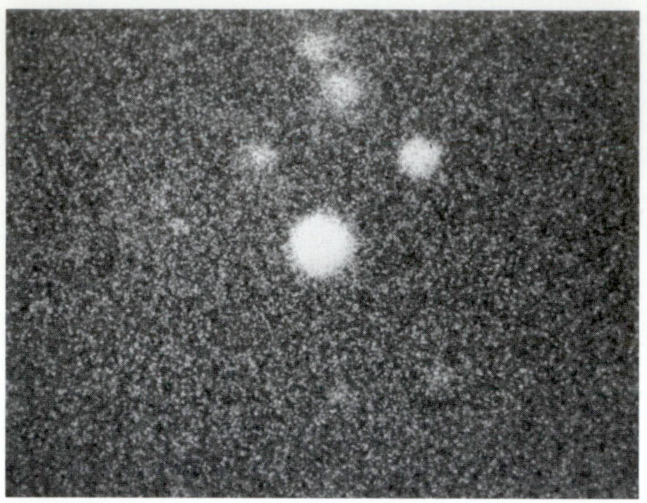

A

B

Figure 12-13. The plaque-forming cell (PFC) assay.

A. Demonstration of plaques (areas of hemolysis) that have formed within the lawn of sheep red blood cells, 310 magnification. *B.* 3100 magnification of a plaque from panel *A* showing the B cell evident in the center of the plaque. (From photos by Dr. Tracey L. Spriggs, with permission.)

1. Bind antigen to plate. Wash.

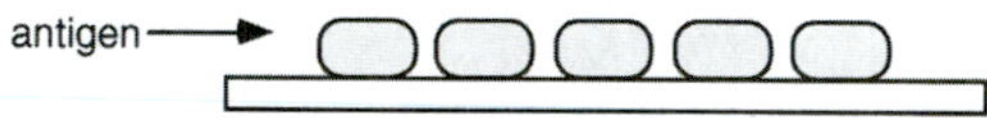

2. Add test sera and incubate. Wash.

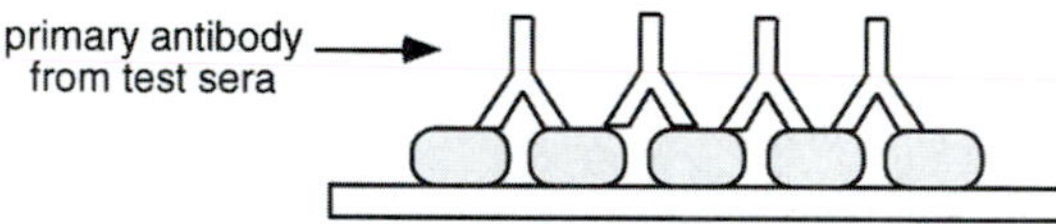

3. Add enzyme-coupled secondary antibody. Wash.

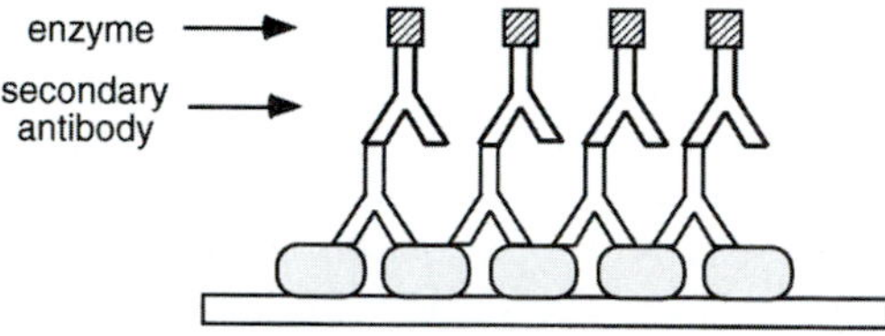

4. Add chromogen and develop color.

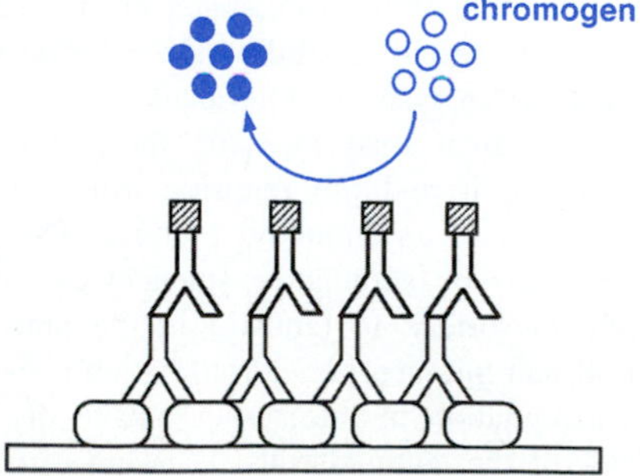

Figure 12-14. Schematic diagram of a standard enzyme-linked immunosorbent assay (ELISA).

ally done in conjunction with T-cell proliferative responses described below.

Humoral Immunity—Cell-Mediated While there are numerous assays used to assess cell-mediated immunity, three primary tests are used routinely in the National Toxicology Program (NTP) test battery: the cytotoxic T-lymphocyte (CTL) assay, the delayed hypersensitivity response (DHR), and the T-cell proliferative responses to antigens (anti-CD3 + IL-2), mitogens (PHA and Con A), and allogeneic cell antigens (mixed lymphocyte responses; MLR).

The CTL assay measures the in vitro ability of splenic T cells to recognize allogeneic target cells by evaluating the ability of the CTLs to proliferate and then lyse the target cells. Splenocytes are incubated with P815 mastocytoma cells, which serve as target cells. These target cells are pretreated with mitomycin C so that they cannot proliferate themselves. During this sensitization phase, the CTLs recognize the targets and undergo proliferation. Five days after sensitization, the CTLs are harvested and incubated in microtiter plates with radiolabeled (^{51}Cr) P815 mastocytoma cells. During this elicitation phase, the CTLs that have acquired memory recognize the foreign MHC class I on the P815 cells and lyse the targets. At the end of the incubation, plates are centrifuged, the supernatant is removed, and radioactivity released into the supernatant is counted on a gamma counter. After correcting for spontaneous release, the percent cytotoxicity is calculated for each effector-to-target ratio and compared to that from control animals.

The DHR evaluates the ability of memory T cells to recognize foreign antigen, proliferate and migrate to the site of the antigen, and secrete cytokines which result in the influx of other inflammatory cells. Like the PFC response, this assay is conducted completely in vivo. The assay itself quantitates the influx of radiolabeled monocytes into the sensitization site. During xenobiotic exposure, mice are sensitized twice with keyhole limpet hemocyanin (KLH) subcutaneously between the shoulders. On the last day of exposure, mononuclear cells are labeled in vivo with an IV injection of ^{125}I-5-iododeoxyuridine (IUdR). One day later, mice are challenged intradermally in one ear with KLH. Twenty-four hours after challenge, animals are euthanized, the ears are biopsied, and radiolabeled cells are counted in a gamma counter. Data are expressed as a stimulation index which represents the cpm in the challenged ear divided by the cpm in the unchallenged ear.

T cells play a central role in cell-mediated immunity and the ability of T cells to undergo blastogenesis and proliferation is critical to this role. Several mechanisms exist to evaluate proliferative capacity. The mixed lymphocyte response (MLR) measures the ability of T cells to recognize foreign MHC class I on splenocytes from an MHC-incompatible mouse (allogeneic cells) and undergo proliferation. For example, splenocytes from B6C3F1 mice (responders) are incubated with splenocytes from mitomycin C-treated DBA/2 mice (stimulators). Proliferation is evaluated 4 to 5 days after stimulation by measuring uptake of ^{3}H-thymidine into the DNA of the cultured responder cells. Cells are collected from each well using a cell harvester and counted in a scintillation counter. Data may be expressed as either the mean cpm for each treatment group or as a stimulation index where the index is calculated by dividing the cpm of wells containing responders and stimulators by the cpm of wells containing responders alone.

General T cell proliferation can be evaluated in a manner similar to that described above for B cells (Table 12-3). Splenocytes are stimulated in microtiter plates with a monoclonal antibody to the CD3 complex of the T-cell receptor (anti-CD3) in the presence of IL-2, or with the T-cell mitogens concanavalin A (Con A) and phytohemagglutinin (PHA). Proliferation is evaluated 2 to 3 days after stimulation by measuring uptake of ^{3}H-thymidine into the DNA of the cultured T cells. Data are usually expressed as mean cpm for each treatment group. These studies are usually done in conjunction with B-cell proliferative responses described above.

Host Resistance Assays Host resistance assays represent a way of assaying how xenobiotic exposure affects the ability of the host to handle infection by a variety of pathogens. Although host resistance studies provide significant insight into the mechanisms by which an immunotoxicant is acting, these assays should not be a first or only choice for evaluating immunocompetence. An example of why this is true is the actions of the semiconductor material gallium arsenide (GaAs) on the immune system. Although GaAs produces profound immunosuppression of nearly all cell types evaluated, this compound was observed to confer varying degrees of protection to challenge with *Listeria monocytogenes* and *Streptococcus pneumoniae*. It was subsequently determined that the circulating blood arsenic concentrations were sufficient to inhibit growth of both of these organisms. In host resistance studies, it is also important to consider the following: (1) strain, route of administration, and challenge size of the pathogen; (2) strain, age, and sex of the host; (3) physiologic state of the host and the pathogen; and (4) time of challenge with the pathogen (prior to, during, or after xenobiotic exposure). All of these can have significant effects on the results from any individual study.

As with other immune function tests, no single host resistance model can predict overall immunocompetence of the host, primarily because each model uses different mechanisms for elimination of various pathogens. A representative list of host resistance models is shown in Table 12-7 as well as some of the cells involved in the immune response to these pathogens. Typically, three challenge levels of pathogen (approximating the LD_{20}, LD_{50}, and LD_{80}) for each concentration of xenobiotic are used in order to be able to detect both increases and decreases in resistance. Endpoint analyses are lethality (for bacterial and viral pathogens), changes in tumor burden, and increased or decreased parasitemia.

Regulatory Approaches to the Assessment of Immunotoxicity

The NTP Tier Approach Luster and colleagues (1988) have described the selection of a battery of tests used by the National Toxicology Program to screen for potential immunotoxic agents. The result was a tier approach to assessing immunotoxicity and is summarized in Table 12-8. Tier I provides assessment of general toxicity (immunopathology, hematology, body and organ weights) as well as endline functional assays (proliferative responses, PFC assay, and NK assay). It was designed to detect potential immunotoxic compounds at concentrations that do not produce overt toxicity. Tier II was designed to further define an immunotoxic effect and includes tests for cell-mediated immunity (CTL and DHR), secondary antibody responses, enumeration of lymphocyte populations, and host resistance models. Subsequently, several testing configurations were defined that would minimize the number of immune tests needed, yet still provide a high degree of sensitivity for detecting potential immunotoxicants. These configurations are depicted in Table 12-9. The FDA has adopted a tier approach in its assessment of the immunotoxicity of food and color additives (*Redbook I*).

Health Effects Test Guidelines After several years of international debate regarding inclusion of functional immunotoxicity assessments in regulatory studies (as opposed to relying on histopathology as an indicator of further testing needs), the Environmental Protection Agency published health effects test guidelines for immunotoxicity testing: TSCA 799.9780 (1997) and

Table 12-7
Models of Host Resistance

PRIMARY FACTORS INVOLVED IN CHALLENGE MODEL	PATHOGEN	HOST RESISTANCE
Bacterial	*Listeria monocytogenes*	Macrophage, T cell, NK cell
	Streptococcus pneumoniae	Complement, PMN, macrophage, B cell
Parasite	*Plasmodium yoelii*	T cell
Viral	Influenza A2	Cytotoxic T cell, antibody, complement
Tumor	B16F10 melanoma	NK cell, macrophage

SOURCE: From Bradley and Morahan (1982), with permission. See also for an extensive review of host resistance models.

Table 12-8
Tier Approach for Immunotoxicology Testing

TESTING LEVEL	PROCEDURES
Tier I	Hematology
	Body weight
	Organ weights (spleen, thymus, kidney, liver)
	Spleen cellularity
	Bone marrow cellularity and CFU
	Immunopathology
	PFC assay
	Proliferative responses
	NK assay
Tier II	Surface marker analysis
	Secondary (IgG) PFC assay
	CTL assay
	DHR assay
	Host resistance studies

OPPTS 870.7800 (1998). These guidelines flow from the configurations depicted in Table 12-8, although conduct of 3 tests is not required by law. Assessment of immunotoxicity begins by exposure for a minimum of 28 days to the chemical followed by assessment of humoral immunity (PFC assay or anti-sRBC ELISA). If the chemical produces significant suppression of the humoral response, surface marker assessment by flow cytometry may be performed. If the chemical produces no suppression of the humoral response, an assessment of innate immunity (NK assay) may be performed. The tests do not represent a comprehensive assessment of immune function but are intended to complement assessment made in routine toxicity testing (hematological assessments, lymphoid organ weights, and histopathology). A phagocytosis assay on pulmonary macrophages obtained by broncheoalveolar lavage was included in TSCA 799.9135 (acute inhalation toxicity with histopathology) to address potential immunological changes in the lung associated with hazardous air pollutants. Although additional tests are not required, these guidelines should be viewed as just that–"guidelines," with both sound science and responsible management of chemicals being the larger guide to determining whether additional tests are needed. These documents are available on the EPA OPPTS Internet web site. In Europe, the OECD has not as yet adopted specific guidelines for immunotoxicity assessment. Instead, functional assessments are included in standard toxicology studies when desired or when suggested by expanded histopathological results on other standard toxicology studies.

Immunotoxicity Testing of Medical Devices Concern over the influence of medical devices on the immune system has grown over the past 10 years (reviewed in Rodgers et al., 1997). Many of these devices may have intimate and prolonged contact with the body. Possible immunologic consequences of this contact could be envisioned to include immunosuppression, immune stimulation, inflammation, and sensitization. In 1999, the Office for Device Evaluation in the Center for Devices and Radiological Health (CDRH) published a guidance document (Immunotoxicity Testing Guidance) to provide FDA reviewers and device manufacturers a systematic approach for evaluating potential adverse immunological effects of medical devices and constituent materials. Because of the complexity of the guidance, the reader is referred to the document itself, which may be located on the FDA CDRH Internet web site.

Animal Models in Immunotoxicology

The mouse has been the animal of choice for studying the actions of xenobiotics on the immune system for several reasons: (1) because there is a vast database available on the immune system of the mouse, (2) mice are less expensive to maintain than larger animals, and (3) a wider variety of reagents (cytokines, antibodies, etc.) are available for the mouse (Vos et al., 1994). Because of the need in the industrial setting to integrate immunotoxicologic assessments with routine toxicology testing, a worldwide effort has been under way to validate the rat as a model for immunotoxicology testing. With the exception of a few functional studies, the rat provides a near equal model to the mouse for assessing immunocompetence. Many reagents that are available for studying the human immune system can also be used in rhesus and cynomolgus monkeys.

Other experimental animals including the chicken and fish are being used to evaluate the immunotoxicity of xenobiotics (reviewed in IPCS, 1996). Development of these animal models and the refinement in methods used to assess immunomodulation in these species is anticipated to grow as pressure continues to build regarding alternative animal models and environmental consciousness, and as the consumer market for poultry and farm-raised fish continues to expand. An understanding of the chicken immune system is well established. Because of the ease in handling the developing embryo, chickens may serve to aid the advancement of the field of developmental immunotoxicology.

There has been significant interest in the teleost immune system over the past 15 years, and equivalents of T, B, NK, and accessory cells have been identified. Fish B cells possess many biochemical and molecular qualities of their mammalian counterparts, and recently T-cell receptor alpha and beta genes have been characterized (reviewed in Miller et al., 1998). The immune systems of several species of fish have been reported to be sensitive to environmental stressors, including chemicals, which produce immunomodulation in mammalian species (reviewed in Zelikoff, 1994; Bly et al., 1997). As a result, teleosts may serve as early indicators of environmental exposure to immunotoxicants (Zelikoff, 1998; Zelikoff et al., 2000). Whether or not fish will eventually

Table 12-9
Suggested Testing Configurations: Three Tests with 100 percent Concordance

PFC	DHR	Surface markers
PFC	NK	DHR
PFC	NK	Thymus:body weight
PFC	DHR	Thymus:body weight
Surface markers	NK	DHR
Surface markers	DHR	T-cell mitogens
Surface markers	DHR	Thymus:body weight
Surface markers	DHR	LPS response

SOURCE: Luster et al. (1988), modified, with permission.

have efficacy as models in immunotoxicology risk assessment for the human population remains uncertain, and more effort will be required before the teleost models are at the current level of the rodent (reviewed in Gogal et al., 1999).

Relationship between Immunotoxicity Data in Animals and Humans

There is a clear association between suppression of immune function and an increased incidence of infectious and neoplastic disease in humans (reviewed in Biagini, 1998). Chemicals that produce immunotoxicity in animals have the potential to produce immune effects in the human population, and these effects may occur in the absence of observable disease (reviewed in Luster et al., 1994). While it would appear relatively straightforward, "the assessment [epidemiologically] of immunotoxicity in humans exposed to potentially immunotoxic chemicals is much more complicated than in experimental animals" (reviewed in IPCS, 1996). Because of this, there is a need and desire to extrapolate from animal data to human health effects. A paralleogram approach has been used to assess relationships between animal data and human data (Fig. 12-15; Selgrade et al., 1999; Van Loveren et al. 1995). In this approach, filled circles represent data which can be readily obtained in vivo or in vitro. Unfilled circles represent data which cannot be obtained experimentally. Data that may occasionally be obtained but must sometimes be extrapolated are represented by circles filled with blue lines. This approach has been used to extrapolate animal to human data in an initial quantitative assessment of risk for deleterious effects of UV radiation (Van Loveren et al. 1995). A dual parallelogram approach has also been used to propose that data for ozone suggest that effects of in vivo human exposure to phosgene on alveolar macrophage phagocytosis may be predicted based on effects of in vitro exposure and in vivo animal data (reviewed in Selgrade et al., 1995).

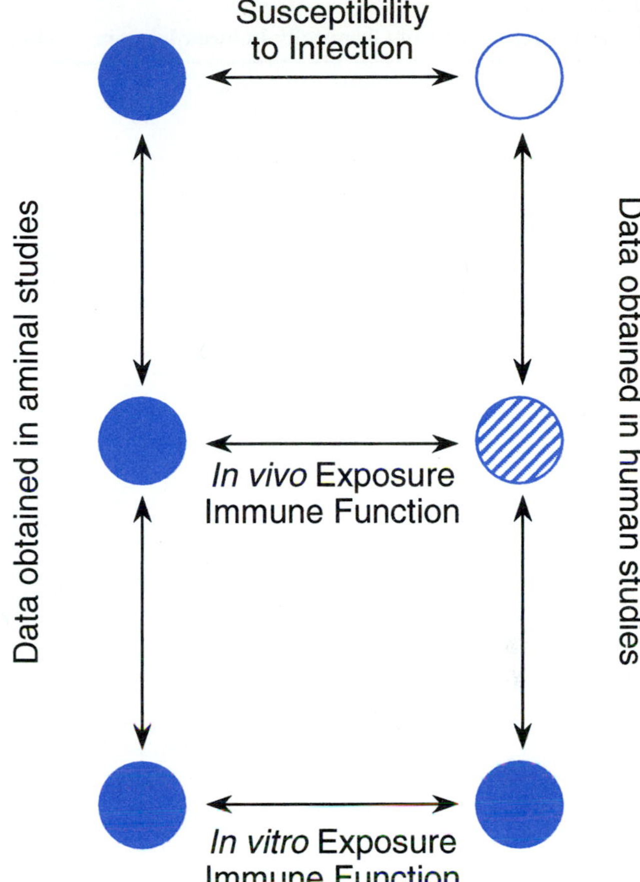

Figure 12-15. Parallelogram approach in immunotoxicology for relating animal data to human data. [Modified from Selgrade (1999), with permission.]

Evaluation of Mechanisms of Action

When we think of the ways chemicals can act on various organ systems we most often think of the direct effects of chemical exposure. Direct effects on the immune system may include chemical effects on immune function, structural alterations in lymphoid organs or on immune cell surfaces, or compositional changes in lymphoid organs or in serum (Table 12-10). Xenobiotics may exert an indirect action on the immune system as well. They may be metabolically activated to their toxic metabolites, may also have effects on other organ systems (e.g., liver damage) which then impacts the immune system, or may induce alterations in hormonal homeostasis.

As mentioned previously, a unique quality of the immune system is the ability to remove immune cells and have them function in vitro. This is particularly important in investigating the mechanisms of action of xenobiotics. For example, it can be determined whether a compound acts either directly or indirectly on immune cells by comparing in vivo to in vitro chemical exposure (refer to Fig. 12-11). Immunotoxic compounds that act indirectly will have no effect on an in vitro—generated immune response. Compounds that require metabolism to reactive metabolites will also have no effect on in vitro—generated immune responses following in vitro exposure. However, this metabolic requirement can be mimicked in vitro by incubating the chemical with a microsomal S9 preparation prior to in vitro exposure of splenocytes. The metabolically activated compound may then be capable of suppressing in vitro—generated immune responses.

Numerous methodologies are available to evaluate cellular and molecular mechanisms of action. Xenobiotic-induced effects on specific cell types of the antibody response can be determined using antigens that require several cell types, such as macrophage, T, and B cells (sRBC), macrophages, and B cells only (DNP-Ficoll), or B cells alone (LPS) for the production of antigen-specific antibody. In addition, splenocytes can be separated into the various cell populations such as adherent cells (primarily macrophages) and nonadherent cells (T and B cells), that can be individually exposed and then reconstituted in cell culture to yield an in vitro—generated immune response equal to that of unseparated cells. This separation/reconstitution analysis is an excellent way to determine specific cell targets of xenobiotic action. In addition, supernatants from in vitro—generated antibody responses can be transferred among themselves in an effort to assess xenobiotic action on soluble factors such as the cytokines, and ELISA methodology and quantitative PCR can be used to quantitate in vitro cytokine production and cytokine gene transcription, respectively, in response to various stimuli. Much of the progress in immunotoxicology research has been the result of the application of advances made in immunology and molecular biology and it is expected that this will continue as these areas of basic science progress by leaps and bounds.

Table 12-10
Possible Mechanisms of Chemically Induced Immune Modulation

TYPE OF EFFECT	MECHANISM	EXAMPLES
Direct	Functional changes	Altered antibody-mediated responses Altered cell-mediated responses Altered release of preformed mediators Altered host resistance Inability of one or more cell types to perform a required activity, e.g., Production of antibody Release of cytokines Processing and presentation of antigen Proliferation and differentiation Receptor-mediated signal transduction
	Structural changes	Alterations in surface receptors or ligands Alteration in expression of receptors or ligands Histopathologic changes in lymphoid organs
	Compositional changes	Alterations in $CD3^+$, $CD4^+$, $CD8^+$, $B220^+$, and/or Ig^+ in spleen Alterations in $CD4^+$, $CD8^+$, $CD4^+/CD8^+$, and/or $CD4^-/CD8^-$ in thymus Changes in hematologic cellular parameters Alterations in circulating Ig Alterations in CFU profile in bone marrow
Indirect	Metabolic Activation	Conversion to a toxic metabolite
	Effects secondary to other target organ toxicity	Induction of acute-phase proteins as a result of liver injury
	Hormonal changes	Increased corticosteroid release from the adrenal gland Alteration in neuroendocrine regulation Alteration in autonomic output from the CNS Altered release of steroids from sex organs

IMMUNOMODULATION BY XENOBIOTICS

Immunosuppression

Halogenated Aromatic Hydrocarbons Few classes of xenobiotics have been as extensively studied for immunotoxicity as the halogenated aromatic hydrocarbons (HAHs; reviewed by Kerkvliet and Burleson, 1994, and Holsapple, 1996). The prototypical and most biologically potent member of this family of chemicals, which includes the polychlorinated biphenyls (PCBs), the polybrominated biphenyls (PBBs), the polychlorinated dibenzofurans (PCDFs), and the polychlorinated dibenzodioxins (PCDDs), is 2,3,7,8-tetrachlorodibenzo-*p*-dioxin (TCDD; dioxin). Substantial evidence has accumulated that demonstrates the immune system to be a target for toxicity for these chemicals. Derived from a variety of animal models, primarily rodents, this evidence includes thymic atrophy, pancytopenia, cachexia, immunosuppression, and tumor promotion. There is also epidemiological evidence suggesting immunotoxicity by the HAHs can also occur in humans; however, significant immunosuppression has not been associated conclusively with specific alterations of human immune function.

Quite possibly the most important advance in recent years in the study of the HAHs has been the determination of a genetic basis for sensitivity to the toxic effects of this family of chemicals. Many of the biochemical and toxic effects of the HAHs appear to be mediated via HAH binding to an intracellular heterodimeric complex between the aryl hydrocarbon receptor (*Ah*-R) and the aromatic receptor nuclear transporter (ARNT; Hoffman et al., 1991). The *Ah*-R–ARNT complex translocates to the nucleus, binds to dioxin-responsive elements (DREs), and directs transcriptional activation (e.g., CYP1A1, PAI-2, *fos/jun*) and mRNA stabilization (e.g., TGFα, IL-1β) (Sutter et al., 1991; Sutter and Greenlee, 1992). In mice, allelic variation at the *Ah* locus has been described. These alleles code for *Ah*-Rs with differential binding affinities for TCDD. For example, the C57Bl/6 mouse represents a strain of mice (Ah^{bb}) which is exquisitely sensitive to TCDD (*TCDD responsive*), while the DBA/2 strain of mice (Ah^{dd}) is much less sensitive to the toxic effects of TCDD (*TCDD nonresponsive* or *TCDD low-responsive*). These allelic differences may ultimately explain the controversial differences in observed toxic responses between animal species and even between individual tissues within the same species.

Polychlorinated Biphenyls PCBs have seen extensive commercial use for over half a century. Their unique physical and chemical properties make PCB mixtures ideal for use as plasticizers, adhesives, and as dielectric fluids in capacitors and transformers. Mixtures of PCBs (e.g., Aroclors) have been commonly used to evaluate the immunotoxicity of PCBs and have been reported to suppress immune responses and decrease host resistance (reviewed by Kerkvliet, 1984). The first indication that PCBs produced immunotoxic effects was the observation of severe atrophy of the primary and secondary lymphoid organs in general toxicity tests and the subsequent demonstration of the reduction in numbers of circulating lymphocytes. Studies to characterize the immunotoxic action of the PCBs have primarily focused on the antibody response. This parameter is by far the one most consistently affected by PCB exposure and effects on antibody response have been demonstrated in guinea pigs, rabbits, mice, and rhesus monkeys. PCB-exposed monkeys exhibit chloracne, alopecia, and facial edema, all classical symptoms of HAH toxicity. In an extensive characterization of the effects of PCBs on nonhuman primates, Tryphonas and colleagues (1991a,b) exposed rhesus monkeys to Aroclor 1254 for 23 to 55 months. The only immune parameter consistently suppressed was the PFC response to sRBC (both IgM and IgG). In addition, after 55 months of exposure, lymphoproliferative responses were dose-dependently suppressed and serum complement levels were significantly elevated. The observed elevation in serum complement has also been reported in PCDD-exposed children from Seveso, Italy (Tognoni and Bonaccorsi, 1982) and in B6C3F1-exposed mice (White et al., 1986).

The effects of PCBs on cell-mediated immunity (CMI) are far less clear and both suppression and enhancement have been reported. Exposure to Aroclor 1260 has been demonstrated to suppress delayed-type hypersensitivity (DTH) responses in guinea pigs, whereas exposure to Aroclor 1254 was reported to enhance lymphoproliferative responses in rats. In a similar study in Fischer 344 rats (Aroclor 1254), thymic weight was decreased, NK cell activity was suppressed, PHA-induced proliferative responses were enhanced, and there was no effect on the MLR proliferative response or CTL activity. Other investigators (Silkworth and Loose, 1978, 1979) have reported enhancement of graft–versus host reactivity and the MLR proliferative response. The augmentation of selected CMI assays may reflect a PCB-induced change in T cell subsets (as described above) and thus in immunoregulation.

Studies on host resistance following exposure to PCBs indicate that the host defenses against hepatitis virus (ducks) and to herpes simplex virus, *Plasmodium berghei, L. monocytogenes,* and *Salmonella typhimurium* (mice) are suppressed (reviewed by Dean et al., 1985). PCB-induced changes in tumor defenses have not been well defined and both augmentation and suppression have been reported. This probably reflects the variability in observed responses in CMI.

Polybrominated Biphenyls The polybrominated biphenyls (PBBs) have been used primarily as flame retardants (Firemaster BP-6 and FF-1). While it is assumed that their profile of activity is similar to that of the PCBs, few studies have actually evaluated the action of the PBBs on immunocompetence. In Michigan (in 1973) Firemaster BP-6 was inadvertently substituted for a nutrient additive in cattle feed, resulting in widespread exposure of animals and humans to PBBs. Studies conducted on livestock following the incident indicated little if any PBB-induced alterations in immunocompetence (Kately and Bazzell, 1978; Vos and Luster, 1989). Like CMI observations involving PCBs, CMI responses in PBB-exposed individuals are not conclusive, showing both a reduction in circulating numbers of T and B cells and a suppression of selected CMI parameters or no effect on CMI at all.

Polychlorinated Dibenzodioxins By far the majority of the investigations into the immunotoxic potential and mechanisms of action of the HAHs have focused on TCDD, primarily because this chemical is the most potent of the HAHs, binding the Ah-R with the highest affinity. The effects of TCDD on immune function have been demonstrated to be among the earliest and most sensitive indicators of TCDD-induced toxicity (reviewed by Holsapple et al., 1991a,b). TCDD is not produced commercially, except in small amounts for research purposes. Rather, it is an environmental contaminant formed primarily as a by-product of the manufacturing process that uses chlorinated phenols or during the combustion of chlorinated materials. It is usually associated with the production of herbicides such as 2,4,5-trichlorophenoxyacetic acid (2,4,5-T), and Agent Orange [a 1:1 combination of 2,4-dichlorophenoxyacetic acid (2,4-D) and 2,4,5-T]. Other sources include pulp and paper manufacturing (chlorine bleaching), automobile exhaust (leaded gasoline), combustion of municipal and industrial waste, and the production of PCBs.

Like other HAHs, exposure to TCDD results in severe lymphoid atrophy. Because thymus-derived cells play an integral role in tumor surveillance and host resistance, the earliest studies on TCDD-induced immunotoxicity focused on changes in cell-mediated immunity. Studies on CMI have shown that this branch of acquired immunity is sensitive to the toxic effects of TCDD. CTL development and activity has been shown by numerous investigators to be significantly decreased after exposure to TCDD, an effect which appeared to be age dependent (e.g., the younger the mice when exposed, the greater the sensitivity to TCDD). In addition to suppression of CTL function, TCDD exposure also results in decreases in PHA- and Con A–induced proliferative responses, DHR, and graft-versus-host responses. Enhanced proliferative responses in juvenile mice have also been observed (Lundberg et al., 1990).

Consistent with the observation that mice exposed perinatally or postnatally (developmentally younger animals) are more sensitive to the effects of TCDD, it has recently been determined that thymic involution is a result of TCDD-induced terminal differentiation of the thymic epithelium and, thus, T cells do not have a proper nutrient-filled microenvironment in which to develop (Greenlee et al., 1984, 1985). This conclusion is supported by previous observations that TCDD significantly decreased the number of immature T cells ($CD4^+/CD8^+$) in the thymus (Kerkvliet and Brauner, 1990).

Numerous investigations have demonstrated the PFC response to be exquisitely sensitive to the toxic effects of TCDD. This effect segregates with the *Ah* locus (Vecchi et al., 1983) and appears to be dependent upon duration and conditions of exposure (Holsapple et al., 1991c). Although TCDD induces profound changes in the PFC assay, no changes have been observed in splenic cellularity (numbers of Ig^+, $CD4^+$, or Thy-1^+ cells) either before or after antigen challenge. In addition, in spite of suppression of antigen-induced antibody production, TCDD has been reported to enhance total serum immunoglobulin concentrations.

Although many labs have defined Th cells as unaffected by TCDD exposure, Kerkvliet has reported suppression of T-cell regulation of immune responses (Kerkvliet and Brauner, 1987; Kerkvliet et al., 1990). However, studies using separation/reconstitution or in vitro exposure techniques have elucidated the B cell as the primary immune cell target for TCDD. In addition, B-cell differentiation was identified as the stage affected. Consistent with these findings, TCDD has a selectively greater effect on immature B cells than on mature B cells. Additionally, the selective effect on

B cells cannot be accounted for by induction of T_s (suppressor T cells).

The information presented so far implicates an effect of TCDD on lymphocyte development/maturation either in the bone marrow, thymus, or after antigenic challenge. In support of this conclusion, TCDD exposure has been shown to suppress bone marrow cellularity and stem cell proliferation in rodent neonates exposed in utero. TCDD also appears to alter homing patterns of lymphocytes after perinatal or postnatal exposure in Fischer 344 rats and can alter development of granulocyte-macrophage colony-forming units (CFU-GM) at concentrations below those that induce thymic atrophy. Using fetal thymic or bone marrow equivalent cells from birds, it has been demonstrated that TCDD severely attenuates proliferation and development of $CD4^+/CD8^+$ cells and of B cells. These data support the conclusions of Greenlee and colleagues (1984,1985) that TCDD alters the microenvironment in which lymphocytes develop.

The effects of TCDD on innate immunity are less well studied. TCDD has been shown to inhibit some functions of polymorphonuclear leukocytes (PMNs), including cytolytic and cytostatic activities. This inhibition has been postulated to be related to PMN development in the bone marrow. Results by several investigators have shown TCDD-induced alterations in serum C3, indicating soluble mediators of innate immunity may also be targeted (White and Anderson, 1985; White et al., 1986). There have been no observed effects on macrophage-mediated cytotoxicity, NK function, or interferon production. In host resistance models, TCDD exposure has been shown to increase susceptibility to several bacterial, viral, and tumor models.

There is little doubt that TCDD and related PCDDs are immunotoxic, particularly in mice. However, extrapolation to human exposure has proven to be difficult. There are a few instances in which accidental human exposure to TCDD and related congeners has afforded the opportunity to study exposure-related human immunologic responses. In children exposed to PCDDs in Seveso, Italy (1976), nearly half of the exposed study group exhibited chloracne (a hallmark of human exposure to PCDDs) 3 years after the accident. Immune parameters measured at that time were unaffected. In a second study conducted 6 years later on different subjects, there was an increase in complement, which correlated with the incidence of chloracne, an increase in circulating T and B cells, and an increase in peripheral blood lymphocyte (PBL) mitogenic responses. A second incident occurred in 1971 in Times Beach, Missouri, when wastes containing TCDD were sprayed on roads to prevent dust formation. Both low-risk and high-risk individuals from this area were examined for DHR responses. Slight, but statistically nonsignificant alterations were observed in high-risk compared to low-risk individuals. In addition, there was a low-level increase in mitogenic responsiveness in high-risk persons. In a second study conducted 12 years later, no alterations were observed in DHR or mitogenic responses between exposed or control individuals. More recently, studies have been undertaken to evaluate the in vitro effects of TCDD on human cells. TCDD suppressed IgM secretion by human B cells in response to the superantigen toxic shock syndrome toxin-1 (TSST-1) and the proliferation and IgG secretion of human tonsillar B cells in response to LPS and cytokines.

Polychlorinated Dibenzofurans Like the PCDDs, polychlorinated dibenzofurans (PCDFs) are not produced commercially but are true environmental contaminants associated with the production of chlorophenoxy acids, pentachlorophenol, and other PCB mixtures. Although higher concentrations are required to achieve observable effects, the immunotoxic profile of the PCDFs is similar in nature to that described for TCDD. In fact, most of what is known regarding the immunotoxicity of the PCDFs in animal models has been learned during structure–activity relationship studies comparing TCDD to congeners of the dibenzofurans. TCDF (tetrachlorodibenzofuran) exposure in most species is associated with thymic atrophy and in guinea pigs it has been shown to suppress the DHR and lymphoproliferative responses to PHA and LPS. Suppression of the PFC response to SRBC after exposure to several PCDF congeners has also been reported.

Two important case studies of human immunotoxicology involved populations accidentally exposed to HAHs. There is evidence that the PCDFs were the primary contributors to the observed toxic effects. Greater than 1850 individuals in Japan (in 1968) and in excess of 2000 people in Taiwan (in 1979) were affected when commercial rice oil was found to be contaminated with HAHs. PCDFs were observed in the tissues of the exposed populations and subsequent studies on immune status revealed a decrease in total circulating T cells, decreased DHR, and enhanced lymphoproliferative responses to PHA and pokeweed mitogen (PWM). In addition, many of the exposed individuals suffered from recurring respiratory infections, suggesting that host resistance mechanisms had been compromised.

Polycyclic Aromatic Hydrocarbons The polycyclic aromatic hydrocarbons (PAHs) are a ubiquitous class of environmental contaminants. They enter the environment through many routes including the burning of fossil fuels and forest fires. In addition to being carcinogenic and mutagenic, the PAHs have been found to be potent immunosuppressants. Effects have been documented on humoral immunity, cell-mediated immunity, and on host resistance (reviewed by Ward et al., 1985, and White et al., 1986). The most extensively studied PAHs are 7,12-dimethylbenz[a]anthracene (DMBA) and benzo[a]pyrene (BaP).

The PAHs suppress the antibody response to a variety of T cell–dependent and T cell–independent antigens. In addition, mice exposed to BaP exhibit suppressed lymphoproliferative responses to mitogens but not alloantigens (Dean et al., 1983). In Dean's studies, host resistance to the PYB6 tumor and to *L. monocytogenes* were unaffected by BaP exposure, as was the DHR response and allograft rejection, suggesting that the T cell (and CMI) was only minimally affected by BaP. Since the PFC response to T cell–dependent and T cell–independent antigens is markedly suppressed by BaP exposure, it would appear that BaP may target the macrophage or the B cell.

In contrast to BaP, DMBA (the more potent PAH) significantly suppresses not only PFC responses but also NK activity, CTL responses, DHR responses, and alloantigen-induced lymphoproliferative responses as well. Therefore DMBA exposure seems to result in long-lasting immunosuppression of humoral immunity (HI), CMI, and tumor resistance mechanisms in mice. Suppression of the immunologic mechanism of tumor resistance by PAHs tends to correlate with their carcinogenic properties and may contribute to their carcinogenicity.

Although it is well established that the PAHs are immunosuppressive in nature, the mechanism or mechanisms by which they elicit this action have remained elusive until recently (reviewed by White et al., 1994). It is generally recognized that PAHs exert carcinogenic and mutagenic effects after being metabolized by P450 enzymes to more toxic metabolites. It has recently been shown that splenocytes from unexposed mice can metabolize exogenously added DMBA via P450 enzymes (Ladics et al., 1991). In addition, Ladics and colleagues (1992a,b) demonstrated that macrophages were the primary cell capable of metabolizing PAHs, and that these cells were capable of generating 7,8-dihydroxy-9,10-epoxy-7,8,9,10-benzo[*a*]pyrene (BPDE), the reactive metabolite proposed to be the ultimate carcinogenic form of BaP. These data are consistent with other studies demonstrating the presence and inducibility of aryl hydrocarbon hydrolase (AHH) in cells of the macrophage lineage and with other data suggesting that the macrophage is the primary target and is functionally compromised (with respect to accessory cell help) following exposure to the PAHs.

Nitrosamines The nitrosamine family comprises the nitrosamines, nitrosamides, and *C*-nitroso compounds. Exposure to nitrosamines, especially *N*-nitrosodimethylamine (DMN, the most prevalent nitrosamine) comes primarily through industrial and dietary means, and minimally through environmental exposure. The toxicity and immunotoxicity of DMN have been extensively reviewed (Myers and Shook, 1996). Single or repeated exposure to DMN inhibits T-dependent humoral immune responses (IgM and IgG), but not T-independent responses. Other symmetrical nitrosamines, such as diethylnitrosamine (DEN), dipropylnitrosamine (DPN), and dibutylnitrosamine (DBN), demonstrated similar effects on humoral immunity but were not as potent as DMN. In fact, as the length of the aliphatic chain increased, the dose required to suppress the anti-sRBC PFC response by 50 percent (ED_{50}) also increased. In contrast, nonsymmetrical nitrosamines suppressed humoral immunity at comparable concentrations. Overall, the rank order of ED_{50} values paralleled their LD_{50} values. T cell–mediated lyphoproliferative responses (mitogens or mixed lymphocyte response) and delayed hypersensitivity response are also suppressed following DMN exposure. In vivo exposure to DMN followed by challenge with several pathogens did not produce a pattern of effects that was consistent (decreased resistance to *Streptococcus zooepidemicus* and influenza, no effects on resistance to herpes simplex types 1 or 2 or *Trichinella spiralis,* increased resistance to *L. monocytogenes*). In contrast, anti-tumor activity in DMN-exposed animals was consistently enhanced. DMN-exposed animals also have altered development of hematopoietic cells (increased macrophage precursors). Together these data suggest the macrophage (or its developmental precursors) as a primary target. Mechanistic studies have demonstrated that DMN alterations in cell-mediated immunity are associated with enhanced macrophage activity, increased myelopoietic activity, and alterations in TNF-α transcriptional activity. It has been postulated that DMN may cause the enhanced production of GM-CSF, which can have autocrine (enhanced tumoricidal and bactericidal activity) and paracrine (induced secretion of T cell–suppressing cytokines by macrophages) activities. Further work is needed to clarify the apparent selectivity of DMN for alteration in macrophage function.

Pesticides Pesticides include all xenobiotics whose specific purpose is to kill another form of life, usually insects or small rodents. These compounds can be divided into four classes: the organophosphates, organotins, carbamates, and organochlorines. While there is increasing evidence that certain pesticides can produce alterations in immune function in animal models (reviewed by Penninks et al., 1990; Barnett and Rodgers, 1994; and Voccia et al., 1999), studies following human exposure are limited and reveal no conclusive results (Thomas et al., 1990).

Organophosphates Occupational exposure to organophosphates has been linked to decreased PMN chemotaxis and increased upper respiratory infection. Overall, relatively little is known about the immunotoxic effects of organophosphates on the immune system. The most extensively studied of these are malathion, parathion, and methyl parathion. Prolonged exposure to low doses of malathion (a cumulative high dose) results in decreased humoral immunity. High doses, which have direct cholinergic effects, also suppress humoral immunity, but whether this is a direct effect of the chemical on the immune system or a stress response elicited by cholinergic effects is unclear. In contrast, acute oral exposure has been shown to enhance humoral immunity and mitogenic proliferative responses with no other immune-related effects. In vitro exposure of either human mononuclear cells or murine splenocytes to malathion results in decreased lymphoproliferative responses, suppressed CTL generation, and a decrease in the stimulus-induced respiratory burst in peritoneal cells. Moreover, after metabolism of malathion by liver S9 preparations, the metabolites of malathion were not immunosuppressive. In addition, separation and reconstitution studies revealed that the adherent population (i.e., the macrophage) is the primary cellular target for malathion. Malathion exposure also induces peritoneal mast cell degranulation and enhances macrophage phagocytosis. In light of the above findings and the fact that mast cell degranulation products can modulate leukocyte activity, it has been suggested that peritoneal mast cell degranulation following acute malathion exposure may subsequently lead to augmentation of leukocyte functions, thereby nonspecifically enhancing the generation of an immune response.

Parathion has attracted more attention than malathion, probably because it is more acutely toxic. This pesticide suppresses both humoral and cell-mediated immunity. Following exposure to methyl parathion, decreased germinal centers after antigen challenge, thymic atrophy, and suppressed DHR responses have been reported. Other experiments have shown suppression of lymphoproliferative responses as well as increased susceptibility to pathogens. In vitro exposure to parathion or paraoxon suppresses CMI in murine splenocytes, IL-2 production in rat splenocytes, and proliferative responses in human lymphocytes. Finally, exposure of human bone marrow cells to organophosphates may result in inhibition of CFU formation.

Organochlorines The organochlorines include chemicals such as chlordane, dichlorodiphenyltrichloroethane (DDT), Mirex, pentachlorophenol, aldrin, dieldrin, and hexachlorobenzene. These are among the longer-lived pesticides and they have an increased propensity for contamination of soil and ground water. The humoral immune response to both T cell–dependent and T cell–independent antigens is suppressed following exposure to dieldrin, and macrophage functions from dieldrin-exposed animals are depressed. The apparent effect of dieldrin on macrophages correlates with the increased susceptibility of dieldrin-exposed animals to murine hepatitis virus, which targets macrophages (Krzystyniak et al., 1985).

Definitive immunosuppression produced by chlordane was first reported in 1982 by Spyker-Cranmer and colleagues. In utero exposure resulted in decreased DHR responses in mice with no deficit in antibody production to sRBC. This correlated with an increase in resistance to influenza infection because the DHR contributes to the pathology of the infection (Menna et al., 1985). As reported for dieldrin, the primary cellular target for chlordane appears to be the macrophage. Although peritoneal exudate cells from mice exposed to chlordane in utero showed normal cytotoxic responses, the response is delayed by 24 to 48 h. Preliminary evidence suggests that prenatal exposure inhibits myeloid progenitor development in bone marrow, but no cause–effect relationship between this and macrophage deficits has been determined. In contrast to observations from mice exposed in utero, exposure of adult mice to chlordane does not result in any changes to several immune parameters, including PFC response to sRBC, MLR, DHR, or mitogenic lymphoproliferation.

DDT is one of the oldest pesticides in use today and one of the first studied for its immunotoxic potential. DDT inhibited antiovalbumin serum antibody titers in rats exposed via the drinking water (Wasserman et al., 1969). In contrast, both rats and guinea pigs fed DDT exhibited no alterations in antitoxin antibody (Gabliks et al., 1973, 1975). These animals did, however, have a suppressed anaphylactic reaction as a result of decreased numbers of mast cells. Studies by Street (1981) indicated that chickens exposed to DDT or Mirex had suppressed levels of circulating IgM and IgG, although specific antibody titers were normal. In addition, DDT exposure resulted in decreased antigen-induced germinal centers, thymic atrophy, and suppressed CMI. While most studies on DDT have focused on humoral immunity, the effects of DDT on CMI, host resistance, and particularly macrophage function remain relatively unexplored.

Organotins Trisubstituted organotins such as TBTO are widely used as biocides and have recently been recognized as producing some immunotoxic effects. The action of these compounds on lymphoid tissue and immunity has been extensively reviewed (Penninks et al., 1990). The most outstanding action of TBTO is the induction of profound but reversible thymic atrophy. In addition, the developing immune system appears to be more sensitive to the effects of TBTO than does the immune system of the adult animal. Studies by Vos et al. (1984) demonstrated a decrease in cellularity in the spleen, bone marrow, and thymus. The decrease in splenic cellularity was associated with a concomitant loss of T lymphocytes. More specifically, oral TBTO exposure resulted in decreased serum IgG, increased serum IgM, and suppression of DHR responses to tuberculin and ovalbumin. In those studies, host resistance to *L. monocytogenes* was diminished. Cytotoxicity by adherent peritoneal cells was suppressed but there was no observed effect on NK cytotoxicity. In contrast, van Loveren et al. (1990) observed suppressed lung NK cytotoxicity in rats exposed orally to TBTO. In addition, the lymphoproliferative response of thymocytes to PHA, Con A, and PWM was significantly suppressed.

Carbamates Carbamate insecticides such as carbaryl (Sevin) and aldicarb have frequently been studied as immunotoxicants. Studies involving oral exposure of chickens to Sevin resulted in acute and sometimes prolonged suppression of germinal centers and antibody production. In addition, carbaryl exposure causes suppression of granulocyte phagocytosis, which may last for up to 9 months. However, other studies have found no indication of immunotoxicity except at near lethal concentrations. In an evaluation of humoral immunity following a 2-week exposure to carbaryl in rats, suppression of the IgM PFC response to sRBC was observed following inhalation exposure but not oral or dermal exposure (Ladics et al., 1994). Conflicting results have also been observed in animals exposed to aldicarb or methyl isocyanate, an intermediate in carbamate pesticide production. Deo and colleagues (1987) reported alterations in T cells and lymphoproliferative responses in humans accidentally exposed to methyl isocyanate. In contrast, mice exposed to the same compound showed no significant alterations in immune status (Luster et al., 1986). More recently, Pruett and coworkers (1992a) evaluated the immunotoxicity of sodium methyldithiocarbamate, a chemical widely used for the control of weeds, fungi, and nematodes in soil. These investigators observed decreased thymus weight, depletion of the $CD4^+/CD8^+$ population of thymocytes, and profound suppression of NK activity following both oral and dermal exposure. Given the number of conflicting reports, currently there is insufficient evidence in either humans or animal models to indicate that carbamate pesticides pose a significant risk to the human population. However, the data by Ladics and colleagues (1994) suggest that immunotoxicologic studies on pesticides should consider relevant exposure routes, as carbaryl was not immunosuppressive by routes through which contact by the general population typically occurs (oral and dermal via residues in water and on food).

Pyrethroids Supermethrin has been demonstrated to decrease the plaque-forming cell response after a single oral administration. However, following repeated exposure (up to 3 mg/kg/day), only slight changes in circulating leukocytes and in nucleated cell numbers in the bone marrow were observed (Siroki et al., 1994). Rabbits administered cypermethrin orally for 7 weeks demonstrated decreased tuberculin skin reactions and a decrease in the antibody titer to *S. typhimurium* (Desi et al., 1985).

Other Pesticides Naphthalene is a bicyclic aromatic hydrocarbon that is used, among other things, as an insect repellent, insecticide, and vermicide. To date, no evidence for immunotoxicity has been demonstrated despite prolonged exposure (Shopp et al., 1984). Recently it has been suggested that this lack of effect may be related to the inability of splenocytes to metabolize naphthalene and/or to relatively low concentrations of metabolites that may be generated in the liver and diffuse to the spleen (Kawabata and White, 1990). Paraquat has been shown to decrease the percentage of circulating neutrophils as a result of their migration to the lungs and propanil can alter immune cell development (myeloid and erythroid progenitors). Thymic atrophy in response to propanil exposure has also been observed, although the contribution of induced glucocorticoids to this effect has not been ascertained (Voccia et al., 1999).

Metals Generally speaking, metals target multiple organ systems and exert their toxic effects via an interaction of the free metal with the target: enzyme systems, membranes, or cellular organelles. Although specific immunotoxic consequences of metal exposure are well documented in the literature (see reviews by Lawrence, 1985; McCabe, 1994; Burns et al., 1994e; and a text edited by Zelikoff and Thomas, 1998), this section focuses on the four best-studied immunotoxic metals: lead, arsenic, mercury, and cadmium. In considering the immunotoxicity of most metals, it is important to remember that at high concentrations, metals usually exert immunosuppressive effects; however, at lower concentrations, immunoenhancement is often observed (Koller, 1980; Vos, 1977).

Lead By far the most consistent finding in studies evaluating the effects of metals on immune responses is increased susceptibility to pathogens. For lead (Pb), decreased resistance to the bacterial pathogens *S. typhimurium, Escherichia coli,* and *L. monocytogenes* has been observed. Enhanced susceptibility to viral challenge has also been reported. Other investigators found no change in virally induced IFN production in Pb-exposed animals.

Studies on the specific effects of Pb on functional cell-mediated immunity have yielded no conclusive results, as reports range from significant suppression to no effect. Currently, these differences cannot be explained by differences in routes of exposure or dose. Suppression of humoral immunity, however, has been demonstrated. In rodents exposed to Pb, lower antibody titers have been observed. In addition, children environmentally exposed to Pb and infected naturally with *Shigella dysenteriae* had prolonged diarrhea, and occupationally exposed persons reported more colds and influenza and exhibited suppressed secretory IgA levels, suggesting Pb-induced suppression of humoral immunity. Pb-induced effects on myeloid cells include an increase in the number of myeloid progenitors in the bone marrow (CFU-GM) with a subsequent decrease in more mature cells. Following in vivo exposure to Pb, splenocytes displayed consistently suppressed IgM PFC responses to sRBC. Separation and reconstitution experiments indicated that this suppression is likely due to an effect on macrophage function.

In recent mechanistic studies (reviewed by McCabe, 1994), an alteration in the ability of the macrophage to process and present antigen to antigen-primed T cells confirmed the previous observation and suggested that Pb alters immune recognition. In contrast to other reports concerning the immunosuppressive action of Pb on PFC responses, enhancement of the in vitro–generated PFC response (in vitro exposure in Mishell-Dutton-type culture) has been reported which appeared to be the result of enhancement of B-cell differentiation. This effect may occur at the level of B-cell activation or cytokine responsiveness. And finally, in vitro addition studies indicate that Pb may have differential effects on Th1 and Th2 cells and can inhibit the production of IL-2. If the production or activity of other cytokines is observed to be suppressed or enhanced by metal exposure, it may be that metals can exert significant effects on immune regulation, which can result in either immunoenhancement or immunosuppression.

Arsenic The literature concerning arsenic (As)-induced immunomodulation is fraught with inconsistencies due to differences in speciation of As (which plays a significant role in arsenic toxicity), the route of administration, the concentrations used, and the various species and strains of animals utilized. As with many other metals, exposure to low concentrations of As often leads to enhanced immune responses while exposure to higher concentrations results in immunosuppression (reviewed by Burns et al., 1994e). Exposure of mice to sodium arsenite ($NaAsO_2$) in the drinking water or subcutaneously was shown to decrease resistance to viral pathogens. Other investigators have shown that exposure to arsenicals offers some degree of protection against tumor incidence, although tumors that did develop grew at a much faster rate. No alterations in CMI were observed in those investigations. Interestingly, host resistance studies, conducted after exposure to the semiconductor material gallium arsenide (GaAs), revealed that GaAs afforded modest protection against infection with both *S. pneumoniae* and *L. monocytogenes,* although resistance to the B16F10 melanoma was reduced. It was subsequently determined that the As concentrations in the blood of these animals was high enough to offer a chemotherapeutic effect against the bacterial pathogens (arsenicals were once widely used as chemotherapeutic agents before the development of drugs with higher efficacy and lower toxicity). These studies are important because they are among the first to demonstrate the intricate interplay between the host, the pathogen, and the xenobiotic.

In addition to these holistic immune alterations, As exposure has been shown to inhibit both the PFC response in animal models and peripheral blood lymphocyte proliferation in humans. Also, substantial mechanistic information exists regarding the immunotoxicity of intratracheally instilled GaAs. Exposure results in suppression of the PFC, CTL, DHR, and MLR responses. Following instillation, both arsenic and gallium can be detected in the blood and tissues for as long as 30 days, suggesting that the lung acts as a depot for prolonged systemic exposure to dissociated gallium and arsenic. Mechanistic studies revealed that all cell types involved in the generation of an antibody response (macrophage, T, and B cells) are affected by GaAs exposure. Decreased expression of Ia and ability to process and present the particulate antigen, sRBC, represent functional deficits of the macrophage, while inhibition of mitogen- or receptor-driven proliferation, expression of the IL-2 receptor, and production of cytokines during the antibody response represent functional deficits of the T cell. A criticism of the studies using GaAs has been that instillation of particulate matter causes a stress response resulting in increased levels of circulating corticosteroids, known to have potent immunosuppressive activity. Studies utilizing the glucocorticoid antagonist RU-486 showed that although GaAs in the lung did increase circulating corticosterone levels, elevated corticosterone was not responsible for suppression of the AFC response. Rather, GaAs exerted direct immunosuppressive effects independent of its ability to increase serum corticosteroid levels.

Mercury Both organic and inorganic mercury (Hg) has been shown to decrease immunologic responses. Specifically, Hg exposure suppresses the PFC response and increases susceptibility to encephalomyocarditis (EMC) virus in addition to decreasing polyclonal activation of lymphocytes by T-cell mitogens. It has also been reported that Hg can activate B cells and augment anaphylaxis by enhancing IgE production. Recently, interest in Hg has focused on the ability of this metal to induce type III hypersensitivity. Hg administration is used to induce glomerulonephritis in brown Norway rats (a model for induction of autoimmune disease; Sapin *et al.,* 1981).

Cadmium Like other metals, cadmium (Cd) exposure increases susceptibility to both bacterial and viral pathogens, although enhanced resistance to tumor and EMC virus has been reported. Exposure to Cd has also been demonstrated to modulate lymphocyte proliferative responses to mitogens and allogeneic cells. Greenspan and Morrow (1984) reported decreased macrophage phagocytic ability, which correlates with changes in host resistance. Humoral immunity (PFC response and serum antibody titer) and NK function have also been demonstrated to be suppressed by Cd exposure, while CTL activity appears to be enhanced.

Other Metals Organotin compounds are used primarily as heat stabilizers and catalytic agents (dialkyltin compounds) and as biocides (trisubstituted organotins). The immunotoxicity of the organotins has been extensively reviewed (Penninks et al., 1990). Since the trisubstituted organotins are examined elsewhere (see "Pesticides," above) discussion here is limited to the dialkyltins, di-*n*-octyltin dichloride (DOTC) and di-*n*-dibutyltin dichloride (DBTC). As in the case of tributyltin oxide (TBTO), the most outstanding action of the dibutyltins is the induction of profound but reversible thymic atrophy. Additionally, there is a preferential loss of $CD4^+$ cells observed in the peripheral blood. The dialkylorganotins have also been observed to decrease resistance to *L. monocytogenes* and to suppress the DHR and allograft rejection responses. Suppression of the PFC response to sRBC and inhibition of T-cell mitogen responses was also observed, while no effect on B-cell mitogenesis or the PFC response to LPS occurred. These data suggest that the T cell may be a primary target for compounds like DOTC and DBTC. Like the trisubstituted organotins and the HAHs, the developing immune system appears to be more sensitive to the effects of these compounds than does the immune system of the adult.

Beryllium is known primarily for its ability to produce beryllium lung disease, a chronic granulomatous inflammation of the lung often observed in persons with occupational contact or environmental exposure to beryllium compounds. This metal produces a T-cell–mediated hypersensitivity and causes the in vitro transformation of PBL (from exposed but not unexposed patients) into large lymphoblasts (Hanifin et al., 1970). In addition, lymphocytes from beryllium oxide–exposed individuals produce migration inhibitor factor (MIF) that inhibits the migration of macrophages (Henderson et al., 1972).

Platinum compounds have been used in cancer chemotherapy and have been shown to suppress macrophage chemotaxis, to inhibit humoral immunity and lymphoproliferation, and to induce hypersensitivity responses. Gold salts, used therapeutically in rheumatic disease, may cause immune complex hypersensitivity and enhance allergic reactions. While nickel has been reported to enhance anaphylaxis, it also inhibits humoral immunity, NK activity, and impairs resistance to pathogenic challenge. Chromium at low doses enhances phagocytic ability and PFC responses but appears to suppress these responses at higher concentrations. Cobalt, a constituent of vitamin B_{12}, has been demonstrated to suppress PMN chemotaxis and host resistance to streptococcal infection and to inhibit the PFC response. Vanadium impairs the activities of macrophages and results in increased susceptibility to disease and bacterial challenge with *L. monocytogenes*.

Inhaled Substances Pulmonary defenses against inhaled gases and particulates are dependent upon both physical and immunologic mechanisms. Immune mechanisms primarily involve the complex interactions between PMNs and alveolar macrophages and their abilities to phagocytize foreign material and produce cytokines, which not only act as local inflammatory mediators but also serve to attract other cells into the airways.

Urethane Urethane (ethyl carbamate) was once widely used as a veterinary anesthetic until its carcinogenic potential was defined in 1948. Exposure to urethane produces severe myelotoxicity, resulting in suppression of NK-cell activity and antibody responses to sRBC (Luster *et al.*, 1982; Gorelik and Heberman, 1981). In addition, urethane exposure leads to increased frequency of spontaneous lung adenomas in susceptible mouse strains and impaired resistance to B16F10 melanoma cells and metastatic tumor growth in the lungs.

Tobacco Smoke Cigarette smoke has been implicated in acute respiratory illness and chronic obstructive lung disease, but the effect of exposure to mainstream cigarette smoke has yielded ambiguous results in humans and in animal models (reviewed by Sopori et al., 1994). In humans, the number of alveolar macrophages is increased three- to fivefold in smokers compared to nonsmokers. This may be a result of increased production of IL-1 by the resident alveolar macrophages, resulting in enhanced influx of other inflammatory cells (PMNs and peripheral blood mononuclear cells) into the lung. In addition to the increased numbers of macrophages, the macrophages present appear to be in an activated state, as evidenced by an increase in cytoplasmic inclusions, increased enzyme levels, altered surface morphology, and enhanced production of oxygen radicals. However, despite their apparent activated state, these macrophages seem to have decreased phagocytic and bactericidal activity. Although the primary site of exposure of the immune system to cigarette smoke is the lung, selected immune parameters have been shown to be altered in smokers. Decreased serum immunoglobulin levels and decreased NK-cell activity have been reported. Concentration-dependent leukocytosis (increased numbers of T and B cells) is well-defined in smokers when compared to nonsmokers. However, the question of whether there is a relationship between smoking and lymphocyte function is debatable.

Numerous immunologic studies conducted in animals exposed to cigarette smoke demonstrate suppression of antibody responses, biphasic lymphoproliferative capacity (enhanced, then suppressed with continued exposure), and enhanced susceptibility to murine sarcoma virus and influenza virus. Animal studies cannot precisely replicate human exposure conditions because of the route of exposure and the rapid chemical changes that occur in the components of tobacco smoke upon its generation.

Particles: Asbestos and Silica It is believed that alterations in both humoral and cell-mediated immunity occur in individuals exposed to asbestos and exhibiting asbestosis. Decreased DHR and fewer T cells circulating in the periphery as well as decreased T-cell proliferative responses have been reported to be associated with asbestosis (reviewed by Miller and Brown, 1985, and Warheit and Hesterberg, 1994). Autoantibodies and increased serum immunoglobulin levels have also been observed. Within the lung, alveolar macrophage activity has been implicated as playing a significant role in asbestos-induced changes in immunocompetence. Fibers of asbestos that are deposited in the lung are phagocytized by macrophages, resulting in macrophage lysis and release of lysosomal enzymes and subsequent activation of other macrophages. Recently it has been hypothesized that the development of asbestosis in animal models occurs by the following mechanism. Fibers of asbestos deposited in the alveolar space recruit macrophages to the site of deposition. Some fibers may migrate to the interstitial space where the complement cascade becomes activated, releasing C5a, a potent macrophage activator and chemoattractant for other inflammatory cells. Recruited interstitial and resident alveolar macrophages phagocytize the fibers and release cytokines, which cause the proliferation of cells within the lung and the release of collagen. A sustained inflammatory response could then contribute to the progressive pattern of fibrosis which is associated with asbestos exposure.

The primary adverse consequence of silica exposure, like that to asbestos, is the induction of lung fibrosis (silicosis). However, several immune alterations have been associated with silica exposure in experimental animals, including decreased antibody- and cell-mediated immune parameters (reviewed in IPCS, 1996). Alterations in both T- and B-cell parameters have been reported, although T cell–dependent responses appear to be more affected than B cell–dependent responses. Dose and route of antigen exposure appear to be important factors in determining silica-induced immunomodulation. Silica is toxic to macrophages and PMNs, and exposure is correlated with increased susceptibility to infectious pathogens. The significance of these immunologic alterations for the pathogenesis of silicosis remains to be determined. The association of this disease with the induction of autoantibodies is covered elsewhere in this chapter.

Pulmonary Irritants Chemicals such as formaldehyde, silica, and ethylenediamine have been classified as pulmonary irritants and may produce hypersensitivity-like reactions. Macrophages from mice exposed to formaldehyde vapor exhibit increased synthesis of hydroperoxide (Dean et al., 1984). This may contribute to enhanced bactericidal activity and potential damage to local tissues. Although silica is usually thought of for its potential to induce silicosis in the lung (a condition similar to asbestosis), its immunomodulatory effects have also been documented (Levy and Wheelock, 1975). Silica decreased reticuloendothelial system (RES) clearance and suppressed both humoral immunity (PFC response) and the cell-mediated response (CTL) against allogeneic fibroblasts. Both local and serum factors were found to play a role in silica-induced alterations in T-cell proliferation. Silica exposure may also inhibit phagocytosis of bacterial antigens (related to RES clearance) and inhibit tumoricidal activity (Thurmond and Dean, 1988).

Oxidant Gases It is becoming increasingly clear that exposure to oxidant gases—such as ozone (O_3), sulfur dioxide (SO_2), nitrogen dioxide (NO_2), and phosgene—alters pulmonary immunologic responses and may increase the susceptibility of the host to bacterial infections (reviewed by Selgrade and Gilmour, 1994). Infiltration of both PMNs and macrophages has been observed, resulting in the release of cellular enzyme components and free radicals, which contribute to pulmonary inflammation, edema, and vascular changes. Exposure to O_3 has been demonstrated to impair the phagocytic function of alveolar macrophages and to inhibit the clearance of bacteria from the lung. This correlated with decreased resistance to *S. zooepidemicus* and suggests that other extracellular bacteriostatic factors may be impaired following exposure to these oxidant gases. Short-term NO_2 exposure decreases killing of several bacterial pathogens and, like O_3, this decreased resistance is probably related to changes in pulmonary macrophage function. A role for the products of aracadonic acid metabolism (specifically, the prostaglandins) has recently been implied. This is supported by the facts that decreased macrophage functions are associated with increased PGE_2 production and that pretreatment with indomethacin inhibits O_3-induced pulmonary hyperresponsiveness and related inflammatory responses.

It is clear that exposure to oxidant gases can also augment pulmonary allergic reactions. This may be a result of increased lung permeability (leading to greater dispersion of the antigen) and to the enhanced influx of antigen-specific IgE-producing cells in the lungs. In studies involving O_3 exposure and challenge with *L. monocytogenes,* decreased resistance to the pathogen correlated not only with changes in macrophage activity, but with alterations in T cell–derived cytokine production (which enhances phagocytosis) as well. In support of an effect on T cells, other cell-mediated changes were observed: changes in the T- to B-cell ratio in the lung, decreased DHR response, enhanced allergic responses, and changes in T-cell proliferative responses. Together, these data suggest that in addition to altering macrophage functions, oxidant gases may also produce an imbalance in the Th1 and Th2 cell populations. Given the different patterns of lymphokine secretion by these T-cell subpopulations (Mosmann and Coffman, 1989) this is a very plausible explanation for some of the observed immune alterations.

Organic Solvents and Related Chemicals ***Aromatic Hydrocarbons*** There is limited but substantive evidence that exposure to organic solvents and their related compounds can produce immunosuppression (reviewed by Snyder, 1994). By far the best-characterized immunotoxic effects are those produced by benzene. In animal models, benzene induces anemia, lymphocytopenia, and hypoplastic bone marrow. In addition, it has recently been suggested that this myelotoxicity may be a result of altered differentiative capacity in bone marrow–derived lymphoid cells. Benzene (oral and inhaled) exposure alters both humoral and cell-mediated immune parameters including suppression of the anti-sRBC antibody response, decreased T- and B-cell lymphoproliferative responses (mitogens and alloantigens), and inhibition of CTL activity. Benzene exposure also appears to increase the production of both IL-1 and TNF-α and to inhibit the production of IL-2. With these dramatic effects on immune responses, it is not surprising that animals exposed to benzene exhibit reduced resistance to a variety of pathogens. More recently, nitrobenzene (an oxidizing agent used in the synthesis of aniline and benzene compounds) has been reported to also produce immunotoxic effects (Burns et al., 1994a), with the primary targets being the peripheral blood erythrocyte and the bone marrow.

Immunomodulating activity has also been observed for toluene, although most effects occur at significantly high concentrations. When compared with benzene, toluene has little to no effect on immunocompetence. However, it should be noted that toluene exposure effectively attenuates the immunotoxic effects of benzene (probably because of competition for metabolic enzymes).

In contrast to the parent toluene, the monosubstituted nitrotoluenes (*para-* and *meta*-nitrotoluene) do significantly alter the immune system (Burns et al., 1994b,c). Exposure to *p*-nitrotoluene has been demonstrated to suppress the antibody response to sRBC, to decrease the number of $CD4^+$ splenic T cells, and to inhibit the DHR to keyhole limpet hemocyanin (KLH). In addition, host resistance to *L. monocytogenes* was impaired, suggesting the T cell as a primary target. Similarly, *m*-nitrotoluene suppresses the antibody response to sRBC, the DHR to KLH, T-cell mitogenesis, and host resistance to *L. monocytogenes,* again suggesting the T cell as the cellular target. The di-substituted nitrotoluene (2,4-dinitrotoluene; DAT) is also immunosuppressive (Burns et al., 1994d), with exposure resulting in suppressed humoral immunity, NK activity, and phagocytosis by splenic macrophages. Host resistance to bacterial challenge was also impaired. It would appear that DAT may perturb the differentiation and maturation of leukocytes.

Haloalkanes and Haloalkenes Carbon tetrachloride (CCl_4) is widely recognized as hepatotoxic. Recent studies have revealed that CCl_4 is also immunotoxic. Mice exposed for 7 to 30 days to CCl_4 (orally or intraperitoneally) exhibit a decreased T cell–dependent antibody response (sRBC), suppressed mixed lymphocyte responses (allogeneic cells), and lower lymphoproliferative capacity (T and B cells). This change in immune status, which primarily affects helper T-cell function, is associated with the serum of treated animals, suggesting specific cytokine involvement. In fact, the CCl_4-dependent induction and release of TGF-β_1 from the liver results in the indirect suppression of these T cell–mediated immunologic responses (Delaney et al, 1994; Jeon *et al.*, 1997). Induction or inhibition of liver P450 activity augmented and blocked, respectively, the immunotoxic actions of CCl_4, suggesting a requirement for metabolism in order for CCl_4 to be immunosuppressive. In contrast, Fischer 344 rats exposed orally for 10 days exhibited no immunotoxic effects, despite signs of liver toxicity. These differences may represent differences in the metabolic capabilities between these two species.

There is relatively little information on other solvents and related chemicals. Exposure to dichloroethylene (in drinking water for 90 days) has been reported to suppress the anti-sRBC antibody response in male CD-1 mice an to inhibit macrophage function in their female counterparts (Shopp et al., 1985). Similarly, exposure to trichloroethylene (in the drinking water for 4 to 6 months) was reported to inhibit both humoral and cell-mediated immunity and bone marrow colony-forming activity (Sanders et al., 1982). In those experiments, females were more sensitive than males. Exposure to 1,1,2-trichloroethane results in suppression of humoral immunity in both sexes. In addition, macrophage function was inhibited (males only; Sanders et al., 1985). Finally, inhalation of dichloroethane, dichloromethane, tetrachloroethane, and trichloroethene has been reported to suppress pulmonary host resistance to *Klebsiella pneumoniae* (Aranyi et al., 1986; Sherwood et al., 1987), suggesting that alveolar macrophages may be affected.

Glycols and Glycol Ethers Exposure to glycol ethers has been associated with adverse effects in laboratory animals, including thymic atrophy and mild leukopenia. Oral administration of ethylene glycol monomethyl ether (EGME) for 1 to 2 weeks (House et al., 1985; Kayama et al., 1991) or its meatabolite methoxyacetic acid (MAA) for 2 weeks (House et al., 1985), produced decreased thymic weight, thymic atrophy, and a selective depletion of immature thymocytes in mice. No alterations in humoral immunity, cell-mediated immunity, macrophage function, or host resistance to *L. monocytogenes* were observed (House et al., 1985). More recently, it has been suggested that perinatal exposure to EGME may produce thymic hypocellularity and inhibition of thymocyte maturation and that it may affect pro-lymphocytes in fetal liver (Holladay et al., 1994).

Oral studies (5 to 10 days) on the glycol ether 2-methoxyethanol (ME) have consistently shown a decrease in thymus weight in the rat (Williams et al., 1995; Smialowicz et al., 1991a). This decrease is often accompanied by alterations in lymphoproliferative responses, although suppression is seen in some cases and stimulation in others, with no clear reason for the differences in response. Alterations in spleen weight and splenic cell populations have also been observed, as well as suppression of TNP-LPS and anti-sRBC plaque-forming-cell responses. Similar results have been obtained following dermal exposure to 2-methoxyethanol (Williams et al., 1995). A decrease in IL-2 production has also been reported (Smialowicz et al., 1991a). Studies using the metabolites of 2-methoxyethanol (methoxyacetaldehyde and methoxyacetic acid) or specific metabolic pathway inhibitors have shown that methoxyacetaldehyde (MAAD) and methoxyacetic acid (MAA) are more immunotoxic than 2-methoxyethanol alone (MAAD>MAA>ME) (Smialowicz et al., 1991a,b; Kim and Smialowicz, 1997), suggesting a role for metabolism in the observed alterations in immunocompetence. Although there was no effect following 10-day oral exposures to 2-methoxyethanol (50 to 200 mg/kg/day) (Smialowicz et al., 1991a), subchronic exposure for 21 days to 2000 to 6000 ppm (males) or 1600 to 4800 ppm (females) did produce an enhanced NK response (Exon et al., 1991) in addition to suppression of the PFC response and a decrease in IFN-γ production. In that study, it was also determined that 2-methoxyethanol produced greater immunotoxic effects than 2-butoxyethanol. 2-Butoxyethanol was observed to enhance NK activity, but only at the low doses.

Mycotoxins The immunotoxicity of mycotoxins, structurally diverse secondary metabolites of fungi that grow on feed, has been reviewed (IPCS, 1996). This class of chemicals comprises such toxins as aflatoxin, ochratoxin, and the tricothecenes, notably T-2 toxin and vomitoxin. As a class, these toxins can produce cellular depletion in lymphoid organs, alterations in T- and B-lymphocyte function, suppression of antibody responses, suppression of NK activity, decreased delayed hypersensitivity responses, and an apparent increase in susceptibility to infectious disease. T-2 toxin has also been implicated as a developmental immunotoxicant, targeting fetal lymphocyte progenitors leading the thymic atrophy often observed with these mycotoxins (Holladay et al., 1993). For ochratoxin, at least, the dose, the route of administration, and the species appear to be critical factors in results obtained in immunotoxicity studies. For the extensively studied tricothecenes, the mechanism of immunoimpairment may be related to inhibition of protein synthesis. The tricothecenes are currently considered among the most potent small-molecule inhibitors of protein synthesis in eukaryotic cells (IPCS, 1996).

Natural and Synthetic Hormones It is well established that a sexual dimorphism exists in the immune system. Females have higher levels of circulating immunoglobulins, a greater antibody response, and a higher incidences of autoimmune disease than do males. Males appear to be more susceptible to the development of sepsis and mortality associated with this following soft tissue trauma and hemorrhagic shock. Specific natural sex hormones in this dichotomy have been implicated. Immune effects of androgens and estrogens appear to be very tightly controlled within the physiologic range of concentrations, and profound changes in immune activity can result for very slight changes in concentrations of hormones.

Estrogens Diethylstilbestrol (DES) is a synthetic nonsteroidal compound possessing estrogenic activity. DES was used in men to treat prostatic cancer and in women to prevent threatened abortions, as an estrogen replacement, and as a contraceptive drug. Extensive functional and host resistance studies on DES (mg/kg/day range) have indicated that exposure to this chemical results in alterations in cell-mediated immunity and/or macrophage function and are believed to be mediated by the presence of the estrogen receptor on immune cells (Kalland, 1980; Luster et al., 1980, 1984a,b; Holsapple et al., 1983). Targeted sites of action include the thymus (thymic depletion, alteration in T-cell maturation process), T cells (decreased MLR, DTH, lymphoproliferative responses), and macrophage (enhanced phagocytic, anti-tumor, and suppressor function). Pre- and neonatal exposures (μg/kg/day dose range) have also demonstrated immunotoxic effects related to T-cell dysfunction. Delayed hypersensitivity and inflammatory responses associated with DES exposure in adult mice have been shown to be reversible upon cessation of exposure (Luster et al., 1980; Holsapple et al., 1983). However, effects from in utero and neonatal exposures appear to have more lasting, possibly permanent effects on immune responses (Luster et al., 1979; Kalland et al., 1979; Ways, 1980).

Exposure to 17β-estradiol in male rats (63 days of age) intraperitoneally for 15 days (1 to 50 μg/kg/day) did not alter spleen weight, spleen cellularity, or the humoral immune response to sRBC (Ladics et al., 1998). As observed with other estrogenic agents, thymic weight was decreased following exposure. Serum androgens and luteinizing hormone and male accessory organ weights were depressed, while serum estradiol and prolactin were increased. Dietary exposure (2.5 to 50 ppm) of male and female rats for 90 days resulted in decreased spleen weights and alterations in hematologic elements suggestive of bone marrow effects. Body weights were also affected. No histological alterations were noted. Decreases in splenic T- and B-cell populations were observed at the higher concentrations. These data suggest the possibility that exposure to 17β-estradiol may have resulted in altered normal immune cell trafficking and distribution, the mechanism of which is not clear. This hypothesis is supported by recent data indicating the observed anti-inflammatory effects of estrogens may be related to combination of alterations in homing and the activation of inflammatory cells and their production of TNF-α and IFN-γ (Salem et al., 2000).

While it appears that estrogens can affect the maturation and function of the thymus and its components, it has recently been observed that estrogen receptor knockout mice have significantly smaller thymi than do their wild-type littermates, apparently due to the lack of the estrogen receptor-alpha (ERα) (Staples et al., 1999). In addition, it has been suggested that the effects of estrogens on the thymus appear to be mediated not only through ERα but also through another pathway.

Androgens Oxymetholone is a synthetic androgen structurally related to testosterone and used in the past in the treatment of pituitary dwarfism and as an adjunctive therapy in osteoporosis. Its current use is limited to treatment of certain anemias. Oxymetholone was administered orally to male mice daily for 14 consecutive days (50 to 300 mg/kg/day). In male mice, oxymetholone exposure resulted in a minimal decrease in cell-mediated immunity (MLR and CTL response) but did not alter the ability of the animals to resist infection in host resistance assays. In contrast, anabolic androgenic steroids have been shown to significantly inhibit the sRBC PFC response and to increase the production of pro-inflammatory cytokines from human peripheral blood lymphocytes.

Exposure to flutamide, an androgen receptor antagonist, in male rats (63 days of age) intraperitoneally for 15 days (0.25 to 20 mg/kg/day) did not alter spleen weight or the humoral immune response to sRBC (Ladics et al., 1998). Relative thymic weight and total spleen cellularity were minimally increased. Serum androgens, estrogens, luteinizing hormone, and follicle-stimulating hormone were increased, while male accessory organ weights were depressed.

No comprehensive studies evaluating the effects of testosterone on immune parameters have been conducted. However, it is clear that testosterone is capable of contributing to the suppression of immune function—in particular, cell-mediated responses and macrophage activity. There are numerous reports in the clinical literature that males are more susceptible than females to infection following soft tissue trauma and hemorrhagic shock (reviewed in Catania and Chaudry, 1999). Treatment of males with agents that block testosterone (e.g., flutamide) can prevent the trauma- and hemorrhage-induced depression of immunity. Similarly, treatment of females with dihydrotestosterone prior to trauma-hemorrhage results in depression of CMI similar to that of males. Furthermore, gonadectomized mice of either sex have elevated immune responses to endotoxin, which can be attenuated in either sex by the administration of testosterone. The mechanisms in these cases, including influences of the neuroendocrine system, are not clear. Other investigators have reported that, like estrogenic agents, testosterone and other androgens are capable of influencing host defense by altering lymphocyte trafficking in the body and altering the ability of the macrophage to participate in immune responses.

Glucocorticoids The immunosuppressive actions of corticosteroids have been known for years. Following binding to an intracellular receptor, these agents produce profound lymphoid cell depletion in rodent models. In nonhuman primates and humans, lymphopenia associated with decreased monocytes and eosinophils and increased PMNs are seen. Corticosteroids induce apoptosis and T cells are particularly sensitive. In addition, these agents inhibit macrophage accessory cell function, the production of IL-1 from the macrophages, and the subsequent synthesis of IL-2 by T cells. In general, corticosteroids suppress the generation of CTL responses, MLR, NK activity, and lymphoproliferation. While it is clear that these drugs inhibit T-cell function, their effects on B cells are not completely clear. Corticosteroids inhibit humoral responses, but this appears to be due to effects on T cells, as antigen-specific antibody production by B cells to T-independent antigens does not appear to be affected by corticosteroid treatment.

Mifepristone (RU-486) is a potent competitive antagonist of both progesterone receptor and glucocorticoid type 1 receptor binding. While use of mifepristone has focused on termination of pregnancy, it may find use as a contraceptive, anti-cancer agent, or inducer of labor. No significant studies could be located examining the immunotoxicity of mifepristone. However, in studies utilizing this compound as a glucocorticoid type 1 receptor antagonist to demonstrate the role of corticosteroids in chemical-induced immunomodulation, some insights can be gleaned. Acute oral administration of mifepristone to mice at 100 mg/kg did elevate circulating levels of corticosterone, presumably by preventing binding to the type 1 glucocorticpoid receptor and thus altering the feedback loop. However, the chemical did not alter humoral immunity or the weights and cellularity of lymphoid organs. Similarly, no effects on thymic or splenocyte cellular subpopulations have been observed.

Therapeutic Agents Historically speaking, very few drugs used today as immunosuppressive agents were actually developed for that purpose. In fact, if one looks closely enough, nearly all therapeutic agents possess some degree of immunomodulatory activity (Descotes, 1986). The recent explosion of knowledge regarding the function and regulation of the immune system (at the cellular, biochemical, and molecular levels) has provided investigators with a relatively new avenue for specific drug development. The following discussion focuses on those drugs used primarily for modulating the immune system: the immunosuppressants (corticosteroids are considered above), AIDS therapeutics, and the recombinant cytokines. Extensive reviews of these drugs can be found elsewhere (Spreafico et al., 1985; Rosenthal and Kowolenko, 1994; Talmadge and Dean, 1994).

Immunosuppressive Drugs Originally developed as an antineoplastic agent, cyclophosphamide (Cytoxan, CYP) is the prototypical member of a class of drugs known as alkylating agents. Upon entering the cell, the inactive drug is cleaved into phosphoramide mustard, a powerful DNA alkylating agent that leads to blockade of cell replication. Clinically, CYP has found use in reducing symptoms of autoimmune disease and in the pretreatment of bone marrow transplant recipients. Experimentally, this drug is often used as a positive immunosuppressive control in immunotoxicology studies because it can suppress both humoral and cell-mediated immune responses. There appears to be preferential inhibition of B-cell responses, possibly due to decreased production and surface expression of immunoglobulins. CMI activities that are suppressed include the DHR, CTL, graft-versus-host (GVH) disease, and the MLR.

Azathioprine (AZA), one of the antimetabolite drugs, is a purine analog that is more potent than the prototype, 6-mercaptopurine, as an inhibitor of cell replication. Immunosuppression likely occurs because of the ability of the drug to inhibit purine biosynthesis. It has found widespread use in the inhibition of allograft rejection, although it is relatively ineffective in attenuating acute rejection reactions. It can also act as an anti-inflammatory drug and can reduce the number of PMNs and monocytes. Clinical use of the drug is limited by bone marrow suppression and leukopenia. AZA inhibits humoral immunity, but secondary responses (IgG) appear more sensitive than primary responses (IgM). A large range of CMI reactivities are also reduced by AZA treatment, including DHR, MLR, and GVH disease. Although T-cell functions are the primary targets for this drug, inhibition of NK function and macrophage activities has also been reported.

Cyclosporin A (Sandimmune, CsA) is a cyclic undecapeptide isolated from fungal organisms found in the soil. Important to its use as an immunosuppressant is the relative lack of secondary toxicity (e.g., myelotoxicity) at therapeutic concentrations (Calne et al., 1981). However, hepatotoxicity and nephrotoxicity are limiting side effects. CsA acts preferentially on T cells by inhibiting the biochemical signaling pathway emanating from the T-cell receptor (TCR). The result is inhibition of IL-2 gene transcription and subsequent inhibition of T-cell proliferation. More specifically, CsA interacts with the intracellular molecule cyclophillin, an intracellular protein with peptidyl proline isomerase activity (although this enzymatic activity probably has nothing to do with the immunosuppressive effect of CsA). The CsA–cyclophillin complex inhibits the serine/threonine phosphatase activity of a third molecule, calcineurin. Calcineurin is proposed to dephosphorylate the cytoplasmic subunit of NF-AT (nuclear factor of activated T cells) and allow the transport of NF-AT into the nucleus, where it can couple with nuclear components and induce the transcription of the IL-2 gene. Inhibition of calcineurin phosphatase activity by the CsA–cyclophillin complex then prevents nuclear translocation of NF-AT and the resulting IL-2 gene transcription.

FK506 is a cyclic macrolide which is structurally distinct from CsA, but which possesses a nearly identical mechanism of action. Like CsA, FK506 binds intracellularly to proteins with peptidyl proline isomerase activity, the most abundant of which is FK506 binding protein-12 (FKBP12). The FK506–FKBP12 complex also binds to and inhibits calcineurin activity, thereby inhibiting IL-2 gene transcription. Clinically, FK506 inhibits T-cell proliferation, lacks myelotoxicity (although, like CsA, it does cause nephrotoxicity), and induces transplantation tolerance. In addition, the minimum effective dose appears to be approximately tenfold lower than that of CsA.

Rapamycin (RAP) is also a cyclic macrolide which is structurally related to FK506. However, the mechanism by which it produces inhibition of proliferation is strikingly distinct. Unlike CsA and FK506, RAP does not inhibit TCR-dependent signaling events and IL-2 gene transcription. Rather, this compound inhibits IL-2–stimulated T-cell proliferation by blocking cell-cycle progression from late G_1 into S phase (Morice et al., 1993; Terada et al., 1993). Like FK506, RAP binds to the intracellular protein FKBP12. But this RAP–FKBP12 complex does not bind calcineurin. Moreover, until very recently, the actual target protein or proteins of this complex have remained elusive. Now it is clear that the RAP–FKBP12 complex binds to the mammalian target of rapamycin, mTOR (Sabers et al., 1995), also referred to as FRAP-1 and RAFT-1 (Brown et al., 1994; Sabatini et al., 1994). This protein, originally identified as two proteins (TOR-1 and TOR-2) in rapamycin-resistant yeast mutants (Kunz et al., 1993), has homology to the lipid kinase domain of the p110 catalytic subunit of phosphatidylinositol 3-kinase (PI3K, a biochemical signaling molecule) and VPS34 (a yeast PI3K). The function of the TOR proteins in cellular regulation (specifically cell-cycle progression) remains unknown at this time. Unlike both CsA and FK506, RAP does not appear to be nephrotoxic.

Leflunomide, an isoxazole derivative, is a relatively new drug that has shown promise as an immunosuppressive agent in the treatment of rheumatic disease and transplantation (Xiao et al., 1994). Experimentally, this agent can block the generation of allospecific antibodies, decrease the mononuclear infiltrate in grafts undergoing rejection, and reverse acute graft rejections. It has been found to be equal to or better than CsA in its ability to inhibit B cell–mediated autoimmune disease. Early mechanistic studies indicate that leflunomide can directly inhibit B-cell proliferation ($IC_{50} \leq 20$ μM), and this may account for the drug's ability to inhibit both T-cell–dependent and T-cell–independent specific antibody production. Leflunomide also can inhibit T-cell proliferation ($IC_{50} = 50$ to 75 μM) induced by mitogens or antibody directed against CD3 or IL-2. IL-2 production is also attenuated, but expression of the IL-2 receptor (CD25) is not altered. Biochemical analyses indicate that this drug can inhibit IL-2–dependent protein tyrosine kinase activity and suggest that the mechanism of T-cell inhibition may be at the level of T-cell responsiveness to IL-2. Although similar in broad terms, this mechanism of action is distinctly different from the mechanism of action of RAP.

Aids Therapeutics Traditionally, antiviral therapies have not been extremely successful in their attempt to rid the host of viral infection. This may be due to the fact that these organisms target the DNA of the host. Thus, eradication of the infection means killing infected cells. Although numerous strategies have been developed to combat the AIDS virus (primarily targeting viral reverse transcriptase or viral protease and up-regulation of other immune responses), no one drug has produced any significant advance. This is possibly because the very nature of the infection has significant immunosuppressive consequences. Without doubt, more basic scientific knowledge about the physiology and biochemistry of the virus is required before rational drug design will yield an effective therapeutic agent.

Zidovudine (3′-azido-3′-deoxythymidine; AZT) is a pyrimidine analog that inhibits viral reverse transcriptase. It was the first drug shown to have any clinical efficacy in the treatment of HIV-1 infection. Unfortunately, its use is limited by myelotoxicity (macrocytic anemia and granulocytopenia). Animal studies have confirmed that the primary action of AZT is on innate immunity, although changes in both humoral and cell-mediated immunity have also been observed. Clinically, AZT increases the number of circulating $CD4^+$ cells and can transiently stimulate cell-mediated immune responses (lymphoproliferation, NK activity, and IFN-γ production).

Stavudine (2′,3′-didehydro-2′,3′-dideoxythymidine; d4T) is another pyrimidine analog currently in clinical trials. Unlike its sister drug AZT, the limiting toxicity appears to be peripheral neuropathy rather than myelotoxicity. In addition, d4T also appears to increase the number of circulating $CD4^+$ cells. Animal studies suggest that d4T does not modulate generation of CTL, NK activity, PFC responses, mitogenicity of lymphocytes, or lymphocyte subsets.

Zalcitabine (2′,3′-dideoxycytidine; ddC) is a third pyrimidine analog which has recently been approved for use. Clinically, there appears to be an increase in circulating $CD4^+$ cells and some restoration of CMI in HIV-infected persons. There also appears to be no significant myelotoxicity and, like d4T, the limiting toxic effect of ddC is peripheral neuropathy. Investigations in animals revealed no significant effect on immune status.

Videx (2′,3′-dideoxyinosine; ddI) is the first purine analog approved for use in HIV infection. In clinical trials, the dose-limiting toxicities were shown to be peripheral neuropathy and pancreatitis. There appears to also be an increase in circulating $CD4^+$ cells, some restoration of CMI, and a reversal of HIV-induced myelotoxicity. Although ddI is converted into ddA-TP, the use of ddA as an antiviral agent was ruled out due to severe nephrotoxic effects. In animal models, both ddI and ddA produce suppression of humoral immunity.

Recombinant DNA–Derived Proteins The development of therapeutic proteins for clinical use is an ever expanding arena for both large and small pharmaceutical and biotechnology companies (reviewed in Warner and Haggerty, 1997). In general, biologics (e.g., blood or vaccine products) and recombinant DNA–derived proteins are derived in some manner from living organisms. Because of the very nature of many of the recombinant DNA–derived proteins, the immune system is often the target not only of therapy but also of toxicity. Manifestations of toxicity include exaggerated pharmacology, effects due to receptor-biochemical cross-talk, and disruptions in immune regulation by cytokine networks. Monoclonal antibodies can bind normal as well as targeted tissues, and any foreign protein may elicit the production of neutralizing antibodies against the therapeutic protein (i.e., the therapeutic protein may be immunogenic). The effects of neutralizing antibodies may also lead to hypersensitivity reactions via either IgE production or immune complex disease, resulting from the activation of the complement cascade and the subsequent release of vasoactive amines that produce anaphylaxis. The majority of recombinant DNA–derived proteins have been used as immunostimulants; these include IFN-α, IFN-γ, GM-CSF, and erythropoietin (EPO). Their immunopharmacology (and toxicity) has been reviewed extensively elsewhere (Talmadge and Dean, 1994). An excellent review of the toxicity associated with CTLA4Ig, anti-CD3, and anti-CD4 (for immunosuppression, transplantation, autoimmunity), and IL-12 (as a cancer therapeutic and an immuno-stimulant), along with other immune related issues in the development of therapeutic proteins is provided in Warner and Haggerty (1997).

Drugs of Abuse Drug abuse is a social issue with far-reaching effects on the abuser as well as on friends and family. While drug paraphernalia has been directly associated with the spread of the AIDS virus, in recent years the actual abuse of some drugs has been linked to the progression, and possibly the onset, of AIDS. Although definitive scientific proof of the hypothesis is lacking, drugs which are often abused have been shown to alter immunocompetence.

Cannabinoids Much attention has been focused on the immunomodulatory effects of the cannabinoids (Δ^9-tetrahydrocannabinol; THC) owing to the therapeutic potential of this drug in the treatment of glaucoma and as an antiemetic in patients undergoing cancer chemotherapy. Early studies showed that exposure to THC decreases host resistance to bacterial and viral pathogens (reviewed by Kaminski, 1994). In addition, cannabinoids alter both humoral and cell-mediated immune responses. Suppression of NK and CTL activity by THC appears to be related to an effect occurring subsequent to target-cell binding. THC exposure also alters macrophage morphology and some nonspecific functions, but the effects on accessory cell activities (e.g., antigen processing and presentation) are only beginning to be elucidated. Recently, it has been shown that THC increases aspartyl cathepsin D proteolytic activity and impairs lysosomal processing in the macrophage (Matveyeva et al., 2000). What is clear, however, is that the suppression of humoral immunity is exquisitely dependent upon the temporal association between exposure and antigen sensitization. Oral exposure to THC during the sensitization process (in vivo antigen administration) suppresses the PFC response to sRBC. In contrast, exposure to THC prior to sensitization (but not during the sensitization time) resulted in no observable effects on the PFC response. This may be one of the most critical factors influencing the reported effects of THC on immune responsiveness.

As in the in vivo situation, for in vitro THC exposure (Mishell-Dutton cultures), the drug must be added within 2 h of the addition of antigen in order to suppress the PFC response (Schatz et al., 1992). Also, humoral responses to T-cell–dependent antigens but not T-cell–independent antigens are suppressed by THC exposure. Together with the fact that T-cell proliferative responses are suppressed after THC exposure in vivo, this suggests that THC affects primarily T cells and may alter early T-cell activation events (e.g., biochemical signaling). Most recently, cannabinoid receptor transcripts have been identified in human spleen, tonsils, peripheral blood lymphocytes, and macrophages (Bouaboula et al., 1993; Munro et al., 1993). Additionally, murine splenocytes exhibit a high degree of saturable, specific binding of THC with a K_d approximating 1 nM and a B_{max} of about 1000 receptors per cell (Kaminski et al., 1992). An understanding of a potential role of this receptor in immune responses awaits identification of the endogenous ligand.

Cocaine Cocaine is a potent local anesthetic and central nervous system (CNS) stimulant. This drug and its derivatives have been shown to alter several measures of immunocompetence, including humoral and cell-mediated immune responses and host resistance (Watson et al., 1983; Ou et al., 1989; Starec et al., 1991). Functions of PMNs—including superoxide production and cell-surface receptor expression as well as inhibition of macrophage killing ability by decreasing the production of reactive oxygen intermediates—have been reported (Haines et al., 1990; Lefkowitz et al., 1993). Cocaine also induces the secretion of TGF-β, which has been linked to the observation that cocaine exposure enhances replication of the HIV-1 virus in human peripheral blood mononuclear cells (PBMC) (Chao et al., 1991; Peterson et al., 1991). Holsapple et al. (1993) evaluated the effect of in vitro cocaine exposure on the generation of an antibody response against sRBCs and found effects only at concentrations that were not clinically relevant (100 μM; lethal blood concentrations are estimated to be around 6 μM). These investigators postulated that the immunosuppressive effects of cocaine in vivo were mediated by P450-generated reactive intermediates; they subsequently demonstrated sex and strain differences in cocaine immunosuppressive activity, which correlated with well-characterized differences in metabolic capability in mice. Male B6C3F1 mice are more sensitive than females and DBA/2 females are more sensitive than B6C3F1 females.

Opioids: Heroin and Morphine Chronic morphine exposure has been associated with increased susceptibility to both bacterial and viral antigens (Arora et al., 1990; Chao et al., 1990), and it is clear that exposure to opioids can suppress immune responses. What is not clear, however, is whether this action is a direct effect of the drug on immune cells or an indirect effect resulting from drug-induced increases in circulating corticosteroids. Evaluation of the immunocompetence of heroin addicts revealed a decrease in total T cells and E-rosette capability (McDonough et al., 1980). In that study, treatment with naloxone reversed these effects, suggesting a role for an opioid receptor in mediating immune suppression.

LeVier and coworkers (1994) reported that chronic morphine exposure decreased serum C3, NK activity, total leukocyte counts, the PFC response to sRBC, and RES clearance. However, because many of these effects were not dose-related (i.e., the dose–response curve was flat), the investigators concluded that these effects were not receptor-mediated but were the result of increased circulating corticosteroids (which were significantly elevated in those animals). This conclusion is supported by the findings of other investigators as well (Pruett et al., 1992b). Morphine-induced suppression of macrophage phagocytosis and cytokine production has also been reported (Eisenstein et al., 1993; Tubaro et al., 1987; LeVier et al., 1993). In the study by LeVier and colleagues (1993), the glucocorticoid antagonist RU-486 was utilized to demonstrate that while suppression of hepatic macrophage function may be due in part to a receptor-mediated event, inhibition of splenic macrophage activity was wholly receptor-independent. A review by Giorgio and colleagues (1996) eloquently describes a likely hypothesis (involving neuroendocrine immunologic mechanisms) for the dual effects observed with opioids as well as a few other compounds with similar effects.

Ethanol Until recently (reviewed by Jerrells and Pruett, 1994), data concerning the immunomodulatory effects of ethanol (EtOH) exposure have largely been based on clinical observations of alcoholic patients. A prime reason for this is that rodents (the animal model of choice for extensive immunologic evaluation) do not voluntarily consume intoxicating quantities of EtOH. Thus, the criteria for the development of animal models for EtOH exposure need to be refined to assure that clinically relevant blood levels are attained and long-term exposure can be assessed. In addition, the effect of acute exposure (binge drinking) needs to be further assessed.

In humans, alcoholism is associated with an increased incidence of pulmonary infection and mortality from it. There is also an increased incidence of bacterial infection and spontaneous bacteremia in alcoholics with cirrhosis of the liver. A consistent finding in abusers of EtOH is the significant change in the mononuclear cells of the peripheral blood. In animal models, this is observed as depletion of T and B cells in the spleen and the T cells in the thymus, particularly $CD4^+/CD8^+$ cells. The latter effect may be related in part to increased levels of corticosteroids.

There are also numerous indications that acute EtOH exposure can have profound immunodepressive consequences: decreased PMN chemotaxis, decreased host resistance, and inhibition of the PFC response. EtOH administration also inhibits mitogen-driven T-cell proliferation and T-cell responsiveness to IL-2. The actions of EtOH exposure on B-cell antibody production and NK-cell activity are still controversial.

Electromagnetic Fields Several epidemiologic studies have suggested an association (albeit very small) between low-frequency (LF) (<300 Hz) electromagnetic fields (EMF) and cancer. Other epidemiologic studies have found no association. In response to growing concern over the effects of LF EMF (<300 Hz) on human health, many studies have been conducted to assess their ability to alter immunocompetence. While some studies, using in vitro exposures of animal or human immune cells, have shown mixed results, a comprehensive evaluation of immunocompetence in mice (using the NTP tier approach) has demonstrated that exposure to LF EMF (60 Hz) for 28 or 90 days does not alter immunocompetence (House et al., 1996).

Ultraviolet Radiation The immunomodulatory effects of ultraviolet radiation (UVR) have been reviewed (IPCS, 1996). UVR has been demonstrated to suppress delayed hypersensitivity responses in both animals and humans and to result in decreased host resistance to infection. The dose of UVR required to suppress the immune response depends on the strain of mouse and the antigen being used. Interestingly, however, it appears that the dose of UVR is not as important to the observed immunosuppression as is the interval between irradiation and antigen exposure (Noonan and De Fabo, 1990). The mechanism of immunosuppression by UVR is not completely clear. Induction of suppressor T cells or alterations in homing patterns have been suggested as possibilities. One plausible explanation is that UVR induces a switch from a predominantly Th1 response (favoring delayed hypersensitivity responses) to a Th2 response (favoring antibody responses). This hypothesis is supported by findings of altered cytokine secretion patterns indicative of a Th1 to Th2 switch (Araneo et al., 1989; Simon et al., 1990). This switch may explain decreased resistance to some infectious pathogens. It may also be related to effects of UVR on Langerhans cells in the skin.

Food Additives Thirty-five food flavoring ingredients (generally recognized as safe) have been screened for potential immunotoxicity. Compounds were administered to mice by oral gavage for 5 consecutive days at multiple dose levels (Gaworski et al., 1994). In addition to body weights, lymphoid organ weights, and cellularity, humoral immunity (sRBC PFC response) and host resistance to *L. monocytogenes* were evaluated. Only two materials gave results suggestive of enhanced susceptibility to infection (peppermint oil and citral dimethyl acetal). Only one material exhibited suppression of humoral immunity (hexanoic acid), and suppression was observed only in the presence of overt toxicity.

Silicon-Based Materials Silicon-based materials have known uses in consumer products such as cosmetics, toiletries, food stuffs, household products, and paints as well as in the medical field (e.g., as lubricants in tubing and syringes and as components in numerous implantable devices). In recent years, significant interest has focused on the biocompatibility of certain silicon-based materials (silicones) and the potential for these products to produce immunotoxic effects. Despite the fact that there has been persistent, unsubstantiated speculation that breast implants made with silicone materials may provoke connective tissue disease, no link between exposure to silicones and human disease has been established. Recently, a committee formed by the Institute of Medicine has concluded that "a review of the toxicology studies of silicones and other substances known to be in breast implant does not provide a basis for health concerns." An extensive report by the IOM Committee, including additional conclusions and recommendations for research, is publicly available (IOM, 2000).

Numerous studies have been conducted that both support and refute the specific actions of various silicon-based materials on the immune system. Two studies have been reported that extensively evaluated immune status following exposure to dimethylpolysiloxanes used in medical practice (Bradley et al., 1944a,b). In the first study, mice were implanted for 10 days with dimethylpolysiloxane fluid, gel, and elastomer as well as polyurethane as a control. There were no observable alterations in innate or acquired immune function. In fact, the materials tested afforded modest protection to an approximate LD_{50} challenge with *L. monocytogenes*. Implantation of the same materials for 180 days resulted in a modest suppression of NK-cell activity that did not correlate with altered susceptibility to challenge with B16F10 melanoma. No alterations in host resistance have been observed.

Studies have also been conducted on two-low molecular-weight cyclic siloxanes: octamethylcyclotetrasiloxane and decamethylcyclotetrasiloxane. One-month inhalation exposures of rats to high concentrations of octamethylcyclotetrasiloxane (up to 540 ppm) and decamethylcyclotetrasiloxane (up to a maximum 160 ppm) did not result in alterations in humoral immunity (Burns-Naas et al., 1998; Klykken et al., 1999). Inhalation exposure of human volunteers to octamethylcyclotetrasiloxane at 10 ppm for 1 h revealed no effects on several immune parameters (Looney et al., 1998). Repeated oral exposure of rodents to octamethylcyclotetrasiloxane at high concentrations has been observed to produce immunomodulatory activity in both humoral and innate immunity; however, as with other chemicals, there are concentrations below which no immunomodulation is observed (LeVier et al., 1995; Wilson et al., 1995; Le and Munson, 1997; Munson et al., 1997; Munson, 1998).

Finally, under highly specific experimental conditions that do *not* mimic human exposure, a few silicon-based materials have been observed to act as immunologic adjuvants (reviewed in Potter and Rose, 1996, and IOM, 2000; Woolhiser et al., 1995). Under typical exposure conditions, neither octamethylcyclotetrasiloxane, a combination of octamethylcyclotetrasiloxane and decamethylcyclotetrasiloxane, nor dimethylpolysiloxane acts as an immunologic adjuvant (Bradley et al., 1994a,b; Klykken and White, 1996; Klykken et al., 1999; Vohr and Bomhard, 2000).

Immune-Mediated Disease

As stated earlier, the purpose of the immune system is to protect the individual from disease states, whether infectious, parasitic, or cancerous—through both cellular and humoral mechanisms. In so doing, the ability to distinguish "self" from "nonself" plays a predominant role. However, situations arise in which the individual's immune system responds in a manner producing tissue damage, resulting in a self-induced disease. These disease states fall into two categories (1) hypersensitivity, or allergy, and (2) autoimmunity. Figure 12-16 is a schematic delineating the possible cascade of effects that can occur when a chemical produces an immune-mediated disease. Hypersensitivity reactions result from the immune system responding in an exaggerated or inappropriate manner. These reactions have been subdivided by Coombs and Gell (1975) into four types, which represent four different mechanisms leading to tissue damage. In the case of autoimmunity, mechanisms of self-recognition break down and immunoglobulins and T-cell receptors react with self-antigens, resulting in tissue damage and disease.

Hypersensitivity ***Classification of Hypersensitivity Reactions*** One characteristic common to all four types of hypersensitivity reactions is the necessity of prior exposure leading to sensitization in order to elicit a reaction upon subsequent challenge. In the case of types I, II and III, prior exposure to antigen leads to the production of specific antibody, IgE, IgM, or IgG, and, in the case of type IV, to the generation of memory T cells. Figure 12-17 illustrates the mechanisms of hypersensitivity reactions as classified by Coombs and Gell. Although not completely understood, regulation of immunoglobulin production is dependent in part on the characteristics of the antigen, the genetics of the individual, and environmental factors. The mechanisms of antibody production in hypersensitivity reactions are identical to those described earlier in the chapter (Fig. 12-7). A brief description of the four types of hypersensitivity reactions is presented below.

Type I (Immediate Hypersensitivity) Using penicillin as an example, Fig. 12-18 depicts the major events involved in a type I hypersensitivity reaction. Sensitization occurs as the result of exposure to appropriate antigens through the respiratory tract, dermally, or by exposure through the gastrointestinal tract. IgE production is highest in lymphatic tissues that drain sites of exposure (i.e., tonsils, bronchial lymph nodes, and intestinal lymphatic tissues, including Peyer's patches). It is low in the spleen. Serum concentration of IgE is low compared to other immunoglobulins, and serum half-life is short (Table 12-4). Once produced, IgE binds to local tissue mast cells before entering the circulation, where it binds to circulating mast cells, basophils, and tissue mast cells at distant sites. Once an individual is sensitized, reexposure to the antigen results in degranulation of the mast cells with the release of preformed mediators and cytokines typical of Th2 cells. Synthesis of leukotrienes and thromboxanes is also induced. These mediators

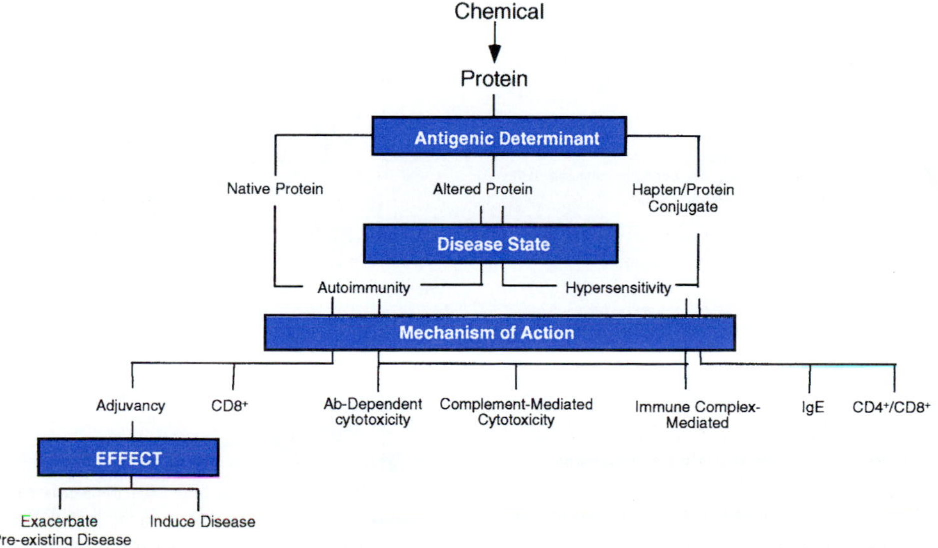

Figure 12-16. Schematic diagram of chemical interaction leading to hypersensitivity reactions or autoimmunity.

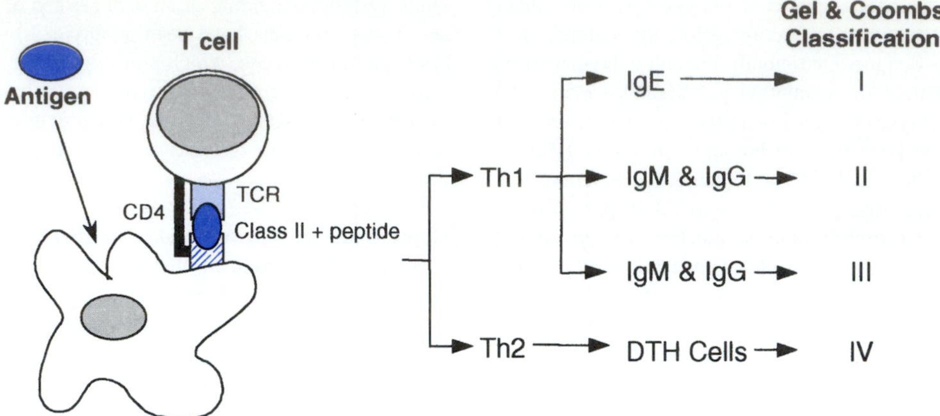

Figure 12-17. Schematic of classification of hypersensitivity reactions.

promote vasodilation, bronchial constriction, and inflammation. Clinical manifestations can vary from urticarial skin reactions (wheals and flares) to signs of hay fever, including rhinitis and conjuctivitis, to more serious diseases, such as asthma and potentially life-threatening anaphylaxis. These responses may begin within minutes of reexposure to the offending antigen; therefore, type I hypersensitivity is often referred to as *immediate hypersensitivity.*

Type II (Antibody-Dependent Cytotoxic Hypersensitivity) Type II hypersensitivity is IgG-mediated. Figure 12-19 shows the mechanisms of action of a complement-independent cytotoxic reaction and complement-dependent lysis. Tissue damage may result from the direct action of cytotoxic cells—such as macrophages, neutrophils, or eosinophils—linked to immunoglobulin-coated target cells through the Fc receptor on the antibody or by antibody activation of the classic complement pathway. Complement activation may result in C3b or C3d binding to the target cell surface. This acts as a recognition site for effector cells. Alternatively, the C5b-9 membrane attack complex may be bound to the target cell surface, resulting in cell lysis (Fig. 12-3).

Type III (Immune Complex–Mediated Hypersensitivity) Type III hypersensitivity reactions also involve IgG immunoglobulins. The distinguishing feature of type III is that, unlike type II, in which immunoglobulin production is against specific tissue-associated antigen, immunoglobulin production is against soluble antigen in the serum (Fig. 12-20). This allows for the formation of circulating immune complexes composed of a lattice of antigen and immunoglobulin, which may result in widely distributed tissue damage in areas where immune complexes are deposited. The most common location is the vascular endothelium in the lung, joints, and kidneys. The skin and circulatory systems may also be involved. Pathology results from the inflammatory response initiated by the activation of complement. Macrophages, neutrophils, and platelets attracted to the deposition site contribute to the tissue damage.

Type IV (Cell-Mediated Hypersensitivity) Type IV, or delayed-type hypersensitivity (DTH) responses, can be divided into two classes: contact hypersensitivity and tuberculin-type hypersensitivity. Contact hypersensitivity is initiated by topical exposure, and the associated pathology is primarily epidermal. It is charac-

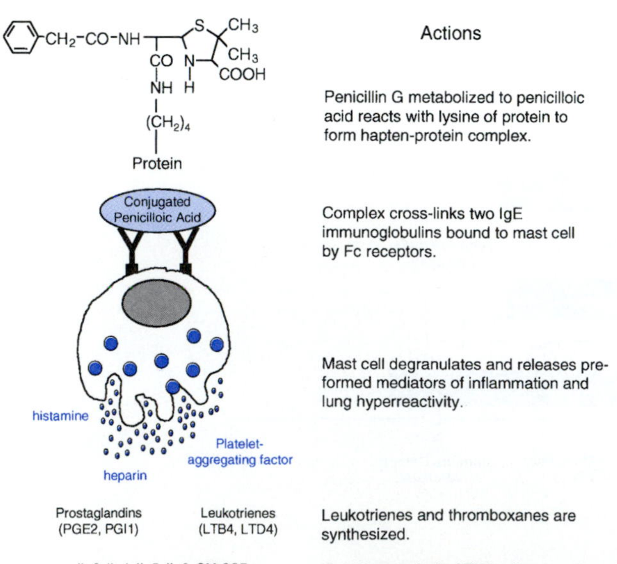

Figure 12-18. Schematic of type I hypersensitivity reaction.

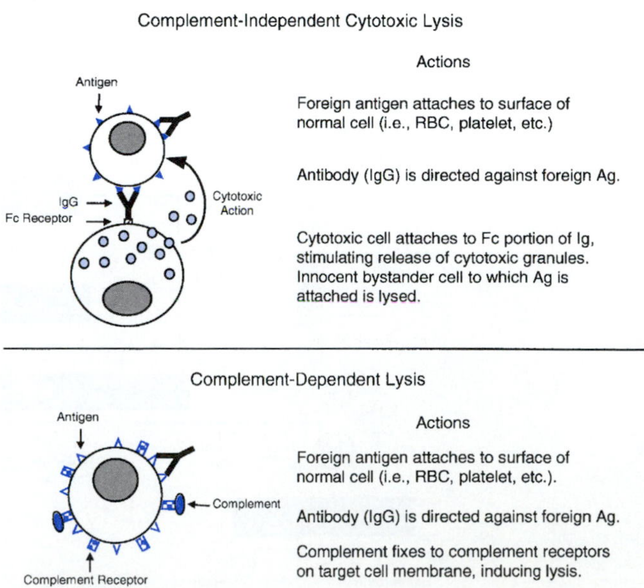

Figure 12-19. Schematic of type II hypersensitivity reactions.

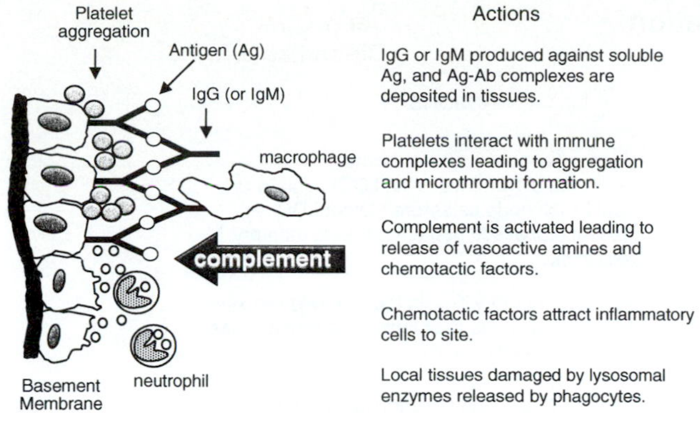

Figure 12-20. Schematic of type III hypersensitivity reaction.

terized clinically by an eczematous reaction at the site of allergen contact and, like type I through III responses, consists of two phases: sensitization and elicitation. However, in this case sensitization is the result of the development of activated and memory T cells as opposed to antibody production (Figs. 12-21 and 12-22). Sensitization occurs when the hapten penetrates the epidermis and forms a complex with a protein carrier. The hapten–carrier complex is processed by Langerhans-dendritic cells that migrate out of the epidermis to the local lymph nodes. There, the APC presents the processed antigen to $CD4^+$ T cells, leading to clonal expansion and the generation of memory T cells.

Upon second contact, Langerhans-dendritic cells present the processed hapten–carrier complex to memory T cells in either the skin or the lymph nodes. These activated T cells then secrete cytokines that bring about further proliferation of T cells and induce the expression of adhesion molecules on the surface of keratinocytes and endothelial cells in the dermis. Both the expression of adhesion molecules and the secretion of proinflammatory cytokines by T cells and keratinocytes facilitate the movement of inflammatory cells into the skin, resulting in erythema and the formation of papules and vesicles. $CD8^+$ cells may play a role in tissue damage. In cases where chemicals are lipid-soluble and can therefore readily cross the cell membrane, they can modify intracellular proteins. These cells then present modified peptides on their cell surface in conjunction with MCH class I molecules. $CD8^+$ cells recognize these foreign peptides and cause tissue damage by either direct cytotoxic action or the secretion of cytokines that further promote the inflammatory response. The description given above has been the accepted dogma for the mechanism of delayed hypersensitivity for years. This is currently an area of intense research; a developing hypothesis for the elicitation phase of contact hypersensitivity involves a greater role for a non-specific inflammatory signal, $CD8^+$ cells, and APCs other than Langerhans cells (Grabbe and Schwarz, 1998).

Tuberculin-type hypersensitivity is primarily a dermal reaction and begins following the intradermal injection of a specific antigen to which the individual has been previously exposed (such as a microbial antigen). Within hours, a cellular infiltrate (primarily $CD4^+$ T cells) begins to appear. This infiltration continues as macrophages and Langerhans-dendritic cells begin to migrate into the area of injection. Circulation of immune cells to and from the local lymph nodes is thought to be like that in contact hypersensitivity. Also, like the contact hypersensitivity response, $CD4^+$ T cells then secrete lymphokines that cause the expression of MHC class II on the surfaces of macrophages and keratinocytes. The result is activation of these cells, the release of proinflammatory mediators, and the generation of an area of firm red swelling in the dermal tissue.

Separation of hypersensitivity responses into the types I to IV as in the classification of Coombs and Gell is helpful in understanding mechanisms involved. It is important, however, to realize that this is a simplification and that often pathology is the result of a combination of these mechanisms. In addition, associated inflammation may be a non-immune acute response and/or the result of an immune-mediated event. For example, if one looks at the pathophysiology of respiratory disease induced by the acid anhy-

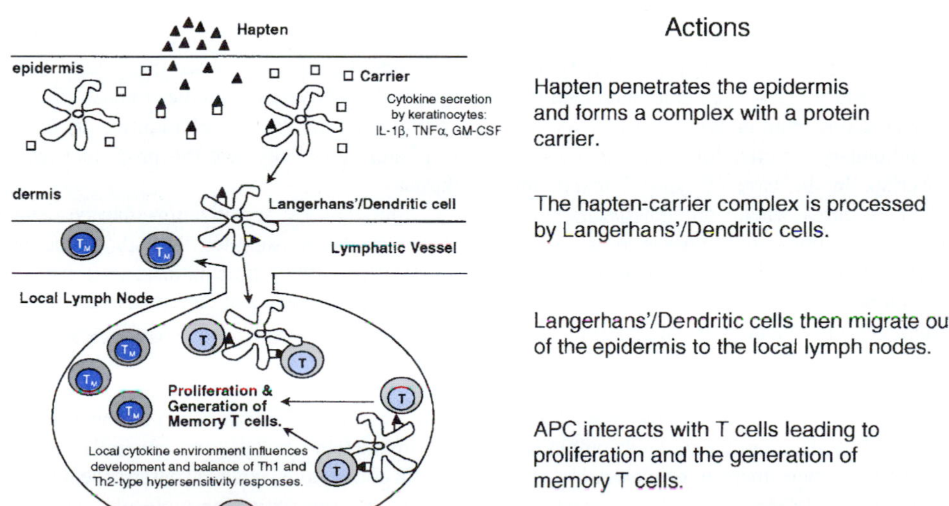

Figure 12-21. Schematic of sensitization phase of type IV hypersensitivity reaction.

Elicitation

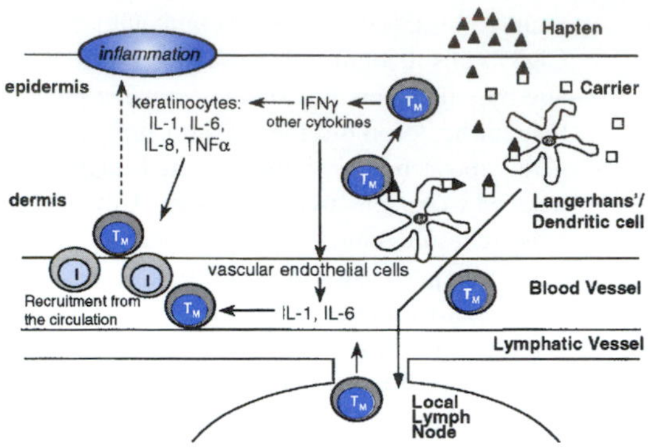

Actions

Upon subsequent contact, some Langerhans'/Dendritic cells (LDC) migrate to local lymph node as before. Other LDC can present processed hapten-carrier to memory T cells in skin.

Activated memory T cells then secrete cytokines which induce release of inflammatory cytokines from other cell types.

Memory T cells and inflammatory cells are recruited from the circulation via local chemoattractant cytokines and expression of adhesion molecules.

These cells migrate to the epidermis and elicit the characteristic local inflammatory response.

Figure 12-22. Schematic of elicitation phase of type IV hypersensitivity reaction.

drides, a mixture of immune and nonimmune events is found to be important. Direct toxic effects of the chemicals may lead to bronchial epithelial damage, causing cells to release cytokines that induce a nonimmune inflammatory response. Damage to epithelial cells may also expose underlying lamina propia, allowing the chemical to exert direct effects on inflammatory cells and to stimulate sensory vagal afferents, leading to reflex bronchoconstriction and hyperresponsiveness. Along with these non-immune mechanisms, all four classes of immune-mediated hypersensitivity responses to acid anhydrides have been shown to occur (Bernstein and Bernstein, 1994).

Assessment of Hypersensitivity Responses One of the most important and challenging problems in the field of immunotoxicology is determining the potential for chemicals to induce immunomodulation and, in the current context, to promote hypersensitivity reactions. Thus, it becomes essential to have validated predictive animal models and to understand the underlying mechanisms of action. The following is a review of the currently used methods of predicting types I and IV, the most frequently occurring hypersensitivity reactions to chemicals.

Assessment of Respiratory Hypersensitivity in Experimental Animals Methods for detecting pulmonary hypersensitivity have been reviewed by Sarlo and Karol (1994) and can be divided into two types: (1) those for detecting immunologic sensitization and (2) those for detecting pulmonary sensitization. In some cases the methodologies may overlap. In the case of types I to III, immunologic sensitization occurs when antigen-specific immunoglobulin is produced in response to exposure to an antigen or, in the case of type IV, when a population of sensitized T lymphocytes is produced. Pulmonary sensitization is determined by a change in respiratory function subsequent to the challenge of a sensitized animal or patient. In certain cases, immunologic sensitization may be confirmed by the detection of antigen-specific antibody; however, subsequent challenge does not produce clinical signs of respiratory distress. It is also possible to detect pulmonary sensitization in animal models where there is no detectable antigen-specific antibody production. In these cases, cell-mediated or other mechanisms may be involved or there may be a difficulty in antibody detection.

Guinea pig models have been most frequently used for detection of pulmonary reactions to chemicals. In the guinea pig, as in the human, the lung is the major shock organ for anaphylactic response. Like humans, the guinea pig also demonstrates immediate- and late-onset allergic reactions as well as bronchial hyperreactivity. The major difference in the mechanism of pulmonary responses between humans and guinea pigs is that the antibody involved in type I reactions in the former is IgE and in the latter is predominantly IgG1. Murine models are becoming more frequently utilized in the evaluation of respiratory hypersensitivity. As in the human, IgE is a major anaphylactogenic antibody in the mouse, and more murine immunologic reagents are available, allowing for more detailed mechanistic studies.

Methods utilized for respiratory exposure to chemicals are inhalation or either intranasal or intratracheal administration. There are advantages and disadvantages to each. Inhalation more closely represents environmental exposure by allowing for chemical contact with the upper as well as the lower respiratory tract. However, the equipment required is expensive and difficult to maintain. Exposure via the intranasal route is easily accomplished and allows for distribution of antigen to the upper and lower respiratory tract; however, studies have shown that a large proportion of the material can be recovered from the stomach (Robinson et al., 1996). In contrast, intratracheal instillation results in exposure to the lower respiratory tract only, and this procedure requires the use of anesthesia.

Immunologic sensitization may be determined by obtaining sequential blood samples throughout the induction period and measuring antibody titer. Pulmonary sensitization is evaluated by detecting the presence of pulmonary reactivity following challenge. This may be accomplished by visual inspection of the animals' respiratory pattern or more quantitatively by plethysmography. With plethysmography, changes in the respiratory rate, tidal volume, and plethysmographic pressure can be measured.

Inhalation models are generally used for low-molecular-weight compounds, whereas intratracheal and intranasal models are frequently used with high-molecular-weight compounds. One of the drawbacks of low-molecular-weight models is that often these compounds must conjugate with body proteins to become antigenic. Often, a challenge with the conjugated chemical is necessary to induce a pulmonary response. Adding this variable can make the analysis of test results more difficult. False negative results may occur due to variability in test article conjugation. Chemical conjugates are also necessary to measure immunologic response.

Assessment of IgE-Mediated Hypersensitivity Responses in Humans Described below are methods of human type I hypersensitivity testing. These test results, in conjunction with a relevant history and physical exam, can be diagnostic of IgE-mediated pulmonary disease. Two skin tests are available for immediate hypersensitivity testing. In both, the measured endpoint is a "wheal and flare" reaction—is the result of edema and erythema subsequent to the release of preformed mediators. The prick-puncture test introduces very small amounts of antigen under the skin and, owing to the reduced chance of systemic reaction, is recommended as a screening test. For test compounds not eliciting a reaction in the less sensitive test, the intradermal test using dilute concentrations of antigen may be used, but there is a higher risk of systemic reactions. For a more detailed description of testing methods see Demoly et al. 1998.

In vitro serologic tests, enzyme-linked immunosorbent assays (ELISAs), and radioallergosorbent tests (RASTs) may also be used to detect the presence of antigen-specific antibody in the patient's serum. These tests do not pose a risk of adverse reactions and may be used in situations where standardized reagents for skin testing are not available. Serologic testing is often used in population-based epidemiologic studies.

Bronchial provocation tests may be performed by having the patient inhale an antigen into the bronchial tree and evaluating his or her pulmonary response. In some cases this may be the only way to demonstrate that a test article is capable of producing an asthmatic response. Care must be taken in these test situations in that it is possible to produce severe asthmatic reactions or anaphylaxis in sensitized individuals.

Assessment of Contact Hypersensitivity in Experimental Animals Classically, the potential for a chemical to produce contact hypersensitivity has been assessed by the use of guinea pig models. These tests vary in their method of application of the test article, in the dosing schedule, and in the utilization of adjuvants. For a description of methods employed in representative tests, see Klecak (1987). The two most commonly utilized guinea pig models, the Büehler test (Büehler, 1965) and the guinea pig maximization test (Magnusson and Kligman, 1969), are described briefly below. In the Büehler test, the test article is applied to the shaven flank and covered with an occlusive bandage for 6 h. This procedure is repeated on days 7 and 14. On day 28, a challenge dose of the test article is applied to a shaven area on the opposite flank and covered with an occlusive dressing for 24 h. At 24 and 48 h after the patch is removed, test animals are compared with vehicle-treated controls for signs of edema and erythema. The guinea pig maximization test differs in that the test article is administered by intradermal injection, an adjuvant is employed, and irritating concentrations are used. Animals are given pairs of intradermal injections at a shaven area on the shoulders. One pair of injections contains adjuvant alone, one pair contains test article alone, and one pair contains the test article mixed with adjuvant. Seven days following injection, after the area is reshaven, the test article is applied topically and an occluded patch is applied for 48 h. In cases where the test article at the given concentration is nonirritating, the area is pretreated with 10% sodium lauryl sulfate 24 h before the patch is applied to produce a mild inflammatory response. Two weeks following topical application, the animals are challenged on the shaven flank with a non-irritating concentration of the test article, which remains under an occluded patch for 24 h. Then, after 24 and 48 h, the test site is examined for signs of erythema and edema. The endpoints for evaluation in the guinea pig assays are subjective and it is difficult to assess irritating or colored compounds using these models.

Over the past 15 years, efforts have been made to develop and validate more quantitative and immunologically based assay methods in other species, focusing mainly on the mouse and in vitro systems. Gad and coworkers (1986) developed the mouse ear-swelling test, which uses a quantitative measurement of ear thickness as an endpoint. Animals are sensitized by topical application of the test article for 4 consecutive days to abdominal skin that has been prepared by intradermal injection of adjuvant and tape stripping. On day 10, the animals are challenged by topical application of the test article to one ear and vehicle to the contralateral ear. Measurements are made of ear thickness 24 and 48 h later. A positive response is considered anything above a 20 percent increase in thickness of the treated ear over the control ear. Thorne and colleagues (1991) showed that dietary supplementation with vitamin A enhanced the mouse ear-swelling assay in the absence of adjuvants, injections, or occlusive patches.

The assays described above evaluate the elicitation phase of the response in previously sensitized animals. The mouse local lymph node assay has recently undergone peer review coordinated by the Interagency Coordinating Committee on the Validation of Alternative Methods and has been accepted by government agencies as a stand-alone alternative to the guinea pig assays for use in hazard identification of chemical sensitizers. In this assay, the induction phase of contact sensitization is measured by the incorporation of ^{3}H-thymidine into proliferating lymphocytes in lymph nodes draining the site where the test article has been applied. Animals are dosed by topical application of the test article to the ears for 3 consecutive days. The animals are rested for 2 days and then injected intravenously with 20 μCi of ^{3}H-thymidine. Five hours later, animals are sacrificed, the draining lymph nodes are dissected out, and single-cell suspensions are made and radioassayed. With consideration of dose response and statistical significance, a threefold increase in ^{3}H-thymidine counts in chemically exposed animals over vehicle control animals is considered to be a positive response. This assay offers several advantages over the guinea pig assays in that (1) has the potential to reduce the number of animals required and reduces animal distress; (2) it provides quantitative data that allow for statistical analysis; (3) and it provides dose–response data. Additionally, the assay evaluates the induction phase of the immune response, making it more applicable to mechanistic studies (NIH publication no. 99-44940). As an example, some compounds capable of producing contact sensitization also induce IgE production and subsequent respiratory hypersensitivity. Using three known allergenic diisocyanates—diphenylmethane-4,4′,-diisocyanate (MDI); dicyclohexylmethane-4,4′-diisocyanate (HMDI); and isophorone diisocyanate (IPDI)—Dearman and coworkers (1992) showed that all three known contact sensitizers induced lymphocyte proliferation in the draining lymph node but that only MDI, a known respiratory sensitizer, induced elevated levels of serum IgE and IgG2b. Attempts have been made to correlate cytokine levels produced by draining lymph node cells with contact and respiratory sensitizing potential.

Antigens, once processed, are presented on the surface of the APC in conjunction with the MHC II antigen. Activation of either

Th1 or Th2 cells stimulates the production of cytokines, which are instrumental in driving the system toward immunoglobulin production or the activation and proliferation of sensitized T cells (delayed-type hypersensitivity). The specific cytokines involved are shown in Fig. 12-23. IL-2, TNF-β, and IFN-γ are produced by Th1 cells and lead to the development of delayed-type hypersensitivity, whereas IL-4, IL-5, IL-6, IL-10, and IL-13 are produced by Th2 cells and lead to the production of IgE (Mosmann et al., 1991). IFN-γ not only promotes the induction of delayed hypersensitivity but also appears to have an inhibitory effect on IgE production (Mosmann and Coffman, 1989). Likewise, IL-10, which promotes IgE production, inhibits the delayed-type hypersensitivity response (Enk et al., 1993; Schwarz et al., 1994). Dearman and Kimber (1999) have demonstrated an elevation in INF-γ but little IL-4 or IL-10 production in draining lymph nodes of animals exposed to contact allergens and, conversely, elevated production of IL-4 or IL-10 and little INF-γ following exposure to chemical respiratory allergens. Measurement of cytokine levels may prove to be an important predictive tool for assessing the potential of chemicals to elicit hypersensitivity reactions.

Assessment of Contact Hypersensitivity in Humans Human testing for contact hypersensitivity reactions is by skin patch testing. Patch testing allows for the diagnostic production of acute lesions of contact hypersensitivity by the application of a suspected allergen to the skin. Patches containing specified concentrations of the allergen in the appropriate vehicle are applied under an occlusive patch for 48 h in most test protocols. Once the patch is removed and enough time elapses for the signs of mechanical irritation to resolve—approximately 30 min—the area is read for signs of erythema, papules, vesicles, and edema. Generally, the test is read again at 72 h and in some cases signs may not appear for up to 1 week or more. For more detailed information on patch testing, the reader is referred to Mydlarski et al. (1998).

Human repeat insult patch tests (HRIPT) are available as predictive tests in humans. Like predictive testing in animal models, there are many variations in attempts to increase the sensitivity of these procedures. These include preparation of the induction site by either stripping, the application of an irritating concentration of sodium lauryl sulfate, or use of high concentrations of the test article for induction of sensitization. In general, the application of multiple occlusive patches, up to ten for 48 h each at the same site, is followed by a rest period and then challenge under an occlusive patch at a different site. Positive reactions are scored in the same manner as for diagnostic patch tests.

Hypersensitivity Reactions to Xenobiotics *Polyisocyanates* Polyisocyanates have a widespread use in industry and are responsible for more cases of occupationally related lung disease than any other class of low-molecular-weight (LMW) compounds. These chemicals are used in the production of adhesives, paint hardeners, elastomers, and coatings. Occupational exposure is by inhalation and skin contact. Members of the group are known to induce the full spectrum of hypersensitivity responses, types I to IV, as well as nonimmune inflammatory and neuroreflex reactions in the lung (Bernstein and Bernstein, 1994; Grammer, 1985). Sensitized individuals have shown cross-reactivity between compounds in this group.

Toluene diisocyanate (TDI) is among the most widely used and most studied members of this group. Pulmonary sensitization to this compound can occur through either topical or inhalation exposure. It is a highly reactive compound that readily conjugates with endogenous protein. Laminin, a 70,000-kDa protein, has been identified as the protein that TDI conjugates in the airways. Studies with guinea pigs have confirmed the need for a threshold level of exposure to be reached in order to obtain pulmonary sensitization. This finding supports the human data in which pulmonary sensitization is frequently the result of exposure to a spill, whereas workers exposed to low levels of vapors for long periods of time fail to develop pulmonary sensitization. Unlike the case in many hypersensitivity reactions, where removal of the antigen alleviates the symptoms of disease, symptoms may persist for as long as years after cessation of exposure in many TDI-induced asthma patients.

Acid Anhydrides The acid anhydrides make up another group of compounds for which nonimmune and IgE, cytotoxic, immune complex, and cell-mediated reactions have been reported (Bernstein and Bernstein, 1994; Grammer, 1985). These reactive organic compounds are used in the manufacturing of paints, varnishes, coating materials, adhesives, and casting and sealing materials. Trimellitic acid anhydride (TMA) is one of the most widely used compounds in this group. Inhaled TMA fumes may conjugate with serum albumin or erythrocytes leading, to type I (TMA-asthma), type II (pulmonary disease–anemia), or type III (hypersensitivity pneumonitis) hypersensitivity reactions upon subsequent exposure. Topical exposure to TMA may lead to type IV hypersensitivity reactions, resulting in contact dermatitis. Also, reexposure by inhalation may lead to a cell-mediated immune response in the lung, which plays a role in the pathology seen in conjunction with type II and III pulmonary disease. Human and animal testing has supported the clinical findings in TMA-exposed workers. Levels of serum IgE can be measured in exposed workers and are predictive of the occurrence of type I pulmonary reactions. Serum titers of IgA, IgG, and IgM have been detected in patients with high levels of exposure to TMA. Similar findings have been reported in studies with rhesus monkeys, in which exposed animals showed IgA, IgG, and IgM titers to TMA-haptenized erythrocytes. Inhalation studies with rats have produced a model corresponding to human TMA-induced pulmonary pneumonitis. Other anhydrides known to induce immune-mediated pulmonary disease

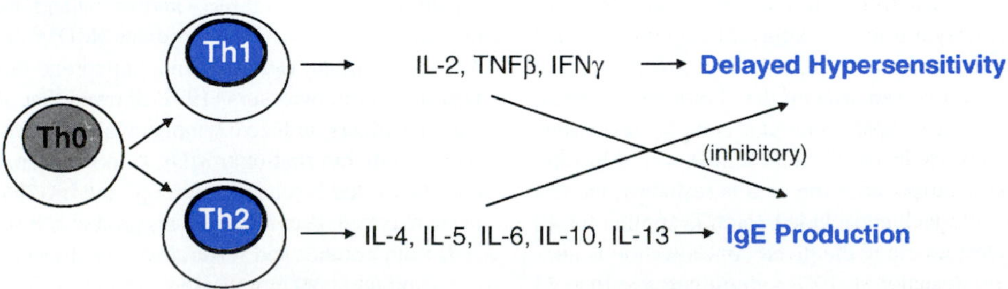

Figure 12-23. Schematic of cytokines involved in hypersensitivity reactions.

include phthalic anhydride, himic anhydride, and hexahydrophthalic anhydride.

Metals Metals and metallic substances, including metallic salts, are responsible for producing contact and pulmonary hypersensitivity reactions. Metallic salts have been implicated in numerous immunologic and nonimmunologic pulmonary diseases. Exposure to these compounds may occur via inhalation or due to their solubility in aqueous media (they can be dissociated and transported into the lungs, where damage due to sensitization or nonimmunologic events takes place). Platinum, nickel, chromium, and cobalt are the most commonly implicated salts. For details the reader is referred to the reviews by Bernstein and Bernstein (1994), Menné (1987), and Marzulli and Maibach (1987).

Platinum Chlorplatinate salts are highly allergenic in comparison to other metalic salts. Exposure may occur in the mining and metallurgic industries, in chemical industries where platinum is used as a catalyst, and in the production of catalytic converters. Exposed workers are at risk of developing allergic rhinitis and asthma secondary to IgE production. Sensitized workers show positive skin tests and antigen-specific IgE by RAST testing.

Cobalt Five percent of workers exposed to cobalt develop occupational asthma. These patients exhibit antigen-specific IgE, and their lymphocytes proliferate in response to free cobalt or cobalt conjugated to human serum albumin.

Nickel Although nickel is a common contact sensitizer, pulmonary hypersensitivity reactions to nickel salts are rare. Occupational exposure to nickel is most common in the mining, milling, smelting, and refinishing industries. When they occur, pulmonary reactions are most frequently due to a direct toxic effect on the CNS and lung tissues. In addition to industrial contact, exposure occurs in the form of jewelry, coins, and fasteners on clothing, making nickel one of the most frequently contacted sensitizers for the general population. Studies have shown nickel sulfate to be the most frequent sensitizer when standard tray sensitizers are used, with positive results being between 6.7 and 11 percent. Nickel appears to require a long sensitization period, and studies have shown that patients may lose their hypersensitivity to nickel after long periods of avoidance.

Chromium Chromium is another metal often associated with dermatoses and less frequently with respiratory disease. Occupational exposure to chromium is most frequent in industries involved in electroplating processes, leather tanning, and paint, cement, and paper pulp production. Chromium eczema (type IV hypersensitivity) is among the most common occupationally associated skin diseases. Predictive tests on normal human subjects have shown sensitization rates to chromium sulfate as high as 48 percent. Occupational asthma from chromium exposure is less well documented, and skin-prick tests have been negative. Evidence of IgE-mediated disease has been supported by immediate bronchial hyperreactivity after challenge and the identification of antigen-specific IgE antibodies. Cell-mediated (type IV) reactions have been postulated to play a role, since late asthmatic reactions following bronchial challenge have been seen.

Beryllium Beryllium is a metal capable of producing both contact and tuberculin type IV hypersensitivity reactions. The role of CMI in beryllium-induced disease has been reviewed by Newman (1994). Beryllium exposure occurs most frequently in the aerospace industry, in high-technology ceramics and dental alloy manufacturing, and in the electronics, nuclear weapons, and nuclear reactors industries. A major source of exposure was in the production of fluorescent light bulbs until the discontinuance of its use for this purpose. Skin contact has been found to produce lesions of contact hypersensitivity, whereas lesions produced by penetration of splinters of beryllium under the skin are granulomatous in nature. Inhalation of beryllium can result in disease ranging from acute pneumonitis, tracheobronchitis, and chronic beryllium disease to an increase in the risk of lung cancer. Environmentally induced berylliosis was evidenced by the incidence of disease in nonfactory workers in communities around beryllium extraction plants. Exposure resulted from emissions from plants and contact with beryllium-contaminated family members' clothing.

In cases of chronic beryllium disease, there is often a latent period of up to 10 years following first exposure. Lung pathology consists of multiple granulomas with mononuclear cell infiltrates—primarily macrophages, lymphocytes, and plasma cells—and fibrosis. Although lesions are usually localized in the lungs and associated lymph nodes, granulomatous involvement of other organs has been seen. As pulmonary disease progresses, effects on pulmonary circulation may lead to right-sided heart failure. Death due to berylliosis may then be due to respiratory or cardiac failure.

Unlike most hypersensitivity reactions in which removal from exposure to the offending agent usually abates the disease, removal from beryllium exposure does little to alter the course of the disease. Although the majority of beryllium is eliminated from the lung soon after inhalation, small amounts of retained beryllium are sufficient to induce and sustain the ongoing cellular immune response. Years after the last exposure, mass absorption data have shown beryllium to be present in lung granulomas.

Owing to the similarities in clinical symptoms and pathology between berylliosis and other granulomatous lung diseases, immunologic testing is important in definitive diagnosis. Patients with beryllium disease tested positive to patch testing with beryllium salt and often showed granulomatous lesions at the patch-test site within 3 weeks. However, these test procedures proved to be unsafe. Patch tests were found to induce sensitization in some patients and often caused exacerbation of lung disease. The beryllium-specific lymphocyte proliferation test (BeLT) has been utilized to detect beryllium sensitization. This test has proven to be a more sensitive indicator of early disease than patient history, physical exam, chest radiographs, or lung function test. Although this disease is not curable, progression of the disease process can be slowed by corticosteriod therapy. BeLT allows for earlier detection of sensitization. This results in improved patient monitoring and permits earlier institution of treatment. In industry, BeLT provides a means of detecting jobs with a high risk of exposure.

Drugs Hypersensitivity responses to drugs are among the major types of unpredictable drug reactions, accounting for up to 10 percent of all adverse effects. Drugs are designed to be reactive in the body and multiple treatments are common. This type of exposure is conducive to producing an immunologic reaction. Immunologic mechanisms of hypersensitivity reactions to drugs include types I through IV. For a detailed review of drug allergy see DeSwarte (1985). Penicillin is the most common agent involved in drug allergy and is discussed here as an example. Exposure to penicillin is responsible for 75 percent of the deaths due to anaphylaxis in the United States. The route of administration, dosage, and length of treatment all appear to play a role in the type and severity of hypersensitivity reaction elicited. Severe reactions are less likely following oral administration as compared to parenteral, and prolonged treatment with high doses increases the risk of acute interstitial nephritis and immune hemolytic anemia. The high incidence of allergic reaction to penicillin is in part due to widespread exposure to the compound. Not only has there been indiscriminant use of the drug, but exposure occurs through food products including milk from treated animals and the use of penicillin as an antimicrobial in the production of vaccines. Efforts have been made to reduce unnecessary exposure.

Reactions to penicillin are varied and may include any of the four types of hypersensitivity reactions. The most commonly seen clinical manifestation of type I reactions is urticaria; however, anaphylactic reactions occur in about 10 to 40 of every 100,000 patients receiving injections. Clinical signs of rhinitis and asthma are much less frequently observed. Blood dyscrasias can occur due to the production of IgG against penicillin metabolites bound to the surface of red blood cells (type II reaction). Penicillin has also been implicated in type III reactions leading to serum-sickness-like symptoms. Owing to the high frequency of type IV reactions when penicillin is applied topically, especially to inflamed or abraded skin, products are no longer available for topical application. Type IV reactions generally result in an eczematous skin reaction, but—infrequently—a life-threatening form of dermal necrosis may result. In these cases there is severe erythema and a separation of the epidermis at the basal layer. This reaction, which gives the clinical appearance of severe scalding, is thought to be a severe delayed reaction.

Pesticides Pesticides have been implicated as causal agents in both contact and immediate hypersensitivity reactions. Definitive diagnosis is often difficult or lacking in reported cases and animal and human predictive data often do not correlate well. Pesticide hypersensitivity responses have been reviewed by Thomas and coworkers (1990) and are described briefly below.

One of the difficulties in obtaining good epidemiologic data to document reactions to pesticides is the nature of exposure. Agricultural workers are among those most commonly exposed, and the fact that workers are exposed to multiple chemicals as well as harsh environmental factors makes diagnosis difficult. Furthermore, diagnostic follow-up among this group is infrequent.

In the case of barban, a carbamate insecticide, the reported incidence of contact sensitivity due to exposure is rare; however, predictive testing with the guinea pig maximization test (GPMT) and the diagnostic human patch test indicates that this pesticide is a potent sensitizer. Likewise, malathion, captan, benomyl, maneb, and naled have been identified as strong to extreme sensitizers using the GPMT. Human predictive data, diagnostic patch testing, and the reported incidence in the literature of toxicity with the use of these compounds are often not in agreement with the animal data.

Pesticides have been implicated in cases of immediate hypersensitivity, including rhinitis, conjunctivitis, asthma, and anaphylaxis. However, there has been no definitive proof of the association. It is possible that observed reactions are of an irritant nature rather than being an immunologic response. It has been shown that the asthmatic response to organophosphate insecticides is not due to the acetylcholinesterase activity, since the administration of atropine, a cholinergic antagonist, failed to block the response. Animal studies show some evidence to support the role of immediate hypersensitivity responses to pesticides. Mice injected intraperitoneally with malathion or 2,4-dichlorophenoxyacetic acid conjugates developed IgE antibody. However, antibody was not detected to these chemicals when they were applied topically. More epidemiologic and mechanistic studies are needed in the area of pesticide hypersensitivity to further define these relationships.

Others *Natural Rubber Latex Products* Allergic reactions to natural rubber latex products have become an important occupational health concern over the past decade. Natural rubber latex is derived from the rubber tree *Hevea brasiliensis* and is used in the manufacture of over 40,000 products including examination and surgical gloves, among other medical products. Dermatologic reactions to latex include irritant dermatitis due to chemical additives or mechanical abrasion and the occlusive conditions caused by wearing gloves; contact dermatitis (which represents approximately 80 percent of the allergic responses) due to the chemical additives used in the glove manufacturing (e.g., thiurams, carbamates, mercapto compounds, and phenylenediamines), and potentially more serious IgE-mediated responses due to residual latex proteins that remained in the finished products. The IgE responses may manifest as urticaria, asthma, or life-threatening anaphylaxis. For a review of latex allergy, see Germolec (1999).

Cosmetics and Personal Hygiene Products Contact dermatitis and dermatoconjuctivitis may result from exposure to many cosmetic and personal hygiene products, including makeup, deodorants, hair sprays, hair dyes and permanent-waving solutions, nail polish, soaps, face creams, and shampoos (Liberman et al., 1985). These agents contain coloring agents, lanolin, paraffin, petrolatum, vehicles, perfumes, and antimicrobials such as paraben esters, sorbic acid, phenolics, organic mercurials, quaternary ammonium compounds, EDTA, and formaldehyde. The devices used to apply these products may also induce allergic reactions. Diagnosis may be accomplished by patch testing; however, in patch testing, it is often necessary to employ products used by the patient in addition to those on a standard test tray. In cases of dermatoconjunctivitis, false-negative testing may occur. The skin of the eyelids may be more sensitive to agents than that of the forearm or back, making patch testing unreliable. Elimination-provocation procedures may be helpful in the diagnosis of difficult cases. All suspect offending agents must be removed from the patient's environment. Once clinical signs have resolved, agents may be reintroduced one at a time while the patient is observed for the recurrence of signs.

Enzymes Enzymes are another group capable of eliciting type I hypersensitivity responses (Gutman, 1985). Subtilin, a proteolytic enzyme derived from *Bacillus subtilis,* is used in laundry detergents to enhance their cleaning ability. Both individuals working in the environment where the product is made and those using the product may become sensitized. Subsequent exposure may produce signs of rhinitis, conjunctivitis, and asthma. An alveolar hypersensitivity reaction associated with precipitation antibodies and an Arthus-type reaction from skin testing has also been seen. Papain is another enzyme known to induce IgE-mediated disease. It is a high-molecular-weight sulfhydryl protease obtained from the fruit of the papaya tree and most commonly used as a meat tenderizer and a clearing agent in the production of beer. However, it is also used in the production of tooth powders, laxatives, and contact-lens cleaning solutions.

Formaldehyde Formaldehyde was discussed above as one of the components of cosmetics capable of causing a contact hypersensitivity reaction. Formaldehyde exposure also occurs in the textile industry, where it is used to improve wrinkle resistance, and in the furniture, auto upholstery, and resins industries. The general public may be exposed to low levels of formaldehyde in products as ubiquitous as newspaper dyes and photographic films and paper. This low-molecular-weight compound is extremely soluble in water and haptenates human proteins easily (Maibach, 1983). Human predictive testing with 1 to 10% formalin (formalin is 37% formaldehyde) for induction and 1% formalin for challenge showed sensitization rates of 4.5 to 7.8 percent (Marzulli and Maibach, 1974). Occupational exposure to formaldehyde has been associated with the occurrence of asthma, although it has been difficult to demonstrate antibodies to formaldehyde in the affected individuals (Hendrick et al., 1982).

For further information and a listing of chemicals known to cause hypersensitivity reactions affecting the respiratory system and skin, see Chaps. 15 and 19.

Autoimmunity In the section on hypersensitivity presented above, we discussed two mechanisms, types II and III, by which host tissues are damaged by the host's own immune system, creating autoimmune-like disease. In these situations, unaltered self antigens are not the target of the immune mechanisms but damage occurs to cells bearing hapten on membranes or to innocent bystander cells in close proximity to antigen-antibody complexes. For example, damage produced in autoimmune Goodpasture's disease is similar to that seen in type III hypersensitivity reactions in the lung due to TMA. Although the resulting pathology may be the same for autoimmune reactions and hypersensitivity, mechanisms of true autoimmune disease are distinguished from hypersensitivity. In cases of autoimmunity, self antigens are the target, and in the case of chemical-induced autoimmunity, is the disease state is induced by a modification of host tissues or immune cells by the chemical and not the chemical acting as an antigen/hapten.

Mechanisms of Autoimmunity The immunopathogenesis of autoimmune disease has been reviewed by Rose (1994) and is described briefly below as background information for understanding how chemicals may induce autoimmunity. Three types of molecules are involved in the process of self-recognition: immunoglobulins (Igs), T-cell receptors (TCRs), and the products of major histocompatibility complex (MHC). Igs and TCRs are expressed clonally on B and T cells, respectively, whereas MHC molecules are present on all nucleated cells. The ability of lymphocytes to distinguish one molecule from another stems from the antigen binding a specific lymphocyte receptor. In B-cell lines, through rearrangement of heavy and light Ig chains, tremendous diversity (10^6 to 10^7 specificities), occurs among Ig recognition structures. Likewise, a similar number of specific TCRs are produced as the result of gene rearrangement in T cells induced by peptide hormones produced by thymic epithelial cells. Two major types of B and T cells are produced. B cells expressing CD5 predominate in embryonic life and are later found mostly in the intestinal mucosa. These cells produce high levels of IgM, and much of it is autoantibody. Although most B cells do not express CD5 prior to class switching, they do express high levels of IgM. Influenced by cytokines produced by interacting T cells following antigen stimulation, these cells produce primarily IgG, IgA, or IgE. Similarly, T cells develop from one of two lineages—those with $\alpha\beta$TCRs and those with $\gamma\delta$TCRs. Although most mature T cells express $\alpha\beta$TCRs, $\gamma\delta$TCRs are predominant on mucosal surfaces. As described earlier in the chapter, $\alpha\beta$TCRs continue differentiation into $CD4^+$ or $CD8^+$ T cells. $CD4^+$ cells have primarily helper and inducer functions and recognize antigens in the context of MHC class II molecules. $CD8^+$ T lymphocytes are mainly cytotoxic cells and recognize antigenic determinants in conjunction with MHC class I molecules.

The process of negative selection against autoreactive T cells in the thymus is important in the prevention of autoimmune disease. T cells expressing $\alpha\beta$TCRs that fit self MHC molecules with high affinity undergo apoptosis (programmed cell death) at an accelerated rate, whereas those with a low affinity for self antigen and a high affinity for foreign antigen undergo positive selection and proliferate in the thymus, eventually migrating to the peripheral lymphatics. Although negative selection greatly reduces the numbers of self-reactive T cells, some of these cells do leave the thymus and remain in circulation in a state of anergy. These cells are able to bind their designated antigen but do not undergo proliferation owing to a lack of necessary second signal. This second signal is generally provided by an APC in the form of a cytokine, IL-2, or a cell surface receptor that interacts with the T cell.

Reactive $CD4^+$ T cells recognize only processed antigen presented by APCs—generally macrophages, B cells, or dendritic cells—in conjunction with MHC class II molecules. These APCs take up exogenous antigens, cleave them with proteolytic enzymes, and express them on their cell surfaces. In contrast, intracellular antigens are processed and presented on cell surfaces in conjunction with MHC class I molecules. These antigens may be the products of malignant or normal cells or may result from infection with bacterial, viral, or other intracellular pathogens. The processed antigen–MHC class I complex is recognized by a specific TCR on a $CD8^+$ lymphocyte.

Several mechanisms are available that may break down self-tolerance, leading to autoimmunity. The first is exposure to antigens not available in the thymus during embryonic development. Therefore, the antigen-specific T cell–reactive lymphocytes not subjected to negative selection could induce an autoimmune reaction. Examples include myelin and organ-specific antigens such as thyroglobulin. Breakdown of self-tolerance to these antigens may be induced by exposure to adjuvants or to another antigenically related protein. The second is the overcoming of T-cell anergy by chronic lymphocyte stimulation. Finally, there is interference with normal immunoregulation by $CD8^+$ T cell suppressor cells, which may create an environment conducive to the development of autoimmune disease.

Effector mechanisms involved in autoimmune disease can be the same as those described earlier for types II and III hypersensitivity or, in the case of pathology associated with solid tissues, including organs, they may involve $CD8^+$ cytotoxic T cells. Tissue damage associated with $CD8^+$ cells may be the result of direct cell-membrane damage and lysis induced by binding or the results of cytokines produced and released by the T cell. TN-β has the ability to kill susceptible cells and IFN-γ may increase the expression of MHC class I on cell surfaces, making them more susceptible to $CD8^+$ cells. Cytokines may also be chemotactic for macrophages, which can cause tissue damage directly or indirectly through the release of proinflammatory cytokines. As is the case with hypersensitivity reactions, autoimmune disease is often the result of more than one mechanism working simultaneously. Therefore, pathology may be the result of antibody-dependent cytotoxicity, complement-dependent antibody-mediated lysis, or direct or indirect effects of cytotoxic T cells.

Genetic and environmental factors appear to affect the susceptibility of individuals to autoimmune disease. Familial predisposition to autoimmune disease has been found, as well as a similarity in MHC genetic traits among individuals involved. Certain chemicals and drugs are known to induce autoimmune disease in genetically predisposed individuals, and examples of these are discussed below. The role of environmental pollutants is uncertain; more study is needed in this area. One point of interest is that in all known cases of drug-induced autoimmunity, the disease has abated once the offending chemical was removed.

Assessment of Autoimmune Responses Few models are available for accessing the potential of a chemical to induce autoimmune disease, and these have major limitations. The most commonly used models include graft-versus-host disease (GVHD), the popliteal lymph node (PLN) model in mice, and human lymphocyte transformation assays. Although these models may have some predictive value, at this point immunohistopathology is the only definitive diagnostic tool.

There are numerous reports of chemicals that have been associated with autoimmunity. These relationships may be causative through direct mechanisms or they may be indirect, acting as an adjuvant. They may also serve to exacerbate a preexisting autoimmune state (reviewed by Kilburn and Warshaw, 1994; Coleman and Sim, 1994). In the area of autoimmunity, exact mechanisms of action are not always known. Table 12-11 lists chemicals known to be associated with autoimmunity, showing the proposed self-antigenic determinant or stating adjuvancy as the mechanism of action. A brief discussion of selected drug and nondrug chemicals is provided.

Autoimmune Reactions to Xenobiotics *Methyldopa* Methyldopa is a centrally acting sympatholytic drug that has been widely used for the treatment of essential hypertension. With the advent of newer antihypertensive drugs, the use of methyldopa has declined. Platelets and erythrocytes are targeted by the immune system in individuals treated with this drug. In the case of thrombocytopenia, antibodies are detected against platelets, which is indicative of immune recognition of a self- or altered self-antigen. Hemolytic anemia occurs in at least 1 percent of individuals treated with methyldopa, and up to 30 percent of these individuals develop antibodies to erythrocytes as manifest in a positive Coombs test. The antibodies are not directed against the chemical or a chemical membrane conjugate.

Hydralazine, Isoniazid, and Procainamide Hydralazine, isoniazid, and procainamide produce autoimmunity, which is manifest as a sytemic lupus erythematosus (SLE)-like syndrome. Antibodies to DNA have been detected in individuals showing this syndrome. Hydralazine is a direct-acting vasodilator drug used in the treatment of hypertension. Isoniazid is an antimicrobial drug used in the treatment of tuberculosis. Procainamide is a drug that selectively blocks Na^+ channels in myocardial membranes, making it useful in the treatment of cardiac arrhythmias. Studies with hydralazine and isoniazid indicate that the antigenic determinant is myeloperoxidase. Immunoglobulins are produced against myeloperoxidase in individuals treated with these drugs. DNA is the apparent antigenic determinant for procainamide. For these three drugs, there is no evidence indicating that the immune system is recognizing the chemical or a chemical conjugate. In addition, these drugs have also been shown to produce hypersensitivity responses not associated with the SLE syndrome.

Halothane Halothane, one of the most widely studied of the drugs inducing autoimmunity, is an inhalation anesthetic that can induce autoimmune hepatitis. The incidence of this iatrogenic disease in humans is about 1 in 20,000. The pathogenesis of the hepatitis results from the chemical altering self (a specific liver protein) to such a degree that the immune system recognizes the altered self and antibodies are produced. Studies using rat microsomes show that halothane has to be oxidized by cytochrome P450 enzymes to trifluoroacetylhalide before it binds to the protein. Investigations indicate that in affected individuals antibodies to specific microsomal proteins are produced.

Vinyl Chloride Vinyl chloride, which is used in the plastics industry as a refrigerant and in the synthesis of organic chemicals, is a known carcinogen and is also associated with a scleroderma-like syndrome. The disease affects multisystemic collagenous tissues, manifesting itself as pulmonary fibrosis, skin sclerosis, and/or fibrosis of the liver and spleen. Ward and coworkers (1976) reported on 320 exposed workers, showing that 58 (18 percent) had a scleroderma-like syndrome. The individuals who showed the disease were in a group genetically similar (i.e., HLA-DR5) to patients with classic idiopathic scleroderma patients. Although the exact mechanism whereby this chemical produces autoimmunity is unclear, it is presumed that vinyl chloride acts as an amino acid and is incorporated into protein. Because this would produce a structurally abnormal protein, which would be antigenic, an immune response would be directed against tissues with the modified protein present.

Table 12-11
Chemical Agents Known to be Associated with Autoimmunity

PROPOSED ANTIGENIC CHEMICAL	CLINICAL MANIFESTATIONS	DEPARTMENT	REFRENCE
Drugs			
Methyl dopa	Hemolytic anemia	Rhesus antigens	Murphy and Kelton (1991)
Hydralazine	SLE-like syndrome	Myeloperoxidase	Cambridge *et al.* (1994)
Isoniazid	SLE-like syndrome	Myeloperoxidase	Jiang *et al.* (1994)
Procainamide	SLE-like syndrome	DNA	Totoritis *et al.* (1988)
Halothane	Autoimmune hepatitis	Liver microsomal proteins	Kenna *et al.* (1987)
Non-drug chemicals			
Vinyl Chloride	Scleroderma-like syndrome	Abnormal protein synthesized in liver	Ward *et al.* (1976)
Mercury	Glomerular neuropathy	Glomerular basement membrane protein	Pelletier *et al.* (1994)
Silica	Scleroderma	Most likely acts as an adjuvant	Pernis and Paronetto (1962)

Mercury This widely used metal is now known to have several target systems, including CNS and renal system. Mercury also has two different actions with respect to the immune system. The first action is direct injury, described previously. Mercury also produces an autoimmune disease demonstrated as glomerular nephropathy. Antibodies produced to laminin are believed to be responsible for damage to the basement membrane of the kidney. Mice and rats exposed to mercury also show antinuclear antibodies. The role of these antibodies in the autoimmune disease is not clear. However, they represent a known biomarker of autoimmunity. Studies in the brown Norway rat point to a mercury-induced autoreactive $CD4^+$ cell as being responsible for the polyclonal antibody response. Mercury chloride induces an increase in the expression of MHC class II molecules on B lymphocytes as well as shifting the T helper cell population along the Th2 line. It is the Th2 cell that promotes antibody production. The imbalance between Th1 and Th2 cells is believed to be caused by the depletion of cysteine and the reduced form of gluthathione in Th1 cells. These chemical groups are known to be important in the synthesis of and responsiveness to IL-2 in T cells. Thus, Th1 cells that synthesize and respond to IL-2 would be at a greater risk than Th2 cells.

Mercury-induced autoimmunity has a strong genetic component. This has been extensively studied in the rat. Some strains of rats, such as the Lewis rat, are completely resistant, while others, such as the brown Norway, are exquisitely sensitive. Susceptibility appears to be linked to three or four genes, one of which is the major histocompatibility complex. An excellent review of mercury and autoimmunity is provided by Pelletier and coworkers. (1994).

Silica Crystalline silica (silicon dioxide) is a primary source of elemental silicon and is used commercially in large quantities as a constituent of building materials, ceramics, concretes, and glasses. Experimental animals as well as humans exposed to silica may have perturbations in the immune system. Depending on the length of exposure, dose, and route of administration of silica, it may kill macrophages or may act as an immunostimulant. Silica has been shown to be associated with an increase in scleroderma in silica-exposed workers (reviewed by Kilburn and Warshaw, 1994). This effect is believed to be mediated via an adjuvant mechanism. Adjuvancy as a mechanism of causing autoimmunity has been implicated with a number of other chemicals, including paraffin and silicones. Inherent in adjuvancy as a mechanism of producing autoimmunity is that the population affected by these chemicals must already be at risk for the autoimmune disease. This is supported by the data indicating a genetic component to many autoimmune diseases.

Table 12-12 shows chemicals that have been implicated in autoimmune reactions, but in these cases the mechanism of autoimmunity has not been as clearly defined or confirmed. The list includes both drug and nondrug chemicals. The heterogeneity of these structures and biological activities illustrate the breadth of potential for the induction of chemically mediated autoimmune disease.

Multiple Chemical Sensitivity Syndrome Multiple chemical sensitivity syndrome (MCS) has been associated with hypersensitivity responses to chemicals. The disease associated with MCS is characterized by multiple subjective symptoms related to more than one system. The more common symptoms are nasal congestion, headaches, lack of concentration, fatigue, and memory loss. Many mechanisms have been suggested to explain how chemicals cause these symptoms; however, there remains considerable controversy as to a cause–effect relationship. Clinical ecologists, the major proponents of MCS, have focused on immunologic mechanisms to explain the etiology. They hypothesize that MCS occurs when chemical exposure sensitizes certain individuals, and, upon subsequent exposure to exceedingly small amounts of these or unrelated chemicals, the individual exhibits an adverse response. Controlled studies on the immunologic status of individuals with MCS have shown no alterations in their immune system or any indication that MCS results from impairment of the immunity, including inappropriate immune response to chemicals. The search for a theoretical basis for MCS is now being focused on the nervous system. Two untested hypotheses have emerged. The first involves a nonspecific inflammatory response to low-level irritants known as "neurogenic inflammation." The second involves induction of lasting changes in limbic and neuronal activity (via kindling) that alter a broad spectrum of behavioral and physiologic functions. The reader is referred to a review by Sikorski and colleagues (1995) for details and references concerning MCS.

NEW FRONTIERS AND CHALLENGES

Immunotoxicology has grown significantly since its beginnings as a recognized subdiscipline of toxicology in the late 1970s. Early work focused on the development of methods that were sensitive and predictive and on an understanding of xenobiotic-induced im-

Table 12-12
Chemicals Implicated in Autoimmunity

MANIFESTATION	IMPLICATED CHEMICAL	REFERENCE
Scleroderma	Solvents (toluene, xylene)	Walder (1983)
	Tryptophan	Silver et al. (1990)
	Silicones	Fock et al. (1984)
Systemic lupus erythrematosus	Phenothiazines	Canoso et al. (1990)
	Penicillamine	Harpey et al. (1971)
	Propylthiouracil	DeSwarte (1985)
	Quinidine	Jiang et al. (1994)
	L-dopa	DeSwarte (1985)
	Lithium carbonate	Ananth et al. (1989)
	Trichloroethylene	Kilburn and Washaw (1992)
	Silicones	Fock et al. (1984)

munomodulation—in particular, immunosuppression. With unprecedented growth in the understanding of immune regulation (brought about in the 1980s as a result of the emergence of AIDS) came investigations into mechanisms of action (including cellular interactions, modulation of transcription factors, and alterations in gene regulation) and in the use of in vitro methods to study these mechanisms and to attempt to predict effects in the whole animal. While these types of investigations continued to grow, the 1990s saw a surge in investigations into the understanding of immune-mediated disease: hypersensitivity and autoimmunity. As understanding of the human genome grows, pharmaceutical companies move faster and deeper into biotechnology, public concern and scientific debate over genetically modified foods increases, concern for the effects of chemicals on children's health grows, concern and debate over the potential impact of chemically induced endocrine disruption continues, the push to use kinetic and mechanistic data in human health risk assessments continues, and increased pressure to reduce the use of animals in testing increases, there is no doubt that immunotoxicology will continue to grow and expand in many ways. The following are a few of the new frontiers and challenges facing the immunotoxicologist of today and tomorrow.

Molecular Biology Methods: Proteomics and Genomics

The use of molecular biology methods in immunotoxicology in the past has been primarily in the understanding of the mechanism of action of identified immunotoxicants. Much research is currently focused on investigating induction of certain mRNAs (e.g., cytokines, transcription factors) in elucidating mechanism or as possible biomarkers of exposure. Proteomics (the study of all expressed proteins in a particular cell, and thus the functional expression of the genome) and genomics (the study of all genes encoded by an organism's DNA), combined with bioinformatics, are making it possible to evaluate chemically induced alterations in entire pathways and signaling networks. The utility of molecular biology tools such as proteomics and genomics in eludicating mechanism of action is obvious. However, can these powerful tools be used to identify new or suspected immunotoxicants? Is it possible that common profiles of gene expression will emerge for classes of structurally related or structurally dissimilar known or suspected immunotoxicants? How is the profile or gene expression related to administered dose, tissue dose, and time course of action of a chemical? Is human gene expression in response to chemical exposure the same as that in the animal or cell culture? If it is determined that these methods are useful tools in the identification of possible immunotoxicants, how should they be validated?

Animal Models: Transgenics and SCID

The developments in molecular biology have not only permitted the evaluation of specific genes or arrays of genes but have also allowed for the manipulation of the embryonic genome, creating transgenic and knockout mice (reviewed in IPCS, 1996). As a consequence of transgenic technology, complex immune responses can be dissected into their components. In this way, the mechanisms by which immunotoxicants act can be better understood. Mice lacking certain receptors, transcription factors, cytokines, etc., can be used for similar mechanistic studies. Severe combined immunodeficient mice (SCID) can easily be engrafted with human or rat immune cells (SCID/hu and SCID/ra) and have been used to study immune regulation, hematopoiesis, hypersensitivity, and autoimmunity. Uses of reconstituted SCID mice have been considered elsewhere (IPCS, 1996), and their use in mechanistic studies is obvious. As with the use of molecular biological techniques, however, there are several questions regarding the broader utility of transgenics and SCID animals in immunotoxicology. Because of their altered biological status, how do they compare with standard animal models with respect to time course of action, dose response, pharmacokinetics, and other factors of chemical toxicity? Are the homing patterns of engrafted cells identical to those in the standard animal (i.e., to the extent possible, how identical are the immune systems of these mice compared to standard mice)? Can these animal models be used to identify new or suspected immunotoxicants, and if so, are they as or more sensitive, predictive, and/or cost-effective as traditional animal models?

Developmental Immunotoxicology

The development (ontogeny) of the mammalian immune system occurs primarily in utero, though some postnatal development or maturation does occur. Developmental immunotoxicology involves investigation into the effects that xenobiotics have on the ontogeny of the immune system and includes prenatal (in utero), perinatal ($<$36 h of age), and neonatal periods of exposure (reviewed in Barnett, 1996). Recent studies suggest that immune development in humans and other species may be altered after perinatal exposure to immunotoxic chemicals, including chemotherapeutics, corticosteroids, polycyclic hydrocarbons, and polyhalogenated hydrocarbons (reviewed in Barnett, 1996, and in Holladay, 1999). It has also been suggested that these effects may be more dramatic or persistent than those following exposure during adult life. With the passage of the Food Quality Protection Act (FQPA), more attention has focused on children's health and thus on this emerging area of immunotoxicology. Specifically, an understanding of the development and functioning of the juvenile immune system and subsequent validated methods (similar to those currently validated in adult animal models) are needed.

Systemic Hypersensitivity

An adverse immune response, in the form of systemic hypersensitivity, is among the most frequent causes for withdrawal of drugs that have made it to the market; such a response can account for approximately 15 percent of adverse reactions to xenobiotics (de Weck, 1983; Guzzie, 1995). These findings are generally unexpected in that they were not predicted in preclinical toxicology and immunotoxicology studies. A primary reason for this is the lack of good preclinical models for predicting systemic hypersensitivity responses, particularly to orally administered chemicals. This concern applies not only to the pharmaceutical industry but also to the food industry (proteins and genetically modified foods). It has been noted that a positive guinea pig hypersensitivity test (any test) has less than a 25 percent chance of predicting human clinical responses with respect to systemic hypersensitivity of drugs (Weaver et al., 1999). Assays are needed that are more predictive of drug antigenicity or hypersensitivity in humans. In the area of food allergy, again there are no validated animal models available, although the brown Norway rat and the Balb/c mouse have been shown to have some promise (Kimber et al., 1999, 2000; Knippels et al., 1999, 2000).

Computational Toxicology

The possibility of ascertaining certain molecular properties of a molecule even before it is synthesized is a highly beneficial use of computational chemistry. In fact, computational chemistry has been a rapidly growing and valued field, particularly in the fast-paced and highly competitive pharmaceutical industry. As a result of the usefulness of this tool, interest has grown in the use of computational toxicology methods to predict the potential biological/toxicologic activity of chemicals. The premise is that the structure of a chemical determines the physiochemical properties and reactivities that underlie its biological and toxicologic properties [quantitative structure-activity relationships (QSAR)]. Being able to predict potential adverse effects cannot only aid in the designed development of new chemicals but also has the potential to reduce the need for animal testing. It may ultimately or potentially lead to better health and environmental protection through the strategic application of limited testing resources and existing information assets to help sort out or identify the most hazardous chemicals. Computational toxicology can also help in screening large numbers of chemicals more efficiently for a variety of toxicologic endpoints. Computational methods will not assure 95 to 100 percent accuracy in the prediction of toxicity, and they will not eliminate the need for testing, but these methods will help reduce and prioritize the testing that is required. The use of computational toxicology cannot replace the need for toxicologists. These individuals will still be needed for their understanding of the relationship between the predicted endpoints and product or component ADME profiles (absorption, distribution, metabolism, and elimination) and the true potential for human exposure as determined by the process, method of application, and end use of the product. Immunotoxicologists studying hypersensitivity have begun to investigate whether computational methods can be used to screen for potential chemical sensitizers (Karol, et al., 1996, 1999; Graham et al., 1997; Gerberick, 1999). Thus, computational toxicology is a tool that may offer promise in the identification/prediction of chemical sensitization. The use of computational methods to predict other aspects of immunotoxicology has not been explored.

Biomarkers

True biomarkers indicate exposure to a specific chemical as well as susceptibility to adverse effect; and/or are predictive of disease associated with chemical exposure. They must be sensitive, specific, relevant, reproducible, and measurable in the population. The most sensitive (and desirable) biomarkers would be those that indicate *exposure* in the absence of immediate adverse effect. Biomarkers of *effect* would indicate subclinical effects of chemical exposure. Various avenues are currently being explored as potential biomarkers, including cytokine gene expression patterns, flow cytometry, and immunomodulation in alternative species such as fish, just to name a few. The International Programme on Chemical Safety (IPCS, 1996) has concluded that, as with other systems in toxicology, few biomarkers are available for immunotoxicity, particularly for assessing immunotoxicity of individual susceptibility. More epidemiologic studies are needed to obtain a better view of the utility of biomarkers for detecting immunotoxic events and, ultimately, possible health risks that may be associated with exposure to chemicals that modulate the immune system.

Risk Assessment

With the demonstration that (1) chemicals can perturb the immune system of animals, (2) perturbation of immune function is correlated with an increased risk of infectious disease, and (3) perturbations in immune function can occur in the absence of any clinically observable effect, attention has focused on the risk to the human population following exposure to chemicals that can alter immune function in animals. However, these initial assessments of the use of immunotoxicology data in animals as predictors of risk for human clinical effects have limitations (reviewed in Luster et al., 1994, and IPCS, 1996). These include the fact that though many were good indicators, no single immune test has been observed to be highly predictive of altered host resistance. Also, to demonstrate chemical-related clinical immune effects in the human population, a significant number of individuals may be required. Variability in the virulence of infectious agents in the human population, the complexity of the immune system, and the redundancy ("immune reserve"; multiple components capable of responding to a foreign challenge) in the immune system may all contribute to the difficulty in quantifying relationships between chemical-induced alterations in immune status and alterations in host resistance in humans. Finally, there is the question of whether the relationship between functional immune changes and susceptibility to disease follows a linear (i.e., any change in immune function may increase the susceptibility to disease) or threshold-like model (i.e., small changes in immune function may be without appreciable changes in host resistance). Although there are suggestions in the literature that this relationship may follow a linear model, the answer to this question in the context of a broad array of chemicals is not clear. Further investigation in this area is warranted.

CONCLUDING COMMENT AND FUTURE DIRECTIONS

Our understanding of the immune system as a target for toxicity, whether it be via xenobiotic-induced immune injury or immune-mediated disease, continues to progress in concert with our knowledge of the biochemistry and physiology of the immune system. The balance between immune recognition and destruction of foreign invaders and the proliferation of these microbes and/or cancer cells can be a precarious one. Xenobiotics that alter the immune system can upset this balance, giving the edge to the invader. Furthermore, new xenobiotics continuously being introduced represent the potential for increased hypersensitivity and/or autoimmune responses. Validated methods are in place to detect xenobiotics that produce adverse effects related to the immune system. Once these are identified, fundamental principles of toxicology can be applied leading to risk assessment and determination of "no-effect" levels. These methods must continually be improved using the latest knowledge and technologies in order to provide a safe environment.

REFERENCES

Ananth J, Johnson R, Kataria P, et al: Immune dysfunctions in psychiatric patients. *Psychiatr J* 14(4):542–546, 1989.

Araneo BAT, Dowell T, Moon HB, Daynes RA: Regulation of murine lymphokine production in vivo: Ultraviolet radiation exposure depresses IL-2 and enhances IL-4 production through an IL-1 independent mechanism. *J Immunol* 143:1737–1745, 1989.

Aranyi C, O'Shea W, Graham J, Miller F: The effects of inhalation of organic chemical air contaminants on murine lung host defenses. *Fundam Appl Toxicol* 6:713–720, 1986.

Arora PK, Fride E, Petitto J, et al: Morphine-induced immune alterations in vivo. *Cell Immunol* 126:343–353, 1990.

Barnett JB: Developmental immunotoxicology, in Smialowicz RJ, Holsapple MP (eds): *Experimental Immunotoxicology.* Boca Raton, FL: CRC Press, 1996, pp 47–62.

Barnett JB, Rodgers KE: Pesticides, in Dean JH, Luster MI, Munson AE, Kimber I (eds): *Immunotoxicology and Immunopharmacology,* 2d ed. New York: Raven Press, 1994, pp 191–212.

Bernstein JA, Bernstein IL: Clinical aspects of respiratory hypersensitivity to chemicals, in Dean JH, Luster MI, Munson AE, Kimber I (eds): *Immunotoxicology and Immunopharmacology,* 2d ed. New York: Raven Press, 1994, pp 617–642.

Biagini RE: Epidemiology studies in immunotoxicity evaluations. *Toxicology* 129:37–54, 1998.

Biegel LB, Flaws JA, Hirshfield AN, et al: 90-day feeding and one-generation reproduction study in Crl:CD BR rats with 17β-estradiol. *Toxicol Sci* 44:116–142, 1998.

Blalock JE: A molecular basis for bidirectional communication between the immune and neuroendocrine systems. *Physiol Rev* 69:1–32, 1989.

Bly JE, Quiniou SM, Clem LW: Environmental effects on fish immune mechanisms. *Dev Biol Stand* 90:33–43, 1997.

Bouaboula M, Rinaldi M, Carayon P, et al: Cannabinoid receptor expression in human leukocytes. *Eur J Biochem* 214:173–180, 1993.

Bradley SG, Morahan PS, Approaches to assessing host resistance. *Environ Health Perspect* 43:61–69, 1982.

Bradley SG, Munson AE, McCay JA, et al: Subchronic 10 day immunotoxicity of polydimethylsiloxane (silicone) fluid, gel and elastomer and polyurethane disks in female B6C3F1 mice. *Drug Chem Toxicol* 17(3):175–220, 1994a.

Bradley SG, White KL Jr, McCay JA, et al: Immunotoxicity of 180 day exposure to polydimethylsiloxane (silicone) fluid, gel and elastomer and polyurethane disks in female B6C3F1 mice. *Drug Chem Toxicol* 17(3):221–269, 1994b.

Brown EJ, Albers MW, Shin TB, et al: A mammalian protein targeted by G_1-arresting rapamycin receptor complex. *Nature* 369:756–758, 1994.

Buehler EV: Delayed contact hypersensitivity in the guinea pig. *Arch Dermatol* 91:171–177, 1965.

Burchiel SW, Krekvliet NI, Gerberick GF, et al: Workshop overview: Assessment of immunotoxicity by multiparameter flow cytometry. *Fundam Appl Toxicol* 38:38–54, 1997.

Burchiel SW, Lauer FT, Gurule, D, et al: Uses and applications of flow cytometry in immunotoxicity testing. *Methods* 19:28–35, 1999.

Burns LA, Bradley SG, White KL, et al: Immunotoxicology of nitrobenzene in female B6C3F1 mice. *Drug Chem Toxicol* 17(3):271–315, 1994a.

Burns LA, Bradley SG, White KL, et al: Immunotoxicology of nitrotoluenes in female B6C3F1 mice. I. Para-nitrotoluene. *Drug Chem Toxicol* 17(3):359–399, 1994b.

Burns LA, Bradley SG, White KL, et al: Immunotoxicology of nitrotoluenes in female B6C3F1 mice. II. Meta-nitrotoluene. *Drug Chem Toxicol* 17(3):401–436, 1994c.

Burns LA, Bradley SG, White KL, et al: Immunotoxicology of 2,4-diaminotoluene in female B6C3F1 mice. *Drug Chem Toxicol* 17(3):317–358, 1994d.

Burns LA, LeVier DG, Munson AE: Immunotoxicology of Arsenic, in Dean JH, Luster MI, Munson AE, Kimber I (eds): *Immunotoxicology and Immunopharmacology,* 2d ed. New York: Raven Press, 1994, pp 213–225.

Burns-Naas LA, Mast RW, Klykken PC, et al: Toxicology and humoral immunity assessment of decamethylcyclopentasiloxane (D_5) following a 1-month whole-body inhalation exposure in Fischer 344 rats. *Toxicol Sci* 43:28–38, 1998.

Calne RY, Rolles K, White DJ, et al: Cyclosporin A in clinical organ grafting. *Transplant Proc* 13:349–358, 1981.

Cambridge G, Wallace H, Bernstein RM, Leaker B: Autoantibodies to myeloperoxidase in idiopathic and drug-induced systemic lupus erythematosus and vasculitis. *Br J Rheumatol* 33(2):109–114, 1994.

Canoso RT, de Oliveira RM, Nixon RA: Neuroleptic-associated autoantibodies. A prevalence study. *Biol Psychiatry* 27(8):863–870, 1990.

Catania RA, Chaudry IH: Immunological consequences of trauma and shock. *Ann Acad Med Singapore* 28(1):120–132, 1999.

Chao CC, Molitor TW, Gekker G, et al: Cocaine-mediated suppression of superoxide production by human peripheral blood mononuclear cells. *J Pharmacol Exp Ther* 256:255–258, 1991.

Chao CC, Sharp BM, Pomeroy C, et al: Lethality of morphine in mice infected with *Toxoplasma gondii. J Pharmacol Exp Ther* 252:605–609, 1990.

Coleman JW, Sim E: Autoallergic responses to drugs: Mechanistic aspects, in Dean JH, Luster MI, Munson AE, Kimber I (eds): *Immunotoxicology and Immunopharmacology,* 2d ed. New York: Raven Press, 1994, pp 553–572.

Coombs RRA, Gell PGH: Classification of allergic reactions responsible for clinical hypersensitivity and disease, in Gell PGH, Coombs RRA, Lachmann PJ (eds): *Clinical Aspects of Immunology,* Oxford, England: Oxford University Press, 1975, p 761.

Dean JH, Luster MI, Boorman GA: Immunotoxicology, in Sirois P, Rola-Pleszcynski M (eds): *Immunopharmacology.* Amsterdam: Elsevier, 1982, pp 349–397.

Dean JH, Luster MI, Boorman GA, et al: Selective immunosuppression resulting from exposure to the carcinogenic congener of benzopyrene in B6C3F1 mice. *Clin Exp Immunol* 52:199–206, 1983.

Dean JH, Lauer LD, House RV, et al: Studies of immune function and host resistance in B6C3F1 mice exposed to formaldehyde. *Toxicol Appl Pharmacol* 72:519–529, 1984.

Dean JH, Luster MI, Munson AE, Amos H (eds): *Immunotoxicology and Immunopharmacology.* New York: Raven Press, 1985.

Dean JH, Luster MI, Munson AE, Kimber I (eds): *Immunotoxicology and Immunopharmacology,* 2d ed. New York: Raven Press, 1994.

Dearman RJ, Kimber I: Cytokine fingerprinting: Characterization of chemical allergens. *Methods* 79(1):56–63, 1999.

Dearman RJ, Kimber I: Differential stimulation of immune function by respiratory and contact chemical allergens. *Immunology* 72:563–570, 1991.

Dearman RJ, Spence LM, Kimber I: Characterization of murine immune responses to allergenic diisocyanates. *Toxicol Appl Pharmacol* 112:190–197, 1992.

Delaney B, Strom SC, Collins S, Kaminski NE: Carbon tetrachloride suppresses T-cell-dependent immune responses by induction to transforming growth factor-β1. *Toxicol Appl Pharmacol* 126:98–107, 1994.

Demoly P, Michel F, Bousquet J: In vivo methods for study of allergy skin tests, techniques and interpretation, in Middleton E Jr, Reed C, Ellis E, et al (eds): *Allergy Principles and Practice.* St. Louis: Mosby, 1998, pp 430–439.

Deo MG, Gangal S, Bhisey AN, et al: Immunological, mutagenic, and genotoxic investigations in gas-exposed population of Bhopal. *Indian J Med Res* 86:63–76, 1987.

Descotes J (ed): *Immunotoxicology and Drugs and Chemicals.* Amsterdam: Elsevier, 1986.

Desi I, Varga L, Dobronyi L, Szklenarik G: Immunotoxicological investigation of the effects of a pesticide: Cypermethrin. *Arch Toxicol* (suppl 8):305–309, 1985.

DeSwarte RD: Drug allergy, in Patterson R (ed): *Allergic Diseases, Diagnosis and Management,* 3d ed. Philadelphia: Lippincott, 1985, pp 505–661.

deWeck AL: Immunopathological mechanisms and clinical aspects of allergic reactions to drugs, in deWeck AL, Bundgaard H (eds): *Handbook of Experimental Pharmacology: Allergic Reactions to Drugs.* New York: Springer-Verlag, 1983, pp 75–133.

Eisenstein TK, Bussiere JL, Rogers TJ, Adler MW: Immunosuppressive effects of morphine on immune responses in mice. *Adv Exp Med Biol* 335:41–52, 1993.

Enk AH, Angeloni VL, Udey MC, Katz SI: Inhibition of Langerhans cell antigen-presenting function by IL-10. *J Immunol* 151:2390–2398, 1993.

Exon JH, Mather GG, Bussiere JL, et al: Effects of subchronic exposure of rats to 2-methoxyethanol or 2-butoxyethanol: Thymic atrophy and immunotoxicity. *Fundam Appl Toxicol* 16(4):830–840, 1991.

Fock KM, Feng PH, Tey BH: Autoimmune disease developing after augmentation mammoplasty: Report of 3 cases. *J Rheumatol* 11:98–100, 1984.

Fuchs BA, Sanders VM: The role of brain-immune interactions in immunotoxicology. *Crit Rev Toxicol* 24(2):151–176, 1994.

Gabliks J, Al-zubaidy T, Askari E: DDT and immunological responses. 3. Reduced anaphylaxis and mast cell population in rats fed DDT. *Arch Environ Health* 30:81–84, 1975.

Gabliks J, Askari EM, Yolen N: DDT and immunological responses. I. Serum antibodies and anaphylactic shock in guinea pig. *Arch Environ Health* 26:305–309, 1973.

Gad SC, Dunn BJ, Dobbs DW, et al: Development and validation of an alternative dermal sensitization test: The mouse ear swelling test (MEST). *Toxicol Appl Pharmacol* 84:93–114, 1986.

Gaworski CL, Vollmuth TA, Dozier MM, et al: An immunotoxicity assessment of food flavouring ingredients. *Fundam Chem Toxicol* 32(5):409–415, 1994.

Gerberick GF: Development, validation, and application of expert systems for predicting skin sensitization. Society of Toxicology Continuing Education course, *The Practice of Structure-Activity Relationships (SAR) in Toxicology,* March, 1999.

Germolec DR, Woolhiser MR, Meade BJ: Allergy to natural rubber latex. Chem Health Saf July: 44–48, 1999.

Giorgio RL, Bongiorno L, Trani E, et al: Review paper: Positive and negative immunomodulation by opioid peptides. *Int J Immunopharmacol* 18(1):1–16, 1996.

Gogal Jr RM, Ahmed SA, Smith SA, Holladay SD: Commentary. Mandates to develop non-mammalian models for chemical immunotoxicity evaluation: Are fish a viable alternate to rodents? *Toxicol Lett* 106:89–92, 1999.

Gorelik E, Heberman R: Susceptibility of various strains of mice to urethane-induced lung tumors and depressed natural killer activity. *J Natl Cancer Inst* 67:1317–1322, 1981.

Grabbe S, Schwarz T: Immunoregulatory mechanisms involved in elicitation of allergic contact hypersensitivity. *Immunol Today* 19:37–44, 1998.

Graham C, Rosenkrantz HS, Karol MH: Structure-activity model of chemicals that cause human respiratory sensitization. *Reg Toxicol Pharmacol* 26:296–306, 1997.

Grammer LC: Occupational immunologic lung disease, in Patterson R (ed): *Allergic Diseases, Diagnosis and Management,* 3d ed. Philadelphia: Lippincott, 1985, pp 691–708.

Greenlee WF, Dold KM, Irons RD, Osborne R: Evidence for a direct action of 2,3,7,8-tetrachlorodibenzo-*p*-dioxin (TCDD) on thymic epithelium. *Toxicol Appl Pharmacol* 79:112–120, 1985.

Greenlee WF, Dold KM, Osborne R: A proposed model for the actions of TCDD on epidermal and thymic epithelial target cells, in Poland A, Kimbrough RD (eds): *Banbury Report 18: Biological Mechanisms of Dioxin Action.* Cold Spring Harbor, NY: Cold Spring Harbor Laboratory, 1984, pp 435ff.

Greenspan BJ, Morrow PE: The effects of in vitro and aerosol exposures to cadmium on phagocytosis by rat pulmonary macrophages. *Fundam Appl Toxicol* 4:48–57, 1984.

Gutman AA: Allergens and other factors important in atopic disease, in Patterson R (ed): *Allergic Diseases, Diagnosis and Management,* 3d ed. Philadelphia: Lippincott, 1985, pp 123–175.

Guzzie PJ: Immunotoxicology in pharmaceutical development. in Gad SC (ed): *Safety Assessment for Pharmaceuticals.* New York: Wiley, 1995, pp 325–385.

Haines KA, Reibman J, Callegari PE, et al: Cocaine and its derivatives blunt neutrophil functions without influencing phosphorylation of a 47-kilodalton component of the reduced nicotinamide-adenine dinucleotide phosphate oxidase. *J Immunol* 144:4757–4764, 1990.

Hanifin JM, Epstein WL, Cline MJ: In vitro studies of granulomatous hypersensitivity to beryllium. *J Invest Dermatol* 55:284–288, 1970.

Harpey JP, Caille B, Moulias R, Goust JM: Lupus-linked syndrome induced by D-penicillamine in Wilson's Disease. *Lancet* 1:292, 1971.

Henderson WR, Fukuyama K, Epstein WL, Spitler LE: In vitro demonstration of delayed hypersensitivity in patients with beryliosis. *J Invest Dermatol* 58:5–8, 1972.

Hendrick DJ, Rando RJ, Lane DJ, Morris MJ: Formaldhyde asthma: Challenge exposure levels and fate after five years. *J Occup Med* 24:893–897, 1982.

Hjorth N: Diagnostic patch testing, in Marzulli FN, Maibach HI (eds): *Dermatotoxicology,* 3d ed. Washington, DC: Hemisphere, 1987, pp 307–317.

Hoffman EC, Reyes H, Chu F-F, et al: Cloning of a factor required for activity of the Ah (dioxin) receptor. *Science* 252:954, 1991.

Holladay SD: Prenatal immunotoxicant exposure and postnatal autoimmune disease. *Environ Health Perspect* 107(suppl 5):687–691, 1999.

Holladay SD, Blaylock BL, Comment CE, et al: Fetal thymic atrophy after exposure to T-2 toxin: Selectivity for lymphoid progenitor cells. *Toxicol Appl Pharmacol* 121(1):8–14, 1993.

Holladay SD, Comment CE, Kwon J, Luster MI: Fetal hematopoietic alterations after maternal exposure to ethylene glycol monomethyl ether: Prolymphoid cell targeting. *Toxicol Appl Pharmacol* 129(1):53–60, 1994.

Holsapple MP: Immunotoxicity of halogenated aromatic hydrocarbons, in Smialowicz R, Holsapple MP (eds): *Experimental Immunotoxicology.* Boca Raton, FL: CRC Press, 1996, pp 257–297.

Holsapple MP, Matulka RA, Stanulis ED, Jordan SD: Cocaine and immunocompetence: Possible role of reactive metabolites. *Adv Exp Med Biol* 335:121–126, 1993.

Holsapple MP, Morris DL, Wood SC, Snyder NK: 2,3,7,8-tetrachlorodibenzo-*p*-dioxin-induced changes in immunocompetence: Possible mechanisms. *Annu Rev Pharmacol Toxicol* 31:73–100, 1991a.

Holsapple MP, Munson AE, Munson JA, Bick PH: Suppression of cell-mediated immunocompetence after subchronic exposure to diethylstilbestrol in female B6C3F1 mice. *J Pharmacol Exp Ther* 227:130–138, 1983.

Holsapple MP, Snyder NK, Gokani V, et al: Role of Ah receptor in suppression of in vivo antibody response by 2,3,7,8-tetrachlorodibenzo-*p*-dioxin (TCDD) is dependent on exposure conditions. *Fed Am Soc Exp Biol J* 5(4):A508, 1991c.

Holsapple MP, Snyder NK, Wood SC, Morris DL: A review of 2,3,7,8-tetrachlorodibenzo-*p*-dioxin-induced changes in immunocompetence. *Toxicology* 69:219–255, 1991b.

House RV, Laurer LD, Murray MJ, et al: Immunological studies in B6C3F1 mice following exposure to ethylene glycol monomethyl ether and its principal metabolite methoxyacetic acid. *Toxicol Appl Pharmacol* 77(2):358–362, 1985.

House RV, Ratajczak HV, Gauger JR, et al: Immune function and host defense in rodents exposed to 60-Hz magnetic fields. *Fundam Appl Toxicol* 34(2):228–239, 1996.

Institute of Medicine (IOM): in Bondurant S, Ernster V, Herdman R (eds): *Safety of Silicone Breast Implants.* Washington, DC: National Academy Press, 2000.

International Life Sciences Institute (ILSI): *Application of Flow Cytometry to Immunotoxicity Testing: Summary of a Workshop.* Washington, DC: ILSI Press, 1999.

International Programme on Chemical Safety (IPCS): *Environmental Health Criteria 180: Principles and Methods for Assessing Direct Immunotoxicity Associated with Exposure to Chemicals.* Geneva, Switzerland: World Health Organization, 1996.

Jeon YJ, Han SH, Yang KH, Kaminski NE: Induction of liver-associated transforming growth factor $\beta1$ (TGF-$\beta1$) mRNA expression by carbon tetrachloride leads to the inhibition of T helper 2 cell-associated lymphokines. *Toxicol Appl Pharmacol* 144:27–35, 1997.

Jerrells TR, Pruett SB: Immunotoxic effects of ethanol, in Dean JH, Luster MI, Munson AE, Kimber I (eds): *Immunotoxicology and Immunopharmacology,* 2d ed. New York: Raven Press, 1994, pp 323–347.

Jiang X, Khursigara G, Rubin RL: Transformation of lupus-inducing drugs to cytotoxic products by activated neutrophils. *Science* 266(5186):810–813, 1994.

Kalland T: Alterations of antibody responses in female mice after neonatal exposure to diethylstilbestrol. *J Immunol* 124:194–198, 1980.

Kalland T, Strand O, Forsberg JG: Long-term effects of neonatal estrogen treatment on mitogen responsiveness of mouse spleen lymphocytes. *J Natl Cancer Inst* 63:413–421, 1979.

Kaminski NE: Mechanisms of immune modulation by cannabinoids, in Dean JH, Luster MI, Munson AE, Kimber I (eds): *Immunotoxicology and Immunopharmacology,* 2d ed. New York: Raven Press, 1994, pp 349–362.

Kaminski NE, Abood ME, Kessler FK, et al: Identification of a functionally relevant cannabinoid receptor on mouse spleen cells involved in cannabinoid-mediated immune modulation. *Mol Pharmacol* 42:736–742, 1992.

Karol MH: Models of contact and respiratory sensitivity and structure-activity relationships, continuing education course, *Chemical Hypersensitivity.* New Orleans: Society of Toxicology, March 1999.

Karol MH, Graham C, Gealy R, et al: Structure-activity relationships and computer-assisted analysis of respiratory sensitization potential. *Toxicol Lett* 86:187–191, 1996.

Kately JR, Bazzell SJ: Immunological studies in cattle exposed to polybrominated biphenyl. *Environ Health Perspect* 23:750, 1978.

Kawabata TT, White KL Jr: Effects of naphthlene metabolites on the in vitro humoral immune response. *J Toxicol Environ Health* 30:53–67, 1990.

Kayama F, Yamashita U, Kawamoto T, Kodama Y: Selective depletion of immature thymocytes by oral administration of ethylene glycol monomethyl ether. *Int J Immunopharmacol* 13(5):531–540, 1991.

Kenna JG, Neuberger J, Williams R: Identification by immunoblotting of three halothane-induced microsomal polypeptide antigens recognized by antibodies in sera from patients with halothane-associated hepatitis. *J Pharmacol Exp Ther* 242:733–740, 1987.

Kerkvliet NI: Halogenated aromatic hydrocarbons (HAH) as immunotoxicants, in Kende M, Gainer J, Chirigos M (eds): *Chemical Regulation of Immunity in Veterinary Medicine.* New York: Liss, 1984, pp 369–387.

Kerkvliet NI, Brauner JA: Flow cytometric analysis of lymphocyte subpopulations in the spleen and thymus of mice exposed to an acute immunosuppressive dose of 2,3,7,8-tetrachlorodibenzo-*p*-dioxin (TCDD). *Environ Res* 52:146–164, 1990.

Kerkvliet NI, Brauner JA: Mechanisms of 1,2,3,4,6,7,8-Heptachlorodibenzo-*p*-dioxin (HpCDD)-induced humoral immune suppression: Evidence of primary defect in T cell regulation. *Toxicol Appl Pharmacol* 87:18–31, 1987.

Kerkvliet NI, Burleson GR: Immunotoxicity of TCDD and related halogenated aromatic hydrocarbons, in Dean JH, Luster MI, Munson AE, Kimber I (eds): *Immunotoxicology and Immunopharmacology,* 2d ed. New York: Raven Press, 1994, pp 97–121.

Kerkvliet NI, Steppan LB, Brauner JA, et al: Influence of the Ah locus on the humoral immunotoxicity of 2,3,7,8-tetrachlorodibenzo-*p*-dioxin: Evidence for Ah receptor-dependent and Ah receptor-independent mechanisms of immunosuppression. *Toxicol Appl Pharmacol* 105:26–36, 1990.

Kilburn KH, Warshaw RH: Chemical-induced autoimmunity, in Dean JH, Luster MI, Munson AE, Kimber I (eds): *Immunotoxicology and Immunopharmacology,* 2d ed. New York: Raven Press, 1994, pp 523–538.

Kilburn KH, Warshaw RH: Prevalence of symptoms of systemic lupus erythematosus (SLE) and of fluorescent antinuclear antibodies associated with chronic exposure to trichlorethylene and other chemicals in well water. *Environ Res* 57:1–9, 1992.

Kim BS, Smialowicz RJ: The role of metabolism in 2-methoxyethanol-induced suppression of in vitro polyclonal antibody responses by rat and mouse lymphocytes. *Toxicology* 123(3):227–239, 1997.

Kimber I, Kerkvliet NI, Taylor SL, et al: Toxicology of protein allergenicity: Prediction and characterization. *Toxicol Sci* 48:157–162, 1999.

Kimber I, Basketter DA, Dearman RJ: Divergent antibody responses induced in mice by food proteins. *Toxicol Sci* 54(1): A1162, 2000.

Kimber IA, Hilton J, Botham PA, et al: The murine local lymph node assay: Results of an inter-laboratory trial. *Toxicol Lett* 55:203–213, 1991.

Kimber IA, Hilton J, Weisenberger C: The murine local lymph node assay for identification of contact allergens: A preliminary evaluation of *in situ* measurement of lymphocyte proliferation. *Contact Dermatitis* 21:215–220, 1989.

Klecak G: Identification of contact allergens: Predicitive tests in animals, in Marzulli FN, Maibach HI (eds): *Dermatotoxicology,* 3d ed. Washington, DC: Hemisphere, 1987, pp 227–290.

Klykken PC, Galbraith TM, Kolesar GB, et al: Toxicology and humoral immunity assessment of octamethylcyclotetrasiloxane (D_4) following a 28-day whole-body vapor inhalation exposure in Fischer 344 rats. *Drug Chem Toxicol* 22(4):655–677, 1999.

Klykken PC, White KL Jr: The adjuvancy of silicones: Dependency on compartmentalization, in Potter M, Rose NR (eds): *Current Topics in Microbiology and Immunology.* Vol 210. New York: Springer-Verlag, 1996, pp 113–121.

Knippels LMJ, Spanhaak S, Pennicks AH: Oral sensitization to peanut proteins: A brown Norway rat food allergy model. *Toxicol Sci* 54(1): A1161, 2000.

Knippels LMJ, Penninks AH, Smit JJ, Houben GF: Immune-mediated effects upon oral challenge of ovalbumin-sensitized brown Norway rats: Further characterization of a rat food allergy model. *Toxicol Appl Pharmacol* 156:161–169, 1999.

Koller LD: Immunotoxicology of heavy metals. *Int J Immunopharmacol* 2:269–279, 1980.

Krzystyniak K, Hugo P, Flipo D, Fournier M: Increased susceptibility to mouse hepatitis virus 3 of peritoneal macrophages exposed to dieldrin. *Toxicol Appl Pharmacol* 80:397–408, 1985.

Kunz J, Henriquez R, Schneider U, et al: Target of rapamycin in yeast, TOR2, is an essential phosphatidylinositol kinase homolog required for G1 progression. *Cell* 73:585–596, 1993.

Ladics GS, Kawabata TT, Munson AE, White KL Jr: Metabolism of benzo[*a*]pyrene by murine splenic cell types. *Toxicol Appl Pharmacol* 116:248–257, 1992a.

Ladics GS, Kawabata TT, Munson AE, White KL Jr: Generation of 7,8-dihydroxy-9,10-epoxy-7,8,9,10-tetrahydrobenzo[*a*]pyrene by murine splenic macrophages. *Toxicol Appl Pharmacol* 115:72–79, 1992b.

Ladics GS, Kawabata TT, White KL Jr: Suppression of the in vitro humoral immune response of mouse splenocytes by 7,12-dimethylbenz[*a*]anthracene metabolites and inhibition of suppression by a-naphthoflavone. *Toxicol Appl Pharmacol* 110:31–44, 1991.

Ladics GS, Smith C, Heaps K, Loveless SE: Evaluation of the humoral immune response to CD rats following a 2-week exposure to the pesticide carbaryl by the oral, dermal, and inhalation routes. *J Toxicol Environ Health* 42:143–156, 1994.

Ladics GS, Smith C, Nicastro S, et al: Evaluation of the primary humoral immune response following exposure of male rats to 17β estradiol or flutamide for 15 days. *Toxicol Sci* 46:75–82, 1998.

Lawrence DA: Immunotoxicity of heavy metals, in Dean JH, Luster MI, Munson AE, Amos H (eds): *Immunotoxicology and Immunopharmacology.* New York: Raven Press, 1985, pp. 341–353.

Lawrence DA (ed), in Sipes IG, McQueen, CA, Gandolfi AJ (eds-in-chief): *Comprehensive Toxicology.* Vol 5. *Toxicology of the Immune System.* New York: Elsevier, 1997.

Lawrence DA, Kim D: Central/peripheral nervous system and immune responses. *Toxicology* 142:189–291, 2000.

Le UL, Munson AE: Differential effects of octamethylcyclotetrasiloxane (D_4) on $CD4^+$ and $CD8^+$-T cell functions in B6C3F1 mice. *Fundam Appl Toxicol Suppl* 36(1):A1346, 1997.

Lefkowitz SS, Vaz A, Lefkowitz DL: Cocaine reduces macrophage killing by inhibiting reactive oxygen intermediates. *Int J Immunopharmacol* 15:717–721, 1993.

LeVier DG, Brown RD, McCay JA, et al: Hepatic and splenic phagocytosis in female B6C3F1 mice implanted with morphine sulfate pellets. *J Pharmacol Exp Ther* 367:357–363, 1993.

LeVier DG, McCay JA, Stern ML, et al: Immunotoxicological profile of morphine sulfate in B6C3F1 mice. *Fundam Appl Toxicol* 22:525–542, 1994.

LeVier DG, Musgrove DL, Munson AE: The effect of octamethylcyclotetrasiloxane (D_4) on the humoral immune response of B6C3F1 mice. *Fundam Appl Toxicol Suppl* 15(1):A1199, 1995.

Levy MH, Wheelock EF: Effects of intravenous silica on immune and non-immune functions of the murine host. *J Immunol* 115:41–48, 1975.

Liberman P, Crawford L, Drewry RD Jr, Tuberville A: Allergic diseases of the eye and ear, in Patterson R (ed): *Allergic Diseases, Diagnosis and Management,* 3d ed. Philadelphia: Lippincott, 1985, pp 374–407.

Looney RJ, Frampton MW, Byam J, et al: Acute respiratory exposure of human volunteers to octamethylcyclotetrasiloxane (D_4): Absence of immunological effects. *Toxicol Sci* 44:214–220, 1998.

Lundberg K, Grovnick K, Goldschmidt TJ, et al: 2,3,7,8-tetrachlorodibenzo-*p*-dioxin (TCDD) alters intrathymic T cell development in mice. *Chem Biol Interact* 74:179, 1990.

Luster MI, Boorman GA, Dean JH, et al: Effect of in utero exposure of diethylstilbestrol on the immune response in mice. *Toxicol Appl Pharmacol* 47:287–293, 1979.

Luster MI, Boorman GA, Dean JH, et al: The effect of adult exposure to diethylstilbestrol in the mouse: Alterations in immunological functions. *J Retic Soc* 28:561–569, 1980.

Luster MI, Boorman GA, Korach KS, et al: Mechanisms of estrogen-induced myelotoxicity: Evidence of thymic regulation. *Int J Immunopharmacol* 6:287–297, 1984a.

Luster MI, Dean JH, Boorman GA, et al: Host resistance and immune functions in methyl and ethyl carbamate treated mice. *Clin Exp Immunol* 50:223–230, 1982.

Luster MI, Hayes HT, Korach K, et al: Estrogen immunosuppression is regulated through estrogenic responses in the thymus. *J Immunol* 133:110–116, 1984b.

Luster MI, Munson AE, Thomas PT, et al: Development of a testing battery to assess chemical-induced immunotoxicity: National Toxicology Program's guidelines for immunotoxicity evaluation in mice. *Fundam Appl Toxicol* 10:2–9, 1988.

Luster MI, Portier C, Pait DG, et al: Risk assessment in immunotoxicology. I. Sensitivity and predictability of immune tests. *Fundam Appl Toxicol* 18:200–210, 1992.

Luster MI, Portier C, Pait DG, and Germolec DR: Use of animal studies in risk assessment for immunotoxicology. *Toxicology* 92:229–243, 1994.

Luster MI, Tucker JA, Germolec DR, et al: Immunotoxicity studies in mice exposed to methyl isocyanate. *Toxicol Appl Pharmacol* 86:140–144, 1986.

Madden KS, Sanders VM, Felten DL: Catecholamine influences and sympathetic neural modulation of immune responsiveness. *Annu Rev Pharmacol Toxicol* 35:417–448, 1995.

Magnusson B, Kligman AM: The identification of contact allergens by animal assay. The guinea pig maximization test. *J Invest Dermatol* 52:268–276, 1969.

Maibach H: Formaldehyde: Effects on animal and human skin, in Gibson J (ed): *Formaldehyde Toxicity.* Washinton, DC: Hemisphere, 1983, pp 166–174.

Marzulli FN, Maibach HI: Contact allergy: Predictive testing in humans, in Marzulli FN, Maibach HI (eds): *Dermatotoxicology,* 3d ed. Washington, DC: Hemisphere, 1987, pp 319–340.

Marzulli FN, Maibach HI: The use of graded concentrations in studying skin sensitizers: Experimental contact sensitization in man. *Food Cosmet Toxicol* 12:219–227, 1974.

Matveyeva M, Hartmann CB, Harrison MT et al: Delta(9)-tetrahydrocannabinol selectively increases aspartyl cathepsin D proteolytic activity and impairs lysozomal processing by macrophages. *Int J Immunopharmacol* 22(5):373–381, 2000.

McCabe MJ Jr: Mechanisms and consequences of immunomodulation by lead, in Dean JH, Luster MI, Munson AE, Kimber I (eds): *Immunotoxicology and Immunopharmacology,* 2d ed. New York: Raven Press, 1994, pp 143–162.

McDonough RJ, Madden JJ, Falck A, et al: Alteration of T and null lymphocyte frequencies in the peripheral blood of human opiate addicts: In vivo evidence for opiate receptor sites on T lymphocytes. *J Immunol* 125:2539–2543, 1980.

Menna JH, Barnett JB, Soderberg LSF: Influenze type A infection of mice exposed in utero to chlordane: Survival and antibody studies. *Toxicol Lett* 24:45–52, 1985.

Menné T: Reactions to systemic exposure to contact allergens, in Marzulli FN, Maibach HI (eds): *Dermatotoxicology,* 3d ed. Washington, DC: Hemisphere, 1987, pp 535–552.

Miller K, Brown RC: The immune system and asbestos-associated disease, in Dean JH, Luster MI, Munson AE, Amos H (eds): *Immunotoxicology and Immunopharmacology.* New York: Raven Press, 1985, pp 429–440.

Miller N, Wilson M, Bengten E, et al: Functional and molecular characterization of teleost leukocytes. *Immunol Rev* 166:187–197, 1998.

Mishell RI, Dutton RW: Immunization of dissociated mouse spleen cell culture from normal mice. *J Exp Med* 126:423–442, 1967.

Morice WG, Brunn GJ, Wiederrecht G, et al: Rapamycin-induced inhibition of $p34^{cdc2}$ kinase activation is associated with G_1/S phase growth arrest in T lymphocytes. *J Biol Chem* 268:3734–3738, 1993.

Mosmann TR, Coffman RL: Heterogeneity of cytokine secretion patterns and function of helper T cells. *Adv Immunol* 46:111–147, 1989.

Mosmann TR, Schumacher JH, Street NF, et al: Diversity of cytokine synthesis and function of mouse $CD4^+$ T cells. *Immunol Rev* 123:209–229, 1991.

Munro S, Thomas KL, Abu-Shaar M: Molecular characterization of peripheral receptor for cannabinoids. *Nature* 365:61–65, 1993.

Munson AE: Immunological evaluation of octamethylcyclotetrasiloxane (D_4) using a twenty-eight day exposure in male and female Fischer 344 rats. Document Control Number 86980000072. Washington, DC: USEPA-OPPT, TSCA Document Processing Center, 1998.

Munson AE, McCay JA, Brown RD, et al: The immune status of Fischer 344 rats administered octamethylcyclotetrasiloxane (D_4) by oral gavage. *Fundam Appl Toxicol Suppl* 36(1):A1347, 1997.

Murphy WG, Kelton JG: Immune haemolytic anaemia and thrombocytopaenia with drugs and antibodies. *Biochem Soc Trans* 19:183–186, 1991.

Myers MJ, Schook LB: Immunotoxicity of nitrosamines, in Smialowicz R, Holsapple MP (eds): *Experimental Immunotoxicology.* Boca Raton, FL: CRC Press, 1996, pp 351–366.

Mydlarski P, Katz A, Sauder D: Contact dermatitis, in Middleton E Jr, Reed C, Ellis E, et al (eds:) *Allergy Principles and Practice.* St. Louis: Mosby, 1998, pp 1141–1143.

Newman LS: Beryllium lung disease: The role of cell-mediated immunity in pathogenesis, in Dean JH, Luster MI, Munson AE, Kimber I (eds): *Immunotoxicology and Immunopharmacology,* 2d ed. New York: Raven Press, 1994, pp 377–394.

NIH Publication No. 99-4494: *The Murine Local Lymph Node Assay: A Test Method for Assessing the Allergic Contact Dermatitis Potential of Chemicals/Compounds.* Washington, DC: National Institute of Environmental Health Sciences, National Institutes of Health, U.S. Public Health Service, Department of Health and Human Services, 1999.

Noonan FP, De Fabo EC: Ultraviolet-B-dose response curves for local and systemic immunosuppression are identical. *Photochem Photobiol* 52:801–810, 1990.

Ou D, Shen ML, Luo YD: Effects of cocaine on the immune system of BALB/c mice. *Clin Immunol Immunopathol* 52:305–312, 1989.

Paul WE (ed): *Fundamental Immunology,* 4d ed. New York: Raven Press, 1999.

Paul WE, Seder RA: Lymphocyte responses and cytokines. *Cell* 76:241–251, 1994.

Pelletier L, Castedo M, Bellon B, Druet P: Mercury and autoimmunity, in Dean JH, Luster MI, Munson AE, Kimber I (eds): *Immunotoxicology and Immunopharmacology,* 2d ed. New York: Raven Press, 1994, pp 539–552.

Penninks AH, Snoeij NJ, Pieters RHH, Seinen W: Effect of organotin compounds on lymphoid organs and lymphoid functions: An overview, in Dayan AD, Hentel RF, Heseltine E, et al (eds): *Immunotoxicity of Metals and Immunotoxicology.* New York: Plenum Press, 1990, pp 191–207.

Pernis B, Paronetto F: Adjuvant effect of silica (tridymite) on antibody production. *Proc Soc Exp Biol Med* 110:390–392, 1962.

Peterson PK, Gekker G, Chao CC, et al: Cocaine potentiates HIV-1 replication in human peripheral blood mononuclear cell cultures. Involvement of transforming growth factor-b. *J Immunol* 146:81–84, 1991.

Potter M, Rose NR (eds): *Immunology of Silicones,* New York: Springer-Verlag, 1996.

Pruett SB, Barnes DB, Han YC, Munson AE: Immunotoxicological characteristics of sodium methyldithiocarbamate. *Fundam Appl Toxicol* 18:40–47, 1992a.

Pruett SB, Han Y, Fuchs BA: Morphine suppresses primary humoral immune responses by a predominantly indirect mechanism. *J Pharmacol Exp Ther* 262:923–928, 1992b.

Quesniaux VFJ: Interleukins 9, 10, 11, and 12, and kit ligand: A brief overview. *Res Immunol* 143:385–400, 1992.

Robinson MK, Babcock LS, Horn PA, Kawabata TT: Specific antibody responses to subtilisin Carlsberg (alcalase) in mice: Development of an intranasal exposure model. *Fundam Appl Toxicol* 34:15–24, 1996.

Rodgers K, Klykken P, Jacobs J, et al: Symposium overview: Immunotoxicity of medical devices. *Fundam Appl Toxicol* 36:1–14, 1997.

Roitt I, Brostoff J, Male D (eds): *Immunology,* 3d ed. London: Mosby, 1993.

Rose RN: Immunopathogenesis of autoimmune diseases, in Dean JH, Luster MI, Munson AE, Kimber I (eds): *Immunotoxicology and Immunopharmacology,* 2d ed. New York: Raven Press, 1994, pp 513–522.

Rosenthal GJ, Kowolenko M: Immunotoxicologic manifestations of AIDS therapeutics, in Dean JH, Luster MI, Munson AE, Kimber I (eds): *Immunotoxicology and Immunopharmacology,* 2d ed. New York: Raven Press, 1994, pp 227–247.

Ruddle NH: Tumor necrosis factor (TNFα) and lymphotoxin (TFNβ). *Curr Opin Immunol* 4:327–332, 1994.

Sabatini DM, Erdjument-Bromage H, Lui M, et al: A mammalian protein that binds to FKBP12 in a rapamycin-dependent fashion and is homologous to yeast TORs. *Cell* 78:35–43, 1994.

Sabers CJ, Martin MM, Brunn GJ, et al: Isolation of a protein target of the FKBP12–rapamycin complex in mammalian cells. *J Biol Chem* 270(2):815–822, 1995.

Salem ML, Hossain MS, Nomoto K: Mediation of the immunomodulatory effect of β-estradiol on inflammatory responses by inhibition of recruitment and activation of inflammatory cells and their gene expression of TNFα and IFNγ. *Int Arch Allergy Immunol* 121(3):235–245, 2000.

Sanders VM: Neuroimmunology, in Sipes IG, McQueen CA, and Gandolfi AJ (eds-in-chief): *Comprehensive Toxicology.* Vol 5. Lawrence DA (ed): *Toxicology of the Immune System.* New York: Elsevier, 1997, pp 175–199.

Sanders VM, Tucker AN, White KL Jr, et al: Humoral and cell-mediated immune status in mice exposed to trichloroethylene in the drinking water. *Toxicol Appl Pharmacol* 62:358–368, 1982.

Sanders VM, White KL Jr, Shopp GM, Munson AE: Humoral and cell-mediated immune status of mice exposed to 1,1,2-trichloroethane. *Drug Chem Toxicol* 8(5):357–372, 1985.

Sapin C, Mandet C, Druet E, et al: Immune complex type disease induced by $HgCl_2$: Genetic control of susceptibility. *Transplant Proc* 13:1404–1406, 1981.

Sarlo K, Karol MH: Guinea pig predictive tests for respiratory allergy, in Dean JH, Luster MI, Munson AE, Kimber I (eds): *Immunotoxicology and Immunopharmacology,* 2d ed. New York: Raven Press, 1994, pp 703–720.

Schatz AR, Kessler FK, Kaminski NE: Inhibition of adenylate cyclase by D9-tetrahydrocannabinol in mouse spleen cells: A potential mechanism for cannabinoid-mediated immunosuppression. *Life Sci* 51:25–30, 1992.

Schwarz A, Grabbe S, Reimann H, et al: In vivo effects of interleukin-10 on contact hypersensitivity and delayed-type hypersensitivity reactions. *J Invest Dematol* 103:211–216, 1994.

Selgrade MJK: Use of immunotoxicity data in health risk assessments: Uncertainties and research to improve the process. *Toxicology* 133:59–72, 1999.

Selgrade MJK, Cooper KD, Devlin RB, et al: Symposium overview: Immunotoxicity—bridging the gap between animal research and human health effects. *Fundam Appl Toxicol* 24:13–32, 1995.

Selgrade MJK, Gilmour MI: Effects of gaseous air pollutants on immune responses and susceptibility to infectious and allergic diseases, in Dean JH, Luster MI, Munson AE, Kimber I (eds): *Immunotoxicology and Immunopharmacology,* 2d ed. New York: Raven Press, 1994, pp 395–411.

Sherwood R, O'Shea W, Thomas P, et al: Effects of inhalation of ethylene dichloride on pulmonary defenses of mice and rats. *Toxicol Appl Pharmacol* 91:491–496, 1987.

Shopp GM, Sanders VM, Munson AE: Humoral and cell-mediated immune status of mice exposed to trans-1,2-dichloroethylene. *Drug Chem Toxicol* 8(5):393–407, 1985.

Shopp GM, White KL Jr, Holsapple MP, et al: Naphthlene toxicity in CD-1 mice: General toxicology and immunotoxicology. *Fundam Appl Toxicol* 4:406–419, 1984.

Sikorski EE, Kipen HM, Selner JC, et al: Roundtable summary: The question of multiple chemical sensitivity. *Fundam Appl Toxicol* 24:22–28, 1995.

Silkworth JB, Loose LD: Cell-mediated immunity in mice fed either Aroclor 1016 or hexachlorobenzene. *Toxicol Appl Pharmacol* 45:326–327, 1978.

Silkworth JB, Loose LD: PCB and HCB induced alteration of lymphocyte blastogenesis. *Toxicol Appl Pharmacol* 49:86, 1979.

Silver RM, Heyes MP, Maize JC, et al: Scleroderma, fasciitis and eosinophilia associated with the ingestion of tryptophan. *N Engl J Med* 322:874–881, 1990.

Simon JC, Cruz PD, Bergstresser PR, Tigelaar RE: Low dose ultraviolet B-irradiated Langerhans cells preferentially activate $CD4^+$ cells of the T helper 2 subset. *J Immunol* 145:2087–2094, 1990.

Siroki O, Institoris L, Tatar F, Desi I: Immunotoxicological investigation of SCMF, a new pyrethroid pesticide in mice. *Hum Exp Toxicol* 13:337–343, 1994.

Smialowicz RJ, Holsapple MP: *Experimental Immunotoxicology* Boca Raton, FL: CRC Press, 1996.

Smialowicz RJ, Riddle MM, Lubke RW, et al: Immunotoxicity of 2-methoxyethanol following oral adminstration in Fischer 344 rats. *Toxicol Appl Pharmacol* 109(3):494–506, 1991a.

Smialowicz RJ, Riddle MM, Rogers RR, et al: Evaluation of the immunotoxicity of orally administered 2-methoxyacetic acid in Fischer 344 rats. *Fundam Appl Toxicol* 17(4):771–781, 1991b.

Snyder CA: Organic solvents, in Dean JH, Luster MI, Munson AE, Kimber I (eds): *Immunotoxicology and Immunopharmacology,* 2d ed. New York: Raven Press, 1994, pp 183–190.

Sopori ML, Goud NS, Kaplan AM: Effects of tobacco smoke on the immune system, in Dean JH, Luster MI, Munson AE, Kimber I (eds): *Immunotoxicology and Immunopharmacology,* 2d ed. New York: Raven Press, 1994, pp 413–434.

Spreafico F, Allegrucci M, Merendino A, Luini W: Chemical immunodepressive drugs: Their action on the cells of the immune system and immune mediators, in Dean JH, Luster MI, Munson AE, Amos H (eds): *Immunotoxicology and Immunopharmacology.* New York: Raven Press, 1985, pp 179–192.

Spyker-Cranmer JM, Barnett JB, Avery DL, Cranmer MF: Immunoteratology of chlordane: Cell-mediated and humoral immune responses in adult mice exposed in utero. *Toxicol Appl Pharmacol* 62:402–408, 1982.

Staples JE, Gasiewicz TA, Fiore NC et al: Estrogen receptor alpha is necessary in thymic development and estradiol-induced thymic alterations. *J Immunol* 162(8):4168–4174, 1999.

Starec M, Rouveix B, Sinet M, et al: Immune status and survival of opiate- and cocaine-treated mice infected with Friend virus. *J Pharmacol Exp Ther* 259:745–750, 1991.

Street JC: Pesticides and the immune system, in Sharma RP (ed): *Immunologic Considerations in Toxicology.* Boca Raton, FL: CRC Press, 1981, pp 46–66.

Sutter TR, Greenlee WF: Classification of members of the Ah gene battery. *Chemosphere* 25:223, 1992.

Sutter TR, Guzman K, Dold KM, Greenlee WF: Targets for dioxin: Genes for plasminogen activator inhibitor-2 and interleukin-1b. *Science* 254:415, 1991.

Talmadge JE, Dean JH: Immunopharmacology of recombinant cytokines, in Dean JH, Luster MI, Munson AE, Kimber I (eds): *Immunotoxicology and Immunopharmacology,* 2d ed. New York: Raven Press, 1994, pp 227–247.

Terada N, Lucas JJ, Szepesi A, et al: Rapamycin blocks cell cycle progression of activated T cells prior to events characteristic of the middle to late G_1 phase of the cycle. *J Cell Physiol* 154:7–15, 1993.

Thomas PT, Busse WW, Kerkvliet NI, et al: Immunologic effects of pesticides, in Baker SR, Wilkinson CF (eds): *The Effects of Pesticides on Human Health.* Vol 18. New York: Princeton Scientific Publishers, 1990, pp 261–295.

Thorne PS, Hawk C, Kaliszewski SD, Guiney PD: The noninvasive mouse ear swelling assay. I. Refinements for detecting weak contact sensitizers. *Fundam Appl Toxicol* 17:790–806, 1991.

Thurmond LM, Dean JH: Immunological responses following inhalation exposure to chemical hazards, in Gardner EE, Crapo JD, Massaro EJ (eds): *Toxicology of the Lung.* Raven Press, New York, 1988, pp 375–406.

Tognoni G, Boniccorsi A: Epidemiological problems with TCDD. A critical review. *Drug Metab Rev* 13:447–469, 1982.

Totoritis MC, Tan EM, McNally EM, Rubin RL: Association of antibody to histone complex H2A-H2B with symptomatic procainamide-induced lupus. *N Engl J Med* 318(22):1431–1436, 1988.

Tryphonas H, Luster MI, Schiffman G, et al: Effect of chronic exposure of PCB (Aroclor 1254) on specific and nonspecific immune parameters in the rhesus (*Macaca mulatta*) monkey. *Fundam Appl Toxicol* 16:773–786, 1991a.

Tryphonas H, Luster MI, White KL Jr, et al: Effect of chronic exposure of PCB (Aroclor 1254) on specific and nonspecific immune parameters in the rhesus (*Macaca mulatta*) monkey. *Int J Immunopharmacol* 13:639–648, 1991b.

Tubaro E, Santiangeli C, Belogi L, et al: Methadone vs morphine: Comparison of their effect on phagocytic functions. *Int J Immunopharmacol* 9:79–88, 1987.

Unanue E: Macrophages, antigen-presenting cells, and the phenomena of antigen handling and presentation, in Paul WE (ed): *Fundamental Immunology,* 3d ed. New York: Raven Press, 1993, pp 111–144.

Van Loveren H, Goettsch W, Slob W, Garssen J: Risk assessment of the harmful effects of UVB radiation on the immunological resistance to infectious diseases. *Arch Toxicol* 18:21–28, 1995.

Van Loveren H, Krajnc E, Rombout PJA, et al: Effects of ozone, hexachlorobenzene and bis(tri-*n*-butyltin)oxide on natural killer activity in the rat lung. *Toxicol Appl Pharmacol* 102:21–33, 1990.

Vecchi A, Sironi M, Canegrati MA, et al: Immunosuppressive effects of 2,3,7,8-tetrachlorodibenzo-*p*-dioxin in strains of mice with different susceptibility to induction of aryl hydrocarbon hydroxylase. *Toxicol Appl Pharmacol* 68:434–441, 1983.

Voccia I, Blakley B, Brousseau P, Fournier M: Immunotoxicity of pesticides: A review. *Toxicol Ind Health* 15:119–132, 1999.

Vohr HW, Bomhard EM: Investigations on the immunostimulating potential of a combination of octamethylcyclotetra and decamethylcycloptentasiloxane in rats and mice. *Toxicol Sci Suppl* 54(1):A734, 2000.

Vos JG: Immune suppression as related to toxicology. *CRC Crit Rev Toxicol* 5:67–101, 1977.

Vos JG, de Klerk A, Krajnc FI, et al: Toxicity of bis(tri-*n*-butyltin)oxide in the rat. II. Suppression of thymus-dependent immune responses and of parameters of non-specific resistance after short-term exposure. *Toxicol Appl Pharmacol* 75:387–408, 1984.

Vos JG, Luster MI: Immune alterations, in Kimbrough RD, Jensen AA (eds): *Halogenated Biphenyls, Terphenyls, Napthalenes, Dibenzodioxins, and Related Products.* Amsterdam: Elsevier, 1989, pp 295–322.

Vos JG, Smialowicz RJ, Van Loveren H: Animal models for assessment, in Dean JH, Luster MI, Munson AE, Kimber I (eds): *Immunotoxicology and Immunopharmacology,* 2d ed. New York: Raven Press, 1994, pp 19–30.

Walder BK: Do solvents cause scleroderma? *Int J Dermatol* 22:157–158, 1983.

Ward AM, Udnoon S, Watkins J, et al: Immunological mechanisms in the pathogenesis of vinyl chloride disease. *Br Med J* 1:936–938, 1976.

Ward EC, Murray MJ, Dean JH: Immunotoxicity of non-halogenated polycyclic aromatic hydrocarbons, in Dean JH, Luster MI, Munson AE, Amos H (eds): *Immunotoxicology and Immunopharmacology.* New York: Raven Press, 1985, pp 291–303.

Warheit DB, Hesterberg TW: Asbestos and other fibers in the lung, in Dean JH, Luster MI, Munson AE, Kimber I (eds): *Immunotoxicology and Immunopharmacology,* 2d ed. New York: Raven Press, 1994, pp 363–376.

Warner GL, Haggerty HG: Immunotoxicology of recombinant DNA-derived therapeutic proteins, in Sipes IG, McQueen CA, Gandolfi AJ (eds-in-chief): *Comprehensive Toxicology.* Vol 5. Lawrence DA (ed): *Toxicology of the Immune System.* New York: Elsevier, 1997, pp 435–450.

Wasserman M, Wasserman D, Gershon Z, Zellermayer L: Effects of organochlorine insecticides on body defense systems. *Ann NY Acad Sci* 160:393–401, 1969.

Watson ES, Murphy JC, El Sohly HN, et al: Effect of the administration of coca alkaloids on the primary immune responses of mice: Interaction with D^9-tetrahydrocannabinol and ethanol. *Toxicol Appl Pharmacol* 71:1–13, 1983.

Ways SC, Blair PB, Bern HA, Staskawicz MO: Immune responsiveness of adult mice exposed neonatally to diethylstilbestrol, steroid hormones, or vitamin A. *J Environ Pathol Toxicol* 3:207–220, 1980.

Weigent DA, Blalock JE: Associations between the neuroendocrine and immune systems. *J Leukocyte Biol* 58:137–150, 1995.

Wester PW, Vethaak AD, van Muiswinkel WB: Fish as biomarkers in immunotoxicology. *Toxicology* 86:213–232, 1994.

White KL Jr: Specific immune function assays, in Miller K, Turk JL, Nicklin S (eds): *Principles and Practice of Immunotoxicology.* Boston: Blackwell, 1992, pp 304–323.

White KL Jr, Anderson AC: Suppression of mouse complement activity by contaminants of technical grade pentachlorophenol. *Agents Actions* 16(5):385, 1985.

White KL Jr, Kawabata TT, Ladics GS: Mechanisms of polycyclic aromatic hydrocarbon immunotoxicity, in Dean JH, Luster MI, Munson AE, Kimber I (eds): *Immunotoxicology and Immunopharmacology,* 2d ed. New York: Raven Press, 1994, pp 123–142.

White KL Jr, Lysy HH, McCay JA, Anderson AC: Modulation of serum complement levels following exposure to polychlorinated dibenzo-*p*-dioxins. *Toxicol Appl Pharmacol* 84:209–219, 1986.

Williams WC, Riddle MM, Copeland CB, et al: Immunological effects of 2-methoxyethanol administered dermally or orally to Fischer 344 rats. *Toxicology* 98(1–3):215–223, 1995.

Wilson SD, LeVier DG, Butterworth LF, Munson AE: Natural killer cell activity is enhanced following exposure to octamethylcyclotetrasiloxane (D_4). *Fund Appl Toxicol Suppl* 15(1):A1198, 1995.

Woolhiser MR, Galbraith TW, Mast RW, Klykken PC: A comparative humoral adjuvancy study of low molecular weight cyclosiloxanes (D_4, D_5, D_6, and D_7) in rats. *Fund Appl Toxicol Suppl* 15(1):A1197, 1995.

Xiao F, Chong AS-F, Bartlett RR, Williams JW: Leflunomide: A promising immunosuppressant in transplantation, in Thomas AW, Starzyl TE (eds): *Immunosuppressive Drugs: Developments in Anti-Rejection Therapy.* Boston: Edward Arnold, 1994, pp 203–212.

Zelikoff JT: Biomarkers of immunotoxicity in fish and other nonmammalian sentinel species: Predictive value for mammals? *Toxicology* 129(1):63–71, 1998.

Zelikoff JT: Fish immunotoxicology. in Dean JH, Luster MI, Munson AE, Kimber I (eds): *Immunotoxicology and Immunopharmacology,* 2d ed. New York: Raven Press, 1994, pp 71–95.

Zelikoff JT, Thomas P (eds): *Immunotoxicology of Environmental and Occupational Metals.* Bristol, PA: Taylor & Francis, 1998.

Zelikoff JT, Raymond A, Carlson E, et al: Biomarkers of immunotoxicity in fish: From the lab to the ocean. *Toxicol Lett* 112–113:325–331, 2000.

Zurawski G, de Vries JE: Interleukin 13, an interleukin 4-like cytokine that acts on monocytes and B cells, but not T cells. *Immunol Today* 15(1):19–26, 1994.

CHAPTER 13

TOXIC RESPONSES OF THE LIVER

Mary Treinen-Moslen

INTRODUCTION

Numerous industrial compounds and therapeutic agents have been found to injure the liver. Consequently, the use of such chemicals has been eliminated or restricted. For example, carbon tetrachloride was commonly used in unventilated garages for degreasing automobile engines. Plastic industry workers without any protective equipment once crawled down into giant vats coated with residue containing vinyl chloride (Kramer, 1974). Now exposures to the potent hepatotoxins carbon tetrachloride and vinyl chloride are tightly regulated. However, each year new chemicals are found to damage the liver, such as the drugs Rezulin (troglitazone), prescribed for type 2 diabetes, and Rimadyl (carprofen), prescribed for dogs with arthritis. Usage of Rezulin in clinical medicine and Rimadyl in veterinary medicine was recently withdrawn or restricted based on reports of hepatic damage in more than 100 humans and over 8000 dogs, respectively (Kohlroser et al., 2000; Adams, 2000). During the 3-year period before the serious and sometimes fatal hepatotoxicity associated with their use was generally recognized, these two drugs were widely prescribed to over 800,000 humans and more than 4 million dogs. Initially promising drugs have been withdrawn during clinical trials when their hepatotoxicity became manifest after weeks or months of exposure. The 1993 clinical trial of fialuridine as a therapy for chronic viral hepatitis was suddenly terminated when some of the participating patients died of liver failure (McKenzie et al., 1995). Humans and animals continue to ingest hepatotoxins in foods, teas, and contaminated water. The serious problem of chemically induced liver damage has inspired excellent monographs (Zimmerman, 1978; Farrell, 1994; McCuskey and Earnest, 1997).

Observations on hepatotoxicants have advanced the understanding of hepatic functions and cell injury. Factors are known that determine why the liver, as opposed to other organs, is the dominant target site of specific toxins. Scientists have identified mechanisms by which chemicals injure specific populations of liver cells. New techniques in molecular biology, immunochemical probes, and the availability of transgenic animals provide new insights into basic physiologic and pathologic processes. Yet many questions remain. Why does end-stage liver disease occur in only 10 to 15 percent of those who chronically consume excess alcohol? How do genetic and acquired factors enhance vulnerability to alcohol and other toxicants?

Toxicologists regard the phrase "produces liver injury" as vague, since liver cells respond in many different ways to acute and chronic insults by chemicals. A basic understanding of chemical hepatotoxicity requires some appreciation of the physiology and anatomy of the liver. Key aspects for such appreciation are (1) major functions of the liver, (2) structural organization of the liver, and (3) processes involved in the excretory function of the liver, namely bile formation. These aspects contribute to the vulnerability of hepatic cells to chemical insults.

PHYSIOLOGY AND PATHOPHYSIOLOGY

Hepatic Functions

The liver's strategic location between intestinal tract and the rest of the body facilitates the performance of its enormous task of maintaining metabolic homeostasis of the body (Table 13-1). Venous blood from the stomach and intestines flows into the portal vein and then through the liver before entering the systemic circulation. Thus the liver is the first organ to encounter ingested nutrients, vitamins, metals, drugs, and environmental toxicants as well as waste products of bacteria that enter portal blood. Efficient scavenging or uptake processes extract these absorbed materials from the blood for catabolism, storage, and/or excretion into bile.

All of the major functions of the liver can be detrimentally altered by acute or chronic exposure to toxicants (Table 13-1). When toxicants inhibit or otherwise impede hepatic transport and synthetic processes, dysfunction can occur without appreciable cell

Table 13-1
Major Functions of Liver and Consequences of Impaired Hepatic Functions

TYPE OF FUNCTION	EXAMPLES	CONSEQUENCES OF IMPAIRED FUNCTIONS
Nutrient homeostasis	Glucose storage and synthesis	Hypoglycemia, confusion
	Cholesterol uptake	Hypercholesterolemia
Filtration of particulates	Products of intestinal bacteria (e.g., endotoxin)	Endotoxemia
Protein synthesis	Clotting factors	Excess bleeding
	Albumin	Hypoalbuminemia, ascites
	Transport proteins (e.g., very low density lipoproteins)	Fatty liver
Bioactivation and detoxification	Bilirubin and ammonia	Jaundice, hyperammonemia-related coma
	Steroid hormones	Loss of secondary male sex characteristics
	Xenobiotics	Diminished drug metabolism Inadequate detoxification
Formation of bile and biliary secretion	Bile acid–dependent uptake of dietary lipids and vitamins	Fatty diarrhea, malnutrition, Vitamin E deficiency
	Bilirubin and cholesterol	Jaundice, gallstones, hypercholesterolemia
	Metals (e.g., Cu and Mn)	Mn-induced neurotoxicity
	Xenobiotics	Delayed drug clearance

damage (Fig. 13-1). Loss of function also occurs when toxicants kill an appreciable number of cells and when chronic insult leads to replacement of cell mass by nonfunctional scar tissue. Alcohol abuse is the major cause of liver disease in most western countries (Crawford, 1999); thus ethanol provides a highly relevant example of a toxin with multiple functional consequences (Lieber, 1994). Early stages of ethanol abuse are characterized by lipid accumulation (fatty liver) due to diminished use of lipids as fuels and impaired ability to synthesize the lipoproteins that transport lipids out of the liver. As alcohol-induced liver disease progresses, appreciable cell death occurs, the functioning mass of the liver is replaced by scar tissue, and hepatic capacity for biotransformation of certain drugs progressively declines. People with hepatic cirrhosis due to chronic alcohol abuse frequently become deficient at detoxifying both the ammonia formed by catabolism of amino acids and the bilirubin derived from breakdown of hemoglobin. Uncontrollable hemorrhage due to inadequate synthesis of clotting factors is a common fatal complication of alcoholic cirrhosis. A consequence of liver injury that merits emphasis is that loss of liver functions can lead to aberrations in other organ systems and to death.

Structural Organization

Two concepts exist for organization of the liver into operational units, namely the lobule and the acinus. Classically, the liver was divided into hexagonal lobules oriented around terminal hepatic venules (also known as central veins). At the corners of the lobule are the portal triads (or portal tracts), containing a branch of the portal vein, a hepatic arteriole, and a bile duct (Fig. 13-2). Blood entering the portal tract via the portal vein and hepatic artery is mixed in the penetrating vessels, enters the sinusoids, and percolates along the cords of parenchymal cells (hepatocytes), eventually flows into terminal hepatic venules, and exits the liver via the hepatic vein. The lobule is divided into three regions known as centrolobular, midzonal, and periportal. Preferred as a concept of a functional hepatic unit is the acinus. The base of the acinus is formed by the terminal branches of the portal vein and hepatic artery, which extend out from the portal tracts. The acinus has three zones: zone 1 is closest to the entry of blood, zone 3 abuts the terminal hepatic vein, and zone 2 is intermediate. Despite the utility of the acinar concept, lobular terminology is still used to describe regions of pathologic lesions of hepatic parenchyma. Fortunately, the three zones of the acinus roughly coincide with the three regions of the lobule (Fig. 13-2).

Acinar zonation is of considerable functional consequence regarding gradients of components both in blood and in hepatocytes (Jungermann and Kietzmann, 2000). Blood entering the acinus consists of oxygen-depleted blood from the portal vein (60 to 70 percent of hepatic blood flow) plus oxygenated blood from the hepatic artery (30 to 40 percent). Enroute to the terminal hepatic venule, oxygen rapidly leaves the blood to meet the high metabolic demands of the parenchymal cells. Approximate oxygen concentrations in zone 1 are 9 to 13 percent, compared with only 4 to 5 percent in zone 3. Therefore hepatocytes in zone 3 are exposed to substantially lower concentrations of oxygen than hepatocytes in zone 1. In comparison to other tissues, zone 3 is hypoxic. Another well-documented acinar gradient is that of bile salts (Groothuis et al., 1982). Physiologic concentrations of bile salts are efficiently extracted by zone 1 hepatocytes with little bile salt left in the blood that flows past zone 3 hepatocytes (Fig. 13-3).

Heterogeneities in protein levels of hepatocytes along the acinus generate gradients of metabolic functions. Hepatocytes in the mitochondria-rich zone 1 are predominant in fatty acid oxidation, gluconeogenesis, and ammonia detoxification to urea. Gradients of

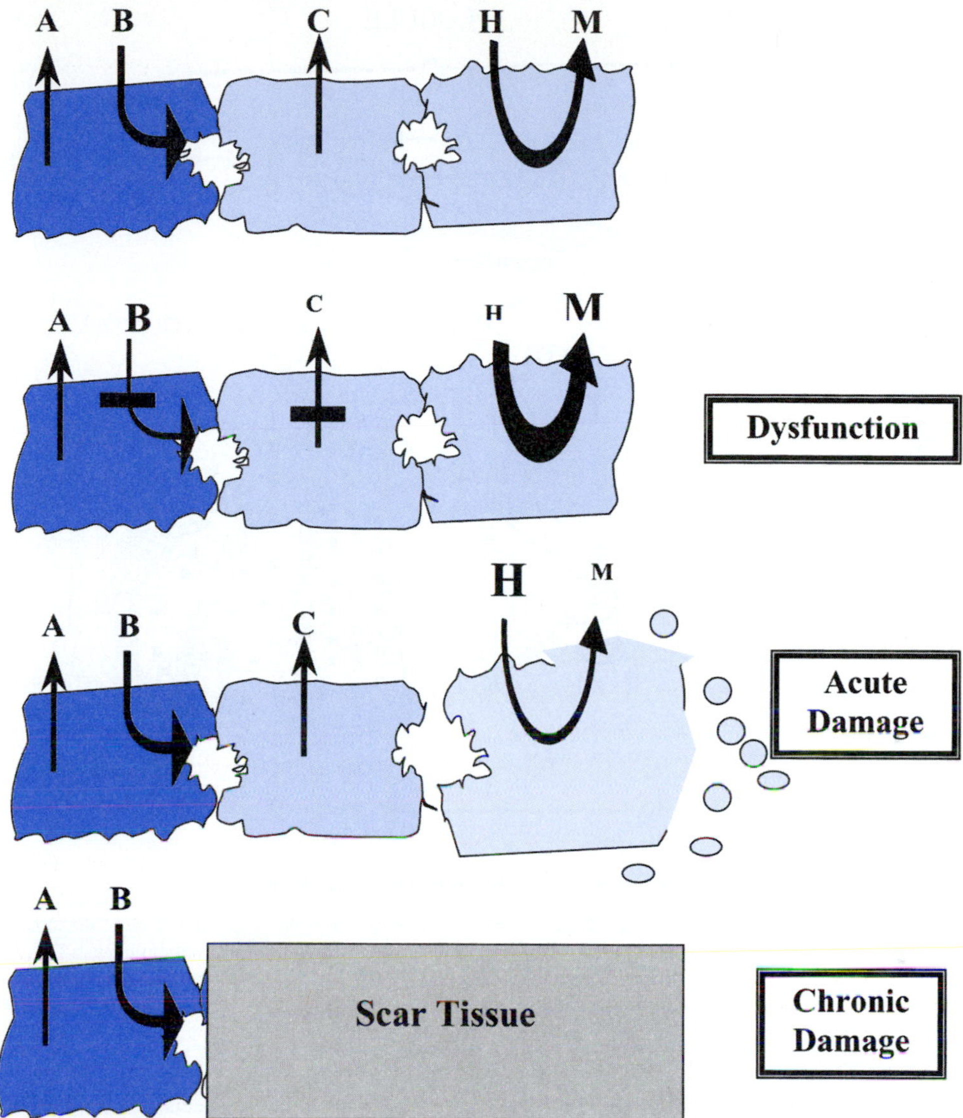

***Figure 13-1.** Cartoon depicting toxicant-mediated events that lead to loss of representative functions of hepatocytes, such as A, albumin secretion; B, bilirubin uptake and export into bile; C, clotting factor secretion; H and M, hormone uptake and bioactivation to metabolites.*

Dysfunction without cell damage can occur when toxicants inhibit uptake and secretion or excessively stimulate bioactivation. The dysfunction can be selective when a toxicant impedes secretion of only some compounds. Acute damage and chronic damage produce a loss of function in the cell population that dies or is replaced by scar tissue.

enzymes involved in the bioactivation and detoxification of xenobiotics have been observed along the acinus by immunohistochemistry (Jungermann and Katz, 1989). Notable gradients for hepatotoxins are the higher levels of glutathione in zone 1 and the greater amounts of cytochrome P450 proteins in zone 3, particularly the CYP2E1 isozyme inducible by ethanol (Tsutsumi, 1989).

Hepatic sinusoids are the channels between cords of hepatocytes where blood percolates on its way to the terminal hepatic vein. Sinusoids are larger and more irregular than normal capillaries. The three major types of cells in the sinusoids are endothelial cells, Kupffer cells, and Ito cells (Fig. 13-4). In addition, there are rare pit cells, a lymphocyte-type cell with anti-tumor activity. Sinusoids are lined by thin, discontinuous endothelial cells with numerous fenestrae (or pores) that allow molecules smaller than 250 kDa to cross the interstitial space (known as the space of Disse) between the endothelium and hepatocytes. Very little if any basement membrane separates the endothelial cells from the hepatocytes. The numerous fenestrae and the lack of basement membrane facilitate exchanges of fluids and molecules, such as albumin, between the sinusoid and hepatocytes but hinder movement of particles larger than chylomicron remnants. Endothelial cells are important in the scavenging of lipoproteins and denatured proteins. Hepatic endothelial cells also secrete cytokines.

Kupffer cells are the resident macrophages of the liver and constitute approximately 80 percent of the fixed macrophages in the body. Kupffer cells are situated within the lumen of the sinusoid. The primary function of Kupffer cells is to ingest and degrade particulate matter. Also, Kupffer cells are a source of cy-

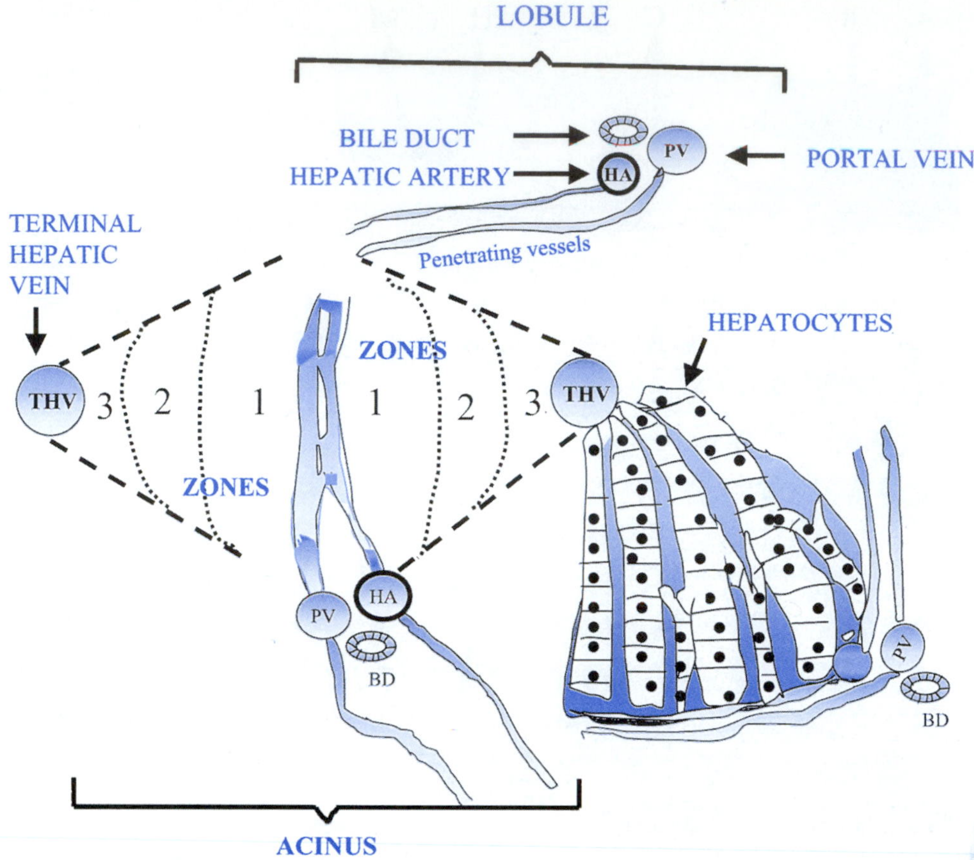

Figure 13-2. Schematic of liver operational units, the classic lobule and the acinus.

The lobule is centered around the terminal hepatic vein (central vein), where the blood drains out of the lobule. The acinus has as its base the penetrating vessels, where blood supplied by the portal vein and hepatic artery flows down the acinus past the cords of hepatocytes. Zones 1, 2, and 3 of the acinus represent metabolic regions that are increasingly distant from the blood supply.

tokines and can act as antigen-presenting cells (Laskin, 1990). Ito cells (also known by the more descriptive terms of *fat-storing cells* and *stellate cells*) are located between endothelial cells and hepatocytes. Ito cells synthesize collagen and are the major site for vitamin A storage in the body.

Bile Formation

Bile is a yellow fluid containing bile salts, glutathione, phospholipids, cholesterol, bilirubin and other organic anions, proteins, metals, ions, and xenobiotics (Klaassen and Watkins, 1984). Formation of this fluid is a specialized function of the liver. Adequate bile formation is essential for uptake of lipid nutrients from the small intestine (Table 13-1), for protection of the small intestine from oxidative insults (Aw, 1994), and for excretion of endogenous and xenobiotic compounds. Hepatocytes begin the process by transporting bile salts, glutathione, and other solutes into the canalicular lumen, which is a space formed by specialized regions of the plasma membrane between adjacent hepatocytes (Fig. 13-4). Tight junctions seal the canalicular lumen from materials in the sinusoid. The structure of the biliary tract is analogous to the roots and trunk of a tree, where the tips of the roots equate to the canalicular lumens. Canaliculi form channels between hepatocytes that connect to a series of larger and larger channels or ducts within the liver. The large extrahepatic bile ducts merge into the common bile duct. Bile can be stored and concentrated in the gallbladder before its release into the duodenum. However, the gallbladder is not essential to life and is absent in several species, including the horse, whale, and rat.

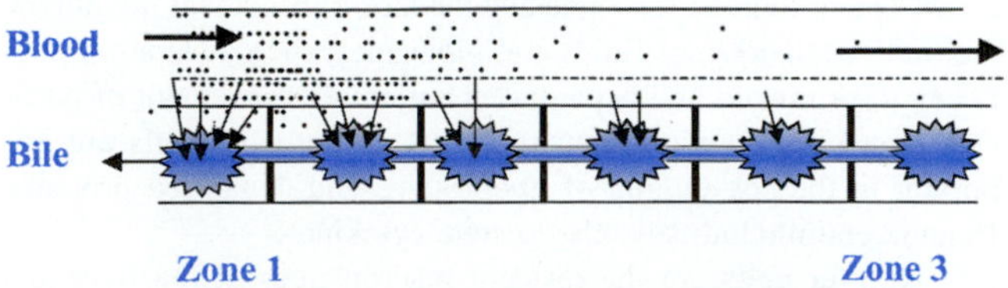

Figure 13-3. Schematic of the acinar gradient of bile salts.

Efficient uptake of bile salts by zone 1 hepatocytes results in very low levels of bile salts in the blood that flows past zone 3 hepatocytes. A less steep gradient exists for the uptake of bilirubin and other organic anions.

Our understanding of bile formation has evolved from a descriptive orientation toward identification of specific cellular and subcellular processes (Trauner et al., 1998). The major driving force is the active transport of bile salts and other osmolytes into the canalicular lumen. Transporters on the sinusoidal and canalicular membranes of hepatocytes are responsible for the uptake of

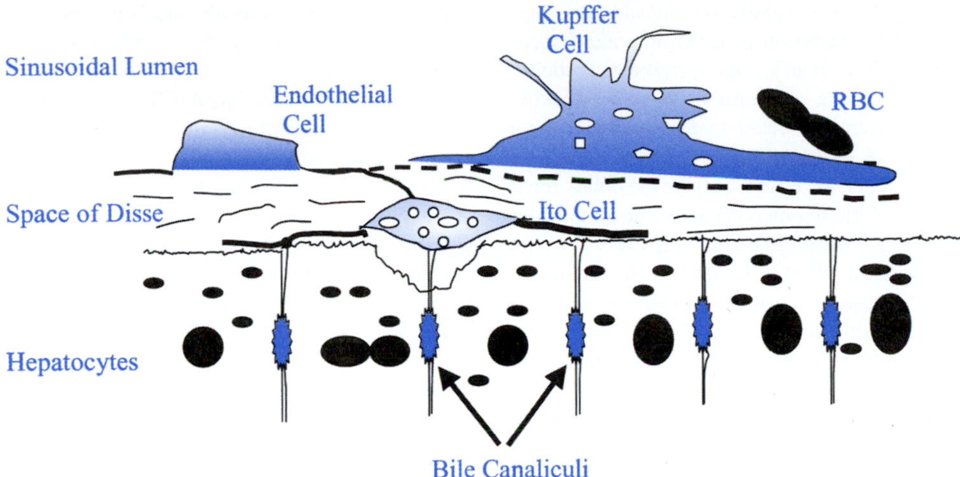

Figure 13-4. Schematic of liver sinusoidal cells.

Note that the Kupffer cell resides within the sinusoidal lumen. The Ito cell is located in the space of Disse between the thin, fenestrated endothelial cells and the cord of hepatocytes.

bile salts and bilirubin from blood and then the secretion of these solutes into the canalicular lumen (Fig. 13-5). Similarly, biliary secretion of drugs, hormones, and xenobiotics involves an extraction from the blood, transcytosis across hepatocytes, and then transport across the canalicular membrane by ATP-dependent exporters. Lipophilic cationic drugs, estrogens, and lipids are exported by the canalicular MDR (multiple-drug resistance) p-glycoproteins, one of which is exclusive for phospholipids (Gosland et al., 1993; Kusuhara et al., 1998). Conjugates of glutathione, glucuronide, and sulfate are exported by the canalicular multiple organic anion transporter (cMOAT), which is also somewhat confusingly known as MRP2, based on similarities of cMOAT with the product of the multidrug-resistance gene.

Metals are excreted into bile by a series of partially understood processes that include (1) uptake across the sinusoidal membrane by facilitated diffusion or receptor-mediated endocytosis; (2) storage in binding proteins or lysosomes; and (3) canalicular secretion via lysosomes, a glutathione-coupled event, or a specific canalicular membrane transporter (Ballatori, 1991). Biliary excretion is important in the homeostasis of multiple metals, notably copper, manganese, cadmium, selenium, gold, silver, and arsenic (Klaassen, 1976; Gregus and Klaassen, 1986). Species differences are known for biliary excretion of several toxic metals; for example, dogs excrete arsenic into bile much more slowly than rats. Inability to export Cu into bile is a central problem in Wilson's disease, a rare genetic disorder characterized by accumulation of Cu in the liver and then in other tissues. The exact nature of the defect in Cu export is uncertain, since the product of the Wilson's disease gene does not localize to the canalicular membrane (Nagano et al., 1998).

Canalicular lumen bile is propelled forward into larger channels by dynamic, ATP-dependent contractions of the pericanalicular cytoskeleton (Watanabe et al., 1991). Bile ducts, once regarded as passive conduits, modify bile by absorption and secretion of solutes (Lira et al., 1992). Biliary epithelial cells also express a variety of phase I and phase II enzymes, which may contribute to the biotransformation of chemical toxicants present in bile (Lakehal et al., 1999).

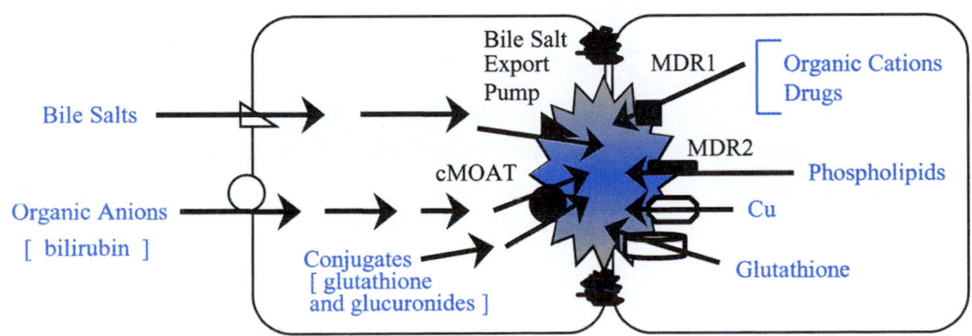

Figure 13-5. Processes involved in hepatocyte uptake and biliary secretion of endogenous solutes and toxicants.

Transporters localized to the sinusoidal membrane extract solutes from the blood. Exporters localized to canalicular membrane move solutes into the lumen of the canaliculus. Exporters of particular relevance to canalicular secretion of toxic chemicals and their metabolites are the canalicular multiple organic anion transporter (MOAT) system and the family of multiple-drug resistant (MDR) P-glycoproteins.

Secretion into biliary ducts is usually but not always a prelude to toxicant clearance by excretion in feces or urine. Exceptions occur when compounds such as arsenic are repeatedly delivered into the intestinal lumen via bile, efficiently absorbed from the intestinal lumen, and then redirected to the liver via portal blood, a processes known as *enterohepatic cycling*. A few compounds, such as methyl mercury, are absorbed from the biliary tract; the extensive reabsorption of methyl mercury from the gallbladder is thought to contribute to the long biological half-life and toxicity of this toxin (Dutczak et al., 1991). Alternatively, secretion into bile of toxicant metabolites can be a critical prelude to the development of injury in extrahepatic tissues. A clinically relevant example of bile as an important delivery route for a proximate toxicant is that of diclofenac, a widely prescribed nonsteroidal anti-inflammatory drug (NSAID) that causes small intestinal ulceration. Convincing experiments with mutant rats lacking a functional canalicular MOAT exporter (Fig. 13-5) have shown that these mutants secrete little of the presumptive proximate toxicant metabolite into bile and are resistant to the intestinal toxicity of diclofenac (Seitz and Boelsterli, 1998).

Toxicant-related impairments of bile formation are more likely to have detrimental consequences in populations with other conditions where biliary secretion is marginal. For example, neonates exhibit delayed development of multiple aspects of bile formation, including synthesis of bile salts and the expression of sinusoidal and canalicular transporters (Arrese et al., 1998). Neonates are more prone to develop jaundice when treated with drugs that compete with bilirubin for biliary clearance. Populations with sepsis are also of concern based on animal studies indicating that sepsis is associated with down-regulation of multiple canalicular exporters (Trauner et al., 1998).

Types of Injury and Toxic Chemicals

Hepatic response to insults by chemicals depends upon the intensity of the insult, the population of cells affected, and whether the exposure is acute or chronic (Fig. 13-1). Acute poisoning with carbon tetrachloride causes rapid lipid accumulation, before necrosis becomes evident. Some chemicals produce a very specific type of damage; others, notably ethanol, produce sequential types of damage or combinations of damage (Table 13-2). Note that the representative hepatotoxins listed in Table 13-2 include pharmaceuticals (valproic acid, cyclosporin A, diclofenac), recreational drugs (ethanol, ecstasy), a vitamin (vitamin A), metals (Fe, Cu, Mn), hormones (estrogens, androgens), industrial chemicals (dimethylformamide, methylene dianiline), compounds found in teas (germander) or foods (phalloidin, pyrrolidine alkaloids), and toxins produced by fungi (sporidesmin) and algae (microcystin). See Fig. 13-6 for the structures of representative hepatotoxic chemicals.

Fatty Liver This change, also known as steatosis, is defined biochemically as an appreciable increase in the hepatic lipid content, which is <5 percent by weight in normal human liver. Histologically, in standard paraffin-embedded and solvent-extracted sections, hepatocytes containing excess fat appear to have multiple round, empty vacuoles that displace the nucleus to the periphery of the cell. Use of frozen sections and special stains is needed to document the contents of the vesicles as fat. Fatty liver can stem from one or more of the following events: oversupply of free fatty acids to the liver, interference with the triglyceride cycle, increases in synthesis or esterification of fatty acids, decreased fatty acid oxidation, decreased apoprotein synthesis, and decreased synthesis or secretion of very low density lipoproteins.

Steatosis is a common response to acute exposure to many but not all hepatotoxins (Farrell, 1994). An exception is acetaminophen. Compounds that produce prominent steatosis associated with lethality include the antiepileptic drug valproic acid (Hall, 1994) and the antiviral agent fialuridine (Honkoop et al., 1997). Often, toxin-induced steatosis is reversible and does not lead to death of hepatocytes. The metabolic inhibitors ethionine, puromycin, and cycloheximide cause fat accumulation without causing death of cells. Many other conditions besides toxin exposure, such as obesity, are associated with marked fat accumulation in the liver. Therefore assumptions about cause-effect relationships in regard to toxins and steatosis need to be made judiciously.

Table 13-2
Types of Hepatobiliary Injury

TYPE OF INJURY OR DAMAGE	REPRESENTATIVE TOXINS
Fatty liver	CCl_4, ethanol, fialuridine, valproic acid
Hepatocyte death	Acetaminophen, Cu, dimethylformamide, ethanol, Ecstasy
Immune-mediated response	Diclofenac, ethanol, halothane, tienilic acid
Canalicular cholestasis	Chlorpromazine, cyclosporin A, 1,1-dichloroethylene, estrogens, Mn, phalloidin
Bile duct damage	Amoxicillin, ANIT, methylene dianiline, sporidesmin
Sinusoidal disorders	Anabolic steroids, cyclophosphamide, microcystin, pyrrolidine alkaloids
Fibrosis and cirrhosis	Arsenic, ethanol, vitamin A, vinyl chloride
Tumors	Aflatoxin, androgens, thorium dioxide, vinyl chloride

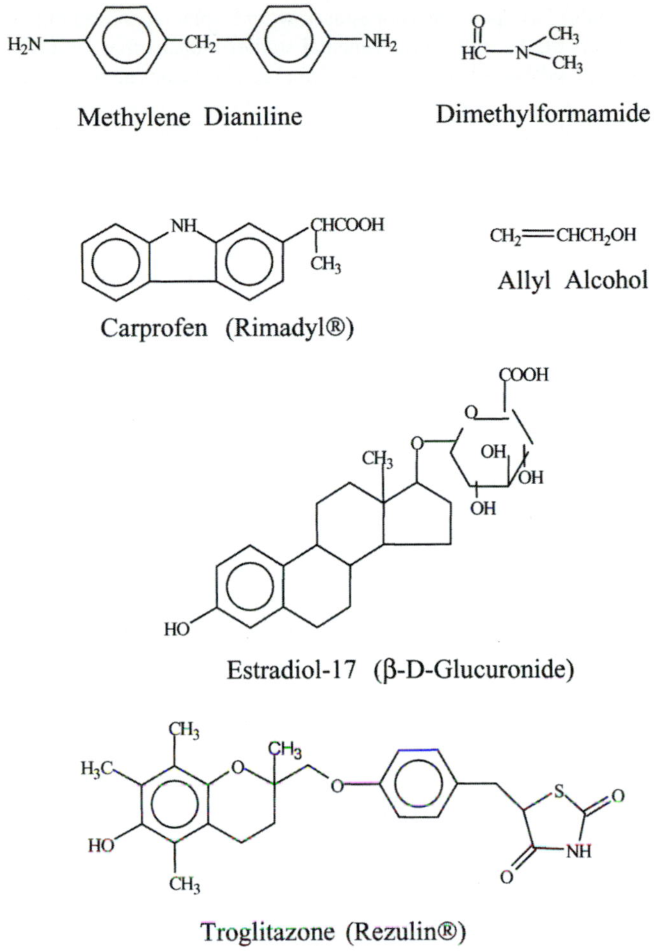

Figure 13-6. Structures of representative hepatotoxic chemicals.

Cell Death Liver cells can die by two different modes, necrosis and apoptosis. Necrosis is characterized by cell swelling, leakage, nuclear disintegration, and an influx of inflammatory cells. Apoptosis is characterized by cell shrinkage, nuclear fragmentation, formation of apoptotic bodies, and a lack of inflammation. Apoptosis is more difficult to detect histologically because of the rapid removal of affected cells (Corcoran et al., 1994). Lysed debris of necrotic cells can persist for days when large numbers of cells die. When necrosis occurs in hepatocytes, the associated plasma membrane leakage can be detected biochemically by assaying plasma (or serum) for liver cytosol-derived enzymes. Particularly informative are the activity levels of alanine aminotransferase (ALT), a predominantly hepatocyte enzyme, unlike lactate dehydrogenase (LDH), which is found in many tissues. Biochemical assays provide a relatively simple way to screen populations for potential hepatocyte necrosis due to occupational or environmental toxins. A careful occupational health study by Redlich et al. (1988; 1990) in a New Haven, Connecticut, plant with primitive systems for worker protection found that exposure to dimethylformamide was associated with liver damage. Serum ALT levels were appreciably elevated in most of the exposed workers; however, liver biopsies indicated that a substantial cause of the liver damage in one of the workers was an infectious agent. Thus a limitation of biochemical indices of hepatocyte necrosis is the inability to distinguish between chemically induced effects and other causes such as hepatitis virus.

Hepatocyte death can occur in a focal, zonal, or panacinar (panlobular) pattern. Focal cell death is characterized by the randomly distributed death of single hepatocytes or small clusters of hepatocytes. Zonal necrosis is death to hepatocytes predominantly in zone 1 (periportal) or zone 3 (centrolobular). Many toxins cause zone 3 necrosis, while fewer agents are known to specifically damage cells in zone 1 or zone 2. Information about the zonal location of injury by a given chemical helps identify a sensitive, noninvasive index of functional change. For example, serum levels of bile salts are more likely to be elevated after damage to zone 1 than to zone 3 due to the direction of the gradient for bile salt uptake from blood (Fig. 13-3).

Some reasons why chemical toxins preferentially damage hepatocytes in specific zones are discussed further on, under "Factors in Liver Injury." Zone 3 necrosis can affect just a narrow rim of cells around the central vein, or it may extend into zone 2. Panacinar necrosis is massive death of hepatocytes with only a few or no remaining survivors. An intermediate form of substantial necrosis is called *bridging necrosis* because the extensive zones of cell lysis become confluent with each other. Mechanisms of toxin-induced injury to liver cells include lipid peroxidation, binding to cell macromolecules, mitochondrial damage, disruption of the cytoskeleton, and massive calcium influx. Progression from injury to death may involve activation of sinusoidal cells and, with repeated toxicant exposure, may lead to an antibody-mediated immune attack.

Canalicular Cholestasis This form of liver injury is defined physiologically as a decrease in the volume of bile formed or an impaired secretion of specific solutes into bile. Cholestasis is characterized biochemically by elevated serum levels of compounds normally concentrated in bile, particularly bile salts and bilirubin. When biliary excretion of the yellowish bilirubin pigment is impaired, this pigment accumulates in the skin and eyes, producing jaundice, and spills into urine, which becomes bright yellow or dark brown. Dyes that are excreted in bile, such as bromsulphalein (BSP), have been used to assess biliary function. The histologic features of cholestasis can be very subtle and difficult to detect without ultrastructural studies. Structural changes include dilation of the bile canaliculus and the presence of bile plugs in bile ducts and canaliculi. Toxin-induced cholestasis can be transient or chronic; when substantial, it is associated with cell swelling, cell death, and inflammation. Many different types of chemicals—including metals, hormones and drugs—cause cholestasis (Table 13-2).

Bile Duct Damage Another name for damage to the intrahepatic bile ducts is *cholangiodestructive cholestasis* (Cullen and Ruebner, 1991). A useful biochemical index of bile duct damage is a sharp elevation in serum activities of enzymes localized to bile ducts, particularly alkaline phosphatase. In addition, serum levels of bile salts and bilirubin are elevated, as observed with canalicular cholestasis. Initial lesions following a single dose of cholangiodestructive agents include swollen biliary epithelium, debris of damaged cells within ductal lumens, and inflammatory cell infiltration of portal tracts. Chronic administration of toxins that cause bile duct destruction can lead to biliary proliferation and fibrosis resembling biliary cirrhosis. Another response is the loss of bile ducts, a condition known as *vanishing bile duct syndrome*. This persisting problem has been reported in patients receiving antibiotics (Davies et al., 1994).

Methylene dianiline, a compound used to make epoxy resins, is a noteworthy cause of bile duct damage. Small doses of methylene dianiline produce selective bile duct injury and thus provide an experimental model to study mechanisms of chemically induced bile duct damage (Kanz et al., 1992). The potent toxicity of methylene dianiline was first recognized in 1966, when an epidemiologic study established this compound as the causal agent of "Epping jaundice"—an outbreak of jaundice and severe hepatobiliary disease in more than 80 residents of the English village of Epping. The affected villagers had eaten bread made from flour contaminated with this compound (Kopelman et al., 1966). A more recent episode of methylene dianiline poisoning occurred at a "technoparty" where six young people ingested this agent due to confusion between its MDA abbreviation and the MDMA abbreviation for the synthetic amphetamine popularly known as Ecstasy (Tillman et al., 1997). All six individuals developed the jaundice, dark urine, abdominal pain, and nausea consistent with bile duct damage. If these young people had ingested the intended drug Ecstasy, they might also have developed liver problems. Although Ecstasy does not target bile ducts, numerous cases of severe liver damage have been reported after single and repeated exposure to this recreational drug (Andreu et al., 1998).

Sinusoidal Damage The sinusoid is, in effect, a specialized capillary with numerous fenestrae for high permeability. The functional integrity of the sinusoid can be compromised by dilation or blockade of its lumen or by progressive destruction of its endothelial cell wall. Dilation of the sinusoid will occur whenever efflux of hepatic blood is impeded. The rare condition of primary dilation, known as *peliosis hepatis,* has been associated with exposure to anabolic steroids and the drug danazol. Blockade will occur when the fenestrae enlarge to such an extent that red blood cells become caught in them or pass through with entrapment in the interstitial space of Disse. Such changes have been illustrated by scanning electron microscopy after large doses of the drug acetaminophen (Walker et al., 1983). A consequence of extensive sinusoidal blockade is that the liver becomes engorged with blood cells while the rest of the body goes into shock. Microcystin produces this effect within hours in rodents (Hooser et al., 1989). Microcystin dramatically deforms hepatocytes by altering cytoskeleton actin filaments, but it does not affect sinusoidal cells (Hooser et al., 1991). Thus the deformities that microcystin produces on the cytoskeleton of hepatocytes likely produce a secondary change in the structural integrity of the sinusoid owing to the close proximity of hepatocytes and sinusoidal endothelial cells (Fig. 13-4).

Progressive destruction of the endothelial wall of the sinusoid will lead to gaps and then ruptures of its barrier integrity, with entrapment of red blood cells. These disruptions of the sinusoid are considered the early structural features of the vascular disorder known as veno-occlusive disease (DeLeve et al., 1999). Well established as a cause of veno-occulsive disease are the pyrrolizidine alkaloids (e.g., monocrotaline, retrorsine, and seneciphylline) found in some plants used for herbal teas and in some seeds that contaminate food grains. Numerous episodes of human and animal poisoning by pyrrolizidine alkaloids have been reported around the world, including massive problems affecting thousands of people in Afghanistan in 1976 and 1993 (Huxtable, 1997). Veno-occlusive disease is also a serious complication in about 15 percent of the patients given high doses of chemotherapy (e.g., cyclophosphamide) as part of bone-marrow transplantation regimens (DeLeve et al., 1999). Experimental studies indicate that toxicant-induced killing of sinusoidal endothelial cells can occur without bioactivation by hepatocytes (DeLeve and Huybrechts, 1996). Depletion of glutathione within sinusoidal endothelial cells precedes the preferential injury to this type of hepatic cell (Wang et al., 2000).

Cirrhosis This form of injury is the end, often fatal, stage of chronic progressive liver injury. Cirrhosis is characterized by the accumulation of extensive amounts of fibrous tissue, specifically collagen fibers, in response to direct injury or to inflammation. Fibrosis can develop around central veins and portal tracts or within the space of Disse, which limits diffusion of material from the sinusoid. With repeated chemical insults, destroyed hepatic cells are replaced by fibrotic scars. With continuing collagen deposition, the architecture of the liver is disrupted by interconnecting fibrous scars. When the fibrous scars subdivide the remaining liver mass into nodules of regenerating hepatocytes, fibrosis has progressed to cirrhosis and the liver has meager residual capacity to perform its essential functions.

Cirrhosis is not reversible, has a poor prognosis for survival, and is usually the result of repeated exposure to chemical toxins. For example, cirrhosis associated with vitamin A has been reported in patients with dermatologic problems on high-dose therapy ($\geq$100,000 IU) for an average of 7 years (Geubel et al., 1991). The risk for cirrhosis in alcoholics increases dramatically in males who consume $\geq$80 g/day and in females who consume $\geq$20 g day for 10 years. Note that the amount of ethanol in 8 beers, 8 glasses of wine, or 7 oz of 80-proof liquor is approximately equivalent to 80 g. The greater vulnerability of females to alcohol can be explained only partially by their smaller body size and lower capacity for ethanol metabolism in the stomach.

Tumors Chemically induced neoplasia can involve tumors that are derived from hepatocytes, bile duct cells, or the rare, highly malignant angiosarcomas derived from sinusoidal lining cells. Hepatocellular cancer has been linked to abuse of androgens and a high prevalence of aflatoxin-contaminated diets. The synergistic effect of co-exposure to aflatoxin and hepatitis virus B was clearly documented by a recent prospective study where the risk for hepatocellular carcinoma was found to be increased threefold in aflatoxin-exposed men with chronic hepatitis B infection (Sun et al., 1999). The investigators monitored urine specimens from the subjects for a metabolite of aflatoxin in order to verify dietary aflatoxin exposure. Angiosarcomas have been tightly associated with occupational exposure to vinyl chloride and arsenic (Farrell, 1994).

Exposure to Thorotrast has been linked to tumors derived from hepatocytes, sinusoidal cells, and bile duct cells (cholangiocarcinoma). The history of Thorotrast (radioactive thorium dioxide) is a sad tale of a useful agent with an unanticipated toxicity due to prolonged retention within the body. Between 1920 and 1950, an estimated 2.5 million people were injected with suspensions of Thorotrast as a contrast medium for radiologic procedures. The compound accumulates in Kupffer cells, the resident macrophage of the sinusoid, and emits radioactivity throughout its very extended half-life. Thus, it is not surprising that multiple types of liver tumors are linked to thorium dioxide exposure. One study of Danish patients exposed to Thorotrast found that the risk for bile duct and gallbladder cancers was increased 14-fold and that for liver cancers more than 100-fold (Andersson and Storm, 1992).

FACTORS IN LIVER INJURY

Why is the liver the target site for so many chemicals of diverse structure? Why do many hepatotoxicants preferentially damage one type of liver cell? Our understanding of these fundamental questions is incomplete. Influences of several factors are of obvious importance (Table 13-3). Location and specialized processes for uptake and biliary secretion produce higher exposure levels in the liver than in other tissues of the body and strikingly high levels within certain types of liver cells. Then the abundant capacity for bioactivation reactions influences the rate of exposure to proximate toxicants. Subsequent events in the pathogenesis appear to be critically influenced by responses of sinusoidal cells and the immune system. Discussion of the evidence for the contributions of these factors to the hepatotoxicity of representative compounds requires commentary about mechanistic events; therefore this section of the chapter is closely related to the next one, entitled "Mechanisms of Liver Injury."

Table 13-4 lists experimental systems useful for defining factors and mechanisms of liver injury. In vitro systems using the isolated perfused liver, isolated liver cells, and cell fraction allow observations at various levels of complexity without the confounding influences of other systems. Models using co-cultures or agents that inactivate a given cell type can document the contributions and interactions between cell types. Whole-animal models are essential for assessment of the progression of injury and responses to chronic insult. Use of agents that induce, inhibit, deplete, or inactivate can define roles of specific processes, although potential influences of nonspecific actions can confound interpretations. Application of molecular biology techniques for gene transfection or repression attenuates some of these interpretive problems. Knockout rodents provided extremely useful models for complex aspects of hepatotoxicity. The reason for the persuasiveness of observations from experiments with knockout rodents is that the gene product of interest is not present and therefore not just inhibited by a nonspecific agent with potential confounding effects on other processes.

Uptake and Concentration

Hepatic "first pass" uptake of ingested toxic chemicals is facilitated by the location of the liver downstream of the portal blood flow from the gastrointestinal tract. Lipophilic compounds, particularly drugs and environmental pollutants, readily diffuse into hepatocytes because the fenestrated epithelium of the sinusoid enables close contact between circulating molecules and hepatocytes. Thus, the membrane-rich liver concentrates lipophilic compounds. Other toxins are rapidly extracted from blood because they are substrates for sinusoidal transporters present exclusively or predominantly in the liver.

Phalloidin and microcystin are illustrative examples of hepatotoxins that target the liver as a consequence of extensive uptake into hepatocytes by sinusoidal transporters (Frimmer, 1982; Runnegar et al., 1995a,b). Ingestion of the mushroom *Amanita phalloides* is a common cause of severe, acute hepatotoxicity in continental Europe and North America. Microcystin has produced numerous outbreaks of hepatotoxicity in sheep and cattle who drank pond water containing the blue-green alga *Microcystis aeruginosa* (Farrell, 1994). An episode of microcystin contamination of the water source used by a hemodialysis center in Brazil led to acute liver injury in 81 percent of the 124 exposed patients and the subsequent death of 50 of these (Jochimsen et al., 1998). Microcystin contamination was verified by analysis of samples from the water-holding tank at the dialysis center and from the livers of patients who died. This episode indicates the vulnerability of the liver to toxicants regardless of the route of administration. Because of

Table 13-3
Factors in the Site-Specific Injury of Representative Hepatotoxicants

SITE	REPRESENTATIVE TOXICANTS	POTENTIAL EXPLANATION FOR SITE-SPECIFICITY
Zone 1 hepatocytes (versus zone 3)	Fe (overload)	Preferential uptake and high oxygen levels
	Allyl alcohol	Higher oxygen levels for oxygen-dependent bioactivation
Zone 3 hepatocytes (versus zone 1)	CCl_4	More P450 isozyme for bioactivation
	Acetaminophen	More P450 isozyme for bioactivation and less GSH for detoxification
	Ethanol	More hypoxic and greater imbalance in bioactivation/detoxification reactions
Bile duct cells	Methylene dianiline, Sporidesmin	Exposure to the high concentration of reactive metabolites in bile
Sinusoidal endothelium (versus hepatocytes)	Cyclophosphamide, Monocrotaline	Greater vulnerability to toxic metabolites and less ability to maintain glutathione levels
Kupffer cells	Endotoxin, $GdCl_3$	Preferential uptake and then activation
Ito cells	Vitamin A	Preferential site for storage and then engorgement
	Ethanol (chronic)	Activation and transformation to collagen-synthesizing cell

Table 13-4
Experimental Systems

In vitro systems
Cell fractions
Primary cell cultures
Primary cell co-cultures
Transfected cell systems
Isolated perfused livers
In vivo systems
Multiple species and strains
Transgenic and knockout rodents

its dual blood supply from both the portal vein and the hepatic artery, the liver is presented with appreciable amounts of all toxicants in the systemic circulation.

An early clue to preferential uptake as a factor in phalloidin's target-organ specificity was the observation that bile duct ligation, which elevates systemic bile salt levels, protects rats against phalloidin-induced hepatotoxicity in association with an 85 percent decrease in hepatic uptake of phalloidin (Walli et al., 1981). Subsequent studies found that co-treatment with substrates (e.g., cyclosporin A, rifampicin) known to prevent the in vivo hepatotoxicity of phalloidin or microcystin would also inhibit their uptake into hepatocytes by sinusoidal transporters for bile acids or organic anions (Ziegler and Frimmer 1984; Runnegar et al., 1995a).

Accumulation within liver cells, by processes that facilitate uptake and storage, is a determining factor in the hepatotoxicity of vitamin A and several metals. Vitamin A hepatotoxicity initially affects the sinusoidal Ito cells, which actively extract and store this vitamin. Early responses to high-dose vitamin A therapy are Ito cell engorgement, activation, increase in number, and protrusion into the sinusoid (Geubel et al., 1991). Cadmium hepatotoxicity becomes manifest when the cells exceed their capacity to sequester cadmium as a complex with the metal-binding protein metallothionein. This protective role for metallothionein was definitively documented by observations with transgenic mice. Specifically, high expression of this metal-binding protein in the transgenic mice rendered them more resistant than wild-type mice to the hepatotoxicity and lethality of cadmium poisoning (Liu et al., 1995).

Iron poisoning will produce severe liver damage. Hepatocytes contribute to the homeostasis of Fe by extracting this essential metal from the sinusoid by a receptor-mediated process and maintaining a reserve of Fe within the storage protein ferritin. Acute Fe toxicity is most commonly observed in young children who accidentally ingest iron tablets. The cytotoxicity of free Fe is attributed to its function as an electron donor for the formation of reactive oxygen species, which initiate destructive oxidative stress reactions. Accumulation of excess Fe beyond the capacity for its safe storage in ferritin is initially evident in the zone 1 hepatocytes, which are closest to the blood entering the sinusoid. Thus the zone 1 pattern of hepatocyte damage after iron poisoning is attributable to location for (1) the preferential uptake of Fe and (2) the higher oxygen concentrations that facilitate the injurious process of lipid peroxidation (Table 13-3). Chronic hepatic accumulation of excess iron in cases of hemochromatosis is associated with a spectrum of hepatic disease including a greater than 200-fold increased risk for liver cancer.

Bioactivation and Detoxification

Hepatocytes have very high constitutive activities of the phase I enzymes that often convert xenobiotics to reactive electrophilic metabolites. Also, hepatocytes have a rich collection of phase II enzymes that add a polar group to a molecule and thereby enhance its removal from the body. Phase II reactions usually yield stable, nonreactive metabolites. In general, the balance between phase I and phase II reactions determines whether a reactive metabolite will initiate liver cell injury or be safely detoxified. The balance can be shifted towards liver injury by acquired or genetic conditions that enhance bioactivation processes or impair detoxification processes. Notable acquired conditions for such a shift in balance are drug or pollutant induction of phase I enzymes and/or depletion of antioxidants.

Ethanol Genetic conditions of high clinical relevance to the bioactivation/detoxification balance are the polymorphisms in the enzymes that control the two-step metabolism of ethanol. Specifically, ethanol is bioactivated by alcohol dehydrogenase to acetaldehyde, a reactive aldehyde, which is subsequently detoxified to acetate by aldehyde dehydrogenase. Both enzymes exhibit genetic polymorphisms that result in higher concentrations of acetaldehyde—a "fast" activity isozyme of alcohol dehydrogenase [ALD2*2] and a physiologically very "slow" mitochondrial isozyme of aldehyde dehydrogenase [ALDH2*2]. Approximately 50 percent of Asian populations but virtually no Caucasians have the slow aldehyde dehydrogenase; alcohol consumption by people with this slow polymorphism leads to uncomfortable symptoms of flushing and nausea due to high systemic levels of acetaldehyde. Thus this slow detoxification polymorphism serves as a strong deterrent for alcoholism. The alcohol dehydrogenase fast polymorphism, which occurs in about 20 percent of Asian and less than 5 percent of Caucasian populations, has also been linked to a lower rate of alcoholism. An extremely low risk for alcoholism has been found in Asians with both polymorphisms that lead to higher levels of acetaldehyde (Chen et al., 1999a).

Allyl alcohol toxicity is also influenced by a balance between the formation and detoxification of its reactive aldehyde metabolite, acrolein, by sequential actions of alcohol dehydrogenase and aldehyde dehydrogenase enzymes. Age and gender differences in allyl alcohol hepatotoxicity can be explained by variations in the balance between these two enzymes (Rikans and Moore, 1987). Allyl alcohol is used in the production of resins, plastics, and fire retardants. The preferential occurrence of allyl alcohol injury in zone 1 hepatocytes (Table 13-3) is due to oxygen-dependent bioactivation. This aspect of its mechanism of hepatotoxicity was demonstrated by creative experiments where the typical decline in the oxygen gradient from zone 1 to zone 3 was reversed by a retrograde (backward) perfusion of isolated perfused livers (Badr et al., 1986).

Cytochrome P450 The importance of cytochrome P450-dependent bioactivation as a mechanism of hepatotoxicity must be emphasized. This common theme can be a factor even for assumedly *safe* compounds since some P450 isozymes generate reactive oxygen species during biotransformation reactions (Albano et al., 1996). Concern about CYP2E1 generation of reactive oxygen species and other free radicals has come largely from efforts to determine why only a fraction of chronic heavy drinkers develop serious, end-stage liver damage. Dietary manipulations that lead to more severe alcohol-associated liver damage in the animal model show a linkage between dietary induction of CYP2E1 and hepatotoxicity (French et al., 1995; Korourian et al., 1999). These manipulation have involved the amount of dietary lipid, the type of fatty acid in the lipid component of the diet, diets deficient in carbohydrates, and co-exposure to inhibitors of CYP2E1. The issue is complex because ethanol is an inducer of P450; heavy drinkers exhibit approximately threefold higher activities of CYP2E1 than nondrinkers. However, the observed modulation of liver injury by dietary manipulations does indicate a role for nutrients in the hepatotoxicity of alcohol.

CYP2E1 is not the only cytochrome P450 isozyme with an impact on hepatotoxicity. An appropriately germane example is the folk medicine plant germander (*Teucrium chamaedrys L.*), which was considered a safe component of herbal teas until widespread consumption of capsules containing large amounts of germander for weight control in France was linked to multiple cases of hepatic damage (Larrey et al., 1992; Loeper et al., 1994). Systematic experimental studies have identified the specific toxic constituent in germander plants, demonstrated a predominant role for the CYP3A isozyme in germander bioactivation to reactive electrophiles, and determined that toxicity can be attenuated by maintenance of glutathione levels (Loeper et al., 1994; Lekehal et al., 1996). This kind of information has practical applications for identifying populations at enhanced risk for germander toxicity due to acquired conditions—such as obesity, sudden weight loss, or concurrent ingestion of other folk medications or pharmaceuticals—that might shift the balance between CYP3A bioactivation and glutathione-dependent detoxification.

Carbon Tetrachloride Cytochrome P450-dependent conversion of CCl_4 to $\bullet CCl_3$ and then to $CCl_3OO\bullet$ is the classic example of xenobiotic bioactivation to a free radical that initiates lipid peroxidation by abstracting a hydrogen atom from the polyunsaturated fatty acid of a phospholipid (Rechnagel, 1967). Experimental studies have identified numerous treatments and conditions that modulate the extent of liver damage produced by CCl_4. Protective situations include baby animals with little cytochrome P450; treatments with compounds that inhibit cytochrome P450; and pretreatment with a small dose of the same toxin that diminishes cytochrome P450 levels (Reynolds and Moslen, 1980). Augmenting situations include hypoxia, diabetes, diets low in vitamin E (since this antioxidant scavenges lipid peroxide radicals), and pretreatment with other chemicals, notably ethanol and acetone, which induce CYP2E1, the isozyme most effective in the activation of CCl_4. Anecdotal reports of human exposures to this toxicant suggest a greater vulnerabilty in individuals who should have high levels of hepatic CYP2E1 due to a history of alcohol abuse (Manno et al., 1996). Uncertainties about the importance of other P450 isozymes have been squelched by documentation of virtual resistance to the hepatotoxicity of CCl_4 in CYP2E1 knockout mice (Wong et al., 1998). Investigations about events in the pathogenesis of carbon tetrachloride hepatotoxicity paved the way for identification of factors important in the toxicity of other insults that also cause lipid peroxidation.

Acetaminophen The hepatotoxicity of this extensively used analgesic is a clinically important problem and an exemplary instance of how acquired factors (e.g., diet, drugs, diabetes, obesity) can enhance hepatotoxicity. Typical therapeutic doses of acetaminophen are not hepatotoxic, since the dominant pathways of biotransformation are conjugation with glucuronide or sulfate with little drug bioactivation. Injury after large doses of acetaminophen is enhanced by fasting and other conditions that deplete glutathione and is minimized by treatments that enhance hepatocyte synthesis of glutathione, particularly cysteine, the rate-limiting amino acid in glutathione synthesis. Introduction of interventive therapy with *N*-acetylcysteine, a well- tolerated source of intracellular cysteine, has saved the lives of many who took overdoses of acetaminophen, usually in suicide attempts (Smilkstein et al., 1988).

Alcoholics are vulnerable to the hepatotoxic effects of acetaminophen at dosages within the high therapeutic range (Lieber, 1994). This acquired enhancement has widely been attributed to accelerated bioactivation of acetaminophen to the electrophilic *N*-acetyl-*p*-benzoquinone imine (NAPQI) intermediate by ethanol induction of CYP2E1 (Fig. 13-7). However, alcoholic beverages also contain higher-chain alcohols, such as isopentanol, in appreciable amounts up to 0.5% (w/v), and alcohol consumption has many effects on the liver besides induction of CYP2E1 (Lieber, 1994). The assumed exclusive role for CYP2E1 bioactivation is controversial, in part because agents used to inhibit this isozyme also inhibit other isozymes of cytochrome P450. Evidence for roles of other alcohols besides ethanol and for other isozymes of P450 is available in the literature. For example, CYP2E1 knockout mice are *not* devoid of a toxic response to acetaminophen (Lee et al., 1996). Particularly convincing evidence is provided by a new report showing (1) synergistic enhancement of acetaminophen hepatotoxicity in rats pretreated with liquid diets containing ethanol plus isopentanol and (2) attenuation of acetaminophen hepatotoxicity when the alcohol-pretreated animals were given a specific inhibitor of CYP3A (Sinclair et al., 2000). This report should heighten suspicion about the potential influences of other CYP3A inducers on acetaminophen toxicity, since hepatic activities of this isozyme are increased by many drugs and by dietary chemicals such as caffeine.

Covalent binding, or adduction, of the reactive NAPQI intermediate of acetaminophen to hepatic proteins is a widely accepted mechanism for the hepatotoxicity of this drug. Adduction of a macromolecule could alter its functional integrity and thus constitute a detrimental molecular change. Early acceptance of the adduction mechanism for acetaminophen stemmed from close parallels found between the magnitude of injury and the extent of covalent binding in livers of animals given labeled acetaminophen (Mitchell et al., 1973). A key variable in these seminal experiments was the availability of glutathione for detoxification. Development of antibodies that recognize adducts of acetaminophen to macromolecules allowed demonstration of adduct formation before cell damage, predominantly in zone 3, where histologic injury occurs (Roberts et al., 1991). Thus adduct formation as a mechanism of injury is plausible temporally and locationally. One difficulty that researchers encountered in looking for a dose-dependent relationship between acetaminophen adducts and liver damage was an appropriate time to measure adduct formation, since damaged cells leak adducted proteins as well as enzymes indicative of tissue-specific injury (e.g., ALT).

A persisting concern about the adduction theory for acetaminophen toxicity is whether adduct formation is the *critical* event in acetaminophen toxicity or a *biomarker* of exposure to electrophilic metabolites. Prompting this concern are questions about how adduction to hepatocyte proteins could explain the importance of macrophages to the toxicity of this drug. A series of studies (Laskin et al., 1990; Gardner et al., 1998) have demonstrated protection by inactivation of hepatic macrophages (Kupffer cells) and contributions of reactive nitrogen species. Pretreatments that inac-

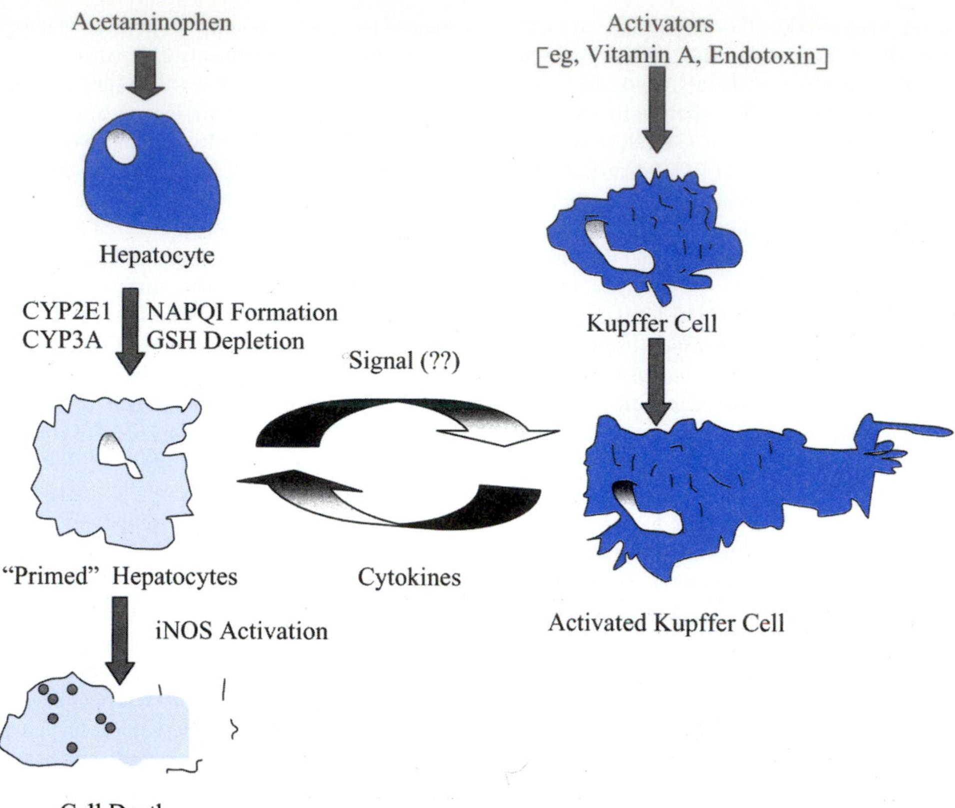

Figure 13-7. Schematic of key events in the bioactivation and hepatotoxicity of acetaminophen.

Bioactivation of acetaminophen by cytochrome P450 isozymes leads to the formation of the reactive intermediate *N*-acetyl-*p*-benzoquinone (NAPQI), which can deplete glutathione or form covalent adducts with hepatic proteins. Experimental observations suggest that such effects "prime" hepatocytes for cytokines released by activated Kupffer cells. Progression to cell death is thought to involve activation of iNOS and other processes that produce reactive nitrogen species and oxidative stress. Agents that activate Kupffer cells exacerbate the toxicity. Exchange of signals between toxicant-primed and activated Kupffer cells is likely a factor in the acute hepatotoxicity produced by many compounds that damage hepatocytes.

tivate macrophages and attenuate toxicity by acetaminophen did *not,* however, diminish the extent of acetaminophen adduct formation (Michael et al., 1999). Yet the pretreatments did diminish the extent of hepatocyte adduction by reactive nitrogen species, an intriguing observation that fits with the reported contributions of reactive nitrogens to acetaminophen toxicity. Michael et al. (1999) have proposed an attractive "two hit" type of revised theory for the hepatotoxicity of acetaminophen. Perhaps adduction by a reactive drug metabolite "primes" the hepatocytes for destructive insults by reactive nitrogen species (e.g., peroxynitrite) (Fig. 13-7).

Activation of Sinusoidal Cells

Four kinds of observations, collectively, indicate roles for sinusoidal cell activation as primary or secondary factors in toxin-induced injury to the liver:

1. Kupffer cells and Ito cells exhibit an activated morphology—enlarged and ruffled—after acute and chronic exposure to hepatotoxicants (Laskin et al., 1990).
2. Pretreatments that activate or inactivate Kupffer cells appropriately modulate the extent of damage produced by classic toxicants (e.g., acetaminophen, carbon tetrachloride, and alcohol). For example, a series of studies by Sipes and colleagues demonstrated that Kupffer cell activation by vitamin A profoundly enhances the acute toxicity of carbon tetrachloride; this enhancement did not occur when animals were also given an inactivator of Kupffer cells (ElSisi et al., 1993).
3. Activated Kupffer cells secrete appreciable amounts of soluble cytotoxins, including reactive oxygen and nitrogen species. Administration of agents that scavenge or inhibit these soluble cytotoxins attenuates the effects of sinusoidal cell enhancement (Gardener et al., 1998; Thurman et al., 1997).
4. Acute and chronic exposure to alcohol directly or indirectly affects sinusoidal cells (Thurman et al., 1997).

Kupffer cells are rapidly activated when the liver is perfused with solutions containing ethanol. Alcoholics have elevated systemic levels of endogenous Kupffer cell activators, notably tumor necrosis factor and the bacterial product endotoxin. The extent of liver injury in animal models of alcoholic hepatitis is consistently diminished by treating animals with antibiotics that lower endotoxin levels or with antibodies to tumor necrosis factor. This antibiotic protection disappears when the animals also receive endotoxin. New animal experiments with knockout mice provide strong evidence for an essential role of tumor necrosis factor in alcohol-induced liver injury (Yin et al., 1999). The knockout mice used in these experiments lacked a receptor for tumor necrosis factor. Observations during the latter phases of chronic alcohol-induced liver disease, when there is an abundance of collagen scarring, show activated, transformed Ito cells; transformed Ito cells are thought to be little factories for collagen synthesis.

Figure 13-8 summarizes information presented in this and earlier sections of this chapter about the multiplicity of toxin-induced interactions with and between various liver cells. The effect on a given cell type can be direct or may result from a cascade of signals and responses between cell types.

Inflammatory and Immune Responses

Migration of neutrophils, lymphocytes, and other inflammatory cells into regions of damaged liver is a well-recognized feature of the hepatotoxicity produced by many chemicals. In fact, the potentially confusing term *hepatitis* refers to hepatocyte damage by any insult where hepatocyte death is associated with an influx of inflammatory cells. The progressive phase of alcohol-induced liver disease (between simple fatty liver and cirrhosis) is called *alcoholic hepatitis.* The liver damage occasionally observed after multiple exposures to the anesthetic halothane is known as *halothane hepatitis.*

A relevant question for chemically induced acute damage to the liver is: Does the influx of inflammatory cells facilitate beneficial removal of debris from damaged liver cells or does the influx contribute in a detrimental way to the extent of liver damage after chemical injury? Detrimental effects are plausible, since activated neutrophils release cytotoxic proteases and reactive oxygen species. Pretreatments with prostaglandins and other compounds with anti-inflammatory activity reduce the acute hepatotoxicity of α-naphthyl-isothiocyanate (ANIT), an extensively studied compound that causes histologic damage to hepatocytes and bile ducts (Dahm et al., 1991); CCl_4; and other compounds (Farrell, 1994). More direct evidence for a detrimental role of neutrophils has come from experiments where depletion of neutrophils diminished the hepatotoxic and cholestatic effects of ANIT. Further insight into the roles of neutrophils in ANIT toxicity has been obtained by use of co-culture techniques for isolated primary hepatocytes, bile duct cells, and neutrophils (Hill et al., 1999). Placement of different types of cells on opposite sides of a permeable chamber indicated a chain reaction of events whereby ANIT-treated bile duct cells release a factor that attracts neutrophils and stimulates them to damage hepatocytes.

Immune responses are considered factors in the hepatotoxicity occasionally observed after repeated exposure to chemicals, usually drugs. Individuals who develop infrequent, unpredictable response are considered to be hypersensitive. An immune-mediated response is considered plausible when the problem subsides after therapy is halted and then recurs on drug challenge or restoration of therapy. Although the concept is generally accepted, compelling evidence for immune-mediated responses is available only for ethanol, halothane, and a few other hepatotoxicants (Pohl, 1990). Some kind of chemical-related molecular change is needed to stimulate an immunological attack, such as the formation of adducts between a reactive metabolite of the drug and hepatocyte proteins. Figure 13-9 depicts key features of the assumed scenario whereby hepatic protein adducts could become antigenic and stimulate the production of antibodies. If on reexposure, more drug-protein adducts are formed, cells with such adducts could be attacked by systemic antibodies. Bioactivation to reactive species capable of forming protein adducts is a commonality for many drugs thought to produce immune-mediated hepatic injury (Selim and Kaplowitz, 1999).

Reports about sporadic instances of apparent immune-mediated injury in individuals taking the widely prescribed NSAID diclofenac have spurred extensive research on this popular and ef-

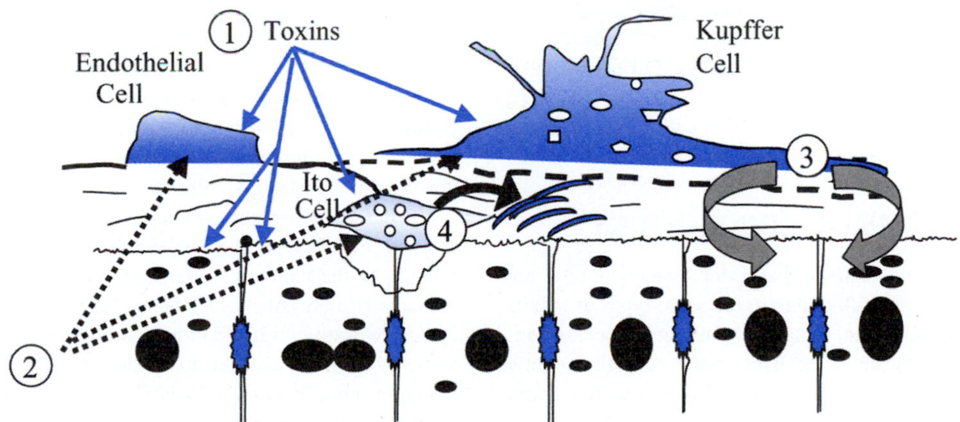

Figure 13-8. Schematic depicting the complex cascade of toxin-evoked interactions between hepatocytes and sinusoidal cells.

Sinusoidal cell responses to toxins can lead to either injury or activation. A scenario could involve (1) toxin injury to hepatocytes, (2) signals from the injured hepatocyte to Kupffer and Ito cells, followed by (3) Kupffer cell release of cytotoxins and (4) Ito cell secretion of collagen. Activation of Kupffer cells is an important factor in the progression of injury evoked by many toxicants. Stimulation of collagen production by activated Ito cells is a proposed mechanism for toxicant-induced fibrosis. [Concept from Crawford JM: The liver and the biliary tract, in Cotran RS, Kumar V, Robbins SL (eds): *Robbins: Pathologic Basis of Disease,* 6th ed. Philadelphia: Saunders, 1999, pp 845–901, with permission.]

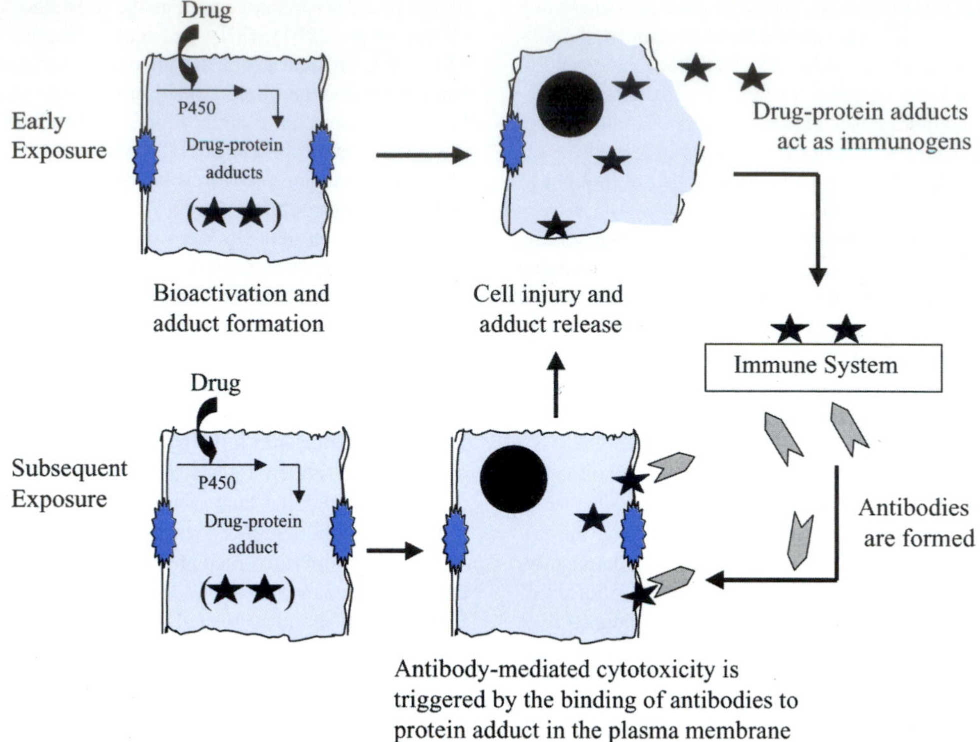

Figure 13-9. Proposed scenario of events leading to immune-mediated hepatotoxicity after repeated exposure to a toxicant that produces drug-protein adducts (★).

fective anti-arthritic drug (Sallie et al., 1991; Farrell, 1994). Hepatic bioactivation of diclofenac leads to the formation of multiple adducts. Some of the diclofenac adducts localize to hepatocyte membrane proteins (Hargus et al., 1994), where recognition by antibodies is feasible. There is considerable evidence for immune-mediated responses as factors in ethanol-induced liver disease. Acetaldehyde, the reactive metabolite of ethanol, forms adducts with hepatic proteins. Circulating antibodies that recognize acetaldehyde-adducted proteins can be found in patients with liver disease related to alcohol, and in some studies the antibody titer is higher in those with more severe disease (Rolla et al., 2000). However, specific contributions of drug-protein adducts and their antibodies to the pathogenesis of diclofenac and alcohol have yet to be defined.

MECHANISMS OF LIVER INJURY

Some aspects of the mechanistic basis for hepatotoxicity are generic, since liver cells are vulnerable to the same types of insults that injure other tissues. Preferential liver damage frequently ensues simply from the location of the liver and/or its high capacity for converting chemicals to reactive entities. Exceptions that merit explanation are the toxins that target the cytoskeleton due to their exclusive uptake by hepatocytes and the drugs that damage hepatic mitochondria due to the potentially fatal systemic consequences. This section emphasizes mechanisms that produce cholestasis, because biliary secretion is a unique and vital function of the liver.

Disruption of the Cytoskeleton

Phalloidin and microcystin disrupt the integrity of hepatocyte cytoskeleton by affecting proteins that are vital to its dynamic nature. The detrimental effects of these two potent hepatotoxicants are independent of their biotransformation and are exclusive for hepatocytes, since there is no appreciable uptake of either toxin into other types of cells. Tight binding of phalloidin to actin filaments prevents the disassembly phase of the normally dynamic rearrangement of the actin filament constituent of the cytoskeleton. Phalloidin uptake into hepatocytes leads to striking alterations in the actin-rich web of cytoskeleton adjacent to the canalicular membrane; the actin web becomes accentuated and the canalicular lumen dilates (Phillips et al., 1986). Experiments using time-lapse video microscopy have documented dose-dependent declines in the contraction of canalicular lumens between isolated hepatocyte couplets after incubation with a range of phalloidin concentrations (Watanabe and Phillips, 1986).

Microcystin uptake into hepatocytes leads to hyperphosphorylation of cytoskeletal proteins secondary to this toxicant's covalent binding to the catalytic subunit of serine/threonine protein phosphatases (Runnegar et al., 1995c). Reversible phosphorylations of cytoskeletal structural and motor proteins are critical to the dynamic integrity of the cytoskeleton. As depicted in Fig. 13-10, extensive hyperphosphorylation produced by large amounts of microcystin leads to marked deformation of hepatocytes due to a unique collapse of the microtubular actin scaffold into a spiny central aggregate (Hooser et al., 1991). Lower doses of microcystin, insufficient to produce the gross structural deformations, diminish uptake and secretory functions of hepatocytes in association with preferential hyperphosphorylation of the cytoplasmic motor protein dynein (Runnegar et al., 1999). Dynein is a mechanicochemical protein that drives vesicles along microtubules using energy from ATP hydrolysis; central to the hydrolysis of the dynein-bound ATP is a cycle of kinase phosphorylation and phosphatase dephosphorylation.

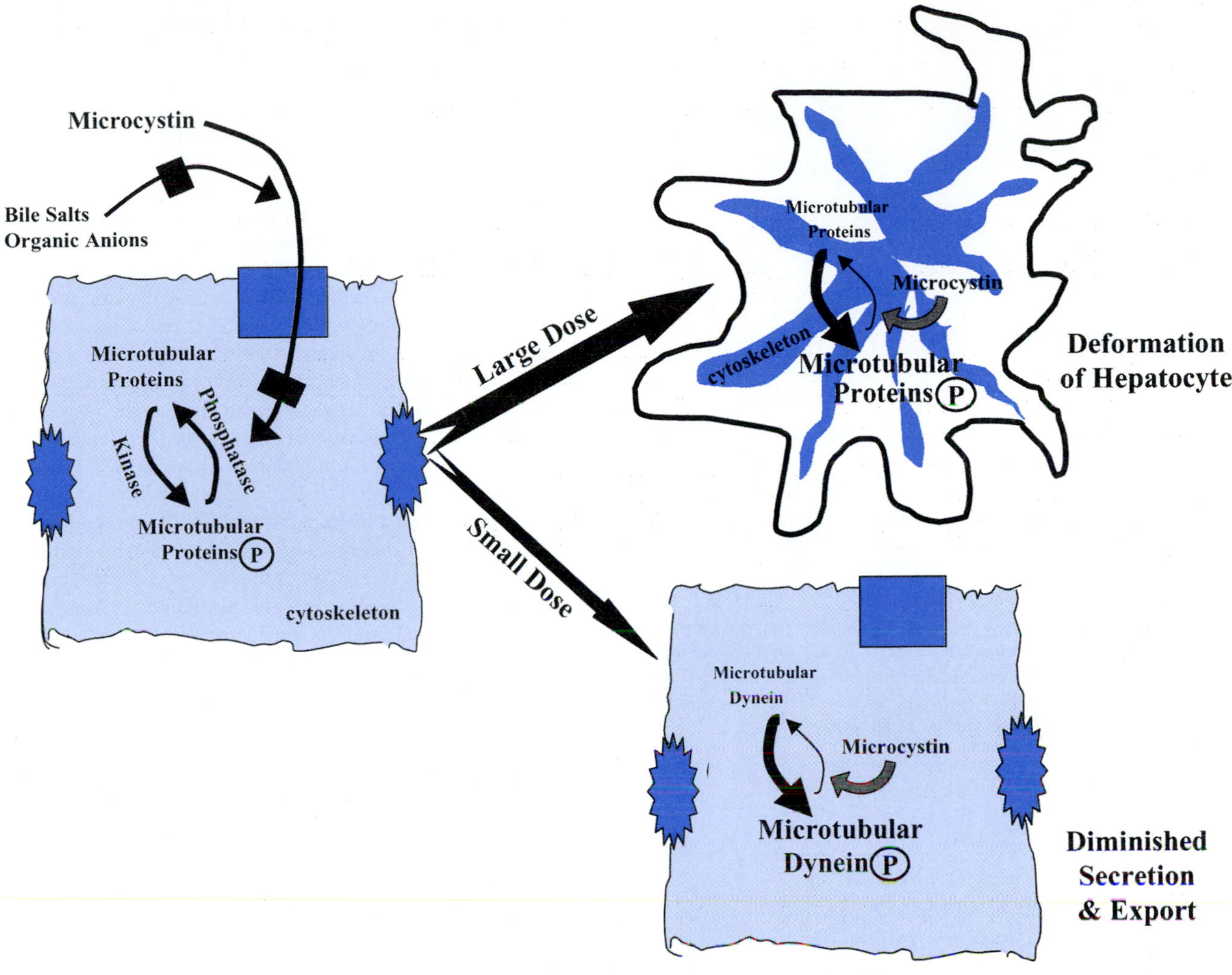

Figure 13-10. Schematic of events in the mechanism by which microcystin damages the structural and functional integrity of hepatocytes.

Microcystin is taken up exclusively into hepatocytes by a sinusoidal transporter in a manner inhibitable by bile salts and organic anions. Then microcystin inhibition of protein phosphatases leads to hyperphosphorylation of cytoskeletal proteins whose dynamic functions are dependent upon reversible phosphorylations. Extensive hyperphosphorylation of microtubular proteins leads to a collapse of the microtubular actin filament scaffold into a spiky aggregate that produces a gross deformation of hepatocytes. More subtle changes in microtubule-mediated transport activities have been linked to hyperphosphorylation of dynein, a cytoskeletal motor protein. (Concept courtesy of Dr. Maria Runnegar, University of Southern California School of Medicine.)

Thus, hyperphosphorylation of dynein freezes this motor pump. New experiments that looked at effects of chronic exposure to low levels of microcystin have raised new concerns about the health effects of this water contaminant. Specifically, low levels of microcystin promote liver tumors and kill hepatocytes in the zone 3 region, where microcystin accumulates (Solter et al., 1998).

Information about the binding of phalloidin and microcystin to specific target molecules is valuable for two reasons. First, the linkages of specific binding to loss of target protein functions provide compelling evidence that such binding constitutes a defined molecular mechanism of injury. Second, the demonstrations of high-affinity binding to a target molecule without confounding effects on other processes or tissues have *translated* into applications of these toxins as tools for cell biology research. For example, phalloidin complexed with a fluorochrome (e.g., rhodamine phalloidin or Texas Red phalloidin) is used to visualize the actin polymer component of the cytoskeleton in all types of permeabilized cells. The collapse of actin filaments into spiny aggregates after microcystin treatment was visualized by fluorescence microscopy of cells stained with rhodamine phalloidin (Hooser et al., 1991). Low levels of microcystin are being used to discriminate the roles of dynein from other cytoskeletal motor proteins (Runnegar et al., 1999).

Cholestasis

Bile formation is vulnerable to toxicant effects on the functional integrity of sinusoidal transporters, canalicular exporters, cytoskeleton-dependent processes for transcytosis, and the contractile closure of the canalicular lumen (Fig. 13-11). Changes that weaken the junctions that form the structural barrier between the blood and the canalicular lumen allow solutes to leak out of the canalicular lumen. These paracellular junctions provide a size and

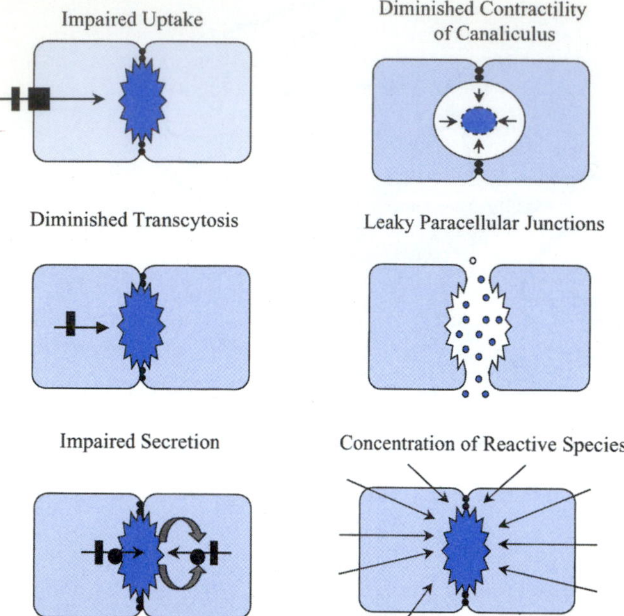

Figure 13-11. Schematic of six potential mechanisms for cholestasis involving inhibited uptake, diminished transcytosis, impaired secretion, diminished contractility of the canaliculus, leakiness of the junctions that seal the canalicular lumen from the blood, and detrimental consequences of high concentrations of toxic entities in the pericanalicular area.

Note that impaired secretion across the canalicular membrane can result from inhibition of a transporter or retraction of a transporter away from the canalicular membrane.

charge barrier to the diffusion of solutes between the blood and the canalicular lumen while water and small ions diffuse across these junctions. One hepatotoxin that causes tight-junction leakage is ANIT (Krell, 1987).

Cholestatic effects of pharmaceuticals present serious complications that often require restrictions in dose or termination of therapy. Such problems are encountered with cyclosporin A, an immunosuppressive drug frequently reported to cause elevated levels of serum bile salts and bilirubin as well as a reductions in bile flow (Farrell, 1994). Careful studies with hepatocyte membrane fractions demonstrated that cyclosporin A is a potent competitive inhibitor of the ATP-dependent bile salt exporter on the canalicular membrane (Bohme et al., 1994). Agents can also impede canalicular export activities by stimulating the retraction of canalicular exporters away from the canalicular membrane or by downregulating their expression (Trauner et al., 1998; Kubitz et al., 1999).

Compounds that produce cholestasis do not necessarily act by a single mechanism or at just one site. Chlorpromazine impairs bile acid uptake and canalicular contractility (Farrell, 1994). Multiple alterations have been well documented for estrogens, a well-known cause of reversible canalicular cholestasis (Vore, 1991; Bossard et al., 1993). Problems occur with both synthetic estrogens and metabolites of endogenous estrogens, particularly D-ring glucuronides. Estrogens decrease bile salt uptake by effects at the sinusoidal membrane including a decrease in the Na^+, K^+-ATPase necessary for Na-dependent transport of bile salts across the plasma membrane and changes in lipid component of this membrane. At the canalicular membrane, estrogens diminish the transport of glutathione conjugates and reduce the number of bile salt transporters.

An additional mechanism for canalicular cholestasis is concentration of reactive forms of chemicals in the pericanalicular area (Fig. 13-11). Most chemicals that cause canalicular cholestasis are excreted in bile. Therefore the proteins and lipids in the canalicular region must encounter a high concentration of these chemicals. Observations consistent with this concentration mechanism have been reported for Mn and 1,1-dicloroethylene. Manganese is a known cholestatic agent in humans and experimental animals (Lustig et al., 1982). Treatments that modify the extent of Mn-induced cholestasis produce consonant changes in the amount of Mn recovered in the canalicular membrane fraction (Ayotte and Plaa, 1985). A postulated mechanism for the canaliculus as the target site of low doses of 1,1-dichloroethylene is the congregation of its reactive thioether glutathione conjugates (Liebler et al., 1988) in the pericanalicular region (Moslen and Kanz, 1993). One striking effect of 1,1-dicloroethylene is a rapid decrease in biliary secretion phospholipids, a function of the MDR2 exporter (Woodard and Moslen, 1998). Concentration within a confined region is also a plausible factor in the target site selectivity of chemicals that damage bile ducts, since all recognized bile duct toxins are excreted in bile. Sporidesmin, a fungus-derived bile duct toxin, is concentrated in bile up to 100-fold (Farrell, 1994).

Mitochondrial Damage

Preferential injury to mitochondrial DNA, as opposed to nuclear DNA, is a plausible mechanistic basis for the structural and functional alterations to hepatic mitochondria associated with nucleoside analog therapy for hepatitis B and AIDS infections and with alcohol abuse. Of particular concern is the lactic acidosis that results when the liver, due to a massive deficit in hepatic mitochondrial function, can no longer maintain systemic lactate homeostasis or even supply its own ATP needs without anaerobic glycolysis.

Mitochondrial DNA codes for several proteins in the mitochondrial electron transport chain. Nucleoside analog drugs cause mitochondrial DNA damage directly when incorporation of the analog base leads to miscoding or early termination of polypeptides. The severe hepatic mitochondrial injury produced by the nucleoside analog fialuridine is attributed to its higher affinity for the polymerase responsible for mitochondrial DNA synthesis than for the polymerases responsible for nuclear DNA synthesis (Honkoop et al., 1997). Mitochondrial DNA is also more vulnerable to miscoding (mutation) due to its limited capacity for repair.

Alcohol abuse can lead to mitochondrial injury by mechanisms involving metabolic imbalance and/or oxidative stress. A shift in the bioactivation/detoxification balance for ethanol can lead to an accumulation of its reactive acetaldehyde metabolite within mitochondria, since mitochondrial aldehyde dehydrogenase is the major enzymatic process for detoxification of acetaldehyde. Bioactivation of large amounts of ethanol by alcohol dehydrogenase hampers the detoxification reaction, since the two enzymes require a common, depletable cofactor—namely, nicotinamide adenine dinucleotide (NAD). Any type of ethanol-induced change that enhances the leakiness of the mitochondrial transport chain would lead to an increased release of reactive oxygen species capable of attacking nearby mitochondrial constituents. Animal experiments have shown that high doses of ethanol lead to adduction of mitochondrial cytochrome oxidase by reactive oxygen species and to declines in the activity of this electron transport chain protein (Chen et al., 1999b). Ethanol-induced damage to mitochondrial DNA by what appears to be oxidative stress pathway is attenuated by antioxidant pretreatment (Mansouri et al., 1999). Too little is known about antioxidant deficiencies as acquired risk factors for alcohol-induced liver damage.

FUTURE DIRECTIONS

Our understanding of mechanisms and critical factors in chemically mediated hepatotoxicity will continue to improve through the application of model systems that allow for the observation of events at the level of the cell, organelle, and molecule. Advances in the area of cholestasis are possible using highly purified canalicular membranes, hepatocyte couplets that secrete bile, and cultures of primary bile duct cells. Consequences of damage to specific parts of the liver will be clarified through experiments with chemicals that have defined target sites. Important interrelationships between sinusoidal cells and other types of liver cells can be identified using coculture systems or treatments that modify functions of each type of sinusoidal cell. Knockout rodents and other applications of molecular biology will provide insight into the roles of bioactivation and excretion processes in hepatotoxicity.

REFERENCES

Monographs

Farrell GC: *Drug-Induced Liver Disease.* Edinburgh: Churchill Livingstone, 1994.

McCuskey RS, Earnest DL: Hepatic and gastrointestinal toxicology, in Sipes, IG, McQueen CA, Gandolfi AJ (eds): *Comprehensive Toxicology.* Vol 9. New York: Pergamon Press, 1997.

Zimmerman HJ: *Hepatotoxicity.* New York: Appleton-Century-Crofts, 1978.

Primary Papers

Adams C: Drug bites man: Most arthritic dogs do great on this pill except those that die. *Wall Street Journal,* March 13, 2000.

Albano E, Clot P, Morimoto M, et al: Role of cytochrome P4502E1-dependent formation of hydroxyethyl free radical in the development of liver damage in rats intragastrically fed with ethanol. *Hepatology* 23:155–163, 1996.

Andersson M, Storm HH: Cancer incidence among Danish thorotrast-exposed patients. *J Natl Cancer Inst* 84:1318–1325, 1992.

Andreu V, Mas A, Brugura M, et al: Ecstasy: A common cause of sever acute hepatotoxicity. *J Hepatol* 29:394–397, 1998.

Arrese M, Ananthananarayanan M, Suchy FJ: Hepatobiliary transport: Molecular mechanisms of development and cholestasis. *Pediatr Res* 44:141–147, 1998.

Aw TY: Biliary glutathione promotes the mucosal metabolism of lumenal peroxidized lipids by rat small intestine in vivo. *J Clin Invest* 94:1218–1225, 1994.

Ayotte P, Plaa GL: Hepatic subcellular distribution of manganese in manganese and manganese-bilirubin induced cholestasis. *Biochem Pharmacol* 34:3857–3865, 1985.

Badr MZ, Belinsky SA, Kauffman FC, Thurman RG: Mechanism of hepatotoxicity to periportal regions of the liver lobule due to allyl alcohol: Role of oxygen and lipid peroxidation. *J Pharmacol Exp Ther* 238:1138–1142, 1986.

Ballatori N: Mechanisms of metal transport across liver cell plasma membranes. *Drug Metab Rev* 23:83–132, 1991.

Bohme M, Muller M, Leier I, et al: Cholestasis caused by inhibition of the adenosine triphosphate-dependent bile salt transport in rat liver. *Gastroenterology* 107:255–265, 1994.

Bossard R, Stieger B, O'Neill B, et al: Ethinylestradiol treatment induces multiple canalicular membrane transport alterations in rat liver. *J Clin Invest* 91:2714–2720, 1993.

Chen C-C, Lu R-B, Chen Y-C, et al: Interaction between the functional polymorphisms of the alcohol metabolism genes in protection against alcoholism. *Am J Hum Genet* 65:795–807, 1999a.

Chen J, Robinson NC, Schenker S, et al: Formation of 4-hydroxynonenal adducts with cytochrome c oxidase in rats following short-term ethanol intake. *Hepatology* 29:1792–1798, 1999.

Crawford JM: The liver and the biliary tract, in Cotran RS, Kumar V, Collins T (eds): *Robbins: Pathologic Basis of Disease.* 6th ed. Philadelphia: Saunders, 1999, pp 845–901.

Cullen JM, Ruebner BH: A histopathologic classification of chemical-induced injury of the liver, in Meeks RG, Harrison SD, Bull RJ (eds): *Hepatotoxicology,* Boca Raton, FL: CRC Press, 1991, pp 67–92.

Dahm LJ, Schultze AE, Roth RA: An antibody to neutrophils attenuates α-napthylisothiocyanate-induced liver injury. *J Pharmacol Exp Ther* 256:412–420, 1991.

Davies MH, Harrison RF, Elias E, Hubscher SG: Antibiotic-associated acute vanishing bile duct syndrome: A pattern associated with severe, prolonged intrahepatic cholestasis. *J Hepatol* 20:112–116, 1994.

DeLeve LD: Cellular target of cyclophosphamide toxicity in the murine liver: Role of glutathione and site of metabolic activation. *Hepatology* 24:830–837, 1996.

DeLeve LD: Dacarbazine toxicity in murine liver cells: A model of hepatic endothelial injury and glutathione defense. *J Pharm Exp Ther* 268:1261–1270, 1994.

DeLeve LD, McCuskey RS, Wang X, et al: Characterization of a reproducible rat model of hepatic veno-occulsive disease. *Hepatology* 29:1779–1791, 1999.

Dutczak WJ, Clarkson TW, Ballatori N: Biliary-hepatic recycling of a xenobiotic: Gallbladder absorption of methyl mercury. *Am J Physiol* 260:G873–G880, 1991.

ElSisi AED, Earnest DL, Sipes IG: Vitamin A potentiation of carbon tetrachloride hepatotoxicity: Role of liver macrophages and active oxygen species. *Toxicol Appl Pharmacol* 119:295–301, 1993.

French SW: Rationale for therapy for alcoholic liver disease. *Gastroenterology* 109:617–620, 1995.

Frimmer M: Organotropism by carrier-mediated transport. *Trends Pharmacol Sci* 3:395–397, 1992.

Gardener CR, Heck DE, Yang CS, et al: Role of nitric oxide in acetaminophen-induced hepatotoxicity in the rat. *Hepatology* 26:748–754, 1998.

Geubel AP, De Galocsy C, Alves N, et al: Liver damage caused by therapeutic vitamin A administration: Estimate of dose-related toxicity in 41 cases. *Gastroenterology* 100:1701–1709, 1991.

Gosland M, Tsuboi C, Hoffman T, et al: 17β-Estradiol glucuronide: An inducer of cholestasis and a physiological substrate for the multidrug resistance transporter. *Cancer Res* 53:5382–5385, 1993.

Gregus Z, Klaassen CD: Disposition of metals in rats: A comparative study of fecal, urinary, and biliary excretion and tissue distribution of eighteen metals. *Toxicol Appl Pharmacol* 85:24–38, 1986.

Groothuis GMM, Hardonk MJ, Keulemans KPT, et al: Autoradiographic and kinetic demonstration of acinar heterogeneity of taurocholate transport. *Am J Physiol* 243:G455–G462, 1982.

Hall PM: Histopathology of drug-induced liver disease. in Farrell GC (ed): *Drug-Induced Liver Disease,* Edinburgh: Churchill Livingstone, 1994, pp 115–151.

Hargus SJ, Amouzedeh HR, Pumford NR, et al: Metabolic activation and immunochemical localization of liver protein adducts of the nonsteroidal anti-inflammatory drug diclofenac. *Chem Res Toxicol* 7:575–582, 1994.

Hill DA, Jean PA, Roth RA: Bile duct epithelial cells exposed to alpha-naththylisothiocyanate produce a factor that causes neutrophil-dependent hepatocellular injury in vitro. *Toxicol Sci* 47:118–125, 1999.

Honkoop P, Scholte HR, de Man RA, Schalm SW: Mitochondrial injury: Lessons from the fialuridine trial. *Drug Saf* 17:1–7, 1997.

Hooser SB, Beasley VR, Lovell RA, et al: Toxicity of microcystin LR, a cyclic heptapeptide hepatotoxin from *Microcystis aeruginosa,* to rats and mice. *Vet Pathol* 26:246–252, 1989.

Hooser SB, Beasley VR, Waite LL, Kuhlenschmidt MS, et al: Actin filament alterations in rat hepatocytes induced in vivo and in vitro by microcystin-LR, a hepatotoxin from the blue green alga *Microcystis aeruginosa. Vet Pathol* 28:259–266, 1991.

Huxtable RJ: Pyrrolizidine alkaloids, in Sipes IG, McQueen CA, Gandolfi AJ (eds): *Comprehensive Toxicology.* Vol 9. New York: Pergamon Press, 1997, pp 423–431.

Ito Y, Kojiro M, Nakashima T, Mori T: Pathomorphological characteristics of 102 cases of thorotrast-related hepatocellular carcinoma, cholangiocarcinoma, and hepatic angiosarcoma. *Cancer* 62:1153–1162, 1988.

Jochimsen EM, Carmichael WW, An J, et al: Liver failure and death after exposure to microcystins at a hemodialysis center in Brazil. *N Engl J Med* 338:873–878, 1998.

Jungermann K, Katz N: Functional specialization of different hepatocyte populations. *Physiol Rev* 69:708–764, 1989.

Jungermann K, Kietzmann T: Oxygen: Modulator of metabolic zonation and disease of the liver. *Hepatology* 31:255–260, 2000.

Kanz MF, Kaphalia L, Kaphalia BS, et al: Methylene dianiline: Acute toxicity and effects on biliary function. *Toxicol Appl Pharmacol* 117:88–97, 1992.

Klaassen CD: Biliary excretion of metals. *Drug Metab Rev* 5:165–193,1976.

Klaassen CD, Watkins JB: Mechanisms of bile formation, hepatic uptake, and biliary excretion. *Pharmacol Rev* 36:1–67, 1984.

Kohlroser J, Mathai J, Reichheld J, et al: Hepatotoxicity due to troglitazone: Report of two cases and review of adverse events reported to the United States Food and Drug Administration. *Am J Gastroenterol* 95:272–276, 2000.

Kopelman H, Scheuer PJ, Williams R: The liver lesion of the Epping jaundice. *Q J Med* 35:553–564, 1966.

Korourian S, Hakkak R, Ronis MJJ, et al: Diet and risk of ethanol-induced hepatotoxicity: Carbohydrate-fat relationships in rats. *Toxicol Sci* 47:110–117, 1999.

Kramer B: Vinyl-chloride risks were known by many before first deaths. *Wall Street Journal,* October 2, 1974.

Krell H, Metz J, Jaeschke H, et al: Drug-induced intrahepatic cholestasis: Characterization of different pathomechanisms. *Arch Toxicol* 60:124–130, 1987.

Kubitz R, Wettstein M, Warskulat U, Haussinger D: Regulation of the multidrug resistance protein 2 in the rat liver by lipopolysaccharides and dexamethasone. *Gastroenterology* 116:401–410, 1999.

Kusuhara H, Suzuki H, Sugiyama Y: The role of P-glycoprotein and canalicular multispecific organic anion transporter in the hepatobiliary excretion of drugs. *J Pharm Sci* 87:1025–1040, 1998.

Lakehal F, Wendum D, Barbu V, et al: Phase I and phase II drug-metabolizing enzymes are expressed and heterogeneously distributed in the biliary epithelium. *Hepatology* 30:1498–1506, 1999.

Larrey D, Vial T, Pauwels A, et al: Hepatitis after germander (*Teucrium chamaedris*) ingestion: Another instance of herbal medicine hepatotoxicity. *Ann Intern Med* 117:129–132, 1992.

Laskin DL: Nonparenchymal cells and hepatotoxicity. *Semin Liver Dis* 10:293–304, 1990.

Lee SS, Buters JT, Pineau T, et al: Role of CYP2E1 in the hepatotoxicity of acetaminophen. *J Biol Chem* 271:12063–12067, 1996.

Lekehal M, Pessayre D, Lereau JM, et al: Hepatotoxicity of the herbal medicine germander: Metabolic activation of its furano diterpenoids by cytochrome P4503A depletes cytoskeleton-associated protein thiols and forms plasma membrane blebs in rat hepatocytes. *Hepatology* 24:212–218, 1996.

Lieber CS: Alcohol and the liver: 1994 update. *Gastroenterology* 106:1085–1105, 1994.

Liebler DC, Latwesen DG, Reeder TC: S-(2-chloroacetyl) glutathione, a reactive glutathione thiol ester and a putative metabolite of 1,1-dichloroethylene. *Biochemistry* 27:3652–3657, 1988.

Lira M, Schteingart CD, Steinbach JH, et al: Sugar absorption by the biliary ductular epithelium of the rat: Evidence for two transport systems. *Gastroenterology* 102:563–571, 1992.

Liu Y, Liu J, Iszard MB, et al: Transgenic mice that overexpress metallothionein-1 are protected from cadmium lethality and hepatotoxicity. *Toxicol Appl Pharmacol* 135:222–228, 1995.

Loeper J, Descatoire V, Letteron P, et al: Hepatotoxicity of germander in mice. *Gastroenterology* 106:464–472, 1994.

Lustig S, Pitlik SD, Rosenfeld JB: Liver damage in acute self-induced hypermanganemia. *Arch Intern Med* 142:405–406, 1982.

Manno M, Rezzadore M, Grossi M, Sbrana C: Potentiation of occupational carbon tetrachloride toxicity by ethanol abuse. *Hum Exp Toxicol* 15:294–300, 1996.

Mansouri A, Gaou I, deKerguenec C, et al: An alcoholic binge causes massive degradation of hepatic mitochondrial DNA in mice. *Gastroenterology* 117:181–190, 1999.

McKenzie R, Fried MW, Salllie R, et al: Hepatic failure and lactic acidosis due to fialuridine (FIAU), an investigational nucleoside analogue for chronic hepatitis B. *N Engl J Med* 333:1099–1105, 1995.

Michael SL, Pumford NR, Mayeu PR, et al: Pretreatment of mice with macrophage inactivators decreases acetaminophen hepatotoxicity and the formation of reactive oxygen and nitrogen species. *Hepatology* 30:186–195, 1999.

Mitchell JR, Jollow DJ, Potter WZ, et al: Acetaminophen-induced hepatic necrosis: IV. Protective role of glutathione. *J Pharmacol Exp Ther* 187:211–217, 1973.

Moslen MT, Kanz MF: Biliary excretion of marker solutes by rats with 1,1-dichloroethylene-induced bile canalicular injury. *Toxicol Appl Pharmacol* 122:117–130, 1993.

Nagano K, Nakamura K, Urakami K-I, et al: Intracellular distribution of the Wilson's disease gene product (ATPase7B) after in vitro and in vivo exogenous expression in hepatocytes from the LEC rat, an animal model of Wilson's disease. *Hepatology* 27:799–807, 1998.

Phillips MJ, Poucell S, Oda M: Mechanisms of cholestasis. *Lab Invest* 54:593–608, 1986.

Pohl LR: Drug induced allergic hepatitis. *Semin Liver Dis* 10:305–315, 1990.

Recknagel RO: Carbon tetrachloride hepatotoxicity. *Pharmacol Rev* 19:145–208, 1967.

Redlich CA, Beckett WS, Sparer J, et al: Liver disease associated with occupational exposure to the solvent dimethylformamide. *Ann Intern Med* 108:680–686, 1988.

Redlich CA, West AB, Fleming L, et al: Clinical and pathological characteristics of hepatotoxicity associated with occupational exposure to dimethylformamide. *Gastroenterology* 99:748–757, 1990.

Reynolds ES, Moslen MT: Environmental liver injury: Halogenated hydrocarbons, in Farber E, Fisher MM (eds): *Toxic Injury of the Liver.* New York: Marcel Dekker, 1980, pp 541–596.

Rikans LE, Moore DR: Effect of age and sex on allyl alcohol hepatotoxicity in rats: Role of liver alcohol and aldehyde dehydrogenase activities. *J Pharmacol Exp Ther* 243:20–26, 1987.

Roberts DW, Bucci TJ, Benson RW, et al: Immunohistochemical localization and quantification of the 3-(cystein-S-yl)-acetaminophen protein adduct in acetaminophen hepatotoxicity. *Am J Pathol* 138:359–371, 1991.

Rolla R, Vay D, Mottaran E, et al: Detection of circulating antibodies against malondialdehyde-acetaldehye adducts in patients with alcohol-induced liver disease. *Hepatology* 31:878–884, 2000.

Runnegar MT, Berndt N, Kaplowitz N: Microcystin uptake and inhibition of protein phosphatases: Effects of chemoprotectants and self-inhibition in relation to known hepatic transporters. *Tox Appl Pharmacol* 134:264–272, 1995a.

Runnegar MT, Berndt N, Kong S-M, et al: In vivo and in vitro binding of microcystin to protein phosphatases 1 and 2A. *Biochem Biophys Res Commun* 216:162–169, 1995c.

Runnegar MT, Maddatu T, DeLeve LD, et al: Differential toxicity of the protein phosphatase inhibitors microcystin and calyculin A. *J Pharm Exp Ther* 273:545–553, 1995b.

Runnegar MT, Wei X, Hamm-Alvarez SF: Increased protein phosphorylation of cytoplasmic dynein results in impaired motor function. *Biochem J* 342:1–6, 1999.

Seitz S, Boelsterli UA: Diclofenac acyl glucuronide, a major biliary metabolite, is directly involved in small intestinal injury in rats. *Gastroenterology* 115:1476–1482, 1998.

Selim K, Kaplowitz N: Hepatotoxicity of psychotrophic drugs. *Hepatology* 29:1347–1351, 1999.

Sinclair JF, Szakac SJG, Wood SG, et al: Acetaminophen hepatotoxicity precipitated by short-term treatment of rats with ethanol and isopentanol. *Biochem Pharmacol* 59:445–545, 2000.

Smilkstein MJ, Knapp GL, Kulig KW, Rumack BH: Efficacy of oral *N*-acetylcysteine in the treatment of acetaminophen overdose: Analysis of the National Multicenter Study (1976–1985). *N Engl J Med* 319:1557–1562, 1988.

Solter PF, Wollenberg, GK, Huang X, et al: Prolonged sublethal exposure to the protein phosphatase inhibitor microcystin-LR results in multiple dose-dependent hepatotoxic effects. *Toxicol Sci* 44: 87–96, 1998.

Sun Z, Lu P, Gail MH, Pee D, et al: Increased risk of hepatocellular carcinoma in male hepatitis B surface antigen carriers with chronic hepatitis who have detectable urinary aflatoxin metabolite M1. *Hepatology* 30:379–383, 1999.

Thurman RG, Bradford BU, Iimuro Y, et al: Role of Kupffer cells, endotoxin and free radicals in mediating hepatotoxicity due to alcohol, in Sipes IG, McQueen CA, Gandolfi AJ (eds): *Comprehensive Toxicology.* Vol 9. New York: Pergamon Press, 1997, pp 309–320.

Tillmann HL, van Pelt RNAM, Martz W, et al: Accidental intoxication with methylene dianiline *p,p′*-diaminophenyl-methane: Acute liver damage after presumed Ecstasy consumption. *Clin Toxicol* 35:35–40, 1997.

Trauner M, Meier PJ, Boyer JL: Mechanisms of disease: Molecular pathogenesis of cholestasis. *N Engl J Med* 339:1217–1227, 1998.

Tsutsumi M, Lasker JM, Shimizu M, et al: The intralobular distribution of ethanol-inducible P450IIE1 in rat and human liver. *Hepatology* 10:437–446, 1989.

Vore M: Mechanisms of cholestasis, in Meeks RG, Harrison SD, Bull RJ (eds): *Hepatotoxicology.* Boca Raton, FL: CRC Press, 1991, pp 525–568.

Walker RM, Racz WJ, McElligott TF: Scanning electron microscopic examination of acetaminophen-induced hepatotoxicity and congestion in mice. *Am J Pathol* 113:321–330, 1983.

Walli AK, Wieland E, Wieland TH: Phalloidin uptake by the liver of cholestatic rats in vivo, in isolated perfused liver and isolated hepatocytes. *Naunyn-Schmiedeberg's Arch Pharmacol* 316:257–261, 1981.

Wang X, Kanel GC, DeLeve LD: Support of sinusoidal endothelial cell glutathione prevents hepatic veno-occlusive disease in the rat. *Hepatology* 31:428–434, 2000.

Watanabe N, Tsukada N, Smith CR, et al: Permeabilized hepatocyte couplets: Adenosine triphosphate-dependent bile canalicular contractions and a circumferential pericanalicular microfilament belt demonstrated. *Lab Invest* 65:203–213, 1991.

Watanabe S, Phillips MJ: Acute phalloidin toxicity in living hepatocytes: Evidence for a possible disturbance in membrane flow and for multiple functions for actin in the liver cell. *Am J Pathol* 122:101–111, 1986.

Wong FW-Y, Chan W-Y, Lee SS-T: Resistance to carbon tetrachloride-induced hepatotoxicity in mice which lack CYP2E1 expression. *Toxicol Appl Pharmacol* 153:109–118, 1998.

Woodard SH, Moslen MT: Decreased biliary secretion of proteins and phospholipids by rats with 1, 1-dichloroethylene-induced bile canalicular injury. *Toxicol Appl Pharmol* 152:295–301, 1998.

Yin M, Wheeler MD, Kono H, et al: Essential role of tumor necrosis factor α in alcohol-induced liver injury in mice. *Gastroenterology* 117:942–952, 1999.

Ziegler K, Frimmer M: Cyclosporin A protects liver cells against phalloidin: Potent inhibition of the inward transport by cholate and phallotoxins. *Biochim Biophys Acta* 805:174–180, 1984.

CHAPTER 14

TOXIC RESPONSES OF THE KIDNEY

Rick G. Schnellmann

The functional integrity of the mammalian kidney is vital to total body homeostasis, as the kidney plays a principal role in the excretion of metabolic wastes and in the regulation of extracellular fluid volume, electrolyte composition, and acid–base balance. In addition, the kidney synthesizes and releases hormones, such as renin and erythropoietin, and metabolizes vitamin D_3 to the active 1,25-dihydroxy vitamin D_3 form. A toxic insult to the kidney therefore could disrupt any or all of these functions and could have profound effects on total-body metabolism. Fortunately, the kidneys are equipped with a variety of detoxification mechanisms and have considerable functional reserve and regenerative capacities. Nonetheless, the nature and severity of the toxic insult may be such that these detoxification and compensatory mechanisms are overwhelmed, and renal failure ensues. The outcome of renal failure can be profound; permanent renal damage may result, requiring chronic dialysis treatment or kidney transplantation.

FUNCTIONAL ANATOMY

Gross examination of a sagittal section of the kidney reveals three clearly demarcated anatomic areas: the cortex, medulla, and papilla (Figs. 14-1 and 14-2). The cortex constitutes the major portion of the kidney and receives a disproportionately higher percentage (90 percent) of blood flow compared to the medulla (~6 to 10 percent) or papilla (1 to 2 percent). Thus, when a blood-borne toxicant is delivered to the kidney, a high percentage of the material will be delivered to the cortex and will have a greater opportunity to influence cortical rather than medullary or papillary functions. However, medullary and papillary tissues are exposed to higher luminal concentrations of toxicants for prolonged periods of time, a consequence of the more concentrated tubular fluid and the more sluggish flow of blood and filtrate in these regions.

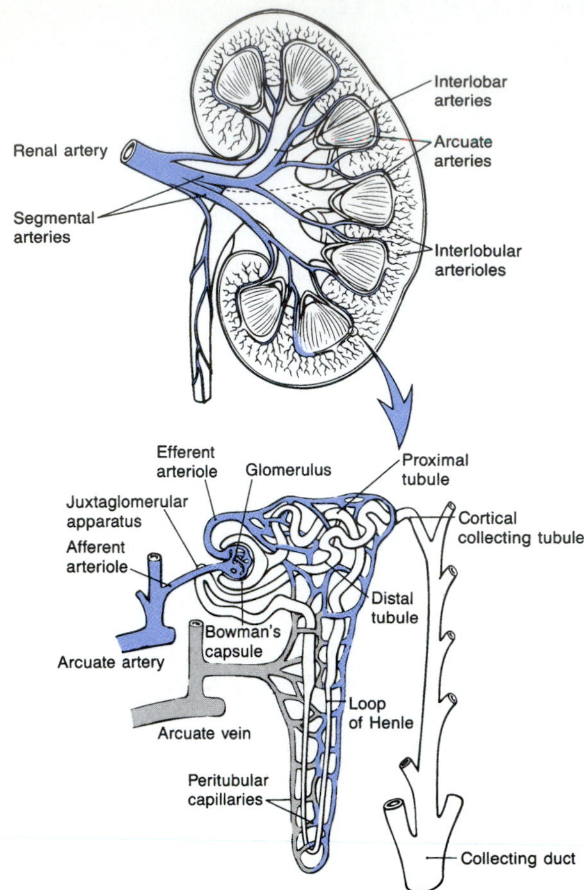

Figure 14-1. Schematic of the human kidney showing the major blood vessels and the microcirculation and tubular components of each nephron. [From Guyton AC, Hall JE (eds): Textbook of Medical Physiology. Philadelphia: Saunders, 1996, p 318, with permission.]

The functional unit of the kidney, the nephron, may be considered in three portions: the vascular element, the glomerulus, and the tubular element.

Renal Vasculature and Glomerulus

The renal artery branches successively into interlobar, arcuate, and interlobular arteries (Fig. 14-1). The last of these give rise to the afferent arterioles, which supply the glomerulus; blood then leaves the glomerular capillaries via the efferent arteriole. Both the afferent and efferent arterioles, arranged in a series before and after the glomerular capillary tuft, respectively, are ideally situated to control glomerular capillary pressure and glomerular plasma flow rate. Indeed, these arterioles are innervated by the sympathetic nervous system and contract in response to nerve stimulation, angiotensin II, vasopressin, endothelin, prostanoids, and cytokines, affecting glomerular pressures and blood flow. The efferent arterioles draining the cortical glomeruli branch into a peritubular capillary network, whereas those draining the juxtamedullary glomeruli form a capillary loop, the vasa recta, supplying the medullary structures. These postglomerular capillary loops provide an efficient arrangement for delivery of nutrients to the postglomerular tubular structures, delivery of wastes to the tubule for excretion, and return of reabsorbed electrolytes, nutrients, and water to the systemic circulation.

The glomerulus is a complex, specialized capillary bed composed primarily of endothelial cells that are characterized by an attenuated and fenestrated cytoplasm, visceral epithelial cells characterized by a cell body (podocyte) from which many trabeculae and pedicles (foot processes) extend, and a glomerular basement membrane (GBM), which is a trilamellar structure sandwiched between the endothelial and epithelial cells (Fig.14-3). A portion of the blood entering the glomerular capillary network is fractionated

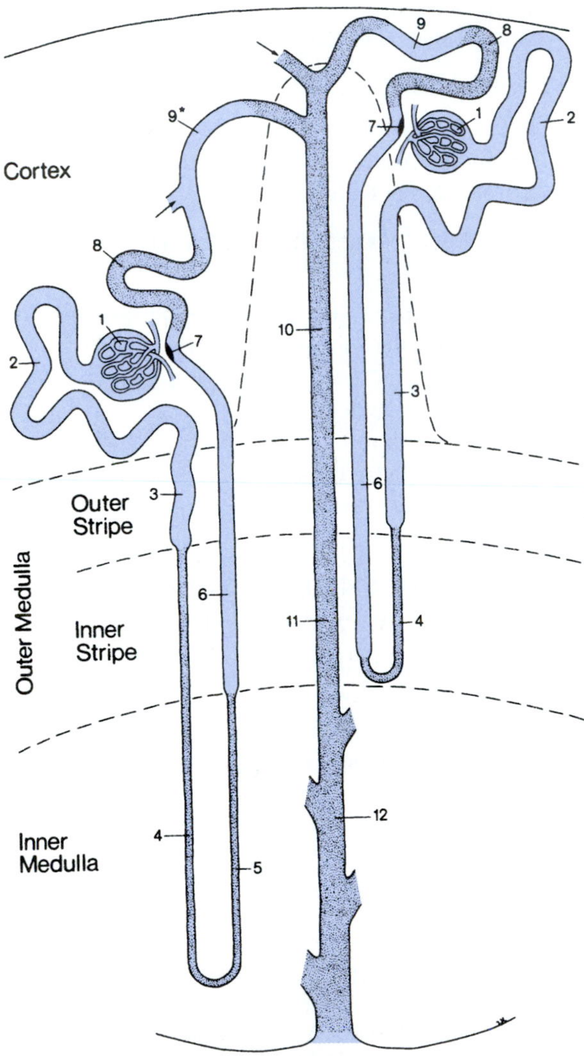

***Figure 14-2.** Schematic of short- and long-looped nephrons and the collecting system.*

A medullary ray is delineated by a dashed line within the cortex. (1) Renal corpuscle including Bowman's capsule and the glomerulus; (2) proximal convoluted tubule; (3) proximal straight tubule; (4) descending thin limb; (5) thin ascending limb; (6) thick ascending limb; (7) macula densa, located within the final portion of the thick ascending limb; (8) distal convoluted tubule; (9) connecting tubule; (9*) connecting tubule of the juxtamedullary nephron, which forms an arcade; (10) cortical collecting duct; (11) outer medullary collecting duct; (12) inner medullary collecting duct. [From Kriz W: Standard nomenclature for structures of the kidney. *Am J Physiol* 254:F1–F8, 1988, with permission.]

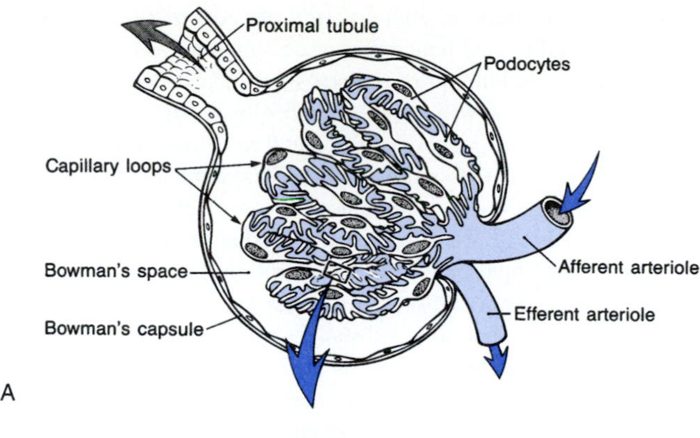

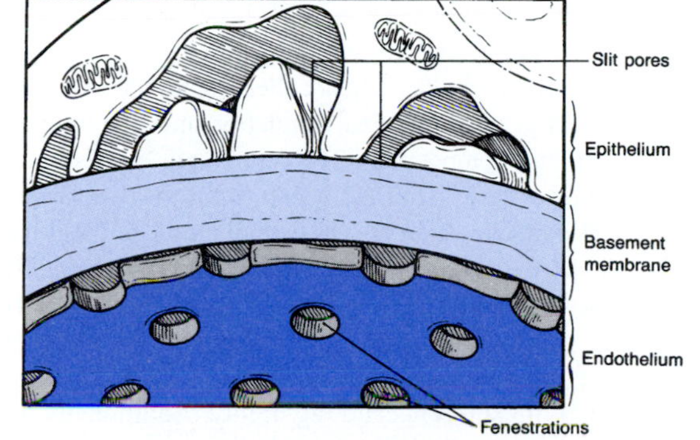

***Figure 14-3.** **A.** Schematic of the ultrastructure of the glomerular capillaries.* ***B.** Cross section of the glomerular capillary membrane with the capillary endothelium, basement membrane, and epithelium podocytes. [From Guyton AC, Hall JE, 1996, p 32, with permission.]*

into a virtually protein-free and cell-free ultrafiltrate, which passes through Bowman's space and into the tubular portion of the nephron. The formation of such an ultrafiltrate is the net result of the Starling forces that determine fluid movement across capillary beds—that is, the balance between transcapillary hydrostatic pressure and colloid oncotic pressure (Maddox and Brenner, 1991). Filtration is therefore favored when transcapillary hydrostatic pressure exceeds plasma oncotic pressure. An additional determinant of ultrafiltration is the effective hydraulic permeability of the glomerular capillary wall, in other words, the ultrafiltration coefficient (K_f), which is determined by the total surface area available for filtration and the hydraulic permeability of the capillary wall. Consequently, chemically induced decreases in glomerular filtration rate (GFR) may be related to decreases in transcapillary hydrostatic pressure and glomerular plasma flow due to increased afferent arteriolar resistance or to decreases in the surface area available for filtration, resulting from decreases in the size and/or number of endothelial fenestrae or detachment or effacement of foot processes.

Although the glomerular capillary wall permits a high rate of fluid filtration (approximately 20 percent of blood entering the glomerulus is filtered), it provides a significant barrier to the transglomerular passage of macromolecules. Experiments using a variety of charged and neutral tracers have established that this barrier function is based on the ability of the glomerulus to act as a size-selective and charge-selective filter (Brenner et al., 1977). In general, the filtration of macromolecules is inversely proportional to the molecular weight of a substance; thus, small molecules, such as inulin (MW 5500), are freely filtered, while large molecules, such as albumin (MW 56,000 to 70,000), are restricted. Filtration of anionic molecules tends to be restricted compared to that of neutral or cationic molecules of the same size. These permselective properties of the glomerulus appear to be directly related to the physicochemical properties of the different cell types within the glomerulus (Kanwar et al., 1991). In particular, charge-selective properties of the glomerulus appear to be related to the anionic groups of the GBM coupled with the anionic coating of the epithelial and endothelial cells (Fig. 14-3). These highly anionic components produce electrostatic repulsion and hinder the circulation of polyanionic macromolecules, thereby markedly retarding passage of these molecules across the filtration barrier. Toxicants that neutralize or reduce the number of fixed anionic charges on glomerular structural elements therefore will impair the charge- and/or size-selective properties of the glomerulus, resulting in urinary excretion of polyanionic and/or high-molecular-weight proteins.

Proximal Tubule

The proximal tubule consists of three discrete segments: the S_1 (pars convoluta), S_2 (transition between pars convoluta and pars recta), and S_3 (the pars recta) segments (Fig. 14-2). The S_1 segment is the initial portion of the proximal convoluted tubule and is characterized by a tall brush border and a well-developed vacuolar lysosomal system. The basolateral membrane is extensively interdigitated and many long mitochondria fill the basal portion of the cell, characteristic of Na^+-transporting epithelia. The S_2 segment comprises the end of the convoluted segment and the initial portion of the straight segment. These cells possess a shorter brush border, fewer apical vacuoles and mitochondria, and less basolateral interdigitation compared to the S_1 cells. The S_3 segment comprises the distal portion of proximal segments and extends to the junction of the outer and inner stripe of the outer medulla. The S_3 cells have a well-developed brush border but fewer and smaller lysosomes and mitochondria than S_1 and S_2 cells.

The formation of urine is a highly complex and integrated process in which the volume and composition of the glomerular filtrate is progressively altered as fluid passes through each of the different tubular segments. The proximal tubule is the workhorse of the nephron, as it reabsorbs approximately 60 to 80 percent of solute and water filtered at the glomerulus. Toxicant-induced injury to the proximal tubule therefore will have major consequences to water and solute balance. Water reabsorption is through a passive iso-osmotic process, driven primarily by Na^+ reabsorption, mediated by the Na^+,K^+-ATPase localized in the basolateral plasma membrane. In addition to active Na^+ reabsorption, the proximal tubule reabsorbs other electrolytes, such as K^+, HCO_3^-, Cl^-, PO_4^{3-}, Ca^{2+}, and Mg^{2+}. The proximal tubule contains numerous transport systems capable of driving concentrative transport of many metabolic substrates, including amino acids, glucose, and citric acid cycle intermediates. The proximal tubule also reabsorbs virtually all of the filtered low-molecular-weight proteins by specific endocytotic protein reabsorption processes. In addition, small linear peptides may be hydrolyzed by peptidases associated with the proximal tubular brush border. An important excretory function of the proximal tubule is secretion of weak organic anions and cations by specialized transporters that drive concentrative movement of these ions from postglomerular blood into proximal tubular cells, followed by secretion into tubular fluid. Toxicant-induced interruptions in the production of energy for any of these active transport mechanisms or the function of critical membrane-bound enzymes or transporters can profoundly affect proximal tubular and whole-kidney function.

The different segments of the proximal tubule exhibit marked biochemical and physiologic heterogeneity (Goldstein, 1993). For example, filtered HCO_3^-, low-molecular-weight proteins, amino acids, and glucose are primarily reabsorbed by the S_1 segment. Transport capacities for these substances in the S_2 and S_3 segments are appreciably less; for example, glucose reabsorption in the S_2 and S_3 segments is about 50 percent and 10 percent of that in the S_1 segment, respectively. In contrast, the principal site of organic anion and cation secretion is in the S_2 and S_1/S_2 segments, respectively. Oxygen consumption, Na^+,K^+-ATPase activity, and gluconeogenic capacity are greater in the S_1 and S_2 segments than in the S_3 segment. Catabolism and apical transport of glutathione (GSH) occurs to a much greater extent in the S_3 segment, where the brush-border enzyme γ-glutamyltranspeptidase (GGT) is present in greater amounts. Chemically induced injury to distinct proximal tubular segments therefore may be related in part to their segmental differences in biochemical properties (see "Site-Selective Injury," below).

Loop of Henle

The thin descending and ascending limbs and the thick ascending limb of the loop of Henle are critical to the processes involved in urinary concentration (Fig. 14-2). Approximately 25 percent of the filtered Na^+ and K^+ and 20 percent of the filtered water are reabsorbed by the segments of the loop of Henle. The tubular fluid entering the thin descending limb is iso-osmotic to the renal interstitium; water is freely permeable and solutes, such as electrolytes and urea, may enter from the interstitium. In contrast, the thin ascending limb is relatively impermeable to water and urea, and Na^+ and Cl^- are reabsorbed by passive diffusion. The thick ascending limb is impermeable to water, and active transport of Na^+ and Cl^- is mediated by the Na^+/K^+-$2Cl^-$ cotransport mechanism, with the energy provided by the Na^+,K^+-ATPase. The relatively high rates of Na^+,K^+-ATPase activity and oxygen demand, coupled with the meager oxygen supply in the medullary thick ascending limb, are believed to contribute to the vulnerability of this segment of the nephron to hypoxic injury. The close interdependence between metabolic workload and tubular vulnerability has been demonstrated, revealing that selective damage to the thick ascending limb in the isolated perfused kidney can be blunted by reducing tubular work and oxygen consumption (via inhibition of the Na^+,K^+-ATPase with ouabain) or by increasing oxygen supply (via provision of an oxygen carrier, hemoglobin) (Brezis and Epstein, 1993). Conversely, increasing the tubular workload (via the ionophore amphotericin B) exacerbates hypoxic injury to this segment (Brezis et al., 1984).

Distal Tubule and Collecting Duct

The macula densa comprises specialized cells located between the end of the thick ascending limb and the early distal tubule, in close proximity to the afferent arteriole (Fig. 14-2). This anatomic arrangement is ideally suited for a feedback system whereby a stimulus received at the macula densa is transmitted to the arterioles of the same nephron. Under normal physiologic conditions, increased solute delivery or concentration at the macula densa triggers a signal resulting in afferent arteriolar constriction leading to decreases in GFR (and hence decreased solute delivery). Thus, increases in fluid/solute out of the proximal tubule, due to impaired tubular reabsorption, will activate this feedback system, referred to as *tubuloglomerular feedback* (TGF) and resulting in decreases in the filtration rate of the same nephron. This regulatory mechanism is viewed as a powerful volume-conserving mechanism, designed to decrease GFR in order to prevent massive losses of fluid/electrolytes due to impaired tubular reabsorption. Humoral mediation of TGF by the renin-angiotensin system has been proposed, and evidence suggests that other substances may be involved. The distal tubular cells contain numerous mitochondria but lack a well-developed brush border and an endocytotic apparatus characteristic of the pars convoluta of the proximal tubule. The early distal tubule reabsorbs most of the remaining intraluminal Na^+, K^+, and Cl^- but is relatively impermeable to water.

The late distal tubule, cortical collecting tubule, and medullary collecting duct perform the final regulation and fine tuning of urinary volume and composition. The remaining Na^+ is reabsorbed in conjunction with K^+ and H^+ secretion in the late distal tubule and cortical collecting tubule. The combination of medullary and papillary hypertonicity generated by countercurrent multiplication and the action of antidiuretic hormone (vasopressin, ADH) serve to enhance water permeability of the medullary collecting duct. Agents that interfere with ADH synthesis, secretion, or action therefore may impair concentrating ability. Additionally, because urinary concentrating ability is dependent upon medullary and papillary hypertonicity, agents that increase medullary blood flow may impair concentrating ability by dissipating the medullary osmotic gradient.

Table 14-1 illustrates the efficiency of the nephrons in the conservation of electrolytes, substrates, and water and excretion of nitrogenous wastes (urea).

PATHOPHYSIOLOGIC RESPONSES OF THE KIDNEY

Acute Renal Failure

One of the most common manifestations of nephrotoxic damage is acute renal failure (ARF), characterized by an abrupt decline in GFR with resulting azotemia. Any decline in GFR is complex and may result from prerenal factors (afferent arteriolar constriction, hypovolemia, insufficient cardiac output, obstruction of renal arteries), postrenal factors (ureteral or bladder obstruction), and intrarenal factors (tubular epithelial cell death/loss, tubular obstruction) resulting in back-leak, glomerular nephritis, and tubulointerstitial nephritis (Fig. 14-4). Figure 14-5 illustrates the pathways that lead to diminished GFR following chemical exposure. As discussed above, pre- and postrenal factors can lead to decreased GFR. If a chemical causes tubular damage directly, then tubular casts can cause tubular obstruction, increased tubular pressure, and decreased GFR. The tubular damage may result in epithelial cell death/loss, leading to back-leak of glomerular filtrate and a decrease in GFR. If a chemical causes intrarenal hemodynamic alterations that lead to vasoconstriction, the resulting medullary hypoxia may cause tubular damage and/or decreases in perfusion pressure, glomerular hydrostatic pressure, and GFR. Finally, a chemical may disrupt glomerular function, resulting in decreased glomerular ultrafiltration and GFR. Table 14-2 provides a partial list of chemicals that produce ARF through these different mechanisms. Importantly, in

Table 14-1
Filtration, Reabsorption, and Excretion Rates of Different Substances by the Kidneys*

	FILTERED, meq/24 h	REABSORBED, meq/24 h	EXCRETED, meq/24 h	REABSORBED, %
Glucose (g/day)	180	180	0	100
Bicarbonate (meq/day)	4,320	4,318	2	>99.9
Sodium (meq/day)	25,560	25410	150	99.4
Chloride (meq/day)	19,440	19260	180	99.1
Water (L/day)	169	167.5	1.5	99.1
Urea (g/day)	48	24	24	50
Creatinine (g/day)	1.8	0	1.8	0

*Glomerular filtration rate: 125 mL/min = 180 L/24h.

most instances ARF is a consequence of tubular damage and/or increased renal vascular resistance.

The maintenance of tubular integrity is dependent on cell-to-cell and cell-to-matrix adhesion; these interactions are mediated in part by integrins and cell adhesion molecules (Fig. 14-6). It has been hypothesized that after a chemical or hypoxic insult, adhesion of non–lethally damaged, apoptotic, and oncotic cells to the basement membrane is compromised, leading to their detachment from the basement membrane and appearance in the tubular lumen (Goligorksy et al., 1993). Morphologically, such an event would lead to gaps in the epithelial cell lining, potentially resulting in back-leak of filtrate and diminished GFR. These detached cells may aggregate in the tubular lumen (cell-to-cell adhesion) and/or adhere or reattach to adherent epithelial cells downstream, resulting

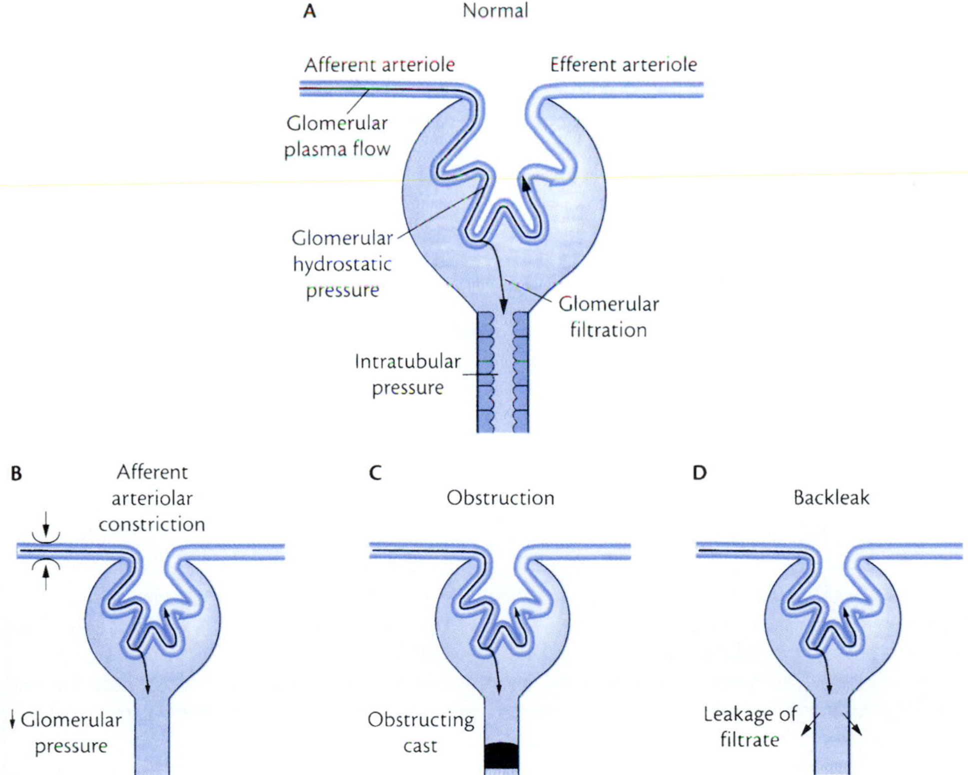

Figure 14-4. Mechanisms of reduction of the glomerular filtration rate (GFR).

A. GFR depends on four factors: (1) adequate blood flow to the glomerulus; (2) adequate glomerular capillary pressure; (3) glomerular permeability; and (4) low intratubular pressure. *B.* Afferent arteriolar constriction decreases GFR by reducing blood flow, resulting in diminished capillary pressure. *C.* Obstruction of the tubular lumen by cast formation increases tubular pressure; when tubular pressure exceeds glomerular capillary pressure, filtration decreases or ceases. *D.* Back-leak occurs when the paracellular space between cells increases and the glomerular filtrate leaks into the extracellular space and bloodstream [From Molitoris BA, Bacallao R: Pathophysiology of ischemic acute renal failure: Cytoskeletal aspects, in Berl T, Bonventre JV (eds): *Atlas of Diseases of the Kidney.* Philadelphia: Current Medicine, 1999, p 13.5, with permission.]

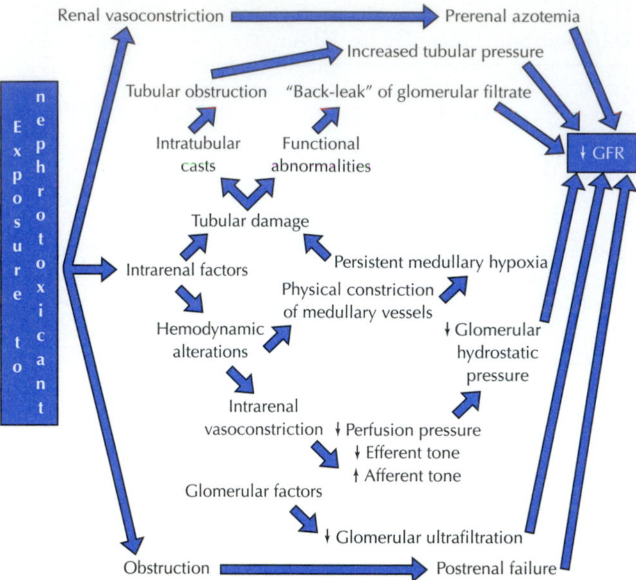

Figure 14-5. Mechanisms that contribute to decreased GFR in acute renal failure.

After exposure to a nephrotoxicant, one or more mechanisms may contribute to a reduction in the GFR. These include renal vasoconstriction resulting in prerenal azotemia and obstruction due to precipitation of a drug or endogenous compound within the kidney. Intrarenal factors include direct tubular obstruction and dysfunction resulting in tubular back-leak and increased tubular pressure. Alterations in the levels of a variety of vasoactive mediators may result in decreased renal perfusion pressure or efferent arteriolar tone and increased afferent arteriolar tone, leading to in decreased glomerular hydrostatic pressure. [Schnellmann RG, Kelly KJ: Pathophysiology of nephrotoxic acute renal failure, in Berl T, Bonventre JV (eds): *Atlas of Diseases of the Kidney*. Philadelphia: Current Medicine, 1999, p 15.4, with permission.]

in tubular obstruction. Further, the loss of expression of integrins on the basolateral membrane may be responsible for the exfoliation of tubular cells, and the redistribution of integrins from the basolateral to the apical membrane facilitates adhesion of detached cells to the in situ epithelium.

Other studies have indicated that leukocyte adhesion molecules play a critical role in ARF, possibly because of the ability of activated leukocytes to release cytokines and reactive oxygen species (ROS), resulting in capillary damage/leakage, which may lead to the vascular congestion often observed in ARF. Bonventre and colleagues have demonstrated that treatment of rats with either monoclonal antibodies against the integrins, CD11a and CD11b, or a monoclonal antibody against ICAM-1 (a ligand for CD11a) conferred significant protection against renal ischemic injury (Kelly et al., 1994; Rabb et al., 1994), suggesting a critical role for leukocyte–endothelial adhesion in the pathophysiology of ischemic ARF.

Whereas chemically induced ARF can be initiated by proximal tubular cell injury, nephrotoxicants also may inhibit cellular proliferation and migration, thereby delaying renal functional recovery. For example, Leonard et al. (1994) demonstrated that cisplatin impaired tubular regeneration resulting in prolonged renal dysfunction, effects that were in contrast to the regenerative response and renal functional recovery following tobramycin-induced nephrotoxicity. Using an in vitro model, Counts et al. (1995) reported that following mechanically induced injury to a proximal tubular monolayer, proliferation and migration were inhibited by the heavy metal $HgCl_2$, the mycotoxin fumonisin B_1, and dichlorovinyl-L-cysteine (DCVC), suggesting that nephrotoxicants may inhibit/delay the regenerative process.

Adaptation Following Toxic Insult

Fortunately, the kidney has a remarkable ability to compensate for a loss in renal functional mass. Micropuncture studies have revealed that following unilateral nephrectomy, GFR of the remnant

Table 14-2
Mechanisms of Chemically Induced Acute Renal Failure

PRERENAL	VASOCONSTRICTION	CRYSTALLURIA	
Diuretics Interleukin-2 Angiotensin-converting enzyme inhibitors Antihypertensive agents	Nonsteroidal anti-inflammatory drugs Radiocontrast agents Cyclosporine Tacrolimus Amphotericin B	Sulfonamides Methotrexate Acyclovir Triamterene Ethylene glycol Protease inhibitors	
TUBULAR TOXICITY	ENDOTHELIAL INJURY	GLOMERULOPATHY	INTERSTITIAL NEPHRITIS
Aminoglycosides Cisplatin Vancomycin Pentamidine Radiocontrast agents Heavy metals Haloalkane- and Haloalkene-cysteine conjugates	Cyclosporine Mitomycin C Tacrolimus Cocaine Conjugated estrogens Quinine	Gold Penicillamine Nonsteroidal anti-inflammatory drugs	Multiple

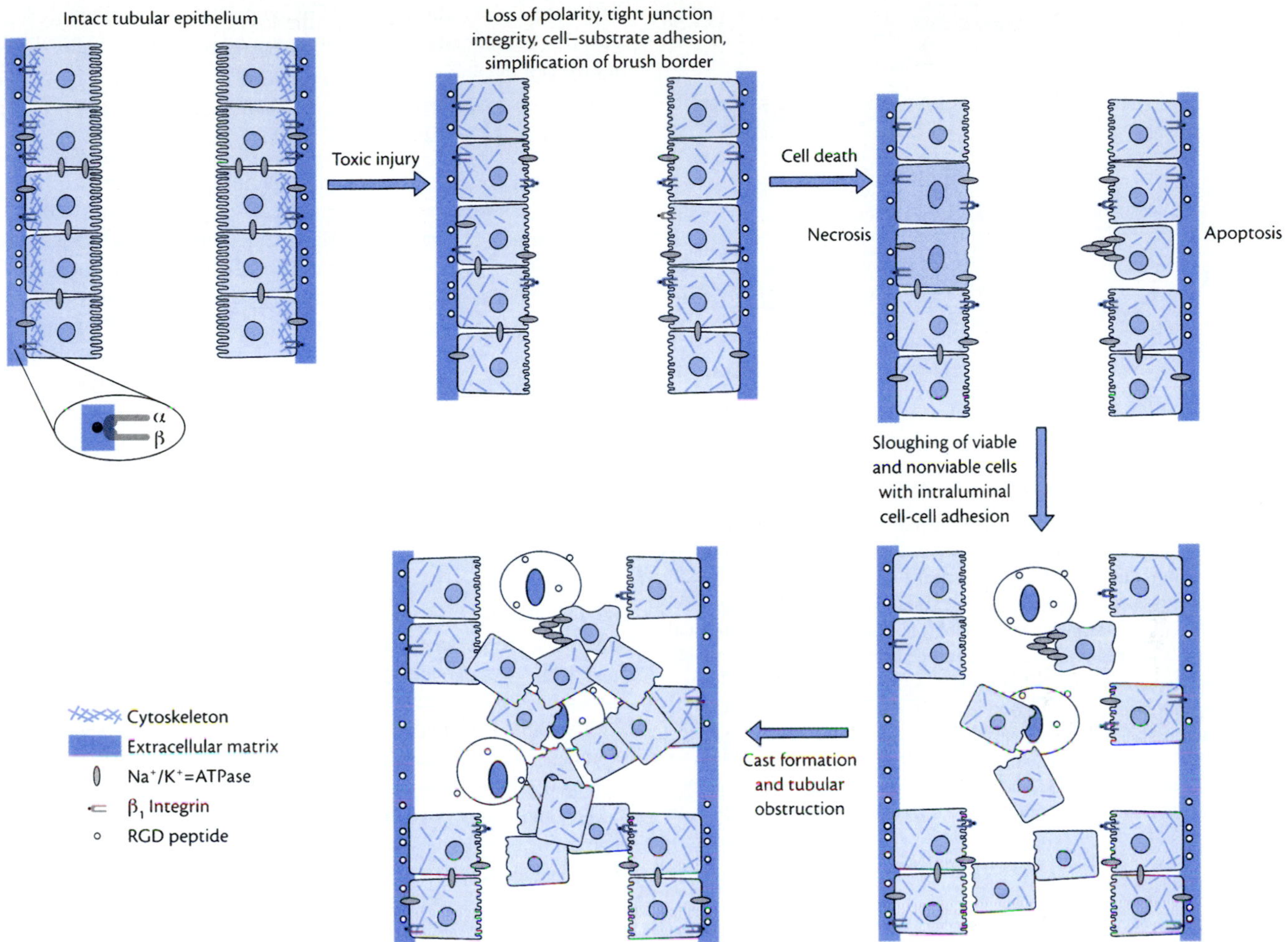

Figure 14-6. After injury, alterations can occur in the cytoskeleton and in the normal distribution of membrane proteins such as Na^+,K^+-ATPase and β_1 integrins in sublethally injured renal tubular cells.

These changes result in loss of cell polarity, tight junction integrity, and cell-substrate adhesion. Lethally injured cells undergo oncosis or apoptosis, and both dead and viable cells may be released into the tubular lumen. Adhesion of released cells to other released cells and to cells remaining adherent to the basement membrane may result in cast formation, tubular obstruction, and further compromise the GFR. [Schnellmann RG, Kelly KJ: Pathophysiology of nephrotoxic acute renal failure, in Berl T, Bonventre JV (eds): *Atlas of Diseases of the Kidney*. Philadelphia: Current Medicine, 1999, p 15.5, with permission.]

kidney increases by approximately 40 to 60 percent, an effect associated with early compensatory increases in glomerular plasma flow rate and glomerular hydraulic pressure. Compensatory increases in single-nephron GFR are accompanied by proportionate increases in proximal tubular water and solute reabsorption; glomerulotubular balance is therefore maintained and overall renal function appears normal by standard clinical tests. Consequently, chemically induced changes in renal function may not be detected until these compensatory mechanisms are overwhelmed by significant nephron loss and/or damage.

There are a number of cellular and molecular responses to a nephrotoxic insult. After a population of renal cells are exposed to a toxicant, a fraction of the cells will be severely injured and undergo cell death by apoptosis or oncosis (see below) (Fig. 14-7). Those cells that are nonlethally injured may undergo cell repair and/or adaptation, which contribute to the structural and functional recovery of the nephron (Fig. 14-8). In addition, there is a population of cells that are uninjured and may undergo compensatory hypertrophy, cellular adaptation, and cellular proliferation. At this time there is little evidence for a stem cell in the kidney; consequently, it is thought that renal cells undergo dedifferentiation, proliferation, migration, and differentiation. The cellular proliferation and compensatory hypertrophy contribute to the structural and functional recovery of the nephron. Growth factors delivered to renal epithelial cells from local and systemic sources may help orchestrate the proliferative response of the nephron. Several growth factors—such as epidermal growth factor (EGF), insulin-like growth factor-1 (IGF-1), hepatocyte growth factor (HGF), fibroblast growth factors, and transforming growth factors α and β have been implicated in proximal tubular regeneration (Hammerman and Miller, 1994). Interestingly, exogenous administration of EGF, HGF, or IGF-1 accelerates renal repair following ischemic-, gen-

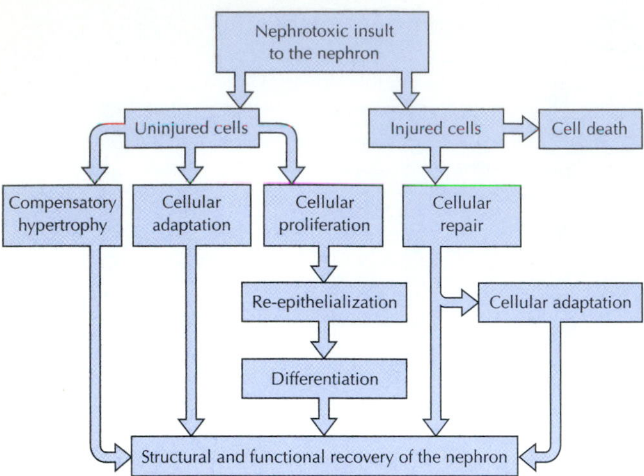

Figure 14-7. The response of the nephron to a nephrotoxic insult.

After a population of cells is exposed to a nephrotoxicant, the cells respond; ultimately the nephron recovers function or, if cell death and loss are extensive, nephron function ceases. Terminally injured cells undergo cell death through oncosis or apoptosis. Cells injured sublethally undergo repair and adaptation in response to the nephrotoxicant. Cells not injured and adjacent to the injured area may undergo dedifferentiation, proliferation, migration or spreading, and differentiation. Cells not injured may also undergo compensatory hypertrophy in response to the cell loss and injury. Finally the uninjured cells also may undergo adaptation in response to a nephrotoxicant exposure. [Schnellmann RG, Kelly KJ: Pathophysiology of nephrotoxic acute renal failure, in Berl T, Bonventre JV (eds): *Atlas of Diseases of the Kidney*. Philadelphia: Current Medicine, 1999, p 15.4, with permission.]

tamicin-, bromohydroquinone-, and/or $HgCl_2$-induced ARF. However, it is not clear which endogenous growth factors are required for tubular regeneration.

Two of the most notable cellular adaptation responses are metallothionein induction (see "Cadmium," below) and stress protein induction. Heat-shock proteins (Hsps) and glucose-regulated proteins (Grps) are two examples of stress protein families that are induced in response to a number of pathophysiologic states such as heat shock, anoxia, oxidative stress, toxicants, heavy metal exposure, and tissue trauma. The distribution of individual stress proteins varies between different cell types in the kidney and within subcellular compartments (Goering et al., 2000). These proteins are believed to play an important housekeeping role in the maintenance of normal protein structure and/or the degradation of damaged proteins and thereby to provide a defense mechanism against toxicity and/or for the facilitation of recovery and repair. Hsp induction in renal tissue has been demonstrated following renal ischemia (Van Why et al., 1992; Enami et al., 1991) and treatment with nephrotoxicants such as gentamicin (Komatsuda et al., 1993), haloalkane cysteine conjugates (Chen et al., 1992), and $HgCl_2$ (Goering et al., 1992). Interestingly, proximal tubular Hsps have been identified as molecular targets of the reactive metabolites of the haloalkane cysteine conjugate tetrafluoroethyl-L-cysteine (TFEC) (Bruschi et al., 1993), an effect that could alter the normal housekeeping functions of the proximal tubule and thereby potentially contribute to and exacerbate TFEC nephrotoxicity. Grp78 is an endoplasmic reticulum stress protein, and recent evidence shows that Grp78 is induced following a cellular stress (Halleck et al., 1997). Prior induction of Grp78 in a renal cell line rendered cells tolerant to a subsequent TFEC exposure. These findings suggest that cellular adaptation is an importance response to renal cell injury and death.

Chronic Renal Failure

Progressive deterioration of renal function may occur with long-term exposure to a variety of chemicals (e.g., analgesics, lithium, cyclosporine). It is generally believed that progression to end-stage renal failure is not simply a function of the primary renal insult per se but rather is related to secondary pathophysiologic processes triggered by the initial injury. The progression of chronic renal disease, for example, has been postulated by Brenner and colleagues (1982) to be a consequence of the glomerular hemodynamic response to renal injury. That is, following nephron loss, there are adaptive increases in glomerular pressures and flows that increase the single-nephron GFR of remnant viable nephrons. Although these compensatory mechanisms serve to maintain whole-kidney GFR, evidence has accumulated to suggest that, with time, these alterations are maladaptive and foster the progression of renal failure. Focal glomerulosclerosis eventually develops and may lead to tubular atrophy and interstitial fibrosis. Consequently, glomerulosclerosis in these nephrons will perpetuate the cycle of triggering further compensatory increases in the hemodynamics of less damaged nephrons, contributing, in turn, to their eventual destruction. Although the underlying mechanisms are not precisely known, compensatory increases in glomerular pressures and flows of the remnant glomeruli may result in mechanical damage to the capillaries due to increased shear stress on the endothelium and damage to the glomerular capillary wall, leading to altered permeabilities, and mesangial thickening due to increased transcapillary flux and local deposition of macromolecules (Dunn et al., 1986). Other

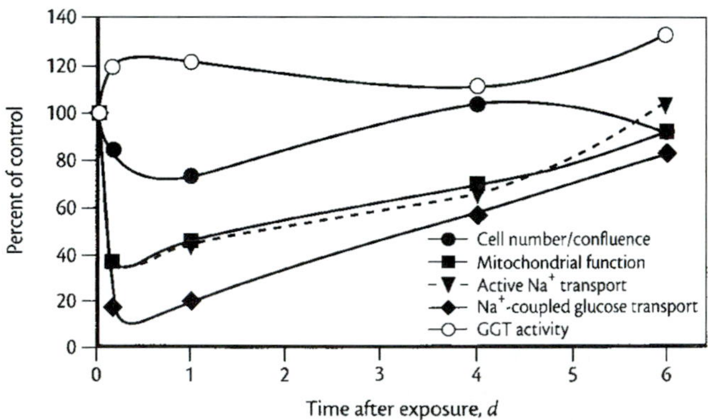

Figure 14-8. Inhibition and repair of renal proximal tubule cellular functions after exposure to the model oxidant t-butylhydroperoxide.

Approximately 25 percent cell loss and marked inhibition of mitochondrial function, active Na^+ transport, and Na^+-coupled glucose transport occurred 24 h after oxidant exposure. The activity of the brush-border membrane enzyme γ-glutamyl transferase (GGT) was not affected by oxidant exposure. Cell proliferation and migration or spreading was complete by day 4, whereas active Na^+ transport and Na^+-coupled glucose transport did not return to control levels until day 6. These data suggest that selective physiologic functions are diminished after oxidant injury and that a hierarchy exists in the repair process. [Schnellmann RG, Kelly KJ: Pathophysiology of nephrotoxic acute renal failure, in Berl T, Bonventre JV (eds): *Atlas of Diseases of the Kidney*. Philadelphia: Current Medicine, 1999, p 15.6, with permission.]

factors likely to play a role in the pathogenesis of chronic renal failure include growth promoters and inhibitors, increased extracellular matrix deposition, ROS, lipid accumulation, and tubulointerstitial injury.

SUSCEPTIBILITY OF THE KIDNEY TO TOXIC INJURY

Incidence and Severity of Toxic Nephropathy

A wide variety of drugs, environmental chemicals, and metals can cause nephrotoxicity (Table 14-2). A large 1-year survey of all patients with ARF admitted to nephrology units revealed that in 18 percent, ARF was considered to be drug-induced (Kleinknecht et al., 1986; Fluery et al., 1990). Nephrotoxicity is a recognized clinical liability of certain classes of drugs; in particular, antibiotics represent the major class of nephrotoxic drugs, followed by angiotensin-converting enzyme inhibitors, glafenin (a European analgesic), nonsteroidal anti-inflammatory drugs (NSAIDs), and radiocontrast media. Approximately 70 percent of the patients presenting with drug-induced ARF were nonoliguric; the pathologic findings revealed acute tubular necrosis in 60 percent. Approximately 50 percent recovered completely. A myriad of risk factors appear to contribute to the incidence/severity of ARF, including genetic/hereditary factors, volume depletion, septic shock, hypotension, multiple chemical insults, age, diabetes, and preexisting renal disease. The consequences of ARF can be profound, as permanent renal damage may result and dialysis or renal transplantation may be required.

Chronic renal failure leading to end-stage renal failure has been associated with long-term abuse of analgesics. The incidence of analgesic nephropathy has been reported to be as high as 20 to 25 percent in certain countries (e.g., Switzerland). Other agents—such as lithium, cyclosporine, NSAIDs, lead, and cadmium—may produce chronic tubulointerstitial nephropathy with progressive loss of renal function.

Reasons for the Susceptibility of the Kidney to Toxicity

The unusual susceptibility of the mammalian kidney to the toxic effects of noxious chemicals can be attributed in part to the unique physiologic and anatomic features of this organ. Although the kidneys constitute only 0.5 percent of total body mass, they receive about 20 to 25 percent of the resting cardiac output. Consequently, any drug or chemical in the systemic circulation will be delivered to these organs in relatively high amounts. The processes involved in forming a concentrated urine also serve to concentrate potential toxicants in the tubular fluid. As water and electrolytes are reabsorbed from the glomerular filtrate, chemicals in the tubular fluid may be concentrated, thereby driving passive diffusion of toxicants into tubular cells. Therefore, a nontoxic concentration of a chemical in the plasma may reach toxic concentrations in the kidney. Progressive concentration of toxicants along the nephron may result in intraluminal precipitation of relatively insoluble compounds, causing ARF secondary to tubular obstruction. Finally, renal transport, accumulation, and metabolism of xenobiotics contribute significantly to the susceptibility of the kidney (and specific nephron segments) to toxic injury (see "Site-Selective Injury," below).

In addition to intrarenal factors, the incidence and/or severity of chemically induced nephrotoxicity may be related to the sensitivity of the kidney to circulating vasoactive substances. For example, nephrotoxicity due to NSAIDs is known to result in ARF if patients are suffering from hypotension, hypovolemia, and/or cardiac insufficiency (Brezis et al., 1991). Under these conditions, vasoconstrictors such as angiotensin II or vasopressin are increased. Normally, the actions of high circulating levels of vasoconstrictor hormones are counterbalanced by the actions of increased vasodilatory prostaglandins; thus, renal blood flow (RBF) and GFR are maintained. However, when prostaglandin synthesis is suppressed by NSAIDs, RBF declines markedly and ARF ensues, due to the unopposed actions of vasoconstrictors. Another example of predisposing risk factors relates to the clinical use of angiotensin-converting enzyme (ACE) inhibitors, such as captopril (De Jong and Woods, 1998). Captopril has been reported to produce ARF in patients with severe hypertension, due either to bilateral renal artery stenosis or to renal artery stenosis in a solitary kidney. Under these conditions, glomerular filtration pressure is dependent on angiotensin II–induced efferent arteriolar constriction. ACE inhibitors will block this vasoconstriction, resulting in a precipitous decline in filtration pressure and ARF.

Site-Selective Injury

Many nephrotoxicants have their primary effects on discrete segments or regions of the nephron. For example, the proximal tubule is the primary target for most nephrotoxic antibiotics, antineoplastics, halogenated hydrocarbons, mycotoxins, and heavy metals, whereas the glomerulus is the primary site for immune complexes, the loop of Henle/collecting ducts for fluoride ions, and the medulla/papilla for chronically consumed analgesic mixtures. The reasons underlying this site-selective injury are complex but can be attributed in part to site-specific differences in blood flow, transport and accumulation of chemicals, physicochemical properties of the epithelium, reactivity of cellular/molecular targets, balance of bioactivation/detoxification reactions, cellular energetics, and/or regenerative/repair mechanisms.

Glomerular Injury

The glomerulus is the initial site of chemical exposure within the nephron, and a number of nephrotoxicants produce structural injury to this segment. In certain instances, chemicals alter glomerular permeability to proteins by altering the size- and charge-selective functions. Both puromycin aminonucleoside and doxorubicin target glomerular epithelial cells, resulting in changes in size and charge selectivity and proteinuria. The decrease in charge selectivity is thought to result from a decrease in negatively charged sites, while the loss of size selectivity is thought to result from focal detachment of podocytes from the glomerular basement membrane.

Cyclosporine, amphotericin B, and gentamicin are examples of chemicals that impair glomerular ultrafiltration without significant loss of structural integrity and decrease GFR. Amphotericin B decreases GFR by causing renal vasoconstriction and decreasing the glomerular capillary ultrafiltration coefficient (K_f), an effect probably mediated through the endothelial cells. Because of its polycationic nature, the aminoglycoside gentamicin interacts with the anionic sites on the endothelial cells, decreasing K_f and GFR. Finally, cyclosporine not only causes renal vasoconstriction and vascular damage but is injurious to the glomerular endothelial cell.

Chemically induced glomerular injury may also be mediated by extrarenal factors. Circulating immune complexes may be trapped within the glomeruli; binding of complement, attraction of neutrophils, and phagocytosis may result. Neutrophils and macrophages are commonly observed within glomeruli in membranous glomerulonephritis, and the local release of cytokines and reactive oxygen species (ROS) may contribute to glomerular injury. Heavy metals (e.g., $HgCl_2$, gold, cadmium), hydrocarbons, penicillamine, and captopril can produce this type of glomerular injury. A chemical may function as a hapten attached to some native protein (e.g., tubular antigens released secondary to toxicity) or as a complete antigen—particularly if it is sequestered within the glomerulus via electrostatic interactions—and elicit an antibody response. Antibody reactions with cell-surface antigens (e.g., GBM) lead to immune deposit formation within the glomeruli, mediator activation, and subsequent injury to glomerular tissue. Volatile hydrocarbons, solvents, and $HgCl_2$ have been implicated in this type of glomerulonephritis.

Proximal Tubular Injury

The proximal tubule is the most common site of toxicant-induced renal injury. The reasons for this relate in part to the selective accumulation of xenobiotics into this segment of the nephron. For example, in contrast to the distal tubule, which is characterized by a relatively tight epithelium with high electrical resistance, the proximal tubule has a leaky epithelium, favoring the flux of compounds into proximal tubular cells. More importantly, tubular transport of organic anions and cations, low-molecular-weight proteins and peptides, GSH conjugates, and heavy metals is localized primarily if not exclusively to the proximal tubule. Thus, transport of these molecules will be greater in the proximal tubule than in other segments, resulting in proximal tubular accumulation and toxicity. Indeed, segmental differences in transport and accumulation appear to play a significant role in the onset and development of proximal tubular toxicity associated with certain drugs such as aminoglycosides, β-lactam antibiotics, and cisplatin; environmental chemicals such as ochratoxin, haloalkene S-conjugates, d-limonene, and 2,4,4-trimethylpentane; and metals such as cadmium and mercury. Although correlations between proximal tubular transport, accumulation, and toxicity suggest that the site of transport is a crucial determinant of the site of toxicity, transport is unlikely to be the sole criterion. For example, the S_2 segment is the primary site of transport and toxicity of cephaloridine, and several lines of evidence suggest a strong correlation between the transport, accumulation, and nephrotoxicity of this antibiotic. However, when a variety of cephalosporins are considered, the rank order of accumulation does not follow the rank order of nephrotoxicity; for example, renal cortical concentrations of the potent nephrotoxicant cephaloglycin are comparable to those of the relatively nontoxic cephalexin. These data suggest that site-specific transport and accumulation are necessary but not sufficient to cause proximal tubular toxicity of cephalosporins. Once taken up and sequestered by the proximal tubular cell, the nephrotoxic potential of these drugs ultimately may be dependent upon the intrinsic reactivity of the drug with subcellular or molecular targets.

In addition to segmental differences in transport, segmental differences in cytochrome P450 and cysteine conjugate β-lyase activity also are contributing factors to the enhanced susceptibility of the proximal tubule. Both enzyme systems are localized almost exclusively in the proximal tubule, with negligible activity in the glomerulus, distal tubules, or collecting ducts. Thus, nephrotoxicity requiring P450 and β-lyase–mediated bioactivation will most certainly be localized in the proximal tubule. Indeed, the site of proximal tubular bioactivation contributes at least in part to the proximal tubular lesions produced by chloroform (via cytochrome P450) and by haloalkene S-conjugates (via cysteine β-lyase).

Finally, proximal tubular cells appear to be more susceptible to ischemic injury than are distal tubular cells. Therefore, the proximal tubule likely will be the primary site of toxicity for chemicals that interfere with renal blood flow, cellular energetics, and/or mitochondrial function.

Loop of Henle/Distal Tubule/Collecting Duct Injury

Chemically-induced injury to the more distal tubular structures, compared to the proximal tubule, is an infrequent occurrence. Functional abnormalities at these sites manifest primarily as impaired concentrating ability and/or acidification defects. Drugs that have been associated with acute injury to the more distal tubular structures include amphotericin B, cisplatin, and methoxyflurane. Each of these drugs induces an ADH-resistant polyuria, suggesting that the concentrating defect occurs at the level of the medullary thick ascending limb and/or the collecting duct. However, the mechanisms mediating these drug-induced concentrating defects appear to be different. Amphotericin B is highly lipophilic and interacts with lipid sterols such as cholesterol, resulting in the formation of transmembrane channels or pores and disrupting membrane permeability (Bernardo and Branch, 1997). Thus, amphotericin effectively transforms the tight distal tubular epithelium into one that is leaky to water and ions and impairs reabsorption at these sites. The mechanisms mediating cisplatin-induced polyuria are not completely understood, but the first phase is responsive to vasopressin and inhibitors of prostaglandin synthesis (Safirstein and Defray, 1998). The second phase is not responsive to vasopressin or prostaglandin synthesis inhibitors but is associated with decreased papillary solute content. Methoxyflurane nephrotoxicity is associated with the inhibitory effects of the metabolite fluoride on solute and water reabsorption (Jarnberg, 1998). Fluoride inhibits sodium chloride reabsorption in the thick ascending limb and inhibits ADH-mediated reabsorption of water, possibly due to disruption in adenylate cyclase.

Papillary Injury

The renal papilla is susceptible to the chronic injurious effects of abusive consumption of analgesics. The intial target is the medullary interstitial cells, followed by degenerative changes in the medullary capillaries, loops of Henle, and collecting ducts (Bach, 1997). Although the exact mechanisms underlying selective damage to the papilla by analgesics are not known, the intrarenal gradient for prostaglandin H synthase activity has been implicated as a contributing factor. This activity is greatest in the medulla and least in the cortex, and the prostaglandin hydroperoxidase component metabolizes phenacetin to reactive intermediates capable of covalent binding to cellular macromolecules. Other factors may contribute to this site-selective injury, including high papillary concentrations of potential toxicants and inhibition of vasodilatory prostaglandins, compromising renal blood flow to the renal medulla/papilla and resulting in tissue ischemia. The lack of animal models that mimic the papillary injury observed in humans has limited mechanistic research in this area (Schnellmann, 1998).

ASSESSMENT OF RENAL FUNCTION

Evaluation of the effects of a chemical on the kidney can be accomplished using a variety of both in vivo and in vitro methods. Initially, nephrotoxicity can be assessed by evaluating serum and urine chemistries following treatment with the chemical in question. The standard battery of noninvasive tests includes measurement of urine volume and osmolality, pH, and urinary composition (e.g., electrolytes, glucose, protein). Although specificity is often lacking in such an assessment, urinalysis provides a relatively easy and noninvasive assessment of overall renal functional integrity and can provide some insight into the nature of the nephrotoxic insult. For example, chemically induced increases in urine volume accompanied by decreases in osmolality may suggest an impaired concentrating ability, possibly via a defect in ADH synthesis, release, and/or action. To determine whether the impaired concentrating ability is due to an altered tubular response to ADH, concentrating ability can be determined before and after an exogenous ADH challenge. Glucosuria may reflect chemically induced defects in proximal tubular reabsorption of sugars; however, because glucosuria also may be secondary to hyperglycemia, measurement of serum glucose concentrations also must be evaluated. Urinary excretion of high-molecular-weight proteins, such as albumin, is suggestive of glomerular damage, whereas excretion of low-molecular-weight proteins, such as β_2-microglobulin, suggests proximal tubular injury (Fig. 14-9). Urinary excretion of enzymes localized in the brush border (e.g., alkaline phosphatase, γ-glutamyl transferase) may reflect brush-border damage, whereas urinary excretion of other enzymes (e.g., lactate dehydrogenase) may

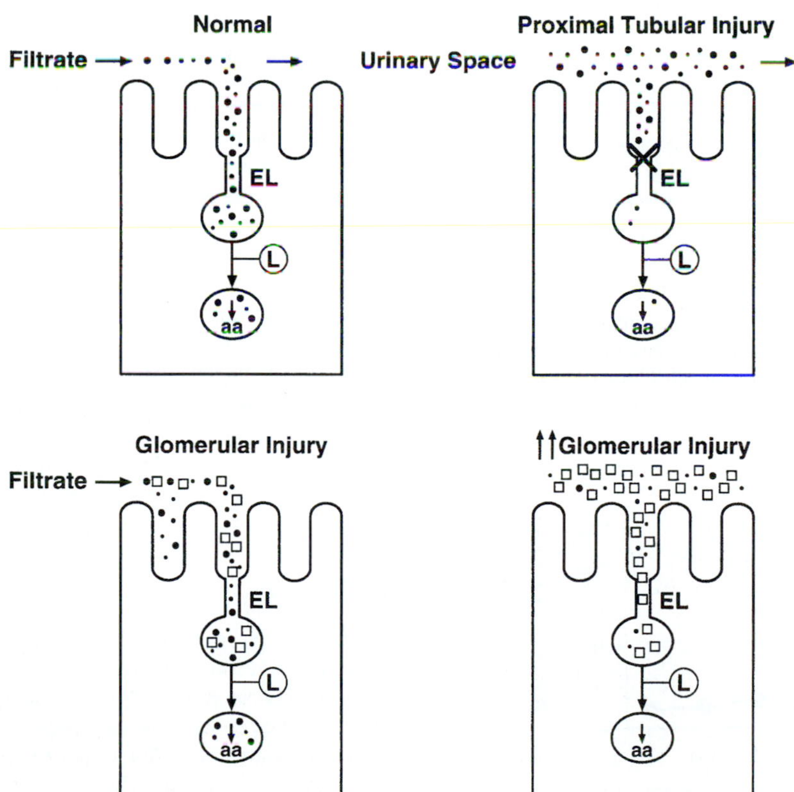

Figure 14-9. Mechanism of glomerular and tubular proteinuria.

In the healthy kidney, low-molecular-weight proteins are filtered by the glomerulus and reabsorbed by an endocytic mechanism to form an endosome (EL), which in turn fuses with lysosomes (L), where proteins are catabolized to their constituent amino acids (aa) (*upper left*). Following proximal tubular injury, formation and internalization of endocytotic vesicles may be impaired, resulting in decreased reabsorption and increased urinary excretion of low-molecular-weight proteins (*upper right*). In mold, glomerular injury, high-molecular-weight proteins, such as albumin, that traverse the glomerular barrier may be taken up by the proximal tubule (*bottom left*); however, with severe glomerular injury, proximal tubular transport of albumin is saturated, resulting in albuminuria (*bottom left*). [Goldstein RS, Schnellmann RG: Toxic responses of the kidney, in Klaassen CD (ed): *Casarett & Doull's Toxicology*. New York: McGraw-Hill, 1996, with permission.]

reflect more generalized cell damage. Enzymuria is often a transient phenomenon, as chemically induced damage may result in an early loss of most of the enzyme available. Thus, the absence of enzymuria does not necessarily reflect an absence of damage.

GFR can be measured directly by determining creatinine or inulin clearance. Creatinine is an endogenous compound released from skeletal muscle at a constant rate under most circumstances. Further, it is completely filtered with limited secretion. Inulin is an exogenous compound that is completely filtered with no reabsorption or secretion. Following the injection of inulin, inulin serum and urinary concentrations and urine volume are determined over time. If creatinine is being used, then serum and urinary creatinine concentrations and urine volume are determined over time. Creatinine or inulin clearance is determined by the following formula:

$$\text{Inulin clearance (mL/min)} = \frac{\text{inulin concentration in urine (mg/L)} \times \text{urine volume (mL/min)}}{\text{Inulin concentration in serum (mg/L)}}$$

Indirect markers of GFR are serial blood urea nitrogen (BUN) and serum creatinine concentrations. However, both serum creatinine and BUN are rather insensitive indices of GFR; a 50 to 70 percent decrease in GFR must occur before increases in serum creatinine and BUN develop (Fig. 14-10). Chemically induced increases in BUN and/or serum creatinine may not necessarily reflect renal damage but rather may be secondary to dehydration, hypovolemia, and/or protein catabolism. These extrarenal events should be taken into consideration in evaluating BUN/serum creatinine as potential endpoints of renal toxicity and/or when correlating these endpoints with renal histopathology.

Histopathologic evaluation of the kidney following treatment is crucial in identifying the site, nature, and severity of the nephrotoxic lesion. Assessment of chemically induced nephrotoxicity therefore should include urinalysis, serum clinical chemistry, and histopathology to provide a reasonable profile of the functional and morphologic effects of a chemical on the kidney. Further, information on the biotransformation and toxicokinetics of the chemical should be used to direct further in vivo and in vitro studies; in particular, what metabolites are found in the kidney and what are the concentrations of parent compound and metabolites in the kidney over time.

Once a chemical has been identified as a nephrotoxicant in vivo, a variety of in vitro techniques may be used to elucidate underlying mechanisms. Tissue obtained from naive animals may be used in the preparation of isolated perfused kidneys, kidney slices, isolated suspensions of renal tubules, cells or subcellular organelles, primary cultures of renal cells, and established renal cell lines. For example, freshly prepared isolated perfused kidneys, kidney slices, and renal tubular suspensions and cells exhibit the greatest degree of differentiated functions and similarity to the in vivo situation. However, these models have limited lifespans of 2 to 24 h. In contrast, primary cultures of renal cells and established renal cell lines exhibit longer life spans (>2 weeks), but—by comparison to the in vivo condition—exhibit differentiated functions and similarity to a lesser degree; this is particularly true of immortalized renal cell lines. The reader is referred to several excellent reviews for further details on the utility and limitations of these preparations (Tarloff and Kinter, 1997; Ford, 1997). Such approaches may be used to distinguish between an effect on the kidney due to a direct chemical insult and one caused by extrarenal effects such as extrarenally generated metabolites, hemodynamic effects, immunologic effects, and so forth. Care must be taken to ensure that the cell type affected in the in vitro model is the same as that affected in vivo. In addition, concentrations of the nephrotoxicant to be used in in vitro preparations must be comparable to those observed in vivo, as different mechanisms of toxicity may be operative at concentrations that saturate metabolic pathways or overwhelm detoxification mechanisms. Once a mechanism has been identified in vitro, the postulated mechanism must be tested in vivo. Thus, appropriately designed in vivo and in vitro studies should provide a complete characterization of the biochemical, functional, and morphologic effects of a chemical on the kidney and an understanding of the underlying mechanisms in the target cell population(s).

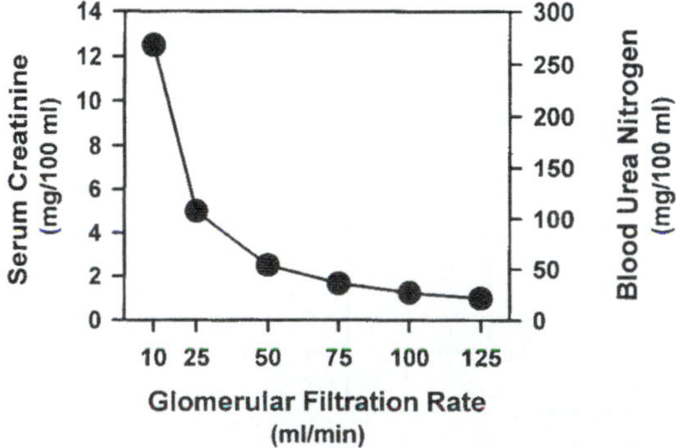

Figure 14-10. Relationships among glomerular filtration rate, serum creatinine, and blood urea nitrogen concentrations in the determination of renal function.

In general, approximately 50 percent of renal function must be lost before serum creatinine or blood urea nitrogen increases.

[From Tarloff JB, Kinter LB: *In vivo* methodologies used to assess renal function, in Sipes IG, McQueen CA, Gandolfi AJ (eds): *Comprehensive Toxicology.* Vol 7. Oxford, England: Elsevier, 1997, pp 99–120, with permission.]

BIOCHEMICAL MECHANISMS/MEDIATORS OF RENAL CELL INJURY

Cell Death

In many cases, renal cell injury may culminate in cell death. In general, cell death is thought to occur through either oncosis or apoptosis (Levin et al., 1999). The morphologic and biochemical characteristics of necrosis and apoptosis are very different. Apoptosis is a tightly controlled, organized process that usually affects scattered individual cells. The organelles retain integrity while cell volume decreases. Ultimately, the cell breaks into small fragments that are phagocytosed by adjacent cells or macrophages without producing an inflammatory response. In some cases DNA fragmentation occurs through an endonuclease-mediated cleavage of the DNA at internucleosomal linker regions, which can be visualized as a ladder-like pattern following agarose gel electrophoresis. In contrast, oncosis often affects many contiguous cells; the organelles swell, cell volume increases, and the cell ruptures with the release of cellular contents, followed by inflammation. With many toxicants, lower but injurious concentrations produce cell

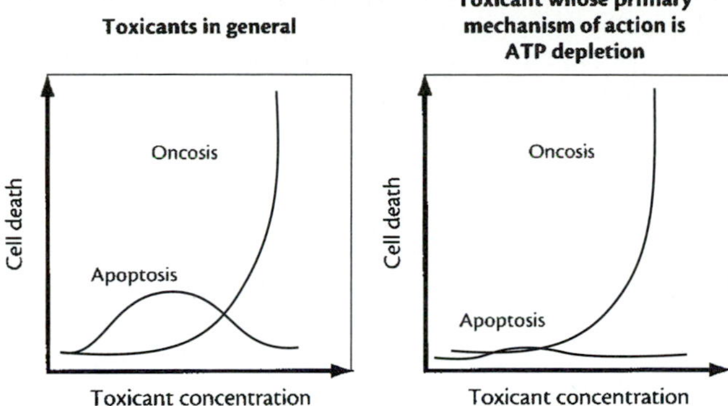

Figure 14-11. The general relationship between oncosis and apoptosis after nephrotoxicant exposure.

For many toxicants, low concentrations primarily cause apoptosis and oncosis occurs principally at higher concentrations. When the primary mechanism of action of the nephrotoxicant is ATP depletion, oncosis may be the predominant cause of cell death, with limited apoptosis occurring. [Schnellmann RG, Kelly KJ: Pathophysiology of nephrotoxic acute renal failure, in Berl T, Bonventre JV (eds): *Atlas of Diseases of the Kidney*. Philadelphia: Current Medicine, 1999, p 15.6, with permission.]

death through apoptosis (Fig. 14-11). As the concentration of the toxicant increases, oncosis plays a predominant role. However, because apoptosis is an ATP-dependent process, for those toxicants that target the mitochondrion, oncosis may be the predominant pathway with only limited apoptosis occurring. In general, while nephrotoxicants produce cell death through apoptosis and oncosis, it is likely that the degree of oncosis leads to renal failure.

Mediators of Toxicity

A chemical can initiate cell injury by a variety of mechanisms (Fig. 14-12). In some cases the chemical may initiate toxicity due to its intrinsic reactivity with cellular macromolecules. For example, amphotericin B reacts with plasma membrane sterols, increasing membrane permeability; fumonisin B_1 inhibits sphinganine (sphingosine) *N*-acyltransferase; and Hg^{2+} binds to sulfhydryl groups on cellular proteins. In contrast, some chemicals are not toxic until they are biotransformed to a reactive intermediate. Biologically reactive intermediates, also known as alkylating agents, are electron-deficient compounds (electrophiles) that bind to cellular nucleophiles (electron-rich compounds) such as proteins and lipids. For example, acetaminophen and chloroform are metabolized in the mouse kidney by cytochrome P450 to the reactive intermediates, *N*-acetyl-*p*-benzoquinonimine and phosgene, respectively (see "Chloroform" and "Acetaminophen," below). The covalent binding of the reactive intermediate to critical cellular macromolecules is thought to interfere with the normal biological activity of the macromolecule and thereby initiate cellular injury. In other instances, extrarenal biotransformation may be required prior to the delivery of the penultimate nephrotoxic species to the proximal tubule, where it is metabolized further to a reactive intermediate.

Finally, chemicals may initiate injury indirectly by inducing oxidative stress via increased production of ROS, such as superoxide anion, hydrogen peroxide, and hydroxyl radicals. ROS can react with a variety of cellular constituents to induce toxicity. For example, ROS are capable of inducing lipid peroxidation, which may result in altered membrane fluidity, enzyme activity, and membrane permeability and transport characteristics; inactivating cellular enzymes by directly oxidizing critical protein sulfhydryl or amino groups; depolymerizing polysaccharides; and inducing DNA strand breaks and chromosome breakage. Each of these events could lead to cell injury and/or death. Oxidative stress has been proposed to contribute, at least in part, to the nephrotoxicity associated with ischemia/reperfusion injury, gentamicin, cyclosporine, cisplatin, and haloalkene cysteine conjugates (Chen et al., 1990; Groves et al., 1991; Ueda et al., 2001).

While nitric oxide is an important second messenger in a number of physiologic pathways, recent studies suggest that in the presence of oxidative stress, nitric oxide can be converted into reactive nitrogen species that contribute to cellular injury and death. For example, in the presence of superoxide anion, nitric oxide can be transformed into peroxynitrite ($ONOO^-$), a strong oxidant and nitrating species (Pryor and Squadrito, 1995). Proteins, lipids, and DNA are all targets of peroxynitrite. The primary evidence for a role of peroxynitrite in renal ischemia/reperfusion injury is the formation of nitrotyrosine-protein adducts and the attenuation of renal dysfunction through the inhibition of the inducible form of nitric oxide synthase (Ueda et al., 2001).

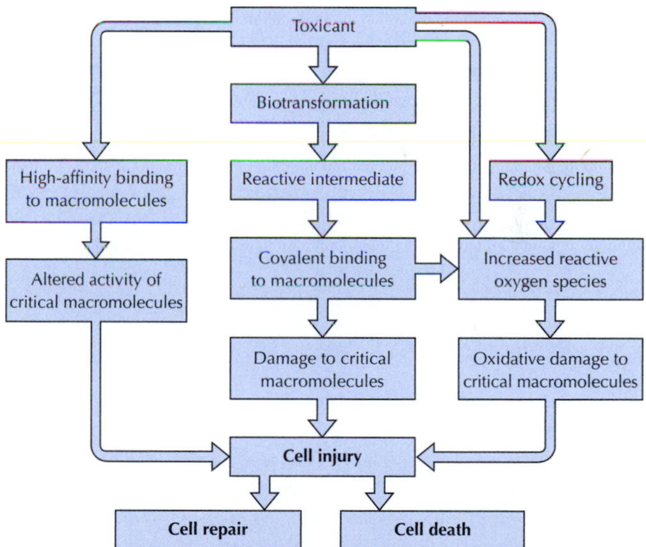

Figure 14-12. Covalent and noncovalent binding versus oxidative stress mechanisms of cell injury.

Nephrotoxicants are generally thought to produce cell injury and death through one of two mechanisms, either alone or in combination. In some cases the toxicant may have a high affinity for a specific macromolecule or class of macromolecules that results in altered activity (increase or decrease) of these molecules and cell injury. Alternatively, the parent nephrotoxicant may not be toxic until it is biotransformed into a reactive intermediate that binds covalently to macromolecules and, in turn, alters their activity, resulting in cell injury. Finally, the toxicant may increase reactive oxygen species in the cells directly, after being biotransformed into a reactive intermediate or through redox cycling. The resulting increase in reactive oxygen species results in oxidative damage and cell injury. [Schnellmann RG, Kelly KJ: Pathophysiology of nephrotoxic acute renal failure, in Berl T, Bonventre JV (eds): *Atlas of Diseases of the Kidney*. Philadelphia: Current Medicine, 1999, p 15.7, with permission.]

Cellular/Subcellular and Molecular Targets

A number of cellular targets have been identified to play a role in cell death. It is generally thought that an intracellular interaction (e.g., an alkylating agent or ROS with a macromolecule) initiates a sequence of events that leads to cell death. In the case of oncosis, a "point of no return" is reached in which the cell will die regardless of any intervention. The idea of a single sequence of events is probably simplistic for most toxicants, given the extensive number of targets available for alkylating species and ROS. Rather, multiple pathways, with both distinct and common sequences of events, may lead to cell death.

Cell Volume and Ion Homeostasis

Cell volume and ion homeostasis are tightly regulated and are critical for the reabsorptive properties of the tubular epithelial cells. Toxicants generally disrupt cell volume and ion homeostasis by interacting with the plasma membrane and increasing ion permeability or by inhibiting energy production. The loss of ATP, for example, results in the inhibition of membrane transporters that maintain the internal ion balance and drive transmembrane ion movement. Following ATP depletion, Na^+,K^+-ATPase activity decreases, resulting in K^+ efflux, Na^+ and Cl^- influx, cell swelling, and ultimately cell membrane rupture. Miller and Schnellmann (1993, 1995) have proposed that ATP depletion in rabbit renal proximal tubule segments initially results in K^+ efflux and Na^+ influx followed by a lag period before Cl^- influx occurs. Cl^- influx occurs during the late stages of cell injury produced by a diverse group of toxicants and does not appear to be due to currently characterized renal Cl^- transporters. Cl^- influx may be a trigger for cell swelling, because decreasing Cl^- influx decreased cell swelling and cell death, and inhibition of cell swelling decreased cell lysis but not Cl^- influx. Meng and Reeves (2000) have reported similar findings using hydrogen peroxide as the toxicant and LLC-PK_1 cells.

Cytoskeleton and Cell Polarity

Toxicants may cause early changes in membrane integrity such as loss of the brush border, blebbing of the plasma membrane, or alterations in membrane polarity. These changes can result from toxicant-induced alterations in cytoskeleton components and cytoskeletal–membrane interactions, or they may be associated with perturbations in energy metabolism or calcium and phospholipid homeostasis. Marked changes in the polarity of tubular epithelium occur following an ischemic insult. Under control conditions, the tubular epithelial cell is polarized with respect to certain transporters and enzymes. During in vivo ischemia and in vitro ATP depletion there is a dissociation of Na^+,K^+-ATPase from the actin cytoskeleton and redistribution from the basolateral membrane to the apical domain in renal proximal tubule cells (Molitoris, 1997). The redistribution of this enzyme has been postulated to explain decreased Na^+ and water reabsorption during ischemic injury.

Mitochondria

Many cellular processes depend on mitochondrial ATP and thus become compromised simultaneously with inhibition of respiration. Conversely, mitochondrial dysfunction may be a consequence of some other cellular process altered by the toxicant. Numerous nephrotoxicants cause mitochondrial dysfunction (Schnellman and Griner, 1994). For example, following an in vivo exposure, $HgCl_2$ altered isolated renal cortical mitochondrial function and mitochondrial morphology prior to the appearance of tubular necrosis (Weinberg et al., 1982a). Furthermore, $HgCl_2$ produced similar changes in various respiratory parameters when added to isolated rat renal cortical mitochondria (Weinberg et al., 1982b). Different toxicants also produce different types of mitochondrial dysfunction. For example, pentachlorobutadienyl-L-cysteine initially uncouples oxidative phosphorylation in renal proximal tubular cells by dissipating the proton gradient, while TFEC does not uncouple oxidative phosphorylation but rather inhibits state 3 respiration by inhibiting sites I and II of the electron transport chain (Schnellmann et al., 1987, 1989; Wallin et al., 1987; Hayden and Stevens, 1990).

Whether toxicants target mitochondria directly or indirectly, it is clear that mitochondria play a critical role in determining whether cells die by apoptosis or oncosis. The mitochondrial permeability transition (MPT) is characterized by the opening of a high-conductance pore that allows solutes of <1500 molecular weight to pass (Lemasters, 1999). It is thought that the MPT occurs during cell injury and ultimately progresses to apoptosis if sufficient ATP is available or oncosis if ATP is depleted. Further, the release of cytochrome c following the MPT plays a key role in activating downstream caspases and executing apoptosis.

Lysosomes

Lysosomes are key subcellular targets of aminoglycosides, unleaded gasoline, and d-limonene and are believed to induce cellular injury via rupture and release of lysosomal enzymes and toxicants into the cytoplasm following excessive accumulation of reabsorbed toxicant(s) and lysosomal overload. α_{2u}-Globulin is normally reabsorbed in the proximal tubule and degraded in the lysosomes. α_{2u}-Nephropathy occurs in male rats when compounds such as d-limonene and constituents of unleaded gasoline bind to α_{2u}-globulin, inhibiting normal lysosomal degradation and resulting in the accumulation of α_{2u}-globulin in the proximal tubule. The size and number of lysosomes increase and a characteristic protein-droplet morphology is observed. Ultimately, this leads to single-cell necrosis and regenerative hyperplasia.

The aminoglycosides also induce lysosomal dysfunction following tubular reabsorption of aminoglycosides and accumulation in lysosomes (Fig. 14-13). The size and number of lysosomes increase and electron-dense lamellar structures called myeloid bodies appear. The myeloid bodies contain undegraded phospholipids and are thought to occur through the inhibition of lysosomal hydrolases and phospholipases by the aminoglycosides.

Ca^{2+} Homeostasis

Ca^{2+} is a second messenger and plays a critical role in a variety of cellular functions. The distribution of Ca^{2+} within renal cells is complex and involves binding to anionic sites on macromolecules and compartmentation within subcellular organelles. The critical cellular Ca^{2+} pool for regulation is the free Ca^{2+} present in the cytosol. The concentration of this pool is approximately 100 nM and is maintained at this level against a large extracellular/intracellular gradient (10,000:1) by a series of pumps and channels lo-

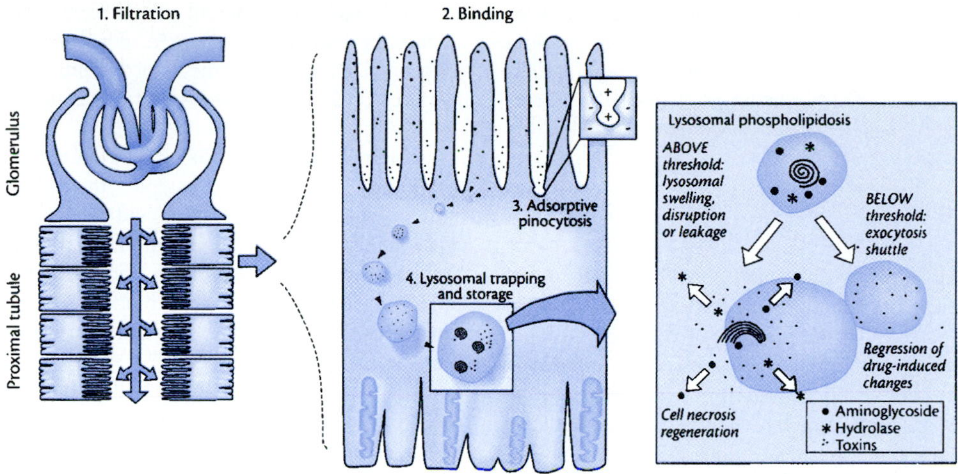

Figure 14-13. Renal handling of aminoglycosides: (1) glomerular filtration, (2) binding to the brush-border membranes of the proximal tubul, (3) pinocytosis, and (4) storage in the lysosomes. [From De Broe ME: Renal injury due to environmental toxins, drugs, and contrast agents, in Berl T, Bonventre JV (eds): Atlas of Diseases of the Kidney. Philadelphia: Current Medicine, 1999, p 11.4, with permission.]

cated on the plasma membrane and endoplasmic reticulum (ER). Because the proximal tubular cells reabsorb approximately 50 to 60 percent of the filtered load of Ca^{2+}, they must maintain low cytosolic Ca^{2+} concentrations during a large Ca^{2+} flux.

Sustained elevations or abnormally large increases in cytosolic free Ca^{2+} can exert a number of detrimental effects on the cell. For example, an increase in cytosolic free Ca^{2+} can activate a number of degradative Ca^{2+}-dependent enzymes, such as phospholipases and proteinases, and can produce aberrations in the structure and function of cytoskeletal elements. While the precise role of Ca^{2+} in toxicant-induced injury remains unclear, release of ER Ca^{2+} stores may be a key step in initiating the injury process and increasing cytosolic free Ca^{2+} concentrations. For example, prior depletion of ER Ca^{2+} stores protects renal proximal tubules from extracellular Ca^{2+} influx and cell death produced by mitochondrial inhibition and hypoxia (Waters et al., 1997b). Mitochondria are known to accumulate Ca^{2+} in lethally injured cells through a low-affinity, high-capacity Ca^{2+} transport system. While this system plays a minor role in normal cellular Ca^{2+} regulation, under injurious conditions the uptake of Ca^{2+} may facilitate ROS formation and damage.

Phospholipases

Phospholipase A_2 (PLA_2) consists of a family of enzymes that hydrolyze the acyl bond at the sn-2 position of phospholipids, resulting in the release of arachidonic acid and lysophospholipid. The enzymes within this family have different biochemical characteristics, substrate preferences, and Ca^{2+} dependencies. PLA_2 activation has been suggested to play a role in various forms of cell injury through a variety of mechanisms (Cummings et al., 2000a). A supraphysiologic increase in PLA_2 activity could result in the loss of membrane phospholipids and consequently impair membrane function. The increase in PLA_2 activity may be secondary to an increase in cytosolic Ca^{2+}, because some PLA_2 enzymes translocate to membranes following increases in cytosolic free Ca^{2+}. Cell membranes are rich with polyunsaturated fatty acids and as such are susceptible to lipid peroxidation. Peroxidized lipids are predisposed to degradation by PLA_2, resulting in increased PLA_2 activity and the formation of peroxidized arachidonic acid metabolites and lysophospholipids. Lysophospholipids can be toxic to cells and alter membrane permeability characteristics and uncouple mitochondrial respiration. Furthermore, the eicosanoid products of arachidonic metabolism are chemotactic for neutrophils, which also may contribute to tissue injury.

The actual role of PLA_2 in renal cell injury has been controversial, as it is unclear whether changes in PLA_2 are a cause or consequence of cell injury or death (Cummings et al., 2000a). Further difficulties arise because inhibitors of PLA_2 are not very selective. However, Sapirstein et al. (1996) showed that cytosolic Ca^{2+}-dependent PLA_2 ($cPLA_2$) contributed to oxidant-induced oncosis by overexpressing $cPLA_2$ or secretory PLA_2 in LLC-PK_1 cells and demonstrating that cells overexpressing $cPLA_2$ were more susceptible to H_2O_2 toxicity, whereas overexpression of $sPLA_2$ did not increase H_2O_2 toxicity. In contrast, Cummings et al. (2000b) demonstrated that inhibition of Ca^{2+}-independent PLA_2 ($iPLA_2$) potentiates *t*-butylhydroperoxide-induced oncosis in rabbit renal proximal tubular cells. Thus, the role of PLA_2s in oncosis depends upon the PLA_2 isoform and stimulus of injury. While the role of PLA_2s in renal cell apoptosis has received minimal attention, it has been reported that inhibition of $iPLA_2$ decreases cisplatin-induced proximal tubular cell apoptosis (Cummings et al., 2000c).

Endonucleases

Endonucleases have been suggested to play a role in renal cell oncosis and apoptosis. Endonuclease activation with the associated DNA cleavage producing a "ladder" pattern following gel elecrophoresis is a well-characterized response of apoptosis. In this case, the observed DNA cleavage is a very late event in the apoptotic process. Ueda et al. (1995) reported DNA damage and the activation of an endonuclease in rat renal proximal tubules undergoing oncosis following hypoxia/reoxygenation. In contrast, DNA cleavage producing a "ladder" pattern was not observed following in vitro exposure of rabbit proximal tubules to mitochondrial inhibitors, the oxidant *t*-butylhydroperoxide, or the calcium ionophore ionomycin (Schnellmann et al., 1993). These studies suggest that endonuclease activation may occur during apoptosis and oncosis, but that endonuclease activation does not uniformly occur following renal cell injury.

Proteinases

Supraphysiologic activation of proteinases could disrupt normal membrane and cytoskeleton function and lead to cell death. One source of proteinases is the lysosomes, where proteins are normally degraded by acid hydrolases. Under conditions of cell injury, the lysosomal membrane could rupture, releasing hydrolases into the cytosol to degrade susceptible proteins. However, several studies suggest that proximal tubular cell death does not necessarily involve lysosomal rupture (Weinberg, 1993). For example, a variety of cysteine and serine proteinase inhibitors were ineffective in protecting rabbit renal proximal tubules from antimycin A, tetrafluoroethyl-L-cysteine, bromohydroquinone, and *t*-butylhydroperoxide (Schnellmann and Williams, 1998). Only E64 demonstrated any cytoprotective properties following exposure to antimycin A and TFEC, and the cytoprotection was not associated with the inhibition of lysosomal cysteine proteinases. These results suggest that nonlysosomal cysteine proteinases play an important role in cell death.

The calpains, calcium-activated neutral proteinases, are likely candidates for a role in cell death because they are cysteine proteinases; they are activated by calcium; and they have cytoskeletal proteins, membrane proteins, and enzymes as substrates. For example, calpain activity increased in rat proximal tubules subjected to hypoxia, and calpain inhibitors were cytoprotective (Edelstein et al., 1996). Further, Schnellmann and coworkers (Waters et al., 1997a) showed that calpain inhibitors with different mechanisms of action decreased cell death produced by a variety of toxicants, suggesting that calpains may play an important role in the cell death produced by a diverse range of toxicants. The mechanisms and targets of calpains in cell injury remain to be determined.

Caspases are another class of cysteine proteinases that play a role in renal cell death. A number of caspases have been identified in the rat kidney (e.g. caspases 1, 2, 3, and 6), and rat kidneys subjected to ischemia/reperfusion injury exhibit differential expression of caspases with marked increases in caspases 1 and 3 (Kaushal et al., 1998). Treatment of LLC-PK_1 cells with cisplatin resulted in caspase 3 activation and apoptosis (Zhan et al., 1999). While the caspase cascade is clearly integral in the initiation and execution of apoptosis, the role of different caspases in chemically induced renal injury requires additional experimentation.

SPECIFIC NEPHROTOXICANTS

Heavy Metals

Many metals—including cadmium, chromium, lead, mercury, platinum, and uranium—are nephrotoxic. It is important to recognize that the nature and severity of metal nephrotoxicity varies with respect to its form. For example, salts of inorganic mercury produce a greater degree of renal injury and a lesser degree of neurotoxicity than do organic mercury compounds, an effect that has been associated with the greater degree of lipophilicity of organic mercury compounds (Conner and Fowler, 1993; Zalups and Lash, 1994). In addition, different metals have different primary targets within the kidney. For example, potassium dichromate primarily affects the S_1 and S_2 segments of the proximal tubule, while mercuric chloride affects the S_2 and S_3 segments (Zalups and Lash, 1994).

Metals may cause toxicity through their ability to bind to sulfhydryl groups. For example, the affinity of mercury for sulfhydryl groups is very high and is about ten orders of magnitude higher than the affinity of mercury for carbonyl or amino groups (Ballatori, 1991). Thus, metals may cause renal cellular injury through their ability to bind to sulfhydryl groups of critical proteins within the cells and thereby inhibit their normal function.

Mercury Humans and animals are exposed to elemental mercury vapor, inorganic mercurous and mercuric salts, and organic mercuric compounds through the environment. Administered elemental mercury is rapidly oxidized in erythrocytes or tissues to inorganic mercury, and thus the tissue distribution of elemental and inorganic mercury is similar. Due to its high affinity for sulfhydryl groups, virtually all of the Hg^{2+} found in blood is bound to cells, albumin, other sulfhydryl containing proteins, glutathione, and cysteine.

The kidneys are the primary target organs for accumulation of Hg^{2+}, and the S_3 segment of the proximal tubule is the initial site of toxicity. As the dose or duration of treatment increases, the S_1 and S_2 segments may be affected. Renal uptake of Hg^{2+} is very rapid with as much as 50 percent of a nontoxic dose of Hg^{2+} found in the kidneys within a few hours of exposure. Considering the fact that virtually all of the Hg^{2+} found in blood is bound to an endogenous ligand, it is likely that the luminal and/or basolateral transport of Hg^{2+} into the proximal tubular epithelial cell is through cotransport of Hg^{2+} with an endogenous ligand such as glutathione, cysteine, or albumin, or through some plasma membrane Hg^{2+}-ligand complex. Current evidence indicates that at least two mechanisms are involved in the proximal tubular uptake of Hg^{2+} (Fig. 14-14) (Zalups, 1997). One mechanism appears to involve the apical activity of γ-glutamyltranspeptidase (γ-GT) and a neutral amino acid transporter. Basolateral membrane transport is likely to be mediated by the organic anion transport system.

The acute nephrotoxicity induced by $HgCl_2$ is characterized by proximal tubular necrosis and ARF within 24 to 48 h after administration (Zalups, 1997). Early markers of $HgCl_2$-induced renal dysfunction include an increase in the urinary excretion of brush-border enzymes such as alkaline phosphatase and γ-GT, suggesting that the brush border may be an initial target of $HgCl_2$. Subsequently, when tubular injury becomes severe, intracellular enzymes such as lactate dehydrogenase and aspartate aminotransferase increase in the urine. As injury progresses, tubular reabsorption of solutes and water decreases and there is an increase in the urinary excretion of glucose, amino acids, albumin, and other proteins. Associated with the increase in injured proximal tubules is a decrease and progressive decline in the GFR. For example, GFR was reduced 35 percent in rats within 6 h of $HgCl_2$ administration and continued to decline to 32 percent and 16 percent of controls at 12 and 24 h, respectively (Eknoyan et al., 1982). The reduction in GFR results from the glomerular injury, tubular injury, and/or vasoconstriction. Interestingly, there is an early decrease in RBF secondary to the vasoconstriction. RBF may return to normal within 24 to 48 h, while GFR continues to decline. If

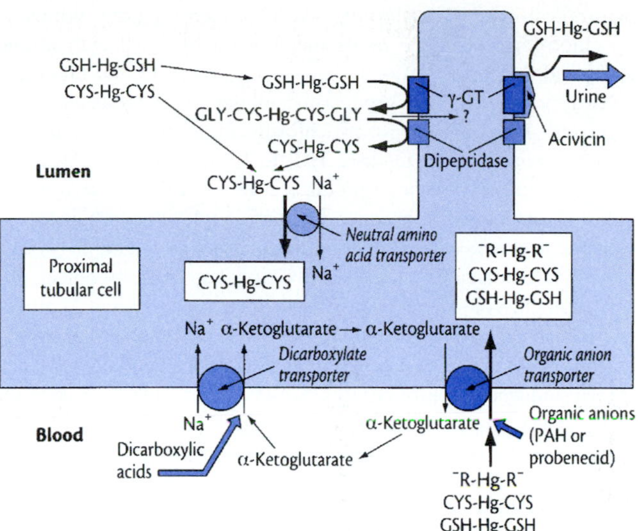

Figure 14-14. Cellular transport of Hg^{2+}.

Proximal tubular uptake of inorganic mercury is thought to be the result of the transport of Hg^{2+} conjugates [e.g., diglutathione-Hg^{2+} conjugate (GSH-Hg-GSH), dicysteine-Hg^{2+} conjugate (CYS-HG-CYS)]. At the luminal membrane, GSH-Hg-GSH is metabolized by γ-GT and a dipeptidase to form CYS-HG-CYS. CYS-HG-CYS may be taken up by an amino acid transporter. At the basolateral membrane, Hg^{2+}-conjugates appear to be transported by the organic anion transporter. Uptake of Hg^{2+}-protein conjugates by endocytosis may play a minor role in the uptake of Hg^{2+}. (Courtesy of Dr. R.K. Zalups.) [Schnellmann RG, Kelly KJ: Pathophysiology of nephrotoxic acute renal failure, in Berl T, Bonventre JV (eds): *Atlas of Diseases of the Kidney*. Philadelphia: Current Medicine, 1999, p 15.7, with permission.]

the decline in renal function is not too severe, the remaining proximal tubular cells undergo a proliferative response and renal function returns over time.

As stated above, inorganic mercury has a very high affinity for protein sulfhydryl groups, and this interaction is thought to play an important role in the toxicity of mercury at the cellular level. Changes in mitochondrial morphology and function are very early events following $HgCl_2$ administration, supporting the hypothesis that mitochondrial dysfunction is an early and important contributor to inorganic mercury–induced cell death along the proximal tubule. Other studies have suggested that oxidative stress plays an important role in $HgCl_2$-induced renal injury. For example, Fukino and colleagues (1984) observed increased thiobarbituric acid–reactive substances, a marker of lipid peroxidation, in renal cortical homogenates following $HgCl_2$ administration, suggesting that oxidative stress did occur. Recent studies by Lund and coworkers (1993) showed that mitochondria isolated from rats treated with $HgCl_2$ exhibited elevated hydrogen peroxide formation and thus were a possible source of ROS. Finally, $HgCl_2$ increases intracellular free calcium in primary cultures of rabbit renal tubular cells (Smith et al., 1987) and may activate a variety of degradative pathways that contribute to proximal tubular injury.

Several animal studies have shown that chronic exposure to inorganic mercury results in an immunologically mediated membranous glomerular nephritis secondary to the production of antibodies against the glomerular basement membrane and the deposition of immune complexes (Zalups, 1997).

Cadmium Chronic exposure of nonsmoking humans and animals to cadmium is primarily through food and results in nephrotoxicity (Kido and Nordberg, 1998). In the workplace, inhalation of cadmium-containing dust and fumes is the major route of exposure. Cadmium has a half-life of greater than 10 years in humans and thus accumulates in the body over time. Approximately 50 percent of the body burden of cadmium can be found in the kidney. Cadmium produces proximal tubule dysfunction (S_1 and S_2 segments) and injury characterized by increases in urinary excretion of glucose, amino acids, calcium, and cellular enzymes. This injury may progress to a chronic interstitial nephritis.

Numerous studies have tried to identify markers to predict the nephrotoxic effects of cadmium in humans. These include but are not limited to urinary cadmium, calcium, amino acids, albumin, β_2-microglobulin, *N*-acetyl-β-D-glucosaminidase, and retinol-binding protein concentrations. Lauwerys and coworkers (1994) have suggested that cadmium concentrations in the urine greater than 5 and 2 nmol/mmol creatinine for adult male workers and the general population, respectively, are associated with tubular dysfunction.

A very interesting aspect of cadmium nephrotoxicity is the role metallothioneins (Klaassen et al., 1999). Metallothioneins are a family of low-molecular-weight, cysteine-rich metal-binding proteins that have a high affinity for cadmium and other heavy metals. In general, the mechanism by which metallothionein is thought to play a role in cadmium and heavy metal toxicity is through its ability to bind to a heavy metal and thereby render it biologically inactive. This assumes that the unbound or "free" concentration of the metal is the toxic species. Metallothionein production can be induced by low, nontoxic concentrations of metals. Subsequently, animals challenged with a higher dose of the metal will not exhibit toxicity compared to naive animals.

Following an oral exposure to $CdCl_2$, Cd^{2+} is thought to reach the kidneys both as Cd^{2+} and as a Cd^{2+}-metallothionein complex formed and released either from intestinal cells or hepatocytes. The Cd^{2+}-metallothionein complex is freely filtered by the glomerulus and is reabsorbed by the proximal tubule. Inside the tubular cells it is thought that lysosomal degradation of the Cd^{2+}-metallothionein results in the release of "free" Cd^{2+}, which, in turn, induces renal metallothionein production. Once the renal metallothionein pool is saturated, "free" Cd^{2+} initiates injury. The mechanism by which Cd^{2+} produces injury at the cellular level is not clear; however, low concentrations of Cd^{2+} have been shown to interfere with the normal function of several cellular signal transduction pathways, including inositol triphosphate, cytosolic free Ca^{2+}, and protein kinase C (Beyersmann et al., 1994; Smith et al., 1989).

Chemically Induced α_{2u}-Globulin Nephropathy

A diverse group of chemicals—including unleaded gasoline, d-limonene, 1,4-dichlorobenzene, tetrachloroethylene, decalin, and lindane—cause α_{2u}-globulin nephropathy or hyaline droplet nephropathy (Lehman-McKeeman, 1997). This nephropathy occurs in male rats, is characterized by the accumulation of protein droplets in the S_2 segment of the proximal tubule, and results in single-cell necrosis, the formation of granular casts at the junction of the proximal tubule and the thin loop of Henle, and cellular regeneration. Chronic exposure to these compounds results in progression of these lesions and ultimately in chronic nephropathy. With compounds such as unleaded gasoline, chronic exposure results in an increased incidence of renal adenomas/carcinomas by nongenotoxic mechanisms.

As the name implies, the expression of this nephropathy requires the presence of the α_{2u}-globulin protein. α_{2u}-Globulin is synthesized in the liver of male rats and is under androgen control. Due to its low molecular weight (18.7 kDa), α_{2u}-globulin is freely filtered by the glomerulus with approximately half being reabsorbed via endocytosis in the S_2 segment of the proximal tubule. Many of the compounds that cause α_{2u}-globulin nephropathy bind to α_{2u}-globulin in a reversible manner and decrease the ability of lysosomal proteases in the proximal tubule to breakdown α_{2u}-globulin (see above). This results in the accumulation of α_{2u}-globulin in the proximal tubule with an increase in the size and number of lysosomes and the characteristic protein-droplet morphology. A proposed mechanism of α_{2u}-globulin nephropathy is that cellular necrosis secondary to lysosomal overload leads to a sustained increase in cell proliferation, which, in turn, results in the promotion of spontaneously or chemically initiated cells to form preneoplastic and neoplastic foci (Lehman-McKeeman, 1997; Melnick, 1992).

α_{2u}-Globulin nephropathy appears to be sex- and species-specific. That is, it occurs in male rats but not female rats and in male or female mice, rabbits, or guinea pigs because they do not produce α_{2u}-globulin (Lehman-McKeeman, 1997). Furthermore, it does not occur in male Black Reiter rats that lack α_{2u}-globulin. Considering the diversity of compounds that cause α_{2u}-globulin nephropathy and renal tumors and the fact that humans are exposed to these compounds regularly, the question arises whether humans are at risk for α_{2u}-globulin nephropathy and renal tumors when exposed to these compounds. Current data suggest that humans are not at risk because (1) humans do not synthesize α_{2u}-globulin, (2) humans secrete less proteins in general and in particular less low-molecular-weight proteins in urine than the rat; (3) the low-molecular-weight proteins in human urine are either not related structurally to α_{2u}-globulin, do not bind to compounds that bind to α_{2u}-globulin, or are similar to proteins in female rats, male Black Reiter rats, rabbits, or guinea pigs that do not exhibit α_{2u}-globulin nephropathy; and (4) mice excrete a low-molecular-weight urinary protein that is 90 percent homologous to α_{2u}-globulin, but they do not exhibit α_{2u}-globulin-nephropathy and renal tumors following exposure to α_{2u}-globulin-nephropathy–inducing agents.

Halogenated Hydrocarbons

Halogenated hydrocarbons are a diverse class of compounds and are used extensively as chemical intermediates, solvents, and pesticides. Consequently, humans are exposed to these compounds not only in the workplace but also through the environment. Numerous toxic effects have been associated with acute and chronic exposure to halogenated hydrocarbons, including nephrotoxicity (Elfarra, 1997). The three examples provided below illustrate the importance of biotransformation in the nephrotoxicity of halogenated hydrocarbons.

Chloroform Chloroform produces nephrotoxicity in a variety of species, with some species being more sensitive than others. The primary cellular target is the proximal tubule, with no primary damage to the glomerulus or the distal tubule. Proteinuria, glucosuria, and increased blood urea nitrogen levels are all characteristic of chloroform-induced nephrotoxicity. The nephrotoxicity produced by chloroform is linked to its metabolism by renal cytochrome P450 and the formation of a reactive intermediate that binds covalently to nucleophilic groups on cellular macromolecules. Cytochrome P450 biotransforms chloroform to trichloromethanol, which is unstable and releases HCl to form phosgene. Phosgene can react with (1) water to produce 2 HCl + CO_2, (2) two molecules of glutathione to produce diglutathionyl dithiocarbonate, (3) cysteine to produce 2-oxothizolidine-4-carboxylic acid, or (4) cellular macromolecules to initiate toxicity. The sex differences observed in chloroform nephrotoxicity appear to be related to differences in renal cytochrome P450 isozyme contents. For example, castration of male mice decreased renal cytochrome P450 and chloroform-induced nephrotoxicity (Smith et al., 1984). Likewise, testosterone pretreatment of female mice increased cytochrome P450 content and rendered female mice susceptible to the nephrotoxic effects of chloroform. Cytochrome P450 isozyme 2E1 is present in male mice and expressed in female mice treated with testosterone (Lock and Reed, 1997). Thus, these isozymes may play a role in chloroform-induced nephrotoxicity.

Tetrafluoroethylene Tetrafluoroethylene is metabolized in the liver by GSH-*S*-transferases to *S*-(1,1,2,2-tetrafluoroethyl)-glutathione. The GSH conjugate is secreted into the bile and small intestine where it is degraded to the cysteine *S*-conjugate (TFEC), reabsorbed, and transported to the kidney. The mercapturic acid may also be formed in the small intestine and reabsorbed. Alternatively, the glutathione conjugate can be transported to the kidney and biotransformed to the cysteine conjugate by γ-GT and a dipeptidase located on the brush border (Fig. 14-15). The mercapturic acid is transported into the proximal tubule cell by the organic anion transporter while cysteine conjugates are transported by the organic anion transporter and the sodium-independent L and T transport systems. The cysteine *S*-conjugate of these compounds is thought to be the penultimate nephrotoxic species. Following transport into the proximal tubule, which is the primary cellular target for haloalkenes and haloalkanes, the cysteine *S*-conjugate is a substrate for the cytosolic and mitochondrial forms of the enzyme cysteine conjugate β-lyase. In the case of the *N*-acetyl-cysteine *S*-conjugate, the *N*-acetyl group must be removed by a deacetylase for it to be a substrate for cysteine conjugate β-lyase. The products of the reaction are ammonia, pyruvate, and a reactive thiol that is capable of binding covalently to cellular macromolecules. There is a correlation between the covalent binding of the reactive thiol of the cysteine conjugate with renal protein and nephrotoxicity. Hayden and colleagues (1991) and Bruschi and coworkers (1993) have shown that biotransformation of TFEC results in difluorothioamidyl-L-lysine-protein adducts in mitochondria and that two of the targeted proteins may belong to the heat-shock family of proteins. Hayden and colleagues (1992) have also shown that halogenated thioamide adducts of phosphatidyl-ethanolamine are formed in mitochondria following cysteine conjugate β-lyase biotransformation of TFEC.

The nephrotoxicity produced by haloalkenes is characterized morphologically by proximal tubular necrosis, primarily affecting the S_3 segment, and functionally by increases in urinary glucose, protein, cellular enzymes, and BUN. Following in vivo and in vitro exposures to TFEC, the mitochondrion appears to be a primary target. In rabbit renal proximal tubules and isolated mitochondria, there is a marked decrease in state 3 respiration (respiration associated with maximal ATP formation) following TFEC exposure

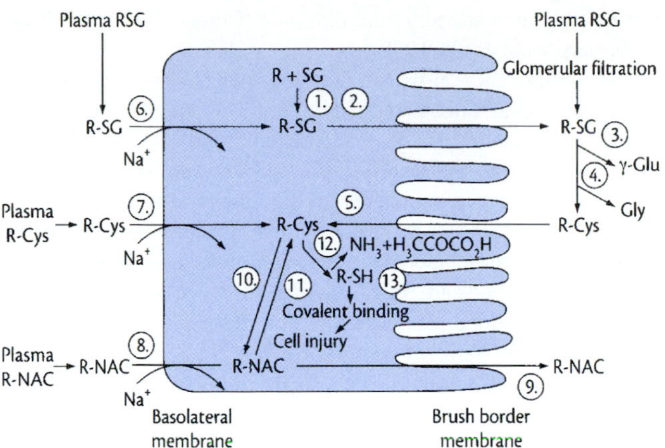

Figure 14-15. Renal tubular uptake and metabolism of GSH conjugates.

(1) Intracellular formation of GSH conjugates (R-SG) catalyzed by renal GSH S-transferase(s); (2) Secretion of the R-SG into the lumen; (3) γ-GT-mediated catabolism of R-SG and formation of the corresponding S-cysteinylglycine conjugate; (4) formation of the corresponding cysteine conjugate (R-Cys); (5) Na^+-coupled transport of R-Cys into the renal proximal tubular cell; (6) Na^+-coupled transport of RSG across the basolateral membrane; (7) Na^+-coupled transport of R-Cys across the basolateral membrane; (8) Na^+-coupled and probenecid-sensitive transport of the mercapturate (R-NAC) across the basolateral membrane; (9) secretion R-NAC into the lumen; (10) deacetylation of R-NAC to R-Cys and (11) acetylation of R-Cys to R-NAC; (12) reactive thiol formation via β-lyase; (13) binding of the reactive thiol to cellular macromolecules and initiation of cell injury. [Schnellmann RG, Kelly KJ: Pathophysiology of nephrotoxic acute renal failure, in Berl T, Bonventre JV (eds): *Atlas of Diseases of the Kidney*. Philadelphia: Current Medicine, 1999, p 15.7, with permission.]

(Groves et al., 1993). Furthermore, the decrease in mitochondrial function occurs prior to the onset of cell death. Oxidative stress may also play a contributing role in TFEC-induced cell death because lipid peroxidation products were formed prior to the onset of cell death, and antioxidants and iron chelators decreased cytotoxicity (Chen et al., 1990; Groves et al., 1991).

Bromobenzene In addition to their hepatotoxic effects, bromobenzene and other halogenated benzenes also produce nephrotoxicity. The biotransformation of these compounds, like that of the haloalkenes, is critical for the expression of the nephrotoxicity. In a series of studies, Lau and Monks demonstrated that bromobenzene must be oxidized by hepatic cytochrome P450 to bromophenol and then further oxidized to bromohydroquinone (BHQ) (Lau and Monks, 1997). BHQ is conjugated to glutathione, forming 2-bromo-*bis*(glutathione-*S*-yl)hydroquinone and three positional isomers of 2-bromo-(glutathione-*S*-yl)hydroquinone. The diglutathione conjugate is approximately a thousandfold more potent than bromobenzene in producing nephrotoxicity, while it produces the same morphologic changes in the S_3 segment and increases the amount of protein, glucose, and cellular enzymes in the urine. The glutathione conjugates of BHQ are substrates for renal γ-GT activity and may ultimately be converted to cysteine and *N*-acetyl-cysteine conjugates of BHQ. Lau and Monks (1997) have proposed a sequence of pathways for the renal disposition of 2-bromo-bis(cystein-*S*-yl)hydroquinone and 2-bromo-(cystein-yl)hydroquinones and identified possible toxic reactive intermediates. While the mechanisms by which these compounds produce proximal tubular cell death remains to be determined, experiments using LLC-PK1 cells as a model suggest that ROS play an important role.

Mycotoxins

The nephrotoxicity of two mycotoxins, ochratoxin A and citrinin, found on a variety of cereal grains have been studied extensively and reviewed by Berndt (1993). Citrinin administration to rats may result in either anuric renal failure and death or nonoliguric renal failure with complete recovery within 8 days. In contrast, ochratoxin A produces renal dysfunction only after repeated injections of small doses—a condition characterized by glucosuria, ketonuria, proteinuria, and polyuria. One or both of these mycotoxins have been implicated in Balkan nephropathy in humans, although the data to support this are less than clear.

Fumonisins (mycotoxins produced by the fungus *Fusarium moniliforme* and other *Fusarium* species) are commonly found on corn and corn products and produce nephrotoxicity in rats and rabbits (Bucci et al., 1998). Histologic examination of the kidney revealed disruption of the basolateral membrane, mitochondrial swelling, increased numbers of clear and electron-dense vacuoles, and apoptosis in proximal tubular cells at the junction of the cortex and medulla. Changes in renal function included increased urine volume, decreased osmolality, and increased excretion of low- and high-molecular-weight proteins. The fumonisins are structurally similar to sphingoid bases and are thought to produce their toxicity through the inhibition of sphinganine (sphingosine) *N*-acyltransferase. Inhibition of this enzyme results in an increase in the ratio of free sphinganine to free sphingosine and a decrease in complex sphingolipids. However, the mechanism by which these sphingolipid alterations results in cell death is unknown.

Therapeutic Agents

Acetaminophen Large doses of the antipyretic and analgesic acetaminophen (APAP) are commonly associated with hepatoxicity. However, large doses of APAP can also cause nephrotoxicity in humans and animals. APAP nephrotoxicity is characterized by proximal tubular necrosis with increases in BUN and plasma creatinine; decreases in GFR and clearance of paraaminohippurate; increases in the fractional excretion of water, sodium, and potassium; and increases in urinary glucose, protein, and brush-border enzymes. There appears to be a marked species difference in the nature and mechanism of APAP nephrotoxicity (Emeigh Hart et al., 1994; Tarloff, 1997). Morphologically, the primary targets in the mouse kidney are the S_1 and S_2 segments of the proximal tubule, while in the rat kidney the S_3 segment is the target. In the mouse, renal cytochrome P450 2E1 has been associated with APAP biotransformation to a reactive intermediate, *N*-acetyl-*p*-amino-benzoquinoneimine, that arylates proteins in the proximal tubule and initiates cell death. Two of the proteins that are targets of *N*-acetyl-*p*-amino-benzoquinoneimine are a selenium-binding protein and a glutamine synthetase (Emeigh Hart et al., 1994; Tarloff, 1997). However, the mechanism by which protein adducts initiate proximal tubular cell death and ultimately nephrotoxicity remains to be determined. While renal cytochrome P450 plays a role in APAP activation and nephrotoxicity, glutathione conjugates of APAP may also contribute to APAP nephrotoxicity. Evidence for this pathway was provided by experiments in which γ-GT or organic anion transport was inhibited and APAP-induced nephrotoxicity decreased (Emeigh Hart et al., 1990).

In contrast to its effects in the mouse, a critical and early step in APAP nephrotoxicity in the rat is the conversion of APAP to *para*-aminophenol (PAP) (Tarloff, 1997). PAP is also a metabolite of phenacetin and aniline and is a known toxicant to the S_3 segment of the proximal tubule in the rat. The steps following PAP formation and the expression of nephrotoxicity are less clear. PAP or a metabolite must be further oxidized to a benzoquinoneimine or other oxidized reactive intermediate for nephrotoxicity to occur, and there is an association between covalent binding of a PAP equivalent to renal protein and nephrotoxicity. Although glutathione conjugates of PAP have been isolated from rats treated with PAP and have been shown to be nephrotoxic when administered, the exact role they play in PAP nephrotoxicity is not clear. For example, inhibition of γ-GT or organic anion transport did not ameliorate PAP-induced nephrotoxicity (Anthony et al., 1993; Fowler et al., 1993), while bile duct cannulation and GSH depletion partially attenuated PAP-induced nephrotoxicity (Gartland et al., 1990).

Nonsteroidal Anti-Inflammatory Drugs (NSAIDs) NSAIDs such as aspirin, ibuprofen, naproxen, and indomethacin are extensively used as analgesics and anti-inflammatory agents and produce their therapeutic effects through the inhibition of prostaglandin synthesis. At least three different types of nephrotoxicity have been associated with NSAID administration (Bach, 1997; Tarloff, 1997; Whelton and Watson, 1998). ARF may occur within hours of a large dose of a NSAID, is usually reversible upon withdrawal of the drug, and is characterized by decreased RBF and GFR and by oliguria. When the normal production of vasodilatory prostaglandins is inhibited by NSAIDs, vasoconstriction induced by circulating catecholamines and angiotensin II are unopposed, resulting in decreased RBF and ischemia.

In contrast, chronic consumption of NSAIDs and/or APAP (>3 years) results in an often irreversible form of nephrotoxicity known as analgesic nephropathy (Bach, 1997; Elseviers and De Broe, 1998). The incidence of analgesic nephropathy varies widely in the western world, ranging from less than 1 to 18 percent of patients who present with end-stage renal disease requiring dialysis. The primary lesion in this nephropathy is papillary necrosis with chronic interstitial nephritis (see above). Initial changes are to the medullary interstitial cells and is followed by degenerative changes to the medullary loops of Henle and medullary capillaries. The mechanism by which NSAIDs produce analgesic nephropathy is not known but may result from chronic medullary/papillary ischemia secondary to renal vasoconstriction. Other studies have suggested that a reactive intermediate is formed in the cells that, in turn, initiates an oxidative stress or binds covalently to critical cellular macromolecules.

The third albeit rare type of nephrotoxicity associated with NSAIDs is an interstitial nephritis (Tarloff, 1997; Whelton and Watson, 1998) characterized by a diffuse interstitial edema with infiltration of inflammatory cells. Patients normally present with elevated serum creatinine and proteinuria. If NSAIDs are discontinued, renal function improves in 1 to 3 months.

Aminoglycosides The aminoglycoside antibiotics are so named because they consist of two or more amino sugars joined in a glycosidic linkage to a central hexose nucleus. While they are drugs of choice for many gram-negative infections, their use is primarily limited by their nephrotoxicity. The incidence of renal dysfunction following aminoglycoside administration ranges from 5 to 25 percent but seldom leads to a fatal outcome (Cojocel, 1997; De Broe, 1999; Verpooten et al., 1998).

Renal dysfunction by aminoglycosides is characterized by a nonoliguric renal failure with reduced GFR and an increase in serum creatinine and BUN. Polyuria is an early event following aminoglycoside administration and may be due to inhibition of chloride transport in the thick ascending limb (Kidwell et al., 1994). Within 24 h, increases in urinary brush-border enzymes, glucosuria, aminoaciduria, and proteinuria are observed. Histologically, lysosomal alterations are noted initially, followed by damage to the brush border, endoplasmic reticulum, mitochondria, and cytoplasm, ultimately leading to tubular cell necrosis. Interestingly, proliferation of renal proximal tubule cells can be observed early after the onset of nephrotoxicity.

Aminoglycosides are highly polar cations; they are almost exclusively filtered by the glomerulus and excreted unchanged. Filtered aminoglycosides undergo proximal tubular reabsorption by binding to anionic phospholipids in the brush border, followed by endocytosis and sequestration in lysosomes of the S_1 and S_2 segments of the proximal tubules (Fig. 14-13). Basolateral membrane binding and uptake also may occur, but this is a minor contribution to the total proximal tubular uptake of aminoglycosides. The earliest lesion observed following clinically relevant doses of aminoglycosides is an increase in the size and number of lysosomes. These lysosomes contain *myeloid bodies,* which are electron-dense lamellar structures containing undergraded phospholipids. The renal phospholipidosis produced by the aminoglycosides is thought to occur through their inhibition of lysosomal hydrolases, such as sphingomyelinase and phospholipases. While phospholipidosis plays an important role in aminoglycoside nephrotoxicity, the steps between the phospholipid accumulation in the lysosomes and tubular cell death are less clear. One hypothesis suggests that the lysosomes become progressively distended until they rupture, releasing lysosomal enzymes and high concentrations of aminoglycosides into the cytoplasm (Fig. 14-13). The released lysosomal contents can interact with various membranes and organelles and trigger cell death. Another mechanism of aminoglycoside nephrotoxicity includes a decrease in K_f and GFR (see above).

Amphotericin B Amphotericin B is a very effective antifungal agent whose clinical utility is limited by its nephrotoxicity (Bernardo and Branch, 1997). Renal dysfunction associated with amphotericin B treatment is dependent on cumulative dose and is due to both hemodynamic and tubular effects. Amphotericin B nephrotoxicity is characterized by ADH-resistant polyuria, renal tubular acidosis, hypokalemia, and either acute or chronic renal failure. Amphotericin B nephrotoxicity is unusual in that it impairs the functional integrity of the glomerulus and of the proximal and distal portions of the nephron.

Amphotericin B administration is associated with decreases in RBF and GFR secondary to renal arteriolar vasoconstriction or activation of TGF. In animals, the calcium channel blocker verapamil blocks the acute amphotericin B–induced renal vasoconstriction, suggesting that the vasoconstriction may be mediated through increased calcium levels in vascular smooth muscle cells (Tolins and Raij, 1988). However, verapamil did not completely block the acute decrease in GFR, suggesting that the decrease in GFR is not exclusively due to vasoconstriction. Thus, renal vasoconstriction is an important component in amphotericin B–induced chronic renal failure.

Some of the renal tubular cell effects of amphotericin B are due to the ability of this polyene to bind to cholesterol in the plasma membrane and form aqueous pores. In the presence of amphotericin B, cells of the turtle and rat distal tubule do not produce a normal net outward flux of protons due to an increase in proton permeability (Steinmetz and Husted, 1982; Gil and Malnic, 1989). This results in impaired proton excretion and renal tubular acidosis. The hypokalemia observed with amphotericin B may be due to an increase in luminal potassium ion permeability in the late distal tubule and the cortical collecting duct and the loss of potassium ions in the urine.

Cyclosporine Cyclosporine is an important immunosuppressive agent and is widely used to prevent graft rejection in organ transplantation. Cyclosporine is a fungal cyclic polypeptide and acts by selectively inhibiting T-cell activation. Nephrotoxicity is a critical side effect of cyclosporine, with nearly all patients who receive the drug exhibiting some form of nephrotoxicity. Clinically, cyclosporine-induced nephrotoxicity may manifest as (1) acute reversible renal dysfunction, (2) acute vasculopathy, and (3) chronic nephropathy with interstitial fibrosis (Mason and Moore, 1997; Dieperink et al., 1998).

Acute renal dysfunction is characterized by dose-related decreases in RBF and GFR and increases in BUN and serum creatinine. These effects are lessened by reducing the dosage or by cessation of therapy. The decrease in RBF and GFR is related to marked vasoconstriction induced by cyclosporine; and it is probably produced by a number of factors, including an imbalance in vasoconstrictor and vasodilatory prostaglandin production. In particular, increased production of the vasoconstrictor thromboxane A_2 appears to play a role in cyclosporine-induced ARF. Endothelin may contribute to constriction of the afferent arteriole because endothelin receptor antagonists inhibit cyclosporine-induced vasoconstriction (Lanese and Conger, 1993). While a number of studies have explored possible direct effects of cyclosporine on tubular cells, it is still not clear whether a direct effect of cyclosporine on tubular cells plays a role in the nephrotoxicity.

Acute vasculopathy or thrombotic microangiopathy is a rather unusual nephrotoxic lesion that affects arterioles and glomerular capillaries, without an inflammatory component, following cyclosporine treatment. Hyaline and/or fibroid changes, often with fibrinogen deposition, is observed in arterioles, while thrombosis with endothelial cell desquamation affects the glomerular capillaries (Racusen and Solez, 1993). The pathogenesis of this lesion is poorly understood. While the characteristics of this lesion differ from the vascular changes of acute rejection, a variety of factors may contribute to this lesion in the clinical transplant setting.

Long-term treatment with cyclosporine can result in chronic nephropathy with interstitial fibrosis. Modest elevations in serum creatinine and decreases in GFR occur along with hypertension, proteinuria, and tubular dysfunction. Histologic changes are profound; they are characterized by arteriolopathy, global and segmental glomerular sclerosis, striped interstitial fibrosis, and tubular atrophy. These lesions may not be reversible if cyclosporine therapy is discontinued and may result in end-stage renal disease. While the mechanism of chronic cyclosporine nephropathy is not known, vasoconstriction probably plays a contributing role. Studies by Wang and Salahudeen (1994, 1995) indicated that rats treated with cyclosporine and an antioxidant lazaroid for 30 days exhibited increased GFR and RBF and less tubulointerstitial fibrosis and lipid peroxidation than rats treated with cyclosporine alone, suggesting that oxidative stress plays a role in cyclosporine nephrotoxicity in rats. The marked interstitial cell proliferation and increased procollagen secretion that occurs following cyclosporine administration may contribute to the interstitial fibrosis (Racusen and Solez, 1993).

Tacrolimus (FK-506) is a new immunosuppressive agent that exhibits nephrotoxicity. At this time, the degree and incidence of nephrotoxicity and morphologic changes associated with tacrolimus exposure are similar to that exhibited with cyclosporine, suggesting similar modes of toxic action.

Cisplatin Cisplatin is a valuable drug in the treatment of solid tumors, with nephrotoxicity limiting its clinical use. The kidney is not only responsible for the majority of cisplatin excretion but is also the primary site of accumulation (Wolfgang and Leibbrant, 1997; Safirstein and Defray, 1998). The effects of cisplatin on the kidney are several, including acute and chronic renal failure, renal magnesium wasting, and polyuria.

ARF—characterized by decreases in RBF and GFR, enzymuria, β_2-microglobulinuria, and inappropriate urinary losses of magnesium—was identified in early clinical trials of cisplatin. Although the primary cellular target associated with ARF is the proximal tubule S_3 segment in the rat, in humans the S_1 and S_2 segments, distal tubule, and collecting ducts can also be affected. The chronic renal failure observed with cisplatin is due to prolonged exposure and is characterized by focal necrosis in numerous segments of the nephron without a significant effect on the glomerulus. Considerable effort has been expended in the development of measures to prevent cisplatin nephrotoxicity. These efforts include the use of extensive hydration and mannitol diuresis and the development of less nephrotoxic platinum compounds such as carboplatin.

The mechanism by which cisplatin produces cellular injury is not known but may involve metabolites of cisplatin. Interestingly, the *trans* isomer of cisplatin is not nephrotoxic even though similar concentrations of platinum are observed in the kidney after dosing. Thus, it is not the platinum atom per se that is responsible for the toxicity but rather the geometry of the complex or a metabolite. The antineoplastic and perhaps the nephrotoxic effects of cisplatin may be due to its intracellular hydrolysis to the reactive mono-chloro-mono-aquo-diammine-platinum or diaquo-diammine-platinum species and the ability of these metabolites to alkylate purine and pyrimidine bases.

In vitro studies using primary cultures of mouse proximal tubular cells revealed that the type of cell death produced by cisplatin is dependent on the concentration (Lieberthal et al., 1996). At cisplatin concentrations less than 100 μM, the primary form of cell death is apoptosis. As the concentration increases above 100 μM, a greater percentage of the cells die by oncosis. Using rabbit renal proximal tubule cells, Courjault et al. (1993) showed that while DNA synthesis, protein synthesis, glucose transport, Na^+, K^+-ATPase activity, and cell viability were all inhibited by cisplatin, DNA synthesis was the most sensitive. These results suggest that cisplatin may produce nephrotoxicity through its ability to inhibit DNA synthesis as well as transport functions. The lack of complete return of renal function following cisplatin treatment in vivo may result from the interference of cisplatin with the normal proliferative response that occurs after injury.

Radiocontrast Agents Iodinated contrast media are used for the imaging of tissues, with two major classes of compounds currently in use. The ionic compounds, diatrizoate derivatives, are (1) ionized at physiologic pH, (2) not significantly bound to protein, (3) restricted to the extracellular space, (4) almost entirely eliminated by the kidney, and (5) freely filtered by the glomerulus and neither secreted nor reabsorbed. These agents have a very high osmolality (>1200 mOsm/L) and are potentially nephrotoxic, particularly in patients with existing renal impairment, diabetes, or heart failure or who are receiving other nephrotoxic drugs. The newer contrast agents (e.g., iotrol, iopamidol) are nonionic owing to the addition of an organic side chain, their low osmolality, and their lower nephrotoxicity. The nephrotoxicity of these agents is due to both hemodynamic alterations (vasoconstriction) and tubular injury (via ROS) (Bakris, 1997; Porter and Kremer, 1998).

REFERENCES

Anthony ML, Beddell CR, Lindon JC, Nicholson JK: Studies on the effects of L(*aS*,5*S*)-*a*-amino-3-chloro-4,5-diphydro-5-isoxazoleacetic acid (AT-125) on 4-aminophenol-induced nephrotoxicity in the Fischer 344 rat. *Arch Toxicol* 67:696–705, 1993.

Bach PH: The renal medulla and distal nephron toxicity, in Sipes IG, McQueen CA, Gandolfi AJ (eds): *Comprehensive Toxicology*. Vol 7. Oxford, England: Elsevier, 1997, pp 279–298.

Bakris GL: The pathogenesis and prevention of radiocontrast-induced renal dysfunction, in Sipes IG, McQueen CA, Gandolfi AJ (eds): *Comprehensive Toxicology*. Vol 7. Oxford, England: Elsevier, 1997, pp 547–566.

Ballatori N: Mechanisms of metal transport across liver cell plasma membrane. *Drug Metab Rev* 23:83–132, 1991.

Bernardo JF, Branch RA: Amphotericin B, in Sipes IG, McQueen CA, Gandolfi,AJ (eds): *Comprehensive Toxicology*. Vol 7. Oxford, England: Elsevier, 1997, pp 475–494.

Berndt WO: Effects of selected fungal toxins on renal function, in Hook JB, Goldstein RS (eds): *Toxicology of the Kidney,* 2d ed. New York: Raven Press, 1993, pp 459–475.

Beyersmann D, Block C, Malviya AN: Effect of cadmium on nuclear protein kinase C. *Environ Health Perspect Suppl* 3:177–180, 1994.

Brenner BM, Bohrer MP, Baylis C, Deen WM: Determinants of glomerular permselectivity: Insights derived from observations in vivo. *Kidney Int* 12:229–237, 1977.

Brenner BM, Meyer TH, Hotstetter TH: Dietary protein intake and the progressive nature of kidney disease: The role of hemodynamically mediated glomerular injury in the pathogenesis of glomerular sclerosis in agina, renal ablation and intrinsic renal disease. *N Engl J Med* 307:652–659, 1982.

Brezis M, Epstein FH: Pathophysiology of acute renal failure, in Hook JB, Goldstein RS (eds): *Toxicology of the Kidney,* 2d ed. New York: Raven Press, 1993, pp 129–152.

Brezis M, Rosen S, Epstein FH: Acute renal failure, in Brenner BM, Rector FJ (eds): *The Kidney,* 4th ed. Philadelphia, Saunders, 1991, pp 993–1061.

Brezis M, Rosen S, Silva P: Transport activity modifies thick ascending limb damage in isolated perfused kidney. *Kidney Int* 25:65–72, 1984.

Bruschi SA, West K, Crabb JW, et al: Mitochondrial HSP60 (P1 protein) and a HSP-70 like protein (mortalin) are major targets for modification during *S*-(1,1,2,2-tetrafluorethyl)-L-cysteine induced nephrotoxicity. *J Biol Chem* 268:23157–23161, 1993.

Bucci TJ, Howard PC, Tolleson WH, et al: Renal effects of fumonisin mycotoxins in animals. *Toxicol Pathol* 26:160–164, 1998.

Chen Q, Jones TW, Brown PC, Stevens JL: The mechanism of cysteine conjugate cytotoxicity in renal epithelial cells. *J Biol Chem* 265:21603–21611, 1990.

Chen Q, Yu K, Stevens JL: Regulation of the cellular stress response by reactive electrophiles: The role of covalent binding and cellular thiols in transcriptional activation of the 70-kDa heat shock protein gene by nephrotoxic cysteine conjugates. *J Biol Chem* 267:24322–24327, 1992.

Cojocel C: Aminoglycoside nephrotoxicity, in Sipes IG, McQueen CA, Gandolfi AJ (eds): *Comprehensive Toxicology.* Vol 7. Oxford, England: Elsevier, 1997, pp 495–524.

Conner EA, Fowler BA: Mechanisms of metal-induced nephrotoxicity, in Hook JB, Goldstein RS (eds): *Toxicology of the Kidney,* 2d ed. New York: Raven Press, pp 437–457, 1993.

Counts RS, Nowak G, Wyatt RD, Schnellmann RG: Nephrotoxicants inhibition of renal proximal tubule cell regeneration. *Am J Physiol* 269:F274–F281, 1995.

Courjault F, Leroy D, Coquery I, Toutain H: Platinum complex–induced dysfunction of cultured renal proximal tubule cells. *Arch Toxicol* 67:338–346, 1993.

Cummings BS, McHowat J, Schnellmann RG: Phospholipase A_2s in cell injury and death. *J Pharmacol Exp Ther* 294(3):793–799, 2000a.

Cummings, BS, McHowat J, Schnellmann RG: Inhibition of a microsomal Ca^{2+}-independent phospholipase A_2 increases oxidant-induced apoptosis in renal proximal tubular cells. *Toxicol Sci* 54:404, 2000b.

Cummings, BS, McHowat, J, Schnellmann, RG: Inhibition of a microsomal Ca^{2+}-independent phospholipase A_2 decreases cisplatin-induced apoptosis in renal proximal tubular cells. *J Am Soc Nephrol* 11:599A, 2000c.

De Broe ME: Renal injury due to environmental toxins, drugs, and contrast agents, in Berl T, Bonventre JV (eds): *Atlas of Diseases of the Kidney.* Philadelphia: Current Medicine, 1999, pp 11.2–11.14.

De Jong PE, Woods LL: Renal injury from angiotensin I converting enzyme inhibitiors, in DeBroe ME, Porter GA, Bennett AM, Verpooten GA (eds): *Clinical Nephrotoxicants, Renal Injury from Drugs and Chemicals.* The Netherlands: Kluwer, 1998, pp 239–250.

Dieperink H, Perico N, Nielsen FT, Remuzzi G: Cyclosporine/tacrolimus (FK-506), in DeBroe ME, Porter GA, Bennett AM, Verpooten GA (eds): *Clinical Nephrotoxicants, Renal Injury from Drugs and Chemicals.* The Netherlands: Kluwer, 1998, pp 275–300.

Dunn RB, Anderson S, Brenner B: The hemodynamic basis of progressive renal disease. *Semin Nephrol* 6:122–138, 1986.

Eknoyan G, Bulger RE, Dobyan DC: Mercuric chloride-induced acute renal failure in the rat: I. Correlation of functional and morphologic changes and their modification by clonidine. *Lab Invest* 46:613–620, 1982.

Elfarra AA: Halogenated hydrocarbons, in Sipes, IG, McQueen, CA, Gandolfi, AJ (eds): *Comprehensive Toxicology.* Vol 7. Oxford, England: Elsevier, 1997, pp 601–616.

Elsevier MM, DeBroe ME: Analgesics, in DeBroe ME, Porter GA, Bennett AM, Verpooten GA (eds): *Clinical Nephrotoxicants, Renal Injury from Drugs and Chemicals.* The Netherlands: Kluwer, 1998, pp 189–202.

Emeigh Hart SG, Wyand DS, Khairallah EA, Cohen SD: A role for the glutathione conjugate and renal cytochrome P450 in acetaminophen (APAP) induced nephrotoxicity in the CD-1 mouse. *Toxicologist* 11:57, 1990.

Emeigh Hart SGE, Beierschmitt WP, Wyand DS, et al: Acetaminophen nephrotoxicity in CD-1 Mice. I. Evidence of a role for in situ activation in selective covalent binding and toxicity. *Toxicol Appl Pharmacol* 126:267–275, 1994.

Enami A, Schwartz JH, Borkan SC: Transient ischemia or heat stress induces a cytoprotectant protein in rat kidney. *Am J Physiol* 260:F479–F485, 1991.

Fluery D, Vanhille P, Pallot JL, Kleinknecht D: Drug-induced acute renal failure: A preventable disease linked to drug misuse. *Kidney Int* 38:1238, 1990.

Ford SM: *In vitro* toxicity systems, in Sipes IG, McQueen CA, Gandolfi AJ (eds): *Comprehensive Toxicology.* Vol 7. Oxford, England: Elsevier, 1997, pp 121–142.

Fowler LM, Foster JR, Lock EA: Effect of ascorbic acid, acivicin and probenecid on the nephrotoxicity of 4-amino-phenol in the Fischer 344 rat. *Arch Toxicol* 67:613–621, 1993.

Fukino H, Hirai M, Hsueh YM, Yamane Y: Effect of zinc pretreatment on mercuric chloride–induced lipid peroxidation in the rat kidney. *Toxicol Appl Pharmacol* 73:395–401, 1984.

Gartland KPR, Eason CT, Bonner FW, Nicholson JK: Effects of biliary cannulation and buthionine sulphoximine pretreatment on the nephrotoxicity of para-aminophenol in the Fischer 344 rat. *Arch Toxicol* 64:14–25, 1990.

Georing, PL: Mercury induces regional and cell-specific stress protein expression in rat kidney. *Toxicol Sci* 53:447–457, 2000.

Gil FZ, Malnic G: Effect of amphotericin B on renal tubular acidification in the rat. *Pflugers Arch* 413:280–286, 1989.

Goering PL, Fisher BR, Chaudhary PP, Dick CA: Relationship between stress protein induction in rat kidney by mercuric chloride and nephrotoxicity. *Toxicol Appl Pharmacol* 113:184–191, 1992.

Goldstein RS: Biochemical heterogeneity and site-specific tubular injury, in Hook JB, Goldstein RS (eds): *Toxicology of the Kidney,* 2d ed. New York: Raven Press, 1993, pp 201–248.

Goligorsky MS, Lieberthal W, Racusen L, Simon EE: Integrin receptors in renal tubular epithelium: New insights into pathophysiology of acute renal failure. *Am J Physiol* 264:F1–F8, 1993.

Groves CE, Hayden PJ, Lock EA, Schnellmann RG: Differential cellular effects in the toxicity of haloalkene and haloalkane cysteine conjugates to rabbit renal proximal tubules. *J Biochem Toxicol* 8:49–56, 1993.

Groves CE, Lock EA, Schnellmann RG: The role of lipid peroxidation in renal proximal tubule cell death induced by haloalkene cysteine conjugates. *J Toxicol Appl Pharmacol* 107:54–62, 1991.

Halleck MM, Liu H, North J, Stevens JL: Reduction of *trans*-4,5-dihydroxy-1,2-dithiane by cellular oxidoreductases activates gadd153/chop an dgrp78 transcription and induces cellular tolerance in kidney epithelial cells. *J Biol Chem* 272:21760–21766, 1997.

Hammerman MR, Miller SB: Therapeutic use of growth factors in renal failure. *J Am Soc Nephrol* 5:1–11, 1994.

Hayden PJ, Stevens JL: Cysteine conjugate toxicity, metabolism and binding to macro-molecules in isolated rat kidney mitochondria. *Mol Pharmacol* 37:468–476, 1990.

Hayden PJ, Welsh CJ, Yang Y, et al: Formation of mitochondrial phospholipid adducts by nephrotoxic cysteine conjugate metabolites. *Chem Res Toxicol* 5:231–237, 1992.

Hayden PJ, Yang Y, Ward AJ, et al: Formation of diflourothionoacetyl-protein adducts by *S*-(1,1,2,2-tetrafluoroethyl)-L-cysteine metabolites: Nucleophilic catalysis of stable lysyl adduct formation by histidine and tyrosine. *Biochemistry* 30:5935–5943, 1991.

Jarnberg P: Renal toxicity of anesthetic agents, in DeBroe ME, Porter GA, Bennett AM, Verpooten GA (eds): *Clinical Nephrotoxicants, Renal Injury from Drugs and Chemicals.* The Netherlands: Kluwer, 1998, pp 413–418.

Kanwar YS, Liu ZZ, Kashihara N, Wallner EI: Current status of the structural and functional basis of glomerular filtration and proteinuria. *Semin Nephrol* 11:390–413, 1991.

Kaushal GP, Singh AB, Shah SV: Identification of gene family cf caspases in rat kidney and altered expression in ischemia-reperfusion injury. *Am J Physiol* 274:F587–F595, 1998.

Kelly KJ, Williams WW, Colvin RB, Bonventre JV: Antibody to intercellular adhesion molecule 1 protects the kidney against ischemic injury. *Proc Natl Acad Sci USA* 91:812–816, 1994.

Kido T, Nordberg G: Cadmium-induced renal effects in the general environment, in DeBroe ME, Porter GA, Bennett AM, Verpooten GA (eds): *Clinical Nephrotoxicants, Renal Injury from Drugs and Chemicals.* The Netherlands: Kluwer, 1998, pp 345–362.

Kidwell DT, KcKeown JW, Grider JS, et al: Acute effects of gentamicin on thick ascending limb function in the rat. *Eur J Pharmaco Environ Toxicol Pharmacol Section* 270:97–103, 1994.

Klaassen, CD, Liu, J, Choudhuri, S. Metallothionein: An intracellular protein to protect cadmium toxicity. *Ann Rev Pharmacol Toxicol* 39:267–294, 1999.

Kleinknecht D, Fillastre JP: Clinical aspects of drug-induced tubular necrosis in man, in Bertani T, Remuzzi G, Garrattini S (eds): *Drugs and Kidney.* New York: Raven Press, 1986, pp 123–136.

Komatsuda A, Wakui H, Satoh K, et al: Altered localization of 73-kilodalton heat shock protein in rat kidneys with gentamicin-induced acute tubular injury. *Lab Invest* 68:687–695, 1993.

Lanese DM, Conger JD: Effects of endothelin receptor antagonist on cyclosporine-induced vasoconstriction in isolated rat renal arterioles. *J Clin Invest* 91:2144–2149, 1993.

Lau SS, Monks TJ: Bromobenzene nephrotoxicity: A model of metabolism-dependent toxicity, in Sipes IG, McQueen CA, Gandolfi AJ (eds): *Comprehensive Toxicology:* Vol 7, Oxford, England: Elsevier, 1997, pp 617–632.

Lauwerys RR, Bernard AM, Roels HA, Buchet JP: Cadmium: Exposure markers as predictors of nephrotoxic effects. *Clin Chem* 40:1391–1394, 1994.

Lehman-McKeeman LD: α_{2u}-globulin nephropathy, in Sipes, IG, McQueen, CA, Gandolfi, AJ (eds): *Comprehensive Toxicology.* Vol 7. Oxford, England: Elsevier, 1997, pp 677–692.

Leiberthal W, Triaca V, Levine J: Mechanisms of death induced by cisplatin in proximal tubular epithelial cells: Apoptosis vs. necrosis. *Am J Physiol* 270:F700–F708, 1996.

Lemasters JJ, Qian T, Bradham CA, et al: Mitochondrial dysfunction in the pathogenesis of necrotic and apoptotic cell death. *J Bioenerg Biomembr* 31:305–319, 1999.

Leonard I, Zanen J, Nonclercq D, et al: Modification of immunoreactive EGF and EGF receptor after acute tubular necrosis induced by tobramycin or cisplatin. *Ren Fail* 16(5):583–608, 1994.

Levin S, Bucci TJ, Cohen SM, et al: The nomenclature of cell death: Recommendations of an *ad hoc* committee of the society of toxicologic pathologists. *Tox Pathol* 27:484–490, 1999.

Lock EA, Reed CJ: Renal xenobiotic metabolism, in Sipes IG, McQueen CA, Gandolfi AJ (eds): *Comprehensive Toxicology.* Vol 7. Oxford, England: Elsevier, 1997, pp 77–98.

Lund BO, Miller DM, Woods JS: Studies in Hg(II)-induced H_2O_2 formation and oxidative stress in vivo and in vitro in rat kidney mitochondria. *Biochem Pharmacol* 45:2017–2024, 1993.

Maddox DA, Brenner BM: Glomerular ultrafiltration, in Brenner BM, Rector FC (eds): *The Kidney,* 4th ed. Philadelphia: Saunders, 1991, pp 205–244.

Mason J, Moore LC: Cyclosporine, in Sipes IG, McQueen CA, Gandolfi AJ (eds): *Comprehensive Toxicology.* Vol 7. Oxford, England: Elsevier, 1997, pp 567–582.

Melnick R: An alternative hypothesis on the role of chemically induced protein droplet (α_{2u}-globulin) nephropathy in renal carcinogenesis. *Reg Toxicol Pharmacol* 16:111–125, 1992.

Meng X, Reeves WB: Effects of chloride channel inhibitors on H_2O_2-induced renal epithelial cell injury. *Am J Physiol Renal Physiol* 278:F83–F90, 2000.

Miller GW, Schnellmann RG: Cytoprotection by inhibition of chloride channels: The mechanism of action of glycine and strychnine. *Life Sci* 53:1211–1215, 1993.

Miller GW, Schnellmann RG: Inhibitors of renal chloride transport do not block toxicant-induced chloride influx in the proximal tubule. *Toxicol Lett* 76:179–184, 1995.

Molitoris BA: Alterations in surface membrane composition and fluidity: role in cell injury, in Sipes IG, McQueen CA, Gandolfi AJ (eds):

Comprehensive Toxicology. Vol 7. Oxford, England: Elsevier, 1997, pp 317–328.

Porter GA, Kremer D: Contrast associated nephropathy: presentation, pathophysiology, and management, in DeBroe ME, Porter GA, Bennett AM, Verpooten GA (eds): *Clinical Nephrotoxicants, Renal Injury from Drugs and Chemicals.* The Netherlands: Kluwer, 1998, pp 317–332.

Pryor WA, Squadrito GL: The chemistry of peroxynitrite: A product from the reaction of nitric oxide with superoxide *Am J Physiol* 268:L699–L722, 1995.

Rabb H, Mendiola CC, Dietz J, et al: Role of CD11a and CD11b in ischemic acute renal failure in rats. *Am J Physiol* 267:F1052–F1058, 1994.

Racusen LC, Solez K: Nephrotoxicity of cyclosporine and other immunotherapeutic agents, in Hook JB, Goldstein RS (eds): *Toxicology of the Kidney,* 2d ed. New York: Raven Press, 1993, pp 319–360.

Safirstein R, Deray G: Anticancer, cisplatin/carboplatin, in DeBroe ME, Porter GA, Bennett AM, Verpooten GA (eds): *Clinical Nephrotoxicants, Renal Injury from Drugs and Chemicals.* The Netherlands: Kluwer, 1998, pp 261–272.

Sapirstein A, Spech RA, Witzgall R, et al: Cytosolic phospholipase A_2 (PLA_2) but not secretory PLA_2, potentiates hydrogen peroxide cytotoxicity in kidney epithelial cells. *J Biol Chem* 271(35):21505–21513, 1996.

Schnellmann RG: Analgesic nephropathy in rodents. *J Toxicol Environ Health, Part B* 1:81–90, 1998.

Schnellmann RG, Cross TJ, Lock EA: Pentachlorabutadienyl-L-cysteine uncouples oxidative phosphorylation by dissipating the proton gradient. *Toxicol Appl Pharmacol* 100:498–505, 1989.

Schnellmann RG, Griner RD: Mitochondrial mechanisms of tubular injury, in Goldstein RS (ed): *Mechanisms of Injury in Renal Disease and Toxicity.* Boca Raton, FL: CRC, 1994, pp 247–265.

Schnellmann RG, Lock EA, Mandel LJ: A mechanism of *S*-(1,2,3,4,4-pentachloro-1,3-butadienyl)-L-cysteine toxicity to rabbit renal proximal tubules. *Toxicol Appl Pharmacol* 90:513–521, 1987.

Schnellmann RG, Swagler AR, Compton MM: Absence of endonuclease activation in acute cell death in renal proximal tubules. *Am J Physiol* 265:C485–C490, 1993.

Schnellmann RG, Williams SW: Proteases in renal cell death: Calpains mediate cell death produced by diverse toxicants. *Ren Fail* 20(5):679–686, 1998.

Smith JB, Dwyer SD, Smith L: Cadmium evokes inositol polyphosphate formation and calcium mobilization. *J Biol Chem* 256:7115–7118, 1989.

Smith JH, Maita K, Sleight SD, Hook JB: Effect of sex hormone status on chloroform nephrotoxicity and renal mixed function oxidases in mice. *Toxicology* 30:305–316, 1984.

Smith MW, Ambudkar IS, Phelps PC, et al: $HgCl_2$-induced changes in cytosolic Ca^{2+} of cultured rabbit renal tubular cells. *Biochem Biophys Acta* 931:130–142, 1987.

Steinmetz PR, Husted RF: Amphotericin B toxicity for epithelial cells, in Porter GA (ed): *Nephrotoxic Mechanisms of Drugs and Environmental Toxins.* New York, London: Plenum, 1982, pp 95–98.

Tarloff JB: Analgesics and nonsteroidal anti-inflammatory drugs, in Sipes IG, McQueen CA, Gandolfi AJ (eds): *Comprehensive Toxicology.* Vol 7. Oxford, England: Elsevier, 1997, pp 583–600.

Tarloff JB, Kinter LB: *In vivo* methodologies used to assess renal function, in Sipes IG, McQueen CA, Gandolfi AJ (eds): *Comprehensive Toxicology.* Vol 7. Oxford, England: Elsevier, 1997, pp 99–120.

Tolins JP, Raij L: Adverse effect of amphotericin B administration on renal hemodynamics in the rat. Neurohumoral mechanisms and influence of calcium channel blockade. *J Pharmacol Exp Ther* 245:594–599, 1988.

Ueda N, Mayeux PR, Baglia R, Shah SV: Oxidant mechanisms in acute renal failure, in Molitoris BA, Finn W (eds): *Acute Renal Failure: A Companion to Brenner's and Rector's The Kidney.* St. Louis: Saunders, 2001. In press.

Ueda N, Walker PD, Hsu SM, Shah SV: Activation of a 15-kDa endonuclease in hypoxia/reoxygenation injury without morphologic features of apoptosis. *Proc Natl Acad Sci USA* 92:7202–7206, 1995.

Van Why SK, Friedhelm H, Ardito T, et al: Induction and intracellular localization of HSP-72 after renal ischemia. *Am J Physiol* 263:F769–F775, 1992.

Verpooten GA, Tulkens PM, Bennett WM: Aminoglycosides and vancomycin, in DeBroe ME, Porter GA, Bennett AM, Verpooten GA (eds): *Clinical Nephrotoxicants, Renal Injury from Drugs and Chemicals.* The Netherlands: Kluwer, 1998, pp 105–120.

Wallin A, Jones TW, Vercesi AE, et al: Toxicity of *S*-pentachorobutadienyl-L-cysteine studied with isolated rat renal cortical mitochondria. *Arch Biochem Biophys* 258:365–372, 1987.

Wang C, Salahudeen AK: Cyclosporine nephrotoxicity: Attenuation by an antioxidant-inhibitor of lipid peroxidation in vitro and in vivo. *Transplantation* 58:940–946, 1994.

Wang C, Salahudeen AK: Lipid peroxidation accompanies cyclosporine nephrotoxicity: effects of vitamin E. *Kidney Int* 47:927–934, 1995.

Waters SL, Sarang SS, Wang KKW, Schnellmann RG: Calpains mediate calcium and chloride influx during the late phase of cell injury. *J Pharmacol Exp Ther* 283:1177–1184, 1997a.

Waters SL. Wong JK. Schnellmann RG. Depletion of endoplasmic reticulum calcium stores protects against hypoxia- and mitochondrial inhibitor–induced cellular injury and death. *Biochem Biophys Res Commun* 240:57–60, 1997b.

Weinberg JM: The cellular basis of nephrotoxicity, in Schrier RW, Gottschalk CW (eds): *Diseases of the Kidney,* 5th ed. Vol 2. Boston, Toronto, London: Little, Brown, 1993, pp 1031–1097.

Weinberg JM, Harding PG, Humes HD: Mitochondrial bioenergetics during the initiation of mercuric chloride-induced renal injury: I. Direct effects of in vitro mercuric chloride on renal cortical mitochondrial function. *J Biol Chem* 257:60–67, 1982b.

Weinberg JM, Harding PG, Humes HD: Mitochondrial bioenergetics during the initiation of mercuric chloride-induced renal injury: II. Functional alterations of renal cortical mitochondria isolated after mercuric chloride treatment. *J Biol Chem* 257:68–74, 1982a.

Whelton A, Watson AJ: Nonsteroidal anti-inflammatory drugs: effects on kidney interstitial nephritis, in DeBroe ME, Porter GA, Bennett AM, Verpooten GA (eds): *Clinical Nephrotoxicants, Renal Injury from Drugs and Chemicals.* The Netherlands: Kluwer, 1998, pp 203–216.

Wolfgang GHI, Leibbrant MEI: Antineoplastic agents, in Sipes IG, McQueen CA, Gandolfi AJ (eds): *Comprehensive Toxicology.* Vol 7. Oxford, England: Elsevier, 1997, pp 525–546.

Zalups RK: Renal toxicity of mercury, in Sipes IG, McQueen CA, Gandolfi AJ (eds): *Comprehensive Toxicology.* Vol 7. Oxford, England: Elsevier, 1997, pp 633–652.

Zalups RK, Lash LH: Advances in understanding the renal transport and toxicity of mercury. *J Toxicol Environ Health* 42:1–44, 1994.

Zhan Y, van de Water B, Wang Y, Stevens JL: The roles of caspase-3 and bcl-2 in chemically induced apoptosis but not necrosis of renal epithelial cells. *Oncogene* 18:6505–6512, 1999.

CHAPTER 15

TOXIC RESPONSES OF THE RESPIRATORY SYSTEM

Hanspeter R. Witschi and Jerold A. Last

Initially, lung injury caused by chemicals was primarily associated with certain professions and occupations. In his classic treatise of 1713, the Italian physician Bernardino Ramazzini provided detailed and harrowing accounts of the sufferings of miners, whose ailments had been known and described since antiquity. Two of Ramazzini's quotations are noteworthy. With regard to miners of metals, he stated that "the lungs and brains of that class of workers are badly affected, the lungs especially, since they take in with the air mineral spirits and are the first to be keenly aware of injury." Ramazzini also was aware of the important concept of exposure: "They (workers who shovel, melt, and cast and refine mined material) are liable of the same diseases, though in less acute form, because they perform their tasks in open air." Thus, exposure to chemicals by inhalation can have two effects: on the lung tissues and on distant organs that are reached after chemicals enter the body by means of inhalation. Indeed, the term *inhalation toxicology* refers to the route of exposure, whereas *respiratory tract toxicology* refers to target-organ toxicity, in this case abnormal changes in the respiratory tract produced by airborne (and on occasion blood-borne) agents. We now know of numerous lung diseases prompted by occupational exposures, many crippling and some fatal. Examples include black lung in coal miners, silicosis and silicotuberculosis in sandblasters and tunnel miners, and asbestosis in shipyard workers and asbestos miners. Occupational exposures to asbestos or metals such as nickel, beryllium, and cadmium can also cause lung cancer. In the twentieth century, it has become obvious that disease caused by airborne agents may not be limited to certain trades. The ubiquitous presence of airborne chemicals is a matter of concern, since "air pollution" adversely affects human health and may be an important contributor to mortality (Zemp et al., 1999).

To better understand environmental lung disease, we need more precise knowledge about the doses of toxic inhalants delivered to specific sites in the respiratory tract and an understanding of the extent to which repeated and often intermittent low-level exposures eventually may initiate and propagate chronic lung disease. Lung tissue can be injured directly or secondarily by metabolic products from organic compounds. However, the most important effect of many toxic inhalants is to place an undue oxidative burden on the lungs. Observations made in humans and animals provide strong evidence that the sequelae of oxidative stress may be instrumental in initiating and propagating ailments such as chronic bronchitis, emphysema, interstitial disorders (fibrosis), and cancer (Crapo et al., 1992).

Respiratory tract toxicology is a field in which collaboration involving epidemiologists, physiologists studying human lung function, toxicologists, and cell and molecular biologists has become close and fruitful. Epidemiologists now use a variety of pulmonary function tests to assess decrements in lung function in workers and populations exposed to air pollutants. These tests have been adapted for animal studies and are used to examine the mechanisms responsible for the pulmonary effects of air pollutants. When similar data can be obtained in both experimental animals and human subjects (for example, studies of mucociliary clearance of particles or responsiveness to bronchoconstrictive agents), these direct comparisons assist in extrapolating from animals to humans. Progress has been made in understanding some of the mechanisms that underlie the response of the lungs to toxic agents. In response to toxic insult, pulmonary cells are known to release a variety of potent chemical mediators that may critically affect lung function. Biochemical data from the study of cells taken from exposed animals and in vitro exposure of cells in culture are also useful in assessing the toxic potential of many agents. Recently, molecular techniques, such as in situ hybridization and immunostains, have been applied to analyze production of chemical mediators and other important macromolecules produced by specific cell types in response to inhaled toxicants. Bronchoalveolar lavage is now widely exploited in experimental animals and human subjects to examine respiratory airways' contents (cellular and acellular) after exposure. This chapter discusses how pulmonary toxicologists profit from these methods to study the biochemical, structural, and functional changes produced by the inhalation of pollutant gases and particles.

LUNG STRUCTURE AND FUNCTION

Nasal Passages

Figure 15-1 shows a schematic overview of the different regions of the respiratory tract. Air enters the respiratory tract through the nasal and oral regions. Many species, particularly small laboratory rodents, are obligatory nose breathers, in whom air passes almost exclusively through the nasal passages. Other species, including humans, monkeys, and dogs, can inhale air both through the nose and through the mouth (oronasal breathers). Air is warmed and humidified while passing through the nose. The nasal passages function as a filter for particles, which may be collected by diffusion or impaction on the nasal mucosa. Highly water-soluble gases are absorbed efficiently in the nasal passages, which reach from the nostril to the pharynx. The nasal turbinates thus form a first defensive barrier against many toxic inhalants.

The nasal passages are lined by distinctive epithelia: stratified squamous epithelium in the vestibule, nonciliated cuboidal/columnar epithelium in the anterior chamber, ciliated pseudostratified respiratory epithelium, and olfactory epithelium. The greater part of the internal nasal passages is covered by respiratory epithelium containing goblet cells, ciliated cells, nonciliated columnar cells, cuboidal cells, brush cells, and basal cells. Located in the superior part is the olfactory epithelium, which contains sensory cells. Nerve endings in the nasal passages are associated mostly with the fifth cranial (trigeminal) nerve.

Nasal epithelia are competent to metabolize foreign compounds (Fanucchi et al., 1999). Nasal tissue has been found to activate nitrosamines to mutagenic compounds. P-450 isozymes 1A1, 2B1, and 4B1 have been localized in the nose of several species by immunohistochemical procedures. The nasal cavity is thus a ready target site for metabolite-induced lesions. The olfactory epithelium appears to be particularly vulnerable. Metabolism by the olfactory epithelium may play a role in providing or preventing access of inhalants directly to the brain; for example, inhaled xylene may be converted to metabolites that move to the brain by axonal transport.

Conducting Airways

The proximal airways—the trachea and bronchi—have a pseudostratified epithelium containing ciliated cells and two types of nonciliated cells: mucous and serous cells. Mucous cells (and glandular structures) produce respiratory tract mucus, a family of high-molecular-weight glycoproteins with a sugar content of 80 percent or more that coat the epithelium with a viscoelastic sticky protective layer that traps pollutants and cell debris. Serous cells produce a fluid in which mucus may be dissolved. The action of the respiratory tract cilia, which beat in synchrony under the control of the central nervous system (CNS), continuously drives the mucous layer toward the pharynx, where it is removed from the respiratory system by swallowing or expectoration. The mucous layer is also thought to have antioxidant, acid-neutralizing, and free radical–scavenging functions that protect the epithelial cells (Cross et al., 1998).

Conducting airways have a characteristic branched bifurcating structure, with successive airway generations containing approximately twice the number of bronchi with a progressively decreasing internal diameter. Thus, the conducting airways contain a continuously increasing total surface area from the trachea to the distal airways. Bifurcations have flow dividers at branch points that serve as sites of impaction for particles, and successively narrower diameters also favor the collection of gases and particles on airway walls. Eventually a transition zone is reached where cartilaginous airways (bronchi) give way to noncartilaginous airways (bronchioles), which in turn give way to gas-exchange regions, respiratory bronchioles, and alveoli. Mucus-producing cells and glands give way to Clara cells in the bronchiolar epithelium. There are important structural and cellular differences between the conductive airways of humans and these of many commonly studied laboratory animals, as discussed later in this chapter.

Gas-Exchange Region

Human lungs are divided into five lobes: the superior and inferior left lobes and the superior, middle, and inferior right lobes. In small laboratory animals such as rats, mice, and hamsters, the left lung consists of a single lobe, whereas the right lung is divided into four lobes: cranial, middle, caudal, and ancillary. In the guinea pig and

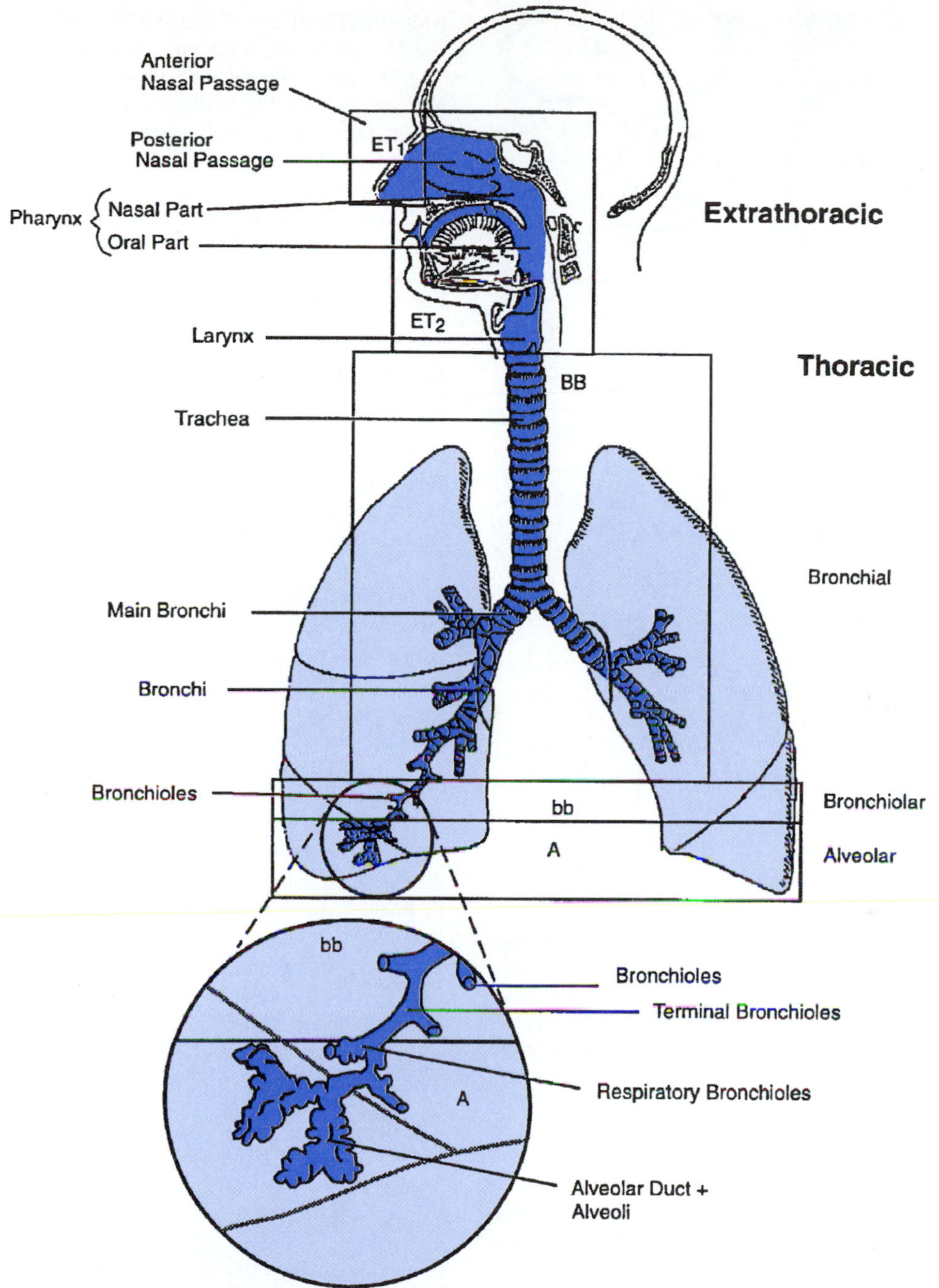

***Figure 15-1.** Schematic drawing of the anatomical regions of the respiratory tract.*

(From International Commission on Radiological Protection, Human Respiratory Tract Model for Radiological Protection. ICRP Publication 66; *Ann ICRP*. Oxford: Pergamon Press, 1994, p 24.)

rabbit, the left lung is divided into two lobes. Dogs have two left and four right lobes. The lung can be further subdivided at the periphery of the bronchial tree into distinct anatomic bronchopulmonary segments, then into lobules, and finally into acini. An acinus includes a terminal bronchiole and all its respiratory bronchioles, alveolar ducts, and alveolar sacs. An acinus may be made up of two to eight ventilatory units. A ventilatory unit is defined as an anatomic region that includes all alveolar ducts and alveoli distal to each bronchiolar-alveolar duct junction (Mercer and Crapo, 1991). The ventilatory unit is important because it represents the smallest common denominator when the distribution of inhaled gases to the gas-exchanging surface of the lung is modeled (Fig. 15-2).

Gas exchange occurs in the alveoli, which represent approximately 80 to 90 percent of the total parenchymal lung volume; adult human lungs contain an estimated 300 million alveoli. The ratio of total capillary surface to total alveolar surface is slightly less than 1. Within the alveolar septum, capillaries are organized

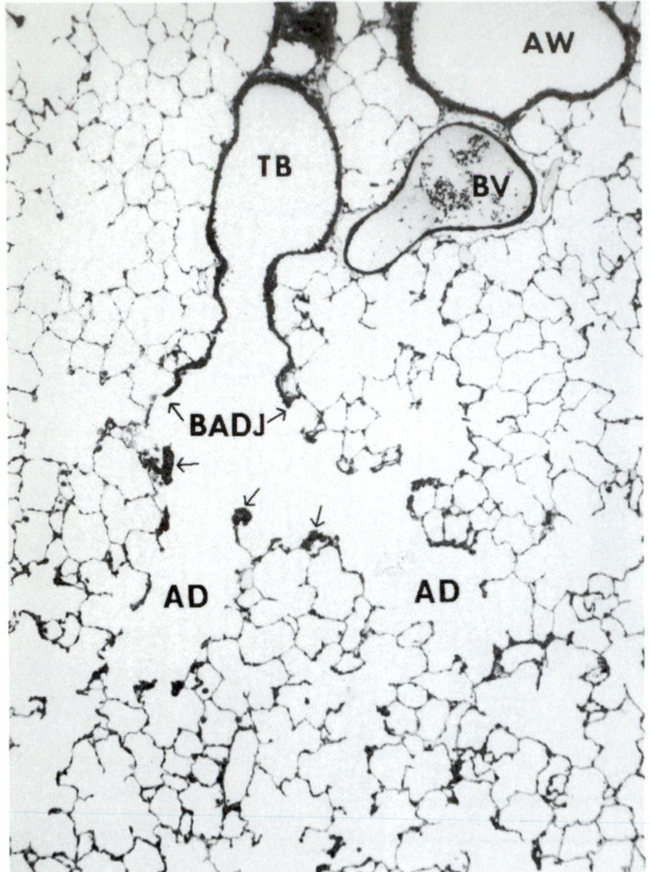

Figure 15-2. Centriacinar region (ventilatory unit) of the lung.

An airway and an arteriole [blood vessel (BV)] are in close proximity to the terminal bronchiole (TB) opening into alveolar ducts (AD) at the bronchiole–alveolar duct junction (BADJ). A number of the alveolar septal tips (*arrows*) close to the BADJ are thickened after a brief (4-h) exposure to asbestos fibers, indicating localization of fiber deposition. Other inhalants, such as ozone, produce lesions in the same locations. (Photograph courtesy of Dr. Kent E. Pinkerton, University of California, Davis.)

in a single sheet. Capillaries, blood plasma, and formed blood elements are separated from the air space by a thin layer of tissue formed by epithelial, interstitial, and endothelial components (Pinkerton et al., 1991).

Type I and type II alveolar cells represent approximately 25 percent of all the cells in the alveolar septum (Fig. 15-3). Type III epithelial cells, also called brush cells, are relatively rare. Type I cells cover a large surface area (approximately 90 percent of the alveolar surface). They have an attenuated cytoplasm and appear to be poor in organelles but probably are as metabolically competent as are the more compact type II cells. Preferential damage to type I cells by various agents may be explained by the fact that they constitute a large percentage of the total target (surface of the epithelium). Type II cells are cuboidal and show abundant perinuclear cytoplasm. They produce surfactant and, in case of damage to the type I epithelium, may undergo mitotic division and replace damaged cells. The shape of type I and type II cells is independent of alveolar size and is remarkably similar in different species. A typical rat alveolus (14,000 μm^2 surface) contains an average of two type I cells and three type II cells, whereas a human alveolus with a surface of 200,000 to 300,000 μm^2 contains 32 type I cells and 51 type II cells (Pinkerton et al., 1991).

The mesenchymal interstitial cell population consists of fibroblasts that produce collagen and elastin, as well as other cell matrix components and various effector molecules. Pericytes, monocytes, and lymphocytes also reside in the interstitium and so do macrophages before they enter the alveoli. Endothelial cells have a thin cytoplasm and cover about one-fourth of the area covered by type I cells. Clara cells are located in the terminal bronchioles and have a high content of xenobiotic metabolizing enzymes.

Gas Exchange

The principal function of the lung is gas exchange, which consists of ventilation, perfusion, and diffusion. The lung is superbly equipped to handle its main task: bringing essential oxygen to the organs and tissues of the body and eliminating its most abundant waste product, CO_2 (Weibel, 1983).

Ventilation During inhalation, fresh air is moved into the lung through the upper respiratory tract and conducting airways and into the terminal respiratory units when the thoracic cage enlarges and the diaphragm moves downward; the lung passively follows this expansion. After diffusion of oxygen into the blood and that of CO_2 from the blood into the alveolar spaces, the air (now enriched in CO_2) is expelled by exhalation. Relaxation of the chest wall and diaphragm diminishes the internal volume of the thoracic cage, the elastic fibers of the lung parenchyma contract, and air is expelled from the alveolar zone through the airways. Any interference with the elastic properties of the lung, for example, the decrease in elastic fibers that occurs in emphysema, adversely affects ventilation, as do decreases in the diameters of or blockage of the conducting airways, as in asthma.

The total volume of air in an inflated human lung, approximately 5700 cm^3, represents the total lung capacity (TLC). After

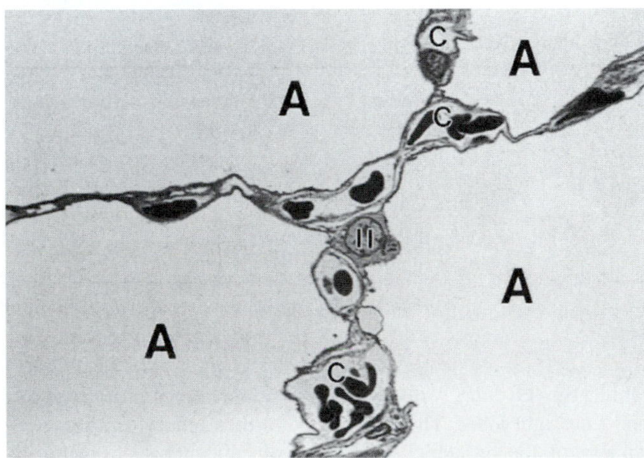

Figure 15-3. Micrograph of four alveoli **(A)** *separated by the alveolar septum.*

The thin air-to-blood tissue barrier of the alveolar septal wall is composed of squamous alveolar type I cells and occasional alveolar type II cells (II), a small interstitial space, and the attenuated cytoplasm of the endothelial cells that form the wall of the capillaries (C). (Photograph courtesy of Dr. Kent E. Pinkerton, University of California, Davis.)

a maximum expiration, the lung retains approximately 1200 cm^3 of air, the residual volume (RV). The air volume moved into and out of the lung with a maximum inspiratory and expiratory movement, which is called the vital capacity (VC), is thus approximately 4500 cm^3. Under resting conditions, only a fraction of the vital capacity, the tidal volume (TV), is moved into and out of the lung. In resting humans, the TV measures approximately 500 cm^3 with each breath (Fig. 15-4). The respiratory frequency, or the number of breaths per minute, is approximately 12 to 20. If an augmented metabolic demand of the body requires the delivery of increased amounts of oxygen—for example, during heavy and prolonged exercise—both the TV and the respiratory rate can be greatly increased. The amount of air moved into and out of the human lung may increase to up to 60 L/min. Increased ventilation in a polluted atmosphere increases the deposition of inhaled toxic material. For this reason, it is often stated that people, particularly children, should not exercise during episodes of heavy air pollution.

The TLC, as well as the ratio of RV to VC, changes when the lung is diseased. In emphysema, the alveoli overextend and more air is trapped. While the TLC may stay the same or even increase, the volume of air that is actually moved during breathing is diminished. This results in decreased VC with a concomitant increase in RV. If part of the lung collapses or becomes filled with edema fluid, TLC and VC are reduced. Pulmonary function tests give quantitative information on such changes.

Perfusion The lung receives the entire output from the right ventricle, approximately 70 to 80 cm^3 of blood per heartbeat, and thus may be exposed to substantial amounts of toxic agents carried in the blood. An agent placed onto or deposited under the skin (subcutaneous injection) or introduced directly into a peripheral vein (intravenous injection) travels through the venous system to the right ventricle and then comes into contact with the pulmonary capillary bed before distribution to other organs or tissues in the body.

Diffusion Gas exchange takes place across the entire alveolar surface. Contact to airborne toxic agent thus occurs over a surface (approximately 140 m^2) that is second only to the small intestine

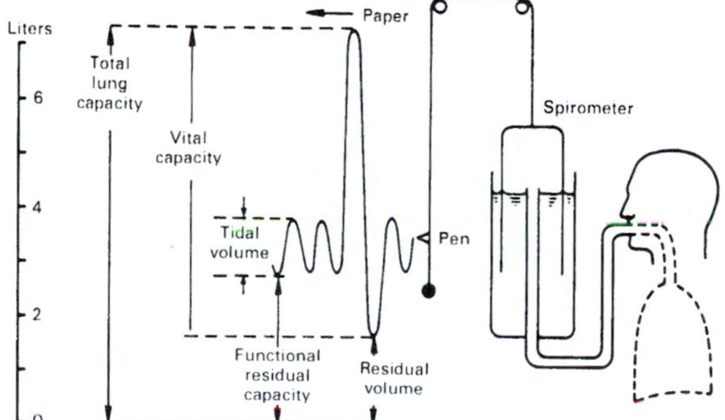

Figure 15-4. Lung volumes.

Note that the functional residual capacity and residual volume cannot be measured with spirometer but require special procedures (e.g., nitrogen or helium outwash). (From West JB: *Respiratory Physiology—The Essentials.* Baltimore: Williams & Wilkins, 1994, with permission.)

(approximately 250 m^2) and considerably larger than the skin (approximately 1.75 m^2), two other organs that are in direct contact with the outside world. A variety of abnormal processes may thicken the alveolar septum and adversely affect the diffusion of oxygen to the erythrocytes. Such processes may include collection of liquid in the alveolar space and an abnormal thickening of the pulmonary epithelium. It is often seen as a result of chronic toxicity because of an abnormal accumulation of tissue constituents in the interstitial space through proliferation of interstitial cells. Increased formation and deposition of extracellular substances such as collagen or because of the interstitial accumulation of edema fluid has similar consequences.

GENERAL PRINCIPLES IN THE PATHOGENESIS OF LUNG DAMAGE CAUSED BY CHEMICALS

Oxidative Burden

An important type of injury to the lung is thought to be caused by an undue oxidative burden that often is mediated by free radicals, such as those generated by ozone, NO_2, tobacco smoke, and lung defense cells (Witschi, 1997a). Evidence for the role of free radicals in lung damage includes a wide variety of observations. Numerous studies have reported increases in the activity of free radical–scavenging enzymes in the lungs of animals exposed to O_3, NO_2, and other toxicants, indirectly supporting this hypothesis. Treatment with various hydroxyl radical scavengers can protect rats from pulmonary edema induced by high doses of thiourea and otherwise lethal levels of gamma irradiation.

Theories of lung oxidant toxicity relate to the formation of reactive and unstable free radicals, with subsequent chain reactions leading to uncontrolled destructive oxidation. Recent work has emphasized the pivotal roles of superoxide, nitric oxide, peroxynitrate, hydroxyl radicals, and perhaps singlet oxygen in mediating tissue damage. Reduction of O_2 to active O_2 metabolites normally occurs as a by-product of cellular metabolism during both microsomal and mitochondrial electron transfer reactions; considerable amounts of superoxide anion are generated by NADPH cytochrome P450 reductase reactions. Because these oxidant species are potentially cytotoxic, they may mediate or promote the actions of various pneumotoxicants. Such mechanisms have been proposed for paraquat- and nitrofurantoin-induced lung injury. When cellular injury of any type occurs, the release of otherwise contained cellular constituents such as microsomes and flavoproteins into the extracellular space may lead to extracellular generation of deleterious reactive O_2 species.

Among mammalian cells, neutrophils, monocytes, and macrophages seem particularly adept at converting molecular O_2 to reactive O_2 metabolites; this probably is related to their phagocytosis and antimicrobial activities. As a by-product of this capability, toxic O_2 species are released (possibly by the plasmalemma itself) into surrounding tissues. As most forms of toxic pulmonary edema are accompanied by phagocyte accumulation in the lung microcirculation (pulmonary leukostasis) and parenchyma, oxidative damage may represent a significant component of all types of pneumotoxic lung injury accompanied by a phagocyte-mediated inflammatory component.

Chemotactic and phagocytic "activation" processes result in a substantial increase in the release of potent oxidants by stimulated phagocytes; these radicals cause oxidative damage to the surrounding tissues. A key role of hydrogen peroxide as the mediator of the extracellular cytotoxic mechanism of "activated" phagocytes has been well documented. Phenomena occurring at the phagocyte surface, such as those which may occur in endogenous lung phagocytes after exposure to dusts and toxic gases, or in circulating phagocytes before their accumulation in the lung or after their attachment to normal or damaged lung endothelium seem to be important in determining their degree of enhanced oxidative activity, which is otherwise at a much lower basal level in the unstimulated cell. It also has been long appreciated that phagocytes may cause lysosomal enzyme release and tissue damage.

The fact that oxidative processes are complex is suggested by the finding that phagocytic production of active oxygen species causes inactivation of proteinase inhibitors and degranulation of mast cells. The production of oxygen radicals by phagocytes is enhanced not only by interactions of cell surface membranes with various appropriate stimuli but also by hyperoxia. Platelets (and platelet microthrombi) also have the ability to generate activated O_2 species.

The lung can respond with specific defense mechanisms that may be acquired over time and may be stimulated by constant exposure to numerous species of airborne microorganisms as well as by a variety of low- and high-molecular-weight antigenic materials. The immune system can mount either cellular or humorally mediated responses to these inhaled antigens. Direct immunologic effects occur when inhaled foreign material sensitizes the respiratory system to further exposure to the same material. The mammalian lung has a well-developed immune system. Lymphocytes reside in the hilar or mediastinal lymph nodes, lymphoid aggregates, and lymphoepithelial nodules as well as in aggregates or as single cells throughout the airways. Bronchoconstriction and chronic pulmonary disease can result from the inhalation of materials that appear to act wholly or partly through an allergic response. In some instances, these reactions are caused by spores of molds or bacterial contaminants. Frequently, chemical components of the sensitizing dusts or gases are responsible for the allergic response. Low-molecular-weight compounds can act as haptens that combine with native proteins to form a complex that is recognized as an antigen by the immune system. Further exposure to the sensitizing compound can result in an allergic reaction that is characterized by the release of various inflammatory mediators that produce an early and/or a late bronchoconstrictor response. Such a response is observed in sensitized workers exposed to toluene diisocyanate (TDI), a chemical widely used in the manufacture of polyurethane plastics (Karol et al., 1994).

Indirect immune effects occur when exposure to air pollutants either suppresses or enhances the immune response to other materials. Both sulfur dioxide (SO_2) and ozone can boost the response of the respiratory system to inhaled foreign material, at least in experimental animals (guinea pigs). It is not known whether these effects occur in humans, but they form the bases for concerns about increased susceptibility of asthmatic individuals to air pollutants such as ozone and sulfur dioxide.

Toxic Inhalants, Gases, and Dosimetry

The sites of deposition of gases in the respiratory tract define the pattern of toxicity of those gases. Water solubility is the critical factor in determining how deeply a given gas penetrates into the lung. Highly soluble gases such as SO_2 do not penetrate farther than the nose and are therefore relatively nontoxic to animals, especially obligatory nose breathers such as the rat. Relatively insoluble gases such as ozone and NO_2 penetrate deeply into the lung and reach the smallest airways and the alveoli (centriacinar region), where they can elicit toxic responses. Mathematical models of gas entry and deposition in the lung that are based solely on the aqueous solubility of a gas predict sites of lung lesions fairly accurately. These models may be useful for extrapolating findings made in laboratory animals to humans (Kimbell and Miller, 1999; Medinsky et al., 1999). Very insoluble gases such as CO and H_2S efficiently pass through the respiratory tract and are taken up by the pulmonary blood supply to be distributed throughout the body.

Particle Deposition and Clearance

The site of deposition of solid particles or droplets in the respiratory tract, along with their chemical makeup, is important. Particle size is usually the critical factor that determines the region of the respiratory tract in which a particle or an aerosol will be deposited. Deposition of particles on the surface of the lung and airways is brought about by a combination of lung anatomy and the patterns of airflow in the respiratory system (Raabe, 1999; Miller, 1999) (Fig. 15–5).

Particle Size Inhaled aerosols are most frequently polydisperse in regard to size. The size distribution of many aerosols approximates a log-normal distribution that may be described by the *median* or *geometric mean* and the *geometric standard deviation.* A plot of the frequency of occurrence of a given size against the log of the size produces a bell-shaped probability curve. Particle data frequently are handled by plotting the cumulative percentage of particles smaller than a stated size on log-probability paper. This results in a straight line that may be fitted by eye or mathematically. In actual practice, it is not unusual to have some deviation

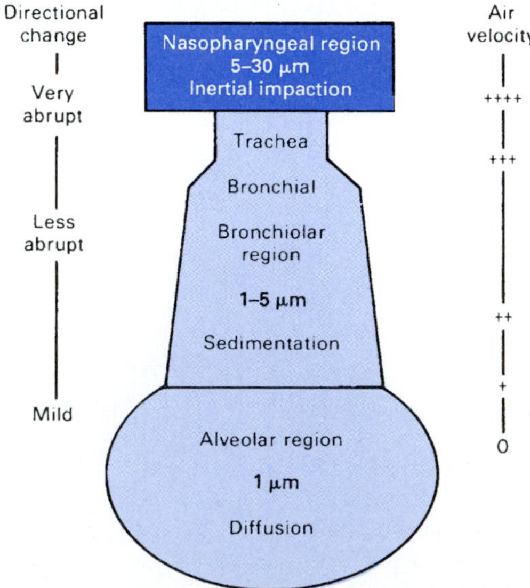

Figure 15-5. Parameters influencing particle deposition.

[From Casarett LJ: The vital sacs: Alveolar clearance mechanisms in inhalation toxicology, in Blood FR (ed): *Essays in Toxicology.* Vol 3. New York: Academic Press, 1972, with permission.]

from a straight line at the largest or smallest particle sizes measured. The geometric mean is the 50 percent size as the mean bisects the curve. The geometric standard deviation (σg) is calculated as

$$\sigma g = 84.1\% \text{ size}/50\% \text{ size}$$

The σg of the particle size distribution is a measure of the polydispersity of the aerosol. In the laboratory, values for σg of 1.8 to 3.0 are encountered frequently. In the field, values for σg may range up to 4.5. An aerosol with a σg below 1.2 may be considered monodisperse.

The median diameter that is determined may reflect the number of particles, as in the count median diameter (CMD), or reflect mass, as in the mass median aerodynamic diameter (MMAD). The larger the number and mass of particles capable of penetrating the lung, the greater the probability of a toxic effect. The size distribution in relation to other factors, such as particle shape and surface area, also may be of interest. Surface area is of special importance when toxic materials are adsorbed on the surfaces of particles and thus are carried to the lung.

Particles that are nonspherical in shape are frequently characterized in terms of equivalent spheres on the basis of equal mass, volume, or aerodynamic drag. The MMAD takes into account both the density of the particle and aerodynamic drag. It represents the diameter of a unit density sphere with the same terminal settling velocity as the particle, regardless of its size, shape, and density. Aerodynamic diameter is the proper measurement for particles that are deposited by impaction and sedimentation. For very small particles, which are deposited primarily by diffusion, the critical factor is particle size, not density. It must be kept in mind that the size of a particle may change before its deposition in the respiratory tract. Materials that are hygroscopic, such as sodium chloride, sulfuric acid, and glycerol, take on water and grow in size in the warm, saturated atmosphere of the lower respiratory tract.

Deposition Mechanisms Deposition of particles occurs primarily by interception, impaction, sedimentation, and diffusion (Brownian movement). Interception occurs only when the trajectory of a particle brings it near enough to a surface so that an edge of the particle contacts the airway surface. Interception is important for the deposition of fibers. Whereas fiber diameter determines the probability of deposition by impaction and sedimentation, interception is dependent on fiber length. Thus, a fiber with a diameter of 1 μm and a length of 200 μm will be deposited in the bronchial tree primarily by interception rather than impaction.

As a result of inertia, particles suspended in air tend to continue to travel along their original path. In a bending airstream, such as at an airway bifurcation, a particle may be impacted on the surface. At relatively symmetrical bifurcations, which typically occur in the human lung, the deposition rate is likely to be high for particles that move in the center of the airway. Generalizations regarding the site of deposition of particles of a given size are problematic. However, in the average adult, most particles larger than 10 μm in aerodynamic diameter are deposited in the nose or oral pharynx and cannot penetrate to tissues distal to the larynx. Recent data have shown that very fine particles (0.01 μm and smaller) are also trapped relatively efficiently in the upper airways by diffusion. Particles that penetrate beyond the upper airways are available to be deposited in the bronchial region and the deeper-lying airways. Therefore, the alveolar region has significant deposition efficiencies for particles smaller than 5 μm and larger than 0.003 μm.

Sedimentation brings about deposition in the smaller bronchi, the bronchioles, and the alveolar spaces, where the airways are small and the velocity of airflow is low. As a particle moves downward through air, buoyancy and the resistance of air act on the particle in an upward direction while gravitational force acts on the particle in a downward direction. Eventually, the gravitational force equilibrates with the sum of the buoyancy and the air resistance, and the particle continues to settle with a constant velocity known as the terminal settling velocity. Sedimentation is not a significant route of particle deposition when the aerodynamic diameter is below 0.5 μm.

Diffusion is an important factor in the deposition of submicrometer particles. A random motion is imparted to these particles by the impact of gas molecules. This brownian motion increases with decreasing particle size, and so diffusion is an important deposition mechanism in the nose and in other airways and alveoli for particles smaller than about 0.5 μm.

An important factor in particle deposition is the pattern of breathing. During quiet breathing, in which the TV is only two to three times the volume of the anatomic dead space (i.e, the volume of the conducting airways where gas exchange does not occur), a large proportion of the inhaled particles may be exhaled. During exercise, when larger volumes are inhaled at higher velocities, impaction in the large airways and sedimentation and diffusion in the smaller airways and alveoli increase. Breath holding also increases deposition from sedimentation and diffusion. Factors that modify the diameter of the conducting airways can alter particle deposition. In patients with chronic bronchitis, the mucous layer is greatly thickened and extended peripherally and may partially block the airways in some areas. Jets formed by air flowing through such partially occluded airways have the potential to increase the deposition of particles by impaction and diffusion in the small airways. Irritant materials that produce bronchoconstriction tend to increase the tracheobronchial deposition of particles. Cigarette smoking has been shown experimentally to produce such an effect.

Particle Clearance The clearance of deposited particles is an important aspect of lung defense. Rapid removal lessens the time available to cause damage to the pulmonary tissues or permit local absorption. The specific mechanisms available for the removal of particles from the respiratory tract vary with the site of the deposition. It is important to emphasize that clearance of particles from the respiratory tract is not synonymous with clearance from the body. Depending on the specific clearance mechanism used, particles are cleared to (1) the stomach and gastrointestinal (GI) tract; (2) the lymphatics and lymph nodes, where they may be dissolved and enter the venous circulation; or (3) the pulmonary vasculature. The only mechanisms by which the respiratory system can truly remove deposited particles from the body are coughing and blowing the nose.

Nasal Clearance Particles deposited in the nose are cleared by various mechanisms, depending on their site of deposition and solubility in mucus. The anterior portion of the nose is lined with relatively dry squamous epithelium, and so particles deposited there are removed by extrinsic actions such as wiping and blowing. The other regions of the nose are largely covered by a mucociliary epithelium that propels mucus toward the glottis, where it is swallowed. Insoluble particles generally are cleared from this region in healthy adults and swallowed within an hour of deposition. Particles that are soluble in mucus may dissolve and enter the epithelium and/or blood before they can be mechanically removed. Uncertainties still remain about the clearance of particles that are deposited on olfactory regions or areas that are damaged by acute infection, chronic illnesses, or toxic injury.

Tracheobronchial Clearance The mucous layer covering the tracheobronchial tree is moved upward by the beating of the underlying cilia. This mucociliary escalator transports deposited particles and particle-laden macrophages upward to the oropharynx, where they are swallowed and pass through the GI tract. Mucociliary clearance is relatively rapid in healthy individuals and is completed within 24 to 48 h for particles deposited in the lower airways. Infection and other injuries can greatly impair clearance.

Pulmonary Clearance There are several primary ways by which particulate material is removed from the lower respiratory tract once it has been deposited:

1. Particles may be directly trapped on the fluid layer of the conducting airways by impaction and cleared upward, in the tracheobronchial tree via the mucociliary escalator.
2. Particles may be phagocytized by macrophages and cleared via the mucociliary escalator.
3. Particles may be phagocytized by alveolar macrophages and removed via the lymphatic drainage.
4. Material may dissolve from the surfaces of particles and be removed via the bloodstream or lymphatics.
5. Small particles may directly penetrate epithelial membranes.

Minutes after particles are inhaled, they may be found in alveolar macrophages. Many alveolar macrophages are ultimately transported to the mucociliary escalator. It is possible that macrophages are carried to the bronchioles with the alveolar fluid that contributes to the fluid layer in the airways. Other particles may be sequestered in the lung for very long periods, often in macrophages located in the interstitium.

ACUTE RESPONSES OF THE LUNG TO INJURY

Airway Reactivity

Large airways are surrounded by bronchial smooth muscles, which help maintain airway tone and diameter during expansion and contraction of the lung. Bronchial smooth muscle tone is normally regulated by the autonomic nervous system. Reflex contraction occurs when receptors in the trachea and large bronchi are stimulated by irritants such as cigarette smoke and air pollutants. Bronchoconstriction can be provoked by cholinergic drugs such as acetylcholine, a phenomenon that serves as the basis for a sensitive measure of whether a toxicant can cause bronchoconstriction in animals or humans primed by a prior dose of an acetylcholinelike agent (bronchoprovocation testing) . These agents bind to cell surface receptors (cholinergic receptors) and trigger an increase in the intracellular concentration of cyclic guanosine monophosphate (cGMP), which in turn facilitates smooth muscle contraction. The actions of cGMP can be antagonized by cyclic adenosine monophospate (cAMP), which has bronchodilatory activity, and can be increased by agents that bind to beta-adrenergic receptors on the cell surface. Other important mediators of airway smooth muscle tone include histamine, various prostaglandins and leukotrienes, substance P, and nitric oxide. The bronchial smooth muscles of individuals with asthma contract with much less provocation than do those of normal subjects. Bronchoconstriction causes a decrease in airway diameter and a corresponding increase in resistance to airflow. Characteristic associated symptoms include wheezing, coughing, a sensation of chest tightness, and dyspnea. Exercise potentiates these problems. A major cause of concern about ambient air pollution is whether asthmatic individuals represent a population that is particularly susceptible to the adverse health effects of sulfur dioxide, ozone, nitrogen dioxide, other respiratory irritant gases, and respirable particles. Since the major component of airway resistance usually is contributed by large bronchi, inhaled agents that cause reflex bronchoconstriction are generally irritant gases with moderate solubility. Demonstrations of the bronchoconstrictive effects of gases in laboratory animals often are performed in guinea pigs, which seem to represent a natural animal model of asthmatic humans with respect to innate airway reactivity.

Pulmonary Edema

Toxic pulmonary edema represents an acute, exudative phase of lung injury that generally produces a thickening of the alveolar-capillary barrier. Edema fluid, when present, alters ventilation-perfusion relationships and limits diffusive transfer of O_2 and CO_2 even in otherwise structurally normal alveoli. Edema is often a sign of acute lung injury.

The biological consequences of toxic pulmonary edema not only induce acute compromise of lung structure and function but also may include abnormalities that remain after resolution of the edematous process. After exposure to some toxic agents in which the alveolar-capillary surface is denuded (such as alloxan), recovery is unlikely, whereas in situations of more modest injury (such as histamine administration), full recovery is readily achievable. Between these two extremes there are forms of severe lung injury accompanied by amplified inflammatory damage and/or exaggerated restorative-reparative processes (e.g., after paraquat ingestion). In these severe forms, the extensive interstitial and intraalveolar inflammatory exudate resolves via fibrogenesis, an outcome that may be beneficial or damaging to the lung. Accumulation and turnover of inflammatory cells and related immune responses in an edematous lung probably play a role in eliciting both mitogenic activity and fibrogenic responses.

Pulmonary edema is customarily quantified in experimental animals by some form of gravimetric measurement of lung water content. Very commonly, the wet (undesiccated) weight of the whole lung or that of a single lung lobe is determined. This value is often normalized to the weight of the animal from which the lung was taken. Alternatively, some investigators determine lung water content by weighing whole lungs or lung slices before and after complete drying in an oven or desiccator. Commonly used methods for expressing such data include (1) percentage water content [$100 \times$ (wet weight − dry weight)/(wet weight)], (2) percentage dry weight [$100 \times$ (dry weight)/(wet weight)], and (3) water content [(milliliters of water)/(dry weight)].

Mechanisms of Respiratory Tract Injury

Airborne agents can contact cells lining the respiratory tract from the nostrils to the gas-exchanging region. The sites of interaction of toxicants in the respiratory tract have important implications for evaluation of the risk to humans posed by inhalants. For example, rats have much more nasal surface on a per body weight basis than do humans. Measurement of DNA-protein cross-links formed in nasal tissue by the highly reactive gas formaldehyde has demonstrated that rats, which readily develop nasal tumors, have many more DNA cross-links per unit of exposure (concentration of formaldehyde × duration of exposure) than do monkeys. Because the breathing pattern of humans resembles that of monkeys more than that of rats, it was concluded that extrapolation of tumor data from rats to humans on the basis of formaldehyde concentration may overestimate doses of formaldehyde to humans. Patterns of animal activity can affect dose to the lung; nocturnally active animals such as rats receive a greater dose per unit of exposure at night than during the day, whereas humans show the opposite diurnal relationships of exposure concentration to dose.

Certain gases and vapors stimulate nerve endings in the nose, particularly those of the trigeminal nerve (Alarie et al., 1998). The result is holding of the breath or changes in breathing patterns, to avoid or reduce further exposure. If continued exposure cannot be avoided, many acidic or alkaline irritants produce cell necrosis and increased permeability of the alveolar walls. Other inhaled agents can be more insidious; inhalation of HCl, NO_2, NH_3, or phosgene may at first produce very little apparent damage in the respiratory tract. The epithelial barrier in the alveolar zone, after a latency period of several hours, begins to leak, flooding the alveoli and producing a delayed pulmonary edema that is often fatal.

A different pathogenetic mechanism is typical of highly reactive molecules such as ozone. It is unlikely that ozone as such can penetrate beyond the layer of fluid covering the cells of the lung. Instead, ozone lesions are propagated by a cascade of secondary reaction products, such as aldehydes and hydroxyperoxides produced by ozonolysis of fatty acids and other substrates in the lung's lining fluid, and by reactive oxygen species arising from free radical reactions. Reactive oxygen species also have been implicated in pulmonary bleomycin toxicity, pulmonary oxygen toxicity, paraquat toxicity, and the development of chronic lesions such as the fibrogenic and carcinogenic effects of asbestos fibers.

Metabolism of foreign compounds can be involved in the pathogenesis of lung injury. The balance of activation and detoxification plays a key role in determining whether a given chemical ultimately will cause damage. The lung contains most of the enzymes involved in xenobiotic metabolism that have been identified in other tissues, such as the liver (Buckpitt et al., 1997). While the overall levels of these enzymes tend to be lower in lung than in liver, they often are highly concentrated in specific cell populations of the respiratory tract. Moreover, their specific content of particular cytochrome P450 isozymes may be much higher in lung. Thus, the turnover of a substrate for a lung P450 may be far more rapid than occurs in liver. Many isozymes of the cytochrome P450 complex have been identified in and isolated from the lungs of rabbits, rats, hamsters and humans. Cytochrome P450 1A1 is present in low amounts in normal rat and rabbit lungs but is highly inducible by polycyclic aromatic hydrocarbons, flavones, and mixtures of polyhalogenated biphenyls. This isozyme also is present in human lungs and is thought to be involved in the metabolic activation of the polycyclic aromatic hydrocarbons that are present in cigarette smoke. By inference, this P450 isozyme may play a role in the pathogenesis of lung cancer. Attempts have been made to use the expression of cytochrome P450 1A1 as a biomarker of exposure and sensitivity to cigarette smoke in humans, although the precise relationships remain unclear. Cytochrome P450 2B1, which is readily inducible in rat liver by phenobarbital, is not inducible in lung tissue. Other isozymes identified in human lung are cytochrome P450 2F1, 4B1, and 3A4. Further microsomal enzymes found in the lung include NADPH cytochrome P450 reductase, epoxide hydrolase, and flavin-containing monoxygenases. Finally, two important cytosolic enzymes involved in lung xenobiotic metabolism are glutathione-*S*-transferase and glutathione peroxidase. Adult human lungs appear to contain several forms of glutathione-*S*-transferase.

Mediators of Lung Toxicity

Advances in cell culture techniques (Leikauf and Driscoll, 1993) have allowed investigators to examine the role of specific signal molecules in toxicant-induced lung damage; this is a very active area of research. Such studies are often guided by results obtained by analysis of cytokines and other mediators in lung lavage fluid from animals or human volunteers exposed to inhaled toxic agents.

For example, interleukin 1 beta (IL-1β), transforming growth factor beta (TGF-β), and tumor necrosis factor alpha (TNF-α) have all been implicated in the cascade of reactions that is thought to be responsible for the pathogenesis of pulmonary fibrosis (Zhang and Phan, 1999). Similarly, several of the nine described members of the interleukin family, especially IL-1, IL-2, IL-5 and IL-8, are thought to be essential components of the lung's response to epithelial cell injury. Various specific prostaglandins, especially PGE_2, and leukotrienes have been implicated in intracellular signaling pathways in the lung. The roles of cell surface adhesion molecules and their interaction with cell matrix components and with control of inflammatory cell migration (particularly neutrophil influx to the lung) have been studied intensively.

Analysis of normal lung homogenates suggests that the lung contains large amounts of endogenous cytokines and inflammatory mediators, far more than enough for these potent compounds to elicit effects. Thus, these agents must be compartmentalized in a healthy lung to control their potent bioactivity. How these processes are regulated normally, what exactly goes wrong with homeostasis in a damaged lung, the temporal and geographic relationship of different cytokines in the amplification of an initial injurious event, and detailed mechanisms of resolution of lung injury are not well understood and represent the current focus of much research on mechanisms of lung injury by toxic agents. The reader is referred to reviews of these topics (Massague, 1998; Barnes et al., 1998) for more details on specific mediators and toxic agents in this rapidly changing research area.

Cell Proliferation

The effects of toxicants on the lung may be reversible or irreversible. Postexposure progression of lung fibrosis has been demonstrated in rats exposed to ozone, mice exposed to cyclophosphamide, and hamsters exposed to bleomycin or bleomycin plus oxygen. The mechanisms for exacerbating lung damage or repairing such damage during a postexposure period in which filtered air alone is inhaled are not obvious. Examination of the time course and cellular components of reepithelialization of the alveolar ducts and walls during the postexposure period would be especially important in this regard. Research on the postexposure effects of inhaled toxicants is an important area for further study.

The normal adult lung is an organ for which under normal circumstances very few cells appear to die and to be replaced. When damaged by a toxic insult, the lung parenchyma is capable to repair itself in an efficient manner. Type I cell damage is followed by proliferation of type II epithelial cells which eventually transform into new type I cells; in the airways, the Clara cells proliferate and divide following injury. The migration of mobile blood cells such as leukocytes across the pulmonary capillaries into the alveolar lumen may also trigger a mitotic response. Other cells in the alveolar zone, such as capillary endothelial cells, interstitial cells, and alveolar macrophages, also proliferate. The result is a normal looking organ again although on occasion excessive proliferation of fibroblasts may result in lung disease. In general, however, the lung appears to have a high capacity to repair itself and thus to deal with the many toxic insults presented by the environment (Witschi, 1997b).

CHRONIC RESPONSES OF THE LUNG TO INJURY

Fibrosis

Defined clinically, lung fibrosis refers to the type of interstitial fibrosis that is seen in the later stages of idiopathic pulmonary fibrosis (also called *cryptogenic fibrosing alveolitis* in the United Kingdom). In this disease, the hallmark of pulmonary fibrosis seen by the pathologist is increased focal staining of collagen fibers in the alveolar interstitium. Fibrotic lungs from humans with acute or chronic pulmonary fibrosis contain increased amounts of collagen as evaluated biochemically, in agreement with the histological findings.

In lungs damaged by toxicants, the response resembles adult or infant respiratory distress syndrome more closely than it resembles chronic interstitial fibrosis. Excess lung collagen is usually observed not only in the alveolar interstitium but also throughout the centriacinar region, including the alveolar ducts and respiratory bronchioles. The relationship between increased collagen deposition around small airways and lung mechanics is not understood either theoretically or empirically.

At least 19 genetically distinct collagen types are known to occur in all mammals, most of which have been found in normal lungs or to be synthesized by isolated lung cells. Two types predominate in the lung, representing about 90 percent or more of the total lung collagen. Type I and type III collagen are major interstitial components and are found in the normal lungs of all mammals in an approximate ratio of 2:1. Type I collagen is the material that stains histologically as "collagen," whereas type III collagen is appreciated histologically as reticulin. Some types of toxicant-induced pulmonary fibrosis, including that induced by O_3, involve abnormalities in the type of collagen made. For example, there is an increase in type I collagen relative to type III collagen in patients with idiopathic pulmonary fibrosis. Similar shifts have been demonstrated in the lungs of adults and infants dying of acute respiratory distress syndrome. It is not known whether shifts in collagen types, compared with absolute increases in collagen content, account for the increased stiffness of fibrotic lungs. Type III collagen is much more compliant than is type I; thus, an increasing proportion of type I relative to type III collagen may result in a stiffer lung, as is observed in pulmonary fibrosis. Changes in collagen cross-linking in fibrotic lungs also may contribute to the increased stiffness. It is unclear whether the observed increase in stainable collagen is due solely to the increase in the collagen content of the lungs observed biochemically or whether altered collagen types or cross-linking might also contribute to the histological changes.

Increased collagen type I:type III ratios also have been observed in newly synthesized collagen in several animal models of acute pulmonary fibrosis. Although the mechanism for this shift in collagen types is unknown, there are many possible explanations. Clones of fibroblasts responsive to recruitment and/or proliferation factors may preferentially synthesize type I collagen compared with the action of the fibroblasts normally present. Alterations in the extracellular matrix resulting from inflammatory mediators secreted by various effector cells also may cause the fibroblasts to switch the collagen phenotype that is synthesized.

Collagen associated with fibrosis also may be abnormal with respect to cross-linking. Alterations in cross-links in experimental silicosis and bleomycin-induced fibrosis have been described. As in the case of alterations in collagen type ratios, it is unclear whether the mechanisms can be ascribed to changes in the clones of fibroblasts that actively synthesize collagen or to changes in the milieu that secondarily affect the nature of the collagen made by a given population of lung fibroblasts.

Emphysema

In many ways emphysema can be viewed as the opposite of fibrosis in terms of the response of the lungs to an insult: the lungs become larger and too compliant rather than becoming smaller and stiffer. Destruction of the gas-exchanging surface area results in a distended, hyperinflated lung that no longer effectively exchanges oxygen and carbon dioxide as a result of both loss of tissue and air trapping. The currently accepted pathological definition of emphysema is "a condition of the lung characterized by abnormal enlargement of the airspaces distal to the terminal bronchiole, accompanied by destruction of the walls, without obvious fibrosis" (Snider et al., 1985). The major cause of human emphysema is, by far, cigarette smoke inhalation, although other toxicants also can elicit this response. A feature of toxicant-induced emphysema is severe or recurrent inflammation, especially alveolitis with release of proteolytic enzymes by participating leukocytes.

A unifying hypothesis that explains the pathogenesis of emphysema has emerged from studies by several investigators. Early clinical research on screening blood protein phenotypes identified a rare mutation giving rise to a hereditary deficiency of the serum globulin alpha$_1$-antitrypsin. Homozygotes for this mutation had no circulating levels of this protein, which can prevent the proteolytic activity of serine proteases such as trypsin. Thus, alpha$_1$-antitrypsin (now called alpha$_1$-antiprotease) is one of the body's main defenses against uncontrolled proteolytic digestion by this class of enzymes, which includes elastase. There is a clinical association between the genetic lack of this important inhibitor of elastase and the development of emphysema at an extraordinarily young age. Further studies in smokers led to the hypothesis that neutrophil (and perhaps alveolar macrophage) elastases can break down lung elastin and thus cause emphysema; these elastases usually are kept in check by alpha$_1$-antiprotease that diffuses into the lung from the blood. As the individual ages, an accumulation of random elastolytic events can cause the emphysematous changes in the lungs that are normally associated with aging. Toxicants that cause inflammatory cell influx and thus increase the burden of neutrophil elastase can accelerate this process. In accordance with this hypothesis are a large number of experimental studies in animals instilled intratracheally with pancreatic or neutrophil elastase or with other proteolytic enzymes that can digest elastin in which a pathological condition develops that has some of the characteristics of emphysema, including destruction of alveolar walls and airspace enlargement in the lung parenchyma.

An additional clue to the pathogenesis of emphysema is provided by the observation that mice with defects in genes that code for elastin and collagen modifying enzymes develop emphysema (O'Byrne and Postma, 1999). These observations suggest that problems with elastin synthesis may play an important role in the pathogenesis of emphysema, and that in its simplest form the elastase-antiprotease model alone cannot fully explain the detailed biochemical mechanisms that underlie the etiology of emphysema.

Asthma

Asthma is becoming increasingly prevalent in the United States and Europe, especially in crowded urban areas. This disease is characterized clinically by attacks of shortness of breath, which may be mild or severe. It is caused by narrowing of the large conducting airways (bronchi) either upon inhalation of provoking agents or for unknown causes. There are well-established links between occupational and environmental exposure to antigens or to chemicals that can act as haptens and in the pathogenesis of asthma. There are histopathologic components that are common between asthma and pulmonary fibrosis, but in this case the disease is centered in and around the large conducting airways rather than the centriacinar region of the lung parenchyma. There may be common mechanisms, especially with regard to the role of inflammatory cells and the cytokines and growth factors they secrete (Barnes et al., 1998). The clinical hallmark of asthma is increased airway reactivity: the smooth muscle around the large airways contract in response to exposure to irritants. The extreme sensitivity of guinea pigs (as opposed to rats or mice) to inhaled irritants such as ozone or SO_2 may be an example of an animal model of the human asthmatic subject (Barnes et al., 1998).

Lung Cancer

Lung cancer, an extremely rare disease around the turn of the century, is now the leading cause of death from cancer among men and women. Retrospective and, more conclusively, prospective epidemiologic studies unequivocally show an association between tobacco smoking and lung cancer. It has been estimated that approximately 80 to 90 percent of lung cancers (and several other cancers, such as cancer of the bladder, esophagus, oral cavity, and pancreas) are caused by cigarette smoking. Average smokers have a 10-fold and heavy smokers a 20-fold increased risk of developing lung cancer compared with nonsmokers. Quitting the habit will reduce the risk (Wingo et al., 1999).

Inhalation of asbestos fibers and metallic dusts or fumes— such as arsenic, beryllium, cadmium, chromium, and nickel, encountered in smelting and manufacturing operations— has been associated with cancer of the respiratory tract. Workers who manufacture chloromethyl ether or mustard gas also have an increased risk of developing lung cancers, as do workers exposed to effluent gases from coke ovens. Radon gas is a known human lung carcinogen. Formaldehyde is a probable human respiratory carcinogen. Silica, human-made fibers, and welding fumes are suspected carcinogens (International Agency for Research on Cancer, 1987, 1993). Smokers who inhale radon or asbestos fibers increase their risk of developing lung cancer severalfold, suggesting a synergistic interaction between the carcinogens. To what extent common air pollutants such as ozone, nitrogen dioxide, sulfur dioxide, and fumes emanating from power plants, oil refineries, and Diesel fuel–powered trucks and cars contribute to the development of lung cancer in the general population remains an open question. Some evidence suggests that respirable particulates suspended in polluted air are a risk factor (Beeson et al., 1998). Indoor air pollution, including environmental tobacco smoke, increases the risk of developing lung cancer in nonsmokers (National Cancer Institute, 1999).

Human lung cancers may have a latency period of 20 to 40 years, making the relationship to specific exposures difficult to establish. Many lung cancers in humans originate from the cells lining the airways (lung cancer originating from such sites is often referred to as bronchogenic carcinoma), but during the last two decades a significant increase in peripheral adenocarcinomas has occurred. Compared with cancer in the lung, cancer in the upper respiratory tract is less common. Malignant lesions of the nasal passages, which are seen frequently in experimental animals, are comparatively rare in humans. They are associated with certain occupations, including work with chromate, nickel, mustard gas, isopropyl alcohol, the manufacture of wooden furniture, and boot and shoe manufacture. Possible carcinogens include hexavalent chromium compounds, metallic nickel and nickel subsulfide, nickel oxide, formaldehyde, and certain wood and leather dusts.

The potential mechanisms of lung carcinogenesis have been studied extensively by means of analysis of tumor material and in studies of human bronchial cells maintained in culture. Damage to DNA is thought to be a key mechanism. An activated carcinogen or its metabolic product, such as alkyldiazonium ions derived from *N*-nitrosamines, may interact with DNA. Persistence of O^6-alkyldeoxyguanosine in DNA appears to correlate with carcinogenicity (Hecht, 1999). However, tumors do not always develop when adducts are present, and adduct formation may be a necessary but not sufficient condition for carcinogenesis. DNA damage caused by active oxygen species is another potentially important mechanism. Ionizing radiation leads to the formation of superoxide, which is converted through the action of superoxide dismutase to hydrogen peroxide. In the presence of Fe and other transition metals, hydroxyl radicals may be formed which then cause DNA strand breaks. Cigarette smoke contains high quantities of active oxygen species and other free radicals. Additional oxidative stress may be placed on the lung tissue of smokers by the release of superoxide anions and hydrogen peroxide by activated macrophages, metabolism of carcinogens, and lipid peroxidation caused by reactive aldehydes.

In laboratory animals, spontaneously occurring malignant lung tumors are uncommon unless the animals reach a very advanced age. Exposure to carcinogens by the inhalation route or by intratracheal instillation or systemic administration readily produces lung tumors in many laboratory species, such as mice, rats, hamsters, and dogs. There are several differences between lung tumors in animals and bronchogenic cancer in humans. In animals, particularly rodents, most tumors are in the periphery rather than arising from the bronchi. The incidence of benign lung tumors such as adenomas is often very high, and carcinomas seem to require more time to develop. Lung tumors in animals do not metastasize as aggressively, if they do so at all, as do human lung cancers (Hahn, 1997). Cancer of the nasal passages is readily induced in experimental animals in inhalation studies.

Because lung tumors in mice and rats are often seen in carcinogenesis bioassays, they deserve special mention. Murine lung tumors are mostly benign-appearing adenomas originating from alveolar type II cells or bronchiolar Clara cells. They can progress to adenocarcinomas and invade lymphatics and blood vessels. Certain mouse strains, such as strain A and the Swiss-Webster mouse, have a high incidence of spontaneously occurring lung tumors. These animals respond with increased numbers of tumors to the inhalation or injection of many carcinogens. Other strains are much more resistant. Lung tumors in strain A mice have become valuable tools for studing the genetic factors that determine susceptibility (Malkinson, 1998). They contain frequent mutations in the K-*ras* gene, a mutation also found frequently in human lung cancers (Graziano et al., 1999). Methylating nitrosamines (NNK and DMN) produce mutations consistent with the formation of O^6-methylguanine and ethylating nitrosamines (ENU and DEN) and mutations consistent with the formation of O^4-ethylthymidine. In strains less susceptible than the A/J mouse, chemicals such as tetranitromethane, 1,3-butadiene, DMN, and NNK generate tumors with mutations consistent with the result of DNA adduct formation, whereas other chemicals (acetylaminofluorene, methylene chloride) do not produce tumors with carcinogen-specific mutations.

Lung tumors in rats exposed to airborne carcinogens consist mostly of peripheral adenocarcinomas and squamous cell carcinomas. In addition, rat lungs on occasion contain lesions that are characterized by an epithelium surrounding a space filled with keratin. The mass may compress the adjacent lung parenchyma and occasionally invades it. These lesions are classified by some pathologists as bona fide tumors, whereas other pathologists characterize this type of lesion as a cyst filled with keratin. Classification of such a lesion as a tumor is important because these lesions often are found in long-term tests in animals that have been exposed to agents that are not considered carcinogens, such as carbon black, titanium dioxide, and certain human-made fibers (ILSI, 2000).

AGENTS KNOWN TO PRODUCE LUNG INJURY IN HUMANS

The prevention and treatment of acute and chronic lung disease will eventually be based on a knowledge of the cellular and molecular events that determine lung injury and repair. During the past 20 years, a large body of evidence has accumulated. Table 15-1 lists common toxicants that are known to produce acute and chronic lung injury in humans. In the following sections, a few examples of our current understanding of lung injury at the mechanistic level are discussed, with emphasis on agents directly responsible for human lung disease.

Airborne Agents That Produce Lung Injury in Humans

Asbestos The term "asbestos" describes silicate minerals in fiber form. The most commonly mined and commercially used asbestos fibers include the serpentine chrysotile asbestos and the amphiboles crocidolite, anthophyllite, amosite, actinolite, and tremolite. Exposure to asbestos fibers occurs in mining operations and in the construction and shipbuilding industries, where asbestos was at one time widely used for its highly desirable insulating and fireproofing properties. During the last few years, concern about asbestos in older buildings has led to the removal of asbestos-based insulating material; abatement workers may now represent an additional population at risk.

Asbestos causes three forms of lung disease in humans: asbestosis, lung cancer, and malignant mesothelioma. Asbestosis is characterized by a diffuse increase of collagen in the alveolar walls (fibrosis) and the presence of asbestos fibers, either free or coated with a proteinaceous material (asbestos bodies). Malignant mesothelioma (a tumor of the cells covering the surface of the visceral and parietal pleura), a tumor that otherwise occurs only extremely rarely in the general population, is unequivocally associated with asbestos exposure. There is some discrepancy between human observations and animal data. In animal experiments, chrysotile produces mesothelioma much more readily than do the amphibole fibers. In humans, amphibole fibers are implicated more often even when the predominant exposure is to chrysotile asbestos. Chrysotile breaks down much more readily than do the amphiboles. It is possible that in small laboratory animals chrysotile fibers, even if broken down, are retained longer relative to the life span of the animal than they are in humans, thus explaining the higher rate of mesothelioma development.

The hazards associated with asbestos exposure depend on fiber length. Fibers 2 μm in length may produce asbestosis; mesothelioma is associated with fibers 5 μm long, and lung cancer with fibers larger than 10 μm. Fiber diameter is another critical feature. Fibers with diameters larger than approximately 3 μm do not readily penetrate into the peripheral lung. For the development of mesothelioma, fiber diameter must be less than 0.5 μm, since thinner fibers may be translocated from their site of deposition via the lymphatics to other organs, including the pleural surface.

Once asbestos fibers have been deposited in the lung, they may become phagocytized by alveolar macrophages. Short fibers are completely ingested and subsequently removed via the mucociliary escalator. Longer fibers are incompletely ingested, and the macrophages become unable to leave the alveoli. Activated by the fibers, macrophages release mediators such as lymphokines and growth factors, which in turn attract immunocompetent cells or stimulate collagen production. Asbestos-related lung disease thus may be mediated through the triggering of an inflammatory sequence of events or the production of changes that eventually lead to the initiation (DNA damage caused by reactive molecular species) or promotion (increased rate of cell turnover in the lung) of the carcinogenic process.

The surface properties of asbestos fibers appear to be an important mechanistic element in toxicity. The protection afforded by superoxide dismutase or free radical scavengers in asbestos-related cell injury in vitro suggests that the generation of active oxygen species and concomitant lipid peroxidation are important mechanisms in asbestos toxicity. The interaction of iron on the surface of asbestos fibers with oxygen may lead to the production of hydrogen peroxide and the highly reactive hydroxyl radical, events that have been associated with asbestos toxicity (Timblin et al., 1999).

Silica Silicosis in humans may be acute or chronic; this distinction is important conceptually because the pathological consequences are manifested quite differently. Acute silicosis occurs only in subjects exposed to a very high level of aerosol containing particles small enough to be respirable (usually less than 5 μm) over a relatively short period, generally a few months to a few years.

Table 15-1
Industrial Toxicants That Produce Lung Disease

TOXICANT	COMMON NAME OF DISEASE	OCCUPATIONAL SOURCE	ACUTE EFFECT	CHRONIC EFFECT
Asbestos	Asbestosis	Mining, construction, shipbuilding, manufacture of asbestos-containing material		Fibrosis, pleural calcification, lung cancer, pleural mesothelioma
Aluminum dust	Aluminosis	Manufacture of aluminum products, fireworks, ceramics, paints, electrical goods, abrasives	Cough, shortness of breath	Interstitial fibrosis
Aluminum abrasives	Shaver's disease, corundum smelter's lung, bauxite lung	Manufacture of abrasives, smelting	Alveolar edema	Interstitial fibrosis, emphysema
Ammonia		Ammonia production, manufacture of fertilizers, chemical production, explosives	Upper and lower respiratory tract irritation, edema	Chronic bronchitis
Arsenic		Manufacture of pesticides, pigments, glass, alloys	Bronchitis	Lung cancer, bronchitis, laryngitis
Beryllium	Berylliosis	Ore extraction, manufacture of alloys, ceramics	Severe pulmonary edema, pneumonia	Fibrosis, progressive dyspnea, interstitial granulomatosis, lung cancer, cor pulmonale
Cadmium oxide		Welding, manufacture of electrical equipment, alloys, pigments, smelting	Cough, pneumonia	Emphysema, cor pulmonale
Carbides of tungsten, titanium, tantalum	Hard metal disease	Manufacture of cutting edges on tools	Hyperplasia and metaplasia of bronchial epithelium	Peribronchial and perivascular fibrosis
Chlorine		Manufacture of pulp and paper, plastics, chlorinated chemicals	Cough, hemoptysis, dyspnea, tracheobronchitis, bronchopneumonia	
Chromium (VI)		Production of Cr compounds, paint pigments, reduction of chromite ore	Nasal irritation, bronchitis	Lung cancer, fibrosis
Coal dust	Pneumoconiosis	Coal mining		Fibrosis
Cotton dust	Byssinosis	Manufacture of textiles	Chest tightness, wheezing, dyspnea	Reduced pulmonary function, chronic bronchitis
Hydrogen fluoride		Manufacture of chemicals, photographic film, solvents, plastics	Respiratory irritation, hemorrhagic pulmonary edema	
Iron oxides	Siderotic lung disease; silver finisher's lung, hematite miner's lung, arc welder's lung	Welding, foundry work, steel manufacture, hematite mining, jewelry making	Cough	Silver finisher's lung: subpleural and perivascular aggregations of macrophages; hematite miner's lung: diffuse fibrosislike pneumoconiosis; arc welder's lung: bronchitis
Isocyanates		Manufacture of plastics, chemical industry	Airway irritation, cough, dyspnea	Asthma, reduced pulmonary function

Table 15-1
Industrial Toxicants That Produce Lung Disease *(Continued)*

TOXICANT	COMMON NAME OF DISEASE	OCCUPATIONAL SOURCE	ACUTE EFFECT	CHRONIC EFFECT
Kaolin	Kaolinosis	Pottery making		Fibrosis
Manganese	Manganese pneumonia	Chemical and metal industries	Acute pneumonia, often fatal	Recurrent pneumonia
Nickel		Nickel ore extraction, smelting, electronic electroplating, fossil fuels	Pulmonary edema, delayed by 2 days (NiCO)	Squamous cell carcinoma of nasal cavity and lung
Oxides of nitrogen		Welding, silo filling, explosive manufacture	Pulmonary congestion and edema	Bronchiolitis obliterans
Ozone		Welding, bleaching flour, deodorizing	Pulmonary edema	Fibrosis
Phosgene		Production of plastics, pesticides, chemicals	Edema	Bronchitis, fibrosis
Perchloro-ethylene		Dry cleaning, metal degreasing, grain fumigating	Edema	Cancer, liver and lung
Silica	Silicosis, pneumoconiosis	Mining, stone cutting, construction, farming, quarrying, sand blasting	Acute silicosis	Fibrosis, silicotuberculosis
Sulfur dioxide		Manufacture of chemicals, refrigeration, bleaching, fumigation	Bronchoconstriction, cough, chest tightness	Chronic bronchitis
Talc	Talcosis	Rubber industry, cosmetics		Fibrosis
Tin	Stanosis	Mining, processing of tin		Widespread mottling of x-ray without clinical signs
Vanadium		Steel manufacture	Airway irritation and mucus production	Chronic bronchitis

These patients have worsening dyspnea, fever, cough, and weight loss. There is rapid progression of respiratory failure, usually ending in death within a year or two. No known treatment modality influences the relentless course of acute silicosis.

Chronic silicosis has a long latency period, usually more than 10 years. Uncomplicated silicosis is almost entirely asymptomatic; little alteration is shown on routine pulmonary function tests even after the disease is radiographically demonstrable. The x-ray picture presents fibrotic nodules, generally in the apical portion of lung. The hilar lymph nodes have peripheral calcifications known as eggshell calcifications. Simple silicosis may progress into complicated silicosis, which is defined as the presence of conglomerate nodules larger than 1 cm in diameter. These nodules usually occur in the upper and midlung zones. At an advanced stage they may be surrounded by emphysematous bullae. Chronic silicosis is associated with an increased incidence of tuberculosis.

Crystalline silica is a major component of the earth's crust; after oxygen, silicon is the most common element. As a pure mineral, silicon exists primarily in the form of its dioxide, silica (SiO_2), which has a crystalline form in which a central silicon atom forms a tetrahedron with four shared oxygen atoms. The three principal crystalline isomeric forms are quartz, tridymite, and cristobalite. The tetrahedral structure is linked to fibrogenic potential. Stishovite, a rare crystalline variant without the tetrahedral conformation, is biologically inert. Amorphous forms of silica such as kieselguhr and vitreous silica have very low fibrogenic potential. The ubiquitous presence of silica has made it an occupational hazard ever since humans began shaping tools from stone, and silicosis remains a significant industrial hazard throughout the world in occupations such as mining and quarrying, sandblasting, and foundry work. The main factors that affect the pathogenicity of silica both in vivo and in vitro, in addition to its structure, are particle size and concentration. Many studies have examined the relationship of silica particle size to fibrogenicity. In studies with humans, the most fibrogenic particle size appears to be about 1 μm (range 0.5 to 3μm). In animal experiments (rats, hamsters), the comparable values appear to be 1 to 2 μm (range 0.5 to 5 μm). In animal models, there appears to be a direct relationship between the concentration of silica dust to which an animal is exposed and the intensity and rapidity of the histologic reaction in the lung.

The pathophysiological basis of pulmonary fibrosis in chronic silicosis is probably better understood than is the etiology of any other form of lung fibrosis. The role of pulmonary alveolar macrophages in the ingestion of silica as an initiating event has been established. Apparently, as part of the cytotoxic response of a macrophage to silica ingestion, the macrophage may release cytokines and other substances that cause fibroblasts to replicate and/or increase their rate of collagen biosynthesis. The role of inflammatory cells other than alveolar macrophages in this process is unknown. Also not understood is the role of the host's immune response and the roles of lymphocyte factors in stimulating fibroblast proliferation and/or collagen synthesis by fibroblasts in lung fibrogenesis (Varani and Ward, 1997).

Lung Overload Caused by Particles Investigators studying the kinetics of the pulmonary clearance of particles have observed a slowing of the rate of alveolar clearance when deposited lung burdens are high. At about the same time, investigators evaluating inhaled particles in carcinogenesis bioassays observed excess tumors in animals that inhaled very high concentrations of apparently inert so-called nuisance dusts, which were included in such experiments as negative controls. From these observations came a unifying hypothesis (Morrow, 1992) that clearance mechanisms in the deep lung depending predominantly if not completely on phagocytosis and migration of pulmonary alveolar macrophages can be overwhelmed by quantities of respirable dusts far in excess of physiologic loads. As a consequence, lung burdens of these dusts persist for months or years, and completely unphysiologic mechanisms of disease pathogenesis may come into play. In rats, lung tumors have been produced by particles such as Diesel exhaust that carry mutagens and carcinogens on their surface, but also by inert carbon black particles. The issue of whether particle overloading defines a threshold in such experiments remains unresolved.

Naphthalene Naphthalene occurs in tars and petroleum and is a widely used precursor chemical for synthetic tanning agents, phthalic acid anhydride, carbaryl, and 2-naphthol. It is present in ambient air. Smokers inhale substantial amounts of naphthalene in cigarette smoke. In experimental animals, inhaled or parenterally administered naphthalene has shown remarkable species and tissue specificity: it produces extensive and selective necrosis in the bronchiolar epithelium of the mouse but much less necrosis in rats and hamsters.

Animals treated with small doses of naphthalene or inhibitors of microsomal oxidases show little or no tissue damage, implicating metabolism in the toxicity of this chemical. Metabolism to the oxide is mediated through cytochrome P450 1A1 and 2F2. Naphthalene epoxides may subsequently be conjugated with glutathione and form adducts that presumably are not toxic. It is also possible that the epoxides undergo rearrangement to 1-naphthol with subsequent metabolism to quinones, which are potentially toxic compounds. In rats and other species, probably including humans, conversion of naphthalene is less stereospecific and rates of formation of the epoxide are much slower than in mice. This may explain the species differences that were noted previously (Franklin et al., 1993).

Oxygen Oxygen toxicity is mediated though increased production of partially reduced oxygen products such as superoxide anion, perhydroperoxy and hydroxyl radicals, peroxynitrite and possibly singlet molecular oxygen. In infants who are given oxygen therapy after birth, a syndrome known as bronchopulmonary dysplasia may develop. Lung pathology is characterized by necrotizing bronchiolitis, fibroblast proliferation, squamous metaplasia of the bronchial lining, and destruction of alveolar ducts. In animals exposed to 95 to 100% oxygen, diffuse pulmonary damage develops and is usually fatal after 3 to 4 days. There is extensive damage to the cells of the alveolar-capillary septum. Type I epithelial cells and capillary endothelial cells develop necrotic changes. Capillary damage leads to leakage of proteinaceous fluid and formed blood elements into the alveolar space. Hyaline membranes formed by cellular debris and proteinaceous exudate are a characteristic sign of pulmonary oxygen toxicity. In animals returned to air after the development of acute oxygen toxicity, there is active cell proliferation (Frank, 1997).

Blood-Borne Agents That Cause Pulmonary Toxicity in Humans

Paraquat The bipyridylium compound paraquat, a widely used herbicide, produces extensive lung injury when ingested by humans. In patients who survive the first few days of acute paraquat poisoning, progressive and eventually fatal lung lesions can develop. Paraquat lung disease is characterized by diffuse interstitial and intraalveolar fibrosis. The initial damage consists of widespread necrosis of both type I and type II epithelial cells of the alveolar region. Extensive proliferation of fibroblasts in the alveolar interstitium and the largely collapsed alveoli follows. Paraquat accumulates in the cells of the lung through the polyamine uptake system. Once inside the cells, paraquat continuously cycles from its oxidized form to the reduced form, with the concomitant formation of active oxygen species. A mechanistic hypothesis to explain paraquat toxicity involves oxidation of cellular NADPH and eventual depletion of the NADPH content of pulmonary cells (Smith, 1997).

Monocrotaline Monocrotaline (MCT) is a pyrrolizidine alkaloid, one of many structurally related naturally occurring products of plants that have been identified in grains, honey and herbal teas. These compounds produce liver toxicity (hepatocellular necrosis and veno-occlusive disease). Although the hepatic metabolism of the pyrrolidine alkaloids is usually completed by 24 h, the administration of a single dose of monocrotaline is known to initiate a delayed lung injury. This pulmonary lesion is characterized by a remodeling of the vascular bed with hyperplasia of capillary endothelial cells, thickening of the arterial media, formation of microthrombi, and eventually capillary occlusion with resulting hypertension of the pulmonary arterial system and hypertrophy of the right side of the heart.

Monocrotaline propagates changes in the contractile response of arterial smooth muscle, changes in smooth muscle Na/K-ATPase activity, release of platelet factors, and decreased serotonin transport by vascular endothelial cells (Wilson et al., 1992). Monocrotaline is metabolized in the liver by cytochrome P450 3A to a highly reactive pyrrole, a bifunctional alkylating agent, where some of the reactive pyrrole forms nontoxic conjugates with either glutathione or cysteine. A percentage of the remaining pyrrole is released from the liver and travels to other organs, such as the lung and possibly the kidney, via red blood cells (RBCs), where it initiates endothelial injury. It had been previously shown that RBCs circulated through an isolated perfused buffer containing [^{14}C]MCT, subsequently washed and recirculated through an isolated lung preparation could transfer electrophiles to pulmonary tissues. Recent evidence has indicated that the pyrrole is conjugated to the RBCs, mainly to the $\beta\beta$-chains of hemoglobin (Laméé et al., 1997) . These pyrrole adducts may be particularly susceptible to removal from globin chains following either enzymatic degradation or environmental changes observed during circulation through hepatic and pulmonary tissues and consequently interact with key target proteins.

Bleomycin Bleomycin, a mixture of several structurally similar compounds, is a widely used cancer chemotherapeutic agent. Pulmonary fibrosis, often fatal, represents the most serious form of toxicity. The sequence of damage includes necrosis of capillary endothelial and type I alveolar cells, edema formation and hemorrhage, delayed (after 1 to 2 weeks) proliferation of type II epithelial cells, and eventually thickening of the alveolar walls by fibrotic changes.

In many tissues, the cytosolic enzyme bleomycin hydrolase inactivates bleomycin. In lung and skin, two target organs for bleomycin toxicity, the activity of this enzyme is low compared with that in other organs. Bleomycin stimulates the production of collagen in the lung. Before increased collagen biosynthesis, steady-state levels of mRNA coding for fibronectin and procollagens are increased, presumably subsequent to a bleomycin-mediated release of cytokines such as TGF-β and TNF. Bleomycin also combines with Fe(II) and molecular oxygen; when it combines with DNA, single- and double-strand breaks are produced by a free radical reaction (Hoyt and Lazo, 1997).

Cyclophosphamide and 1,3-Bis-(2-Chloroethyl)-1-Nitrosourea (BCNU) Cyclophosphamide is widely used as an anticancer and immunosuppressive agent. The undesirable side effects include hemorrhagic cystitis and pulmonary fibrosis. Cyclophosphamide is metabolized by the cytochrome P450 system to two highly reactive metabolites: acrolein and phosphoramide mustard. In the lung, cooxidation with the prostaglandin-H synthase system, which has high activity in the lung, is a possibility. Although the exact mechanism of action for causing lung damage has not been established, studies with isolated lung microsomes have shown that cyclophosphamide and its metabolite acrolein initiate lipid peroxidation. Carmustine (BCNU) is an effective chemotherapeutic agent that exerts its antitumor properties by reacting with cellular macromolecules and forms inter- and intrastrand cross-links with DNA. In humans, a dose-related pulmonary toxicity is often noticed first by a decrease in diffusion capacity. Pulmonary fibrosis caused by this drug can be fatal. The mechanism of action is not entirely clear. It is possible that BCNU inhibits pulmonary glutathione disulfide reductase, an event that may lead to a disturbed GSH/GSSG state in pulmonary cells. Eventually, this state leaves the cell unable to cope with oxidant stress. High concentrations of oxygen in the inspired air may enhance the pulmonary toxicity of BCNU and also that of the other anticancer drugs known to affect lung tissue: cyclophosphamide and bleomycin. Several other chemotherapeutic agents can produce lung damage and pulmonary toxicity in patients treated with these drugs can be a significant problem (Ramu and Kehrer, 1997).

Cationic Amphophilic Drugs Several drugs with similar structural characteristics that are called cationic amphophilic drugs (CADs) produce pulmonary lipidosis. The antiarrhythmic amiodarone and the anorexic chlorphentermine elicit such changes in humans. Pulmonary lipidosis is characterized by the intracellular presence, particularly in macrophages, of large concentric membranous structures now known to be secondary lysosomes. CADs inhibit phospholipases A and B, presumably because these drugs combine with phospholipids and form indigestible complexes. Degradation of pulmonary surfactant is impaired, and the material accumulates in phagocytic cells. In humans, amiodarone may cause dyspnea and cough. In animals and humans, the condition is fully reversible on drug withdrawal (Reasor, 1997).

METHODS FOR STUDYING LUNG INJURY

Inhalation Exposure Systems

The generation of a gas available in high purity as a compressed "tank gas," for example, SO_2, O_2, or NO_2, is relatively straightforward, and metering and dilution produce appropriate concentrations for exposure. Monitoring and quantifying gaseous pollutants require either expensive detectors that need frequent calibration (and usually a computer to process the tremendous amount of data generated) or very labor intensive wet chemical analysis procedures after sampled gases from the chambers are bubbled through traps. Particle generation is difficult, and specialized references must be consulted (Wong, 1999).

Exposure chambers must allow for the rapid attainment of the desired concentrations of toxicants, maintenance of desired levels homogeneously throughout the chamber, adequate capacity for experimental animals, and minimal accumulation of undesired products associated with animal occupancy (usually ammonia, dander, heat, and carbon dioxide). Modern chambers tend to be fabricated from inert materials (usually glass, stainless steel, and Teflon) and have flow patterns that are designed to promote mixing and homogeneity of the chamber atmosphere and prevent a buildup of undesirable contaminants. A major concern with regard to exposure to acid aerosols has been the putative buildup of ammonia in chambers because of microbial action on animal excreta. Thus, maximal loading factors and sanitation also must be considered in chamber usage. As a general rule, the total body volume of the animals should not exceed 5 percent of the chamber volume. Nose-only exposure chambers avoid some of these problems. Finally, concern for the environment and the safety of facility personnel suggest prudence in how chambers are exhausted.

In inhalation studies, selection of animals with a respiratory system similar to that of humans is particularly desirable. The respiratory system of monkeys most closely resembles that of humans. However, the availability and cost of animals and the necessity for special facilities for housing monkeys and performing long-term exposures, along with ethical considerations, including the confinement of primates in small exposure chambers for prolonged periods, severely limit the use of primates. Rats are widely used, although fundamental differences in respiratory anatomy (for example, lack of respiratory bronchioles) and function (rats are obligate nose breathers) can complicate the extrapolation of effects to humans. Guinea pigs and rabbits have been used to predict the response of humans to sulfuric acid (Amdur, 1989).

Pulmonary Function Studies

Numerous tests are available with which to study pulmonary function and gas exchange in humans and experimental animals. Commonly used tests include measurement of VC, TLC, functional residual volume, TV, airway resistance, and maximum flow (Fig. 15-6). Additional tests evaluate the distribution of ventilation,

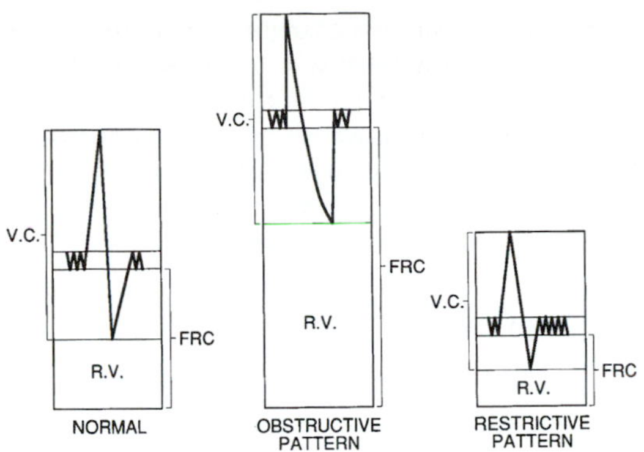

Figure 15-6. Typical lung volume measurements from individuals with normal lung function, obstructive airways disease, or restrictive lung disease.

Note that there is (1) a slowing of forced expiration in addition to gas trapping (an increase in residual volume) in obstructive disease and (2) a general decrease in lung volumes in restrictive disease. Note that the measurements read from left to right.

lung and chest wall compliance, diffusion capacity, and the oxygen and carbon dioxide content of the arterial and venous blood (Costa et al., 1991).

Many pulmonary function tests require active collaboration by the subject examined, for example, the so-called FEV_1 (forced expiratory volume) during the first second of an active exhalation. This is an easy test to administer to humans, does not require sophisticated equipment or a hospital setting, and is completely noninvasive. The subject is asked first to inhale deeply and then to exhale the air as quickly as possible. The test is often used in epidemiological studies or controlled clinical studies designed to assess the potential adverse effects of air pollutants. A reduction in FEV_1 is usually indicative of impaired ventilation such as that found in restrictive (increased lung stiffness) or obstructive (obstructed airflow) lung disease. Experimental animals, by contrast, cannot be made to maximally inhale or exhale at the investigator's will. In experimental animals, FEV_1 can be obtained, but the test is done under anesthesia. Expiration is forced by applying external pressure to the thorax or negative pressure to the airways.

Analysis of breathing patterns has been widely used to assess the effects of irritants. This technique allows one to differentiate between sensory or upper airway irritants and "pulmonary" irritants. Highly water soluble irritants such as ammonia, chlorine, and formaldehyde produce upper respiratory tract irritation, whereas less soluble gases such as nitrogen dioxide and ozone generate pulmonary irritation. The sensory irritant pattern has been described as slowing down respiratory frequency while increasing TV. Pulmonary irritants usually increase respiratory frequency and decrease minute volume. The result is rapid, shallow breathing.

Analysis of volume-pressure curves of the lung provides some indication of lung compliance. Compliance (volume/ pressure) is measured as the slope of the volume-pressure curve; it gives some indication of the intrinsic elastic properties of the lung parenchyma and, when measured in vivo, the thoracic cage. This is a comparatively easy test to perform in animals, requiring little specialized apparatus. Cannulation of the excised lungs and attachment to a syringe and manometer to measure volume and pressure are all that is needed. Volume-pressure curves can be obtained from lungs filled with air or physiological saline. The latter test is much more sensitive to structural changes in lung parenchyma, as the effects of surfactant are eliminated in a saline-filled lung.

To accomplish proper oxygenation of venous blood and elimination of CO_2, the gases have to diffuse across the air-blood barrier. Gas exchange may be hindered by the accumulation of fluids or cellular elements in the alveoli (edema, pneumonic infiltrates), thickening of the alveolar wall (fibrosis), insufficient ventilation of the alveolar region (emphysema), or insufficient presence of oxygen transport elements (reduced alveolar blood volume or reduced amount of hemoglobin in the blood). Gas exchange can be evaluated by measuring the arterial partial pressure of both oxygen and CO_2. In experimental animals, the collection of arterial blood may require the presence of indwelling catheters.

In general, blood gas analysis is a comparatively insensitive assay for disturbed ventilation because of the organism's buffering and reserve capacities. While it is a useful tool in clinical medicine, only the most severe obstructive or restrictive pulmonary alterations cause signs of impaired gas exchange in animals. Measurement of diffusion capacity with CO, a gas that binds with 250 times higher affinity to hemoglobin than does oxygen, is more sensitive. The test is comparatively easy to perform in both humans and laboratory animals and is widely used in toxicology studies.

Morphologic Techniques

The pathology of acute and chronic injury may be described after examination of the respiratory tract by gross inspection and under the microscope. Morphologic evaluation should not be limited to the peripheral lung; nasal passages, the larynx, and major airways must be examined as carefully as is the lung parenchyma. For example, formaldehyde produces nasal tumors but not deep lung tumors in the rat. In hamsters exposed to cigarette smoke, cancerous changes are found in the larynx but not in the more distal airways.

Careful consideration must be given to tissue fixation and preparation. Nasal passages must be flushed with fixative. After decalcification, cross sections should be cut at multiple levels; the regional distribution of lesions may vary from agent to agent. Proper fixation of the lung is done by vascular perfusion with fixative through the pulmonary artery or by instillation of fixative through the trachea. Perfusion fixation does not dislodge material (lining fluid, deposited particles) or cells in the lumen of the airways or the alveoli from their original position. Fixation by instillation does this, but it also keeps the alveoli open. It is done under controlled pressure, usually 30 cm H_2O, and is required if semiquantitative or quantitative measurements will be made. The choice of fixative depends on how the lung will be further analyzed. Formalin-based fixatives are satisfactory for routine histopathology, whereas the use of more sophisticated techniques such as electron microscopy, immunohistochemistry, and in situ hybridization require careful selection of the fixative.

Ordinary paraffin sections of respiratory tract tissue are suitable for routine histopathologic analysis; gross pathological changes such as inflammation and the presence of cancerous tissue can be detected easily. Plastic or epon sections about 1 μm thick are required for proper identification of different cell types lining the airways or alveoli and for recognition of cytoplasmic changes in damaged Clara cells. Other structural alterations, such as degenerative changes or necrosis of type I epithelial cells or capillary endothelial cells, usually are detected by transmission electron microscopy (TEM). TEM is essential for an unequivocal identification of cells in the alveolar interstitium and is used mainly in morphometric analysis of the lung. Scanning electron microscopy allows visualization of the surface of interior lung structures, reveals alterations in the tissue surface, and detects rearrangement of the overall cell population. Confocal microscopy, consisting of a laser microscope coupled to a computer, allows examination of thick sections and discovery of specific cell types deep within the tissue; it is an ideal tool for three-dimensional reconstruction of normal and damaged lung.

Morphometry, the quantitative description of structure, refers to a quantitative analysis of tissue (Gehr et al., 1993). Measurements made in two dimensions on photographs taken under the microscope allow one to measure areas, the thickness of a structure, and numerical density. With the help of appropriate formulas, values such as the volume occupied by a specific cell population in the entire lung parenchyma can be calculated. The method is particualry useful for the detection of subtle toxic effects in the lung parenchyma (Witschi et al., 1999).

Additional tools for the study of toxic lung injury include immunohistochemistry, in situ hybridization, and analysis of cell kinetics. Antibodies to a variety of enzymes, mediators, and other proteins are available. It is possible to identify cell types that carry certain enzymes and their anatomic locations. This information is important for mechanistic studies. In situ hybridization allows one to visualize anatomic sites where a specific gene product is expressed, for example, collagen production in a fibrotic lung. This technique is especially important in an organ such as the lung where there are more than 40 morphologically distinct cell types present. Ascribing a given metabolic capability to a specific cell type requires evaluation of gene expression and/or protein production in specific cells in situ. Flow cytometry is valuable in the study of cell populations prepared from the lung. The technique requires dissociation of the lung parenchyma into its individual cell populations. Different lung cells then can be identified and isolated.

Pulmonary Lavage

Pulmonary edema and/or pulmonary inflammation appear to be obligatory early events in acute and chronic lung injury. Markers of these processes generally are chosen to reflect lung edema or cellular changes in the lung. The most popular of these types of assays have quantified various parameters in lung lavage fluid from animals exposed to pneumotoxic substances. Generally, the lungs of exposed and control animals are washed with multiple small volumes of isotonic saline This technique has the further advantage of allowing direct comparisons with data accessible from normal human volunteers or patients undergoing bronchopulmonary lavage for therapeutic purposes. Current emphasis seems to be on the measurement of polymorphonuclear leukocytes, macrophages, and monocytes (and their phagocytotic capabilities) in the cellular fraction and the measurement of lactate dehydrogenase (and its substituent isoenzymes), *N*-acetylglucosaminidase, acid or alkaline phosphatase, other lysosomal hydrolases, lavageable total protein and/or albumin, and sialic acid. Although such measurements have often formed the basis of mechanistic interpretations, we really do not have a rigorous theoretical understanding of the exact source of any of these parameters.

Measurement of apparent changes in the permeability of the air-blood barrier by quantification of intravenously injected tracer in lung lavage fluid is another useful index of lung damage. The movement of low-molecular-weight tracers such as [^{51}Cr] EDTA across the blood-air barrier occurs rapidly (within 10 min of IV injection). High-molecular-weight tracers such as radiolabeled albumin also have been used for this purpose.

In Vitro Approaches

In vitro systems are particularly suited for the study of mechanisms that cause lung injury. The following systems are widely used (Postlethwait and Bidani, 1997).

Isolated Perfused Lung The isolated perfused lung method is applicable to lungs from many laboratory animal species (rabbit, rat, mouse, guinea pig). The lung, in situ or excised, is perfused with blood or a blood substitute through the pulmonary arterial bed. At the same time, the lung is actively (through rhythmic inflation-deflation cycles with positive pressure) or passively (by creating negative pressure with an "artificial thorax" in which the lung is suspended) ventilated. Toxic agents can be introduced into the perfusate or the inspired air. Repeated sampling of the perfusate allows one to determine the rate of metabolism of drugs and the metabolic activity of the lung.

Lung Explants and Slices Slices and explants from the conducting airways or the lung parenchyma allow one to examine biochemical and morphologic changes in the lung parenchyma without intervening complications from cells migrating into the tissue (e.g., leukocytes). If the lung is first inflated with agar, the alveolar spaces remain open in the explant. Slices prepared in this way can be kept viable for several weeks, and the mechanisms of development of chronic lesions can be studied.

Microdissection Many inhalants act in circumscribed regions of the respiratory tract, such as the terminal bronchioles, a region especially rich in metabolically highly competent Clara cells. Microdissection of the airways consists of the stripping of small bronchi and terminal bronchioli from the surrounding parenchyma and maintenance of the isolated airways in culture. Specific biochemical reactions predominantly located in the cells of the small airways can then be studied with biochemical or morphologic techniques.

Organotypic Cell Culture Systems Tissue culture systems have been developed in which epithelial cells maintain their polarity, differentiation, and normal function similar to what is observed in vivo. Epithelial cell surfaces are exposed to air (or a gas phase containing an airborne toxic agent), while the basal portion is bathed by a tissue culture medium. Epithelial cells may be seeded on top of a suitable supporting material (e.g., collagen or nitrocellulose membranes) with mesenchymal cells seeded on the other side to observe epithelial cell–fibroblast interactions.

Isolated Lung Cell Populations Many specific lung cell types have been isolated and maintained as primary cultures in vitro. Alveolar macrophages are easily obtained from human and animal lungs by lavage. Their function can be examined in vitro with or without exposure to appropriate toxic stimuli. Type II alveolar epithelial cells are isolated after digestion of the lung. Direct isolation of type I epithelial cells has also been successful. Systems for the isolation and culture of Clara cells and neuroepithelial cells are available. Lung fibroblasts are easily grown and have been studied in coculture with epithelial cells. Multiple primary cell cultures and cell lines have been established from lung tumors found in experimental animals and humans. Isolated cell techniques suffer from possible enzymatic digestion of critical cellular components. Caution should be exercised in the final interpretation of experiments utilizing this approach.

REFERENCES

Alarie Y, Nielsen GD, Abraham MD: A theoretical approach to the Ferguson principle and its use with nonreactive and reactive airborne chemicals. *Pharmacol Toxicol* 83:270–279, 1998.

Amdur MO: Sulfuric acid: The animals tried to tell us. 1989 Herbert Stokinger Lecture. *Appl Ind Hyg* 4:189–197, 1989.

Barnes PJ, Chung KF, Page CP: Inflammatory mediators of asthma: An update. *Pharmaco. Rev* 50:575–596, 1998.

Beeson WL, Abbey DE, Knutsen SF: Long-term concentrations of ambient air pollutants and incident lung cancer in California adults: Results from the ASHMOG study. *Environ Health Perspect* 106:813–823, 1998.

Buckpitt AR, Cruikshank MK: Biochemical function of the respiratory tract: Metabolism of xenobiotics, in Sipes IG, McQueen CA, Gandolfi JA (eds): *Comprehensive Toxicology.* Vol 8. Roth RA (ed): *Toxicology of the Respiratory System.* Oxford, England: Elsevier, 1997, pp 159–186.

Costa DL, Tepper JS, Raub JA: Interpretations and limitations of pulmonary function testing in small laboratory animals, in Parent RA (ed): *Comparative Biology of the Normal Lung.* Vol 1. *Treatise on Pulmonary Toxicology.* Boca Raton, FL: CRC Press, 1991, pp 367–399.

Crapo J, Miller FJ, Mossman B, et al: Relationship between acute inflammatory responses to air pollution and chronic lung disease. *Am Rev Respir Dis* 145:1506–1512, 1992.

Cross DE, van der Vliet A, Louie S, et al: Oxidative stress and antioxidants at biosurfaces: Plants, skin, and respiratory tract surfaces. *Environ Health Perspect* 106(suppl 5):1241–1251, 1998.

Fanucchi MV, Harkema JR, Plopper CG, Hotchkiss JA: In vitro culture of microdissected rat nasal airway tissues. *Am J Respir Cell Mol Biol* 20:1274–1285, 1999.

Frank L: Oxygen toxicity, in Sipes IG, McQueen CA, Gandolfi JA (eds): *Comprehensive Toxicology.*Vol 8. Roth RA (ed): *Toxicology of the Respiratory System.* Oxford, England: Elsevier, 1997, pp 275–302.

Franklin RB, Plopper CG, Buckpitt AR: Naphthalene and 2-methylnaphthalene-induced pulmonary bronchiolar epithelial cell necrosis: Metabolism and relationship to toxicity, in Gram TE (ed): *International Encyclopedia of Pharmacology and Therapeutics.* Sec 138: *Metabolic Activation of Toxicity of Chemical Agents to Lung Tissue and Cells.* New York: Pergamon Press, 1993, pp 123–144.

Gehr P, Geiser M, Stone KC, Crapo JD: Morphometric analysis of the gas exchange region of the lung, in: Gardner DE, Crapo JD, McClellan RO (eds): *Toxicology of the Lung,* 2d ed. New York: Raven Press, 1993, pp 111–154.

Graziano SL, Gamble GP, Newman NB, et al: Prognostic significance of K-*ras* codon 12 mutations in patients with resected stage I and II non-small-cell lung cancer. *J Cli Oncol* 17:668–675, 1999.

Hahn FF: Carcinogenic responses of the respiratory tract, in Sipes IG, McQueen CA, Gandolfi JA (eds): *Comprehensive Toxicology.* Vol 8. Roth RA (ed): *Toxicology of the Respiratory System.* Oxford, England: Elsevier, 1997, pp 187–202.

Hecht SS: Tobacco smoke carcinogens and lung cancer. *J Natl Cancer Inst* 91:1194–1210, 1999.

Hoyt DG, Lazo JS: Bleomycin-induced pulmonary fibrosis, in Sipes IG, McQueen CA, Gandolfi JA (eds): *Comprehensive Toxicology.* Vol 8. Roth RA (ed): *Toxicology of the Respiratory System.* Oxford, England: Elsevier, 1997, pp 543–554.

ILSI Risk Science Institute Workshop: The relevance of the rat lung response to particle overload for human risk assessment. *Inhalat Toxicol* 12:1–148, 2000.

International Agency for Research on Cancer: *Overall evaluations of carcinogenicity.* An updating of IARC monograph vols 1–47, suppl 7. Lyons, France: IARC, 1987.

International Agency for Research on Cancer: *Iarc Monographs on the Evaluation of Carcinogenic Risks to Humans: Beryllium, Cadmium, Mercury and Exposures in the Glass Manufacturing Industry.* Vol 58. Lyons, France: IARC, 1993.

Karol MH, Tollerud DJ, Campbell TP, et al: Predictive value of airways hyperresponsiveness and circulating IgE for identifying types of responses to toluene diisocyanate inhalation challenge. *Am J Respir Crit Care Med* 149:611–615, 1994.

Kimball JS, Miller F: Regional respiratory-tract absorption of inhaled reactive gases: A modeling approach, in Gardner DE, Crapo JD, McClellan RO (eds): *Toxicology of the Lung,* 3d ed. Philadelphia: Taylor & Francis, 1999, pp 557–597.

Laméé MW, Jones AD, Morin DW, et al: Association of dehydromonocrotaline with rat red blood cells. *Chem Res Toxicol* 10:694–701, 1997.

Leikauf G, Driscoll K: Cellular approaches in respiratory tract toxicology, in Gardner DE, Crapo JD, McClellan RO (eds): *Toxicology of the Lung,* 2d ed. New York: Raven Press, 1993, pp 335–370.

Malkinson AM: Molecular comparison of human and mouse pulmonary adenocarcinomas. *Exp Lung Res* 24:541–555, 1998.

Massague J. TGF-β signal transduction. *Annu Rev Biochem* 67:753–791, 1998.

Medinsky MA, Bond JA, Schlosser PM, Morris JB: Mechanisms and models for respiratory-tract uptake of volatile organic chemicals, in Gardner DE, Crapo JD, McClellan RO (eds): *Toxicology of the Lung,* 3d ed. Philadelphia: Taylor & Francis, 1999, pp 483–512.

Mercer RR, Crapo JD: Architecture of the acinus, in Parent RA (ed): *Treatise on Pulmonary Toxicology: Comparative Biology of the Normal Lung.* Boca Raton, FL: CRC Press, 1991, pp 109–120.

Miller F: Dosimetry of particles in laboratory animals and humans, in Gardner DE, Crapo JD, McClellan RO (eds): *Toxicology of the Lung,* 3d ed. Philadelphia: Taylor & Francis, 1999, pp 513–555.

Morrow PE: Dust overloading in the lungs: Update and appraisal. *Toxicol Appl Pharmacol* 113:1–12, 1992.

National Cancer Institute: *Health Effects of Exposure to Environmental Tobacco Smoke: The Report of the California Environmental Protection Agency.* Smoking and Tobacco Control Monograph No. 10. NIH Pub. No. 99-4645. Bethesda, MD: U.S. Department of Health and Human Services, National Institutes of Health, National Cancer Institute, 1999.

O'Byrne PM, Postma DS: The many faces of airway inflammation. *Am Respir Crit Care Med* 159:541–566, 1999.

Pinkerton KE, Gehr P, Crapo JD: Architecture and cellular composition of the air-blood barrier, in Parent RA (ed): *Treatise on Pulmonary Toxicology: Comparative Biology of the Normal Lung.* Boca Raton, FL: CRC Press, 1991, pp 121–128.

Postlethwait EM, Bidani A: In vitro systems for studying respiratory system toxicology, in Sipes IG, McQueen CA Gandolfi JA (eds): *Comprehensive Toxicology.* Vol 8. Roth RA (ed): *Toxicology of the Respiratory System.* Oxford England: Elsevier, 1997, pp 249–264.

Raabe OG: Respiratory exposure to air pollutants, in Swift DL, Foster WM (eds): *Air Pollutants and the Respiratory Tract.* New York: Marcel Dekker 1999, pp 39–73.

Ramazzini B: *Disease of Workers.* Translated from the Latin text *De Morbis Artificum* by Wright WC. New York and London: Hafner, 1964.

Ramu K, Kehrer JP: The pulmonary toxicity of chemotherapeutic agents, in Sipes IG, McQueen CA, Gandolfi JA (eds): *Comprehensive Toxicology.* Vol 8. Roth RA (ed): *Toxicology of the Respiratory System.* Oxford, England: Elsevier, 1997, pp 521–541.

Reasor M: Cationic amphophilic drugs, in Sipes IG, McQueen CA, Gandolfi JA (eds): *Comprehensive Toxicology.* Vol 8. Roth RA (ed): *Toxicology of the Respiratory System.* Oxford, England: Elsevier, 1997, pp 555–566.

Smith LL: Paraquat, in Sipes IG, McQueen CA, Gandolfi JA (eds): *Comprehensive Toxicology.* Vol 8. Roth RA (ed): *Toxicology of the Respiratory System.* Oxford, England: Elsevier, 1997, pp 581–590.

Snider GL, Kleinerman J, Thurlbeck WM, Bengali ZH: The definition emphysema: Report of a National Heart, Lung, and Blood Institute Workshop. *Am Rev Respir Dis* 132:182–185, 1985.

Timblin C, Janssen-Heininger Y, Mossmann BT: Pulmonary reactions and mechanisms of toxicity of inhaled fibers, in Gardner DE, Crapo JD, McClellan RO (eds): *Toxicology of the Lung,* 3d ed. Philadelphia: Taylor & Francis, 1999, pp 221–240.

Varani J, Ward PA: Activation of the inflammatory response by asbestos and silicate mineral dusts, in Wallace KB (ed): *Free Radical Toxicology.* New York: Taylor & Francis 1997, pp 295–322.

Weibel ER: Is the lung built reasonably? The 1983 J. Burns Anderson lecture. *Am Rev Respir Dis* 128:752–760, 1983.

Wilson DW, Segall HJ, Pan LC, et al: Mechanism and pathology of monocrotaline pulmonary toxicity. *CRC Crit Rev Toxicol* 22:307–325, 1992.

Wingo PA, Ries LA, Giovino GA, et al: Annual report to the nation on the status of cancer, 1973–1996, with a special section lung cancer and tobacco smoking. *J Natl Cancer Inst* 91:675–690, 1999.

Witschi HP: Selected examples of free-radical-mediated lung injury, in Wallace KB (ed): *Free Radical Toxicology.* New York: Taylor & Francis, 1997a, pp 279–294.

Witschi HP: Cell damage and cell renewal in the lung, in Sipes IG, McQueen CA, Gandolfi JA (eds): *Comprehensive Toxicology.* Vol 8. Roth RA (ed): *Toxicology of the Respiratory System.* Oxford, England: Elsevier, 1997b, pp 231–248.

Witschi HP, Espiritu I, Pinkerton KE, et al: Ozone carcinogenesis revisited. *Toxicol Sci* 52:62–167, 1999.

Wong BA: Inhalation exposure systems design, methods, and operation, in Gardner DE, Crapo JD, McClellan RO (eds): *Toxicology of the Lung,* 3d ed. Philadelphia:Taylor & Francis 1999, pp 1–53.

Zemp E, Elsasser S, Schindler C, et al: Long-term ambient air pollution and respiratory symptoms in adults (SAPALDIA study). The SAPALDIA Team. *Am J Respir Crit Care Med* 159:1257–1266, 1999.

Zhang HY, Phan S: Inhibition of myofibroblast apoptosis by transforming growth factor β_1. *Am J Respir Cell Mol Biol* 21:658–665, 1999.

CHAPTER 16

TOXIC RESPONSES OF THE NERVOUS SYSTEM

Douglas C. Anthony, Thomas J. Montine, William M. Valentine, and Doyle G. Graham

OVERVIEW OF THE NERVOUS SYSTEM

Neurotoxicants and toxins have been extensively studied, both because of their toxic effects on humans and because of their utility in the study of the nervous system (NS). Many insights into the organization and function of the NS are based on observations derived from the action of neurotoxicants. The binding of exogenous compounds to membranes has been the basis for the definition of specific receptors within the brain; an understanding of the roles of different cell types in the function of the NS has stemmed from the selectivity of certain toxicants in injuring only certain cell types; and important differences in basic metabolic requirements of different subpopulations of neurons have been inferred from the effects of toxicants.

It is estimated that millions of people worldwide are exposed to known neurotoxicants each year, a fact underscored by repeated outbreaks of neurologic disease (Federal Register, 1994). An even larger potential problem is the incomplete information on many compounds that may have neurotoxic effects. Unknown is the extent to which neurologic disability may be related to chronic low-level exposures, nor do we understand the overall impact of environmental contaminants on brain function.

In order to study neurotoxicologic diseases, one must understand some of the anatomy, physiology, development, and regenerative capacity of the NS. These complex functions can be reduced to several generalities that allow a basic understanding of the actions of neurotoxicants. These general principles include (1) the privileged status of the NS with the maintenance of a biochemical barrier between the brain and the blood, (2) the importance of the high energy requirements of the brain, (3) the spatial extensions of the NS as long cellular processes and the requirements of cells with such a complex geometry, (4) the maintenance of an environment rich in lipids, and (5) the transmission of information across extracellular space at the synapse. Each of these features of the NS carries with it specialized metabolic requirements and unique vulnerabilities to toxic compounds.

Blood-Brain Barrier

The NS is protected from the adverse effects of many potential toxicants by an anatomic barrier. In 1885, Ehrlich, while studying the distribution of dyes in the body, noticed that although other tissues became stained, the brain and spinal cord did not develop the color of the dyes. This observation pointed to the existence of an interface between the blood and the brain, or a "blood-brain barrier." Most of the brain, spinal cord, retina, and peripheral NS maintain this barrier with the blood, with a selectivity similar to the interface between cells and extracellular space. The principal basis of the blood-brain barrier is thought to be specialized endothelial cells in the brain's microvasculature, aided, at least in part, by interactions with glia (Kniesel and Wolburg, 2000).

Among the unique properties of endothelial cells in the NS is the presence of tight junctions between cells (Kniesel and Wolburg, 2000; Rubin and Staddon, 1999), compared to the 4-nm gaps between endothelial cells outside the NS. To gain entry to the NS, molecules must pass through the cell membranes of endothelial cells of the brain rather than between endothelial cells, as they do in other tissues (Fig. 16-1). The blood-brain barrier also contains xenobiotic transporters, such as the multidrug-resistant protein, which transports some xenobiotics that have diffused through endothelial cells back into the blood. Aside from molecules that are actively transported in the brain, the penetration of toxicants or their metabolites into the NS is largely related to their lipid solubility and to their ability to pass through the plasma membranes of the cells forming the barrier (Pardridge, 1999; Stewart, 2000). There are important exceptions to this general rule. In the mature NS, the spinal and autonomic ganglia as well as a small number of other sites within the brain, called *circumventricular organs,* do not contain specialized endothelial tight junctions and are not protected by blood-tissue barriers. This discontinuity of the barrier allows entry of the anticancer drug doxorubicin into the sensory ganglia and forms the basis for the selective neurotoxicity of this compound to ganglionic neurons (Spencer, 2000). The blood-brain barrier is incompletely developed at birth and even less so in premature infants. This predisposes the premature infant to brain injury by toxins, such as unconjugated bilirubin, that later in life are excluded from the NS (Lucey et al., 1964).

In addition to this interface with blood, the brain, spinal cord, and peripheral nerves are also completely covered with a continuous lining of specialized cells that limits the entry of molecules from adjacent tissue. In the brain and spinal cord, this surface is the meningeal surface; in peripheral nerves, each fascicle of nerve is surrounded by perineurial cells.

Energy Requirements

Neurons and cardiac myocytes are highly dependent upon aerobic metabolism. These cells share the property of conduction of electrical impulses, and their dependence on aerobic respiration emphasizes the high metabolic demand associated with the maintenance and repetitive reinstitution of ion gradients. Membrane depolarizations and repolarizations occur with such frequency that these cells must be able to produce large quantities of high-energy phosphates even in a resting state. That the energy requirements of the brain are related to membrane depolarizations is supported by the fact that hyperactivity, as in epileptic foci, increases the energy requirements by as much as five times (Plum and Posner, 1985). The dependence on a continual source of energy, in the absence of energy reserves, places the neuron in a vulnerable position. To meet these high energy requirements, the brain utilizes aerobic glycolysis and, therefore, is extremely sensitive to even brief interruptions in the supply of oxygen or glucose.

The systemic exposure to toxicants that inhibit aerobic respiration, such as cyanide, or to conditions that produce hypoxia, such as carbon monoxide (CO) poisoning, leads to the earliest signs of dysfunction in the myocardium and neurons. Damage to the NS under these conditions is a combination of direct toxic effects on neurons and secondary damage from systemic hypoxia or ischemia. For example, acute CO poisoning damages those structures in the central nervous system (CNS) that are most vulnerable to hypoxia: the neurons in specific regions of the basal ganglia and hippocampus, certain layers of the cerebral cortex, and the cerebellar Purkinje cells. Experiments utilizing several different laboratory animal species have shown that systemic hypotension is the best predictor of these lesions following CO poisoning; however, CO poisoning also may produce white matter damage, and this

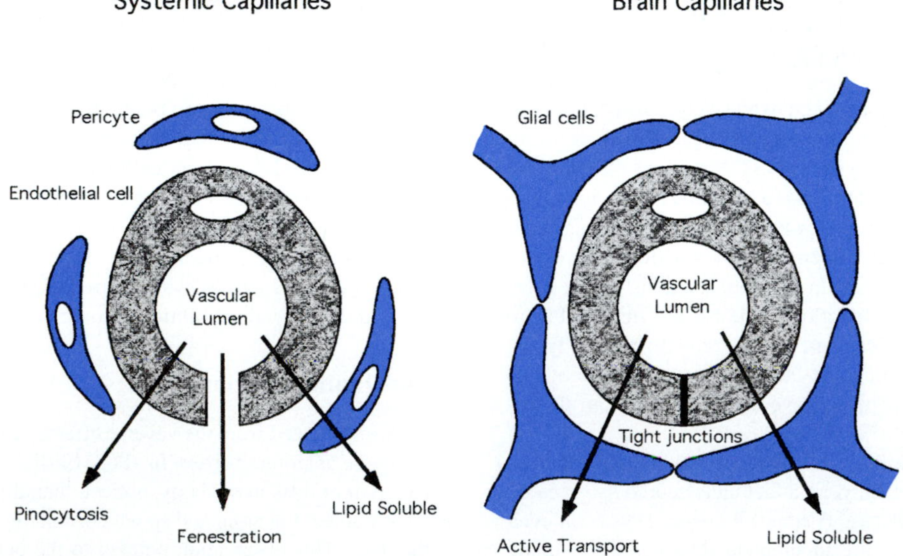

Figure 16-1. Schematic diagram of the blood-brain barrier.

Systemic capillaries are depicted with intercellular gaps, or fenestrations, which permit the passage of molecules incapable of crossing the endothelial cell. There is also more abundant pinocytosis in systemic capillaries, in addition to the transcellular passage of lipid soluble compounds. In brain capillaries, tight junctions between endothelial cells and the lack of pinocytosis limit transport to compounds with active transport mechanisms or those which pass through cellular membranes by virtue of their lipid solubility.

leukoencephalopathy may result from a primary effect of CO in the CNS (Penny, 1990). As in the case of acute CO intoxication, survivors of cyanide poisoning may develop lesions in the CNS that are characteristic of systemic hypoxic or ischemic injury, and experiments in rats and monkeys have led to the conclusion that global hypoperfusion, rather than direct histotoxicity, is the major cause of CNS damage (Auer and Benveniste, 1997). 3-Nitropropionic acid (3-NP), a naturally occurring mycotoxin, is an irreversible inhibitor of succinate dehydrogenase that produces adenosine triphosphate (ATP) depletion in cerebral cortical explants and is associated with motor disorders in livestock and humans that have ingested contaminated food (Ludolf et al., 1991, 1992). Some investigators removed the complication of systemic toxicity by directly injecting 3-NP into specific regions of the brain. They have observed neuron degeneration mediated in part by excitotoxic mechanisms (Brouillet et al., 1993). These examples demonstrate the exquisite sensitivity of neurons to energy depletion and also underscore the complex relationships between direct neurotoxicity and the effects of systemic toxicity on the NS.

Axonal Transport

Some forms of intercellular communication are conducted through the vascular system as hormones, which transmit information to remote sites through the bloodstream. Some information, however, is too vital to be conducted in such a diffuse and slow manner, and the NS can be envisioned as a remedy to the obstacle of space in intercellular communication. Impulses are conducted over great distances at rapid speed and provide information about the environment to the organism in a coordinated manner that allows an organized response to be carried out at a specific site. However, the intricate organization of such a complex network places an unparalleled demand on the cells of the NS. Single cells, rather than being spherical and a few micrometers in diameter, are elongated and may extend over a meter in length!

The anatomy of such a complex cellular network creates features of metabolism and cellular geometry that are peculiar to the NS. The two immediate demands placed on the neuron are the maintenance of a much larger cellular volume and the transport of intracellular materials over great distances. Although the length of neurons may exceed 200,000 times the dimensions of most other cells, the cellular volume has not undergone a similar increase due to the unique attribute of very fine cylindrical extensions of the cell to span the long distances. In the form of long delicate axons, the neuron spans large distances but maintains less cytoplasmic volume and cell surface. Even so, the volume of the axon is much greater than the volume of the cell body. If one considers the lower motor neuron in humans, the cell body is located in the spinal cord and the axon extends to the site of innervation of a muscle at a distant location. In spite of the smaller diameter of the axon, the tremendous distances traversed by the axon translate to an axonal volume that is hundreds of times greater than that of the cell body itself (Schwartz, 1991). This places a great burden on the neuron to provide protein synthetic machinery for such a cytoplasmic volume. The cellular machinery is readily visible in large neurons through the light microscope as the Nissl substance, which is formed by clusters of ribosomal complexes for the synthesis of proteins (Parent, 1996). That this is a reflection of an unusual protein synthetic burden may be surmised from the fact that neurons are the only cell type with such a Nissl substance.

In addition to the increased burden of protein synthesis, the neuron is dependent on the ability to distribute materials over the distances encompassed by its processes. While analogous systems exist in all cell types and are referred to as cytoplasmic streaming, in the NS this process occurs over much greater distances and is referred to as axonal transport. Protein synthesis occurs in the cell body, and the protein products are then transported to the appropriate site through the process of axonal transport. The assembly of the cytoskeleton at tremendous distances from their site of synthesis in the cell body represents a formidable challenge (Nixon, 1998). Through studies of the movement of radiolabeled amino acid precursors, several major components of axonal transport are known (Grafstein, 1995). The fastest component is referred to as *fast axonal transport* and carries a large number of proteins from their site of synthesis in the cell body into the axon. Many of these proteins are associated with vesicles (Grafstein, 1995) and migrate through the axon at a rate of 400 mm/day (Fig. 16-2). This process has been known for some time to be dependent on ATP, but it was

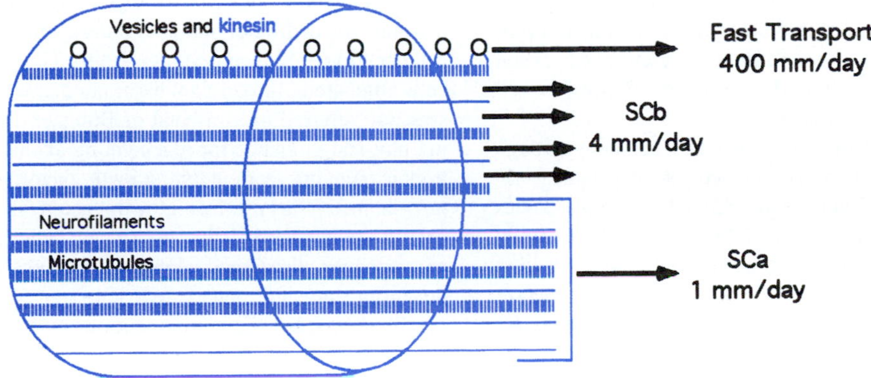

Figure 16-2. Schematic diagram of axonal transport.

Fast axonal transport is depicted as spherical vesicles moving along microtubules with intervening microtubule-associated motors. The slow component A (SCa) represents the movement of the cytoskeleton, composed of neurofilaments and microtubules. Slow component b (SCb) moves at a faster rate than SCa and includes soluble proteins, which are apparently moving between the more slowly moving cytoskeleton.

not until the description of a microtubule-associated ATPase activity that there rapidly emerged the concept of microtubule-associated motor proteins. These proteins, kinesin and dynein being the prototypes of a class of microtubule-associated motors, provide both the mechanochemical force in the form of a microtubule-associated ATPase and the interface between microtubules as the track and vesicles as the cargo. Vesicles are transported rapidly in an anterograde direction by kinesin, and they are transported in a retrograde direction by dynein (Schnapp and Reese, 1989). While this mechanism of cytoplasmic transport toward the cell periphery and back toward the nucleus appears to be a general feature of cells, the process is amplified within the NS by the distances encompassed by the axonal extensions of neurons. In the axon, multiple waves of transport can be detected in the fast component of axonal transport (Mulugeta et al., 2000).

The transport of some organelles, including mitochondria, constitutes an intermediate component of axonal transport, moving at 50 mm/day (Grafstein, 1995). As with the fast component, the function is apparently the continuous replacement of organelles within the axon. The slowest component of axonal transport represents the movement of the cytoskeleton itself, rather than the movement of enzymes or organelles through the cytosol (Fig. 16-2). The cytoskeleton is composed of structural elements, including microtubules formed by the association of tubulin subunits and neurofilaments formed by the association of three neurofilament protein subunits. Dynamic exchange of subunits of the filamentous structure has now been observed with high-resolution microscopy of living cells, indicating that stationary filamentous structures exchange subunits that move rapidly once dissociated (Wang et al., 2000). Each of the elements of the cytoskeleton moves along the length of the axon at a specific rate. Overall, slow component A (SCa), so named to distinguish this wave of movement from another slow component of axonal transport, slow component B (SCb) (Hoffman and Lasek, 1975), is composed of the movement of the axonal cytoskelton in an anterograde direction.

Neurofilaments and microtubules move at a rate of approximately 1 mm/day and make up the majority of SCa, the slowest-moving component of axonal transport. Subunit structures appear to migrate and reassemble in a process that is dependent on nucleoside triphosphates, kinases, and phosphatases (Koehnle and Brown, 1999; Nixon, 1998). Moving at only a slightly more rapid rate of 2 to 4 mm/day is SCb, which is composed of many proteins (Grafstein, 1995). Included in SCb are several structural proteins, such as the component of microfilaments (actin) and several microfilament-associated proteins (M2 protein and fodrin), as well as clathrin and many soluble proteins.

This continual transport of proteins from the cell body through the various components of forward-directed, or anterograde, axonal transport is the mechanism through which the neuron provides the distal axon with its complement of functional and structural proteins. Some vesicles are also moving in a retrograde direction and undoubtedly provide the cell body with information concerning the status of the distal axon. The evidence for such a dynamic interchange of materials and information stems not only from the biochemical detection of these components of axonal transport but also from the observations of the effects of terminating this interchange by severing the axon from its cell body. The result of transection of an axon is that the distal axon is destined to degenerate, a process known as axonal degeneration which is unique to the NS. The cell body of the neuron responds to the transection of the axon as well and undergoes a process of chromatolysis, a response of the cell body to degeneration of the axon.

Axonal Degeneration Current concepts of axonal degeneration were initially derived from the transection of nerve, first reported by Augustus Waller over a hundred years ago. Accordingly, the recognized sequence of events that occur in the distal stump of an axon following transection are referred to as *Wallerian degeneration*. Because the axonal degeneration associated with chemical agents and some disease states is thought to occur through a similar sequence of events, it is often referred to as *Wallerian-like* axonal degeneration.

Following axotomy, there is degeneration of the distal nerve stump, followed by generation of a microenvironment supportive of regeneration. This process proceeds through a sequence of changes involving the distal axon, ensheathing glial cells and the blood nerve barrier. Initially there is a period during which the distal stump survives and maintains relatively normal structural, transport, and conduction properties. The duration of survival is proportional to the length of the axonal stump (Chaudry and Cornblath, 1992), and this relationship appears to be maintained across species. An exception has been noted in the C57/BL6/01a mouse, in which transected nerve fibers function electrically for 14 to 28 days (Lunn et al., 1989). Although the underlying reason for slow degeneration in this mutant is unknown, the trait is transmitted by a dominant gene on chromosome 4 (Lyon et al., 1993) and is an intrinsic property of the neuron that does not involve macrophages or Schwann cells (Glass et al., 1993). Terminating the period of survival is an active proteolysis that digests the axolemma and axoplasm, leaving only a myelin sheath surrounding a swollen degenerate axon (Fig. 16-3). Digestion of the axon appears to be an all-or-none event effected through endogenous proteases (Schaefler and Zimmerman, 1984) that appear to be activated through increased levels of intracellular free Ca^{2+} (George et al., 1995). Although it is established that degeneration of the most terminal portion of the axon occurs first, whether degeneration of the remainder of the stump occurs from proximal to distal, distal to proximal, or simultaneously along its entire length remains a matter of debate. The active proteolysis phase occurs so rapidly in mammals that it has been difficult to define a spatial distribution.

Schwann cells respond to loss of axons by decreasing synthesis of myelin lipids, down-regulating genes encoding myelin proteins, and dedifferentiating to a premyelinating mitotic Schwann cell phenotype (Stoll and Muller, 1999). The proliferating Schwann cells align along the original basal lamina, which creates a tubular structure referred to as a band of Bungner. In addition to providing physical guidance for regenerating axons, these tubes provide trophic support from nerve growth factor, brain-derived nerve growth factor, insulin-like growth factor, and corresponding receptors produced by the associated Schwann cells. Resident macrophages distributed along the endothelium within the endoneurium and the denervated Schwann cells assist in clearing myelin debris, but the recruitment of hematogenous macrophages accounts for the removal of the majority of myelin. Infiltrating macrophages express complement receptor 3, and the presence of complement 3 on the surface of degenerating myelin sheaths facilitates opsonization. In contrast to the proteolysis of the axon, processing of myelin breakdown products proceeds in an established proximal-to-distal progression. Another essential role of recruited circulating macrophages is the secretion of interleukin-1,

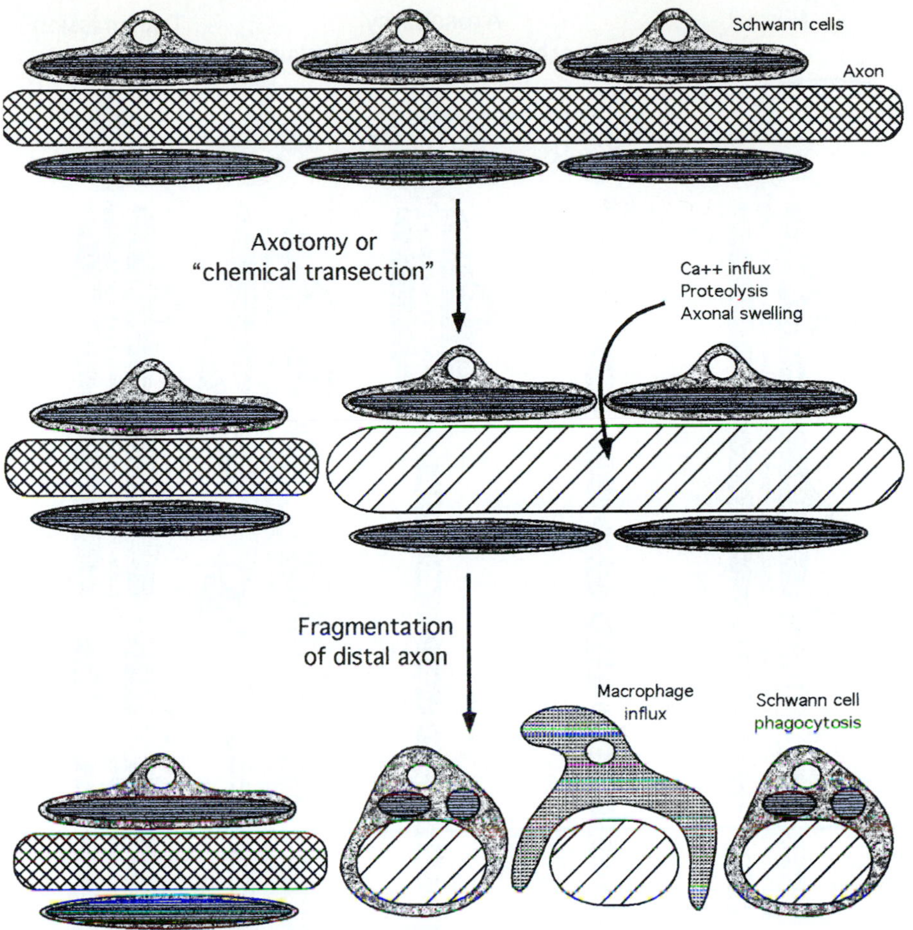

Figure 16-3. Schematic diagram of axonal degeneration.

Following axotomy, or chemical injury of an axon, the distal portion of the axon undergoes a process of axonal degeneration. Initial stages of axonal swelling are followed by fragmentation of the distal axon and phagocytosis by resident Schwann cells and an influx of macrophages, which are largely derived from the circulation.

which is responsible for stimulating production of nerve growth factor by Schwann cells.

Investigations have shown that degeneration of the distal axonal stump after transection is an active, synchronized process that can be delayed experimentally through decreasing temperature, preventing the entry of extracellular Ca^{2+} or inhibiting proteolysis by calpain II (George et al., 1995). Accompanying events in glial cells and macrophages direct and facilitate the sprouting neurite originating from the surviving proximal axon that also undergoes changes in protein expression resembling a less differentiated state. The facilitation of regeneration in the peripheral nervous system by Schwann cells distinguishes it from the central nervous system (CNS), in which oligodendrocytes secrete inhibitory factors that impede neurite outgrowth. Eventually, though, even in the peripheral nervous system (PNS), if axonal contact is not restored, Schwann cell numbers will decrease, bands of Bungner will disappear, and increased fibroblast collagen production will render regeneration increasingly unlikely.

These dynamic relationships between the neuronal cell body and its axon are important in understanding the basic pathological responses to axonal and neuronal injuries caused by neurotoxicants. When the neuronal cell body has been lethally injured, it degenerates, along with all of its cellular processes. This process is a *neuronopathy* and is characterized by the loss of the cell body and all of its processes, with no potential for regeneration. However, when the injury is at the level of the axon, the axon may degenerate while the neuronal cell body continues to survive, a condition known as an "axonopathy" (Fig. 16-4). In this setting, there is a potential for regeneration and recovery from the toxic injury as the axonal stump sprouts and regenerates. Since axonal transport is the process by which the neuron supplies proteins to the distal portions of the axon, axonal transport systems have become of major interest in attempts to understand the toxic degeneration of axons.

Myelin Formation and Maintenance

Myelin is formed in the CNS by oligodendrocytes and in the PNS by Schwann cells. Both of these cell types form concentric layers of lipid-rich myelin by the progressive wrapping of their cytoplasmic processes around the axon in successive loops (Fig. 16-5). Ultimately, these cells exclude cytoplasm from the inner surface of their membranes to form the major dense line of myelin (Quarles et al., 1997; Monuki and Lemke, 1995; Parent, 1996). In a similar process, the extracellular space is reduced on the extra-

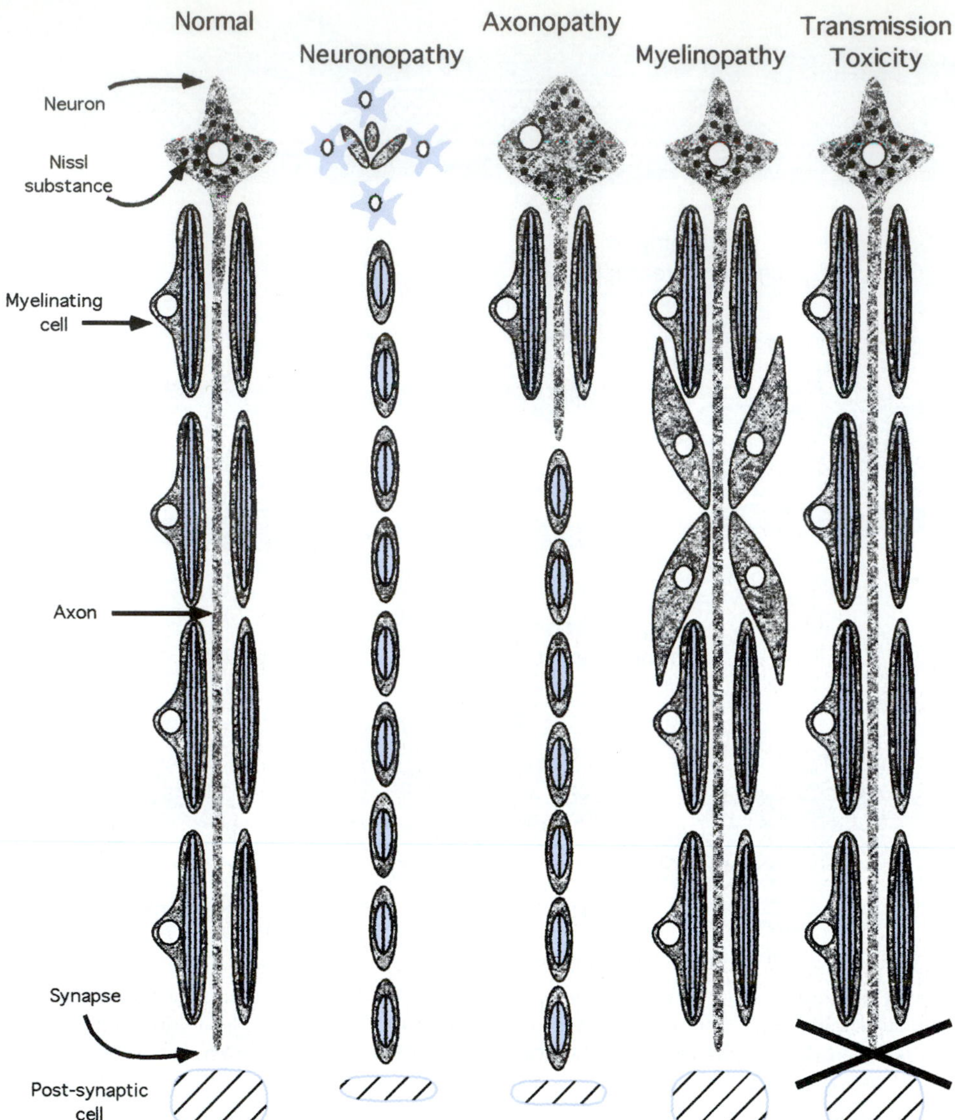

Figure 16-4. Patterns of neurotoxic injury.

A neuronopathy results from the death of the entire neuron. Astrocytes often proliferate in response to the neuronal loss, creating both neuronal loss and gliosis. When the axon is the primary site of injury, the axon degenerates, while the surviving neuron shows only chromatolysis with margination of its Nissl substance and nucleus to the cell periphery. This condition is termed an axonopathy. Myelinopathies result from disruption of myelin or from selective injury to the myelinating cells. To prevent cross-talk between adjacent axons, myelinating cells divide and cover the denuded axon rapidly; however, the process of remyelination is much less effective in the CNS than in the PNS. Some compounds do not lead to cell death but exert their toxic effects by interrupting the process of neurotransmission, either through blocking excitation or by excessive stimulation.

cellular surface of the bilayers, and the lipid membranes stack together, separated only by a proteinaceous intraperiod line existing between successive layers.

The formation and maintenance of myelin requires metabolic and structural proteins that are unique to the NS. Myelin basic protein, an integral protein of CNS myelin, is closely associated with the intracellular space (at the major dense line of myelin) (Quarles et al., 1997; Monuki and Lemke, 1995), and an analogous protein, P1 protein, is located in the PNS. On the extracellular surface of the lipid bilayers is the CNS protein, proteolipid protein, at the intraperiod line of myelin. Mutation of this protein in several species, including humans, or overexpression of the wild-type gene in transgenic mice, results in disorders in which myelin of the CNS does not form normally (Pham-Dinh et al., 1991; Readhead et al., 1994).

There are a variety of hereditary disorders in which myelin is either poorly formed from the outset or is not maintained after its formation. In addition to mutation of proteolipid protein, there are a variety of inherited abnormalities of myelin proteins and myelin-specific lipid catabolism. These genetic defects have provided some insight into the special processes required to maintain the lipid-rich environment of myelin. It is now known that the maintenance of myelin is dependent on a number of membrane-associated proteins and on metabolism of specific lipids present in myelin bi-

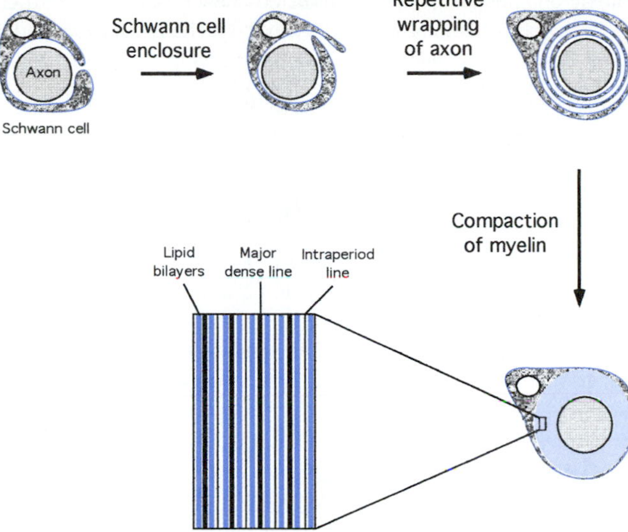

Figure 16-5. Schematic diagram of myelination.

Myelination begins when a myelinating cell encircles an axon, either Schwann cells in the peripheral nervous system or oligodendrocytes in the central nervous system. Simple enclosure of the axon persists in unmyelinated axons. Myelin formation proceeds by a progressive wrapping of multiple layers of the myelinating cell around the axon, with extrusion of the cytoplasm and extracellular space to bring the lipid bilayers into close proximity. The intracellular space is compressed to form the major dense line of myelin, and the extracellular space is compressed to form the intraperiod line.

layers. In the context of toxic exposures, it is easy to imagine how some toxic compounds interfere with this complex process of the maintenance of myelin and result in the toxic "myelinopathies" (Fig. 16-4). In general, the loss of myelin, with the preservation of axons is referred to as *demyelination*.

Neurotransmission

Intercellular communication is achieved in the NS through the synapse. Neurotransmitters released from one axon act as the first messenger. Binding of the transmitter to the postsynaptic receptor is followed by modulation of an ion channel or activation of a second messenger system, leading to changes in the responding cell. In the case of neuromuscular transmission, acetylcholine crosses the synaptic cleft to bind the cholinergic receptor of the myocyte and leads to muscle contraction.

The process of neurotransmission is targeted by a variety of therapeutic drugs and is a major component of the science of neuropharmacology. In addition, there are a variety of toxic compounds that interact directly with the process of neurotransmission, hence forming the basis of neurotransmitter-associated toxicity. To a certain extent, many of the toxic effects associated with neurotransmitters is related to the dose. While a desirable effect may occur, with some agonists or antagonists acting at a neurotransmitter receptor site, excessive effect may result in neurotoxicity. The therapeutic index, in general, is a measure of the margin between the desirable and toxic effects of a compound. Thus, the very processes targeted by many clinical neuropharmacologic strategies and drug designs are also the targets of certain neurotoxic compounds.

Development of the Nervous System

Replication, migration, differentiation, myelination, and synapse formation are the basic processes that underlie development of the NS. Both neuronal and glial precursors replicate in a discrete zone near the inner surface of the neural tube (Fig. 16-6). This germinal mantle, a collection of cells near the ventricular system, gives rise to successive waves of neurons, which migrate toward the outer surface of the brain to form the cerebral cortex, as well as other neurons, supportive astrocytes, and myelinating oligodendrocytes. Each wave of cells migrates from the germinal mantle in a precisely ordered sequence both in utero and in early postnatal life. Myelination begins in utero and continues through childhood (Kinney and Armstrong, 1997). Synaptic connectivity, the basis of neurologic function, is a dynamic process throughout life.

Development of the brain during childhood provides a certain resilience toward injuries. Much of this is due to the fact that the younger brain has greater plasticity, an ability of one portion of the NS to assume the function of an injured area. The brain of a child may compensate partially for an injury that would result in much greater disability in an adult (Goldberger and Murray, 1985). This plasticity of the immature NS appears to derive from the ability of

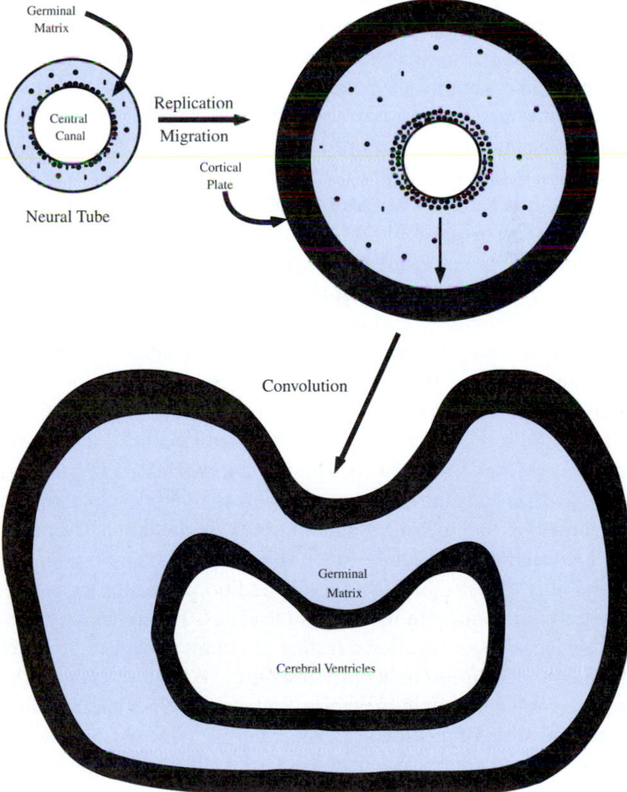

Figure 16-6. Development of the central nervous system.

Initially a tube of committed neuroepithelial cells around a central lumen (the neural tube), the central nervous system develops by replication of cells within the periventricular germinal matrix and migration of waves of neurons toward the surface. The basic tube structure persists in the spinal cord with its central canal. However, in the forebrain, the tube becomes extensively convoluted to form the gyrations of the brain.

dendrites to arborize and form new synapses. It is both curious and tragic that this capacity wanes with age.

This regenerative ability notwithstanding, the immature NS is especially vulnerable to certain agents. Ethanol exposure during pregnancy can result in abnormalities in the fetus, including abnormal neuronal migration, abnormal facial development, and diffuse abnormalities in the development of neuronal processes, especially the dendritic spines (Stoltenburg-Didinger and Spohre, 1983). While the exposure may be of little consequence to the mother, it can be devastating to the fetus. There is an effect on NMDA glutamate receptors and excessive activation of GABA receptors, with induction of apoptosis throughout the brain (Ikonomidou et al., 2000). The clinical result of fetal alcohol exposure is often mental retardation, with malformations of the brain and delayed myelination of white matter (Riikonen et al., 1999). Although there remains a great deal of uncertainty concerning the molecular basis of this developmental aberration, it occurs in a variety of experimental animals, and it appears that acetaldehyde, a product of ethanol catabolism, can produce migration defects in developing animals similar to those that occur in the fetal alcohol syndrome (O'Shea and Kaufman, 1979).

FUNCTIONAL MANIFESTATIONS OF NEUROTOXICITY

A variety of methods are available to investigate the deleterious effects of neurotoxicants. A complete biochemical or molecular mechanism for all toxicants is the ultimate goal of neurotoxicology, and it is from this perspective that the remainder of this chapter presents specific neurotoxic agents. One hastens to note that a vast ignorance lies between our current knowledge and this objective. The foremost priority is the identification of potential neurotoxicants. It is here that behavioral methods continue to make great achievements. In most instances, mechanistic data have accrued following functional assessment of exposed populations.

The strength of functional assessment has been exploited by many investigators and regulatory agencies that now employ functional test batteries as a means for screening potentially neurotoxic compounds (Tilson, 1993). A group or "battery" of behavioral tests is typically performed to evaluate a variety of neurologic functions, and its validity has been established with collaborative intergroup measures (Moser et al., 1997a). These *functional observational batteries* (FOBs) have the advantage over biochemical and pathologic measures that they permit evaluation of a single animal over longitudinal studies to determine the onset, progression, duration, and reversibility of a neurotoxic injury. In addition, repeated exposures may lead to tolerance in behavioral measures. Tilson has proposed two distinct tiers of functional testing of neurotoxicants: a first tier in which FOBs or motor activity tests may be used to identify the presence of a neurotoxic substance, and a second tier that involves characterization of the effects of the compound on sensory, motor, autonomic, and cognitive functions (Tilson, 1993). The second tier is critical, since it is in this phase that the validity of behavioral tests is established, and behavioral changes are correlated with physiologic, biochemical, and pathologic identification of neurotoxic injury (Becking et al., 1993). Problems exist in the cross-species extrapolation of behavioral abnormalities from experimental animals to humans (Winneke, 1992). Nonetheless, comparisons of defined protocols of FOBs with limited numbers of compounds (Moser et al., 1997b,c) suggest that these methods can identify neurotoxic compounds reliably. Ultimately, neurotoxicants identified by behavioral methods are evaluated at a cellular and molecular level to provide an understanding of the events in the NS that cause the neurologic dysfunction detected by observational tests.

MECHANISMS OF NEUROTOXICITY

Efforts to understand the mechanism of action of individual neurotoxic compounds have begun with the identification of the cellular target. In the nervous system, this has most often been one of four targets: the neuron, the axon, the myelinating cell, or the neurotransmitter system. As a result, neurotoxic compounds may be identified which cause neuronopathies, axonopathies, myelinopathies, or neurotransmitter-associated toxicity (Fig. 16-4). This is the classification system that is utilized here to organize the discussion of neurotoxic compounds and their mechanisms of action.

Neuronopathies

Certain toxicants are specific for neurons, or sometimes a particular group of neurons, resulting in their injury or, when intoxication is severe enough, their death. The loss of a neuron is irreversible and includes degeneration of all of its cytoplasmic extensions, dendrites and axons, and of the myelin ensheathing the axon (Fig. 16-4). Although the neuron is similar to other cell types in many respects, some features of the neuron are unique, placing it at risk for the action of cellular toxicants. Some of the unique features of the neuron include a high metabolic rate, a long cellular process that is supported by the cell body, and an excitable membrane that is rapidly depolarized and repolarized. Because many neurotoxic compounds act at the site of the cell body, when massive loss of axons and myelin are discovered in the PNS or CNS, the first question is whether the neuronal cell bodies themselves have been destroyed.

Although a large number of compounds are known to result in toxic neuronopathies (Table 16-1), all of these toxicants share certain features. Each toxic condition is the result of a cellular toxicant that has a predilection for neurons, most likely due to one of the neuron's peculiar vulnerabilities. The initial injury to neurons is followed by apoptosis or necrosis, leading to permanent loss of the neuron. These agents tend to be diffuse in their action, although they may show some selectivity in the degree of injury of different neuronal subpopulations or at times an exquisite selectivity for such a subpopulation. The expression of these cellular events is often a diffuse encephalopathy, with global dysfunctions; however, the symptomatology reflects the injury to the brain, so neurotoxicants that are selective in their action and affect only a subpopulation of neurons may lead to interruption of only a particular functionality.

Doxorubicin Although it is the cardiac toxicity that limits the quantity of doxorubicin (Adriamycin) that can be given to cancer patients, doxorubicin also injures neurons in the PNS, specifically those of the dorsal root ganglia and autonomic ganglia (Spencer, 2000). This selective vulnerability of peripheral ganglion cells is particularly dramatic in experimental animals, where it has been well documented. Doxorubicin is an anthracycline antibiotic derivative whose antineoplastic properties derive from its ability to intercalate in double-stranded DNA, interfering with transcription.

Table 16-1

Compounds Associated with Neuronal Injury (Neuronopathies)

NEUROTOXICANT	NEUROLOGIC FINDINGS	CELLULAR BASIS OF NEUROTOXICITY	REFERENCE
Aluminum	Dementia, encephalopathy (humans), learning deficits	Spongiosis cortex, neurofibrillary aggregates, degenerative changes in cortex	*a–c*
6-Amino-nicotinamide	Not reported in humans; hind limb paralysis (experimental animals)	Spongy (vacuolar) degeneration in spinal cord, brainstem, cerebellum; axonal degeneration of the peripheral nervous system (PNS)	*b, c*
Arsenic	Encephalopathy (acute), peripheral neuropathy (chronic)	Brain swelling and hemorrhage (acute), axonal degeneration in PNS (chronic)	*b, c*
Azide	Insufficient data (humans); convulsions, ataxia (primates)	Neuronal loss in cerebellum and cortex	
Bismuth	Emotional disturbances, encephalopathy, myoclonus	Neuronal loss, basal ganglia and Purkinje cells of cerebellum	*b, c*
Carbon monoxide	Encephalopathy, delayed parkinsonism/dystonia	Neuronal loss in cortex, necrosis of globus pallidus, focal demyelination; blocks oxygen binding site of hemoglobin and iron-binding sites of brain	*c*
Carbon tetrachloride	Encephalopathy (probably secondary to liver failure)	Enlarged astrocytes in striatum, globus pallidus	*c*
Chloramphenicol	Optic neuritis, peripheral neuropathy	Neuronal loss (retina), axonal degeneration (PNS)	*c*
Cyanide	Coma, convulsions, rapid death; delayed parkinsonism/dystonia	Neuronal degeneration, cerebellum and globus pallidus; focal demyelination; blocks cytochrome oxidase/ATP production	*b, c*
Doxorubicin	Insufficient data (humans); progressive ataxia (experimental animals)	Degeneration of dorsal root ganglion cells, axonal degeneration (PNS)	*b, c*
Ethanol	Mental retardation, hearing deficits (prenatal exposure)	Microcephaly, cerebral malformations	*b*
Lead	Encephalopathy (acute), learning deficits (children), neuropathy with demyelination (rats)	Brain swelling, hemorrhages (acute), axonal loss in PNS (humans)	*a–c*
Manganese	Emotional disturbances, parkinsonism/dystonia	Degeneration of striatum, globus pallidus	*a, b*
Mercury, inorganic	Emotional disturbances, tremor, fatigue	Insufficient data in humans (may affect spinal tracts; cerebellum)	*a–c*
Methanol	Headache, visual loss or blindness, coma (severe)	Necrosis of putamen, degeneration of retinal ganglion cells	*b, c*
Methylazoxymethanol acetate	Microcephaly (rats)	Developmental abnormalities of fetal brain (rats)	*d*
Methyl bromide	Visual and speech impairment; peripheral neuropathy	Insufficient data	*c*
Methyl mercury (organic mercury)	Ataxia, constriction of visula fields, paresthesias (adult)	Neuronal degeneration, visual cortex, cerebellum, ganglia	*a–c*
	Psychomotor retardation (fetal exposure)	Spongy disruption, cortex and cerebellum	*b, c*
1-Methyl-4-phenyl-1,2,3,6-tetrahydropyridine (MPTP)	Parkinsonism, dystonia (acute exposure)	Neuronal degeneration in substantia nigra	*b, c*
	Early onset parkinsonism (late effect of acute exposure)	Neuronal degeneration in substantia nigra	*b, c*
3-Nitropropionic acid	Seizures, delayed dystonia/grimacing	Necrosis in basal ganglia	*b, c*
Phenytoin (diphenylhydantoin; Dilantin)	Nystagmus, ataxia, dizziness	Degeneration of Purkinje cells (cerebellum)	*b, c*
Quinine	Constriction of visual fields	Vacuolization of retinal ganglion cells	*c*
Streptomycin (aminoglycosides)	Hearing loss	Degeneration of inner ear (organ of Corti)	*c*
Thallium	Emotional disturbances, ataxia, peripheral neuropathy	Brain swelling (acute), axonal degeneration in PNS	*b, c*
Trimethyltin	Tremors, hyperexcitability (experimental animals)	Loss of hippocampal neurons, amygdala pyriform cortex	*b*

[a]Chang LW, Dyer RS, eds: *Handbook of Neurotoxicology*. New York: Marcel Dekker, 1995.

[b]Graham DI, Lantos PL, eds: *Greenfield's Neuropathology*, 6th ed. New York: Arnold, 1997.

[c]Spencer PS, Schaumburg HH, eds: *Experimental and Clinical Neurotoxicology*, 2d ed. New York: Oxford University Press, 2000.

[d]Abou-Donia MB, ed: *Neurotoxicology*. Boca Raton, FL: CRC Press, 1993.

Because all neurons are dependent on the ability to transcribe DNA, it is quite interesting that the neurotoxicity of doxorubicin is so limited in its extent. The particular vulnerability of sensory and autonomic neurons appears to reflect the lack of protection of these neurons by a blood-tissue barrier within ganglia. If the blood-brain barrier is temporarily opened by the use of mannitol, the toxicity of doxorubicin is expressed in a much more diffuse manner, with injury of neurons in the cortex and subcortical nuclei of the brain (Spencer, 2000).

Methyl Mercury The neuronal toxicity of organomercurial compounds, such as methyl mercury, was tragically revealed in large numbers of poisonings in Japan and Iraq. The residents of Minamata Bay in Japan, whose diet was largely composed of fish from the bay, were exposed to massive amounts of methyl mercury when mercury-laden industrial effluent was rerouted into the bay (Kurland et al., 1960; Takeuchi et al., 1962). Methyl mercury injured even more people in Iraq, with more than 400 deaths and 6000 people hospitalized. In this epidemic, as well as in several smaller ones, the effects occurred after the consumption of grain that had been dusted with methyl mercury as an inexpensive pesticide (Bakir et al., 1973).

The clinical picture varies both with the severity of exposure and the age of the individual at the time of exposure. In adults, the most dramatic sites of injury are the neurons of the visual cortex and the small internal granular cell neurons of the cerebellar cortex, whose massive degeneration results in blindness and marked ataxia. In children, particularly those exposed to methyl mercury in utero, the neuronal loss is widespread, and in settings of greatest exposure, it produces profound mental retardation and paralysis (Reuhl and Chang, 1979). Studies on primates exposed in utero also have demonstrated abnormal social development (Burbacher et al., 1990). Recent studies in rats show that the neurons that are most sensitive to the toxic effects of methyl mercury are those that reside in the dorsal root ganglia, perhaps again reflecting the vulnerability of neurons not shielded by blood-tissue barriers (Schionning et al., 1998).

The mechanism of methyl mercury toxicity has been the subject of intense investigation. However, it remains unknown whether the ultimate toxicant is methyl mercury or the liberated mercuric ion. While Hg^{2+} is known to bind strongly to sulfhydryl groups, it is not clear that MeHg results in cell death through sulfhydryl binding. A variety of aberrations in cellular function have been noted, including impaired glycolysis, nucleic acid biosynthesis, aerobic respiration, protein synthesis (Cheung and Verity, 1985), and neurotransmitter release (Atchison and Hare, 1994). In addition, there is evidence for enhanced oxidative injury (LeBel et al., 1992) and altered calcium homeostasis (Marty and Atchison, 1997). It seems likely that MeHg toxicity is mediated by numerous reactions and that no single critical target will be identified. As these toxic events occur, the injured neurons eventually die. Exposure to methyl mercury leads to widespread neuronal injury and subsequently to a diffuse encephalopathy. However, there is relative selectivity of the toxicant for some groups of neurons over others. The distribution of neuronal injury does not appear to be related to the tissue distribution of either methyl mercury or ionic mercury but rather to particular vulnerabilities of these neurons.

Trimethyltin Organotins are used industrially as plasticizers, antifungal agents, or pesticides. Intoxication with trimethyltin has been associated with a potentially irreversible limbic-cerebellar syndrome in humans and similar behavioral changes in primates (Besser et al., 1987; Reuhl et al., 1985). Trimethyltin gains access to the nervous system where, by an undefined mechanism, it leads to diffuse neuronal injury. Many neurons of the brain begin to accumulate cytoplasmic bodies composed of Golgi-like structures, followed by cellular swelling and necrosis (Bouldin et al., 1981). The hippocampus is particularly vulnerable to this process. Following acute intoxication, the cells of the fascia dentata degenerate; with chronic intoxication, the cells of the corpus ammonis are lost. Ganglion cells and hair cells of the cochlea are similarly sensitive (Liu and Fechter, 1996). Several hypotheses seek the mechanism of trimethyltin neurotoxicity, including energy deprivation and excitotoxic damage. The role of stannin, a protein present in trimethyltin-sensitive neurons (Toggas et al., 1992), remains to be established, though the gene has been sequenced and is highly conserved between species (Dejneka et al., 1998).

Dopamine, 6-Hydroxydopamine, and Catecholamine Toxicity The progressive loss of catecholaminergic neurons that occurs with age has been postulated to derive from the toxicity of the oxidation products of catecholamines, especially dopamine, as well as from the products of the partial reduction of oxygen. The oxidation of catecholamines by monoamine oxidase (MAO) yields H_2O_2, a known cytotoxic metabolite. The metal ion–catalyzed autoxidation of catecholamines, especially dopamine, results in the production of catecholamine-derived quinones as well as superoxide anion ($O_2^{\bar{\cdot}}$), H_2O_2 from $O_2^{\bar{\cdot}}$ dismutation, and the hydroxyl radical (·OH) from the Fenton reaction (Fig. 16-7) (Cohen and Heikkila, 1977; Graham et al., 1978). Cellular glutathione affords protection from the flux of quinones, glutathione peroxidase from H_2O_2, and superoxide dismutase from $O_2^{\bar{\cdot}}$. Among the naturally occurring catecholamines, dopamine is the most cytotoxic, because of both its greater ease of autoxidation and the greater reactivity of its orthoquinone oxidation product (Graham, 1978). There is evidence that the mercapturate of dopamine may play a major role in dopaminergic neurodegeneration (Zhang et al., 2000b).

An analog of dopamine, 6-hydroxydopamine, is extremely potent in leading to a chemical sympathectomy. This compound fails to cross the blood-brain barrier, so its site of action is limited to the periphery after systemic administration. In addition, it does not cross into peripheral nerves and gains access to nerves only at their terminals. 6-Hydroxydopamine is actively transported into nerve terminals, employing the uptake mechanism utilized by the structurally similar catecholamines in sympathetic terminals. The uptake of 6-hydroxydopamine results in an injury to sympathetic neurons due to oxidation of this catecholamine analog similar to what occurs with dopamine (Fig. 16-7) (Graham, 1978). The result is selective destruction of sympathetic innervation (Malmfors, 1971). The sympathetic fibers degenerate, resulting in an uncompensated parasympathetic tone, a slowing of the heart rate, and hypermotility of the gastrointestinal system. It is noteworthy that neurobiologists employ 6-hydroxydopamine to destroy specific groups of catecholaminergic neurons. For example, stereotaxic injection of 6-hydroxydopamine into the caudate nucleus, which is rich in dopaminergic synapses, leads to neurite degeneration; if it is injected into the substantia nigra, the cell bodies of the dopamine neurons are destroyed (Marshall et al., 1983). The mechanism of toxicity of 6-hydroxydopamine appears to derive from its autoxidation and production of reactive oxygen species (Storch et al., 2000). Support for this mechanism is provided in the observation that overexpression of either Cu,Zn-superoxide dismutase or glu-

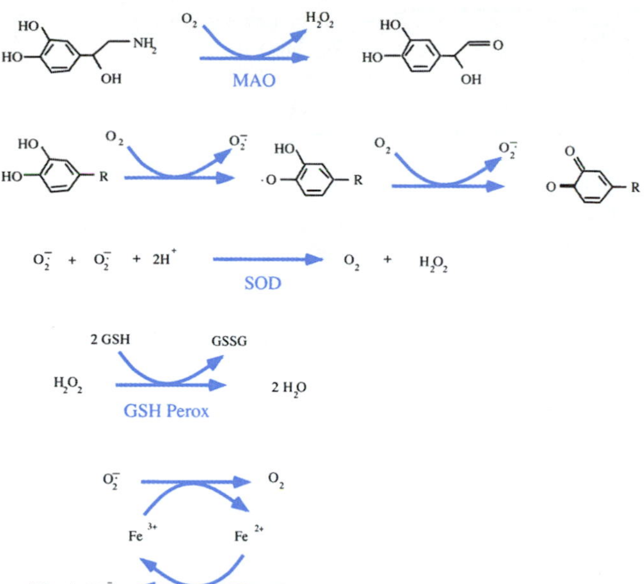

Figure 16-7. Catecholamine oxidation and activated oxygen species.

Both the enzyme-catalyzed oxidation of catecholamines, here illustrating the action of monoamine oxidase (MAO) on norepinephrine, and the nonenzymatic oxidation of catecholamines generate activated oxygen species, including hydrogen peroxide and superoxide. There are intracellular enzymes that handle the flux of superoxide (superoxide dismutase, SOD) and hydrogen peroxide (glutathione peroxidase, GSH Perox). The hydroxyl radical (OH·) is a highly reactive molecule that may react with lipids, proteins, and nucleic acids. Although originally thought to arise through the direct reaction of peroxide (H_2O_2) and superoxide (O2·), it appears that the only likely source of hydroxyl radical is through the metal-catalyzed Fenton reaction (with cycling of Fe^{3+} and Fe^{2+}). In addition, the autoxidation of catecholamines generates the semiquinone and the catecholamine-derived quinone, which is a strong electrophile and reacts with available sulfhydryls.

tathione peroxidase in transgenic mice provides protection from the toxicity of 6-hydroxydopamine (Bensadoun et al., 1998; Asanuma et al., 1998).

MPTP Because of a chemist's error, people who injected themselves with a meperidine derivative, or synthetic heroin, also received a contaminant, 1-methyl-4-phenyl-1,2,3,6-tetrahydropyridine (MPTP). Over hours to days, dozens of these patients developed the signs and symptoms of irreversible Parkinson's disease (Langston and Irwin, 1986), some becoming almost immobile with rigidity. Autopsy studies have demonstrated marked degeneration of dopaminergic neurons in the substantia nigra, with degeneration continuing many years after exposure (Langston et al., 1999).

It is surprising not only that a compound like MPTP is neurotoxic but also that MPTP is a substrate for the B isozyme of monoamine oxidase (MAO-B). It appears that MPTP, an uncharged species at physiologic pH, easily crosses the blood-brain barrier and diffuses into cells, including astrocytes. The MAO-B of astrocytes catalyzes the two-electron oxidation to yield $MPDP^+$, the corresponding dihydropyridinium ion. A further two-electron oxidation yields the pyridinium ion, MPP^+ (Fig. 16-8). MPP^+ enters dopaminergic neurons of the substantia nigra via the dopamine uptake system, resulting in injury or death of the neuron. Noradrenergic neurons of the locus ceruleus are also vulnerable to repeated exposures of MPTP (Langston and Irwin, 1986), although they are less affected by single exposures than the dopaminergic neurons. Once inside neurons, MPP^+ acts as a general mitochondrial toxin, blocking respiration at complex I (DiMonte and Langston, 2000). MPP^+ may also lead to the production of activated oxygen species, and MPP^+ results in the release of dopamine from vesicles to the higher pH environment of the cytosol where it undergoes autoxidation (Lotharius and O'Malley, 2000). Mice deficient in either Cu,Zn-superoxide dismutase or glutathione peroxidase show increased vulnerability to MPTP neurotoxicity (Zhang et al., 2000a), while overexpression of manganese superoxide dismutase attenuates the toxicity (Klivenyi et al., 1998). Metallothionein-I and -II, by contrast, do not play a role in protecting against MPTP (Rojas and Klaassen, 1999). It should be noted that the general toxicity of MPP^+ itself is great when it is administered to animals, although systemic exposure to MPP^+ does not result in neurotoxicity because it does not cross the blood-brain barrier.

Although not identical, MPTP neurotoxicity and Parkinson's disease are strikingly similar. The symptomatology of each reflects a disruption of the nigrostriatal pathway: masked facies, difficulties in initiating and terminating movements, resting "pill-rolling" tremors, rigidity, and bradykinesias are all features of both conditions. Pathologically, there is an unusually selective degeneration of neurons in the substantia nigra and depletion of striatal dopamine in both diseases (Di Monte and Langston, 2000). However, PET studies employing [$^{(18)}$F]-fluorodopa show that while patients with idiopathic Parkinson's disease demonstrate greater loss of dopaminergic function in the putamen than the caudate nucleus, the loss from these two nuclei was the same in patients who had taken MPTP (Snow et al., 2000).

Environmental Factors Relevant to Neurodegenerative Diseases It has been observed that individuals exposed to insufficient MPTP to result in immediate parkinsonism have developed early signs of the disease years later (Calne et al., 1985). This observation presents the possibility that the onset of a neurotoxic problem may follow toxic exposure by many years. It does not seem likely that an early sublethal injury to dopaminergic neurons later becomes lethal. Rather, smaller exposures to MPTP may cause a decrement in the population of neurons within the substantia nigra. Such a loss would most likely be silent, because the symptoms of Parkinson's disease do not develop until approximately 80 percent of the substantia nigra neurons are lost. These individuals with a diminished number of neurons may be more vulnerable to further loss of dopaminergic neurons. The neurologic picture of Parkinson's disease develops at an earlier age than in unexposed individuals, as a further loss of catecholaminergic neurons occurs during the process of aging.

The relationship between MPTP intoxication and parkinsonism has stimulated investigations into the role that environmental and occupational exposures may play in the pathogenesis of Parkinson's disease. While several families with early-onset Parkinson's disease demonstrate autosomal dominant inheritance, with identification of candidate genes (Polymeropoulos et al., 1997; Agundez et al., 1995; Kurth et al., 1993), twin studies indicate that environmental exposures play a more significant role than genetics in the vast majority of Parkinson's disease patients, particularly those with late-onset disease (Tanner et al., 1999; Kuopio et al., 1999). Epidemiologic studies implicate exposure to herbicides, pesticides, and metals as risk factors for Parkinson's disease (Gorell et al., 1998, 1999; Liou et al., 1997). Several studies suggest that dithiocarbamates also play an important role (Miller, 1982; Ferraz et al., 1988; Bachurin et al., 1996).

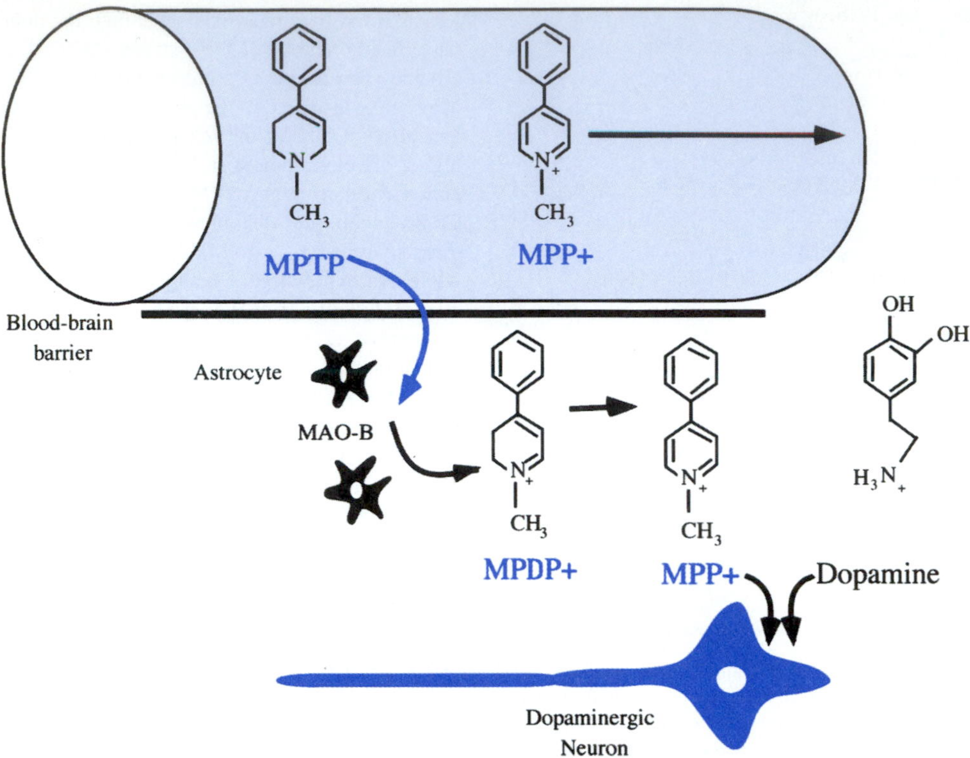

Figure 16-8. Diagram of MPTP toxicity.

MPP+, either formed elsewhere in the body following exposure to MPTP or injected directly into the blood, is unable to cross the blood-brain barrier. In contrast, MPTP gains access and is oxidized in situ to MPDP+ and MPP+. The same transport system that carries dopamine into the dopaminergic neurons also transports the cytotoxic MPP+.

Some studies suggest that cigarette smoking may have a protective effect against both Alzheimer's disease and Parkinson's disease, but alternative explanations have been offered (Riggs, 1992). An epidemic of dialysis-related dementia with some pathologic resemblance to Alzheimer's disease appears to have been related to aluminum in the dialysate, and its removal has prevented further instances of dialysis dementia. However, there is no substantial evidence to date that aluminum is in any way related to sporadic Alzheimer's disease in the general population (Letzel et al., 2000).

Axonopathies

The neurotoxic disorders termed *axonopathies* are those in which the primary site of toxicity is the axon itself. The axon degenerates, and with it the myelin surrounding that axon; however, the neuron cell body remains intact (Fig. 16-4). John Cavanagh coined the term *dying-back neuropathy* as a synonym for *axonopathy* (Cavanagh, 1964). The concept of "dying back" postulated that the focus of toxicity was the neuronal cell body itself and that the distal axon degenerated progressively from the synapse, back toward the cell body with increasing injury. It now appears that, in the best-studied axonopathies, a different pathogenetic sequence occurs; the toxicant results in a "chemical transection" of the axon at some point along its length, and the axon distal to the transection, biologically separated from its cell body, degenerates.

Because longer axons have more targets for toxic damage than shorter axons, one would predict that longer axons would be more affected in toxic axonopathies. Indeed, such is the case. The involvement of long axons of the CNS, such as ascending sensory axons in the posterior columns or descending motor axons, along with long sensory and motor axons of the PNS, prompted Spencer and Schaumburg (1976) to suggest that the toxic axonopathies in which the distal axon was most vulnerable be called *central peripheral distal axonopathies,* which, though cumbersome, accurately depicts the pathologic sequence.

A critical difference exists in the significance of axonal degeneration in the CNS compared with that in the PNS: peripheral axons can regenerate whereas central axons cannot. In the PNS, glial cells and macrophages create an environment supportive of axonal regeneration, and Schwann cells transplanted to the CNS maintain this ability. In the CNS, release of inhibitory factors from damaged myelin and astrocyte scarring actually interfere with regeneration (Qui, 2000). Interestingly, when this glial interference is removed through transplantation of CNS neurons to the PNS, the neurons are capable of extending neurites. But there appears to be more than just glial interference to account for the lack of CNS regeneration. The observation that embryonic neurons can overcome glial interference when placed into the adult NS is consistent with the development of an intrinsic sensitivity to inhibitory factors during maturation. Therefore, the inability of the CNS to regenerate appears to be due to both unfavorable environmental glial factors and properties of the mature neuron. The clinical relevance of the disparity between the CNS and PNS is that partial recovery—or, in mild cases, complete recovery—can occur after axonal degeneration in the PNS, whereas the same event is irreversible in the CNS.

Axonopathies can be considered to result from a chemical transection of the axon. The number of axonal toxicants is large and increasing in number (Table 16-2); however, they may be viewed as a group, all of which result in the pathologic loss of distal axons with the survival of the cell body. Because the axonopathies pathologically resemble the actual physical transection of the axon, axonal transport appears to be a likely target in many of the toxic axonopathies. Furthermore, as these axons degenerate, the result is most often the clinical condition of peripheral neuropathy, in which sensations and motor strength are first impaired in the most distal extent of the axonal processes, the feet and hands. With time and continued injury, the deficit progresses to involve more proximal areas of the body and the long axons of the spinal cord. The potential for regeneration is great when the insult is limited to peripheral nerves and may be complete in axonopathies in which the initiating event can be determined and removed.

Gamma-Diketones Since the late 1960s and early 1970s, it has been appreciated that humans develop a progressive sensorimotor distal axonopathy when exposed to high concentrations of a simple alkane, *n*-hexane, day after day in work settings (Yamamura, 1969) or after repeated intentional inhalation of hexane-containing glues. This axonopathy can be reproduced in its entirety in rats and larger species after weeks to months of exposure to *n*-hexane or its oxidative metabolites (Krasavage et al., 1980).

The subsequent observation that methyl *n*-butyl ketone (2-hexanone) resulted in a neuropathy identical to that caused by *n*-hexane prompted elucidation of the metabolism of these two 6-carbon compounds. The ω-1 oxidation of the carbon chain (Fig. 16-9) results ultimately in the γ-diketone, 2,5-hexanedione (HD). That HD is the ultimate toxic metabolite of both *n*-hexane and methyl *n*-butyl ketone is shown by the fact that other γ-diketones or γ-diketone precursors are similarly neurotoxic, while α- and β-diketones are not (Krasavage et al., 1980).

The elucidation of the pathogenetic mechanism of γ-diketone neuropathy has come from an understanding of the biology of the axon and the chemistry of γ-diketone reactivity. The γ-diketones react with amino groups in all tissues to form pyrroles (Amarnath et al., 1991a). That pyrrole formation is an actual step in the pathogenesis of this axonopathy has been established by two observations. First, 3,3-dimethyl-2,5-hexanedione, which cannot form a pyrrole, is not neurotoxic (Sayre et al., 1986). Second, the d,l-diastereomer of 3,4-dimethyl-2,5-hexanedione (DMHD) both forms pyrroles faster than meso-DMHD and is more neurotoxic than meso-DMHD (Genter et al., 1987).

While all proteins are derivatized by γ-diketones, the cytoskeleton of the axon, and especially the neurofilament, are very stable proteins, making it the toxicologically significant target in γ-diketone intoxication. The cellular changes are identical in rats and humans: the development of neurofilament aggregates in the distal, subterminal axon, which, as they grow larger, form massive swellings of the axon, often just proximal to nodes of Ranvier. The neurofilament-filled axonal swellings result in marked distortions of nodal anatomy, including the retraction of paranodal myelin. Following labeling of neurofilament proteins with radioactive precursors, the neurofilament transport is impaired in the γ-diketone model (Griffin et al., 1984; Pyle et al., 1994). With continued intoxication, swellings are seen more proximally and there is degeneration of the distal axon along with its myelin. Long axons in the CNS also develop neurofilament-filled swellings distally, but axonal degeneration is seen much less often. The attribute of the neurofilament that seemingly determines it as the toxicologically relevant target is its slow rate of transport down the axon (Nixon and Sihag, 1991), predisposing it to progressive derivatization and cross-linking.

Hexane neuropathy is one of the best understood of the toxic neuropathies, and much of this understanding has stemmed from controversy over whether pyrrole formation alone is the injury (an arylation reaction) or whether subsequent oxidation of pyrroles leading to covalent protein cross-linking is a necessary step (Amarnath et al., 1994). The question was apparently resolved in experiments with a novel γ-diketone, 3-acetyl-2,5-hexanedione (AcHD) (St. Clair et al., 1988). AcHD results in very rapid pyrrole formation both in vitro and in vivo. However, the electron-withdrawing acetyl group renders the resulting pyrrole essentially inert, so that it does not undergo oxidation. Despite massive pyrrole derivatization, AcHD results in neither clinical nor morphologic evidence of neurotoxicity. Thus, pyrrole derivatization is not sufficient to produce the neurofilamentous swellings; pyrrole oxidation, followed by nucleophilic attack and neurofilament cross-linking, seems to be necessary for neurotoxicity. The extent to which the accumulation is directly responsible for impaired fast axonal transport and axonal degeneration is unclear. Recent observations from transgenic animals lacking axonal neurofilaments suggest that HD impairs fast axonal transport even in the absence of neurofilaments (Stone et al., 1999).

The pathologic processes of neurofilament accumulation and degeneration of the axon are followed by the emergence of a clinical peripheral neuropathy. Experimental animals become progressively weak, beginning in the hind limbs. With continued exposure, the axonopathy may progress, leading to successive weakness in more proximal muscle groups. This is precisely the sequence of events in humans as well, and the initial stocking-and-glove distribution of sensory loss progresses to involve more proximal segments of sensory and motor axons.

Carbon Disulfide The most significant exposures of humans to CS_2 have occurred in the vulcan rubber and viscose rayon industries. Manic psychoses were observed in the former setting and were correlated with very high levels of exposure (Seppaleinen and Haltia, 1980). In recent decades, interest in the human health effects has been focused on the NS and the cardiovascular system, where injury has been documented in workers exposed to much higher levels than those that are allowed today.

What is clearly established is the capacity of CS_2 to cause a distal axonopathy that is identical pathologically to that caused by hexane. There is growing evidence that covalent cross-linking of neurofilaments also underlies CS_2 neuropathy through a series of reactions that parallel the sequence of events in hexane neuropathy. While hexane requires metabolism to 2,5-hexanedione, CS_2 is itself the ultimate toxicant, reacting with protein amino groups to form dithiocarbamate adducts (Lam and DiStefano, 1986). The dithiocarbamate adducts of lysyl amino groups undergo decomposition to isothiocyanate adducts, electrophiles that then react with protein nucleophiles to yield covalent cross-linking (Fig. 16-9). The reaction of the isothiocyanate adducts with cysteinyl sulfhydryls to form *N,S*-dialkyldithiocarbamate ester cross-links is reversible, while the reaction with protein amino functions forms thiourea cross-links irreversibly. Over time, the thiourea cross-links predominate and are most likely the most biologically significant (Amar-

Table 16-2
Compounds Associated with Axonal Injury (Axonopathies)

NEUROTOXICANT	NEUROLOGIC FINDINGS	CELLULAR BASIS OF NEUROTOXICITY	REFERENCE
Acrylamide	Peripheral neuropathy (often sensory)	Axonal degeneration, axon terminal affected in earliest stages	*b, c*
p-Bromophenylacetyl urea	Peripheral neuropathy	Axonal degeneration in the peripheral nervous system (PNS) and central nervous system (CNS)	*c*
Carbon disulfide	Psychosis (acute), peripheral neuropathy (chronic)	Axonal degeneration, early stages include neurofilamentous swelling	*b, c*
Chlordecone (Kepone)	Tremors, incoordination (experimental animals)	Insufficient data (humans); axonal swelling and degeneration	*c*
Chloroquine	Peripheral neuropathy, weakness	Axonal degeneration, inclusions in dorsal root ganglion cells; also vacuolar myopathy	*b, c*
Clioquinol	Encephalopathy (acute), subacute myelooptic neuropathy (subacute)	Axonal degeneration, spinal cord, PNS, optic tracts	*b, c*
Colchicine	Peripheral neuropathy	Axonal degeneration, neuronal perikaryal filamentous aggregates; vacuolar myopathy	*b, c*
Dapsone	Peripheral neuropathy, predominantly motor	Axonal degeneration (both myelinated and unmyelinated axons)	*b*
Dichlorophenoxyacetate	Peripheral neuropathy (delayed)	Insufficient data	*c*
Dimethylaminopropionitrile	Peripheral neuropathy, urinary retention	Axonal degeneration (both myelinated and unmyelinated axons)	*c*
Ethylene oxide	Peripheral neuropathy	Axonal degeneration	*b*
Glutethimide	Peripheral neuropathy (predominantly sensory)	Insufficient data	*c*
Gold	Peripheral neuopathy (may have psychiatric problems)	Axonal degeneration, some segmental demyelination	*b, c*
Hexane	Peripheral neuropathy, severe cases have spasticity	Axonal degeneration, early neurofilamentous swelling, PNS and spinal cord	*b, c*
Hydralazine	Peripheral neuropathy	Insufficient data	*c*
3,3′-Iminodipropionitrile	No data in humans; excitatory movement disorder (rats)	Axonal swellings, degeneration of olfactory epithelial cells, vestibular hair cells	*b*
Isoniazid	Peripheral neuropathy (sensory), ataxia (high doses)	Axonal degeneration	*b, c*
Lithium	Lethargy, tremor, ataxia (reversible)	Insufficient data	*c*
Methyl *n*-butyl ketone	Peripheral neuropathy	Axonal degeneration, early neurofilamentous swelling, PNS and spinal cord	*b, c*
Metronidazole	Sensory peripheral neuropathy, ataxia, seizures	Axonal degeneration, mostly affecting myelinated fibers; lesions of cerebellar nuclei	*b, c*
Misonidazole	Peripheral neuropathy	Axonal degeneration	*b, c*
Nitrofurantoin	Peripheral neuropathy	Axonal degeneration	*c*
Organophosphorus compounds	Headache, abdominal pain (acute; anticholinesterase)	No anatomic changes (neurotransmitter effect)	*a–c*
	Delayed peripheral neuropathy (motor), spasticity	Axonal degeneration (delayed after single exposure), PNS and spinal cord	*a–d*
Paclitaxel (taxoids)	Peripheral neuropathy	Axonal degeneration; microtubule accumulation in early stages	*b, c*
Platinum (cisplatin)	Ototoxicity with tinnitus, sensory peripheral neuropathy	Axonal degeneration, axonal loss in posterior columns of spinal cord	*b*
Pyrethroids	Movement disorders (tremor, choreoathetosis)	Axonal degeneration (variable)	*a, c*
Pyridinethione (pyrithione)	No reported human toxicity; weakness (experimental animals)	Axonal degeneration, early stages with membranous arrays in axon terminals	*c*
Trichloroethylene	Cranial (most often trigeminal) neuropathy	Insufficient data	*c*
Vincristine (vinca alkaloids)	Peripheral neuropathy, variable autonomic symptoms	Axonal degeneration (PNS), neurofibrillary changes (spinal cord, intrathecal route)	*b, c*

[a]Chang LW, Dyer RS, eds: *Handbook of Neurotoxicology*. New York: Marcel Dekker, 1995.
[b]Graham DI, Lantos PL, eds: *Greenfield's Neuropathology*, 6th ed. New York: Arnold, 1997.
[c]Spencer PS, Schaumburg HH, eds: *Experimental and Clinical Neurotoxicology*, 2d ed. New York: Oxford University Press, 2000.
[d]Abou-Donia MB, ed: *Neurotoxicology*. Boca Raton, FL: CRC Press, 1993.

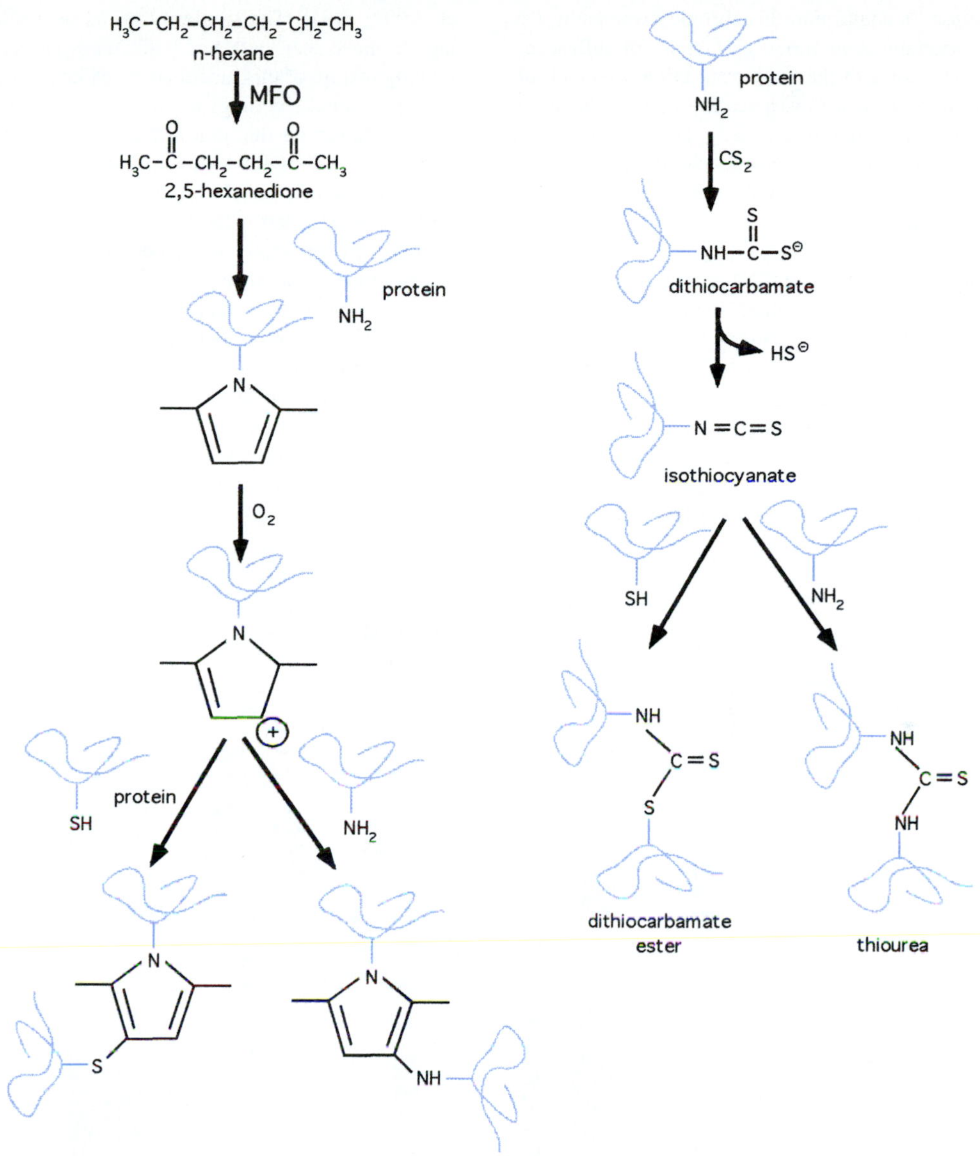

Figure 16-9. Molecular mechanisms of protein cross-linking in the neurofilamentous neuropathies.

Both 2,5-hexanedione, produced from hexane via ω-1 oxidation function of mixed function oxidase (MFO), and CS_2 are capable of cross-linking proteins. Pyrrole formation from 2,5-hexanedione is followed by oxidation and reaction with adjacent protein nucleophiles. Dithiocarbamate formation from CS_2 is followed by formation of the protein-bound isothiocyanate and subsequent reaction with adjacent protein nucleophiles.

nath et al., 1991b; Valentine et al., 1992, 1995; Graham et al., 1995).

As with hexane neuropathy, it has been postulated that the stability and long transport distance of the neurofilament determine that this protein is the toxicologically relevant target in chronic CS_2 intoxication. Nonetheless, proteins throughout the organism are derivatized and cross-linked as well. Cross-linking has been identified in erythrocyte-associated proteins including spectrin and globin as well as in the putative neurotoxic target neurofilament subunits (Valentine et al., 1993, 1997). Analysis of cross-linking in erythrocyte proteins has verified that cross-linking occurs through thiourea bridges that accumulate with continuing exposure (Erve et al., 1998a,b). Neurofilament cross-linking involves all three subunits and also demonstrates a cumulative dose response and temporal relationship consistent with a contributing event in the development of the axonal neurofilamentous swellings. The correlation of protein cross-linking in erythrocyte proteins and axonal proteins together with the ability to detect covalent modifications on peripheral proteins at subneurotoxic levels and at preneurotoxic time points suggests that modifications on peripheral proteins can be used as biomarkers of effect for CS_2 exposure. These biomarkers together with morphologic changes have been used to establish CS_2 as the ultimate neurotoxic species in the peripheral neuropathy produced by oral administration of *N,N*-diethyldithiocarbamate (Johnson, 1998).

The clinical effects of exposure to CS_2 in the chronic setting are very similar to those of hexane exposure, with the development of sensory and motor symptoms occurring initially in a stocking-

and-glove distribution. In addition to this chronic axonopathy, CS_2 can also lead to aberrations in mood and signs of diffuse encephalopathic disease. Some of these are transient at first and subsequently become more long-lasting, a feature that is common in vascular insufficiency in the nervous system. This fact, in combination with the knowledge that CS_2 may accelerate the process of atherosclerosis, suggests that some of the effects of CS_2 on the CNS are vascular in origin.

IDPN β,β'-Iminodipropionitrile (IDPN) is a bifunctional nitrile that causes a bizarre "waltzing syndrome," which appears to result from degeneration of the vestibular sensory hair cells (Llorens et al., 1993). In addition, administration of IDPN is followed by massive neurofilament-filled swellings (Griffin and Price, 1980) of the proximal, instead of the distal, axon (Fig. 16-10). The possibility that the nitrile groups undergo bioactivation to generate a bifunctional cross-linking reagent is suggested by the effects of deuterium substitution on the potency and metabolism of IDPN (Denlinger et al., 1992, 1994). The similarity of the neurofilament-filled swellings to those seen with the γ-diketones and carbon disulfide is a striking feature of this model neurotoxicant, underscoring this possibility. Axonal swellings do not occur in neurofilament-deficient quails, supporting the notion that the disorder is caused by a selective effect of IDPN on neurofilaments (Mitsuishi et al., 1993).

Understanding of the similarities between the γ-diketones and IDPN was extended when the potency of the γ-diketones was increased through molecular modeling. DMHD (3,4-dimethyl-2,5-hexanedione) is an analog of 2,5-hexanedione that accelerates the rates of both pyrrole formation and oxidation of the pyrrole. DMHD is 20 to 30 times more potent as a neurotoxicant and, in addition, the neurofilament-filled swellings occur in the proximal axon (Anthony et al., 1983a), as in IDPN intoxication. In these models of proximal neurofilamentous axonopathies, there is a block of neurofilament transport down the axon; thus, in this situation, the accumulation of neurofilaments results from blockage of the slow component A of axonal transport (Griffin et al., 1978, 1984). De-

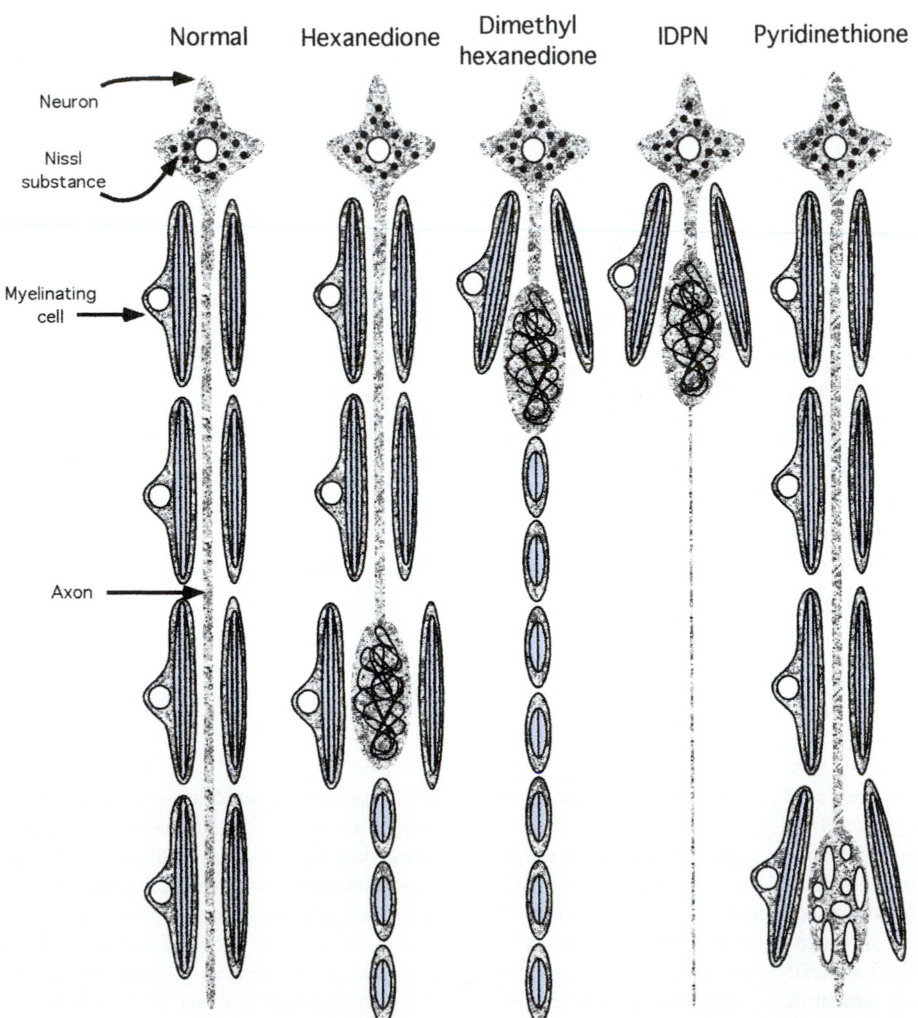

Figure 16-10. Diagram of axonopathies.

While 2,5-hexanedione results in the accumulation of neurofilaments in the distal regions of the axon, 3,4-dimethyl-2,5-hexanedione results in identical accumulation within the proximal segments. These proximal neurofilamentous swellings are quite similar to those that occur in the toxicity of β,β'-iminodipropionitrile (IDPN), although the distal axon does not degenerate in IDPN axonopathy but becomes atrophic. Pyridinethione results in axonal swellings that are distended with tubulovesicular material, followed by distal axonal degeneration.

creasing the rate of intoxication with DMHD changes the location of the swellings to more distal locations, suggesting that the neurofilamentous axonopathies have a common mechanism and that the position of the neurofilamentous swellings along the axon reflects the rate at which this process occurs (Anthony et al., 1983b).

An important difference is seen between the two proximal neurofilamentous axonopathies caused by IDPN and DMHD, however. After DMHD intoxication, animals become progressively paralyzed in all four limbs, corresponding with marked degeneration of the axon distal to the swellings. By contrast, the axon distal to IDPN-induced swellings undergoes atrophy, not degeneration, and the animal does not experience the same muscle weakness or paralysis. This observation suggests not only that axonal degeneration is required before muscle weakness develops but also that the presence of neurofilamentous aggregates in the proximal axon is not incompatible with the survival of the distal axon.

Acrylamide Acrylamide is a vinyl monomer used in the manufacture of paper products, as a flocculant in water treatment, as a soil-stabilizing and waterproofing agent, and for making polyacrylamide gels in the research laboratory. While cautious handling of acrylamide in the laboratory should be encouraged, human poisonings have been largely limited to factory and construction workers exposed to high doses (Kesson et al., 1977; Myers and Macun, 1991; Collins et al., 1989).

The neuropathy induced by acrylamide is a toxic distal axonopathy, beginning with degeneration of the nerve terminal. Continued intoxication results in degeneration of the more proximal axon, a sequence of events that recapitulates what one would expect in "dying back" process. The neuropathy appears identical whether acrylamide is administered in a single dose or in multiple smaller doses (Crofton et al., 1996). The earliest changes are seen in pacinian corpuscles, then in muscle spindles and motor nerve terminals. Within nerve terminals, early events include decreased densities of synaptic vesicles and mitochondria and accumulations of neurofilaments and tubulovesicular profiles (DeGrandechamp et al., 1990), along with evidence for terminal sprouting (DeGrandechamp and Lowndes, 1990). Multifocal accumulations of membranous bodies, mitochondria, and neurofilaments are observed in the distal axon, suggesting abnormal axonal transport. Indeed, retrograde fast transport has been shown to be impaired by acrylamide exposure (Padilla et al., 1993) and appears to occur before any morphologic changes are evident in axons or their terminals. Abnormalities in fast axonal transport have been observed in peripheral nerve axons from transgenic animals lacking neurofilaments when exposed in vitro to acrylamide (Stone et al., 1999).

Studies employing chick or rat embryo neuron cultures have demonstrated that both anterograde and retrograde fast axonal transport are inhibited by acrylamide (Harris et al., 1994). These effects are clearly not the result of ATP depletion. In addition, specific alterations of growth cone structure, including loss of filopodial elements, follow exposure to acrylamide, and these are separable from the effects of ATP depletion and sulfhydryl alkylation (Martenson et al., 1995). Because the growth cone of growing neurites in culture has many similarities to the axon terminal in vivo, it has been suggested that the growth cone alterations are a good model for the initial reactions of acrylamide with its axon terminal target(s).

Organophosphorus Esters Many toxicologists and most physicians who practice in rural areas are aware of the acute cholinergic poisoning induced by certain organophosphorus esters. These compounds, which are used as pesticides and as additives in plastics and petroleum products, inhibit acetylcholinesterase and create a cholinergic excess. However, as tens of thousands of humans could attest, tri-ortho-cresyl phosphate (TOCP) may also cause a severe central peripheral distal axonopathy without inducing cholinergic poisoning. An epidemic of massive proportion occurred during Prohibition in the United States, when a popular drink (Ginger Jake) was contaminated with TOCP. Another outbreak occurred in Morocco when olive oil was adulterated with TOCP. Human cases of paralysis have also occurred after exposure to the herbicides and cotton defoliants EPN (*O*-ethyl *O*-4-nitrophenyl phenylphosphonothionate) and leptophos [*O*-(4-bromo-2,5-dichlorophenyl) *O*-methyl phenylphosphonothionate] (Abou-Donia and Lapadula, 1990).

The hydrophobic organophosphorus compounds readily enter the NS, where they alkylate or phosphorylate macromolecules and lead to delayed-onset neurotoxicity. There are probably multiple targets for attack by organophosphorus esters, but which targets are critically related to axonal degeneration is not clear. Not all of the organophosphorus esters that inhibit acetylcholinesterase lead to a delayed neurotoxicity. While these "nontoxic" organophosphorus esters inhibit most of the esterase activity of the NS, there is another esterase activity, or *neuropathy target esterase* (NTE), that is inhibited by the neurotoxic organophosphorus esters. Furthermore, there is a good correlation between the potency of a given organophosphorus ester as an axonal toxicant and its potency as an inhibitor of NTE, both in vivo and in culture systems (Funk et al., 1994). Neither the normal function for this enzyme activity nor its relation to axonal degeneration is understood (Lotti et al., 1993). Certain neurotoxic esterase inhibitors—including phosphonates, carbamates, thiocarbamates and sulfonyl fluorides—that do not cause significant neurotoxicity can protect against organophosphate-induced delayed neurotoxicity when given before neurotoxic organophosphates. It has been proposed that these compounds protect through partial inhibition of neurotoxic esterase. In contrast, when these protective neurotoxic esterase inhibitors are administerd up to 12 days following exposure to a neurotoxic organophosphate, the delayed neurotoxicity is enhanced, such that lower initial levels of neurotoxic esterase inhibition are required to produce a delayed neuropathy (Moretto, 2000). Although the promoting agents inhibit neurotoxic esterase, this enzyme is not thought to be the target of promotion. The level of neurotoxic esterase inhibition produced by the promoter is not related to the level of promotion observed, and these promoters appear to exacerbate axonopathies from other etiologic agents as well, such as trauma and 2,5-hexanedione exposure.

The degeneration of axons does not commence immediately after acute organophosphorus ester exposure but is delayed for 7 to 10 days between the acute high-dose exposure and the clinical signs of axonopathy. The axonal lesion in the PNS appears to be readily repaired, and the peripheral nerve becomes refractory to degeneration after repeated doses. By contrast, axonal degeneration in the long tracks of the spinal cord is progressive, resulting in a clinical picture that may resemble multiple sclerosis.

Pyridinethione Zinc pyridinethione has antibacterial and antifungal properties and is a component of shampoos that are effective in the treatment of seborrhea and dandruff. Because the compound is directly applied to the human scalp, it caused some concern when it was discovered that zinc pyridinethione is neurotoxic in rodents. Rats, rabbits, and guinea pigs all develop a distal axonopathy when zinc pyridinethione is a contaminant of their food

(Sahenk and Mendell, 2000). Fortunately, however, zinc pyridinethione does not penetrate skin well, and it has not resulted in human injury to date.

Although the zinc ion is an important element of the therapeutic action of the compound, only the pyridinethione moiety is absorbed following ingestion, with the majority of zinc eliminated in the feces. In addition, sodium pyridinethione is also neurotoxic, establishing that it is the pyridinethione that is responsible for the neurotoxicity. Pyridinethione chelates metal ions and, once oxidized to the disulfide, may lead to the formation of mixed disulfides with proteins. However, which of these properties, if either, is the molecular mechanism of its neurotoxicity remains unknown.

Although these molecular issues remain to be resolved, pyridinethione appears to interfere with the fast axonal transport systems. While the fast anterograde system is less affected, pyridinethione impairs the turnaround of rapidly transported vesicles and slows the retrograde transport of vesicles (Sahenk and Mendell, 1980). This aberration of the fast axonal transport systems is the most likely physiologic basis of the accumulation of tubular and vesicular structures in the distal axon (Fig. 16-10). As these materials accumulate in one region of the axon, they distend the axonal diameter, resulting in axonal swellings filled with tubulovesicular profiles. As in many other distal axonopathies, the axon degenerates in its more distal regions beyond the accumulated structures. The earliest signs are diminished grip strength and electrophysiologic changes of the axon terminal, with normal conduction along the proximal axon in the early stages of exposure (Ross and Lawborn, 1990). Ultimately, the functional consequence of the axonal degeneration in this exposure is similar to that of other axonopathies—namely, a peripheral neuropathy.

Microtubule-Associated Neurotoxicity The role of microtubules in axonal transport and in the maintenance of axonal viability is still being elucidated; however, the biochemistry and toxicity of several alkaloids isolated from plants have greatly aided the understanding of these processes. The first of these historically are the vinca alkaloids and colchicine, which bind to tubulin and inhibit the association of this protein subunit to form microtubules. Vincristine, one of the vinca alkaloids, has found clinical use in the treatment of leukemia due to the antimitotic activity of its microtubule-directed action. Colchicine, in contrast, is used primarily in the treatment of gout. Both of these microtubule inhibitors also have been the cause of peripheral neuropathies in patients (Verity, 1997).

Much more recently another plant alkaloid, paclitaxel (Taxol) has been described that has a significantly different interaction with microtubules. Paclitaxel binds to tubules when they are assembled and stabilizes the polymerized form of tubules, so that they remain assembled even in the cold or in the presence of calcium, conditions under which microtubules normally dissociate into tubulin subunits (Schiff and Horwitz, 1981). Paclitaxel has also found its way into clinical usage as a treatment of certain cancers and has resulted in sensorimotor axonopathy—in patients receiving large doses of this compound (Lipton et al., 1989; Sahenk et al., 1994)—or in autonomic neuropathy (Jerian et al., 1993).

It is fascinating that both the depolymerization of tubules by colchicine and the vinca alkaloids and the stabilization of tubules by paclitaxel lead to an axonopathy. It has been known for some time that microtubules are in a state of dynamic equilibrium in vitro, with tubules existing in equilibrium with dissociated subunits. This process almost certainly occurs in vivo as well, even as tubulin migrates down the axon. Thus, the tubules are constantly associating and dissociating. It is within this dynamic equilibrium that paclitaxel and the vinca alkaloids exert their toxic effects, preventing the interchange of the two pools of tubulin (Fig. 16-11).

The morphology of the axon is, of course, different in the two situations. In the case of colchicine, the axon appears to undergo atrophy and there are fewer microtubules within the axons. In contrast, following exposure to paclitaxel, microtubules are present in great numbers and are aggregated to create arrays of microtubules (Roytta et al., 1984; Roytta and Raine, 1986). Both situations probably interfere with the process of fast axonal transport, although this has not yet been demonstrated definitively with paclitaxel. In both situations, the resultant clinical condition is a peripheral neuropathy.

Myelinopathies

Myelin provides electrical insulation of neuronal processes, and its absence leads to a slowing of conduction and aberrant conduction of impulses between adjacent processes, so-called ephaptic transmission. Toxicants exist that result in the separation of the myelin lamellae, termed *intramyelinic edema,* and in the selective loss of myelin, termed *demyelination* (Fig. 16-4). Intramyelinic edema may be caused by alterations in the transcript levels of myelin basic protein-mRNA (Veronesi et al., 1991) and early in its evolution is reversible. However, the initial stages may progress to demyelination, with loss of myelin from the axon. Demyelination may also result from direct toxicity to the myelinating cell. Remyelination in the CNS occurs to only a limited extent after demyelination. However, Schwann cells in the PNS are capable of remyelinating the axon after a demyelinating injury. Interestingly, remyelination after segmental demyelination in peripheral nerve involves multiple Schwann cells and results, therefore, in internodal lengths (the distances between adjacent nodes of Ranvier) that are much shorter than normal and a permanent record of the demyelinating event.

The compounds in Table 16-3 all lead to a myelinopathy. Some of these compounds have created problems in humans, and

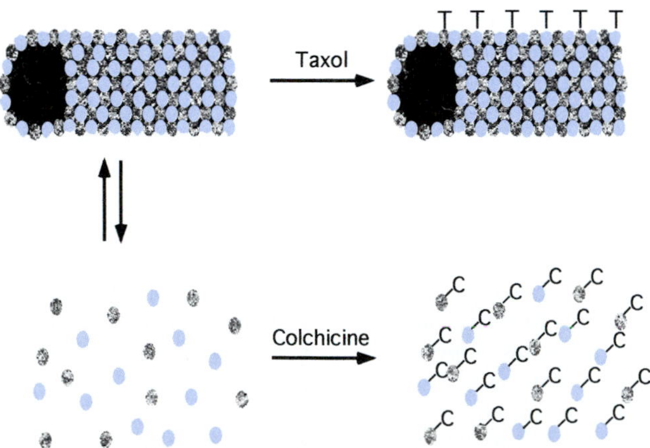

Figure 16-11. Neurotoxicants directed toward microtubules.

Colchicine leads to the depolymerization of microtubules by binding to the tubulin monomers and preventing their association into tubules. Paclitaxel stabilizes the microtubules, preventing their dissociation into subunits under conditions in which they would normally dissociate. Both compounds interfere with the normal dynamic equilibrium that exists between tubulin monomers and microtubules, and both are neurotoxic.

Table 16-3

Compounds Associated with Injury of Myelin (Myelinopathies)

NEUROTOXICANT	NEUROLOGIC FINDINGS	CELLULAR BASIS OF NEUROTOXICITY	REFERENCE
Acetylethyltetramethyl tetralin (AETT)	Not reported in humans; hyperexcitability, tremors (rats)	Intramyelinic edema; pigment accumulation in neurons	*b, c*
Amiodarone	Peripheral neuropathy	Axonal degeneration and demyelination; lipid-laden lysosomes in Schwann cells	*b, c*
Cuprizone	Not reported in humans; encephalopathy (experimental animals)	Status spongiosis of white matter, intramyelinic edema (early stages); gliosis (late)	*b, c*
Disulfiram	Peripheral neuropathy, predominantly sensory	Axonal degeneration, swellings in distal axons	*b*
Ethidium bromide	Insufficient data (humans)	Intramyelinic edema, status spongiosis of white matter	*c*
Hexachlorophene	Irritability, confusion, seizures	Brain swelling, intramyelinic edema in CNS and PNS, late axonal degeneration	*b, c*
Lysolecithin	Effects only on direct injection into peripheral nervous system (PNS) or central nervous system (CNS) (experimental animals)	Selective demyelination	*b*
Perhexilene	Peripheral neuropathy	Demyelinating neuropathy, membrane-bound inclusions in Schwann cells	*b, c*
Tellurium	Hydrocephalus, hind-limb paralysis (experimental animals)	Demyelinating neuropathy, lipofuscinosis (experimental animals)	*b*
Triethyltin	Headache, photophobia, vomiting, paraplegia (irreversible)	Brain swelling (acute) with intramyelinic edema, spongiosis of white matter	*a–c*

[a]Chang LW, Dyer RS, eds: *Handbook of Neurotoxicology*. New York: Marcel Dekker, 1995.

[b]Graham DI, Lantos PL, eds: *Greenfield's Neuropathology,* 6th ed. New York: Arnold, 1997.

[c]Spencer PS, Schaumburg HH, eds: *Experimental and Clinical Neurotoxicology,* 2d ed. New York: Oxford University Press, 2000.

many have been used as tools to explore the process of myelination of the NS and the process of remyelination following toxic disruption of myelin. In general, the functional consequences of demyelination depend on the extent of the demyelination and whether it is localized within the CNS or the PNS or is more diffuse in its distribution. Those toxic myelinopathies in which the disruption of myelin is diffuse generate a global neurologic deficit, whereas those that are limited to the PNS produce the symptoms of peripheral neuropathy.

Hexachlorophene Hexachlorophene, or methylene 2,2′-methylenebis(3,4,6-trichlorophenol), resulted in human neurotoxicity when newborn infants, particularly premature infants, were bathed with the compound to avoid staphylococcal skin infections (Mullick, 1973). Following skin absorption of this hydrophobic compound, hexachlorophene enters the NS and results in intramyelinic edema, splitting the intraperiod line of myelin in both the CNS and the PNS. The intramyelinic edema leads to the formation of vacuoles, creating a "spongiosis" of the brain (Purves et al., 1991). Experimental studies with erythrocyte membranes show that hexachlorophene binds tightly to cell membranes, resulting in the loss of ion gradients across the membrane (Flores and Buhler, 1974). It may be that hexachlorophene results in loss of the ability to exclude ions from between the layers of myelin and that, with ion entry, water also separates the myelin layers as "edema." Another, perhaps related effect is the uncoupling of mitochondrial oxidative phosphorylation by hexachlorophene (Cammer and Moore, 1974), because this process is dependent on a proton gradient. Intramyelinic edema is reversible in the early stages, but with increasing exposure, hexachlorophene causes segmental demyelination. Swelling of the brain causes increased intracranial pressure, which may be fatal in and of itself. With high-dose exposure, axonal degeneration is seen, along with degeneration of photoreceptors in the retina. It has been postulated that the pressure from severe intramyelinic edema may also injure the axon, leading to axonal degeneration, and endoneurial pressure measurements support this idea (Myers et al., 1982). The toxicity of hexachlorophene expresses itself functionally in diffuse terms that reflect the diffuse process of myelin injury. Humans exposed acutely to hexachlorophene may have generalized weakness, confusion, and seizures. Progression may occur, to include coma and death.

Tellurium Although human cases have not been reported, neurotoxicity of tellurium has been demonstrated in animals. Young rats exposed to tellurium in their diet develop a severe peripheral neuropathy. Within the first 2 days of beginning a diet containing tellurium, the synthesis of myelin lipids in Schwann cells displays some striking changes (Harry et al., 1989). There is a decreased synthesis of cholesterol and cerebrosides, lipids richly represented in myelin, whereas the synthesis of phosphatidylcholine, a more ubiquitous membrane lipid, is unaffected. Myelin protein mRNA steady-state levels are down-regulated (Morell et al., 1994). The synthesis of free fatty acids and cholesterol esters increases to some degree, and there is a marked elevation of squalene, a precursor of cholesterol. These biochemical findings demonstrate that there are a variety of lipid abnormalities, and the simultaneous increase in squalene and decrease in cholesterol suggest that tellurium or one of its derivatives may interfere with the normal conversion of squalene to cholesterol. Squalene epoxidase, a microsomal monooxygenase that utilizes NAPDH cytochrome P450 reductase, has been strongly implicated as the target of tellurium. It is specifically inhibited by tellurium (Wagner et al., 1995), and its inhibition also occurs with certain organotellurium compounds, with a correlation between the potency of enzyme inhibition and demyelination in vivo (Goodrum, 1998).

At the same time as these biochemical changes are occurring, lipids accumulate in Schwann cells within intracytoplasmic vacuoles; shortly afterwards, these Schwann cells lose their ability to maintain myelin. Axons and the myelin of the CNS are impervious to the effects of tellurium. However, individual Schwann cells in the PNS disassemble their concentric layers of myelin membranes, depriving the adjacent intact axon of its electrically insulated status. Not all Schwann cells are equally affected by the process; rather, those Schwann cells that encompass the greatest distances appear to be the most affected. These cells are associated with the largest-diameter axons, encompass the longest intervals of myelination, and provide the thickest layers of myelin. Thus, it appears that the most vulnerable cells are those with the largest volume of myelin to support (Bouldin et al., 1988).

As the process of remyelination begins, several cells cooperate to reproduce the myelin layers that were previously formed by a single Schwann cell. Perhaps this diminished demand placed upon an individual cell is the reason that remyelination occurs even in the presence of continued exposure to tellurium (Bouldin et al., 1988). The expression of the neurologic impairment is also short in duration, reflecting the transient cellular and biochemical events. The animals initially develop severe weakness in the hind limbs but then recover their strength after 2 weeks on the tellurium-laden diet.

Lead Lead exposure in animals results in a peripheral neuropathy with prominent segmental demyelination, a process that bears a strong resemblance to tellurium toxicity (Dyck et al., 1977). However, the neurotoxicity of lead is much more variable in humans than in rats, and there are also a variety of manifestations of lead toxicity in other organ systems.

The neurotoxicity of lead has been appreciated for centuries. In current times, adults are exposed to lead in occupational settings through lead smelting processes and soldering and in domestic settings through lead pipes or through the consumption of "moonshine" contaminated with lead. In addition, some areas contain higher levels of environmental lead, resulting in higher blood levels in the inhabitants. Children, especially those below 5 years of age, have higher blood levels of lead than adults in the same environment, due to the mouthing of objects and the consumption of substances other than food. The most common acute exposure in children, however, has been through the consumption of paint chips containing lead pigments (Perlstein and Attala, 1966), a finding that has led to public efforts to prevent the use of lead paints in homes with children.

In young children, acute massive exposures to lead result in severe cerebral edema, perhaps from damage to endothelial cells. Children seem to be more susceptible to this lead encephalopathy than adults (Johnston and Goldstein, 1998); however, adults may also develop an acute encephalopathy in the setting of massive lead exposure.

Chronic lead intoxication in adults results in peripheral neuropathy, often accompanied by manifestations outside the NS, such as gastritis, colicky abdominal pain, anemia, and the prominent deposition of lead in particular anatomic sites, creating lead lines in the gums and in the epiphyses of long bones in children. The effects of lead in the peripheral nerve of humans (lead neuropathy) is not entirely understood. Electrophysiologic studies have demonstrated a slowing of nerve conduction. While this observation is consistent with the segmental demyelination that develops in experimental animals, pathologic studies in humans with lead neuropathy typically have demonstrated an axonopathy. Another finding in humans is the predominant involvement of motor axons, creating one of the few clinical situations in which patients present with predominantly motor symptoms. The basis for the effect on the brain (lead encephalopathy) is also unclear, although an effect on the membrane structure of myelin and myelin membrane fluidity has been shown (Dabrowski-Bouta et al., 1999).

Although the manifestations of acute and chronic exposures to lead have been long established, it is only in recent years that the concept has emerged that extremely low levels of exposure to lead in "asymptomatic" children may have an effect on their intelligence. Initial reports noted a relationship between mild elevations of blood lead in children and school performance; more recently, correlations between elevated lead levels in decidual teeth and performance on tests of verbal abilities, attention, and behavior (nonadaptive) have been demonstrated (Needleman and Gatsonis, 1990; Needleman, 1994). Although there is a clear association between lead level and intellectual performance, there has been some discussion as to whether lead is causal. Children with higher blood levels tend to share certain other environmental factors, such as socioeconomic status and parental educational level. However, in spite of these complex social factors, it appears that lead exposure has an adverse effect on the intellectual abilities of children (Needleman, 1994), an association between lead exposure and brain dysfunction that has received experimental support in animal models (Gilbert and Rice, 1987) and has prompted screening for lead in children (Benjamin and Platt, 1999).

Neurotransmission-Associated Neurotoxicity

Many neurotoxicants destroy cellular structures within the NS, providing anatomic footprints of their toxicity. In some instances, however, dysfunction of the NS may occur without evidence of altered cellular structures; rather, the neurotoxicity expresses itself in terms of altered behavior or impaired performance on neurologic tests. In fact, many of the neurotoxic agents that lead to anatomic evidence of cellular injury were first demonstrated to be neurotoxic through the detection of neurologic dysfunction.

Molecular mechanisms are not understood for some of these agents; however, there is a group of such compounds in which the chemical basis of their action is clear. These are the toxicants that impair the process of neurotransmission. A wide variety of naturally occurring toxins as well as synthetic drugs interact with specific mechanisms of intercellular communication. At times, interruption of neurotransmission is beneficial to an individual, and the process may be viewed as neuropharmacology. However, excessive or inappropriate exposure to compounds that alter neurotransmission may be viewed as one of the patterns of neurotoxicology.

This group of compounds may interrupt the transmission of impulses, block or accentuate transsynaptic communication, block reuptake of neurotransmitters, or interfere with second-messenger systems. In general, the acute effects of these compounds are directly related to the immediate concentration of the compound at the active site, which bears a direct relationship to the level of the drug in the blood. The structural similarity of many compounds with similar actions has led to the recognition of specific categories of drugs and toxins. For example, some mimic the process of neurotransmission of the sympathetic nervous system and are termed the sympathomimetic compounds. As the targets of these drugs are located throughout the body, the responses are not localized; however, the responses are stereotyped in that each member of a class tends to have similar biological effects. In terms of toxicity, most of the side effects of these drugs may be viewed as short-term interactions that are easily reversible with time or that may be counteracted by the use of appropriate antagonists. However, some of the toxicity associated with long-term use is irreversible. For example, phenothiazines, which have been used to treat chronic schizophrenia for long periods of time, may lead to the condition of tardive dyskinesia, in which the patient is left with a permanent disability of prominent facial grimaces (DeVeaugh-Geiss, 1982). Both reversible acute high-dose toxicity and sustained effects following chronic exposure are common features of the agents that interact with the process of neurotransmission. Some compounds which have neurotransmitter-associated toxicity are listed in Table 16-4.

Nicotine Widely available in tobacco products and in certain pesticides, nicotine has diverse pharmacologic actions and may be the source of considerable toxicity. These toxic effects range from acute poisoning to more chronic effects. Nicotine exerts its effects by binding to a subset of cholinergic receptors, the nicotinic receptors. These receptors are located in ganglia, at the neuromuscular junction, and also within the CNS, where the psychoactive and addictive properties most likely reside. Smoking and "pharmacologic" doses of nicotine accelerate heart rate, elevate blood pressure, and constrict blood vessels within the skin. Because the majority of these effects may be prevented by the administration of α- and β-adrenergic blockade, these consequences may be viewed as the result of stimulation of the ganglionic sympathetic nervous system (Benowitz, 1986). At the same time, nicotine leads to a sensation of "relaxation" and is associated with alterations of electroencephalographic (EEG) recordings in humans. These effects are probably related to the binding of nicotine with nicotinic receptors within the CNS, and the EEG changes may be blocked with mecamylamine, an antagonist.

Acute overdose of nicotine has occurred in children who accidentally ingest tobacco products, in tobacco workers exposed to wet tobacco leaves (Gehlbach et al., 1974), and in workers exposed to nicotine-containing pesticides. In each of these settings, the rapid rise in circulating levels of nicotine leads to excessive stimulation of nicotinic receptors, a process that is followed rapidly by ganglionic paralysis. Initial nausea, rapid heart rate, and perspiration are followed shortly by marked slowing of heart rate with a fall in blood pressure. Somnolence and confusion may occur, followed by coma; if death results, it is often the result of paralysis of the muscles of respiration.

Such acute poisoning with nicotine fortunately is uncommon. Exposure to lower levels for longer duration, in contrast, is very common, and the health effects of this exposure are of considerable epidemiologic concern. In humans, however, it has been impossible so far to separate the effects of nicotine from those of other components of cigarette smoke. The complications of smoking include cardiovascular disease, cancers (especially malignancies of the lung and upper airway), chronic pulmonary disease, and attention deficit disorders in children of women who smoke dur-

Table 16-4
Compounds Associated with Neurotransmitter-Associated Toxicity

NEUROTOXICANT	NEUROLOGIC FINDINGS	CELLULAR BASIS OF NEUROTOXICITY	REFERENCE
Amphetamine and methamphetamine	Tremor, restlessness (acute); cerebral infarction and hemorrhage; neuropsychiatric disturbances	Bilateral infarcts of globus pallidus, abnormalities in dopaminergic, serotonergic, cholinergic systems Acts at adrenergic receptors	*b, c*
Atropine	Restlessness, irritability, hallucinations	Block cholinergic receptors (anticholinergic)	*b, c*
Cocaine	Increased risk of stroke and cerebral atrophy (chronic users); increased risk of sudden cardiac death; movement and psychiatric abnormalities, especially during withdrawal Decreased head circumference (fetal exposure)	Infarcts and hemorrhages; alteration in striatal dopamine neurotransmission (binds to voltage-gated sodium channels) Structural malformations in newborns	*b, c*
Domoic acid	Headache, memory loss, hemiparesis, disorientation, seizures	Neuronal loss, hippocampus and amygdala, layers 5 and 6 of neocortex Kainate-like pattern of excitotoxicity	*a, b*
Kainate	Insufficient data in humans; seizures in animals (selective lesioning compound in neuroscience)	Degeneration of neurons in hippocampus, olfactory cortex, amygdala, thalamus Binds AMPA/kainate receptors	*a*
β-*N*-Methylamino-L-alanine (BMAA)	Weakness, movement disorder (monkeys)	Degenerative changes in motor neurons (monkeys) Excitotoxic probably via NMDA receptors	*a, b*
Muscarine (mushrooms)	Nausea, vomiting, headache	Binds muscarinic receptors (cholinergic)	*c*
Nicotine	Nausea, vomiting, convulsions	Binds nicotinic receptors (cholinergic) low-dose stimulation; high-dose blocking	*b, c*
β-*N*-Oxalylamino-L-alanine (BOAA)	Seizures	Excitotoxic probably via AMPA class of glutamate receptors	*a, b*

[a]Graham DI, Lantos PL, eds: *Greenfield's Neuropathology,* 6th ed: New York: Arnold, 1997.
[b]Spencer PS, Schaumburg HH, eds: *Experimental and Clinical Neurotoxicology,* 2d ed. New York: Oxford University Press, 2000.
[c]Hardman JG, Limbird LE, Molinoff PB, Ruddon RW, eds: *Goodman and Gilman's The Pharmacologic Basis of Therapeutics,* 9th ed. New York: McGraw-Hill, 1996.

ing pregnancy. Nicotine may be a factor in some of these problems. For example, an increased propensity for platelets to aggregate is seen in smokers, and this platelet abnormality correlates with the level of nicotine. Nicotine also places an increased burden on the heart through its acceleration of heart rate and blood pressure, suggesting that nicotine may play a role in the onset of myocardial ischemia (Benowitz, 1986). In addition, nicotine also inhibits apoptosis and may play a direct role in tumor promotion and tobacco-related cancers (Wright et al., 1993).

It seems more clear that chronic exposure to nicotine has effects on the developing fetus. Along with decreased birth weights, attention deficit disorders are more common in children whose mothers smoke cigarettes during pregnancy, and nicotine has been shown to lead to analogous neurobehavioral abnormalities in animals exposed prenatally to nicotine (Lichensteiger et al., 1988). Nicotinic receptors are expressed early in the development of the NS, beginning in the developing brainstem and later expressed in the diencephalon. The role of these nicotinic receptors during development is unclear; however, it appears that prenatal exposure to nicotine alters the development of nicotinic receptors in the CNS (van de Kamp and Collins, 1994)—changes that may be related to subsequent attention and cognitive disorders in animals and children.

Cocaine and Amphetamines Cocaine differs from nicotine in the eyes of the law, a feature of the compound that affects the willingness of users to discuss their patterns of use. Nonetheless, it has been possible to obtain estimates of the number of users. In 1972, approximately 9 million college-age adults were using the drug; in 1982, it was approximately 33 million (Fishburne et al., 1983). In urban settings, from 10 to 45 percent of pregnant women take cocaine (Volpe, 1992), and cocaine metabolites can be detected in as many as 6 percent of babies born at suburban hospitals (Schutzman et al., 1991).

The euphoric and addictive properties of cocaine derive from alterations in catecholaminergic neurotransmission, especially enhanced dopaminergic neurotransmission, by blocking the dopamine reuptake transporter (DAT) (Giros et al., 1996). Acute toxicity due to excessive intake, or overdose, may result in unanticipated deaths. While the tragic accounts of celebrities' overdoses may attract media attention, it is the chronic "recreational" consumption of cocaine that is of greatest epidemiologic concern.

Although cocaine increases maternal blood pressure during acute exposure in pregnant animals, the blood flow to the uterus actually diminishes. Depending on the level of the drug in the mother, the fetus may develop marked hypoxia as a result of the diminished uterine blood flow (Woods et al., 1987). In a study of women who used cocaine during pregnancy, there were more miscarriages and placental hemorrhages (abruptions) than in drug-free women (Chasnoff et al., 1985). Impaired placental function may be the cause for the increase in infarctions and hemorrhages in the newborn infant who has been exposed to cocaine (Volpe, 1992). In addition, the newborn infants of cocaine users were less interactive than normal newborns and exhibited a poor response to stimuli in the environment (Chasnoff et al., 1985). Evidence for other forms of structural damage to brain in newborns exposed to cocaine is mixed (Behnke et al., 1998).

In addition to deleterious effects on fetal growth and development, cocaine abuse is associated with an increased risk of cerebrovascular disease, cerebral perfusion defects, and cerebral atrophy in adults (Filley and Kelly, 1993; Freilich and Byrne, 1992; Kaku and Lowenstein, 1990). While the mechanisms for these effects are not known, imaging studies have demonstrated increased cerebrovascular resistance in cocaine abusers (Herning et al., 1999). Chronic cocaine abuse has been associated with neurodegenerative changes in the striatum, and these changes are thought to underlie some of the neurologic and psychiatric outcomes in chronic cocaine abusers (Wilson et al., 1996b).

Like cocaine, amphetamines exert their effects in the CNS by altering catecholamine neurotransmission; however, unlike cocaine, the actions of amphetamines are not limited to plasma membrane transporters but also appear to involve disruption of vesicular storage of dopamine. Analogous to cocaine, amphetamines have been associated with an increased risk of abnormal fetal growth and development, increased risk of cerebrovascular disease, and increased risk of psychiatric and neurologic problems in chronic abusers that may be related to dopaminergic neurodegeneration (Wilson et al., 1996a).

Excitatory Amino Acids Glutamate and certain other acidic amino acids are excitatory neurotransmitters within the CNS. The discovery that these excitatory amino acids can be neurotoxic at concentrations that can be achieved in the brain has generated a great amount of interest in these "excitotoxins." In vitro systems have established that the toxicity of glutamate can be blocked by certain glutamate antagonists (Rothman and Olney, 1986), and the concept has emerged that the toxicity of excitatory amino acids may be related to such divergent conditions as hypoxia, epilepsy, and neurodegenerative diseases (Meldrum, 1987; Choi, 1988; Lipton and Rosenberg, 1994; Beal, 1992, 1995, 1998).

Glutamate is the main excitatory neurotransmitter of the brain and its effects are mediated by several subtypes of receptors (Fig. 16-12) called *excitatory amino acid receptors* (EAARs) (Schoepfer

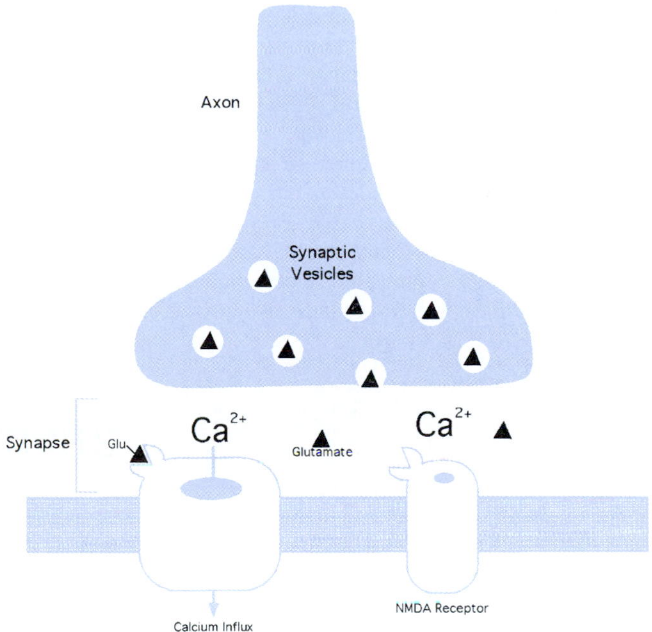

Figure 16-12. Schematic diagram of a synapse.

Synaptic vesicles are tranported to the axonal terminus, and released across the synaptic cleft to bind to the postsynaptic receptors. Glutamate, as an excitatory neurotransmitter, binds to its receptor and opens a calcium channel, leading to the excitation of the postsynaptic cell.

et al., 1994; Hollmann and Heinemann, 1994; Lipton and Rosenberg, 1994). The two major subtypes of glutamate receptors are those that are ligand-gated directly to ion channels (ionotropic) and those that are coupled with G proteins (metabotropic). Ionotropic receptors may be further subdivided by their specificity for binding kainate, quisqualate, and α-amino-3-hydroxy-5-methylisoxazole-4-propionic acid (AMPA), and *N*-methyl-D-aspartate (NMDA). The entry of glutamate into the CNS is regulated at the blood-brain barrier and, following an injection of a large dose of glutamate in infant rodents, glutamate exerts its effects in the area of the brain in which the blood-brain barrier is least developed, the circumventricular organ. Within this site of limited access, glutamate injures neurons, apparently by opening glutamate-dependent ion channels, ultimately leading to neuronal swelling and neuronal cell death (Olney, 1978; Coyle, 1987). The toxicity affects the dendrites and neuronal cell bodies but seems to spare axons. The only known related human condition is the "Chinese restaurant syndrome," in which consumption of large amounts of monosodium glutamate as a seasoning may lead to a burning sensation in the face, neck and chest.

The cyclic glutamate analog kainate was initially isolated from a seaweed in Japan as the active component of an herbal treatment of ascariasis. Kainate is extremely potent as an excitotoxin, being a hundredfold more toxic than glutamate and is selective at a molecular level for the kainate receptor (Coyle, 1987). Like glutamate, kainate selectively injures dendrites and neurons and shows no substantial effect on glia or axons. As a result, this compound has found use in neurobiology as a tool. Injected into a region of the brain, kainate can destroy the neurons of that area without disrupting all of the fibers that pass through the same region. Neurobiologists, with the help of this neurotoxic tool, are able to study the role of neurons in a particular area independent of the axonal injuries that occur when similar lesioning experiments are performed by mechanical cutting.

Development of permanent neurologic deficits in individuals accidentally exposed to high doses of an EAAR agonist has underscored the potential importance of EAAs in disease (Perl et al., 1990; Teitelbaum et al., 1990). A total of 107 individuals in the Maritime Provinces of Canada were exposed to domoic acid, an analog of glutamate, and suffered an acute illness that most commonly presented as gastrointestinal disturbance, severe headache, and short-term memory loss. A subset of the more severely afflicted patients was subsequently shown to have chronic memory deficits and motor neuropathy. Neuropathologic investigation of patients who died within 4 months of intoxication showed neurodegeneration that was most prominent in the hippocampus and amygdala but also affected regions of the thalamus and cerebral cortex.

Other foci of unusual neurodegenerative diseases also have been evaluated for being caused by dietary exposure to EAARs. Perhaps the best known of these is the complex neurodegenerative disease in the indigenous population of Guam and surrounding islands that shares features of amyotrophic lateral sclerosis, Parkinson's disease, and Alzheimer's disease. Early investigations of this Guamanian neurodegenerative complex suggested that the disorder may be related to an environmental factor, perhaps consumption of seeds of *Cycas circinalis* (Kurland, 1963). Subsequently, α-amino-methylaminopropionic acid (or B-*N*-methylamino-L-alanine, BMAA) was isolated from the cycad and was shown to be neurotoxic in model systems. The toxicity of BMAA is similar to that of glutamate in vitro and can be blocked by certain EAAR antagonists (Nunn et al., 1987). Studies in vivo, however, have not demonstrated a relationship between BMAA and the Guamanian neurodegenerative complex (Spencer et al., 1987; Hugon et al., 1988; Seawright et al., 1990; Duncan, 1992). Therefore, it remains unresolved what role cycad consumption and environmental factors play in this cluster of atypical neurodegenerative disease.

The expanding field of the excitotoxic amino acids embodies many of the same attributes that characterize the entire discipline of neurotoxicology. Neurotoxicology is generally viewed as the study of compounds that are deleterious to the NS, and the effects of glutamate and kainate may be viewed as examples of this type of deleterious toxicity. Exposure to these excitotoxic amino acids leads to neuronal injury and—when of sufficient degree—may kill neurons. However, the implications of these findings, as with the entire field of neurotoxicology, extend beyond the direct toxicity of the compounds in exposed populations. With kainate, as with many other neurotoxic compounds, has come a tool for neurobiologists who seek to explore the anatomy and function of the NS. Kainate, through its selective action on neuronal cell bodies, has provided a greater understanding of the functions of cells within a specific region of the brain, while previous lesioning techniques addressed only regional functions. Finally, the questions surrounding domoic acid poisoning and the Guamanian neurodegenerative complex serve to remind the student of neurotoxicology that the causes of many neurologic diseases remain unknown. This void in understanding and the epidemiologic evidence that some neurodegenerative diseases may have environmental contributors provide a heightened desire to appreciate more fully the effects of elements of our environment on the NS.

REFERENCES

Abou-Donia MB, Lapadula DM: Mechanisms of organophosphorus ester-induced delayed neurotoxicity: Type I and type II. *Annu Rev Pharmacol Toxicol* 30:405–440, 1990.

Agundez JA, Jimenex JF, Luengo A, et al: Association between the oxidative polymorphism and early onset of Parkinson's disease. *Clin Pharmacol Ther* 57:291–298, 1995.

Amarnath V, Anthony DC, Amarnath K, et al: Intermediates in the Paal-Knorr synthesis of pyrroles. *J Org Chem* 56:6924–6931, 1991a.

Amarnath V, Anthony DC, Valentine WM, et al: The molecular mechanism of the carbon disulfide mediated crosslinking of proteins. *Chem Res Toxicol* 4:148–150, 1991b.

Amarnath V, Valentine WM, Amarnath K, et al: The mechanism of nucleophilic substitution of alkylpyrroles in the presence of oxygen. *Chem Res Toxicol* 7:56–61, 1994.

Anthony DC, Boekelheide K, Anderson CW, et al: The effect of 3,4-dimethyl substitution on the neurotoxicity of 2,5-hexanedione: II. Dimethyl substitution accelerates pyrrole formation and protein crosslinking. *Toxicol Appl Pharmacol* 71:372–382, 1983a.

Anthony DC, Boekelheide K, Graham DG: The effect of 3,4-dimethyl substitution on the neurotoxicity of 2,5-hexanedione: I. Accelerated clinical neuropathy is accompanied by more proximal axonal swellings. *Toxicol Appl Pharmacol* 71:362–371, 1983b.

Asanuma M, Hirata H, Cadet JL: Attenuation of 6-hydroxydopamine nigrostriatal lesions in superoxide dismutase transgenic mice. *Neuroscience* 85:907–917, 1998.

Atchison WD, Hare MF: Mechanisms of methylmercury-induced neurotoxicity. *FASEB J* 8:622–629, 1994.

Auer RN, Benveniste H: Hypoxia and related conditions, in Graham DI, Lantos PL (eds): *Greenfield's Neuropathology,* 6th ed. New York: Arnold, 1997, pp 263–314.

Bachurin SO, Shevtzove EP, Lermontova NN, et al: The effect of dithiocarbamates on neurotoxic action of 1-methyl-4-phenyl-1,2,3,6-tetrahydropyridine (MPTP) and on mitochondrial respiration chain. *Neurotoxicology* 17:897–903, 1996.

Bakir F, Damluji SF, Amin-Zaki L, et al: Methylmercury poisoning in Iraq. *Science* 181:230–241, 1973.

Beal MF: Does impairment of energy metabolism result in excitotoxic neuronal death in neurodegenerative illnesses? *Ann Neurol* 31:119–130, 1992.

Beal MF: Aging, energy, and oxidative stress in neurodegenerative diseases. *Ann Neurol* 38:357–366, 1995.

Beal MF: Excitotoxicity and nitric oxide in Parkinson's disease pathogenesis. *Ann Neurol* 44:S110–S114, 1998.

Becking GC, Boyes WK, Damstra T, et al: Assessing the neurotoxic potential of chemicals: A multidisciplinary approach. *Environ Res* 61:164–175, 1993.

Behnke M, Eyler F, Conlon M, et al: Incidence and description of structural brain abnormalities in newborns exposed to cocaine. *J Pediatr* 132:291–294, 1998.

Benjamin JT, Platt C: Is universal screening for lead in children indicated? An analysis of lead results in Augusta, Georgia in 1997. *J Med Assoc Georgia* 88:24–26, 1999.

Benowitz NL: Clinical pharmacology of nicotine. *Annu Rev Med* 37:21–32, 1986.

Bensadoun JC, Mirochnitchenko O, Innouye M, et al: Attenuation of 6-OHDA-induced neurotoxicity in glutathione peroxidase transgenic mice. *Eur J Neurosci* 10:3231–3236, 1998.

Besser R, Kramer G, Thumler R, et al: Acute trimethyltin limbic-cerebellar syndrome. *Neurology* 37:945–950, 1987.

Bouldin TW, Goines ND, Bagnell CR, Krigman MR: Pathogenesis of trimethyltin neuronal toxicity: Ultrastructural and cytochemical observations. *Am J Pathol* 104:237–249, 1981.

Bouldin TW, Samsa G, Earnhardt TS, et al: Schwann cell vulnerability to demyelination is associated with internodal length in tellurium neuropathy. *J Neuropathol Exp Neurol* 47:41–47, 1988.

Brouillet E, Jenkins BG, Hyman BT, et al: Age-dependent vulnerability of the striatum to the mitochondrial toxin 3-nitropropionic acid. *J Neurochem* 60:356–359, 1993.

Burbacher TM, Sackett GP, Mottet NK: Methylmercury effects on the social behavior of Macaca fascicularis. *Neurotoxicol Teratol* 12:65–71, 1990.

Calne DB, Langston JW, Martin WR, et al: Positron emission tomography after MPTP: Observations relating to the cause of Parkinson's disease. *Nature* 317:246–248, 1985.

Cammer W, Moore CL: The effect of hexachlorophene on the respiration of brain and liver mitochondria. *Biochem Biophys Res Commun* 46:1887–1894, 1972.

Cavanagh JB: The significance of the "dying-back" process in experimental and human neurological disease. *Int Nat Rev Exp Pathol* 7:219–267, 1964.

Chasnoff IJ, Burns WJ, Schnoll SH, et al: Cocaine use in pregnancy. *N Engl J Med* 313:666–669, 1985.

Chaudry, V, Cornblath, DR: Wallerian degeneration in human nerves: Serial electrophysiological studies. *Muscle Nerve* 15:687–693, 1992.

Cheung MK, Verity MA: Experimental methyl mercury neurotoxicity: Locus of mercurial inhibition of brain protein synthesis in vivo and in vitro. *J Neurochem* 44:1799–1808, 1985.

Choi DW: Glutamate neurotoxicity and diseases of the nervous system. *Neuron* 1:623–634, 1988.

Cohen G, Heikkila RE: In vivo scavenging of superoxide radicals by catecholamines, in Michelson AM, McCord JM, Fridovich I (eds): *Superoxide and Superoxide Dismutases.* London: Academic Press, 1977, pp 351–365.

Collins JJ, Swaen GMH, Marsh GM, et al: Mortality patterns among workers exposed to acrylamide. *J Occup Med* 31:614–617, 1989.

Coyle JT: Kainic acid: Insights into excitatory mechanisms causing selective neuronal degeneration, in Bock G, O'Connor M (eds): *Selective Neuronal Death.* New York: Wiley, 1987, pp 186–203.

Crofton KM, Padilla S, Tilson HA, et al: The impact of dose rate on the neurotoxicity of acrylamide: The interaction of administered dose, target tissue concentrations, tissue damage, and functional effects. *Toxicol Appl Pharmacol* 139:163–176, 1996.

Dabrowska-Bouta G, Sulkowski G, Bartosz G, et al: Chronic lead intoxication affects the myelin membrane status in the central nervous system of adult rats. *J Mol Neurosci* 13:127–139, 1999.

DeGrandchamp RL, Lowndes HE: Early degeneration and sprouting at the rat neuromuscular junction following acrylamide administration. *Neuropathol Appl Neurobiol* 16:239–254, 1990.

DeGrandchamp RL, Reuhl KR, Lowndes HE: Synaptic terminal degeneration and remodeling at the rat neuromuscular junction resulting from a single exposure to acrylamide. *Toxicol Appl Pharmacol* 105:422–433, 1990.

Dejneka NS, Polavarapu R, Deng X, et al: Chromosomal localization and characterization of the stannin (Snn) gene. *Mamm Genome* 9:556–564, 1998.

Denlinger RH, Anthony DC, Amarnath K, et al: Metabolism of 3,3′-iminodipropionitrile and deuterium-substituted analogs: Potential mechanisms of detoxification and activation. *Toxicol Appl Pharmacol* 124:59–66, 1994.

Denlinger RH, Anthony DC, Amarnath V, et al: Comparison of location, severity, and dose response of proximal axonal lesions induced by 3,3′-iminodipropionitrile and deuterium substituted analogs. *J Neuropathol Exp Neurol* 51:569–576, 1992.

DeVeaugh-Geiss J: Tardive dyskinesia: Phenomenology, pathophysiology, and pharmacology, in *Tardive Dyskinesia and Related Involuntary Movement Disorders.* Boston: John Wright PSG, 1982, pp 1–18.

Di Monte DA, Langston JW: MPTP and analogs, in Spencer PS, Schaumburg HH (eds): *Experimental and Clinical Neurotoxicology.* New York: Oxford University Press, 2000, pp 812–818.

Duncan MW: β-Methylamino-L-alanine (BMAA) and amyotrophic lateral sclerosis-parkinsonism dementia of the western Pacific. *Ann NY Acad Sci* 648:161–168, 1992.

Dyck PJ, O'Brien PC, Ohnishi A: Lead neuropathy: 2. Random distribution of segmental demyelination among "old internodes" of myelinated fibers. *J Neuropathol Exp Neurol* 36:570–575, 1977.

Erve JCL, Amarnath V, Graham D, et al: Carbon disulfide and *N,N*-diethyldithiocarbamate generate thiourea cross-links on erythrocyte spectrin. *Chem Res Toxicol* 11:544–549, 1998a.

Erve JCL, Amarnath V, Sills RC, et al: Characterization of a valine-lysine thiourea cross-link on rat globin produced by carbon disulfide or *N,N*-diethyldithiocarbamate in vivo. *Chem Res Toxicol* 11:1128–1136, 1998b.

Federal Register: *Principles of Neurotoxicity Risk Assessment. Environmental Protection Agency Final Report,* vol 59, no 158. Washington, DC: U.S. Government Printing Office, 1994, pp 42360–42404.

Ferraz HB, Bertolucci PH, Pereira JS, et al: Chronic exposure to the fungicide maneb may produce symptoms and signs of CNS manganese intoxication. *Neurology* 38:550–553, 1988.

Filley CM, Kelly JP: Alcohol- and drug-related neurotoxicity. *Curr Opin Neurol Neurosurg* 6:443–447, 1993.

Fishburne PM, Abelson HI, Cisin I: *National Household Survey on Drug Abuse: National Institute of Drug and Alcohol Abuse Capsules, 1982.* Washington, DC: Department of Health and Human Services, 1983.

Flores G, Buhler DR: Hemolytic properties of hexachlorophene and related chlorinated biphenols. *Biochem Pharmacol* 23:1835–1843, 1974.

Freilich RJ, Byrne E: Alcohol and drug abuse. *Curr Opin Neurol Neurosurg* 5:391–395, 1992.

Funk KA, Liu CH, Higgins RJ, et al: Avian embryonic brain reaggregate culture system. II. NTE activity discriminates between effects of a single neuropathic or nonneuropathic organophosphorus compound exposure. *Toxicol Appl Pharmacol* 124:159–163, 1994.

Gehlbach SH, Williams WA, Perry LD, et al: Green-tobacco sickness: An illness of tobacco harvesters. *JAMA* 229:1880–1883, 1974.

Genter MB, Szkal-Quin G, Anderson CW, et al: Evidence that pyrrole formation is a pathogenetic step in γ-diketone neuropathy. *Toxicol Appl Pharmacol* 87:351–362, 1987.

George EB, Glass JD, Griffin JW: Axotomy-induced axonal degeneration is mediated by calcium influx through ion-specific channels. *J Neurosci* 15:6445–6452, 1995.

Gilbert SG, Rice DC: Low-level lifetime lead exposure produces behavioral toxicity (spatial discrimination reversal) in adult monkeys. *Toxicol Appl Pharmacol* 91:484–490, 1987.

Giros B, Jaber SR, Wightman RM, et al: Hyperlocomotion and indifference to cocaine and amphetamine in mice lacking the dopamine transporter. *Nature* 379:606–612, 1996.

Glass JD, Brushart TM, George EB, et al: Prolonged survival of transected fibers in C57BL/Ola mice is intrinsic characteristic of the axon. *J Neurocytol* 22:311–321, 1993.

Goldberger ME, Murray M: Recovery of function and anatomical plasticity after damage to the adult and neonatal spinal cord, in Cotman CW (ed): *Synaptic Plasticity.* New York: Guilford Press, 1985, pp 77–110.

Goodrum JF: Role of organotellurium species in tellurium neuropathy. *Neurochem Res* 23:1313–1319, 1998.

Gorell JM, Johnson CC, Rybicki BA, et al: Occupational exposure to manganese copper, lead, iron, mercury and zinc and the risk of Parkinson's disease. *Neurotoxicology* 20:239–247, 1999.

Gorell JM, Johnson CC, Rybicki BA, et al: The risk of Parkinson's disease with exposure to pesticides, farming, well water and rural living. *Neurology* 59:1346–1350, 1998.

Grafstein B: Axonal transport: Function and mechanisms, in Waxman SG, Kocsis JD, Stys PK (eds): *The Axon: Structure, Function, and Pathophysiology.* New York: Oxford University Press, 1995, pp 185–199.

Graham DG, Oxidative pathways for catecholamines in the genesis of neuromelanin and cytotoxic quinones. *Mol Pharmacol* 14:633–643, 1978.

Graham DG, Amarnath V, Valentine WM, et al: Pathogenetic studies of hexane and carbon disulfide neurotoxicity. *CRC Crit Rev Toxicol* 25: 91–112, 1995.

Graham DG, Tiffany SM, Bell WR Jr, Gutknecht WF: Autoxidation versus covalent binding of quinones as the mechanism of toxicity of dopamine 6-hydroxydopamine and related compounds for C1300 neuroblastoma cells in vitro. *Mol Pharmacol* 14:644–653, 1978.

Griffin JW, Anthony DC, Fahnestock KE, et al: 3,4-Dimethyl-2,5-hexanedione impairs the axonal transport of neurofilament proteins. *J Neurosci* 4:1516–1526, 1984.

Griffin JW, Hoffman PN, Clark AW, et al: Slow axonal transport of neurofilament proteins: Impairment by β,β'-iminodipropionitrile administration. *Science* 202:633–635, 1978.

Griffin JW, Price DL: Proximal axonopathies induced by toxic chemicals, in Spencer PS, Schaumburg HH (eds): *Experimental and Clinical Neurotoxicology.* Baltimore: Williams & Wilkins, 1980, pp 161–178.

Harris CH, Gulati AK, Friedman MA, et al: Toxic neurofilamentous axonopathies and fast axonal transport: V. Reduced bidirectional vesicle transport in cultured neurons by acrylamide and glycidamide. *J Toxicol Environ Health* 42:343–456, 1994.

Harry GJ, Goodrum JF, Bouldin TW, et al: Tellurium-induced neuropathy: Metabolic alterations associated with demyelination and remyelination in rat sciatic nerve. *J Neurochem* 52:938–945, 1989.

Herning R, King D, Better W, et al: Neurovascular deficits in cocaine abusers. *Neuropsychopharmacology* 21:110–118, 1999.

Hoffman PN, Lasek RJ: The slow component of axonal transport: Identification of major structural polypeptides of the axon and their generality among mammalian neurons. *J Cell Biol* 66:351–366, 1975.

Hollmann M, Heinemann S: Cloned glutamate receptors. *Annu Rev Neurosci* 17:31–108, 1994.

Hugon J, Ludolph A, Roy DN, et al: Studies on the etiology and pathogenesis of motor neuron diseases: II. Clinical and electrophysiologic features of pyramidal dysfunction in macaques fed *Lathyrus sativus* and IDPN. *Neurology* 38:435–442, 1988.

Ikonomidou C, Bittigau P, Ishimaru MJ, et al: Ethanol-induced apoptotic neurodegeneration and fetal alcohol syndrome. *Science* 287:1056–1060, 2000.

Jerian SM, Sarosy GA, Link CJ Jr, et al: Incapacitating autonomic neuropathy precipitated by Taxol. *Gynecol Oncol* 51:277–280, 1993.

Johnson DJ, Graham DG, Amarnath V, et al: Release of carbon disulfide is a contributing mechanism in the axonopathy produced by *N,N*-diethyldithiocarbamate. *Toxicol Appl Pharmacol* 148:288–296, 1998.

Johnston MV, Goldstein GW: Selective vulnerability of the developing brain to lead. *Curr Opin Neurol* 11:689–693, 1998.

Kaku DA, Lowenstein DH: Emergence of recreational drug abuse as a major risk factor for stroke in young adults. *Ann Intern Med* 113:821–827, 1990.

Kesson CM, Baird AW, Lawson DH: Acrylamide poisoning. *Postgrad Med J* 53:16–17, 1977.

Kinney HK, Armstrong DD: Perinatal neuropathology, in Graham DI, Lantos PL (eds): *Greenfield's Neuropathology,* 6th ed. New York: Arnold, 1997, pp 535–599.

Klivenyi P, Clair D, Wermer M, et al: Manganese superoxide dismutase overexpression attenuates MPTP toxicity. *Neurobiol Dis* 5:253–258, 1998.

Kniesel U, Wolburg H: Tight junctions of the blood-brain barrier. *Cell Mol Neurobiol* 20:57–76, 2000.

Koehnle TJ, Brown A: Slow axonal transport of neurofilament protein in cultured neurons. *J Cell Biol* 144:447–458, 1999.

Krasavage WJ, O'Donoghue JL, DiVincenzo GD, et al: The relative neurotoxicity of MnBk, *n*-hexane, and their metabolites. *Toxicol Appl Pharmacol* 52:433–441, 1980.

Kuopio AM, Marttila RJ, Helenius H, et al: Changing epidemiology of Parkinson's disease in southwestern Finland. *Neurology* 52:302–308, 1999.

Kurland LT: Epidemiological investigations of neurological disorders in the Mariana islands, in Pemberton J (ed): *Epidemiology Reports on Research and Teaching.* Oxford and New York: Oxford University Press, 1963, pp 219–223.

Kurland LT, Faro SN, Siedler J: Minamata disease. *World Neurol* 1:370–395, 1960.

Kurth MC, Kurth JH: Variant cytochrome P450 CYP2D6 allelic frequencies in Parkinson's disease. *Am J Med Genet* 48:166–168, 1993.

Lam G-W, DiStefano V: Characterization of carbon disulfide binding in blood and to other biological substances. *Toxicol Appl Pharmacol* 86:235–242, 1986.

Langston JW, Forno LS, Tetrud J, et al: Evidence of active nerve cell degeneration in the substantia nigra of humans years after 1-methyl-4-phenyl-1,2,3,6-tetrahydropyridine exposure. *Ann Neurol* 46:598–605, 1999.

Langston JW, Irwin I: MPTP: Current concepts and controversies. *Clin Neuropharmacol* 9:485–507, 1986.

LeBel CP, Ali SF, Bondy SC: Deferoxamine inhibits methyl mercury-induced increases in reactive oxygen species formation in rat brain. *Toxicol Appl Pharmacol* 112:161–165, 1992.

Letzel S, Lang CJ, Schaller KH, et al: Longitudinal study of neurotoxicity with occupational exposure to aluminum dust. *Neurology* 54:997–1000, 2000.

Lichensteiger W, Ribary U, Schlumpf M, et al: Prenatal adverse effects of nicotine on the developing brain, in Boer GJ, Feenstra MGP, Mirmiran M, et al (eds): *Progress in Brain Research.* Vol 73. Amsterdam: Elsevier, 1988, pp 137–157.

Liou HH, Tsai MC, Chen CJ, et al: Environmental risk factors and Parkinson's disease: A case-control study in Taiwan. *Neurology* 48:1583–1588, 1997.

Lipton RB, Apfel SC, Dutcher JP, et al: Taxol produces a predominantly sensory neuropathy. *Neurology* 39:368–373, 1989.

Lipton SA, Rosenberg PA: Excitatory amino acids as a final common pathway for neurologic disorders. *N Engl J Med* 330:613–622, 1994.

Liu Y, Fechter LD: Comparison of the effects of trimethyltin on the intracellular calcium levels in spiral ganglion cells and outer hair cells. *Acta Otolaryngol* 116:417–421, 1996.

Llorens J, Dememes D, Sans A: The behavioral syndrome caused by 3,3′-iminodipropionitrile and related nitriles in the rat is associated with degeneration of the vestibular sensory hair cells. *Toxicol Appl Pharmacol* 123:199–210, 1993.

Lotharius J, O'Malley KL: The parkinsonian-inducing drug 1-methyl-4-phenylpyridinium triggers intracellular dopamine oxidation. *J Biol Chem* 275:38581–38588, 2000.

Lotti M, Moretto A, Capodicasa E, et al: Interactions between neuropathy target esterase and its inhibitors and the development of polyneuropathy. *Toxicol Appl Pharmacol* 122:165–171, 1993.

Lucey JF, Hibbard E, Behrman RE, et al: Kernicterus in asphyxiated newborn rhesus monkeys. *Exp Neurol* 9:43–58, 1964.

Ludolf AC, He F, Spencer PS, et al: 3-Nitropropionic acid: Exogenous animal neurotoxin and possible human striatal toxin. *Can J Neurol Sci* 18:492–498, 1991.

Ludolf AC, Seelig M, Ludolf A, et al: 3-Nitropropionic acid decreases cellular energy levels and causes neuronal degeneration in cortical explants. *Neurodegeneration* 1:155–161, 1992.

Lunn ER, Perry VH, Brown MC, et al: Absence of Wallerian degeneration does not hinder regeneration in peripheral nerve. *Eur J Neurosci* 1:27–33, 1989.

Lyon MF, Ogunkolade BW, Brown MC, et al: A gene affecting Wallerian nerve degeneration maps distally on mouse chromosome 4. *Proc Nat Acad Sci USA* 90:9717–9720, 1993.

Malmfors T: The effects of 6-hydroxydopamine on the adrenergic nerves as revealed by fluorescence histochemical method, in Malmfors T, Thoenen H (eds): *6-Hydroxydopamine and Catecholaminergic Neurons.* Amsterdam: North-Holland, 1971, pp 47–58.

Marshall JF, Drew MC, Neve KA: Recovery of function after mesotelencephalic dopaminergic injury in senescence. *Brain Res* 259:249–260, 1983.

Martenson CH, Sheetz MP, Graham DG: In vitro acrylamide exposure alters growth cone morphology. *Toxicol Appl Pharmacol* 131:119–129, 1995.

Marty MS, Atchison WD: Pathways mediating Ca^{2+} entry in rat cerebellar granule cells following in vitro exposure to methyl mercury. *Toxicol Appl Pharmacol* 147:319–330, 1997.

Meldrum B: Excitatory amino acid antagonists as potential therapeutic agents, in Jenner P (ed): *Neurotoxins and Their Pharmacological Implications.* New York: Raven Press, 1987, pp 33–53.

Miller DB: Neurotoxicity of the pesticidal carbamates. *Neurobehav Toxicol Teratol* 4:779–787, 1982.

Mitsuishi K, Takahashi A, Mizutani M, et al: Beta,beta′-iminodipropionitrile toxicity in normal and congenitally neurofilament-deficient Japanese quails. *Acta Neuropathol* 86:578–581, 1993.

Monuki ES, Lemke G: Molecular biology of myelination, in Waxman SG, Kocsis JD, Stys PK (eds): *The Axon: Structure, Function, and Pathophysiology.* New York: Oxford University Press, 1995, pp 144–163.

Morell P, Toews AD, Wagner M, et al: Gene expression during tellurium-induced primary demyelination. *Neurotoxicology* 15:171 – 180, 1994.

Moretta A: Promoters and promotion of axonopathies. *Toxicol Lett* 112: 17–21, 2000.

Moser VC, Becking GC, Cuomo V, et al.: The IPCS collaborative study on neurobehavioral screening methods. III. Results of proficiency studies. *Neurotoxicology* 18:939–946, 1997a.

Moser VC, Becking GC, Cuomo V, et al: The IPCS collaborative study on neurobehavioral screening methods: IV. Control data. *Neurotoxicology* 18:947–967, 1997b.

Moser VC, Becking GC, Cuomo V, et al: The IPCS collaborative study on neurobehavioral screening methods: V. Results of chemical testing. *Neurotoxicology* 18:969–1055, 1997c.

Mullick FG: Hexachlorophene toxicity: Human experience at the AFIP. *Pediatrics* 51:395–399, 1973.

Mulugeta S, Ciavarra RP, Maney RK, et al: Three subpopulations of fast axonally transported retinal ganglion cell proteins are differentially trafficked in the rat optic pathway. *J Neurosci Res* 59:247–258, 2000.

Myers JE, Macun I: Acrylamide neuropathy in a South African factory: An epidemiologic investigation. *Am J Indust Med* 19:487–493, 1991.

Myers RR, Mizisin AP, Powell HC, et al: Reduced nerve blood flow in hexachlorophene neuropathy: Relationship to elevated endoneurial pressure. *J Neuropathol Exp Neurol* 41:391–399, 1982.

Needleman HL: Childhood lead poisoning. *Curr Opin Neurol* 7:187–190, 1994.

Needleman HL, Gatsonis CA: Low-level lead exposure and the IQ of children. A meta-analysis of modern studies. *JAMA* 263:673–678, 1990.

Nixon RA: Dynamic behavior and organization of cytoskeleton proteins in neurons: Reconciling old and new findings. *Bioessays* 20:798–807, 1998.

Nixon RA, Sihag RK: Neurofilament phosphorylation: A new look at regulation and function. *TINS* 14:501–506, 1991.

Nunn PB, Seelig M, Zagoren JC, et al: Stereospecific acute neurotoxicity of "uncommon" plant amino acids linked to human motor system diseases. *Brain Res* 410:375–379, 1987.

Olney JW: Neurotoxicity of excitatory amino acids, in McGeer EG, Olney JW, McGeer PL (eds): *Kainic Acid as a Tool in Neurobiology.* New York: Raven Press, 1978, pp 95–122.

O'Shea KS, Kaufman MH: The teratogenic effect of acetaldehyde: Implications for the study of fetal alcohol syndrome. *J Anat* 128:65–76, 1979.

Padilla S, Atkinson MB, Breuer AC: Direct measurement of fast axonal organelle transport in the sciatic nerve of rats treated with acrylamide. *J Toxicol Environ Health* 39:429–445, 1993.

Pardridge WM: Blood-brain barrier biology and methodology. *J Neurovirol* 5:556–569, 1999.

Parent A: *Carpenter's Human Neuroanatomy,* 9th ed. Baltimore: Williams & Wilkins, 1996, pp 131–198.

Penny DG: Acute carbon monoxide poisoning: Animal models: A review. *Toxicology* 62:123–160, 1990.

Perl TM, Bedard L, Kosatsky T, et al: An outbreak of toxic encephalopathy caused by eating mussels contaminated with domoic acid. *N Engl J Med* 322:1775–1780, 1990.

Perlstein MA, Attala R: Neurologic sequelae of plumbism in children. *Clin Pediatr* 5:292–298, 1966.

Pham-Dinh D, Popot JL, Boespflug-Tanguy O, et al: Pelizaeus-Merzbacher disease: A valine to phenylalanine point mutation in a putative extracellular loop of myelin proteolipid. *Proc Natl Acad Sci USA* 88: 7562–7566, 1991.

Plum F, Posner JB: Neurobiologic essentials, in Smith LH Jr, Thier SO (eds): *Pathophysiology: The Biological Principles of Disease.* Philadelphia: Saunders, 1985, pp 1009–1036.

Polymerpoulos MH, Lavedan C, Leroy E, et al: Mutation in the alpha-synuclein gene identified in families with Parkinson's disease. *Science* 276:2045–2047, 1997.

Purves DC, Garrod IJ, Dayan AD: A comparison of spongiosis induced in the brain by hexachlorophene, cuprizone, and triethyl tin in the Sprague-Dawley rat. *Hum Exp Toxicol* 10:439–444, 1991.

Pyle SJ, Graham DG, Anthony DC: Dimethylhexanedione impairs the movement of neurofilament protein subunits, NFM and NFL, in the optic system. *Neurotoxicology* 15:279–286, 1994.

Quarles RH, Farrer RG, Yim SH: Structure and function of myelin, an extended and biochemically modified cell surface membrane, in Juurlink BHJ, Devon RM, Doucette JR, et al. (eds): *Cell Biology and Pathology of Myelin: Evolving Biological Concepts and Therapeutic Approaches.* New York: Plenum Press, 1997, pp 1–12.

Qiu J, Cai D, Filbin MT: Glial inhibition of nerve regeneration in mature mammalian CNS. *Glia* 29:166–174, 2000.

Readhead C, Schneider A, Griffiths I, et al: Premature arrest of myelin formation in transgenic mice with increased proteolipid protein gene dosage. *Neuron* 12:583–595, 1994.

Reuhl KR, Chang LW: Effects of methylmercury on the development of the nervous system: A review. *Neurotoxicology* 1:21–55, 1979.

Reuhl KR, Gilbert SG, Mackenzie BA, et al: Acute trimethyltin intoxication in the monkey *(Macaca fascicularis)*. *Toxicol Appl Pharmacol* 79:436–452, 1985.

Riggs JE: Cigarette smoking and Parkinson's disease: The illusion of a neuroprotective effect. *Clin Neuropharmacol* 15:88–99, 1992.

Riikonen R, Salonen I, Partanen K, et al: Brain perfusion SPECT and MRI in foetal alcohol syndrome. *Dev Med Child Neurol* 41:652–659, 1999.

Rojas P, Klaassen CD: Metallothionein-I and -II knock-out mice are not more sensitive than control mice to 1-methyl-1,2,3,6-tetrahydropyridine neurotoxicity. *Neurosci Lett* 273:113–116, 1999.

Ross JF, Lawhorn GT: ZPT-related distal axonopathy: Behavioral and electrophysiologic correlates in rats. *Neurotoxicol Teratol* 12:153–159, 1990.

Rothman SM, Olney JM: Glutamate and the pathophysiology of hypoxic-ischemic brain damage. Ann Neurol 19:105–111, 1986.

Roytta M, Horwitz SB, Raine CS: Taxol-induced neuropathy: Short-term effects of local injection. *J Neurocytol* 13:685–701, 1984.

Roytta M, Raine CS: Taxol-induced neuropathy: Chronic effects of local injection. *J Neurocytol* 15:483–496, 1986.

Rubin LL, Staddon JM: The cell biology of the blood-brain barrier. *Annu Rev Neurosci* 22:11–28, 1999.

Sahenk Z, Barohn R, New P, Mendell JR: Taxol neuropathy: Electrodiagnostic and sural nerve biopsy findings. *Arch Neurol* 51:726–729, 1994.

Sahenk Z, Mendell JR: Pyrithione, in Spencer PS, Schaumburg HH (eds): *Experimental and Clinical Neurotoxicology.* New York: Oxford University Press, 2000, pp 1050–1054.

Sahenk Z, Mendell JR: Axoplasmic transport in zinc pyridinethione neuropathy: Evidence for an abnormality in distal turn-around. *Brain Res* 186:343–353, 1980.

St. Clair MBG, Amarnath V, Moody MA, et al: Pyrrole oxidation and protein crosslinking are necessary steps in the development of γ-diketone neuropathy. *Chem Res Toxicol* 1:179–185, 1988.

Sayre LM, Shearson CM, Wongmongkolrit T, et al: Structural basis of γ-diketone neurotoxicity: Non-neurotoxicity of 3,3-dimethyl-2,5-hexanedione a γ-diketone incapable of pyrrole formation. *Toxicol Appl Pharmacol* 84:36–44, 1986.

Schiff PB, Horwitz SB: Taxol assembles tubulin in the absence of exogenous guanosine 59-triphosphate or microtubule-associated proteins. *Biochemistry* 20:3242–3252, 1981.

Schionning JD, Larsen JO, Tandrup T, et al.: Selective degeneration of dorsal root ganglia and dorsal nerve roots in methyl mercury–intoxicated rats: A stereological study. *Acta Neuropathol* 96:191–201, 1998.

Schlafer WW, Zimmerman U-JP: Calcium-activated protease and the regulation of the axonal cytoskeleton, in Elam JS, Cancalon P (eds): *Advances in Neurochemistry*. New York: Plenum Press, 1984, pp 261–273.

Schnapp BJ, Reese TS: Dynein is the motor for retrograde axonal transport of organelles. *Proc Natl Acad Sci USA* 86:1548–1552, 1989.

Schoepfer R, Monyer H, Sommer B, et al: Molecular biology of glutamate receptors. *Prog Neurobiol* 42:353–357, 1994.

Schutzman DL, Frankenfield-Chernicoff M, Clatterbaugh HE, et al: Incidence of intrauterine cocaine exposure in a suburban setting. *Pediatrics* 88:825–827, 1991.

Schwartz JH: The cytology of neurons, in Kandel ER, Schwartz JH, Jessell TM (eds): *Principles of Neural Science.* 3d ed. Norwalk, CT: Appleton & Lange, 1991, pp 37–48.

Seawright AA, Brown AW, Nolan CC, et al: Selective degeneration of cerebellar cortical neurons caused by cycad neurotoxin, L-beta-methylaminoalanine (L-BMAA), in rats. *Neuropathol Appl Neurobiol* 16:153–164, 1990.

Seppaleinen AM, Haltia M: Carbon disulfide, in Spencer PS, Schaumburg HH (eds): *Experimental and Clinical Neurotoxicology.* Baltimore: Williams & Wilkins, 1980, pp 356–373.

Snow BJ, Vingerhoets FJ, Langston JW, et al: Pattern of dopaminergic loss in the striatum of humans with MPTP induced parkinsonism. *J Neurol Neurosurg Psychiatry* 68:313–316, 2000.

Spencer PS: Doxorubicin and related anthracyclines, in Spencer PS, Schaumburg HH (eds): *Experimental and Clinical Neurotoxicology.* New York: Oxford University Press, 2000, pp 529–533.

Spencer PS, Nunn PB, Hugon J, et al: Guam amyotrophic lateral sclerosis-parkinsonism-dementia linked to a plant excitant neurotoxin. *Science* 237:517–522, 1987.

Spencer PS, Schaumburg HH: Central-peripheral distal axonopathy: The pathology of dying-back polyneuropathies, in Zimmerman H (ed): *Progress in Neuropathology,* vol 3. New York: Grune & Stratton, 1976, pp 253–295.

Stewart PA: Endothelial vesicles in the blood-brain barrier: Are they related to permeability? *Cell Mol Neurobiol* 20:149–163, 2000.

Stoll G, Muller HW: Nerve injury, axonal degeneration and neural regeneration: Basic insights. *Brain Pathol* 9:313–325, 1999.

Stoltenburg-Didinger G, Spohr HL: Fetal alcohol syndrome and mental retardation: Spine distribution of pyramidal cells in prenatal alcohol exposed rat cerebral cortex. *Brain Res* 11:119–123, 1983.

Stone JD, Peterson AP, Eyer J, et al: Axonal neurofilaments are nonessential elements of toxicant-induced reductions in fast axonal transport: Video-enhanced differential interference microscopy in peripheral nervous system axons. *Toxicol Appl Pharmacol* 161:50–58, 1999.

Storch A, Kaftan A, Burkhardt K, et al: 6-Hydroxydopamine toxicity towards human SH-SY5Y dopaminergic neuroblastoma cells: Independent of mitochondrial energy metabolism. *J Neural Transm* 107: 281–293, 2000.

Takeuchi T, Morikawa H, Matsumoto H, et al: A pathological study of Minamata disease in Japan. *Acta Neuropathol* 2:40–57, 1962.

Tanner CM, Ottman R, Goldman SM, et al: Parkinson disease in twins: An etiologic study. *JAMA* 281:341–346, 1999.

Teitelbaum JS, Zatorre RJ, Carpenter S, et al: Neurologic sequelae of domoic acid intoxication due to the ingestion of contaminated mussels. *N Engl J Med* 322:1781–1787, 1990.

Tilson HA: Neurobehavioral methods used in neurotoxicological research. *Toxicol Lett* 68:231–240, 1993.

Toggas SM, Krady JK, Billingsley ML: Molecular neurotoxicology of trimethyltin: Identification of stannin, a novel protein expressed in trimethyltin-sensitive cells. *Mol Pharmacol* 42:44–56, 1992.

Valentine WM, Amarnath V, Amarnath K, et al: Carbon disulfide-mediated protein cross-linking by *N,N*-diethyldithiocarbamate. *Chem Res Toxicol* 8:96–102, 1995.

Valentine WM, Amarnath V, Graham DG, et al: CS_2 mediated cross-linking of erythrocyte spectrin and neurofilament protein: Dose response and temporal relationship to the formation of axonal swellings. *Toxicol Appl Pharmacol* 142:95–105, 1997.

Valentine WM, Amarnath V, Graham DG, et al: Covalent cross-linking of proteins by carbon disulfide. *Chem Res Toxicol* 5:254–262, 1992.

Valentine WM, Graham DG, Anthony DC: Covalent cross-linking of erythrocyte spectrin in vivo. *Toxicol Appl Pharmacol* 121:71–77, 1993.

Van de Kamp JL, Collins AC: Prenatal nicotine alters nicotinic receptor development in the mouse brain. *Pharmacol Biochem Behav* 47:889–900, 1994.

Verity MA: Toxic disorders, in Graham DI, Lantos PL (eds): *Greenfield's Neuropathology,* 6th ed. New York: Arnold, 1997, pp 755–811.

Veronesi B, Jones K, Gupta S, et al: Myelin basic protein-messenger RNA (MBP-mRNA) expression during triethyltin-induced myelin edema. *Neurotoxicology* 12:265–276, 1991.

Volpe JJ: Effect of cocaine use on the fetus. *N Engl J Med* 327:399–407, 1992.

Wagner M, Toews AD, Morell P: Tellurite specifically affects squalene epoxidase: Investigations examining the mechanism of tellurium-induced neuropathy. *J Neurochem* 64:2169–2176, 1995.

Wang L, Ho CL, Sun D, et al: Rapid movement of axonal neurofilaments interrupted by prolonged pauses. *Nature Cell Biol* 2:137–141, 2000.

Williamson AM: The development of a neurobehavioral test battery for use in hazard evaluations in occupational settings. *Neurotoxicol Teratol* 12:509–514, 1990.

Wilson JM, Kalasinsky K, Levey A, et al: Striatal dopamine nerve terminal markers in human, chronic methamphetamine users. *Nat Med* 2:699–703, 1996a.

Wilson JM, Levey AI, Bergeron C, et al: Striatal dopamine, dopamine transporter, and vesicular monoamine transporter in chronic cocaine users. *Ann Neurol* 40:428–439, 1996b.

Winneke G: Cross species extrapolation in neurotoxicology: Neurophysiological and neurobehavioral aspects. *Neurotoxicology* 13:15–25, 1992.

Woods JR, Plessinger MA, Clark KE: Effect of cocaine on uterine blood flow and fetal oxygenation. *JAMA* 257:957–961, 1987.

Wright SC, Zhong J, Zheng H, et al: Nicotine inhibition of apoptosis suggests a role in tumor production. *FASEB J* 7:1045–1051, 1993.

Yamamura Y: n-Hexane polyneuropathy. *Folia Psychiatr Neurol* 23:45–57, 1969.

Zhang J, Graham DG, Montine TS, et al: Enhanced N-methyl-4-tetrahydropyridine toxicity in mice deficient in CuZn-superoxide dismutase or glutathione peroxidase. *J Neuropathol Exp Neurol* 59:53–61, 2000a.

Zhang J, Kravtsov V, Amarnath V, et al: Enhancement of dopaminergic neurotoxicity by the mercapturate of dopamine: Relevance to Parkinson's disease. *J Neurochem* 74:970–978, 2000b.

CHAPTER 17

TOXIC RESPONSES OF THE OCULAR AND VISUAL SYSTEM

Donald A. Fox and William K. Boyes

INTRODUCTION TO OCULAR AND VISUAL SYSTEM TOXICOLOGY*

Environmental and occupational exposure to toxic chemicals, gases, and vapors as well as side effects resulting from therapeutic drugs frequently result in structural and functional alterations in the eye and central visual system (Grant, 1986; Anger and Johnson, 1985; Grant and Shuhman, 1993; Otto and Fox, 1993; Jaanus et al., 1995; Fox, 1998). It has been estimated that almost half of all neurotoxic chemicals affect some aspect of sensory function (Crofton and Sheets, 1989). The most frequently reported sensory system alterations occur in the visual system (Anger and Johnson, 1985; Crofton and Sheets, 1989; Fox, 1998). Grant (1986) lists approximately 2800 substances that are reportedly toxic to the eye. In many cases, alterations in visual function are the first symptoms following chemical exposure (Hanninen et al., 1978; Damstra, 1978; Baker et al., 1984; Mergler et al., 1987). Even more relevant is the fact that these alterations often occur in the absence of any clinical signs of toxicity (Baker et al., 1984; Anger and Johnson, 1985). This suggests that sensory systems, and in particular the retina and central visual system, may be especially vulnerable to toxic insult. In fact, alterations in the structure and/or function of the eye or central visual system are among the criteria utilized for setting permissible occupational exposure levels for 33 different chemicals in the United States (Anger, 1984). Moreover, subtle alterations in visual processing of information (e.g., visual perceptual, visual motor) can have profound immediate, long-term, and—in some cases—delayed effects on the mental, social, and physical health and performance of an individual. Finally, ocular and visual system impairments can lead to increased occupational injuries, loss of productive work time, costs for providing medical and social services, lost productivity, and a distinct decrease in the overall quality of life.

The overall goal of this chapter is to review the structural and functional alterations in the mammalian eye and central visual system commonly produced by environmental and workplace chemicals, gases, and vapors and by therapeutic drugs. Except where noted, all these compounds are referred to as chemicals and

*This chapter has been reviewed by the National Health and Environmental Effects Research Laboratory, U.S. EPA, and approved for publication. Mention of trade names and commercial products does not constitute endorsement or recommendation for use.

Table 17-1
Ocular and Central Visual System Sites of Action of Selected Xenobiotics following Systemic Exposure

XENOBIOTIC	CORNEA	LENS	OUTER RETINA: RPE	OUTER RETINA: RODS AND CONES	INNER RETINA: BCs, ACs, IPCs	RGCs AND OPTIC NERVE OR TRACT	LGN, VISUAL CORTEX
Acrylamide				–	–	++	++
Amiodarone	+	+				+	
Carbon disulfide				+	–	++	+
Chloroquine	+		+	+		+	
Chlorpromazine	+	+	+	+			
Corticosteroids		++				+	
Digoxin and digitoxin	+	+	+	++		+	+
Ethambutol				+		++	
Hexachlorophene				+		+	+
Indomethacin	+		+	+			
Isotretinoin	+						
Lead	+		+	++	+	+	+
Methanol			+	++	–	++	+
Methyl mercury, mercury				+	–	–	++
n-Hexane			+	+		+	
Naphthalene		+		+			
Organic solvents				+			+
Organophosphates		+		+		+	+
Styrene				+			
Tamoxifen	+			+		+	

KEY: RPE = retinal pigment epithelium; BC = bipolar cell; AC = amacrine cell; IPC = interplexiform cell; RGC = retinal ganglion cell; LGN = lateral geniculate nucleus.

drugs. The adverse effects of these agents on the different compartments of the eye [i.e., cornea, lens, retina, and retinal pigment epithelium (RPE)], central visual pathway [i.e., optic nerve (ON) and optic tract (OT)], and the central processing areas [i.e., lateral geniculate nucleus (LGN), visual cortex] are addressed (Table 17-1). To further understand the disposition and effects of these chemicals and drugs on the eye and central visual system, the pharmacodynamics and pharmacokinetics of these compartments are briefly reviewed (Table 17-2). Furthermore, the ophthalmologic evaluation of the eye and the testing of visual function are discussed, as the results from these clinical, behavioral, and electrophysiologic studies form the basis of our diagnosis and under-

Table 17-2
Distribution of Ocular Xenobiotic-Biotransforming Enzymes

	ENZYMES	TEARS	CORNEA	IRIS/CILIARY BODY	LENS	RETINA	CHORIOD
Phase I reactions	Acetylcholinesterase (AChE)	+		+		+	+
	Alcohol dehydrogenase		+		–	+	+
	Aldehyde dehydrogenase		+		+	+	+
	Aldehyde reductase		+	+	+	+	+
	Aldose reductase		+		+	+	
	Carboxylesterase	+	+	+		+	+
	Catalase	–	+	+	+	+	+
	Cu/Zn superoxide dismutase	+	+		–/+	+	
	CYP1A1 or CYP1A2	+	+	+	–	+	+
	CYP4A1 or CYP4B2		+				
	MAO-A or B	+		+		+	+
Phase II reactions	Glutathione peroxidase	–	+	+	+	+	+
	Glutathione reductase		+		+	+	
	Glutathione-*S*-transferase		+	+	+	+	
	N-Acetyltransferase		+	+	+	+	+

standing of adverse visual system effects in patients and animals. Many of the chemicals discussed below initially appear to have a single site and, by inference, mechanism of action, whereas others have several sites and corresponding mechanisms of action. However, a more in-depth examination often reveals that, depending upon dose (concentration), many of these chemicals have multiple sites of action. Two examples illustrate the point. First, as described below in more detail, carbon disulfide produces ON and OT degeneration and also adversely affects the neurons and vasculature of the retina, resulting in photoreceptor and retinal ganglion cell (RGC) structural and functional alterations (Hotta et al., 1971; Raitta et al., 1974; Palacz et al., 1980; Seppalainen et al., 1980; Raitta et al., 1981; De Rouck et al., 1986; Eskin et al., 1988; Merigan et al., 1988; Fox, 1998). Second, inorganic lead clearly affects rod photoreceptors in developing and adult mammals, resulting in rod-mediated (or scotopic) vision deficits; however, structural and functional deficits at the level of the RGCs, visual cortex, and oculomotor system are also observed (Fox and Sillman, 1979; Costa and Fox, 1983; Fox, 1984; Glickman et al., 1984; Lilienthal et al., 1988, 1994; Reuhl et al., 1989; Ruan et al., 1994; Fox et al., 1997; Rice, 1998; Rice and Hayward, 1999; He et al., 2000; and see reviews by Otto and Fox, 1993; Fox, 1998). Finally, some environmental and occupational neurotoxicants (e.g., acrylamide, lead) have been utilized for in vivo and in vitro animal models to examine the pathogenesis of selected retinal, neuronal, or axonal diseases; the basic functions of the retinocortical pathways; and/or the molecular mechanisms of apoptosis (Fox and Sillman, 1979; Vidyasagar, 1981; Lynch et al., 1992; He et al., 2000).

The conceptual approach, format, and overall organization of this entirely new chapter on ocular and visual system toxicology for the 6th edition of Casarett and Doull's *Toxicology: The Basic Science of Poisons* were designed by the authors of this chapter in anticipation that our main audience would be graduate and medical school students, ophthalmologists and occupational physicians, basic and applied science researchers interested in ocular and visual system toxicology, and those interested in having a basic reference source. To write this chapter we synthesized and condensed the information contained in several excellent resources on different aspects of ocular, retinal, and visual system anatomy, biochemistry, cell and molecular biology, histology, pharmacology, physiology, and toxicology (Hogan et al., 1971; Merigan and Weiss, 1980; Fox et al., 1982; Sears, 1984; Dayhaw-Barker et al., 1986; Grant, 1986; Dowling, 1987; Fraunfelder and Meyer, 1989; Ogden and Schachat, 1989; Davson, 1990; Berman, 1991; Boyes, 1992; Chiou, 1992; Hart, 1992; Hockwin et al., 1992; Bartlett and Jaanus, 1995; Herr and Boyes, 1995; Potts, 1996; Fox, 1998; Rodieck, 1998; Ballantyne, 1999). The interested reader should consult these sources for more detail than is provided below. We gratefully acknowledge the use of the information in these sources as well as those cited in the text below.

EXPOSURE TO THE EYE AND VISUAL SYSTEM

Ocular Pharmacodynamics and Pharmacokinetics

Toxic chemicals and systemic drugs can affect all parts of the eye (Fig. 17-1; Table 17-1). Several factors determine whether a chemical can reach a particular ocular site of action, including the physiochemical properties of the chemical, concentration and duration of exposure, route of exposure, and the movement of the chemical into and across the different ocular compartments and barriers. The cornea and external adnexa of the eye (i.e., conjunctiva and eyelids) are often exposed directly to chemicals (i.e., acids, bases, solvents), gases and particles, and drugs. The first site of action is the tear film—a three-layered structure with both hydrophobic and hydrophilic properties. The outermost tear film layer is a thin (0.1-μm) hydrophobic layer that is secreted by the meibomian (sebaceous) glands. This superficial lipid layer protects the underlying thicker (7-μm) aqueous layer that is produced by the lacrimal glands. The third layer, which has both hydrophobic and hydrophilic properties, is the very thin (0.02 to 0.05 μm) mucoid layer. It is secreted by the goblet cells of the conjunctiva and acts as an interface between the hydrophilic layer of the tears and the hydrophobic layer of the corneal epithelial cells. Thus, water-soluble chemical compounds more readily mix with the tears and gain access to the cornea. However, a large proportion of the compounds that are splashed into the eyes are washed away by the tears and thus are not absorbed.

The cornea, an avascular tissue, is considered the external barrier to the internal ocular structures. Once a chemical interacts with the tear film and subsequently contacts the cornea and conjunctiva, the majority of what is absorbed locally enters the anterior segment by passing across the cornea. In contrast, a greater systemic absorption and higher blood concentration occurs through contact with the vascularized conjunctiva (Sears, 1984; Pepose and Ubels, 1992; Fig. 17-2). The human cornea, which is approximately 500 μm thick, has several distinct layers, or barriers, through which a chemical must pass in order to reach the anterior chamber (see discussion on the cornea, below). The first is the corneal epithelium. It is a stratified squamous, nonkeratinized, multicellular hydrophobic layer. These cells have a relatively low ionic conductance through apical cell membranes, and due to the tight junctions (desmosomes), they have a high resistance paracellular pathway. The primary barrier to chemical penetration of the cornea is tight junctions at the superficial layer of the corneal epithelial cells. Thus, the permeability of the corneal epithelium as a whole is low and only lipid soluble chemicals readily pass through this layer. The corneal stroma makes up 90 percent of the corneal thickness and is composed of water, collagen, and glycosaminoglycans. It contains approximately 200 lamellae, each about 1.5 to 2.0 μm thick. Due to the composition and structure of the stroma, hydrophilic chemicals easily dissolve in this thick layer, which can also act as a reservoir for these chemicals. The inner edge of the corneal stroma is bounded by a thin, limiting basement membrane, called Descemet's membrane, which is secreted by the corneal endothelium. The innermost layer of the cornea, the corneal endothelium, is composed of a single layer of large diameter hexagonal cells connected by terminal bars and surrounded by lipid membranes. The endothelial cells have a relatively low ionic conductance through apical cell surface and a high-resistance paracellular pathway. Although the permeability of the corneal endothelial cells to ionized chemicals is relatively low, it is still 100 to 200 times more permeable than the corneal epithelium. The Na^+,K^+-pump is located on the basolateral membrane while the energy-dependent Na^+,HCO_3^--transporter is located on the apical membrane (Sears, 1984; Pepose and Ubels, 1992).

There are two separate vascular systems in the eye: (1) the uveal blood vessels, which include the vascular beds of the iris, ciliary body, and choroid, and (2) the retinal vessels (Hogan, 1971; Alm, 1992). In humans, the ocular vessels are derived from the

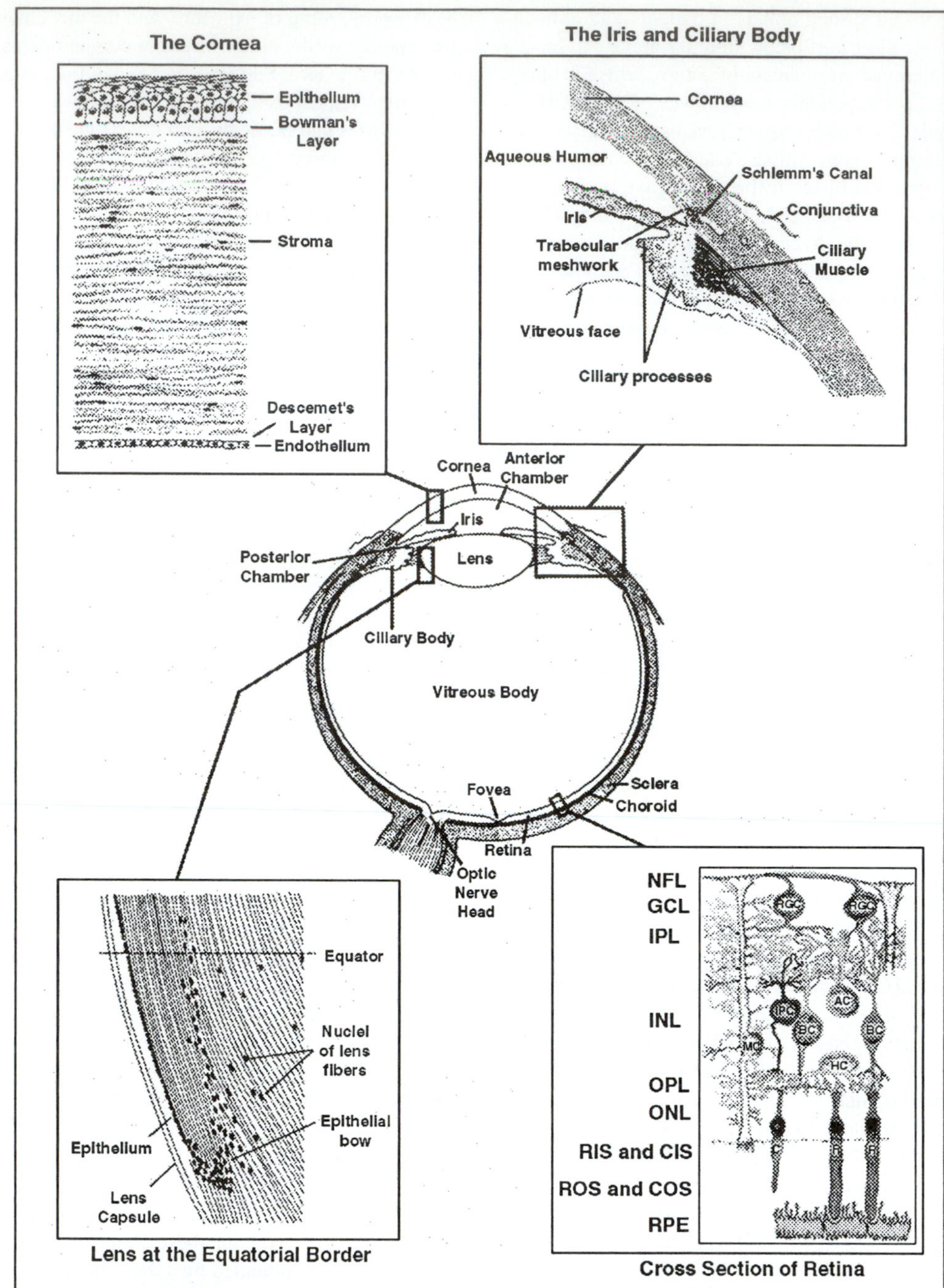

Figure 17-1. Diagrammatic horizontal cross section of the eye, with medium-power enlargement of details for the cornea, iris and ciliary body, lens, and retina.

The morphologic features, their role in ocular pharmacodynamics, pharmacokinetics, drug metabolism, and the adverse effects of drugs and chemical agents on these sites are discussed in the text.

ophthalmic artery, which is a branch of the internal carotid artery. The ophthalmic artery branches into (1) the central retinal artery, which enters the eye and then further branches into four major vessels serving each of the retinal quadrants; (2) two posterior ciliary arteries; and (3) several anterior arteries. In the anterior segment of the eye, there is a blood-aqueous barrier that has relatively tight junctions between the endothelial cells of the iris capillaries and nonpigmented cells of the ciliary epithelium (Hogan, 1971; Alm, 1992). The major function of the ciliary epithelium is the production of aqueous humor from the plasma filtrate present in the stroma of the ciliary processes.

In humans and several widely used experimental animals (e.g., monkeys, pigs, dogs, rats, mice), the retina has a dual circulatory supply: choroidal and retinal. The retinal blood vessels are distributed within the inner or proximal portion of the retina, which consists of the outer plexiform layer (OPL), inner nuclear layer

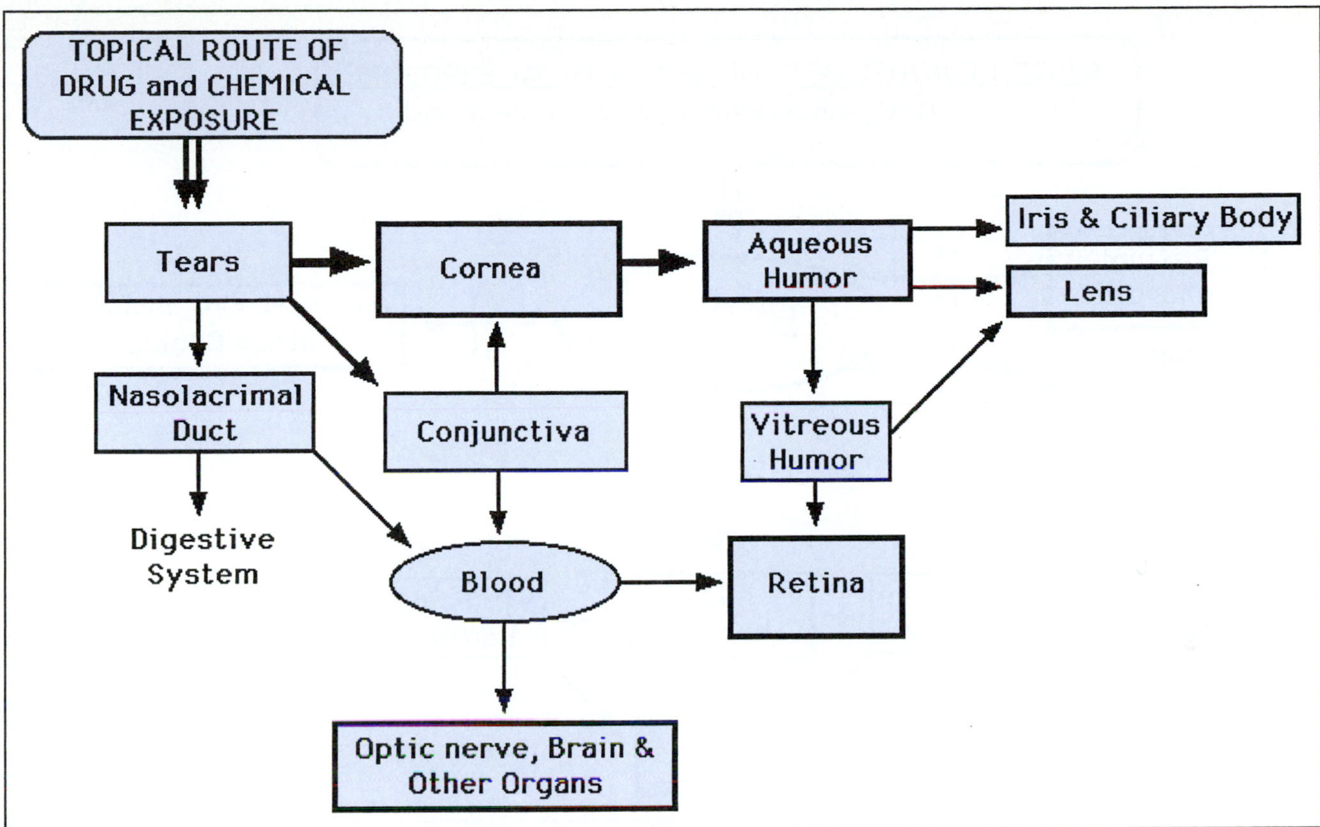

Figure 17-2. Ocular absorption and distribution of drugs and chemicals following the topical route of exposure.

The details for movement of drugs and chemicals between compartments of the eye and subsequently to the optic nerve, brain, and other organs are discussed in the text. The conceptual idea for this figure was obtained from Lapalus and Garaffo (1992).

(INL), inner plexiform layer (IPL), and ganglion cell layer (GCL). The endothelial cells of capillaries of the retinal vessels have tight junctions similar to those that form the blood-brain barrier in the cerebral capillaries. These continuous types of capillaries form the blood-retinal barrier and under normal physiologic conditions they are largely impermeable to chemicals such as glucose and amino acids (Alm, 1992). However, at the level of the optic disk the blood-retinal barrier lacks these continuous type of capillaries and thus hydrophilic molecules can enter the optic nerve (ON) head by diffusion from the extravascular space (Alm, 1992) and cause selective damage at this site of action. The outer or distal retina, which consists of the retinal pigment epithelium (RPE), rod, and cone photoreceptor outer segments (ROS, COS) and inner segments (RIS, CIS), and the photoreceptor outer nuclear layer (ONL), are avascular. These areas of the retina are supplied by the choriocapillaris: a dense, one-layered network of fenestrated vessels formed by the short posterior ciliary arteries and located next to the RPE. Consistent with their known structure and function, these capillaries have loose endothelial junctions and abundant fenestrae; they are highly permeable to large proteins. Thus, the extravascular space contains a high concentration of albumin and γ-globulin (Sears, 1992).

Following systemic exposure to drugs and chemicals by the oral, inhalation, dermal, or parenteral route, these compounds are distributed to all parts of the eye by the blood in the uveal blood vessels and retinal vessels (Fig. 17-3). Most of these drugs and chemicals can rapidly equilibrate with the extravascular space of the choroid where they are separated from the retina and vitreous body by the RPE and endothelial cells of the retinal capillaries, respectively. Hydrophilic molecules with molecular weights less than 200 to 300 Da can cross the ciliary epithelium and iris capillaries and enter the aqueous humor (Sears, 1992). Thus, the corneal endothelium—the cells responsible for maintaining normal hydration and transparency of the corneal stroma—could be exposed to chemical compounds by the aqueous humor and limbal capillaries. Similarly, the anterior surface of the lens also can be exposed as a result of its contact with the aqueous humor. The most likely retinal target sites following systemic drug and chemical exposure appear to be the RPE and photoreceptors in the distal retina because the endothelial cells of the choriocapillaris are permeable to proteins smaller than 50 to 70 kDa. However, the cells of the RPE are joined on their basolateral surface by tight junctions—zonula occludens—that limit the passive penetration of large molecules into the neural retina.

The presence of intraocular melanin plays a special role in ocular toxicology. First, it is found in several different locations in the eye: pigmented cells of the iris, ciliary body, RPE, and uveal tract. Second, it has a high binding affinity for polycyclic aromatic hydrocarbons, electrophiles, calcium, and toxic heavy metals such as aluminum, iron, lead, and mercury (Meier-Ruge, 1972; Potts

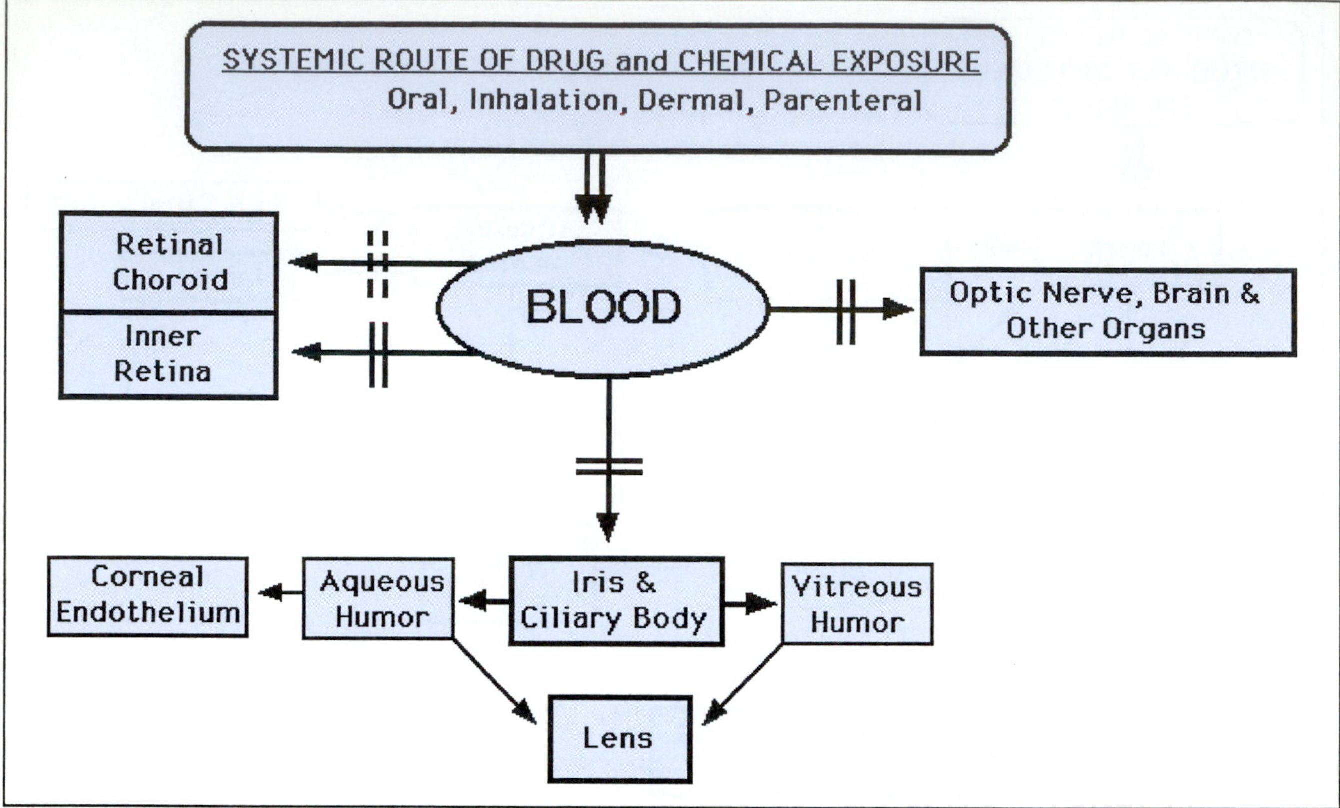

Figure 17-3. Distribution of drugs and chemicals in the anterior and posterior segments of the eye, optic nerve, brain, and other organs following the systemic route of exposure.

The details for movement of drugs and chemicals between compartments of the eye are discussed in the text. The conceptual idea for this part of the figure was obtained from Lapalus and Garaffo (1992). The solid and dotted double lines represent the different blood-tissue barriers present in the anterior segment of the eye, retina, optic nerve, and brain. The solid double lines represent tight endothelial junctions, whereas the dotted double lines represent loose endothelial junctions.

and Au, 1976; Dräger, 1985; Ulshafer et al., 1990; Eichenbaum and Zheng, 2000). Although this initially may play a protective role, it also results in the excessive accumulation, long-term storage, and slow release of numerous drugs and chemicals from melanin. For example, atropine binds more avidly to pigmented irides and thus its duration of action is prolonged (Bartlett and Jaanus, 1995). In addition, the accumulation of chloroquine in the RPE produces an 80-fold higher concentration of chloroquine in the retina relative to liver (Meier-Rouge, 1972). Similarly, lead accumulates in the human retina such that its concentration is 5 to 750 times that in other ocular tissues (Eichenbaum and Zheng, 2000).

Ocular Drug Metabolism

Metabolism of xenobiotics occurs in all compartments of the eye by well known phase I and II xenobiotic-biotransforming enzymes. Drug metabolizing enzymes such as acetylcholinesterase, carboxylesterase (also known as pseudocholinesterase: see Chap. 6, "Biotransformation of Xenobiotics"), alcohol and aldehyde dehydrogenase, aldehyde and aldose reductase, catalase, monoamine oxidase A and/or B, and Cu^{2+}/Zn^{2+} superoxide dismutase as well as several types of proteases are present in the tears, iris-ciliary body, choroid, and retina of many different species (Shanthaverrappa and Bourne, 1964; Waltmann and Sears, 1964; Bausher, 1976; Anderson, 1980; Puro, 1985; Atalla et al., 1998; Berman, 1991; Crouch et al., 1991; Watkins et al., 1991; Gondhowiardjo and van Haeringen, 1993; Downes and Holmes, 1995; Gaudet et al., 1995; Behndig et al., 1998; King et al., 1999; Table 17-2). Compared to other tissues, there is only limited data on the type, number, and activity of cytochrome P450 (CYP) isoforms (phase I metabolism) and phase II conjugating enzymes in ocular tissues (Shichi et al., 1975; Shichi and Nebert, 1982; Sears, 1992; Zhao and Shichi, 1995; Srivastava et al., 1996; Schwartzman, 1997; Singh and Shichi, 1998; Mastyugin et al., 1999). CYP1A1 and CYP1A2—previously known as aryl hydrocarbon hydroxylase activity—are found in all bovine and mouse ocular tissues except the lens and can be induced by 3-methylcholanthrene and β-naphthoflavone (Shichi et al., 1975; Shichi et al., 1982; Zhao and Shichi, 1995). Moreover, a CYP4 family member—CYP4A1 in the mouse and CYP4B1 in the rabbit—is present in corneal epithelium and can be induced by phenobarbital and the peroxisome proliferator clofibrate (Zhao et al., 1996; Mastyugin et al., 1999). This corneal epithelial CYP monooxygenase metabolizes arachidonic acid to two of its major metabolites: 12(R)-HETE [12(R)-hydroxy-5,8,10,14-eicosatrienoic acid] and 12(R)-HETrE [12(R)-hydroxy-5,8,14-eicosatrienoic acid] (Schwartzman, 1987; Asakura et al., 1994; Mastyugin et al., 1999). In the corneal epithelium, 12(R)-HETE is a potent inhibitor of Na^{+},K^{+}-ATPase, whereas 12(R)-

HETrE is a potent angiogenic and chemotactic factor (Schwartzman, 1997).

The phase II conjugating enzymes found in bovine, rabbit, and rat ocular tissues include UDP glucuronosyltransferase, glutathione peroxidase, glutathione reductase, glutathione *S*-transferase, and *N*-acetyltransferase (Awasthi et al., 1980; Shichi and Nebert, 1982; Penn et al., 1987; Watkins et al., 1991: Srivastava et al., 1996; Singh and Shichi, 1998; see Table 17-2). The activity of these enzymes varies between species and ocular tissues, however, the whole lens appears to have low biotransformational activity. It was subsequently found that the glutathione *S*-transferase activity was in the lens epithelium and not in the lens cortex or nucleus (Srivastava et al., 1996). Overall, these findings suggest that ocular tissues that contact the external environment or have a blood supply that possess both CYPs and phase II conjugating enzymes, especially those related to glutathione conjugation. The presence and need for a competent glutathione conjugation system is clearly understandable in ocular tissues that directly interact with UV radiation, light, and xenobiotics and that have high rates of metabolism and high lipid content. Finally, further work is needed to determine the presence and activity of other CYP family members in ocular tissue, the various factors (i.e., age, gender, tissue-specific, xenobiotics, etc.) that regulate their expression, and their endogenous and exogenous substrates.

Central Visual System Pharmacokinetics

The penetration of potentially toxic compounds into visual areas of the central nervous system (CNS) is governed, like other parts of the CNS, by the blood-brain barrier (Fig. 17-3). The blood-brain barrier is formed through a combination of tight junctions in brain capillary endothelial cells and foot processes of astrocytic glial cells that surround the brain capillaries. Together these structures serve to limit the penetration of blood-borne compounds into the brain. The concept of an absolute barrier is not correct, however, because the blood-brain barrier is differentially permeable to compounds depending on their size, charge, and lipophilicity. Compounds that are large, highly charged, or otherwise not very lipid soluble tend to be excluded from the brain, whereas smaller, uncharged, and lipid-soluble compounds more readily penetrate into the brain tissue. In addition to entering the CNS through this nonspecific semipermeable diffusion barrier, some specific nutrients including, ions, amino acids, and glucose enter the CNS through selective transport mechanisms. In some cases, toxic compounds may be actively transported into the brain by mimicking the natural substrates of active transport systems. A few areas of the brain lack a blood-brain barrier; consequently blood-borne compounds readily penetrate into the brain tissue in these regions. Interestingly, one such area is the ON near the lamina cribrosa (Alm, 1992), which could cause this part of the central visual system to be vulnerable to exposures that do not affect much of the remainder of the brain.

TESTING VISUAL FUNCTION

Testing for potential toxic effects of compounds on the eye and visual system can be divided into tests of ocular toxicity and tests of visual function. Alternatively, such tests could be grouped according to the professional training of the individual conducting the evaluation. Such a categorization might include tests of contact irritancy or toxicity akin to dermatologic procedures, ophthalmologic evaluations, neurophysiologic studies of the function of the visual system, and behavioral or psychophysical evaluations of visual thresholds and aspects of perception.

Evaluation of Ocular Irritancy and Toxicity

Standard procedures for evaluating ocular irritation have been based on a method originally published by Draize et al. over a half a century ago (Draize et al., 1944). The Draize test, with some additions and revisions, has formed the basis of procedures employed for safety evaluations in data submitted to several government regulatory bodies including the European Economic Community and several federal agencies within the United States. Traditionally, albino rabbits are the subjects evaluated in the Draize test, although the Environmental Protection Agency (EPA) protocol allows different test species to be used if sufficient justification is provided. The standard procedure involves instillation of 0.1 mL of a liquid or 100 mg of a solid into the conjunctival sac of one eye and then gently holding the eye closed for 1 s. The untreated eye serves as a control. Both eyes are evaluated at 1, 24, 48, and 72 h after treatment. If there is evidence of damage in the treated eye at 72 h, the examination time may be extended. The cornea, iris, and conjunctiva are evaluated and scored according to a weighted scale. The cornea is scored for both the degree of opacity and area of involvement, with each measure having a potential range from 0 (none) to 4 (most severe). The iris receives a single score (0 to 2) for irritation, including degree of swelling, congestion, and degree of reaction to light. The conjunctiva is scored for the redness (0 to 3), chemosis (swelling: 0 to 4), and discharge (0 to 3). The individual scores are then multiplied by a weighting factor: 5 for the cornea, 2 for the iris, and 5 for the conjunctiva. The results are summed for a maximum total score of 110. Photographic examples of lesions receiving each score are provided in Datson and Freeberg (1991). In this scale, the cornea accounts for 80 (73 percent) of the total possible points, in accordance with the severity associated with corneal injury.

The Draize test, although a standard for decades, has been criticized on several grounds, including high interlaboratory variability, the subjective nature of the scoring, poor predictive value for human irritants, and—most significantly—for causing undue pain and distress to the tested animals. These criticisms have spawned a concerted effort to develop alternative methods or strategies to evaluate compounds for their potential to cause ocular irritation. These alternatives include modifications of the traditional Draize test to reduce the number of test animals required, reduce the volume of the compound administered, and increase objectivity of scoring (e.g., Kennah et al., 1989; Bruner et al., 1992; Lambert et al., 1993). In addition, several alternative test procedures have been proposed, including the use of skin irritancy tests as substitutes for ocular irritancy and the use of in vitro assays (Datson and Freeberg, 1991; Chamberlain et al., 1997; Kruszewski et al., 1997). Additional research efforts are developing quantitative structure activity relationships to better predict ocular irritancy (Barratt, 1995; Sugai et al., 1990; Kulkarni and Hopfinger, 1999). To date, there is no general consensus as to which of these alternatives, alone or in combination, provides a suitable alternative to the Draize procedure. The Interagency Coordinating Committee on the Validation of Alternative Methods (ICCVAM), a committee with representatives from 14 agencies of the U.S. federal government, however, has established criteria for validating methods to substitute for whole animals tests of ocular corrosiveness or irritancy (NIEHS, 1997). In June of 1999, ICCVAM found that a nonanimal test product developed under the trade name of Corrositex was useful in determining whether compounds have a potential to corrode or burn the skin or eyes (NIEHS, 1999).

The Corrositex assay is an in vitro procedure in which compounds are tested for the ability to penetrate a biological barrier, a hydrated collagen matrix, and cause a color change in an underlying liquid chemical detection system. The chemical detection system is composed of water and pH indicator dyes; it changes color when contact with the test chemical or mixture causes the pH of the solution to become either less than 5 or greater than 8.5. Chemicals that do not cause a color change in the chemical detection system when added directly in the absence of the biological barrier are not eligible for evaluation with this system. The relative corrosivity of test compounds or mixtures is determined by measuring the penetration time. The ICCVAM peer-review panel reported that in comparison with in vivo testing of rabbit skin for corrosivity, the Corrositex assay had an overall sensitivity of 85 percent (76 of 89 compounds tested), a specificity of 70 percent (52 of 74 compounds tested), and an accuracy of 79 percent (128 of 163 compounds tested). The committee concluded that use of Corrositex as a stand alone procedure in some applications, or in a tiered testing approach in other applications, could help to refine, reduce, or replace the use of whole animal testing procedures. Application of the test is limited, however, by the fact that a number of potential test compounds do not cause a change in color when added directly to the fluid chemical detection system and therefore do not qualify for testing. The test also has a rate of false positive results (30 percent) that may be too high for some applications. These limitations emphasize that it is unlikely for any single simple alternative procedure to serve as an adequate substitute for in vivo animal testing, due to the complexity of the living ocular tissue and the number of tissues and processes that must be reproduced (Bruner et al., 1991).

Ophthalmologic Evaluations

There are many ophthalmologic procedures for evaluating the health of the eye. These should be conducted by a trained ophthalmologist or optometrist experienced in evaluating the species of interest. Procedures available range from fairly routine clinical screening evaluations to sophisticated techniques for very targeted purposes, the later of which are beyond the scope of this chapter. A clinical evaluation of the eye addresses the adnexa and both the anterior and posterior structures in the eye. Examination of the adnexa includes evaluating the eyelids, lacrimal apparatus, and palpebral (covering the eyelid) and bulbar (covering the eye) conjunctiva. The anterior structures or anterior segment include the cornea, iris, lens, and anterior chamber. The posterior structures, referred to as the *ocular fundus,* include the retina, retinal vasculature, choroid, ON, and sclera. The adnexa and surface of the cornea can be examined initially with the naked eye and a hand-held light. Closer examination requires a slit-lamp biomicroscope, using a mydriatic drug (causes pupil dilation) if the lens is to be observed. The width of the reflection of a thin beam of light projected from the slitlamp is an indication of the thickness of the cornea and may be used to evaluate corneal edema. Lesions of the cornea can be better visualized with the use of fluorescein dye, which is retained where there is an ulceration of the corneal epithelium. Examination of the fundus requires use of a mydriatic drug. Fundoscopic examination is conducted using a direct or an indirect ophthalmoscope, as described (Gelatt, 1981; Harroff, 1991; Hockwin et al., 1992). Several recently developed techniques are described in Peiffer et al. (2000).

An ophthalmologic examination of the eye may also involve, prior to introducing mydriatics, an examination of the pupillary light reflex. The direct pupillary reflex involves shining a bright light into the eye and observing the reflexive pupil constriction in the same eye. The consensual pupillary reflex is observed in the eye not stimulated. Both the direct and consensual pupillary light reflexes are dependent on function of a reflex arc involving cells in the retina, which travel through the ON, optic chiasm, and optic tract (OT) to project to neurons in the pretectal area. Pretectal neurons travel to both ipsilateral (for the direct reflex) and contralateral (for the consensual reflex) parasympathetic neurons of the midbrain accessory oculomotor (Edinger-Westphal) nucleus. Preganglion neurons from the Edinger-Westphal nucleus project through the oculomotor nerve to the ciliary ganglion. Postganglionic neurons from the ciliary ganglion then innervate the smooth muscle fibers of the iridal pupillary sphincter. The absence of a pupillary reflex is indicative of damage somewhere in the reflex pathway, and differential impairment of the direct or consensual reflexes can indicate the location of the lesion. The presence of a pupillary light reflex, however, is not synonymous with normal visual function. Pupillary reflexes can be maintained even with substantial retinal damage. In addition, lesions in visual areas outside of the reflex pathway, such as in the visual cortex, may also leave the reflex function intact.

Electrophysiologic Techniques

Many electrophysiologic or neurophysiologic procedures are available for testing visual function in a toxicologic context. In a simple sense, most of these procedures involve stimulating the eyes with visual stimuli and electrically recording potentials generated by visually responsive neurons. Different techniques and stimuli are used to selectively study the function of specific retinal or visual cortical neurons. In the study of the effects of potential toxic substances on visual function, the most commonly used electrophysiologic procedures are the flash-evoked electroretinogram (ERG), visual-evoked potentials (VEPs), and, less often, the electrooculogram (EOG).

ERGs are typically elicited with a brief flash of light and recorded from an electrode placed in contact with the cornea. A typical ERG waveform (see Fox and Farber, 1988) includes an initial negative-going waveform, called the a-wave, that reflects the activation of photoreceptors, and a following positive b-wave that reflects the activity of retinal bipolar cells and associated membrane potential changes in Müller cells, a type of retinal glial cell that buffers extracellular potassium ions and glutamate (Dowling, 1987; Rodieck, 1998). In addition, a series of oscillatory potentials can be observed overriding the b-wave, of which the neural generators are somewhat uncertain, but they presumably reflect various stages of intraretinal signal processing. A standard set of ERG procedures has been recommended and updated for screening assessments of human clinical patients (Marmor et al., 1989; Marmor and Zrenner, 1995). These procedures include the recording of (1) a response reflective of only rod photoreceptor function in the dark-adapted eye, (2) the maximal response in the dark-adapted eye, (3) a response developed by cone photoreceptors, (4) oscillatory potentials, and (5) the response to rapidly flickered light. These recommendations were used to create a protocol for screening the retinal function of dogs in toxicologic studies (Jones et al., 1994). For testing retinal function beyond a screening level evaluation, ERG amplitude and latency versus log stimulus intensity functions are very useful (e.g., Fox and Farber, 1988). Although flash-evoked ERGs do not reflect the function of the RGC layer, ERGs elicited with pattern-reversal stimuli (PERGs) do reflect the activation of RGCs. To date, PERGs have not been used widely in toxicological evaluations.

VEPs are elicited with stimuli similar to those used to evoke ERGs; however, VEPs are recorded from electrodes overlying visual (striate) cortex. Consequently VEPs reflect the activity of the retinogeniculostriate pathway and the activity of cells in the visual cortex. Flash-elicited VEPs have been used in a number of studies of potentially neurotoxic compounds in laboratory animals (Fox et al., 1977, 1982; Dyer et al., 1982; Rebert, 1983; Dyer, 1985; Boyes, 1992; Mattsson et al., 1992; Herr and Boyes, 1995). Pattern-elicited VEPs (PEPs) are more widely used in human clinical evaluations because of their diagnostic value. However, they are infrequently used in laboratory animals because albino rats do not produce usable PEPs (Boyes and Dyer, 1983). Recording PEPs and conducting psychophysic studies with pigmented Long-Evans hooded rats, Fox (1984) found that the PEP spatial frequency functions yielded almost the same visual acuity values (1.4 cycles per degree) as the psychophysically determined spatial resolution limit values (1.8 cycles per degree). These values are in good agreement with those obtained by others using single-cell electrophysiologic and behavioral techniques (Powers and Green, 1978; Birch and Jacobs, 1979; Dean, 1981). Moreover, PEPs and flash-elicited VEPs have exhibited differential sensitivity to some neurotoxic agents (Boyes and Dyer, 1984; Fox, 1984). The U.S. Environmental Protection Agency has published guidelines for conducting visual evoked potential testing in a toxicological context, along with analogous sensory evoked potential procedures for evaluating auditory and somatosensory function (EPA, 1998a).

The EOG is generated by a potential difference between the front and back of the eye, which originates primarily within the RPE (Berson, 1992). Metabolic activity in the RPE generates a light-insensitive potential (the standing potential) and a light-sensitive potential; the difference in amplitude between these two potentials is easily measured as the EOG. The magnitude of the EOG is a function of the level of illumination and health status of the RPE. Electrodes placed on the skin on a line lateral or vertical to the eye measure potential changes correlated with eye movements as the relative position of the ocular dipole changes. Thus, the EOG finds applications in assessing both RPE status and measuring eye movements. The EOG is also used in monitoring eye movements during the recording of other brain potentials, so that eye movement artifacts are not misinterpreted as brain generated electrical activity (Berson, 1992).

As noted in the introduction to this chapter, there is a clear need for testing visual function as a component of the toxicologic evaluation of commercial chemicals. The magnitude of the potential threat posed by visual system toxicity is not known, because sensory function has not been evaluated in a systematic fashion. Currently the EPA screening batteries for neurotoxicologic evaluation of laboratory animals include only minimal evaluations of visual function. Standard screening procedures such as those included in EPA's neurotoxicity screening battery (EPA, 1998b) include a functional observational battery (FOB)—an automated measurement of motor activity and neuropathology. Of the screening procedures, only the FOB evaluates visual function and the extent of these measures is very limited. The entire assessment of visual function includes observing the animal's response to an approaching object such as a pencil and observing the pupil's response to a light. These procedures are limited in not exploring responsiveness over a range of stimulus features such as luminance, color, spatial frequency, and temporal frequency. In addition, they do not evaluate rod or cone sensory thresholds, nor do they isolate potential motor or integrative contributions to task performance. Despite these shortcomings, the FOB has been successful at detecting visual deficits produced by exposure to 3,3′-iminodipropionitrile (Moser and Boyes, 1993) or carbon disulfide (Moser et al., 1998), which illustrates the importance of conducting at least this level of visual function screening in routine testing programs. Some studies include ophthalmologic and/or ocular pathologic evaluations. Comprehensive visual toxicity studies should include ophthalmologic and pathologic evaluation of ocular tissues and assessments of visual function.

Another potentially limiting problem in product safety testing is the routine use of albino animals, whose capacity for visual function is limited at best. The toxicity of many polycyclic aromatic compounds are mediated through interactions with melanin (Potts, 1964, 1996; Meier-Ruge, 1972; see discussion of the retina, below), which is absent in the eyes of albino strains. Furthermore, light-related ocular lesions, including cataracts and retinal degeneration, are often observed in control albino rats and mice used in 2 year product-safety evaluations. It is well known that normal photoreceptor physiology and susceptibility to chemical damage in rats and mice are mediated by light (LaVail, 1976; Williams et al., 1985; Williams, 1986; Penn and Williams, 1986; LaVail et al., 1987; Penn et al., 1987, 1989; Rapp et al., 1990; Backstrom et al., 1993). For example, one study showed that the proportion of Fisher 344 rats in the control group with photoreceptor lesions ranged from less than 10 percent of rats housed on the bottom row of the cage racks to over 55 percent of rats housed on the top row, where the luminance was greater (Rao, 1991). Even under reduced light levels, the incidence of these effects was as high as 15 percent. If albino animals are used as the test subjects, it is important to control the overall level of illumination in the animal colony and also to periodically rotate the animals among the rows of the cage racks. Even under these conditions, it is extremely difficult to interpret pathologic changes in albino rats and mice exposed to test compounds against such high rates of background retinal lesions.

Sensory dysfunction can confound other measures of neurotoxicity. Many behavioral and observational evaluations of neurotoxicity involve presentation of sensory stimuli to human or animal subjects followed by the observation or measurement of a behavioral or motor response. In many cases, the inferences drawn from such measures are stated in terms of the cognitive abilities of the test subject, such as whether learning or memory have been compromised as a function of exposure to the test compound. If the subject was unable to clearly and precisely perceive the test stimuli, which are often complex patterns or contain color, task performance may be affected independently of any effect on cognition. Controlling for visual deficits may alter the interpretation of performance of ostensibly cognitive tasks (Anger et al., 1994; Hudnell et al., 1996; Walkowiak et al., 1998; Cestnick and Coltheart, 1999).

Behavioral and Psychophysical Techniques

Behavioral and psychophysical testing procedures typically vary the parameters of the visual stimulus and then determine whether the subject can discriminate or perceive the stimulus (Woodhouse and Barlow, 1982; Maurissen, 1995). Many facets of visual function in humans and laboratory animals have been studied using these procedures. Often, the goal of these procedures is to resolve the spatial or temporal limits of visual discrimination; however, most visual scenes and targets in our daily life involve discrimination of objects with low to middle spatial and temporal frequencies (Woodhouse and Barlow, 1982). Contrast sensitivity functions are used to assess these parameters. In addition, as discussed below, other visual parameters also have been investigated.

Contrast sensitivity refers to the ability to resolve small differences in luminance contrast, such as the difference between subtle shades of gray. Contrast sensitivity should be measured for a series of visual patterns that differ in pattern size. Typically, such patterns are a series of sine-wave gratings (striped patterns where the luminance changes across the pattern in a sinusoidal profile) where the spatial frequency of the sinusoidal pattern (i.e., the width of the bars in the pattern) varies in log steps. The contrast of the patterns (i.e., the difference between the brightest and darkest parts of the pattern that is adjusted for mean luminance) also varies. The resulting data, when plotted on log/log coordinates, forms a contrast sensitivity function that is representative of the ability to detect visual patterns over the range of visible pattern sizes. Contrast sensitivity functions are dependent primarily on the neural as opposed to the optical properties of the visual system. The contrast sensitivity functions generally form an inverted U-shaped profile with highest sensitivity to contrast at intermediate spatial frequencies. The peak of the function as well as the limits of resolution on both the spatial frequency and contrast axes vary across species. For example, at relatively mesopic (rod- and cone-mediated) luminance levels, the peak of the spatial contrast sensitivity function for the albino rat, hooded rat, cat, and human are 0.1, 0.3, 0.3, and 2 cycles per degree, respectively (Birch and Jacobs, 1979; Fox, 1984).

Some of the visual parameters that have been investigated include (1) the absolute luminance threshold, which is the threshold value for detecting an illuminated target by a dark-adapted subject in a dark-adapted environment; (2) visual acuity, which is the spatial resolution of the visual system [approximately 50 cycles per degree in humans (Woodhouse and Barlow, 1982) and 1.1 to 1.8 cycles per degree in albino and hooded rats (Fox, 1984; Birch and Jacobs, 1979; Dean, 1981)]; (3) color and spectral discriminations (Porkony et al., 1979); (4) critical flicker fusion frequency, which is the threshold value for detecting a flickering light at different luminance intensities; and (5) the peak of the spatial and temporal contrast sensitivity functions at different luminance levels (Woodhouse and Barlow, 1982). Most of these tests are dependent upon the quality of the ocular optics and the ability to obtain a sharply focused visual image on the retina. Thresholds for detecting luminance, contrast, flicker, and color are primarily dependent on retinal and central mechanisms of neural function, although optical impairments (e.g., cataracts) interfere with these functions. The assessment of visual acuity and contrast sensitivity has been recommended for field studies of humans potentially exposed to neurotoxic substances (ATSDR, 1992).

Color vision deficits are either inherited or acquired. Hereditary red-green color deficits occur in about 8 percent of males (X-linked), while only about 0.5 percent of females show similar congenital deficits (Porkony et al., 1979). Inherited color deficiencies take two common forms: protan, a red-green confusion caused by abnormality or absence of the long-wavelength (red) sensitive cones; and deutan, concomitant confusion of red-green and blue-yellow caused by abnormality or absence of the middle-wavelength (green) sensitive cones. Congenital loss of short-wavelength cones, resulting in a blue-yellow confusion (tritanopia, or type III), is extremely rare. Most acquired color vision deficits, such as those caused by drug and chemical exposure, begin with a reduced ability to perform blue-yellow discriminations (Porkony et al., 1979; Jaanus et al., 1995). With increased or prolonged low-level exposure, the color confusion can progress to the red-green axis as well. Because of the rarity of inherited tritanopia, it is generally assumed that blue-yellow deficits, when observed, are acquired deficits. Köllner's rule of thumb is that disorders of the outer retina produce blue-yellow deficits, whereas disorders of the inner retina and ON produce red-green perceptual deficits (Porkony et al., 1979). Bilateral lesions in the area V4 of visual cortex can also lead to color blindness (prosopagnosia). Several reviews discuss and/or list the effects of drugs and chemicals on color vision (Lyle, 1974; Porkony, 1979; Grant, 1986; Mergler, 1990; Grant and Shuhman, 1993; Jaanus et al., 1995; Lessel, 1998).

Recently, the assessment of color vision by rapid screening procedures has been used to evaluate occupationally and environmentally exposed populations (Mergler, 1990; Geller and Hudnell, 1997; see discussion below of the retina and optic nerve/tract for specific references and details). Color vision may be evaluated using several different testing procedures. Commonly used procedures in human toxicologic evaluations include the Ishihara color plates and chip arrangement tests such as the Farnsworth-Munson 100 Hue (FM-100) test and the simplified 15-chip tests using either the saturated hues of the Farnsworth D-15 or the desaturated hues of the Lanthony Desaturated Panel D-15. The Ishihara plates involve a series of colored spots arranged in patterns that take advantage of perceived difference in shades resulting from either protan or deutan anomalies. Normal observers perceive different sets of embedded numbers than do those with color vision deficits. The Farnsworth-Munson procedure involves arrangement of 85 chips in order of progressively changing color. The relative chromatic value of successive chips induces those with color perception deficits to abnormally arrange the chips. The pattern is indicative of the nature of the color perception anomaly. The FM-100 is considered more diagnostically reliable but takes considerably longer to administer than the similar but more efficient Farnsworth and Lanthony tests. The desaturated hues of the Lanthony D-15 are designed to better identify subtle acquired color vision deficits. For this reason, and because it requires only a few minutes to administer, the Lanthony D-15 was recommended as the procedure for color vision screening of potentially occupationally and environmentally exposed populations (ATSDR, 1992). A critical review of this procedure and its use in toxicologic applications can be found in Geller and Hudnell (1997).

TARGET SITES AND MECHANISMS OF ACTION: CORNEA

The cornea provides the anterior covering of the eye and as such must provide three essential functions. First, it must provide a clear refractive surface. The air-to-fluid/tissue interface at the cornea is the principal refractive surface of the eye, providing approximately 48 diopters of refraction. The curvature of the cornea must be correct for the visual image to be focused at the retina. Second, the cornea provides tensile strength to maintain the appropriate shape of the globe. Third, the cornea protects the eye from external factors, including potentially toxic chemicals. The anatomy is reviewed in the discussion of ocular pharmacodynamics and pharmacokinetics above.

The cornea is transparent to wavelengths of light ranging between 310 (UV) to 2500 nm (IR) in wavelengths. Exposure to UV light below this range can damage the cornea. It is most sensitive to wavelengths of approximately 270 nm. Excessive UV exposure leads to photokeratitus and corneal pathology, the classic example being welder's-arc burns.

The cornea can be damaged by topical or systemic exposure to drugs and chemicals. Reports of such adverse reactions have been catalogued and reviewed by Diamante and Fraunfelder (1998). One summary analysis, of approximately 600 agricultural and industrial chemicals (raw materials, intermediates, formulation components, and sales products), evaluated using the Draize procedure, reported that over half of the materials tested caused no (18 to 31 percent) or minimal (42 to 51 percent) irritation. Depending on the chemical category, between 9 to 17 percent of compounds were graded as slightly irritant, whereas 1 to 6 percent were graded as strong or extreme irritants (Kobel and Gfeller, 1985).

Direct chemical exposure to the eye requires emergency medical attention. Acid and alkali chemicals that come into contact with the cornea can be extremely destructive. Products at pH extremes ≤ 2.5 or ≥ 11.5 are considered as extreme ocular irritants (Potts, 1996). They can cause severe ocular damage and permanent loss of vision. Damage that extends to the corneal endothelium is associated with poor repair and recovery. The most important therapy is immediate and adequate irrigation with large amounts of water or saline, whichever is most readily available. The extent of damage to the eye and the ability to achieve a full recovery are dependent upon the nature of the chemical, the concentration and duration of exposure, and the speed and magnitude of the initial irrigation.

Acids

Strong acids with a pH ≤ 2.5 can be highly injurious. Among the most significant acidic chemicals in terms of the tendency to cause clinical ocular damage are hydrofluoric acid, sulfurous acid, sulfuric acid, and chromic acid, followed by hydrochloric and nitric acid and finally acetic acid (McCulley, 1998). Injuries may be mild if contact is with weak acids or with dilute solutions of strong acids. Compounds with a pH between 2.5 and 7 produce pain or stinging; but with only brief contact, they will cause no lasting damage (Grant and Shuhman, 1993). Following mild burns, the corneal epithelium may become turbid as the corneal stroma swells (chemosis). Mild burns are typically followed by rapid regeneration of the corneal epithelium and full recovery. In more severe burns, the epithelium of the cornea and conjunctiva become opaque and necrotic and may disintegrate over the course of a few days. In severe burns, there may be no sensation of pain because the corneal nerve endings are destroyed (Grant, 1986; Potts, 1996).

Acid chemical burns of the cornea occur through hydrogen ion–induced denaturing and coagulation of proteins. As epithelial cell proteins coagulate, glycosaminoglycans precipitate and stromal collagen fibers shrink. These events cause the cornea to become cloudy. The protein coagulation and shrinkage of the collagen is protective in that it forms a barrier and reduces further penetration of the acid. The collagen shrinkage, however, contracts the eye and can lead to a dangerous acute increase in intraocular pressure. The pH of the acid is not the only determinant of the severity of injury; however, as equimolar solutions of several chemicals adjusted to the same pH of 2 produce a wide range of outcomes. Both the hydrogen ion and anionic portions of the acid molecules contribute to protein coagulation and precipitation. The tissue proteins also tend to act as buffers (Grant, 1986; Potts, 1996).

Bases or Alkalies

Compounds with a basic pH are potentially even more damaging to the eye than are strong acids. Among the compounds of clinical significance in terms of frequency and severity of injuries are ammonia or ammonium hydroxide, sodium hydroxide (lye), potassium hydroxide (caustic potash), calcium hydroxide (lime), and magnesium hydroxide (McCulley, 1998). One of the reasons that caustic agents are so dangerous is their ability to rapidly penetrate the ocular tissues. This is particularly true for ammonia, which has been measured in the aqueous humor just seconds after application to the cornea. The toxicity of these substances is a function of their pH, being more toxic with increasing pH values. As with acid burns, the concentration of the solution and the duration of contact with the eye are important determinants of the eventual clinical outcome. Rapid and extensive irrigation after exposure and removal of particles, if present, is the immediate therapy of choice (Grant, 1986; Potts, 1996).

A feature of caustic burns that differentiates them from acid burns is that two phases of injury may be observed. There is an acute phase from exposure up to 1 week. Depending on the extent of injury, direct damage from exposure is observed in the cornea, adnexia, and possibly in the iris, ciliary body, and lens. The presence of strong hydroxide ions causes rapid necrosis of the corneal epithelium and, if sufficient amounts are present, penetration through and/or destruction of the successive corneal layers. Strong alkali substances attack membrane lipids, causing necrosis and enhancing penetration of the substance to deeper tissue layers. The cations also react with the carboxyl groups of glycosaminoglycans and collagen, the latter reaction leading to hydration of the collagen matrix and corneal swelling. The cornea may appear clouded or become opaque immediately after exposure as a result of stromal edema and changes to, or precipitation of, proteoglycans. The denaturing of the collagen and loss of protective covering of the glycosoaminoglycans is thought to make the collagen fibrils more susceptible to subsequent enzymatic degradation. Intraocular pressure may increase as a result of initial hydration of the collagen fibrils and later through the blockage of aqueous humor outflow. Conversely, if the alkali burn extends to involve the ciliary body, the intraocular pressure may decrease due to reduced formation of aqueous humor. The acute phase of damage is typically followed by initiation of corneal repair. The repair process may involve corneal neovascularization along with regeneration of the corneal epithelium. Approximately 2 to 3 weeks after alkali burns, however, damaging ulceration of the corneal stroma often occurs. The formation of these lesions is related to the inflammatory infiltration of polymorphonuclear leukocytes and fibroblasts and the release of degratory proteolytic enzymes. Clinically, anti-inflammatory therapy limits ulcerative damage. Stromal ulceration usually stops when the corneal epithelium is restored (Grant, 1986; Potts, 1996).

Organic Solvents

When organic solvents are splashed into the eye, the result is typically a painful immediate reaction. As in the case of acids and bases, exposure of the eye to solvents should be treated rapidly with abundant water irrigation. Highly lipophilic solvents can damage the corneal epithelium and produce swelling of the corneal stroma. Most organic solvents do not have a strongly acid or basic pH and therefore cause little in the way of chemical burns to the cornea. In most cases, the corneal epithelium will be repaired over the course of a few days and there will be no residual damage. Exposure to solvent vapors may produce small transparent vacuoles in the corneal epithelium, which may be asymptomatic or associated with moderate irritation and tearing (Grant, 1986; Potts, 1996).

Surfactants

These compounds have water-soluble (hydrophilic) properties at one end of the molecule and lipophilic properties at the other end that help to dissolve fatty substances in water and also serve to reduce water surface tension. The widespread use of these agents in soaps, shampoos, detergents, cosmetics, and similar consumer products leads to abundant opportunities for exposure to ocular tissues. Many of these agents may be irritating or injurious to the eye. The hydrophilic portion of these compounds may be anionic, cationic, or neutral. In general the cationic substances tend to be stronger irritants and more injurious that the other types, and anionic compounds more so than neutral ones (Grant, 1986; Potts, 1996). Because these compounds are by design soluble in both aqueous and lipid media, they readily penetrate the sandwiched aqueous and lipid barriers of the cornea (see discussion of ocular pharmacodynamics and pharmacokinetics, above). This property has implications in drug delivery; for example, low concentrations of the preservative benzalkonium chloride to ophthalmic solutions enhances ocular penetration of topically applied medications (Jaanus et al., 1995).

TARGET SITES AND MECHANISMS OF ACTION: LENS

The lens of the eye plays a critical role in focusing the visual image on the retina. While the cornea is the primary refractive surface for bending incoming light rays, the lens is capable of being reshaped to adjust the focal point to adapt for the distance of visual objects. The lens is a biconvex transparent body, encased in an elastic capsule, and located between the pupil and the vitreous humor (Fig. 17-1). The mature lens has a dense inner nuclear region surrounded by the lens cortex. The high transparency of the lens to visible wavelengths of light is a function of its chemical composition, approximately two-thirds water and one-third protein, and the special organizational structure of the lenticular proteins. The water-soluble crystallins are a set of proteins particular to the lens that, through their close intermolecular structure, give the lens both transparency and the proper refractive index. The lens fibers are laid down during development, as the epithelial cells grow and elongate along meridian pathways between the anterior and posterior poles of the lens. As the epithelial cells continue to grow, the nuclei recede and, in the central portions of the lens, disappear, such that the inner lens substance is composed of nonnucleated cells that form long proteinaceous fibers. The lens fibers are arranged within the lens in an onion-like fashion of concentric rings that have a prismatic arrangement in cross section. The regular geometric organization of the lens fibers is essential for the refractive index and transparency of the lens. At birth, the lens has no blood supply and no innervation. Nutrients are provided from the aqueous and vitreous fluids and are transported into the lens substance through a system of intercellular gap-type junctions. The lens is a metabolically active tissue that maintains careful electrolyte and ionic balance. The lens continues to grow throughout life, with new cells added to the epithelial margin of the lens as the older cells condense into a central nuclear region. The dramatic growth of the lens is illustrated by increasing its weight, from approximately 150 mg at 20 years of age to approximately 250 mg at 80 years of age (Patterson and Delamere, 1992).

Cataracts are decreases in the optical transparency of the lens that ultimately can lead to functional visual disturbances. They are the leading cause of blindness worldwide, affecting an estimated 30 to 45 million people. In the United States, approximately 400,000 people develop cataracts each year, which accounts for about 35 percent of existing visual impairments (Patterson and Delamere, 1992). Cataracts can occur at any age; they can also be congenital (Rogers and Chernoff, 1988). However, they are much more frequent with advancing age. Senile cataracts develop most frequently in the cortical or nuclear regions of the lens and less frequently in the posterior subcapsular region of the lens. Senile cataracts in the cortical region of the lens are associated with disruptions of water and electrolyte homeostasis, while nuclear cataracts are characterized by an increase in the water-insoluble fraction of lens proteins (Patterson and Delamere, 1992).

Recent studies indicate that both genetic and environmental factors contribute to age-related and environmentally mediated cataracts and that these involve several different mechanisms of action (Hammond et al., 2000; Ottonello et al., 2000; Spector, 2000). Risk factors for the development of cataracts include aging, diabetes, low antioxidant levels, and exposure to a variety of environmental factors. Environmental factors include exposure to UV radiation and visible light, trauma, smoking, and exposure to a large variety of topical and systemic drugs and chemicals (e.g., Grant, 1986; Leske et al., 1991; Taylor and Nowell, 1997; Spector, 2000). Several different mechanisms of action have been hypothesized to account for the development of cataracts. These include the disruption of lens energy metabolism, hydration and/or electrolyte balance, the occurrence of oxidative stress due to the generation of free radicals and reactive oxygen species, and the occurrence of oxidative stress due a decrease in antioxidant defense mechanisms (Giblin, 2000; Ottonello et al., 2000; Spector, 2000). The antioxidants include glutathione, superoxide dismutase, catalase, ascorbic acid, and vitamin E. The generation of reactive oxygen species leads to oxidation of lens membrane proteins and lipids. A critical pathway in the development of high-molecular-weight aggregates involves the oxidation of protein thiol groups, particularly in methionine or cysteine amino acids, that leads to the formation of polypeptide links through disulfide bonds, and in turn, high-molecular-weight protein aggregates (Patterson and Delamere, 1992; Ottonello et al., 2000; Spector, 2000). These large aggregations of proteins can attain a size sufficient to scatter light, thus reducing lens transparency. Oxidation of membrane lipids and proteins may also impair membrane transport and permeability.

Corticosteroids

Topical or systemic treatment with corticosteroids causes cataracts (Urban and Cotlier, 1986). Observable opacities begin in the posterior subcapsular region of the lens and progress into the cortical region as the size of the lesion increases. Development of cataracts in individuals varies as a function of total dose of the drug, age, and the nature of the individual's underlying disease. Recently it was estimated that 22 percent of patients receiving corticosteroid immunosuppressive therapy for renal transplants experienced cataracts as a side effect of therapy (Veenstra et al., 1999). The use of inhaled corticosteroids—commonly prescribed asthma therapy—was once thought to be without this risk, but recent epidemiologic evidence documents a significant association between inhaled steroidal therapy and development of nuclear and posterior subcapsular cataracts (Cumming et al., 1997; Cumming and Mitchell, 1999). There are two proposed mechanisms through which corticosteroids might cause cataracts. One proposal involves disruption of the lens epithelium electrolyte balance through inhibition of Na^+,K^+-ATPase. The regular hexagonal array structure of normal lens epithelial cells is disrupted and appears reticulated, while gaps appear between the lateral epithelial cell borders in lenses of humans with steroid-induced cataracts (Karim et al., 1989). Another theory is that corticosteroid molecules react with lens crystallin proteins through Schiff base reactions between the carbonyl group of the steroid and protein amino groups, with subsequent rearrangement into stable products (Urban and Cotlier, 1986). The resulting covalent corticosteroid-crystallin adducts would be high-molecular-weight light-scattering complexes. Whichever mechanism is responsible, these results illustrate the importance of routine ophthalmologic screening of patients receiving chronic corticosteroid therapy.

Light

The most important oxidizing agents are visible light and UV radiation, particularly UV-A (320 to 400 nm) and UV-B (290 to 320 nm), and other forms of electromagnetic radiation. Light- and UV-induced photooxidation leads to generation of reactive oxygen species, and oxidative damage that can accumulate over time. Higher-energy UV-C (100 to 290 nm) is even more damaging. At sea level, the atmosphere filters out virtually all UV-C and all but a small fraction of UV-B derived from solar radiance (AMA Report, 1989). The cornea absorbs about 45 percent of light with wavelengths below 280 nm, but only about 12 percent between 320 and 400 nm. The lens absorbs much of the light between 300 and 400 nm and transmits 400 nm and above to the retina (Patterson and Delamere, 1992). Absorption of light energy in the lens triggers a variety of photoreactions, including the generation of fluorophores and pigments that lead to the yellow-brown coloration of the lens. Sufficient exposure to infrared radiation, as occurs to glassblowers, or microwave radiation will also produce cataracts through direct heating of the ocular tissues.

Naphthalene

Accidental exposure to naphthalene results in cortical cataracts and retinal degeneration (Grant, 1986; Potts, 1996). Naphthalene itself is not cataractogenic; instead, the metabolite 1,2-dihydro-1,2-dihydroxynaphthalene (naphthalene dihydrodiol) is the cataract-inducing agent (van Heyningen and Pirie, 1967). Subsequent studies using biochemical and pharmacologic techniques, in vitro assays, and transgenic mice showed that aldose reductase in the rat lens is a major protein associated with naphthalene dihydrodiol dehydrogenase activity and that lens aldose reductase is the enzyme responsible for the formation of naphthalene dihydrodiol (Sato, 1993; Lee and Chung, 1998; Sato et al., 1999). In addition, in vivo and in vitro studies have shown that aldose reductase inhibitors prevent naphthalene-induced cataracts (Lou et al., 1993; Sato et al., 1999). Finally, there is a difference in naphthalene-induced cataract formation between albino and pigmented rats, with the latter showing a faster onset and more uniform cataract (Murano et al., 1993).

Phenothiazines

It has been known since the 1950s that schizophrenics receiving phenothiazine drugs as anti-psychotic medication develop pigmented deposits in their eyes and skin (Grant, 1986; Potts, 1996). The pigmentation begins as tiny deposits on the anterior surface of the lens and progresses, with increasing dose, to involve the cornea as well. The phenothiazines combine with melanin to form a photosensitive product that reacts with sunlight, causing formation of the deposits. The amount of pigmentation is related to the dose of the drug, with the annual yearly dose being the most predictive dose metric (Thaler et al., 1985). More recent epidemiologic evidence demonstrates a dose-related increase in the risk of cataracts from use of phenothiazine-like drugs, including both antipsychotic drugs such as chlorpromazine and nonantipsychotic phenothiazines (Issac et al., 1991).

TARGET SITES AND MECHANISMS OF ACTION: RETINA

The adult mammalian retina is a highly differentiated tissue containing nine distinct layers plus the RPE, ten major types of neurons, and three cells with glial functions (Fig. 17-1). The nine layers of the neural retina, which originate from the cells of the inner layer of the embryonic optic cup, are the nerve fiber layer (NFL), ganglion cell layer (GCL), inner plexiform layer (IPL), inner nuclear layer (INL), outer plexiform layer (OPL), outer nuclear layer (ONL), rod and cone photoreceptor inner segment layer (RIS; CIS), and the rod and cone photoreceptor outer segment layer (ROS; COS). The RPE, which originates from the cells of the outer layer of the embryonic optic cup, is a single layer of cuboidal epithelial cells that lies on Bruch's membrane adjacent to the vascular choroid. Between the RPE and photoreceptor outer segments lies the subretinal space, which is similar to the brain ventricles. The ten major types of neurons are the rod (R) and cone (C) photoreceptors, ON-rod and ON-cone bipolar cells (BC), OFF-cone bipolar cells, horizontal cells (HC), numerous subtypes of amacrine cells (AC), an interplexiform cell (IPC), and ON-RGCs and OFF-RGCs. The three cells with glial functions are the Müller cells (MC), fibrous astrocytes, and microglia. The somas of the MCs are in the INL. The end feet of the MCs in the proximal or inner retina along with a basal lamina form the internal limiting membrane (ILM) of the retina, which is similar to the pial surface of the brain. In the distal retinal, the MC end feet join with the photoreceptors and zonula adherens to form the external limiting membrane (ELM), which is located between the ONL and RIS/CIS. The interested reader is referred to the excellent references in the Introduction as well as to numerous outstanding websites devoted exclusively to the retina (e.g., http://webvision.umh.es/webvision/intro.html; http://cvs.anu.edu.au/; http://retina.anatomy.upenn.edu/~lance/retina/retina.html) for basic information on the anatomic, biochemical, cell and molecular biological, and physiologic aspects of retinal structure and function.

The mammalian retina is highly vulnerable to toxicant-induced structural and/or functional damage due to (1) the presence of a highly fenestrated choriocapillaris that supplies the distal or outer retina as well as a portion of the inner retina; (2) the very high rate of oxidative mitochondrial metabolism, especially that in the photoreceptors (Linsenmeier, 1986; Ahmed et al., 1993; Medrano and Fox, 1994, 1995; Braun et al., 1995; Winkler, 1995; Shulman and Fox, 1996); (3) high daily turnover of rod and cone outer segments (LaVail, 1976; Rodieck, 1998); (4) high susceptibility of the rod and cones to degeneration due to inherited retinal dystrophies as well as associated syndromes and metabolic disorders (Ogden and Schachat, 1989; Hart, 1992; von Soest et al., 1999); (5) presence of specialized ribbon synapses and synaptic contact sites (Dowling, 1987; Ogden and Schachat, 1989; Cohen, 1992; Rodieck, 1998); (6) presence of numerous neurotransmitter and neuromodulatory systems, including extensive glutamatergic, GABAergic and glycinergic systems (Rauen et al., 1996; Brandstätter et al., 1998; Rodieck, 1998; Kalloniatis and Tomisich, 1999; Winkler et al., 1999); (7) presence of numerous and highly specialized gap junctions used in the information signaling process (Cohen, 1992; Cook and Becker, 1995; Rodieck, 1998); (8) presence of melanin in the choroid and RPE and also in the iris and pupil (Meier-Rouge, 1972; Potts, 1996); (9) a very high choroidal blood flow rate, as high as ten times that of the gray matter of the brain (Alm, 1992; Cohen, 1992); and (10) the additive or synergistic toxic action of certain chemicals with ultraviolet and visible light (Dayhaw-Barker et al., 1986; Backstrom et al., 1993).

The retina is also an excellent model system for studying the effects of chemicals on the developing and mature CNS. Its structure-function relations are well established. The neurogenetic steps of development of the neurons and glial components are well characterized. The development of the CNS and most retinal cells occurs early during gestation in humans (Hendrickson, 1992; Hendrickson and Drucker, 1992) and continues for an additional 7 to 14 days postnatally in the rat (Dobbing and Sands, 1979; Raedler and Sievers, 1975). Therefore, the rodent retina has relevance for chemical exposure during the early gestation period in humans as well as during early postnatal development. The retina contains a wide diversity of synaptic transmitters and second messengers whose developmental patterns are well described. Moreover, the rodent retina is easily accessible, it has most of the same anatomical and functional features found in the developing and mature human retina, and the rat rod pathway is similar to that in other mammals (Dowling, 1987; Finlay and Sengelbaub, 1989; Berman, 1991; Chun et al., 1993). Finally, rat rods have similar dimensions, photochemistry, and photocurrents as human and monkey rods (Baylor et al., 1984; Schnapf et al., 1988). These general and specific features underscore the relevance and applicability of using the rodent retina to investigate the effects of chemicals on this target site as well as a model to investigate the neurotoxic effects of chemicals during development.

Each of the retinal layers can undergo specific as well as general toxic effects. These alterations and deficits include but are not limited to visual field deficits, scotopic vision deficits such as night blindness and increases in the threshold for dark adaptation, cone-mediated (photopic) deficits such as decreased color perception, decreased visual acuity, macular and general retina edema, retinal hemorrhages and vasoconstriction, and pigmentary changes. The list of chemicals and drugs that cause retinal alterations is extensive, as evidenced by an examination of Grant's *Toxicology of the Eye* (Grant, 1986) and Dr. Potts' chapter entitled "Toxic Responses of the Eye" in an earlier edition of the present work (1996). In addition, the review chapter by Jaanus et al. (1995) discusses the adverse retinal effects of therapeutic systemic drugs. The main aim of this section is to discuss in detail several chemicals and drugs (1) that are currently used pharmacological agents or environmentally relevant neurotoxicants; (2) whose behavioral, physiologic, and/or pathologic effects on retina are known; and (3) whose retinal site(s) and/or mechanism of action are well characterized. In addition, the effects of organic solvents and organophosphates on retinal function and vision are discussed, as these are emerging areas of concern.

The chemical- and drug-induced alterations in retinal structure and function are grouped into two major categories. The first category focuses on retinotoxicity of systemically administered therapeutic drugs. Four major drugs are discussed in detail: chloroquine/hydroxychloroquine, digoxin/digitoxin, indomethacin, and tamoxifen. The second category focuses on well-known neurotoxicants that produce retinotoxicity: inorganic lead, methanol, selected organic solvents, and organophosphates. See Chap. 16, "Toxic Responses of the Nervous System," and Chap. 23, "Toxic Effects of Metals," for information on the effects of lead on the brain and other target organs. See Chap. 16 and Chap. 24, "Toxic Effects of Solvents and Vapors," for additional information on methanol and the organic solvents discussed below.

Retinotoxicity of Systemically Administered Therapeutic Drugs

Chloroquine and Hydroxychloroquine Two of the most extensively studied retinotoxic drugs are chloroquine (Aralen) and hydroxychloroquine (Plaquenil). The first cases of chloroquine-induced retinopathy were reported more than 40 years ago (Jaanus et al., 1995; Potts, 1996). These 4-aminoquinoline derivatives are used as antimalarial and anti-inflammatory drugs. The low-dose therapy used for malaria is essentially free from toxic side effects; however, the chronic, high-dose therapy used for rheumatoid arthritis, and discoid and systemic lupus erythematosus (initially 400 to 600 mg/day for 4 to 12 weeks and then 200 to 400 mg day; Ellsworth et al., 1999) can cause irreversible loss of retinal function. Chloroquine, its major metabolite desethylchloroquine, and hydroxychloroquine have high affinity for melanin, which results in very high concentrations of these drugs accumulating in the choroid and RPE, ciliary body, and iris during and following drug administration (Rosenthal et al., 1978; Potts, 1996). Prolonged exposure of the retina to these drugs, especially chloroquine, may lead to an irreversible retinopathy. In fact, small amounts of chloroquine and its metabolites were excreted in the urine years after cessation of drug treatment (Bernstein, 1967). Approximately 20 to 30 percent of patients who received high doses of chloroquine exhibited some type of retinal abnormality, while 5 to 10 percent showed severe changes in retinal function (Burns, 1966; Potts, 1996; Shearer and Dubois, 1967; Sassaman et al., 1970; Krill et al., 1971). Hydroxychloroquine is now the drug of choice for treatment of rheumatic diseases because it has fewer side effects and less ocular toxicity. Doses less than 400 mg per day appear to produce little or no retinopathy even after prolonged therapy (Johnson and Vine, 1987).

The clinical findings accompanying chloroquine retinopathy can be divided into early and late stages. The early changes include (1) the pathognomonic "bull's-eye retina" visualized as a dark, central pigmented area involving the macula, surrounded by a pale ring of depigmentation, which, in turn, is surrounded by another ring of pigmentation; (2) a diminished EOG; (3) possible granular pigmentation in the peripheral retina; and (4) visual complaints such as blurred vision and problems discerning letters or words. Late-stage findings, which can occur during or even following cessation of drug exposure, include (1) a progressive scotoma, (2) constriction of the peripheral fields commencing in the upper temporal quadrant, (3) narrowing of the retinal artery, (4) color and night blindness, (5) absence of a typical retinal pigment pattern, and (6) very abnormal EOGs and ERGs. These late-stage symptoms are irreversible. Interestingly, dark adaptation is relatively normal even during the late stages of chloroquine retinopathy, which helps distinguish the peripheral retinal changes from those observed in patients with retinitis pigmentosa (Bernstein, 1967).

In humans and monkeys, long-term chloroquine administration results in sequential degeneration of the RGCs, photoreceptors, and RPE and the eventual migration of RPE pigment into the ONL and OPL. In addition, in the RPE there is a thickening of the RPE layer, an increase in the mucopolysaccharide and sulfhydryl group content, and a decrease in activity of several enzymes (Potts, 1996; Ramsey and Fine, 1972; Rosenthal et al., 1978). Although the molecular mechanism of action is unknown, it has been suggested that the primary biochemical mechanism is inhibition of protein synthesis (Bernstein, 1967).

Digoxin and Digitoxin The cardiac glycosides digoxin (Lanoxin) and digitoxin (Crystodigin) are digitalis derivatives used in the treatment of congestive heart disease and in certain cardiac arrhythmias. As part of the extract of the plant foxglove, digitalis was recommended for heart failure (dropsy) over 200 years ago. Digitalis-induced visual system abnormalities such as decreased vision, flickering scotomas, and altered color vision were documented during that time (Withering, 1785). Approximately 20 to 60 percent of patients with cardiac glycoside serum levels in the therapeutic range and 50 to 80 percent of the patients with cardiac glycoside serum levels in the toxic range complain of visual system disturbances within 2 weeks after the onset of therapy (Robertson et al., 1966a; Aronson and Ford, 1980; Rietbrock and Alken, 1980; Haustein et al., 1982; Piltz et al., 1993; Duncker et al., 1994). Digoxin produces more toxicity than digitoxin due to its greater volume of distribution and plasma protein binding (Haustein and Schmidt, 1988). The most frequent visual complaints are color vision impairments and hazy or snowy vision, although complaints of flickering light, colored spots surrounded by bright halos, blurred vision, and glare sensitivity also are reported. The color vision disturbances have been confirmed with the Farnsworth-Munsell 100 Hue Test (Aronson and Ford, 1980; Rietbrock and Alken, 1980; Haustein et al., 1982; Haustein and Schmidt, 1988; Duncker and Krastel, 1990). Clinical examinations show that these patients have decreased visual acuity and central scotomas but no funduscopic changes. ERG analysis revealed a depressed critical flicker fusion frequency function, reduced rod and cone amplitudes, increased rod and cone implicit times, and elevated rod and cone thresholds (Robertson et al., 1966a; Robertson et al., 1966b; Alken and Belz, 1984; Duncker and Krastel, 1990; Madreperla et al., 1994). Taken together, these ophthalmologic, behavioral, and electrophysiologic findings demonstrate that the photoreceptors are a primary target site of the cardiac glycosides digoxin and digitoxin.

The above results suggest that cone photoreceptors are more susceptible to the effects of cardiac glycosides than rod photoreceptors. To directly test this hypothesis, Madreperla et al. (1994) conducted electrophysiologic (suction electrode) experiments with isolated tiger salamander (*Ambystoma tigrinum*) rods and cones exposed to different physiologically and toxicologically relevant concentrations of digoxin in the bathing solution. Following a single light flash of saturating intensity, rods and cones exhibited concentration-dependent decreases in the peak light (current) response. The cones, however, were about 50 times more sensitive to digoxin and were impaired to a greater degree at the same digoxin concentration than the rods. Neither the rods or cones recovered to their dark-adapted baseline following the short-duration saturating light flash. The rods, however, appeared to recover faster and more completely than the cones. Moreover, following a return to control Ringer's solution, the photoreceptors still did not recover to their dark-adapted baseline response level. This latter finding correlates with the slow recovery of the ERG seen in patients following termination of digoxin exposure (Robertson et al., 1966b; Duncker and Krastel, 1990; Madreperla et al., 1994) and is most likely due to the high affinity and slow off-rate of digoxin binding to the cardiac glycoside site located on the extracellular side of the catalytic α-subunit of the Na^+,K^+-ATPase enzyme (Sweadner, 1989).

Digitalis glycosides, like ouabain, are potent inhibitors of retinal Na^+,K^+-ATPase (Winkler and Riley, 1977; Fox et al., 1991b; Ottlecz et al., 1993; Shulman and Fox, 1996). Digoxin binding studies show that the retina has the highest number of Na^+,K^+-ATPase sites of any ocular tissue, even higher than those of brain (Lissner et al., 1971; Lufkin et al., 1967). There are three different isoforms of the α subunit of Na^+,K^+-ATPase (i.e., $\alpha 1$, $\alpha 2$, and $\alpha 3$), and they differ most significantly in their sensitivity to cardiac glycoside inhibition (Sweadner, 1989). In the rat retina, the $\alpha 1$-low and $\alpha 3$-high ouabain affinity isoforms of the enzyme account for $\geq$97 percent of the Na^+,K^+-ATPase mRNA. The $\alpha 3$ isoform is localized to rat photoreceptors, horizontal cells, and bipolar cells. Photoreceptors predominantly express the $\alpha 3$ mRNA ($\sim$85 percent), a small amount of $\alpha 1$ mRNA ($\sim$15 percent), and almost no detectable $\alpha 2$ mRNA. Electron microscopic immunocytochemistry studies reveal that the $\alpha 3$ isoform is localized exclusively to the plasma membrane of the rat photoreceptor inner segments (McGrail and Sweadner, 1989; Schneider and Kraig, 1990; Schneider et al., 1990). The $\alpha 3$ isozyme accounts for most of the rod Na^+,K^+-ATPase activity (Shulman and Fox, 1996). The rat rod photoreceptor Na^+,K^+-ATPase–specific activity is approximately threefold higher than whole retinal (Fox et al., 1991b; Shulman and Fox, 1996) or whole brain values (Marks and Seeds, 1978). This is also reflected in the two- to threefold greater ouabain-sensitive oxygen consumption in the dark-adapted outer retina relative to the whole or inner retina, respectively (Medrano and Fox, 1995; Shulman and Fox, 1996). The rod Na^+,K^+-pump maintains the dark current responsible for the light response and operates near V_{max} in the dark-adapted or depolarized state, due to the high flux of Na^+ ions into the rod outer segments through the cGMP gated nonselective cation channels. In addition, light adaptation in mammalian rods is critically dependent upon Na^+,K^+-ATPase activity (Demontis et al., 1995). During constant illumination, the rod Na^+,K^+-pump is slowed in response to a decrease in intracellular Na^+ (Demontis et al., 1995) and a dopamine-mediated inhibition that is independent of the intracellular Na^+ concentration (Shulman and Fox, 1996). Presently there is no such information on the role of Na^+,K^+-ATPase in cones or on cone Na^+,K^+-ATPase–specific activity.

Indomethacin Indomethacin is a nonsteroidal anti-inflammatory drug with analgesic and antipyretic properties that is frequently used for the management of arthritis, gout, and musculoskeletal discomfort. It inhibits prostaglandin synthesis by inhibiting cyclooxygenase. The first cases of indomethacin-induced retinopathy were reported approximately 30 years ago (Jaanus et al., 1995; Potts, 1996). Chronic administration of 50 to 200 mg per day of indomethacin for 1 to 2 years has been reported to produce corneal opacities, discrete pigment scattering of the RPE perifoveally, paramacular depigmentation, decreases in visual acuity, altered visual fields, increases in the threshold for dark adaptation, blue-yellow color deficits, and decreases in ERG and EOG amplitudes (Burns, 1966; Burns, 1968; Henkes et al., 1972; Koliopoulos and Palimeris, 1972; Palimeris et al., 1972). Decreases in the ERG a- and b-wave amplitudes, with larger changes observed under scotopic dark-adapted than light-adapted conditions, have been reported. Upon cessation of drug treatment, the ERG waveforms and color vision changes return to near normal, although the pigmentary changes are irreversible (Burns, 1968; Henkes et al., 1972; Palimeris et al., 1972). The mechanism of retinotoxicity is unknown; however, it appears likely that the RPE is a primary target site.

Tamoxifen Tamoxifen (Nolvadex, Tamoplex), a triphenylethylene derivative, is a nonsteroidal antiestrogenic drug that competes with estrogen for its receptor sites. It is a highly effective antitumor agent used for the treatment of metastatic breast carcinoma in postmenopausal women. Tamoxifen-induced retinopathy following chronic high-dose therapy (180 to 240 mg per day for ~2 years) was first reported 20 years ago (Kaiser-Kupfer et al., 1981). At this dose, there is widespread axonal degeneration in the macular and perimacular area, as evidenced by the presence of different sized yellow-white refractile opacities in the IPL and NFL observed during fundus examination. Macular edema may or may not be present. Clinical symptoms include a permanent decrease in visual acuity and abnormal visual fields, as the axonal degeneration is irreversible (reviewed by Jaanus et al., 1995; Potts, 1996; Ah-Song and Sasco, 1997). Several prospective studies, with sample sizes ranging from 63 to 303 women with breast cancer, have shown that chronic low-dose tamoxifen (20 mg per day) can result in a small but significant increase in the incidence (≤10 percent) of keratopathy (Pavlividis et al., 1992; Gorin et al., 1998; Lazzaroni et al., 1998; Noureddin et al., 1999). In addition, these studies showed that retinopathy is much less frequently observed than with high-dose therapy and, except for a few reports of altered color vision and decreased visual acuity, there were no significant alterations in visual function. Following cessation of low-dose tamoxifen therapy, most of the keratopathy and retinal alterations except the corneal opacities and retinopathy were reversible (Pavlividis et al., 1992; Gorin et al., 1998; Noureddin et al., 1999).

Retinotoxicity of Known Neurotoxicants

Inorganic Lead Inorganic lead is probably the oldest known and most studied environmental toxicant. For almost 100 years, it has been known that overt lead poisoning [mean blood lead (BPb) ≥80 μg/dL] in humans produces visual system pathology and overt visual symptoms (Grant, 1986; Otto and Fox, 1993; Fox, 1998). Clinical symptoms include amblyopia, blindness, optic neuritis or atrophy, peripheral and central scotomas, paralysis of eye muscles, and decreased visual function. More recently, it has been shown that low-(BPb from 10 to 20 μg/dL) to moderate-(BPb from 21 to 60 μg/dL) level lead exposure produces scotopic and temporal visual system deficits in occupationally exposed factory workers and developmentally lead-exposed monkeys and rats (Bushnell et al., 1977; Guguchkova, 1972; Cavelleri et al., 1982; Betta et al., 1983; Signorino et al., 1983; Campara et al., 1984; Jeyaratnam et al., 1986; Fox and Farber, 1988; Lilienthal et al., 1988; Fox et al., 1991a; Fox and Katz, 1992; Otto and Fox, 1993; Lilienthal et al., 1994; Fox, 1998; Rice, 1998). Interestingly, relatively little effort has been made to understand the impact of lead-induced alterations in the visual system of children, although recent preliminary studies suggest that scotopic deficits are present (Rothenberg et al., 1999). Moreover, relatively little effort has been made to understand the impact of lead-induced alterations on retinal and central visual information processing on learning and memory in children, although these types of visual deficits can adversely affect learning and memory as well as experimental procedures used to assess these cognitive parameters (Anger et al., 1994; Hudnell et al., 1996; Walkowiak et al., 1998; Cestnick and Coltheart, 1999).

Studies in Occupationally Exposed Workers Clinical and electrophysiologic studies in lead-exposed factory workers have assessed both the site of action and extent of injury. Several cases of retrobulbar neuritis and ON atrophy have been observed following chronic moderate-level or acute high-level lead exposure (Sherer, 1935; Baghdassarian, 1968; Baloh et al., 1979; Karai et al., 1979). Most of these cases presented with fundus lesions, peripheral or paracentral scotomas while the most severe cases also had a central scotoma. Generally, the scotomas were not observed until approximately 5 years of continuous lead exposure. Interestingly, the earliest observable scotomas were not detected under standard photopic viewing conditions but became evident only under scotopic or mesopic (rod- and cone-mediated) viewing conditions. These ophthalmologic findings correlate directly with the ERG data observed in similarly exposed lead workers. No alterations in the critical flicker fusion threshold (i.e., temporal resolution) were observed when the test was conducted under photopic conditions or when using red lights but consistent decreases in temporal resolution were observed when the test was conducted under scotopic conditions or when green lights were used (Cavelleri et al., 1982; Betta et al., 1983; Signorino et al., 1983; Campara et al., 1984; Jeyaratnam et al., 1986). Moreover, in occupationally lead-exposed workers with or without visual acuity deficits or no observable alterations following ophthalmologic examination, the sensitivity and amplitude of the a-wave and/or b-wave of the dark-adapted ERG were decreased (Guguchkova, 1972; Scholl and Zrenner, 2000). In other lead-exposed workers, one funduscopic study noted the presence of a grayish lead pigmentary deposit in the area peripheral to the optic disk margins (Sonkin, 1963).

In addition to the retinal deficits, occulomotor deficits occur in chronically lead-exposed workers who have no observable ophthalmologic abnormalities. Results from three independent studies, including a follow-up, show that the mean accuracy of saccadic eye movements is lower in lead-exposed workers and the number of overshoots are increased (Baloh et al., 1979; Spivey et al., 1980; Specchio et al., 1981; Glickman et al., 1984). In addition, these studies also revealed that the saccade maximum velocity was decreased. Moreover, one study also observed abnormal smooth pursuit eye movements in lead-exposed workers (Specchio et al., 1981). Although the site and mechanism of action underlying these alterations are unknown, they most likely result from CNS-mediated deficits.

In summary, these results suggest that occupational lead exposure produces concentration- and time-dependent alterations in the retina such that higher levels of lead directly and adversely affect both the retina and ON, whereas lower levels of lead appear to primarily affect the rod photoreceptors and the rod pathway. Interestingly, these latter clinical findings showing preferential lead-induced rod-selective deficits in sensitivity and temporal resolution are observed in both in vivo and in vitro animal studies (see below). Furthermore, these retinal and oculomotor alterations were, in most cases, correlated with the blood lead levels and occurred in the absence of observable ophthalmologic changes, CNS symptoms, and abnormal performance test scores. Thus, these measures of temporal visual function may be among the most sensitive for the early detection of the neurotoxic effects of inorganic lead.

In Vivo and in Vitro Animal Studies Lead exposure to adult and developing animals produces retinal damage and functional deficits. The degree and extent of these alterations depends upon the dose, age, and duration of lead exposure. High-level lead exposure to adult rabbits for 60 to 300 days (Hass et al., 1964; Brown, 1974; Hughes and Coogan, 1974) and to newborn rats for 60 days (Santos-Anderson et al., 1984) resulted in focal necrosis of the rod inner and outer segments, necrosis in the inner nuclear layer and Müller cells, and lysosomal inclusions in the RPE. In addition, high-level lead exposure to mice and rats from birth to weaning resulted in hypomyelination of the ON and a reduction in its diameter; but, interestingly, there were no changes in the sciatic nerve (Tennekoon et al., 1979; Toews et al., 1980). Newborn monkeys exposed to high levels of lead for 6 years had no changes in ON diameter or myelination, although visual cortex neuronal volume and branching were decreased (Reuhl et al., 1989). Rhesus monkeys exposed prenatally and postnatally to moderate or high levels of lead for 9 years, followed by almost 2 years of no lead exposure, had decreased tyrosine hydroxylase immunoreactivity in the large dopaminergic amacrine cells and a complete loss of tyrosine hydroxylase immunoreactivity in small subset of amacrine cells (Kohler et al., 1997). These results suggest that long-term lead exposure produces a decrease in tyrosine hydroxylase synthesis, a finding consistent with other studies (Lasley and Lane, 1988; Jadhav and Ramesh, 1997), and/or a loss of a subset of tyrosine hydroxylase–positive amacrine cells, a finding consistent with recent in vitro work (Scortegagna and Hanbauer, 1997). In contrast to these studies, 6 weeks of moderate-level lead exposure to adult rats (Fox et al., 1997) and 3 weeks of low- or moderate-level lead exposure to neonatal rats from birth to weaning produces rod- and bipolar cell–selective apoptotic cell death (Fox and Chu, 1988; Fox et al., 1997). Moreover, recent results reveal that brief (15-min) exposure of isolated adult rat retinas to nanomolar to micromolar Pb^{2+}, concentrations regarded as pathophysiologically relevant (Cavalleri et al., 1984; Al-Modhefer et al., 1991), resulted in rod-selective apoptosis (He et al., 2000). By extension, these results suggest that the triggering event (initiating phase) and the execution phase of rod and bipolar cell death share common underlying biochemical mechanisms.

Results from several studies suggest that an elevated level of rod photoreceptor Ca^{2+} and/or Pb^{2+} plays a key role in the process of apoptotic rod cell death in humans and animals during inherited retinal degenerations, retinal diseases and injuries, chemical exposure, and lead exposure. These include patients with retinitis pigmentosa and cancer-associated retinopathy (Thirkill et al., 1987; van Soest et al., 1999), retinal degeneration (*rd*) mice (Chang et al., 1993; Fox et al., 1999), rats injected with antirecoverin monoclonal antibodies (Adamus et al., 1998), rats with hypoxic-ischemic injury (Crosson et al., 1990), rats with light-induced damage (Edward et al., 1991), and lead-exposed rats (Fox and Chu, 1988; Fox et al., 1997, 1999). In addition, moderate-level Pb^{2+} exposure produces apoptotic neuronal cell death in primary cultured cells (Oberto et al., 1996; Scortegagna et al., 1997). In vivo and in vitro data suggest that Pb^{2+} produces a dose (concentration)-dependent inhibition of rod cGMP phosphodiesterase (PDE), a resultant elevation of rod cGMP (Fox and Farber, 1988; Fox et al., 1991a; Srivastava et al., 1995a; Srivastava et al., 1995b; Fox et al., 1997), which gates the nonselective cation channel of the rod photoreceptor outer segments (Yau and Baylor, 1989), and an elevation of the rod Ca^{2+} concentration (Fox and Katz, 1992; Medrano and Fox, 1994; He et al., 2000). Detailed kinetic analysis revealed that picomolar Pb^{2+} competitively and directly inhibits rod cGMP PDE relative to millimolar concentrations of Mg^{2+} (Srivastava et al., 1995a, 1995b). In addition, nanomolar Pb^{2+} can elevate the rod Ca^{2+} (and Pb^{2+}) concentration via its competitive inhibition of retinal Na^{+},K^{+}-ATPase relative to MgATP (Fox et al., 1991b). Once inside the rod, both Ca^{2+} and Pb^{2+} enter the mitochondria via the ruthenium red-sensitive Ca^{2+} uniporter and induce mitochondrial depolarization [as measured by the mitochondrial membrane potential sensitive dye JC-1 (5,5′,6,6′,-tetrachloro- 1,1′,3,3′,-tetraethylbenzimidazolycarbocyanine iodide)], swelling, and cytochrome *c* release (He et al., 2000). The effects of Ca^{2+} and Pb^{2+} were additive and blocked completely by the mitochondrial permeability transition pore inhibitor cyclosporin A, whereas the calcineurin inhibitor FK506 had no effect. Following cytochrome *c* release, caspase-9 and caspase-3 are sequentially activated. The caspase-9 inhibitor LEHD-fmk (carbobenzoxy-Leu-Glu-His-Asp-CH_2F) and caspase-3 inhibitor DEVD-fmk (carbobenzoxy-Asp-Glu-Val-Asp-CH_2F)—but not the caspase-8 inhibitor IETD-fmk (carbobenzoxy-Ile-Glu-Thr-Asp-CH_2F)—blocked the postmitochondrial events. There was no evidence of oxidative stress or lipid peroxidation in this model, as the levels of reduced and oxidized glutathione and pyridine nucleotides as well as several lipid parameters in rods were unchanged. These results demonstrate that rod mitochondria are the target site for Ca^{2+} and Pb^{2+}. This is consistent with numerous studies from different tissues demonstrating that lead is preferentially associated with mitochondria and particularly with the inner membrane and matrix fractions (Barltrop et al., 1971; Bull, 1980; Pounds, 1984). Taken together, the results suggest that Ca^{2+} and Pb^{2+} bind to the internal divalent metal binding site of the mitochondrial permeability transition pore (Szabo et al., 1992) and subsequently open it, which initiates the cytochrome *c*–caspase cascade of apoptosis in rods (He et al., 2000).

In vitro extracellular and intracellular electrophysiologic recordings in isolated whole retinas or photoreceptors reveal that nanomolar to micromolar concentrations of lead chloride selectively depress the amplitude and absolute sensitivity of the rod but not cone photoreceptor potential (Fox and Sillman, 1979; Sillman et al., 1982; Tessier-Lavigne et al., 1985; Frumkes and Eysteinsson, 1988). These electrophysiologic results are similar to the ERG alterations observed in occupationally lead-exposed workers (Cavelleri et al., 1982; Betta et al., 1983; Signorino et al., 1983; Campara et al., 1984; Jeyaratnam et al., 1986) and in adult rats exposed to low and moderate levels of lead only during development (Fox and Farber, 1988; Fox and Rubinstein, 1989; Fox et al., 1991a; Fox and Katz, 1992). In addition, these developmentally lead-exposed rats exhibit rod-mediated increases in dark and light adaptation time, decreases in critical flicker fusion frequency (i.e., temporal resolution), decreases in relative sensitivity, and increases in a- and b-wave latencies (Fox and Farber, 1988; Fox and Rubinstein, 1989; Fox et al., 1991a; Fox and Katz, 1992) and decreases in the temporal response properties of both sustained (X-type) and transient (Y-type) RGCs, such as decreased optimal temporal frequency and temporal resolution (Ruan et al., 1994). By extension, these results suggest that there is a common underlying biochemical mechanism responsible for these rod-mediated deficits. In vivo and in vitro data suggest that lead-induced inhibition of cGMP PDE and resultant elevation of rod Ca^{2+} underlies the ERG deficits (Fox and Katz, 1992; Medrano and Fox, 1994; Fox et al., 1997; He et al., 2000). Finally, rod-mediated alterations in dark adaptation and b-wave amplitude are also observed in adult rats and monkeys with prenatal and lifetime moderate- and high-level lead exposure (Hennekes et al., 1987; Lilienthal et al., 1988; Lilienthal et al., 1994). In the lead-exposed monkeys, the amplitude of the scotopic b-wave was increased—an effect hypothesized to result from the loss of dopaminergic amacrine cells or their processes (Lilienthal et al., 1994; Kohler et al., 1997). If rods and blue-sensitive cones in humans exhibit the same sensitivity to a lead-induced inhibition of cGMP-PDE as they do to the drug-induced inhibition of cGMP-PDE (Zrenner and Gouras, 1979; Zrenner et al., 1982). Fox and Farber (1998) predicted that blue-cone color vision deficits as well as scotopic deficits may be found in adults and children exposed to lead. Recently, S- (or blue-) cone deficits were observed in an occupationally lead-exposed worker (Scholl and Zrenner, 2000).

Methanol Methanol is a low-molecular-weight (32), colorless and volatile liquid that is widely used as an industrial solvent; a chemical intermediate; a fuel source for picnic stoves, racing cars, and soldering torches; an antifreeze agent; and an octane booster for gasoline. The basic toxicology and references can be found in two thorough reviews (Tephly and McMartin, 1984; Eells, 1992). Briefly, methanol is readily and rapidly absorbed from all routes of exposure (dermal, inhalation, and oral), easily crosses all membranes, and thus is uniformly distributed to organs and tissues in direct relation to their water content. Following different routes of exposures, the highest concentrations of methanol are found in the blood, aqueous and vitreous humor, and bile as well as the brain, kidneys, lungs, and spleen. In the liver, methanol is oxidized sequentially to formaldehyde by alcohol dehydrogenase in human and nonhuman primates or by catalase in rodents and then to formic acid. It is excreted as formic acid in the urine or oxidized further to carbon dioxide and then excreted by the lungs. Formic acid is the toxic metabolite that mediates the metabolic acidosis as well as the retinal and ON toxicity observed in humans, monkeys, and rats with a decreased capacity for folate metabolism (Tephly and McMartin, 1984; Murray et al., 1991; Eells, 1992; Lee et al., 1994a; Lee et al., 1994b; Garner et al., 1995a; Garner et al., 1995b; Eells et al., 1996; Seme et al., 1999).

Human and nonhuman primates are highly sensitive to methanol-induced neurotoxicity due to their limited capacity to oxidize formic acid. The toxicity occurs in several stages. It first occurs as a mild CNS depression, followed by an asymptomatic 12- to 24-h latent period, followed by a syndrome consisting of formic acidemia, uncompensated metabolic acidosis, ocular and visual toxicity, coma, and possibly death (Tephly and McMartin, 1984; Eells, 1992). The treatment of methanol poisoning involves both combating acidosis and preventing methanol oxidation, but it is not discussed further here. Experimental rats have been made as sensitive to acute methanol exposure as primates by using two different, but related, procedures that effectively reduce the levels of hepatic tetrahydrofolate. One study used a brief (4 h) conditioning and then continuous exposure (60 h) to subanesthetic concentrations of nitrous oxide to inhibit methionine synthase and reduce the level of hepatic tetrahydrofolate (Murray et al., 1991; Eells et al., 1996; Seme et al., 1999). The other fed rats a folate-deficient diet for 18 weeks (Lee et al., 1994a; Lee et al., 1994b). Administration of methanol to these rats with a decreased capacity for folate metabolism resulted in toxic blood formate concentrations of 8 to 16 mM (Murray et al., 1991; Lee et al., 1994a; Lee et al., 1994b; Garner et al., 1995a; Garner et al., 1995b; Eells et al., 1996; Seme et al., 1999). Permanent visual damage occurs in humans and monkeys when the blood folate levels exceed 7 mM (Tephly and McMartin, 1984; Eells, 1992).

Acute methanol poisoning in humans, monkeys, and experimental rats results in profound and permanent structural alterations in the retina and ON and visual impairments ranging from blurred vision to decreased visual acuity and sensitivity to blindness. Ophthalmologic studies of exposed humans and monkeys reveal varying degrees of edema of the papillomacular bundle, ON head, and entire optic disk (Benton and Calhoun, 1952; Potts, 1955; Baumbach et al., 1977; Hayreh et al., 1980). Histopathologic and ultrastructural investigations in methanol-exposed monkeys and folate-modified rats show retinal edema, swollen and degenerated photoreceptors, degenerated RGCs, swollen retinal pigment epithelial cells, axonal (ON) swelling, and mitochondrial swelling and disintegration in each of these cells but especially in the photoreceptors and ON (Baumbach et al., 1977; Hayreh et al., 1980; Murray et al., 1991; Seme et al., 1999). Considering the differences in species, methanol exposures, time course of analysis, and procedures utilized, the overall data for the acute effects of methanol on the ERG are remarkably consistent. Following methanol exposure, the ERG b-wave amplitude in humans, monkeys, and folate-modified rats starts to decrease significantly when the blood formate concentration exceeded 7 mM (Potts, 1955; Ruedeman, 1961; Ingemansson, 1983; Murray et al., 1991; Lee et al., 1994b). These ERG b-wave alterations, as well as flicker-evoked ERG alterations (Seme et al., 1999), occur at lower formate concentrations than those associated with structural changes in the retina and ON, as discussed above. Decreases in the a-wave amplitude are delayed, relative to the b-wave and occur when blood formate concentrations further increase (Ruedeman, 1961; Ingemansson, 1983; Murray et al., 1991; Eells et al., 1996). In addition, it has been shown that intraretinal metabolism of methanol is necessary for the formate-mediated alterations in the ERG (Garner et al., 1995a), although intravenous infusion of formate in monkeys does induce ON edema (Martin-Amat et al., 1978). Finally, in the folate-modified rats, it appears that photoreceptors that respond to a 15-Hz flicker/510-nm wavelength mesopic-photopic stimulus [i.e., rods and middle wavelength–sensitive (M) cones] are more sensitive to methanol than the ultraviolet-sensitive (UV) cones (Seme et al., 1999).

The retinal sources of the ERG a-wave and b-wave are discussed in the beginning of this chapter. Thus, the data from the ERG b-wave methanol studies suggests that the initial effect of formate is directly on the depolarizing (ON-type) rod bipolar cells, Müller glial cells, and/or synaptic transmission between the photoreceptors and bipolar cells. A well-designed series of pharmacologic, ERG, and potassium-induced Müller cell depolarization studies using several controls and folate-modified rats revealed a direct toxic effect of formate on Müller glial cell function (Garner et al., 1995a; Garner et al., 1995b). These studies also provided evidence that formate does not directly affect depolarizing rod bipolar cells or synaptic transmission between the photoreceptors and bipolar cells. Formate also appears to directly and adversely affect the rod and cone photoreceptors as evidenced by the markedly decreased ERG a-wave and flicker response data (Ruedeman, 1961; Ingemansson, 1983; Murray et al., 1991; Eells et al., 1996; Seme et al., 1999).

Although there are no direct data on the underlying molecular mechanism responsible for the toxic effects of formate on Müller glial cells and photoreceptors, several findings suggest that the mechanism involves a disruption in oxidative energy metabolism. First, the whole retinal ATP concentration is decreased in folate-deficient rats 48 h following methanol exposure, the time point when the b-wave was lost (Garner et al., 1995b). Second, both formate-(10 to 200 mM) and formaldehyde-(0.5 to 5 mM)inhibited oxygen consumption in isolated ox retina, and formaldehdye was considerably more potent (Kini and Cooper, 1962). Third, similar concentrations of formaldehyde inhibited oxidative phosphorylation of isolated ox retinal mitochondria, with greater effects observed using FAD-linked than NADH-linked substrates (Kini and Cooper, 1962). Unfortunately the effects of formate were not examined. Fourth, and consistent with the above results, formate inhibits succinate-cytochrome *c* reductase and cytochrome oxidase activity (Ki = 5 to 30 mM), but not NADH-cytochrome *c* reductase activity in isolated beef heart mitochondria and/or submitochondrial particles (Nicholls, 1976). Fifth, ultrastructural studies reveal swollen mitochondria in rat photoreceptor inner segment and ON 48 to 72 h after nitrous oxide/methanol exposure (Murray et al., 1991; Seme et al., 1999). To date, there are no such studies conducted on the Müller glial cells. Taken together, these results suggest formate is a mitochondrial poison that inhibits oxidative phosphorylation of photoreceptors, Müller glial cells, and ON. The evidence for this hypothesis and establishment of subsequent steps resulting in retinal and ON cell injury and death remain to be elucidated.

Organic Solvents ***Trichloroethylene, Xylene, Toluene, n-Hexane and Mixtures*** The neurotoxicity of organic solvents is well established; however, there are not many reports concerning the adverse effects of organic solvents on the retina and visual system despite findings of structural alterations in rods and cones as well as functional alterations such as color vision deficits, decreased contrast sensitivity, and altered visual-motor performance (Raitta et al., 1978; Odkvist et al., 1983; Baker and Fine, 1986; Larsby et al., 1986; Mergler, 1990; Arlien-Söborg, 1992; Backstrom and Collins, 1992; Backstrom et al., 1993; Broadwell et al., 1995; Fox, 1998; also see Chap. 24, "Toxic Effects of Solvents and Vapors").

Dose-response color vision loss (acquired dyschromatopsia) and decreases in the contrast sensitivity function occur in workers exposed to organic solvents such as trichlorethylene, alcohols, xylene, toluene, *n*-hexane, mixtures of these and others. Adverse effects usually occur only at concentrations above the occupational exposure limits (Raitta et al., 1978; Baird et al., 1994; Mergler et al., 1987, 1988, 1991; Nakatsuka et al., 1992). A large percentage of workers in microelectronic plants, print shops, and paint manufacturing facilities, who were exposed to concentrations of solvents that exceeded the threshold limit values, had acquired dyschromatopsia as assessed by the Lanthony D-15 desaturated color arrangement panel (Mergler et al., 1987, 1988, 1991). These workers had no observable clinical abnormalities as assessed by biomicroscopy, funduscopy, and peripheral visual field tests. The color vision losses were mainly blue-yellow losses, although more severe red-green losses were reported. As a rule, acquired blue-yellow losses generally result from lens opacification or outer retinal alterations, whereas red-green losses are associated with inner retinal, retrobular, or central visual pathway alterations (Porkony et al., 1979). Moreover, these occupationally exposed workers also exhibited intermediate spatial frequency losses in their contrast sensitivity function, which reflect alterations in neural function (Mergler et al., 1991). The data from the Mergler et al. (1987, 1988, 1991) studies appear to show gender differences in these adverse visual effects. For example, one recent comprehensive color vision study on male workers exposed to only toluene shows that even high concentration of this solvent had no effect on color vision (Muttray et al., 1995). However, one study on female workers, where the Lanthony D-15 desaturated test was used to assess color vision, showed a trend toward increased prevalence of color vision impairment following exposure to low to moderate concentrations of toluene (Zavalic et al., 1996). Similar blue-yellow deficits as well as macular changes were observed in workers exposed to *n*-hexane for 5 to 21 years (Raitta et al., 1978). These findings correlate with the rod and cone degeneration observed in rats exposed to 2,5-hexanedione (Backstrom and Collins, 1992; Backstrom et al., 1993). Clearly more detailed, well-designed, and well-executed studies are needed to determine (1) which solvent(s) cause alterations in color vision, (2) are spatial and temporal contrast sensitivity affected, (3) the dose(concentration)-response relations between exposure and effects, (4) possible gender differences, and (5) whether these deficits are reversible.

Styrene Five independent studies report that workers exposed to mean atmospheric concentrations of styrene ranging from 20 to 70 ppm exhibit concentration-dependent alterations in color vision (Gobba et al., 1992; Fallas et al., 1992; Chia et al., 1994; Eguchi et al., 1995; Campagna et al., 1995). A combined data analysis from two of the above studies (Gobba et al., 1991; Campagna et al., 1995) suggests that the threshold for color visual impairments is ≤4 ppm styrene (Campagna et al., 1996). This is well below the threshold limit value–time weighted average (TLV-TWA) value for any country: range 20 to 50 ppm. The findings of similar blue-yellow color vision deficits by five different groups of investigators in different countries argues convincingly for the reproducibility and validity of these styrene-induced color vision deficits. The reversibility of these impairments is unknown, however, in one study no recovery was found after a 1-month period of no exposure (Gobba et al., 1991). The findings reveal the sensitivity of the visual system and especially the photoreceptors to toxicant exposure. Moreover, the results demonstrate that the Lanthony D-15 desaturated test can be a sensitive and reliable test for detecting color vision abnormalities in solvent-exposed workers. In summary, the evidence indicates that organic solvents can produce color vision deficits in occupationally exposed workers.

Organophosphates The neurotoxicity of organophosphates is well established (see Chap. 16, "Toxic Responses of the Nervous System"); however, the link between organophosphate exposure and retinotoxicity is presently unresolved. Clinical studies conducted in Japan, reports on ocular toxicity from laboratory animals exposed to organophosphates, and reports to the EPA by pesticide manufacturers suggest that various organophosphates produce retinotoxicity and chronic ocular damage (Ishikawa, 1973; Plestina and Piukovic-Plestina, 1978; Dementi, 1994). However, many of the early clinical reports were poorly designed and remain unconfirmed. The evidence for organophosphate-induced retinal toxicity is strongest for fenthion (dimethyl 3-methyl-4-methylthiophenyl phosphorothionate) (Imai et al., 1983; Misra et al., 1985; Boyes et al., 1994; Tandon et al., 1994). A recent epidemiologic study of licensed pesticide applicators in two states, North Carolina and Iowa, did not find a statistically increased risk of retinal degeneration from use of organophosphate insecticides as a class, but risks were increased for some individual members of the chemical class (Kamel et al., 2000). Interestingly this study did identify an increased risk of retinal degeneration in workers using fungicides. One unexplained report in the Japanese studies was a high incidence of myopia in children exposed to organophosphates. A recent report found that visual control of ocular growth was impaired in the eyes of chicks exposed to the organophosphate insecticide chlorpyrifos (Geller et al., 1998). Until further detailed, well-designed, and replicated clinical and basic science studies are conducted, an adequate discussion of the sites and mechanisms of action of organophosphates must be delayed. In the interim, the references noted above will provide the interested reader with a synopsis of the current status in this area.

TARGET SITES AND MECHANISMS OF ACTION: OPTIC NERVE AND TRACT

The ON consists primarily of RGC axons carrying visual information from the retina to several distinct anatomic destinations in the CNS. Both myelinated and nonmyelinated axons are present and grouped into bundles of axons that maintain a topographic distribution with respect to the site of origin in the retina. At the optic chiasm, the fibers split, so that, in humans and other primates, those fibers originating from the temporal retina continue in the OT toward the ipsilateral side of the brain, while those fibers originating in the nasal half of the retina cross the midline and project to the contralateral side of the brain. In species with sideward-facing eyes such as the rat, a larger proportion of the ON fibers (up to 90 percent) cross the midline. Fibers from the ON terminate in the dorsal LGN, the superior colliculus, and pretectal areas. Information passing through the LGN to visual cortex gives rise to conscious visual perception. Information traveling to the superior colliculus is used to generate eye movements. Pathways leading to the pretectal areas subserve the pupil response. The LGN of primates contains six histologic layers that are alternately innervated by cells from the contralateral and ipsilateral eyes. The cells projecting to and from the ventral two layers of the LGN have large cell bodies and consequently this pathway is referred to as the magnocellular system. Retinal ganglion cells projecting to the magnocellular layers of the LGN are referred to as either M-type or P_α cells. Magnocellular neurons are sensitive to fast moving stimuli and to low levels of luminance contrast, but are insensitive to differences in color. The cells from the magnocellular pathway are involved in motion perception. On the dorsal side of the LGN, the cells are smaller and form the parvocellular pathway. Retinal ganglion cells projecting to the parvocellular layers of the LGN are referred to as P-type or P_β cells. Parvocellular neuron are sensitive to color and to fine detailed patterns, have slower conduction velocities, and are involved in perception of color and form (Horton, 1992; Rodieck, 1998).

Disorders of the ON may be termed *optic neuritis, optic neuropathy,* or *ON atrophy,* referring to inflammation, damage or degeneration, respectively, of the ON. *Retrobulbar neuritis* refers to inflammation or involvement of the orbital portion of the ON posterior to the globe. Among the symptoms of ON disease are reduced visual acuity, contrast sensitivity, and color vision. Toxic effects observed in the ON may originate from damage to the ON fibers themselves or to the RGC somas that provide axons to the ON. A number of toxic and nutritional disorders can adversely affect the ON. Deficiency of thiamine, vitamin B_{12}, or zinc results in degenerative changes in ON fibers. Occasional toxic and nutritional and toxic factors interact to produce ON damage. A condition referred to as *alcohol-tobacco amblyopia* or simply as *toxic amblyopia* is observed in habitually heavy users of these substances and is associated nutritional deficiency. Dietary supplementation with vitamin B_{12} is therapeutically helpful, even when patients continue to consume large amounts of alcohol and tobacco (Grant, 1986; Anderson and Quigley, 1992; Potts, 1996).

Acrylamide

Acrylamide monomer is used in a variety of industrial and laboratory applications, where it serves as the basis for the production of polyacrylamide gels and other polyacrylamide products. Exposure to acrylamide produces a distal axonopathy in large-diameter axons of the peripheral nerves and spinal cord that is well documented in humans and laboratory animals (Spencer and Schaumburg, 1974a, 1974b). Visual effects of acrylamide exposure occur at dose levels sufficient to cause substantial peripheral neuropathy, but the selective nature of the visual deficits and associated neuropathology is very instructive. While the large-diameter and long axons are most vulnerable to acrylamide in the peripheral nerve and spinal cord, this is not the case in the OT. The middle diameter axons of the P_β-type RGCs that project to the parvocellular layers of the LGN of New- and Old-World primates degenerate after prolonged treatment with acrylamide (Eskin and Merigan, 1986; Lynch et al., 1989). The larger-diameter P_α-type RGCs that project to the magnocellular layers of the LGN are apparently spared. Visual function testing in these primates, without a functional parvocellular system, revealed selective perceptual deficits in detecting visual stimuli with high spatial-frequency components (i.e., fine visual patterns) and low temporal-frequency components (i.e., slowly modulating sine waves) (Merigan and Eskin, 1986). On the other hand, the monkeys' perception of larger visual patterns, modulated at higher temporal rates, was not impaired. These toxicologic experiments helped elucidate the functional differentiation of primate parvocellular and magnocellular visual systems. Why the axons of the ON and OT show a different size-based pattern of vulnerability than do axons of the peripheral nerve and spinal cord is not currently understood.

Carbon Disulfide

Carbon disulfide (CS_2) is used in industry to manufacture viscose rayon, carbon tetrachloride, and cellophane. The neurotoxicity of CS_2 is well known and involves damage to the peripheral and central nervous systems as well as profound effects on vision (Beauchamp et al., 1983). The peripheral neuropathy results from a distal axonal degeneration of the large-caliber and long axons of the peripheral nerves and spinal cord, probably through the reactions with the sulfhydryl groups of axonal neurofilament proteins, yielding covalent cross linkages that lead to filamentous tangles and axonal swellings (Graham and Valantine, 2000). The mechanism of action through which inhalation of high concentrations of CS_2 vapors leads to psychotic mania is not currently established but may result from alterations in catecholamine synthesis or neuronal degeneration in several brain areas (Beauchamp et al., 1983). In the visual system, workers exposed to CS_2 experience loss of visual function accompanied by observable lesions in the retinal vasculature. Among the changes in visual function reported in viscose rayon workers are central scotoma, depressed visual sensitivity in the peripheral visual field, optic atrophy, pupillary disturbances, blurred vision, and disorders of color perception. A recent workplace study of 123 Belgian viscose rayon workers found a statistical association between a weighted cumulative CS_2 exposure score, deficits in color vision measured using the Farnsworth-Munsell 100-HUE test, and observations of excess microaneurysms observed ophthalmoscopically and in fundus photographs (Vanhoorne et al., 1996). This association was not observed in the 42 workers who were never exposed to levels above the TLV value of 31 mg/m^3. The coexistence of retinal microaneurysms with functional loss has led to the presumption that the visual deficits were a secondary consequence of vascular disease and perhaps of retinal hemorrhages. This association was addressed in carbon disulfide–exposed macaque monkeys used in visual psychophysical, fluorescein angiography, and fundus photography studies as well as postmortem neuropathologic evaluations (Merigan et al., 1988; Eskin et al., 1988). They observed markedly decreased contrast sensitivity functions, decreased visual acuity, and degeneration of the RGCs, all of which occurred in the absence of retinal microaneurysms or hemorrhages. There was little evidence of effects on the other retinal neurons. These findings indicate that the retinal and ON pathology produced by CS_2 are likely a direct neuropathologic action and not the indirect result of vasculopathy. Interestingly, and importantly, after cessation of exposure, the visual acuity measures recovered temporarily in two of the CS_2-treated monkeys; however, the contrast sensitivity measures did not recover. This demonstrates the independence of these two measures and the utility and importance of independent evaluations of contrast sensitivity and visual acuity.

Cuban Epidemic of Optic Neuropathy

During 1992 and 1993, an epidemic occurred in Cuba in which over 50,000 people suffered from optic neuropathy, sensory and autonomic peripheral neuropathy, high-frequency neural hearing loss, and myelopathy. This is thought to be the largest epidemic of neurologic disease in the twentieth century (Roman, 1998). The affected individuals were characterized as having bilateral low visual acuity, impaired color perception, impaired visual contrast sensitivity, central scotoma, optic disk pallor, and, in particular, loss of nerve fibers from the papillomacular bundle (Sadun et al., 1994a; Hedges et al., 1997). Individuals with neurologic findings demonstrated stocking-glove sensory deficits, leg cramps, sensory ataxia, altered reflexes, and complaints of memory loss (Mojon et al., 1997). Various authors noticed similarities between the Cuban cases and nutritional or alcohol-tobacco amblyopia, Leber's hereditary optic neuropathy, and Strachan's disease (Hedges et al., 1994; Hirano et al; 1994; Espinosa et al., 1994; Sadun et al., 1994b; Mojon et al., 1997). The optic neuropathy resembled methanol poisoning (Roman, 1998; Sadun, 1998). The outbreak of the epidemic was linked to nutritional deficiencies from food shortages after a combination of reduced aid from the former Soviet Union and continued economic sanctions that included shipments of food and medicines imposed by the United States (Hedges et al., 1997; Mojon et al., 1997; Roman, 1998). Aggressive supplementation of the diet with B vitamins and folic acid led to a significant clinical improvement in most identified cases (Mojon et al., 1997). Nutritional deficiencies were a primary contributor to the epidemic; however, it was not clear whether they were solely responsible or whether dietary insufficiency served to make individuals more susceptible to other factors. Genetic susceptibility factors and viral exposures have been considered (Johns et al., 1994; Johns and Sadun, 1994; Newman et al., 1994; Mas et al., 1997; Hedges et al., 1997). One likely contributing factor was coexposure to low levels of neurotoxic compounds that would otherwise have been tolerated (Sadun, 1998). In addition to low food intake, risk factors for the development of optic neuropathy included use of tobacco, in particular the frequent smoking of cigars, and high cassava consumption (Roman, 1998). The mitochondrial toxicant cyanide may be a contaminant of both cassava and tobacco products. Moderate to severe folic acid deficiency was observed in more than half of the cases (Roman, 1998). Samples of local home-brewed rum showed approximately 1 percent contamination with methanol, a level that would not produce ON toxicity in normal healthy individuals (Sadun et al., 1994). However, one-quarter of the Cuban patients showed elevated serum formate concentrations, probably a result of folic acid deficiency. The maximum serum formate concentrations observed (approximately 4 mM) were equivalent to levels that produce retinal and ON toxicity in a rodent model of methanol toxicity (Eells et al., 1996). Sadun (1998) postulated that mitochondrial impairment, created by the combination of low nutritional status and toxic exposures, was responsible for the neurologic impairments. The nutritional deficiency would lead to ATP depletion. Exposure to either cyanide or formic acid, the toxic metabolite of methanol, causes inhibition of cytochrome oxidase, which further depletes ATP levels (Nicholls, 1976; also see retinal section for additional references and details). Because axoplasmic transport of new mitochondria from nerve cell bodies to distal axonal segments is energy-dependent (Vale et al., 1992), the lowered ATP levels would be expected to impair mitochondrial transport and start a vicious cycle of further ATP depletion and reduced mitochondrial transport to the nerve terminal regions. Sadun proposed that the nerve fibers most sensitive to this type of damage would be the long peripheral nerve axons, which have high transport demands, and the small caliber fibers of the ON, in particular at the papillomacular bundle, which have physical constrictions to transporting mitochondria. Exposure to toxicants could not be documented in most of the people identified late in the epidemic, suggesting nutritional deficit as the principal cause. However, co-exposure to low levels of mitochondrial toxicants or other factors may have pushed individuals over a threshold for causing nerve damage.

Ethambutol

The dextro isomer of ethambutol is widely used as an antimycobacterial agent for the treatment of tuberculosis. It is well known that ethambutol produces dose-related alterations in the visual system, such as blue-yellow and red-green dyschromatopsias, decreased contrast sensitivity, reduced visual acuity, and visual field loss. The earliest visual symptoms appear to be a decrease in contrast sensitivity and color vision, although impaired red-green color vision is the most frequently observed and reported complaint. However, the loss of contrast sensitivity may explain why some patients with normal visual acuity and color perception still complain of visual disturbance. These visual system alterations can occur with a few weeks of doses equal to or greater than 20 mg/kg body weight; however, they usually become manifest after several months of treatment (Koliopoulos and Palimeris, 1972; Polak et al., 1985; Salmon et al., 1987; Jaanus et al., 1995). The symptoms are primarily associated with one of two forms of retrobulbar neuritis (i.e., optic neuropathy). The most common form, seen in almost all cases, involves the central ON fibers and typically results in a central or paracentral scotoma in the visual field and is associated with impaired red-green color vision and decreased visual acuity, whereas the second form involves the peripheral ON fibers and typically results in a peripheral scotoma and visual field loss (Jaanus et al., 1995; Lessell, 1998).

In experimental animals, ethambutol causes RGC and ON degeneration, discoloration of the tapetum lucidum (in dogs), retinal detachment (in cats), and possibly amacrine and bipolar cell alterations (van Dijk and Spekreijse, 1983; Grant and Shuhman, 1995; Sjoerdsma et al., 1999). Although the mechanism responsible for producing the RGC and ON degeneration is unknown, recent in vivo studies in rats and in vitro rat RGC cell culture experiments suggest that ethambutol causes RGC death secondary to glutamate-induced excitotoxicity (Heng et al., 1999). Pharmacologic studies, using the in vivo and in vitro models, show that although ethambutol is not a direct NMDA-receptor agonist, it makes RGCs more sensitive to endogenous levels of glutamate. Using the fluorescent Ca^{2+} dyes calcium green 1-AM and rhod-2, Heng et al. (1999) showed that following application of ethambutol in the presence, but not absence, of glutamate to isolated RGCs, there was a decrease in cytosolic Ca^{2+} and a subsequent increase in mitochondrial Ca^{2+}. Interestingly, the increase in mitochondrial Ca^{2+} resulted in an increase in the mitochondrial membrane potential as measured by the mitochondrial membrane potential sensitive dye JC-1. The authors (Heng et al., 1999) postulate that this latter phenomenon occurs as a result of an ethambutol-mediated chelation of Zn^{2+} from the mitochondrial ATPase inhibitor protein IF1 (Rouslin et al., 1993) that subsequently results in the inhibition of mitochondrial ATP synthesis and elevation of mitochondrial membrane potential. These intriguing ideas have merit; however, many additional experiments will be needed to prove this hypothesis. In addition, the authors suggest that some glutamate antagonists may be useful in decreasing the side effects of ethambutol—a practical suggestion that appears worthy of clinical investigation.

TARGET SITES AND MECHANISMS OF ACTION: THE CENTRAL VISUAL SYSTEM

Many areas of the cerebral cortex are involved in the perception of visual information. The primary visual cortex—called V1, Brodmann's area 17, or striate cortex—receives the primary projections of visual information from the LGN and also from the superior colliculus. Neurons from the LGN project to visual cortex maintaining a topographic representation of the receptive field origin in the retina. The receptive fields in the left and right sides of area 17 reflect the contralateral visual world and representations of the upper and lower regions of the visual field are separated below and above, respectively, the calcarine fissure. Cells in the posterior aspects of the calcarine fissure have receptive fields located in the central part of the retina. Cortical cells progressively deeper in the calcarine fissure have retinal receptive fields that are located more and more peripherally in the retina. The central part of the fovea has tightly packed photoreceptors for resolution of fine detailed images, and the cortical representation of the central fovea is proportionately larger than the peripheral retina in order to accommodate a proportionately larger need for neural image processing. The magnocelluar and parvocellular pathways project differently to the histologically defined layers of primary striate visual cortex and then to extrastriate visual areas. The receptive fields of neurons in visual cortex are more complex than the circular center-surround arrangement found in the retina and LGN. Cortical cells respond better to lines of a particular orientation than to simple spots. The receptive fields of cortical cells are thought to represent computational summaries of a number of simpler input signals. As the visual information proceeds from area V1 to extrastriate visual cortical areas, the representation of the visual world reflected in the receptive fields of individual neurons becomes progressively more complex (Horton, 1992).

Lead

In addition to the well-documented retinal effects of lead (see above), lead exposure during adulthood or perinatal development produces structural, biochemical, and functional deficits in the visual cortex of humans, nonhuman primates, and rats (Fox et al., 1977; Winneke, 1979; Costa and Fox, 1983; Sborgia et al., 1983; Fox, 1984; Otto et al., 1985; Lilienthal et al., 1988; Reuhl et al., 1989; Otto, 1990; Murata et al., 1993; Otto and Fox, 1993; Altmann et al., 1994, 1998; Winneke et al., 1994). Quantitative morphometric studies in monkeys exposed to either high levels of lead from birth or infancy to 6 years of age revealed a decrease in visual cortex (areas V1 and V2), cell volume density, and a decrease in the number of initial arborizations among pyramidal neurons (Reuhl et al., 1989). The former results may be due to an absolute decrease in total cell numbers, possibly resulting from lead-induced apoptosis as observed in the retina (Fox et al., 1997; He et al. 2000). This may also account for the decreased density of cholinergic muscarinic receptors found in the visual cortex of adult rats following moderate level developmental lead exposure (Costa and Fox, 1983). The morphometric results on neuronal branching are reminiscent of earlier findings in the neocortex of rats following high level developmental lead exposure (Petit and LeBoutillier, 1979), and recent findings in the somatosensory cortex of rats following low or moderate level developmental lead exposure (Wilson et al., 2000). These alterations could partially contribute to the decreases in contrast sensitivity observed in lead-exposed rats and monkeys (Fox, 1984; Rice, 1998), the alterations in the amplitude and latency measures of the flash and pattern-reversal evoked potentials in lead-exposed children, workers, monkeys, and rats (Fox et al., 1977; Winneke, 1979; Sborgia et al., 1983; Otto et al., 1985; Lilienthal et al., 1988; Otto, 1990; Murata et al., 1993; Altmann et al., 1994, 1998; Winneke et al., 1994), and the alterations in tasks assessing visual function in lead-exposed children (Winneke et al., 1983; Hansen et al., 1989; Muñoz et al., 1993).

Methyl Mercury

Methyl mercury became notorious in two episodes of mass poisoning (see Chap. 16, "Toxic Responses of the Nervous System"). In the 1950s industrial discharges of mercury into Minamata Bay in Japan became biomethylated to form methyl mercury, which then accumulated in the food chain and reached toxic concentrations in the fish and shellfish consumed in the surrounding communities. Hundreds of people were poisoned, showing a combination of sensory, motor, and cognitive deficits. A more widespread episode of methyl mercury poisoning affected thousands of Iraqi citizens who mistakenly ground wheat grain into flour that had been treated with methyl mercury as a fungicide and that was intended for planting and not for direct human consumption.

Visual deficits are a prominent feature of methyl mercury intoxication in adult humans, along with several other neurologic manifestations such as difficulties with sensation, gait, memory, and cognition. Methyl mercury poisoned individuals experienced a striking and progressive constriction of the visual field (peripheral scotoma) as patients became progressively less able to see objects in the visual periphery (Iwata, 1977). The narrowing of the visual world gives impression of looking through a long tunnel, hence the term *tunnel vision.* Visual field constrictions also have been observed in methyl mercury–poisoned monkeys (Merigan, 1979). On autopsy of some of the Minamata patients, focal neurologic degeneration was observed in several brain regions including motor cortex, cerebellum, and calcarine fissure of visual cortex (Takeuchi and Eto, 1977). The histopathologic feature was a destruction of the cortical neural and glial cells, with sparing of the subcortical white matter, optic radiations, and LGN. Monkeys and dogs that were treated experimentally with methyl mercury showed greater damage in the calcarine fissure, associated with higher regional concentrations of protein-bound mercury, than in other brain regions (Yoshino et al., 1966; Berlin et al., 1975). In the Minamata patients there was a regional distribution of damage observed within striate cortex, such that the most extensive damage occurred deep in the calcarine fissure and was progressively less in the more posterior portions. Thus, the damage was most severe in the regions of primary visual cortex that subserved the peripheral visual field, with relative sparing of the cortical areas representing the central vision. This regional distribution of damage corresponded with the progressive loss of peripheral vision while central vision was relatively preserved. Methyl mercury–poisoned individuals also experienced poor night vision (i.e., scotopic vision deficits), also attributable to peripheral visual field losses. Similar changes were observed in adult monkeys exposed to methyl mercury (Berlin et al., 1975). Interestingly, mercury also accumulates in the retina of animals exposed to methyl mercury (DuVal et al., 1987) and produces rod-selective electrophysiologic and morphologic alterations (Fox and Sillman, 1979; Braekevelt, 1982). The neurologic damage in adult cases of Minamata disease was focally localized in the calcarine cortex and other areas but was more globally distributed throughout the brain in those developmentally exposed.

The levels of methyl mercury exposure experienced by people in Minamata Bay were undoubtedly high. Studies of visual function in nonhuman primates exposed to methyl mercury during perinatal development demonstrate a decrease in visual contrast sensitivity, visual acuity, and temporal flicker resolution at dose levels lower than those associated with constriction of the visual fields (Rice and Gilbert, 1982; Rice and Gilbert, 1990; Rice, 1996). Monkeys exposed to methyl mercury from birth onward or in utero plus postnatally exhibited spatial vision deficits under both high and low luminance conditions, although the deficits were greater under scotopic illumination (Rice and Gilbert, 1982; Rice, 1990). The effects on temporal vision were different. That is, monkeys exposed from birth displayed superior low-luminance temporal vision, while high-luminance temporal vision was not impaired. In contrast, monkeys exposed to methyl mercury in utero plus postnatally exhibited deficits in low-frequency high-luminance temporal vision, while low-luminance temporal vision was superior to that of control monkeys (Rice, 1990). These data indicate that the spatial and temporal vision deficits produced by developmental exposure to methyl mercury are different from those produced during adulthood. The underlying mechanisms have yet to be determined.

REFERENCES

Adamus G, Machnicki M, Elerding H, et al: Antibodies to recoverin induce apoptosis of photoreceptor and bipolar cells in vivo. *J Autoimmun* 11:523–533, 1998.

Agency for Toxic Substances and Disease Registry (ATSDR). *Neurobehavioral Test Batteries for Use in Environmental Health Field Studies.* Atlanta, GA: U.S. Department of Health, Public Health Service 1992.

Ahmed J, Braun RD, Dunn R Jr, Linsenmeier RA: Oxygen distribution in the macaque retina. *Invest Ophthalmol Vis Sci* 34:516–521, 1993.

Ah-Song R, Sasco AJ: Tamoxifen and ocular toxicity. *Cancer Detect Prev* 21:522–531, 1997.

Al-Modhefer AJA, Bradbury MWB, Simons TJB: Observations on the chemical nature of lead in human blood serum. *Clin Sci* 81:823–829, 1991.

Alken RG, Belz GG: A comparative dose-effect study with cardiac glycosides assessing cardiac and extracardiac responses in normal subjects. *J Cardiovasc Pharmacol* 6:634–640, 1984.

Alm A: Ocular circulation, in Hart WM (ed): *Adler's Physiology of the Eye,* 9th ed. St. Louis: Mosby–Year Book, 1992, pp 198–227.

Altmann L, Bottger A, Wiegand H: Neurophysiological and psychophysical measurements reveal effects of acute low-level organic solvent exposure in humans. *Int Arch Occup Environ Health* 62:493–499, 1990.

Altmann L, Gutowski M, Wiegand H: Effects of maternal lead exposure on functional plasticity in the visual cortex and hippocampus of immature rats. *Brain Res Dev Brain Res* 81:50–56, 1994.

Altmann L, Sveinsson K, Kramer U, et al: Visual functions in 6-year-old children in relation to lead and mercury levels. *Neurotoxicol Teratol* 20:9–17, 1998.

American Medical Association, Council on Scientific Affairs: Harmful effects of ultraviolet radiation. *JAMA* 262:380–384, 1989.

Anderson DR, Quigley HA: The optic nerve, in Hart WM (ed): *Adler's Physiology of the Eye,* 9th ed. St. Louis: Mosby–Year Book, 1992, pp 616–640.

Anderson JA, Davis WL, Wei CP: Site of ocular hydrolysis of a prodrug, dipivefrin, and a comparison of its ocular metabolism with that of the parent compound, epinephrine. *Invest Ophthalmol Vis Sci* 19:817–823, 1980.

Anger WK: Neurobehavioral testing on chemicals: Impact on recommended standards. *Neurobehav Toxicol Teratol* 6:147–153, 1984.

Anger WK, Johnson BL: Chemicals affecting behavior, in O'Donoghue JL (ed): *Neurotoxicity of Industrial and Commercial Chemicals.* Boca Raton, FL: CRC Press, 1985, pp 51–148.

Anger WK, Letz R, Chrislip DW, et al: Neurobehavioral test methods for environmental health studies of adults. *Neurotoxicol Teratol* 16:489–497, 1994.

Arlien-Söborg P: *Solvent Neurotoxicity.* Boca Raton, FL: CRC Press, 1992.

Aronson JK, Ford AR: The use of colour vision measurement in the diagnosis of digoxin toxicity. *Q J Med* 49:273–282, 1980.

Asakura T, Matsuda M, Matsuda S, Shichi H: Synthesis of 12(R)- and 12(S)-hydroxyeicosatetraenoic acid by porcine ocular tissues. *J Ocul Pharmacol* 10:525–535, 1994.

Atalla LR, Sevanian A, Rao NA: Immunohistochemical localization of glutathione peroxidase in ocular tissue. *Curr Eye Res* 7:1023–1027, 1988.

Awasthi YC, Saneto RP, Srivastava SK: Purification and properties of bovine lens glutathione *S*-transferase. *Exp Eye Res* 30:29–39, 1980.

Backstrom B, Collins VP: The effects of 2,5-hexanedione on rods and cones of the retina of albino rats. *Neurotoxicology* 13:199–202, 1992.

Backstrom B, Nylen P, Hagman M, et al: Effect of exposure to 2,5-hexanediol in light or darkness on the retina of albino and pigmented rats. I. Morphology. *Arch Toxicol* 67:277–283, 1993.

Baghdassarian SA: Optic neuropathy due to lead poisoning. *Arch Ophthalmol* 80:721–723, 1968.

Baird, B, Camp J, Daniell W, Antonelli J: Solvents and color discrimination ability. *J Occup Med* 36:747–751, 1994.

Baker EL, Feldman RG, White RA, et al: Occupational lead neurotoxicity: A behavioral and electrophysiological evaluation. *Br J Ind Med* 41:352–361, 1984.

Baker EL, Fine LJ: Solvent neurotoxicity. The current evidence. *J Occup Med* 28:126–129, 1986.

Ballantyne B: Toxicology related to the eye, in Ballantyne B, Marrs TC, Syversen T (eds): *General and Applied Toxicology,* New York: McGraw-Hill, 1999, pp 737–774.

Baloh RW, Langhofer L, Brown CP, Spivey GH: Quantitative tracking tests in lead workers. *Am J Med* 1:109–113, 1980.

Baloh RW, Spivey GH, Brown CP, et al: Subclinical effects of chronic increased lead absorption—A prospective study. II. Results of baseline neurologic testing. *J Occup Med* 21:490–496, 1979.

Barltrop D, Barrett AJ, Dingle JT: Subcellular distribution of lead in the rat. *J Lab Clin Med* 77:705–712, 1971.

Barratt MD: A quantitative structure-activity relationship for the eye irritation potential of neutral organic chemicals. *Toxicol Lett* 80:69–74, 1995.

Bartlett JD, Jaanus SD: *Clinical Ocular Pharmacology.* Boston: Butterworth-Heinemann, 3d ed. 1995.

Baumbach GL, Cancilla PA, Martin-Amat G, et al: Methyl alcohol poisoning: IV. Alterations of the morphological findings of the retina and optic nerve. *Arch Ophthalmol* 95:1859–1865, 1977.

Bausher LP: Identification of A and B forms of monoamine oxidase in the iris-ciliary body, superior cervical ganglion, and pineal gland of albino rabbits. *Invest Ophthalmol* 15:529–537, 1976.

Baylor DA, Nunn BJ, Schnapf JL: The photocurrent, noise and spectral sensitivity of rods of the monkey *Macaca fascicularis. J Physiol* 357:575–607, 1984.

Beauchamp RO Jr, Bus JS, Popp JA, et al: A critical review of the literature on carbon disulfide toxicity. *CRC Crit Rev Toxicol* 11:168–277, 1983.

Behndig A, Svensson B, Marklund SL, Karlsson K: Superoxide dismutase isoenzymes in the human eye. *Invest Ophthalmol Vis Sci* 39:471–475, 1998.

Benton CD, Calhoun FP: The ocular effects of methyl alcohol poisioning: Report of a catastrophe involving three hundred and twenty persons. *Trans Am Acad Ophthalmol* 56:875–883, 1952.

Berlin M, Grant CA, Hellberg J, et al: Neurotoxicity of methyl mercury in squirrel monkeys. Cerebral cortical pathology, interference with scotopic vision, and changes in operant behavior. *Arch Environ Health* 30:340–348, 1975.

Berman ER: *Biochemistry of the Eye.* New York: Plenum Press, 1991.

Bernstein HN: Chloroquine ocular toxicity. *Surv Ophthalmol* 12:415–477, 1967.

Berson EL: Electrical phenomena in the retina, in Hart WM (ed): *Adler's Physiology of the Eye,* 9th ed. St. Louis: Mosby–Year Book, 1992, pp 641–707.

Betta A, De Santa A, Savonitto C, D'Andrea F: Flicker fusion test and occupational toxicology performance evaluation in workers exposed to lead and solvents. *Hum Toxicol* 2:83–90, 1983.

Birch D, Jacobs GH: Spatial contrast sensitivity in albino and pigmented rats. *Vision Res* 19:933–937, 1979.

Boyes WK: Testing visual system toxicity using visual evoked potential technology, in Isaacson RL, Jensen KF (eds): *The Vulnerable Brain and Environmental Risk: Malnutrition and Hazard Assessment.* Vol 1. New York: Plenum Press, 1992, pp 193–222.

Boyes WK, Dyer RS: Chlordimeform produces profound but transient changes in visual evoked potentials of hooded rats. *Exp Neurol* 86:434–447, 1984.

Boyes WK, Dyer RS: Pattern reversal visual evoked potentials in awake rats. *Brain Res Bull* 10:817–823, 1983.

Boyes WK, Tandon P, Barone S Jr, Padilla S: Effects of organophosphates on the visual system of rats. *J Appl Toxicol* 14:135–143, 1994.

Braekevelt CR: Morphological changes in rat retinal photoreceptors with acute methyl mercury intoxication, in Hollyfield JG (ed): *The Structure of the Eye.* New York: Elsevier, 1982, pp 123–131.

Brandstätter JH, Koulen P, Wässle H: Diversity of glutamate receptors in the mammalian retina. *Vision Res* 38:1385–1397, 1998.

Braun RD, Linsenmeier RA, Goldstick TK: Oxygen consumption in the inner and outer retina of the cat. *Invest Ophthalmol Vis Sci* 36:542–554, 1995.

Broadwell DK, Darcey DJ, Hudnell HK, et al: Worksite clinical and neurobehavioral assessment of solvent-exposed workers. *Am J Indust Med* 27:677–698, 1995.

Brown DVL: Reaction of the rabbit retinal pigment epithelium to systemic lead poisoning. *Tr Am Ophthalmol Soc* 72:404–447, 1974.

Bruner LH, Parker RD, Bruce RD: Reducing the number of rabbits in the low-volume eye test. *Fundam Appl Toxicol* 19:330–335, 1992.

Bruner LH, Shadduck J, Essex-Sorlie D: Alternative methods for assessing the effects of chemicals in the eye, in Hobson DW (ed): *Dermal and Ocular Toxicity: Fundamentals and Methods.* Boca Raton, FL: CRC Press, 1991, pp 585–606.

Bull RJ: Lead and energy metabolism, in Singhal RL, Thomas JA (eds): *Lead Toxicity.* Baltimore: Urban and Schwarzenberg, 1980, pp 119–168.

Burns CA: Indomethacin, reduced retinal sensitivity and corneal deposits. *Am J Ophthalmol* 66:825–835, 1968.

Burns CA: Ocular effects of indomethacin. Slit lamp and electroretinographic: ERG study. *Invest Ophthalmol* 5:325–331, 1966.

Bushnell PJ, Bowman RE, Allen JR, Marlar RJ: Scotopic vision deficits in young monkeys exposed to lead. *Science* 196:333–335, 1977.

Campagna D, Gobba F, Mergler D, et al: Color vision loss among styrene-exposed workers: Neurotoxicological threshold assessment. *Neurotoxicology* 17:367–373, 1996.

Campagna D, Mergler D, Huel G, et al: Visual dysfunction among styrene-exposed workers. *Scand J Work Environ Health* 21:382–390, 1995.

Campara P, D'Andrea F, Micciolo R, et al: Psychological performance of workers with blood-lead concentration below the current threshold limit value. *Int Arch Occup Environ Health* 53:233–246, 1984.

Cavalleri A, Minoia C, Ceroni A, Poloni M: Lead in cerebrospinal fluid and its relationship to plasma lead in humans. *J Appl Toxicol* 4:63–65, 1984.

Cavelleri A, Trimarchi F, Gelmi C, et al: Effects of lead on the visual system of occupationally exposed subjects. *Scand J Work Environ Health* 8(suppl 1):148–151, 1982.

Cestnick L, Coltheart M: The relationship between language-processing and visual-processing deficits in developmental dyslexia. *Cognition* 71:231–255, 1999.

Chamberlain M, Gad SC, Gautheron P, Prinsen MK: IRAG working group 1. Organotypic models for the assessment/prediction of ocular irritation. Interagency Regulatory Alternatives Group. *Food Chem Toxicol* 35:23–37, 1997.

Chang GQ, Hao Y, Wong F: Apoptosis: Final common pathway of photoreceptor death in rd, rds, and rhodopsin mutant mice. *Neuron* 11:595–605, 1993.

Chia SE, Jeyaratnam J, Ong CN, et al: Impairment of color vision among workers exposed to low concentrations of styrene. *Am J Ind Med* 26:481–488, 1994.

Chiou GCY: *Ophthalmic Toxicology.* New York: Raven Press, 1992.

Chun MH, Han SH, Chung JW, Wässle H: Electron microscopic analysis of the rod pathway of the rat retina. *J Comp Neurol* 332:421–432, 1993.

Cohen AI: The retina, in Hart WM (ed): *Adler's Physiology of the Eye,* 9th ed. St. Louis: Mosby–Year Book, 1992, pp 579–615.

Cook JE, Becker DL: Gap junctions in the vertebrate retina. *Microsc Res Tech* 31:408–419, 1995.

Costa LG, Fox DA: A selective decrease in cholinergic muscarinic receptors in the visual cortex of adult rats following developmental lead exposure. *Brain Res* 276:259–266, 1983.

Crofton KM, Sheets LP: Evaluation of sensory system function using reflex modification of the startle response. *J Am Coll Toxicol* 8:199–211, 1989.

Crosson CE, Willis JA, Potter DE: Effect of the calcium antagonist, nifedipine, on ischemic retinal dysfunction. *J Ocul Pharmacol* 6:293–299, 1990.

Crouch RK, Goletz P, Snyder A, Coles WH: Antioxidant enzymes in human tears. *J Ocul Pharmacol* 7:253–258, 1991.

Cumming RG, Mitchell P: Alcohol, smoking, and cataracts: The Blue Mountains Eye Study. *Arch Ophthalmol* 115:1296–1303, 1997.

Cumming RG, Mitchell P: Inhaled corticosteroids and cataract: Prevalence, prevention and management. *Drug Safety* 20:77–84, 1999.

Cumming RG, Mitchell P, Leeder SR: Use of inhaled corticosteroids and the risk of cataracts. *N Engl J Med* 337:8–14, 1997.

Damstra T: Environmental chemicals and nervous system dysfunction. *Yale J Biol Med* 51:457–468, 1978.

Datson GP, Freeberg FE: Ocular irritation testing, in Hobson DW (ed): *Dermal and Ocular Toxicity: Fundamentals and Methods.* Boca Raton, FL: CRC Press, 1991, pp 509–539.

Davson H: *Adler's Physiology of the Eye,* 5th ed. New York: Pergamon Press, 1990.

Dayhaw-Barker P, Forbes D, Fox DA, et al: Drug photoxicity and visual health, in Waxler M, Hitchins VM (eds): *Optical Radiation and Visual Health.* Boca Raton, FL: CRC Press, 1986, pp 147–175.

Dean P: Visual pathways and acuity hooded rats. *Behav Brain Res* 3:239–271, 1981.

Delcourt C, Carriere I, Ponton-Sanchez A, et al: Light exposure and the risk of cortical, nuclear, and posterior subcapsular cataracts: The Pathologies Oculaires Liees a l'Age (POLA) study. *Arch Ophthalmol* 118:385–392, 2000.

Dementi B: Ocular effects of organophosphates: A historical perspective of Saku disease. *J Appl Toxicol* 14:119–129, 1994.

Demontis GC, Ratto GM, Bisti S, Cervetto L: Effect of blocking the Na^+/K^+ ATPase on Ca^{2+} extrusion and light adaptation in mammalian rods. *Biophys J* 69:439–450, 1995.

De Rouck A, De Laey JJ, Van Hoorne M, et al: Chronic carbon disulfide poisoning: A 4-year follow-up study of the ophthalmological signs. *Int Ophthalmol* 9:17–27, 1986.

Diamante GG, Fraunfelder FT: Adverse effects of therapeutic agents on cornea and conjunctiva, in Leibowitz HM, Waring GO (eds): *Corneal Disorders, Clinical Diagnosis and Management,* 2d ed. Philadelphia: Saunders, 1998, pp 736–769.

Dobbing J, Sands J: Comparative aspects of the brain growth spurt. *Early Hum Dev* 3:79–91, 1979.

Dowling JE: *The Retina: An Approachable Part of the Brain.* Cambridge, MA: Belknap Press, 1987.

Downes JE, Holmes RS: Purification and properties of murine corneal alcohol dehydrogenase. Evidence for class IV ADH properties. *Adv Exp Med Biol* 372:349–354, 1995.

Dräger UC: Calcium binding in pigmented and albino eyes. *Proc Natl Acad Sci USA* 82:6716–6720, 1985.

Draize JH, Woodard G, Calvery HO: Methods for the study of irritation and toxicity of substances applied topically to the skin and mucous membranes. *J Pharmacol Exp Ther* 82:377–389, 1944.

Duncker G, Krastel H: Ocular digitalis effects in normal subjects. *Lens Eye Tox Res* 7:281–303, 1990.

Duncker GI, Kisters G, Grille W: Prospective, randomized, placebo-controlled, double-blind testing of colour vision and electroretinogram at therapeutic and subtherapeutic digitoxin serum levels. *Ophthalmologica* 208:259–261, 1994.

DuVal G, Grubb BR, Bentley PJ: Mercury accumulation in the eye following administration of methyl mercury. *Exp Eye Res* 44:161–164, 1987.

Dyer RS: The use of sensory evoked potentials in toxicology. *Fundam Appl Toxicol* 5:24–40, 1985.

Dyer RS, Howell WE, Wonderlin WF: Visual system dysfunction following acute trimethyltin exposure in rats. *Neurobehav Toxicol Teratol* 4:191–195, 1982.

Edward DP, Lam TT, Shahinfar S, et al: Amelioration of light-induced retinal degeneration by a calcium overload blocker: flunarizine. *Arch Ophthalmol* 109:554–562, 1991.

Eells, JT: Methanol, in Thurman RG, Kauffman FC (eds): *Browning's Toxicity and Metabolism of Industrial Solvents: Alcohols and Esters.* Vol 3. Amsterdam: Elsevier, 1992, pp 3–20.

Eells JT, Salzman MM, Lewandowski MF, Murray TG: Formate-induced alterations in retinal function in methanol-intoxicated rats. *Toxicol Appl Pharmacol* 140:58–69, 1996.

Eguchi T, Kishi R, Harabuchi I, et al: Impaired colour discrimination among workers exposed to styrene: Relevance of a urinary metabolite. *Occup Environ Med* 52:534–538, 1995.

Eichenbaum JW, Zheng W: Distribution of lead and transthyretin in human eyes. *Clin Toxicol* 38:371–381, 2000.

Ellsworth AJ, Witt DM, Dugdale DC, Oliver LM: *Mosby's 1999–2000 Medical Drug Reference.* St. Louis: Mosby, 1999, pp 184–185.

Eskin TA, Merigan WH, Wood RW: Carbon disulfide effects on the visual system: II. Retinogeniculate degeneration. *Invest Ophthalmol Vis Sci* 29:519–527, 1988.

Espinosa A, Alvarez F, Vazquez L, Ordunez PO: Optic and peripheral neuropathy in Cuba. *JAMA* 271:664, 1994.

Fallas C, Fallas J, Maslard P, Dally S: Subclinical impairment of colour vision among workers exposed to styrene. *Br J Ind Med* 49:679–682, 1992.

Finlay BL, Sengelaub DR: *Development of the Vertebrate Retina.* New York: Plenum Press, 1989.

Fox DA: Psychophysically and electrophysiologically determined spatial vision deficits in lead-exposed rats have a cholinergic component, in Narahashi T (ed): *Cellular and Molecular Basis of Neurotoxicity.* New York: Raven Press, 1984, pp 123–140.

Fox DA: Sensory system alterations following occupational exposure to chemicals, in Manzo L, Costa LG (eds): *Occupational Neurotoxicology.* Boca Raton, FL: CRC Press, 1998, pp 169–184.

Fox DA, Campbell ML, Blocker YS: Functional alterations and apoptotic cell death in the retina following developmental or adult lead exposure. *Neurotoxicology* 18:645–665, 1997.

Fox DA, Chu LWF: Rods are selectively altered by lead: II. Ultrastructure and quantitative histology. *Exp Eye Res* 46:613–625, 1988.

Fox DA, Farber DB: Rods are selectively altered by lead: I. Electrophysiology and biochemistry. *Exp Eye Res* 46:579–611, 1988.

Fox DA, Katz LM: Developmental lead exposure selectively alters the scotopic ERG component of dark and light adaptation and increases rod calcium content. *Vision Res* 32:249–252, 1992.

Fox DA, Katz LM, Farber DB: Low-level developmental lead exposure decreases the sensitivity, amplitude and temporal resolution of rods. *Neurotoxicology* 12:641–654, 1991a.

Fox DA, Lewkowski JP, Cooper GP: Acute and chronic effects of neonatal lead exposure on the development of the visual evoked response in rats. *Toxicol Appl Pharmacol* 40:449–461, 1977.

Fox DA, Lowndes HE, Bierkamper GG: Electrophysiological techniques in neurotoxicology, in Mitchel CL (ed): *Nervous System Toxicology.* New York: Raven Press, 1982, pp 299–335.

Fox DA, Poblenz AT, He L: Calcium overload triggers rod photoreceptor apoptotic cell death in chemical-induced and inherited retinal degenerations. *Ann NY Acad Sci* 893:282–286, 1999.

Fox DA, Rubinstein SD: Age-related changes in retinal sensitivity, rhodopsin content and rod outer-segment length in hooded rats following low level lead exposure during development. *Exp Eye Res* 48:237–249, 1989.

Fox DA, Rubinstein SD, Hsu P: Developmental lead exposure inhibits adult rat retinal, but not kidney, Na^+,K^+-ATPase. *Toxicol Appl Pharmacol* 109:482–493, 1991b.

Fox DA, Sillman AJ: Heavy metals affect rod, but not cone photoreceptors. *Science* 206:78–80, 1979.

Fraunfelder FT, Meyer SM: *Drug-Induced Ocular Side Effects and Drug Interactions,* 3d ed. Philadelphia: Lea & Febiger, 1989.

Frumkes TE, Eysteinsson T: The cellular basis for suppressive rod-cone interaction. *Vis Neurosci* 1:263–273, 1988.

Garner CD, Lee EW, Louis-Ferdinand RT: Muller cell involvement in methanol-induced retinal toxicity. *Toxicol Appl Pharmacol* 130:101–107, 1995b.

Garner CD, Lee EW, Terzo TS, Louis-Ferdinand RT: Role of retinal metabolism in methanol-induced retinal toxicity. *J Toxicol Environ Health* 44:43–56, 1995a.

Gaudet SJ, Razavi P, Caiafa GJ, Chader GJ: Identification of arylamine *N*-acetyltransferase activity in the bovine lens. *Curr Eye Res* 14:873–877, 1995.

Gelatt KN: *Veterinary Ophthalmology.* Philadelphia: Lea & Febiger, 1981.

Geller AM, Abdel-Rahman AA, Abou-Donia MB, et al: The organophosphate pesticide chlorpyrifos affects form deprivation myopia. *Invest Ophthalmol Vis Sci* 39:1290–1294, 1998.

Geller AM, Hudnell HK: Critical issues in the use and analysis of the Lanthony desaturate color vision test. *Neurotoxicol Teratol* 19:455–465, 1997.

Giblin FJ: Glutathione: A vital lens antioxidant. *J Ocul Pharmacol Ther* 16:121–135, 2000.

Glickman L, Valciukas JA, Lilis R, Weisman I: Occupational lead exposure. Effects on saccadic eye movements. *Int Arch Occup Environ Health* 54:115–125, 1984.

Gobba F, Galassi C, Imbriani M, et al: Acquired dyschromatopsia among styrene-exposed workers. *J Occup Med* 33:761–765, 1991.

Gondhowiardjo TD, van Haeringen NJ: Corneal aldehyde dehydrogenase, glutathione reductase, and glutathione *S*-transferase in pathologic corneas. *Cornea* 12:310–314, 1993.

Gorin MB, Day R, Costantino JP, et al: Long-term tamoxifen citrate use and potential ocular toxicity. *Am J Ophthalmol* 125:493–501, 1998.

Graham DG, Valentine WM: Carbon disulfide, in Spencer PS, Schaumburg HH (eds): *Experimental and Clinical Neurotoxicology,* 2d ed. New York: Oxford University Press, 2000, pp 315–317.

Grant WM: *Toxicology of the Eye,* 3d ed. Springfield, IL: Charles C Thomas, 1986.

Grant WM, Shuhman JS: *Toxicology of the Eye,* 4th ed. Springfield, IL: Charles C Thomas, 1993.

Guguchkova PT: Electroretinographic and electrooculographic examinations of persons occupationally exposed to lead. *Vestnik Oftalmolog* 85:60–65, 1972.

Hammond CJ, Snieder H, Spector TD, Gilbert CE: Genetic and environmental factors in age-related nuclear cataracts in monozygotic twins. *N Engl J Med* 342:1786–1790, 2000.

Hanninen H, Nurminen M, Tolonen M, Martelin T: Psychological tests as indicators of excessive exposure to carbon disulfide. *Scand J Work Environ* 19:163–174, 1978.

Hansen ON, Trillingsgaard A, Beese I, et al: A neuropsychological study of children with elevated dentine lead level: Assessment of the effect of lead in different socioeconomic groups. *Neurotoxicol Teratol* 11:205–213, 1989.

Harroff HH: Pathological processes of the eye related to chemical exposure, in Hobson DW (ed): *Dermal and Ocular Toxicity: Fundamentals and Methods.* Boca Raton, FL: CRC Press, 1991, pp 493–508.

Hart WM: *Adler's Physiology of the Eye,* 9th ed. St. Louis: Mosby–Year Book, 1992.

Hass GM, Brown DVL, Eisenstein R, Hemmens A: Relation between lead poisoning in rabbit and man. *Am J Pathol* 45:691–727, 1964.

Haustein KO, Oltmanns G, Rietbrock N, Alken RG: Differences in color vision impairment caused by digoxin, digitoxin, or pengitoxin. *J Cardiovasc Pharmacol* 4:536–541, 1982.

Haustein KO, Schmidt C: Differences in color discrimination between three cardioactive glycosides. *Int J Clin Pharmacol Ther Toxicol* 26:517–520, 1988.

Hayreh MM, Hayreh SS, Baumbach GL, et al: Ocular toxicity of methanol: An experimental study, in Merigan WH, Weiss B (eds): *Neurotoxicity of the Visual System.* New York: Raven Press, 1980, pp 33–53.

He L, Poblenz AT, Medrano CJ, Fox DA: Lead and calcium produce photoreceptor cell apoptosis by opening the mitochondrial permeability transition pore. *J Biol Chem* 275:12175–12184, 2000.

Hedges TR III, Hirano M, Tucker K, Caballero B: Epidemic optic and peripheral neuropathy in Cuba: A unique geopolitical public health problem. *Surv Ophthalmol* 41:341–353, 1997.

Hedges TR III, Sokol S, Tucker K: Optic and peripheral neuropathy in Cuba. *JAMA* 271:662–663, 1994.

Hendrickson A: A morphological comparison of foveal development in man and monkey. *Eye* 6:136–144, 1992

Hendrickson A, Drucker D: The development of parafoveal and mid-peripheral human retina. *Behav Brain Res* 49:21–31, 1992.

Heng JE, Vorwerk CK, Lessell E, et al: Ethambutol is toxic to retinal ganglion cells via an excitotoxic pathway. *Invest Ophthalmol Vis Sci* 40:190–196, 1999.

Henkes HE, van Lith GHM, Canta LR: Indomethacin retinopathy. *Am J Ophthalmol* 73:846–856, 1972.

Hennekes R, Janssen K, Munoz C, Winneke G: Lead-induced ERG alterations in rats at high and low levels of exposure. *Concepts Toxicol* 4:193–199, 1987.

Herr DW, Boyes WK: Electrophysiological analysis of complex brain systems: Sensory evoked potentials and their generators, in Chang LW, Slikker W (eds): *Neurotoxicology: Approaches and Methods.* New York: Academic Press, 1995, pp 205–221.

Herr DW, Boyes WK, Dyer RS: Alterations in rat flash and pattern evoked potentials after acute or repeated administration of carbon disulfide. *Fund Appl Toxicol* 18:328–342, 1992.

Hirano M, Odel JG, Lincoff NS: Optic and peripheral neuropathy in Cuba. *JAMA* 271:663, 1994.

Hockwin O, Green K, Rubin LF: *Manual of Oculotoxicity Testing of Drugs.* Stuttgart, Germany: Gustav Fischer Verlag, 1992.

Hogan MJ, Alvarado JA, Weddell JE: *Histology of the Human Eye.* Philadelphia: Saunders, 1971.

Horton JC: The central visual pathways, in Hart WM (ed): *Adler's Physiology of the Eye,* 9th ed. St. Louis: Mosby–Year Book, 1992, pp 728–772.

Hotta R, Gotto S: A fluorescein angiographic study on micro-angiopathia sulfocarbonica. *Jpn J Ophthalmol* 15:132–139, 1971.

Hudnell HK, Otto DA, House DE: The influence of vision on computerized neurobehavioral test scores: A proposal for improving test protocols. *Neurotoxicol Teratol* 18:391–400, 1996.

Hughes WF, Coogan PS: Pathology of the pigment epithelium and retina in rabbits poisoned with lead. *Am J Pathol* 77:237–254, 1974.

Imai H, Miyata M, Uga S, Ishikawa S: Retinal degeneration in rats exposed to an organophosphate pesticide (fenthion). *Environ Res* 30:453–465, 1983.

Ingemansson SO: Studies on the effect of 4-methylpyrazole on retinal activity in the methanol poisoned monkey by recording the electroretinogram. *Acta Ophthalmol Suppl* 158:1–24, 1983.

Isaac NE, Walker AM, Jick H, Gorman M: Exposure to phenothiazine drugs and risk of cataract. *Arch Ophthalmol* 109:256–260, 1991.

Ito M, Nishibe Y, Inoue YK: Isolation of Inoue-Melnick virus from cerebrospinal fluid of patients with epidemic neuropathy in Cuba. *Arch Pathol Lab Med* 122:520–522, 1998.

Iwata K: Neuro-ophthalmological findings and a follow-up study in the Agano area, Niigata Pref, in Tsubaki T, Irukayama K (eds): *Minamata Disease: MethylMercury poisoning in Minamata and Niigata, Tokyo.* Tokyo: Kodansha, 1977, pp 166–185.

Jaanus SD, Bartlett JD, Hiett JA: Ocular effects of systemic drugs, in Bartlett JD, Jaanus SD (eds): *Clinical Ocular Pharmacology,* 3d ed. Boston: Butterworth-Heinemann, 1995, pp 957–1006.

Jadhav AL, Ramesh GT: Pb-induced alterations in tyrosine hydroxylase activity in rat brain. *Mol Cell Biochem* 175:137–141, 1997.

Jeyaratnam J, Boey KW, Ong CN, et al: Neuropsychological studies on lead workers in Singapore. *Br J Ind Med* 43:626–629, 1986.

Johns DR, Neufeld MJ, Hedges TR III: Mitochondrial DNA mutations in Cuban optic and peripheral neuropathy. *J Neuroophthalmol* 14:135–140, 1994.

Johns DR, Sadun AA: Cuban epidemic optic neuropathy. Mitochondrial DNA analysis. *J Neuroophthalmol* 14:130–134, 1994.

Johnson MW, Vine AK: Hydroxychloroquine therapy in massive total doses without retinal toxicity. *Am J Ophthalmol* 104:139–144, 1987.

Jones RD, Brenneke CJ, Hoss HE, Loney ML: An electroretinogram protocol for toxicological screening in the canine model. *Toxicol Lett* 70:223–234, 1994.

Kaiser-Kupfer MI, Kupfer C, Rodriques MM: Tamoxifen retinopathy. A clinocopathologic report. *Ophthalmology* 88:89–93, 1981.

Kalloniatis M, Tomisich G: Amino acid neurochemistry of the vertebrate retina. *Prog Retinal Eye Res* 18:811–866, 1999.

Kamel F, Boyes WK, Gladen BC, et al: Retinal degeneration in licensed pesticide applicators. *Am J Ind Med* 37:618–628, 2000.

Karai I, Horiguchi SH, Nishikawa N: Optic atrophy with visual field defect in workers occupationally exposed to lead for 30 years. *J Toxicol Clin Toxicol* 19:409–418, 1982.

Karim AKA, Jacob TJC, Thompson GM: The human lens epithelium, morphological and ultrastructural changes associated with steroid therapy. *Exp Eye Res* 48:215–224, 1989.

Kennah HE II, Hignet S, Laux PE, Dorko JD, Barrow CS: An objective procedure for quantitating eye irritation based upon changes of corneal thickness. *Fundam Appl Toxicol* 12:258–268, 1989.

King G, Hirst L, Holmes R: Human corneal and lens aldehyde dehydrogenases. Localization and function(s) of ocular ALDH1 and ALDH3 isozymes. *Adv Exp Med Biol* 463:189–198, 1999.

Kini MM, Cooper JR: Biochemistry of methanol poisoning. 4. The effect of methanol and its metabolites on retinal metabolism. *Biochem J* 82:164–172, 1962.

Klein BE, Klein RE, Lee KE: Incident cataract after a five-year interval and lifestyle factors: The Beaver Dam eye study. *Ophthalm Epidemiol* 6:247–255, 1999.

Kobel W, Gfeller W: Distribution of eye irritation scores of industrial chemicals. *Food Chem Toxicol* 23:311–312, 1985.

Kohler K, Lilienthal H, Guenther E, et al: Persistent decrease of the dopamine-synthesizing enzyme tyrosine hydroxylase in the rhesus monkey retina after chronic lead exposure. *Neurotoxicology* 18:623–632, 1997.

Koliopoulos J, Palimeris G: On acquired colour vision disturbances during treatment with ethambutol and indomethacin. *Mod Probl Ophthalmol* 11:178–184, 1972.

Krill AE, Potts AM, Johanson CE: Chloroquine retinopathy. Investigation of discrepancy between dark adaptation and electroretinographic findings in advanced stages. *Am J Ophthalmol* 71:530–543, 1971.

Kruszewski FH, Walker TL, DiPasquale LC: Evaluation of a human corneal epithelial cell line as an in vitro model for assessing ocular irritation. *Fundam Appl Toxicol* 36:130–140, 1997.

Kulkarni AS, Hopfinger AJ: Membrane-interaction QSAR analysis: Application to the estimation of eye irritation by organic compounds. *Pharm Res* 16:1245–1253, 1999.

Lambert LA, Chambers WA, Green S, et al: The use of low-volume dosing in the eye irritation test. *Food Chem Toxicol* 31:99–103, 1993.

Lapalus P, Garaffo RG: Ocular pharmacokinetics, in Hockwin O, Green K, Rubin LF (eds): *Manual of Oculotoxicity Testing of Drugs.* Stuttgart, Germany: Gustav Fischer Verlag, 1992, pp 119–136.

Larsby B, Tham R, Eriksson B, et al: Effects of trichloroethylene on the human vestibulo-oculomotor system. *Acta Otololaryngol (Stockholm)* 101:193–199, 1986.

Lasley SM, Lane JD: Diminished regulation of mesolimbic dopaminergic activity in rat after chronic inorganix lead exposure. *Toxicol Appl Pharmacol* 95:474–483, 1988.

LaVail MM: Rod outer segment disk shedding in rat retina: Relationship to cyclic lighting. *Science* 194:1071–1074, 1976.

LaVail MM, Gorrin GM, Repaci MA, Yasumura D: Light-induced retinal degeneration in albino mice and rats: Strain and species differences. *Prog Clin Biol Res* 247:439–454, 1987.

Lazzaroni F, Scorolli L, Pizzoleo CF, et al: Tamoxifen retinopathy: Does it really exist? *Graefes Arch Clin Exp Ophthalmol* 236:669–673, 1998.

Lee AY, Chung SS: Involvement of aldose reductase in naphthalene cataract. *Invest Ophthalmol Vis Sci* 39:193–197, 1998.

Lee EW, Garner CD, Terzo TS: A rat model manifesting methanol-induced visual dysfunction suitable for both acute and long-term exposure studies. *Toxicol Appl Pharmacol* 128:199–206, 1994b.

Lee EW, Garner CD, Terzo TS: Animal model for the study of methanol toxicity: Comparison of folate-reduced rat responses with published monkey data. *J Toxicol Environ Health* 41:71–82, 1994a.

Leske MC, Chylack LT Jr, Wu SY: The lens opacities case-control study. Risk factors for cataract. *Arch Ophthalmol* 109:244–251, 1991.

Lessell S: Toxic and deficiency optic neuropathies, in Miller NR, Newman NJ (eds): *Walsh and Hoyt's Clinical Neuro-Ophthalmology,* 5th ed. Baltimore: Williams & Wilkins, 1998.

Lilienthal H, Kohler K, Turfeld M, Winneke G: Persistent increases in scotopic b-wave amplitudes after lead exposure in monkeys. *Exp Eye Res* 59:203–209, 1994.

Lilienthal H, Lenaerts C, Winneke G, Hennekes R: Alteration of the visual evoked potential and the electroretinogram in lead-treated monkeys. *Neurotoxicol Teratol* 10:417–422, 1988.

Linsenmeier RA: Effects of light and darkness on oxygen distribution and consumption in the cat retina. *J Gen Physiol* 88:521–542, 1986.

Lissner W, Greenlee JE, Cameron JD, Goren SB: Localization of tritiated digoxin in the rat eye. *Am J Ophthalmol* 72:608–614, 1971.

Lou MF, Xu GT, Zigler S Jr, York B Jr: Inhibition of naphthalene cataract in rats by aldose reductase inhibitors. *Curr Eye Res* 15:423–432, 1996.

Lufkin MW, Harrison CE, Henderson JW, Ogle KN: Ocular distribution of digoxin-^{3}H in the cat. *Am J Ophthalmol* 64:1134–1140, 1967.

Lyle WM: Drugs and conditions which may affect color vision: Part 1. Drugs and chemicals. *J Am Ophthalmol Soc* 45:47–60, 1974.

Lynch JJ III, Silveira LC, Perry VH, Merigan WH: Visual effects of damage to P ganglion cells in macaques. *Vis Neurosci* 8:575–583, 1992.

Madreperla SA, Johnson MA, Nakatani K: Electrophysiological and electroretinographic evidence for phototreceptor dysfunction as a toxic effect of digoxin. *Arch Ophthalmol* 112:807–812, 1994.

Marks MJ, Seeds NW: A heterogeneous ouabain-ATPase interaction in mouse brain. *Life Sci* 23:2735–2744, 1978.

Marmor MF, Arden GB, Nilsson SEG, Zrenner E: International standardization committee. Standards for clinical electroretinography. *Arch Ophthalmol* 107:816–819, 1989.

Marmor MF, Zrenner E: Standard for clinical electroretinography (1994 update). *Doc Ophthalmol* 89:199–210, 1995.

Martin-Amat G, McMartin KE, Hayreh SS, et al: Methanol poisoning: Ocular toxicity produced by formate. *Toxicol Appl Pharmacol* 45:201–208, 1978.

Mas P, Pelegrino JL, Guzman MG, et al: Viral isolation from cases of epidemic neuropathy in Cuba. *Arch Pathol Lab Med* 121:825–833, 1997.

Mastyugin V, Aversa E, Bonazzi A, et al: Hypoxia-induced production of 12-hydroxyeicosanoids in the corneal epithelium: Involvement of a cytochrome P-4504B1 isoform. *J Pharmacol Exp Ther* 289:1611–1619, 1999.

Mattsson JL, Boyes WK, Ross JF: Incorporating evoked potentials into neurotoxicity test schemes, in Tilson HA, Mitchell CL (eds): *Target Organ Toxicology Series: Neurotoxicity.* New York: Raven Press, 1992, pp 125–145.

Maurer JK, Parker RD: Light microscopic comparison of surfactant-induced eye irritation in rabbits and rats at three hours and recovery at day 35. *Toxicol Pathol* 24:403–411, 1996.

Maurer JK, Parker RD, Carr GJ: Ocular irritation: Microscopic changes occurring over time in the rat with surfactants of known irritancy. *Toxicol Pathol* 26:217–225, 1998.

Maurissen JPJ: Neurobehavioral methods for the evaluation of sensory functions, in Chang LW, Slikker W (eds): *Neurotoxicology: Approaches and Methods.* New York: Academic Press, 1995, pp 239–264.

McCulley JP: Chemical injuries of the eye, in Leibowitz HM, Waring GO (eds): *Corneal Disorders, Clinical Diagnosis and Management,* 2d ed. Philadelphia: Saunders, 1998, pp 770–790.

McGrail KM, Sweadner KJ: Complex expression patterns for Na^+,K^+-ATPase isoforms in retina and optic nerve. *Eur J Neurosci* 2:170–176, 1989.

Medrano CJ, Fox DA: Oxygen consumption in rat outer and inner retina: Light- and pharmacologically induced inhibition. *Exp Eye Res* 61:273–284, 1995.

Medrano CJ, Fox DA: Substrate-dependent effects of calcium on rat retinal mitochondria respiration: Physiological and toxicological studies. *Toxicol Appl Pharmacol* 125:309–321, 1994.

Meier-Ruge W: Drug induced retinopathy. *CRC Toxicol* 1:325–360, 1972.

Mergler D: Color vision loss: A sensitive indicator of the severity of optic neuropathy, in Anger WK (ed): *Advances in Neurobehavioral Toxicology: Applications in Environmental and Occupational Health.* Chelsea, MI: Lewis Publishers, 1990, pp 175–183.

Mergler D, Belanger S, Grosbois S, Vachon N: Chromal focus of acquired chromatic discrimination loss and slovent exposure among printshop workers. *Toxicology* 49:341–348, 1988.

Mergler D, Blain L, Lagace JP: Solvent related colour vision loss: An indicator of damage? *Int Arch Occup Environ Health* 59:313–321, 1987.

Mergler D, Huel G, Bowler R, et al: Visual dysfunction among former microelectronics assembly workers. *Arch Environ Health* 46:326–334, 1991.

Merigan WH: Effects of toxicants on visual systems. *Neurobehav Toxicol* 1(suppl 1):15–22, 1979.

Merigan WH, Weiss B: *Neurotoxicity of the Visual System.* New York: Raven Press, 1980.

Merigan WH, Wood RW, Zehl D, Eskin TA: Carbon disulfide effects on the visual system: I. Visual thresholds and ophthalmoscopy. *Invest Ophthalmol Vis Sci* 29:512–518, 1988.

Misra UK, Nag D, Misra NK, et al: Some observations on the macula of pesticide workers. *Hum Toxicol* 4:135–145, 1985.

Mojon DS, Kaufmann P, Odel JG, et al: Clinical course of a cohort in the Cuban epidemic optic and peripheral neuropathy. *Neurology* 48:19–22, 1997.

Möller C, Odkvist L, Larsby B, et al: Otoneurological findings in workers exposed to styrene. *Scand J Work Environ Health* 16:189–194, 1990.

Moser VC, Boyes WK: Prolonged neurobehavioral and visual effects of short-term exposure to 3,3′-iminodipropionitrile (IDPN) in rats. *Fund Appl Toxicol* 21:277–290, 1993.

Moser VC, Phillips PM, Morgan DL, Sills RC: Carbon disulfide neurotoxicity in rats: VII. Behavioral evaluations using a functional observational battery. *Neurotoxicology* 19:147–158, 1998.

Muñoz H, Romiew I, Palazuelos E, et al: Blood lead level and neurobehavioral development among children living in Mexico City. *Arch Environ Health* 48:132–139, 1993.

Murano H, Kojima M, Sasaki K: Differences in naphthalene cataract formation between albino and pigmented rat eyes. *Ophthalm Res* 25:16–22, 1993.

Murata K, Araki S, Yokoyama K, et al: Assessment of central, peripheral, and autonomic nervous system functions in lead workers: Neuroelectrophysiological studies. *Environ Res* 61:323–336, 1993.

Murray TG, Burton TC, Rajani C, et al: Methanol poisoning. A rodent model with structural and functional evidence for retinal involvement. *Arch Ophthalmol* 109:1012–1016, 1991.

Muttray A, Wolters V, Mayer-Popken O, et al: Effect of subacute occupational exposure to toluene on color vision. *Int J Occup Med Environ Health* 8:339–345, 1995.

Nakatsuka H, Watanabe T, Takeuchi Y, et al: Absence of blue-yellow color vision loss among workers exposed to toluene or tetrachloroethylene, mostly at levels below occupational exposure limits. *Int Arch Occup Environ Health* 64:113–117, 1992.

National Institute of Environmental Health Sciences (NIEHS): Corrositex: *An In Vitro Test Method for Assessing Dermal Corrosivity Potential of Chemicals: The Results of an Independent Peer Review Evaluation.* NIH Publication No. 99-4495. Research Triangle Park, NC: NIEHS, 1999. Also at: *http://iccvam.niehs.nih.gov/corprrep.htm.*

National Institute of Environmental Health Sciences (NIEHS): *Validation and Regulatory Acceptance of Toxicological Test Methods: A Report of the ad hoc Interagency Coordinating Committee on the Validation of Alternative Methods.* NIH Publication No. 97-3981. Research Triangle Park, NC: NIEHS, 1997. Also at: *http://ntp-server.niehs.nih.gov/htdocs/ICCVAM/iccvam.html.*

Newman NJ, Torroni A, Brown MD, et al: Epidemic neuropathy in Cuba not associated with mitochondrial DNA mutations found in Leber's hereditary optic neuropathy patients. Cuba Neuropathy Field Investation Team. *Am J Ophthalmol* 118:158–168, 1994.

Nicholls P: The effect of formate on cytochrome aa3 and on electron transport in the intact respiratory chain. *Biochim Biophys Acta* 430:13–29, 1976.

Niklasson M, Tham R, Larsby B, Eriksson B: Effects of toluene, styrene, trichloroethylene, and trichloroethane on the vestibulo- and opto-oculomotor system in rats. *Neurotoxicol Teratol* 15:327–334, 1993.

Noureddin BN, Seoud M, Bashshur Z, et al: Ocular toxicity in low-dose tamoxifen: A prospective study. *Eye* 13:729–733, 1999.

Oberto A, Marks N, Evans HL, Guidotti A: Lead promotes apoptosis in newborn rat cerebellar neurons: Pathological implications. *J Pharmacol Exp Ther* 279:435–442, 1996.

Odkvist L, Larsby B, Tham R, Hyden D: Vestibulo-oculomotor disturbances caused by industrial solvents. *Otololaryngol Head Neck Surg* 91:537–539, 1983.

Ogden TE, Schachat AP: *Retina. Basic Science and Inherited Diseases.* Vol 1. St. Louis: Mosby, 1989.

Ottlecz A, Garcia CA, Eichberg J, Fox DA: Alterations in retinal Na^+,K^+-ATPase in diabetes: Streptozotocin-induced and Zucker diabetic fatty rats. *Curr Eye Res* 12:1111–1121, 1993.

Otto DA: The assessment of neurotoxicity in children. Electrophysiological methods. *Monogr Am Assoc Ment Defic* 8:139–158, 1987.

Otto DA, Fox DA: Auditory and visual dysfunction following lead exposure. *Neurotoxicology* 14:191–208, 1993.

Otto DA, Robinson G, Baumann S, et al: 5-year follow-up study of children with low-to-moderate lead absorption: Electrophysiological evaluation. *Environ Res* 38:168–186, 1985.

Ottonello S, Foroni C, Carta A, et al: Oxidative stress and age-related cataract. *Ophthalmologica* 214:78–85, 2000.

Palacz O, Szymanska K, Czepita D: Studies on the ERG in subjects with chronic exposure to carbon disulfide: I. Assessment of the condition of the visual system taking into account ERG findings depending on the duration of exposure to CS_2. *Klin Oczna* 82:65–68, 1980.

Palimeris G, Koliopoulos J, Velissaropoulos P: Ocular side effects of indomethacin. *Ophthalmologica* 164:339–353, 1972.

Patterson CA, Delamere NA: The lens, in Hart WM (ed): *Adler's Physiology of the Eye,* 9th ed. St. Louis: Mosby–Year Book, 1992, pp 348–390.

Pavlidis NA, Petris C, Briassoulis E, et al: Clear evidence that long-term, low-dose tamoxifen treatment can induce ocular toxicity. A prospective study of 63 patients. *Cancer* 69:2961–2964, 1992.

Peiffer RL, McCary B, Bee W, et al: Contemporary methods in ocular toxicology. *Toxicol Methods* 10:17–39, 2000.

Penn JS, Naash MI, Anderson RE: Effect of light history on retinal antioxidants and light damage susceptibility in the rat. *Exp Eye Res* 44:779–788, 1987.

Penn JS, Thum LA, Naash MI: Photoreceptor physiology in the rat is governed by the light environment. *Exp Eye Res* 49:205–215, 1989.

Penn JS, Williams TP: Photostasis: Regulation of daily photon-catch by rat retinas in response to various cyclic illuminances. *Exp Eye Res* 43:915–928, 1986.

Pepose JS, Ubels JL: The Cornea, in Hart WM (ed): *Adler's Physiology of the Eye,* 9th ed. St. Louis: Mosby–Year Book, 1992, pp 29–70.

Petit TL, LeBoutillier JC: Effects of lead exposure during development on neocortical dendritic and synaptic structure. *Exp Neurol* 64:482–492, 1979.

Piltz JR, Wertenbaker C, Lance SE, et al: Digoxin toxicity. Recognizing the varied visual presentations. *J Clin Neuroophthalmol* 13:275–280, 1993.

Polak BC, Leys M, van Lith GH: Blue-yellow colour vision changes as early symptoms of ethambutol oculotoxicity. *Ophthalmologica* 191:223–226, 1985.

Porkony J, Smith VS, Verriest G, Pinckers A: *Congenital and Acquired Color Vision Defects.* New York: Grune & Stratton, 1979.

Potts AM: The reaction of uveal pigment in vitro with polycyclic compounds. *Invest Ophthalmol* 3:405–416, 1964.

Potts AM: The visual toxicity of methanol: VI. The clinical aspects of experimental methanol poisoning treated with base. *Am J Ophthalmol* 39:76–82, 1955.

Potts AM: Toxic responses of the eye, in Klaassen CD (ed): *Casarett and Doull's Toxicology: The Basic Science of Poisons,* 5th ed. New York: McGraw-Hill, 1996, pp 583–615.

Potts AM, Au PC: The affinity of melanin for inorganic ions. *Exp Eye Res* 22:487–491, 1976.

Pounds, JG: Effect of lead intoxication on calcium homeostasis and calcium-mediated cell function: A review. *Neurotoxicology* 5:295–332, 1984.

Powers MK, Green DG: Single retinal ganglion cell responses in the dark-reared rat: Grating acuity, contrast sensitivity, and defocusing. *Vision Res* 18:1533–1539, 1978.

Puro DG: Cholinergic systems, in Morgan WW (ed): *Retinal Transmitters and Modulators: Models for the Brain.* Vol 1. Boca Raton, FL: CRC Press, 1985.

Raedler A, Sievers J: The development of the visual system of the albino rat. *Adv Anat Embryol Cell Biol* 50:7–87, 1975.

Raitta C, Seppalainen AN, Huuskonen MS: *n*-hexane maculopathy in industrial workers. *Von Graefes Arch Klin Exp Ophthalmol* 209:99–110, 1978.

Raitta C, Teir H, Tolonen M, Nurminen M, Helpio E, Malmstrom S: Impaired color discrimination among viscose rayon workers exposed to carbon disulfide. *J Occup Med* 23:189–192, 1981.

Raitta C, Tolonen M, Nurminen M: Microcirculation of ocular fundus in viscose rayon workers exposed to carbon disulfide. *Arch Klin Exp Ophthalmol* 191:151–164, 1974.

Ramsey MS, Fine BS: Chloroquine toxicity in the human eye. Histopathologic observations by electron microscopy. *Am J Ophthalmol* 73:229–235, 1972.

Rao GN: Light intensity-associated eye lesions of Fisher 344 rats in long-term studies. *Toxicol Pathol* 19:148–155, 1991.

Rapp LM, Tolman BL, Koutz CA, Thum LA: Predisposing factors to light-induced photoreceptor cell damage: Retinal changes in maturing rats. *Exp Eye Res* 51:177–184, 1990.

Rauen T, Rothstein JD, Wässle H: Differential expression of three glutamate transporters subtypes in the rat retina. *Cell Tissue Res* 286:325–336, 1996.

Rebert CS: Multisensory evoked potentials in experimental and applied neurotoxicology. *Neurobehav Toxicol Teratol* 5:659–671, 1983.

Reuhl KR, Rice DC, Gilbert SG, Mallett J: Effects of chronic developmental lead exposure on monkey neuroanatomy: Visual system. *Toxicol Appl Pharmacol* 99:501–509, 1989.

Rice DC: Effects of lifetime lead exposure on spatial and temporal visual function in monkeys. *Neurotoxicology* 19:893–902, 1998.

Rice DC: Sensory and cognitive effects of developmental methylmercury exposure in monkeys, and a comparison to effects in rodents. *Neurotoxicology* 17:139–154, 1996.

Rice DC, Gilbert SG: Early chronic low-level methylmercury poisoning in monkeys impairs spatial vision. *Science* 216:759–761, 1982.

Rice DC, Gilbert SG: Effects of developmental exposure to methylmercury on spatial and temporal visual function in monkeys. *Toxicol Appl Pharmacol* 102:151–163, 1990.

Rice DC, Hayward S: Comparison of visual function at adulthood and during aging in monkeys exposed to lead or methylmercury. *Neurotoxicology* 20:767–784, 1999.

Rietbrock N, Alken RG: Color vision deficiencies: A common sign of intoxication in chronically digoxin-treated patients. *J Cardiovasc Pharmacol* 2:93–99, 1980.

Robertson DM, Hollenhorst RW, Callahan JA: Ocular manifestations of digitalis toxicity. *Arch Ophthalmol* 76:640–645, 1966a.

Robertson DM, Hollenhorst RW, Callahan JA: Receptor function in digitalis toxicity. *Arch Ophthalmol* 76:852–857, 1966b.

Rodieck RW: *The First Steps in Seeing.* Sunderland, MA: Sinuaer, 1998.

Rogers JM, Chernoff N: Chemically induced cataracts in the fetus and neonate, in Kacew S and Lock S (eds): *Toxicologic and Pharmacologic Principles in Pediatrics.* New York: Hemisphere, 1988, pp 255–275.

Roman G: Tropical myeloneuropathies revisited. *Curr Opin Neurol* 11:539–544, 1998.

Rosenthal AR, Kolb H, Bergsma D, et al: Chloroquine retinopathy in the Rhesus monkey. *Invest Ophthalmol Vis Sci* 17:1158–1175, 1978.

Rothenberg SJ, Schnaas L, Salgado M, et al: Reduction of electroretinogram amplitude in the dark-adapted eye of children associated with prenatal and postnatal blood lead level. *Toxicologist* 48:50, 1999.

Ruan DY, Tang LX, Zhao C, Guo YJ: Effects of low-level lead on retinal ganglion sustained and transient cells in developing rats. *Neurotoxicol Teratol* 16:47–53, 1994.

Ruedeman AD: The electroretinogram in chronic methyl alcohol poisoning in human beings. *Trans Am Ophthalmol Soc* 59:480–529, 1961.

Sadun AA, Martone JF, Muci-Mendoza R, et al: Epidemic optic neuropathy in Cuba. Eye findings. *Arch Ophthalmol* 112:691–699, 1994a.

Sadun AA, Martone JF, Reyes L, et al: Optic and peripheral neuropathy in Cuba. *JAMA* 271:663–664, 1994b.

Sadun AA: Acquired mitochondrial impairment as a cause of optic nerve disease. *Trans Am Ophthalmol Soc* 96:881–923, 1998.

Salmon JF, Carmichael TR, Welsh NH: Use of contrast sensitivity measurement in the detection of subclinical ethambutol toxic optic neuropathy. *Br J Ophthalmol* 71:192–196, 1987.

Santos-Anderson RM, Tso MOM, Valdes JJ, Annau Z: Chronic lead administration in neonatal rats. Electron microscopy of the retina. *J Neuropathol Exp Neurol* 43:175–187, 1984.

Sassaman FW, Cassidy JT, Alpern M, Maaseidvaag F: Electroretinography in patients with connective tissue diseases treated with hydroxychloroquine. *Am J Ophthalmol* 70:515–523, 1970.

Sato S: Aldose reductase the major protein associated with naphthalene dihydrodiol dehydrogenase activity in rat lens. *Invest Ophthalmol Vis Sci* 34:3172–3178, 1993.

Sato S, Sugiyama K, Lee YS, Kador PF: Prevention of naphthalene-1,2-dihydrodiol-induced lens protein modifications by structurally diverse aldose reductase inhibitors. *Exp Eye Res* 68:601–608, 1999.

Sborgia G, Assennato G, L'Abbate N, et al: Comprehensive neurophysiological evaluation of lead-exposed workers, in Gilioli R, Cassito M, Foa V (eds): *Neurobehavioral Methods in Occupational Health.* New York: Pergamon Press, 1983, pp 283–294.

Schnapf JL, Kraft TW, Nunn BJ, Baylor DA: Spectral sensitivity of primate photoreceptors. *Vis Neurosci* 1:255–261, 1988.

Schneider BG, Kraig E: Na^+,K^+-ATPase of the photoreceptor: Selective expression of $\alpha3$ and $\beta2$ isoforms. *Exp Eye Res* 51:553–564, 1990.

Schneider BG, Shygan AW, Levinson R: Co-localization and polarized distribution of Na,K-ATPase: $\alpha3$ and $\beta2$ subunits in photoreceptor cells. *J Histochem Cytochem* 39:507–517, 1991.

Scholl HPN, Zrenner E: Electrophysiology in the investigation of acquired retinal disorders. *Surv Ophthalmol* 45:29-47, 2000.

Schwartzmann ML: Cytochrome P450 and arachidonic acid metabolism in the corneal epithelium, in Green K, Edelhauser HF, Hackett RB, et al (eds): *Advances in Ocular Toxicology.* New York: Plenum Press, 1997, pp 3–20.

Schwartzman ML, Balazy M, Masferrer J, et al: 12(R)-hydroxyicosatetraenoic acid: A cytochrome-P450–dependent arachidonate metabolite that inhibits Na^+,K^+-ATPase in the cornea. *Proc Natl Acad Sci USA* 84:8125–8129, 1987.

Scortegagna M, Hanbauer I: The effect of lead exposure and serum deprivation on mesencephalic primary cultures. *Neurotoxicology* 18:331–340, 1997.

Sears ML: *Pharmacology of the Eye.* Berlin: Springer-Verlag, 1984.

Seme MT, Summerfelt P, Henry MM, et al: Formate-induced inhibition of photoreceptor function in methanol intoxication. *J Pharmacol Exp Ther* 289:361–370, 1999.

Seppalainen AM, Haltia M: Carbon disulfide, in Spencer PS, Schaumberg HH (eds): *Experimental and Clinical Neurotoxicology.* Baltimore: William & Wilkins, 1980, pp 356–373.

Shanthaverrappa TR, Bourne GH: Monoamine oxidase distribution in the rabbit eye. *J Histochem Cytochem* 12:281–287, 1964.

Shearer RV, Dubois EL: Ocular changes induced by long-term hydroxychloroquine (Plaqenil) therapy. *Am J Ophthalmol* 64:245–252, 1967.

Sherer JW: Lead ablyopia with cataract from the same source. *J Missouri State Med Assoc* 32:275–277, 1935.

Shichi H, Atlas SA, Nebert DW: Genetically regulated aryl hydrocarbon hydroxylase induction in the eye: Possible significance of the drug-metabolizing enzyme system for the retinal pigmented epithelium-choroid. *Exp Eye Res* 21:557–567, 1975.

Shichi H, Nebert DW: Genetic differences in drug metabolism associated with ocular toxicity. *Environ Health Perspect* 44:107–117, 1982.

Shulman LM, Fox DA: Dopamine inhibits mammalian photoreceptor Na^+,K^+-ATPase activity via a selective effect on the $\alpha3$ isozyme. *Proc Natl Acad Sci USA* 93:8034–8039, 1996.

Signorino M, Scarpino O, Provincialli L, et al: Modification of the electroretinogram and of different components of the visual evoked potentials in workers exposed to lead. *Ital Electroencephalogr J* 10:51P, 1983.

Sillman AJ, Bolnick DA, Bosetti JB, et al: The effects of lead and cadmium on the mass photoreceptor potential the dose-response relationship. *Neurotoxicology* 3:179–194, 1982.

Singh AK, Shichi H: A novel glutathione peroxidase in bovine eye. Sequence analysis, mRNA level, and translation. *J Biol Chem* 273:26171–26178, 1998.

Sjoerdsma T, Kamermans M, Spekreijse H: Effect of the tuberculostaticum ethambutol and stimulus intensity on chromatic discrimination in man. *Vision Res* 39:2955–2962, 1999.

Sonkin N: Stippling of the retina: A new physical sign in the early dignosis of lead poisoning. *N Engl J Med* 269:779–780, 1963.

Specchio LM, Bellomo R, Dicuonzo F, et al: Smooth pursuit eye movements among storage battery workers. *Clin Toxicol* 18:1269–1276, 1981.

Spector A: Oxidative stress and disease. *J Ocul Pharmacol Ther* 16:193–201, 2000.

Spencer PS, Schaumburg HH: A review of acrylamide neurotoxicity: Part I. Properties, uses and human exposure. *Can J Neurol Sci* 1:145–150, 1974a.

Spencer PS, Schaumburg HH: A review of acrylamide neurotoxicity: Part II. Experimental animal neuorotoxicity and pathologic mechanisms. *Can J Neurol Sci* 1:152–169, 1974b.

Spivey GH, Baloh RW, Brown CP, et al: Subclinical effects of chronic increased lead absorption—a prospective study: III. Neurologic findings at follow-up examination. *J Occup Med* 22:607–612, 1980.

Srivastava D, Fox DA, Hurwitz RL: Effects of magnesium on cyclic GMP hydrolysis by the bovine retinal rod cyclic GMP phosphodiesterase. *Biochem J* 308:653–658, 1995a.

Srivastava D, Hurwitz RL, Fox DA: Lead- and calcium-mediated inhibition of bovine rod cGMP phosphodiesterase: Interactions with magnesium. *Toxicol Appl Pharmacol* 134:43–52, 1995b.

Srivastava SK, Singhal SS, Awasthi S, et al: A glutathione *S*-transferases isozyme (bGST 5.8) involved in the metabolism of 4-hydroxy-2-trans-nonenal is localized in bovine lens epithelium. *Exp Eye Res* 63:329–337, 1996.

Sugai S, Murata K, Kitagaki T, Tomita I: Studies on eye irritation caused by chemicals in rabbits—1. A quantitative structure-activity relationships approach to primary eye irritation of chemicals in rabbits. *J Toxicol Sci* 15:245–262, 1990.

Sweadner KJ: Isozymes of Na^+/K^+-ATPase. *Biochem Biophys Acta* 989:185–220, 1989.

Szabo I, Bernardi P, Zoratti M: Modulation of the mitochondrial megachannel by divalent cations and protons. *J Biol Chem* 267:2940–2946, 1992.

Takeuchi T, Eto K: Pathology and pathogenesis of Minamata disease, in Tsubaki T, Irukayama K (eds): *Minamata Disease: Methylmercury poisoning in Minamata and Niigata, Japan.* Tokyo: Kodansha; Amsterdam: Elsevier, 1977, pp 103–141.

Tandon P, Padilla S, Barone S Jr, et al: Fenthion produces a persistent decrease in muscarinic receptor function in the adult rat retina. *Toxicol Appl Pharmacol* 125:271–280, 1994.

Taylor A, Nowell T: Oxidative stress and antioxidant function in relation to risk for cataract. *Adv Pharmacol* 38:515–536, 1997.

Tennekoon G, Aitchison CS, Frangia J, et al: Chronic lead intoxication: Effects on developing optic nerve. *Ann Neurol* 5:558–564, 1979.

Tephly TR, McMatin KE: Methanol metabolism, in Stegnik LD, Filer LJ Jr (eds): *Aspartame: Physiology and Biochemistry.* New York: Marcel Dekker, 1984, pp 111–140.

Tessier-Lavigne M, Mobbs P, Attwell D: Lead and mercury toxicity and the rod light response. *Invest Ophthalmol Vis Sci* 26:1117–1123, 1985.

Thaler JS, Curinga R, Kiracofe G: Relation of graded ocular anterior chamber pigmentation to phenothiazine intake in schizophrenics—Quantification procedures. *Am J Optom Physiol Ophthalmol* 62:600–604, 1985.

Tham R, Bunnfors I, Eriksson B, et al: Vestibulo-ocular disturbances in rats exposed to organic solvents. *Acta Pharmacol Toxicol* 54:58–63, 1984.

Thirkill CE, Roth AM, Keltner JL: Cancer-associated retinopathy. *Arch Ophthalmol* 105: 372–375, 1987.

Toews AD, Krigman MR, Thomas DJ, Morell P: Effect of inorganic lead exposure on myelination in the rat. *Neurochem Res* 5:605–616, 1980.

Ulshafer RJ, Allen CB, Rubin ML: Distributions of elements in the human retinal pigment epithelium. *Arch Ophthalmol* 108:113–117, 1990.

United States Environmental Protection Agency (EPA): *Prevention, Pesticides and Toxic Substances* (7101). EPA 712-C-98–242. *Health Effects Test Guideline.* OPPTS 870.6855. *Neurophysiology: Sensory Evoked Potentials.* August 1998a. Also at: http:/www.epa.gov/docs/OPPTS_Harmonized/870_Health_Effects_Test_Guidelines/Series/.

United States Environmental Protection Agency (EPA): *Prevention, Pesticides and Toxic Substances* (7101). EPA 712–C–98–238. *Health Effects Test Guideline.* OPPTS 870.6200. *Neurotoxicity Screening Battery.* August 1998b. Also at: http:/www.epa.gov/docs/OPPTS_Harmonized/870_Health_Effects_Test_Guidelines/Series/.

Urban RC, Cotlier E: Corticosteroid-induced cataracts. *Surv Ophthalmol* 31:102–110, 1986.

Vale RD, Banker G, Hall ZW: The neuronal cytoskeleton, in Hall ZW (ed): *An Introduction to Molecular Neurobiology.* Sunderland, MA: Sinauer, 1992, pp 247–280.

van Dijk BW, Spekreijse H: Ethambutol changes the color coding of carp retinal ganglion cells reversibly. *Invest Ophthalmol Vis Sci* 24:128–133, 1983.

van Heyningen R, Pirie A: The metabolism of naphthalene and its toxic effect on the eye. *Biochem J* 102:842–852, 1967.

Vanhoorne M, De Rouck A, Bacquer D: Epidemiological study of the systemic ophthalmological effects of carbon disulfide. *Arch Environ Health* 51:181–188, 1996.

van Soest S, Westerveld A, de Jong PT, et al: Retinitis pigmentosa: Defined from a molecular point of view. *Surv Ophthalmol* 43:321–334, 1999.

Veenstra DL, Best JH, Hornberger J, et al: Incidence and long-term cost of steroid-related side effects after renal transplantation. *Am J Kidney Dis* 33:829–839, 1999.

Vidyasagar TR: Optic nerve components may not be equally susceptible to damage by acrylamide. *Brain Res* 224:452–455, 1981.

Walkowiak J, Altmann L, Kramer U, et al: Cognitive and sensorimotor functions in 6-year-old children in relation to lead and mercury levels: Adjustment for intelligence and contrast sensitivity in computerized testing. *Neurotoxicol Teratol* 20:511–521, 1998.

Waltman S, Sears ML: Catechol-*O*-methyltransferase and monoamine oxidase activity in the ocular tissues of albino rabbits. *Invest Ophthalmol* 3:601–605, 1964.

Watkins JB III, Wirthwein DP, Sanders RA: Comparative study of phase II biotransformation in rabbit ocular tissues. *Drug Metab Dispos* 19:708–713, 1991.

Williams RA, Howard AG, Williams TP: Retinal damage in pigmented and albino rats exposed to low levels of cyclic light following a single-mydriatic treatment. *Curr Eye Res* 4:97–102, 1985.

Wilson MA, Johnston MV, Goldstein GW, Blue ME: Neonatal lead exposure impairs development of rodent barrel field cortex. *Proc Natl Acad Sci USA* 97:5540–5545, 2000.

Winkler BS, Kapousta-Bruneau N, Arnold MJ, Green DG: Effects of inhibiting glutamine synthetase and blocking glutamate uptake on b-wave generation in the isolated rat retina. *Vis Neurosci* 16:345–353, 1999.

Winkler BS, Riley MV: Na^+,K^+ and HCO_3 ATPase activity in retina: Dependence on calcium and sodium. *Invest Ophthalmol Vis Sci* 16:1151–1154, 1977.

Winkler BS: A quantitative assessment of glucose metabolism in the rat retina, in Christen Y, Doly M, Droy-Lefaix MT (eds): *Vision and Adaptation, Les Seminaires Ophtamologiques d'IPSEN.* Vol 6. Paris: Elsevier, 1995, pp 78–96.

Winneke G: Modification of visual evoked potentials in rats after long-term blood lead elevation. *Act Nerv Sup* (*Praha*) 4:282–284, 1979.

Winneke G, Beginn U, Ewert T, et al: Study to determine the subclinical effects of lead on the nervous system in children with known prenatal exposure in Nordenham. *Schr-Reine Verein Wabolu* 59:215–230, 1984.

Winneke G, Kramer U, Brockhaus A, et al: Neuropsychological studies in children with elevated tooth-lead concentrations: II. Extended study. *Int Arch Occup Environ Health* 51:231–252, 1983.

Withering W: *An Account of the Foxglove and Some of Its Medicinal Uses: With Practical Remarks on Dropsy and Other Diseases.* London: Broomsleigh Press, 1785.

Woodhouse JM, Barlow HB: Spatial and temporal resolution and analysis, in Barlow HB, Mollon JD (eds): *The Senses.* Cambridge: Cambridge University Press, 1982, pp 133–164.

Yau KW, Baylor DA: Cyclic GMP-activated conductance of retinal photoreceptor cells. *Annu Rev Neurosci* 12:289–327, 1989.

Yoshino Y, Mozai T, Nako K: Distribution of mercury in the brain and its subcellular units in experimental organic mercury poisonings. *J Neurochem* 13:397–406, 1966.

Zavalic M, Turk R, Bogadi-Sare A, Skender L: Colour vision impairment in workers exposed to low concentrations of toluene. *Arh Hig Rada Toksikol* 47:167–175, 1996.

Zhao C, Schwartzman ML, Shichi H: Immunocytochemical study of cytochrome P450 4A induction in mouse eye. *Exp Eye Res* 63:747–751, 1996.

Zhao C, Shichi H: Immunocytochemical study of cytochrome P450 (1A1/1A2) induction in murine ocular tissues. *Exp Eye Res* 60:143–152, 1995.

Zrenner E, Gouras P: Blue-sensitive cones of the cat produce a rod like electroretinogram. *Invest Ophthalmol Vis Sci* 18:1076–1081, 1979.

Zrenner E, Kramer W, Bittner C, et al: Rapid effects on colour vision following intravenous injection of a new, non-glycoside positive ionotropic substance (AR-L 115BS). *Doc Ophthalmol Proc Ser* 33:493–507, 1982.

CHAPTER 18

TOXIC RESPONSES OF THE HEART AND VASCULAR SYSTEMS

Kenneth S. Ramos, Russell B. Melchert, Enrique Chacon, and Daniel Acosta, Jr.

INTRODUCTION

The cardiovascular system has two major components: the myocardium and a diverse network of vascular vessels consisting of arteries, capillaries, and veins. Both units of the cardiovascular system have important functions in supplying the tissues and cells of the body with appropriate nutrients, respiratory gases, hormones, and metabolites and removing the waste products of tissue and cellular metabolism as well as foreign matter such as invading microorganisms. In addition, the cardiovascular system, through its circulation of blood and fluids to every tissue in the body, is responsible for maintaining the optimal internal homeostasis of the body as well as for critical regulation of body temperature and maintenance of tissue and cellular pH. Thus, the cardiovascular system plays a critical role in the well-being and survival of the other major organs of the body, especially highly vascularized organs that are dependent on nutrients and oxygen carried by the blood. If the cardiovascular system is injured by disease or toxic chemicals, this damage has a far-reaching impact on the survival of the organism.

The discipline of cardiovascular toxicology is concerned with the adverse effects of drugs, chemicals, and xenobiotics on the heart and circulatory system of a living organism. The introduction of drugs or xenobiotics into the body eventually leads to their absorption into the bloodstream and transport to the heart; toxic interactions with the cardiovascular system usually are determined by the concentration of a xenobiotic in contact with the myocardium or vasculature and by the duration of exposure. A wide spectrum of xenobiotics—including drugs, natural products, industrial chemicals, and environmentally introduced agents—may interact directly with the cardiovascular system to cause structural and/or functional changes. There may also be indirect actions secondary to changes in other organ systems, especially the central and autonomic nervous systems and selective actions of the endocrine system. Functional alterations that affect the rhythmicity of the heart, if severe enough, may lead to lethal arrhythmias without major evidence of structural damage to the myocardium. Structural alterations such as degenerative necrosis and inflammatory reactions are often caused by direct effects of chemicals on the myocardium.

This chapter presents a major review on general mechanisms of cardiotoxicity and injury to the vasculature and provides a systematic examination of major categories of cardiovascular toxicants. Specifically, the authors have highlighted the roles of ion homeostasis, altered blood flow, oxidative stress, organelle dysfunction, and apoptosis and oncosis in the production of injury to the heart by prototypic myocardial toxicants. The discussion of injury to the vascular system focuses on mechanisms that involve vascular reactivity, bioactivation and erratic detoxification, and molecular genetic alterations. Several major classes of cardiovascular toxicants are described: (1) pharmaceutical agents, such as antineoplastics, antibiotics, autonomic and centrally acting drugs, antihistamines, immunosuppressants, cardiovascular-acting pharmacologic drugs, local anesthetics, and other miscellaneous drugs; (2) natural products, such as steroids, cytokines, vitamins, and animal/plant toxins; and (3) industrial chemicals, such as solvents, alcohols, heavy metals, gases, alkylamines, halogenated amines, and other miscellaneous agents. In order to provide a clearer picture of the toxic responses of the heart and vascular systems, an overview of the physiology of the myocardium and vasculature is also presented.

OVERVIEW OF CARDIAC PHYSIOLOGY

A clear grasp of the normal anatomy and physiology of the heart provides the basis for understanding the effects of xenobiotics on cardiac function. Figure 18-1 illustrates the basic anatomy of the heart. The main purpose of the heart is to pump blood to the lungs and the systemic arteries so as to provide oxygen and nutrients to all the tissues of the body. The heart consists of four pumping chambers: the right and left atria and the right and left ventricles. Venous blood from the systemic circulation enters the right atrium and right ventricle, from which it is then pumped into the lungs to become oxygenated. The left atrium and ventricle then receive the oxygenated blood via the pulmonary veins and pump it to the systemic arteries via the aorta. In addition, the heart receives oxygenated blood flow from the right and left coronary arteries, which begin at the root of the aorta. Each contraction cycle consists of an orchestrated series of events that result in the blood-pumping action of the heart.

Review of Cardiac Structure

The structural organization of myocardial tissue is shown in Fig. 18-2. The primary contractile unit within the heart is the cardiac muscle cell, or cardiac myocyte. Cardiac myocytes are composed of several major structural features and organelles. A primary component is the contractile elements known as the myofibril. Each myofibril consists of a number of smaller filaments (the thick and thin myofilaments). The thick filaments are special assemblies of the protein myosin, whereas the thin filaments are made up primarily of the protein actin. Cardiac myosin is a hexamer composed of one pair of myosin heavy chains (MHC) and two pairs of myosin light chains (MLC). Two isoforms of MHC, α and β, are expressed in cardiac muscle; the expression of these is under developmental control and may be altered by a variety of physiologic, pathologic, and pharmacologic stimuli (Martin et al., 1996; Metzger et al., 1999). Furthermore, the predominant isoform expressed in normal adult cardiac tissue also depends upon the species examined. Similarly, two isoforms of actin are expressed in the heart (cardiac and skeletal α-actin), and, as with MHC, actin isoform expression is influenced by developmental, physiologic, pathologic, and pharmacologic stimuli. Again, the primary isoform of actin found in normal adult cardiac muscle also depends upon the species examined.

Under electron microscopy, these essential structural components of myocardial contractile proteins display alternating dark bands (A bands, predominantly composed of myosin) and light bands (I bands, predominantly composed of actin). Visible in the middle of the I band is a dense vertical Z line. The area between two Z lines is called a sarcomere, the fundamental unit of muscle contraction. Although cardiac and skeletal muscle share many similarities, a major difference lies in the organization of cardiac myocytes into a functional syncytium where cardiac myocytes are joined end-to-end by dense structures known as intercalated disks. Within these, there are tight gap junctions that facilitate action potential propagation and intercellular communication. About 50 percent of each cardiac myocyte is composed of myofibrils. The rest of the intracellular space contains the remaining major components of the cell: mitochondria (33 percent), one or more nuclei (5 percent), the sarcoplasmic reticulum (2 percent), lysosomes (very

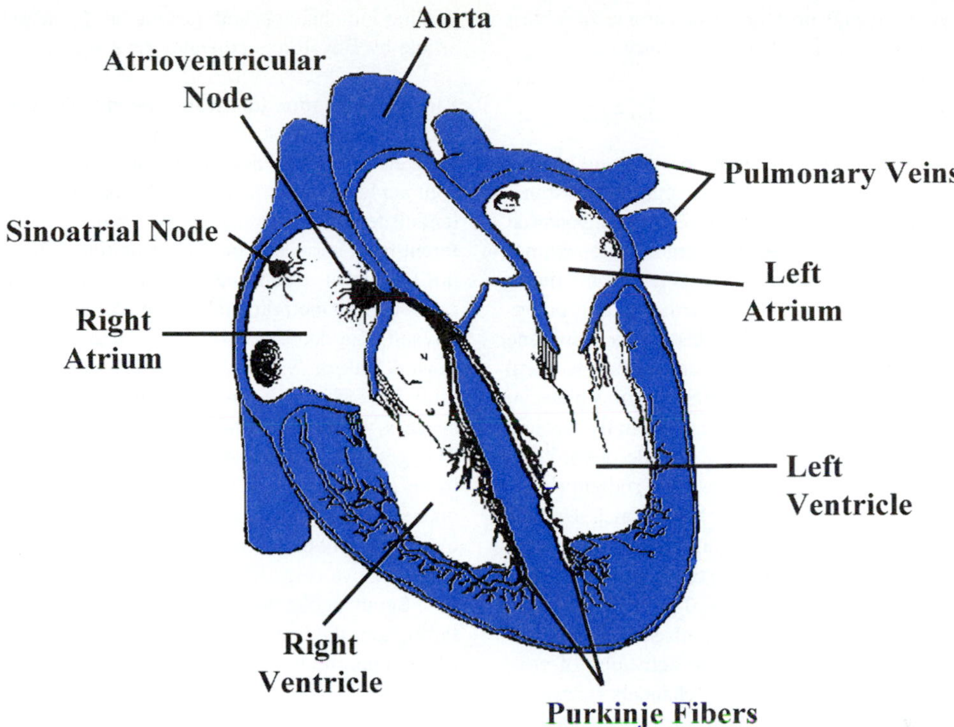

Figure 18-1. Diagram illustrating the basic anatomy of the heart.

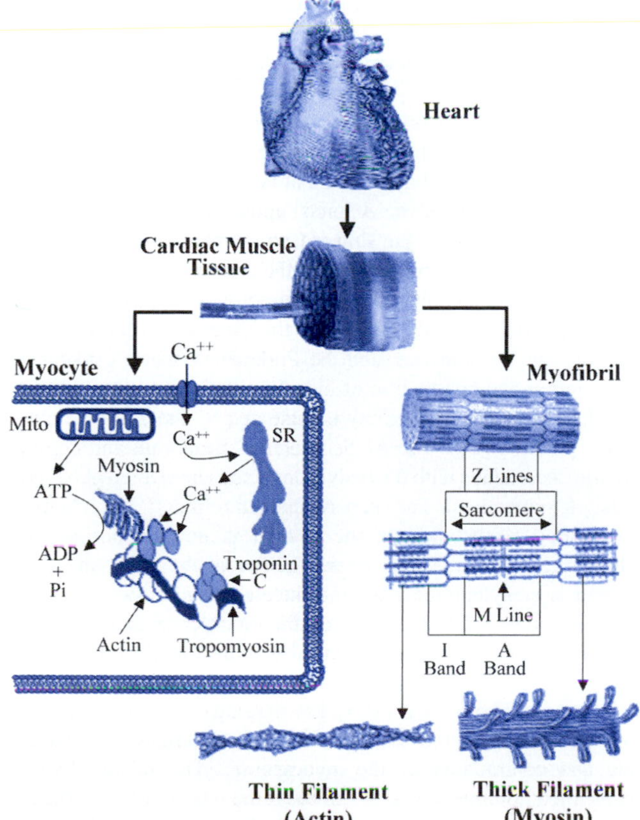

Figure 18-2. Structural organization of cardiac muscle tissue.

low), glycogen granules, a Golgi network, and cytosol (12 percent) (Opie, 1986a).

Cellular Phenotypes within the Heart

The major cellular phenotype in the heart is the cardiac myocyte, which is the largest cell in the heart and contributes to the majority of cardiac mass. However, cardiac myocytes make up only about one-quarter of all the cells in the heart. Cardiac fibroblasts, vascular cells, Purkinje cells, and other connective tissue cells make up the majority of cell number in the heart. Cardiac fibroblasts make up approximately 90 percent of these "nonmuscle" cells. Cardiac myocytes are generally considered to be terminally differentiated. That is, although these cells may be multinucleated, they normally do not divide after birth. The heart undergoes a significant increase in size and mass throughout growth of the organism, but the increase in heart size and mass is produced by enlargement (or hypertrophy) of pre-existing cardiac myocytes (Li et al., 1996). With regard to this developmental period, cardiac hypertrophy is considered to be a normal physiologic process. Although cardiac myocyte division has been debated for some time, the clear lack of significant regeneration of cardiac tissue and subsequent hypertrophy of remaining myocytes following myocardial infarction suggests, at best, a very limited proliferative capacity of mature cardiac myocytes. Moreover, hypertrophy of remaining cardiac myocytes is a hallmark of cardiac remodeling following myocardial infarction. In contrast, cardiac fibroblasts may continue to proliferate after birth, particularly in response to injury. Cardiac fibroblasts also contribute to cardiac remodeling following myocardial infarction and are believed to promote fibrosis and scarring of injured cardiac tissue. Thus, from a toxicological perspective, the heart is vulnerable to injury because of limited proliferative capacity of cardiac myocytes, and promotion of cardiac fibroblast proliferation and cardiac remodeling following injury.

Cardiac Electrophysiology

Review of the Action Potential The ionic basis of membrane activity is reflected by and dependent upon changes in the transmembrane potential. At any given time, the electrical potential across the cardiac myocyte cytoplasmic membrane (sarcolemma) is a reflection of the ion concentration gradients across the membrane. The characteristic appearance of the cardiac action potential demonstrates how ion currents result in changes in membrane potential (Fig. 18-3). In a resting cell, the density of the electrical charge on both sides of the sarcolemma is referred to as phase 4, or diastolic membrane potential, which is normally around −90 mV (inside negative with respect to the outside of the cell). When an action potential is initiated, voltage-gated sodium (Na^+) channels open, and there is a rapid influx of Na^+, which depolarizes the cell from approximately −90 mV (nonpacemaker cardiac cells) to greater than 0 mV, thus giving rise to the Na^+ current (I_{Na}) and the upstroke of the action potential (phase 0). The initial, brief, and rapid depolarization that occurs following phase 0 is produced by closure of voltage-gated Na^+ channels and activation of voltage-gated transient outward potassium (K^+) channels (phase 1). During the rapid influx of Na^+ and resulting membrane depolarization, voltage-gated calcium (Ca^{2+}) channels open and Ca^{2+} begins a slower but prolonged inward flux at approximately −30 to −40 mV, giving rise to Ca^{2+} current (I_{Ca}). As the Na^+ current dissipates, Ca^{2+} continues to enter the cell, giving rise to the characteristic plateau appearance of phase 2. Final repolarization (phase 3) of the cell results from closure of voltage-gated Ca^{2+} channels and K^+ efflux through two major types of K^+ channels: a channel responsible for inward rectifier current (I_{K1}) and a channel responsible for delayed rectifier current (I_K). Thus the normal resting potential is restored, but the cell must continue to normalize the Na^+ and K^+ concentration gradients through activity of the Na^+,K^+-ATPase that actively extrudes intracellular Na^+ in exchange for extracellular K^+. For further detailed information regarding ion channels and currents in the heart, refer to the review article by Boyett and colleagues (1996).

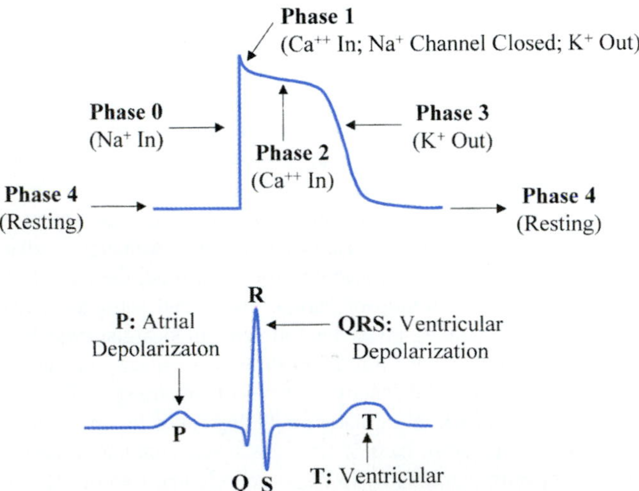

Figure 18-3. Characteristic cardiac action potential and electrocardiogram (ECG).

Electrical Conduction in the Heart The cardiac cycle begins in pacemaker cells that spontaneously depolarize and pass a depolarizing electrical current to neighboring cells. Pacemaker cells do not contract but are responsible for initiating and conducting action potentials to the cardiac myocytes. Spontaneous depolarization is different from nerve and muscle excitation in that pacemaker cells do not remain at a constant resting potential. Instead, a pacemaker cell's membrane potential slowly depolarizes toward threshold as a result of a decreased K^+ efflux that is superimposed on a slow inward leak of Na^+ and Ca^{2+}. Overall, there is a gradual accumulation of positive ions inside the cells, causing the intracellular space to become less negative relative to the extracellular space. This gradual depolarization toward threshold eventually gives rise to an action potential. Once threshold is reached, Na^+ channels open and then Ca^{2+} channels open, leading to a rapid influx of Ca^{2+} and production of the characteristic action potential, as discussed above (Fig. 18-3).

Spontaneous depolarization can be found in various regions throughout the heart: the sinoatrial (SA) node, the atrioventricular (AV) node, the bundle of His (atrioventricular bundle), and Purkinje fibers. Under physiologic conditions, SA nodal cells exhibit the fastest rate of action potential discharge and thus set the pace of the heart (hence the term *pacemaker*). If the SA node is damaged or inhibited, the next fastest depolarizing cells (AV node) assume the pacemaking activity. AV nodal cells spontaneously depolarize at a slower rate than SA nodal cells, and the bundle of His and Purkinje fibers spontaneously fire at yet a slower rate. The non-SA nodal pacemaker cells are referred to as latent pacemakers and can take over to set the cardiac pace if the normal pacemaker cells fail. However, because of decreased rates of firing in the latent pacemaker cells, normal cardiac function is compromised as a result of slower spontaneous depolarization rates.

Normally, the cardiac cycle begins with spontaneous depolarization of cells in the SA node. The electrical impulse propagates through the atrial muscle and converges on the AV node. The dense fibrous tissue of the AV node causes the electrical impulse to slow down owing to the slower Ca^{2+}-dependent upstroke. This delayed transfer of current between the atria and the ventricles allows the atria to complete contraction before depolarization of the ventricles. The AV node impulse is then sent down the bundle of His, the bundle branches, and the Purkinje network, causing depolarization and contraction of muscle cells in the ventricles.

Electrical cardiac activity is regulated by the autonomic nervous system (ANS). The ANS influences heart rate and contractility in accordance with the body's demand. The efferent ANS consists of sympathetic and parasympathetic fibers. The chemical transmitter of the sympathetic system is norepinephrine (noradrenaline), and the chemical transmitter of the parasympathetic system is acetylcholine (ACh). Sympathetic activation alters SA and AV nodal function as well as atrial and ventricular contractility. Parasympathetic fibers (vagal fibers) are found in the SA and AV nodes as well as in atrial muscle. Thus, norepinephrine and similar sympathomimetics stimulate the rate of depolarization and the rate of impulse transmission, resulting in an increase in cardiac rate and contractility of the myocardium. The major effect of parasympathomimetics is to enhance the vagal tone of the SA and AV nodes and the atrial muscle and thus decrease the rate of depolarization with only a slight decrease in ventricular contractility.

Excitation-Contraction Coupling The key to conversion of electrical activity to mechanical work in the heart lies in the coupling of cardiac myocyte excitation (depolarization) to mechanical contraction. An overview of the process of excitation-contraction coupling is presented in Fig. 18-4. For contraction to occur, both energy (in the form of ATP) and Ca^{2+} must be readily available. Energy for contraction is obtained from the splitting of adenosine triphosphate (ATP) by hydrolysis via an ATPase site on myosin. Each mole of ATP hydrolyzed liberates about 30 kilojoules (kJ) of energy. The ATP necessary for contraction is derived from three major sources: oxidative phosphorylation in the mitochondria, substrate-level phosphorylation in glycolysis and the citric acid cycle, and ADP phosphorylation by creatine phosphokinase. However, oxidative phosphorylation is the most significant source of ATP in the heart, accounting for more than 90 percent of total ATP production (Vary et al., 1981). The heart contains about 3 mg of ATP per gram of wet weight (5 μmol/g) and a pool of creatine phosphate that is approximately three times larger; this accounts for a minimal reserve sufficient to last only about 50 to 75 beats (Opie, 1986b). Since the majority of ATP for contraction is provided by the mitochondria, it is not surprising that mitochondria occupy a large portion of each cardiac myocyte and maintain integrity to support myocardial function.

The Ca^{2+} necessary for contraction comes largely from two sources: extracellular Ca^{2+} and intracellular Ca^{2+} stores. Beginning in phase 0 (rapid depolarization) and persisting in the plateau of the action potential (phase 2), voltage-gated Ca^{2+} channels (L type) are open, allowing influx of extracellular Ca^{2+} down the electrochemical gradient. Furthermore, some extracellular Ca^{2+}, albeit likely a small amount, enters the cell through the Na^+/Ca^{2+} exchanger (in reverse mode) during depolarization, whereby intracellular Na^+ is exchanged for extracellular Ca^{2+}. Although uptake of external Ca^{2+} during this process is necessary and contributes to contraction and in some cases may be sufficient for contraction, the majority of Ca^{2+} required for contraction comes from the sarcoplasmic reticulum (SR). Ryanodine receptors (RyRs), closely related to inositol trisphosphate (IP_3) receptors, reside on the surface of the SR, and serve as Ca^{2+} release channels. Although IP_3 receptors may release some of the Ca^{2+} required for contraction, RyRs are thought to contribute the majority of Ca^{2+} release from the SR. When intracellular free Ca^{2+} rises subsequent to opening of L-type Ca^{2+} channels, RyRs are activated to release Ca^{2+} from the SR. This process is known as Ca^{2+}-induced Ca^{2+} release (CICR), and CICR contributes the majority of Ca^{2+} necessary for contraction. Following CICR, a transient increase in intracellular free Ca^{2+} concentration (Ca^{2+} transient) occurs allowing contraction to proceed. Mechanical contraction of cardiac myocytes occurs when Ca^{2+} binds to the protein troponin C (located on a complex with tropomysin), which under resting conditions inhibits the interaction of myosin and actin. Following a Ca^{2+}-induced conformational change in troponin C and tropomysin, the ATPase catalytic site and myosin binding site on actin are exposed. Then, ATP is hydrolyzed, inducing a conformational change in myosin and subsequently allowing myosin to bind actin, thus producing "cross-bridge cycling" and contraction.

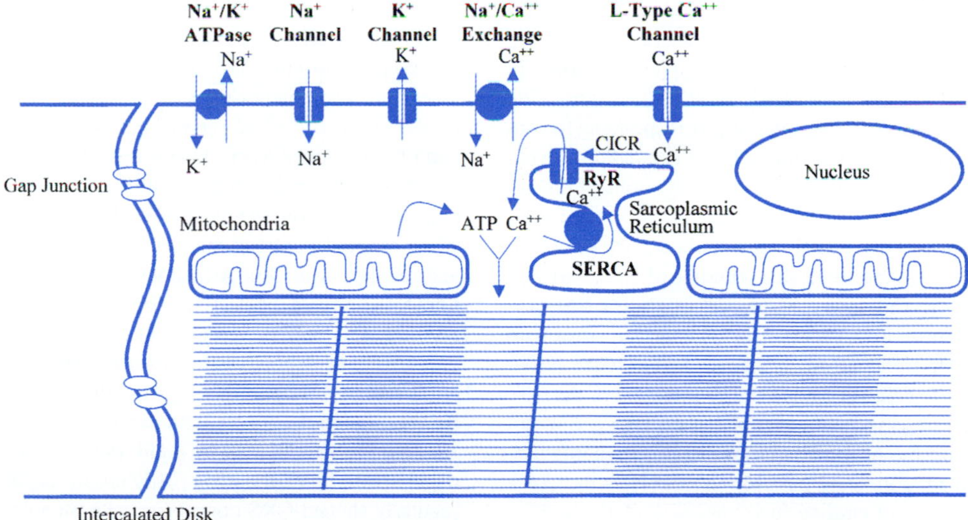

Figure 18-4. Overview of excitation-contraction coupling in cardiac myocytes.

Upon rapid depolarization (rapid influx of Na^+ through fast channels; phase 0 of the action potential), L-type Ca^{2+} channels are opened allowing a slower but sustained influx of Ca^{2+} down the electrochemical gradient (phase 2 of the action potential). During the process of Ca^{2+}-induced Ca^{2+} release (CICR), slight elevation in intracellular free Ca^{2+} stimulates Ca^{2+} release from the sarcoplasmic reticulum (SR) through ryanodine receptors (RyR). The SR provides the majority of Ca^{2+} required for contraction. The mitochondria provide energy for contraction in the form of ATP. Repolarization of the cell occurs largely by activation of K^+ channels and efflux of K^+ (phase 3 of the action potential). For relaxation, the SR Ca^{2+} ATPase (SERCA) actively pumps Ca^{2+} back into the SR, although some Ca^{2+} may be removed by the Na^+/Ca^{2+} exchanger or by sarcolemmal Ca^{2+} pumps.

Relaxation of cardiac myocytes requires reductions in cytoplasmic free Ca^{2+} and consequently reductions in the free Ca^{2+} pool available for interaction with troponin C. Several ion pumps and exchangers facilitate removal or sequestration of Ca^{2+}. The sarcolemmal Na^+/Ca^{2+} exchange (in forward mode) may extrude Ca^{2+} from the cell by exchanging intracellular Ca^{2+} for extracellular Na^+. In addition, a uniporter exists on the mitochondrial membrane, which acts to sequester Ca^{2+} into the mitochondria. Furthermore, a sarcolemmal Ca^{2+} ATPase can actively extrude Ca^{2+} from the cell. However, the majority of Ca^{2+} available for interaction with troponin C is removed by the active ion pump SR Ca^{2+} ATPase (SERCA), which actively pumps Ca^{2+} back into the SR, whereas the other ion pumps and exchangers make significantly less contributions to Ca^{2+} reduction (Bers, 1997). The SERCA requires energy in the form of ATP; therefore, ATP is required for both contraction and relaxation. As SERCA reduces cytoplasmic free Ca^{2+}, and consequently Ca^{2+} available for interaction with troponin C, the actin-myosin interaction ceases and the cell relaxes.

Cardiac Function

Electrocardiogram Electrical currents generated during depolarization and repolarization spread throughout the heart, body fluids, and body surface. Therefore electrical activity of the heart is monitored by recording electrodes placed on the skin surface, resulting in the characteristic electrocardiogram (ECG). Examination of ECG patterns is useful for diagnosing abnormal heart rates, arrhythmias, and damage to heart muscle. On the ECG shown in Fig. 18-3, deflections (or waves) are recorded that correspond to atrial depolarization (P wave), ventricular depolarization (QRS complex), and ventricular repolarization (T wave); however, atrial repolarization is not normally observed on the ECG because it is obscured by the large QRS complex. Several useful intervals are noted on the ECG, such as the PR interval, corresponding primarily to conduction through the AV node; QRS duration, corresponding to ventricular depolarization; the ST interval, corresponding to ventricular repolarization; and the QT interval, corresponding to ventricular depolarization and repolarization. Prolongations of the PR interval may indicate disturbances of AV nodal conduction; whereas prolongations of QRS duration may indicate blocks in conduction pathways through the ventricles (bundles of His). Any significant deviations of the ST interval from the isoelectric line may indicate ischemic damage to the heart. The QT interval varies with heart rate and is often corrected for heart rate (QTc) when possibly abnormal ECGs are being considered. Prolongation of the QTc interval is frequently observed with agents that prolong action potential duration within the heart. Therefore the ECG records useful information that may indicate possible mechanisms by which xenobiotics adversely affect cardiac function.

Cardiac Output The primary indicator of cardiac function is cardiac output (i.e. the volume of blood pumped by the ventricles per minute). Cardiac output is dependent on heart rate and stroke volume (the amount of blood ejected by the ventricles during systole). If stroke volume were easily and noninvasively measured, then the monitoring of cardiac output would be routine because heart rate is readily acquired, and cardiac output would be equivalent to heart rate (beats per minute) times stroke volume (milliliters per beat). However, stroke volume is not routinely obtained, and accurate measurement of cardiac output requires either echocardiography with Doppler techniques or indicator-dilution techniques. Normal cardiac output at rest is approximately 5 L/min in an average adult human (Sherwood, 1993), and this value may increase three- to four-fold during strenuous exercise. Measurement of cardiac output in animals is useful for determining potential adverse effects of xenobiotics on cardiac function, because the primary concern regarding cardiotoxicity is how an agent affects the pumping action of the heart. Reflecting the ability of the heart to meet the demands of the body (e.g., exercise), numerous factors affect cardiac output either by altering heart rate or stroke volume: autonomic regulation of heart rate or contractility, preload (muscle stretch from ventricular filling), afterload (arterial pressure and peripheral vascular resistance), and left ventricular size. Therefore toxicants may alter cardiac output though numerous mechanisms and effects on the heart, vasculature, and/or nervous system.

DISTURBANCES IN CARDIAC FUNCTION

Abnormal Heart Rhythm

Typical chemically induced disturbances in cardiac function consist of effects on heart rate (chronotropic), contractility (inotropic), conductivity (dromotropic), and/or excitability (bathmotropic). The normal human heart rate at rest is approximately 70 beats per minute. A rapid resting heart rate (i.e., above 100 beats per minute) is known as tachycardia (Greek *tachys,* meaning "rapid"), whereas a slow heart rate (i.e., below 60 beats per minute) is known as bradycardia (Greek *bradys,* meaning "slow"). Any variation from normal rhythm is termed an arrhythmia, and arrhythmias are often complications secondary to other on-going disturbances in cardiac function, such as ischemic heart disease or cardiac hypertrophy (as described below). Arrhythmias are classified on the basis of their origin (supraventricular or ventricular).

Supraventricular arrhythmias (atrial in origin) are further divided into two categories: (1) supraventricular tachycardia based on defects in AV nodal reentry circuits or anatomic bypass tracts and (2) atrial fibrillation, where there is some form of atrial muscle injury. Although often symptomatic, atrial arrhythmias are seldom fatal, largely because the ventricles will fill even in the absence of atrial contraction. *Atrial flutter* is characterized by rapid and regular atrial depolarizations between 200 and 380 beats per minute. However, because of the longer refractory period of the AV node and ventricles, the ventricles typically are unable to synchronize their depolarization with the rapidly firing atria. During atrial flutter, only one of every two to three atrial depolarizations passes through the AV node to depolarize the ventricles. *Atrial fibrillation* is characterized by rapid, randomized, and uncoordinated depolarizations of the atria. This erratic depolarization results in regularly shaped QRS complexes without a definite P wave (atrial repolarization). Atrial contractions are unsynchronized, and AV conduction is also irregular. The AV irregularity causes irregular ventricular rhythm and subsequent inefficiency in ventricular filling. Less ventricular filling time results in diminished blood pumping to the extent that the pulse rate may be depressed. Under normal circumstances, pulse rate coincides with heart rate.

In contrast to atrial arrhythmias, ventricular arrhythmias are almost always symptomatic and will lead to loss of consciousness within a few seconds and even to death if they are unresolved or untreated. Therefore most ventricular arrhythmias are considered at least potentially life-threatening. Frequently, ventricular arrhythmias arise from muscle injury secondary to ischemia, infarction, and subsequent scarring and fibrosis or by ventricular hypertrophy. Such arrhythmias may begin as *ventricular tachycardia* and progress to more severe complications such as ventricular fibrillation. *Ventricular fibrillation* is characterized by repetitive, rapid, and randomized excitation of the ventricles, usually as a result of ectopic foci in the ventricles. Impulses travel chaotically around the ventricles. Hence, the ventricles become inefficient as pumps and death is inevitable unless normal rhythm is reestablished through the use of electrical defibrillation or cardiac compression.

Heart block is due to impairments in the cardiac conducting system. Typically, the atria maintain regular beating rates, but the ventricles occasionally fail to depolarize. For example, only every second or third atrial impulse may pass to depolarize the ventricles. Heart blocks are classified on the basis of their degree of depression of the conduction system. Complete heart block is characterized by complete block of conduction between the atria and ventricles. Under complete heart block, the atria beat regularly but the ventricles begin their own pacemaker activity at a much slower rate. Thus, the P wave (atrial depolarization) exhibits normal rhythm, while the QRS and T waves exhibit a slower rhythm that is independent of the P wave rhythm.

Xenobiotics may alter normal heart rate or rhythm. Those that are particularly prone to produce arrhythmias are compounds that interfere with ion channel function, alter action potential, or disturb conductance through the heart. As extensions of the mechanisms of action or lack of specificity, many antiarrhythmic drugs carry the risk of promoting arrhythmias. Examples of these drugs are included later in the chapter. Far too frequently, however, drugs used to treat non-cardiac-related illness are later found to alter ion homeostasis and/or flux in cardiac myocytes. Examples of such compounds include some antibacterial agents and antihistamines, as discussed later in the chapter. Therefore monitoring of heart rhythm with ECG is important in testing the cardiotoxic potential of drugs or chemicals.

Ischemic Heart Disease

Ischemic heart disease (IHD) is a major leading cause of death for men and women in the United States and other industrialized nations. IHD may be produced by a variety of pathologic conditions and/or xenobiotics that disturb the balance of myocardial perfusion and myocardial oxygen and nutrient demand. Pathologic conditions and/or compounds that reduce myocardial perfusion may induce ischemia and subsequent oxygen and nutrient deficiency as well as inadequate removal of metabolic products. A major cause of IHD is coronary artery atherosclerosis and resulting arterial obstruction. Several major syndromes comprise the clinical manifestations of IHD, including myocardial infarction, angina pectoris (pain radiating to the chest, left shoulder and/or arm, or neck) and its three variants (stable angina, unstable angina and Prinzmetal angina), and chronic ischemia with heart failure. Many of these syndromes may end in sudden cardiac death, but the severity of symptoms and progression of disease vary dramatically between affected individuals. Unfortunately, an alarming number of cases of myocardial infarction and/or sudden cardiac death fail to present symptoms and are assumed to be "silent" or asymptomatic ischemia. IHD may be produced by pathologic conditions other than atherosclerosis. For example, cardiac hypertrophy (discussed below) may contribute to IHD through increased myocardial oxygen demand, decreased perfusion of the hypertrophic wall, and increased risk of arrhythmias. In some cases, coronary vasospasm not associated with atherosclerotic plaques may contribute to IHD. Xenobiotics that have been associated with ischemic heart disease include cocaine, sympathomimetics, and anabolic-androgenic steroids (as reviewed later in the chapter).

Whatever the cause of IHD and its clinical syndromes, the end results when left unresolved or untreated share some common effects on cardiac myocyte function and viability. Because the myocardium derives the majority of the ATP required for contraction from the aerobic metabolism of glucose, pathologic conditions or xenobiotics that reduce myocardial perfusion, and thus oxygen and nutrient delivery, will force the cardiac myocytes to derive ATP from creatine phosphate and anaerobic glycolysis until stores are depleted. Therefore, ATP depletion begins almost immediately in ischemic cardiac myocytes, and within 20 to 40 min, ATP is significantly depleted and irreversible injury begins. Undoubtedly, large numbers of cardiac myocytes within the ischemic or infarcted zone will undergo nonapoptotic (oncocytic necrosis, or *oncosis*) cell death (discussed below). However, more recent research has demonstrated that significant numbers of myocytes will undergo programmed cell death, or *apoptosis* (discussed below), following ischemia or infarction (Haunstetter and Izumo, 1998). Interestingly, the apoptotic regions of myocyte death following ischemia appear to be near the border zone, perhaps extending into adjacent perfused myocardium, which suggests the release of local factors (e.g., cytokines) in necrotic regions that alter viability of surrounding regions. The size of the ischemic or infarcted zone will depend on a number of factors including the duration and severity of ischemia, position of obstruction or size of the myocardial bed at risk, and collateral blood flow capabilities (Buja, 1998). Following myocyte death, cytosolic contents may eventually enter the systemic circulation, where they may be detected as markers of IHD. For example, serum levels of cardiac-specific isoforms of lactate dehydrogenase (LDH), creatine kinase (CK), and troponin are elevated several hours following acute myocardial infarction (AMI). Eventually, permanently damaged zones are replaced with scar tissue contributed by connective tissue cells such as cardiac fibroblasts. Furthermore, surviving cardiac myocytes compensate for increased workload by increasing in size (hypertrophy). The *cardiac remodeling* process thus includes initial myocyte loss and subsequent connective tissue cell activation and scar production, hypertrophy of remaining myocytes, altered cardiac geometry, and microcirculatory changes within the heart.

Cardiac Hypertrophy and Heart Failure

As mentioned above, cardiac hypertrophy is an important component to cardiac remodeling following IHD. However, cardiac hypertrophy is a growth response during development of the organism and is often a compensatory response of the heart to increased workload. For example, prolonged hypertension contributes to load-induced left ventricular hypertrophy. Therefore, cardiac hypertrophy in and of itself does not necessarily result in a disturbance in cardiac function. With regard to cardiac remodeling following injury, hypertrophy of surviving myocytes may be necessary to sustain cardiac output for life support. At some point in the progression of IHD, however, the hypertrophic myocardium may "decompensate," resulting in failure. During failure, ventricular contractility and/or compliance are reduced, such that cardiac output is diminished. Failure may present as left- or right-sided failure or both. When left-sided failure is the primary pathology, blood pools in the lungs and pulmonary edema develops. When right-sided failure is the primary pathology, blood pools in the extremities and pitting edema is found in the lower legs.

Unfortunately, the mechanisms responsible for the transition from cardiac hypertrophy to failure are not understood. Likely possibilities include ischemia (resulting from larger myocytes, increased oxygen demand, and limited capillary density), synthesis of defective contractile proteins or Ca^{2+} handling proteins, and/or increased deposition of collagen with resulting fibrosis. Thus, scientists are challenged with attempting to determine the point at which hypertrophy becomes pathologic and the mechanisms responsible for the conversion of hypertrophy to overt failure. To this end, significant advancements have occurred in the understanding of stimuli for and signaling pathways of cardiac myocyte hypertrophy (discussed below) and death (discussed under "General Mechanisms of Cardiotoxicity," further on). For toxicologists, these findings may have considerable impact on the understanding of xenobiotic-induced cardiotoxicity. Chronic exposure to some xenobiotics may promote hypertrophic growth of cardiac myocytes by serving as direct stimuli or by altering signaling pathways associated with hypertrophic growth.

Hypertrophic Stimuli Sustained hypertension may induce compensatory left ventricular hypertrophy. Similarly, when neonatal rat cardiac myocytes are grown in culture and subjected to stretch, a hypertrophic growth response is observed where cell size and/or protein synthesis is stimulated while DNA content remains unchanged. Thus, mechanical load or stretch serves as a hypertrophic stimulus, perhaps through secretion of autocrine or paracrine growth factors such as angiotensin II. Furthermore, several other growth factors, hormones, and pharmacologic agents will stimulate hypertrophic growth of cardiac myocytes in vitro (Hefti et al., 1997). These hypertrophic stimuli include $alpha_1$ adrenergic agonists (epinephrine, norepinephrine, phenylephrine), growth factors (endothelin-1 and transforming growth factor beta), cytokines (leukemia inhibitor factor, interleukin-1β, and cardiotrophin-1), prostaglandins (prostaglandin $F_{2\alpha}$), and hormones (thyroid hormone and testosterone). Many of these stimuli may promote growth of cardiac myocytes in vivo, providing necessary stimulation for cardiac hypertrophy during development or compensatory hypertrophy during cardiac remodeling.

Hypertrophic Signal Transduction Following interactions of hypertrophic stimuli with receptors, a multitude of enzyme systems and second messengers are activated: phospholipases A_2, C, and D (PLA_2, PLC, PLD), protein kinase C (PKC), three subfamilies of mitogen-activated protein kinases (MAPKs) [extracellular signal-regulated kinases (ERK 1/2), c-jun NH_2-terminal kinase/stress-activated protein kinases (JNK/SAPK), and p38 reactivating kinase (p38 RK)], receptor tyrosine kinases (RTKs), S6 kinases, and increases in intracellular free Ca^{2+} and subsequent activation of the calcineurin pathway (Sugden, 1999). Importantly, considerable cross-talk between these general pathways exists. For example, increases in PLC and PLD activity stimulate increases in PKC activity and Ca^{2+} through increased formation of diacylglycerol (DG) and inositol trisphosphate (IP_3). Receptor tyrosine kinases may activate PLC, PKC, and MAPKs. In addition, PKC activates MAPKs and may activate JNK/SAPK in cardiac myocyte cultures exposed to mechanical stretch. The common downstream effectors in these cross-talk schemes seem to be PKC, ERK 1/2, JNK/SAPK, and calcineurin; and in cardiomyocyte cultures, various hypertrophic stimuli are coupled to these enzyme systems. Figure 18-5 summarizes the various signaling pathways known to be involved in hypertrophic growth of cardiac myocytes. Many of these signaling enzymes serve as potential targets for pharmacologic intervention in hypertrophic growth and may also serve as target enzymes whereby xenobiotics may alter cardiac myocyte function. Importantly, variations in these signaling pathways should be expected depending upon species and developmental stage of the cardiac tissue or cells used.

Cardiomyopathies

The term *cardiomyopathy* essentially refers to any disease state that alters myocardial function. Therefore, causes of cardiomyopathy include IHD (ischemic cardiomyopathy), cardiac hypertrophy, infectious diseases (e.g., viral cardiomyopathy), drug- or chemical-induced cardiomyopathy, and unknown causes (idiopathic cardiomyopathy). Regardless of exact cause, the cardiomyopathies can be divided into two major categories: dilated cardiomyopathy and hypertrophic cardiomyopathy. *Dilated cardiomyopathy* is produced by progressive cardiac hypertrophy, decompensation, ventricular dilation, and eventual systolic dysfunction or impaired contractility. Some drugs or chemicals may produce dilated cardiomyopathy, including chronic alcohol consumption (alcoholic cardiomyopathy) and doxorubicin (discussed later in the chapter). *Hypertrophic cardiomyopathy* is produced by progressive cardiac hypertrophy, with diastolic dysfunction including impaired compliance of the ventricular walls and reduced diastolic ventricular filling. Many cases of hypertrophic cardiomyopathy are due to inherited diseases with mutations in contractile proteins such as β-myosin heavy chain, troponin, or tropomysin, while other cases are idiopathic.

GENERAL MECHANISMS OF CARDIOTOXICITY

Interference with Ion Homeostasis

As discussed above, the cardiac action potential and excitation-contraction coupling are dependent upon tight regulation of ion channel activity and ion homeostasis. Therefore any xenobiotic that disrupts ion movement or homeostasis may induce a cardiotoxic reaction composed principally of disturbances in heart rhythm. The most notorious agents that disrupt ion channel activity and promote arrhythmia are, ironically, the drugs used to treat arrhythmias and other cardiac diseases.

Inhibition of Na^+,K^+-ATPase

Because Na^+,K^+-ATPase is responsible for reducing intracellular Na^+ in exchange for extracellular K^+, agents that inhibit cardiac Na^+,K^+-ATPase will increase resting intracellular Na^+ concentrations. This, in turn, will increase intracellular Ca^{2+} concentrations through Na^+/Ca^{2+} exchange in reverse mode, and the elevated intracellular Ca^{2+} and Ca^{2+} stores thus contribute to the inotropic actions of these agents. These properties in part lead to the clinical usefulness of the cardiac glycosides (digoxin and digitoxin) in the treatment of heart failure. These drugs are also useful for slowing conduction velocity in the treatment of atrial fibrillation. However, excessive inhibition by high doses of cardiac glycosides can lead to Ca^{2+} overload (sustained elevated intracel-

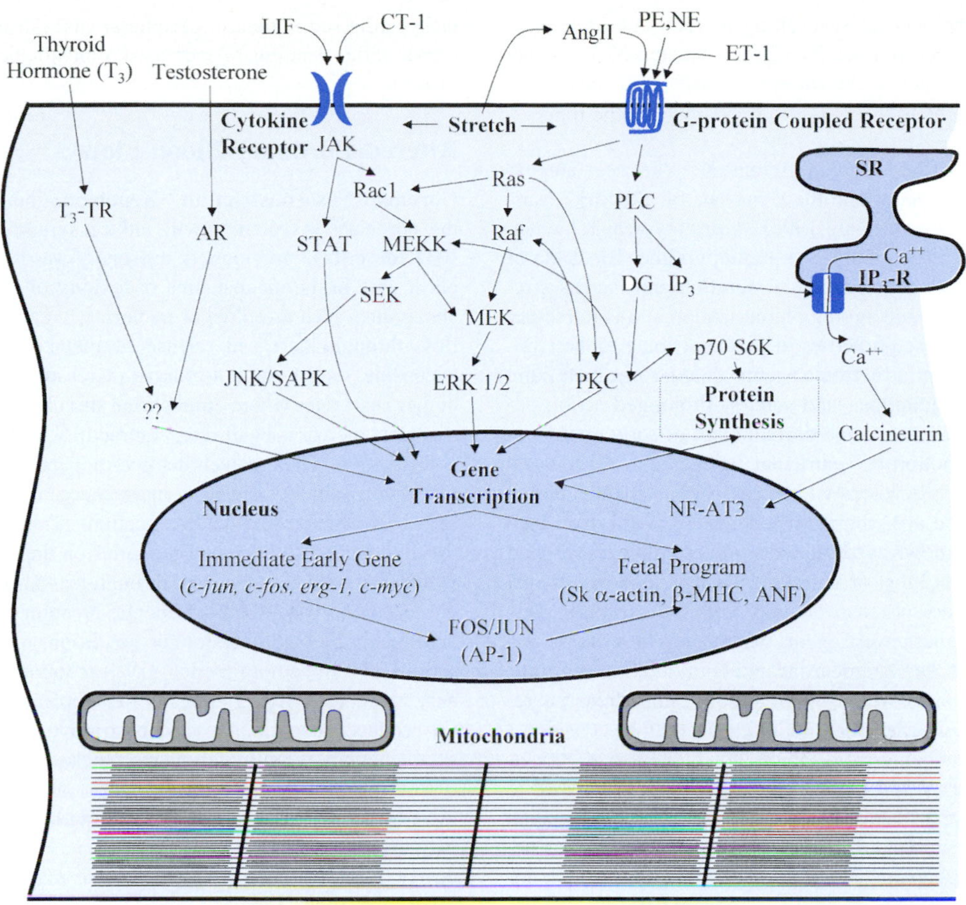

Figure 18-5. Signal transduction pathways involved in hypertrophic growth of cardiac myocytes.

The figure represents a simplistic view of the signaling pathways involved in hypertrophic growth of cardiac myocytes. Significant "cross-talk" between various pathways is present, and opposing pathways are not shown. Arrows represent activation or increases in second messengers. Question marks represent additional steps leading to the response have not been identified. *Abbreviations for stimuli:* AngII, angiotensin II; ANP, atrial natriuretic peptide; CT-1, cardiotrophin 1; ET-1, endothelin-1; LIF, leukemia inhibitor factor; NE, norepinephrine; PE, phenylephrine; T_3, thyroid hormone, triiodothyronine. *Abbreviations for growth pathways:* AR, androgen receptor; Ca^{2+}, intracellular free calcium; DG, diacylglycerol; ERK $1/2$, extracellular signal–regulated kinases 1 and 2; IP_3, inositol-1,4,5-trisphosphate; JAK, Janus kinase; JNK/SAPK, c-Jun N-terminal kinase/stress-activated protein kinase; MEK, mitogen-activated protein kinase effector kinase; MEKK, MEK kinase; p70 S6K, ribosomal S6 kinase; PKC, protein kinase C; PLC, phospholipase C; Rac, a member of the Ras superfamily; Raf, a mitogen-activated protein kinase kinase kinase; Ras, a GTPase; SEK, SAPK effector kinase; STAT, signal transducer and activator of transcription; TR, thyroid hormone receptor. *Abbreviations for nuclear components:* ANF, atrial natriuretic factor; AP-1, heterodimeric transcription factor consisting of FOS and JUN; β-MHC, β-myosin heavy chain; JUN, protein product of *c-jun;* FOS, protein product of *c-fos;* NF-AT3, nuclear factor and activator of T-cells 3; Sk α-actin, skeletal α-actin.

lular free Ca^{2+} concentration) through Na^+/Ca^{2+} exhange in reverse mode. Perhaps related to elevated intracellular Ca^{2+}, cardiac glycosides will increase the incidence and magnitude of afterdepolarizations thus contributing ectopic arrhythmias.

Na^+ Channel Blockade Agents that bind to and inhibit Na^+ channels in cardiac cells will alter cardiac excitability by requiring greater membrane depolarization for opening of Na^+ channels. Effects of Na^+ channel blockade include reduction of conduction velocity, prolonged QRS duration, decreased automaticity, and inhibition of triggered activity from delayed or early afterdepolarizations (Roden, 1996). These properties lead to the clinical usefulness of the class I antiarrhythmic agents disopyramide, flecainide, lidocaine, mexiletine, moricizine, phenytoin, procainamide, propafenone, quinidine, and tocainide (as discussed later in the chapter). However, excessively slowed conduction may facilitate reentry arrhythmias, thus providing a proarrhythmic effect, particularly when the drugs are used in the setting of AMI or previous history of AMI (Nattel, 1998). An example of how slowed conduction velocity may induce proarrhythmic effects is supraventricular tachycardia arising from atrial flutter. In atrial flutter, atrial depolarizations may rise as high as 200 and 380 beats per minute, yet only one of every two to three atrial depolarizations passes through the AV node to depolarize the ventricles. Use of a Na^+ channel blocker would slow conduction velocity and reduce atrial depolarization rate but may actually increase the rate of depolarizations reaching the ventricles, resulting in ventricular tachycardia (Roden, 1996). As discussed later in the chapter, Na^+ channel blockade also contributes to the cardiotoxic effects of local anesthetics such as cocaine.

K^+ Channel Blockade Many different K^+ channels are expressed in the human heart, and these may be blocked by a variety of compounds (Boyett et al., 1996). A prototypical K^+ channel blocker used experimentally is 4-aminopyridine. Blockade of K^+ channels increases action potential duration and increases refractoriness (the cell is undergoing repolarization and is refractory to depolarization). These properties in part contribute to the clinical usefulness of the antiarrhythmic agents amiodarone, bretylium, dofetilide, ibutilide, quinidine, and sotalol. Prolonged action potential duration contributes to the development of early afterdepolarizations and promotion of ventricular tachycardia. An unusual tachycardia frequently develops with excessive K^+ channel blockade. On the ECG, the arrhythmia presents as a polymorphic ventricular tachycardia known as torsades de pointes or twisting around the isoelectric points. Most of the clinically available agents that block K^+ channels do so nonspecifically with the exception, perhaps, of dofetilide, the newest agent, which may be a more specific K^+ channel blocker. Amiodarone and quinidine, for example, also block Na^+ channels, while sotalol inhibits beta-adrenergic receptors in the heart. Consequently, these agents may be considered potentially arrhythmogenic from effects not related to K^+ channels. Moreover, unexpected blockade of K^+ channels has lead to the removal of several "noncardiac" drugs from the U.S. market (e.g., astemizole, cisapride, grepafloxacin, and terfenadine, as described later in the chapter). Blockade of K^+ channels is also implicated in the mechanism of cardiotoxicity of tricyclic antidepressants (as discussed later in the chapter). Toxicities stemming from inhibition of K^+ channels likely result from disproportionate prolongation of action potential duration during slow heart rates, thus predisposing the myocardium to early afterdepolarizations and triggered activity (Roden, 1996) and subsequent "quinidine syncope" (Jackman et al., 1988).

Ca^{2+} Channel Blockade The primary Ca^{2+} channel expressed in the human heart is the L-type voltage-gated Ca^{2+} channel, although T-type Ca^{2+} channels are also expressed. As described previously, the L-type Ca^{2+} channels contribute to excitation-contraction coupling; whereas, the T-type Ca^{2+} channels contribute to pacemaker potential in the SA node (Boyett et al., 1996). L-type Ca^{2+} channels are also expressed in vascular smooth muscle. A variety of agents inhibit these channels. Bepridil, verapamil, and diltiazem inhibit L-type Ca^{2+} channels throughout the vasculature and in the heart. Although the dihydropyridines may also block Ca^{2+} channels in the heart, they exert more profound effects on the vasculature and are often referred to as "vascular selective." Therefore both groups of Ca^{2+} blockers receive significant use for the treatment of hypertension. Verapamil and diltiazem are also used for the treatment of angina and cardiac arrhythmias. Blockade of Ca^{2+} channels in the heart produces a negative inotropic effect due to reductions in Ca^{2+}-induced Ca^{2+} release. Furthermore, verapamil and diltiazem decrease the rate of the SA-nodal pacemaker cell depolarizations and slow AV conduction; they are useful for the treatment of supraventricular tachycardia. As a consequence of these effects, verapamil and diltiazem exert a negative chronotropic effect and may produce bradycardia. Interestingly, the dihydropyridine Ca^{2+} channel blockers typically induce a reflex tachycardia subsequent to peripheral vascular dilation and baroreceptor reflex leading to increased sympathetic outflow from the medulla.

Altered Coronary Blood Flow

Coronary Vasoconstriction Xenobiotic-induced constriction of the coronary vasculature will induce symptoms consistent with IHD (described previously). Coronary vasospasm is thought to participate in the mechanisms of toxicity of several agents. Catecholamines such as epinephrine normally enhance coronary blood flow through increased release of metabolic vasodilators (e.g., adenosine) and through a relative increase in diastolic duration at higher heart rates where epinephrine stimulation of beta-adrenergic receptors increases heart rate, contractility, and myocardial oxygen consumption. Thus, catecholamine-induced increases in coronary blood flow largely stem from indirect actions of these agents—effects that largely override direct actions of the agents. In constrast, the direct effect of sympathomimetics on the coronary vasculature includes coronary vasospasm through activation of alpha-adrenergic receptors. When beta-adrenergic receptors are blocked or during underlying pathophysiologic conditions of the heart, the direct actions of sympathomimetics may predominate leading to coronary vasoconstriction. In dogs, for example, coronary artery stenosis produced a coronary vasoconstrictive response mediated by sympathetic nerve stimulation and blocked by alpha-adrenergic receptor antagonists (Heusch and Duessen, 1983). In addition, release of autocoids during underlying pathophysiologic conditions may enhance coronary vasoconstriction. For example, histamine, thromboxane A_2, and some leukotrienes may exert direct coronary vasoconstriction. Finally, some cardiotoxic agents may induce coronary vasoconstriction and subsequent myocardial ischemia as a part of a multicomponent mechanism of toxicity. For example, coronary vasoconstriction has been implicated in cocaine-induced cardiotoxicity (discussed later in the chapter).

Ischemia-Reperfusion Injury As described previously, IHD is a leading cause of morbidity and mortality in the United States and other industrialized nations. Relief of the offending cause of ischemia (e.g., thrombolytic therapy following acute myocardial infarction) provides reperfusion of the myocardium. However, depending on the duration of ischemia, a reversible contractile dysfunction remains for one to several days following reperfusion—a condition referred to as myocardial stunning. Thus, reperfusion of the myocardium leads to subsequent tissue damage that may be reversible or permanent, and this phenomenon is known as ischemia-reperfusion (I/R) injury.

Intracellular acidosis, inhibition of oxidative phosphorylation, and ATP depletion are consequences of myocardial ischemia. Reperfusion of ischemic tissue results in cell death. Several mechanisms have been proposed to account for the reperfusion injury, including the generation of toxic oxygen radicals (O_2 paradox), Ca^{2+} overload (Ca^{2+} paradox), uncoupling of mitochondrial oxidative phosphorylation, and physical damage to the sarcolemma. However, none of these mechanisms adequately explains the cell injury associated with I/R.

A more recent hypothesis to explain the mechanism of cell death associated with I/R injury is the pH paradox (Lemasters et al., 1995). Following reperfusion of the myocardium, reoxygenation, Ca^{2+} loading, and a return to physiologic pH occur. These changes correspond with the onset of cell death. Inhibition of

Na^+/H^+ exchange across the sarcolemma during reperfusion maintains intracellular acidosis and prevents cell killing despite reoxygenation or Ca^{2+} overload. The pH paradox suggests that the acidosis of ischemia is generally protective and that a return to physiologic pH precipitates cell injury. Thus, rescue of ischemic myocardium may be possible to a much greater extent than is generally assumed, provided that the tissue is reperfused at acidic pH, followed by a gradual return of pH to normal levels.

Ischemic Preconditioning An interesting phenonomen related to I/R injury is the paradoxical protection from long-term ischemic injury provided by single or multiple brief periods of ischemia and/or hypoxia (preconditioning). Ischemic preconditioning prior to a longer-term ischemic insult will reduce infarct size, risk of I/R related arrhythmias, and severity of myocardial stunning. Although cardiac myocyte death may be delayed by ischemic preconditioning, cell death is not necessarily prevented. The mechanisms responsible for the paradoxical protection provided by preconditioning are not fully understood, but several likely mechanisms have been proposed. Adenosine may be a major mediator of preconditioning. Acting through its G protein–coupled receptors, adenosine utilizes a wide variety of signaling pathways including phospholipase C, protein kinase C, tyrosine kinases, and MAPK. Subsequently, at least one of the downstream effectors of adenosine receptor activation is the ATP-sensitive K^+ channel, which is phosphorylated after adenosine exposure. Opening of ATP-sensitive K^+ channels residing on the sarcolemmal membrane and/or in the mitochondrial membrane may provide the subsequent protection from I/R injury. At the sarcolemmal membrane level, opening ATP-sensitive K^+ channels would shorten phase 3 of the action potential, hyperpolarize the membrane, reduce Ca^{2+} entry and overload, and spare ATP (Gross and Fryer, 1999). At the mitochondrial membrane level, opening of ATP-sensitive K^+ channels would depolarize the mitochondrial membrane, produce matrix swelling, enhanced respiration, and reduced Ca^{2+} overload in the mitochondria (Gross and Fryer, 1999). Therefore compounds that block ATP-sensitive K^+ channels (e.g., glibenclamide) abolish the protection provided by ischemic preconditioning. Moreover, whether ischemic preconditioning protects the myocardium from xenobiotic-induced injury remains largely unknown.

Oxidative Stress

If a reactive molecule contains one or more unpaired electrons, the molecule is termed a free radical. For many years, much interest has been focused on the biochemistry of oxygen activation and the biological significance of reactive oxygen species. Highly reactive oxygen species are intermediates formed as a normal consequence of a variety of essential biochemical reactions. For example, the univalent stepwise reduction of molecular oxygen to water results in the formation of several potentially toxic intermediates, including superoxide anion radical, hydrogen peroxide, and hydroxyl radical (i.e., prooxidants). Furthermore, superoxide anion can interact with nitric oxide to produce peroxynitrite, which is now recognized as a major contributing radical to oxidative stress-induced damage. Oxidases and electron transport systems are prime and continuous sources of intracellular reactive oxygen species.

An intracellular oxidative environment denotes a shift in the prooxidant/antioxidant balance in favor of the prooxidants; thus oxidative damage inflicted by reactive oxygen species has been called oxidative stress (Sies, 1991). The extent of tissue damage depends on the balance between the free oxygen radicals generated and the antioxidant protective defenses of the tissue. Antioxidant enzymes such as superoxide dismutase, catalase, and glutathione peroxidase are preventive antioxidants because they inactivate or remove the oxygen species involved in lipid peroxidative damage of membranes, inactivation of sulfhydryl-containing enzymes, and cross-linking of integral proteins. Small-molecule antioxidants such as glutathione, ascorbate, and the tocopherols interact directly with free oxygen radicals to detoxify them. Under normal conditions, reactive oxygen species are broken down rapidly by these tissue defensive mechanisms to protect cells against their deleterious effects. The toxic effects of reactive oxygen species are observed only when their rates of formation exceed their rates of inactivation. Figure 18-6 depicts the formation of these reactive oxygen species and their inactivation by specific enzyme systems.

A number of studies have indicated that reactive oxygen species are generated during myocardial ischemia and at the time of reperfusion (Simpson and Lucchesi, 1987; Bolli, 1988). In cardiovascular diseases such as atherosclerosis, oxidative alteration of low-density lipoprotein is thought to be involved in the formation of atherosclerotic plaques. Among the major reactive oxygen species, peroxynitrite and hydroxyl radical are thought to be the most toxic, reacting with membrane phospholipids and proteins and leading to increased membrane fluidity and permeability and loss of membrane integrity. Upon reperfusion of ischemic myocardium, the production of oxygen free radicals has been associated with arrhythmias, myocardial stunning, and cardiac myocyte death. However, it is controversial whether oxygen free radicals contribute significantly to cardiac myocyte death in the clinical setting (Kloner and Przyklenk, 1992). At the subcellular and biochemical levels, reactive oxygen species have been shown to alter

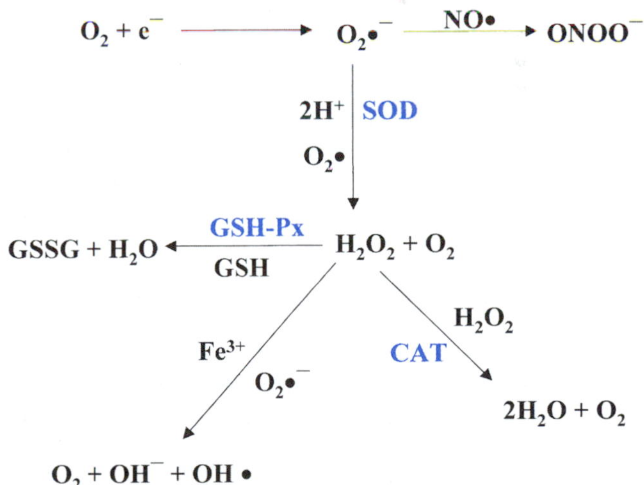

Figure 18-6. Formation and inactivation of reactive oxygen species.

Single-electron reduction of oxygen (O_2) results in the formation of superoxide anion radical ($O_2\bullet^-$). Although $O_2\bullet^-$ is normally maintained at low intracellular concentrations by spontaneous dismutation and/or catalytic breakdown by the enzyme superoxide dismutase (SOD) to form hydrogen peroxide (H_2O_2), it may react with nitric oxide (NO•) to form peroxynitrite ($ONOO^-$). Three possible events may occur with H_2O_2: (1) in the presence of $O_2\bullet^-$ or transition metals such as iron (Fe^{2+}) and copper, it is reduced to the hydroxyl radical (OH•); (2) it may be catalyzed by catalase (CAT) to form water and oxygen; and/or (3) it may be detoxified by glutathione peroxidase (GSH-Px) in the presence of glutathione (GSH) to form water and oxidized glutathione (GSSG).

the activities of enzymes such as Na^+,K^+-ATPase, phospholipase D, glucose-6-phosphatase, and cytochrome oxidase. Calcium homeostasis is also altered by reactive oxygen species, as reflected by modifications in Na^+/Ca^{2+} exchange, sarcoplasmic reticular Ca^{2+} transport, and mitochondrial Ca^{2+} uptake. Figure 18-7 summarizes the adverse effects of reactive oxygen radicals generated during myocardial ischemia and reperfusion.

Xenobiotics may induce cardiotoxicity through generation of reactive oxygen species. For example, two drugs—doxorubicin and ethanol—have been shown to have prominent cardiotoxic effects which have been associated with the production of reactive oxygen species. The role of reactive oxygen species in doxorubicin- and ethanol-induced cardiotoxicity is discussed later in the chapter.

Organellar Dysfunction

Sarcolemmal Injury, SR Dysfunction, and Ca^{2+} Overload Investigations into Ca^{2+} regulation of various cellular functions have been an area of productive research for many years (Carafoli, 1987). The role of Ca^{2+} as a second messenger may be considered an integral function of several systems (not limited to excitation-contraction coupling) and is highly influenced by homeostatic mechanisms. All cells contain elaborate systems for the regulation of intracellular Ca^{2+}. Because of the large concentration gradient of Ca^{2+} (extracellular Ca^{2+} concentrations are typically several orders of magnitude higher than resting intracellular free Ca^{2+}), the sarcolemmal membrane must maintain integrity to prevent a rapid influx of Ca^{2+} and subsequent Ca^{2+} overload (sustained elevated intracellular free Ca^{2+} concentration). As discussed previously, the principal Ca^{2+} regulatory organelle in cardiac myocytes is the sarcoplasmic reticulum (SR), and the SR provides the majority of Ca^{2+} required for contraction. This intricate reliance on the SR serves as a protective mechanism from Ca^{2+} overload allowing tight regulation of Ca^{2+} release instead of a veritable flood of extracellular Ca^{2+} that may activate a variety of proteases, endonucleases, and signaling pathways of apoptotic cell death (Marks, 1997). Thus, prevention of Ca^{2+}-induced cell death is dependent upon sarcolemmal membrane integrity and SR function.

Homeostatic regulation of Ca^{2+} is complicated in the cardiac myocyte, primarily because the cell must allow transient increases in intracellular free Ca^{2+} concentration (Ca^{2+} transients) for contraction to occur. Nonetheless, alterations of cardiac Ca^{2+} homeostasis by toxicants may perturb the regulation of cellular functions beyond the normal range of physiologic control. Intracellular Ca^{2+} overload has been proposed to result in a breakdown of high-energy phosphates. Other cytotoxic effects induced by Ca^{2+} overload include blebbing of the plasma membrane, activation of Ca^{2+}-dependent phospholipases, stimulation of Ca^{2+}-dependent neutral proteases, Ca^{2+}-activated DNA fragmentation, and Ca^{2+} activation of oncocytic and apoptotic cell death as described below.

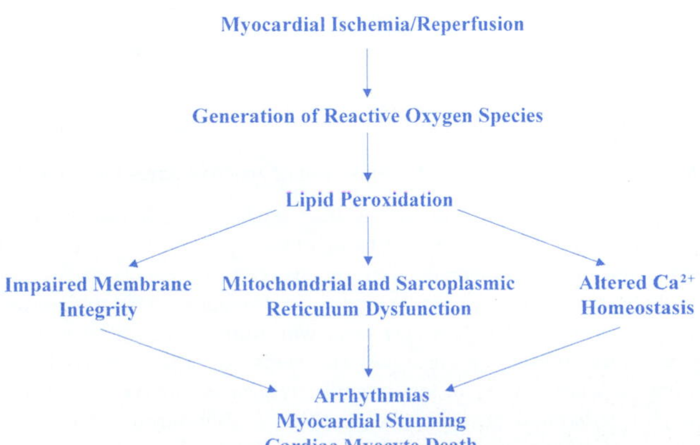

Figure 18-7. Deleterious effects of reactive oxygen species in myocardial ischemia and reperfusion.

A variety of xenobiotics may alter Ca^{2+} homeostasis in the heart. As discussed in further detail later in the chapter, doxorubicin may alter Ca^{2+} homeostasis through several mechanisms including altered sarcolemmal integrity through lipid peroxidation, altered mitochondrial Ca^{2+} handling (Chacon and Acosta, 1991), and/or altered expression of RyR in the SR (Marks, 1997). Catecholamines may also alter Ca^{2+} homeostasis by producing altered sarcolemmal integrity through lipid peroxidation or altered Ca^{2+} permeability. Pharmacological modulation of Ca^{2+} homeostasis has been useful for experiments aimed at delineating sites of potential toxicant-induced alterations in Ca^{2+} homeostasis. High concentrations (i.e., millimolar) of caffeine, for example, activate RyR to release SR Ca^{2+} stores resulting in a massive Ca^{2+} transient and subsequent refractory period to contraction. Yet, in the absence of underlying SR dysfunction, the SR will eventually reload the Ca^{2+} that must be released for contraction. In contrast, ryanodine will block RyR channels thus inhibiting SR Ca^{2+} release. In addition, the immunosuppressant drugs FK506 and rapamycin are known to bind to a regulatory protein associated with RyRs: FK506 binding protein (FKBP). When FK506 or rapamycin bind, FKBP dissociates from the RyR, and sensitivity of the RyR to caffeine is enhanced; consequently, these immunosuppressants may exert a cardiotoxic effect associated with leakage of Ca^{2+} from the SR (Marks, 1997).

Mitochondrial Injury Cells are continuously engaged in various biochemical reactions. In particular, the synthesis of the major cell components requires energy. The energy required for work (e.g., contraction in a cardiac myocyte) is derived from food by oxidizing the nutrients and channeling them into the formation of high-energy phosphate compounds such as adenosine triphosphate (ATP). ATP is the immediate energy source required for work in most biological systems and is obtained mainly through the oxidative phosphorylation of adenine diphosphate (ADP). Oxidative phosphorylation (ATP formation) occurs as a function of cellular respiration. Mitochondria possess an inner membrane and an outer membrane and are subcellular organelles in aerobic eukaryotic cells that are sites of cellular respiration. In essence, mitochondria are the energy producers within a cell. In a highly energy demanding organ such as the heart, mitochondria occupy a large proportion of the cell.

Cellular respiration which gives rise to the formation of ATP is dependent on electron transfer reactions and is measured as oxygen consumption (Scarpa, 1979). Various oxidative pathways in a cell utilize coenzymes such as nicotinamide adenine dinucleotide (NAD^+) and flavin adenine dinucleotide (FAD^+) as electron acceptors, giving rise to their reduced states (NADH and $FADH_2$, respectively). The availability of oxidized coenzymes (NAD^+ and FAD^+) for use as electron acceptors depends on reoxidation of the reduced coenzymes. Molecular oxygen functions as the terminal electron acceptor for coenzyme oxidation. However, the free-energy change for the direct oxidation of NADH or $FADH_2$ by oxygen is larger than that which is usually encountered in biological reactions, and so the electrons are not passed directly to oxygen. The electrons are transferred in a stepwise fashion by means of a series of reversible oxidizable electron acceptor proteins in the inner mitochondrial membrane. These proteins make up the mitochondrial respiratory chain (electron transport chain). Hence, the total free energy available between reduced coenzymes and oxygen is distributed along the respiratory chain. More specifically, the energy of electron transport is used to build up and maintain an electrochemical potential across the inner membrane, establishing the mitochondrial membrane potential.

The process of electron transfer coupled with oxidative phosphorylation is a phenomenon described as coupling (Scarpa, 1979). Electron flow and consequently the rate of oxygen consumption in the presence of substrate and ADP are maximally stimulated (state 3 respiration). After the ADP has been consumed, electron flow and rates of oxygen consumption are low (state 4 respiration). The respiratory control ratio (RCR), which is calculated as the ratio of state 3 to state 4 respiration, can be used to determine the extent of coupling, which provides an index of mitochondrial function and integrity. Mitochondria that show no difference between state 3 and state 4 respiration are termed *uncoupled*. The synthesis of ATP occurs at the expense of the free energy available at three distinct sites (shown in Fig. 18-8) designated as site I (between NADH and coenzyme Q), site II (between cytochrome *b* and cytochrome *c*), and site III (between cytochrome oxidase and oxygen). Because oxygen consumption and ATP synthesis proceed in parallel, substrates entering the respiratory chain at site I give rise to the formation of three molecules of ATP (P/O ratio of 3). Hence, substrates entering the respiratory chain at complex II produce only two molecules of ATP (P/O ratio of 2). The P/O ratio can be calculated by the amount of ATP synthesized (nmoles of ADP added) divided by the nano atoms of oxygen in state 3 respiration.

Oxidative phosphorylation can be affected by several chemical agents (Scarpa, 1979). Respiration can be inhibited at various sites along the respiratory chain by using different chemical inhibitors (Fig. 18-8). Rotenone is an inhibitor that blocks electron transfer between NADH and coenzyme Q (site I). Antimycin A blocks electron transport between coenzyme Q and cytochrome *c* (site II). Cyanide and carbon monoxide block the final step of electron transfer from cytochrome oxidase to oxygen (site III). Conversely, uncouplers stimulate electron flow and respiration but prevent the formation of ATP by short-circuiting the proton current. Uncouplers such as 2,4-dinitrophenol are lipophilic weak acids that may migrate through the lipid membrane and shuttle protons across the membrane, bypassing the normal flow of protons through the ATP synthetase.

In the evaluation of the various cardiac toxicants discussed below (see "Cardiotoxicants," below), mitochondrial injury or dysfunction may be an important element in explaining the mechanism of cardiotoxicity. For a recent review of mitochondrial targets of drug toxicity, see the review article by Wallace and Starkov (2000).

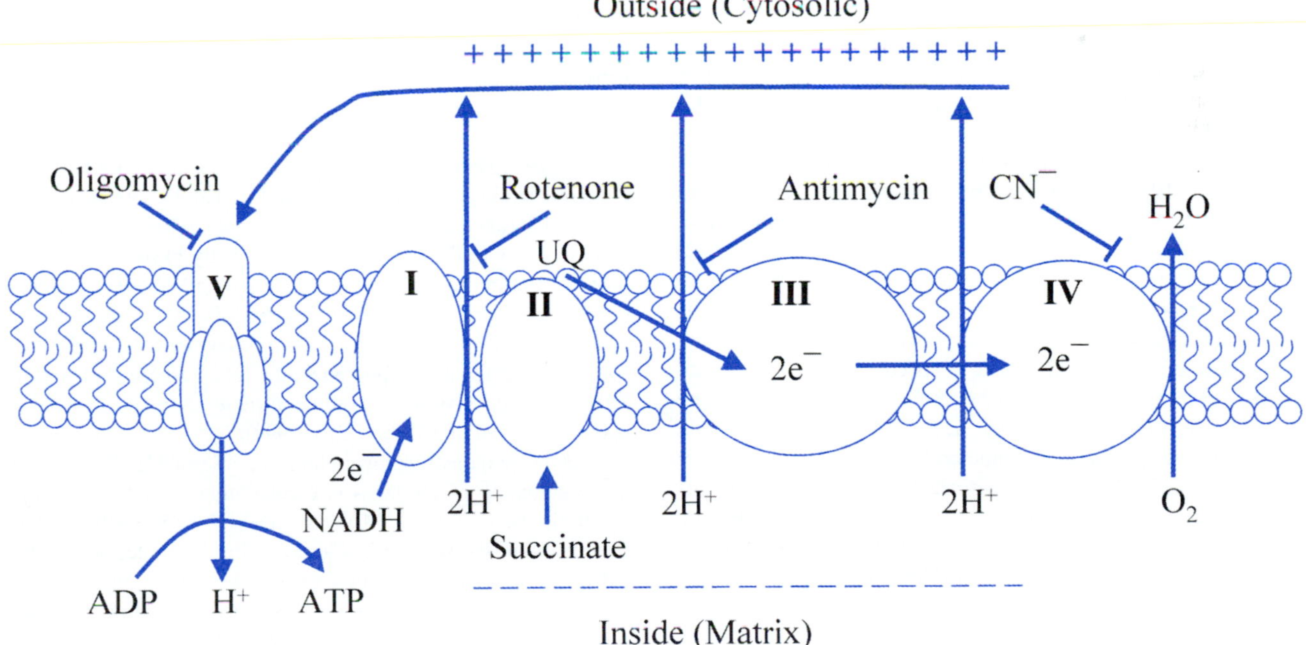

Figure 18-8. Diagram of the electron-transferring complexes I, II, III, and IV and the ATPase (V) present in the inner mitochondrial membrane.

The respective complexes are I, NADH: ubiquinone oxidoreductase; II, succinate: ubiquinone oxidoreductase; III, ubiquinol: ferrocytochrome *c* oxidoreductase; IV, ferrocytochrome *c*: oxygen oxidoreductase; V, ATP synthesase. UQ 5 ubiquinone or coenzyme Q. The mitochondrial electron transport chain is coupled at three points so that the electron transfer between carriers is sufficiently exergonic to drive the transport of protons and to establish an electrochemical proton gradient upon which ATP formation depends. Various inhibitors and their sites are also noted.

Apoptosis and Oncosis

The processes of apoptosis and oncosis are described in numerous places throughout this textbook with regard to basic mechanisms of toxicity and other target organs. Therefore, the mechanisms known to precipitate these processes in numerous cell types are not reviewed in detail in this chapter; rather, focus is on known events occurring within cardiac myocytes. Apoptosis and oncosis are both described as "prelethal" forms of injury, where cell death may eventually occur through necrosis (Trump et al., 1997). Apoptosis is characterized by cellular shrinkage, cytoplasmic blebbing, nuclear chromatin condensation, redistribution of phosphatidylethanolamine and phosphatidylserine from the inner leaflet to outer leaflet of the lipid bilayer, and DNA fragmentation; whereas, oncosis is characterized by cellular swelling, cytoplasmic blebbing, chromatin clumping, and mitochondrial condensation followed by mitochondrial swelling (Haunstetter and Izumo, 1998; Trump et al., 1997). Cardiac myocyte death associated with apoptosis may occur in the heart following ishemic injury, I/R injury, or toxicant-induced injury. In the early periods following myocardial infarction, cardiac myocyte death likely occurs predominantly through apoptotic pathways, whereas necrosis occurs at later time points following the insult (MacLellan and Schneider, 1997). Moreover, apoptotic cardiac myocyte death was found to be a consistent feature of end-stage heart failure in humans, and was quantitatively associated with the clinical severity of deterioration in dilated cardiomyopathy (Saraste et al., 1999). Because IHD is a leading cause of morbidity and mortality in the United States and other industrialized nations, stimuli and signaling pathways responsible for cardiac myocyte apoptosis are currently under intense laboratory investigation.

Apoptotic Stimuli Several peptides and cytokines directly activate apoptotic signaling pathways and death of cardiac myocytes in vitro. These substances include atrial natriuretic peptide (ANP), angiotensin II (also a hypertrophic growth stimulus), tumor necrosis factor alpha (TNF-α), and Fas ligand (Kajstura et al., 1997; Krown et al., 1996; Wu et al., 1997). Furthermore, other proinflammatory cytokines may induce the synthesis and/or release of TNF-α including interleukin-1 (IL-1) and interleukin-2 (IL-2) (Pulkki, 1997). Interestingly, these cytokines and peptides are elevated in the blood and myocardium during the progression of various cardiac diseases, and cardiac myocytes may synthesize and secrete them as well (Pulkki, 1997). As discussed later in the chapter, many of these cytokines depress cardiac function, some acting through production of nitric oxide. Lipid stimuli of apoptosis in cardiac myocytes include ceramide and saturated fatty acids (de Vries et al., 1997). Xenobiotics associated with induction of cardiac myocyte apoptosis in vitro include cocaine, daunorubicin, doxorubicin, isoproterenol (and norepinephrine), and staurosporine (Sawyer et al., 1999; Shizukuda et al., 1998; Umansky et al., 1997). Although the list of known apoptotic stimuli in cardiac myocytes is currently limited, on-going research will undoubtedly identify more stimuli in addition to evaluating the role of apoptosis in the mechanisms of toxicity of previously established cardiotoxicants.

Apoptotic Signal Transduction The literature regarding signaling pathways associated with apoptosis in mammalian cells is colossal. Much less, however, is known about signaling pathways responsible for cardiac myocyte apoptosis. Although these pathways may be relatively conserved among eukaryotes, a greater likelihood of variations of these pathways within cardiac myocytes seems plausible because of the terminally differentiated nature of these cells. As a result, consideration of signaling pathways of apoptosis will be limited to findings in cardiac myocytes. Figure 18-9 is an overview of the known signaling pathways of cardiac myocyte apoptosis. The information in this figure was obtained from investigations spanning 1997–2000. Importantly, variations in these signaling pathways should be expected depending upon species and developmental stage of the cardiac tissue or cells used.

The first central concept of apoptotic signaling in the heart is that generation of reactive oxygen species (ROS) is intimately involved in many of the pathways. Exposure of cardiac myocytes to cytokines, anthracyclines, cocaine, hypoxia, or I/R injury will lead to production of ROS. In cardiac myocytes, ROS are known to upregulate expression of the mitochondrial protein Bax, upregulate and/or activate the tumor suppressor protein p53, upregulate and/or activate nuclear factor-kappa B (NF-κB), activate MAPKs (ERK 1/2, JNK/SAPK, and p38), and for superoxide anion (O_2^-) interact with nitric oxide (NO) to produce peroxynitrite ($ONOO^-$) which subsequently leads to upregulation of Bax expression (Maulik et al., 1999; Turner et al., 1998; von Harsdorf et al., 1999).

The second central concept of apoptotic signaling in the heart is that the mitochondria are critical regulators of apoptotic death. Several members of the Bcl-2 family of proteins are localized on the outer membrane of mitochondria including proapoptotic proteins that facilitate the release of mitochondrial cytochrome *c* (i.e., Bax, Bad, Bak) and antiapoptotic proteins that inhibit the release of mitochondrial cytochrome *c* (i.e., Bcl-2, Mcl-1, Bcl-X_L). Under physiologic conditions, cardiac myocytes express significant quantities of Bcl-2 and other antiapoptotic members of the Bcl-2 family; however, when Bax expression is upregulated, the cells will be at risk of apoptotic death (O'Rourke, 1999). Thus, the Bcl-2/Bax expression ratio has become an indicator of susceptibility to and activation of apoptosis. Release of cytochrome *c* occurs, at least theoretically, through the opening of an inner mitochondrial membrane permeability transition pore and perhaps other ion channels (O'Rourke, 1999). Subsequently, cytochrome *c* in conjuction with apoptotic protease activating factor-1 (Apaf-1) activates the cytosolic aspartate-specific cysteine protease (caspase 9). Caspase 9 then activates caspase 3 which subsequently cleaves a variety of proteins leading to inactivation of poly (ADP-ribose) polymerase (PARP) and protein kinase C-δ (PKC-δ). Although somewhat controversial, PARP is a DNA repair enzyme that is believed to participate as an antiapoptic enzyme; thus, caspase 3 cleavage of PARP to an inactive form would contribute to the development of apoptosis (Reed and Paternostro, 1999).

Much remains unknown about the role of MAPKs and PKC in the signaling of apoptosis in cardiac myocytes; however, many apoptotic stimuli activate MAPKs (ERK 1/2, JNK/SAPK, and p38) during apoptosis of cardiac myocytes. For example, doxorubicin, I/R injury, and ROS are known to activate MAPKs in cardiac myocytes undergoing apoptosis. Increasing evidence suggests that activation of ERK 1/2 is a protective mechanism in cardiac myocytes (see signaling pathways of hypertrophic growth) because inhibitors of ERK 1/2 activation have been shown to exacerbate apoptosis while inhibitors of JNK/SAPK and p38 have been shown to inhibit apoptosis from a number of different stimuli (Yue et al., 2000). Therefore, activation of JNK/SAPK and p38 may be actively involved in promoting apoptotic death of cardiac myocytes.

Other signaling pathways of apoptosis in cardiac myocytes include effects arising from beta-adrenergic receptor stimulation and activation of cytokine receptors. In cardiac myocytes, stimu-

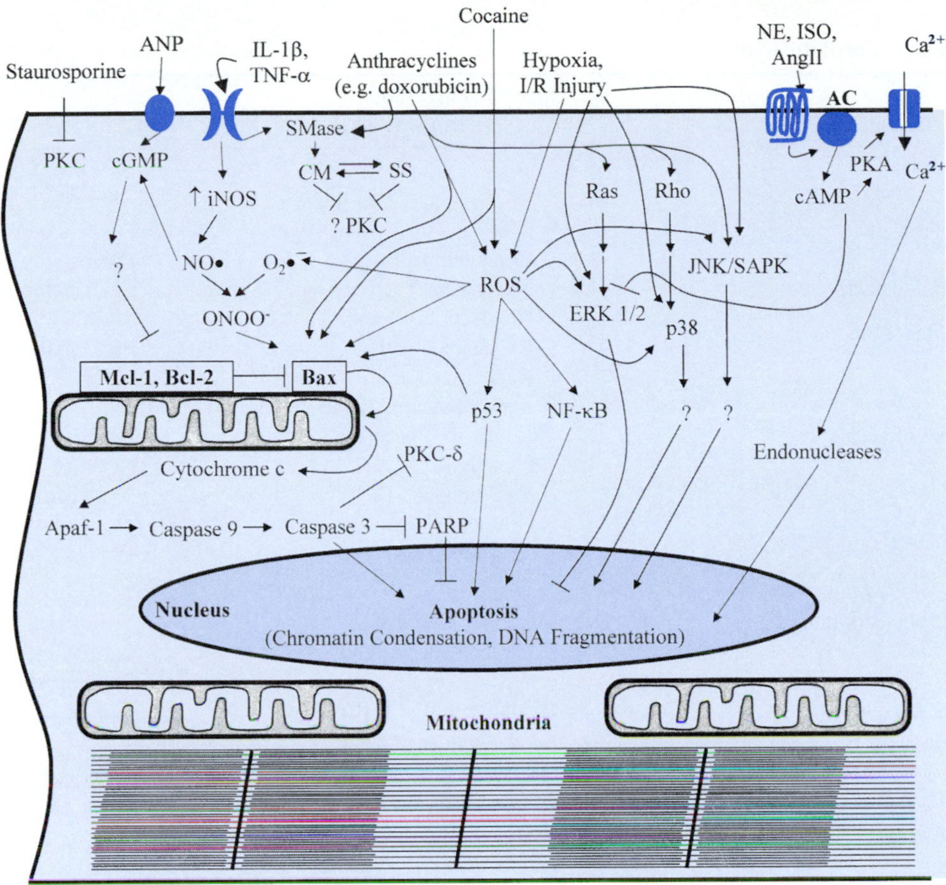

Figure 18-9. Signal transduction pathways involved in apoptotic death of cardiac myocytes.

The figure represents a simplistic view of the signaling pathways involved in apoptotic death of cardiac myocytes. The pathways presented in the figure are from the literature referenced throughout the text, and only those pathways where evidence has demonstrated the presence in cardiac myocytes or heart tissue are presented. Significant "cross-talk" between various pathways is present, and opposing pathways are not shown. Arrows represent activation or increases in second messengers. Question marks represent additional steps leading to the response have not been identified. Abbreviations for stimuli: AngII, angiotensin II; ANP, atrial natriuretic peptide; Ca^{2+}, calcium; IL-1β, interleukin-1β; I/R, ischemia/reperfusion injury; ISO, isoproterenol; NE, norepinephrine. *Abbreviations for pathways:* AC, adenylyl cyclase; Apaf-1, apoptotic protease activating factor-1; Bax, homolog of Bcl-2, a protein originally identified in B cell lymphoma; Ca^{2+}, intracellular free calcium; cAMP, cyclic adenosine monophosphate; cGMP, cyclic guanosine monophosphate; CM ceramide; ERK $\frac{1}{2}$ extracellular signal-regulated kinases 1 and 2; iNOS, inducible nitric oxide synthase; JNK/SAPK, c-Jun N-terminal kinase/stress activated protein kinase; Mcl-1, homolog of Bcl-2; NF-κB, nuclear factor-κB; NO•, nitric oxide; $O_2•^-$, superoxide anion radical; $ONOO^-$, peroxynitrite; PARP, poly ADP-ribose polymerase; p38, 38-kDa member of the mitogen-activated protein kinase family; p53, 53-kDa tumor suppressor protein; PKA, protein kinase A; PKC, protein kinase C; Ras, a GTPase; Rho, a GTPase; ROS, reactive oxygen species; Smase, sphingomyelinase; SS, sphingosine.

lation of beta-adrenergic receptors (e.g. from norepinephrine or isoproterenol) leads to activation of adenylyl cyclase with resulting increases in cyclic AMP, activation of protein kinase A (PKA), and phosphorylation and activation of L-type Ca^{2+} channels (Communal et al., 1998). Entry of Ca^{2+} then may lead to activation of Ca^{2+}-dependent proteases and endonucleases culminating in apoptosis. In contrast, cytokine receptor stimulation (e.g., by IL-1β) in cardiac myocytes leads to upregulation of inducible nitric oxide synthase (iNOS), increased production of NO, formation of $ONOO^-$ and upregulation of Bax (Arstall et al., 1999). Furthermore, TNF-α receptor stimulation activates sphingomyelinase (SMase) to increase ceramide (CM) and sphingosine (SS) which subsequently induce apoptosis (Krown et al., 1996).

Often, no single biochemical event can explain the process by which a chemical agent is cardiotoxic. Thus, several of the biochemical mechanisms discussed in this section may be interrelated and may help explain the cardiotoxicity of selected chemical agents. Table 18-1 summarizes the general mechanisms of cardiotoxicity including some of the cellular perturbations involved and organ manifestations.

CARDIOTOXICANTS

For simplicity, the cardiotoxicants have been classified into three major groups: (1) pharmaceutical agents including drugs of social use and abuse; (2) natural occurring substances including hor-

Table 18-1
General Mechanisms of Cardiotoxicity

MECHANISM	CELLULAR PERTURBATIONS	ORGAN MANIFESTATIONS
Interference with ion homeostasis		
Inhibition of Na^+/K^+ ATPase	↑ $[Ca^{2+}]_i$, ↓ Conduction velocity	Positive inotropic effect Proarrhythmic
Na^+ channel blockade	↓ Na^+ channel activity ↓ Conduction velocity	Proarrhythmic
K^+ channel blockade	↓ K^+ channel activity ↓ Repolarization ↑ Action potential duration	Proarrhythmic
Ca^{2+} channel blockade	↓ L-type Ca^{2+} channel activity ↓ Ca^{2+}-induced-Ca^{2+} release ↓ AV Conduction	Negative inotropic effect Negative chronotropic effect Bradycardia
Altered coronary blood flow		
Coronary vasoconstriction or obstruction	Ischemia (ATP depletion, intracellular acidosis)	Myocardial infarction Cardiac myocyte death Cardiac remodeling
Ischemia/reperfusion injury	Oxidative stress, ↑ $[Ca^{2+}]_i$ Intracellular pH change	Cardiac myocyte death
Oxidative stress	Lipid peroxidation DNA damage Mitochondrial dysfunction, Altered $[Ca^{2+}]_i$ homeostasis	Cardiac myocyte death
Organellar dysfunction		
Sarcolemmal injury	Altered membrane integrity	Cardiac myocyte death
Sarcoplasmic reticulum dysfunction	Altered $[Ca^{2+}]_i$ homeostasis	Cardiac myocyte death
Mitochondrial injury	ATP depletion Cytochrome *c* release Altered mitochondrial $[Ca^{2+}]_i$ homeostasis	Cardiac myocyte death
Apoptosis	Cellular shrinkage Sarcolemmal blebbing Chromatin condensation Redistribution of membrane phospholipids DNA fragmentation	Cardiac myocyte death
Oncosis	Cellular swelling Sarcolemmal blebbing Chromatin clumping Mitochondrial swelling	Cardiac myocyte death

mones, cytokines, and animal and plant toxins; and (3) industrial chemicals and other miscellaneous agents. Wherever possible, the major biochemical mechanisms of cardiotoxicity proposed for the agents under discussion are emphasized.

Pharmaceutical Agents

The cardiotoxicity of a pharmacologically active cardiovascular drug often represents an overexpression of its principal pharmacologic effect on the heart (Sperelakis, 1992). For example, digitalis, quinidine, and procainamide may induce cardiac arrhythmias as an exaggerated pharmacologic action of the drugs. In contrast, other cardiovascular drugs may produce cardiotoxicity by actions that are not necessarily related to their intended therapeutic use and principal pharmacologic effects. For instance, in addition to their pharmacologic actions on the myocardium and because of their pronounced sympathomimetic actions, the catecholamines may exert cardiotoxicity through their biochemical effects on certain cellular and subcellular processes (e.g., oxidative stress and calcium overload). Furthermore, other pharmaceutical agents, such as antibacterial agents, anthracyclines, and other antineoplastic agents, may produce myocardial injury and other cardiotoxic effects that are not related to their therapeutic and pharmacologic uses. The agents chosen for discussion do not necessarily encompass a comprehensive list of compounds that are potentially cardiotoxic; however, major classes of each group of compounds are discussed, and in many cases cardiotoxicity may be at least a potential concern with similar agents in the same class. Table 18-2 provides a summary of key pharmaceutical agents with their prominent cardiotoxic effects and proposed mechanisms of toxicity.

Alcohol Ethanol cardiotoxicity can be divided into two categories: acute and chronic (associated with alcoholism). The acute toxicity of ethanol includes a negative dromotropic effect (reduced conductivity) and a decreased threshold for ventricular fibrillation. However, arrhythmias are prominent only after long-term or chronic exposure. The chronic consumption of ethanol by humans has been associated with myocardial abnormalities and dysfunction, a condition or syndrome known as alcoholic cardiomyopathy that may present similar symptoms as congestive heart failure.

Alcoholic Cardiomyopathy Chronic ethanol consumption and its implications in cardiac disease were first reported in the early 1960s. However, for many decades the role of ethanol in the pathogenesis of alcoholic cardiomyopathy was not widely understood, mainly because heart dysfunction was attributed to thiamine deficiency secondary to alcoholism (beriberi heart disease) and other types of malnutrition or to specific additives found in alcoholic beverages, such as cobalt (beer drinker's cardiomyopathy). However, more recent studies have clearly demonstrated that cardiac dysfunction in alcoholics can be dissociated from nutritional deficiencies and beriberi heart disease. In addition, the withdrawal of ethanol from patients with myocardial dysfunction may reverse many of the clinical symptoms, providing more evidence that ethanol is involved in the pathogenesis of the cardiomyopathy.

After years of investigation, it was proposed that the metabolite acetaldehyde is responsible for some of the cardiac injury associated with ethanol consumption. The metabolic enzyme responsible for the conversion of ethanol to acetaldehyde is alcohol dehydrogenase, which is absent in cardiac myocytes. Oxidation of ethanol to acetaldehyde proceeds at a rate that is independent of blood concentration. Studies have indicated that the impaired liver function of alcoholics may be sufficient to generate quantities of acetaldehyde that can reach the heart. The direct effects of acetaldehyde on the myocardium include inhibition of protein synthesis, inhibition of Ca^{2+} sequestration by the SR, alterations in mitochondrial respiration, and disturbances in the association of actin and myosin. The exact mechanism of alcoholic cardiomyopathy is unresolved. It has been suggested that a combination of multiple factors is involved and that certain conditions may predispose an individual to cardiac injury from ethanol. Factors such as chronic ethanol consumption, malnutrition, cigarette smoking, systemic hypertension, and beverage additives have all been implicated as potential contributors that can result in alcoholic cardiomyopathy (Ahmed and Regan, 1992).

Mechanisms of Alcohol-Induced Cardiotoxicity There is suggestive evidence that the generation of reactive oxidative metabolites from the metabolism of ethanol may lead to lipid peroxidation of cardiac myocytes or oxidation of cytosolic and membraneous protein thiols (Ribiere et al., 1992). Additional evidence that reactive oxidative metabolites derived from ethanol may be involved in the pathogenesis of alcoholic cardiomyopathy is provided by the report by Redetzki et al. (1983), who showed that pretreatment of rodents with α-tocopherol (vitamin E) before an acute dose of ethanol prevented increases in lactate dehydrogenase isoenzymes in the plasma and reduced ultrastructural evidence of myocardial injury. Because α-tocopherol can serve as an antioxidant and a free radical scavenger, this study suggested that ethanol-induced heart injury was mediated by the generation of free radicals from ethanol metabolism. Other investigations have shown that ethanol administration may increase the conversion of xanthine dehydrogenase to xanthine oxidase, an enzyme involved in the generation of superoxide anions, and may enhance the activity of peroxisomal acyl-CoA oxidase and catalase in rat myocardium. These two enzymes may increase the production of hydrogen peroxide and acetaldehyde, which may contribute to myocardial lipid peroxidation by ethanol treatment.

Antiarrhythmic and Inotropic Agents Antiarrhythmic agents have historically been classified based upon a primary mechanism of action: Na^+ channel blockers (class I), beta-adrenergic blockers (class II), agents that prolong action potential duration especially K^+ channel blockers (class III), and Ca^{2+} channel blockers (class IV). However, this classification scheme is somewhat confusing given the lack of specificity of most of the agents with one particular channel or receptor. Most of the antiarrhythmic drugs have cardiotoxic actions as a result of their pharmacologic effects. A review of the proarrhythmic mechanisms of antiarrhythmic drugs is provided by Nattel (1998). Inotropic agents include the cardiac glycosides, Ca^{2+} sensitizing agents, catecholamines, and other sympathomimetic agents. As with the antiarrhythmic drugs, inotropic agents may exert cardiotoxic effects through extensions of their pharmacologic mechanism. A brief review of antiarrhythmic and inotropic drug-induced cardiotoxicity is included; however, a wealth of literature regarding the proarrhythmic effects of these agents exists, and where appropriate, review articles have been suggested.

Na^+ Channel Blockers The class I antiarrhythmic agents are primarily Na^+ channel blockers and include disopyramide, encainide, flecainide, lidocaine, mexiletine, moricizine, phenytoin, procainamide, propafenone, quinidine, and tocainide. Blockade of cardiac Na^+ channels results in reduction of conduction velocity, prolonged QRS duration, decreased automaticity, and inhibition of triggered activity from delayed afterdepolarizations or early afterdepolarizations (Roden, 1996). Excessively slowed conduction may facilitate re-entry arrhythmias thus providing a proarrhythmic effect. As mentioned previously, the primary concern of Na^+ channel blocker toxicity is that proarrhythmic effects are seen at a much higher incidence in those patients with a previous history of myocardial infarction or with acute myocardial ischemia (Nattel, 1998). Furthermore, the possibility is likely that proarrhythmic effects of these agents would also be more prevalent in patients with other cardiovascular diseases. Importantly, encainide, flecainide, propafenone, and quinidine are all substrates for gastrointestinal and hepatic cytochrome P450 3A4. Therefore, concomitant use of these class I antiarrhythmic agents with other drugs that inhibit cytochrome P450 3A4 is contraindicated because of increased serum concentrations of the antiarrhythmic agents. As discussed throughout this chapter, substrates and/or inhibitors of cytochrome P450 3A4 include, but are not limited to, the macrolide antibacterials, azole antifungals, benzodiazepines, human immunodeficiency virus (HIV) protease inhibitors, non-nucleoside reverse transcriptase inhibitors, astemizole, terfenadine, and cisapride.

Table 18-2
Cardiotoxicity of Key Pharmaceutical Agents

AGENTS	CARDIOTOXIC MANIFESTATIONS	PROPOSED MECHANISMS OF CARDIOTOXICITY
Ethanol	↓ Conductivity (acute) Cardiomyopathy (chronic)	Acetaldehyde (metabolite) Altered $[Ca^{2+}]_i$ homeostasis Oxidative stress Mitochondrial injury
Antiarrhythmic drugs		
Class I (disopyramide, encainide, flecainide, lidocaine, mexiletine, moricizine, phenytoin, procainamide, propafenone, quinidine, tocainide)	↓ Conduction velocity Proarrhythmic	Na^+ channel blockade
Class II (acebutolol, esmolol, propranolol, sotalol)	Bradycardia, heart block	β-adrenergic receptor blockade
Class III (amiodarone, bretylium, dofetilide, ibutilide, quinidine, sotalol)	↑ Action potential duration QTc interval prolongation Proarrhythmic	K^+ channel blockade
Class IV (diltiazem, verapamil)	↓ AV Conduction Negative inotropic effect Negative chronotropic effect Bradycardia	Ca^{2+} channel blockade
Inotropic drugs and related agents		
Cardiac glycosides (digoxin, digitoxin)	Action potential duration AV conduction Parasympathomimetic (low doses) Sympathomimetic (high doses)	Inhibition of Na^+,K^+-ATPase, ↑ $[Ca^{2+}]_i$
Ca^{2+} sensitizing agents (adibendan, levosimendan, pimobendan)	↓ Diastolic function? Proarrhythmic?	↑ Ca^{2+} sensitivity, Inhibition of phosphodiesterase
Other Ca^{2+} sensitizing agents (allopurinol, oxypurinol)	?	Inhibition of xanthine oxidase
Catecholamines (dobutamine, epinephrine, isoproterenol, norepinephrine)	Tachycardia Cardiac myocyte death	β_1-adrenergic receptor activation Coronary vasoconstriction Mitochondrial dysfunction ↑ $[Ca^{2+}]_i$ Oxidative stress Apoptosis
Bronchodilators (albuterol, bitolterol, fenoterol, formeterol, metaproterenol, pirbuterol, procaterol, salmeterol, terbutaline)	Tachycardia	Non-selective activation of β_1-adrenergic receptors
Nasal decongestants (ephedrine, ephedrine	Tachycardia	Non-selective activation of β_1-adrenergic receptors

(continued)

Table 18-2 Cardiotoxicity of Key Pharmaceutical Agents (*continued*)

AGENTS	CARDIOTOXIC MANIFESTATIONS	PROPOSED MECHANISMS OF CARDIOTOXICITY
alkaloids, ma huang, phenylephrine, phenylpropanolamine, pseudoephedrine)		
Appetite suppressants (amphetamines, fenfluramine, phentermine)	Tachycardia, Pulmonary hypertension Valvular disease	↑ Serotonin? Na^+ channel blockade?
Antineoplastic drugs		
Anthracyclines (daunorubicin, doxorubicin, epirubicin)	Cardiomyopathy Heart failure	Altered $[Ca^{2+}]_i$ homeostasis Oxidative stress Mitochondrial injury Apoptosis
5-Fluorouracil	Proarrhythmic	Coronary vasospasm?
Cyclophosphamide	Cardiac myocyte death	4-Hydroxycyclophosphamide (metabolite) Altered ion homeostasis
Antibacterial drugs		
Aminoglycosides (amikacin, gentamicin, kanamycin, netilmicin, streptomycin, tobramycin)	Negative inotropic effect	↓ $[Ca^{2+}]_i$
Macrolides (azithromycin, clarithromycin, dirithromycin, erythromycin)	↑ Action potential duration QTc interval prolongation Proarrhythmic	K^+ channel blockade
Fluoroquinolones (grepafloxacin, moxifloxacin, sparfloxacin)	↑ Action potential duration QTc interval prolongation Proarrhythmic	K^+ channel blockade
Tetracycline	Negative inotropic effect	↓ $[Ca^{2+}]_i$
Chloramphenicol	Negative inotropic effect	↓ $[Ca^{2+}]_i$
Antifungal drugs		
Amphotericin B	Negative inotropic effect	Ca^{2+} channel blockade? Na^+ channel blockade? ↑ Membrane permeability?
Flucytosine	Proarrhythmic Cardiac arrest	5-fluorouracil metabolite Coronary vasospasm?
Antiviral drugs		
Nucleoside analog reverse transcriptase inhibitors (stavudine, zalcitabine, zidovudine)	Cardiomyopathy	Mitochondrial injury Inhibition of mitochondrial DNA polymerase Inhibition of mitochondrial DNA synthesis Inhibition of mitochondrial ATP synthesis
Centrally acting drugs		
Tricyclic antidepressants (amitriptyline,	ST segment elevation QTc interval prolongation	Altered ion homeostasis Ca^{2+} channel blockade

(continued)

Table 18-2 Cardiotoxicity of Key Pharmaceutical Agents (*continued*)

AGENTS	CARDIOTOXIC MANIFESTATIONS	PROPOSED MECHANISMS OF CARDIOTOXICITY
desipramine, doxepin, imipramine, protriptyline)	Proarrhythmic Cardiac arrest	Na^+ channel blockade K^+ channel blockade
Selective serotonin reuptake inhibitors (fluoxetine)	Bradycardia, Atrial fibrillation	Ca^{2+} channel blockade Na^+ channel blockade
Phenothiazine antipsychotic drugs (chlorpromazine, thioridazine) Other antipsychotic drugs (clozapine)	Anticholinergic effects Negative inotropic effect QTc interval prolongation PR interval prolongation Blunting of T waves ST segment depression	Ca^{2+} channel blockade?
General inhalational anesthetics (enflurane, desflurane, halothane, isoflurane, methoxyflurane, sevoflurane)	Negative inotropic effect Decreased cardiac output Proarrhythmic	Ca^{2+} channel blockade Altered Ca^{2+} homeostasis β-adrenergic receptor sensitization
Other general anesthetics (propofol)	Negative inotropic effect	Ca^{2+} channel blockade Altered Ca^{2+} homeostasis, β-adrenergic receptor sensitization
Local anesthetics		
Cocaine	Sympathomimetic effects Ischemia/myocardial infarction Proarrhythmic Cardiac arrest Cardiac myocyte death	Na^+ channel blockade Coronary vasospasm, Altered Ca^{2+} homeostasis Mitochondrial injury Oxidative stress Apoptosis
Other local anesthetics (bupivacaine, etidocaine, lidocaine, procainamide)	Decreased excitability ↓ Conduction velocity Proarrhythmic	Na^+ channel blockade
Antihistamines		
(astemizole, terfenadine)	↑ Action potential duration QTc interval prolongation Proarrhythmic	K^+ channel blockade
Immunosuppressants		
(rapamycin, tacrolimus)	Cardiomyopathy Heart failure	Altered Ca^{2+} homeostasis
Miscellaneous drugs		
Cisapride	↑ Action potential duration QTc interval prolongation Proarrhythmic	K^+ channel blockade
Methylxanthines (theophylline)	↑ Cardiac ouput Tachycardia Proarrhythmic	Altered Ca^{2+} homeostasis, Inhibition of phosphodiesterase
Sildenafil	?	Inhibition of phosphodiesterase
Radiocontrast agents (diatrizoate-meglumine, iohexol)	Proarrhythmic Cardiac arrest	Apoptosis?

K^+ Channel Blockers The class III antiarrhythmic agents are drugs which prolong action potential duration, primarily by blockade of cardiac K^+ channels. These agents include amiodarone, bretylium, dofetilide, ibutilide, quinidine, and sotalol. Blockade of K^+ channels increases action potential duration and increases refractoriness (cell is undergoing repolarization and is refractory to depolarization). Prolonged action potential duration contributes to the development of early afterdepolarizations and promotion of tachycardia, especially polymorphic ventricular tachycardia (torsades de pointes). Most of the agents in this class also affect other ion channels and/or receptors. Amiodarone and quinidine also block Na^+ channels while sotalol inhibits beta-adrenergic receptors in the heart. Amiodarone prolongs action potential duration and effective refractory period of Purkinje fibers and ventricular myocytes, and the most common adverse cardiovascular effect of amiodarone is bradycardia. However, amiodarone may have cardiotoxic effects by stimulating excessive Ca^{2+} uptake, especially in the presence of procaine (Gotzsche and Pederson, 1994). In addition, amiodarone induces a variety of other adverse effects at relatively high incidence including pulmonary toxicity (interstitial pneumonitis), thyroid toxicity, hepatotoxicity, neurotoxicity, ocular toxicity, and dermatologic toxicity. As with the Na^+ channel blockers, the proarrhythmic effects of K^+ channels blockers is enhanced in those patients with other forms of cardiac dysfunction include myocardial infarction and cardiac hypertrophy. Amiodarone and quinidine are substrates for cytochromes P450 3A4. Therefore, the concomitant use of amiodarone or quinidine is contraindicated with other drugs that inhibit cytochromes P450 3A4 (e.g., macrolides, azole antifungals, HIV protease inhibitors, nonnucleoside reverse transcriptase inhibitors, and many other drugs). With the multitude of K^+ channels expressed in human heart, it seems possible that improved antiarrhythmic agents in this class could be developed.

Ca^{2+} Channel Blockers The class IV antiarrhythmic agents are Ca^{2+} channel blockers and include diltiazem and verapamil. The dihydropyridine Ca^{2+} channel blocking agents are not used to treat arrhythmias because they have a greater selectivity for vascular cells; however, these agents may also alter cardiac ion homeostasis when plasma concentrations of the drugs are elevated. The dihydropyridines interact with Ca^{2+} channels in the inactivated state of the channel, and because vascular smooth muscle resting potentials are lower than cardiac cells, the time spent in the inactivated state is relatively longer in vascular smooth muscle thus providing some preference of dihydropyridines for the vasculature (Galan et al., 1998). As described previously, bepridil, verapamil, and diltiazem exert negative inotropic and chronotropic effects (see "General Mechanisms of Cardiotoxicity," above). As discussed previously, these drugs exert a negative chronotropic effect and may produce bradycardia. In contrast, the dihydropyridine Ca^{2+} channel blockers typically induce a reflex tachycardia subsequent to peripheral vascular dilation and baroreceptor reflex leading to increased sympathetic outflow from the medulla. Verapamil and diltiazem are substrates for cytochrome P450 3A4; therefore, use of these drugs is cautioned in patients who are taking drugs that inhibit cytochrome P450 3A4. Moreover, verapamil and diltiazem may increase serum digoxin concentrations during concomitant use. These drug interactions do not involve inhibition of cytochrome P450 3A4 because digoxin is not significantly metabolized, but rather, altered renal elimination or volume of distribution.

Beta-Adrenergic Receptor Blocking Agents The class II antiarrhythmic agents are beta-adrenergic receptor blocking agents, and those used to treat arrhythmias include acebutolol, esmolol, propranolol, and sotalol. The catecholamines increase contractility, heart rate, and conduction through activation of beta-adrenergic receptors in the heart. These effects can be explained by increased adenylyl cyclase activity, increased cyclic AMP, activation of protein kinase A, and phosphorylation and activation of L-type Ca^{2+} channels thereby increasing intracellular Ca^{2+}, and particularly the amplitude of the Ca^{2+} transient (see "Catecholamines and sympathomimetics," below). Therefore, antagonists of beta-adrenergic receptors in the heart lead to effects that are opposite that of catecholamines and are useful for the treatment of supraventricular tachycardia. The main adverse cardiovascular effect of beta-adrenergic receptor antagonists is hypotension. However, these drugs may exacerbate AV conduction deficits (e.g., heart block) and promote arrhythmias during bradycardia. As discussed previously, sotalol also inhibits K^+ channels in the heart, thus carrying the proarrhythmic effects of class III antiarrhythmic drugs. Propranolol may also block Na^+ channels (often described as a "membrane stabilizing" effect of propranolol) thereby carrying the proarrhythmic effects of class I antiarrhythmic drugs.

Cardiac Glycosides Cardiac glycosides (digoxin and digitoxin) are inotropic agents used for the treatment of congestive heart failure. Ouabain is a cardiac glycoside commonly used in the laboratory for electrophysiologic experiments in cardiac myocytes. As previously described, the mechanism of inotropic action of cardiac glycosides involves inhibition of Na^+,K^+-ATPase, elevation of intracellular Na^+, activation of Na^+/Ca^{2+} exchange, and increased availability of intracellular Ca^{2+} for contraction. Consequently, cardiotoxicity may result from Ca^{2+} overload, and arrhythmias may occur. However, the cardiovascular effects of cardiac glycosides are complex because of direct and indirect actions. As to the direct effects in addition to inhibition of Na^+,K^+-ATPase, cardiac glycosides initially prolong and then shorten action potential duration, perhaps through Ca^{2+}-induced activation of K^+ channels. Cardiac glycosides may also reduce resting membrane potential (less negative), induce delayed afterdepolarizations perhaps due to Ca^{2+} overload, and induce premature ventricular contraction or ectopic beats when membrane potential is reduced to threshold. As to the indirect effects, cardiac glycosides exhibit parasympathomimetic activity through vagal stimulation and facilitation of muscarinic transmission; however, at higher doses, sympathomimetic effects may occur as sympathetic outflow is enhanced. The principal adverse cardiac effects of cardiac glycosides include slowed AV conduction with potential block, ectopic beats, and bradycardia; however, during overdose, when resting membrane potential is significantly altered and ectopic beats are prevalent, ventricular tachycardia may develop and could progress to ventricular fibrillation. Importantly, a wide variety of drug interactions with digoxin have been reported, including both pharmacokinetic interactions (drugs that alter serum concentrations of digoxin) and pharmacodynamic interactions (drugs that alter the cardiac effects of digoxin).

Ca^{2+}-Sensitizing Agents The newest class of agents that may be useful inotropic drugs for the treatment of heart failure have been designated as Ca^{2+}-sensitizing agents (e.g., adibendan, levosimendan, and pimobendan). The main mechanism by which clinically available inotropic agents work is elevating intracellular free Ca^{2+} ($[Ca^{2+}]_i$) during the Ca^{2+} transient (i.e., increase the amplitude of the Ca^{2+} transient). Several pharmacologic means exist to achieve this effect: Na^+,K^+-ATPase inhibitors increase $[Ca^{2+}]_i$ by elevating intracellular Na^+ and activating Na^+/Ca^{2+} exchange;

beta-adrenergic receptor agonists elevate $[Ca^{2+}]_i$ by activating adenylyl cyclase (to increase cyclic AMP) and protein kinase A which phosporylate and activate L-type Ca^{2+} channels in the plasma membrane; and phosphodiesterase inhibitors reduce the degradation of cyclic AMP. However, these mechanisms carry the risk of inducing Ca^{2+} overload. Therefore, considerable effort has gone into a search for compounds that increase Ca^{2+} sensitivity of cardiac myocytes, thereby obviating the need to increase $[Ca^{2+}]_i$ (Lee and Allen, 1997). Several compounds have been identified that increase the sensitivity of cardiac myocyte contractions to Ca^{2+} without increasing $[Ca^{2+}]_i$, but the mechanism(s) responsible remain elusive and may include inhibition of cardiac phosphodiesterase. Although cardiotoxicity from the Ca^{2+} overload mechanism would not be expected following administration of these new agents, some experimental data suggests that they may still exert proarrhythmic effects—isolated working rat heart models demonstrated enhanced ventricular arrhythmias from some of these compounds (Lee and Allen, 1997). The possibility that such Ca^{2+}-sensitizing agents interfere with diastolic function (relaxation) requires further investigation but may contribute to the ventricular arrhythmias associated with these drugs. Other Ca^{2+}-sensitizing agents include the xanthine oxidase inhibitors allopurinol and oxypurinol, which have been shown to increase contractile force but decrease Ca^{2+} transient amplitude (Perez et al., 1998). The long clinical history of allopurinol use suggests that cardiotoxicity would be minimal if these drugs were used as inotropic agents.

Catecholamines and Sympathomimetics Catecholamines represent a chemical class of neurotransmitters synthesized in the adrenal medulla (epinephrine and norepinephrine) and in the sympathetic nervous system (norepinephrine). These neurotransmitters exert a wide variety of cardiovascular effects. Because of their ability to activate alpha- and beta-adrenergic receptors, especially in the cardiovascular system, a number of synthetic catecholamines have been developed for the treatment of cardiovascular disorders and other conditions such as asthma and nasal congestion. Inotropic and chronotropic catecholamines used to treat bradycardia, cardiac decompensation following surgery, or to increase blood pressure (e.g. hypotensive shock) include epinephrine, isoproterenol, and dobutamine, and these drugs typically display non-selective activation of adrenergic receptors. More selective $beta_2$-adrenergic receptor agonists used for bronchodilatory effects in asthma include albuterol, bitolterol, fenoterol, formoterol, metaproterenol, pirbuterol, procaterol, salmeterol, and terbutaline. High oral doses of albuterol or terbutaline or inhalational doses (i.e., enhanced delivery to the stomach instead of the lungs with subsequent systemic absorption) of these agents may lead to non-selective activation of $beta_1$-adrenergic receptors in the heart with subsequent tachycardia. Sympathomimetic drugs that are more selective for alpha-adrenergic receptors include the nasal decongestants ephedrine, phenylephrine, phenylpropanolamine, and pseudoephedrine. As with the asthma drugs, at high doses of nasal decongestants can produce tachycardia, and a number of deaths have been reported. Of particular interest is the high concentration of ephedra alkaloids that may be present in some herbal remedies or "neutraceuticals," especially in products containing ma huang (Gurley et al., 1998). Tachycardia may occur from the consumption of large amounts of ephedra alkaloids, which may predispose the myocardium to ventricular arrhythmias. Some catecholamine derivatives (e.g., amphetamines, fenfluramine, phentermine) are used for their CNS-stimulant properties to reduce appetite. Significant concern has arisen regarding the potential for these drugs to induce pulmonary hypertension and cardiac valvular disease perhaps related to elevated serotonin levels in the blood (Fishman, 1999). Recently, however, fenfluramine was found to block Na^+ current in guinea pig heart tissue (Rajamani et al., 2000). Therefore these drugs may also exert a direct cardiotoxic effect, but the mechanisms responsible are not fully understood.

Mechanisms of Catecholamine-Induced Cardiotoxicity High circulating concentrations of epinephrine (adrenaline) and norepinephrine (noradrenaline) and high doses of synthetic catecholamines such as isoproterenol may induce toxic effects on the heart, including cardiac myocyte death. Furthermore, many of the catecholamines and related drugs have been shown to induce cardiac myocyte hypertrophic growth in vitro. The pathogenesis of catecholamine-induced cardiotoxicity is, however, unclear. Dhalla and colleagues (1992) have written a comprehensive review of the cardiotoxicity of catecholamines and related agents. Some of the more important hypotheses that explain the cardiotoxicity of catecholamines are discussed below.

A prominent early hypothesis regarding catecholamine-induced cardiotoxicity involved the pronounced pharmacologic effects of high concentrations of these compounds on the cardiovascular system, including increased heart rate, enhanced myocardial oxygen demand, and an overall increase in systolic arterial blood pressure. In the case of isoproterenol, there is a fall in blood pressure. These actions may cause myocardial hypoxia and, if severe enough, lead to the production of necrotic lesions in the heart. Because isoproterenol has greater cardiotoxic potential than does epinephrine or norepinephrine, it was suggested that the hypotension produced by isoproterenol is a major factor in lesions produced in the myocardium. However, subsequent investigations revealed that hypotension is not essential for the production of cardiac myocyte death by isoproterenol.

Other possible mechanisms for the cardiotoxicity of high concentrations of catecholamines include coronary insufficiency resulting from coronary vasospasm, decreased levels of high-energy phosphate stores caused by mitochondrial dysfunction, increased sarcolemmal permeability leading to electrolyte alterations, altered lipid metabolism resulting in the accumulation of fatty acids, and intracellular Ca^{2+} overload. Although these mechanisms have received support through the years, there are conflicting studies that argue against one or more of these proposed mechanisms (Dhalla et al., 1992).

As discussed under "General Biochemical Mechanisms of Cardiotoxicity," above, oxidative stress is a major factor in cardiac myocyte injury induced by several xenobiotics, and oxidative stress has been implicated in catecholamine-induced cardiotoxicity (Dhalla et al., 1992). Because the oxidation of catecholamines may result in the formation of aminochromes and oxygen free radicals, oxidative stress may play a significant role in catecholamine-induced cardiotoxicity. Antioxidants such as vitamin E and ascorbic acid have been shown to provide protection against the cardiotoxicity of isoproterenol and other catecholamines.

Sarcolemmal Injury and Ca^{2+} Alterations Induced by Catecholamines Another hypothesis to explain the cardiotoxicity of catecholamines such as isoproterenol is derangement of electrolyte homeostasis of cardiac myocytes at the level of the sarcolemma and other subcellular membrane sites. Electrolyte shifts in magnesium (Mg^{2+}) and K^+ have been suggested as possible factors in the myocardial dysfunction and cardiac myocyte death associated with isoproterenol administration. For example, Mg^{2+} may serve as a cofactor in the regulation of phosphate transfers and may cause a decrease in the uptake of Ca^{2+} by isolated respiring mitochondria.

The use of the concept of Ca^{2+} overload to explain isoproterenol-induced cardiac necrosis has generated much interest (Fleckenstein et al., 1973). These investigators showed that there was a six- to sevenfold increase in the rate of Ca^{2+} uptake and a doubling of the net myocardial Ca^{2+} content. It was suggested that this excessive Ca^{2+} overload may initiate a loss of high-energy phosphates through increased activation of Ca^{2+}-dependent intracellular ATPase and impaired mitochondrial oxidative phosphorylation. Accumulation of large amounts of Ca^{2+} in cardiac myocytes may alter the integrity and function of several membrane systems. In addition to affecting mitochondrial energy production, Ca^{2+} may activate neutral proteases, phospholipases, and endonucleases. Activation of these degradative enzymes may inhibit membrane-bound enzymes such as Na^+,K^+-ATPase. As a result, there is an increase in Na^+ levels and a loss of cytoplasmic K^+. The increased Na^+ content would further enhance Ca^{2+} accumulation through the Na^+/Ca^{2+} exchanger. Recently, it has been suggested that oxidative degeneration of membrane lipids results in increased sarcolemmal Ca^{2+} permeability. Because isoproterenol may form oxidative by-products, these metabolites could interact with the lipid bilayer, cause sarcolemmal injury, and alter Ca^{2+} regulatory mechanisms. The summation of these alterations likely contributes to the cellular dysfunction and cardiotoxicity induced by catecholamines.

Apoptosis and Catecholamine-Induced Cardiotoxicity Catecholamines have recently been found to induce apoptosis of cardiac myocytes. Norepinephrine and isoproterenol stimulated apoptosis (as defined by DNA fragmentation and flow cytometry) of adult rat ventricular myocytes (Communal et al., 1998). Furthermore, catecholamine-induced apoptosis was inhibited by a beta-adrenergic receptor antagonist (the non-selective beta-blocker propranolol), protein kinase A inhibitor (H-89), and L-type Ca^{2+} channel blocker (diltiazem); whereas, an adenylyl cyclase activator (forskolin) mimicked the effects of norepinephrine and isoproterenol. Activation of beta-adrenergic receptors increases cyclic AMP and phosphorylates L-type Ca^{2+} channels, leading to Ca^{2+} influx. Subsequent studies by the same group demonstrated that catecholamine-induced apoptosis in this model was mediated by $beta_1$-adrenergic receptor stimulation, while $beta_2$-adrenergic receptor stimulation inhibited apoptosis (Communal et al., 1999). Furthermore, transgenic mice overexpressing $Gs\alpha$ (GTP binding protein coupling beta-adrenergic receptors to adenylyl cyclase) developed cardiomyopathy, and evidence of cardiac myocyte apoptosis was found (Geng et al., 1999). Therefore at least part of the mechanism of catecholamine-induced cardiotoxicity may involve stimulation of $beta_1$-adrenergic receptors, activation of adenylyl cyclase and protein kinase A, phosphorylation of L-type Ca^{2+} channels, increased intracellular Ca^{2+}, and activation of endonucleases, proteases, and/or other enzymes and proteins involved in apoptosis.

Anthracyclines and Other Antineoplastic Agents Cardiotoxicity is recognized as a serious side effect of chemotherapy for malignant cancers, especially with well-known antitumor agents such as doxorubicin, daunorubicin, 5-fluorouracil, and cyclophosphamide. Havlin (1992) has published an excellent review of some of these important antitumor agents and their cardiotoxic effects.

Anthracyclines The anthracyclines—doxorubicin and daunorubicin—are widely used antineoplastic agents for the treatment of breast cancer, leukemias, and a variety of other solid tumors. Unfortunately, the clinical usefulness of these agents is limited because of cardiotoxicity manifest by ECG changes and dose-dependent cardiomyopathy (Doroshow, 1991; Havlin, 1992). Both acute and chronic cardiotoxic effects of anthracyclines have been described. The acute effects mimic anaphylactic-type responses, such as tachycardia and various arrhythmias. These effects are usually manageable and most likely are due to the potent release of histamine from mast cells sometimes observed in acute dosing. Acutely, large doses can also cause left ventricular failure, which responds to inotropic agents (e.g., digitalis, isoproterenol) and high perfusions of Ca^{2+}, suggesting an acute mechanism of toxicity that involves altered Ca^{2+} homeostasis. The greatest limiting factor of the anthracyclines is associated with long-term exposure, which usually results in the development of cardiomyopathies and, in severe stages, congestive heart failure (Havlin, 1992). Morphologically, there is vacuolization of the SR, myofibrillar loss, and swelling of the mitochondria.

Two new anthracyclines were introduced to the U.S. market in 1999, and a lipid formulation of doxorubicin (liposomal doxorubicin) is under development. *Valrubicin* is a semisynthetic derivative of doxorubicin approved for treatment of carcinoma in situ of the bladder. It is administered locally for bladder cancer and therefore induces only mild systemic toxicities; however, systemic absorption from the bladder may occur, but valrubicin seems to exhibit a lower propensity for cardiotoxicity than doxorubicin (Hussar, 2000). *Epirubicin* is a semisynthetic derivative of daunorubicin approved for treatment of breast cancer. Like doxorubicin, epirubicin is given systemically and may induce cardiotoxicity. However, epirubicin is more lipophilic than doxorubicin and is significantly metabolized by the conjugative pathways in the liver, resulting in a shorter half-life and a lower incidence of cardiotoxicity than with doxorubicin (Hussar, 2000).

Mechanisms of Anthracycline-Induced Cardiotoxicity Several major hypotheses have been suggested to account for the onset of anthracycline-induced cardiomyopathy: (1) oxidative stress from redox cycling or mitochondrial Ca^{2+} cycling, (2) defects in mitochondrial integrity and subsequent deterioration of myocardial energetics, (3) alterations in both SR Ca^{2+} currents and mitochondrial Ca^{2+} homeostasis, and (4) altered cardiac myocyte gene expression and induction of apoptosis. The cause-and-effect relationships of the proposed mechanisms of cardiotoxicity have not been determined, and no single theory adequately explains the exact mechanism for anthracycline-induced cardiomyopathy.

Reactive Oxygen Species and Doxorubicin-Induced Cardiotoxicity Although several hypotheses have been proposed to explain the mechanism of the cardiotoxicity of doxorubicin, the free radical hypothesis has received the most attention. The formation of reactive oxygen species by doxorubicin (schematically shown in Fig. 18-10) has been attributed to redox cycling of the drug (Powis, 1989). Doxorubicin can undergo futile redox cycling that results in the production of oxygen free radicals; these reactive oxygen species may then oxidize proteins, lipids, and nucleic acids and potentially cause DNA strand scission.

The quinone-like structure of doxorubicin permits this molecule to accept an electron and form a semiquinone radical. Oxidation of the semiquinone back to the parent quinone by molecular oxygen results in superoxide radical ions that are believed to initiate oxidative stress. The enzymatic reduction that is believed to be responsible for the generation of superoxide by doxorubicin (at

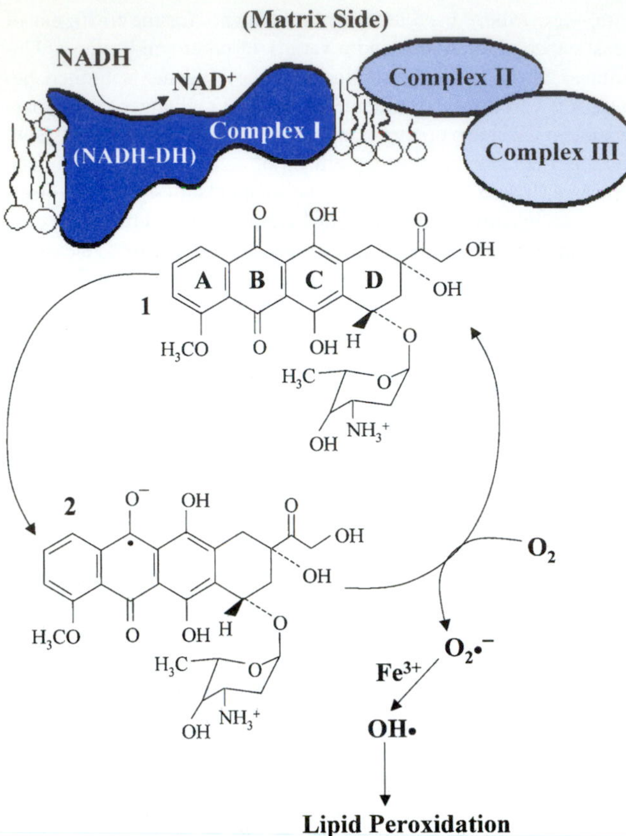

Figure 18-10. Production of superoxide radical anions by oxidation-reduction cycling of doxorubicin at the level of the mitochondria.

NADH dehydrogenase (NAD-DH), which is located within complex I, has been proposed as the enzyme that catalyzes the one-electron reduction of doxorubicin (1) to a semiquinone radical (2). The semiquinone then may be reoxidized back to the parent compound by means of the reduction of molecular oxygen (O_2) to the superoxide anion ($O_2\bullet^-$).

the level of the mitochondria) has been proposed to occur between complexes I and III of the mitochondrial respiratory chain. Doxorubicin has high affinity for cardiolipin, a phospholipid found on the inner mitochondrial membrane, where NADH dehydrogenase converts the drug to a semiquinone radical (Marcillat et al., 1989). In the presence of oxygen, this radical is responsible for the generation of reactive oxygen species, which then may peroxidize unsaturated membrane lipids and initiate myocardial cell injury. Nonetheless, several observations appear to be inconsistent with the free radical–induced cardiotoxicity of doxorubicin (Olson and Mushlin, 1990).

Mitochondrial Ca^{2+} Homeostasis and Doxorubicin-Induced Cardiotoxicity An alternate hypothesis to explain the cardiotoxicity of doxorubicin implicates a disruption of mitochondrial Ca^{2+} homeostasis without necessarily involving pronounced Ca^{2+} overload (Chacon and Acosta, 1991; Chacon et al., 1992; Solem et al., 1994). This hypothesis suggests that doxorubicin induces a cycling of mitochondrial Ca^{2+} that is associated with the production of reactive oxygen species and dissipation in the mitochondrial membrane potential, which in turn may result in depletion of cellular ATP. Ruthenium red, an inhibitor of the mitochondrial Ca^{2+} uniport, decreased doxorubicin production of reactive oxygen species in mitochondria and isolated cardiac myocytes and protected the cells from doxorubicin-induced cell killing. Therefore, disruption of mitochondrial Ca^{2+} homeostasis may be an important mechanism responsible for the cardiotoxicity of doxorubicin. Furthermore, cyclosporin A, an inhibitor of the Ca^{2+}-dependent Ca^{2+} release channel in mitochondria, inhibited the Ca^{2+}-induced depolarization of membrane potential of mitochondria isolated from rats chronically treated with doxorubicin. These results suggest that doxorubicin may induce futile cycling of Ca^{2+} across the mitochondrial membrane and that this may be responsible for the formation of reactive oxygen species rather than or in addition to redox cycling of the quinone moiety.

Apoptosis and Anthracycline-Induced Cardiotoxicity Increasing evidence suggests that at least part of the mechanism of anthracycline-induced cardiotoxicity includes induction of apoptosis. As described under "General Mechanisms of Cardiotoxicity," generation of reactive oxygen species, altered mitochondrial function or permeability, and altered Ca^{2+} homeostasis serve as important stimuli of cardiac myocyte apoptosis. Therefore, apoptosis may be an extension of the previously described possible mechanisms of anthracycline-induced cardiotoxicity. For example, daunorubicin induced apoptosis of cultured neonatal and adult rat cardiac myocytes, and induction of apoptosis was prevented by dexrazoxane, an iron chelator, suggesting that reactive oxygen species were involved with daunorubicin-induced apoptosis (Sawyer et al., 1999). Furthermore, doxorubicin induced Bax expression, activated caspase 3, and induced apoptosis in cultured fetal cardiac myocytes (Wang et al., 1998). In cultured neonatal rat cardiac myocytes, daunorubicin activated the MAPKs, an effect that was inhibited by free radical scavengers and Ca^{2+} chelators (Zhu et al., 1999). In these experiments, ERK 1/2 activation likely occurred through Ras activation and appeared protective; whereas JNK/SAPK and p38 activation (likely through Rho activation) contributed to daunorubicin-induced apoptosis. Ceramide may also be involved in doxorubicin-induced apoptosis, as adult rat ventricular myocytes developed signs of apoptosis associated with increased sphingomyelinase activity and ceramide production (Andrieu-Abadie et al., 1999). Doxorubicin-induced apoptosis has also been demonstrated in whole-animal studies, where intraperitoneal injection in adult Wistar rats produced histologic signs of apoptosis in the heart (Arola et al., 2000).

Other Possible Mechanisms of Doxorubicin-Induced Cardiotoxicity Other possible mechanisms to explain the cardiotoxicity of doxorubicin include Ca^{2+} overload that overwhelms intracellular homeostatic processes, increased production of prostaglandins and platelet-activating factor, increased release of histamine, and the formation of a toxic metabolite of doxorubicin (Olson and Mushlin, 1990).

5-Fluorouracil Clinical evidence of 5-fluorouracil cardiotoxicity ranges from mild precordial pain and ECG abnormalities (ST segment elevation, high peaked T waves, T-wave inversions, and sinus tachycardia) to severe hypotension, atrial fibrillation, and abnormalities of ventricular wall motion. A principal mechanism proposed for the cardiotoxicity of fluorouracil is myocardial ischemia precipitated by coronary vasospasm, but this finding has been disputed because of the short half-life of fluorouracil. More recent studies suggest that the cardiotoxicity of fluorouracil can be attributed to impurities present in commercial products of the drug, one of which is metabolized to fluoroacetate, a compound that might also participate in fluorouracil-induced cardiotoxicity.

Cyclophosphamide High doses of cyclophosphamide given to cancer or transplant patients may lead to severe hemorrhagic cardiac necrosis. The mechanism of the cardiotoxicity of this agent is not clear, but there is suggestive evidence that the toxic metabolite of cyclophosphamide, 4-hydroperoxycyclophosphamide (4-HC), may alter the ion homeostasis in cardiac myocytes, resulting in increased Na^+ and Ca^{2+} content and reduced K^+ levels (Levine et al., 1993). Furthermore, the same investigators showed that the cytotoxicity of 4-HC is markedly altered by the cellular glutathione concentration, suggesting a role for oxidative stress in 4-HC–induced cardiotoxicity.

Antimicrobial and Antiviral Agents Although the clinical use of antimicrobial and antiviral agents usually presents limited cardiovascular problems in routine therapy for uncomplicated infections, the use of some of these agents may result in adverse cardiac effects, especially in instances of overdosage and in patients with preexisting cardiovascular dysfunction. Keller and associates (1992) have presented an excellent review of key antibacterial agents that may have adverse cardiovascular effects.

Aminoglycosides The aminoglycoside class of antibiotics—which includes agents such as amikacin, gentamicin, kanamycin, netilmicin, streptomycin, and tobramycin—is associated with direct cardiodepressant actions in a number of species, although these effects are clinically rare in humans. Gentamicin, a representative aminoglycoside, has been thoroughly investigated for its Ca^{2+}-related myocardial depressant actions. Gentamicin's negative inotropic actions can be antagonized by excess Ca^{2+}, and gentamicin has an inhibitory action on slow inward Ca^{2+} channels in heart muscle. It has been proposed that aminoglycosides inhibit the uptake or binding of Ca^{2+} at sarcolemmal sites, thus reducing the concentration of membrane-bound Ca^{2+} available for movement into the myoplasm during depolarization of the sarcolemma. Other investigators have confirmed these observations and have reported other data that suggest that gentamicin's principal mechanism of cardiodepression is the dislocation of Ca^{2+} from slow-channel binding sites on the external surface of the sarcolemma, which results in a blockade of the channels (Hino et al., 1982).

Macrolides Macrolide antibacterial agents include azithromycin, clarithromycin, dirithromycin, and erythromycin. Erythromycin has been associated, although rarely, with QT interval prolongation and with cardiac dysrhythmias characterized by polymorphic ventricular tachycardia (torsades de pointes). These effects occur primarily in patients with underlying cardiac disease. The clinical findings of erythromycin-induced cardiotoxicity suggest that the drug blocks delayed rectifier K^+ channels. Importantly, erythromycin and other macrolides (most of which are significantly metabolized by and are competitive inhibitors of gastrointestinal and hepatic cytochrome P450 3A4) inhibit the elimination of other agents that are cytochrome P450 3A4 substrates and also inhibit delayed rectifier K^+ current in the heart (as discussed below). Consequently, macrolides were contraindicated for use in patients also taking astemizole, terfenadine, and cisapride (although all three of these drugs have been removed from the market).

Fluoroquinolones In recent years (i.e.,1997–2000), no other class of antibacterial agents has experienced as rapid growth in terms of numbers of new agents released on the market in the United States than the fluoroquinolones. Fluoroquinolone antibacterial agents include ciprofloxacin, enoxacin, gatifloxacin, gemifloxacin, grepafloxacin, levofloxacin (levo-rotatory isomer of ofloxacin), lomefloxacin, moxifloxacin, norfloxacin, ofloxacin, sparfloxacin, and trovafloxacin (Pickerill et al., 2000). These drugs exhibit a wide variety of toxicities including CNS stimulation from inhibition of γ-aminobutyric acid receptors, photosensitivity, hepatotoxicity, arthropathy, and QT interval prolongation. Of the numerous fluoroquinolones, grepafloxacin, moxifloxacin, and sparfloxacin have been associated with QT interval prolongation in perhaps a higher incidence than macrolides. In fact, grepafloxacin was voluntarily removed from the U.S. market because of the relatively high incidence of QT interval prolongation and risk of torsades de pointes. As with erythromycin, the signs of fluoroquinolone-induced cardiotoxicity are consistent with inhibition of delayed rectifier K^+ channels in the heart.

Other Antibacterial Agents Tetracycline and chloramphenicol have been reported to depress myocardial contractility by direct cardiac myocyte interaction or an indirect effect that lowers Ca^{2+} concentrations in the plasma or extracellular spaces, respectively. Indeed, the tetracylcines are Ca^{2+} chelating agents. However, tetracycline or chloramphenicol-induced cardiotoxicity is a rare clinical findings.

Antifungal Agents Some of the polyene group of antifungal agents (e.g., amphotericin B) may depress myocardial contractility by blocking activation of slow Ca^{2+} channels and inhibiting the influx of Na^+. Very high concentrations of amphotericin B increase the permeability of the sarcolemmal membrane, and electrophysiologists use the drug to create perforated patch-clamp models. Ventricular tachycardia and cardiac arrest have been reported in patients treated with amphotericin B. However, the incidence of amphotericin B–induced cardiotoxicity pales in comparison with its prominent toxicity in the kidney (see Chap. 14, "Toxic Responses of the Kidney"). Flucytosine is another antifungal agent that has been associated with cardiotoxicity. In fungal cells, flucytosine is converted to 5-fluorouracil, which then exerts antifungal effects. However, flucytosine may be converted to 5-fluorouracil by gastrointestinal microflora in humans, which then may be absorbed systemically and induce cardiotoxicity (see 5-fluorouracil above, under "Anthracyclines and Other Antineoplastic Agents"). Cardiac arrest has been reported in individuals receiving flucytosine. Finally, concern about azole antifungal drug interactions with astemizole, terfenadine, and cisapride was prevalent, and coadministration of azoles with these drugs was contraindicated. The azole antifungals itraconazole and ketoconazole are not potent cardiotoxicants in humans; however, they are substrates and competitive inhibitors of gastrointestinal and hepatic cytochrome P450 3A4. Because itraconazole and ketoconazole reduce clearance and increase plasma concentrations of astemizole, terfenadine, and cisapride when used concomitantly, these azoles may predispose individuals to astemizole-, terfenadine-, or cisapride-induced QT interval prolongation and risk of torsades de pointes.

Antiviral Agents Antiviral agents that are potentially cardiotoxic include the nucleoside analog reverse transcriptase inhibitors (NRTIs) used for the treatment of human immunodeficiency virus (HIV) infections. However, direct cardiotoxicity of these agents is rare in HIV patients and clinical studies are complicated by the findings that cardiomyopathy is related to disease progression. Nonetheless, zidovudine (AZT) was recently found to induce cardiomyopathy in transgenic mice expressing replication-incompetent HIV (Lewis et al., 2000). Cardiac function was depressed in these mice and accompanied by depressed SERCA mRNA expression, increased atrial natriuretic factor mRNA expression, left ventricular hypertrophy, and damaged mitochondria (swelling, dissolution of cristae, and fragmentation). Therefore, AZT-induced cardiotoxicity in this model may be produced by altered Ca^{2+} homeostasis and/or mitochondrial toxicity. The mitochondrial toxicity of AZT has been shown in skeletal muscle biopsy samples from AIDS patients (Dalakas, et al., 1990). Furthermore, mitochondrial toxicity from the NRTIs has been implicated as a cause of NRTI-induced hepatotoxicity, lipodystrophy, and pancreatic toxicity, and, at least in vitro, several NRTIs (zalcitabine, ddc; stavudine, d4T; and AZT) inhibited mitochondrial DNA polymerase while also decreasing mitochondrial DNA synthesis, DNA content, and ATP production—effects that may be related to the therapeutic mechanism yet resulting in incorporation of NRTIs into mitochondrial DNA (Brinkman et al., 1998).

As with macrolides and azole antifungal agents, some antiviral agents participate in drug interactions with agents that exhibit cardiotoxicity. The HIV protease inhibitors are substrates and competitive inhibitors of cytochromes P450 3A4; therefore amprenavir, indinavir, nelfinavir, ritonavir, and saquinavir are contraindicated for coadministration with astemizole, terfenadine, cisapride, or other drugs that prolong the QT interval and are substrates for cytochrome P450 3A4. Finally, the nonnucleoside reverse transciptase inhibitor (NNRTIs) delaviridine is also an inhibitor of cytochromes P450 3A4 and would produce similar interactions with astemizole, terfenadine, and cisapride. However, the NNRTI nevirapine (and perhaps efavirenz) is an inducer of cytochromes P450 3A4 and would not be expected to interact with these drugs.

Centrally Acting Drugs There are numerous examples of CNS-acting drugs that have considerable effects on the cardiovascular system. Some of the more cardiotoxic agents that have a major pharmacologic action on the brain and nervous system include tricyclic antidepressants, general anesthetics, some of the opioids, and antipsychotic drugs. Other drugs, such as cocaine and ethanol, are discussed in separate sections.

Tricyclic and Other Antidepressants Standard tricyclic antidepressants (TCAs, including amitriptyline, desipramine, doxepin, imipramine, and protriptyline) have significant cardiotoxic actions, particularly in cases of overdose. The effects of TCAs on the heart include ST segment elevation, QT interval prolongation, supraventricular and ventricular arrhythmias (including torsades de pointes), and sudden cardiac death. In addition, as a result of peripheral alpha-adrenergic blockade, they may cause postural hypotension —probably the cardiovascular effect of TCAs that is the most prevalent. Although many of these adverse effects are related to the quinidine-like actions, anticholinergic effects, and adrenergic actions of these agents, the tricyclics also may have direct cardiotoxic actions on cardiac myocytes and Purkinje fibers, including depression of inward Na^+ and Ca^{2+} and outward K^+ currents (Pacher et al., 1998). Furthermore, the risk of TCA-induced cardiotoxicity is significantly enhanced in children and by concomitant administration of other agents that alter ion movement or homeostasis in the heart (e.g., the Na^+ channel–blocking class I antiarrhythmic agents), or use in patients with underlying cardiovascular disease.

In contrast, the selective serotonin reuptake inhibitors (SSRIs including fluoxetine, fluvoxamine, paroxetine, sertraline, and venlafaxine) carry a lower risk of cardiotoxicity than the TCAs. Moreover, the SSRIs have fewer anticholinergic and antihistaminergic effects than the TCAs. Indeed, clinical studies have not revealed any fluoxetine-induced conduction delays in the heart, nor have clinical studies shown any significant effects of fluoxetine on the electrocardiogram (Pacher et al., 1998). Nonetheless, some case reports of atrial fibrillation and bradycardia secondary to fluoxetine administration have surfaced; in animal models, fluoxetine may block Na^+ and/or Ca^{2+} channels (Pacher et al., 1998).

Antipsychotic Agents Many antipsychotic agents exert profound cardiovascular effects, particularly orthostatic hypotension. Currently used antipsychotic agents include the phenothiazines (acetophenazine, chlorpromazine, fluphenazine, mesoridazine, perphenazine, thioridazine, and trifluoperazine), chlorprothixene, thiothixene, and other heterocyclic compounds (clozapine, haloperidol, loxapine, molindone, pimozide, and risperidone). The mechanisms responsible for the cardiovascular effects of antipsychotics are extremely complex because the drugs may alter cardiovascular function through indirect actions on the autonomic and central nervous systems and through direct actions on the myocardium. As with TCAs, the most prominent adverse cardiovascular effect of antipsychotic agents is orthostatic hypotension. However, the phenothiazines (e.g., chlorpromazine and thioridazine) may exert direct effects on the myocardium, including negative inotropic actions and quinidine-like effects (Baldessarini, 1996). Some ECG changes induced by these agents include prolongation of the QT and PR intervals, blunting of T waves, and depression of the ST segment. Through anticholinergic actions, clozapine can produce substantial elevations in heart rate (tachycardia), but the most prominent adverse cardiovascular effect is orthostatic hypotension.

General Anesthetics The inhalational general anesthetics, as exemplified by enflurane, desflurane, halothane, isoflurane, methoxyflurane, and sevoflurane may have adverse cardiac effects, including reduced cardiac output by 20 to 50 percent, depression of contractility, and production of arrhythmias (generally benign in healthy myocardium but more serious in cardiac disease). These anesthetics may sensitize the heart to the arrhythmogenic effects of endogenous epinephrine or to beta-receptor agonists. Investigations suggest that halothane, as a prototype, may block the L-type Ca^{2+} channel by interacting with dihydropyridine binding sites, may disrupt Ca^{2+} homeostasis associated with the SR, and may modify the responsiveness of the contractile proteins to activation by Ca^{2+} (Bosnjak, 1991). Propofol is an intravenously administered general anesthetic that has also been shown to decrease cardiac output and blood pressure. Several investigations have demonstrated that propofol exerts direct actions on cardiac myocytes resulting in a negative inotropic effect. As to the mechanism(s) involved, propofol has been shown to antagonize beta-adrenergic receptors, inhibit L-type Ca^{2+} current, and reduce Ca^{2+} transients (Zhou et al., 1997; Zhou et al., 1999; Guenoun et al., 2000). These effects have been observed in vitro at concentrations that could be achieved following bolus administration of propofol. Furthermore, the adverse cardiovascular effects of propofol may be enhanced in patients with underlying cardiovascular disease.

Local Anesthetics Because of their ability to block conduction in nerve axons, local anesthetics interfere with the conduction or transmission of impulses in other excitable organs, including the heart and circulatory system. In general, local anesthetics such as lidocaine and mepivacaine have few undesirable cardiovascular effects. However, when high systemic concentrations of cocaine and procainamide are attained, these agents may have prominent adverse effects on the heart. Because cocaine is abused by a significant number of individuals, its adverse effects on the myocardium are described in more detail.

Cocaine The cardiotoxicity of cocaine is usually explained by its general pharmacologic effects on excitable tissues, which include its ability to act as a local anesthetic and block conduction in nerve fibers by reversibly inhibiting Na^+ channels and stopping the transient rise in Na^+ conductance. In the heart, cocaine decreases the rate of depolarization and the amplitude of the action potential, slows conduction speed, and increases the effective refractory period. The other major pharmacologic action of cocaine is its ability to inhibit the reuptake of norepinephrine and dopamine into sympathetic nerve terminals (sympathomimetic effect). Cocaine will, indirectly through its actions on catecholamine reuptake, stimulate beta- and alpha-adrenergic receptors, leading to increased cyclic AMP and inositol triphosphate levels. These second messengers will, in turn, provoke a rise in cytosolic Ca^{2+}, which causes sustained action potential generation and extrasystoles. The local anesthetic action, as described above, impairs conduction and creates a condition for reentrant circuits. The net effect of these two pharmacologic actions is to elicit and maintain ventricular fibrillation.

Whereas the sympathomimetic and local anesthetic actions of cocaine are plausible mechanisms to explain the cardiac arrhythmias experienced by some cocaine abusers, it is still not clear how cardiac myocyte death and myocardial infarction may develop with cocaine use. One explanation is that the increased levels of catecholamines caused by cocaine's inhibition of reuptake leads to myocardial ischemia resulting from coronary artery vasoconstriction by the catecholamines (as described under "General Mechanisms of Cardiotoxicity," above). While the adverse actions of cocaine have been documented in humans with advanced coronary artery disease, cocaine users are often young and have normal coronary arteries. Whether coronary vasoconstriction by cocaine and the catecholamines is sufficient to lead to myocardial ischemia and/or myocardial infarction in the normal population is not known.

A third explanation for the cardiotoxicity of cocaine is that it may be directly toxic to the myocardium beyond the direct effects on the Na^+ channel. Peng and coworkers (1989) ultrastructurally examined endomyocardial biopsy specimens from seven patients with a history of cocaine abuse and found that more than 70 percent of these showed multifocal myocyte necrosis. There was extensive loss of myofibrils, and marked sarcoplasmic vacuolization was observed. Peng and coworkers suggested that these toxic manifestations were not secondary to myocardial ischemic events because the amount of myocardial necrosis was small and focal and usually involved individual cells that were occasionally surrounded by inflammatory cell infiltrates—changes that are not associated with myocardial ischemia. In addition, these cardiotoxic manifestations produced by cocaine are similar to those seen in cardiotoxicity due to doxorubicin, an agent known for its direct toxicity to myocardial cells.

The mechanism by which cocaine directly injures myocardial cells is not clear. However, this drug may significantly inhibit mitochondrial electron transport, especially in the NADH dehydrogenase region (Fantel et al., 1990). Alterations in Ca^{2+} homeostasis by excess catecholamine release induced by cocaine or by the direct effects of cocaine on sarcolemmal integrity may also be involved in myocyte necrosis. For example, in neonatal rat cardiac myocyte cultures, cocaine inhibited Ca^{2+} mobilization from the SR, and in adult rat ventricular myocytes, cocaine depressed Ca^{2+} transients and inhibited excitation-contraction coupling (Yuan and Acosta, 1994; Stewart et al., 1991). More recent investigations have found that repeated administration of cocaine to rats decreased cardiac concentrations of glutathione (GSH), GSH peroxidase, GSH *S*-transferase, catalase, and ATP, and it increased cardiac concentrations of oxidized glutathione (GSSG), protein carbonyls, manganese superoxide disumutase, and malondialdehyde (Devi and Chan, 1999). Therefore repeated cocaine administration may promote oxidative stress in the heart.

Given these changes in cardiac myocytes of the heart following cocaine administration, it is perhaps not surprising that cocaine has also been shown to induce apoptosis of cardiac myocytes. In fetal cardiac myocyte cultures, cocaine exposure induced redistribution of phosphatidylserine from the inner leaflet to the outer leaflet of the sarcolemmal membrane, DNA fragmentation, and release of cytochrome *c* from the mitochondria (Xiao et al., 2000). Furthermore, inhibitors of caspase 9 and caspase 3 reduced the percentage of apoptotic cells in these experiments, consistent with cocaine-induced cytochrome *c* release from the mitochondria and activation of these caspases. Other studies have shown that cocaine induces apoptosis of adult rat cardiac myocytes as well (Zhang et al., 1999a). However, chronic cocaine administration to rats has also been shown to induce left ventricular hypertrophy while blood pressure remained normal (Besse et al., 1997). Thus, a combination of actions involving inhibition of Na^+ channels, altered Ca^{2+} homeostasis, promotion of oxidative stress, inhibition of mitochondrial function, and induction of hypertrophy and apoptosis may contribute to direct injury of the myocardium by cocaine. Overlying ethanol consumption may exacerbate all of the effects of cocaine on the heart. In the presence of ethanol, cocaine is converted to a benzoylecgonine ethyl ester called cocaethylene (Dean et al., 1992), which may also exert cardiotoxic effects. However, little is known about mechanisms of cocaethylene-induced cardiotoxicity and whether this metabolite contributes to cocaine associated morbidity and mortality.

Other Local Anesthetics Other local anesthetic drugs include benzocaine, bupivacaine, etidocaine, lidocaine, mepivacaine, pramoxine, prilocaine, procaine, procainamide, proparacaine, ropivacaine, and tetracaine. Two of these local anesthetic agents are also used as antiarrhythmic agents (discussed previously): lidocaine and procainamide. In general and with the exception of bupivacaine, etidocaine, lidocaine and procainamide, direct cardiotoxic effects of the remaining local anesthetics are rare. However, extremely high doses of these other agents may result in direct cardiotoxicity where decreases in electrical excitability, conduction rate, and force of contraction occur likely through inhibition of cardiac Na^+ channels (Catterall and Mackie, 1996). Bupivacaine and etidocaine are more potent cardiotoxicants than lidocaine, and high dose intravenous administration can produce severe ventricular arrhythmias. The more potent cardiotoxic effects of these agents may be related to slower dissociation from the Na^+ channel and more prolonged block in comparison with lidocaine (Catterall and Mackie, 1996).

Antihistamines The second-generation histamine H_1 receptor antagonists (antihistamines) have been associated with life-threatening ventricular arrhythmias and sudden cardiac death (Simons, 1994). For example, terfenadine and astemizole have been shown to have a number of adverse effects on the electrophysiology of the heart, including altered repolarization, notched inverted T waves, prominent TU waves, prolonged QT interval, first- and second-degree AV block, ventricular tachycardia or fibrillation, and torsades de pointes. Numerous studies have demonstrated that these antihistamines produce cardiac arrhythmias by blocking the delayed rectifier K^+ channel and prolonging action potential duration in cardiac myocytes. The prolonged action potential duration promotes early afterdepolarizations and predisposes the myocardium to ventricular arrhythmias. However, terfenadine also inhibits L-type Ca^{2+} channels in rat ventricular myocytes at concentrations near or below that required to inhibit delayed rectifier K^+ current (Liu et al., 1997). Therefore, both inhibition of Ca^{2+} and K^+ current likely contribute to the cardiotoxic actions of terfenadine. As a result of cardiotoxicity, both astemizole and terfenadine have been removed from the United States market. However, the understanding of astemizole- and terfenadine-induced cardiotoxicity continues to be an important consideration in drug development, and other drugs have demonstrated similar clinical limitations (e.g., cisapride and fluoroquinolone antibacterial agents).

As mentioned previously, drug interactions with astemizole and terfenadine have been important components to the case reports of severe cardiotoxicity from these antihistamines. Both astemizole and terfenadine are substrates for gastrointestinal and hepatic cytochrome P450 3A4. First-pass metabolism of astemizole and terfenadine is high, so much so that in a normal patient, serum concentrations of the parent agent terfenadine are extremely low and risk of cardiotoxicity is also low. The active P450 metabolite of terfenadine is terfenadine carboxylate (now sold under the generic name fexofenadine). While terfenadine carboxylate is the active antihistamine following terfenadine administration, it exhibits little to no inhibition of cardiac delayed rectifier K^+ current (Rampe et al., 1993). However, in patients with hepatic dysfunction or in those receiving concomitant inhibitors of cytochrome P450 3A4 (e.g., macrolides, azole antifungals, HIV protease inhibitors, and nonnucleoside reverse transriptase inhibitors), metabolism of astemizole or terfenadine may be significantly impaired, such that plasma concentrations of parent drug rises and risk of cardiotoxicity is enhanced. Furthermore, accidental overdose of astemizole or terfenadine in adults or children with no hepatic dysfunction or concomitant inhibitors of cytochrome P450 3A4 has been associated with cardiotoxicity.

Immunosuppressants The immunosuppressants, including the cyclic polypeptide cyclosporin A and the macrolide tacrolimus (FK506), are potent nephrotoxicants and are discussed elsewhere in this textbook (see Chap. 14). However, rapamycin and tacrolimus (both macrolides) may also produce adverse cardiovascular effects, including hypertension, hypokalemia, and hypomagnesemia. All three of these agents alter signal transduction in cardiac myocytes. Specifically, rapamycin and tacrolimus interact with a protein that associates with ryanodine receptors (RyRs), and the protein carries the name FK506-binding protein (FKBP). When rapamycin or tacrolimus binds to FKBP in cardiac myocytes, RyR may become destabilized, resulting in Ca^{2+} leak from the SR (Marks, 1997). Clinically, tacrolimus has been associated with hypertrophic cardiomyopathy in pediatric patients, a condition that was reversed by discontinuation of tacrolimus and administration of cyclosporin A; some of these patients developed severe heart failure (Atkinson et al., 1995). Interestingly, cyclosporin A has been shown to inhibit cardiac myocyte hypertrophy and cardiotoxicity from a number of different stimuli, including doxorubicin.

Miscellaneous Drugs ***Cisapride*** Cisapride has been used as a prokinetic agent for gastrointestinal hypomotility. However, cisapride has been removed from the U.S. market because of risk of potentially life-threatening arrhythmias (torsades de pointes) associated with its use. Like astemizole and terfenadine, cisapride inhibits delayed rectifier K^+ current, prolongs action potential duration, prolongs the QT interval, and predisposes the heart to ventricular arrhythmias.

Methylxanthines The methylxanthines include caffeine, theobromine, and theophylline, all of which can be found in significant quantities in coffee, tea, chocolate, soft-drinks, and other foods. The methylxanthines are rather potent CNS stimulants but exert a wide variety of effects in the body and within the cardiovascular system. Theophylline has been used for many decades for the treatment of asthma, yet the bronchodilatory mechanisms responsible for the clinical benefits of theophylline in asthmatics are still not fully understood. Similarly, whether methylxanthines contribute significant adverse cardiovascular effects in humans is controversial. At the cardiac myocyte level, high concentrations of caffeine stimulate massive release ("dumping") of Ca^{2+} from the SR, an effect that is often utilized experimentally to determine SR function. Yet caffeine consumption by humans has not been clearly associated with any serious arrhythmias. This is likely explained by pharmacokinetics and stimulation of the chemoreceptor trigger zone (CTZ). For example, enormous amounts of caffeine would have to be consumed to achieve myocardial concentrations sufficient to dump SR Ca^{2+}, and prior to achieving those concentrations, absorption would likely be impaired because of caffeine stimulation of the CTZ and vomiting. Nonetheless, caffeine-associated ventricular arrhythmias have been reported. In contrast, overdose of theophylline or rapid intravenous administration of therapeutic doses of aminophylline (theophylline complexed with ethylenediamine to increase water solubility) may produce life-threatening ventricular arrhythmias; these effects may in part be explained by direct actions of theophylline on cardiac myocyte SR or by inhibition of phosphodiesterase and elevation of cyclic AMP. Moreover, the cardiac effects of methylxanthines observed in vivo (including increases in cardiac output and heart rate) may be explained by elevated catecholamines, as theophylline has been shown to increase plasma epinephrine concentrations (Vestal et al., 1983).

Sildenafil Sildenafil is a relatively specific inhibitor of phosphodiesterase 5 (PDE5), which is responsible for the degradation of cyclic GMP (a vasodilatory second messenger). Interestingly, sildenafil was originally developed as a potential drug for treating angina; however, it was not very effective for this purpose and was subsequently developed for treatment of erectile dysfunction, where it produces vasodilation and filling of the corpus cavernosum. The primary concern regarding adverse effects of sildenafil is nonspecific inhibition of PDE3 in the heart and vasculature (Hussar, 1999). In vitro studies have revealed that sildenafil increases cyclic AMP in cardiac tissue without significant effects on cyclic GMP (Stief et al., 2000); however, whether these effects are associated with cardiotoxicity is not known. Sildenafil will potentiate the vasodilatory effects of nitroglycerin and other organic nitrates or nitric oxide donors; therefore, sildenafil is contraindicated in patients using these drugs. Postmarketing surveillance has found numerous deaths associated with the use of sildenafil, but many of these individuals may have been experiencing underlying cardiovascular disease. Furthermore, sildenafil is a cytochrome P450 3A4 substrate (the primary means of sildenafil metabolism), so concomitant use of sildenafil with drugs that are inhibitors of cytochrome P450 3A4 (e.g., macrolides, azole antifungals, HIV protease inhibitors, nonnucleoside reverse transcriptase inhibitors) is contraindicated.

Radiocontrast Agents Many radiocontrast agents have long been associated with anaphylactic reactions and nephrotoxicity. Recently, however, two iodinated radiocontrast agents (diatrizoate meglumine and iohexol) were shown to induce cardiac myocyte apoptosis and apoptosis of kidney cells (as determined by DNA fragmentation and morphology) in spontaneously hypertensive rats (Zhang et al., 1999b). Furthermore, radiocontrast agent-induced apoptosis in the kidney was associated with increased expression of Bax and p53 while Bcl-2 was down-regulated. Cardiac myocyte apoptosis related to diatrizoate meglumine may contribute to the clinical cardiotoxicity when the dye is inadvertently injected into the myocardium (cardiac arrhythmias, cardiac arrest, and death have been reported).

Naturally Occurring Substances

The compounds discussed in this section are chemical agents that are synthesized by humans, animals, or plants and have significant cardiotoxic effects. These natural products include steroid hormones and some synthetic steroid hormone–like compounds, cytokines, animal toxins, and plant toxins. Because of the diverse nature of these natural compounds, representative examples will be used to illustrate key toxicological actions on the cardiovascular system. Limited discussion will be provided on plant and animal toxins; the reader is directed to the chapters "Toxic Effects of Animal Toxins" and "Toxic Effects of Plants" for more detailed information on the toxicities of these natural products. Table 18-3 summarizes the cardiotoxicity of various naturally occurring substances, including cardiotoxic manifestations and proposed mechanisms of toxicity.

Steroids and Related Hormones The principal steroid hormones produced by humans are estrogens, progestins, androgens, and adrenocortical steroids. First, it is important to realize that the myocardium expresses steroid receptors; therefore the heart serves as a target organ for steroid effects. Based upon autoradiography, radioligand binding, immunoblotting, ribonuclease protection assay, and reverse transcriptase polymerase chain reaction, numerous research articles have demonstrated expression of cardiac receptors for estrogens (both alpha and beta), androgens, progestins, mineralocorticoids, and glucocorticoids. These data suggest the presence of these receptors (at least at the mRNA level) in nearly every species examined regardless of sex or age. Moreover, receptors for thyroid hormones are also found in cardiac tissue. Evidence also suggests that cardiac tissue can synthesize steroid hormones, although the capacity for synthesis may be much lower than more classic steroid synthesizing tissue. Steroid and related hormone receptors (e.g., vitamin D and retinoic acid receptors) belong to a superfamily of transcription factors; therefore the hormones exert their effects primarily by altered gene transcription (genomic mechanisms). However, increasing evidence suggests that steroids and/or steroid and receptor complexes may exert nongenomic mechanisms that alter signaling pathways of growth or death, modulate actions of membrane-bound growth factor receptors, or alter ion channel function (Christ and Wehling, 1998). The possibility seems likely that steroid and related hormones participate in development of the heart; however, many questions remain unanswered regarding the effects of these hormones on the fully developed, adult myocardium and their potential roles in cardiac pathogenesis and protection.

Estrogens Estrogens are synthesized in the ovaries, testes, and adrenal glands, and estrogen is an active metabolite of testosterone. Endogenous estrogens include 17β-estradiol (E_2), estrone, and estriol. Synthetic estrogens include diethylstilbestrol (nonsteroidal), equilin, esterified versions of E_2, ethinyl estradiol, mestranol, and quinestrol. Importantly, many other synthetic chemicals have been shown to exert estrogenic activity, including the pesticides DDT and methoxychlor, the plasticizer bisphenol A, other industrial chemicals including polychlorinated biphenyls, and some compounds found in soybeans and tofu (e.g., phytoestrogens). Estrogens (frequently in combination with progestins) have been used for over forty years as oral contraceptive agents. The initial "pill" included relatively high doses of estrogens in comparison with the modern birth control pill. The older versions of estrogenic oral contraceptives were associated with increased risk of coronary thrombosis and myocardial infarction; however, lower doses of estrogens have been found by numerous investigators to impart protective effects on the cardiovascular system, including beneficial effects on lipid metabolism [decreased low-density lipoproteins (LDL cholesterol) and increased high-density lipoproteins (HDL cholesterol)] and direct beneficial actions on cardiac tissue. Interestingly, the well-known gender differences in cardiovascular mortality are not entirely explained by protective effects of estrogens on lipid metabolism. Therefore significant ongoing work is focused on the direct protective effects of estrogens on the heart. Estrogens alter cardiac fibroblast proliferation; they have been shown to both increase and decrease proliferation of these cells. Some data suggest that E_2 inhibits L-type Ca^{2+} current in cardiac myocytes (Meyer et al., 1998), while other studies suggest that E_2 stimulates Na^+,K^+-ATPase activity (Dzurba et al., 1997) and may exert some antioxidant activity. Furthermore, antiapoptotic effects of estrogen in cardiac myocytes have been reported. Cultured cardiac myocytes exposed to staurosporine exhibited signs of apoptosis (nuclear staining, DNA fragmentation, and activation of caspase 3 and nuclear factor kappa B) that were inhibited when cells were also treated with E_2 (10 nanomolar) (Pelzer et al., 2000). Whether E_2 inhibits apoptosis from other stimuli such as xenobiotics, oxidative stress, I/R injury, etc., is unknown. Also important to realize is that E_2 may alter cardiac gene expression with deleterious consequences. For example, women have longer QT intervals than men and are at higher risk of torsades de pointes after exposure to antiarrhythmic agents such as quinidine. Currently, the consequences and mechanisms of direct actions of estrogens on the heart are an area of intense research, and clarification is pending.

Progestins Like estrogens, progestins are synthesized in the ovaries, testes, and adrenal glands. Naturally occurring and synthetic progestins include desogestrel, hydroxyprogesterone, medroxyprogesterone, norethindrone, norethynodrel, norgestimate, norgestrel, and progesterone. As part of hormone replacement therapy, progestins serve an opposing role to estrogens. Unfortunately, estrogen treatment opposed with progestins may negate the cardiovascular benefits of estrogens on lipid metabolism (Kalin and Zumoff, 1990). Thus, the effects of progestins on lipid metabolism are similar to those of androgens (see below), particularly those protestins that are similar in structure to 19-nortestosterone (desogestrel, norethindrone, norethynodrel, norgestimate, and nor-

Table 18-3
Cardiotoxicity of Naturally Occurring Substances

AGENTS	CARDIOTOXIC MANIFESTATIONS	PROPOSED MECHANISMS OF CARDIOTOXICITY
Estrogens		
Natural estrogens (17β-estradiol, estrone, estriol)	QTc interval prolongation?	Gender differences in K^+ channel expression?
Synthetic estrogens (diethylstilbestrol, equilin, ethinyl estradiol, mestranol, quinestrol)	Cardioprotection?	Antiapoptotic effects? Antioxidant activity? ↑ Na^+,K^+-ATPase activity? Ca^{2+} channel blockade? Other mechanisms?
Nonsteroidal estrogens (bisphenol A, diethylstilbestrol, DDT, genistein)		
Progestins		
(desogestrel, hydroxyprogesterone, medroxyprogesterone, norethindrone, norethynodrel, norgestimate, norgestrel, progesterone)	Enhanced toxicity of cocaine?	Mechanisms?
Androgens		
Natural androgens (androstenedione, dehydroepi-androsterone, dihydrotestosterone, testosterone)	Myocardial infarction Cardiac hypertrophy	Mitochondrial injury? Altered Ca^{2+} homeostasis? Other mechanisms?
Synthetic androgens (boldenone, danazol, fluoxymesterone, methandrostenolone, methenolone, methyltestosterone, nandrolone, oxandrolone, oxymetholone, stanozolol)		
Glucocorticoids		
Natural glucocorticoids (corticosterone, cortisone, hydrocortisone)	Cardiac hypertrophy Cardiac fibrosis	Increased collagen expression Other mechanisms?
Synthetic glucocorticoids (e.g., dexamethasone, methylprednisolone, prednisolone, prednisone)		
Mineralocorticoids		
(aldosterone)	Cardiac fibrosis, Heart failure	Increased collagen expression, Other mechanisms?

(continued)

Table 18-3 Cardiotoxicity of Naturally Occurring Substances (*continued*)

AGENTS	CARDIOTOXIC MANIFESTATIONS	PROPOSED MECHANISMS OF CARDIOTOXICITY
Thyroid hormones		
(thyroxine, triiodothyronine)	Tachycardia, Positive inotropic effect, Increased cardiac output, Cardiac hypertrophy, Proarrhythmic	Altered Ca^{2+} homeostasis
Cytokines		
Interleukin-1β	Negative inotropic effect Cardiac myocyte death	↑ Nitric oxide synthase expression Apoptosis
Interleukin-2	Negative inotropic effect	↑ Nitric oxide synthase expression
Interleukin-6	Negative inotropic effect	↑ Nitric oxide synthase expression
Interferon-γ	Cardomyopathy Proarrhythmic	↑ Nitric oxide synthase expression Altered ion homeostasis
Tumor necrosis factor-α	Negative inotropic effect Cardiac myocyte death	↑ Nitric oxide synthase expression ↑ Sphingosine production ↓ Ca^{2+} transients Apoptosis

gestrel). Very little is known about the direct effects of progestins on the heart. Interestingly, the progesterone receptor antagonist mifepristone (RU-486) was shown to decrease the cardiotoxicity of cocaine as determined in cocaine-exposed papillary muscle preparations from progesterone- and progesterone plus mifepristone–treated rats (Sharma et al., 1993). In rats treated only with progesterone, cocaine-induced contractile dysfunction in papillary muscle was enhanced. These data suggest that progesterone could exert deleterious direct effects on the heart, but more studies are required to investigate mechanisms.

Androgens The adverse cardiovascular effects of anabolic-androgenic steroids have been reviewed (Rockhold, 1993; Melchert and Welder, 1995). The principal androgens are testosterone—which is synthesized in the testes, ovaries, and adrenal glands—and its active metabolite dihydrotestosterone, which serves as an intracellular mediator of most androgen actions. Precursors of testosterone synthesis include androstenedione and dehydroepiandrosterone. Synthetic anabolic-androgenic steroids include the alkylated and orally available drugs danazol, fluoxymesterone, methandrostenolone, methenolone, methyltestosterone, oxandrolone, oxymetholone, and stanozolol. The nonalkylated drugs with poor oral bioavailability include androstenedione and dehydroepiandrosterone (both sold in various "nutraceutical" formulations), boldenone (veterinary product), nandrolone (19-nortestosterone), and testosterone. Very limited clinical indications exist for these drugs—with the exception, of course, for use in hypgonadal males. However, nearly all of these agents have received significant illicit use, particularly in extremely high doses with attempts to improve physical appearance or performance. Anabolic-androgenic steroids have been associated with alterations in lipid metabolism, including increased LDL cholesterol and decreased HDL cholesterol; therefore these agents may predispose individuals to atherosclerosis (Melchert and Welder, 1995). Increasing evidence suggests that the anabolic-androgenic steroids may exert direct cardiotoxic actions. Initial studies demonstrated that methandrostenolone given intramuscularly to rats produced mitochondrial (swollen and elongated) and myofibrillar lesions (dissolution of sarcomeric contractile units) (Behrendt and Boffin, 1977). Subsequent studies demonstrated rapid Ca^{2+} fluxes (both directions) in cardiac myocytes induced by testosterone (Koenig et al., 1989), suggesting that androgens may produce nongenomic actions in cardiac myocytes. In more recent studies, testosterone and dihydrotestosterone stimulated hypertrophic growth of neonatal rat cardiac myocytes; this growth effect was blocked by the androgen receptor antagonist cyproterone (Marsh et al., 1998). In humans, high-dose anabolic-androgenic steroid use has been associated with cardiac hypertrophy (case reports and some clinical echocardiography studies) and myocardial infarction (case reports). However, the mechanisms responsible for the cardiotoxic effects of anabolic-androgenic steroids remain poorly understood.

Glucocorticoids and Mineralocorticoids Glucocorticoids and mineralocorticoids are primarily synthesized in the adrenal glands. Endogenous glucocorticoids include corticosterone, cortisone, and hydrocortisone (cortisol), and the endogenous mineralocorticoid is aldosterone. A large number of synthetic glucocorticoids are used for treatment of various autoimmune and inflammatory diseases. These drugs include alclometasone, amcinonide, beclomethasone, betamethasone, clobetasol, desonide, desoximetasone, dexamethasone, diflorasone, fludrocortisone, flunisolide, fluocinolone, fluocinonide, fluorometholone, flurandrenolide, halcinonide, medrysone, methylprednisolone, mometasone, paramethasone, prednisolone, prednisone, and triamcinolone. Most of these agents are primarily used topically, intranasally, or inhalationally. The primary glucocorticoids used systemically include cortisone, hydrocortisone, dexamethasone, methylprednisolone, prednisolone, and prednisone. The mineralocorticoid aldosterone is not used clinically; however, the aldosterone receptor antagonist spironolactone has been used for years to treat hypertension and is now thought to decrease morbidity and mortality associated with congestive heart failure. Chronic administration of these glucocorticoids is associated with a wide variety of adverse effects. For example, chronic glucocorticoid therapy often results in elevated total, LDL, and HDL cholesterol. Furthermore, glucocorticoids are known to cause Na^+ and water retention through mineralocorticoid receptor activation, which could produce hypertension during chronic therapy. Similarly, aldosterone exerts profound effects on Na^+ and water retention and is associated with the pathogenesis of congestive heart failure. In terms of direct effects on the heart, both aldosterone and glucocorticoids appear to stimulate cardiac fibrosis by regulating cardiac collagen expression independently of hemodynamic alterations (Robert et al., 1995; Young et al., 1994). Furthermore, aldosterone and glucocorticoids have been found to induce hypertrophic growth and alter expression of Na^+,K^+-ATPase, Na^+/H^+ antiporter, and chloride/bicarbonate exchanger of cardiac myocytes in vitro. Clinically relevant cardiac hypertrophy has been observed in premature infants undergoing dexamethasone treatment. Therefore, glucocorticoids and mineralocorticoids have the ability to alter cardiac gene expression, and complications from direct effects of these agents on the heart have been observed clinically. The mechanisms responsible for the direct effects of these agents remain, however, poorly understood.

Thyroid Hormones The adverse effects of excessive thyroid hormones are reviewed in an article by Williams (1997). The principal thyroid hormones include thyroxine (T_4) and triiodothyronine (T_3), and these hormones exert profound effects on the cardiovascular system. Hypothyroid states are associated with decreased heart rate, contractility, and cardiac output; whereas hyperthyroid states are associated with increased heart rate, contractility, cardiac output, ejection fraction, and heart mass, peripheral vascular resistance is either unchanged or decreases regardless of thyroid status. In those patients with underlying cardiovascular disease, the effects of thyroid hormones may promote arrhythmias. Thyroid hormones are known to promote hypertrophic growth of cardiac myocytes (Hefti et al., 1997). Furthermore, thyroid hormones alter expression of cardiac sarcoplasmic reticulum (SR) Ca^{2+} handling proteins. For example, thyroid hormones increased cardiac expression of SR Ca^{2+} ATPase (SERCA) and decreased the expression of phospholamban, an inhibitory protein of SERCA, and these changes in protein expression corresponded to functional alterations in Ca^{2+} homeostasis (Kaasik et al., 1997).

Cytokines Cytokines represent a diverse and heterogeneous group of proteins with important functions in cellular and humoral immune responses. More than 100 different cytokines have been found, and the cardiovascular effects of these substances can be classified as proinflammatory, anti-inflammatory, or cardioprotective (Pulkki, 1997). Members of the proinflammatory class include tumor necrosis factor-alpha (TNF-α) interleukin-1β (IL-1β), interleukin-2 (IL-2), interleukin-6 (IL-6), interleukin-8 (IL-8), Fas ligand, and chemokines (e.g., C-C chemokines such as MCP-1, macrophage chemoattractant protein-1; MIP-1α, macrophage inflammatory protein-1α; and RANTES, regulated on activation normally T cell–expressed and secreted). Members of the anti-inflammatory class typically down-regulate expression of proinflammatory cytokines and include interleukin-4 (IL-4), interleukin-10 (IL-10), interleukin-13 (IL-13), and transforming growth factor-beta (TGF-β). The cardioprotective cytokines include cardiotrophin-1 (CT-1) and leukemia inhibitor factor (LIF), which have been shown to inhibit cardiac myocyte apoptosis from a number of different stimuli. For a review of the cardiovascular effects of these cytokines, see the article by Pulkki (1997). Many of these cytokines are elevated during cardiovascular diseases such as I/R injury, myocardial infarction, and congestive heart failure. In addition, it is now recognized that cardiac myocytes may serve as the synthetic source of many of these cytokines. Therefore, significant research effort is now aimed at understanding the direct effects of these cytokines on the heart. The clinical impact of the direct effects of individual cytokines on cardiac myocyte viability and function is difficult to predict given the pleiotrophic actions of most of these cytokines and the fact that cardiac myocytes would be exposed to multiple cytokines during disease states.

Interleukin-1β IL-1β is known to exert negative inotropic actions and induce apoptosis of cardiac myocytes. The effects of IL-1β on cardiac myocytes are likely mediated through induction of nitric oxide synthase and/or increased production of nitric oxide. For example, induction of nitric oxide synthase is associated with negative inotropic effects that could be mediated by activation of guanylyl cyclase, in increased cyclic GMP, inhibition of electron transport, nitrosylation of thiol residues on vital proteins, or production of reactive oxygen species such as peroxynitrite (Arstall et al., 1999). Superoxide anion and peroxynitrite formation was associated with reduced left ventricular ejection fraction in dogs treated with microspheres containing IL-1β, and nitrotyrosine residues were found suggesting that several proteins were affected by peroxynitrite (Cheng et al., 1999). Overall, however, little else is known regarding the mechanisms of IL-1β–induced cardiotoxic effects. Complicating the understanding of direct actions of IL-1β on cardiac myocytes is the observation that IL-1β induces cardiac myocyte expression of mRNA encoding for IL-6, and IL-6 may have subsequent deleterious effects on cardiac myocyte function (Gwechenberger et al., 1999).

Tumor Necrosis Factor Alpha TNF-α induces apoptotic death of target cells including cardiac myocytes (Krown et al., 1996). The mechanisms responsible for TNF-α–induced apoptosis of cardiac myocytes are not entirely clear. For example, TNF-α increased ceramide and sphingosine production in cardiac myocytes, and sphingosine exposure also induced apoptotic death (Krown et al., 1996). However, TNF-α also exerts negative inotropic effects on cardiac myocytes at least potentially through increased production of sphingosine (Sugishita et al., 1999). In the studies by Sugishita and colleagues, TNF-α reduced the amplitude of Ca^{2+} transients without detectable changes in L-type Ca^{2+} current in guinea pig ventricular myocytes (although TNF-α did depress isoproterenol-stimulated L-type Ca^{2+} current), and the effects of TNF-α were mimicked by sphingosine. As with IL-1β, complicating the understanding of direct actions of TNF-α on cardiac myocytes is the observation that TNF-α induces cardiac myocyte expression of IL-6, which may have subsequent deleterious effects on cardiac myocyte function (Gwechenberger et al., 1999).

Other Cytokines IL-6 has been shown to induce negative inotropic effects on cardiac myocytes, possibly through induction of nitric oxide synthase expression and increased nitric oxide production (Sugishita et al., 1999). IL-2 may decrease the mechanical performance and metabolic efficiency of the heart, and these myocardial effects may be related to changes in nitric oxide synthesis and Na^+/H^+ exchange. Interferon administration may result in cardiac arrhythmias, dilated cardiomyopathy, and signs of myocardial ischemia. Furthermore, IL-1β and interferon-γ act synergistically to increase nitric oxide formation in the heart, and when combined, induce Bax expression and apoptosis in cardiac myocyte cultures (Arstall et al., 1999). Although the mechanisms of cytokine-induced cardiotoxicity are not clearly defined, significant new information is forthcoming.

Animal and Plant Toxins Animal toxins in the venom of snakes, spiders, scorpions, and marine organisms have profound effects on the cardiovascular system. There are also a number of plants—such as foxglove, oleander, and monkshood—that contain toxic constituents and have adverse effects on the cardiovascular system. A description of these toxic cardiovascular effects is found in subsequent chapters.

Industrial Agents

Table 18-4 provides a summary of selected industrial agents with their prominent cardiotoxic effects and proposed mechanisms of cardiotoxicity. For a more comprehensive review of industrial agents and their cardiotoxic potential, the reader is referred to Zakhari (1992).

Solvents Cardiotoxicity from industrial solvents can involve multiple mechanisms. Their inherent lipohilicity allows them to act on the nervous system, which in turn is responsible for regulating cardiac electrical activity. In addition, because of high lipid solubility, solvents may disperse into cell membranes and affect membrane fluidity, which is crucial for cellular functions such as signal transduction and oxidative phosphorylation. Hence, solvents may affect physiologic functions such as contraction and energy production. Solvents may disrupt sympathetic and parasympathetic control of the heart either directly or indirectly. Their influence on cardiac function may also involve the release of circulating hormones such as catecholamines, vasopressin, and serotonin. From a more general perspective, industrial solvents typically produce a depressant effect on the CNS and an attenuation of myocardial contractility. Moreover, chronic exposure to solvents in sublethal doses may result in subtle toxicities that may be apparent only after prolonged exposure.

Alcohols and Aldehydes On a molar basis, there is a relationship between increased carbon chain length of the alcohol and cardiotoxicity. Metabolic oxidation of alcohols yields aldehydes. Aldehydes have sympathomimetic activity as a result of their effect on releasing catecholamines. Unlike alcohols, the sympathomimetic activity of aldehydes decreases with increased chain length. The acute cardiodepressant effects of alcohols and aldehydes may be related to inhibition of intracellular Ca^{2+} transport and/or generation of oxidative stress (see "Alcohol," above).

Methanol Methanol (methyl alcohol or wood alcohol) is a common industrial solvent whose effects on the heart are similar to those of ethanol. Methanol is metabolized by alcohol dehydrogenase and aldehyde dehydrogenase to formaldehyde and formic acid. As with ethanol, oxidation of methanol proceeds at a rate that is independent of blood concentration. However, the rate of oxidation is about one-seventh that of ethanol, and complete elimination requires several days. Clinically, blood pressure is usually unaffected but heart rate may be reduced.

Isopropyl Alcohol Isopropyl alcohol (isopropanol) is a common industrial and household solvent whose effects on the heart are similar to those of ethanol. Isopropyl alcohol–induced toxicity typically occurs from ingestion or inhalation. Isopropanol is a potent CNS depressant that causes cardiovascular depression in large doses. Isopropanol is metabolized to acetone, which is also believed to potentiate and lengthen the duration of CNS depression. Acetone is metabolized to formic acid and acetic acid, which have the potential to induce mild acidosis. Tachycardia is the most prominent clinical finding.

Acetaldehyde Acetaldehyde, a hepatic metabolite of ethanol, has negative inotropic effects at concentrations that can be obtained with moderate alcohol consumption. At higher blood levels, acetaldehyde has sympathomimetic effects.

Halogenated Alkanes Halogenated alkanes encompass a wide range of industrial and pharmaceutical agents. Their highly lipophilic nature allows them to cross the blood-brain barrier readily. This action, coupled with their CNS-depressant activity, makes these compounds ideally suited for anesthetics (halothane, methoxyfluorane, and enflurane). Halogenated hydrocarbons depress heart rate, contractility, and conduction. In addition, some of these agents sensitize the heart to the arrhythmogenic effects of beta-adrenergic receptor agonists such as endogenous epinephrine. Fluorocarbons (freons) have been reported to have this sensitizing effect on the myocardium. Trichlorofluoromethane is one of the most toxic fluorocarbons. Table 18-4 summarizes some halogenated hydrocarbons that have been reported to have arrhythmogenic properties. Chronic exposure to halogenated hydrocarbons has been postulated to have degenerative cardiac effects.

Recent interest in halogenated hydrocarbons has focused on the development of more "environmentally friendly" replacements for the fire suppressant halon, which has come under "fire" as an ozone-depleting compound. Ironically, several of the lead agents that have lower ozone depletion potential have proven to be less friendly to the cardiovascular systems of animals. Trifluoroiodomethane (CF3I) and heptafluoro-1-iodopropane (C37I) are two such lead agents. These compounds have been shown to produce cardiac sensitization to adrenergic agonists such as epinephrine. When epinephrine was administered to dogs before and during inhalation of CF3I and C37I, significant ventricular arrhythmias occurred (Dodd and Vinegar, 1998). The mechanisms responsible for halogenated hydrocarbon–induced sensitization of the myocardium to adrenergic agonists are not fully understood.

Heavy Metals The most common heavy metals that have been associated with cardiotoxicity are cadmium, lead, and cobalt. These metals exhibit negative inotropic and dromotropic effects and also can produce structural changes in the heart. Chronic exposure to cadmium has been reported to cause cardiac hypertrophy. Lead has an arrhythmogenic sensitizing effect on the myocardium. In addition, lead has been reported to cause degenerative changes in the heart. Cobalt has been reported to cause cardiomyopathy. The cardiotoxic effects of heavy metals are attributed to their ability to form complexes with intracellular macromolecules and their ability to antagonize intracellular Ca^{2+}.

Other metals that have been reported to affect cardiac function are manganese, nickel, and lanthanum. Their mechanism of action appears to be the blocking of Ca^{2+} channels. However, high concentrations are required to block Ca^{2+} channels (e.g., millimolar range). Barium is another metal that can affect cardiac func-

Table 18-4
Cardiotoxicity of Selected Industrial Agents

AGENTS	CARDIOTOXIC MANIFESTATIONS	PROPOSED MECHANISMS OF CARDIOTOXICITY
Solvents		
Toluene (paint products)	Proarrhythmic	↓ Parasympathetic activity ↑ Adrenergic sensitivity Altered ion homeostasis
Halogenated hydrocarbons		
(carbon tetrachloride, chloroform, chloropentafluoroethane, 1,2-dibromotetra-fluoromethane, dichlorodifluoromethane, *cis*-dichloroethylene *trans*-dichloroethylene dichlortetrafluorethane, difluoroethane, ethyl bromide, ethyl chloride, fluorocarbon 502, heptafluoro-1-iodo-propane 1,2-hexafluoroethane, isopropyl chloride, methyl bromide, methyl chloride, methylene chloride, monochlorodifluoro-ethane, monochlorodifluoro-methane, octafluorcyclobutane, propyl chloride, 1,1,1-trichloroethane, trichloroethane, trichloroethylene, trichlorofluoromethane, trichloromonofluoro-ethylene, trichlorotrifluoroethane, trifluoroiodomethane, trifluorobromomethane)	Proarrhythmic Negative inotropic effect Decreased cardiac output	↓ Parasympathetic activity ↑ Adrenergic sensitivity Altered ion homeostasis Altered coronary blood flow
Ketones		
(e.g., acetone, methyl ethyl ketone)	Proarrhythmic	↓ Parasympathetic activity ↑ Adrenergic sensitivity Altered ion homeostasis
Heavy metals		
(cadmium, cobalt, lead)	Negative inotropic effect Cardiac hypertrophy Proarrhythmic	Complex formation, Altered Ca^{2+} homeostasis
(barium, lanthanum, manganese, nickel)	Proarrhythmic	Ca^{2+} channel blockade

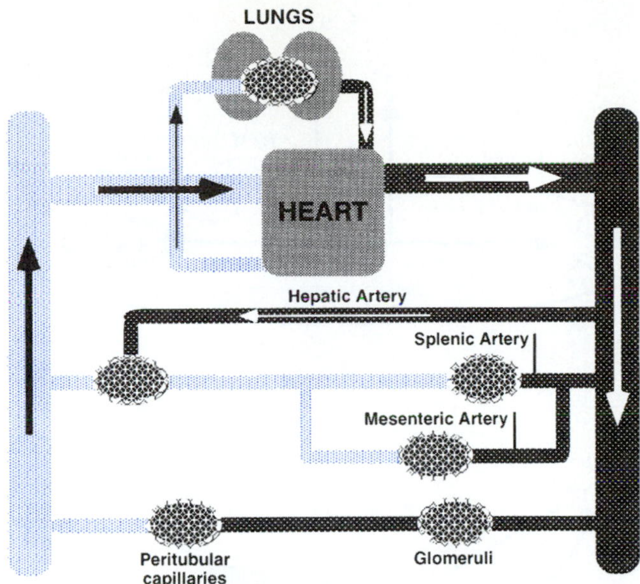

Figure 18-11. Schematic diagram of vascular supply to selected organs.

The capillary beds represented by a meshwork connnecting the arteries (*right*) with the veins (*left*); the distribution of the vasculature in several organs (liver, kidney, lung) indicates the importance of the vascular system in toxicology.

tion. Barium chloride given intravenously in high doses to laboratory animals has been reported to induce arrhythmias. This arrhythmogenic effect of barium chloride has been utilized to screen antirrhythmic agents.

OVERVIEW OF VASCULAR PHYSIOLOGY

The vascular system consists of a complex network of vessels of varying size and complexity that serve as the circuitry for the delivery of oxygen and nutrients to tissues throughout the body and for the removal of the waste products of cellular metabolism. Oxygenated blood returning from the lungs to the heart is emptied into the aorta, a large conduit vessel, which gradually branches off, giving rise to smaller vessels that reach individual organs (Fig. 18-11). Although the distribution of the cardiac output among different organs depends on their relative resistance to blood flow, in most instances the blood flow to critical regions such as the brain and the kidney remains constant despite changes in arterial pressure or cardiac output. The general laws of hemodynamics govern the movement of blood through the vascular network, although the properties of the blood and those of the vessels impose some modifications. Blood returns to the heart for reoxygenation through the venous system before the reinitiation of subsequent cycles.

Large and medium-size blood vessels in mammals are organized into three morphologically distinct layers (Fig.18-12). The innermost layer is referred to as the tunica intima and consists of a single layer of endothelial cells resting on a thin basal lamina and a subendothelial layer. Luminal endothelial cells are flat and elongated, with the long axis parallel to blood flow. These cells act as a semipermeable barrier between the blood and underlying components of the vessel wall. The subendothelial layer is formed by connective tissue bundles and elastic fibrils, in which a few cells of smooth muscle origin may be oriented parallel to the long axis of the vessel. The subendothelial layer is seen only in large elastic arteries such as the human aorta and is not clearly defined in smaller species. The medial layer, or tunica media, is composed of elastin and collagen interwoven between multiple layers of smooth muscle cells. In the majority of vascular beds, smooth muscle cells dominate the media, but these cells may also be present in the intima of some arteries and veins and in the adventitia of veins. The media is separated from the outermost layer, the tunica adventitia, by a poorly defined external lamina. The adventitial layer consists of a loose layer of fibroblasts, collagen, elastin, and glycosaminoglycans. With the exception of capillaries, the walls of smaller vessels also have three distinct layers. However, in smaller vessels the tunica media is less elastic and consists of fewer layers of smooth muscle cells. As described for the muscular arteries, venules are structurally similar to their arteriolar counterparts. Because muscular venules are larger than arterioles, a large fraction of blood is contained in these so-called capacitance vessels. Capillaries are endothelial tubes measuring 4 to 8 mm in diameter that rest on a thin

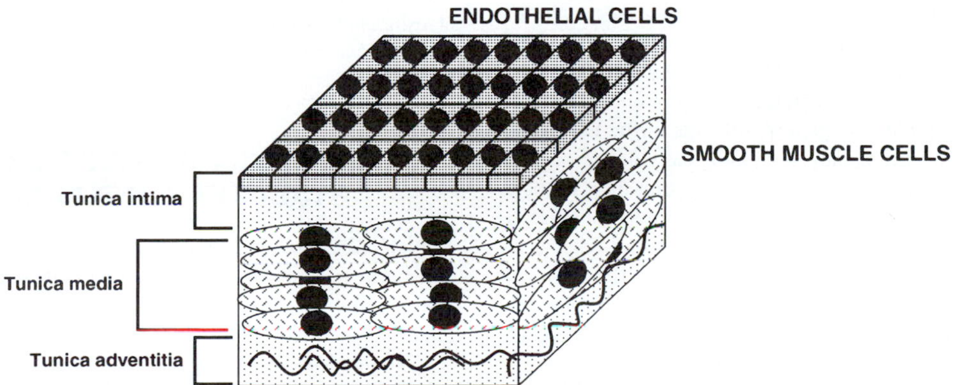

Figure 18-12. Cross-sectional representation of the vascular wall of large and medium-size blood vessels.

The tunica intima is composed of endothelial cells, facing the vessel lumen, which rest on a thin basal lamina. The tunica media consists mainly of vascular smooth muscle cells interwoven with collagen and elastin. The tunica adventia is a layer of fibroblasts, collagen, elastin, and glycosaminoglycans.

basal lamina to which pericytes are often are attached. When one capillary converges with another, the vessel formed is referred to as a postcapillary venule. The capillary and the pericytic venule are the principal sites of exchange between the blood and tissues.

Vascular endothelial cells play an integral role in the regulation of hemostasis, vascular tone, and angiogenesis. Angiogenesis involves the formation of blood vessels secondary to the migration, proliferation, and differentiation of vascular cells. The process of angiogenesis is subject to regulation by hypoxia and has been identified as a likely target for selective toxicity by newly developed antineoplastic agents. Endothelial cells also are involved in the regulation of macromolecular transport across the vessel wall, attachment and recruitment of inflammatory cells, synthesis of connective tissue proteins, and generation of reactive oxygen species. Medial smooth muscle cells are responsible for the regulation of vascular tone. The contractile response of blood vessels is mediated by receptors located primarily on the plasma membrane of smooth muscle cells. Activation of these receptors brings about changes in calcium conductance that lead to activation of the contractile apparatus. Calcium homeostasis is controlled by the interplay of multiple regulatory mechanisms (Fig. 18-13). In contrast to cardiac myocytes, where relatively large stores of calcium are found, vascular smooth muscle depends primarily on extracellular calcium sources for contraction. Increases in cytoplasmic calcium often involve the influx of calcium through either receptor- or voltage-operated channels. Cytoplasmic Ca^{2+} activates a calmodulin-dependent protein kinase that in turn phosphorylates myosin to allow the interaction of myosin and actin and the shortening of the sarcomere.

Catecholamines influence vascular function through the activation of surface receptors, among which the $alpha_1$ and $beta_2$ receptors have been the most extensively characterized. Activation of $alpha_1$ receptors in smooth muscle cells increases contractility, while activation of $beta_2$ receptors decreases it. Two $alpha_1$-adrenergic receptor subtypes—$alpha_{1A}$ and the $alpha_{1B}$—have been identified. $Alpha_{1B}$-adrenergic stimulation elicits smooth muscle contraction by activating phospholipase-mediated hydrolysis of phosphatidylinositol-4,5-bisphosphate to yield diacylglycerol and inositol-1,4,5-trisphosphate (Fig. 18-14). Diacylglycerol binds to and activates protein kinase C, while inositol-1,4,5-trisphosphate binds to an intracellular receptor on the sarcoplasmic reticulum to initiate the release of calcium stores. The $alpha_{1A}$-adrenergic receptor mediates extracellular calcium entry through voltage-sensitive L-type calcium channels. Activation of $beta_2$ receptors leads to G protein-mediated activation of adenylyl cyclase and the production of cyclic AMP (Fig. 18-15). $Beta_2$ agonists induce a conformational change in the receptor, resulting in dissociation of the alpha subunit from the beta-gamma subunits of the G protein. The alpha subunit, in turn, achieves a biologically active conformation that modulates adenylyl cyclase activity after displacement of GDP by GTP. Inactivation occurs through hydrolysis of GTP by the intrinsic GTPase activity of the G protein. Several other neurohormones—such as acetylcholine, angiotensin II, arginine-vasopressin, histamine, thrombin, and endothelin—modulate contractile events by activation of G protein–coupled receptors. Smooth muscle cells are also responsible for the synthesis of extracellular matrix proteins during arterial repair, the metabolism and/or secretion of bioactive substances, and the regulation of monocyte function. Fibroblasts in the adventitial layer secrete some of the collagen and glycosaminoglycans needed to give structural support to the vessel wall.

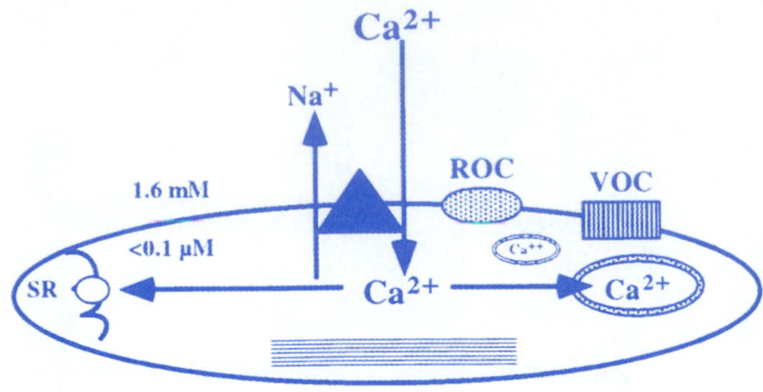

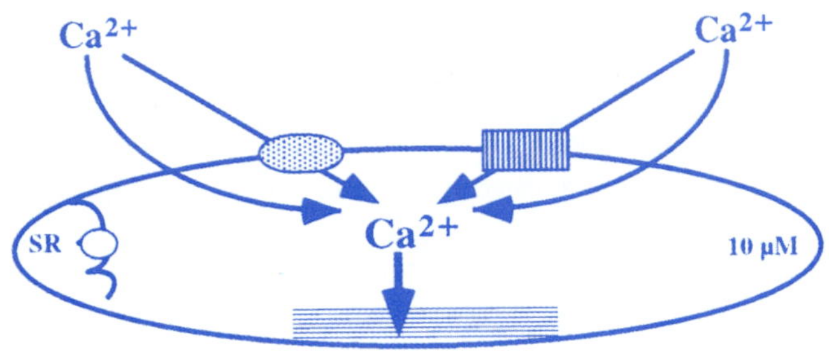

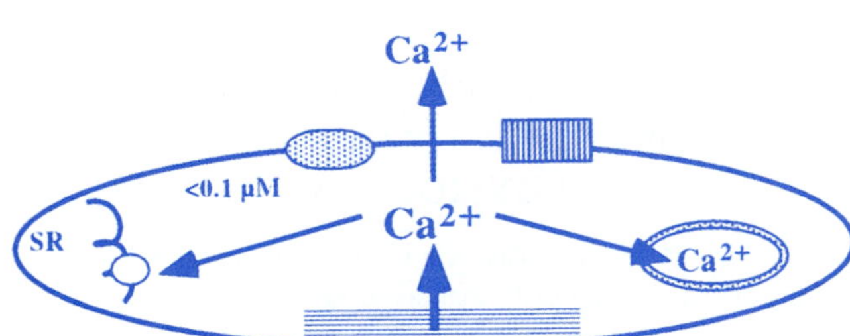

Figure 18-13. Calcium regulation and homeostasis in vascular smooth muscle cells.

Intracellular calcium is sequestered primarily in the sarcoplasmic reticulum (SR), but contraction of smooth muscle cells is initiated by an influx of extracellular calcium through receptor-operated channels (ROC) or voltage-operated channels (VOC).

DISTURBANCES OF VASCULAR STRUCTURE AND FUNCTION

Human epidemiologic studies have established a positive correlation between injury to a blood vessel wall and the occurrence of vascular diseases such as atherosclerosis and hypertension (Rosenman, 1990). Atherosclerosis is a major structural change in the vessel wall that leads to deleterious consequences to the vessel as well as the other organs involved. This disease is a degenerative process involving focal intimal thickenings formed after migration of smooth muscle cells to the intima and uncontrolled proliferation. Extracellular matrix components such as collagen and elastin, intra- and extracellular lipids, complex carbohydrates, blood products,

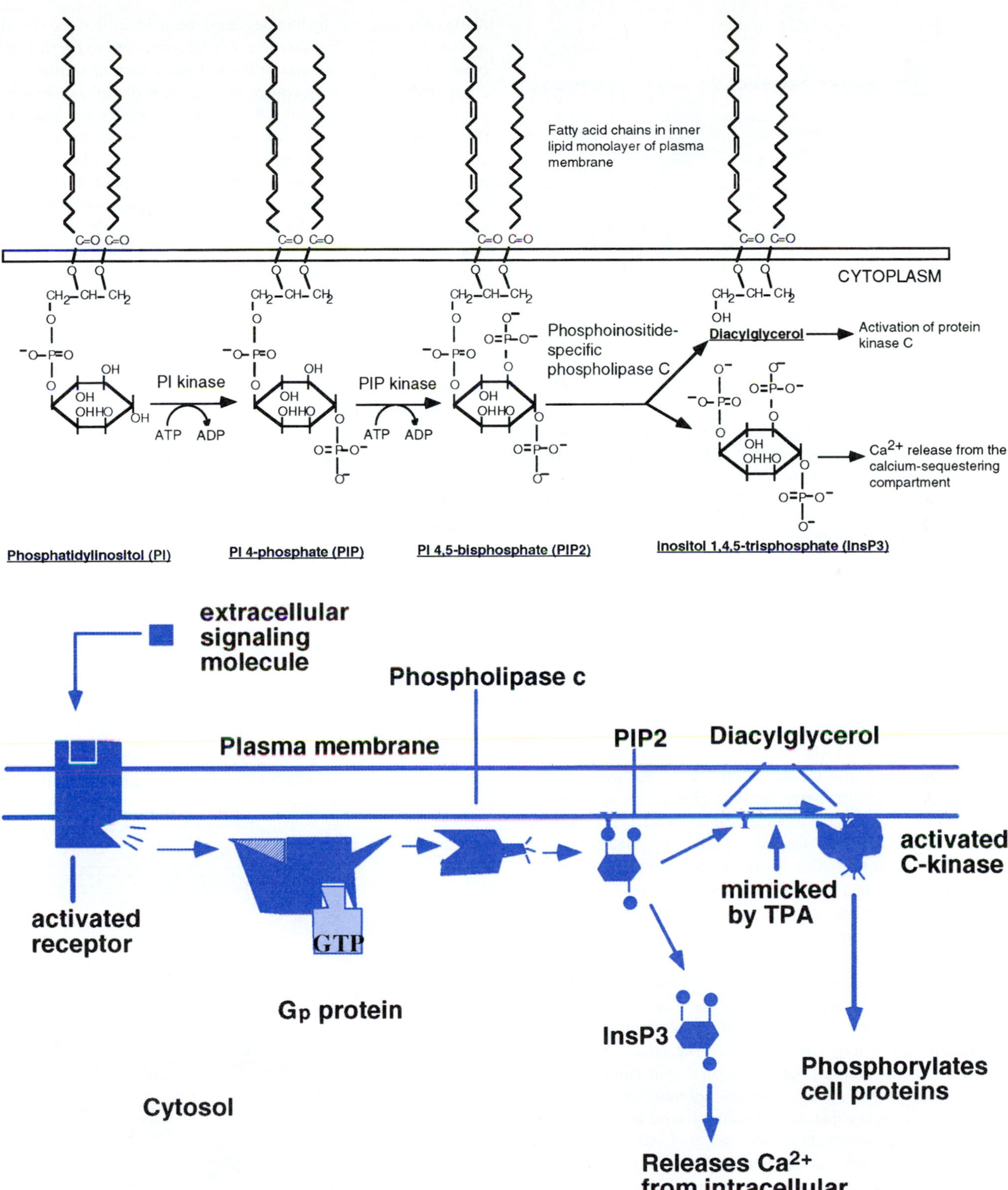

Figure 18-14. Phosphatidylinositol metabolism and subsequent production of intracellular second messengers in vascular smooth muscle cells.

Inositol 1,4,5-trisphosphate (InsP3), which elicits intracellular Ca^{2+} release, is generated from phosphatidylinositol (PI) by the sequential actions of PI kinase, PIP kinase, and phospholipase C (*A*). PI 4,5-bisphosphate (PIP2) can also be cleaved by phospholipase C to form diacylglycerol, which activates protein kinase C (*B*).

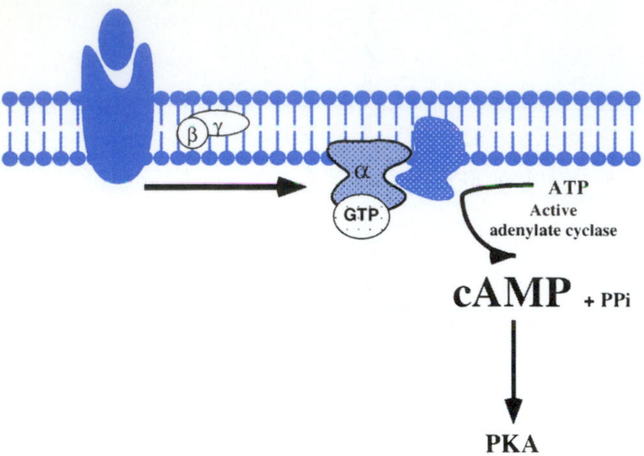

Figure 18-15. Depiction of the activation of adenyl cyclase through the activation of a beta$_2$-adrenergic receptor.

Ligand binding results in a conformational change in the receptor, leading to GTP displacement of GDP on the *a* subunit of the receptor-linked G protein. The binding of GTP elicits the release of the *b* and *c* subunits and the binding of the *a* subunit to adenyl cyclase, activating the enzyme. Cyclic AMP (cAMP) is produced, and this can lead to various events, including the activation of protein kinase A.

and calcium accumulate to varying degrees as the lesion advances. The plaque also contains inflammatory cells, such as infiltrated monocytes and leukocytes, which participate in the progression of the pathologic response. Figure 18-16 shows two pathways that can mediate the initiation and/or promotion of the atherosclerotic process by toxic chemicals. Lesions generally occur in large and medium-sized blood vessels such as the aorta and the coronary, carotid, and femoral arteries. In young human subjects, atherosclerotic lesions are distributed in the region of the aortic valve ring. The aortic arch and the thoracic and abdominal aorta become more severely affected as a function of age. The principal consequence of atheroma formation is progressive narrowing of the arterial lumen that leads to a restricted blood supply to distal sites. Such changes can result in renal hypertension, stroke, and myocardial ischemia and infarction.

Toxic chemicals can induce or enhance atheroma formation by several mechanisms involving injury to luminal endothelial cells and/or medial smooth muscle cells (Ramos et al., 1994). Such lesions often result from chronic cycles of vascular injury and repair and typically require long latency periods. Mechanical or toxic injury to the endothelium has been associated with initiation of the atherogenic response. Agents such as acrolein, butadiene, cyclophosphamide, heavy metals, and homocysteine have been identified as endothelial toxins. In a wide variety of animal species (including rabbits and rats), vascular endothelial cell injury potentiates the atherogenic process and in some instances precedes the development of atherosclerotic plaques. In humans and animals, a hypercholesterolemic diet causes an increase in plasma lipoproteins, damages the endothelium, and results in proliferation of smooth muscle cells. Recent evidence implicates oxidized forms of LDL in the induction of atherosclerotic lesions by hyperlipoproteinemia. As part of the repair process, smooth muscle cell mitogens and chemotatic agents are released from one or more cell types. Atherosclerotic lesions can also develop as a result of injury to medial smooth muscle cells. Agents such as allylamine, benzo[*a*]pyrene, dinitrotoluenes, and hydrazines have been identified as smooth muscle cell toxins. Proliferation may be secondary to regenerative repair or to genetic changes in a small population of medial cells. After studying the monotypism of glucose-6-phosphate dehydrogenase, Benditt and Benditt (1973) proposed over twenty years ago that smooth muscle cells in the atherosclerotic plaque are the progeny of a single smooth muscle cell. Thus, the atherosclerotic process would resemble benign neoplastic growth of smooth muscle tumors (leiomyomas) (Fig. 18-17). Upon exposure to a toxic agent, smooth muscle cells may exist in a genetically altered state that gives rise to lesions after exposure to chemotatic/growth-promoting factors. Alternatively, mutations could induce the constitutive production of growth factors in smooth muscle cells, resulting in autocrine stimulation of growth. DNA isolated from human atherosclerotic plaques is capable of transforming NIH3T3 cells and producing tumors in nude mice, a finding that suggests that atherosclerotic cells possess intrinsic transforming potential.

Changes in blood pressure are often seen during acute poisonings. Hypotension—a sustained reduction of systemic arterial pressure—is common in poisonings with CNS depressants or antihypertensive agents as well as during anaphylactic reactions. Postural hypotension, particularly in elderly people, can be induced by therapeutic agents such as drugs that lower cardiac output or decrease blood volume. These agents include depressants of the va-

A. Response to Injury

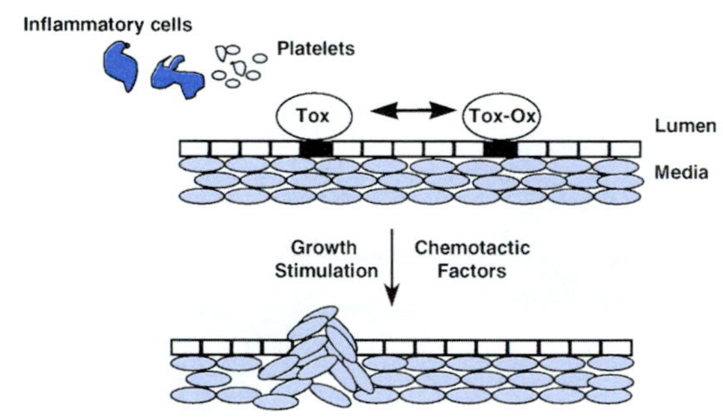

B. Somatic Mutation

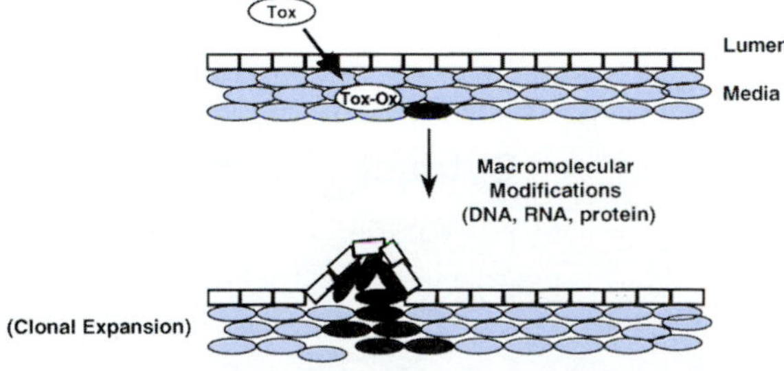

Figure 18-16. Representation of the two major hypotheses for the molecular and cellular events that lead to atherosclerosis.

The response to injury hypothesis (*A*) initially proposed by Ross and subsequently modified (1993) states that injury of endothelial cells triggers a response involving recruitment of platelets and inflammatory cells that stimulate smooth muscle cell migration and proliferation. In contrast, Benditt and Benditt (1973) proposed that atherosclerotic lesions are a result of the monoclonal expansion of a mutated smooth muscle cell (*B*).

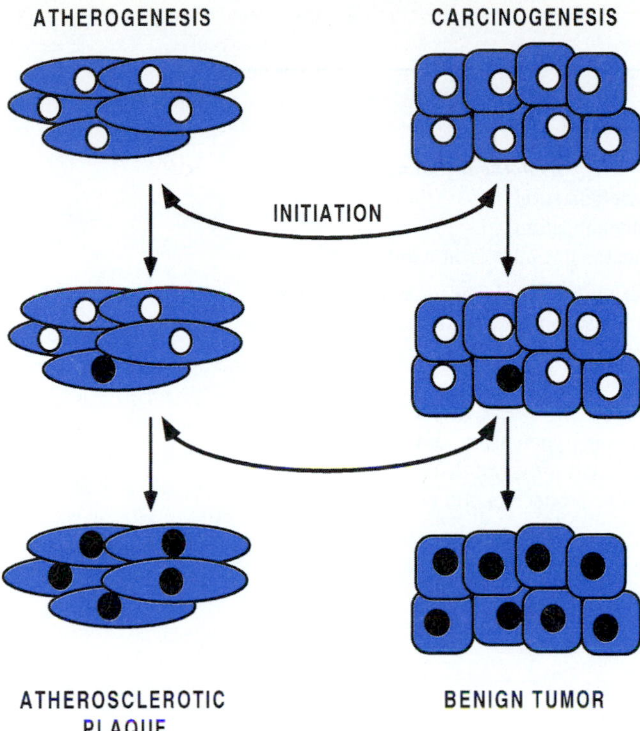

Figure 18-17. Representation of the links between atherogenesis and carcinogenesis.

Both disease processes may involve the initiation of a target cell and subsequent promotional events to result in a full response.

somotor center such as morphine-like compounds, antihypertensive agents, sedatives, neuroleptics, and antiparkinsonian agents. In addition, agents that inhibit noradrenaline production and reuptake, such as methyldopa or antidepressants, respectively, also induce postural hypotension. Circulatory insufficiency can be delayed or even prevented by increased sympathoadrenal activity. However, poisonings associated with extreme loss of body fluids caused by persistent vomiting or diarrhea and conditions resulting in marked reductions in plasma, such as hemorrhage, lead to a state of circulatory insufficiency (shock). Other causes of shock include inadequate myocardial contraction resulting from severe arrhythmia and inadequate peripheral circulation brought about by altered vasomotor tone resulting from the effects of chemical mediators, such as histamine, leukotriene, and kinins. Vasodilation, which is mediated by activation of H_1 and H_2 receptors located throughout the resistance vessels, is the most prominent action of histamine in humans. Histamine tends to constrict the larger blood vessels.

Hypertension may result from an increased concentration of circulating vasoconstrictors such as angiotensin II and catecholamines or from disturbances of local regulation mediated by metabolic, myogenic, or angiogenic mechanisms. Increased vascular resistance has been associated with an overall increase in wall thickness caused at least in part by hypertrophy and proliferation of smooth muscle cells. A sustained elevation in blood pressure has also been associated with destruction of capillaries at the tissue level and compensatory angiogenesis. Arterial hypertension may occur in the course of an overdose of sympathomimetic and anticholinergic drugs. Sudden drug-induced hypertension can cause cerebrovascular accidents when diseased blood vessels cannot adapt to high perfusion pressures. Mineralocorticoids can cause excessive sodium retention and lead to sustained elevation of blood pressure by increasing circulatory volume. Licorice, which contains glycyrrhizin, an aldosterone-like substance that exerts mineralocorticoid activity, can cause sustained hypertension. Agents that cause hyperreninemia, such as cadmium, can raise blood pressure through the generation of angiotensinogen II. Depletion of renomedullary vasodilator substances has been implicated in the hypertensive episodes associated with analgesic drug-induced nephropathy. Increased synthesis of angiotensinogen has been considered an important factor in the hypertension produced by high doses of estrogen-containing oral contraceptives. Sustained hypertension is the most important risk factor predisposing a person to coronary and cerebral atherosclerosis. The mechanisms by which hypertension produces vascular degenerative lesions involve increased vascular permeability that leads to entry of blood constituents into the vessel wall.

The vascular toxicity of some therapeutic agents, including antimicrobial drugs and anticoagulants, often involves vasculitis secondary to hypersensitivity reactions. Some chemicals can cause hemorrhage by damaging the large vessels, such as the aneurysms produced by lathyrogens. Damage to capillaries by cytotoxic chemicals leading to petechial hemorrhages is seen in several organs after acute poisonings. A chemically induced defect in the blood-clotting mechanism increases the probability that a hemorrhage will occur. Thrombosis—the formation of a semisolid mass from blood constituents in the circulation—can occur in both arteries and veins as a result of toxicant exposure. Predisposition to thrombosis occurs by means of induction of platelet aggregation, an increase in their adhesiveness, or creation of a state of hypercoagulability through an increase in or activation of clotting factors, as seen with large doses of epinephrine. Other chemicals may lead to thrombosis by interfering with antithrombin III (oral contraceptive steroids) or inhibiting fibrinolysis (corticosteroids, mercurials). Sudden changes in blood flow brought about by excessive vasoconstriction or decreased peripheral resistance can trigger arterial thrombosis. Venous stasis contributes to the development of venous thrombosis. Table 18-5 provides a partial list of thrombogenic agents and their putative mechanisms of action. Injury to the vessel wall by intravenous infusion of an irritating drug produces generalized endothelial damage and leads to thromboses at the sites of lesions. Portions of a thrombus may be released and travel in the vascular system until arrested as an embolus in a vessel with a caliber even smaller than that of its origin. The consequence depends on the site of arrest, but a thrombus can result in death. The most important drugs known to produce thromboembolisms are the contraceptive steroids.

GENERAL BIOCHEMICAL MECHANISMS OF VASCULAR TOXICITY

Epidemiologic and experimental evidence has established a correlation between exposure to toxic chemicals and the incidence of cardiovascular morbidity and mortality. Such a correlation is best exemplified by the role of tobacco smoke as a major contributor to myocardial infarction, sudden cardiac death, arteriosclerotic peripheral vascular disease, and atherosclerotic aneurysm of the aorta. Angiotoxic chemicals are found in the ambient environment as a result of anthropogenic activity or occur as natural variations in the

Table 18-5
Compounds Producing Thrombosis

AGENT	MECHANISM OF ACTION / SPECIFIC EFFECTS
	Endothelial damage
Homocysteine	Deendothelialization
Endotoxin	Deendothelialization
Sodium acetriozate	Disseminated thrombosis in capillaries and veins
	Pathophysiologic circulatory dynamics
Ergotamine	Profound vasoconstriction in peripheral arteries
Pitressin	Profound vasoconstriction in coronary and mesenteric arteries
Oral contraceptives	Venous stasis in lower extremities
ACh and autonomic blockers	Hypovolemic hypotension and stasis
Sympathomimetic agents	Elevated blood pressure; distentions of vessels to produce endothelial damage
	Effects on platelets
Serotonin	Increase in platelet count (above $10^6/mm^3$)
Progesterone	
Testosterone	
Somatotropic hormone	
Vinblastine	
Vincristine	
Congo Red	
Ristocetin	
Thrombin	
Epinephrine	
Adenosine diphosphate	Increase in platelet adhesiveness
Thrombin	
Evans blue	
	Effects on clotting factors
Epinephrine	Increase in factors VIII and IX
Guanethidine	Secondary effects due to release of epinephrine
Debrisoquin	
Tyramine	
Lactic acid (IV infusion)	Activation of Hageman factor
Long-chain fatty acids (IV infusion)	Activation of contact factors
Catecholamines	Elevation in circulating levels of fatty acids
ACTH	
Thymoleptics	
Nicotine	
Oral contraceptives	Decrease in antithrombin III levels
Mercuric chloride	Inhibition of fibrinolysis
Corticosteroids	
ε-Aminocaproic acid	Plasminogen antiactivator
Aprotinine	Proteinase inhibitors

environment, such as fungal toxins in food supplies. Chemicals absorbed through the respiratory, cutaneous, gastrointestinal, and intravenous routes by necessity come in contact with vascular cells before reaching other sites in the body. This property alone puts the vascular system at increased risk of toxic insult. Although this relationship has largely been ignored, the recognition that many target organ toxicities involve a significant microvascular component has become more prevalent.

Chemicals can produce degenerative or inflammatory changes in blood vessels as a consequence of an excessive pharmacologic effect. For example, ergotamine, a naturally occurring alkaloid, causes sustained arterial vasoconstriction that leads to peripheral arterial lesions involving intimal proliferation and medial degenerative changes. Degenerative or inflammatory changes can also occur secondary to the interaction of chemicals or their reactive metabolites with a structural and/or functional component of the vessel wall. For example, endothelial cell death and atherosclerosis can be induced by homocysteine, a sulfur-containing amino acid produced in the biosynthesis of cysteine from methionine. The reactivity of the sulfhydryl group of homocysteine has been implicated in the atherogenic response. Injury to the endothelium leads to recruitment of white blood cells into the affected sites as part of the inflammatory response. The inflammatory response is directed by a variety of signaling molecules that are produced locally by mast cells, nerve endings, platelets, and white blood cells as well as by the activation of complement. In the case of medial smooth muscle cells, injury is associated with degenerative changes in the media of blood vessels. For example, allylamine toxicity is associated primarily with medial changes, but changes in endothelial cells also have been noted. Repeated cycles of vascular injury by this amine result in smooth muscle hyperplasia and coronary artery and aortic lesions which mimic those found in atherosclerotic vessels. Changes in the collagen of large arteries leading to localized dilation (aneurysms) occur in lathyrism and can be reproduced experimentally by administration of beta-aminopropionitrile.

Angiotoxicity may be expressed at the mechanical, metabolic, or genetic level and in general involves interactions of multiple cellular elements (Table 18-6). Endothelial cells represent the first cellular barrier to the movement of blood-borne toxins from the lumen of the vessel to deeper layers of the wall. This location makes these regions particularly susceptible to toxic insult. Endothelial injury also occurs as a result of the production of oxygen free radicals during reperfusion injury in transplanted organs. Toxic chemicals reaching the subendothelial space may cause injury to medial smooth muscle cells and/or adventitial fibroblasts. Adventitial and medial cells in large elastic arteries such as the human aorta also may be reached via the vasa vasorum, the intrinsic blood supply to the vessel wall. The vasculotoxic response is also dependent on the influence of (1) extracellular matrix proteins that influence cell behavior, (2) coagulation factors that dictate the extent of hemostatic involvement, (3) hormones and growth factors that regulate vascular function, and (4) plasma lipoproteins, some of which modulate cellular metabolism and facilitate the transport and delivery of hydrophobic substances (Ferrario et al., 1985).

Common mechanisms of vascular toxicity include (1) selective alterations of vascular reactivity mediated by alterations in membrane structure and function; (2) in certain forms of chemically induced vascular toxicity, chemical exposure may be associated redox stress leading to disruption of gene regulatory mechanisms, compromised antioxidant defenses, and generalized loss of homeostasis; (3) vessel-specific bioactivation of protoxicants; (4) preferential accumulation of the active toxin in vascular cells (Fig. 18-18). Multiple mechanisms often operate simultaneously in the course of the toxic response. Interestingly, although vascular injury by toxic chemicals often involves different mechanisms, the modulation of growth and differentiation in vascular cells is a common endpoint of vasculotoxic injury.

Vascular reactivity is regulated by the transfer of signals from the surface to the interior of the cell and/or direct modulation of the structure and function of contractile protein. Usually, disorders of vascular reactivity involve generalized disturbances of ionic regulation. Nontoxic chemicals can be converted by vascular enzymes to reactive species that cause injury to both intra- and extracellular targets. Enzyme systems that are present in vascular cells and are involved in the bioactivation of vascular toxins include amine oxidases, cytochrome P450 monooxygenases, and prostaglandin synthetase. Amine oxidases are copper-containing enzymes that catalyze the oxidative removal of biogenic amines from blood plasma, the cross-linking of collagen and elastin in connective tissue, and the regulation of intracellular spermine and spermidine levels. These microsomal enzyme systems are involved in the bioactivation of allylamine to acrolein and hydrogen peroxide. The occurrence of several cytochrome P450 metabolites of arachidonic

Table 18-6
Cell Types Implicated in the Vasculotoxic Response

CELL TYPE	FUNCTION
Endothelial cells	First barrier to blood-borne toxins; synthesis and release of endothelium-derived relaxing factor; synthesis of pro- and antiaggregatory factors; attachment and recruitment of inflammatory cells; synthesis of connective tissue proteins; generation of oxygen-derived free radicals and other radical moeities.
Smooth muscle cells	Maintenance of vasomotor tone; synthesis of extracellular matrix proteins including collagen and elastin; synthesis of prostaglandins and other biologically active lipids; regulation of monocyte function; formation of free radicals.
Fibroblasts	Synthesis of extracellular matrix proteins including collagens, structural support to the vessel wall.
Monocytes/macrophages	Scavenger potential; synthesis of macrophage-derived growth factor; generation of reactive oxygen species; lymphocyte activation, progenitor of foam cells.
Platelets	Synthesis of proaggregatory substances and smooth muscle mitogens such as platelet-derived growth factor.
Lymphocytes	Release of activated oxygen species; cellular immunity; production of immunoglobulins.

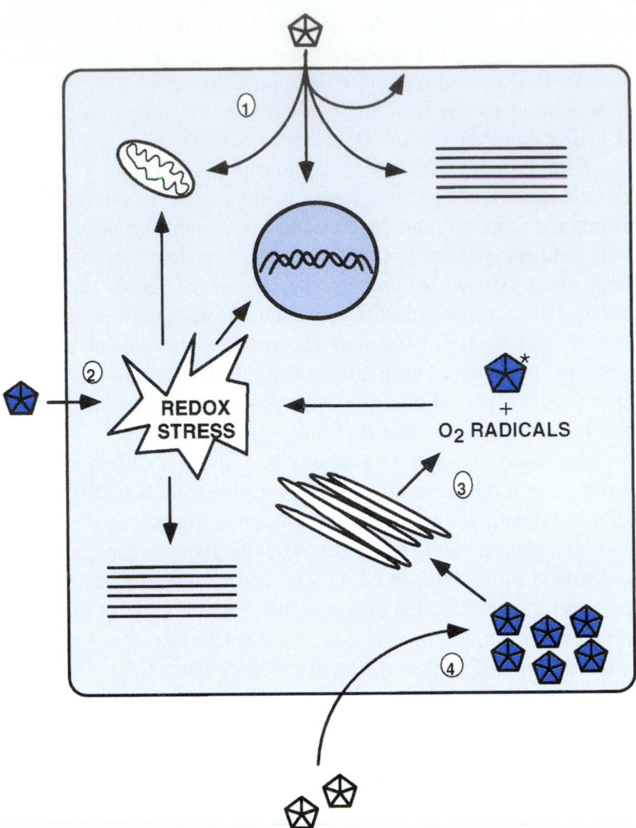

Figure 18-18. Toxic injury to vascular cells may involve four common mechanisms.

(1) Vascular injury may involve disruption of cellular membranes or the contractile apparatus of smooth muscle cells by a toxicant. (2) In certain forms of chemically induced vascular toxicity, chemical exposure is associated with redox stress, leading to disruption of gene regulatory mechanisms, compromised antioxidant defenses, and generalized loss of homeostasis. (3) Additionally, vascular cells may bioactivate protoxicants in a vessel-specific manner to generate reactive intermediates and/or oxygen derived free radicals that induce cell injury. (4) Vascular cells also may preferentially accumulate potential toxins.

acid involved in the regulation of vascular tone and sodium pump activity has also been noted. For instance, cytochrome P450 1A1 in endothelial and smooth muscle cells metabolizes benzo[*a*]pyrene and other polycyclic aromatic hydrocarbons to toxic and genotoxic intermediates. A complex of microsomal enzymes collectively referred to as prostaglandin synthetase catalyzes the formation of biologically active lipids, including prostacyclin and thromboxane A_2. Prostacyclin, the major arachidonic acid metabolite in blood vessels, is a strong vasodilator and an endogenous inhibitor of platelet aggregation, while thromboxane A_2, the major arachidonic acid metabolite in platelets, is a potent vasoconstrictor and a promoter of platelet aggregation. The bioactivation of vascular toxins need not be confined to vascular tissue. Evidence that angiotoxic chemicals can be bioactivated by the liver and lung, with the activated metabolites leaving the metabolizing sites and reaching vascular targets through the systemic circulation, has been presented. Vascular toxicity also may be due to deficiencies in the capacity of target cells to detoxify the active toxin or handle prooxidant states. Key components of the endogenous antioxidant defense system—including the glutathione/glutathione reductase/glutathione peroxidase system, superoxide dismutase—and catalase, are operative in vascular cells.

Oxidative metabolism is critical to the preservation of vascular function, as is best exemplified by the role of oxidation in the metabolism and cytotoxicity of plasma lipoproteins. LDLs are oxidized by oxygen free radicals released by arterial cells, and this reaction is considered to be critical in the initiation and progression of the atherosclerotic process (Fig. 18-19). Modified LDLs attract macrophages and prevent their migration from the tissues (Ross, 1993). Oxidation of low-density lipoproteins generates activated oxygen species, which can directly injure endothelial cells and increase adherence and the migration of monocytes and T lymphocytes into the subendothelial space. Subsequent release of growth modulators from endothelial cells and/or macrophages can promote smooth muscle cell proliferation and the secretion of extracellular matrix proteins. In the vasculature, free radicals in vivo can be generated secondary to anoxic/reoxygenation injury, metabolism of xenobiotics, neutrophil/monocyte-mediated inflammation, and oxidative modification of low-density lipoproteins. Superoxide anions inactivate endothelium-derived relaxing factor, while hydrogen peroxide and hydroxyl radicals cause direct vasodilation and stimulate the synthesis and release of relaxation factors. Oxygen radicals are considered important mediators of vascular damage in acute arterial hypertension and experimental brain injury (Wei et al., 1985). Acute exposure of rats to angiotensin II results in a hypertensive episode that results from irregular constriction patterns and in vascular hyperpermeability in small arteries and arterioles (Wilson, 1990). The treatment of hypertensive rats with free radical scavengers inhibits the vascular hyperpermeability and cellular damage associated with angiotensin II–induced hypertension. The release of superoxide from endothelial cells may modulate endothelial functions as well as the functions of other constituents of the vascular wall. In this context, activated endothelial cells have been reported to produce and secrete proteases

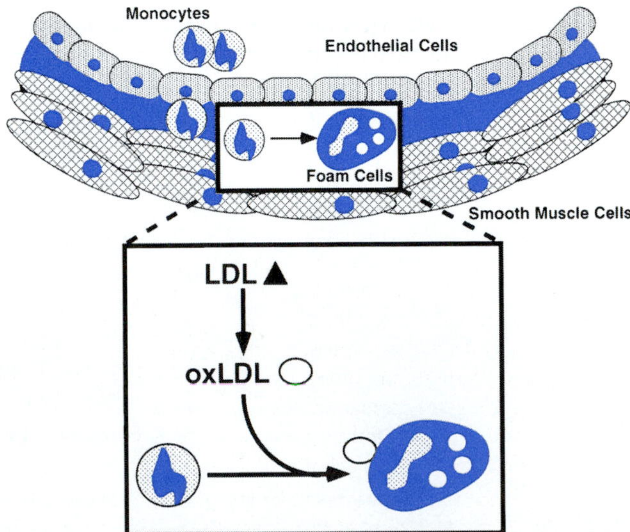

Figure 18-19. Oxidized lipoproteins participate in the progression of atherosclerosis.

Low-density lipoproteins (LDL) are oxidized within the vasculature. The uptake of oxidized LDL by macrophage scavenger receptors results in the formation of foam cells, an important cell type found in atherosclerotic plaques.

in association with vessel penetration into surrounding connective tissue in response to angiogenic stimuli (Gross et al., 1983).

Vascular toxicity may be due to selective accumulation of chemicals in the vascular wall. Although the mechanisms responsible for preferential accumulation of toxins in the vessel wall are not known, receptor-mediated internalization of LDLs may be critical in this process. This process appears to be critical in the deposition of aromatic hydrocarbons and other ubiquitous environmental contaminants, including organic acids, aldehydes, alcohols, and esters, in the vessel wall (Ferrario et al., 1985). Agents such as nonenal, naphthalene, propylfuranacetaldehyde, DDT, and hexachlorobenzene have been identified in atherosclerotic plaques. The deposition of these toxicants could be accounted for by chemical partitioning into the lipid phase of the atherosclerotic plaques. The consequences of vasculotoxic insult are dictated by the interplay between vascular and nonvascular cells and by noncellular factors such as extracellular matrix proteins, coagulation factors, hormones, immune complexes, and plasma lipoproteins. Furthermore, the toxic response can be modulated by mechanical and hemodynamic factors such as arterial pressure, shear stress, and blood viscosity. An additional consideration is the fact that kinetic and pharmacodynamic differences among different animal species also may alter the toxicological profile of a toxicant.

CLASSIFICATION OF VASCULOTOXIC AGENTS

Pharmaceutical Agents

Autonomic Agents ***Sympathomimetic Amines*** The sympathomimetic amines—including epinephrine, norepinephrine, dopamine, and isoproterenol—can damage the arterial vasculature by a variety of mechanisms. Amphetamine, a noncatecholamine sympathomimetic, damages cerebral arteries in experimental animal models. Large doses of norepinephrine produce toxic effects on the endothelium of the thoracic aorta of rabbits. Degenerative changes in the aortic arch have taken the form of increased numbers of microvilli and many focal areas of unusual endothelial cytoarchitecture. Repeated exposure to catecholamines induces atherosclerotic lesions in several animal species. The atherosclerotic effect of catecholamines probably is related to their ability to induce endothelial cell injury and/or modulate the proliferation of vascular cells. Evidence is available suggesting that the proliferative disturbances induced by catecholamines are mediated via alpha-receptors because prazocin, an alpha-receptor antagonist, effectively prevents the toxic response (Nakaki et al., 1989). However, potentiation of the atherosclerotic process by sympathetic activation is inhibited by beta-adrenergic receptor blockade. Smooth muscle cells subjected to increased stress by diabetes, hypertension, and balloon injury are more susceptible to the effects of catecholamines. Thus, the formation of arteriosclerotic lesions in certain forms of hypertension may be initiated and/or supported by high levels of circulating catecholamines.

Nicotine Nicotine, an alkaloid found in various plants, mimics the actions of acetylcholine at nicotinic receptors throughout the body. At pharmacologic concentrations, nicotine increases heart rate and blood pressure as a result of stimulation of sympathetic ganglia and the adrenal medulla. Epidemiologic and experimental studies have suggested that nicotine is a causative or aggravating factor in myocardial and cerebral infarction, gangrene, and aneurysm. Bull and associates (1985) have shown that repeated subcutaneous infusion of nicotine for 7 days is associated with reduced prostacyclin production in aortic segments. Reduced prostacyclin production has been observed in isolated rabbit hearts, rabbit aortas, human veins, rat aortas, and rat umbilical arteries when incubated with nicotine in vitro. It has been suggested that the effects of nicotine are due to competitive inhibition of cyclooxygenase, which precludes the formation of prostaglandin endoperoxides in vivo.

Cocaine Cardiovascular disorders are among the most common complications associated with cocaine abuse. The central actions of cocaine trigger an increase in the circulating levels of catecholamines and a generalized state of vasoconstriction. Hypertension and cerebral strokes are common vascular complications. In pregnant women, cocaine-induced vascular changes have been associated with abortions and abruptio placentae. Recent studies have shown that cocaine enhances leukocyte migration across the cerebral vessel wall during inflammatory conditions. This effect is exerted through a cascade of augmented expression of inflammatory cytokines and endothelial adhesion molecules and may in fact underlie the cerebrovascular complications associated with cocaine abuse (Gan et al., 1999).

Psychotropic Agents Several agents in the psychotropic class of drugs have been identified as potential atherogens. For instance, trifluoperazine and chlorpromazine have been shown to cause intracellular cholesterol accumulation in cultured cells of the aortic intima (Iakushkin et al., 1992). Enalapril has been shown to cause angioedema in humans. Aside from the atherogenic effects, postural hypotension has been identified as the most common cardiovascular side effect of tricyclic antidepressants.

Antineoplastic Agents The vasculotoxic responses elicited by antineoplastic agents range from asymptomatic arterial lesions to thrombotic microangiopathy. Pulmonary veno-occlusive disease has been reported after the administration of various agents, including 5-fluorouracil, doxorubicin, and mitomycin. Long latencies characterize the occurrence of this disorder. Cyclophosphamide causes cerebrovascular and viscerovascular lesions, resulting in hemorrhages. In studies with 5-fluoro-2-deoxyuridine in dogs, chronic infusions into the hepatic artery resulted in gastrointestinal hemorrhage and portal vein thrombosis.

Analgesics and Nonsteroidal Anti-Inflammatory Agents Aspirin can produce endothelial damage as part of a pattern of gastric erosion. Studies in rats have shown early changes in the basement membrane of endothelial cells of the capillaries and postcapillary venules, leading to obliteration of small vessels and ischemic infarcts in the large intestine. Regular use of analgesics containing phenacetin has been associated with an increased risk of hypertension and cardiovascular morbidity. Nonsteroidal anti-inflammatory drugs may induce glomerular and vascular renal lesions.

Oral Contraceptives Oral contraceptive steroids can produce thromboembolic disorders. An increased incidence of deep vein phlebitis and pulmonary embolism has been reported in young women who use oral contraceptives. Intracranial venous thrombosis and secondary increases in the risk of stroke have also been noted. A combination of cholesterol and estradiol given to experimental animals produced severe degenerative atherosclerotic effects on coronary arteries as well as lipid deposition along the ascending aorta. In an epidemiologic review, Stolley and colleagues (1989) summarized the risks of vascular disease associated with the use of oral contraceptives. Oral contraceptive users have an increased risk of myocardial infarction relative to nonusers, a correlation that is markedly exacerbated by smoking. Oral contraceptive users experience an increased risk of cerebral thrombosis, hemorrhage, venous thrombosis, and pulmonary embolism. Although this has not been established with certainty, several groups have proposed that an immunologic mechanism mediates the vasculotoxic actions of oral contraceptives. However, the mechanism by which oral contraceptives increase the risk of vascular disease is unclear.

Radiologic Contrast Dyes The iodinated radio contrast dyes used for visualization of blood vessels in angiography can cause thrombophlebitis. The cyanoacrylate adhesives used in repairing blood vessels and other tissues have produced degenerative changes in the arteries of dogs. Certain rapidly polymerizing polyurethane preparations used for transcatheter embolization techniques in surgery have produced dissolution of arterial walls. Dermal microvascular lesions have been reported after plastic film wound dressings were applied in various animal species.

Phosphodiesterase Inhibitors The class of compounds that includes phosphodiesterase inhibitors is associated with toxicity in medium-size arteries of the mesentery, testis, and myocardium. Other reports showing that theophylline, an inhibitor of phosphodiesterase, causes cardiovascular lesions in mesenteric arterioles and that isomazole and indolidan cause periarteritis of the media and adventitia of small and medium-size arteries have been presented (Sandusky et al., 1991).

Miscellaneous Agents Interleukin-2 therapy has been associated with a spectrum of cardiovascular toxicities and hemodynamic alterations often indistinguishable from septic shock. Many of these effects may be mediated by overproduction of nitric oxide via cytokine-inducible nitric oxide pathway (Shahidi and Kilbourn, 1998).

Natural Products

Bacterial Endotoxins Bacterial endotoxins produce a variety of toxic effects in many vascular beds. In the liver, they cause swelling of endothelial cells and adhesion of platelets to sinusoid walls. In the lung, endotoxins produce increased vascular permeability and pulmonary hypertension. Infusion of endotoxin into experimental animals produces thickening of endothelial cells and the formation of fibrin thrombi in small veins. In piglets, severe coronary artery damage has been demonstrated. These changes include disappearance of endothelial cells (exfoliation) followed by necrosis of medial smooth muscle cells. The terminal phase of the effects of endotoxin on the systemic vasculature results in marked hypotension. The ability of vitamin E to prevent disseminated intravascular coagulation induced by bacterial endotoxins in the rat suggests that this disorder is related to free radical–mediated mechanisms.

Homocysteine Moderately elevated levels of homocysteine have been associated with atherosclerosis and venous thrombosis. Toxicity may involve oxidative injury to vascular endothelial and/or smooth muscle cells, leading to deregulation of vascular smooth muscle growth, synthesis and deposition of matrix proteins, and adverse effects on anticoagulant systems (Harpel, 1997).

Hydrazinobenzoic Acid Hydrazinobenzoic acid is a nitrogen-nitrogen bonded chemical that is present in the cultivated mushroom *Agaricus bisporus*. McManus and associates (1987) reported that this hydrazine derivative causes smooth muscle cell tumors in the aorta and large arteries of mice when administered over the life span of the animals. These tumors had the characteristic appearance and immunocytochemical features of vascular leiomyomas and leiomyosarcomas. Smooth muscle cell lysis with vascular perforation apparently precedes malignant transformation. The ability of hydrazinobenzoic acid to cause vascular smooth muscle cell tumors is shared by other synthetic and naturally occurring hydrazines. Although angiomyomas (or vascular leiomyomas) derived histogenetically from the media of blood and lymph vessels occur most commonly in the oral cavity and skin, primary leiomyosarcomas occur in the abdominal aorta.

T-2 Toxin Trichothecene mycotoxins, commonly classified as tetracyclic sesquiterpenes, are naturally occurring cytotoxic metabolites of *Fusarium* species. These mycotoxins—including T-2 toxin [4β,15-diacetoxy-8α-(3-methylbutyryloxy)-3α-hydroxy-12,13-epoxytrichothec-9-ene]—are major contaminants of foods and animal feeds and may cause illness in animals and humans. Acute parenteral administration of T-2 toxin to laboratory animals induces shock, hypothermia, and death from cardiovascular and respiratory failure. Wilson and coworkers (1982) reported that intravenous infusion of T-2 toxin in rats causes an initial decrease in heart rate and blood pressure, followed by tachycardia and hypertension and finally by bradycardia and hypotension. These actions may be related to a central effect on blood pressure and catecholamine release. Acute T-2 toxin exposure causes extensive destruction of myocardial capillaries, while repeated dosing promotes thickening of large coronary arteries.

Vitamin D Vitamin D hypervitaminosis causes medial degeneration, calcification of the coronary arteries, and smooth muscle cell proliferation in laboratory animals. The toxic effects of vitamin D may be related to its structural similarity to 25-hydroxycholesterol, a potent vascular toxin.

A summary of selected agents and their vascular effects can be found in Tables 18-7 through 18-9.

Miscellaneous Recent evidence has implicated vascular dysfunction as a contributing factor to Alzheimer's dementia. Thomas et al. (1997) have shown that administration of β-amyloid produces extensive vascular disruption, including endothelial and smooth muscle damage, adhesion and migration of leukocytes across arteries and venules. Most importantly, the vascular actions of β-amyloid appear to be distinct from the neurotoxic properties of the peptide.

Industrial Agents

Alkylamines Aliphatic amines such as allylamine (3-aminopropene) are utilized in the synthesis of pharmaceutical and commercial products. Several allylamine analogs are being developed as antifungal agents for human and veterinary use. Allylamine is more toxic than are other unsaturated primary amines of higher molecular weight. Exposure to allylamine by a variety of routes in

Table 18-7
Vasculotoxic Agents: Industrial and Environmental Agents

AGENT	SOURCES	PROMINENT VASCULAR EFFECTS	ASSOCIATED DISEASES
Allylamine	Synthetic precursor	Bioactivation of parent compound by amine oxidase to acrolein and hydrogen peroxide results in smooth muscle cell injury; intimal smooth muscle cell proliferation in large arteries	Atherosclerosis
β-Aminopropionitrile		Damage to vascular connective tissue; aortic lesions; atheroma formation, aneurysm	
Boron		Hemorrhage; edema; increase in microvascular permeability of the lung	Pulmonary edema
Butadiene	Synthetic precursor	Hemangiosarcomas in several organs	
Carbamylhydrazine		Tumors of pulmonary blood vessels	Cancer
Carbon disulfide	Fumigant/solvent	Microvascular effect on ocular fundus and retina; direct injury to endothelial cells; atheroma formation	Coronary vascular disease Atherosclerosis
Chlorophenoxy herbicides			Hypertension
Dimethylnitrosamine		Decreased hepatic flow; hemorrhage; necrosis	Occlusion of veins
Dinitrotoluenes	Synthetic precursor		
4-Fluoro-10-methyl-12-benzyanthracene		Pulmonary artery lesions; coronary vessel lesion	
Glycerol		Strong renal vasoconstriction	Acute renal failure
Hydrogen fluoride		Hemorrhage; edema in the lungs	Pulmonary edema
Hydrazinobenzoic acid	Constituent of *A. bisporus*		
Paraquat		Vascular damage in lungs and brain	Cerebral purpura
Polycyclic aromatic hydrocarbons	Environmental tobacco smoke		
Pyrrolidine alkaloids		Pulmonary vasculitis; damage to vascular smooth muscle cells; proliferation of endothelium and vascular connective tissue in the liver	Pulmonary hypertension; hepatic venoocclusive disease
Organophosphate pesticides			Cerebral arteriosclerosis
T-2 toxin	*Fusarium* mycotoxin		
Vinyl chloride		Portal hypertension; tumors of hepatic blood vessels	Cancer

various animal species is associated with selective cardiovascular toxicity (Boor et al., 1979; Ramos and Thurlow, 1993). Hines and associates (1960) reported that acute intragastric administration of allylamine causes congestion of blood vessels in rats. The multiple organ toxicities observed after chronic inhalation of allylamine are characterized by a prominent vascular component (Lalich, 1969) involving mesenteric, pancreatic, testicular, and pulmonary artery hypertrophy and occasional alveolar hemorrhage and pulmonary edema. The specificity of the vasculotoxic response may be related to the accumulation of allylamine in elastic and muscu-

Table 18-8
Vasculotoxic Agents: Gases

AGENT	SOURCES	PROMINENT VASCULAR EFFECTS	ASSOCIATED DISEASE
Auto exhaust		Hemorrhage and infarct in cerebral hemispheres; atheroma formation in aorta	Atherosclerosis
Carbon monoxide	Environmental	Damage to intimal layer; edema; atheroma formation	Atherosclerosis
Nitric oxide		Vacuolation of arteriolar endothelial cells; edema, thickening of alveolar-capillary membranes	Pulmonary edema
Oxygen		Vasoconstriction—retinal damage; increased retinal vascular permeability—edema; increased pulmonary vascular permeability—edema	Blindness in neonate; shrinking of visual field in adults; edema
Ozone		Arterial lesion in the lung	Pulmonary edema

lar arteries upon administration in vivo. Gross lesions are evident in the myocardium, aorta, and coronary arteries of animals exposed to allylamine. Chronic administration is associated with the development of atherosclerotic-like lesions characterized by proliferation of smooth muscle cells and fibrosis.

Boor and associates (1990) first proposed that allylamine toxicity results from bioactivation of the parent compound to a toxic aldehyde. The oxidative deamination of allylamine results in the formation of acrolein and hydrogen peroxide, metabolites that mediate the acute and long-term toxic effects of allylamine (Fig. 18-20). Vascular-specific bioactivation of allylamine is a prerequisite for toxicity (Ramos et al., 1988). Benzylamine oxidase, also known as semicarbazide-sensitive amine oxidase, is believed to catalyze the oxidative deamination of allylamine. This enzyme is found in cardiovascular tissue in higher concentrations than is any other tissue. Methylamine and aminoacetone are believed to be endogenous substrates for semicarbize-sensitive amine oxidase (Yu, 1998). Although the endogenous substrates and physiologic function of this enzyme have not been fully characterized, recent studies have shown that chronic enzyme inhibition is associated with disorganization of elastin architecture within the aortic media of weanling rats, degenerative medial changes, and metaplastic changes in vascular smooth muscle cells (Langford et al., 1999). Therefore, excessive deamination reactions may initiate endothelial injury and atherosclerotic plaque formation, induce oxidative stress, and potentiate oxidative injury to the vascular wall by glycation products and oxidized lipoproteins. Allylamine preferentially injures smooth muscle cells relative to other cell types in the vascular wall. Mitochondria have been identified as early targets of allylamine toxicity—an observation that is consistent with the enrichment of amine oxidase activity in this subcellular compartment. Because the cytotoxic response also involves alterations in cellular glutathione status that compromise the integrity of membrane compartments (Ramos and Thurlow, 1993), modulation of glutathione status by acrolein and/or hydrogen peroxide may also disrupt mitochondrial function. Pretreatment of cultured vascular smooth muscle cells with sulfasalazine, a glutathione *S*-transferase inhibitor, potentiates allylamine and acrolein cytotoxicity, indicating a protective role of this enzyme in vascular injury by α,β unsaturated carbonyls (He et al., 1999). Acrolein is a highly reactive aldehyde that disrupts the thiol balance of target cells, including vascular cells (Ramos and Cox, 1987); denatures proteins; and interferes with nucleic acid synthesis. Although many molecules react with acrolein under physiologic conditions, the main reaction products result from nucleophilic addition at the terminal ethylenic carbon. Acrolein toxicity also may involve conversion by NADPH-dependent microsomal enzymes to glycidaldehyde, a known mutagen and carcinogen. Acrolein is a ubiquitous toxic chemical that is found in engine exhaust and cigarette smoke. Using Dahl hypertension-resistant and hypertension-sensitive rat strains, Kutzman and colleagues (1984) demonstrated that exposure to acrolein for 62 days is more toxic to hypertension-sensitive animals than to their hypertension-resistant counterparts. The indirect sympathomimetic activity of aldehydes, including acrolein, acetaldehyde, and formaldehyde, may contribute to the enhanced sensitivity of hypertension-prone animals.

Repeated cycles of vascular injury upon in vivo exposure of rats to allylamine modulate medial aortic smooth muscle cells from a quiescent to a proliferative state (Cox and Ramos, 1990). Because cells from allylamine-treated rats maintain this altered phenotype after serial propagation in vitro, phenotypic modulation is believed to involve genotypic alterations secondary to chemical insult. The enhanced capacity for proliferation in allylamine cells is associated with modulation of phospholipid metabolism, enhanced protein kinase C activity, increased *c-Ha-ras* proto-oncogene expression, and differential secretion and deposition of extracellular matrix components (Ramos et al., 1993). Enhanced secretion of osteopontin characterizes the proliferative phenotype induced by allylamine (Parrish and Ramos, 1995). Osteopontin is a secreted phosphoprotein that has effects on gene expression, Ca^{2+} regulation, and nitric oxide production, presumably mediated through the α_{vb3} integrin. Osteopontin has been associated with arterial smooth muscle cell proliferation and migration and is present in atherosclerotic lesions. Although a major contributory role in adhesion and migration has been established with a fair degree of certainty, its role in the regulation of vascular smooth muscle cell proliferation has not yet been fully elucidated. Recent studies established that allylamine treatment in vivo modulates the relative expression of integrin receptors and integrin-coupled NF-kB signaling in vascular smooth muscle cells (Parrish and Ramos, 1995).

Table 18-9
Vasculotoxic Agents: Therapeutic Agents and Related Compounds

CLASS (AGENT)	SOURCES	PROMINENT VASCULAR EFFECTS	ASSOCIATED DISEASES
Antibiotics/antimitotics			
Cyclophosphamide		Lesions of pulmonary endothelial cells	
5-Fluorodeoxyuridine		GI tract hemorrhage; portal vein thrombosis	
Gentamicin		Long-lasting renal vasoconstriction	Renal failure
Vasoactive agents			
Amphetamine		Cerebrovascular lesions secondary to drug abuse	Disseminated arterial lesions similar to periarteritis nodosa
Dihydroergotamine		Spasm of retinal vessels	
Ergonovine		Coronary artery spasm	Angina
Ergotamine		Vasospastic phenomena with and without medial atrophy	Gangrene of the thrombosis; peripheral tissues
Epinephrine		Peripheral arterial thrombi in hyperlipemic rats	Participates in thrombogenesis
Histamine		Coronary spasm; damage to endothelial cells in hepatic portal vein	
Methysergide		Intimal proliferation; vascular occlusion of coronary arteries	Coronary artery disease
Nicotine	Tobacco	Alteration of cytoarchitecture of aortic endothelium; increase in microvilli	
Nitrites and nitrates		"Aging" of coronary arteries	Repeated vasodilation
Norepinephrine		Spasm of coronary artery; endothelial damage	
Metabolic affectors			
Alloxan		Microvascular retinopathy	Diabetes; blindness
Chloroquine		Retinopathy	
Fructose		Microvascular lesions in retina	Diabetes-like condition
Iodoacetates		Vascular changes in retina	
Anticoagulants			
Sodium warfarin: warfarin		Spinal hematoma; subdural hematoma; vasculitis	Uncontrolled bleeding; hemorrhage
Radiocontrast dyes			
Metrizamide; metrizoate		Coagulation; necrosis in celiac and renal vasculature	
Cyanoacrylate adhesives			
2-Cyano-acrylate-*n*-butyl		Granulation of arteries with fibrous masses	
Ethyl-2-cyanoacrylate		Degeneration of vascular wall with thrombosis	
Methyl-2-cyanoacrylate		Vascular necrosis	
Miscellaneous			
Aminorex fumarate		Intimal and medial thickening of pulmonary arteries	Pulmonary hypertension
Aspirin		Endothelial damage, gastric erosion obliteration of small vessels, ischemic infarcts	
Cholesterol; oxygenated		Atheroma formation; arterial damage	Atherosclerosis derivatives of cholesterol: noncholesterol steroids
Homocysteine		Increase of vascular fragility, loss of endothelium, proliferation of smooth muscle cells promotion of atheroma formation	Atherosclerosis; synthesis

(continued)

Table 18-9 Vasculotoxic Agents: Therapeutic Agents and Related Compounds (*continued*)

CLASS (AGENT)	SOURCES	PROMINENT VASCULAR EFFECTS	ASSOCIATED DISEASES
Oral contraceptives		Thrombosis in cerebral and peripheral vasculature	Thromboembolic disorders
Penicillamine		Vascular lesion in connective tissue matrix of arterial wall, glomerular immune complex deposits, inhibits synthesis of vascular connective tissue	Glomerulonephritis
Talc and other silicates		Pulmonary arteriolar thrombosis, emboli	
Tetradecylsulfate Na		Sclerosis of veins	
Thromboxane A_2		Extreme cerebral vasoconstriction	Cerebrovascular ischemia
Vitamin D	Dietary		

*Based on information gathered from sources listed in references.

Heavy Metals The vascular toxicity of food- and water-borne elements (selenium, chromium, copper, zinc, cadmium, lead, and mercury) as well as airborne elements (vanadium and lead) involves reactions of metals with sulfhydryl, carboxyl, or phosphate groups. Metals such as cobalt, magnesium, manganese, nickel, cadmium, and lead also interact with and block calcium channels. Evidence suggesting that intracellular calcium-binding proteins such as calmodulin are biologically relevant targets of heavy metals, including mercury and lead, has been presented. The contribution of this mechanism to the toxic effects of metals has been questioned because of the inability of beryllium, barium, cobalt, zinc, and cadmium to bind readily to calmodulin in vitro.

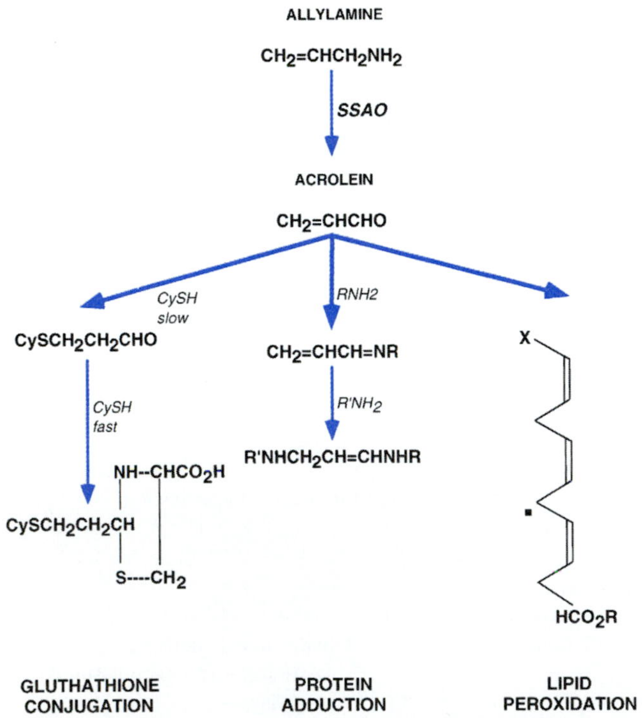

The vascular effects of cadmium have been studied in the greatest detail. Although cadmium is not preferentially localized in blood vessels relative to other tissues, when present, cadmium is localized in the elastic lamina of large arteries, with particularly high concentrations at arterial branching points (Perry et al., 1989). A large portion of the cadmium that accumulates in the body is tightly bound to hepatic and renal metallothionein, a known detoxification mechanism. The low metallothionein levels in vascular tissue may actually predispose a person to the toxic effects of cadmium (Perry et al., 1989). Long-term exposure of laboratory animals to low levels of cadmium has been associated with the development of atherosclerosis and hypertension in the absence of other toxic effects. Selenium and zinc inhibit, while lead potentiates, the hypertensive effects of cadmium. Concentrations of cadmium that increase blood pressure do not raise blood pressure in the presence of calcium. In contrast, the protective effects of zinc and selenium may be related to their ability to increase the synthesis of cadmium-binding proteins and thus enhance detoxification. Cadmium increases sodium retention, induces vasoconstriction, increases cardiac output, and produces hyperreninemia. Any one of these mechanisms could account for the putative hypertensive effects of cadmium. In rats, chronic administration of cadmium caused renal arteriolar thickening as well as diffuse fibrosis of capillaries. Low levels of cadmium have been associated with a higher frequency of atherosclerosis in humans (Houtman, 1993). Similar vascular changes are also responsible for the development of testicular damage and atrophy. The hypertensive effects of cadmium remain questionable, since population studies in humans have not confirmed the associations made in studies with laboratory animals. Kaji and coworkers have recently shown that the sensitivity of cultured bovine aortic smooth muscle cells to cadmium is considerably greater than that of aortic endothelial cells and renal epithelial cells (1996). In related studies, this group showed that the regulation of fibrinolysis mediated by vascular smooth muscle cells and fibroblasts during hemostasis may be disturbed by cadmium (Yamamoto et al., 1996).

Less work has been conducted to evaluate the vasculotoxic effects of other heavy metals. Because hypertension is not commonly observed during clinical lead intoxication, many investigators consider the existing evidence to be conflicting and inconclusive. Epidemiologic studies have shown that a large percentage of

Figure 18-20. Metabolism of allylamine to acrolein by semicarbazide-sensitive amine oxidase in vascular smooth muscle cells.

Acrolein may be conjugated to gluthathione by the action of glutathione-*S*-transferase or may interact with intracellular proteins to form protein adducts. In addition, acrolein may initiate intracellular lipid peroxidation, which may lead to genotoxic or cell damage.

patients with essential hypertension have increased body stores of lead (Batuman et al., 1983). Elevated blood pressure also has been observed during childhood lead poisoning. Although in these children the level of lead burden was not severe, a significant increase in blood pressure was seen on the tenth day of poisoning and persisted for the remainder of the study. The direct vasoconstrictor effect of lead may be related to the putative hypertensive response. This effect can be complemented by the ability of lead to activate the renin-angiotensin-aldosterone system. Recent investigations have shown direct effects of lead in vascular endothelial and smooth muscle cells. For instance, lead has been shown to inhibit repair process in damaged endothelial cells (Fujiwara et al., 1997) and to modulate spontaneous release of fibrinolytic proteins from subendothelial cells is disturbed by lead through intracellular calcium-independent pathways (Yamamoto et al., 1997).

Inorganic mercury produces vasoconstriction of preglomerular vessels. In addition, the integrity of the blood-brain barrier may be disrupted by mercury. The opening of the blood-brain barrier results in extravasation of plasma protein across vascular walls into adjoining brain tissues. Mercury added to platelet-rich plasma causes a marked increase in platelet thromboxane B_2 production and platelet responsiveness to arachidonic acid. Although it is unlikely that mercury and lead compete with calcium for intracellular binding sites, their accessibility to the intracellular compartment appears to be calcium-dependent (Tomera and Harakal, 1986). Acute lead-induced neuropathy may be due to cerebral capillary dysfunction. Inorganic lead alters arterial elasticity and causes sclerosis of renal vessels. Lead intoxication has been linked to hypertension in humans, but its exact role is questionable.

Acute arsenic poisoning causes vasodilation and capillary dilation. These actions have been associated with extravasation, transudation of plasma, and decreased intravascular volume. It has been proposed that high levels of arsenic in the soil and water of Taiwan are responsible for blackfoot disease, a severe form of arteriosclerosis. Blackfoot disease is an endemic peripheral vascular occlusive disease that exhibits arteriosclerosis obliterans and thromboangiitis. The ability of arsenic to induce these changes has been attributed to its effects on vascular endothelial cells. Arsenic has been reported to cause noncirrhotic portal hypertension in humans. Chromium appears to play an important role in the maintenance of vascular integrity. A deficiency of this metal in animals results in elevated serum cholesterol levels and increased atherosclerotic aortic plaques. Autopsies of humans have revealed virtually no chromium in the aortas of individuals who died of atherosclerotic heart disease compared with individuals dying of other causes.

Nitroaromatics Dinitrotoluene is used as a precursor in the synthesis of polyurethane foams, coatings, elastomers, and explosives. The manufacture of dinitrotoluene generates a technical-grade mixture that consists of 75.8 percent 2,4-dinitrotoluene, 19.5 percent 2,6-dinitrotoluene, and 4.7 percent other isomers. Several chronic toxicity studies in laboratory animals have shown that 2,4- and/or 2,6-dinitrotoluene can cause cancers of the liver, gallbladder, and kidney as well as benign tumors of the connective tissues. In humans, however, retrospective mortality studies in workers exposed daily to dinitrotoluene have shown that dinitrotoluenes cause circulatory disorders of atherosclerotic etiology. As with other chronic occupational illnesses, increased mortality from cardiovascular disorders upon exposure to dinitrotoluenes has been related to the duration and intensity of exposure.

The atherogenic effects of dinitrotoluenes have been examined experimentally. Repeated in vivo exposure of rats to 2,4- or 2,6-dinitrotoluene is associated with dysplasia and rearrangement of aortic smooth muscle cells (Ramos et al., 1990). Dinitrotoluenes are metabolized in the liver to dinitrobenzylalcohol, which is then conjugated to form a glucuronide conjugate that is excreted in bile or urine. This conjugate is hydrolyzed by intestinal microflora and subsequently reduced to a toxic metabolite or the precursor of a toxic metabolite. Dent and colleagues (1981) have shown that rat cecal microflora convert dinitrotoluene to nitrosonitrotoluenes, aminonitrotoluenes, and diaminotoluenes. In vitro exposure of rat aortic smooth muscle cells to 2,4- or 2,6-diaminotoluene inhibited DNA synthesis, a response comparable to that seen in medial smooth muscle cells isolated from dinitrotoluene-treated animals.

Aromatic Hydrocarbons Aromatic hydrocarbons, including polycyclic aromatic hydrocarbons and polychlorinated dibenzo-*p*-dioxins, are persistent toxic environmental contaminants. Several aromatic hydrocarbons have been identified as vascular toxins that can initiate and/or promote the atherogenic process in experimental animals (Ou and Ramos, 1992a, b). Much of the work involved in investigations of aromatic hydrocarbon toxicity have focused on the polycyclic aromatic hydrocarbons, of which benzo[*a*]pyrene has been examined in the greatest detail. Exposure of avian species to benzo[*a*]pyrene and 7,12-dimethylbenz[*a*]anthracene causes atherosclerosis without altering serum cholesterol levels. The atherogenic effect is associated with cytochrome P450–mediated conversion of the parent compound to toxic metabolic intermediates. The majority of the activity responsible for the biotransformation of these chemicals is associated with the smooth muscle layers of the aorta, although cytochrome P450–dependent monoxygenase activity that can bioactivate carcinogens also has been localized in the aortic endothelium. Interestingly, the activity of aortic aryl hydrocarbon hydroxylase has been correlated with the degree of susceptibility to atherosclerosis in avian species, and Ah-responsive mice are more susceptible to atherosclerosis than are Ah-resistant mice. Recent studies have demonstrated that CYP1B1 is the predominant cytochrome P450 isoform expressed in human (Zhao et al., 1998), as well as rodent (Kerzee and Ramos, 2000) vascular cells.

3-Methylcholantrene increases both the number and the size of lipid-staining lesions in the aorta of animals that are fed an atherogenic diet for 8 weeks, suggesting that aromatic hydrocarbons can also initiate the atherogenic process. Furthermore, focal proliferation of intimal smooth muscle cells can be produced by an initiation-promotion sequence using 7,12-dimethylbenz[*a*]anthracene and the alpha_1 selective adrenergic agonist methoxamine. In contrast, Albert and coworkers (1977) and Penn and Snyder (1988) have reported that treatment with several polycylic hydrocarbons increases the size but not the frequency of atherosclerotic lesions. These observations suggest that polycyclic aromatic hydrocarbons act as promoters of the atherosclerotic process. Although additional studies are required to define the "initiating" versus "promotional" actions of polycyclic aromatic hydrocarbons, their ability to readily associate with plasma lipoproteins may play a critical role in vascular toxicity. In fact, the localization of these and other lipophilic chemicals in blood vessels may depend on lipoprotein-mediated transport.

The enhanced proliferative and migratory potential of smooth muscle cells induced by benzo[*a*]pyrene may involve a mutagenic process, as predicted by the monoclonal theory of atherogenesis

(Benditt and Benditt, 1973). Thus, "initiation" of the atherogenic process by benzo[*a*]pyrene and related chemicals would involve mutation of target genes, while promotion would involve modulation of mitogenic signaling, including growth-related gene expression and protein phosphorylation. Because a promotional mechanism of atherogenesis implies the existence of an "initiated" resident cell population in the vessel wall, information about the cellular heterogeneity of vascular smooth muscle cells in the vessel wall is needed.

Benzo[*a*]pyrene modulates protein kinase C signal transduction in aortic smooth muscle cells of atherosclerosis-susceptible (quail) and atherosclerosis-resistant (rat) species (Ou et al., 1995). Other aromatic hydrocarbons, such as 2,3,7,8-tetrachlorodibenzo-*p*-dioxin, share with benzo[*a*]pyrene the ability to inhibit protein kinase C in aortic smooth muscle cells, but the mechanisms appear to be different. As atherogenesis ultimately involves enhanced smooth muscle cell proliferation, the role of protein kinase C inhibition and the associated suppression of cell growth may involve phosphorylation-dependent changes in DNA repair efficiency. Genotoxic actions of metabolites formed in situ probably contribute to the growth inhibitory response of benzo[*a*]pyrene because sister chromatid exchanges, mutations, and unscheduled DNA synthesis in cultured aortic smooth muscle cells have been noted (Zwijsen et al., 1990; Lu et al., 2000). Benzo[*a*]pyrene modulates the expression of genes involved in the regulation of coordinated cell cycle progression (Kerzee and Ramos, 2000), antioxidant defense mechanisms (Chen and Ramos, 2000), and genomic stability (Lu et. al., 2000).

In summary, benzo[*a*]pyrene elicits alterations of smooth muscle cell proliferation through several mechanisms, including enhanced transcription of growth-related genes through aryl hydrocarbon receptor–mediated pathways, interaction and inactivation of protein kinase C, and conversion of the parent molecule to metabolites that can form covalent DNA adducts (Fig. 18-21).

Gases ***Carbon Monoxide*** Carbon monoxide induces focal intimal damage and edema in laboratory animals at 180 ppm, a concentration to which humans may be exposed from environmental sources such as automobile exhaust, tobacco smoke, and fossil fuels. Because most sources of carbon monoxide are complex mixtures of chemicals, attempts to distinguish the direct effects of carbon monoxide from those of chemicals such as sulfur oxides, nitrogen oxides, aldehydes, and hydrocarbons have not yielded clear results. This is exemplified by the prominent vasculotoxic effects observed upon exposure of laboratory animals to other complex gas mixtures. For instance, automobile exhaust causes structural changes in the myocardium and aorta of guinea pigs and hemorrhage and infarct in the hemispheres and basal ganglia of spontaneously hypertensive rats. In addition, composition and deposition of lipids in the wall of the aorta of rats can be affected. However, it is not clear which of the many chemicals present in these mixtures mediate the atherogenic effect. Degenerative changes of myocardial arterioles have been produced experimentally in dogs forced to smoke. Similar changes have also been detected in humans who were heavy smokers and died of noncardiac causes (Wald and Howard, 1975; Auerbach and Carter, 1980). Tobacco smoke not only exerts a direct atherogenic effect (endothelial injury, changes in lipid profiles, and proliferation of smooth muscle cells) but also facilitates thrombosis by modulation of platelet function and vascular spasm.

Short-term exposure to carbon monoxide has been associated with direct damage to vascular endothelial and smooth muscle cells. Injury to endothelial cells increases intimal permeability and allows the interaction of blood constituents with underlying components of the vascular wall. This response may account in part for the ability of carbon monoxide to induce atherosclerotic lesions in several animal species. Although carbon monoxide enhances total arterial deposition of cholesterol in animals fed a lipid-rich diet, its vascular effects appear to be independent of serum cholesterol levels. The toxic effects of carbon monoxide have been attributed to its reversible interaction with hemoglobin. The formation of carboxyhemoglobin in vivo is favored because binding of carbon monoxide to hemoglobin is more cooperative than the binding of oxygen. As a result of this interaction, carboxyhemoglobin decreases the oxygen-carrying capacity of blood and shifts the oxyhemoglobin saturation curve to the left. These actions make it more difficult to unload oxygen and eventually cause functional anemia resulting from reduced oxygen availability. More recently, evidence has been presented that carbon monoxide interacts with cellular proteins such as myoglobin and cytochrome *c* oxidase and that carbon monoxide elicits a direct vasodilatory response of the coronary circulation.

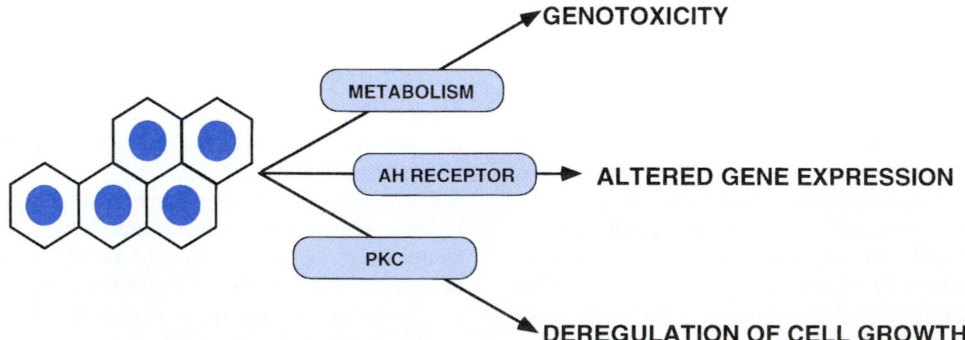

Figure 18-21. Cellular and molecular targets of benzo[a]pyrene in vascular smooth muscle cells.

Benzo[*a*]pyrene may be metabolized to reactive intermediates that bind covalently to DNA. Additionally, benzo[*a*]pyrene may bind to cytosolic receptors that act as ligand-activated transcription factors to regulate gene expression. Benzo[*a*]pyrene and/or its metabolites also may interact with protein kinase C to deregulate cell growth.

Oxygen The administration of oxygen to a premature newborn can cause irreversible vasoconstriction and obliteration of retinal vasculature, resulting in permanent blindness. In squirrel monkeys, exposure to 100% oxygen for 50 to 117 h increases vascular permeability, with leakage and edema of the retina, but these effects are largely reversible. In the pulmonary capillary bed, the volume and thickness of capillary endothelium decrease and perivascular edema is present. Exposure to high oxygen pressures for relatively short periods (less than 8 h) damages pulmonary endothelial cells in several species. Ozone affects the pulmonary vasculature; the injuries usually take the form of pulmonary arterial lesions that lead to thickening of the artery walls.

Carbon Disulfide Carbon disulfide (dithiocarbonic anhydride) occurs in coal tar and crude petroleum and is commonly utilized in the manufacture of rayon and soil disinfectants. This chemical has been identified as an atherogenic agent in laboratory animals. In humans, a two- to threefold increase in coronary heart disease has been reported. Although the mechanism of toxicity is not known, alterations of glucose and/or lipid metabolism and blood coagulation have been suggested. The mechanism for CS_2-atheroma production also may involve direct injury to the endothelium coupled with hypothyroidism, because thiocarbamate (thiourea), a potent antithyroid substance, is a principal urinary metabolite of CS_2. More recently, evidence has been presented that carbon disulfide modifies low density lipoprotein in vitro and enhances arterial fatty deposits induced by a high-fat diet in C57BL/6 mice (Lewis et al., 2000).

1,3-Butadiene Studies have shown that 1,3-butadiene, a chemical used in the production of styrene-butadiene, increases the incidence of cardiac hemangiosarcomas, which are tumors of endothelial origin (Miller and Boorman, 1990). Although hemangiosarcomas have also been observed in the liver, lung, and kidney, cardiac tumors are a major cause of death in animals exposed to this chemical. The toxic effects of 1,3-butadiene are dependent on its metabolic activation by cytochrome P450 to toxic epoxide metabolites. The ultimate outcomes of exposure probably are influenced by the rates of glutathione-mediated detoxification of oxidative metabolites. Although 1,3-butadiene is a carcinogen in rats and mice, mice are considerably more sensitive than are rats to this carcinogenicity. This difference in susceptibility has been attributed to differences in the formation of the toxic mono- and diepoxide metabolites.

REFERENCES

Ahmed SS, Regan TJ: Cardiotoxicity of acute and chronic ingestion of various alcohols, in Acosta D (ed): *Cardiovascular Toxicology,* 2d ed. New York: Raven Press, 1992, pp 345–407.

Albert RE, Vanderlaan M, Burns FJ, Nishiizumi M: Effects of carcinogens on chicken atherosclerosis. *Cancer Res* 37:2232, 1977.

Andrieu-Abadie N, Jaffrezou JP, Hatem S, et al: L-carnitine prevents doxorubicin-induced apoptosis of cardiac myocytes: Role of inhibition of ceramide generation. *FASEB J* 13:1501–1510, 1999.

Arola OJ, Saraste A, Pulkki K, et al: Acute doxorubicin cardiotoxicity involves cardiomyocyte apoptosis. *Cancer Res* 60:1789–1792, 2000.

Arstall MA, Sawyer DB, Fukazawa R, Kelly RA: Cytokine-mediated apoptosis in cardiac myocytes: The role of inducible nitric oxide synthase induction and peroxynitrite generation. *Circ Res* 85:829–840, 1999.

Atkinson P, Joubert G, Barron A, et al: Hypertrophic cardiomyopathy associated with tacrolimus in paediatric transplant patients. *Lancet* 345:894–896, 1995.

Auerbach O, Carter HW: Smoking and the heart, in Bristow MR (ed): *Drug-Induced Heart Disease.* Amsterdam: Elsevier North-Holland, 1980, p 359.

Baldessarini RJ: Drugs and the treatment of psychiatric disorders, in Hardman JG, Limbird LE, Molinoff PB, et al (eds): *Goodman & Gilman's The Pharmacological Basis of Therapeutics.* 9th ed. New York: McGraw-Hill, 1996, pp 399–430.

Batuman V, Landy E, Maesaka JK, Wedeen RP: Contribution of lead to hypertension with renal impairment. *N Engl J Med* 309:17, 1983.

Behrendt H, Boffin H: Myocardial cell lesions caused by anabolic hormone. *Cell Tissue Res* 181:423–426, 1977.

Benditt EP, Benditt JM: Evidence for a monoclonal origin of human atherosclerotic plaques. *Proc Natl Acad Sci USA* 70:1753, 1973.

Bers DM: Ca transport during contraction and relaxation in mammalian ventricular muscle. *Basic Res Cardiol* 92:1–10, 1997.

Besse S, Assayag P, Latour C, et al: Molecular characteristics of cocaine-induced cardiomyopathy in rats. *Eur J Pharmacol* 338:123–129, 1997.

Bolli R: Oxygen-derived free radicals and postischemic myocardial dysfunction ("stunned myocardium"). *J Am Coll Cardiol* 12:239–249, 1988.

Boor PJ, Hysmith RM, Sanduja R: A role for a new vascular enzyme in the metabolism of xenobiotic amines. *Circ Res* 66(1):249, 1990.

Boor PJ, Moslen MJ, Reynolds ES: Allylamine cardiotoxicity: I. Sequence of pathologic events. *Toxicol Appl Pharmacol* 50:581, 1979.

Bosnjak ZJ: Cardiac effects of anesthetics, in Blanck TJJ, Wheeler DM (eds): *Mechanisms of Anesthetic Action in Skeletal, Cardiac, and Smooth Muscle.* New York: Plenum Press, 1991, pp 91–96.

Boyett MR, Harrison SM, Janvier NC, et at: A list of vertebrate ionic currents: Nomenclature, properties, function, and cloned equivalents. *Cardiovasc Res* 32:455–481, 1996.

Brinkman K, ter Hofstede HJM, Burger DM, et al: Adverse effects of reverse transcriptase inhibitors: Mitochondrial toxicity as common pathway. *AIDS* 12:1735–1744, 1998.

Buja LM: Modulation of the myocardial response to ischemia. *Lab Invest* 78:1345–1373, 1998.

Bull HA, Pittilo RM, Blow DJ, et al: The effects of nicotine on PGI_2 production by rat aortic endothelium. *Thromb Haemost* 54(2):472, 1985.

Carafoli E: Intracellular calcium homeostasis. *Annu Rev Biochem* 56: 395–433, 1987.

Catterall W, Mackie K: Local anesthetics, in Hardman JG, Limbird LE, Molinoff PB, et al (eds): *Goodman & Gilman's The Pharmacological Basis of Therapeutics,* 9th ed. New York: McGraw-Hill, 1996, pp 331–347.

Chacon E, Acosta D: Mitochondrial regulation of superoxide by Ca^{2+}: An alternate mechanism for the cardiotoxicity of doxorubicin. *Toxicol Appl Pharmacol* 107:117–128, 1991.

Chacon E, Ulrich R, Acosta D: A digitized-fluorescence-imaging study of mitochondrial Ca^{2+} increase by doxorubicin in cardiac myocytes. *Biochem J* 281:871–878, 1992.

Chen Y-H, Ramos KS: A CCAAT/enhancer binding protein (C/EBP) site within antioxidant/electrophile response elements (ARE/EpRE) along with CREB binding protein (CBP) participate in the negative regulation of rat GSTYa gene in vascular smooth muscle cells. *J Bio Chem* 2000. In press.

Cheng X-S, Shimokawa H, Momii H, et al: Role of superoxide anion in the pathogenesis of cytokine-induced myocardial dysfunction in dogs in vivo. *Cardiovasc Res* 42:651–659, 1999.

Christ M, Wehling M: Cardiovascular steroid actions: Swift swallows or sluggish snails? *Cardiovasc Res* 40:34–44, 1998.

Communal C, Singh K, Pimentel DR, Colucci WS: Norepinephrine stimulates apoptosis in adult rat ventricular myocytes by activation of the β-adrenergic pathway. *Circulation* 98:1329–1334, 1998.

Communal C, Singh K, Sawyer DB, Colucci WS: Opposing effects of β_1- and β_2-adrenergic receptors on cardiac myocyte apoptosis: role of a pertussis toxin-sensitive G protein. *Circulation* 100:2210–2212, 1999.

Cox LR, Ramos K: Allylamine-induced phenotypic modulation of aortic smooth muscle cells. *J Exp Pathol* 71:11, 1990.

Dalakas MC, Illa I, Pezeshkpour GH, et al: Mitochondrial myopathy caused by long-term zidovudine therapy. *N Engl J Med* 322:1098–1105, 1990.

Dean RA, Harper ET, Dumaual N, et al: Effects of ethanol on cocaine metabolism: Formation of cocaethylene and norcocaethylene. *Toxicol Appl Pharmacol* 117:1–8, 1992.

Dent JG, Schnell SR, Guest D: Metabolism of 2,4-dinitrotoluene in rat hepatic microsomes and cecal flora, in Snyder R, Park DV, Kocsis JJ, et al (eds): *Proceedings of the Second International Symposium on Biologically Reactive Intermediates: Chemical Mechanisms and Biologic Effects.* New York: Plenum Press, 1981, p 431.

Devi BG, Chan AW: Effect of cocaine on cardiac biochemical functions. *J Cardiovasc Pharmacol* 33:1–6, 1999.

de Vries JE, Vork MM, Roemen THM, et al: Saturated but not monounsaturated fatty acids induce apoptotic cell death in neonatal rat ventricular myocytes. *J Lipid Res* 38:1384–1394, 1997.

Dhalla NS, Yates JC, Naimark B, et al: Cardiotoxicity of catecholamines and related agents, in Acosta D (ed): *Cardiovascular Toxicology,* 2d ed. New York: Raven Press, 1992, pp 239–282.

Dodd DE, Vinegar A: Cardiac sensitization testing of the halon replacement candidates trifluoroiodomethane (CF3I) and 1,1,2,2,3,3,3-heptafluoro-1-iodopropane (C3F7I). *Drug Chem Toxicol* 21:137–149, 1998.

Doroshow JH: Doxorubicin-induced cardiac toxicity. *N Engl J Med* 324:843–845, 1991.

Dzurba A, Ziegelhoffer A, Vrbjar N, et al: Estradiol modulates the sodium pump in the heart sarcolemmal. *Mol Cell Biochem* 176:113–118, 1997.

Fajiwara T, Kaji T, Sakurai S, et al: Inhibitory effect of lead on the repair of wounded monolayers of cultured vascular endothelial cells. *Toxicology* 117:193, 1997.

Fantel AG, Person RE, Burroughs-Gleim CJ, Mackler B: Direct embryotoxicity of cocaine in rats: Effects on mitochondrial activity, cardiac function, and growth and development in vitro. *Teratology* 42:35–43, 1990.

Ferrario JB, DeLeon IR, Tracy RE: Evidence for toxic anthropogenic chemicals in human thrombogenic coronary plaques. *Arch Environ Contam Toxicol* 14:529, 1985.

Fishman AP: Aminorex to fen/phen: An epidemic foretold. *Circulation* 99:156–161, 1999.

Fleckenstein A, Janke J, Doring HJ, Pachinger O: Calcium overload as the determinant factor in the production of catecholamine-induced myocardial lesions, in Bajusz E, Rona G (eds): *Recent Advances in Studies on Cardiac Structure and Metabolism.* Baltimore: University Park Press, 1973, pp 455–460.

Galan L, Talavera K, Vassort G, Alvarez JL: Characteristics of Ca^{2+} channel blockade by oxodipine and elgodipine in rat cardiomyocytes. *Eur J Pharmacol* 357:93–105, 1998.

Gan X, Zhang L, Berger O, et al: Cocaine enhances brain endothelial adhesion molecules and leukocyte migration. *Clin Immunol* 91:68, 1999.

Geng Y-J, Ishikawa Y, Vatner DE, et al: Apoptosis of cardiac myocytes in Gs alpha transgenic mice. *Circ Res* 84:34–42, 1999.

Gotzsche LS, Pederson EM: Dose-dependent cardiotoxic effect of amiodarone in cardioplegic solutions correlates with loss of dihydropyridine binding sites: In vitro evidence for a potentially lethal interaction with procaine. *J Cardiovasc Pharmacol* 23:13–23, 1994.

Gross GJ, Fryer RM: Sarcolemmal versus mitochondrial ATP-sensitive K^+ channels and myocardial preconditioning. *Circ Res* 84:973–979, 1999.

Gross JL, Moscatelli D, Rifkin DB: Increased capillary endothelial cell protease activity in response to angiogenic stimuli in vitro. *Proc Natl Acad Sci USA* 80:2623, 1983.

Guenoun T, Montagne O, Laplace M, Crozatier B: Propofol-induced modifications of cardiomyocyte calcium transient and sarcoplasmic reticulum function in rats. *Anesthesiology* 92:542–549, 2000.

Gurley BJ, Gardner SF, White LM, Wang PL: Ephedrine pharmacokinetics after the ingestion of nutrional supplements containing *Ephedra sinica* (ma huang). *Ther Drug Monit* 20:439–445, 1998.

Gwechenberger M, Mendoza LH, Youker KA, et al: Cardiac myocytes produce interleukin-6 in culture and in viable border zone of reperfused infarctions. *Circulation* 99:546–551, 1999.

Harpel PC: Homocysteine, atherogenesis and thrombosis. *Fibrinolysis Proteolysis* 11 (suppl. 1):77, 1997.

Haunstetter A, Izumo S: Apoptosis: Basic mechanisms and implications for cardiovascular disease. *Circ Res* 82:1111–1129, 1998.

Havlin KA: Cardiotoxicity of anthracyclines and other antineoplastic agents, in Acosta D (ed): *Cardiovascular Toxicology,* 2d ed. New York: Raven Press, 1992, pp 143–164.

He N, Singhal SS, Awasthi S, et al: Role of glutathione S-transferase 8-8 in allylamine resistance of vascular smooth muscle cells in vitro. *Toxicol Appl Pharmacol* 158:177, 1999.

Hefti MA, Harder BA, Eppenberger HM, Schaub MC: Signaling pathways in cardiac myocyte hypertrophy. *J Mol Cell Cardiol* 29:2873–2892, 1997.

Heusch G, Duessen A: The effects of cardiac sympathetic nerve stimulation on perfusion of stenotic coronary arteries in the dog. *Circ Res* 53:8–15, 1983.

Hines CH, Kodama JK, Guzman RJ, Loquvam GS: The toxicity of allylamines. *Arch Environ Health* 1:343, 1960.

Hino N, Ochi R, Yanagisawa T: Inhibition of the slow inward current and the time-dependent outward current of mammalian ventricular muscle by gentamicin. *Pflugers Arch* 394:243–249, 1982.

Houtman JP: Prolonged low-level cadmium intake and atherosclerosis. *Sci Total Environ* 138:31, 1993.

Hussar D. New drugs of 1999. *J Am Pharm Assoc* 40:181–221, 2000.

Hussar D. New drugs of 1998. *J Am Pharm Assoc* 39:151–206, 1999.

Iakushkin VV, Baldenov GN, Tertov VV, Orekhov AN: Atherogenic properties of phenothiazine drugs manifesting in cultured cells of the human aortic intima. *Kardiologiia* 32:66, 1992.

Jackman WM, Friday KJ, Anderson JL, et al: The long QT syndromes: A critical review, new clinical observations and a unifying hypothesis. *Prog Cardiovasc Dis* 31:115–172, 1988.

Kaasik A, Minajeva A, Paju K, et al: Thyroid hormones differentially affect sarcoplasmic reticulum function in rat atria and ventricles. *Mol Cell Biochem* 176:119–126, 1997.

Kaji T, Suzuki M, Yamamoto C, et al: Sensitive response of cultured vascular smooth muscle cells to cadmium cytotoxicity: Comparison with cultured vascular endothelial cells and kidney epithelial LLC-PK1 cells. *Toxicol Lett* 89:131, 1996.

Kajstura J, Cigola E, Malhotra A, et al: Angiotensin II induces apoptosis of adult ventricular myocytes in vitro. *J Mol Cell Cardiol* 29:859–870, 1997.

Kalin MF, Zumoff B: Sex hormones and coronary disease: A review of the clinical studies. *Steroids* 55:330–352, 1990.

Keller RS, Parker JL, Adams HR: Cardiovascular toxicity of antibacterial antibiotics, in Acosta D (ed): *Cardiovascular Toxicology,* 2d ed. New York: Raven Press, 1992, pp 165–195.

Kerzee JK, Ramos KS: Activation of C-Ha-ras by benzo[*a*]pyrene in vascular smooth muscle cells involves redox stress and aryl hydrocarbon receptor. *Mol Pharmacol* 58:152–158, 2000.

Kloner RA, Przyklenk K: Reperfusion injury to the heart. Is it a phenomenon? in Acosta D (ed): *Cardiovascular Toxicology,* 2d ed. New York: Raven Press, 1992, pp 131–140.

Koenig H, Fan C-C, Goldstone AD, et al: Polyamines mediate androgenic stimulation of calcium fluxes and membrane transport in rat heart myocytes. *Circ Res* 64:415–426, 1989.

Krown KA, Page MT, Nguyen C, et al: Tumor necrosis factor alpha-induced apoptosis in cardiac myocytes. *J Clin Invest* 98:2854–2865, 1996.

Kutzman RS, Wehner RW, Haber SB: Selected responses of hypertension-sensitive and resistant rats to inhaled acrolein. *Toxicology* 31:53, 1984.

Lalich JJ: Coronary artery hyalinosis in rats fed allylamine. *Exp Mol Pathol* 10:14, 1969.

Langford SD, Trent MB, Balakumaran A, Boor PJ: Developmental vasculotoxicity associated with inhibition of semicarbazide-sensitive amine oxidase. *Toxicol Appl Pharmacol* 155:237, 1999.

Lee JA, Allen DG: Calcium sensitizers: Mechanisms of action and potential usefulnes as inotropes. *Cardiovasc Res* 36:10–20, 1997.

Lemasters JJ, Bond JM, Harper IS, et al: The pH paradox in reperfusion injury to heart cells, in Lemasters JJ, Oliver C (eds): *Cell Biology of Trauma.* Boca Raton, FL: CRC Press, 1995, pp 149–162.

Levine ES, Friedman HS, Griffith OW, et al: Cardiac cell toxicity by 4-hydroperoxycyclophosphamide is modulated by glutathione. *Cardiovasc Res* 27:1248–1253, 1993.

Lewis JG, Graham DG, Valentine WM, et al: Exposure of C57BL/6 mice to carbon disulfide induces early lesions of atherosclerosis and enhances arterial fatty deposits induced by high fat diet. *Toxicol Sci* 49:124,1999.

Lewis W, Grupp IL, Grupp G, et al: Cardiac dysfunction occurs in the HIV-1 transgenic mouse treated with zidovudine. *Lab Invest* 80:187–197, 2000.

Li F, Wang X, Capasso JM, Gerdes AM: Rapid transition of cardiac myocytes from hyperplasia to hypertrophy during postnatal development. *J Mol Cell Cardiol* 28:1737–1746, 1996.

Liu S, Melchert RB, Kennedy RH: Inhibition of L-type Ca^{2+} channel current in rat ventricular myocytes by terfenadine. *Circ Res* 81:202–210, 1997.

Lu KP, Hallberg LM, Tomlinson J, Ramos KS: Benzo[*a*]pyrene activates LlMd retrotransposon and inhibits DNA repair in vascular smooth muscle cells. *Mutat Res* 454:35–44, 2000.

MacLellan WR, Schneider MD: Death by design: Programmed cell death in cardiovascular biology and disease. *Circ Res* 81:137–144, 1997.

Marcillat O, Zhang Y, Davies KJA: Oxidative and non-oxidative mechanisms in the Inactivation of cardiac mitochondrial electron transport chain components by doxorubicin. *Biochem J* 259:181–189, 1989.

Marks AR: Intracellular calcium-release channels: Regulators of cell life and death. *Am J Physiol* 272:H597–H605, 1997.

Marsh JD, Lehmann MH, Ritchie RH, et al: Androgen receptors mediate hypertrophy in cardiac myocytes. *Circulation* 98:256–261, 1998.

Martin XJ, Wynne DG, Glennon PE, et al: Regulation of expression of contractile proteins with cardiac hypertrophy and failure. *Mol Cell Biochem* 157:181–189, 1996.

Maulik N, Engelman RM, Rousou JA, et al: Ischemic preconditioning reduces apoptosis by upregulating anti-death gene Bcl-2. *Circulation* 100:II369–II375, 1999.

McManus BM, Toth B, Patil KD: Aortic rupture and aortic smooth muscle tumors in mice: Induction by *p*-hydrazinobenzoic acid hydrochloride of the cultivated mushroom *Agaricus bisporus. Lab Invest* 57(1):78, 1987.

Melchert RB, Welder AA: Cardiovascular effects of androgenic-anabolic steroids. *Med Sci Sports Exerc* 27:1252–1262, 1995.

Metzger JM, Wahr PA, Michele DE, et al: Effects of myosin heavy chain isoform switching on Ca^{2+}-activated tension and development in single adult cardiac myocytes. *Circ Res* 84:1310–1317, 1999.

Meyer R, Linz KW, Surges R, et al: Rapid modulation of L-type calcium current by acutely applied oestrogens in isolated cardiac myocytes from human, guinea-pig and rat. *Exp Physiol* 83:305–321, 1998.

Miller RA, Boorman GA: Morphology of neoplastic lesions induced by 1,3-butadiene in $B6C3F_1$ mice. *Environ Health Perspect* 86:37, 1990.

Nakaki T, Nakayama M, Yamamoto S, Kato R: α_1-Adrenergic stimulation and β_2-adrenergic inhibition of DNA synthesis in vascular smooth muscle cells. *Mol Pharmacol* 37:30, 1989.

Nattel S: Experimental evidence for proarrhythmic mechanisms of antiarrhythmic drugs. *Cardiovasc Res* 37:567–577, 1998.

Olson RD, Mushlin PS: Doxorubicin cardiotoxicity: Analysis of prevailing hypothesis. *FASEB J* 4:3076–3086, 1990.

Opie L: Heart cells and organelles, in Opie L (ed): *The Heart.* New York: Harcourt Brace Jovanovich, 1986a, pp 15–29.

Opie L: The mechanism of myocardial contraction, in Opie L (ed): *The Heart.* New York: Harcourt Brace Jovanovich, 1986b, pp 98–107.

O'Rourke B: Apoptosis: Rekindling the mitochondrial fire. *Circ Res* 85:880, 1999.

Ou X, Weber TJ, Chapkin RS, Ramos KS: Interference with protein kinase C-related signal transduction in vascular smooth muscle cells by benzo[*a*]pyrene. *Arch Biochem Biophys* 760:354, 1995.

Pacher P, Ungvai Z, Kecskemeti V, Furst S: Review of cardiovascular effects of fluoxetine, a selective serotonin reuptake inhibitor, compared to tricyclic antidepressants. *Curr Med Chem* 5:381–390, 1998.

Parrish AR, Ramos KS: Differential processing of osteopontin characterizes the proliferative vascular smooth muscle phenotype induced by allylamine. *J Cell Biochem* 65:267–275, 1997.

Parrish AR, Ramos KS: Osteopontin mRNA expression in a chemically induced model of atherogenesis. *Proc NY Acad Sci* 760:354, 1995.

Pelzer T, Schumann M, Neumann M, 17β-estradiol prevents programmed cell death in cardiac myocytes. *Biochem Biophys Res Commun* 268:192–200, 2000.

Peng SK, French WJ, Pelikan PCD: Direct cocaine cardiotoxicity demonstrated by endomyocardial biopsy. *Arch Pathol Lab Med* 113:842–845, 1989.

Penn A, Snyder C: Arteriosclerotic plaque development is "promoted" by polynuclear aromatic hydrocarbons. *Carcinogenesis* 9(12):2185, 1988.

Perez NG, Gao WD, Marban E: Novel myofilament Ca^{2+}-sensitizing property of xanthine oxidase inhibitors. *Circ Res* 83:423–430, 1998.

Perry MH, Erlanger MW, Gustafsson TO, Perry EF: Reversal of cadmium-induced hypertension by D-myo-inositol-1,2,6-trisphosphate. *J Toxicol Environ Health* 28:151, 1989.

Pickerill KE, Paladino JA, Schentag JJ: Comparison of the fluorquinolones based on pharmacokinetic and pharmacodynamic parameters. *Pharmacotherapy* 20:417–428, 2000.

Powis G: Free radical formation by antitumor quinones. *Free Radic Biol Med* 6:63–101, 1989.

Pulkki KJ: Cytokines and cardiomyocyte death. *Ann Med* 29:339–343, 1997.

Rajamani S, Studenick C, Lemmens-Gruber R, Heistracher P: Cardiotoxic effects of fenfluramine hydrochloride on isolated cardiac preparations and ventricular myocytes of guinea-pigs. *Br J Pharmacol* 129:843–852, 2000.

Ramos KS: Redox regulation of c-Ha-ras and osteopontin signaling in vascular smooth muscle cells: Implications in chemical atherogenesis. *Annu Rev Pharmacol Toxicol* 29:243, 1999.

Ramos KS, Bowes RC III, Ou X, Weber TJ: Responses of vascular smooth muscle cells to toxic insult: Cellular and molecular perspectives for environmental toxicants. *J Toxicol Environ Health* 43:419, 1994.

Ramos KS, Combs AB, Acosta D: Role of calcium in isoproterenol cytotoxicity to cultured myocardial cells. *Biochem Pharmacol* 33:1989, 1984.

Ramos K, Cox LR: Primary cultures of rat aortic endothelial and smooth muscle cells: I. An in vitro model to study xenobiotic-induced vascular cytotoxicity. *In Vitro Cell Dev Biol* 21:495, 1987.

Ramos K, Grossman SL, Cox LR: Allylamine-induced vascular toxicity in vitro: Prevention by semicarbizide-sensitive amine oxidase inhibitors. *Toxicol Appl Pharmacol* 96:61, 1988.

Ramos K, McMahon KK, Alipui C, Demick D: Modulation of smooth muscle cell proliferation by dinitrotoluene, in Witmer CM, Snyder RR, Jollow DJ, et al (eds): *Biologic Reductive Intermediates.* Vol V. New York: Plenum Press, 1990, p 805.

Ramos KS, Thurlow CH: Comparative cytotoxic responses of cultured avian and rodent aortic smooth muscle cells to allylamine. *J Toxicol Environ Health* 40:61, 1993.

Ramos KS, Weber TJ, Liau G: Altered protein secretion and extracellular matrix deposition is associated with the proliferative phenotype induced by allylamine in aortic smooth muscle cells. *Biochem J* 289:57, 1993.

Rampe D, Wible B, Brown AM, Dage RC: Effects of terfenadine and its metabolites on a delayed rectifier K^+ channel cloned from human heart. *Mol Pharmacol* 44:1240–1245, 1993.

Redetzki JE, Guiswold KE, Nopajaroonsei C, Redetzki HM: Amelioration of cardiotoxic effects of alcohol by vitamin E. *J Toxicol Clin Toxicol* 20:319–331, 1983.

Reed JC, Paternostro G: Postmitochondrial regulation of apoptosis during heart failure. *Proc Natl Acad Sci USA* 96:7614–7616, 1999.

Ribiere C, Hininger I, Rouach H, Nordmann R: Effects of chronic ethanol administration on free radical defence in rat myocardium. *Biochem Pharmacol* 44:1495–1500, 1992.

Robert V, Silvestre J-S, Charlemagne D, et al: Biological determinants of aldosterone-induced cardiac fibrosis in rats. *Hypertension* 26:971–978, 1995.

Rockhold RW: Cardiovascular toxicity of anabolic steroids. *Annu Rev Pharmacol Toxicol* 33:497–520, 1993.

Roden DM: Antiarrhythmic drugs, in Hardman JG, Limbird LE, Molinoff PB, et al (eds): *Goodman & Gilman's The Pharmacological Basis of Therapeutics.* 9th ed. New York, McGraw-Hill, 1996, pp 839–874.

Rosenman KD: Environmentally related disorders of the cardiovascular system. *Med Clin North Am* 74:361, 1990.

Sandusky GE, Vodicnik MJ, Tamura RN: Cardiovascular and adrenal proliferative lesions in Fischer 344 rats induced by long-term treatment with type III phosphodiesterase inhibitors (positive inotropic agents), isomazole and indolidan. *Fundam Appl Toxicol* 16:198, 1991.

Saraste A, Pulkki K, Kallajoki M, et al: Cardiomyocyte apoptosis and progression of heart failure to transplantation. *Eur J Clin Invest* 29:380–386, 1999.

Sawyer DB, Fukazawa R, Arstall MA, Kelly RA: Daunorubicin-induced apoptosis in rat cardiac myocytes is inhibited by dexrazoxane. *Circ Res* 84:257–265, 1999.

Scarpa A: Transport across mitochondrial membranes, in Giebisch G, Tosteson DC, Ussing HH (eds): *Membrane Transport in Biology.* New York: Springer, 1979, pp 263–355.

Shahidi H, Kilbourn RG: The role of nitric oxide in interleukin-2 therapy induced hypotension. *Cancer Metast Rev* 17(1):119, 1998.

Sharma A, Plessinger MA, Miller RK, Woods JR: Progesterone antagonist mifepristone (RU486) decreases cardiotoxicity of cocaine. *Proc Soc Exp Biol Med* 202:2279–2287, 1993.

Sherwood L: Cardiac physiology, in Sherwood L (ed): *Human Physiology.* Minneapolis/St. Paul: West Publishing, 1993, pp 258–298.

Shizukuda Y, Buttrick PM, Geenen DL, et al: Beta-adrenergic stimulation causes cardiocyte apoptosis: Influence of tachycardia and hypertrophy. *Am J Physiol* 275:H961–H968, 1998.

Sies H: Oxidative stress: From basic research to clinical application. *Am J Med* 91:315–385, 1991.

Simons FER: The therapeutic index of newer H_1-receptor antagonists. *Clin Exp Allergy* 24:707–723, 1994.

Simpson PJ, Lucchesi BR: Free radicals and myocardial ischemia and reperfusion injury. *J Clin Lab Med* 110:13–30, 1987.

Solem LE, Henry TR, Wallace KB: Disruption of mitochondrial calcium homeostasis following chronic doxorubicin administration. *Toxicol Appl Pharmacol* 129:214–222, 1994.

Sperelakis N: Chemical agent actions on ion channels and electrophysiology of the heart, in Acosta D (ed): *Cardiovascular Toxicology,* 2d ed. New York: Raven Press, 1992, pp 283–338.

Stewart G, Rubin E, Thomas AP: Inhibition by cocaine of excitation-contraction coupling in isolated cardiomyocytes. *Am J Physiol* 260:H50–H57, 1991.

Stief CG, Uckert S, Becker AJ, et al: Effects of sildenafil on cAMP and cGMP levels in isolated human cavernous and cardiac tissue. *Urology* 55:146–150, 2000.

Stolley PD, Strom BL, Sartwell PE: Oral contraceptives and vascular disease. *Epidemiol Rev* 11:241, 1989.

Sugden PH: Signaling in myocardial hypertrophy: Life after calcineurin? *Circ Res* 84:633–646, 1999.

Sugishita K, Kinugawa K-I, Shimizu T, et al: Cellular basis for the acute inhibitory effects of IL-6 and TNF-α on excitation-contraction coupling. *J Mol Cell Cardiol* 31:1457–1467, 1999.

Thomas T, Sutton ET, Bryant MW, Rhodin JA: In vivo vascular damage, leukocyte activation and inflammatory response induced by beta-amyloid. *J Submicrosc Cytol Pathol* 29:293, 1997.

Tomera JF, Harakal C: Mercury and lead-induced contraction of aortic smooth muscle in vitro. *Arch Int Pharmacodyn Ther* 283:295, 1986.

Trump BF, Berezesky IK, Chang SH, Phelps PC: The pathways of cell death: Oncosis, apoptosis, and necrosis. *Toxicol Pathol* 25:82–88, 1997.

Turner NA, Zia F, Azhar G, et al: Oxidative stress induces DNA fragmentation and caspase activation via the c-Jun NH_2-terminal kinase pathway in H9c2 cardiac muscle cells. *J Mol Cell Cardiol* 30:1789–1801, 1998.

Umansky SR, Shapiro JP, Cuenco GM, et al: Prevention of rat neonatal cardiomyocyte apoptosis induced by simulated *in vitro* ischemia and reperfusion *Cell Growth Differ* 4:608–616, 1997.

Vary TC, Reibel DK, Neely JR: Control of energy metabolism of heart muscle *Annu Rev Physiol* 43:419–430, 1981.

Vestal RE, Eriksson CE, Musser B, et al: Effect of intravenous aminophylline on plasma levels of catecholamines and related cardiovascular and metabolic responses in man. *Circulation* 67:162–171, 1983.

von Harsdorf R, Li PF, Dietz R: Signaling pathways in reactive oxygen species-induced cardiomyocyte apoptosis. *Circulation* 99:2934–2941, 1999.

Wald N, Howard S: Smoking, carbon monoxide and disease. *Ann Occup Hyg* 18:1, 1975.

Wallace KB, Starkov AA: Mitochondrial targets of drug toxicity. *Annu Rev Pharmacol Toxicol* 40:353–388, 2000.

Wang L, Weiqiong M, Markovich R, et al: Regulation of cardiomyocyte apoptotic signaling by insulin-like growth factor I. *Circ Res* 83:516–522, 1998.

Wei EP, Christman CW, Kontos HA, Povlishock JT: Effects of oxygen radicals on cerebral arterioles. *Am J Physiol* 248:H157, 1985.

Williams JB: Adverse effects of thyroid hormones. *Drugs Aging* 11:460–469, 1997.

Wilson CA, Everard DM, Schoental R: Blood pressure changes and cardiovascular lesions found in rats given T-2 toxin, a trichothecene secondary metabolite of certain *Fusarium microfungi. Toxicol Lett* 10:35, 1982.

Wilson SK: Role of oxygen-derived free radicals in acute angiotensin II-induced hypertensive vascular disease in the rat. *Circ Res* 66:722, 1990.

Wu C-F, Bishopric NH, Pratt RE: Atrial natriuretic peptide induces apoptosis in neonatal rat cardiac myocytes. *J Biol Chem* 272:14860–14866, 1997.

Xiao Y, He J, Gilbert RD, Zhang L: Cocaine induces apoptosis in fetal myocardial cells through a mitochondria-dependent pathway. *J Pharmacol Exp Ther* 292:8–14, 2000.

Yamamoto C, Kaji T, Sakamoto M, Kozuka H: Effects of cadmium on the release of tissue plasminogen activator and plasminogen activator inhibitor type 1 from cultured human vascular smooth muscle cells and fibroblasts. *Toxicology* 106:179, 1996.

Yamamoto C, Miyamoto A, Sakamoto M, et al: Lead perturbs the regulation of spontaneous release of tissue plasminogen activator inhibitor-1 from vascular smooth muscle cells and fibroblasts in culture. *Toxicology* 117:153, 1997.

Young M, Fullerton M, Dilley R, Funder J: Mineralocorticoids, hypertension, and cardiac fibrosis. *J Clin Invest* 93:2578–2583, 1994.

Yu PH: Deamination of methylamine and angiopathy: Toxicity of formaldehyde, oxidative stress and relevance to protein glycooxidation in diabetes. *J Neural Transm Suppl* 52:201, 1998.

Yuan C, Acosta D: Inhibitory effect of cocaine on calcium mobilization in cultured rat myocardial cells. *J Mol Cell Cardiol* 26:1415–1419, 1994.

Yue TL, Wang C, Gu JL, et al: Inhibition of extracellular signal-regulated kinase enhances ischemia/reoxygenation-induced apoptosis in cultured cardiac myocytes and exaggerates reperfusion injury in isolated perfused heart. *Circ Res* 86:692–699, 2000.

Zakhari S: Cardiovascular toxicology of halogenated hydrocarbons and other solvents, in Acosta D (ed): *Cardiovascular Toxicology.* New York: Raven Press, 1992, pp 409–454.

Zhang J, Duarte CG, Ellis S: Contrast medium- and mannitol-induced apoptosis in heart and kidney of SHR rats. *Toxicol Pathol* 27:427–435, 1999b.

Zhang L, Xiao Y, He J: Cocaine and apoptosis in myocardial cells. *Anat Rec* 257:208–216, 1999a.

Zhao W, Parrish AR, Ramos KS: Constitutive and inducible expression of cytochrome P4501A1 and 1B1 in human vascular endothelial and smooth muscle cells. *In Vitro Cell Dev Biol* 34:671, 1998.

Zhou W, Fontenot HJ, Liu S, Kennedy RH: Modulation of cardiac calcium channels by propofol. *Anesthesiology* 86:670–675, 1997.

Zhou W, Fontenot HJ, Wang S-N, Kennedy RH: Propofol-induced alterations in myocardial b-adrenoceptor binding and responsiveness. *Anesth Analg* 89:604–608, 1999.

Zhu, W, Zou Y, Aikawa R, et al: MAPK superfamily plays an important role in daunomycin-induced apoptosis of cardiac myocytes. *Circulation* 100:2100–2107, 1999.

Zwijsen RML, van Kleef EM, Alink GM: A comparative study on the metabolic activation of 3,4-benzo[*a*]pyrene to mutagens by aortic smooth muscle cells of rat and rabbit. *Mutat Res* 230:111, 1990.

CHAPTER 19

TOXIC RESPONSES OF THE SKIN

David E. Cohen and Robert H. Rice

As the body's first line of defense against external insult, the skin's enormous surface area (1.5 to 2 m^2) is exposed routinely to chemical agents and may inadvertently serve as a portal of entry for topical contactants. Recognizing the potential hazards of skin exposure, the National Institute of Occupational Safety and Health (NIOSH) characterized skin disease as one of the most pervasive occupational health problems in the United States. In 1982 NIOSH placed skin disease in the top ten leading work-related diseases based on frequency, severity, and the potential for prevention. Data from the Bureau of Labor Statistics indicate that skin disease attributed to workplace exposures accounts for more than 30 percent of all reported occupational disease. Incidence data from 1990 indicate a rate of 7.9 cases per 10,000 or about 61,000 new cases per year. Exposures in the agricultural and manufacturing industries were responsible for the greatest volume of disease, with incidence rates of 86 and 41 per 10,000, respectively. Skin conditions resulting from exposures to consumer products or occupational illnesses not resulting in lost work time are poorly recorded and tracked. Hence the incidence of such skin diseases is grossly underestimated.

SKIN AS A BARRIER

A large and highly accessible human organ, the skin protects the body against external insults in order to maintain internal homeostasis. Its biological sophistication allows it to perform a myriad of functions above and beyond that of a suit of armor. Physiologically, the skin participates directly in thermal, electrolyte, hormonal, metabolic, and immune regulation, without which a human being would perish. Rather than merely repelling noxious physical agents, the skin may react to them with a variety of defensive mechanisms that serve to prevent internal or widespread cutaneous damage. If an insult is severe or intense enough to overwhelm the protective function of the skin, acute or chronic injury becomes readily manifest in a variety of ways. The specific presentation depends on a variety of intrinsic and extrinsic factors including body site, duration of exposure, and other environmental conditions (Table 19-1).

Skin Histology

The skin consists of two major components: the outer epidermis and the underlying dermis, which are separated by a basement membrane (Fig. 19-1). The junction ordinarily is not flat but has an undulating appearance (rete ridges). In addition, epidermal appendages (hair follicles, sebaceous glands, and eccrine glands) span the epidermis and are embedded in the dermis. In thickness, the dermis makes up approximately 90 percent of the skin and has largely a supportive function. It has a high content of collagen and elastin, secreted by scattered fibroblasts, thus providing the skin with elastic properties. Separating the dermis from underlying tissues is a layer of adipocytes, whose accumulation of fat has a cushioning action. The blood supply to the epidermis originates in the capillaries located in the rete ridges at the dermal-epidermal junction. Capillaries also supply the bulbs of the hair follicles and the secretory cells of the eccrine (sweat) glands. The ducts from these glands carry a dilute salt solution to the surface of the skin, where its evaporation provides cooling.

The interfollicular epidermis is a stratified squamous epithelium consisting primarily of keratinocytes. These cells are tightly attached to each other by desmosomes and to the basement membrane by hemidesmosomes. Melanocytes are interspersed among the basal cells and distributed sparsely in the dermis, with occasional concentrations beneath the basal lamina and in the papillae of hair follicles. In the epidermis, these cells are stimulated by ultraviolet light to produce melanin granules. The granules are ex-

Table 19-1
Factors Influencing Cutaneous Responses

VARIABLE	COMMENT
Body site	
Palms/soles	Thick stratum corneum—good physical barrier Common site of contact with chemicals Occlusion with protective clothing
Intertriginous areas (axillae, groin, neck, finger webs, umbilicus, genitalia)	Moist, occluded areas Chemical trapping Enhanced percutaneous absorption
Face	Exposed frequently Surface lipid interacts with hydrophobic substances Chemicals frequently transferred from hands
Eyelids	Poor barrier function—thin epidermis Sensitive to irritants
Postauricular region	Chemical trapping Occlusion
Scalp	Chemical trapping Hair follicles susceptible to metabolic damage
Predisposing cutaneous illnesses	
Atopic dermatitis	Increased sensitivity to irritants Impaired barrier function
Psoriasis	Impaired barrier function
Genetic factors	Predisposition to skin disorders Variation in sensitivity to irritants Susceptibility to contact sensitization
Temperature	Vasodilation—improved percutaneous absorption Increased sweating—trapping
Humidity	Increased sweating—trapping
Season	Variation in relative humidity Chapping and wind-related skin changes

SOURCE: Adapted from Fitzpatrick et al. (1993).

truded and taken up by the surrounding epidermal cells, which thereby become pigmented. Migrating through the epidermis are numerous Langerhans cells, which are important participants in the immune response of skin to foreign agents.

Keratinocytes of the basal layer make up the germinative compartment. When a basal cell divides, one of the progeny detaches from the basal lamina and migrates outward. As cells move toward the skin surface, they undergo a remarkable program of terminal differentiation. They gradually express new protein markers and accumulate keratin proteins, from which the name of this cell type is derived. The keratins form insoluble intermediate filaments, accounting for nearly 40 percent of the total cell protein in the spinous layer. At the granular layer, the cells undergo a striking morphologic transformation, becoming flattened and increasing in volume nearly 40-fold. Lipid granules fuse with the plasma membrane, replacing the aqueous environment in the intercellular space with their contents. Meanwhile, the plasma membranes of these cells become permeable, resulting in the loss of their reducing environment and consequently in extensive disulfide bonding among keratin proteins. Cell organelles are degraded, while a protein envelope is synthesized immediately beneath the plasma membrane. The membrane is altered characteristically by the loss of phospholipid and the addition of sphingolipid.

This program of terminal differentiation, beginning as keratinocytes leave the basal layer, produces the outermost layer of the skin, the stratum corneum. No longer viable, the mature cells (called *corneocytes*) are approximately 80 percent keratin in content. They are gradually shed from the surface and replaced from beneath. The process typically takes 2 weeks for basal cells to reach the stratum corneum and another 2 weeks to be shed from the surface. In the skin disease psoriasis, the migration of cells to the surface is nearly tenfold faster than normal, resulting in a stratum corneum populated by cells that are not completely mature. In instances in which the outer layer is deficient due to disease or physical or chemical trauma, the barrier to the environment that the skin provides is inferior to that provided by normal, healthy skin.

Percutaneous Absorption

Until the turn of the century, the skin was believed to provide an impervious barrier to exogenous substances. Gradually, the ability of substances to penetrate the skin, though this process generally is very slow, became appreciated. During the past 50 years, the stratum corneum has been recognized as the primary barrier (Scheuplein and Blank, 1971). Diseases (e.g., psoriasis) or other conditions (e.g., abrasion, wounding) in which this barrier is com-

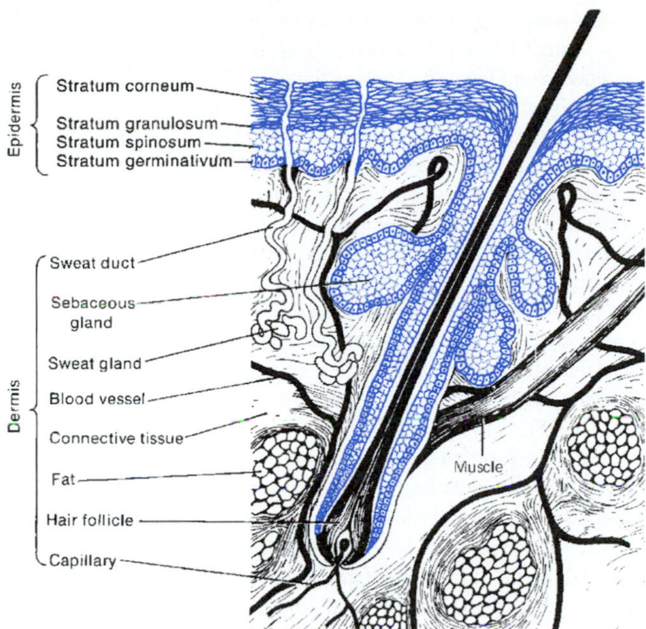

Figure 19-1. Diagram of a cross section of human skin.

The epidermis and pilosebaceous unit are shown in blue.

promised can permit greatly increased uptake of poorly permeable substances, as does removal of the stratum corneum by tape stripping. The viable layer of epidermis provides a much less effective barrier, because hydrophilic agents readily diffuse into the intercellular water, while hydrophobic agents can partition into cell membranes, and each can diffuse readily to the blood supply in the rete ridges of the dermis.

Probably the best-known biological membrane barrier for this purpose, the stratum corneum, prevents water loss from underlying tissues by evaporation. Its hydrophobic character reflects the lipid content of the intercellular space, approximately 15 percent of the total volume (Elias, 1992). The lipids, a major component being sphingolipids, have a high content of long-chain ceramides, removal of which seriously compromises barrier function as measured by transepidermal water loss. The stratum corneum is ordinarily hydrated (typically 20 percent water), the moisture residing in corneocyte protein, but it can take up a great deal more water upon prolonged immersion, thereby reducing the effectiveness of the barrier to agents with a hydrophilic character. Indeed, occlusion of the skin with plastic wrap, permitting the retention of perspiration underneath, is a commonly employed technique to enhance uptake of agents applied to the skin surface. Although penetration from the air is generally too low to be of concern, protection from skin uptake may be advisable for some compounds (e.g., nitrobenzene) at concentrations high enough to require respirator use.

Finding the rate at which the uptake of agents through the skin occurs is important for estimating the consequences of exposure to many agents we encounter in the environment. Indeed, a regulatory strategy permitting bathing in water considered barely unfit for drinking was revised when it was realized that exposure from dermal/inhalation uptake during bathing could be comparable to that from drinking 2 L of the water (Brown et al., 1984). Uptake through the skin is now incorporated in pharmacokinetic modeling to estimate potential risks from exposures. The degree of uptake depends upon the details of exposure conditions, being proportional to solute concentration (assuming it is dilute), time, and the amount of skin surface exposed. In addition, two intrinsic factors contribute to the absorption rate of a given compound: its hydrophobicity, which affects its ability to partition into epidermal lipid, and its rate of diffusion through this barrier. A measure of the first property is the commonly used octanol/water partitioning ratio (K_{ow}). This is particularly relevant for exposure to contaminated water, such as occurs during bathing or swimming. However, partitioning of an agent into the skin is greatly affected by its solubility in or adhesion to the medium in which it is applied (including soil). The second property is an inverse function of molecular weight (MW) or molecular volume. Thus, hydrophobic agents of low MW permeate the skin better than those of high MW or those that are hydrophilic. For small molecules, hydrophobicity is a dominant factor in penetration.

Although only small amounts of agents may penetrate the stratum corneum, those of high potency may still be very dangerous. For example, hydrophobic organophosphorus pesticides can be neurotoxic by skin contact to humans and domestic animals. Conditions of topical treatment of the latter for pest control must take into consideration not only the tolerance of the animals but also residues in meat and milk resulting from skin penetration. High level skin exposure to agents considered safe at low levels can be dangerous, evident from the nervous system toxicity and deaths of babies exposed to hexachlorophene mistakenly added to talcum powder for their diapers (Martin-Bouyer et al., 1982). Previous findings of *N*-nitrosamines that penetrate skin well (such as *N*-nitrosodiethanolamine) in cutting oils and cosmetics raised concern and led to their monitoring and to reduction of exposure.

Considerable empiric information has been collected on some compounds of special interest (including pharmaceuticals, pesticides, and pollutants) for use in quantifying structure/penetration relationships. From such information, relations can be obtained for skin penetration (P_{cw}) using empirically derived constants (C_1, C_2, C_3) that have the form shown below (Potts and Guy, 1992). Such

$$\log P_{cw} = C_1 - C_2(\text{MW}) + C_3 \log K_{ow}$$

relations describe steady-state conditions, in which an agent leaves the stratum corneum at the same rate it enters. Because rates of transfer of very hydrophobic agents into the aqueous phase of the spinous layer are slow, saturation of the stratum corneum provides a depot, leading to continued penetration into the body for relatively long time periods after external exposure to an agent stops.

Diffusion through the epidermis is considerably faster at some anatomic sites than others. A list in order of decreasing permeability under steady state conditions gives the following hierarchy: foot sole > palm > scrotum > forehead > abdomen (Scheuplein and Blank, 1971). Under ordinary circumstances, absorption through the epidermal appendages is generally neglected, despite the ability of agents to bypass the stratum corneum by this route, because the combined appendageal surface area is such a small fraction of the total available for uptake. However, because loading of the stratum corneum is slow, penetration through the appendages can constitute an appreciable fraction of the total for short exposures. In some cases, the effects of appendages can even be dominant. For instance, benzo(a)pyrene penetrates the skin of haired mice severalfold faster than that of hairless strains (Kao et al., 1988).

Transdermal Drug Delivery The ability of the stratum corneum to serve as a reservoir for exogenously applied agents is well illustrated by the recent development of methods to exploit this property for the delivery of pharmaceuticals. Application of drugs to the skin can produce systemic effects, a phenomenon observed fortuitously before the ability of the skin to serve as a delivery system was appreciated. For example, topical exposure of young girls to estrogens has led to reports of pseudoprecocious puberty, while in young or adult males, such exposure has produced gynecomastia (reviewed in Amin et al., 1998). Specially designed patches are currently in use to deliver estradiol, testosterone, nitroglycerin, scopolamine, clonidine, fentanyl, and nicotine for therapeutic purposes, and others are under development. The advantages of this approach over oral dosing include providing a steady infusion for extended periods (typically 1 to 7 days), thereby avoiding large variations in plasma concentration, preventing exposure to the acidic pH of the stomach, and avoiding biotransformation in the gastrointestinal tract or from first-pass removal by the liver. The contrast in plasma concentration kinetics between different methods of delivery is particularly evident for agents that are rapidly metabolized, such as nitroglycerin, which has a half-life of minutes.

Measurements of Penetration For many purposes, including risk assessment and pharmaceutical design, the most useful subject for experimentation is human skin. Volunteers are dosed, plasma and/or urine concentrations are measured at suitable intervals, and amounts excreted from the body are estimated. Past measurements of penetration, for example of pesticides (Feldman and Maibach, 1974), often used ^{14}C-labeled agents. For most compounds, this approach is not preferred, but use of isotopic labels is now readily feasible when coupled to ultrasensitive detection by accelerator mass spectrometry (Buchholz et al., 1999). For in vitro work, excised split-thickness skin can be employed in special diffusion chambers, though care is needed to preserve the viability of the living layer of epidermis. The agent is removed for measurement from the underside by a fluid into which it partitions, thereby permitting continued penetration. Commonly employed is a simpler setup using cadaver skin with the lower dermis removed. This lacks biotransformation capability but retains the barrier function of the stratum corneum. The pharmacokinetic approach with intact subjects is most commonly employed with experimental animals. Without verification using human skin, such measurements are subject to large uncertainties due to species differences in density of epidermal appendages, stratum corneum properties (e.g., thickness, lipid composition), and biotransformation rates. Because penetration through rodent skin is usually faster than through human skin, the former provides a conservative estimate for behavior of the latter. To simplify determination of penetration kinetics, skin flaps may be employed and the capillary blood flow monitored to measure penetration. For this purpose, pig skin has particular utility (Riviere, 1993). A promising variation minimizing species differences is to use skin grafts on experimental animals for these measurements. Human skin persists well on athymic mice and retains its normal barrier properties (Kreuger and Pershing, 1993).

Biotransformation

The ability of the skin to metabolize agents that diffuse through it contributes to its barrier function. This influences the potential biological activity of xenobiotics and topically applied drugs, leading to their degradation or their activation as skin sensitizers or carcinogens (for a comprehensive review see Hotchkiss, 1998). To this end, the epidermis and pilosebaceous units are the most relevant and indeed are the major sources of such activity in the skin. On a body-weight basis, phase I metabolism in this organ usually is only a small fraction (≈2 percent) of that in the liver, but its importance should not be underestimated. For example, when the epidermis of the neonatal rat is treated with benzo(a)pyrene or Aroclor 1254, the arylhydrocarbon hydroxylase (P450) activity in the skin can exceed 20 percent of that in the whole body (Mukhtar and Bickers, 1981). As illustrated in this example, cytochrome P4501A1 is inducible in the epidermis by agents that are inducers in other tissues—TCDD (tetrachlorodibenzo-*p*-dioxin), polycyclic aromatic hydrocarbons, PCBs (polychlorinated biphenyls), and crude coal tar, which is used in dermatologic therapy. Thus, exposure to such inducers could influence skin biotransformation and even sensitize epidermal cells to other agents that are not good inducers themselves, a phenomenon observable in cell culture (Walsh et al., 1995).

Biotransformation of a variety of compounds in the skin has been detected, including arachidonic acid derivatives, steroids, retinoids, and 2-amino-anthracene, suggesting that multiple P450 activities are expressed. Evidence has been presented for P4502A1 and 2B1 in rat skin, for example, using specific substrates, immunoblotting of the protein, and polymerase chain reaction techniques. These and other P450s are expressed in murine skin, and at least some of them are stimulated by glucocorticoids, commonly used therapeutic agents on human skin (Jugert et al., 1994). Novel cytochrome P450 isozymes 2B12 and 2B19, which use arachidonic acid as a substrate and thus likely participate in signaling pathways, have been detected in the epidermis and pilosebaceous units (Keeney et al., 1998). The TCDD-inducible isozyme P4501B1 has been reported in human keratinocytes and is expressed in a variety of other tissues as well (Sutter et al., 1994). Species differences are apparent in the amounts of P450 activities detectable. For example, measured ethoxycoumarin-*O*-deethylase activity is 20-fold higher in mouse than human (or rat) skin. Differences of such magnitude help rationalize the observation that the rate of penetration of ethoxycoumarin is sufficient to saturate its metabolism in some species (e.g., the human) but not in others (e.g., the mouse or guinea pig) (Storm et al., 1990).

Enzymes participating in phase II metabolism are expressed in skin. For example, multiple forms of epoxide hydrolase and UDP–glucuronosyl transferase have been detected in human and rodent skin. In general, this activity occurs at a much lower rate than observed in the liver, but exceptions are evident, as in the case of quinone reductase (Khan et al., 1987). Human and rodent skin exhibit qualitatively similar phase II reactions, but rodent skin often has a higher level of activity. An additional consideration is that different species express different relative amounts of the various isozymes, which could alter resulting target specificities or degree of responsiveness. Glutathione transferase, for instance, catalyzes the reaction of glutathione with exogenous nucleophiles or provides intracellular transport of bound compounds in the absence of a reaction. It also facilitates the reaction of glutathione with endogenous products of arachidonate lipoxygenation (leukotrienes) to yield mediators of anaphylaxis and chemotaxis, which are elements of the inflammatory response in the skin. Of the three major transferase forms characterized in the liver, the major form in the skin of humans and rodents is the π isozyme. Human skin also expresses the α isozyme, while rat and mouse skin express the μ isozyme and, in much smaller amounts, the α isozyme (Raza et al., 1992).

A variety of other metabolic enzyme activites have also been detected in human epidermal cells, including sulfatases,

β-glucuronidase, *N*-acetyl transferases, esterases, and reductases (Hotchkiss, 1998). The intercellular region of the stratum corneum has catabolic activities (e.g., proteases, lipases, glycosidases, phosphatase) supplied by the lamellar bodies along with their characteristic lipid (Elias, 1992). Such activities can have major effects on agents that penetrate the skin. For example, methyl salicylate readily diffuses through the epidermis and is detected in the dermis, but only as deesterified salicylate, illustrating first-pass metabolism (Cross et al., 1997). The influence of hydroxysteroid dehydrogenases and microsomal reductase activities during percutaneous absorption is evident in studies on mouse skin in organ culture. In one study (Kao and Hall, 1987), 8 h after topical application of testosterone, 59 percent of the permeated steroid was collected unchanged and the rest was transformed into metabolites. In parallel, estrone was converted substantially to estradiol (67 percent), while only 23 percent was collected as the parent compound. By contrast, estradiol was metabolized to a much lower extent (21 percent).

CONTACT DERMATITIS

Of all occupational skin disease, contact dermatitis accounts for over 90 percent of reported causes (American Academy of Dermatology, 1994; Beltrani, 1999). As the single most prevalent occupational skin disease, it is one of the most important occupational illnesses affecting American workers. It comprises two distinct inflammatory processes caused by adverse exposure of the skin, irritant and allergic contact dermatitis. These syndromes have indistinguishable clinical characteristics. Classically, erythema (redness), induration (thickening and firmness), scaling (flaking), and vesiculation (blistering) are present on areas directly contacting the chemical agent. Paraffin-embedded biopsies from affected sites reveal a mixed-cell inflammatory infiltrate of lymphocytes and eosinophils and the hallmark finding of spongiosis (intercellular edema). Unfortunately, these histopathologic features are not sufficient to differentiate allergic from irritant contact dermatitis, atopic dermatitis, or certain other common syndromes. Since their etiology is different, as supported by subtle but clear differences in the inflammatory responses, the two syndromes are presented separately here.

Irritant Dermatitis

Irritant dermatitis is a non-immune-related response caused by the direct action of an agent on the skin. Despite the "nonsensitization" pathways responsible for the genesis of irritant contact dermatitis, specific cytokines have been identified in the pathophysiology of the eruption (Corsini et al., 2000; Morhenn, 1999). Extrinsic variables such as concentration, pH, temperature, duration, repetitiveness of contact, and occlusion impact significantly on the appearance of the eruption. Suffice it to say that chemicals like strong acids, bases, solvents, and unstable or reactive chemicals rank high among the many possible human irritants.

Strongly noxious substances such as those with extreme pH can produce an immediate irreversible and potentially scarring dermatitis following a single exposure. This acute irritant phenomenon is akin to a chemical burn and has been described as an "etching" reaction (Bjornberg, 1987). More commonly, single exposures to potentially irritating chemicals will not produce significant reactions; repeated exposures are necessary to elicit clinically noticeable changes. Such repeated exposures eventually result in either an eczematous dermatitis with clinical and histopathologic changes characteristic of allergic contact dermatitis or a fissured, thickened eruption without a substantial inflammatory component. Chemicals inducing the latter two reactions are termed *marginal irritants.*

Because the thresholds for irritant reactions vary greatly from person to person, a genetic component to the response has been considered. Monozygotic twins have shown greater concordance than dizygotic twins in their reactions to irritant chemicals like sodium lauryl sulfate and benzalkonium chloride (Holst and Moller, 1975). While young individuals with fair complexion appear more sensitive to irritant chemicals than older individuals with dark complexion, sex does not appear to be a significant factor. Attempts to predict the relative irritancy of substances based upon their chemical relatedness to other irritants have been unsuccessful.

Divergent etiologies make it difficult to assign a specific mechanism for the pathophysiology of irritant dermatitis. Direct corrosives, protein solvents, oxidizing and reducing agents, and dehydrating agents act as irritants by disrupting the keratin ultrastructure or directly injuring critical cellular macromolecules or organelles. Marginal irritants require multifactorial variables to create disease and may not be capable of producing reactions under all circumstances. The varying time courses necessary to produce dermatitis by different known irritants result not merely from differing rates of percutaneous absorption but also depend on the specific agent selected. Thus, "chemicals do not produce skin irritation by a common inflammatory pathway" (Patrick et al., 1987). Supporting this view, tetradecanoylphorbol acetate (the major active ingredient of croton oil, a potent irritant) induced a tenfold increase in prostaglandin E_2 (PGE_2) in cultured human keratinocytes, whereas another irritant, ethylphenyl propriolate, induced no change in PGE_2 (Bloom et al., 1987). Elevation of prostaglandins and leukotriene B4 in blister fluids correlated with the induction of erythema and the impairment of the epidermal barrier secondary to specific irritants such as benzalkonium chloride and sodium lauryl sulfate. This cytokine and eicosanoid profile was considered important for irritant dermatitis from surfactants but was not characteristic of other common skin irritants like triethanolamine and Tween 80 (Muller-Decker et al., 1998). Forsey demonstrated sodium lauryl sulfate induced keratinocyte proliferation after a 48-h exposure with no effect on Langerhans cell (LC) number or distribution, and keratinocyte apoptosis after 24- and 48-h exposure. Conversely, nonanoic acid decreased keratinocyte proliferation after a 24-h exposure and induced epidermal cell apoptosis after only a 6-h exposure. More significantly, LC number decreased after 24- and 48-h exposures, and induced apoptosis in over half of the LCs present after 24- and 48-h exposures (Forsey et al., 1998). The expression of soluble adhesion molecules, sICAM-1, sVCAM-1, and sE-selectin have been shown to be selectively expressed when comparing irritant contact dermatitis (CD) and the induction and elicitation phases of allergic CD. Allergic contact dermatitis produces a tripling of soluble adhesion molecule output compared to no change in the irritant CD variety (Ballmer-Weber et al., 1997).

No single testing method has been successful in determining the irritancy potential of specific chemicals. Several tests exploit various contributory factors necessary to elicit irritant contact dermatitis. These tests involve either a single or repeated application of the same material to the skin. As discussed below, the single-application patch test has been in use for over 100 years in the United States and is utilized for the determination of allergic-type reactions. The use of animals in the testing of potentially irritant chemicals is based on a variety of epicutaneous (epidermal surface) methods and has continued for decades. Generally, both intact and abraded skin of albino rabbits is tested with various materials under occluded patches. The patches are removed in 24 h and the tested areas of the skin are evaluated at this time and again in 1 to 3 days.

In the Repeat Insult Patch Test, used primarily in humans for the evaluation of potential allergic sensitization, chemicals are placed on the skin under occlusion for 3 to 4 weeks. The test materials are replaced every 2 to 3 days to maintain an adequate reservoir in the patch site. The test is functionally similar to the Cumulative Irritancy Test, where daily patches are applied under occlusion for 2 weeks in parallel with control substances. The Chamber Scarification Test modifies the aforementioned tests by abrading the skin to expose the upper dermis. All of these provocative tests rely on overt clinical changes such as erythema and induration at the site of challenge with a potential irritant. Recent work suggests that patch-test chamber size may influence the ability to assess test sites visually, and using a midsize chamber of 12 mm may provide optimal results (Nicholson et al., 1999).

Transepidermal water loss, which is not visually observable, can increase as an early response to irritation and be directly measured with an evaporometer. Hence, subtle changes can be documented even if overt clinical changes cannot be induced (Lammintausta et al., 1988).

Chemical Burns

Extremely corrosive and reactive chemicals may produce immediate coagulative necrosis that results in substantial tissue damage, with ulceration and sloughing. This is distinct from irritant dermatitis, since the lesion is the direct result of the chemical insult and does not rely heavily on secondary inflammation to manifest the cutaneous signs of injury. In addition to the direct effects of the chemical, necrotic tissue can act as a chemical reservoir resulting in either continued cutaneous damage or percutaneous absorption and systemic injury after exposure. Table 19-2 lists selected corrosive chemicals that are important clinically.

Table 19-2
Selected Chemicals Causing Skin Burns

CHEMICAL	COMMENT
Ammonia	Potent skin corrosive Contact with compressed gas can cause frostbite
Calcium oxide (CaO)	Severe chemical burns Extremely exothermic reaction—dissolving in water can cause heat burns
Chlorine	Liquid and concentrated vapors cause cell death and ulceration
Ethylene oxide	Solutions and vapors may burn Compressed gas can cause frostbite
Hydrogen chloride (HCl)	Severe burning with scar formation
Hydrogen fluoride (HF)	Severe, painful, slowly healing burns in high concentration Lower concentration causes delayed cutaneous injury Systemic absorption can lead to electrolyte abnormalities and death Calcium containing topical medications and quaternary ammonium compounds are used to limit damage
Hydrogen peroxide	High concentration causes severe burns and blistering
Methyl bromide	Liquid exposure produces blistering, deep burns
Nitrogen oxides	Moist skin facilitates the formation of nitric acid causing severe yellow-colored burns
Phosphorus	White phosphorus continues to burn on skin in the presence of air
Phenol	Extremely corrosive even in low concentrations Systemic absorption through burn sites may result in cardiac arrhythmias, renal disease, and death
Sodium hydroxide	High concentration causes deep burns, readily denatures keratin
Toluene diisocyanate	Severe burns with contact Skin contact rarely may result in respiratory sensitization

SOURCE: Adapted from *Managing Hazardous Materials Incidents, Medical Management Guidelines for Acute Chemical Exposures.* Vol III. Washington, DC: U.S. Department of Health and Human Services, Agency for Toxic Substances and Disease Registry, 1991.

Allergic Contact Dermatitis

Allergic contact dermatitis represents a delayed (type IV) hypersensitivity reaction (Landsteiner and Jacobs, 1935). Since this is a true allergy, only minute quantities of material are necessary to elicit overt reactions. This is distinct from irritant contact dermatitis, where the intensity of the reaction is proportional to the dose applied. An estimated 20 percent of all contact dermatitis is allergic in nature. Currently 3700 chemicals have been described as potential allergens (de Groot, 1994).

For allergic contact dermatitis to occur, one must first be sensitized to the potential allergen. Subsequent contact elicits the classic clinical and pathologic findings. Evidence dating back to the 1940s indicates that the ability to be sensitized to specific agents has a genetic component (Chase, 1941). Recent work has linked the presence of specific HLA alleles to allergy to nickel, chromium, and cobalt (Emtestam et al., 1993; Vollmer et al., 1999; Onder et al., 1995). Thus, to mount an immune reaction to a sensitizer, one must be genetically prepared to become sensitized, have a sufficient contact with a sensitizing chemical, and then have repeated contact later.

In general, low-molecular-weight chemicals (haptens) are responsible for causing allergic contact dermatitis. Most are less than 1000 Da and are electrophilic or hydrophilic. Some of these molecules are not inherently allergenic and must undergo metabolic transformation before participating in an allergic response (Andersen and Maibach, 1989). Since the skin has substantial metabolic capabilities, including many phase I and phase II enzymes, such biotransformation may occur in the skin at the site of contact with the chemical. Haptens, which are not intrinsically allergenic, must penetrate the stratum corneum and link to epidermal carrier proteins to form a complete allergen. The linkage between haptens and epidermal proteins is usually covalent, although metallic haptens may form stable noncovalent linkages with carrier proteins (Belsito, 1989). These binding proteins are probably cell surface molecules on the Langerhans cell (LC), most likely class II antigens encoded by genes of the HLA-DR locus (Weller et al., 1995).

For sensitization to occur, the hapten/carrier protein complex is incorporated into the cytoplasm of an LC by pinocytosis for intracellular processing. Following antigen presentation there are phenotypic changes in the LC including the up-regulation of class II molecules, lymphocyte function–associated antigen (LFA) 3 (CD58), and trafficking molecules including intercellular adhesion molecule-1 (ICAM-1). The LC then migrates to a regional lymph node to present the processed antigen to T-helper cells (CD4 cells). An LC bearing HLA-DR antigen and the hapten on its surface may present this package to a T-helper cell that also must bear an antigen-specific receptor (CD3-Ti) and the cell surface molecule CD4. These virgin T cells also bear the cell surface molecule CD45RA and are referred to as TH0 cells. Concurrent with the antigen presentation, the LC produces interleukins-1 and -12 (IL-1 and IL-12), which directly stimulate the T cell to produce interleukin-2 (IL-2) and interferon gamma. IL-12 probably promotes differentiation of TH0 to the classical allergic contact dermatitis effector cell bearing TH1/CD45RO on their surface (Dilulio et al, 1996). IL-2 activates and causes proliferation of T cells specifically sensitized to that antigen.

Circulating sensitized T cells will slow and egress the vascular compartment when passing activated endothelial cells. These vascular cells will present trafficking surface molecules such as selectins and ICAMS in areas where antigen has contacted the skin, facilitating this outlet. Concurrently keratinocytes themselves play an active role in the pathogenesis of allergic contact dermatitis. They are capable not only of producing a legion of cytokines—including IL-1 , IL-2, IL-3, vascular permeability factor (VPF), and granulocyte-macrophage colony-stimulating factor (GM-CSF)—but also of expressing HLA-DR antigen under certain circumstances. The end result is the production of IL-2 and interferon gamma, which ultimately leads to an interplay of recruited lymphocytes and macrophages that creates the vascular and infiltrative changes classic for allergic contact dermatitis. This scheme admittedly simplifies a complex loop of events. Once induction of sensitization occurs, subsequent contact with the identical antigen initiates a similar cascade of events as the aforementioned sensitization process. At that point, however, specifically sensitized T cells are abundant and may present in the skin, so that the immune response occurs with great alacrity.

Contact dermatitis may occur upon exposure to any number of the thousands of allergens that people are potentially exposed to in the course of a day. Table 19-3 lists frequent allergens based on common exposure patterns, and Fig. 19-2 illustrates some potent sensitizers. Typical nonoccupational sources of exposure include the use of topical medications, personal hygiene products, rubber materials, textiles, surfactants, cosmetics, glues, pesticides, and plastics. Contact with esoteric allergens frequently occurs in the workplace. Table 19-4 lists the index of sensitivity for many common allergens in a group of 3974 individuals who were recently patch tested by the North American Contact Dermatitis Group. Such individuals are generally evaluated because they are already affected by contact dermatitis. Thus, the epidemiologic data generated, not based on blinded cross-sectional evaluations, may not be representative of the general population. Nevertheless, such data permit recognition of allergens with high sensitizing potential and strategies for their replacement by substances with low sensitizing potential.

Inspection of the chemicals listed in Tables 19-3 and 19-4 indicates that common causes of allergic contact dermatitis are ubiquitous in the materials that touch human skin regularly. There are, however, several allergens—like nickel, chromium, cobalt, and some food flavorings—that are also ingested with great frequency. In cases where an individual has a contact sensitivity to an agent that is systemically administered (orally), a generalized skin eruption with associated symptoms such as headache, malaise, and arthralgia may occur. Less dramatic eruptions may include flaring of a previous contact dermatitis to the same substance, vesicular hand eruptions, and an eczematous eruption in flexural areas. One unusual clinical presentation has been termed the "baboon syndrome," where a pink to dark-violet eruption occurs around the buttocks and genitalia. Systemic contact dermatitis may produce a delayed-type hypersensitivity reaction and/or deposition of immunoglobulins and complement components in the skin. Such deposits are potent inducers of a secondary inflammatory response and are responsible for the initial pathophysiology of many blistering and connective tissue diseases of the skin (Menne et al., 1994).

Cross-reactions between chemicals may occur if they share similar functional groups critical to the formation of complete allergens (hapten plus carrier protein). These reactions may cause difficulties in controlling contact dermatitis, since avoidance of known allergens and potentially cross-reacting substances are necessary for improvement. Table 19-5 lists common cross-reacting

Table 19-3
Common Contact Allergens

SOURCE	COMMON ALLERGENS	
Topical medications/ hygiene products	**Antibiotics**	**Therapeutics**
	Bacitracin	Benzocaine
	Neomycin	Fluorouracil
	Polymyxin	Idoxuridine
	Aminoglycosides	α-Tocopherol (vitamin E)
	Sulfonamides	Corticosteroids
	Preservatives	**Others**
	Benzalkonium chloride	Cinnamic aldehyde
	Formaldehyde	Ethylenediamine
	Formaldehyde releasers	Lanolin
	Quaternium-15	*p*-Phenylenediamine
	Imidazolidinyl urea	Propylene glycol
	Diazolidinyl urea	Benzophenones
	DMDM Hydantoin	Fragrances
	Methylchloroisothiazolone	Thioglycolates
Plants and trees	Abietic acid	Pentadecylcatechols
	Balsam of Peru	Sesquiterpene lactone
	Rosin (colophony)	Tuliposide A
Antiseptics	Chloramine	Glutaraldehyde
	Chlorhexidine	Hexachlorophene
	Chloroxylenol	Thimerosal (Merthiolate)
	Dichlorophene	Mercurials
	Dodecylaminoethyl glycine HCl	Triphenylmethane dyes
Rubber products	Diphenylguanidine	Resorcinol monobenzoate
	Hydroquinone	Benzothiazolesulfenamides
	Mercaptobenzothiazole	Dithiocarbamates
	p-Phenylenediamine	Thiurams
Leather	Formaldehyde	Potassium dichromate
	Glutaraldehyde	
Paper products	Abietic acid	Rosin (colophony)
	Formaldehyde	Triphenyl phosphate
	Nigrosine	Dyes
Glues and bonding agents	Bisphenol A	Epoxy resins
	Epichlorohydrin	*p*-(*t*-Butyl)formaldehyde resin
	Formaldehyde	Toluene sulfonamide resins
	Acrylic monomers	Urea formaldehyde resins
	Cyanoacrylates	
Metals	Chromium	Mercury
	Cobalt	Nickel

substances, and Fig. 19-3 illustrates three cross-reactors. Proper diagnosis can be hampered by concomitant sensitization to two different chemicals in the same product or simultaneous sensitization to two chemicals in different products.

Testing Methods

Predictive As with irritant dermatitis, animals have been used to determine the allergenicity of chemicals with the hope of correlating the data to humans. The Draize test is an intradermal test where induction of sensitization is accomplished by 10 intracutaneous injections of a specific test material. Subsequent challenges are performed by the same method and local reactions are graded by their clinical appearance. The Guinea Pig Maximization Test attempts to induce allergy by serial intradermal injections of an agent with the addition of Freund's complete adjuvant, an immune enhancer consisting of mycobacterial proteins. Subsequent challenge with the agent alone under an occluded chamber is graded clinically. Variations on this form of provocative testing have been done as well as performing many of them in human volunteers. It should be noted that Freund's adjuvant is not approved for use in humans; however, other techniques, such as use of higher induction con-

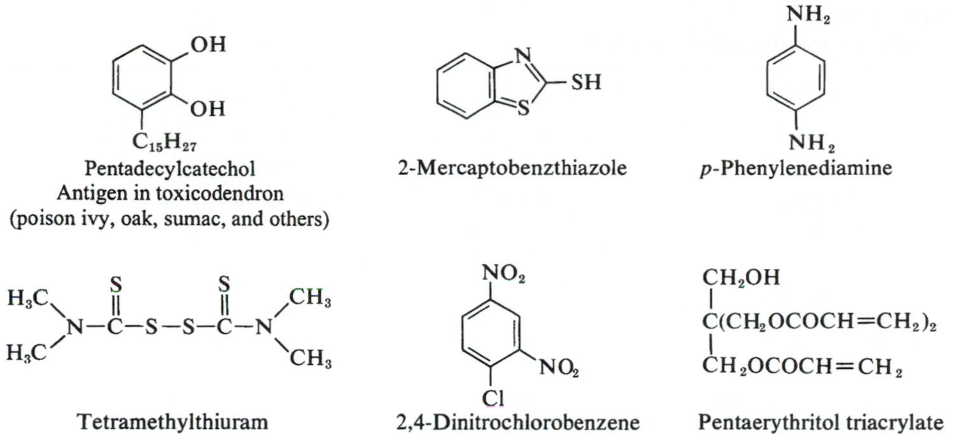

Pentadecylcatechol
Antigen in toxicodendron
(poison ivy, oak, sumac, and others)

2-Mercaptobenzthiazole

p-Phenylenediamine

Tetramethylthiuram

2,4-Dinitrochlorobenzene

Pentaerythritol triacrylate

Figure 19-2. Structural formulas of some potent contact sensitizers.

centrations, can be used to boost sensitization. For chemicals with higher allergenicity, epicutaneous skin testing can be performed, thus obviating the need for percutaneous (through the epidermis) sensitization. A variety of animal models have been described utilizing intact and abraded skin to induce sensitization and subsequent elicitation upon rechallenge. The Buehler test, Guinea Pig Maximization Test, and Epicutaneous Maximization Test utilize this form of testing and may occasionally add Freund's complete adjuvant to enhance sensitization (Guillot and Gonnet, 1985). The aforementioned tests have been used successfully to predict the allergenicity of strongly sensitizing substances in human beings. However, weaker allergens are often not discovered until they reach a large human population.

Table 19-4
Prevalence of Positive Reactions in Patch Test Patients

ALLERGEN	PATIENTS WITH POSITIVE PATCH TESTS (%)
Nickel sulfate	14.2
Neomycin	13.1
Balsam of Peru	11.8
Fragrance mix	11.7
Thimerosal	10.9
Sodium gold thiosulfate	9.5
Formaldehyde	9.3
Quaternium-15	9.0
Cobalt chloride	9.0
Bacitracin	8.7
Methyldibromoglutaronitrile/ phenoxy ethanol	7.6
Carba mix	7.3
Ethyleneurea melamine formaldehyde resin	7.2
Thiuram mix	6.9
p-Phenylenediamine	6.0
Propylene glycol	3.8
Diazolidinyl urea	3.7
Lanolin	3.3
Imidazolidinyl urea	3.2
2-Bromo-2-nitropropane	3.2

SOURCE: Marks et al. (2000).

Diagnostic Determining the cause of a contact dermatitis requires a careful evaluation of possible chemical exposures, history of the illness, and distribution of lesions. This alone will only home in on groups or classes of allergens, but it will be insufficient to identify the specific offending chemical. Such evaluation is imperative, since without strict avoidance, the dermatitis will continue. Diagnostic patch testing has been utilized in the United States for almost 100 years. Since its introduction, little has changed in the procedure and its usefulness (Sulzberger, 1940). Standardized concentrations of material dissolved or suspended in petrolatum or water are placed on stainless steel chambers adhering to acrylic tape. Most testing material is commercially available, and the concentrations have been tested in a sufficiently large population to establish a nonirritancy threshold. Chambers are left in place for 48 h, and an initial reading is performed at the time the patches are removed. A subsequent reading 24 to 96 h later is also made, since delayed reactions commonly occur. Reactions are graded as positive if erythema (redness) and induration (skin thickening) occur at the test site. Strict adherence to established protocols are necessary to draw conclusions about the clinical relevance of the reactions (Cronin, 1980). Mere redness without infiltration of the site or the presence of an irritant morphology is not considered a significant reaction. Assigning relevance to a positive reaction is difficult in some situations, but it is vital, since many positive reactions may have a meaningless correlation to the dermatitis being tested. Relevance is determined through history of chemical contactants, distribution of the eruption, and provocative use tests. Use tests or open epicutaneous tests simulate everyday exposures better than other skin tests. Here a product containing a suspect allergen is applied to the same area of the skin for several days. Erythema with induration of the area denotes a positive test and contributes to the determination of relevance. Avoidance and substitution of the offending agent will lead to improvement in the majority of cases in a few weeks.

The adequate predictive and diagnostic abilities of all of the aforementioned tests rest on the use of a human or animal with an intact immune system. In vitro models such as the macrophage migration inhibition assay and the lymphocyte transformation/blastogenesis assay have been of some value for a few strong allergens

Table 19-5
Common Cross-Reacting Chemicals

CHEMICAL	CROSS REACTOR
Abietic acid	Pine resin (colophony)
Balsam of Peru	Pine resin, cinnamates, benzoates
Bisphenol A	Diethylstilbestrol, hydroquinone monobenzyl ether
Canaga oil	Benzyl salicylate
Chlorocresol	Chloroxylenol
Diazolidinyl urea	Imidazolidinyl urea, formaldehyde
Ethylenediamine di-HCl	Aminophylline, piperazine
Formaldehyde	Arylsulfonamide resin, chloroallyl-hexaminium chloride
Hydroquinone	Resorcinol
Methyl hydroxybenzoate	Parabens, hydroquinone monobenzyl ether
p-Aminobenzoic acid	*p*-Aminosalicylic acid, sulfonamide
Phenylenediamine	Parabens, *p*-aminobenzoic acid
Propyl hydroxybenzoate	Hydroquinone monobenzyl ether
Phenol	Resorcinol, cresols, hydroquinone
Tetramethylthiuram disulfide	Tetraethylthiuram mono- and disulfide

like dinitrochlorobenzene (Kashima et al., 1993), but their use in predicting chemical allergenicity or their role as diagnostic tools is quite limited at this time.

PHOTOTOXICOLOGY

In the course of life, the skin is exposed to radiation that spans the electromagnetic spectrum, including ultraviolet, visible, and infrared radiation from the sun, artificial light sources, and heat sources. In general, the solar radiation reaching the earth that is most capable of inducing skin changes extends from 290 to 700 nm, the ultraviolet and visible spectra. Wavelengths on the extremes of this range are either significantly filtered by the earth's atmosphere or are insufficiently energetic to cause cutaneous pathology. Adequate doses of artificially produced radiation such as UV-C (<290 nm) or x-ray can produce profound physical and toxicologic skin changes. For any form of electromagnetic radiation to produce a biological change, it must first be absorbed. The absorption of light in deeper, more vital structures of the skin is dependent on a variety of optical parameters (chromophores, epidermal thickness, water content) that differ from region to region on the body. Melanin is a significant chromophore in the skin since it is capable of absorbing a broad range of radiation from UV-B (290 to 320 nm) through the visible spectrum. Other chromophores in the skin include amino acids and their breakdown products, such as tryptophan and urocanic acid, that are able to absorb light in the UV-B band. Biologically, the most significant chromophore is DNA, because the resultant damage from radiation will have lasting effects on the structure and function of the tissue.

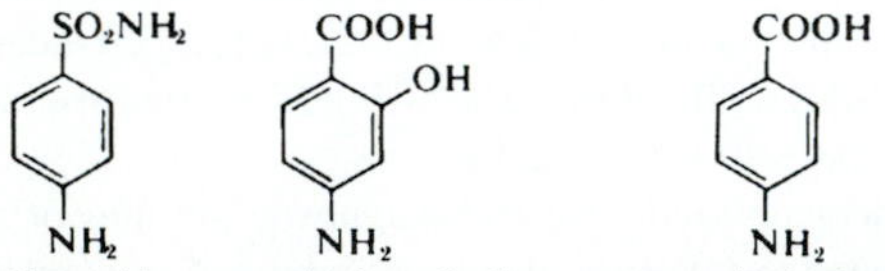

SO_2NH_2 / NH_2 — Sulfonamide; COOH / OH / NH_2 — *para*-Aminosalicylic acid; COOH / NH_2 — *para*-Aminobenzoic acid

Figure 19-3. Structural formulas of selected para-amino compounds that show cross-reactions in allergic contact sensitization.

Adverse Responses to Electromagnetic Radiation

After exposure, the skin manifests injury in a variety of ways, including both acute and chronic responses. The most evident acute feature of UV radiation exposure is erythema (redness or sunburn). The minimal erythema dose (MED), the smallest dose of UV light needed to induce an erythematous response, varies greatly from person to person. The vasodilation responsible for the color change is accompanied by significant alterations in inflammatory mediators such as prostaglandins D2, E2, and F2a, leukotriene B4, and prostacyclin I2 (Soter, 1993). Also, IL-1 activity is elevated within hours of exposure to UVB and may be responsible for several of the systemic symptoms associated with sunburn, such as fever, chills, and malaise. This cytokine may be released from local inflammatory cells as well as directly from injured keratinocytes. UV-B (290 to 320 nm) is the most effective solar band to cause erythema in human skin. Environmental conditions that affect UV-induced injury include duration of exposure, season, altitude, body site, skin pigmentation, and previous exposure. A substantially greater dosage of UV-A (320 to 400 nm) reaches the earth compared to UV-B (up to 100-fold); however, its efficiency in generating erythema in humans is about 1000-fold less than that of UV-B (Morrison, 1991). Overt pigment darkening is another typical response to UV exposure. This may be accomplished by enhanced melanin production by melanocytes or by photooxidation of melanin. Tanning or increased pigmentation usually occurs within 3 days of UV light exposure, while photooxidation is evident immediately. The tanning response is most readily produced by exposure in the UV-B band, although broader wavelengths of light are also capable of eliciting this response to a lesser degree. Immediate pigment darkening is characteristic of UV-A and visible light exposure. The tanning response serves to augment the protective effects of melanin in the skin; however, the immediate photooxidation darkening response does not confer improved photoprotection.

Commensurate with melanogenesis, UV radiation will provoke skin thickening primarily in the stratum corneum. For light-skinned individuals where melanin is not a major photoprotectant, or in situations where melanin is completely absent (i.e., albinism or vitiligo), this response lends significant defense against subsequent UV insult. Chronic exposure to radiation may induce a variety of characteristic skin changes. For UV light, these changes depend greatly on the baseline skin pigmentation of the individual as well as the duration and location of the exposure. Lighter-skinned people tend to suffer from chronic skin changes with greater frequency than darker individuals, and locations such as the head, neck, hands, and upper chest are more readily involved due to their routine exposures. Pigmentary changes—such as freckling and hypomelanotic areas, wrinkling, telangiectasias (fine superficial blood vessels), actinic keratoses (precancerous lesions), and malignant skin lesions such as basal and squamous cell carcinomas and malignant melanomas—are all consequences of chronic exposure to UV light. One significant pathophysiologic response of chronic exposure to UV light is the pronounced decrease of epidermal Langerhans cells (LCs). Chronically sun-exposed skin may have up to 50 percent fewer LCs compared to photoprotected areas. This decrease may result in lessened immune surveillance of neoantigens on malignant cells and thus allow such transformation to proceed unabated. Exposures to ionizing radiation may produce a different spectrum of disease, depending upon the dose delivered. Large acute exposures will result in local redness, blistering, swelling, ulceration, and pain. After a latent period or following subacute chronic exposures, characteristic changes such as epidermal thinning, freckling, telangiectasias, and nonhealing ulcerations may occur. Also, a variety of skin malignancies have been described years after the skin's exposure to radiation.

Aside from the toxic nature of electromagnetic radiation, natural and environmental exposures to certain bands of light are vital for survival. Ultraviolet radiation is critical for the conversion of 7-dehydrocholesterol to previtamin D3, without which normal endogenous production of vitamin D would not take place. Blue light in the 420- to 490-nm range can be lifesaving due to its capacity to photoisomerize bilirubin (a red blood cell breakdown product) in the skin. Infants with elevated serum bilirubin have difficulty clearing this by-product because of its low water solubility. Its presence in high serum concentrations can be neurotoxic. The photoisomerization by blue light renders bilirubin more water-soluble; hence, excretion in the urine is markedly augmented. In addition, the toxic effects of UV light have been exploited for decades through artificial light sources for treatment of hyperproliferative skin disorders like psoriasis.

Photosensitivity

An abnormal sensitivity to UV and visible light, photosensitivity may result from endogenous or exogenous factors. Illustrating the former, a variety of genetic diseases impair the cell's ability to repair UV light–induced damage. The autoimmune disease lupus erythematosus also features abnormal sensitivity to UV light. In hereditary or chemically induced porphyrias, enzyme abnormalities disrupt the biosynthetic pathways producing heme—the prosthetic building block for hemoglobin, myoglobin, catalases, peroxidases, and cytochromes—leading to accumulation of porphyrin precursors or derivatives throughout the body, including the skin. These compounds in general fluoresce when exposed to light of 400 to 410 nm (Soret band), and in this excited state interact with cellular macromolecules or with molecular oxygen to generate toxic free radicals (Lim and Sassa, 1993). Chlorinated aromatic hydrocarbons such as hexachlorobenzene and TCDD are known to induce this syndrome (Goldstein et al., 1977).

Phototoxicity Phototoxic reactions from exogenous chemicals may be produced by systemic or topical administration or exposure. In acute reactions, the skin may appear red and blister within minutes to hours after ultraviolet light exposure and resemble a bad sunburn. Chronic phototoxic responses may result in hyperpigmention and thickening of the affected areas. UV-A (320 to 400 nm) is most commonly responsible; however, UV-B may occasionally be involved (Johnson and Ferguson, 1990).

Agents most often associated with phototoxic reactions are listed in Table 19-6. These chemicals readily absorb UV light and assume a higher-energy excited state, as described for porphyrins. The oxygen-dependent photodynamic reaction is the most common as these excited molecules return to the ground state. Here, excited triplet-state molecules transfer their energy to oxygen, forming singlet oxygen, or become reduced and form other highly reactive free radicals. These reactive products are capable of damaging cellular components and macromolecules and causing cell death. The resulting damage elaborates a variety of immune mediators from keratinocytes and local white blood cells that recruit more inflammatory cells to the skin and thus yield the clinical signs of phototoxicity.

Table 19-6
Selected Phototoxic Chemicals

Chemical
Furocoumarins
8-Methoxypsoralen
5-Methoxypsoralen
Trimethoxypsoralen
Polycyclic aromatic hydrocarbons
Anthracene
Fluoranthene
Acridine
Phenanthrene
Tetracyclines
Demethylchlortetracycline
Sulfonamides
Chlorpromazine
Nalidixic acid
Nonsteroidal antiinflammatory drugs
Benoxaprofen
Amyl *O*-dimethylaminobenzoic acid
Dyes
Eosin
Acridine orange
Porphyrin derivatives
Hematoporphyrin

Nonphotodynamic mechanisms have been described in the pathogenesis of phototoxicity, with psoralens being prime examples. Upon entering the cell, psoralens intercalate with DNA in a non-photo-dependent interaction. Subsequent excitation with UV-A provokes a photochemical reaction that ultimately results in a covalently linked cycloadduct between the psoralen and pyrimidine bases. This substantially inhibits DNA synthesis and repair, resulting in clinical phototoxic reactions (Laskin, 1994). Psoralens may be found in sufficiently high concentrations in plants (e.g., limes and celery) that contact with their fruit and leaves in the presence of sunlight can cause a significant blistering eruption called phytophotodermatitis. Psoralen-induced phototoxicity may be harnessed and controlled pharmacologically. Topically and orally administered psoralens are used therapeutically to enhance the effects of controlled delivery of UV-A. PUVA (psoralens plus UV-A) is administered to control keratinocyte and lymphocyte hyperproliferative diseases such as psoriasis, eczema, and cutaneous T-cell lymphomas.

The photosensitive nature of porphyrins can also be tempered and utilized therapeutically. Some extraneously administered porphyrins can selectively accumulate in specific target tissues such as neoplasms. Subsequent administration of light of 600- to 700 nm wavelength (absorption spectra of currently available sensitizers) results in the formation of oxygen singlets and cell death (Regula et al., 1994).

Table 19-7
Photoallergen Series for Photo Patch Testing

p-Aminobenzoic acid
Bithionol (thiobis-dichlorophenol)
Butyl methoxydibenzoylmethane
Chlorhexidine diacetate
Chlorpromazine hydrochloride
Cinoxate
Dichlorophen
4,5-Dibromosalicylanide
Diphenhydramine hydrochloride
Eusolex 8020 (1-(4-Isopropylphenyl)-3-phenyl-1,3-propandione)
Eusolex 6300 (3-(4-Methylbenzyliden)-camphor)
Fenticlor (thiobis-chlorophenol)
Hexachlorophene
Homosalate
Menthyl anthranilate
6-Methylcoumarin
Musk ambrette
Octyl dimethyl *p*-aminobenzoic acid
Octyl methoxycinnamate
Octyl salicylate
Oxybenzone
Petrolatum control
Promethazine
Sandalwood oil
Sulfanilamide
Sulisobenzone
Tetrachlorocarbanilide
Thiourea
Tribromosalicylanilide
Trichlorocarbanilide
Triclosan

SOURCE: New York University Medical Center (January 2000).

Photoallergy In contrast to phototoxicity, photoallergy represents a true type IV delayed hypersensitivity reaction. Hence, while phototoxic reactions can occur with the first exposure to the offending chemical, photoallergy requires prior sensitization. Induction and subsequent elicitation of reactions may result from topical or systemic exposure to the agent. If topical, the reactions are termed *photocontact dermatitis,* while systemic exposures are termed *systemic photoallergy.* In most situations, systemic photoallergy is the result of the administration of medications. Photocontact dermatitis was described over 50 years ago following the use of topical antibacterial agents. Thousands of cases were reported in the 1960s after halogenated salicylanilides were used in soaps as antibacterial additives. Tetrachlorosalicylanilide and tribromosalicylamide were quickly withdrawn from the market after numerous reports of photoallergy surfaced (Cronin, 1980). Generally, the mechanisms of photocontact dermatitis and even that of systemic photoallergy are the same as that described above for allergic contact dermatitis. In this context, however, UV light is necessary to convert a potential photosensitizing chemical into a hapten that elicits an allergic response.

Testing for photoallergy is similar to patch testing for allergic contact dermatitis. Duplicate allergens are placed on the back under occlusion with stainless steel chambers. Approximately 24 h later, one set of patches is removed and irradiated with UV-A. All patches are removed and clinical assessments of patch-test sites are made 48 h and 4 to 7 days following placement. A reaction to an allergen solely on the irradiated side is termed photocontact dermatitis. Reactions occurring simultaneously on the irradiated and nonirradiated sides are consistent with an allergic contact dermatitis. There is disagreement about the presence of coexisting allergic contact and photocontact dermatitis to the same agent since a photopatch test may occasionally exhibit greater reactivity on the irradiated side compared to the nonirradiated side. Table 19-7 lists potential photoallergens used in photo patch testing at New York University Medical Center.

ACNE

"Acne is the pleomorphic disease par excellence. Its expressions are multifarious and eloquent" (Plewig and Kligman, 1993). Despite the multifactorial etiology of acne, the influence of sebum, hormones, bacteria, genetics, and environmental factors is well known. In many situations, one of these factors has an overwhelmingly greater influence in the genesis of lesions than the others. Among the literally dozens of different kinds of acne that have been described over the decades, this section concentrates on acne venenata (in Latin, *venenum* means "poison").

Chemicals able to induce lesions of acne are termed *comedogenic.* The clinical hallmark of acne is the comedone, which may be open or closed (blackhead or whitehead, respectively, in the vernacular). Additionally papules, pustules, cysts, and scars may complicate the process. Hair follicles and associated sebaceous glands become clogged with compacted keratinocytes that are bathed in sebum. The pigmentary change most evident in open comedones is from melanin (Plewig and Kligman, 1993). Most commonly, lesions are present on the face, back, and chest, but for acne venenata the location of the lesions may be characteristic, based on the route of topical or systemic exposure.

Oil acne is caused by a variety of petroleum, coal tar, and cutting-oil products. In animal models the application of comedogenic oil will result in biochemical and physiologic alteration in the hair follicle and cell structure leading to the development of comedones. In practical situations, the skin is contaminated with oil that is permitted to remain long enough for adequate penetration into the hair follicle resulting in acneiform alterations.

Chloracne

Chloracne, one of the most disfiguring forms of acne in humans, is caused by exposure to halogenated aromatic hydrocarbons. Table 19-8 lists several chloracnegens, and Fig. 19-4 illustrates some structures. Chloracne is a relatively rare disease; however, its recalcitrant nature and preventability make it an important occupational and environmental illness. Typically, comedones and straw-colored cysts are present behind the ears, around the eyes, and on the shoulders, back, and genitalia. In addition to acne, hypertrichosis (increased hair in atypical locations), hyperpigmentation, brown discoloration of the nail, conjunctivitis, and eye discharge may be present. Since chloracnegens commonly affect many organ systems, concurrent illness in the liver and nervous system may accompany the integumentary findings (U.S. Department of Health and Human Services, 1993). Histologically, chloracne is distinct from other forms of acne with progressive degeneration of sebaceous units, transition of sebaceous gland cells to keratinizing cells, and prominent hyperkeratosis in the follicular canal (Moses and Prioleau, 1985).

The effects of chloracnegens on humans have become well recognized over the past four decades through a series of industrial disasters. In 1953 a chemical plant in Ludwigshafen exploded, discharging 2,4,5 trichlorophenol; in 1976 in Seveso, Italy, a reactor explosion liberated tetrachlorodibenzo-*p*-dioxin (TCDD); in 1968 and 1979 in Japan and Taiwan, respectively, rice cooking oil was contaminated with polychlorinated biphenyls (PCBs), polychlorinated dibenzofurans (PCDFs), and polychlorinated quaterphenyls; and in 1973 in Michigan, cattle were inadvertently fed a hexabrominated biphenyl flame retardant. These incidents represent only a few of the dozens relating to human poisonings (Wolff et al., 1982). Chloracne was noted soon after exposure and has remained manifest even decades after exposure ceased (Urabe and Asahi, 1985). While reports from such events have indicated that these halogenated hydrocarbons may affect a variety of organs—such as the gastrointestinal, central nervous, reproductive, immune, and cardiovascular systems—epidemiologic studies have failed reproducibly to demonstrate organ-specific illness. Similarly, evidence pointing to human carcinogenicity of the multitude of PCB and TCDD species is also inconclusive. In contrast, chloracne has been an extremely reliable indicator of PCB and TCDD exposure in the large populations that have been studied (Caputo et al., 1988; James et al., 1993). Several incidents of accidental exposure to PCBs probably included other polyhalogenated species, since PCDFs and dioxins may be formed during the combustion of PCBs in fires and explosions.

Table 19-8
Causes of Chloracne

Polyhalogenated dibenzofurans
Polychlorodibenzofurans (PCDFs), especially tri-, tetra- (TCDFs), penta- (PCDFs), and hexachlorodibenzofuran
Polybromodibenzofurans (PBDFs), especially tetrabomodibenzofuran (TBDF)
Polychlorinated dibenzodioxins (PCDDs)
2,3,7,8-Tetrachlorodibenzo-*p*-dioxin (TCDD)
Hexachlorodibenzo-*p*-dioxin
Polychloronaphthalenes (PCNs)
Polyhalogenated biphenyls
Polychlorobiphenyls (PCBs)
Polybromobiphenyls (PBBs)
3,3′,4,4′-Tetrachloroazoxybenzene (TCAOB)
3,3′,4,4′-Tetrachloroazobenzene (TCAB)

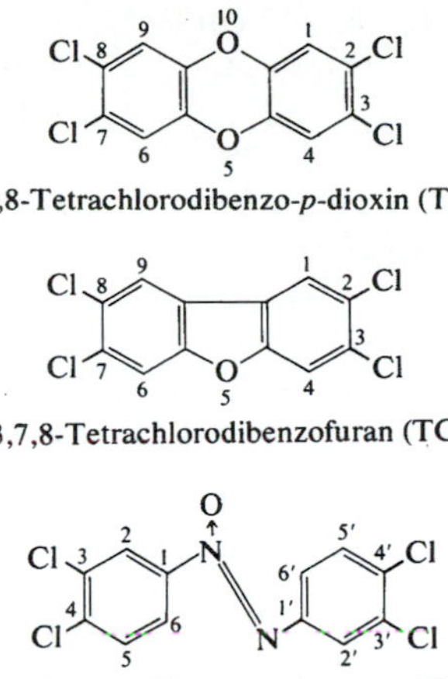

2,3,7,8-Tetrachlorodibenzo-*p*-dioxin (TCDD)

2,3,7,8-Tetrachlorodibenzofuran (TCDF)

3,3′4,4′-Tetrachloroazoxybenzene (TCAB)

Figure 19-4. Structural formulas of certain potent chloracnegens.

Chlorinated dioxins and PCBs have significant and reproducible effects on cellular function. TCDD is one of the most potent known inducers of certain cytochrome P450 isozymes (arylhydrocarbon hydroxylase) by virtue of its high affinity for the Ah receptor controlling their expression. Some studies have suggested a more frequent association of chloracne with the more highly chlorinated congeners of PCBs than with the less chlorinated ones. Most levels of chlorination, however, have been associated with this skin problem to some degree. Given the high lipid solubility of these chemicals and their recalcitrance to metabolic clearance, their half-life in humans is quite long. Highly chlorinated PCBs can have a serum half-life of 15 years and less chlorinated PCBs of 5 to 9 years (Wolff et al., 1992). Serum concentrations of PCBs in patients with chloracne are elevated, but the degree of elevation cannot be correlated directly with disease activity.

PIGMENTARY DISTURBANCES

Several factors influence the appearance of pigmentation on the skin. Melanin is produced through a series of enzymatic pathways beginning with tyrosine. Errors in this pathway from genetically deranged enzymes (i.e., albinism) or through tyrosine analogs result in abnormal pigmentation (Fig. 19-5). Other factors—such as the thickness of the epidermis and regional blood flow—impact greatly on the appearance of skin color. Hyperpigmentation results from increased melanin production or deposition of endogenous or exogenous pigment in the upper dermis. Endogenous materials are usually melanin and hemosiderin (breakdown product of hemoglobin), while exogenous hyperpigmentation can arise from

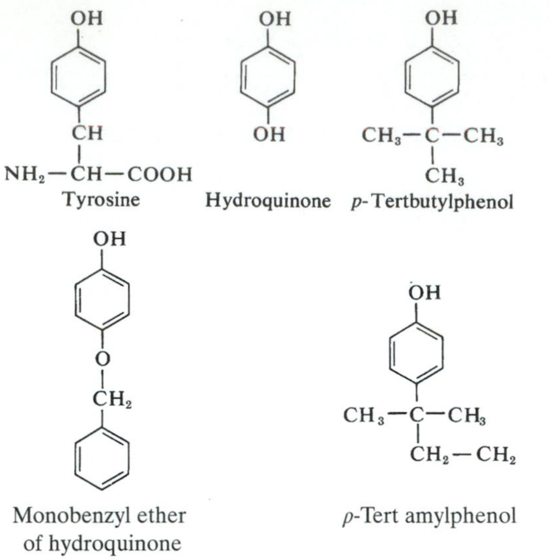

Tyrosine Hydroquinone *p*-Tertbutylphenol

Monobenzyl ether of hydroquinone *p*-Tert amylphenol

Figure 19-5. Chemical structure of tyrosine and of selected hypopigmenting and depigmenting agents.

deposition of metals and drugs in dermal tissue. Conversely, hypopigmentation is a loss of pigmentation from either melanin loss, melanocyte damage, or vascular abnormalities. Leukoderma and depigmentation denote complete loss of melanin from the skin, imparting a porcelain-white appearance. Many drugs and chemicals are capable of interfering with the normal formation and clearance of pigments as well as being directly toxic to melanocytes. The phenols and catechols are particularly potent melanocidal chemicals and can produce disfiguring depigmented regions. Table 19-9 lists common chemicals capable of causing alterations in pigmentation.

GRANULOMATOUS DISEASE

A variety of dermatologic illnesses produce the histopathologic findings of granulomatous inflammation. In general, a granuloma is an immune mechanism to "wall off" an adverse injury. It is seen in the skin in infectious diseases (i.e. leprosy, tuberculosis), foreign-body reactions, and idiopathic illnesses. Foreign-body reactions may be secondary to a primary irritant phenomenon such as traumatic introduction of talc, silica, or wood into the dermis. More rarely, sensitization may drive a granulomatous reaction, as is the case for beryllium, zirconium, cobalt, mercury, and chromium, sometimes occurring in response to tattoo dyes. The pathophysiology of these granulomatous reactions is not dissimilar to those occurring in other organ systems like berylliosis in the lung (Lever and Schaumburg-Lever, 1990).

URTICARIA

Urticaria (hives) represents an immediate type I hypersensitivity reaction primarily driven by histamine and vasoactive peptide release from mast cells. The mechanism of release may be immune-mediated through IgE allergen binding or by nonimmune mechanisms. Potential nonimmune releasers of histamine from mast cells include curare, aspirin, azo dyes, benzoates, and toxins from plants and animals. The majority of generalized or nonspecific urticarial responses occur either from systemically ingested substances to which the person has a specific allergy or from completely

Table 19-9
Selected Causes of Cutaneous Pigmentary Disturbances

- I. Hyperpigmentation
  - Ultraviolet light exposure
  - Postinflammatory changes (melanin and/or hemosiderin deposition)
  - Hypoadrenalism
  - Internal malignancy
  - Chemical exposures
    - Coal tar volatiles
    - Anthracene
    - Picric acid
    - Mercury
    - Lead
    - Bismuth
    - Furocoumarins (psoralens)
    - Hydroquinone (paradoxical)
  - Drugs
    - Chloroquine
    - Amiodarone
    - Bleomycin
    - Zidovudine (AZT)
    - Minocycline
- II. Hypopigmentation/depigmentation/leukoderma
  - Postinflammatory pigmentary loss
    - Vitiligo
    - Chemical leukoderma/hypopigmentation
      - Hydroquinone
      - Monobenzyl, monoethyl, and monomethyl ethers of hydroquinone
      - *p*-(*t*-Butyl)phenol
      - Mercaptoamines
      - Phenolic germicides
      - *p*-(*t*-Butyl)catechols
      - Butylated hydroxytoluene

idiopathic mechanisms. Localized urticaria may be elicited by certain substances in the area of epicutaneous contact and is referred to as *contact urticaria.* Some reported causes are described in Table 19-10. Often patients experiencing this phenomenon may describe itching or stinging at the contact site, with clinical manifestations ranging from minimal redness to frank edematous urticarial plaques.

A syndrome of contact urticaria, rhinitis, conjunctivitis, asthma, and rarely anaphylaxis and death has been associated with latex proteins found in rubber. This observation became apparent shortly after the emergence and recognition of the human immunodeficiency virus (HIV) and the escalating incidence of hepatitis. Universal precautions, a systematic process of personal protection, charged health care personnel to handle all blood and body fluids as if they were infected with a serious transmissible agent. As a result, the use of protective gloves made of latex and, more recently, synthetic materials became widespread. This resulted in a tremendous increase in the number of gloves being used by over 5 million health care workers (Centers for Disease Control, 1987). For workers with occupational exposures to rubber, the newly recognized syndrome proved useful in providing an etiology for their symptoms (Cohen, 1998).

Table 19-10
Selected Substances Reported to Elicit Contact Urticaria

CHEMICALS	FOODS
Anhydrides	Animal viscera
Methylhexahydrophthalic anhydride	Apple
Hexahydrophthalic anhydride	Artichoke
Antibiotics	Asparagus
Bacitracin	Beef
Streptomycin	Beer
Cephalosporins	Carrot
Penicillin	Chicken
Rifamycin	Deer
Benzoic acid	Egg
Cobalt chloride	Fish
Butylhydroxyanisol (BHA)	Lamb
Butylhydroxytoluene (BHT)	Mustard
Carboxymethylcellulose	Paprika
Cyclopentolate hydrochloride	Potato
Diphenyl guanidine	Pork
Epoxy resin	Rice
Formaldehyde	Strawberry
Fragrances	Turkey
Balsam of Peru	
Cinnamic aldehyde	
Isocyanates	
Diphenylmethane-4,4-diisocyanate	
Maleic anhydride	
Menthol	
Plants, woods, trees, and weeds	
Latex	
Phenylmercuric acetate	
Xylene	

SOURCES: Maibach (1995); Odom and Maibach (1977).

The allergens in natural latex rubber are incompletely characterized water-soluble proteins that perform a variety of cellular functions in the living tree (Table 19-11). These protein are capable of inducing type I allergic responses in sensitized individuals. Contact with rubber products like gloves can cause hives solely in the area of contact with the skin; however, more allergic individuals may experience generalized hiving, asthma, anaphylaxis, and death. This syndrome is distinct from allergic contact dermatitis to rubber components like accelerators and antioxidants, which cause delayed-type hypersensitivity/contact dermatitis. Risk factors have been elucidated in epidemiologic studies and are enumerated in Table 19-12.

Table 19-11
Natural Rubber Latex Allergens

ALLERGEN	WEIGHT	SOURCE
Hev b1	14 kDa	Rubber elongation factor
Hev b2	35 kDa	Beta-glucanase
Hev b3	23 kDa	Rubber particle protein
Hev b4	50–57 kDa	Microhelix
Hev b5	≤60 kDa	Homology with some fruit
Hev b6	21 kDa	Prohevein
Hev b7	46 kDa	Potatin
Hev b8	?	Profilin

SOURCE: Petsonk (2000).

Table 19-12
Risk Factors for Latex Allergy

Atopy (history of eczema, hay fever, asthma)
Spina bifida (highest risk factor)
Multiple surgical procedures
History of hand dermatitis
Frequent exposure to latex products
Female gender
Fruit allergy

SOURCE: Warshaw (1998).

Powders used to assist in glove donning can bind latex protein allergens and jettison them when gloves are removed. Subsequently inhaled (mucosal exposure) latex protein can trigger more severe allergic reactions than typical epicutaneous ones. Diagnosis is accomplished through determination of antilatex immunoglobulin E via serum RAST test or through clinical challenge with glove materials.

TOXIC EPIDERMAL NECROLYSIS

Toxic epidermal necrolysis (TEN) represents one of the most immediately life-threatening dermatologic diseases and is most often caused by drugs and chemicals. It is characterized by full-thickness necrosis of the epidermis accompanied by widespread detachment of this necrotic material. After the epidermis has sloughed, only dermis remains, thus severely compromising heat, fluid, and electrolyte homeostasis. Though controversy exists as to their relationship, TEN and severe erythema multiforme (Stevens-Johnson syndrome), another serious reaction to drugs and infections, are often considered part of the same spectrum of disease (Roujeau and Revuz, 1994). The etiology of TEN has remained elusive, with immunologic and metabolic mechanisms popularly entertained. A study evaluating TEN induced by carbamazepine (an anticonvulsive drug) revealed reduced lymphocyte capacity to metabolize cytotoxic carbamazepine intermediates. Lymphocyte toxicity was not demonstrated to native carbamazepine but was shown to carbamazepine metabolized by liver microsomes. Abnormalities in epoxide hydrolase and glutathione transferase may be responsible for the metabolism of the purported toxin, which may be an arene oxide. The inflammatory reaction of CD8 lymphocytes in TEN has suggested that a cytotoxic immune mediated reaction is induced by the abnormal presence of this drug intermediate (Friedmann et al., 1994). Recent work has demonstrated a role of nitric oxide metabolites as mediators of epidermal necrosis in TEN, again suggesting a metabolic pathogenesis over a strictly immunologic one (Lerner et al., 2000).

CARCINOGENESIS

Radiation

Skin cancer is the most common neoplasm in humans, accounting for nearly one-third of all cancers diagnosed each year. At present the major cause of skin cancer (half a million new cases per year in the United States) is sunlight, which damages epidermal-cell

DNA. UV-B (290 to 320 nm) induces pyrimidine dimers, thereby eliciting mutations in critical genes (reviewed in Grossman and Leffell, 1997). The *p*53 tumor suppressor gene is a major target in which damage occurs early and is detectable in nearly all resulting squamous cell carcinomas. Because the *p*53 protein arrests cell cycling until DNA damage is repaired and may induce apoptosis, its loss destabilizes the genome of initiated cells and gives them a growth advantage. UV light also has immunosuppressive effects that may help skin tumors survive. Skin cancer incidence is highest in the tropics and in pale-complexioned whites, particularly at sites on the head and neck that receive the most intense exposure. Individuals with xeroderma pigmentosum, who are deficient in repair of pyrimidine dimers, must scrupulously avoid sun exposure to prevent the occurrence of premalignant lesions that progress with continued exposure. Even when it does not cause cancer in normal individuals, sun exposure leads to premature aging of the skin. For this reason, sunbathing is discouraged and the use of sun-block lotions is encouraged, especially those that remove wavelengths up to 400 nm. In a mouse model, sun-block preparations have been shown capable of preventing *p*53 mutations and development of UV light–induced skin carcinomas (Ananthaswamy et al., 1999).

In the recent past, ionizing radiation was an important source of skin cancer. With the discovery of radioactive elements at the turn of the century came the observation that x-rays can cause severe burns and squamous cell carcinomas of the skin. By the 1920s, basal cell carcinomas were also noted. For several decades thereafter, ionizing radiation was used to treat a variety of skin ailments (acne, atopic dermatitis, psoriasis, and ringworm) and for hair removal. The levels of exposure led to an increased risk of skin cancer and sometimes produced atrophy of the dermis (radiodermatitis) from the death or premature aging of fibroblasts that secrete elastic supporting fibrous proteins.

Polycyclic Aromatic Hydrocarbons

A landmark epidemiologic investigation by Percival Pott in 1775 connected soot with the scrotal cancer prevalent among chimney sweeps in England. Since that time, substances rich in polycyclic aromatic hydrocarbons (coal tar, creosote, pitch, and soot) have become recognized as skin carcinogens in humans and animals. The polycyclic aromatic compounds alone are relatively inert chemically, but they tend to accumulate in membranes and thus perturb cell function if they are not removed. They are hydroxylated by a number of cytochrome P450 isozymes, primarily 1A1 and 1B1 in epidermal cells, and conjugated for disposal from the body. Oxidative biotransformation, however, produces electrophilic epoxides that can form DNA adducts. Phenols, produced by rearrangement of the epoxides, can be oxidized further to quinones, yielding active oxygen species, and they are also toxic electrophiles. Occupations at risk of skin cancer from exposure to these compounds (e.g., roofing) often involve considerable sun exposure, an additional risk factor. The combination of coal tar and UV light is useful in treating severe psoriasis, since the toxicity reduces the excessive turnover rate of keratinocytes that characterizies this disease. Repeated treatments are necessary, however, and they carry with them an elevated risk of skin cancer. Using longer-wave UV-A with phototoxic psoralen derivatives in place of coal tar in such protocols is much less messy and avoids UV-B but produces DNA adducts and an elevation of skin cancer risk as well.

Arsenic

An abundant element in the earth's crust, arsenic is encountered routinely in small doses in the air, water, and food. High exposures from smelting operations and from well water derived from rock strata with a high arsenic content are associated with arsenical keratoses (premalignant lesions), blackfoot disease (a circulatory disorder reflecting endothelial cell damage), and squamous cell carcinoma of the skin and several other organs (bladder, lung, liver). In earlier times, high exposures occurred from the medication Fowler's solution (potassium arsenite) and from certain pesticides. Arsenite (+3 oxidation state) avidly binds vicinal thiols and is thought to inhibit DNA repair, while arsenate (+5 oxidation state) can replace phosphate in macromolecules such as DNA, but the resulting esters are unstable. By such means, both forms give chromosomal breaks and gene amplification (Lee et al., 1988), a plausible basis for their ability to cause transformation of cultured cells and to assist tumor development. Arsenic has also been found to alter DNA methylation (Goering et al., 1999), suppress keratinocyte differentiation markers (Kachinskas et al., 1997), and enhance growth factor secretion in the epidermis (Germolec et al., 1998).

The mechanism of arsenic carcinogenicity remains an enigma, and regulation of human exposure presents challenges from difficulties in estimating carcinogenic risk (reviewed in Goering et al., 1999). Much of the data on carcinogenicity of arsenic to skin comes from populations exposed at high levels for decades in Taiwan. Similarly high exposures have been occurring recently in Bangladesh and India, where skin lesions are now in evidence. Although high exposure levels in drinking water are effective in causing cancer, considerable uncertainty exists regarding the shape of the dose–response curve, an important issue in view of the estimated 100,000 Americans whose water supplies contain arsenic near the 50 ppb standard for drinking water in the United States. This value, set in 1942 and currently under review, has been proposed to entail substantial lifetime risk of skin and other cancer. However, suggestions have been made that the carcinogenic response at lower doses may not be approximated well by linear extrapolation from the known response to high dose levels. Indeed, low doses may be less dangerous than expected and a threshold could even exist. Methylation has been considered the most likely detoxification method, since the observed mono- and dimethyl arsenate isolated in urine from exposed humans and animals are indeed much less toxic. Wide species differences in methylation capability, however, have raised the possibility other detoxification pathways exist. In the absence of a normal animal model showing carcinogenic effects, pharmacokinetic and mechanistic studies are directed to reducing the uncertainty of such speculations.

Mouse Skin Tumor Promotion

Through the work of numerous investigators over the past 50 years, mouse skin has been developed as an important target for carcinogenicity testing. The observed incidence of squamous cell carcinomas has been helpful in providing a biological basis for conclusions from epidemiologic studies. For instance, mouse skin carcinogenicity of tobacco smoke condensate and constituents (Wynder and Hoffman, 1967) strongly supported the conclusion that tobacco smoke is carcinogenic in humans (Report of the Surgeon General, 1979). Carcinogenicity in mouse skin is taken as evidence of a more general carcinogenic risk for humans. Much has been learned about the pathogenesis of squamous cell carcinomas in mouse skin that does have general applicability to human squamous cell carcinomas of the skin and other anatomic sites (Yuspa, 1998).

A complete carcinogen induces tumors by itself at high doses but not at sufficiently low doses. One explanation for the commonly observed nonlinear response is that a large dose does more than initiate carcinogenesis by damaging the DNA in cells. It is also toxic, killing some cells and thereby stimulating a regenerative response in the surviving basal cells. Tumor promoters are agents that do not cause cancer themselves but induce tumor development in skin that has been initiated by a low dose of a carcinogen. Their promoting power is generally parallel to their ability to give sustained hyperplasia of the epidermis with continued treatment. Selective stimulation of tumor growth is envisioned to occur from differential stimulation of initiated cells or due to the insensitivity of initiated cells to toxicity or to terminal differentiation induced by the promoter (DiGiovanni, 1992).

An advantage of the experimental model of mouse skin carcinogenesis is the ability to separate the neoplastic process into stages of initiation, promotion, and progression. With this model, the skin is treated once with a low dose of an initiator—a polycyclic aromatic hydrocarbon, for example. The skin does not develop tumors unless it is subsequently treated with a promoter, which must be applied numerous times at frequent intervals (e.g., twice a week for 3 months). Application of the promoter need not start immediately after initiation; but if it is not continued long enough or if it is applied before or without the initiator, tumors do not develop. A consequence of promotion then is a tendency to linearize the dose–response curve for the initiator. Although an important aspect of promotion is its epigenetic nature, papillomas are characteristically aneuploid. Mutations in the *c-Ha-ras* gene are commonly found in papillomas, particularly those initiated by polycyclic aromatic hydrocarbons. Eventually some of the resulting papillomas become autonomous, continuing to grow without the further addition of the promoter. Genetic damage accumulates in the small fraction of tumors that progress to malignancy.

A number of natural products are tumor promoters, many of which alter phosphorylation pathways. The best-studied example, and one of the most potent, is the active ingredient of croton oil, 12-*O*-tetradecanoylphorbol-13-acetate. This is a member of a diverse group of compounds that give transitory stimulation followed by chronic depletion of protein kinase C in mouse epidermis (Fournier and Murray, 1987). Another group of agents, an example of which is okadaic acid, consists of phosphatase inhibitors. Compounds acting by other routes are known, including thapsigargin (calcium channel modulator) and benzoyl peroxide (free radical generator). Sensitivity to tumor promotion is an important factor in the relative sensitivity to skin carcinogenesis among different mouse strains and even among other laboratory animal species. To cite an intriguing example, TCDD is 100-fold more potent than tetradecanoylphorbol acetate in certain hairless mouse strains but virtually inactive in nonhairless strains (Poland et al., 1982). By elucidating the genetic basis for this difference, we may improve our understanding of TCDD's activity as a promoter.

The desire to reduce the cost and improve the effectiveness of cancer testing in animals has led to development of transgenic mice with useful properties (Spalding et al., 2000). The Tg.AC strain, for example, exhibits a genetically initiated epidermis. Integrated in this mouse genome is a *v-Ha-ras* oncogene driven by part of the ζ-globin promoter, which in this context fortuitously drives expression only in epidermis that is wounded or treated with tumor promoters (Leder et al., 1990). The mice display enhanced skin sensitivity to a number of genotoxic and nongenotoxic carcinogens and have low backgrounds of spontaneous tumors over a 26-week treatment period. Tg.AC mice can be employed for testing in combination with a different strain that has one of its *p*53 alleles inactivated and thus has enhanced sensitivity to genotoxic carcinogens in other tissues in addition to the skin. These genetically modified mice promise to speed up testing using fewer animals and to reduce false-positive results arising from strain or species-specific idiosyncrasies. Trials to validate use of these modified strains are well under way (Spalding et al., 2000).

REFERENCES

American Academy of Dermatology: *Proceedings of the National Conference on Environmental Hazards to the Skin.* Schaumburg, IL: American Academy of Dermatology, 1994, pp 61–79.

Amin S, Freeman S, Maibach HI: Systemic toxicity in man secondary to percutaneous absorption, in Roberts MS, Walters KA (eds): *Dermal Absorption and Toxicity Assessment.* New York: Marcel Dekker, 1998, pp 103–125.

Ananthaswamy HN, Ullrich SE, Mascotto RE, et al: Inhibition of solar simulator-induced p53 mutations and protection against skin cancer development in mice by sunscreens. *J Invest Dermatol* 112:763-768, 1999.

Andersen KE, Maibach HI: (1989). Utilization of guinea pig sensitization data in office practice. *Immunol Allergy Clin North Am* 9:563–577, 1989.

Ballmer-Weber BK, Braathen LR, Brand CU: sE-selectin and sVCAM-1 are constitutively present in human skin lymph and increased in allergic contact dermatitis sICAM-1. *Arch Dermatol Res* 289:251–255, 1997.

Belsito DV: Mechanisms of allergic contact dermatitis. *Immunol Allergy Clin North Am* 9:579–595, 1989.

Beltrani VS: Occupational dermatoses. *Ann Allergy Asthma Immunol* 83:607–613, 1999.

Bjornberg A: Irritant dermatitis, in Maibach HI (ed): *Occupational and Industrial Dermatology,* 2d ed. Chicago: Year Book, 1987, pp 15–21.

Bloom E, Goldyne M, Maibach HI, et al: In vitro effects of irritants using human skin cell and organ culture models. *J Invest Dermatol* 88:478, 1987.

Brown HS, Bishop DR, Rowan CA: The role of skin absorption as a route of exposure for volatile organic compounds (VOCs) in drinking water. *Am J Public Health* 74:479–484, 1984.

Buchholz BA, Fultz E, Haack KW, et al: HPLC-accelerator MS measurement of atrazine metabolites in human urine after dermal exposure. *Anal Chem* 71:3519–3525, 1999.

Caputo R, Monti MD, Ermacora E, et al: Cutaneous manifestations of tetrachlorodibenzo-*p*-dioxin in children and adolescents. *J Am Acad Dermatol* 19:812–819, 1988.

Centers for Disease Control: Recommendations for prevention of HIV transmission in health-care settings. *MMWR* 36(suppl 2):1S–18S, 1987.

Chase MW: Inheritance in guinea pigs of the susceptibility to skin sensitization with simple chemical compounds. *J Exp Med* 73:711–726, 1941.

Cohen DE, Scheman A, Stewart L, et al: American Academy of Dermatology's position paper on latex allergy. *J Am Acad Dermatol* 39:98–106, 1998.

Corsini E, Galli CL: Epidermal cytokines in experimental contact dermatitis. *Toxicolgy* 142:203, 2000.

Cronin E: *Contact Dermatitis.* New York: Churchill-Livingstone, 1980.

Cross SE, Anderson C, Thompson MJ, Roberts MS: Is there tissue penetration after application of topical salicylate formulations? *Lancet* 350:636, 1997.

de Groot AC: *Patch Testing: Test Concentrations and Vehicles for 3700 Chemicals,* 2d ed. Amsterdam, New York: Elsevier, 1994.

DiGiovanni, J: Multistage carcinogenesis in mouse skin. *Pharmacol Ther* 54:63–128, 1992.

Dilulio NA, Xu H, Fairchild RL: Diversion of CD4 + T cell development from regulatory T helper to effector T helper cells alters the contact hypersensitivity response. *Eur J Immunol* 26:2606, 1996.

Elias PM: Role of lipids in barrier function of the skin, in Mukhtar H (ed): *Pharmacology of the Skin.* Boca Raton, FL: CRC Press, 1992, pp 29–38.

Emtestam L, Zetterquist H, Olerup O: HLA-DR, -DQ, and -DP alleles in nickel, chromium, and/or cobalt-sensitive individuals: Genomic analysis based on restriction fragment length polymorphisms. *J Invest Dermatol* 100:271–274, 1993.

Feldman RJ, Maibach HI: Percutaneous penetration of some pesticides and herbicides in man. *Toxicol Appl Pharmacol* 28:126–132, 1974.

Fitzpatrick, TB, Eisen AZ, Wolff K, et al: *Dermatology in General Medicine,* 4th ed. New York: McGraw-Hill, 1993.

Forsey RJ, Shahidullah H, Sands C, et al: Epidermal Langerhans cell apoptosis is induced in vivo by nonanoic acid but not by sodium lauryl sulphate. *Br J Dermatol* 139:453–461, 1998.

Fournier A, Murray AW: Application of phorbol ester to mouse skin causes a rapid and sustained loss of protein kinase C. *Nature* 330:767–769, 1987.

Friedmann PS, Strickland I, Pirmohamed M, Park BK: Investigation of the mechanisms in toxic epidermal necrolysis induced by carbamazepine. *Arch Dermatol* 130:598–604, 1994.

Germolec DR, Spalding J, Yu HS, et al: Arsenic enhancement of skin neoplasia by chronic stimulation of growth factors. *Am J Pathol* 153:1775–1785, 1998.

Goering PL, Aposhian HV, Mass MJ, et al: The enigma of arsenic carcinogenesis: Role of metabolism. *Toxicol Sci.* 49:5–14, 1999.

Gold M, Swartz JS, Braude BM, et al: Intraoperative anaphylaxis: An association with latex sensitivity. *J Allergy Clin Immunol* 87:662–666, 1991.

Goldstein JA, Friesen M, Linder RE, et al: Effects of pentachlorophenol on hepatic drug-metabolizing enzymes and porphyria related to contamination with chlorinated dibenzo-p-dioxins and dibenzofurans. *Biochem Pharmacol* 26:1549–1557, 1977.

Grossman D, Leffell DJ: The molecular basis of nonmelanoma skin cancer. New understanding. *Arch Dermatol* 133:1263–1270, 1997.

Guillot JP, Gonnet JF: The epicutaneous maximization test. *Curr Probl Dermatol* 14:220–247, 1985.

Holst R, Moller H: One hundred twin pairs patch tested with primary irritants. *Br J Dermatol* 93:145–149, 1975.

Hotchkiss SAM: Dermal metabolism, in Roberts MS, Walters KA (eds): *Dermal Absorption and Toxicity Assessment.* New York: Marcel Dekker, 1998, pp 43–101.

James RC, Busch H, Tamburro CH, et al: Polychlorinated biphenyl exposure and human disease. *J Occup Med* 35:136–148, 1993.

Johnson BE, Ferguson J: Drug and chemical photosensitivity. *Semin Dermatol* 9:39–46, 1990.

Jugert FK, Agarwal R, Kuhn A, et al: Multiple cytochrome P450 isozymes in murine skin: Induction of P450 1A, 2B, 2E, and 3A by dexamethasone. *J Invest Dermatol* 102:970–975, 1994.

Kachinskas DJ, Qin Q, Phillips MA, Rice RH: Arsenate suppression of human keratinocyte programming. *Mutat Res* 386:253–261, 1997.

Kao J, Hall J: Skin absorption and cutaneous first pass metabolism of topical steroids: In vitro studies with mouse skin in organ culture. *J Pharmacol Exp Ther* 241:482–487, 1987.

Kao J, Hall J, Helman G: In vitro percutaneous absorption in mouse skin: Influence of skin appendages. *Toxicol Appl Pharmacol* 94:93–103, 1988.

Kashima R, Okada J, Ikeda Y, Yoshizuka N: Challenge assay in vitro using lymphocyte blastogenesis for the contact hypersensitivity assay. *Food Chem Toxicol* 31:759–766, 1993.

Keeney DS, Skinner C, Travers JB, et al: Differentiating keratinocytes express a novel cytochrome P450 enzyme, CYP2B19, having arachidonate monooxygenase activity. *J Biol Chem* 273:32071–32079, 1998.

Khan WA, Das M, Stick S, et al: Induction of epidermal NAD(P)H:quinone reductase by chemical carcinogens: A possible mechanism for the detoxification. *Biochem Biophys Res Commun* 146:126–133, 1987.

Kreuger GG, Pershing LK: Human skin xenografts to athymic rodents as a system to study toxins delivered to or through skin, in Wang RGM, Knaak JB, Maibach HI (eds): *Health Risk Assessment. Dermal and Inhalation Exposure and Absorption of Toxicants.* Boca Raton, FL: CRC Press, 1993, pp 413–452.

Lammintausta K, Maibach HI, Wilson D: Susceptibility to cumulative and acute irritant dermatitis: An experimental approach in human volunteers. *Contact Dermatitis* 19:84–90, 1998.

Landsteiner K, Jacobs J: Studies on the sensitization of animals with simple chemical compounds: II. *J Exp Med* 61:625–639, 1935.

Laskin JD: Cellular and molecular mechanisms in photochemical sensitization: Studies on the mechanism of action of psoralens. *Food Chem Toxicol* 32:119–127, 1994.

Leder A, Kuo A, Cardiff RD, et al: v-Ha-ras transgene abrogates the initiation step in mouse skin tumorigenesis: Effects of phorbol esters and retinoic acid. *Proc Natl Acad Sci USA* 87:9178–9182, 1990.

Lee TC, Tanaka N, Lamb PW, et al: Induction of gene amplification by arsenic. *Science* 241:79–81, 1988.

Lerner LH, Qureshi AA, Reddy BV, Lerner EA: Nitric oxide synthase in toxic epidermal necrolysis and Stevens-Johnson syndrome. *J Invest Dermatol* 114:196–199, 2000.

Lever WF, and Schaumburg-Lever G: *Histopathology of the Skin.* New York: Lippincott, 1990, pp 243–248.

Lim HW, Sassa S: The porphyrias, in Lim HW, Soter NA (eds): *Clinical Photomedicine.* New York: Marcel Dekker, 1993, pp 241–268.

Maibach HI: Contact urticaria syndrome from mold on salami casing. *Contact Dermatitis* 32:120–121, 1995.

Marks JG Jr, Belsito DV, DeLeo VA, et al: North American Contact Dermatitis Group patch-test results, 1996–1998. *Arch Dermatol* 136:272–273, 2000.

Martin-Bouyer G, Lebreton R, Toga M, et al: Outbreak of accidental hexachlorophene poisoning in France. *Lancet* 1:91–95, 1982.

Menne T, Veien N, Sjolin KE, Maibach, HI: Systemic contact dermatitis. *Am J Contact Dermatitis* 5:1–12, 1994.

Morhenn VB, Chang EY, Rheins LA: A noninvasive method for quantifying and distinguishing inflammatory skin reactions. *J Am Acad Dermatol* 41:687–692, 1999.

Morrison WL: *Phototherapy and Photochemotherapy of Skin Disease,* 2d ed. New York: Raven Press, 1991.

Moses M, Prioleau PG: Cutaneous histologic findings in chemical workers with and without chloracne with past exposure to 2,3,7,8-tetrachlorodibenzo-*p*-dioxin. *J Am Acad Dermatol* 12:497–506, 1985.

Mukhtar H, Bickers DR: Comparative activity of the mixed function oxidases, epoxide hydratase, and glutathione-*S*-transferase in liver and skin of the neonatal rat. *Drug Metab Dispos* 9:311–314, 1981.

Muller-Decker K, Heinzelmann T, Furstenberger G, et al: Arachidonic acid metabolism in primary irritant dermatitis produced by patch testing of human skin with surfactants. *Toxicol Appl Pharmacol* 153:59–67, 1998.

Nicholson M, Willis CM: The influence of patch test size and design on the distribution of erythema induced by sodium lauryl sulfate. *Contact Dermatitis* 41:264–267, 1999.

Odom RB, Maibach HI: Contact urticaria: A different contact dermatitis in dermatotoxicology and pharmacology, in Marzulli FN, Maibach HI, (eds): *Advances in Modern Toxicology.* Vol. 4. Washington, DC: Hemisphere, 1977.

Onder M, Aksakal B, Gulekon A, et al: HLA DR, DQA, DQB and DP antigens in patients allergic to nickel. *Contact Dermatitis* 33:434–435, 1995.

Patrick E, Burkhalter A, Maibach HI: Recent investigations of mechanisms of chemically induced skin irritation in laboratory mice. *J Invest Dermatol* 88:124S–131S, 1987.

Petsonk EL: Couriers of asthma: Antigenic proteins in natural rubber latex. *Occup Med* 15:421–430, 2000.

Plewig G, Kligman AM: *Acne and Rosacea.* New York: Springer-Verlag, 1993, pp 3–121.

Poland A, Palen D, Glover E: Tumor promotion by TCDD in skin of HRS/J hairless mice. *Nature* 300:271–273, 1982.

Potts RO, Guy RH: Predicting skin permeability. *Pharmacol Res* 9:663–669.

Raza H, Agarwal R, Mukhtar H: Cutaneous glutathione *S*-transferases, in Mukhtar H (ed): *Pharmacology of the Skin.* Boca Raton, FL: CRC Press, 1992.

Regula J, Ravi B, Bedwell J, et al: Photodynamic therapy using 5-aminoaevulinic acid for experimental pancreatic cancer—Prolonged animal survival. *Br J Cancer* 70:248–254, 1994.

Report of the Surgeon General: *Smoking and Health.* Washington, DC: U.S. DHEW, 1979.

Riviere JE: The isolated perfused porcine skin flap, in Wang RGM, Knaak JB, Maibach HI (eds): *Health Risk Assessment: Dermal and Inhalation Exposure and Absorption of Toxicants.* Boca Raton, FL: CRC Press, 1993, pp 439–452.

Roujeau JC, Revuz J: Toxic epidermal necrolysis: An expanding field of knowledge. *J Am Acad Dermatol* 31:301–302, 1994.

Scheuplein RJ, Blank IH: Permeability of the skin. *Physiol Rev* 51: 702–747, 1971.

Soter NA: Acute effects of ultraviolet radiation on the skin, in Lim HW, Soter NA (eds): *Clinical Photomedicine.* New York: Marcel Dekker, 1993, pp 73–94.

Spalding JW, French JE, Stasiewicz S, et al: Responses of transgenic mouse lines $p53^{+/-}$ and Tg.AC to agents tested in conventional carcinogenicity bioassays. *Toxicol Sci* 53:213–223, 2000.

Storm JE, Collier SW, Stewart RF, Bronaugh RL: Metabolism of xenobiotics during percutaneous penetration: Role of absorption rate and cutaneous enzyme activity. *Fundam Appl Toxicol* 15:132–141, 1990.

Sulzberger MB: *Dermatologic Allergy.* Springfield, IL: Charles C Thomas, 1940, pp 87–128.

Sutter TR, Tang YM, Hayes CL, et al: Complete cDNA sequence of a human dioxin-inducible mRNA identifies a new gene subfamily of cytochrome P450 that maps to chromosome 2. *J Biol Chem* 269:13092–13099, 1994.

U.S. Department of Health and Human Services: Skin lesions and environmental exposures, in *Case Studies in Environmental Medicine,* Vol 28. Atlanta: Agency for Toxic Substances and Disease Registry, May 1993.

Urabe H, Asahi M: Past and current dermatological status of Yusho patients. *Environ Health Perspect* 59:11–15, 1985.

Vollmer J, Weltzien HU, Dormoy A, et al: Functional expression and analysis of a human HLA-DQ restricted, nickel-reaction T cell receptor in mouse hybridoma cells. *J Invest Dermatol* 113:175–181, 1999.

Walsh AA, deGraffenried LA, Rice RH: 2,3,7,8-Tetrachlorodibenzo-*p*-dioxin sensitization of cultured human epidermal cells to carcinogenic heterocyclic amine toxicity. *Carcinogenesis* 16:2187–2191, 1995.

Warshaw EM: Latex allergy. *J Am Acad Dermatol* 39:1–24, 1998.

Weller FR, De Jong MC, Weller MS, et al: HLA-DR expression in induced on keratinocytes in delayed hypersensitivity but not in allergen induced late-phase reactions. *Clin Exp Allergy* 25:252–259, 1995.

Wolff MS, Anderson HA, Selikoff IJ: Human tissue burdens of halogenated aromatic chemical in Michigan. *JAMA* 247:2112–2116, 1982.

Wolff MS, Fischbein A, Selikoff IJ: Changes in PCB serum concentrations among capacitor manufacturing workers. *Environ Res* 59:202–216, 1992.

Wynder EL, Hoffman D: *Tobacco and Tobacco Smoke: Studies in Experimental Carcinogenesis.* New York: Academic Press, 1967, pp 138–143.

Yuspa SH: The pathogenesis of squamous cell cancer: Lessons learned from studies of skin carcinogenesis. *J Dermatol Sci* 17:1–7, 1998.

CHAPTER 20

TOXIC RESPONSES OF THE REPRODUCTIVE SYSTEM

Michael J. Thomas and John A. Thomas

INTRODUCTION

History

The endocrine function of the gonads is primarily concerned with perpetuation of the species. The survival of any species depends on the integrity of its reproductive system. Sexual reproduction involves a very complex process for the gonads. Genes located in the chromosomes of the germ cells transmit genetic information and modulate cell differentiation and organogenesis. Germ cells ensure the maintenance of structure and function in the organism in its own lifetime and from generation to generation.

The twentieth century has undergone an industrial renaissance; through scientific and technical advances, there has been a significant extension in life expectancy and generally an enhanced quality of life. Concomitantly with this industrial renaissance, an estimated 50,000 to 60,000 chemicals have come into common use. Approximately 600 or more new chemicals enter commerce each year. The production of synthetic organic chemicals has risen from less than 1 billion lb in 1920 to over 20 billion lb in 1945, to 75 billion lb in 1960, and to over 200 billion lb in the late 1980s (cf. Lave and Ennever, 1990). Several endocrine disorders are associated with industrial chemicals (cf. Barsano and Thomas, 1992). Overall, occupational diseases in the United States may be responsible for about 60,000 deaths per year (Baker and Landrigan, 1991). The impact of new chemicals (or drugs) on the reproductive system was tragically accentuated by the thalidomide disaster in the 1960s (cf. Fabrio, 1985). This episode led to increased awareness on a worldwide basis and brought forth laws and guidelines pertaining to reproductive system safety and testing protocols. This new awareness of reproductive hazards in the workplace has led to corporate policies and legal considerations (Bond, 1986; McElveen, 1986). In 1985, the American Medical Association (AMA) Council on Scientific Affairs of charged its Advisory Panel on Reproductive Hazards in the Work Place to consider over 100 chemicals with the intent of estimating their imminent hazards (AMA Council on Scientific Affairs, 1985).

Endocrine Disruptors

Large numbers and large quantities of endocrine-disrupting chemicals (e.g., *o,p*-DDT) have been released into the environment since World War II (cf. Colborn, et al., 1993). Exposure to endocrine-disrupting chemicals has been linked with abnormal thyroid function in birds and fish; diminished fertility in birds, fish, shellfish, and mammals; and demasculatinization and feminization in fish, gastropods, and birds (Vos et al., 2000). The significance of endocrine-disrupting chemicals, also known as environmental estrogens or xenoestrogens, is unknown at this time. In general, the mechanism(s) of endocrine disruption caused by non-heavy metal agents is due to competition for receptors or inhibition of steroidogenesis.

Concern for reproductive hazards is not new; it dates back to the Roman Empire. Lead, found in high concentration in pottery and water vessels, probably played a role in the increased incidence of stillbirths. Lead is now known to be an abortifacient as well as capable of producing teratospermias. In the United States, male factory workers occupationally exposed to 1,2-dibromo-3-chloropropane (DBCP) became sterile, as evidenced by oligospermia, azoospermia, and germinal cell aplasia. Factory workers in battery plants in Bulgaria, lead mine workers in the U.S. state of Missouri, and workers in Sweden who handle organic solvents (toluene, benzene, and xylene) suffer from low sperm counts, abnormal sperm, and varying degrees of infertility. Diethylstilbestrol (DES), lead, chlordecone, methyl mercury, and many cancer chemotherapeutic agents have been shown to be toxic to the male and female reproductive systems and possibly capable of inflicting genetic damage to germ cells (cf. Barlow and Sullivan, 1982; Office of Technology Assessment Report, 1985).

In the past few years, there has been an ongoing debate about a decline in human sperm counts (Carlsen et al., 1992). Carlsen and coworkers (1992) reported that there has been a decline in semen quality over the past 50 years. Additionally, they reported an increased incidence in genitourinary abnormalities, including testicular cancer, cryptorchidism, and hypospadias. The outcome of these studies has been challenged by several groups of investigators (Bromwich et al., 1994; Lipshultz, 1996; Thomas, 1998). The original evidence using meta-analysis failed to support the hypothesis that sperm counts declined significantly between 1940 and 1990 (Bromwich et al., 1994). Sharpe and Skakkeback (1993) have hypothesized that the increasing incidence of reproductive abnormalities in the human male may be related to increased estrogen exposure in utero. Their hypothesis includes an increased exposure to DES and the possible presence of environmental estrogen mimics (e.g., DDT). A number of natural and anthropogenic substances exhibit weak estrogen properties (Muller et al., 1995; Cooper and Kavlock, 1997). There are many naturally occurring phytoestrogens (e.g., coumestans and isoflavonoids) that possess weak estrogen-binding properties (Thomas, 1997). Many botanically derived substances possess estrogen-like activity, including soy proteins. Not only are there compounds in the environment that possess estrogenic properties, but there are also environmental antiandrogens (e.g., vinclozolin) (Kelce and Wilson, 1997).

The etiology of many adverse reproductive outcomes among humans is poorly understood. Generally, studies of epidemiologic and reproductive outcomes have focused upon maternal factors (Olshan and Faustman, 1993). Relatively speaking, only recently have studies begun to examine the role of chemical perturbation of paternal exposures. Male-mediated developmental toxicity has received some recent attention. It has become increasingly clear that reproductive toxicity involves both the male and female (Mattison et al., 1990). Also noteworthy is the fact that nonreproductive endocrine organs can be adversely affected by drugs and chemicals (Thomas, 1994).

Reproductive Hazards

The potential hazard of chemicals to reproduction and the risks to humans from chemical exposure are difficult to assess because of the complexity of the reproductive process, the unreliability of laboratory tests, and the quality of human data. In the human, it is estimated that one in five couples are involuntarily sterile; over one-third of early embryos die, and about 15 percent of recognized pregnancies abort spontaneously. Among the surviving fetuses at birth, approximately 3 percent have developmental defects (not always anatomic); with increasing age, over twice that many become detectable. It should be obvious that even under normal physiologic conditions, the reproductive system does not function in a very optimal state. Not surprisingly, the imposition of chemicals (or drugs) on this system can further interfere with a number of biological processes or events.

GENERAL REPRODUCTIVE BIOLOGY

The developing gonad is very sensitive to chemical insult, with some cellular populations being more vulnerable than others to an agent's toxic actions. Further, the developing embryo is uniquely sensitive to changes in its environment, whether such changes are caused by exposure to foreign chemicals or certain viruses. The toxicologist must be mindful of the teratogenic potential of a chemical as well as be aware of its potential deleterious actions on maternal biochemical processes. The development of normal reproductive capacity may offer particularly susceptible targets for toxins. Environmental factors might alter the genetic determinants of gonadal sex, the hormonal determinants of phenotypic sex, fetal gametogenesis, and reproductive tract differentiation as well as postnatal integration of endocrine functions and other processes essential for the propagation of the species. The effects of environmental agents on sexual differentiation and development of reproductive capacity are largely unknown. Of the chemicals that have been studied, it is noteworthy that they possess a wide diversity in molecular structure and that they may affect specific cell populations within the reproductive system.

Sexual Differentiation

An understanding of reproductive physiology requires consideration of the process of sexual differentiation or the pattern of development of the gonads, genital ducts, and external genitalia (cf. Simpson, 1980; De La Chapelle, 1987; Goldberg, 1988).

The transformation of androgens into estrogens through the aromatization occurs in the hypothalamus during fetal life; this is one of the key events leading to sexual differentiation. During the last decade, the increased evidence of disorders of male sexual differentiation (e.g., hypospadias, cryptorchidism, micropenis) has raised the possibility that certain environmental chemicals might be detrimental to normal male genital development in utero. Male sexual differentiation is critically dependent on the physiologic action of androgens. Thus, an imbalance of the androgen/estrogen ratio can affect sexual differentiation. Environmental xenoestrogens that mimic estrogens (e.g., certain herbicides, pesticides, plasticizers, nonylphenols, etc.) or environmental antiandrogens [e.g., *p,p'*-DDE (the major metabolite of DDT) vinclozolin, linuron, etc.] that perturb endocrine balance might cause demasculinizing and feminizing effects in the male fetus. Disturbed male sexual differentiation has, in some instances, been purported to be caused by increased exposure to environmental xenoestrogens and/or antiandrogens.

Gonadal Sex A testes-determining gene [sex-determining region of the Y chromosome (SRY)] on the Y chromosome is responsible for determining gonadal sex (cf. De La Chapelle, 1987, Swain and Lovell-Badge, 1999). It converts undifferentiated gonads into a testes. The organization of the gonadal anlage into the seminiferous or spermatogenic tubules of the male may be mediated by the SRY gene. The testes produces two separate hormones: the müllerian inhibiting factor (MIF) and testosterone. Testosterone-induced masculine differentiation is modulated by androgen receptors regulated by genes on the X chromosome. Alterations of the sex chromosomes may be transmitted by either one of the parents (gonadal dysgenesis) or may occur in the embryo itself. Failure of the sex chromosomes of either of the parents to separate during gametogenesis is called nondisjunction and can result in gonadal agenesis. Klinefelter's syndrome is characterized by testicular dysgenesis with male morphology and an XXY karyotype; Turner's syndrome includes ovarian agenesis with female morphology (XO karyotype).

Hermaphroditism (true and pseudo) may occur secondary to nondisjunction of sex chromosomes during the initial cleavage mitosis of the egg. Such a condition is usually due to an XY karyotype and sometimes to sex mosaics of XY/XX or XY/XO. Pseudohermaphrodites are characterized by secondary sex characteristics that differ from those predicted by genotype.

Chemically induced nondisjunction is a common genetic abnormality. Nondisjunction of Y chromosomes may be detected by the presence or absence of fluorescent bodies on the chromatin of sperm (YFF spermatozoa). YFF sperm are increased in patients treated with certain antineoplastic agents and irradiation.

Genotypic Sex The normal female chromosome complement is 44 autosomes and 2 sex chromosomes, XX. The two X chromosomes contained in the germ cells are necessary for the development of a normal ovary. Autosomes are also involved in ovarian development, differentiation of the genital ducts, and external genitalia characteristic of a normal female. This requires the involvement of a single X chromosome with genetic cellular events. Generally, the second X chromosome of a normal XX female is genetically inactive in nongonadal cells, although it has been shown that the tip of the short arm of the chromosome is genetically active.

The Y chromosome is consistent with the male determinant. The normal male has a chromosome complement of 44 autosomes and 2 sex chromosomes, X and Y. An additional X chromosome does not change the male phenotype conferred by the Y chromosome, but the gonads are often dysfunctional (Klinefelter's syndrome, XXY genotype). Genetic coding on the X chromosome may be involved in transforming the gonad into a testis.

The presence of chromatin material on the short (p) arm of the (Y_p) chromosome directs the development of the testes. Chromatin material (Y_q) on the long (q) arm directs the development of spermatogenesis.

Phenotypic (Genital) Sex During the early stages of fetal development, sexual differentiation does not require any known hormonal products. The differentiation of the genital ducts and the external genitalia, however, requires hormones. The onset of testosterone synthesis by the male gonad is necessary for the initiation of male differentiation. Although the testes are required in male differentiation, the embryonic ovaries are not needed to attain the female phenotype. Female characteristics develop in the absence of androgen secretion.

Two principal types of hormones are secreted by the fetal testes—an androgenic steroid responsible for male reproductive tract development and a nonsteroid factor that causes regression of the mullerian ducts. Sertoli cells are the likely source of MIF or antimüllerian hormone (AMH). Leydig cell differentiation and regression correspond well with the onset and subsequent decline in testosterone synthesis by the fetal testis. Thus, the embryonic testis suppresses the development of the mullerian ducts, allows the development of the wolffian duct and its derivatives, and thereby imposes the male phenotype on the embryo.

Three periods for testosterone production are important to sexual differentiation. The first period occurs on days 14 to 17 of gestation in the rat and weeks 4 to 6 in the human. The second period occurs about day 17 of gestation to about 2 weeks postnatal age in the rat and from month 4 of pregnancy to 1 to 3 months of postnatal age in the human. The third period follows a long period of testicular inactivity in both species until testosterone production is reinitiated between 40 and 60 days of age in the rat and between 12 to 14 years of age in the human.

The dynamics of testosterone and dihydrotestosterone production and cellular interactions are an important prerequisite to knowing which chemicals might affect sexual differentiation. Factors that reduce the ability of testosterone to be synthesized and activated, to enter the cell, and/or to affect the cell nucleus's ability to regulate the synthesis of androgen-dependent proteins would have a potential to alter sexual differentiation. Some chemicals are capable of exerting a testosterone-depriving effect on the developing systems. These include effects on the feedback regulation of gonadotropin secretion, gonadotropin effectiveness, testosterone and dihydrotestosterone synthesis, and plasma binding as well as cytoplasmic receptor and nuclear chromatin binding.

Insufficient amounts of androgens can feminize the male fetus with otherwise normal testes and an XY karyotype. Slight deficiencies affect only the later stages of differentiation of the external genital organs and result in microphallus, hypospadias (the urethra opens on undersurface of penis), and a valviform appearance of the scrotum with masculine general morphology. However, a severe androgen deficiency (or resistance) allows the mullerian system to persist and results in external genital organs of a female type (vagina and uterus) that coexist with ectopic testes and normal male efferent ducts. A lack of androgen receptors can also lead to a testicular feminization type of syndrome even when normal levels of testosterone are present. Finally, sexual behavior also appears to be "imprinted" in the central nervous system by androgens from the testis and could be affected by endogenous and exogenous chemicals.

Estrogens exert an important developmental effect. Nearly 30 years have elapsed since the association between maternal DES administration and vaginal adenocarcinoma in female offspring was reported. DES, a synthetic estrogen, was used extensively in the treatment of both humans and livestock. Other nonsteroidal estrogens, namely, the insecticides chlordecone and DDT (and its metabolites) exhibit uterotropic actions in experimental animals (cf. Thomas, 1975). The estrogenicity of chlordecone was first described in workers at a pesticide-producing plant (Cohn et al., 1978). Several so-called xenoestrogens—including herbicides, fungicides, insecticides, and nematocides—have been identified (cf. Colborn, et al., 1993). Similarly, polychlorinated biphenyls (PCBs) are uterotropic. Zearalenone, a plant mycotoxin, also exhibits female sex hormone properties. The effects of environmental hormone-disrupters (namely xenoestrogens) are not restricted to females. Indeed, vinclozolin, a dicarboximide fungicide, has metabolites that can act as androgen antagonists (Kelce et al., 1994).

GONADAL FUNCTION

Central Modulation

Regardless of gender, the gonads possess a dual function: an endocrine function involving the secretion of sex hormones and a nonendocrine function or the production of germ cells (gametogenesis). The testes secrete male sex steroids, including testosterone and dihydrotestosterone. The testes also secrete small amounts of estrogens. The ovaries, depending on the phase of the menstrual cycle, secrete various amounts of estrogens and progesterone. Estradiol is the principal steroid estrogen secreted by the ovary in most mammalian species. The ovary is also the chief source of progesterone. The corpus luteum and the placenta are also primary sites of secretion of progesterone.

Gametogenic and secretory functions of either the ovary or testes are dependent on the secretion of adenohypophyseal gonadotropins, follicle stimulating hormone (FSH), and luteinizing hormone (LH). In the male, LH is also referred to as ICSH (interstitial cell–stimulating hormone). FSH in the female stimulates follicular development and maturation in the ovary. FSH in the male stimulates the process of spermatogenesis. Sertoli cells are the target cells for the action of FSH in the testes of mammals. FSH receptors are present on the Sertoli cells, and the gene for the FSH receptor is predominantly expressed in these cells (cf. Heckert and Griswold, 1993). The secretion of pituitary FSH and LH is modulated by gonadal hormones. Sex steroids secreted by the testes or ovaries regulate the secretion of pituitary gonadotropins. The Sertoli cell of the testes secretes small amounts of estrogen and a proteinaceous hormone called inhibin. Inhibin aids in the modulation of spermatogenesis. ICSH (LH) provokes the process of steroidogenesis in the testes (cf. Herbert et al., 1995).

The onset of puberty results in the cyclic secretion of pituitary gonadotropins in the female. This establishes the normal menstrual cycle. In males, puberty is advanced by the continuous and noncyclic secretion of gonadotropins.

Testicular Function

There are several subpopulations of cells in the mammalian testes, all of which are subject to some degree of local regulation (cf. Maddocks, et al., 1990; Spiteri-Grech and Nieschlag, 1993). These local regulatory factors include peptide growth factors, proopiomelanocortin derivatives, neuropeptides, and steroids (Table 20-1). There are many complex cell-to-cell communications, any one of which could serve as a site for chemical or heavy metal perturbation. Many agents that can affect either spermatogenesis or steroidogenesis can also affect leukocytes and other testes-regulating factors produced by cells of the immune system (cf. Murdoch, 1994). The paracrine or local regulation of testicular function is an interesting concept, yet the nature of the testicular architecture and the multiple interactions that can occur at various cellular levels renders this biological system not only complex, but very difficult to study from both a physiologic or a toxicologic standpoint. Nevertheless, these local testicular factors are very important in modulating the paracrine control of the male gonad (Table 20-2). Paracrine and autocrine factors from Sertoli and germ cells are important in the functioning of both cell types (Griswold, 1995).

Apoptosis Apoptosis and necrosis constitute two distinct forms of cell death that differ in morphology, mechanism, and incidence (Fig. 20-1) (see also Chap. 10, "Developmental Toxicology"). Necrosis includes membrane disruption, respiratory hypovia, membrane collapse, cell swelling, and rupture in pathologic tissue. Apoptosis, on the other hand, describes the scattered, apparently random cell deaths in normal cells (cf. Nakano, 1997). The ca-

Table 20-1
Growth Factors Isolated from the Testis

GROWTH FACTOR	TESTICULAR ORIGIN	PROPOSED MITOGENIC TARGET IN THE TESTIS
IGF-I	Sertoli cells	NI
IGF-II	Germ cells	NI
TGF-β	Sertoli cells Peritubular cells	NI
Inhibin	Sertoli cells	NI
SGF	Sertoli cells	Sertoli cells?
*b*FGF	NI	NI
TGF-α	Sertoli cells Peritubular cells	NI
SCSGF (=TGF-α?) EGF	Sertoli cells	Germ cells?
RTFGF	Rete testis fluid	NI
tIL-I	Sertoli cells	Germ cells
NGF-β	Germ cells	NI

KEY: IGF I and II, insulin-like growth factors I and II; TGF, transforming growth factor; SCSGF, Sertoli cell secreted growth factor; EGF, epidermal growth factor; RTFGF, rete testis fluid–derived growth factor; tIL-1, testicular interleukin-1–like factor; NGF, nerve growth factor. NI, no information available.

SOURCES: Derived from Maddocks et al., 1990; Spiteri-Grech and Nieschlag, 1993; and Shioda et al., 1994.

pacity for cell "suicide" appears to be present in most, if not all tissues to maintain a homeostatic state.

During the fertile phase of the life span of mammals, the function of the gonads is hormonally controlled. In addition to the proliferation of somatic and germ cells in the ovary and in the testes during normal gonadal development, degeneration of gonadal cells plays an important physiologic role and leads to a depletion of a majority of germ cells in both sexes (cf. Billig, et al., 1996; Robertson and Orrenius, 2000). In the testes, morphologic signs of germ cell degeneration during spermatogenesis were recognized nearly 100 years ago (Regaud, 1900).

The biochemical pathway(s) that cause apoptosis are not known, but DNA lysis is involved (Thompson, 1994). Several specific genes/gene products have been associated with the apoptosis that follows androgen depletion. For example, one prominent marker is TRPM-2 (a sulfated glycoprotein-2, or "clusterin"), which increases shortly after androgen removal. Likewise, transforming growth factor beta (TGF-β) increases after androgen removal. In the female, the role of TGF-β in uterine apoptosis is unclear.

There is increasing evidence suggesting that apoptosis rather than necrosis predominates in many cytolethal toxic injuries (Raffray and Cohen, 1997). Tissue selectivity of toxicants can stem from the apoptotic or necrotic thresholds at which different cells die.

Physiologically, apoptosis serves to limit the number of germ cells in the seminiferous epithelium (cf. Billig et al., 1995). During the process of spermatogenesis, clonal proliferation of germ cells occurs during the many mitotic divisions, leading to a significantly expanding germ cell population. Left unchecked, the number of germ cells would quickly outgrow the supportive capacity of the Sertoli cell. Hence, a delicate balance exists in the testes between proliferation and apoptosis. About three-fourths of the potential population of mature germ cells in the testes may be lost by active elimination (DeRooÿ and Lok, 1987).

The Sertoli cell of the testes has been suggested to be a controlling factor in germ cell apoptosis (cf. Roberts, et al., 1997). Further, germ cell viability depends on Sertoli cell factors as well as the intimate contact between these two testicular cell types. Sertoli cells appear to regulate germ cell apoptosis directly through a paracrine mechanism. The Sertoli cell may mediate the death of *fas*-bearing germ cells via the expression of *fasL* on its cell membrane.

A number of chemicals reportedly increase the incidence of apoptosis in the rodent testes (Ku et al., 1995; Billig et al., 1995; Richburg and Boekelheide, 1996; Nakagawa et al., 1997). In rats, the Sertoli cell toxicant mono-2-ethylhexyl phthalate (MEHP) causes an early and progressive detachment of germ cells from the seminiferous epithelium (Richburg and Boekelheide, 1996). This MEHP-induced distruption of the Sertoli cell–germ cell physical interaction has been suggested to alter normal Sertoli cell–directed regulation of germ cell apoptosis. Mitomycin C, an antibiotic that inhibits DNA synthesis, induces apoptosis with fragmentation of nuclear DNA in mouse spermatogenic cells, especially spermatogonia (Nakagawa et al., 1997). Why spermatogenic germ cells have a relatively high level of apoptosis is unknown, but it could be a mechanism for eliminating cells with abnormal chromosomes.

Spermatogenesis *Spermatogenesis* is a unique process in which the timing and stages of differentiation are known with a considerable degree of certainty. The dynamics of the process of spermatogenesis as well as the kinetics have been studied extensively and have recently been reviewed by Foote and Berndtson (1992). In producing spermatozoa by the process of spermatogenesis, the germinal epithelium plays a dual role: It must produce millions of spermatozoa each day and also continuously replace the popula-

Table 20-2
Local Factors Modulating the Function of Testicular Cells

MODULATING FACTORS	CELL OF ORIGIN	ACTION*	SECRETORY FACTORS	CELL OF ORIGIN	ACTION*
Germ Cell (GC)					
IGF-1	(SC)†	—	NGF	(SC)	—
IL-1	(SC)	—			
Inhibin	(SC)	Inhibits			
SCF	(SC)	—			
Activin	(LC)	Stimulates			
Leydig Cell (LC)‡					
IGF-1	(SC)	Stimulates	β-Endorphin	(SC)	Inhibits
IL-1	(SC)	Stimulates/inhibits?	ACTH	(SC)	Stimulates
Inhibin	(SC)	Stimulates	CRF	(SC)	—
SCF	(SC)	Stimulates	Testosterone	(SC)	Stimulates
TGF-α	(SC)	Inhibits	Activin	(SC)	?
IGF-1	(PT)	Stimulates	Testosterone	(PT)	Stimulates
TGF-α	(PT)	Inhibits	Oxytocin	(PT)	Stimulates
TGF-β	(PT)	Inhibits	Activin	(PT)	Stimulates
Peritubular Cell (PT)					
TGF-α	(SC)	Stimulates	P-MOD-S	(SC)	Stimulates
Testosterone	(LC)	Stimulates			
Oxytocin	(LC)	Stimulates			
IGF-1	(Serum)	—			
Sertoli Cell (SC)§					
NGF	(GC)	Stimulates	TGF-α	(PT)	Stimulates
P-MOD-S	(PT)	Stimulates	TGF-β	(PT)	Inhibits
ACTH	(LC)	Stimulates	NGAG	(PT)	Inhibits
MSN	(LC)	Stimulates	IGF-1	(GC)	—
CRH	(LC)	—	IL-1α	(GC)	—
Testosterone	(LC)	Stimulates	SGF	(GC)	Stimulates
β-endorphin	(LC)	Inhibits	LHRH	(LC)	Stimulates/inhibits?
			SCF	(LC)	Stimulates
			TGF-β	(LC)	Inhibits
			IL-1-α	(LC)	Stimulates/inhibits?
			IGF-1	(LC)	Stimulates
			Inhibin	(LG)	Stimulates
			β-FGF	(LC)	Stimulates
			Estrogen	(LC)	Inhibits

**Stimulates* denotes known stimulatory action; *inhibits* denotes known inhibitory action on respective cell(s).

†Letters in parentheses denote cell of origin of the various factor (e.g., SC, Sertoli cell; GC, germ cell, etc.).

‡Leydig cells (LC) are also influenced by serum-derived factors (e.g., glucocorticoids, ANF, etc.), ICSH, and autoregulatory factors (e.g., estrogen, angiotensis II, β-endorphin, CRF, etc.).

§Sertoli cells (SC) are also influenced by serum-derived factors (e.g., retinol, EGF, insulin, etc.), FSH, and autoregulatory factor (e.g., IGF-1, β-FGF, etc.).

SOURCE: Thomas, 1995a, with permission.

tion of cells that give rise to the process, the spermatogonia (cf. Amann, 1989).

Sperm are among the smallest cells in humans, where its length is about 50 μm or only about one-half the diameter of the ovum, the largest cell of the female organism. The relative volume of a sperm is about 1/100,000 that of the egg. The sperm has a head, a middle piece, and a tail, which correspond, respectively, to the following functions: activation and genetics, metabolism, and motility.

Whereas only a few hundred human ova are released as cells ready for fertilization in a life-time, millions of motile sperm are formed in the spermatogenic tubules each day. Several physiologic factors affect the regulation of sperm motility (e.g., spermine, spermidine, "quiescence" factor, cAMP, motility stimulating factor) (Lindemann and Kanous, 1989).

Spermatogenesis starts at puberty and continues almost throughout life. The primitive male germ cells are spermatogonia, which are situated next to the basement membrane of the seminif-

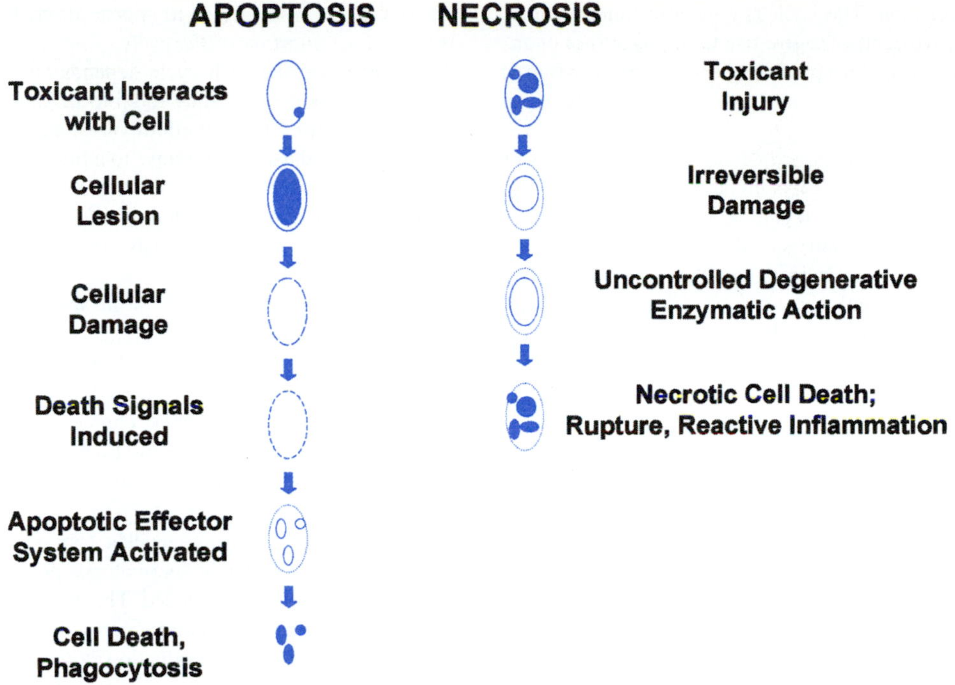

Figure 20-1. Comparison of cellular events during apoptosis and necrosis. (Modified from Raffray and Cohen, 1997, with permission.)

erous tubules. Following birth, spermatogonia are dormant until puberty, when proliferative activity begins again. The onset of spermatogenesis accompanies functional maturation of the testes. Two major types of spermatogonia are present—type A, which generates other spermatogonia, and type B, which becomes a mature sperm. The latter type develops into primary spermatocytes, which undergo meiotic divisions to become secondary spermatocytes. The process of meiosis results in the reduction of the normal complement of chromosomes (diploid) to half this number (haploid) (Fig. 20-2). Meiosis ensures the biologic necessity of evolution through the introduction of controlled variability. Each gamete must receive one of each pair of chromosomes. Whether it receives the maternal or paternal chromosome is a matter of chance. In the male, meiosis is completed within several days. In the female, meiotic division begins during fetal life but is then suspended until puberty. Meiosis may be the most susceptible stage for chemical insult (cf. Herbert, et al., 1995).

Secondary spermatocytes give rise to spermatids. Spermatids complete their development into sperm by undergoing a period of transformation (spermiogenesis) involving extensive nuclear and

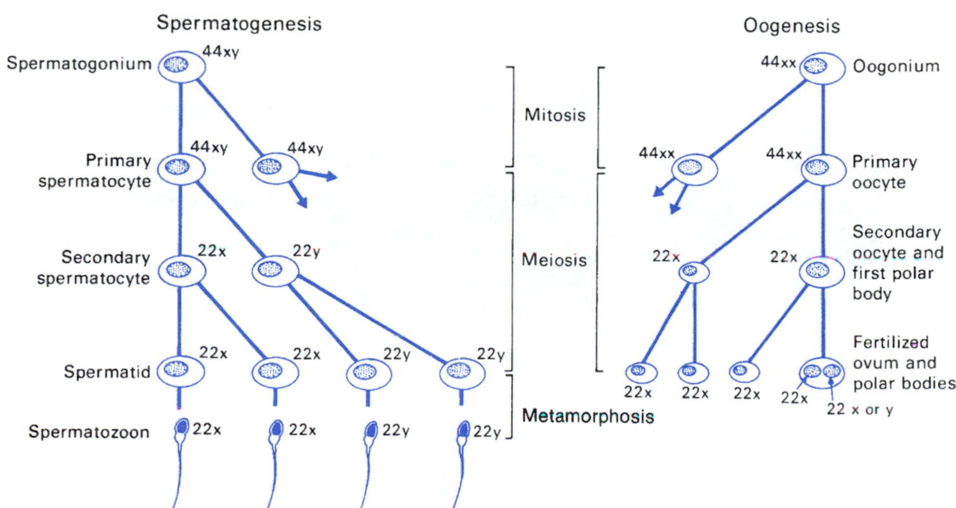

Figure 20-2. Cellular replication (mitosis) and cellular reductive divisions (meiosis) involved in spermatogenesis, oogenesis, and fertilization.

cytoplasmic reorganization. The nucleus condenses and becomes the sperm head; the two centrioles give rise to the flagellum or axial filament. Part of the Golgi apparatus becomes the acrosome, and the mitochondria concentrate into a sheath located between two centrioles.

Seminiferous tubules contain germ cells at different stages of differentiation and also Sertoli cells. In a cyclic fashion, spermatogonia A of certain areas of a tubule become committed to divide synchronously, and the cohorts of the resulting cells differentiate in unison. Thus, a synchronous population of developing germ cells occupies a defined area within a seminiferous tubule. Cells within each cohort are connected by intercellular bridges.

The anatomic relationships of the mammalian testes reveal that the process of spermatogenesis occurs within the seminiferous tubules (Fig. 20-3). The germ cells, along with the Sertoli cells, are contained within the membranous boundaries of the seminiferous tubules. Conversely, the Leydig cells are situated in the interstitium or outside the seminiferous tubules. Several different species display a single cellular association of the seminiferous tubules; in humans, however, such cellular associations differ and are intermingled in a mosaic-like pattern. Several cellular associations, varying among species, may be detected. Each cellular association contains four or five types of germ cells organized in a specific, layered pattern. Each layer represents one cellular generation. Fourteen cellular associations are observed in the seminiferous epithelium in the rat (LeBlond and Clermont, 1952; Heller and Clermont, 1964).

Presuming a fixed point within the seminiferous tubule could be viewed in the developing germ cell, there would be a sequential appearance of each of these cellular associations that would be characteristic of the particular species. This progression through the series of cellular associations would continue to repeat itself in a predictable fashion. The interval required for one complete series of cellular associations to appear at one point within a tubule is termed *the duration of the cycle of the seminiferous epithelium.* The duration of one such cycle depends on the cell turnover rate of spermatogonia and is thus equal to it. Thus, the duration of the cycle of seminiferous epithelium varies among mammals, being a low of about 9 days in the mouse to a high of about 16 days in humans (Table 20-3) (Galbraith, et al., 1982). Spermatids, emanating from spermatogonia committed to differentiate approximately 4.5 cycles earlier, are continuously released from the germinal epithelium.

Maturation changes occur in the sperm as they traverse along the tubules of the testes and the epididymides. During this passage, sperm acquire the capacity for fertilization and become more motile. There is a progressive dehydration of the cytoplasm, decreased resistance to cold shock, changes in metabolism, and variations in membrane permeability. Each ejaculate contains a spectrum of normal sperm as well as those that are either abnormal or immature.

Normalcy of spermatogenesis can be evaluated from two standpoints: the number of spermatozoa produced per day and the quality of spermatozoa produced. The number of spermatozoa produced per day is defined as daily sperm production (Amann, 1981). The efficiency of sperm production is the number of sperm produced per day per gram of testicular parenchyma. The efficiency of sperm production in humans is only about 20 to 40 percent of that in other mammals (Amann, 1986). Sperm production in a young man is about 7 million sperm per day per gram; by the fifth to ninth decade of life, it drops to approximately one-half or about 3.5 million per day per gram (cf. Johnson, 1986).

Blazak et al. (1985)—using several parameters including sperm production, sperm number, sperm transit time, and sperm motility—have provided an assessment of the effects of chemicals on the male reproductive system. These authors concluded that

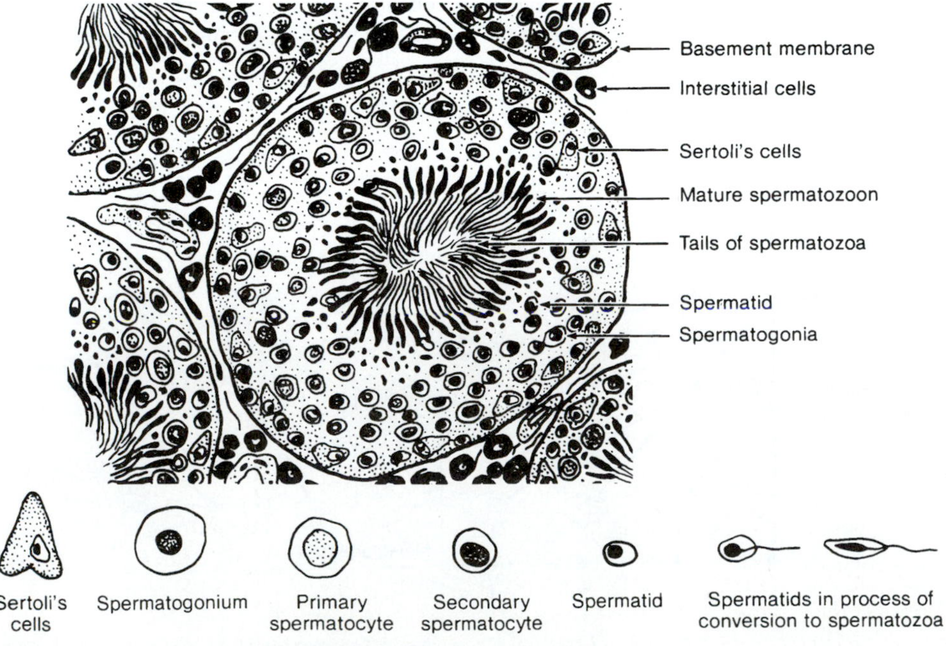

Figure 20-3. Schematic cross section of seminiferous tubules of testes.

Morphology of the Sertoli cell along with the cellular events involved in spermatogenesis (spermatogonium through spermatid).

Table 20-3
Criteria for Spermatogenesis in Laboratory Animals and Humans

	MOUSE	RAT	RABBIT (NEW ZEALAND WHITE)	DOG (BEAGLE)	MONKEY (RHESUS)	HUMAN
Duration of cycle of seminiferous epithelium (days)	8.6	12.9	10.7	13.6	9.5	16.0
Life span of:						
B-type spermatogonia (days)	1.5	2.0	1.3	4.0	2.9	6.3
L + Z spermatocytes (days)	4.7	7.8	7.3	5.2	6.0	9.2
P + D spermatocytes (days)	8.3	12.2	10.7	13.5	9.5	15.6
Golgi spermatids (days)	1.7	2.9	2.1	6.9	1.8	7.9
Cap spermatids (days)	3.5	5.0	5.2	3.0	3.7	1.6
Fraction of a lifespan as:						
B-type spermatogonia	0.11	0.10	0.08	0.19	0.19	0.25
Primary spermatocyte	1.00	1.00	1.00	1.00	1.00	1.00
Round spermatid	0.41	0.40	0.43	0.48	0.35	0.38
Testes weight (g)	0.2	3.7	6.4	12.0	49	34
Daily sperm production:						
Per gram testis (10^6/g)	28	24	25	20	23	4.4
Per male (10^6)	5	86	160	300	1100	125
Sperm reserves in caudia (at sexual rest: only 10^6)	49	440	1600	?*	5700	420
Transit time (days) through (at sexual rest):						
Caput + corpus epididymides	3.1	3.0	3.0	?	4.9	1.8
Cauda epididymides	5.6	5.1	9.7	?	5.6	3.7

KEY: L, leptotene; Z, zygotene; P, pachytene; D, diplotene.
*A question mark indicates unclear or inadequate data.
SOURCE: Galbraith WM, Voytek P, Ryon MG: *Assessment of Risks to Human Reproduction and to Development of the Human Conceptus from Exposure to Environmental Substances.* Oak Ridge, TN: Oak Ridge National Laboratory, U.S. Environmental Protection Agency, 1982. Available as order number DE82007897 from the National Technical Information Service, Springfield, VA.

testes weights and epididymal sperm numbers were unreliable indicators of sperm production.

Sertoli Cells The Sertoli cell is now recognized as playing an important role in the process of spermatogenesis (cf. Foster, 1992; Griswold, 1995). In early fetal life, the Sertoli cells secrete antimüllerian hormone (AMH). Their exact physiologic role is not understood, but after puberty, these cells begin to secrete the hormone inhibin, which may aid in modulating pituitary FSH.

Germ cell development occurs in close association with the Sertoli cells, which provide them with structural support, nutrients, and regulatory/paracrine factors. Brinster and Zimmerman (1994) described the interaction between germ cells and Sertoli cells within the seminiferous tubules. Recent experiments indicate that spermatogenesis can be restored in infertile testes through germ cell tranplantation (Ogawa et al., 1999).

The Sertoli cell junctions form the blood-testis barrier that partitions the seminiferous epithelium into a basal compartment containing spermatogonia and early spermatocytes and an adluminal compartment containing more fully developed spermatogenic cells. An ionic gradient is maintained between the two tubular compartments. Nutrients, hormones, and other chemicals must pass either between or through Sertoli cells in order to diffuse from one compartment to another. Germinal cells are found either between adjacent pairs of Sertoli cells or inside their luminal margin (see Fig. 20-4).

Sertoli cells secrete a number of hormones and/or proteins. These secretory products can be used to measure Sertoli function in the presence of chemical insult. The Sertoli cells secrete tissue plasminogen activator, androgen-binding protein (ABP), inhibin, AMH, transferrin, and other proteases. ABP is a protein similar to plasma sex steroid–binding globulin (SSBG). In rodents, ABP acts as a carrier for testosterone and dihydrotestosterone. Sertoli cells probably synthesize estradiol and estrone in response to FSH stimulation.

Normal spermatogenesis requires Sertoli cells. Many chemicals affecting spermatogenesis act indirectly through their effect on the Sertoli cell [e.g., dibromochloropropane (DBCP), monoethylhexyl phthalate (MEHP)] rather than directly on the germ cells. Tetrahydrocannabinol (THC) acts at several sites in the reproductive system, including the Sertoli cell, where it acts by inhibiting FSH-stimulated cAMP accumulation (Heindel and Keith, 1989).

Interstitium (Leydig Cells) The Leydig or interstitial cells are the primary sites of testosterone synthesis (Fig. 20-5) (cf. Ewing, 1992). These cells are closely associated with the testicular blood vessels and the lymphatic space. The spermatic arteries to the testes

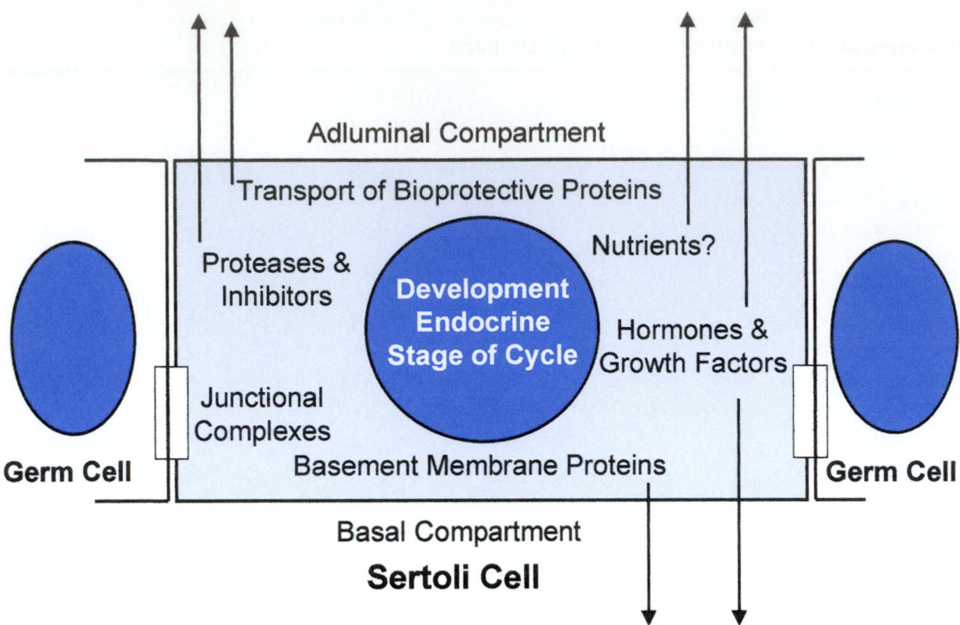

Figure 20-4. Cellular sites of action of chemical or drugs in the testes.

Secretion may occur to both the adluminal and basal compartments in the seminiferous tubules. The type, amount, and detection of Sertoli cell secretion may be influenced by the stage of testicular development endocrine status and the stage of cycle of the seminiferous epithelium (Griswold, 1995). Note the anatomic proximity of the Sertoli cell and the germ cell. See also Tables 20-1 and 20-2 for various hormonal and growth factor interactions between the various subpopulations of testicular cells.

are tortuous; their blood flows parallel to blood in the pampiniform plexus of the spermatic veins but in the opposite direction (Fig. 20-5). This anatomic arrangement seems to facilitate a countercurrent exchange of heat, androgens, and other chemicals.

LH stimulates testicular steroidogenesis (Zirkin and Chen, 2000). Androgens are essential to spermatogenesis, epididymal sperm maturation, the growth and secretory activity of accessory sex organs, somatic masculinization, male behavior, and various metabolic processes. Surprisingly, there are a large number of diverse chemicals/drugs that can cause Leydig cell hyperplasia/neoplasia. This chemically induced proliferation of Leydig cells is particularly evident in the rodent (Table 20-4) (Thomas, 1995b; Cook et al., 1999).

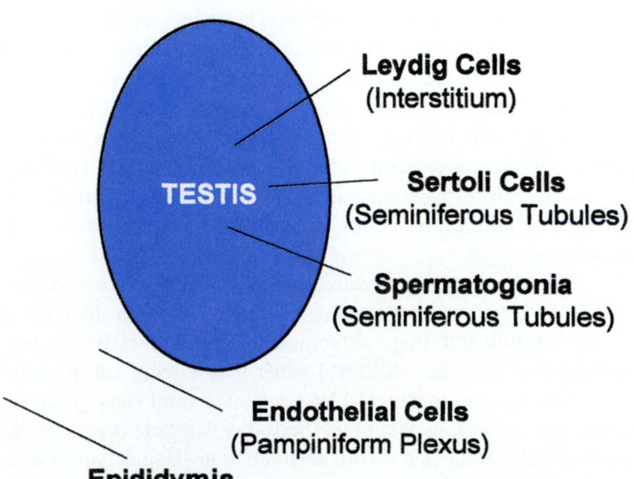

Figure 20-5. Schematic representation of secretory elements from the Sertoli cell.

Extratesticular sites include the epididymis and the endothelial cells of the pampiniform plexus.

A number of nongenotoxic agents can produce Leydig cell hyperplasia in rats, mice, and dogs (Cook et al., 1999). Androgen receptor antagonists (e.g., flutamide), 5α-reductase inhibitors (e.g., finasteride), testosterone biosynthesis inhibitors (e.g., cimetidine, metronidazole, vinclozolin, etc.), aromatase inhibitors (e.g., formestane), dopamine agonists (e.g., mesulergine), estrogen agonists/antagonists (e.g., DES, tamoxifen, etc.), and GnRH agonists (e.g., leuprolide, etc.) are all capable of producing Leydig cell hyperplasia. It is obvious that they exhibit vastly different modes of action. Agents that produce Leydig cell hyperplasia in experimental animals can also be grouped according to their chemical activity (e.g., antihypertensives, calcium channel blockers, fungicides, goitrogens, etc.) as well as by their chemical class (e.g., flurochemicals, nitroaromatics, organochlorines, etc.). Nongenotoxic compounds that induce Leydig cell tumors in rats most likely have little relevance to humans under most exposure conditions because humans are quantitatively less sensitive than rats (Cook et al., 1999).

Posttesticular Processes

The end product of testicular gametogenesis is immature sperm. Posttesticular processes involve ducts that move maturing sperm from the testis to storage sites where they await ejaculation. A number of secretory processes exist that control fluid production and ion composition; secretory organs contribute to the chemical composition (including specific proteins) of the semen.

Table 20-4
Chemicals/Drugs Causing Leydig Cell Hyperplasia/Neoplasia in Rodents

AGENT/CHEMICAL/DRUG	AGENT CLASS OR BIOLOGIC ACTIVITY
Cadmium	Heavy metal
Estrogen	Hormone
Linuron	Herbicide
S0Z-200-110, isradine	Calcium channel blocker
Flutamide	Antiandrogen
Gemfibrozil	Hypolidemic agent
Finasteride	5α-reductase inhibitor
Cimetidine	Histamine (H_2) receptor blocker
Hydralazine	Antihypertensive agent
Carbamazepine	Anticonvulsant/analgesic
Vidarabine	Antiviral agent
Mesulegine	Dopamine (D_2) agonist-antagonist
Clomiphene	Treatment of infertility
Perfluoroctanoate	Industrial ingredient (plasticizers, lubricant/wetting agent(s)
Dimethylformide	Industrial use (tannery & leathergoods, metal dyes)
Diethylstilbestrol	Synthetic hormone
Nitrosamine	Industrial uses
Methoxychlor	Pesticide with estrogenic properties
Oxolinic acid	Antimicrobial agent
Reserpine	Antihypertensive
Metronidazole	Antiprotozoal
Cyclophosphamide	Antineoplastic
Methylcholanthrene	Experimental carcinogen

SOURCES: Ewing, 1992; Bosland, 1994; Prentice et al., 1992; Thomas, 1995b; Cook et al., 1999.

Efferent Ducts The fluid produced in the seminiferous tubules moves into a system of spaces called the rete testis. The chemical composition of the rete testis fluid is unique and has a total protein concentration much lower than that of the blood plasma. The efferent ducts open into the caput epididymis.

Although the rete testis fluid normally contains inhibin, ABP, transferrin, myoinositol, steroid hormones, amino acids, and various enzymes, only ABP and inhibin appear to be specific products and useful indicators of the functional integrity of the seminiferous epithelium or Sertoli cells (Mann and Lutwak-Mann, 1981). However, relative concentrations of other constituents may indicate alterations in membrane barriers or active transport processes. The concentration of chemicals in the rete testis fluid relative to unbound plasma concentration has been used to estimate the permeability of the blood-testis barrier for selected chemicals (Okumura et al., 1975).

Epididymides The epididymis is a single, highly coiled duct measuring approximately 5 m in humans. It is arranged anatomically into three parts called the caput, the corpus, and the cauda epididymides (cf. Cooper, 1986).

From the rete testis, testicular fluid first enters efferent ducts and then the epididymides. Here the sperm are subjected to a changing chemical environment as they move through the organ.

The first two sections together (the caput and the corpus) are regarded as making up that part of the epididymis involved with sperm maturation, whereas the terminal segment (the cauda) is regarded as the site of sperm storage. There are, however, differences in the position and extent of the segments in various species of mammals.

From 1.8 to 4.9 days are required for sperm to move through the caput to the corpus epididymis, where maturation takes place. In contrast, the transit time for sperm through the cauda epididymis in sexually rested males differs greatly among species and ranges from 3.7 to 9.7 days. Average sperm transit time for a 21- to 30-year-old man is 6 days. The number of sperm in the caput and corpus epididymis is similar in sexually rested males and in males ejaculating daily. The number of sperm in the cauda epididymis is more variable, being lower in sexually active males.

Active transport processes affect the amount of fluid flowing through the epididymis. Because much of the fluid produced by the testis is apparently absorbed in the epididymis, the relative concentration of sperm is increased.

Hence, important functions of the epididymis are reabsorption of rete testis fluid, metabolism, epithelial cell secretions, sperm maturation, and sperm storage. The chemical composition of the epididymal plasma plays an important role in both sperm maturation and sperm storage. Environmental chemicals perturb these processes and can produce adverse effects.

Accessory Sex Organs The anatomic relationship of accessory sex organs in the male rodent is depicted in Fig. 20-6. Most mammals possess seminal vesicles (exceptions: cats and dogs) and most have prostate glands. However, the physiologic and anatomic characteristics of the prostate gland may vary considerably among mammals (Wilson, 1995).

The seminal plasma functions as a vehicle for conveying the ejaculated sperm from the male to the female reproductive tract. This plasma is produced by the secretory organs of the male reproductive system, which, along with the epididymides, include the

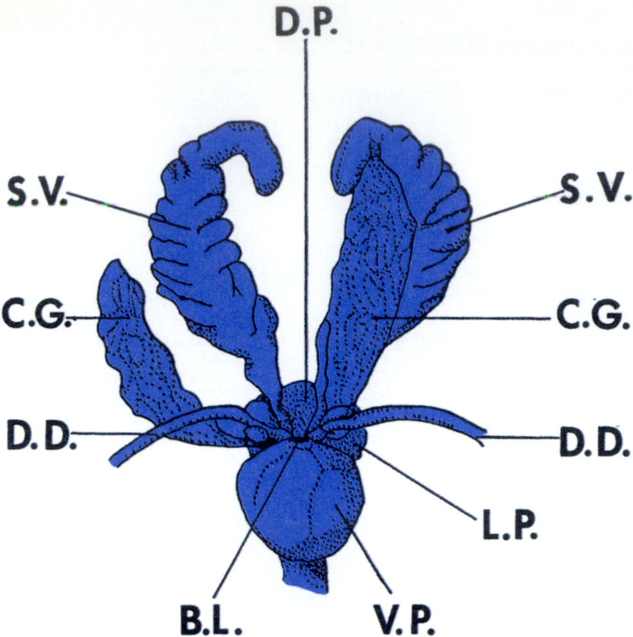

Figure 20-6. Anatomic relation of components of rodent sex accessory glands.

D.D., ductus deferens; B.L., bladder; V.P., ventral prostate; L.P., lateral prostate; C.G., coagulating gland (also called the anterior prostate); S.V., seminal vesicle; D.P., dorsal prostate. (From Hayes, 1982, with permission.)

prostate, seminal vesicles, bulbourethral (Cowper's) glands, and urethral (Littre's) glands. Any abnormal function of these organs can be reflected in altered seminal plasma characteristics. Seminal plasma is normally an isotonic, neutral medium, which, in many species, contains sources of energy such as fructose and sorbitol, that are directly available to sperm. Functions of the other constituents, such as citric acid and inositol, are not known. In general, the secretions from the prostate and seminal vesicles contribute little to fertility (Mann and Lutwak-Mann, 1981).

The accessory sex organs are androgen-dependent. They serve as indicators of the Leydig cell function and/or androgen action. The weights of the accessory sex glands are an indirect measure of circulating testosterone levels. The ventral prostate of rats has been used to study the actions of testosterone and to investigate the molecular basis of androgen-regulated gene function.

Human semen emission initially involves the urethral and Cowper's glands, with the prostatic secretion and sperm coming next and the seminal vesicle secretion delivered last. There is a considerable overlap between the presperm, sperm-rich, and postsperm fractions. Therefore even if an ejaculate is collected in as many as six (split ejaculate) fractions, it is rarely possible to obtain a sperm-free fraction consisting exclusively of prostatic or vesicular secretions.

Acid phosphatase and citric acid are markers for prostatic secretion; fructose is an indicator for seminal vesicle secretion. It is estimated that about one-third of the entire human ejaculate is contributed by the prostate and about two-thirds by the seminal vesicles. Both the vas deferens and the seminal vesicles apparently synthesize prostaglandins. Semen varies both in volume and composition between species. Human, bovine, and canine species have a relatively small semen volume (1 to 10 mL); semen of stallions and boars is ejaculated in much larger quantities. Sperm move from the distal portion of the epididymis through the vas deferens (ductus deferens) to the urethra. Vasectomy is the surgical removal of the vas deferens or a portion of it. The semen of some animals, including rodents and humans, tends to coagulate on ejaculation. The clotting mechanism (e.g., "copulatory plug") involves enzymes and substrates from different accessory organs.

Although all male mammals have prostates, the organ differs anatomically, physiologically, and chemically among species, and lobe differences in the same species may be pronounced. The rat prostate is noted for its complex structure and its prompt response to castration and androgen stimulation. The human prostate is a tubuloalveolar gland made up of two prominent lateral lobes that contribute about one-third of the ejaculate.

Prostatic secretion in humans and many other mammalian species contains acid phosphatase, zinc, and citric acid. The prostatic secretion is the main source of acid phosphatase in human semen; its concentration provides a convenient method for assessing the functional state of the prostate. The human prostate also produces spermine. Prostate-specific antigen (PSA) is a 33-kDa protein synthesized primarily by the prostatic epithelium (Polascik et al., 1999). It is a tumor marker for prostate cancer. Certain proteins and enzymes (acid phosphatase, γ-glutamyl transpeptidase, glutamicoxaloacetic transaminase), cholesterol, inositol, zinc, and magnesium have also been proposed as indicators of prostatic secretory function. Radioactive zinc (^{65}Zn) uptake by rodent prostate glands has been used as an index for androgenic potency (Gunn and Gould, 1956). An ionic antagonism exists between zinc and cadmium. Cadmium can induce metallothionein in the prostate glands of experimental animals (Waalkes et al., 1982; cf. Waalkes, et al., 1992).

The anatomic structure of the seminal vesicle varies among animals. The seminal vesicle is a compact glandular tissue arranged in the form of multiple lobes that surround secretory ducts. Like the prostate, the seminal vesicle is responsive to androgens and is a useful indicator of Leydig cell function. The vesicular glands can be used as a gravimetric indicator for androgens.

In humans, the seminal vesicle contributes about 60 percent of the seminal fluid. The seminal vesicles also produce more than half of the seminal plasma in laboratory and domestic animals such as the rat, guinea pig, and bull. In the human, bull, ram, and boar (but not the cat), most of the seminal fructose is secreted by the seminal vesicles; consequently, in these species the chemical assay of fructose in semen is a useful indicator of the relative contribution of the seminal vesicles to whole semen. Seminal vesicle secretion is also characterized by the presence of proteins and enzymes, phosphorylcholine, and prostaglandins. PSA occurs in high concentration in seminal fluid.

Erection and Ejaculation These physiologic processes are controlled by the central nervous system (CNS) but are modulated by the autonomic nervous system. Parasympathetic nerve stimulation results in dilatation of the arterioles of the penis, which initiates an erection. Erectile tissue of the penis engorges with blood, veins are compressed to block outflow, and the turgor of the organ increases. In the human, afferent impulses from the genitalia and descending tracts, which mediate erections in response to erotic psychic stimuli, reach the integrating centers in the lumbar segments of the spinal cord. The efferent fibers are located in the pelvic splanchnic nerves (Andersson and Wagner, 1995).

Ejaculation is a two-stage spinal reflex involving emission and ejaculation. Emission is the movement of the semen into the urethra; ejaculation is the propulsion of the semen out of the urethra at the time of orgasm. Afferent pathways involve fibers from receptors in the glans penis that reach the spinal cord through the internal pudendal nerves. Emission is a sympathetic response effected by contraction of the smooth muscle of the vas deferens and seminal vesicles. Semen is ejaculated out of the urethra by contraction of the bulbocavernosus muscle. The spinal reflex centers for this portion of the reflex are in the upper sacral and lowest lumbar segments of the spinal cord; the motor pathways traverse the first to third sacral roots of the internal pudendal nerves.

Little is known concerning the effects of chemicals on erection or ejaculation (Woods, 1984). Pesticides, particularly the organophosphates, are known to affect neuroendocrine processes involved in erection and ejaculation. Many drugs act on the autonomic nervous system and affect potency (Table 20-5) (see also Papadopoulas, 1980; Buchanan and Davis, 1984; Stevenson and Umstead, 1984; Keene and Davies, 1999). Impotence, the failure to obtain or sustain an erection, is rarely of endocrine origin; more often, the cause is psychological. The occurrence of nocturnal or early-morning erections implies that the neurologic and circulatory pathways involved in attaining an erection are intact and suggests the possibility of a psychological cause.

Normal penile erection depends upon the relaxation of smooth muscles in the corpora cavernosa. In response to sexual stimuli, cavernous nerves and endothelial cells release nitric oxide, which stimulates the formation of cyclic guanosine monophosphate (GMP) by guanylate cyclase. The drug sildenafil (Viagra) is used to treat erectile dysfunction; its mechanism of action resides in its ability to selectively inhibit cGMP-specific phosphodiesterase type 5. By selectively inhibiting cGMP catabolism in cavernosal smooth muscle cells, sildenafil restores the natural erectile response (cf. Goldstein, et al., 1998; Lu, 2000).

Ovarian Function

Oogenesis Ovarian germ cells with their follicles have a dual origin; the theca or stromal cells arise from fetal connective tissues of the ovarian medulla, the granulosa cells from the cortical mesenchyme (Fig, 20-7).

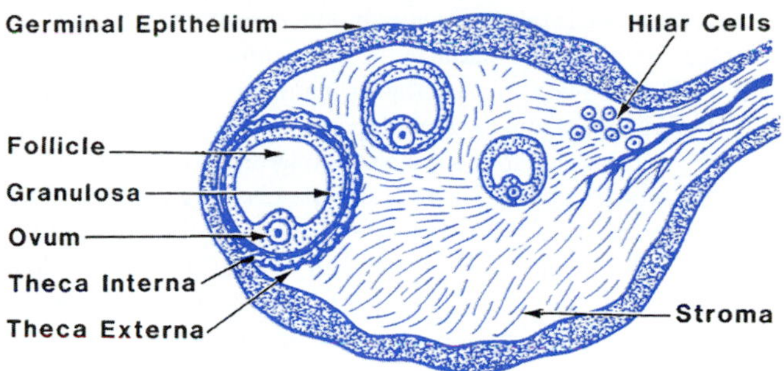

Figure 20-7. Schematic representation of ovarian morphology.

About 400,000 follicles are present at birth in each human ovary. After birth, many undergo atresia, and those that survive are continuously reduced in number. Any agent that damages the oocytes will accelerate the depletion of the pool and can lead to reduced fertility in females. About one-half of the number of oocytes present at birth remain at puberty; the number is reduced to about 25,000 by 30 years of age. About 400 primary follicles will yield mature ova during a woman's reproductive life span. During the approximately three decades of fecundity, follicles in various stages of growth can always be found. After menopause, follicles are no longer present in the ovary.

Follicles remain in a primary follicle stage following birth until puberty, when a number of follicles start to grow during each ovarian cycle. However, most fail to achieve maturity. For the follicles that continue to grow, the first event is an increase in size of the primary oocytes. During this stage, fluid-filled spaces appear among the cells of the follicle, which unite to form a cavity or antrum, otherwise known as the graafian follicle.

Primary oocytes undergo two specialized nuclear divisions, which result in the formation of four cells containing one-half the

Table 20-5
Drug-Induced Impotence

	AGENT	CNS	ANS	ENDO
Narcotics	Morphine	+	+	?
	Ethanol	+		
Psychotropics	Chlorpromazine		+	
	Diazepam	+		
	Tricyclic antidepressants		+	?
	MAO inhibitors		+	
Hypotensives	Methyldopa	+	+	+
	Clonidine	+	+	
	Reserpine	+	+	
	Guanethidine		++	
Hormones/antagonists	Estrogens			+
	Cyproterone			+

KEY: CNS, central nervous system; ANS, autonomic nervous system; ENDO, endocrine.
SOURCES: Millar, 1979, Buchanan and Davis, 1984.

number of chromosomes (Fig. 20-2). The first meiotic division occurs within the ovary just before ovulation, and the second occurs just after the sperm fuses with the egg. In the first stage of meiosis, the primary oocyte is actively synthesizing DNA and protein in preparation for entering prophase. The DNA content doubles as each of the prophase chromosomes produces its mirror image. Each doubled chromosome is attracted to its homologous mate to form tetrads. The members of the tetrads synapse or come to lie side by side. Before separation, the homologous pairs of chromosomes exchange genetic material by a process known as crossing over. Thus, qualitative differences occur between the resulting gametes. Subsequent meiotic stages distribute the members of the tetrads to the daughter cells in such a way that each cell receives the haploid number of chromosomes. At telophase, one secondary oocyte and a polar body have been formed, which are no longer genetically identical.

The secondary oocyte enters the next cycle of division very rapidly; each chromosome splits longitudinally; the ovum and the three polar bodies now contain the haploid number of chromosomes and half the amount of genetic material. Although the nuclei of all four eggs are equivalent, the cytoplasm is divided unequally. The end products are one large ovum and three rudimentary ova (polar bodies), which subsequently degenerate. The ovum is released from the ovary at the secondary oocyte stage; the second stage of meiotic division is triggered in the oviduct by the entry of the sperm.

Ovarian Cycle The cyclic release of pituitary gonadotropins involving the secretion of ovarian progesterone and estrogen is depicted in Fig. 20-8. These female sex steroids determine ovulation and prepare the female accessory sex organs to receive the male sperm. Sperm, ejaculated into the vagina, must make their way through the cervix into the uterus, where they are capacitated. Sperm then migrate into the oviducts, where fertilization takes place. The conceptus then returns from the oviducts to the uterus and implants into the endometrium.

Postovarian Processes

Female accessory sex organs function to bring together the ovulated ovum and the ejaculated sperm. The chemical composition and viscosity of reproductive tract fluids, as well as the epithelial morphology of these organs, are controlled by ovarian (and trophoblastic) hormones.

Oviducts The oviducts provide the taxis of the fimbria, which is under muscular control. The involvement of the autonomic nervous system in this process, as well as in oviductal transport of both the male and female gametes, raises the possibility that pharmacologic agents known to alter the autonomic nervous system may alter function and therefore fertility.

Uterus Uterine endometrium reflects the cyclicity of the ovary as it is prepared to receive the conceptus. The myometrium's major role is contractile. In primates, at the end of menstruation, all but the deep layers of the endometrium are sloughed. Under the influence of estrogens from the developing follicle, the endometrium increases rapidly in thickness. The uterine glands increase in length but do not secrete to any degree. These endometrial changes are called proliferative. After ovulation, the endometrium becomes slightly edematous, and the actively secreting glands become tightly coiled and folded under the influence of estrogen and progesterone from the corpus luteum. These are secretory (progestational) changes (Fig. 20-8).

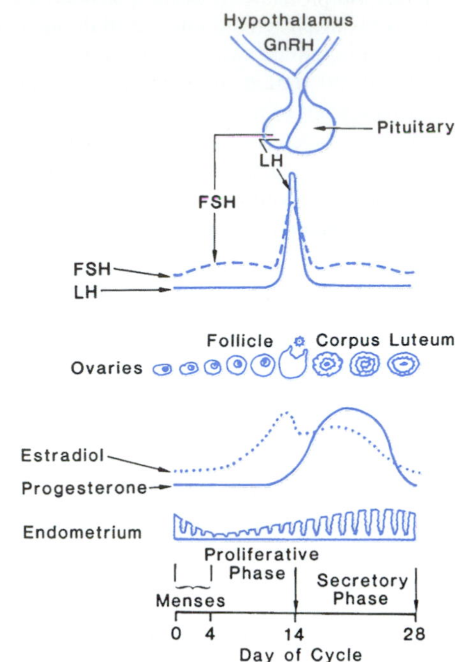

Figure 20-8. Hormonal regulation of menstrual function.

FSH, follicle stimulating hormone; *GnRH*, gonadotropin releasing hormone: *LH*, luteinizing hormone.

When fertilization fails to occur, the endometrium is shed and a new cycle begins. Only primates menstruate. Other mammals have a sexual or estrus cycle. Female animals come into "heat" (estrus) at the time of ovulation. This is generally the only time during which the female is receptive to the male. In spontaneously ovulating species (e.g., rodents), the endocrine events are comparable with those in the menstrual cycle. In the rabbit, ovulation is a reflex produced by copulation.

Cervix The mucosa of the uterine cervix does not undergo cyclic desquamation, but there are regular changes in the cervical mucus. Estrogen, which makes the mucus thinner and more alkaline, promotes the survival and transport of sperm. Progesterone makes the mucus thick, tenacious, and cellular. The mucus is thinnest at the time of ovulation and dries in an arborizing, fernlike pattern on a slide. After ovulation and during pregnancy, it becomes thick and fails to form the fern pattern. Disruptions of the cervix may be expressed as disorders of differentiation (including neoplasia), disturbed secretion, and incompetence. Exfoliative cytologic (Papanicolaou's stain) and histologic techniques are currently used to assess disorders of differentiation. Various synthetic steroids (e.g., oral contraceptives) can affect the extent and pattern of cervical mucus.

Vagina Estrogen produces a growth and proliferation of vaginal epithelium. The layers of cells become cornified and can be readily identified in vaginal smears. Vaginal cornification has been used as an index for estrogens. Progesterone stimulation produces a thick mucus and the epithelium proliferates, becoming infiltrated with leukocytes. The cyclic changes in the vaginal smear in rats are easily recognized. The changes in humans and other species are similar but less apparent. Analysis of vaginal fluid or cytologic studies of desquamated vaginal cells (quantitative cytochemistry) reflects ovarian function. Vaginal sampling of cells and fluid might offer a reliable and easily available external monitor of internal function and dysfunction. Alteration in vaginal flora can indicate a toxicologic condition associated with the use of vaginal tampons [namely toxic shock syndrome (TSS)].

Fertilization During fertilization, the ovum contributes the maternal complement of genes to the nucleus of the fertilized egg and provides food reserves for the early embryo. The innermost of the egg is the vitelline membrane. Outside the ovum proper lies a thick, tough, and highly refractile capsule termed the zona pellucida, which increases the total diameter of the human ovum to about 0.15 mm. Beyond the zona pellucida is the corona radiata, derived from the follicle; it surrounds the ovum during its passage in the oviduct.

Formation, maturation, and union of a male and female germ cell are all preliminary events leading to a combined cell or zygote. Penetration of ovum by sperm and the coming together and pooling of their respective nuclei constitute the process of fertilization.

Only minutes are required for the sperm to penetrate the zona pellucida after passing through the cumulus oophorus in vitro, and probably less in vivo. The sperm traverse along a curved oblique path. Entering the perivitelline space, the sperm head immediately lies flat on the vitellus; its plasma membrane fuses with that of the vitellus and then embeds into the ovum. The cortical granules of the egg disappear, the vitellus shrinks, and the second maturation division is reinitiated, which results in extrusion of the second polar body. A specific factor in the ovum appears to trigger the development of the male pronucleus; the chromatin of the ovum forms a female pronucleus.

As syngamy approaches, the two pronuclei become intimately opposed but do not fuse. The nuclear envelopes of the pronuclei break up; nucleoli disappear, and chromosomes condense and promptly aggregate. The chromosomes mingle to form the prometaphase of the first spindle, and the egg divides into two blastomeres. From sperm penetration to first cleavage usually requires about 12 h in laboratory animals.

From a single fertilized cell (the zygote), cells proliferate and differentiate until more than a trillion cells of about a hundred different types are present in the adult organism.

Implantation The developing embryo migrates through the oviduct into the uterus. Upon contact with the endometrium, the blastocyst becomes surrounded by an outer layer or syncytiotrophoblast, a multinucleated mass of cells with no discernible boundaries, and an inner layer of individual cells, the cytotrophoblast. The syncytiotrophoblast erodes the endometrium, and the blastocyst implants. Placental circulation is then established and trophoblastic function continues. The blastocysts of most mammalian species implant about day 6 or 7 following fertilization. At this stage, the differentiation of the embryonic and extraembryonic (trophoblastic) tissues is apparent.

Trophoblastic tissue differentiates into cytotrophoblast and syncytiotrophoblast cells. The syncytiotrophoblast cells produce chorionic gonadotropin, chorionic growth hormones, placental lactogen, estrogen, and progesterone, which are needed to achieve independence from the ovary in maintaining the pregnancy. Rapid proliferation of the cytotrophoblast serves to anchor the growing placenta to the maternal tissue.

The developing placenta consists of proliferating trophoblasts, which expand rapidly and infiltrate the maternal vascular channels. Shortly after implantation, the syncytiotrophoblast is bathed by maternal venous blood, which supplies nutrients and permits an exchange of gases. Histotrophic nutrition involves yolk sac circulation; hemotrophic nutrition involves the placenta. Placental circulation is established quite early in women and primates and relatively much later in rodents and rabbits. Interestingly, placental dysfunction due to vascular compromise caused by cocaine leads to increased fetal risk, causing growth retardation and prematurity. Fetal loss due to abruptio placentae may occur (cf. Doering, et al., 1989).

Placentation Morphologically, the placenta may be defined as the fusion or opposition of fetal membranes to the uterine mucous membrane (cf., Slikker and Miller, 1994). In humans, the placenta varies considerably throughout gestation. The integral unit of the placenta is the villous tree. The core of the villous tree contains the fetal capilaries and associated endothelium.

Placentation varies considerably among various domestic animals, experimental animals, and primates (Slikker and Miller, 1994). Humans and monkey possess a hemochorial placenta. Pigs, horses, and donkeys have an epitheliochorial type of placenta, whereas sheep, goats, and cows have a syndesmochorial type of placenta. In laboratory animals (e.g., rat, rabbit, and guinea pig), the placenta is termed a hemoendothelial type. Among the various species, the number of maternal and fetal cell layers ranges from six (e.g., pig, horse) to a single one (e.g., rat, rabbit). Primates, including humans, have three layers of cells in the placenta that a substance must pass across. Thus, the placentas of some species are "thicker" than others.

Generally, the placenta is quite impermeable to chemicals/drugs with molecular weights of 1000 Da or more. Most medications have molecular weights of 500 Da or less. Hence, molecular size is rarely a factor in denying a drug's entrance across the placenta and into the embryo/fetus. Placental permeability to a chemical is affected by placental characteristics including thickness, surface area, carrier systems, and lipid-protein concentration of the membranes. The inherent characteristics of the chemical itself, such as its degree of ionization, lipid solubility, protein binding, and molecular size also affect its transport across the placenta.

INTEGRATIVE PROCESSES

Hypothalamo-Pituitary-Gonadal Axis

FSH and LH are glycoproteins synthesized and released from a subpopulation of the basophilic gonadotropic cells of the pituitary gland. Hypothalamic neuroendocrine neurons secrete specific releasing or release-inhibiting factors into the hypophyseal portal system, which carries them to the adenohypophysis, where they act to stimulate or inhibit the release of anterior pituitary hormones. Luteinizing hormone-releasing hormone (LHRH) acts on gonadotropic cells, thereby stimulating the release of FSH and LH. LHRH and follicle stimulating hormone-releasing hormone (FSHRH) appear to be the same substance. Native and synthetic forms of LHRH stimulate the release of both gonadotrophic hormones; thus, it has been proposed to call this compound gonadotropin-releasing hormone (GnRH).

The neuroendocrine neurons have nerve terminals containing monoamines (norepinephrine, dopamine, serotonin) that impinge on them. Reserpine, chlorpromazine, and monoamine oxidase (MAO) inhibitors modify the content or actions of brain monoamines that affect gonadotropins.

FSH probably acts primarily on the Sertoli cells, but it also appears to stimulate the mitotic activity of spermatogonia. LH stimulates steroidogenesis. A defect in the function of the testis (in the production of spermatozoa or testosterone) will tend to be reflected in increased levels of FSH and LH in serum because of the lack of the "negative feedback" effect of testicular hormones (Fig. 20-9).

The hypothalamo-pituitary-gonadal feedback system is a very delicately modulated hormonal process. Several sites in the endocrine process can be perturbed by drugs (e.g., oral contraceptives) and by different chemicals (Fig. 20-9). Gonadotoxic agents may act on neuroendocrine processes in the brain or they may act directly on the target organ (e.g., gonad). Toxicants that adversely or otherwise alter the hepatic and/or renal biotransformation of endogenous sex steroid might be expected to interfere with the pituitary feedback system (cf. Cooper, et al., 1998).

Puberty

From the early newborn period to the onset of puberty, the testes remain hormonally dormant. After birth, the androgen-secreting Leydig cells in the mammalian fetal testes become quiescent, and a period follows in which the gonads of both sexes await final maturation of the reproductive system.

The onset of puberty begins with secretion of increasing levels of gonadotropins. The physiologic trigger for puberty is poorly understood, but somehow a hypothalamic gonadostat changes the rate of secretion of LHRH, resulting in increases in LH. As puberty approaches, a pulsatile pattern of LH and FSH secretion is observed. The gonad itself is not required for activating FSH or LH at the onset of puberty. It is a CNS phenomenon. Female puberty is affected by a wide range of influences including climate, race, heredity, athletic activity, and degree of adiposity.

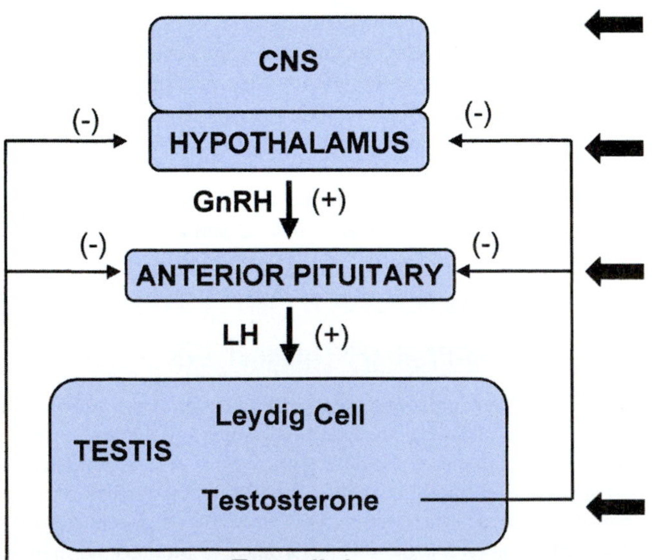

Figure 20-9. Hormonal relationship between the adenohypopyseal-hypothalamic-gonadal axis.

Inhibitory actions (−) and stimulatory actions (+) are depicted along with sites of chemical/drug perturbation (*Large black arrows*).

SEXUAL BEHAVIOR AND LIBIDO

Physiologic processes that account for sexual behavior are poorly understood. The external environment greatly affects sexual behavior, and libido components of reproductive activity depend on a close interplay between neural and endocrine events. For example, a correlation of behavior and receptivity for insemination is attained by complex neuroendocrine mechanisms involving the brain, the pituitary, and sex steroid hormones. This complexity varies even among higher vertebrates. Thus, in reproductive studies involving rodents, the investigator must determine whether the animals actually mate. In the rat, this can be determined by inspecting females each day for vaginal plugs. The number of mountings, thrusts, and ejaculations each can be quantified as indicators of reproductive behavior. It is also important to determine whether the male animal mounts females or other males. If the male copulates and is still sterile, indicators of male fertility such as testicular function should be considered. Failure to copulate suggests either a neuromuscular and/or behavioral defect in the experimental animal.

GENERAL TOXICOLOGIC/ PHARMACOLOGIC PRINCIPLES

Many of the principles that govern absorption, distribution, metabolism, and excretion of a chemical or drug also apply to the reproductive system. There are, however, some rather unique barriers that affect a chemical's action on the mammalian reproductive system. The maternal-fetal interface occurring at the placenta represents a barrier to chemicals coming in contact with the developing embryo. Unfortunately, the placenta is not so restrictive as to prevent most chemicals from crossing the placenta. Most chemicals are not denied entrance into a number of compartments or secretions of the reproductive tract. Indeed, xenobiotic and certain drugs can be readily detected in uterine secretions, in milk of the lactating mother, and in seminal fluid (Mann and Lutwak-Mann, 1981). No specialized barriers appear to prevent chemicals or drugs from acting on the ovary. Several drugs are known to interfere with ovarian function (Table 20-6) (Gorospe and Reinhard, 1995). Unlike the female gonad, the male gonad has a somewhat specialized barrier. This specialized biological barrier is referred to as the blood–testis barrier.

Blood–Testis Barrier

There are a number of specialized anatomic barriers in the body. Tissue permeability barriers include the blood–brain barrier, the blood–thymus barrier, and the blood–bile barrier. Important barriers within the endocrine system are the placental barrier and the blood–testis barrier. The blood–testis barrier is situated somewhere between the lumen of an interstitial capillary and the lumen of a seminiferous tubule (Neaves, 1977). Several anatomically related features intervene between the two luminal spaces, including the

Table 20-6
Inhibitors of Steroidogenic Enzymes

ENZYME	INHIBITOR
Cholesterol side chain cleavage	Aminoglutethimide, 3-methoxybenzidine, cyanoketone, estrogens, azastene, danazol
Aromatase	4-Acetoxy-androstene-3,17-dione, 4-hydroxy-androstene-3,17-dione, 1,4,6-androstatriene-3,17-dione, 6-bromoandrostene-3,17-dione, 7α(4′amino)phenylthioandrostenedione, δ′-testolactone, fenarimol,* MEHP†
11-Hydroxylase	Danazol, metyrapone, furosemide and other diuretics‡
21-Hydroxylase	Danazol, spironolactone
17-Hydroxylase	Danazol, spironolactone
17,20-Desmolase	Danazol, spironolactone
17-Hydroxysteroid dehydrogenase	Danazol
3-Hydroxysteroid dehydrogenase	Danazol
c-17-L-20-lyase	Ketoconozole§

**See* Hirsch et al., 1987.
†*See* Davis et al., 1989.
‡See Bicikova et al., 1996.
§*See* Effendy and Krause, 1989.
SOURCE: Modified from Haney, 1985, with permission.

capillary endothelium, capillary basal lamina, lymphatic endothelium, myoid cells, basal lamina of the seminiferous tubule, and Sertoli cells. The barrier that impedes or denies the free exchange of chemicals/drugs between the blood and the fluid inside the seminiferous tubules is located in one or more of these structures. The apparent positioning of distances relative to transepithelial permeability can affect the passage (or blockage) of a substance through the blood–testis barrier. These epithelial cell anatomic relationships can affect the tightness of fit between cells and the extent to which a chemical's passage can occur. Such junctions or cell unions are often leaky and may allow for a substance's passage. These so-called gap junctions may even be less developed in the immature or young mammalian testes, hence affording greater opportunities for foreign chemicals to permeate the seminiferous tubule. Steinberger and Klinefelter (1993) have developed a two-compartment model for culturing testicular cells that similates a blood–testis barrier. This culture model has been proposed to study Sertoli cell and Leydig cell dysfunction in vitro.

Setchell and coworkers (1969) first demonstrated that immunoglobulins and iodinated albumin, inulin, and a number of small molecules were excluded from the seminiferous tubules by the blood–testis barrier. Dym and Fawcett (1970) suggested that the primary permeability barrier for the seminiferous tubules was composed of the surrounding layers of myoid cells while specialized Sertoli cell-to-Sertoli cell junctions within the seminiferous epithelium constituted a secondary cellular barrier. Certain classes of adhesive molecules (e.g., E- and N-cadherin, α- and β-catenin, plakoglobin, etc.) may act to promote Sertoli-to-Sertoli cell adhesion and tight junction formation (Byers, et al., 1994) (see also Fig. 20-4).

Okumura and coworkers (1975) quantified permeability rates for nonelectrolytes and certain chemicals/drugs. Low-molecular-weight molecules (e.g., water, urea) can readily cross the blood–testis barrier; larger-sized substances (e.g., inulin) are impeded. The degree of lipid solubility and ionization are important determinants as to whether a substance can permeate the blood–testis barrier. A number of factors are known to affect the permeability of the blood–testis barrier, including ligation of the efferent ductules, autoimmune orchiditis, and vasectomy (cf. Sundaram and Witorsch, 1995).

Biotransformation of Exogenous Chemicals

Testes The mammalian gonad is capable of metabolizing a host of foreign chemicals that have traversed the blood–testis barrier. While mixed-function oxidases and epoxide-degrading enzymes may not be as active as hepatic systems, they are nevertheless present in the testes. Cytochrome P450, in general, is quite sensitive to the effects of a number of chemicals. Gonadal cytochrome P450 is no exception. Arylhydrocarbon hydroxylase (AHH) is present in testicular microsomes (Lee et al., 1981). Consequently, the pathways for steroidogenesis contain a number of enzymes that are affected by chemicals or drugs (Table 20-6). Like the process of steroidogenesis in the gonads, the adrenal cortex is also vulnerable to chemical insult (cf. Colby, 1988). Both the parent compound and its metabolite(s) can adversely affect the gonad (Table 20-7). Whether biotransformation occurs gonadally or extragonadally, the end result can be interference with spermatogenesis and/or steroidogenesis. Their mechanisms of toxicity vary considerably.

The microsomal ozidation of *n*-hexane yields 2,5-hexanedione (2,5-HD). *N*-hexane, an environmental toxicant, causes peripheral polyneuropathy and testicular atrophy (Boekelheide, 1987, 1988).

Table 20-7
Biotransformation of Drugs, Chemicals, and Their Metabolites—Ability to Exert Toxic Actions on the Male Gonad

PARENT COMPOUND	METABOLITE	REFERENCE
Amiodarone (antiarrhythmic drug)	Desethylamiodarone	Holt et al., 1984
Cephalosporin analogs (antimicrobial drug)	*N*-Methyletetrazolethiol*	Comereski et al., 1987
Valproic acid (antiepileptic drug)	Isomers of 2-ethyl hexanol (?)†	Ritter et al., 1987
Diethylhexyl phthalate (DEHP; plasticizer)	Mono-ethylhexyl phthalate and 2-ethyl hexanol (?)†	Thomas et al., 1982
Dibromochloropropane‡ (DBCP; fungicide)	Dichloropropene(s) derivatives (?)†	Torkelson *et al.*, 1961
Ethylene glycol monoethyl ether (industrial solvent)	2-Methoxyacetaldehyde	Foster et al., 1986
n-Hexane (environmental toxicant)	2,5-Hexanedione	Boekelheide, 1987
Acrylamide (industrial use)	*N*-Methylacrylamide, *N*-isopropylacrylamide	Sakamoto and Hashimoto, 1986
Vinclozolin (fungicide)	Butanoic acid derivative and an enanilide metabolite	Kelce et al., 1994

*Only substituent is a testicular toxin, not cephalosporin.
†Questionable testicular toxin but probably teratogenic.
‡Radiometabolites of (^{3}H)-DBCP are not preferentially labeled in the testes.
SOURCES: Modified from Thomas and Ballantyne, 1990; Shemi et al., 1987.

The testicular toxicity is separate from its neurotoxicity. 2,5-HD produces gonadal toxicity by altering testicular tubulin. The HD testicular toxicity results from alterations in Sertoli cell microtubules and the altered microtubules result from pyrole-dependent cross-linking (cf. Li and Heindel, 1998). HD toxicity is slow in onset. Initially, HD affects the cross-linking of cytoskeletal elements leading to altered protein secretions and trafficking in the Sertoli cell. Consequently, there is altered Sertoli cell–germ cell contacts and a loss of Sertoli cell paracrine support of the germ cells (Richburg, et al., 1994; Li and Heindel, 1998).

Ethylene glycol monoethyl ether, along with its metabolites, is a gonadal toxin (Nagano et al., 1979; Wang and Chapin, 2000). Metabolites such as 2-methoxy-ethanol (2-ME) and 2-ethoxyethanol (2-EE) induce testicular toxicity. They may cause testicular atrophy, decreased sperm motility, and an increased incidence of abnormal sperm. Most likely, the metabolism of monoalkyl glycol ethers occurs via alcohol and aldehyde dehydrogenases, leading to the formation of methoxyacetic acid (MAA). MAA is believed to be the ultimate toxic metabolite of 2-ME. However, methoxyacetaldehyde (MALD), an intermediate metabolite of 2-ME, can also produce testicular lesions (Foster et al., 1986; Feuston et al., 1989). Although the site of action was thought to be upon the late spermatocyte, it now appears that the Sertoli cells are the prime target for 2-ME (cf. Li and Heindel, 1998). It is unclear whether the mechanism of testicular toxicity of 2-ME induces germ cell death by reducing the available purine bases causing decreased RNA synthesis in spermatocytes or that 2-ME induces germ cell death by interfering with interregulating signal transduction pathways within either Sertoli cells or germ cells, causing a disruption of cell-to-cell communication (Li and Heindel, 1998).

Dinitrobenzene (DNB) or 1,3 dinitrobenzene can cause testicular toxicity in rats. The toxicity is species- and age-dependent and can be partially reversible (cf. Li and Heindel, 1998). DNB causes vacuolization of the Sertoli cells and the detachment of germ cells (Foster et al., 1992). The mechanism of toxicity of DNB is unclear, but both Sertoli cells and germ cells may be affected.

Several heavy metals are known to adversely affect testicular function (cf. Thomas, 1995a). Cadmium causes testicular toxicity, which consists of a loss of endothelial tight junctional barriers, leading to edema, increased fluid pressure, ischemia, and tissue necrosis. Cadmium's effect on Sertoli cell tight junctions (namely the blood–tubule barriers) may be due to its actions on the actin filaments associated with these junctions (cf. Li and Heindel, 1998). Like other Sertoli toxicants (e.g., HD, DNB, 2-ME, and phthalates), testicular toxicity is age-related. Some species are more sensitive than others. Cadmium-induced capillary toxicity (e.g., pampiniform plexus) leads to necrosis and ischemia. Cadmium, at least at low doses, appears to be a stage-specific Sertoli cell toxicant.

Esters of *o*-phthalic acid (phthalate esters or PAEs) are used extensively in medical devices and other consumer products as plasticizers. Because the PAEs are not convalently bound to the plastic, they can leach into the environment (cf. Thomas and Thomas, 1984). There are several different PAEs exhibiting varying degrees of testicular toxicity, particularly in rats and mice. Diethyl hexyl phthalate (DEHP) and its metabolite monoethyhexyl phthalate (MEHP) cause early sloughing of spermatids and spermatocytes and severe vacuolization of Sertoli cell cytoplasm. Gray and Beamand (1984) proposed that the mechanism of DEHP-induced testicular atrophy involves a membrane alteration leading to separation of germ cells (spermatocytes and spermatids) from the underlying Sertoli cells. The action of MEHP has been attributed to its ability to reduce FSH binding to Sertoli cell membranes (Grasso, et al., 1993). The separation of spermatocytes and spermatids interferes with the transfer of nutrients from the Sertoli cells, leading to death and disintegration of the germ cells. MEHP, and not DEHP, is most likely the proximate testicular toxicant (Albro, et al., 1989). MEHP increases germ cell detachment from the Sertoli cell. MEHP is the only phthalate monoester that reduced Sertoli cell ATP levels. It specifically inhibits FSH-stimulated cAMP accumulation in Sertoli cell cultures (cf. Li and Heindel, 1998). The collapse of vimentin filaments in Sertoli cells by MEHP appears to lead to a loss of Sertoli–germ cell contacts (Richburg and Boekelheide, 1996). Finally, DEHP is not only a reproductive toxicant in the male (e.g., rodents) but it can significantly suppress preovulatory follicle granulosa cell estradiol production (Davis et al., 1994a).

Many other chemicals can produce testicular toxicity, but less information is generally available about their mechanism(s) than some of the more well-studied Sertoli cell toxicants (e.g., HD, DNB, PAE, cadmium, and glycol ethers). Vinclozolin, a fungicide that undergoes biotransformation, produces at least two major metabolites that can effectively act as antagonists to the androgen receptor (Kelce et al., 1994). Epichlorohydrin, a highly reactive electrophile used in the manufacture of glycerol and epoxy resins, produces spermatozoal metabolic lesions (cf. Toth et al., 1989). Tri-*o*-cresyl phosphate (TOCP), an industrial chemical used as a plasticizer in lacquers and varnishes, decreases epididymal sperm motility and density. TOCP interferes with spermatogenic processes and sperm motility directly and not via an androgenic mechanism or decreased vitamin E (Somkuti et al., 1987).

The male reproductive system can be adversely affected by 2,3,7,8-tetrachlorodibenzo-*p*-dioxin (TCDD) (cf. Bjerke and Peterson, 1994; Zacharewski and Safe, 1998). TCDD can alter germ cells at all developmental stages in the testes (Chahoud et al., 1992). Dioxin can reduce Leydig cell volume, but at doses that do not appear to affect spermatogenesis (Johnson et al., 1992). In rodents, TCDD is both embryotoxic and teratogenic (cf. Dickson and Buzik, 1993). TCDD has an avidity for the estrogen receptor (cf. Hruska and Olson, 1989) and other receptors (e.g., Ah receptor). Recently, the safety assessment of the polychlorinated biphenyls (PCBs), with particular reference to reproductive toxicity, has been reviewed (Battershill, 1994; Birnbaum, 1998).

2-Methoxylethanol (2-ME), an industrial solvent, is toxic to both the male and female reproductive system (Mebus et al., 1989). 2-ME must be metabolized to 2-methoxyacetic acid (2-MAA) by alcohol and aldehyde dehydrogenases in order to attain its testicular toxicity. All stages of spermatocyte development and some stages of spermatid development are affected by 2-ME, but it seems to be more selective in destroying early- and late-stage pachytene primary spermatocytes. 2-ME is also embryotoxic and teratogenic in several species (Hanly et al., 1984). 2-ME (also known as methyl cellosolve) when applied dermally can produce a decline in epididymal sperm and testicular spermatid counts in rats (Feuston et al., 1989). Ethanol also causes delayed testicular development and may affect the Sertoli cell and/or the Leydig cell (Anderson et al., 1989). Trifluoroethanol and trifluoroacetaldehyde produce specific damage to pachytene and dividing spermatocytes and round spermatids in rats (Lloyd et al., 1988). Ethane dimethane sulfonate (EDS) effectively eradicates Leydig cells and endogenous testosterone (cf. Bremner, et al., 1994).

Metabolites of cephalosporin reportedly cause testicular toxicity in rats (Comereski et al., 1987). Testicular degeneration from analogs of cephalosporin is most likely to occur with cefbuperazone, cefamandole, and cefoperazone. Cyclosporine can also inhibit testosterone biosynthesis in the rat testes (Rajfer et al., 1987). Amiodarone and its desethyl metabolite can be detected in high concentrations in the testes and semen, but their effects on spermatogenesis or sperm motility are not known (Holt et al., 1984).

Ovary Like the testes, the ovary has the metabolic capability to biotransform certain exogenous substrates. Furthermore, the process of ovarian steroidogenesis, like that of the testes and the adrenal cortex (cf. Colby, 1988), is susceptible to different agents that interfere with the biosynthesis of estrogens (see Table 20-6). Less is known about how chemicals or drugs interfere with ovarian metabolism. The ovary has not been studied as extensively because of its more difficult and complex hormonal relationships. Nevertheless, several chemotherapeutic agents can inhibit ovarian function (Table 20-8). Recently, Faustman et al. (1989) have studied the toxicity of direct-acting alkylating agents on rodent embryos. Their findings failed to reveal any specific structure/activity patterns among various alkylating agents. Like the testes, mixed-function oxidases and various cytochrome systems are found in the ovary. Primordial oocyte toxicity as well as toxicity at other sites can be affected by certain chemicals or drugs (Haney, 1985).

DNA Repair

Alkylating Agents Depending on the species, there are varying degrees of capacity for spermatogenic cells to repair DNA damage due to environmental toxicants (Lee, 1983). It is well known that ultraviolet and x-rays can damage DNA molecules; lethal mutation (i.e., cell deaths) and mutation resulting from transformed cells can also occur. Spermatogenic cells can be used to study unscheduled DNA synthesis (Dixon and Lee, 1980). Unscheduled DNA repair in spermatogenic cells is dose- and time-dependent. Spermiogenic cells are less able to repair DNA damage resulting from alkylating agents. This DNA repair system provides a protective mechanism from certain toxicants; it is also a sensitive index of chromosome damage.

Drug-induced unscheduled DNA synthesis in mammalian oocytes reveals that female gametes possess an excision repair capacity (Pedersen and Brandriff, 1980). Unlike mature sperm, the

Table 20-8
Chemotherapeutic Agents and Ovarian Dysfunction

Prednisone	Busulfan
Vincristine	Methotrexate
Vinblastine	Cytosine arabinoside
6-Mercaptopurine	L-Asparginase
Nitrogen mustard	5-Fluorouracil
Cyclophosphamide	Adriamycin
Chlorambucil	

SOURCES: Haney, 1985, with permission. See also Gorospe and Reinhard, 1995.

mature oocyte maintains a DNA repair ability. However, this ability decreases at the time of meiotic maturation.

Lead Different occupations can result in varying degrees of chromosomal aberration (Table 20-9). In particular, lead toxicity can induce a variety of chromatid and chromosome breaks. Lead is one of the earliest substances associated with deleterious effects on the reproductive system (Thomas and Brogan, 1983). Lead poisoning has been associated with reduced fertility, miscarriages, and stillbirth since antiquity (Lancranjan et al., 1975). Lead salts are among the oldest known spermicidal agents; lead has long been known to be an abortifacient *(cf.* Hildebrand et al., 1973). Lead exposure results in a general suppression of the hypothalamic-pituitary-testicular axis in rats (Klein et al., 1994) and possibly in men occupationally exposed to this heavy metal (Rodamilans et al., 1988) (Table 20-10).

TARGETS FOR CHEMICAL TOXICITY

CNS

There are several sites of interference by chemicals upon the mammalian reproductive system (Fig. 20-9). Drugs and chemicals can act directly on the CNS, particularly the hypothalamus and the adenohypophysis (cf. Cooper et al., 1998). A number of drugs (e.g., tranquilizers, sedatives, etc.) can modify the CNS, leading to alterations in the secretion of hypothalamic-releasing hormones and/or gonadotropins. Synthetic steroids (namely 19-nortestosterones) are very effective in suppressing gonadotropin secretion and hence block ovulation.

Gonads

The gonads are also targets for a host of drugs and chemicals (Table 20-11) (Chapman, 1983; Thomas and Keenan, 1986). The majority of these agents are representatives of major chemical classes of cancer chemotherapeutic agents, particularly the alkylating agents. A number of endocrine agents are of value in the treatment of certain cancers. Antiestrogens (e.g., tamoxifen), aromatase inhibitors (e.g., aminoglutethimide), GnRH agonists and antagonists, and antiandrogens (e.g., flutamide) can interfere with the endocrine system (cf., Lonning and Lien, 1993). Procarbazine, an antineoplastic drug, causes severe damage to the acrosomal plasma membrane and the nucleus of the sperm head in hamsters (Singh et al., 1989). Alkylating agents are effective against rapidly dividing cells. Not surprisingly, the division of germ cells is also affected, leading to arrest of spermatogenesis.

Different cell populations of the mammalian testis exhibit somewhat different thresholds of sensitivity to different toxicants (Fig. 20-5). Thus, the germ cells are most sensitive to chemical insult (i.e., spermatogenesis). The Sertoli cells possess a somewhat intermediate sensitivity to chemical inhibition; Leydig cells are quite resistant to environmental toxicants. Cell-specific testicular toxicants have been employed to evaluate the distribution of creatine in the rete testis (Moore et al., 1992). Creatine is associated with cells of the seminiferous epithelium: elevated urinary excretion of creatine may provide a noninvasive marker for testicular toxicity in vivo.

Sertoli Cells (See also "Biotranformation of Exogenous Chemicals—Testes," above.) Dibromochloropropane (DBCP), a fungicide, causes infertility in a number of species, including hu-

Table 20-9
Occupational Exposure to Lead and Its Relationship to Chromosomal Aberrations

EXPOSED SUBJECTS	TYPE OF ABERRATION
Positive findings	
Lead oxide factory workers	Chromatid and chromosome breaks
Chemical factory workers	Chromatid gaps, breaks
Zinc plant workers	Gaps, fragments, rings, exchanges, dicentrics
Blast-furnace workers, metal grinders, scrap workers	Gaps, breaks, hyperploidy, structural abnormalities
Battery plant workers and lead foundry workers	Gaps, breaks, fragments
Lead oxide factory workers	Chromatid and chromosome aberrations
Battery melters, tin workers	Dicentrics, rings, fragments
Ceramic, lead, and battery workers	Breaks, fragments
Smelter workers	Gaps, chromatid and chromosome aberrations
Battery plant workers	Chromatid and chromosome aberrations
Negative findings	
Policemen	
Lead workers	
Shipyard workers	
Smelter workers	
Volunteers (ingested lead)	
Children (near a smelter)	

SOURCE: Thomas and Brogan, 1983, with permission.

Table 20-10
Some Actions of Lead on the Male Reproductive System

SPECIES	EFFECT
Rat	Infertility
Rat	Germinal epithelial damage
Rat	Oligospermia and testicular degeneration
Rat	Decreased sperm motility and prostate hyperplasia
Mouse	Infertility
Mouse	Abnormal sperm
Human	Teratospermia, hypospermia, and asthenospermia

SOURCE: Bell and Thomas, 1980, with permission.

mans. DBCP causes sterility, but it may do so by acting through the Sertoli cell. DBCP may also inhibit sperm carbohydrate metabolism at the NADH dehydrogenase step in the mitochondrial electron transport chain (Greenwell et al., 1987). Despite DBCP's propensity to cause degeneration of the seminiferous tubules, toxicokinetic studies fail to reveal any preferential uptake by the testes (Shemi et al., 1987). DBCP gonadotoxicity appears to be gender-specific, since only testicular injury has been reported; it does not cause comparable adverse effects in the female rat (Shaked et al., 1988). Analogs of DBCP cause testicular necrosis as well as DNA damage in the rat (Soderlund, et al., 1988).

The production of lactate and pyruvate are indicators of Sertoli cell function (Williams and Foster, 1988). Either dinitrobenzene (DNB) or mono-(2-ethylhexyl)phthalate (MEHP) can affect lactate (and pyruvate) production by rat Sertoli cell cultures. The Sertoli cell appears to be a prime target for the toxic actions of DNB (Blackburn, et al., 1988). Chapin et al. (1988) have also indicated that MEHP adversely affects the mitochondria of the Sertoli cell in vitro. Likewise, dinitrotoluene (DNT) has a locus of toxic action that is the Sertoli cell (Bloch et al., 1988). Dinitrobenzene initially damages Sertoli cells with a subsequent degeneration and exfoliation of germ cells.

Steroidogenesis Steroid biosynthesis can occur in several endocrine organs including the adrenal cortex, ovary, and the testes. Other peripheral tissues and the CNS contain enzymatic systems also capable of steroid synthesis. Pregnenolone is the common precursor of all steroid hormones produced by the adrenal cortex (e.g., mineratocorticoids and glucocorticoids), the ovary (e.g., estrogens and progesterone), and the testes (e.g., androgens). Specific subpopulations of cells in the mammalian gonad are capable of synthesizing steroids. In the ovary, the granulosa cells secrete estrogens in response to FSH. The thecal cells of the ovary secrete progesterone (as does the corpus luteum) (see Fig. 20-7). In the testes, the Leydig cell (or the interstitial cell) in response to LH (or ICSH) secretes androgens (e.g., testosterone and dihydrotestosterone).

Several drugs, hormones, and chemicals can affect steroidogenesis (see Table 20-7) by interfering or inhibiting specific enzymes (see also "Biotransformaton of Exogenous Chemicals," above). Also, anti-LH peptides can affect Leydig cell steroidogenesis. LHRH analogs (e.g., buserelin) can interfere with both ovarian and testicular function (Donaubauer et al., 1987).

The liver and the kidney contain enzyme systems that affect the biological half-life of steroids and other hormones. Hence, xenobiotics that interfere with excretory processes might be expected to alter the endocrine system. For example, a number of hepatic steroid hydroxylases can be induced by either organophosphates or organochlorine pesticides. Such hydroxylation reactions can be expected to render the endogenous steroid more polar and hence more readily excreted by the kidney.

Table 20-11
Drugs That Are Gonadotoxic in Humans

MALES	FEMALES
Busulfan	Busulfan
Chlorambucil	Chlorambucil
Cyclophosphamide	Cyclophosphamide
Nitrogen mustard	Nitrogen mustard
Doxorubicin	
Corticosteroids	
Cytosine-arabinoside	
Methotrexate	
Procarbazine	
Vincristine	
Vinblastine	Vinblastine

SOURCE: Chapman, 1983, with permission.

EVALUATING REPRODUCTIVE CAPACITY

A number of hormone assays are available to assess endocrine function (Thomas and Thomas, 2001). The endocrine system of the female is more complex and dynamic than that of the male. Hence, evaluating reproductive function in the female is more difficult. Immediate distinctions must also be made between the pregnant and the nonpregnant female. Regardless of gender, both behavioral and physiologic factors must be considered in evaluating reproductive toxicity. The physiologic events involved in reproduction involve inherent time factors that are species-specific. Often, evaluating the potential of a chemical or drug to affect the reproductive system is costly and time-consuming. Furthermore, many of the endpoints used to evaluate the reproductive system are not always reliable and have limitations (Table 20-12).

The fact that such a wide variety of chemicals and drugs can perturb the reproductive system adds another dimension of difficulty in attempting to evaluate reproductive toxicity. Not only is there considerable diversity in chemical configuration of the toxicant, but sites and mechanisms of action can be very different. It is obvious that several classes of therapeutic agents can affect both the male and the female reproductive systems.

TESTING MALE REPRODUCTIVE CAPACITY

General Considerations

A host of tests have been used or proposed for evaluating the male reproductive system (Table 20-13). Several cellular sites or processes are vulnerable to chemical and/or drug insult. Perturbation of many of the endocrine or biochemical events associated with the male reproductive system seldom occurs after a single exposure to a toxicant(s). Rather, multiple exposure extended over

Table 20-12
Advantages and Limitations of Standard Reproductive Procedures

ENDPOINT	LIMITATIONS	VALUE
Fertility	Insensitive	Integrates all reproductive functions
Testicular histology	Subjective; not quantitative	Information on target cell
Testis weights	Less sensitive than sperm counts; affected by edema	Rapid; quantitative

SOURCE: Meistrich, 1989, with permission.

Table 20-13
Potentially Useful Tests of Male Reproductive Toxicity for Laboratory Animals and/or Humans*

Testis
- Size in situ
- Weight
- Spermatid reserves
- Gross and histologic evaluation
- Nonfunctional tubules (%)
- Tubules with lumen sperm (%)
- Tubule diameter
- Counts of leptotene spermatocytes

Epididymis
- Weight and histology
- Number of sperm in distal half
- Motility of sperm, distal end (%)
- Gross sperm morphology, distal end (%)
- Detailed sperm morphology, distal end (%)
- Biochemical assays

Accessory sex glands
- Histology
- Gravimetric

Semen
- Total volume
- Gel-free volume
- Sperm concentration
- Total sperm/ejaculate
- Total sperm/day of abstinence
- Sperm motility, visual (%)
- Sperm motility, videotape (% and velocity)
- Gross sperm morphology
- Detailed sperm morphology

Endocrine
- Luteinizing hormone
- Follicle stimulating hormone
- Testosterone
- Gonadotropin-releasing hormone

Fertility
- Ratio exposed: pregnant females
- Number of embryos or young per pregnant female
- Ratio viable embryos: corpora lutea
- Number 2–8 cell eggs
- Sperm per ovum

In vitro
- Incubation of sperm in agent
- Hamster egg penetration test

Other tests considered
- Tonometric measurement of testicular consistency
- Qualitative testicular histology
- Stage of cycle at which spermiation occurs
- Quantitative testicular histology

Sperm motility
- Time-exposure photography
- Multiple-exposure photography
- Cinemicrography
- Videomicrography
- Sperm membrane characteristics
- Evaluation of sperm metabolism
- Fluorescent Y bodies in spermatozoa
- Flow cytometry of spermatozoa
- Karyotyping human sperm pronuclei
- Cervical mucus penetration test

**See* Galbraith et al., 1982, for complete table and discussion of the relative usefulness of these tests.
SOURCE: Dixon, 1986, with permission.

Table 20-14
Dietary Deficiency(s) and Spermatogenic Arrest

DEFICIENCY	SPECIES
Manganese	Rats and rabbits
Vitamin A	Mice, rats, and guinea pigs
Vitamin B (pyridoxine)	Rats
Vitamine E	Rats, hamsters, and guinea pigs
Zinc	Mice, rats, dogs, and sheep

SOURCE: Mann and Lutwak-Mann, 1981, with permission.

some length of time are most likely required to detect male reproductive toxicity. Most of the tests are invasive and hence limited to animals and not generally acceptable for use in humans. Indeed, in humans, the noninvasive approaches involve sperm counts, blood gonadotrophin levels, and a nonbarren marriage. Testicular biopsy can be used in selected circumstances to evaluate spermatogenesis (i.e., infertility/sterility), but this procedure is obviously invasive. Azoospermia can be caused by certain chemical agents, genetic disorders (e.g., Klinefelter's syndrome), infections (e.g., mumps), irradiation, and hormonal defects. Dietary deficiencies are well known to cause spermatogenic arrest (Table 20-14). Similarly, lead can produce infertility, sterility, and varying abnormalities in sperm function and morphology (Table 20-10). Pogach et al., (1989) have reported that cisplatin causes Sertoli cell dysfunction in rodents. These changes in Sertoli cell function appear to be responsible for cisplatin-induced impairment in spermatogenesis. Other heavy metals such as cobalt, iron, cadmium, mercury, molybdenum, and silver can adversely affect spermatogenesis and accessory sex organ function. Dietary zinc deficiency can produce sterility (Prasad et al., 1967). Likewise, chemically induced zinc depletion (e.g., phthalates) can produce testicular damage, as evidenced by sterile seminiferous tubules (Thomas et al., 1982). In experimental animals, zinc prevents cadmium carcinogenicity in the rat testes (Koizumi and Waalkes, 1989). The major preventive effect of zinc against cadmium-induced testicular tumors may be due to its ability to reduce the cytotoxicity of cadmium in interstitial cells. Different heavy metals seem to exert their toxic effects upon different subpopulations of testicular cells (Table 20-15). Mechanisms of heavy metal toxicity vary and include not only different cell sensitivities but also direct versus indirect actions. Furthermore, it appears that primary damage to one cell type may secondarily affect other cell types in the testes.

The sensitivity of the various parameters used to evaluate the male reproductive system varies considerably. There are advantages as well as limitations to a number of standard reproductive procedures. Testicular weight is a rapid quantitative index, but this measurement is less sensitive than sperm counts and is affected by water imbibition (edema). In normal males, the number of sperm produced per day per testis is largely determined by testicular size. In many mammals, testis size is correlated to daily sperm production. Fertility as an index is quite insensitive, although it does incorporate all reproductive functions. Fertility profiles using serial mating studies to assess the biological status of sperm cells have been a useful test for both dominant lethal mutations (Epstein et al., 1972) and male reproductive capacity (Lee and Dixon, 1972). Testicular histology provides information on target cell morphology, although it too is subjective and not particularly quantitative. Histologic evaluation of the seminiferous tubules can establish cellular integrity and provide information about the process of spermatogenesis (Fig. 20-10). Good tissue fixation is essential for detecting the more subtle changes in the seminiferous epithelium (cf. Creasy, 1997). It is more difficult to detect morphologic changes in Leydig cells and to some extent Sertoli cells. Leydig cell function is better determined by evaluating androgen levels (or gonadotropins) or, in the case of Sertoli cells, by the measurement of androgen-binding protein (ABP).

In order to undertake a meaningful histologic evaluation of the testes, it is necessary to understand the spermatogenic cycle and to identify its various stages. The use of seminiferous tubule staging is very important to the evaluation of testicular injury (Creasy, 1997). If damage is detected, it must be characterized. For example, Sertoli cell damage is frequently recognized by inter- or intracellular vacuoles or by swelling of the basal Sertoli cell cyto-

Table 20-15
Summary of Cellular Site(s) of Action of Excess Heavy Metals on the Male Reproductive System

		Evidence for Testicular Toxicity (Primary or Secondary)			
METAL	EVIDENCE FOR HYPOTHALAMIC/ ADENOHYPOPHYSIAL EFFECTS	GC	LC	SC	MECHANISM/COMMENT
Cadmium	None	◑	◑	◑	Hypoxia/ischemia (Endothelial Cells)
Zinc	None	⊙	◑	⊙	Toxicity due to deficiency
Lead	Possible suppression of FSH and LH	•	•	◑?	Endocrine and paracrine toxicity
Chromium	None	•			Unknown?
Cobalt	None	◑		◑	Toxicity due to general hypoxia
Platinum	None	•	•	•	Inhibits DNA synthesis
Vanadium	None	•?			

•-Evidence for *direct* cellular action
◑-Evidence for *some direct* action, but possibly *secondarily* mediated
⊙-Deficiency of metal causes cellular toxicity
SOURCE: Thomas, 1995a, with permission.

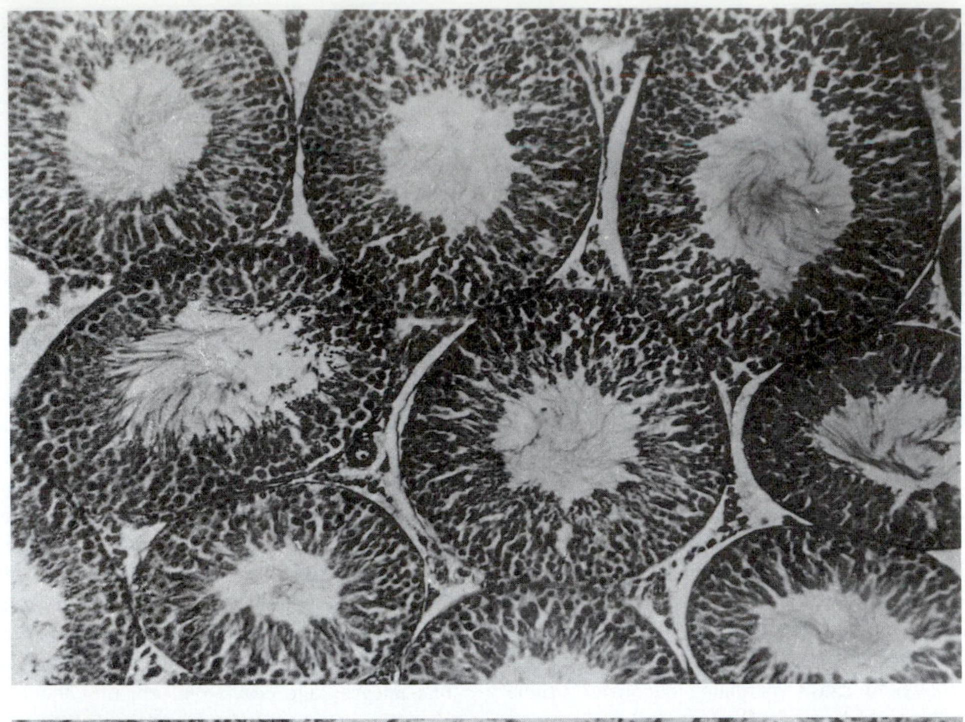

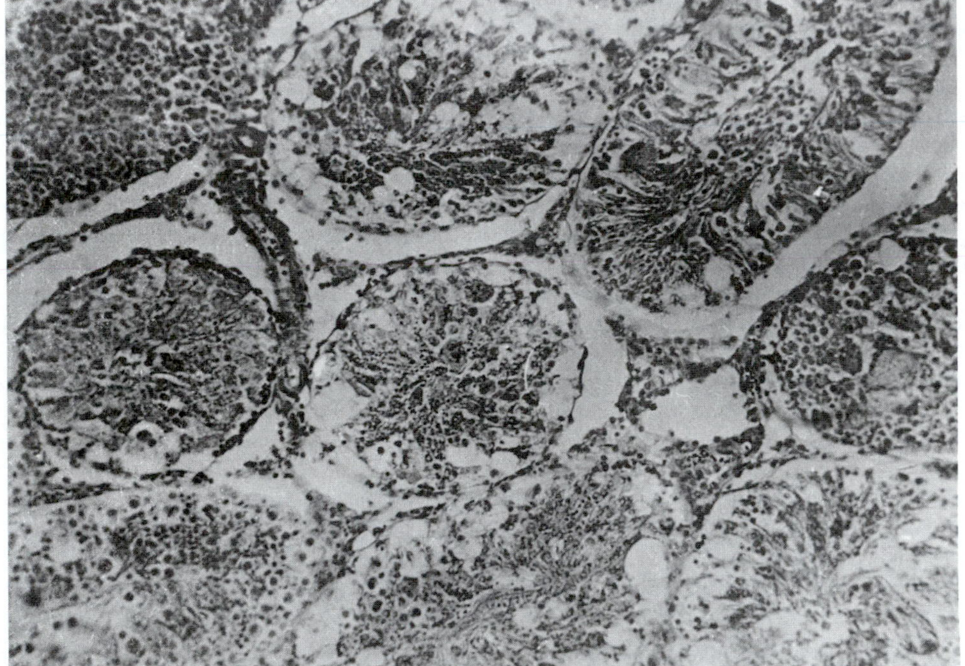

Figure 20-10. Histology section of rat testes.

Above: Normal H&E section revealing morphologic integrity of seminiferous tubules. Below: Chemically induced testicular damage resulting in vacuolation of seminiferous tubules. Note partially sterile tubules. (From Thomas and Thomas, 1994, with permission.)

plasm. Morphologic changes in the Leydig cell may be more difficult to detect. Degeneration and necrosis of germ cells can be recognized by the normal criteria of nuclear pyknosis and cytoplasmic eosinophilia. Some quantitative assessment of the histology of the testes includes measuring tubular diameter and cell counts of spermatocytes or round spermatids.

Thus, there are essentially two approaches to establishing whether or not a chemical is able to exert an adverse effect on spermatogenesis: (1) evaluation of testicular morphology (i.e., pathology) and (2) functional evaluation of spermatogenesis (Sharpe, 1998). Included in the assessment are the detection of abnormalities in spermatogenesis/testicular morphology, stage-dependent germ cell degeneration, and impairment of normal sperm release.

Flow Cytometry

Flow cytometric analyses of the testes can be used to evaluate specific cell populations (Selden et al., 1989). This technique has the advantage of being able to assess simultaneously multiple characteristics on a cell-to-cell basis, with the results being rapidly correlated for each cell type or property. Cell size, cell shape, cytoplasmic granularity and pigmentation, along with measurements of surface antigens, lectin binding, DNA/RNA, and chromatin structure are among some of the intrinsic and extrinsic parameters that can be evaluated. The toxic effects of thiotepa on mouse spermatogenesis have been determined using dual-parameter flow cytometry. The dual parameters of DNA stainability versus RNA content provide excellent resolution of testicular cell types (Evenson et al., 1986). Flow cytometry has also been used to study the effects of methyl-benzimidazol-2-yl-carbamate (MBC) on mouse germ cells. MBC exposure results in an altered ratio of testicular cell types, abnormal sperm head morphology, and altered sperm chromatin structure (Evenson et al., 1987).

Oxidative damage to spermatogenic cells has also been associated with reproductive dysfunction in laboratory animals, and this too can provide an index for assessing risk. Angioli et al., (1987) have proposed an in vitro spermatogenic cell model for assessing reproductive toxicity; it involves the ability of bleomycin to reduce oxidative changes in male germ cell populations.

Penetration of zona-free hamster eggs by human sperm has also been suggested as a useful chemical test to assess male fertility. Recently, this assay has also been recommended as a prognostic indicator in in vitro fertilization programs (Nahhas and Blumenfeld, 1989).

Sex Accessory Organs

The epididymis and the sex accessory organs can also be used to evaluate the status of male reproductive processes. While the epididymis has an important physiologic role in the male reproductive tract, it is less useful as a parameter for assessing gonadotoxins. Its histologic integrity may be examined, but the most meaningful determinations are the number of sperm stored within the cauda epididymis and a measure of sperm motility and morphology. Epididymal sperm may be extruded onto a glass slide and viewed under the microscope for motility and abnormalities. Sex accessory organs, usually the prostate (e.g., ventral lobes in the rodent) and the seminal vesicles (empty), provide a rapid and quantitative measure of the male reproductive processes that are androgen-dependent. Chemical indicators in sex accessory glands such as fructose and citric acid have also been used to evaluate male sex hormone function (cf. Mann and Lutwak-Mann, 1981).

Semen Analyses

Semen analysis can be used as an index of testicular and posttesticular organ function. Semen can be collected from a number of experimental and domestic animals using an artificial vagina. Electroejaculatory techniques and chemically induced ejaculations have also been employed to produce semen samples, particularly in animal husbandry. In humans, several trace elements—including Ca, Cd, Co, Cr, Cu, Fe, Mg, Mn, Mo, Ni, Pb, Rb, Se, Vd and Zn—can be detected in seminal plasma (Abou-Shakra et al., 1989).

Both quantitative and qualitative characteristics of more than one ejaculate must be evaluated to ensure that conclusions concerning testicular function are valid. Since semen represents contributions from accessory sex glands as well as the testes and epididymides, only the total number of sperm in an ejaculate is a reliable estimate of sperm production. The number of sperm introduced into the pelvic urethra during emission and the volume of fluid from the accessory sex glands are independent. The potential sources of error in measuring ejaculate volume, concentration, and the seminal characteristics necessary to calculate total sperm per ejaculate must be considered (Amann, 1981).

There have been recent advances in the automation of semen analysis. Semiautomated measures of sperm motility may be categorized as indirect or direct methods. Indirect methods of sperm analysis estimate mean swimming speed of cells by measuring properties of the whole sperm suspension. Spectrometry or turbidimetric methods record changes in optical density. Direct methods involve visual assessment of individual sperm cells and stem from early efforts to quantitate sperm swimming speed. Such direct measurements may include photographic methods like timed-exposure photography, multiple-exposure photography, and cinematography. Computer-aided sperm motion analysis (CASMA) may be applied to morphology, physiology, motility, or flagellar analysis. CASMA allows visualization of both digitized static and dynamic sperm images. Semen analysis and fertility assessment should recognize statistical power and experimental design for toxicologic studies (Williams et al., 1990).

Sperm Counts and Motility

Several factors affect the number of sperm in an ejaculate, including age, testicular size, frequency, degree of sexual arousal, and seasons (particularly in domestic animals) (cf. Thomas, 1996). Although ejaculatory frequency or the interval since the last ejaculation alters the total number of sperm per ejaculate, ejaculation frequency does not influence daily sperm production. However, because of epididymal storage, frequent ejaculation is necessary if the number of sperm counted in ejaculated semen is to reflect sperm production accurately. If only one or two ejaculates are collected weekly, a 50 percent reduction in sperm production probably would remain undetected. Ejaculates should be collected daily (or every other day) over a period of time. The analysis of isolated ejaculate or even several ejaculates collected at irregular intervals cannot estimate sperm production or output. The first several ejaculates in each series contain more sperm than subsequent ejaculates because the number of sperm available for ejaculation is being reduced.

In experimental animals (e.g., rodents), epididymal sperm may be extruded, diluted with saline in a hemocytometer, and counted. Sperm motility may also be assessed. Sperm morphology may be evaluated using either wet preparations or properly prepared stained smears, which require an appropriate classification scheme (Wyrobek, 1983; Wyrobek et al., 1983). Chromosomal analyses can be used in the laboratory or the clinic to diagnose certain genetic diseases.

Androgens and Their Receptors

The androgen receptor (AR) is a member of the steroid/nuclear receptor superfamily, all members of which share a basic and functional homology. AR action is highly specific in spite of the homology between AR and other steroid receptors. The AR is composed of three functional domains. The two predominant naturally occurring ligands of the AR are testosterone and dihydrotestosterone. AR exists as a phosphoprotein in different cell types (cf. MacLean et al., 1997).

Androgen receptors for testosterone and dihydrotestosterone (DHT) have also been used to evaluate the effects of various gonadotoxins. A number of divalent metal ions (Zn, Hg, Cu, Cd, etc.) can inhibit androgen-receptor binding in rodent prostate glands (Donovan et al., 1980). In addition to heavy metals interfering with androgen binding, DDT and *p,p′*-DDE are potent androgen receptor antagonists and can affect male reproduction (Kelce et al., 1995). The major metabolite of DDT, namely, *p,p′*-DDE, inhibits androgen binding to the androgen receptor as well as androgen-induced transcriptional activity. Hydroxyflutamide and *p,p′*-DDE were equally effective in inhibiting androgen-induced transcriptional activity.

Hormonally active androgens promote reproductive and anabolic (myotropic) functions. Both reproductive and anabolic effects of androgens are mediated by their interaction with AR (cf. Roy et al., 1999). Hormonally active androgens are C-19 steroids with an oxo-functional group at the C-3 position and a hydroxy group at 17β. Androgen target cells (e.g., prostate gland, seminal vesicles) contain steroid-modifying enzymes that can activate, inactivate, and alter the receptor specificity of androgens. For example, steroid 5α-reductase converts testosterone to 5α-dihydrotestosterone, which is a more potent androgenic ligand. Many factors can affect androgenic actions (Table 20-16).

Other Secretory Biomarkers

Efforts have been made to identify so-called testicular marker enzymes as indicators of normal or abnormal cellular differentiation in the gonad (Hodgen, 1977; Shen and Lee, 1977; Chapin et al., 1982). At least eight enzymes—hyaluronidase (H), lactate dehydrogenase isoenzyme-X (LDH-X), and the dehydrogenases of sorbitol (SDH), α-glycerophosphate (GPDH), glucose-6-phosphate (G6PDH), malate (MDH), glyceraldehyde-3-phosphate (G3PDH), and isocitrate (ICDH)—have been studied with regard to their usefulness as predictors of gonadal toxicity. Several genes are expressed exclusively in male germ cells (cf. Heckert and Griswold, 1993).

A number of secretory products of the Sertoli cell hold some potential for evaluating male reproductive function. Of the several secretory products of the Sertoli cell (e.g., transferrin, ceruloplasmin, tissue plasminogen activator, sulfated glycoproteins), androgen-binding protein (ABP) has perhaps received the most attention

Table 20-16
Factors Affecting Androgen Effectiveness

TARGET	EFFECT	EXAMPLE
Hypothalamic-pituitary interaction	Feedback control of LHRH-mediated gonadotropin secretion	Estrogens, progestins
Gonadotropin action	Disrupt reproductive control processes involving gonadotropins	LH-FSH antibodies
Androgen synthesis	Inhibit key enzymes, e.g., cholesterol desmolase, 17α-hydroxylase, 3 β-hydroxysteroid oxidoreductase, 5α-reductase	Steroid analogues, diphenylmethylanes (amphenone B,DDD), pyridine derivatives (SU series), disubstituted glutaric acid imides (glutethimides), triazines, hydrazines, thiosemicarbazones
DHT synthesis	Inhibit 5α-reductase in target tissue	Androstene-17-carboxylic acid, progesterone
Plasma binding	Alter ratio of bound and free androgen in systemic circulation	Estrogens
Cytoplasmic receptors	Alter effect on target tissue by affecting binding to cytoplasmic receptors	Cyproterone acetate, 17α-methyl-β-testosterone, flutamide
DHT cellular binding	Block DHT effect on target tissue	Cyproterone acetate, spironolactone, dihydroprogesterone, RU-22930

SOURCE: Dixon, 1982, with permission.

as a potential indicator for detecting gonadal injury. Sertoli cell ABP and testicular transferrin may be affected by similar regulatory agents (e.g., FSH, insulin) (Skinner et al., 1989). Leydig cell cultures can also be considered as a potential indicator to evaluate endocrine function of the gonad (Brun et al., 1991). Pig Leydig cell culture can be used to discriminate between specific and nonspecific inhibitors of steroidogenesis. Leydig cells, like Sertoli cells, secrete a number of proteins, peptides, and other substances [e.g., β-endorphin, corticotropin-releasing factor (CRF)] (Eskeland et al., 1989). The testes contain various neuropeptides and growth factors. These include LHRH, TRH, POMC, oxytocin, vasopressin and still other peptide precursors (cf. Shioda et al., 1994; Spiteri-Grech and Nieschlag, 1993). Many of these factors are involved in the autocrine or paracrine regulation of the testes (Table 20-2). Other than the inhibitory actions of DBCP on Sertoli cell ABP secretions, neither this cell and its secretions nor the Leydig cell has been used in reproductive toxicology evaluation.

TESTING FEMALE REPRODUCTIVE CAPACITY

General Considerations

The evaluation of mammalian reproductive processes is far more complex in the female than in the male. Female reproductive processes involve oogenesis, ovulation, the development of sexual receptivity, coitus, gamete and zygote transport, fertilization, and implantation of the concepters. All these processes or events offer potential opportunities for chemical or drug interference.

Evaluation of the female reproductive tract for toxicologic perturbations not surprisingly may overlap with testing methods for assessing teratogenicity and mutagenicity. Indeed, reproductive endpoints that indicate dysfunction in the female (Table 20-17), including perinatal parameters, often overlap with developmental toxicity endpoints (Table 20-18). The neonate is particularly sensitive to a variety of drugs and chemicals (Thomas, 1989).

Gross pathology (e.g., gravimetric responses—ovary, uterus, etc.) and histopathology are important to reproductivity and should be evaluated (Ettlin and Dixon, 1985). Both light microscopy and electron (transmission and scanning) microscopy may be useful in assessing ovarian and pituitary ultrastructure. As in the male (Table 20-13), there are a number of useful tests to evaluate the female reproductive system (Table 20-17). These tests can be performed on a wide variety of endpoints, at different anatomic sites, and can include biochemical, hormonal, or morphologic parameters.

Oogenesis/Folliculogenesis

Methods to assess directly the effects of test compounds on oogenesis and/or folliculogenesis include histologic determination of oocytes and/or follicle number (Dobson et al., 1978). Chemical effects on oogenesis can be measured indirectly by determining the fertility of the offspring (McLachlan et al., 1981; Kimmel et al., 1995; Davis and Heindel, 1998). Other indirect measures of ovarian toxicity in animals include assessment of age at vaginal opening, onset of reproductive senescence, and total reproductive capacity (Gellert, 1978; Khan-Dawood and Satyaswaroop, 1995).

Morphologic tests can quantify and assess primordial germ cell number, stem cell migration, oogonial proliferation, and urogenital ridge development. In vitro techniques can be used to evaluate primordial germ cell proliferation, migration, ovarian differentiation, and folliculogenesis (Ways et al., 1980; Thompson, 1981).

Serial oocyte counts can monitor oocyte and/or follicle destruction in experimental animals (Pedersen and Peters, 1968). This approach is a reliable means of quantifying the effects of chemicals on oocytes and follicles.

Follicular growth may be assayed in experimental animals using (^{3}H)-thymidine uptake, ovarian response to gonadotropins, and follicular kinetics (Hillier et al., 1980). These approaches identify both direct and indirect effects on follicular growth and identify drugs and other environmental chemicals that are ovotoxic (Mattison and Nightingale, 1980).

Estrogens and Their Receptors

The rat, mouse, and human estrogen receptor (ER) exists as two subtypes, ERα and ERβ, which differ in the C-terminal ligand-binding domain and in the N-terminal transactivation domain (Kuiper et al., 1998). Estrogen influences the growth, differentiation, and functioning of several target organs. Such organs include the mammary gland, uterus, vagina, ovary, and several male reproductive system organs (e.g., testes, prostate gland, etc.). Estrogens affect osteogenesis and the CNS and seem to play a role in the cardiovascular system's homeostasis. Estrogens migrate in and out of cells but are retained with high affinity and specificity in certain target tissues by an intranuclear binding protein called the estrogen receptor (ER). The newly discovered ERβ is an important sex hormone receptor not only in the female, but also in the male. It has been suggested that a possible physiologic ligand for ERβ in the male is 5α-androstane-3β,17β-diol. This testosterone metabolite binds more firmly to ERβ than to ERα. ERα and ERβ are differentially expressed along the length of the male reproductive tract. ER are expressed in the Sertoli cell, the Leydig cell, and the epididymis and accessory sex organs. ERβ is expressed in Sertoli cells and in most germ cells. The presence of aromatase activity in these two cells suggests that estrogens may be involved in the modulation of spermatogenesis. ERβ is expressed in the rodent and human testes (van Pelt et al., 1999). ERα is localized in the nuclei of Leydig cells in fetal and adult rodent testes.

The biological activity of estrogens (and progesterone) is manifest through high-affinity receptors located in the nuclei of specific target cells (Vegeto et al., 1996). The receptors for estrogen (and progesterone) are members of a large superfamily of nuclear proteins. Nuclear hormone receptors are single polypeptides organized into discrete functional domains (i.e., regions A through F).

It is understood that the activation of steroid hormone receptors (e.g., estrogen) regulates the transcriptional activity of specific genes, hence mediating classic or genomic actions of steroid hormones. However, not all steroid effects can be explained by such a classic model of steroid-target cell interaction. Instead, signal-generating steroid receptors on the cell surface have been referred to as nonclassic, nongenomic steroid effects (Revelli et al., 1998). There are several cell types within the reproductive system wherein estrogens exert early physiologic effects that are too rapid to be mediated by the sequence of genomic activation. Signal transduction mechanisms involving nongenomic steroid effects are particularly evident in spermatozoa. Most nongenomic actions of steroids seem to involve Ca^{2+} as a second messenger. It is possible that nongenomic and genomic actions may synergize, resulting in both rapid onset and long-lasting or persistent actions.

Table 20-17
Potentially Useful Tests of Female Reproductive Toxicity

Body Weight	*Oviduct*
Ovary	Histology
Organ weight	Gamete transport
Histology	Fertilization
Number of oocytes	Transport of early embryo
Rate of follicular atresia	*Uterus*
Follicular steroidogenesis	Cytology and histology
Follicular maturation	Luminal fluid analysis (xenobiotics, proteins)
Oocyte maturation	Decidual response
Ovulation	Dysfunctional bleeding
Luteal function	*Cervix/vulva/vagina*
Hypothalamus	Cytology
Histology	Histology
Altered synthesis and release of neurotransmitters, neuromodulators, and neurohormones	Mucus production
Pituitary	Mucus quality (sperm penetration test)
Histology	*Fertility*
Altered synthesis and release of trophic hormones	Ratio exposed: pregnant females
Endocrine	Number of embryos or young per pregnant female
Gonadotropin	Ratio viable embryos: corpora lutea
Chorionic gonadotropin levels	Ratio implantation: corpora lutea
Estrogen and progesterone	Number 2–8 cell eggs
	In Vitro
	In vitro fertilization of superovulated eggs, either exposed to chemical in culture or from treated females

SOURCE: Modified from Dixon, 1986, with permission.

Table 20-18
Developmental Toxicity Endpoints

Type I changes
(Outcomes permanent, life-threatening, and frequently associated with gross malformations)
Reduction of number of live births (litter size)
Increased number of stillbirths
Reduced number of live fetuses (litter size)
Increased number of resorptions
Increased number of fetuses with malformations
Type II changes
(Outcomes nonpermanent, non-life-threatening, and not associated with malformations)
Reduced birth weights
Reduced postnatal survival
Decreased postnatal growth, reproductive capacity
Increased number of fetuses with retarded development

SOURCES: Frankos, 1985; Collins et al., 1998.

Serum levels of estrogen or estrogenic effects on target tissues are indicators of normal follicular function. Tissue and organ responses include time of vaginal opening in immature rats, uterine weight, endometrial morphology, and/or serum levels of FSH and LH. Granulosa cell culture techniques provide direct screens of the ability of chemicals to inhibit cell proliferation and/or estrogen production (Zeleznik et al., 1979). The biosynthesis of estradiol and its metabolism to estrone and estriol by the ovary constitutes another indicator of the reproductive process. The peripheral catabolism of these steroids is principally a function of the liver.

Nuclear and cytoplasmic estrogen/progesterone may provide important toxicologic applications. Estradiol and progesterone receptors are especially important since chemicals (e.g., DDT and other organochlorine pesticides) compete for these receptors and perhaps alter their molecular conformation (Thomas, 1975).

Ovulation/Fertilization/Implantation

Ovulation differs among various mammalian species. Some animals ovulate spontaneously upon copulation (e.g., the rabbit), whereas other species (e.g., humans and subhuman primates) have a hormonally dependent cycle. Several steroidal and nonsteroidal agents can interfere with this neuroendocrine process of ovulation. In the estrus cycle of rodents, ovulation occurs at intervals of 4 to 5 days. Ovulation occurs during estrus and can be readily detected by cornification of vaginal epithelium. The rat's estrus cycle can be divided into four stages and can be recognized by changes in vaginal cytology: proestrus, estrus, metestrus, and diestrus.

The processes of fertilization and implantation can be affected by both chemicals and drugs. The formation, maturation, and union of germ cells compose a complex physiologic event that is sensitive to foreign substances. Fertilization can also be achieved in vitro with sperm and ova extradited from a variety of different mammalian species including humans.

Reproductive performance is best assessed by pregnancy, and this represents a successful index for evaluating endocrine toxicity (or lack thereof). The mating study using rats is a fundamental procedure that determines total reproductive capacity.

REPRODUCTIVE TESTS AND REGULATORY REQUIREMENTS

General Considerations

The history of reproductive guidelines has recently been reviewed (Collins et al., 1998). Over the years several attempts have been made to standardize testing methods. Testing procedures to simulate human exposure have taken two different paths. One is based on the premise that specific injury from a chemical/drug can be more readily established by administering it only during certain periods of gestation. The second path was devised for compounds likely to involve chronic exposure and for which there may be a concentration factor when administered during several generations. Over the years, many efforts have been undertaken to harmonize testing guidelines (Christian, 1992; 2001.)

Guidelines

Testing guidelines for evaluating reproductive and developmental toxicity in females are outlined in Table 20-19 (Collins et al., 1998) (see also Chap. 10, "Developmental Toxicology"). It may be seen that there is reasonable harmonization between the various regulatory agencies. This condensed table (Table 20-19) does not reveal the protocol for mating procedures, F1 mating, second mating, and other experimental design conditions, but they too are similar among the various regulatory agencies. The reproductive study guidelines of the U.S. Food and Drug Administration (FDA) harmonize with those of the Environmental Protection Agency (EPA) and the [OECD (Organization for Economic Cooperation and Development)]. Some of the guidelines of the [ICH (International Conference on Harmonization)] are blank because these guidelines are intended to be generic (Collins et al., 1998). While guidelines are reviewed periodically to keep abreast of changing science and technology, the FDA's *Redbook II* has reduced the number of generations from three to two. The number of litters/generations has been decreased from two to one. Monitoring of estrous cycle, time of vaginal opening, and time of preputial separation are new requirements. The amount of histopathology, particularly of the pups, has been increased (Collins et al., 1998).

Reproduction (multigenerational) study test guidelines have also undergone some revisions (Collins et al., 1998). The FDA prefers that either the rat or the rabbit be used, with the choice of species based on pharmacokinetic differences. The EPA, OECD, and ICH recommend the most relevant species, but again the rat or the rabbit is often preferred. At least three dose levels are recommended. All adults must undergo necropsy with examination of the uterus and placenta.

The minimal reproductive study recommended consists of two generations, with one litter per generation (Collins et al., 1999). The guideline contains optional procedures for inclusion of additional litters per generation, additional generations, a test for teratogenic and developmental toxicity effects, optional neurotoxicity screening, and optional immunotoxicity screening.

Endpoints—Females

Endpoints in studies of female reproductive toxicity include the following:

- Female fertility index
  [(number of pregnancies/number of matings) × 100]
- Gestation index
  [(number of litters—live pups/number of pregnancies) × 100]
- Live-born index
  [(number of pups born alive/total number of pups born) × 100]
- Weaning index
  [(number of pups alive at day 21/number of pups alive and kept on day 4) × 100]
- Sex ratio and percentage by sex
- Viability index
  [(number of pups alive on day 7/number of pups alive and kept on day 4) × 100]

Endpoints—Males

The endpoints of male reproductive toxicity include the following:

- Evaluation of testicular spermatid numbers
- Sperm evaluation for motility, morphology and numbers

Table 20-19
Comparison of Reproductive Guidelines

	U.S. FDA (1993)	U.S. EPA (1996)	OECD (1996)	ICH (U.S. FDA, 1994)
Number of generations	Two, one litter/generation	Two	Two	Two
Animal species	Rodent	Rat (preferred)	Rat (preferred)	Rat (preferred)
Age of animals	5–9 weeks	5–9 weeks	6–9 weeks	
Number of animals	30/sex	At least 20 pregnant	At least 20 pregnant	Sufficient to allow meaningful interpretation
Dose levels	Minimum three dose levels	Minimum three dose levels	Minimum three dose levels	Minimum three dose levels
Route of administration	Oral (preferred) diet, drinking water, gavage	Oral (preferred) diet, drinking water, gavage	Oral (preferred) diet, drinking water, gavage	Determined by intended human usage
Dosing schedule	8–11 weeks before mating, throughout mating and pregnancy	10 weeks before mating; dosing continued during mating and pregnancy	10 weeks before mating; dosing continued during mating and pregnancy	Treat males and females before mating, during mating and through implantation. Other treatment regimens required.

SOURCE: Condensed and modified from Collins et al., 1998, with permission. See original table for more detailed information.

Sperm motility can be assessed by microscopic techniques or with a computer-assisted sperm analysis (CASA) system (Seed et al., 1996). Sperm (minimum 200 per sample) from the cauda epididymis or proximal vas deferens should be examined as a fixed wet preparation and classified as either normal or abnormal (Clegg et al., 2001). Total sperm counts in the cauda epididymis can be assessed (Robb et al., 1978).

Both the FDA and the EPA have established study protocols to assess the reproductive risks of chemicals and drugs. The FDA imposes guidelines for drugs that includes three different protocols (namely segments) on development, fertility, and general reproductive performance:

Segment I: Fertility and Reproduction Function in Males and Females
Segment II: Developmental Toxicology and Teratology
Segment III: Perinatal and Postnatal Studies

Segment I studies are initial studies often leading to additional protocols such as developmental protocols. By using pregnant animals (e.g., segment III) that are treated for the last third of their period of gestation, including lactation and weaning, assessment can be made about the effects of chemical and/or drug exposure on late fetal development, particularly lactation and offspring survival.

The National Toxicology Program (NTP) adopted the Fertility Assessment by Continuous Breeding (FACB) protocol in the early 1980s. The FACB protocol was introduced by McLachlan et al. (1981) and was designed to reduce the time for reproductive toxicity testing yet still provide data comparable with those obtained from other testing systems. FACB tests take no longer than the improved and shortened EPA test designs. The FACB protocol uses more animals per group and in general increases the statistical power of the assay. Morrissey et al. (1988) have evaluated the effectiveness of continuous breeding reproduction studies. This subtle modification of increasing the statistical power of the assay is important, since fertility is an especially important indicator of reproductive toxicity and is one of the least sensitive indicators in the assessment of the reproductive system (Schwetz et al., 1980). Experimental design for toxicologic studies, particularly in studies involving semen analysis and fertility assessment, must recognize statistical power (Williams et al., 1990).

Reproductive toxicity studies extending over multiple generations are scientifically and logistically difficult to manage, interpret, and finance (Johnson, 1986). While the FDA segment tests are collectively very meaningful in assessing reproductive toxicity (or safety), none of these batteries of tests can replace the other, and the multigeneration evaluation has considerable scientific merit for justifying their expense. However, current multigeneration protocols could be revised in order to improve on the toxicologic information collected. FDA reproductive testing guidelines require preclinical animal testing for each new drug depending on how women might be exposed to the drug itself. The FDA further categorizes drugs on five different levels, depending on potential risk (e.g., category A, no evidence of human development toxicity, to category D or X, demonstrated birth defects) (cf. Frankos, 1985).

It is evident that a number of test systems are available to assess the degree of change in the reproductive system. Some such tests employ many animals and follow their reproductive histories for more than one generation, whereas others employ cell systems that are perhaps representative of a molecular approach to determining mechanisms of toxicologic action.

HUMAN RISK FACTORS AFFECTING FERTILITY

General Considerations

Most humans are exposed to a vast number of chemicals that may be hazardous to their reproductive capacity (Faber and Hughes, 1995). Many chemicals have been identified as reproductive hazards in laboratory studies (Clegg et al., 1986; 2001; Working, 1988). Although the extrapolation of data from laboratory animals to humans is inexact, a number of these chemicals have also been shown to exert detrimental effects on human reproductive performance. The list includes drugs, especially steroid hormones and chemotherapeutic agents; metals and trace elements; pesticides; food additives and contaminants; industrial chemicals; and consumer products.

Fertility in humans, like that in experimental animals, is susceptible to toxic effects from environmental and/or industrial chemicals. Infertility is a problem of increasing concern in several industrialized countries. Levine (1983) has suggested methods for detecting occupational causes of male infertility. The decrease in sperm quality purportedly having occurred over the past 50 years (Carlsen et al., 1992) has been refuted as being due to the lower reference standards (cf. Bromwich et al., 1994). Furthermore, a comparison of the production of spermatozoa from the testes of different species reveals that the output of sperm in humans is approximately four times less than that in other mammals in terms of the number of sperm produced per gram of tissue (Amann and Howard, 1980).

Male

It has also been suggested that the human male is more vulnerable to environmental and occupational toxins than other mammals (Overstreet, 1984; Overstreet et al., 1988). Reproductive hazards and reproductive risks have led to the formulation of protection policies in certain occupations (Perrolle, 1993; Sattler, 1992; Thomas and Barsano, 1994). The somewhat fragile nature of the male reproductive system to occupational exposure to the fungicide DBCP was reaffirmed when Whorton et al. (1977) described its injurious effects on the testes. Fortunately, recovery from severe oligospermia after DBCP exposure has been reported by Lantz et al. (1981). Levine et al. (1983), however, have indicated that reproductive histories are superior to sperm counts in assessing male infertility caused by DBCP.

It has been extremely difficult to directly correlate human exposure to occupational chemicals with alterations in the reproductive system. A particularly complicating factor in this lack of correlation is that the normal reproductive processes seldom operate at a physiologic optimum. For example, as many as 15 percent of all married couples in the United States are defined as being clinically infertile (MacLeod, 1971), whereas another 25 percent of the women exhibit impaired fecundity (Mosher, 1981). At least 30 percent of early human conceptions and up to 15 percent of recognized pregnancies are terminated by spontaneous abortion (cf. Haney, 1985). Of the 15 percent of spontaneous abortions that terminate recognized pregnancies, about 25 percent involve abnormalities related to genetic etiologies and another 7 percent are caused by so-called environmental agents. By far, most of these abortions are due to unknown factors, and this constitutes about 7 percent of the cases of spontaneous abortions.

It is noteworthy that chronic illness may have a profound affect on gonadal function (Turner and Wass, 1997). Several systemic illnesses can reduce spermatogenesis, including thyrotoxicosis, hypothyroidism, renal failure, mumps, and Crohn's disease. A large number of nonhormonal diseases can likewise decrease serum testosterone as well as gonadotrophins. Aging, nutritional deficiencies, and obesity can affect fertility. Thus, a host of both endocrine and nonendocrine diseases can affect male fertility.

Female

Many factors can affect the normalcy of the female reproductive system, as evidenced by variations in the menstrual process. Hence, physiologic, sociologic, and psychological factors have been linked with menstrual disorders. Factors that are known to affect menstruation yet are for the most part completely unrelated to occupational settings include age, body weight extremes, liver disease, thyroid dysfunction, intrauterine contraceptive devices, stress, exercise, and marital status. It is, therefore, obvious that a number of factors can affect menstruation and that these factors do not even include such things as therapeutic drugs (Selevan et al., 1985), so-called recreational drugs, or potentially toxic substances present in occupational environments. Even the choice of control populations in studies involving the adverse effects on the reproductive system can affect the risk estimates.

EXTRAPOLATION OF ANIMAL DATA TO HUMANS

The exclusive use of animal experimental results to predict outcomes in humans still represents an uncertainty. This uncertainty can be somewhat relieved if findings from multiple species are known, particularly subhuman primates, and there are epidemiologic studies that help substantiate laboratory experiments. While there are many general similarities among mammals with respect to their response to drugs and/or chemicals, there are nevertheless some notable differences. Many of these species differences can be attributed to toxicokinetics, especially biotransformation. Greater predictability can be seen in results from well-validated animal models. Clegg et al. (2001), Buiatti et al. (1984), and Paul (1988) have reviewed several factors that are important in assessing risk to the male reproductive system. It is considerably easier to extrapolate controlled drug studies in animals to exact therapeutic regimens in humans than it is to simulate a chemical's exposure in an animal to a presumed environmental exposure in humans. Occupational exposures are inexact, and environmental levels are even more difficult to document (cf. Lemasters and Selevan, 1984). Exposures usually involve mixtures of chemicals, and individuals may not be aware of all the chemicals with which they come into contact. Thus, the effect of individual chemicals is difficult to assess, and cause-and-effect relationships are nearly impossible to establish.

Ulbrich and Palmer (1995) have undertaken a large survey of medicinal products in an effort to match human (male) and several experimental animals with respect to reproductive endpoints (e.g., spermatogenesis, sperm counts, sperm motility, etc.). The survey included a wide range of medicinal products, both hormonal and nonhormonal formulations. Sperm analysis results were comparable to results obtained by histopathology and/or organ weight changes following drug administration. Validation of sperm analyses is problematic but provides a realistic alternative to histopathology and organ weight when the latter are impractical.

EPIDEMIOLOGIC STUDIES

Epidemiology is increasingly important in establishing cause-and-effect relationships (Scialli and Lemasters, 1995). Epidemiology and risk assessment are inextricably related. Reproductive surveillance programs are important underpinnings for monitoring endocrine processes. By closely monitoring worker exposures to industrial/environmental toxicants, safer conditions will be established.

If exposure to a chemical has occurred in a human population or if concern surrounds the use of a certain chemical, epidemiologic studies may be used to identify effects on reproduction. Sheikh (1987) has pointed out factors that are important in selecting control populations for studying adverse reproductive effects on occupational environments. The design of epidemiologic studies may involve either retrospective or prospective gathering of data. Statistical aspects to be considered in epidemiologic studies include power, sample size, significance level, and magnitude of effect.

REFERENCES

Abou-Shakra FR, Ward NI, Everard DM: The role of trace elements in male infertility. *Fertil Steril.* 52:307–310, 1989.

Albro PW, Chapin RE, Corbett JT, et al: Mono-2-ethylhexyl phthalate, a metabolite of di-(2-ethylhexyl) phthalate, causally linked to testicular atrophy in rats. *Toxicol Appl Pharmacol* 100:193–200, 1989.

AMA Council on Scientific Affairs: Effects of toxic chemicals on the reproductive system. *JAMA* 253:3431–3437, 1985.

Amann RP: A critical review of methods for evaluation of spermatogenesis from seminal characteristics. *J Androl* 2:37–58, 1981.

Amann RP: Detection of alterations in testicular and epididymal function in laboratory animals. *Environ Health Perspect* 70:149–158, 1986.

Amann RP: Structure and function of the normal testis and epididymis. *J Am Coll Toxicol* 8:457–471, 1989.

Amann RP, Howard SS: Daily spermatozoal production and epididymal spermatozoal reserves of the human male. *J Urol,* 124:211–219, 1980.

Anderson RA Jr, Berryman SH, Phillips JF, et al: Biochemical and structural evidence for ethanol-induced impairment of testicular development: Apparent lack of Leydig cell involvement. *Toxicol Appl Pharmacol,* 100:62–85, 1989.

Andersson, KE, Wagner G: Physiology of penile erection. *Physiol Rev* 75:191–236, 1995.

Angioli MP, Ramos K, Rosenblum IY: Interactions of bleomycin with reduced and oxidized ion in rat spermatogenic cells. *In Vitro Toxicol* 1:45–54, 1987.

Baker DB, Landrigan PJ: Occupationally related disorders. *Med Clin North Am,* 74:441–460, 1990.

Barlow SM, Sullivan FM: *Reproductive Hazards of Industrial Chemicals.* London: Academic Press, 1982.

Barsano CP, Thomas JA: Endocrine disorders of occupational and environmental origin. *Occup Med* 7:479–502, 1992.

Battershill JM: Review of the safety assessment of polychlorinated biphenlyls (PCBs) with particular reference to reproductive toxicity. *Hum Exp Toxicol* 13:581–587, 1994.

Bell JU, Thomas JA: Effects of lead on the reproductive system, in Singhal RL, Thomas JA (eds): *Basic and Clinical Toxicity of Lead.* Baltimore: Urban & Schwarzenberg, 1980, pp 169–189.

Biciková M, Hill M, Hampl R, et al: Inhibition of rat renal and testicular 11β-hydroxysteroid dehydrogenase by some antihypertensive drugs, diuretics, and epitestosterone. *Horm Metab Res* 29:465–468, 1997.

Billig H, Chun SY, Eisenhauer K, et al: Gonadal cell apoptosis: Hormone-regulated cell demise. *Hum Reprod Update* 2:2, 103–117, 1996.

Billig H, Furuta I, Rivier C, et al: Apoptosis in testis germ cells: Developmental changes in gonadotropin dependence and localization to selective tubule stages. *Endocrinology* 136:5–12, 1995.

Birnbaum LS: Developmental effects of dioxins, in Korach K (ed): *Reproductive and Developmental Toxicology.* New York: Marcel Dekker, 1998, pp 87–112.

Bjerke DJ, Peterson RE: Reproductive toxicity of 2,3,7,8-Tetrachlorodibenzo-*p*-dioxin in male rats: Different effects of *in utero* versus lactational exposure. *Toxicol Appl Pharmacol* 127:241–249, 1994.

Blackburn DM, Gray AJ, Lloyd SC, et al: A comparison of the effects of the three isomers of dinitrobenzene on the testis in the rat. *Toxicol Appl Pharmacol* 92:54–64, 1988.

Blazak WF, Ernest TL, Stewart BE: Potential indicators of reproductive toxicity: Testicular sperm production and epididymal sperm number, transit time, and motility in Fischer 344 rats. *Fund Appl Toxicol* 5:1097–1103, 1985.

Bloch E, Gondos B, Gatz M, et al: Reproductive toxicity of 2,4-dinitrobenzene in the rat. *Toxicol Appl Pharmacol,* 94:466–472, 1988.

Boekelheide, K: 2,5-Hexanedione alters microtubule assembly: I. Testicular atrophy, not nervous system toxicity, correlates with enhanced tubulin polymerization. *Toxicol Appl Pharmacol,* 88:370–382, 1987.

Boekelheide, K: Rat testis during 2,5-hexanedione intoxication and recovery: II. Dynamic of pyrrole reactivity, tubulin content, and microtubule assembly. *Toxicol Appl Pharmacol* 92:28–33, 1988.

Bond MB: Role of corporate policy on reproductive hazards of the workplace. *J Occup Med* 28:193–199, 1986.

Bremner WJ, Millar MR, Sharpe RM, et al: Immunohistochemical localization of androgen receptors in the rat testis: Evidence for stage-dependent expression and regulation by androgens. *Endocrinology* 135:1227–1353, 1994.

Brinster RL, Zimmerman JW: Spermatogenesis following male germ-cell transplantation. *Proc Natl Acad Sci USA* 91:11298–11302, 1994.

Bromwich P, Cohen J, Stewart J, et al: Decline in sperm counts: An artifact of changed reference range of "normal"? *Br Med J* 309:10–20, 1994.

Brun HP, Leonard JF, Moronvalle V, et al: Pig Leydig cell culture: A useful *in vitro* test for evaluating the testicular toxicity of compounds. *Toxicol Appl Pharmacol* 108:307–320, 1991.

Buchanan JF, Davis LJ: Drug-induced infertility. *Drug Intell Clin Pharm* 18:122–132, 1984.

Buiatti E, Barchielli A, Geddes M, et al: Risk factors in male infertility: A case-control study. *Arch Environ Health* 39:266–270, 1984.

Byers SW, Sujarit S, Jegou B, et al: Cadherins and cadherin-associated molecules in the developing and maturing rat testis. *Endocrinology* 134:630–639, 1993.

Carlsen E, Giwercman A, Keiding N, et al: Evidence for decreasing quality of semen during past 50 years. *Br Med J* 305:609–612, 1992.

Chahoud I, Hartmann J, Rune GM, et al: Reproductive toxicity and toxicokinetics of 2,3,7,8-tetrachlorodibenzo-*p*-dioxin. *Arch Toxicol* 66:567–572, 1992.

Chapin RE, Gray TJB, Phelps JL, et al: The effects of mono-(2-ethylhexyl)-phthalate on rat Sertoli cell-enriched primary cultures. *Toxicol Appl Pharmacol* 92:467–479, 1988.

Chapin RE, Norton RM, Popp JA, et al: The effects of 2,5-hexanedione on reproductive hormones and testicular enzyme activities in the F-344 rat. *Toxicol Appl Pharmacol* 62:262–272, 1982.

Chapman RM: Gonadal injury resulting from chemotherapy. *Am J Ind Med* 4:149–161, 1983.

Christian MS: Harmonization of reproductive guidelines: Perspective from the International Federation of Teratology Societies. *J Am Coll Toxicol* 11:299–302, 1992.

Christian, MS: Test methods for assessing female reproductive and developmental toxicity, in Hayes AW (ed): *Principles and Methods of Toxicology*, 4th ed. Philadelphia: Taylor & Francis, 2001, pp 1301–1381.

Clegg ED, Sakai CS, Voytek PE: Assessment of reproductive risks. *Biol Reprod* 34:5–16, 1986.

Clegg ED, Perreault, SD, Klinefelter GR: Assessment of male reproductive toxicity, in Hayes AW (ed): *Principles and Methods of Toxicology*, 4th ed. Philadelphia: Taylor & Francis, 2001, pp 1263–1300.

Colborn T, vom Saal FS, Soto AM: Developmental effects of endocrine-disrupting chemicals in wildlife and humans. *Environ Health Perspect* 101:378–384, 1993.

Colby H: Adrenal gland toxicity: Chemically-induced dysfunction. *J Am Coll Toxicol* 7:45–69, 1988.

Collins TFX, Sprando RL, Hansen DL, et al: Testing guidelines for evaluation of reproductive and developmental toxicity of food additives in females. *Int J Toxicol* 17:299–325, 1998.

Collins TFX, Sprando RL, Shackelford ME, et al: Food and Drug Administration proposed testing guidelines for reproduction studies. *Regul Toxicol Pharmacol* 30:29–38, 1999.

Comereski CR, Bergman CL, Buroker RA: Testicular toxicity of *N*-methyltetrazolethiol cephalosporin analogues in the juvenile rat. *Fund Appl Toxicol* 8:280–289, 1987.

Cook JC, Klinefelter GR, Hardisty JF, et al: Rodent Leydig cell tumorigenesis: A review of the physiology, pathology, mechanisms, and relevance to humans. *Crit Rev Toxicol* 29:2, 169–261, 1999.

Cooper RL, Goldman JM, Tyrey L: The hypothalamus and pituitary as targets for reproductive toxicants, in Korach KS (ed): *Reproductive and Developmental Toxicology.* New York: Marcel Dekker, 1998, pp 195–210.

Cooper RL, Kavlock RJ: Endocrine disruptors and reproductive development: A weight-of-evidence overview. *J Endocrinol* 152:159–166, 1997.

Cooper TG: *The Epididymis, Sperm Maturation and Fertilization.* Berlin: Springer-Verlag, 1986.

Creasy DM: Evaluation of testicular toxicity in safety evaluation studies: The appropriate use of spermatogenic staging. *Toxicol Pathol* 25:119–131, 1997.

Davis BJ, Heindel JJ: Ovarian toxicants: multiple mechanisms of action, in Korach KS (ed): *Reproduction and Developmental Toxicology.* New York: Marcel Dekker, 1998, pp 375–398.

Davis BJ, Maronpot RR, Heindel JJ: Di-(2-ethylhexyl) Phthalate suppresses estradiol and ovulation in cycling rats. *Toxicol Appl Pharmacol* 128:216–223, 1994a.

Davis BJ, Weaver R, Gaines LJ, et al: Mono-(2-ethylhexyl) phthalate suppresses estradiol production independent of FSH-cAMP: Stimulation in rat granulosa cells. *Toxicol Appl Pharmacol* 128:224–228, 1994b.

De La Chapelle A: The Y-chromosomal and autosomal testis-determining genes, in Goodfellow PN, Craig IW, Smith JC, Wolfe J (eds): The sex-determining factor. *Development* 101 (suppl):33–38, 1987.

De Rooij D, Lok D: Regulation of the density of spermatogonia in the seminiferous epitheliium of the Chinese hamster, II. *Anat Rec* 217:131–136, 1987.

Dickson LC, Buzik SC: Health risks of "dioxins": A review of environmental and toxicological considerations. *Vet Hum Toxicol* 35:68–77, 1993.

Dixon RL: Potential of environmental factors to affect development of reproductive system. *Fund Appl Toxicol* 2:5–12, 1982.

Dixon RL: Toxic responses of the reproductive system, in, Klaassen CD, Amdur MO, Doull J (eds): *Casarett and Doull's Toxicology: The Basic Science of Poisons,* 3d ed. New York: Macmillian, 1986.

Dixon RL, Lee IP: Pharmacokinetic and adaptation factors in testicular toxicity. *Fed Proc* 39:66–72, 1980.

Dobson RL, Koehler CG, Felton JS, et al: Vulnerability of female germ cells in developing mice and monkeys to tritium, gamma rays, and polycyclic aromatic hydrocarbons, in Mahlum DD, Sikor MR, Hackett PL, Andrew FD (eds): *Developmental Toxicology of Energy-Related Pollutants. Conference 771017.* Washington, DC: U.S. Department of Energy Technical Information Center, 1978.

Doering PL, Davidson CL, LaFauce L, et al: Effects of cocaine on the human fetus: A review of clinical studies. *Drug Intellig Clin Pharm* 23:639–645, 1989.

Donaubauer AH, Kramer M, Krein K, et al.: Investigations of the carcinogenicity of the LH-RH analog buserelin (HOE 766) in rats using the subcutaneous route of administration. *Fund Appl Toxicol* 9:738–752, 1987.

Donovan MP, Schein LG, Thomas JA: Inhibition of androgen-receptor interaction in mouse prostate gland cytosol by divalent metal ions. *Mol Pharmacol* 17:156–162, 1980.

Dym M, Fawcett DW: The blood-testis barrier in the rat and the physiological compartmentation of the seminiferous ephithelium. *Biol Reprod* 3:300–326, 1970.

Eckols K, Williams J, Uphouse L: Effects of chlordecone on progesterone receptors in immature and adult rats. *Toxicol Appl Pharmacol* 100:506–516, 1989.

Effendy I, Krause W: In vivo effects of terbinafine and ketoconazole on testosterone plasma levels in healthy males. *Dermatologica* 178:103–106, 1989.

Epstein SS, Arnold E, Andrea J, et al: Detection of chemical mutagens by the dominant lethal assay in mice. *Toxicol Appl Pharmacol* 23:288–325, 1972.

Eskeland NL, Lugo DI, Pintar JE, et al: Stimulation of beta-endorphin secretion by corticotropin-releasing factor in primary rat Leydig cell cultures. *Endocrinology* 124:2914–2919, 1989.

Ettlin RA, Dixon RL: Reproductive toxicology, in Mottet NK (ed): *Environmental Pathology, Chemicals.* New York: Oxford University Press, 1985.

Evenson DP, Baer RK, Jost LK, et al: Toxicity of thiotepa on mouse spermatogenesis as determined by dual-parameter flow cytometry. *Toxicol Appl Pharmacol* 82:151–163, 1986.

Evenson DP, Janca FC, Jost LK: Effects of the fungicide methyl-benzimidazol-2-yl carbamate (MBC) on mouse germ cells as determined by flow cytometry. *J Toxicol Environ Health* 20:387–399, 1987.

Ewing LL: The Leydig cell, in Scialli AR, Clegg ED (eds): *Reversibility in Testicular Toxicity Assessment.* Boca Raton, FL: CRC Press, 1992.

Faber KA, Hughes CL Jr: Clinical aspects of reproductive toxicology, in Witorsch RJ (ed): *Reproductive Toxicology* 2d ed. New York: Raven Press, 1995, pp 217–240.

Fabrio S: On predicting environmentally-induced human reproductive hazards: An overview and historical perspective. *Fund Appl Toxicol* 5:609–614, 1985.

Faustman EM, Kirby Z, Gage D, et al: In vitro developmental toxicity of five direct acting alkylating agents in rodent embryos: Structure-activity patterns. *Teratology* 40:199–210, 1989.

Feuston MH, Bodnar, KR, Kerstetter SL, et al: Reproductive toxicity of 2-methoxyethanol applied dermally to occluded and nonoccluded sites in male rats. *Toxicol Appl Pharmacol* 100:145–161, 1989.

Foote RH, Berndtson WE: The germinal cells, in Scialli AR, Clegg ED (eds): *Testicular Toxicity Assessment.* Boca Raton, FL: CRC Press, 1992.

Foster PMD: The Sertoli cell, in Scialli AR, Clegg ED (eds): *Reversibility in Testicular Toxicity Assessment.* Boca Raton, FL: CRC Press, 1992.

Foster PMD, Blackburn DM, Moore RB, et al: Testicular toxicity of 2-methoxyacetaldehyde, a possible metabolite of ethylene glycol monomethyl ether in the rat. *Toxicol Lett* 32:73–80, 1986.

Frankos VH: FDA perspectives on the use of teratology data for human risk. *Fund Appl Toxicol* 5:615–625, 1985.

Galbraith WM, Voytek P, Ryon MG: *Assessment of Risks to Human Reproduction and to Development of the Human Conceptus from Exposure to Environmental Substances.* Soringfield, VA: Oak Ridge National Laboratory, U.S. Environmental Protection Agency, National Technical Information Service, 1982.

Gellert RJ: Uterotrophic activity of polychlorinated biphenyls (PCB) and induction of precocious reproductive aging in neonatally treated female rats. *Environ Res* 16:123–130, 1978.

Gilfillan SC: Lead poisoning and the fall of Rome. *J Occup Med* 7:53–60, 1965.

Goldberg EH: H-Y antigen and sex determination. *Philos Trans R Soc Lond [Biol]* 322:73–81, 1988.

Goldstein I, Lue TF, Padma-Nathan H, et al: Oral sildenafil in the treatment of erectile dysfunction. *N Engl J Med* 338:1397–1404, 1998.

Gorospe WC, Reinhard M: Toxic effects on the ovary of the nonpregnant female, in Witorsch RJ (ed): *Reproductive Toxicology,* 2d ed. New York: Raven Press, 1995, pp 141–157.

Grasso P, Heindel JJ, Powell, CJ, et al: Effects on mono(2-ethylhexyl) phthalate, a testicular toxicant, on follicle-stimulating hormone binding to membranes from cultured rat sertoli cells. *Biol Reprod* 48:454–459, 1993.

Gray TJB, Beamand JA: Effect of some phthalate esters and other testicular toxins on primary cultures of testicular cells. *Food Cosmet Toxicol* 22:123–131, 1984.

Greenwell A, Tomaszewski KE, Melnick RL: A biochemical basis for 1,2-dibromo-3-chloropropane-induced male infertility: Inhibition of sperm mitochondrial electron transport activity. *Toxicol Appl Pharmacol* 91:274–280, 1987.

Griswold MD: Interactions between germ cells and Sertoli cells in the testis. *Biol Reprod* 52:211–216, 1995.

Gunn SA, Gould TC: Difference between dorsal and lateral components of dorsolateral prostate in Zn^{65} uptake. *Proc Soc Exp Biol Med* 92:17–20, 1956.

Haney AF: Effects of toxic agents on ovarian function, in Thomas JA, Korach KS, McLachlan JA (eds): *Endocrine Toxicology.* New York: Raven Press, 1985.

Hanly JR Jr, Yano BL, Nitschke KD, et al: Comparison of the teratogenic potential of inhaled ethylene glycol monomethyl ether in rats, mice and rabbits. *Toxicol Appl Pharmacol* 75:409–422, 1984.

Hayes AW: *Principles and Methods of Toxicology.* New York: Raven Press, 1982.

Heckert L, Griswold MD: Expression of the FSH receptor in the testis. *Rec Progr Horm Res* 48:61–82, 1993.

Heindel JJ, Keith WB: Specific inhibition of FSH-stimulated cAMP accumulation by delta-9 tetrahydro-cannabinol in cultures of rat Sertoli cells. *Toxicol Appl Pharmacol* 101:124–134, 1989.

Heller CG, Clermont Y: Kinetics of the germinal epithelium in man. *Recent Progr Horm Res* 20:545–575, 1964.

Herbert DC, Supakar PC, Roy AR: Male reproduction, in Witorsch RJ (ed): *Reproductive Toxicology,* 2d ed. New York: Raven Press, 1995, pp 3–21.

Hildebrand DC, Der R, Griffin WT, et al: Effect of lead acetate on reproduction. *Am J Obstet Gynecol* 115:1058–1065, 1973.

Hillier SG, Zeleznik AJ, Knazek RA, et al: Hormonal regulation of preovulatory follicle maturation in the rat. *J Reprod Fertil* 60:219–229, 1980.

Hirsch KS, Weaver DE, Black LJ, et al: Inhibition of central nervous system aromatase activity: A mechanism for Fenarinol-induced infertility in the male rat. *Toxicol Appl Pharmacol* 91:235–245, 1987.

Hodgen GD: Enzyme markers of testicular function, in Johnson AD, Gomes WR (eds): *The Testis.* Vol 4. *Advances in Physiology, Biochemistry, and Function.* New York: Academic Press, 1977.

Holt DW, Adams PC, Campbell RWJ, et al: Amiodarone and its desethyl metabolite: Tissue distribution and ultrastructural changes in amiodarone-treated patients. *Br J Clin Pharmacol* 17:195–196, 1984.

Hruska RE, Olson JR: Species differences in estrogen receptors and in response to 2,3,7,8-tetrachlorodibenzo-*p*-dioxin exposure. *Toxicol Lett* 48:289–299, 1989.

Johnson EM: The scientific basis for multigeneration safety evaluations. *J Am Coll Toxicol* 5:197–201, 1986.

Johnson L, Dickerson R, Safe SH, et al: Reduced Leydig cell volume and function in adult rats exposed to 2,3,7,8-tetrachlorodibenzo-*p*-dioxin without a significant effect on spermatogenesis. *Toxicology* 76:103–118, 1992.

Keene LC, Davies PH: Drug-related erectile dysfunction. *Adverse Drug React Toxicol Rev* 18:1, 5–24, 1999.

Keke WR, Stone CR, Laws SL, et al: Persistent DDT metabolite *p,p′*-DDE is a potent androgen receptor antagonist. *Nature* 375, 581–585, 1995.

Kelce WR, Monosson E, Gamcsik MP, et al: Environmental hormone disruptors: Evidence that vinclozolin developmental toxicity is mediated by antiandrogenic metabolites. *Toxicol Appl Pharmacol* 126:276–285, 1994.

Kelce WR, Wilson EM: Clinical, functional and molecular implications of environmental antiandrogens. *J Mol Med* 75:198–207, 1997.

Khan-Dawood FS, Satyaswaroop PG: Toxic effects of chemicals and drugs on the sex accessory organs in the nonpregnant female, in Witorsch RJ (ed): *Reproductive Toxicology,* 2d ed. New York: Raven Press, 1995, pp 159–173.

Kimmel GL, Clegg ED, Crisp TM: Reproductive toxicity testing: A risk assessment perspective, in Witorsch RJ (ed): *Reproductive Toxicology,* 2d ed. New York: Raven Press, 1995, pp 75–98.

Klein D, Wan YY, Kamyab S, et al: Effects of toxic levels of lead on gene regulation in the male axis: Increase in messenger ribonucleic acids and intracellular stores on gonadotrophs within the central nervous system. *Biol Reprod* 50:802–811, 1994.

Koizumi T, Waalkes MP: Effects of zinc on the distribution and toxicity of cadmium in isolated interstitial cells of the rat testis. *Toxicology* 56:137–146, 1989.

Ku WW, Wine RN, Chae BY, et al: Spermatocyte toxicity of 2-methoxyethanol (ME) in rats and guinea pigs: Evidence for the induction of apoptosis. *Toxicol Appl Pharmacol* 134:100–110, 1995.

Kuiper GGJM, Lemmen JG, Carlsson B, et al: Interaction of estrogenic chemicals and phytoestrogens with estrogen receptor *β*. *Endocrinology* 139:4252–4263, 1998.

Lancranjan I, Papescu HI, Gavanescu O, et al: Reproductive ability of workmen occupationally exposed to lead. *Arch Environ Health* 30:396–401, 1975.

Lantz GD, Cunningham GR, Huckins C, et al: Recovery from severe oligospermia after exposure to dibromochloropropane. *Fertil Steril* 35:46–53, 1981.

Lave LB: Toxic substances control in the 1990s: Are we poisoning ourselves with low-level exposures? *Annu Rev Public Health* 11:69–87, 1990.

LeBlond CP, Clermont Y: Definition of the stages of the cycle of the seminiferous epithelium of the rat. *Ann NY Acad Sci* 55:548–571, 1952.

Lee IP, Dixon RL: Effects of procarbazine on spermatogenesis studied by velocity sedimentation cell separation and serial mating. *J Pharmacol Exp Ther* 181:219–226, 1972.

Lee IP, Suzuki K, Nagayama J: Metabolism of benzo(*a*)pyrene in rat prostate glands following 2,3,7,8-tetrachlorodibenzo-*p*-dioxin exposure. *Carcinogenesis* 2:823–831, 1981.

Lee JP: Adaptive biochemical repair response toward germ cell DNA damage. *Am J Ind Med* 4:135–147, 1983.

Lemasters GK, Selevan SG: Use of exposure data in occupational reproductive studies. *Scand J Work Environ Health* 10:1–6, 1984.

Levine RJ: Methods for detecting occupational causes of male infertility. *Scand J Work Environ Health* 9:371–376, 1983.

Levine RJ, Blunden PB, DalCorso RD, et al: Superiority of reproductive histories to sperm counts in detecting infertility at a DBCP manufacturing plant. *J Occup Med* 25:591–597, 1983.

Li LH, Heindel JJ: Sertoli cell toxicants, in Korach KS (ed): *Reproduction and Developmental Toxicology.* New York: Marcel Dekker, 1998, pp 655–691.

Lindemann CB, Kanous KS: Regulation of mammalian sperm motility. *Arch Androl* 23:1–22, 1989.

Lipshultz L: "The debate continues" —The continuing debate over the possible decline in semen quality. *Am Soc Reprod Med* 65:909–911, 1996.

Lloyd SC, Blackburn DM, Foster PMD: Trifluoroethanol and its oxidative metabolites: Comparison of in vivo and in vitro effects in rat testis. *Toxicol Appl Pharmacol* 92:390–401, 1988.

Lonning PE, Lien EA: Pharmacokinetics of anti-endocrine agents. *Cancer Surv* 17:343–370, 1993.

Lu T: Erectile dysfunction *N Engl J Med* 348:1802–1813, 2000.

MacLean HE, Warne GL, Zajac JD: Localization of functional domains in the androgen receptor. *J Steroid Biochem Mol Biol* 62:4, 233–242, 1997.

MacLeod J: Human male infertility. *Obstet Gynecol Surv* 26:335–351, 1971.

Maddocks S, Parvinen M, Soder O, et al: Regulation of the testis. *J Reprod Immunol* 18:33–50, 1990.

Mann T, Lutwak-Mann C: *Male Reproductive Function and Semen: Themes and Trends in Physiology, Biochemistry, and Investigative Andrology.* New York: Springer-Verlag, 1981.

Mattison DR, Nightingale MS: The biochemical and genetic characteristics of murine ovarian aryl hydrocarbon (benzo*[a]*pyrene)hydroxylase activity and its relationship to primordial oocyte destruction by polycyclic aromatic hydrocarbons. *Toxicol Appl Pharmacol* 56:399–408, 1980.

Mattison DR, Plowchalk DR, Meadows MJ, et al: Reproductive toxicity: Male and female reproductive systems as targets for chemical injury. *Med Clin North Am* 74:391–411, 1990.

McElveen JC Jr: Reproduction hazards in the workplace: Some legal considerations. *J Occup Med* 28:103–110, 1986.

McLachlan JA, Newbold RR, Korach KS, et al: Transplacental toxicology: Prenatal factors influencing postnatal fertility, in Kimmel CA, Buelke-Sam J (eds): *Developmental Toxicology.* New York: Raven Press, 1981.

Mebus CA, Welsch F, Working PK: Attenuation of 2-methoxyethanol-induced testicular toxicity in the rat by simple physiological compounds. *Toxicol Appl Pharmacol* 99:110–121, 1989.

Meistrich ML: Evaluation of reproductive toxicity by testicular sperm head counts. *J Am Coll Toxicol* 8:551–567, 1989.

Millar JGB: Drug-induced impotence. *Practitioner* 223:634–639, 1979.

Moore NP, Creasy DM, Gray TJB: Urinary creatine profiles after administration of cell-specific testicular toxicants to the rat. *Arch Toxicol* 66:435–442, 1992.

Morrissey RE, Lamb IV JC, Schwetz BA, et al: Association of sperm, vaginal cytology, and reproductive organ weight data with results of continuous breeding reproduction studies in Swiss (CD-1) mice. *Fundam Appl Toxicol* 11:359–371, 1988.

Mosher WD: Contraceptive utilization: United States. *Vital Health Stat* 23:1–58, 1981.

Müller AMF, Makropoulos V, Bolt HM: Toxicological aspects of pestrogen-mimetic xenobiotics present in the environment. *Toxicol Environ News* 2:68–73, 1995.

Murdoch WJ: Immunoregulation of mammalian fertility. *Life Sci* 55:1871–1886, 1994.

Nagano K, Nakayama E, Koyano M, et al: Testicular atrophy of mice induced by ethylene glycol monoakyl ethers. *Jpn J Ind Health* 21:29–35, 1979.

Nahhas F, Blumenfeld F: Zona-free hamster egg penetration assay and prognostic indicator in an IVF program. *Arch Androl* 23:33–37, 1989.

Nakagawa S, Nakamura N, Fujioka M, et al: Spermatogenic cell apoptosis induced by mitomycin C in the mouse testis. *Toxicol Appl Pharmacol* 147. 204–213, 1997.

Nakano R: Apoptosis: Gene-directed cell death. *Horm Res* 48(suppl 3):2–4, 1997.

Neaves WB: The blood-testis barrier, in Johnson AD, Gomes WR (eds): *The Testis.* Vol 6. New York: Academic Press, 1977, pp.125–153.

Nisbet IC, Karch NJ: *Chemical Hazards to Human Reproduction.* Park Ridge, NJ: Noyes Data, 1983.

Office of Technology Assessment Report. *Reproductive Health Hazards in the Workplace.* Washington, DC: U.S. Government Printing Office, 1985.

Ogawa T, Dobrinski I, Avarbock MR, Brinster RL: Transplantation of male germ line stem cells restores fertility in infertile mice. *Nature Med* 5:29–34, 1999.

Okumura K, Lee IP, Dixon RL: Permeability of selected drugs and chemicals across the blood-testis barrier of the rat. *J Pharmacol Exp Ther* 194:89–95, 1975.

Olshan AF, Faustman EM: Male-mediated developmental toxicity. *Annu Rev Public Health* 14:159–181, 1994.

Overstreet JW: Reproductive risk assessment. *Teratogenesis Carcinog Mutagen* 4:67–75, 1984.

Overstreet JW, Samuels SJ, Day P, et al: Early indicators of male reproductive toxicity. *Risk Anal* 8:21–26, 1988.

Papadopoulas C: Cardiovascular drugs and sexuality. *Arch Intern Med* 140:1341–1345, 1980.

Paul ME: Reproductive fitness and risk. *Occup Med* 3:323–340, 1988.

Pedersen I, Peters H: Proposal for a classification of oocytes and follicles in the mouse ovary. *J Reprod Fertil* 17:555–557, 1968.

Pedersen RA, Brandriff B: Radiation- and drug-induced DNA repair in mammalian oocytes and embryos, in Generoso WM, Shelby MD, DeSerres FJ (eds): *DNA Repair and Mutagenesis in Eukaryotes.* New York: Plenum Press, 1980.

Perrolle JA: Reproductive hazards: A model protection policy for the chemical industry. *Occup Med* 8:755–786, 1993.

Pogach LM, Lee Y, Gould S, et al: Characterization of *cis*-platinum-induced Sertoli cell dysfunction in rodents. *Toxicol Appl Pharmacol* 98:350–361, 1989.

Polascik TJ, Osterling JE, Partin AW: Prostate specific antigen: A decade of discovery—What we have learned and where we are going. *J Urol* 162:293–306, 1999.

Prasad AS, Obeleas D, Wolf P, et al: Studies on zinc deficiency: Changes in trace element and enzyme activities in tissues of zinc-deficient rats. *J Clin Invest* 46:549–557, 1967.

Raffray M, Cohen GM: Apoptosis and necrosis in toxicology: A continuum of distinct modes of cell death? *Pharmacol Ther* 75:3, 153–177, 1997.

Rajfer J, Sikka SC, Lemmi C, et al: Cyclosporine inhibits testosterone biosynthesis in the rat testis. *Endocrinology* 121:586–589, 1987.

Regaud CP: Degenerescence des cellules seminales chez mammiferes en l'abscence de tout etat pathologique. *CR Séances Soc Biol* 52:268–270.

Revelli A, Massobrio M, Tesarik J: Nongenomic actions of steroid hormones in reproductive tissues. *Endocrinol Rev* 19:3–17, 1998.

Richburg JH, Boekelheide K: Mono-(2-ethylhexyl) phthatate rapidly alters both Sertoli cell vimentin filaments and germ cell apoptosis in young rat testes. *Toxicol Appl Pharmacol* 137:42–50, 1996.

Richburg JH, Redenbach DM, Boekelheide K: Seminferous tubule fluid secretion is a Sertoli cell microtubule-dependent process inhibited by 2,5-Hexanedione exposure. *Toxicol Appl Pharmacol* 128:302–309, 1994.

Ritter EJ, Scott WJ Jr, Randall JL, et al: Teratogenicity of di(ethylhexyl) phthalate, 2-ethylhexanol, 2-ethylhexanoic acid, and valproic acid, and potentiation by caffeine. *Teratology* 35:41–46, 1987.

Robb GW, Amann RP, Killian GJ: Daily sperm production and epididymal sperm reserve of pubertal and adult rats. *J Reprod Fertil* 54:103–107, 1978.

Roberts RA, Nebert DW, Hickman JA, et al: Perturbation of the mitosis/apoptosis balance: A fundamental mechanism in toxicology. *Fundam Appl Toxicol* 38:107–115, 1997.

Robertson JD, Orrenius S: Molecular mechanisms of apoptosis induced by cytotoxic chemicals. *Crit Rev Toxicol* 30:609–627, 2000.

Rodamilans M, Osaba MJ Mtz, To-Figueras J, et al: Lead toxicity on endocrine testicular function in an occupationally exposed population. *Hum Toxicol* 7:125–128, 1988.

Roy AK, Lavrovsky CS, Song S, et al: Regulation of androgen action. *Vitam Horm* 55:309–352, 1999.

Safe SH: Dietary and environmental estrogens and antiestrogens and their possible role in human disease. *Environ Sci Pollut Res* 1(1):29–33, 1994.

Sakamoto J, Hashimoto K: Reproductive toxicity of acrylamide and related compounds in mice—Effects on fertility and sperm morphology. *Arch Toxicol* 59:201–205, 1986.

Sattler B: Rights and realities: A critical review of the accessibility of information on hazardous chemicals. *Occup Med* 7:189–196, 1992.

Schrag SD, Dixon RL: Occupational exposure associated with male reproductive dysfunction. *Annu Rev Pharmacol Toxicol* 25:567–592, 1985.

Schwetz BA, Roa KS, Park CN: Insensitivity of tests for reproductive problems. *J Environ Pathol Toxicol* 3:81–98, 1980.

Scialli AR, Lemasters GK: Epidemiologic aspects of reproductive toxicology, in Witorsch RJ (ed): *Reproductive Toxicology,* 2d ed. New York: Raven Press, 1995, pp 241–263.

Seed J, Chapin RE, Clegg ED, et al: Consensus report: Methods for assessing sperm motility, morphology, and counts in the rat, rabbit and dog. *Reprod Toxicol* 10:237–244, 1996.

Selden JR, Robertson RT, Miller JE, et al: The rapid and sensitive detection of perturbations in spermatogenesis: Assessment by quantitative dual parameter (DNA/RNA) flow cytometry. *J Am Coll Toxicol* 8:507–523, 1989.

Selevan SG, Lindhohm ML, Hornung RW, et al: A study of occupational exposure to antineoplastic drugs and fetal loss in nurses. *N Engl J Med* 313:1173–1178, 1985.

Setchell BP, Vogimayr JK, Waites GMH: A blood-testis barrier restricting passage from blood lymph into rete testis fluid but not into lymph. *J Physiol* 200:73–85, 1969.

Shaked I, Sod-Moriah UA, Kaplanski J, et al: Reproductive performance of dibromochloropropane-treated female rats. *Int J Fertil* 33:129–133, 1988.

Sharpe RM: Toxicity of spermatogenesis and its detection, in Korach K (ed): *Reproductive and Developmental Toxicology.* New York: Marcel Dekker, 1998, pp 625–654.

Sharpe RM, Shakkenback NE: Are oestrogens involved in falling sperm counts and disorders of the male reproductive tract? *Lancet* 341:1392–1395, 1993.

Sheikh K: Choice of control population in studies of adverse reproductive effects of occupational exposures and its effect on risk estimates. *Br J Ind Med* 44:244–249, 1987.

Shemi D, Sod-Moriah UA, Kaplanski J, et al: Gonadotoxicity and kinetics of dibromochloropropane in male rats. *Toxicol. Lett* 36:209–212, 1987.

Shen RS, Lee IP: Developmental patterns of enzymes in mouse testis. *J Reprod Fertil* 48:301–305, 1977.

Shioda S, Legradi G, Leung W, et al.: Localization of pituitary adenylate cyclase-activating polypeptide and its messenger ribonucleic acid in the rat testis by light and electron microscopic immunocytochemistry and *in situ* hybridization. *Endocrinology* 135:818–825, 1994.

Simpson JL: Genes, chromosomes, and reproductive failure. *Fertil Steril* 33:107–116, 1980.

Singh H, Kozel T, Jackson S: Effect of procarbazine on sperm morphology in Syrian hamsters. *J Toxicol Environ Health* 27:107–121, 1989.

Skinner MK, Schlitz SM, Anthony CA: Regulation of Sertoli cell differentiated function: Testicular transferrin and androgen-binding protein expression. *Endocrinology* 124:3015–3024, 1989.

Slikker W Jr, Miller RK: Placental metabolism and transfer role in developmental toxicology, in Kimmel CA, Buelke JS (eds), *Developmental Toxicology,* 2d ed. New York: Raven Press, 1994.

Soderlund EJ, Brunborg G, Omichinski JG, et al: Testicular necrosis and DNA damage caused by deuterated and methylated analogues of 1,2-dibromo-3-chloropropane in the rat. *Toxicol Appl Pharmacol* 94:437–447, 1988.

Somkuti SG, Lapadula DM, Chapin RE, et al: Reproductive tract lesions resulting from subchronic administration (63 days) of tri-*o*-cresyl phosphate in male rats. *Toxicol Appl Pharmacol* 89:49–63, 1987.

Spiteri-Grech J, Nieschlag E: Paracrine factors relevant to the regulation of spermatogenesis. *J Reprod Fertil* 98:1–4, 1993.

Stevenson JG, Umstead, GS: Sexual dysfunction due to antihypertensive agents. *Drug Intell Clin Pharm* 18:113–121, 1984.

Sullivan FM: The European Community classification of chemicals for reproductive toxicity. *Toxicol Lett* 64/65:183–189.

Sundaram K, Witorsch RJ: Toxic effects on the testes, in Witorsch RJ (ed): *Reproductive Toxicology,* 2d ed. New York: Raven Press, 1995, pp 99–121.

Swain, A., Lovell-Badge, R. Mammalian sex determination: A molecular drama. *Genes Dev* 13:755:767, 1999.

Thomas JA: Actions of chemicals and other factors on Leydig cell growth and proliferation, in *Endocrine Toxicology.* New York: Raven Press, 1995b.

Thomas JA: Actions of drugs/chemicals on nonreproductive endocrine organs. *Toxic Subst J* 13:187–200, 1994.

Thomas JA: Effects of chemicals/drugs on spermatogenesis, in Hamamah S, Mieusset R (eds): *Male Gametes: Production and Quality.* Paris: INSERM, 1996, pp 151–158.

Thomas JA: Effects of pesticides on reproduction, in Thomas JA, Singhal RL (eds): *Molecular Mechanisms of Gonadal Hormone Action.* Baltimore: University Park Press, 1975, pp 205–223.

Thomas JA: Phytoestrogens and hormonal modulation: A mini-review. *Environ Nutr Int eract* 1:5–12, 1997.

Thomas JA: Reproductive hazards and environmental chemicals: A review. *Toxic Subst J* 2:318–348, 1981.

Thomas JA: Sperm counts, phytoestrogens, and estrogen-mimic substances, in Dunaif GE, Olin SS, Scimeca, et al (eds): *Human Diet and Endocrine Modulation (Estrogenic and Androgenic Effects).* Washington DC: ILSI Press, 1998, pp 257–263.

Thomas JA: Testes-specific metal toxicology, in Goyer RA, Waalkes MP, Klassen CD (eds): *Organ Specific Metal Toxicology.* Orlando, FL: Academic Press, 1995a.

Thomas JA, Barsano CP: Occupational reproductive risks, in *Encyclopedia of Environmental Control Technology.* 1994, pp 195–215.

Thomas JA, Barsano CP: Pharmacologic and toxicologic responses in the neonate. *J Am Coll Toxicol* 5:957–962, 1989.

Thomas JA, Barsano CP: Survey of reproductive hazards. *J Am Coll Toxicol* 5:203–207, 1986.

Thomas JA, Brogan WC: Some actions of lead on the sperm and on the male reproductive system. *Am J Ind Med* 4:127–134, 1983.

Thomas JA, Curto KA, Thomas MJ: MEHP/DEHP gonadal toxicity and effects on rodent accessory sex organs. *Environ Health Perspect* 45:85–92, 1982.

Thomas JA, Keenan EJ: *Principles of Endocrine Pharmacology.* New York: Plenum Press, 1986.

Thomas JA, Thomas MJ: Biological effects of di-(2-ethylhexyl) phthalate and other phthalic acid esters. *Crit Rev Toxicol* 13:283–317, 1984.

Thomas MJ, Thomas JA: Hormone assays and endocrine function, in Hayes AW (ed), *Principles and Methods of Toxicology.* Philadelphia: Taylor & Francis, 2001, pp 1383–1414.

Thompson E Jr: The effects of estradiol upon the thymus of the sexually immature female mouse. *J Steroid Biochem* 14:167–174, 1981.

Thompson EB: Apoptosis and steroid hormones. *Mol Endocrinol* 8:665–673, 1994.

Torkelson RR, Sadek SE, Rowe VK: Toxicologic investigations of 1,2-dibromo-3-chlorpropane. *Toxicol Appl Pharmacol* 3:545–557, 1961.

Toth GP, Zenick H, Smith MK: Effects of epichlorohydrin on male and female reproduction in Long-Evan rats. *Fundam Appl Pharmacol* 13:16–25, 1989.

Tuchmann-Duplessis H, David G, Haegel P: *Illustrated Human Embryology.* Vol I. New York: Springer-Verlag, 1972.

Turner HE, Wass JAH: Gonadal function in men with chronic illness. *Clin Endocrinol* 47:379–403, 1997.

Ulbrich B, Palmer AK: Detection of effects on male reproduction—A literature survey. *J Am Coll Toxicol* 14:293–327, 1996.

Van Pelt AMM, de Rooij DG, van der Burg B, et al: Ontogeny of estrogen receptor-β expression in rat testis. *Endocrinology* 140:478–483, 1999.

Vegeto E, Wagner BL, Imhof MO, et al: The molecular pharmacology of ovarian steroid receptors. *Vitam Horm* 52:99–128, 1996.

Vos, JG, Dybing, E., Greim, HA, et al: Health effects of endocrine-disrupting chemicals on wildlife, with special reference to the European situation. *Crit Rev Toxicol* 30:71–133, 2000.

Waalkes MP, Coogan TP, Barter RA: Toxicological principles of metal carcinogenesis with special emphasis on cadmium. *Crit Rev Toxicol* 22:175–201, 1992.

Waalkes MP, Donovan MP, Thomas JA: Cadmium-induced prostate metallothionein in the rabbit. *Prostate* 3:23–25, 1982.

Wang W, Chapin RE: Differential gene expression detected by suppression substractive hybridization in ethylene glycol monomethyl ether-induced testicular lesion. *Toxicol Sci* 56:165–174, 2000.

Ways SC, Blair PB, Bern HA, et al: Immune responsiveness of adult mice exposed neonatally to diethylstilbestrol, steroid hormones, or vitamin A. *J Environ Pathol* 3:207–227, 1980.

Whorton DM, Kraus RM, Marshall S, et al: Infertility in male pesticide workers. *Lancet* 2:1259–1267, 1977.

Williams J, Foster PMD: The production of lactate and pyruvate as sensitive indices of altered rat Sertoli cell function in vitro following the addition of various testicular toxicants. *Toxicol Appl Pharmacol* 94:160–170, 1988.

Williams J, Gladen BC, Schrader, SM, et al: Semen analysis and fertility assessment in rabbits: Statistical power and design considerations for toxicology studies. *Fundam Appl Toxicol* 15, 651–665, 1990.

Wilson MJ: Toxicology of the male accessory sex organs and related glands, in Witorsch RJ (ed): *Reproductive Toxicology,* 2d ed. New York: Raven Press, 1995, 123–139.

Woods JS: Drug effects on human sexual behavior, in Woods NF (ed): *Human Sexuality in Health and Illness,* 3d ed. St. Louis: Mosby, 1984.

Working PK: Male reproductive toxicology: Comparison of the human to animal models. *Environ Health Perspect* 77:37–44, 1988.

Wyrobek AJ: Methods for evaluating the effects of environmental chemicals on human sperm production. *Environ Health Perspect* 48:53–59, 1983.

Wyrobek AJ, Gordon LA, Burkhart JG, et al: An evaluation of the mouse sperm morphology test and other sperm tests in nonhuman mammals. A report of the U.S. Environmental Protection Agency Gene-Tox Program. *Mutat Res* 115:1–72, 1983.

Zacharewski T, Sate SH: Antiestrogenic activity of TCDD and related compounds, in Korach KS (ed): *Reproduction and Developmental Toxicology.* New York: Marcel Dekker, 1998, pp 431–448.

Zeleznik AJ, Hillier SG, Knazek RA, et al: Production of long-term steroid producing granulosa cell cultures by cell hybridization. *Endocrinology* 105:156–162, 1979.

Zenick H, Clegg ED: Tissues in risk assessment in male reproduction toxicology. *J Am Coll Toxicol* 5:249–261, 1986.

Zirkin BR, Chen H: Regulation of Leydig cell steroidogenic function during aging. *Biol Reprod* 63:977–981, 2000.

CHAPTER 21

TOXIC RESPONSES OF THE ENDOCRINE SYSTEM

Charles C. Capen

INTRODUCTION

Endocrine glands are collections of specialized cells that synthesize, store, and release their secretions directly into the bloodstream. They are sensing and signaling devices located in the extracellular fluid compartment and are capable of responding to changes in the internal and external environments to coordinate a multiplicity of activities that maintain homeostasis.

Endocrine cells that produce polypeptide hormones have a well-developed rough endoplasmic reticulum that assembles hormone and a prominent Golgi apparatus for packaging hormone into granules for intracellular storage and transport. Secretory granules are unique to polypeptide hormone- and catecholamine-secreting endocrine cells and provide a mechanism for intracellular storage of substantial amounts of preformed active hormone. When the cell receives a signal for hormone secretion, secretory granules are directed to the periphery of the endocrine cell, probably by the contraction of microfilaments.

Steroid hormone-secreting cells are characterized by prominent cytoplasmic lipid bodies that contain cholesterol and other precursor molecules. The lipid bodies are in close proximity to an extensive tubular network of smooth endoplasmic reticulum and large mitochondria which contain hydroxylase and dehydrogenase enzyme systems. These enzyme systems function to attach various side chains to the basic steroid nucleus. Steroid hormone-producing cells lack secretory granules and do not store significant amounts of preformed hormone. They are dependent on continued biosynthesis to maintain the normal secretory rate for a particular hormone.

Many diseases of the endocrine system are characterized by dramatic functional disturbances and characteristic clinicopathologic alterations affecting one or several body systems. The affected animal or human patient may have clinical signs that primarily involve the skin (hair loss caused by hypothyroidism), nervous system (seizures caused by hyperinsulinism), urinary system (polyuria caused by diabetes mellitus, diabetes insipidus, and hyperadrenocorticism), or skeletal system (fractures induced by hyperparathyroidism).

The literature suggests that chemically induced lesions of the endocrine organs are most commonly encountered in the adrenal glands, followed in descending order by the thyroid, pancreas, pituitary, and parathyroid glands. In the adrenal glands, chemically induced lesions are most frequently found in the zona fasciculata/zona reticularis and to a lesser extent in either the zona glomerulosa or medulla. In a recent survey, conducted by the Pharmaceutical Manufacturers Association, of tumor types developing in carcinogenicity studies, endocrine tumors developed frequently in rats, with the thyroid gland third in frequency (behind the liver and mammary gland), followed by the pituitary gland (fourth), and adrenal gland (fifth). Selected examples of commonly encountered toxic endpoints involving endocrine organs in laboratory animals are discussed in this chapter. Mechanistic data is included whenever possible to aid in the interpretation of findings in animal toxicology studies and to determine their significance in risk assessment.

PITUITARY GLAND

Normal Structure and Function

The pituitary gland (hypophysis) is divided into two major compartments: (1) the adenohypophysis (anterior lobe), composed of the pars distalis, pars tuberalis, and pars intermedia, and (2) the neurohypophyseal system, which includes the pars nervosa (posterior lobe), infundibular stalk, and hypothalamic nuclei (supraoptic and paraventricular) containing the neurosecretory neurons, which synthesize and package the neurohypophyseal hormones into secretory granules. The pars intermedia forms the thin cellular zone between the adenohypophysis and neurohypophysis. The pituitary gland lies within the sella turcica of the sphenoid bone. The gland receives its blood supply via the posterior and anterior hypophyseal arteries, which originate from the internal carotid arteries. Arteriolar branches penetrate the pituitary stalk near the median eminence, lose their muscular coat, and form a capillary plexus. These vessels drain into the hypophyseal portal veins, which supply the adenohypophysis. The hypothalamic-hypophyseal portal system functionally is important as it transports the hypothalamic releasing- and release-inhibiting hormones directly to the adenohypophysis, where they interact with their specific populations of trophic hormone-producing cells.

The adenohypophysis in many animal species completely surrounds the pars nervosa of the neurohypophyseal system, in contrast to its position in human beings, where it is situated on the anterior surface. The pars distalis is the largest portion and is composed of the multiple populations of endocrine cells that secrete the pituitary trophic hormones. The secretory cells are surrounded by abundant capillaries derived from the hypothalamic-hypophyseal portal system. The pars tuberalis consists of dorsal projections of supportive cells along the infundibular stalk. It functions primarily as a scaffold for the capillary network of the hypophyseal portal system during its course from the median eminence to the pars distalis. The pars intermedia is located between the pars distalis and pars nervosa and lines the residual lumen of Rathke's pouch. It contains two populations of endocrine cells in certain species. One of these cell types (B cells) in the dog synthesizes and secretes adrenocorticotropic hormone (ACTH).

A specific population of endocrine cells is present in the pars distalis (and in the pars intermedia of dogs for ACTH) that synthesizes, processes, and secretes each of the pituitary trophic hormones. Secretory cells in the adenohypophysis formerly were classified either as acidophils, basophils, or chromophobes based on the reactions of their secretory granules with pH-dependent histochemical stains. Based upon contemporary specific immunocytochemical procedures, acidophils can be further subclassified functionally into somatotrophs that secrete growth hormone (GH; somatotrophin) and luteotrophs that secrete luteotropic hormone (LTH; prolactin). Their granules contain simple protein hormones. Basophils include both gonadotrophs, which secrete luteinizing hormone (LH) and follicle-stimulating hormone (FSH), and thyrotrophs, which secrete thyrotropic hormone [thyroid-stimulating hormone (TSH)]. Chromophobes are pituitary cells that, by light microscopy, do not have stainable cytoplasmic secretory granules. They include the pituitary cells involved with the synthesis of ACTH and melanocyte-stimulating hormone (MSH) in some species, nonsecretory follicular (stellate) cells, degranulated chromophils (acidophils and basophils) in the actively synthesizing phase of the secretory cycle, and undifferentiated stem cells of the adenohypophysis.

Each type of endocrine cell in the adenohypophysis is under the control of a specific releasing hormone from the hypothalamus (Fig. 21-1). These releasing hormones are small peptides that are synthesized and secreted by neurons of the hypothalamus. They are transported by short axonal processes to the median eminence, where they are released into capillaries and are conveyed by the

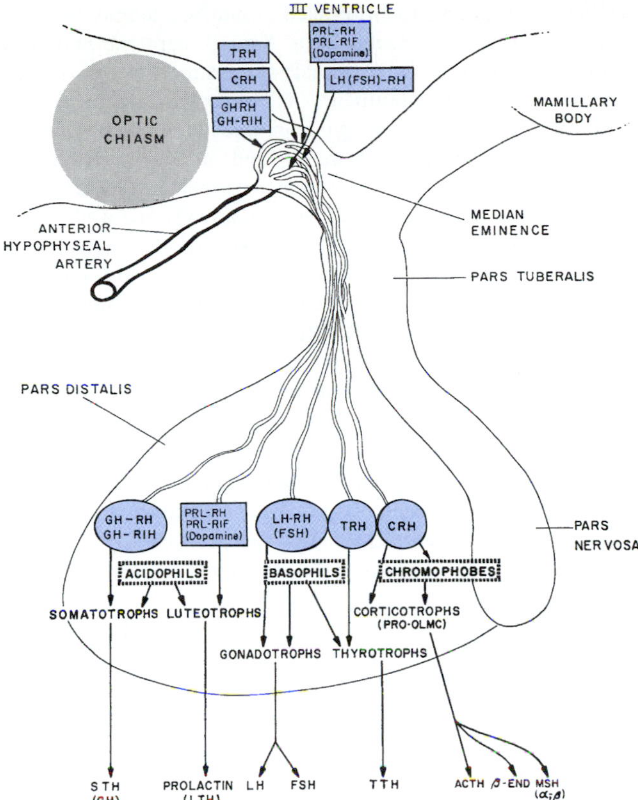

Figure 21-1. Control of trophic hormone secretion from the adenohypophysis by hypothalamic releasing hormones (RH) and release-inhibiting hormones (RIH).

The releasing and release-inhibiting hormones are synthesized by neurons in the hypothalamus, transported by axonal processes, and released into capillary plexus in the median eminence. They are transported to the adenohypophysis by the hypothalamic-hypophyseal portal system, where they interact with specific populations of trophic hormone–secreting cells to govern the rate of release of preformed hormones, such as growth hormone (GH), somatotropic hormone (STH), luteotropic hormone (LTH), luteinizing hormone (LH), follicle-stimulating hormone (FSH), thyrotropic hormone (TTH), adrenocorticotropic hormone (ACTH), and melanocyte-stimulating hormone (MSH). There are RIHs for those trophic hormones (e.g., prolactin and growth hormone) that do not directly influence the activity of target cells and result in production of a final endocrine product (hormone) that could exert negative feedback control.

hypophyseal portal system to specific trophic hormone-secreting cells in the adenohypophysis. Each hormone stimulates the rapid release of preformed secretory granules containing a specific trophic hormone. Specific releasing hormones have been identified for TSH, FSH and LH, ACTH, and GH. Prolactin (PRL) secretion is stimulated by a number of factors, the most important of which appears to be thyrotropin-releasing hormone (TRH). Dopamine serves as the major prolactin-inhibitory factor and suppresses prolactin secretion and also inhibits cell division and DNA synthesis of luteotrophs. Dopamine also suppresses ACTH production by corticotrophs in the pars intermedia of some species. Another hypothalamic release-inhibiting hormone is somatostatin (somatotropin-release inhibiting hormone, SRIH). This tetradecapeptide inhibits the secretion of both growth hormone and TSH. Control of pituitary trophic hormone secretion also is affected by negative feedback by the circulating concentration of target organ (thyroid, adrenal cortex, and gonad) hormones.

The neurohypophysis is subdivided into three anatomic parts. The pars nervosa (posterior lobe of the human pituitary) represents the distal component of the neurohypophyseal system. The infundibular stalk joins the pars nervosa to the overlying hypothalamus and is composed of long axonal processes from neurosecretory neurons in the hypothalamus. It is made up of numerous capillaries, supported by modified glial cells (pituicytes), which are termination sites for the nonmyelinated axonal processes of neurosecretory neurons. The neurohypophyseal hormones (i.e., oxytocin and antidiuretic hormone) are synthesized in the cell body of hypothalamic neurons, packaged into secretory granules, transported by long axonal processes, and released into the bloodstream in the pars nervosa.

Antidiuretic hormone (ADH or vasopressin) and oxytocin are nonapeptides synthesized by neurons situated either in the supraoptic (primarily ADH) or paraventricular (primarily oxytocin) nuclei of the hypothalamus. ADH and its corresponding neurophysin are synthesized as part of a common larger biosynthetic precursor molecule, termed propressophysin. The hormones are packaged with a corresponding binding protein (i.e., neurophysin) into membrane-limited neurosecretory granules and transported by axons to the pars nervosa for release into the circulation. As the biosynthetic precursor molecules travel along the axons in secretion granules from the neurosecretory neurons, the precursors are cleaved into the active hormones and their respective neurophysins. These secretory products can be detected immunocytochemically. In Brattleboro rats with hereditary hypothalamic diabetes insipidus, nerve cells in the hypothalamus that normally produce ADH and neurophysin-I are negative immunocytochemically for both proteins whereas neurosecretory stain positive for cells that produce vasopressin and neurophysin-II are positive.

In addition to the specific trophic hormone-secreting cells, a population of supporting cells is also present in the adenohypophysis. These cells are referred to as stellate (follicular) cells and can be stained selectively with antibodies to S-100 protein. The stellate cells typically have elongate processes and prominent cytoplasmic filaments. These cells appear to provide a phagocytic or supportive function in addition to producing a colloid-like material that accumulates in follicles.

Mechanisms of Toxicity

Pituitary tumors can be induced readily by sustained uncompensated hormonal derangements leading to increased synthesis and secretion of pituitary hormones. The absence of negative feedback inhibition of pituitary cells leads to unrestrained proliferation (hyperplasia initially, neoplasia later). This effect can be potentiated by the concurrent administration of ionizing radiation or chemical carcinogens.

In the pituitary-thyroid axis, thyroxine (T_4) and triiodothyronine (T_3) normally regulate the pituitary secretion of TSH by a classic negative feedback control system. Surgical removal or radiation-induced ablation of the thyroid or interference with the production of thyroid hormones by the use of specific chemical inhibitors of thyroid hormone synthesis leads to a stimulation of TSH synthesis and secretion with elevated blood levels. The thyrotrophic cells in the adenohypophysis undergo prominent hypertrophy. Subsequently, hyperplasia of the thyrotrophs occurs concurrently with hypertrophy as a consequence of the lack of normal negative feedback control. In rodents foci of hyperplasia may progress to the formation of adenomas in the pituitary gland. The role of gonadectomy in pituitary tumor induction has been studied most intensively in mice. The pituitary tumors induced by gonadectomy in mice are markedly strain-dependent and may contain FSH, LH, or both.

The administration of estrogens is a reproducible method for inducing pituitary tumors in certain experimental animals. The effect of exogenous estrogen on the rat pituitary includes stimulation of prolactin secretion and the induction of prolactin-secreting tumors. The administration of estrogens in susceptible strains results in elevated serum prolactin levels, increased numbers of prolactin cells within the pituitary, enhanced incorporation of tritiated thymidine within the gland, and increased mitotic activity. The pituitary of the ovariectomized F344 female rat is more responsive to the tumorigenic effect of diethylstilbestrol than the intact female; however, there is considerable variation in the induction of pituitary tumors by estrogens in different rat strains. For example, F344 and Holtzman rats respond to an initial estrogen stimulus by increasing the rate of DNA synthesis in the pituitary within 2 to 4 days. The rate of DNA synthesis declines after 7 to 10 days of treatment to unstimulated levels in the Holtzman strain but remains elevated in F344 rats.

Sarkar and coworkers (1982) have reported that estrogen-induced pituitary adenomas derived from prolactin-secreting cells are associated with loss of hypothalamic dopaminergic neurons, which normally inhibit the function of prolactin-secreting cells. Prolactin-producing tumors, when transplanted subcutaneously, also were associated with degenerative changes in hypothalamic dopaminergic neurons. The tumorigenic action of estrogen may not be due exclusively to its effect on the hypothalamus, since estrogen can produce prolactinomas in pituitaries grafted beneath the renal capsule. The effects of estrogens on prolactin cells have been studied in hypophysectomized rats bearing transplanted pituitaries beneath the kidney capsule. The studies of El Etreby and coworkers (1988) using this model have shown that dopamine agonists, including lisuride and bromocriptine, antagonize the direct stimulatory effects of estrogens on the prolactin cells. These dopamine agonists may act directly on dopaminergic receptors within the transplanted pituitaries.

Other agents, including caffeine, have been implicated in the development of pituitary adenomas in rats. The administration of *N*-methylnitrosourea also is associated with the development of pituitary adenomas in Wistar rats. The neuroleptic agent sulpiride has been reported to cause the release of prolactin from the anterior pituitary in the rat and to stimulate DNA replication. The administration of clomiphene prevents the stimulation of DNA synthesis produced by sulpiride, but does not affect prolactin release from the gland. These findings suggest that the intracellular prolactin content of the pituitary plays a role in the regulation of DNA synthesis through a mechanism mediated by estrogens.

Morphologic Alterations and Proliferative Lesions of Pituitary Cells

Jameson et al. (1992) reported that the administration of salmon calcitonin for 1 year to Sprague-Dawley and Fisher 344 rats was associated with an increased incidence of focal hyperplasia and adenomas in the pituitary. The association of calcitonin treatment and pituitary tumors was dose-dependent and was more pronounced with salmon calcitonin than with porcine calcitonin. Using both immunohistochemical analysis and measurements of serum hormone levels, they provided evidence that prolonged administration of calcitonin resulted in pituitary tumors that produced the common α-subunit of the glycoprotein hormones [luteinizing hormone (LH), follicle-stimulating hormone (FSH) and thyroid-stimulating hormones (TSH)], a type of tumor that has been reported to compose a significant fraction of pituitary tumors in humans. Immunohistochemistry and in situ hybridization demonstrated that most pituitary tumors associated with the chronic administration of high doses of calcitonin expressed a glycoprotein hormone α-subunit, whereas expression of the α-subunit was identified infrequently in hyperplastic lesions of control rats.

Serum levels of each of the major pituitary hormones were measured in both sexes of Sprague-Dawley and Fisher rats administered calcitonin. There were no significant alterations in the circulating levels of growth hormone, prolactin, or ACTH and the tumors were negative by immunohistochemical and in situ hybridization assessment for these hormones. Serum LH and FSH levels were unaffected by the treatment with calcitonin; however, TSH levels were elevated 2.1-fold after calcitonin treatment in Sprague-Dawley but not Fischer rats of both sexes (Fig. 21-2). Interestingly, thyroid weights were decreased by 43 percent in

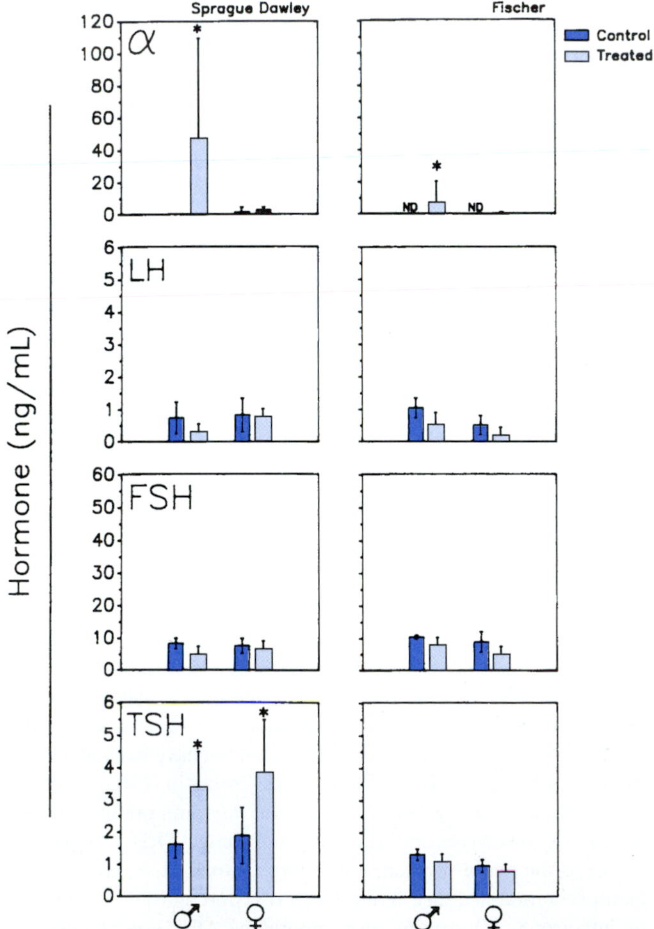

Figure 21-2. Serum glycoprotein hormone levels in rats treated chronically with salmon calcitonin.

Sprague-Dawley (*left panels*) or Fischer rats (*right panels*) were treated for 52 weeks with vehicle (*dark blue bars*) or calcitonin (80 IU/kg/day) (*light blue bars*). Results are the mean ± SD; *$p < 0.05$. (From Jameson et al., 1992, with permission.)

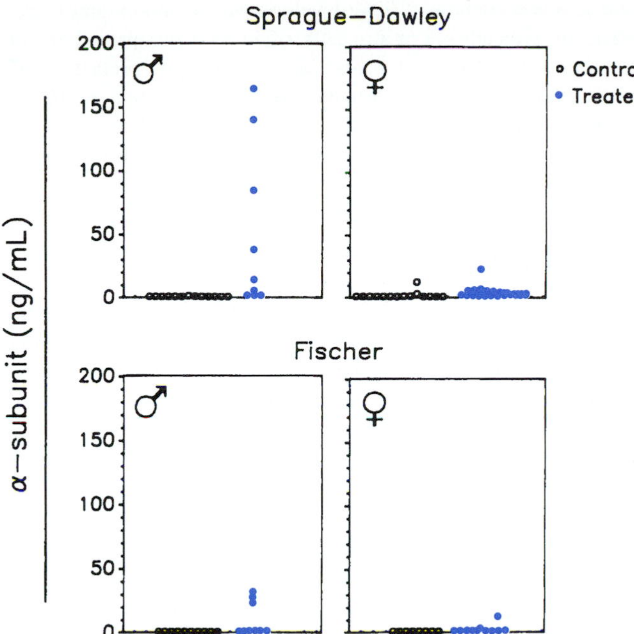

Figure 21-3. Serum α-subunit levels in individual male rats treated chronically with calcitonin.

The serum levels for individual animals are denoted. ○ = vehicle; ● = calcitonin-treated. (From Jameson et al., 1992, with permission.)

calcitonin-treated male rats and there was atrophy of thyroid follicular cells in some treated rats, suggesting that the immunoreactivity detected by the TSH assay was not biologically active. After treatment with calcitonin, serum α-subunit levels were increased by at least 20-fold in Sprague-Dawley males and 4-fold in male Fischer rats (Figs. 21-3 and 21-4). There was a good correlation between histopathologic evidence of α-subunit–producing pituitary tumors and elevated serum levels. In each of the calcitonin-treated rats that had adenomas, the tumors were positive for α-

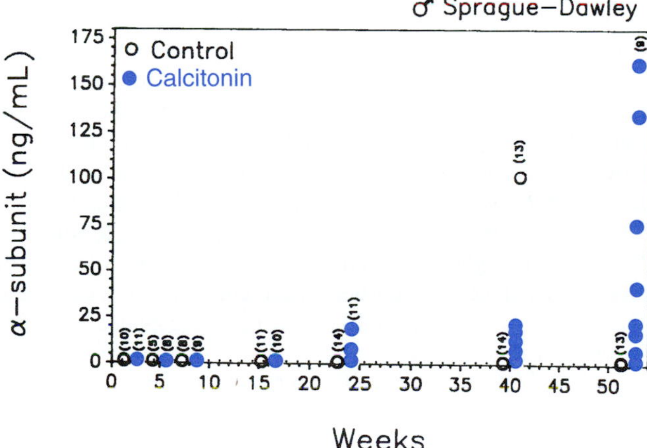

Figure 21-4. Time course for the increase in serum α-subunit levels in male Sprague-Dawley rats.

Symbols in the undetectable range represent values for more than one animal. The number of animals in each group is shown in parenthesis. ○ = control; ● = calcitonin-treated. (From Jameson et al., 1992, with permission.)

subunit by immunohistochemistry and in situ hybridization for expression of α-subunit mRNA.

Serum levels of α-subunit were elevated in male Sprague-Dawley rats after 2, 5, 8, 16, 24, 40, and 52 weeks to determine the time course for hormone elevation. Elevated levels of α-subunit were detected as early as 24 weeks in rats treated with calcitonin and the majority of animals had increased α-subunit levels by 40 weeks of treatment (Fig. 21-4), suggesting that pituitary tumors developed only after several months of exposure to calcitonin. Levels of α-subunit in vehicle-treated rats were below the detection limits of the assay at each time point.

The studies reported by Jameson et al. (1992) did not determine whether the effects of calcitonin on the pituitary were direct or indirect. Calcitonin is known to be produced in large amounts in the posterior hypothalamus and median eminence where it may normally exert an effect on the hypothalamus-pituitary axis. Calcitonin receptors have been identified in the hypothalamus and lower numbers of receptors are found in the pituitary gland. A striking feature of the calcitonin-induced pituitary tumors and elevated serum α-subunit levels was the predilection for male compared with female rats. The basis for the sex- and species-specific effects of calcitonin was not determined. The relevance of the effects of calcitonin in the rat pituitary gland to human pathophysiology is uncertain at present. However, neither the treatment of patients with calcitonin nor patients with the multiple endocrine neoplasia syndrome II with medullary thyroid cancer and elevated serum calcitonin levels have resulted in the development of pituitary tumors. The doses of calcitonin used in rats were from 25- to 50-fold greater on a per-weight basis than doses administered to patients. In addition, several strains of rats are known to be highly predisposed to develop pituitary tumors compared to humans.

The high frequency of spontaneous pituitary adenomas in laboratory rats is a well-recognized phenomenon which must be considered in any long-term toxicological study. The incidence of pituitary tumors is determined by many factors including strain, age, sex, reproductive status, and diet. Studies from the National Toxicology Program (NTP) historical database of 2-year-old F344 rats have shown that the incidence of pituitary adenomas was 21.7 and 44 percent for males and females, respectively. Corresponding figures for carcinomas arising in the adenohypophysis were 2.4 and 3.5 percent for males and females, respectively. Numerous hypotheses have been invoked to explain the high incidence of pituitary adenomas in certain inbred rat strains. Both hereditary factors and the levels of circulating sex steroids have been suggested as important etiological mechanisms. The hypothalamus has also been incriminated in the development of these tumors. Age-related hypothalamic changes may result in diminished activity of dopamine, the major prolactin-inhibitory factor.

Numerous studies have demonstrated the striking degree of strain variation in the incidence of pituitary tumors in rats, which has been reported to range from 10 to more than 90 percent. Particularly high incidences of pituitary adenomas have been reported in Wistar, WAG/Rij, Osborne-Mendel, Long-Evans, Amsterdam, and Columbia-Sherman rats. In the BN/Bi strain, pituitary adenomas have been found in 26 percent of females and 14 percent of males. Adenomas were identified in 95 percent of females and 96 percent of males in the WAG/Rij strain while (WAG/Rij 3 BN) F_1 rats had incidences of 83 percent for females and 64 percent for males. Rapid body growth rates and high levels of conversion of feed to body mass in early life or high protein intake in early adult life predispose any strain of rat to the development of pituitary adenomas. In rats fed a low protein diet (less than 12.7 percent crude protein) the overall tumor incidence, the numbers of multifocal tumors, and the degree of cellular atypia within tumors are significantly lower than in rats fed a standard diet.

"Cystoid degeneration" has been used to describe foci of parenchymal cell loss in the adenohypophysis. Foci of cystoid degeneration (50 to 150 mm in diameter) have margins composed of normal secretory cells of the pars distalis. Cystoid degeneration also may occur in hyperplastic foci and in neoplasms of the pituitary. The frequency of cystoid degeneration is increased by feeding diets containing diethylstilbestrol to female C3H HeN (MTV+) mice.

The separation between focal hyperplasia, adenoma, and carcinoma utilizing histopathologic techniques is difficult in the pituitary gland. However, criteria for their separation have been established and should be applied in a consistent manner in the evaluation of proliferative lesions of the pituitary gland. For the specific trophic hormone–secreting cells of the adenohypophysis, there appears to be a continuous spectrum of proliferative lesions between diffuse or focal hyperplasia and adenomas derived from a specific population of secretory cells. It appears to be a common feature of endocrine glands that prolonged stimulation of a population of secretory cells predisposes to the subsequent development of a higher than expected incidence of focal hyperplasia and tumors. Long-continued stimulation may lead to the development of clones of cells within the hyperplastic foci that grow more rapidly than the rest and are more susceptible to neoplastic transformation when exposed to the right combination of promoting carcinogens.

Focal ("nodular") hyperplasia in the adenohypophysis appears as multiple small areas that are well demarcated but not encapsulated from adjacent normal cells. Cells in areas of focal hyperplasia closely resemble the cells of origin; however, the cytoplasmic area may be slightly enlarged and the nucleus more hyperchromatic than in the normal cells. Adenomas usually are solitary nodules that are larger than the often multiple areas of focal hyperplasia. They are sharply demarcated from the adjacent normal pituitary glandular parenchyma and there often is a thin, partial to complete, fibrous capsule. The adjacent parenchyma is compressed to varying degrees depending on the size of the adenoma. Cells composing an adenoma closely resemble the cells of origin morphologically and in their architectural pattern of arrangement.

Carcinomas usually are larger than adenomas in the pituitary and usually result in a macroscopically detectable enlargement. Histopathologic features that are suggestive of malignancy include extensive intraglandular invasion, invasion into adjacent structures (e.g., dura mater, sphenoid bone), formation of tumor cell thrombi within vessels, and particularly the establishment of metastases at distant sites. The growth of neoplastic cells subendothelially in highly vascular benign tumors of the pituitary should not be mistaken for vascular invasion. Malignant cells often are more pleomorphic than normal, but nuclear and cellular pleomorphism are not a consistent criterion to distinguish adenoma from carcinoma in the adenohypophysis of rodents.

The vast majority of pituitary adenomas in humans and rodents have been described as chromophobic in type by light microscopy; however, many of these tumors have been found to stain for prolactin by immunohistochemistry. Of the prolactin-producing tumors, most are sparsely granulated with low levels of prolactin immunoreactivity by immunohistochemistry and having small numbers of secretory granules by electron microscopy. Diffuse hyperplasia of the prolactin cells has been observed adjacent to some adenomas. The development of tumors and hyperplasia of prolactin-secreting cells often is accompanied by increasing serum levels of prolactin. Occasionally, prolactin cells within adenomas may be admixed with FSH/LH-, TSH-, or ACTH-positive cells in the rat pituitary.

ADRENAL CORTEX

Introduction

The adrenal cortex of animals is prone to develop degenerative and proliferative lesions, the etiology of which may be either spontaneous in nature or experimentally induced. Therefore, testing of xenobiotic chemicals using various laboratory animal species is a valid means of assessing the toxic potential for humans exposed to various xenobiotic chemicals. The choice of test animal species also is critical, as a number of studies have demonstrated that there often is a variable species susceptibility to chemical toxicity. This suggests that interspecies differences in metabolism plays a role in the development of adrenal cortical toxicity and in the inhibition of steroidogenesis. The age of the test animal, to a lesser degree, can be a factor in the development of chemically induced adrenal cortical lesions.

Normal Structure and Function

The adrenal (suprarenal) glands in mammals are flattened bilobed organs located in close proximity to the kidneys. The adrenal glands receive arterial blood from branches of the aorta or from the phrenic, renal, and lumbar arteries resulting in a subcapsular sinusoidal vascular plexus that drains through the cortex into the medulla. The ratio of cortex:medulla is approximately 2:1 in healthy laboratory-reared animals.

The cortex is histologically characterized by defined regions or zones. The cortical zones consist of the zona glomerulosa (multiformis), zona fasciculata, and zona reticularis. The zones are not always clearly delineated, as in the normal rat adrenal cortex. The mineralocorticoid-producing zona glomerulosa (multiformis) (approximately 15 percent of the cortex) contains cells aligned in a sigmoid pattern in relationship to the capsule. Degeneration of this zone or an interference in the ability to produce mineralocorticoids (namely, aldosterone) results in a life-threatening retention of potassium and hypovolemic shock associated with the excessive urinary loss of sodium, chloride, and water. The largest part of the cortex is the zona fasciculata comprising >70 percent of the cortical width. Cells in this zone are arranged in long anastomosing columns separated by vascular sinusoids and are responsible for the secretion of glucocorticoid hormones (e.g., corticosterone or cortisol). The innermost portion of the cortex is the zona reticularis (>15 percent of the cortex), which secretes minute quantities of adrenal sex hormones.

The adrenal cortical cells contain large cytoplasmic lipid droplets consisting of cholesterol and other steroid hormone precursors. The lipid droplets are in close proximity to the smooth endoplasmic reticulum and large mitochondria, which contain the specific hydroxylase and dehydrogenase enzyme systems required to synthesize the different steroid hormones. Unlike polypeptidehormone-secreting cells, there are no secretory granules in the cytoplasm, since there is direct secretion without significant storage of preformed steroid hormones.

Steroid hormone-producing cells of the adrenal cortex synthesizes a major parent steroid with one to four additional carbon atoms added to the basic 17-carbon steroid nucleus. Since steroid hormones are not stored in any significant amount, a continued rate of synthesis is required to maintain a normal secretory rate. Once in the circulation, cortisol or corticosterone are bound reversibly to plasma proteins (such as transcortin, albumin). Under normal conditions 10 percent of the glucocorticoids are in a free unbound state.

Adrenal steroids are synthesized from cholesterol by specific enzyme-catalyzed reactions and involve a complex shuttling of steroid intermediates between mitochondria and endoplasmic reticulum. The specificity of mitochondrial hydroxylation reactions in terms of precursor acted upon and the position of the substrate which is hydroxylated is confined to a specific cytochrome P450. The common biosynthetic pathway from cholesterol is the formation of pregnenolone, the basic precursor for the three major classes of adrenal steroids. Pregnenolone is formed after two hydroxylation reactions at the carbon 20 and 22 positions of cholesterol and a subsequent cleavage between these two carbon atoms. In the zona fasciculata, pregnenolone is first converted to progesterone by two microsomal enzymes. Three subsequent hydroxylation reactions occur involving, in order, carbon atoms at the 17, 21, and 11 positions. The resulting steroid is cortisol, which is the major glucocorticoid in teleosts, hamsters, dogs, nonhuman primates, and humans. Corticosterone is the major glucocorticoid produced in amphibians, reptiles, birds, rats, mice, and rabbits. It is produced in a manner similar to the production of cortisol, except that progesterone does not undergo 17α-hydroxylation and proceeds directly to 21-hydroxylation and 11β-hydroxylation.

In the zona glomerulosa, pregnenolone is converted to aldosterone by a series of enzyme-catalyzed reactions similar to those involved in cortisol formation; however, the cells of this zone lack the 17α-hydroxylase and thus cannot produce 17α-hydroxyprogesterone, which is required to produce cortisol. Therefore, the initial hydroxylation product is corticosterone. Some of the corticosterone is acted on by 18-hydroxylase to form 18-hydroxycorticosterone, which in turn interacts with 18-hydroxysteroid dehydrogenase to form aldosterone. Since 18-hydroxysteroid dehydrogenase is found only in the zona glomerulosa, it is not surprising that only this zone has the capacity to produce aldosterone. In addition to the aforementioned steroid hormones, cells in the zona reticularis also produces small amounts of sex steroids including progesterone, estrogens, and androgens.

The mineralocorticoids (e.g., aldosterone) are the major steroids secreted from the zona glomerulosa under the control of the renin–angiotensin II system. The mineralocorticoids have their effects on ion transport by epithelial cells, particularly renal cells, resulting in conservation of sodium (chloride and water) and loss of potassium. In the distal convoluted tubule of the mammalian nephron, a cation exchange exists that promotes the resorption of sodium from the glomerular filtrate and the secretion of potassium into the lumen.

Under conditions of decreased blood flow or volume, the enzyme renin is released into the circulation at an increased rate by cells of the juxtaglomerular apparatus of the kidney. Renin release has also been associated with potassium loading or sodium depletion. Renin in the peripheral circulation acts to cleave a plasma globulin precursor (angiotensinogen produced by the liver) to angiotensin I. An angiotensin converting enzyme (ACE), subsequently hydrolyzes angiotensin I to angiotensin II, which acts as a trophic hormone to stimulate the synthesis and secretion of aldosterone. Under normal conditions negative feedback control to inhibit further renin release is exerted by the elevated levels of angiotensin (principally angiotensin II) as well as the expanded extracellular fluid volume resulting from the increased electrolyte (sodium and chloride) and water reabsorption by the kidney.

The principal control for the production of glucocorticoids by the zona fasciculata and zona reticularis is exerted by adrenocorticotropin (ACTH), a polypeptide hormone produced by corticotrophs in the adenohypophysis of the pituitary gland. ACTH release is largely controlled by the hypothalamus through the secretion of corticotropin-releasing hormone (CRH). An increase in ACTH production results in an increase in circulating levels of glucocorticoids and under certain conditions also can result in weak stimulation of aldosterone secretion. Negative feedback control normally occurs when the elevated blood levels of cortisol act either on the hypothalamus, anterior pituitary, or both to cause a suppression of ACTH secretion.

Mechanisms of Toxicity

The reason the adrenal cortex is predisposed to the toxic effects of xenobiotic chemicals appears to be related to at least two factors. *First,* adrenal cortical cells of most animal species contain large stores of lipids used primarily as substrate for steroidogenesis. Many adrenal cortical toxic compounds are lipophilic and therefore can accumulate in these lipid-rich cells. *Second,* adrenal cortical cells have enzymes capable of metabolizing of xenobiotic chemicals, including enzymes of the cytochrome P450 family. Many of these enzymes function in the biosynthesis of endogenous steroids and are localized in membranes of the endoplasmic reticulum or mitochondria. A number of toxic xenobiotic chemicals serve as pseudosubstrates for these enzymes and can be metabolized to reactive toxic compounds. These reactive compounds result in direct toxic effects by covalent interactions with cellular macromolecules or through oxygen activation with the generation of free radicals.

Classes of chemicals known to be toxic for the adrenal cortex include short-chain (three- or four-carbon) aliphatic compounds, lipidosis-inducers, and amphiphilic compounds. A variety of other compounds also may affect the medulla. The most potent aliphatic compounds are of three-carbon length with electronegative groups at both ends. These compounds frequently produce necrosis, particularly in the zonae fasciculata and reticularis. Examples include acrylonitrile, 3-aminopropionitrile, 3-bromopropionitrile, 1-butanethiol, and 1,4-butanedithiol. By comparison, lipidosis-inducers can cause the accumulations, often coalescing, of neutral fats, which may be of sufficient quantity to cause a reduction or loss of organellar function and eventual cell destruction. Cholesterol is the precursor substrate required to synthesize steroid hormones. Steroidogenic cells obtain cholesterol exogenously from serum lipoproteins and endogenously from de novo synthesis via the acetyl coenzyme A pathway (Fig. 21-5). The adrenal cortical cells and OI cells in the rat preferentially utilize serum high-density lipoproteins (HDLs) for their primary source of cholesterol and resort to de novo synthesis if HDL does not meet the demand of steroidogenesis. This is in contrast to Leydig cells of the testis, which preferentially utilizes de novo synthesis of cholesterol and uses an exogenous source only when intracellular synthesis does not meet the demand and the cholesterol pool has been depleted (Payne et al., 1985).

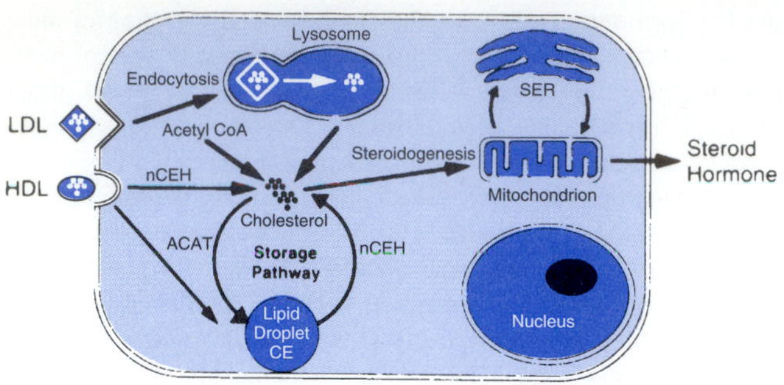

Figure 21-5. Cholesterol metabolism and steroid biosynthesis in adrenocortical and ovarian interstitial cells.

Cholesterol is the substrate for steroid biosynthesis. Conversion of cholesterol to pregnenolone occurs in the mitochondria, and oxidative reactions catalyzed by P450 enzymes occur in the smooth endoplasmic reticulum and mitochondria. Sources of cholesterol include lipoprotein uptake from serum (LDL and HDL), de novo synthesis from acetate via the acetyl coenzyme A pathway, and hydrolysis of cholesteryl ester (CE) by neutral CE hydrolase (nCEH). The storage pool in the form of lipid droplets is derived principally from the conversion of free cholesterol to CE catalyzed by acyl coenzyme A: cholesterol acyltransferase (ACAT). Direct uptake of CE from serum to the storage pool is minimal in the rat. (From Latendresse et al., 1993, with permission.)

The zonae reticularis and fasciculata appear to be the principal targets of xenobiotic chemicals in the adrenal cortex. Examples of the compounds causing lipidosis include aminoglutethimide, amphenone, and anilines. Tricresyl phosphate (TCP) and other triaryl phosphates cause a defect in cholesterol metabolism by blocking both the uptake from serum and storage pathways. An inhibition of cytosolic neutral cholesteryl ester hydroxylase (nCEH) by triaryl phosphate (97 percent inhibition compared to controls) results in the progressive accumulation of cholesteryl ester in the form of lipid droplets in the cytoplasm of adrenal cortical and ovarian interstitial (OI) cells (Fig. 21-6) but not in testicular Leydig cells of rats (Latendresse et al., 1993). Acyl coenzyme A: cholesterol acyl

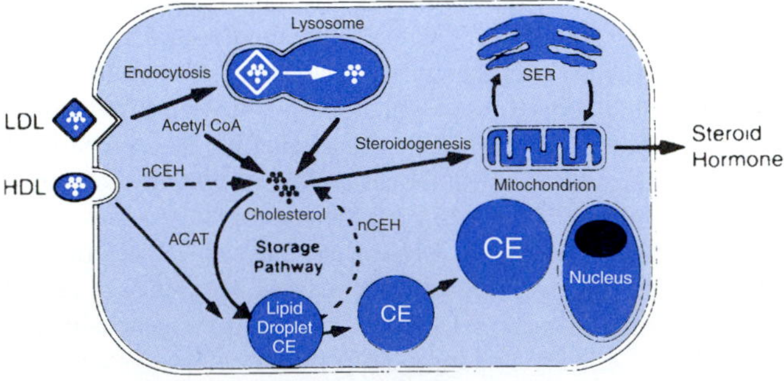

Figure 21-6. Pathogenesis of cholesteryl lipidosis in adrenocortical cells and ovarian interstitial cells.

The defect in cholesterol metabolism occurs in the uptake from serum and storage pathways. An inhibition of neutral cholesteryl ester hydrolase (nCEH) by a xenobiotic chemical results in the accumulation of CE in the form of lipid droplets in the cytoplasm. Acyl coenzyme A:cholesterol acyltransferase (ACAT) (catalyzes the formation of CE from cholesterol) activity remains near normal levels. (From Latendresse et al., 1993, with permission.)

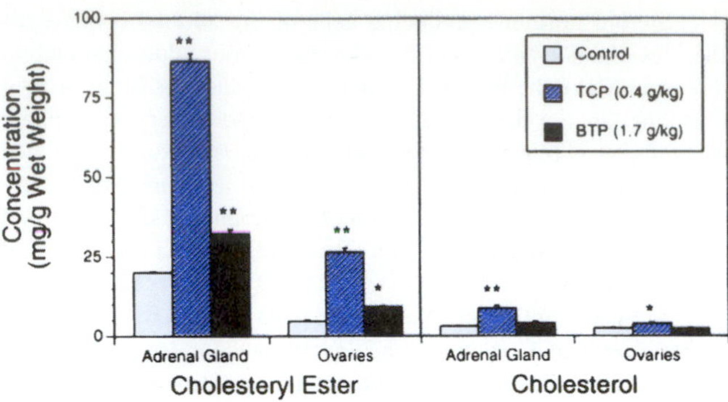

Figure 21-7. The effects of tricresyl phosphate (TCP) and butylated triphenyl phosphate (BTH) on concentration of cholesteryl ester (CE) and cholesterol in adrenal gland and ovary of rats.

Mean ± SEM ($n = 8$–9)mg/g wet weight of adrenal gland and ovary. ***Different ($p \leq 0.01$, $p \leq 0.05$, respectively) from control. (From Latendresse et al., 1993, with permission.)

transferase (ACAT), an enzyme that esterifies cholesterol to make cholesteryl ester, was depressed only 27 percent (compared to controls) resulting in elevated intracellular storage of cholesterol in the form of lipid droplets (Fig. 21-7).

Biologically active cationic amphiphilic compounds produce a generalized phospholipidosis that involves primarily the zonae reticularis and fasciculata and produce microscopic phospholipid-rich inclusions. These compounds affect the functional integrity of lysosomes, which appear ultrastructurally to be enlarged and filled with membranous lamellae or myelin figures. Examples of compounds known to induce phospholipidosis include chloroquine, triparanol, and chlorphentermine.

Another class of compounds that affect the adrenal cortex are hormones, particularly natural and synthetic steroids. The administration of exogenous steroid hormones such as corticosteroids may cause functional inactivity and trophic atrophy following prolonged use. Other steroid hormones such as natural and synthetic estrogens and androgens have been reported to cause proliferative lesions in the adrenal cortex of laboratory animals.

In addition, there is a miscellaneous group of chemicals that affect hydroxylation and other functions of mitochondrial and microsomal fractions (e.g., smooth endoplasmic reticulum) in the adrenal cortex. Examples of these compounds include *o,p*'-DDD and α-(1,4-dioxido-3-methylquinoxalin-2-yl)-*N*-methylnitrone (DMNM). Other compounds in this miscellaneous category cause their effects by means of cytochrome P450 metabolism and the production of toxic metabolites. A classic example is the activation of carbon tetrachloride, resulting in lipid peroxidation and covalent binding to cellular macromolecules of the adrenal cortex.

Many of the chemicals that cause morphologic changes in the adrenal glands also affect cortical function. Chemically induced changes in adrenal function result either from blockage of the action of adrenocorticoids at peripheral sites or by inhibition of synthesis and/or secretion of hormone. In the first mechanism, many antisteroidal compounds (antagonists) act by competing with or binding to steroid hormone–receptor sites; thereby, either reducing the number of available receptor sites or by altering their binding affinity. Cortexolone (11α-deoxycortisol) an antiglucocorticoid and spironolactone, an antimineralocorticoid, are two examples of peripherally acting adrenal cortical hormone antagonists.

Xenobiotic chemicals affecting adrenal function often do so by altering steroidogenesis and result in histologic and ultrastructural changes in adrenal cortical cells. For example, chemicals causing increased lipid droplets often inhibit the utilization of steroid precursors, including the conversion of cholesterol to pregnenolone. Chemicals that affect the fine structure of mitochondria and smooth endoplasmic reticulum often impair the activity of 11α-, 17α-, and 21-hydroxylases, respectively, and are associated with lesions primarily in the zonae reticularis and fasciculata. Atrophy of the zona glomerulosa may reflect specific inhibition of aldosterone synthesis or secretion, either directly (e.g., inhibition of 18α-hydroxylation) or indirectly (e.g., suppression of the renin–angiotensin system II) by chemicals such as spironolactone and captopril.

It is well documented that synthetic and naturally occurring corticosteroids are potent teratogens in laboratory animals. The principal induced defect is cleft lip or palate; however, there is a paucity of information on the direct effect of xenobiotic chemicals on the development of the adrenal cortex. For example, adrenal aplasia occurred in 7.6 of 9.8 percent of white Danish rabbits when thalidomide was given to their dams.

Pathologic Alterations and Proliferative Lesions in Cortical Cells

Macroscopic lesions of chemically affected adrenal glands are characterized either by enlargement or reduction in size that often is bilateral. Cortical hypertrophy due to impaired steroidogenesis or hyperplasia due to long-term stimulation often is present when the adrenal cortex is increased in size. Small adrenal glands often are indicative of degenerative changes or trophic atrophy of the adrenal cortex. Midsagittal longitudinal sections of adrenal glands under the above conditions will reveal either a disproportionately wider cortex relative to the medulla or vice versa, resulting in an abnormal cortical:medullary ratio. Nodular lesions that distort and enlarge one or both adrenal glands suggest that a neoplasm is present. A single well-demarcated nodular lesion suggests a cortical adenoma, whereas widespread incorporation of the entire adrenal gland by a proliferative mass is suggestive of cortical carcinoma, especially if there is evidence of local invasion into periadrenal connective tissues or into adjacent blood vessels and the kidney.

Nonneoplastic lesions of the adrenal cortex induced by xenobiotic chemicals are characterized by changes ranging from acute progressive degeneration to reparative processes such as multifocal hyperplasia. Early degenerative lesions characterized by enlarged cortical cells filled with cytoplasmic vacuoles (often lipid) may result in a diffuse hypertrophy of the cortex. A lesion of this type has been observed in rats treated with an antibacterial compound α-(1,4-dioxido-3-methylquinoxalin-2-yl)-*N*-methylntrone (DMNM). This type of vacuolar degeneration is a reflection of impaired steroidogenesis resulting in an accumulation of steriod precursors. More destructive lesions such as hemorrhage and/or necrosis are associated with an inflammatory response in the cortex. If the zona glomerulosa remains functional there will be no life-threatening electrolyte disturbances and no signs of hypoadrenocorticism (Addison's disease). While many chemical agents that affect the adrenal cortex initially involve the zona reticularis and inner zona fasciculata, certain chemicals such as DMNM can cause a progressive degeneration of the entire adrenal cortex. Occasionally, a chemical's effect is limited to a specific zone of the adrenal cortex and may be species-specific.

Ultrastructural alterations of adrenal cortical cells associated with chemical injury are quite diverse in nature. The zonae reticularis and fasciculata typically are most severely affected, although eventually the lesions involve the zona glomerulosa. These lesions may be classified as follows: endothelial damage (e.g., acrylonitrile), mitochondrial damage (e.g., DMNM, *o,p*'-DDD, amphenone), endoplasmic reticulum disruption (e.g., triparanol), lipid aggregation (e.g., aniline), lysosomal phospholipid aggregation (e.g., chlorophentermine), and secondary effects due to embolization by medullary cells (e.g., acrylonitrile). Mitochondrial damage with vacuolization and accompanying changes in the endoplasmic reticulum and autophagocytic responses appear to be among the most common ultrastructural changes observed following chemical injury in the adrenal cortex. Since mitochondria and smooth endoplasmic reticulum form an intimate subcellular organellar network in cortical cells with important hydroxylases and dehydrogenase enzymes, it is not surprising that many chemical agents altering the ultrastructural morphology of cortical cells inhibit steroidogenesis.

Chemically induced proliferative lesions of the adrenal cortex are less frequently reported and include hyperplasia, adenoma, and carcinoma. Unlike the diffuse cortical hyperplasia/hypertrophy associated with excess ACTH stimulation, chemically induced hyperplasia usually is nodular in type, often multiple in distribution, and composed of increased numbers of normal or vacuolated cortical cells.

A variety of different chemicals are associated with an increased incidence of adrenal cortical neoplasia. Most of the reported tumors tend to be benign (adenomas) although an occasional tumor may be malignant (carcinomas). The zonae reticularis and fasciculata are more prone to develop tumors following chemical injury whereas the zona glomerulosa is spared unless invaded by an expanding tumor in the adjacent zones of the cortex. The tumorigenic agents of the adrenal cortex have a diverse chemical nature and use.

Spontaneous proliferative lesions may be found in all zones of the adrenal cortex but in adult rats are found most frequently in the zona fasciculata. Spontaneous nodular hyperplasia of the adrenal cortex is common in the rabbit, golden hamster, rat, mouse, dog, cat, horse, and baboon. Naturally occurring adrenal cortical tumors are found infrequently in domestic animals except adult dogs and castrated male goats. However, cortical adenomas and (to a lesser extent) cortical carcinomas have been reported in moderately high incidence in certain strains of laboratory hamsters (e.g., BIO 4.24 and BIO 45.5 strains) and rat (e.g., Osborne Mendel, WAG/Rij, BUF, and BN/Bi strains). The incidence often increases markedly in rats over 18 months of age. Adrenal cortical neoplasms in mice are uncommon but the incidence may be increased by gonadectomy.

ADRENAL MEDULLA

Normal Structure and Function

The medulla constitutes approximately 10 percent of the volume of the adrenal gland. In the normal rodent adrenal gland and in most other laboratory animal species, the medulla is sharply demarcated from the surrounding cortex. The bulk of the medulla is composed of chromaffin cells, which are the sites of synthesis and storage of the catecholamine hormones. In the rat and mouse, norepinephrine and epinephrine are stored in separate cell types that can be distinguished ultrastructurally after fixation in glutaraldehyde and postfixation in osmium tetroxide. The norepinephrine-containing core of the secretory granules appears electron-dense and is surrounded by a wide submembranous space, whereas epinephrine-containing granules are less dense; they have a finely granular core and a narrow space beneath the limiting membrane. Granules of varying densities may be found in the same cell types in the adrenal medulla of immature rats. Human adrenal medullary cells may contain both norepinephrine and epinephrine within a single chromaffin cell.

The adrenal medulla contains variable numbers of ganglion cells in addition to chromaffin cells. A third cell type has been described in the medulla and designated the small granule–containing (SGC) cell or small intensely fluorescent (SIF) cell. These cells morphologically appear intermediate between chromaffin cells and ganglion cells, and may function as interneurons. The adrenal medullary cells also contain serotonin and histamine, but it has not been determined if these products are synthesized in situ or taken up from the circulation. A number of neuropeptides also are present in rat chromaffin cells, including enkephalins, neurotensin, and neuropeptide Y.

In the catecholamine biosynthetic pathway, tyrosine is acted on by tyrosine hydroxylase to produce dopa, which is converted to dopamine by dopa decarboxylase. Dopamine in turn, is acted on by dopamine beta-hydroxylase to form norepinephrine, which is converted to epinephrine by phenylethanolamine-*N*-methyltransferase (PNMT). Tyrosine hydroxylase and PNMT are the principal rate-limiting steps in catecholamine synthesis. The conversion of tyrosine into dopa and dopamine occurs within the cytosol of chromaffin cells. Dopamine then enters the chromaffin granule, where it is converted to norepinephrine. Norepinephrine leaves the granule and is converted into epinephrine in the cytosol, and epinephrine reenters and is stored in the chromaffin granule. In contrast to the synthesis of catecholamines, which occurs in the cytosol, neuropeptides and chromogranin-A proteins are synthesized in the granular endoplasmic reticulum and are packaged into granules in the Golgi apparatus.

Innervation plays an important role in regulating the functions of chromaffin cells. During adult life, stresses such as insulin-induced hypoglycemia or reserpine-induced depletion of catecholamines produces a reflex increase in splanchnic nerve discharge, resulting both in catecholamine secretion and transsynaptic induction of catecholamine biosynthetic enzymes, including tyrosine hydroxylase. These effects become apparent during the first week of life, following an increase in the number of nerve terminals in the adrenal medulla. Other environmental influences including growth factors, extracellular matrix, and a variety of hormonal signals that generate cyclic AMP also may regulate the function of chromaffin cells.

Mechanisms of Toxicity

Proliferative lesions of the medulla, particularly in the rat, have been reported to develop as a result of a variety of different mechanisms. Warren and coworkers (1966) studied over 700 pairs of rats with parabiosis and found that more than 50 percent of male irradiated rats developed adrenal medullary tumors. A relationship exists between adenohypophyseal (anterior pituitary) hormones and the development of adrenal medullary proliferative lesions. For example, the long-term administration of growth hormone is associated with an increased incidence of pheochromocytomas as well as the development of tumors at other sites. Prolactin-secreting pituitary tumors, which occur commonly in many rat strains, also play a role in the development of proliferative medullary lesions. In addition, several neuroleptic compounds that increase prolactin secretion by inhibiting dopamine production have been associated with an increased incidence of proliferative lesions of medullary cells in chronic toxicity studies in rats.

Both nicotine and reserpine have been implicated in the development of adrenal medullary proliferative lesions in rats. Both agents act by a shared mechanism, since nicotine directly stimulates nicotinic acetylcholine receptors whereas reserpine causes a reflex increase in the activity of cholinergic nerve endings in the adrenal. A short dosing regimen of reserpine administration in vivo stimulates proliferation of chromaffin cells in the adult rat, and the mechanism may involve a reflex increase in neurogenic stimulation via the splanchnic nerve. Several other drugs have been reported to increase the incidence of adrenal medullary proliferative lesions. These include zomepirac sodium (a nonsteroidal anti-inflammatory drug), isoretinoin (a retinoid), and nafarelin (LHRH analog), atenolol (beta-adrenergic blocker), terazosin (alpha-adrenergic blocker), ribavirin (antiviral), and pamidronate (bisphosphonate) (Davies and Monro, 1995).

Lynch et al. (1996) have reported that nutritional factors have an important modulating effect on the spontaneous incidence of adrenal medullary proliferative lesions in rats. Several sugars and sugar alcohols have produced adrenal medullary tumors at high dosages (concentrations of 10 to 20 percent in the diet), including xylitol, sorbitol, lacitol, and lactose. Although the exact mechanism involved is not completely understood, an important role for calcium has been suggested. High doses of slowly absorbed sugars and starches increase the intestinal absorption and urinary excretion of calcium. Hypercalcemia is known to increase catecholamine synthesis in response to stress, and low-calcium diets will reduce the incidence of adrenal medullary tumors in xylitol-treated rats. Other compounds that may act by a similar mechanism of altered calcium homeostasis include the retinoids (which will produce hypercalcemia) and conditions such as progressive nephrocalcinosis in aging male rats treated with nonsteroidal anti-inflammatory agents.

Roe and Bar (1985) have suggested that environmental and dietary factors may be more important than genetic factors as determinants of the incidence of adrenal medullary proliferative lesions in rats. The incidence of adrenal medullary lesions can be reduced by lowering the carbohydrate content of the diet. Several of the agents that increase the incidence of adrenal medullary lesions, including sugar alcohols, increase absorption of calcium from the gut. Calcium ions as well as cyclic nucleotides and prostaglandins may act as mediators capable of stimulating both hormonal secretion and cellular proliferation.

Tischler et al. (1999) recently presented data that vitamin D is the most potent in vivo stimulus yet identified for chromaffin cell proliferation in the adrenal medulla. Vitamin D_3 (5000; 10,000; or 20,000 IU/kg/day in corn oil) resulted in a four- to fivefold increase in bromodeoxyuridine (BrdU) labeling at week 4 that diminished to a twofold increase by week 26 (Fig. 21-8). An initial preponderance of epinephrine-labeled (PNMT-positive cells) subsequently gave way to norepinephrine-labeled cells. By week 26, a total of 89 percent of rats receiving the two highest doses of vitamin D_3 had focal medullary proliferative lesions (BrdU-labeled focal hyperplasia, or "hot spots") and pheochromocytomas in contrast to absence of proliferative lesions in controls. This increase in medullary cell proliferation was associated with a significant increase in circulating levels of both calcium and phosphorus after

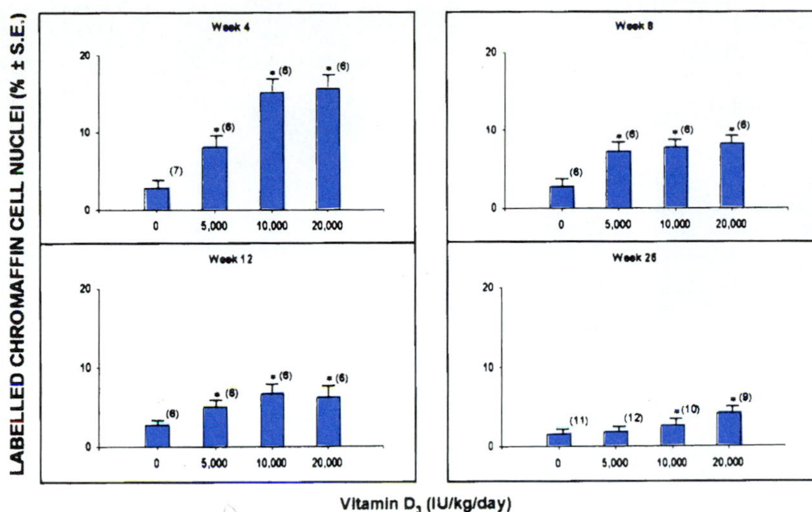

Figure 21-8. Effects of vitamin D_3 on percent of chromaffin cells labeled with BrdU during weeks 4, 8, 12, and 26 of dietary supplementation.

Asterisks indicate statistically significant increases over corn oil controls. Numbers in parentheses indicate numbers of rats scored for each point. Premature deaths or euthanasia caused loss of three animals from the group receiving 20,000 IU/kg/day, two from the group receiving 10,000 IU/kg/day, and one control. Histologic examination of these animals' adrenal glands showed no detectable abnormalities. One extra animal at the start of the experiment was assigned to the control group at week 1. At least 2500 chromaffin cells were scored for each rat. (From Tischler et al., 1999, with permission.)

vitamin D administration (Fig. 21-9). The nuclei of hyperplastic chromaffin cells labeled by BrdU but were phenylethanolamine-*N*-methyl transferase-negative indicating they most likely were norepinephrine-producing cells of the rat medulla (Fig. 21-10). The proliferative lesions usually were multicentric, bilateral, and peripheral in location in the medulla; nearly all were PNMT negative, and they appeared to represent a morphologic continuum rather than separate entities. Earlier studies reported by the same research group had demonstrated that the vitamin D_3 (20,000; 40,000 IU/kg/day) increase in chromaffin cell proliferation was observed as early as 1 week and had declined by 4 weeks. These findings support the hypothesis that altered calcium homeostasis is involved in the pathogenesis of pheochromocytomas in rodents, most likely via effects on increasing chromaffin cell proliferation (Fig. 21-11). Vitamin D_3, calcitriol (active metabolite of D_3), lactose, and xylitol all failed to stimulate directly the proliferation of rat chromaffin cells in vitro.

In summary, three dietary factors have been suggested to lead to an increased incidence of adrenal medullary proliferative lesions in chronic toxicity studies in rats (Roe and Bar, 1985). These are (1) excessive intake of food associated with feeding ad libitum; (2) excessive intake of calcium and phosphorus, since commercial diets contain two to three times more calcium and phosphorus than needed by young rats; and (3) excessive intake of other food components (e.g., vitamin D and poorly absorbable carbohydrates), which increase calcium absorption.

Pathologic Alterations and Proliferative Lesions in Medullary Cells

The adrenal medulla undergoes a series of proliferative changes ranging from diffuse hyperplasia to benign and malignant neoplasia. The latter neoplasms have the capacity to invade locally and to metastasize to distant sites. Diffuse hyperplasia is characterized by symmetrical expansion of the medulla with maintenance of the usual sharp demarcation between the cortex and the medulla. The medullary cell cords often are widened, but the ratio of norepinephrine to epinephrine cells is similar to that of normal glands. Focal hyperplastic lesions are often juxtacortical but may occur within any area of the medulla. The small nodules of hyperplasia in general are not associated with compression of the adjacent medulla; however, the larger foci may be associated with limited medullary compression. The foci of adrenal medullary hyperplasia are typically composed of small cells with round to ovoid nuclei and scanty cytoplasm. At the ultrastructural level, the cells composing these focal areas of hyperplasia contain small numbers of dense core secretory granules resembling the granules of SIF or SGC cells.

Larger benign adrenal medullary proliferative lesions are designated as pheochromocytomas. These lesions may be composed of relatively small cells similar to those found in smaller hyperplastic foci or larger chromaffin cells or a mixture of small and large cells. According to some authors, the lack of a positive chromaffin reaction in these focal proliferative lesions precludes the diagnosis of pheochromocytoma; however, the chromaffin reaction is quite insensitive and catecholamines (particularly norepinephrine) can be demonstrated in these proliferative lesions by biochemical extraction studies and by the formaldehyde- or glyoxylic-acid-induced fluorescence methods. Even in some of the larger medullary lesions, the chromaffin reaction is equivocal but catecholamines can be demonstrated both biochemically and histochemically. Malignant pheochromocytomas invade the adrenal capsule and often grow in the periadrenal connective tissues with or without distant metastases.

Proliferative lesions occur with high frequency in many strains of laboratory rats. The incidence of these lesions varies with strain, age, sex, diet, and exposure to drugs, and a variety of environmental agents. Studies from the NTP historical data base of 2-year-old

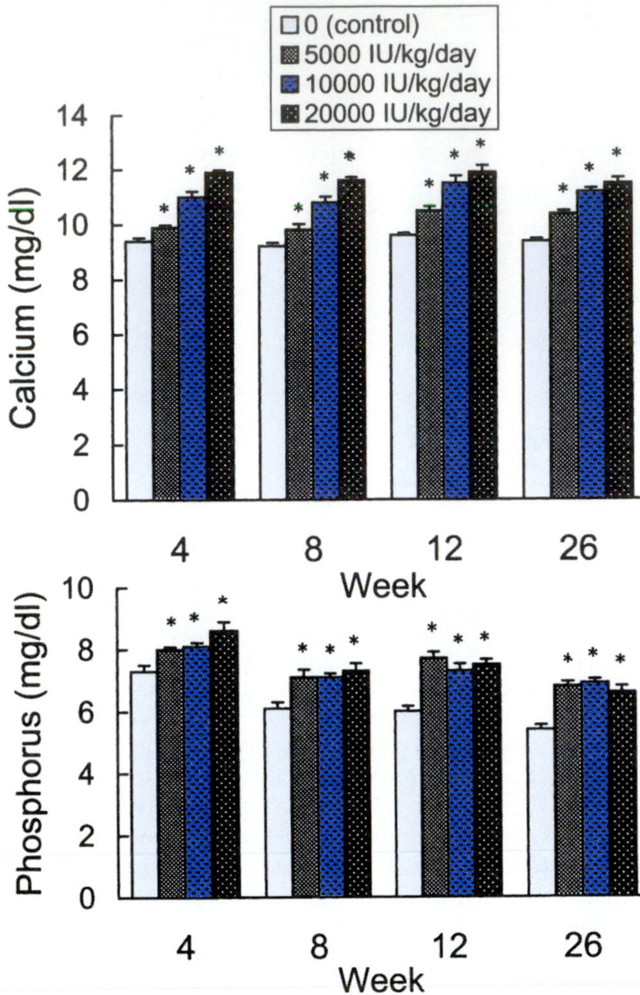

Figure 21-9. Effects of vitamin D_3 on serum calcium and phosphorus levels at weeks 4, 8, 12, and 26.

Sustained perturbation of both Ca^{2+} and PO_4 concentrations persisted throughout the time course. (From Tischler et al., 1999, with permission.)

F344 rats have reported that the incidence of pheochromocytomas was 17.0 percent and 3.1 percent for males and females, respectively. Malignant pheochromocytomas were detected in 1 percent of males and 0.5 percent of females. In addition to F344 rats, other strains with a high incidence of pheochromocytomas include Wistar, NEDH (New England Deaconess Hospital), Long-Evans, and Sprague-Dawley. Pheochromocytomas are considerably less common in Osborne-Mendel, Charles River, Holtzman, and WAG/Rij rats. Most studies have revealed a higher incidence in males than in females (Figs. 21-12 and 21-13). Crossbreeding of animals with high and low frequencies of adrenal medullary proliferative lesions results in F_1 animals with an intermediate tumor frequency. Pheochromocytomas are less common in the mouse than in most strains of rats.

There is a conspicuous relationship between increasing age and the frequency, size, and bilateral occurrence of adrenal medullary proliferative lesions in the rat. In the Long-Evans strain, medullary nodules have been found in less than 1 percent of animals under twelve months of age. The frequency increases to almost 20 percent in 2-year-old animals and to 40 percent in animals

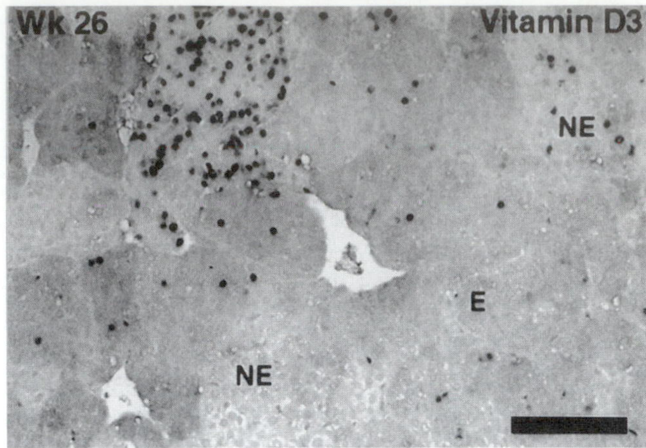

Figure 21-10. Photomicrographs of adrenal medullary sections stained for BrdU **(dark nuclei)** *and PNMT* **(dark cytoplasm)** *to compare BrdU labeling of epinephrine (E) and norepinephrine (NE) cells.*

Vitamin D_3 (20,000 IU/kg/day) caused a dramatic increase in BrdU labeling of predominantly E cells at week 4. The response was greatly reduced at week 26 and there was no longer an E-cell predominance. A representative hyperplasic nodule in the vitamin D_3–stimulated adrenal medulla at week 26 (*top left*) is densely labeled with BrdU and is PNMT-negative (bar = 100 μm). (From Tischler et al., 1999, with permission.)

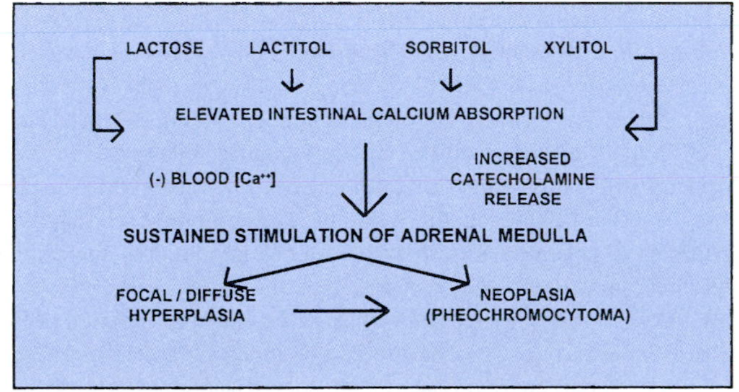

Figure 21-11. Pathogenesis of adrenal medullary proliferative lesions associated with ingestion of polyols resulting in elevation of the blood calcium concentration. (Modified from Lynch et al., 1996, with permission.)

RAT STRAIN	INCIDENCE (%) MALES (%)	FEMALES (%)	REFERENCE
CHARLES RIVER-CD	109/1211 (9.0)	24/1204 (2.0)	SHER *et al.* (1982)
F344 (NTP)	158/1794 (8.8)	55/1754 (3.1)	GOODMAN *et al* (1979)
HOLTZMAN	4/806 (0.5)	3/618 (0.5)	SCHARDIEN *et al* (1968)
F344	76/448 (17.0)	14/450 (3.1)	SHER *et al.* (1982)

Figure 21-12. Rat strains with a high incidence of pheochromocytomas. (Modified from Lynch et al., 1996, with permission.)

RAT STRAIN	INCIDENCE (%) MALES (%)	FEMALES (%)	REFERENCE
OSBORNE-MENDEL (NTP)	21/975 (2.2)	9/970 (0.9)	GOODMAN et al. (1980)
SPRAGUE-DAWLEY (CIBA-GEIGY)	121/578 (20.9)	36/585 (6.2)	McMARTIN et al. (1992)
WISTAR (BOR:WISW [SPF Cpb])	131/445 (29.4)	16/447 (3.6)	BOMHARD (1992) (30 mo.)
WISTAR (BOR:WISW [SPF Cpb])	133/1230 (10.6)	27/1242 (2.1)	BOMHARD & RINKE (1994) (24 mo.)
WISTAR (LOBUND)	46/66 (69.2)	NO DATA	POLLARD & LUCKERT (1989)

Figure 21-13. Rat strains with a low incidence of pheochromocytomas. (Modified from Lynch et al., 1996, with permission.)

BrdU INCORPORATION *IN VITRO*

	CONTROL	NGF	FGF	FORSKOLIN	PMA
RAT	<1%	UP TO 40%	UP TO 40%	UP TO 40%	UP TO 10%
HUMAN	<0.1%	<0.1%	<0.1%	<0.1%	<0.1%
BOVINE	0	0	0	0	0
MOUSE	<0.1%	0	UP TO 5%	UP TO 1 %	UP TO 1%

PM = PHORBOL MYRISTATE; NGF = NERVE GROWTH FACTOR; FGF = FIBROBLAST GROWTH FACTOR; BrdU = BROMODEOXYURIDINE

[1] RAT (3- TO 9-MONTH-OLD MALE AND FEMALE F344 OR CHARLES RIVER SPRAGUE-DAWLEY); [2] BOVINE (ADULT FEMALE); [3] MOUSE (12/SVJ x C57 L/6J; 3-MONTH-OLD FEMALES)

FROM: TISCHLER AND RISEBERG. ENDOCRINE PATH 4:1993, 15-19

Figure 21-15. Species differences in mitogenic responses of chromaffin cells in vitro from adult rat, human, bovine, and mouse adrenals. (From Tischler and Riseberg, 1993, with permission.)

between 2 and 3 years of age. The mean tumor size increases progressively with age, as does the frequency of bilateral and multicentric occurrence.

A variety of techniques may be used for the demonstration of catecholamines in tissue sections. The chromaffin reaction is the oxidation of catecholamines by potassium dichromate solutions and results in the formation of a brown-to-yellow pigment in medullary tissue. The chromaffin reaction as traditionally performed possesses a low level of sensitivity and should not be used for the definitive demonstration of the presence of catecholamines in tissues. Similarly, both the argentaffin and argyrophil reactions, which have been used extensively in the past for the demonstration of chromaffin cells, also possess low sensitivity and specificity. Fluorescence techniques using formaldehyde or glyoxylic acid represent the methods of choice for the demonstration of catecholamines at the cellular level. These aldehydes form highly fluorescent derivatives with catecholamines, which can be visualized by ultraviolet microscopy. Immunohistochemistry provides an alternative approach for the localization of catecholamines in chromaffin cells and other cell types. Antibodies are available that permit epinephrine- and norepinephrine-containing cells to be distinguished in routinely fixed and embedded tissue samples. Several of the important enzymes involved in the biosynthesis of catecholamine hormones also may be demonstrated by immunohistochemical procedures. Antibodies to chromogranin-A can be used for the demonstration of this unique protein in chromaffin cells.

CHARACTERISTICS	RATS	HUMANS
TUMOR CELLS	SMALLER THAN NORMAL	SMALL OR LARGE
SECRETORY GRANULES	OFTEN SMALL	VARIABLE (E + NOR E)
HORMONE CONTENT	NOR E	E + NOR E
FUNCTIONAL STATUS	INACTIVE	CATECHOLAMINE EXCESS
INCIDENCE	HIGH (STRAIN DIFFERENCE)	LOW (MEN SYNDROME)
RESPONSE OF AM TO MITOGENIC STIMULI	SENSITIVE	RESISTANT

Figure 21-14. Characteristics of pheochromocytomas in rats compared to humans. (Modified from Lynch et al., 1996, with permission.)

Pheochromocytomas in rats and human beings are both composed of chromaffin cells with variable numbers of hormone-containing secretory granules (Fig. 21-14). The incidence is high in many strains of rats by comparison to human patients, where pheochromocytomas are uncommon except in patients with inherited clinical syndromes of multiple endocrine neoplasia (MEN). These tumors in rats usually do not secrete excess amounts of catecholamines, whereas human pheochromocytomas episodically secrete increased amounts of catecholamines leading to hypertension and other clinical disturbances. There appears to be a striking species difference in the response of medullary chromaffin cells to mitogenic stimuli with rats being very sensitive compared to humans (Fig. 21-14).

Tischler and Riseberg (1993) reported that adult rat chromaffin cells had a marked increase (from not more than 10 to 40 percent) in bromodeoxyuridine (BrdU)–labeled nuclei in vitro following the addition of the following mitogens: nerve growth factor (NGF), fibroblast growth factor (FGF), forskolin, and phorbol myristate (PMA), whereas human chromaffin cells had a minimal (<0.1 percent) response to the same mitogens (Fig. 21-15). This striking difference in sensitivity to mitogenic stimuli may explain the lower frequency of adrenal medullary proliferative lesions in humans compared to many rat strains (Tischler and Riseberg, 1993). The mouse adrenal medulla, which, as in humans, has a low spontaneous incidence of proliferative lesions of chromaffin cells, also failed to respond to a variety of mitogenic stimuli (Fig. 21-15). These findings and others suggest that chromaffin cells of the rat represent an inappropriate model to assess the potential effects of xenobiotic chemicals on chromaffin cells of the human adrenal medulla (Lynch et al., 1996).

THYROID GLAND (FOLLICULAR CELLS)

Species Differences in Thyroid Hormone Economy

Long-term perturbations of the pituitary-thyroid axis by various xenobiotics or physiologic alterations (e.g., iodine deficiency, partial thyroidectomy, and natural goitrogens in food) are more likely to predispose the laboratory rat to a higher incidence of proliferative lesions [e.g., hyperplasia and benign tumors (adenomas) of fol-

Table 21-1
Thyroxine (T_4) Binding to Serum Proteins in Selected Vertebrate Species

SPECIES	T_4 BINDING GLOBULIN	POSTALBUMIN	ALBUMIN	PREALBUMIN
Human being	++*	—	++	+
Monkey	++	—	++	+
Dog	++*	—	++	—
Mouse	—*	++	++	—
Rat	—	+	++	+
Chicken	—	—	++	—

KEY: +, ++, Degree of T_4 binding to serum proteins; —, absence of binding of T_4 to serum proteins.
SOURCE: Döhler et al., 1979, with permission.

licular cells] in response to chronic TSH stimulation than in the human thyroid (Capen and Martin, 1989; Curran and DeGroot, 1991). This is particularly true in the male rat which has higher circulating levels of TSH than in females. The greater sensitivity of the rodent thyroid to derangement by drugs, chemicals, and physiologic perturbations also is related to the shorter plasma half-life of thyroxine T_4 in rats than in humans due to the considerable differences in the transport proteins for thyroid hormones between these species (Döhler et al., 1979).

The plasma T_4 half-life in rats is considerably shorter (12 to 24 h) than in humans (5 to 9 days). In human beings and monkeys circulating T_4 is bound primarily to thyroxine-binding globulin (TBG), but this high-affinity binding protein is not present in rodents, birds, amphibians, or fish (Table 21-1).

The binding affinity of TBG for T_4 is approximately a thousand times higher than for prealbumin. The percent of unbound active T_4 is lower in species with high levels of TBG than in animals in which T_4 binding is limited to albumin and prealbumin. Therefore, a rat without a functional thyroid requires about 10 times more T_4 (20 μg/kg body weight) for full substitution than an adult human (2.2 μg/kg body weight). Triiodothyronine (T_3) is transported bound to TBG and albumin and transthyretin in the human being, monkey, and dog but only to albumin in the mouse, rat, and chicken (Table 21-2). In general, T_3 is bound less avidly to transport proteins than T_4, resulting in a faster turnover and shorter plasma half-life in most species. These differences in plasma half-life of thyroid hormones and binding to transport proteins between rats and human beings may be one factor in the greater sensitivity of the rat thyroid to developing hyperplastic and/or neoplastic nodules in response to chronic TSH stimulation.

Thyroid-stimulating hormone levels are higher in male than female rats and castration decreases both the baseline serum TSH and response to thyrotropin-releasing hormone (TRH) injection. Follicular cell height often is higher in male than in female rats in response to the greater circulating TSH levels. The administration of exogenous testosterone to castrated male rats restores the TSH level to that of intact rats. Malignant thyroid tumors (carcinomas or "cancer") develop at a higher incidence following irradiation in males than females (2:1) and castration of irradiated male rats decreases the incidence to that of intact irradiated female rats. Testosterone replacement to castrated male rats restores the incidence of irradiation-induced thyroid carcinomas in proportion to the dose of testosterone and, similarly, serum TSH levels increase proportionally to the dose of replacement hormone. Likewise, higher incidence of follicular cell hyperplasia and neoplasia has been reported in males compared to female rats following the administration of a wide variety of drugs and chemicals in chronic toxicity/carcinogenicity testing.

There also are marked species differences in the sensitivity of the functionally important peroxidase enzyme to inhibition by xenobiotics. Thioamides (e.g., sulfonamides) and other chemicals can selectively inhibit the thyroperoxidase and significantly interfere with the iodination of tyrosyl residues incorporated in the thyroglobulin molecule, thereby disrupting the orderly synthesis of T_4

Table 21-2
Triiodothyronine (T_3) Binding to Serum Proteins in Selected Vertebrate Species

SPECIES	T_4 BINDING GLOBULIN	POSTALBUMIN	ALBUMIN	PREALBUMIN
Human being	+	—	+	—
Monkey	+	—	+	—
Dog	+	—	+	—
Mouse	—	+	+	—
Rat	—	—	+	—
Chicken	—	—	+	—

KEY: +, T_3 binding to serum proteins; —, absence of binding of T_3 to serum proteins.
SOURCE: Döhler et al., 1979, with permission.

and T_3. A number of studies have shown that the long-term administration of sulfonamides results in the development of thyroid nodules frequently in the sensitive species (such as the rat, dog, and mouse) but not in species resistant (e.g., monkey, guinea pig, chicken, and human beings) to the inhibition of peroxidase in follicular cells.

Mechanisms of Thyroid Tumorigenesis

Numerous studies have reported that chronic treatment of rodents with goitrogenic compounds results in the development of follicular cell adenomas. Thiouracil and its derivatives have this effect in rats (Napolkov, 1976) and mice (Morris, 1955). This phenomenon also has been observed in rats that consumed brassica seeds (Kennedy and Purves, 1941), erythrosine (FD&C Red No. 3) (Capen and Martin, 1989; Borzelleca et al., 1987), sulfonamides (Swarm et al., 1973), and many other compounds (Hill et al., 1989; Paynter et al., 1988). The pathogenetic mechanism of this phenomenon has been understood for some time (Furth, 1954) and are widely accepted by the scientific community. These goitrogenic agents either directly interfere with thyroid hormone synthesis or secretion in the thyroid gland, increase thyroid hormone catabolism and subsequent excretion into the bile, or disrupt the peripheral conversion of thyroxine (T_4) to triiodothyronine (T_3). The ensuing decrease in circulating thyroid hormone levels results in a compensatory increased secretion of pituitary thyroid stimulating hormone (TSH). The receptor-mediated TSH stimulation of the thyroid gland leads to proliferative changes of follicular cells that include hypertrophy, hyperplasia, and ultimately, neoplasia in rodents.

Excessive secretion of TSH alone (i.e., in the absence of any chemical exposure) also has been reported to produce a high incidence of thyroid tumors in rodents (Ohshima and Ward, 1984, 1986). This has been observed in rats fed an iodine-deficient diet (Axelrod and Leblond, 1955) and in mice that received TSH-secreting pituitary tumor transplants (Furth, 1954). The pathogenetic mechanism of thyroid follicular cell tumor development in rodents involves a sustained excessive stimulation of the thyroid gland by TSH. In addition, iodine deficiency is a potent promoter of the development of thyroid tumors in rodents induced by intravenous injection of *N*-methyl-*N*-nitrosurea (Fig. 21-16) (Ohshima and Ward, 1984). The subsequent parts of thyroid section discuss specific mechanisms by which xenobiotic chemicals disrupt thyroid hormone synthesis and secretion, induce hepatic microsomal enzymes that enhance thyroid hormone catabolism or inhibit enzymes involved in monodeiodination in peripheral tissues that result in perturbations of thyroid hormone economy which in rodents predisposes to the development of follicular cell tumors in chronic studies.

Chemicals that Directly Inhibit Thyroid Hormone Synthesis

Blockage of Iodine Uptake The biosynthesis of thyroid hormones is unique among endocrine glands because the final assembly of the hormones occurs extracellularly within the follicular lumen. Essential raw materials, such as iodide, are trapped efficiently at the basilar aspect of follicular cells from interfollicular capillaries, transported rapidly against a concentration gradient to the lumen, and oxidized by a thyroid peroxidase in microvillar membranes to reactive iodine (I_2) (Fig. 21-17). The mechanism of active transport of iodide has been shown to be associated with a sodium-iodide (Na^+-I^-) symporter (NIS) present in the basolateral membrane of thyroid follicular cells. Transport of iodide ion across the thyroid cell membrane is linked to the transport of Na^+. The ion gradient generated by the Na^+, K^+-ATPase appears to be the driving force for the active cotransport of iodide. The transporter protein is present in the basolateral membrane of thyroid follicular cells (thyrocytes) and is a

PROMOTING EFFECT OF IODINE DEFICIENCY (ID) ON THYROID CARCINOGENESIS INDUCED BY N-NITROSOMETHYLUREA (NMU) AT 33 WEEKS

GROUP	THYROID WEIGHT ($\bar{x}$ mg + SD)	DIFFUSE FC HYPERPLASIA (%)	FOLLICULAR CELL (FC) ADENOMA (%)	FOLLICULAR CELL (FC) CARCINOMA (%)	TOTAL FOCAL FC LESIONS (no./cm2)
NMU + ID DIET	632 ± 208*	100x	100xx	100xxxx	11 ± 6
NMU + IODINE ADEQUATE (IA) DIET	46 ± 13**	0	70xxx	10	14 ± 14
NMU + CONTROL DIET	29 ± 4***	0	50	0	17 ± 20
ID DIET	109 ± 12****	100x	0	0	0.4 ± 0.8
IODINE ADEQUATE DIET	40 ± 16	0	0	0	0
CONTROL DIET	36 ± 4	0	0	0	0

* P<0.01 vs. GROUPS 2, 3, 4, 5, or 6
** P<0.05 vs. GROUPS 3 or 4
*** P<0.01 vs. GROUP 4
**** P<0.01 vs. GROUPS 5 or 6

x P<0.001 vs. GROUPS 2, 3, 5 or 6
xx P<0.001 vs. GROUPS 4, 5, or 6
xxx P<0.01 vs. GROUPS 4, 5, or 6
xxxx P<0.001 vs. GROUPS 2, 3, 4, 5, or 6

CONTROL DIET = STERILIZABLE WAYNE BLOX DIET; IODINE ADEQUATE = ID (REMINGTON) DIET + 0.01 gm/kg K IODATE.
NMU 41 mg/kg IV AT 6 WK OF AGE (2 WK BEFORE DIETS STARTED).

Figure 21-16. Data demonstrating the potent promoting effects of iodine deficiency (ID) *in rats administered a single intravenous dose of a known initiator* [N = *nitrosomethylurea* (NMU)] *of thyroid neoplasms. (From Ohshima and Ward, 1984, with permission.)*

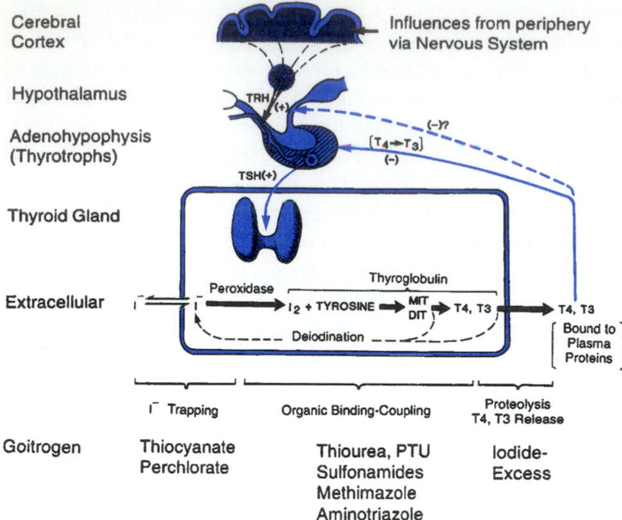

Figure 21-17. Mechanism of action of goitrogenic chemicals on thyroid hormone synthesis and secretion. (From Capen and Martin, 1989, with permission.)

large protein containing 643 amino acids with 13 transmembrane domains.

Immunohistochemical staining using a polyclonal antibody against the human NIS fusion protein (hNIS) revealed that expression of the protein is heterogenous in the normal human thyroid and detected only in occasional thyrocytes of a follicle (Jhiang et al., 1998). The hNIS-positive thyrocytes usually were detected in small follicles composed of cuboidal to columnar cells but rarely were detected in large follicles composed of flattened thyrocytes. The heterogeneity of hNIS expression among thyroid follicles is consistent with the finding that iodide concentrating ability also varies between follicles in the thyroid gland (Spitzweg et al., 2000).

Other tissues such as the salivary gland, gastric mucosa, choroid plexus, ciliary body of the eye, and lactating mammary gland also have the capacity to actively transport iodide, albeit at a much lower level than the thyroid. In the salivary glands the hNIS protein was detected in ductal cells but not in acinar cells. Only the thyroid follicular cells accumulate iodide in a TSH-dependent manner. The NIS gene is complex (15 exons, 14 introns) and its expression in the thyroid is up-regulated by TSH. The functionally active iodine transport system in the thyroid gland has important clinical applications in the evaluation, diagnosis, and treatment of several thyroid disorders, including cancer. The NIS and active transport of iodide can be selectively inhibited by competitive anion inhibitors, thereby effectively blocking the ability of the gland to iodinate tyrosine residues in thyroglobulin and synthesize thyroid hormones.

The initial step in the biosynthesis of thyroid hormones is the uptake of iodide from the circulation and transport against a gradient across follicular cells to the lumen of the follicle. A number of anions act as competitive inhibitors of iodide transport in the thyroid, including perchlorate (ClO_4^-), thiocyanate (SCN^-), and pertechnetate (Fig. 21-17). Thiocyanate is a potent inhibitor of iodide transport and is a competitive substrate for the thyroid peroxidase, but it does not appear to be concentrated in the thyroid. Blockage of the iodide trapping mechanism has a disruptive effect on the thyroid-pituitary axis, similar to iodine deficiency. The blood levels of T_4 and T_3 decrease, resulting in a compensatory increase in the secretion of TSH by the pituitary gland. The hypertrophy and hyperplasia of follicular cells following sustained exposure results in an increased thyroid weight and the development of goiter.

Inhibition of Thyroid Peroxidase Resulting in an Organification Defect A wide variety of chemicals, drugs, and other xenobiotics affect the second step in thyroid hormone biosynthesis (Fig. 21-17). The stepwise binding of iodide to the tyrosyl residues in thyroglobulin requires oxidation of inorganic iodide (I^2) to molecular (reactive) iodine (I_2) by the thyroid peroxidase present in the luminal aspect (microvillar membranes) of follicular cells and adjacent colloid. Classes of chemicals that inhibit the organification of thyroglobulin include (1) the thionamides (such as thiourea, thiouracil, propylthiouracil, methimazole, carbimazole, and goitrin); (2) aniline derivatives and related compounds (e.g., sulfonamides, paraaminobenzoic acid, paraaminosalicylic acid, and amphenone); (3) substituted phenols (such as resorcinol, phloroglucinol, and 2,4-dihydroxybenzoic acid); and (4) miscellaneous inhibitors [e.g., aminotriazole, tricyanoaminopropene, antipyrine, and its iodinated derivative (iodopyrine)] (Fig. 21-18).

Many of these chemicals exert their action by inhibiting the thyroid peroxidase, which results in a disruption both of the iodination of tyrosyl residues in thyroglobulin and also the coupling reaction of iodotyrosines [e.g., monoiodothyronine (MIT) and di-iodothyronine (DIT)] to form iodothyronines (T_3 and T_4) (Fig. 21-19). Propylthiouracil (PTU) has been shown to affect each step in thyroid hormone synthesis beyond iodide transport in rats. The order of susceptibility to the inhibition by PTU is the coupling reaction (most susceptible), iodination of MIT to form DIT, and iodination of tyrosyl residues to form MIT (least susceptible). Thiourea differs from PTU and other thioamides in that it neither inhibits guaiacol oxidation (the standard assay for peroxidase) nor inactivates the thyroid peroxidase in the absence of iodine. Its ability to inhibit organic iodinations is due primarily to the reversible reduction of active I_2 to $2I^-$.

The goitrogenic effects of sulfonamides have been known for more than fifty years, since the reports of the action of sulfaguanidine on the rat thyroid. Sulfamethoxazole and trimethroprim exert a potent goitrogenic effect in rats, resulting in marked decreases in circulating T_3 and T_4, a substantial compensatory increase in TSH, and increased thyroid weights due to follicular cell hyperplasia.

- THIOUREA
- PROPYLTHIOUREA (PTU)
- ANILINE DERIVATIVES: SULFONAMINDES
  - SULFAMETHAZINE
  - MANY OTHERS, NOT ALL
- METHIMAZOLE, CARBIMAZOLE
- AMINOTRIAZOLE
- ACETOACETAMIDE

Figure 21-18. Chemicals disrupting thyroid function (decreased synthesis of thyroid hormones) by inhibiting thyroperoxidase.

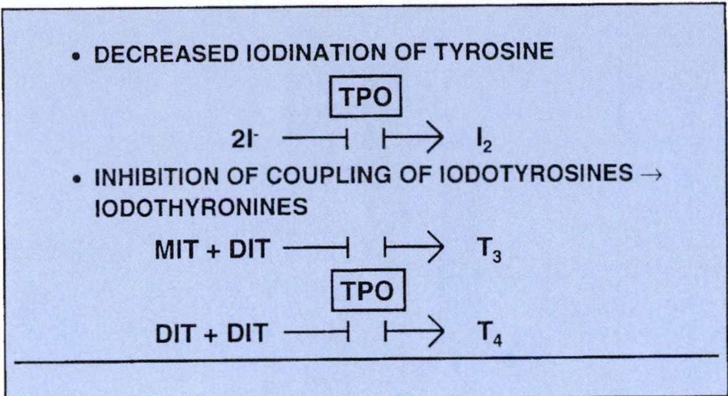

Figure 21-19. Mechanisms by which xenobiotic chemicals decrease thyroid hormone synthesis by inhibiting thyroperoxidase (TPO) in follicular cells.

The dog also is a species sensitive to the effects of sulfonamides, resulting in markedly decreased serum T_4 and T_3 levels, hyperplasia of thyrotrophic basophils in the pituitary gland, and increased thyroid weights.

By comparison, the thyroids of monkeys and human beings are resistant to the development of changes that sulfonamides produce in rodents (rats and mice) and the dog. Rhesus monkeys treated for 52 weeks with sulfamethoxazole (doses up to 300 mg/kg/day) with and without trimethroprim had no changes in thyroid weights and the thyroid histology was normal. Takayama and coworkers (1986) compared the effects of PTU and a goitrogenic sulfonamide (sulfamonomethoxine) on the activity of thyroid peroxidase in the rat and monkey using the guaiacol peroxidation assay. The concentration required for a 50 percent inhibition of the peroxidase enzyme was designated as the inhibition constant_{50} (IC_{50}). When the IC_{50} for PTU was set at 1 for rats it took 50 times the concentration of PTU to produce a comparable inhibition in the monkey. Sulfamonomethoxine was almost as potent as PTU in inhibiting the peroxidase in rats. However, it required about 500 times the concentration of sulfonamide to inhibit the peroxidase in the monkey compared to the rat. Studies such as these with sulfonamides demonstrate distinct species differences between rodents and primates in the response of the thyroid to chemical inhibition of hormone synthesis. It is not surprising that the sensitive species (e.g., rats, mice, and dogs) are much more likely to develop follicular cell hyperplasia and thyroid nodules after long-term exposure to sulfonamides than the resistant species (e.g., subhuman primates, human beings, guinea pigs, and chickens) (Fig. 21-20).

Recent evidence suggests that propylthiouracil (PTU) or feeding a low-iodine diet markedly increase thyroid follicular cell proliferation in rats by disrupting the movement of low-molecular-weight ions and molecules through gap junctions (Kolaja et al., 2000). Inhibition of gap-junction intercellular communication (GJIC) prior to induction of cell proliferation has been reported with several tumor promoters and in proliferative diseases. After 14 days of either PTU or a low iodine diet (plus 1 percent $KClO_4$ in water) serum T_3 and T_4 were decreased to undetectable levels, serum TSH was increased significantly and thyroid follicular cell proliferation was increased nearly threefold. This was accompanied by a 30 to 35 percent decrease in GJIC [determined by an ex vivo method with Lucifer yellow—a low-molecular-weight (457) fluorescent dye] and a twofold increase in apoptosis in both treated groups. Therefore, inhibition of GJIC by PTU or a low-iodine diet may result in increased thyroid follicular cell proliferation, similar to other tissues, possibly by disrupting the passage of regulatory substance(s) through these highly permeable intercellular channels.

A contemporary example of a chemical acting as a thyroperoxidase inhibitor is sulfamethazine. This is a widely used antibacterial compound in food-producing animals with a current permissible tissue residue level of 100 ppb. Recently completed carcinogenicity studies at NCTR reported a significant increase of thyroid tumors in male Fischer 344 rats administered the high dose (2400 ppm) of sulfamethazine (McClain, 1995). The incidence of thyroid tumors was increased in both male and female $B_6C_3F_1$ mice after two years in the high-dose (4800 ppm) group but not in the lower-dose groups. Quantitative risk assessment based upon these new carcinogenicity findings, using low-dose linear extrapolation, yielded a 1×10^6 lifetime risk of 90 ppb in female rats and 40 ppb in male rats. A consideration of the ratio of intact drug to metabolites further reduced the tissue residue level to 0.4 ppb, which would be unachievable in practice (McClain, 1995).

A number of mechanistic studies have been performed in collaboration with Dr. McClain and others with the objective of developing a database that would support the hypothesis that the thyroid tumors observed in rats and mice from chronic studies were secondary to hormonal imbalances following the administration of high doses of sulfamethazine. In a 4-week mechanistic study, the effects of 10 dose levels ($0 > 12{,}000$ ppm) of sulfamethazine, spanning the range that induced thyroid tumors in rodents, were evaluated on thyroid hormone economy in Sprague-Dawley rats. There was a characteristic log-dose response relationship in all parameters of thyroid function evaluated. There were no significant changes at the six lower doses ($20 > 800$ ppm) of sulfamethazine, followed by sharp relatively linear changes at the four higher dose levels ($1600 > 12{,}000$ ppm) in percent decrease of serum T_3 and T_4, increase in serum TSH, and increase in thyroid weight. A similar, nonlinear dose response was present in the morphologic changes of thyroid follicular cells following the feeding of varying levels of sulfamethazine. Follicular cell hypertrophy was observed at lower doses of sulfamethazine than hyperplasia, which was increased only at dose levels of 3300 ppm and above (Fig. 21-21).

Other mode-of-action studies have demonstrated sulfamethazine to be a potent inhibitor of thyroperoxidase in rodents with a IC_{50} of 1.2×10^{-6} M. The morphologic effects on the thyroid

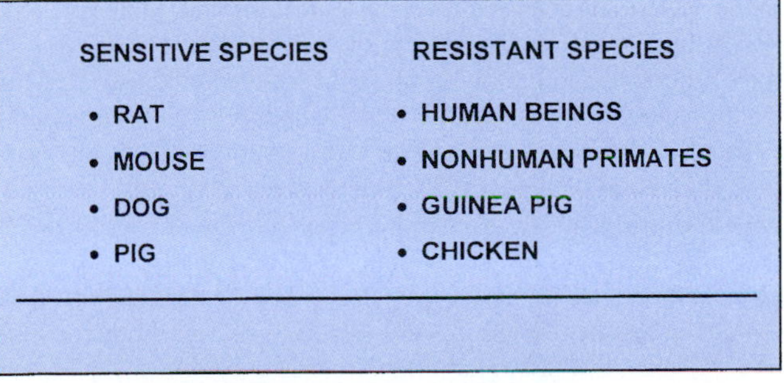

Figure 21-20. Variable species sensitivity of thyroperoxidase (TPO) inhibition by sulfonamides. (From Takayama et al., 1986, with permission.)

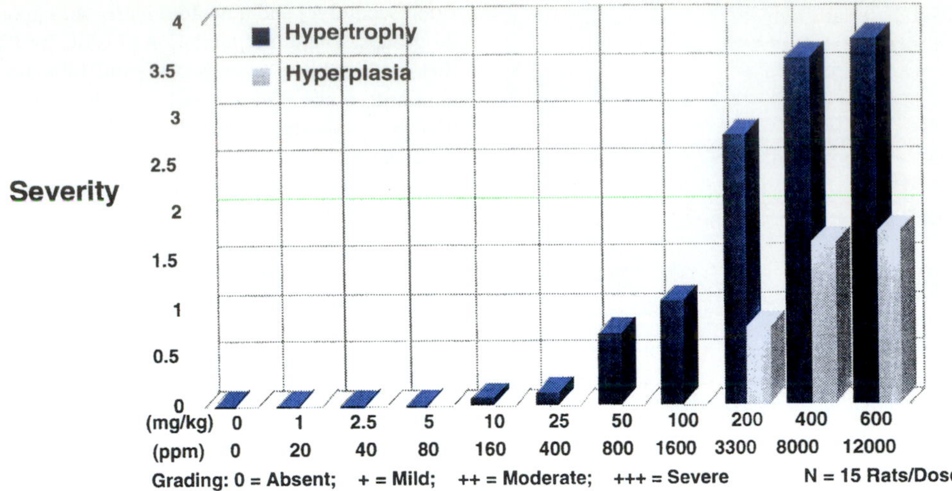

Figure 21-21. Nonlinear dose-response in morphologic changes in thyroid follicular cells in response to 10 dose levels of sulfamethazine administered in the feed to male Sprague-Dawley rats. (From Capen, 1997, with permission.)

were reversible after withdrawal of compound and addition of supplemental T_4 to the diet inhibited the development of the functional and morphologic changes in thyroid follicular cells (McClain, 1995). Hypophysectomized rats (with no TSH) administered sulfamethazine did not develop morphologic changes in the thyroid. Sulfamethazine did not increase thyroid cell proliferation in vitro in the absence of TSH and there was no effect on thyroid structure/function in cynomolgus monkeys administered sulfamethazine. Nonhuman primates and human beings are known to be more resistant than rodents to the inhibition of thyroperoxidase.

Chemicals that Disrupt Thyroid Hormone Secretion

Blockage of Thyroid Hormone Release by Excess Iodide and Lithium Relatively few chemicals selectively inhibit the secretion of thyroid hormone from the thyroid gland (Fig. 21-17). An excess of iodine has been known for years to inhibit secretion of thyroid hormone and occasionally can result in goiter and subnormal function (hypothyroidism) in animals and human patients. High doses of iodide have been used therapeutically in the treatment of patients with Graves' disease and hyperthyroidism to lower circulating levels of thyroid hormones. Several mechanisms have been suggested for this effect of high iodide levels on thyroid hormone secretion, including a decrease in lysosomal protease activity (in human glands), inhibition of colloid droplet formation (in mice and rats), and inhibition of TSH-mediated increase in cAMP (in dog thyroid slices). Studies in my laboratory demonstrated that rats fed an iodide-excessive diet had a hypertrophy of the cytoplasmic area of follicular cells with an accumulation of numerous colloid droplets and lysosomal bodies (Collins and Capen, 1980). However, there was limited evidence ultrastructurally of the fusion of the membranes of these organelles and of the degradation of the colloid necessary for the release of active thyroid hormones (T_4 and T_3) from the thyroglobulin. Circulating levels of T_4, T_3, and rT_3 all would be decreased by an iodide-excess in rats.

Lithium also has been reported to have a striking inhibitory effect on thyroid hormone release (Fig. 21-17). The widespread use of lithium carbonate in the treatment of manic states occasionally results in the development of goiter with either euthyroidism or occasionally hypothyroidism in human patients. Lithium inhibits colloid droplet formation stimulated by cAMP in vitro and inhibits the release of thyroid hormones.

Xenobiotic-Induced Thyroid Pigmentation or Alterations in Colloid The antibiotic minocycline produces a striking black discoloration of the thyroid lobes in laboratory animals and humans with the formation of brown pigment granules within follicular cells. The pigment granules stain similarly to melanin and are best visualized on thyroid sections stained with the Fontana-Masson procedure. Electron-dense material first accumulates in lysosome-like granules and in the rough endoplasmic reticulum. The pigment appears to be a metabolic derivative of minocycline and the administration of the antibiotic at high dose to rats for extended periods may result in a disruption of thyroid function and the development of goiter. The release of T_4 from perfused thyroids of minocycline-treated rats was significantly decreased but the follicular cells retained the ability to phagocytose colloid in response to TSH and had numerous colloid droplets in their cytoplasm.

Other xenobiotics [or metabolite(s)] selectively localize in the thyroid colloid of rodents resulting in abnormal clumping and increased basophilia to the colloid. Brown to black pigment granules may be present in follicular cells, colloid, and macrophages in the interthyroidal tissues resulting in a macroscopic darkening of both thyroid lobes. The physiochemically altered colloid in the lumen of thyroid follicles appears to be less able than normal colloid either of reacting with organic iodine in a stepwise manner to result in the orderly synthesis of iodothyronines or being phagocytized by follicular cells and enzymatically processed to release active thyroid hormones into the circulation. Serum T_4 and T_3 are decreased, serum TSH levels are increased by an expanded population of pituitary thyrotrophs, and thyroid follicular cells undergo hypertrophy and hyperplasia. As would be expected, the incidence of thyroid follicular cell tumors in 2-year carcinogenicity studies is significantly increased at the higher dose levels, usually with a greater effect in males than females. Autoradiographic studies often demonstrate tritiated material to be preferentially localized in the colloid and not within follicular cells. Tissue distribution studies with ^{14}C-labeled compound may reveal preferential uptake and persistence in the thyroid gland compared to other tissues. However, thyroperoxidase activity is normal and the thyroid's ability to take up radioactive iodine often is increased compared to controls in response to the greater circulating levels of TSH. Similar thyroid changes and/or functional alterations usually do not occur in dogs, monkeys, or humans.

Hepatic Microsomal Enzyme Induction

Hepatic microsomal enzymes play an important role in thyroid hormone economy because glucuronidation is the rate-limiting step in the biliary excretion of T_4 and sulfation primarily by phenol sulfotransferase for the excretion of T_3. Long-term exposure of rats to a wide variety of different chemicals may induce these enzyme pathways and result in chronic stimulation of the thyroid by disrupting the hypothalamic-pituitary-thyroid axis (Curran and DeGroot, 1991). The resulting chronic stimulation of the thyroid by increased circulating levels of TSH often results in a greater risk of developing tumors derived from follicular cells in 2-year or lifetime chronic toxicity/carcinogenicity studies with these compounds in rats (Fig. 21-22). Recent studies have suggested that glucuronidation and enhanced biliary excretion of T_3 may be the reason why serum TSH is increased in short-term (7 days) studies with some microsomal enzyme inducing chemicals (e.g., phenobarbital, pregnenolone-16α-carbonitrile) but is less affected with others (3-methylcholanthrene, PCB) (Hood and Klaassen, 2000). However, microsomal enzyme inducers are more effective in reducing serum T_4 than serum T_3 (Hood and Klaassen, 2000). Outer-ring deiodinase (ORD) activity, an enzyme involved in the peripheral conversion of T_4 (major secretory product of the thyroid) to T_3, was reduced (not increased as would be expected if this was the mechanism) following the administration of four well-characterized enzyme inducers in rats. Type I ORD was measured in thyroid, kidney, and liver whereas type II ORD was quantified in brown adipose tissue, pituitary gland, and brain.

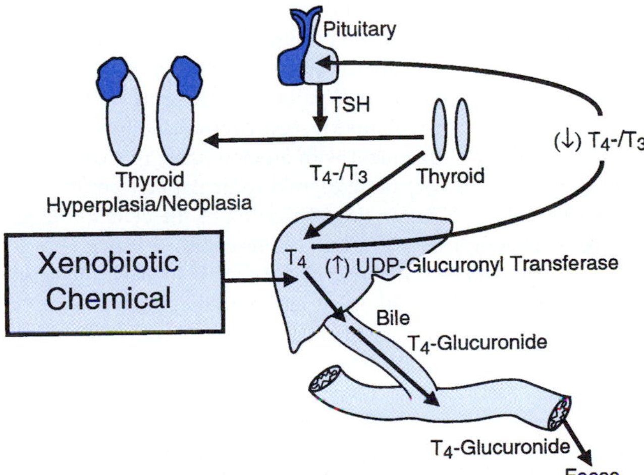

Figure 21-22. Hepatic microsomal enzyme induction by the chronic administration of xenobiotic chemicals, leading to thyroid follicular cell hyperplasia and neoplasia.

Xenobiotics that induce liver microsomal enzymes and disrupt thyroid function in rats include CNS-acting drugs (e.g., phenobarbital, benzodiazepines); calcium channel blockers (e.g., nicardipine, bepridil); steroids (spironolactone); retinoids; chlorinated hydrocarbons (e.g., chlordane, DDT, TCDD), polyhalogenated biphenyls (PCB, PBB), among others. Most of the hepatic microsomal enzyme inducers have no apparent intrinsic carcinogenic activity and produce little or no mutagenicity or DNA damage. Their promoting effect on thyroid tumors usually is greater in rats than in mice, with males more often developing a higher incidence of tumors than females. In certain strains of mice these compounds alter liver cell turnover and promote the development of hepatic tumors from spontaneously initiated hepatocytes.

Phenobarbital has been studied extensively as the prototype for hepatic microsomal inducers that increase a spectrum of cytochrome P450 isoenzymes (McClain et al., 1988). McClain and associates (1989) reported that the activity of uridine diphosphate glucuronyltransferase (UDP-GT), the rate limiting enzyme in T_4 metabolism, is increased in purified hepatic microsomes of male rats when expressed as picomoles/min/mg microsomal protein (1.3-fold) or as total hepatic activity (threefold). This resulted in a significantly higher cumulative (4-h) biliary excretion of ^{125}I-labeled T_4 and bile flow than in controls.

Phenobarbital-treated rats develop a characteristic pattern of changes in circulating thyroid hormone levels (McClain et al., 1988, 1989). Plasma T_3 and T_4 are markedly decreased after 1 week and remain decreased for 4 weeks. By 8 weeks T_3 levels return to near normal due to compensation by the hypothalamic-pituitary-thyroid axis. Serum TSH values are elevated significantly throughout the first month but often decline after a new steady state is attained. Thyroid weights increase significantly after 2 to 4 weeks of phenobarbital, reach a maximum increase of 40 to 50 percent by 8 weeks, and remain elevated throughout the period of treatment.

McClain and coworkers (1988) in a series of experiments have shown that supplemental administration of thyroxine (at doses that returned the plasma level of TSH to the normal range) blocked the thyroid tumor-promoting effects of phenobarbital and that the promoting effects were directly proportional to the level of plasma TSH in rats. The sustained increase in circulating TSH levels results initially in hypertrophy of follicular cells, followed by hyperplasia, and ultimately places the rat thyroid at greater risk to develop an increased incidence of benign tumors.

Phenobarbital has been reported to be a thyroid gland tumor promoter in a rat initiation-promotion model. Treatment with a nitrosamine followed by phenobarbital has been shown to increase serum TSH concentrations, thyroid gland weights, and the incidence of follicular cell tumors in the thyroid gland (McClain 1988; McClain et al., 1989). These effects could be decreased in a dose-related manner by simultaneous treatment with increasing doses of exogenous thyroxine. McClain et al. (1989) have demonstrated that rats treated with phenobarbital have a significantly higher cumulative biliary excretion of ^{125}I-labeled thyroxine than controls (Fig. 21-23). Most of the increase in biliary excretion was accounted for by an increase in T_4-glucuronide due to an increased metabolism of thyroxine in phenobarbital-treated rats. This is consistent with enzymatic activity measurements which result in increased hepatic T_4-UDP-glucuronyl transferase activity in phenobarbital-treated rats (Fig. 21-24). Results from these experiments are consistent with the hypothesis that the promotion of thyroid tumors in rats was not a direct effect of phenobarbital on the thyroid gland but rather an indirect effect mediated by TSH secretion from

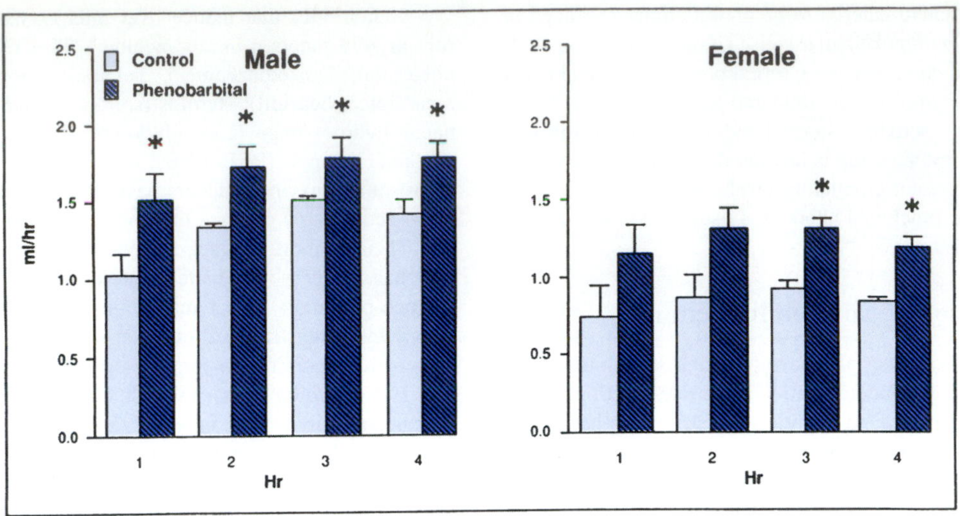

Figure 21-23. Cumulative biliary excretion of ^{125}I-thyroxine (percentage of administered dose) in control and phenobarbital treated rats (100 mg/kg/day in the diet for 4 to 6 weeks).

Phenobarbital treatment resulted in an increase in the cumulative excretion of thyroxine over a 4-h period. Thin-layer chromatography of bile samples indicated that most of the increase in biliary excretion was accounted for by an increase in the fraction corresponding to thyroxine-glucuronide. (From McClain, 1989, with permission.)

the pituitary secondary to the hepatic microsomal enzyme-induced increase of T_4 excretion in the bile.

The activation of the thyroid gland during the treatment of rodents with substances that stimulate thyroxine catabolism is a well-known phenomenon and has been investigated extensively with phenobarbital and many other compounds (Curran and DeGroot, 1991). It occurs particularly with rodents, first because UDP-glucuronyl transferase can easily be induced in rodent species, and second because thyroxine metabolism takes place very rapidly in rats in the absence of thyroxine-binding globulin. In humans a lowering of the circulating T_4 level but no change in TSH and T_3 concentrations has been observed only with high doses of very powerful enzyme-inducing compounds, such as rifampicin with and without antipyrine.

Although phenobarbital is the only UDP-glucuronyl transferase (UDP-GT) inducer that has been investigated in detail to act as a thyroid tumor promoter, the effects of other well-known UDP-GT inducers on the disruption of serum T_4 TSH and thyroid gland have been investigated. For example, pregnenolone-16α-carbonitrile (PCN), 3-methylcholanthrene (3MC) and aroclor 1254 (PCB) induce hepatic microsomal UDP-GT activity towards T_4 (Barter and Klaassen, 1992a). These UDP-GT inducers reduce serum T_4 levels in both control as well as in thyroidectomized rats that are infused with T_4, indicating that reductions in serum T_4 levels are not due to a direct effect of the inducers on the thyroid gland (Barter and Klaassen, 1992b, 1994). However, serum TSH levels and the thyroid response to reductions in serum T_4 levels by UDP-GT inducers is not always predictable. While PCN increased serum TSH and resulted in thyroid follicular cell hyperplasia similar to that observed with phenobarbital, 3MC and PCB in these short-duration experiments and at the dose levels used did not increase serum TSH levels or produce thyroid follicular cell hyperplasia (Liu et al., 1995; Hood et al., 1995). These findings support the overall hypothesis that UDP-GT inducers can adversely affect the thyroid gland by a secondary mechanism, but this applies only to those UDP-GT inducers that increase serum TSH in addition to reducing serum T_4.

Additional investigations by this research group demonstrated that hepatic microsomal enzyme inducing xenobiotic chemicals [e.g., phenobarbital and pregnenolone-16α-carbontrile (PCN)] increased serum TSH ($0 > 75$ percent) much less than the thyroperoxidase inhibitor propylthiouracil (PTU) (830 percent) (Hood et al., 1999). Phenobarbital and PCN administration increased thyroid weight approximately 80 percent compared to a 500 percent increase in PTU-treated rats. Thyroid follicular cell proliferation (determined by BrdU labeling) was increased 260, 330, and 850 percent in rats treated with phenobarbital, PCN, and PTU, respectively, for 7 days but the labeling index had returned to control levels by the 45th day of treatment. These findings demonstrate that certain hepatic microsomal enzyme-inducing chemicals that result in mild to modest elevations in serum TSH lead to dramatic increases in thyroid follicular cell proliferation that peak after 7 days of treatment and then rapidly return to control values. These findings are similar to those of Wynford-Thomas et al. (1982), who reported a maximal proliferative response (evaluated by mitotic index) after 7 days of treatment with aminotriazole (a thyroperoxidase inhibitor). The decline in thyroid follicular cell proliferation was suggested to be due to desensitization of the cells to the mitogenic actions of TSH (Wynford-Thomas et al., 1982a).

Hood et al. (1999) reported that moderate increases in serum TSH of between 10 and 20 ng/ml increased the number of proliferating thyroid follicular cells but had no effect on thyroid weight, emphasizing that small increases in serum TSH can be sufficient to stimulate proliferation. These important findings suggest that quantitation of follicular cell proliferation may be more useful than thyroid weights for assessing alterations in thyroid growth in rats administered xenobiotic chemicals that produce only small to moderate increases in serum TSH.

There is no convincing evidence that humans treated with drugs or exposed to chemicals that induce hepatic microsomal

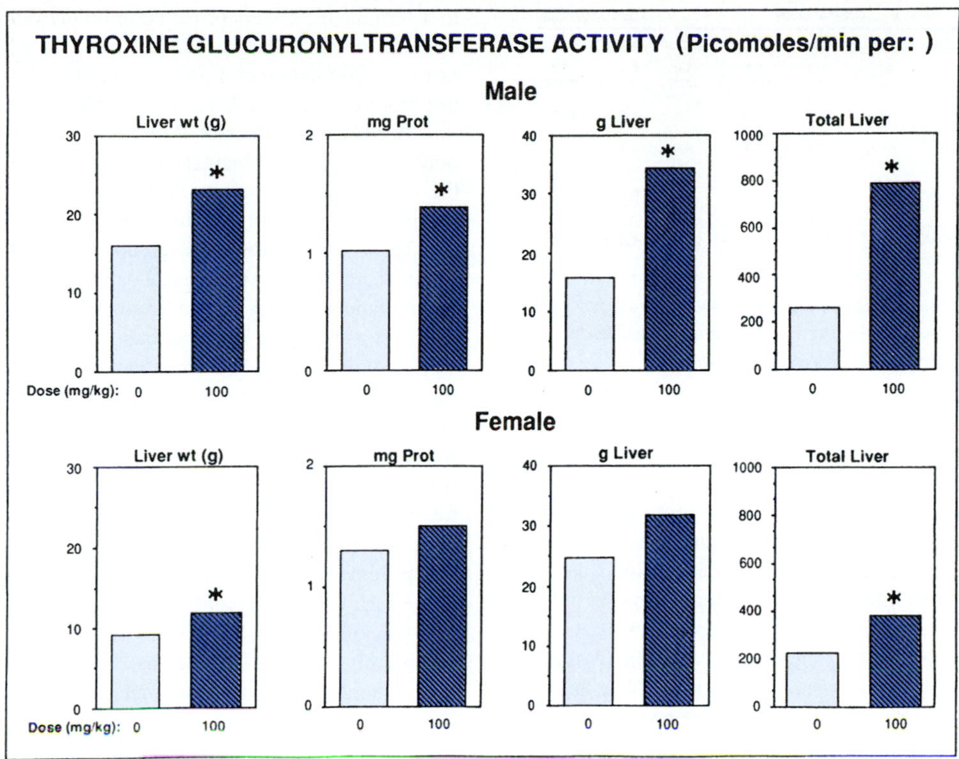

Figure 21-24. Hepatic thyroxine glucuronyltransferase activity in control and phenobarbital-treated rats (100 mg/kg/day in the diet for 4 weeks).

Glucuronyltransferase activity was measured in hepatic microsomes using thyroxine as a substrate. Phenobarbital treatment induced thyroxine-glucuronyltransferase in male and female rats; however, the effect in male rats was quantitatively larger. (From McClain, 1989, with permission.)

enzymes are at increased risk for the development of thyroid cancer (Curran and DeGroot, 1991). In a study on the effects of microsomal enzyme–inducing compounds on thyroid hormone metabolism in normal healthy adults, phenobarbital (100 mg daily for 14 days) did not affect the serum T_4, T_3, or TSH levels (Ohnhaus et al., 1981). A decrease in serum T_4 levels was observed after treatment with either a combination of phenobarbital plus rifampicin or a combination of phenobarbital plus antipyrine; however, these treatments had no effect on serum T_3 or TSH levels (Ohnhaus and Studer, 1983). Epidemiologic studies of patients treated with therapeutic doses of phenobarbital have reported no increase in risk for the development of thyroid neoplasia (Clemmesen et al., 1974; Clemmesen and Hualgrim-Jensen, 1977, 1978, 1981; White et al., 1979; Friedman, 1981; Shirts et al., 1986; Olsen et al., 1989). Highly sensitive assays for thyroid and pituitary hormones are readily available in a clinical setting to monitor circulating hormone levels in patients exposed to chemicals potentially disruptive of pituitary-thyroid axis homeostasis.

Likewise, there is no substantive evidence that humans treated with drugs or exposed to chemicals that induce hepatic microsomal enzymes are at increased risk for the development of liver cancer. This is best exemplified by the extensive epidemiologic information on the clinical use of phenobarbital. Phenobarbital has been used clinically as an anticonvulsant for more than eighty years. Relatively high microsomal enzyme-inducing doses have been used chronically, sometimes for lifetime exposures, to control seizure activity in human beings. A study of over 8000 patients admitted to a Danish epilepsy center from 1933 to 1962 revealed no evidence for an increased incidence of hepatic tumors in phenobarbital-treated humans when patients receiving thorotrast, a known human liver carcinogen, were excluded (Clemmesen and Hjalgrim-Jensen, 1978). A follow-up report on this patient population confirmed and extended this observation (Clemmesen and Hjalgrim-Jensen, 1981; Olsen et al., 1989). The results of two other smaller studies (2099 epileptics and 959 epileptics) also revealed no hepatic tumors in patients treated with phenobarbital (White et al., 1979).

Chemical Inhibition of 5′-Monodeiodinase

FD&C Red No. 3 (erythrosine) is an example of a well-characterized xenobiotic that results in perturbations of thyroid function in rodents and in long-term studies is associated with an increased incidence of benign thyroid tumors. Red No. 3 is a widely used color additive in foods, cosmetics, and pharmaceuticals. A chronic toxicity/carcinogenicity study revealed that male Sprague-Dawley rats fed a 4 percent dietary concentration of Red No. 3 beginning in utero and extending over their lifetime (30 months) developed a 22 percent incidence of thyroid adenomas derived from follicular cells compared to 1.5 percent in control rats and a historical incidence of 1.8 percent for this strain (Borzelleca et al., 1987; Capen, 1989) (Fig. 21-25). There was no significant increase in follicular cell adenomas in the lower-dose groups of male rats or an increase in malignant thyroid follicular cell tumors. Female rats fed similar amounts of the color did not develop a significant increase in

Groups	Original Study					High-Dose Study	
	I_A	I_B	II	III	IV	I_C	V
Red No. 3 (%) (mg/kg/day)	0 —	0 —	0.1 (49)	0.5 (251)	1.0 (507)	0 —	4.0 (2.464)
F.C. Adenoma (%)	0	0	0	2.9	1.5	1.5	21.8
F.C. Carcinoma (%)	0	0	4.5	1.5	4.4	2.9	4.4
Cystic follicular hyperplasia (%)	2.9	1.5	12	16.2	7.3	0	23.2
Diffuse or focal F.C. hyperplasia (%)	1.4	0	7.5	7.4	26.1	5.8	87.0
Follicular cysts (%)	10	14.5	9.0	11.8	11.6	2.9	14.5

Figure 21-25. Thyroid lesions in male Sprague-Dawley rats fed varying doses of FD&C Red No. 3 beginning in utero and for a lifetime of 30 months. (From Borzelleca et al., 1987, with permission.)

either benign or malignant thyroid tumors. Feeding of the color at the high dose (4 percent) level provided male rats with 2464 mg/kg of Red No. 3 daily; by comparison human consumption in the United States is estimated to be 0.023 mg/kg/day.

The results of mechanistic studies with FD&C Red No. 3 have suggested that a primary (direct) action on the thyroid is unlikely to result from (1) failure of the color (^{14}C-labeled) to accumulate in the gland, (2) negative genotoxicity and mutagenicity assays, (3) lack of an oncogenic response in mice and gerbils, (4) a failure to promote thyroid tumor development at dietary concentrations of 1.0 percent or less in male and female rats (Capen, 1989), and (5) no increased tumor development in other organs. Investigations with radiolabeled compound have demonstrated that the color does not accumulate in the thyroid glands of rats following the feeding of either 0.5 percent or 4.0 percent FD&C Red No. 3 for 1 week prior to the oral dose of ^{14}C-labeled material.

Mechanistic investigations with FD&C Red No. 3 included, among others, a 60-day study of male Sprague-Dawley rats fed either 4 percent (high dose) or 0.25 percent (low dose) Red No. 3 compared to controls, whose food was without the color, in order to determine the effects of the color on thyroid hormone economy. The experimental design of the study was to sacrifice groups of rats ($n = 20$ rats/interval and dose) fed Red No. 3 and their control groups after 0, 3, 7, 10, 14, 21, 30, and 60 days.

A consistent effect of Red No. 3 on thyroid hormone economy was the striking increase in serum reverse T_3 (Fig. 21-26). In the rats fed high doses, reverse T_3 was increased at all intervals compared to controls and this also held for rats killed at 10, 14, and 21 days in the low-dose group. The mechanisms responsible for the increased serum reverse T_3 appear to be, first, substrate (T_4) accumulation due to 5′-monodeiodinase inhibition with subsequent conversion to reverse T_3 rather than active T_3; and, second, reverse T_3 accumulation due to 5′-monodeiodinase inhibition resulting in an inability to degrade reverse T_3 further to diiodothyronine (T_2). Serum triiodothyronine (T_3) was decreased significantly at all intervals in rats of the high-dose group compared to interval controls (Fig. 21-27). The mechanism responsible for the reduced serum T_3 following feeding of Red No. 3 was decreased monodeiodination of T_4 due to an inhibition of the 5′-monodeiodinase by the color.

Serum TSH was increased significantly at all intervals in rats of the high-dose (4 percent) group compared to controls. Rats fed 0.25 percent Red No. 3 had increased serum TSH only at days 21, 30, and 60 (Fig. 21-28). The mechanism responsible for the increased serum TSH following ingestion of Red No. 3 was a compensatory response by the pituitary gland to the low circulating levels of T_3 that resulted from an inhibition of the 5′-monodeiodinase. Serum T_4 also was increased significantly at all intervals in rats fed 4 percent Red No. 3 compared to controls (Fig. 21-29). The mechanism responsible for the increased serum T_4 was, first, accumulation due to an inability to monodeiodinate T_4 to T_3 in the liver and kidney from the inhibition of 5′-monodeiodinase by the color; and, second, TSH stimulation of increased T_4 production by the thyroid gland.

^{125}I-labeled T_4 metabolism was significantly altered in liver homogenates prepared from rats fed 4 percent FD&C Red No. 3. Degradation of labeled T_4 was decreased to approximately 40 percent of the values in control homogenates (Fig. 21-30). This was associated with a 75 percent decrease in percent generation of ^{125}I and an approximately 80 percent decrease in percent generation of

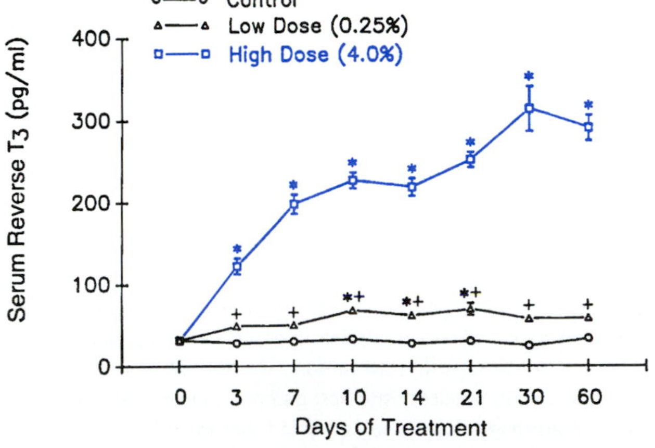

***Figure 21-26.** Rapid and significant increase in serum reverse triiodothyronine (rT_3) levels in Sprague-Dawley rats (N = 20 per group and interval) administered a high (4 percent) and low (0.25 percent) dose of FD&C Red No. 3.*

The significant increase in rT3 was detected at the initial interval of 3 days and persisted during the 60-day experiment in the high-dose group. (Courtesy of the Certified Color Manufacturers Association, Inc., and Dr. L.E. Braverman and Dr. W.J. DeVito, University of Massachusetts Medical School.)

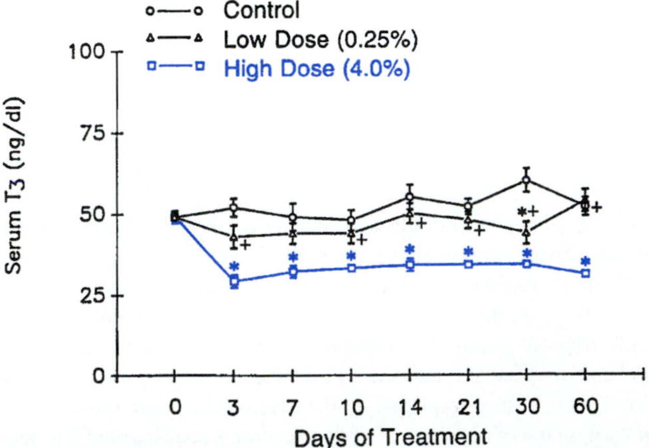

Figure 21-27. Changes in serum triiodthyronine (T_3) following administration of a high (4 percent) and low (0.25 percent) dose of FD&C Red No. 3 in the diet to Sprague-Dawley rats. (Courtesy of the Certified Color Manufacturers Association, Inc., and Dr. L.E. Braverman and Dr. W.J. DeVito, University of Massachusetts Medical School.)

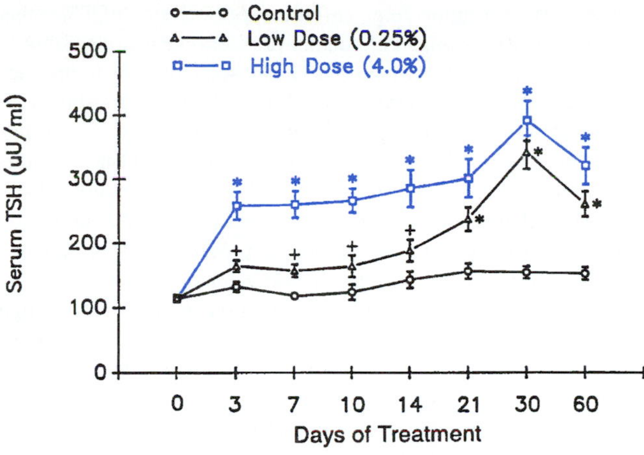

Figure 21-28. Changes in serum thyroid stimulating hormone (TSH) following administration of a high (4 percent) and low (0.25 percent) dose of FD&C Red No. 3 in the diet to Sprague-Dawley rats. (Courtesy of the Certified Color Manufacturers Association, Inc., and Dr. L.E. Braverman and Dr. W.J. DeVito, University of Massachusetts Medical School.)

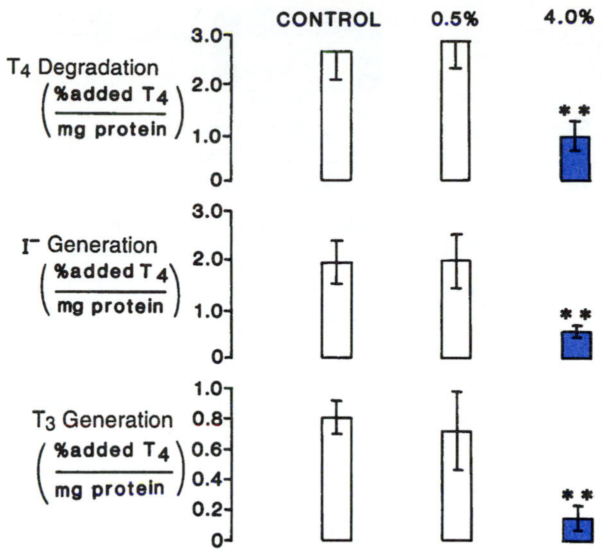

Figure 21-30. Effects of dietary FD&C Red No. 3 on the hepatic metabolism of ^{125}I-labeled thyroxine in male Sprague-Dawley rats fed diets containing 0.5 and 4.0 percent color compared to controls. (Courtesy of the Certified Color Manufacturers Association, Inc., and the late Sidney H. Ingbar, M.D.)

^{125}I-labeled T_3 from radiolabeled T_4 substrate. These mechanistic investigations suggested that the color results in a perturbation of thyroid hormone economy in rodents by inhibiting the 5'-monodeiodinase in the liver, resulting in long-term stimulation of follicular cells by TSH, which over their lifetime predisposed to an increased incidence of thyroid tumors (Capen and Martin, 1989; Borzelleca et al., 1987). The color tested negative in standard genotoxic and mutagenic assays, and it did not increase the incidence of tumors in other organs.

Morphometric evaluation was performed on thyroid glands from all rats at each interval during the 60-day study. Four levels of exposure of rat thyroid to Red No. 3 were evaluated, with 25 measurements from each rat. The direct measurements included the diameter of thyroid follicles, area of follicular colloid, and height of follicular cells. Thyroid follicular diameter was decreased significantly in both low- and high-dose groups at 3, 7, 10, and 14 days compared to interval controls. The area of follicular colloid generally reflected the decrease in thyroid follicular diameter and was decreased significantly at days 3 and 10 in high-dose rats and days 7 and 10 in the low-dose group compared to interval controls. These reductions in thyroid follicular diameter and colloid area were consistent with morphologic changes expected in response to an increased serum TSH concentration.

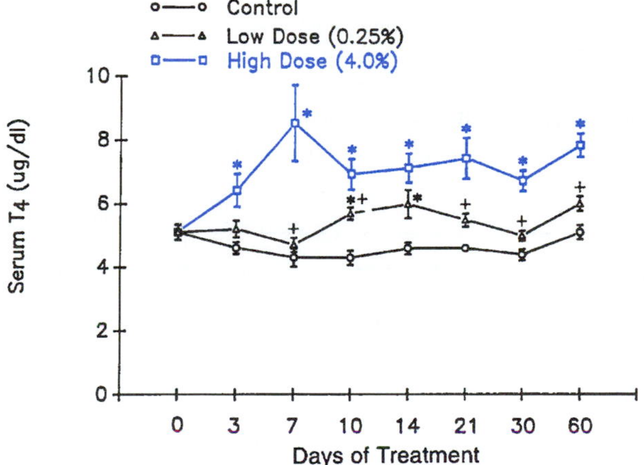

Figure 21-29. Changes in serum thyroxine (T_4) following administration of a high (4 percent) and low (0.25 percent) dose of FD&C Red No. 3 in the diet to Sprague-Dawley rats. (Courtesy of the Certified Color Manufacturers Association, Inc., and Dr. L.E. Braverman and Dr. W.J. DeVito, University of Massachusetts Medical School.)

Thyroid follicular height was increased significantly only after feeding FD&C Red No. 3 for 60 days in both the high- and low-dose groups compared to interval controls. The absence of morphometric evidence of follicular cell hypertrophy at the shorter intervals was consistent with the modest increase (15.8 percent) in thyroid gland:body weight ratio after this relatively short exposure to the color. The lack of follicular cell hypertrophy at the shorter intervals of feeding Red No. 3 in rats with severalfold elevations in serum TSH levels may be related, in part, to the high iodine content (58 percent of molecular weight) interfering with the receptor-mediated response of thyroid follicular cells to TSH. The thyroid responsiveness to TSH is known to vary inversely with iodine content (Ingbar, 1972; Lamas and Ingbar, 1978). Thyroid glands of rats fed FD&C Red No. 3 would be exposed to an increased iodine concentration primarily from sodium iodide contamination of the color and, to a lesser extent, from metabolism of the compound and release of iodide.

Secondary Mechanisms of Thyroid Tumorigenesis and Risk Assessment

Understanding the mechanism of action of xenobiotics on the thyroid gland provides a rational basis for extrapolation findings from long-term rodent studies to the assessment of a particular compound's safety for humans. Many chemicals and drugs disrupt one

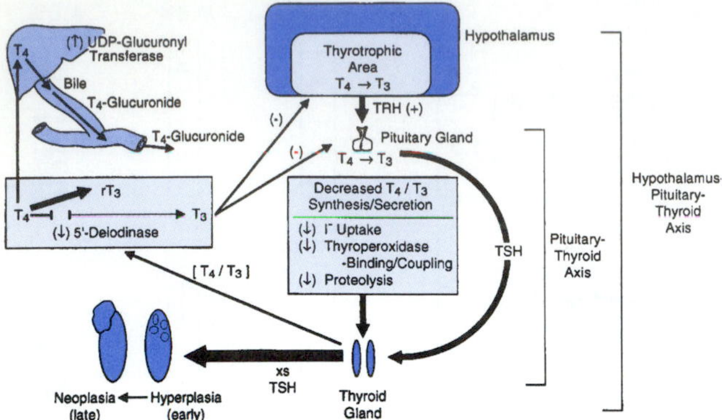

Figure 21-31. Multiple sites of disruption of the hypothalamic-pituitary-thyroid axis by xenobiotic chemicals.

Chemicals can exert direct effects by disrupting thyroid hormone synthesis or secretion and indirectly influence the thyroid through an inhibition of 5'-deiodinase or by inducing hepatic microsomal enzymes (e.g., T_4-UDP glucuronyltransferase). All of these mechanisms can lower circulating levels of thyroid hormones (T_4 and/or T_3), resulting in a release from negative-feedback inhibition and increased secretion of thyroid stimulating hormone (TSH) by the pituitary gland. The chronic hypersecretion of TSH predisposes the sensitive rodent thyroid gland to develop an increased incidence of focal hyperplastic and neoplastic lesions (adenomas) by a secondary (epigenetic) mechanism.

or more steps in the synthesis and secretion of thyroid hormones, resulting in subnormal levels of T_4 and T_3, associated with a compensatory increased secretion of pituitary TSH (Fig. 21-31). When tested in highly sensitive species, such as rats and mice, early on these compounds resulted in follicular cell hypertrophy/hyperplasia and increased thyroid weights, and in long-term studies they produced an increased incidence of thyroid tumors by a secondary (indirect) mechanism associated with hormonal inbalances.

Review of the *Physicians' Desk Reference* (PDR) reveals a number of marketed drugs that result in a thyroid tumorigenic response when tested at high concentrations in rodents, primarily in rats. A broad spectrum of product classes are represented including antibiotics, calcium-channel blockers, antidepressants, hypolipidemic agents, among others (Fig. 21-32). Amiodarone (an antiarrhythmic drug) and iodinated glycerol (an expectorant) are highly iodinated molecules that disrupt thyroid hormone economy by mechanisms similar to the food color FD&C Red No. 3 (Fig. 21-33).

In the secondary mechanism of thyroid oncogenesis in rodents, the specific xenobiotic chemical or physiologic perturbation evokes another stimulus (e.g., chronic hypersecretion of TSH) that promotes the development of nodular proliferative lesions (initially hypertrophy, followed by hyperplasia, subsequently adenomas, infrequently carcinomas) derived from follicular cells. Thresholds for "no effect" on the thyroid gland can be established by determining the dose of xenobiotic that fails to elicit an elevation in the circulating level of TSH. Compounds acting by this indirect (secondary) mechanism with hormonal imbalances usually show little or no evidence for mutagenicity or for producing DNA damage.

In human patients who have marked changes in thyroid function and elevated TSH levels, as is common in areas with a high incidence of endemic goiter due to iodine deficiency, there is little if any increase in the incidence of thyroid cancer (Doniach, 1970; Curran and DeGroot, 1991). The relative resistance to the development of thyroid cancer in humans with elevated plasma TSH levels is in marked contrast to the response of the thyroid gland to chronic TSH stimulation in rats and mice. The human thyroid is much less sensitive to this pathogenetic phenomenon than rodents (McClain, 1989).

Human patients with congenital defects in thyroid hormone synthesis (dyshormonogenetic goiter) and markedly increased circulating TSH levels have been reported to have an increased incidence of thyroid carcinomas (Cooper et al., 1981; McGirr et al., 1959). Likewise, thyrotoxic patients with Graves' disease, in which follicular cells are autonomously stimulated by an immunoglobulin (long-acting thyroid stimulator, or LATS) also appear to be at greater risk of developing thyroid tumors (Pendergrast et al., 1961; Clements, 1954). Therefore, the literature suggests that prolonged stimulation of the human thyroid by TSH will induce neoplasia only in exceptional circumstances, possibly by acting together with some other metabolic or immunologic abnormality (Curran and DeGroot, 1991).

THYROID C CELLS

Normal Structure and Function

Calcitonin (CT) has been shown to be secreted by a second population of endocrine cells in the mammalian thyroid gland that are much less numerous than follicular cells. C cells (parafollicular or light cells) are distinct from follicular cells in the thyroid that secrete T_4 and T_3 (Kalina and Pearse, 1971). They are situated either within the follicular wall immediately beneath the basement membrane or between follicular cells and as small groups of cells between thyroid follicles. C cells do not border the follicular colloid directly and their secretory polarity is oriented toward the in-

DRUG	PRODUCT CLASS	SPECIES
• MINOCYCLINE	ANTIBIOTIC	R
• OXAZEPAM	ANTIANXIETY	R
• NICARDIPINE	Ca-CHANNEL BLOCKER	R
• SERTRALINE	ANTIDEPRESSANT	R
• SIMVASTATIN	HYPOLIPIDEMIC	R
• SPIRONOLACTONE	DIURETIC	R
• VIDARABINE	ANTIVIRAL	R

Figure 21-32. Examples of marketed drugs with a tumorigenic response in the thyroid gland of rats. (Modified from Davis and Monro, 1995, with permission.)

DRUG	PRODUCT CLASS	SPECIES
• AMIODARONE	ANTIARRHYTHMIC	R
• ATENOLOL	β-ADRENERGIC BLOCKER	R
• BEPRIDIL	Ca-CHANNEL BLOCKER	R
• DAPSONE	ANTINEOPLASTIC	R
• GRISEOFULVIN	ANTIBIOTIC	R
• IODINATED GLYCEROL	EXPECTORANT	R
• METHINAZOLE	ANTI-THYROID	R
• MIDAZOLAM	SEDATIVE	R

Figure 21-33. Marketed drugs with a thyroid tumorigenic response. (Modified from Davis and Monro, 1995, with permission.)

terfollicular capillaries. The distinctive feature of C cells, compared to thyroid follicular cells, is the presence of numerous small membrane-limited secretory granules in the cytoplasm. Immunocytochemical techniques have localized the calcitonin activity of C cells to these secretory granules (DeGrandi et al., 1971).

Calcitonin-secreting thyroid C cells have been shown to be derived embryologically from cells of the neural crest. Primordial cells from the neural crest migrate ventrally and become incorporated within the last (ultimobranchial) pharyngeal pouch (Fig. 21-34). They move caudally with the ultimobranchial body to the point of fusion with the midline thyroglossal duct primordia that gives rise to the thyroid gland. The ultimobranchial body fuses with and is incorporated into the thyroid near the hilum in mammals, and C cells subsequently are distributed throughout the

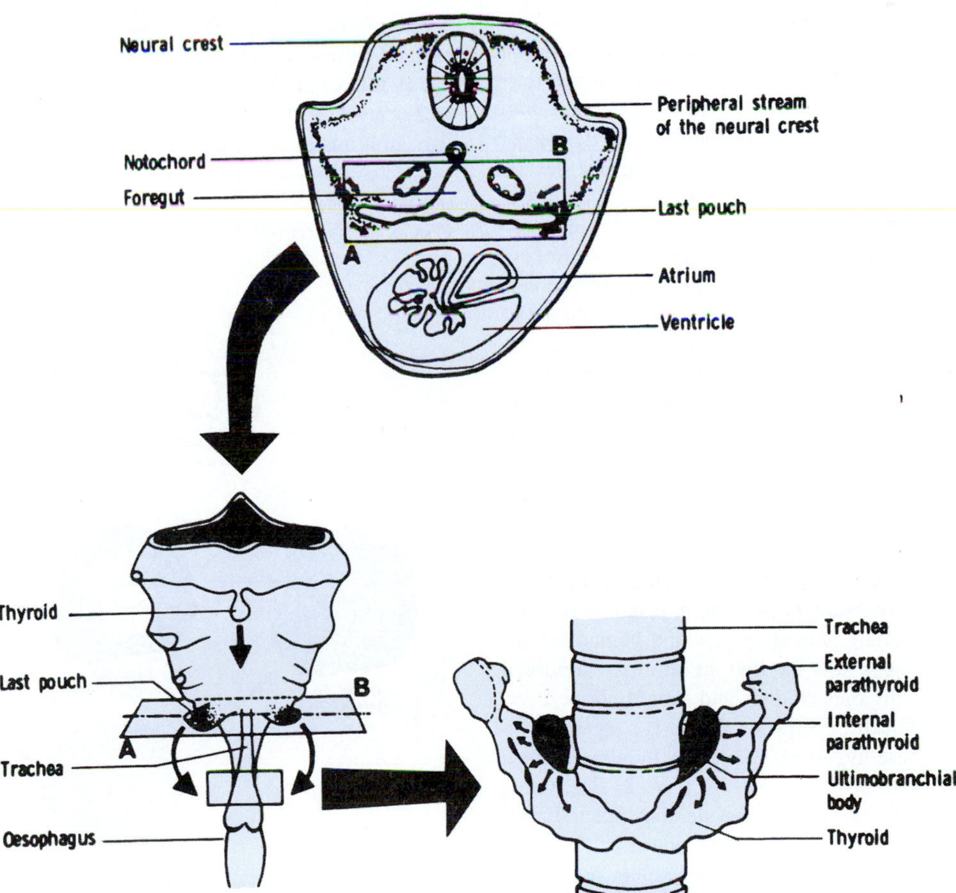

Figure 21-34. Schematic representation of neural crest origin of calcitonin-secreting C cells.

Primordial cells arising from the neural crest migrate ventrally during embryonic life to become incorporated in the last (ultimobranchial) pharyngeal pouch. The ultimobranchial body fuses with primordia of the thyroid and distributes C cells to varying degrees throughout the mammalian thyroid gland. (From Foster, 1972, with permission.)

gland. Although C cells are present throughout the thyroid gland of humans and most other mammals in postnatal life, they often remain more numerous near the hilum and point of fusion with the ultimobranchial body. Under certain conditions colloid-containing follicles lined by follicular cells also can differentiate from cells of ultimobranchial origin (Takayama et al., 1986).

In contrast to the iodothyronines (T_4 and T_3) produced by follicular cells, calcitonin is a polypeptide hormone composed of 32 amino acid residues arranged in a straight chain (Copp, 1970). The concentration of calcium ion in plasma and extracellular fluids is the principal physiological stimulus for the secretion of CT by C cells. CT is secreted continuously under conditions of normocalcemia, but the rate of secretion of CT is increased greatly in response to elevations in blood calcium. C cells store substantial amounts of CT in their cytoplasm in the form of membrane-limited secretory granules. In response to hypercalcemia there is a rapid discharge of stored hormone from C cells into interfollicular capillaries. The hypercalcemic stimulus, if sustained, is followed by hypertrophy of C cells and an increased development of cytoplasmic organelles concerned with the synthesis and secretion of CT. Hyperplasia of C cells occurs in response to long-term hypercalcemia. When the blood calcium is lowered, the stimulus for CT secretion is diminished and numerous secretory granules accumulate in the cytoplasm of C cells.

Calcitonin exerts its function by interacting with target cells, primarily in bone and kidney. The action of calcitonin is antagonistic to that of parathyroid hormone on mobilizing calcium from bone but synergistic on decreasing the renal tubular reabsorption of phosphorus. The storage of large amounts of preformed hormone in C cells and rapid release in response to moderate elevations of blood calcium are a reflection of the physiologic role of calcitonin as an "emergency" hormone to protect against the development of hypercalcemia. Calcitonin and parathyroid hormone, acting in concert, provide a dual negative feedback control mechanism to maintain the life-sustaining concentration of calcium ion in extracellular fluids within narrow limits. Calcitonin secretion is increased in response to a high-calcium meal often before a significant rise in plasma calcium can be detected. Gastrin, pancreozymin, and glucagon are examples of gastrointestinal hormones whose secretion is stimulated by an oral calcium load which, in turn, act as secretagogues for calcitonin release from the thyroid gland.

Mechanisms of Toxicity

Nodular and/or diffuse hyperplasia of C cells occurs with advancing age in many strains of laboratory rats and in response to long-term hypercalcemia in certain animal species and human beings. Focal aggregation of C cells near the thyroid hilum are a normal anatomic finding in the thyroids of dogs and should not be overinterpreted as areas of C-cell hyperplasia. There is suggestive evidence that focal or diffuse hyperplasia precedes the development of C-cell neoplasms (DeLellis et al., 1977) (Fig. 21-35). Other studies (Triggs and Williams, 1977) have demonstrated significantly elevated circulating levels of immunoreactive calcitonin in rats with C-cell neoplasms compared to either young or old rats without C-cell tumors. Neither consistent changes in total blood calcium and phosphorus nor bone lesions have been reported in rats with calcitonin-secreting C-cell neoplasms.

Triggs and Williams (1977) reported that radiation (5 or 10 μCi ^{131}I) increased the incidence of C-cell (as well as follicular cell) thyroid tumors in Wistar rats but that high dietary calcium intake (2,000 mg/100 g) did not further incease the incidence of C cell tumors in irradiated rats. Further studies by Thurston and Williams (1982) found that irradiated rats receiving diets high in vitamin D that developed hypercalcemia had a higher incidence of C-cell tumors than rats fed diets adequate or deficient in vitamin D. Stoll et al. (1978) reported that the antithyroid drug thiamazole can result in proliferative lesions (hyperplasia and adenoma) in thyroid C cells as well as in follicular cells in rats.

Morphologic Alterations and Proliferative Lesions of Thyroid C Cells

C-cell proliferative lesions occur commonly in many rat strains but are uncommon in the mouse. Rat strains with high incidences of these lesions include WAG/Rij, Sprague-Dawley, Fisher, Wistar, Buffalo, and Osborne-Mendel. The incidence varies from 19 to 33 percent with no obvious sex differences. Burek (1978) reported that cross-breeding of high- (WAG/Rij) and low- (BN/Bi) incidence strains results in F_1 animals with intermediate tumor incidences. As with proliferative lesions of other endocrine organs, there is a correlation between the age of the animal and the presence of the entire spectrum of C-cell proliferative lesions. For example, Long-Evans rats under 1 year of age rarely have C-cell neoplasms in the thyroid. Rats that were between 12 and 24 months of age had a 10 percent incidence, whereas approximately 20 percent of 2- to 3-year-old rats had C-cell tumors. Similarly, the frequency of focal and diffuse C-cell hyperplasia increased progressively with age in this strain of rat. According to the NTP historical database of 2-year-old F344 rats, the incidence of C-cell neoplasms was 8.9 percent in males and 8.5 percent in females.

There are two types of C-cell hyperplasia: diffuse and focal (nodular) (Fig. 21-35). In diffuse hyperplasia, the numbers of C cells are increased throughout the thyroid lobe to a point where

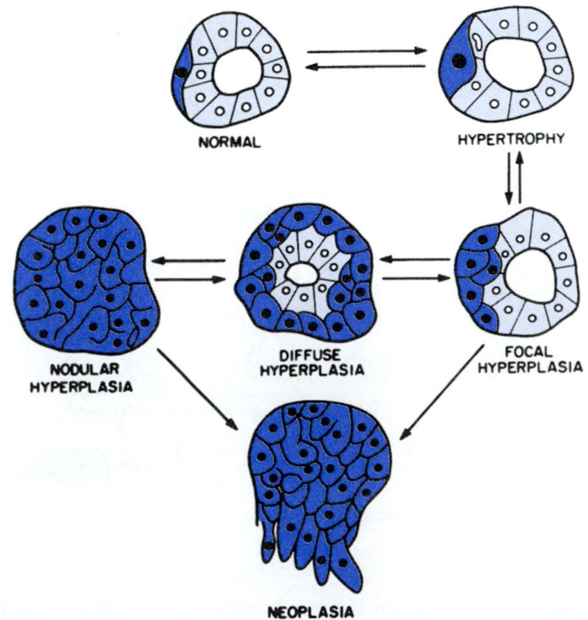

Figure 21-35. Focal and nodular hyperplasia of C cells in the thyroid often precedes the development of C-cell neoplasms. (From DeLellis et al., 1977, with permission.)

they may be more numerous than follicular cells. In contrast to the predominantly central distribution of C cells in thyroids from young rats, C cells in the more severe forms of hyperplasia extend to the extreme upper and lower poles as well as the peripheral regions of the lobes. Focal (nodular) hyperplasia of C cells often occurs concurrently with diffuse hyperplasia in the thyroid glands of rats. Follicular cells adjacent to the proliferating C cells often are compressed and atrophic with prominent supranuclear accumulations of lipofuscin. In the later stages, follicles with intense C-cell hyperplasia often assume irregular, twisted, and elongated configurations. Occasional colloid-filled thyroid follicles are entrapped among the proliferating C cells.

The histologic distinction between focal hyperplasia and adenoma of C cells is indistinct and somewhat arbitrary. The diagnosis of C-cell hyperplasia refers to a focal or diffuse increase of C cells between thyroid follicles and/or within the follicular basement membrane. The C cells appear normal with an abundant, lightly eosinophilic, granular cytoplasm and a round-to-oval nucleus with finely stippled chromatin. In focal C-cell hyperplasia the accumulations of proliferating C cells are of a lesser diameter than five average colloid-containing thyroid follicles, with minimal evidence of compression of adjacent follicles. Hyperplastic C cells within the follicular basement membrane may compress individual thyroid follicles.

The ultimobranchial body (last, usually fifth, pharyngeal pouch) that delivers the neural crest–derived C cells to the postnatal thyroid gland fuses with each thyroid lobe at the hilum during embryonic development and distributes C cells throughout each lobe to varying degrees in different species (Fig. 21-34). In the dog nodular aggregations of C cells frequently persist along the course of the major vessels to the thyroid; therefore, C-cell hyperplasia in dogs should be diagnosed only when there is a definite increase in C cells throughout each thyroid lobe compared to age-matched controls. Both thyroid lobes should be sectioned longitudinally in a consistent manner for microscopic evaluation. This will minimize the prominent regional differences of C cells in the thyroid glands of normal dogs that can result in the overinterpretation of these focal aggregations of C cells as a significant lesion. There are occasional ultimobranchial-derived, colloid-containing follicles within the focal accumulations of microscopically normal C cells along the course of vessels within the thyroid lobe or in the connective tissues of the thyroid hilum in dogs.

By comparison, C-cell adenomas are discrete, expansive masses of C cells larger than five average colloid-containing thyroid follicles. Adenomas either are well circumscribed or partially encapsulated from adjacent thyroid follicles that often are compressed to varying degrees. C cells composing an adenoma may be subdivided by fine connective tissue septae and capillaries into small neuroendocrine packets. Some C-cell adenomas are composed of larger pleomorphic cells with amphophilic cytoplasm, large nuclei with coarsely clumped chromatin, and prominent nucleoli; histologically, they resemble ganglion cells. Occasional amyloid deposits may be found both in nodular hyperplasia and in adenomas.

C-cell carcinomas often result in macroscopic enlargement of one or both thyroid lobes due to the extensive proliferation and infiltration of C cells. There is evidence of intrathyroidal and/or capsular invasion by the malignant C cells, often with areas of hemorrhage and necrosis within the neoplasm. The malignant C cells are more pleomorphic than those making up benign proliferative lesions. Immunoperoxidase reactions for calcitonin generally are more intense in diffuse or nodular hyperplasia, whereas in adenomas and carcinomas calcitonin immunoreactivity is much more variable between tumors and in different regions of a tumor. Hyperplastic C cells adjacent to adenomas and carcinomas usually are intensely positive for calcitonin. In addition to calcitonin, some of the tumor cells and adjacent hyperplastic C cells have positive staining for somatostatin or bombesin.

PARATHYROID GLAND

Introduction

Calcium plays a key role as an essential structural component of the skeleton and also in many fundamental biological processes. These processes include neuromuscular excitability, membrane permeability, muscle contraction, enzyme activity, hormone release, and blood coagulation, among others. The precise control of calcium in extracellular fluids is vital to health. To maintain a constant concentration of calcium, despite marked variations in intake and excretion, endocrine control mechanisms have evolved that primarily consist of the interactions of three major hormones—parathyroid hormone (PTH), calcitonin (CT), and cholecalciferol (vitamin D) (Fig. 21-36).

Normal Structure and Function of Chief Cells

Biosynthesis of Parathyroid Hormone Parathyroid chief cells in humans and many animal species store relatively small amounts of preformed hormone, but they respond quickly to variations in the need for hormone by changing the rate of hormone synthesis. Parathyroid hormone, like many peptide hormones, is first synthesized as a larger biosynthetic precursor molecule that undergoes posttranslational processing in chief cells. Preproparathyroid hormone (preproPTH) is the initial translation product synthesized on ribosomes of the rough endoplasmic reticulum in chief cells. It is composed of 115 amino acids and contains a hydrophobic signal or leader sequence of 25 amino acid residues that facilitates the penetration and subsequent vectorial discharge of the nascent peptide into the cisternal space of the rough endoplasmic reticulum (Kronenberg et al., 1986) (Fig. 21-37). PreproPTH is rapidly converted within 1 min or less of its synthesis to proparathyroid hormone (ProPTH) by the proteolytic cleavage of 25 amino acids from the NH_2-terminal end of the molecule (Habener, 1981). The intermediate precursor, proPTH, is composed of 90 amino acids and moves within membranous channels of the rough endoplasmic reticulum to the Golgi apparatus (Fig. 21-37). Enzymes within membranes of the Golgi apparatus cleave a hexapeptide from the NH_2-terminal (biologically active) end of the molecule, forming active PTH. Active PTH is packaged into membrane-limited, macromolecular aggregates in the Golgi apparatus for subsequent storage in chief cells. Under certain conditions of increased demand (e.g., a low calcium ion concentration in the extracellular fluid compartment), PTH may be released directly from chief cells without being packaged into secretion granules by a process termed bypass secretion.

Although the principal form of active PTH secreted from chief cells is a straight-chain peptide of 84 amino acids (molecular weight 9500), the molecule is rapidly cleaved into amino- and carboxy-terminal fragments in the peripheral circulation and especially in the liver. The purpose of this fragmentation is uncertain

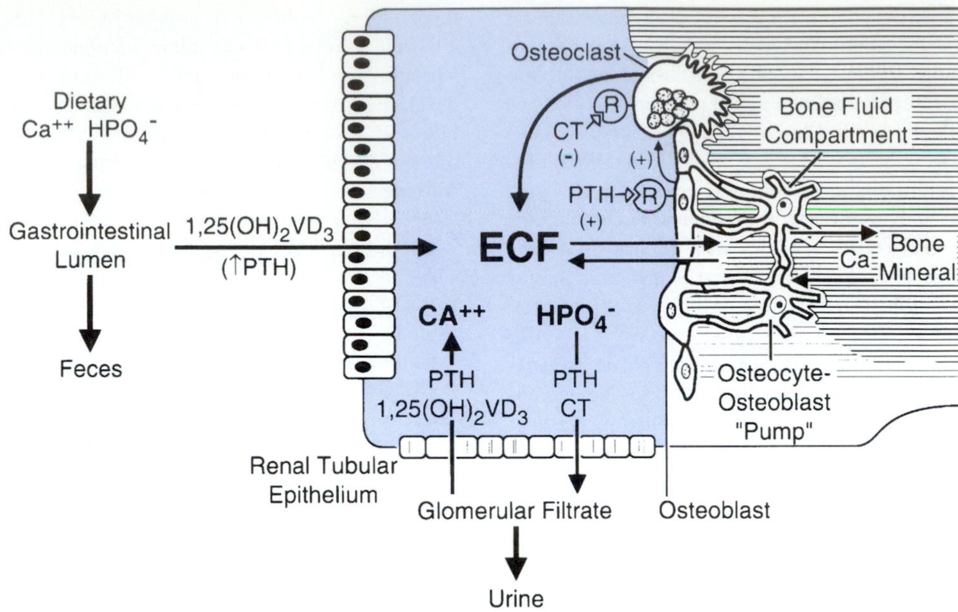

Figure 21-36. Interrelationship of parathyroid hormone (PTH), calcitonin (CT), and 1,25-dihydroxycholecalciferol (1,25(OH)$_2$VD$_3$) in the regulation of calcium (Ca) and phosphorus in extracellular fluids.

Receptors for PTH are on osteoblasts and for CT on osteoclasts in bone. PTH and CT are antagonistic in their action on bone but synergistic in stimulating the renal excretion of phosphorous. Vitamin D exerts its action primarily on the intestine to enhance the absorption of both calcium and phosphorus.

because the biologically active amino-terminal fragment is no more active than the entire PTH molecule (amino acids 1 to 84). The plasma half-life of the *N*-terminal fragment is considerably shorter than that of the biologically inactive carboxy-terminal fragment of parathyroid hormone. The C terminal and other portions of the PTH molecule are degraded primarily in the kidney and tend to accumulate with chronic renal disease.

Control of Parathyroid Hormone Secretion Secretory cells in the parathyroid gland store small amounts of preformed hormone

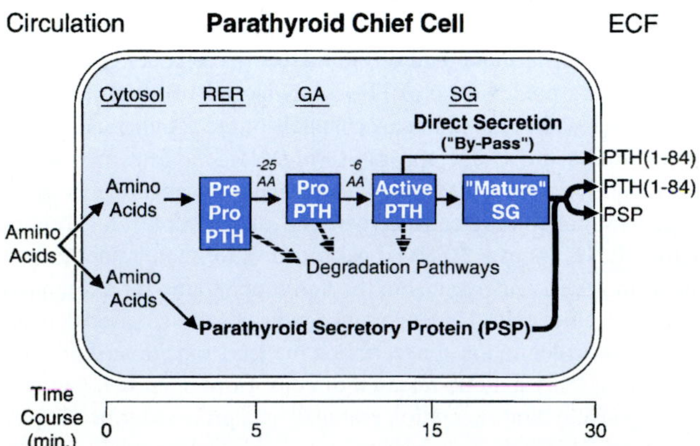

Figure 21-37. Biosynthesis of parathyroid hormone (PTH) and parathyroid secretory protein (PSP) by parathyroid chief cells.

Active PTH is synthesized as a larger biosynthetic precursor molecule (preproPTH) that undergoes rapid posttranslational processing to proPTH prior to secretion from chief cells as active PTH (amino acids 1 to 84).

but are capable of responding to minor fluctuations in calcium concentration by rapidly altering the rate of hormonal secretion and more slowly by altering the rate of hormonal synthesis. In contrast to most endocrine organs that are under complex controls involving both long and short feedback loops, the parathyroids have a unique feedback controlled by the concentration of calcium (and to a lesser extent magnesium) ion in serum. The concentration of blood phosphorus has no direct regulatory influence on the synthesis and secretion of PTH; however, several disease conditions with hyperphosphatemia in both animals and humans are associated clinically with secondary hyperparathyroidism. An elevated blood phosphorus level may lead indirectly to parathyroid stimulation by virtue of its ability to lower blood calcium, primarily by suppressing the 1α-hydroxylase in the kidney and decreasing the production of the active form of vitamin D [1,25-(OH)$_2$-cholecalciferol] thereby diminishing the rate of intestinal calcium absorption. Magnesium ion has an effect on parathyroid secretion rate similar to that of calcium, but its effect is not equipotent to that of calcium.

Serum Ca^{2+} binds to a recently identified Ca receptor on the chief cell, which permits the serum Ca^{2+} to regulate chief cell function (Pollak et al., 1993). The receptor is present on the plasma membranes of parathyroid chief cells, renal epithelial cells, and other cells that respond to extracellular Ca^{2+}. Mutations in one or both of the Ca^{2+}-sensing receptor genes in humans results in familial hypocalciuric hypercalcemia or neonatal severe hypercalcemia, respectively. Interaction of serum Ca^{2+} with its receptor on chief cells results in the formation of an inverse sigmoidal relationship between serum Ca^{2+} and PTH concentrations (Cloutier et al., 1993; Silver, 1992).

The serum [Ca^{2+}] that results in half maximal PTH secretion is defined as the serum calcium "set point" and is stable for an individual animal. The sigmoidal relationship between serum [Ca^{2+}] and PTH secretion permits the chief cells to respond rapidly to a reduction in serum Ca^{2+}. The major inhibitors of PTH synthesis and secretion are increased serum [Ca^{2+}] and 1,25-dihydroxyvitamin D. Inhibition of PTH synthesis by 1,25-dihydroxyvitamin D completes an important endocrine feedback loop between the parathyroid chief cells and the renal epithelial cells since PTH stimulates renal production of 1,25-dihydroxyvitamin D.

Chief cells synthesize and secrete another major protein termed parathyroid secretory protein (I), or chromogranin A. It is a higher-molecular-weight molecule (70 kDa) composed of from 430 to 448 amino acids that is stored and secreted together with PTH. A similar molecule has been found in secretory granules of a wide variety of peptide hormone–secreting cells and in neurotransmitter secretory vesicles. An internal region of the parathyroid secretory protein or chromogranin A molecule is identical in sequence to pancreastatin, a C terminal amidated peptide, which inhibits glucose-stimulated insulin secretion. This 49–amino acid proteolytic cleavage product (amino acids number 240 to 280) of parathyroid secretory protein has been reported to inhibit low calcium-stimulated secretion of parathyroid hormone and chromogranin A from parathyroid cells. These findings suggest that chromogranin A–derived peptides may act locally in an autocrine manner to inhibit the secretion of active hormone by endocrine cells, such as chief cells of the parathyroid gland (Barbosa et al., 1991; Cohn et al., 1993; Fasciotto et al., 1990) (Fig. 21-38).

Xenobiotic Chemical-Induced Toxic Injury of Parathyroids

Ozone Inhalation of a single dose of ozone (0.75 ppm) for 4 to 8 h has been reported to produce light and electron microscopic changes in parathyroid glands (Atwal and Wilson, 1974). Subsequent studies have utilized longer (48-h) exposure to ozone in order to define the pathogenesis of the parathyroid lesions (Atwal et al., 1975; Atwal, 1979). Initially (1 to 5 days after ozone exposure), many chief cells undergo compensatory hypertrophy and hyperplasia with areas of capillary endothelial cell proliferation, interstitial edema, degeneration of vascular endothelium, formation of platelet thrombi, leukocyte infiltration of the walls of larger vessels in the gland, and disruption of basement membranes. Chief cells had prominent Golgi complexes and endoplasmic reticulum, aggregations of free ribosomes, and swelling of mitochondria (Atwal and Pemsingh, 1981).

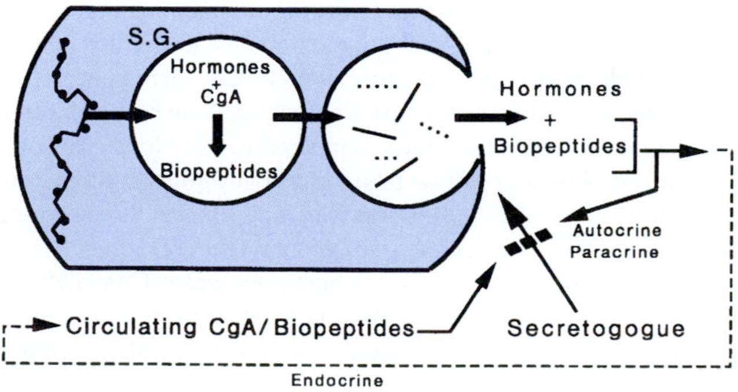

Figure 21-38. Autocrine/paracrine action of chromogranin A (CgA)-derived peptides. PTH and CgA are coreleased from chief cells in response to a low calcium ion signal.

Pancreastatin (PST) is a 49–amino acid peptide derived from CgA that exerts local negative feedback on chief cells and decreases PTH secretion from chief cells. (Modified from Cohn et al., 1993, with permission.)

Inactive chief cells with few secretory granules predominate in the parathyroids in the later stages of exposure to ozone. There was evidence of parathyroid atrophy from 12 to 20 days after ozone exposure, with mononuclear cell infiltration and necrosis of chief cells. The reduced cytoplasmic area contained vacuolated endoplasmic reticulum, a small Golgi apparatus, and numerous lysosomal bodies. Plasma membranes of adjacent chief cells were disrupted, resulting in coalescence of the cytoplasmic area. Fibroblasts with associated collagen bundles were prominent in the interstitium, and the basal lamina of the numerous capillaries often was duplicated.

The parathyroid lesions in ozone-exposed animals are similar to isoimmune parathyroiditis in other species (Lupulescu et al., 1968). Antibody against parathyroid tissue was localized near the periphery of chief cells by indirect immunofluorescence, especially 14 days following ozone injury (Atwal et al., 1975).

Aluminum Evidence for a direct effect of aluminum on the parathyroid was suggested from studies of patients with chronic renal failure treated by hemodialysis with aluminum-containing fluids or orally administered drugs containing aluminum. These patients often had normal or minimal elevations of immunoreactive parathyroid hormone (iPTH), little histologic evidence of osteitis fibrosa in bone, and a depressed response by the parathyroid gland to acute hypocalcemia (Bourdeau et al., 1987). Studies by Morrissey and coworkers (1983) have reported that an increase in aluminum concentration in vitro over a range of 0.5 to 2.0 mM in a low-calcium medium (0.5 mM) progressively inhibited the secretion of PTH. At 2.0 mM aluminum, PTH secretion was inhibited by 68 percent, while a high-calcium medium (2.0 mM) without aluminum maximally inhibited PTH secretion by only 39 percent. The inhibition of PTH secretion by aluminum does not appear to be related to an irreversible toxic effect because normal secretion was restored when parathyroid cells were returned to the 0.5 mM calcium medium without aluminum. The incorporation of [^{3}H] leucine into total cell protein, parathyroid secretory protein, proparathyroid hormone, or PTH was not affected by aluminum; however, the secretion of radiolabeled protein by dispersed parathyroid cells was inhibited by aluminum (Morrissey et al., 1983).

The molecular mechanism by which aluminum inhibits PTH secretion, reducing diglyceride levels in chief cells (Morrissey and Slatopolsky, 1986), appears to be similar to that of the calcium ion. Aluminum appears to decrease diglyceride synthesis, which is reflected in a corresponding decrease in synthesis of phosphatidylcholine and possible triglyceride; however, phosphatidylinositol synthesis was not affected by aluminum. The mechanism by which aluminum decreases diglycerides and maintains phosphatidylinositol synthesis in parathyroid cells is not known.

L-Asparaginase Tettenborn and colleagues (1970) and Chisari et al. (1972) reported that rabbits administered L-asparaginase develop severe hypocalcemia and tetany characterized by muscle tremors, opisthotonos, carpopedal spasms, paralysis, and coma. This drug was of interest in cancer chemotherapy because of the beneficial effects of guinea pig serum against lymphosarcoma in mice.

Parathyroid chief cells appeared to be selectively destroyed by L-asparaginase (Young et al., 1973). Chief cells were predominately inactive and degranulated, with large autophagic vacuoles present in the cytoplasm of degenerating cells. Cytoplasmic organelles concerned with synthesis and packaging of secretory products were poorly developed in chief cells. Rabbits developed hyperphosphatemia, hypomagnesemia, hyperkalemia, and azotemia in addition to acute hypocalcemia. Rabbits with clinical hypocalcemic tetany did not recover spontaneously; however, administration of parathyroid extract prior to or during treatment with L-asparaginase decreased the incidence of hypocalcemic tetany.

The development of hypocalcemia and tetany has not been observed in other experimental animals administered L-asparaginase (Oettgen et al., 1970). However, this response may not be limited to the rabbit, because some human patients receiving the drug also have developed hypocalcemia (Jaffe et al., 1972). The L-asparaginase-induced hypoparathyroidism in rabbits is a valuable model for investigating drug–endocrine cell interactions, somewhat analogous to the selective destruction of pancreatic beta cells by alloxan with production of experimental diabetes mellitus.

Proliferative Lesions of Parathyroid Chief Cells

Chief Cell Adenoma ***Introduction*** Parathyroid adenomas in adult-aged rats vary in size from microscopic to unilateral nodules several millimeters in diameter; they are located in the cervical region by the thyroids or infrequently in the thoracic cavity near the base of the heart. Parathyroid neoplasms in the precardiac mediastinum are derived from ectopic parathyroid tissue displaced into the thorax with the expanding thymus during embryonic development. Tumors of parathyroid chief cells do not appear to be a sequela of long-standing secondary hyperparathyroidism of either renal or nutritional origin. The unaffected parathyroid glands may be atrophic if the adenoma is functional, normal if the adenoma is nonfunctional, or enlarged if there is concomitant hyperplasia. In functional adenomas, the normal mechanism by which PTH secretion is regulated—changes in the concentration of blood calcium ion—is lost and hormone secretion is excessive in spite of an increased level of blood calcium.

Adenomas are solitary nodules that are sharply demarcated from adjacent parathyroid parenchyma. Because the adenoma compresses the rim of surrounding parathyroid to varying degrees depending upon its size, there may be a partial fibrous capsule, resulting either from compression of existing stroma or from proliferation of fibrous connective tissue.

Adenomas are usually nonfunctional (endocrinologically inactive) in adult-aged rats from chronic toxicity/carcinogenicity studies. Chief cells in nonfunctional adenomas are cuboidal or polyhedral and arranged either in a diffuse sheet, in lobules, or in acini with or without lumens. Chief cells from functional adenomas often are closely packed into small groups by fine connective tissue septa. The cytoplasmic area varies from normal size to an expanded area. There is a much lower density of cells in functional parathyroid adenoma compared to the adjacent rim with atrophic chief cells.

Larger parathyroid adenomas, such as those that are detected macroscopically, often nearly incorporate the entire affected gland. A narrow rim of compressed parenchyma may be detected at one side of the gland, or the affected parathyroid may be completely incorporated by the adenoma. Chief cells in this rim often are compressed and atrophic due to pressure and the persistent hypercalcemia. Peripherally situated follicles in the adjacent thyroid lobe may be compressed to a limited extent by larger parathyroid adenomas. The parathyroid glands that do not contain a functional adenoma also undergo trophic atrophy in response to the hypercalcemia and become smaller.

Influence of Age on Development of Parathyroid Tumors There are relatively few chemicals or experimental manipulations reported in the literature that significantly increase the incidence of parathyroid tumors. Long-standing renal failure with intense diffuse hyperplasia does not appear to increase the development of chief cell tumors in rats. The historical incidence of parathyroid adenomas in untreated control male F344 rats in studies conducted by the NTP was 4/1315 (0.3 percent); for female F344 rats, it was 2/1330 (0.15 percent). However, parathyroid adenomas are an example of a neoplasm in F344 rats whose incidence increases dramatically when life-span data are compared to 2-year studies. Solleveld and coworkers (1984) reported that the incidence of parathyroid adenomas increased in males from 0.1 percent at 2 years to 3.1 percent in lifetime studies. Corresponding data for female F344 rats was 0.1 percent at 2 years and 0.6 percent in lifetime studies. Hexachlorobenzene (40ppm) fed to Sprague-Dawley rats (F_0 rats for 3 months and until weaning of F_1 rats that subsequently were fed for the rest of their life of 130 weeks) has been reported to increase the incidence of parathyroid adenomas in the male rats (24.5 percent; 12 of 49 rats) (Arnold et al., 1985).

Influence of Gonadectomy Oslapas and colleagues (1982) reported an increased incidence of parathyroid adenomas in female (34 percent) and male (27 percent) rats of the Long-Evans strain administered 40 μCi sodium ^{131}I and saline at 8 weeks of age. There were no significant changes in serum calcium, phosphorus, and parathyroid hormone compared to controls. Gonadectomy performed at 7 weeks of age decreased the incidence of parathyroid adenomas in irradiated rats (7.4 percent in gonadectomy versus 27 percent in intact controls), but there was little change in the incidence of parathyroid adenomas in irradiated females. X-irradiation of the thyroid-parathyroid region also increased the incidence of parathyroid adenomas. When female Sprague-Dawley rats received a single absorbed dose of x-rays at 4 weeks of age, they subsequently developed a 24 percent incidence of parathyroid adenomas after 14 months (Oslapas et al., 1981).

Influence of Xenobiotic Chemicals Parathyroid adenomas have been encountered infrequently following the administration of a variety of chemicals in 2-year bioassay studies in Fischer rats. In a study with the pesticide rotenone in F344 rats, there appeared to be an increased incidence of parathyroid adenomas in high-dose (75 ppm) males (4 of 44 rats) compared to low-dose (38 ppm) males, control males (1 of 44 rats), or NTP historical controls (0.3 percent) (Abdo et al., 1988). It was uncertain whether the increased incidence of this uncommon tumor was a direct effect of rotenone feeding or the increased survival in high-dose males. Chief cell hyperplasia was not present in parathyroids that developed adenomas.

Influence of Irradiation and Hypercalcemia Induced by Vitamin D Wynford-Thomas and associates (1982) reported that irradiation significantly increases the incidence of parathyroid adenomas in inbred Wistar albino rats and that the incidence could be modified by feeding diets with variable amounts of vitamin D. Neonatal Wistar rats were given either 5 or 10 μCi radioiodine (^{131}I) within 24 h of birth. In rats 12 months of age and older, parathyroid adenomas were found in 33 percent of rats administered 5 μCi ^{131}I and in 37 percent of rats given 10 μCi ^{131}I compared to 0 percent in unirradiated controls. The incidence of parathyroid adenomas was highest (55 percent) in normocalcemic rats fed a low vitamin D diet and lowest (20 percent) in irradiated rats fed a diet high in vitamin D (40,000 IU/kg) that had a significant elevation in plasma calcium.

Age-Related Changes in Parathyroid Function

Serum immunoreactive parathyroid hormone (iPTH) [as well as calcitonin (iCT)] has been reported to be different in young compared to aged Fischer 344 (F344) rats; however, the serum calcium concentration does not change with age (Wongsurawat and Armbrecht, 1987). This suggests that the regulation of iPTH (and iCT) secretion may be affected by the process of aging. The decreased responsiveness of chief cells to calcium may be due to age-related changes in the regulation of the secretory pathway. This could include age-related changes in the effect of calcium on release of stored PTH, intracellular degradation of PTH, or modification of adenylate cyclase activity as observed in other tissues that utilize calcium as an intermediary signal (Brown, 1982). Therefore, the sensitivity of parathyroid chief cells to circulating calcium ion concentration appears not to be fixed but may change during development, aging, and in response to certain disease processes.

The increased secretion of iPTH with advancing age in rats could be due to several factors: *first,* an increased number of parathyroid secretory cells with age; or, *second,* an altered regulation of chief cells in response to calcium ion associated with the process of aging. For example, a decreased sensitivity of chief cells to negative feedback by calcium ion could result in the higher blood levels of iPTH in aged F344 rats. Wada et al. (1992) reported that the early age-related rise in plasma PTH in F344 rats was neither a consequence of low plasma calcium nor of renal insufficiency. Age-related changes in the responsiveness of chief cells to circulating levels of other factors that modulate iPTH secretion, particularly 1,25-dihydroxycholecalciferol and alpha- and beta-adrenergic catecholamines, also could contribute to the variations in blood levels of iPTH in rats of different ages. In addition, target cell responsiveness to PTH also decreases with advancing age in rats. PTH does not increase the renal production of 1,25-dihydroxyvitamin D in adult (13-month-old) male F344 rats compared to young (2-month-old) rats, where its production was increased 61 percent (Armbrecht et al., 1982). Older rats have a decreased calcemic response and decreased renal production of 1,25-dihydroxycholecalciferol compared to young rats (Armbrecht et al., 1982; Kalu et al., 1982).

TESTIS

Introduction

Leydig (interstitial) cell tumors are among the more frequently occurring endocrine tumors in rodents in chronic toxicity/carcinogenicity studies, and a great deal of research has been published investigating their pathogenesis and implications for safety assessment. Rodent testicular tumors are classified into five general categories, including tumors derived from cells of the gonadal stroma, neoplasms of germ cell origin, tumors derived from adnexal structures or serous membranes, and, last, a group of tumors derived from the supporting connective tissues and vessels of the testis.

Neoplasms of the gonadal stroma include benign and malignant tumors derived from Leydig (interstitial) cells, Sertoli cells of the seminiferous tubules, as well as a rare mixed tumor with an admixture of both cell types. The Leydig cell tumor is the most common tumor developing in the rodent testis and frequently presents a problem in separating between focal hyperplasia and early neoplastic growth (i.e., adenoma formation).

The incidence of Leydig cell tumors in old rats varies considerably depending upon the strain. In general, Sprague-Dawley, Osborne-Mendel, and Brown-Norway strains have a much lower incidence than other strains frequently used in chronic toxicity/carcinogenicity studies, including the Fischer 344 and Wistar strains. The spontaneous incidence of Leydig cell tumors in three different strains of rats is illustrated in Fig. 21-39 (Bär, 1992). The actual incidence of Leydig cell tumors in old rats is lowest in Sprague-Dawley, highly variable in Wistar rats, and highest in Fischer rats (in which the incidence at 2 years of age often approaches 100 percent). The specific numerical incidence of benign Leydig cell tumors in rats also will vary considerably depending upon the histologic criteria used by the pathologist in the separation of focal hyperplasia from adenomas.

The incidence of Leydig cell tumors in human patients, in comparison to rodents, is extremely rare, something on the order of 1 in 5 million, with age peaks at approximately 30 and 60 years.

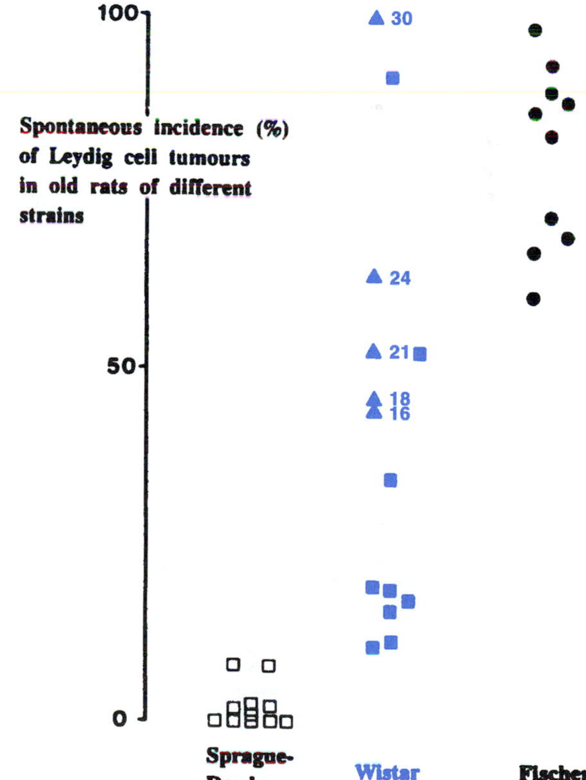

Figure 21-39. Spontaneous incidence of Leydig cell tumors of the testis in Sprague-Dawley, Wistar, and Fischer rats. (From Bär, 1992, with permission.)

Ninety or more percent of Leydig cell tumors in humans are benign and some appear to be endocrinologically active and associated clinically with gynecomastia.

Structure and Endocrinologic Regulation of Leydig (Interstitial) Cells

Although the numbers of Leydig cells vary somewhat among different animal species and humans, the basic structural arrangement is similar. In the rat, there are small groups of Leydig cells clustered around blood vessels in the interstitium, between seminiferous tubules with an incomplete layer of endothelial cells around the groups of Leydig cells. In humans, the Leydig cells are present as small groups in the interstitium near blood vessels or in loose connective tissue but without the surrounding layer of endothelial cells. Leydig cells are much more numerous in some animal species, such as the domestic pig. Microscopic evaluation of the normal rat testis reveals the inconspicuous clusters of Leydig cells in the interstitium between the much larger seminiferous tubules composed of spermatogonia and Sertoli cells. The close anatomic association of Leydig cells and interstitial blood vessels permits the rapid exchange of materials between this endocrine cell population and the systemic circulation.

The endocrinologic regulation of Leydig cells involves the coordinated activity of the hypothalamus and adenohypophysis (anterior pituitary) with negative feedback control exerted by the blood concentration of gonadal steroids (Fig. 21-40). Hypothalamic gonadotrophin-releasing hormone (GnRH) stimulates the pulsatile release of both luteinizing hormone (LH) and follicle-stimulating hormone (FSH) from gonadotrophs in the adenohypopthysis. Luteinizing hormone is the major trophic factor controlling the activity of Leydig cells and the synthesis of testosterone. The blood levels of testosterone exert negative feedback on the hypothalamus and, to a lesser extent, on the adenohypophysis. Follicle-stimulating hormone binds to receptors on Sertoli cells in the seminiferous tubules and, along with the local concentration of testosterone, plays a critical role in spermatogenesis. Testosterone, by controlling GnRH release, is one important regulator of FSH secretion by the pituitary gland. The seminiferous tubules also produce a glycopeptide, designated as inhibin, which exerts negative feedback on the release of FSH by the gonadotrophs.

Leydig cells have a similar ultrastructural appearance as other endocrine cells that synthesize and release steroid hormones. The abundant cytoplasmic area contains numerous mitochondria, abundant profiles of smooth endoplasmic reticulum, prominent Golgi apparatuses associated with lysosomal bodies, and occasional lipofucsin inclusions. However, they lack the hormone-containing secretory granules that are found characteristically in peptide hormone–secreting endocrine cells.

The hormonal control of testicular function is largely the result of the coordinated activities of LH and FSH from the pituitary gland. LH binds to high-affinity, low-capacity receptors on the surface of Leydig cells and activates adenylate cyclase in the plasma membrane resulting in the generation of an intracellular messenger, cyclic AMP (Fig. 21-41). The cyclic AMP binds to a protein kinase, resulting in the phosphorylation of a specific set of proteins in the cytosol, which increases the conversion of cholesterol to pregnenolone by making more substrate available and increasing the activity of an enzyme that cleaves the side chain of cholesterol. The pregnenolone in Leydig cells is rapidly converted to testosterone, which is released into interstitial blood vessels or taken up by adjacent Sertoli cells. Testosterone in the Sertoli cells binds to nuclear receptors, where it increases genomic expression and transcription of mRNAs that direct the synthesis of proteins (e.g., androgen-binding protein and others) involved in spermatogenesis. In the rat, the mitotic phase of gametogenesis can occur without hormonal stimulation but testosterone is necessary for meiosis of spermatocytes to spermatids. FSH is required for the later stages for spermatid maturation to spermatazoa (Fig. 21-41). Once FSH and testosterone initiate spermatogenesis at puberty in the rat, testosterone alone is sufficient to maintain sperm production.

Pathology of Leydig (Interstitial) Cell Tumors

Before discussing the pathology of focal proliferative lesions of Leydig cells, a few points should be made about the importance of

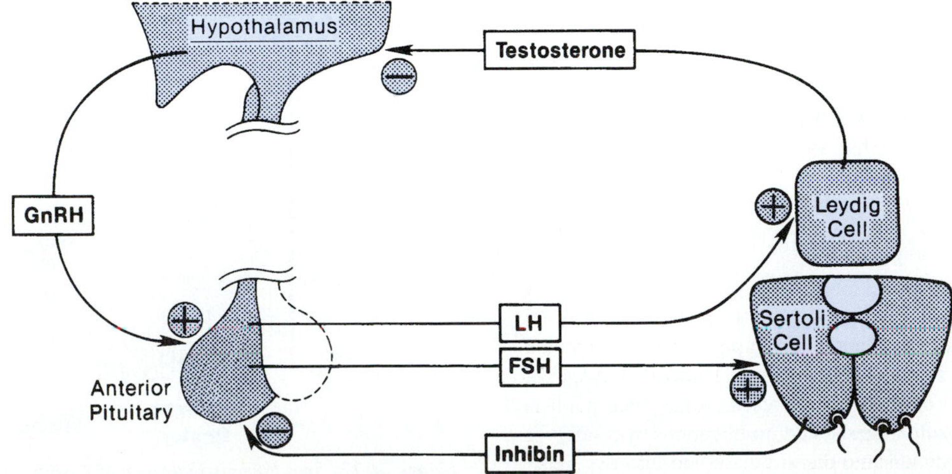

Figure 21-40. Hypothalamus–anterior pituitary gland–gonad axis in the endocrine control of Leydig and Sertoli cells by luteinizing hormone (LH) and follicle stimulating hormone (FSH). (From Hedge et al. 1987, with permission.)

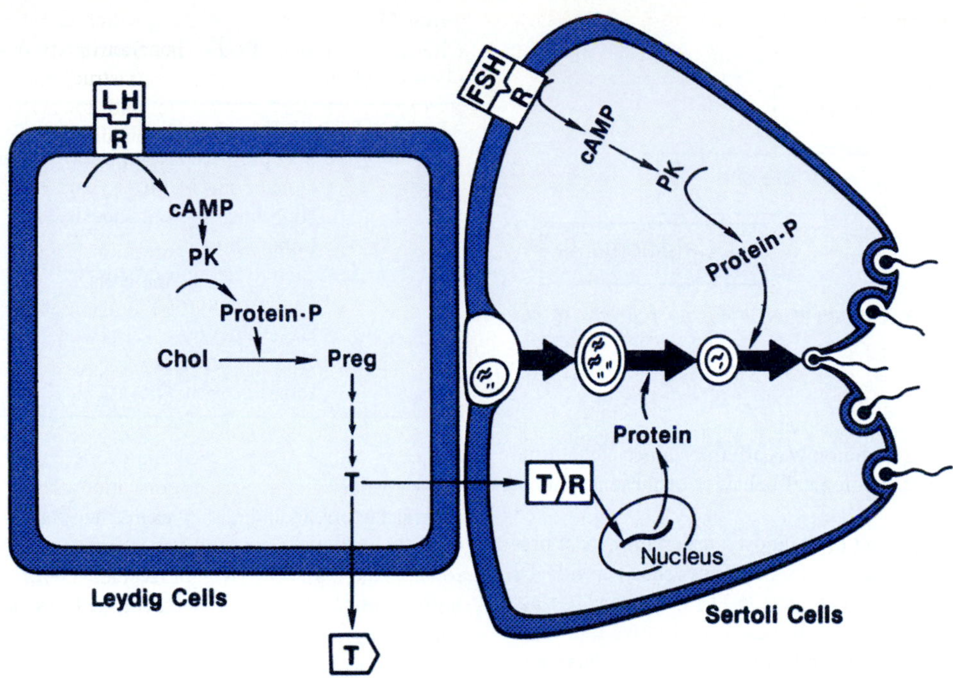

Figure 21-41. Hormonal control of testicular function.

Luteinizing hormone (LH) stimulates testosterone (T) release by binding to its receptor (R) and increasing the conversion of cholesterol (chol) to pregnenolone (preg) via a cAMP-protein kinase (PK) cascade. Spermatogenesis (*bold arrows*) is controlled by both FSH and testosterone acting via Sertoli cells. (From Hedge et al., 1987, with permission.)

standardized sectioning methods for the complete evaluation of the rodent testis. It is not unusual to have less than optimal sections to evaluate, due either to a lack of a consistent plane of section or to inadequate fixation. The goal should be to include the largest testicular area containing all anatomic features on a mid-sagittal section along the long axis of the testis, including spermatic vessels, attachment sites of the epididymis, the tubulus rectus, and the intratesticular rete testis. It is also important to emphasize the need to cut the thick outer covering (tunica albuginea) of the testis at several points prior to immersion in the fixative in order to permit more rapid penetration of the formalin or other fixing solution.

The major issue in the interpretation of focal proliferative lesions of Leydig cells in the rodent testis is the accurate and consistent separation of focal hyperplasia from benign tumors (adenomas) that possess autonomous growth. The separation of focal hyperplasia from adenomas derived from Leydig cells is arbitrary based upon current methods of evaluation and often is based primarily on the size of the focal lesion, since cytologic features usually are similar between focal hyperplastic and benign neoplastic lesions derived from Leydig cells.

In the multistage model of carcinogenesis, proliferative lesions are designated as beginning with hyperplasia, often progressing to benign tumors (adenomas); infrequently, a few assume malignant potential and form carcinomas ("cancer") (Fig. 21-42). Although this terminology often is applied to focal proliferative lesions in rodent endocrine tissues for convenience and standardization, it is essential to understand that the separation, especially between focal hyperplasia and adenoma, is based primarily on size and morphologic changes in the proliferating Leydig cells. It is important to emphasize that focal proliferative lesions associated with hormonal imbalances in rodent endocrine tissues—also including Leydig cells, adrenal medullary cells, thyroid follicular cells, and C cells, among others—represent a morphologic continuum that begins with hyperplasia and progresses often but not always to the formation of adenomas that grow autonomously and only occasionally undergo a malignant transformation to form carcinomas ("cancer") (Fig. 21-43).

The National Toxicology Program (NTP), in an attempt to standardize the classification of focal proliferative lesions of Leydig cells between studies with different xenobiotic chemicals and different testing laboratories, established the following diagnostic criteria (Boorman, 1987): (1) Hyperplasia was defined as a focal collection of Leydig cells with little atypia and a diameter of less than 1 seminiferous tubule. (2) An adenoma was defined as a mass of Leydig cells larger in diameter than 1 seminiferous tubule with some cellular atypia and compression of adjacent tubules. (3) It

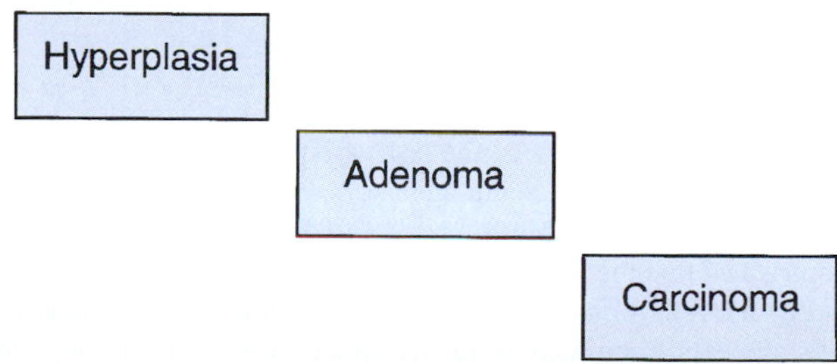

Figure 21-42. Multistage model of carcinogenesis of proliferative lesions in endocrine tissues of rodents.

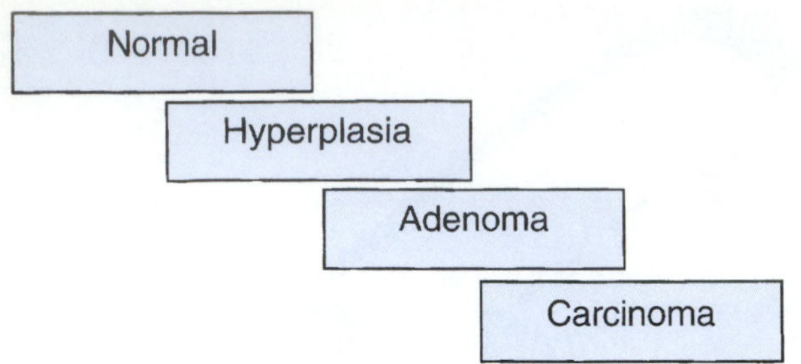

Figure 21-43. Morphologic continuum of proliferative lesions in endocrine tissues of rodents.

was emphasized that the separation was arbitrary, since at that time little was known about the biological behavior of these lesions in rodents.

A more contemporary set of diagnostic criteria for focal proliferative lesions of Leydig cells has been published recently by the Society of Toxicologic Pathologists (STP) (McConnell et al., 1992). Recognizing that many small focal proliferative lesions of Leydig cells (i.e., between one and three tubule diameters) will regress following removal of the inciting stimulus, they recommend the diagnosis of Leydig cell adenoma be used for a mass of interstitial cells equal to or greater than the diameter of three adjacent seminiferous tubules plus one or more of the following criteria: symmetrical peripheral compression of adjacent tubules, evidence of cellular pleomorphism or an increase in the nuclear:cytoplasmic ratio, an endocrine sinusoidal vascular network, increased mitotic activity, or coalescence of adjacent cell masses.

Leydig cell neoplasms in laboratory rats associated with hormonal imbalances rarely undergo malignant transformation with progression to the development of carcinomas ("cancer"). Histologic features of malignancy include invasion into the epididymis, spermatic cord, or tunica albuginea. The most definitive criteria of malignancy is the demonstration of metastases in extratesticular sites. Leydig cell carinomas are large and often distort the overall contour of the affected testis, with extensive areas of both hemorrhage and necrosis. The cytology of Leydig cell carcinomas usually is more pleomorphic than with adenomas consisting of an admixture of poorly differentiated cells with an increased nuclear:cytoplasmic ratio and larger, more differentiated cells with an abundant vacuolated eosinophilic cytoplasmic area. The frequency of mitotic figures may be increased either in focal areas or throughout the Leydig cell carcinomas. The most convincing evidence of malignancy in carcinomas is the establishment of foci of growth outside of the testis, such as multiple foci of tumor cell emboli growing within and distending vessels of the lung.

Mechanisms of Leydig (Interstitial) Cell Tumor Development

Leydig (interstitial) cells of the testis frequently undergo proliferative changes with advancing age and following chronic exposure to large doses of xenobiotic chemicals. In addition, it should be emphasized that the "sensitivity" of rodent endocrine tissues, such as Leydig cells of the testis and other populations of endocrine cells, appears to be increasing over time particularly if one compares data generated in the 1970s to that gathered in the 1990s for the same compound (Table 21-3). This appears to be the result of several factors, including (1) animal husbandry practices, such as specific pathogen-free conditions, that result in a greater survival for 2 years, high body weight related to over feeding, and immobility; and (2) the genetic selection process for high productivity and rapid growth.

Table 21-3

Changes in Rodent Endocrine Sensitivity over Time (1970s–1990s)

1. Animal husbandry practices
Specific pathogen-free (SPF) conditions
Greater survival to 2 years+
High body weight (obesity)
Immobility
2. Genetic selection process
High productivity
Large litters
High lactation yield
Rapid growth

Pathogenic mechanisms reported in the literature to be important in the development of proliferative lesions of Leydig cells include irradiation, the species and strain differences mentioned previously, and exposure to certain chemicals such as cadmium salts and 2-acetoaminofluorene (Prentice and Meikle, 1995) (Table 21-4). Other pathogenic mechanisms include physiologic perturbations such as cryptorchidism, a compromised blood supply to the testis, or heterotransplantation into the spleen. Hormonal imbalances also are important factors in the development of focal proliferative lesions of Leydig cells, including increased estrogenic steroids in mice and hamsters and elevated pituitary gonadotrophins resulting from the chronic administration of androgen receptor antagonists, 5α-reductase inhibitors, testosterone biosynthesis inhibitors, GnRH agonists, and aromatase inhibitors (Fig. 21-44) (Clegg et al., 1997; Cook et al., 1999). Many xenobiotic chemicals administered chronically to rats disrupt the hypothalamic-pituitary-testis axis at one of several possible sites, interfering with negative feedback control and resulting in an overproduction of luteinizing hormone (LH), which causes the proliferative changes

Table 21-4

Pathogenic Mechanisms for Development of Leydig (Interstitial) Cell Proliferative Lesions in Rodents

Physiologic perturbations
Cryptorchidism
Compromised blood supply
Heterotransplantation (spleen)
Hormonal imbalances
Decreased testosterone
Increased estrogens (mice, hamsters)
Increased pituitary gonadotropins (e.g., LH)
Irradiation
Species/strain differences
Chemicals
Cadmium salts
2-Acetoaminofluorene

- **ANDROGEN RECEPTOR ANTAGONISTS (RATS)**
- **5α-REDUCTASE INHIBITORS (RAT, MOUSE)**
- **TESTOSTERONE BIOSYNTHESIS INHIBITORS (RAT)**
- **AROMATASE INHIBITORS (DOG, RAT)**
- **DOPAmine AGONISTS (RAT)**
- **GnRH AGONISTS (RAT)**
- **ESTROGEN AGONISTS / ANTAGONISTS (MOUSE)**

Figure 21-44. Model of action of nongenotoxic compounds that produce Leydig cell hyperplasia/adenoma in rodents.

(hyperplasia, adenoma) in Leydig cells (Fig. 21-45). For example, chronic exposure to chemicals with antiandrogenic activity, such as procymidone due to binding to the androgen receptor, increases circulating levels of LH and results in stimulation of Leydig cells leading to an increased incidence of hyperplasia and adenomas in rats (Murakami et al., 1995).

Data from several studies in the recent literature emphasize the importance of several of these pathogenetic factors in the frequent development of Leydig cell tumors in rats. Thurman and colleagues (1994) reported the effects of food restriction on the development of Leydig cell adenomas in the high incidence strain of Fischer 344 rats (Table 21-5). Beginning at 13 weeks of age, rats were either continued on an ad libitum feeding or were food-restricted 40 percent (NIH-31 diet with 1.673 fat-soluble and B vitamins) over their lifetime until they died or became moribund due to spontaneous disease. The incidence of Leydig cell adenomas was decreased to 19 percent in food-restricted rats compared to 49 percent in the ad libitum–fed group (Table 21-5). In another group from the food restriction study reported by Thurman and coworkers (1994), rats were periodically removed for serial sacrifice at 6-month intervals. Food restriction resulted in a similar marked reduction in Leydig cell adenomas (23 percent compared to 60 percent in ad libitum–fed rats) (Table 21-6). Examination of the serially sacrificed F344 rats in this study also demonstrated that feed restriction delayed the onset of development as well as decreasing the incidence of Leydig cell adenomas compared to the ad libitum–fed group (Table 21-7). For example, at the 30-month sacrifice, only 17 percent of feed-restricted F344 rats had developed Leydig cell adenomas, compared to 100 percent in the ad libitum group.

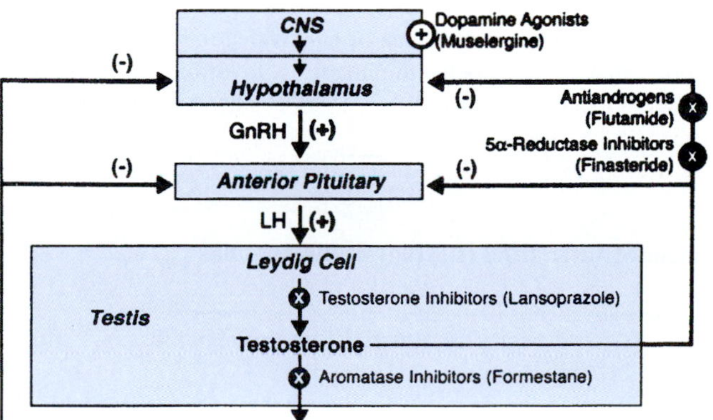

Figure 21-45. Regulation of the hypothalamic-pituitary-testis (HPT) axis and control points for potential disruption by xenobiotic chemicals. Symbols: (+) feedback stimulation; (−) feedback inhibition; ⊕ receptor stimulation; ⊗ enzyme or receptor inhibition. (Modified from Cook et al., 1999, with permission.)

Investigations reported by Chatani and associated (1990) documented the importance of hormonal imbalances on the incidence of Leydig cell adenomas and hyperplasia in Fischer rats (Table 21-8). The incidence of adenomas was 70 percent and of hyperplasia 100 percent in control rats killed at 70 weeks of age. In rats administered testosterone for 28 weeks (by silastic tubes implanted subcutaneously at 42 weeks of age), the incidence of Leydig cell adenomas and hyperplasias was decreased to 0 percent for both at 70 weeks of age. This dramatic reduction in the incidence of focal proliferative lesions of Leydig cells was associated with a significant lowering in circulating levels of LH, through negative feedback exerted by testosterone on the pituitary gland.

The important studies reported by Chatani and coworkers (1990) also demonstrated that hormones other than testosterone could markedly decrease the development of Leydig cell adenomas in F344 rats (Table 21-9). The administration of estradiol-17β for 28 weeks (by silastic tubes implanted subcutaneously) decreased the incidence of Leydig cell adenomas to 0 percent (compared to 100 percent in controls) and significantly reduced serum LH, due to negative feedback control on the pituitary gland. An LH-releasing hormone agonist administered continuously for 28 weeks (injection of microcapsules every 4 weeks at a dose of 5 mg/2 mL/kg) also decreased the incidence of Leydig cell adenomas to 0 percent and significantly decreased circulating LH levels, most likely a result of the known-down regulation of LH-RH receptors on pituitary gonadotrophs (Table 21-9).

The studies of Bartke and colleagues (1985) demonstrated that hyperprolactinemia also markedly decreased the incidence of Leydig cell adenomas in Fischer rats (Table 21-10). Pituitaries transplanted beneath the renal capsule (four per rat) resulted in a chronic elevation of circulating prolactin levels, owing, most likely, to the lack of dopamine inhibition of prolactin secretion, which occurs when the pituitary gland is in its normal anatomic location in close proximity to the hypothalamus. In this interesting experiment, 83 percent of sham-operated rats developed Leydig cell adenomas at 21 to 24 months of age, whereas 0 percent of rats developed tumors in animals with ectopic pituitaries and elevated serum prolactin levels.

The administration of a calcium-channel blocker (SVZ 200-110) at high doses (62.5 mg/kg/day for 2 years) significantly increased the incidence of Leydig cell adenomas in Sprague-Dawley rats. Endocrinologic studies demonstrated that increased serum levels of LH and FSH were present only after 52 and 66 weeks, respectively, and persisted to week 104 for LH. This compound is unusual in that most xenobiotic chemicals that cause hormonal imbalances result in earlier significant changes in circulating hormone levels.

Another important mechanism by which xenobiotics increase the incidence of Leydig cell tumors in rats is by inhibition of testosterone synthesis by cells in the testis. For example, lansoprazole is a substituted benzimidazole, which inhibits the hydrogen-potassium ATPase (proton pump) responsible for acid secretion by the parietal cells in the fundic mucosa of the stomach (Fort et al., 1995). The presence of the imidazole moiety in lansoprazole was suggestive of an effect on testosterone synthesis, since several imidazole compounds (e.g., ketoconazole and miconazole) are known

Table 21-5
Effect of Food Restriction on the Development of Interstitial (Leydig) Cell Adenomas in F344 Rats*

		Interstitial Cell Adenomas	
FEEDING	NO. OF RATS	NUMBER	PERCENT
Ad libitum	49	24	49
Food-restricted (40%)	52	10	19

*Lifetime study without periodic sacrifice removals (died from spontaneous disease).
SOURCE: Thurman et al., 1994, with permission.

to inhibit testosterone synthesis. Lansoprazole resulted in decreased circulating levels of testosterone, increased levels of LH, and an increased incidence of Leydig cell hyperplasia and benign neoplasia (adenomas) in chronic studies in rats (Fort et al., 1995). The most sensitive site for inhibition of testosterone synthesis by lansoprazole was the transport of cholesterol to the cholesterol side chain cleavage enzyme.

Although several hormonal imbalances result in an increased incidence of Leydig cell tumors in rodents, several disease conditions associated with chronic elevations in serum LH (including Klinefelter's syndrome and gonadotroph adenomas of the pituitary gland) in human patients have not been associated with an increased development of this type of rare testicular tumor.

There are a number of reports in the literature of xenobiotic chemicals (many of which are marketed drugs) that increase the incidence of proliferative lesions of Leydig cells in chronic toxicology/carcinogenicity in rats. These include indomethacin, lactitol, muselergine, cimetidine, gemfibrozil, and flutamide, among many others (Table 21-11).

Flutamide is a potent nonsteroidal, antiandrogen compound that displaces testosterone from specific receptors in target cells and decreases negative feedback on the hypothalamus-pituitary gland, resulting in elevated circulating levels of LH and FSH. The chronic administration of flutamide is known to result in a striking increase in the incidence of Leydig cell adenomas in rats. The Schering-Plough Research Institute's Department of Drug Safety and Metabolism completed an important reversibility study in which Sprague-Dawley rats were administered flutamide daily either for 1 year, 1 year followed by a 1-year recovery period, or continuously for 2 years (Table 21-12). This important study emphasizes the lack of autonomy of many focal proliferative lesions of Leydig cells in rats and their continued dependence upon compound administration for stimulation of growth. There was a reduction in the incidence of Leydig cell adenomas (using the conservative NTP criteria of greater than 1 tubule diameter) in rats administered three dose levels of flutamide daily for 1 year followed by a 1-year recovery prior to termination compared to rats given flutamide for 1 year and immediately evaluated (Table 21-12). Conversely, in rats administered flutamide for 2 years the numbers of adenomas continued to increase until 95 percent of animals in the mid- and high-dose groups (30 and 50 μg/kg, respectively) had developed Leydig cell tumors. There also was a marked reduction in the incidence of focal hyperplasia (focus less than 1 tubule diameter) after 1 year of recovery, compared to rats terminated immediately following 1 year of flutamide administration, a finding that emphasizes the frequent reversibility of these small proliferative lesions of Leydig cells.

Although a number of xenobiotics have been reported to increase the incidence of Leydig cell adenomas in chronic studies in rats, similar compounds such as cimetidine, ketoconazole, and certain calcium channel blocking agents have not resulted in an increased incidence of Leydig cell neoplasia in humans. In summary, Leydig cell tumors are a frequently occurring tumor in rats, often associated mechanistically with hormonal imbalances; however, they are not an appropriate model for assessing the potential risk to human males of developing this rare testicular tumor.

OVARY

Introduction

Ovarian tumors in rodents can be subdivided into five broad categories, including epithelial tumors, sex cord–stromal tumors, germ cell tumors, tumors derived from nonspecialized soft tissues of the

Table 21-6
Effect of Food Restriction on the Development of Interstitial (Leydig) Cell Adenomas in F344 Rats*

		Interstitial Cell Adenomas	
FEEDING	NO. OF RATS	NUMBER	PERCENT
Ad libitum	98	59	60
Food-restricted (40%)	112	26	23

*Lifetime study with periodic removal of serially sacrificed rats (died from spontaneous disease).
SOURCE: Thurman et al., 1994, with permission.

Table 21-7

Effects of Food Restriction on the Development of Interstitial (Leydig) Cell Adenoma (ICA) in F344 Rats at Different Ages

	ICA [Tumors/No. Rats (%)]	
AGE AT SACRIFICE (MONTHS)	AD LIBITUM	FEED-RESTRICTED (40%)
12	0/12 (0)	0/12 (0)
18	5/12 (42)	0/12 (0)
24	10/12 (83)	1/12 (8)
30	9/9 (100)	2/12 (17)
36	—	4/9 (44)

SOURCE: Thurman et al., 1994, with permission.

ovary, and tumors metastatic to the ovary from distant sites. The epithelial tumors of the ovary include cystadenomas and cystadenocarcinomas, tubulostromal adenomas, and mesothelioma. The tubular (or tubulostromal) adenomas are the most important of the ovarian tumors in mice, and they are the tumors whose incidence often is increased by various endocrine perturbations associated with exposure to xenobiotics, senescence, or inherited genic deletion (Murphy and Beamer, 1973). Tubular adenomas are a unique lesion that develops frequently in the mouse ovary, accounting for approximately 25 percent of naturally occurring ovarian tumors in this species (Alison and Morgan, 1987; Rehm et al., 1984). They are uncommon in rats, rare in other animal species, and not recognized in the ovaries of women. In some ovarian tumors of this type in mice, there is an intense proliferation of stromal (interstitial) cells of sex cord origin. These tumors often are designated tubulostromal adenomas or carcinomas to reflect the bimorphic appearance.

The tubulostromal adenomas in mice are composed of numerous tubular profiles derived from the surface epithelium, plus abundant large luteinized stromal cells from the ovarian interstitium. The differences in histologic appearance of this type of unique ovarian tumor in mice are interpreted to represent a morphologic spectrum with variable contributions from the surface epithelium and sex cord–derived ovarian interstitium rather than being two distinct types of ovarian tumors. The histogenic origin of this unique ovarian tumor in mice has been a controversial topic in the literature, but most investigators currently agree that it is derived from the ovarian surface epithelium, with varying contributions from stromal cells of the ovarian interstitium. However, some early reports suggested an origin from the rete ovarii or thecal/granulosal cells of the ovary.

Another important group of ovarian tumors are those derived from the sex cords and/or ovarian stroma. These include the granulosal cell tumors, luteoma, thecoma, Sertoli cell tumor, tubular adenoma (with contributions from ovarian stroma), and undifferentiated sex cord–stromal tumors. The granulosal cell tumor is the most common of this group which, according to Alison and Morgan (1987), accounts for 27 percent of naturally occurring ovarian tumors in mice. Granulosal cell tumors may develop within certain tubular or tubulostromal adenomas following a long-term perturbation of endocrine function associated with genic deletion, irradiation, oocytotoxic chemicals, and neonatal thymectomy (Frith et al., 1981; Li and Gardner, 1949; Hummel, 1954).

Mechanisms of Ovarian Tumorigenesis in Rodents

Five model systems of ovarian tumorigenesis in mice have been reported in the literature. The first model system identified was the production of ovarian neoplasms by radiation (Furth and Boon, 1947; Gardner, 1950). After acute radiation exposure, the initial change was a rapid loss of oocytes and a destruction of graafian follicles. There was proliferation and down-growth of the ovarian epithelium into the stroma within 10 weeks after radiation exposure. The first ovarian tumors developed approximately 1 year after exposure. The tubular adenomas that develop following radiation often were bilateral, endocrinologically inactive, and not lethal unless they reached a very large size. Some irradiated mice also developed endocrinologically active granulosal cell tumors, which transplantation experiments have shown to be different from the tubular adenomas. Granulosal cell tumors were transplantable into the spleen and often grew rapidly, whereas tubular adenomas grew slowly after transplantation, most successfully in castrated animals.

Table 21-8

Effect of Aging and Testosterone on the Incidence of Interstitial Cell Adenomas (ICA) and Hyperplasia (ICH) in Fischer 344 Rats*

TREATMENT (23 WEEKS)	TERMINAL AGE (WEEKS)	ICA %(NO./NO. TESTES)	ICH % TESTES	ICH† (NODULES/ TESTES)	SERUM LH (ng/mL)†
0	42	0 (0/20)	10	0.3 ± 0.8	20.9 ± 19.5
0	50	0 (0/20)	95	5.0 ± 2.3	N.D.
0	60	0 (0/10)	90	8.3 ± 7.0	48.7 ± 16.7
0	70	70 (14/20)	100	11.1 ± 6.2	22.1 ± 8.4
Testosterone§	70	0 (0/10)‡	0‡	0.0 ± 0.0‡	8.4 ± 8.8‡

*NTP criteria: ICA greater and ICH less than one normal seminiferous tubule diameter.

†Mean ± SD.

‡$p < 0.05$ compared to controls.

§Silastic tubes implanted subcutaneously at 42 weeks.

SOURCE: Chatani et al., 1990, with permission.

Table 21-9

Effect of Testosterone, Estradiol, and LH-RH Agonist on Incidence of Interstitial Cell Adenoma (ICA) in F344 Rats*

TREATMENT (28 WEEKS)	TERMINAL AGE (WEEKS)	ICA % (NO./NO. TESTES)	SERUM LH (ng/mL)†
Control	88	100 (18/18)	12.9 ± 11.7
Testosterone‡	88	0 (0/18)§	1.7 ± 1.6§
Estradiol-17β‡	88	0 (0/18)§	4.7 ± 2.4§
LH-RH Agonist¶	88	0 (0/16)§	4.9 ± 3.5§

*NTP criteria: ICA greater than one normal seminiferous tubule diameter.

†Mean ± SD.

‡Silastic tubes implanted subcutaneously.

§$p < 0.05$ compared to controls.

¶Injected subcutaneously at 60 weeks of age.

SOURCE: Chatani et al., 1990, with permission.

Table 21-10

Effect of Hyperprolactinemia from Ectopic Pituitary Transplants on the Incidence of Interstitial Cell Adenoma (ICA) and Testicular/Seminal Vesicle Weights in Fischer 344 Rats

RAT GROUP	ICA % (NO./NO. RATS)	WEIGHT OF TESTES (g)*	WEIGHT OF SEMINAL VESICLES (g)†
Sham-operated			
With tumors	83 (20/24)	4.88 ± 0.22‡	0.55 ± 0.08‡
Without tumors	17 (4/24)	2.66 ± 0.48	1.35 ± 0.14
Pituitary-grafted†			
With tumors	0 (0/0)	—	—
Without tumors	100 (24/24)	2.79 ± 0.05	1.26 ± 0.07

*Pituitary transplants (four per rat) beneath renal capsule or sham-operated at 2 to 5 months of age; terminated at 21 to 24 months of age.

†Mean ± SE.

‡$p < 0.05$ compared to other two groups.

SOURCE: Bartke et al., 1985, with permission.

Table 21-11

Selected Examples of Drugs that Increase the Incidence of Proliferative Lesions of Leydig Cells in Chronic Exposure Studies in Rats or Mice

NAME	SPECIES	CLINICAL INDICATION	REFERENCE
Indomethacin	R	Anti-inflammatory	Roberts et al., 1989
Lactitol	R	Laxative	Bär, 1992
Metronidazole	R	Antibacterial	Rustia and Shubik, 1979
Muselergine	R	Parkinson's disease	Prentice et al., 1992
Buserelin	R	Prostatic and breast carcinoma, endometriosis	Donaubauer et al., 1989
Cimetidine	R	Reduction of gastric acid secretion	PDR, 1992
Flutamide	R	Prostatic carcinoma	PDR, 1992
Gemfibrozil	R	Hypolipidemia	Fitzgerald et al., 1981
Spironolactone	R	Diuretic	PDR, 1994
Nararelin	R	LH-RH analog	PDR, 1994
Tamoxifen	M	Antiestrogen	PDR, 1994
Vidarabine	R	Antiviral	PDR, 1994
Clofibrate	R	Hypolipidemia	PDR, 1994
Finasteride	M	Prostatic hyperplasia	Prahalada et al., 1994

Table 21-12
Flutamide: Incidence of Interstitial Cell (IC) Adenoma in Sprague-Dawley Rats after Various Dosing Intervals

	1-Year Dosing				*1-Year Dosing 1-Year Recovery*				*2-Year Dosing*			
DOSE	0	10	30	50	0	10	30	50	0	10	30	50
Number/group	58	57	57	57	52	53	53	53	55	55	55	55
IC adenoma (>1 tubule)	0	28	43	40	6	25	23	25	6	50	52	52
IC hyperplasia (<1 tubule)	6	39	44	48	8	7	10	17	5	12	9	12

SOURCE: Courtesy of Schering Plough Research Institute, Department of Drug Safety and Metabolism, Lafayette, NJ.

The second model of ovarian tumorigenesis arose out of the work published by Biskind and Biskind (1944). They transplanted ovaries into the spleen of castrated rats to prevent negative feedback by circulating sex hormones on the hypothalamus and pituitary gland because estrogen is degraded as it circulates through the liver. Transplantation resulted in a rapid loss of ovarian follicles as well as an interference with estrogen feedback on the hypothalamus. Following the loss of graafian follicles, the epithelial covering of the ovary began to proliferate and invaginate into the ovary, with an accompanying increase in stromal tissue, which ultimately resulted in the formation of tubular adenomas and, occasionally, granulosal cell tumors (Guthrie, 1957). The presence of a single functioning gonad prevented the development of the proliferative lesions in the ovary, suggesting that the lack of negative feedback from estrogen was necessary for the changes to develop. Administration of exogenous estrogen or testosterone after transplantation completely suppressed development of the proliferative changes in the ovarian cortex.

The third model of ovarian tumorigenesis was described by Marchant (1957, 1960), who reported that ovarian tumors developed in mice exposed to dimethylbenzanthracene. This chemical is a reproductive toxicant that is cytotoxic to oocytes, resulting in the loss of graafian follicles from the ovary. This was followed by a proliferation of the interstitial (stromal) tissue, invaginations of the surface epithelium, and subsequent development of tubular adenomas and occasionally granulosal cell tumors of the ovary (Taguchi et al., 1988). Support for an endocrinologic mechanism of hormonal imbalance included the observation that the xenobiotic chemical first must cause sterility, because the presence of a single normal gonad prevented the development of the hyperplastic lesions and tumors of the ovary. The administration of estrogen prevented tumor formation even in sterile mice, and hypophysectomy also prevented the development of ovarian tumors.

The fourth model of ovarian tumorigenesis was described by Nishizuki and associates (1979). They reported that removal of the thymus from neonatal mice resulted in ovarian dysgenesis and the development of ovarian tumors. Thymectomy prior to 7 days of age resulted in an immune-mediated destruction of follicles in the ovary. Because estrogen was not produced by the follicles, these mice also developed hormone-mediated proliferative lesions and ovarian tumors identical to those in the previously described models. After the immune-mediated destruction of follicles, there was a proliferation of the interstitial (stromal) and surface epithelial cells of the ovary, resulting in the formation of tubular adenomas. If the mice survived for longer periods, some animals developed granulosal cell tumors and luteomas in the ovary. Because this model also did not involve exposure to any carcinogen, it is another indication that the prerequisite for ovarian tumor response in mice is the production of sterility, which results in hormonal imbalances that lead to stimulation of the sensitive populations of target cells (Michael et al., 1981).

Case Study: Ovarian Tumors Associated with Xenobiotic Chemicals

Nitrofurantoin Nitrofurantoin is an example of a chemical that, when fed at high doses to mice for 2 years in a NTP study, increased the incidence of ovarian tumors of the tubular or tubulostromal type (Table 21-13). Nitrofurantoin fed at both low (1300 ppm) and high (2500 ppm) doses to $B_6C_3F_1$ mice caused sterility due to the destruction of ovarian follicles, leading to hormonal imbalances, which resulted in the development of an increased incidence of this unique type of ovarian tumor.

Mice administered nitrofurantoin had a consistent change in the ovarian cortex, termed *ovarian atrophy.* This lesion was characterized by an absence of graafian follicles, developing ova, and corpora lutea; by focal or diffuse hyperplasia with localized or diffuse down-growth of surface epithelium into the ovary; and by varying numbers of polygonal, often vacuolated, sex cord–derived stromal (interstitial) cells between the tubular profiles. The ovaries were small, had irregular surfaces due to the tubular down-growths into the cortex, and had scattered eosinophilic stromal cells between tubular profiles. In addition, there was a lack of graafian follicles and corpora lutea throughout the ovarian cortex.

The benign ovarian tumors in this study were classified either as tubular adenomas (5 of 50 mice) or as tubulostromal tumors (4 of 50 mice) (Table 21-13). In tubulostromal adenomas, the proliferating stromal (interstitial) cells between the tubules were considered to represent a significant component of the lesion. However, the separation between these two types of proliferating ovarian lesions in mice was not distinct and both appeared to be part of a continuous morphologic spectrum. Because all treated mice in the NTP nitrofurantoin feeding study were sterile due to ovarian atrophy, an indirect mechanism secondary to a disruption of endocrine function leading to hormonal imbalances was suggested to explain the development of the ovarian tubular adenomas.

The results of an investigative study demonstrated that nitrofurantoin had an effect on graafian follicles in the ovary of $B_6C_3F_1$ mice. Female mice of the same strain were fed 350 or 500

Table 21-13
NTP Nitrofurantoin Study of Treatment-Related Ovarian Lesions in $B_6C_3F_1$ Mice (50/Group Exposed for 2 Years in Feed)

LESION	CONTROL	LOW DOSE (0.13%)	HIGH DOSE (0.25%)
Tubular adenoma	0	0	5*
Tubulostromal adenoma	0	0	4†
Benign GCT	0	3	2
Malignant GCT	0	0	1
Cystadenoma	2	1	1
Cysts	14	15	10
Abscess	18	0	0
Ovarian atrophy	0	49	48
Survival at 2 Years	19	37	37

KEY: NTP, National Toxicology Program; GCT, granulosa cell tumor.
*Trend test positive ($p \leq 0.05$).
†Fischer exact test positive ($p \leq 0.05$).

mg/kg/day of nitrofurantoin beginning at 7 weeks of age. These levels approximate the low (1300 ppm) and high (2500 ppm) doses used in the NTP study with nitrofurantoin. Ten female mice per group were sacrificed at 4, 8, 13, 17, 43, and 64 weeks of feeding nitrofurantoin. The numbers of follicles were quantified from nitrofurantoin-treated and control mice on serial sections of the ovary. The morphometric data revealed that the numbers of small, medium, and large follicles in nitrofurantoin-treated mice were numerically decreased at 17 weeks compared with controls and were significantly decreased in rats fed 350 and 500 mg/kg/day nitrofurantoin after 43 and 64 weeks (Fig. 21-46). All mice in the treated groups were sterile by 43 weeks of feeding nitrofurantoin.

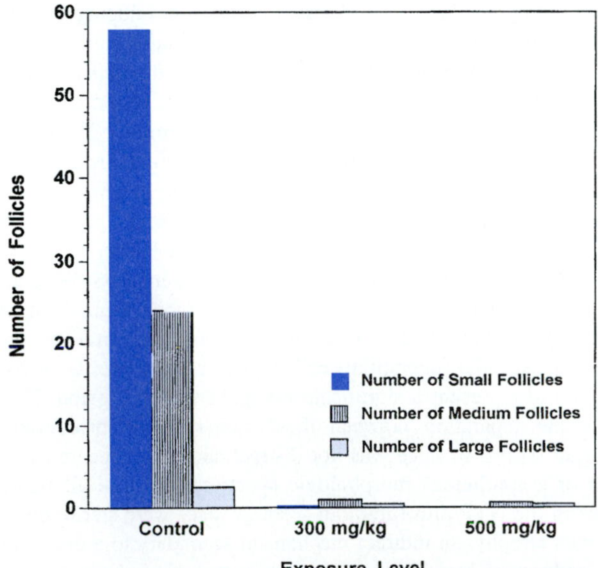

Figure 21-46. Morphometric evaluation of ovaries of mice following the administration of 350 and 500 mg/kg/day of nitrofurantoin.

The numbers of small, medium, and large ovarian follicles were decreased after 17 weeks and significantly decreased after 43 and 64 weeks due to a direct action of the nitrofurantoin.

Selective Estrogen Receptor Modulators Selective estrogen receptor modulators (SERMs) are compounds that have estrogen agonist effects on some tissues and estrogen antagonist actions on other tissues (Cohen et al., 2000). The triphenylethylene SERMs tamoxifen and toremifene have estrogen antagonist effects in the breast and currently are used in the medical management of breast cancer. The benzothiophene SERM raloxifene has estrogen agonist effects on bone and serum lipids but estrogen antagonist actions on the uterus and breast. This is in contrast to tamoxifen, which has an estrogen agonist effect on bone and also may stimulate the uterine endometrium. These SERMs (e.g., tamoxifen, toremifene, and raloxifene) all have been reported to increase the incidence of ovarian tumors when administered chronically to mice. For example, CD_1 mice administered raloxifene (9, 50, 225 mg/kg) per day for 21 months developed an increased incidence of granulosa/theca cell tumors (benign and malignant) and tubular/papillary adenomas of the ovary. However, there is no evidence of an increased risk for ovarian cancer in women administered SERMs, since tamoxifen has been used clinically since 1978 (Fisher et al., 1994; Cook et al., 1995).

Raloxifene binds to the estrogen receptor (Yang et al., 1996) and appears to block the negative feedback of circulating levels of estrogen on the hypothalamus, resulting in a sustained increase in circulating levels of LH. Mice (CD_1) administered raloxifene (233 or 236 mg/kg) daily for 2 and 4 weeks had a dose-dependent significant elevation of serum LH levels (4- to 7-fold and 4.4-fold compared to controls, respectively) (Cohen et al., 2000). Raloxifene-treated mice had sustained elevations in serum LH over a 24-h period and did not have the preovulatory LH surge present in many control mice. Histomorphologic changes in the ovary were indicative of arrested follicular maturation including anovulatory hemorrhagic follicles, some developing follicles, and few corpora lutea. Following a recovery period of 3 weeks during which no raloxifene was administered, serum LH concentrations were indistinguishable from controls and follicular maturation and corpora lutea distribution were normal (Long et al., 2001). Raloxifene binding to the estrogen receptor resulted in an elevation of serum LH and ovarian tumor development similar to those in estrogen receptor-α knockout mice with genetic deletion of the estrogen receptor (Korach, 1994), suggesting that the tumors in both instances develop secondary to the hormonal imbalances.

Ovarian Tumors in Mutant Strains of Mice

W^x/W^v Strain with Genetic Deletion of Germ Cells in Ovarian Cortex In an attempt to arrive at further mechanistic explanations for the development of tubular adenomas in $B_6C_3F_1$ mice fed high doses of nitrofurantoin, ovaries were evaluated from several mutant mouse strains not exposed to any xenobiotic chemicals but known to develop ovarian tumors. In this mutant mouse strain, referred to as W^x/W^v, few germ cells migrate into the ovary during development. Murphy (1972) reported that less than 1 percent of the normal complement of oocytes were present in the ovary at 1 day of age and the numbers of graafian follicles decrease progressively until none were present at 13 weeks of age. In this mutant mouse strain (W^x/W^v), a mutant allele at the C-kit locus encodes for a defective protein kinase receptor, resulting in an inability to respond to stem cell growth factor encoded by the Steel locus (Witte, 1990; Majumder et al., 1988). A failure of proliferation of primordial germ cells during gonadogenesis leads to the marked reduction of graafian follicles in the ovarian cortex.

Ovaries from mutant mice at age 13 weeks were small, had an irregular surface, were devoid of graafian follicles, and had numerous hyperplastic tubules growing into the cortex. These tubules were lined by a hyperplastic cuboidal epithelium similar to that on the surface of the ovary. Interspersed between the tubular profiles were luteinized stromal cells of the ovarian interstitium with a lightly eosinophilic, often vacuolated, cytoplasm. The proliferative changes observed in the ovary of these mutant (W^x/W^v) mice at 13 weeks of age were similar morphologically to the ovarian atrophy lesions in the NTP nitrofurantoin study.

The ovaries of heterozygous controls (1/1) of this strain were larger than in the mutant mice and had a histologic appearance similar to normal mouse ovaries. The ovarian cortex in control mice had plentiful graafian follicles with developing ova. The surface epithelium covering the ovary consisted of a single layer of cuboidal cells without the down-growth of tubules into the underlying cortex.

The ovaries of mutant (W^x/W^v) mice at 22 weeks of age had a more intense proliferation of surface epithelium, either with extensive down-growths of hyperplastic tubules into the cortex or the formation of small tubular adenomas. The tubular adenomas in the mutant (W^x/W^v) mice with genetic deletion of graafian follicles but without any exposure to xenobiotic chemicals were composed of proliferating tubules of surface epithelium that replaced much of the ovary. They were similar microscopically to the smaller tubular adenomas in the $B_6C_3F_1$ mice fed the high dose (2500 ppm) of nitrofurantoin in the 2-year NTP feeding study. Interspersed between the hyperplastic profiles of surface epithelium in the tubular adenomas were scattered luteinized stromal cells with varying degrees of vacuolation of the eosinophilic cytoplasm. In mutant (W^x/W^v) mice, age 22 weeks, whose ovaries had been under long-term intense gonadotrophin stimulation, there appeared to be a morphologic continuum between ovarian atrophy and tubular adenomas.

At age 20 months, ovaries of the mutant (W^x/W^v) mice without any exposure to xenobiotic chemicals consistently had large tubular adenomas that incorporated all of the ovarian parenchyma and greatly enlarged the ovary. These neoplasms were similar histologically to the larger tubular adenomas in the high-dose (2500 ppm) mice of the NTP study. Several of the larger ovarian neoplasms of the 20-month-old mutant mice had evidence of malignancy with invasion of tumor cells through the ovarian capsule into the periovarian tissues, often accompanied by a localized desmoplastic response. Histopathologic evidence of malignancy was not observed in the ovarian tubular adenomas from the high-dose (2500 ppm) female mice in the NTP study. An occasional mutant mouse at 20 months of age also had developed focal areas of hyperplasia of granulosal cells or small granulosa cell tumors.

Hypogonadal (hpg/hpg) Mice Unable to Synthesize Hypothalamic Gonadotrophin-Releasing Hormone (GnRH) Mutant hypogonadal mice, designated hpg/hpg, are unable to synthesize normal amounts of hypothalamic GnRH (Tennent and Beamer, 1986). They have low circulating levels of pituitary gonadotrophins (both FSH and LH); however, hypogonadal mice have a normal complement of ovarian follicles (Cattanach et al., 1977).

In the studies of Tennent and Beamer (1986), both genetically normal littermates and hypogonadal (hpg/hpg) mice were irradiated at age 30 days to destroy the oocytes. The irradiated control mice of this strain produced normal amounts of pituitary gonadotrophic hormones and developed ovarian tubular adenomas at age 10 to 15 months. The tumors that developed in the absence of any exposure to xenobiotic chemicals had similar histological characteristics as tubular adenomas in the high-dose (2500 ppm) females of the nitrofurantoin study. They either were small nodules involving only a portion of the ovary or large masses that completely incorporated the affected gonad. They were composed predominantly of tubular profiles, some of which were dilated, with interspersed stromal cells.

The irradiated hypogonadal (hpg/hpg) mice failed to develop tubular adenomas or to have intense hyperplasia of the ovarian surface epithelium and interstitial (stromal) cells in the absence of GnRH and with low circulating levels of pituitary gonadotrophins. The ovaries of irradiated hypogonadal mice were small and had single- or multiple-layered follicles, without oocytes, scattered throughout the ovary. There also was an absence of stromal cell hypertrophy and hyperplasia, a change frequently observed in ovaries of the irradiated normal littermates.

The experiments reported by Tennent and Beamer (1986) demonstrated that a normal secretion of hypothalamic GnRH and pituitary gonadotrophins was necessary for the intense proliferation of ovarian surface epithelium and stromal cells, leading to the formation of tubular adenomas in mice, which develop subsequent to irradiation-induced loss of ovarian follicles and decreased ability to produce gonadal steroids (especially estradiol-17β).

Genetically Engineered Mouse Models of Ovarian Tumors Transgenic mice expressing a chimeric lutenizing hormone (LH) β submit (LHβ) in pituitary gonadotrophs have increased pituitary expression of LH mRNA and elevated circulating levels of LH (as well as estradiol and testosterone) but are infertile (Risma et al. 1995 and 1997). They ovulate infrequently, maintain a prolonged luteal phase, and develop a variety of ovarian lesions including cyst (blood and fluid filled) formation and ovarian tumors. A subset of LHβ transgenic mice developed ovarian granulosa and theca–interstitial cell tumors by 4 to 8 months of age as a result of the chronic stimulation by the elevated gonadotropin (LH) lev-

- TUMORS DEVELOP ONLY IN STERILE MICE
- REQUIRES AN INTACT HYPOTHALAMUS-PITUITARY-OVARIAN AXIS
- EXOGENOUS ESTROGEN PREVENTS OVARIAN TUMOR DEVELOPMENT

Figure 21-47. Secondary mechanisms of ovarian oncogenesis in mice.

els. The findings of granulosa and stromal cell tumors in transgenic mice whose only genetic alteration is the addition of a gene encoding a chimeric gonadotropin suggest that abnormal gonadotropin stimulation is tumorigenic to the ovary in mice. In addition, genetically altered mice deficient in inhibin (hormone which suppresses the secretion of follicle stimulating hormone [FSH]) have elevated blood concentrations of FSH (two- to threefold) and develop granulosa cell tumors and mixed or incompletely differentiated gonadal stromal tumors of the ovary (Matzuk et al., 1992).

Another example of hormonal dysregulation leading to the induction of ovarian tumors are the estrogen receptor knockout (ERKO) mice that lack the alpha estrogen receptors and are unable to regulate gonadotropin secretion due to a lack of negative feedback control by the blood estrogen level (Lubahan et al., 1993; Korach, 1994). Female mice are infertile with hypoplastic uteri and hyperemic ovaries with no detectable corpora lutea. There was no uterine stimulation (uterotropic response) when these animals were treated with tamoxifen (an estrogen agonist in mice). ERKO mice also develop ovarian granulosa cell tumors in response to the chronic elevations in circulating gonadotropin levels.

Summary: Ovarian Tumorigenesis in Rodents

A review of studies on mutant mice and the NTP study of nitrofurantoin support an interpretation that the unique intense hyperplasia of ovarian surface epithelium and stromal cells, leading eventually to an increased incidence of tubular adenomas and occasionally granulosa cell tumors, develops secondary to chronic pituitary gonadotrophic hormone stimulation. Factors that destroy or greatly diminish the numbers of ovarian follicles—such as senescence, genetic deletion of follicles, x-irradiation, drugs, and chemicals such as nitrofurantoin, and early thymectomy with the development of autoantibodies to oocytes—are known to diminish sex steroid hormone secretion by the ovary. This results in elevated circulating levels of gonadotrophins, especially LH, due to decreased negative feedback on the hypothalamic-pituitary axis by estrogens and possibly other humoral factors produced by the graafian follicles (Carson et al., 1989). The long-term stimulation of stromal (interstitial) cells, which have receptors for LH (Beamer and Tennent, 1986), and, indirectly, the ovarian surface epithelium appears to place the mouse ovary at increased risk for developing the unique tubular or tubulostromal adenomas.

The finding of similar tubular adenomas in the ovaries of the xenobiotic-treated and genetically sterile mice not exposed to exogenous chemicals supports the concept of a secondary (hormonally mediated) mechanism of ovarian oncogenesis associated with hormonal imbalances (Fig. 21-47). The ovarian tumors developed only in sterile mice in which the pituitary-hypothalamic axis was intact; administration of exogenous estrogen early in the course will prevent ovarian tumor development. The intense proliferation of ovarian surface epithelium and stromal (interstitial) cells with the development of unique tubular adenomas in response to sterility does not appear to have a counterpart in the ovaries of human adult females.

Experimental ovarian carcinogenesis has been investigated in inbred and hybrid strains of mice and induced by a diversity of

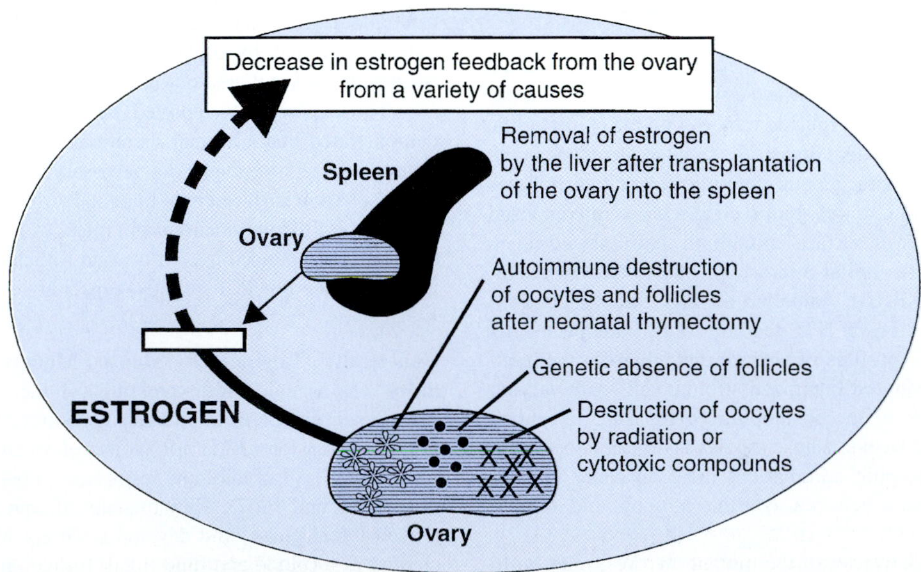

Figure 21-48. Multiple pathogenic mechanisms in ovarian tumorigenesis of mice resulting in decreased negative feedback by diminished levels of gonadal steroids, particularly estrogen.

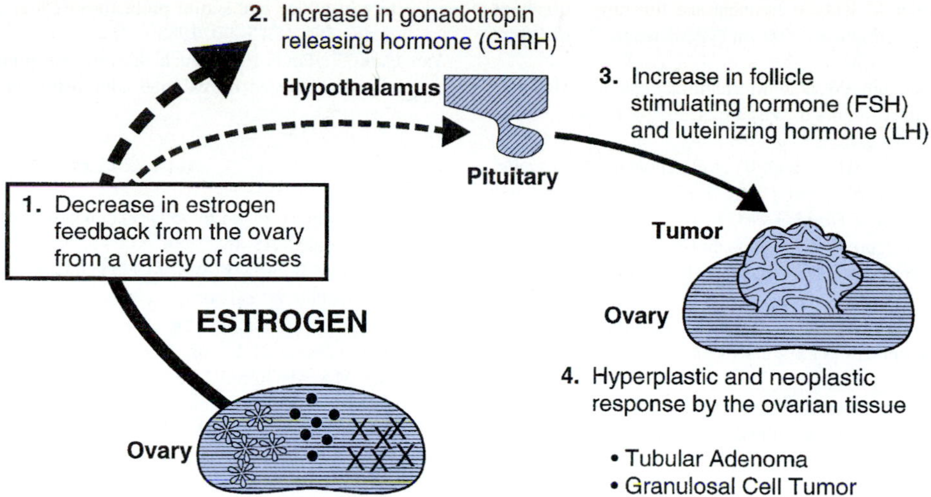

Figure 21-49. Decreased circulating estrogens release the hypothalamus-pituitary gland from negative feedback inhibition.

The increased gonadotrophin levels (LH and FSH) result in the mouse ovary being at greater risk of developing tubular adenomas in chronic studies.

mechanisms, including x-irradiation, oocytotoxic xenobiotic chemicals, ovarian grafting to ectopic or orthotopic sites, neonatal thymectomy, mutant genes reducing germ cell populations, and aging (Fig. 21-48). Disruptions in the function of graafian follicles by a variety of mechanisms results in a spectrum of ovarian proliferative lesions, including tumors. The findings in mutant mice support the concept of a secondary (hormonally mediated) mechanism of ovarian carcinogenesis in mice associated with sterility. Multiple pathogenetic factors that either destroy or diminish the numbers of graafian follicles in the ovary result in decreased sex hormone secretion (especially estradiol-17β), leading to a compensatory overproduction of pituitary gonadotrophins (particularly LH) (Fig. 21-48), which places the mouse ovary at an increased risk for developing tumors (Fig. 21-49). The intense proliferation of ovarian surface epithelium and stromal (interstitial) cells with the development of unique tubular adenomas in response to sterility does not appear to have a counterpart in the ovaries of human adult females.

REFERENCES

General

Alison RH, Capen CC, Prentice DE: Neoplastic lesions of questionable significance to humans. *Toxicol Pathol* 22:179–186, 1994.

Capen CC: Correlation of mechanistic data and histopathology in the evaluation of selected toxic endpoints of the endocrine system. *Toxicol Lett* 102–103:405–409, 1998.

Davies TS, Monro A: Marketed human pharmaceuticals reported to be tumorigenic in rodents. *J Am Coll Toxicol* 14:90–107, 1995.

Doss JC, Gröne A, Capen CC, et al: Immunohistochemical localization of chromogranin A in endocrine tissues and endocrine tumors of dogs. *Vet Pathol* 35:312–315, 1998.

Frith CH, Botts S, Jokinen MP, et al: Non-proliferative lesions of the endocrine system in rats, in *Guides for Toxicologic Pathology.* Washington, DC: STP/ARP/AFIP, 2000, pp 1–22.

Haseman JK, Hailey JR, Morris RW: Spontaneous neoplasm incidences in Fischer 344 rats and $B_6C_3F_1$ mice in two-year carcinogenicity studies: A national toxicology program update. *Toxicol Pathol* 26:428–441, 1998.

Keenan KP, Smith PF, Hertzog P, et al: The effects of overfeeding and dietary restriction of Sprague-Dawley rat survival and early pathology biomarkers of aging. *Toxicol Pathol* 22:300–315, 1994.

Keenan KP, Soper KA, Smith PF: Diet, overfeeding, and moderate dietary restriction in control Sprague-Dawley rats: I. Effects on spontaneous neoplasms. *Toxicol Pathol* 23:269–286, 1995.

McClain RM: Mechanistic considerations in the regulation and classification of chemical carcinogens, in Kotsonis FN, Mackey M, Hjelle J (eds): *Nutritional Toxicology.* New York: Raven Press, 1994, pp 273–304.

Roe FJC, Lee PN, Conybeare G, et al: The biosure study: Influence of composition of diet and food consumption on longevity, degenerative diseases and neoplasia in Wistar rats studied for up to 30 months post weaning. *Food Chem Toxicol* 33 (suppl 1): 1S–100S, 1995.

Solleveld HA, Haseman JK, McConnell EE: National history of body weight gain, survival and neoplasia in the F344 rat. *J Natl Cancer Inst* 72:929–940, 1984.

Thurman JD, Bucci TJ, Hart RW, et al: Survival, body weight, and spontaneous neoplasms in ad libitum-fed and food-restricted Fischer-344 rats. *Toxicol Pathol* 22:1–9, 1994.

Pituitary Gland

Attia MA: Neoplastic and nonneoplastic lesions in aging female rats with special reference to the functional morphology of the hyperplastic and neoplastic changes in the pituitary gland. *Arch Toxicol* 57:77–83, 1985.

Azad N, Nayyar R, Tentler J, et al: Anatomical and functional effects of estrogen-induced prolactinomas on the rat hypothalamus. *J Exp Pathol* 4:237–249, 1989.

Barsoum NJ, Moore JD, Gough AW, et al: Morphofunctional investigations on spontaneous pituitary tumors in Wistar rats. *Toxicol Pathol* 13:200–208, 1985.

Berkvens JM, van Nesselrooy JHJ, Kroes R, et al: Spontaneous tumours in the pituitary gland of old Wistar rats. A morphological and immunocytochemical study. *J Pathol* 130:179–191, 1980.

Berry PH: Effect of diet or reproductive status on the histology of spontaneous pituitary tumors in female Wistar rats. *Vet Pathol* 23:606–618, 1986.

Brown WR, Fetter AD, Van Ryzin RJ, et al: Proliferative pituitary lesions in rats treated with salmon or porcine calcitonin. *Toxicol Pathol* 21:81–86, 1993.

Capen CC: Functional and pathologic interrelationships of the pituitary gland and hypothalamus in animals, in Jones TC, Capen CC, Mohr U (eds): *Endocrine System. Series II. Monographs on Pathology of Laboratory Animals,* 2d ed. International Life Sciences Institute Series. Berlin, Heidelberg, New York: Springer-Verlag, 1996, pp 3–32.

El Etreby MF, Lorenz B, Habenicht UF: Immunocytochemical studies on the pituitary gland and spontaneous pituitary tumors of Sprague-Dawley rats. *Pathol Res Pract* 183:645–650, 1988.

Furth J, Boon MC: Induction of ovarian tumors in mice by x-rays. *Cancer Res* 7:241–245, 1947.

Gunnison AF, Bowers A, Nadziejko C, et al: Modulation of the inflammatory effects of inhaled ozone in rats by subcutaneous prolactin-secreting, pituitary-derived tumors. *Fundam Appl Toxicol* 37:88–94, 1997.

Jameson JL, Weiss J, Polak JM, et al: Glycoprotein hormone alpha-subunit-producing pituitary adenomas in rats treated for one year with calcitonin. *Am J Pathol* 140:75–84, 1992.

McComb DJ, Kovacs K, Beri J, et al: Pituitary gonadotroph adenomas in old Sprague-Dawley rats. *J Submicrosc Cytol* 17:517–530, 1985.

McComb DJ, Kovacs K, Beri J, et al: Pituitary adenomas in old Sprague-Dawley rats: A histologic, ultrastructural, and immunocytochemical study. *J Natl Cancer Inst* 73:1143–1166, 1984.

Osamura RY, Komatsu N, Izumi S, et al: Ultrastructural localization of prolactin in the rat anterior pituitary glands by preembedding peroxidase-labeled antibody method: Observations in normal, castrated, or estrogen-stimulated specimen. *J Histochem Cytochem* 30:919–925, 1982.

Parkening TA, Collins TJ, Smith ER: A comparative study of prolactin levels in five species of aged female laboratory rodents. *Biol Reprod* 22:513–518, 1980.

Pickering CE, Pickering RG: The effect of repeated reproduction on the incidence of pituitary tumours in Wistar rats. *Lab Anim* 18:371–378, 1984.

Sandusky GE, Van Pelt CS, Todd GC, et al: An immunocytochemical study of pituitary adenomas and focal hyperplasia in old Sprague-Dawley and Fischer 344 rats. *Toxicol Pathol* 16:376–380, 1988.

Sarkar DK, Gottschall PE, Meites J: Damage to hypothalamic dopaminergic neurons is associated with development of prolactin-secreting pituitary tumors. *Science* 218:684–686, 1982.

Satoh H, Kajimura T, Chen C-J, et al: Invasive pituitary tumors in female F344 rats induced by estradiol dipropionate. *Toxicol Pathol* 25:462–469, 1997.

Sher SP, Jensen RD, Bokelman DL: Spontaneous tumors in control F344 and Charles River-CD rats and Charles River CD-1 and $B_6C_3HF_1$ mice. *Toxicol Lett* 11:103–110, 1982.

van Putten LJA, van Zwieten MJ: Studies on prolactin-secreting cells in aging rats of different strains: II. Selected morphological and immunocytochemical features of pituitary tumors correlated with serum prolactin levels. *Mech Ageing Dev* 42:115–127, 1988.

van Putten LJA, van Zwieten MJ, Mattheij JAM, et al: Studies on prolactin-secreting cells in aging rats of different strains. I. Alterations in pituitary histology and serum prolactin levels as related to aging. *Mech Ageing Dev* 42:75–90, 1988.

Yamagami T, Handa H, Takeuchi J, et al: Rat pituitary adenoma and hyperplasia induced by caffeine administration. *Surg Neurol* 20:323–331, 1983.

Adrenal Cortex

Colby HD: Adrenal gland toxicity: chemically induced dysfunction. *J Am Coll Toxicol* 7:45–69, 1988.

Dominick MA, Bobrowski WA, MacDonald JR, et al: Morphogenesis of a zone-specific adrenocortical cytotoxicity in guinea pigs administered PD 132301-2, an inhibitor of acyl-CoA; cholesterol acyltransferase. *Toxicol Pathol* 21:54–62, 1993.

Dominick MA, McGuire EJ, Reindel JF, et al: Subacute toxicity of a novel inhibitor of acyl-CoA: cholesterol acyltransferase in beagle dogs. *Fundam Appl Toxicol* 20:217–224, 1993.

Hart MM, Swackhamer ES, Straw JA: Studies on the site of action of *o,p*'-DDD in the dog adrenal cortex: II. TPNH- and corticosteroid precursor-stimulation of *o,p*'-DDD inhibited steroidogenesis. *Steroids* 17:575–586, 1971.

Latendresse JR, Azhar S, Brooks CL, Capen CC: Pathogenesis of cholesteryl lipidosis of adrenocortical and ovarian interstitial cells in F344 rats caused by tricresyl phosphate and butylated triphenyl phosphate. *Toxicol Appl Pharmacol* 122:281–289, 1993.

Latendresse JR, Brooks CL, Capen CC: Pathologic effects of butylated triphenyl phosphate-based hydraulic fluid and tricresyl phosphate on the adrenal gland, ovary and testis in the F344 rat. *Toxicol Pathol* 22:341–352, 1994.

Latendresse JR, Brooks CL, Capen CC: Toxic effects of butylated triphenyl phosphate-based hydraulic fluid and tricresyl phosphate in female F344 rats. *Vet Pathol* 32:394–402, 1995.

Latendresse JR, Brooks CL, Fleming CD, Capen CC: Reproductive toxicity of butylated triphenyl phosphate (BTP) and tricresyl phosphate (TCP) fluids in F344 rats. *Fundam Applied Toxicol* 22:392–399, 1994.

Reindel JF, Dominick MA, Bocan TM, et al: Toxicologic effects of a novel acyl-CoA: Cholesterol acyltransferase (ACAT) inhibitor in cymomolgus monkeys. *Toxicol Pathol* 22:510–518, 1994.

Ribelin WE: The effects of drugs and chemicals upon the structure of the adrenal gland. *Fundam Appl Toxicol* 4:105–119, 1984.

Rothuizen J, Reul JM, Fijnberk A, et al: Aging and the hypothalamus-pituitary-adrenocortical axis, with special reference to the dog. *Acta Endocrinol* 125(suppl):73–76, 1991.

Szabo S, Huttner I, Kovacs K, et al: Pathogenesis of experimental adrenal hemorrhagic necrosis ("apoplexy"). Ultrastructural, biochemical, neuropharmacologic, and blood coagulation studies with acrylonitrate in the rat. *Lab Invest* 42:533–546, 1980.

Vilar O, Tullner WW: Effects of *o,p*'-DDD on histology and 17-hydroxycorticosteroid output of the dog adrenal cortex. *Endocrinology* 65:80–86, 1959.

Yarrington JT, Huffman KW, Gibson JP: Adrenocortical degeneration in dogs, monkeys, and rats treated with α-(1,4-dioxido-3-methylquinoxalin-2-yl)-*N*-methylnitrone. *Toxicol Lett* 8:229–234, 1981.

Yarrington JT, Huffman KW, Leeson GA, et al: Comparative toxicity of the hematinic MDL 80,478 effects on the liver and adrenal cortex of the dog, rat and monkey. *Fundam Appl Toxicol* 3:86–94, 1983.

Yarrington JT, Johnston JO: Aging in the adrenal cortex, in Mohr U, Dungworth DL, Capen CC (eds): *Pathobiology of the Aging Rat.* Washington, DC: ILSI Press, 1994, pp 227–244.

Yarrington JT, Loudy DE, Sprinkle DJ, et al: Degeneration of the rat and canine adrenal cortex caused by α-(1,4-dioxido-3-methylquinoxalin-2-yl)-*N*-methylnitrone (DMNM). *Fundam Appl Toxicol* 5:370, 1985.

Adrenal Medulla

Baer A: Sugars and adrenomedullary proliferative lesions: The effects of lactose and various polyalcohols. *J Am Coll Toxicol* 7:71–81, 1988.

Lynch BS, Tischler AS, Capen C, et al: Low digestible carbohydrates (polyols and lactose): Significance of adrenal medullary proliferative lesions in the rat. *Regul Toxicol Pharmacol* 23:256–297, 1996.

Manger WM, Hulse MC, Forsyth MS, et al: Effect of pheochromocytoma and hypophysectomy on blood pressure and catecholamines in NEDH rats. *Hypertension* 4(suppl 2):200–202, 1982.

Mosher AH, Kircher CH: Proliferative lesions of the adrenal medulla in rats treated with Zomepirac sodium. *J Am Coll Toxicol* 7:83–93, 1988.

Nyska A, Haseman JK, Hailey JR, et al: The association between severe nephropathy and pheochromocytoma in the male F344 rat—The national toxicology program experience. *Toxicol Pathol* 27:456–462, 1999.

Puchacz E, Stumpf WE, Stachowiak EK, et al: Vitamin D increases expression of the tyrosine hydroxylase gene in adrenal medullary cells. *Mol Brain Res* 36:193–196, 1996.

Reznik G, Ward JM, Reznik-Shuller H: Ganglioneuromas in the adrenal medulla of F344 rats. *Vet Pathol* 17:614–621, 1980.

Roe FJC, Bär A: Enzootic and epizootic adrenal medullary proliferative disease of rats: Influence of dietary factors which affect calcium absorption. *Hum Toxicol* 4:27–52, 1985.

Tischler AS, DeLellis RA: The rat adrenal medulla: I. The normal adrenal. *J Am Coll Toxicol* 7:1–21, 1988.

Tischler AS, DeLellis RA: The rat adrenal medulla: II. Proliferative lesions. *J Am Coll Toxicol* 7:23–44, 1988.

Tischler AS, DeLellis RA, Nunnemacher G, et al: Acute stimulation of chromaffin cell proliferation in the adult rat adrenal medulla. *Lab Invest* 58:733–735, 1988.

Tischler AS, DeLellis RA, Perlman RL, et al: Spontaneous proliferative lesions of the adrenal medulla in aging Long-Evans rats: Comparison to PC12 cells, small granule-containing cells, and human adrenal medullary hyperplasia. *Lab Invest* 53:486–498, 1985.

Tischler AS, McClain RM, Childers H, et al: Neurogenic signals regulate chromaffin cell proliferation and mediate the mitogenic effect of reserpine in the adult rat adrenal medulla. *Lab Invest* 65:374–376, 1991.

Tischler AS, Powers JF, Downing JC, et al: Vitamin D_3, lactose, and xylitol stimulate chromaffin cell proliferation in the rat adrenal medulla. *Toxicol Appl Pharmacol* 140:115–123, 1996.

Tischler AS, Powers JF, Pignatello M, et al: Vitamin D_3-induced proliferative lesions in the rat adrenal medulla. *Toxicol Sci* 51:9–18, 1999.

Tischler AS, Riseberg J: Different responses to mitogenic agents by adult rat and human chromaffin cells *in vitro*. *Endocr Pathol* 4:15–19, 1993.

Tischler AS, Riseberg J, Cherington V: Multiple mitogenic signaling pathways in chromaffin cells: A model for cell cycle regulation in the nervous system. *Neurosci Lett* 168:181–184, 1994.

Tischler AS, Ruzicka LA, Van Pelt CS, et al: Catecholamine-synthesizing enzymes and chromogranin proteins in drug-induced proliferative lesions of the rat adrenal medulla. *Lab Invest* 63:44–51, 1990.

Tischler AS, Ziar J, Downing JC, et al: Sustained stimulation of rat adrenal chromaffin cell proliferation by reserpine. *Toxicol Appl Pharmacol* 135:254–257, 1995.

Warren S, Gruzdev L, Gates O, et al: Radiation induced adrenal medullary tumors in the rat. *Arch Pathol* 82:115–118, 1966.

Thyroid Gland (Follicular Cells)

Atterwill CK, Collins P, Brown CG, et al: The perchlorate discharge test for examing thyroid function in rats. *J Pharmacol Methods* 18:199–203, 1987.

Axelrod AA, Leblond CP: Induction of thyroid tumors in rats by low iodine diet. *Cancer* 8:339–367,1955.

Barter RA, Klaassen CD: Rat liver microsomal UDP-glucuronosyltransferase activity toward thyroxine: Characterization, induction, and form specificity. *Toxicol Appl Pharmacol* 115:261–267, 1992.

Barter RA, Klaassen CD: Reduction of thyroid hormone levels and alteration of thyroid function by four representative UDP-glucuronosyltransferase inducers in rats. *Toxicol Appl Pharmacol* 128:9–17, 1994.

Barter RA, Klaassen CD: UDP-glucuronosyltransferase inducers reduce thyroid hormone levels in rats by an extrathyroidal mechanism. *Toxicol Appl Pharmacol* 113:36–42, 1992.

Borzelleca JF, Capen CC, Hallagan JB: Lifetime toxicity carcinogenicity study of FC&C Red No. 3 (erythrosine) in rats. *Food Chem Toxicol* 25:723–733, 1987.

Capen C, Sagartz J: A Ret transgenic mouse model of thyroid carcinogenesis. *Lab Anim Sci* 48:580–583, 1998.

Capen CC, DeLellis RA, Williams ED: Experimental thyroid carcinogenesis: Role of radiation and xenobiotic chemicals, in: *Proceedings of the First International Conference on Radiation and Thyroid Cancer.* St. John's College, Cambridge, UK, 20-23 July 1998; and in Thomas G, Karaoglou A, Williams ED (eds): *Radiation and Thyroid Cancer.* Singapore, New Jersey, London, Hong Kong: World Scientific Publishing, 1999, pp 167–176.

Capen CC: Comparative anatomy and physiology of the thyroid, in Braverman LE, Utiger RD (eds): *Werner and Ingbar's The Thyroid: A Fundamental and Clinical Text,* 8th ed. Philadelphia: Lippincott-Raven, 2000, pp 20–44.

Capen CC: Thyroid and parathyroid toxicology, in Harvey PW, Rush K, Cockburn A (eds): *Endocrine and Hormonal Toxicology.* Sussex, England: Wiley, 1999, pp 33–66.

Capen CC: Mechanistic data and risk assessment of selected toxic end points of the thyroid gland. *Toxicol Pathol* 25:39–48, 1997.

Capen CC: Mechanistic considerations for thyroid gland neoplasia with FD&C Red No. 3 (erythrosine), in *The Toxicology Forum.* Proceedings of the 1989 Annual Winter Meeting, Washington, DC, 1989; pp 113–130.

Capen CC, Martin SL: The effects of xenobiotics on the structure and function of thyroid follicles and C cells. *Toxicol Pathol* 17:266–293, 1989.

Clements FW: Relationship of thyrotoxicosis and carcinoma of thyroid to endemic goiter. *Med J Aust* 2:894–899, 1954.

Clemmesen J, Fuglsang-Frederiksen V, Plum CM: Are anticonvulsants oncogenic? *Lancet* 1:705–707, 1974.

Clemmesen J, Hjalgrim-Jensen S: Does phenobarbital cause intracranial tumors? A follow-up through 35 years. *Ecotoxicol Environ Saf* 5:255–260, 1981.

Clemmesen J, Hjalgrim-Jensen S: Is phenobarbital carcinogenic? A follow-up of 8078 epileptics. *Ecotoxicol Environ Saf* 1:255–260, 1978.

Clemmesen J, Hjalgrim-Jensen S: On the absence of carcinogenicity to man of phenobarbital, in *Statistical Studies in the Aetiology of Malignant Neoplasms. Acta Pathol Microb Scand* 261 (suppl):38–50, 1977.

Collins WT Jr, Capen CC: Ultrastructural and functional alterations in thyroid glands of rats produced by polychlorinated biphenyls compared with the effects of iodide excess and deficiency, and thyrotropin and thyroxine administration. *Virchows Arch B Cell Pathol* 33:213–231, 1980.

Cooper DS, Axelrod L, DeGroot LJ, et al: Congenital goiter and the development of metastatic follicular carcinoma with evidence for a leak of non-hormonal iodide: Clinical, pathological, kinetic, and biochemical studies and a review of the literature. *J Clin Endocrinol Metab* 52:294–306, 1981.

Copp DH: Endocrine regulation of calcium metabolism. *Annu Rev Physiol* 32:61–86, 1970.

Curran PG, DeGroot LJ: The effect of hepatic enzyme-inducing drugs on thyroid hormones and the thyroid gland. *Endocr Rev* 12:135–150, 1991.

Döhler K-D, Wong CC, von zut Mühlen A: The rat as model for the study of drug effects on thyroid function: consideration of methodological problems. *Pharmacol Ther* 5:305–313, 1979.

Doniach I: Aetiological consideration of thyroid carcinoma, in Smithers D (ed): *Tumors of the Thyroid Gland.* London: E & S Livingstone, 1970; pp 55–72.

Friedman GD: Barbiturates and lung cancer in humans. *J Natl Cancer Inst* 67:291–295, 1981.

Gutshall DM, Pilcher GD, Langley AE: Effect of thyroxine supplementation on the response to perfluoro-*n*-decanoic acid (PFDA) in rats. *J Toxicol Environ Health* 24:491–498, 1988.

Hard GC: Recent developments in the investigation of thyroid regulation and thyroid carcinogenesis. *Environ Health Perspect* 106:427–436, 1998.

Hiasa Y, Kitahori Y, Kato Y, et al: Potassium perchlorate, potassium iodide, and propylthiouracil: Promoting effect on the development of thyroid tumors in rats treated with *N*-Bis(2-hydroxypropyl)-nitrosamine. *Jpn J Cancer Res* 78:1335–1340, 1987.

Hill RN, Crisp TM, Hurley PM, et al: Risk assessment of thyroid follicular cell tumors. *Environ Health Perspect* 106:447–457, 1998.

Hill RN, Erdreich LS, Paynter O, et al: Assessment of thyroid follicular cell tumors: Risk Assessment Forum. Washington, DC: U.S. Environmental Protection Agency, March 1998, pp 1–43.

Hill RN, Erdreich LS, Paynter O, et al: Thyroid follicular cell carcinogenesis. *Fundam Appl Toxicol* 12:629–697, 1989.

Hood A, Harstad E, Klaassen CD: Effects of UDP-glucuronosyltransferase (UDP-GT) inducers on thyroid cell proliferation. *Toxicologist* 15:229, 1995.

Hood A, Hashmi R, Klaassen CD: Effects of microsomal enzyme inducers on thyroid-follicular cell proliferation, hyperplasia, and hypertrophy. *Toxicol Appl Pharmacol* 160:163–170, 1999.

Hood A, Klaassen CD: Differential effects of microsomal enzyme inducers on *in vitro* thyroxine (T_4) and triiodothyronine (T_3) glucuronidation. *Toxicol Sci* 55:78–84, 2000.

Hood A, Klaassen CD: Effects of microsomal enzyme inducers on outer-ring deiodinase activity toward thyroid hormones in various rat tissues. *Toxicol Appl Pharmacol* 163:240–248, 2000.

Hood A, Liu YP, Gattone VH II, et al: Sensitivity of thyroid gland growth to thyroid stimulating hormone (TSH) in rats treated with antithyroid drugs. *Toxicol Sci* 49:263–271, 1999.

Hood A, Liu YP, Klaassen CD: Effects of phenobarbital, pregnenolone-16α-carbonitrile, and propylthiouracil on thyroid follicular cell proliferation. *Toxicol Sci* 50:45–53, 1999.

Hotz KJ, Wilson AGE, Thake DC, et al: Mechanism of thiazopyr-induced effects on thyroid hormone homeostasis in male Sprague-Dawley rats. *Toxicol Appl Pharmacol* 142:133–142, 1997.

Hurley PM, Hill RN, Whiting RJ: Mode of carcinogenic action of pesticides inducing thyroid follicular cell tumors in rodents. *Environ Health Perspect* 106:437–445, 1998.

Ingbar SH: Autoregulation of the thyroid. Response to iodide excess and depletion. *Mayo Clin Proc* 47:814, 1972.

Jhiang SM, Cho J-Y, Furminger TL, et al: Thyroid carcinomas in RET/PTC transgenic mice, in Schwab M, Rabes H, Munk K, Hofschneider PH (eds): *Genes and Environment in Cancer. Recent Results in Cancer Research Vol 154,* Berlin: Springer-Verlag, 1998, pp 265–270.

Jhiang SM, Cho J-Y, Ryu K-Y, et al: An immunohistochemical study of Na^+/I^- symporter in human thyroid tissues and salivary gland tissues. *Endocrinology* 139:4416, 1998.

Jhiang SM, Sagartz JE, Tong Q, et al: Targeted expression of the *ret*/PTC1 oncogene induces papillary thyroid carcinomas. *Endocrinology* 137:375–378, 1996.

Kanno J, Nemoto T, Kasuga T, et al: Effects of a six-week exposure to excess iodide on thyroid glands of growing and nongrowing male Fischer-344 rats. *Toxicol Pathol* 22:23–28, 1994.

Kennedy TH, Purves HD: Studies on experimental goiter: Effect of *Brassica* seed diets on rats. *Br J Exp Pathol* 22:241–244, 1941.

Kolaja KL, Klaassen CD: Dose-response examination of UDP-glucuronosyltransferase inducers and their ability to increase both TGF-β expression and thyroid follicular cell apoptosis. *Toxicol Sci* 46:31–37, 1998.

Kolaja KL, Petrick JS, Klaassen CD: Inhibition of gap-junctional-intercellular communication in thyroid-follicular cells by propylthiouracil and low iodine diet. *Toxicology* 143:195–202, 2000.

Lamas L, Ingbar SH: The effect of varying iodine content on the susceptibility of thyroglobulin to hydrolysis by thyroid acid protease. *Endocrinology* 102:188–197, 1978.

Lamm SH, Braverman LE, Li FX, et al: Thyroid health status of ammonium perchlorate workers: A cross-sectional occupational health study. *J Occup Environ Med* 41:248–260.

Lamm SH, Doemland M: Has perchlorate in drinking water increased the rate of congenital hypothyroidism? *J Occup Environ Med* 41:409–411, 1999.

Li Z, Li FX, Byrd D, et al: Neonatal thyroxine level and perchlorate in drinking water. *J Occup Environ Med* 42:200–205, 2000.

Liu J, Liu Y, Barter RA, et al: Alteration of thyroid homeostasis by UDP-glucuronosyltransferase inducers in rats: A dose-response study. *J Pharmacol Exp Ther* 273:977–985, 1995.

Many M-C, Denef J-F, Haumont S, et al: Morphological and functional changes during thyroid hyperplasia and involution in C3H mice: Effects of iodine and 3,5,38-triiodothyronine during involution. *Endocrinology* 116:798, 1985.

McClain RM: The use of mechanistic data in cancer risk assessment: Case example sulfonamides, in *Low-Dose Extrapolation of Cancer Risk: Issues and Perspectives.* International Life Sciences Institute Series. Washington, DC: ILSI Press, 1995, pp 163–173.

McClain RM: The significance of hepatic microsomal enzyme induction and altered thyroid function in rats: Implications for thyroid gland neoplasia. *Toxicol Pathol* 17:294–306, 1989.

McClain RM, Levin AA, Posch R, et al: The effects of phenobarbital on the metabolism and excretion of thyroxine in rats. *Toxicol Appl Pharmacol* 99:216–228, 1989.

McClain RM, Posch RC, Bosakowski T, et al: Studies on the mode of action for thyroid gland tumor promotion in rats by phenobarbital. *Toxicol Appl Pharmacol* 94:254–265, 1988.

McGirr EM, Clement WE, Currie AR, et al: Impaired dehalogenase activity as a cause of goiter with malignant changes. *Scott Med J* 4:232–242, 1959.

Morris HP: The experimental development and metabolism of thyroid gland tumors. *Adv Cancer Res* 3:51–115, 1955.

Napalkov NP: Tumours of the thyroid gland, in Turusov VS (ed): *Pathology of Tumors in Laboratory Animals:* Part 2. Vol 1. *Tumors of the Rat.* IARC Scientific Publication No. 6. Lyons, France: IARC, 1976, pp 239–272.

Nilsson M, Engström G, Ericson LE: Graded response in the individual thyroid follicle cell to increasing doses of TSH. *Mol Cell Endocrinol* 44:165, 1986.

Ohnhaus EE, Burgi H, Burger A, et al: The effect of antipyrine, phenobarbital, and rifampicin on the thyroid hormone metabolism in man. *Eur J Clin Invest* 11:381–387, 1981.

Ohnhaus EE, Studer H: A link between liver microsomal enzyme activity and thyroid hormone metabolism in man. *Br J Clin Pharmacol* 15:71–76, 1983.

Ohshima M, Ward JM: Dietary iodine deficiency as a tumor promoter and carcinogen in male F344/NCr rats. *Cancer Res* 46:877–883, 1986.

Ohshima M, Ward JM: Promotion of *N*-methyl-*N*-nitrosourea-induced thyroid tumors by iodine deficiency in F344/NCr rats. *J Natl Cancer Inst* 73:289–296, 1984.

Olsen JH, Boice JD, Jensen JP, et al: Cancer among epileptic patients exposed to anticonvulsant drugs. *J Natl Cancer Inst* 81:803–808, 1989.

Ozaki A, Sagartz JE, Capen CC: Phagocytic activity of FRTL-5 rat thyroid follicular cells as measured by ingestion of fluorescent latex beads. *Exp Cell Res* 219:547–554, 1995.

Paynter OH, Burin GJ, Jaeger RB, et al: Goitrogens and thyroid follicular cell neoplasmia: Evidence for a threshold process. *Reg Toxicol Pharmacol* 8:102–119, 1988.

Pendergrast WJ, Milmore BK, Marcus SC: Thyroid cancer and toxicosis in the United States: Their relation to endemic goiter. *J Chronic Dis* 13:22–38, 1961.

Poirier LA, Doerge DR, Gaylor DW, et al: An FDA review of sulfamethazine toxicity. *Regul Toxicol Pharmacol* 30:217–222, 1999.

Sagartz JE, Jhiang SM, Tong Q, Capen CC: Thyroid stimulating hormone promotes growth of thyroid carcinomas in transgenic mice with targeted expression of ret/PTC_1 oncogene. *Lab Invest* 76:307–318, 1997.

Sagartz JE, Ozaki A, Capen CC: Phagocytosis of fluorescent beads by rat thyroid follicular (FRTL-5) cells: Comparison with iodine uptake as an index of functional activity of thyrocytes *in vitro. Toxicol Pathol* 23:635–643, 1995.

Shirts SB, Annegers JF, Hauser WA, et al: Cancer incidence in a cohort of patients with seizure disorders. *J Natl Cancer Inst* 77:83–87, 1986.

Spitzweg C, Heufelder AE, Morris JC: Review: Thyroid iodine transport. *Thyroid* 10:321–330, 2000.

Swarm RL, Roberts GKS, Levy AC: Observations on the thyroid gland in rats following the administration of sulfamethoxazole and trimethoprim. *Toxicol Appl Pharmacol* 24:351–363, 1973.

Tajima K, Miyagawa J-I, Nakajima H, et al: Morphological and biochemical studies on minocycline-induced black thyroid in rats. *Toxicol Appl Pharmacol* 81:393–400, 1985.

Takayama S, Aihara K, Onodera T, et al: Antithyroid effects of propylthiouracil and sulfamonomethoxine in rats and monkeys. *Toxicol Appl Pharmacol* 82:191–199, 1986.

Waritz RS, Steinberg M, Kinoshita FK, et al: Thyroid function and thyroid tumors in toxaphene-treated rats. *Regul Toxicol Pharmacol* 24:184–192, 1996.

White SJ, McLean AEM, Howland C: Anticonvulsant drugs and cancer. A cohort study in patients with severe epilepsy. *Lancet* 2:458–461, 1979.

Wynford-Thomas D, Smith P, Williams ED: Proliferative response to cyclic AMP elevation of thyroid epithelium in suspension culture. *Mol Cell Endocrinol* 51:163, 1987.

Wynford-Thomas D, Stringer BM, Williams ED: Desensitisation of rat thyroid to the growth-stimulating action of TSH during prolonged goitrogen administration. Persistence of refractoriness following withdrawal of stimulation. *Acta Endocrinol Copenh* 101:562–569, 1982.

Wynford-Thomas D, Stringer BM, Williams ED: Dissociation of growth and function in the rat thyroid during prolonged goitrogen administration. *Acta Endocrinol Copenh* 101:210–216, 1982.

Wynford-Thomas V, Wynford-Thomas D, Williams ED: Experimental induction of parathyroid adenomas in the rat. *J Natl Cancer Inst* 70:127–134, 1982.

Zbinden G: Hyperplastic and neoplastic responses of the thyroid gland in toxicological studies. *Arch Toxicol Suppl* 12:98–106, 1988.

Thyroid C Cells

Burek JD: *Pathology of Aging Rats.* West Palm Beach, FL: CRC Press, 1978.

DeGrandi PB, Kraehenbuhl JP, Campiche MA: Ultrastructural localization of calcitonin in the parafollicular cells of the pig thyroid gland with cytochrome c-labeled antibody fragments. *J Cell Biol* 50:446–456, 1971.

DeLellis RA, Dayal Y, Tischler AS, et al: Multiple endocrine neoplasia syndromes. Cellular origins and interrelationships. *Int Rev Exp Pathol* 28:163–215, 1986.

DeLellis RA, Nunnemacher G, Bitman WR, et al: C cell hyperplasia and medullary thyroid carcinoma in the rat: An immunohistochemical and ultrastructural analysis. *Lab Invest* 40:140–154, 1979.

DeLellis RA, Nunnemacher G, Wolfe HJ: C cell hyperplasia, an ultrastructural analysis. *Lab Invest* 36:237–248, 1977.

Foster GV, Byfield PGH, Gudmundsson TV: Calcitonin, in MacIntyre I (ed): *Clinics in Endocrinology and Metabolism.* Vol. 1. Philadelphia: Saunders, 1972, pp 93–124.

Kalina M, Pearse AGE: Ultrastructural localization of calcitonin in C cells of dog thyroid: An immunocytochemical study. *Histochemie* 26:1–8, 1971.

Leblanc B, Paulus G, Andreu M, et al: Immunocytochemistry of thyroid C-cell complexes in dogs. *Vet Pathol* 27:445–452, 1990.

Nonidez José F: The origin of the "parafollicular" cell, A second epithelial component of the thyroid gland of the dog. *Am J Anat* 49:479–505, 1931–1932.

Stoll R, Faucounau N, Maraud R: Les adenomes a cellules folliculaires et parafolliculaires de la thyroide du rat soumis au thiamazole. [Development of follicular and parafollicular adenomas in the thyroid of rats treated with thiamazole.] *Ann Endocrinol (Paris),* 39, 179–189, 1978.

Teitelbaum SL, Moore KE, Shieber W: C cell follicles in the dog thyroid: Demonstration by in vivo perfusion. *Anat Rec* 168:69–78, 1970.

Thurston V, Williams ED: Experimental induction of C-cell tumours in thyroid by increased dietary content of vitamin D2. *Acta Endocrinol* 100:41–45, 1982.

Triggs SM, Williams ED: Experimental carcinogenesis in the rat thyroid follicular and C cells. *Acta Endocrinol* 85:84–92, 1977.

Parathyroid Gland

Abdo KM, Eustis SL, Haseman J, et al: Toxicity and carcinogenicity of rotenone given in the feed to F344/N rats and $B_6C_3F_1$ mice for up to two years. *Drug Chem Toxicol* 11:225–235, 1988.

Armbrecht HJ, Wongsurawat N, Zenser TV, et al: Differential effects of parathyroid hormone on the renal 125-dihydroxyvitamin D3 and 24,25-dihydroxyvitamin D3 production of young and adult rats. *Endocrinology* 111:1339–1344, 1982.

Arnold DL, Moodie CA, Charbonneau SM, et al: Long-term toxicity of hexachlorobenzene in the rat and the effect of dietary vitamin A. *Chem Toxicol* 23:779–793, 1985.

Atwal OS: Ultrastructural pathology of ozone-induced experimental parathyroiditis: IV. Biphasic activity in the chief cells of regenerating parathyroid glands. *Am J Pathol* 95:611–632, 1979.

Atwal OS, Pemsingh RS: Morphology of microvascular changes and endothelial regeneration in experimental ozone-induced parathyroiditis: III. Some pathologic considerations. *Am J Pathol* 102:297–307, 1981.

Atwal OS, Samagh BS, Bhatnagar MK: A possible autoimmune parathyroiditis following ozone inhalation: II. A histopathologic, ultrastructural, and immunofluorescent study. *Am J Pathol* 80:53–68, 1975.

Atwal OS, Wilson T: Parathyroid gland changes following oxone inhalation. A morphologic study. *Arch Environ Health* 28:91–100, 1974.

Barbosa JA, Gill BM, Takiyyuddin MA, et al: Chromogranin A: Posttranslational modifications in secretory granules. *Endocrinology* 128:174–190, 1991.

Bourdeau AM, Plachot JJ, Cournot-Witmer G, et al: Parathyroid response to aluminum in vitro: Ultrastructural changes and PTH release. *Kidney Int* 31:15–24, 1987.

Brown EM: PTH secretion in vivo and in vitro. Regulation by calcium and other secretagogues. *Miner Electrolyte Metab* 8:130–150, 1982.

Capen CC: Age-related changes in structure and function of the parathyroid gland in laboratory rats, in Mohr U, Dungworth DL, Capen CC (eds): *Pathobiology of the Aging Rat.* Vol. II. Washington, DC: International Life Sciences Press (ILSI), 1994, pp 199–226.

Capen CC: Pathobiology of parathyroid gland structure and function in animals, in Jones TC, Capen CC, Mohr U (eds): *Endocrine System. Series II. Monographs on Pathology of Laboratory Animals,* 2d ed. International Life Sciences Institute Series. Berlin, Heidelberg, New York: Springer-Verlag, 1996, pp 293–327.

Capen CC, Gröne A, Bucci TJ, et al: Changes in structure and function of the parathyroid gland, in Mohr U, Dungworth D, Capen C, Sundberg J (eds): *Pathobiology of the Aging Mouse.* Washington, DC: International Life Sciences (ILSI) Press, 1996, pp 109–124.

Chisari FV, Hochstein HD, Kirschstein RL: Parathyroid necrosis and hypocalcemic tetany induced in rabbits by L-asparaginase. *Am J Pathol* 69:461–476, 1972.

Cloutier M, Rousseau L, Gascon-Barré M, et al: Immunological evidences for post-translational control of the parathyroid function by ionized calcium in dogs. *Bone Miner* 22:197–207, 1993.

Cohn DV, Fasciotto BH, Zhang J-X, et al: Chemistry and biology of chromogranin A (secretory protein-I) of the parathyroid and other endocrine glands, in Bilezikian JP, Marcus R, Levine MA (eds): *The Parathyroids: Basic and Clinical Concepts.* New York: Raven Press, 1993, pp 107–119.

Fasciotto BH, Gorr S-U, Bourdeau AM, et al: Autocrine regulation of parathyroid secretion: Inhibition of secretion by chromogranin-A (secretory protein-I) and potentiation of secretion by chromogranin-A and pancreastatin antibodies. *Endocrinology* 127:1329–1335, 1990.

Goltzman D, Bennett HPJ, Koutsilieris M, et al: Studies of the multiple molecular forms of bioactive parathyroid hormone and parathyroid hormone-like substances. *Recent Prog Horm Res* 42:665–703, 1986.

Habener JF: Recent advances in parathyroid hormone research. *Clin Biochem* 14:223–229, 1981.

Jaffe N, Traggis D, Lakshmi D, et al: Comparison of daily and twice-weekly schedule of L-asparaginase in childhood leukemia. *Pediatrics* 49:590–595, 1972.

Kalu DN, Hardin RR, Murata I, et al: Age-dependent modulation of parathyroid hormone action. *Age* 5:25–29, 1982.

Kronenberg HM, Igarashi T, Freeman MW, et al: Structure and expression of the human parathyroid hormone gene. *Recent Prog Horm Res* 42:641–663, 1986.

Lupulescu A, Potorac E, Pop A: Experimental investigation on immunology of the parathyroid gland. *Immunology* 14:475–482, 1968.

Morrissey J, Rothstein M, Mayor G, et al: Suppression of parathyroid hormone secretion by aluminum. *Kidney Int* 23:699–704, 1983.

Morrissey J, Slatopolsky E: Effect of aluminum on parathyroid hormone secretion. *Kidney Int* 29:S41–S44, 1986.

Oettgen HF, Old LJ, Boyse EA, et al: Toxicity of *E. coli* L-asparaginase in man. *Cancer* 25:253–278, 1970.

Oslapas R, Prinz R, Ernst K, et al: Incidence of radiation-induced parathyroid tumors in male and female rats. *Clin Res* 29:734A, 1981.

Oslapas R, Shah KH, Hoffman, et al: Effect of gonadectomy on the incidence of radiation-induced parathyroid tumors in male and female rats. *Clin Res* 30:401A, 1982.

Pollak MR, Brown EM, Chou YW, et al: Mutations in the human Ca^{2+}-sensing receptor gene cause familial hypocalciuric hypercalcemia and neonatal severe hypercalcemia. *Cell* 75:1297–1303, 1993.

Silver J: Regulation of parathyroid hormone synthesis and secretion, in Coe FL, Favus MJ (eds): *Disorders of Bone and Mineral Metabolism.* New York: Raven Press, 1992, pp 83–106.

Tettenborn D, Hobik HP, Luckhaus G: Hypoparathyroidismus beim Kaninchen nach Verabreichung von L-asparaginase. *Arzneimittelforschung* 20:1753–1755, 1970.

Wada L, Daly R, Kern D, et al: Kinetics of 1,25-dihydroxyvitamin D metabolism in the aging rat. *Am J Physiol* 262 (*Endocrinol Metab,* 25): E906–E910, 1992.

Wongsurawat N, Armbrecht HJ: Comparison of calcium effect on in vitro calcitonin and parathyroid hormone release by young and aged thyroparathyroid glands. *Exp Gerontol* 22:263–269, 1987.

Young DM, Olson HM, Prieur DJ, et al: Clinicopathologic and ultrastructural studies of L-asparaginase-induced hypocalcemia in rabbits. An experimental animal model of acute hypoparathyroidism. *Lab Invest* 29:374–386, 1973.

Testis

Bär A: Significance of Leydig cell neoplasia in rats fed lactitol or lactose. *J Am Coll Toxicol* 11:189–207, 1992.

Bartke A, Sweeney CA, Johnson L, et al: Hyperprolactinemia inhibits development of Leydig cell tumors in aging Fischer rats. *Exp Aging Res* 11:123–128, 1985.

Boorman GA, Hamlin MH, Eustis SL: Focal interstitial cell hyperplasia, testis, rat, in Jones TC, Möhr U, Hunt RD (eds): *Monographs on Pathology of Laboratory Animals.* Berlin: Springer-Verlag, 1987; pp 200–220.

Chatani F, Nonoyama T, Katsuichi S, et al: Stimulatory effect of luteinizing hormone on the development and maintenance of 5α-reduced steroid-producing testicular interstitial cell tumors in Fischer 344 rats. *Anticancer Res* 10:337–342, 1990.

Clegg ED, Cook JC, Chapin RE, et al: Leydig cell hyperplasia and adenoma formation: Mechanisms and relevance to humans. *Reprod Toxicol* 11:107–121, 1997.

Cook JC, Klinefelter GR, Hardisty JF, et al: Rodent Leydig cell tumorigenesis: A review of the physiology, pathology, mechanisms, and relevance to humans. *Crit Rev Toxicol* 29:169–261, 1999.

Cook JC, Murray SM, Frame SR, et al: Induction of Leydig cell adenomas by ammonium perfluorooctanoate: A possible endocrine-related mechanism. *Toxicol Appl Pharmacol* 113:209–217, 1992.

Fort FL, Miyajima H, Ando T, et al: Mechanism for species-specific induction of Leydig cell tumors in rats by lansoprazole. *Fundam Appl Toxicol* 26:191–202, 1995.

McConnell RF, Westen HH, Ulland BM, et al: Proliferative lesions of the testes in rats with selected examples from mice, in *Guides for Toxicologic Pathology.* Washington, DC: STP/ARP/AFIP, 1992, pp 1–32.

Murakami M, Hosokawa S, Yamada T, et al: Species-specific mechanism in rat Leydig cell tumorigenesis by procymidone. *Toxicol Appl Pharmacol* 131:244–252, 1995.

Prahalada S, Majka JA, Soper KA, et al: Leydig cell hyperplasia and adenomas in mice treated with finasteride, a 5α-reductase inhibitor: A possible mechanism. *Fundam Appl Toxicol* 22:211–219, 1994.

Prentice DE, Meikle AW: A review of drug-induced Leydig cell hyperplasia and neoplasia in the rat and some comparisons with man. *Hum Exp Toxicol* 14:562–572, 1995.

Waalkes MP, Rehm S, Devor DE: The effects of continuous testosterone exposure on spontaneous and cadmium-induced tumors in the male Fischer (F344/NCr) rat: Loss of testicular response. *Toxicol Appl Pharmacol* 142:40–46, 1997.

Ovary

Alison RH, Morgan KT: Ovarian neoplasms in F344 rats and $B_6C_3F_1$ mice. *Environ Health Perspect* 73:91–106, 1987.

Amsterdam A, Selvaraj N: Control of differentiation, transformation, and apoptosis in granulosa cells by oncogenes, oncoviruses, and tumor suppressor genes. *Endocr Rev* 18:435–461, 1997.

Biskind MS, Biskind JR: Development of tumors in the rat ovary after transplantation into the spleen. *Proc Soc Exp Biol Med* 55:176–179, 1944.

Blaakaer J, Baeksted M, Micic S, et al: Gonadotrophin-releasing hormone agonist suppression of ovarian tumorigenesis in mice of the W^x/W^v genotype. *Biol Reprod* 53:775–779, 1995.

Capen CC, Beamer WG, Tennent BJ, et al: Mechanisms of hormone-mediated carcinogenesis of the ovary in mice. *Mutat Res* 333:143–151, 1995.

Carson RS, Zhang Z, Hutchinson LA, et al: Growth factors in ovarian function. *J Reprod Fertil* 85:735–746, 1989.

Cattanach BM, Iddon A, Charlton HM, et al: Gonadotropin releasing hormone deficiency in a mutant mouse with hypogonadism. *Nature* 269:238–240, 1977.

Cohen IR, Sims ML, Robbins MR, et al: The reversible effects of raloxifene on luteinizing hormone levels and ovarian morphology in mice. *Reprod Toxicol* 14:37–44, 2000.

Cook LS, Weiss NS, Schwartz SM, et al: Population-based study of tamoxifen therapy and subsequent ovarian, endometrial, and breast cancers. *J Natl Cancer Inst* 87:1359–1364, 1995.

Davis BJ, Maronpot RR: Chemically associated toxicity and carcinogenicity of the ovary, in Huff J, Boyd J, Barrett J (eds): *Cellular and Molecular Mechanisms of Hormonal Carcinogenesis: Environmental Influences,* New York, Wiley-Liss, 1996, pp 285–309.

Delmas PD, Bjarnason NH, Mitlak BH, et al: Effects of raloxifene on bone mineral density, serum cholesterol concentrations, and uterine endometrium in postmenopausal women. *N Engl J Med* 337:23:1641–1647, 1997.

Evista Package Insert. Indianapolis, IN: Eli Lilly, 1997.

Fisher B, Costantino JP, Redmond CK, et al: Endometrial cancer in tamoxifen-treated breast cancer patients: Findings from the National Surgical Adjuvant Breast and Bowel Project (NSABP) B-14. *J Natl Cancer Inst* 86:527–537, 1994.

Frith CH, Zuna RF, Morgan K: A morphologic classification and incidence of spontaneous ovarian neoplasms in three strains of mice. *J Natl Cancer Inst* 67:693–702, 1981.

Furth J: Morphologic changes associated with thyrotropin-secreting pituitary tumors. *Am J Pathol* 30:421–463, 1954.

Gardner WU: Ovarian and lymphoid tumors in female mice subsequent to

Roentgen-ray irradiation and hormone treatment. *Proc Soc Exp Biol Med* 75:434–436, 1950.

Guthrie MJ: Tumorigenesis in intrasplenic ovaries in mice. *Cancer* 10:190–203, 1957.

Hart JE: Endocrine pathology of estrogens: Species differences. *Pharmacol Ther* 47:203–218, 1990.

Hsu SY, Hsueh AJW: Hormonal regulation of apoptosis: An ovarian perspective. *Trends Endocrinol Metab* 8:207–213, 1997.

Hummel KP: Induced ovarian tumors. *J Natl Cancer Inst* 15:711–715, 1954.

Korach KS: Insights from the study of animals lacking functional estrogen receptor. *Science* 266:1524–1527, 1994.

Li MH, Gardner WU: Further studies on the pathogenesis of ovarian tumors in mice. *Cancer Res* 9:35–44, 1949.

Long GG, Cohen IR, Gries CL, et al: Proliferative lesions of ovarian granulosa cells induced in rats by a selective estrogen-receptor modulator. *Toxicol Pathol* 27, in press.

Lubahn DB, Moyer JS, Golding TS, et al: Alteration of reproductive function but not prenatal sexual development after insertional disruption of the mouse estrogen receptor gene. *Proc Natl Acad Sci USA* 90:11162–11166, 1993.

Majumder S, Brown K, Qiu F-H, et al: *c-kit* Protein, a transmembrane kinase: Identification in tissues and characterization. *Mol Cell Biol* 8:4896–4903, 1988.

Marchant J: The chemical induction of ovarian tumours in mice. *Br J Cancer* 11:452–464, 1957.

Marchant J: The development of ovarian tumors in ovaries grafted from mice treated with dimethylbenzanthracene. Inhibition by the presence of normal ovarian tissue. *Br J Cancer* 14:514–519, 1960.

Matzuk MM, Finegold MJ, Su JG, et al: Alpha-inhibin is a tumour-suppressor gene with gonadal specificity in mice. *Nature* 360:313–319, 1992.

Michael SD, Taguchi O, Nishizuka Y: Changes in hypophyseal hormones associated with accelerated aging and tumorigenesis of the ovaries in neonatally thymectomized mice. *Endocrinology* 108:2375–2380, 1981.

Murphy ED, Beamer WG: Plasma gonadotrophin levels during early stages of ovarian tumorigenesis in mice of the W^x/W^v genotype. *Cancer Res* 33:721–723, 1973.

Murphy ED: Hyperplastic and early neoplastic changes in the ovaries of mice after genic deletion of germ cells. *J Natl Cancer Inst* 48:1283–1295, 1972.

Nishizuki Y, Sakakura T, Taguchi O: Mechanism of ovarian tumorigenesis in mice after neonatal thymectomy. *J Natl Cancer Inst Monogr* 51:89–96, 1979.

Payne AH, Quinn PG, Stalvey JRD: The stimulation of steroid biosynthesis by luteinizing hormone, in Ascoli M (ed): *Luteinizing Hormone Action and Receptors.* Boca Raton, FL: CRC Press, 1985, pp 136–173.

Rao AR: Effects of carcinogen and/or mutagen on normal and gonadotrophin-primed ovaries of mice. *Int J Cancer* 28:105–110, 1981.

Rehm S, Dierksen D, Deerberg F: Spontaneous ovarian tumors in Han:NMRI mice: Histologic classification, incidence, and influence of food restriction. *J Natl Cancer Inst* 72:1383–1395, 1984.

Risma KA, Clay CM, Nett TM, et al: Targeted overexpression of luteinizing hormone in transgenic mice leads to infertility, polycystic ovaries, and ovarian tumors. *Proc Natl Acad Sci USA* 92:1322–1326, 1995.

Risma KA, Hirshfield AN, Nilson JH: Elevated luteinizing hormone in prepubertal transgenic mice causes hyperandrogenemia, precocious puberty, and substantial ovarian pathology. *Endocrinology* 138:3540–3547, 1997.

Taguchi O, Michael SD, Nishizuka Y: Rapid induction of ovarian granulosa cell tumors by 7,12-dimethylbenz[*a*]anthracene in neonatally estrogenized mice. *Cancer Res* 48:425–429, 1988.

Tennent BJ, Beamer WG: Ovarian tumors not induced by irradiation and gonadotropins in hypogonadal (*hpg*) mice. *Biol Reprod* 34:751–760, 1986.

Willemsen W, Kruitwagen R, Bastiaans B, et al: Ovarian stimulation and granulosa-cell tumour. *Lancet* 341:986–988, 1993.

Witte ON: Steel locus defines new multipotent growth factor. *Cell* 63:5–6, 1990.

Yang NN, Venugopalan M, Hardikar S, et al: Identification of an estrogen response element activated by metabolites of 17β-estradiol and raloxifene. *Science* 273:1222–1225, 1996.

UNIT 5

TOXIC AGENTS

CHAPTER 22

TOXIC EFFECTS OF PESTICIDES

Donald J. Ecobichon

INTRODUCTION

The U.S. Environmental Protection Agency (U.S. EPA) defines a pesticide as any substance or mixture of substances intended for preventing, destroying, repelling, or mitigating any pest. A pesticide may also be described as any physical, chemical, or biological agent that will kill an undesirable plant or animal pest. The term *pest* includes harmful, destructive, or troublesome animals, plants, or microorganisms. *Pesticide* is a generic name for a variety of agents that are classified more specifically on the basis of the pattern of use and organism killed. In addition to the major agricultural classes that encompass insecticides, herbicides, and fungicides, one finds pest-control agents grouped as acaricides, larvacides, miticides, molluscides, pediculicides, rodenticides, scabicides, plus attractants (pheromones), defoliants, desiccants, plant growth regulators, and repellants.

HISTORICAL DEVELOPMENT

Over the centuries, humans have developed many ingenious methods in their attempts to control the invertebrates, vertebrates, and microorganisms that constantly threatened the supply of food and fiber as well as posing a threat to health. The historical literature is replete with descriptions of plant diseases and insect plagues and the measures taken to control them. Sulfur was used as a fumigant by the Chinese before 1000 B.C. and as a fungicide in the 1800s in Europe against powdery mildew on fruit; it is still the major pesticide used in California today. In sixteenth-century Japan, poor-quality rendered whale oil was mixed with vinegar and sprayed on paddies and fields to prevent the development of insect larvae by weakening the cuticle. The Chinese applied moderate amounts of arsenic-containing compounds as insecticides in the sixteenth century. As early as 1690, water extracts of tobacco leaves (*Nicotiana tabacum*) were sprayed on plants as insecticides, and nux vomica, the seed of *Strychnos nux-vomica* (strychnine), was introduced to kill rodents. In the mid-1800s, the pulverized root of *Derris eliptica,* containing rotenone, was used as an insecticide, as was pyrethrum extracted from the flowers of the chrysanthemum (*Chrysanthemum cineariaefolum*). In the late 1800s, arsenic trioxide was used as a weed killer, particularly for dandelions. Bordeaux mixture—copper sulfate, lime [$Ca(OH)_2$], and water—was introduced in 1882 to combat vine downy mildew (*Plasmopara viti-*

cola), a disease introduced into France from the United States when phylloxera-resistant vine rootstocks were imported. Sulfuric acid, at a concentration of 10% v/v, was used in the early 1900s to destroy dicotyledonous weeds that would absorb the acid, whereas cereal grains and substitute plants, having a smooth and waxy monocotyledon, were protected. Paris Green (copper arsenite) was introduced to control the Colorado beetle in the late 1800s; calcium arsenate replaced Paris Green and lead arsenate was a major cornerstone in the agriculturalist's armamentarium against insect pests in the early 1900s. By the 1900s, the widespread use of arsenical pesticides caused considerable public concern because some treated fruits and vegetables were found to have toxic residues. Although some of these early pesticides caused only minimal harm to the humans exposed, other agents were exceedingly toxic, and the medical literature of the era is sprinkled with anecdotal reports of poisonings. Looking back over the early years of pesticide development, before the 1930s, it is somewhat surprising to realize just how few pesticides were available (Cremlyn, 1978).

The 1930s ushered in the era of modern synthetic chemistry, including the development of a variety of agents such as alkyl thiocyanate insecticides, dithiiocarbamate fungicides, ethylene dibromide, methyl bromide, and ethylene oxide (Cremlyn, 1978). By the beginning of World War II, there were a number of pesticides, including dichlorodiphenyltrichloroethane (DDT), dinitrocresol, 4-chloro-2-methyloxyacetic acid (MCPA), and 2.4-dichlorophenoxyacetic acid (2,4-D) under experimental investigation, much of this activity being kept under wraps during the war (Kirby, 1980). In the postwar era, there was rapid development in the agrochemical field, with a plethora of insecticides, fungicides, herbicides, and other chemical agents being introduced. In no other field of chemistry has there been such a diversity of structures arising from the application of the principles of chemistry to the mechanism(s) of action in pests to develop selectivity and specificity in agents toward certain species while reducing toxicity to other forms of life.

Despite the modern-day development of second- and third-generation derivatives of the early chemical pesticides, all pesticides possess an inherent degree of toxicity to some living organism, otherwise they would be of no practical use. Unfortunately, the target-species selectivity of pesticides is not as well developed as might be hoped for, and nontarget species frequently are affected because they have physiologic and/or biochemical systems similar to those of the target organisms. There is no such thing as a completely safe pesticide. There are, however, pesticides that can be used safely and/or that present a low level of risk to human health when applied with proper attention to the label's instructions. Despite the current controversy over pesticide use and the presence of low levels of residues in food, groundwater, and air, these agents are integral components of our crop- and health-protection programs. As long as pesticides continue to be used, accidental and/or intentional poisoning of wildlife, domestic stock, and humans can be anticipated and will require treatment.

On a worldwide basis, intoxications attributed to pesticides have been estimated to be as high 3 million cases of acute, severe poisoning annually, with as many or more unreported cases and some 220,000 deaths (WHO, 1990). These estimates suffer from inadequate reporting of data for developing countries, but they may not be too far off the mark. From estimations based on California data, a total of some 25,000 cases of pesticide-related illness occur annually among agricultural workers in that state, with national estimate for the United States as a whole being on the order 80,000 cases per year (Coye et al., 1986). Results from California, a state that uses a vast amount of chemical pesticides, revealed that 1087 occupationally related exposures occurred in 1978. A breakdown of these poisonings by job category, as shown in Fig. 22-1, revealed that ground applicators were at greatest risk, whereas aerial applicators and workers involved in mosquito-abatement programs had the least pesticide-related illness (Kilgore, 1980, 1988). Of 1211 cases of pesticide-related illness reported to California physicians in 1986, a total of 1065 were occupational in nature (Edmiston and Maddy, 1987). However, in other countries, the incidence of poisoning is very low; for example, in the United Kingdom, fewer than 20 agricultural incidents with organophosphates are reported each year (Weir et al., 1992). Such data are not representative of the rest of the agricultural world.

The incidence of poisoning is 13-fold higher in developing countries than in highly industrialized nations, which consume 85 percent of world's pesticide production (Forget, 1989). A recently published proceedings gives a good overview of the situation in developing nations, where there are few regulations controlling the importation, registration, and sale of pesticides (Forget, 1993). Many countries in Central and South America, Africa, and Southeast Asia are becoming "breadbaskets" for countries of more temperate climate, being sources of fresh fruits, vegetables, cut flowers, and so on in the off-season, since they are capable of growing two or three crops of export produce each year. Figure 22-2 shows the quantities of pesticidal active ingredients used in a number of countries in 1994 (UN FAO, 1994). A more complete listing can be found in O'Malley (1997). In developed countries, more herbicides are used than any other class of pesticides, whereas in tropical, developing nations, there is a predominant use of insecticides. As other developing nations explore the global export produce market, pesticide consumption—now around 3000 to 10,000 metric tons—will increase dramatically. Most developing nations have yet

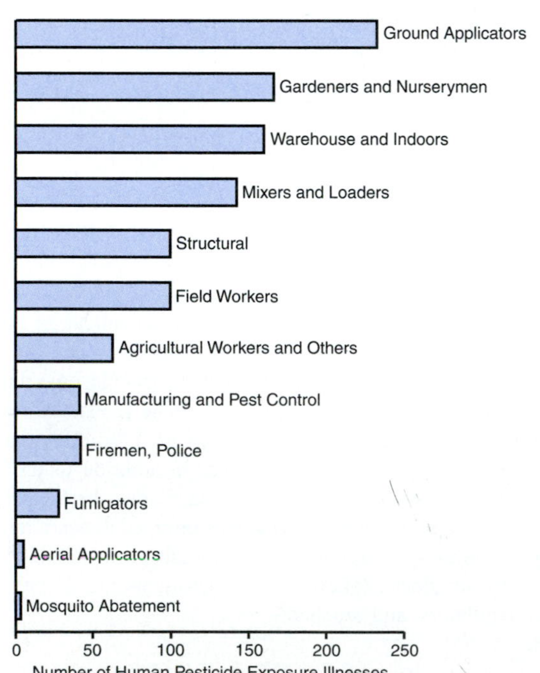

Figure 22-1. Frequency of pesticide poisoning related to occupation and potential for exposure. [From the records of the California Department of Public Health (Kilgore, 1988)].

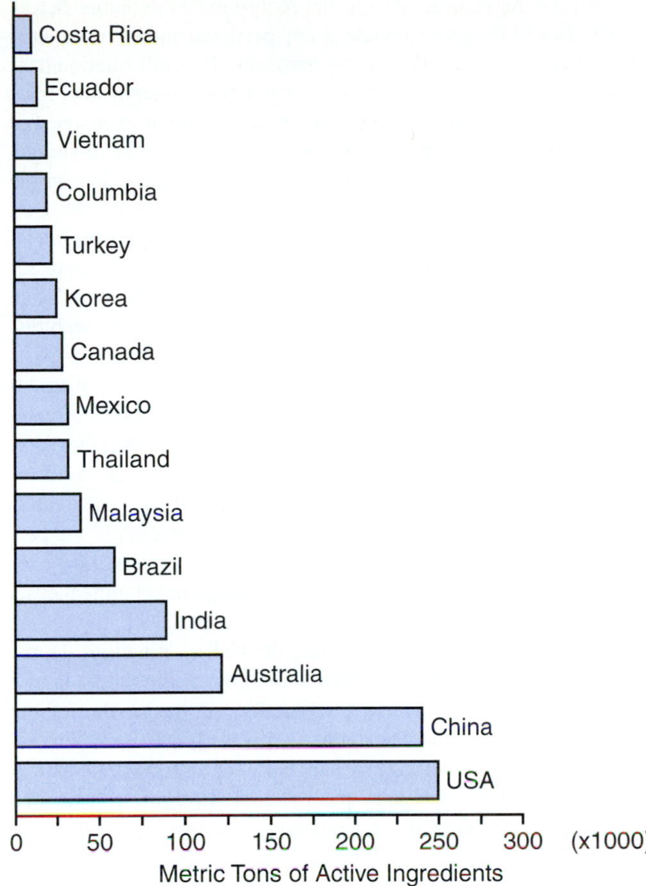

Figure 22-2. Quantities of pesticides (active ingredients) used in representative countries around the world in 1994. (From O'Malley, 1997, with permission.)

to develop stringent "philosophies" concerning pesticide control and usage (Mbiapo and Youovop, 1993).

Most pesticide-related poisonings in developing nations can be attributed to inexperience with such chemicals, negligible training in their use, and the absence of appropriate personal protective equipment. In 1983 in Thailand, 117 incidents per 100,000 agricultural workers were reported for compensation claims by companies having more than 20 employees; by comparison, hospital admissions/deaths due to pesticide poisonings totaled 8268 per 100,000 individual farmers, cooperative members, and workers for small companies (Boon-Long et al., 1986). In 1981 in Sri Lanka, approximately 10,000 to 13,000 persons were admitted to hospitals for acute poisoning annually, with almost 1000 deaths (Jeyaratnam, 1993; Jeyaratnam et al., 1982). In Taiwan, for the years 1985 to 1993, some 7386 out of a total of 23,436 chemical-related poisonings involved pesticides (Yang et al., 1996). In Costa Rica in 1996, some 920 out of a total of 1274 pesticide-related poisonings were due to occupational or accidental exposure (Leveridge, 1998). Poisonings by organophosphorus and carbamate insecticides represented 38.5 percent of the total (438 out of 1274), while only 8 intoxications were associated with organochlorine insecticides (Leveridge, 1998). None of the above values included affected individuals who either did not seek medical attention or could not afford the time away from work to do so.

No one can doubt the efficacy of pesticides for the protection of crops in the field, thereby providing us with abundant, inexpensive, wholesome, and attractive fruits and vegetables. It has been estimated that in 1830 it took 58 person-hours to tend and harvest an acre of grain, whereas today it takes approximately 2 person-hours (Kirby, 1980). Over this time period, the price of cereal grain has not risen proportionally to the costs of the labor to produce it. Along with improved strains of crops, an important role in crop improvements and yields has been played by insecticides, fungicides, and herbicides. Even with such advances, it is estimated that up to 50 percent of harvested crops can be damaged by postharvest infestation by insects, fungi, rodents, and the like (Table 22-1).

The medical miracles accomplished by pesticides have been documented: the suppression of a typhus epidemic in Naples, Italy, by DDT in the winter of 1943–1944 (Brooks, 1974); the control of river blindness (onchocerciasis) in West Africa by killing of the insect vector (black fly) carrying the filariae for this disease (WHO, 1977; Calamari et al., 1988); and the control of malaria in Africa, the Middle East, and Asia by elimination of the plasmodium-bearing mosquito populations with a variety of insecticides (Matsumura, 1985). There is still a great need for advancement in the control of disease vector with pesticides: 600 million people are at risk from schistosomiasis in the Middle East and Asia; 200 million suffer from filariasis in tropical Africa, Asia, Indonesia, and the Caribbean region; 20 million people in tropical Africa, the Middle East, Mexico, and Guatemala are infected by the filarium causing onchocerciasis; and 1000 million people worldwide harbor pathologic intestinal worm infestations (Albert, 1987). Although the benefits of pesticides are recognized by those who re-

Table 22-1
Worldwide Harvest Losses in Five Important Crops

CROP	POTENTIAL HARVEST (1000 TONS)	HARVEST 1978 (1000 TONS)	*Losses Through* WEEDS %	DISEASES %	INSECTS %
Rice	715,800	378,645	10.6	9.0	27.5
Maize	563,016	362,582	13.0	9.6	13.0
Wheat	578,400	437,236	9.8	9.5	5.1
Sugarcane	1,603,200	737,483	15.1	19.4	19.5
Cotton	63,172	41,757	5.8	12.1	16.0

SOURCE: GIFAP: International Group of National Association of Agrochemical Manufacturers. Brussels. *GIFAP Bulletin*, vol 12, March/April 1986.

quire them, certain parts of the world are experiencing an environmentalist- and media-evoked backlash toward all pesticide use because of the carelessness, misuse, and/or abuse of some agents by a relatively few individuals in a limited number of well-publicized incidents. Without bearing any direct responsibility for planning or involvement in health care or food or fiber production, some environmental and consumer advocacy groups propose a total ban on pesticide use. Between the two extremes of overwhelming use and total ban lies a position advocating the careful and rational use of the beneficial chemicals.

REGULATORY MANDATE

The widespread use and misuse of the early, toxic pesticides created an awareness of the potential health hazards posed by them and the need to protect the consumer from residues in foods. It was not until 1906 that the Wiley or Sherman Act was passed, creating the first Federal Food and Drugs Act. This was replaced by the Federal Food, Drug and Cosmetic Act (FDCA) in 1938, with specific pesticide amendments being passed in 1954 and 1958; these required that pesticide tolerances be established for all agricultural commodities. The 1958 amendment contained the famous Delaney clause (Section 409), which states that "no additive shall be deemed safe if it is found to induce cancer when ingested by man or animal or, if it is found, after tests which are appropriate for the evaluation of the safely of food additives, to induce cancer in man or animals" (National Academy of Sciences, 1987). It should be noted that the Delaney clause does not require proof of carcinogenicity in humans. Pesticides fall under this "additive" legislation.

The Federal Insecticide, Fungicide, and Rodenticide Act (FIFRA) was originally passed by Congress in 1947 as a labeling statute that would group all pest control products—initially only insecticides, fungicides, rodenticides, and herbicides—under one law to be administered by the U.S. Department of Agriculture (USDA). Amendments in 1959 and 1961 added nematicides, plant growth regulators, defoliants, and desiccants to FIFRA jurisdiction, plus the authorizations to deny, suspend, or cancel registrations of products, although it assured the registrant's right to appeal. In 1972, FIFRA was reorganized and administrative authority was turned over to the newly formed Environmental Protection Agency (EPA). The new law, along with subsequent amendments in 1975, 1978, 1980, and 1984, defines the registration requirements and appropriate chemical, toxicologic, and environmental impact studies, label specifications, use restrictions, tolerances for pesticide residues on raw agricultural products, and the responsibility to monitor pesticide residue levels in foods. FIFRA is not all-encompassing because the Food and Drug Administration (FDA) retains the basic responsibility for both monitoring residue levels and for seizure of foods not in compliance with the regulations; what is more, the USDA continues to be the authority responsible for the monitoring of meat and poultry for pesticides as well as for other chemicals. The Food Quality Protection Act (FQPA), passed by the U.S. Congress in 1996, amended federal laws regarding pesticides to give special consideration for children by (1) providing additional protection when allowable levels of pesticides for foods are set (data providing children's food consumption patterns, recognition of all possible routes of exposure in risk assessment); and (2) considering whether infants and children are disproportionally susceptible to pesticides. Where data on the pesticides are not adequate, pesticide tolerances for children must incorporate an additional 10-fold safety factor.

FIFRA regulations set out the requirements essential before EPA-Office of Programs review of any pesticide and/or formulated product can occur for registration purposes. This information base includes product and residue chemistry, environmental fate, toxicology, biotransformation/degradation, occupational exposure and reentry protection, spray drift, environmental impact on nontarget species, and product performance and efficacy. Depending on the proposed use pattern of the pesticide, results from different "groups" or toxicologic studies are required to support the registration. The typical spectrum of basic pesticide toxicity data required under FIFRA regulations is summarized in Table 22-2. Extensive ancillary studies of environmental impact on birds, mammals, aquatic organisms, plants, soils, environmental persistence, and bioaccumulation are also required. A schematic diagram showing the "information package" required in support of a registration and the appropriate time span required to develop this database—from the point of patenting the newly synthesized chemical until its registration, production, marketing, and user acceptability—is shown in Fig. 22-3. Although the ultimate uses of the particular chemical will govern the extent of the information base required prior to registration, estimates of average development costs on the order of \$30 to \$80 million are not unrealistic.

Other nations including Canada, the United Kingdom, Japan, and, more recently, the European Economic Community (EEC) have promulgated harmonizing legislation similar to that of the United States as safeguards in human exposure to pesticides in food commodities. Some developing nations, with a shortage of trained technical, scientific, and legal professionals to develop their own legislation, have adopted the regulatory framework of one or another of the industrialized nations, permitting the sale and use of

Table 22-2

Basic Requirements Regarding Toxicity Data for New Pesticide Registrations

Acute	
Oral (rat)	
Dermal (rabbit)	
Inhalation (usually rat)	
Irritation studies	
Eye (rabbit)	
Skin (rabbit, guinea pig)	
Dermal sensitization (guinea pig)	
Delayed neurotoxicity (hen)	
Subchronic	
90-Day feeding study	
Rodent (rat, mouse)	
Nonrodent (dog)	
Dermal	Dependent upon use pattern and potential for occupational exposure
Inhalation	
Neurotoxicity	
Chronic	
One- or two-year oral study	
Rodent (usually rat)	
Nonrodent (dog)	
Oncogenicity study (rat or mouse)	
Reproductive	
In vitro mutagenicity (microorganisms, etc.)	
Fertility/reproduction (rat, mouse, rabbit)	
Teratogenicity (rat, mouse, rabbit)	

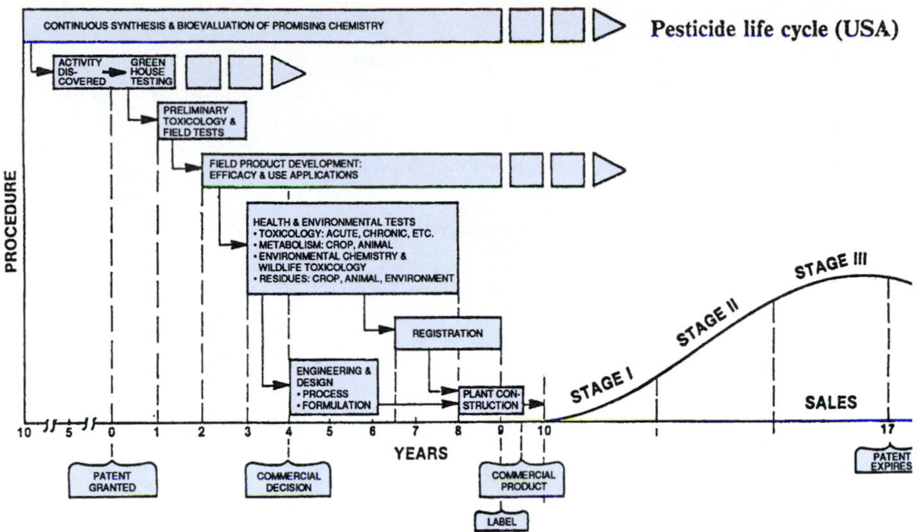

Figure 22-3. A schematic diagram depicting the generation of an appropriate toxicity database, the time frame for data acquisition and the significant milestones in the life cycle of a pesticide in the United States. Stages I to III represent the sales of the pesticide once the commercial product enters the marketplace. (GI-FAP Bulletin, Sept. 1983, with permission.)

pesticides registered under the legislation of that country but prohibiting the use of agents unable to meet the stringent requirements. In still other countries, almost any pesticide ever manufactured is available, no legislation having been introduced to curb adverse effects to the environment and human health.

Exposure

The evaluation of the hazards of pesticides to human health begins with the development of a dose-effect relationship based on documented and anecdotal information on human exposure (Fig. 22-4). Several populations of individuals may be identified as having exposure to a range of concentrations of a particular agent, including: (1) accidental and/or suicidal poisonings that no amount of legislation or study can prevent; (2) occupational (manufacturing, mixing/loading, application, harvesting, and handling of crops) exposure (Albertson and Cross, 1993; Edmiston and Maddy, 1987); (3) bystander exposure to off-target drift from spraying operations with, in some cases, the development of hypersensitivity (Bartle, 1991); (4) the general public who consume food items containing pesticide residues as a consequence of the illegal use of an agent (e.g., aldicarb on melons and cucumbers) or its misuse, in terms of an incorrect application rate or picking and shipping a crop too soon after pesticide application, resulting in residue concentrations above established tolerance levels. The media are replete with documented incidents of environmental contamination by pesticides: (1) of surface and/or groundwater essential as sources of potable drinking water; (2) of commercial fish stock as well as sporting fish; (3) of wildlife upon which native peoples depend as a major source of dietary protein; and (4) of long-distance aerial transport of undeposited and/or revolatilized pesticide.

The shape of the dose-effect curve is dependent on a detailed knowledge of the amount of exposure received by each of these groups. Within each group, variability will be considerable. Frequently, exposure evaluations begin at the top of the relationship where exposure is greatest, more easily estimated, and, in most cases, the acute biological effects are clearly observed and may be associated with a specific agent or a class of chemicals over a relatively narrow dosage range. If no discernible adverse health effects are seen at high levels of exposure, it is unlikely that anything will be observed at lower levels of exposure. Although this hypothesis may be true for acute systemic effects, it is not applicable to chronic effects (changes in organ function, mutagenicity, teratogenicity, carcinogenicity) that may develop after some latent period following either a single high-level exposure, repeated moderate or high-level exposure, or annual exposure to low levels of the agents for decades.

There is sufficiently detailed documentation on many pesticidal poisonings to permit an estimation of exposure (Hayes, 1982). In some 48 suicide attempts by ingestion of the herbicide glyphosate, the average volume of product (concentrate containing active ingredient and a surfactant) ingested was 120 mL [range of 104 mL (nonfatal) to 206 mL (fatal)] (Swada et al., 1988). In other cases, such as one involving the insecticide fenitrothion, where the individual experienced dermal exposure to a 7.5% solution of the agent in corn oil wiped up with facial tissues by a bare hand, exposure was more difficult to assess (Ecobichon et al., 1977). It is imperative that forensic and clinical toxicologists and emergency service personnel attempt to ascertain how much of the material was involved in the poisoning.

Worker exposure can be estimated within reason by considering the various job functions performed (e.g., diluting concentrated formulations, loading diluted end-use formulations into tanks, spray application, harvesting sprayed crops, postharvest handling of sprayed crops, etc.). The potential level(s) of pesticide encountered in each job category and the route(s) of exposure can be estimated. The majority of occupational illnesses arising from pesticides involve dermal exposure enhanced, in certain job categories, by acquisition of a portion of the dosage by the inhalation of the aerosolized spray. Many exposures appear to be entirely dermal in character (Vercruysse et al., 1999). The surface areas of the unclothed parts of the body of an unprotected worker are shown in

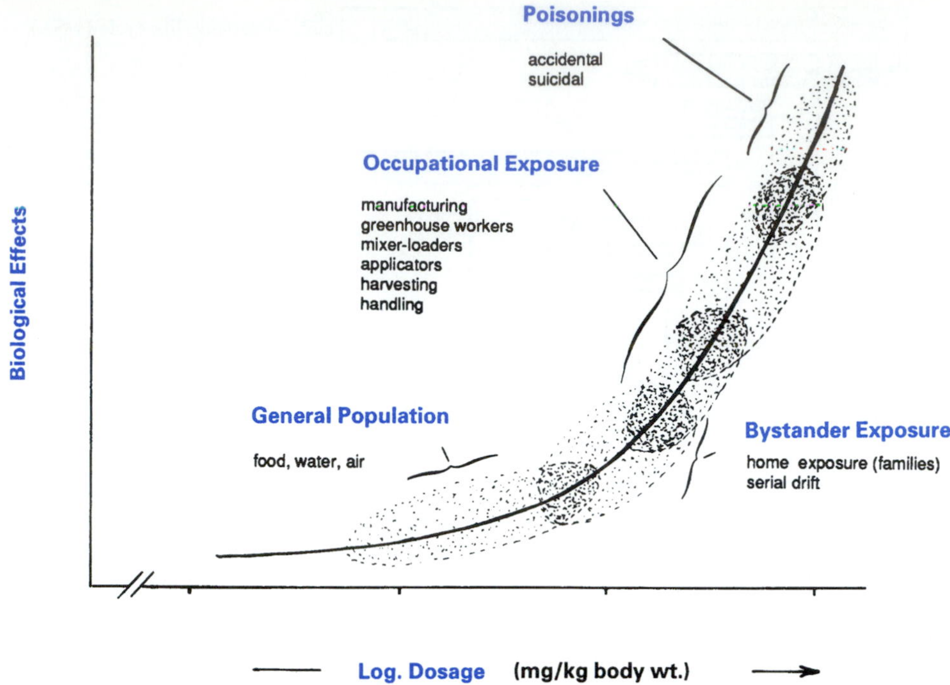

Figure 22-4. A theoretical dose–effect relationship for acute toxicity, comparing the potential for exposure in terms of occupation, level of exposure and possible biological effects.

Table 22-3, being derived from the U.S. EPA (1987). Data for the entire surface area of a "50 percentile man," as determined by Spear and coworkers (1977), are shown in Table 22-4. With surface patch (gauze, fabric) testing on various parts of the body, accurate estimates of dermal exposure can be obtained. The reader is referred to the following studies for details: Wolfe and colleagues (1967, 1972), Wojeck and coworkers (1981), and Franklin and coworkers (1981). Where inhalation can be considered to contribute significantly to the total exposure, as in greenhouse and other structural spraying operations in enclosed environments, drivers in tractor cabs, operators of rotary fan mist sprayers, and other operations, measurements of aerial concentrations in the working environment can be made and related to respiratory rates and length of time spent in that environment. Assessment of the inhalation component of an exposure can be obtained with personal air sampling monitors worn during the day (Trumbull et al., 1985; Grover et al., 1986).

In the past, direct exposure was estimated by measuring deposition (on skin, clothing, or surrogate patch) or by ambient air concentrations of the potentially toxic agent (Durham and Wolfe, 1962). In reality, direct exposure should be attributed only to pesticide residues gaining entry into the body by systemic absorption following ingestion, inhalation, and/or transdermal penetration. Total exposure can be estimated by measuring excretory products (the parent chemical, degradation products) in urine and feces over a suitable postexposure time interval (Durham et al., 1972; Kolmodin-Hedmann et al., 1983; Frank et al., 1985; Grover et al., 1986; Takamiya, 1994; Azaroff, 1999). Potential biological effects of exposure can be monitored, including plasma and erythrocytic cholinesterase measurements, δ-aminolevulinic dehydratase (ALAD), superoxide dismutase (SOD) activities, cytogenic analy-

Table 22-3
Estimated Surface Area of Exposed Portions of a Body of a Casually Dressed Individual

UNCLOTHED SURFACE	SURFACE AREA (SQ FT)	PERCENT OF TOTAL
Face	0.70	22.0
Hands	0.87	27.6
Forearms	1.30	41.3
Back of neck	0.12	3.8
Front of neck and "v" of chest	0.16	5.1

SOURCE: Batchelor and Walker, 1954.

Table 22-4
Percent of Total Body Surface Area Represented by Body Regions*

BODY REGION	SURFACE AREA (% OF TOTAL)
Head	5.60
Neck	1.20
Upper arms	9.70
Forearms	6.70
Hands	6.90
Chest, back, shoulders	22.80
Hips	9.10
Thighs	18.00
Calves	13.50
Feet	6.40

*Estimated proportions from the "50 percentile man" having a surface area of 1.92 m^2, height of 175 cm, and body weight of 78 kg.

SOURCE: Spear et al., 1977.

sis of lymphocytic micronuclei, semen quality, fertility, etc. (Lopez-Carillo and Lopez-Cervantes, 1993; Ciesielski et al., 1994; Davies et al., 1998; Panemangalore et al., 1998; Venegas et al., 1998; Larsen et al., 1999). A more complete discussion of the topic of occupational exposure can be found in Ecobichon (1998a).

Minimal protection of certain parts of the body can markedly reduce exposure to an agent. Protection of the hands (5.6 percent of the body surface) by appropriate chemical-resistant gloves may reduce contamination by 33 percent (in forest spraying with a knapsack sprayer having a single-nozzle lance), by 66 percent (in weed control using tractor-mounted booms equipped with hydraulic nozzles), or by 86 percent (involving filling tanks on tractor-powered sprayers) (Bdonsall, 1985). Studies monitoring the absorption of pesticides applied to the skin of different areas of the human body have revealed marked regional variations in per cutaneous absorption, with the greatest uptake being in the scrotal region, followed by the axilla, forehead, face, scalp, the dorsal aspect of the hand, the palm of the hand, and the forearm in decreasing order (Feldman and Maiback, 1974).

The exposure of a bystander, where an individual is accidentally sprayed directly or exposed to aerial off-target drifting aerosol, is considerably more difficult to assess. The levels encountered may be severalfold lower than those in the occupational setting, making the analysis of residue and the detection of meaningful biological changes more difficult. Greater variation in exposure estimates and biological effects can be anticipated. The adverse health effects may be subtle in appearance and nonspecific, reflecting a slow deterioration of physiologic function clouded by the individual's adjustment or adaptation to the changes, taking many years to develop to the point of detection. The identification of pesticide-related adverse health effects in the general population, who inadvertently acquire low levels of pesticides daily via food and water, is extremely difficult. The residue levels in these media are often orders of magnitude lower than those encountered in occupational or bystander exposure and are at or near the limits of analytical detection by sophisticated techniques. Any biological effects resulting from such low-level exposure are unlikely to be distinctive and any causal association with a particular chemical or class of agents is likely to be tenuous and confounded by many other factors of a given lifestyle.

Many of the public concerns about pesticides are related to "older" chemicals, these having entered the market in the 1950s and 1960s without the benefit of the extensive toxicity and environmental impact studies demanded prior to the registration of chemicals today. It must also be pointed out that many of these older pesticides have received little reassessment using the more definitive techniques and protocols required today. Although government agencies and industry have been slow in their reevaluation of a vast array of pesticides in use, reassessment often comes in the wake of or concomitant with some recently disclosed adverse environmental or health effect. Given the above-mentioned costs of conducting a full range of studies (introductory section, this chapter), the time frame required, and the limited market for some of these chemicals in North America or even worldwide, the registration of many of these pesticides will be withdrawn voluntarily by industry, and the answers to some of the public's concerns will never be obtained. Hazardous chemicals will be removed from use but, unfortunately, it is possible that some very beneficial and essential pesticides will be lost. The problems of today's situation, created by the last generation and inherited by the present one, still must be dealt with.

INSECTICIDES

The literature pertaining to the chemistry and development of the various classes of insecticides over the past 45 years is extensive and the reader is referred to the monographs of O'Brien (1960, 1967), Melnikov (1971), Fest and Schmidt (1973), Brooks (1974), Eto (1974), Hayes (1982), Kuhr and Dorough (1976), Buchel (1983), Leahey (1985), Chambers and Levi (1992), and Ecobichon and Joy (1994) for detailed discussions of the chemistry, nomenclature (chemical, common, and trade names), biotransformation and degradation, and environmental effects as well as target and nontarget species toxicity. Compilations of LD_{50} values in the laboratory rat may be found in Gaines (1969), Frear (1969), and Worthing (1987). Acute toxicity data for laboratory animals, fish, and wildlife are recorded in a number of reports (Pickering et al., 1962; Tucker and Crabtree, 1970; Worthing, 1987). Several compilations of pesticide monographs exist, giving brief but succinct profiles of the physical and chemical properties of various pesticides as well as their environmental persistence and toxicity to wildlife, domestic animals, and humans (Kamrin, 1997; Montgomery, 1997; Tomlin, 1997). Only selected examples of the classes of insecticides are discussed in this chapter, with emphasis on their toxicity to humans.

All of the chemical insecticides in use today are neurotoxicants and act by poisoning the nervous systems of the target organisms. The central nervous system (CNS) of insects is highly developed and not unlike that of the mammal (O'Brien, 1960). While the peripheral nervous system (PNS) of insects is not as complex as that of mammals, there are striking similarities (O'Brien, 1960). The development of insecticides has been based on specific structure-activity relationships requiring the manipulation of a basic chemical structure to obtain an optimal shape and configuration for specificity toward a unique biochemical or physiologic feature of the nervous system. Given the fact that insecticides are not selective and affect nontarget species as readily as target organisms, it is not surprising that a chemical that acts on the insect's nervous system will elicit similar effects in higher forms of life. The target sites and/or mechanism(s) of action may be similar in all species; only the dosage (level of exposure and duration) will dictate the intensity of biological effects. It is sufficient at this stage to indicate the potential sites of action of the insecticide classes (Fig. 22-5) and their interference with the membrane transport of sodium, potassium, calcium, or chloride ions; inhibition of selective enzymatic activities; or contribution to the release and/or the persistence of chemical transmitters at nerve endings.

Organochlorine Compounds

No longer considered an important class of insecticides in North America and Europe, the organochlorine insecticides see continued use in developing, tropical countries because they are effective, inexpensive, essential chemicals in agriculture, forestry, structural protection, and public health. The risk-benefit ratio is highly weighted in favor of their continued use for the control of insects causing devastation to crops and human health. For example, technical-grade hexachlorocyclohexane (HCH), banned in Canada, the United States, China, the Soviet Union, and Australia in 1971, 1976, 1983, 1990 and 1994, respectively, still sees extensive use in a number of African nations, Brazil, India, and others (Li, 1999). While banned in the early 1970s, DDT was still being manufactured in the United States and exported at the rate of 1 ton per day

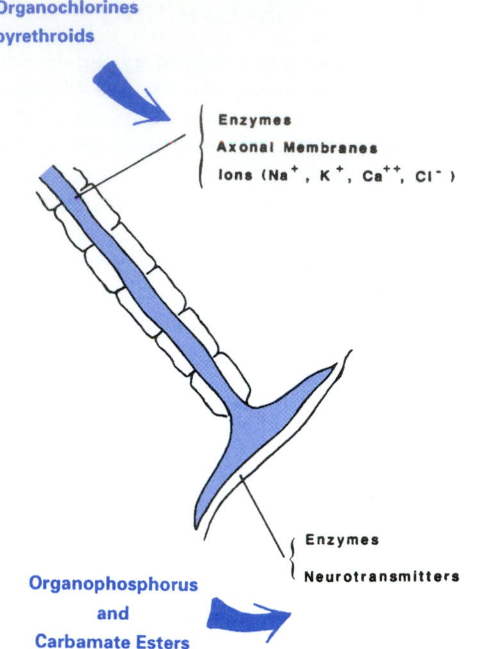

Figure 22-5. Potential sites of action of classes of insecticides on the axon and terminal portions of the nerve.

in 1994 (Smith, 1995). Global transport of such chemicals from equatorial regions to Arctic and Antarctic regions, with contamination of wildlife food sources, suggests that these agents are still toxicologically important. Currently, major concerns are centered on the indigenous people living in Arctic regions, where the sources of dietary protein (fish, seals, walruses, whales, etc.) have proven to be major depositories of organochlorine insecticides and other chlorinated hydrocarbons (PCBs, PBBs, PCDDs, PSDFs) (Berti et al., 1998; Chan, 1998).

The properties (low volatility, chemical stability, lipid solubility, slow rate of biotransformation and degradation) that made these chemicals such effective insecticides also brought about their demise because of their persistence in the environment, bioconcentration and biomagnification in food chains, and the acquisition of biologically active body burdens at higher trophic levels (Carson, 1962). Definitive studies in wild, domestic, and laboratory species demonstrated potent enzyme-inducing and/or estrogenic properties, with interference indirectly or directly with fertility and reproduction (Stickel, 1968; McFarland and Lacy, 1969; Peakall, 1970; Longcore et al., 1971; McBlain et al., 1977; Crum et al., 1993).

The organochlorine (chlorinated hydrocarbon) insecticides are a diverse group of agents belonging to three distinct chemical classes including the dichlorodiphenylethane-, chlorinated cyclodiene- and chlorinated benzene- and cyclohexane-related structures (Table 22-5). The historical development of these chemicals from the mid-1940s and their impact on agriculture and human health can be found in O'Brien (1967), Metcalf (1973), and Brooks (1974).

Signs and Symptoms of Poisoning Given the diversity of chemical structures, it is not surprising that the signs and symptoms of toxicity and the mechanisms of action are somewhat different (Table 22-6).

Exposure of humans and animals to high oral doses of DDT results in paresthesia of the tongue, lips, and face; apprehension; hypersusceptibilty to external (light, touch, sound) stimuli; irritability, dizziness, and vertigo; tremor and tonic and clonic convulsions. Motor unrest and fine tremors associated with voluntary movements progress to coarse tremors without interruption in moderate to severe poisonings. Symptoms generally appear several hours (6 to 24 h) after exposure to large doses. Little toxicity is seen following the dermal exposure to DDT, presumably because the agent is poorly absorbed through the skin, a physiologic phenomenon that has contributed to the fairly good safety record of DDT despite careless handling by applicators and formulators (Hayes, 1971). It has been estimated that a dose of 10 mg/kg will cause signs of poisoning in humans. Chronic exposure to moderate concentrations of DDT causes somewhat milder signs to toxicity, as listed in Table 22-6.

Table 22-5
Structural Classification of Organochlorine Insecticides

Class	Structure	Examples
Dichlorodiphenylethanes	Cl—(ring)—CH—(ring)—Cl, —C—	DDT, DDD Dicofol Perthane Methoxychlor Methlochlor
Cyclodienes	Cl, Cl, C(CCl)$_2$, Cl, Cl, Cl	Aldrin, Dieldrin Heptachlor Chlordane Endosulfan
Chlorinated benzenes Cyclohexanes	(Cl)$_6$; Cl, Cl, Cl, Cl, Cl, Cl	HCB, HCH Lindane (α-BHC)

Table 22-6
Signs and Symptoms of Acute and Chronic Toxicity Following Exposure to Organochlorine Insecticides

INSECTICIDE CLASS	ACUTE SIGNS	CHRONIC SIGNS
Dichlorodiphenylethanes		
DDT	Parethesia (oral ingestion)	Loss of weight, anorexia
DDD (Rothane)	Ataxia, abnormal stepping	Mild anemia
DMC (Dimite)	Dizziness, confusion, headache	Tremors
Dicofol (Kelthane)	Nausea, vomiting	Muscular weakness
Methoxychlor	Fatigue, lethargy	EEG pattern changes
Methiochlor	Tremor (peripheral)	Hyperexcitability, anxiety
Chlorbenzylate		Nervous tension
Hexachlorocyclohexanes		
Lindane (γ-isomer)		
Benzene hexachloride (mixed isomers)		
Cyclodienes		
Endrin	Dizziness, headache	Headache, dizziness, hyperexcitability
Telodrin	Nausea, vomiting	Intermittent muscle twitching and myoclonic jerking
Isodrin	Motor hyperexcitability	Psychological disorders including insomnia, anxiety, irritability
Endosulfan	Hyperreflexia	EEG pattern changes
Heptachlor	Myoclonic jerking	Loss of consciousness
Aldrin	General malaise	Epileptiform convulsions
Dieldrin	Convulsive seizures	
Chlordane	Generalized convulsions	
Toxaphene		
Chlordecone (Kepone)		Chest pains, arthralgia
Mirex		Skin rashes
		Ataxia, incoordination, slurred speech, opsoclonus
		Visual difficulty, inability to focus and fixate
		Nervousness, irritability, depression
		Loss of recent memory
		Muscle weakness, tremors of hands
		Severe impairment of spermatogenesis

Although the functional injury of DDT poisoning can be associated with effects on the CNS in humans, few pathologic changes can be demonstrated in CNS tissue in animals. However, following exposure to moderate or high nonfatal doses or subsequent to subacute or chronic feeding, major pathologic changes are observed in the liver and reproductive organs. Morphologic changes in mammalian liver include hypertrophy of hepatocytes and subcellular organelles such as mitochondria, proliferation of smooth endoplasmic reticulum and the formation of inclusion bodies, centrolobular necrosis following exposure to high concentrations, and an increase in the incidence of hepatic tumors (Hayes, 1959; Hansell and Ecobichon, 1974; IARC, 1974). However, there has yet to be conclusive epidemiologic evidence linking DDT to carcinogenicity in humans (Hayes, 1982; Baris et al., 1998; Takayama et al., 1999). When technical-grade DDT (20 percent *o,p′*-DDT plus 80 percent *p,p′*-DDT) was administered to male cockerels or rats, reduced testicular size was observed and, in female rats, the estrogenic effects of the *o,p′*-isomer were observed in the edematous, blood-engorged uteri (Hayes, 1959; Ecobichon and MacKenzie, 1974). The *o,p′*-isomer has been shown to compete with estradiol for binding the estrogen receptors in rat uterine cytosol (Kupfer and Bulger, 1976). The DDT analog methoxychlor [1,1,1-trichloro-2,2-bis(4-methoxyphenyl) ethane] is estrogenic in the mouse; problems in initiating and/or maintaining a pregnancy are seen, due possibly to alterations in preimplantation embryonic development and estrogenic effects on the oviduct and uterus (Hall et al., 1997; Swartz and Eroschenko, 1998).

Dicofol (*p-p′*-dichlorodiphenyl-2,2,2-trichloroethanol)—an analog of DDT still registered as an agricultural miticide for cotton, beans, citrus, and grapes—has been associated with acute toxicity (nausea, dizziness, double vision, ataxia, confusion, disorientation) in a 12-year-old male whose clothing because saturated in an accident (Lessenger and Riley, 1991). These acute effects progressed to chronic signs (headaches, blurred vision, horizontal nystagmus, numbness/tingling in the legs with shooting pains, clumsiness, memory loss and decreasing academic performance, impulsive behavior, restlessness and fatigue), which persisted in some fashion for up to 4 months. Continuing emotional and academic difficulties, impairment of certain cognitive skills, poor self-esteem and depression, all of which were subtle cognitive and psychological changes, persisted for over 18 months. Dicofol is known to be contaminated by a small percentage of *p-p′*-DDT, showing estrogenicity in birds (Peakall, 1970).

Unlike the situation with DDT, in which there have been few recorded fatalities following poisoning, there have been a number of fatalities following poisoning by the cyclodiene- and hexachlorocyclohexane-type insecticides. The chlorinated cyclodiene insecticides are among the most toxic and environmentally persistent pesticides known (Hayes, 1982). One recent study of two patients, one with a history of chronic exposure to aldrin and the other with a chronic exposure to lindane/heptachlor, reported death within 2 years of developing clinical and electromyographic signs and symptoms of chronic motor disease with aggravation of dysphagia and weight loss resulting in the mobilization of adipose tissue and stored insecticide to enhance the neuronal toxicity (Fonseca et al., 1993). Even at low doses, these chemicals tend to induce convulsions before less serious signs of illness occur. Although the sequence of signs generally follows the appearance of headaches, nausea, vertigo, and mild clonic jerking, motor hyperexcitability, and hyperreflexia, some patients have convulsions without warning symptoms (Hayes, 1982). An important difference between DDT and the chlorinated cyclodienes is that the latter are efficiently absorbed through the skin and therefore pose an appreciable hazard to occupationally exposed individuals. Chronic exposure to low or moderate concentrations of these agents elicits a spectrum of signs and symptoms, involving both sensory and motor components of the CNS (Table 22-6). In addition to the recognized neurotoxicity, aldrin and dieldrin interfere with reproduction, with increased pup losses (vitality, viability) being reported in studies in rats and dogs (Kitselman, 1953; Treon and Cleveland 1955). Treatment with dieldrin during pregnancy caused a reduction in fertility and increased pup mortality (Treon and Cleveland, 1955). The treatment of pregnant mice with dieldrin resulted in teratologic effects (delayed ossification, increases in supernumerary ribs) (Chernoff et al., 1975).

Exposure to lindane (the γ-isomer of hexachlorocyclohexane, HCH) produces signs of poisoning that resemble those caused by DDT (e.g., tremors, ataxia, convulsions, stimulated respiration, and prostration). In severe cases of acute poisoning, violent tonic and clinic convulsions occur and degenerative changes in the liver and renal tubules have been noted. Technical-grade HCH used in insecticidal preparations contains a mixture of isomers: the γ- and α-isomer are convulsant poisons; the β- and δ-isomers are CNS depressants. The mechanisms of action remain unknown. Lifetime feeding studies in mice have revealed that technical-grade HCH and some of the isomers caused an increase in hepatocellular tumors (IARC, 1974). Only the γ-isomer (lindane) sees any medicinal use today, as a component of a pediculicide shampoo for head lice. One undocumented case of lindane toxicity, known to the author, resulted in mild tremors in a child on whose head the shampoo was used vigorously and repeatedly for more than a week. The symptoms disappeared rapidly when the treatment was terminated.

Industrial carelessness during the manufacture of an organochlorine compound chlordecone (Kepone) brought this agent and mirex, the closely related insecticide, to the attention of toxicologists in 1975, when 76 of 148 workers in a factory in Hopewell, Virginia, developed a severe neurologic syndrome (Cannon et al., 1978; Taylor et al., 1978; Guzelian, 1982). This condition, known as the "Kepone shakes," was characterized by tremors, altered gait, behavioral changes, ocular flutter (opsoclonus), arthralgia, headache, chest pains, weight loss, hepatomegaly, splenomegaly, and impotence, the onset of symptoms generally occurring with a latency of approximately 30 days from the initiation of exposure and persisting for many months after the termination of exposure (Joy, 1994a). Laboratory tests showed a reduced sperm count and reduced sperm motility. Routine neurologic studies showed nothing untoward, but microscopic examination of biopsies of the sural nerve revealed relative decreases in the populations of small myelinated and unmyelinated axons. With electron microscopy, a number of abnormalities were visible; the significant findings included damage to Schwann cells (membranous inclusions, cytoplasmic folds), prominent endoneural collagen pockets, vacuolization of unmyelinated fibers, focal degeneration of axons with condensations of neurofilaments and neurotubules, focal interlamellar splitting of myelin sheaths, and the formation of myelin bodies and a complex infolding of inner mesaxonal membranes into axoplasm (Martinez et al., 1977). The involvement of unmyelinated fibers and small myelinated fibers may partially explain the clinical picture. It has been suggested that chlordecone may interfere with metabolic processes in Schwann cells. However, it should be noted that all of these degenerative changes are nonspecific in nature and are commonly seen in other toxic polyneuropathies. Many of the toxic manifestations of chlordecone poisoning in these workers have been confirmed in animal studies, the major target organs being the CNS, liver, adrenals, and testes, as summarized by Joy (1994a). As with other organochlorine insecticides, chlordecone is an excellent inducer of hepatic microsomal monooxygenase enzymes and, in rats and mice, has been associated with the formation of hepatomas and malignant tumors in organs other than the liver, female animals being more susceptible than male (Guzelian, 1982). In many ways, mirex behaves like chlordecone, and there is evidence for the oxidative biotransformation of mirex to chlordecone in vivo. Mirex causes hepatomegaly and a dose-dependent increase in neoplastic nodules and hepatocellular carcinomas, particularly in male animals (Innes et al., 1969; Waters et al., 1977).

Site and Mechanism of Toxic Actions Essential to the action of organochlorine insecticides is an intact reflex are consisting of afferent (sensory) peripheral neurons impinging on interneurons in the spinal cord, with accompanying ramifications and interconnections up and down the CNS and interactions with efferent motor neurons, as shown schematically in Fig. 22-6. In terms of the mechanism of action of the DDT-type insecticides, the most striking observation in a poisoned insect or mammal is the display of periodic sequences of persistent tremoring and/or convulsive seizures suggestive of repetitive discharges in neurons. These characteristic episodes of hyperactivity interspersed with normal function were recognized as early as 1946. The second most striking observation is that these repetitive tremors, seizures, and electrical activity can be initiated by tactile and auditory stimuli, suggesting that the sensory nervous system appears to be much more responsive to stimuli. An examination of the sequence of electrical events in normal and DDT-poisoned nerves reveals that, in the latter, a characteristic prolongation of the falling phase of the action potential (the negative afterpotential) occurs (Fig. 22-7). The nerve membrane remains in a partially depolarized state and is extremely sensitive to complete depolarization again by very small stimuli (Joy, 1994a). Thus, following exposure to DDT, the repetitive stimulation of the peripheral sensory nerves by touch or sound is mag-

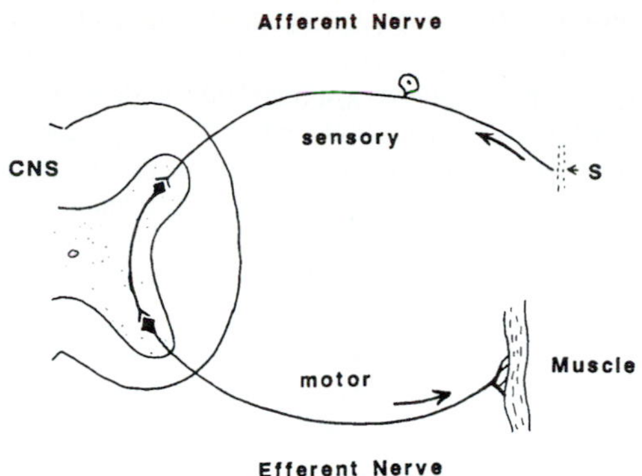

Figure 22-6. A simple, intact reflex arc involving a peripheral, afferent (sensory) neuron, interneurons, and a peripheral, efferent (motor) neuron that innervates a muscle.

nified in the CNS, causing generalized tremoring throughout the body.

How does DDT elicit this effect? There are at least four mechanisms, possibly all functioning simultaneously (Matsumura, 1985), as seen in Fig. 22-8. At the level of the neuronal membrane, DDT affects the permeability to potassium ions, reducing potassium transport across the membrane. DDT alters the porous channels through which sodium ions pass. These channels activate (open) normally, but, once open, are inactivated (closed) slowly, thereby interfering with the active transport of sodium out of the nerve axon during repolarization. DDT inhibits neuronal adenosine triphosphatase (ATPase), particularly the Na^+,K^+-ATPase and Ca^{2+}-ATPase, which play vital roles in neuronal repolarization. DDT also inhibits the ability of calmodulin, a calcium mediator in nerves, to transport calcium ions essential for the intraneuronal release of neurotransmitters. All of these inhibited functions reduce the rate at which depolarization occurs and increase the sensitivity of the neurons to small stimuli that would not elicit a response in a fully depolarized neuron.

The chlorinated cyclodiene-, benzene-, and cyclohexane-type insecticides are different from DDT in many respects, both in the appearance of the intoxicated individual and possibly also in the mechanism(s), which appear to be localized more in the CNS than

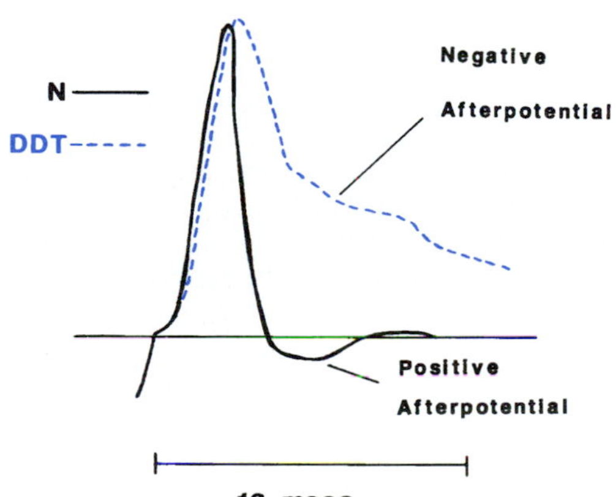

Figure 22-7. A schematic diagram of an oscilloscope recording of the depolarization and repolarization of a normal neuron (——) and one from a DDT-treated (---) animal, showing the prolonged, negative afterpotential (AP).

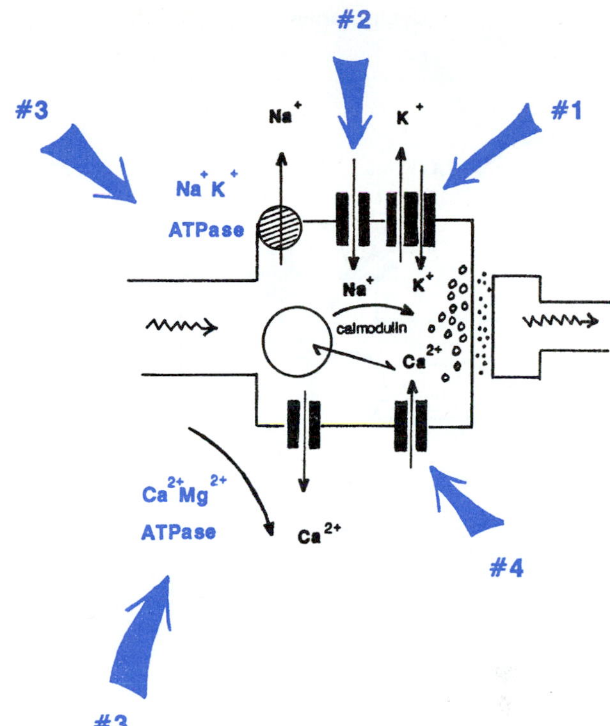

Figure 22-8. Proposed sites of action of DDT on (1) reducing potassium transport through pores, (2) inactivating sodium channel closure, (3) inhibiting sodium-potassium and calcium-magnesium ATPases, and (4) calmodulin-calcium binding with the release of neurotransmitter.

in the sensory division of the PNS (Table 22-6). The overall appearance of the intoxicated individual is one of CNS stimulation. As shown in Fig. 22-9, the cyclodiene compounds antagonize the action of the neurotransmitter gamma-aminobutyric acid (GABA) acting at the $GABA_A$ receptors in rat dorsal root ganglia and effectively blocking the GABA-induced uptake of chloride ions by desensitizing the current in the receptor-channel complex (Nagata and Narahashi, 1994). A more recent paper explains the fact that dieldrin has a dual effect on the $GABA_A$ receptor-channel: an initial enhancement of the GABA-induced chloride ion current (with an EC_{50} of 754 nM) followed by a suppression (Narahashi et al., 1995). Two types of chloride currents exist, one having a high sensitivity to dieldrin ($IC_{50} = 5$ nM) and the other having a lower sensitivity to dieldrin ($IC_{50} = 92$ nM). The dieldrin-suppressive action is responsible for the hyperactivity observed in poisoned animals. The nature of the $GABA_A$ receptor-channel is still being explored. The cyclodienes are also potent inhibitors of Na^+,K^+-ATPase and, more importantly, of the enzyme Ca^{2+}, Mg^{2+}-ATPase essential for the transport (uptake and release) of calcium across membranes (Matsumura, 1985; Wafford et al., 1989). Evidence suggests that gamma-hexachlorocyclohexane (γ-HCH, lindane) neurotoxicity is primarily related to the blockade of chloride ion flux through the inotropic $GABA_A$ receptors, resulting in depolarization and hyperexcitation of post-synaptic membranes (Matsumura and Tanaka, 1984). There is also evidence that γ-HCH can alter calcium homeostasis, elevating free calcium ion levels intracellularly with the release of neurotransmitters (Joy, 1994a). The inhibition of Ca^{2+}, Mg^{2+}-ATPase, located in the terminal ends of neurons in synaptic membranes, results in an accumulation of intracellular free calcium ions with the promotion of calcium-induced

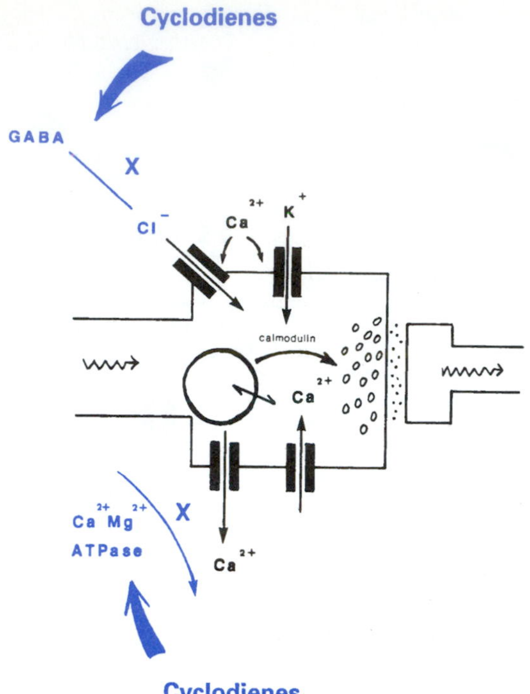

Figure 22-9. Proposed sites of action of cyclodiene-type organochlorine insecticides on chloride ion transport through inhibition of the $GABA_A$ receptor channel as well as inhibition of calcium-magnesium ATPase.

release of neurotransmitters from storage vesicles and the subsequent depolarization of adjacent neurons and the propagation of stimuli throughout the CNS.

Biotransformation, Distribution, and Storage The phenomenon of bioconcentration and biomagnification of the organochlorine insecticides in food chains has been mentioned. Once acquired, biotransformation/degradation proceeds at an exceptionally slow pace, in part due to the complex aromatic ring structures and the number of the chlorine substituents, the latter being exceedingly difficult to remove by the enzymatic processes available in tissues. The biotransformation of the various organochlorines has been extensively studied—for example, DDT (Ecobichon and Saschenbrecker, 1968), aldrin and heptachlor conversion to dieldrin and heptachlor epoxide, respectively (Keane and Zavon, 1969; Matthews and Matsumura, 1969); chlordane (Menzie, 1969); hexachlorocyclohexane (Egan et al., 1965; O'Brien, 1967; Abbott et al., 1969); and toxaphene (Saleh et al., 1977; Turner et al., 1977). With the exception of aldrin, chlordane, and heptachlor, most biotransformation reactions reduce the neurotoxicant activities but marginally affect the weak estrogenicity of the agents.

Slow biotransformation, in addition to the highly lipophilic nature of the organochlorine compounds, guarantees that these agents will be sequestered in body tissue having a high lipid content, where some biological action may result. In the case of adipose tissue, the agents will remain stored and undisturbed, only small amounts equilibrating with the blood and being degraded and/or excreted (Dale and Quinby, 1963; Davies et al., 1972). The depuration of these chemicals from systems occurs slowly, in a matter of a few weeks for chlordane, and months to years for aldrin/dieldrin, DDT, and others (Laben et al., 1965; Ecobichon and Saschenbrecker, 1969; Craan and Haines, 1998; Delorme et al., 1999).

It is not surprising that humans acquired body burdens of these chemicals during the 1950s and 1960s, when they were used on almost all food crops. Depending on the region of the world, the intensity of use, the extent of occupational and accidental exposure, and dietary habits, the bioconcentration/bioaccumulation of DDT in human adipose tissue resulted in levels on the order of 5 ppm DDT and approximately 15 ppm of total DDT-derived material (Quinby et al., 1965; Fiserova-Bergerova et al., 1967; Abbott et al., 1968; Morgan and Roan, 1970). The levels of other organochlorine insecticides sequestered in body fat were never as high as those of DDT. With declining use and the eventual ban of this class on insecticides from the North American market, body burdens of these insecticides declined slowly. By the late 1960s, adipose levels of 2 ppm DDT(0 ppm of total DDT-derived material) were detectable. Whereas the daily intake of DDT in the United States was approximately 0.2 mg/day in 1958, this had decreased to about 0.04 mg/day by 1970 (Hayes, 1971). Today, only trace levels of DDT, less than 2.0 ppm of total DDT-derived material, are detectable in human adipose tissue (Mes et al., 1982; Redetzke and Applegate, 1993; Stevens et al., 1993).

Treatment of Poisoning The life-threatening situation in organochlorine insecticide poisoning is associated with tremors, motor seizures, and interference with respiratory function (hypoxemia and resulting acidosis) arising from repetitve stimulation of the CNS. In addition to general decontamination and supportive treatment, diazepam (0.3 mg/kg IV; maximum dose of 10 mg) or phenobarbital (15 mg/kg IV; maximum dose of 1.0 g) may be administered by slow injection to control the convulsions. It may be necessary to repeat the treatment.

Anticholinesterase Agents

The agents comprising this type of insecticide have a common mechanism of action but arise from two distinctly different chemical classes, the esters of phosphoric or phosphorothioic acid and those of carbamic acid (Fig. 22-10). The anticholinesterase insecticides are represented by a vast array of structures that have demonstrated the ultimate in structure-activity relationships in attempts to produce potent and selective insect toxicity while minimizing the toxicity toward nontarget species. Today, there are some 200 different organophosphorus ester insecticides and approximately 25 carbamic acid ester insecticides in the marketplace, formulated into literally thousands of products. For detailed discussions on the nomenclature, chemistry, and development of these insecticides, the reader is referred to the books of O'Brien (1960), Heath (1961), Melnikov (1971), Fest and Schmidt (1973), Eto (1974), Kuhr and Dorough (1976), Ecobichon and Joy (1994), and Matsumura (1985) and a review by Holmstedt (1959).

The organophosphorus ester insecticides were first synthesized in 1937 by a group of German chemists led by Gerhard Schrader at Farbenfabriken Bayer AG (Schrader and Kukenthal, 1937). Many of their trial compounds proved to be exceedingly toxic and unfortunately, under the management of the Nazis in World War II, some were developed as potential chemical warfare agents. It is unwise to dismiss the chemical warfare nerve gases completely as the weapons of a past, more barbaric era, because it is known that at least one country has stocks of a number of these

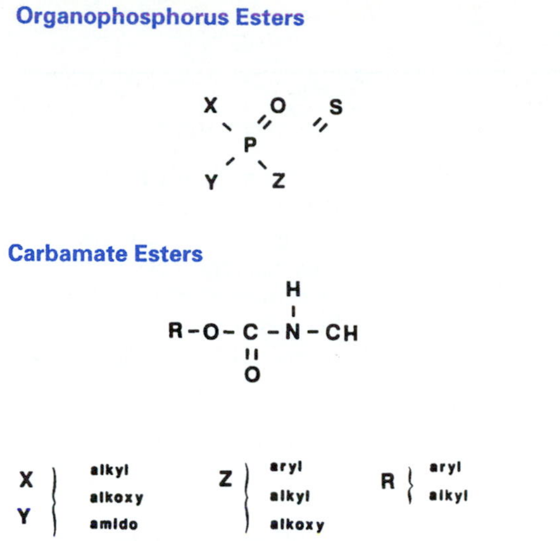

Organophosphorus Esters

Carbamate Esters

Figure 22-10. *The basic backbone structures of the two types of anticholinesterase-class insecticides, the organophosphorus and carbamate esters.*

agents (Fig. 22-11) (Clement, 1994; Gee, 1992). The physicochemical and toxicologic properties of these agents have been reviewed (Sidell, 1992; Somani et al., 1992). Sarin (*O*-isopropyl methylphosphonofluoridate) was used in Iraq against Kurdish villages in northern Iraq in 1988 and residues of isopropyl methylphosphonic acid were found in soil samples along with minute traces of sarin (Webb, 1993). These potent agents should not be ignored, since they are relatively easy to manufacture in small amounts and have been the toxicants of choice of terrorists in at least two documented attacks in Japan, in Matsumoto on June 27, 1994 (Morita et al., 1995), and in the Tokyo subway on March 20, 1995 (Masuda et al., 1995; Nazaki and Aikowa, 1995; Nazaki et al., 1995; Suzuki et al., 1995). The acute and chronic toxicologic effects of these incidents are discussed below.

Although it is true that all of the organoposphorus esters were derived from "nerve gases" (chemicals such as soman, sarin, and tabun), a fact that the media continually emphasizes, the insecticides used today are at least four generations of development away from those highly toxic chemicals. The first organophosphorus ester insecticide to be used commercially was tetraethylpyrophosphate (TEPP); although effective, it was extremely, toxic to all forms of life and chemical stability was a major problem in that TEPP hydrolyzed readily in the presenced of moisture. Further development was directed toward the synthesis of more stable chemicals having moderate environmental persistence, giving rise to parathion (*O,O*-diethyl-*O*-*p*-nitrophenyl phosphorothioate, E-605) in 1944 and the oxygen analog paraoxon (*O,O*-diethyl-*O*-*p*-nitrophenyl phosphate) at a later date. Although these two chemicals had the properties desired in an insecticide (low volatility, chemical stability in sunlight and in the presence of water, environmental persistence for efficacy), they both exhibited a marked mammalian toxicy and were unselective with respect to target and nontarget species. The replacement of DDT with parathion in the 1950s resulted in a series of fatal poisonings and bizarre accidents arising from the fact that workers did not appreciate that this agent was far different from the relatively innocuous organochlorine insecticides with which they were familiar (Ecobichon, 1994a). The number of severe poisonings attributed to parathion provided the stimulus for a search for analogs more selective in their toxicity to target species and less toxic to nontarget organisms, including wildlife, domestic stock, and humans.

The first pesticidal carbamic acid esters were synthesized in the 1930s and were marketed as fungicides. Since these aliphatic esters possessed poor insecticidal activity, interest lay dormant until the mid-1950s, when renewed interest in insecticides having anticholinesterase activity but reduced mammalian toxicity led to the synthesis of several potent aryl esters of methylcarbamic acid. The insecticidal carbamates were synthesized on purely chemical grounds as analogs of the drug physostigmine, a toxic anticholinesterase alkaloid extracted from the seeds of the plant *Physostigma venenosum,* the Calabar bean.

Signs and Symptoms of Poisoning Although their structures are diverse in nature, the mechanism by which the organophosphorus and carbamate ester insecticides elicit their toxicity is idential and is associated with the inhibition of the nervous tissue acetylcholinesterase (AChE), the enzyme responsible the the destruction and termination of the biological activity of the neurotransmitter acetylcholine (ACh). With the accumulation of free, unbound ACh at the nerve endings of all cholinergic nerves, there is continual stimulation of electrical activity. The signs of toxicity include those resulting from stimulation of the muscarinic receptors of the parasympathetic autonomic nervous system (increased secretions, bronchoconstriction, miosis, gastrointestinal cramps, diarrhea, urination, bradycardia); those resulting from the parasympathetic divisions of the autonomic nervous system as well as the junctions between nerves and muscles (causing tachycardia, hypertension, muscle fasciculation, tremors, muscle weakness, and/or flaccid paralysis); and those resulting from effects on the CNS (restlessness, emotional liability, ataxia, lethargy, mental confusion, loss of memory, generalized weakness, convulsion, cyanosis, coma) (Table 22-7).

The classic picture of anticholinesterase insecticide intoxication, first described by DuBois (DuBois, 1948; DuBois et al., 1949), has become more complicated in recent years by the recognition of additional and persistent signs of neurotoxicity not previously associated with these chemicals. First, and frequently associated with exposure to high concentrations of the insecticides (resulting from suicide attempts or drenching with dilute or concentrated

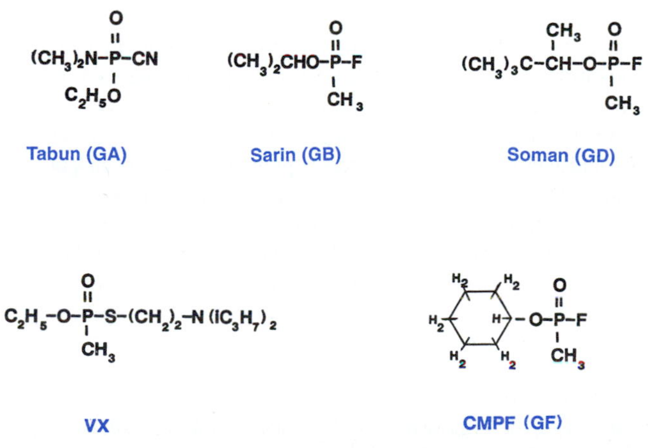

Tabun (GA)

Sarin (GB)

Soman (GD)

VX

CMPF (GF)

Figure 22-11. *Structures of the organophosphorus ester chemical warfare nerve gases, the forerunners of the organophosphorus ester insecticides.*

Table 22-7
Signs and Symptoms of Anticholinesterase Insecticide Poisoning

NERVOUS TISSUE AND RECEPTORS AFFECTED	SITE AFFECTED	MANIFESTATIONS
Parasympatheic autonomic (muscarinic receptors) postganglionic nerve fibers	Exocrine glands	Increased salivation, lacrimation, perspiration
	Eyes	Miosis (pinpoint and nonreactive), ptosis, blurring of vision, conjunctival injection, "bloody tears"
	Gastrointestinal tract	Nausea, vomiting, abdominal tightness, swelling and cramps, diarrhea, tenesmus, fecal incontinence
	Respiratory tract	Excessive bronchial secretions, rhinorrhea, wheezing, edema, tightness in chest, bronchospasms, bronchoconstriction, cough, bradypnea, dyspnea
	Cardiovascular system	Bradycardia, decrease in blood pressure
	Bladder	Urinary frequency and incontinence
Parasympathetic and sympathetic autonomic fibers (nicotinic receptors)	Cardiovascular system	Tachycardia, pallor, increase in blood pressure
Somatic motor nerve fibers (nicotine receptors)	Skeletal muscles	Muscle fasciculations (eyelids, fine facial muscles), cramps, diminished tendon reflexes, generalized muscle weakness in peripheral and respiratory muscles, paralysis, flaccid or rigid tone
		Restlessness, generalized motor activity, reaction to acoustic stimuli, tremulousness, emotional lability, ataxia
Brain (acetylcholine receptors)	Central nervous system	Drowsiness, lethargy, fatigue, mental confusion, inability to concentrate, headache, pressure in head, generalized weakness
		Coma with absence of reflexes, tremors, Cheyne-Stokes respiration, dyspnea, convulsions, depression of respiratory centers, cyanosis

SOURCE: Ecobichon and Joy, 1982.

chemicals), are effects that may persist for several months following exposure and may involve neurobehavioral, cognitive, and neuromuscular functions (Marrs, 1993; Ecobichon, 1994a; Jamal, 1997; Ecobichon, 1998b). One author describes this as a chronic organophosphate-induced neuropsychiatric disorder (COPIND) (Jamal, 1997). The first evidence of this type of syndrome, delayed psychopathologic-neurologic lesions, was reported by Spiegelberg (1963), who had been studying workers involved in the production and handling of the highly toxic nerve gases in Germany during World War II. The characteristic symptomatology subdivided these patients into two distinct groups. The first and largest group was characterized by persistently lowered vitality and ambition; defective autonomic regulation leading to cephalalgia and gastrointestinal and cardiovascular symptoms; premature decline in potency and libido; intolerance to alcohol, nicotine, and various medicines; and an impression of premature aging. The second group, in addition to the above symptoms, showed one or more of the following: depressive or subdepressive disorders of vital function; cerebral vegetative (syncopal) attacks; slight or moderate amnestic or demential effects; and slight organoneurologic defects. These symptoms developed and persisted for some 5 to 10 years following exposure to these most toxic organophosphorus esters during the war years. The controversial paper of Gershon and Shaw (1961), a study of 16 cases of pesticide applicators exposed primarily to organophosphorus ester insecticides for 10 to 15 years, reported a wide range of persistent signs of toxicity, including tinnitus, nystagmus, pyrexia, ataxia, tremor, paresthesia, polyneuritits, paralysis, speech difficulty (slurring), loss of memory, insomnia, somnambulism, excessive dreaming, drowsiness, lassitude, generalized weakness, emotional liability, mental confusion, difficulty in concentration, restlessness, anxiety, depression, dissociation, and schizophrenic reactions. Although the results of other studies have been equivocal in their support of such an array of long-term signs and symptoms, there is a persistent recurrence of the symptomatology in a number of anecdotal and documented reports (Ecobichon, 1994a; Marrs, 1993; Jamal, 1997). The literature on potential, suspected, and established sequelae of organophosphorus ester insecticide intoxications does not confirm the frequently seen statement that clinical recovery from nonfatal poisoning is always complete in a few days. Continuous and close observation of acutely intoxicated patients for some weeks following their recovery from the initial toxicity and treatment thereof would be necessary to identify the subtle changes indicated above. The emergency service physician rarely sees the patient following stabilization and initial "recovery." Definitive examples in which such observation has been possible are few, but one such fortuitous case illustrates what can be achieved if there is close follow-up (Ecobichon et al., 1977).

While most clinical manifestations of acute poisoning are resolved within days to weeks, some symptoms, particularly those of a neuropsychological nature, appear to persist for months or longer. Complete reviews of this aspect have been published recently (Ecobichon, 1994a; Jamal, 1997). A 4-month surveillance of 19 acutely poisoned farm workers revealed many subjective signs and symptoms (blurred vision, muscle weakness, nausea, headaches, night sweats) to persist through the study period, accompanied by a slow recovery of plasma and erythrocytic cholinesterases (Whorton and Obrinsky, 1983). Rosenstock and coworkers (1991) described the neuropsychological testing of 36 poisoned Nicaraguan agricultural workers some 2 years postexposure, reporting that the poisoned group did much worse than controls on all subtests, with significantly worse performance on five of six subtests in the World Health Organization (WHO) neuropsychological test battery and on three of six additional tests that assessed verbal and visual attention, visual memory, visuomotor speed, sequencing and problem solving, motor steadiness, and dexterity (Ecobichon, 1998b). More recent examples of acute intoxications—e.g. "dippers' flu" from repeated exposure to organophosphorus esters (diazinon, propetamphos, chlorfenvinphos) used in sheep dip—have revealed persistent adverse neurophysiological and psychological/behavioral effects that can be evaluated by suitable test batteries (Cook, 1992; Murray et al., 1992; Sims, 1992; Stephens et al., 1995; Beach et al., 1996; Stephens et al., 1996). As has been seen with signs and symptoms in acute intoxications, those afflicted did not show adverse responses to all test battery parameters; only some responses were significantly different from normal-range values. However, such poisoning incidents have progressed from an anecdotal stage to a testable basis, with refined test parameters revealing subtle but distinct changes in memory, academic and motor skills, abstraction, and flexibility in thinking (Ecobichon, 1998b).

A second distinct manifestation of exposure to organophosphorus ester insecticides has been described by clinicians in Sri Lanka involved in the treatment of suicide attempts (Senanayake and Karalliedde, 1987). This paralytic condition, called the *intermediate syndrome,* consisted of a sequence of neurologic signs that appeared some 24 to 96 h after the acute cholinergic crisis but before the expected onset of delayed neuropathy, the major effect being muscle weakness, primarily affecting muscles innervated by the cranial nerves (neck flexors, muscles of respiration) as well as those of the limbs. Cranial nerve palsies were common. There was a distinct risk of death during this time interval because of respiratory depression and distress that required urgent ventilatory support and was not responsive to atropine or oximes. The chemicals involved in these distinctive intoxications included fenthion, dimethoate, monocrotophos, and methamidophos. There were no obvious clinical differences during the acute intoxication phase in those patients who developed the intermediate syndrome and others who did not, and all patients were treated in the same manner.

A third syndrome, that of organophosphate-induced delayed neurotoxicity (OPIDN), is caused by some phosphate, phosphonate, and phosphoramidate esters, very few of which have ever been used as insecticides (Fig. 22-12). Historically, this syndrome has been known for almost 100 years and has been associated with the chemical tri-*o*-tolyl phosphate (TOTP) (Ecobichon, 1994a). The first major epidemic of OPIDN occurred during the prohibition years in the United States, resulting from the consumption of a particular brand of alcoholic extract of Jamaican ginger contaminated or adulterated with mixed tolyl phosphate esters. The syndrome, affecting some 20,000 individuals to varying degrees, was known as *ginger jake paralysis* or *jake leg* and was studied in detail by Maurice Smith of the U.S. Public Health Service. He not only confirmed that the condition could be reproduced in animals (e.g., rabbits, dogs, monkeys, calves) but also demonstrated that only one of the three isomers found in commercial tri-tolyl phosphate, the ortho-isomer, was responsible for the toxicity (Smith and Lillie, 1931). The initial flaccidity, characterized by muscle weakness in the arms and legs—giving rise to a clumsy shuffling gait—was replaced by spasticity, hypertonicity, hyperreflexia, clonus, and abnormal reflexes, indicative of damage to the pyramidal tracts and a permanent upper motor neuron syndrome (Ecobichon, 1994a). In many patients, recovery was limited to the arms and hands and damage to the lower extremities (foot drop, spasticity, and hyperactive reflexes) was permanent, suggesting damage to the spinal cord (Moregan and Penovich 1978), Recent studies have demonstrated that other commercial triarylphosphates (flame retardants in lubricants and plastics) did not elicit significant OPIDN-type neurotoxicity at the maximum dose of 2000 mg/kg (Weiner and Jortner, 1999). An OPIDN-type neuropathy occurred with an experimental organophosphorus ester insecticide, mipafox, following an accident in a manufacturing pilot plant. Details of the effects on two of the workers were described by Bidstrup and coworkers (1953) and Ecobichon (1994a). The poisoning of water buffalo in the early 1970s in Egypt by a phosphonate insecticide, leptophos, revealed a neurologic syndrome similar to that observed following exposure to TOTP (Abou-Donia, 1981). There was also evidence of leptophos-induced neuropathies among workers in a manufacturing plant in the United States, but the controversial observations were obscured by concomitant exposure of the workers to *n*-hexane, another neurotoxic chemical (Xintaris et al., 1978).

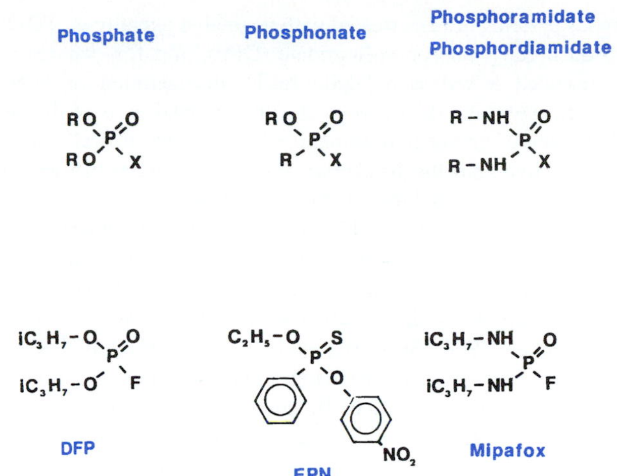

Figure 22-12. The basic structures and nomenclature of organophosphorus esters, with examples, capable of causing organophosphate-induced delayed neurotoxicity (OPIDN).

A number of organophosphorus insecticides—including omethoate, trichloronate, trichlorfon, parathion, methamidophos, fenthion, and chlorpyrifos—have been implicated in causing OPIDN in humans (Abou-Donia and Lapadula, 1990). However, it should be emphasized that these incidents all involved accidental or suicidal exposure to excessively high levels. Concern that many of the over 200 organophosphorus ester insecticides in use might cause this unique neuropathy has resulted in an intensive study of the syndrome, the identification of the most susceptible species (the hen and the cat), the development of standard protocols to test all insecticides, and at least a partial elucidation of the mechanisms by which agents elicit this condition. Histologic examination of the nervous systems of hens treated with a suitable agent [e.g., TOTP, *O,O*-diisopropyl phosphorofluoridate (DFP), mipafox, leptophos] has revealed a wallerian "dying-back" degeneration of large-diameter axons and their myelin sheaths in distal parts of the peripheral nerves and of long spinal cord tracts—the rostral ends of ascending tracts and the distal ends of descending tracts (Cavanagh, 1954; Sprague and Bickford, 1981). At autopsy, examination of an unfortunate victim who died 15 months after the sarin attack in the Tokyo subway revealed moderate-to-severe fiber loss in the sural and sciatic nerves with little effect in the CNS, results consistent with the dying-back degeneration of the PNS described above (Himuro et al., 1998). Surviving victims also showed a higher frequency of sister chromatid exchanges (SCEs) in peripheral blood lymphocytes (Li et al., 1998). Biochemical studies have demonstrated that the above-mentioned agents inhibit a neuronal, nonspecific carboxylesterase, neuropathic target esterase (NTE), which appears to have some, as yet unknown, role in lipid metabolism in neurons (Johnson, 1982). If acute exposure to an appropriate organophosphorus ester results in >70 percent inhibition of NTE, the characteristic OPIDN usually follows, with ataxia being observed some 7 to 14 days following treatment and progression to moderate to severe muscular weakness and paralysis with concomitant changes in neuronal morphology (Johnson, 1982; Slott and Ecobichon, 1984). It is the considered opinion of many investigators that many of the commonly used phosphate and phosphorothioate ester insecticides might be capable of causing this syndrome if only sufficient concentrations of the agents could be attained in vivo. However, taking paraoxon as an example of such a phosphate ester, the animal(s) would either die as a consequence of other acute toxic effects or would rapidly detoxify the agent, thereby preventing the acquisition of sufficient paraoxon to inhibit NTE. There also appear to be subtle structure-activity relationships between organophosphorus esters and the active site on the NTE protein, because many phosphate esters are not good inhibitors of NTE (Ohkawa et al., 1980; Abou-Donia, 1981). Conversely, while the nerve gases cause a marked inhibition of NTE, the exposed animals do not develop OPIDN, suggesting that NTE inhibition may not be obligatory (Johnson et al., 1985, Lotti, 1992; Marrs, 1993; Jamal, 1997). It should be emphasized that although NTE inhibition remains a useful function for monitoring the potential of organophosphorus esters to induce OPIDN, the role of this enzyme in the initiation of the syndrome remains unknown and histopathologic evidence is a requirement of the U.S. EPA protocol. However, a recently reported poisoning by methamidophos proved that lymphocyte NTE inhibition was predictive of the subsequent OPIDN, the level of activity increasing from 3.1 to 13.3 nmol/min/mg protein between day 3 after poisoning and day 52 (McConnell et al., 1999). Interestingly, serum autoantibodies (IgM, IgG) to glial fibrillary acidic protein (GFAP), myelin basic protein (MBP), and cytoskeletal elements increased immediately after poisoning in this case and persisted to day 52, suggesting that these parameters might be useful markers. Two noninsecticidal organophosphorus esters, the tri-*S*-alkyl defoliant *S,S,S*-tributyl phosphorotrithioite (Merphos) and its oxidation product, *S,S,S*-tributyl phosphorotrithioate (DEF), have been implicated in producing OPIDN in at least one agricultural worker and cause a characteristic delayed neurotoxicity in hens (Abou-Donia and Lapadula, 1990).

The signs and symptoms of acute intoxication by carbamate insecticides are similar to those described for organophosphorus compounds, differing only in the duration and intensity of the toxicity. The most apparent reasons are that (1) carbamate insecticides are reversible inhibitors of nervous tissue AChE, unlike most of the organophosphorus esters (see below, "Mechanism of Toxic Action") and (2) they are rapidly biotransformed in vivo. Despite the extensive toxicologic short-term toxicity following acute administration, carbamate insecticide toxicity has been reported in humans and fatalities have occurred (Ecobichon, 1994b; Hayes, 1982, Feldman, 1999). Invariably, these serious poisonings have involved carbaryl and have occurred as a consequence of accidental or purposeful (suicidal) exposure to high concentrations (Hayes, 1982; Cranmer, 1986). Information on the incidences of human intoxication by carbaryl can be found in the Carbaryl Decision Document (EPA, 1980). For the period 1966–1980, a total of 195 human intoxication cases were reported (3 fatalities, 16 hospitalizations, and 176 cases receiving medical attention). A single oral dose of 250 mg of carbaryl (2.8 mg/kg body weight) is sufficient to elicit moderately severe poisoning in an adult man (Cranmer, 1986). Moderate but transient toxicity has also been observed following exposure to a few of the more potent carbamate ester insecticides methomyl (Lannate) and propoxur (Baygon) (Fandekar et al., 1968, 1971; Liddle et al., 1979). More recently the illegal use of aldicarb (Temik), a very acutely toxic carbamate ester, on watermelons in California and on English cucumbers in British Columbia, Canada, resulted in moderate to severe toxicity in consumers of these products, with signs and symptoms including nausea, vomiting, gastrointestinal cramps, and diarrhea (Goldman et al., 1990a,b).

While there is little evidence of prolonged neurotoxicity after exposure to carbamate ester insecticides, this statement should be made cautiously because the signal danger appears to involve acute single exposures to massive doses or at least repeated exposures to large doses. Examining a number of carbamate (aldicarb, methomyl) intoxications in children and adults, Lifshitz et al. (1997) discovered that the predominant symptoms in adults were miosis and muscle fasciculations, while the children were more likely to reveal CNS effects (stupor and/or coma) in addition to diarrhea and hypotension. The authors suggested that the blood-brain barrier was more permeable in the children.

Bizarre anecdotal cases exist that are contrary to everything that we know about carbamates. One case, that of a farmer who hand-sprayed a vegetable garden with a water-wettable formulation of carbaryl, drenching himself in the process, developed a chronic polyneuropathy, persistent photophobia and paresthesia, recent memory loss, muscular weakness, fatigue, and lassitude (Ecobichon, 1994b). The case study presented by Branch and Jacqz (1986) developed into a persistent, stocking-and-glove peripheral neuropathy accompanied by mental confusion and weakness in major skeletal muscle groups, with fasciculations and cerebral atrophy. Grendon et al. (1994) presented long-term observations of a group of men who had been exposed acutely to aldicarb, several experiencing symptoms 3 years after the initial severe intoxication. Feldman (1999) conducted extensive neurologic and psychological investigations on three individuals exposed accidentally to aerially applied carbaryl some three to five years before. Their persisting subjective symptoms were confirmed by peripheral nerve conduction studies, electromyography, and neuropsychological assessment, both peripheral and central impairment being documented.

There is evidence in animal studies, albeit at near toxic doses, of a wallerian-type degeneration of spinal cord tracts in rabbits and hens following treatment with sodium diethyldithiocarbamate

(Edingon and Howell, 1969). Carbaryl, when fed to hogs (150 mg/kg per day for 72 or 83 days), caused a rear leg paralysis, minimal at rest but, when the animals were forced to move, resulting in marked incoordination, ataxia, tremors, clonic muscle contractions, and prostration, with histologic evidence of lesions in the CNS and in skeletal muscle (Smalley et al., 1969). Carbamate ester insecticides do no inhibit NTE or elicit OPIDN-type neurotoxicity. Behavioral changes have been noted in a number of animal studies following the subchronic or chronic administration of different carbamate insecticides (Santalucito and Morrison, 1971; Desi et al., 1974).

Mechanism of Toxic Action Although the anticholinesterase-type insecticides have a common mode of action, there are significant difference between organophosphorus and carbamate esters. The reaction between and organophosphorus ester and the active site in the AChE protein (a serine hydroxyl group) results in the formation of a transient intermediate complex that partially hydrolyzes with the loss of the "Z" substituent group, leaving a stable, phosphorylated, and largely unreactive inhibited enzyme that, under normal circumstances, can be reactivated only at a very slow rate (Fig. 22-13). With many organophosphorus ester insecticides, an irreversibly inhibited enzyme is formed, and the signs and symptoms of intoxication are prolonged and persistent, requiring vigorous medical intervention including the reactivation of the enzyme with specific chemical antidotes (see "Treatment of Poisoning," below, this section). Without intervention, the toxicity will persist until sufficient quantities of "new" AChE are synthesized in 20 to 30 days to destroy efficiently the excess neurotransmitter. The nature of the substituent groups at "X," "Y," and "Z" plays an important role in the specificity for the enzyme, the tenacity of binding to the active site, and the rate at which the phosphorylated enzyme dissociates to produce free enzyme. More recently introduced organophosphorus esters (acephate, temephos, dichlorvos, trichlorfon) are less tenacious inhibitors of nervous tissue AChE, the phosphorylated enzyme being more readily and spontaneously dissociated.

In contrast, carbamic acid esters, which attach to the reactive site of the AChE, undergo hydrolysis in two stages: the first stage is the removal of the "X" substituent (an aryl or alkyl group) with the formation of a carbamylated enzyme; the second stage is the

Organophosphorus Ester

E-OH + (XO)(YO)P(=O)Z ⟶ E-O-P(=O)(XO)(YO) + ZH ⟶ E-OH + (XO)(YO)P(=O)OH

Carbamate Ester

E-OH + XOC(=O)-NHCH$_3$ ⟶ E-O-C(=O)-NHCH$_3$ + XOH ⟶ E-OH + HO-C(=O)-NHCH$_3$

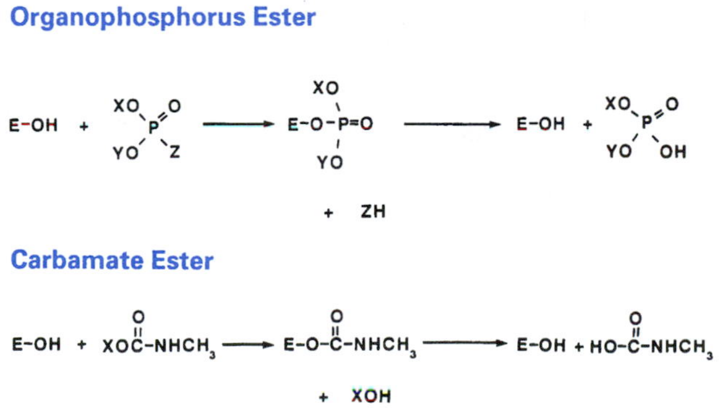

Figure 22-13. The interaction between an organophosphorus or carbamate ester with the serine hydroxyl groups in the active site of the enzyme acetylcholinesterase (E-OH). The intermediate, unstable complexes formed before the release of the "leaving" groups (ZH and XOH) are not shown. The dephosphorylation or decarbamoylation of the inhibited enzyme is the rate-limiting step to forming free enzymes.

decarbamylation of the inhibited enzyme with the generation of free, active enzyme (Fig. 22-13). Carbamic acid esters are nothing more than poor substrates for the cholinesterase-type enzymes.

When the concept of the interaction between organophosphorus and carbamic esters with AChE is presented in another manner (Table 22-8), one can see that the only distinctive difference between the two anticholinesterase-type insecticides lies in the rate at which the dephosphorylation or decarbamylation takes place. The rate is exceedingly slow for organophosphorus esters, so much so that the enzyme is frequently considered to be irreversibly inhibited. The rate of decarbamylation is sufficiently rapid that these esters are often considered to be reversible inhibitors with low turnover rates. The characteristics of the various rate constants for the natural substrate (ACh), organophosphorus, and carbamylation esters are shown in Table 22-8. It is important to appreciate that the rate at which step 3 proceeds is thousands of times slower with carbamate esters than with ACh, whereas with organophosphorus esters it is several orders of manitude slower (Ecobichon, 1979). This subject has been extensively reviewed by Aldridge and Reiner (1972). A number of organophosphorus (phosphate, phosphonate, and phosphoramidate) esters (Fig. 22-12)—the chemical warfare agents sarin, soman, and tabun, and a few other compounds such as DFP, mipafox, and leptophos—have the ability to bind tenaciously to the active site of AChE and NTE to produce an irreversibly inhibited enzyme by a mechanism known as *aging*. The aging process is dependent on the size and configuration of the alkyl (R) substituent, with the potency of the ester increasing in the order of diethyl, dipropyl, and dibutyl for such analogs as DFP and mipafox (Aldridge and Johnson, 1971). The aging process is generally accepted as being caused by the dealkylation of the intermediate dialkylphosphorylated enzymes by one of two possible mechanisms (Fig. 22-14). The first involves the hydrolysis of a P–O bond following a nucleophile (base) attack on the phosphorus atom. The second mechanism involves the hydrolysis of an O–C bond by an acid catalysis, resulting in the formation of a carbonium ion as the leaving group (O'Brien, 1960; Eto, 1974; Johnson, 1982). The aging process is believed to fix an extra charge to the protein, causing some perturbation to the active site and thereby preventing dephosphorylation. While the exact nature of this reaction has not been demonstrated for AChE and NTE, evidence from experiments with saligenin cyclic phosphorus esters (derivatives of TOTP) and α-chymotrypsin points to the possibility of two stabilized forms of "aged" enzyme (Toia and Casida, 1979). Both of the reactions utilize the imidazole group of a neighboring histidine. In one reaction, the hydroxylated substituent is released and the phosphorylated enzyme is stabilized by a hydrogen on the imidazole group. In the other reaction, the leaving substituent becomes attached to the imidazole, yielding a N–C-hydroxylated derivative of the phospyhorylated enzyme. Johnson (1982) proposed that, in the case of NTE, if one or two of the P–R bonds were P–O–C (as in phosphates and phosphonates), aging would occur rapidly, whereas if the P–R bonds were P–C (as in phosphinates), aging would not be possible.

A number of acute, high-level exposures and intoxications by organophosphorus and carbamate esters have resulted in persistent CNS effects as well as debilitating muscle weakness, particularly in the legs, that cannot be explained on the basis of nervous tissue AChE inhibition alone. One hypothesis has been put forward that the excessive amount of undestroyed acetylcholine (ACh) may be involved by an action at nicotinic (nAChR) and muscarinic (mAChR) acetylcholine receptors (Ecobichon, 1994a). As shown

Table 22-8
Kinectics of Ester Hydrolysis

	EH + AB ⇄ EHAB → BH + EA → EH + AOH		
ESTERS	COMPLEX FORMATION ($K_A = k_{-1}/k_{+1}$)	ACYLATION (k_2)	DEACYLATION (k_3)
Substrates	Small	Extremely fast	Extremely fast
Organophosphorus esters	Small	Moderately fast	Slow or extremely slow
Carbamate esters	Small	Slow	Slow

SOURCE: Ecobichon, 1979.

in Fig. 22-15, the ACh accumulating at nAChR would elicit stimulation of the neuromuscular junctions, causing fasciculations (repetitive stimulation) followed by a depolarizing blockade if the ACh levels remained elevated, leading subsequently to a desensitization process with a more or less permanent reduction in nAChR numbers and causing the persistent muscle weakness observed through a lack of response to stimuli. Support for this hypothesis has been seen in studies revealing chronic abnormal electromyographic (EMG) activity in human intoxications by anticholinesterase insecticides, the details of which can be found in Ecobichon (1994a) and Feldman (1999). An alternative theory bears examination.

In an acute tabun study in rats, necrotic diaphragmatic muscle was observed, the effect being prevented by sectioning the phrenic nerve to a portion of the diaphragm (Ariens et al., 1969). Similar diaphragmatic damage has been observed in human poisonings (DeRueck and Willens, 1975; Wecker et al., 1986). Early work by Dettbarn and colleagues demonstrated that close intramuscular injections of parathion or paraoxon resulted in a skeletal myopathy accompanied by necrosis of the nerve terminal membrane and of the underlying muscle (summarized in Ecobichon, 1994a). There is evidence that organophosphate-induced AChE inhibition causes muscle hyperactivity as an initial step that triggers free radical–induced lipid peroxidation before muscle injury (Yang and Dettbarn, 1996; Yang et al., 1996). More recent studies, conducted at the level of brain mAChR and nAChR, have demonstrated that organophosphorus esters (soman, VX, DFP, parathion, paraoxon, chlorpyrifos) bind to both receptor types, particularly if the circulatory concentrations are in the micromolar range as would be encountered in poisoning cases, resulting in desensitization (Bakry et al., 1988; Eldefrawi et al., 1988; Huff et al., 1994; Katz et al., 1997). There is also evidence of differential down-regulation of nAChR subtypes through reduction of messenger RNA expression in rat brain following repeated injections of parathion (Jett et al., 1993, 1994; Ward and Mundy, 1996). Adult mice, exposed to DFP on postnatal day 3 or 10, showed decreases in brain nAChR

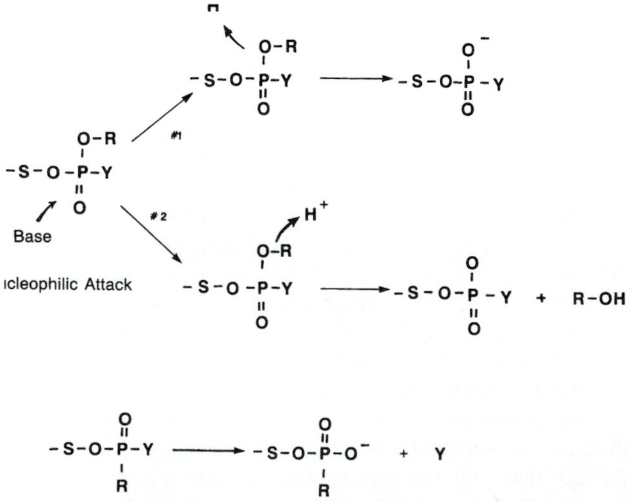

Figure 22-14. A schematic diagram illustrating two mechanisms by which the "aging" of organophosphorus ester–inhibited acetylcholinesterase may occur. See text for details.

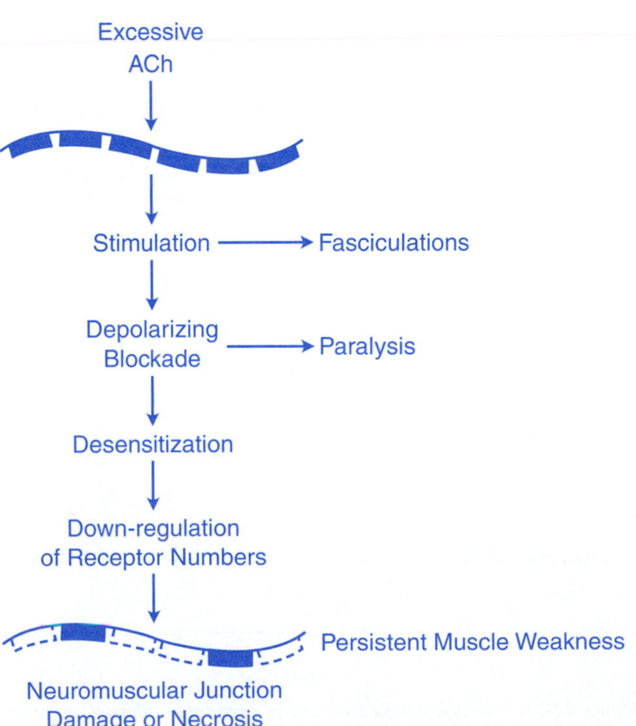

Figure 22-15. A schematic diagram illustrating the impact of excessive concentrations of acetylcholine (ACh) on muscarinic and nicotinic acetylcholine receptors in order to explain neuromuscular weakness and damage.

density as well as significant alterations in spontaneous motor behavior (Ahlbom et al., 1995).

Can the carbamate esters induce muscle damage and receptor alterations through mechanisms involving ACh, direct binding to receptors, or through receptor expression? The repeated injection of such reversible anticholinesterase carbamates as physostigmine or neostigmine has produced myopathies qualitatively similar to those produced by paraoxon, possibly supporting the ACh-related theory (Wecker et al., 1978). Skeletal muscle lesions (myodegeneration, vacuolization) were observed in swine fed carbaryl over a period of 80+ days (Smalley et al., 1969). The peripheral neuropathy of a carbaryl-exposed elderly male has been described (Branch and Jacqz, 1986). Some interesting experiments could be performed with some of the more potent carbamate insecticides.

Biotransformation, Distribution, and Storage Both the organophosphorus and carbamate ester insecticides undergo extensive biotransformation in all forms of life. Both the route(s) and the rate(s) of metabolism are highly species-specific and dependent on the substituent chemical groups attached to the basic "backbone" structure of these esters (Fig. 22-10). Tissue enzymes of both phase I (oxidative, reductive, hydrolytic) and phase II (transfer or conjugative reactions with glutathione, glucuronic acid, glycine, and so forth) types are founds in a widespread pattern in plant, invertebrate, and vertebrate species and, indeed, are responsible for some aspects of the species sensitivity and/or both natural and acquired restance to many of these insecticides. The phase I detoxification processes usually form reactive metabolites, whereas phase II processes conjugate the polar phase I metabolites with some natural body substituent to form a product with enhanced water solubility and excretability. The biotransformation of anticholinesterase-type insecticides has been extensively reviewed in the literature and the reader is referred to such sources as O'Brien (1967), Menzie (1969), Eto (1974), Kulkarni and Hodgson (1984), and Matsumura (1985) for details on the various mechanisms involved.

Organophosphorus esters undergo simultaneous oxidative biotransformation at a number of points in the molecule (Fig. 22-16), the enzymes utilizing the ubiquitous cytochrome P450 isoenzyme system. One reaction, that of oxidative desulfuration of phosphorothioate (parathion, methyl parathion, fenitrothion, etc.) and phosphorodithioate (azinophos methyl, malathion, etc.) esters, results in a significant increase in the toxicity of the biotransformation products, oxygen analogs (mechanism 1). This reaction is a major obligatory pathway in ester detoxification in mammals equipped with tissue aryl and aliphatic hydrolases (mechanism 8), whereas insects are deficient in these enzymes, making them more susceptible. Dealkylation with the formation of an aldehyde occurs readily (mechanism 2), but this pathway does not function efficiently when the alkyl group becomes longer. Dearylation occurs with the formation of a phenol and either a dialkylphosphoric or dialkylphosphorothioic acid (mechanism 3). The cytochrome system can also catalyze (1) aromatic ring hydroxylation (mechanism 4); (2) thioether oxidation (mechanism 5); (3) deamination; (4) alkyl and *N*-hydroxylation; (5) *N*-oxide formation; and (6) *N*-dealkylation. A number of transferases use glutathione (gamma-glutamyl-

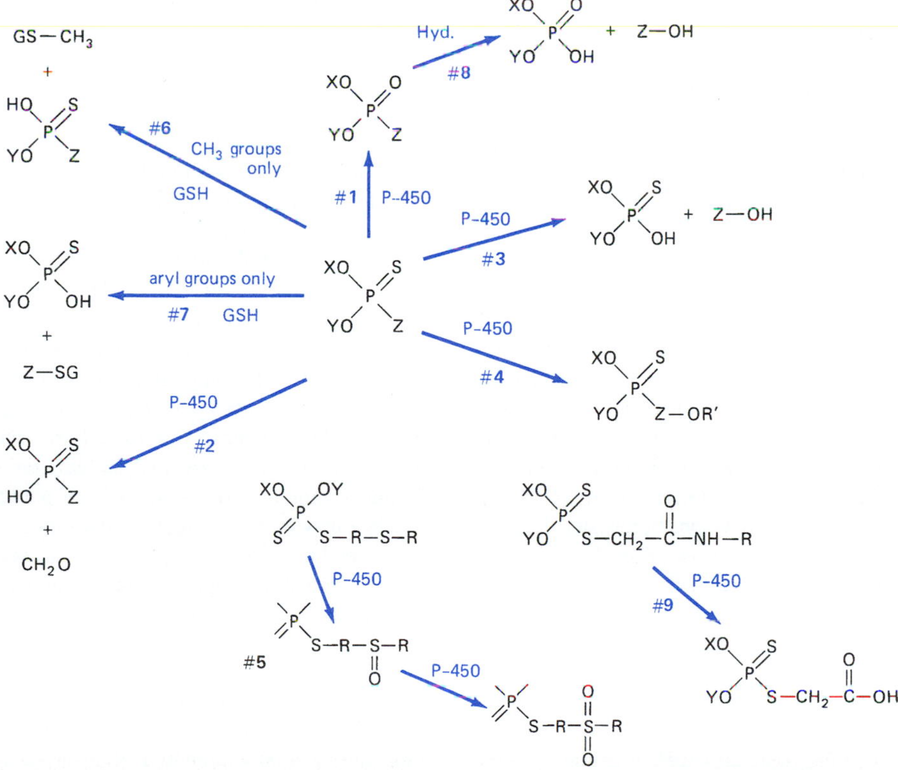

Figure 22-16. A schematic diagram depicting the various phase I and II biotransformation pathways of an organophosphorus ester and the nature of the products formed as a consequence of oxidative, hydrolytic, GSH-mediated transfer and conjugation of intermediates in mammals. See text for details.

L-cysteinyl glycine, GSH) as a cofactor and acceptor for *O*-alkyl (methyl) and *O*-aryl groups (mechanisms 6 and 7) to yield monodesmethyl products plus *S*-methylglutathione or aryl-glutathione derivatives plus the respective phosphoric or phosphorothioic acids.

Hydrolysis of phosphoric and phosphorothioic acid ester occurs via a number of different tissue hydrolases (nonspecific carboxylesterases, arylesterases, phosphorylphosphatases, phosphotriesterases, carboxyamidases) scattered ubiquitously throughout the plant and animal kingdoms, with activity being highly dependent on the nature of the substituents (Ecobichon, 1979). Slight structural modifications to substituents on the insecticide molecule can dramatically alter the specificity of these enzymes toward an agent and affect species selectivity. The arylesterases [aromatic or A-esterases (ArE), EC 3.1.1.2] preferentially hydrolyze aryl (phenol, naphtol, indole) esters of short-chain aliphatic or phosphorus acids, particulary if there is a double bond present in the alcohol moiety in position α with respect to the ester bond (mechanism 8). Carboxylesterases [carboxylic acid ester hydrolases (CE), EC 3.1.1.] are capable of hydrolyzing a variety of aliphatic and aryl esters of short-chain fatty acids. The most important example of this reaction involving organophosphorus ester insecticides is with malathion [*O,O*-dimethyl-*S*-(1,2-dicarbethoxyethyl) phosphorodithioate], in which one of the two available ethylated carboxylic ester groups is hydrolyzed to yield malathion (or malaoxon) α-monoacids that are biologically inactive (Dauterman and Main, 1966). This CE-catalyzed reaction is an important feature of resistance to this insecticide in insects and to tolerance in mammals. Potentiation of anticholinergic effects can be produced by the combined administration of certain pairs of organophosphate ester insecticides, such as EPN (*O*-ethyl-*O*-*p*-nitrophenylbenzenethiophosphonate) and malathion (Frawley et al., 1957). The mechanism for this effect involves the inhibition of carboxyesterases by EPN (Murphy, 1969, 1972, 1980). Carboxyamidases (acylamide amdiohydrolase, EC 3.5.1.4), found extensively in plant, insect, and vertebrate tissues, are of limited current interest in the degradation of insecticides; dimethoate (*O,O*-dimethyl-*S*-(*N*-methylcarbamoylmethyl) phosphorodithioate] is the only organophosphorus ester insecticide shown to be hydrolyzed by mammalian tissue amidases (mechanism 9). Phosphorylphosphatases and phosphotriesterases have limited involvement in the biotransformation of organophosphorus ester insecticides but play a role in the detoxification of some of the chemical warfare agents.

Phase II conjugative reactions are of limited use in the biotransformation of organophosphorus ester insecticides, and they are usually relegated to the task of glucuronidating or sulfating the aromatic phenols, cresols, and other substances hydrolyzed from the ester (Yang, 1976). However, one must be wary of these enzyme systems because metabolism studies of chlorfenvinphos (2-chloro-1-(29,49-dichlorophenyl)vinyl diethylphosphate) revealed the presence of glucuronide and glycine conjugates of several products, whereas studies with trichlorfon (*O,O*-dimethyl-1-hydroxy-2,2,2-trichloroethyl phosphonate) revealed direct glucuronidation of the insecticide without prior biotransformation (Hutson et al., 1967; Bull, 1972).

Carbamate ester insecticides can undergo simultaneous attack at several points in the molecule, depending on the nature of the substituents attached to the basic structure. In addition to the hydrolysis of the carbamate ester group by tissue CE and the release of a substituted phenol, carbon dioxide, and methylamine (Fig. 22-10), (mechanism 1), several oxidative and reductive reactions involving cytochrome P450–related monooxygenases can proceed, the ultimate products being considerably more polar than the parent insecticide. The extent of hydrolysis of carbamate ester insecticides varies greatly between species, ranging from 30 to 95 percent hydrolysis. The type of oxidative reactions observed with carbamate esters can be simplified into two main groups: (1) direct ring hydroxylation (mechanism 2) and (2) oxidation of appropriate side chains as is shown for this "mythical" methylcarbamate, resulting in the hydroxylation of *N*-methyl groups or methyl groups to form hydroxymethyl groups (mechanism 3), *N*-demethylation of secondary and tertiary amines (mechanism 4), *O*-dealkylation of alkoxy side chains (mechanism 5), thioether oxidation (mechanism 6), and so forth. Phase II conjugative reactions can occur at any free reactive grouping with glucuronide and sulfate derivatives (mechanism 7), and GSH conjugates (mercapturates) may be formed (mechanism 8). For a comprehensive exposition of the various mechanisms involved, the reader is referred to those reviews mentioned above, this section, as well as to pertinent articles by Ryan (1971), Fukuto (1972), and Kuhr and Dorough (1976).

Treatment of Poisoning Despite the qualitative and quantitative differences between organophosphorus and carbamate insecticide intoxications, all cases of anticholinesterase poisoning should be treated as serious medical emergencies and the patient should be hospitalized as quickly as possible. The status of the patient should be monitored by repeated analysis of the plasma (serum) cholinesterase and the erythrocyte AChE; the inhibition of the activities of these two enzymes is a good indicator of the severity of organophosphorus ester poisoning, because only the erythrocytic AChE is inhibited by carbamate esters (except at excessively high levels of exposure). As a consequence of the extensive involvement of the entire nervous system, the life-threatening signs (respiratory depression, bronchospasm, bronchial secretions, pulmonary edema, muscular weakness) resulting in hypoxemia will require immediate artificial respiration and suctioning via an endotracheal tube to maintain a patent airway. Arterial blood gases and cardiac function should be monitored.

The regimen for the treatment of organophosphorus ester insecticide intoxication, based on the analysis of serum pseudocholinesterase, is described in Table 22-9 (Namba et al., 1971; Ecobichon et al., 1977; Marrs, 1993). Atropine is used to counteract the initial muscarinic effects of the accumulating neurotransmitter. However, atropine is a highly toxic antidote and great care must be taken. Frequent small doses of atropine (subcutaneously or intravenously) are indicated for mild signs and symptoms following a brief, intense exposure. Large cumulative doses of atropine, up to 50 mg daily, may be essential to control severe muscarinic symptoms. The status of the patient must be monitored continuously by examining for the disappearance of secretions (dry mouth and nose) and sweating, facial flushing, and mydriasis (dilatation of pupils). Supplementary treatment to offset moderate to severe nicotinic and CNS signs and symptoms usually takes the form of one of the specific antidotal chemicals, the oximes (pralidoxime chloride or 2-PAM, pralidoxime methanesulfonate or P2S), administered intravenously to reactivate the inhibited nervous tissue AChE. The use of oximes may not be necessary for cases of mild intoxication and should be reserved for moderate to severe poisonings. Treatment by slow intravenous infusion of doses of 1.0 g should be initiated as soon as possible, because the longer the interval between exposure and treatment, the less effective the

Table 22-9
Classification and Treatment of Organophosphorus Insecticide Poisoning Based on Plasma Pseudocholinesterase Activity Measurement

CLASSIFICATION OF POISONING	ENZYME ACTIVITY (% OF NORMAL)	TREATMENT	
		ATROPINE	PRALIDOXIME
Mild	20–50	1.0 mg SC	1.0 g IV over 20 to 30 min
Moderate	10–20	1.0 mg IV every 20 to 30 min until sweating and salivation disappear and slight flush and mydriasis appear	1.0 g IV over 20 to 30 min
Severe	10	5.0 mg IV every 20 to 30 min until sweating and salivation disappear and slight flush and mydriasis appear	1.0 g IV as above. If no improvement, administer another 1.0 g IV. If no improvement, start IV infusion at 0.5 g/h

SOURCE: Ecobichon et al., 1977.

oxime will be. In many poisonings, a single treatment with pralidoxime will be sufficient to elicit a reversal of the signs and symptoms and to reduce the amount of atropine needed. In severe poisoning cases, a prodigious amount of pralidoxime may be needed. If absorption, distribution, and/or metabolism of the organophosphorus ester is delayed in the body, pralidoxime may be administered repeatedly over several days after the initial treatment. Care should be taken with repeated dosing because pralidoxime effectively binds calcium ions and causes muscle spasms not unlike those elicited by the organophosphorus esters. Severe muscle cramping, particularly in the extremities, may be alleviated by oral or intravenous calcium solutions (Ecobichon et al., 1977).

The therapeutic action of the oxime compounds resides in their capacity to reactivate AChE without contributing markedly toxic actions of their own. Those organophosphorus esters that possess good "leaving groups" (i.e., the "X" moiety) phosphorylate the nervous tissue AChE by a mechanism similar to that of acetylation by the substrate ACh. These esters are frequently called *irreversible inhibitors* because the hydrolysis of the phosphorylated enzyme by water is exceedingly slow (Table 22-8). However, various nucleophilic agents containing a substituted ammonium group will dephosphorylate the phosphorylated enzyme at a much more rapid rate than water. The basic requirements for a reactivating molecule consist of a rigid structure containing a quaternary ammonium group and an acidic nucleophile, which would be complementary with the phosphorylated enzyme, in such a way that the nucleophilic oxygen would be positioned close to the electrophilic phosphorus atom. These structure-activity requirements led to the development of the pralidoxime compounds, with the *syn*-isomer of 2-PAM (2-formyl-*N*-methylpyridinium chloride oxime) being particularly active (Childs et al., 1955; Askew, 1956; Kewitz and Wilson, 1956; Namba and Hiraki, 1958). The reaction of 2-PAM with the phosphorylated enzyme proceeds as shown in Fig. 22-17.

The reactivation is an equilibrium reaction, the oxime reacting either with the phosphorylated enzyme or with free, unbound organophosphorus ester, and the product is a phosphorylated oxime which in itself can be a potent cholinesterase inhibitor if it is stable in an aqueous medium (Schoene, 1972). In general, the phosphorylated oxime degrades quickly in water.

A practical limitation on the usefulness of oxime reactivators lies in the inability of these agents to reactivate "aged" AChE, that enzyme in which the phosphorylated enzyme has been further dealkylated and the phosphoryl group becomes tightly bound to the reactive site (see Fig. 22-14). Success with the pyridinium analogs led to an intensive search for more effective oximes and the discovery of the bispyridinium compounds toxogonin or obidoxime [bis(4-formyl-*N*-methylpyridinium oxime) ether dichloride], TMB-4 [*N,N*-trimethylene bis(pyridine-4-aldoxime) bromide], and, more recently, the H-series compounds. However, these agents are not without toxicity and only pralidoxime and toxogonin have seen extensive antidotal use (Engelhard and Erdmann, 1964; Steinberg et al., 1977).

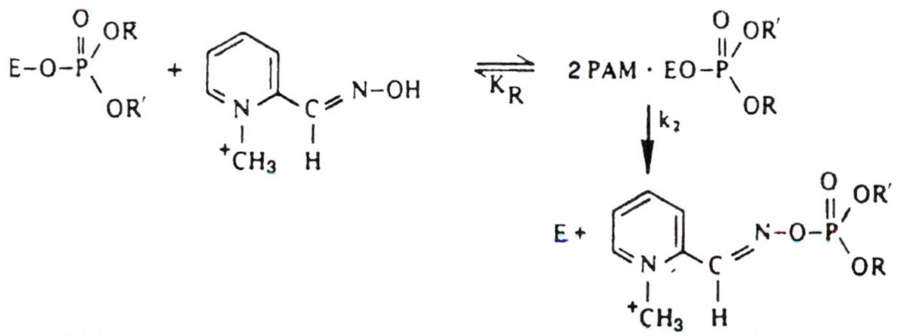

Figure 22-17. The pralidoxime-catalyzed reactivation of an organo-phosphate-inhibited molecule of acetylcholinesterase, showing the release of active enzyme and the formation of an oxime-phosphate complex.

With the apparent availability of organophosphorus nerve gases and their known ability to form rapidly aging complexes with AChE, the relative ineffectiveness of atropine and pralidoxime in such poisonings must be taken into account when the treatment of individuals exposed to these agents is confronted (Koplovitz et al., 1992; Webb, 1993; Clement, 1994). Toxogonin (obidoxime chloride) appears to be effective in tabun poisoning while, of the H-series of bis-pyridinium monooximes, HI-6 appears to be efficacious in soman and cyclohexylmethyl phosphorofluoridate (CMPF, or CF) poisonings. However, despite striking therapeutic effects, the issue is clouded by the fact that little reactivation of erythrocytic or brain AChE occurs (Kusic et al., 1991; Shih, 1993).

The clinical treatment of carbamate toxicity is similar to that for organophosphorus ester insecticide intoxication with the exception that the use of oximes is contraindicated. Early reports, in which pralidoxime or toxogonin was used in treating carbaryl intoxications, revealed that the oxime enhanced the carbaryl-induced toxicity (Sterri et al., 1979; Ecobichon and Joy, 1994). However, the oximes appear to offer some antidotal properties in patients exposed to aliphatic oxime carbamates (aldicarb, methomyl) (Feldman, 1999).

Diazepam (10 mg SC or IV) may be included in the treatment regimen of all but the mildest cases of organophosphorus and/or carbamate intoxications. In addition to relieving any mental anxiety associated with the exposure, diazepam counteracts some aspects of the CNS and neuromuscular signs that are not affected by atropine. Doses of 10 mg (SC or IV) are appropriate and may be repeated. Other centrally acting drugs that may depress respiration are not recommended in the absence of artificial respiration.

It is important to appreciate that vigorous treatment of anticholinesterase-type insecticide intoxications does not offer protection against the possibility of delayed-onset neurotoxicity or the persistent sensory, cognitive, and motor defects discussed earlier. These deficits, albeit reversible over a long time interval, appear consistently in intoxications and are caused by mechanisms as yet unknown. Certain evidence points to severe damage to the neuromuscular junctions in skeletal muscle, resulting in a persistent peripheral muscular weakness (Wecker et al., 1978).

Pyrethroid Esters

A major class of insecticides comprises the synthetic pyrethroids, a group of chemicals that entered the marketplace in 1980 but, by 1982, accounted for more than 30 percent of worldwide insecticide usage (Anon., 1977; Vijverberg and van den Bercken, 1982). However, these synthetics arise from a much older class of botanical insecticides, pyrethrum, a mixture of six insecticidal esters (pyrethrins, cinerins, and jasmolins) extracted from dried pyrethrum or chrysanthemum flowers (*Chrysanthemum cinerariaefolium, Chrysanthemum coccineum*) (Hartley and West, 1969). Although it is believed that the natural pyrethroids were discovered by the Chinese in the first century A.D., the first written accounts of these agents are found in the seventeenth-century literature and commercial preparations made their appearance in the mid-1800s (Neumann and Peter, 1987). Japanese woodblock prints from the early 1800s exist in which one can see smoldering insecticide coils of pressed pyrethrum powder not unlike those manufactured and used today.

In 1965, the world output of pyrethrum was approximately 20,000 tons, with Kenya alone producing some 10,000 tons (Cremlyn, 1978). The ever-increasing demand for this product has far exceeded the limited world production, leading chemists to focus attention on the synthesis of new analogs, hopefully with better stability in light and air, better persistence, more selectivity in target species, and low mammalian toxicity. In addition to extensive agricultural use, the synthetic pyrethroids are components of household sprays, flea preparations for pets, plant sprays for home and greenhouse use, and other applications. For an in-depth discussion of the development of the pyrethroid ester insecticides, their chemistry, and their biological activity, the reader is referred to Elliott (1976), Cremlyn (1978), Casida et al. (1983), Leahey (1985), Matsumura (1985), Narahashi (1985), Narahashi et al. (1985), and Joy (1994b).

Natural pyrethrum consists of a mixture of six esters derived from two acids (chrysanthemic, pyrethric) and three alcohols (pyrethrolol, cinerolol, jasmolol), producing an effective contact and stomach poison mixture having both knockdown and lethality. When the complex structure was identified, the synthetic esters were marketed (Fig. 22-18). Distinctive molecular structures convey selectivity toward certain insect species and in some cases to toxicity in mammals. Several of the pyrethroid esters exist in isomeric forms around the cyclopropane nucleus, resulting in distinctly different toxicities and potencies (Casida et al., 1983).

Signs and Symptoms of Poisoning Based on the symptoms produced in animals receiving acute toxic doses, the pyrethroids fall into two distinct classes of chemicals (Table 22-10). The type I poisoning syndrome or *T syndrome* is produced by esters lacking the α-cyano substituent and is characterized by restlessness, incoordination, prostration, and paralysis in the cockroach, as compared with the rat, which exhibits such signs as sparring and aggressive behavior, enhanced startle response, whole-body tremor, and prostration. The type II syndrome, also known as the *CS syndrome,* is produced by those esters containing the α-cyano substituent and elicits intense hyperactivity, incoordination, and convulsions in cockroaches, in contrast to rats, which display burrowing behavior, coarse tremors, clonic seizures, sinuous writhing (choreoathetosis), and profuse salivation without lacrimation; hence the

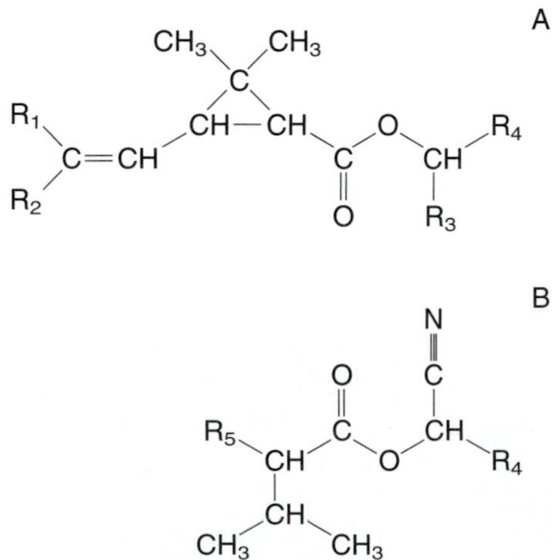

Figure 22-18. The basic structures of the synthetic pyrethroid ester insecticides showing (A) the intact cyclopropane ring in type I esters, with R_1 and R_2 (methyl, bromine, chlorine, etc.), R_3 (hydrogens or cyano) and R_4 (3-phenoxybenzoate, other) substituents; and (B) the "open" structure of type II esters with R_4 (3-phenoxybenzoate, other) and R_5 (substituted phenyl substituents).

Table 22-10
Classification of Pyrethroid Ester Insecticides on the Basis of Chemical Structure and Observed Biological Activity

	Signs and Symptoms		
SYNDROME	COCKROACH	RAT	CHEMICALS
Type I ("T" syndrome)	Restlessness Incoordination Prostration Paralysis	Hyperexcitation Sparring Aggressiveness Enhanced startle response Whole-body tremor Prostration	Allethrin Cismethrin Phenothrin Pyrethrin I Resmethrin Tetramethrin
Type II ("CS" syndrome)	Hyperactivity Incoordination Convulsions	Burrowing Dermal tingling Clonic seizures Writhing Profuse salivation	Acrinathrin Cycloprothrin Cyfluthrin Cyhalothrin Cyphenothrin Cypermethrin Deltamethrin Esfenvalerate Fenvalerate Flucynthrate Fluvalinate

term *CS* (choreoathetosis/salivation) *syndrome*. A few of these agents, fenpropanthrin, for example, cause a mixture of type I and II effects, depending on the species (rat or mouse) treated and possibly on the route of administration (Verschoyle and Aldridge, 1980; Gammon et al., 1981; Lawrence and Casida, 1982). The bulk of evidence points to the fact that the type II syndrome involves primarily an action in the mammalian CNS, whereas with the type I syndrome, peripheral nerves are also involved. This hypothesis was based initially on the observed symptomatology, but more recent evidence has revealed a correlation between the severity of type II responses and brain concentrations of deltamethrin in mice, regardless of the route of administration (Barnes and Verschoyle, 1974; Ruzo et al., 1979). Agents eliciting the type II syndrome have greater potency when injected intracerebrally, relative to intraperitoneal injection, than those causing type I syndrome effects (Lawrence and Casida, 1982). There is no indication of a fundamental difference between the mode of action of pyrethroids on neurons of target and nontarget species, and the neurotoxicologic responses depend on a combination of physicochemical properties of the particular pyrethroid ester, the dose applied, the time interval after treatment, and the physiologic properties of the particular model used (Leaks et al., 1985).

Although these insecticides cannot be considered to be highly toxic to mammals, their use indoors in enclosed and poorly ventilated spaces has resulted in some interesting signs and symptoms of toxicity to humans. Exposure to the natural pyrethrum mixture is known to cause contact dermatitis; descriptions of the effects range from localized erythema to a severe vesicular eruption (McCord et al., 1921). The allergenic nature of this natural product is not surprising, with asthma-like attacks and anaphylactic reactions and peripheral vascular collapse among the responses observed. Human toxicity associated with the natural pyrethrins stems from their allergenic properties rather than from direct neurotoxicity. There has been little evidence of the allergic-type reactions in humans exposed to synthetic pyrethroid esters.

One notable form of toxicity associated with synthetic pyrethroids has been a cutaneous paresthesia observed in workers spraying esters containing an α-cyano substituent (deltamethrin, cypermethrin, fenvalerate). The paresthesia developed several hours following exposure and was described as a stinging or burning sensation on the skin which, in some cases, progressed to a tingling and numbness, the effects lasting some 12 to 24 h (LeQuesne et al., 1980; Tucker and Flannigan, 1983; Zhang et al., 1991).

Reports have appeared in the literature from the People's Republic of China, where synthetic pyrethroids have been used on a large scale on cotton crops since 1982 (Stuart-Harte, 1988; He et al., 1988, 1989). Associated with the sloppy handling of deltamethrin and fenvalerate, both of which are type II compounds, some 573 cases of acute poisoning have occurred with some 229 cases of occupational exposure. Some 45 cases of intoxication involved cypermethrin. Occupational exposure resulted in some dizziness plus a burning, itching, or tingling sensation of the exposed skin, which was exacerbated by sweating and washing with warm water. The signs and symptoms disappeared by 24 h after exposure. Spilling these agents on the head, face, and eyes resulted in pain, lacrimation, photophobia, congestion, and edema of the conjunctiva and eyelids. Ingestion of pyrethroid esters caused epigastric pain, nausea and vomiting, headache, dizziness, anorexia, fatigue, tightness in the chest, blurred vision, paresthesia, palpitations, coarse muscular fasciculations in the large muscles of the extremities, and disturbances of consciousness. In severe poisonings, convulsive attacks persisting from 30 to 120 s were accompanied by flexion of the upper limbs and extension of the lower limbs, with opisthotonos and loss of consciousness. The frequency of these seizures was on the order of 10 to 30 times a day in the first week after exposure, gradually decreasing in incidence, with recovery within 2 to 3 weeks (He et al., 1989). The signs and symptoms of acute intoxication appear to be reversible and no chronic toxicity has been reported to date.

Site and Mechanism of Toxicity Several mechanisms of action of pyrethroid esters exist in the sensory, motor, and central nervous systems of insects and vertebrates, many of these actions being studied in vitro using cockroach, crayfish, and squid giant axon preparations or various cultured cell systems (Narahashi, 1971, 1976, 1985; Casida et al., 1983; Forshaw et al., 1993; Narahashi, 1998; Ray, 2000).

Both type I and type II esters modify the gating kinetics of sodium channels involved in the inward flow of sodium ions, producing the action potential in cells that are normally closed at the resting potential (Marban et al., 1998). The pyrethroids affect both the activation (opening) and inactivation (closing) of the channel, resulting in a hyperexcitable state as a consequence of a prolonged negative afterpotential that is raised to the threshold membrane potential and producing abnormal repetitive discharges (Ginsburg and Narahashi, 1993; Narahashi et al., 1998). The observed differences between type I and type II esters lie in the fact that the former hold sodium channels open for a relatively short time period (milliseconds), whereas type II esters keep the channel open for a prolonged time period (up to seconds) (Joy, 1994b). Although the repetitive discharges could occur in any region of the nervous system, those at presynaptic nerve terminals would have the most dramatic effect on synaptic transmission (i.e., on the CNS and peripheral sensory and motor ganglia), giving rise to the signs documented in Table 22-10. The depolarizing action would have a dramatic effect on the sensory nervous system because such neurons tend to discharge when depolarized even slightly, resulting in an increased number of discharges and accounting for the tingling and/or burning sensation felt on the skin and observed in particular with type II esters (van den Bercken and Vijverberg, 1983). The biological actions of different pyrethroid esters at sodium channels is highly variable in that (1) *cis* and *trans* stereospecificity exists, the *cis* isomers being as much as 10-fold more toxic than *trans* isomers (Soderlund, 1985); (2) an additional chiral center is produced if a cyano-substituent is added to the alcohol (Fig. 22-18), giving rise to eight possible isomers; (3) the binding of *cis* and *trans* isomers differs, being competitive at one site and noncompetitive at another (Narahashi, 1986); (4) tetrodotoxin-resistant sodium channels are 10-fold more sensitive to pyrethroids than are tetrodotoxin-sensitive channels (Ginsburg and Narahashi, 1993; Song and Narahashi, 1996); (5) affinity to sodium channels is dependent on the variable α-subunit composition of the 10 or more different channels identified to date (Marban et al., 1998); (6) insect sodium channels are 100-fold more sensitive than mammalian channels, thereby in part explaining species susceptibility (Warmke et al., 1997); (7) low temperature (25°C) exerts a greater inhibitory effect of pyrethroid esters (on sodium channels) than a higher (37°C) temperature due to increased current flow at low temperature (Narahashi et al., 1998). According to Narahashi et al. (1998), the most important factor that causes differential toxicity is the sodium channel of the nervous system.

Other sites of action have been noted for pyrethroid esters, as shown in Fig. 22-19. Calcium channels have been proposed targets, particularly in insects at levels of 10^{-7} M (Duce et al., 1999). Mammalian calcium channels appear to be less sensitive, with effects being seen only with type I esters. However, many of these

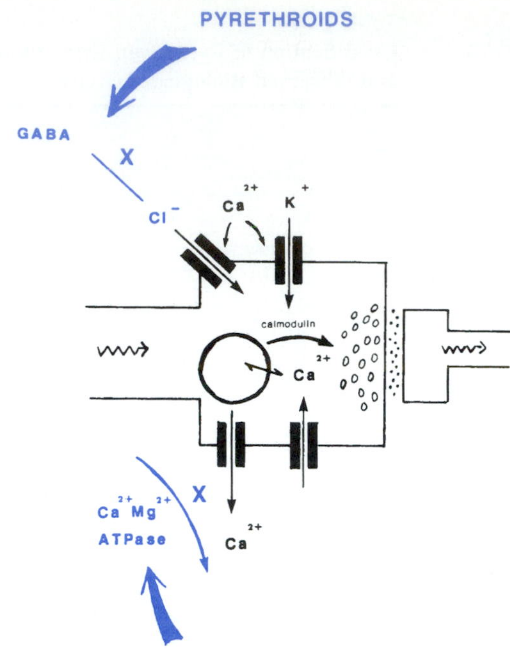

Figure 22-19. Other proposed cellular mechanisms by which pyrethroid esters interfere with neuronal function.

experiments were conducted on cultured neuroblastoma cells, sinoatrial node cells, and so on, with results difficult to reconcile with neuronal actions. Several agents (permethrin, cypermethrin, deltamethrin) inhibit Ca^{2+}, Mg^{2+}-ATPase, the effect of which would result in increased intracellular calcium levels accompanied by increased neurotransmitter release and postsynaptic depolarization (Clark and Matsumura, 1982).

Type II esters at relatively high concentrations act on the GABA-gated chloride channels in mammalian brain, this action perhaps being related to the seizures seen with type II ester intoxication (Abalis et al., 1986; Bloomquist et al., 1986). However, other studies have shown pyrethroids to have no GABA-antagonistic activity (Joy and Albertson, 1991; Ray, 2000).

Voltage-sensitive calcium-independent chloride channels in nervous tissue control cell excitability and exist in functionally different kinds, those sensitive to pyrethroid esters belonging to the maxi-chloride channel type (Franciolini and Petris, 1990; Forshaw and Ray, 1993). The pyrethroid-induced decrease in chloride ion current would result in cell excitability, synergizing with the pyrethroid effect on sodium channels. Only type II esters affect maxi-chloride channels and may be responsible for the generation of salivation and myotonia along with those effects elicited on sodium channels (Joy, 1994; Ray et al., 1997; Ray, 2000).

Biotransformation, Distribution, and Storage Evidence to date suggests that pyrethroid esters elicit little chronic toxicity in either in animals or humans. Chronic animal feeding studies yield high "no effect" levels, suggesting that there is little storage or accumulation of a body burden of these agents and, perhaps, an efficient detoxification of the chemicals.

Two ester linkages exist in pyrethroid esters, a terminal methyl ester (pyrethrin II) and one more centrally located ester adjacent to the cyclopropane moiety (allethrin, tetramethrin, phenothrin, deltamethrin) and/or the α-cyano substituent (deltamethrin, cypermethrin, fenvalerate, cyphenothrin). Pyrethroid esters are susceptible to degradation by hydrolytic enzymes, possibly by nonspecific carboxylesterases found associated with the microsomal fraction of tissue homogenates in various species (Ecobichon, 1979; Casida et al., 1983). Hydrolysis of the methoxycarbonyl group in pyrethrin II by an esterase in rat liver has been reported, but the major site of hydrolytic activity would appear to be at the central ester linkage (Elliott et al., 1972; Shono et al., 1979; Glickman and Casida, 1982). The importance of ester hydrolysis as a route of detoxification is verified by the fact that many organophosphorus esters that are capable of inhibiting tissue esterases potentiate pyrethroid ester toxicity in a variety of species (Casida et al., 1983). Species susceptibility to pyrethroid ester toxicity would appear to be highly dependent on the nature of the tissue esterase, the level of activity detected, the substrate specificity, and rate of hydrolysis encountered in target and nontarget species. The microsomal monooxygenase system found in the tissues of almost all species is extensively involved in the detoxification of every pyrethroid ester in mammals and of some of these agents in insect and fish species. Much of the research in this field has been summarized by Shono et al. (1979), Kulkami and Hodgson (1984), and Casida et al., (1983). The importance of the oxidative mechanisms in detoxification is demonstrated by the inclusion of the synergist piperonyl butoxide, a classic monooxygenase inhibitor, in preparations toxic to houseflies and other insects, in order to enhance the potency of pyrethroid esters in the 10- to 300-fold range (Casida et al., 1983; Matsumura, 1985).

Treatment of Poisoning Limited experience with pyrethroid intoxications has restricted the development of acceptable protocols for treatment. Removal from exposure and lavage with vegetable and/or vitamin E cream will alleviate dermal paresthesia, presumably by binding the lipophilic pyrethroids (Flannigan et al., 1985). Most other therapies have been symptom-related topical steroids for contact dermatitis, antihistaminics, decongestants, and steroid nasal spray for rhinitis and inhaled steroids for asthma (O'Malley, 1997). Systemic poisoning is more difficult to treat, symptomatic and supportive measures being appropriate (He et al., 1989). Experimental therapies in animals have included local anesthetics, phenytoin, phenobarbitone, valproate, diazepam, mephenesin, and urethane, all at exceptionally high doses with interfering side effects (Ray, 2000). Only the chloride channel agonists ivermectin and pentobarbitone appeared to be of any benefit, particularly in type II ester intoxications (Forshaw, 2000).

Avermectins

The avermectins were discovered in 1975, isolated from a culture of the actinomycete *Streptomyces avermitilis* in a soil sample made available to Merck and Co. by the Kitisato Institute in Japan (Campbell et al., 1983; Campbell, 1989; Fisher and Mrozik, 1992). Avermectins are derived from 16-member macrocyclic lactones, three of which—avermectin B1a, the homolog B1b (abamectin), and the semisynthetic ivermectin—have come into wide use in veterinary medicine as potent insecticidal, acaricidal, and anthelmintic agents (Fisher and Mrozik, 1992) (Fig. 22-20). Ivermectin is used for a wide range of ecto- and endoparasites of domestic and wild animals. Potent anthelmintic activity against most gastrointestinal and systemic nematodes has been identified at exceptionally low (0.001 to 0.05 mg/kg body weight) dose levels, but this efficacy does not extend to tapeworms or flukes (Campbell et al., 1983). Administered topically or subcutaneously (systemically), ivermectin controls grubs, lice, mites, certain ticks, and biting flies on cattle, horses, sheep, swine, and dogs (except the collie breed, which appears to be uniquely susceptible) (Fisher and Mrozik, 1992). Ivermectin treatment does not result in the rapid death of biting insects but appears to disrupt engorgement, molting, and reproduction (Campbell et al., 1983). A mixture of avermectins B1a and B1b is also used currently as a foliar spray on crops against various mites, Colorado potato beetle, tomato hornworm, Mexican bean beetle, pea aphid, cabbage looper, corn earworm, and southern army worm (Fisher and Mrozik, 1992). Emamectin (MK-244), a derivative of avermectin B1, is more effective against Lepidoptera larvae.

The discovery that ivermectin was efficacious against the skin-dwelling microfilaria of *Onchocerca* species in cattle and horses suggested that it might be of use in treating onchocerciasis (river blindness) in humans, a debilitating disease caused by the organism *Onchocerca volvulus* (Taylor and Green, 1989). It has become the drug of choice in treating lightly infected individuals, markedly reducing the number of microfilaria in the skin though without effect on the adult worms (Aziz et al., 1982; Taylor and Greene, 1989). It is a safe, long-acting microfilaricide, an applied single dose (150 ug/kg body weight) killing the immature microfilaria and keeping the numbers of reappearing microfilaria well below pretreatment levels for up to 1 year (Fisher and Mrozik, 1992). Ivermectin treatment can significantly reduce the incidence of onchocerciasis by limiting the source of infection.

While the avermectins are highly lipid soluble, dermal absorption is less than 1.0 percent of the applied dose (Fisher and Mrozik, 1992). Minimal oxidative biotransformation occurs, 2,4-hydroxymethyl ivermectin and 3′-*O*-desmethyl ivermectin being formed. Regardless of the route of administration, urinary excretion accounts for only 0.5 to 2.0 percent of the dose, the remainder being excreted slowly in the feces (Campbell et al., 1983). While the liver and adipose tissue took up the agent(s), very little residue was found in muscle, kidney or brain. In the case of the brain, presumably the agent could not penetrate the blood-brain barrier. In 28 days, almost complete elimination of ivermectin occurred from the tissues of treated cattle with the exception of the liver and body fat (Fisher and Mrozik, 1992).

Toxicologically, ivermectin is acutely toxic to rodents and other species, the oral and intraperitoneal LD_{50} values being of the order of 25 to 80 mg/kg body weight (Fisher and Mrozik, 1992). Dermal toxicity is low, the LD_{50} for rats and rabbits being >660 and 406 mg/kg body weight, respectively. In subchronic studies, no treatment-related effects were observed in rats, dogs, and monkeys at the usual therapeutic dosage range (0.1 to 1.2 mg/kg body weight per day). Ivermectin showed no positive genotoxic effects in microbial assays, in a forward mutation assay (mouse lymphoma), or in an unscheduled DNA synthesis assay. In developmental/reproductive studies, offspring abnormalities were observed only at maternotoxic doses in mice, rats, and rabbits. Oncogenic effects were not found in studies with abamectin.

Mechanism of Action Early studies, with a variety of invertebrate species and model systems, resulted in a number of possible mechanisms of action on neuronal transmission, chloride channels,

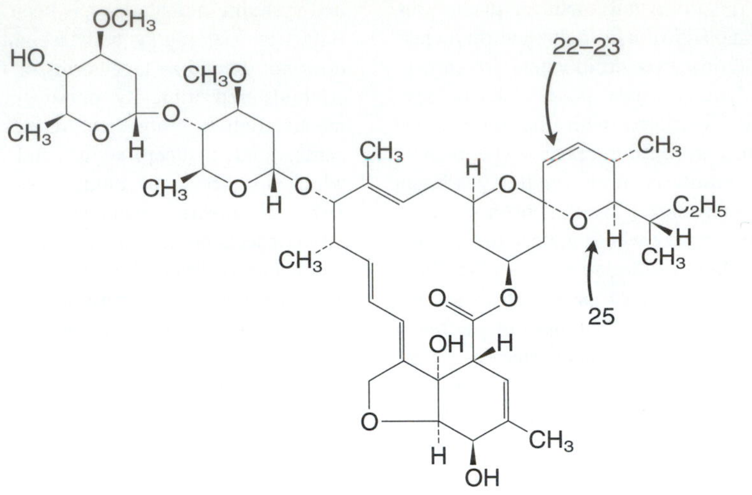

Common Name	Structural Positions	
	22–23	25
Avermectin Bla	As above	As above
Avermectin Blb Abamectin	As above	$—CH(CH_3)_2$
Ivermectin	$—CH_2—CH_2—$	80% As above 20% $—CH(CH_3)_2$

Figure 22-20. ***A structural representation of the macrocyclic lactone avermectin (B1a), abamectin (B1b), and the semisynthetic insecticide ivermectin showing the structural differences at positions 22 to 23 and 25 of the ring.***

and GABA-like effects, summarized in Fisher and Mrozik (1992). However, care must be taken in interpreting such results, since interneuronal and neuromuscular junctions are known to differ considerably between species (Gerschenfeld, 1973). The low water solubility and extensive (nonspecific) binding of avermectins preclude accurate estimations of target-site concentrations, overestimating the actual target-site concentrations (Fisher and Mrozik, 1992). More recent binding affinity studies in rat brain and in insect and nematode nerve tissue preparations have revealed that, in invertebrates, biological activity occurred at nanomolar and picomolar concentrations (Schaeffer et al., 1989; Fisher and Mrozik, 1992). Higher concentrations appear to cause secondary events and/or artifacts. While there may be different species-specific avermectin "receptors," this insecticide class has a high binding affinity to chloride-channel proteins, opening the channels, reducing membrane resistance, and increasing conductance inward. Such binding sites appear to be distinct from those of other effector molecules and involve GABA-insensitive chloride channels (Arena et al., 1991; Payne and Soderlund, 1991). Explaining the selective specificity of avermectins (wide range of nematodes, arthropods, insects but not tapeworms, flukes, and adult filaria) must await the molecular study of the receptor proteins in these species. In mammals, in the nematode *Caenorhabditis elegans,* and the house fly, avermectins interact with the GABA-receptor complex, as has been shown by avermectin-induced changes in GABA receptor–directed ligands (Deng and Casida, 1992; Arena et al., 1995; Lankas et al., 1997).

Newer Chemical Insecticides

With the development of insect resistance to various classes of chemical insecticides, new approaches to insect control are needed. Utilizing a better understanding of insect neurobiology, some new and highly specific agents have been developed, capitalizing on the recognition that various receptors in insect nervous systems are significantly different from those in mammals. Shown in Fig. 22-21 are the structures of three types of new agents entering or available in the marketplace: (1) the nitromethylene heterocycles, developed from the cyclodienes and cyclohexanes; (2) the nitroimino derivatives (chloronicotinyl or neonicotinoids), similar to nicotine; and (3) the phenylpyrazoles. These chemicals are effective at low application rates (8 to 10 g/ha), are not environmentally persistent, and show negligible toxicity toward vertebrates. They possess unique and selective mechanisms of action and perhaps point the way to future insecticide development. To date, there have been no reports of toxicity in humans.

Nitromethylenes A search for new classes of insecticides led to a study of various aromatic heterocycles containing a nitromethylene substituent, only those containing a pyridine system being insecticidal (Fig. 22-21*A* and *B*) (Soloway et al., 1979). The nitromethylene heterocycle (NMH) insecticides are fast-acting neurotoxicants, effective by both contact or oral ingestion; they are relatively safe to vertebrates and degrade rapidly in the environment (Schroeder and Flattum, 1984).

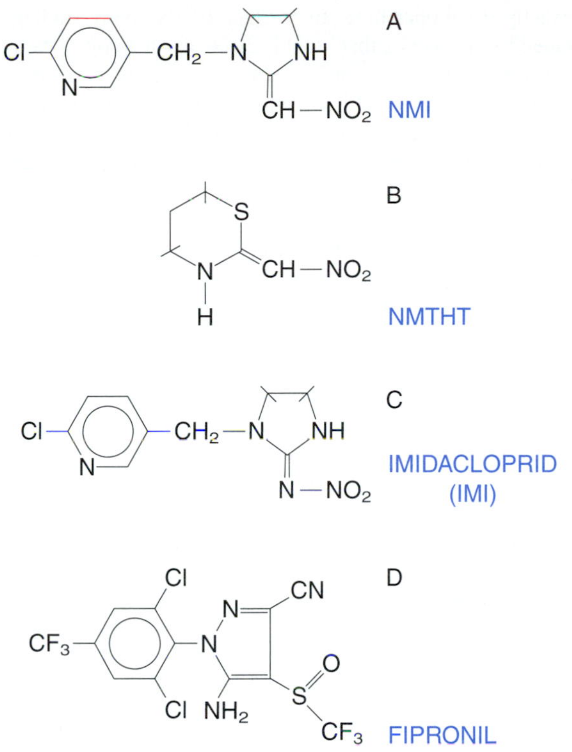

Figure 22-21. Representative structures of the nitromethylene, chloronicotinyl, and phenylpyrazole insecticides.

Using the cockroach ventral nerve cord (the sixth abdominal ganglion nerve) preparation, various NMHs at micromolar concentrations produced a biphasic effect characterized by an initial increase in the frequency of spontaneous discharges followed by a blockade of nerve impulse conduction (Schroeder and Flattum, 1984). Elegant, classic neuropharmacologic experiments conducted by these authors demonstrated that the NMHs acted as neurotransmitter mimics and had both excitatory depressant effects, eventually blocking postsynaptic nicotinic receptors (nAChR). More recent experiments with 2(nitromethylene)tetrahydro-1,3-thiazine (NMTHT) (Fig. 22-21*B*) confirmed the biphasic action at nAChRs in several insect species and suggested that a binding site resided on the α-subunits of insect nAChRs (Leech et al., 1991).

Chloronicotinyl An outgrowth of studies of the nitromethylene-type insecticides was the discovery of the nitroimino heterocycles best known by the compound imidacloprid (Fig. 22-21*C*), developed in Japan in the mid-1980s. This agent combines high potency to insects with exceptionally low mammalian toxicity and a favorable persistence (Liu et al., 1993; Bayer Corp., 1994). The potency of imidacloprid and several analogs can be correlated with the binding affinity to house fly head membranes and mouse brain membranes, these agents having a low affinity to the latter (Liu et al., 1993, 1995; Chao and Casida, 1997). Extensive studies have demonstrated that imidacloprid binds specifically to nAChRs in various insects' nervous systems (Liu and Casida, 1993; Nishimura et al., 1994; Liu et al., 1995). Imidacloprid acts as a partial agonist at the nAChR channel, generating subconductance-state currents (Nagata et al., 1997). Characterization of cloned nAChRs from insects (*Myzus persicae,* peach aphid) revealed that imidacloprid affinity was influenced strongly by the α-subunit content of the receptor (Huang et al., 1999). Investigations of a nAChR structure and function will prove to be a boon to further insecticide development.

Phenylpyrazoles The phenylpyrazole derivatives show extensive biological activity, including insecticidal, herbicidal, and miticidal properties. The compound fipronil (Fig. 22-21*D*) is insecticidal and has been shown to be highly effective against a broad range of insect pests at low-level foliar or soil application. It was first studied by Rhone-Poulenc Agro in 1987 and is now available commercially (Gant et al., 1998). It is considered to be a second generation removed from the earlier organochlorine insecticides (lindane, α-endosulfan) acting at the GABA receptor to block the chloride channel (Damgaard et al., 1999).

Fipronil has a unique mode of action in that it blocks the passage of chloride ions through the GABA-regulated chloride channel, disrupting CNS activity, since GABA is an inhibitory neurotransmitter. Fipronil is a noncompetitive inhibitor of GABA-induced effects, the effects in neurons being an increase in rapid bursts of electrical activity (Gant et al., 1998). Fipronil, a sulfoxide, is biotransformed to the corresponding sulfone in biological systems, the latter compound still being a potent insecticide. This conversion can be blocked by piperonyl butoxide, the cytochrome-P450 inhibitor. There is also a photoproduct, desulfinyl fipronil. Fipronyl and the sulfone selctively bind with high affinity to insect GABA receptors and with much lower affinity to vertebrate brain receptors (Cole et al., 1993; Hainzl et al., 1998). Comparing fipronil and its derivatives to earlier chloride-channel blockers, the IC_{50} vertebrate/IC_{50} insect ratios are 158 for fipronil, 140 for lindane, 31 for the desulfinyl product, 19 for fipronil sulfone, and 4 for α-endosulfan (Hainzl et al., 1998). The selectivity ratios relative to human GABA receptor are 135 for fipronil, 17 for the sulfone, and 16 for the desulfinyl photoproduct (Hainzl et al., 1998).

All of the above receptor-specific insecticides have provided new ligand probes for neurotransmitter receptors as well as a new approach to insecticide development. The only worrisome concern is that, with increasing use and reliance on such agents, target insects may develop resistance to these new compounds through mechanisms similar to those seen for other neurotransmitters. In the meantime, the high insect selectivity, low mammalian toxicity, and low rates of application may provide a breathing space in the ongoing search for efficacious, nontoxic chemical insecticides.

BOTANICAL INSECTICIDES

Naturally occurring agents of plant origin have been used to control insect pests. These chemicals ranged from highly toxic agents (to both target and nontarget species), such as nicotine, to relatively innocuous substances, such as derris root. Interestingly, despite the overwhelming number of synthetic insecticide formulations on the market, the two above-mentioned agents can still be purchased and are still considered effective insecticides.

Nicotine

Nicotine, first used as an insecticide in 1763, has been used as a contact insecticide, stomach poison, and fumigant in the form of nicotine alkaloid, the sulfate salt, or in the form of other derivatives. Commercially, nicotine is extracted from the leaves of *Nicotiana tabacum* and *Nicotiana rustica* by alkali treatment and steam distillation or by extraction with benzene, trichloroethylene, or diethyl ether. Nicotine makes up some 97 percent of the alkaloid content of commercial tobacco. It is marketed under the trade name of Black Leaf 40, an aqueous solution of the sulfate salt of nicotine, containing 40 percent nicotine.

Nicotine is extremely toxic, the acute oral LD_{50} in rats being on the order of 50 to 60 mg/kg. It is readily absorbed through the skin, and any contact with nicotine solutions should be washed off immediately. Anecdotal accounts of experiences by people who sprayed this chemical as an agricultural insecticide make an interesting collection of stories, all pointing to the fact that nicotine mimics the action of acetylcholine at all ganglionic synapses and at neuromuscular junctions, causing muscular fasciculations, convulsions, and death from paralysis of the respiratory muscles via blockade of the neuromuscular junctions (see Table 22-7). It functions as an insecticide in much the same manner, causing a blockade of synapses associated with motor nerves in insects.

Rotenoids

Six rotenoid esters occur naturally and are isolated from the plant *Derris eliptica* found in Southeast Asia or from the plant *Lonchocarpus utilis* or *Lonchocarpus urucu,* native to South America. Rotenone, one of the alkaloids, is the most potent and can be purified by solvent extraction and recrystallization. It can be used either as a contact or a stomach poison. However, it is unstable in light and heat and almost all toxicity can be lost after 2 to 3 days during the summer. Rotenone is very toxic to fish, and one of its main uses by native people over the centuries was to paralyze fish for capture and consumption. The mammalian toxicity varies greatly with the species exposed, the method of administration, and the type of formulation. Crystalline rotenone has an acute oral LD_{50} of 60, 132, and 3000 mg/kg for guinea pigs, rats, and rabbits, respectively (Matsumura, 1985). Because the toxicity of derris powders exceeds that of the equivalent content of rotenone, it is obvious that the other esters in crude preparations have significant biological activity. Acute poisoning in animals is characterized by an initial respiratory stimulation followed by respiratory depression, ataxia, convulsions, and death by respiratory arrest (Shimkin and Anderson, 1936). The anesthetic-like action on nerves appears to be related to the ability of rotenone to block electron transport in mitochondria by inhibiting oxidation linked to $NADH_2$, this resulting in nerve conduction blockade (O'Brien, 1967; Corbett, 1974). Although toxicity in laboratory and domestic animals has been reported with acute LD_{50} values of 10 to 30 mg/kg, human intoxications are rare. The estimated fatal oral dose for a 70-kg man is of the order of 10 to 100 g. Rotenone has been used topically for treatment of head lice, scabies, and other ectoparasites, but the dust is highly irritating to the eyes (potentially causing conjunctivitis), the skin (causing contact dermatitis), and the upper respiratory tract (causing rhinitis) and throat (linked with pharyngitis).

HERBICIDES

A herbicide, in the broadest definition, is any compound that is capable of either killing or severely injuring plants; it may be used for the elimination of plant growth or the killing off of plant parts (Jager, 1983). Many of the early chemicals—such as sulfuric acid, sodium chlorate, arsenic trioxide, sodium arsenite, petroleum oils, iron and copper sulfate, or sodium borate—were frequently hard to handle and/or were very toxic, relatively nonspecific, or phytotoxic to the crop as well as the unwanted plant life if not applied at exactly the proper time. In the late 1930s, many studies were initiated to find agents that would selectively destroy certain plant species. Many of these early chemicals were more effective but still possessed considerable mammalian toxicity. However, a few compounds served as prototype chemicals for further development. Summaries of the early days of herbicide development are presented by Cremlyn (1978), McEwen and Stephenson (1979), Kirby (1980), and Jager (1983).

In the past two decades, the herbicides have represented the most rapidly growing section of the agrochemical pesticide business due in part to (1) movement into monocultural practices, where the risk of weed infestation has increased because fallowing and crop rotation, which would change weed species, are no longer in vogue; and (2) mechanization of agricultural practices (planting, tending, harvesting) because of increased labor costs. The annual rate of growth of herbicide production on a worldwide basis between 1980 and 1985 was 1.9 percent per year, more than double the rate of growth for insecticides during the same period (Marquis, 1986). The result has been a plethora of chemically diverse structures rivaling the innovative chemistry of the insecticides, the aim being to protect desirable crops and obtain high yields by selectively eliminating unwanted plant species, thereby reducing the competition for nutrients.

Herbicides may be classified by chemical structure, although this is not very enlightening because of overlapping biological effects for a variety of chemical structures. The second method of classification pertains to how and when the agents are applied. *Preplanting* herbicides are applied to the soil before a crop is seeded. *Preemergent* herbicides are applied to the soil before the usual time of appearance of the unwanted vegetation. *Postemergent* herbicides are applied to the soil or foliage after the germination of the crop and/or weeds. Plant biochemists classify herbicides according to their mechanism of toxicity in plants; their action is referred to as *selective* (toxic to some species), *contact* (act when impinging on the plant foliage), or *translocated* (being absorbed via the soil or through the foliage into the plant xylem and phloem).

In this chapter, herbicides are classified by their ability to interfere with specific biochemical processes essential for normal growth and development—interactions that result in severe injury to the plant and its eventual death. In Table 22-11, the various mechanisms by which herbicides exert their biological effects are shown, along with the generic and chemical names of the classes of herbicides and some examples of each class. The claim has been made that, because the modes of action involve biochemical phytoprocesses having no counterparts in mammalian systems, no risk of mammalian toxicity is associated with these chemicals. With the exception of a few chemicals, the herbicides have demonstrated low toxicity in mammals.

However, the current controversy around these chemicals centers on demonstrated or suspected mutagenicity, teratogenicity, and/or carcinogenicity associated either with the agent(s) or with contaminants and by-products of manufacture found in trace amounts in technical-grade material. The presence of some of these contaminants has been largely ignored without any recognition that the toxicities associated with them are different from those observed with the herbicidal chemical and frequently occur at far lower dosages.

In terms of general toxicity, because the major route of exposure to herbicides is dermal and these agents tend to be strong acids, amines, esters, and phenols, they are dermal irritants, causing skin rashes and contact dermatitis even when exposure involves

Table 22-11
Mechanisms of Action of Herbicides

MECHANISM(S)	CHEMICAL CLASSES
Inhibition of photosynthesis by disruption of light reactions and blockade of electron transport	Ureas, 1,3,5-triazines, 1,4-triazines, uracils, pyridazones, 4-hydroxybenzonitriles, *N*-arylcarbamates, acylanilides
Inhibition of respiration by blockade of electron transfer from NADH or blocking the coupling of electron transfer to ADP to form ATP	Dinitrophenols Halophenols
Growth stimulants, "auxins"	Aryloxyalkylcarboxylic acids, benzoic acids
Inhibitors of cell and nucleus division	Alkyl *N*-arylcarbamates
Inhibitors of protein synthesis	Dinitroanilines
Inhibition of carotenoid synthesis, protective pigments in chloroplasts to prevent chlorophyll from being destroyed by oxidative reactions	Chloracetamide, hydrazines, *o*-substituted diphenyl ethers
Inhibition of lipid synthesis	*S*-alkyl dialkylcarbamodithioates Aliphatic chlorocarboxylic acids
Inhibition of acetolase synthase	Sulfonylureas, imidazolines, triazolopyrimidines, sulfonamides
Inhibition of protoporphyrinogen oxidase	Diphenyl ethers, heterocyclic phenyl ethers (benzotriazoles, indolinones, benzisoxazoles, quinoxalindones, benzoxazines)
Inhibition of enolpyruvylshikimate-3-phosphate synthetase	Glyphosate
Inhibition of glutamine synthetase	Glufosinate
Unknown mechanisms, nonselective chemicals	Inorganic agents (copper sulfate, sulfuric acid, sodium chlorate, sodium borate) Organic agents (dichlobenil, benzoylpropethyl, chlorthiamid, bentazone)

diluted formulations. There appear to be subpopulations of individuals who are hypersensitive to dermal contact with solutions or aerosolized mists of certain types of herbicides, and moderate to severe urticaria has been observed to persist for 5 to 10 days following exposure. Certain individuals, particularly those prone to allergic reactions, may experience severe contact dermatitis, asthma-like attacks, and even anaphylactic reactions following dermal or inhalation contact with formulated herbicides. Whether these effects are chemical-specific for the herbicide or for emulsifiers, cosolvents, and so-called inerts found in formulations has not been established. One such example is discussed below. Although skin patch testing of herbicidal chemicals has usually proven to be negative, it is possible that patients' responses may be associated with a generalized, nonspecific irritant effect of the formulation. Many of these dermal and pulmonary reactions respond satisfactorily to treatment with antihistaminic agents.

In contrast, there are other herbicides that can elicit a range of acute and chronic effects following exposure, and it is on these chemicals that attention is focused here.

Chlorophenoxy Compounds

During World War II, considerable effort was directed toward the development of effective, broad-spectrum herbicides in both the United States and the United Kingdom with a view to both increasing food production and finding potential chemical warfare agents (Kirby, 1980). The chlorophenoxy compounds (Fig. 22-22)—including the acids, salts, amines, and esters—were the first commercially available products evolving from this research in 1946. This class of herbicides has seen continuous, extensive, and uninterrupted use since 1947 in agriculture for broadleafed weeds and in the control of woody plants along roadside, railway, and utilities' rights of way and in reforestation programs. In plants, these chemicals mimic the action of auxins, hormones chemically related to indoleacetic acid, that stimulate growth. No hormonal activity is observed in mammals and other species, and beyond target organ toxicity that can be associated with the pharmacokinetics, biotransformation, and/or elimination of these chemicals, their mechanisms of toxic action are poorly understood. The chlorophenoxy herbicides are no longer the agents of choice because of concerns over the formation of chlorinated dibenzofurans and dibenzodioxins, particularly 2,3,7,8-tetrachlorodibenzo-*p*-dioxin (TCDD), as a consequence of poorly monitored manufacturing practices or improper product storage in steel drums sitting beside

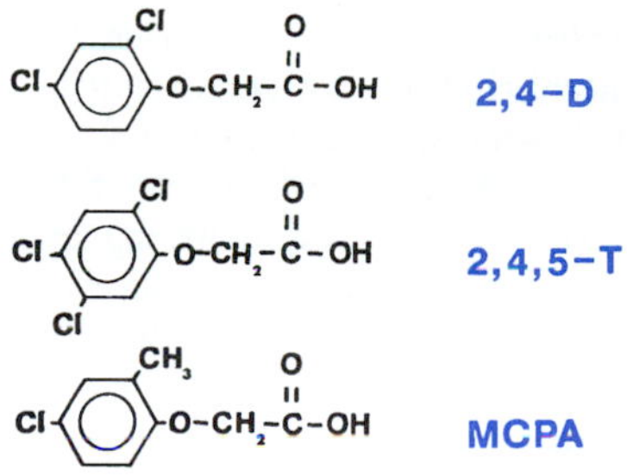

2,4-D

2,4,5-T

MCPA

Figure 22-22. The molecular structure of the three most common chlorophenoxyacetic acid herbicides: 2,4-dichlorophenoxyacetic acid (2,4-D), 2,4,5-trichlorophenoxyacetic acid (2,4,5-T), and 4-chloro-o-toloxyacetic acid (MCPA). Ester and amine salt derivatives are also marketed.

runways under the tropical sun. However, since they are still used in developing nations around the world, their toxicology cannot be ignored.

A tremendous volume of mammalian toxicity data has been collected over the past 42 years from both animal studies and incidents of human exposure (Hayes, 1982; Stevens and Sumner, 1991). It is of interest to note that, in a recent toxicologic reevaluation of 2,4-D for the purposes of providing the U.S. EPA with a new toxicity database for the chemical, an industry task force discovered nothing of toxicologic significance that was not already known about the chemical, with one exception (Mullison, 1986). The exceptional finding was the appearance of astrocytomas in the brains of male Fischer 344 strain rats exposed to the highest (45 mg/kg per day) dosage. A subsequent review of the findings suggested that this tumor incidence was not treatment-related (Koestner, 1986; Solleveld et al., 1984). The acute toxicity elicited by chlorophenoxy herbicides has been described by Hayes (1982). The oral LD_{50} values ranged from 300 to >1000 mg/kg in different animal species, and only the dog appeared to be particularly sensitive, possibly on the basis that it has considerable difficulty in the renal elimination of such organic acids (Gehring et al., 1976).

Accidental and/or occupational intoxications have been reviewed (Hayes, 1982; Stevens and Sumner, 1991; Ecobichon, 1996). An industrial accident in 1949 in a 2,4,5-T manufacturing plant in Nitro, West Virginia, presented the first large occupational exposure, with acute symptoms of exposure to the reaction products, including skin, eye, and respiratory tract irritation; headache; dizziness; nausea; acneiform eruptions; severe muscle pain in the thorax, shoulders and extremities; fatigue; nervousness; irritability; dyspnea; complaints of decreased libido; and intolerance to cold (Ashe and Suskind, 1953). In an epidemiologic study of these same workers conducted in 1984, clinical evidence of chloracne persisted in some 55.7 percent of those exposed (113 out of 204), and an association was found between the persistence of chloracne and the presence and severity of actinic elastosis of the skin (Suskind and Hertzberg, 1984). There was no evidence of increased risk of cardiovascular, hepatic, or renal disease or of central or peripheral nervous tissue damage. One study documented neurotoxicity, decreased peripheral conduction velocities being observed in workers employed in the manufacture of 2,4-D and 2,4,5-T (Singer et al., 1982). Earlier literature reported significant peripheral neuropathies in three sprayers using 2,4-D ester, signs and symptoms progressing from muscle pain and paresthesias to severe paralysis, all of which was supported by electromyographic analysis (Goldstein et al., 1959). Chloracne, or "weed bumps," has been the most persistent effect observed in almost all incidents of chlorophenoxy herbicide exposure, although this is not a specific effect, being caused by a number of halogenated aromatic compounds including polyhalogenated biphenyls, dibenzo-*p*-dioxins, dibenzofurans, and naphthalenes (Schultz, 1968; Poland et al., 1971).

A wide range of human lethal dosages of 2,4-D has been reported, the average being in excess of 300 mg/kg, although it may be as low as 80 mg/kg. The oral dose required to elicit symptoms is of the order of 50 to 60 mg/kg. Since these chemicals are irritants, oral ingestion has caused focal submucosal hemorrhage, moderate congestion, and edema as well as necrosis of the intestinal tract, fatty infiltration and necrosis of the liver, degeneration of the convoluted tubules of the kidney, and pneumonitis and inflammation in the terminal bronchioles (Hayes, 1982).

In hindsight, many of the above-mentioned signs and symptoms might be attributed to contaminants found in chlorophenoxy herbicides from early production times, principally from a mixture of polychlorinated dibenzo-*p*-dioxins, the main one being TCDD, found in samples of 2,4,5-T at levels of 30 to 50 ug/g (Hay, 1982; Gough, 1986). The teratogenicity (cleft palate, renal anomalies) produced by commercial, TCDD-contaminated (30 ug/g) 2,4,5-T was not reproduced when highly purified 2,4,5-T was used (Courtney et al., 1970; Courtney and Moore, 1971). Recent in vitro and in vivo genotoxicity studies of 2,4-D have proven negative (Charles et al., 1999a, b; Gollapudi et al., 1999). Recent accidental/occupational exposures to chlorophenoxy herbicides have not resulted in peripheral neuropathies, a fact confirmed in animal studies using purified 2,4-D dimethylamine salt (Mattsson et al., 1986). While the carcinogenicity of purified 2,4-D and 2,4,5-T has not been established in rodent studies, that of TCDD has (Van Miller et al., 1977; Kociba et al., 1978). The toxicology of the polychlorinated dioxins and furans is discussed in other chapters.

Public concerns about the chlorophenoxy herbicides have focused on birth defects, cancers, and the spurious illnesses reported among military personnel exposed to the defoliant Agent Orange (a 50:50 mixture of the *n*-butyl esters of 2,4-D and 2,4,5-T) sprayed extensively during the Vietnam conflict and found to be contaminated with TCDD to a maximum of 47 ug/g (Hay, 1982; Greenwald et al., 1984; Gough, 1986; CDC, 1988; Stellman et al., 1988; Tamburro, 1992). While exposure to this persistent contaminant can be verified by blood analysis of veterans, the multifaceted nature of the adverse effects has precluded a definitive association (Ketchum et al., 1999). Epidemiologic studies of cancer in farmers and others occupationally exposed to chlorophenoxy herbicides for long periods of time have suggested an association with soft tissue sarcomas, non-Hodgkin's lymphoma (NHL), and Hodgkin's lymphoma (HL) without any definitive conclusions (Hardell and Sandstrom, 1979; Ott et al., 1980; Eriksson et al., 1981; Hardell et al., 1981; Cantor, 1982; Theiss et al., 1982; Lynge, 1985; Schumacher, 1985; Hoar et al., 1986; Pearce et al., 1986; Bond et al., 1988; Bond and Rossbacher, 1993). A study of wheat farmers in western Canada, where 2,4-D has been used almost exclusively from 1947, showed an overall lower mortality and cancer rate than expected (Wigle et al., 1990). A review of published studies presented evidence of an association between occupational exposure to chlorophenoxy herbicides and an increased risk of NHL (Morrison et al., 1992). The study of an international database set up by IARC/NIEHS revealed no clearly detectable excess for NHL and HL but a sixfold excess of soft tissue sarcomas in the cohort and a ninefold excess among sprayers (Saracci et al., 1991). An increase in prostate cancer mortality among Canadian farmers has been reported (Morrison et al., 1993). Other studies of databases have suggested that the carcinogenic impact of chlorophenoxy compounds was negligible (Munro et al., 1992; Bond and Rossbacher, 1993). Lacking the ideal "definitive, clean" study, this controversy will continue in the literature. In the meantime, the chlorophenoxy herbicides have been phased out of use in developed nations, being replaced by other agents. However, the concerns persist, particularly in developing countries where use continues and in Vietnam, where exposure was so heavy.

Animals will tolerate repeated oral exposure to doses of chlorophenoxy herbicides marginally below the single, toxic oral dose without showing significant signs of toxicity, an observation suggesting that there is little cumulative effect on target organs. At dosages causing toxicity, few specific signs other than muscular and neuromuscular involvement were observed in animals, although tenseness, stiffness in extremities, muscular weakness, ataxia, and paralysis have been reported. Hepatic and renal injury in addition to irritation of the gastrointestinal mucosa have been observed in acute lethality studies in animals.

Bipyridyl Derivatives

One chemical class of herbicides deserving of particular attention is the bipyridyl group, specifically paraquat (1,1′-dimethyl-4,4′-bipyridylium dichloride, methyl viologen) and diquat (1,1′-ethylene-2,2′-bipyridylium dibromide) (Fig. 22-23). Paraquat was first synthesized in 1882, but its pesticidal properties were not discovered until 1959 (Haley, 1979). This agent, a nonselective contact herbicide, is one of the most specific pulmonary toxicants known and has been the subject of intensive investigation because of the startling toxicity observed in humans. A high mortality rate is encountered in poisoning cases. Many countries have banned or severely restricted the use of paraquat because of the debilitating or life-threatening hazards from occupational exposure and the large number of reported accidental and suicidal fatalities (Campbell, 1968; Davies et al., 1977; Haley, 1979; Tinoco et al., 1993). However, paraquat is still used in some 130 countries and, in third-world nations, is available to 98 percent of the agricultural workers (WHO, 1984; Ramasamy et al., 1988). In Taiwan, paraquat accounted for 54 percent of the pesticide-related poisonings in the years 1985 to 1993 (Yang et al., 1996). The toxicology of this class of herbicides should not be ignored.

In animals, paraquat shows moderate acute toxicity, the oral LD_{50} values for various species ranging from 22 to 262 mg/kg. Intoxication involves a combination of signs and symptoms that include lethargy, hypoxia, dyspnea, tachycardia, hyperpnea, adipsia, diarrhea, ataxia, hyperexcitability, and convulsions, depending on the dosage and the species studied (Smith and Heath, 1976; Haley, 1979). Necropsy reveals hemorrhagic and edematous lungs, intraalveolar hemorrhage, congestion and pulmonary fibrosis, centrilobular hepatic necrosis, and renal tubular necrosis. Lung weights of intoxicated animals increase significantly despite marked losses in body weight. From a catalog of all the signs and symptoms, it is obvious that the lung is the most susceptible target organ, and the same histopathologic picture of pulmonary lesions is observed in mice, rats, dogs, and humans (Clark et al., 1966). In poisonings, immediate effects are usually not seen in animals; within 10 to 14 days, however, respiration becomes impaired, rapid, and shallow and the morphologic changes seen include degeneration and vacuolization of pneumocytes, damage to type I and type II alveolar epithelial cells, destruction of the epithelial membranes, and proliferation of fibrotic cells.

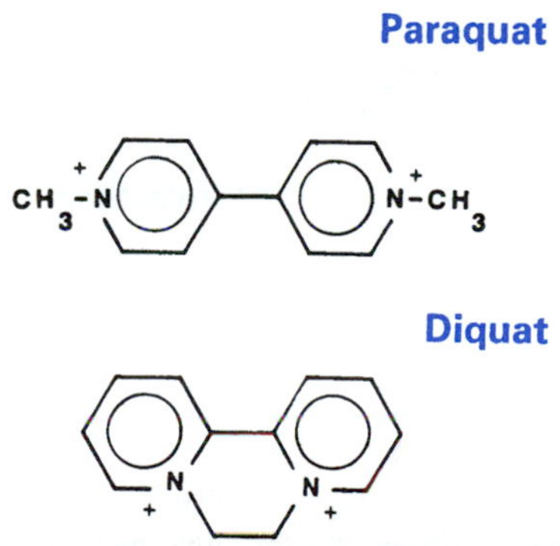

Paraquat

CH_3-N^+ … N^+-CH_3

Diquat

N N + +

Figure 22-23. The chemical structures of paraquat and diquat, marketed as the dichloride and dibromide salts, respectively.

Paraquat, a highly polar compound, is poorly absorbed from the gastrointestinal tract (5 to 10 percent) (Haley, 1979). Experiments in rats showed that 52 percent of the administered oral dose was still localized in the intestine some 32 h postadministration, although 45 percent of the dose had been excreted in the urine and feces within 48 h, with some detected in urine for up to 21 days (Murray and Gibson, 1974). Intoxication by the ingestion of formulation concentrates may be enhanced by increased absorption due to the presence of emulsifiers and cosolvents. Metabolism by mammalian tissue is not extensive, although intestinal microflora may account for 30 percent of the excreted metabolites in animal studies (Daniel and Gage, 1966). Elevated levels of paraquat in renal tissue suggest the kidney as a primary route of excretion (Rose et al., 1976).

Pulmonary tissue, both in vivo and in vitro, acquires much higher concentrations of paraquat than other tissues with the exception of the kidney. Over a 30-h posttreatment period, disproportionately high levels are found in the lung (Sharp et al., 1972; Rose et al., 1976). Acquisition is due to a unique diamine/polyamine transport system in the alveolar cells. Upon uptake, paraquat undergoes a NADPH-dependent one-electron reduction to a free radical that reacts with molecular oxygen to regenerate the paraquat cation plus a reactive superoxide anion ($O_2^{\bar{\cdot}}$), which is converted into hydrogen peroxide (H_2O_2) by the enzyme superoxide dismutase. Both O_2 and H_2O_2 can attack polyunsaturated lipids, forming lipid hydroperoxides that, in turn, react with unsaturated lipids to form more lipid-free radicals, perpetuating the destructive reaction (Smith, 1987). Alveolar cell membrane damage results in alveolitis, the destruction of alveolar cells, invasion of the space by fibrotic cells accompanied by a loss of pulmonary elasticity and respiratory impairment, with an inefficient gas (O_2, CO_2) exchange. Cellular events can be modulated by the availability of oxygen, animals kept in air with only 10% oxygen faring better than those kept in room air (Rhodes, 1974).

Paraquat poisonings in children and adults have been described in detail in the literature (Almog and Tal, 1967; Davies et al., 1977; Haley, 1979; Hayes, 1982; Tinoco et al., 1993). Paraquat is a favored agent in suicide attempts in many parts of the world (Wesseling et al., 1993, 1997; Yang et al., 1996). Paraquat-induced intoxications should be divided into two categories: (1) poisonings by accidental or intentional ingestion, usually involving formulation concentrates containing up to 20 percent active ingredient, and (2) functional intoxications, associated with dermal and/or inhalation exposure of diluted spray formulations.

The ingestion of commercial paraquat concentrates is invariably fatal and runs a time course of 3 to 4 weeks. The initial irritation and burning of the mouth and throat, the necrosis and sloughing of the oral mucosa, severe gastroenteritis with esophageal and gastric lesions, abdominal and substernal chest pains, and bloody stools give way to the characteristic dominant pulmonary symptoms, including dyspnea, anoxia, opacity in the lungs seen in chest x-rays, progressive fibrosis, coma, and death. While the pulmonary lesions are the most life-threatening, paraquat induces multiorgan toxicity with necrotic damage to the liver, kidneys, and myocardial muscle plus extensive hemorrhagic incidents throughout the body.

Survivors of moderate-to-severe paraquat poisonings showed significant impairment in respiratory function tests, which improved dramatically or partially with time (Lin et al., 1995). However, it is as yet unknown whether long-term respiratory health effects occur with repeated and/or seasonal inhalation and/or dermal exposure to diluted paraquat aerosols (Wesseling et al., 1997). Swan (1969) found no detectable changes in workers exposed to sprays 6 days per week for 12 weeks. Senanayake et al. (1993) found no changes in standard spirometric tests in Sri Lankan tea plantation workers continually exposed to paraquat aerosols. More recent studies have confirmed that no correlation exists between exposure and parameters such as $FEV_{1.0}$, FVC, etc. (Castro-Gutierrez et al., 1997; Dalvie et al., 1999). However, in one study, severity of dyspnea and a threefold increase in episodic wheezing accompanied by shortness of breath was found among the most highly exposed workers (Castro-Gutierrez et al., 1997). Perhaps the standard, spirometric, functional tests are not sensitive enough since, in the second study, there was a significant relationship between long-term exposure and arterial oxygen desaturation measured by oximetry during an exercise test (Dalvie et al., 1999). More sensitive tests may be needed to assess long-term respiratory disabilities.

Treatment of paraquat poisoning should be vigorous and initiated as quickly as possible. Gastric lavage should be followed by the administration of mineral adsorbents such as Fuller's earth (kaolin), bentonite clay, or activated charcoal to bind any unabsorbed paraquat remaining in the gastrointestinal tract. Purgatives may be given. Absorbed paraquat may be removed from the bloodstream by aggressive, lengthy hemoperfusion through charcoal or by hemodialysis. To avoid excessive pulmonary damage, supplemental oxygen should be reduced to a level just sufficient to maintain acceptable arterial oxygen tension (>40 to 50 mmHg) (Haley, 1979; Hayes, 1982). Even though these patients may suffer from hypoxia and respiratory insufficiency, hyperbaric oxygen is contraindicated because it appears to promote cellular toxicity.

Diquat is a rapid-acting contact herbicide used as a desiccant, for the control of aquatic weeds, and to destroy potato halums before harvesting. Diquat is slightly less toxic than paraquat; the oral LD_{50} values in various species are on the order of 100 to 400 mg/kg. Part of the reduced toxicity may be related to the fact that it is poorly absorbed from the gastrointestinal tract; only 6 percent of an ingested dose is excreted in the urine, whereas 90 to 98 percent of the dose is eliminated via the urine following subcutaneous administration (Daniel and Gage, 1966). A latency period of 24 h is seen prior to visible toxic effects.

Following acute, high-dose exposure or chronic exposure of animals to diquat, the major target organs were the gastrointestinal tract, the liver, and the kidneys (Hayes, 1982; Morgan, 1982). Chronic feeding studies resulted in an increased incidence of cataracts in both dogs and rats (Clark and Hurst, 1970). It is considered that diquat can form free radicals and that the tissue necrosis is associated with the same mechanism(s) of superoxide-induced peroxidation as observed with paraquat. Unlike paraquat, diquat shows no special affinity for the lung and does not appear to involve the same mechanism that selectively concentrates paraquat in the lung (Rose and Smith, 1977).

Few diquat-related human intoxications have been reported to date (Schonborn et al., 1971; Narita et al., 1978; Hayes, 1982). In the few cases of suicidal intent described, ulceration of mucosal membranes, gastrointestinal symptoms, acute renal failure, hepatic damage, and respiratory difficulties were observed. CNS effects were more severe. Interestingly, no fibrosis was evident in the lungs. One individual died of cardiac arrest.

Chloroacetanilides

Alachlor (Lasso) (Fig. 22-24) is an aniline herbicide used to control annual grasses and broad-leaf weeds in a number of crops (corn, soybeans, peanuts) as a systemic herbicide absorbed by the germinating shoots and roots by interfering with protein synthesis and root elongation. It is a slightly toxic (EPA class III) herbicide, the oral LD_{50} (rat) being 930 to 1350 mg/kg, and is a slight-to-moderate skin irritant (WSSA, 1994; Kamrin, 1997). Subchronic studies in rats and dogs, with doses of 1 to 100 mg/kg/day, showed no adverse effects, but a 6-month dog study showed hepatic toxicity at all doses above 5 mg/kg/day, while a year-long study revealed hepatic, renal, and splenic effects above a dosage of 1 mg/kg/day. In reproductive studies, maternal and fetal toxicity was observed at the high oral doses used (150 and 400 mg/kg/day), but there was no effect on reproduction. Neither were teratogenic effects seen in rats and rabbits, confirming the negative results in microbial mutagenicity studies. Revisiting the toxicity database and providing replacement studies for carcinogenicity revealed thyroid tumors and adenocarcinomas of the stomach and nasal turbinates of Long-Evans rats and in the lungs of CD-1 mice receiving relatively high doses (126 and 260 mg/kg/day for rats and mice, respectively (Alachlor Review Board, 1987). Alachlor is considered to be a category 2B (probable) human carcinogen by the U.S. EPA, a risk to agricultural workers during mixing and loading, with levels of exposure ranging from 0.00038 to 2.7 mg/kg/day depending on the exposure model used. The putative carcinogen metabolite, 2.6-diethylbenzoquinonimine (DEBQ1), is formed by oxidative and nonoxidative reactions in mice, rats, and monkeys but not in humans (Coleman et al., 1999). However, the human may form DEBQ1 via another route. Studies of thyroid tumors in rats suggest that alachlor-induced follicular cell tumors were related to increased metabolism of thyroxine via hepatic enzyme conjugation (Wilson et al., 1996). To date, there has been no evidence of an appreciable effect of alachlor exposure on worker mortality or cancer rates (Acquavella et al., 1996).

The discovery of alachlor in well water at levels of 0.11 to 2.11 μg/L, the highest being 9.1 μg/L, led to the cancellation of its registration in Canada in 1985. Concerns about one analog of a series has led to the examination of other chloracetanilides and closely related agents—e.g., acetochlor, amidochlor, butachlor,

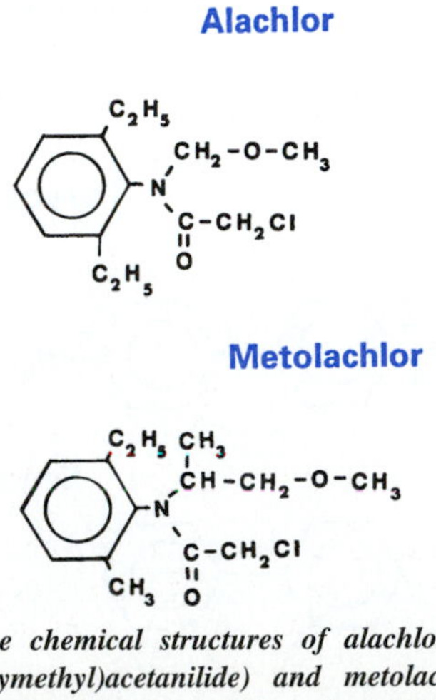

Alachlor

C_2H_5, CH_2-O-CH_3, N, C-CH_2Cl, O, C_2H_5

Metolachlor

C_2H_5, CH_3, CH-CH_2-O-CH_3, N, C-CH_2Cl, O, CH_3

Figure 22-24. The chemical structures of alachlor (2-chloro-2′, 6′-diethyl-N-(methoxymethyl)acetanilide) and metolachlor (2-chloro-6′-ethyl-ethyl-N-(2-methoxy-1-methylethyl) acet-o-toluidide.

metalaxyl, metolachlor (Fig. 22-24), propachlor, etc.—all of the agents showing a consistent pattern of mutagenic activity mediated via metabolites, possibly even species-specific intermediates (Dearfield et al., 1999). One example acetochlor is converted into a rat-specific metabolite that may be related to the nasal tumors, thus posing no genetic or carcinogenic hazard to humans (Ashby et al., 1996). However, changes in leopard frog metamorphosis by acetochlor appears to be related to an interaction with thyroid hormone via a nonthyroid receptor mechanism (Cheek et al., 1999). No doubt, detailed mechanistic studies will reveal one or more modes of action.

Phosphonomethyl Amino Acids

Two agents, *N*-phosphonomethyl glycine (glyphosate, Roundup, Vision) and *N*-phosphonomethyl homoalanine (glufosinate, Basta) must be considered because of their use in attempted suicides in southeastern Asia (Fig. 22-25). Both agents are broad-spectrum nonselective systemic herbicides for postemergent control of annual and perennial plants (grasses, sedges, broad-leaf weeds) and woody plants. While they exist as free acids, these agents are marketed as the isopropylamine or trimethylsulfonium salts of glyphosate and the ammonium salt of glufosinate in formulation concentrates of 41 percent and 18.5 percent, respectively. In considering any toxicity data, one must make the distinction whether the data pertain to the acid, the salt, or the complete formulation(s) containing what appear to be biologically active surfactants (Kamrin, 1997; Watanabe and Sano, 1998).

Glyphosate Glyphosate binds to and inhibits the enzyme 5-enolpyruvyl-shikimate-3-phosphate synthetase (EPSPS), an enzyme of the aromatic amino acid biosynthesis pathway essential for protein synthesis in plants (Haslam, 1993). In mammals, ingestion, with oral LD_{50} values in the rat being 5600 mg/kg, although that of the trimethylsulfonium salt is 750 mg/kg (WSSA, 1994). Formulations of glyphosate show moderate toxicity, LD_{50} values being between 1000 and 5000 mg/kg (Monsanto, 1985; WSSA, 1994). Glyphosate is nontoxic by the dermal route, with dermal LD_{50} values being in excess of 5000 mg/kg for the acid and the isopropylamine salt. While glyphosate is not a dermal irritant in animals and does not induce photosensitization, formulations can cause severe occupational contact dermatitis, although patch testing in humans resulted in no visible skin changes or sensitization (WSSA, 1994; Maibach, 1986). Glyphosate is an ocular irritant in the rabbit and human (Acquavella et al., 1999). Chronic studies with rats, dogs, and rabbits resulted in no glyphosate-related effects up to the highest doses tested (400 to 500 mg/kg/day) (WSSA, 1994). Reproductive problems were observed in test animals only at very high (150 mg/kg/day) doses that elicited maternal toxicity. Glyphosate was not teratogenic at elevated doses in rabbits (350 mg/kg/day) or rats (175 mg/kg/day), although other signs of toxicity in dams and fetuses were observed. Glyphosate was not mutagenic in standard tests (Ames and other bacterial assays, dominant lethal test in mouse) (Li and Long, 1998; WSSA, 1994). However, one study, with glyphosate isopropylamine salt and Roundup formulation, showed weak mutagenic activity in the Ames test and a significant increase in chromosomal aberrations in the *Allium* root cell when Roundup was tested (Rank et al., 1993). Carcinogenicity was not observed in mice, rats or dogs, glyphosate being classified by the U.S. EPA as a class E agent. Moses (1989) has reported tumors in the pituitary and mammary glands in glyphosate-treated rats. Glyphosate does not inhibit cholinesterases.

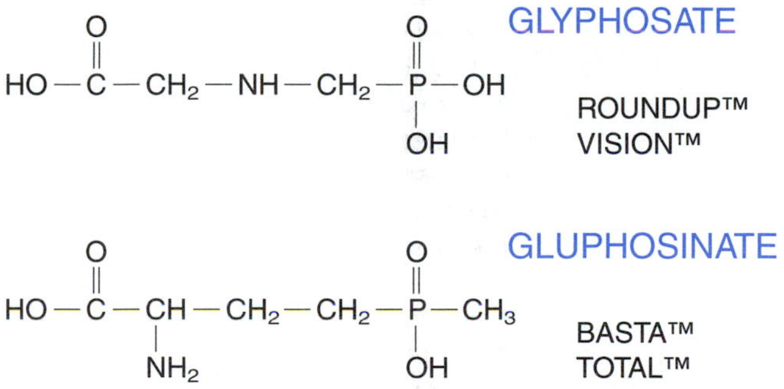

Unfortunately, glyphosate has become the agent of choice to replace paraquat as a suicidal agent in many countries, the incidence of such poisonings increasing as paraquat is banned or is more tightly controlled (Talbot et al., 1991; Tominack et al., 1991; Mendes et al., 1991; Leveridge, 1996; Yang et al., 1996). The formulation concentrate is used. Mild intoxications are characterized by gastrointestinal symptoms (nausea, vomiting, diarrhea, abdominal pain) due to mucosal irritation and injury, with resolution within 24 h (Talbot et al., 1991). In moderate intoxications, more severe and persistent intestinal symptoms (ulceration, esophagitis, hemorrhage) are seen, along with hypotension, some pulmonary dysfunction, acid-base disturbance, and evidence of hepatic and renal damage. Severe poisoning is characterized by pulmonary dysfunction requiring intubation, renal failure requiring dialysis, hypotension and vascular shock, cardiac arrest, repeated seizures, coma, and death (Talbot et al., 1991; Tominack et al., 1991). A reasonable dose-effect relationship was established by Talbot et al. (1991), who estimated the volume(s) of formulation (concentrate) ingested causing asymptomatic, mild, moderate or severe poisoning in humans to be 17, 58, 128 and 184 mL, respectively. This could be converted to glyphosate concentrations of 87, 298, 658, and 946 mg/kg based on the formulation containing 360 g/L of free glyphosate and a 70-kg body weight.

Several reviews of intoxication cases, particularly the Japanese and Taiwanese series, have raised suspicions about the toxicity of the surfactant polyoxyethyleneamine (POEA) in the formulations used currently (Sawada and Nagai, 1987; Sawada et al., 1988; Talbot et al., 1991; Tominack et al. 1991). The median lethal dose of POEA is less than one-third that of the formulation or glyphosate (Sawada et al., 1988). Tai et al. (1990) found that POEA was responsible for the hypotensive effect in dogs. This class of surfactants has been associated with hemolysis and with gastrointestinal and CNS effects (Grugg et al., 1960; Sawada et al., 1988). As of 1999, efforts were being made to reformulate the Roundup product to replace POEA (personal communication).

GLYPHOSATE

HO—C(=O)—CH_2—NH—CH_2—P(=O)(OH)—OH

ROUNDUP™
VISION™

GLUPHOSINATE

HO—C(=O)—CH(NH_2)—CH_2—CH_2—P(=O)(OH)—CH_3

BASTA™
TOTAL™

Figure 22-25. The chemical structures of glyphosate (N-phosphonomethyl glycine) and glufosinate (N-phosphonomethyl homoalanine).

Glufosinate *N*-phosphonomethyl homoalanine acts as a suicide substrate, interfering with glutamate synthesis in plants by irreversibly inhibiting the enzyme glutamine synthetase, which plays an important role in ammonia detoxification and amino acid metabolism (Ebert et al., 1990). The herbicidal effect is caused by cytotoxicity from increased ammonia levels and impairment of photorespiration and photosynthesis (Hack et al., 1994).

The acute oral toxicity of glufosinate in mice, rats, and rabbits was low, the oral LD_{50} lying between 1500 and 2000 mg/kg (Ebert et al., 1990; Hack et al., 1994). In subchronic feeding studies in rats, no agent-related deaths occurred, although body weight gains in males were retarded in the 5000-ppm group. Food consumption was reduced and water consumption increased and, at this high dose, signs of CNS excitation and hypothermia were noted (Hack et al., 1994). Glufosinate was not considered to be mutaginic, teratogenic, or carcinogenic in animal studies, although in more recent studies using whole-embryo culture, teratogenic effects in mice have been observed, the effect being induced apoptosis in the neuroepithelium of developing embryos (Watanabe and Iwase, 1996; Watanabe, 1997). While glufosinate did not inhibit brain cholinesterase, reductions in erythrocytic and serum cholinesterases have been seen in 7 of 16 patients affected by this herbicide (Watanabe and Iwase, 1998). In contrast to plant metabolism, glufosinate ammonium inhibited glutamine synthetase in animals, but this did not lead to a problem in ammonia metabolism, the mammal obviously compensating by using other metabolic pathways (Hack et al., 1994).

Glufosinate ammonium has been involved in a number of poisoning cases, particularly in Japan (Koyama et al., 1994; Watanabe and Sano, 1998; Tanaka et al., 1998). Early clinical symptoms included nausea, vomiting, and diarrhea associated with intestinal mucosal irritation but were followed in 24 h by neurologic signs, including impaired respiration, seizures, muscle weakness (post–status epileptic myopathy), convulsions, and death within 4 days in 6 of 31 patients (Koyama, 1995). Some survivors showed either a brief loss of memory or amnesia for 7 to 10 days after intoxication (Koyama, 1995). Any significant role of glutamate in the neurologic events has not been confirmed. Limited information is available regarding glufosinate persistence in vivo, but urinary levels higher than concomitant blood levels have been reported and urinary excretion persisted for 3 to 5 days after ingestion (Watanabe and Iwase, 1998).

Once again, concerns have been raised about the role of the surfactant. The direct cause of death seemed to be circulatory disturbance, especially cardiac insufficiency, possibly related to the surfactant in the formulation involved in the intoxications (Koyama et al., 1995; Watanabe and Sano, 1998). The absorption of glufosinate in animals was 25 to 30 percent higher than the absorption rate of the agent when given alone (Watanabe and Sano, 1998). This suggested that the glufosinate-related effects might be enhanced by surfactant-induced penetration of the CNS, while the cardiovascular system effects were surfactant-related.

Many herbicides representative of several chemical classifications and diverse structures have recently been introduced into agricultural practice (Table 22-11). In general, these chemicals have relatively low acute toxicity, the oral LD_{50} values in rats being of the order of 100 to 10,000 mg/kg, and they are toxicologically uninteresting, since—in subchronic and chronic studies—large doses can be administered without eliciting significant biological effects. Many of these newer chemicals are applied to crops or soil at exceedingly low application rates, minimizing nontarget species toxicity and avoiding environmental contamination. Present concerns focus on groundwater contamination and closer scrutiny of minor contaminants for mutagenic, teratogenic, and carcinogenic effects. Poisonings in humans have usually been associated with occupational exposure or with a few atypical but sometimes well-publicized incidents (Stevens and Sumner, 1991).

FUNGICIDES

Fungicidal chemicals are derived from a variety of structures ranging from simple inorganic compounds, such as sulfur and copper sulfate, through the aryl- and alkyl-mercurial compounds and chlorinated phenols to metal-containing derivatives of thiocarbamic acid (Fig. 22-26). The chemistry of fungicides and their properties have been discussed by Cremlyn (1978), Kramer (1983), and Edwards et al. (1991). *Foliar fungicides* are applied as liquids or powders to the aerial green parts of plants, producing a protective barrier on the cuticular surface and systemic toxicity in the developing

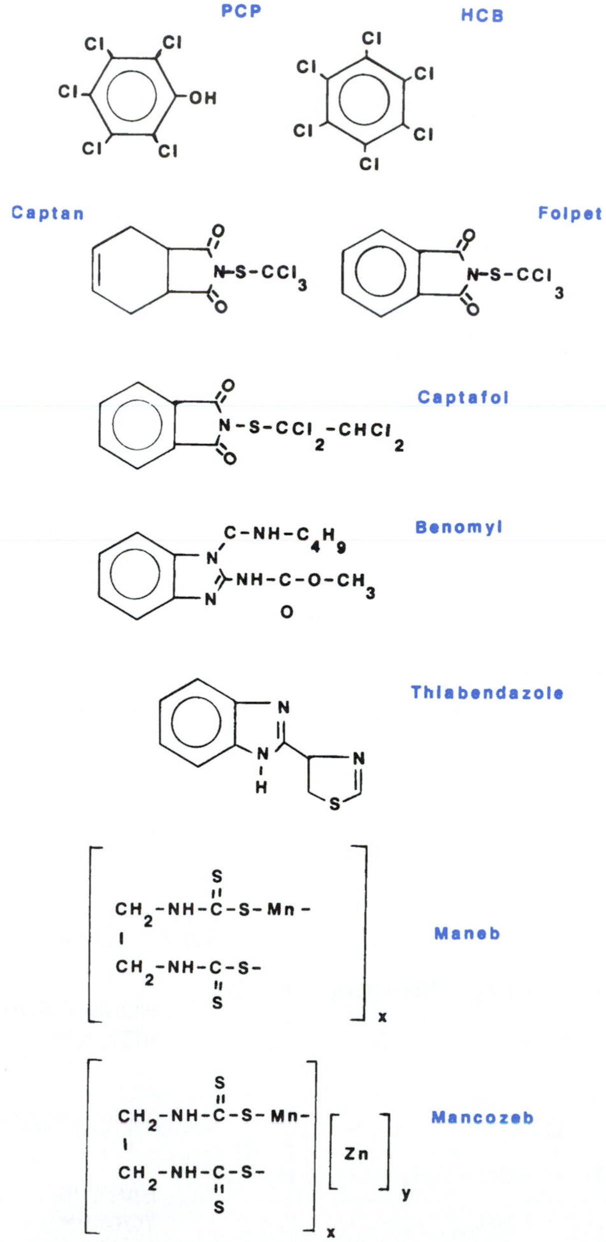

Figure 22-26. Chemical structures of fungicides representative of various chemical classifications.

fungus. *Soil fungicides* are applied as liquids, dry powders, or granules, acting either through the vapor phase or by systemic properties. *Dressing fungicides* are applied to the postharvest crop (cereal grains, tubers, corms, etc.) as liquids or dry powders to prevent fungal infestation of the crop, particularly if it may be stored under less than optimum conditions of temperature and humidity. The postharvest loss of food crops to disease is a serious worldwide problem (Table 22-1). Fungicides may be described as protective, curative, or eradicative, according to their mode of action. *Protective fungicides,* applied to the plant before the appearance of any phytopathic fungi, prevent infection by either sporicidal activity or by changing the physiologic environment on the leaf surface. *Curative fungicides* are used when an infestation has already begun to invade the plant, and these chemicals function by penetrating the plant cuticle and destroying the young fungal mycelium (the hyphae) growing in the epidermis of the plant, preventing further development. *Eradicative fungicides* control fungal development following the appearance of symptoms, usually after sporulation, by killing both the new spores and the mycelia and by penetrating the cuticle of the plant to the subdermal level (Kramer, 1983).

An effective fungicide must possess the following properties: (1) low toxicity to the plant but high toxicity to the particular fungus; (2) activity per se or ability to convert itself (by plant or fungal enzymes) into a toxic intermediate; (3) ability to penetrate fungal spores or the developing mycelium to reach a site of action; and (4) formation of a protective, tenacious deposit on the plant surface that will be resistant to weathering by sunlight, rain, and wind (Cremlyn, 1978). This list of properties is never fulfilled entirely by any single fungicide, and all commercially available compounds show some phytotoxicity, lack of persistence due to environmental degradation, and so forth. Thus, the timing of the application is critical in terms of the development of the plant as well as the fungus.

The topic of fungicidal toxicity has been extensively reviewed by Hayes (1982) Edwards et al. (1991), and Kamrin (1997). With a few exceptions, most of these chemicals have a low order of toxicity to mammals (Table 22-12). However, all fungicides are cytotoxic and most produce positive results in the usual in vitro microbial mutagenicity test systems. Such results are not surprising because the microorganisms (*Salmonella,* coliforms, yeasts, and

Table 22-12
Acute Toxicity of Fungicides

COMMON NAME	CLASS	IRRITATION* (EYE/SKIN)	ORAL LD_{50}, RAT (mg/kg)
Anilazine	Triazine	I	2,710
Benomyl	Imidazole	I	>10,000
Captan	Phthalimide	I	8,400–15,000
Carboxin	Oxathiin	NI	3,820
Chinomethionate	Quinomethionate	NI	2,500–3,000
Chlorothalonil	Organochlorine	I	>10,000
Dichloropropene	Chlorinated alkene	I	130–713
Dinocap	Dinitrophenol	NI	980
Dodine	Aliphatic nitrogen	I	1,000
EPTC	Thiocarbamate	I	1,632
Etridiazole	Thiadiazole	NI	>1,000
Fenarimol	Pyrimidine	I	2,500
Hexachloroben-	Organochlorine	I	3,500
Imazalil	Imidazole	I	227–334
Iprodione	Dicarboximide	I	3,500
Maneb	Dithiocarbamate	I	5,000–8,000
Mancozeb	Dithiocarbamate	I	5,000–>11,200
Metalaxyl	Benzenoid	I	669
Metiram	Dithiocarbamate	I	6,180–>10,000
Nabam	Dithiocarbamate	I	395
Oxycarboxin	Oxathiin	NI	2,000
Pyrazophos	Phosphorothionate	NI	151–632
Quintozene	Organochlorine	I	1,710
Thiabendazole	Imidazole	NI	3,100–3,600
Thiophanate–Me	Dithiocarbamate	I	10,000
Thiram	Thiocarbamate	I	800–>1,900
Triallate	Thiocarbamate	I	800–2,165
Vinclozolin	Dicarboximide	I	>10,000
Zineb	Dithiocarbamate	I	7,600–8,900
Ziram	Dithiocarbamate	I	1,400

*KEY: I, irritant properties; NI, nonirritation.

fungi) used in these test systems are not dissimilar from those cell systems that fungicides are designed to kill, either through a direct lethal effect or via lethal genetic mutations (Lukens, 1971). A safe fungicide (nonmutagenic in test cell systems) would be useless for the protection of food and health. Public concern has focused on the positive mutagenicity tests obtained with many fungicides and the predictive possibility of both teratogenic and carcinogenic potential. The fact that nearly 90 percent of all agricultural fungicides are carcinogenic in animal models has not reassured the public, especially when this is translated into the fact that some 75 million pounds of the fungicides used annually fall into this category (NAS, 1987). An evaluation of 11 fungicides concluded that, although the areas treated with these chemicals represented only 10 percent of the acreage treated annually with pesticides, they could account for 60 percent of the total estimated dietary carcinogenic risk.

While a number of different chemicals are shown in Fig. 22-26 to illustrate the diversity of structures, agents such as pentachlorophenol (PCP), hexachlorobenzene (HCB), captafol, and folpet have been deregistered or banned in many countries but still see some use in other, less regulated parts of the world. Other fungicides are undergoing reevaluation because of suspected toxicity, particularly as teratogens or carcinogens and incomplete or outdated toxicity databases.

Hexachlorobenzene

From the 1940s through the 1950s, HCB saw extensive use as a fungidical dressing applied to seed grain as a dry powder. Between 1955 and 1959, an epidemic of poisoning occurred in Turkey, ultimately involving some 4000 individuals who consumed treated grain during times of crop failure. The syndrome, called *black sore,* was characterized by dermal blistering and epidermolysis, pigmentation and scarring, alopecia, photosensitivity, hepatomegaly, porphyria, suppurative arthritis, osteomyelitis, and osteoporosis of the bones of the hands (Cam and Nigogosyan, 1963). Both adults and children were afflicted, young children and nursing infants being at particular risk (Schmid, 1960; Wray et al., 1962; Hayes, 1982). While this agent has largely fallen by the wayside, it is still being used in developing countries and still presents a health hazard.

The mammalian toxicity of HCB has been reviewed by Hayes (1982) and Hayes and Laws (1991). Like other organochlorine compounds, HCB possesses all of the properties of chemical stability, slow degradation and biotransformation, environmental persistence, bioaccumulation in adipose tissue and organs containing a high content of lipid membranes, and the ability to induce a range of tissue cytochrome-P450 as well as conjugative enzymes. Repeated exposure of animals results in hepatomegaly and porphyria as well as focal alopecia with itching and eruptions, followed by pigmented scars, anorexia, and neurotoxicity expressed as irritability, ataxia, and tremors. Immunosuppression was observed in both mice and rats and a dose-dependent increase in hepatic and thyroid tumors was observed in hamsters (Lambrecht et al., 1982). While not mutagenic in microbial test systems and negative in dominant lethal studies, HCB was teratogenic in mice (renal and palate malformations) and in rats (increased incidence of 14th rib). Hexachlorobenzene was particularly toxic to developing perinatal animals, acquisition transplacentally and via the milk causing hepatomegaly, enlarged kidneys, hydronephrosis, and possible effects on the immune system.

Pentachlorophenol

Once used in tremendous volumes as a biocide in leather tanning, wood preservation, the paper and cellulose industry, and in paints, this chemical has been phased out of use because many commercial products were contaminated by polychlorinated dibenzodioxins and dibenzofurans, predominantly by hexachlorinated, heptachlorinated, and octachlorinated congeners. While these congeners are considerably less toxic than TCDD, evidence from animal studies has pointed to the fact that the contaminants in commercial- or technical-grade PCP were responsible for the toxicity observed. Technical-grade PCP fed to rats caused altered plasma enzymes, increased hepatic and renal weights, and caused hepatocellular degeneration in addition to changes in blood biochemistry (decreased erythrocyte count, decreased hemoglobin and serum albumin). The administration of purified PCP resulted only in increased liver and kidney weight. Prolonged treatment of female rats with technical PCP caused hepatic porphyria, increased microsomal monooxygenase activity, and increased liver weight, whereas purified PCP caused no changes over the dosage range studied (Goldstein et al., 1977). Pentachlorophenol was not teratogenic in rats and is not considered to be carcinogenic in mice or rats (Innes et al., 1969; Johnson et al., 1973; Schwetz et al., 1977). A number of environmental problems have been associated with PCP (Eisler, 1989).

Human poisoning by commercial PCP has occurred, usually associated with occupational exposure and instances of sloppy handling and neglect of hygienic principles (Jorens and Schepens, 1993). The chemical is absorbed readily through the skin, the most usual route of acquisition, with several products, including PCP, detected in the urine.

High-level exposure can result in death, preceded by an elevated body temperature (42°C or 108°F), profuse sweating and dehydration, marked loss of appetite, decrease in body weight, tightness in the chest, dyspnea following exercise, rapid pulse, nausea and vomiting, headache, incoordination, generalized weakness, and early coma (Hayes, 1982). Pentachlorophenol acts cellularly to uncouple oxidative phosphorylation, the target enzyme being Na^{+},K^{+}-ATPase (Desaiah, 1977). Survivors frequently display dermal irritation and exfoliation, irritation of the upper respiratory tract, and possible impairment of autonomic function and circulation.

Phthalimides

Of this class of chemicals, folpet and captofol, true phthalimides, have been deregistered and only captan, being structurally different with a cyclohexene ring (Fig. 22-26), sees any use today. All of the agents were embroiled in a prolonged controversy concerning mutagenic and possible teratogenic and carcinogenic properties. All three chemicals were recognized as effective, persistent foliar fungicides for rusts and smut, for *Botrytis* mold on soft fruit, apple and pear scab, black spot on roses, and as seed dressings (Cremlyn,1978). All three chemicals have high oral LD_{50} values of approximately 10,000 mg/kg in the rat. Mutagenicity associated with these agents was confirmed, but—because of the exceptionally high doses (up to 500 mg/kg) required to elicit biological effects—teratogenicity was not proven or was masked by maternal toxicity and possible nutritional deficits.

Although the mechanism(s) by which captan and its analogs exerted their cellular toxicity has never been established, captan is known to react with cellular thiols to produce thiophosgene, a potent and unstable chemical capable of reacting with sulfhydryl-, amino-, or hydroxyl-containing enzymes (Cremlyn, 1978). Thiols reduce the potency of captan. A volatile breakdown product of captan was responsible for mutagenic activity, the intermediate being short-lived and forming more quickly at higher levels at an alkaline pH. It is possible that there may be several mechanisms by which these chemicals can induce cellular toxicity.

Dithiocarbamates

Dimethyl- and ethylene-bisdithiocarbamate (EBDC) compounds have been employed since the early 1950s as fungicides, and the EBDC chemicals saw widespread use on a large variety of small fruits and vegetables. The nomenclature of these agents arises from the metal cations with which they are associated; for instance, dimethyldithio-carbamic acid bound to iron or zinc are ferbam and ziram, respectively, whereas EBDC compounds associated with sodium, manganese, or zinc are nabam, maneb, and zineb, respectively. As is shown in Fig. 22-24, these chemicals are polymeric structures that possess environmental stability and yield good foliar protection as well as a low order of acute toxicity, with LD_{50} values in excess of 6000 mg/kg with the exception of nabam (395 mg/kg). Mancozeb is a polymeric mixture of a zinc salt and the chemical maneb.

Although toxicity is negligible in animal feeding trials even at high doses, acceptance of these agents has been marred by reported adverse health effects. Maneb, nabam, and zineb have been reported to be teratogenic (Petrova-Vergieva and Ivanova-Chemischanka, 1973). Mancozeb has not been demonstrated to be teratogenic in the rat but has been associated with abnormally shaped sperm (Hemavathi and Ratiman, 1993). Maneb has been associated with adverse reproductive outcomes (embryotoxicity: changes in usual number of offspring per litter, pregnancy rate, estrous cycle, and fetal development) (Lu and Kennedy, 1986). Maneb caused pulmonary tumors in mice, but studies in the rat have been equivocal (IARC, 1976). Environmental and mammalian degradation of the EBDC compounds into ethylene thiourea (ETU), a known mutagen, teratogen, and carcinogen, as well as an antithyroid compound, has raised suspicions about these agents and fostered requests for more in-depth studies (IARC, 1976). Recent chronic studies of mancozeb administered to rats at high (500 to 1500 mg/kg/day) doses demonstrated increased thyroid weight, reduced iodine uptake, reduced protein-bound iodine and thyroxine, as well as a dose-related decrease in thyroid peroxidase activity (Kackar et al., 1997). Significant histopathologic changes were observed, including thyroid hyperplasia and hypertrophy of the follicular mass with a loss of colloid mass. A study of EBDC fungicide–exposed backpack sprayers in Mexico demonstrated that ETU was formed in vivo and excreted in the urine and that thyroid-stimulating hormone levels were increased, although there was a nonsignificant reduction in thyroxine and significant increases in sister chromatic exchanges and chromosomal translocations in blood lymphocytes (Steenland et al., 1997).

Neurotoxicity has not been attributed to EBDC fungicides in either experimental animals or humans except at excessively high doses (Ecobichon, 1994c). A double (within 2 weeks) acute occupational, dermal exposure to Mandizan (mixture of maneb and zineb) resulted in initial complaints of muscle weakness, dizziness, and fatigue, with disorientation, slurred speech, muscle incoordination, loss of consciousness, and tonic/clonic convulsions appearing rapidly following the second exposure (Israeli et al., 1983). A recent report from Brazil on two apparent Parkinson patients revealed that, as sprayers, they had experienced significant annual exposure to maneb over 4 to 5 years (Ferraz et al., 1988). Signs and symptoms included inability to walk, difficulty in talking, tremors in hands and feet, a short-stepped gait with cogwheeling, and bradykinesia. An extended study of 50 rural workers, 84 percent of whom admitted to using maneb improperly or carelessly, revealed milder but similar signs and symptoms. It was suggested that the effects might be related to the manganese content, although blood manganese levels were not elevated. Other evidence might point to breakdown products of EBDC, such as carbon disulfide, as the neurotoxicant, although it is hard to accept such a high level of absorption. It is also known that dithiocarbamates can bind various divalent metals to form more lipophilic complexes capable of entering the CNS (Ecobichon, 1994c).

FUMIGANTS

Such agents are used to kill insects, nematodes, weed seeds, and fungi in soil as well as in silo-stored cereal grains, fruits and vegetables, clothes, and other consumables, generally with the treatment carried out in enclosed spaces because of the volatility of most of the products. Fumigants range from acrylonitrile and carbon disulfide to carbon tetrachloride, ethylene dibromide, chloropicrin, and ethylene oxide; their toxicologic properties are discussed under other headings because many have other uses. Attention in this section is directed only to a very few agents, although all of the chemicals mentioned have the potential for inhalation exposure and, for some of them, dermal and ingestion exposure.

Fumigants may be liquids (ethylene dibromide, dibromochloropropane, formaldehyde) that readily vaporize at ambient temperature, solids that can release a toxic gas on reacting with water (Zn_2P_3, AlP) or with acid [NACN, $Ca(CN)_2$], or gases (methylbromide, hydrogen cyanide, ethylene oxide). These chemicals are nonselective, highly reactive, and cytotoxic. The physicochemical properties of these agents and hence their pattern(s) of use vary considerably (Cremlyn, 1978). With proper attention to use and appropriate safety precautions, there should be little effect other than occasional occupational exposure, because the volatility of the agents is such that, when the enclosed space is opened, the gas or vapor escapes readily. However, reports in the literature have indicated the presence of low residual levels of ethylene dibromide, methylbromide, and other chemicals in various samples of treated foods. More extensive descriptions of fumigant toxicity can be found in Hayes (1982), Morgan (1982), and Hayes and Laws (1991).

Phosphine

Used extensively as a grain fumigant, phosphine (PH_3) is released from aluminum phosphide (AlP) by the natural moisture in the grain over a long period of time, giving continual protection during transhipment of the grain. One serious accident with this chemical has been reported, in which this author played a small role in identifying the causative agent, as the problem originated in the port of Montreal, Canada (Wilson et al., 1980). Grain leaving Canada for European destinations is fumigated by adding a certain number of sachets of AlP per ton of grain in the hold of the ship while loading. Phosphine (PH_3), being heavier than air, sinks slowly through the grain. The particular ship in question ran into a bad storm off Nova Scotia and began to leak, hastening the breakdown of the AlP to form PH_3. The toxicant penetrated the quarters of the crew and officers, where 29 out of 31 crew members became acutely ill and two children, family members of one of the officers, were seriously affected, one dying before reaching a hospital in Boston. Symptoms of PH_3 intoxication in the adults included shortness of breath, cough and pulmonary irritation, nausea, headache, jaundice, and fatigue. The highest concentrations of PH_3 (20 to 30 ppm) were measured in a void space on the main deck near the air intake for the ship's ventilation system. In some of the living quarters, PH_3 levels of 0.5 ppm were detected. Although this could be considered a bizarre situation, it does illustrate an apparent problem with the use of this type of agent in an atmosphere of excess moisture.

Ethylene Dibromide/ Dibromochloropropane

When inhaled at relatively high (>200 ppm) concentrations, ethylene dibromide can cause pulmonary edema and inflammation in the exposed animals. As one might expect, repeated exposures to lower concentrations produced hepatic and renal damage visualized as morphologic changes. Centrolobular hepatic necrosis and proximal tubular damage in the kidneys were observed in one fatal poisoning in which the individual ingested 4.5 ml of ethylene dibromide. This chemical, along with 1,2-dibromo-3-chloropropane (DBCP), was found to elicit malignant gastric squamous cell carcinomas in mice and rats (IARC, 1977). DBCP was also found to cause sterility in male animals, and concentrations as low as 5 ppm had an adverse effect on testicular morphology and spermatogenesis. However, these results in animals came to light only when a similar situation was detected in workers who manufactured the agent. Equivocal results have been reported for the mutagenicity of DBCP, the agent that causes base-pair substitution but not a frame-shift mutation in *Salmonella* strains. In animal studies of the dominant lethal assay, DBCP was positive (mutagenic) in rats but not in mice. DBCP was a reproductive toxicant in rabbits and rats but not in mice (IARC, 1977).

RODENTICIDES

Many vertebrates—including rats, mice, squirrels, bats, rabbits, skunks, monkeys, and even elephants—on occasion can be considered to be pests. Rodents, the most important of which are the black rat (*Rattus rattus*), the brown or Norway rat (*Rattus norvegicus*), and the house mouse (*Mus musculus*), are particularly serious problems because they act as vectors for several human diseases. They can consume large quantities of postharvest stored food and/or foul or contaminate even greater amounts of foodstuffs with urine, feces, hair, and bacteria that cause diseases.

To be effective yet safe, a rodenticide must satisfy the following criteria: (1) it must not be unpalatable to the target species and therefore must be potent; (2) it must not induce bait shyness, so that the animal will continue to eat it; (3) death should occur in a manner that does not raise the suspicions of the survivors; (4) it should make the intoxicated animal go out into the open to die (otherwise the rotting corpses create health hazards); and (5) it should be species-specific, with considerably lower toxicity to other animals that might inadvertently consume the bait or eat the poisoned rodent (Cremlyn, 1978). The agents used constitute a diverse range of chemical structures having a variety of mechanisms of action for at least partially successful attempts to attain species selectivity (Fig. 22-27). With some chemicals, advantage has been taken of the physiology and biochemistry unique to rodents. With other rodenticides, the sites of action are common to most mammals but advantage is taken of the habits of the pest animal and/or the dosage, thereby minimizing toxicity to nontarget species.

Although most rodenticides are formulated in baits that are unpalatable to humans, thereby minimizing the potential hazard, there are surprising numbers of rodenticide intoxications each year. With only a few exceptions, the accidental or intentional ingestion of most rodenticides poses a serious, acute toxicologic problem because the dosage ingested is invariably high and the signs and symptoms of intoxication are generally well advanced and severe when the patient is seen by a physician. As with other household products, rodenticide poisoning is more frequently seen in children, whose added hazard is a small body weight in relation to the dosage ingested. The toxicology of the various classes of rodenticides has been extensively reviewed and the reader is referred to Hayes and Laws (1991) and to Ellenhorn and Barceloux (1988) for in-depth coverage of the subject.

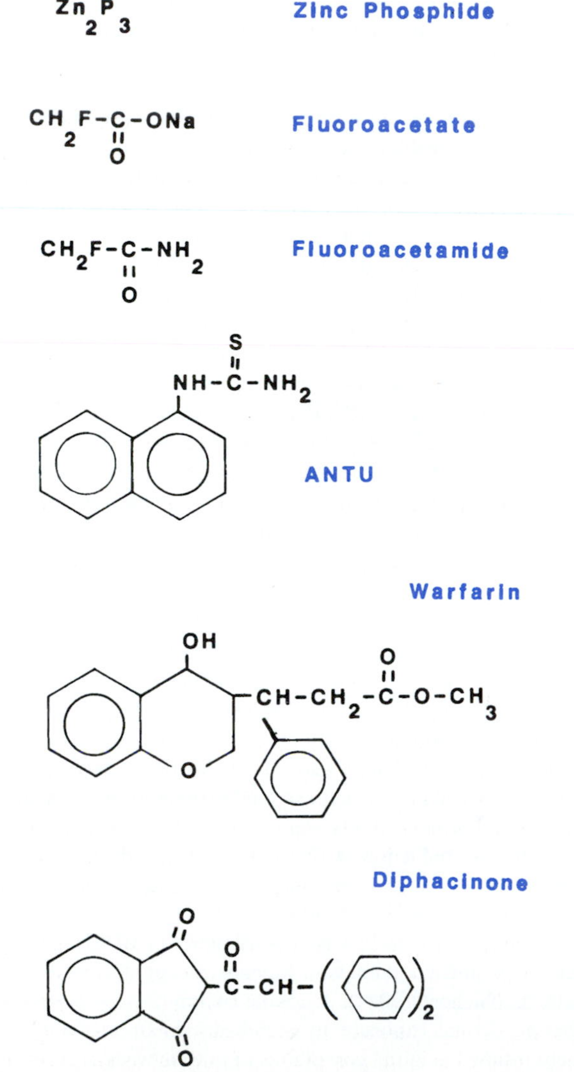

Figure 22-27. Representative structures of inorganic and organic rodenticides from various chemical classifications.

A number of inorganic compounds—including thallium sulfate, arsenious oxide, other arsenic salts, barium carbonate, yellow phosphorus, aluminum phosphide, and zinc phosphide—have been used as rodenticides. A mixture of sodium cyanide with magnesium carbonate and anhydrous magnesium sulfate has been used in rabbit and mole burrows, causing hydrogen cyanide gas to be liberated slowly on contact with moisture. Natural or synthetic organic chemicals, including strychnine, red squill (scillaren glycosides), and DDT have been used in the past. All of these agents are nonselective, highly toxic, and hazardous to other forms of life and, with the exception of zinc phosphide, have been abandoned in favor of target-specific, selective chemicals.

Zinc Phosphide

This agent is used in developing nations because it is both cheap and effective. The toxicity of the chemical can be accounted for by the phosphine (PH_3) formed following a hydrolytic reaction with water in the stomach on ingestion. Phosphine causes widespread cellular toxicity with necrosis of the gastrointestinal tract and injury to other organs, such as the liver and kidneys. Although moist zinc phosphide emits an unpleasant, rotten-fish odor, it is accepted by rodents at concentrations of 0.5 or 1.0 percent in baits.

Accidental poisonings are rare in adults but a definite problem in children. Hayes (1982) recounts a poisoning attributed to the inhalation of zinc phosphide dust from treated grain, with signs of intoxication that included vomiting, diarrhea, cyanosis, tachycardia, rhales, restlessness, fever, and albuminuria several hours following exposure. It is a favorite chemical in suicides in Egypt (A. Amr, personal communication). The signs and symptoms include nausea, vomiting, headache, light-headedness, dyspnea, hypertension, pulmonary edema, dysrrhythmias, and convulsions. Doses of the order of 4000 to 5000 mg have been fatal, but other individuals have survived doses of 25,000 to 100,000 mg if early vomiting has occurred. The usual decontamination measures and supportive therapy are often successful if initiated early.

Fluoroacetic Acid and Derivatives

Sodium fluoroacetate (compound 1080) and fluoroacetamide (compound 1081) are white in color, odorless, and tasteless. The extreme toxicity of these two chemicals has restricted their use to prepared baits. Both agents are well absorbed from the gastrointestinal tract. Acute oral toxicity of fluoroacetate in the rat is of the order of 0.2 mg/kg, whereas that of fluoroacetamide is 4 to 15 mg/kg. The mechanism of action involves the incorporation of the fluoroacetate into fluoroacetyl–coenzyme A, which condenses with oxaloacetate to form fluorocitrate, which inhibits the enzyme aconitase and prevents the conversion of citrate to isocitrate in the tricarboxylic (Krebs) cycle. Inhibition of this system by fluorocitrate results in reduced glucose metabolism and cellular respiration and affects tissue energy stores. These chemicals are uniquely effective in mice and rats because of the high metabolic rate in the tissues susceptible to inhibition.

Estimates of the lethal dose of fluoroacetate in humans lie in the range of 2 to 10 mg/kg. Gastrointestinal symptoms are seen initially at some 30 to 100 min following ingestion. Initial nausea, vomiting, and abdominal pain are replaced by sinus tachycardia, ventricular tachycardia or fibrillation, hypotension, renal failure, muscle spasms, and such CNS symptoms as agitation, stupor, seizures, and coma. Histopathologic examination of postmortem samples has revealed cerebellar degeneration and atrophy. There are no known antidotes to fluoroacetate intoxication, although glycerol monoacetate has proved beneficial in the treatment of poisoned monkeys.

α-Naphthyl Thiourea

Following the discovery that phenylthiourea was lethal to rats but not toxic to humans, α-naphthyl thiourea (ANTU) was introduced as a relatively selective rodenticide (Richter, 1946). A wide range of acute oral LD_{50} values has been reported for different species, the rat being the most sensitive at 3 mg/kg and the monkey the least susceptible at 4 g/kg. The exact mechanism of action is not known, but it is suspected that ANTU must be biotransformed in vivo into a reactive intermediate. Young rats are resistant to the chemical, whereas older rats become tolerant to it, suggesting that perhaps microsomal monooxygenases in young rats metabolize the agent too rapidly into nontoxic products, whereas in older rats either the lower levels of monooxygenases or the inhibition of these enzymes results in less activation and affords protection (Boyd and Neal, 1976). ANTU causes extensive pulmonary edema and pleural effusion as a consequence of action on the pulmonary capillaries. Studies with ^{35}S- and ^{14}C-labeled ANTU revealed that covalent binding to macromolecules in the lung and liver occurred following treatment (Boyd and Neal, 1976). Following exposure to ANTU, there are a number of biochemical effects, such as alterations in carbohydrate metabolism, adrenal stimulation, and interaction of the chemical with sulfhydryl groups, but none of these appear to bear any relationship to the observed signs of toxicity.

Although it would appear that the human is very resistant to ANTU intoxication, probably because insufficient quantities are ingested, poisonings have occurred, with tracheobronchial hypersecretion of a white, nonmucous froth containing little protein, pulmonary edema, and respiratory difficulty (Hayes, 1982).

Anticoagulants

With the discovery that coumadin [3-(α-acetonylbenzyl)-4-hydroxycoumarin, warfarin), isolated from spoiled sweet clover, acted as an anticoagulant by antagonizing the actions of vitamin K in the synthesis of clotting factors (factors II, VII, IX, and X), it was introduced as a rodenticide. The onset of anticoagulation is delayed 8 to 12 h after the ingestion of warfarin, with this latent period of onset dependent on the half-lives of the various clotting factors (Katona and Wason, 1986). The safety of warfarin as a rodenticide rests with the fact that multiple doses are required before toxicity develops and that single doses have little effect. However, the development of resistance to warfarin in rats in the 1950s prompted research into newer compounds, and the exploration of structure-activity relationships led to the development of the superwarfarins (brodifacoum, bromadiolone, coumachlor, diphencoumarin) and the indanediones (diphacinone, chlorophacinone, pindone), a new class of anticoagulant compounds that are more water-soluble. All of these newer agents differ from one another in terms of acute toxicity, rapidity of action, and acceptance by the rodent.

Human poisonings by these agents are rare because they are dispensed in grain-based baits. However, there are sufficient numbers of suicide attempts, attempted murders, and a famous classic case of the inadvertent consumption of warfarin-laden cornmeal bait by an unsuspecting Korean family to provide adequate docu-

Table 22-13
The WHO Recommended Classification of Pesticides by Hazard

		LD_{50} FOR THE RAT (mg/kg BODY WEIGHT)			
		ORAL		DERMAL	
CLASS		SOLIDS	LIQUIDS	SOLIDS	LIQUIDS
Ia	Extremely hazardous	≤5	≤20	≤10	≤40
Ib	Highly hazardous	5–50	20–200	10–100	40–400
II	Moderately hazardous	50–500	200–2000	100–1000	400–4000
III	Slightly hazardous	>500	>2000	>1000	>4000
III+	Unlikely to present hazard in normal use	>2000	>3000	—	—

mentation of the signs and symptoms of poisoning (Lange and Terveer, 1954; Hayes, 1982; Jones, 1984; Lipton, 1984; Katona and Wason, 1986). Following consumption over a period of days, bleeding of the gingiva and nose occurs, with bruising and hematomas developing at the knee and elbow joints and on the buttocks, gastrointestinal bleeding with dark tarry stools, hematuria accompanied by abdominal or low back (flank) pain, epistaxis, and cerebrovascular accidents. The signs and symptoms will persist for many days after cessation of exposure, particularly so in the case of the superwarfarins, which have prolonged biological half-lives (e.g., brodifacoun with 156 h compared to 37 h for warfarin) (Katona and Wason, 1986). In the Korean episode, consumption of warfarin was estimated to be on the order of 1 to 2 mg/kg/day for a period of 15 days, and signs and symptoms appeared 7 to 10 days after initial exposure; 2 out of the 14 affected individuals died as a consequence of not receiving any treatment (Lange and Terveer, 1954).

CONCLUSIONS

With the advent of the chemical pesticides with their diverse nature, structures, and biological activity, the problem of ranking the hazard that each one poses to health has arisen. Should a classification system be based on acute toxicity alone or should some numerical scoring system be used to evaluate other endpoints of toxicity? Should the classification scheme be based on the oral, dermal, or inhalation routes of exposure to the active ingredient or to a formulation concentrate? If one chooses acute toxicity and a definitive endpoint expressed as the LD_{50}, one must be cognizant of the fact that the LD_{50} is an estimate, with the range and confidence limits for any particular chemical possibly overlapping a class boundary. To establish a classification system on the basis of other toxicologic endpoints would be impossible given the variability of biological effects, the dosages required to attain them, and the significance of such results in terms of human exposure.

In 1972, the WHO Expert Committee on Insecticides recommended the preparation of a classification of pesticides that would serve as a guide for developing countries (WHO, 1973). The classification was to distinguish between the more and the less hazardous forms of each pesticide and was meant to permit formulations to be classified according to the percentage of the active ingredient and its physical state. Only acute hazards to health were considered, meaning those resulting from single or multiple exposures over a relatively short period of time, from handling the product in accordance with the manufacturer's directions. In 1975, the categories of the classification were established and, with only one modification to class 111, they are essentially the same as those that appear in Table 22-13. It is important to appreciate that the LD_{50} value quoted for any pesticide is not the median value but the lower confidence limit value for the most sensitive sex, thereby ensuring that a large safety factor has been built into the classification. A recent paper by Copplestone (1988) discusses the advantages and disadvantages of the system and the placement of problem chemicals such as rodenticides (highly toxic to rats but not presenting the same hazard to humans) and paraquat (having a low dermal toxicity but causing fatal effects if ingested).

From experience, the WHO is of the opinion that this classification scheme has worked well in practice, faithfully reflecting the toxicity of these chemicals for humans. Only a few changes in classification have been made for chemicals and/or their formulations since the introduction of the scheme, signifying that the system functions effectively. It would appear that acute toxicity is the most effective parameter by which to judge the hazard to human health. With the move away from animal experimentation to in vitro testing, this classification system can be modified to reflect other endpoints of toxicity if they can be quantitated, correlated, and validated to be equivalent to the LD_{50} results. As Dr. Copplestone described it, "the classification has been a meeting point between science and administration and a useful tool in the armamentarium of preventive medicine" (Copplestone, 1988).

REFERENCES

Abalis IM, Eldefrawi EM, Eldefrawi AT: Effects of insecticide on GABA-induced chloride flux into rat brain microsacs. *J Toxicol Environ Health* 18:13–23, 1986.

Abbott DC, Goulding R, Tatton JO'G: Organochlorine pesticide residues in human fat in Great Britain. *Br Med J* 3:146–149, 1968.

Abou-Donia MB: Organophosphorus ester-induced delayed neurotoxicity. *Annu Rev Pharmacol Toxicol* 21:511–548, 1981.

Abou-Donia MB, Lapadula D: Mechanisms of organophosphorus ester-induced delayed neurotoxicity: Type 1 and type 11. *Annu Rev Pharmacol Toxicol* 30:405–440, 1990.

Acquavella JF, Riordan SG, Anne M, et al: Evaluation of mortality and cancer incidence among alachlor manufacturing workers. *Environ Health Perspect* 104:728–733, 1996.

Acquavella JF, Weber JA, Cullen MR, et al: Human ocular effects from self-reported exposures to Roundup herbicides. *Hum Exp Toxicol* 18:479–486, 1999.

Ahlbom J, Fredriksson A, Eriksson P: Exposure to an organophosphate (DFP) during a defined period in neonatal life induces permanent changes in brain muscarinic receptors and behavior in adult mice. *Brain Res* 677:13–19, 1995.

Alachlor Review Board: *Report of the Alachlor Review Board.* Ottawa, Canada: Agriculture Canada, Canadian Government Publishing Centre, 1987.

Albert A: *Xenobiosis, Food, Drugs and Poisons in the Human Body.* London: Chapman and Hall, 1987, pp 113–116.

Albertson TE, Cross CE: Pesticides in the workplace: A worldwide issue. *Arch Environ Health* 48:364–365, 1993.

Aldridge WN, Johnson MK: Side effects of organophosphorus compounds: Delayed neurotoxicity. *Bull WHO* 44:259–263, 1971.

Aldridge WN, Reiner E: *Enzyme Inhibitors as Substrates.* Amsterdam and New York: North-Holland/American Elsevier, 1972.

Almog C, Tal E: Death from paraquat after subcutaneous injection. *Br Med J* 3:721, 1967.

Anon.: A look at world pesticide markets. *Farm Chem* 141:38–42, 1977.

Arena J, Liu K, Paress PS, et al: Avermectin-sensitive chloride currents induced by *Caenorhabditis elegans* RNA in *Xenopus* oocytes. *Mol Pharmacol* 40:368–374, 1991.

Arena J, Liu K, Paress P, et al: The mechanism of action of avermectins in *Caenorhabditis elegans*: Correlation between activation of glutamate-sensitive chloride current, membrane binding and biological activity. *J Parasitol* 81:286–294, 1995.

Ariens ATh, Meeter E, Wolthius OL, et al: Reversible necrosis at the end-plate region in striated muscle of the rat poisoned with cholinesterase inhibitors. *Experientia* 25:57–59, 1969.

Ashby J, Kier L, Wilson AG, et al: Evaluation of the potential carcinogenicity and genetic toxicity to humans of the herbicide acetochlor. *Hum Exp Toxicol* 15:702–735, 1996.

Ashe W, Suskind RR: Chloracne cases of the Monsanto Chemical Company, Nitro, West Virginia, in *Reports of the Kettering Laboratory.* Cincinnati, OH: University of Cincinnati, October 1949, April 1950, July 1953.

Askew BM: Oximes and hydroxamic acids as antidotes in anticholinesterase poisoning. *Br J Pharmacol Chemother* 11:417–423, 1956.

Azaroff LS: Biomarkers of exposure to organophosphorus insecticides among farmers' families in rural El Salvador: Factors associated with exposure: *Environ Res A* 80:138–147, 1999.

Aziz MA, Diallo S, Diopp IM, et al: Efficacy and tolerance of ivermectic in human onchocerciasis. *Lancet* 2:171–173, 1982.

Bakry NM, El-Rashidy AH, Eldefrawi AT, et al: Direct actions of organophosphate anticholinesterases on nicotinic and muscarinic acetylcholine receptors. *J Biochem Toxicol* 3:235–259, 1988.

Baris D, Zahm SH, Cantor KP, et al: Agricultural use of DDT and the risk of non-Hodgkin's lymphoma: Pooled analysis of three case-control studies in the United States. *Occup Environ Med* 55:522–527, 1998.

Barnes JM, Verschoyle RD: Toxicity of new pyrethroid insecticides. *Nature* 248:711, 1974.

Bartle H: Quiet sufferers of the silent spring. *New Scientist* 130:30–35, 1991.

Batchelor GS, Walker KC: Health hazards involved inuse of parathion in fruit orchards on north central Washington. *AMA Arch Ind Hyg Occup Health* 10:522, 529,1954.

Bayer Corp: Material Safety Data Sheet—Admire™. Bayer Corp Agriculture Division, 1994.

Beach JR, Spurgeon A, Stephens R, et al: Abnormalities on neurological examination among sheep farmers exposed to organophosphorus pesticides. *Occup Environ Med* 53:520–525, 1996.

Berti PR, Receveur O, Chan H-M, et al: Dietary exposure to chemical contaminants from traditional food among adult Dene/Metis in the western Northwest Territories, Canada. *Environ Res A* 76:131–142, 1998.

Bidstrup PL, Bonner JA, Beckett AG: Paralysis following poisoning by a new organic phosphorus insecticide (Mipafox). *Br Med J* 1:1068–1072, 1953.

Bloomquist JR, Adams PM Soderlund DM: Inhibition of gamma-aminobutyric acid–stimulated chloride flux in mouse brain vesicles by polychloroalkane and pyrethroid insecticides. *Neurotoxicology* 7:11–20, 1986.

Bond GG, Rossbacher R: A review of potential human carcinogenicity of the chlorophenoxy herbicides MCPA, MCPP and 2,4-DP. *Br J Ind Med* 50:340–348, 1993.

Bond GG, Wetterstroem NH, Roush GJ, et al: Cause specific mortality among employees engaged in the manufacture, formulation or packaging of 2,4-dichlorophenoxyacetic acid and related salts. *Br J Ind Med* 45:98–105, 1988.

Bonsall JL: Measurement of occupational exposure to pesticides, in Turnbull GS (ed): *Occupational Hazards of Pesticide Use.* London: Taylor & Francis, 1985, pp 13–33.

Boon-Long J, Glinsukon T, Pothisiri P, et al: Toxicological problems in Thailand, in Ruchirawat M, Shank RC (eds): *Environmental Toxicity and Carcinogenesis.* Bangkok: Text and Journal Corp, 1986, pp 283–293.

Boyd MR, Neal RA: Studies on the mechanism of toxicity and of development of tolerance to the pulmonary toxic α-naphthylthiourea (ANTU). *Drug Metab Dispos* 4:314–322, 1976.

Branch RA, Jacqz E: Subacute neurotoxicity following long-term exposure to carbaryl. *Am J Med* 80:741–746, 1986.

Brooks GT: *Chlorinated Insecticides. Technology, and Application.* Vol 1. Cleveland, OH: CRC Press, 1974, pp 12–13.

Büchel KH (ed): *Chemistry of Pesticides.* New York: Wiley, 1983.

Bull DL: Metabolism of organophosphorus insecticides in animals and plants. *Residue Rev* 43:1–22, 1972.

Calamari D, Yameogo L, Hougard J-M, et al: Environmental assessment of larvacide use in the onchocerciasis control programme. *Parasitol Today* 14:485–489, 1998.

Cam C, Nigogosyan G: Acquired toxic porphyria cutanea tarda due to hexachlorobenzene. *JAMA* 183:88–91, 1963.

Campbell S: Paraquat poisoning. *Clin Toxicol* 1:245–249, 1968.

Campbell WC: *Ivermectin and Abamectin.* New York, Springer-Verlag, 1989.

Campbell WC, Fisher MH, Stapley EO, et al: Ivermectin: A potent antiparasitic agent. *Science* 221:823–828, 1983.

Cannon SB, Veasey JM Jr, Jackson RS, et al: Epidemic kepone poisoning in chemical workers. *Am J Epidemiol* 107:529–537, 1978.

Cantor KP: Farming and mortality from non-Hodgkin's lymphoma: A case-control study. *Int J Cancer* 29:239–247, 1982.

Carson R: *Silent Spring.* Boston: Houghton Mifflin, 1962.

Casida JE, Gammon DW, Glockman AH, Lawrence LJ: Mechanisms of selective action of pyrethroid insecticides. *Annu Rev Pharmacol Toxicol* 23:413–438, 1983.

Castro-Gutierrez N, McConnell R, Andersson K, et al: Respiratory symptoms, spirometry and chronic occupational paraquat exposure. *Scand J Work Environ Health* 23:421–427, 1997.

Cavanagh JB: The toxic effects of tri-ortho-cresyl phosphate on the nervous system, an experimental study in hens. *J Neurol Neurosurg Psychiatry* 17:163–172, 1954.

Centers for Disease Control Veterans Health Studies: Serum 2,3,7,8-tetrachlorodibenzo-*p*-dioxin levels in U.S. Army Vietnam-era veterans. *JAMA* 260:1249–1254, 1988.

Chambers JE, Levi PE: *Organophosphates. Chemistry, Fate and Effects.* New York: Academic Press, 1992.

Chan H-M: A database for environmental contaminants in traditional foods in northern and arctic Canada. *Food Add Contam* 15:127–134, 1998.

Chao SL, Casida JE: Interaction of imidacloprid metabolites and analogs with the nicotinic acetylcholine receptor of mouse brain in relation to toxicity. *Pestic Biochem Physiol* 58:77–88, 1997.

Charles JM, Cunny HC, Wilson RD, et al: Ames assays and unscheduled DNA synthesis assays on 2,4-dichloro-phenoxyacetic acid and its derivatives. *Mutat Res* 444:207–216, 1999a.

Charles JM, Cunny HC, Wilson RD, et al: *In vivo* micronucleus assay on 2,4-dichlorophenoxyacetic acid and its derivatives. *Mutat Res* 444:227–234, 1999b.

Cheek AO, Ide CF, Bollinger JE, et al: Alteration of leopard frog (*Rana pipiens*) metamorphosis by the herbicide acetochlor. *Arch Environ Contam Toxicol* 37:70–77, 1999.

Chernoff N, Kavlock RJ, Kathrein JR, et al: Prenatal effects of dieldrin and photodieldrin in mice and rats. *Toxicol Appl Pharmacol* 31:302–308, 1975.

Childs AF, Davies DR, Green AL, Rutland JP: The reactivation by oximes and hydroxamic acids of cholinesterase inhibited by organophosphorus compounds. *Br J Pharmacol Chemother* 10:462–465, 1955.

Ciesielski S, Loomis DP, Mims SR, et al: Pesticide exposures, cholinesterase depression and symptoms among North Carolina migrant farmworkers. *Am J Pub Health* 84:446–451, 1994.

Clark DG, Hurst EW: The toxicity of diquat. *Br J Ind Med* 27:51–55, 1970.

Clark DG, McElligott TF, Hurst EW: The toxicity of paraquat. *Br J Ind Med* 23:126–132, 1966.

Clark JM, Matsumura F: Two different types of inhibitory effects of pyrethroids on nerve Ca and Ca-Mg-ATPase activity in the squid, *Loligo pealei*. *Pestic Biochem Physiol* 18:180–190, 1982.

Clement JG: Toxicity of the combined nerve agents GB/GF in mice: Efficacy of atropine and various oximes as antidotes. *Arch Toxicol* 68:64–66, 1994.

Cole LM, Nicholson RA and Casida JE: Action of phenylpyrazole insecticides in the GABA-gated chloride channel. *Pestic Biochem Physiol* 46:47–54, 1993.

Coleman S, Liu S, Linderman R, et al: *In vitro* metabolism of alachlor by human liver microsomes and human cytochrome P450 isoforms. *Chemico-Biol Int* 122:27–39, 1999.

Committee on Scientific and Regulatory Issues Underlying Pesticide Use Patterns and Agricultural Innovation: *Regulating Pesticides in Food.* Washington, DC: National Academy Press, 1987.

Cook RR: Health effects of organophosphate sheep dips. *Br Med J* 305:1502–1503, 1992.

Copplestone JF: The development of the WHO Recommended Classification of Pesticides by Hazard. *Bull WHO* 66:545–551, 1988.

Corbett JR: *The Biochemical Mode of Action of Pesticides.* New York: Academic Press, 1974.

Courtney KD, Gaylor DW, Hogan MD, et al: Teratogenic evaluation of 2,4,5-T. *Science* 168:864–866, 1970.

Courtney KD, Moore JA: Teratology studies with 2,4,5-trichlorophenoxyacetic acid and 2,3,7,8-tetra-chlorodibenzo-dioxin. *Toxicol Appl Pharmacol* 20:396–403, 1971.

Coye MJ, Lowe IA, Maddy KT: Biological monitoring of agricultural workers exposed to pesticides: I. Cholinesterase activity determinators. *J Occup Med* 28:619–627, 1986.

Craan AG, Haines DA: Twenty-five years of surveillance for contaminants in human breast milk. *Arch Environ Cont Toxicol* 35:702–710, 1998.

Cranmer MF: Carbaryl. A toxicological review and risk analysis. *Neurotoxicology* 1:247–332, 1986.

Cremlyn R: *Pesticides. Preparation and Mode of Action.* New York: Wiley, 1978.

Crum JA, Bursian SJ, Aulerich RJ, Brazelton WE: The reproductive effects of dietary heptachlor in mink *(Mustela vison). Arch Environ Contam Toxicol* 24:156–164, 1993.

Dale WE, Quinby GE: Chlorinated insecticides in the body fat of people in the United States. *Science* 142:593–595, 1963.

Dalvie MA, White N, Raine R, et al: Long term respiratory health effects of the herbicide paraquat among workers in the Western Cape. *Occup Environ Med* 56:391–396, 1999.

Damgaard I, Nyitrai G, Kovacs I, et al: Possible involvement of $GABA_A$ and $GABA_B$ receptors in the inhibitory action of lindane on transmitter release from cerebellar granule neurons. *Neurochem Res* 24:1189–1193, 1999.

Daniel JW, Gage JC: Absorption and excretion of diquat and paraquat in rats, *Br J Ind Med* 23:133–136, 1966.

Dauterman WC, Main AR: Relationship between acute toxicity and m vitro inhibition and hydrolysis of a serves of homologs of malathion. *Toxicol Appl Pharmacol* 9:408–418, 1966.

Davies DS, Hawksworth GM, Bennett PN: Paraquat poisoning. *Proc Eur Soc Toxicol* 18:21–26, 1977.

Davies HW, Kennedy SM, Teschke K, et al: Cytogenetic analysis of South Asian berry pickers in British Columbia using the micronucleus assay in peripheral lymphocytes. *Mutat Res* 416:101–113, 1998.

Davies JE, Edmundson WF, Schneider NJ, Cassady JC: Problems of prevalence of pesticide residues in humans, in Davies JE, Edmondson WF (eds): *Epidemiology of DDT.* Mount Kisco, NY: Futura, 1972, pp 27–37.

Dearfield KL, McCarroll NE, Protzel A, et al: A survey of EPA/OPP and open literature on selected pesticide chemicals: II Mutagenicity and carcinogenicity of selected chloro-acetanilides and related compounds. *Mutat Res* 443:183–221, 1999.

Delorme PD, Lockhart WL, Mills KH, et al: Long-term effects of toxaphene and depuration in lake trout and white sucker in a natural ecosystem. *Environ Toxicol Chem* 18:1992–2000, 1999.

Deng Y, Casida JE: House fly GABA-gated chloride channel: Toxicologically relevant binding site for avermectins coupled to site for ethynylbicycloorthobenzoate. *Pestic Biochem Physiol* 43:116–122, 1992.

DeRueck J, Willems J: Acute parathion poisoning: myopathic changes in the diaphragm. *J Neurol* 208:309–314, 1975.

Desaiah D: Effects of pentachlorophenol on the ATPases in rat tissue, in Rao KR (ed): *Pentachlorophenol.* New York: Plenum Press, 1977, pp 277–283.

Desi I, Gonczi L, Simon G, et al: Neurotoxicologic studies of two carbamate pesticides in subacute animal experiments. *Toxicol Appl Pharmacol* 27:465–476, 1974.

DuBois KP: New rodenticidal compounds. *J Am Pharm Assoc* 37:307–310, 1948.

DuBois KP, Doull J, Salerno PR, Coon JM: Studies on the toxicity and mechanisms of action of *p*-nitrophenyl-diethyl-thionophosphate (Parathion). *J Pharmacol Exp Ther* 95:75–91, 1949.

Duce IR, Khan TR, Green AC, et al: Calcium channels in insects, in Beadle JD (ed): *Progress in Neuropharmacology and Neurotoxicology of Pesticides and Drugs.* London: Royal Society of Chemistry, 1999, pp 55–66.

Durham WF, Wolfe HR: Measurement of the exposure of workers to pesticides. *Bull WHO* 26:75–91, 1962.

Durham WF, Wolfe HR, Elliott JW: Absorption and excretion of parathion by spraymen. *Arch Environ Health* 24:381–387, 1972.

Ebert E, Leist KH, Mayer D: Summary of safety evaluation of toxicity studies of glufosinate ammonium. *Food Chem Toxicol* 28:339–349, 1990.

Ecobichon DJ: Biological monitoring: Neurophysiological and behavioral assessments, in Ecobichon DJ (ed): *Occupational Hazards of Pesticide Exposure. Sampling, Monitoring, Measuring.* Philadelphia, Taylor & Francis, 1998b, pp 209–230.

Ecobichon DJ: Carbamic acid ester insecticides, in Ecobichon DJ, Joy RM: *Pesticides and Neurological Diseases,* 2d ed. Boca Raton, FL: CRC Press, 1994b, pp 251–289.

Ecobichon DJ: Fungicides, in Ecobichon DJ, Joy RM: *Pesticides and Neurological Diseases,* 2d ed. Boca Raton, FL: CRC Press, 1994c, pp 313–351.

Ecobichon DJ: Hydrolytic mechanisms of pesticide degradation, in Geissbuhler H (ed): *Advances in Pesticide Science. Biochemistry of Pests and Mode of Action of Pesticides, Pesticide Degradation, Pesticide Residues and Formulation Chemistry.* New York: Pergamon, 1979, part 3, pp 516–524.

Ecobichon DJ (ed): *Occupational Hazards of Pesticide Exposure. Sampling, Monitoring, Measuring.* Philadelphia, Taylor & Francis, 1998a.

Ecobichon DJ: Organophosphorus ester insecticides, in Ecobichon DJ, Joy RM: *Pesticides and Neurological Diseases,* 2d ed. Boca Raton, FL: CRC Press, 1994a, pp 171–249.

Ecobichon DJ: Toxic effects of pesticides, in Klaassen CD (ed): *Casarett and Doull's Toxicology. The Basic Science of Poisons*. 5th ed. New York, McGraw-Hill, 1996; pp 643–689.

Ecobichon DJ, Joy RM: *Pesticides and Neurological Diseases,* 2d ed. Boca Raton, FL: CRC Press, 1994.

Ecobichon DJ, MacKenzie DO: The uterotropic activity of commercial and isomerically pure chlorobiphenyls in the rat. *Res Commun Chem Pathol Pharmacol* 9:85–95, 1974.

Ecobichon DJ, Ozere RL, Reid E, Crocker JFS: Acute fenitrothion poisoning. *Can Med Assoc J* 116:377–379, 1977.

Ecobichon DJ, Saschenbrecker PW: Pharmacodynamic study of DDT in cockerels. *Can J Physiol Pharmacol* 46:785–794, 1968.

Ecobichon DJ, Saschenbrecker PW: The redistribution of stored DDT in cockerels under the influence of food deprivation. *Toxicol Appl Pharmacol* 5:420–432, 1969.

Edington N, Howell JM: The neurotoxicity of sodium diethyl-diethiocarbamate in the rabbit. *Acta Neuropathol* 12:339–346, 1969.

Edmiston S, Maddy KT: Summary of illnesses and injuries reported in California by physicians in 1986 as potentially related to pesticides. *Vet Hum Toxicol* 29:391–397, 1987.

Edwards R, Ferry DG, Temple WA: Fungicides and related compounds, in Hayes WJ Jr, Laws ER Jr (eds): *Handbook* of *Pesticide Toxicology. Classes of Pesticides.* Vol 3. New York: Academic Press, 1991, pp 1409–1470.

Egan H, Goulding R, Toburn J, Tatton JO'G: Organochlorine residues in human fat and human milk. *Br Med J* 2:66–69, 1965.

Eldefrawi ME, Schweizer C, Bakry NM, et al: Desensitization of the nicotinic acetylcholine receptor by diisopropyl-fluorophosphate. *J Biochem Toxicol* 3:21–32, 1988.

Ellenhorn MJ, Barceloux DG: Pesticides, in *Medical Toxicology. Diagnosis and Treatment of Human Poisoning.* New York: Elsevier, 1988, pp 1081–1108.

Elliott M: Future use of natural and synthetic pyrethroids, in Metcalf RL, McKelvey JJ Jr (eds): *The Future for Insecticides: Needs and Prospects.* New York: Wiley, 1976, pp 163–193.

Elliott M, Janes NF, Kimmel EC, Casida JE: Metabolic fate of pyrethrin 1, pyrethrin II and allethrin administered orally to rats. *J Agric Food Chem* 20:300–313, 1972.

Englehard H, Erdmann WD: Beziehangen zwischen chemischer struktur und cholinesterase reaktivierendes wirksamkeit bei einen reihe neuer bisquartarer pyridin-4-aldoxime. *Arznem Forsch* 14:870–875, 1964.

EPA: *Carbaryl Decision Document.* Washington, DC: U.S. Environmental Protection Agency. Government Printing Office, 1980.

Eriksson M, Hardell L, Berg NO, et al: Soft-tissue sarcomas and exposure to chemical substances: a case-referent study. *Br J Ind Med* 38:27–33, 1981.

Eto M: *Organophosphorus Pesticides: Organic and Biological Chemistry.* Cleveland, OH: CRC Press, 1974.

Feldman RC: *Carbamates. Occupational and Environmental Neurotoxicology.* Philadelphia: Lippincott-Raven, 1999, pp 442–465.

Feldman RJ, Maiback HI: Percutaneous penetration of some pesticides and herbicides in man. *Toxicol Appl Pharmacol* 28:126–132, 1974.

Ferraz HB, Bertolucci PHF, Pereira JS, et al: Chronic exposure to the fungicide maneb may produce symptoms and signs of CNS manganese intoxication. *Neurology* 38:550–553, 1988.

Fest C, Schmidt K-J: *The Chemistry of Organophosphorus Pesticides.* New York: Springer-Verlag, 1973.

Fiserova-Bergerova V, Radomski JL, Davies JE, Davis JH: Levels of chlorinated hydrocarbon pesticides in human tissues. *Ind Med Surg* 36:65–70, 1967.

Fisher MH, Mrozik H: The chemistry and pharmacology of avermectins. *Annu Rev Pharmacol Toxicol* 32:537–553, 1992.

Flannigan SA, Tucker SB, Key MM., et al: Synthetic pyrethroid insecticides: A dermatological evaluation. *Br J Ind Med* 42:363–372, 1985.

Fonseca RG, Resende LAL, Silva MD, Camargo A: Chronic motor neuron disease possibly related to intoxication with organochlorine insecticides. *Acta Neurol Scand* 88:56–58, 1993.

Forget G: Pesticides: Necessary but dangerous poisons. *IDRC Rep* 18:4–5, 1989.

Forget G, Goodman T, deVilliers A (eds): *Impact of Pesticide Use on Health in Developing Countries.* Ottawa, Canada: International Development Research Centre, 1993.

Forshaw PJ, Lister T, Ray DE: Inhibition of a neuronal voltage-dependent chloride channel by the type II pyrethroid, deltamethrin. *Neuropharmacology* 32:105–111, 1993.

Forshaw PJ, Ray DE: A voltage-dependent chloride channel in NIE115 neuroblastoma cells is activated by protein-kinase-C and also by the pyrethroid deltamethrin. *J Physiol* 467:252P, 1993.

Franciolini F, Petris A: Chloride channels of biological membranes. *Biochim Biophys Acta* 1031:247–259, 1990.

Frank R, Campbell RA, Sirons GJ: Forestry workers involved in aerial application of 2,4-dichlorophenoxyacetic acid (2,4-D): Exposure and urinary excretion. *Arch Environ Contam Toxicol* 14:427–435, 1985.

Franklin CA, Fenske RA, Greenhalgh R, et al: Correlation of urinary pesticide metabolite excretion with estimated dermal contact in the course of occupational exposure to guthion. *J Toxicol Environ Health* 7:715–731, 1981.

Frawley JP, Fuyat HN, Hagan EC, et al: Marked potentiation in mammalian toxicity from simultaneous administration of two anticholinesterase compounds. *J Pharmacol Exp Ther* 121:96–106, 1957.

Frear DEH: *Pesticide Index,* 4th ed. State College, PA: College Science, 1969.

Fukuto TR: Metabolism of carbamate insecticides. *Drug Metab Rev* 1:117–147, 1972.

Gaines TB: Acute toxicity of pesticides. *Toxicol Appl Pharmacol* 14:515–534, 1969.

Gammon DW, Brown MA, Casida JE: Two classes of pyrethroid action in the cockroach. *Pestic Biochem Physiol* 15:181–191, 1981.

Gant DB, Chalmers AE, Wolff MA, et al: Fipronil: Action at the GABA receptor. *Rev Toxicol* 2:147–156, 1998.

Gee J: Iraqui declarations of chemical weapons: How much did they really have and what is it? Fourth International Symposium on Protection Against Chemical Warfare Agents, Stockholm, June 8–12, 1992.

Gehring PJ, Watanabe PG, Blau GE: Pharmacokinetic studies in evaluation of the toxicological and environmental hazard of chemicals, in Mehlman MA, Shapiro RE, Blumenthal LL (eds): *New Concepts in Safety Evaluation.* New York: Wiley, 1976, pp 195–270.

Gershenfeld HM: Chemical transmission in invertebrate central nervous systems and neuromuscular junctions. *Physiol Rev* 53:1–119, 1973.

Gershon S, Shaw FH: Psychiatric sequelae of chronic exposure to organophosphorus insecticides. *Lancet* 1:1371–1374, 1961.

Ginsburg KS, Narahashi T: Differential sensitivity of tetrodotoxin-sensitive and tetrodotoxin-resistant sodium channels to the insecticide allethrin in rat dorsal root ganglion neurons. *Brain Res* 627:239–248, 1993.

Glickman Ali, Casida JE: Species and structural variations affecting pyrethroid neurotoxicity. *Neurobehav Toxicol Teratol* 4:793–799, 1982.

Gochfeld M: New light on the health of Vietnam veterans. *Environ Res* 47:109–111, 1988.

Goldman LR, Better M, Jackson RJ: Aldicarb food poisonings in California, 1985–1988: Toxicity estimates for humans. *Arch Environ Health* 45:141–148, 1990a.

Goldman LR, Smith DF, Neutra RR, et al: Pesticide food poisoning from contaminated watermelons in California, 1985. *Arch Environ Health* 45:229–236, 1990b.

Goldstein JA, Fridsen M, Linder PE, et al: Effects of pentachlorophenol on hepatic drug-metabolizing enzymes and porphyria related to contamination with chlorinated dibenzo p-dioxins and dibenzofurans. *Biochem Pharmacol* 26:1549–1557, 1977.

Goldstein NP, Jones PH, Brown JR: Peripheral neuropathy after exposure to an ester of dichlorophenoxyacetic acid. *JAMA* 171:1306–1309, 1959.

Gollapudi BB, Charles JM, Linscombe VA, et al: Evaluation of the genotoxicity of 2,4-dichlorophenoxyacetic acid and its derivatives in mammalian cell cultures. *Mutat Res* 444:217–225, 1999.

Gough M: *Dioxin, Agent Orange. The Facts.* New York: Plenum Press, 1986.

Greenwald W, Kovasznay B, Collins DN, Therriault G: Sarcomas of soft tissues after Vietnam service. *J Natl Cancer Inst* 73:1107–1109, 1984.

Grendon J, Frost F, Baum L: Chronic health effects among sheep and humans surviving an aldicarb poisoning incident. *Vet Hum Toxicol* 36:218–223, 1994.

Grover R, Cessna AJ, Muir NI, et al: Factors affecting the exposure of ground-rig applicators to 2,4-D dimethylamine salt. *Arch Environ Contam Toxicol* 15:677–686, 1986.

Grubb TC, Dick LC, Oser M: Studies on the toxicity of polyoxyethylene dodecanol. *Toxicol Appl Pharmacol* 2:133–143, 1960.

Guzelian PS: Comparative toxicology of chlordecone (kepone) in humans and experimental animals. *Annu Rev Pharmacol Toxicol* 22:89–113, 1982.

Hack R, Ebert E, Ehling G, et al: Glufosinate ammonium—Some aspects of its mode of action in mammals. *Food Chem Toxicol* 32:461–470, 1994.

Hainzl D, Cole LM, Casida JE: Mechanisms for selective toxicity of fipronil insecticide and its sulfone metabolite and desulfinyl photoproduct. *Chem Res Toxicol* 11:1529–1535, 1998.

Haley TJ: Review of the toxicology of paraquat (1,19-dimethyl-4,49-bipyridinium chloride). *Clin Toxicol* 14:1–46, 1979.

Hall R, Payne LA, Putnam JM, et al: Effect of methoxychlor on implantation and embryo development in the mouse. *Reprod Toxicol* 11:703–708, 1997.

Hardell L, Eriksson M, Lenner P, Lundgren E: Malignant lymphoma and exposure to chemicals, especially organic solvents, chlorophenols and phenoxy acids: A case-control study. *Br J Cancer* 43:169–176, 1981.

Hardell L, Sandstrom A: Case-control study: Soft-tissue sarcomas and exposure to phenoxyacetic acids or chlorophenols. *Br J Cancer* 39:711–717, 1979.

Hartley GS, West TF: *Chemicals for Pest Control.* Oxford, England: Pergamon Press, 1969, p 26.

Haslam E: *Shikimic Acid: Metabolism and Metabolites.* Chichester, UK: Wiley, 1993.

Hay A: *The Chemical Scythe. Lessons of 2,4,5,-T and Dioxin.* New York: Plenum Press, 1982.

Hayes WJ Jr: *Pesticides Studied in Man.* Baltimore: Williams & Wilkins, 1982.

Hayes WJ Jr: The pharmacology and toxicology of DDT, in Muller P (ed): *The Insecticide DDT and Its Importance.* Vol 2. Basel: Birkhauser Verlag, 1959, pp 9–247.

Hayes WJ Jr, Dale WE, Pirkle CI: Evidence of the safety of long-term, high, oral doses of DDT for man. *Arch Environ Health* 22:19–35, 1971.

He F, Sun J, Han K, et al: Effects of pyrethroid insecticides on subjects engaged in packaging pyrethroids. *Br J Ind Med* 45:548–551, 1988.

He F, Wang S, Liu L, et al: Clinical manifestations and diagnosis of acute pyrethroid poisoning. *Arch Toxicol* 63:54–58, 1989.

Heath DF: *Organophosphorus Poisons. Anticholinesterases and Related Compounds.* London: Pergamon Press, 1961.

Hemavathi E, Rahiman MA: Toxicological effects of ziram, thiram and Dithane M-45 assessed by sperm shape abnormalities in mice. *J Toxicol Environ Health* 38:393–398, 1993.

Himuro K, Murayame S, Nishiyama K, et al: Distal sensory axonopathy after sarin intoxication. *Neurology* 51:1195–1197, 1998.

Hoar SK, Blair A, Holmes FF, et al: Agricultural herbicide use and risk of lymphoma and soft-tissue sarcoma. *JAMA* 256:1141–1147, 1986.

Holmstedt B: Pharmacology of organophosphorus cholinesterase inhibitors. *Pharmacol Rev* 11:567–688, 1959.

Huang Y, Williamson MS, Devonshire AL, et al: Molecular characterization and imidacloprid selectivity of nicotinic acetylcholine receptor subunits from the peach-potato aphid *Myzus persicae. J Neurochem* 73:380–389, 1999.

Huff RA, Corcoran JJ, Anderson JK, et al: *Chlorpyrifos oxon* binds directly to muscarinic receptors and inhibits cAMP accumulation in rat striatum. *J Pharmacol Exp Ther* 269:329–335, 1994.

Hutson DH, Akintonwa DAA, Hathway DE: The metabolism of 2-chloro-l-(29,49-dichlorophenyl) vinyl diethylphosphate (chlorfenvinphos) in the dog and rat. *Biochem J* 102:133–142, 1967.

IARC: *Monograph on the Evaluation of Carcinogenic Risk of Chemicals to Man. Some Organochlorine Pesticides.* Vol 5. Lyons, France: International Agency for Research on Cancer, 1974.

IARC: *Monographs on the Evaluation of Carcinogenic Risk of Chemicals to Man. Some Carbamates, Thiocarbamates and Carbazines.* Vol 12. Lyons, France: International Agency for Research on Cancer, 1976.

IARC: *Monographs on the Evaluation of Carcinogenic Risk of Chemicals to Man. Some Fumigants, the Herbicides 2,4-D and 2,4,5-T, Chlorinated Dibenzodioxins and Miscellaneous Industrial Chemicals.* Vol 15. Lyons, France: International Agency for Research on Cancer, 1977.

Innes JRM, Ulland BM, Valerio MG, et al: Bioassay of pesticides and industrial chemicals for tumorigenicity in mice: a preliminary note. *J Natl Cancer Inst* 42:1101–1114, 1969.

Israeli R, Sculsky M, Tiberin P: Acute intoxication due to exposure to maneb and zineb. A case with behavioral and central nervous system changes. *Scand J Work Environ Health* 9:47–51, 1983.

Jager G: Herbicides, in Buchel KH (ed): *Chemistry of Pesticides.* New York: Wiley, 1983, pp 322–392.

Jamal GA: Neurological syndromes of organophosphorus compounds. *Adverse Drug React Toxicol Rev* 16:133–170, 1997.

Jett DA, Fernando JC, Eldefrawi ME, et al: Differential regulation of muscarinic receptor subtypes in rat brain regions by repeated injections of parathion. *Toxicol Lett* 73:33–41, 1994.

Jett DA, Hill EF, Fernando JC, et al: Down-regulation of muscarinic receptors and the m_3 subtype in white-footed mice by dietary exposure to parathion. *J Toxicol Environ Health* 39:395–415, 1993.

Jeyaratnam J: Occupational health issues in developing countries. *Environ Res* 60:207–212, 1993.

Jeyaratnam J, De Alwis Senevirathe RS, Copplestone JF: Survey of pesticide poisoning in Sri Lanka. *Bull WHO* 60:615–619, 1982.

Johnson MK: The target for initiation of delayed neurotoxicity by organophosphorus esters: Biochemical studies and toxicological applications, in Hodgson E, Bend JR, Philpot RM (eds): *Reviews of Biochemical Toxicology.* Vol 4. New York: Elsevier, 1982, pp 141–212.

Johnson MK, Willems JL, DeBisschop HC, et al: Can soman cause delayed neuropathy? *Fundam Appl Toxicol* 5:SI80–SI81, 1985.

Johnson RL, Gehring PJ, Kociba RJ, Schwetz BA: Chlorinated dibenzodioxins and pentachlorophenol. *Environ Health Perspect* 5:171–175, 1973.

Jones EC, Growe GH, Naiman SC: Prolonged anticoagulation in rat poisoning. *JAMA* 252:3005–3007, 1984.

Jorens PG, Schepens PJC: Human pentachlorophenol poisoning. *Hum Exp Toxicol* 12:479–495, 1993.

Joy RM: Chlorinated hydrocarbon insecticides, in Ecobichon DJ, Joy RM: *Pesticides and Neurological Diseases,* 2d ed. Boca Raton, FL: CRC Press, 1994a, pp 81–170.

Joy RM: Pyrethrins and pyrethroid insecticides, in Ecobichon DJ, Joy RM: *Pesticides and Neurological Diseases,* 2d ed. Boca Raton, FL: CRC, 1994b, pp 291–312.

Joy RM, Albertson TE: Interactions of GABA-A antagonists with deltamethrin, diazepam, phenobarbital and SKF 100330A in the rat dentate gyrus. *Toxicol Appl Pharmacol* 109:251–262, 1991.

Kackar R, Srivastava MK, Raizada RB: Studies on rat thyroid after oral administration of mancozeb: Morphological and biochemical evaluations. *J Appl Toxicol* 17:369–375, 1997.

Kamrin MA (ed): *Pesticide Profiles. Toxicity, Environmental Impact and Fate.* Boca Raton, FL: Lewis Publishers, 1997.

Katona B, Wason S: Anticoagulant rodenticides. *Clin Toxicol Rev* 8:1–2, 1986.

Katz EJ, Cortes VI, Eldefrawi ME: Chlorpyrifos, parathion and their oxons bind to and desensitize a nicotinic acetylcholine receptor: Relevance to their toxicities. *Toxicol Appl Pharmacol* 146:227–236, 1997.

Keane WT, Zavon MR: The total body burden of dieldrin. *Bull Environ Contam Toxicol* 4:1–16, 1969.

Ketchum NS, Michalek JE, Burton JE: Serum dioxin and cancer in veterans of Operation Ranch Hand. *Am J Epidemiol* 149:630–639, 1999.

Kewitz H, Wilson IB: A specific antidote against lethal alkylphosphate intoxication. *Arch Biochem Biophys* 60:261–263, 1956.

Kilgore W: Human exposure to pesticides, in Newberne PM, Shank RC, Ruchirawat M (eds): *International Toxicology Seminar: Environmental Toxicology.* Bangkok: Chulabhorn Research Institute and Mahidol University, 1988.

Kilgore WW, Akesson NB: Minimizing occupational exposure to pesticides; populations at exposure risk. *Residue Rev* 75:21–31, 1980.

Kirby C: *The Hormone Weedkillers.* Croydon, UK: BCPC Publications, 1980.

Kitselman CH: Long-term studies on dogs fed aldrin and dieldrin in sublethal dosages with reference to the histopathological findings and reproduction. *J Am Vet Med Assoc* 123:28–36, 1953.

Kociba RI, Keyes DG, Beyer JE: Results of a two year chronic toxicity and oncogenicity study of 2,3,7,8-tetrechlorodibenzo-*p*-dioxin in rats. *Toxicol Appl Pharmacol* 46:279–303, 1978.

Koestner A: The brain-tumor issue in long-term toxicity studies in rats. *Food Chem Toxicol* 24:139–143, 1986.

Kolmodin-Hedman B, Hoglund S, Ak-erblom M: Studies on phenoxy acid herbicides. 1. Field Study. Occupational exposure to phenoxy acid herbicides (MCPA, dichlorprop, mecoprop and 2,4-D) in agriculture. *Arch Toxicol* 54:257–275, 1983.

Koos BJ, Longo LD: Mercury toxicity in the pregnant woman, fetus and newborn infant. *Am J Obstet Gynecol* 126:390–409, 1976.

Koplovitz I, Gresham VC, Dochterman LW, et al: Evaluation of the toxicity, pathology and treatment of cyclohexylmethylphosphonofluoridate (CMPF) poisoning in rhesus monkeys. *Arch Toxicol* 66:622–628, 1992.

Koyama K: Acute oral poisoning caused by a herbicide containing glufosinate. *Jpn J Toxicol* 8:391–398, 1995.

Koyama K, Andou Y, Saruki K, et al: Delayed and severe toxicities of a herbicide containing glufosinate and a surfactant. *Vet Hum Toxicol* 36:17–18, 1994.

Kramer W: Fungicides and bacteriocides, in Buchel KH (ed): *Chemistry of Pesticides.* New York: Wiley, 1983, pp 227–321.

Kuhr RJ, Dorough HW: *Carbamate Insecticides: Chemistry, Biochemistry and Toxicology.* Boca Raton, FL: CRC Press, 1976.

Kulkami AP, Hodgson E: The metabolism of insecticides: The role of monooxygenase enzymes. *Annu Rev Pharmacol* 24:19–42, 1984.

Kupfer D, Bulger WH: Studies on the mechanism of estrogenic actions of *o,p*-DDT: Interactions with the estrogen receptor. *Pestic Biochem Physiol* 6:461–470, 1976.

Kusic R, Jovanovic D, Randjelovic S, et al: HI-6 in man: Efficacy of the oxime in poisoning by organophosphorus insecticides. *Human Exp Toxicol* 10:113–118, 1991.

Laben RC, Archer TE, Crosby DG, Peoples SA: Lactational output of DDT fed postpartum to dairy cattle. *J Dairy Sci* 48:701–708, 1965.

Lambrecht RW, Erturk E, Grunden E, et al: Hepatotoxicity and tumorigenicity of hexachlorobenzene (HCB) in Syrian golden hamsters after subchronic administration. *Fed Proc* 41:329, 1982.

Lange PF, Terveer J: Warfarin poisoning. US *Armed Forces J* 5:872–877, 1954.

Lankas GR, Cartwright ME, Umbenhauer D: P-glycoprotein deficiency in a subpopulation of CF-1 mice enhances avermectin-induced neurotoxicity. *Toxicol Appl Pharmacol* 143:357–365, 1997.

Larsen SB, Spano M, Giwercman A, et al: Semen quality and sex hormones among organic and traditional Danish farmers. *Occup Environ Med* 56:139–144, 1999.

Lawrence LJ, Casida JE: Pyrethroid toxicology: Mouse intracerebral structure-toxicity relationships. *Pestic Biochem Physiol* 18:9–14, 1982.

Leahey JP: *The Pyrethroid Insecticides.* London: Taylor & Francis, 1985.

Leake LD, Buckley DS, Ford MG, Salt DW: Comparative effects of pyrethroids on neurones of target and non-target organisms. *Neurotoxicology* 6:99–116, 1985.

Leech CA, Jewess P, Marshall J, et al: Nitromethylene actions on in situ and expressed insect nicotinic acetylcholine receptors. *FEBS Lett* 290:90–94, 1991.

LeQuesne PM, Maxwell IC, Butterworth ST: Transient facial sensory symptoms following exposure to synthetic pyrethroids: A clinical and electrophysiological assessment. *Neurotoxicology* 2:1–11, 1980.

Lessenger JE, Riley N: Neurotoxicities and behavioral changes in a 12-year-old male exposed to dicofol, an organochlorine pesticide. *J Toxicol Environ Health* 33:255–261, 1991.

Leveridge YR: Pesticide poisoning in Costa Rica during 1996. *Vet Hum Toxicol* 40:42–44, 1998.

Li AP, Long TJ: An evaluation of the genotoxic potential of glyphosate. *Fundam Appl Toxicol* 10:537–546, 1988.

Li Q, Minami M, Clement JG, et al: Elevated frequency of sister chromatid exchanges in lymphocytes of victims of the Tokyo sarin disaster and in experiments exposing lymphocytes to by-products of sarin synthesis. *Toxicol Lett* 98:95–103, 1998.

Li Y-F: Global technical hexachlorocyclohexane usage and its contamination consequences in the environment from 1948 to 1997. *Sci Total Environ* 232:121–158, 1999.

Liddle JA, Kimbrough RD, Needham LL, et al: A fatal episode of accidental methomyl poisoning. *Clin Toxicol* 15:159–167, 1979.

Lifshitz M, Shahak E, Bolotin A, et al: Carbamate poisoning in early childhood and in adults. *Clin Toxicol* 53:25–27, 1997.

Lin J-L, Liu L, Leu M-L: Recovery of respiratory function in survivors with paraquat intoxication. *Arch Environ Health* 50:432–439, 1995.

Lipton RA, Klass EM: Human ingestion of a "superwarfarin" rodenticide resulting in prolonged anticoagulant effect. *JAMA* 252:3004–3005, 1984.

Liu M-Y, Casida JE: High affinity binding of [^{3}H] imidacloprid in the insect acetylcholine receptor. *Pestic Biochem Physiol* 46:40–46, 1993.

Liu M-Y, Lanford J, Casida JE: Relevance of [^{3}H] imidacloprid binding site in house fly head acetylcholine receptor to insecticidal activity of 2-nitromethylene and 2-nitroimino-imidazolines. *Pestic Biochem Physiol* 46:200–206, 1993.

Lui M-Y, Latli B, Casida JE: Imidacloprid binding site in Musca nicotinic acetylcholine receptor: Interactions with physostigmine and a variety of nicotinic agonists with cloropyridyl and chlorothiazolyl substituents. *Pestic Biochem Physiol* 52:170–181, 1995.

Longcore JR, Samson FB, Whittendale TW Jr: DDE thins eggshells and lowers reproductive success of captive black ducks. *Bull Environ Contamin Toxicol* 6:485–490, 1971.

Lopez-Carillo L, Lopez-Cervantes M: Effect of exposure to organophosphate pesticides on serum cholinesterase levels. *Arch Environ Health* 48:359–363, 1993.

Lotti M: The pathogenesis of organophosphate polyneuropathy. *Crit Rev Toxicol* 21:465–487, 1992.

Lu M-H, Kennedy GL Jr: Teratogenic evaluation of mancozeb in the rat following inhalation exposure. *Toxicol Appl Pharmacol* 84:355–368, 1986.

Lukens RJ: *Chemistry of Fungicidal Action.* New York: Springer-Verlag, 1971.

Lynge E: A follow-up study of cancer incidence among workers in manufacture of phenoxy herbicides in Denmark. *Br J Cancer* 52:259–270, 1985.

Maibach H: Irritation, sensitization, photoirritation and photosensitization assays with a glyphosate herbicide. *Contact Dermatitis* 15:152–156, 1986.

Marban E, Yamagishi T, Tomaselli GF: Structure and function of voltage-gated sodium channels. *J Physiol* 508:647–657, 1998.

Marquis JK: *Contemporary Issues in Pesticide Toxicology and Pharmacology.* Basel: Karger, 1982, pp 87–95.

Marrs TC: Organophosphate poisoning. *Pharmacol Ther* 58:51–66, 1993.

Martinez AJ, Taylor JR, Houff SA, Isaacs ER: Kepone poisoning: Cliniconeuropathological study, in Roizin L, Shiraki H, Greevic N (eds): *Neurotoxicology.* New York: Raven Press, 1977, pp 443–156.

Masuda N, Takatsu M, Morinari H, et al: Sarin poisoning in Tokyo subway. *Lancet* 345:1446, 1995.

Matsumura F: *Toxicology of Insecticides.* New York: Plenum Press, 1985, pp 122–128.

Matthews HB, Matsumura F: Metabolic fate of dieldrin in the rat. *J Agric Food Chem* 17:845–852, 1969.

Mattsson JL, Johnson KA, Albee RR: Lack of neuropathologic consequences of repeated dermal exposure to 2,4-dichloro-phenoxy acid in rats. *Fundam Appl Toxicol* 6:175–181, 1986.

Mbiapo F, Youovop G: Regulation of pesticides in Cameroon. *J Toxicol Environ Health* 39:1–10, 1993.

McBlain WA, Lewin V, Wolfe FH: Estrogenic effects of the enantiomers of *o,p′* -DDT in Japanese quail. *Can J Zool* 55:562–568, 1977.

McConnell R, Delgado-Tellez E, Cuadra R, et al: Organophosphate neuropathy due to methamidophos: Biochemical and neurophysiological markers. *Arch Toxicol* 73:296–300, 1999.

McCord CP, Kilker CH, Minster DK: Pyrethrum dermatitis: A record of the occurrence of occupational dermatoses among workers in the pyrethrum industry. *JAMA* 77:448–449, 1921.

McEwen FL, Stephenson GR: *The Use and Significance of Pesticides in the Environment.* New York: Wiley, 1979, pp 91–154.

McFarland LZ, Lacy PB: Physiologic and endocrinologic effects of the insecticide kepone in the Japanese quail. *Toxicol Appl Pharmacol* 15:441–450, 1969.

Melnikov NN: Chemistry of pesticides. *Residue Rev* 36:1–480, 1971.

Menkes DB, Temple WA, Edwards IR: Intentional self-poisoning with glyphosate-containing herbicides. *Hum Exp Toxicol* 10:103–107, 1991.

Menzie CM: *Metabolism of Pesticides.* Special Scientific Report. Wildlife No. 127. Washington, DC: Bureau of Sport Fisheries and Wildlife, 1969.

Mes J, Davies DJ, Turton D: Polychlorinated biphenyl and other chlorinated hydrocarbon residues in adipose tissue of Canadians. *Bull Environ Contam Toxicol* 28:97–104, 1982.

Metcalfe RL: A century of DDT. *J Agric Food Chem* 21:511–519, 1973.

Metcalfe RL: Development of selective and biodegradable pesticides, in *Pest Control Strategies for the Future.* Washington, DC: Agriculture Board, Division of Biology and Agriculture, National Research Council, National Academy of Science, 1972, pp 137–156.

Monsanto Company: *Toxicology of Glyphosate and Roundup Herbicide.* St Louis, 1985.

Montgomery JH: *Agrochemicals Desk Reference,* 2d ed. Boca Raton, FL: CRC Press, 1997.

Morgan DP: *Recognition and Management of Pesticide Poisonings,* 3d ed. Publication EPA-540/9-80-005. Washington, DC: U.S. Environmental Protection Agency, 1982.

Morgan DP, Roan CC: Chlorinated hydrocarbon pesticide residue in human tissues. *Arch Environ Health* 20:452–457, 1970.

Morgan JP, Penovich P: Jamaica ginger paralysis. Forty-seven year follow-up. *Arch Neurol* 35:530–532, 1978.

Morita H, Yanagisawa N, Nakajima T, et al: Sarin poisoning in Matsumoto, Japan. *Lancet* 346:290–293, 1995.

Morrison HI, Wilkins K, Semenciw R, et al: Herbicides and cancer. *J Natl Cancer Inst* 84:1866–1874, 1992.

Moses M: Glyphosate herbicide toxicity. *JAMA* 261:2549, 1989.

Mullison WR: *An Interim Report Summarizing 2,4-D Toxicological Research Sponsored by the Industry Task Force on 2,4-D Research Data and a Brief Review of 2,4-D Environmental Effects.* Technical and Toxicology Committees of the Industry Task Force on 2,4-D Research Data, 1986.

Munro IC, Carlo GL, Orr JC, et al: A comprehensive, integrated review and evaluation of the scientific evidence relating to the safety of the herbicide 2,4-D. *J Am Coll Toxicol* 11:559–664, 1992.

Murphy SD: Mechanisms of pesticide interactions in vertebrates. *Residue Rev* 25:201–221, 1969.

Murphy SD: The toxicity of pesticides and their metabolites, in *Degradation of Synthetic Organic Molecules in the Biosphere.* Proceedings of a Conference. Washington, DC: National Academy of Sciences, 1972, pp 313–335.

Murray V, Wiseman HM, Dawling S, et al: Health effects of organophosphate sheep dips. *Br Med J* 305:1090, 1992.

Nagata K, Iwanaga Y, Shono T, et al: Modulation of the neuronal nicotinic acetylcholine receptor channel by imidacloprid and cartap. *Pestic Biochem Physiol* 59:119–128, 1997.

Nagata K, Narahashi T: Dual action of the cyclodiene insecticide dieldrin on the aminobutyric acid receptor chloride ion channel complex of rat dorsal root ganglion neurons. *J Pharmacol Exp Ther* 269:164–171, 1994.

Narahashi T: Mechanisms of action of pyrethroids on sodium and calcium channel gating, in Ford MG, Lunt GG, Reay RC, Usherwood PN (eds): *Neuropharmacology of Pesticide Action.* Chichester, UK: Ellis Horwood, 1986, pp 36–40.

Narahashi T, Ginsburg KS, Nagata K, et al: Ion channels as targets for insecticides. *Neurotoxicology* 19:581–590, 1998.

Nishimura K, Kanda Y, Okazawa A, et al: Relationship between insecticidal and neurophysiological activities of imidacloprid and related compounds. *Pestic Biochem Physiol* 50:51–59, 1994.

Nozaki H, Aikawa N: Sarin poisoning in Tokyo subway. *Lancet* 345:1446–1447, 1995.

Nozaki H, Aikawa N, Shinozawa Y, et al: Sarin poisoning in Tokyo subway. *Lancet* 345:980–981, 1995.

O'Malley M: Clinical evaluation of pesticide exposure and poisonings. *Lancet* 349:1161–1166, 1997.

Panemangalore M, Dowla HA, Byers ME: Occupational exposure to agricultural chemicals: Effect on the activities of some enzymes in the blood of farm workers. *Int Arch Occup Environ Health* 72:84–88, 1999.

Payne GT, Soderlund DM: Activation of γ-aminobutyric acid insensitive chloride channels in mouse brain synaptic vesicles by avermectin B1a. *J Biochem Toxicol* 6:283–292, 1991.

Ramasamy S, Tajol Akos NM: A survey of pesticide use and associated incidences of poisoning in Peninsular Malaysia. *J Plant Protect Trop* 5:1–9, 1988.

Rank J, Jensen A-G, Skov B, et al: Genotoxicity testing of the herbicide Roundup and its active ingredient glyphosate isopropylamine using the mouse bone marrow micronucleus test, *Salmonella* mutagenicity test and *Allium* anaphase-telophase test. *Mutat Res* 300:29–36, 1993.

Ray DE: Pyrethroid insecticides: Mechanisms of toxicity, systemic poisoning syndromes, paresthesia and therapy, in Krieger R (ed.): *Hayes' and Laws' Handbook of Pesticide Toxicology,* 3d ed. San Diego, CA: Academic Press, 2000.

Ray DE, Sutharsan S, Forshaw PJ: Actions of pyrethroid insecticides on voltage-gated chloride channels in neuroblastoma cells. *Neurotoxicology* 18:755–760, 1997.

Sawada Y, Nagai Y: Roundup poisoning—its clinical observation: Possible involvement of surfactant. *J Clin Exp Med* 143:25–27, 1987.

Schaeffer JM, Haines HW: Avermectin binding in *Caenorhabditis elegans.* A two-state model for the avermectin-binding site. *Biochem Pharmacol* 38:2329–2338, 1989.

Shroeder ME, Flattum RF: The mode of action and neurotoxic properties of the nitromethylene heterocycle insecticides. *Pestic Biochem Physiol* 22:148–160, 1984.

Sims P: Letter to the Editor. *Br Med J* 305:1503, 1992.

Smith K: *Pesticides exported from the U.S., 1992–1994.* Los Angeles: Foundation for Advancement in Sciences and Education, 1995.

Soderlund DM: Pyrethroid-receptor interactions: Stereo-specific binding and effects on sodium channels in mouse brain preparation. *Neurotoxicology* 6:35–46, 1985.

Soloway SB, Henry AC, Kollmeyer WD, et al: Nitromethylene insecticides, in Geissbuhler H, Brooks GT, Kearney PC (eds): *Advances in Pesticide Science,* Part 2. New York: Pergamon Press, 1978, pp 206–217.

Song J-H, Narahashi T: Differential effects of the pyrethroid tetramethrin on tetrodotoxin-sensitive and tetrodotoxin-resistant single sodium channels. *Brain Res* 712:258–264, 1996.

Spiegelberg U: Psychopathologisch-neurologische spat und dauerschaden nach gewerblicher Intoxikation durch Phosporsaureester (alkylphosphate). *Proc l4th Int Congr Occup Health Exerpta Med Found Int Congr Ser* 62, 1963, pp 1778–1780.

Steenland K, Cedillo L, Tucker J, et al: Thyroid hormones and cytogenetic outcomes in backpack sprayers using ethylenebis(dithiocarbamate) (EBDC) fungicides in Mexico. *Environ Health Perspect* 105:1126–1130, 1997.

Stephens R, Spurgeon A, Berry H: Organophosphates. The relationship between chronic and acute exposure effects. *Neurotoxicol Teratol* 18:449–453, 1996.

Stephens R, Spurgeon IA, Calvert J, et al: Neuro-psychological effects of long-term exposure to organophosphates in sheep dip. *Lancet* 345:1135–1139, 1995.

Stevens MF, Ebell GF, Psaila-Savona P: Organochlorine pesticides in Western Australia nursing mothers. *Med J Aust* 158:238–241, 1993.

Stickel LF: *Organochlorine Pesticides in the Environment.* Special Scientific Report-Wildlife No. 119. Washington, DC: United States Department of the Interior, Fish and, Wildlife Service. 1968.

Suskind RR, Hertzberg VS: Human health effects of 2,4,5-T and its toxic contaminants. *JAMA* 251:2372–2380, 1984.

Suzuki T, Morita H, Ono K, et al: Sarin poisoning in Tokyo subway. *Lancet* 345:980, 1995.

Swan AAB: Exposure of spray operators to paraquat. *Br J Ind Med* 26:322–329, 1969.

Swartz WJ, Eroschenko VP: Neonatal exposure to technical methoxychlor alters pregnancy outcome in female mice. *Reprod Toxicol* 12:565–573, 1998.

Tai T, Yamashita M, Wakimori H: Hemodynamic effects of Roundup, glyphosate and surfactant in dogs. *Jpn J Toxicol* 3:63–68, 1990.

Takamiya K: Monitoring of urinary alkyl phosphates in pest control operators exposed to various organophosphorus insecticides. *Bull Environ Contam Toxicol* 52:190–195, 1994.

Takayama S, Sieber SM, Dalgard DW, et al: Effects of long-term oral administration of DDT on nonhuman primates. *J Cancer Res Clin Oncol* 125:219–225, 1999.

Talbot AR, Shiaw M-H, Huang J-S, et al: Acute poisoning with a glyphosate-surfactant herbicide (Roundup): A review of 93 cases. *Hum Exp Toxicol* 10:1–8, 1991.

Tamburro CH: Chronic liver injury in phenoxy herbicide-exposed Vietnam veterans. *Environ Res* 59:175–188, 1992.

Tanaka J, Yamashita M, Yamashita M, et al: Two cases of glufosinate poisoning with late onset convulsions. *Vet Hum Toxicol* 40:219–222, 1998.

Taylor HR, Greene BM: The status of ivermectin in the treatment of onchocerciasis. *Am J Trop Med* 41:460–466, 1989.

Thiess AM, Frentzel-Beyme R, Link R: Mortality study of persons exposed to dioxin in a trichlorophenol process accident that occurred in the BASF AG on November 17, 1953. *Am J Ind Med* 3:179–189, 1982.

Tinoco R, Halperin D, Tinoco R, Parsonhet J: Paraquat poisoning in southern Mexico: A report of 25 cases. *Arch Environ Health* 48:78–80, 1993.

Toia RF, Casida JE: Phosphorylation, "aging" and possible alkylation reactions of saligenin cyclic phosphorus esters with α-chymotrypsin. *Biochem Pharmacol* 28:211–216, 1979.

Tominack RL, Yang G-Y, Tsai W-J, et al: Taiwan National Poison Center survey of glyphosate-surfactant herbicide ingestions. *Clin Toxicol* 29:91–109, 1991.

Tomlin CD (ed), *The Pesticide Manual,* 11th ed. Farnham, UK, British Crop Protection Council, 1997.

Treon JF, Cleveland FP: Toxicity of certain chlorinated hydrocarbon insecticides for laboratory animals with special reference to aldrin and dieldrin. *J Agric Food Chem* 3:402–408, 1955.

Tucker RK, Crabtree DG: *Handbook of Toxicity of Pesticides to Wildlife.* Resource Publication No. 84. Washington, DC: US Department of Interior, Fish and Wildlife Service, U.S. Government Printing Office, 1970.

Tucker SB, Flannigan SA: Cutaneous effects from occupational exposure to fenvalerate. *Arch Toxicol* 54:195–202, 1983.

Turnbull GJ, Sanderson DM, Crome SJ: Exposure to pesticides during application, in Turnbull GJ (ed): *Occupational Hazards of Pesticide Use.* London: Taylor & Francis, 1985, pp 35–49.

Turner WA, Engel JL, Casida JE: Toxaphene components and related compounds: Preparation and toxicity of some hepta-, octa- and nonachlorobomanes, hexa- and heptachlorobomenes and a hexachlorobomadiene. *J Agric Food Chem* 25:1394–1401, 1977.

Vandekar M, Heyadat S, Plestina R, Ahmady G: A study of the safety of *o*-isopropoxyphenylmethylcarbamate in an operational field-trial in Iran. *Bull WHO* 38:609–623, 1968.

Vandekar M, Plestina R, Wilhelm K: Toxicity of carbamates for mammals. *Bull WHO* 44:241–248, 1971.

Van den Bercken J, Vijverberg HPM: Interaction of pyrethroids and DDT-like compounds with the sodium channels in the nerve membrane, in Miyamoto J, Kearney PC (eds): *Pesticide Chemistry. Human Welfare and the Environment. Mode of Action, Metabolism and Toxicology.* Vol 3. Oxford, England: Pergamon Press, 1983, pp 115–121.

Van Miller JP, Lalich JJ, Allen JR: Increased incidence of neoplasm in rats exposed to low levels of 2,3,7,8-tetrachlorodibenzo-*p*-dioxin. *Chemosphere* 6:537–544, 1977.

Venegas W, Zapata I, Carbonell E, et al: Micronuclei analysis in lymphocytes of pesticide sprayers from Concepcion, Chile. *Teratogenesis Carcinog Mutagen* 18:123–129, 1998.

Vercruysse F, Driegne S, Steurbaut W, et al: Exposure assessment of professional pesticide users during treatment of potato fields. *Pestic Sci* 55:467–473, 1999.

Verschoyle RD, Aldridge WN: Structure-activity relationships of some pyrethroids in rats. *Arch Toxicol* 45:325–329, 1980.

Wafford KA, Sattelle DB, Gant DB, et al: Non competitive inhibition of GABA receptors in insect and vertebrate CNS by endrin and lindane. *Pestic Biochem Physiol* 33:213–219, 1989.

Ward TR, Mundy WR: Organophosphorus compounds preferentially affect second messenger systems coupled to M2/M4 receptors in rat frontal cortex. *Brain Res Bull* 39:49–55, 1996.

Warmke JW, Reenan RA, Wang P, et al: Functional expression of *Drosophila para* sodium channels. Modulation by the membrane protein TipE and toxin pharmacology. *J Gen Physiol* 110:119–138, 1997.

Watanabe T: Apoptosis induced by glufosinate ammonium in the neuroepithelium of developing mouse embryos in culture. *Neurosci Lett* 222:17–20, 1997.

Watanabe T, Iwase T: Developmental effects of glufosinate ammonium on mouse embryos in culture. *Teratogenesis Carcinog Mutagen* 16:287–299, 1996.

Watanabe T, Sano T: Neurological effects of glufosinate poisoning with a brief review. *Hum Exp Toxicol* 17:35–39, 1998.

Waters EM, Huff JE, Gerstner HB: Mirex. An overview. *Environ Res* 14:212–222, 1977.

Webb J: Iraq caught out over nerve gas attack. *New Scientist* 138: May 1, p 4, 1993.

Wecker L, Kiauta T, Dettbarn W-D: Relationship between acetylcholinesterase inhibition and the development of a myopathy. *J Pharmacol Exp Ther* 206:97–104, 1978.

Wecker L, Mrak RE, Dettbarn WD: Evidence of necrosis in human intercostal muscle following inhalation of an organophosphate insecticide. *Fundam Appl Toxicol* 6:172–174, 1986.

Weed Science Society of America (WSSA): *Herbicide Handbook,* 7th ed. Champaign, IL: WSSA, 1994.

Weiner ML, Jortner BS: Organophosphate-induced delayed neurotoxicity of triarylphosphates. *Neurotoxicology* 20:653–674, 1999.

Weir S, Minton N, Murray V: Organophosphate poisoning: The UK National Poisons Unit experience during 1984–1987, in Ballantyne B, Barrs TC (eds): *Clinical and Experimental Toxicology* of *Organophosphates and Carbamates.* Oxford, England: Butterworth-Heinemann, 1992, pp 463–470.

Wesseling C, Castillo L, Elinder CC: Pesticide poisonings in Costa Rica. *Scand J Work Environ Health* 19:227–235, 1993.

Wesseling C, Hogstedt C, Picado, et al: Unintentional fatal paraquat poisonings among agricultural workers in Costa Rica: Report of 15 cases. *Am J Ind Med* 32:433–441, 1997.

Whorton MD, Obrinsky DL: Persistence of symptoms after mild to moderate acute organophosphate poisoning among 19 farm field workers. *J Toxicol Environ Health* 11:347–354, 1983.

Wigle DT, Semenciw RM, Wilkins K, et al: Mortality study of Canadian male farm operators: Non-Hodgkin's lymphoma mortality and agricultural practices in Saskatchewan. *J Natl Cancer Inst* 82:575–582, 1990.

Wilson AG, Thake DC, Heydens WE, et al: Mode of action of thyroid tumor formation in the male Long-Evans rat administered high doses of alachlor. *Fundam Appl Toxicol* 33:16–23, 1996.

Wilson R, Lovejoy FH, Jaeger RJ, Landrigan PL: Acute phosphine poisoning aboard a grain freighter. *JAMA* 244:148–150, 1980.

Wojeck GA, Nigg FfN, Stamper JH, Bradway DE: Worker exposure to ethion in Florida citrus. *Arch Environ Contam in Toxicol* 10:725–735, 1981.

Wolfe HR, Armstrong JF, Staiff DC, Comer SW: Exposure of spraymen to pesticides. *Arch Environ Health* 25:29–31, 1972.

Wolfe HR, Durham WF, Armstrong JF: Exposure of workers to pesticides. *Arch Environ Health* 14:622–633, 1967.

World Health Organization (WHO): *International Programme on Chemical Safety: Environmental Health Criteria 39. Paraquat and Diquat.* Geneva: WHO, 1984.

World Health Organization (WHO): *Public Health Impact of Pesticides Used in Agriculture.* Geneva: WHO, 1990.

World Health Organization (WHO): *Twenty Years of Onchocerciasis Control in West Africa. Review of the Work of the Onchocerciasis Control Programme in West Africa 1974–1994.* Geneva: WHO, 1997.

World Health Organization (WHO): *WHO Technical Report Series* 513 *(Safe Use of Pesticides: Twentieth Report of the WHO Expert Committee on Insecticides).* Geneva: WHO, 1973, pp 43–44.

Worthing CR (ed): *The Pesticide Manual. A World Compendium,* 8th ed. British Crop Protection Council. Lavenham, UK: Lavenham Press, 1987.

Wray JE, Mufti Y, Dogramaci I: Hexachlorobenzene as a cause of porphyria turcica. *Turk J Pediatr* 4:132–137, 1962.

Xintaris C, Burg JR, Tanaka S, et al: *Occupational Exposure to Leptophos and Other Chemicals.* DHEW (NIOSH) Publication No. 78-136. Washington, DC: DHEW, U.S. Government Printing Office, 1978.

Yang C-C, Wu J-F, Ong H-C, et al: Taiwan national poison control center: Epidemiologic data. 1985–1993. *Clin Toxicol* 34:651–663, 1996.

Yang RSH: Enzymatic conjugation and insecticide metabolism, in Wilkinson CF (ed): *Insecticide Biochemistry and Physiology.* New York: Plenum Press, 1976, pp 177–225.

Yang ZP, Dettbarn WD: Diisopropylphosphorofluoridate-induced cholinergic hyperactivity and lipid peroxidation. *Toxicol Appl Pharmacol* 138:48–53, 1996.

Yang ZP, Morrow J, Wu A, et al: Diisopropylphosphoro-fluoridate induced muscle hyperactivity associated with enhanced lipid peroxidation *in vivo. Biochem Pharmacol* 52:357–361, 1996.

Zhang Z, Sun J, Chen S, et al: Levels of exposure and biological monitoring of pyrethroids in spraymen. *Br J Indus Med* 48:82–86, 1991.

CHAPTER 23

TOXIC EFFECTS OF METALS

Robert A. Goyer and Thomas W. Clarkson

INTRODUCTION

Metals differ from other toxic substances in that they are neither created nor destroyed by humans. Nevertheless, their utilization by humans influences the potential for health effects in at least two major ways: first, by environmental transport, that is, by human or anthropogenic contributions to air, water, soil, and food, and second, by altering the speciation or biochemical form of the element (Beijer and Jernelov, 1986).

Metals are probably the oldest toxins known to humans. Lead usage may have begun prior to 2000 B.C., when abundant supplies were obtained from ores as a by-product of smelting silver. Hippocrates is credited in 370 B.C. with the first description of abdominal colic in a man who extracted metals. Arsenic and mercury are cited by Theophrastus of Erebus (370–287 B.C.) and Pliny the Elder (A.D. 23–79). Arsenic was obtained during the melting of copper and tin, and an early use was for decoration in Egyptian tombs. In contrast, many of the metals of toxicologic concern today are only recently known to humans. Cadmium was first recognized in ores containing zinc carbonate in 1817. About 80 of the 105 elements in the periodic table are regarded as metals, but less than 30 have been reported to produce toxicity in humans. The importance of some of the rarer or lesser known metals such as indium or gallium might increase with new applications in microelectronics, antitumor therapy, or other new technologies.

Metals are redistributed naturally in the environment by both geologic and biological cycles (Fig. 23-1). Rainwater dissolves rocks and ores and physically transports material to streams and rivers, depositing and stripping materials from adjacent soil and eventually transporting these substances to the ocean to be precipitated as sediment or taken up in rainwater to be relocated elsewhere on earth. The biological cycles include bioconcentration by plants and animals and incorporation into food cycles. These natural cycles may exceed the anthropogenic cycle, as is the case for mercury. Human industrial activity, however, may greatly shorten the residence time of metals in ore, may form new compounds, and may greatly enhance worldwide distribution not only by discharge to land and water but also to the atmosphere. When discharged in gaseous or fine particulate forms, metal may be trans-

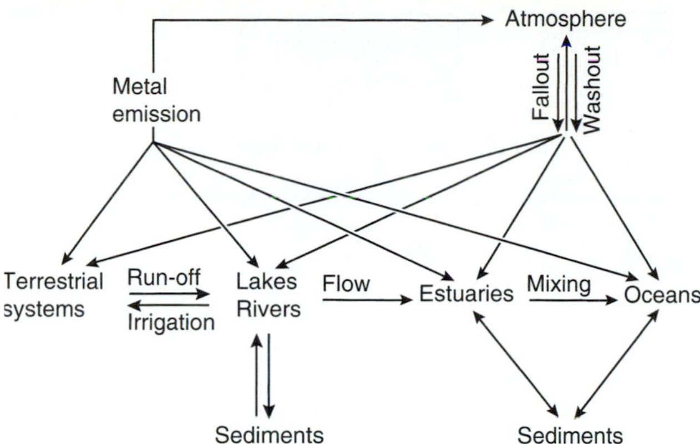

Figure 23-1. Routes for transport of trace elements in the environment. [From Beijer and Jernelõv (1986).]

ported in the atmosphere over global distances. The role of human activity in the redistribution of metals is demonstrated by the 200-fold increase in lead content of Greenland ice, beginning with a natural low level (about 800 B.C.) and continuing with a gradual rise in lead content of ice through the evolution of the industrial age and finally a nearly precipitous rise in lead corresponding to the period when lead was added to gasoline in the 1920s (Ng and Patterson, 1981). Metal contamination of the environment therefore reflects both natural sources and a contribution from industrial activity.

The conceptual boundaries of what is regarded as the toxicology of metals continue to broaden. Historically, metal toxicology largely concerned acute or overt effects, such as abdominal colic from lead toxicity or the bloody diarrhea and suppression of urine formation from ingestion of corrosive (mercury) sublimate. There must continue to be knowledge and understanding of such effects, but they are uncommon with present-day occupational and environmental standards. There is, however, growing interest in, and inquiry into, subtle, chronic, or long-term effects in which cause-and-effect relationships are not obvious or may be subclinical. These might include a level of effect that causes a change in an important index of affected individuals' performance—that is, lower than expected IQs due to childhood lead exposure. Assigning responsibility for such toxicologic effects is extremely difficult and sometimes impossible, particularly when the endpoint in question lacks specificity, in that it may be caused by a number of agents or even combinations of substances. The challenges for the toxicologist, therefore, are many. The major ones include the need for quantitative information regarding dose and tissue levels as well as greater understanding of the metabolism of metals, particularly at the tissue and cellular levels, where specific effects may occur. Depending on the dose, most metals affect multiple organ systems; but at the lowest dose where effects occur, each metal tends to effect first a specific organ or tissue.

There is increasing emphasis on the use of biomarkers of exposure, toxicity, and suseptiblity to toxic metals. Biomarkers of exposure, also called biological monitors, such as metal concentrations in blood, and urine, have a long history of use, but the advent of molecular biology has greatly expanded the possiblities for all three types of biomarkers. Thus in the case of chromium, DNA-protein complexes may serve as a biomarker of both exposure and carcinogenic potential. The induction of genes known to play a protective role against metal toxicity—for example, the metallothionein and heme oxygenase genes—show promise as markers of both effect and susceptiblity. The use of such biomarkers provides guidelines for preventive measures or therapeutic intervention.

DOSE–EFFECT RELATIONSHIPS

Estimates of the relationship of dose or level of exposure to toxic effects for a particular metal are in many ways a measure of the dose–response relationships discussed in greater detail in Chap. 2. Relationships between sources of exposure, transport, and distribution to various organs and excretory pathways are shown in Fig. 23-2. The dose or estimate of exposure to a metal may be a multidimensional concept and is a function of time as well as the concentration of metal. The most precise definition of dose is the amount of metal within cells of organs manifesting a toxicologic effect. Results from single measurements may reflect recent exposure or longer-term or past exposure, depending on retention time in the particular tissue.

A critical determinant of retention of a metal is its biological half-life, that is, the time it takes for the body or organ to excrete half of an accumulated amount. The biological half-life varies according to the metal as well as the organ or tissue; in the case of many metals, more than one half-life is needed to fully describe the retention time. For example, the biological half-lives of cadmium in kidney and lead in bone are 20 to 30 years, whereas for some metals, such as arsenic or lithium, they are only a few hours or days. The half-life of lead in blood is only a few weeks, as compared to the much longer half-time in bone. After inhalation of mercury vapor, at least two half-lives describe the retention in brain—one of the order of a few weeks and the other measured in years.

Blood, urine, and hair are the most accessible tissues in which to measure an exposure or dose; they are sometimes referred to as *indicator tissues.* In vivo, the quantitation of metals within organs is not yet possible, although techniques such as neutron activation and x-ray fluorescence spectroscopy are emerging technologies. Indirect estimates of quantities of toxic metals in specific organs may be calculated from metabolic models derived from autopsy data. Blood and urine concentrations usually reflect recent exposure and correlate best with acute effects. An exception is urinary cadmium, which may reflect renal damage related to an accumulation of cadmium in the kidney. Partitioning of metal between cells and plasma and between filterable and nonfilterable components of plasma should provide more precise information regarding the presence of biologically active forms of a particular metal. For example, most of the methyl mercury in blood is protein-bound, whereas the transportable species—believed to be a complex with low-molecular-weight thiol amino acids—accounts for a tiny fraction. Such partitioning is now standard laboratory practice for blood calcium; ionic calcium is by far the most active form of the metal. Other specific metal complexes, such as chromate and arsenate anions, have now been shown to be the species transported into cells. Speciation of toxic metals in urine may also provide diagnostic insights. For example, cadmium metallothionein in plasma or urine may be of greater toxicologic significance than total cadmium.

Hair might be useful in assessing variations in exposure to metals over the long term. Analyses may be performed on segments of the hair, so that metal content of the newest growth can be compared with past exposures. Hair levels of mercury have been found to be a reliable measure of exposure to alkyl or methyl mercury. For most other metals, however, hair is not a reliable tissue

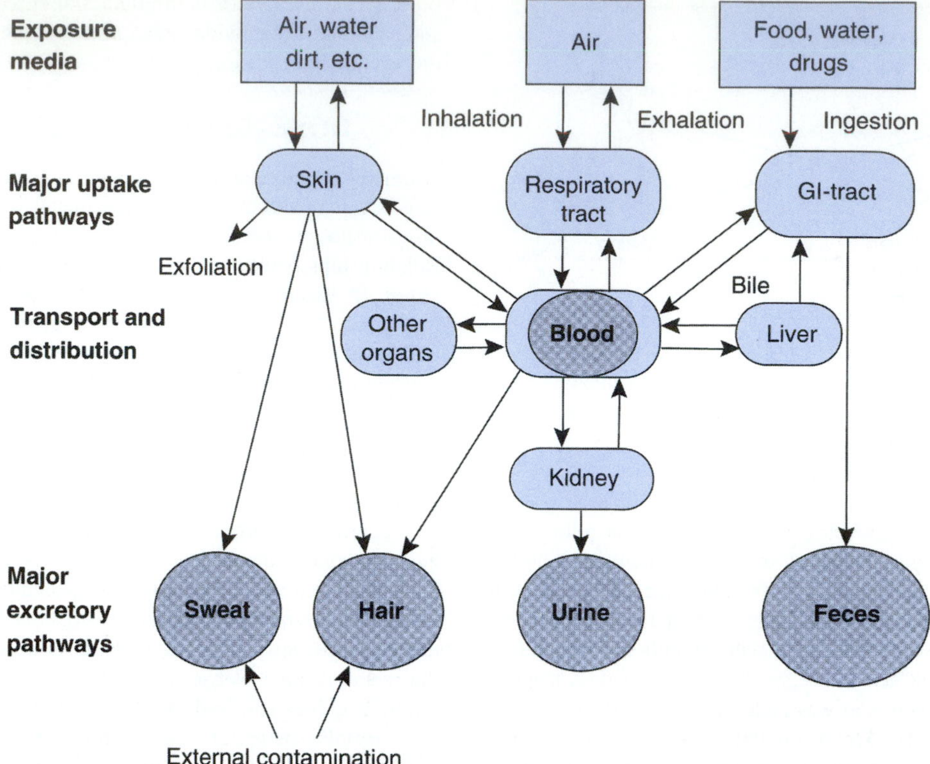

Figure 23-2. Metabolism after exposure to metals via skin absorption, inhalation and ingestion.

The arrows indicate how the metals are transported and distributed. Tissues that are particularly useful for biological monitoring are identified in shaded areas. [From Elinder et al. (1994), with permission.]

for measuring exposure because of metal deposits from external contamination that complicate analyses, in spite of washing.

Cellular targets for toxicity are specific biochemical processes (enzymes) and/or receptors on membranes of cells and organelles. The proximate toxic action of the metal may involve an interaction between the free metal ion and the toxicologic target—for example, in the case of alkali and alkaline earth metals such as lithium and barium. Other metals that bind with high affinities to cellular ligands may transfer from a ligand involved in transport of the metal directly to the target ligand. For example, methyl mercury is believed to transfer from one thiol group to another without any intermediary free mercury ion.

Toxicity is determined by dose at the cellular level as well as such factors as valence state and ligand binding. Hexavalent chromium is highly toxic, whereas the trivalent form functions as an essential trace element. Ligand binding is probably the most fundamental chemical process in metal toxicity and in cellular defense against metals. The thiol ligands of metallothionein avidly bind a number of toxic metals as part of a defense system. Lead attaches to thiol ligands on enzymes involved in heme synthesis, trivalent arsenic to the thiol groups of alpha lipoic acid, and uranium to phosphate groups on glucose transporters, all metal ligand interactions underlying toxic action.

Certain metals can form organometallic compounds involving covalent metal-carbon bonds. These "organic" forms differ in toxic properties from the inorganic counterparts. Nonionized alkyl compounds such as tetraethyl lead and dimethyl mercury are lipid soluble and pass readily across biological membranes unaltered by their surrounding medium. They are dealkylated or transformed ultimately to inorganic species. Hence, the patterns of disposition and toxicity of organic forms tend to differ from those of inorganic forms. For example, alkyl mercury is primarily a neurotoxin, whereas mercuric chloride is toxic to the kidneys.

HOST FACTORS INFLUENCING THE TOXICITY OF METALS

Recognition of factors that influence toxicity of a particular level of exposure to a toxic metal are important in determining the risk of toxicity, particularly in susceptible populations. A number of factors influencing the toxicity of metals are shown in Table 23-1. The interaction of toxic with essential metals occurs when the metabolism of a toxic metal is similar to that of the essential element (Goyer, 1995). Absorption of toxic metals from the lung or gastrointestinal tract may be influenced by an essential metal, partic-

Table 23-1
Factors Influencing Toxicity of Metals

Interactions with essential metals
Formation of metal–protein complexes
Age and stage of development
Lifestyle factors
Chemical form or speciation
Immune status of host

ularly if the toxic metal shares or influences a homeostatic mechanism, as occurs for lead and calcium and iron, and for cadmium and iron. There is an inverse relationship between the protein content of the diet and cadmium and lead toxicity. Vitamin C reduces lead and cadmium absorption, probably because of increased absorption of ferrous ion. Toxic metals may influence the role of essential metals as cofactors for enzymes or other metabolic processes (e.g., lead interferes with the calcium-dependent release of neurotransmitters). Lead, calcium, and vitamin D have a complex relationship affecting mineralization of bone, and they have a more direct one involving impairment of 1-25-dihydroxy vitamin D synthesis in the kidney.

Metalloprotein complexes involved in detoxification or protection from toxicity have now been described for a few metals (Goyer, 1984). Morphologically discernible cellular inclusion bodies are present with exposures to lead, bismuth, and a mercury-selenate mixture. Metallothioneins form complexes with cadmium, zinc, copper, and other metals, and ferritin and hemosiderin are intracellular iron-protein complexes. None of these proteins or metal-protein complexes have any known enzymatic activity. The nature and influences of these complexes are discussed below (this chapter) in the discussion of the toxicology of the particular metals involved.

Persons at either end of the life span, whether they are young children or elderly people, are believed to be more susceptible to toxicity from exposure to a particular level of metal than most adults (NRC, 1993). The major pathway of exposure to many toxic metals in children is food, and children consume more calories per pound of body weight than adults. Moreover, children have higher gastrointestinal absorption of metals, particularly lead. Experimental studies have extended these observations to many metals, and a milk diet, probably because of its lipid content, seems to increase metal absorption. The rapid growth and rapid cell division that children's bodies experience represent opportunities for genotoxic effects. Intrauterine toxicity to methyl mercury is well documented. There is no impediment to the transplacental transport of lead, so that fetal blood lead levels are similar to maternal levels.

Lifestyle factors such as smoking or alcohol ingestion may have indirect influences on toxicity. Cigarette smoke by itself contains some toxic metals, such as cadmium, and cigarette smoking may also influence pulmonary effects. Alcohol ingestion may influence toxicity indirectly by altering diet and reducing essential mineral intake.

For metals that produce hypersensitivity reactions, the immune status of an individual becomes an additional toxicologic variable. Metals that provoke immune reactions include mercury, gold, platinum, beryllium, chromium, and nickel. Clinical effects are varied but usually involve any of four types of immune responses. In anaphylactic or immediate hypersensitivity reactions, the antibody IgE reacts with the antigen on the surface of mast cells, releasing vasoreactive amines. Clinical reactions include conjunctivitis, asthma, urticaria, or even systemic anaphylaxis. Cutaneous, mucosal, and bronchial reactions to platinum have been attributed to this type of hypersensitivity reaction. Cytotoxic hypersensitivity is the result of a complement-fixing reaction of IgG immunoglobulin with antigen or hapten bound to the cell surface. The thrombocytopenia sometimes occurring with exposure to organic gold salts may be brought about in this manner. Immune complex hypersensitivity occurs when soluble immune complex forms deposits (antigen, antibody, and complement) within tissues, producing an acute inflammatory reaction. Immune complexes are typically deposited on the epithelial (subepithelial) side of glomerular basement membrane, resulting in proteinuria following exposure to mercury vapor or gold therapy. Cell-mediated hypersensitivity, also known as the *delayed hypersensitivity reaction,* is mediated by thymus-dependent lymphocytes and usually occurs 24 to 48 h after exposure. The histologic reaction consists of mononuclear cells and is the typical reaction seen in the contact dermatitis following exposure to chromium or nickel. The granuloma formation occurring with beryllium and zirconium exposure may be a form of cell-mediated immune response.

METAL-BINDING PROTEINS

Protein binding of metals has been the subject of a recent major review on the molecular biology of metal toxicology (Zalups and Koropatnick, 2000). Several kinds of metal-protein interactions may be considered. A protein may be the target of toxicity. Enzymes are the best-documented targets. The protein may play a protective role, reducing the activity (toxicity of the metal). The metallothioneins are the best-known example.

Many different classes of proteins are known to play a role in the disposition of metals in the body. Nonspecific binding to proteins, such as serum albumin or hemoglobin, plays a role in metal transport in the bloodstream and in the distribution of metals between red cells and plasma. Metals bound to albumin may be carried into cells by endocytotic mechanisms. The distribution of methyl mercury between red cells and plasma depends upon genetically determined species of hemoglobin molecules differing in their content of cysteine residues. In addition, proteins with specific metal binding properties play a special role in both the transport of metals from plasma to tissues and in the transport of metals across cell membranes and within the cell.

Specific Metal-Binding Proteins

The metallothioneins, discovered over 40 years ago, may have several diverse functions, including essential metal homeostasis and protection against metal toxicity. They have low molecular weights (about 6000 Da) and are rich in thiol ligands. These ligands provide the basis for high-affinity binding of several essential and nonessential but toxic metals such as Cd, Cu, Hg, Ag, and Zn. In most cases but not all, the metallothioneins are highly inducible by a number of metals and other stimulants. Metallothioneins can interact with metals in complex physiologic and biochemical pathways, as illustrated in the discussion of cadmium, below.

Transferrin is a glycoprotein that binds most of ferric iron in plasma. Transport of iron across cell membranes occurs by receptor-mediated endocytosis of ferric transferrin. The receptor is a disulfide-linked membrane glycoprotein whose affinity for apotransferrin is two orders of magnitude lower than that for ferric transferrin. Once inside the cell, iron is separated from transferrin by an acidification process within the endosomes. This protein also transports Al^{3+} and Mn^{2+}.

Ferritin is primarily a storage protein for iron in the reticuloendothelial cells of liver, spleen, and bone. It plays a major role in hepatic turnover of iron. Kupffer cells release iron acquired from the phagocytosis of red cells in the form of ferritin, which is efficiently internalized by hepatocytes via their ferritin receptors. It has been suggested that ferritin may serve as a general metal detoxicant, since it binds a variety of toxic metals including Cd, Zn, Be and Al.

Ceruloplasmin is a copper-containing glycoprotein oxidase in plasma that converts ferrous to ferric iron, which then binds to transferrin. This protein also stimulates iron uptake by a transferrin-independent mechanism.

Membrane Carrier Proteins

In addition to the cases discussed above, a rapidly increasing number of carrier proteins are being discovered that transport metals across cell membranes and organelles inside the cells. Although certain metals may be transported in the free ionic forms, as through calcium channels, many metals are transported as complexes with endogenous ligands on transport systems intended for the ligand itself. This is made possible because many of these carriers are generally multispecific, accepting substrates that differ considerably in their chemical structure and are not able to discriminate between substrates whose only modification is the attachment of a metal ion.

The phosphate and sulfate transporters can carry a number of metal oxyanions across the plasma membrane. Vanadate and arsenate are structurally similar to phosphate and can compete with phosphate for transport as well as intracellular binding sites. In fact, their toxicity may be related to this competition. Similarly, chromate, molybdate, and selenate are structurally similar to sulfate and are carried on the sulfate transporter.

Amino acid and peptide transporters and organic solute carriers also accept metals as complexes with endogenous molecules such as amino acids, peptides, and bicarbonate. Cellular uptake of copper or zinc may occur as complexes with the amino acid histidine. Methyl mercury crosses cell membranes as a complex with cysteine on the large neutral amino acid carrier and is exported from hepatocytes into bile as a complex with glutathione. Zinc appears to be taken up into red blood cells as an anionic complex with bicarbonate, $Zn(HCO_3)_2$, through the anion exchanger. Bicarbonate complexes of lead may follow a similar route.

Other examples of metal transporters have been the subject of a recent review (Ballatori, 2000a). These include divalent cation transporters and ATP-activated membrane pumps. For example, Wilson's and Menke's diseases are due to genetic errors in copper metabolism related to ATP-activated copper carriers. It has been estimated (Ballatori, 2000b) that the human genome may contain upwards of 9000 genes coding for transporter proteins, of which 2000 are concerned with the transport of drugs and other xenobiotics. This rapidly expanding field is still not sufficiently developed to identify polymorphisms of these protein carriers. The future holds promise that identification and measurement of expression of these carriers in cells and tissues will result in valuable biomarkers of metal effects and of individual susceptibility to metal toxicity.

COMPLEXATION AND CHELATION THERAPY

Treatment of poisoning from toxic metals is sometimes warranted to prevent or reverse toxicity and therefore remains an important topic, particularly for those metals that are cumulative and persistent (e.g., lead). It must be emphasized, however, that treatment is only a secondary alternative to reduction or prevention of exposures to toxic metals.

Complexation is the formation of a metal ion complex in which the metal ion is associated with a charged or uncharged electron donor, referred to as a *ligand.* The ligand may be monodentate, bidentate, or multidentate; that is, it may attach or coordinate using one, two or more donor atoms. *Chelation* occurs when bidentate ligands form ring structures (*chelate* comes from the Greek word for claw) that include the metal ion and the two ligand atoms attached to the metal (Williams and Halstead, 1982). Metals may react with O-, S-, and N-containing ligands present in the form of OH, COOH, SH, NH_2, NH, and N. A resultant metal complex is formed by coordinate bonds (coordination compound), in which both electrons are contributed by the ligand (Klaassen, 1990).

Chelating[1] agents (drugs) vary in their specificity for toxic metals. Ideal chelating agents should be water-soluble, resistant to biotransformation, able to reach sites of metal storage, capable of forming nontoxic complexes with toxic metals, and of being excreted from the body; they should also have a low affinity for essential metals, particularly calcium and zinc (Klaassen, 1990). The challenge in the development of safer and more effective chelating agents is to design all of the desirable chemical, physiologic, and pharmacologic properties into the drug (Jones, 1992).

The general properties of chelating agents that are of current interest are briefly described below. Additional details and comments are provided later in the chapter with discussions of specific metals.

BAL (British Anti-Lewisite)

BAL (2,3-dimercaptopropanol) was the first clinically useful chelating agent. It was developed during World War II as a specific antagonist to vesicant arsenical war gases, based on the observation that arsenic has an affinity for sulfhydryl-containing substances. BAL, a dithiol compound with two sulfur atoms on adjacent carbon atoms, competes with the critical binding sites responsible for the toxic effects. These observations led to the prediction that the "biochemical lesion" of arsenic poisoning would prove to be a thiol with sulfhydryl groups separated by one or more intervening carbon atoms. This prediction was borne out a few years later with the discovery that arsenic interferes with the function of 6,8-dithiooctanoic acid in biological oxidation (Gunsalus, 1953).

BAL has been found to form stable chelates in vivo with many toxic metals, including inorganic mercury, antimony, bismuth, cadmium, chromium, cobalt, gold, and nickel. However, it is not necessarily the treatment of choice for toxicity to these metals. BAL has been used as an adjunct in the treatment of the acute encephalopathy of lead toxicity. It is a potentially toxic drug, and its use may be accompanied by multiple side effects. Although treatment with BAL will increase the excretion of cadmium, there is a

[1]Chelating agents are a subset of the more general class of complexing agents. However, the terms *chelation* and *chelating agents* are now used to cover all types of metal complexation therapy even though some agents cannot form ring structures—for example, penicillamine, to be discussed later. Also, bidentate complexing agents such as BAL that have the capacity to form ring structures with metals; in fact, they may form complexes without ring structures, depending on the molar ratio of metal to BAL (for further discussion, see Clarkson and DiStefano, 1971). In this text we follow the common practice of using the terms *chelation* and *chelating agent* to cover all types of complexation therapy.

concomitant increase in renal cadmium concentration, so that its use in case of cadmium toxicity is to be avoided. It does, however, remove inorganic mercury from the kidney, but it is not useful in the treatment of alkyl mercury or phenyl mercury toxicity. BAL also enhances the toxicity of selenium and tellurium, so it is not to be used to remove these metals from the body.

DMPS

DMPS (2,3-dimercapto-1-propanesulfonic acid) is a water-soluble derivative of BAL developed in response to BAL's toxicity and unpleasant side effects. DMPS has been shown to reduce blood lead levels in children (Chisholm and Thomas, 1985). It has the advantage over ethylene diamine tetraacetic acid (EDTA) in that it is administered orally and does not appear to have toxic side effects. It has been widely used in the former Soviet Union to treat many different metal intoxications. DMPS has been used experimentally to estimate the renal burden of lead (Twarog and Cherian, 1984) and inorganic mercury (Cherian et al., 1988). Its effectiveness in mobilizing metals from the kidney may be due to the fact that it is transported into kidney cells on the organic anion transport system (Zalups et al., 1998). It increases the urinary excretion of mercury in persons with an increased body burden from industrial exposure, from dentists and dental technicians, from persons with dental amalgams, from those exposed to mercurous chloride in skin creams (Aposhian et al., 1992; Gonzalez-Ramirez et al., 1998). This agent has also been used to assess body burdens of inorganic mercury from dental amalgams and of arsenic ingested from drinking water (Aposhian, 1998).

DMSA

DMSA (meso-2.3.-dimercaptosuccinic acid; succimer), like DMPS, is a chemical analog of BAL. More than 90 percent of DMSA is in the form of a mixed disulfide in which each of the sulfur atoms is in disulfide linkage with a cysteine molecule (Aposhian and Aposhian, 1992). The drug is of current interest clinically because of its ability to lower blood lead levels. It has advantages over EDTA because it is given orally and has greater specificity for lead. It may be safer than EDTA in that it does not enhance excretion of calcium and zinc to the same degree. Studies in rodents showed that a single dose of DMSA primarily removes lead from soft tissues (Smith and Flegal, 1992). A lead mobilzation test with DMSA does not appear to give better information on body burden than measurements of lead in blood, plasma, or urine (Gerhardsson et al., 1999).

The drug has been licensed recently by the U.S. Food and Drug Administration (FDA) specifically for the treatment of lead poisoning in children whose blood lead levels are ≥45 μg/dL, and it has been used in Europe. However its effectiveness in improving long-term blood lead levels in children has been questioned (O'Connor and Rich, 1999), nor, according to studies on primates, does it appear effective in removing lead from the brain (Cremin et al., 1999). Its ability to reverse some of the toxic outcomes of lead poisoning, such as negative effects on cognitive and behavioral development, has not been demonstrated.

EDTA

Calcium salt of ethylene diamine tetraacetic acid (EDTA) must be used for clinical purposes because the sodium salt has greater affinity for calcium and will produce hypocalcemic tetany. However, the calcium salt will bind lead, with displacement of calcium from the chelate. EDTA is poorly absorbed from the gastrointestinal tract so it must be given parenterally, which distributes it rapidly throughout the body. It has long been the method of choice for the treatment of lead toxicity. The peak excretion point is within the first 24 h and represents the excretion of lead from soft tissues. Removal of lead from the skeletal system occurs more slowly, with the restoration of equilibrium with soft tissue compartments. Animal experiments indicate that EDTA is not effective in reducing total brain lead (Seaton et al., 1999). Calcium EDTA does have the potential for nephrotoxicity, so it should be administered only when clinically indicated (EPA, 1986). Combination therapy of EDTA with other chelating agents, such as BAL and DMSA, has been used to reduce the risk of side effects from either agent alone, as each agent can be given at a lower dose in combined therapy. Whether BAL or DMSA is used as the second agent, the results are equally effective in reducing blood lead in children (Besunder et al., 1997).

DTPA

DTPA, or diethylenetriaminepentaacetic acid, has chelating properties similar to those of EDTA. The calcium salt ($CaNa_2DTPA$) must be used clinically because of DTPA's high affinity for calcium. It has been used for the chelation of plutonium and other actinide elements, but with mixed success. Experimental studies have shown that various multidentate hydroxypyridinonate ligands are more effective than $CaNa_2DTPA$ for promoting excretion of Pu and other actinides (Durbin et al., 2000).

Desferrioxamine

Desferrioxamine is a hydroxylamine isolated as the iron chelate of *Streptomyces pilosus* and is used clinically in the metal-free form (Keberle, 1964). It has a remarkable affinity for ferric iron and a low affinity for calcium, and it competes effectively for iron in ferritin and hemosiderin but not in transferrin and not for the iron in hemoglobin or heme-containing enzymes. It is poorly absorbed from the gastrointestinal tract, so it must be given parenterally. Clinical usefulness is limited by a variety of toxic effects, including hypotension, skin rashes, and possibly cataract formation. It seems to be more effective in hemosiderosis due to blood transfusion but is less effective in treatment of hemochromatosis. A high-molecular-weight derivative in which desferrioxamine is chemically coupled to hydroxyethyl starch shows promise in human tests as an effective iron chelator, with lower toxicity than the parent compound (Dragsten et al., 2000).

Dithiocarbamate (DTC)

Dithiocarb (diethyldithiocarbamate), or DTC, has been recommended as the drug of choice in the treatment of acute nickel carbonyl poisoning. The drug may be administered orally for mild toxicity and parenterally for acute or severe poisoning (Sunderman, 1979). However, no adequately controlled clinical studies have been performed (Bradberry and Vale, 1999).

DTC has also been used experimentally for removal of cadmium bound to metallothionein (Kojima et al., 1990). A number of DTC compounds with various substitutions of nonpolar, nonionizing groups have been synthesized by Jones and Cherian (1990). Sodium, *N*-(4-methoxybenzyl)-D-glucamine dithiocarbamate (MeOBGDTC), is among the most effective in removing cadmium from tissues. The CdMeOBGDTC complex is excreted in the bile rather than by the kidney, avoiding the nephrotoxicity characteristic of cadmium chelates. To date the use of this compound has been limited to experimental studies in rodents.

Penicillamine and *N*-Acetylcysteine

Penicillamine (β, β-dimethylcysteine), a hydrolytic product of penicillin, has been used for the removal of copper in persons with Wilson's disease and for the removal of lead, mercury, and iron (Walshe, 1964). It is also important to note that penicillamine removes other physiologically essential metals, including zinc, cobalt, and manganese. Attached to its use is the risk of inducing a hypersensitivity reaction with a wide spectrum of undesirable immunologic effects, including skin rash, blood dyscrasia, and possibly proteinuria and nephrotic syndrome. It has cross-sensitivity with penicillin, so it should be avoided by persons with penicillin hypersensitivity. For persons who have developed a sensitivity to penicillamine, an orally active chelating agent, triethylene tetramine 2HCl (Trien), is an alternative for the removal of copper (Walshe, 1983). Reducing the commonly used dose from 25 to 30 mg/kg/day to 15 mg/kg/day maintains the efficacy of d-penicillamine at reducing blood lead with reduced side effects in lead-exposed children (Shannon and Townsend, 2000).

N-acetylcysteine has been widely used clinically as a mucolytic agent (e.g., for cystic fibrosis) and to protect against the toxic effects of a number of chemicals. It is a free-radical scavenger, a precursor to glutathione, and it can form stable water-soluble complexes with mercury and other metals. Its ease of administration (oral), low toxicity, and wide availability in the clinical setting makes it an attractive therapeutic agent. It is effective in accelerating the removal of methyl mercury in animal tests (Ornaghi et al., 1993; Ballatori et al., 1998). It was also effective in extracorporeal complexation hemodialysis (see below) in one case of human exposure to methyl mercury (Lund et al., 1984).

Hemodialysis with Chelation

Hemodialysis is usually not effective in removing metals from the bloodstream because many metals are associated with red blood cells and/or bound to plasma proteins (for example, Sauder et al., 1988). However a chelating agent may transform the metal into a diffusible form amenable to removal by hemodialysis (Kostyniak and Clarkson, 1981). The chelating agent may be given systemically, as in the application of desferrioxamine to remove aluminum in conjunction with hemodialysis (Nakamura et al., 2000). Extracorporeal complexation hemodialysis avoids systemic application of the complexing agent by introducing the agent into the blood as it enters the dialyzer. Hemodialysis then removes the metal chelate and as well as the excess chelating agent. The method was first successfully used to remove methyl mercury from intoxicated patients (Al-Abbasi et al., 1978), and it has subsequently been applied to a case of inorganic poisoning (Kostyniak et al., 1990). The most effective complexing agent appears to be DMSA for mercury removal with hemodialysis (Kostyniak, 1982). The method has been successfully tested in dogs to remove cadmium using a combination of EDTA and glutathione as complexing agents (Sheabar et al., 1989).

MAJOR TOXIC METALS WITH MULTIPLE EFFECTS

Arsenic (As)

Arsenic[1] is particularly difficult to characterize as a single element because its chemistry is so complex and there are many different arsenic compounds. It may be trivalent or pentavalent and is widely distributed in nature. The most common inorganic trivalent arsenic compounds are arsenic trioxide, sodium arsenite, and arsenic trichloride. Pentavalent inorganic compounds are arsenic pentoxide, arsenic acid, and arsenates, such as lead arsenate and calcium arsenate. Organic compounds may also be trivalent or pentavalent, such as arsanilic acid, or may even occur in methylated forms as a consequance of biomethylation by organisms in soil, fresh water, and seawater.

A summary of environmental sources of arsenic as well as their potential health effects is contained in the National Research Council's is report on arsenic in drinking water (NRC, 1999). Inorganic arsenic is released into the environment from a number of anthropogenic sources, which include primary copper, zinc, and lead smelters, glass manufacturers that add arsenic to raw materials, and chemical manufacturers. The National Air Sampling Network tests conducted by the EPA indicate that in areas not influenced by copper smelters, maximum 24-h concentrations do not exceed 0.1 $\mu g/m^3$.

Drinking water usually contains a few micrograms per liter or less. Most major U.S. drinking water supplies contain levels lower than 5 μg/L. It has been estimated that about 350,000 people might drink water containing more than 50 μg/L (Smith et al., 1992). While seafoods contain several times the amount of arsenic in other foods, about 90 percent or more is organic arsenic that is unabsorbed (NRC, 1999). According to the 1991–1997 FDA Total Diet Market Basket Study conducted by the FDA for the 1991–1997 period, daily intake of arsenic from food is less than 10 μg/day (Tao and Bulger, 1998). Assuming consumption of 2000 mL/day of drinking water containing as much as 5 μg/L of arsenic, drinking water also contributes 10 μg/day for a total of 20 μg/day from food and water. Youst et al. (1998) estimated that daily dietary intake of inorganic arsenic ranges from 8.3 to 14 μg/day in the United States and 4.8 to 12.7 μg/day in Canada. Major sources of occupational exposure to arsenic in the United States include the manufacture of pesticides, herbicides, and other agricultural products. High exposure to arsenic fumes and dust may occur in the smelting industries; the highest concentrations most likely are among roaster workers.

Toxicokinetics About 80 to 90 percent of a single dose of arsenite [As(III) or arsenate As(V)] has been shown to be absorbed from the gastrointestinal tract of humans and experimental animals. Arsenic compounds of low solubility (e.g., arsenic selenide, lead arsenide, and gallium arsenide) are absorbed less efficiently than dissolved arsenic. Skin can be a route of exposure to arsenic, and systemic toxicity has been reported in persons having extensive acute dermal contact with solutions of inorganic arsenic (Hostynek et al., 1993). Airborne arsenic is largely trivalent arsenic oxide, but deposition in airways and absorption from lungs is dependent on particle size and chemical form (Morrow et al.,

[1]Atomic weight, 74.92; periodic table group, VA; valence, −3, +3 or +5; discovered in A.D. 1250.

1980). Excretion of absorbed arsenic is mainly via urine. The biological half-life of ingested inorganic arsenic is about 10 h, and 50 to 80 percent is excreted in about 3 days. The biological half-life of methylated arsenic is about 30 h. Arsenic has a predilection for skin and is excreted by desquamation of skin and in sweat, particularly during periods of profuse sweating. It also concentrates in nails and hair. Arsenic in nails produces Mees' lines (transverse white bands across fingernails), which appear about 6 weeks after the onset of symptoms of toxicity. The time of exposure may be estimated from measuring the distance of the line from the base of the nail and the rate of nail growth, which is about 0.3 cm per month or 0.1 mm per day. Arsenic in hair may also reflect past exposure, but intrinsic or systematically absorbed arsenic in hair must be distinguished from arsenic that is deposited from external sources.

Biotransformation The metabolism and potential for toxicity of arsenic is complicated by in vivo transformation of inorganic forms by methylation to monomethyl arsenic (MMA) and dimethyl arsenic (DMA). The methylation of arsenic compounds involves both oxidation states of the element. The liver is the major site for methylation. A substantial fraction of absorbed As(V) is rapidly reduced to AS(III), most of which is then methylated to MMA or DMA. The probable mechanisms of in vivo methylation involve a two-electron process that probably involves thiol oxidation. As(V) is reduced to As(III). The resulting As(III) then reacts with *S*-adenosylmethionine (SAM) in an oxidative addition resulting in the transfer of a methyl group from sulfur to arsenic (Abernathy et al., 1999). Compared with inorganic arsenic, the methylated metabolites are less reactive with tissue constituents, less acutely toxic, less cytotoxic, and more readily excreted in the urine (NRC, 1999). This is presumed to be a process of detoxification of the more toxic inorganic forms, and dimethyl arsenic appears to be a terminal metabolite, which is rapidly formed and rapidly excreted. The liver is the major site for methylation of inorganic arsenic. Studies using primary cultures of normal human hepatocytes have shown that the total methylation yield (MMA and DMA) increased in a dose-dependent manner, but the methylation process is saturable. DMA production was inhibited by As(III) in a concentration-dependent manner and DMA/MMA ratio decreased. At higher concentrations of As(III), both methylated forms of arsenic decreased (Styblo et al., 1999). There are major differences in the biotransformation of inorganic arsenic in different mammalian species (Vahter, 1994; Vahter et al., 1995). For most animal species, DMA is the main metabolite. Studies of marmoset monkeys and chimpanzees show no methylation of inorganic arsenic.

A number of studies in humans in which metabolites of inorganic arsenic in urine have been speciated consistently show average values of 10 to 30 percent inorganic arsenic, 10 to 20 percent MMA, and 55 to 76 percent DMA. Those results were found in human subjects in the general environment and in those exposed at work. However, there are variations in arsenic methylation due to such factors as possible genetic polymorphisms, age, and sex. Studies of native peoples and people of Spanish descent in northern Argentina and Chile exposed to arsenic in drinking water showed that urinary arsenic consisted of only 2 to 4 percent MMA on average (Concha et al., 1998a). On the other hand, a study of exposure to arsenic in drinking water in northeastern Taiwan showed 27 percent MMA in urine—an unusually high percentage (Chiou et al., 1997).

Mechanisms of Toxicity It has been known for some years that trivalent compounds of arsenic are the principal toxic forms and that pentavalent arsenic compounds have little effect on enzyme activity. A number of sulfhydryl-containing proteins and enzyme systems have been found to be altered by exposure to arsenic. Some of these can be reversed by addition of an excess of a monothiol such as glutathione. Effects on enzymes containing two thiol groups can be reversed by dithiols such as 2,3-dimercapto-propanol (British anti-Lewisite, or BAL) but not by monothiol. Arsenic affects mitochondrial enzymes and impairs tissue respiration (Brown et al., 1976), which seems to be related to the cellular toxicity of arsenic. Mitochondria accumulate arsenic, and respiration mediated by NAD-linked substrates is particularly sensitive to arsenic; this is thought to result from a reaction between the arsenite ion and the dihydrolipoic acid cofactor, which is necessary for oxidation of the substrate. Arsenite also inhibits succinic dehydrogenase activity and uncouples oxidative phosphorylation, which results in stimulation of mitochondrial ATPase activity. Arsenic inhibits energy-linked functions of mitochondria in two ways: competition with phosphate during oxidative phosphorylation and inhibition of energy-linked reduction of NAD. Inhibition of mitochondrial respiration results in decreased cellular production of ATP and increased production of hydrogen peroxide, which might cause oxidative stress, and production of reactive oxygen species (ROS). Intracellular production of ROS results in observed induction of major stress protein families (NRC, 1999).

Arsenic compounds induce metallothionein in vivo. Potency is dependent on the chemical form of arsenic. As(III) is most potent, followed by As(V), monomethylarsenate, and dimethylarsenate (Kreppel et al., 1993). Metallothionein is thought to have a protective effect against arsenic toxicity and may be responsible at least in part for its self-induced tolerance. Metallothionein-null mice are more sensitive than wild-type mice to the hepatotoxic and nephrotoxic effects of chronic or injected inorganic arsenicals (Liu et al., 1998). The role of asenical-induced oxidative stress and ROS may play a role in mediating DNA damage and initiating the carcinogenic process (NRC, 1999).

Toxicology Ingestion of large doses (70 to 180 mg) of arsenic may be fatal. Symptoms of acute illness, possibly leading to death, consist of fever, anorexia, hepatomegaly, melanosis, and cardiac arrhythmia, with changes in electrocardiograph results that may point to eventual cardiovascular failure. Other features include upper respiratory tract symptoms, peripheral neuropathy, and gastrointestinal, cardiovascular, and hematopoietic effects. Acute ingestion may be suspected from damage to mucous membranes, such as irritation, vesicle formation, and even sloughing. Sensory loss in the peripheral nervous system is the most common neurologic effect, appearing 1 or 2 weeks after large exposures and consisting of wallerian degeneration of axons, a condition that is reversible if exposure is stopped. Anemia and leukopenia, particularly granulocytopenia, occur a few days following exposure and are reversible. The hematologic consequences of chronic exposure to arsenic are similar to effects from acute exposure. There may also be disturbances in heme synthesis, with an increase in urinary porphyrin excretion.

Chronic exposure to inorganic arsenic compounds may lead to neurotoxicity of both the peripheral and central nervous systems. Neurotoxicity usually begins with sensory changes, paresthesia, and muscle tenderness followed by weakness, progressing from proximal to distal muscle groups. Peripheral neuropathy may be progressive, involving both sensory and motor neurons leading to demyelination of long axon nerve fibers, but effects are dose-related. Acute exposure to a single high dose can produce the onset of paresthesia and motor dysfunction within 10 days. More chronic occupational exposures producing more gradual, insidious effects may occur over a period of years, and it has been difficult to establish dose–response relationships (Murphy et al., 1981; Donorio et al., 1987).

Liver injury, characteristic of longer-term or chronic exposure, manifests itself initially in jaundice and may progress to cirrhosis and ascites. Toxic effects on hepatic parenchymal cells result in the elevation of liver enzymes in the blood, and studies in experimental animals show granules and alterations in the ultrastructure of mitochondria as well as nonspecific manifestations of cell injury, including loss of glycogen.

The relationship between the prevalence of ingestion of inorganic arsenic in drinking water and cardiovascular disease has been shown in studies in the United States (Engel and Smith, 1994) and in Taiwan (Chiou et al., 1997). Peripheral vascular disease has been observed in persons with chronic exposure to arsenic in drinking water in Taiwan and Chile; it is manifest by acrocyanosis and Raynaud's phenomenon and may progress to endarteritis obliterans and gangrene of the lower extremities (blackfoot disease). This specific effect seems to be related to the cumulative dose of arsenic, but the prevalence is uncertain because of difficulties in separating arsenic-induced peripheral vascular disease (NRC, 1999). Recent studies in southwestern Taiwan (Lai et al., 1994) and cohorts with occupational exposure in Sweden (Rahman and Axelson, 1995) were associated with chronic arsenic ingestion in drinking water and an increase risk of diabetes mellitus. Immunomodulating and immunotoxic effects of arsenic have been suggested from studies in experimental animals, while human studies have shown some effect on lymphocyte replicating ability (Gonsebatt et al., 1994).

Reproductive Effects and Teratogenicity High doses of inorganic arsenic compounds given to pregnant experimental animals produced various malformations, somewhat dependent on time and route of administration, in fetuses and offspring. However, no such effects have been noted in humans with excessive occupational exposures to arsenic compounds. Arsenic readily crosses the placenta in women without known exposure to arsenic. In a fetus and suckling infant in an Andean village where the arsenic content of drinking water was about 200 μg/L, the concentration of arsenic in cord blood was almost as high as that in maternal blood (Concha et al., 1998b). However, more than 90 percent of the arsenic in plasma and urine was in the form of DMA, a percentage that is higher than the percentage in nonpregnant women, suggesting that there is increased methylation during pregnancy. Animal data indicate that less developmental toxicity is caused by the methylated metabolites than by arsenite (NRC, 1999).

Carcinogenicity The potential carcinogenicity of arsenic compounds was recognized over 100 years ago by Hutchinson (1887), who observed an unusual number of skin cancers occurring in patients treated with arsenicals. The IARC (1987) and EPA (1988) classify arsenic as a carcinogen, for which there is sufficient evidence from epidemiologic studies to support a causal association between exposure and skin cancer and lung cancer via inhalation. There is now evidence that arsenic causes cancer of internal organs from oral ingestion (Bates et al., 1992). In humans, chronic exposure to arsenic induces a series of characteristic changes in skin epithelium, proceeding from hyperpigmentation to hyperkeratosis. Diffuse or spotted hyperpigmentation, the initial nonmalignant cutaneous effect, can first appear within 6 months to 3 years of chronic ingestion at concentrations in excess of approximately 0.4 mg/kg/day. Lower exposure rates, on the order of 0.01 mg/kg/day or longer, can result in pigmentation after intervals as long as 5 to 15 years. Palmar-plantar hyperkeratosis usually follows the initial appearance of arsenical hyperpigmentation within a period of years. There may actually be two cell types of arsenic-induced skin cancer—basal cell carcinomas and squamous cell carcinomas—arising in keratotic areas. The basal cell cancers are usually only locally invasive, but squamous cell carcinomas may have distant metastases. The skin cancers related to arsenic differ from ultraviolet light–induced tumors in that they generally occur on areas of the body not exposed to sunlight (e.g., on palms and soles), and they occur as multiple lesions.

The NRC report (1999), utilizing various statistical approaches, cites lifetime cancer risks for bladder cancer from exposure at different levels of arsenic in drinking water. The current EPA maximum contaminant level for arsenic in drinking water is under revision.

Occupational exposure to airborne arsenic may also be associated with lung cancer, usually a poorly differentiated form of epidermoid bronchogenic carcinoma. The time period between initiation of exposure and occurrence of arsenic-associated lung cancer has been found to be on the order of 35 to 45 years. Enterline and Marsh (1980) report a latency period of 20 years in their study of copper smelter workers.

In contrast to most other human carcinogens, it has been difficult to confirm the carcinogenicity of arsenic in experimental animals. Intratracheal installations of arsenic trioxide produced an increased incidence of pulmonary adenomas, papillomas, and adenomatoid lesions, suggesting that arsenic trioxide can induce lung carcinomas (Pershagan et al., 1984), but other studies testing As(III) and As(V) compounds by oral administration or skin application have not shown potential for either promotion or initiation of carcinogenicity. Similarly, experimental studies for carcinogenicity of organic arsenic compounds have been negative.

The mode of action of arsenic carcinogenicity has not been established. Inorganic arsenic and its metabolites have been shown to induce deletion mutations and chromosomal aberrations but not point mutations. Arsenic has also been shown to be comutagenic. Other modes of action that have been suggested include effects on DNA methylation, oxidative stress, and cell proliferation, but that data are not sufficient to draw firm conclusions (NRC, 1999).

Arsine

Arsine gas (AsH_3) is formed by the reaction of hydrogen with arsenic and is generated as a by-product in the refining of nonferrous metals. Arsine is a potent hemolytic agent, producing acute symptoms of nausea, vomiting, shortness of breath, and headache accompanying the hemolytic reaction. Exposure may be fatal and may be accompanied by hemoglobinuria and renal failure and even jaundice and anemia in nonfatal cases when exposure persists (Fowler et al., 1989).

Biomarkers Biomarkers of arsenic exposure are arsenic concentrations in urine, blood, and hair (Table 23-2). Urinary arsenic is the best indicator of exposure because it is the main route of ex-

Table 23-2
Biomarkers of Arsenic Exposure

	NORMAL	EXCESSIVE EXPOSURE
Urine μg/L	5–50	>100 (without seafood)
Blood μg/L	1–4	50
Hair μg/kg	<1	

cretion for most arsenic compounds. The half-time of inorganic arsenic in humans is about 4 days. Urine arsenic level in persons in the general population without seafood intake is usually in the range of 10 μg/L (5 to 50 μg/L). Some marine organisms may contain very high concentrations of organoarsenicals, which do not have significant toxicity and are rapidly excreted in urine without transformation. One serving of seafood might give rise to urinary arsenic concentrations of 1000 μg/L (Norin and Vahter, 1981). Individuals should be advised not to ingest seafood for a day or two before measurement of urinary arsenic. Most of the absorbed inorganic or organic arsenic has a short half-time in blood, so that arsenic concentrations in blood are increased only a short time following absorption. Like lead, arsenic is measured in whole blood, not serum, because most of the arsenic is in red blood cells. Levels are usually very low and expressed per liter of whole blood. High levels of arsenic in drinking water (wells) will increase urine and blood arsenic. In studies carried out in California and Nevada, a water concentration of 400 μg/L corresponded to about 75 μg/L in the urine and about 14 μg/L in the blood (Valentine et al., 1979). Compared with urine, blood is a much less sensitive indicator of arsenic exposure. Hair or even fingernail concentrations of arsenic may be helpful in evaluating past exposures, but interpretation is made difficult because of the problem of differentiating external contamination.

There are no specific biomarkers of arsenic toxicity, and evaluation of clinical effects must be interpreted with knowledge of exposure history.

Treatment For acute toxicity, treatment is symptomatic, with particular attention to fluid volume replacement and support of blood pressure with pressor agents. For acute symptoms, dimercaprol may be given (3 mg/kg intramuscularly every 4 hours) until symptoms subside, followed by oral penicillamine. Succimer (2,3-dimercaptosuccinic acid) is also thought to be effective. For chronic exposures, dimercaprol and/or penicillamine may also be used (Klaassen, 1990).

Beryllium (Be)

Beryllium[1] is an uncommon metal with a few specific industrial uses. Environmental sources and toxicologic effects of beryllium are reviewed in detail in health criteria documents (EPA, 1987; WHO, 1990). Release of beryllium to the environment largely results from coal combustion. The combustion of coal and oil contributes about 1250 or more tons of beryllium to the environment each year (mostly from coal), which is about five times the annual production from industrial use. The major industrial processes that release beryllium into the environment are beryllium extraction plants, ceramic plants, and beryllium alloy manufacturers. These industries also provide the greatest potential for occupational exposure. Currently, the major use for beryllium is as an alloy, but about 20 percent of world production is for applications utilizing the free metal in nuclear reactions, x-ray windows, and other special applications related to space optics, missile fuel, and space vehicles. It is also present in cigarette smoke (Smith et al., 1997). The mean urinary levels of beryllium in the general population are reported as 0.26 μg/L (Apostoli et al., 1989).

[1]Atomic weight, 9.01; periodic table group, IIA; valence, +2; discovered in 1828.

Toxicokinetics Knowledge of the toxicokinetics of beryllium has largely been obtained from experimental animals, particularly the rat. Clearance of inhaled beryllium is multiphasic; half is cleared in about 2 weeks, the remainder is removed slowly, and a residuum becomes fixed in the tissues probably within fibrotic granulomata. Gastrointestinal absorption of ingested beryllium probably occurs only in the acidic milieu of the stomach, where it is in the ionized form, but beryllium passes through the intestinal tract as precipitated phosphate. Removal of radiolabeled beryllium chloride from rat blood is rapid, whereas beryllium has a half-life of about 3 h. It is distributed to all tissues, but most goes to the skeleton. High doses go predominantly to the liver, but it is gradually transferred to the bone. The half-life in tissues is relatively short except in the lungs, and a variable fraction of an administered dose is excreted in the urine, where it has a long biological half-life.

Skin Effects Contact dermatitis is the commonest beryllium-related toxic effect. Exposure to soluble beryllium compounds may result in papulovesicular lesions on the skin, which is a delayed-type hypersensitivity reaction. The hypersensitivity is cell-mediated, and passive transfer with lymphoid cells has been accomplished in guinea pigs. If contact is made with an insoluble beryllium compound, a chronic granulomatous lesion develops, which may be necrotizing or ulcerative. If insoluble beryllium-containing material becomes embedded under the skin, the lesion will not heal and may progress in severity. Use of a beryllium patch test to identify beryllium-sensitive individuals may in itself be sensitizing, so any use of this procedure as a diagnostic test is discouraged.

Pulmonary Effects ***Acute Chemical Pneumonitis*** Acute pulmonary disease from inhalation of beryllium is a fulminating inflammatory reaction of the entire respiratory tract, involving the nasal passages, pharynx, tracheobronchial airways, and the alveoli; in the most severe cases, it produces an acute fulminating pneumonitis. This occurs almost immediately following inhalation of aerosols of soluble beryllium compounds, particularly fluoride, an intermediate in the ore extraction process. Severity is dose-related. Fatalities have occurred, although recovery is generally complete after a period of several weeks or even months.

Chronic Granulomatous Disease, Berylliosis Chronic beryllium disease (CBD) was first described among fluorescent lamp workers exposed to insoluble beryllium compounds, particularly beryllium oxide. CBD is an antigen-stimulated, cell-mediated immune response that leads to granulomatous lung disease (Tinkle and Newman, 1997). The major symptom is shortness of breath, which in severe cases may be accompanied by cyanosis and clubbing of fingers (hypertrophic osteoarthropathy, a characteristic manifestation of chronic pulmonary disease). Chest x-rays show miliary mottling. Histologically, the alveoli contain small interstitial granulomas resembling those seen in sarcoidosis. In the early stages, the lesions are composed of fluid, lymphocytes, and plasma cells.

Multinucleated giant cells are common. Later, the granulomas become organized with proliferation of fibrotic tissue, eventually forming small fibrous nodules. As the lesions progress, interstitial fibrosis increases, with loss of functioning alveoli, impairment of effective air–capillary gas exchange, and increasing respiratory dysfunction. CD4+ cells are believed to be involved in the pathogenesis of CBD (Fontenot et al., 1999). The alpha subunit of the soluble IL-2 receptor is elevated in serum and bronchiolar lavage cells of individuals with CBD and correlates with the degree of clinical severity. This soluble receptor may be a useful biomarker for progression of the disease (Tinkle et al., 1997).

Carcinogenicity Evidence for the carcinogenicity of beryllium was first observed in experimental studies beginning in 1946, before the establishment of carcinogenicity in humans. Epidemiologic confirmation in humans has been evolving. Studies of humans with occupational exposure to beryllium prior to 1970 were negative. However, reports of two worker populations and a registry of berylliosis cases studied earlier show a small excess of lung cancer, although the total number of cases is small. These findings of excess cancer risk in humans are supported by a clear demonstration of carcinogenicity in animals (Hayes, 1997). The IARC (1994) states there is sufficient evidence in humans and animals for the carcinogenicity of beryllium and its compounds. In vitro studies of genotoxicity have shown that beryllium will induce morphologic transformation in mammalian cells (Dipaolo and Casto, 1979). Beryllium will also decrease the fidelity of DNA synthesis but is negative when tested as a mutagen in bacterial systems.

Cadmium (Cd)

Cadmium[1] is a modern toxic metal. It was discovered as an element only in 1817, and industrial use was minor until about 50 years ago. But now it is a very important metal with many applications. Because of its noncorrosive properties, its main use is in electroplating or galvanizing. It is also used as a color pigment for paints and plastics and as a cathode material for nickel-cadmium batteries. Cadmium is a by-product of zinc and lead mining and smelting, which are important sources of environmental pollution. The toxicology of cadmium is extensively reviewed by Friberg et al. (1986), WHO (1992), EPA (1997), and ATSDR (1998).

Exposure For persons in the general population, the major source of cadmium is food. Plants readily take up cadmium from soil contaminated by fallout from the air, cadmium-containing water used for irrigation and cadmium-containing fertilizers. Another source of concern about potential sources of cadmium toxicity is the use of commercial sludge to fertilize agricultural fields. Commercial sludge may contain up to 1500 mg of cadmium per kilogram of dry material. Studies from Sweden have shown a slow but steady increase in the cadmium content of vegetables over the years. Shellfish, such as mussels, scallops, and oysters, may be a major source of dietary cadmium and contain 100 to 1000 μg/kg. Shellfish accumulate cadmium from the water in the form of cadmium-binding peptides. Meat, fish, and fruit contain 1 to 50 μg/kg, grains contain 10 to 150 μg/kg, and the greatest concentrations are in the liver and kidney of animals. Total daily intake of cadmium from food, water, and air in North America and Europe varies considerably but is estimated to be about 10 to 40 μg/day.

[1]Atomic weight, 112.41; periodic table group, IIB; valence, +2; discovered in 1817.

Workplace exposure to cadmium is particularly hazardous in the presence of cadmium fumes or airborne cadmium. Airborne cadmium in the present-day workplace environment is generally 0.05 or $\mu g/m^3$ or less. Occupations at risk include electrolytic refining of lead and zinc and other industries that employ thermal processes—e.g., iron production, fossil fuel combustion, and cement manufacture—all of which release airborne cadmium, the metal being a constituent of the natural raw material. Other occupations include the manufacture of paint pigments, cadmium-nickel batteries, and electroplanting (WHO, 1992). A major nonoccupational source of respirable cadmium is cigarettes.

Toxicokinetics Gastrointestinal absorption of cadmium is about 5 to 8 percent. Absorption is enhanced by dietary deficiencies of calcium and iron and by diets low in protein. Low dietary calcium stimulates synthesis of calcium-binding protein, which enhances cadmium absorption. In general, women have higher blood cadmium concentrations than men. This is most likely due to increased gastrointestinal absorption because of low iron stores in women of childbearing age. Women with low serum ferritin levels have been shown to have twice the normal absorption of cadmium (Flanagan et al., 1978; Berglund et al., 1994). Respiratory absorption of cadmium is greater than gastrointestinal absorption and independent on solubility of cadmium compound, but it ranges from about 15 to 30 percent. As much as 50 percent of cadmium fumes, as in cigarette smoke, may be absorbed. One cigarette contains 1 to 2 μg of cadmium, and 10 percent of the cadmium in a cigarette is inhaled (0.1 to 0.2 μg). Smoking one or more packs of cigarettes a day may double the daily absorbed burden of cadmium.

Absorbed cadmium is excreted in urine. While gastrointestinal excretion is possible, particularly in bile as a glutathione complex, there are no available data to indicate net gastrointestinal excretion in humans. Cadmium excretion in urine increases proportionally with body burden (Friberg et al., 1986; ATSDR, 1998).

Cadmium is transported in blood by binding to red blood cells and high-molecular-weight proteins in plasma, particularly albumin; it is distributed primarily to liver and kidney (Fig. 23-3).

In the liver, cadmium induces the synthesis of metallothionein and is then either stored in the liver as Cd-MT complex or transported via blood to the kidney, where it may accumulate in lysosomes. cd-MT complex in lysosomes is slowly catabolized to non-metallothionein-bound cadmium but may again be complexed with metallothionein or may induce renal toxicity (see "Nephrotoxicity," below).

Blood cadmium levels in adults without excessive exposure is usually less than 1 μg/dL. Newborns have a low body content of cadmium, usually less than 1 mg total body burden. The placenta synthesizes metallothionein and may serve as a barrier to maternal cadmium, but the fetus may be exposed with increased maternal exposure. Human breast milk and cow's milk are low in cadmium, with less than 1 μg/kg of milk. About 50 to 75 percent of the body burden of cadmium is in the liver and kidneys; its half-life in the body is not known exactly, but it may be as long as 30 years. With continued retention, there is progressive accumulation in the soft tissues, particularly in the kidneys, through ages 50 to 60, when the cadmium burden in soft tissues begins to decline slowly (Fig. 23-4).

Because of the potential for renal toxicity, there is considerable concern about the levels of dietary cadmium intake for the general population (Nordberg, 1984).

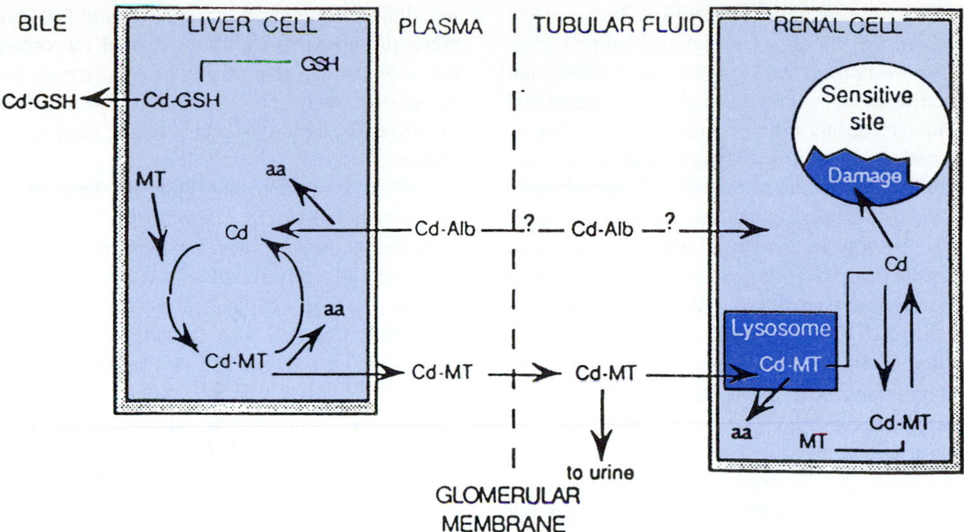

Figure 23-3. A schematic representation of the role of metallothionein in the disposition of cadmium in the liver and kidney. [Adapted from Jarup et al. (1998).]

Acute Toxicity Acute toxicity may result from the ingestion of relatively high concentrations of cadmium, as may occur from contaminated beverages or food. Nordberg (1972) relates an instance in which nausea, vomiting, and abdominal pain occurred from consumption of drinks containing approximately 16 mg/L cadmium. Recovery was rapid, without apparent long-term effects. Inhalation of cadmium fumes or other heated cadmium-containing materials may produce an acute chemical pneumonitis and pulmonary edema. Inhalation of large doses of cadmium compounds may be lethal for humans and experimental animals (ATSDR, 1998). Experimental studies have shown that the chemical form of cadmium can affect its toxicity, probably related to solubility. In acute exposures, the relatively more soluble cadmium chloride, cadmium oxide fume, and cadmium carbonate are more toxic that than the relatively less soluble cadmium sulfide (Klimisch, 1993).

Chronic Toxicity The principal long-term effects of low-level exposure to cadmium are chronic obstructive pulmonary disease and emphysema and chronic renal tubular disease. There may also be effects on the cardiovascular and skeletal systems.

Chronic Pulmonary Disease Toxicity to the respiratory system is proportional to the time and level of exposure. Obstructive lung

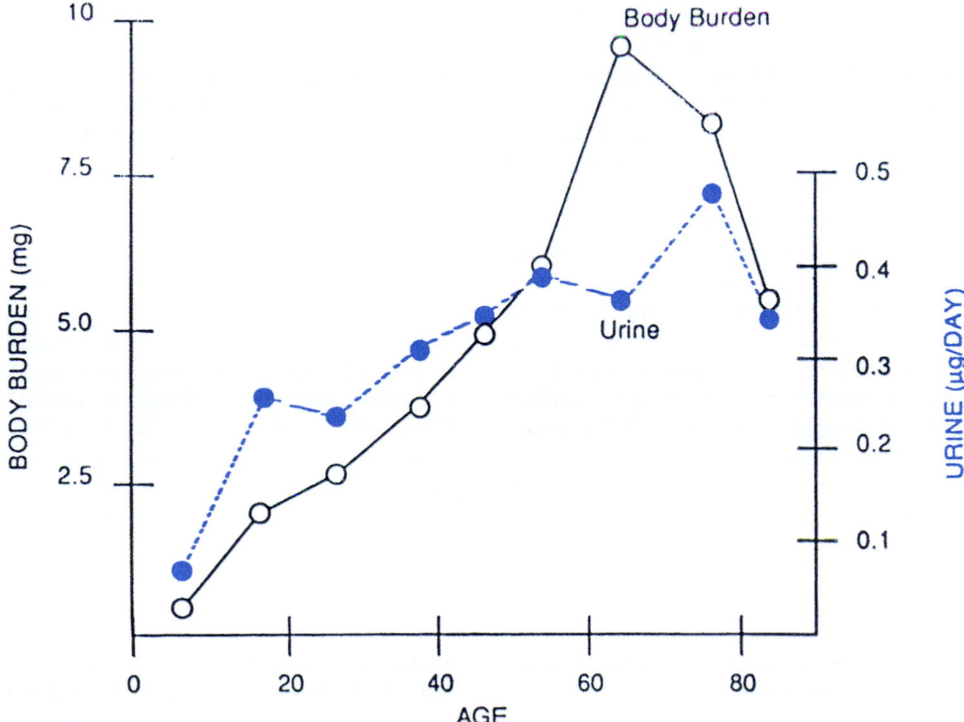

Figure 23-4. Illustration of the accumulation of cadmium with age.

disease results from chronic bronchitis, progressive fibrosis of the lower airways, and accompanying alveolar damage leading to emphysema. The lung disease is manifest by dyspnea, reduced vital capacity, and increased residual volume. The pathogenesis of the lung lesion is the turnover and necrosis of alveolar macrophages. Released enzymes produce irreversible damage to alveolar basement membranes, including the rupture of septa and interstitial fibrosis (Davison, 1988). It has been found that cadmium reduces a_1-antitrypsin activity, perhaps enhancing pulmonary toxicity. However, no difference in plasma a_1-antitrypsin activity could be found between cadmium-exposed workers with and without emphysema (Lauwerys et al., 1979).

Nephrotoxicity Cadmium is toxic to renal tubular cells and glomeruli as reflected by impairment of renal tubular and glomerular function. Morphologic changes are nonspecific and consist of tubular cell degeneration in the initial stages, progressing to an interstitial inflammatory reaction and fibrosis. Analysis of kidney cadmium levels by in vivo neutron activation analysis and x-ray fluorescence has made it possible to study the relationship between renal cadmium levels and the occurrence of effects (Skerfving et al., 1987). The critical concentration of cadmium in the renal cortex that produces tubular dysfunction in 10 percent of the population is about 200 μg/g and about 300 μg/g in 50 percent of the population. There is a pattern in which liver and kidney cadmium levels increase simultaneously until the average cadmium concentration in the renal cortex is about 300 μg/g and the average level in the liver is about 60 μg/g. At higher cadmium liver levels, the level in the renal cortex is disproportionately low, as cadmium is lost from the kidney (Ellis et al., 1984). Daily intake in food of 140 to 260 μg of cadmium per day for more than 50 years or exposure in workroom air of 50 $\mu g/m^3$ for more than 10 years has produced renal dysfunction (Thun et al., 1989; WHO, 1992). An epidemiologic study of the dose–response relationship of cadmium intake from historical data, rice consumption, and β_2-microglobulin as an index of renal tubular dysfunction, found that the total cadmium intake over a lifetime that produced an adverse health effect was 2000 mg for both men and women (Nogawa et al., 1989).

Renal tubular dysfunction is reflected by proteinuria. The proteinuria is principally tubular, consisting of low-molecular-weight proteins whose tubular reabsorption has been impaired by cadmium injury to proximal tubular lining cells. The predominant protein is a β_2-microglobulin (β_2-m), but a number of other low-molecular-weight proteins have been identified in the urine of workers with excessive cadmium exposure, such as retinol-binding protein (RBP), lysozyme, *N*-acetyl-β-D-glucosaminidase (NAG), ribonuclease, α_1-microglobulin, and immunoglobulin light chains (Lauwerys et al., 1980; Buchet et al., 1990). The presence of high-molecular-weight proteins in the urine, such as albumin and transferrin, indicates that some workers may actually have a mixed proteinuria and suggests a glomerular effect as well. The pathogenesis of the glomerular lesion in cadmium nephropathy is not presently understood.

Role of Metallothionein The accumulation of cadmium in the kidneys to some extent without apparent toxic effect is possible because of the formation of cadmium-thionein or metallothionein, a metal–protein complex with a low molecular weight (see "Metal-Binding Proteins," above). Metallothionein is primarily a tissue protein and is ubiquitous in most organs, but it exists in the highest concentration in the liver, particularly following recent exposure to cadmium, and in the kidneys, where it accumulates with age in proportion to cadmium concentration. Cadmium bound to metallothionein within tissues is thought to be nontoxic. However, when the levels of cadmium exceed the critical concentration, it becomes toxic. The protective role of metallothionein is supported by an experiment showing that metallothionein-null mice are more sensitive to cadmium nephrotoxicity than control mice (Liu et al., 1998).

The factors that determine the level of cadmium or of cadmium-metallothionein complex that is toxic are not clear, but experimental studies have shown that repeated injections of low levels of cadmium-metallothionein over several weeks result in a chronic and irreversible nephrotoxicity with renal accumulations of cadmium of only 40 μg/g, less than the 200 μg/g in the renal cortex, which is suggested as the critical level in humans (Wang et al., 1993). Also, renal tubular necrosis occurs in non-cadmium-exposed rats following transplantation of livers from cadmium-toxic animals (Chan et al., 1993). These studies suggest that cadmium nephrotoxicity follows the slow release and renal excretion of cadmium-metallothionein from liver and other soft tissues. Cadmium-metallothionein is toxic when taken up by the proximal tubular cell complex, whereas cadmium chloride at even greater concentrations in proximal tubular cells is not toxic (Dorian et al., 1995).

Skeletal Effects Cadmium toxicity affects calcium metabolism, and individuals with severe cadmium nephropathy may have renal calculi and excess excretion of calcium, probably related to increased urinary loss. With chronic exposure, however, urinary calcium may be less than normal. Associated skeletal changes are probably related to calcium loss and include bone pain, osteomalacia, and/or osteoporosis. Bone changes are part of Itai-Itai disease, a syndrome recognized in postmenopausal multiparous women living in the Fuchu area of Japan prior to and during World War II. The syndrome consists of severe bone deformities and chronic renal disease. Excess cadmium exposure has been implicated in the pathogenesis of the syndrome, but vitamin D and perhaps other nutritional deficiencies are thought to be cofactors. Itai-Itai translates to "ouch-ouch," reflecting the accompanying bone pain. Also, cadmium can affect calcium, phosphorus, and bone metabolism in both industrial workers and people exposed in the general environment. These effects may be secondary to the cadmium effects on the kidneys and/or the direct toxic effect of cadmium on bone metabolism, but there has been little study of calcium metabolism in people with excess exposure to cadmium (Friberg, 1986).

Whether the skeletal effects from cadmium exposure are a product of cadmium toxicity per se or the result of cadmium toxicity plus renal disease and nutritional deficiencies, particularly calcium deficiency, has been debated (Nogawa et al., 1999). Cadmium in bone may interfere with calcification, decalcification, and bone remodeling. Anderson and Danylchuk (1979) found that exposure of beagle dogs for 6 months to cadmium (25 mg/wL) reduced bone turnover rate, consistent with calcium deficiency or osteomalacia. Wang and Battachharyya (1993) showed that cadmium increased release of ^{45}Ca from skeletons of mice and dogs as early as 72 h after the start of dietary cadmium.

A proposed mechanism for the decreased calcium absorption and negative calcium balance in cadmium-exposed rats is that cadmium inhibits activation of vitamin D in the renal cortex (Feldman and Cousins, 1974). Nogawa and colleagues (1987) reported that serum $1,25(OH)_2$ vitamin D levels were lower in Itai-Itai disease patients and in cadmium-exposed subjects with renal damage than in nonexposed subjects. A decrease in serum $1,25(OH)_2$ vitamin D levels was closely related to serum concentrations of parathyroid hormone, β_2-microglobulin, and the percentage of tubular reabsorption, suggesting that cadmium-induced bone effects were mainly due to a disturbance in vitamin D and parathyroid hormone metabolism. Friberg et al. (1986) suggest that cadmium in the proximal tubular cells depresses cellular functions, which may be followed by the depressed conversion of 25(OH) vitamin D to $1,25(OH)_2$ vitamin D. This is likely to lead to decreased calcium absorption and mineralization of bone, which in turn may lead to osteomalacia. Bhattacharyya and coworkers (1988) found, in studies of mice, that multiparity enhanced cadmium's toxicity to bone. Hypercalciuria is a sensitive indicator for cadmium exposure (Buchet, 1990).

Hypertension and Cardiovascular Effects Epidemiologic studies suggest that cadmium is an etiologic agent for essential hypertension. A study of blood pressures in cadmium workers found an increase in systolic but not diastolic blood pressure (Thun et al., 1989). Studies from Japan have found that the rate of cerebrovascular disease mortality among people who had cadmium-induced renal tubular proteinuria was twice as high as among people in cadmium-polluted areas without proteinuria (Nogawa et al., 1979). Although the population-based U.S. NHANES II study and studies in Belgium (Staessen et al., 1995) have not supported a role for cadmium in the etiology of hypertension and cardiovascular disease in humans, animal studies indicate that cadmium may be toxic to myocardial function. Rats exposed to cadmium in drinking water (Kopp et al., 1983) developed electrocardiographic and biochemical changes in the myocardium and impairment of the functional status of the myocardium. These effects may be related to (1) decreased high-energy phosphate stored in the myocardium, (2) reduced myocardial contractility, and (3) diminished excitability of the cardiac conduction system. Jamall and Sprowls (1987) found that rats whose diets were supplemented with copper, selenium, and cadmium had a marked reduction in heart cytosolic glutathione peroxidase, superoxide dismutase, and catalase. They suggest that heart mitochondria may be the site of the cadmium-induced biochemical lesion in the myocardium.

Neurologic Disorders Epidemiologic studies in humans have suggested a relationship between abnormal behavior and/or decreased intelligence in children and adults exposed to cadmium. However such studies are typically complicated by exposure to other toxic metals. Furthermore, the blood-brain barrier and circumventricular epithelial cells with tight junctions limit the pathways of entrance for cadmium into the central nervous system. In addition, the choroid plexus epithelium accumulates high levels of toxic metals from the blood or cerebrospinal fluid (Murphy, 1997). Metallothionein in glial cells and ependymal cells near circumventricular organs also serves to minimize cadmium diffusion into other parts of the brain.

Carcinogenicity Epidemiologic studies have shown a relationship between occupational (respiratory) exposure to cadmium and lung cancer and possibly prostate cancer. An increase in respiratory cancers was also found in a restudy of a cohort in a U.S. cadmium recovery plant (Thun et al., 1985). Concern has been expressed regarding the influence of confounding factors in the work environment, particularly coexposure to arsenic (Sorahan and Lancashire, 1997). Cadmium has recently been accepted by the International Agency for Research on Cancer as a category 1 (human) carcinogen, based primarily on its relationship to pulmonary tumors (IARC, 1994). There are few studies that examine a relationship between oral intake of cadmium and cancer in humans. A study of cancer incidence among inhabitants with renal tubular dysfunction in a cadmium-polluted area of Japan was negative. The potential relationship between cadmium exposure and prostate cancer in humans remains controversial (Waalkes, 1995).

Cadmium chloride exposure by inhalation produced a dose-dependent increase in the incidence of lung carcinomas in rats (Takenaka et al., 1983; Oldiges, 1989). In rats, cadmium will produce a variety of tumors, including malignant tumors at the site of injection and in the lungs after inhalation. Cadmium chloride, oxide, sulfate, and sulfide produced local sarcomas in rats after their subcutaneous injection, and cadmium powder and cadmium sulfide produced local sarcomas in rats following their intramuscular administration. Other studies have found that oral cadmium exposure was associated with tumor of the prostate, testes, and hematopoietic system in rats. The incidence of lesions was less in zinc-deficient rats, but there was no dose–response relationship (Waalkes, 1995). Other studies have produced cancer in the ventral lobe of the rat prostate by oral or parenteral exposures as well as by direct injection. The lobular structure of the prostate is absent in humans; it is thought that the ventral prostate in rats has no human analog and that tumors of the dorsolateral lobe are more comparable to the human disease (Waalkes and Rehm, 1994). However, subcutaneous injection of cadmium in a particularly cancer-sensitive strain of rat (Noble/Cr) did produce proliferative lesions of the dorsolateral prostate as well as tumors of the testes, pituitary adenomas, and injection-site sarcomas (Waalkes et al., 1999).

Biomarkers of Cadmium Effects Urinary Beta$_2$-microglobulin (β_2m), retinal-binding protein (RBP), *N*-acetyl-β-glucosaminidase (NAG), and metallothionein have been used in conjunction with urinary cadmium levels as a measure of cadmium exposure to cadmium renal tubular dysfunction. Other sensitive indicators include α_1-m, trehalase, and calcium (ATSDR, 1998). The relationship of these indicators to urine cadmium levels were determined in a large population study in Belgium (Buchet, 1990). It was estimated that more than 10 percent of values would be abnormal when urine cadmium excretion rate exceeded 2.87 μg/24 h for RBP, 3.05 μg/24 h for β_2-m, 4.29 μg/24 h for amino acids, and 1.92 μg/24 h for calcium.

Increased excretion of β_2-m is an early indicator of tubular proteinuria, but samples must be controlled for pH. RBP measurements may be a more practical and reliable test of proximal tubular function than β_2-m because sensitive immunologic analytic methods are now available, and β_2-m is less stable in urine (Lauwerys et al., 1984). Activity of the enzyme NAG in urine may be a sensitive indicator of cadmium-induced renal tubular dysfunction, but a dose–response relationship has not been established (Kawada et al., 1998). None of the biomarkers of tubular dysfunction are specific indicators of cadmium effects and their levels must be interpreted in association with a corresponding increase in urinary cadmium. Minor increases in excretion of biomarkers of renal tubular dysfunction may not in themselves indicate an adverse health effect but are indicators of likely possible progression of renal disease if cadmium exposure is continued.

Increase in urinary calcium excretion is a sensitive effect of cadmium-induced renal tubular dysfunction and may contribute to the age-related decline in bone mass (Aoshima et al., 1997). Roels et al. (1993) identified three main groups of thresholds for increased excretion of biomarkers of cadmium effect on the kidney. When calcium levels are at around 2 μg/g creatinine, there was increased excretion 6-keto prostaglandin and sialic acid; at around 4 μg/g creatinine, there were increases in NAG, albumin, and transferrin; and at around 10 μg/g creatinine, there were increases in excretion of β_2-m, RBP, and antiglomerular basement membrane antibodies.

Biomarkers of Cadmium Exposure The most important measure of excessive cadmium exposure is increased cadmium excretion in urine. In persons in the general population without excessive cadmium exposure, urinary cadmium excretion is both small and constant. Ninety-five percent of U.S. residents excrete less than 2 μg/L in urine and less than 1 percent excrete 4 μg/L (Gunter, 1997). With excessive exposure to cadmium, as might occur in workers, an increase in urinary cadmium may not occur until all of the available cadmium binding sites are saturated. However, when the available binding sites (e.g., metallothionein) are saturated, increased urinary cadmium reflects recent exposure, body burden, and renal cadmium concentration, so that urinary cadmium measurement does provide a good index of excessive cadmium exposure. Most of the cadmium in urine is bound to metallothionein, and there is good correlation between metallothionein and cadmium in urine in cadmium workers with normal or abnormal renal function (Shaikh et al., 1989). Therefore, the measurement of metallothionein in urine provides the same toxicologic information as the measurement of cadmium, and it does not have the problem of external contamination. Radioimmunoassay techniques for measurement of metallothionein are available (Chang et al., 1980) but are not as practical as other biomarkers of cadmium effect.

There is debate as to whether the threshold for preventing cadmium nephropathy is 5 μg/g or 10 μg/g creatinine. Changes in urinary excretion of low-molecular-weight proteins were consistently observed in workers excreting more than 10 μg cadmium per gram of creatinine (Buchet et al., 1980). The American Conference of Governmental Industrial Hygienists biological exposure indexes for cadmium are 5 μg/g creatinine in the urine and 5 μg/L cadmium in the blood (ACGIH, 1996). Roels et al. (1999), recommends that, on the basis of increased excretion of a number of biomarkers (cited above) at urinary cadmium levels ranging from 2.4 to 11.5 μg/g creatinine, occupational exposure to cadmium should not exceed 5 μg of cadmium per gram of creatinine.

Blood cadmium levels generally reflect recent exposure rather than accumulated body burden and are usually in the range of 0.4 to 1.0 μg/L for nonsmokers and somewhat higher for smokers (Lauwerys et al., 1994). Workers with cumulative cadmium exposure equivalent to a blood cadmium concentration of 10 μg/L for 20 years have been shown to have a 14 percent incidence of renal dysfunction (Jarup et al., 1988).

Reversibility of Renal Effects Follow-up studies of persons with renal tubular dysfunction (β_2-microglobulinuria) from occupational exposure to cadmium have shown that the proteinuria is irreversible and that there is a significant increase of creatinine in serum with time, suggesting a progressive glomerulopathy (Roels et al., 1989). Also, persons with renal tubular dysfunction from excess dietary ingestion of cadmium (cadmium-polluted rice) do not have a reversal of the defect as long as 10 years after reduced exposure in cases when the β_2-m exceeds 1000 μg/g of creatinine (Kido et al., 1988). Ellis (1985) has shown, however, that liver cadmium in workers no longer exposed to cadmium gradually declines. Persistence of renal tubular dysfunction after cessation of exposure may reflect the level of body burden and the shifting of cadmium from liver to kidney.

Treatment At the present time, there is no chelation therapy for cadmium toxicity approved for clinical use in humans. Experimentally, DMSA and CaEDTA best reduce acute mortality from cadmium exposure in combination with glutathione. Some DMSA analogs acutely increase biliary excretion of cadmium. However, each of these therapies may result in significant adverse effects (Angle, 1995).

Chromium (Cr)

Chromium[1] is a generally abundant element in the earth's crust and occurs in oxidation states ranging from Cr^{2+} to Cr^{6+}, but only trivalent and hexavalent forms are of biological significance. The trivalent is the more common form. However, hexavalent forms such as chromate compounds are of greater industrial importance. Sodium chromate and dichromate are the principal substances for the production of all chromium chemicals. The major source of chromium is from chromite ore. Metallurgic-grade chromite is usually converted into one of several types of ferrochromium or other chromium alloys containing cobalt or nickel. Ferrochrome is used for the production of stainless steel. Chromates are produced by a smelting, roasting, and extraction process. The major uses of sodium dichromate are for the production of chrome pigments; for the production of chrome salts used for tanning leather, mordant dying, wood preservatives; and as an anticorrosive in cooking systems, boilers, and oil-drilling muds. Overviews of chromium exposures and health effect have been reviewed (Fishbein, 1981; WHO, 1988; O'Flaherty, 1995).

Chromium in ambient air originates from industrial sources, particularly ferrochrome production, ore refining, chemical and refractory processing, the manufacture of cement, and combustion of fossil fuels. Chromium precipitates and fallout are deposited on land and water; land fallout is eventually carried to water by runoff, where it is deposited in sediments. A controllable source of chromium is wastewater from chrome-plating and metal-finishing industries, textile plants, and tanneries. Cobalt-chromium alloy hip replacements lead to elevated blood levels of chromium (Habbab et al., 2000). The daily intake by humans is under 100 μg, mostly from food, with trivial quantities from most water supplies and ambient air.

Human Body Burden Tissue concentrations of chromium in the general population have considerable geographic variation; concentrations as high as 7 μg/kg occur in the lungs of persons in New York or Chicago, with lower concentrations in liver and kidney. In persons without excess exposure, blood chromium concentration is between 20 and 30 μg/L and is evenly distributed between erythrocytes and plasma. With occupational exposure, an increase in blood chromium is related to increased chromium in red blood cells. Chromates readily cross cell membranes on anion carriers as they are isostructural with sulfate and phosphate anions. Urinary excretion is independent of the oxidation state of chromium administered to animals and is less than 10 μg/day for humans in the absence of excess exposure.

[1]Atomic weight, 52; periodic table group, VIB; valence, +6, +3 +2, rare +1, +4, +5; discovered in 1797; isolated in 1798.

Essentiality See the discussion of trivalent chromium—Cr(III)—under "Essential Metals with Potential for Toxicity," below.

Toxicity Systemic toxicity to chromium compounds occurs largely from accidental exposures, occasional attempts to use chromium as a suicidal agent, and from previous therapeutic uses. The major effect from ingestion of high levels of Cr(VI) is acute tubular and glomerular damage. Evidence of kidney damage from lower-level chronic exposure is equivocal (Wadeen 1991). Animal studies of chronic exposure to Cr(VI) have not shown evidence of toxicity (O'Flaherty, 1995). Cr(VI) is corrosive and causes chronic ulceration and perforation of the nasal septum. It also causes chronic ulceration of other skin surfaces, which is independent of hypersensitivity reactions on skin. Allergic chromium skin reactions readily occur with exposure and are independent of dose (Proctor et al., 1998). Occupational exposure to chromium may be a cause of asthma (Bright et al., 1997). The known harmful effects of chromium in humans have been attributed to the hexavalent form, and it has been speculated that the biological effects of Cr(VI) may be related to the reduction to Cr(III) and the formation of complexes with intracellular macromolecules. Cr(III) compounds are considerably less toxic than the hexavalent compounds and are neither irritating nor corrosive. Nevertheless, nearly all industrial workers are exposed to both forms of chromium compounds, and at present there is no information as to whether there is a gradient of risk from predominant exposure to hexavalent or insoluble forms of chromium to exposure to soluble trivalent forms.

Carcinogenicity Exposure to chromium, particularly in the chrome production and chrome pigment industries, is associated with cancer of the respiratory tract (Langard and Norseth, 1986). The mechanism of Cr(VI) carcinogenicity in the lung is believed to be its reduction to Cr(III) and its generation of reactive intermediates.

Animal studies support the notion that the most potent carcinogenic chromium compounds are the slightly soluble hexavalent compounds. Studies on in vitro bacterial systems, however, show no difference between soluble and slightly soluble compounds. Trivalent chromium salts have little or no mutagenic activity in bacterial systems. Because there is preferred uptake of the hexavalent form by cells and it is the trivalent form that is metabolically active and binds with nucleic acids within the cell, it has been suggested that the causative agent in chromium mutagenesis is trivalent chromium bound to genetic material after reduction of the hexavalent form. The intracellular reduction of Cr(VI) involves the oxidation of both small (acorbate and glutathione) and large (macromolecules—DNA and protein) forms and probably plays a role in the carcinogenic process. In fact chromium elicits a variety of effects: (1) at the biochemical level, the formation of coordination covalent interaction of Cr(V) and Cr(III) with DNA and of DNA-DNA and DNA-protein complexes; (2) at the genomic level, the induction of gene expression (oxidant stress and metallothionein and tumor supressor genes), gene mutations, DNA lesions, and inhibition of protein synthesis and arrest of DNA replication; (3) at the cellular level, cell cycle arrest, apoptosis, and neoplastic transformation (Bridgewater et al., 1998; Singh et al., 1998; Klatreider et al., 1999; Dubrovskaya and Wetterhahn, 1998; Solis-Heredia et al., 2000).

Costa and coworkers (1993) have shown that detection of DNA-protein complexes may serve as a biomarker of exposure and of carcinogenic potential from occupational exposure to chromium. There is suggestive evidence that chromium compounds cause cancer at sites other than the respiratory tract (Costa 1997).

Lead (Pb)

If we were to judge of the interest excited by any medical subject by the number of writings to which it has given birth, we could not but regard the poisoning by lead as the most important to be known of all those that have been treated of, up to the present time (Orfila, 1817).

Lead[1] is a ubiquitous toxic metal and is detectable in practically all phases of the inert environment and in all biological systems. Because it is toxic to most living things at high exposures and there is no demonstrated biological need for it, the major issue regarding lead is determining the dose at which it becomes toxic. Specific concerns vary with the age and circumstances of the host, and the major risk is toxicity to the nervous system. The most susceptible populations are children, particularly toddlers, infants in the neonatal period, and the fetus. Several reviews and multiauthored books on the toxicology of lead are available (Goyer and Rhyne, 1973; EPA, 1986; Goyer, 1993; NRC, 1993; ATSDR, 1999).

Exposure The principal route of exposure for people in the general population is food, and sources that produce excess exposure and toxic effects are usually environmental and presumably controllable. These sources include lead-based indoor paint in old dwellings, lead in dust from environmental sources, lead in contaminated drinking water, lead in air from combustion of lead-containing industrial emissions, hand-to-mouth activities of young children living in polluted environments, lead-glazed pottery, and—less commonly—lead dust brought home by industrial workers on their shoes and clothes. Dietary intake of lead has decreased since the 1940s, when estimates of intake were 400 to 500 μg/day for U.S. populations to present levels of under 20 μg/day. One factor reducing the lead content of food has been a reduction in the use of lead-soldered cans for food and beverages. Most municipal water supplies measured at the tap contain less than 0.05 μg/mL, so that daily intake from water is usually about 10 μg; it is unlikely to be more than 20 μg. Corrosive water (pH 6.4) will leach lead from soldered joints and lead-containing brass fittings (NRC, 1993). The introduction of lead-free gasoline and awareness of the hazards of indoor leaded paint has been credited with a decline in blood lead levels for persons ages 1 to 74 from 12.8 to 2.8 μg/day for 1988 to 1991 (Pirkle et al., 1994). Blood lead levels among people in the general population have continued to decline in the United States to <5 μg/dL (Pirkle, 1998). Nevertheless, the most current national survey (N-HANES IV) shows that nearly a million U.S. children are at risk from lead poisoning (blood lead levels >10 μg/dL) and that specific groups of children are at greatest risk (Fig. 23-5).

The geometric mean blood lead level of African-American children living in central portions of cities with more than 1 million people is 13.9 μg/dL, and about 35 percent of these children have blood lead levels greater than 10 μg/dL—that is, above the guideline recommended by the U.S. Centers for Disease Control (CDC, 1991). Major risk factors for these children are housing containing lead-based paint and exposure to urban dust (CDC, 1997).

[1]Atomic weight, 207.2; periodic table group, IVA; valence, +2 or + 4; discovery uncertain—known since early times.

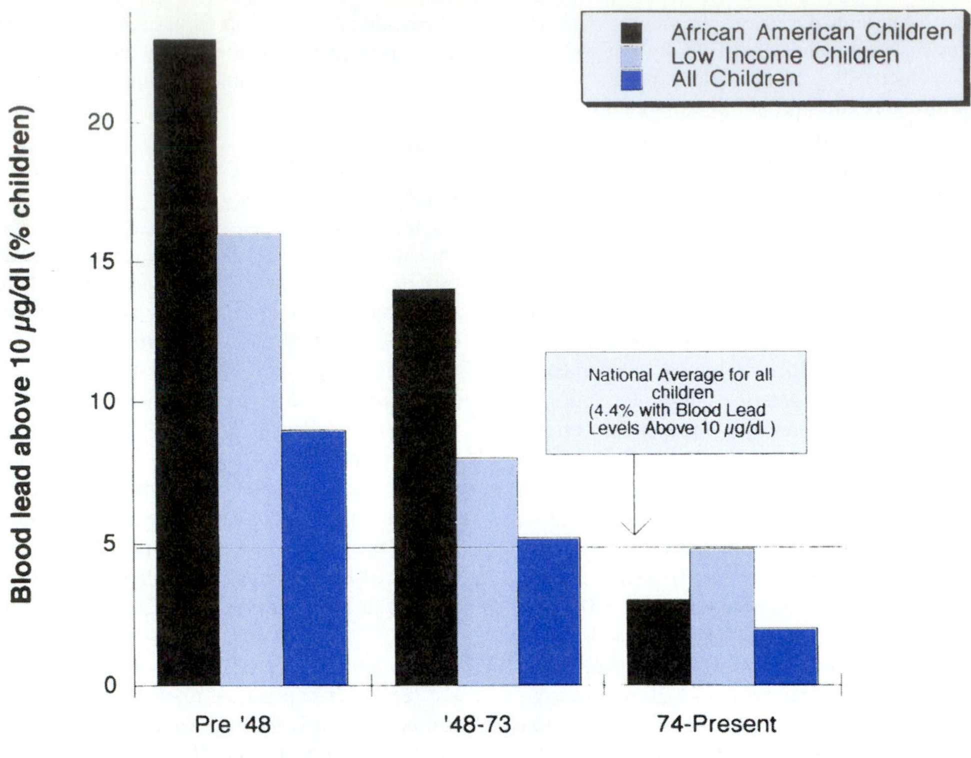

Figure 23-5. National blood lead levels. National Health and Nutrition Examination Survey. Phase 2, 1991–1994. [Adapted from CDC (2000).]

Utilizing radioisotope techniques, Manton et al. (2000) determined that major environmental sources of lead for infants and toddlers up to 4 years of age were hand-to-mouth transfer from floors, the lead being derived from dust sills and exterior surfaces. Seasonal influences, or increases in childhood lead exposure during the hot summer months, were previously thought to be due to effect of sunlight and mobilization of lead from bone. It has now been shown that seasonal variation in blood lead levels in children is related to dust lead levels in the home (Yin et al., 2000).

Other potential sources of exposure to lead are recreational shooting on indoor ranges, hand-loading of ammunition, soldering, jewelry making, pottery making, gunsmithing, glass polishing, painting, and stained glass crafting, all of which involve some exposure to lead. Workplace exposure is gradually being reduced. Overt or clinical lead poisoning among workers in lead industries was common in the 1930s, 1940s, and even in the early 1950s, but it is far less frequently observed today (Wegman and Fine, 1990). Nevertheless, lead continues to be one of the metals presenting a hazardous occupational exposure. Children of workers with occupational exposure to lead may have higher blood lead levels than children in the general population (Whelan et al., 1997). In addition, there are several nutritional and dietary factors that influence lead toxicity (Mahaffey, 1985). In a study of effects of lifestyle factors on blood lead levels, alcohol consumption has been shown to account for the large proportion of variability in blood lead levels, followed by age and smoking (Weyermann and Brenner, 1997). Wine had a greater effect on blood lead levels than beer. Other significant contributing factors were gender, hematocrit, calcium intake, and consumption of milk products.

Toxicokinetics Toxicokinetics of lead are reviewed in reports by the NRC (1993), and ATSDR (1999). Adults absorb 5 to 15 percent of ingested lead and usually retain less than 5 percent of what is absorbed. Children are known to have a greater absorption of lead than adults; one study found an average net absorption of 41.5 percent and 31.8 percent net retention in infants on regular diets. Lead absorption in children is related to age and development of the gastrointestinal tract (Ziegler et al., 1978). Nutritional problems—such as low dietary iron and calcium—enhance lead absorption (Wassermann et al., 1994; Bruening et al., 1999). Lead in water and other beverages is absorbed to a greater degree than lead in food. Lead ingested between meals is absorbed more than lead with meals, and increasing frequency of food intake minimizes lead absorption.

Concentrations of lead in air vary due to point-source emissions but are now usually less than 1.0 $\mu g/m^3$. Since the introduction of lead-free gasoline in the United States, airborne lead is only a minor component of total daily lead exposure. Lead in the atmosphere exists either in solid forms, dust or particulates of lead dioxide, or in the form of vapors. Lead absorption by the lungs also depends on a number of factors in addition to concentration. These include volume of air respired per day, whether the lead is in particle or vapor form, and size distribution of lead-containing particles. Only a very minor fraction of particles over 0.5 μm in mean maximal external diameter are retained in the lung, but they are then cleared from the respiratory track and swallowed. However, the percentage of particles less than 0.5 μm retained in the lung increases with reduction in particle size. About 90 percent of lead particles in ambient air that are deposited in the lungs are small enough to be retained. Absorption of retained lead through alveoli is relatively efficient and complete.

More than 90 percent of the lead in blood is in red blood cells. There seem to be at least two major compartments for lead in the red blood cell, one associated with the membrane and the other with hemoglobin and other blood cell components. Blood lead is in equilibrium between plasma and erythrocytes with 1 percent or less in the plasma, for blood lead levels up to 100 μg/dL. The relationship between blood and plasma lead is stable and nearly linear for blood lead levels up to 50 μg/dL. Above this level the relationship becomes curvilinear, with rapid increase in plasma levels (Manton et al., 1984). Because of analytic difficulties in the accurate measurement of the low levels of lead in plasma and the complicating potential of lead from hemolysis, measurement of plasma lead seems to be of limited usefulness for monitoring persons with occupational exposure.

The total body burden of lead may be divided into at least two kinetic pools, which have different rates of turnover (O'Flaherty, 1998). The largest and kinetically slowest pool is the skeleton, with a half-life of more than 20 years; the soft tissue pool is much more labile. Lead in trabecular bone is more labile than that in cortical bone, and trabecular bone has a shorter turnover time. Lead in bone may contribute as much as 50 percent of blood lead, so that it may be a significant source of internal exposure to lead. Lead in maternal bone is of particular concern during pregnancy and lactation, and it may be mobilized in later years in persons with osteoporosis (Silbergeld et al., 1988). The fraction of lead in bone increases with age from about 70 percent of body lead in childhood to as much as 95 percent of the body burden with advancing years. The total lifetime accumulation of lead may be as much as 200 mg to over 500 mg for a worker with heavy occupational exposure. The largest soft tissue accumulations of lead are in liver and kidney, but lead is present in most tissues of the body. Animal studies have shown that lead in the central nervous system tends to concentrate in gray matter and certain nuclei.

The major route of excretion of absorbed lead is the kidney. Renal excretion of lead is usually with glomerular filtrate with some renal tubular absorption. With elevated blood lead levels, excretion may be augmented by transtubular transport. Lead is also excreted to a lesser degree with other body fluids, including milk during lactation (Gulson et al., 1998). Lead crosses the placenta, so that cord blood lead levels generally correlate with maternal blood lead levels but are slightly lower. Maternal blood lead decreases slightly during pregnancy, probably due to hemodilution. Lead accumulation in fetal tissues, including brain, is proportional to maternal blood lead levels (Goyer, 1996).

Toxicity The toxic effects from exposures to inorganic lead form a continuum from subtle or biochemical effects to clinical or overt effects (Goyer, 1990). These effects involve several organ systems and biochemical activities. The critical effects or most sensitive effects in infants and children involve the nervous system (NRC, 1993; ATSDR, 1999). For adults with excess occupational exposure or even accidental exposure, the concerns are peripheral neuropathy and/or chronic nephropathy. However, the critical effect or most sensitive effect for adults in the general population may be hypertension. Effects on the heme system provide biochemical indicators of lead exposure in the absence of chemically detectable effects, but anemia due to lead exposure is uncommon without other detectable effects or other synergistic factors. Other target organs are the gastrointestinal, reproductive, and skeletal systems.

Neurologic, Neurobehavioral, and Developmental Effects in Children Clinically overt lead encephalopathy may occur in children with high exposure to lead, probably at blood lead levels of 80 μg/dL or higher. Symptoms of lead encephalopathy begin with lethargy, vomiting, irritability, loss of appetite, and dizziness progressing to obvious ataxia and a reduced level of consciousness, which may progress to coma and death. The pathologic findings at autopsy are severe edema of the brain due to extravasation of fluid from capillaries in the brain. This is accompanied by the loss of neuronal cells and an increase in glial cells. Recovery is often accompanied by sequelae including epilepsy, mental retardation, and, in some cases, optic neuropathy and blindness (Perlstein and Attala, 1966).

Over the past 20 or more years there have been a number of cross-sectional and prospective epidemiologic studies relating blood lead levels at the time of birth, during infancy, and through early childhood with measures of psychomoter, cognitive, and behavioral outcomes. These studies have been summarized by NRC (1993) and ATSDR (1999). Despite differences in the ranges of blood lead represented in a cohort, most studies report a 2- to 4-point IQ deficit for each 10 microgram-per-deciliter increase in blood lead within the range of 5 to 35 μg/dL. A threshold is not evident from these studies.

It has been difficult to discern whether there are specific neuropsychological deficits associated with increased lead exposures. To date there are no specific indicators of the neurologic effects of lead. The most sensitive indicators of adverse neurologic outcomes are psychomotor tests or mental development indices, such as the Bayley Scales for infants, and broad measures of IQ, such as full-scale WISC-R IQ scores for older children. Blood lead levels at 2 years of age are more predictive of a longer-term adverse neurologic outcome than umbilical cord blood lead concentration. Children in the lower socioeconomic strata may begin to manifest language deficits by the second year of life, which may be prevented in children with greater academic advantages. Increased blood lead levels in infancy and early childhood may be manifest in older children and adolescents as decreased attention span, reading disabilities, and failure to graduate from high school (Needleman et al., 1990).

The public health significance of small deficits in IQ may be considerable. When the actual cumulative frequency distribution of IQ between high- and low-lead subjects are plotted and compared, there is an increase in the number of children with a severe deficit, that is, IQ scores below 80. Also, the same shift truncates the upper end of the curve, where there is a 5 percent reduction in children with superior function (IQ 125 or greater). There is presently no estimate of the cost of this effect at the high end of the curve, but it may be of considerable importance to both society and to the individual. Small changes in IQ have been associated with differences in measures of socioeconomic status, such as income and educational achievement (Needleman, 1989).

An association between hearing thresholds and blood lead greater than 20 μg/dL has been found in teenagers (Schwartz et al., 1991).

Adults with occupational exposure may demonstrate abnormalities in a number of measures in neurobehavior, with cumulative exposures resulting from blood lead levels <40 μg/dL (Lindgren et al. 1996). Payton et al. (1998) performed a number of cognitive tests and measured tibial lead concentration on a cohort of men with mean age of 66.8 years and mean blood lead level of 55 μg/dL. They found those men with higher blood lead levels performed less well than men with lower blood lead levels. They also found that men with higher blood lead and tibeal lead showed a slower response for pattern memory.

Mechanisms of Effects on the Developing Nervous System Studies to date suggest that the primary anatomic site for lead effect on the brain is the endothelial cell of the blood-brain barrier leading to entry of lead into the brain, followed by morphologic and pharmacologic effects (summarized by Goyer, 1996). Possible mechanisms for lead effects on the nervous system are summarized in Table 23-3.

A highly significant morphologic effect during development is the result of lead impairment of timed programming of cell:cell connections, resulting in modification of neuronal circuitry. Lead also induces precocious differentiation of the glia, whereby cells migrate to their eventual positions during structuring of the central nervous system. Within the catecholaminergic nervous system, lead exposure causes alterations in the concentrations of the transmitters noradrenaline and dopamine in addition to changes in the activities of the enzymes tyrosine hydroxylase and phenylethanolamine-*N*-methyl transferase. The activity of the cholinergic biosynthetic enzyme choline acetyltransferase is also affected (McIntosh et al., 1987).

Calcium is a critical component of numerous biochemical and metabolic functions in the brain, and lead may act as a surrogate for calcium, resulting in subtle disruptions of essential functions. Lead impairs normal calcium homeostasis and uptake by calcium membrane channels and substitutes for calcium in calcium-sodium ATP pumps. Lead also blocks entry of calcium into nerve terminals; it inhibits calcium uptake in brain mitochondria, with a decrease in energy production to perform brain functions. Probably the most critical interaction between lead and calcium is in cells where lead interferes with calcium receptors that are coupled with second-messenger functions. Intracellular calcium signals are received by a variety of calcium receptor proteins. The two that have received the most attention are calmodulin and protein kinase C. Calmodulin serves as a sensor for the concentration of calcium within cells. Lead acts by displacing calcium ions bound to calmodulin. Protein kinase C–mediated responses include cell division and proliferation, cell-cell communications, and organization of the cytoskeleton. Markovac and Goldstein (1988) found that lead activates protein kinase C in microvessels which may be a factor in altering the normally tight blood-brain barrier.

Table 23-3
Mechanisms for Lead Effects on the Nervous System

Morphologic effects (neurodevelopmental)
- Impairment of timed programming of cell–cell connections
- Interference with neural cell adhesion molecules
- Altered migration of neurons during development

Pharmacologic effects (functional)
- Interferes with neurotransmitter function

Disrupts calcium metabolism
- Blocks voltage-dependent calcium membrane channels
- Substitutes for calcium in calcium–sodium ATP pump
- Competes for uptake by mitochondria
- Binds to second messenger calcium receptors (e.g., calmodulin, protein kinase C)

SOURCE: Modified from Goyer (1996).

Peripheral Neuropathy Peripheral neuropathy is a classic manifestation of lead toxicity, particularly the footdrop and wristdrop that characterized the house painter and other workers with excessive occupational exposure to lead more than a half-century ago. Segmental demyelination and possibly axonal degeneration follow lead-induced Schwann cell degeneration. Wallerian degeneration of the posterior roots of sciatic and tibial nerves is possible, but sensory nerves are less sensitive to lead than motor nerve structure and function. Motor nerve dysfunction, assessed clinically by electrophysiologic measurement of nerve conduction velocities, has been shown to occur with blood lead levels as low as 40 μg/dL (ATSDR, 1999).

Hematologic Effects Lead has multiple hematologic effects. In lead-induced anemia, the red blood cells are microcytic and hypochromic, as in iron deficiency, and there are usually increased numbers of reticulocytes with basophilic stippling. The anemia results from two basic defects: shortened erythrocyte life span and impairment of heme synthesis. Shortened life span of the red blood cell is thought to be due to increased mechanical fragility of the cell membrane. The biochemical basis for this effect is not known, but the effect is accompanied by inhibition of sodium- and potassium-dependent ATPases.

A schematic presentation of the effects of lead on heme synthesis is shown in Fig. 23-6.

Probably the most sensitive effect is inhibition of δ-aminolevulinic acid dehydratase (ALA-D), resulting in a negative exponential relationship between ALA-D and blood lead. There is also depression of coproporphyrinogen oxidase, resulting in increased coproporphyrin activity. Lead also decreases ferrochelatase activity. This enzyme catalyzes the incorporation of the ferrous ion into the porphyrin ring structure. Failure to insert iron into protoporphyrin results in depressed heme formation. The excess protoporphyrin takes the place of heme in the hemoglobin molecule and, as the red blood cells containing protoporphyrin circulate, zinc is chelated at the center of the molecule at the site usually occupied by iron. Red blood cells containing zinc-protoporphyrin are intensely fluorescent and may be used to diagnose lead toxicity. Depressed heme synthesis is thought to be the stimulus for increasing the rate of activity of the first step in the heme synthetic pathway. Delta-aminolevulinic acid synthetase is subject to negative feedback control. As a consequence, the increased production of δ-aminolevulinic acid (ALA) and decreased activity of ALA-D result in a marked increase in circulating blood levels and urinary excretion of ALA. Prefeeding of lead to experimental animals also raises heme oxygenase activity, resulting in some increase in bilirubin formation. The change in rates of activity of these enzymes by lead produces a dose-related alteration in the activity of the affected enzymes, but anemia only occurs in very marked lead toxicity. The changes in enzyme activities, particularly ALA-D in peripheral blood and excretion of ALA in urine, correlate very closely with actual blood lead levels and serve as early biochemical indices of lead exposure (ATSDR, 1999).

A genetic polymorphism for the heme pathway enzyme was identified by Granick et al. in 1973, but the molecular characteristics and potential clinical implications have received attention only

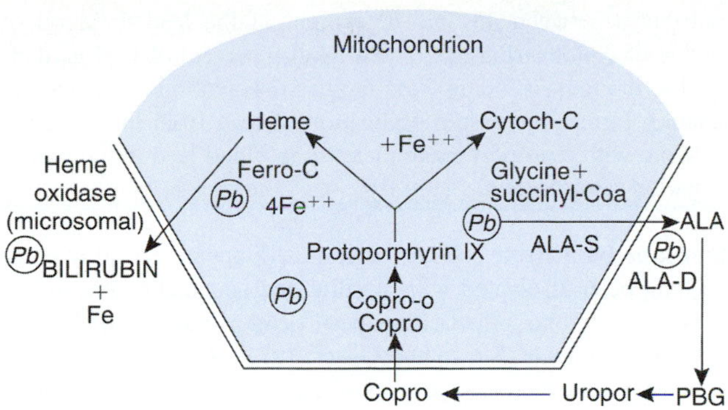

Figure 23-6. Scheme of heme synthesis showing sites where lead has an effect.

CoA, coenzyme A; *ALA-S*, aminolevulinic acid synthetase; *ALA*, δ-aminolevulinic acid; *ALA-D*, aminolevulinic acid dehydratase; *PBG*, porphobilinogen; *Uropor*, urorporphyrinogen; *Copro*, coproporphyrinogen; *Copro-O*, coproporphyrinogen oxidase; *Ferro-C*, ferrochelatase; *Cytoch-C*, cytoachrome-*C*; *Pb*, site for lead effect.

recently. Battistuzzi et al. (1981) identified two common alleles, ALAD-1 and ALAD-2, with frequencies of 0.9 and 0.1 in European-based populations, giving rise to three phenotypes, 1-1, 1-2, and 2-2. Heterozygotes have ALAD-2 activity that is 50 percent normal, whereas severely deficient homozygous (2-2) people have ALA-D activity that is approximately 2 percent of homozygous normal. Doss et al. (1982) reported that those workers with moderate workplace exposure to lead and high free erythrocyte protoporphyrin (FEP) concentrations were heterozygous for ALAD deficiency. Fleming and coworkers (1998) found that lead workers with the ALAD-2 allele had higher blood serum levels than ALAD-1 homozygotes and that the cumulative blood lead index based on blood lead histories and in vivo x-ray fluorescent (XRF) measurements of bone lead was greater in workers homozygous for ALAD-1. This finding suggested a greater transfer of blood lead to bone in this group than in workers with the ALAD-1/2 genotype. It is suggested, therefore, that the ALAD-2 allele affects the metabolism of lead, possibly leaving workers with this genotype more susceptible to soft tissue accumulation of lead. Smith et al. (1998) suggests a potential link between the ALAD variant and the subclinical indices of renal function (elevated BUN, uric acid, and creatinine).

Renal Toxicity Lead nephropathy is one of the oldest recognized health effects of lead (Oliver, 1902). It has been a major hazard from industrial exposure. However, with progressive reduction of exposure in the workplace and more sensitive biological indicators of renal toxicity, lead nephropathy should be a vanishing disease. The pathogenesis of lead nephropathy is described in stages, or as acute (reversible) or chronic (irreversible). Lead is a renal carcinogen in rodents, but whether it is carcinogenic to people is unclear. Acute lead nephrotoxicity is limited to functional and morphologic changes in proximal tubular cells (Goyer and Rhyne, 1973). It is manifest clinically by decrease in energy-dependent transport functions, including aminoaciduria, glycosuria, and ion transport. The functional changes are thought to be related to a lead effect on mitochondrial respiration and phosphorylation. In experimental models and biopsies from children with lead toxicity, there are ultrastructural changes in mitochondria consisting of swelling with distorted cristae. Mitochondria isolated from lead-poisoned rats show decreased state III respiration. These changes are reversible by treatment with a chelating agent.

A characteristic microscopic change is the formation of a lead–protein complex which appears in renal tubular cells as inclusion bodies. By light microscopy the inclusions are dense, homogeneous eosinophilic bodies. The bodies are composed of a lead–protein complex. The protein is acidic and contains large amounts of aspartic and glutamic acids and little cystine. It is suggested that lead binds loosely to the carboxyl groups of the acidic amino acids (Moore et al., 1973). Lead will form inclusion bodies in the cytoplasm of kidney cells grown in culture and tends to migrate into nuclei secondarily (McLaughlin et al., 1980). Renal biopsies from a group of shipwreckers with heavy exposure to lead have shown that the histologic features of early and chronic exposure to lead are similar in experimental animals and humans, suggesting similar pathogenetic mechanisms. Nuclear inclusion bodies become less common as renal tubules atrophy and as interstitial fibrosis increases in severity.

Proximal tubular dysfunction is usually not demonstrable in the chronic phase of lead nephropathy, but interstitial fibrosis is usually associated with asymptomatic renal azotemia and reduced glomerular filtration rate. In workers without azotemia but with decreased inulin clearance, there is decreased maximum reabsorption of glucose. Although progression from acute reversible to chronic irreversible lead nephropathy has not been clearly shown to occur in humans, this progression has been demonstrated in rodent models.

There is no specific biomarker for lead-induced renal disease. Lead may produce a chronic interstitial nephropathy, most commonly with prolonged exposure to blood lead levels greater than 60 μg/dL, but biochemical indicators may respond as low as 40 μg/dL. In a mortality study of 4519 battery plant workers and 2300 lead production workers by Cooper and coworkers (1985), there was excess mortality from chronic nephritis. The mean blood concentration of 1326 of the battery workers in this study with three or more analyses was 62.7 μg/100 g. Gennart and colleagues (1992), found that none of the indicators of renal function, including red blood plasma (RBP), β_2-microglobulin, albumin and NAG in urine, and creatinine differed from controls and did not correlate with blood lead levels (mean 51 μg/dL, range 40 to 75) or duration of exposure. This finding is consistent with the observation of Buchet and coworkers (1980) that workers who do not have recorded blood lead levels over 62 or 63 μg/dL for up to 12 years do not have lead nephropathy. However, depressed glomerular filtration rates have been reported in a group of lead-exposed workers whose blood lead levels were as low as 40 μg/dL. Some studies report correlations of blood lead levels as low as 30 μg/dL with urinary levels of NAG and urinary and serum β_2-microglobulin, but these findings are not confirmed by others (Buchet et al., 1980; Gennart et al., 1992). Increase in urinary β_2-microglobulin is not a characteristic finding in lead-induced nephropathy and there is no meaningful correlation with blood lead levels (Bernard and Lauwerys, 1989). Also, Ong et al. (1987) were not able to find a dose–response relationship between blood lead levels and urinary excretion of NAG. Urinary excretion of NAG might occur at an early stage of lead nephropathy, perhaps reflecting increased urinary leakage from damaged renal tubular epithelium. There is evidence that lead impairs heme-containing enzyme systems in the kidney that are involved in vitamin D metabolism. Vitamin D synthesis requires a heme-containing hydroxylase enzyme in the kidney for the hydroxylation of 25-hydroxyvitamin D to 1,25-dehydroxy-vitamin D, which is important in the gastrointestinal absorption of calcium. These effects may occur with lead levels as low as 30 μg/dL, below the levels of lead that alters other biomarkers for nephrotoxicity (Rosen et al., 1985).

Lead and Gout The relationship between chronic lead exposure and gouty nephropathy was suggested more than a hundred years ago. The tubular or metabolic mechanism for the elevated blood uric acid levels is not known. However, patients with gout and renal disease have a greater chelate-provoked lead excretion than do renal patients without gout (Batuman et al., 1981).

Effects on Cardiovascular System There is considerable debate regarding the causal relationship between lead exposure and hypertension. Many of the studies are summarized in review literature (NRC, 1993; WHO, 1995; ATSDR, 1999). Epidemiologic studies on the effects of lead on blood pressure are inconclusive or contradictory and the WHO (1995) and ATSDR (1999) reviews conclude that the evidence to date is not sufficient to support causal relationship between blood lead levels and increases in blood pressure. Hu et al. (1996) related lead accumulation in bone with blood pressure in a cohort of 590 men, mean age 66.6 years, with hypertension (BP > 160/90 mmHg). Results indicated an increase in odds ratio of 1.5 for hypertension for individuals with elevated bone lead.

The largest populations have been studied in the second National Health and Nutrition Examination Survey (NHANES II) for the U.S. population, performed during the years 1976 to 1980. These studies included blood lead levels and blood pressure measurements in a general population sample of 5803 men and women aged 12 to 74. Analysis of the data (Harlan et al., 1988) found a correlation between blood lead and blood pressure. Possible mechanisms for a lead effect on blood pressure include changes in plasma renin and in urinary kallikrein; alterations in calcium-activated functions of vascular smooth muscle cells, including contractility, by decreasing Na^+/K^+-ATPase activity and stimulation of the Na/Ca exchange pump; and changes in responsiveness to catecholamines (Victery, 1988; ATSDR, 1999).

Immunotoxicity Studies of workers with occupational exposures to lead suggest that lead is an immunosuppressive. McCabe and Lawrence (1991) suggest that decreases in immunoglobulins as well as other components of the immunologic system may be affected by lead. Changes in chemotaxis have been found in polymorphonuclear lymphocytes in workers with blood lead levels < 33 μg/dL (Valentino et al., 1991). Also, numbers of peripheral B lymphocytes may be decreased (Jaremin, 1983).

Bone Effects The regulation of skeletal mass, including lead in bone, are determined by four different types of cells; osteoblasts, lining cells, osteoclasts, and osteocytes. These cells line and penetrate the mineralized matrix of bone and are responsible for matrix formation, mineralization, and bone resorption. Lead toxicity directly and indirectly alters many aspects of bone cell function. Retention and mobilization of lead in bone occur by the same mechanisms involved in regulating calcium influx and efflux, namely parathyroid hormone, calcitonin, vitamin D, and other hormones that influence calcium metabolism (Pounds et al., 1991). Lead also competes with calcium for gastrointestinal absorption (Fullmer et al., 1992). The interrelationship of vitamin D and calcium is complex and involves interactions with parathyroid hormone. Lead in bone readily exchanges with blood lead. Using stable isotope techniques, Gulson and coworkers (1995) have shown that lead in bone contributes between 45 and 70 percent of the lead in blood of women of childbearing age, and a similar percent of lead is identified in the fetus as being from mother's skeleton. Pregnancy and lactation further increase mobilization of lead from the maternal skeleton, with a proportionate increase in blood lead in the prenatal period (Gulson et al., 1998).

Reproductive Effects Overt or clinically apparent lead toxicity has long been associated with sterility and neonatal deaths in humans. Gametotoxic effects have been demonstrated in both male and female animals (Stowe and Goyer, 1971). A few clinical studies have found increased chromosomal defects in workers with blood lead levels above 60 μg/dL; reduction in sperm counts and abnormal sperm motility and morphology are found in lead battery workers with blood lead levels as low as 40 μg/dL (Assenato et al., 1986). Decreases in testicular endocrine function were found to be related to duration of lead exposure of smelter workers with mean blood lead level of 60 μg/dL (Rodamilans et al., 1988). An effect of chronic exposure to low levels of lead on female reproduction including abortion has not been demonstrated (Murphy et al., 1990).

Birth Outcomes The early literature on toxicology of lead focused on an increased incidence of spontaneous abortion and stillbirth, but these outcomes are rare today. Andrews et al. (1994) reviewed 25 epidemiologic studies to determine the relationship of prenatal lead exposure and birth outcomes. They concluded that prenatal lead exposure is unlikely to increase the risk of premature rupture of membranes but does appear to increase the risk of preterm delivery. An increase in the maternal blood lead level may also contribute to reducing gestational duration and birth weight (McMichael et al., 1988; Borschein et al., 1989).

Carcinogenicity Lead is classified as a 2B carcinogen by the IARC (1987). A study of workmen with occupational exposure to lead in England many years ago did not show an increased incidence of cancer (Dingwall-Fordyce and Lane, 1963). Causes of mortality in 7000 lead workers in the United States showed a slight excess of deaths from cancer (Cooper and Gaffey, 1975), but the statistical significance of these findings has been debated (Kang et al., 1980). The most common tumors found were of the respiratory and digestive systems, not the kidney. However, case reports of renal adenocarcinoma in workmen with prolonged occupational exposure to lead have appeared (Baker et al., 1980; Lilis, 1981).

Epidemiologic studies suggest a relationship between occupational lead exposure and cancer of the lung and brain. Anttila et al. (1995) correlated blood lead levels and mortality rates and cancer incidence for a cohort of 20,700 workers coexposed to lead and engine exhausts. Blood lead levels were monitored for over 10 years. A 1.4-fold increase in the overall cancer incidence was found, as well as a 1.8-fold increase in lung cancer among those who had ever a blood-lead level over 1.0 μmol/dL. Another epidemiologic study provides evidence for a potential link between occupational exposure to lead and brain cancer (Cocco et al., 1998). A job-exposure matrix for lead to occupation and industry codes was applied to information on death certificates of 27,060 brain cancer cases and 108,240 controls who died of nonmalignant disease in 24 U.S. states in 1984 to 1992. Brain cancer risk increased by probability of exposure to lead among Caucasian men and women with high-level exposure. Fu and Boffetta (1995) performed a meta-analysis of published data on cancer incidence among various industries. They focused the analysis on overall cancer, stomach cancer, kidney cancer, and bladder cancer. The meta-analysis indicates a significant excess of cancer deaths from stomach cancer, lung cancer, and bladder cancer among workers exposed to lead. There was also a non-statistically-significant excess of deaths from kidney cancer. The investigators concluded that most of the studies lacked data on the level of cumulative exposure. Suggested relationships between high occupational exposure are from multimedia exposure, largely from inhalation, and often in association with potential toxins and/or cocarcinogens, so that the role of lead is generally nonconclusive.

Lead induction of renal adenocarcinoma in rats and mice is dose related and has not been reported at levels below that which produces nephrotoxicity. Lead-induced tumors may be a consequence of increased cellular proliferation (Calabrese, 1992). Lead compounds have been shown to stimulate the proliferation of renal tubular epithelial cells (Choie and Richter, 1980), and similar effects have been noted in the livers of rats (Columbano et al., 1983). Lead compounds induce cell transformation in Syrian hamster embryo cells (Zelikoff et al., 1988). Lead-related renal tumors may be a nonspecific response to epithelial hyperplasia, as has been noted in other experimental nephropathies and human diseases where renal tubular cysts and hyperplasia occur (Goyer, 1992).

Other Effects Lead lines (Burton's lines) or purple-blue discoloration of gingiva is a classic feature of severe lead toxicity in children with lead encephalopathy. However, this feature of lead toxicity, as well as the presence of lead lines at the epiphyses margins of long bones, is uncommon today.

Dose Response The toxic effects of lead and the minimum blood lead level at which the effect is likely to be observed are shown in Table 23-4. A detailed compilation of lowest observed effect levels in humans and animals from individual reports is available (ATSDR, 1999). Levels provided in this table are meant to be guidelines recognizing variation in susceptibility between individuals.

Table 23-4
Summary of Lowest Observed Effect Levels for Lead-Related Health Effects

EFFECT	*Blood Lead Levels, μg/dL* ADULT	CHILDREN
Neurologic		
Encephalopathy (overt)	80–100	100–120
Hearing deficits	20	—
IQ deficits	10–15	—
In utero effects	10–15	—
Nerve conduction velocity ↓	40	40
Hematologic		
Anemia	80–100	80–100
U-ALA ↑	40	40
B-EP ↑	15	15
ALA-D inhibition	10	10
Renal		
Nephropathy	40	40–60
Vitamin D metabolism	<30?	—
Blood pressure		30?
Reproduction		
Males		40
Females		?

SOURCE: Modified from NIOSH (1997) and ATSDR (1999).

Treatment Foremost in the treatment of increased blood lead levels and lead toxicity is removal of the subject from source(s) of exposure. The blood lead levels at which treatment with chelating drugs should begin are debatable. Certainly chelation usually has a role in the treatment of the symptomatic worker or child. Institution of chelation therapy is probably warranted in workers with blood lead levels over 60 μg/dL, but this determination must be made after an assessment of exposure factors, including biological estimates of clinical and biochemical parameters of toxicity. For children, criteria have been established that may serve as guidelines to assist in evaluating the individual case (CDC, 1991). For children with severe lead poisoning, including encephalopathy, chelation therapy is standard practice. Even then, the mortality rate may be 25 to 38 percent when EDTA or BAL is used singly, whereas combination therapy of EDTA and BAL has been shown to be effective in reducing mortality.

The decision to chelate children with blood lead levels above 45 μg/dL is a matter of clinical judgment. The oral chelating agent succimer [dimercaptosuccinic acid, (DMSA)] has been licensed by the U.S. Food and Drug Administration (FDA) for reduction of blood lead levels of 45 μg/dL or greater. DMSA has an advantage over EDTA in that it can be administered orally and is effective in temporarily reducing blood lead levels. Studies in rats suggest it may be effective in the treatment of acute lead poisoning (Kostial et al., 1999). However, DMSA does not seem to improve long-term blood lead levels in children with blood lead levels between 30 and 45 μg/dL. (O'Connor and Rich, 1999). Studies in monkeys suggest that DMSA does not reduce brain lead beyond the effect of cessation of exposure of lead alone (Cremin et al., 1999).

Organic Lead Compounds Tetraethyl lead (TEL) was used for many years as a gasoline additive, but production and use have now stopped in the United States. While the importance of TEL as a potential toxin for workers and the general population has lessened, it is still produced and used in some other countries. The potential use of gasoline as a recreational drug (gasoline sniffing) for a psychedelic high is an additional reason for concern about its potential toxicity.

Toxicokinetics Organic lead compounds have a special affinity for lipoid and nerve tissue, resulting in rapid metabolism and toxicity to the brain. Within 24 h of exposure, 50 percent of TEL is metabolized by P450 metabolizing enzymes to trimethyl lead (TML). The second metabolic product of TEL is inorganic lead, which is distributed to various tissues and excreted in urine. Most TEL is excreted from the body in about 20 days. Mechanisms of toxicity include damage to membranes, impairment of energy metabolism, and direct interference with neurotransmitter synthesis. Exposure to TEL is usually by inhalation, and about 60 to 80 percent is absorbed. The liquid is readily absorbed by the gastrointestinal tract and skin (Bolanowska et al., 1968; Bondy, 1991; Audesirk et al., 1995).

Toxicity Symptoms of acute intoxication include nausea, vomiting, and diarrhea associated with nervous system symptoms of irritability, headache, and restlessness. These symptoms progress rapidly to severe signs of central nervous system toxicity, including convulsions and coma. The mortality rate for acute intoxication is about 29 percent. Chronic exposure may result in milder symptoms. An immediate effect among recreational users may be euphoria, followed by violent excitement and then coma. Chronic, heavy sniffing of leaded gasoline results in signs of dementia and encephalopathy, with cerebellar and corticospinal symptoms. Which aspects of these symptoms are due to TEL per se or other components of gasoline is unknown. Chelating agents are not thought to be a rational aspect of treatment and experience with gasoline sniffers has shown that chelation does not benefit these patients (Tenenbein, 1997). A case-control study of former workers in a TEL-producing plant found a strong association between exposure to the TEL manufacturing process and colorectal cancer (Fayerweather et al., 1997).

Mercury (Hg)

No other metal better illustrates the diversity of effects caused by different chemical species than does mercury.[1] There have been several major reviews (ATSDR, 1999; WHO, 1990; WHO, 1991; Goyer, 1996).

Mercury is unique as being the only metal that is in a liquid state at room temperature. The vapor from this liquid, usually referred to as *mercury vapor,* is much more hazardous than the liquid form. This element exists in three oxidation states. In the zero oxidation state (Hg^0) mercury exists in its metallic form or as the vapor. The mercurous and mercuric states are the two higher-oxidation states where the mercury atom has lost one (Hg^+) and two electrons (Hg^{2+}), respectively. In addition, mercuric mercury can form a number of stable organic mercury compounds by attaching to one or two carbon atoms. Methyl mercury (CH_3Hg^+) is the most important organic form from the point of view of human exposure. Each oxidation state and each organic species has characteristic toxicokinetics and health effects.

Exposure The major source of mercury (as mercury vapor) in the atmosphere is the natural degassing of the earth's crust. It is difficult to assess what quantities of mercury come from human activities, but these are believed to be approximately similar in magnitude to natural sources. Calculations based on the mercury content of the Greenland ice cap show an increase from the year 1900 to the present.

Mercury vapor in the atmosphere represents the major pathway of global transport of mercury. It resides there unchanged for periods of a year or so. Thus there is time for it to be distributed globally even from a point source of pollution. Eventually it is converted to a water-soluble form and returned to the earth's surface in rainwater.

At this stage, two important chemical changes may occur. The metal may be reduced back to mercury vapor and returned to the atmosphere, or it may be methylated by microorganisms present in sediments of bodies of fresh and ocean water. The main product of this natural biomethylation reaction is monomethyl mercury compounds, usually referred to generically as "methyl mercury." Some of the oldest organisms on an evolutionary scale, the methanogenic bacteria, carry out this methylation reaction.

Once produced, methyl mercury enters an aquatic food chain involving plankton, herbivorous fish, and finally carnivorous fish. In the tissues of fish consuming sea mammals, mercury can rise to levels a millionfold higher than those in the surrounding water. The sequence of biomethylation and bioconcentration can result in human dietary exposure to methyl mercury, whether the latter originated from natural or anthropogenic sources of inorganic mercury. Methyl mercury is found in most if not all fish tissues but most importantly in edible tissue, mainly muscle, in a water-soluble protein-bound form. Unlike the case of PCBs, which are deposited in fat, cooking the fish does not lower the methyl mercury content.

Inorganic compounds of mercury are also found in food. The source is unknown and the amount ingested is far below known toxic intakes.

Other sources of human exposure to mercury are occupational, where the main route is inhalation of mercury vapor from the working environment. Mercury has numerous uses, as in the chlor-alkali industry, where it is used as a cathode in the electrolysis of brine; in making a variety of scientific instruments and electrical control devices; in dentistry, as amalgam tooth filling; and in the extraction of gold. The last has now become a widespread activity in developing countries, where large quantities of metallic mercury are used to form an amalgam with gold. The amalgam is heated to drive off the mercury, resulting in a substantial release to the atmosphere.

Mercury vapor emitted from amalgam dental fillings is the major source of mercury vapor affecting the general public. Chewing increases the rate of release. Although the amount inhaled is low compared to known toxic levels, some individuals with a history of excessive chewing might attain levels that could pose a health risk.

Mercury levels in the general atmosphere and in drinking water are so low that they do not constitute an important source of exposure to the general population.

Disposition and Toxicokinetics Liquid metallic mercury, such as may be swallowed from a broken thermometer, is only slowly absorbed by the gastrointestinal tract (0.01 percent) at a rate related to the vaporization of the elemental mercury and is generally thought to be of no toxicologic consequence.

The vapor from metallic mercury is readily absorbed in the lungs, and, in mercury's dissolved form in the bloodstream, diffuses to all tissues in the body. Its high mobility is due to the fact that it is a monatomic gas, highly diffusible and lipid-soluble. It is rapidly oxidized to mercuric mercury, as discussed below.

Since human exposure to compounds of mercurous mercury now occurs rarely if at all, we have little information on its disposition in the body. Compounds of mercurous mercury, especially the chloride salt, have a low solubility in water and are poorly absorbed from the gastrointestinal tract. In the presence of protein, the mercurous ion disproportionates to one atom of metallic mercury (Hg^0) and one of mercuric mercury (Hg^{2+}). The latter will probably be absorbed into the bloodstream and distributed to tissues, as discussed below.

Gastrointestinal absorption of compounds of mercuric mercury from food is about 15 percent in a study of human volunteers, whereas absorption of methyl mercury is on the order of 90 to 95 percent. Distribution between red blood cells and plasma also differs. For inorganic mercury the cell-to-plasma ratio ranges from a high of 2 with high exposure to less than 1 but for methyl mercury it is about 10. The distribution ratio of the two forms of mercury between hair and blood also differs; much higher concentrations of methyl mercury are accumulated from blood.

Kidneys contain the greatest concentrations of mercury following exposure to inorganic salts of mercury and mercury vapor, whereas organic mercury has a greater affinity for the brain, particularly the posterior cortex. Mercury vapor also has a greater predilection for the central nervous system than do inorganic mercury salts.

[1]Atomic weight, 200.5; periodic table group, IIB; valence, +1 or +2; discovered before 1500 B.C.

Excretion of mercury from the body is by way of urine and feces, again differing with the form of mercury, size of the dose, and time after exposure. Exposure to mercury vapor is followed by exhalation of a small fraction, but fecal excretion is the major and predominant route of excretion initially after exposure to inorganic mercury. Renal excretion increases with time. About 90 percent of methyl mercury is excreted in feces after acute or chronic exposure, and this figure does not change with time (Miettinen, 1973).

All forms of mercury cross the placenta to the fetus, but most of what is known has been learned from experimental animals. Fetal uptake of elemental mercury in rats has been shown to be 10 to 40 times higher than uptake after exposure to inorganic salts. Concentrations of mercury in the fetus after exposure to alkylmercuric compounds are twice those found in maternal tissues, and levels of methyl mercury in fetal red blood cells are 30 percent higher than those in maternal red cells. Although maternal milk may contain only 5 percent of the mercury concentration of maternal blood, neonatal exposure to mercury may be increased by nursing (Grandjean et al., 1994).

Metabolic Transformation Elemental or metallic mercury is oxidized to divalent mercury after absorption to tissues in the body and is probably mediated by catalases. Inhaled mercury vapor absorbed into red blood cells is transformed to divalent mercury, but a portion is also transported as metallic mercury to more distal tissues, particularly the brain, where biotransformation may occur.

Methyl mercury undergoes biotransformation to divalent mercury compounds in tissues by cleavage of the carbon mercury bond. There is no evidence of formation of any organic form of mercury in mammalian tissues. The aryl (phenyl) compounds are converted to inorganic mercury more rapidly than the shorter-chain alkyl (methyl) compounds.

Biological half-lives are available for a limited number of mercury compounds. Elimination of methyl mercury from the body is adequately described by a single half-life. The most recent estimate is 44 days. More complex kinetics describe the elimination of mercury after inorganic salts or exposure to mercury vapor. The half-lives vary between tissues and sometimes more than one half-life is needed to characterize the kinetics of elimination. Generally, the half-lives are in the range of 20 to 90 days.

Cellular Metabolism Within cells, mercury may bind to a variety of enzyme systems including those of microsomes and mitochondria, producing nonspecific cell injury or cell death. It has a particular affinity for ligands containing sulfhydryl groups. In liver cells, methyl mercury forms soluble complexes of glutathione, which are secreted in bile and reabsorbed from the gastrointestinal tract. Inorganic mercury is also secreted in bile as a glutathione complex. The cysteine complex of methyl mercury enters the endothelial cells of the blood-brain barrier on the large neutral amino acid transporter.

Mercuric mercury, but not methyl mercury, induces synthesis of metallothionein in kidney cells; but unlike cadmium-metallothionein, it does not have a long biological half-life. Mercury within renal cells becomes localized in lysosomes (Madsen and Christensen, 1978).

Toxicology ***Mercury Vapor*** Inhalation of mercury vapor at extremely high concentrations may produce an acute, corrosive bronchitis and interstitial pneumonitis and, if not fatal, may be associated with symptoms of central nervous system effects such as tremor or increased excitability. With chronic exposure to mercury vapor, the major effects are on the central nervous system. Early signs are nonspecific, and this condition has been termed the *asthenic-vegetative syndrome* or *micromercurialism.* Identification of the syndrome requires neurasthenic symptoms and three or more of the following clinical findings: tremor, enlargement of the thyroid, increased uptake of radioiodine in the thyroid, labile pulse, tachycardia, dermographism, gingivitis, hematologic changes, or increased excretion of mercury in urine. With increasing exposure, the symptoms become more characteristic, beginning with tremors of muscles that perform fine-motor functions (highly innervated)—such as fingers, eyelids, and lips—and may progress to generalized trembling of the entire body and violent chronic spasms of the extremities. This is accompanied by changes in personality and behavior, with loss of memory, increased excitability (erethism), severe depression, and even delirium and hallucination. Another characteristic feature of mercury toxicity is severe salivation and gingivitis.

The triad of increased excitability, tremors, and gingivitis has been recognized historically as the major manifestation of mercury poisoning from inhalation of mercury vapor and exposure to mercury nitrate in the fur, felt, and hat industries (Goldwater, 1972).

Sporadic instances of proteinuria and even nephrotic syndrome may occur in persons with exposure to mercury vapor, particularly with chronic occupational exposure. The pathogenesis is probably immunologically similar to that which may occur following exposure to inorganic mercury.

There is growing concern that the toxic potential of mercury vapor released from dental amalgams may cause various health effects. Estimates of absorption of mercury by an adult with the average number of amalgams (8 per adult) is 30 to 40 percent of the total mercury exposure of 5 to 6 μg per day (Richardson et al., 1995). An increase in urinary mercury and accumulation in several organs, including the central nervous system and kidneys, has been related to the release of mercury from dental amalgams (Clarkson et al., 1988; Langworth et al., 1988). Aposhian and coworkers (1992) found a highly positive correlation between mercury excreted in urine following the administration of dimercapto-succinic acid (DMPS) and numbers of dental amalgams. However, this level of mercury exposure is believed to be below that which will produce any discernible health effect except for highly sensitive people.

Mercuric Salts Bichloride of mercury (corrosive sublimate) is the best-known mercuric salt of mercury from a toxicologic standpoint. Even the trivial name suggests its most apparent toxicologic effect when the salt is ingested in concentrations greater than 10 percent. A reference from the Middle Ages in Goldwater's book on mercury describes oral ingestion of mercury as causing severe abdominal cramps, bloody diarrhea, and suppression of urine (Goldwater, 1972). This is an accurate report of the effects following accidental or suicidal ingestion of mercuric chloride or other mercuric salts. Corrosive ulceration, bleeding, and necrosis of the gastrointestinal tract are usually accompanied by shock and circulatory collapse. If the patient survives the gastrointestinal damage, renal failure occurs within 24 h owing to necrosis of the proximal tubular epithelium, followed by oliguria, anuria, and uremia. If the patient can be maintained by dialysis, regeneration of the tubular lining cells is possible. These changes may be followed by ultrastructural changes consistent with irreversible cell injury, including actual disruption of mitochondria, release of lysosomal enzymes, and rupture of cell membranes.

Injection of mercuric chloride produces necrosis of the epithelium of the pars recta kidney (Gritzka and Trump, 1968). Cellular changes include fragmentation and disruption of the plasma membrane and its appendages, vesiculation and disruption of the endoplasmic reticulum and other cytoplasmic membranes, dissociation of polysomes and loss of ribosomes, mitochondrial swelling with appearance of amorphous intramatrical deposits, and condensation of nuclear chromatin. These changes are common to renal cell necrosis due to various causes. Slight tubular cell injury, manifest by enzymuria and low-molecular-weight proteinuria may occur in workers with low-level exposure to metallic mercury vapor (Roels et al., 1985).

Although a high dose of mercuric chloride is directly toxic to renal tubular lining cells, chronic low-dose exposure to mercuric salts or even elemental mercury vapor levels may induce an immunologic glomerular disease. Exposed persons may develop a proteinuria that is reversible after workers are removed from exposure.

Experimental studies have shown that the pathogenesis has two phases: an early phase characterized by an anti–basement membrane glomerulonephritis, followed by a superimposed immune-complex glomerulonephritis with transiently raised concentrations of circulating immune complexes (Henry et al., 1988). The pathogenesis of the nephropathy in humans appears similar, although antigens have not been characterized. Also, the early glomerular nephritis may progress in humans to an interstitial immune-complex nephritis (Pelletier and Druet, 1995).

Mercurous Mercury Mercurous compounds of mercury are less corrosive and less toxic than mercuric salts, presumably because they are less soluble. Calomel, a powder containing mercurous chloride, has a long history of use in medicine. Perhaps the most notable modern usage has been in teething powder for children, and this powder is now known to be responsible for acrodynia or "pink disease." This is most likely a hypersensitivity response to the mercury salts in skin, producing vasodilation, hyperkeratosis, and hypersecretion of sweat. Children develop fever, a pink-colored rash, swelling of the spleen and lymph nodes, and hyperkeratosis and swelling of the fingers. The effects are thought to be a hypersensitivity reaction (Matheson et al., 1980).

Methyl Mercury Methyl mercury is the most important form of mercury in terms of toxicity and health effects from environmental exposures. Many of the effects produced by short-term alkyls are unique in terms of mercury toxicity but nonspecific in that they may be found in other disease states. Most of what is known about the clinical signs and symptoms and neuropathology of high-level or overt methyl mercury toxicity has been learned from studies of epidemics in Japan and Iraq (WHO, 1990; Berlin, 1986) and from published reports of occupational exposures (Hunter et al., 1940). Observations of changes in nonhuman primates studied experimentally are consistent with findings in humans and therefore provide additional information about the relationship between time, dose, and tissue burden, particularly for subclinical and subtle low-level effects (Mottet et al., 1985).

The major human health effects from exposure to methyl mercury are neurotoxic effects in adults (Bakir et al., 1973) and toxicity to the fetuses of mothers exposed to methyl mercury during pregnancy (Cox et al., 1989). The major source of exposure for people in the general population is from the consumption of fish, and in this instance the brain is the critical organ.

Clinical manifestations of neurotoxic effects are (1) paresthesia, a numbness and tingling sensation around the mouth, lips, and extremities, particularly the fingers and toes; (2) ataxia, a clumsy, stumbling gait, difficulty in swallowing and articulating words; (3) neurasthenia, a generalized sensation of weakness, fatigue, and inability to concentrate; (4) vision and hearing loss; (5) spasticity and tremor; and finally (6) coma and death.

Neuropathologic observations have shown that the cortex of the cerebrum and cerebellum are selectively involved with focal necrosis of neurons, lysis and phagocytosis, and replacement by supporting glial cells. These changes are most prominent in the deeper fissures (sulci), as in the visual cortex and insula. The overall acute effect is cerebral edema; but with prolonged destruction of gray matter and subsequent gliosis, cerebral atrophy results (Takeuchi, 1977).

The mechanisms of damage to the mature brain are not known. Inhibition of protein synthesis is among the earliest biochemical effects seen in animals. Syversen (1982) has proposed that all neuronal cells may be affected initially, but those cells having the least repair capacity eventually succumb whereas cells with more repair capacity survive. This mechanism may account for the highly localized focal pathology seen in the adult brain.

Experimental studies on the mechanisms of methyl mercury toxicity provide some insight into the basis for the clinical observations as well as the greater sensitivity of the developing brain (Clarkson, 1983). Exposure of the fetus in utero to high levels of mercury result in abnormal neuronal migration and deranged organization of brain nuclei (clusters of neurons) and layering of neurons in the cortex. Studies in mice have demonstrated an effect of methyl mercury on the microtubules of neurons. These observations may provide the cellular basis for the observed neuropathologic changes in the migration pattern of neurons during development, which is thought to be the basis for the developmental effects in the central nervous system. Male mice are more sensitive than females, consistent with the findings in humans (Sager et al., 1984; Choi et al., 1978).

Biological Indicators ***Inorganic Mercury*** The recommended standard (time-weight average) for permissible exposure limits for inorganic mercury in air in the workplace is 0.05 mg/m^3 (DHEW, 1977) and is equivalent to an ambient air level of 0.015 mg/m^3 for the general population (24-h exposure) (Table 23-5). The U.S. federal standard for alkyl mercury exposure in the workplace is 0.01 mg/m^3 as an 8-h time-weighted average with an acceptable ceiling of 0.04 mg/m^3. A study of the Iraq epidemic has provided estimates of the body burden of mercury and the onset and frequency of occurrence of symptoms (Fig. 23-7).

Table 23-5

The Time-Weighted Average Air Concentrations Associated with the Earliest Effects in the Most Sensitive Adults following Long-Term Exposure to Elemental Mercury Vapor

*Equivalent Concentrations**			
AIR, mg/m^3	BLOOD, μg/100 mL	URINE, μg/L	EARLIEST EFFECTS
0.05	3.5	150	Nonspecific symptoms
0.1–0.2	7–14	300–600	Tremor

*Blood and urine values may be used only on a group basis owing to gross individual variations. These average values reflect exposure for a year or more. After shorter periods of exposure, air concentrations would be associated with lower concentrations in blood and urine.

SOURCE: WHO (1976).

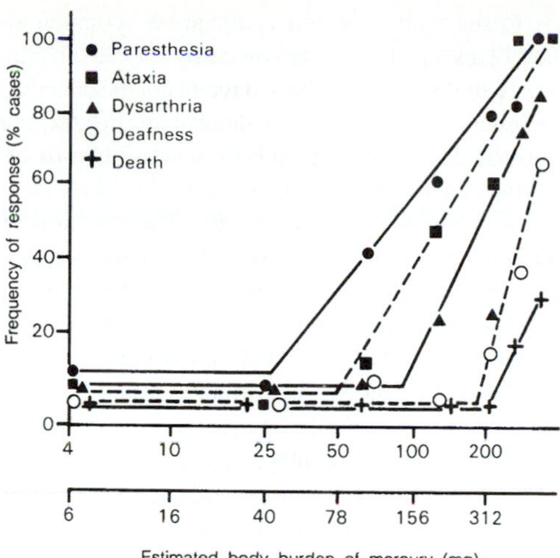

Figure 23-7. Dose–response relationships for methyl mercury.

The upper scale of estimated body burden of mercury was based on the author's actual estimate of intake. The lower scale is based on the body burden, which was calculated based on the concentration of mercury in the blood and its relationship to intake derived from radioisotopic studies of methyl mercury kinetics in human volunteers. [From Bakir et al. (1973).]

Methyl Mercury The relationship between health risks and intake of methyl mercury has been developed from toxicologic data obtained from studies of epidemics due to accidental poisoning in Minamata and Niigata, Japan, in the 1950s and 1960s and from studies of the episode in Iraq in 1972 (Berlin, 1986).

The critical or lowest level of observed adverse health effect in adults is paresthesia. By combining two relationships, body burden versus intake and effect versus body burden, a Swedish Expert Group (1971) was able to calculate the average long-term daily intake associated with health effects in the most susceptible individual. This was estimated to be about 300 μg/day for an adult or 4.3 μg/kg/day and would correspond to a steady-state blood level of 200 μg/L or a hair level of 50 μg/g.

Treatment Therapy for mercury poisoning should be directed toward lowering the concentration of mercury at the critical organ or site of injury. For the most severe cases, particularly with acute renal failure, hemodialysis may be the first measure, along with infusion of chelating agents for mercury, such as cysteine or penicillamine. For less severe cases of inorganic mercury poisoning, chelation with BAL may be effective.

However, chelation therapy is not very helpful for alkyl mercury exposure. Biliary excretion and reabsorption by the intestine and the enterohepatic cycling of mercury may be interrupted by surgically establishing gallbladder drainage or by the oral administration of a nonabsorbable thiol resin, which binds mercury and enhances intestinal excretion (Berlin, 1986).

Nickel (Ni)

Nickel[1] is a respiratory tract carcinogen in workers in the nickel-refining industry. Other serious consequences of long-term exposure to nickel are not apparent, but severe acute and sometimes fatal toxicity may follow exposure to nickel carbonyl. Allergic contact dermatitis is common among the general population.

Metallic nickel is produced from sulfide and silcate-oxide ores. In the United States approximately 200,000 metric tons of nickel (primary plus secondary use) are utilized per year. Nickel is included in various metal alloys, stainless steels, and electroplating. Major properties are strength, corrosion resistance, and good thermal and electrical conductivity (NIDI, 1997).

Exposure Nickel is ubiquitous in nature, occurring mainly in the form of sulfide, oxide, and silicate minerals. Very low levels of nickel can be found in ambient air as a result of industrial uses, combustion of fossil fuels, and sludge and waste incineration. Human exposure may be by inhalation, ingestion, and dermal contact. The main route of occupational exposure to nickel is through inhalation and to a lesser degree skin contact. Nickel refinery dust contains a mixture of many chemical species. Occupational exposures may contain elemental nickel, nickel compounds, complexes and alloys, and fumes from alloys used in welding and brazing. While there are no refineries in operation in the United States at present, there is still concern regarding effects on former workers from past exposures. Exposure to individuals in the general environment may result from contact with everyday items such as nickel-containing jewelry, cooking utensils, and clothing fasteners. Food is a major source of exposure for most people. The Environmental Protection Agency (EPA) estimates that an average adult consumes 100 to 300 μg of nickel per day. Drinking water contains very small amounts of nickel (ATSDR, 1997).

Toxicokinetics In the workplace, inhalation is the most serious toxicologic concern, followed by dermal exposure. Almost 35 percent of inhaled nickel is absorbed into the blood from the respiratory tract (WHO, 1991). Deposition, absorption, and elimination of nickel particles in the respiratory tract depend largely on the particle size and concentration of nickel. Only about half of particles larger than 30 μm are inhalable. Particles less than 10 μm may be deposited in the lower respiratory tract. Half-lives of 1 to 3 days for nickel sulfate, 5 days for nickel subsulfide, and more than 100 days for nickel oxide have been reported for inhaled or intratracheally instilled nickel compounds (Benson et al., 1987; Dunnick, 1989). Nickel has a half-life ranging from 30 to 53 h in the urine of workers exposed to insoluble nickel particles of small diameter (Raithel et al., 1982). Urinary nickel ranges from approximately 0.2 to 10 μg/L in unexposed individuals but from 2.6 μg/L in high nickel alloy production to 222 μg Ni/L in electrolyte refinery workers (Bernacki et al., 1978). In human volunteers exposed orally to soluble nickel sulfate hexahydrate, a half-life of 11 h was observed (Christensen and Lagesson, 1981). Nickel concentrations in the serum of unexposed individuals ranged from 0.05 to 1.1 μg/L (Sunderman et al., 1986). Urinary nickel has been shown to correlate closely with airborne levels of insoluble nickel compounds. It is not influenced by duration of exposure and may serve as a suitable measure of current nickel exposure (White and Boran, 1988).

The rate of dermal absorption depends on the rate of penetration of the epidermis, which differs for different chemical species of nickel. Nickel chloride penetrates in amounts ranging from 0.23 to 3.5 percent of the applied dose, whereas nickel sulfate may penetrate at rates 50 times lower (NIDI, 1997).

Nickel administered parenterally to animals is rapidly distributed to the kidneys, pituitary, lungs, skin, adrenals, ovaries, and

[1]Atomic weight, 58.69; periodic table group, VIII; valence, +0, +1, +2, +3; discovered in 1751.

testes (Sunderman, 1981). The intracellular distribution and binding of nickel is not well understood. Ultrafilterable ligands seem to be of major importance in the transport in serum and bile and urinary excretion as well as in intracellular binding. The ligands are not well characterized, but Sunderman (1981) suggests that cysteine, histidine, and aspartic acid form nickel complexes either singly or as nickel–ligand species. In vivo binding with metallothionein has been demonstrated, but nickel at best induces metallothionein synthesis in liver or kidney only slightly. A nickel-binding metalloprotein, called nickeloplasmin, has also been identified in plasma with properties suggesting that it is an α_1-glycoprotein complex and is important in the extracellular transport, intracellular binding, and urinary and biliary excretion of nickel (Niebor et al., 1988; Tabata et al., 1992).

Essentiality Evidence has accumulated over the past few years indicating that nickel is a nutritionally essential trace metal for some plant life, bacteria, and invertebrates (summarized by Nielson, 1996). Jackbean urease has been identified as a nickel metalloenzyme, and nickel is required for urea metabolism in cell cultures of soybean. However, a nickel-containing metalloenzyme has not yet been recovered from animal tissues. Nickel deficiency in rats is associated with retarded body growth and anemia, probably secondary to impaired absorption of iron from the gastrointestinal tract. In addition, there is a significant reduction in serum glucose concentration. An interaction of nickel with copper and zinc is also suspected because anemia-induced nickel deficiency is only partially corrected with nickel supplementation in rats receiving low dietary copper and zinc (Spears, 1978). A defined biochemical function in higher animals and humans has not been described, and human nutritional requirements have not been established (WHO, 1996).

Toxicity *Carcinogenicity* The IARC working group for consideration of nickel and nickel compounds concluded that nickel compounds are carcinogenic to humans (IARC, 1990). The respiratory tract is the main site of chronic effects reported in relation to nickel and its compounds. Risks were highest for lung and nasal cancers among workers heavily exposed to nickel sulfide, nickel oxide, and to metallic nickel. A cohort of 418 workers employed in a Finnish refinery reported a twofold increased incidence of lung cancer and a large increase in sinonasal cancers (Karjalainen et al., 1992). A follow-up of this study, including a total of 1155 workers, confirmed an elevated risk of lung and nasal cancers among refinery workers, with a greater risk among workers with a longer latency (greater than 20 years), (Anttila et al., 1998).

Because the refining of nickel in the plants that were studied involved the Mond process, with the formation of nickel carbonyl, it was believed for some time that nickel carbonyl was the principal carcinogen. However, additional epidemiologic studies of workers in refineries that do not use the Mond process also showed an increased risk of respiratory cancer, suggesting that the source of the increased risk is the mixture of nickel sulfides present in molten ore. Studies with experimental animals have shown that the nickel subsulfide (Ni_3S_2) produces local tumors at injection sites and by inhalation in rats, and in vitro mammalian cell tests demonstrate that Ni_3S_2 and $NiSO_4$ compounds give rise to mammalian cell transformation (IARC, 1990). Differences in the carcinogenic activities of nickel compounds may be attributable to variations in their capacities to provide nickel ion at critical sites within target cells (Sunderman, 1989; Costa, 1995). The order of lung toxicity corresponds to the water solubility of various compounds, with nickel sulfate being most toxic, followed by nickel subsulfide and nickel oxide (Dunick et al., 1989). However, nickel compounds lose their original chemical identity upon entering the blood, so that it is not possible to identify the original source of exposure (Grant and Mushak, 1989).

Mechanisms For Nickel Carcinogenesis The carcinogenicity of nickel is thought to be due to the ionic nickel species, but it has been difficult to explain the differences in carcinogenic potency between different nickel compounds. Some studies have suggested that water-insoluble crystalline nickel compounds were responsible for lung and nasal cancers seen in animal and human studies (IARC, 1990). However, not all water-insoluble crystalline nickel compounds induce tumors, so it was assumed that factors other than solubility were involved. More recently, Costa (1995) has proposed an epigenetic model suggesting that tumor induction is related to the ability of the cell to incorporate the crystalline compound into the cell by phagocytosis. Costa showed that Syrian hamster cells undergoing transformation selectively phagocytosed the negatively charged crystalline nickel sulfide compounds and not the positively charged amorphous nickel sulfide particles. When a negative charge was induced on the amorphous nickel sulfide particles, they too were phagocytosed and were able to exhibit transformation potency equivalent to that of crystalline nickel sulfide particles. Inside the cell, the particles dissolved in the intracellular space, a process enchanced by the acidic pH of the cytoplasm. Therefore, transformation appeared to directly relate to the ability of the particle to enter the cell and increase intracellular nickel concentrations. The model is based upon the known ability of nickel compounds to enhance DNA chromatin condensation. DNA found in heterochromatin is hypermethylated for direct protein binding for increased condensation. Another theory is that nickel damages DNA indirectly through reactive oxygen species (McCoy and Kenny, 1992). This proposal is supported by evidence that the antioxidant vitamin E inhibits some chromosomal condensation caused by nickel (Lin et al., 1991).

Sunderman and Barber (1988) proposed that nickel interacts with DNA by replacement of Zn^{2+} with Ni^{2+} on the Zn^{2+} binding sites of DNA-binding proteins. Ni^{2+} has a similar ionic radius to Zn^{2+}. DNA-binding proteins or "finger loop domains" have been identified on some proto-oncogenes and are thought to be likely targets for metal toxicity.

Nickel Carbonyl Poisoning Metallic nickel combines with carbon monoxide to form nickel carbonyl ($Ni[CO]_4$), which decomposes to pure nickel and carbon monoxide on heating to 200°C (the Mond process). This reaction provides a convenient and efficient method for the refinement of nickel. However, nickel carbonyl is extremely toxic, and many cases of acute toxicity have been reported. The illness begins with headache, nausea, vomiting, and epigastric or chest pain, followed by cough, hyperpnea, cyanosis, gastrointestinal symptoms, and weakness. The symptoms may be accompanied by fever and leukocytosis and the more severe cases progress to pneumonia, respiratory failure, and eventually to cerebral edema and death (WHO, 1991).

Dermatitis Nickel dermatitis is one of the most common forms of allergic dermatitis: 4 to 9 percent of persons with contact dermatitis react positively to nickels patch tests. Sensitization might occur from any of the metal products in common use, such as coins and jewelry. The notion that increased ingestion of nickel-containing food increases the probability of external sensitization to nickel is supported by the finding that increased urinary nickel excretion is associated with episodes of acute nickel dermatitis (Liden et al., 1995).

Indicators of Nickel Toxicity Blood nickel levels immediately following exposure to nickel carbonyl provide a guideline as to the severity of exposure and indication for chelation therapy (Sunderman, 1979). Sodium diethyldithiocarbamate is the preferred drug, but other chelating agents, such as D-penicillamine and DMPS, provide some degree of protection from clinical effects.

ESSENTIAL METALS WITH POTENTIAL FOR TOXICITY

This group includes eight metals generally accepted as essential: cobalt, copper, iron, magnesium, manganese, molybdenum, selenium, and zinc. The traditional criteria for nutritionally essential metals is that deficiency produces either functional or structural abnormalities and that the abnormalities are related to or a consequence of specific biochemical changes that can be reversed by the presence of the essential metal (WHO, 1996). There are other metals in this chapter that may be nutritionally essential for vegetative life and may have beneficial health effects in humans but have not met the criteria for essentiality for human health. For essential trace elements, risk assessment requires consideration of both toxicity from excess exposures and health consequences as a result of deficiencies. There is increasing use of various standards that are designed to protect human health from excess exposure but provide risk for health effects from deficiency. Recognition of this problem prompted conferences in the United States and Scandinavia to address aspects of this problem (Mertz et al., 1994; Oskarsson et al., 1995). A methodology has been proposed to determine an acceptable level of oral intake for these metals (Nordberg et al., 1999).

Cobalt (Co)

Cobalt[1] is a relatively rare metal produced primarily as a by-product of other metals, chiefly copper. It is used in high-temperature alloys and in permanent magnets. Its salts are useful in paint dryers, as catalysts, and in the production of numerous pigments. Cobalt, in the form of cobalamin, is an essential component of vitamin B_{12} required for the production of red blood cells and prevention of pernicious anemia. Cobalamin is actually synthesized by intestinal flora, so that in actuality the nutritional requirement for cobalt in humans is as cobalamin produced by intestinal bacteria and not for colbalt ion per se. This consideration has led nutritionists not to regard cobalt as an essential element for humans. However, insufficient natural levels of cobalt in feed stock of sheep and cattle result in cobalt deficiency disease, characterized by anemia and loss of weight or retarded growth. If other requirements for cobalt exist, they are not well understood (WHO, 1996; Herbert, 1996).

The toxicokinetics and possible health effects of cobalt are summarized by Elinder and Friberg (1986), and Schrauzer (1995). Cobalt salts are generally well absorbed after oral ingestion, probably in the jejunum. Despite this fact, increased levels tend not to cause significant accumulation. About 80 percent of the ingested cobalt is excreted in the urine. Of the remaining portion, about 15 percent is excreted in the feces by an enterohepatic pathway, while the milk and sweat are other secondary routes of excretion. The total body burden has been estimated as 1.1 mg. Muscle contains the largest total fraction, but fat has the highest concentration. The liver, heart, and hair have significantly higher concentrations than other organs, but the concentration in these organs is relatively low. The normal levels in human urine and blood are about 1.0 and 0.18 μg/L, respectively. The blood level is largely associated with the concentration in red cells. Significant species differences have been observed in the excretion of radiocobalt. In rats and cattle, 80 percent is eliminated in the feces.

Cobalt has an erythropoietic effect when an excessive amount of cobalt is ingested by most mammals, including humans. High levels of chronic oral administration of cobalt for treatment of anemia may result in the production of goiter, and epidemiologic studies suggest that the incidence of goiter is higher in regions containing increased levels of cobalt in the water and soil. The goitrogenic effect has been elicited by the oral administration of 3 to 4 mg/kg to children in the course of treatment of sickle cell anemia. Toxicity resulting from overzealous therapeutic administration has been reported to produce vomiting, diarrhea, and a sensation of warmth. Intravenous administration leads to flushing of the face, increased blood pressure, slowed respiration, giddiness, tinnitus, and deafness due to nerve damage. Cardiomyopathy has been caused by an excessive intake of cobalt, >10 mg day, particularly from the drinking of beer to which cobalt was added to enhance its foaming qualities. The signs and symptoms were those of congestive heart failure. Autopsy findings have found a tenfold increase in the cardiac levels of cobalt.

Occupational inhalation of cobalt-containing dust in the cemented tungsten carbide industry may cause respiratory irritation at air concentrations of 0.002 to 0.01 mg/m^3. Higher concentrations (0.1 mg Co/m^3 or higher) may be a cause of "hard metal" pneumoconiosis, a progressive form of interstitial fibrosis. Skin contact is sometimes associated with an allergic dermatitis of an erythematous papular type. Affected persons may have positive skin tests.

Injection of cobalt in animal models produces myocardial degeneration. Also, hyperglycemia due to β-cell pancreatic damage has been reported after injection of cobalt into rats. Single and repeated subcutaneous or intramuscular injection of cobalt powder and salts in rats may cause sarcomas at the site of injection. Cobalt is only weakly mutagenic and there is no evidence of carcinogenicity from any other route of exposure.

Trivalent Chromium, Cr(III)

Chromium,[1] the most common form found in nature and chromium in biological materials, is probably always trivalent. There is no evidence that trivalent chromium is converted to hexavalent forms in biological systems. However, hexavalent chromium readily crosses cell membranes and is reduced intracellularly to trivalent chromium.

Essentiality Cr (III) is considered an essential trace nutrient serving as a component of the "glucose tolerance factor." Evidence for the physiologic role of chromium is summarized by Stoecker (1996). It is thought to be a cofactor for insulin action and to have a role in the peripheral activities of this hormone by forming a ter-

[1] Atomic weight, 58.93; periodic table group, VIII; valence, +2 or +3; discovered in 1735.

[1] Atomic weight, 52; periodic table group, VIB; valence, +3; discovered in 1797.

nary complex with insulin receptors, facilitating the attachment of insulin to these sites. The role for chromium in carbohydrate metabolism is based on epidemiologic studies showing that chromium supplementation improved the efficiency of insulin effects on blood lipid profiles. Of 15 controlled studies, only three found no effect on glucose, insulin, or lipids. Subjects with some degree of impaired glucose tolerance were more responsive to chromium supplementation than others. In studies of patients whose total parenteral nutrition solutions contained no chromium, chromium supplementation reduced insulin requirements and glucose intolerance. Other evidence for a physiologic role for chromium is from animal studies. Decreased weight gain has been reported for rats, mice, and guinea pigs whose diets were depleted of chromium. Also, chromium in mouse liver is concentrated in the nuclei 48 h after intraperitoneal injection. Also, Cr(III) bound to DNA in vitro, thus enhancing RNA synthesis. Chromium supplementation in diets of "travel-stressed cattle" significantly decreased serum cortisol and increased serum immunoglobulin. It is recognized, however, that further research is needed to resolve questions about the structure and function of the glucose tolerance factor and other possible physiologic functions of Cr(III). The Food and Nutrition Board of the United States Academy of Sciences has established that an estimated safe and adequate daily intake for chromium in adults ranges from 50 to 200 μg (NRC, 1989).

Copper (Cu)

Copper[1] is widely distributed in nature and is a nutritionally essential element. Ambient air levels are generally low in the United States; for the general population, food, beverages, and drinking water are potential sources of excess exposure. Daily intake of copper in adults varies between 0.9 and 2.2 mg. Intake in children has been estimated to be 0.6 to 0.8 mg/day (0.07 to 0.1 mg/kg body weight per day) (WHO, 1998). The EPA's maximum contaminant level for copper in drinking water is 1.3 mg/L, but this is under revision (EPA, 1994). The provisional WHO guideline for copper in drinking water is 2 mg/L (WHO, 1993). Copper exposures in industry are to particulates in miners or to metal fumes in smelting operations, welding, and related activities.

Toxicokinetics The metabolism and health effects of copper are reviewed by WHO (1996), Sheinberg and Sternlieb (1996), Chan et al. (1998), Harris (1997), and NRC (2000). An overview of copper metabolism is shown in Fig. 23-8.

Gastrointestinal absorption of copper is normally regulated by homeostatic mechanisms. It is transported in serum bound initially to albumin and later more firmly to ceruloplasmin and transcuprein. The normal serum level of copper is 120 to 145 μg/L. The bile is the normal excretory pathway and plays a primary role in copper homeostasis. Most copper is stored in liver and bone marrow, where it may be bound to metallothionein. Copper as Cu(II) entering into hepatocytes is initially reduced and complexed by glutathione prior to binding with metallothionein. Alternatively, copper entering the cell may be exported by a copper ATPase translocase. Copper is not an effective inducer of metallothionein relative to zinc or cadmium. Nevertheless, copper bound to metallothionein is thought to be a normal storage form of copper, particularly in infancy and childhood. Isolated hepatic cells are protected from copper toxicity by prior induction of metallothionein with zinc. Copper-metallothionein accumulates in lysosomes, facilitating the biliary excretion of copper.

The newborn is dependent on stored copper, which may not be adequate in premature infants. The amount of copper in milk is not enough to maintain adequate copper levels in the liver, lungs, and spleen of the newborn. Tissue levels gradually decline up to about 10 years of age, remaining relatively constant thereafter. Brain levels, on the other hand, tend to almost double from infancy to adulthood. The ratio of newborn to adult liver copper levels shows considerable species difference: human, 15:4; rat, 6:4, and rabbit, 1:6. Since urinary copper levels may be increased by soft water, concentrations of approximately 60 μg/L under these conditions are not uncommon.

Essentiality Copper is a component of all living cells and is associated with many oxidative processes. It is an essential component of several metalloenzymes, including type A oxidases and type b monamine oxidases. Of the type B oxidases, cytochrome *c*-oxidase is probably the most important because it catalyzes a key reaction in energy metabolism. Of the type A oxidases, lysyl oxidase plays a major role in elastin and collagen synthesis. There are two forms of superoxide dismutase. The copper/zinc superoxide dismutase is present in the cytosol of most cells, particularly brain, thyroid, liver, and erythrocytes. Both dismutases scavenger superoxide radical by reducing them to hydrogen peroxide. Impairment of the function of these enzymes is responsible for the various diseases associated with copper deficiency (Chan et al., 1998).

Deficiency Copper deficiency is uncommon in humans. The most susceptibile are low-birth-weight infants and infants who were malnourished after birth. Copper deficiency is manifest clinically by hypochromic, microcytic anemia refractory to iron as well as susceptibility to infections. This deficiency is sometimes accompanied by bone abnormalities. Less frequent manifestations are hypopigmentation of the hair and hypotonia. Molybdenum also influences tissue levels of copper. Biomarkers of copper deficiency include ceruloplasmin and serum copper levels, levels of low-density lipoproteins, and cytochrome oxidase activity.

Toxicity Experimental studies in humans suggest that ingestion of drinking water with >3 mg Cu/L will produce gastrointestinal symptoms including nausea, vomiting, and diarrhea (Pizzaro et al., 1999). Ingestion of large amounts of copper salts, most frequently copper sulfate, may produce hepatic necrosis and death. Epidemiologic studies have not found any relation between copper exposure and cancer (WHO, 1998). Individuals with glucose-6-phosphate deficiency may be at increased risk for the hematologic effects of copper, but there is uncertainty as to the magnitude of the risk (Goldstein et al., 1985).

Wilson's Disease Wilson's disease is characterized by the excessive accumulation of copper in liver, brain, kidneys, and cornea. Serum ceruloplasmin is low and serum copper that is not bound to ceruloplasmin is elevated. Urinary excretion of copper is high. Clinical abnormalities of the nervous system, liver, kidneys, and cornea are related to copper accumulation. The disorder is sometimes referred to as *hepatolenticular degeneration* in reference to effects of copper accumulation in the brain. Patients with Wilson's disease have impaired biliary excretion of copper, which is believed to be the fundamental cause of copper overload. Reversal of abnormal copper metabolism is achieved by liver transplantation, con-

[1]Atomic weight, 63.5; periodic table group, IB; valence, +1 or +2; discovered 5000 years ago.

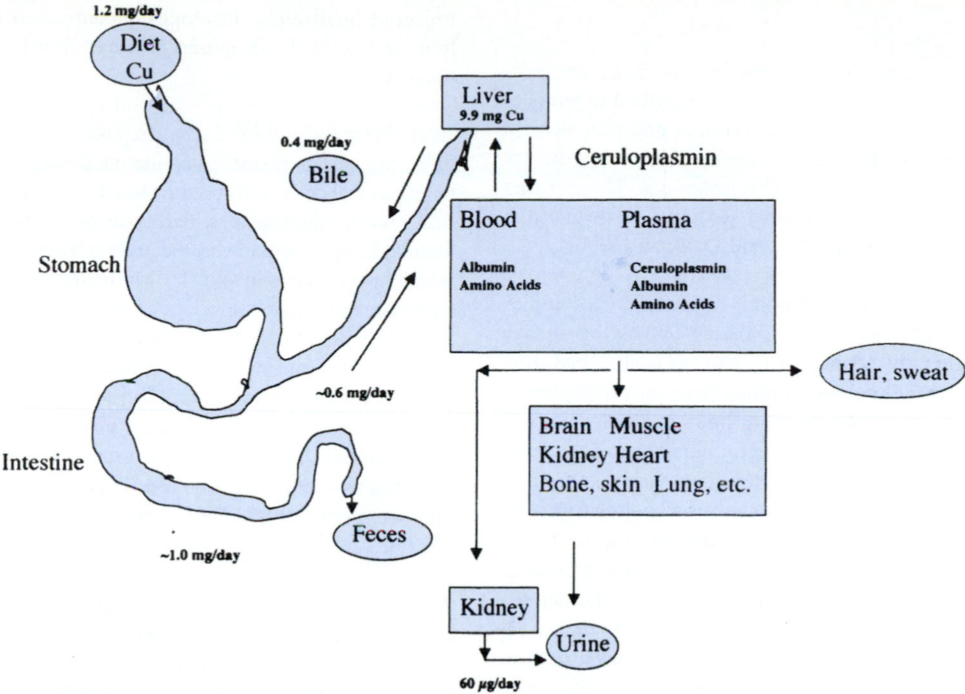

Figure 23-8. Overview of copper absorption, transport, and excretion.

The liver receives copper from the intestine via the portal circulation and redistributes the copper to the tissue via ceruloplasmin, albumin, and amino acids. Approximately half the copper consumed is not absorbed and passes into the feces. Another two-thirds of the daily intake is returned to the liver and released into the bile. Consequently fecal excretion accounts quantitatively for nearly all of the copper consumed as the systems endeavor to stay in balance. A small amount, 60 μg/day, is excreted by the kidney via the urine, and still lesser amounts appear in hair and sweat. This interplay among the various systems maintains homeostasis and balance throughout the organism. The values in the figure are based on a dietary input of 1.2 mg/day. [Adapted from Harris (1997).]

firming that the basic defect is in the liver. Genetic studies have identified a linkage between the Wilson's disease locus (WND) and the erythrocyte enzyme esterase D, establishing that the defect is on chromosome 13 (Frydman et al., 1985). The abnormal gene product, WND protein, converts the energy from ATP hydrolysis to cation transport and is responsible for copper secretion from the liver cell into the biliary canaliculus (Tanzi et al., 1993). However, there appears to be several polymorphisms of the defect, which may explain the clinical variability in the disorder. Diagnosis may be suspected with elevated serum copper but must be confirmed by liver biopsy and elevated liver copper (normal 15 to 55 μg/g; Wilson's disease, >250 μg/g to as high as 300 μg/g). Fibroblasts from persons with Wilson's disease have increased intracellular copper when cultured in Eagle's minimum essential medium with fetal bovine serum (Chan et al., 1983). Clinical improvement can be achieved by chelation of copper with penicillamine (Walshe, 1964). Trien [triethylene tetramine (2HCl)] is also effective and has been used in patients with Wilson's disease who have toxic reactions to penicillamine. The antagonistic effect of zinc on copper absorption may also be useful in the treatment of Wilson's disease (Brewer, 1993). An animal model of Wilson's disease, the Long-Evans cinnamon (LEC) rat, has excessive liver copper and diminished biliary excretion (Schilsky et al., 1994).

Menke's Disease Menke's disease, or Menke's "kinky-hair syndrome," is a sex-linked trait characterized by peculiar hair, failure to thrive, severe mental retardation, neurologic impairment, and death usually by 5 years of age. Bones are osteoporotic with flared metaphases of the long bones and bones of the skull. There is extensive degeneration of the cerebral cortex and of white matter. The symptoms result from copper deficiency and effects on copper-containing enzymes. The gene responsible for Menke's disease produces a cation transporting ATPase and has some homologies with the gene responsible for Wilson's disease (Mercer et al., 1993).

Indian Childhood Cirrhosis (ICC) ICC is a peculiar disorder occurring in young children; it is characterized by jaundice due to an insidious but progressive liver disease. Diagnosis is by liver biopsy. Two distinguishing features are a widespread brown orcein staining (copper) and intralobular fibrosis progressing to portal cirrhosis and inflammation (Pradham et al., 1983). Etiology is not known but suspected to be related to bottle feeding of copper contaminated from storage in brass vessels. However, epidemiologic studies suggest an autosomal recessive genetic component because of strong familial occurrence and high consanguinity among affected children (Sethi et al., 1993).

Idiopathic Copper Toxicosis or Non-Indian Childhood Cirrhosis There are scattered reports of a disorder in children similar to ICC occurring in some western countries (WHO, 1998). The largest non-Indian series of cases are reported by Muller et al. (1996) from the Tyrol region of Austria. This group also used copper vessels to store milk, and the incidence of the disorder has declined since replacement of the copper vessels. A number of other cases have been reported from other parts of the world, some with increased amounts of copper in drinking water (Fewtrell et al., 1996).

Iron (Fe)

The major scientific and medical interest in iron[1] is as an essential metal, but toxicologic considerations are important in terms of iron deficiency and accidental acute exposures and chronic iron overload due to idiopathic hemochromatosis or as a consequence of excess dietary iron or frequent blood transfusions. The complex metabolism of iron and mechanisms of toxicity are detailed by Spivey Fox and Rader (1988) and Yip and Dallman (1996).

Toxicokinetics The disposition of iron is regulated by a complex mechanism to maintain homeostasis, mainly involving intake, stores, and loss. Generally, about 2 to 15 percent is absorbed from the gastrointestinal tract, whereas elimination of absorbed iron, is only about 0.01 percent per day (percent body burden or amount absorbed). Iron absorption is influenced by quantity and bioavailability of dietary iron, amount of storage iron, and rate of erythrocyte production. The best-known enhancer is vitamin C (ascorbic acid). Dietary inhibitors of nonheme iron absorption include calcium phosphate, bran, phytic acid, and polyphenols present in some plants. During periods of increased iron need (childhood, pregnancy, or blood loss), absorption of iron is greatly increased. Absorption occurs in two steps: (1) absorption of ferrous ions from the intestinal lumen into the mucosal cells and (2) transfer from the mucosal cell to plasma, where it is bound to transferrin for transfer to storage sites. Transferrin is a β_1-globulin with a molecular weight of 75,000 and is produced in the liver. As ferrous ion is released into plasma, it becomes oxidized by oxygen in the presence of ferroxidase I, which is identical to ceruloplasmin. There are 3 to 5 g of iron in the body. About two-thirds is bound to hemoglobin, 10 percent in myoglobin and iron-containing enzymes, and the remainder is bound to the iron storage proteins ferritin and hemosiderin. Exposure to iron induces synthesis of apoferritin, which then binds ferrous ions. The ferrous ion becomes oxidized, probably by histidine and cysteine residues and carbonyl groups. Iron may be released from ferritin by reducing agents. Ascorbic acid, cysteine, and reduced glutathione release iron slowly. Normally, excess ingested iron is excreted, and some is contained within shed intestinal cells and in bile and urine and in even smaller amounts in sweat, nails, and hair. Total iron excretion is usually on the order of 0.5 mg/day.

Iron Deficiency Iron deficiency is the most common nutritional deficiency in the United States and worldwide, affecting older infants, young children, and women of childbearing age. The third National Health and Nutrition Examination Survey 1991–1994 identified about 5 percent of children 1 to 2 years of age as iron-deficient. Infants are born with stores of iron roughly proportional to birth weight. Low-birth-weight infants have less stores than full-term infants, so that iron stores are depleted earlier, often by 2 to 3 months of age. The critical period for iron deficiency is between the ages of 6 months and 2 years. The major manifestation of iron deficiency is anemia, diagnosed in the presence of microcytic hypochromic red blood cells and laboratory evidence of iron deficiency. Iron status is determined by measurement of parameters of iron metabolism. For example, low serum ferritin is evidence of iron deficiency. A rise in hemoglobin levels should occur promptly after iron administration. Other effects of iron deficiency include impaired intellectual development, decreased resistance to infection, and possibly increased susceptibility to lead and cadmium toxicity.

Iron Overload With excess exposure to iron or iron overload, there may be a further increase in ferritin synthesis in hepatic parenchymal cells. In fact, the ability of the liver to synthesize ferritin exceeds the rate at which lysosomes can process iron for excretion. Lysosomes convert the protein from ferritin to hemosiderin, which then remains in situ. The formation of hemosiderin from ferritin is not well understood, but it seems to involve denaturation of the apoferritin molecule. With increasing iron loading, ferritin concentration appears to reach a maximum, and a greater portion of iron is found in hemosiderin. Both ferritin and hemosiderin are, in fact, storage sites for intracellular metal and are protective in that they maintain intracellular iron in bound form. A portion of the iron taken up by cells of the reticuloendothelial system enters a labile iron pool available for erythropoiesis and becomes stored as ferritin.

Toxicity Acute iron poisoning from accidental ingestion of iron-containing medicines is the most common cause of acute iron toxicity. It most often occurs in children. A decrease in occurrences of this type followed the use of "childproof" lids on prescription medicines. Severe toxicity occurs after the ingestion of more than 0.5 g of iron or 2.5 g of ferrous sulfate. Toxicity becomes manifest with vomiting 1 to 6 h after ingestion. This is followed by signs of shock and metabolic acidosis, liver damage, and coagulation defects within the next couple of days. Late effects may include renal failure and hepatic cirrhosis. The mechanism of the toxicity is thought to begin with acute mucosal cell damage and absorption of ferrous ions directly into the circulation, which causes capillary endothelial cell damage in the liver.

Chronic iron toxicity or iron overload in adults is a more common problem. There are three basic ways in which excessive amounts of iron can accumulate in the body. The first circumstance is hereditary hemochromatosis due to abnormal absorption of iron from the intestinal tract. The frequency of homozygosity is approximately 3 to 4 per 1000 in populations of European extraction. The heterozygote (incidence about 1 in 10) may also have a lesser degree of increased iron absorption. A second possible cause of iron overload is excess dietary iron. The African Bantu who prepares their daily food and brew fermented beverages in iron pots are classic subjects for this form of iron overload. Sporadic other cases occur owing to excessive ingestion of iron-containing tonics or medicines. The third circumstance in which iron overload may occur is from the regular requirement for blood transfusion for some form of refractory anemia and is sometimes referred to as *transfusional siderosis.* The pathologic consequences of iron overload are similar regardless of basic cause. The body iron content is increased to between 20 and 40 g. Most of the extra iron is hemosiderin. The greatest concentrations are in the parenchymal cells of liver and pancreas as well as in endocrine organs and the heart. Iron in reticuloendothelial cells (in the spleen) is greatest in transfusional siderosis. Further clinical effects may include disturbances in liver function, diabetes mellitus, and even endocrine disturbances and cardiovascular effects. At the cellular level, increased lipid peroxidation occurs, with consequent membrane damage to mitochondria, microsomes, and other cellular organelles. There is epidemiologic evidence for a relationship between iron levels and cardiovascular disease (Sa-

[1]Atomic weight, 56; periodic table group, VIII; valence, +2, +3, +4, or +6; discovered in prehistoric times.

lomen et al., 1992). It has also been suggested that women who are heterozygous for hereditary hemochromatosis are at increased risk for cardiovascular disease (Roest et al., 1999). Experimental evidence suggests that iron may contribute to lipid peroxidation in an early step in the formation of atherosclerotic lesions. Macrophages and endothelial cells are involved, but the details of the mechanism are only speculative (de Valk et al., 1999). Iron loading in mice can alter and damage cellular organelles in heart muscle, including mitochondria, lysosomes, and endoplasmic reticulum (Bartfay et al., 1999).

Treatment of acute iron poisoning is directed toward removal of the ingested iron from the gastrointestinal tract by inducing vomiting or gastric lavage and providing corrective therapy for systemic effects such as acidosis and shock. Desferrioxamine is the chelating agent of choice for the treatment of iron overload absorbed from acute exposure as well as for removal of tissue iron in hemosiderosis. Repeated phlebotomy can remove as much as 20 g of iron per year. Inhalation of iron oxide fumes or dust by workers in metal industries may result in deposition of iron particles in lungs, producing an x-ray appearance resembling silicosis. These effects are seen in hematite miners, iron and steelworkers, and arc welders. Hematite is the most important iron ore (mainly Fe_2O_3).

Magnesium (Mg)

Magnesium[1] is a nutritionally essential metal that can be responsible for adverse health effects due to deficiency or excess (Birch, 1995; Shils, 1996). Nuts, cereals, seafoods, and meats are high dietary sources of magnesium. The drinking water content of magnesium increases with the hardness of the water. Magnesium citrate, oxide, sulfate, hydroxide, and carbonate are widely taken as antacids or cathartics. Magnesium hydroxide, or milk of magnesia, is one of the constituents of the universal antidote for poisoning. Topically, the sulfate also is used widely to relieve inflammation. Magnesium sulfate may be used as a parenterally administered central nervous system depressant. Its most frequent use for this purpose is in the treatment of seizures associated with eclampsia of pregnancy and acute nephritis.

Toxicokinetics Magnesium is a cofactor of many enzymes involved in intermediary metabolism. In the glycolytic cycle converting glucose to pyruvate, there are seven key enzymes that require Mg^{2+}. It is also involved in the citric acid cycle and in the beta oxidation of fatty acids. Magnesium salts are poorly absorbed from the intestine. In cases of overload, this may be due in part to their dehydrating action. Magnesium is absorbed mainly in the small intestine; the colon also absorbs some. Calcium and magnesium are competitive with respect to their absorptive sites, and excess calcium may partially inhibit the absorption of magnesium. Magnesium is excreted into the digestive tract by the bile and pancreatic and intestinal juices. A small amount of radiomagnesium given intravenously appears in the gastrointestinal tract. The serum levels are remarkably constant. There is an apparent obligatory urinary loss of magnesium, which amounts to about 12 mg/day, and the urine is the major route of excretion under normal conditions. Magnesium found in the stool is probably not absorbed. Magnesium is filtered by the glomeruli and reabsorbed by the renal tubules. In the blood plasma, about 65 percent is in the ionic form while the remainder is bound to protein. The former is that which appears in the glomerular filtrate. Excretion also occurs in the sweat and milk. As in the case of other essential elements, physiologic homeostatic mechanisms prevent large fluctuations in blood through changes in absorption and excretion. Approximately 70 percent of serum magnesium is ultrafilterable, and about 95 percent of filtered magnesium is reabsorbed, an important factor in maintaining magnesium homeostasis. Endocrine activity—particularly of the adrenocortical hormones, aldosterone, and parathyroid hormone—also has an effect on magnesium levels, although this may be related to the interaction of calcium and magnesium. Tissue distribution studies indicate that of the 20-g body burden, the majority is intracellular in the bone and muscle including the myocardium, but some magnesium is present in every cell of the body. Bone concentration of magnesium decreases as calcium increases.

Deficiency Deficiency may occur and, in humans, is usually a complication of various disease states that cause intake of magnesium to be impaired (malabsorption syndromes), renal dysfunction with excessive losses, and endocrine disorders. Deficiency in humans causes neuromuscular irritability, frank tetany, and even convulsions. There is a decrease in the magnesium content of ischemic hearts, but the cause and significance are not known.

Deficiency in animals may result from ingestion of grasses grown in magnesium-poor soil. The deficiency is called *grass staggers* in cattle and *magnesium tetany* in calves.

Toxicity Magnesium toxicity can occur when magnesium-containing drugs, usually antacids, are ingested chronically by individuals with serious renal insufficiency. The toxic effects may progress from nausea and vomiting to hypotension, electrocardiograph abnormalities, and secondary central nervous system effects. Magnesium toxicity can be counteracted with calcium infusion.

With industrial exposures, increases of serum magnesium up to twice the normal levels have failed to produce ill effects but were accompanied by calcium increases. Freshly generated magnesium oxide can cause metal fume fever if inhaled in sufficient amounts, analogous to the effect caused by zinc oxide. Both zinc and magnesium exposure of animals produced similar effects.

Manganese (Mn)

Manganese[1] is a transitional metal and can exist in 11 oxidation states, from -3 to $+7$. The most common valences are $+2$, $+4$, and $+7$. The most common valence in biological systems is $+2$; $+4$ is present as MnO_2. Mn^{3+} is also important in biological systems. It is the oxidative state of manganese in superoxide dismutase and is probably the form that interacts with Fe^{3+}. Cycling between Mn^{2+} and Mn^{3+} may be potentially deleterious to biological systems because it can involve the generation of free radicals. Manganese is an essential element and is a cofactor for a number of enzymatic reactions, particularly those involved in phosphorylation, cholesterol, and fatty acids synthesis. Manganese is present in all living organisms. The principal source of intake is food. Veg-

[1]Atomic weight, 55; periodic table group, IIA; valence, +2; discovered in 1831.

[1]Atomic weight, 55; periodic table group, VIIB; valence, +1, +4, +6, or +7; isolated in 1774.

etables, the germinal portions of grains, fruits, nuts, tea, and some spices are rich in manganese (Keen and Zidenberg-Cherr, 1996). Daily manganese intake ranges from 2 to 9 mg. There is current interest in the toxicology of manganese because of potential exposure from the use of the manganese-containing fuel additive MMT (methylcyclopentadienyl Mn tricarbonyl) as a replacement for lead containing additives in gasoline.

The industrial use of manganese has also expanded in recent years as a ferroalloy in the iron industry and as a component of alloys used in welding (Apostoli et al., 2000).

Toxicokinetics Gastrointestinal absorption is less than 5 percent and occurs throughout the length of the small intestine. Manganese is transported in plasma bound to a β_1-globulin, thought to be transferrin, and is widely distributed in the body. Manganese concentrates in mitochondria, so that tissues rich in these organelles—including the pancreas, liver, kidneys, and intestines—have the highest concentrations of manganese. The biological half-life in the body is 37 days. Manganese readily crosses the blood-brain barrier and its half-life in the brain is longer than in the whole body. Manganese is eliminated in the bile and is reabsorbed in the intestine, but the principal route of excretion is with feces.

Deficiency Manganese deficiency has been produced in many species of animals, but so far there are questions about whether deficiency has actually been demonstrated in humans (WHO, 1996). Deficiency in animals results in impaired growth, skeletal abnormalities, and disturbed reproductive function.

Toxicity There are few reported cases of manganese toxicity from oral ingestion. Homeostatic mechanisms involving the liver and biliary excretion, gastrointestinal mechanisms for excreting excess manganese, and perhaps the adrenal cortex, plus the tendency for extremely large doses of manganese salts to cause gastrointestinal irritation, account for the lack of systemic toxicity following oral administration or dermal application. The most common form of manganese toxicity is the result of chronic inhalation of airborne manganese in mines, steel mills, and some chemical industries (ATSDR, 1997). Industrial toxicity from inhalation exposure, generally to manganese dioxide in mining or manufacturing, is of two types: The first, manganese pneumonitis, is the result of acute exposure. Men working in plants with high concentrations of manganese dust show an incidence of respiratory disease 30 times greater than normal. Pathologic changes include epithelial necrosis followed by mononuclear proliferation.

The second and more serious type of disease resulting from chronic inhalation exposure to manganese dioxide, generally over a period of more than 2 years, involves the central nervous system. Chronic manganese poisoning (manganism) produces a neuropsychiatric disorder characterized by irritability, difficulty in walking, speech disturbances, and compulsive behavior that may include running, fighting, and singing. If the condition persists, a mask-like face, retropulsion or propulsion, and a Parkinson-like syndrome develop. The outstanding feature of manganese encephalopathy has been classified as severe selective damage to the subthalamic nucleus and pallidum. These symptoms and the pathologic lesions—degenerative changes in the basal ganglia—make the analogy to Parkinson's disease feasible. In addition to the central nervous system changes, liver cirrhosis is frequently observed. Victims of chronic manganese poisoning tend to recover slowly, even when removed from the excessive exposure. Metal-sequestering agents have not produced remarkable recovery; L-dopa, which is used in the treatment of Parkinson's disease, has been more consistently effective in the treatment of chronic manganese poisoning than in Parkinson's disease (Cotzias et al., 1971).

The oral absorption of manganese is increased by iron deficiency, which may contribute to variations in individual susceptibility. The syndrome of chronic nervous system effects has been duplicated only in squirrel monkeys by inhalation or intraperitoneal injection.

Molybdenum (Mo)

Molybdenum[1] is an essential element and may exist in multiple oxidation states, +3, +4, +5, and +6, facilitating electron transfer. Molybdenum concentration of food varies considerably, depending on the environment in which the food was grown. Molybdenum is added in trace amounts to fertilizers to stimulate plant growth. The average daily human intake in food ranges from 120 to 240 μg/day. The human requirement for molybdenum is low and easily provided by a common U.S. diet; the provisional recommended range for the dietary intake of molybdenum is based on average reported intakes. The concentration of molybdenum in urban air is minimal. Most public water supplies contribute between 2 and 8 μg/day. Excess exposure can result in toxicity to animals and humans (NRC, 1989).

The most important mineral source of molybdenum is molybdenite (MoS_2). The United States is the major world producer of molybdenum. The industrial uses of this metal include the manufacture of high temperature–resistant steel alloys for use in gas turbines and jet aircraft engines and in the production of catalysts, lubricants, and dyes.

Toxicokinetics The soluble hexavalent compounds are well absorbed from the gastrointestinal tract into the liver (Nielson, 1996). It is a component of xanthine oxidase, which has a role in purine metabolism and has been shown to be a component of aldehyde oxidase and sulfite oxidase. In plants, it is necessary for the fixing of atmospheric nitrogen by bacteria at the start of protein synthesis. Increased molybdenum intake in experimental animals has been shown to increase tissue levels of xanthine oxidase. In humans, molybdenum is contained principally in the liver, kidneys, fat, and blood. Of the approximate total of 9 mg in the body, most is concentrated in the liver, kidneys, adrenal, and omentum. More than 50 percent of molybdenum in the liver is contained in a nonprotein cofactor bound to the mitochondrial outer membrane and can be transferred to an apoenzyme, transforming it into an active enzyme molecule. The molybdenum level is relatively low in the newborn and increases until age 20, declining in concentration thereafter. More than half of the molybdenum excreted is in the urine. The blood level is in association with the level in red blood cells. The excretion of molybdenum is rapid, mainly as molybdate. Excesses may be excreted also by the bile, particularly the hexavalent forms.

Deficiency Molybdenum deficiency has been described in various animal species and consists of disturbances in uric acid metabolism and sulfite metabolism, but the clinical manifestation of molybdenum deficiency in humans is still evolving. Molybdenum is a component of sulfite oxidase, which converts sulfite to sulfates.

[1]Atomic weight, 96; periodic table group, VIB; valence, +2, +3, +4, +5(?), or +6.

Molybdenum deficiency resulting from parenteral methionine therapy has been described and is characterized by mouth and gum disorders as well as hypouricemia, hyperoxypurinemia, mental disturbances, and coma. The symptoms are indicative of a defect in sulfur-containing amino acid metabolism; supplementation with ammonium molybdate improved the clinical condition, reversed the sulfur handling defect, and normalized uric acid production. A rare genetic disease characterized by a deficiency of sulfite oxidase has been identified in humans and is characterized by severe brain damage; mental retardation; dislocation of the ocular lenses; increased output of sulfite, *S*-sulfocysteine, and thiosulfate; and decreased output of sulfate (Nielson, 1996).

Toxicity Chronic exposure to excess molybdenum in humans is characterized by high uric acid levels in serum and urine, loss of appetite, diarrhea, anemia, and slow growth. A gout-like disease has been observed in inhabitants of a high-molybdenum area of a province of Russia (Chan et al., 1998). Experimental studies have revealed differences in toxicity of molybdenum salts. In nonruminants, intake of 100 to 5000 mg/kg in food and water was required to produce clinical toxicity. In rats, molybdenum trioxide at a dose of 100 mg/kg/day by inhalation was irritating to the eyes and mucous membranes and subsequently lethal. After repeated oral administration at sufficient levels, fatty degeneration of the liver and kidney was induced (Nielson, 1996).

Selenium (Se)

The availability as well as the toxic potential of selenium[1] and selenium compounds is related to their chemical form and, most importantly, to solubility. Selenium occurs in nature and biological systems as selenate (Se^{6+}), selenite (Se^{4+}), elemental selenium (Se^{0}), and selenide (Se^{22}); deficiency leads to a cardiomyopathy in mammals, including humans (WHO, 1987; Levander and Burk, 1996).

Foodstuffs are a daily source of selenium. Seafoods, especially shrimp, and meat, milk products, and grains provide the largest amounts in the diet. Levels of selenium in river water vary, depending on environmental and geological factors; 0.02 ppm has been reported as a representative estimate. Selenium has also been detected in urban air, presumably from sulfur-containing materials.

Toxicokinetics Absorption of selenium does not appear to be regulated and appears to be very high, above 50 percent, whereas selenites and elemental selenium are virtually insoluble. Because of their insolubility, these forms may be regarded as a form of inert selenium sink. Elemental selenium is probably not absorbed from the gastrointestinal tract. Absorption of selenite is from the duodenum. Monogastric animals have a higher intestinal absorption than ruminants, probably because selenite is reduced to an insoluble form in rumen. Over 90 percent of milligram doses of sodium selenite may be absorbed by humans and widely distributed in organs, with the highest accumulation initially in the liver and kidneys, but appreciable levels remain in the blood, brain, myocardium, skeletal muscle, and testes. Selenium is transferred through the placenta to the fetus, and it also appears in milk. Levels in milk are dependent on dietary intake. Selenium in red cells is associated with glutathione peroxidase and is about three times more concentrated than in plasma. The excretion pattern of a single exposure to selenite appears to have at least two phases, the first being rapid, with as much as 15 to 40 percent of the absorbed dose excreted in the urine the first week. During the second phase there is an exponential excretion of the remainder of the dose, with a half-life of 103 days. The half-life of Se-methionine is 234 days. In the steady state, urine contains about twice as much as feces, and increased urinary levels provide a measure of exposure. Urinary selenium is usually less than 100 μg/L. Excretory products appear in sweat and expired air. The latter may have a garlicky odor due to dimethyl selenide (WHO, 1987).

[1]Atomic weight, 79; periodic table group, VIA; valence, −2, +4, or +6; discovered in 1817.

Essentiality Selenates are relatively soluble compounds, similar to sulfates, and are readily taken up by biological systems. Selenium metabolism is regulated to meet several metabolic needs and is outlined in Fig. 23-9.

Selenophosphate is an anabolic form of selenium involved in the synthesis of selenoproteins and seleno-tRNAs. Selenoprotein synthesis is regulated transcriptionally by tissue specificity, cell development, and environmental factors. Most selenium in animal tissues is present in two forms, selenomethionein, which is incorporated in place of methionine in a variety of proteins, and selenocysteine, a cofactor for both glutathione peroxidase, an enzyme of the antioxidant defense system and type 1 iodothyronine deiodinase, and selenoprotein P. Both enzymes contain one unit of selenocysteine at each of four catalytic sites. Glutathione peroxidase uses glutathione to reduce peroxides in cells and, in this way, protects membrane lipids and possibly proteins and nucleic acids from damage by oxidants or free radicals. It is present in many tissues and in high concentrations in liver, lung, stomach mucosa, erythrocytes and skeletal muscle and has both extracellular and intracellular forms. Type 1 iodothyronine is present in liver, kidney, and skeletal muscle and catalyzes the conversion of thyroxine (T_4) to triodothyronine (T_3). Deficiency of the cofactor may lead to hypothyroidism in the elderly. Selenoprotein P is an abundant extracellular selenoprotein that contains multiple selenocysteine residues and may have an antioxidant functioning in the extracellular space. Biologically active selenium can be assessed by measuring glutathione peroxidase and selenoprotein P concentration. The requirement for selenium is related to the degree of oxidant activity and the supply of nutrients such as zinc, copper, manganese, iron, and vitamin E, so that increased amounts of these elements increase the need for selenium.

Selenium Deficiency The most extensively documented deficiency of selenium in humans is Keshan disease. This is an endemic cardiomyopathy first discovered in Keshan county in the People's Republic of China in 1935. It occurs most frequently in children under 15 years of age and in women of childbearing age. The disease is characterized clinically by various degrees of cardiomegaly and cardiac decompensation, and the histopathology of the myocardium consists of the degeneration and necrosis of myocardial fibers and their replacement by fibrosis and scar formation (Chen et al., 1980). Occurrence of the disease was invariably associated with a lower content of selenium in the diet of maize and rice than that in grain grown in unaffected areas. The average selenium concentration in the hair of residents of affected areas was 0.122 ± 0.010 ppm versus 0.270 ± 0.066 ppm in the hair of people in unaffected areas. Also, low glutathione peroxidase activities of whole blood in the affected population coincided with low blood selenium levels in affected areas. It was suggested that

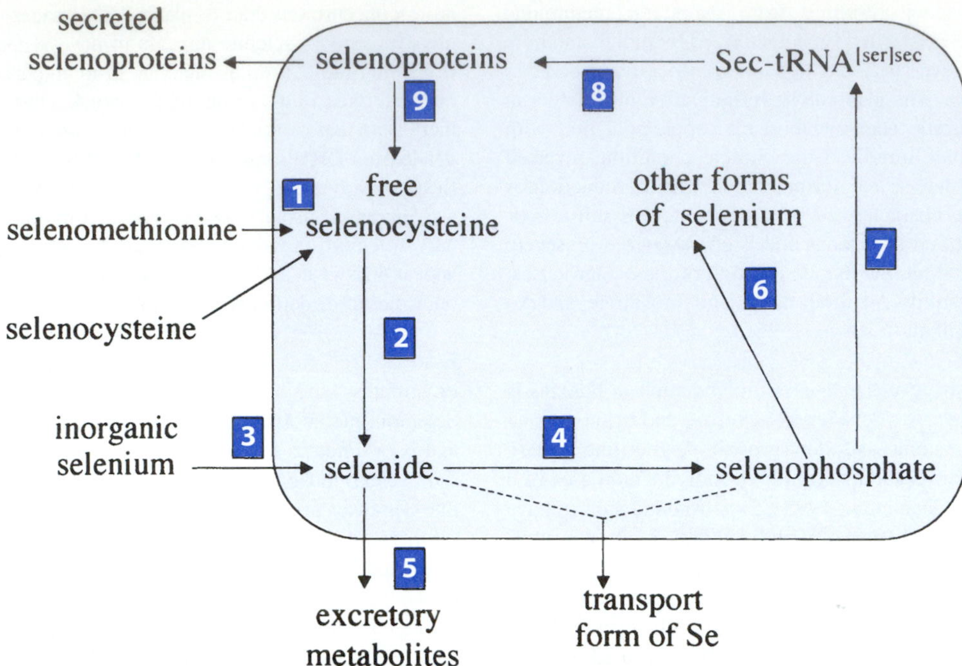

Figure 23-9. Regulated selenium metabolism.

The box represents the cell. The numbers in the squares indicate (1) the transulfuration pathway, (2) selenocysteine β-lyase, (3) reduction by glutathione, (4) selenophosphate synthetase, (5) methylation, (6) replacement of sulfur in tRNA by selenium, (7) replacement of oxygen in serine with selenium to produce selenocysteine, (8) decoding of UGA in mRNA with insertion of selenocysteine into primary structure of protein, and (9) proteolytic breakdown of proteins. The origin and identity of the transport form of selenium is unknown. It might arise from selenide or selenophosphate, as indicated by the broken lines. [Adapted from Levander and Burk

the low blood selenium content and low blood glutathione peroxidase activity might play a role in the myocardial lesions. Administration of sodium selenite greatly reduced the incidence of the disease—a fact that provides additional support for the role of selenium deficiency in the etiology of the disorder.

Deficiency of selenium in lambs and calves produces congenital "white muscle disease," a form of nutritionally induced muscular dystrophy. Deficiency of selenium produces liver necrosis in rats, a bleeding disorder in poultry, and cellular necrosis in the liver, kidneys, and skeletal and heart muscle in mice, resulting in cardiac failure and death. In each of these entities the health effect is prevented by adding selenium to the diet, so that now there are well-defined dietary requirements for selenium for livestock and poultry (WHO, 1987).

Toxicity Selenium toxicity occurs when the intake exceeds the excretory capacity. The potential toxicity of selenium was first suspected over 50 years ago and, through the years, well-defined syndromes of toxicity have been described in animals and humans living in seminiferous areas where the soil content is relatively rich in selenium, contributing to relatively high selenium in vegetation. Plants vary in their ability to accumulate selenium. Grasses, grains, and most weeds do not accumulate selenium even when grown in high-selenium areas, so that these plants add very little to the selenium content of livestock feed. But there are several plant species that are classified as "selenium accumulators" and they may contain selenium levels of 100 to 10,000 mg/kg. These plants, however, usually grow in nonagricultural areas and when consumed by livestock may, within a few weeks, cause a disease syndrome described as the *blind staggers.* Early symptoms are impaired vision, depressed appetite, and a tendency to wander in circles. This may progress to various degrees of paralysis and death from respiratory failure (Alexander et al., 1987). A more chronic syndrome described in livestock and horses is *alkali disease,* characterized by the loss of vitality, emaciation, deformity and shedding of hoofs, loss of long hair, and erosion of joints of long bones. Similar syndromes have been described in sheep and dogs. The areas of the world where human toxicity has been noted include several areas of China, areas of Venezuela, and parts of the state of South Dakota in the United States. A study of 70 families living in three counties of South Dakota and in one county of northern Nebraska, from farms where alkali disease in cattle had been recognized, found bad teeth, a yellowish discoloration of the skin, skin eruptions, and diseased nails of the fingers and toes in various family members. A syndrome now believed to be the result of selenium intoxication was discovered in 1961 to affect about 50 percent of 248 inhabitants of five villages in the Hubei province of China (Yang et al., 1983). There are similarities between this syndrome and the chronic effects in livestock and horses. The main symptoms were brittle hair with intact follicles, brittle nails with spots and streaks, and skin lesions on the backs of hands and feet and on the forearms, legs, and the back of the neck. These areas were red and swollen and contained blisters. In addition, 13 of 22 people in one village had neurologic symptoms, including peripheral anesthesia, pain, and hyperreflexia. In some individuals, these symptoms progressed to numbness, convulsions, paralysis, and altered motor function. Selenium has produced loss of fertility and congenital defects and is considered embryotoxic and teratogenic on the basis of animal experiments (WHO, 1987).

Biological Interactions Selenium has various biological interactions, which may affect the toxicity or deficiency of selenium as well as toxicity of another metal. If the intake of vitamin E is low, susceptibility to selenium toxicity is increased in experimental animals, whereas resistance is increased if vitamin E intake is increased. Selenium also forms insoluble complexes with silver, copper, cadmium, and mercury. Feeding silver to experimental animals results in tissue accumulations of both metals and symptoms of selenium deficiency may occur. Selenium forms complexes with copper, and toxicity to either selenium or copper is influenced by the intake of both metals. Selenium may prevent the toxic effects of cadmium on rat testicular tissue and dietary selenium can reduce the toxic effects of methyl mercury. Workers in a mercury mine and local inhabitants accumulate equimolar amounts of mercury and selenium in the pituitary and thyroid glands and in the brain. And finally, arsenite increases the biliary excretion of selenium, enhancing selenium excretion in urine. The mechanisms for these interactions are only partially understood, but their occurrence certainly influences the determination of safe and toxic levels of selenium for persons in the general population (WHO, 1987, 1996).

Anticarcinogenicity Selenium has been suspected of being a human carcinogen, but further studies have shown that it has anticarcinogenic properties (WHO, 1987).

Epidemiologic investigations have indicated a decrease in human cancer death rates (age- and sex-adjusted) correlated with an increasing selenium content of forage crops. In addition, experimental evidence supports the antineoplastic effect of selenium with regard to benzo[a]pyrene- and benzanthracene-induced skin tumors in mice, *N*-2-fluorenylacetamide- and diethylaminoazobenzene-induced hepatic tumors in rats, and spontaneous mammary tumors in mice. A possible mechanism of the protective effects of selenium has been postulated to involve inhibition of the formation of malonaldehyde, a product of peroxidative tissue damage, which is carcinogenic. In addition to the apparent protective effect against some carcinogenic agents, selenium is an antidote to the toxic effects of other metals, particularly arsenic, cadmium, mercury, copper, and thallium. The mechanism underlying these interactions is unknown.

Dose Effect in Humans Because of the potential for producing adverse health effects from both selenium excess and from deficiency, risk assessment must include both possible effects. The National Research Council's Food and Nutrition Board (NAS, 1980) recommends 200 μg/day as the maximum safe upper limit for an adult human's intake. Metabolic balance studies on North American adults showed that 70 μg/day for the standard human (70 kg body weight) appears to be required to maintain selenium balance and presumably to satisfy selenium requirements in these subjects. Chinese data indicate that daily intake of less than 20 μg can cause Keshan disease. Countries such as New Zealand have areas where daily intake is around 30 μg, but there is no evidence that this has a significant effect on the health of the people living in these areas. The critical level for prevention of deficiency, therefore, is 20 μg/day.

Zinc (Zn)

Zinc[1] is a nutritionally essential metal, and a deficiency results in severe health consequences. At the other extreme, excessive exposure to zinc is relatively uncommon and occurs only at very high levels. Zinc is ubiquitous in the environment, so that it is present in most foodstuffs, water, and air. The zinc content of substances in contact with galvanized copper or plastic pipes may be increased. Seafoods, meats, whole grains, dairy products, nuts, and legumes are high in zinc, while vegetables are lower, although zinc applied to soil is taken up by growing vegetables. Atmospheric zinc levels are higher in industrial areas (NRC, 2000).

[1]Atomic weight, 65; periodic table group, IIB; valence, +2; discovered in the thirteeth century.

Essentiality and Metabolism More than 200 metalloenzymes belonging to six major categories—including oxidoreductases, transferases, hydrolases, lyases, isomerases, and ligases—require zinc as a cofactor (Cousins, 1996). Zinc induces the synthesis of metallothionein, which is a factor in regulating the metabolism of zinc, including absorption and storage (Nordberg, 1998; Miles et al., 2000). Zinc is a functional component of several proteins that contribute to gene expression and regulation of genetic activity. Zinc chelates with cysteine and/or histidine in a tetrahedral configuration forming looped structures, called "zinc fingers," which bind to specific DNA regions and are bound in various transcription factors such as steroid hormone receptors and polymerase (Berg and Shi, 1996; Wang et al., 1997). Zinc has a normal physiologic role in membrane stabilization by binding ligands in membranes for maintenance of the normal structural geometry of the protein and lipid components (Cousins, 1996). Zinc is essential for the development and normal function of the nervous system.

Zinc has a role in immune function and the cytokines, primarily interleukin-1 (IL-1) and IL-6, influence zinc metabolism (Cousins, 1996). Zinc is required for optimal vitamin A metabolism. Although the mechanisms for intestinal absorption of iron and zinc differ, they appear to be inverse. There is a reciprocal relationship between plasma levels of zinc and copper, to the degree that massive zinc ingestion may produce copper deficiency and large doses of elemental zinc result in negative copper balance in patients with Wilson's disease. The metabolisms of zinc and calcium are interrelated in that zinc is required for normal calcification of bone (Leek et al., 1988).

Toxicokinetics The average daily intake for Americans is approximately 12 to 15 mg, mostly from food. Gastrointestinal absorption of zinc is homeostatically controlled and is probably a carrier-mediated process (Cousins, 1996; WHO, 1996). It is influenced by prostaglandins E_2 and F_2 and is chelated by picolinic acid, a tryptophan derivative. A deficiency of pyridoxine or tryptophan depresses zinc absorption. Within the mucosal cell, zinc induces metallothionein synthesis and, when the cell is saturated, this may depress zinc absorption. In the blood, about two-thirds of the zinc is bound to albumin and most of the remainder is complexed with β_2-macroglobulin. Zinc enters the gastrointestinal tract as a component of metallothionein secreted by the salivary glands, intestinal mucosa, pancreas, and liver. The normal basic physiologic requirement for absorbed zinc is 1.4 mg/day. Assuming 20 percent absorption, a daily diet of 7 mg will meet the basic requirement for males, but the requirement for females is greater during pregnancy and lactation. Adaptation to low dietary zinc will increase gastrointestinal absorption to as much as 50 percent. Bile is the major route of zinc excretion. Homeostatic control of zinc is maintained primarily by fecal excretion of endogenous zinc. Urinary excretion of zinc is low and not significantly influenced by dietary zinc. Zinc concentration in tissues varies widely. The liver receives up to about 40 percent of a tracer dose, declining to about 25 dto cent within 5 days. Liver concentration is influenced by humoral factors, including adrenocorticotropic hormone, parathyroid hormone, and endotoxin. In the liver as well as in other tissues, zinc is bound to metallothionein. The greatest concentration of zinc in the body is in the prostate, probably related to the rich content of zinc-containing enzyme acid phosphatase.

Assessment of Zinc Status The concentration of zinc in the plasma is not a sensitive indicator of zinc status and does not reflect the dose-response relationship between zinc levels in the body and effects at various target sites. Other approaches include measurement of zinc levels in hair and nails and in urine and zinc in shed teeth from children. The most reliable index of zinc status is the determination of zinc balance—that is, the relationship between intake and excretion—but these measurements require the facilities of a metabolic research unit in order to control dietary zinc intake while measuring excretion. An alternative approach is to identify a biomarker sensitive to changes in zinc status, such as metallothionein, serum alkaline phosphatase, and erythrocyte superoxide dismutase. The thymic hormone thymulin, which is involved in the differentiation of T cells, is zinc-dependent (Prasad et al., 1988). Reduced activity of this hormone may provide an early indication of mild zinc deficiency.

Deficiency Zinc deficiency results in a wide spectrum of clinical effects depending on age, stage of development, and deficiencies of related metals. Zinc deficiency in humans was first characterized by Prasad (1983) in adolescent Egyptian boys with growth failure and delayed sexual maturation accompanied by protein-calorie malnutrition, pellegra, and iron and folate deficiency. Zinc deficiency in the newborn may be manifest by dermatitis, loss of hair, impaired healing, susceptibility to infections, and neuropsychological abnormalities. Dietary inadequacies coupled with liver disease from chronic alcoholism may be associated with dermatitis, night blindness, testicular atrophy, impotence, and poor wound healing. Other chronic clinical disorders— such as ulcerative colitis and the malabsorption syndromes, chronic renal disease, and hemolytic anemia — are also associated with zinc deficiency. Many drugs affect zinc homeostasis, particularly metal-chelating agents and some antibiotics, such as penicillin and isoniazid. Less common zinc deficiency may occur with myocardial infarction, arthritis, and even hypertension (Walshe et al., 1994). Latent zinc deficiency is the most common zinc deficiency syndrome, implying marginally adequate zinc status. This may be the result of zinc-deficient dietary habits, particularly among young children or the elderly, or may occur as a consequence of a disease state (USDA, 1986). Zinc deficiency in growing children may result in poor growth performance, which has been shown to be improved with zinc supplementation (Prentice, 1997).

Zinc in Neurologic Disorders Because of its requirement as a cofactor for numerous enzymes and proteins, zinc has been implicated in various degenerative diseases of the nervous system (Prasad, 1995). It has been suggested that zinc modulates the solubility of β-amyloid in the brain and contributes to the formation of degenerative plaques in brains of patients with Alzheimer's disease. Also, zinc deficiency may alter activity of the antioxidant enzyme Cu-Zn-superoxide dismutase (SOD), resulting in excess free radicals that are damaging to cell membranes (Cuajungco and Lees, 1997). A genetic abnormality of one of the forms of Cu-Zn SOD may be the basis of a familial form of amyotrophic lateral sclerosis (Lyons, 1996).

Toxicity Acute zinc toxicity from excessive ingestion is uncommon, but gastrointestinal distress and diarrhea have been reported following ingestion of beverages standing in galvanized cans or from the use of galvanized utensils. However, evidence of hematologic, hepatic, or renal toxicity has not been observed in individuals ingesting as much as 12 g of elemental zinc over a 2-day period.

With regard to industrial exposure, metal fume fever resulting from inhalation of freshly formed fumes of zinc presents the most significant effect. This disorder has been most commonly associated with inhalation of zinc oxide fumes, but it may be seen after inhalation of the fumes of other metals, particularly magnesium, iron, and copper. Attacks usually begin after 4 to 8 h of exposure—chills and fever, profuse sweating, and weakness. Attacks usually last only 24 to 48 h and are most common on Mondays or after holidays. The pathogenesis is not known, but it is thought to result from endogenous pyrogen release due to cell lysis. Extracts prepared from tracheal mucosa and from the lungs of animals with experimentally induced metal fume fever produce similar symptoms when injected into other animals. Exposure of guinea pigs for 3 h/day for 6 consecutive days to 5 mg/m^3 of freshly formed ultrafine zinc oxide (the recommended threshold limit value) produced decrements in lung volumes and carbon monoxide diffusing capacity that persisted for 72 h after exposure. These functional changes were correlated with microscopic evidence of interstitial thickening and cellular infiltrate in alveolar ducts and alveoli (Lam et al., 1985).

Carcinogenicity Epidemiologic studies of workers in lead industries have not found any evidence of a relationship between zinc and cancer (Logue et al., 1982). Testicular tumors have been produced by direct injection in rats and chickens. This effect is probably related to the concentration of zinc normally in the gonads and may be hormonally dependent (Walshe et al., 1994).

METALS RELATED TO MEDICAL THERAPY

Metals considered in this group include aluminum, bismuth, gold, lithium, and platinum. Metals at one time were used to treat a number of human ills, particularly heavy metals like mercury and arsenic. Gold salts are still useful for the treatment of forms of rheumatism, and organic bismuth compounds are used to treat gastrointestinal disturbances. Lithium has become an important aid in the treatment of depression. The toxicologic hazards from aluminum are not from its use as an antacid but rather from the accumulations that occur in bone and from neurotoxicity in patients with chronic renal failure receiving hemodialysis therapy. A more recent concern regarding the potential neurotoxicity of aluminum involves its relationship to Alzheimer's dementia and its increase in bioavailability from changes in soil and water pH from acid rain. Platinum is receiving attention as an antitumor agent. Barium and gallium are used as radiopaque and radiotracer materials, respectively, and gallium is used for treating hypercalcemia.

Aluminum (Al)

Aluminum[1] is the most abundant metal and the third most abundant element in the earth's crust. Due to its high reactivity, aluminum is not found in the free state in nature. All the chemical

[1]Atomic weight, 26.98; periodic table group, III; valence, +3; first isolated in 1825.

compounds involve aluminum in the +3 valence state (Al^{3+}). As a hard trivalent ion, Al^{3+} binds strongly to oxygen-donor ligands such as citrate and phosphate. The chemistry of aluminum compounds is complicated by a tendency to hydrolyze and form polynuclear species, many of which are sparingly soluble (Harris et al., 1996).

Aluminum has, until recently, existed predominantly in forms that are not available to humans and most other species. Acid rain, however, has dramatically increased the amount of aluminum appearing in biological ecosystems, resulting in well-described destructive effects on fish and plant species. However, it is not bioaccumulated to any significant extent except in the tea plant.

Aluminum has many uses, mainly in the form of alloys in packaging, building, construction, transportation, and electrical applications. Over 95 percent of beer and carbonated drinks are packaged in two-piece aluminum cans. Cooking in aluminum utensils results in the transfer of aluminum to food. Human exposure to aluminum comes from food and drinking water as well as from pharmaceuticals. The normal average daily intake is 1 to 10 mg for adults (Greger, 1992).

Toxicokinetics Aluminum is poorly absorbed following either oral or inhalation exposure and is essentially not absorbed dermally. Inhalation of particulate aluminum may result in direct transfer to brain tissue via the olfactory system (Roberts 1986; Perl and Good, 1987). Approximately 0.1 percent of aluminum in the diet is absorbed, but this figure may rise to 1 percent depending on speciation. Absorption from the gut depends largely on pH and the presence of complexing ligands, particularly carboxylic acids, which are absorbable. For example, intestinal absorption is enhanced in the presence of citrate. However, the citrate complex is not itself absorbed. Apparently citrate makes aluminum available to other transport pathways across the gastrointestinal (GI) tract (Jouhanneau et al., 1997). Silicon is a potent inhibitor of GI absorption of aluminum and may also accelerate urinary excretion (Flaten et al, 1993). It probably interacts with aluminum to form poorly absorbed hydroxyalumino-silicates.

Biological speciation is also of major importance in distribution, and excretion of aluminum in mammals. In plasma, 80 to 90 percent of aluminum binds to transferrin, an iron-transport protein for which there are receptors in many body tissues. Based on potentiometric and nuclear magnetic resonance studies, it is predicted that the remainder of aluminum in plasma is in the form of small-molecule hydroxy species and small complexes with carboxylic acids, phosphate, and, to a lesser degree, amino acids (DeVoto and Yokel, 1994).

Bone and lung have the highest concentrations of aluminum, suggesting that bone may be a sink for aluminum. It does not normally accumulate in blood to any great extent (Ganrote, 1986). It is removed from blood by the kidneys and excreted in urine. Uremic animals and humans have higher-than-normal levels of aluminum in spite of increased urinary clearance.

Aluminum compounds can affect absorption of other elements in the gastrointestinal tract and alter intestinal function. Aluminum inhibits fluoride absorption and may decrease the absorption of calcium and iron compounds and salicylic acid, which, in turn, may affect the absorption of aluminum (Exley et al., 1996). The absorption of cholesterol may be inhibited by forming an aluminum pectin complex that binds fats to nondigestible vegetable fibers (Nagyvary and Bradbury, 1977). The binding of phosphorus in the intestinal tract can lead to phosphate depletion and osteomalacia. Aluminum may alter gastrointestinal tract motility by inhibition of acetylcholine-induced contractions and may be the explanation of why aluminum-containing antacids often produce constipation.

Toxicity In cases of human toxicity, the target organs are the lung, bone, or central nervous system. Aluminum affects the same target organs in animals as well as producing developmental effects. In addition, aluminum released into bodies of fresh water via the action of acid rain kills fish by damaging the gills (Flaten et al., 1993).

Lung and Bone Toxicity Occupational exposure to aluminum dusts can produce lung fibrosis in humans. The effects are probably due to lung overload caused by excessive deposits of dust (Morrow, 1992). Osteomalacia has been associated with excessive intake of aluminum-containing antacids in otherwise healthy individuals; this is assumed to be due to interference with intestinal phosphate absorption. Osteomalacia also can occur in uremic patients exposed to aluminum in the dialysis fluid. In these patients, osteomalacia may be a direct effect of aluminum on bone mineralization as bone levels are high.

Neurotoxicity Aluminum has markedly different effects on animals at different points in their life span and in different species. The normal concentration of aluminum in the mammalian brain is approximately 1 to 2 $\mu g/g$. In certain aluminum-sensitive species, such as cats and rabbits, increased aluminum by intrathecal infusion so that brain concentration is greater than 4 $\mu g/g$ induces a characteristic clinical and pathologic response. Initially, animals show subtle behavioral changes, including learning and memory deficits and poor motor function. These changes progress to tremor, incoordination, weakness, and ataxia. This is followed by focal seizures and death within 3 or 4 weeks of initial exposure. With lesser doses, there is longer survival but no recovery (DeBoni et al., 1976).

The most prominent early pathologic change is an accumulation of neurofibrillary tangles (NFT) in cell body, proximal axons, and dendrites of neurons of many brain regions. This is associated with loss of synapses and atrophy of the dendritic tree. Not all species show this reaction to aluminum, however. The rat fails to develop NFTs or encephalopathy and the monkey develops these only after more than a year following aluminum infusion. NFTs are found primarily in large neurons such as Purkinje cells of the cerebellum and large neurons of the cerebral cortex. There is marked reduction in the numbers of neurotubules and the rate of cytoplasmic transport with impairment of intracellular transport. Aluminum also interacts with neuronal chromatin or DNA and is associated with a decreased rate of DNA synthesis. RNA polymerase activity is also reduced.

Aluminum competes with or alters calcium metabolism in several organ systems including the brain. Brain tissue calcium rises following aluminum exposure. Aluminum also binds to calmodulin and induces changes in its structure, leading to the suggestion that aluminum impairs the function of calmodulin as a calcium regulator. While these studies in animals have provided some insights into the mechanisms of the neurotoxicity of aluminum in experimental models, the relationship to human disease is presently uncertain (Siegel and Hagu, 1983; Bizzi and Gambetti, 1986; Birchall and Chappel, 1988).

Human Dementia Syndromes ***Dialysis Dementia*** A progressive, fatal neurologic syndrome has also been reported in patients on long-term intermittent hemodialysis treatment for chronic renal failure (Alfrey, 1993). The first symptom in these patients is a speech disorder followed by dementia, convulsions, and myoclonus. The disorder, which typically arises after 3 to 7 years of dialysis treatment, may be due to aluminum intoxication. The aluminum content of brain, muscle, and bone tissues increases in these patients. Sources of the excess aluminum may be from oral aluminum hydroxide commonly given to these patients or from aluminum in dialysis fluid derived from the tap water used to prepare the dialysate fluid. The high serum and aluminum concentrations may be related to increased parathyroid hormone, which is due to the low blood calcium and osteodystrophy common in patients with chronic renal disease. The syndrome may be prevented by avoidance of the use of aluminum-containing oral phosphate binders and by monitoring of aluminum in the dialysate. Chelation of aluminum may be achieved with use of desferrioxamine, and progression of the dementia may be arrested or slowed (Wills and Savory, 1983).

Amyotrophic Lateral Sclerosis and Parkinsonism-Dementia Syndromes of Guam (Guam ALS-PD Complex) The Chamorro peoples of the Marina Islands in the western Pacific Ocean, particularly Guam and Rota, have an unusually high incidence of neurodegenerative diseases associated with nerve cell loss and neurofibrillary degeneration of the Alzheimer's type. Garruto et al. (1984) noted that the volcanic soils of the regions of Guam with a high incidence of ALS-PD contained high concentrations of aluminum and manganese and were low in calcium and magnesium. They postulated that a low intake of calcium and magnesium induced secondary hyperparathyroidism, resulting in an increase in calcium, aluminum, and other toxic metals, resulting in neuronal injury and death. How and why aluminum enters the brain of these people is unclear. A recent study of mineral content of food did not indicate high exposure to aluminum or low dietary calcium (Crapper-McLachlan et al., 1989). These authors suggest that the diet of the inhabitants of Guam may be the source of the aluminum, particularly through the respiratory tract. Perl and Good (1987) have shown that aluminum may be taken up through nasal-olfactory pathways. On the other hand, the consumption of the neurotoxic seed of the false sago palm tree may also play a role in the prevalence of ALS in these areas.

Alzheimer's Disease A possible relationship between aluminum and Alzheimer's disease has been a matter of speculation for many decades. The basis for this relationship is the finding of increased aluminum levels in Alzheimer brains, neurofibrillary lesions in experimental animals, and the fact that aluminum is associated with various components of the pathologic lesions in Alzheimer brain tissue. However, elevated aluminum levels in Alzheimer brains may be a consequence and not a cause of the disease. The reduced blood-brain barrier in Alzheimer's might allow more aluminum into the brain (Banks et al., 1988; Liss and Thornton, 1986; Shore and Wyatt, 1983). Also, recent studies have raised the possibility that the staining methods in earlier studies may have lead to aluminum contamination (Makjanic et al., 1998). Furthermore, the neurofibrillary tangles seen in aluminum encephalopathy differ structurally and chemically from those in Alzheimer's (Goyer, 1996).

Epidemiologic and case-control studies examining the role of aluminum exposure in Alzheimer's disease arrive at conflicting conclusions. Some studies have found significant associations (Martyn et al., 1989; McLachlan et al., 1996; Michel et al., 1990) whereas other studies did not find a significant relationship (Forster et al., 1995; Martyn et al., 1997; Wettstein et al., 1991).

In conclusion, whereas a causative role for aluminum in the etiology of Alzheimer's and other neurodegenerative diseases has not been established, observations on dialyzed patients provide convincing evidence that aluminum is the causative agent of "dialysis dementia."

Bismuth (Bi)

Bismuth[1] has a long history of use in pharmaceuticals in Europe and North America. Both inorganic and organic salts have been used, depending on the specific application. Trivalent insoluble bismuth salts are used medicinally to control diarrhea and other types of GI distress. Various bismuth salts have been used externally for their astringent and slight antiseptic properties. Bismuth salts have also been used as radiocontrast agents. Further potential for exposure comes from the use of insoluble bismuth salts in cosmetics. Injections of soluble and insoluble salts, suspended in oil to maintain adequate blood levels, have been used to treat syphilis. Bismuth sodium thioglycollate, a water-soluble salt, was injected intramuscularly for malaria (*Plasmodium vivax*). Bismuth glycolyarsanilate is one of the few pentavalent salts that have been used medicinally. This material was formerly used for treatment of amebiasis (Fowler and Vouk, 1986). Exposure to various bismuth salts for medicinal use has decreased with the advent of newer therapeutic agents.

Recently there has been an increased interest in bismuth to treat peptic ulcer disease. This interest was prompted by the discovery in 1982 of a gram-negative bacterium from the gastric mucosa of patients suffering from gastritis. The bacterium, *Helicobacter pylori,* is now thought to predispose patients with chronic gastritis to peptic ulcer formation and duodenal ulceration. Antacids containing bismuth compounds have been effective in promoting healing of peptic ulcers, which is now thought to be due to the antibacterial action of bismuth.

Toxicokinetics Most bismuth compounds are insoluble and poorly absorbed from the GI tract or when applied to the skin, even if the skin is abraded or burned. The three compounds used clinically, colloidal tripotassium dicitrato bismuthate, bismuth subsalicylate (Pepto Bismol) and bismuth citrate are also poorly absorbed (less than 1 percent of an oral dose) (Tillman et al., 1996). Binding in blood is thought to be due largely to a plasma protein with a molecular weight greater than 50,000. In vitro studies have shown the Bi^{3+} binds to serum transferrin (Li et al., 1996). Tissue distribution, omitting injection depots, reveals the kidney as the site of the highest concentration (Zidenberg et al., 1989), probably due to its capacity to induce metallothionein (Tanaka-Kagawa et al., 1993). Passage of bismuth into the amniotic fluid and into the fetus has been demonstrated. The urine is the major route of excretion. It is also secreted in bile in association with glutathione (Gyurasics et al., 1992). Traces of bismuth can be found in milk and saliva. The elimination half-life is reported to be about 21 days (Froomes et al., 1989); but after injection, elimination of total bismuth may be slow, depending on its mobilization from the injection site.

Toxicity Acute renal failure can occur following oral administration of such compounds as bismuth sodium triglycocollamate or thioglycollate, particularly in children (Urizar and Vernier, 1966). The tubular epithelium is the primary site of toxicity, producing degeneration of renal tubular cells and nuclear inclusion bodies

[1]Atomic weight, 209; periodic table group, VA; valence, +3 or +5; discovered in 1753.

composed of a bismuth-protein complex analogous to those found in lead toxicity (Fowler and Goyer, 1975).

The symptoms of chronic toxicity in humans consist of decreased appetite, weakness, rheumatic pain, diarrhea, fever, metal lines on the gums, foul breath, gingivitis, and dermatitis. Jaundice and conjunctival hemorrhage are rare but have been reported. Bismuth nephropathy with proteinuria may occur. In the 1970s reports appeared from France and Australia of a unique encephalopathy occurring in colostomy and ileostomy patients using bismuth subgallate, subnitrate, and subcarbonate for control of fecal odor and consistency (Slikkerveer and de Wolff, 1989). The symptoms included progressive mental confusion, irregular myoclonic jerks, a distinctive pattern of disordered gait, and a variable degree of dysarthria. The disorder was fatal to patients who continued use of the bismuth compounds, but full recovery was rapid in those in whom therapy was discontinued. The severity of the disorder seemed to be independent of dose and duration of therapy (Thomas et al., 1977). Bismuth-containing paste dressings have produced encephalopathy when applied to brain tissues after neurosurgery (Sharma et al., 1994).

Chelation therapy using dimercaprol (BAL) is said to be helpful in the removal of bismuth from children with acute toxicity (Arena, 1974).

Gallium (Ga)

The main valence state of gallium[1] is +3 (gallic), but the +2 (gallous) also can form stable compounds. Gallium is of interest because of the use of radiogallium as a diagnostic tool for the localization of bone lesions and the use of nonradioactive gallium nitrate, $Ga(NO_3)_3$ as an antitumor agent. Also, it has recently been approved in the United States for the treatment of hypercalcemia. Gallium is obtained as a by-product of copper, zinc, lead, and aluminum refining and is used in high-temperature thermometers, as a substitute for mercury in arc lamps, as a component of metal alloys, and as a seal for vacuum equipment. It is the only metal other than mercury that is liquid at or near room temperature.

Toxicokinetics Gallium is sparsely absorbed from the GI tract, but concentrations of less than 1 ppm can be localized radiographically in bone lesions. Higher doses will allow one to visualize the liver, spleen, and kidney as well (Hayes, 1988). Gallium binds to plasma transferrin and enters cells on iron (Fe^{3+}) transport mechanisms. Urine is the major route of excretion. The half-life in the body is about 4 to 5 days.

Toxicity Clinical studies on $Ga(NO_3)_3$ as an antitumor agent, reveal that it accumulates in metabolically active regions of bone and increases the calcium and phosphate content. It inhibits osteoclastic bone resorption without poisoning the osteoclast cells (Bockman, 1991). Therapeutic trials with intravenous doses indicate that nephrotoxicity is dose-limiting. Other effects include nausea, vomiting, and anemia with mild leukopenia. Less frequent are neurologic, pulmonary, and dermatologic effects. It can elicit a variety of biochemical and hormonal changes. The mechanism of bone uptake and inhibition of bone resorption is not known, but the gallate anion, $Ga(OH)_4^-$, may be the active species. Uptake by and effects on other cells may be explained by Ga^{3+} competition with Fe^{3+} for transferrin and other iron-binding proteins leading the depletion of intracellular iron and apoptosis. [For a detailed review, see Bernstein (1998).]

Administration of gallium arsenide to experimental animals results in arsenic intoxication (Webb et al., 1984). There are no reported adverse effects of gallium following industrial exposure.

[1]Atomic weight, 69.72; periodic table group, IIIA; valence, +2 or +3; discovered in 1875.

Gold (Au)

Gold[1] is widely distributed in small quantities, but economically usable deposits occur as the free metal in quartz veins or alluvial gravel. Gold is almost always found in association with silver. Seawater contains 3 or 4 mg/ton and small amounts, 0.03 to 1 percent, have been reported in many foods. Gold has a number of industrial uses because of its electrical and thermal conductivity. While gold and its salts have been used for a wide variety of medicinal purposes, their present uses are limited to the treatment of rheumatoid arthritis and rare skin diseases such as discoid lupus.

Toxicokinetics Gold salts are poorly absorbed from the gastrointestinal tract. The upper limit of normal levels can be considered to be 0.5 μg/L for both whole blood and urine (Perelli and Piolotto, 1992). After injection of most of the soluble salts, gold is excreted via the urine, while the feces account for the major portion of insoluble compounds. Gold seems to have a long biological half-life, and detectable blood levels can be demonstrated for 10 months after cessation of treatment. Trivalent gold binds strongly to metallothionein (Saito and Kuraski, 1996).

Toxicity Dermatitis is the most frequently reported toxic reaction to gold and is sometimes accompanied by stomatitis probably involving allergic mechanisms (Hostynek, 1997). The use of gold in the form of organic salts to treat rheumatoid arthritis may be complicated by the development of proteinuria and the nephrotic syndrome, which morphologically consists of an immune-complex glomerulonephritis, with granular deposits along the glomerular basement membrane and in the mesangium (Bigazzi, 1994). The pathogenesis of the immune-complex disease is not certain, but gold may behave as a hapten and generate the production of antibodies with subsequent disposition of gold protein-antibody complexes in the glomerular subepithelium. Another hypothesis is that antibodies are formed against damaged tubular structures, particularly mitochondria, providing immune complexes for the glomerular deposits (Voil et al., 1977).

The pathogenesis of the renal lesions induced by gold therapy also has a direct toxicity to renal tubular cell components. From experimental studies it appears that gold salts have an affinity for mitochondria of proximal tubular lining cells, which is followed by autophagocytosis and accumulation of gold in amorphous phagolysosomes (Stuve and Galle, 1970). Gold particles can be identified in degenerating mitochondria in tubular lining cells and in glomerular epithelial cell by x-ray microanalysis (Ainsworth et al., 1981).

[1]Atomic weight, 197; periodic table group, IB; valence, +1 or +3; discovered in earliest times.

Lithium (Li)

Lithium[1] (carbonate) is used in the treatment of depression. There must be careful monitoring of usage to provide optimal therapeutic value and to avoid toxicity. The therapeutic index is narrow (0.6 to 1.5 meq/L). Lithium is present in many plant and animal tissues. It has some industrial uses, in alloys, as a catalytic agent, and as a lubricant. Lithium hydride produces hydrogen on contact with water and is used in manufacturing electronic tubes, in ceramics, and in chemical synthesis.

Toxicokinetics The physiology, pharmacology, and toxicology of lithium compounds have been reviewed in detail by Timer and Sands (1999). Daily intake is about 2 mg. It is readily absorbed from the GI tract. Distribution is to total body water with higher levels in kidney, thyroid, and bone as compared to other tissues. Excretion is chiefly through the kidneys with 80 percent of the filtered load reabsorbed. The usual elimination half-life is 12 to 27 h, but it may rise to nearly 60 h if renal excretion is compromised. Lithium can substitute for sodium or potassium on several transport proteins. It enters cells via the amiloride-sensitive sodium channel or the Na/H^+ exchanger. The greater part of lithium is contained in the cells, perhaps at the expense of potassium. In general it may be competing with sodium at certain sites—for example, in renal tubular reabsorption.

Toxicity From the industrial point of view, except for lithium hydride, none of the other salts is hazardous, nor is the metal itself. Lithium hydride is intensely corrosive and may produce burns on the skin because of the formation of hydroxides (Cox and Singer, 1981). The therapeutic use of lithium carbonate may produce unusual toxic responses. These include neuromuscular changes (tremor, muscle hyperirritability, and ataxia), central nervous system changes (blackout spells, epileptic seizures, slurred speech, coma, psychosomatic retardation, and increased thirst), cardiovascular changes (cardiac arrhythmia, hypertension, and circulatory collapse), GI changes (anorexia, nausea, and vomiting), and renal damage (albuminuria and glycosuria). The last is believed to be due to temporary hypokalemic nephritis. Long-term sequelae from acute lithium poisoning include cognitive losses such as impaired memory, attention and executive functions, and visuospatial deficits (Brumm et al., 1998).

Chronic lithium nephrotoxicity and interstitial nephritis can occur with long-term exposure even when lithium levels remain within the therapeutic range (Singer, 1981). Animal studies have shown a similarity between lithium and sodium handling and that lithium may cause an antidiuretic hormone (ADH)–resistant polyuria and secondary polydipsia. This abnormality appears to be mediated by a central pituitary effect that reduces ADH release (Carney et al., 1996). Treatment with lithium salts has also been associated with nephrotic syndrome with minimal glomerular changes. The cardiovascular and nervous system changes may be due to the competitive relationship between lithium and potassium and may thus produce a disturbance in intracellular metabolism. The effects of lithium on neurotransmitter, neuropeptide, and signal transduction systems have been reviewed by Lenox et al. (1998).

Thyrotoxic reactions, including goiter formation, have also been suggested (Davis and Fann, 1971). While there has been some indication of adverse effects on fetuses following lithium treatment, none was observed in rats (4.05 meq/kg), rabbits (1.08 meq/kg), or primates (0.67 meq/kg). This dose to rats was sufficient to produce maternal toxicity and effects on the pups of treated, lactating dams.

Lithium overdosage and toxicity may be treated by the administration of diuretics (amiloride) and lowering of blood levels (via hemodialysis). Treatment with diuretics must be accompanied by replacement of water and electrolytes (Steele, 1977).

[1]Atomic weight, 6.94; periodic table group, 1; valence, +1; discovered in 1817.

Platinum (Pt) and Related Metals

Platinum-group metals include a relatively light triad of ruthenium, rhodium, and palladium, and the heavy metals osmium, iridium, and platinum.[1] They are found together in sparsely distributed mineral deposits or as a by-product of refining other metals, chiefly nickel and copper. Osmium and iridium are not important toxicologically. Osmium tetroxide, however, is a powerful eye irritant. The other metals are generally nontoxic in their metallic states but have been noted to have toxic effects in particular circumstances. Toxicologic information for ruthenium is limited to references in the literature indicating that fumes may be injurious to eyes and lungs (Browning, 1969). Palladium chloride is not readily absorbed from subcutaneous injection, and no adverse effects have been reported from industrial exposure. Colloid palladium ($Pd[OH]_2$) is reported to increase body temperature, produce discoloration and necrosis at the site of injection, decrease body weight, and cause slight hemolysis.

Allergenic Effects of Platinum Salts Platinum is interesting because of its extensive industrial applications and because of the use of certain complexes as antitumor agents. Higher platinum levels are found in roadside dust where traffic density is high because of its use in catalytic converters. Mean levels of platinum in whole blood and urine in nonoccupationally exposed adults are reported as 0.13 μg/L of blood and 0.11 μg/g of creatinine, respectively (Farago et al., 1998). Platinum metal itself is generally harmless, but an allergic dermatitis can be produced in susceptible individuals (Hunter, 1969). Skin changes are most common between the fingers and in the antecubital fossae. Symptoms of respiratory distress, ranging from irritation to an asthmatic syndrome—with coughing, wheezing, and shortness of breath—have been reported following exposure to platinum dust. The skin and respiratory changes are termed *platinosis*. They are mainly confined to persons with a history of industrial exposure to soluble compounds such as sodium chloroplatinate, although cases resulting from the wearing of platinum jewelry have been reported (WHO, 1991). The complex salts of platinum may act as powerful allergens, particularly ammonium hexachloroplatinate and hexachloroplatinic acid. Platinum salt sensitization may persist for years after cessation of exposure (Brooks et al., 1990). In general, platinum allergy is confined to a small group of charged compounds that contain reactive ligands, the most effective of which are chloride ligands (Farago et al., 1998).

Antitumor Effects of Platinum Complexes Major consideration for this group of metals are the potential antitumor and carcinogenic effects of certain neutral complexes such as *cis*-dichlorodiammine platinum (II) (or cisplatin), and various analogs

[1]Atomic weight, 195.08; periodic table group, VIII; valence, +1?, +2, +3, or +4; discovered in 1735.

(Kazantzis, 1981). Other metals in the group give complexes that are inactive or less active than the platinum analog. They can inhibit cell division and have antibacterial properties as well. These compounds can react selectively with specific chemical sites in proteins such as disulfide bonds and terminal NH_2 groups, with functional groups in amino acids and, in particular, with receptor sites in nucleic acids. These compounds also exhibit neuromuscular toxicity and nephrotoxicity. Platinum complexes, particularly cisplatin, are effective antitumor agents and are used clinically for the treatment of cancers of the head and neck, certain lymphomas, and testicular and ovarian tumors. For antitumor activity, the complexes should be neutral and should have a pair of *cis*-leaving groups. At dosages that are therapeutically effective (antitumor), these complexes produce severe and persistent inhibition of DNA synthesis and little inhibition of RNA and protein synthesis. DNA polymerase activity and transport of DNA precursors through plasma membranes are not inhibited. The complexes are thought to react directly with DNA in regions that are rich in guanosine and cytosine (Abrams and Murrer, 1993).

Mutagenic and Carcinogenic Effects of Platinum Complexes Cisplatin is a strong mutagen in bacterial systems and has been shown to form both intrastrand and interstrand cross-links. There is also a correlation between antitumor activity of cisplatin and its ability to bind DNA and induce phage from bacterial cells. It also causes chromosomal aberrations in cultured hamster cells and a dose-dependent increase in sister chromosome exchanges. Although cisplatin has antitumorigenic activity, it also seems to increase the frequency of lung adenomas and give rise to skin papillomas and carcinomas in mice. These observations are consistent with the activity of other alkylating agents used in cancer chemotherapy. There are no reports of increased risk of cancer from occupational exposure to platinum compounds.

Nephrotoxicity Cisplatin is also a nephrotoxin, which compromises its usefulness as a therapeutic agent. Platinum compounds with antitumor activity produce proximal and distal tubular cell injury, mainly in the corticomedullary region, where the concentration of platinum is highest (Madias and Harrington, 1978). Although 90 percent of administered cisplatin becomes tightly bound to plasma proteins, only unbound platinum is rapidly filtered by the glomerulus and has a half-life of only 48 min. Within tissues, platinum is protein-bound, with the largest concentrations in kidney, liver, and spleen, and it has a half-life of 2 or 3 days. Tubular cell toxicity seems to be directly related to dose, and prolonged weekly injection in rats causes atrophy of the cortical portions of nephrons, cystic dilatation of inner cortical or medullary tubules, and chronic renal failure due to tubulointerstitial nephritis (Choie et al., 1981). Experimental studies suggest that the preadministration of bismuth subnitrate, a potent inducer of metallothionein in the kidney, reduces the nephrotoxicity of cisplatin without interfering with its anticancer effect (Kondo et al., 1992).

MINOR TOXIC METALS

Antimony (Sb)

Antimony[1] belongs to the same periodic group as arsenic and has the same oxidation states. Most compounds of antimony involve the tri- and pentavalent states. Antimony is included in alloys in the metals industry and is used for producing fireproofing chemicals, ceramics, glassware, and pigments. Antimony has been used medicinally in the treatment of schistosomiasis and leishmaniasis. Antimony is a common air pollutant from industrial emissions, but exposure for the general population is largely from food. The average daily intake from food and water is about 5 μg (ATSDR, 1992).

[1]Atomic weight, 121.75; periodic table group, VA; valence; −2, +3, or +5; discovered in about 1450.

The disposition of antimony in the body resembles that of arsenic. Most antimony compounds can be absorbed from the lung and GI tract, but no quantitative data are available on humans. Clearance from the lung is estimated to be on the order of days to weeks and GI absorption from most compounds has been estimated to be about 1 percent (ICRP, 1981). Many antimony compounds are GI irritants. Trivalent antimony is concentrated in red blood cells and liver, whereas the pentavalent form is mostly in plasma. The pentavalent form is predominantly excreted in urine, whereas the trivalent is found mainly in feces after injection into animals. [For detailed review, see ATSDR (1992).]

Most information about antimony toxicity has been obtained from industrial experiences. Occupational exposures are usually by inhalation of dust containing antimony compounds, such as the pentachloride and trichloride, trioxide, and trisulfide. Effects may be acute, particularly from the pentachloride and trichloride exposures, producing a rhinitis and even acute pulmonary edema. Chronic exposures by inhalation of other antimony compounds result in rhinitis, pharyngitis, tracheitis, and, over the longer term, bronchitis and eventually pneumoconiosis with obstructive lung disease and emphysema. Transient skin eruptions (antimony spots) may occur in workers with chronic exposure (Elinder and Friberg, 1986). Antimony-containing compounds may also produce alterations in cardiac function, and autopsy studies have shown that cardiac toxicity was the cause of death in patients treated with antimonial drugs (Winship, 1987).

A recent review by Léonard and Garber (1996) concluded that evidence that antimony compounds have mutagenic properties is insufficient. In most studies claiming to find carcinogenic properties, exposure to antimony compounds has been accompanied by other proven or likely carcinogens. Two exceptions are antimony trioxide and trisulfide, for which evidence for carcinogenicity was described as sufficient and limited respectively by the IARC (1989). In general, the mutagenic, carcinogenic, and teratogenic risks of antimony compounds, if they exist at all, are not very important in relation to such metals as arsenic, chromium, and nickel.

The metal hydride of antimony, stibine (H_3Sb), is a highly toxic gas that can be generated when antimony is exposed to reducing acids or when batteries are overcharged. High-purity stibine is also used in the production of semiconductors. Stibine, like arsine, causes hemolysis.

Barium (Ba)

Barium[1] is used in various alloys; in paints, soap, paper, and rubber; and in the manufacture of ceramics and glass. Barium fluorosilicate and carbonate have been used in pesticides. Barium sulfate, an insoluble compound, is used as a radiopaque aid to x-ray diagnosis. Barium is relatively abundant in nature and is found in plants and animal tissue. Brazil nuts have very high concentrations

[1]Atomic weight, 137.33; periodic table group, II; valence, +2; discovered in 1808.

(3000 to 4000 ppm). Barium from natural sources may exceed federal safety standards in some bodies of freshwater. Daily intake is about 750 μg coming mainly from the diet.

The toxicity of barium compounds depends on their solubility. Aerosols of soluble barium compounds are well absorbed in the lung. Ingested soluble compounds are absorbed similarly to calcium to the extent of about 8 percent of the dose. Bone and teeth are the major sites of deposition, up to 90 percent of the body burden. The lung has an average concentration of 1 ppm (dry weight). The kidney, spleen, muscle, heart, brain, and liver concentrations are 0.10, 0.08, 0.05, and 0.03 ppm, respectively. Barium is reabsorbed by the renal tubules with only minor amounts appearing in the urine. The major route of excretion is the feces. The elimination half-life is about 3 to 4 days.

Occupational poisoning to barium is uncommon, but a benign pneumoconiosis (baritosis) may result from inhalation of barium sulfate (barite) dust and barium carbonate. It is not incapacitating and is usually reversible with cessation of exposure. Accidental poisoning from ingestion of an acute toxic dose (over 200 mg) of soluble barium salt results first in perioral paresthesia, intractable vomiting, and severe diarrhea. Hypertension and cardiac dysrhythmias may ensue. Profound hypokalemia and weakness progressing to flaccid paralysis are the hallmarks of barium poisoning (Johnson and VanTassell, 1991). Experimental studies indicate that barium directly stimulates muscle cells. Its basic mechanism of action probably involves the blocking of calcium activated potassium channels responsible for the cellular efflux of potassium. As a result, intracellular potassium rises and extra cellular levels fall leading to hypokalemia. Treatment with intravenous potassium appears beneficial. The lethal dose is between 1 to 15 g as barium carbonate. [For more detailed reviews, see Reeves (1986), ATSDR (1992).]

Germanium (Ge)

The chemical and physical properties of germanium[1] are intermediate between a metal and a nonmetal. It has two stable oxidation states, divalent and tetravalent. It forms organometallic compounds such as dimethyl germanium and a hydride (GeH_4). It was widely used in the semiconductor industry up to the mid-1970s, when it was replaced by silicon. Its current uses are in infrared lenses, optic fibers, as a catalyst, and in alloys with other metals. Some organogermanium compounds such as spirogermanium have antineoplastic properties but so far have not achieved therapeutic applications.

The diet is the dominant source of exposure to the general population. Germanium concentrations in most foods are similar to the natural abundance level of about 0.6 to 1.0 ppm in soils. But some canned foods are higher (tuna 2.2; baked beans 5.8 ppm). The daily intake from food is reported in the range of 370 to 3700 μg. Intake from drinking water and ambient air (except for occupational exposures) is negligible.

Inorganic germanium compounds are well absorbed from the diet. It is widely distributed throughout the body with the highest concentrations occurring in the spleen. Germanium is excreted mainly via the kidneys. The whole-body half-lives are between 1 and 4 days. Hair and nails may be useful media for biological monitoring.

[1]Atomic weight, 72.59; periodic table group, IVA; valence, +2 and +4; discovered in 1886.

The gas germane (GeH_4) is highly toxic to the cardiovascular system, liver and kidneys. It causes hemolysis of red cells and probably acts in the same way as stibine (SbH_3). The inorganic compounds exhibit low toxicity when taken orally. The LD_{50} values in animals are above 100 mg/kg body weight of germane. Ingestion of germanium dioxide (GeO_2) in an elixir, according to a case report on 18 people, resulted in renal damage that did not completely disappear after cessation of exposure. Approximately 16 to 328 g of germanium were ingested over a period of 4 to 36 months.

Germanium is not carcinogenic and may even inhibit carcinogenesis. The organo derivative, spirogermanium, selectively kills cancer cells. It is not mutagenic and can inhibit the action of other mutagens. High doses can cause embryonic resorption and the organo derivative, dimethyl germanium oxide, can produce fetal malformations in animal tests. [For references and details see the review by Gerber and Leonard (1997).]

Indium (In)

Indium[1] is a rare metal whose principal valence state is +3. In its metallic form, it is used in alloys, solders, and as a hardening agent for bearings. Its compounds such as indium phosphide (InP) are widely used in the electronics industry for production of semiconductors and photovoltaic. It is currently being used in medicine for the scanning of organs and the treatment of tumors. The average human intake of indium has been estimated in the range of 8 to 10 μg/day (Smith et al., 1978).

Indium compounds, specially InP, are poorly absorbed from the gastrointestinal tract or after intratracheal instillation (Zheng et al., 1994). It is excreted in the urine and feces. Its tissue distribution is relatively uniform.

There are no meaningful reports of human toxicity to indium. From animal experiments it is apparent that toxicity is related to the chemical form. Indium chloride given intravenously to mice produces renal toxicity and liver necrosis. Intratracheal instillation of the trichloride can produce severe pulmonary damage with fibrosis (Blazka et al., 1994). The phosphide appears less toxic (Oda, 1997). No evidence could be found for reproductive toxicity of $InCl_3$ in animal tests (Chapin et al., 1995) and teratogenic effects were found only when maternal toxicity occurred (Ungvary et al., 2000).

Silver (Ag)

Silver[2] forms only a +1 valence state, Ag^+, from which all its chemical compounds are formed. It occurs naturally as a silver ore often in association with gold and copper deposits. Silver mines are known to have been worked in Asia Minor before 2500 BC. Its principal industrial use is as silver halide in the manufacture of photographic plates. Other uses are for jewelry, coins, and eating utensils. Silver nitrate is used for making indelible inks and for medicinal purposes. The use of silver nitrate for prophylaxis of ophthalmia neonatorum is a legal requirement in some states. Other medicinal uses of silver salts are as an antiseptic and astringent.

[1]Atomic weight, 114.82; periodic table group, IIIA; valence, +1, +2, or +3; discovered in 1863.

[2]Atomic weight, 107.86; periodic table group, IB; valence, +2; discovered in ancient times.

Silver sulfadiazine is widely used in the treatment of burn injuries. Dietary intake including fluids is in the range of 70 to 90 μg/day.

Silver compounds can be absorbed orally, by inhalation, and through damaged skin. In the unexposed general population, average blood levels of silver are about 2.4 μg/L, urinary excretion is 2 μg/day, and tissue levels are about 0.05 μg/g (Wan et al., 1991). Dental amalgam fillings lead to higher tissue levels (Drasch et al., 1995). Complexes with serum albumin accumulate in the liver, from which a fractional amount is excreted. In animals parenterally dosed with silver salts, silver is widely distributed to most tissues. It can cross the blood-brain barrier and produce long-lasting deposits in many structures of the nervous system (Rungby, 1990). It is located exclusively in lysosomes of neuronal cells (Stoltenberg et al., 1994). A specific transporter protein may be involved (Havelaar et al., 1998). Autopsy findings after treatment of burn injuries indicated highest levels in skin, gingiva, cornea, liver, and kidneys (Wan et al., 1991). Excretion is via the GI tract and kidneys. Specific transport proteins are responsible for secretion of silver from liver cells to bile (Dijkstra et al., 1996).

The major effect of excessive absorption of silver is local or generalized impregnation of the tissues, where it remains as silver sulfide, which forms an insoluble complex in elastic fibers, resulting in argyria. The complexes also contain selenium (Matsumura et al., 1992). Industrial argyria, a chronic occupational disease, has two forms, local and generalized. The local form involves the formation of gray-blue patches on the skin or may manifest itself in the conjunctiva of the eye. In generalized argyria, the skin shows widespread pigmentation, often spreading from the face to most uncovered parts of the body. In some cases the skin may become black, with a metallic luster. The eyes may be affected to such a point that the lens and vision are disturbed. The respiratory tract may also be affected in severe cases. Large oral doses of silver nitrate cause severe gastrointestinal irritation due to its caustic action. Lesions of the kidneys and lungs and the possibility of arteriosclerosis have been attributed to both industrial and medicinal exposures. Chronic bronchitis has also been reported to result from medicinal use of colloidal silver (Browning, 1969). Animal experiments indicate that silver disturbs copper metabolism (Hirasawa et al., 1994) and that metallothionein may protect against the toxic action of silver (Shinogi and Maeizumi, 1993).

Tellurium (Te)

Tellurium[1] is a semimetallic element in the sulfur and selenium family. It is found in various sulfide ores along with selenium and is produced as a by-product of metal refineries. Its industrial uses include applications in the refining of copper and in the manufacture of rubber. Tellurium vapor is used in "daylight" lamps and in various alloys as a catalyst and as a semiconductor frequently in combination with other metals.

Tellurium in food is probably in the form of tellurates. Condiments, dairy products, nuts, and fish have high concentrations of tellurium. Food packaging contains some tellurium; higher concentrations are found in aluminum cans than in tin cans. Some plants, such as garlic, accumulate tellurium from the soil. Potassium tellurate has been used to reduce sweating. The average body burden in humans is about 600 mg, mainly in bone.

The biochemistry and toxicity of the metal has been reviewed recently by Taylor (1996). Soluble tetravalent tellurates, absorbed into the body after oral administration, are reduced to tellurides, partly methylated, and then exhaled as dimethyl telluride. The latter is responsible for the garlic odor in persons exposed to tellurium compounds. The kidney has the highest content among the soft tissues. Tellurium may also accumulate in the liver (Schroeder and Mitchener, 1972). The urine and bile are the principal routes of excretion. Sweat and milk are secondary routes of excretion.

Tellurates and tellurium are of low toxicity, but tellurites are generally more toxic. Acute inhalation exposure results in sweating, nausea, a metallic taste, and sleeplessness. A typical garlic breath is an indicator of exposure to tellurium by the dermal, inhalation, or oral route. Serious cases of tellurium intoxication from industrial exposure have not been reported. One of the few serious recorded cases of tellurium toxicity resulted from accidental poisoning by injection of tellurium into the ureters during retrograde pyelography. Two of the three victims died. Garlic breath, renal pain, cyanosis, vomiting, stupor, and loss of consciousness were observed in this unlikely incident. The amount of sodium telluride used was about 2 g (Hunter, 1969).

In rats, chronic exposure to high doses of tellurium dioxide has produced decreased growth and necrosis of the liver and kidney (Cerwenka and Cooper, 1961; Browning, 1969). Rats fed 1 percent of metallic tellurium in the diet developed demyelination of peripheral nerve (Goddrum, 1998), probably due to the inhibition of squalene monooxygenase, a key enzyme in cholesterol biosynthesis (Laden et al., 2000). Cadmium telluride is a novel compound used in semiconductors. On inhalation this compound was shown to cause severe pulmonary inflammation and fibrosis in rats (Morgan et al., 1997). Tellurium compounds can produce hydrocephalus in experimental animals. Dimercaprol treatment for tellurium toxicity increases the renal damage. While ascorbic acid decreases the characteristic garlic odor, it may also adversely affect the kidneys in the presence of increased amounts of tellurium (Fishbein, 1977).

Thallium (Tl)

Thallium[1] is one of the more toxic metals. The thallium ion, Tl^+, has a similar charge and ionic radius as the potassium ion. Some of its toxic effects (see below) may result from interference with the biological functions of potassium. It is obtained as a by-product of the refining of iron, cadmium, and zinc. It is used as a catalyst in certain alloys, optical lenses, jewelry, low-temperature thermometers, semiconductors, dyes and pigments, and scintillation counters. Industrial poisoning is a special risk in the manufacture of fused halides for the production of lenses and windows. It has been used medicinally as a depilatory. Thallium compounds, chiefly thallous sulfate, have been used as rat poison and insecticides. This is one of the commonest sources of human thallium poisoning.

Thallium is absorbed through the skin and gastrointestinal tract. The highest concentrations after poisoning are in the kidney. Following the initial exposure, large amounts are excreted in urine during the first 24 h, but after that period excretion is slow and the feces may be an important route of excretion. The half-life in humans has been reported in the range of 1 to 30 days and may be dose-dependent. Thallium undergoes enterohepatic circulation.

[1]Atomic weight, 127.6; periodic table group, VIA; valence, +2, +4, or +6; discovered in 1792.

[1]Atomic weight, 204; periodic table group, IIIA; valence, +1 or +3; discovered in 1861.

Prussian blue, the most commonly used antidote, is given orally to break the enterohepatic cycle by trapping thallium secreted in bile and carrying it into the feces. For major reviews, see Malkey and Oehme (1993), Galván-Arzate and Santamaría (1998).

There are numerous clinical reports of acute thallium poisoning in humans characterized by GI irritation, acute ascending paralysis, psychic disturbances, and alopecia. The estimated acute lethal dose in humans is 8 to 12 mg/kg. Epilation begins about 10 days after ingestion and complete hair loss in about 1 month. Thallium targets the epithelial cells of the hair papillae. The turnover of these cells allows complete restoration of the hair in about 2 to 3 months. The growth of fingernails is impaired and transverse white stripes appear in the nails.

The acute cardiovascular effects of thallium ions probably result from competition with potassium for membrane transport systems, inhibition of mitochondrial oxidative phosphorylation, and disruption of protein synthesis. It also alters heme metabolism.

In humans, fatty infiltration and necrosis of the liver, nephritis, gastroenteritis, pulmonary edema, degenerative changes in the adrenals, degeneration of the peripheral and central nervous system, alopecia, and in some cases death have been reported as a result of long-term systemic thallium intake. These cases usually are caused by the contamination of food or the use of thallium as a depilatory. Loss of vision plus the other signs of thallium poisoning have been related to industrial exposures (Browning, 1969).

Studies on animals suggest that the mitochondrion is an important intracellular target. Thallium, besides competing with potassium, may combine with the sulfhydryl groups in the mitochondria and thereby interfere with oxidative phosphorylation. Its affinity for sulfydryl groups may also explain its ability to induce lipid peroxidation and deplete intracellular glutathione levels.

Evidence is scanty that thallium is mutagenic or carcinogenic (Leonard and Gerber, 1997). On the other hand, it may be teratogenic, especially with regard to cartilage and bone formation, but most of the evidence comes from chicks, not mammals. A teratogenic response to thallium salts characterized as achondroplasia (dwarfism) has been described in rats (Nogami and Terashima, 1973). Prenatal exposure of humans has resulted in skin and nail dystrophy, alopecia, and low body weight in newborns.

Tin (Sn)

Tin[1] has two higher valence states: stannous, Sn^{2+} and stannic, Sn^{4+}, tin. Both form stable inorganic compounds. In addition, stannic tin can form a volatile hydride, SnH_4 and a number of toxicologically important organometallic compounds in which the stannic atom form is covalently attached to one or more carbon atoms. Tin has a long history of use dating back to ancient Egypt. Currently it is used in the manufacture of tinplate, in food packaging, and in solder, bronze, and brass. Stannous and stannic chlorides are used in dyeing textiles. Organic tin compounds have been used in fungicides, bactericides, and slimicides, as well as in plastics as stabilizers. The daily intake is about 3.5 mg of tin, considerably lower than the 17 mg estimated in previous decades thanks to better food packaging methods. [The disposition and possible health effects of inorganic and organic tin compounds have been summarized in a number of reviews (WHO (1980), Alessio and Dell'Orto (1998), and Winship (1988).]

[1]Atomic weight, 118.7; periodic table group, IVA; valence, +2, +4; discovered in ancient times.

There is only limited absorption of even soluble inorganic compounds after oral administration. Ninety percent of the tin administered in this manner is recovered in the feces. The small amounts absorbed are reflected by increases in the liver and kidneys. Injected tin is excreted by the kidneys, with smaller amounts in bile. A mean normal urine level of 16.6 μg/L or 23.4 μg/day has been reported. The majority of inhaled tin remains in the lungs, most extracellularly, with some in the macrophages, in the form of SnO_2.

The organic tins, particularly the trimethyltin and triethyltin compounds, are better absorbed than inorganic species of tin. The tissue distribution of tin from these compounds shows the highest concentrations in the blood and liver, with smaller amounts in the muscle, spleen, heart, or brain. Tetraethyltin is converted to triethyltin in vivo.

Chronic inhalation of tin in the form of dust or fumes leads to benign pneumoconiosis. Tin hydride (SnH_4) is more toxic to mice and guinea pigs than is arsine; however, its effects appear mainly in the central nervous system and no hemolysis is produced. Orally, tin or its inorganic compounds require relatively large doses (500 mg/kg for 14 months) to produce toxicity. Inorganic tin salts given by injection produce diarrhea, muscle paralysis, and twitching. Studies on animals reveal that administration of inorganic tin compounds disturbs copper, zinc, and iron metabolism [Yu and Beynen (1995), Reicks and Rader (1990)]. The stannous ion also interacts with N-type calcium channels enhancing calcium transport into neurons (Hattori and Maehashi, 1991, 1992). Stannous is a more potent inducer than stannic tin of hemeoxygenase (HO-1), the rate determining enzyme in the catabolism of the heme ring (Neil et al., 1995). Tin also inhibits aminolevulinic dehydratase, a key enzyme in the synthesis of the heme ring, but not as potently as lead (Zareba and Chmielnicka, 1992). This action may be another example of tin displacing an essential metal cofactor, in this case zinc (Chmielnicka et al., 1992). Experimental studies have failed to find any evidence of mutagenicity, carcinogenicity, or teratogenicity of inorganic tin compounds. In fact some anticarcinogenic properties have been detected (Winship, 1988).

Some organic tin compounds are highly toxic, particularly triethyltin. Trimethyltin and triethyltin cause encephalopathy and cerebral edema. Toxicity declines as the number of carbon atoms in the chain increases. An outbreak of almost epidemic nature took place in France due to the oral ingestion of a preparation (Stalinon) containing diethyltin diodide for the treatment of skin disorders. Excessive industrial exposure to triethyltin has been reported to produce headaches, visual defects, and electroencephalographic (EEG) changes that were very slowly reversed (Prull and Rompel, 1970). Experimentally, triethyltin produces depression and cerebral edema. The resulting hyperglycemia may be related to the centrally mediated depletion of catecholamines from the adrenals. Acute burns or subacute dermal irritation has been reported among workers as a result of tributyltin. Triphenyltin has been shown to be a potent immunosuppressant (Verschuuren et al., 1970). Inhibition on the hydrolysis of adenosine triphosphate and an uncoupling of the oxidative phosphorylation taking place in the mitochondria have been suggested as the cellular mechanisms of tin toxicity (WHO, 1980).

Some butyl and methyl compounds of tin were positive in the Ames mutagenicity test (Hamasaki et al., 1993). Tributyl tin can suppress natural killer cells in mice. This inhibition may predispose animals to malignancy (Ghoneum et al., 1990).

Titanium (Ti)

Most titanium compounds are in the oxidation state +4 (titanic), but oxidation state +3 (titanous) and oxidation state +2 compounds as well as several organometallic compounds do occur. Because of its resistance to corrosion and inertness, metallic titanium[1] has many metallurgic applications, particularly as a component of surgical implants and prostheses. Titanium dioxide, the most widely used compound, is a white pigment used in paints and plastics; as a food additive to whiten flour, dairy products, and confections; and as a whitener in cosmetic products. It occurs widely in the environment; in urban air, rivers, and drinking water and is detectable in many foods. Titanium in feces is sometimes used as a measure of soil ingestion.

Approximately 3 percent of an oral dose of titanium is absorbed. The majority of that absorbed is excreted in the urine. The normal urinary concentration has been estimated at 10 μg/L (Schroeder et al., 1963; Kazantzis, 1981). The estimated body burden of titanium is about 15 mg. Most of it is in the lungs, probably as a result of inhalation exposure, as it tends to remain in the lungs for long periods. Lung burdens increase with age and vary according to geographic location. Mean concentrations of 8 and 6 ppm for the liver and kidney, respectively, were reported in the United States. Titanium IV may circulate in plasma bound to transferrin (Messori et al., 1999). Newborns have little titanium.

Occupational exposure to titanium, usually in the form of titanium dioxide, (TiO_2) may be heavy, and concentrations in air up to 50 mg/m^3 have been recorded. TiO_2 has been classified as a nuisance particulate with a TLV of 10 mg/m^3. Nevertheless, slight fibrosis of lung tissue has been reported following inhalation exposure to titanium dioxide pigment, but the injury was not disabling. Ultrafine particles of TiO_2 are more likely to produce pulmonary inflammation than larger particles (Baggs et al., 1997). Excessive deposits in the lung will cause pulmonary overload, impairing the clearance mechanism (Warheit et al., 1997). Otherwise, titanium dioxide has been considered physiologically inert by all routes (ingestion, inhalation, dermal, and subcutaneous). Titanium dioxide was found not to be carcinogenic in a bioassay study in rats and mice (NCI, 1979).

The metal and other salts are also relatively nontoxic except for titanic acid, which, as might be expected, will produce irritation (Berlin and Nordberg, 1986). A titanium coordination complex, titanocene, suspended in trioctanoin and administered by intramuscular injection to rats and mice produced fibrosarcomas at the site of injection and hepatomas and malignant lymphomas (Furst and Haro, 1969). A titanocene is a sandwich arrangement of titanium between two cyclopentadiene molecules.

Uranium (U)

The chief raw material of uranium[2] is pitchblende or carnotite ore. This element is largely limited to use as a nuclear fuel and, as a spent fuel in military ordinance. It is present naturally in air, water, food, and soil. The average daily intake from food is 1 to 2 μg and about 1.5 μg from 1 L of drinking water. This metal has five oxidation states but only the +4 and +6 forms are stable enough to be of practical importance. The +6 forms the uranyl ion (UO_2^{2+}), which forms water-soluble compounds and is an important species of uranium in body fluids.

The uranyl ion is rapidly absorbed from the GI tract. About 60 percent is carried as a soluble bicarbonate complex, while the remainder is bound to plasma protein. Sixty percent is excreted in the urine within 24 h. About 25 percent may be fixed in the bone (Chen et al., 1961).

Naturally occurring depleted uranium, although radioactive, presents predominantly a toxicologic rather than radiologic health risk. Following inhalation of the insoluble salts, retention by the lungs is prolonged. Uranium tetrafluoride and uranyl fluoride can produce toxicity because of hydrolysis to hafnium. For example, they will burn skin on contact.

The soluble uranium present in plasma as the uranyl ion complexed with bicarbonate produces systemic toxicity in the form of acute renal damage and renal failure, which may be fatal. However, if exposure is not severe enough, the renal tubular epithelium is regenerated and recovery occurs. Renal toxicity with the classic signs of impairment—including albuminuria, elevated blood urea nitrogen, and loss of weight—is brought about by filtration of the bicarbonate complex through the glomerulus, bicarbonate reabsorption by the proximal tubule, liberation of uranyl ion, and subsequent damage to the proximal tubular cells. Uranyl ion is most likely concentrated intracellularly in lysosomes (Ghadially et al., 1982). A study of uranium mill workers suggested that workers' long-term low level exposure is associated with β_2-microglobulinuria and amino aciduria (Thun et al., 1985).

In those studies where a higher incidence of lung cancer has been found in uranium miners, the cancer is probably due to radon and its daughter products, not to uranium itself (ATSDR, 1999). In fact, there is no convincing evidence that uranium is carcinogenic.

The threshold limit for uranium in the workroom (TWA) is 200 $\mu g/m^3$ and the EPA-established limit in drinking water is 100 μg/L. [For a detailed review of uranium, see ATSDR (1999).]

Vanadium (V)

Vanadium[1] may be an essential trace element, but a deficiency disease has not yet been defined in humans. It has several oxidation states, the most common being +3, +4, and +5. It is a by-product of petroleum refining, and vanadium pentoxide is used as a catalyst in the reactions of various chemicals including sulfuric acid. It is used in the hardening of steel, in the manufacture of pigments, in photography, and in the formulation of insecticides. Food is the major source of human exposure. Significant amounts are found in milk, seafood, cereals, and vegetables. The daily intake in the U.S. population ranges from 10 to 60 μg. The normal blood and urine levels are estimated to be around 1 and 10 nmol/L respectively (Sabbioni et al., 1996).

Metallic vanadium does not occur in nature, but human tissues come into long-term contact in medical implants. The lungs absorb soluble vanadium compounds well, but the absorption of vanadium salts from the gastrointestinal tract is poor. In the body, the pentavalent form (VO_3^-) is the predominant species in extracellular fluid whereas quadrivalent form (VO^{2+}) is most common inside the cell. The largest single compartment is the fat. Bone and teeth stores contribute to the body burden. The principal route of

[1]Atomic weight, 47.9; periodic table group, IVB; valence, +2, +3, or +4; discovered in 1791.

[2]Atomic weight, 238; periodic table group, V; valence, +2, +3, +4, and +6; discovered in 1841.

[1]Atomic weight, 50.93; periodic table group, VA; valence, +2, +3, +4, or +5; discovered in 1801.

excretion of vanadium is the urine with a biological half-life of 20 to 40 h.

The pentavalent compounds are the most toxic. The toxicity of vanadium compounds usually increases as the valence increases. The toxic action of vanadium is largely confined to the respiratory tract. Bronchitis and bronchopneumonia are more frequent in workers exposed to vanadium compounds. In industrial exposures to vanadium pentoxide dust, a greenish-black discoloration of the tongue is characteristic. Irritant activity with respect to skin and eyes has also been ascribed to industrial exposure. Gastrointestinal distress, nausea, vomiting, abdominal pain, cardiac palpitation, tremor, nervous depression, and kidney damage, too, have been linked with industrial vanadium exposure (Waters, 1977; Wennig and Kirsch, 1988; Goyer, 1996; Barceloux, 1999).

REFERENCES

Abrams M, Murrer BA: Metal compounds in therapy and diagnosis. *Science* 261:725–730, 1993.

ACGIH: *Threshold Limit Values for Chemicals and Physical Agents and Biological Exposure Indices for 1995–1996.* Cincinnati, OH: American Conference of Governmental Industrial Hygienists, 1996.

Agency for Toxic Substances and Disease Registry (ATSDR): *Toxicological Profile for Antimony,* TP-91/02. Washington, DC: U.S. Department of Health and Human Services, Public Health Service, 1992.

Agency for Toxic Substances and Disease Registry (ATSDR): *Toxicological Profile for Barium.* Washington, DC: U.S. Department of Health and Human Services, U.S. Public Health Services, July 1992.

Agency for Toxic Substances and Disease Registry (ATSDR): *Mercury.* Washington, DC: U.S. Department of Health and Human Services, March 1999.

Ainsworth SK, Swain RP, Watabe N, et al: Gold nephropathy, ultrastructural fluorescent and energy-dispersive x-ray microanalysis study. *Arch Pathol Lab Med* 105:373–378, 1981.

Al-Abbasi AH, Kostyniak PJ, Clarkson TW: An extracorporeal complexing hemodialysis system for the treatment of methylmercury poisoning: III. Clinical applications. *J Pharmacol Exp Ther* 207(1):249–254, 1978.

Alessio L, Dell'Orto A: Biological monitoring of tin, in Clarkson TW, Friberg L, Nordberg G, Sager PR (eds): *Biological Monitoring of Toxic Metals.* New York: Plenum Press, 1988, pp 419–425.

Alexander J, Hogberg J, Thomassen Y, et al: Selenium, in Seiler HG, Sigel H (eds): *Handbook on Toxicity of Inorganic Compounds.* New York: Marcel Dekker, 1988, pp 581–588.

Alfrey AC: Aluminum toxicity in patients with chronic renal failure. *Ther Drug Monit* 15:593–597, 1993.

Anderson C, Danylchuk KD: Effect of chronic low-level cadmium intoxication on the Haversian remodeling system in dogs. *Calcif Tiss Res* 26:143–148, 1978.

Andrews KW, Savitz DA, Hertz-Picciotto I: Prenatal lead exposure in relation to gestational age and birth weight: A review of epidemiological studies. *Am J Ind Med* 26:13–32, 1994.

Angle CR: Organ-specific therapeutic intervention, in Goyer RA, Klaassen CD, Waalkes MP (eds): *Metal Toxicology.* San Diego, CA: Academic Press, 1995, pp 71–110.

Anttila A, Pukkala A, Aiti T, et al: Update of cancer incidence among workers at a copper/nickel smelter and nickel refinery. *Int Arch Occup Environ Health* 71:245–250, 1998.

Aoshima K, Fan J, Kawanishi Y, et al: Changes in bone density in women with cadmium-induced renal tubular dysfunction: A six-year follow-up study. *Arch Complex Environ Studies* 9:1–8, 1997.

Aposhian HV: Mobilization of mercury and arsenic in humans by sodium 2.3-dimercapto-1-propane sulfonate (DMPS). *Environ Health Perspect* 106(suppl 4):1017–1025, 1998.

Aposhian HV, Aposhian MM: Meao-2,3 dimercaptosuccinic acid: Chemical, pharmacological and toxicological properties of an orally effective metal chalting agent. *Annu Rev Pharmacol Toxicol* 30:279–306, 1992.

Aposhian HV, Bruce DC, Alter W, et al: Urinary mercury after administration of 2-3 dimercaptopropane-1-sulfonic acid: Correlation with dental amalgam score. *FASEB J* 6:2472–2476, 1992.

Apostoli P, Lucchini R, Alessi L: Are current biomarkers suitable for the assessment of manganese exposure in individual workers? *Am J Ind Med* 37:283–290, 2000.

Apostoli P, Porru S, Alessio L: Behavior of urinary beryllium in general population and in subjects with low-level occupational exposure. *Med Lav* 80(5):390–396, 1989.

Arena JM: *Poisoning,* 3d ed. Springfield, IL: Charles C Thomas, 1974.

Armstrong RA, Winsper SJ, Blair JA: Aluminium and Alzheimer's disease: Review of possible pathogenic mechanisms. *Dementia* 7:1–9, 1996.

Assenato G, Pac C, Molinini R, et al: Sperm count suppression without endocrine dysfunction in lead-exposed men. *Arch Environ Health* 41:387–390, 1986.

ATSDR: *Cadmium (Update).* Washington, DC: U.S. Department of Health and Human Services, 1998.

ATSDR: *Manganese.* Atlanta: Agency for Toxic Substances and Disease Registry, 1997, pp 1–199.

ATSDR: *Toxicological Profile for Lead.* Washington, DC: U.S. Department of Health and Human Services, Agency for Toxic Substances and Disease Registry, 1999.

ATSDR: *Toxicological Profile for Nickel.* Atlanta, GA: Public Health Service, U.S. Department of Health and Human Services, 1997, pp 1–262.

ATSDR: *Toxicological Profile for Uranium.* Atlanta, GA: Agency for Toxic Substances and Disease Control, Division of Toxicology, 1999.

Audesirk T, Shugarts D, Cabell-Kluch L: The effects of triethyl lead on the development of hippocampal neurons in culture. *Cell Biol Toxicol* 11:1–10, 1995.

Baggs RB, Ferin J, Oberdorster G: Regression of pulmonary lesions produced by inhaled titanium dioxide in rats. *Vet Pathol* 34:592–597, 1997.

Baker EL, Goyer RA, Fowler BA, et al: Occupational lead exposure, nephropathy, and renal cancer. *Am J Ind Med* 1:139–148, 1980.

Bakir F, Damluji SF, Amin-Zaki L, et al: Methylmercury poisoning in Iraq. *Science* 181:230–241, 1973.

Ballatori N: Molecular mechanisms of hepatic metal transport, in Zalups RK, Koropatnick J (eds): *Molecular Biology and Toxicology of Metals.* New York: Taylor & Francis, 2000a, pp 346–381.

Ballatori N, Lieberman MW, Wang W: *N*-acetylcysteine as an antidote in methyl mercury poisoning. *Environ Health Perspect* 106:267–271, 1998.

Ballatori N: Personal communication, 2000b.

Banks WA, Kasin AJ, Fasold MB: Differential effect of aluminum on the blood-brain barrier transport of peptides, technetium and albumin. *J Pharmacol Exp Ther* 244:579–585, 1988.

Barceloux DG: Vanadium. *Clin Toxicol* 37:265–278, 1999.

Bartfay WJ, Butany J, Lehotay DC, et al: A biochemical, histochemical, and electron microscopic study on the effects of iron-loading on the hearts of mice. *Cardiovascul Pathol* 8:305–315, 1999.

Bates MN, Smith AH, Hopenhayn-Rich C: Arsenic ingestion and internal cancers: A review. *Am J Epidemiol* 135:462–476, 1992.

Battistuzzi G, Petrucci R, Silvagni L, et al: Delta-aminolevulinate dehydrase: A new genetic polymorphism in man. *Ann Hum Genet* 45:223–229, 1981.

Batuman V, Maesaka JK, Haddad B, et al: The role of lead in gout nephropathy. *N Engl J Med* 304:520–523, 1981.

Beijer K, Jernelov A: Sources, transport and transformation of metals in the environment, in Friberg L, Nordberg GF, Vouk VB (eds): *Handbook on the Toxicoloy of Metals,* 2d ed. *General Aspects.* Amsterdam: Elsevier, 1986, pp 68–74.

Benson JM, Carpenter RL, Hahn FF, et al: Comparative toxicity of nickel subsulfide to F344/N rats and B6C3F1 mice exposed for 12 days. *Fundam Appl Toxicol* 9:251–265, 1987.

Berg JM, Shi Y: The galvanization of biology: A growing appreciation for the roles of zinc. *Science* 271:1081–1085, 1996.

Berglund M, Askesson A, Nermell B, et al: Intestinal absorption of dietary cadmium in women depends on body iron stores and fiber intake. *Environ Health Perspect* 102:1058–1066, 1994.

Berlin M, Nordberg G: Titanium, in Friberg L, Nordberg GF, Vouk VB (eds): *Handbook on the Toxicology of Metals.* Vol 2. *Specific Metals.* Amsterdam: Elsevier, 1986, pp 594–609.

Berlin M: Mercury, in Friberg L, Nordberg GF, Nordman C (eds): *Handbook on the Toxicology of Metals,* 2d ed. Vol 2. *Specific Metals.* Amsterdam: Elsevier, 1986, pp 386–445.

Bernacke EG, Parsons B, Roy B, et al: Urine concentrations in nickel-exposed workers. *Ann Clin Lab Med* 8:184–189, 1978.

Bernard A, Lauwerys R: Epidemiological application of early markers of nephrotoxicity. *Toxicol Lett* 46:293–306, 1989.

Bernstein LR: Mechanisms of therapeutic activity for gallium. *Pharmacol Rev* 50:665–681, 1998.

Besunder JB, Super DM, Anderson RL: Comparison of dimercaptosuccinic acid and calcium disodium ethylenediaminetetraacetic acid versus dimercaptopropanol and ethylenediaminetetraacetic acid in children with lead poisoning. *J Pediatr* 130:966–971, 1997.

Bhattacharyya MH, Whelton BD, Peterson DP, et al: Skeletal changes in multiparous mice fed a nutrient-sufficient diet containing cadmium. *Toxicology* 50:193–204, 1988.

Bigazzi PE: Autoimmunity and heavy metals. *Lupus* 3:449–453, 1 994.

Birch NJ: Magnesium and calcium, in Berthon G (ed): *Handbook of Metal-Ligand Interactions in Biological Fluids: Bioinorganic Medicine.* New York: Marcel Dekker, 1995, pp 679–682.

Birchall J, Chappel J: The chemistry of aluminum and silicon in relation to Alzheimer's disease. *Clin Chem* 34:265–267,1988

Bizzi A, Gambetti P: Phosphorylation of neurofilaments is altered in aluminum intoxication. *Acta Neuropathol* 71:154–158, 1986.

Blazka ME, Dixon D, Haskins E, et al: Pulmonary toxicity to intratracheally administered indium trichloride in Fischer 344 rats. *Fundam Appl Toxicol* 22:231–239, 1994.

Bockman RS: Studies on the mechanisms of action of gallium nitrate. *Semin Oncol* 18(suppl 5):21–25, 1991.

Bolanowska W: Distribution and excretion of triethyllead in rats. *Br J Ind Med* 25:203–208, 1968.

Bondy SC: The neurotoxicity of organic and inorganic lead, in Tilson HA, Sparber SB (eds): *Neurotoxicants and Neurobiological Function: Effects of Organoheavy Metals.* New York: Wiley, 1991, pp 1–17.

Borschein RL, Grote J, Mitchell T: Effects of prenatal lead exposure on infant sized at birth, in Smith M, Grant LD, Sors A (eds): *Lead Exposure and Child Development: An International Assessment.* Lancaster, UK: Kluwer, 1989, pp 307–319.

Bradberry SM, Vale JA: Therapeutic review: Do diethelydiothiocarmate and disufiram have a role in acute nickel carbonyl poisoning. *J Toxicol Clin Toxicol* 37:259–264, 1999.

Brewer GJ, Hill GM, Prasad AS, et al: Oral zinc therapy for Wilson's disease. *Ann Intern Med* 99:314–320, 1993.

Bridgewater LC, Manning FC, Patierno SR: Arrest of replication of mammalian DNA polymerase alpha and beta caused by Cr-DNA lesions. *Mol Carcinogern* 23:201–206, 1998.

Bright P, Burge PS, O'Hickey SP, et al: Occupational asthma due to chrome and nickel electroplating. *Thorax* 52:28–32, 1997.

Brooks SM, Baker DB, Gann PH, et al: Cold air challenge and platinum skin reactivity in platinum refinery workers: Bronchial reactivity precedes skin prick response. *Chest* 97:1401–1407, 1990.

Brown MM, Rhyne BC, Goyer RA, et al: The intracellular effects of chronic arsenic exposure on renal proximal tubule cells. *J Toxicol Environ Health* 1:505–514, 1976.

Browning E: *Toxicity of Industrial Metals,* 2d ed. London: Butterworth, 1969.

Bruening K, Kemp FW, Simone N, et al: Dietary calcium intakes in urban children at risk of lead poisoning (abstr). *Environ Health Perspect* 107:431–436, 1999.

Brumm VL, van Gorp WG, Wirshing W: Chronic neuropsychological sequelae in a case of severe lithium intoxication. *Neuropsychiatry Neuropsychol Behav Neurol* 11:245–249, 1998.

Buchet JP, Lauwerys R, Roels H, et al: Renal effects of cadmium body burden of the general population. *Lancet* 336:699–702, 1990.

Buchet JP, Roels H, Bernard A, et al: Assessment of renal function of workers exposed to inorganic lead, cadmium or mercury vapor. *J Occup Med* 22:741–750, 1980.

Calabrese EJ, Baldwin LA: Lead-induced cell proliferation and organ-specific tumorigenicity. *Drug Metab Rev* 24:409–416, 1992.

Carney SL, Ray C, Gillies AH: Mechanism of lithium-induced polyuria in the rat. *Kidney Int* 50:377–383, 1996.

CDC: Blood lead levels—United States, 1988–1991. *MMWR* 46:141–146, 1997.

CDC: *Eliminating Childhood Lead Poisoning: A Federal Strategy Targeting Lead Paint Hazards.* Atlanta: Centers for Disease Control, 2000, pp 1–46.

CDC: *Preventing Lead Poisoning in Young Children: A Statement by the Centers for Disease Control.* Atlanta: U.S. Department of Health and Human Services/Public Health Service/Centers for Disease Control, 1991.

Cerwenka EA, Cooper WC: Toxicology of selenium and tellurium and their compounds. *Arch Environ Health* 3:189–200, 1961.

Chan HM, Tease LA, Liu HC, et al: Cell cultures in Wilson's disease, in Sarkar B (ed): *Biological Aspects of Metals and Metal-Related Diseases.* New York: Raven Press, 1983, pp 147–158.

Chan HM, Zhu L, Zhong R, et al: Nephrotoxicity in rats following liver transplantation from cadmium-exposed rats. *Toxicol Appl Pharmacol* 123:89–96, 1993.

Chan S, Gerson B, Subramanian S: The role of copper, molybdenum, selenium and zinc in nutrition and health. *Clin Lab Med* 18:673–685, 1998.

Chang CC, Vander Maillie RJ, Garvey JS: A radioimmunoassay for human metallothionein. *Toxicol Appl Pharmacol* 55:94–102, 1980.

Chapin RE, Harris MW, Hunter ES III, et al: The reproductive and developmental toxicity of indium in the Swiss mouse. *Fundam Appl Toxicol* 27:140–148, 1995.

Chen PS, Terepka R, Hodge HC: The pharmacology and toxicology of the bone seekers. *Annu Rev Pharmacol* 2:369–396, 1961.

Chen X, Yang G, Chen J, et al: Studies on the relations of selenium and Keshan disease. *Biol Tr Elem Res* 2:91–107, 1980.

Cherian MG, Miles EF, Clarkson TW, et al: Estimation of mercury burdens in rats by chelation with dimercaptopropane sulfonate. *J Pharmacol Exp Ther* 245:479–484, 1988.

Chiou HY, Hsueh YM, Hsu LL, et al: Arsenic methylation capacity, body retention, and null genotypes of glutathione S-transferase M1 and T1 among current arsenic-exposed residents in Taiwan. *Mutat Res* 386:197–207, 1997.

Chisholm JJ Jr, Thomas D: Use of 2,3-dimercaptopropane-1-sulfonate in treatment of lead poisoning in children. *J Pharmacol Exp Ther* 235:665–660, 1985.

Chmielnicka J, Zareba G, Grabowska U: Protective effect of zinc on heme biosynthesis disturbances in rabbits after administration per os of tin. *Ecotoxicol Environ Saf* 24:266–274, 1992.

Choi BH, Laspham LW, Amin-Zaki L, et al: Abnormal neuronal migration, deranged cerebral cortical organization and diffuse white matter astrocytosis of human fetal brain. *J Neuropathol Exp Neurol* 37:719–733, 1978.

Choie DD, Longenecker DS, Del Campo AA: Acute and chronic cisplatin nephropathy in rats. *Lab Invest* 44:397–402, 1981.

Choie DD, Richter GW: Effects of lead on the kidney, in Singhall RL, Thomas JA (eds): *Lead Toxicity.* Baltimore: Urban and Schwarzenberg, 1980, pp 187–212.

Christensen OB, Lagesson V: Nickel concentration of blood and urine after oral administration. *Ann Clin Lab Med* 11:119–125, 1981.

Clarkson TW: Methylmercury toxicity to the mature and developing nervous system: Possible mechanisms, in Sarkar B (ed): *Biological Aspects of Metals and Metal-Related Diseases.* New York: Raven Press, 1983, pp 183–187.

Clarkson TW, DiStefano V: Lead, mercury arsenic and chelating agents, in Dipalma JR (ed): *Drill's Pharmacology in Medicine.* New York: McGraw-Hill, 1971, chap 53.

Clarkson TW, Friberg L, Hursh JB, et al: The prediction of intake of mercury vapor from amalgams, in Clarkson TW, Friberg L, Nordberg GF, Sager PR (eds): *Biological Monitoring of Toxic Metals.* New York: Plenum Press, 1988, pp 247–264.

Cocco P, Dosemeci M, Heineman EF: Brain cancer and occupational exposure to lead. *J Occup Environ Med* 40:937–942, 1998.

Columbano A, Ledda GM, Sirigu P, et al: Liver cell proliferation induced by a single dose of lead nitrate. *Am J Pathol* 110:83–88, 1983.

Concha GG, Nermell B, Vahtera M: Metabolism of inorganic arsenic in children with chronic high arsenic exposure in northern Argentina. *Environ Health Perspect* 106:355–359, 1998a.

Concha GG, Vogbler D, Lezeano D, et al: Exposure to inorganic arsenic metabolites during early development. *Toxicol Sci* 44:185–190, 1998b.

Cooper WC, Gaffey WR: Mortality of lead workers. *J Occup Med* 17:100–107, 1975.

Cooper WC, Wong O, Kheifets L: Mortality among employees of lead battery plants and lead-producing plants, 1947–1980. *Scand J Work Environ Health* 11:331–345, 1985.

Costa M: Model for the epigenetic mechanism of action of nongenotoxic carcinogens. *Am J Clin Nutr* 61:6666S–6669S, 1995.

Costa M: Toxicity and carcinogenicity of Cr (VI) in animal models and humans. *Crit Rev Toxicol* 27:431–442, 1997.

Costa M, Zhitkovich A, Toniolo P: DNA-protein cross-links in welders: Molecular implications. *Cancer Res* 53:460–463, 1993.

Cotzias GC, Papavasiliou PS, Ginos J: Metabolic modification of Parkinson's disease and of chronic manganese poisoning (abstr). *Annu Rev Med* 22:305–336, 1971.

Cousins RJ: Zinc, in Ziegler EE, Filer LJ (eds): *Present Knowledge in Nutrition.* Washington, DC: ILSI Press, 1996, pp 293–306.

Cox C, Clarkson TW, Marsh DO, et al: Dose-response analysis of infants prenatally exposed to methyl mercury: An application of a single compartment model to single-strand hair analysis. *Environ Res* 49:318–332, 1989.

Cox M, Singer I: Lithium, in Bronner F, Coburn JW (eds): *Disorders of Mineral Metabolism.* New York: Academic Press, 1981, pp 369–438.

Crapper-McLachlan DR: Aluminum neurotoxicity: Criteria for assigning a role in Alzheimer's disease, in Spencer PS, Schaumburg HH (eds): *Environmental Chemistry and Toxicology of Aluminum.* Chelsea, MI: Lewis, 1989, pp 299–315.

Cremin JD Jr, Luck ML, Laughlin NK, et al: Efficacy of succimer for reducing brain lead in a primate model of human lead exposure. *Toxicol Appl Pharmacol* 161:283–293, 1999.

Cuajungco MP, Lees GJ: Zinc and Alzheimer's disease: Is there a direct link? *Brain Res Rev* 23:219–236, 1998.

Davis JW, Fann WE: Lithium. *Annu Rev Pharmacol* 11:285–298, 1971.

Davison AG, Taylor AJN, Darbyshire J, et al: Cadmium fume inhalation and emphysema. *Lancet* 26:663–667, 1988.

DeBoni U, Otavos A, Scott JW, et al.: Neurofibrillary degeneration induced by systemic aluminum. *Acta Neuropathol* 35:285–294, 1976.

De Valk B, Marx JJ: Iron, atherosclerosis, and ischemic heart disease. *Arch Int Med* 159:1542–1548, 1999.

DeVoto E, Yokel RA: The biological speciation and toxicokinetics of aluminum. *Environ Health Perspect* 102:940–951, 1994.

Dijkstra M, Havinga R,Vonk RJ, et al: Bile secretion of cadmium, silver, zinc and copper in the rat: Involvement of various transport systems. *Life Sci* 59:1237–1246, 1996.

Dingwall-Fordyce I, Lane RE: A follow-up study of lead workers. *Br J Ind Med* 20:313–315, 1963.

Dipaolo JA, Casto BC: Quantitative studies of in vitro morphologic transformation of Syrian hamster cells by inorganic metal salts. *Cancer Res* 39:1008–1019, 1979.

Donoffrio PD, Wilbourn AJ, Alberrs JW, et al: Acute arsenical intoxication presenting as Guillian-Barré-like syndrome. *Muscle Nerve* 10:114–120, 2000.

Dorian C, Gattone VH, Klaassen CD: Renal cadmium deposition and injury as a result of accumulation of cadmium-metallothionein (CdMT) by the proximal convoluted tubules—A light microscopic study with 109Cd. *Toxicol Appl Pharmacol* 114:173–181, 1992.

Doss M, Beacker U, Sixel F, et al: Persistent protoporphyrinemia in hereditary porphobilinogen synthase (delta-aminolevulinic acid dehydrase) deficiency under low lead exposure: A molecular basis for the pathogenesis of lead intoxication. *Klin Wochenschr* 60:599–606, 1982.

Dragsten PR, Hallaway PE, Hanson GJ, et al: First human studies with a high-molecular-weight iron chelator. *J Lab Clin Med* 135:57–65, 2000.

Drasch G, Gath HJ, Heissler E, et al: Silver concentrations in human tissues: Their dependence on dental amalgam and other factors. *J Trace Elem Med Biol* 9:82–87, 1995.

Dubrovskaya VA, Wetterhahn KE: Effects of Cr(VI) on the expression of the oxidative stress genes in human lung cells. *Carcinogenesis* 19: 1401–1407, 1998.

Dunnick JK, Elwell MR, Benson JM, et al: Lung toxicity after 13-week inhalation exposure to nickel oxide, nickel subsulfide, or nickel sulfate hexahydrate in F344/N rats and $B6C3F_1$ mice. *Fundam Appl Toxicol* 12:584–594, 1989.

Durbin PW, Kullgren B, Xu J, et al: Multidentate hydroxypyridninonate ligands for Pu(IV) chelation in vivo: Comparative efficiency and toxicity in mouse of ligands containing 1.2-HOPO of Me-3,2 HOPH. *Int J Radiat Biol* 76:199–214, 2000.

Elinder C-G, Friberg L: Antimony, in Friberg L, et al. (eds): *Handbook on the Toxicology of Metals,* 2d ed. Vol II. Amsterdam: Elsevier, 1986, pp 26–42.

Elinder C-G, Friberg L: Cobalt, in Friberg L, Nordberg GF, Vouk VB (eds): *Handbook on the Toxicology of Metals.* Amsterdam: Elsevier, 1986, pp 212–232.

Elinder C-G, Friberg L, Kjellstrom T, et al: *Biological Monitoring of Metals.* Geneva: World Health Organization, 1994.

Ellis KJ, Cohn SH, Smith TJ: Cadmium inhalation exposure estimates: Their significance with respect to kidney and liver cadmium burden. *J Toxicol Environ Health* 15:173–187, 1985.

Enterline PE, Marsh GM: Mortality studies of smelter workers. *Am J Ind Med* 1:251–259, 1989.

EPA: *Air Quality Criteria for Lead.* Vol I–IV. EPA-600/8-83/02aF. Washington, DC: U.S. Environmental Protection Agency, 1986.

EPA: Drinking water maximum contamination level goal and national primary water regulation for lead and copper. *Fed Reg* 59:33860–33864, 1994.

EPA: *Air Quality Criteria for Lead.* Vol I–IV, EPA-600/8-83/028f. Washington, DC: U.S. Environmental Protection Agency, 1986.

EPA: *Integrated Risk Information System (IRIS) for Cadmium.* Washington, DC: Office of Health and Environmental Assessment, U.S. Environmental Protection Agency, 1997.

EPA: *Special Report on Ingested Arsenic, Risk Assessment Forum.* EPA/625/3-87/013, Washington, DC: U.S. Environmental Protection Agency, 1988.

EPA: *Health Assessment for Beryllium.* EPA/600/8-84/026F. Washington, DC: U.S. Environmental Protection Agency, 1987.

Exley C, Brugess E, Day JP, et al: Aluminum toxicokinetics. *J Toxicol Environ Health* 48:569–584, 1996.

Farago ME, Kavanagh P, Blanks R, et al: Platinum concentrations in urban road dust and soil, and in blood and urine in the United Kingdom. *Analyst* 123:451–454, 1998.

Fayerweather WE, Karns ME, Nuwayhid IA: Case-control study of cancer risk in tetraethyl lead manufacturing. *Am J Ind Med* 31:28–35, 1997.

Fewtrell L, Kay D, Jones F, et al: Copper in drinking water—An investigation into possible health effects (abstr). *Public Health* 110:175–177, 1996.

Fishbein L: Sources, transport and alteration of metal compounds: An overview: Arsenic, beryllium, cadmium, chromium and nickel. *Environ Health Perspect* 40:43–64, 1981.

Fishbein L: Toxicology of selenium and tellurium, in Goyer RA, Mehlman MA (eds): *Toxicology of Trace Metals.* New York: Wiley, 1977, pp 191–240.

Flanagan PR, McLellan JS, Hais J, et al: Increased dietary cadmium absorption in mice and human subjects with iron deficiency. *Gastroenterology* 74:841–846, 1978.

Flaten TP, Wakayama I, Sturm MJ, et al: Natural models of aluminum toxicity in fish from acid-rain lakes, in Nicolini M, Zatta PF, Corain B, (eds): *Alzheimer's Disease and Related Disorders.* Oxford: Pergamon Press, 1993, pp 253–254.

Fleming DEB, Chettle DR, Wetmur JG, et al: Effect of the delta-aminolevulinate dehydratase polymorphism on the accumulation of lead in bone and blood in lead smelter workers. *Environ Res* 77:49–61, 1998.

Fontenot AP, Falta MT, Freed BM, et al: Identification of pathogenic T cells in patients with beryllium-induced lung disease. *J Immunol* 163:1091–1026, 1999.

Forster DP, Newens AJ, Kay DWK, et al: Risk factors in clinically diagnosed presenile dementia of the Alzheimer type: A case-control study in northern England. *J Epidemiol Commun Health* 49:253–258, 1995.

Fowler BA, Goyer RA: Bismuth localization within nuclear inclusions by x-ray microanalysis. *J Histochem Cytochem* 23:722–726, 1975.

Fowler BA, Moorman B, Atkins WE, et al: Toxicity data from acute and short-term inhalation exposures, in American Conference of Governmental Industrial Hygenists (eds): *Hazard Assessment amd Control Technology in Semiconductor Manufacturing.* Boca Raton, FL: American Conference of Governmental Industrial Hygienists, 1989, pp 85–89.

Fowler BA, Vouk V: Bismuth, in Friberg L, Nordberg GF, Vouk VB (eds): *Handbook on the Toxicology of Metals.* 2d ed. Vol II. Amsterdam: Elsevier, 1986, pp 117–129.

Friberg L, Eliner CF, Kjellstrom T, et al: *Cadmium and Health: A Toxicological and Epidemiological Appraisal.* Vol II. *Effects and Response.* Boca Raton, FL: CRC Press, 1986, pp 1–307.

Friberg L, Lener J: Molybdenum, in Friberg L, Nordberg G, Vouk VB (eds): *Handbook on the Toxicology of Metals,* 2d ed. Vol 1: *Specific Metals.* Amsterdam: Elsevier, 1986, pp 446–461.

Froomes PR, Wan AT, Keech AC, et al: Absorption and elimination of bismuth from oral doses of tripotassium dicitrato bismuthate. *Eur J Clin Pharmacol* 37:533–536, 1989.

Frydman M, Bonne-Tamir B, Farrer LA, et al: Assignment of the gene for Wilson's disease to chromosome 13: Linkage to the esterase D locus. *Proc Natl Acad Sci USA* 82:1819–1821, 1985.

Fu H, Boffetta P: Cancer and occupational exposure to inorganic lead compounds: A meta-analysis of published data. *Occup Environ Med* 52:73–81, 1995.

Fullmer CS: Intestinal interactions of lead and calcium. *Neurotoxicology* 13:799–808, 1992.

Furst A, Haro RT: A survey of metal carcinogenesis. *Prog Exp Tumour Res* 12:102–133, 1969.

Galván-Arzate S, Santamaría A: Thallium toxicity. *Toxicol Lett* 99:1–13, 1998.

Ganrote PO: Metabolism and possible health effects of aluminum. *Environ Health Perspect* 65:363–441, 1986.

Garruto RM, Fukatsu R, Yanagihara R, et al: Imaging of calcium and aluminum in neurofibrillary tangle–bearing neurons in parkinsonism-dementia of Guam. *Proc Natl Acad Sci USA* 81:1875, 1984.

Gennart JP, Bernard A, Lauwerys R: Assessement of thyroid, testis, kidney, and autonomic nervous system function in lead-exposed workers. *Int Arch Occup Health* 64:49–58, 1992.

Gerber GB, Léonard A: Mutagenicity, carcinogenicity and teratogenicity of germanium compounds. *Mutat Res* 387:141–146, 1997.

Gerhardsson L, Borjesson J, Mattson S, et al: Chelated lead in relation to lead in bone and ALAD genotype. *Environ Res* 80:389–398, 1999.

Ghadially FN, Lalonde JA, Yang-Steppuhn S: Uraniosomes produced in cultured rabbit kidney cells by uranyl acetate. *Virchows Arch* (*Cell Pathol*) 39:21–30, 1982.

Ghoneum M, Hussein E, Gill G, et al: Suppression of murine natural killer cell activity by tributyltin: In vivo and in vitro assessment. *Environ Res* 52:178–186, 1990.

Goddrum JF: Role of organotellurium species in tellurium neuropathy. *Neurochem Res* 23:1313–1319, 1998.

Goldwater LJ: *Mercury: A History of Quicksilver.* Baltimore: York Press, 1972.

Gonsebatt ME, Vega L, Montero R, et al: Lymphocyte replicating ability in individuals exposed to arsenic via drinking water. *Mutat Res* 313:293–299, 2000.

Gonzalez D, Zuniga-Charles M, Narro-Juarez A, et al: DMPS (2,3 dimercaptopropane-1-sulfonate, dimaval) decreases the body burden of mercury in humans exposed to mercurous chloride. *J Pharmacol Exp Ther* 287(1):8–12, 1998.

Goyer RA: Lead toxicity: Current concerns. *Environ Health Perspect* 100:177–187, 1993.

Goyer RA: Lead toxicity: From overt to subclinical to subtle health effects. *Environ Health Perspect* 86:177–181, 1990.

Goyer RA: Metal-protein complexes in detoxification process, in Brown SS (ed): *Clinical Chemistry and Clinical Toxicology.* Vol 2. London: Academic Press, 1984, pp 199–209.

Goyer RA: Nephrotoxicity and carcinogenicity of lead, in Beck BD (ed): An update on exposure and effects of lead. *Fundam Appl Toxicol* 18:4–7, 1992.

Goyer RA: Nutrition and metal toxicity. *Am J Clin Nutr* 61(suppl):646S–650S, 1995.

Goyer RA: Results of lead research: Prenatal exposure and neurological consequences. *Environ Health Perspect* 104:1050–1054, 1996.

Goyer RA: Toxic effects of metals, in Klaassen CD (ed): *Casarett & Doull's Toxicology: The Basic Science of Poisons.* New York: McGraw-Hill, 1996, pp 691–736.

Goyer RA, Rhyne BC: Pathological effects of lead. *Int Rev Exp Pathol* 12:1–77, 1973.

Grandjean P, Jorgensen PJ, Weihe P: Human milk as a source of methylmercury exposure in infants. *Environ Health Perspect* 102:74–77, 1994.

Granick JL, Sassa S, Granick RD, et al: Studies in lead poisoning: II. Correlation between the ratio of activated to inactivated aminolevulinic acid dehydratase of whole blood and the blood lead level. *Biochem Med* 8:149–159, 1973.

Grant L, Mushak P: Speciation of metals and metal compounds: Implications for biological monitoring and development of regulatory approaches. *Toxicol Ind Health* 5:891–908, 1989.

Greger JL: Dietary and other sources of aluminum intake, in *Aluminum in Biology and Medicine.* New York: Wiley, 1992, pp 26–49.

Gritzka TL, Trump BF: Renal tubular lesions caused by mercuric chloride. *Am J Pathol* 52:1225–1277, 1968.

Gulson BL, Mahaffey KR, Jameson CW, et al: Mobilization of lead from the skeleton during the postnatal period is larger than during pregnancy. *J Lab Clin Med* 131:324–329, 1998.

Gulson BL, Mahaffey KR, Mizon KJ, et al: Contribution of tissue lead to blood lead in adult female subjects based on stable lead isotope methods. *J Lab Clin Med* 125:703–712, 1995.

Gunsalus IC: The chemistry and function of the pyruvate oxidation factor (lipoic acid). *J Cell Comp Physiol* 41(suppl 1):113–136, 1953.

Gunter E: Urine cadmium levels in general U.S. population from NHANES III. *Chemosphere* 34:1945–1953, 1997.

Gyurasies A, Koszorus L, Varga F, et al: Increased biliary excretion of glutathione is generated by the glutathione-dependent hepatobiliary transport of antimony and bismuth. *Biochem Pharmacol* 44:1275–1281, 1992.

Hallab NJ, Jacobs JJ, Skipor A, et al: Systemic metal-protein binding associated with total joint replacement arthroplasty. *J Biomed Mater Res* 49:353–361, 2000.

Hamasaki T, Sato T, Nagase H, et al: The mutagenicity of organotin compounds as environmental pollutants. *Mutat Res* 300:265–271, 1993.

Harlan WR: The relationship of blood lead levels to blood pressure in the U.S. population. *Environ Health Perspect* 78:9–13, 1988.

Harris ED: Copper, in O'Dell BL, Sunde RA (eds): *Handbook of Nutritionally Essential Mineral Elements.* New York: Marcel Dekker, 1997, pp 231–273.

Harris WR, Berthon G, Day JP, et al: Speciation of aluminum in biological systems. *J Toxicol Environ Health* 48:543–568, 1996.

Hattori T, Maehahsi H: Activation of N-type calcium channels by stannous chloride at frog motor nerve terminals. *Res Commun Chem Pathol Pharmacol* 74:125–128, 1991.

Hattori T, Maehahsi H: Interaction between stannous chloride and calcium channel blockers in frog neuromuscular transmission. *Res Commun Chem Pathol Pharmacol* 75:243–246, 1992.

Havelaar AC, de Gast IL, Snijders S, et al: Characterization of a heavy metal ion transporter in the lysosomal membrane. *FEBS Lett* 436:223–227, 1998.

Hayes RB: The carcinogenicity of metals in humans. *Cancer Causes Control* 8:371–385, 1997.

Hayes RJ: Gallium, in Seiler HG, Sigel N (eds): *Handbook on the Toxicity of Inorganic Compounds.* New York: Marcel Dekker, 1988, pp 297–300.

Henry GA, Jarnot BM, Steinhoff MM, et al: Mercury-induced autoimmunity in the MAXX rat. *Clin Immunol Immunopathol* 49:187–203, 1988.

Herbert V: Vitamin B_{12}, in Ziegler EE, Filer LJ (eds): *Present Knowledge in Nutrition.* Washington, DC: ILSI, 1996, pp 191–205.

Hirasawa F, Sato M, Takizawa Y: Organ distribution of silver and the effect of silver on copper status in rats. *Toxicol Lett* 70:193–201, 1994.

Holt D, Webb M: Teratogenicity of ionic cadmium in the Wistar rat. *Arch Toxicol* 59:443–447, 1987.

Hostynek JJ: Gold: An allergen of growing significance. *Food Chem Toxicol* 35:839–844, 1997.

Hostynek JJ, Hinz RS, Lorence CR, et al: Metals and the skin. *Crit Rev Toxicol* 23:171–235, 1993.

Hu H, Aro A, Payton M, et al: The relationship of bone and blood lead to hypertension. *JAMA* 275:1171–1176, 1996.

Hunter D, Bomford RR, Russell DS: Poisoning by methyl mercury compounds. *Q J Med* 9:193–197, 1940.

Hunter D: *Diseases of Occupations,* 4th ed. Boston: Little, Brown, 1969.

Hutchinson J: Arsenic cancer. *Br Med J* 2:1280–1281, 1887.

IARC: *IARC Monographs on the Evaluation of Carcinogenic Risks to Humans: Overall Evaluations of Carcinogenicity: An Updating of IARC Monographs.* Vols 1 to 42. Suppl 7. Lyons, France: IARC, 1987, pp 230–232.

IARC: *IARC Monographs on the Evaluation of Risks to Humans.* Vol 58. *Cadmium, Mercury, Beryllium and the Glass Industry.* Lyons, France: IARC, 1993.

IARC: *Monograph on the Evaluation of Risks to Humans.* Vol 58. *Cadmium, Mercury, Beryllium and the Glass Industry.* Lyons, France: IARC, 1994.

IARC: *Monographs on the Evaluation of Carcinogenic Risks to Humans.* Vol 47. Lyons, France: IARC, 1989.

ICRP (International Commission on Radiological Protection): Limited of intakes of radionuclides by workers. Metabolic data for antimony. ICRP Publication 30. Part 3. *Ann ICRP* 1981.

IPCS: *Environmental Health Criteria.* Vol 108. *Nickel.* Geneva: World Health Organization, 1991, pp 1–383.

Jamall IS, Sorowls JJ: Effects of cadmium and dietary selenium on cytoplasmic and mitochondrial antioxidant defense systems in the heart of rats fed high dietary copper. *Toxicol Appl Pharmacol* 87:102–110, 1987.

Jaremin B: Blast lymphocyte transformation (LTT), rosette (E-RFC) and leukocyte migration inhibition(MIF) tests in persons exposed to lead during work. Report II. *Bull Inst Marit Trop Med (Gdynia)* 34:187–197, 1983.

Jarup L, Berglund M, Elinder CG, et al: Health effects of cadmium exposure: A review of its literature and a risk estimation. *Scand J Work Environ Health* 24:1–51, 1998.

Jarup L, Elinger C-G, Spang G: Cumulative blood-cadmium and tubular proteinuria: A dose-response relationship. *Int Arch Occup Environ Health* 60:223–229, 1988.

Johnson CH, Van Tassell VJ: Acute barium poisoning with respiratory failure and rhabdomyolysis. *Ann Emerg Med* 20:1138–1142, 1991.

Jones MM, Cherian MG: The search for chelate antagonists for chronic cadmium intoxication. *Toxicology* 62:1–25, 1990.

Jones MM: Newer chelating agents for in vivo toxic metal mobilization. *Comments Inorg Chem* 13:91–110, 1992.

Jouhanneau P, Raisbeck GM, Viou F, et al: Gastrointestinal absorption, tissue retention and urinary excretion of dietary levels of aluminum in rats as determined by using ^{26}Al. *Clin Chem* 43(pt 1):1023–1028, 1997.

Kaltreider RC, Pesce CA, Ihnat MA, et al: Differential effects of arsenic (III) and Cr(VI) on nuclear transcription factor binding. *Mol Carcinogen* 25:219–229, 1999.

Kang HK, Infante PF: Occupational lead exposure and cancer. *Science* 207:935–936, 1980.

Kanzantzis G: Role of cobalt, iron, lead, manganese, mercury, platinum, selenium and titanium in carcinogenesis. *Environ Health Perspect* 40:143–161, 1981.

Karjalainen SR, Kerttula R, Pukkala E: Cancer risk among workers at a copper/nickel smelter and nickel refinery. *Int Arch Occup Environ Health* 63:547–551, 1992.

Kawada T: Indicators of renal effects of exposure to cadmium: *N*-acetyl-β-D-glucosaminidase and others. *J Occup Med* 17:69–73, 1998.

Kazantzis G: Role of cobal, iron, lead, manganese, mercury, platinum, selenium and titanium in carcinogenesis. *Environ Health Perspect* 40:143–161, 1981.

Keberle H: The biochemistry of desferrioxamine and its relation to iron metabolism. *Ann NY Acad Sci* 119:758–768, 1964.

Keen CL, Zidenberg-Cherr S: Manganese, in Ziegler EE, Filer LJ Jr (eds): *Present Knowledge in Nutrition.* Washington, DC: ILSI, 1996, pp 334–343.

Kido T, Honda R, Tsuritani I, et al: Progress of renal dysfunction in inhabitants environmentally exposed to cadmium. *Arch Environ Health* 43:213–217, 1988.

Kjellstrom T: Exposure and accumulation of cadmium in populations from Japan, the United States, and Sweden. *Environ Health Perspect* 28:169–197, 1979.

Klaassen CD: Heavy metal and heavy-metal antagonists, in Gilman AG, Rall TW, Nies AS, Taylor P (eds): *Goodman and Gilman's The Pharmacological Basis of Therapeutics.* New York: Pergamon Press, 1990, pp 1592–1614.

Klimisch HJ: Lung deposition, lung clearance and renal accumulation of inhaled cadmium chloride. *Toxicology* 84:103–124, 1993.

Kojima S, Ono H, Furukuawa A, et al: Effect of *N*-benzyl-D-glucamine dithiocarbamate on renal toxicity induced by cadmium-metallothionein. *Arch Toxicol* 64:91–96, 1990.

Kondo Y, Satoh M, Imura N, et al: Tissue-specific induction of metallothionein by bismuth as a promising protocol for chemotherapy with repeated administration of *cis*-diaminedichlorplatinum(II) against bladder cancer. *Anticancer Res* 12:2303–2308, 1992.

Kopp SJ: Cadmium and the cardiovascular system, in Foulkes EC (ed): *Handbook of Experimental Pharmacology.* New York: Springer-Verlag, 1986, pp 195–280.

Kostial K, Blanusa M, Piasek M, et al: Combined chelation therapy in reducing tissue lead concentration in suckling rats. *J Appl Toxicol* 19:143–147, 1999.

Kostyniak PJ: Mobilization and removal of methyl mercury in the dog during extracorporeal complexing hemodialysis with 2,3-dimercaptosuccinic acid (DMSA). *J Pharmacol Exp Ther* 221:63–68, 1982.

Kostyniak PJ, Clarkson TW: Role of chelating agents in metal toxicity. *Fund Appl Toxicol* 1:376–380, 1981.

Kostyniak PJ, Greizerstein HB, Goldstein J, et al: Extracorporeal regional complexing haemodialysis treatment of acute inorganic mercury intoxication. *Hum Exp Toxicol* 9:137–141, 1990.

Kreppel H, Liu J, Reichl FX, et al: Zinc-induced arsenite tolerance in mice. *Fundam Appl Toxicol* 23:32–37, 1993.

Laden BP, Tang Y, Porter TD: Cloning, heterologous expression and enzymological characterization of human squalene monooxygenase. *Arch Biochem Biophys* 374:381–388, 2000.

Lai MS, Hsueh CJ, Chen MP, et al: Ingested inorganic arsenic and prevalence of diabetes mellitus. *Am J Epidemiol* 138:484–492, 1994.

Lam HF, Conner MW, Rogers AE: Functional and morphological changes in the lungs of guinea pigs exposed to freshly generated ultrafine zinc oxide. *Toxicol Appl Pharmacol* 78:29–38, 1985.

Langard S, Norseth T: Chromium, in Friberg L, Nordberg GF, Vouk VB (eds): *Handbook on Toxicology of Metals,* 2d ed. Amsterdam: Elsevier, 1986, pp 185–210.

Langworth S, Elinder CG, Akesson A: Mercury exposure from dental fillings. I. Moving concentration in blood and urine. *Swed Dent J* 12:69–70, 1988.

Lauwerys R, Hardy R, Job M, et al: Environmental pollution by cadmium and cadmium body burden: An autopsy study. *Toxicol Lett* 23:287–289, 1984.

Lauwerys RR, Bernard AM, Roels HA: Cadmium: Exposure markers as predictors of nephrotoxic effects. *Clin Chem* 40:1391–1394, 1994.

Lauwerys RR, Roels H, Bernard A, et al: Renal response to cadmium in a population living in a nonferrous smelter area in Belgium. *Int Arch Occup Environ Health* 45:271–274, 1980.

Lauwerys RR, Roels H, Buchet JP, et al: Investigations on the lung and kidney functions in workers exposed to cadmium. *Environ Health Perspect* 28:137–145, 1979.

Leek JC, Keen CL, Vogler JP, et al: Long-term marginal zinc deprivation in rhesus monkeys: IV. effects on skeletal growth and mineralization. *Am J Clin Nutr* 47:889–895, 1988.

Lenox RH, McNamara RK, Papke RL, et al: Neurobiology of lithium. *J Clin. Psychiatry* 58:37–47, 1998.

Léonard A, Gerber GB: Mutagenicity, carcinogenicity and teratogenicity of antimony compounds. *Mutat Res* 366:1–8, 1996.

Léonard A, Gerber GB: Mutagenicity, carcinogenicity and teratogenicity of thallium compounds. *Mutat Res* 387:47–53, 1997.

Levander OA, Burk RF: Selenium, in Ziegler EE, Filer LJ (eds): *Present Knowledge in Nutrition.* Washington, DC: ILSI, 1996, pp 320–328.

Li H, Sadler PJ, Sun H: Unexpectedly strong binding of a large metal ion (Bi^{3+}) to human serum transferrin. *J Biol Chem* 271:9483–9489, 1996.

Liden C, Maibach HJ, Wahlberg JE: Skin, in Goyer RA, Klaassen CD, Waalkes MP (eds): *Metal Toxicology.* San Diego, CA: Academic Press, 1995, pp 447–464.

Lilis R: Long-term occupational lead exposure, chronic nephropathy, and renal cancer: A case report. *Am J Ind Med* 2:293–297, 1981.

Lin XH, Sugiyama M, Costa M: Differences in the effect of vitamin E on nickel sulfide or nickel chloride-induced chromosomal alterations in mammalian cells. *Mutat Res* 260:159–164, 1991.

Lindgren KN, Masten VL, Ford DP: Relation of cumulative exposure to inorganic and neuropsychological test performance. *Occup Environ Med* 53:472–477, 1996.

Liss L, Thornton DJ: The rationale for aluminum absorption control in early stages of Alzheimer's disease. *Neurobiol Aging* 7:552–554, 1986.

Liu J, Liu Y, Habeebu SS, et al: Susceptibility of MT-Null mice to chronic CdCl2-induced nephrotoxicity indicates that renal injury is not (only) mediated by the CdMt complex. *Toxicol Sci* 46:197–203, 1998.

Logue J, Koontz M, Hattwick A: Historical prospective mortality study of workers in copper and zinc refineries. *J Occup Med* 24:398–408, 1982.

Lund ME, Banner W Jr, Clarkson TW, et al: Treatment of acute methyl mercury ingestion by hemodialysis with *N*-acetylcysteine (Mucomyst) infusion and 2.3-dimercaptopropane sulfonate. *J Toxicol Clin Toxicol* 22:31–49, 1984.

Lyons TJ, Liu H, Goto JJ, et al: Mutations in copper-zinc superoxide dismutase that cause amyotrophic lateral sclerosis alter the zinc binding site and redox behavior of the protein. *Proc Natl Acad Sci USA* 93:12240–12244, 1996.

Madias NE, Harrington JT: Platinum nephrotoxicity. *Am J Med* 65:307–314, 1978.

Madsen KM, Christensen EF: Effects of mercury on lysosomal protein digestion in the kidney proximal tubule. *Lab Invest* 38:165–171, 1978.

Mahaffey KR: Factors modifying susceptibility to lead toxicity, in Mahaffey KR (ed): *Dietary and Environmental Lead: Human Health Effects.* New York: Elsevier, 1985, pp 373–420.

Malkey JP, Oehme FW: A review of thallium toxicity. *Vet Hum Toxicol* 35:445–453, 1993.

Manton WI, Angle CR, Stanek KL, et al: Acquisition and retention of lead by young children. *Environ Res* 82:60–80, 2000.

Manton WI, Cook JD: High accuracy (stable isotope dilution) measurements of lead in serum and cerebrospinal fluid. *Br J Ind Med* 41:313–319, 1984.

Markjanic J, McDonald B, Chen CPLH, et al: Absence of aluminum in neurofibrillary tangles in Alzheimer's disease. *Neurosci Lett* 240:123–125, 1998.

Markovac J, Goldstein GW: Lead activates protein kinase C in immature rat brain microvessels. *Toxicol Appl Pharmacol* 96:14–23, 1988.

Martyn CN, Coggin DN, Inskip H, et al. Aluminum concentrations in drinking water and risk of Alzheimer's disease. *Epidemiology* 8:281–286, 1997.

Martyn CN, Osmond C, Edwardson JA, et al: Geographical relation between Alzheimer's disease and aluminium in drinking water. *Lancet* 1:59–62, 1989.

Matheson DS, Clarkson TW, Gelfand EW: Mercury toxicity (acrodynia) induced by long-term injection of gamma globulin. *J Pediatr* 97:153–155, 1980.

Matsumura T, Kumakiri M, Obkawara A, et al: Detection of selenium in generalized and localized argyria: Report of four cases with x-ray microanalysis. *J Dermatol* 19:87–93, 1992.

McCabe MJ, Lawrence DA: Lead, a major environmental pollutant, is immunomodulatory by its different effects on CD4+T cell subsets. *Toxicol Appl Pharmacol* 111:13–23, 1991.

McCoy H, Kenney M: A review of biointeractions of Ni and Mg: II. Immune system and oncology. *Magnes Res* 5:223–232, 1992.

McIntosh MJ, Meredith PA, Moore MR, et al: Action of lead on neurotransmission in rats. *Xenobiotica* 19:101–113, 1989.

McLachlan DRC, Bergeron C, Smith JE, et al: Risk for neuropathologically confirmed Alzheimer's disease and residual aluminum in municipal drinking water employing weighted residential histories. *Neurology* 46:401–405, 1996.

McLachlin JR, Goyer RA, Cherian MG: Formation of lead-induced inclusion bodies in primary rat kidney epithelial cell cultures: Effect of actinomycin D and cycloheximide. *Toxicol Appl Pharmacol* 56:418–431, 1980.

McMichael AJ, Vimpani GV, Robertson EF, et al: The Port Pirie study: Maternal blood lead and pregnancy outcome. *J Epidemiol Commun Health* 40:18–25, 1986.

Mercer JF, Livingston J, Hall B, et al: Isolation of a partial candidate gene for Menkes disease by positional cloning. *Nat Genet* 3:20–25, 1993.

Mertz W: Chromium occurrence and function in biological systems. *Physiol Rev* 49:163–239, 1969.

Mertz W, Abernathy CO, Olin SS: *Risk Assessment of Essential Elements.* Washington, DC: ILSI, 1994.

Messori L, Orioli P, Banholzer V, et al: Formation of titanium (IV) transferrin by reaction of human serum apotransferrin with titanium complexes. *FEBS Lett* 442:157–161, 1999.

Michel P, Commenges D, Dartigues JF, et al: Study of the relationship between Alzheimer's disease and aluminum in drinking water. *Neurobiol Aging* 11:264, 1990.

Miettinen JK: Absorption and elimination of dietary mercury (Hg^{++}) and methyl mercury in man, in Miller MW, Clarkson TW (eds): *Mercury, Mercurials and Mercaptans.* Springfield, IL: Charles C Thomas, 1973.

Miles AT, Hawksworth GM, Beattie JH, et al: Induction, regulation, degradation and biological significance of mammalian metallothioneins (abstr). *Crit Rev Biochem Mol Biol* 35:35–75, 2000.

Moore JF, Goyer RA, Wilson MH: Lead-induced inclusion bodies: Solubility, amino acid content and relationship to residual acidic nuclear proteins. *Lab Invest* 29:488–494, 1973.

Morgan DL, Shines CJ, Jeter SP, et al: Comparative pulmonary absorption, distribution and toxicity of copper gallium diselenide, copper indium diselenide and cadmium telluride in Spague-Dawley rats. *Toxicol Appl Pharmacol* 147:399–410, 1997.

Morrow PE: Dust overloading of the lungs: Update and appraisal. *Toxicol Appl Pharmacol* 113:1–12, 1992.

Morrow PE, Beiter H, Amato F, et al: Pulmonary retention of lead: An experimental study in man. *Environ Res* 21:373–384, 1980.

Mottet NK, Shaw C-M, Burbacher TM: Health risks from increases in methylmercury exposure. *Environ Health Perspect* 63:133–140, 1985.

Muller T, Feichtinger H, Berger H, et al: Endemic Tyrolean Infantile cirrhosis: An ecogenetic genetic disorder. *Lancet* 347:877–880, 1996.

Murphy MJ, Graziano JH, Popovac D, et al: Past pregnancy outcomes among women living in the vicinity of a lead smelter in Kosovo, Yugoslavia. *Am J Public Health* 80:33–35, 1990.

Murphy MJ, Lyon L, Taylor JW: Subacute arsenic neuropathy: Clinical and electrophysiological observations. *J Neurol Neurosurg Psychiatry* 44:896–900, 1981.

Murphy V: Cadmium: Acute and chronic neurological disorders, in Yasui M, Strong M, Ota K, Verity MA (eds): *Mineral and Metal Neurotoxicology.* Boca Raton, FL: CRC Press, 2000, pp 229–240.

Nagyvary J, Bradbury EL: Hypocholesterolemic effects of Al^{3+} complexes. *Biochem Res Commun* 2:592–598, 1977.

Nakamura H, Rose PG, Blumer JL, et al: Acute encephalopathy due to aluminum toxicity successfully treated by combined intravenous defroxamine and hemodialysis. *J Clin Pharmacol* 40:296–300, 2000.

NCI: *Bioassay of Titanium Dioxide for Possible Carcinogenicity.* National Cancer Institute Carcinogenesis Technical Report No. 97. DHEW Publ No. (NIH) d79-1347. Washington, DC: NCI/DHEW, 1979.

Needleman HL: The persistent threat of lead: A singular opportunity. *Am J Public* 79:643–645, 1989.

Needleman HL, Schell A, Bellinger D, et al: Long-term effects of childhood exposure to lead at low dose: An eleven-year follow-up report. *N Engl J Med* 322:82–88, 1990.

Neil TK, Abraham NG, Levere RD, et al: Differential heme oxygenase inducation by stannouse and stannic ions in the heart. *J Cell Biochem* 57:409–414, 1995.

Ng A, Patterson C: Natural concentrations of lead in ancient Arctic and Antarctic ice. *Geochim Cosmochim Acta* 45:2109–2121, 1981.

NIDI. *Safe Use of Nickel in the Workplace,* 2d ed. Ontario, Canada: Nickel Development Institute, 1997.

Niebor E, Nriagu JO: *Nickel and Human Health—Current Perspectives.* New York: Wiley, 1992, pp 1–680.

Nielson F: Other trace elements, in Ziegler EE, Filer LJ (eds): *Present Knowledge in Nutrition.* Washington, DC: ILSI, 1996, pp 353–377.

NIOSH. *Protecting Workers Exposed to Lead-Based Paint Hazards: A Report to Congress.* Washington, DC: U.S. Department of Health and Human Services, 1997, pp 1–74.

Nogami H, Terashima Y: Thallium-induced achondroplasia in the rat. *Teratology* 8:101–102, 1973.

Nogawa K, Honda R, Kido T, et al: A dose-response analysis of cadmium in the general environment with special reference to total cadmium. *Environ Res* 48:7–16, 1989.

Nogawa K, Tsuritani I, Kido T, et al: Mechanism for bone disease found in inhabitants environmentally exposed to cadmium: Decreased serum 1α,25-dihydroxyvitamin D level. *Int Arch Occup Environ Health* 59:21–30, 1987.

Nordberg G, Sandstrom B, Becking G, et al: Essentiality and toxicity of trace elements: Principles and methods for assessment of risk from human exposure to essential trace elements. *J Trace Elem Exp Med* 13:593–597, 2000.

Nordberg GF: Cadmium metabolism and toxicity. *Environ Physiol* 2:7–36, 1972.

Nordberg M: Metallothioneins: Historical review and state of knowledge. *Talanta* 46:243–254, 1998.

Norin H, Vahter M: A rapid method for the selective analysis of total urinary metabolites of inorganic arsenic. *Scand J Work Environ Health* 7:38–44, 1981.

NRC: *Arsenic in Drinking Water.* Washington, DC: National Academy Press, 1999, pp 1–308.

NRC: *Copper in Drinking Water.* Washington, DC: National Academy of Sciences, 2000, pp 1–145.

NRC: *Measuring Lead Exposure in Infants, Children and Other Sensitive Populations.* Washington, DC: National Academy Press, 1993.

NRC: *Recommended Dietary Allowances,* 10th ed. Washington DC: National Academy Press, 1989, pp 1–285.

O'Connor ME, Rich D: Children with moderately elevated lead levels: Is chelation with DMSA helpful? *Clin Pediatr (Phila)* 38:325–331, 1999.

O'Conner ME, Rich D: Children with moderately elevated lead levels: Is chelation helpful? (Abstr) *Clin Pediatr* 38:325–331, 1999.

Oda K: Toxicity of a low level of indium phosphide (InP) in rats after intratracheal instillation. *Ind Health* 35:61–68, 1997.

O'Flaherty EJ: Chromium toxicokinetics, in Goyer RA, Çherian MG (eds): *Toxicology of Metals: Biochemical Aspects.* Heidelberg, Germany: Springer-Verlag, 1995, pp 315–328.

O'Flaherty EJ: Physiologically based models of metal kinetics. *Crit Rev Toxicol* 28:271–317, 1998.

Oldiges H, Hochrainer D, Takenaka S, et al: Lung carcinomas in rats after low-level cadmium inhalation. *Toxicol Environ Chem* 9:41–51, 1984.

Oliver T: *Lead Poisoning: From the Industrial, Medical and Social Points of View.* London: Lewis, 1914, pp 1–294.

Ong CN, Endo G, Chia KS, et al: Evaluation of renal function in workers with low blood lead levels, in Foa V, Emmett EA, Maroni M, Colombi A (eds): *Occupational and Environmental Chemical Hazards: Cellular and Biochemical Indices for Monitoring Toxicity.* New York: Halsted Press, 1987, pp 327–333.

Orfila MP: *A General System of Toxicology.* Philadelphia: Carey, 1817.

Ornaghi F, Ferrini S, Prati M, et al: The protective effects of *N*-acetyl-L-cysteine against methyl mercury embryotoxicity in mice. *Fundam Appl Toxicol* 20:437–445, 1993.

Oskarsson A: *Risk Evaluation of Essential Elements—Essential Versus Toxic Levels of Intake.* Copenhagen: Nord, 1995.

Payton M, Riggs KM, Spiro AI: Relations of bone and blood lead to cognitive function: The VA normative study. *Neurotoxicol Teratol* 20:19–27, 1998.

Pelletier L, Druet P: Immunotoxicology of metals, in Goyer RA, Cherian MG (eds): *Handbook of Experimental Pharmacology.* Vol 115. Heidelberg, Germany: Springer-Verlag, 1995, pp 77–92.

Perelli G, Piolatto G: Tentative reference values for gold, silver and platinum: Literature data analysis. *Sci Total Environ* 120:93–96, 1992.

Perl DP, Good PF: Uptake of aluminum into central nervous system along nasal olfactory pathways. *Lancet* 1:1028–1029, 1987.

Perlstein MA, Attila R: Neurologic sequelae of plumbism in children. *Clin Pediatr* 5:292–298, 1966.

Pershagan G, Nordberg G, Bjorklund N: Carcinoma of the respiratory tract in hamsters given arsenic trioxide and/or benzoapyrene by the pulmonary route. *Environ Res* 227–241, 1984.

Pirkle JL, Brody DJ, Gunter EW, et al: The decline in blood lead levels in the United States. *JAMA* 272:284–291, 1994.

Pirkle JL, Kaufmann RB, Brody DJ, et al: Exposure of the U.S. population to lead, 1991–1994. *Environ Health Perspect* 106:745–750, 1998.

Pizzaro FM, Olivares M, Uauy R, et al: Acute gastrointestinal effects of graded levels of copper in drinking water. *Environ Health Perspect* 107:117–121, 1999.

Pounds JG, Long GJ, Rosen JF: Cellular and molecular toxicity of lead in bone. *Environ Health Perspect* 91:17–32, 1991.

Pradham AM, Talbot IC, Tanner MS: Indian childhood cirrhosis and other cirrhosis of Indian children. *Pediatr Res* 17:435–438, 2000.

Prasad AS: Clinical, biochemical and nutritional spectrum of zinc deficiency in human subjects: An update. *Nutr Rev* 41:197–208, 1983.

Prasad AS: Functional roles of zinc, in Berthon G (ed): *Handbook of Metal-Ligand Interactions in Biological Fluids*. Vol I. New York: Marcel Dekker, 1995, pp 232–241.

Prasad AS, Meftah S, Abdulla JD, et al: Serum thymulin in human zinc deficiency. *J Clin Invest* 82:1202–1210, 1988.

Prentice A: Does mild zinc deficiency contribute to pooor growth performance? *Nutr Rev* 51:268–277, 1997.

Proctor DM, Fredrick MM, Scott PK, et al: The prevalence of chromium allergy in the United States and its implications for setting soil cleanup: A cost-effectiveness case study. *Regul Toxicol Pharmacol* 28:27–37, 1998.

Prull G, Rompel K: EEG changes in acute poisoning with organic tin compounds. *Electroencephalog Clin Neurophysiol* 29:215–222, 1970.

Rahman M, Axelson O: Diabetes mellitus and arsenic exposure: A second look at case-control data from a Swedish copper smelter. *Occup Environ Med* 52:773–774, 1995.

Raithel HJ, Schaller KH, Kraus T, et al: Biomonitoring of nickel and chromium in human pulmonary tissue (abstr). *Int Arch Occup Environ Health* 65:S197–S200, 2000.

Reeves AL: Barium, in Friberg L, Nordberg GF, Vouk VB (eds): *Handbook on the Toxicology of Metals*. 2d ed. New York: Elsevier, 1986, pp 84–94.

Reicks M, Rader JI: Effects of dietary tin and copper on rat hepatocellular antioxidant protection. *Proc Soc Exp Biol Med* 195:123–128, 1990.

Richardson GM, Mitchell M, Coad S, et al: Exposure to mercury in Canada: A multimedia analysis. *Water Air Soil Pollut J* 80:21–30, 1995.

Roberts E: Alzheimer's disease may begin in the nose and may be caused by aluminosilicates. *Neurobiol Aging* 7:561–567, 1986.

Rodamilans M, Martinez-Osaba MJ, To-Figueras J, et al: Lead toxicity on endocrine testicular function in an occupationally exposed population. *Hum Toxicol* 7:125–128, 1988.

Roels H, Bernard AM, Cardenas A, et al: Markers of early renal changes induced by industrial pollutants: III. Application to workers exposed to cadmium. *Br J Ind Med* 50:37–48, 1993.

Roels H, Gennart J-P, Lauwerys R, et al: Surveillance of workers exposed to mercury vapor: Validation of a previously proposed biological threshold limit value for mercury concentration in urine. *Am J Ind Med* 7:45–71, 1985.

Roels HA, Hoet P, Lison D: Usefulness of biomarkers of exposure to inorganic mercury, lead, or cadmium in controlling occupational and environmental risks of nephrotoxicity. *Renal Failure* 3–4:251–262, 1999.

Roest M, van der Schouw YT, de Valk B, et al: Heterozygosity for a hereditary hemochromatosis gene is associated with cardiovascular death in women (comment). *Circulation* 100:1268–1273, 1999.

Rosen JF: Metabolic and cellular effects of lead: A guide to low level lead toxicity in children, in Mahaffey KR (eds): *Dietary and Environmental Lead: Human Health Effects*. Amsterdam: Elsevier, 1985, pp 157–181.

Rungby J: An experimental study on silver in the nervous system and on aspects of its general cellular toxicity. *Dan Med Bull* 37:442–449, 1990.

Sabbioni E, Kueera J, Pietra R, et al: A critical review on normal concentrations of vanadium in human blood, serum, and urine. *Sci Total Environ* 188:49–58, 1996.

Sager PR, Aschner M, Rodier PM: Persistent differential alterations in developing cerebellar cortex of male and female mice after methylmercury exposure. *Dev Brain Res* 12:1–11, 1984.

Saito S, Kuraski M: Gold replacement of cadmium, zinc-binding metallothionein. *Res Commun Mol Pathol Pharmacol* 93:101–107, 1996.

Salomen JY, Nyysson K, Korpela H: High stored iron levels are associated with excess risk of myocardial infarction in Western Finnish men. *Circulation* 86:803–811, 1992.

Sauder P, Livardjani F, Kaeger A, et al: Acute mercury chloride intoxication: Effects of hemodialysis and plasma exchange on mercury kinetic. *J Toxicol Clin Toxicol* 26:189–197, 1998.

Scheinberg JH, Sternlieb I: Wilson disease and idiopathic copper toxicosis. *Am J Clin Nutr* 63:842S–845S, 1996.

Schilsky ML, Sternlieb I: Animal models of copper toxicosis. *Adv Vet Sci Comp Med* 37:357–377, 1993.

Schrauzer GN: Functional roles of cobalt, in Berthon G (ed): *Handbook of Metal-Ligand Interactions in Biological Fluids*. New York: Marcel Dekker, 1995, pp 244–247.

Schroeder HA, Balassa JJ, Tipton IH: Abnormal trace metals in man: Titanium. *J Chronic Dis* 16:55–69, 1963.

Schroeder HA, Mitchener M: Selenium and tellurium in mice. *Arch Environ Health* 24:66–71, 1972.

Schwartz J, Otto D: Lead and minor hearing impairment. *Arch Environ Health* 46:300–306, 1991.

Seaton CL, Lasman J, Smith DR : The effects of CaNa (2) EDTA on brain lead mobilization in rodents determined using a stable isotope tracer. *Toxicol Appl Pharmacol* 159:153–160, 1999.

Sethi S, Grover S, Khodaskar MB: Role of copper in Indian childhood cirrhosis. *Ann Trop Paediatr* 14:3–6, 1993.

Shaikh ZA, Harnett KM, Perlin SA: Chronic cadmium intake results in dose-related excretion of metallothionein in urine. *Experientia* 45:146–148, 1989.

Shannon MW, Tornsend MK: Adverse effects of reduced-dose D-penicillamine in children with mild-to-moderate lead poisoning. *Ann Pharmacother* 34:15–18, 2000.

Sharma RR, Cast IP, Refern RM, et al: Extradural application of bismuth iodoform paraffin paste causing relapsing bismuth encephalopathy: A case report with CT and MRI studies. *J Neurol Neurosurg Psychiatry* 57:990–993, 1994.

Sheabar FZ, Yanni S, Taitelman U: Extracorporeal complexation hemodialysis for the treament of cadmium poisoning: II. In vivo mobilization and removal. *Pharmacol Toxicol* 65:13–16, 1989.

Shils ME: Magnesium, in Ziegler EE, Filer LJ (eds): *Present Knowledge in Nutrition*. Washington, DC: ILSI, 2000, pp 256–264.

Shinogi M, Maeizumi S: Effect of preinduction of metallothionein on tissue distribution of silver and hepatic lipid peroxidation. *Biol Pharm Bull* 16:372–374, 1993.

Shore D, Wyatt RJ: Aluminum and Alzheimer's disease. *J Nerve Ment Dis* 171:553–558, 1983.

Siegel N, Hagu A: Aluminum interaction with calmodulin: Evidence for altered structure and function from optical enzymatic studies. *Biochem Biophys Acta* 744:36–45, 1983.

Silbergeld EK, Schwartz J, Mahaffey K: Lead and osteoporosis: Mobilization of lead from bone in postmenopausal women. *Environ Res* 47:79–94, 1988.

Singer I: Lithium and the kidney. *Kidney Int* 19:374–387, 1981.

Singh J, Carlisle DL, Pritchard DE, et al: Cr-induced genotoxicity and apoptosis: Relationship to Cr carcinogenesis (review). *Oncol Rep* 5:1307–1318, 1998.

Skerfving S, Christoffersson J-O, Schutz A, et al: Biological monitoring by in vivo XRF measurements, of occupational exposure to lead, cadmium and mercury. *Biol Trace Elem Res* 13:241–251, 1987.

Slikkerveer A, de Wolff FA: Pharmacokinetics and toxicity of bismuth compounds. *Med Toxicol Adverse Drug Exp* 4:303–323, 1989.

Smith AH, Hopenhayn-Rich C, Bates MN, et al: Cancer risks from arsenic in drinking water. *Environ Health Perspect* 97:259–267, 1992.

Smith CJ, Livingston SD, Doolittle DJ: An international literature survey of "IARC group I carcinogens" reported in mainstream cigarette smoke. *Food Chem Toxicol* 35:1107–1130, 1997.

Smith CM, Wang X, Hu H, et al: A polymorphism in the delta-aminolivulinic acid dehydratase gene may modify the pharmacokinetics of lead. *Environ Health Perspect* 103:248–253, 1998.

Smith DR, Flegal AR: Stable isotopic tracers of lead mobilized by DMSA chelation in low lead-exposed rats. *Toxicol Appl Pharmacol* 116:85–91, 1992.

Smith IC, Carson BC, Hoffmeister F: Indium, in *Trace Elements in the Environment*. Vol 5. Ann Arbor, MI: Ann Arbor Science Publishers, 1978, p 562.

Solis-Heredia MJ, Quintanilla-Vega B, Sierra-Santoyo A, et al: Chromium increases pancreatic metallothionein in the rat. *Toxicology* 142:111–117, 2000.

Sorahan T, Lancashire RJ: Lung cancer mortality in a cohort of workers employed at a cadmium recovery plant in the United States: An analysis with detailed job histories. *Occup Environ Med* 54:194–201, 1997.

Spears JW, Hatfield EE, Forbes RM, et al: Studies on role of nickel in the ruminant. *J Nutr* 108:313–320, 1978.

Spivey Fox MR, Rader JI: Iron, in Seiler HG, Sigel H (eds): *Handbook on Toxicity of Inorganic Compounds*. New York: Marcel Dekker, 1988, pp 346–358.

Staessen JA, Bilpitt CJ, Fagard R: Hypertension caused by low-level lead exposure: Myth or fact. *J Cardiovasc Risk* 1:87–97, 1994.

Steele TN: Treatment of lithium intoxication with diuretics, in Brown SS (ed): *Clinical Chemistry and Chemical Toxicology of Metals*. Amsterdam: Elsevier, 1977, pp 289–292.

Stoecker BJ: Chromium, in Ziegler EE, Filer LJ (eds): *Present Knowledge in Nutrition*. Washington, DC: ILSI, 1996, pp 344–352.

Stoltenberg M, Juyl S, Poulsen EG, et al: Autometallographic detection of silver in hypothalamic neurons of rats exposed to silver nitrate. *J Appl Toxicol* 14:275–280, 1994.

Stowe HD, Goyer RA: The reproductive ability and progeny of F1 lead-toxic rats. *Fertil Steril* 22:755–760, 1971.

Stuve J, Galle P: Role of mitochondria in the renal handling of gold by the kidney. *J Cell Biol* 44:667–676, 1970.

Styblo M, Del Razo L, LeCluyse EL, et al: Metabolism of arsenic in primary cultures of human and rat hepatocytes. *Chem Res Toxicol* 12:560–565, 1999.

Sunderman F Jr, Aito A, Morgan LO, et al: Biological monitoring of nickel. *Toxicol Ind Health* 2:77–78, 1986.

Sunderman FW Sr: Efficacy of sodium diethyldithiocarbamate (dithiocarb) in acute nickel carbonyl poisoning. *Ann Clin Lab Sci* 9:1–10, 1979.

Sunderman FW Sr: Efficacy of sodium diethyldithiocarbamate (dithiocarb) in acute nickel carbonyl poisoning. *Ann Clin Lab Sci* 9:1–10, 1979.

Sunderman FW: Mechanisms of nickel carcinogenesis. *Scand J Work Environ Health* 15:1–12, 1989.

Sunderman FW Jr, Barber AM: Finger-loops, oncogenes, and metals. *Ann Clin Lab Sci* 18:267–288, 1988.

Swedish Expert Group: Methylmercury in fish: A toxicological–epidemiological evaluation of risks. *Nord Hyg Tidskr* 4(suppl):19–364, 1971.

Syversen TL: Changes in protein and RNA synthesis in rat brain neurons after a single dose of methyl mercury. *Toxicol Lett* 10:31–34, 1982.

Tabata M, Sarkar B: Specific nickel (II)-transfer process between the native sequence peptide representing the nickel (ii) transport site of human albumin and L-histidine (abstr). *J Inorg Biochem* 45:93–104, 1992.

Takenaka S, Oldiges H, Konig H, et al: Carcinogenicity of cadmium chloride aerosols in Wistar rats. *J Natl Cancer Inst* 70:367–373, 1983.

Takeuchi T: Neuropathology of Minamata disease in Kumamoto: Especially at the chronic stage, in Roisin L, Shiaki H, Greevic N (eds): *Neurotoxicology*. New York: Raven Press, 1977, pp 235–246.

Tanaka-Kagawa T, Naganuma A, Imura N: Tubular section and reabsorption of mercury compounds in mouse kidney. *J Pharmacol Exp Ther* 264:776–782, 1993.

Tanzi RE, Petrukhin K, Cherov I: The Wilson gene is a copper transporting ATPase with homology to the Menkes disease gene. *Nat Genet* 5:344–350, 1993.

Tao SS, Bolger PM: Dietary arsenic intakes in the United States: FDA Total Diet Study, September 1991–December 1996. *Food Addit Contam* 16:465–472, 1999.

Taylor A: Biochemistry of tellurium. *Biol Trace Elem Res* 55:231–239, 1996.

Tenenbein M: Does lead poisoning occur in Canadian children? *Can Med Assoc J* 142:40–41, 1990.

Thomas DW, Hartly TF, Sobecki S: Clinical and laboratory investigations of the metabolism of bismuth containing pharmaceuticals by man and dogs, in Brown SS (ed): *Clinical Chemistry and Clinical Toxicology of Metals*. Amsterdam: Elsevier, 1977, pp 293–296.

Thun MJ, Baker DB, Steenland K, et al: Renal toxicity in uranium mill workers. *Scand J Work Environ Health* 11:83–90, 1985.

Thun MJ, Osorio AM, Schober S, et al: Nephropathy in cadmium workers: Assessment of risk from airborne occupational exposure to cadmium. *Br J Ind Med* 46:689–697, 1989.

Thun MJ, Schnorr TM, Smith AB, et al: Mortality among a cohort of U.S. cadmium production workers—An update. *J Natl Cancer Inst* 74:325–333, 1985.

Tillman LA, Drake FM, Dixon JS, et al: Review article: Safety of bismuth in the treatment of gastrointestinal diseases. *Aliment Pharmacol Ther* 10:459–467, 1996.

Timer RT, Sands JM: Lithium intoxication. *J Am Soc Nephrol* 10:666–674, 1999.

Tinkle SS, Kittle LA, Schumacher BA: Beryllium induces IL-2 and IFN-gamma in berylliosis. *J Immunol* 158: 518–526, 1997.

Tinkle SS, Newman LS: Beryllium-stimulated release of tumor necrotising factor alpha, interleukin-6, and their soluble receptors in chronic beryllium disease. *Am J Respir Crit Care Med* 156:1884–1891, 1997.

Toxicological Profile for Antimony. TP-91/02. Washington, DC: U.S. Department of Health and Human Services, Public Health Service, 1992.

Twarog T, Cherian MG: Chelation of lead by dimercaptopropane sulfonate and a possible diagnosis. *Toxicol Appl Pharmacol* 72:550–556, 1984.

Ungvary G, Szakmary E, Tatrai E, et al: Embryotoxic and teratogenic effects of indium trichloride in rats and rabbits. *J Toxicol Environ Health* 59:27–42, 2000.

Urizar R, Vernier RL: Bismuth nephropathy. *JAMA* 198:187–189, 1966.

Vahter, M: Species differences in the metabolism of arsenic compounds. *Appl Organometal Chem* 8:175–182, 1984.

Vahter M, Couch G, Nermell B, et al: Lack of methylation of inorganic arsenic in the chimpanzee. *Toxicol Appl Pharmacol* 133:262–268, 1995.

Valentine JL, Kang HK, Spivey G: Arsenic levels in human blood, urine and hair in response to exposure via drinking water. *Environ Res* 20:24–32, 1979.

Valentino M, Governa M, Marchiseppe I, et al: Effects of lead on polymorphonuclear leukocyte (PMN) functions in occupationally exposed workers. *Arch Toxicol* 65:685–688, 1991.

Verschuuren HG, Ruitenberg EJ, Peetoom F, et al: Influence of triphenyltin acetate on lymphatic tissue and immune response in guinea pigs. *Toxicol Appl Pharmacol* 16:400–410, 1970.

Victery W: Evidence for effects of chronic lead exposure on blood pressure in experimental animals: An overview. *Environ Health Perspect* 78:71–76, 1988.

Voil GW, Minielly JA, Bisricki T: Gold nephropathy tissue analysis by x-ray fluorescent spectroscopy. *Arch Pathol Lab Med* 101:635–640, 1977.

Waalkes MP, Anver M, Diwan BA: Carcinogenic effects of cadmium in the Noble (NBL/Cr) rat: Induction of pituitary, testicular, and injection site tumors and intraepithelial proliferative lesions of the dorsolateral prostate. *Toxicol Sci* 52:154–161, 1999.

Waalkes MP, Bhalchandra AD, Ward JM, et al: Renal tubular tumors and atypical hyperplasias in B6C3F1 mice exposed to lead acetate during gestation and lactation occur with minimal chronic nephropathy. *Cancer Res* 55:5265–5271, 1995.

Waalkes MP, Rehm S: Cadmium and prostate cancer. *J Toxicol Environ Health* 43:251–269, 1994.

Walshe JM: Endogenous copper clearance in Wilson's disease: A study of the mode of action of penicillamine. *Clin Sci* 26:461–469, 1964.

Walshe CT, Sandstead HH, Prasad AS, et al: Zinc: Health effects and research priorities for the 1990s. *Environ Health Perspect* 102(suppl 2):5–46, 1994.

Walshe JM: Assessment of treatment of Wilson's disease with triethylene tetramine 2HCl (trien 2HCl), in Sarkar B (ed): *Biological Aspects of Metals and Metal-Related Diseases.* New York: Raven Press, 1983, pp 243–261.

Wan AT, Conyers RA, Coombs CJ, et al: Determination of silver in blood, urine, and tissues of volunteers and burn patients. *Clin Chem* 37(10 pt 1):1683–1687, 1991.

Wang C, Bhattacharyya MH: Effect of cadmium on bone calcium and 45Ca in mouse dams on calcium deficient diet: Evidence of a direct effect of cadmium on bone. *Toxicol Appl Pharmacol* 120:228–239, 1993.

Wang R, Hwang DM, Cukerman E, Liew CC: Identification of genes encoding zinc finger motifs in the cardiovascular system. *J Mol Cell Cardiol* 86:281–287, 1997.

Wang X, Cahn HN, Goyer RA, et al: Nephrotoxicity of repeated injections of cadmium-metallothionein in rats. *Toxicol Appl Pharmacol* 119:11–16, 1993.

Warheit DB, Hansen JF, Yuen IS, et al: Inhalation of high concentrations of low toxicity dusts in rats results in impaired pulmonary clearance mechanisms and persistent inflammation. *Toxicol Appl Pharmacol* 145:10–22, 1997.

Wasserman GA, Graziano JH, Factor-Litvak P, et al: Consequences of lead exposure and iron supplementation on childhood development at age 4 years. *Neurotoxicol Teratol* 16:233–240, 1994.

Waters MD: Toxicology of vanadium, in Goyer RA, Mehlman MA (eds): *Toxicology of Trace Metals.* New York: Wiley, 1977, pp 147–189.

Webb DR, Sipes IG, Carter DE: In vitro solubility and in vivo toxicity of gallium arsenide. *Toxicol Appl Pharmacol* 76:96–104, 1984.

Wedeen RP, Qian LF: Cr induced kidney disease. *Environ Health Perspect* 92:71–74, 1991.

Wegman DH, Fine LJ: Occupational health in the 1990s. *Annu Rev Public Health* 11:89–103, 1990.

Wennig R, Kirsch N: Vanadium, in Seiler Hg, Siegel H (eds): *Toxicity of Inorganic Compounds.* New York: Marcel Dekker, 1988, pp 749–758.

Wettstein A, Aeppli J, Gautschi K, et al: Failure to find a relationship between amnestic skills of octogenarians and aluminum in drinking water. *Int Arch Occup Environ Health* 63:97–103, 1991.

Weyermann M, Brenner H: Alcohol consumption and smoking habits as determinants of blood lead levels in a national population sample from Germany. *Arch Environ Health* 52:233–240, 1997.

Whelan EA, Piacitelli GM, Gerwel B, et al: Elevated blood lead levels in children of construction workers. *Am J Public Health* 87:1352–1355, 1997.

White M, Boran A: Urinary excretion of nickel in nickel-chromium electroplaters, in Niebor E, Nriagu JO (eds): *Nickel and Human Health.* New York: Wiley, 1998, pp 89–96.

WHO: *Guidelines for Drinking Water Quality*, 2d ed. Vol 1. *Recommendations*. Geneva: World Health Organization, 1993.

WHO: *IARC Monographs on the Evaluation of Carcinogenic Risks to Humans*. Lyons, France: WHO/IARC, 1990, pp 1–445.

WHO: *IPCS Environmental Health Criteria:Copper*. Geneva: World Health Organization, 1998.

WHO: *IPCS Environmental Health Criteria.* Vol 134. *Cadmium.* Geneva: World Health Organization, 1992.

WHO: *IPCS Environmental Health Criteria.* Vol 61. *Chromium.* Geneva: World Health Organization, 1988.

WHO: *IPCS Environmental Health Criteria for Inorganic Lead.* Vol 165. *Geneva:* World Health Oraganization, 1995.

WHO: *Selenium: Environmental Health Criteria.* Vol 58. Geneva: World Health Organization, 1987, pp 1–238.

WHO: *WHO/FAO/IASEA Report on Trace Elements in Human Nutrition and Human Health.* Geneva: World Health Organization, 1996.

WHO/FAO/IAEA: Manganese, in *Trace Elements in Human Nutrition and Health.* Geneva: World Health Organization, 1996, pp 163–167.

WHO: *IPCS Environmental Health Criteria.* Vol 125. *Platinum.* Geneva: World Health Organization, 1991.

WHO: *IPCS Environmental Health Criteria.* Vol 13. *Tin and Organotin Compounds: A Preliminary Review.* Geneva: World Health Organization, 1980.

WHO: *IPCS Environmental Health Criteria.* Vol 101. *Methylmercury.* Geneva: World Health Organization, 1990.

WHO: *IPCS Environmental Health Criteria.* Vol 106. *Beryllium.* Geneva: World Health Organization, 1990.

WHO: *IPCS Environmental Health Criteria.* Vol 118. *Inorganic Mercury.* Geneva: World Health Organization, 1991.

Williams DR, Halstead BW: Chelating agents in medicine. *Clin Toxicol* 19:1081–1115, 1982.

Wills MR, Savory J: Aluminum poisoning: Dialysis encephalopathy, osteomalacia and anemia. *Lancet* 2:29–33, 1983.

Winge DR, Mehra RK: Host defenses against copper toxicity. *Int Rev Exp Pathol* 31:47–83, 1990.

Winship KA: Toxicity of antimony and its compounds. *Adv Drug React Acute Poison Rev* 2:67–90, 1987.

Winship KA: Toxicity of tin and its compounds. *Adv Drug React Acute Poison Rev* 7:19–38, 1988.

Yang G, Wang S, Zhou R: Endemic selenium intoxication of humans in China. *Am J Clin Nutr* 37:872–881, 1983.

Yin L, Rhoads GC, Lioy PJ: Seasonal influences on childhood lead exposure. *Environ Health Perspect* 108:177–182, 1999.

Yip R, Dallman PR: Iron, in Ziegler EE, Filer LJ (eds): *Present Knowledge in Nutrition.* Washington, DC: ILSI, 1996, pp 277–292.

Youst LJ, Schoof RA, Aucoin R: Intake of inorganic arsenic in the North American diet. *Hum Ecol Risk Assess* 4:137–152, 1998.

Yu S, Beynen AC: High tin intake reduces copper status in rats through inhibition of copper absorption. *Br J Nutr* 73:863–869, 1995.

Zalups RK, Koropatnick J: *Molecular Biology and Toxicology of Metals.* New York: Taylor & Francis, 2000.

Zalups RK, Parks LD, Cannon VT, et al.: Mechanism of action of 2.3 dimercaptopropane-1-sulfonate and transport, disposition and toxicity of inorganic mercury in isolated perfused segments of rabbit proximal tubules. *Mol Pharmacol* 54:353–363, 1998.

Zareba G, Chmielnicka J: Disturbances in heme biosynthesis in rabbits after administration per os of low doses of tin or lead. *Biol Trace Elem Res* 34:115–122, 1992.

Zelikoff JT, Li JH, Hartwig A, et al: Genetic toxicology of lead compounds. *Carcinogen* 9:1727–1732, 1988.

Zheng W, Winter SM, Kattnig MJ, et al: Tissue distribution and elimination of indium in male Fischer 344 rats following oral and intratracheal administration of indium phosphide. *J Toxicol Environ Health* 43:483–494,1994.

Zidenberg-Cherr S, Clegg MS, Parks NJ, et al: Localization of bismuth radiotracer in rat kidney following exposure to bismuth. *Biol Trace Elem Res* 19:185–194, 1989.

Ziegler EE, Edwards BB, Jensen RL, et al: Absorption and retention of lead by infants. *Pediatr Res* 12:29–34, 1978.

CHAPTER 24

TOXIC EFFECTS OF SOLVENTS AND VAPORS

James V. Bruckner and D. Alan Warren

INTRODUCTION

The term *solvent* refers to a class of liquid organic chemicals of variable lipophilicity and volatility. These properties, coupled with small molecular size and lack of charge, make inhalation the major route of solvent exposure and provide for ready absorption across the lung, gastrointestinal (GI) tract, and skin. In general, the lipophilicity of solvents increases with increasing molecular weight, while volatility decreases. Solvents are frequently used to dissolve, dilute, or disperse materials that are insoluble in water. As such, they are widely employed as degreasers and as constituents of paints, varnishes, lacquers, inks, aerosol spray products, dyes, and adhesives. Other uses are as intermediates in chemical synthesis, and as fuels and fuel additives. Most solvents are refined from petroleum. Many such as naphthas and gasoline are complex mixtures, often consisting of hundreds of compounds. Early in the twentieth century, there were perhaps a dozen or so known and commonly used solvents. By 1981, this number had climbed to approximately 350 (OSHA, 2000).

Solvents are classified largely according to molecular structure or functional group. Classes of solvents include aliphatic hydrocarbons, many of which are chlorinated (i.e., halocarbons); aromatic hydrocarbons; alcohols; ethers; esters/acetates; amides/amines; aldehydes; ketones; and complex mixtures that defy classification. The main determinants of a solvent's inherent toxicity are (1) its number of carbon atoms; (2) whether it is saturated or has double or triple bonds between adjacent carbon atoms; (3) its configuration (i.e., straight-chain, branched-chain, or cyclic); and (4) the presence of functional groups. Some class-wide generalizations regarding toxicity can be made. For example, amides/amines tend to be potent sensitizers; aldehydes are particularly irritating; hydrocarbons that are extensively metabolized tend to be more cytotoxic/mutagenic; and many unsaturated, short-chain halocarbons are animal carcinogens. The toxicity of solvents within the same class may vary dramatically. For example, 1,1,1-trichloroethane (TRI) and 1,1,2-trichloroethylene (TCE) are both halocarbons, yet the unsaturated TCE is carcinogenic in the rat and mouse, but TRI is not. Similar results have been reported for 2,4- and 2,6-diaminotoluene in rodents, as only the 2,4 isomer is capable of inducing significant hepatocyte proliferation and liver tumors. Slight structural differences in solvent metabolites are also of toxicologic consequence. The peripheral neuropathy induced by *n*-hexane and 2-hexanone is dependent on the production of the γ-diketone metabolite, 2,5-hexanedione. Diketones lacking the gamma structure are not neurotoxic. Thus, subtle differences in chemical structure can translate into dramatic differences in solvent toxicity.

Nearly everyone is exposed to solvents in the conduct of their normal daily activities. Consider, for example, a person who works in an aircraft factory as a metal degreaser (TCE exposure); drives to the neighborhood bar after work and has a few drinks (ethanol exposure) and a cigarette (benzene and styrene exposure); stops on the way home at a self-service filling station for gasoline (benzene, toluene, 1,3-butadiene exposure) and the dry cleaner's for laundry [tetrachloroethylene (PERC) exposure]; and after dinner enjoys his hobby of model shipbuilding that requires the use of glue (toluene exposure). While everyone may not identify with the above scenario, detailed surveys of indoor and outdoor air such as EPA's Total Exposure Assessment Methodology (TEAM) and National Human Exposure Assessment Survey (NHEXAS) studies, indicate that airborne solvent exposure is unavoidable (Wallace, 1990; Clayton et al., 1999). Drinking water is also a common source of solvent exposure due to discharge of solvents and the presence of disinfection by-products, such as the animal carcinogens, chloroform ($CHCl_3$), trichloroacetic acid (TCA), and dichloroacetic acid (DCA). TCA and DCA are metabolites of TCE and PERC.

Environmental exposures to solvents in air and groundwater are frequent subjects of toxic tort litigation, despite concentrations typically in the low parts per billion (ppb) range. Multiple exposure pathways frequently exist (Fig. 24-1). Though not reflected in Fig. 24-1, household use of solvent-contaminated water may result in solvent intake from inhalation and dermal absorption as well as ingestion. In many cases, environmental risk assessment requires that risks be determined for physiologically diverse individuals who are exposed to several solvents by multiple exposure pathways. As an aid to the risk assessment process, the EPA has derived toxicity factors for many of the most toxic solvents. These toxicity factors are referred to as Reference Concentrations (RfCs), Reference Doses (RfDs), and Cancer Slope Factors (CSFs). Values for these are available from the EPA's on-line Integrated Risk Information System (IRIS). Additional sources of exposure guidelines for noncancer endpoints are found in the toxicologic profiles of the U.S. Agency for Toxic Substances and Disease Registry (ATSDR). These profiles often contain Minimal Risk Levels (MRLs) that are derived in a similar manner to EPA's RfCs and RfDs, but are frequently based on different critical studies or derived with the use of different uncertainty factors.

Occupational solvent exposures involve situations ranging from a secretary using typewriter correction fluid to the loading and offloading of tanker trucks with thousands of gallons of gasoline. The greatest industrial use of solvents is as metal degreasers. The work environment is typically where the highest exposures occur, mainly via inhalation and dermal contact. An estimated 10 million people are potentially exposed to organic solvents in the workplace (OSHA, 2000). Many of the most severe exposures to solvents have occurred as a result of their use in confined spaces with inadequate ventilation. While the Occupational Safety and Health Administration (OSHA) has established legally enforceable Permissible Exposure Limits (PELs) for over 100 solvents, most PELs are outdated. The majority of existing PELs were adopted from the list of Threshold Limit Values (TLVs) published by the

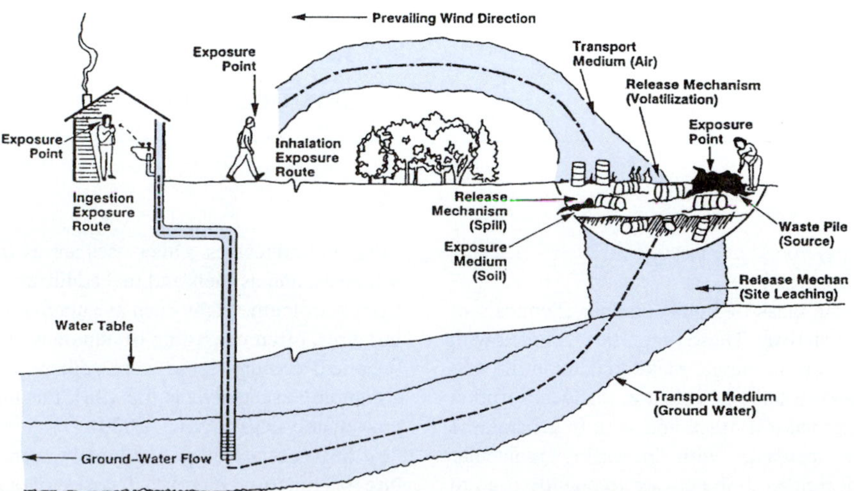

Figure 24-1. Solvent exposure pathways and media. [From **EPA Risk Assessment Guidance for Superfund.** *Human Health Evaluation Manual Part A, Interim Final. Washington, DC: Office of Emergency and Remedial Response, 1989.]*

American Conference of Governmental Industrial Hygienists (ACGIH) in 1968, and have not been updated. Many current TLVs are more stringent than the PELs but do not carry the weight of law. (See appendix of this book for TLV and PEL.) While the ACGIH's TLVs for an 8-h work day, 40-h work week are designed to be protective for a working lifetime, its Short-Term Exposure Limits (STELs) and ceiling values are designed to protect against the acute effects of high-level, short-term solvent exposures. If warranted, the ACGIH will assign a skin notation to a solvent, indicating that a significant contribution to overall exposure is possible by the dermal route, either by contact with vapors or direct skin contact with the liquid. Biological monitoring in the workplace should find increasing use as technologic advances are made, since it often provides a better measure of exposure than classic industrial hygiene monitoring. The ACGIH has published several Biological Exposure Indices (BEIs), on which basis the safety of internal measures of exposure can be judged (ACGIH, 1999).

Most solvent exposures involve a mixture of chemicals, rather than a single compound. Our knowledge of the toxicity of solvent mixtures is rudimentary relative to the toxicology of individual solvents. While the assumption is frequently made that the toxic effects of multiple solvents are additive, solvents may also interact synergistically or antagonistically. For example, repetitive alcohol consumption induces P450 activities, and may therefore induce the metabolic activation of other solvents to cytotoxic metabolites. Ethanol intake near the time of exposure to such solvents, on the other hand, may inhibit their metabolism and be protective. Another well-characterized example of solvent antagonism is the interaction between benzene and toluene (Medinsky et al., 1994). Coexposure to these chemicals results in diminished benzene metabolism, genotoxicity, and erythropoietic toxicity relative to that which follows benzene exposure alone. It is now recognized that significant data gaps exist in the area of mixtures toxicology, and these can preclude accurate risk assessments.

Although some solvents are less hazardous than others, all solvents can cause toxic effects. Provided that the dose is sufficient, most all have the potential to induce a state of narcosis and cause dermal and mucous membrane irritation. A number of solvents are animal carcinogens, but only a handful have been classified as known human carcinogens. Herein lies a major challenge for toxicology—determining the human relevance of tumors observed in high-dose rodent studies. As with other chemicals, whether health effects occur from solvent exposure is dependent upon several factors: (1) toxicity of the solvent, (2) exposure route, (3) amount or rate of exposure, (4) duration of exposure, (5) individual susceptibility, and (6) interactions with other chemicals. Adverse health effects may occur acutely and be readily discernible, or they may be the result of chronic exposure with insidious onset. Numerous epidemiologic studies of environmentally and occupationally exposed populations have been conducted for some solvents, but human risk assessment remains heavily reliant upon extrapolation from animal studies. One must bear in mind that the toxic effects and their underlying mechanisms discussed herein may be operative only in certain animal species or strains and under certain exposure conditions. Care must therefore be taken in generalizing beyond the experimental conditions under which data were collected. While a relatively small number of commercially available solvents is discussed in this chapter, those selected for discussion are thought to best demonstrate principles of solvent toxicology, are of particular commercial importance, and/or are currently garnering significant attention from the toxicologic and regulatory communities. A recent book chapter that examines solvents from an organ systems standpoint, in contrast to the discussion of individual solvents herein, is that of Gerr and Letz (1998).

IS THERE A SOLVENT-INDUCED CHRONIC ENCEPHALOPATHY?

The central nervous system (CNS)–depressant effects of acute, high-level exposures and the potential for permanent neurologic damage in chronic solvent abusers are not a matter of debate. It is also clear that chronic, moderate- to high-level exposure to a few solvents such as *n*-hexane and carbon disulfide can cause specific degenerative changes in the CNS or peripheral nervous system (PNS). Far less clear is whether chronic, low-level exposure to virtually any solvent or solvent mixture can produce a pattern of neurologic dysfunction referred to as *painter's syndrome, organic solvent syndrome, psychoorganic syndrome,* and *chronic solvent encephalopathy* (CSE). CSE is characterized by nonspecific symptoms (e.g., headache, fatigue, sleep disorders) with or without changes in neuropsychological function. There is a reversible form of CSE referred to as *neuroasthenic syndrome* that consists of symptoms only, and both "mild" and "severe" forms accompanied by objective signs of neuropsychological dysfunction that may or may not be fully reversible. This syndrome was first described in the Scandinavian occupational literature in the late 1970s among solvent-exposed painters (Axelson et al., 1976; Arlien-Soborg et al., 1979). Since that time, numerous studies from Scandinavia have been published suggesting that solvents as a class have chronic neurotoxic properties. These countries have actually passed legislation recognizing CSE as a compensable occupational disability. Scientists outside of Scandinavia, including those in the United States, have generally been less willing to recognize CSE as a legitimate disease state and have published studies to the contrary (Triebig et al., 1988; Bleecker et al., 1991; Spurgeon et al., 1994).

In response to the numerous reports of CSE, two conferences were convened in 1985. The first was held in Copenhagen by the Nordic Council of the World Health Organization (WHO, 1985). The second in Raleigh, NC, was attended by an international group of scientists from academia, industry, and government (Cranmer, 1986). The categorization scheme that resulted from the Raleigh meeting is presented in Table 24-1. The WHO scheme is similar. Among those who utilize the categorization scheme, it is generally believed that the most severe CSE category, type 3, results from repeated, severe intoxications like those experienced by solvent abusers. CSE types 1 and 2, on the other hand, are thought to be associated with prolonged, low-level exposure common to work environments. A major criticism of the categorization scheme is the lack of consideration of inhaled solvent concentration and exposure duration. While no consensus exists, even most CSE proponents believe that solvent exposure must occur for $\geq$10 years before clinical symptoms are manifest.

CSE researchers typically rely upon self-reported symptoms and a clinical neuropsychological evaluation (Table 24-2), and to a much lesser extent on diagnostic tests such as electroencephalography and computerized brain tomography. It has been argued that the neuropsychological tests are of questionable validity, sensitivity, specificity, and predictive value. It has also been noted that many investigations of CSE are fraught with methodologic flaws that render their results unreliable. For example, CSE investigators frequently fail to measure premorbid function or intellect; to employ a reference population; to control adequately for the po-

Table 24-1
Proposed Categories of Solvent-Induced Encephalopathy

CATEGORY	CLINICAL MANIFESTATIONS
Type 1	**Symptoms Only.** The patient complains of nonspecific symptoms such as fatigability, memory impairment, difficulty in concentration, and loss of initiative. These symptoms are reversible if exposure is discontinued, and there is no objective evidence of neuropsychiatric dysfunction.
Type 2A	**Sustained Personality or Mood Change.** There is a marked and sustained change in personality involving fatigue, emotional lability, impulse control, and general mood and motivation.
Type 2B	**Impairment in Intellectual Function.** There is difficulty in concentration, impairment of memory, and a decrease in learning capacity. These symptoms are accompanied by objective evidence of impairment. There may also be minor neurologic signs. The complete reversibility of type 2B is questionable.
Type 3	**Dementia.** In this condition, marked global deterioration in intellect and memory is often accompanied by neurologic signs and or neuroradiologic findings. This condition is, at best, poorly reversible, but is generally nonprogressive once exposure has ceased.

SOURCE: Reproduced with permission from Cranmer (1986).

tential confounders of age, alcohol use, and other CNS diseases; to corroborate functional deficits with objective evidence of brain disease; and/or examine the exposure-response relationship. Gade et al. (1988), for example, reanalyzed individuals originally reported by Arlien-Soborg et al. (1979) to have "painter's syndrome." When the influences of age, education, and intelligence were considered, the previously reported reduction in neuropsychological test scores disappeared. Another example is that of Cherry et al. (1985), who demonstrated the importance of matching solvent-exposed and control groups for preexposure intellect before making a diagnosis of CSE.

It is evident that resolution of the controversial issue of CSE will come only through the conduct of well-designed and controlled clinical epidemiologic studies, especially considering the absence of an appropriate animal model. Brief, but insightful reviews of CSE by Rosenberg (1995) and Schaumburg and Spencer (2000) can be found in recent texts. These reviews conclude that the current literature, including the "landmark" North American study of 187 paint manufacturing workers (Bleecker et al., 1991), does not support chronic, low-level solvent exposure as a cause of *symptomatic* CNS or PNS dysfunction. This does not preclude, however, the possibility that such exposure can be associated with *subclinical* cognitive dysfunction in the form of slight psychomotor and attentional deficits. For the viewpoint of CSE proponents, readers are directed to texts by Arlien-Soborg (1992) and Kilburn (1998).

Table 24-2
Functions That May Be Assessed in a Neuropsychological Evaluation

Psychomotor functions
Reaction time
Motor speed and dexterity
Eye-hand coordination
Sustained attention/concentration and perceptual speed
Verbal and nonverbal memory
Immediate memory
Delayed memory
Learning
Visual constructive ability
Conceptual ability
Evaluation of personality and affect

SOURCE: Adapted from Cranmer (1986).

SOLVENT ABUSE

Many solvents are intentionally inhaled in order to achieve a state of intoxication (Dinwiddie, 1994; Marelich, 1997). Solvent inhalation can rapidly produce euphoria, delusions, and sedation as well as visual and auditory hallucinations (Fig. 24-2). Solvent abuse is a unique exposure situation in that participants repeatedly subject themselves to vapor concentrations high enough to produce effects as extreme as unconsciousness. Solvents can be addicting and are often abused in combination with other drugs. The practice may be continued for years. Various solvents are present in a wide variety of household and commercial products including glue, model cement, paint thinner and stripper, aerosols, typewriter correction fluid, dry-cleaning fluid, and gasoline. These products are relatively inexpensive and readily available to children and adolescents (NIDA, 1977).

Nearly all hydrocarbon solvents cause CNS depression, but residual organ damage is chemical-dependent. It is important to recognize the distinction between reversible CNS depression and neurotoxicity. Neurotoxicity is usually considered to be residual damage (i.e., dysfunction after elimination of the solvent). There is concern that chronic solvent abuse can lead to long-term neurologic and psychological sequelae (Ron, 1986; Marelich, 1997). Some solvents, such as *n*-hexane and methyl-*n*-butyl ketone, cause peripheral neuropathies. Chronic abuse of solvents such as toluene, which were previously thought to be relatively innocuous, may be responsible for diffuse cerebral and cerebellar atrophy (Ron, 1986; Caldemeyer et al., 1996). Blood dyscrasias, liver damage, kidney injury, and other toxicities are seen in patients who have abused

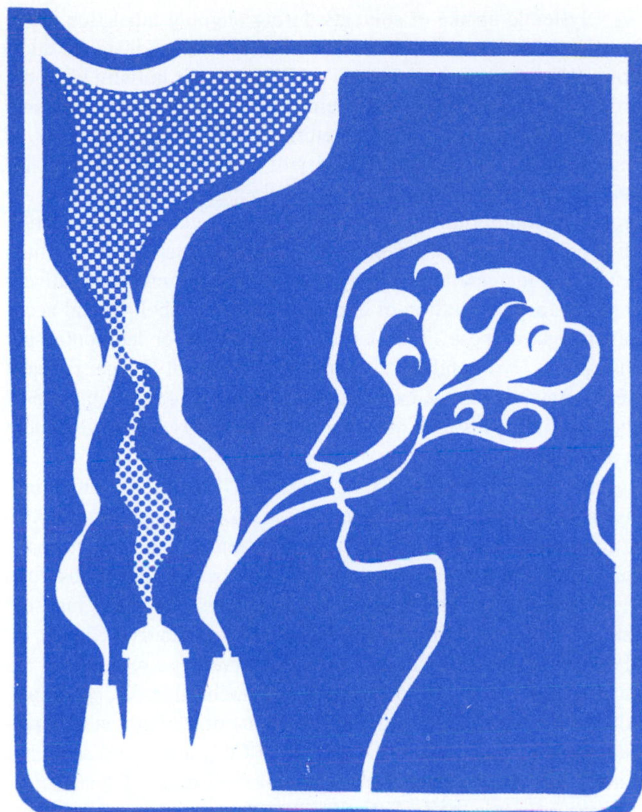

Figure 24-2. Solvent abuse: Euphoria to dysfunction. [Reproduced from NIDA (1977).]

solvents known to be injurious to those organs. Death, frequently due to arrhythmogenic effects of high concentrations of some solvents (e.g., 1,1,1-trichloroethane, freons, benzene), is sometimes a consequence of solvent abuse.

ENVIRONMENTAL CONTAMINATION

Widespread use of solvents has resulted in their dissemination throughout the environment (Fig. 24-1). Most everyone is exposed daily to solvents, albeit in minute amounts (Ashley et al., 1994). Since solvents as a chemical class are volatile, the preponderance of solvents entering the environment do so by evaporation. The majority of the more volatile organic compounds (VOCs) volatilize when products containing them (e.g., aerosol propellants, paint thinners, cleaners, soil fumigants) are used as intended. Solvent loss into the atmosphere also occurs during production, processing, storage and transport activities, resulting in elevated concentrations in air in the proximity of point sources. Winds dilute and disperse solvent vapors across the world. Atmospheric concentrations of most VOCs are usually extremely low (i.e., nondetectable to nanograms or a few micrograms per cubic millimeter of air). Higher concentrations of certain solvents (e.g., 10 to 520 $\mu g/m^3$, or 3 to 163 ppb of benzene) have been measured in urban areas, around petrochemical plants, and in the immediate vicinity of hazardous waste sites (Bennett, 1987; Kelly et al., 1993).

Solvent contamination of drinking water supplies has become a major health concern. Although the majority of a solvent spilled onto the ground evaporates, some may permeate the soil and migrate through it until reaching groundwater or impermeable material. In years past, the more lipophilic solvents were generally regarded as water-insoluble. It is now recognized that all solvents are soluble in water to some extent. Some (e.g., alcohols, ketones, glycols) are freely soluble. Maximum solubilities of some common hydrocarbon solvents range from 10 mg/L (ppm) for *n*-hexane to 24,000 mg/L for bromochloromethane. High concentrations of VOCs are sometimes found in the effluent of facilities of rubber producers, chemical companies, petrochemical plants, and paper mills (Comba et al., 1994). Concentrations diminish rapidly after VOCs enter bodies of water, due primarily to dilution and evaporation. VOCs in surface waters rise to the surface or sink to the bottom, according to their density. VOCs on the surface will largely evaporate. VOCs on the bottom must depend on solubilization in the water or upon mixing by current or wave action to reach the surface. VOCs in groundwater tend to remain trapped until the water reaches the surface. Concentrations in well water are rarely high enough for acute or subacute toxicity to be of concern. The very low levels of some solvents typically found in water have, however, caused a great deal of concern and debate about their potential for carcinogenicity.

Potential health effects of solvent contaminants of water have received considerable attention for over 30 years. A report by Mason and McKay (1974), of an increased incidence of cancer in persons who drank water from the Mississippi River, prompted the EPA to analyze the water supply of New Orleans. The finding of some 76 synthetic organic chemicals, many of which were solvents, prompted passage of the Safe Drinking Water Act in 1974. $CHCl_3$ is the most frequently found VOC in finished drinking water supplies in the U.S. (ATSDR, 1997b). It and certain other trihalomethanes are formed by reaction of the chlorine added as a disinfectant with natural organic compounds present in the water. Levels of solvents found in drinking water in the U.S. are typically in the ng/L (ppt) to μg/L (ppb) range, though concentrations in the low mg/L (ppm) range are found in water from wells situated in solvent plumes from hazardous waste sites and other point discharges (Barbash and Roberts, 1986; Salanitro, 1993; Mushrush et al., 1994). Of the thousands of chemicals found at hazardous waste sites, 6 of the 10 most commonly present are solvents (Fay and Mumtaz, 1996).

People are subjected to solvents in environmental media by inhalation, ingestion, and skin contact. Considerable effort was devoted by the EPA, from 1979 to 1985, to assess personal exposure to solvents in different locales of the United States. TRI, PERC, benzene, xylenes, and ethylbenzene were most frequently found in highest concentrations ($\sim$1-32 $\mu g/m^3$) in air (Wallace et al., 1987). Exhaled breath levels of some chemicals (e.g., $CHCl_3$, ethylbenzene) corresponded to indoor air levels. Personal activities (e.g., smoking, visiting dry cleaner's and service stations) and occupational exposures were believed to be largely responsible for relatively high exposures to other VOCs (e.g., benzene, toluene, xylenes, PERC) (Ashley et al., 1994). Subsequent studies, accounting for all pertinent exposure pathways, were conducted by the EPA in the mid-1990s (Gordon et al., 1999). Toluene and benzene were the most commonly found VOCs in indoor air. $CHCl_3$ was most prevalent in drinking water. It should be recognized that $CHCl_3$ and other VOCs volatilize to some degree during home water usage, particularly when the water is heated. Thus, a significant proportion of one's total exposure to VOCs in tap water can occur via inhalation. Weisel and Jo (1996) estimated that inhalation and ingestion contribute equally to the internal dose of TCE a person receives when using TCE-contaminated tap water.

TOXICOKINETICS

Toxicokinetic (TK) studies are playing an increasingly important role in reducing uncertainties in risk assessments of solvents (Leung and Paustenbach, 1995; Andersen, 1995). The fundamental goal of TK studies is to delineate the uptake and disposition of chemicals in the body. It is now recognized that toxicity is a dynamic process, in which the degree and duration of injury of a target tissue are dependent upon the net effect of toxicodynamic (TD) and TK processes including systemic absorption, tissue deposition, metabolism, interaction with cellular components, elimination, and tissue repair. Estimation of risk of toxicity from TK data is based on the fundamental concept that the intensity of response from an administered dose is dependent upon the amount(s) of biologically active chemical moiety(ies) present in a target tissue (i.e., the tissue dose). A related concept is that the tissue dose in a given target organ in one species will have the same degree of effect as an equivalent target organ dose in a second species. This concept of tissue dose equivalence appears to be applicable in many cases to solvents (Andersen, 1987). Gaining understanding of how the processes that govern solvent kinetics vary with dose, species, and even different individuals greatly reduces the number of assumptions that have to be made in assessment of health risks from toxicity data.

Volatility and lipophilicity are two of the most important properties of solvents which govern their absorption and deposition in the body. Most solvents are volatile under normal usage conditions, though volatility varies from compound to compound. Lipophilicity also can vary substantially, from quite water soluble (e.g., glycols and alcohols) to quite lipid soluble (e.g., halocarbons and aromatic hydrocarbons). Many solvents of particular concern at present are relatively lipid soluble and volatile, hence their designation as VOCs. These compounds have a relatively low molecular weight and are uncharged. Thus, they pass freely through membranes from areas of high to low concentration by passive diffusion.

Absorption

The majority of systemic absorption of inhaled VOCs occurs in the alveoli, although some absorption has been demonstrated to occur in the upper respiratory tract (Stott and McKenna, 1984). Gases in the alveoli are thought to equilibrate almost instantaneously with blood in the pulmonary capillaries (Goldstein et al., 1974). Blood: air partition coefficients (PCs) of VOCs are important determinants of the extent of their uptake. A PC is defined by Gargas et al. (1989) as the ratio of concentration of VOC achieved between two different media at equilibrium. As blood is largely aqueous, the more hydrophilic solvents have relatively high blood:air PCs, which favor extensive uptake. Gargas and colleagues (1989) determined PCs for 55 VOCs in F344 rats. Human blood:air values were measured for 36 of the compounds. Since VOCs diffuse from areas of high to low concentration, increases in respiration (to maintain a high alveolar concentration) and in cardiac output/pulmonary blood flow (to maintain a large concentration gradient by removing capillary blood containing the VOC) enhance pulmonary absorption.

Systemic uptake of solvents during ongoing inhalation exposures is dependent upon tissue loading and metabolism, in addition to the factors noted above. Percent uptake is initially high, but progressively declines as the chemical accumulates in tissues, and the level of chemical in blood returning to the lungs increases. A near steady-state, or equilibrium will soon be reached with inhalation of a fixed concentration of lipophilic solvents. The approach to equilibrium is asymptotic. Despite continued inhalation of lipophilic solvents, levels in the blood and tissues (other than fat) do not increase appreciably. Percent uptake remains relatively constant for the duration of exposure, with metabolism and accumulation in adipose tissue largely responsible for the continuing absorption. Hydrophilic solvents take considerably longer to reach steady-state, due to the extended time required for equilibration of chemical in the inspired air with that in the body water (Goldstein et al., 1974).

Solvents are well absorbed from the GI tract. Peak blood levels are observed within minutes of dosing, although the presence of food in the GI tract can delay absorption. It is now usually assumed that 100 percent of an oral dose of most solvents is absorbed systemically. The vehicle or diluent in which a solvent is ingested can affect the absorption and TK of the compound. Kim et al. (1990a, b) found that a corn oil vehicle served as a reservoir in the gut to delay GI absorption of carbon tetrachloride (CCl_4) in rats. Although bioavailability of CCl_4 given in corn oil and in an aqueous emulsion was the same, peak blood CCl_4 levels and acute hepatotoxicity were much lower in the corn oil group. Other factors that can influence the oral absorption of other classes of chemicals have relatively little influence on most solvents.

Absorption of solvents through the skin can result in both local and systemic effects. Skin contact with vapors and concentrated solutions of solvents is a common occurrence in the workplace. Dermal contact with solvent contaminants of water can also occur in the home and in recreational settings (Weisel and Jo, 1996). Solvents penetrate the stratum corneum, the skin's barrier to absorption, by passive diffusion. Important determinants of the rate of dermal absorption of solvents include the chemical concentration, surface area exposed, exposure duration, integrity and thickness of the stratum corneum, and lipophilicity and molecular weight of the solvent (EPA, 1998). Skin penetration can be measured in laboratory animals and humans by a variety of in vitro and in vivo techniques (Morgan et al., 1991; Nakai et al., 1999). Although absorption rates measured by these methods may vary quantitatively, there is often good agreement in their relative ranking of chemicals for ability to penetrate the skin. Dermal permeability constants are typically two to four times lower for human than for rodent skin (McDougal et al., 1990). The extent of dermal absorption in occupational and environmental exposure settings should be taken into account when conducting risk assessments of solvents.

Transport and Distribution

Chemicals and nutrients absorbed into portal venous blood from the GI tract can be removed from the bloodstream by first-pass, or presystemic elimination. Blood in the portal venous circulation passes through the liver before entering the pulmonary circulation. Thus, solvents are subject to uptake/elimination by the liver and exhalation by the lungs during their first pass along this absorption pathway. Those solvents that are well metabolized and quite volatile are most efficiently eliminated before they enter the arterial blood. The efficiency of the hepatic first-pass elimination is thus dependent upon the chemical, as well as the rate at which it arrives in the liver. Pulmonary first-pass elimination, in contrast, is believed to be a first-order process irrespective of the chemical concentration in the blood. Lee et al. (1996) demonstrated in rats that pulmonary first-pass elimination of TCE was relatively constant over a range of doses, but that hepatic elimination was inversely related to dose. Andersen (1981) has concluded that the liver is capable of removing "virtually all" of a VOC, if the amount in the blood is not great enough to saturate metabolism. This hypothesis, if proven, could have a profound effect on cancer and noncancer risk estimates of environmentally encountered levels of solvents.

Solvents are transported by the arterial blood and taken up according to tissue blood flow and mass and tissue:blood PCs (Astrand, 1983). Relatively hydrophilic solvents solubilize to different extents in plasma. Nevertheless, as much as 50 percent of such compounds is still carried by erythrocytes (Lam et al., 1990). These researchers found that 90 to 95 percent of the more lipophilic solvents is transported by erythrocytes. Lipophilic solvents do not bind to plasma proteins or hemoglobin, but partition into hydrophobic sites in the molecules. Lipophilic solvents also partition into phospholipids, lipoproteins and cholesterol present in the blood. Initial uptake into organs is largely dependent upon their rate of blood flow and the tissue:blood PC of the solvent. The brain is an example of a rapidly perfused tissue with a relatively high lipid content. Lipophilic solvents quickly accumulate in the brain after the initiation of exposures, producing CNS effects as profound as surgical anesthesia within as little as 1 to 2 min. Redistribution to poorly perfused, lipoidal tissues will subsequently occur. Adipose tissue accumulates relatively large amounts of VOCs.

Route of exposure can significantly influence target organ deposition and toxicity of solvents. Much of the toxicology database for solvents, before 1980, was comprised of results of inhalation studies. Inhalation is the major route of occupational exposure to these chemicals. Since then, much attention has been focused on potential health effects of VOC contaminants of drinking water. Due to the initial paucity of oral data, regulatory agencies sometimes extrapolated directly from inhalation data to predict risks of ingestion of VOCs. Such a practice does not appear to be scientifically valid when physiologic differences in the absorption pathways are taken into account. For example, all of the cardiac output passes through the pulmonary circulation versus ~20 percent for the GI tract. Also, the alveolar surface area for absorption is approximately 20 times that of the entire GI tract. VOCs absorbed in the lungs directly enter the arterial circulation and are transported throughout the body. In contrast, VOCs absorbed from the GI tract largely enter the portal circulation and are subject to first-pass elimination by the liver and lungs. It is not surprising then that extrahepatic organs receive a greater dose following inhalation of VOCs . The liver should take up and metabolize more of a VOC following ingestion. This has been demonstrated in rats receiving the same systemic dose of CCl_4 by inhalation and gastric infusion (Sanzgiri et al., 1997).

The pattern of ingestion of solvents can significantly influence their TK and health effects. For convenience, test chemicals are often given to animals as a single bolus by gavage in short- and long-term oral toxicity studies. Actual human exposures to solvents in drinking water are quite different, in that people typically ingest water in divided doses. High gavage doses of $CHCl_3$ and other halocarbons have produced hepatocellular carcinoma in B6C3F1 mice. No evidence of hepatic tumorigenesis was seen, however, when these mice were given the same doses of the chemicals in their drinking water (Jorgenson et al., 1985; Klaunig et al., 1986). The maximum blood level of CCl_4 was found to be 35 times higher and hepatotoxicity more severe in rats dosed with CCl_4 by gavage, than in those given the same dose over 2 h by gastric infusion (Sanzgiri et al., 1995). Oral bolus doses of solvents can cause damage by exceeding the capacity of hepatic and pulmonary first-pass elimination, as well as other protection and repair processes.

The rate of systemic elimination of different solvents varies considerably. The two major routes of systemic elimination of VOCs are metabolism and exhalation. The rate and extent of metabolic clearance are dose- and compound-dependent. Exhalation is determined largely by the rate of pulmonary blood flow, the chemical's air:blood PC, and the alveolar ventilation rate. The more volatile, lipophilic VOCs are exhaled the most readily, since they have the higher air:blood PCs (Gargas et al., 1989). A good "case in point" is comparison of toluene with acetone. The extent of CNS depression caused by each chemical is dependent upon the concentration of the parent compound present in the brain (Bruckner and Peterson, 1981). As can be seen in Fig. 24-3, recovery of rats from toluene anesthesia occurs within minutes of cessation of exposure. This can be attributed to redistribution of toluene from the brain to body fat and other tissues, as well as to relatively rapid metabolism and exhalation. In contrast, recovery from acetone narcosis does not occur for ~9 h. Acetone is water soluble and is distributed in the considerable volume of the blood and other body water. Clearance of acetone is low due to its large volume of distribution and its relatively slow metabolism and exhalation. Acetone's water solubility is responsible for its relatively low air:blood PC and retention in the pulmonary blood. Thus, acetone is available for diffusion into the brain and induction of a modest degree of CNS depression for a prolonged time.

Body fat plays an important role in the elimination of lipophilic solvents. Blood levels of such solvents drop very rapidly during the initial elimination phase. This so-called redistribution

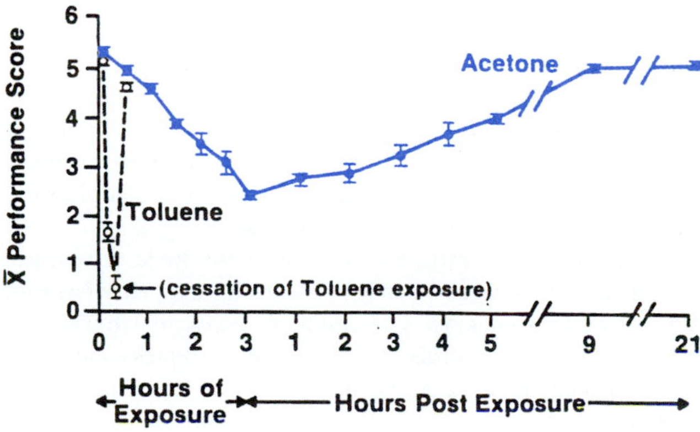

Figure 24-3. Comparison of the induction of and recovery from toluene and acetone narcosis.

Rats inhaled 45 mg/L of toluene or acetone for 20 min or 3 h, respectively. Animal performance/reflexes were monitored periodically as measures of the degree of CNS depression. [Used with permission of Bruckner and Peterson (1981).]

phase is characterized by rapid diffusion of solvent from the blood into most tissues. Equilibration of adipose tissue is prolonged due to the small fraction of cardiac output (~3 percent) supplying fat depots (Goldstein et al., 1974). Body fat increases the volume of distribution and total body burden of lipophilic solvents. Deequilibration from adipose tissue during the terminal elimination phase is prolonged due to slow blood flow and high fat:blood PC.

Metabolism

Biotransformation plays a key role in modulating the toxicities of solvents. Many solvents are poorly soluble in water. Certain cellular enzymes can convert them to relatively water-soluble derivatives, which may be more readily eliminated in the largely aqueous urine and/or bile. Conversion of a bioactive parent compound to less bioactive or inactive metabolite(s) that (is/are) efficiently eliminated is termed *metabolic inactivation,* or *detoxification.* Toluene, for example, accumulates in neuronal membranes and inhibits their functions. Toluene is metabolized to hydroxyl and carboxyl metabolites, which are too polar to accumulate in substantial quantities in membranes. Thus, metabolism serves to detoxify and to accelerate the elimination of toluene. Metabolism of other solvents can produce reactive metabolites that are cytotoxic and/or mutagenic. This phenomenon is known as *metabolic activation,* or *bioactivation.* Benzene, for example, is oxidized to a variety of quinones and semiquinones that can produce hematopoietic toxicities and leukemias (Snyder et al., 1993). Benzene and many other VOCs are converted via multiple metabolic pathways to products of varying toxicity. Some of these competing pathways are considered bioactivation, others detoxification pathways. A variety of factors can influence the prominence of the different pathways and hence alter toxicity outcomes.

Biotransformation of relatively lipophilic solvents is catalyzed largely by cytochrome P450s. The cytochrome P450s, are a "superfamily" of hemoproteins that act as terminal oxidases of the mixed-function oxidase (MFO) system. Their mode of action is described in Chap. 6. The P450s can catalyze a number of oxidative reactions as well as certain reductive reactions (Omiecinski et al., 1999). More than 20 different human P450 isozymes have been identified to date, but 6 (2D6, 2C9, 3A4, 1A2, 2C19, and 2E1) account for the majority of xenobiotic metabolism (Smith et al., 1998). Although the P450s have generally been thought to have broad, overlapping substrate specificities, it is now believed that enzyme kinetics under physiologic conditions may favor one or two isozymes as the primary catalysts for a given chemical (Wrighton and Stevens, 1992). Different isozymes can predominate at different doses of the same chemical.

The outcome of exposure to a potentially toxic solvent can depend on the relative abundance of P450 isozymes. Expression of P450s varies considerably as a result of genetic polymorphisms and exposure to chemicals which induce or repress individual isozymes. Inheritable gene alterations, such as base changes and deletions, can result not only in functionally deficient enzymes but in the absence of certain P450s (Daly et al., 1993). As P450s have different modes of regulatory control, their expression in response to various inducers and inhibitors varies. It should also be recognized that there are interspecies differences in the presence, regulation, and catalytic activities of P450s (Lewis et al., 1998).

There has been a focus on identification of P450 isozymes which participate in the metabolism of individual solvents. Nakajima et al. (1992a) found that low concentrations of TCE in rat liver were metabolized primarily by cytochrome P450IIE1 (CYP2E1), a constitutive high-affinity, low-capacity isozyme. CYP2B1/2, a low-affinity, high-capacity form, predominated under high dose (substrate) conditions. CYP2E1 was observed to be a major contributor to the metabolism of TCE and benzene, but not toluene. CYP1A1 catalyzed the formation of *o*-cresol, but not benzyl alcohol from toluene. CYP1A1 biotransformed TCE in mice but not in rats. Thus, P450 isozymes exhibit species-, substrate-, and regioselectivity for solvents (Nakajima, 1997).

CYP2E1 has been shown to be a major catalyst of the oxidation of a variety of low-molecular-weight compounds, including many solvents. CYP2E1 is found in the liver, kidneys, and other extrahepatic tissues of rodents and humans (Lieber, 1997a). Guengerich et al. (1991) demonstrated that human CYP2E1 was primarily responsible for oxidation of some 16 halogenated and aromatic hydrocarbons, including benzene, styrene, $CHCl_3$, TCE, and vinyl chloride. These compounds are oxidized to electrophilic metabolites, capable of causing cytotoxicity and/or mutagenicity (Raucy et al., 1993). The isozyme is also responsible for reduction of CCl_4 to free radicals (see the discussion of CCl_4 in this chapter). CYP2E1 activity is associated with the pathogenesis of alcoholic cirrhosis, through formation of highly reactive oxygen radicals and acetaldehyde from ethanol (Lieber, 1997a). CYP2E1 is inducible by ethanol, acetone, and other of its substrates. Activity of the isozyme varies from species to species (Nakajima, 1997) and from human to human (Lipscomb et al., 1997). Such differences in CYP2E1 may play an important role in susceptibility to solvent toxicity and carcinogenesis (Gonzalez and Gelboin, 1994; Raunio et al., 1995).

A number of environmental factors can predispose people to harmful effects of solvents by altering P450s (Lof and Johanson, 1998). Ethanol is an effective CYP2E1 inducer when ingested repeatedly in substantial amounts. The person who drinks in such a manner may be subject to potentiation of solvent toxicity, due to increased solvent metabolic activation (Manno et al., 1996). Conversely, ethanol consumed at about the same time as a solvent exposure can be protective by competitively inhibiting metabolic activation of the solvent (Lieber, 1997a). Thus, the timing of exposures is important. Folland et al. (1976) report severe CCl_4-induced hepatorenal injury in workers at an isopropyl alcohol bottling plant. These subjects' preexposure to the alcohol, which is metabolized to acetone, caused marked CYP2E1 induction. Their induced condition resulted in a substantial increase in the metabolic activation and cytotoxicity of CCl_4, upon inhalation of a normally nontoxic concentration of the halocarbon.

The metabolic basis of solvent interactions receives considerable attention. The consequence of CYP2E1 induction by one solvent depends upon the nature of the second solvent. Kaneko et al. (1994) report that ethanol pretreatment of rats has a more profound effect on the TK of 1,1,1-trichloroethane (poorly metabolized) than TCE (well metabolized). Similarly, ethanol pretreatment of rats results in a greater increase in metabolism and hepatotoxicity of CCl_4 (poorly metabolized) than $CHCl_3$ (well metabolized) (Wang et al., 1997). These investigators reason that alterations in the metabolism of low doses of well-metabolized compounds are of little consequence, since their metabolism is perfusion- (i.e., hepatic blood flow–) limited. Capacity- (i.e., metabolic capacity of the liver) limited metabolism prevails for poorly metabolized compounds, irrespective of dose. Although chemical/solvent interactions can be toxicologically significant in occupational settings, it is not clear whether exposures to trace levels of solvents in the environment result in metabolic interactions of consequence.

Physiologic Modeling

Physiologically based toxicokinetic (PBTK) models have been developed to provide predictions of chemical concentrations in blood and tissues as a function of time. PBTK models are thus used to relate the administered dose to the tissue dose of bioactive moiety or moieties. If there is sufficient knowledge of the physiology of the test animal/tissue, interactions of the bioactive moiety with cellular components and ensuing responses, physiologically based toxicodynamic (PBTD) models can be developed (Conolly and Andersen, 1991). PBTD models describe the relationship between the tissue dose, early chemical-tissue interactions, and resulting toxic effect(s). Development of PBTK models for anesthetic gases and other pharmaceutical agents was initially undertaken in the 1920s and 1930s. Modeling enjoyed widespread use in the design of experiments and dosage regimens for drugs, but the practice was not extended to industrial chemicals until the 1970s and 1980s. A "benchmark" paper by Ramsey and Andersen (1984) described the development of a PBTK model for styrene. By 1995, PBTK models had been developed for ~50 chemical environmental contaminants (Leung and Paustenbach, 1995). Some 28 of these 50 chemicals were solvents.

PBTK/TD models are being used with increasing frequency to incorporate dosimetry and mechanistic data into noncancer and cancer risk assessments. Physiologic modeling accounts for species- and dose-dependent shifts from linear to nonlinear kinetics, which impact tissue doses of bioactive moiety or moieties. The models are well suited for species-to-species extrapolations, since human physiologic and metabolic parameter values can be input and simulations of target tissue doses and effects in humans generated. Thus, solvent exposures necessary to produce the same target organ dose in humans, as that found experimentally to cause an unacceptable cancer or noncancer incidence in test animals, can be determined in some cases with reasonable certainty (Andersen, 1995). Modeling is now even being used for individual-specific dosimetry (Pierce et al., 1996). In a limited number of cases where there may be species differences in tissue sensitivity, PBTD models may be used to forecast toxicologically effective target organ doses.

POTENTIALLY SENSITIVE SUBPOPULATIONS

There is considerable variability in responses of humans to solvents and other xenobiotics (Hattis et al., 1987). Although information on interindividual differences in the kinetics and toxicity of solvents is limited, some significant differences are reported and should be taken into account in risk assessments (Grassman et al., 1998). Current EPA cancer and noncancer risk assessment practices are generally considered to be protective of potentially vulnerable subgroups, because of the conservative default assumptions upon which the practices are based.

Endogenous Factors

Children Currently there is considerable interest in regulatory and scientific issues related to protection of children's health. The potential sensitivity of infants and children to pesticides and other chemicals was brought to the public's attention by a National Academy of Sciences report (NAS, 1993; Bruckner, 2000). The ensuing Executive Order 13045, in 1997, directed all federal agencies to make protection of children a high priority and to consider risks to children when making policies and setting standards.

Very limited information is available on the toxic potential of solvents and other chemicals in children. The most comprehensive data sets available are compilations of LD_{50} values from studies of immature and mature laboratory animals (Done, 1964; Goldenthal, 1971). Results of these experiments and other investigations of systemic toxicity reveal that immature animals are more sensitive to some but not all chemicals. Most reported age-dependent differences are less than an order of magnitude, usually varying no more than two- to threefold. The younger and more immature the subject, the more different its response from that of an adult. Substantial anatomical, physiologic, and biochemical changes occur during infancy, childhood, and puberty. There may be developmental periods, or "windows of vulnerability" when the endocrine, reproductive, immune, audiovisual, nervous, and other organ systems are particularly sensitive to certain chemicals. Maturational changes may also substantially affect the kinetics and ensuing toxicity of solvents and other agents (Hein, 1987; ILSI, 1992; Bruckner and Weil, 1999).

Despite a virtual "data vacuum," logical assumptions can be made about age-dependent changes in the kinetics and toxicity of solvents. GI absorption of solvents would not be expected to vary with age, since most solvents are rapidly and completely absorbed by passive diffusion. Systemic absorption of inhaled VOCs may be greater in infants and children than in adults. Infants' and children's cardiac output and respiratory rates are relatively high, although their alveolar surface area is lower than that of adults (Snodgrass, 1992). Reduced plasma protein binding capacity in neonates and infants may be of consequence for solvent metabolites. Extracellular water, expressed as percentage of body weight, is highest in newborns and gradually diminishes through childhood. Body fat content is high from ~1/2 to 3 years of age, then steadily decreases until adolescence, when it increases again in females. Lipophilic solvents accumulate in adipose tissue, so more body fat would result in greater body burdens and slower clearance of the chemicals.

Changes in xenobiotic metabolism during maturation may have the greatest impact on susceptibility to solvent toxicity and carcinogenicity. Poisonings of premature and term newborns exposed to benzyl alcohol, hexachlorobenzene, chloramphenicol, and other compounds are primarily attributable to initial deficits in metabolic conjugation capacity. Studies of human liver reveal that P450 isoforms are age-dependent and develop asynchronously, possibly by different mechanisms (Treluyer et al., 1996; Cresteil, 1998). Levels of CYP2E1, the principal catalyst of oxidation of a variety of solvents, are very low at birth but "surge" within hours and then steadily increase during the first year of life (Vieira et al., 1996; Treluyer et al., 1996). Systemic clearance of many drugs is higher in children than in adults. Although Blanco et al. (2000) recently failed to find an age-related difference in the maximal activity of CYP2E1 or other hepatic P450 isozymes in vitro, it is generally believed that P450 activities are higher in infants and children than in adults. It should be recognized that increased metabolic activation does not necessarily mean increased toxicity in children. Cyclophosphamide, for example, is metabolically activated to acrolein and phosphoramide mustard. Children are less susceptible to cyclophosphamide toxicity than adults (Crom et al., 1987), due to more rapid detoxification and elimination of these reactive intermediates. Increased rates of metabolism, urinary excretion of metabolites, and exhalation by children should hasten elimination and reduce body burdens of solvents.

The net effect of immaturity on solvent disposition and toxicity is difficult to predict. An age-related change in one parameter may be offset or augmented by concurrent changes in other parameters. Susceptibility of immature subjects may be age-, organ-, chemical- and species-dependent. Newborn mice and rats are less mature at birth than are humans, though maturation of rodents is much more rapid. A few days of age can result in a marked disparity in toxicity test results in rodents (Done, 1964). Organs and their functions mature at different rates in different species. Thus interspecies extrapolations in immature animals are difficult, and selection of an appropriate animal model for a particular phase of human development can be difficult. PBTK models may be useful here. Physiologic and metabolic parameter values will need to be measured in healthy children of different ages by noninvasive methods for input into the models.

Elderly A number of factors would appear to be involved in differential sensitivities of the elderly to solvents (Dawling and Chrome, 1989; Birnbaum, 1991). With aging, body fat usually increases substantially at the expense of lean mass and body water. Thus, relatively polar solvents tend to reach higher blood levels during exposures. Relatively lipid-soluble solvents accumulate in adipose tissue and are released slowly to sites of action, metabolism, and elimination. Cardiac output diminishes 30 to 40 percent between the ages of 25 and 65, as do renal and hepatic blood flows (Cody, 1993; Woodhouse and Wynne, 1992). The latter two researchers concluded that reduced clearance of flow- and capacity-limited drugs in the elderly was due primarily to reductions in liver blood flow and liver size. Schmucker et al. (1990) did not find a relationship between aging and P450 activities and content in human liver. McMahon et al. (1994) used a PBTK model to demonstrate that reduced urinary elimination of benzene metabolites in geriatric mice was due to decreased renal blood flow rather than altered formation of metabolites.

The elderly, like infants and children, may be more or less sensitive to the toxicity of solvents than young adults. Data are lacking on age-dependent susceptibility of humans to solvents and other industrial chemicals. Older people do appear to be more sensitive to CNS-depressant effects of ethanol, due in part to lower gastric alcohol dehydrogenase activity (Seitz et al., 1993). Experiments have shown that aged rodents are more vulnerable to hepatocellular injury by some solvents including allyl alcohol, ethanol, and CCl_4. Rikans et al. (1999) have suggested that the greater liver damage could be due to increased inflammatory damage, due to age-related dysregulation of cytokines. Other major sources of variability and complexity in responses of geriatric populations to solvents include toxicodynamic (TD) changes, inadequate nutrition, the prevalence of disease states, and the concurrent use of multiple medications.

Gender Women may differ from men in some respects in their responses to solvents, but the differences do not appear to be too great. Most men have more muscle mass and larger body size. Women typically have more body fat and smaller volumes of distribution for polar solvents. Nomiyama and Nomiyama (1974) found that women retained less inhaled acetone and ethyl acetate than men. Levels of toluene and TCE in expired air were lower in females, reflecting greater fat deposition. The major sex differences in P450-mediated metabolism in rats are not seen in humans or most other mammals (Nakajima, 1997). No marked gender differences in P450-dependent enzyme activities have been identified in humans (Mugford and Kedderis, 1998). Gender differences in responses to ethanol are well recognized and described in this chapter under "Ethanol." Relatively little is known about potential influences of contraceptives, hormone replacement therapy, or pregnancy on the metabolism and kinetics of xenobiotics (Gleiter and Gundert-Remy, 1996).

Genetics A variety of genetic polymorphisms for biotransformation have been found to occur at different frequencies in different ethnic groups (Daly et al., 1993). Polymorphisms for xenobiotic metabolizing enzymes may affect the quantity and quality of enzymes and the outcomes of exposures to solvents (Ingelman-Sundberg et al., 1994). It is important to note that culturally linked environmental factors also contribute to ethnic differences in metabolism and disposition of solvents and other chemicals. It is difficult to disentangle the influences of genetic traits from those of different lifestyles, socioeconomic status, and geographic setting.

Ethnic differences in regulation of the expression of P450 isozymes and other enzymes appear to be associated with variations in drug and solvent metabolism (Ingelman-Sundberg et al., 1994; Weber, 1999). Shimada et al. (1994) found that Caucasians had higher total hepatic P450 levels than Japanese. Caucasians exhibited higher CYP2E1 activities, as reflected by aniline *p*-hydroxylation and 7-ethoxycoumarin *O*-deethylation. Individuals with two linked polymorphisms in the transcription regulatory region of the CYP2E1 gene exhibited greater expression of the isoform. Reported frequencies of these rare alleles were 2 percent in Caucasians, 2 to 5 percent in African Americans, and 24 to 27 percent in Japanese. Kawamoto et al. (1995) found that a CYP2E1 polymorphism in Japanese workers did not affect metabolism of toluene to benzoic acid, but that CYP1A1 and aldehyde dehydrogenase (ALDH2) polymorphisms did. About half of the Japanese population lacks ALDH2 due to a structural point mutation in the ALDH2 gene. Pronounced interethnic differences in rates of ethanol metabolism have been associated with a number of ADH and ALDH polymorphisms. Ethnic differences have also been demonstrated for some phase II biotransformation reactions. Glutathione *S*-transferases (GSTs) are a family of enzymes which promote the detoxification of electrophilic metabolites by catalyzing their conjugation with reduced glutathione (GSH). Some individuals with a null/null genotype for GST theta lack the ability to conjugate and detoxify metabolites of methyl chloride and methylene chloride. The prevalence of this genotype ranges from 10 percent in Mexican Americans to 60 to 65 percent in Chinese and Koreans (Nelson et al., 1995).

Increased susceptibility to different cancers has been reported to be associated with certain genetic polymorphisms, which occur with different frequencies in different ethnic groups (Daly et al., 1993). Significant variations in allelic distributions for isozymes including CYP2E1, 2D6, 1A1, and GSTM1 have been observed in different racial groups. Results of investigations of a relationship between occurrence of defective alleles for CYP2E1 and cancer incidence have been contradictory. Studies with more statistical power of selected ethnic groups need to be conducted to clarify the roles of P450 polymorphisms in cancers. Although molecular markers clearly indicate variances in P450 genes, biologically plausible mechanisms linking specific genotypes with specific outcomes are lacking at present.

Exogenous Factors

P450 Inducers Considerable effort has been devoted to the study of effects of inducers of solvent metabolism. Preexposure to chemicals that induce CYP2E1 and/or CYP2B1/2 can potentiate the toxicity of high doses of solvents that undergo metabolic activation (Fig. 24-4). Induction of these P450s may be of little consequence, however, for low doses of well metabolized solvents (Kaneko et al., 1994; Wang et al., 1997). Notable inducers include ethanol and other alcohols, acetone and other ketones, polycyclic aromatic hydrocarbons, and certain drugs (e.g., phenobarbital, phenytoin, diazepam, rifampicin). Nitcotine and some of the polycyclic hydrocarbons in cigarette smoke are P450 inducers. Smoking, however, has not been clearly shown to influence the TK of VOCs (Sato, 1991). It is important to recognize that many compounds that induce P450s are also inducers of detoxifying enzymes (e.g., epoxide hydratase, glucuronyl- and sulfotransferases). A comprehensive compilation and account of solvent-solvent interactions is presented by Lof and Johanson (1998).

P450 Inhibitors A number of drugs and other compounds inhibit P450s. Such agents would generally be anticipated to enhance the toxicity of solvents that are metabolically inactivated. Conversely, P450 inhibitors should protect from solvents that undergo metabolic activation. Compounds including disulfiram (Antabuse®), 3-amino-1,2,4-triazole, and several constituents of foods (e.g., diallyl sulfide, dihydrocapsaicin, phenylethyl isothiocyanate) inhibit CYP2E1 and protect animals from some carcinogens (Lieber, 1997a). Although quite high doses of the natural products were used in these studies, consumption of such foods may be shown to aid in prevention of some tumors in humans. Certain drugs and solvents are categorized as noncompetitive inhibitors, in that they bind so strongly to P450s that the amount of functional P450 is diminished. Solvents, which in the course of their own metabolism destroy P450s, are known as suicide inhibitors. *Trans-* and *cis*-1,2-dichloroethylene, for example, are potent suicide inhibitors of CYP2E1 in rat liver, but TCE is not (Lilly et al., 1998).

Physical Activity Exercise can significantly affect the kinetics of xenobiotics (van Baak, 1990) but is often not considered in occupational risk assessments of solvents. Exercise increases two of the major determinants of VOC uptake, alveolar ventilation and cardiac output/pulmonary blood flow. Polar solvents with relatively high blood:air PCs (e.g., acetone, ethanol, ethylene glycol) are very rapidly absorbed into the pulmonary circulation. Alveolar ventilation is rate-limiting for these chemicals. In contrast, pulmonary blood flow and metabolism are rate-limiting for uptake of the more lipophilic solvents (Johanson and Filser, 1992). Heavy exercise can increase pulmonary uptake of relatively polar solvents as much as fivefold in human subjects (Astrand, 1983). Light exercise doubles uptake of relatively lipid-soluble solvents, but no further increase occurs at higher workloads. Blood flow to the liver and kidneys diminishes with exercise, so biotransformation of well-metabolized solvents and urinary elimination of polar metabolites may be diminished (Lof and Johnanson, 1998). Dankovic and Bailer (1994) modified the human PBTK model of Reitz et al. (1988) for methylene chloride to reflect light work conditions. The modified model predicted that light exercise would result in a twofold increase in

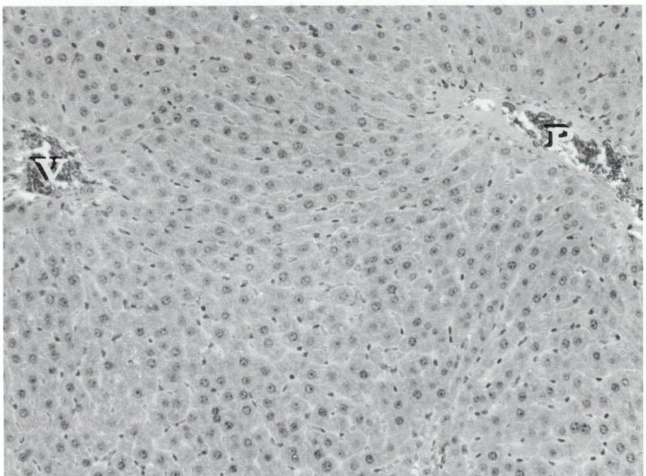

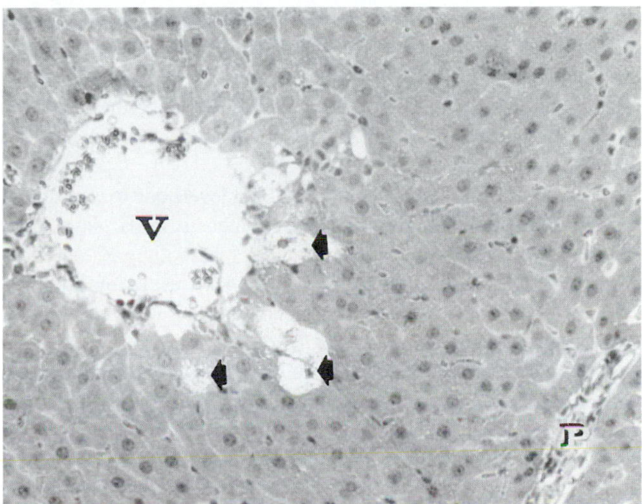

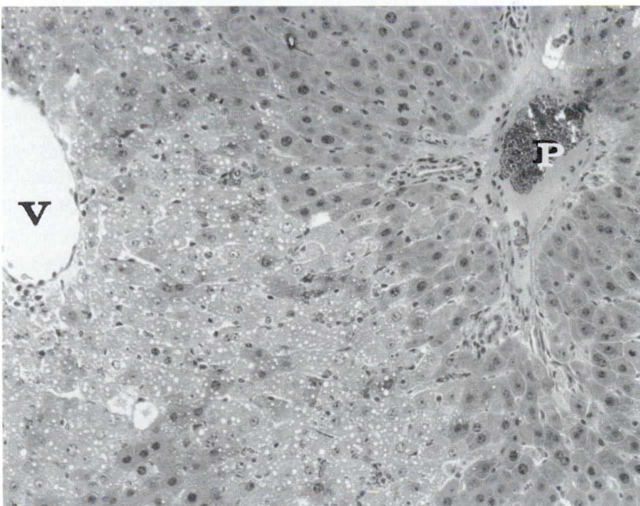

Figure 24-4. Potentiation of CCl_4 hepatotoxicity by 2-butanol.

Rats were (*A*) untreated; (*B*) given 0.1 mL CCl_4/kg IP; or (*C*) pretreated with 2-butanol (2.2 mL/kg PO) 16 h before 0.1 mL CCl_4 IP. Central veins and portal triads are designated V and P, respectively. Occasional hepatocytes adjacent to the central vein are vacuolated in (*B*). Note the demarcation between vacuolated/necrotic centrilobular and midzonal cells, and normally appearing periportal cells in (*C*). Hematoxylin and eosin stain. (*A*) and (*C*) ×315; (*B*) ×480. [Used with permission of Traiger and Bruckner (1976).]

hepatic methylene chloride deposition and in metabolite formation via P450- and GSH-dependent pathways.

Diet Dietary habits can influence the TK and toxicity of solvents in several ways. The mere bulk of food in the stomach and intestines can inhibit systemic absorption of ingested chemicals. VOCs in the GI tract partition into dietary lipids, largely remaining there until the lipids are emulsified and digested. This serves to substantially delay absorption of VOCs such as CCl_4, resulting in lower blood levels and diminished acute hepatotoxicity in rats (Kim et al., 1990a). Food intake results in increased splanchnic blood flow, which favors GI absorption. The accompanying increase in hepatic blood flow would be expected to enhance the biotransformation of low doses of well-metabolized solvents, but to have little effect on first-pass metabolism of relatively high (i.e., saturating) doses (Tam, 1993). Consumption of a high-fat diet can result in an increase in CYP2E1 in the liver of obese rats, possibly due to induction of the isozyme by acetone and other ketone bodies (Raucy et al., 1991). Increased incidences of several types of cancer have been observed in obese humans (Moller et al., 1994). Caloric restriction has clearly been shown to reduce the incidence of several chemically induced tumors in rodents (Kritchevsky, 1999).

Fasting results in decreased liver GSH levels due to interrupted intake of amino acids required for its synthesis. GSH plays a key role in the detoxification of electrophilic metabolites of a number of solvents. Short-term fasting ($\sim$18 to 24 h) results in induction of liver CYP2E1 and increase in metabolism of a number of aromatic hydrocarbons and halocarbons (Nakajima et al., 1982). The hepatotoxicity of CCl_4, which requires CYP2E1-catalyzed metabolic activation, is more severe in fasted animals (Nakajima et al., 1982). In contrast, long-term food deprivation (i.e, starvation) results in decreased synthesis and activity of P450s. Foods may contain certain natural constituents, pesticides, and other chemicals which may enhance or reduce solvent metabolism.

Clock Time Many physiologic and biochemical processes that impact solvent TK exhibit circadian or diurnal rhythms. Investigations have revealed circadian rhythms in susceptibility of rats to liver damage by several VOCs, including CCl_4, $CHCl_3$, 1,1-dichloroethylene, ethanol, and styrene (Labrecque and Belanger, 1991). In each instance, the chemicals were most toxic when given during the initial part of the rodents' dark/active cycle. Low hepatic GSH levels at this time were an important contributing factor to the increased liver injury by 1,1-dichloroethylene and $CHCl_3$. Restricted food intake during sleep resulted in lipolysis and formation of acetone, which contributed to the diurnal induction of CYP2E1 and the ensuing increases in hepatic metabolic activation and cytotoxicity of CCl_4 in rats (Bruckner et al., 2001). Furukawa et al. (1999) attributed high hepatic microsomal 7-alkoxycoumarin *O*-dealkylase activity during male rats' active cycle to diurnal secretion of growth hormone. Hepatic blood flow and acetone levels in expired air of humans peak before breakfast. Clearance rates for a number of well metabolized compounds, including ethanol (Sturtevant et al., 1978) and nicotine (Gries et al., 1996), are maximal in human subjects during the first part of their active/wake cycle. Thus, humans may also be more susceptible at this time to the toxicity of solvents that undergo metabolic activation.

Diseases Illness can be a major source of variability in response to solvents. Impaired drug metabolism and clearance are commonly seen in patients with cirrhosis and hepatitis (Welling and Pool, 1996). Reduced metabolism of solvents may result from decrease in hepatic mass, diminished enzymatic activity, and/or decreased portal blood flow (McLean and Morgan, 1991). Lower levels of CYP2E1, CYP1A2, and GSH are seen in livers of patients with cirrhosis (Murray, 1992). Reduced P450-catalyzed metabolic activation of certain solvents could be protective, but diminished capacity to conjugate electrophilic metabolites with GSH would have the opposite effect. Plasma levels of albumin and α_1-acid glycoprotein fall in cirrhotic patients. Thus, plasma protein binding of many drug metabolites decreases and their elimination increases (McLean and Morgan, 1991). Definitive information is lacking, however, on the net effect of liver diseases on solvents.

Little is known about the influence of kidney disease on the TK of solvents and their metabolites. The protein binding of many drugs is reduced in patients with compromised renal function. The binding and urinary elimination of relatively polar metabolites of solvents may also be diminished, resulting in accumulation of high concentrations of metabolites. Findings in studies of the influence of impaired renal function on hepatic drug metabolism are conflicting. Hepatic clearance of therapeutic agents may be increased, decreased, or unaffected (Elston et al., 1993). The mechanisms of these changes are unclear, as is their applicability to solvents.

Diabetics may be at increased risk of injury by solvents which undergo metabolic activation. Metabolic ketosis in diabetics results in elevated concentrations of acetone, an inducer of hepatic CYP2E1. Hormonal perturbations, including decreases in circulating thyroid hormone, plasma growth hormone, and testosterone, are associated with uncontrolled diabetes. These and other hormones are involved in regulation of P450 isoforms. CYP2E1 and CYP2B1, for example, are induced in diabetic rats, while other isoforms are diminished (Waxman and Chang, 1995). Thus, diabetes may predispose individuals to increased risk of cell injury and/or mutation by solvents which are metabolically activated by CYP2E1 and/or CYP2B1/2.

Persons with bacterial infections may be more sensitive to cytotoxic actions of solvents. Endotoxin, which includes a lipopolysaccharide, is released from the cell wall of gram-negative organisms. The lipopolysaccharide causes the release of inflammatory mediators, which alter cell membranes, intercellular signaling, and gene expression (Roth et al., 1997). These effects may render cells more susceptible to damage by solvents and other chemicals. Exposure of animals to small amounts of endotoxin potentiates liver injury by CCl_4, halothane, allyl alcohol, ethanol, and other solvents (Roth et al., 1997). Endotoxin apparently activates Kupffer cells to release inflammatory mediators and cytotoxic moieties to hepatocytes (Thurman, 1998).

CHLORINATED HYDROCARBONS

Trichloroethylene

1,1,2-Trichloroethylene (TCE) is a widely used solvent for metal degreasing that has been identified at more than one-half of the 1416 hazardous waste sites proposed for inclusion on the EPA's National Priority List (Fay and Muntaz, 1996). TCE has received a great deal of attention from the scientific and regulatory communities recently, due to the EPA's effort to update its more than decade-old risk assessment for TCE. Moderate to high doses of TCE, like other halocarbons, are associated with a number of noncancer toxicities (Barton and Das, 1996). Cancer is the dominant issue for TCE, however. Testament to this includes Germany's recent classification of TCE as a known human carcinogen (Bruning and Bolt, 2000) and the National Toxicology Program's reconsideration of its classification status (NTP, 2000). Attempts to understand the mechanistic underpinnings of TCE's carcinogenicity have resulted in a body of work of massive proportion, that—while providing significant insights—has not eliminated many of the uncertainties that plague the risk-assessment process. Nonetheless, TCE provides a stellar example of how research methods can be applied to generate experimental and epidemiologic data for use in a regulatory context. A 16-article series of state-of-the-science papers, upon which the EPA will heavily rely in its new risk assessment, has been recently published (Scott and Cogliano, 2000).

Cancer Epidemiology As pointed out by Wartenberg et al. (2000), there is no shortage of published studies examining cancer incidence and mortality among TCE-exposed human populations. Examples include those of Morgan et al. (1998), Blair et al. (1998), Boice et al. (1999), and Ritz (1999), of whom all but the last examined cancer mortality or incidence among aircraft manufacturing or maintenance workers. In addition to these U.S. studies, the mortality experience of smaller Swedish, Finnish, and German worker cohorts has been examined (Axelson et al., 1978; Tola et al., 1980; Axelson et al., 1994; Anttila et al., 1995; Henschler et al., 1995). All of the studies mentioned above constitute what Wartenberg and colleagues refer to as tier I studies, meaning that exposure was better characterized than in cohort studies in lower tiers. Thus, tier I studies received a greater weighting from these authors when making causal inferences than lower-tier cohort studies, case-control studies, and community-based studies. An average relative cancer risk was calculated by Wartenberg et al. (2000) for studies within each tier using a meta-analysis-like approach for both mortality and incidence data. Among the tier I studies, evidence for an excess incidence of cancer was strongest for the kidney (relative risk (RR) = 1.7, 95 percent confidence interval (CI) = 1.1 to 2.7), liver (RR = 1.9, 95 percent CI = 1.0 to 3.4), and non-Hodgkin's lymphoma (RR = 1.5, 95 percent CI = 0.9 to 2.3). These investigators also contend that the data support weak associations between TCE exposure and multiple myeloma, Hodgkin's disease, and cancers of the prostate, skin, and cervix.

While not as comprehensive as that of Wartenberg et al. (2000), other reviews of occupational epidemiologic studies have been conducted. Weiss (1996) concluded that the evidence for the carcinogenicity of TCE was "quite limited." He acknowledged that there was some suggestive evidence that TCE could possibly be associated with non-Hodgkin's lymphoma and cancers of the liver, biliary tract, and kidney, with evidence for the kidney coming solely from the study of German cardboard workers by Henschler et al. (1995). Another review of cohort and case-control studies (McLaughlin and Blot, 1997) concluded that the totality of the evidence did not support a role for TCE in renal cell cancer (RCC). Morgan et al. (1998) combined their data with that of others in a meta-analysis-like approach that resulted in slight, statistically insignificant elevations in meta-standardized mortality ratios for cancers of the liver, prostate, kidney, bladder, and non-Hodgkin's lymphoma. The IARC (1995) concluded that TCE is "probably carcinogenic to humans," based on its assessment of sufficient evidence in animals and limited evidence in humans.

The report of Henschler et al. (1995) was the first in a series of German studies that has provided the strongest evidence to date for an association between TCE and RCC. These authors reported on a cohort of male cardboard factory workers who were exposed to moderate to extremely high concentrations of TCE. By the closing date of the study, five of 169 exposed workers had been diagnosed with kidney cancer versus none of the 190 controls. This resulted in standardized incidence ratios (SIRs) of 7.97 (95 percent CI = 2.59 to 18.59) and 9.66 (95 percent CI = 3.14 to 22.55) using Danish and German Cancer Registry data for comparison, respectively. Two additional kidney cancers were diagnosed after the end of the observation period that further increased the SIRs. A single U.S. study had reported a weaker, but significantly elevated SIR for RCC (SIR = 3.7, 95 percent CI = 1.4 to 8.1) among paperboard workers exposed to TCE (Sinks et al., 1992). German researchers also conducted a hospital-based case-control study with 58 RCC patients and 84 patients from accident wards who served as controls. Of the 59 RCC patients, 19 had histories of occupational TCE exposure for at least 2 years, compared to only 5 of the controls. After adjustment for potential confounders, an association between RCC and long-term exposure to TCE was reported (odds ratio = 10.80, 95 percent CI = 3.36 to 34.75) (Vamvakas et al., 1998).

The two German studies detailed above provide some evidence of a link between kidney cancer and TCE, although the link may be operative only under extreme exposure conditions. As will be discussed later, the application of molecular biology techniques to the issue of TCE and kidney cancer has strengthened the argument for a causal association. Controversy surrounds the German studies, as indicated in a critical review (Green and Lash, 1999), to which the researchers responded (Vamvakas et al., 2000).

Metabolism With rare exception, the toxicities associated with TCE are thought to be mediated by metabolites rather than by the parent compound. Even the CNS-depressant effects of TCE are due in part to the sedative properties of the metabolite trichloroethanol (TCOH). As is often the case in risk assessment, a detailed knowledge of metabolism is a prerequisite to an accurate assessment of human risk from TCE exposure. To this end, the enormous amount of information on the subject is summarized in a state-of-the-science paper by Lash et al. (2000).

TCE is rapidly absorbed into the systemic circulation via the oral and inhalation routes. The majority of TCE undergoes oxidation via cytochrome P450s, with a small proportion being conjugated with glutathione (GSH) via glutathione *S*-transferases (GSTs). Thus, two distinct metabolic pathways exist for TCE, the GSH pathway as shown to the left in Fig. 24-5, and the oxidative pathway as shown to the right.

TCE is first oxidized to chloral in a step that may or may not involve an epoxide intermediate. Chloral is then oxidized to trichloroacetic acid (TCA) or reduced to TCOH. TCOH, in turn, is either oxidized to TCA or glucuronidated. TCOH glucuronide may undergo enterohepatic recirculation by hydrolysis to TCOH in the gut, with reabsorption and the possibility of further conversion to TCA. TCA accumulates in the body due to strong protein binding and slow excretion. In contrast, blood levels of dichloroacetic acid (DCA), formed by TCA dechlorination or from TCOH, are very low or nondetectable in humans.

Relatively small amounts of TCE can be conjugated in the liver with GSH to form *S*-(1,2-dichlorovinyl)glutathione (DCVG).

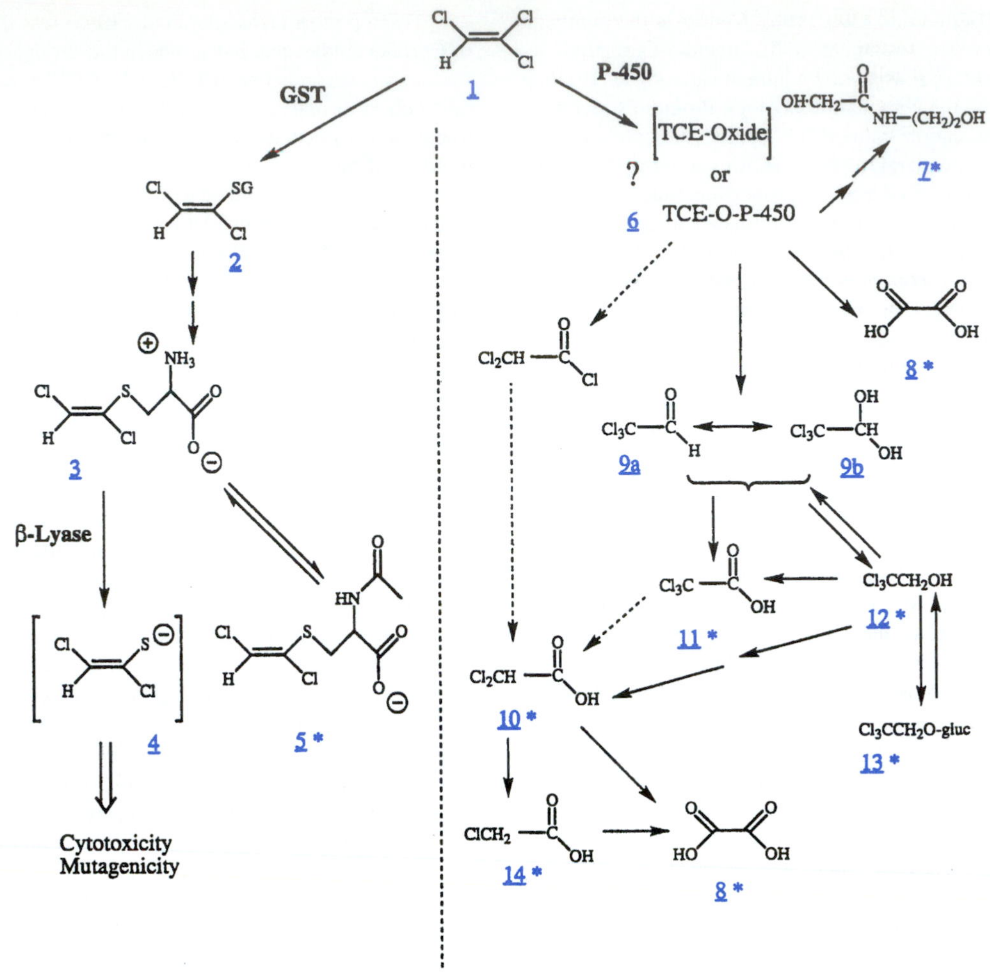

Figure 24-5. Scheme of metabolism of TCE.

Metabolites marked with an asterisk are known urinary metabolites. 1 = TCE; 2 = DCVG; 3 = DCVC; 4 = 1,2-dichlorovinylthiol; 5 = NacDCVC; 6 = TCE-P450 or TCE-oxide intermediate; 7 = *N*-(hydroxyacetyl)-aminoethanol; 8 = oxalic acid; 9a = chloral; 9b = chloral hydrate; 10 = dichloroacetic acid; 11 = trichloroacetic acid; 12 = trichloroethanol; 13 = trichloroethanol glucuronide; 14 = monochloroacetic acid. [Used with permission of Lash et al. (2000).]

DCVG is then effluxed from the hepatocyte into plasma and bile for translocation to the kidney and small intestine, respectively. The plasma DCVG is intrarenally converted by γ-glutamyltransferase and dipeptidases to the cysteine conjugate *S*-(1,2-dichlorovinyl)-L-cysteine (DCVC). The DCVG effluxed into bile can undergo extrarenal processing to DCVC, that is subsequently delivered to the kidney by enterohepatic recirculation. DCVC represents a branch point in the pathway. It may be detoxified through *N*-acetylation or bioactivated to reactive thiols via renal β-lyase located in renal proximal tubular cells.

Modes of Action in Target Tissues The goal of much of the TCE research conducted to date has been to understand the relevance of positive rodent cancer bioassays to humans. Both metabolic pathways are implicated in the carcinogenicity of TCE: reactive metabolite(s) of the GSH pathway in kidney tumors in rats, and oxidative metabolites in liver and lung tumors in mice. That tumor formation in many cases is species-, strain-, sex-, and route of exposure–dependent has provided understanding of TCE's modes of carcinogenic action. While substantial progress has been made toward this end, the reader should not infer from the following discussions that the modes of action are known with absolute certainty. Rather, they should be considered working hypotheses that await further experimental confirmation.

Liver Cancer TCE induces liver cancer in B6C3F1 mice but not in rats. This differential susceptibility can be explained by the greater capacity of the mouse to metabolize TCE via the oxidative pathway. B6C3F1 mice also develop liver tumors when chloral hydrate (CH), TCA, and DCA are administered in very high doses, suggesting that one or more of these metabolites is ultimately responsible for TCE-induced liver cancer. Of the three, TCA and/or DCA are/is most likely responsible, since TCE metabolism results in extremely low blood levels of CH due to its rapid oxidation to TCA or reduction to TCOH. The proposed mechanisms by which TCE induces liver cancer have been reviewed in a recent state-of-the-science paper (Bull, 2000), upon which the following discussion is based.

The sensitivity of B6C3F1 mice to TCE suggests that liver tumor formation might be related to the abnormally high frequency of spontaneously initiated cells in this mouse strain, which manifests itself as an unusually high background liver tumor incidence. While TCA and/or DCA might induce liver tumors in B6C3F1 mice by simply promoting preexisting initiated cells, the finding that DCA (but not TCA) also induces liver tumors in F344 rats suggests that another mechanism might also be operable.

As for a promotional mechanism for TCE, overt cytotoxicity and reparative cell proliferation are unlikely, especially at tumorigenic doses. Peroxisome proliferation represents a more viable promotional mechanism. As peroxisomes contain a variety of peroxidative enzymes, their proliferation results in an increased potential for oxidative DNA damage and decreased gap junctional intercellular communication, both of which have been implicated in neoplastic transformation. At tumorigenic doses, TCA induces sustained peroxisome proliferation in B6C3F1 mice. The peroxisome proliferative response to DCA is transient however, and requires a dose higher than that capable of inducing tumors. Therefore, a primary role for TCA is likely if liver tumor promotion occurs via peroxisome proliferation.

An alternative promotional mechanism is suggested by evidence that TCA and DCA depress replication rates of normal hepatocytes, conferring a selective growth advantage to initiated tumorigenic cells. This is referred to as *negative selection.* At high tumorigenic doses, DCA (but not TCA) is thought to stimulate cell replication within tumors. Interestingly, DCA tumors overexpress the insulin receptor relative to surrounding normal tissue. As overexpression of the insulin receptor is associated with the suppression of transforming growth factor β1–induced apoptosis in human liver cells, it is conceivable that DCA could promote cancer by a dual mechanism: enhanced mitotic activity and decreased apoptotic activity of preneoplastic cells.

DCA-promoted liver tumors differ phenotypically from those of TCA in that they express c-*jun* and c-*fos,* TGF-α, *GST* pi, and two P450s, CYP2E1 and CYP4A1. The expression of CYP2E1 raises the possibility that oxidative metabolites could be produced within targeted hepatocytes, which could be important in tumor induction. DCA- and TCA-induced tumors also differ with respect to the reversibility of the depression of cytosine methylation upon cessation of treatment. The simplest explanation for these differences is that DCA and TCA selectively modify growth and death rates of different clones of liver cells.

Kidney Cancer TCE exposure by inhalation or the oral route results in kidney tumors in male but not female rats. The susceptibility of the male rat can be explained by its greater capacity for TCE metabolism via the GSH pathway. TCE-induced kidney tumors are believed to result from reactive metabolite(s) of this pathway, particularly DCVC. DCVC is bioactivated in proximal tubular cells to a reactive thiol, *S*-(1,2-dichlorovinyl)thiol, which is chemically unstable and rearranges to reactive species capable of alkylating cellular nucleophiles, including DNA. The resulting DNA mutations lead to alterations in gene expression, which in turn lead to neoplastic transformation and tumorigenesis via a genotoxic pathway.

Alternatively, there are many processes that can lead to proximal tubular cell cytotoxicity and subsequent tumor formation via a nongenotoxic mode of action. Reactive metabolites formed within proximal tubular cells exposed to high doses of DCVC result in oxidative stress, alkylation of cytosolic and mitochondrial proteins, marked ATP depletion, and perturbations in Ca^{2+} homeostasis. Tubular necrosis ensues, with subsequent reparative proliferation that can alter gene expression and, in turn, alter the regulation of cell growth and differentiation. Modes of action for TCE-induced kidney tumor formation are discussed in greater detail by Lash et al. (2000) in their state-of-the-science paper.

Animal studies typically provide insight on mode of action, but in the case of TCE-induced RCC, human studies have been of significant value. Bruning et al. (1997a) analyzed tumor tissues from 23 RCC patients with occupational histories of long-term, high-level TCE exposure. Tumor cell DNA was isolated and analyzed for somatic mutations in the von-Hippel Lindau (VHL) tumor suppressor gene. Compared to VHL gene mutation rates of 33 to 55 percent in TCE-unexposed RCC patients, all 23 TCE-exposed RCC patients exhibited aberrations of the VHL gene. In a follow-up study, Brauch et al. (1999) sought to determine whether TCE produced a specific mutational effect in the VHL gene. These investigators analyzed VHL gene sequences in DNA isolated from renal cell tumors of patients exposed to high levels of TCE in metal-processing factories. Renal cell tumors of TCE-exposed patients showed somatic VHL mutations in 33 of 44 cases (75 percent). Of the 33 cases with VHL mutations, a specific mutational hot spot at VHL nucleotide 454 was observed in 13. The nucleotide 454 mutation was not found in any of the 107 RCC patients without TCE exposure or among 97 healthy subjects, 47 of whom had a history of TCE exposure. These data suggest that the VHL gene might be a specific and susceptible target of TCE.

Considering the implications of a genotoxic mode of action for the cancer risk assessment of TCE, the question of whether chronic tubular damage occurs in renal tumor formation is an important one. Answers have come from the use of electrophoresis to examine protein excretion patterns in the urine of RCC patients with and without a history of chronic high-level TCE exposure (Bruning et al., 1996). Protein excretion patterns indicative of tubular damage were identified in all 17 of the TCE-exposed cases but in only about half of the 35 controls. This observation suggests that chronic tubular damage may be a prerequisite to TCE-induced RCC. Bruning and colleagues (1999) recently published a larger but similar study that also supported this concept.

Bruning and Bolt (2000) suggest that reactive metabolite(s) of the GSH pathway may have a genotoxic effect on the proximal tubule of the human kidney, but that full development of a malignant tumor requires a promotional effect such as cell proliferation in response to tubular damage. If this is true, then RCC secondary to TCE exposure would be a threshold response, something supported by the occurrence of human RCC only among cases with unusually high and prolonged TCE exposure. Factors other than the intensity and duration of exposure may determine one's susceptibility to TCE-induced RCC, however. Bruning et al. (1997b) have investigated the influence of GST isoenzyme polymorphisms on RCC risk using long-term, highly exposed workers with or without RCC. These investigators reported an unequal distribution of GSTμ1 and GSTθ1 polymorphisms among RCC cases and controls, which suggested a higher risk for RCC in TCE-exposed persons carrying either the GSTθ1 or GSTμ1 polymorphic gene. GSTμ is thought to function to detoxify reactive electrophiles, while GSTθ is primarily involved in conjugation reactions.

Lung Cancer As discussed in the state-of-the science paper by Green (2000), inhaled TCE is carcinogenic to the mouse lung but not to that of the rat. Oral TCE is not carcinogenic to the lung, probably due to hepatic metabolism that limits the amount of TCE reaching the organ. The primary target of TCE within the mouse lung is the nonciliated Clara cell. Toxicity to these cells is characterized by vacuolization and increases in cell replication in the bronchiolar epithelium. A dose-dependent reduction in the CYP450 activity of Clara cells is observed as well. This loss of metabolic capacity is thought to be an adaptive response, since Clara cells recover morphologically during repeated daily inhalation exposures to TCE.

Chloral is the putative toxicant responsible for pulmonary tumor formation. Clara cells of the mouse efficiently metabolize TCE to TCA and chloral. Chloral accumulates, due to its efficient production and the low activity of alcohol dehydrogenase, the enzyme responsible for the metabolism of chloral to TCOH. The lack of glucuronosyltransferase, the enzyme that normally catalyzes the formation of TCOH glucuronide, has also been implicated in chloral accumulation. This mechanism explains the species difference in susceptibility of the lung to TCE. Mouse lung Clara cells have a much higher concentration of CYP2E1 than those of the rat and thus a much higher capacity to metabolize TCE to chloral. Also, Clara cells in mice are much more numerous than in rats. The critical role for chloral is supported by the finding that its administration to mice, but not that of TCA or TCOH, causes Clara cell toxicity identical to that of TCE. Chloral does appear to have some genotoxic potential, especially in regard to inducing aneuploidy. However, the fact that tumors are not seen in species where cytotoxicity does not occur strongly implicates cytotoxicity and reparative proliferation in tumor formation.

Risk Assessment The human relevance of TCE-induced rodent tumors is an unresolved issue. For liver tumors, humans appear to be more similar to rats than mice in their capacity for oxidative TCE metabolism. For kidney tumors, evidence exists that TCE bioactivation via the GSH pathway is greater in rats than in humans. As for promotional mechanisms, rodent liver is much more responsive to the action of peroxisome proliferators than human liver, and α_{2u}-globulin nephropathy is thought to be specific to the male rat. With regard to lung cancer, the CYP450 content and the number of Clara cells in the human lung are but a fraction of those in the mouse. This suggests that the risk of chloral accumulation in humans is minimal. Based on the above, it appears that direct extrapolation from rodent data would overstate human TCE cancer risk.

Most mechanistic cancer research over the last decade on TCE has been focused on the liver and metabolites of TCE in mice. The most compelling mechanistic studies to date, however, are associated with kidney cancer in TCE-exposed workers. In two recent state-of-the-science papers, rodent and human PBPK models for TCE (and its metabolites) were used for cancer dose–response analyses in rodents and for extrapolation of rodent dose metrics to humans (Clewell et al., 2000; Fisher, 2000). The EPA is expected to use PBPK models in its risk assessment update, because compelling hypotheses are available concerning the mode of action (and appropriate dose metrics) for cancer in the liver, lung, and kidney of rodents.

Tetrachloroethylene

Tetrachloroethylene (perchloroethylene, PERC) is commonly used as a dry cleaner, fabric finisher, degreaser, rug and upholstery cleaner, paint and stain remover, solvent, and chemical intermediate. The highest exposures usually occur in occupational settings via inhalation. Much attention is now focused on adverse health effects experienced by dry cleaners and other persons living in the proximity of such facilities (Garetano and Gochfeld, 2000). PERC is frequently detected in the low ppt range in the breath and blood of the general populace (Wallace et al., 1987; Ashley et al., 1994; Clayton et al., 1999). Although releases are primarily to the atmosphere, PERC enters surface and groundwaters by accidental and intentional discharges (ATSDR, 1997d). Levels of 18 ppb are reported in municipal water in areas of New England, where PERC was used in a process to treat plastic water pipe (Paulu et al., 1999). Fay and Mumtaz (1996) report that PERC is the third most frequently found chemical in water at hazardous waste sites.

The systemic disposition and metabolism of *PERC* and trichloroethylene (TCE) are quite similar. Both chemicals are well absorbed from the lungs and GI tract, distributed to tissues according to their lipid content, partially exhaled unchanged, and metabolized by P450s. PERC is oxidized by hepatic P450s to a much lesser degree than TCE, though the two have a common major metabolite, trichloroacetic acid. GSH conjugation is a minor metabolic pathway, quantitatively, for TCE and PERC. The resulting conjugates of TCE and PERC are *S*-(dichlorovinyl)glutathione (DCVG) and *S*-(trichlorovinyl)glutathione (TCVG), respectively. These are cleaved to *S*-(dichlorovinyl)-L-cysteine (DCVC) and *S*-(trichlorovinyl)-L-cysteine (TCVC) (Birner et al., 1994). TCVC can be detoxified by acetylation and excretion in the urine, or metabolically activated by cleavage by a β-lyase in the kidney to dichlorothioketene. The latter compound can covalently bind to proteins and other macromolecules, or react with water to form dichloroacetic acid (DCA), a mutagen and high-dose animal carcinogen. DCA is also believed to be formed from TCE (see discussion of trichloroethylene, above). Dichlorothioketene is purported to be the ultimate PERC metabolite responsible for nephrotoxicity and mutagenicity (Volkel et al., 1998).

PERC has very limited capacity to produce acute or chronic hepatorenal toxicity in laboratory animals. Near-lethal IP doses of PERC were required to cause acute liver or kidney injury in mice (Klaassen and Plaa, 1966). Liver injury was not seen in B6C3F1 mice or Osborne-Mendel rats gavaged with up to $\sim$1000 mg/kg daily for 78 weeks (NCI, 1977). Dose-dependent karyomegaly was observed in the renal proximal tubular epithelium of mice and rats exposed to PERC for 103 weeks (NTP, 1986). This change was most prominent in the male rats. Green et al. (1990) found increases in protein droplets and cell proliferation in the proximal tubular epithelium of male F344 rats gavaged with 1500 mg PERC/kg daily for up to 42 days. These changes are accompanied by an increase in α_{2u}-globulin, a male rat–specific protein (Fig. 24-6).

PERC's potential for causing cancer in humans continues to be a subject of controversy. Male and female B6C3F1 mice, gavaged with very high doses of PERC for up to 78 weeks, exhibited an increase in hepatocellular carcinoma (NCI, 1977). No increase in tumor incidence was seen in Osborne-Mendel rats. Hepatocellular carcinoma was seen again in B6C3F1 mice inhaling 100 or 200 ppm PERC over a 2-year period (NTP, 1986). There was a low incidence of renal adenomas and carcinomas in male F344 rats exposed to 200 or 400 ppm PERC. Such tumors are *rare* in this species. There was also a significant increase over controls in mononuclear cell leukemia in the male and female rats, but $\sim$50 percent of the controls had this disease. There have been many epidemiologic studies of cancer incidence and mortality in groups of

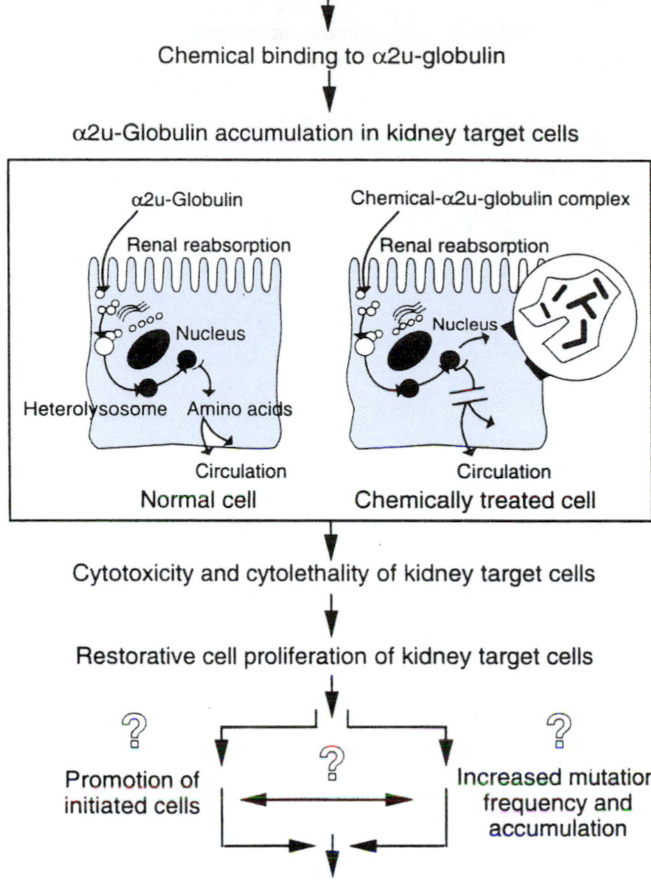

Figure 24-6. Proposed mechanism of solvent-induced kidney cancer in male rats involving α_{2u}-globulin.

[Used with permission of Borghoff et al: *CIIT Activities* 16(10):1–8, 1996.]

dry cleaners and other persons occupationally exposed to PERC (ATSDR, 1997d). Some researchers have reported findings of excess risks of different cancers, while others have not. Frequently, there was not a determination of the degree or duration of PERC exposure, or consideration of major confounding factors (e.g., exposure to other solvents/chemicals, smoking, alcohol, socioeconomic status). Nevertheless, there was sufficient information for Weiss (1995) to conclude that cigarette smoking and alcohol consumption could only partially account for an increased rate of esophageal cancer in dry cleaners. Kidney cancer incidences did not appear to be elevated. McLaughlin and Blot (1997) concluded that epidemiologic evidence gathered to date clearly does not support a cause-and-effect relationship between either PERC or TCE and kidney cancer.

The relevance of the male rat kidney tumor findings to humans has received considerable attention. Several mechanisms have been proposed for the development of renal cell carcinoma in PERC-exposed male rats. Chronic exposure to high doses of PERC can cause ongoing cell death, regenerative hyperplasia, and the opportunity for spontaneous errors in replication during repair. Increased cell replication, protein droplet accumulation, and enhanced α_{2u}-gobulin levels in the P2 segment of renal proximal tubules appear to be unique to male rats (Green et al., 1990). Melnick et al. (1999), however, have pointed out that the association between α_{2u}-globulin accumulation and kidney cancer is unknown, and that quantitative relationships between key biological processes have yet to be demonstrated. They offered an alternative hypothesis, namely the α_{2u}-globulin may bind to and thereby increase the renal concentration and action of approximate carcinogen. As described above, a limited amount of PERC can be metabolized to TCVC, which in turn is cleaved in the kidneys to the cytotoxin and mutagen dichlorothioketene. Upon equivalent inhalation exposures of Wistar rats and humans to PERC, the rats excreted substantially larger amounts of DCA and acetylated TCVC (Volkel et al., 1998). These observations were consistent with in vitro findings of greater conversion of PERC to TCVC by rat liver cytosol and of a 10-fold higher cysteine conjugate β-lyase activity in rat kidney (Cooper, 1994). Thus, Volkel et al. (1998) concluded that humans are much less susceptible than rats to PERC-induced renal tumors. Such metabolic and physiologic differences between species can be input into PBTK models and used to predict risks of cancer in PERC-exposed humans (Reitz et al., 1996; Lash et al., 1998).

Methylene Chloride

Methylene chloride (dichloromethane, MC) enjoys widespread use as a solvent in industrial processes, food preparation, degreasing agents, aerosol propellants, and agriculture. Thus, large numbers of people are exposed occupationally and in the home. The primary route of exposure to this very volatile solvent is inhalation. The preponderance of MC escaping into the environment does so by volatilization (ATSDR, 1998b). The VOC is also frequently found in wastewater discharges and in air and water at hazardous-waste sites (Fay and Mumtaz, 1996).

The TK of MC has been well characterized in humans and rodents. Inhaled MC was extensively absorbed and reached near steady state in the blood of human subjects within 1 to 2 h of continuous exposure (DiVincenzo and Kaplan, 1981). Less than 5 percent of the absorbed dose was exhaled unchanged. Some 25 to 34 percent was exhaled as carbon monoxide, the major end-metabolite of MC. Exposure of the volunteers to 50, 100, 150, and 200 ppm for 7.5 h produced peak blood carboxyhemoglobin saturations of 1.9, 3.4, 5.3, and 6.8 percent, respectively. MC was very rapidly eliminated from the body and did not accumulate over 5 days of exposure. Metabolism of MC in humans and rodents is believed to occur via three pathways (Andersen et al., 1987). One entails CYP2E1-catalyzed oxidation to carbon monoxide via formyl chloride, a reactive intermediate. The second, a glutathione (GSH)-mediated pathway, involves a theta-class glutathione *S*-transferase, GSTT1-1. The P450 pathway is a high-affinity, low-capacity pathway that predominates at MC concentrations present in occupational and environmental settings. The GST pathway is a low-affinity, high-capacity pathway operative at the high exposure levels used in cancer bioassays (Green, 1997). With the third, it is postulated that CO_2 is also formed via the oxidative pathway by reaction of formyl chloride with a nucleophile such as GSH (Fig. 24-7).

MC has only a limited systemic toxicity potential. High, repeated inhalation exposures are required to produce slight, reversible changes in the livers of rodents. Centrilobular vacuolization and focal necrosis occur in the livers of rats exposed 6 h/day,

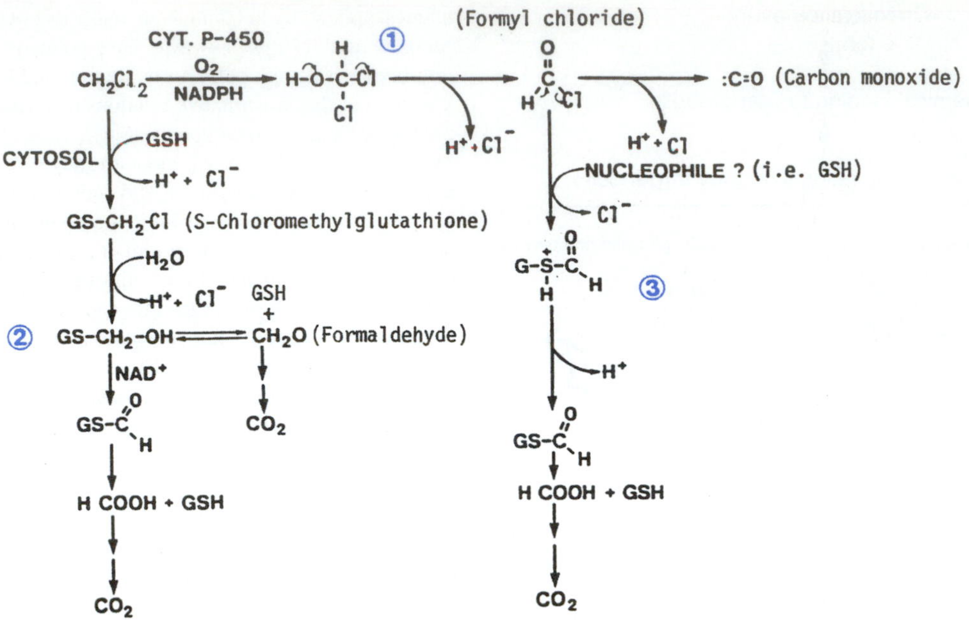

Figure 24-7. Proposed pathways for methylene chloride (CH_2Cl_2) metabolism.

(1) Mixed function oxidase pathway; (2) glutathione transferase pathway; and (3) nucleophile pathway. [Modified and used with permission from Andersen et al. (1987).]

5 days/week for 2 years to 500 to 4000 ppm MC (Burek et al., 1984; Mennear et al., 1988). Manifestations of kidney injury are infrequent in laboratory animals but are occasionally reported in persons subjected to high vapor levels. As described above, the carbon monoxide that is formed from MC binds to hemoglobin to produce dose-dependent increases in carboxyhemoglobin. It is generally accepted that tissue hypoxia can contribute to acute CNS effects of MC. There are few reports of residual neurologic dysfunction in MC-exposed employees (Lash et al., 1991; ATSDR, 1998b).

Occupational and environmental MC exposures are of concern primarily because of MC's carcinogenicity in rodents and its potential as a human carcinogen. Burek et al. (1984) saw increased numbers of salivary gland sarcomas in male rats and benign mammary tumors in female rats exposed to very high MC vapor levels five times weekly over 2 years. Hamsters were not affected. Benign mammary tumors in female rats were also seen in subsequent inhalation bioassays (Nitschke et al., 1988; Mennear et al., 1988). Dose-dependent increases in lung and liver tumors in male and female B6C3F1 mice were also found in the latter investigation. Epidemiology studies of workers exposed to MC have not revealed increases in mortality from lung or liver tumors (ATSDR, 1998b). There have been occasional reports of cancer excess in other organs, including the pancreas (Hearne et al., 1990) and the prostate and cervix (Gibbs et al., 1996). Upon a comprehensive review of the epidemiology literature, Dell et al. (1999) recently concluded that cancer risks from occupational exposure to MC, if any, are quite small.

There has been a great deal of research to define mechanisms of MC carcinogenicity, in order to more clearly understand the relevance of the murine tumors to humans (Green, 1997). Liver and lung tumors in mice do not seem to be associated with overt cytotoxicity or increased replicative DNA synthesis (Maronpot et al., 1995). Induction of the tumors in mice is generally believed to be due to a reactive intermediate generated via the GST pathway (Andersen et al., 1987). GSTT1-1 in liver and lung catalyzes conversion of MC to *S*-chloromethylglutathione ($GSCH_2Cl$), which apparently breaks down rapidly to GSH and formaldehyde. $GSCH_2Cl$ has yet to be isolated and quantified. Metabolism of MC via the GST pathway is an order of magnitude greater in mouse than in rat liver. Metabolic rates in hamster and human liver are even lower (Reitz et al., 1989; Thier et al., 1998). High GSTT1-1 activity was measured in the nuclei of mouse centrilobular hepatocytes. Mice may be unique in that extensive metabolic activation of MC to an unstable intermediate occurs in the proximity of the DNA. GSTT1-1 was also detected in relatively high levels in mouse lung Clara cells and ciliated cells at alveolar/bronchiolar junctions. $GSCH_2Cl$ apparently causes single-strand breaks in vivo and in vitro in DNA of mouse liver and lung (Graves et al., 1995). No DNA breaks were detected in hamster or human hepatocytes in vitro. Casanova and coworkers have proposed an alternate mechanism of MC carcinogenicity, namely formation of DNA-protein cross-links (DPX) by formaldehyde. Upon incubation of MC with hepatocytes from mice, rats, hamsters, and humans, DPX were found only in the mouse samples (Casanova et al., 1996). Formaldehyde-RNA adducts, a more sensitive marker than DPX, were subsequently found in human hepatocytes incubated with MC, though the adducts were seven times more prevalent in mouse hepatocytes (Casanova et al., 1997).

We now have a substantial amount of information on the TK and mechanism(s) of carcinogenicity of MC. Considerable time and money have been spent on MC research by federal agencies and academia as well as by industry. MC was one of the first chemicals for which PBTK modeling was employed by the EPA in cancer risk estimation. Although uncertainties remain, species differences appear to be largely quantitative rather than qualitative. Persons with a GSTT1-1 null genotype (Nelson et al., 1995) may not be at risk from certain MC-induced tumors. This concept was recently incorporated into a cancer risk assessment based upon PBTK estimation of DPX formation in humans (El-Masri et al., 1999).

Carbon Tetrachloride

Carbon tetrachloride (CCl_4) previously enjoyed widespread use as a solvent, cleaning agent, fire extinguisher, synthetic intermediate, grain fumigant, and anthelmintic for humans. Its use has steadily declined since the 1970s, due to its hepatorenal toxicity, carcinogenicity, and contribution to ozone depletion in the atmosphere (ATSDR, 1994). Nevertheless, CCl_4 appears to be ubiquitous in ambient air in the United States, and it is still found in groundwater from some wells and waste sites. CCl_4 is a classic hepatotoxin, but kidney injury is often more severe in humans. There does not appear to be a good animal model for kidney toxicity.

The time course of CCl_4-induced acute liver injury has been well characterized (ATSDR, 1994). Early signs of hepatocellular injury in rats include dissociation of polysomes and ribosomes from rough endoplasmic reticulum, disarray of smooth endoplasmic reticulum, inhibition of protein synthesis, and triglyceride accumulation. Ingested CCl_4 reaches the liver, undergoes metabolic activation, produces lipoperoxidation, covalently binds, and inhibits microsomal ATPase activity within minutes in rats. Single cell necrosis, evident 5 to 6 h postdosing, progresses to maximal centrilobular necrosis within 24 to 48 h. Most microsomal enzyme activities are significantly depressed (Recknagel et al., 1989). A variety of cytoplasmic enzymes are released from dead and dying hepatocytes into the bloodstream. The activity of these enzymes in serum generally parallels the extent of necrosis in the liver. Cellular regeneration, manifest by increased DNA synthesis and cell cycle progression, is maximal 36 to 48 h postdosing (Rao et al., 1997). The rate and extent of tissue repair are important determinants of the ultimate outcome of toxic liver injury.

It is likely that the mechanism of liver injury by CCl_4 has received more attention than that of any other chemical. Nevertheless, there is still considerable debate about the relative importance of different actions of CCl_4, notably covalent binding and lipid peroxidation. CCl_4 is known to be metabolized by P450-dependent reductive dehalogenation to a trichloromethyl radical ($CCl_3\cdot$). This radical can bind covalently to lipids and proteins, causing structural damage of membranes and inhibition of a variety of enzymes. $CCl_3\cdot$ may also react with O_2 to produce $Cl_3COO\cdot$, the trichloromethylperoxy radical. $CCl_3\cdot$ can also attack enoic fatty acids, leading to organic free radicals, which may in turn react with O_2 to form peroxides and other cytotoxic metabolites (Recknagel et al., 1989). This process is known as lipid peroxidation. Numerous studies have shown various antioxidants to ameliorate CCl_4 cytotoxicity in vitro and in vivo. Agents that inhibit CCl_4 covalent binding are also protective. In vivo experiments in rats by Padron et al. (1996) demonstrated that both of these degenerative processes (i.e., covalent binding and lipid peroxidation) were necessary for CCl_4 cytotoxicity. Liu et al. (1995) have proposed that CCl_4 oxidative stress in the liver enhances nuclear factor kappa B activity, which, in turn, promotes expression of proinflammatory cytotoxic cytokines. Shi et al. (1998) have even proposed apoptosis as an additional/alternate mechanism of CCl_4-induced cell death.

Perturbation of intracellular calcium (Ca^{2+}) homeostasis appears to be an integral part of CCl_4 cytotoxicity (Stoyanovsky and Cederbaum, 1996). Increased cytosolic Ca^{2+} levels may result from influx of extracellular Ca^{2+} due to plasma membrane damage and from decreased intracellular Ca^{2+} sequestration. Elevation of intracellular Ca^{2+} in hepatocytes can cause activation of phospholipase A_2 and exacerbation of membrane damage (Glende and Recknagel, 1992). Elevated Ca^{2+} may also be involved in alterations in calmodulin and phosphorylase activity as well as changes in nuclear protein kinase C activity (Omura et al., 1999). Increased Ca^{2+} may stimulate the release of cytokines and eicosanoids from Kupffer cells. Edwards et al. (1993) demonstrated that destruction of Kupffer cells prior to CCl_4 dosing of rats resulted in significant reductions in neutrophil infiltration and in hepatocellular injury. CCl_4 hepatotoxicity is obviously a complex, multifactorial process, which is likely to continue to receive considerable attention.

CCl_4 has frequently been used as a model hepatotoxic compound with which to examine the influence of various factors that alter P450s. CYP2E1 is primarily responsible for catalyzing the bioactivation of low doses of CCl_4 in humans. CYP3A contributes to the metabolism of higher doses (Zangar et al., 2000). The preeminent role of CYP2E1 in animals is clearly demonstrated by the protection afforded CCl_4-treated rodents by 2E1 antibody (Castillo et al., 1992), the 2E1 inhibitor 3-amino-1,2,4-triazole (Padron et al., 1996), and the absence of 2E1 expression (Wong et al., 1998). As discussed previously, a variety of conditions which induce 2E1 potentiate CCl_4 hepatotoxicity in test animals and humans. Sufficient doses of 2E1 inhibitors, including several natural constituents of foods, can prevent CCl_4 toxicity (Lieber, 1997a).

Chloroform

The primary use of chloroform ($CHCl_3$, trichloromethane) at present is in the production of the refrigerant chlorodifluoromethane. $CHCl_3$ was among the first inhalation anesthetics, but its use was eventually discontinued. Under certain conditions $CHCl_3$ is hepatotoxic and nephrotoxic. These toxicities are potentiated by aliphatic alcohols, ketones, and di- and trichloroacetic acid (Davis, 1992). The latter two chemicals are produced along with $CHCl_3$ as by-products of drinking water chlorination. Concentrations of $CHCl_3$ in municipal drinking water supplies as high as several hundred parts per billion (ppb) have been measured, although levels are usually less than 50 ppb. $CHCl_3$ has also been found in ppb concentrations in swimming pool water and surrounding air (Aggazzotti et al., 1995). $CHCl_3$ can invoke CNS symptoms at subanesthetic concentrations similar to those of alcohol intoxication. Like many other halocarbons, extremely high $CHCl_3$ exposures can sensitize the myocardium to catecholamines.

The reproductive and developmental toxicities of $CHCl_3$ are rather unremarkable. The EPA's IRIS profile characterizes $CHCl_3$ as fetotoxic but not teratogenic. Schwetz et al. (1974) found that inhalation of 100 to 300 ppm $CHCl_3$ by pregnant rats caused a high incidence of fetal resorption and retardation of fetal development as well as a low incidence of fetal anomalies. Murray et al. (1979) reported that gestational exposure to just 100 ppm $CHCl_3$ resulted in the decreased ability of females to maintain pregnancy—as well as cleft palate, decreased fetal weight and length, and decreased ossification in pups. Very high $CHCl_3$ concentrations retarded development and induced diffuse cell death in cultured rat embryos (Brown-Woodman et al., 1998). These studies support $CHCl_3$ as a weak teratogen, but negative studies employing maternally toxic doses argue against this characterization (Thompson et al., 1974; NTP, 1997a).

Potentiation by cytochrome P450 inducers and protection by GSH and by P450 inhibitors suggest that a metabolite, presumably phosgene, is responsible for $CHCl_3$'s hepatorenal toxicity. Both target organs metabolize $CHCl_3$ to phosgene. By using an irreversible cytochrome CYP2E1 inhibitor and CYP2E1-knockout mice, Constan et al. (1999) have demonstrated that metabolism of $CHCl_3$ by CYP2E1 is required for liver and kidney necrosis and cell proliferation. Nakajima et al. (1995) published results indicating that CYP2E1 is responsible for metabolic activation at low doses, whereas CYP2B1/2 is more important at high doses, such as those used in cancer bioassays. Preexposure to low doses of $CHCl_3$ induces resistance to a higher dose, presumably by suicidal inhibition of P450s responsible for $CHCl_3$ activation (Pereira and Grothaus, 1997).

There is ample experimental evidence for the generation of an electrophilic intermediate (i.e., phosgene) that is initially detoxified by covalently binding cytosolic GSH. Once GSH is depleted, phosgene is free to covalently bind hepatic and renal proteins and lipids. Such binding damages membranes and other intracellular structures, leading to necrosis and subsequent reparative cellular proliferation that promotes tumor formation in rodents by irreversibly "fixing" spontaneously altered DNA and clonally expanding initiated cells. The expression of certain genes, including *myc* and *fos,* is altered during regenerative cell proliferation in response to $CHCl_3$-induced cytotoxicity (Sprankle et al., 1996; Kegelmeyer et al., 1997).

The identity of the intracellular targets of phosgene is largely unknown, but Guastadisegni et al. (1999) reported that phosgene reacts with phosphatidylethanolamine (PE). The adduct formed appears to consist of two PE moieties cross-linked at the amino head groups by the carbonyl moiety of phosgene. $CHCl_3$-modified PE preferentially accumulates on inner mitochondria membranes, inducing ultrastructural modifications and inhibiting functions of the organelle. These researchers observed the induction of hepatic apoptosis and necrosis in rats and pointed out that apoptosis may be initiated by the release of regulatory components normally sequestered in mitochondria. Evidence that Ca^{2+} perturbation plays a role in $CHCl_3$ toxicity comes from a recent report of Ca^{2+} mobilization in Madin-Darby canine kidney cells using Fura-2 as a Ca^{2+} probe. $CHCl_3$, albeit at millimolar concentrations, increased the cytosolic Ca^{2+} levels by releasing Ca^{2+} from multiple stores within the cell (Jan et al., 2000).

The status of $CHCl_3$ as a rodent carcinogen is indisputable. It causes liver and kidney tumors that are species-, strain-, sex-, and route of exposure–dependent. $CHCl_3$-induced liver tumors in mice and their dependence on ongoing liver necrosis were reported near the end of World War II (Eschenbrenner and Miller, 1945). These same authors observed that male but not female mice suffered kidney necrosis. This observation was supported by the report of Roe et al. (1979) that $CHCl_3$ ingested in a toothpaste base resulted in renal tumors in male but not female mice. This sex difference is thought to be attributable to testosterone-mediated differences in renal MFO activity (Smith et al., 1984; Wolf, 1991). The NCI (1976) cancer bioassay, on which the EPA has based its inhalation cancer potency factor, demonstrated renal tumors in male rats and an extremely high incidence of liver tumors in both sexes of B6C3F1 mice gavaged with $CHCl_3$ in corn oil. In 1985, Jorgenson and colleagues reported that daily doses of $CHCl_3$ in drinking water comparable to those in the NCI gavage assay also produced renal tumors, but failed to cause liver tumors in B6C3F1 mice. This finding provided evidence that the dose rate of $CHCl_3$ was a determinant of liver tumor formation, supporting the existence of a threshold mechanism. Hard et al. (2000) have reevaluated the kidneys from the Jorgenson et al. (1985) study and have confirmed the presence of chronic renal tubule injury, indicative of renal tumor formation via an epigenetic mechanism. In what may be a "landmark" study, Larson et al. (1994) compared cytotoxicity and cell proliferation in female B6C3F1 mice given $CHCl_3$ by gavage in corn oil versus ad libitum ingestion in drinking water. As seen in Fig. 24-8, the hepatocyte labeling index, a measure of the proliferative response, differed between the two dosage regimens at comparable doses. This suggests that ingestion of $CHCl_3$ in small increments, similar to drinking water patterns of humans, fails to produce a sufficient amount of cytotoxic metabolite(s) per unit time to overwhelm detoxification mechanisms.

Currently, the EPA classifies $CHCl_3$ as a probable human carcinogen (group B2), meaning that there is sufficient evidence for carcinogenicity in animals and inadequate or no evidence in humans. Experimental evidence, such as that of Larson et al. (1994),

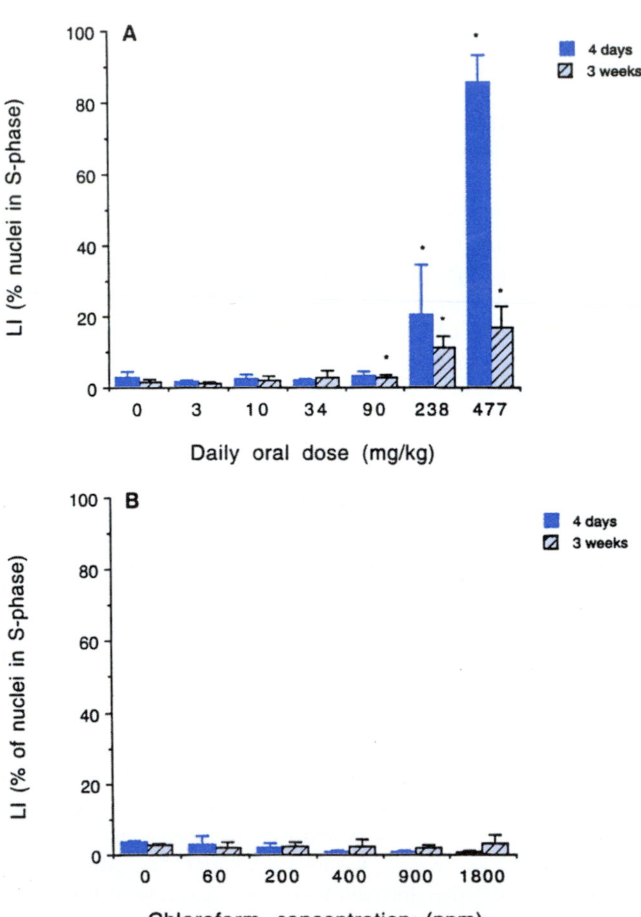

Figure 24-8. Hepatocyte liver LI in female B6C3F1 mice given $CHCl_3$ in corn oil (A) or drinking water (B) for 4 days or 3 weeks.

The LI is defined as the percent of hepatocyte nuclei positive for 5-bromo-2′-deoxyuridine immunohistochemical staining (i.e., percent of cells in the S phase, the period of DNA synthesis during the cell cycle). Values represent the mean ±SD for 5 mice. Asterisks (*) denote a significant difference from similarly treated control mice ($p < 0.05$). Note that 1800 ppm $CHCl_3$ in water corresponds to a cumulative uptake of 329 mg/kg/day. [Reproduced with permission of Larson et al. (1994).]

and the prevailing opinion that $CHCl_3$ is nongenotoxic, indicates that the relationship between $CHCl_3$ dose and tumor formation is nonlinear or threshold, meaning that there is a dose of $CHCl_3$ below which cytotoxicity is insufficient to produce a significant cancer risk. The EPA has, however, derived oral and inhalation cancer toxicity factors by applying the linearized multistage model to animal bioassay data. This model assumes there is no threshold. This has created controversy over EPA's approach to carcinogen regulation, a debate in which proponents of an epigenetic mechanism for $CHCl_3$ point toward EPA's recently *Proposed Guidelines for Carcinogen Risk Assessment* (EPA, 1999), that emphasize consideration of mode of action in the determination of cancer risk. The issues surrounding this debate have been summarily articulated in an article by Golden et al. (1997).

AROMATIC HYDROCARBONS

Benzene

Benzene produced commercially in the United States is derived primarily from petroleum. Benzene has been utilized as a general purpose solvent, but it is now used principally in the synthesis of other chemicals (ATSDR, 1997a). The percentage by volume of benzene in gasoline is 1 to 2 percent. Benzene plays an important role in unleaded gasoline due to its antiknock properties. Inhalation is the primary route of exposure in industrial and in everyday settings. Cigarette smoke is the major source of benzene in the home (Wallace, 1996). Smokers have benzene body burdens which are 6 to 10 times greater than those of nonsmokers. Passive smoke can be a significant source of benzene exposure to nonsmokers. Gasoline vapor emissions and auto exhaust are the other key contributors to exposures of the general populace.

The most important toxic effect of benzene is hematopoietic toxicity. Chronic exposure to benzene can lead to bone marrow damage, which may be manifest initially as anemia, leukopenia, thrombocytopenia, or a combination of these. Bone marrow depression appears to be dose-dependent in both laboratory animals and humans. Continued exposure may result in marrow aplasia and pancytopenia, an often fatal outcome. Survivors of aplastic anemia frequently exhibit a preneoplastic state, termed *myelodysplasia,* which may progress to myelogenous leukemia (Snyder et al., 1993; Rangan and Snyder, 1997).

There is strong evidence from epidemiologic studies that high-level benzene exposures result in an increased risk of acute myelogenous leukemia (AML) in humans (ATSDR, 1997a; Bergsagel et al., 1999). Evidence of increased risks of other cancers in such populations is less compelling. Only AML incidence was significantly elevated in the largest cohort study to date, in which ~75,000 benzene-exposed workers in 12 cities in China were evaluated (Yin et al., 1996). Marginal, nonsignificant increases were seen for lung cancer and chronic myelogenous leukemia. Some investigations of persons exposed to engine exhausts have reported a significant association with multiple myeloma. Bezabeth et al. (1996) and Bergsagel et al. (1999) have concluded, however, that there is no scientific evidence to support a causal relationship between benzene exposure and multiple myeloma. Increased incidences of malignant lymphomas and a variety of solid tumors were found in male and female B6C3F1 mice dosed orally with high doses of benzene for up to 103 weeks (Huff et al., 1989). Male and female F344 rats in this bioassay exhibited excesses of Zymbal gland, skin, and oral cavity carcinomas. Thus, benzene is clearly an animal and human carcinogen, but major species differences exist.

It is essential to understand the metabolism of benzene in order to address its mechanisms of toxicity. The initial metabolic step (Fig. 24-9), oxidation of benzene to an epoxide (i.e., benzene oxide), is catalyzed primarily by hepatic CYP2E1. Valentine et al. (1996) demonstrated that benzene-treated transgenic CYP2E1 knockout mice had relatively low levels of all benzene metabolites in their urine. A 5-day, 200 ppm benzene inhalation regimen produced severe genotoxicity and cytotoxicity in wild-type and B6C3F1 mice, but no adverse effects in the knockout mice. Benzene oxide, which is in equilibrium with its oxepin form, is further metabolized by three pathways: (1) conjugation with GSH to form a premercapturic acid, which is converted to phenyl-mercapturic acid; (2) rearrangement nonenzymatically to form phenol; and (3) hydration by epoxide hydratase to benzene dihydrodiol, which in turn can be oxidized by dihydrodiol dehydrogenase to catechol. If phenol is hydroxylated in the *ortho* position, more catechol will be formed. Catechol can be converted to *o*-benzoquinone. If benzene is hydroxylated in the *para* position, *p*-hydroquinone is formed. It can be oxidized to *p*-benzoquinone. The *o*- and *p*-benzoquinones are believed to be among the ultimate toxic metabolites of benzene. Another potentially toxic metabolite, muconaldehyde, may arise from ring opening of benzene oxide. Muconaldehyde undergoes a series of reactions that ultimately lead to *t,t*-muconic acid, an end-metabolite found in the urine (Snyder and Hedli, 1996; Golding and Watson, 1999).

Metabolism of benzene occurs primarily in the liver, though metabolism in bone marrow is *also* believed to play an important role in myelotoxicity. It has been generally accepted that phenolic conjugates are formed in the liver and transported via the blood to the bone marrow, where they are hydrolyzed and oxidized to quinones. Researchers have been unable to reproduce benzene toxicity, however, by giving individual phenolic metabolites to animals. The quinones are believed to be too reactive to be transported in the bloodstream. Lindstrom et al. (1997) have recently reported that benzene oxide has an estimated half-life of 7.9 min in rat blood, and thus may be able to travel from the liver to the bone marrow. Ring-opened metabolites of muconaldehyde, which are less reactive, could be transported to bone marrow and reoxidized. Bernauer et al. (1999) measured activity and levels of CYP2E1 in the liver and bone marrow of five strains of mice of varying sensitivity to benzene. CYP2E1 amounts and activity were considerably greater in the liver than the marrow, but no interstrain differences were seen in either tissue. It is likely that noncytochrome P450 enzymes (e.g., peroxidase, myeloperoxidase, cyclooxygenase) play an important role in generation of semiquinones and quinones in bone marrow (Ross et al., 1996). It has been proposed that both benzene and an array of its metabolites are necessary to elicit myelotoxicity (Snyder and Hedli, 1996; Witz et al., 1996).

Benzene's metabolic pathways appear to be qualitatively similar in all species studied to date (Henderson, 1996). Mice have a greater overall capacity to metabolize benzene than do rats or primates. Mani et al. (1999) report good correlation between protein/DNA adduct levels in bone marrow and susceptibility to benzene genotoxicity and carcinogenesis in F344 rats and three strains of mice. The B6C3F1 mouse shows the highest adduct levels and is the most sensitive of the animals tested. Powley and Carlson (1999) report similar findings upon measurement of benzene me-

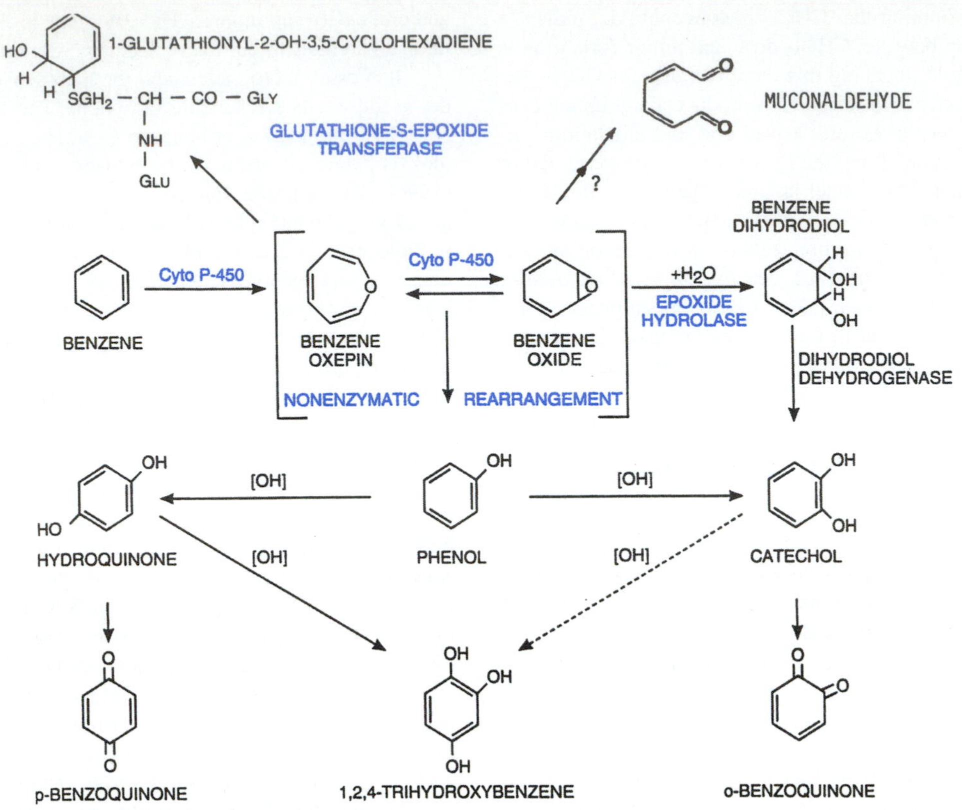

Figure 24-9. Biotransformation of benzene.

A question mark leads from the oxepin-oxide compartment to muconaldehyde because the substrate for the ring opening has yet to be identified. The dotted line leading to 1,2,4-trihydroxybenzene (1,2,4-T) indicates that it is not clear what the relative contributions of hydroquinone and catechol are to 1,2,4-T. [Modified and used with permission of Rangan and Snyder (1997).]

tabolism in mouse, rat, rabbit, and human lung and liver microsomes.

Factors that alter the metabolism of benzene have the potential to influence the hematopoietic toxicity and carcinogenicity of the VOC. Nakajima et al. (1985) demonstrated that pretreatment of rats with ethanol, a CYP2E1 inducer, enhanced metabolism of benzene, and potentiated its acute myelotoxicity. Phenobarbital had a negligible effect. Pretreatment of male B6C3F1 mice with acetone, another CYP2E1 inducer, increased benzene oxidation about five times (Kenyon et al., 1996). Pretreatment with diethyldithiocarbamate, a CYP2E1 inhibitor, completely abolished benzene oxidation. Metabolism of benzene by hepatic microsomes from 10 human donors was directly proportional to CYP2E1 activity in the samples (Seaton et al., 1994). Thus, it would be anticipated that CYP2E1 polymorphisms may significantly influence susceptibility to benzene toxicity. Male mice have consistently been found to be more sensitive than females to genotoxic effects of benzene. PBTK analysis of data from gas uptake experiments with B6C3F1 mice of both sexes revealed that the optimized maximum rate of benzene metabolism was twice as high in males (Kenyon et al., 1996). It is not clear whether there is a sex-dependent difference in benzene metabolism in humans. Sato et al. (1975) saw a more rapid rate of pulmonary elimination of benzene in men than in women following inhalation of 25 ppm for 2 h. Benzene was retained longer in the females due to their higher body-fat content. Unfortunately, most epidemiology studies of benzene-exposed workers have not provided a gender comparison. Li et al. (1994) did not see a statistically significant difference in cancer mortality between male and female workers exposed to benzene, though risks tended to be somewhat higher for males.

There are a number of cell populations in the bone marrow that may serve as targets for benzene metabolites. Benzene exposure in vivo results in inhibited growth and development of pluripotential bone marrow stem cells. More mature precursors, such as stromal cells and erythroid and myeloid colony-forming units, are also affected. Trush et al. (1996) point out that hydroquinone-induced inhibition of interleukin-1 synthesis by stromal macrophages results in altered differentiation of myeloid and lymphoid cells, which are normally active in immune responses. These investigators also note that killing of stromal macrophages and fibroblasts could result in such a pronounced reduction of cytokines and growth factors that immature and committed hematopoietic progenitors would die from apoptosis. The erythroid series is more susceptible than the myeloid series to benzene-induced cytotoxicity. Immature myeloid cells can proliferate when the development of erythroid cells is restricted and acquire neoplastic characteristics upon dedifferentiation. The end result is acute myelogenous leukemia (Golding and Watson, 1999).

Investigations of benzene toxicity/leukemogenesis have uncovered a variety of potential mechanisms (Golding and Watson, 1999). As mentioned before, experimental evidence indicates that the complementary actions of benzene and several of its metabolites are required for toxicity. It has been recognized for 20 years that a number of benzene metabolites can bind covalently to GSH, proteins, DNA and RNA. This can result in disruption of the functional hematopoietic microenvironment by inhibition of enzymes, destruction of certain cell populations, and alteration of the growth of other cell types. Covalent binding of hydroquinones to spindle-fiber proteins will inhibit cell replication (Smith, 1996). In vitro studies have established that reactive benzene metabolites bind covalently to DNA of several tissues of different species. Results of studies of formation of DNA adducts in vivo have been more difficult to interpret, due to benzene's low covalent binding index and the complexity of bone marrow (Snyder and Hedli, 1996). Through the use of accelerator mass spectrophotometry, Creek et al. (1997) could demonstrate DNA binding in mice exposed to extremely low ^{14}C-benzene levels. The binding was dose-dependent over a wide range of doses. DNA adduct levels were so low, however, that this mechanism alone seems insufficient to fully account for leukemogenic effects.

It appears likely that oxidative stress contributes to benzene toxicity. As the bone marrow is rich in peroxidase activity, phenolic metabolites of benzene can be activated there to reactive quinone derivatives. Ross et al. (1996) discovered that myeloperoxidase present in murine and human progenitor cells could bioactivate hydroquinone to *p*-benzoquinone. Electron spin resonance experiments by Hiraku and Kawanishi (1996) revealed the formation of a semiquinone radical in *p*-benzoquinone-treated HL-60 cells (a human myeloid cell line). This suggested that reactive oxygen moieties (e.g., $O_2^{\cdot-}$ and H_2O_2) are produced via the formation of the semiquinone radicals. These active oxygen species can cause DNA strand breakage or fragmentation, leading to cell mutation or apoptosis, respectively. Ross et al. (1996), however, pointed out that quinones can also inhibit proteases involved in induction of apoptosis. These authors noted that modulation of apoptosis may lead to aberrant hematopoiesis and neoplastic progression.

A number of biomarkers of exposure to benzene have been developed and carefully evaluated. Concentrations of the parent compound in exhaled breath parallel blood concentrations. Clayton et al. (1999) recently reported a high correlation between extent of smoking-related activities and levels of benzene in exhaled breath of humans. Urinary excretion of a variety of benzene metabolites (i.e., phenol, catechol, hydroquinone, 1,2,4-trihydroxybenzene, *S*-phenylmercapturic acid and *t,t*-muconic acid) have been shown to be correlated with benzene exposure in occupational settings. Phenol, catechol, and hydroquinone, however, are neither sensitive nor specific, since relatively high levels are found in nonexposed individuals (Medeiros et al., 1997). Similarly, *t,t*-muconic acid is not specific, since it is a metabolite of sorbic acid, a common food additive. Boogaard and van Sittert (1996) conclude that *S*-phenylmercapturic acid, an end-product of the conjugation of benzene oxide and GSH, is a suitable urinary biomarker of low-level benzene exposure because of its specificity and relatively long half-life. Adducts to hemoglobin and cysteine groups of proteins have been demonstrated in rodents, but not in humans. DNA damage has been detected in benzene-exposed workers (Liu et al., 1996; Andreoli et al., 1997), though such measures have not yet found widespread acceptance as biomarkers of effect.

PBTK models have been developed to aid in predicting risks of myelotoxicity and leukemia posed to humans by benzene. Medinsky et al. (1989) published one of the first models for benzene. They assumed that benzene metabolism followed Michaelis-Menten kinetics and occurred via benzene oxide. B6C3F1 mice, which are more sensitive than F344 rats to benzene myelotoxicity, were predicted to metabolize two to three times more inhaled benzene. This and other PBTK models do not accurately simulate some laboratory data sets. Modeling benzene metabolism and disposition is difficult because of its inherent complexity and variability. In light of intricate dose–response relationships, Medinsky et al. (1996) emphasized the importance of considering competitive metabolic interactions between benzene and its metabolites as well as the balance between enzymatic activation and inactivation processes.

Toluene

Toluene is present in paints, lacquers, thinners, cleaning agents, glues, and many other products. Toluene is also used in the production of other chemicals. Gasoline, which contains 5 to 7 percent toluene by weight, is the largest source of atmospheric emissions and exposure of the general populace (ATSDR, 1998c). Inhalation is the primary route of exposure, though skin contact occurs frequently. Toluene is a favorite of solvent abusers, who intentionally inhale high concentrations of the VOC. Large amounts of toluene enter the environment each year by volatilization. Relatively small amounts are released in industrial wastewater. Toluene is frequently found in water, soil, and air at hazardous waste sites (Fay and Mumtaz, 1996).

Toluene TK has been thoroughly characterized in humans and laboratory animals. Toluene is well absorbed from the lungs and GI tract. It rapidly accumulates in and affects the brain, due to that organ's high rate of blood perfusion and high lipid content. Toluene subsequently is deposited in other tissues according to their lipid content, with adipose tissue attaining the highest levels. Toluene is well metabolized, but a portion is exhaled unchanged. Hepatic P450s catalyze metabolism of toluene to benzyl alcohol and lesser amounts of cresols. The benzyl alcohol is converted by alcohol dehydrogenase (ADH) to benzoic acid, which is conjugated and eliminated in the urine. Nakajima et al. (1992a) report that CYP2E1 and CYP2C11 are primarily responsible for catalyzing the initial hydroxylation step in rat liver at low and high toluene levels, respectively. CYP2E1 is most active in humans (Nakajima et al., 1997).

The CNS is the primary target organ of toluene and other alkylbenzenes. Manifestations of exposure range from slight dizziness and headache to unconsciousness, respiratory depression, and death. Occupational inhalation exposure guidelines are established to prevent significant decrements in psychomotor functions. Acute CNS effects are rapidly reversible upon cessation of exposure (Fig. 24-3). Subtle neurologic effects have been reported in some groups of occupationally exposed individuals. Exposure to ~100 ppm toluene for years may result in subclinical effects, as evidenced by altered brainstem auditory evoked potentials (Abbate et al., 1993) and changes in visual evoked potentials (Vrca et al., 1995). Foo et al. (1990) reported good correlation between toluene exposure and poor scores on neurobehavioral tests of 30 female rotogravure workers. Severe neurotoxicity is sometimes diagnosed in persons who have abused toluene for a prolonged period. Clinical signs include abnormal electroencephalographic (EEG) activity, tremors, nystagmus, and cerebral atrophy as well as impaired hearing, vision, and speech (Ron, 1986; Dinwiddie, 1994). Magnetic resonance imaging has revealed permanent changes in brain structure, which correspond to the degree of brain dysfunction (Filley et al., 1990; Caldemeyer et al., 1996).

Little is known about mechanisms by which toluene and similar solvents produce acute or residual CNS effects (Balster, 1998). The Meyer-Overton theory of partitioning of the parent compounds into membrane lipids has been widely accepted for a century. Recently it has been proposed that the presence of solvent molecules in cholesterol-filled interstices between phospholipids and sphingolipids changes membrane fluidity, thereby altering intercellular communication and normal ion movements (Engelke et al., 1996). Such a process is reversible. An alternate hypothesis is that toluene partitions into hydrophobic regions of proteins and interacts with them, thereby altering membrane-bound enzyme activity and/or receptor specificity (Balster, 1998). Other evidence suggests that toluene and other VOCs may act by enhancing $GABA_A$ receptor function (Mihic et al., 1994), attenuating NMDA receptor-stimulated calcium flux (Cruz et al., 1998), and/or activating dopaminergic systems (von Euler, 1994).

As toluene is metabolized by P450s and ADH, the chemical can interact with other xenobiotics metabolized by these enzymes. Concurrent exposure to solvents metabolized by the same P450 isozymes can result in competitive metabolic inhibition. Inoue et al. (1988) observed that benzene and toluene suppressed one another's metabolism in humans. Thus, the risk of leukopenia in workers exposed to benzene and toluene should be less than that in workers exposed to benzene alone. Pryor and Rebert (1992) found that toluene greatly reduced manifestations of peripheral neuropathy caused by *n*-hexane in rats. Although no interaction between toluene and xylenes was seen in humans inhaling low levels of each, simultaneous exposure to higher levels resulted in mutual metabolic suppression (Tardif et al., 1991). Prior exposure to P450 inducers can result in increased rates of toluene metabolism/elimination and more rapid recovery from toluene-induced CNS depression. Nakajima and Wang (1994) observed that toluene induced four of the six P450 isozymes that metabolize it, but inhibited the other two in rat liver. The influence of toluene on the metabolism of other P450 substrates is usually modest.

Xylenes and Ethylbenzene

Large numbers of people are exposed to xylenes and ethylbenzene occupationally and environmentally (Wallace et al., 1987). Xylenes and ethylbenzene, like benzene and toluene, are major components of gasoline and fuel oil. The primary uses of xylenes industrially are as solvents and synthetic intermediates. Most of the aromatics released into the environment evaporate into the atmosphere. They may also enter groundwater from oil and gasoline spills and discharge, leakage of storage tanks, and migration from waste sites (ATSDR, 1995, 1999).

The TK and acute toxicity of toluene, xylenes, and other aromatic solvents are quite similar. Xylenes and the others are well absorbed from the lungs and GI tract, distributed to tissues according to tissue blood flow and lipid content, exhaled to some extent, well metabolized by hepatic P450s, and largely excreted as urinary metabolites (Lof and Johanson, 1998). Nielsen and Alarie (1982) state that the potency of benzene and a series of alkylbenzenes, as sensory irritants of the upper respiratory tract of mice, increases with increasing lipophilicity. Acute lethality of hydrocarbons (i.e., CNS depressant potency) also varies directly with lipophilicity (Swann et al., 1974). There is limited evidence that chronic occupational exposure to xylenes is associated with residual neurological effects (ATSDR, 1995). Exposure conditions, including the presence of other solvents, have usually not been characterized in such reports. Uchida et al. (1993), for example, reported increased subjective CNS symptoms in workers exposed for ~7 years to a mean of 21 ppm xylenes. The prevalence of symptoms was not dose-dependent. This vapor concentration is significantly lower than current occupational exposure standards in the United States, which are established on the basis of acute irritancy or CNS effects.

Xylenes and ethylbenzene appear to have very limited capacity to adversely affect organs other than the CNS. Mild, transient liver and/or kidney toxicity have/has occasionally been reported in humans exposed to high vapor concentrations of xylenes. Little evidence of hepatorenal injury is typically manifest in laboratory animals (ATSDR, 1995). Generally, hepatic P450s are moderately induced by alkylbenzenes (Gut et al., 1993). Many investigators have reported xylenes to increase liver weight and to induce liver P450s in rats and other rodents. The *o*, *p* and *m* isomers of xylene vary somewhat in their capacity to induce different P450 isozymes in different organs of rats (Backes et al., 1993). Concurrent exposure to an alkylbenzene and another compound metabolized by P450s generally results in their competitive metabolic inhibition. Preexposure to an alkylbenzene or another P450-inducing compound, conversely, can result in increased metabolism of the other chemical.

The majority of alkylbenzenes do not appear to be genotoxic or carcinogenic. Ethylbenzene and styrene are two exceptions. Kidney injury and an increased incidence of renal adenoma and carcinoma (combined) were found in male F344 rats exposed to 750 ppm ethylbenzene for up to 2 years (NTP, 1997b). Styrene's carcinogenic potential is discussed below.

Styrene

Styrene is primarily used in the production of polystyrene, rubbers, resins, and insulators (Gibbs and Mulligan, 1997). Worker exposures in the rubber industry are of greatest concern toxicologically. Styrene is sometimes found in indoor air of buildings and homes (Wallace et al., 1987). Sources include tobacco smoke and emissions from building materials. Discharges from industry are the major source of environmental pollution (ATSDR, 1993).

There is considerable debate as to whether styrene is a human carcinogen. Styrene is metabolized principally by P450-catalyzed side-chain oxidation to styrene oxide (Linhart et al., 2000). This epoxide is detoxified by the actions of epoxide hydratase and glutathione *S*-transferase. Styrene oxide can bind covalently to proteins and nucleic acids. Results of in vitro and in vivo mutagenicity and genotoxicity studies of styrene have been mixed (ATSDR, 1993). Chromosomal aberrations have been found in employees in some occupational exposure studies, but not in others. Increased rates of different cancers have been reported in workers exposed to 1,3-butadiene and styrene in the synthetic rubber industry. The excesses of cancers have largely been attributed to 1,3-butadiene, though styrene may modify the actions of 1,3-butadiene and/or be implicated itself (Matonoski et al., 1997). Styrene oxide is carcinogenic to the forestomach of orally dosed mice and rats (Roe, 1994). The activity of epoxide hydratase relative to P450 oxidation is much greater in human than in mouse liver (Mendrala et al., 1993). Carcinogenicity bioassays of inhaled styrene in rats, conducted some 20 years ago, yielded equivocal findings (McConnell and Swenberg, 1994). Recently, Cruzan et al. (1998) reported the negative results of a 104-week styrene inhalation cancer study in CD rats. Nevertheless, the question of whether styrene should be considered a human carcinogen remains highly controversial.

ALCOHOLS

Ethanol

Many humans experience greater exposure to ethanol (ethyl alcohol, alcohol) than to any other solvent. Not only is ethyl alcohol used as a solvent in industry and in many household products and pharmaceuticals, but it is heavily consumed in intoxicating beverages. Frank toxic effects are less important occupationally than injuries resulting from psychomotor impairment. Driving under the influence of alcohol is, of course, the major cause of fatal auto accidents. In many states a blood alcohol level of 100 mg/100 mL blood (100 mg %) is prima facie evidence of "driving while intoxicated." One's blood alcohol level and the time necessary to achieve it are controlled largely by the rapidity and extent of consumption of the chemical. Ethanol is distributed in body water and to some degree in adipose tissue. The alcohol is eliminated by urinary excretion, exhalation, and metabolism. The blood level in an average adult decreases by ~15 to 20 mg % per h. Thus, a person with a blood alcohol level of 120 mg % would require 6 to 8 h to reach negligible levels.

Ethanol is metabolized to acetaldehyde by three enzymes: (1) The major pathway involves alcohol dehydrogenase (ADH)–catalyzed oxidation to acetaldehyde. ADHs are present in high concentrations in the cytoplasm of hepatocytes (Yin et al., 1999). The oxidation they catalyze is reversible, but the acetaldehyde that is formed is rapidly oxidized by acetaldehyde dehydrogenase (ALDH) to acetate. (2) A second enzyme, catalase, utilizes H_2O_2 supplied by the actions of NADPH oxidase and xanthine oxidase. There is usually little H_2O_2 available in hepatocytes to support the reaction, so it is unlikely that catalase will normally account for more than 10% of ethyl alcohol metabolism. (3) The third enzyme, CYP2E1, is the principle component of the hepatic microsomal ethanol oxidizing system (MEOS).

Ethanol interacts with other solvents which are also metabolized by ADH and CYP2E1. Ethanol can be an effective antidote for poisoning by methanol, ethylene glycol, and diethylene glycol. As ethyl alcohol has a relatively high affinity for ADH, it competitively inhibits the metabolic activation of the other alcohols. Preexposure to a single high dose or multiple doses of ethanol can induce CYP2E1, thereby enhancing the metabolic activation and potentiating the toxicity of a considerable number of other solvents and drugs (Lieber, 1997a; Klotz and Ammon, 1998). Manno et al. (1996), for example, describe heavy drinkers who developed severe hepatorenal toxicity from CCl_4 exposures, which caused no ill effects in nondrinkers. Other alcohols, such as 2-butanol (Fig. 24-4), can have analogous effects (Traiger and Bruckner, 1976). Such interactions are also described under "Metabolism" and "Exogenous Factors" in this chapter.

Modulation of ALDH activity can influence adverse effects experienced by drinkers. Acetaldehyde is acutely toxic. It is reactive and binds covalently to proteins and other macromolecules (Niemela, 1999). Fortunately, ALDH activity is usually sufficiently high to metabolize large amounts of acetaldehyde to acetate. Caucasians, blacks, and Asians have varying percentages of different ALDH isozymes, which impact the efficiency of acetaldehyde metabolism. Some 50 percent of Asians have inactive ALDH, due to a single base change in the gene that encodes for the enzyme (Schuckit, 1986). These persons may experience flushing, headache, tachycardia, nausea, vomiting, and hyperventilation upon ingestion of ethanol. Disulfiram, an ALDH inhibitor, is used to treat alcoholism, since it acts similarly if alcohol is consumed.

Gender differences in responses to ethanol are well recognized. Females exhibit slightly higher blood ethanol levels than men following ingestion of equivalent doses of ethanol (Pikaar et al., 1988). This phenomenon appears to be due in part to more extensive ADH-catalyzed metabolism of ethanol by the gastric mucosa of males (Seitz et al., 1993). Sex differences in ethanol metabolism in the remainder of the body appear to be small or nonexistent (Frezza et al., 1990). A second factor contributing to the higher blood ethanol levels and greater CNS effects in women is their smaller volume of distribution for relatively polar solvents such as alcohols. It is well known that women are more susceptible to alcohol-induced hepatotoxicity (Thurman, 1998). A postulated mechanism for this sex difference is described below.

Fetal alcohol syndrome (FAS) is the most common preventable cause of mental retardation. Diagnostic criteria for FAS include (1) heavy maternal alcohol consumption during gestation; (2) pre- and postnatal growth retardation; (3) craniofacial malformations including microcephaly; and (4) mental retardation. Less complete manifestations of gestational ethanol exposure also occur and are referred to as fetal alcohol effects or alcohol-related neurodevelopmental disorder. FAS is estimated to affect 4000 infants per year in the United States, with an additional 7000 cases of fetal alcohol effects (Shibley and Pennington, 1997). Although the total amount of alcohol consumed and the pattern of drinking are both important factors, peak maternal blood alcohol level is the most important determinant of the likelihood and severity of effects. Overconsumption during all three trimesters of pregnancy can result in certain manifestations, with the particular manifestations dependent upon the period of gestation during which insult occurs.

Despite an intensive research effort, the mechanisms underlying FAS remain unclear. Exposure of embryonic tissue to ethanol adversely affects many cellular functions critical to development, including protein and DNA synthesis, uptake of critical nutrients such as glucose and amino acids, and changes in several kinase-mediated signal transduction pathways (Shibley and Pennington, 1997). Some studies have suggested that oxidative stress in fetal tissues is responsible (Henderson et al., 1999), while others have implicated ethanol's effects on neurotransmitter-gated ion channels, particularly the *N*-methyl-D-aspartate receptor (Costa et al., 2000). Others have reported that ethanol produces a long-lasting reduction in synaptic efficacy (Bellinger et al., 1999) and alters the fetal expression of developmentally important genes such as Msx2 and insulin-like growth factors (Singh et al., 1996; Rifas et al., 1997). Ethanol triggers widespread apoptotic neurodegeneration in the developing brain (Ikonomidou et al., 2000). A role for CYP2E1 in the induction of FAS has been hypothesized, given its expression in human cephalic tissues during embryogenesis (Boutelet-Bochan et al., 1997).

CYP2E1 plays a key role in alcoholic liver disease and associated oxidative stress (Baker and Cramer, 1999). Results of in vitro experiments indicate that human CYP2E1 is effective in production of reactive oxygen intermediates (e.g., hydroxy radicals, superoxide anion, H_2O_2) and in causation of lipid peroxidation (Dai et al., 1993). Membrane lipids and a variety of enzymes, including CYP2E1, are targets for free radical attack. Albano and coworkers (1999) have demonstrated a marked increase in covalent binding of hydroxyethyl radicals to hepatic microsomal proteins from rats following chronic ethanol administration. There is not yet direct evidence that hydroxyethyl radicals contribute to lipid peroxidation, but they do readily react with α-tocopherol, GSH, and ascorbic acid, thereby potentially lowering liver antioxidant levels in vivo. Albano et al. (1999) also describe evidence that hydroxyethyl radical-protein adducts in hepatocytes induce immune responses, which may contribute to chronic ethanol hepatotoxicity.

Alcohol-induced hepatotoxicity is postulated to be caused by elevation of endotoxin in the bloodstream. Endotoxin, released by the action of ethanol on gram-negative bacteria in the gut, is believed to be taken up by Kupffer cells, causing the release of mediators which are cytotoxic to hepatocytes and chemoattractants for neutrophils (Bautista and Spitzer, 1999). These mediators include interleukins, prostaglandins, free radicals, and tumor necrosis factor α. Kupffer cells of female rats are more sensitive to endotoxin than cells of males. Estrogen increases the sensitivity of Kupffer cells of rats to endotoxin. This phenomenon is believed to account in part for the more severe hepatitis and cirrhosis commonly seen in female alcoholics (Thurman, 1998).

Alcohol-induced tissue damage is believed to result from nutritional disturbances as well as direct toxic effects (Lieber, 1997b). Lack of money, poor judgment, prolonged inebriation, and appetite loss contribute to poor nutrition and weight loss in alcoholics. A high percentage of calories in the alcoholic's diet are furnished by alcohol. Malabsorption of thiamine, diminished enterohepatic circulation of folate, degradation of pyridoxal phosphate, and disturbances in the metabolism of vitamins A and D can occur (Mezey, 1985). Prostaglandins released from endotoxin-activated Kupffer cells may be responsible for a hypermetabolic state in the liver. With the increase in oxygen demand, the viability of centrilobular hepatocytes would be most compromised due to their relatively poor oxygen supply (Thurman, 1998). Metabolism of ethanol via ADH and ALDH results in a shift in the redox state of the cell. The metabolites and the more reduced state can result in hyperlactacidemia, hyperuricemia, and hyperglycemia (Lieber, 1997b).

Alcoholism can result in damage of extrahepatic tissues. Cardiomyopathy is one of the more serious consequences. Alcoholic cardiomyopathy is a complex process that is believed to result from decreased synthesis of cardiac contractile proteins, attack of oxygen radicals, and antibody response to acetaldehyde-protein adducts (Richardson et al., 1998). Interestingly, light to moderate drinking is reported to protect against atherosclerosis in the carotid artery, a major cause of ischemic stroke (Hillbom, 1999). It is hypothesized that ethanol metabolism in the vascular wall may inhibit oxidation of low density lipoproteins (LDL), a requisite for atherogenesis. Phenolic antioxidants in wines may also inhibit LDL oxidation as well as reduce platelet aggregation. Conversely, heavy drinking appears to deplete antioxidants and have the opposite effects (Camargo, 1996; Hillbom, 1999). Recent heavy drinking increases the risk of both hemorrhagic and ischemic strokes. Other organ systems can be adversely affected in alcoholics including the brain and pancreas (Preedy et al., 1997; Kril et al., 1997).

There is concern about the role of ethyl alcohol in carcinogenesis, due to the frequent consumption of alcoholic beverages by millions of people. IARC (1988) concluded that there was "sufficient evidence" for causation of tumors of the oral cavity, pharynx and larynx, esophagus, and liver of humans. The associations between alcohol and cancers came primarily from epidemiologic case-control and cohort studies. One such cohort study of 276,000 American men showed increase in total cancer risk with increasing ethanol consumption (Boffeta and Garfinkel, 1990). Ethanol and smoking act synergistically to cause oral, pharyngeal, and laryngeal cancers. It is generally believed that alcohol induces liver cancer by causing cirrhosis or other liver damage and/or by enhancing the bioactivation of carcinogens. Hypotheses of Ahmed (1995) for possible mechanisms of causation of cancers are included in Table 24-3.

Methanol

Methanol (methyl alcohol, wood alcohol) is found in a host of consumer products including windshield washer fluid, and is used in the manufacture of formaldehyde and methyl *tert*-butyl ether (MTBE). Methanol is being promoted as a gasoline additive and alternative automotive fuel. Risks of low-level, chronic exposures will be at issue if the latter uses become commonplace.

Like most hydrocarbon solvents, methanol can produce reversible sensory irritation and narcosis at airborne concentrations below those producing organ system pathology. Serious methanol toxicity is most commonly associated with ingestion. Left untreated, acute methanol poisoning in humans is characterized by an asymptomatic latent period of 12 to 24 h followed by formic acidemia, ocular toxicity, coma, and in extreme cases death. Visual disturbances generally develop between 18 and 48 h after ingestion and range from mild photophobia and misty or blurred vision to markedly reduced visual acuity and complete blindness (Eells et al., 1996). Although there is considerable variability among individuals in susceptibility to methanol toxicity, a frequently cited lethal oral dosage is 1 mL/kg. Blindness and death have been reported with dosages as low as 0.1 mL/kg (ATSDR, 1993).

The target of methanol within the eye is the retina, specifically the optic disk and optic nerve. Optic disk edema and hyperemia are seen, along with morphological alterations in the optic nerve head and the intraorbital portion of the optic nerve. Both axons and glial cells exhibit altered morphologies (Kavet and Nauss, 1990). Evidence is accumulating that Müller cells, neuroglia that function in the maintenance of retinal structure and in intra- and intercellular transport, are early targets of methanol (Garner et al., 1995a). Rods and cones, the photoreceptors of the retina, are also altered functionally and structurally (Seme et al., 1999). There are indications of mitochondrial disruption in Müller and photoreceptor cells. This is consistent with the long-held view that cytochrome

Table 24-3
Possible Mechanisms of Ethanol Carcinogenicity

Congeners, additives and contaminants in alcoholic beverages influence carcinogenicity.
CYP2E1 induction by ethanol increases metabolic activation of procarcinogens.
Ethanol acts as a solvent for carcinogens, enhancing their absorption into tissues of the upper GI tract.
Ethanol affects the actions of certain hormones on hormone-sensitive tissues.
Immune function is suppressed by alcohol.
Absorption and bioavailability of nutrients are reduced by alcohol.

SOURCE: Adapted with permission of Ahmed (1995).

oxidase activity in mitochondria is inhibited, resulting in a reduction in ATP. This mechanism would explain, at least in part, the selective toxicity to photoreceptors and other highly metabolically active cells (Eells et al. 1996).

Elucidation of the mechanism of acute toxicity of methanol was hampered for years by species differences in susceptibility and the lack of appropriate animal models. Largely based on the work of Gilger and Potts (1955), it became apparent that only nonhuman primates respond to methanol similarly to humans. The severe metabolic acidosis frequently seen in humans does not occur in rodents. In all mammalian species studied, methanol is metabolized in the liver to formaldehyde (HCOH), which in turn is very rapidly converted to formate. The conversion of formate to CO_2 then occurs via a two-step, tetrahydrofolate (THF)-dependent pathway. First, formate is converted to 10-formyl-THF by formyl-THF synthetase, after which 10-formyl-THF is oxidized to CO_2 by formyl-THF dehydrogenase (F-THF-DH). The species differences in susceptibility to methanol are thought to result primarily from differences in the rate of THF-dependent oxidation of formate to CO_2. Since rodents have higher hepatic THF levels than primates, formate does not accumulate as it does in humans and monkeys (Medinsky and Dorman, 1995; Martinasevic et al., 1996). Another possible explanation is the lower F-THF-DH activity in primate liver (Johlin et al., 1989). Thus, susceptibility to methanol toxicity is dependent upon the relative rate of formate clearance. Dietary and chemical depletion of endogenous folate cofactors in rats have been shown to increase formate accumulation following methanol, resulting in the development of metabolic acidosis and ocular toxicity similar to that observed in humans (Eells et al., 1996). A simplified scheme of methanol metabolism is presented in Fig. 24-10.

For years there was considerable debate about whether HCOH or formate was responsible for methanol's ocular toxicity. The finding that HCOH does not accumulate following methanol treatment, even in folate-deficient monkeys profoundly sensitive to methanol, argues against a role for HCOH. Also, species of differing susceptibility exhibit comparable blood HCOH half-lives (~1 to 2 min). In contrast, formate has been shown to accumulate in the human and monkey following methanol treatment, and to induce ocular toxicity in monkeys after an infusion where normal blood pH was maintained (Martin-Amat et al., 1978). Eells et al. (1996), using a rat model in which formate oxidation had been selectively

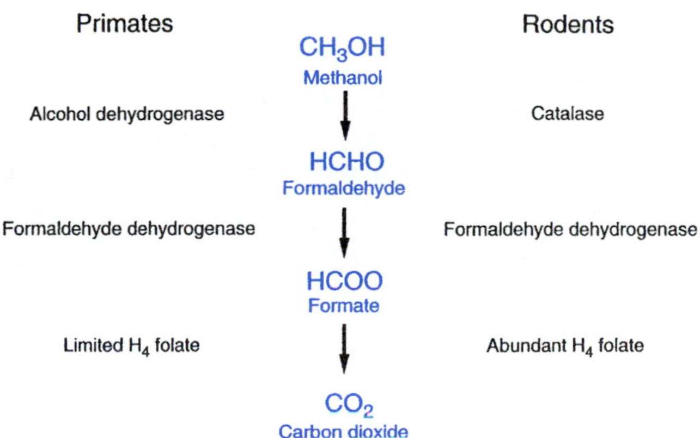

Figure 24-10. Scheme for the metabolism of methanol.

Major enzymes are listed for primates (*left*) and rodents (*right*). Conversion of formate to CO_2 is rapid in rodents, but relatively slow in primates. (Used with permission of Dorman DC, Welsch F: *CIIT Activities* 16:1–7, 1996.)

inhibited with nitrous oxide, have also shown that methanol-induced retinal dysfunction can be produced in the absence of metabolic acidosis. In this same publication, methanol-derived formate was quantified in the vitreous humor, retina, and to a lesser extent in the optic nerve. Moreover, these authors demonstrated that methanol-induced retinal dysfunction, as indicated by diminution of the amplitude of electroretinogram (ERG) *a* and *b* waves, was negatively correlated in a linear fashion with blood formate concentrations. Others have reported similar relationships between blood formate and ERG responses indicative of photoreceptor dysfunction (Seme et al., 1999). Thus, formate appears to act as a direct ocular toxin and not indirectly through the induction of an acidotic state, though acidosis may potentiate formate toxicity since the inhibition of cytochrome oxidase increases as pH decreases.

The question has been raised as to whether ocular toxicity is simply a function of circulating formate reaching the visual tract, or whether metabolism in retinal or optic nerve tissues generates toxic metabolites locally. This is a legitimate question considering that metabolism of methanol to formaldehyde via peroxisomal enzymes (catalase) has been demonstrated in rat retina in vitro (Garner et al., 1995a), and the presence of cytoplasmic aldehyde dehydrogenase activity has been demonstrated in several regions of the rat and mouse eye, including the retina (Messiha and Price, 1983; McCaffery et al., 1991). By use of a folate-deficient rat model that mimics human methanol toxicity, Garner et al. (1995b) showed that a level of blood formate generated by IV infusion of pH-buffered formate did not diminish the ERG *b*-wave amplitude generated by Müller cells of the retina, as did a comparable level of blood formate derived from methanol. This suggests that the intraretinal metabolism of methanol is necessary for the initiation of retinal toxicity by formate. Not only are the enzymes necessary to produce formate present in the retina, but so too are folate and formyl-THF dehydrogenase, both necessary for formate oxidation. Formyl-THF dehydrogenase was found to be localized in the mitochondria of Müller cells, prompting the suggestion that formyl-THF dehydrogenase may serve a dual role, one protective of the Müller cell and the other toxic. Protection would come in the form of formate oxidation; toxicity from the overconsumption of ATP required for formate metabolism via the folate pathway (Martinasevic et al., 1996). These findings raise new questions about the safety of methanol exposure. For example, chamber studies of human volunteers exposed to 200 ppm methanol for 4 or 6 h showed no blood formate accumulation above background (Lee et al., 1992; d'Alessandro et al., 1994). While this might be considered as evidence that exposure at the current ACGIH TLV and OSHA PEL of 200 ppm poses no risk for ocular toxicity, such an interpretation may not be valid given that ocular toxicity may be a function of intraretinal methanol metabolism rather than circulating formate levels.

While there is still much to be learned about mechanisms of methanol toxicity, what is known allows for effective therapies, if they are applied in a timely manner. Sodium bicarbonate is usually given iv to correct severe acidosis. Metabolic blockade is usually achieved with ethanol or 4-methylpyrazole, both acting as effective competitive inhibitors of ADH by virtue of their greater affinities than methanol for ADH. Folate therapy is also indicated to increase the efficiency of formate oxidation. Methanol exemplifies the benefits of knowing a chemical's mode of action when treating the poisoned patient. This knowledge also aids in identifying potentially sensitive subpopulations, such as those suffering from dietary folate deficiency.

GLYCOLS

Ethylene Glycol

Ethylene glycol (EG) is a major constituent of antifreeze, deicers, hydraulic fluids, drying agents, and inks, and is used to make plastics and polyester fibers. The most important routes of exposure are dermal and accidental or intentional ingestion. Workers may also be exposed by inhalation in situations where solutions containing EG are heated or sprayed. EG enters the environment as a result of disposal of industrial and consumer products containing the chemical (ATSDR, 1997c). It partitions into and is transported by surface waters and groundwater. EG is rapidly degraded in environmental media.

EG is acutely toxic to humans and is believed to cause over 100 deaths annually in the United States (LaKind et al., 1999). It appears to be two to five times more acutely toxic to humans and cats than to other species. LaKind et al. (1999) estimate the minimum lethal oral dose in humans to be ~1.4 mL/kg. Acute poisoning (Egbert and Abraham, 1999) entails three clinical stages after an asymptomatic period, during which EG is metabolized: (1) a period of inebriation, the duration and degree depending upon dose; (2) the cardiopulmonary stage 12 to 24 h after exposure, characterized by tachycardia and tachypnea, which may progress to cardiac failure and pulmonary edema; and (3) the renal toxicity stage 24 to 72 h postexposure. Metabolic acidosis can become progressively more severe during stages 2 and 3.

The TK of EG in humans and in laboratory animals is well understood. Absorption from the GI tract of rodents is very rapid and virtually complete (Frantz et al., 1996). Dermal absorption in humans appears to be less extensive. EG is distributed throughout the body extracellular fluid. As illustrated in Fig. 24-11, EG is metabolized by NAD$^+$-dependent alcohol dehydrogenase (ADH) to glycolaldehyde and on to glycolic acid (Wierner and Richardson, 1988). Ethanol is frequently given as an antidote in EG poisoning, because the alcohol effectively competes for ADH, thereby blocking the metabolic activation of EG. 4-Methylpyrazole, an ADH inhibitor, may be even more efficacious (Egbert and Abraham, 1999). Glycolic acid is oxidized to glyoxylic acid by glycolic acid oxidase and lactic dehydrogenase. Glyoxylic acid may be converted to formate and CO_2, or oxidized by glyoxylic acid oxidase to oxalic acid (Frantz et al., 1996). Metabolic acidosis in humans appears to be due largely to accumulation of glycolic acid (Jacobsen et al., 1984). Hypocalcemia can result from calcium chelation by oxalic acid to form calcium oxalate crystals. Deposition of these crystals in tubules of the kidney and small blood vessels in the

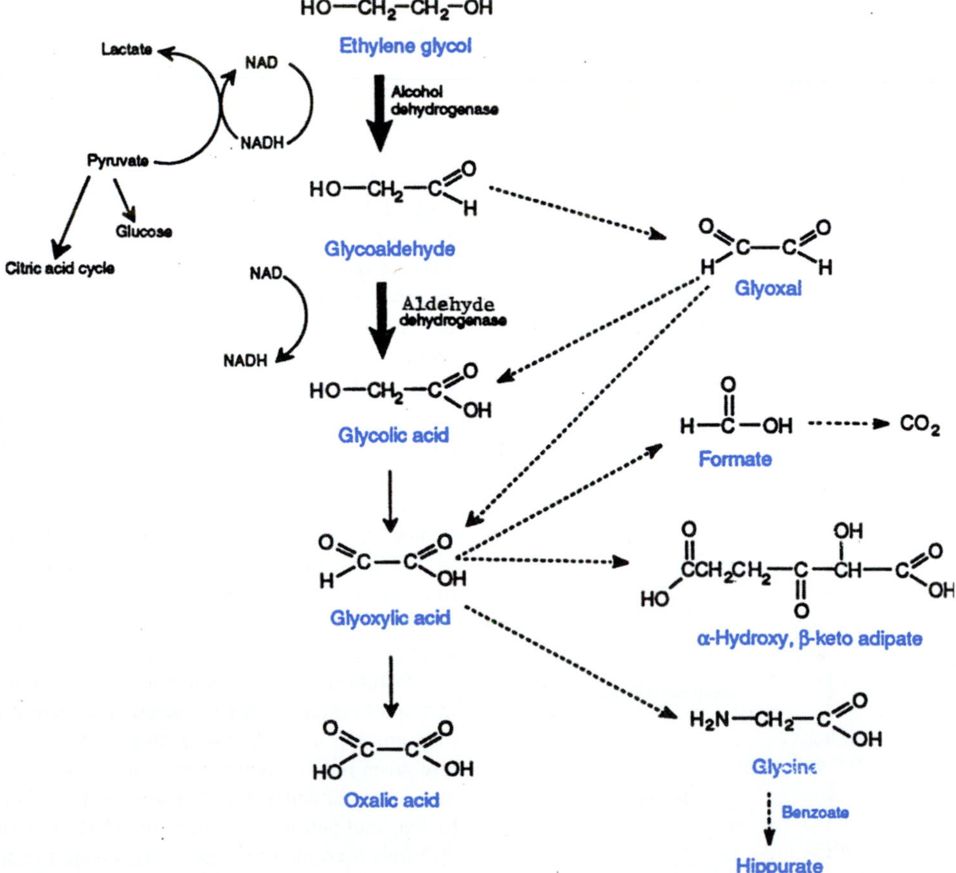

Figure 24-11. Metabolic pathway for oxidation of ethylene glycol.

Solid arrows represent steps that are quantitatively the most important in humans. Broken arrows indicate minor conversions. [Modified with permission from Wiener and Richardson (1988).]

brain is associated with damage of these organs. The actual mechanisms of cytotoxicity are poorly understood.

EG appears to have limited chronic toxicity potential. TK studies in mice and rats have shown that EG is rapidly metabolized and eliminated (Frantz et al., 1996), so bioaccumulation should not occur upon repetitive exposures. DePass et al. (1986) observed that male F344 rats were more susceptible to nephrotoxicity than female rats or B6C3F1 mice of either sex fed EG at 1000 mg/kg/day for 2 years. Renal toxicity was not seen in animals ingesting 40 or 200 mg/kg/day. NTP (1993) found oxalate crystals in the renal tubules, urethra and/or bladder of male B6C3F1 mice consuming EG at 6000 mg/kg/day for 103 weeks. NOAELs were estimated to be 1500 and 6000 mg/kg/day for the male and female mice, respectively. There was no evidence of carcinogenicity in two lifetime dietary studies of EG in mice or rats (DePass et al., 1986; NTP, 1993).

EG does not appear to be a reproductive toxicant, but it can cause adverse developmental effects in rodents. Certain skeletal and soft tissue malformations, delayed ossification, and reduced body weight have been consistently observed in fetuses and pups of rodents given ≥1000 mg/kg/day during gestation. Neeper-Bradley et al. (1995) reported oral NOAELs for developmental toxicity of 150 mg/kg for CD-1 mice and 500 mg/kg for CD rats. Dermal application of as much as ~3500 mg/kg/day under an occlusive dressing on days 6 to 15 of gestation was without observable maternal or fetal toxicity in CD-1 mice (Tyl et al., 1995). This lack of effect was attributed to the relatively poor percutaneous absorption of EG. Carney et al. (1999b) recently concluded that glycolic acid was the proximate developmental toxicant in EG-dosed rats. Metabolic acidosis was believed to exacerbate the teratogenicity of high doses of EG. The mechanism of the teratogenic action of glycolate is unknown.

Diethylene Glycol

Diethylene glycol (DEG) is used in industry as a solvent; a deicer; an additive for inks, lacquers, cosmetics and brake fluids; and as a textile finishing agent. DEG's use as an excipient in a liquid sulfanilamide preparation resulted in 105 deaths in the United States in 1937. This incident prompted passage of the Food, Drug and Cosmetic Act of 1938 (Wax, 1995). DEG is sometimes present as a contaminant of components of pharmaceuticals. Use of propylene glycol or glycerin contaminated with DEG has caused multiple fatalities from renal failure in Nigeria, Bangladesh, India, and Haiti. In the last incident, 109 cases of acute renal failure (with 88 deaths) were identified in children who received a locally manufactured acetaminophen syrup containing DEG-contaminated glycerin (O'Brien et al., 1998). The median lethal dose of DEG was estimated to be 1.34 mL/kg, with some victims receiving less than 1 mL/kg. Renal failure was the "hallmark" finding in these cases, but hepatitis, pancreatitis, and severe neurologic manifestations (e.g., encephalopathy, optic neuritis with retinal edema, unilateral facial paralysis) were frequently seen.

DEG toxicological data are limited. Oliguria or polyuria, proteinuria, and other manifestations of kidney injury were reported in rats given 5.0 or 7.5 mL DEG/kg ip (Kraul et al., 1991). The nephrotoxicity was maximally expressed 4 to 8 days after the single dose. Rats that consumed diets containing 1, 2, or 4 percent DEG (~1, 2, or 4 g/kg/day) exhibited dose-dependent hepatorenal injury (Fitzhugh and Nelson, 1946). Hellwig et al. (1995) did not find signs of maternal or fetal toxicity in rabbits given up to 1 g DEG/kg PO on days 7 to 19 postinsemination. Swiss CD-1 mice had to ingest as much as 6.1 g/kg/day for 14 weeks before their reproductive performance was diminished (Williams et al., 1990).

Relatively little information was located on the TK or mechanism of action of DEG. Heilmair et al. (1993) did find that doses of 1 and 5 mL/kg PO were rapidly and almost completely absorbed by male Sprague-Dawley (S-D) rats. ^{14}C-DEG was quickly distributed throughout the animals' bodies, and largely eliminated in the urine within 12 to 16 h. Wiener and Richardson (1989) identified a single urinary metabolite in DEG-dosed male Wistar rats, namely (2-hydroxyethoxy) acetic acid (HEAA). DEG, like EG, is oxidized in turn by alcohol dehydrogenase (ADH) and by aldehyde dehydrogenase. The ether linkage of DEG is not cleaved, as no EG or EG metabolites are formed from DEG. Lenk et al. (1989) observed that unchanged DEG, recovered in the urine of male S-D rats, constituted the majority (61 to 68 percent) of orally administered doses of 1, 5, and 10 mL/kg. HEAA accounted for 16 to 31 percent of these doses. DEG accelerated its own elimination by inducing osmotic diuresis at the two highest dosage levels. DEG's nephrotoxic moiety(ies) has (have) not been positively identified. Pretreatment of rats with pyrazole, an ADH inhibitor, did reduce the lethality of DEG in rats (Wiener and Richardson, 1989). Brophy et al. (2000) recently reported utilizing 4-methylpyrazole, an ADH inhibitor, and hemodialysis in the successful treatment of a 17-month-old girl who ingested DEG.

Propylene Glycol

Propylene glycol (PG) is used extensively as a solvent, coolant, antifreeze, and component of hydraulic fluids. As PG is "generally recognized as safe" by the FDA, it is a constituent of many cosmetics and processed foods. Furthermore, it serves as a solvent/diluent for a substantial number of oral, dermal, and intravenous drug preparations (ATSDR, 1997c).

PG has a very low order of acute and chronic toxicity (ATSDR, 1997c; LaKind et al., 1999). Extremely high doses can cause CNS depression, metabolic acidosis, encephalopathy, and hemolysis in humans and laboratory animals. No accounts of human fatalities were located. Glover and Reed (1996) reported a typical clinical case in which a 2-year-old child experienced CNS depression and anion-gap acidosis after ingesting a hair gel containing PG. Christopher et al. (1990) noted that cats ingesting 1.6 g PG/kg/day exhibited increases in serum anion gap acidosis and in D-lactate over a period of 35 days. Cats fed 8 g/kg/day for 35 days developed depression and ataxia, consistent with their progressively elevated plasma lactate levels. No organ system has apparently been identified as a target for acute or chronic injury by PG (LaKind et al., 1999). Carcinogenic or non-carcinogenic effects have not been seen in chronic bioassays in a number of species (ATSDR, 1997c). PG has not been shown to be mutagenic or teratogenic, or to adversely affect fertility or reproduction in CD-1 mice (Morrissey et al., 1989).

The explanation for PG's low toxicity lies in its metabolism. PG is metabolized by alcohol dehydrogenase to lactaldehyde, which in turn is oxidized by aldehyde dehydrogenase to lactate (Morshed et al., 1988). Excessive lactic acid is primarily responsible for systemic metabolic acidosis. Lactate, of course, can be converted to pyruvate and glucose through gluconeogenic pathways. PG is readily absorbed from the GI tract and distributed throughout total body water. PG accumulation is reported to differ significantly among people maintained on a repetitive oral dosing schedule, due to intersubject variability in clearance (Yu et al., 1985).

GLYCOL ETHERS

If one of the alcohol residues of ethylene glycol (HO—CH_2—CH_2—OH) is replaced by an ether, the resulting compound is a monoalkyl glycol ether such as ethylene glycol monomethyl ether, also called 2-methoxyethanol (2-ME; **CH_3—O**—CH_2—CH_2—OH). If both alcohols are replaced by ethers, the result is a dialkyl glycol ether such as ethylene glycol dimethyl ether (**CH_3—O**—CH_2—CH_2—**O—CH_3**). The alkyl group at the end of the ether linkage may be a straight or branched short chain moiety (e.g., methyl, ethyl, *n*-propyl, isopropyl, or butyl). The latter results in one of the most widely used glycol ethers, 2-butoxyethanol (2-BE; **CH_3—CH_2—CH_2—CH_2—O**—CH_2—CH_2—OH). Acetates of monoalkyl ethers such as 2-ME acetate (**CH_3—CO—O**—CH_2—CH_2—O—CH_3) are also common solvents that undergo rapid ester hydrolysis in vivo, and are thus likely to exhibit the same toxicity profile as unesterified glycols. Glycol ethers exhibit properties of both alcohols and ethers and are thus soluble in water and most organic solvents. This dual solubility, along with a favorable evaporation rate, make glycol ethers very popular as solvents for surface coatings such as lacquers, varnishes, and latex paints. Glycol ethers also find use as solvents in paint thinners and strippers, inks, metal cleaning products, liquid soaps, household cleaners, and in the fabrication of semiconductors.

Although the metabolism of glycol ethers varies with the chemical structure, some generalizations are possible (Fig. 24-12). For ethylene glycol monoalkyl ethers, the major metabolic pathway is oxidation via alcohol and aldehyde dehydrogenases to alkoxyacetic acids. For example, 2-ME and 2-BE are metabolized to methoxyacetic acid (MAA; **CH_3—CO—O**—CH_2—O—CH_3) and butoxyacetic acid (BAA; **CH_3—CO—O**—CH_2—O—CH_2—CH_2—CH_2—CH_3), respectively. The competing *O*-dealkylase pathway results in the cleavage of the ether linkage to form ethylene glycol and an alkyl aldehyde. Medinsky et al. (1990) reported that the relative contribution of the oxidative pathway to metabolism of ethylene glycol ethers increases with increasing alkyl chain length, while that of the *O*-dealkylase pathway decreases. In contrast, the propylene series (e.g., propylene glycol monomethyl ether; PGME) is predominantly biotransformed to propylene glycol via *O*-dealkylation. Glycol ethers may also be conjugated with glucuronide or sulfate, but this is thought to occur mainly after saturation of the other metabolic pathways.

The metabolism of glycol ethers is considered a prerequisite for their toxicity, as the alkoxyacetic acids are regarded as the ultimate toxicants. Their acetaldehyde precursors have also been implicated on occasion. Evidence for this comes from numerous in vitro and in vivo toxicity studies demonstrating that glycol ethers and their oxidative metabolites are reproductive, developmental, hematologic, and immunologic toxicants by all exposure routes. Additional evidence comes from: protection from toxicity afforded by inhibition of alcohol and aldehyde dehydrogenases; similar toxicity profiles of ethylene glycol ethers and their alkoxyacetic acid metabolites; and the differential toxicities of those glycol ethers metabolized via the oxidative and *O*-dealkylase pathways (Miller et al., 1984; Ghanayem et al., 1987).

Like glycol ether metabolism, glycol ether toxicity varies with chemical structure. With increasing alkyl chain length, reproductive and developmental toxicity decrease, whereas hematotoxicity increases (Ghanayem et al., 1989; Carney et al., 1999a). This

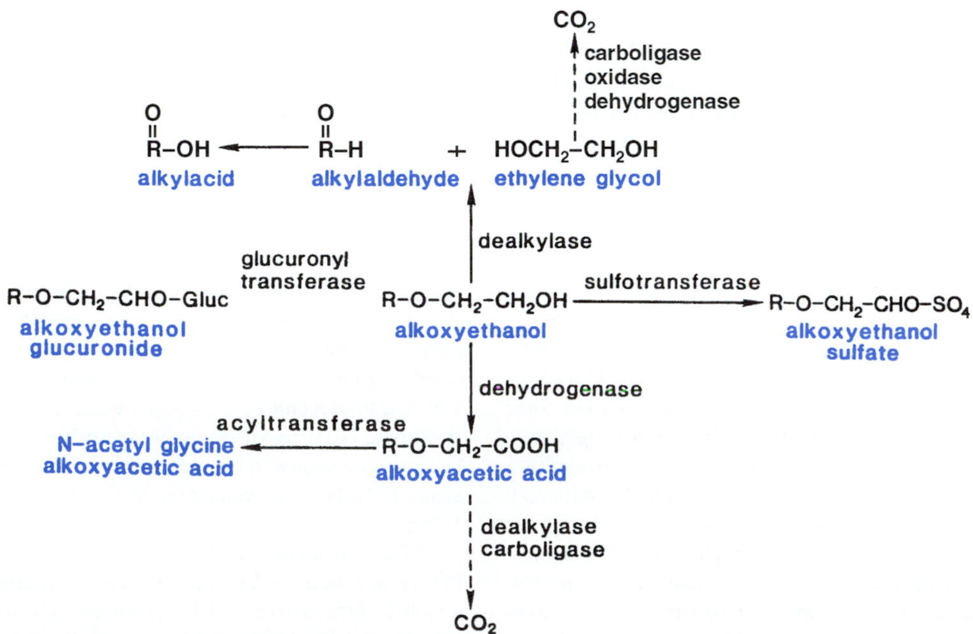

Figure 24-12. Metabolism of glycol ethers.

R denotes alkyl group of —CH_3, —CH_2—CH_3, or —CH_2—CH_2—CH_2—CH_3 for methoxy-, ethoxy-, or butoxyethanol, respectively. The formation of alkoxy glucuronide or sulfate conjugates has been identified only for butoxyethanol. [Reproduced with permission of Medinsky et al. (1990).]

demonstrates that structure-activity relationships are universally applicable across multiple toxicologic endpoints. Metabolic activation does not appear to be the sole determinant of the acute, oral lethality of ethylene glycol ethers. This was demonstrated by Tanii and coworkers (1992), who determined that LD_{50}s for ethylene glycol ethers in mice were highly correlated with their hydrophobicities. These researchers speculated that increasing hydrophobicity simply allowed the glycol ethers to more readily gain access to critical cellular targets.

Reproductive Toxicity

The reproductive toxicity of the glycol ethers is almost exclusively limited to reversible spermatotoxicity in males. Typical responses include testicular and seminiferous tubule atrophy, abnormal sperm head morphology, necrotic spermatocytes, decreased sperm motility and count, and infertility (Nolen et al., 1985; Heindel, 1990). Creasy and Foster (1984) noted a consistent order of spermatocyte susceptibility following oral administration of 2-ME or 2-EE to rats: dividing spermatocytes > early-pachytene spermatocytes > late-pachytene spermatocytes > mid-pachytene spermatocytes. Spermatocytes in the leptotene/zygotene stages of cell division, late-stage spermatids, and spermatogonia can be affected if the dose is increased and exposure prolonged. As for a mechanism of action, Beattie et al. (1984) reported that rates of lactate accumulation in cultured rat Sertoli cells were significantly decreased by MAA. Lactate is the preferred metabolic substrate of spermatocytes. Also, 2-EE has been shown to increase oxygen consumption and decrease ATP levels in pachytene spermatocytes in a manner consistent with an uncoupled oxidative state (Oudiz and Zenick, 1986). Mebus et al. (1989) demonstrated that serine, acetate, sarcosine, and glycine attenuated the spermatotoxicity of 2-ME in the rat, suggesting that MAA may interfere with the availability of one-carbon units for incorporation into purine and pyrimidine bases necessary for nucleic acid synthesis in pachytene spermatocytes. A mechanistic role for Ca^{2+} has been promoted by Ghanayem and Chapin (1990) who observed that a Ca^{2+} channel blocker afforded protection against 2-ME-induced pachytene spermatocyte cell death. These authors hypothesized that 2-ME perturbed Ca^{2+} homeostasis, which is consistent with observations of spermatocyte mitochondrial disruption. Involvement of Ca^{2+} is further suggested by observations that 2-ME induces spermatocyte apoptosis in both the rat and guinea pig, and activates or induces an endogenous endonuclease. An increase in intracellular Ca^{2+} is thought by many to be the trigger for endonuclease activation/induction and subsequent apoptotic cell death (Ku et al., 1995).

Testicular effects similar to those in rodents have been described for humans, in some cases at concentrations well below current OSHA PELs for 2-ME and 2-EE of 25 and 200 ppm, respectively. Men exposed to a mean level of 6.6 ppm 2-EE in a foundry had decreased numbers of sperm per ejaculate (Ratcliffe et al., 1989). Similarly, Welch et al. (1988) found that painters exhibited oligospermia and azoospermia following exposure to 2-EE and 2-ME at 2.7 ppm and 0.8 ppm on average, respectively. A large case-control study of male fertility clinic patients revealed a highly significant association between a diagnosis of impaired fertility and the detection of ethoxyacetic acid in urine (Veulemans et al., 1993). Significant associations between potential exposure to mixtures containing ethylene glycol ethers and increased risk for spontaneous abortion and subfertility have been observed in females. These results are interesting in light of findings that MAA increases progesterone production in human luteal cells (Almekinder et al., 1997).

Developmental Toxicity

Developmental toxicity has been described for several glycol ethers. Structural anomalies in rodents have included a variety of minor skeletal variations, hydrocephalus, exencephaly, cardiovascular malformations, dilatation of the renal pelvis, craniofacial malformations, and digit malformations (Hardin et al., 1986; Tyl et al., 1989). Electrocardiograms of fetal rats from dams treated with 2-ME during gestation showed persistent, aberrant QRS waves in the absence of structural defect, suggestive of an intraventricular conduction delay (Toraason and Breitenstein, 1988). Neurobehavioral changes and regional brain alterations of several neurotransmitters in the offspring of rats treated with 2-ME or 2-EE have been reported (Nelson and Brightwell, 1984). Ambroso et al. (1998) applied confocal laser scanning microscopy, classical histopathology, and in situ immunohistochemistry to demonstrate that 2-ME caused a dose-dependent increase and expansion of apoptosis in gestation day 8 mouse embryos that could underly 2-ME-induced neural tube defects. Such a mechanism has also been hypothesized for malformations induced by the prototypical teratogens, retinoic acid and ethanol.

A case-control study was conducted in Europe to determine whether maternal occupational exposure to glycol ethers in the first trimester was associated with congenital malformations (Cordier et al., 1997). The overall odds ratio of congenital malformations was 1.44 (95 percent CI = 1.10 to 1.90), with significant associations for glycol ether exposure with cleft lip and neural tube defects such as spina bifida. PBTK models have been applied to estimate inhaled concentrations of 2-EE, its acetate ester, and 2-ME in humans that would result in blood levels equivalent to those observed at the rat NOAELs and LOAELs for developmental effects (Gargas et al., 2000a, b). It is worthy of note that 2-ME has been largely removed from commerce due to its teratogenic potency.

Hematotoxicity

Some glycol ethers are hemolytic to red blood cells (RBCs). Typically, the osmotic balance of the cells is disrupted, they imbibe water and swell, their ATP concentration decreases, and hemolysis occurs. The swelling suggests that the erythrocyte membrane is the ultimate target (Ghanayem, 1989). Nyska et al. (1999) report that subchronic exposure to 2-BE causes disseminated thrombosis and bone infarction in female, but not male rats, likely due to the impedance of blood flow by intravascular hemolysis. It is thought that females might be susceptible, since they are less efficient at eliminating BAA and exhibit higher peak blood BAA levels. Young rats are more resistant to the hematologic effects of 2-BE than older rats, an observation attributed to depressed degradation and renal clearance of BAA in older rats. Hoflack et al. (1997) have shown 2-BE capable of inducing apoptosis in a human leukemia cell line and have hypothesized that the hematopoietic toxicity of 2-BE may be the result of its ability to induce cell death.

Species differ dramatically in their sensitivities to glycol ether–induced RBC deformity and hemolysis. Humans are less susceptible than rodents. This lower susceptibility applies even to RBCs from potentially sensitive subpopulations, such as the elderly and persons with hereditary blood disorders (Udden, 1994; Udden and Patton, 1994). A good example of using PBTK models in human risk assessment has been published by Corley et al. (1997). Based on comparisons of the model output with data collected by Udden et al. on levels of 2-BE required to affect osmotic fragility of human RBCs, Corley et al. (1997) concluded that humans are unlikely to achieve hemolytic blood levels of BAA, unless very large volumes of 2-BE are intentionally ingested.

Immunotoxicity/Carcinogenicity

It also appears that the immune system is a sensitive target of glycol ether oxidative metabolites. Exon et al. (1991) exposed male and female rats to high concentrations of 2-ME in drinking water for 21 days. Among the effects seen were thymic atrophy, increased natural killer cell cytotoxic activity, decreased antibody production, decreased splenocyte production of interferon-γ, and a reduction in spleen cellularity. 2-ME-induced immunosuppression has also been reported by Kim and Smialowicz (1997). Interestingly, 2-methoxyacetaldehyde proved more immunotoxic than MAA in this study.

Chronic inhalation bioassays were recently conducted on 2-BE in F344 rats (0 to 125 ppm) and B6C3F1 mice (0 to 250 ppm) (NTP, 1998). Conclusions from the 2-year bioassay included: no evidence of carcinogenicity in male F344 rats; equivocal evidence of carcinogenicity in female F344 rats, based on the combined incidences of benign and malignant pheochromocytoma (mainly benign) of the adrenal medulla; and some evidence of carcinogenicity in male and female B6C3F1 mice, based on increased incidences of hemangiosarcoma of the liver and forestomach squamous cell papilloma or carcinoma (mainly papilloma), respectively. The genotoxicity of some of the glycol ethers and their metabolites has been evaluated, with most studies indicating a lack of genotoxic potential and with others yielding positive responses in certain tests. Therefore, the role of genetic toxicology in the toxicities discussed above cannot be summarily dismissed but is of unknown significance (Elliot and Ashby, 1997).

FUELS AND FUEL ADDITIVES

Automotive Gasoline

Automotive gasoline is a complex mixture of hundreds of hydrocarbons predominantly in the range of C_4 to C_{12}. The sheer number of people exposed in the manufacture, distribution, and use of gasoline make the characterization of its acute and chronic toxicities important. Generalizations regarding the toxicity of gasoline must be made with care, since its composition varies with the crude oil from which it is refined, the refining process, and the use of specific additives. Experiments conducted with fully vaporized gasoline may not be predictive of actual risk, since humans are exposed primarily to the more volatile components in the range of C_4 to C_5. These hydrocarbons are generally regarded as less toxic than their higher-molecular-weight counterparts. Concern for gasoline is fueled in part by the toxicities of its individual components, some of which are classified by the EPA as known or probable human carcinogens (e.g., benzene and 1,3-butadiene). The ACGIH has established a threshold limit value (TLV) for gasoline of 300 ppm to prevent ocular and upper respiratory tract irritation and a short-term exposure limit (STEL) of 500 ppm to avoid acute CNS depression.

Inhalation exposure to gasoline has been measured for service station attendants and self-service customers, for truck drivers and distribution workers, and for workers removing leaking underground storage tanks (Kearney and Dunham, 1986; Shamsky and Samimi, 1987). In one survey, short-term exposures to self-service customers averaged about 6 ppm. The TLV is rarely exceeded in occupationally exposed individuals, due in part to the use of vapor scavenging systems. Brief exposures in excess of the STEL have, however, been documented for workers engaged in bulk handling operations (Phillips and Jones, 1978). The most extreme exposures occur to those intentionally sniffing gasoline for its euphoric effects. Several case reports of acute and chronic encephalopathies, expressed as both motor and cognitive impairment, are testament to the dangers of this habit (Valpey et al., 1978; Fortenberry, 1985). In these cases, the identity of the offending agent(s) is often unclear. An all too common occurrence is the ingestion of gasoline during siphoning events. This is typically followed by a burning sensation in the mouth and pharynx, as well as nausea, vomiting, and diarrhea resulting from GI irritation. If aspirated into the lungs, gasoline may produce pulmonary epithelial damage, edema, and pneumonitis. Thus, emetic therapy for gasoline ingestion is usually contraindicated.

Reese and Kimbrough (1993), as well as Caprino and Togna (1998), have reviewed the acute toxicity of gasoline and its additives. Like some other solvents, gasoline can sensitize the heart to catecholamines, defat the skin upon repeated contact, and induce hepatic MFO and UDP-glucuronyltransferase activities (Poon et al., 1995). The issue of whether there is a "fetal gasoline syndrome" has been raised, although case reports offered in support of the affirmative are confounded by tetraethyl lead, alcohol abuse, and the possibility that an aberrant gene is distributed within the small Amerindian population where the cases reside (Hunter et al., 1979). There is a paucity of data on the reproductive toxicity of gasoline, but reports of enhanced estrogen metabolism and uterine atrophy among unleaded gasoline-treated mice suggest that this endpoint warrants investigation (Standeven et al., 1994a). The study of Lykke and Stewart (1978) is of interest, in the rats exposed to the modest concentration of 100 ppm leaded gasoline (one-third the current ACGIH TLV) 40 h/week for 6 to 12 weeks were observed to have a progressive interstitial fibrosis of the lungs associated with irregular alveolar collapse.

Prior to the identification of α_{2u}-globulin as the principal accumulating protein in the syndrome referred to as α_{2u}-globulin nephropathy, Kuna and Ulrich (1984) reported regenerative epithelium and dilated tubules in the kidneys of male rats exposed to 1552 ppm unleaded gasoline for 90 days. At about the same time, a chronic inhalation study reported not only the nephropathy, but increased renal tumors in male rats (MacFarland et al., 1984). Subsequent studies by Halder et al. (1986) and Aranyi et al. (1986) showed that such nephropathy could not be produced by exposure of rats to a mixture of the butane and pentane components of gasoline or the 0° to 145°F gasoline distillation fraction. These are thought to be more representative of human occupational exposures than wholly vaporized gasoline. In addition, the authors of a gavage screening study of 15 pure hydrocarbons and gasoline fractions concluded that branched aliphatic alkane components were primarily responsible for the nephropathy (Halder et al., 1985).

Investigations of mechanisms of the nephropathy and renal tumors included an assessment of unscheduled (a measure of genotoxicity) and replicative DNA synthesis (a measure of cell proliferation) in rat kidney cells exposed in vitro and in vivo to unleaded gasoline. No unscheduled DNA synthesis occurred, even at a tumorigenic dose, while a five- to eightfold increase in cell proliferation was observed (Loury et al., 1987). In a publication the same year by Olson et al. (1987), unleaded gasoline was reported to result in an increase in hyaline droplets harboring large accumulations of α_{2u}-globulin within proximal convoluted tubule epithelial cells. It was hypothesized that α_{2u}-globulin accumulated secondary to a defect in renal lysosomal degradation of the protein (Fig. 24-6). Supportive evidence for this hypothesis came from Olson et al. (1988), who demonstrated that inhibition of the lysosomal peptidase cathepsin B caused a rapid accumulation of phagolysosomes and α_{2u}-globulin in the kidney similar to that of gasoline.

Further progress in elucidating the mechanism of α_{2u}-globulin nephropathy came from the demonstration that the unleaded gasoline component, 2,2,4-trimethylpentane (TMP), itself an inducer of α_{2u}-globulin nephropathy, was metabolized to 2,4,4-trimethyl-2-pentanol (TMPOH), which was selectively retained by the kidney of male rats. Subsequently, it was demonstrated that the sex-specific retention of TMPOH in the kidney was due to reversible binding with α_{2u}-globulin. This binding rendered the protein less digestible by lysosomal enzymes, which accounted for its accumulation (Charbonneau and Swenberg, 1988). This accumulation, in turn, led to cellular degeneration and necrosis, primarily in the P_2 segment of the proximal tubule. In response, regenerative proliferation occurs and promotes formation of renal cell tumors by irreversibly "fixing" spontaneously altered DNA and clonally expanding initiated cells. The promotional effects of gasoline and TMP on atypical cell foci and renal cell tumors have been demonstrated in male rats following initiation with *N*-ethyl-*N*-hydroxyethylnitrosamine (Short et al., 1989). NCI-Black-Reiter male rats, the only rat strain not to synthesize α_{2u}-globulin, are resistant to gasoline- and TMP-induced nephropathy (Dietrich and Swenberg, 1991). Thus, gasoline and TMP have been of great value in elucidating the mechanism of α_{2u}-globulin nephropathy and shedding light on its implications for renal tumorigenesis. Most toxicologists, and indeed the EPA, have concluded that renal tumors secondary to α_{2u}-globulin nephropathy are of little relevance, because humans do not synthesize α_{2u}-globulin.

Chronic inhalation of gasoline has also resulted in increased hepatocellular adenomas and carcinomas in B6C3F1 female mice (MacFarland et al., 1984). This increase may have been due to the promotion of spontaneously initiated cells that occur with unusually high frequency in this mouse strain. Unleaded gasoline is a liver tumor promoter in *N*-nitrosodiethylamine–initiated female B6C3F1 mice (Standeven and Goldsworthy, 1993). Gasoline has been shown to induce cytochrome P450 activity and to produce hepatomegaly and a transient increase in hepatocyte proliferation, all of which are considered relevant to tumor-promoting activity (Moser et al., 1996a). An effort has been made to link gasoline's promoting effect to its antiestrogenicity (Standeven et al., 1994a, b). Unleaded gasoline has also been shown to induce unscheduled DNA synthesis in hepatocytes from male and female mice treated in vivo and in cultured mouse, rat and human hepatocytes (IARC, 1989). The epidemiologic evidence for an association between gasoline exposure and cancer in humans is inconclusive. IARC (1989) provides perhaps the best and least biased epidemiologic overview, from which they conclude that there is inadequate evidence for the carcinogenicity of gasoline in humans.

Methyl Tertiary-Butyl Ether

Methyl tertiary-butyl ether's (MTBE's) high octane rating made it a logical replacement for tetraethyl lead as an octane booster for gasoline, and later as a gasoline oxygenator. As an oxygenator, MTBE makes fuel combustion more complete, thereby reducing pollutant emissions from automobile exhaust. MTBE may be added to gasoline at levels up to 15 percent by volume in order to comply with the 1990 Amendments to the Clean Air Act. By 1997, it was being used at the rate of 10 million gal/day, with more than one-third of the usage in California. While routine, low-level exposure of customers occurs at self-service stations, heightened concern about MTBE has resulted primarily from its contamination of groundwater by leaking underground gasoline tanks. Water containing MTBE has an unpleasant taste and odor, which may alert consumers to the fact that their water is contaminated. Based on the results of studies of taste and odor thresholds for humans, an advisory guidance range of 20 to 40 μg/L has been set by the EPA to assure consumer acceptance and provide a large margin of safety from toxicity and carcinogenicity.

Comprehensive reviews of MTBE toxicity include those of the EPA and State of California in their Drinking Water Advisory and Public Health Goal documents, respectively (EPA, 1997; Wang et al., 1999). Scientists from three different federal government agencies have published a comprehensive review (Melnick et al., 1997), while the review of Borak et al. (1998) focuses upon the acute human health effects of MTBE. The conclusion of this latter work, based on 19 reports of inhalation exposure to MTBE alone or in gasoline and 12 reports of parenteral MTBE administration to dissolve cholesterol gallstones, is that no significant association exists between MTBE exposure and the acute symptoms commonly attributed to MTBE. These symptoms include headache, eye, nose and throat irritation, cough, nausea, dizziness, and disorientation. The ATSDR has published a Toxicological Profile for MTBE (ATSDR, 1996b).

In 1988, the EPA and industry developed a Testing Consent Order for MTBE under the Toxic Substances Control Act that precipitated investigations of MTBE's potential two-generation reproductive toxicity, developmental toxicity, in vivo mutagenicity, subchronic inhalation toxicity, oncogenicity, and neurotoxicity. Results of these studies are a major addition to the toxicity literature on MTBE and define several NOAELs (Bevan et al., 1997a, b; Bird et al., 1997; Daughtrey et al., 1997; Lington et al., 1997; McKee et al., 1997). The publication of Bird and colleagues is actually a recapitulation of reports by Chun et al. (1992) and Burleigh-Flayer et al. (1992), both of which are of particular value, as they represent two of only three MTBE cancer bioassays. In the Chun et al. study, male and female F344 rats were exposed to 0, 400, 3000, or 8000 ppm MTBE vapor 6 h/day, 5 days/week for 24 months. In the other inhalation study, Burleigh-Flayer et al. (1992) subjected male and female CD-1 mice to the same exposure regimen for 18 months. The only oral chronic bioassay is that by Belpoggi et al. (1995, 1997), who subjected male and female S-D rats by olive oil gavage to 0, 250, or 1000 mg/kg MTBE 4 days/week for 2 years. The results of the three MTBE animal cancer bioassays are presented in Table 24-4.

Taken at face value, one might interpret these cancer bioassay findings as ample evidence of carcinogenicity in animals and suggestive of a cancer risk for humans. The relevance of these findings to humans, however, has been a source of debate among toxicologists. Critics have questioned these studies on the basis of (1) the appropriateness of a combined incidence category for leukemias and lymphomas; (2) the possibility that renal tumors were secondary to male rat–specific α_{2u}-globulin nephropathy; (3) the possibility that Leydig cell tumors were a function of abnormally low testicular tumor rates in control animals or increased survival time of treated rats; (4) the questionable relevance of testicular tumors in rats to humans, given the species' differential re-

Table 24-4
Summary Results of MTBE Cancer Bioassays

AUTHORS	ANIMAL STRAIN/SPECIES	EXPOSURE ROUTE	POSITIVE RESULTS
Chun et al. (1992)	Fischer 344 rats	Inhalation	Kidney and testicular tumors (males)
Burleigh-Flayer et al. (1992)	CD-1 mice	Inhalation	Liver adenomas (females)
Belpoggie et al. (1995)	Sprague-Dawley rats	Oral	Testicular tumors (males)
			Leukemia + lymphoma (females)

sponses of Leydig cells to proliferative stimuli; (5) the possibility that liver and kidney tumors are the result of high dose-induced chronic cytotoxicity, cell death, and reparative cell proliferation; (6) the relevance of inhalation bioassays to prediction of drinking water risks; and (7) the use of an oil rather than a water dosing vehicle, which could unduly influence MTBE's oral TK. Some of these issues are discussed in more detail in Mennear's (1997) review and interpretation of the MTBE carcinogenicity studies.

As an outgrowth of the uncertainties surrounding MTBE's carcinogenicity, several mechanistic studies have been published. For example, after only 10 days of MTBE inhalation exposure, a strong positive linear relationship between renal α_{2u}-globulin concentration and cell proliferation was seen in the male F344 rat (Prescott-Matthews et al., 1997). This study, unlike the chronic bioassay of Chun et al. (1992), definitively identified the accumulating protein as α_{2u}-globulin (Fig. 24-6). The concentration of α_{2u}-globulin in kidney cytosol was measured with an enzyme-linked immunosorbent assay. MTBE has been shown to be a hepatic mitogen in the female mouse, but not a promoter of tumor formation in *N*-nitrosodiethylamine (DEN)-initiated female mouse liver (Moser et al., 1996b). It has been suggested in light of these findings, that MTBE may promote the growth of spontaneously initiated cell populations having genetic lesions different from those produced by DEN. Studies also indicate that MTBE causes endocrine dysregulation in rodents at high doses, suggesting that consideration be given to the possibility that MTBE-induced tumor formation is hormonally mediated (Moser et al., 1998; Williams et al., 2000). Although it has generally been accepted that MTBE's carcinogenicity in animals occurs through a non-genotoxic mechanism, MTBE has been shown to be moderately mutagenic in the Ames assay in the requisite presence of a functional excision repair system (Williams-Hill et al., 1999).

Several mechanistic issues, including the contribution of MTBE's metabolites, *tert*-butyl alcohol and formaldehyde, to MTBE's toxicity have yet to be resolved. To this end, Casanova and Heck (1997) have reported a lack of concentration-, species-, and sex-dependence in the formation of formaldehyde-induced DNA-protein crosslinks and RNA-formaldehyde adducts in isolated female CD-1 mouse hepatocytes incubated with MTBE. As the cancer bioassay data suggest that hepatocarcinogenicity varies with all of these factors, these results do not support a role for formaldehyde in MTBE-induced liver tumor formation.

As a reflection of the paucity of data available, IARC (1999) has concluded that MTBE is not classifiable as to its carcinogenicity to humans (group 3), and the EPA has classified MTBE as a possible human carcinogen (group C), meaning limited evidence from animal studies and inadequate or no data in humans. Despite data limitations, the EPA Office of Water has calculated three cancer slope factors, one for each of the cancer bioassays, all using the linearized multistage model that assumes the absence of a threshold for tumor formation. California has derived both a cancer potency estimate and adopted a Public Health Goal of 13 ppb for MTBE in drinking water (Wang et al., 1999). There are advocates for the suspension of MTBE's use in reformulated gasoline, but such a decision should weigh the benefits against the risks associated with increased auto emissions of carcinogenic VOCs and the public health impact of increased CO_2 emissions and ozone formation. Two articles that discuss this subject in considerable detail are those of Spitzer (1997) and Erdal et al. (1997).

Jet Fuel

Jet propellant-8 (JP-8 jet fuel) is a complex, kerosene-like mixture of hundreds of aliphatic and aromatic hydrocarbons. It is now the recognized battlefield fuel for all NATO ground and air forces. Owing to slight differences in hydrocarbon composition and additives, JP-8's chemicophysical properties differ from those of its predecessor fuels in ways that impart added safety, enhance combat aircraft survivability, simplify battlefield logistics, and promote standardization with commercial jet fuel. Both civilian and military personnel are exposed to JP-8. For instance, ground crews have identified highly visible aerosol emissions during jet aircraft "cold starts," resulting in some crew members working behind the aircraft becoming "drenched" in fuel. Jet fuel can also be released into the environment by in-flight jettisoning and by spills or leaks to soil or water during use, storage, or transportation. In many cases, the United States Department of Defense (DoD) is ultimately responsible for the cost of remediating contaminated military sites and contractor facilities. Since toxicity is a primary determinant of the extent to which contaminated sites must be remediated, it is in DoD's interest to accurately characterize the toxicity of JP-8. Thus, much of the recent research on jet fuel toxicity has been conducted and/or funded by the military.

Toxicity data on jet fuels have recently been summarized (ATSDR, 1998a; IARC, 1989). There is no evidence that JP-8 or other jet fuels are a genetic risk. JP-8 was not teratogenic, based on a single study that identified a NOAEL of 1000 mg/kg/day for reduction in fetal body weight of rats (Cooper and Mattie, 1996). In a 90-day continuous inhalation study of JP-8 vapor, no treatment-related adverse effects other than α_{2u}-globulin nephropathy were seen in mice or rats (Mattie et al., 1991). Bruner et al. (1993) exposed rats and mice of each sex 6 h/day, 5 days/week to JP-4 vapors for 12 months. The main finding was renal toxicity and neoplasia in male rats consistent with α_{2u}-globulin nephropathy. Data suggest that the chronic dermal application of jet fuels can be carcinogenic to the skin of mice. It has been effectively argued, however, that the tumorigenic effect is secondary to chronic irritation (Nessel, 1999).

Some of the most interesting toxicity data on jet fuel have been published on the subject of JP-8-induced lung and immune dysfunction. In the first of this series of studies (Pfaff et al., 1995), the pulmonary effects of an aerosol/vapor mixture of JP-8 jet fuel (495–520 mg/m^3) were investigated in rats with nose only exposures for 1 h/day for 7 or 28 days to simulate military flightline exposures. Changes in pulmonary function, in the form of increases in pulmonary resistance and alveolar permeability, were accompanied by a decrease in the concentration of Substance P (SP) in bronchoalveolar lavage fluid. Pfaff et al. (1996) published another study in which reductions in SP were accompanied by pathological changes in lower pulmonary structures such as inflammation of the terminal bronchioles, degeneration of alveolar type II cells, disruption of terminal bronchial airway epithelium, interstitial and perivascular edema, thickened epithelium of the bronchioles, and minute irregular microvilli. Most interestingly, however, neutral endopeptidase (NEP), the enzyme most responsible for the metabolism of tachykinins such as SP in the lung, was increased by exposure and a significant inverse relationship between SP and NEP activity was demonstrated. Thus, JP-8 appears to exhibit a rather novel mechanism of lung injury that involves the reduction or depletion of SP due to its enhanced metabolism by NEP.

Because SP participates in the maintenance of airway epithelial cell competency, the effect of JP-8 and *n*-tetradecane (C_{14}), a primary constituent of JP-8, on epithelial barrier integrity was examined in vitro using paracellular mannitol flux in BEAS-2B human bronchial epithelial cells. Noncytotoxic concentrations of JP-8 and C_{14} dose-dependently increased transepithelial mannitol flux that spontaneously reversed to control values over a 48-hr recovery period. This suggests that JP-8 and C_{14} compromise the integrity of intercellular tight junctions that may precede and initiate the pathologic alterations observed in whole animal studies (Robledo et al., 1999). These same authors also have collected evidence that SP's protective affect on the lung is largely mediated through the plasma membrane bound neurokinin receptor, NK1, that is present on airway epithelium from the trachea to the respiratory bronchioles (Robledo and Witten, 1999). Further insight into the effects of JP-8 have come from the use of high resolution two-dimensional electrophoresis applied to samples of lung and kidney cytosol collected from JP-8 exposed mice. Both qualitative and quantitative changes were apparent in proteins, many of which were identified and related to impaired processes that could underlie the pathophysiological changes induced by JP-8 in the lung (Witzmann et al., 1999; Witzmann et al., 2000). It is conceivable that these altered proteins could one day serve as biomarkers of JP-8 exposure and effect in humans.

The immune system appears to be susceptible to insult at lower JP-8 concentrations than the lung. As reported by Harris et al. (1997a), mice were exposed nose-only to several concentrations of JP-8 aerosol/vapor mix (0-2500 mg/m^3) for 1 h/day for 7 days and sacrificed 24 h after the last exposure for immune assays. JP-8 exposure decreased spleen and thymus organ weights and cellularities and altered the number of viable immune cells of the lymph nodes, bone marrow, and peripheral blood. Depending upon the immune organ examined, different immune cell subpopulations were lost, including T and B cells and macrophages. In addition, JP-8 was found to affect immune function as demonstrated by a concentration-dependent suppression of T cell proliferation upon stimulation with the mitogen concanavalin A. As a follow-up study, Harris et al. (1997b) determined that JP-8-induced immunotoxicity persisted for at least 1 month after insult. Recently, these same authors have expanded the number of immune parameters examined and report that JP-8 exposure to mice (1 h/day for 7 days, 1000 mg/m^3) nearly completely ablated NK cell function, suppressed the generation of lymphokine-activated killer cell activity and cytotoxic T lymphocyte generation from precursor T cells, and inhibited helper T cell activity (Harris et al., 2000). Ullrich (1999) has demonstrated that the dermal application of JP-8 to mice also induces immune suppression. Ullrich found interleukin-10, a cytokine with potent immune suppressive activity, in the serum of JP-8 treated mice. He interpreted this as suggestive of an immune suppressive mechanism involving the upregulation of cytokine release. As in the case of JP-8-induced pulmonary toxicity, aerosolized SP afforded protection against JP-8 induced immunotoxicity, suggesting a key mechanistic role for the neuropeptide (Harris et al., 1997c).

The ATSDR has derived an intermediate MRL for JP-5 and JP-8 of 3 mg/m^3 from a study in which hepatocellular fatty vacuolization was observed in mice exposed to JP-5 at 150 mg/m^3 continuously for 5 days (ATSDR, 1998a). EPA has not verified a RfD or RfC for JP-5 or JP-8, but an EPA memorandum has detailed the derivation of provisional RfDs for JP-4 and JP-5 of 8×10^{-2} and 2×10^{-2} mg/kg/day, respectively (EPA, 1992).

Kerosene

In contrast to automobile gasoline and jet fuels that together account for about 60 percent of all United States refinery output, kerosene accounts for just 0.3 percent. Since the late 1970s, the demand for kerosene and its production have sharply declined. As a middle distillate consisting of C_9 to C_{16} hydrocarbons, its makeup is very similar to that of jet fuel. Therefore, one might predict that its toxicity would resemble that of jet fuel. The majority of published literature on kerosene deals with localized effects at the portals of entry, mainly the skin and the lung. A comprehensive evaluation of the carcinogenic potential of middle distillate fuels has been recently published that focused on skin tumors secondary to chronic skin irritation (Nessel, 1999). A discussion of the toxicology of dermally applied middle distillates is also a recent addition to the literature (Koschier, 1999). For the most comprehensive review, see IARC's (1989) discussion of jet fuels and kerosene.

CARBON DISULFIDE

The majority of carbon disulfide (CS_2) is used in the production of viscose rayon and cellophane, CCl_4 and pesticides, and as a solubilizer for waxes and oils (ATSDR, 1996a). Exposure is predominantly occupational, but CS_2 has been identified at ~200 current or former EPA National Priority List hazardous waste sites (ATSDR, 1996a). As discussed in EPA's IRIS profile, a RfC of 0.7 mg/m^3 ($\sim$0.22 ppm) is based on reduced maximum motor conduction velocity in the peroneal nerves of viscose rayon workers exposed to CS_2. The RfD of 0.1 mg/kg/day is based on the teratogenic potential of CS_2 in rats and rabbits. For the protection of workers, OSHA has established a PEL of 20 ppm as an 8-h time-weighted average (TWA) and an acceptable ceiling concentration of 30 ppm. The ACGIH TLV is 10 ppm as an 8-h TWA.

At present, the relative contributions of parent compound and metabolites to most CS_2-induced toxicities are unknown. Two distinct metabolic pathways for CS_2 exist: (1) the direct interaction of CS_2 with free amine and sulfhydryl groups of amino acids and polypeptides to form dithiocarbamates and trithiocarbonates and (2) microsomal metabolism of CS_2 to reactive sulfur intermediates capable of covalently binding to tissue macromolecules (Fig. 24-13). The conjugation of CS_2 with GSH results in the formation of 2-thiothiazolidine-4-carboxylic acid (TTCA), which is excreted in urine and has been frequently used as a biomarker of CS_2 exposure, especially among viscose rayon workers (Riihimaki et al., 1992; Lee et al., 1995). Several limitations of TTCA as a biomarker have been noted, and covalently cross-linked erythrocyte spectrin and hemoglobin have been discussed as potential alternatives (Valentine et al., 1993, 1998). Nonetheless, the current ACGIH Biological Exposure Index (BEI) for CS_2 is 5 mg of TTCA per g of creatinine for a urine sample collected at the end of a workshift. Commentary on the derivation of this BEI has been published by Cox et al. (1992).

A few reviews of CS_2 toxicity appear in the literature (WHO, 1979; Beauchamp et al., 1983; ATSDR, 1996a). CS_2 targets multiple organ systems and has been associated with toxicities as diverse as ocular/auditory toxicity and spermatotoxicity. Two target organs have garnered the majority of attention, the nervous and cardiovascular systems. With regard to the former, CS_2 is associated with the following clinical syndromes as stated by Rosenberg (1995):

> (1) acute and chronic encephalopathy (often with prominent psychiatric manifestations), (2) polyneuropathy (both peripheral and cranial), (3) Parkinsonism, and (4) asymptomatic CNS and PNS dysfunction....Pathologic changes occur in both the CNS and PNS...CNS pathology consists of neuronal degeneration throughout the cerebral hemispheres, wth maximal diffuse involvement in the frontal regions. Cell loss is also noted in the globus pallidus, putamen, and cerebellar cortex, with loss of Purkinje cells. Vascular abnormalities with endothelial proliferation of arterioles may be seen, sometimes associated with focal necrosis or demyelination. PNS changes consist primarily of myelin swelling and fragmentation and large focal axonal swellings, characteristic of distal axonopathy.

For those interested in the nervous system, the classic paper by Richter (1945), detailing his observations of chronic CS_2 poisoning in monkeys, is recommended. Much more recently, collaborative research by the NIEHS, EPA, and two universities was conducted. Studies were conducted to assess multiple biological and mechanistic endpoints at various times during subchronic exposure of F344 rats to a range of CS_2 concentrations. The endpoints included (1) TK in blood and urine; (2) assessment of covalently modified hemoglobin and nerve growth factor receptor mRNA as biomarkers of exposure and effect; (3) alterations in axon/Schwann cell interactions; (4) morphology of distal axonopathy; (5) nerve conduction velocity and compound nerve action potentials; and (6) a functional observational battery. The findings have been published as a series (Harry et al., 1998; Sills et al., 1998).

Neither the concentration nor the exposure duration required for CS_2-induced neurotoxicity in humans is known, although frequent and prolonged exposures over a course of months are likely required. Studies indicate that CS_2, like *n*-hexane, causes neurofilament-filled swellings proximal to nodes of Ranvier of distal axons. Distortions of nodal anatomy and demyelination occur, and some axons undergo degeneration distal to the neurofilamentous swellings. The success of regeneration of peripheral nerves is related to the severity of the loss of motor and sensory function, with greater degrees of recovery in those individuals with milder symptoms. While the primary clinical manifestations reflect changes in peripheral nerves, the axonopathy also involves the long axons in the CNS that cannot regenerate, particularly the ascending and descending tracks of the spinal cord and the visual pathways.

Several mechanisms for the disruption of neurofilament transport that underlies CS_2 axonopathy have been proposed including impaired energy metabolism, metal ion chelation by CS_2's dithiocarbamate derivatives, the induction of vitamin deficiency, neurofilament derivatization, and the disruption of cytoskeletal protein association by the increased phosphorylation of neurofilaments (Wilmarth et al., 1993; Graham et al., 1995). One mechanism has emerged as more plausible than the others, however, that of progressive cross-linking of neurofilaments by the reaction of elec-

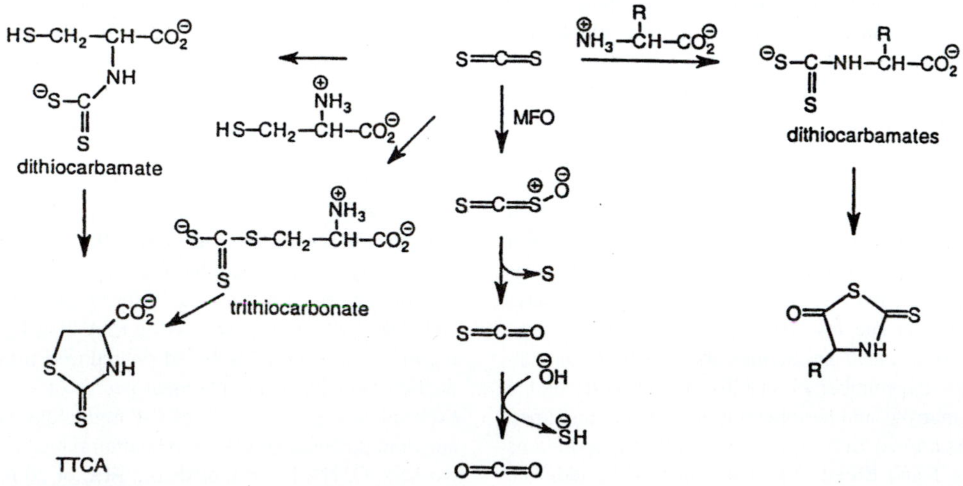

Figure 24-13. Metabolism of carbon disulfide (CS_2).

CS_2 is metabolized by the MFO system to carbonyl sulfide, atomic sulfur and HS^-. Reaction of CS_2 with sulfhydryls of cysteine or GSH yields trithiocarbonates, which can cyclize to form thiazolidine-2-thione-4-carboxylic acid (TTCA). Reaction of CS_2 with amino groups of amino acids results in dithiocarbamate derivatives, which can cyclize to yield 2-thio-5-thiazolidinones; reaction of cysteine amine could also produce TTCA. CS_2 is also metabolized in the liver by P450s to an unstable oxygen intermediate, which spontaneously generates atomic sulfur, carbonyl sulfide (COS), and CO_2. [Reproduced with permission of Graham et al. (1995).]

trophilic CS_2 metabolites with protein nucleophiles (Valentine et al., 1997).

Some epidemiology studies support an association between CS_2 exposure and cardiovascular disease in viscose rayon workers (Sweetnam et al., 1987; Peplonska et al., 1996; Kuo et al., 1997), but others do not (Drexler et al., 1996; Omae et al., 1998). Wronska-Nofer (1979) conducted studies in rats supporting a role for CS_2 in the elevation of blood cholesterol, and more recently Lewis et al. (1999) demonstrated that high doses of CS_2 in mice can induce the early lesions of atherosclerosis. Data were also presented in this study that suggest protein cross-linking may be involved in the atherosclerotic process. Egeland et al. (1992) reported a significant and positive linear trend in elevation of low-density lipoprotein cholesterol and diastolic blood pressure with increasing CS_2 exposure in a group of workers with average 8-h exposures from 0.6 to 11.8 ppm. This study seems contradictory to the conclusion of Price et al. (1997), that an association between CS_2 and ischemic heart disease mortality is meaningful only for workers exposed to extreme levels for many years. The general public may be exposed to low background concentrations of CS_2, as demonstrated by detection of CS_2 in all samples of breath and indoor and outdoor air surveyed in and around New York City (Phillips, 1992).

REFERENCES

Abbate C, Giorgianni C, Munao F, Brecciaroli R: Neurotoxicity induced by exposure to toluene. An electropyhysiologic study. *Int Arch Occup Environ Health* 64:389–392, 1993.

ACGIH (American Conference of Governmental Industrial Hygienists): *1999 TLVs and BEIs. Threshold Limit Values for Chemical Substances and Physical Agents, Biological Exposure Indices.* Cincinnati, OH: ACGIH, 1999.

Aggazzotti G, Fantuzzi G, Righi E, Predieri G: Environmental and biological monitoring of chloroform in indoor swimming pools. *J Chromatogr A* 710:181–190, 1995.

Ahmed FE: Toxicological effects of ethanol on human health. *Crit Rev Toxicol* 25:347–367, 1995.

Albano E, French SW, Ingelman-Sundberg M: Hydroxyethyl radicals in ethanol hepatotoxicity. *Front Biosci* 4:533–540, 1999.

Almekinder JL, Lennard DE, Walmer DK, et al: Toxicity of methoxyacetic acid in cultured human luteal cells. *Fundam Appl Toxicol* 38:191–194, 1997.

Ambroso JL, Stedman DB, Elswick BA, Welsch F: Characterization of cell death induced by 2-methoxyethanol in CD-1 mouse embryos on gestation day 8. *Teratology* 58:231–240, 1998.

Andersen ME: A physiologically based toxicokinetic description of the metabolism of inhaled gases and vapors: Analysis at steady state. *Toxicol Appl Pharmacol* 60:509–526, 1981.

Andersen, ME: Development of physiologically based pharmacokinetic and physiologically based pharmacodynamic models for applications in toxicology and risk assessment. *Toxicol Lett* 79:35–44, 1995.

Andersen, ME: Tissue dosimetry in risk assessment, or What's the problem here anyway? in Gillette JR, Jollow P (Chairs): *Drinking Water and Health.* Vol 8. Washington, DC: National Academy Press, 1987, pp 8–26.

Andersen, ME, Clewell HJ III, Gargas ML, et al: Physiologically based pharmacokinetics and the risk assessment process for methylene chloride. *Toxicol Appl Pharmacol* 87:185–205, 1987.

Andreoli C, Leopardi P, Crebelli R: Detection of DNA damage in human lymphocytes by alkaline single cell gel electrophoresis after exposure to benzene or benzene metabolites. *Mutat Res* 377:95–104, 1997.

Anttila A, Pukkala E, Sallmen M, et al: Cancer incidence among Finnish workers exposed to halogenated hydrocarbons. *J Occup Environ Med* 37:797–806, 1995.

Aranyi C, O'Shea WJ, Halder CA, et al: Absence of hydrocarbon-induced nephropathy in rats exposed subchronically to volatile hydrocarbon mixtures pertinent to gasoline. *Toxicol Ind Health* 2:85–98, 1986.

Arlien-Soborg P: *Solvent Neurotoxicity*. Boca Raton, FL: CRC Press, 1992.

Arlien-Soborg P, Bruhn P, Gyldensted P, Melgaard, B: Chronic painters' syndrome: Chronic toxic encephalopathy in house painters. *Acta Neurol Scand* 60:149–156, 1979.

Ashley DL, Bonin MA, Cardinali FL, et al: Blood concentrations of volatile organic compounds in a nonoccupationally exposed US population and in groups with suspected exposure. *Clin Chem* 40:1401–1404, 1994.

Astrand I: Effect of physical exercise on uptake, distribution and elimination of vapors in man, in Fiserova-Bergerova V (ed): *Modeling of Inhalation Exposure to Vapors: Uptake, Distribution, and Elimination.* Vol II. Boca Raton, FL: CRC Press, 1983, pp 107–130.

ATSDR (Agency for Toxic Substances and Disease Registry). Methanol toxicity. *Am Fam Physician* 47:163–171, 1993.

ATSDR (Agency for Toxic Substances and Disease Registry): *Toxicological Profile for Styrene.* Atlanta, GA: Public Health Service, 1993.

ATSDR (Agency for Toxic Substances and Disease Registry): *Toxicological Profile for Carbon Tetrachloride.* Atlanta, GA: Public Health Service, 1994.

ATSDR (Agency for Toxic Substances and Disease Registry): *Toxicological Profile for Xylenes.* Atlanta, GA: Public Health Service, 1995.

ATSDR (Agency for Toxic Substances and Disease Registry): *Toxicological Profile for Carbon Disulfide.* Atlanta, GA: Public Health Service, 1996a.

ATSDR (Agency for Toxic Substances and Disease Registry): *Toxicological Profile For Methyl T-Butyl Ether.* Atlanta, GA: Public Health Service, 1996b.

ATSDR (Agency for Toxic Substances and Disease Registry): *Toxicological Profile for Benzene.* Atlanta, GA: Public Health Service, 1997a.

ATSDR (Agency for Toxic Substances and Disease Registry): *Toxicological Profile for Chloroform.* Atlanta, GA: Public Health Service, 1997b.

ATSDR (Agency for Toxic Substances and Disease Registry): *Toxicological Profile for Ethylene Glycol and Propylene Glycol.* Atlanta, GA: Public Health Service, 1997c.

ATSDR (Agency for Toxic Substances and Disease Registry): *Toxicological Profile for Tetrachloroethylene.* Atlanta, GA: Public Health Service, 1997d.

ATSDR (Agency for Toxic Substances and Disease Registry): *Toxicological Profile for Trichloroethylene.* Atlanta, GA: Public Health Service, 1997e.

ATSDR (Agency for Toxic Substances and Disease Registry): *Toxicological Profile for Jet Fuels (JP-5 and JP-8).* Atlanta, GA: Public Health Service, 1998a.

ATSDR (Agency for Toxic Substances and Disease Registry): *Toxicological Profile for Methylene Chloride.* Atlanta, GA: Public Health Service, 1998b.

ATSDR (Agency for Toxic Substances and Disease Registry): *Toxicological Profile for Toluene.* Atlanta, GA: Public Health Service, 1998c.

ATSDR (Agency for Toxic Substances and Disease Registry): *Toxicological Profile for Ethylbenzene.* Atlanta, GA: Public Health Service, 1999.

Axelson O, Andersson K, Hogstedt C, et al: A cohort study on trichloroethylene exposure and cancer mortality. *J Occup Med* 20:194–196, 1978.

Axelson O, Hane M, Hogstedt C: A case-referent study of neuropsychiatric disorders among workers exposed to solvents. *Scand J Work Environ Health* 2:14–20, 1976.

Axelson O, Selden A, Andersson K, et al: Updated and expanded Swedish cohort study of trichloroethylene and cancer risk. *J Occup Med* 36:556–562, 1994.

Backes WL, Sequeira DJ, Cawley GF, Eyer CS: Relationship between hydrocarbon structure and induction of P450: Effects on protein levels and enzyme activities. *Xenobiotica* 23:1353–1366, 1993.

Baker RC, Kramer RE: Cytotoxicity of short-chain alcohols. *Annu Rev Pharmacol Toxicol* 39:127–150, 1999.

Balster, RL: Neural basis of inhalant abuse. *Drug Alcohol Dep* 512:207–214, 1998.

Barbash J, Roberts PV: Volatile organic chemical contamination of groundwater resources in the U.S. *J Water Pollut Control Fed* 58:343–348, 1986.

Barton HA, Creech JR, Godin CS, et al: Chloroethylene mixtures: Pharmacokinetic modeling and in vitro metabolism of vinyl chloride, trichloroethylene, and *trans*-1,2-dichloroethylene in rat. *Toxicol Appl Pharmacol* 130:237–247, 1995.

Barton HA, Das S: Alternative for a risk assessment on chronic non-cancer effects from oral exposure to trichloroethylene. *Regul Toxicol Pharmacol* 24:269–285, 1996.

Bautista AP, Spitzer JJ: Role of Kupffer cells in ethanol-induced oxidative stress in the liver. *Front Biosci* 4:589–595, 1999.

Beattie PJ, Welsh MJ, Brabec MJ: The effect of 2-methoxyethanol and methoxyacetic acid on Sertoli cell lactate production and protein synthesis in vitro. *Toxicol Appl Pharmacol* 76:56–61, 1984.

Beauchamp RO, Bus JS, Popp JA, et al: A critical review of the literature on carbon disulfide toxicity. *Crit Rev Toxicol* 11:169–278, 1983.

Bellinger FP, Bedi KS, Wilson P, Wilce PA: Ethanol exposure during the third trimester equivalent results in long-lasting decreased synaptic efficacy but not plasticity in the CA1 region of the rat hippocampus. *Synapse* 31:51–58, 1999.

Belpoggi F, Soffritti M, Filippini F, Maltoni C: Results of long-term experimental studies on the carinogenicity of methyl *tert*-butyl ether. *Ann NY Acad Sci* 837:77–95, 1997.

Bennett GF: Air quality aspects of hazardous waste landfills. *Haz Waste Haz Mater* 4:119–138, 1987.

Bergsagel DE, Wong O, Bergsagel PL, et al: Benzene and multiple myeloma: Appraisal of the scientific evidence. *Blood* 94:1174–1182, 1999.

Bernauer U, Vieth B, Ellrich R, et al: CYP2E1-dependent benzene toxicity: The role of extrahepatic benzene metabolism. *Arch Toxicol* 73: 189–196, 1999.

Bevan C, Neeper-Bradley TL, Tyl RW, et al: Two-generation reproductive toxicity study of methyl tertiary-butyl ether (MTBE) in rats. *J Appl Toxicol* 17(S1):S13–S19, 1997a.

Bevan C, Tyl RW, Neeper-Bradley TL, et al: Developmental toxicity evaluation of methyl tertiary-butyl ether (MTBE) by inhalation in mice and rabbits. *J Appl Toxicol* 17(S1):S21–S29, 1997b.

Bezabeth S, Engel A, Morris CB, Lamm SH: Does benzene cause multiple myeloma? An analysis of the published case-control literature. *Environ Health Perspec* 104(suppl 6):1393–1398, 1996.

Birnbaum LS: Pharmacokinetic basis of age-related changes in sensitivity to toxicants. *Annu Rev Pharmacol* 31:101–128, 1991.

Birner G, Richling C, Henschler D, et al: Metabolism of tetrachloroethylene in rats: Identification of *N*-(dichloroacetyl)-L-cysteine and *N*-(trichloroacetyl)-L-lysine as protein adducts. *Chem Res Toxicol* 7:724–732, 1994.

Blair A, Hartge P, Stewart PA, et al: Mortality and cancer incidence of aircraft maintenance workers exposed to trichloroethylene and other organic solvents and chemicals: Extended follow-up. *Occup Environ Med* 55:161–171, 1998.

Blanco, JG, Harrison PL, Evans WE, Relling MV: Human cytochrome P450 maximal activities in pediatric versus adult liver. *Drug Metab Dispos* 28:379–382, 2000.

Bleecker ML, Bolla KI, Agnew J, et al: Dose-related subclinical neurobehavioral effects of chronic exposure to low levels of organic solvents. *Am J Ind Med* 19:715–728, 1991.

Boffeta P, Garfinkel L: Alcohol drinking and mortality among men enrolled in an American Cancer Society prospective study. *Epidemiology* 1:342–348, 1990.

Boice JD, Marano DE, Fryzek JP, et al: Mortality among aircraft manufacturing workers. *Occup Environ Med* 56:581–597, 1999.

Boogaard PJ, van Sittert NJ: Suitability of *S*-phenylmercapturic acid and *trans-trans*-muconic acid as biomarkers for exposure to low concentrations of benzene. *Environ Health Perspec* 104 (suppl 6):1151–1157, 1996.

Borak J, Pastides H, Van Ert M, et al: Exposure to MTBE and acute human health effects: A critical literature review. *Hum Ecol Assess* 4:177–200, 1998.

Boutelet-Bochan H, Huang Y, Juchau MR: Expression of CYP2E1 during embryogenesis and fetogenesis in human cephalic tissues: Implications for the fetal alcohol syndrome. *Biochem Biophys Res Commun* 238:443–447, 1997.

Brauch H, Weirich G, Hornauer MA, et al: Trichloroethylene exposure and specific somatic mutations in patients with renal cell carcinoma. *J Natl Cancer Inst* 91:854–861, 1999.

Brophy PD, Tenebein M, Gardner J, et al: Childhood diethylene glycol poisoning treated with alcohol dehydrogenase inhibitor Fomepizole and hemodialysis. *Am J Kidney Dis* 35:958–962, 2000.

Brown-Woodman, PDC, Hayes LC, Huq F, et al: In vitro assessment of the effect of halogenated hydrocarbons: Chloroform, dichloromethane, and dibromoethane on embryonic development of the rat. *Teratology* 57:321–333, 1998.

Bruckner, JV: Differences in sensitivity of children and adults to chemical toxicity: The NAS panel report. *Reg Toxicol Pharmacol* 31:280–285, 2000.

Bruckner JV, Davis BD, Blancato JN: Metabolism, toxicity, and carcinogenicity of trichloroethylene. *Crit Rev Toxicol* 20:30–51, 1989.

Bruckner JV, Peterson RG: Evaluation of toluene and acetone inhalant abuse. I. Pharmacology and pharmacodynamics. *Toxicol Appl Pharmacol* 61:27–38, 1981.

Bruckner JV, Weil WB: Biological factors which may influence an older child's or adolescent's responses to toxic chemicals. *Reg Toxicol Pharmacol* 29:158–164, 1999.

Bruckner JV, Ramanathan R, Lee KM, Muralidhara S: Mechanisms of circadian rhythmicity of carbon tetrachloride hepatotoxicity. *J Pharmacol Exp Ther* 2001. In press.

Bruner RH, Kinkead ER, O'Neill TP, et al: The toxicologic and oncogenic potential of JP-4 jet fuel vapors in rats and mice: 12-Month intermittent inhalation exposures. *Fundam Appl Toxicol* 20:97–110, 1993.

Bruning T, Bolt HM: Renal toxicity and carcinogenicity of trichloroethylene: Key results, mechanisms, and controversies. *Crit Rev Toxicol* 30:253–285, 2000.

Bruning T, Golka K, Makropoulos V, Bolt HM: Preexistence of chronic tubular damage in cases of renal cell cancer after long and high exposure to trichloroethylene. *Arch Toxicol* 70:259–260, 1996.

Bruning T, Lammert M, Kempkes M, et al: Influence of polymorphisms of GSTM1 and GSTT1 for risk of renal cell cancer in workers with long-term high occupational exposure to trichloroethene. *Arch Toxicol* 71: 596–599, 1997b.

Bruning T, Mann H, Melzer H, et al: Pathological excretion patterns of urinary proteins in renal cell cancer patients exposed to trichloroethylene. *Occup Med* 49:299–305, 1999.

Bruning T, Weirich G, Hornauer MA, et al: Renal cell carcinomas in trichloroethene (TRI) exposed persons are associated with somatic mutations in the von Hippel-Lindau (VHL) tumour suppressor gene. *Arch Toxicol* 71:332–335, 1997a.

Bull RJ: Mode of action of liver tumor induction by trichloroethylene and its metabolites, trichloroacetate and dichloroacetate. *Environ Health Perspect* 108(suppl 2):241–259, 2000.

Burek JD, Nitschke KD, Bell TJ, et al: Methylene chloride: A two-year inhalation toxicity and oncogenicity study in rats and hamsters. *Fund Appl Toxicol* 4:30–47, 1984.

Burleigh-Flayer HD, Chun JS, Kintigh WJ: *Methyl tertiary butyl ether: Vapor Inhalation Oncogenicity Study in CD Mice*. Export, PA: Bushy Run Research Center, 1992.

Caldemeyer KS, Armstrong SW, George KK, et al: The spectrum of neuroimaging abnormalities in solvent abuse and their clinical correlation. *J Neuroimaging* 6:167–173, 1996.

Camargo CA Jr: Case-control and cohort studies of moderate alcohol consumption and stroke. *Clin Chim Acta* 246:107–119, 1996.

Caprino L, Togna GI: Potential health effects of gasoline and its constituents: A review of current literature (1990–1997) on toxicological data. *Environ Health Perspect* 106:115–125, 1998.

Carney EW, Crissman JW, Liberacki AB, et al: Assessment of adult and neonatal reproductive parameters in Sprague-Dawley rats exposed to propylene glycol monomethyl ether vapors for two generations. *Toxicol Sci* 50:249–258, 1999a.

Carney EW, Freshour NL, Dittenber DA, Dryzga MD: Ethylene glycol developmental toxicity: Unraveling the roles of glycolic acid and metabolic acidosis. *Toxicol Sci* 50:117–126, 1999b.

Casanova M, Bell DA, Heck H d'A: Dichloromethane metabolism to formaldehyde and reaction of formaldehyde with nucleic acids in hepatocytes of rodents and humans with and without glutathione S-transferase *T1* and *M1* genes. *Fund Appl Toxicol* 37:168–180, 1997.

Casanova M, Conolly RB, Heck H d'A: DNA-protein cross-links (DPX) and cell proliferation in B6C3F1 mice but not Syrian golden hamsters exposed to dichloromethane: Pharmacokinetics and risk assessment with DPX as dosimeter. *Fund Appl Toxicol* 31:103–116, 1996.

Casanova M, Heck H d'A: Lack of evidence for the involvement of formaldehyde in the hepatocarcinogenicity of methyl *tertiary*-butyl ether in CD-1 mice. *Chem Biol Interact* 105:131–143, 1997.

Castillo T, Koop DR, Kamimura S, et al: Role of cytochrome P-450 2E1 in ethanol-, carbon tetrachloride- and iron-dependent microsomal lipid peroxidation. *Hepatology* 16:992–996, 1992.

Charbonneau M, Swenberg JA: Studies on the biochemical mechanism of α_{2u}-globulin nephropathy in rats. *CIIT Activities* 8:1–5, 1988.

Cherry NH, Hutchins H, Pace T, Waldron JA: Neurobehavioral effects of repeated occupational exposure to toluene and paint solvents. *Br J Ind Med* 42:291–300, 1985.

Christopher MM, Eckfeldt JH, Eaton JW: Propylene glycol ingestion causes D-lactic acidosis. *Lab Invest* 62:114–118, 1990.

Chun JS, Burleigh-Flayer HD, Kintigh WJ: *Methyl tertiary butyl ether: Vapor Inhalation Oncogenicity Study in Fisher 344 Rats*. Export, PA: Bushy Run Research Center, 1992.

Clayton CA, Pellizzari ED, Whitmore RW, et al: National Human Exposure Assessment Survey (NHEXAS): Distributions and associations of lead, arsenic and volatile organic compounds in EPA Region 5. *J Expos Anal Environ Epidemiol* 9:381–392, 1999.

Clewell HJ, Gentry PR, Covington TR, Gearhart JM: Development of a physiologically based pharmacokinetic model of trichloroethylene and its metabolites for use in risk assessment. *Environ Health Perspect* 108(suppl 2):283–305, 2000.

Cody RJ: Physiological changes due to age. Implications for drug therapy of congestive heart failure. *Drugs Aging* 3:320–334, 1993.

Comba ME, Palabrica VS, Kaiser KLE: Volatile halocarbons as tracers of pulp mill effluent plumes. *Environ Toxicol Chem* 13:1065–1074, 1994.

Conolly RB, Andersen ME: Biologically based pharmacodynamic models: Tools for toxicological research and risk assessment. *Annu Rev Pharmacol Toxicol* 31:503–523, 1991.

Constan AA, Sprankle CS, Peters JM, et al: Metabolism of chloroform by cytochrome P4502E1 is required for induction of toxicity in the liver, kidney, and nose of male mice. *Toxicol Appl Pharmacol* 160:120–126, 1999.

Cooper AJL: Enzymology of cysteine *S*-conjugate β-lyases. *Adv Pharmacol* 27:71–113, 1994.

Cooper JR, Mattie DR: Developmental toxicity of JP-8 jet fuel in the rat. *J Appl Toxicol* 16:197–200, 1996.

Cordier S, Bergeret A, Goujard J, et al: Congenital malformations and maternal occupational exposure to glycol ethers. *Epidemiology* 8:355–363, 1997.

Corley RA, Markham DA, Banks C, et al: Physiologically based pharmacokinetics and the dermal absorption of 2-butoxyethanol vapor by humans. *Fundam Appl Toxicol* 39:120–130, 1997.

Costa ET, Savage DD, Valenzuela CF: A review of the effects of prenatal or early postnatal ethanol exposure on brain ligand-gated ion channels. *Alcohol Clin Exp Res* 24:706–715, 2000.

Cox C, Lowry LK, Que Hee SS: Urinary 2-thiothiazolidine-4-carboxylic acid as a biological indicator of exposure to carbon disulfide: Derivation of a biological exposure index. *Appl Occup Environ Hyg* 7:672–676, 1992.

Cranmer JM: Proceedings of the workshop on neurobehavioral effects of solvents. *Neurotoxicology* 7:1–95, 1986.

Creasy DM, Foster PMD: The morphological development of glycol ether-induced testicular atrophy in the rat. *Exp Mol Pathol* 40:169–176, 1984.

Creek MR, Mani C, Vogel JS, Turteltaub KW: Tissue distribution and macromolecular binding of extremely low doses of [^{14}C]-benzene in B6C3F1 mice. *Carcinogenesis* 18:2421–2427, 1997.

Cresteil T: Onset of xenobiotic metabolism in children: Toxicological implications. *Food Add Contam* 15(suppl.):45–51, 1998.

Crom WR, Glynn-Barnhart AM, Rodman JH, et al: Pharmacokinetics of anticancer drugs in children. *Clin Pharmacokinet* 12:168–213, 1987.

Cruz SL, Mirshahi T, Thomas B, et al: Effects of the abused solvent toluene on recombinant *N*-methyl-D-aspartate and non-*N*-methyl-D-aspartate receptors expressed in *Xenopus* oocytes. *J Pharmacol Exp Ther* 286:334–340, 1998.

Cruzan CG, Cushman JR, Andrews LS, et al: Chronic toxicity/oncogenicity study of styrene in CD rats by inhalation exposure for 104 weeks. *Toxicol Sci* 46:266–281, 1998.

Dai Y, Rashba-Step J, Cederbaum AI: Stable expression of human cytochrome P4502E1 in HepG2 cells: Characterization of catalytic activities and production of reactive oxygen intermediates. *Biochemistry* 32:6928–6937, 1993.

d'Alessandro A, Osterloh JD, Chuwers P, et al: Formate in serum and urine after controlled methanol exposure at the threshold limit value. *Environ Health Perspect* 102:178–181, 1994.

Daly AK, Cholerton S, Gregory W, Idle JR: Metabolic polymorphisms. *Pharmacol Ther* 57:129–160, 1993.

Dankovic, DA, Bailer AJ: The impact of exercise and intersubject variability on dose estimates for dichloromethane derived from a physiologically based pharmacokinetic model. *Fund Appl Toxicol* 22:20–25, 1994.

Daughtrey WC, Gill MW, Pritts IM, et al: Neurotoxicological evaluation of methyl tertiary-butyl ether in rats. *J Appl Toxicol* 17(S1):S57–S64, 1997.

Davis ME: Dichloroacetic acid and trichloroacetic acid increase chloroform toxicity. *J Toxicol Environ Health* 37:139–148, 1992.

Dawling S, Crome P: Clinical pharmacokinetic considerations in the elderly. An update. *Clin Pharmacokinet* 17:236–263, 1989.

Dell LD, Mundt KA, McDonald M, et al: Critical review of the epidemiology literature on the potential cancer risks of methylene chloride. *Int Arch Occup Environ Health* 72:429–442, 1999.

DePass LR, Garman RH, Woodside MD, et al: Chronic toxicity and oncogenicity studies of ethylene glycol in rats and mice. *Fund Appl Toxicol* 7:547–565, 1986.

Dietrich DR, Swenberg JA: NCI-Black-Reiter (NBR) male rats fail to develop renal disease following exposure to agents that induce α-2u-globulin (α_{2u}) nephropathy. *Fund Appl Toxicol* 16:749–762, 1991.

Dinwiddie SH: Abuse of inhalants: A review. *Addiction* 89:925–939, 1994.

DiVincenzo GD, Kaplan CJ: Uptake, metabolism, and elimination of methylene chloride vapor by humans. *Toxicol Appl Pharmacol* 59:130–140, 1981.

Done AK: Developmental pharmacology. *Clin Pharmacol Ther* 5:432–479, 1964.

Drexler H, Ulm K, Hardt R, et al: Carbon disulphide: IV. Cardiovascular function in workers in the viscose industry. *Int Arch Occup Environ Health* 69:27–32, 1996.

Edwards MJ, Keller BJ, Kauffman FC, Thurman RG: The involvement of Kupffer cells in carbon tetrachloride toxicity. *Toxicol Appl Pharmacol* 119:275–279, 1993.

Eells JT, Salzman MM, Lewandowski MR, Murray TG: Formate-induced alterations in retinal function in methanol-intoxicated rats. *Toxicol Appl Pharmacol* 140:58–69, 1996.

Egbert PA, Abraham K: Ethylene glycol intoxication: Pathophysiology, diagnosis, and emergency management. *ANNA J* 26:295–302, 1999.

Egeland GM, Burkhart GA, Schnorr TM, et al: Effects of exposure to carbon disulphide on low density lipoprotein cholesterol concentration and diastolic blood pressure. *Br J Ind Med* 49:287–293, 1992.

Elliot BM, Ashby J: Review of the genotoxicity of 2-butoxyethanol. *Mutat Res* 387:89–96, 1997.

El-Masri HA, Bell DA, Portier CJ: Effects of glutathione transferase theta polymorphism on the risk estimates of dichloromethane to humans. *Toxicol Appl Pharmacol* 158:221–230, 1999.

Elston AC, Bayliss MK, Park GR: Effect of renal failure on drug metabolism by the liver. *Br J Anaesth* 71:282–290, 1993.

Engelke M, Tahti H, Vaalavirta L: Perturbation of artificial and biological membranes by organic compounds of aliphatic, alicyclic and aromatic structure. *Toxicol in Vitro* 10:111–115, 1996.

EPA (U.S. Environmental Protection Agency): Memorandum from Joan S. Dollarhide, Associate Director, Surperfund Health Risk Technical Support Center, Chemical Mixtures Assessment Branch to Carol Sweeney, U.S. EPA, Region X. Subject: Oral Reference Doses and Oral Slope Factors for JP-4, JP-5, and Gasoline. March 24, 1992.

EPA (U.S. Environmental Protection Agency). *Proposed Guidelines for Carcinogen Risk Assessment*. Office of Research and Development. NCEA-F-0644, 1999.

EPA (U.S. Environmental Protection Agency): *Drinking Water Advisory: Consumer Acceptability Advice and Health Effects Analysis on Methyl Tertiary-Butyl Ether (MtBE).* Washington, DC: Office of Water, December 1997.

EPA (U.S. Environmental Protection Agency): *Risk Assessment Guidance for Superfund*. Vol. I. *Human Health Evaluation Manual Supplemental Guidance, Dermal Risk Assessment, Interim Guidance.* Washington, DC: Office of Emergency and Remedial Response, 1998.

EPA (U.S. Environmental Protection Agency): *Draft Trichloroethylene Health Risk Assessment*. Vol. 2. *Synthesis and Characterization*. Washington, DC: National Center for Environmental Assessment, 1999a.

EPA (U.S. Environmental Protection Agency): *Draft Risk Assessment Issue Paper for: Revised Update Quantifying the Uncertainty Bounding the Inhalation Unit Risk for Tetrachloroethylene.* Report 99-003/04-07-99. Cincinnati, OH: Prepared for the Superfund Technical Support Center, 1999b.

EPA (U.S. Environmental Protection Agency): *Toxicological Review for 1,3-Dichloropropene.* Review Draft. Washington, DC: IRIS, 1999c.

EPA (U.S. Environmental Protection Agency): On-line Integrated Risk Information System (IRIS) Substance file—carbon disulfide. Washington, DC: May 20, 2000. http://www.epa.gov/iris/subst/0217.htm

Erdal S, Gong H, Linn WS, Rykowski R: Projection of health benefits from ambient ozone reduction related to the use of methyl tertiary butyl ether (MTBE) in the reformulated gasoline program. *Risk Anal* 17:693–704, 1997.

Eschenbrenner AB, Miller E: Induction of hepatomas in mice by repeated oral administration of chloroform, with observations on sex differences. *J Natl Cancer Inst* 5:251–255, 1945.

Exon JH, Mather GG, Bussiere JL: Effects of subchronic exposure of rats to 2-methoxyethanol of 2-butoxyethanol: Thymic atrophy and immunotoxicity. *Fundam Appl Toxicol* 16:830–840, 1991.

Fay, RM, Mumtaz MM: Development of a priority list of chemical mixtures occurring at 1188 hazardous waste sites, using the HazDat database. *Food Chem Toxicol* 34:1163–1165, 1996.

Filley CM, Heaton RK, Rosenberg NL: White matter dementia in chronic toluene abuse. *Neurology* 40:532–534, 1990.

Fisher JW: Physiologically based pharmacokinetic models for trichloroethylene and its oxidative metabolites. *Environ Health Perspect* 108 (suppl 2):265–273, 2000.

Fitzhugh OG, Nelson AA: Comparison of the chronic toxicity of triethylene glycol with that of diethylene glycol. *J Ind Hyg Toxicol* 28:40–43, 1946.

Folland DS, Schaffner W, Ginn EH, et al: Carbon tetrachloride toxicity potentiated by isopropyl alcohol. *JAMA* 236:1853–1856, 1976.

Foo SC, Jeyaratnam J, Koh D: Chronic neurobehavioral effects of toluene. *Br J Ind Med* 47:480–484, 1990.

Fortenberry JD: Gasoline sniffing. *Am J Med* 79:740–744, 1985.

Frantz SW, Beskitt JL, Grosse CM, et al: Pharmacokinetics of ethylene glycol II. Tissue distribution, dose-dependent elimination, and identification of urinary metabolites following single intravenous, peroral or percutaneous doses in female Sprague-Dawley rats and CD-1 mice. *Xenobiotica* 26:1195–1220, 1996.

Frezza M, di Padova C, Pozzato G, et al: High blood alcohol levels in women. The role of decreased gastric alcohol dehydrogenase activity and first-pass metabolism. *N Engl J Med* 322:95–99, 1990.

Furukawa T, Manabe S, Watanabe T, et al: Sex differences in the daily rhythm of hepatic P450 monooxygenase activities in rats is regulated by growth hormone release. *Toxicol Appl Pharmacol* 161:219–224, 1999.

Gade A, Mortensen EL, Bruhn P: "Chronic painter's syndrome." A reanalysis of psychological test data in a group of diagnosed cases, based on comparisons with matched controls. *Acta Neurol Scand* 77:293–306, 1988.

Garetano G, Gochfeld M: Factors affecting tetrachloroethylene concentrations in residences above dry cleaning establishments. *Arch Environ Health* 55:59–68, 2000.

Gargas ML, Burgess RJ, Voisard, DE, et al: Partition coefficients of low-molecular-weight volatile chemicals in various liquids and tissues. *Toxicol Appl Pharmacol* 98:87–99, 1989.

Gargas ML, Tyler TR, Sweeney LM, et al: A toxicokinetic study of inhaled ethylene glycol monomethyl ether (2-ME) and validation of a physiologically based pharmacokinetic model for the pregnant rat and human. *Toxicol Appl Pharmacol* 165:53–62, 2000a.

Gargas ML, Tyler TR, Sweeney LM, et al: A toxicokinetic study of inhaled ethylene glycol ethyl ether acetate and validation of a physiologically based pharmacokinetic model for rat and human. *Toxicol Appl Pharmacol* 165:63–73, 2000b.

Garner CD, Lee EW, Louis-Ferdinand RT: Muller cell involvement in methanol-induced retinal toxicity. *Toxicol Appl Pharmacol* 130:101–107, 1995a.

Garner CD, Lee EW, Terzo TS, Louis-Ferdinand RT: Role of retinal metabolism in methanol-induced retinal toxicity. *J Toxicol Environ Health* 44:43–56, 1995b.

Gerr F, Letz R: Organic solvents, in Rom WD (ed): *Environmental and Occupational Medicine,* 3rd ed. Philadelphia: Lippincott-Raven, 1998, pp 1091–1108.

Ghanayem BI: Metabolic and cellular basis of 2-butoxyethanol-induced hemolytic anemia in rats and assessment of human risk in vitro. *Biochem Pharmacol* 38:1679–1684, 1989.

Ghanayem BI, Burka LT, Matthews HB: Metabolic basis of ethylene glycol monobutyl ether (2-butoxyethanol) toxicity: Role of alcohol and aldehyde dehydrogenases. *J Pharmacol Exp Ther* 242:222–231, 1987.

Ghanayem BI, Burka LT, Matthews HB: Structure-activity relationships for the *in vitro* hematotoxicity of *n*-alkoxyacetic acids, toxic metabolites of glycol ethers. *Chem Biol Interact* 70:339–352, 1989.

Ghanayem BI, Chapin RE: Calcium channel blockers protect against ethylene glycol monomethyl ether (2-methoxyethanol)-induced testicular toxicity. *Exp Mol Pathol* 52:279–290, 1990.

Gibbs BF, Mulligan CN: Styrene toxicity: An ecotoxicological assessment. *Ecotoxicol Environ Saf* 38:181–194, 1997.

Gibbs GW, Amsel J, Soden K: A cohort mortality study of cellulose triacetate-fiber workers exposed to methylene chloride. *J Occup Environ Med* 38:693–697, 1996.

Gilger AP, Potts AM: Studies on the visual toxicity of methanol: V. The role of acidosis in experimental methanol poisoning. *Am J Ophthalmol* 39:63–86, 1955.

Gleiter CH, Gundert-Remy U: Gender differences in pharmacokinetics. *Eur J Drug Metab Pharmacokinet* 21:123–128, 1996.

Glende EA Jr, Recknagel RO: Phospholipase A_2 activation and cell injury in isolated rat hepatocytes exposed to bromotrichloromethane, chloroform and 1,1-dichloroethylene as compared to effects of carbon tetrachloride. *Toxicol Appl Pharmacol* 113:159–162, 1992.

Glover ML, Reed MD: Propylene glycol: The safe diluent that continues to cause harm. *Pharmacotherapy* 16:690–693, 1996.

Golden RJ, Holm SE, Robinson DE, et al: Chloroform mode of action: Implications for cancer risk assessment. *Reg Toxicol Pharmacol* 26:142–155, 1997.

Goldenthal EI: A compilation of LD50 values in newborn and adult animals. *Toxicol Appl Pharmacol* 18:185–207, 1971.

Golding BT, Watson WP: Possible mechanisms of carcinogenesis after exposure to benzene, in Singer B, Bartsch H (eds): *Exocyclic DNA Adducts in Mutagenesis and Carcinogenesis*. IARC Publ No. 150. Lyons, France: ARC, 1999, pp 75–88.

Goldstein A, Aronow L, Kalman, SM: Kinetics of the uptake and distribution of drugs administered by inhalation, in Pratt WB, Taylor P (eds): *Principles of Drug Action. The Basis of Pharmacology,* 2nd ed. New York: Wiley, 1974, pp 338–355.

Gonzalez FJ, Gelboin HV: Role of human cytochromes P450 in the metabolic activation of chemical carcinogens and toxins. *Drug Metab Rev* 26:165–183, 1994.

Gordon SM, Callahan PJ, Nishioka MG, et al: Residential environmental measurements in the National Human Exposure Assessment Survery (NHEXAS) pilot study in Arizona: Preliminary results for pesticides and VOCs. *J Expos Anal Environ Epidemiol* 9:456–470, 1999.

Gottfried MR, Graham DG, Morgan M, et al: The morphology of carbon disulfide neurotoxicity. *Neurotoxicology* 6:89–96, 1985.

Graham DG, Amarnath V, Valentine WM, et al: Pathogenetic studies of hexane and carbon disulfide neurotoxicity. *Crit Rev Toxicol* 25:91–112, 1995.

Grassman JA, Kimmel CA, Neumann DA: Accounting for variability in responsiveness in human risk assessment, in Neumann DA, Kimmel CA (eds): *Human Variability in Response to Chemical Exposures.* Washington, DC: International Life Sciences Institute, 1998, pp 1–26.

Graves RJ, Coutts C, Green T: Methylene chloride-induced DNA damage: An interspecies comparison. *Carcinogenesis* 16:1919–1926, 1995.

Green LC, Lash TL: Renal cell cancer correlated with occupational exposure to trichloroethylene. *J Cancer Res Clin Oncol* 125:430–432, 1999.

Green T: Methylene chloride induced mouse liver and lung tumors: An overview of the role of mechanistic studies in human safety assessment. *Hum Exp Toxicol* 16:3–13, 1997.

Green T: Pulmonary toxicity and carcinogenicity of trichloroethylene: Species differences and modes of action. *Environ Health Perspect* 108(suppl 2):261–264, 2000.

Green T, Odum J, Nash JA, et al: Perchloroethylene-induced rat kidney tumors: An investigation of the mechanisms involved and their relevance to humans. *Toxicol Appl Pharmacol* 103:77–89, 1990.

Gries J-M, Benowitz N, Verotta D: Chronopharmacokinetics of nicotine. *Clinical Pharmacol Ther* 60:385–395, 1996.

Guastadisegni C, Balduzzi M, Mancuso MT, Di Consiglio E: Liver mitochondria alterations in chloroform-treated Sprague-Dawley rats. *J Toxicol Environ Health* 57:415–429, 1999.

Guengerich FP, Kim DH, Iwasaki M: Role of human cytochrome P-450 IIE1 in the oxidation of many low molecular weight cancer suspects. *Chem Res Toxicol* 4:168–179, 1991.

Gut I, Terelius Y, Frantik E, et al: Exposure to various benzene derivatives differently induces cytochromes P450 2B1 and P450 2E1 in rat liver. *Arch Toxicol* 67:237–243, 1993.

Halder CA, Holdsworth CE, Cockrell BY, Piccirillo VJ: Hydrocarbon nephropathy in male rats: Identification of the nephrotoxic components of unleaded gasoline. *Toxicol Ind Health* 1:67–87, 1985.

Halder CA, Van Gorp GS, Hatoum NS, Warne TM: Gasoline vapor exposures. Part II. Evaluation of the nephrotoxicity of the major C_4/C_5 hydrocarbon components. *Am Ind Hyg Assoc J* 47:173–175, 1986.

Hard GC, Boorman GA, Wolf DC: Re-evaluation of the 2-year chloroform drinking water carcinogenicity bioassay in Osborne-Mendel rats supports chronic renal tubule injury as the mode of action underlying the renal tumor response. *Toxicol Sci* 53:237–244, 2000.

Hardin BD, Goad PT, Burg JR: Developmental toxicity of diethylene glycol monomethyl ether (diEGME). *Fundam Appl Toxicol* 6:430–439, 1986.

Harris DT, Sakiestewa D, Robledo RF, Witten M: Immunotoxicological effects of JP-8 jet fuel exposure. *Toxicol Ind Health* 13:43–55, 1997a.

Harris DT, Sakiestewa D, Robledo RF, Witten M: Short-term exposure to JP-8 jet fuel results in long-term immunotoxicity. *Toxicol Ind Health* 13:559–570, 1997b.

Harris DT, Sakiestewa D, Robledo RF, Witten M: Protection from JP-8 jet fuel induced immunotoxicity by administration of aerosolized substance P. *Toxicol Ind Health* 13:571–588, 1997c.

Harris DT, Sakiestewa D, Robledo RF, et al: Effects of short-term JP-8 jet fuel exposure on cell-mediated immunity. *Toxicol Ind Health* 16:78–84, 2000.

Harry GJ, Graham DG, Valentine WM, et al: Carbon disulfide neurotoxicity in rats: VIII. Summary. *Neurotoxicology* 19:159–162, 1998.

Hattis D, Erdreich L, Ballew M: Human variability in susceptibility to toxic chemicals—A preliminary analysis of pharmacokinetic data from normal volunteers. *Risk Anal* 7:415–426, 1987.

Hearne FT, Pifer JW, Grose F: Absence of adverse mortality effects in workers exposed to methylene chloride: An update. *J Occup Med* 32:234–240, 1990.

Heilmair R, Lenk W, Lohr D: Toxicokinetics of diethylene glycol (DEG) in the rat. *Arch Toxicol* 67:655–666, 1993.

Hein K: The use of therapeutics in adolescence. *J Adoles Health Care* 8:8–35, 1987.

Heindel JJ, Gulati DK, Russell VS, et al: Assessment of ethylene glycol monobutyl and monophenyl ether reproductive toxicity using a continuous breeding protocol in Swiss CD-1 mice. *Fund Appl Toxicol* 15:683–696, 1990.

Hellwig J, Klimisch H-J, Jackh R: Investigation of the prenatal toxicity of orally administered diethylene glycol in rabbits. *Fund Appl Toxicol* 28:27–33, 1995.

Henderson GI, Chen JJ, Schenker S: Ethanol, oxidative stress, reactive aldehydes, and the fetus. *Front Biosci* 4:D541–D550, 1999.

Henderson RF: Species differences in the metabolism of benzene. *Environ Health Perspect* 104(suppl 6):1173–1175, 1996.

Henschler D, Vamvakas S, Lammert M, et al: Increased incidence of renal cell tumors in a cohort of cardboard workers exposed to trichloroethene. *Arch Toxicol* 69:291–299, 1995.

Hillbom M: Oxidants, antioxidants, alcohol and stroke. *Front Biosci* 4:67–71, 1999.

Hiraku Y, Kawanishi S: Oxidative DNA damage and apoptosis induced by benzene metabolites. *Cancer Res* 56:5172–5178, 1996.

Hoflack J-C, Vasseur P, Poirier GG: Glycol ethers induce death and necrosis in human leukemia cells. *Biochem Cell Biol* 75:415–425, 1997.

Huff JE, Haseman JK, DeMarini DM, et al: Multiple-site carcinogenicity of benzene in Fischer 344 rats and B6C3F1 mice. *Environ Health Perspect* 82:125–163, 1989.

Hunter AGW, Thompson D, Evans JA: Is there a fetal gasoline syndrome? *Teratology* 20:75–80, 1979.

IARC (International Agency for Research on Cancer): *IARC Monographs on the Evaluation of Carcinogenic Risks to Humans: Alcohol Drinking.* Vol 44. Lyons, France: World Health Organization, 1988, pp 251–259.

IARC (International Agency for Research on Cancer): *IARC Monographs on the Evaluation of Carcinogenic Risks to Humans. Occupational Exposures in Petroleum Refining: Crude Oil and Major Petroleum Fuels.* Vol 45. Lyons, France: World Health Organization, 1989.

IARC (International Agency for Research on Cancer): *IARC Monographs on the Evaluation of Carcinogenic Risks to Humans. Drycleaning, Some Chlorinated Solvents, and Other Industrial Chemicals.* Vol 63. Lyons, France: World Health Organization, 1995.

IARC (International Agency for Research on Cancer): *IARC Monographs on the Evaluation of Carcinogenic Risks to Humans. Some Chemicals That Cause Tumours of the Kidney or Urinary Bladder in Rodents and Some Other Substances.* Vol 73. Lyons, France: World Health Organization, 1999.

Ikonomidou C, Bittigau P, Ishimaru MJ, et al: Ethanol-induced apoptotic neurodegeneration and fetal alcohol syndrome. *Science* 287:1056–1060, 2000.

ILSI (International Life Sciences Institute): Characterization of similarities and differences, Part 1, in Guzelian PS, Henry CJ, Olin SS (eds): *Similarities and Differences Between Children and Adults:Implications for Risk Assessment.* Washington, DC: ILSI Press, 1992.

Ingelman-Sundberg M, Johansson I, Persson I, et al: Genetic polymorphism of cytochrome P450. Functional consequences and possible relationship to disease and alcohol toxicity, in Jansson B, Jornvall H, Rydberg U, et al (eds): *Toward a Molecular Basis of Alcohol Use and Abuse.* Basel, Switzerland: Birkhauser Verlag, 1994, pp 197–207.

Inoue, O, Seiji K, Watanabe T, et al: Mutual metabolic suppression between benzene and toluene in man. *Int Arch Occup Environ Health* 60:15–20, 1988.

Jacobsen D, Ovrebo S, Ostborg J, Sejersted OM: Glycolate causes the acidosis in ethylene glycol poisoning and is effectively removed by hemodialysis. *Acta Med Scand* 216:409–416, 1984.

Jan CR, Chen LW, Lin MW: Ca(2+) mobilization evoked by chloroform in Madin-Darby canine kidney cells. *J Pharmacol Exp Ther* 292:995–1001, 2000.

Jansson B, Jornvall H, Rydberg U, et al (eds): *Toward a Molecular Basis of Alcohol Use and Abuse.* Basel, Switzerland: Birkhauser Verlag, 1994, pp 197–207.

Johanson G, Filser JG: Experimental data from closed chamber gas uptake studies in rodents suggest lower uptake rate of chemical than calculated from literature values on alveolar ventilation. *Arch Toxicol* 66:291–295, 1992.

Johlin FC, Swain E, Smith C, Tephly TR: Studies on the mechanism of methanol poisoning: Purification and comparison of rat and human liver 10-formyltetrahydrofolate dehydrogenase. *Mol Pharmacol* 35:745–750, 1989.

Jorgenson TA, Meierhenry EF, Rushbrook CJ, et al: Carcinogenicity of chloroform in drinking water to male Osborne-Mendel rats and female B6C3F1 mice. *Fund Appl Toxicol* 5:760–769, 1985.

Kaneko T, Wang P-Y, Sato A: Enzymes induced by ethanol differently affect the pharmacokinetics of trichloroethylene and 1,1,1-trichloroethane. *Occup Environ Med* 51:113–119, 1994.

Kavet R, Nauss KM: The toxicity of inhaled methanol vapors. *Crit Rev Toxicol* 21:21–50, 1990.

Kawamoto T, Koga M, Murata K, et al: Effects of ALDH2, CYP1A1, and CYP2E1 genetic polymorphisms and smoking and drinking habits on toluene metabolism in humans. *Toxicol Appl Pharmacol* 133:295–304, 1995.

Kearney CA, Dunham DB: Gasoline vapor exposures at a high volume service station. *Am Ind Hyg Assoc J* 47:535–539, 1986.

Kegelmeyer AE, Sprankle CS, Horesovsky GJ, Butterworth BE: Differential display identified changes in mRNA levels in regenerating livers from chloroform-treated mice. *Mol Carcinogen* 20:288–297, 1997.

Kelly TJ, Callahan PJ, Pleil J, Evans GF: Method development and field measurements for polar volatile organic compounds in ambient air. *Environ Sci Technol* 27:1146–1152, 1993.

Kenyon EM, Kraichely RE, Hudson KT, Medinsky MA: Differences in rates of benzene metabolism correlate with observed genotoxicity. *Toxicol Appl Pharmacol* 136:49–56, 1996.

Kilburn KH: *Chemical Brain Injury.* New York: Van Nostrand Reinhold, 1998.

Kim B-S, Smialowicz RJ: The role of metabolism in 2-methoxyethanol-induced suppression of in vitro polyclonal antibody responses by rat and mouse lymphocytes. *Toxicology* 123:227–239, 1997.

Kim HJ, Bruckner JV, Dallas CE, Gallo JM: Effect of dosing vehicles on the pharmacokinetics of orally administered carbon tetrachloride in rats. *Toxicol Appl Pharmacol* 102:50–60, 1990b.

Kim HJ, Oden'hal S, Bruckner JV: Effect of oral dosing vehicles on the acute hepatotoxicity of carbon tetrachloride in rats. *Toxicol Appl Pharmacol* 102:34–49, 1990a.

Kinkead ER, Salins SA, Wolfe RE: Acute irritation and sensitization potential of JP-8 jet fuel. *J Am Col Toxicol* 11:700, 1992.

Klaassen CD, Plaa GL: Relative effects of various chlorinated hydrocarbons on liver and kidney function in mice. *Toxicol Appl Pharmacol* 9:139–151, 1966.

Klaunig JE, Ruch RJ, Pereira MA: Carcinogenicity of chlorinated methane and ethane compounds administered in drinking water to mice. *Environ Health Perspect* 69:89–95, 1986.

Klotz U, Ammon E: Clinical and toxicological consequences of the inductive potential of ethanol. *Eur J Clin Pharmacol* 54:7–12, 1998.

Koschier FJ: Toxicity of middle distillates from dermal exposure. *Drug Chem Toxicol* 22:155–164, 1999.

Kraul H, Jahn F, Braunlich H: Nephrotoxic effects of diethylene glycol (DEG) in rats. *Exp Pathol* 42:27–32, 1991.

Kril JJ, Halliday GM, Svoboda MD, Cartwright H: The cerebral cortex is damaged in chronic alcoholics. *Neuroscience* 79:983–998, 1997.

Kritchevsky D: Caloric restriction and experimental carcinogenesis. *Toxicol Sci* 52(suppl):13–16, 1999.

Ku WW, Wine RN, Chae BY, et al: Spermatocyte toxicity of 2-methoxyethanol (ME) in rats and guinea pigs: Evidence for the induction of apoptosis. *Toxicol Appl Pharmacol* 134:100–110, 1995.

Kuna RA, Ulrich CE: Subchronic inhalation toxicity of two motor fuels. *J Am Col Toxicol* 3:217–229, 1984.

Kuo HW, Lai JS, Lin M, Su ES: Effects of exposure to carbon disulfide (CS2) on electrocardiographic features of ischaemic heart disease among viscose rayon factory workers. *Int Arch Occup Environ Health* 70:61–66, 1997.

Labrecque G, Belanger PM: Biological rhythms in the absorption, distribution, metabolism and excretion of drugs. *Pharmacol Ther* 52:95–107, 1991.

LaKind JS, McKenna EA, Hubner RP, Tardiff RG: A review of the comparative mamalian toxicity of ethylene glycol and propylene glycol. *Crit Rev Toxicol* 29:331–365, 1999.

Lam C-W, Galen TJ, Boyd JF, Pierson DL: Mechanism of transport and distribution of organic solvents in blood. *Toxicol Appl Pharmacol* 104:117–129, 1990.

Larson JL, Wolf DC, Butterworth BE: Induced cytotoxicity and cell proliferation in the hepatocarcinogenicity of chloroform in female B6C3F1 mice: Comparison of administration by gavage in corn oil vs ad libitum in drinking water. *Fundam Appl Toxicol* 22:90–102, 1994.

Lash AA, Becker CE, So Y, Shore M: Neurotoxic effects of methylene chloride: Are they long lasting in humans? *Br J Ind Med* 48:418–426, 1991.

Lash LH, Fisher JW, Lipscomb JC, Parker JC: Metabolism of trichloroethylene. *Environ Health Perspect* 108(suppl 2):177–200, 2000.

Lash LH, Parker JC, Scott CS: Modes of action of trichloroethylene for kidney tumorigenesis. *Environ Health Perspect* 108(suppl 2):225–240, 2000.

Lash LH, Qian W, Putt DA, et al: Glutathione conjugation of perchloroethylene in rats and mice in vitro: Sex-, species-, and tissue-dependent differences. *Toxicol Appl Pharmacol* 150:49–57, 1998.

Lee BL, Yang XF, New AL, Ong CN: Liquid chromatographic determination of urinary 2-thiothiazlidine-4-carboxylic acid, a biomarker of carbon disulphide exposure. *J Chromatogr B* 668:265–272, 1995.

Lee EW, Terzo TS, D'Arcy JB, et al: Lack of blood formate accumulation in humans following exposure to methanol vapor at the current permissible exposure limit of 200 ppm. *Am Ind Hyg Assoc J* 53:99–104, 1992.

Lee, KM, Bruckner, JV, Muralidhara S, Gallo JM: Characterization of presystemic elimination of trichloroethylene and its nonlinear kinetics in rats. *Toxicol Appl Pharmacol* 139:262–271, 1996.

Lenk W, Lohr D, Sonnenbichler J: Pharmacokinetics and biotransformation of diethylene glycol and ethylene glycol in the rat. *Xenobiotica* 19:961–979, 1989.

Leung H-W, Paustenbach DJ: Physiologically based pharmacokinetic and pharmacodynamic modeling in health risk assessment and characterization of hazardous substances. *Toxicol Lett* 79:55–65, 1995.

Lewis DFV, Ioannides C, Parke DV: Cytochrome P450 and species differences in xenobiotic metabolism and activation of carcinogen. *Environ Health Perspect* 106:633–641, 1998.

Lewis JG, Graham DG, Valentine WM, et al: Exposure of C57BL/6 mice to carbon disulfide induces early lesions of atherosclerosis and enhances arterial fatty deposits induced by a high fat diet. *Toxicol Sci* 49:124–132, 1999.

Li G-L, Linet MS, Hayes RB et al: Gender differences in hematopoietic and lymphoproliferative disorders and other cancer risks by major occupational group among workers exposed to benzene in China. *J Occup Med* 36:875–881, 1994.

Lieber CS: Cytochrome P4502E1: Its physiological and pathological role. *Physiol Rev* 77:517–544, 1997a.

Lieber CS: Ethanol metabolism, cirrhosis and alcoholism. *Clin Chem Acta* 257:59–84, 1997b.

Lilly PD, Thorton-Manning JR, Gargas ML, et al: Kinetic characterization of CYP2E1 inhibition in vivo and in vitro by the chloroethylenes. *Arch Toxicol* 72:609–621, 1998.

Lindstrom AB, Yeowell-O'Connell K, Waidyanatha S, et al: Measurement of benzene oxide in the blood of rats following administration of benzene. *Carcinogenesis* 18:1637–1641, 1997.

Lington AW, Dodd DE, Ridlon SA, et al: Evaluation of 13-week inhalation toxicity study on methyl *t*-butyl ether (MTBE) in Fischer 344 rats. *J Appl Toxicol* 17(S1):S37–S44, 1997.

Linhart I, Gut I, Smejkal J, Novak J: Biotransformation of styrene in mice. Stereochemical aspects. *Chem Res Toxicol* 13:36–44, 2000.

Lipscomb JC, Garrett CM, Snawder JE: Cytochrome P450-dependent metabolism of trichloroethylene: Interindividual differences in humans. *Toxicol Appl Pharmacol* 142:311–318, 1997.

Liu L, Zhang Q, Feng J, et al: The study of DNA oxidative damage in benzene-exposed workers. *Mutation Res* 370:145–150, 1996.

Liu S-L, Esposti SD, Yao T, et al: Vitamin E therapy of acute CCl_4-induced hepatic injury in mice is associated with inhibition of nuclear factor kappa B binding. *Hepatology* 22:1474–1481, 1995.

Lof A, Johanson G: Toxicokinetics of organic solvents: A review of modifying factors. *Crit Rev Toxicol* 28:571–650, 1998.

Loury DJ, Smith-Oliver T, Butterworth BE: Assessment of unscheduled DNA and replicative DNA synthesis in rat kidney cells exposed in vitro or in vivo to unleaded gasoline. *Toxicol Appl Pharmacol* 87:127–140, 1987.

Lykke AWJ, Stewart BW: Fibrosing alveolitis (pulmonary interstitial fibrosis) evoked by experimental inhalation of gasoline vapours. *Experientia* 34:498, 1978.

MacFarland HN, Ulrich CE, Holdsworth CE, et al: A chronic inhalation study with unleaded gasoline vapor. *J Am Col Toxicol* 3:231–248, 1984.

Mainwaring GW, William SM, Foster JR, et al: The distribution of theta-class transferases in the liver and lung of mouse, rat and human. *Biochem J* 318:297–303, 1996.

Mani C, Freeman S, Nelson DO, et al: Species and strain comparisons in the macromolecular binding of extremely low doses of [^{14}C] benzene in rodents using accelerator mass spectrophotometry. *Toxicol Appl Pharmacol* 159:83–90, 1999.

Manno M, Rezzadore M, Grossi M, Sbrana C: Potentiation of occupational carbon tetrachloride toxicity by ethanol abuse. *Hum Exp Toxicol* 15:294–300, 1996.

Marelich GP: Volatile substance abuse. *Crit Rev Allergy Immunol* 15:271–289, 1997.

Maronpot RR, Devereux TR, Hegi M, et al. Hepatic and pulmonary carcinogenicity of methylene chloride in mice: A search for mechanisms. *Toxicology* 102:73–81, 1995.

Martin-Amat G, McMartin KE, Hayreh SS, et al: Methanol poisoning: Ocular toxicity produced by formate. *Toxicol Appl Pharmacol* 45:201–208, 1978.

Martinasevic K, Green MD, Baron J, Tephly TR: Folate and 10-formyltetrahydrofolate dehydrogenase in human and rat retina: Relation to methanol toxicity. *Toxicol Appl Pharmacol* 141:373–381, 1996.

Mason TJ, McKay FW: *U.S. Cancer Mortality by County:1950–1969.* DHEW Publ No NIH 74-615. Bethesda, MD: National Institutes of Health, 1974.

Matonoski G, Elliott E, Tao X, et al: Lymphohematopoietic cancers and butadiene and styrene exposure in synthetic rubber manufacture. *Ann NY Acad Sci* 837:157–169, 1997.

Mattie DR, Alden CL, Newell TK, et al: A 90-day continuous vapor inhalation toxicity study of JP-8 jet fuel followed by 20–21 months of recovery in Fischer 344 rats and C57BL/6 mice. *Toxicol Pathol* 19:77–87, 1991.

Mattie DR, Marit GB, Flemming CD, et al: The effects of JP-8 jet fuel on male Sprague-Dawley rats after a 90-day exposure by oral gavage. *Toxicol Ind Health* 11:423–435, 1995.

McCaffery P, Tempst P, Lara G, Drager U: Aldehyde dehydrogenase as a positional marker in the retina. *Development* 112:693–702, 1991.

McConnell EE, Swenberg JA: Styrene and styrene oxide long-term animal studies. *Crit Rev Toxicol* 24 (suppl 1):S49–S55, 1994.

McDougal JN, Jepson GW, Clewell HJ III, et al: Dermal absorption of organic chemical vapors in rats and humans. *Fund Appl Toxicol* 14:299–308, 1990.

McKee RH, Vergnes JS, Galvin JB, et al: Assessment of the in vivo mutagenic potential of methyl tertiary-butyl ether. *J Appl Toxicol* 17(S1):S31–S36, 1997.

McLaughlin JK, Blot WJ: A critical review of epidemiology studies of trichloroethylene and perchloroethylene and risk of renal-cell cancer. *Int Arch Occup Environ Health* 70:222–231, 1997.

McLean, AJ, Morgan DJ: Clinical pharmacokinetics in patients with liver disease. *Clin Pharmacokinet* 21:42–69, 1991.

McMahon TF, Medinsky MA, Birnbaum LS: Age-related changes in benzene disposition in male C57BL/6N mice described by a physiologically based model. *Toxicol Lett* 74:241–253, 1994.

Mebus CA, Welsch F, Working PK: Attenuation of 2-methoxyethanol-induced testicular toxicity in the rat by simple physiological compounds. *Toxicol Appl Pharmacol* 99:110–121, 1989.

Medeiros AM, Bird MG, Witz G: Potential biomarkers of benzene exposure. *J Toxicol Environ Health* 51:519–539, 1997.

Medinsky MA, Dorman DC: Recent developments in methanol toxicity. *Toxicol Lett* 82/83:707–711, 1995.

Medinsky MA, Kenyon EM, Seaton MJ, Schlosser PM: Mechanistic considerations in benzene physiological model development. *Environ Health Perspect* 104 (suppl 6):1399–1404, 1996.

Medinsky MA, Sabourin PJ Lucier G, et al: A physiological model for simulation of benzene metabolism by rats and mice. *Toxicol Appl Pharmacol* 99:193–206, 1989.

Medinsky MA, Schlosser PM, Bond JA: Critical issues in benzene toxicity and metabolism: The effect of interactions with other organic chemicals on risk assessment. *Environ Health Perspect* 102(suppl 9):119–124, 1994.

Medinsky MA, Singh G, Bechtold WE, et al: Disposition of three glycol ethers administered in drinking water to male F344/N rats. *Toxicol Appl Pharmacol* 102:443–455, 1990.

Melnick RL, Kohn MC: Possible mechanisms of induction of renal tubule cell neoplasms in rats associated with $\alpha 2\mu$-globulin: Role of protein accumulation versus ligand delivery to the kidney, in Cappen CC, Dybing E, Rice JM, Wilbourn JD (eds): *Species Differences in Thyroid, Kidney and Urinary Bladder Carcinogenesis.* Publ No 147. Lyons. France: IARC, 1999, pp 119–137.

Melnick RL, White MC, Davis JM, et al: Potential health effects of oxygenated gasoline in *Interagency Assessment of Oxygenated Fuels,* Washington, DC: National Science and Technology Council, Committee on Environment and Natural Resources, June 1997, chap 4.

Mendrala AL, Langvardt PW, Nitschke KD, et al: In vitro kinetics of styrene and styrene oxide metabolism in rat, mouse and human. *Arch Toxicol* 67:18–27, 1993.

Mennear JH: Carcinogenicity studies on MTBE: Critical review and interpretation. *Risk Anal* 17:673–681, 1997.

Mennear JH, McConnell EE, Huff JE, et al: Inhalation and carcinogenesis studies of methylene chloride (dichloromethane) in F344/N rats and B6C3F1 mice. *Ann NY Acad Sci* 534:343–351, 1988.

Messiha FS, Price J: Properties and regional distribution of ocular aldehyde dehydrogenase in the rat. *Neurobehav Toxicol Teratol* 5:251–254, 1983.

Mezey E: Metabolic effects of ethanol. *Fed Proc* 44:134–138, 1985.

Mihic SJ, McQuilkin SJ, Eger EI, et al: Potentiation of γ-aminobutyric acid type A receptor-mediated chloride currents by novel halogenated compounds correlated with their abilities to induce general anesthesia. *Mol Pharmacol* 46:851–857, 1994.

Miller RR, Ayres JA, Young JT, McKenna MJ: Ethylene glycol monomethyl ether. I. Subchronic vapor inhalation study with rats and rabbits. *Fund Appl Toxicol* 3:49–54, 1983.

Miller RR, Hermann EA, Young JT, et al: Ethylene glycol monomethyl ether and propylene glycol monomethyl ether: Metabolism, disposition, and subchronic inhalation toxicity studies. *Environ Health Perspect* 57:233–239, 1984.

Moller H, Mellemgaard A, Lindvig K, Olsen JH: Obesity and cancer risk: A Danish record-linkage study. *Eur J Cancer* 30A:344–350, 1994.

Morgan DL, Cooper SW, Carlock DL, et al: Dermal absorption of neat and aqueous volatile organic chemicals in the Fischer 344 rat. *Environ Res* 55:51–63, 1991.

Morgan RW, Kelsh MA, Zhao K, Heringer S: Mortality of aerospace workers exposed to trichloroethylene. *Epidemiology* 9:424–431, 1998.

Morrissey RE, Lamb JC IV, Morris JW, et al: Results and evaluations of 48 continuous breeding reproduction studies conducted in mice. *Fund Appl Toxicol* 13:747–777, 1989.

Morshed KM, Nagpaul JP, Majumdar S et al: Kinetics of propylene glycol elimination and metabolism in the rat. *Biochem Med Metab Biol* 39:90–97, 1988.

Moser GJ, Wong BA, Wolf DC, et al: Comparative short-term effects of methyl tertiary butyl ether and unleaded gasoline vapor in B6C3F1 mice. *Fundam Appl Toxicol* 31:173–183, 1996a.

Moser GJ, Wong BA, Wolf DC, et al: Methyl tertiary butyl ether lacks tumor-promoting activity in *N*-nitrosodiethylamine-initiated B6C3F1 female mouse liver. *Carcinogenesis* 17:2753–2761, 1996b.

Moser GJ, Wolf DC, Sar M, et al: Methyl tertiary butyl ether-induced endocrine alterations in mice are not mediated through the estrogen receptor. *Toxicol Sci* 41:77–87, 1998.

Mugford CA, Kedderis GL: Sex-dependent metabolism of xenobiotics. *Drug Metab Rev* 30:441–498, 1998.

Murray FJ, Schwetz BA, McBride JG, Staples RE: Toxicity of inhaled chloroform in pregnant mice and their offspring. *Toxicol Appl Pharmacol* 50:515–522, 1979.

Murray M: P450 enzymes. Inhibition mechanisms, genetic regulation and effects of liver disease. *Clin Pharmacokinet* 23:132–146, 1992.

Mushrush GW, Mose DG, Sullivan KT: Soil vapor and groundwater analysis from a recent oil spill. *Bull Environ Contam Toxicol* 52:31–38, 1994.

Nakai JS, Stathopulos PB, Campbell GL, et al: Penetration of chloroform, trichloroethylene, and tetrachloroethylene through human skin. *J. Toxicol Environ Health* 58:157–170, 1999.

Nakajima T: Cytochrome P450 isoforms and the metabolism of volatile hydrocarbons of low relative molecular mass. *J Occup Health* 39:83–91, 1997.

Nakajima T, Elovaara E, Okino T, et al: Different contributions of cytochrome P450 2E1 and P450 2B1/2 to chloroform hepatotoxicity in rat. *Toxicol Appl Pharmacol* 133:215–222, 1995.

Nakajima T, Koyama Y, Sato A: Dietary modification of metabolism and toxicity of chemical substances—with special reference to carbohydrate. *Biochem Pharmacol* 31:1005–1011, 1982.

Nakajima T, Okuyama S, Yonekura I, Sato A: Effects of ethanol and phenobarbital administration on the metabolism and toxicity of benzene. *Chem Biol Interact* 55:23–38, 1985.

Nakajima T, Wang R-S: Induction of cytochrome P450 by toluene. *Int J Biochem* 26:1333–1340, 1994.

Nakajima T, Wang R-S, Elovaara E, et al: A comparative study on the contribution of cytochrome P450 isozymes to metabolism of benzene, toluene and trichloroethylene in rat liver. *Biochem Pharmacol* 43:251–257, 1992a.

Nakajima T, Wang R-S, Elovaara E, et al: Toluene metabolism by cDNA-expressed human hepatic cytochrome P450. *Biochem Pharmacol* 53:271–277, 1997.

Nakajima T, Wang R-S, Katakura Y, et al: Sex-, age- and pregnancy-induced changes in the metabolism of toluene and trichloroethylene in rat liver in relation to the regulation of cytochrome P450IIE1 and P450IIC11 content. *J Pharmacol Exp Ther* 261:869–874, 1992b.

NAS (National Academy of Sciences): *Pesticides in the Diets of Infants and Children.* National Research Council, Washington, DC: National Academy Press, 1993, pp 1–12.

NCI (National Cancer Institute): *Carcinogenesis Bioassay of Chloroform.* National Technical Information Service No. PB264018/AS. Bethesda, MD: NCI, 1976.

NCI (National Cancer Institute): *Bioassay of Tetrachloroethylene for Possible Carcinogenicity.* NCI: DHEW Publ. No. NIH 77-813, Bethesda, MD: NCI, 1977.

Neeper-Bradley TL, Tyl RW, Fisher LC, et al: Determination of a no-observed-effect level for developmental toxicity of ethylene glycol administered by gavage to CD rats and CD-1 mice. *Fund Appl Toxicol* 27:121–130, 1995.

Nelson BK, Brightwell WS: Behavioral teratology of ethylene glycol monomethyl and monoethyl ethers. *Environ Health Perspect* 57:43–46, 1984.

Nelson HH, Wiencke JK, Christiani DC, et al: Ethnic differences in the prevalence of the homozygous deleted genotype of glutathione *S*-transferase theta. *Carcinogenesis* 16:1243–1245, 1995.

Nessel CS: A comprehensive evaluation of the carcinogenic potential of middle distillate fuels. *Drug Chem Toxicol* 22:165–180, 1999.

NIDA (National Institute on Drug Abuse): in Sharp CW, Brehm, ML (eds): *Review of Inhalants: Euphoria to Dysfunction.* Research Monograph 15. Rockville, MD: Public Health Service, 1977.

Nielsen GD, Alarie Y: Sensory irritation, pulmonary irritation, and respiratory stimulation by airborne benzene and alkylbenzenes: Prediction of safe industrial exposure levels and correlation with their thermodynamic properties. *Toxicol Appl Pharmacol* 65:459–477, 1982.

Niemela O: Aldehyde-protein adducts in the liver as a result of ETH induced oxidative stress. *Front Biosci* 4:506–513, 1999.

Nitschke KD, Burek JD, Bell TJ, et al: Methylene chloride: A 2-year inhalation toxicity and oncogenicity study in rats. *Fund Appl Toxicol* 11:48–59, 1988.

Nolen GA, Gibson WB, Benedict JH, et al: Fertility and teratogenic studies of diethylene glycol monobutyl ether in rats and rabbits. *Fundam Appl Toxicol* 5:1137–1143, 1985.

Nomiyama K, Nomiyama H: Respiratory retention, uptake and excretion of organic solvents in man. *Int Arch Arbeitsmed* 32:75–83, 1974.

NTP (National Toxicology Program): *Toxicology and Carcinogenesis Stud-*

ies of Tetrachloroethylene (Perchloroethylene) in F344/N Rats and B6C3F1 Mice. Research Triangle Park, NC: NTP, 1986.

NTP (National Toxicology Program): *Toxicology and Carcinogenesis Studies of Ethylene Glycol in B6C3F1 Mice (Feed Studies).* NIH Publ. No 93-3144. Research Triangle Park, NC: NTP, 1993.

NTP (National Toxicology Program): Chloroform. NTP reproductive assessment by continuous breeding study. *Environ Health Perspect* 105(suppl 1):285–286, 1997a.

NTP (National Toxicology Program): *Toxicology and Carcinogenesis Studies of Ethylbenzene in F344/N Rats and B6C3F1 Mice. (Inhalation Studies).* Research Triangle Park, NC: NTP, 1997b.

NTP (National Toxicology Program): TR-484 *Toxicology and Carcinogenesis Studies of 2-Butoxyethanol (CAS NO. 111-76-2) in F344/N Rats and B6C3F1 Mice (Inhalation Studies).* http://ntpserver.niehs.nih.gov /htdocs/LT-studies/tr484.html, 1998.

NTP (National Toxicology Program): *Report on Carcinogens. What Is Under Consideration for the 10th RoC?* http://ntp-server.niehs.nih.gov/NewHomeRoc/10thConsideration.html, July 16, 2000.

Nyska A, Maronpot RR, Long PH, et al: Disseminated thrombosis and bone infarction in female rats following inhalation exposure to 2-butoxyethanol. *Toxicol Pathol* 27:287–294, 1999.

O'Brien KL, Selanikio JD, Hecdivert C, et al: Epidemic of pediatric deaths from acute renal failure caused by diethylene glycol poisoning. *JAMA* 279:1175–1180, 1998.

Olson MJ, Garg BD, Murty CVR, Roy AK: Accumulation of α_{2u}-globulin in the renal proximal tubules of male rats exposed to unleaded gasoline. *Toxicol Appl Pharmacol* 90:43–51, 1987.

Olson MJ, Mancini MA, Garg BD, Roy AK: Leupeptin-mediated alteration of renal phagolysosomes: Similarity to hyaline droplet nephropathy of male rats exposed to unleaded gasoline. *Toxicol Lett* 41:245–254, 1988.

Omae K, Takebayashi T, Nomiyama T, et al: Cross sectional observation of the effects of carbon disulphide on arteriosclerosis in rayon manufacturing workers. *Occup Environ Med* 55:468–472, 1998.

Omiecinski CJ, Remmel RP, Hosagrahara VP: Concise review of the cytochrome P450s and their roles in toxicology. *Toxicol Sci* 4:151–156, 1999.

Omura M, Katsumata T, Misawa H, Yamaguchi M: Decreases in protein kinase and phosphatase activities in the liver nuclei of rats exposed to carbon tetrachloride. *Toxicol Appl Pharmacol* 160:192–197, 1999.

OSHA (Occupational Safety and Health Administration): Solvents. http://www.osha.gov/oshinfo/priorities/solvents.html, July 8, 2000.

Oudiz D, Zenick H: In vivo and in vitro evaluations of spermatotoxicity induced by 2-ethoxyethanol treatment. *Toxicol Appl Pharmacol* 84:576–583, 1986.

Padron AG, de Toranzo EGD, Castro JA: Depression of liver microsomal glucose 6-phosphatase activity in carbon tetrachloride-poisoned rats. Potential synergistic effects of lipid peroxidation and of covalent binding of haloalkane-derived free radicals to cellular components in the process. *Free Radic Biol Med* 21:81–87, 1996.

Paulu C, Aschengrau A, Ozonoff D: Tetrachloroethylene-contaminated drinking water in Massachusetts and the risk of colon-rectum, lung, and other cancers. *Environ Health Perspect* 107:265–271, 1999.

Peplonska B, Szeszenia-Dabrowska N, Sobala W, Wilczynska U: A mortality study of workers with reported chronic occupational carbon disulfide poisoning. *Int J Occup Med Environ Health* 9:291–299, 1996.

Pereira MA, Grothaus M: Chloroform in drinking water prevents hepatic cell proliferation induced by chloroform administered by gavage in corn oil to mice. *Fundam Appl Toxicol* 37:82–87, 1997.

Pfaff J, Parton K, Lantz RC, et al: Inhalation exposure to JP-8 jet fuel alters pulmonary function and substance P levels in Fischer 344 rats. *J Appl Toxicol* 15:249–256, 1995.

Pfaff JK, Tollinger BJ, Lantz RC, et al: Neutral endopeptidase (NEP) and its role in pathological pulmonary change with inhalation exposure to JP-8 jet fuel. *Toxicol Ind Health* 12:93–103, 1996.

Phillips CF, Jones RK: Gasoline vapor exposures during bulk handling operations. *Am Ind Hyg Assoc J* 39:118–128, 1978.

Phillips M: Detection of carbon disulfide in breath and air: A possible new risk factor for coronary artery disease. *Int Arch Occup Environ Health* 64:119–123, 1992.

Pierce CH, Dills RL, Morgan MS, et al: Interindividual differences in 2H8-toluene toxicokinetics assessed by a semiempirical physiologically based model. *Toxicol Appl Pharmacol* 139:49–61, 1996.

Pikaar NA, Wedel M, Hermus RJJ: Influence of several factors on blood alcohol concentrations after drinking alcohol. *Alcohol Alcoholism* 23:289–297, 1988.

Poon R, Chu IH, Bjarnason S, et al: Short-term inhalation toxicity of methanol, gasoline, and methanol/gasoline in the rat. *Toxicol Ind Health* 11:343–361, 1995.

Powley MW, Carlson GP: Species comparison of hepatic and pulmonary metabolism of benzene. *Toxicology* 139:207–217, 1999.

Preedy VR, Peters TJ, Why H: Metabolic consequences of alcohol dependency. *Adverse Drug React Toxicol Rev* 16:235–256, 1997.

Prescott-Matthews JS, Wolf DC, Wong BA, Borghoff SJ: Methyl *tert*-butyl ether causes α_{2u}-globulin nephropathy and enhanced renal cell proliferation in male Fischer-344 rats. *Toxicol Appl Pharmacol* 143:301–314, 1997.

Price B, Bergman TS, Rodriguez M, et al: A review of carbon disulphide exposure data and the association between carbon disulfide exposure and ischemic heart disease mortality. *Reg Toxicol Pharmacol* 26:119–128, 1997.

Pryor GT, Rebert CS: Interactive effects of toluene and hexane on behavior and neurophysiologic responses in Fischer-344 rats. *Neurotoxicology* 13:225–234, 1992.

Ramsey JC, Andersen ME: A physiologically based description of the inhalation pharmacokinetics of styrene in rats and humans. *Toxicol Appl Pharmacol* 73:159–175, 1984.

Rangan U, Snyder R: An update on benzene. *Ann NY Acad Sci* 837:105–113, 1997.

Rao PS, Mangipudy RS, Mehendale HM: Tissue injury and repair as parallel and opposing responses to CCl_4 hepatotoxicity: A novel dose–response. *Toxicology* 118:181–193, 1997.

Rasheed A, Hines RN, McCarver-May DG: Variation in induction of human placental CYP2E1: Possible role in susceptibility to fetal alcohol syndrome. *Toxicol Appl Pharmacol* 144:396–400, 1997.

Ratcliffe JM, Schrader SM, Clapp DE, et al: Semen quality in workers exposed to 2-ethoxyethanol. *Br J Ind Med* 46:399–406, 1989.

Raucy JL, Kraner JC, Lasker JM: Bioactivation of halogenated hydrocarbons by cytochrome P4502E1. *Crit Rev Toxicol* 23:1–20, 1993.

Raucy JL, Lasker JM, Kraner JC, et al: Induction of cytochrome P450IIE1 in the obese overfed rat. *Mol Pharmacol* 39:275–280, 1991.

Raunio H, Husgafvel-Pursiainen K, Anttila S, et al: Diagnosis of polymorphisms in carcinogen-activating and inactivating enzymes and cancer susceptibility: A review. *Gene* 159:113–121, 1995.

Recknagel RO, Glende EA Jr, Dolak JA, Waller RL: Mechanisms of carbon tetrachloride toxicity. *Pharmacol Ther* 43:139–154, 1989.

Reese E, Kimbrough RD: Acute toxicity of gasoline and some additives. *Environ Health Perspect* 101(suppl 6):115–131, 1993.

Reitz RH, Gargas ML, Mendrala AL, Schumann AM: In vivo and in vitro studies of perchloroethylene metabolism for physiologically based pharmacokinetic modeling in rats, mice, and humans. *Toxicol Appl Pharmacol* 136:289–306, 1996.

Reitz RH, McDougal JN, Himmelstein MW, et al: Physiologically-based pharmacokinetic modeling with methylchloroform: Implications for interspecies, high dose/low dose, and dose route extrapolations. *Toxicol Appl Pharmacol* 95:185–199, 1988.

Reitz RH, Mendrala AL, Guengerich FP: In vitro metabolism of methylene chloride in human and animal tissues: Use in physiologically based pharmacokinetic models. *Toxicol Appl Pharmacol* 97:220–246, 1989.

Richardson PJ, Patel VB, Preedy VR: Alcohol and the myocardium. *Novartis Found Symp* 216:35–45, 1998.

Richter, R: Degeneration of the basal ganglia in monkeys from chronic carbon disulfide poisoning. *J Neuropathol Exp Neurol* 4:324–353, 1945.

Rifas L, Towler DA, Avioli LV: Gestational exposure to ethanol suppresses msx2 expression in developing mouse embryos. *Proc Natl Acad Sci USA* 94:7549–7554, 1997.

Riihimaki V, Kivisto H, Peltonen K, et al: Assessment of exposure to carbon disulfide in viscose production workers from urinary 2-thiothiazolidine-4-carboxylic acid determinations. *Am J Ind Med* 22:85–97, 1992.

Rikans LE, DeCicco LA, Hornbrook KR, Yamano T: Effect of age and carbon tetrachloride on cytokine concentrations in rat liver. *Mech Age Dev* 108:173–182, 1999.

Ritz B: Cancer mortality among workers exposed to chemicals during uranium processing. *J Occup Environ Med* 41:556–566, 1999.

Robledo RF, Witten ML: NK_1-receptor activation prevents hydrocarbon-induced lung injury in mice. *Am J Physiol* 276:L229–L238, 1999.

Roe FJ: Styrene: Toxicity studies–What do they show? *Crit Rev Toxicol* 24 (suppl 1):S117–S125, 1994.

Roe FJC, Palmer AK, Worden AN, Van Abbe NJ: Safety evaluation of toothpaste containing chloroform. I. Long-term studies in mice. *J Environ Pathol Toxicol* 2:799–819, 1979.

Ron MA: Volatile substance abuse: A review of possible long-term neurological, intellectual and psychiatric sequelae. *Br J Psychiatr* 148:235–246, 1986.

Rosenberg NL: Neurotoxicity of organic solvents, in Rosenberg NL (ed): *Occupational and Environmental Neurology*. Newton, MA: Butterworth-Heinemann, 1995, pp 71–113.

Ross D, Siegel D, Schattenberg DG, et al: Cell-specific activation and detoxification of benzene metabolites in mouse and human bone marrow: Identification of target cells and potential role for modulation of apoptosis in benzene toxicity. *Environ Health Perspect* 104 (suppl 6):1177–1182, 1996.

Roth, RA, Harkema JR, Pestka JP, Ganey PE: Is exposure to bacterial endotoxin a determinant of susceptibility to intoxication from xenobiotic agents? *Toxicol Appl Pharmacol* 147:300–311, 1997.

Salanitro JP: The role of bioattenuation in the management of aromatic hydrocarbon plumes in aquifers. *Ground Water Monit Rem* 13:150–161, 1993.

Sanzgiri UY, Kim HJ, Muralidhara S, et al: Effect of route and pattern of exposure on the pharmacokinetics and acute hepatotoxicity of carbon tetrachloride. *Toxicol Appl Pharmacol* 134:148–154, 1995.

Sanzgiri UY, Srivatsan V, Muralidhara S, et al: Uptake, distribution, and elimination of carbon tetrachloride in rat tissues following inhalation and ingestion exposures. *Toxicol Appl Pharmacol* 143:120–129, 1997.

Sato A: The effect of environmental factors on the pharmacokinetic behavior of organic solvent vapours. *Ann Occup Hyg* 35:525–541, 1991.

Sato A, Nakajima T: A structure-activity relationship of some chlorinated hydrocarbons. *Arch Environ Health* 34:69–75, 1979.

Sato A, Nakajima T, Fujiwara Y, Murayama N: Kinetic studies on sex difference in susceptibility to chronic benzene intoxication with special reference to body fat content. *Br J Ind Med* 32:321–328, 1975.

Schaumburg HH, Spencer PS: Organic solvent mixtures, in Spencer PS, Schaumburg HH (eds): *Experimental and Clinical Neurotoxicology,* 2d ed. New York: Oxford University Press, 2000, pp 894–897.

Schmucker DL, Woodhouse KW, Wang RK, et al: Effects of age and gender on in vitro properties of human liver microsomal monooxygenases. *Clin Pharmacol Ther* 48:365–374, 1990.

Schuckit MA: Genetic aspects of alcoholism. *Ann Intern Med* 15:991–996, 1986.

Schwetz BA, Leong BK, Gehring PJ: Embryo- and fetotoxicity of inhaled chloroform in rats. *Toxicol Appl Pharmacol* 28:442–451, 1974.

Seaton MJ, Schlosser PM, Bond JA, Medinsky MA: Benzene metabolism by human liver microsomes in relation to cytochrome P450 2E1 activity. *Carcinogenesis* 15:1799–1806, 1994.

Seitz HK, Egerer G, Simanowski UA, et al: Human gastric alcohol dehydrogenase activity: Effect of age, sex, and alcoholism. *Gut* 34:1433–1437, 1993.

Seme MT, Summerfelt P, Henry MM, et al: Formate-induced inhibition of photoreceptor function in methanol intoxication. *J Pharmacol Exp Ther* 289:361–370, 1999.

Shamsky S, Samimi B: Organic vapors at underground gasoline tank removal sites. *Appl Ind Hyg* 2:242–245, 1987.

Shi J, Aisaki K, Ikawa Y, Wake K: Evidence of hepatocyte apoptosis in rat liver after the administration of carbon tetrachloride. *Am J Pathol* 153:515–525, 1998.

Shibley IA, Pennington SN: Metabolic and mitotic changes associated with the fetal alcohol syndrome. *Alcohol Alcoholism* 32:423–434, 1997.

Shimada T, Yamazaki H, Mimura M, et al: Interindividual variations in human liver P-450 enzymes involved in the oxidation of drugs, carcinogens and toxic chemicals: Studies with liver microsomes of 30 Japanese and 30 Caucasians. *J Pharmacol Exp Ther* 270:414–423, 1994.

Short BG, Steinhagen WH, Swenberg JA: Promoting effects of unleaded gasoline and 2,2,4-trimethylpentane on the development of atypical cell foci and renal tubular cell tumors in rats exposed to *N*-ethyl-*N*-hydroxyethylnitrosamine. *Cancer Res* 49:369–378, 1989.

Sills RC, Morgan DL, Harry GJ: Carbon disulfide neurotoxicity in rats: I. Introduction and study design. *Neurotoxicology* 19:83–88, 1998.

Singh SP, Ehmann S, Snyder AK: Ethanol-induced changes in insulin-like growth factors and IGF gene expression in the fetal brain. *Proc Soc Exp Biol Med* 212:349–354, 1996.

Sinks T, Lushniak B, Haussler BJ, et al: Renal cell cancer among paperboard printing workers. *Epidemiology* 3:483–489, 1992.

Smith DA, Abel SM, Hyland R, Jones BC: Human cytochromes P450s: Selectivity and measurement in vivo. *Xenobiotica* 28:1095–1128, 1998.

Smith JH, Maita K, Sleight SD, Hook JB: Effect of sex hormone status on chloroform nephrotoxicity and renal mixed function oxidases in mice. *Toxicology* 30:305–316, 1984.

Smith MT: The mechanism of benzene-induced leukemia: A hypothesis and speculations on the causes of leukemia. *Environ Health Perspect* 104(suppl 6):1219–1225, 1996.

Snodgrass WR: Physiological and biochemical differences between children and adults as determinants of toxic response to environmental pollutants, in Guzelian PS, Henry CJ, Olin SS (eds): *Similarities and Differences Between Children and Adults: Implications for Risk Assessment.* Washington, DC: International Life Sciences Institute Press, 1992, pp 35–42.

Snyder R, Hedli CC: An overview of benzene metabolism. *Environ Health Perspect* 104(suppl 6):1165–1171, 1996.

Snyder R, Witz G, Goldstein BD: The toxicology of benzene. *Environ Health Perspect* 100:293–306, 1993.

Spitzer HL: An analysis of the health benefits associated with the use of MTBE reformulated gasoline and oxygenated fuels in reducing atmospheric concentrations of selected volatile organic compounds. *Risk Anal* 17:683–691, 1997.

Sprankle CS, Larson JL, Goldsworthy SM, Butterworth BE: Levels of *myc, fos,* Ha-*ras, met* and hepatocyte growth factor mRNA during regenerative cell proliferation in female mouse liver and male rat kidney after a cytotoxic dose of chloroform. *Cancer Lett* 101:97–106, 1996.

Spurgeon A Glass DC, Calvert IA, et al: Investigation of dose related neurobehavioral effects in paintmakers exposed to low levels of solvents. *Occup Environ Med* 51:626–630, 1994.

Standeven AM, Blazer DG, Goldsworthy TL: Investigation of antiestrogenic properties of unleaded gasoline in female mice. *Toxicol Appl Pharmacol* 127:233–240, 1994a.

Standeven AM, Goldsworthy TL: Promotion of preneoplastic lesions and induction of CYP2B by unleaded gasoline vapor in female B6C3F1 mouse liver. *Carcinogenesis* 14:2137–2141, 1993.

Standeven AM, Wolf DC, Goldsworthy TL: Interactive effects of unleaded gasoline and estrogen on liver tumor promotion in female B6C3F1 mice. *Cancer Res* 54:1198–1204, 1994b.

Stott WT, McKenna MJ: The comparative absorption and excretion of chemical vapors by the upper, lower and intact respiratory tract of rats. *Fund Appl Toxicol* 4:594–602, 1984.

Stoyanovsky DA, Cederbaum AI: Thiol oxidation and cytochrome P450-

dependent metabolism of CCl_4 triggers Ca^{+2} release from liver microsomes. *Biochemistry* 35:15839–15845, 1996.

Sturtevant RP, Sturtevant FM, Pauly JE, Scheving LE: Chronopharmacokinetics of ethanol. *Int J Clin Pharmacol* 16:594–599, 1978.

Swann HE Jr, Kwon BK, Hogan GK, Snellings WM: Acute inhalation toxicology of volatile hydrocarbons. *Am Ind Hyg Assoc J* 35:511–518, 1974.

Sweetnam PM, Taylor SW, Elwood PC: Exposure to carbon disulphide and ischaemic heart disease in a viscose rayon factory. *Br J Ind Med* 44:220–227, 1987.

Tam, YK: Individual variation in first-pass metabolism. *Clin Pharmacokinet* 25:300–328, 1993.

Tanii H, Saito S, Hashimoto K: Structure-toxicity relationship of ethylene glycol ethers. *Arch Toxicol* 66:368–371, 1992.

Tardif R, Lapare S, Plaa GL, Brodeur J: Effect of simultaneous exposure to toluene and xylene on their respective biological exposure indices in humans. *Int Arch Occup Environ Health* 63:279–284, 1991.

Thier R, Wiebel FA, Hinkel A, et al: Species differences in the glutathione transferase GSTT1-1 activity towards the model substrates methyl chloride and dichloromethane in liver and kidney. *Arch Toxicol* 72:622–629, 1998.

Thompson DJ, Warner SD, Robinson VB: Teratology studies on orally administered chloroform in the rat and rabbit. *Toxicol Appl Pharmacol* 29:348–357, 1974.

Thurman RG: Mechanisms of hepatic toxicity II. Alcoholic liver injury involves activation of Kupffer cells by endotoxin. *Am J Physiol* 275:G605–G611, 1998.

Tola S, Vilhunen R, Jarvinen E, Korkala ML: A cohort study on workers exposed to trichloroethylene. *J Occup Med* 22:737–740, 1980.

Toraason M, Breitenstein M: Prenatal ethylene glycol ether (EGME) exposure produces electrocardiographic changes in the rat. *Toxicol Appl Pharmacol* 95:321–327, 1988.

Traiger GJ, Bruckner JV: The participation of 2-butanone in 2-butanol-induced potentiation of carbon tetrachloride hepatotoxicity. *J Pharmacol Exp Ther* 196:493–500, 1976.

Treluyer JM, Cheron G, Sonnier M, Cresteil T: Cytochrome P-450 expression in sudden infant death syndrome. *Biochem Pharmacol* 52:497–504, 1996.

Triebig G, Claus D, Csuzda I, et al: Cross-sectional epidemiological study on neurotoxicity of solvents in paints and lacquers. *Int Arch Occup Environ Health* 60:233–241, 1988.

Trush MA, Twerdok LE, Rembish SJ, et al: Analysis of target cell susceptibility as a basis for the development of a chemoprotective strategy against benzene-induced hematotoxicities. *Environ Health Perspect* 104(suppl 6):1227–1234, 1996.

Tyl RW, Ballantyne B, France KA, et al: Evaluation of the developmental toxicity of ethylene glycol monohexyl ether vapor in Fischer 344 rats and New Zealand white rabbits. *Fund Appl Toxicol* 12:269–280, 1989.

Tyl RW, Fisher LC, Kubena MF, et al: Assessment of the developmental toxicity of ethylene glycol applied cutaneously to CD-1 mice. *Fund Appl Toxicol* 27:155–166, 1995.

Uchida Y, Nakatsuka H, Ukai H, et al: Symptoms and signs in workers exposed predominantly to xylenes. *Int Arch Occup Environ Health* 64:597–605, 1993.

Udden MM: Hemolysis and deformability of erythrocytes exposed to butoxyacetic acid, a metabolite of 2-butoxyethanol: II. Resistance in red blood cells from humans with potential susceptibility. *J Appl Toxicol* 14:97–102, 1994.

Udden MM, Patton CS: Hemolysis and deformability of erythrocytes exposed to butoxyacetic acid, a metabolite of 2-butoxyethanol: I. Sensitivity in rats and resistance in normal humans. *J Appl Toxicol* 14:91–96, 1994.

Ullrich SE: Dermal application of JP-8 jet fuel induces immune suppression. *Toxicol Sci* 52:61–67, 1999.

Valentine JL, Lee SS-T, Seaton MJ, et al: Reduction of benzene metabolism and toxicity in mice that lack CYP2E1 expression. *Toxicol Appl Pharmacol* 141:205–213, 1996.

Valentine WM, Amarnath V, Graham DG, et al: CS2-mediated cross-linking of erythrocyte spectrin and neurofilament protein: Dose response and temporal relationship to the formation of axonal swellings. *Toxicol Appl Pharmacol* 142:95–105, 1997.

Valentine WM, Amarnath V, Amarnath K, et al: Covalent modification of hemoglobin by carbon disulfide: III. A potential biomarker of effect. *Neurotoxicology* 19:99–108, 1998.

Valentine WM, Graham DG, Anthony DC: Covalent cross-linking of erythrocyte spectrin by carbon disulfide in vivo. *Toxicol Appl Pharmacol* 121:71–77, 1993.

Valpey R, Sumi SM, Copass MK, Goble GJ: Acute and chronic progressive encephalopathy due to gasoline sniffing. *Neurology* 28:507–510, 1978.

Vamvakas S, Bruning T, Bolt HM, et al: Renal cell cancer correlated with occupational exposure to trichloroethylene. *J Cancer Res Clin Oncol* 126:178–180, 2000.

Vamvakas S, Bruning T, Thomasson B, et al: Renal cell cancer correlated with occupational exposure to trichloroethene. *J Cancer Res Clin Oncol* 124:374–382, 1998.

van Baak MA: Influence of exercise on the pharmacokinetics of drugs. *Clin Pharmacokinet* 19:32–43, 1990.

Veulemans H, Steeno O, Maschelein R, Groeseneken D: Exposure to ethylene glycol ethers and spermatogenic disorders in man: A case-control study. *Br J Ind Med* 50:71–78, 1993.

Vieira I, Sonnier M, Cresteil T: Developmental expression of *CYP2E1* in human liver. Hypermethylation control of gene expression during the neonatal period. *Eur J Biochem* 238:476–483, 1996.

Volkel W, Friedewald M, Lederer E, et al: Biotransformation of perchloroethene: Dose-dependent excretion of trichloroacetic, dichloroacetic acid, and *N*-acetyl-*S*-(trichlorovinyl)-L-cysteine in rats and humans after inhalation. *Toxicol Appl Pharmacol* 153:20–27, 1998.

von Euler G: Toluene and dopaminergic transmission, in Isaacon RL, Jensen KF (eds): *The Vulnerable Brain and Environmental Risk. Toxins in Air and Water*. Vol 3. New York: Plenum Press, 1994, pp 301–321.

Vrca A, Bozicevic D, Karacic V, et al: Visual evoked potentials in individuals exposed to long-term low concentrations of toluene. *Arch Toxicol* 69:337–340, 1995.

Wallace L: Environmental exposure to benzene: An update. *Environ Health Perspect* 104(suppl 6):1129–1136, 1996.

Wallace L: Major sources of exposure to benzene and other volatile organic chemicals. *Risk Anal* 10:59–64, 1990.

Wallace LA, Pellizzari ED, Hartwell TD, et al: A TEAM study: Personal exposures to toxic substances in air, drinking water, and breath of 400 residents of New Jersey, North Carolina, and North Dakota. *Environ Res* 43:290–307, 1987.

Wang PY, Kaneko T, Tsukada H, et al: Dose- and route-dependent alterations in metabolism and toxicity of chemical compounds in ethanol-treated rats: Difference between highly (chloroform) and poorly (carbon tetrachloride) metabolized hepatotoxic compounds. *Toxicol Appl Pharmacol* 142:13–21, 1997.

Wang YY, Brown JP, Sandy MS: *Public Health Goal for Methyl Tertiary Butyl Ether (MTBE) in Drinking Water.* Oakland, CA: California Environmental Protection Agency, Office of Environmental Health Hazard Assessment, March, 1999.

Warner A: Drug use in the neonate: Interrelationships of pharmacokinetics, toxicity, and biochemical maturity. *Clin Chem* 32:721–727, 1986.

Wartenberg D, Reyner D, Scott CS: Trichloroethylene and cancer: Epidemiologic evidence. *Environ Health Perspect* 108(suppl. 2):161–176, 2000.

Wax PM: Elixirs, diluents, and the passage of the 1938 Federal Food, Drug and Cosmetic Act. *Ann Intern Med* 122:456–461, 1995.

Waxman DJ, Chang TKH: Hormonal regulation of liver cytochrome P450 enzymes, in Ortiz de Montellano PR (ed): *Cytochrome P450: Structure, Mechanism, and Biochemistry,* 2d ed. New York: Plenum Press, 1995, pp 391–394.

Weber, WW: Populations and genetic polymorphisms. *Mol Diagn* 4:299–307, 1999.

Weisel CP, Jo WK: Ingestion, inhalation, and dermal exposures to chloroform and trichloroethene from tap water. *Environ Health Perspec* 104:48–51, 1996.

Weiss NS: Cancer in relation to occupational exposure to perchloroethylene. *Cancer Causes Control* 6:257–266, 1995.

Weiss NS: Cancer in relation to occupational exposure to trichloroethylene. *Occup Environ Med* 53:1–5, 1996.

Welch LS, Schrader SM, Turner TW, Cullen MR: Effects of exposure to ethylene glycol ethers on shipyard painters: II. Male reproduction. *Am J Ind Med* 14:509–526, 1988.

Welling PG, Pool WF: Effect of liver disease on drug metabolism and pharmacokinetics, in Cameron RG, Feuer G, De la Iglesia FA (eds): *Drug Induced Hepatotoxicity.* Berlin: Springer-Verlag, 1996, pp 367–394.

WHO (World Health Organization): *Environmental Health Criteria 10. Carbon Disulfide.* Geneva: WHO, 1979, pp 1–101.

WHO (World Health Organization)/Nordic Council of Ministers: *Chronic Effects of Organic Solvents on the Central Nervous System and Diagnostic Criteria.* Copenhagen: WHO, 1985.

Wiener HL, Richardson KE: The metabolism and toxicity of ethylene glycol. *Res Commun Subst Abuse* 9:77–87, 1988.

Wiener HL, Richardson KE: Metabolism of diethylene glycol in male rats. *Biochem Pharmacol* 38:539–541, 1989.

Williams J, Reel JR, George JD, Lamb JC IV: Reproductive effects of diethylene glycol and diethylene glycol monethyl ether in Swiss CD-1 mice assessed by a continuous breeding protocol. *Fund Appl Toxicol* 14:622–635, 1990.

Williams TM, Cattley RC, Borghoff SJ: Alterations in endocrine responses in male Sprague-Dawley rats following oral administration of methyl *tert*-butyl ether. *Toxicol Sci* 54:168–176, 2000.

Williams-Hill D, Spears CP, Prakash S, et al: Mutagenicity studies of methyl-*tert*-butylether using the Ames tester strain TA102. *Mutat Res* 446:15–21, 1999.

Wilmarth KR, Viana ME, Abou-Donia MB: Carbon disulfide inhalation increases Ca^{2+}/calmodulin-dependent kinase phosphorylation of cytoskeletal proteins in the rat central nervous system. *Brain Res* 628:293–300, 1993.

Witz G, Zhang Z, Goldstein BD: Reactive ring-opened aldehyde metabolites in benzene hematotoxicity. *Environ Health Perspec* 104 (suppl 6):1195–1199, 1996.

Witzmann FA, Bauer MD, Fieno AM, et al: Proteomic analysis of simulated jet fuel exposure in the lung. *Electrophoresis* 20:3659–3669, 1999.

Witzmann FA, Bauer MD, Fieno AM, et al: Proteomic analysis of the renal effects of simulated occupational jet fuel exposure. *Electrophoresis* 21:976–984, 2000.

Wolf CR: Individuality in cytochrome P450 expression and its association with the nephrotoxic and carcinogenic effects of chemicals. *IARC Sci Publ* 115:281–287, 1991.

Wong FW-Y, Chan W-Y, Lee SS-T: Resistance to carbon tetrachloride-induced hepatotoxocity in mice which lack CYP2E1 expression. *Toxicol Appl Pharmacol* 153:109–118, 1998.

Woodhouse K, Wynne HA: Age-related changes in hepatic function. Implications for drug therapy. *Drugs Aging* 2:243–255, 1992.

Wrighton SA, Stevens JC: The human cytochromes P450 involved in drug metabolism. *Crit Rev Toxicol* 22:1–21, 1992.

Wronska-Nofer T: Various disorders of cholesterol metabolism and their effect on the development of experimental arteriosclerosis in rats exposed to carbon disulfide. *Med Proc* 30:121–134, 1979.

Yin SJ, Han CL, Lee AI, Wu CW: Human alcohol dehydrogenase family. Functional classification, ethanol/retinol metabolism, and medical implications. *Adv Exp Med Biol* 463:265–274, 1999.

Yin, S-N, Hayes RB, Linet MS, et al: A cohort study of cancer among benzene-exposed workers in China: Overall results. *Am J Ind Med* 29:227–235, 1996.

Yu DK, Elmquist WF, Sawchuck RJ: Pharmacokinetics of propylene glycol in humans during multiple dosing regimens. *J Pharm Sci* 74:876–879, 1985.

Zangar RC, Benson JM, Burnett VL, Springer DL: Cytochrome P450 2E1 is the primary enzyme responsible for low-dose carbon tetrachloride metabolism in human liver microsomes. *Chem Biol Interact* 125:233–243, 2000.

CHAPTER 25

TOXIC EFFECTS OF RADIATION AND RADIOACTIVE MATERIALS

Naomi H. Harley

INTRODUCTION

Among all the branches of toxicology, ionizing radiation provides the most quantitative estimates of health detriments for humans. Five large studies provide data on the health effects of radiation on people. These effects include those due to external x-rays and gamma-ray radiation and internal alpha radioactivity. The studies encompass radium exposures, including those sustained by radium dial painters, atom bomb survivors, patients irradiated with x-rays for ankylosing spondylitis, children irradiated with x-rays for tinea capitis (ringworm), and uranium miners exposed to radon and its short-lived daughter products. The only health effect subsequent to radiation exposure seen with statistical significance to date is cancer. The various types and the quantitative risks are described in subsequent sections.

All the studies provide a consistent picture of the risk of exposure to ionizing radiation. There are sufficient details in the studies of atom bomb, occupational, and medical exposures to estimate the risk from lifelong low-level environmental exposure. Natural background radiation is substantial, and only within the past two decades has the extent of the radiation insult to the global population from natural radiation and radioactivity been appreciated.

BASIC RADIATION CONCEPTS

The four main types of radiation are due to alpha particles, electrons (negatively charged beta particles or positively charged positrons), gamma rays, and x-rays. An atom can decay to a product element through the loss of a heavy (mass = 4) charged (+2) alpha particle (He^{+2}) that consists of two protons and two neutrons. An atom can decay by loss of a negatively or positively charged electron (beta particle or positron). Gamma radiation results when the nucleus releases excess energy, usually after an alpha, beta, or positron transition. X-rays occur whenever an inner-shell orbital electron is removed and rearrangement of the atomic electrons results, with the release of the element's characteristic x-ray energy.

There are several excellent textbooks describing the details of radiologic physics (Evans, 1955; Andrews, 1974; Turner, 1986, Cember 1996).

Energy

Alpha particles and beta rays (or positrons) have kinetic energy as a result of their motion. The energy is equal to

$$E = 1/2\, mV^2 \tag{1}$$

where m = mass of the particle
V = velocity of the particle

Alpha particles have a low velocity compared with the speed of light, and calculations of alpha particle energy do not require any corrections for relativity. Most beta particles (or positrons) have high velocity, and the basic expression must be corrected for their increased relativistic mass (the rest mass of the electron is 0.511 MeV). The total energy is equal to

$$E = 0.511/(1 - v^2/c^2) + 0.511 \tag{2}$$

where v = velocity of the beta particle
c = speed of light

Gamma rays and x-rays are pure electromagnetic radiation with energy equal to

$$E = hv \tag{3}$$

where h = Planck's constant (6.626×10^{-34} J s)
v = frequency of radiation

The conventional energy units for ionizing radiation are the electron volt (eV) or multiples of this basic unit, kiloelectron volts (keV) and million electron volts (MeV). The conversion to the international system of units, the Système Internationale (SI), is currently taking place in many countries, and the more fundamental energy unit of the Joule (J) is slowly replacing the older unit. The relationship is

$$1 \text{ eV} = 1.6 \times 10^{-19} \text{ J}$$

Authoritative tables of nuclear data such as those of Browne and Firestone (1986) contain the older but more widely accepted units of MeV for energy.

Alpha Particles

Alpha particles are helium nuclei (consisting of two protons and two neutrons), with a charge of +2, that are ejected from the nucleus of an atom. When an alpha particle loses energy, slows to the velocity of a gas atom, and acquires two electrons from the vast sea of free electrons present in most media, it becomes part of the normal background helium in the environment. All helium in nature is the result of alpha particle decay. The formula for alpha decay is

$$\begin{matrix} A & & A-4 & \\ & X \rightarrow & & Y + He^{2+} + \text{gamma} + Q_\alpha \\ Z & & Z-2 & \end{matrix}$$

where Z = atomic number
A = atomic weight

The energy available in this decay is Q_α and is equal to the mass difference of the parent and the two products. The energy is shared among the particles and the gamma ray if one is present.

An example of alpha decay is given by the natural radionuclide radium (^{226}Ra):

$$\begin{matrix} 226 & & 222 & \\ & Ra \rightarrow & & Rn + \text{alpha (5.2 MeV)} \\ 86 & & 84 & \end{matrix}$$

The energy of alpha particles for most emitters lies in the range of 4 to 8 MeV. More energetic alpha particles exist but are seen only in very short-lived emitters such as those formed by reactions occurring in particle accelerators. These particles are not considered in this chapter.

Although there may be several alpha particles with very similar energy emitted by a particular element such as radium, each particular alpha particle is monoenergetic, i.e., no continuous spectrum of energies exists, only discrete energies.

Beta Particles, Positrons, and Electron Capture

Beta particle decay occurs when a neutron in the nucleus of an element is effectively transformed into a proton and an electron. Subsequent ejection of the electron occurs, and the maximum energy of the beta particle equals the mass difference between the parent and the product nuclei. A gamma ray may also be present to share the energy, Q_β:

$$\begin{matrix} A & & A & \\ & X \rightarrow & & Y + \text{beta} + Q_\beta \\ Z & & Z+1 & \end{matrix}$$

An example of beta decay is given by the natural radionuclide lead (^{210}Pb):

$$\begin{matrix} 210 & 210 & \\ Pb \rightarrow & & Bi + \text{beta (0.015 MeV)} + \text{gamma (0.046 MeV)} \\ 82 & 83 & \end{matrix}$$

Unlike alpha particles in alpha decay, in which each alpha particle is monoenergetic, beta particles are emitted with a continuous spectrum of energy from zero to the maximum energy available for the transition. The reason for this is that the total available energy is shared in each decay or transition by two particles: the beta particle and an antineutrino. The total energy released in each transition is constant, but the observed beta particles then appear as a spectrum. The residual energy is carried away by the antineutrino, which is a particle with essentially zero mass and charge that cannot be observed without extraordinarily complex instrumentation. The beta particle, by contrast, is readily observed with conventional nuclear counting equipment.

Positron emission is similar to beta particle emission but results from the effective nucleon transformation of a proton to a neutron plus a positively charged electron. The atomic number decreases rather than increases, as it does in beta decay.

An example of positron decay is given by the natural radionuclide copper (^{64}Cu), which decays by beta emission 41 percent of the time, positron emission 19 percent of the time, and electron capture 40 percent of the time:

$$^{64}_{29}\mathrm{Cu} \rightarrow {}^{64}_{28}\mathrm{Ni} + \text{positron (0.66 MeV)} \qquad \text{19 percent}$$

$$^{64}_{29}\mathrm{Cu} \rightarrow {}^{64}_{30}\mathrm{Zn} + \text{beta (0.57 MeV)} \qquad \text{41 percent}$$

$$^{64}_{29}\mathrm{Cu} \rightarrow {}^{64}_{28}\mathrm{Ni}\ \text{electron capture} \qquad \text{40 percent}$$

The energy of the positron appears as a continuous spectrum, similar to that in beta decay, where the total energy available for decay is again shared between the positron and a neutrino. In the case of positron emission, the maximum energy of the emitted particle is the mass difference of the parent and product nuclide minus the energy needed to create two electron masses (1.02 MeV), whereas the maximum energy of the beta particle is the mass difference itself. This happens because in beta decay, the increase in the number of orbital electrons resulting from the increase in atomic number of the product nucleus cancels the mass of the electron lost in emitting the beta particle. This does not happen in positron decay, and there is an orbital electron lost as a result of the decrease in atomic number of the product and the loss of the electron mass in positron emission.

Electron capture competes with positron decay, and the resulting product nucleus is the same nuclide. In electron capture, an orbiting electron is acquired by the nucleus, and the transformation of a proton plus the electron to form a neutron takes place. In some cases the energy available is released as a gamma-ray photon, but this is not necessary, and a monoenergetic neutrino may be emitted. If the 1.02 MeV required for positron decay is not available, positron decay is not kinetically possible and electron capture is the only mode observed.

Gamma-Ray (Photon) Emission

Gamma-ray emission is not a primary process except in rare instances, but it occurs in combination with alpha, beta, or positron emission or electron capture. Whenever the ejected particle does not utilize all the available energy for decay, the nucleus contains the excess energy and is in an excited state. The excess energy is released as photon or gamma-ray emission coincident with the ejection of the particle.

One of the rare instances of pure gamma-ray emission is technetium 99m (^{99m}Tc), which has a 6.0-h half-life and is widely used in diagnostic medicine for various organ scans. Its decay product, ^{99}Tc, has a very long half life (2.13×10^5 years), and as all ^{99}Tc is ultimately released to the environment, a background of this nuclide is emerging.

$$^{99m}_{43}\mathrm{Tc} \rightarrow {}^{99}_{43}\mathrm{Tc} + \text{gamma (0.14 MeV)}$$

In many cases, the photon will not actually be emitted by the nucleus but the excess excitation energy will be transferred to an orbital electron. This electron is then ejected as a monoenergetic particle with energy equal to that of the photon minus the binding energy of the orbital electron. This process is known as internal conversion. In tables of nuclear data such as those of Browne and Firestone (1986), the ratio of the conversion process to the photon is given as e/v. For example, the e/v ratio for ^{99m}Tc is 0.11, and therefore the photon is emitted 90 percent of the time and the conversion electron is emitted 10 percent of the time.

INTERACTION OF RADIATION WITH MATTER

Ionizing radiation, by definition, loses energy when passing through matter by producing ion pairs (an electron and a positively charged atom residue). A fraction of the energy loss raises atomic electrons to an excited state. The average energy needed to produce an ion pair is given the notation W and is numerically equal to 33.85 eV. This energy is roughly two times the ionization potential of most gases or other elements because it includes the energy lost in the excitation process. It is not clear what role the excitation plays, for example, in damage to targets in the cellular DNA. Ionization, by contrast, can break bonds in DNA, causing strand breaks and easily understood damage.

All particles and rays interact through their charge or field with atomic or free electrons in the medium through which they are passing. There is no interaction with the atomic nucleus except at energies above about 8 MeV, which is required for interactions that break apart the nucleus (spallation). Very high energy cosmic-ray particles, for example, produce ^{3}H, ^{7}Be, ^{14}C, and ^{22}Na in the upper atmosphere by spallation of atmospheric oxygen and nitrogen.

Alpha and beta particles and gamma rays lose energy by ionization and excitation in somewhat different ways, as described in the following sections.

Alpha Particles

The alpha particle is a heavy charged particle with a mass that is 7300 times that of the electrons with which it interacts. A massive particle interacting with a small particle has the interesting property that it can give a maximum velocity during energy transfer to the small particle of only two times the initial velocity of the heavy particle. In terms of the maximum energy that can be transferred per interaction, this is

$$E_{(\text{maximum electron})} = 4/7300\ E_{(\text{alpha particle})} \qquad (4)$$

Although alpha particles can lose perhaps 10 to 20 percent of their energy in traveling 10 μm in tissue (1 cm in air), each interaction can impart only the small energy, given in the maximum, in Eq. (4). Thus, alpha particles are characterized by a high energy loss per unit path length and a high ionization density along the track length. This is called a *high linear-energy-transfer* (LET) or *high-LET* particle.

Hans Bethe (1953) derived an exact expression for the energy loss in matter, dE/dx or stopping power, with later modifications added by Bloch and others. For alpha energies between 0.2 and 10 MeV, the Bethe-Bloch expression can be simplified to

$$dE/dx = 3.8 \times 10^{-25}\ C\ NZ/E \ln\{548\ E/I\}\ \text{MeV} / \mu\text{m}^{-1} \quad (5)$$

where N = number of atoms cm^{-3} in medium
Z = atomic number of medium
I = ionization potential of medium
E = energy of alpha particle
C = charge correction for alpha particles with energy below
1.6 MeV

A simple rule of thumb derived by Bloch may be used to estimate the ionization potential of a compound or element,

$$I = 10(Z) \quad (6)$$

or the Bragg additivity rule (Attix et al., 1968) may be used for compounds when the individual values of ionization potential for the elements are available. A tabulation of values of ionization potential is given in ICRU 37 (ICRU, 1984), and the stopping power in all elements has been calculated in ICRU 49 (ICRU, 1993) and by Ziegler (Ziegler, 1977).

When alpha particles are near the end of their range, the charge is not constant at +2 but can be +1 or even zero as the particle acquires or loses electrons. A correction factor, C, is needed for energies between 0.2 and 1.5 MeV to account for this effect. Whaling (1958) published values for the correction factor by which Eq. (4) should be multiplied. These factors vary from 0.24 at 0.2 MeV, 0.75 at 0.6 MeV, 0.875 at 1.0 MeV, up to 1.0 at 1.6 MeV.

For the case of tissue, Eq. (5) reduces to

$$dE/dx_{\text{tissue}} = [0.126C/E] \ln\{7.99\ E\}\ \text{MeV} / \mu\text{m}^{-1} \quad (7)$$

Example 1 Find the energy loss (stopping power) of a 0.6 and a 5-MeV alpha particle in tissue.

$$\begin{aligned} dE/dx &= 0.126\ (0.75)/0.6 \ln(7.99 \times 0.6) \\ &= 0.25\ \text{MeV} / \mu\text{m}^{-1} \\ &= 0.126\ (1.0)/5.0 \ln(7.99 \times 5.0) \\ &= 0.093\ \text{MeV} / \mu\text{m}^{-1} \end{aligned}$$

The significance of this energy loss is seen in that it requires 33.85 eV to produce an ion pair; therefore, a 5-MeV alpha particle can produce $(0.25 \times 10^6\ \text{eV}/\mu\text{m}^{-1})$ / (33.86 ev / ion pair) = 7400 ion pairs in 1 μm, or enough damage to cause a double-strand break.

Beta Particles

The equations for beta particle energy loss in matter cannot be simplified, as in the case of alpha particles, because of three factors:

1. Even at low energies of a few tenths of an MeV, beta particles are traveling near the speed of light and relativistic effects (mass increase) must be considered.
2. Electrons are interacting with particles of the same mass in the medium (free or orbital electrons), so large energy losses per collision are possible.
3. Radiative or bremsstrahlung energy loss occurs when electrons or positrons are slowing down in matter. Such a loss also occurs with alpha particles, but the magnitude of this energy loss is negligible.

Including the effects of these three factors, the energy loss for electrons and positrons has been well quantitated. Tabulations of energy loss in various media have been prepared with the ionization energy loss and the radiative loss detailed. Tables of energy loss for electrons in tissue and many other substance as a function of electron energy can be found in ICRU 37 (1984).

Gamma Rays

Photons do not have a mass or charge, as do alpha and beta particles. The interaction between a photon and matter therefore is controlled not by the electrostatic Coulomb fields but by interaction of the electric and magnetic field of the photon with the electron in the medium. There are three modes of interaction with the medium.

The Photoelectric Effect The photon interaction with an orbital electron in the medium is complete, and the full energy of the photon is given to the electron.

The Compton Effect Part of the photon energy is transferred to an electron, and the photon scatters (usually at a small angle from its original path) (Evans, 1955) with reduced energy. The governing expressions are

$$\begin{aligned} E' &= E\ 0.511/(1 + 1/a - \cos\theta) \quad (8) \\ T &= E\ a(1 - \cos\theta)/[1 + a(1 - \cos\theta)] \end{aligned}$$

where E, E' = initial and scattered photon energy in MeV
T = kinetic energy of electron in MeV
$a = E/0.511$
θ = angle of photon scatter from its original path

Pair Production Pair production occurs whenever the photon energy is greater than the rest mass of two electrons, 2(0.511 MeV) = 1.02 MeV. The electromagnetic energy of the photon can be converted directly to an electron-positron pair, with any excess energy above 1.02 MeV appearing as kinetic energy given to these particles.

The loss of photons and energy loss from a photon beam as it passes through matter are described by two coefficients. The attenuation coefficient determines the fractional loss of photons per unit distance (usually in normalized units of g/cm^2, which is the linear distance times the density of the medium). The mass energy absorption coefficient determines the fractional energy deposition per unit distance traveled. The loss of photons from the beam is given by

$$I/I_0 = \exp(-\mu/\rho\ d) \quad (9)$$

where I = intensity of photon beam (numbers of photons)
I_0 = beam intensity
μ/ρ = attenuation coefficient in medium for energy considered (in $m^2\ kg^{-2}$)
d = thickness of medium in superficial density units kg m^{-2} (thickness in m times density in kg m^{-3})

Superficial density is convenient in that it normalizes energy absorption in different media. For example, air and tissue have approximately the same energy absorption per kg m^{-2}, whereas in linear dimension, the energy absorption, say, per meter, is vastly different. The energy actually deposited in the medium per unit distance is calculated using the mass energy absorption coefficient as opposed to the overall attenuation coefficient and the energy loss is given by

$$\Delta E = (\mu_{en}/\rho)E_0 \tag{10}$$

where ΔE = energy loss in medium per unit distance (in MeV $m^2\ kg^{-1}$)
μ_{en}/ρ = mass energy absorption coefficient ($m^2\ kg^{-2}$)
E_0 = initial photon energy

The values for μ_{en}/ρ as a function of gamma-ray energy are shown in Table 25-1 for air and muscle. Energy loss can then be expressed per unit linear distance by multiplying by the density of the medium (kg m^{-3}).

Table 25-1
Mass Energy Absorption Coefficients for Air and Water

PHOTON ENERGY, MeV	AIR, $\mu_{en}/\rho(m^2\ kg^{-1})$	MUSCLE, STRIATE (ICRU), $\mu_{en}/\rho(m^2\ kg^{-1})$
0.01	0.46	0.49
0.015	0.13	0.14
0.02	0.052	0.055
0.03	0.015	0.016
0.04	0.0067	0.0070
0.05	0.0040	0.0043
0.06	0.0030	0.0032
0.08	0.0024	0.0026
0.10	0.0023	0.0025
0.15	0.0025	0.0027
0.20	0.0027	0.0029
0.30	0.0029	0.0032
0.40	0.0029	0.0032
0.50	0.0030	0.0033
0.60	0.0030	0.0033
0.80	0.0029	0.0032
1.00	0.0028	0.0031
1.50	0.0025	0.0028
2.00	0.0023	0.0026
3.00	0.0021	0.0023

SOURCE: Hubbell, 1982, with permission.

ABSORBED DOSE

Dose and Dose Rate

Absorbed dose is defined as the mean energy, e, imparted by ionizing radiation to matter of mass m (ICRU, 1993):

$$D = e/m \tag{11}$$

where D = absorbed dose
e = mean energy deposited in mass
m = mass

The unit for absorbed dose is the gray (Gy), which is equal to 1 J kg^{-1}. The older unit of dose is the rad, which is equal to 100 erg g^{-1}, a value numerically equal to 100 times the dose in gray. The conversion between the two units is 100 rad = 1 Gy.

For uncharged particles (gamma rays and neutrons), kerma (kinetic energy released in matter) is sometimes used. It is the sum of the initial kinetic energies of all the charged ionizing particles liberated in unit mass. The units of kerma are the same as those for dose.

Exposure often is confused with absorbed dose. Exposure is defined only in air for gamma rays or photons and is the charge of the ions of one sign when all electrons liberated by photons are completely stopped in air of mass m:

$$X = Q/m \tag{12}$$

where X = exposure
Q = total charge of one sign
m = mass of air

The unit of exposure is coulombs per kilogram of air. The older unit of exposure is the roentgen, which is equal to 2.58×10^{-4} C kg^{-1} of air.

Exposure and dose are used interchangeably in some publications, even though this is not correct. The reason is that the older numerical values of dose in rad and exposure in roentgen are similar. Although they are similar numerically, they are fundamentally different in that exposure is ionization (only in air) and dose is absorbed energy in any specified medium:

$$1 \text{ roentgen} = 0.87 \text{ rad (in air)}$$

The SI units are not numerically similar:

$$1 \text{ C kg}^{-1} = 33.85 \text{ Gy}$$

Dose Rate

Dose rate is the dose expressed per unit time interval. The dose rate delivered to the thyroid by ^{99m}Tc for a nuclear medicine scan, for example, diminishes with time because of the 6.0-h half-life of the nuclide. The total dose is a more pertinent quantity in this case because it can be related directly to risk and compared with the benefit of the thyroid scan. The total dose over all time is expressed by

$$D = D_0 \times \{T_{eff})/\ln 2$$

where D_0 = dose rate at time zero
T_{eff} = effective half-life = $\{T_r + T_b) / \{T_r \times T_b\}$
T_r = radiologic half-life
T_b = biological half-life

In general, substances in the body are removed through biological processes as well as by radioactive decay; therefore the effective half-life is shorter than the radiologic half-life.

The dose rate from natural body ^{40}K in all living cells, by contrast, is relatively constant throughout life and is usually expressed as the annual dose rate.

Equivalent Dose

Ionizing radiation creates ion pairs in a substance such as air or tissue in relatively dense or sparse distribution depending upon the particle. Alpha particles with large mass produce relatively intense ionization tracks per unit distance relative to beta particles, and beta particles produce more dense ionization than gamma-rays. The ability to produce more or less ionization per unit path in a medium is quantitated by the LET. The linear energy transfer in a substance such as water is readily calculated.

The calculated LET from alpha and beta particles is therefore much greater than it is for gamma rays. In considering the health or cellular effects of each particle or ray, it is necessary to normalize the various types of radiation. For a particular biological endpoint, such as cell death in an experiment with mouse fibroblasts, it is common to calculate a relative biological effectiveness (RBE). This is defined as the ratio of gamma ray dose that yields the same endpoint to the dose from the radiation under study, for example, cell death.

Although giving the same dose to an organ from alpha particles as opposed to gamma rays would result in greater effects from the alpha particles, such refinement in the normalization of endpoints (cancer) in the human is not possible with the available data. An attempt to normalize human health effects from different types of radiation, i.e., to calculate an "equivalent" dose is made through the values for LET of the various types of radiation in water. The ratio of the LET for gamma to the radiation in question is defined as a *radiation weighting factor,* w_r (formerly Q), and the normalized (or weighted) dose is called the *equivalent dose*. The unit for the equivalent dose is the sievert (Sv), and the older unit is the rem:

$$H = Dw_r \tag{13}$$

where H = equivalent dose in sievert (older unit rem)
D = dose in gray (older unit rad)
w_r = radiation weighting factor

Table 25-2 gives the values of LET for different particles or rays and is reproduced from the National Council on Radiation Protection (NCRP, 1993) and the International Commission on Radiation Protection (ICRP, 1990).

Example 2 Find the equivalent dose (in sievert) for a dose to lung from an internal emitter of 0.01-Gy alpha particles and 0.01 Gy from external gamma-ray radiation.

$$\text{Alpha, } H = 0.01\ (20) = 0.20 \text{ Sv}$$
$$\text{Gamma, } H = 0.01\ (1) = 0.01 \text{ Sv}$$

Effective Dose and Cancer Risk

The term *effective dose* (ED) (formerly *effective dose equivalent*) was introduced formally by the ICRP in 1977 to allow addition or direct comparison of the cancer and genetic risk from different partial-body or whole-body doses. A partial-body gamma-ray dose to the lung, for example, is thought to give 0.0064 cancers over a lifetime per sievert, whereas a whole-body dose of 1 Sv would result in 0.056 total cancers and early genetic effects over the same lifetime interval. Both values are derived from the human A-bomb follow-up data. The ratio 0.0064/0.056 was defined as a tissue weighting factor, w_t, for lung and is numerically equal to 0.12.

The effective dose, H_E, is defined as a doubly weighted dose, weighted for radiation type and the tissue at risk.

$$H_E = w_t \times (Dw_r) \tag{14}$$

Table 25-2
Recommended Values of W_r for Various Types of Radiation

TYPE OF RADIATION	APPROXIMATE W_r
X-rays, gamma rays, beta particles, and electrons	1
Thermal neutrons	5
Neutrons (other than thermal ≫100 kev to 2 Mev), protons, alpha particles, charged particles of unknown energy	20

SOURCE: NCRP, 1993, and ICRP, 1990.

Table 25-3
Recommended Values of the Weighting Factors, w_t, for Calculating Effective Dose

TISSUE OR ORGAN	TISSUE WEIGHTING FACTOR, w_t
Gonads	0.20
Bone marrow (red)	0.12
Colon	0.12
Lung	0.12
Stomach	0.12
Bladder	0.05
Breast	0.05
Liver	0.05
Esophagus	0.05
Thyroid	0.05
Skin	0.01
Bone surface	0.01
Remainder	0.05*†

NOTE: The values have been developed from a reference population of equal numbers of both sexes and a wide range of ages. In the definition of effective dose, they apply to workers, to the whole population, and to either sex.

*For purposes of calculation, the remainder is composed of the following additional tissues and organs: adrenals, brain, upper large intestine, small intestine, kidney, muscle, pancreas, spleen, thymus, and uterus. The list includes organs that are likely to be selectively irradiated. Some organs in the list are known to be susceptible to cancer induction. If other tissues and organs subsequently become identified as having a significant risk of induced cancer, they will then be included either with a specific w_t or in this additional list constituting the remainder. The latter also may include other tissues or organs selectively irradiated.

†In exceptional cases in which a single one of the remainder tissues or organs receives an equivalent dose in excess of the highest dose in any of the 12 organs for which a weighting factor is specified, a weighting factor of 0.025 should be applied to that tissue or organ and a weighting factor of 0.025 should be applied to the average dose in the rest of the remainder as defined above.

SOURCES: NCRP, 1987, and ICRP, 1990.

This concept is useful in the case of occupational exposure, because H_E values from different sources to different organs can be summed to yield a direct estimate of total cancer and genetic risk.

Table 25-3 is taken from ICRP (1990) and gives the values of w_t for various organs.

The occupational guideline for H_E is 20 mSv per annum (NCRP, 1987; ICRP, 1990). This requires that the sum of all H_E be less than or equal to this value:

$$H_E = \sum w_t H \leq 20 \text{ mSv} \tag{15}$$

In 1990, the ICRP revised its 1977 estimates of risk and adopted and published Publication 60. This document includes new estimates of risk for both fatal and nonfatal cancer and new guidelines for the exposure of workers to external and internal radiation. The risk estimates are based largely on the analysis of Japanese A-bomb survivors. The occupational guidelines for radiation protection developed from the 1990 document are 100 mSv in 5 years (average, 20 mSv per year) with a limit of 50 mSv in any single year. This is compared with the 1977 limit of 50 mSv per year.

The ICRP document (ICRP, 1990) is a response to the increase in lifetime cancer risk from ionizing radiation observed in A-bomb survivors. Mental retardation for those exposed in utero is a finding in the A-bomb survivor cohort and is now included in the risk estimates.

The overall risk per unit exposure for adult workers and the risk for the whole population given in the ICRP (1990) are shown in Table 25-4. The risk of fatal cancer is adopted as 0.04 per sievert [4 percent per sievert (100 rem)] for adult workers and 0.05 per sievert [5 percent per sievert (100 rem)], for the whole adult population.

The NCRP (1993) chose to limit exposure to 20 mSv per year with a lifetime limit of (age × 10 mSv). The ICRP had been criticized for excluding the effects of nonfatal cancer in previous documents. An attempt to correct this omission was made in ICRP 60 (1990). An attempt was made to calculate the total detriment and is given the notation *aggregated detriment*. The aggregated detriment is the product of four factors: the probability of attributable fatal cancer, the weighted probability of nonfatal cancer, the weighted probability of severe hereditary effects, and the relative length of life lost. The nominal probability of fatal cancer per sievert, F, and the aggregated detriment are shown in Table 25-4. The computation of the aggregated detriment proceeds as follows. A cancer lethality fraction, K (the fraction of total cancer that is lethal), is used as a weighting factor for nonfatal cancers. The total number of cancers (fatal plus nonfatal) Sv^{-1} will be F/K. The total number of nonfatal cancers is $(1 - K)F/K$. The total weighted detriment is then

$$F + K(1 - K)F/K = F(2 - K)$$

The aggregated detriment is then the product of $F(2 - K)$ times the relative length of life lost, $1/l_{av}$, for a particular cancer. The average length of life lost, l_{av}, is 15 years per cancer. The aggregated detriment is tabulated as 7.3×10^{-2} Sv^{-1} for the whole adult population and $\times 10^{-2}$ 5.6 Sv^{-1} for the working population.

In assessing radiation risk from low-dose, low-dose-rate, low-LET radiation using risk coefficients derived from high-dose, high-dose-rate exposures, a dose rate–reduction factor (DREF) must be applied. NCRP (1980) and the United Nations Scientific Committee on the Effects of Atomic Radiation (UNSCEAR) (1988, 1993) have shown that the human data cover a range for the DREF of 2 to 10. That is, the original risk coefficients derived from the high-

Table 25-4
Nominal Probability Coefficients for Individual Tissues and Organs

	Probability of Fatal Cancer 10^{-2} Sv^{-1}		*Aggregated Detriment* 10^{-2} Sv^{-1}	
TISSUE OR ORGAN	WHOLE POPULATION	WORKERS	WHOLE POPULATION	WORKERS
Bladder	0.30	0.24	0.29	0.24
Bone marrow	0.50	0.40	1.04	0.83
Bone surface	0.05	0.04	0.07	0.06
Breast	0.20	0.16	0.36	0.29
Colon	0.85	0.68	1.03	0.82
Liver	0.15	0.12	0.16	0.13
Lung	0.85	0.68	0.80	0.64
Esophagus	0.30	0.24	0.24	0.19
Ovary	0.10	0.08	0.15	0.12
Skin	0.02	0.02	0.04	0.03
Stomach	1.10	0.88	1.00	0.80
Thyroid	0.08	0.06	0.15	0.12
Remainder	0.50	0.40	0.59	0.47
Total	5.00	4.00	5.92	4.74
	Probability of Severe Hereditary Disorders			
Gonads	1.00	0.6	1.33	0.80
Grand total (rounded)			7.3	5.6

NOTE: The values relate to a population of equal numbers of both sexes and a wide range of ages.
SOURCE: ICRP, 1990.

dose data are divided by the DREF factor to obtain the best estimate of effects at typical low-dose exposures. ICRP has used 2.5 as the adopted DREF; however, in ICRP (1990) a DREF of 2.0 was used, and this is incorporated in the nominal probability coefficients in Table 25-4. Table 25-4 is used universally to assess the effects of occupational exposure.

The overall objective of both NCRP and ICRP dose limitation recommendations is to control the lifetime risk to maximally exposed individuals. ICRP (1990) limits the lifetime occupational effective dose to (20 mSv × 50 years) = 1000 mSv. In 1993, NCRP (1993) reduced the U.S. Recommendation for Lifetime Exposure to (age × 10 mSv) or approximately 700 mSv, with an average annual limit of 20 mSv and a maximum annual limit of 50 mSv.

The dose to members of the public is also considered by ICRP and NCRP. For continuous exposure to human-made sources, i.e., other than medical or natural, it is recommended that the annual effective dose not exceed 1 mSv (100 mrem), and for infrequent exposures the annual effective dose should not exceed 5 mSv (500 mrem).

Committed Equivalent Dose

A problem arises with internal emitters in that once they are ingested, there is an irreversible dose that is committed because of the biokinetics of the particular element. The absorbed dose depends on the biological and physical half-times of the element in the body. For this reason, the concepts of committed equivalent dose and committed effective dose were derived to accommodate the potential for the dose to be delivered over long periods after incorporation in the body. The committed dose is taken over a 50-year interval after exposure and is equal to

$$H_{\mathrm{t},50} = \int_{t_0}^{t_0+50} H_\mathrm{t}\,\mathrm{d}t \tag{16}$$

where $H_{\mathrm{t},50}$ = 50-year dose to tissue T for a single intake at time t_0

H_t = equivalent dose rate in organ or tissue T at time t

The NCRP (1987, 1993) recognizes that for radionuclides with half-lives ranging up to about 3 months, the committed equivalent dose is equal to the annual dose for the year of intake. For longer-lived nuclides, the committed equivalent dose will be greater than the annual equivalent dose and must be calculated on an individual basis. ICRP Publication 30 (ICRP, 1978) provides the details of this calculation for all nuclides.

Negligible Individual Risk Level (Negligible Dose)

The current radiobiologic principle commonly accepted is that of linear, nonthreshold cancer induction from ionizing radiation. Thus, regardless of the magnitude of the dose, a numerical cancer risk can be calculated. For this reason, the NCRP proposed the negligible individual risk level (NIRL) and defined it as "a level of annual excess risk of fatal health effects attributable to irradiation below which further effort to reduce radiation exposure to the individual is unwarranted."

The NCRP emphasized that the NIRL is not to be confused with an acceptable risk level, a level of significance, or a limit.

The NCRP recommended an annual effective equivalent dose limit for continuous exposure of members of the public of 1 mSv (0.1 rem). This value is in addition to that received from natural background radiation (about 2 mSv). In this context, the NIRL was taken to be 0.01 mSv (1 mrem). In NCRP (1993) the notation used currently is negligible individual dose (NID).

MECHANISMS OF DNA DAMAGE AND MUTAGENESIS

Energy Deposition in the Cell Nucleus

DNA is a double-helical macromolecule consisting of four repeating units: the purine bases adenine (A) and guanine (G) and the pyrimidine bases thymine (T) and cytosine (C). The bases are arranged in two linear arrays (or strands) held together by hydrogen bonds centrally and linked externally by covalent bonds to sugar-phosphate residues (the DNA "backbone"). The adenine base pairs naturally with thymine (A:T base pair), while guanine pairs with cytosine (G:C base pair), so that one DNA strand has the complementary sequence of the other. The sequence of the bases defines the genetic code; each gene has a unique sequence, but certain common sequences exist in control and structural DNA elements. Damage to DNA may affect any one of its components, but it is the loss or alteration of base sequence that has genetic consequences (UNSCEAR, 2000).

Ionizing radiation loses energy and slows down by forming ion pairs (a positively charged atom and an electron). Different ionization densities result from gamma rays, beta particles, and alpha particles. Their track structure is broadly characterized as from sparsely ionizing, (or low-LET), to densely ionizing (high-LET) radiation. Each track of low-LET radiation, resulting from x-rays or gamma rays, consists of a few ionizations across an average-sized cell nucleus (e.g., an electron set in motion by a gamma ray crossing an 8-μm-diameter nucleus gives an average of about 70 ionizations, equivalent to about 5 mGy (500 mrad) absorbed dose. Individual tracks vary widely about this value because of the stochastic nature of energy deposition, i.e., variability of ion pars per μm and path length through the nucleus. A high-LET alpha particle produces many thousands of ionizations and gives a relatively high dose to the cell. For example, a 4-MeV alpha-particle track yields on average, about 30,000 ionizations (3 Gy, 300 rad) in an average-sized cell nucleus. However, within the nucleus even low-LET gamma radiation will give some microregions of relatively dense ionization over the dimensions of DNA structures due to the low-energy electrons set in motion (UNSCEAR, 2000).

Direct and Indirect Ionization

Radiation tracks may deposit energy directly in DNA (direct effect) or may ionize other molecules closely associated with DNA, hydrogen or oxygen, to form free radicals that can damage DNA (indirect effect). Within a cell, the indirect effect occurs over very short distances, of the order of a few nanometers. The diffusion distance of radicals is limited by their reactivity. Although it is difficult to measure accurately the different contributions made by the direct and indirect effects to DNA damage caused by low-LET radiation, evidence from radical scavengers introduced into cells suggests that about 35 percent is exclusively direct and 65 percent has an indirect (scavengeable) component (Reuvers et al., 1973).

It has been argued that both direct and indirect effects cause similar early damage to DNA; this is because the ion radicals produced by direct ionization of DNA may react further to produce DNA radicals similar to those produced by water-radical attack on DNA (Ward, 1975).

DNA Damage

Ionization frequently disrupts chemical bonding in cellular molecules such as DNA. If the majority of ionizations occur as single isolated events (low-LET radiation), the disruptions are readily repaired by cellular enzymes. The average density of ionization by high-LET radiations is such that several ionizations may occur as the particle traverses a DNA double helix. Therefore, much of the damage from high-LET radiations, as well as a minority of the DNA damage from low-LET radiations, will derive from localized clusters of ionizations that can severely disrupt the DNA structure (Goodhead, 1992; Ward, 1994). While the extent of local clustering of ionizations in DNA from single tracks of low and high-LET radiations will overlap, high-LET radiation tracks are more efficient at inducing larger clusters and hence more complex damage. Also, high-LET radiations will induce some very large clusters of ionizations that do not occur with low-LET radiations; the resulting damage may be irreparable and may also have unique cellular consequences (Goodhead, 1994). When a cell is damaged by high-LET radiation, each track will give large numbers of ionizations, so that the cell will receive a relatively high dose, as noted in the calculation above, and there will be a greater probability of correlated damage within a single DNA molecule. As a consequence, the irradiation of a population of cells or a tissue with a "low dose" of high-LET radiation results in a few cells being hit with a relatively high dose (one track) rather than in each cell receiving a small dose. In contrast, low-LET radiation is more uniformly distributed over the cell population. At doses of low-LET radiation in excess of about 1 mGy (for an average-size cell nucleus of 8 μm in diameter), each cell nucleus is likely to be traversed by more than one sparsely ionizing track.

The interaction of ionizing radiation with DNA produces numerous types of damage; the chemical products of many of these have been identified and classified according to their structure. These products differ according to which chemical bond is attacked, which base is modified, and the extent of the damage within a given segment of DNA. Table 25-5 lists some of the main damage products that can be measured following low-LET irradiation of DNA, with a rough estimate of their abundance (UNSCEAR, 2000). Attempts have also been made to predict the frequencies of different damage types from the knowledge of radiation track structure, with certain assumptions about the minimum energy deposition (number of ionizations) required. Interactions can be classified according to the probability they will cause a single-strand DNA alteration (e.g., a break in the backbone or base alteration) or alterations in both strands in close proximity in one DNA molecule (e.g., a double-strand break), or a more complex type of DNA damage (e.g., a double-strand break with adjacent damage). Good agreement has been obtained between these predictions and direct measurements of single-strand breaks, but there is less agreement for other categories of damage. While complex forms of damage are difficult to quantify with current experimental techniques, the

Table 25-5
Estimated Yields of DNA Damage in Mammalian Cells Caused by Low-LET Radiation Exposures

TYPE OF DAMAGE	YIELD (NUMBER OF DEFECTS PER CELL Gy^{-1})
Single-strand breaks	1000
Base damage*	500
Double-strand breaks	40
DNA protein cross-links	150

*Base excision enzyme-sensitive sites or antibody detection of thymine glycol.
SOURCE: UNSCEAR, 2000.

use of enzymes that cut DNA at sites of base damage suggests that irradiation of DNA in solution gives complex damage sites consisting mainly of closely spaced base damage (measured as oxidized bases of abasic sites); double-strand breaks were associated with only 20 percent of the complex damage sites (Sutherland et al., 2000). It is expected that the occurrence of more complex types of damage will increase with increasing LET, and that this category of damage will be less repairable than the simpler forms of damage. Theoretical simulations have predicted that about 30 percent of DNA double-strand breaks from low-LET radiation are complex because of additional breaks (Nikjoo et al., 1977) and that this proportion rises to more than 70 percent, and the degree of complexity increases, for high-LET particles (Goodhead and Nikjoo, 1997).

Some of the DNA damage caused by ionizing radiation is chemically similar to damage that occurs naturally in the cell. This "spontaneous" damage arises from the thermal instability of DNA as well as endogenous oxidative and enzymatic processes. Several metabolic pathways produce oxidative radicals within the cell, and these radicals can attack DNA to give both DNA base damage and breakage, mostly as isolated events. The more complex types of damage caused by radiation may not occur spontaneously, since localized concentrations of endogenous radicals are less likely to be generated in the immediate vicinity of DNA (UNSCEAR, 2000).

HUMAN STUDIES OF RADIATION TOXICITY

There have been five major studies of the health detriment resulting from exposure of humans to ionizing radiation. Other studies of large worker populations exposed to very low levels of radiation and environmental populations exposed to radon are ongoing, but they are not expected to provide new data on the risk estimates from ionizing radiation. These worker or environmental populations are studied to ensure that there is no inconsistency in the radiation risk data in extrapolating from the higher exposures. The basic studies on which the quantitative risk calculations are founded include radium exposures, A-bomb survivors, underground miners exposed to radon, patients irradiated with x-rays for ankylosing spondylitis, and children irradiated with x-rays for tinea capitis (ringworm).

Radium Exposures ($^{226,228}Ra$)

Radium was discovered in the early part of the twentieth century. Its unique properties suggested a potential for the healing arts. It was incorporated into a wide variety of nostrums, medicines, and artifacts. The highest exposure occurred in the United States among radium dial painters who ingested from 10s to 1000s of micrograms (microcuries). These exposed groups, including patients, chemists, and dial painters, have been studied for over 60 years to determine the body retention of radium and the health effects of long-term body burdens.

The only late effect of ingestion of $^{226,228}Ra$ seen is osteogenic sarcoma. It is significant that no study has identified a statistically significant excess of leukemia after even massive doses of radium. This implies that the target cells for leukemia residing in bone marrow are outside the short range of the radium series alpha particles (70 μm). Several thousand people were exposed to radium salts either as part of the modish therapies using radium in the era from 1900 to 1930 or occupationally in the radium dial–painting industry around 1920. Radium therapy was accepted by the American Medical Association, and in around 1915 advertisements were common for radium treatment of rheumatism and as a general tonic and in the treatment of mental disorders. Solutions were available for drinking containing 2 μg/60 cm^3 as well as ampoules for intravenous injection containing 5 to 100 μg radium (Woodard, 1980). Luminous paint was developed before World War I, and in 1917 there were many plants in New England and New Jersey painting watch dials, clocks, and military instruments (Woodard, 1980).

The first large studies on osteogenic sarcoma in radium-exposed people were done by Martland (1931) and Aub and associates (1952), who found 30 cases of bone sarcoma; Evans and associates (1969) with 496 cases of sarcoma out of 1064 studied at the Massachusetts Institute of Technology; and Rowland et al. (1978), with 61 cases out of 1474 female dial painters (Woodard 1980).

Radium, once ingested, is somewhat similar to calcium in its metabolism and is incorporated on bone surfaces into the mineralized portion of bone. The long half-life of ^{226}Ra (1600 y) allows distribution throughout the mineral skeleton over life. The target cells for osteogenic sarcoma reside in marrow on endosteal surfaces at about 10 μm from the bone surface. At long times after exposure, target cells are beyond the range of alpha particles from radium not on bone surfaces.

The loss of radium from the body by excretion was determined to follow a relatively simple power function (Norris et al., 1955):

$$R = 0.54\, t^{-0.52} \tag{17}$$

where R = total body retention
t = time in days

Other models to fit the data were developed as more information became available, the most recent being that of Marshall et al. (1972). The entire body of radium data and the various models are shown in Fig. 25-1. It can be seen that the Norris function fits the observed data well except at very long times after exposure. A simplified form of the more complex later model of Marshall and associates (1972) which fits the human data over all observed times is

$$R = 0.8t^{-0.5}\,(0.5e^{-\lambda t} + 0.5e^{-4\lambda t}) \tag{18}$$

where R = whole body retention
λ = rate of bone apposition or resorption = 0.0001 day^{-1}
t = time in days

For most purposes, the Norris formula is applicable. It can be seen from Fig. 25-1 for the Norris equation that even 1 year after exposure, only about 2 percent of the radium is retained in the body but that after 30 years, about 0.5 percent still remains. The risk of osteogenic bone cancer after radium exposure has been summa-

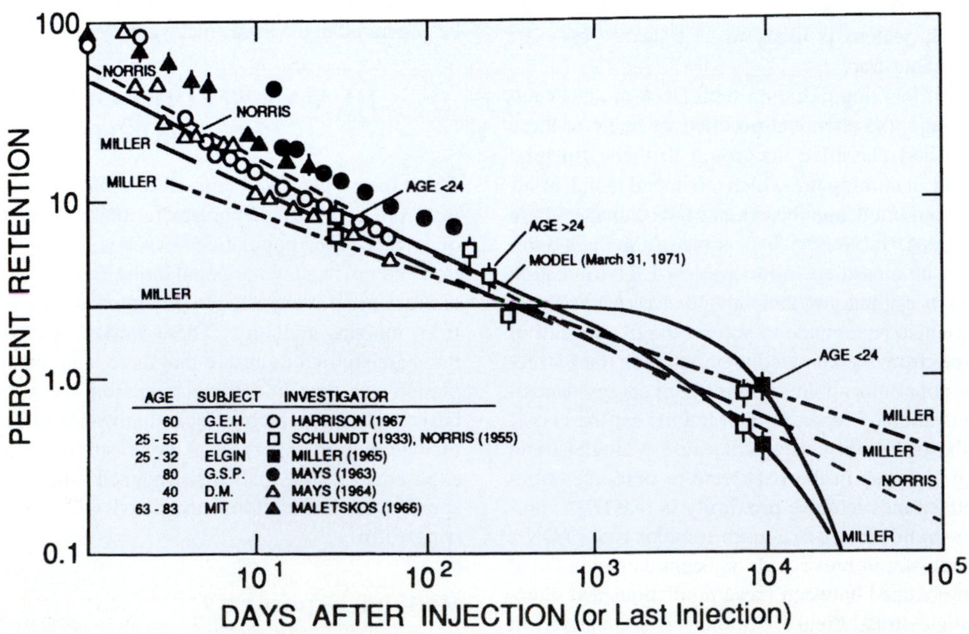

Figure 25-1. Whole-body radium retention in humans. Summary of all available data for adult humans. (From Marshall et al., 1972, with permission.)

rized in the National Academy of Sciences report BEIR IV (NAS, 1988).

Equations were proposed by Rowland and coworkers (1978) for the annual risk of sarcoma (including the natural risk), and expressed as a function of either radium intake or dose from $^{226,228}Ra$. Risk per unit intake is

$$I = [0.7 \times 10^{-5} + (7 \times 10^{-8})\, D^2]\, \exp[-(1.1 \times 10^{-3})\, D] \quad (19)$$

where I = total bone sarcomas per person year at risk
D = total systemic intake of ^{226}Ra plus 2.5 times total systemic intake of ^{228}Ra, both in microcuries

Risk per unit dose is

$$I = [10^{-5} + (9.8 \times 10^{-6})D^2]\, \exp(-1.5 \times 10^{-2}\, D) \quad (20)$$

where I = total bone sarcomas per person year at risk
D = total mean skeletal dose in Gray from ^{226}Ra plus 1.5 times mean skeletal dose from ^{228}Ra

Raabe and associates (1980) modeled bone sarcoma risk in the human, dog, and mouse and determined that there is a practical threshold dose and dose rate (a dose low enough so that bone cancer will not appear within the human life span). The dose rate is 0.04 Gy per day or a total dose of 0.8 Gy to the skeleton. This practical threshold for bone cancer has useful implications in considering health effects from exposures to environmental radioactivity.

Radium Exposure (^{224}Ra)

In Europe, ^{224}Ra was used for more than 40 years in the treatment of tuberculosis and ankylosing spondylitis. The treatment of children was abandoned in the 1950s, but the ability to relieve debilitating pain from ankylosing spondylitis in adults has prolonged its use. ^{224}Ra is different from ^{226}Ra in that it has a short half-life (3.62 days) and the alpha dose is delivered completely while the radium is still on bone surfaces.

Spiess and Mays (1970) and Mays (1988) studied the health of 899 German patients given ^{224}Ra therapeutically. The calculated average mean skeletal dose was 30 Gy (range, 0.06 to 57.5 Gy) with injection time spans ranging from 1 to 45 months. There were two groups—juveniles and adults—and the bone sarcoma response was not significantly different for the two. There were 60 patients who developed bone sarcoma (Gossner 1999), 46 have been studied for histologic type. Further study of this group revealed other solid tumors with statistically significant excesses of male and female breast cancer, thyroid cancer and liver cancer (Nekolla et al., 1999).

In a second cohort, Wick and colleagues (1986, 1999) studied 1432 adult patients treated for ankylosing spondylitis with an average skeletal dose of 0.65 Gy. This study was originally started by Otto Hug and Fritz Schales and has been continued since their deaths. Four patients in this group have developed osteogenic sarcoma, and one in the control group.

Spiess and Mays (1973) found that the observed effectiveness of the ^{224}Ra in their cohort in producing bone sarcomas increased if the time span of the injections was long. Injections were given in 1, 10, or 50 weekly fractions. They developed an empiric expression to estimate the added risk from this protracted injection schedule:

$$I = \{0.003 + 0.014\, [1 - \exp(0.09m)]D \quad (21)$$

where I = cumulative incidence of bone sarcomas after most tumors have appeared (25 years)
m = span of injections in months
D = average skeletal dose in Gy

Chemelevsky and coworkers (1986) analyzed the Spiess data and developed an equation for the total cumulative sarcoma risk from ^{224}Ra:

$$R = (0.0085D + 0.0017D^2)\exp(-0.025D) \quad (22)$$

where R = cumulative risk of bone sarcoma
D = average skeletal dose in Gy

These two equations for risk predict 5.7 and 5.8 bone sarcomas in the second series of (spondylitis) patients, with 2 actually observed.

Chemelevsky and coworkers (1986) also showed that in the Spiess study, linearity (sarcoma response with dose) could be rejected. For example, equation 22 results in a lifetime risk of sarcoma of 0.02 Gy^{-1} at an average skeletal dose of 10 Gy but 0.01 Gy^{-1} at 1 Gy. Also, there was no difference in sarcoma response between juveniles and adults. These data are presented in Fig. 25-2. Again, no excess leukemia was found in either series of ^{224}Ra patients.

Atomic Bomb Survivors

On August 6, 1945, the U.S. military dropped an atomic bomb on the city of Hiroshima, Japan. Three days later a second bomb was dropped on Nagasaki which effectively ended World War II. The weapons were of two different types, the first being ^{235}U and the second a ^{239}Pu device.

Within 1 km of the explosions in both cities, a total of 64,000 people were killed by the blast and the thermal effects and as a result of the instantaneous gamma and neutron radiation released by the weapons. Others between 1 and 2 km from the hypocenter (the

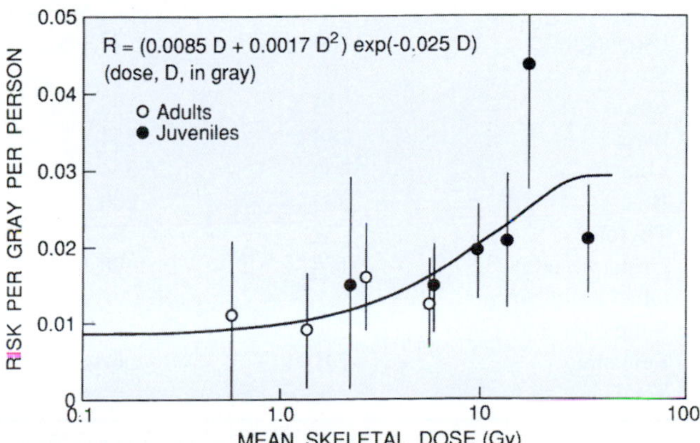

Figure 25-2. Lifetime risk per gray versus mean skeletal dose in ^{224}Ra-exposed subjects. (From Chemelevsky et al., 1986, with permission.)

point on earth directly below the detonation point in air) received radiation doses up to several gray.

Within a few years it was decided to follow the health of the people in both cities over their lifetime to determine quantitatively the effects of external ionizing radiation. The study of prospective mortality of A-bomb survivors was initiated by the Atomic Bomb Casualty Commission (ABCC) in 1950 and is ongoing by the Radiation Effects Research Foundation (RERF). The main study, called the Life Span Study (LSS), included 92,228 people within 10,000 m of the hypocenter and 26,850 people who were not in either city at the time of bombing (ATB). The most recent reports of the RERF (1987) are follow-up of the cancer mortality of a subcohort (DS86 subcohort) of 75,991 persons over the periods 1950–1985, and 1950–1990 (Pierce and Preston 1993).

In 1978, questions arose that the original dose estimates for persons in the LSS might be somewhat in error and that an effort should be made to improve the dose estimates. This study was published in a United States–Japan joint reassessment of dose called DS86—Dosimetry System 1986 (RERF, 1987).

Dose estimation by reconstruction of the event is always problematic, but direct computation of dose to about 18,500 persons in the LSS with detailed shielding information is complete. The remaining DS86 dose values for 57,000 individuals without detailed shielding information are also incorporated into the mortality study by various estimation techniques. Of the 75,991 persons in the DS86 subcohort, 16,207 were within 2000 m of the hypocenter, and these are the individuals who received a substantial exposure.

Previous reports of cancer risk estimates were based on the air dose (gamma ray plus neutron tissue kerma in air) adjusted for shielding by structures or terrain. The 1987 and 1988 reports also include DS86 organ dose estimates, and these are about 80 percent of the shielded kerma (Shimizu et al., 1988).

The dose from fallout at Hiroshima and Nagasaki has not been included in the health effects studies. Fallout was found in certain restricted localities in Nagasaki and Hiroshima. The absorbed dose from gamma rays at Nagasaki for persons continuously in the fallout area from 1 h on ranged from 0.12 to 0.24 Gy. The absorbed doses at Hiroshima ranged from 0.006 to 0.02 Gy. Because the region of fallout was quite limited, the total contribution of fallout to survivor dose was probably negligible in Hiroshima but may have been significant for a limited number of survivors in Nagasaki, where an exposure of one-fifth the maximum extends over some 1000 hectares. Estimates of internal dose from ingested ^{137}Cs yield about 0.0001 Gy integrated over 40 years (Harley, 1987; RERF, 1987).

Complete mortality data and the dose estimates are reported in RERF Technical Reports 5-88 (RERF, 1988) and were updated by Pierce and Preston (1993) and in UNSCEAR (2000). The projected lifetime cancer risks as of the follow-up through 1990 are reported in UNSCEAR (2000), and these data are summarized in Table 25-6.

No statistically significant excess cancer of the gallbladder, bone, pancreas, uterus, or prostate or of malignant lymphoma has been seen in the LSS to date.

It is of interest to consider the effect of smoking, as it is the most important factor in assessing lung cancer risk. The analysis performed by Shimuzu and associates (1988) examined the interaction of smoking and radiation in detail. The results showed no interaction indicating that smoking and the atom bomb radiation act independently rather than multiplicatively in lung cancer induction.

It is also possible to model the risk over the full life if a projection model is assumed. RERF has preferred a constant relative risk model (radiation mortality is a constant fraction of the baseline age-specific mortality per gray) for this purpose. There is evidence in the atom bomb mortality and in several other studies discussed later (ankylosing spondylitis patients, uranium miners) that the constant relative risk model is not appropriate but that the risk coefficient decreases with time subsequent to exposure. In most cases this also means that the absolute excess cancer risk (risk above that expected) declines with time. This is a biologically plau-

Table 25-6

Observed and Expected Cases of Cancer in A-Bomb Survivors with DS86 Dose Estimate and Projections of Lifetime Cancer Incidence from Radiation for a Dose of 0.1 Sv

				*Projection of Lifetime Cancer Incidence (%) for a Dose of 0.1 Sv**	
CANCER TYPE	OBSERVED CASES	EXPECTED CASES	MEAN DOSE (Sv)	MALES	FEMALES
Esophagus	84	77.4	0.23	0.04	0.02
Stomach	1307	1222	0.23	0.17	0.17
Colon	223	193.7	0.23	0.13	0.19
Liver	284	254.5	0.24	0.23	0.41
Lung	456	364.7	0.25	0.23	0.07
Breast	295	200	0.27	0.0	0.52
Thyroid	132	94.3	0.26	0.07	0.04
Urinary bladder	115	98.1	0.23	0.03	0.13
Other solid cancer				0.26	0.15
Solid cancer				1.16	1.70
Leukemia	141	67.4	0.25	0.05	0.05
Total				1.21	1.75

*Projection of cancer incidence based on the attained age model, UNSCEAR (2000), and a whole-body exposure of 0.1 Sv at age 30. Mortality projections for total cancer 0.67 and 0.99 percent per 0.1 Sv, for males and females respectively.

sible model suggesting the loss or repair of the damaged stem cell population.

The estimates of lifetime risk of cancer may increase somewhat with time, but given the present age of the population, the final values are unlikely to be significantly higher than the values in Table 25-6.

Tinea Capitis (Ringworm) Irradiation

During the period 1905–1960, x-ray epilation in the treatment of tinea capitis was performed regularly in children. The treatment was introduced by Sabouraud in 1904 and was standardized by Kienbock (1907) and Adamson (1909). Over the half century it was used, as many as 200,000 children worldwide may have been irradiated (Albert et al., 1986).

No follow-up studies of the long-term effects of irradiation were performed until Albert and Omran (1968) reported on 2200 children irradiated at the Skin and Cancer Unit of New York University Hospital during 1940–1959. Subsequent publications on this group have appeared at regular intervals (Shore et al., 1976, 1984, 1990).

Since the New York University (NYU) study, a follow-up of 11,000 children irradiated in Israel was performed (Ron and Modan, 1984; Ron et al. 1991).

The mean age of children irradiated in both the New York and Israeli studies was between 7 and 8 years. Dose reconstruction in the NYU series was performed using a head phantom containing the skull of a 7-year-old child covered with tissue-equivalent material (Schulz and Albert, 1963; Harley et al., 1976, 1983). The doses to organs in the head and neck for a typical Adamson-Kienbock five-field treatment of the scalp are shown in Table 25-7, and the dose to the skin is shown in Fig. 25-3.

In the NYU series there were 2 thyroid cancers with 1.4 expected cases. In the Israeli series there were 43 thyroid cancers with 10.7 expected cases. In the NYU series there are 83 skin lesions, predominantly basal cell carcinoma, with 24 expected cases, in 41 persons. Fairness of skin is an important factor in the appearance of skin cancer (Shore et al., 1984, 1990). Skin cancer was found only in whites even though 25 percent of the study population consisted of blacks. This and the fact that there appears to be a much lower dose response on the hair-covered scalp than on the face and neck (Harley et al., 1983) suggest that the promotional effects of UV radiation play an important role in skin cancer.

The dose estimate for the thyroid in the Israeli study is 0.09 Gy compared with 0.06 Gy in the NYU study.

A risk projection model was used to estimate the lifetime risk of basal cell carcinoma (BCC) for facial skin and for the hair-covered scalp after x-ray epilation in whites. The model used was a cumulative hazard plot which assumes that the BCC appearance rate in the exposed population remains constant over time (Harley et al., 1983). The result of this risk projection for BCC is shown in Table 25-8.

The small numbers of tumors other than skin cancers in the NYU study make it of dubious value in estimating the lifetime risk per Gy although an excess is appearing. The tinea capitis studies are prospective, and sound numerical values are forthcoming as these populations age. These are particularly important studies because children were the exposed group and because only partial body irradiation was involved. The temporal pattern of appearance of these tumors is also important. The dose was delivered over a short time interval (minutes at NYU and 5 days in Israel), and lifetime patterns will be indicative of the underlying carcinogenic mechanisms.

Skin and thyroid cancers are of importance in documenting health effects from ionizing radiation. However, both types of cancer are rarely fatal. NCRP (1985) reported that about 10 percent of thyroid cancer is lethal. It is estimated that the fatality rate of skin cancer is 1 percent (NCRP, 1990). The lifetime risk per gray derived by NCRP for total thyroid cancer incidence (0.003 for females and 0.0014 for males for external x-ray or gamma radiation for persons under 18 years of age) is about a factor of 10 lower than that reported by Ron and Modan (1984, 1991) in tinea capitis irradiations. However, the tinea irradiations were given to children with a mean age of about 7 years, also in the Israeli study there is apparently an increased sensitivity resulting from ethnicity.

The effect of ethnicity and sex is also suggested by NCRP (1985) for thyroid cancer. The incidence rates of spontaneous thyroid cancer for persons of Jewish origin in Europe and North America are three to four times that for other racial groups. There is an obvious susceptibility of women for thyroid cancer and adenomas in both the NYU and Israeli tinea capitis studies.

Table 25-7
Average Dose to Organs in the Head and Neck from Measurements Performed with a Phantom for a Child's Head

ORGAN	AVERAGE DOSE AT 25 cm TREATMENT DISTANCE, rad
Scalp	220–540
Brain	140
Eye	16
Internal ear	71
Cranial marrow	385
Pituitary	49
Parotid gland	39
Thyroid	6
Skin (eyelid)	16
Skin (nose)	11
Skin (midneck)	9

Chernobyl and Radioactive Iodine (^{131}I)–Induced Thyroid Cancer

The Chernobyl accident (April 26, 1986) was the result of efforts to conduct a test on the electrical control system, which allows power to be provided in the event of a station blackout. The details of the accident have been published in a report of the International Atomic Energy Agency (IAEA 1992), and UNSCEAR (2000). Basically, there was a rapid increase in the reactor power. Part of the fuel in the pressurized water reactor was vaporized, resulting in an explosion that blew the reactor core apart and destroyed much of the containment building. The estimates of the significant radionuclides for health effects released during the accident are 1800 PBq (4.9×10^7 Ci) ^{131}I and 85 PBq (2.3×10^6 Ci) ^{137}Cs, and 10 PBq (2.7×10^5 Ci) ^{90}Sr (UNSCEAR, 2000).

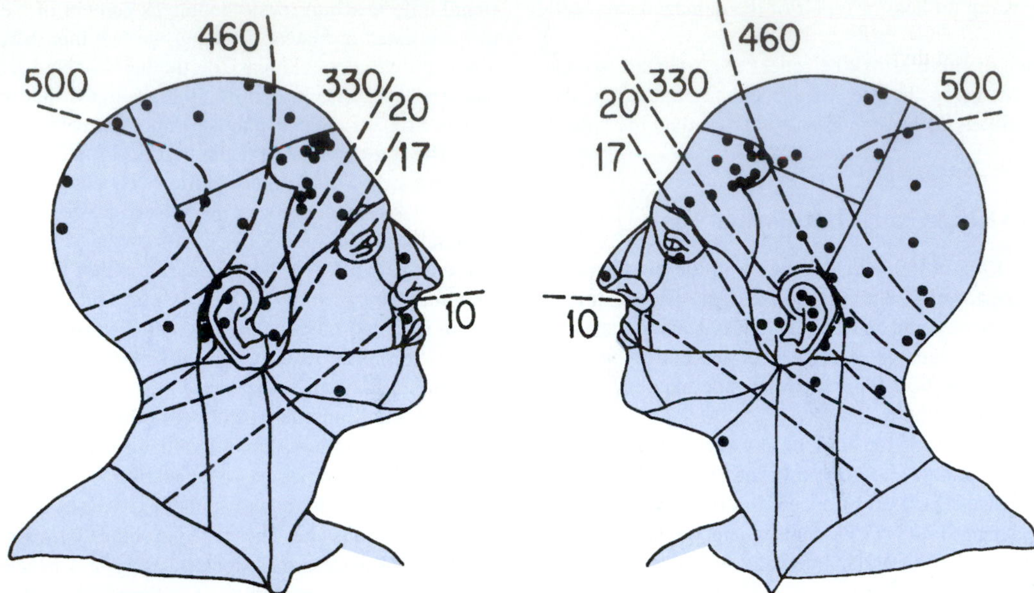

Figure 25-3. X-ray dose in rads for the Adamson-Kienbock five-field tinea capitis treatment and locations of basal cell lesions. (From Shore et al., 1984, with permission.)

The accident caused the deaths within days or weeks of 30 power plant employees and firemen (including 28 deaths that were due to radiation exposure). During 1986, 220,000 people were evacuated from areas surrounding the reactor, and, after 1986, of about 250,000 people were relocated from what were at that time three constituent republics of the Soviet Union: Belarus, the Russian Federation, and Ukraine. Large areas in these three republics were contaminated, and deposition of fission product radionuclides was measurable in all countries of the northern hemisphere. In addition, about 240,000 workers, termed "liquidators," were mobilized in 1986 and 1987 to take part in major mitigation activities at the reactor and within the 30-km zone surrounding the reactor. Residual mitigation activities continued until 1990. In all, about 600,000 persons received the special status of "liquidator."

The radiation exposures resulting from the Chernobyl accident were due initially to ^{131}I and short-lived radionuclides and subsequently to radiocesium (^{134}Cs and ^{137}Cs) from both external exposure and the consumption of foods contaminated with these radionuclides. UNSCEAR (1988) estimated that, outside the regions of Belarus, the Russian Federation, and Ukraine, thyroid doses averaged over large portions of European countries were 25 mGy for 1-year-old infants. However, the dose distribution was very heterogeneous, especially in countries near the reactor site. For example, in Poland, although the countrywide population-weighted average thyroid dose was estimated to be 8 mGy, the mean thyroid doses for the populations of particular districts ranged from 0.2 to 64 mGy. Individual dose values for about 5 percent of the children were 200 mGy. UNSCEAR (1988) estimates that effective dose averaged over large portions of European countries were 1 mSv or less in the first year after the accident and approximately two to five times the first-year dose over a full lifetime.

To date there is a significant increase in the number of thyroid cancers in the three territories. Approximately 1600 thyroid cancers have been identified in children under the age of 17 at the

Table 25-8
Estimated Lifetime Risk Estimates for Basal Cell Carcinoma (BCC) and Thyroid Cancer after X-Ray Irradiation for Tinea Capitis

	TOTAL INCIDENCE, RISK Gy^{-1}	MORTALITY, RISK Gy^{-1}
Skin malignancies (NYU study)		
BCC (facial skin)	0.32	
BCC (hair-covered scalp)	0.01	
Thyroid malignancies (Israeli study)		
Male	0.01	0.001
Female	0.04	0.004

time of the accident. The expected number of thyroid cancer cases is not known, but is evidently a small fraction of those observed. No solid tumors other than thyroid cancer have been identified resulting from the accident. Figure 25-4 shows the sequential increase in the number of thyroid cancers in children under the age of 14 at the time of the accident. It is well established that release of ^{131}I presents the major health effect in a nuclear accident. Many countries prepare for such accidents and have ready a large supply of potassium iodide (KI), which effectively blocks the thyroid uptake of radioactive iodine. Had this been available in time, it is questionable whether the large number of tumors seen would have occurred.

Medical Administration of ^{131}I Iodine-131 is given medically in three ways. Very large quantities, 3.7×10^9 Bq (100 mCi) or more are administered to ablate the thyroid in thyroid cancer, lesser quantities (about 10 mCi or 3.7×10^8 Bq) are given for hyperthyroidism, and the lowest quantity given (0.1 mCi or 3.7×10^6) is for diagnostic purposes (UNSCEAR, 1993). Individuals have also been exposed to ^{131}I as a result of nuclear weapons testing. Very few thyroid cancers have been found subsequent to these exposures, with the exception of the 243 Marshall Island inhabitants who received a large dose from a mixture of radionuclides (^{131}I, ^{132}I, ^{133}I, ^{134}I, and ^{135}I), tellurium, and gamma-ray radiation from the 1954 Bravo thermonuclear test (Conard, 1984) in the Pacific. The mean thyroid dose was estimated as 3 to 52 Gy in children and 1.6 to 12 Gy in adults. Over a 32-year follow-up period, 7 of 130 women and 2 of 113 men developed thyroid cancer.

Attempts have been made to relate external gamma-ray radiation and ^{131}I exposure. The NCRP (NCRP, 1985) estimated from human data that the effectiveness ratio of ^{131}I/gamma-ray radiation is between 0.1 and 1.0. In a more recent review of the human data, Shore (1992) found 8.3 observed excess cancers derived from all ^{131}I studies and 37 cases based on risk estimates from external exposure. The ratio 8.3/37 yields an estimate for the effectiveness ratio of 0.22. The protracted dose to the thyroid during the decay of ^{131}I may explain the difference; however, the nonuniform distribution of ^{131}I in the thyroid also may be a factor (Sinclair et al., 1956).

It is evident that ^{131}I can expose large populations after nuclear weapons testing or nuclear accidents. Generally, it is the ingestion

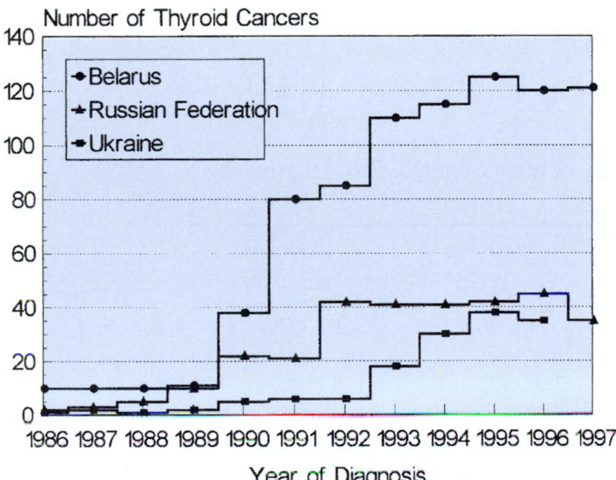

Figure 25-4. Thyroid cancer in children under 14 at the time of the Chernobyl accident. (From UNSCEAR, 2000.)

pathway that is most significant. Iodine is ingested quickly either from surface deposition on edible plants or from pasture grass to the cow, to milk, and to the thyroid. A large body of data exists on the transfer coefficients, P_{24} (intake to the body per unit deposition), P_{45} (effective dose per unit intake), and P_{25} ($P_{25} = P_{24} \times P_{45}$) = effective dose per unit deposition). UNSCEAR (1993) reported the transfer coefficients for ^{131}I to be

$P_{24} = 0.07$ Bq per Bq m^{-2}
$P_{45} = 61$ nSv per Bq intake (effective dose for the thyroid)
$P_{25} = P_{24} \times P_{45} = 4.2$ nSv per Bq m^{-2} (effective dose for the thyroid)

Ankylosing Spondylitis

About 14,000 persons, mostly men, were treated with x-rays for ankylosing spondylitis at 87 radiotherapy centers in Great Britain and Northern Ireland between 1935 and 1954. Court Brown and Doll (1957) were the first to report that these patients had a leukemia risk substantially in excess of that for the general population. Subsequent publications have developed the time pattern of appearance not only of leukemia but also of solid tumors (Court Brown and Doll, 1959, 1965; Smith and Doll, 1978, 1982; Smith, 1984; Darby et al., 1985, 1987; Weiss et al., 1994).

A group was selected consisting of 11,776 men and 2335 women all of whom had been treated with x-rays either once or twice. About half the total group received a second x-ray treatment or treatment with thorium. The reports on the ankylosing spondylitis patients attempt to consider health effects from only the first x-ray treatment. For this reason, an individual receiving a second treatment is included in their follow-up only until 18 months after the second course (a short enough time so that any malignancies in this interval cannot be ascribed to the second x-ray treatment).

The appearance of excess leukemia is now well documented, and solid tumors are also apparent in the population. The part of the body in the direct x-ray beam (spine) received the highest dose, but it is thought that other sites received substantial radiation from scatter or from the beam itself.

The importance of this study lies in the health effects of partial body exposure and in the temporal pattern of appearance of solid tumors in irradiated adults. Smith and Doll (1978, 1982), Darby et al. (1985, 1987), and Weiss et al. (1994, 1995), in the most recent follow-up publications concerning these patients, have shown that the excess risk for solid tumors diminishes with time since exposure, with maximum appearance 5 to 20 years after exposure. This has significant implications for risk projection modeling. Many projection models assume a constant rate of appearance either as an absolute number of tumors per person per unit exposure (constant absolute risk) or as a fraction of the baseline age-specific cancer mortality rate (constant relative risk). The emerging pattern is that constant risk models, either absolute or relative, are not correct for certain cancers, such as lung cancer. Thirty-five years after the first treatment, excess lung cancer had completely disappeared.

The dosimetry was redone in 1988 (Lewis et al., 1988), and although better estimates of dose are now available, it is still the dose that is most uncertain for the cohort. No details about the x-ray machines used to deliver the exposures, such as output, kilovoltage, and half-value layer, are reported.

The excess cancers and the estimate of lifetime cancer risk at three sites in the ankylosing spondylitis cohort are shown in

Table 25-9. For the purpose of calculating lifetime risks as of the time of follow-up, the number of persons used here as the individuals at risk is the number actually receiving only one x-ray treatment (6158). This assumes that those followed for 18 months after the second treatment do not contribute significantly to the malignancies.

The relatively low risk for leukemia (compared with atom bomb survivors) has been suggested to be due to cell sterilization at the high dose delivered. It is also possible that the low risk is due to partial irradiation of the skeletal red marrow. The volume of bone marrow irradiated in the spine, rib, and pelvis is much less than 50 percent of that in whole-body irradiation.

The deaths resulting from causes other than neoplasms in the total cohort are about 30 percent higher than expected. This higher total mortality is of significance in risk modeling as the premature deaths resulting from competing causes decrease the observed fractional cancer mortality. Thus, the lifetime risk in this population probably underestimates the risk when projecting the effects of exposure in a healthy population.

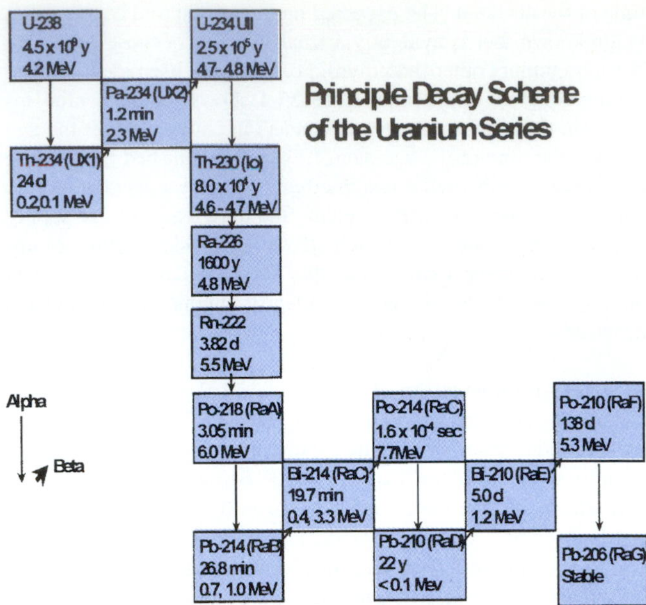

Figure 25-5. Uranium-238 decay series. (From NCRP, 1987.)

Uranium Miners

Radon is ubiquitous on earth. It is found outdoors and in all dwellings as a result of the decay of the parent ^{226}Ra, which is present in all of earth's minerals.

Although the risk of developing lung cancer from radon exposure among underground miners is firmly documented and quantitative risk estimates are available, the current interest lies in whether this risk carries over into environmental situations. Radon levels in homes that are comparable to those in mines surely confer risks to the residents. The question remains: Can the risks in mines for exposures at higher concentrations over short time periods be used to model risks at lower environmental levels over a lifetime?

Radon Exposure in Underground Mines There are 11 large follow-up studies of underground miners exposed to high concentrations of radon and radon decay products, and the documentation of excess lung cancer is convincing (NCRP, 1984; NAS, 1988; NIH, 1994; NAS, 1998). The carcinogen in the case of radon is actually the alpha-emitting short-lived decay products of radon, ^{218}Po, and ^{214}Po. The decay scheme for the entire uranium series, including radon and the daughter species, is shown in Fig. 25-5. The decay products or daughter products are solids and are deposited on the bronchial airways during inhalation and exhalation according to the laws of diffusion. As the airway lining (bronchial epithelium) is only 40 μm thick, the alpha particles emitted are able to reach and transfer a significant amount of energy to all the cells implicated in lung cancer induction. Although the daughters are the carcinogen, the term *radon* is here used interchangeably for *radon decay products,* because without the parent radon, the daughters could not exist longer than a few hours. The measurements in mines were usually of the daughter species rather than radon, and the term *working level* (WL) was adopted for occupational exposure. It indicated the total potential energy content in 1 L of air for complete decay of the short-lived daughters.* The exposure attributed to miners was developed in working-level months (WLMs), which is the

*One working level (WL) is any combination of short-lived daughters in 1 L of air that will result in 1.3×10^5 MeV of alpha energy when complete decay occurs. One working level is approximately equal to 7400 Bq m^{-3} (200 pCi/L) in a home and 11,000 Bq m^{-3} (300 pCi/L) in a mine.

Table 25-9

Excess Cancer in 6158 Ankylosing Spondylitis Patients Given a Single X-Ray Treatment as of the Last Follow-up

SITE	OBS	EXP	DOSE, Gy	LIFETIME, RISK Gy^{-1}
Leukemia	53	17	4.8	0.0011
Lung*	563	469	2.5	0.0027
Esophagus	74	38	5.6	0.0007

*Lung cancer appearing less than 5 years after exposure is not included as less than the minimum latency for tumor expression. The doses to the pulmonary lung and main bronchi were estimated as 1.8 and 6.8 Gy, respectively. The majority of lung cancer is bronchogenic, and the dose estimates for the main bronchi are probably most pertinent. Lifetime risk calculated as 30-year risk.

SOURCE: UNSCEAR, 2000.

numerical value of WL times the time exposed in multiples of a working month of 170 h (Holaday et al., 1957).

$$\text{WLM} = \text{WL (hours exposed/170)}.$$

Estimating Lung Cancer Risk from Underground Miner Epidemiology The follow-up studies from 11 large underground mining cohorts in Australia, Canada, Czechoslovakia, France, Sweden, and the United States have all produced data that show that the excess lung cancer risk from exposure to radon is about 1 to 3 per 10,000 persons per WLM exposure (Radford and Renard, 1984; Hornung and Meinhardt, 1987; Sevc et al., 1988; Muller et al., 1989; Howe et al., 1986, 1987; Tirmarche et al., 1993; Woodward et al., 1991; NCRP 1984, NIH, 1994, NAS 1998). Expressed another way, radon exposure increases the normal age-specific lung cancer risk by about 0.5 percent for each WLM exposure. This way of expressing risk leads to the concept that many epidemiologists prefer—that the lung cancer risk is proportional to the normal baseline risk. This means, for example, that the lifetime excess lung cancer risk from radon is different for smokers and nonsmokers (NAS, 1988; NIH, 1994).

The actual data from the underground studies are not clear-cut with regard to the effect of smoking, and it is apparent from more recent analyses that radon exposure does not simply multiply the baseline risks of the population by a constant factor. This is considered in the discussion of risk, earlier in this chapter. The excess lung cancer risk in each of the exposure cohorts for the 11 major mining populations as of the date of the last published follow-up is summarized in Fig. 25-6. It can be seen in the figure that the range of risks for the same exposure varies by about a factor of 10 among the different studies. The differences are likely accounted for by errors in measuring and estimating total exposure. However, the Czech mine atmosphere contained arsenic as well as radon, and the arsenic contributed to the excess lung cancers observed. A maximum value of 50 percent lung cancer risk is the highest value ever observed in a mining population and was reported in mines in Saxony at the turn of the century (Muller, 1989). These mines are thought to have had about 100,000 Bq m^{-3} of radon. It is noteworthy that concentrations this high have been reported in a few homes in the United States. In Fig. 25-6, the lowest (well-documented) exposures were in the Ontario mines, and a mean exposure of 29 WLM has given an excess lung cancer risk of about 1 percent.

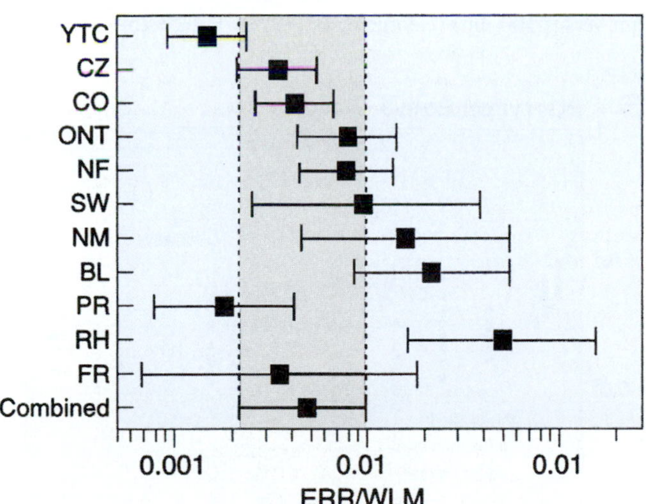

Figure 25-6. Excess relative risk (ERR) of lung cancer per working-level month (WLM) for each of the 11 cohorts studied.

RRs plotted per WLM exposure. YTC, Yunnan China Tin miners; CZ, Chechoslovakian uranium miners; CO, Colorado uranium miners; ONT, Ontario uranium miners; NF, Newfoundland fluorspar miners; SW, Swedish iron miners; NM, New Mexico uranium miners; BL, Beaverlodge, Canada, uranium miners; PR, Port Radium, Canada, uranium miners; RH, Radium Hill, Australia, uranium miners; FR, French uranium miners. (From NIH, 1994.)

To date, the most comprehensive epidemiologic analysis of underground miners exposed to high concentrations of ^{222}Rn is a joint analysis of 11 underground mining studies conducted by the National Cancer Institute (NIH, 1994), and updated by NAS (1998). The study encompasses the Chinese, Czechoslovakian, Colorado, Ontario, Newfoundland, Swedish, New Mexico, Beaverlodge, Port Radium, Radium Hill, and French mining data. Domestic studies do not prove useful in obtaining risk estimates for radon. This is because the effects of ^{222}Rn in the environment are obscured by typical low exposure rates and the large numbers of lung cancers caused by smoking. In mines, the average concentration can be thousands of Bq m^{-3} compared with less than 100 Bq m^{-3} in a typical domestic environment. The occupational exposure in mines is relatively short compared with that over a full life in homes. Although the time exposed in mines is shorter, the cumulative exposure in mines is generally many times that in homes. The joint analysis of the 11 cohorts (NIH, 1994) focused on 10 variables:

1. The estimation of excess relative risk per working level month (ERR/WLM) and the form of the exposure response
2. The variation of ERR/WLM with attained age
3. The variation of ERR/WLM with duration of exposure, considering total exposure as well as exposure rate
4. The variation of ERR/WLM with age at first exposure
5. The variation of ERR/WLM as a function of time after exposure ceased
6. The evaluation of an optimal exposure lag interval, that is, the interval before lung cancer death during which ^{222}Rn exposure has no effect
7. The consistency among the 11 cohorts
8. The joint effect of smoking and ^{222}Rn exposure
9. The role of exposure to other airborne contaminants in mines
10. The direct modeling of the relative risk of lung cancer with duration and rate of exposure

The relative risk of lung cancer for the Colorado uranium miners is shown in Fig. 25-7 and that for all 11 cohorts—showing only the data for exposures below 400 WLM—is shown in Fig. 25-8.

The pooled cohorts included 2620 lung cancer deaths among 60,570 exposed miners, accumulating 1.2 million person-years of observation. The excess relative risk of lung cancer is seen in Fig. 25-7 to be linearly related to the cumulative radon decay product exposure in units of WLM. The exception is at the highest exposures, where a clear reduction in excess relative risk is evident. This is often noted as an *inverse dose rate effect*. Confusion exists concerning the inverse dose rate effect in that the relative risk is not *higher at lower dose rates* but is *lower at higher dose rates,* in agreement with cell killing and removal of damaged cells from

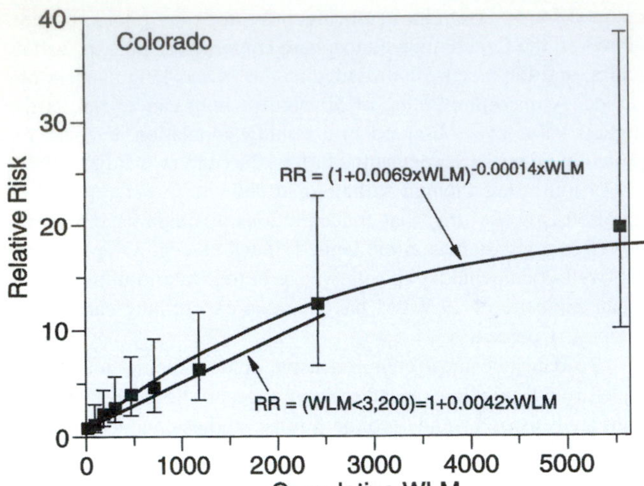

Figure 25-7. Excess relative risk per unit exposure for the Colorado mining cohort. (From NIH, 1994.)

the pool of cells that are potential sites of malignant transformation. This effect is seen in all studies of radiation damage at high dose.

Data on tobacco use were available in six of the cohorts. The ERR/WLM was not related to age at first exposure in this analysis. The joint effect of smoking and ^{222}Rn exposure did not show a clear pattern except that the risk was consistent with a relationship that was intermediate between additive and multiplicative.

Lung (Bronchial) Dose from Radon Exposure When radon gas decays to its solid decay products, some 8 to 15 percent of the ^{218}Po atoms do not attach to the normal aerosol particles. This ultrafine species (unattached fraction) is deposited with 100 percent efficiency on the upper bronchial airways. In mines the unattached fraction is low (4 to 5 percent) because of the normal aerosol loading. The rest of the decay products attach to the ambient aerosol of about 100-nm average diameter (George and Breslin, 1980) and only a few percent of this aerosol is deposited on these airways. Measurements in mines have mostly involved the short-lived radon daughters, as they are the easiest to measure rapidly. The alpha dose from radon gas itself is very low in comparison with that from the daughters, as the daughters deposit and accumulate on the airway surfaces. The upper airways of the bronchial tree are the region where almost all the lung cancers appear. This is true in general, not only for miners exposed to radon daughters but also for smokers.

The alpha dose from radon daughters therefore must be calculated in these airways, not in the pulmonary or gas-exchange regions. Although the dose to the pulmonary region should not be neglected, it is about 15 percent of that to the airways (Saccomanno et al., 1995). Several calculations regarding the absorbed alpha dose exist for radon daughters (NCRP, 1984; ICRP, 1987; Harley, 1987, 1989; Harley et al., 1996, NRC, 1991). The authors make different assumptions about the atmospheric and biological parameters that go into the dose calculation, and this can cause discrepancies among the models. The most significant variables are the particle size of the ambient aerosol, the assumed breathing rate, and the target cells considered.

Very small particles deposit more efficiently in the airways. Therefore if small particles, such as those from open burning flame (Tu and Knutson, 1988), contribute to the atmosphere, the dose delivered to the bronchial epithelium can be higher per unit WLM exposure than is the dose predicted from an average particle size. Conversely, a hygroscopic particle can increase in size in the humid environment of the bronchial airways, and deposition will be diminished. The particle size of the aerosol in mines is somewhat larger than that for environmental conditions (200 to perhaps 600 nm versus 100 nm) (George et al., 1975). Figure 25-9 shows the

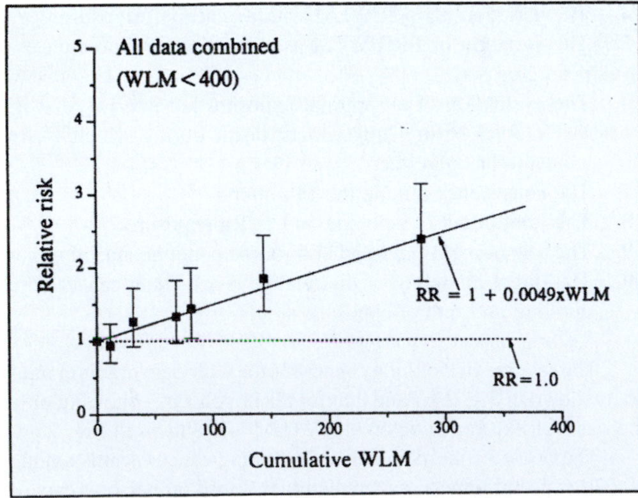

Figure 25-8. Relative risk (RR) of lung cancer by cumulative working-level month (WLM) and fitted linear excess RR model for each cohort and for all data combined (WLM < 400).

RRs are plotted at mean WLM for category. When the referent category for RRs is not zero exposure, a fitted exposure-response line is adjusted to pass through the mean of the referent category. For the China, Ontario, and Beaverlodge cohorts, the excess RR model was fitted with a free intercept. (From NIH, 1994.)

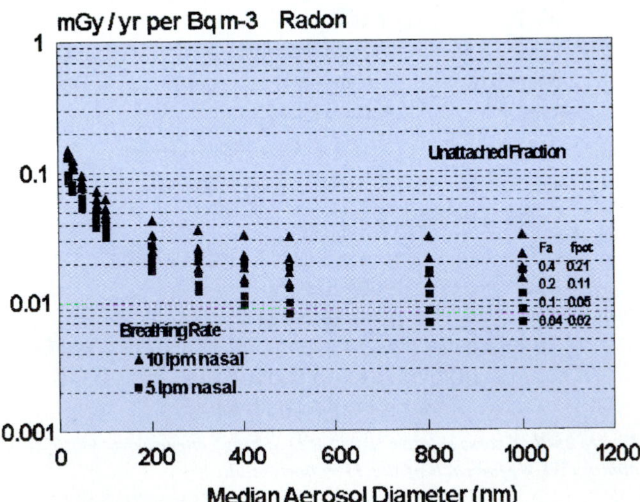

Figure 25-9. Radon decay product bronchial dose as a function of inhaled aerosol diameter, breathing rate, and unattached fraction. (Breathing rates from Ruzer et al., 1995; target cells from Robbins and Meyers, 1995, with permission.)

alpha dose per unit exposure as it is related to the variables (particle size, unattached fraction, breathing rate) known to affect dose.

As carcinogenesis is related to absorbed alpha dose, Fig. 25-9 shows that particle size is an important determinant of risk. The average dose per unit exposure in WLM for miners in Fig. 25-9 is about the same as that for average environmental conditions, assuming 100 nm aerosol in homes and 200 to 600 nm aerosol in mines.

Radon can deliver a greater or lesser carcinogenic potential by about a factor of 2 over the range of realistic indoor conditions (average particle size ranging from 80 to 300 nm). The allowable effective dose for continuous exposure of the population in the United States is 1 mSv/year (100 mrem/year) (NCRP, 1993). This limit would be delivered by exposure to 10 Bq m^{-3} of radon, or one-quarter the actual average measured indoor concentration in most countries where measurements have been made. Thus, the guidelines for exposure to radon cannot be set in the usual way from dosimetric considerations.

LIFETIME ENVIRONMENTAL LUNG CANCER RISK PROJECTIONS FOR RADON EXPOSURE

There are at present six sets of models based on the underground miner epidemiology that provide risk projection calculations for exposure to radon daughters in the home. The following sections describe each in detail.

National Council on Radiation Protection and Measurements

In 1984, the NRCP on Protection and Measurements (NCRP, 1984) developed a model to project the risk derived from miner studies to whole-life risk in the environment. It is a modified absolute risk model that reduces the risk subsequent to exposure with a half-life of 20 years. Risk is not accumulated until after age 40, the time when lung cancer normally appears in the population. There is no indication that early exposure produces any significant shift to younger ages, even for young miners exposed at significantly higher concentrations. This model was the first to incorporate a time since exposure reduction in risk.

National Academy of Sciences

The National Academy of Sciences report in 1988 (BEIR IV) developed a model based on examination of the raw data from five mining cohorts (NAS, 1988). The data indicated that the highest risk appears from 5 to 15 years after exposure. After 15 years, the risk is one-half that of the 5- to 15-year risk (per unit exposure), and this risk was assumed to persist to the end of life. Again, no significant risk appears before 40, the usual age for the appearance of lung cancer. The NAS model also included a correction for attained age (at age 65, the risk is 0.4 of that for ages 55 to 64). The BEIR IV committee assumed a relative risk model (risk is proportional to the normal age-specific lung cancer risk per unit radon exposure), but with risk dependent on time from exposure. This was the first modified relative risk model. This means that the risk for smokers and nonsmokers differs because of their different baseline lung cancer values. Although the miners' epidemiology did not support this strictly multiplicative relationship, the NAS chose the relative risk model as a conservative one. Its analysis supported the risk reduction subsequent to exposure by using a two-step risk reduction window.

NAS 1998 (BEIR VI) expanded on the models developed in NAS (1988) using 11 underground mining cohorts rather than 4. The models for the 11 cohorts were developed first by NIH (1994), see below, and updated for the NAS report.

International Commission on Radiation Protection

The IRCP (ICRP, 1987) developed two risk projection models: one was based on a constant relative risk and the other was a constant absolute risk model. Although neither risk model is correct because of the temporal reduction pattern of lung cancer subsequent to the cessation of exposure, the numerical values obtained for the lifetime risk of lung cancer from radon exposure are not significantly different from those in other models. Later follow-up of the Czechoslovakian underground uranium miners presented by Kunz and Sevc (1988) indicates that the excess lung cancer risk may actually be reduced to zero 35 years after exposure. If this factor were included in the NAS model (zero risk after 35 years), it would reduce those values by about a factor of 2. The risk values obtained from the various models are shown in Table 25-10. In 1993, ICRP simply adopted a lifetime lung cancer fatality coefficient of 3×10^{-4} per WLM.

NIH Joint Analysis of 11 Underground Mining Cohorts

The pooled analysis from the 11 underground mining cohorts was used to develop two models for full-life risk projection (NIH, 1994). The models are similar to the model used by the NAS (1988), utilizing time since exposure reduction and reduction with attained age. Three time windows for reduction of risk with time since exposure are used instead of two. Also, an additional parameter is incorporated; one model decreases the risk with increasing exposure rate, and the other decreases the risk with decreasing exposure duration. The lifetime domestic risk for lifetime exposure to unit concentration was not reported. However, the ratio of the relative risk of lung cancer for the BEIR IV and joint analysis model was given as 0.9 for continuous exposure to 4 $pCiI^{-1}$ (1 WLM per year) for the model incorporating exposure duration as a parameter. The joint analysis estimated that there are 15,000 lung cancer deaths in the United States attributable to ^{222}Rn: 10,000 in smokers and 5000 in those who have never smoked.

BEIR VI (NAS 1998) updated these two models and increased the calculated risk in the United States to 15,400 or 21,800 per year for ever smokers and never smokers for the two model values. The BEIR VI best annual estimate of deaths for ever smokers is stated to be 11,000 per year with 2100 or 2900 calculated deaths for never smokers, depending upon the model chosen.

ENVIRONMENTAL EPIDEMIOLOGY

The Environmental Studies

There are at least 24 published studies that attempt to define or detect the effect of radon exposure in the environment. Most are summarized by Borak and Johnson (1988), Neuberger (1989, 1992),

Table 25-10
Lung Cancer Risk for Continuous Whole-life Exposure to 4 pCi/L (150 Bq m^{-3} or 0.58 WLM per year at Indoor Conditions) as Predicted by Various Models of Domestic Exposure*

MODEL	LIFETIME RISK %	MODEL TYPE	COMMENT
NCRP (1984a)	0.50	Modified absolute risk. Two parameter model.	Risk decreases with time since exposure.
ICRP (1987)	0.90	Constant relative risk.	
ICRP (1987)	0.62	Constant additive risk.	
ICRP (1993)	0.56	Single-value risk per WLM.	Adopted lifetime risk per WLM exposure.
BEIR IV (NRC 1988)	1.1	Modified relative risk. Two-time windows. Two-parameter model.	Risk decreases with time since exposure.
NIH (1994)	1.8	Modified relative risk, three-time windows, age and exposure rate. Three parameter model.	Risk decreases with time since exposure and decreases with very high exposures.
BEIR VI (NRC 1998)	2.0	Modified relative risk. Three time windows, age and exposure rate. Three parameter model.	Risk decreases with time since exposure and decreases with very high exposures.
Meta-analysis of eight domestic case-control studies (Lubin and Boice, 1997)	0.7	Observed mortality.	Linear regression fit to data from eight domestic studies.

*Exposure assumes a home concentration of 148 Bq m^{-3} (4 pCi l^{-1} or 0.56 WLM), calculated with 40 percent decay product equilibrium, and actual exposure is 70 percent of the home exposure.
SOURCE: NAS, 1999.

and Samet and associates (1991). A study in the United States was performed in 1989 by the New Jersey Department of Health (NJDOH) (Schoenberg and Klotz, 1989; Schoenberg et al., 1990). This is a case-control study of women, 433 lung cancer cases and 402 controls with yearlong measurements of radon in the homes where the individuals lived for 10 or more years. This study devoted considerable effort to quality control concerning the exposure measurements. The results of this study are slightly positive, suggesting an association of radon and lung cancer even at concentrations of 80 Bq m^{-3}, but the results are not statistically significant. A case-control study of 538 nonsmoking women (1183 controls) in Missouri with an average exposure of 70 Bq m^{23} also showed no statistically significant increase in lung cancer (Alavanja et al., 1994).

The largest case-control study to date concerning the effects of residential ^{222}Rn exposure was conducted nationwide in 109 municipalities in Sweden. It included all subjects 35 to 74 years old who had lived in one of the 109 municipalities at some time between January 1980 and December 31, 1984, and who had been living in Sweden on January 1, 1947. Fifty-six of the municipalities were known to have elevated ^{222}Rn concentrations on the basis of earlier measurements.

Thus, an attempt was made to study a large group of persons living in a known area of greater than average ^{222}Rn and to estimate their exposure over a large fraction of life (34 years). The primary aim of the study was to narrow the uncertainty in the estimation of lung cancer risk.

The environmental epidemiologic studies conducted before this study suffered from the small numbers of persons observed and relatively low ^{222}Rn exposures. For this reason, although the risk in underground miners was seen clearly, the outcome regarding the lung cancer risk from residential exposure has been ambiguous. All the existing domestic studies, including the measurement protocols, have been reviewed (Neuberger, 1992, 1994; Samet, 1989; Samet et al., 1991, 1989; Lubin et al., 1990).

Pershagen and coworkers (1994) included 586 women and 774 men with lung cancer diagnosed between 1980 and 1984. For a comparison control population, 1380 women and 1467 men were studied.

The ^{222}Rn concentration in 8992 homes was measured for 3 months during the heating season. The geometric and arithmetic mean concentrations were 1.6 and 2.9 pCi L^{21} (60 and 106 Bq m^{-3}). The cumulative exposure since 1947 was estimated for each subject by the addition of the products of concentration by the length of time the subject lived in each residence.

The data were reported in terms of the relative risk (RR) of lung cancer (ratio of observed to expected lung cancer) normalized to a relative risk of 1.0 for persons who never smoked and who had radon exposure below 50 Bq m^{-3}. The excess risk due to smoking could be seen easily. Smokers smoking less than or more than 10 cigarettes per day with a radon concentration of $\ll$50 Bq m^{-3} had RR of 6.2 (with a confidence interval from 4.2 to 9.2) and 12.6 (CI from 8.7 to 18.4), respectively.

The only statistically significant lung cancer excess resulting from ^{222}Rn was seen in those who smoked fewer than 10 cigarettes per day and had a time-weighted mean ^{222}Rn concentration $>$400 Bq m^{-3}. Their relative risk was 25.1 (CI 7.7 to 82.4). For those smoking more than 10 cigarettes per day, the relative risk compared with those who had never smoked and had ^{222}Rn concentrations <50 Bq m^{-3} was 32.5 (CI 10.3 to 23.7). Although this relative risk appears higher than that for those smoking <10 cigarettes per day, the result is not statistically signficant. If the effect of ^{222}Rn alone is examined by comparing the risk only among smokers, that is, those with <50 Bq m^{-3} against smokers having >400 Bq m^{-3}, the relative risk due to ^{222}Rn alone is 3.7 (CI 1.1 to 11.7) for those smoking less than 10 cigarettes per day and 2.5 (CI 0.8 to 7.9) for those smoking more than 10 cigarettes per day (Pershagen et al., 1994). Because the confidence interval includes 1.0, it cannot be stated with statistical certainty that there was increased lung cancer caused by ^{222}Rn exposure although the point estimate RR = 2.5 suggests at least an upper bound of risk.

The analysis was done for the combined group of men and women (Pershagen et al., 1994). There were no details given concerning lung cancer and sex difference. However, the preliminary report (Pershagen et al., 1994) suggested that women may indeed have had less lung cancer than men for the same exposure conditions. Also of interest in the study of Pershagen and associates (1994) was the relative risk of lung cancer by histological type. In the >400 Bq m^{-3} group, only small cell carcinoma and adenocarcinoma had a statistically significant increased risk.

The pattern emerging from the domestic studies indicates that the lung cancer risk from ^{222}Rn exposure is difficult to determine with accuracy or precision. This is mostly due to the high background lung cancer mortality caused by smoking.

Among the 24 published domestic studies, 13 are ecologic and 11 are case-control (Neuberger 1989). Ecologic studies depend on relating the disease response of a population to some measure of a suspected causative agent. There usually are not enough data on all the variables involved in the disease to infer any reliable associations. Ecologic studies are the weakest type of epidemiologic exploration. Unless a biological marker for radon-induced lung cancer is found, it is unlikely that environmental epidemiology will be effective in assessing risk. The effects of radon in the environment are subtle compared with the overwhelming lung cancer mortality that results from smoking.

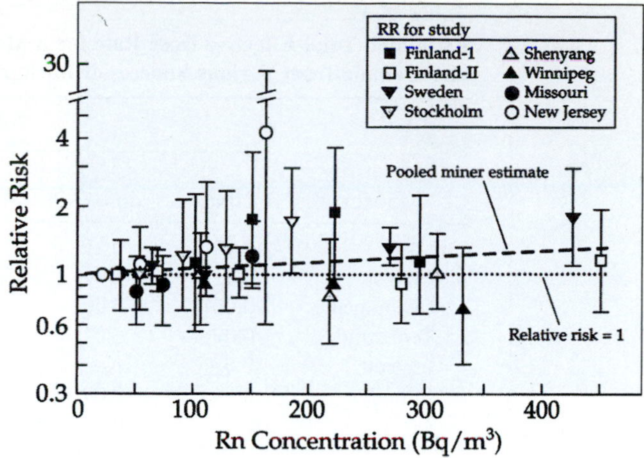

Figure 25-10. Meta-analysis of eight domestic radon case-control studies. σg = 2 for size distributions. (From Harley et al., 1993, with permission.)

Meta-analysis of Environmental Epidemiology

In an attempt to combine the largest domestic studies to determine whether any risk from radon exposure in the home was apparent, Lubin and Boice (1997) performed a meta-analysis of 8 domestic case control studies. A meta-analysis combines the published information from several studies into one study without actually having the raw data available. The results are shown in Fig. 25-10. The data showed that essentially no study found statistically significant cancer deaths due to radon, but the authors state that the combined trend in the relative risk with increasing exposure was

Table 25-11

Equivalent Dose Rates to Various Tissues from Natural Radionuclides Contained in the Body

	Equivalent Dose Rate, mSv yr^{-1}			
RADIONUCLIDE	BRONCHIAL EPITHELIUM	SOFT TISSUE	BONE SURFACES	BONE MARROW
^{14}C	—	0.10	0.08	0.30
^{40}K	—	1.80	1.40	2.70
^{87}Rb	—	0.03	0.14	0.07
^{238}U-^{234}Th	—	0.046	0.03	0.004
^{230}Th	—	0.001	0.06	0.001
^{226}Ra	—	0.03	0.90	0.15
^{222}Rn	—	0.07	0.14	0.14
^{222}Rn daughters	24	—	—	—
^{210}Pb-^{210}Po	—	1.40	7.00	1.40
^{232}Th	—	0.001	0.02	0.004
^{228}Ra-^{224}Ra	—	0.0015	1.20	0.22
^{220}Rn	—	0.001	—	—
Total	24	3.50	11.00	5.00

Table 25-12

Estimated Total Effective Dose Rate for a Member of the Population in the United States and Canada from Various Sources of Background Radiation

	Total Effective Dose Rate, mSv yr^{-1}					
SOURCE	LUNG	GONADS	BONE SURFACE	BONE MARROW	OTHER TISSUES	TOTAL
w_t*	0.12	0.25	0.03	0.12	0.48	1.0
Cosmic	0.03	0.07	0.008	0.03	0.13	0.27
Cosmogenic	0.001	0.002	—	0.004	0.003	0.01
Terrestrial	0.03	0.07	0.008	0.03	0.14	0.28
Inhaled	2.0	—	—	—	—	2.0
In body	0.04	0.09	0.03	0.06	0.17	0.40
Total	2.1	0.23	0.05	0.12	0.44	3.0

*Tissue weighting factor–see Table 25.3
SOURCE: NCRP, 1987.

statistically significant, with an estimated RR of 1.14 (95 percent CI = 1.0 to 1.3) at an exposure of 150 Bq m^{-3} (4 pCil^{-1}).

What Is Known about Radon Exposure in the Home

Four concepts have emerged from the radon research so far:

1. The mining epidemiology indicates that short exposure to high levels of radon and daughters produces a clear excess of lung cancer.
2. Particle size can change the actual dose delivered by radon to bronchial tissue, with small particles giving a substantially higher dose per unit exposure. The use of open flames, electric motors, and the like indoors produces a higher dose per unit exposure.
3. Smokers are at higher risk from radon per unit exposure than are nonsmokers. The relative risk for nonsmokers is about three times that for smokers, but their age-specific lung cancer mortality is about ten times lower than that for smokers. Thus, the overall lifetime lung cancer risk is three times higher for smokers.
4. Urban areas almost universally have low radon, and apartment dwellers removed from the ground source have particularly low radon exposure at home.

The miners' data show clearly that there is a risk of lung cancer from exposure to high concentrations of radon delivered over short periods. Comparable exposures delivered over a lifetime in the home have not produced statistically significant increases in lung cancer mortality except among smokers in one large study in Sweden. The risk can still exist, but the confounding effects of other carcinogens, such as smoking and urbanization, make it impossible to extract the more subtle impact of radon in existing studies.

Table 25-13

Lifetime Effective Dose (in mSv from Birth to Age 85) from Natural Radionuclide Exposure

	LUNG	BONE MARROW	WHOLE BODY
Effective dose	180	10	260

SOURCE: NCRP, 1987.

NATURAL RADIOACTIVITY AND RADIATION BACKGROUND

The occupational, accidental, and wartime experiences detailed in the preceding sections have provided the bases for all the current radiation risk estimates. For many years, the radioisotopes deposited internally were compared with ^{226}Ra to evaluate the maximum permissible body burden for a particular emitter. The present limits for external and internal radiation are based on dose estimates that, in turn, can be related to cancer risks. One standard of comparison has always been the exposure from natural background, and this source is assessed here.

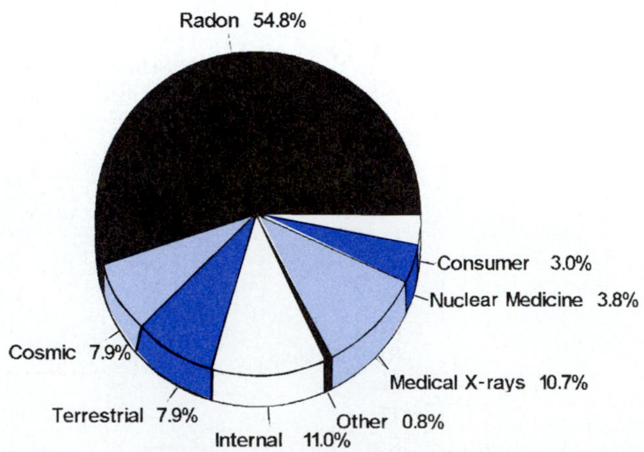

Figure 25-11. Contribution from natural background to effective dose of radiation in the U.S. population. Annual average effective dose, 3.6 mSv. (From NCRP, 1987.)

Background radiation from all sources is described in detail in NCRP report 94 (1987b), and some of the information is summarized here.

The risk estimates in the previous sections must be placed in context with the radiation dose received by all humans from natural background radiation. A substantial dose is received annually from cosmic radiation and from external terrestrial radiation present from uranium, thorium, and potassium in the earth's crust. Internal emitters are present in the body as a consequence of dietary consumption and inhalation. For example, potassium is a necessary element in the body and is under homeostatic control. Radioactive ^{40}K constitutes a constant fraction of all natural potassium. Potassium delivers the largest internal dose from the diet of 0.15 mSv per year. However, the data are scanty on the dietary intake of other radionuclides in the U.S. population. Given the usual distribution of intakes across a large population, it is probable that

Table 25-14
Estimates of Radionuclide Released and Collective Effective Dose from Human-Made Environmental Sources of Radiation

	Release (PBq)						*Collective Effective Dose* Person Sv*	
SOURCE	^{3}H	^{14}C	NOBLE GASES	^{90}Sr	^{131}I	^{137}Cs	LOCAL AND REGIONAL	GLOBAL
Atmospheric nuclear testing	240,000	220		604	650,000	910		2,230,000
Local								
Semipalatinsk							4600	
Nevada							500†	
Australia							700	
Pacific test site							160†	
Underground nuclear testing			50		15		200	
Nuclear weapons fabrication								
Early practice								
Hanford							8000‡	
Chelyabinsk							15,000§	
Later practice							1000 30,000¶	10,000
Nuclear power production								
Milling and mining							2700	
Reactor operation	140	1.1	3,200		0.04		3700	
Fuel reprocessing	57	0.3	1,200	6.9	0.004	40	4600	
Fuel cycle							300,000¶	100,000
Radioisotope production and use	2.6	1.0	52		6.0		2000	80,000
Accidents								
Three Mile Island			370		0.0006		40	
Chernobyl					630	70		600,000
Kyshtym				5.4		0.04	2500	
Windscale			1.2		0.7	0.02	2000	
Palomares							3	
Thule							0	
SNAP 9A								2100
Cosmos 954				0.003	0.2	0.003		20
Ciudad Juarez							150	
Mohammedia							80	
Goiania						0.05	60	
Total							380,000	23,100,000
Total collective effective dose (Person Sv)								23,500,000

*Truncated at 10,000 years.
†External dose only.
‡From release of ^{131}I to the atmosphere.
§From releases of radionuclides into the Techa River.
¶Long-term collective dose from release of ^{222}Rn from tailings.
SOURCE: UNSCEAR, 1993.

other emitters, notably ^{210}Pb, could deliver a significant dose to a fraction of the population.

The largest dose received by the population is from the inhaled short-lived daughters of radon. These are present in all atmospheres because radon is released rather efficiently from the ^{226}Ra in rock and soil. The short-lived daughters, ^{218}Po, ^{214}Pb, ^{214}Bi-^{214}Po, have an effective half-life of 30 min, but the 3.8-day parent radon supports their presence in the atmosphere. Figure 25-5 shows the entire uranium series decay.

Average outdoor concentrations in every state in the United States have been measured and summarized as 15 Bq m^{-3}, and indoors, as 40 Bq m^{-3} (NAS, 1999). A structure such as a house prevents the rapid upward distribution of radon into the atmosphere, and substantial levels can be built up indoors. The source of radon is the ground; therefore levels in living areas above the ground are generally one-third to one-fifth the concentrations measured in basements. An effective barrier across the soil-building interface also inhibits the entry of radon to buildings. Ventilation with outdoor air reduces indoor radon. For this reason, industrial buildings with more substantial foundations and higher ventilation rates tend to have lower radon concentrations than do single-family (or detached) houses. Apartments above ground level have radon concentrations about half the average of those in single-family dwellings.

It is of significance that an average radon concentration indoors of 40 Bq m^{-3} results in an equivalent dose to bronchial epithelium of 24 mSv/year or an effective dose of 2 mSv per year.

The equivalent doses for the major natural internal emitters are shown in Table 25-11. These are reproduced from NCRP (1987).

The annual effective dose equivalents for all the external and internal emitters from natural background are summarized in NCRP Report 94 (1987) and are shown in Table 25-12.

The lifetime dose from natural emitters is shown in Table 25-13, assuming an average exposure from birth to a full life of 85 years. It should be recognized that the actual dose accumulated by an individual depends on dietary habits, location (Denver, for example, at an altitude of 1.6 km, has double the average cosmic-ray exposure), and the dwelling. An apartment dweller would accumulate approximately half the dose from inhaled radon daughters as would a person living in a single-family dwelling. Table 25-13 is informative in considering the effects of radiation exposure from other than natural sources. For example, in assessing an occupational dose, which might add, say, 10 mSv effective dose equivalent, natural background would be a strong confounder. Any health detriment would have to be calculated rather than observed directly. No study would be able to detect an increase in health effects from 10 mSv above the average whole-life natural background of 260 mSv.

Figure 25-11 shows the average components of natural background in the United States, and Harley (2000) gives a detailed summary of background radiation and internal radioactivity.

LOCAL ENVIRONMENTAL RELEASES

Large- and small-scale accidents will undoubtedly occur that release radioactivity into the environment. The accident at the Windscale nuclear power reactor in 1957 was a local incident in Great Britain. The nearby population has been studied for over 30 years without the appearance of significant health effects.

The nuclear power accident at Three Mile Island caused enormous financial damage, but the containment vessel was not breached and virtually no radioactivity escaped.

The accident at the Chernobyl nuclear power plant was another such occasion, and in this case containment did not exist and some of the radioactivity was widespread over Europe. The United Nations Scientific Committee on the Effects of Atomic Radiation

Table 25-15
Lifetime Cancer Mortality per Gray from Five Major Epidemiologic Studies (in parentheses, risk per sievert for alpha emitters, $w_r = 20$)*

STUDY	ALL SITES	LEUKEMIA	LUNG	FEMALE BREAST	BONE	THYROID	SKIN
Atom bomb whole-body, gamma	0.05	0.005	0.0085	0.002	0.0005	0.0008	0.0002
Uranium miner bronchial epithelium, alpha			(0.04) 0.0020				
Ankylosing spondylitis, spincal x-ray		0.0011	0.0008 0.0028	0.0015			
Tinea capitis, head x-ray						0.0010§	0.0030‡
Radium ingestion, bone,* alpha (^{226}Ra)					0.004 (0.0002)		
Radium ingestion, bone,† alpha (^{224}Ra)					0.02 (0.0010)		

*The lifetime risk is calculated for an average skeletal dose of 10 Gy, assuming that the risk persists for 50 years and using Eq. (20). The risk is nonlinear and is about 0.01 Gy^{-1} at 100 Gy, for example.

†The lifetime risk is calculated for an average skeletal dose of 10 Gy using equation 22. The risk is nonlinear and is about 0.01 Gy^{-1} for a skeletal dose of 1 Gy.

‡The mortality for skin cancer is estimated as 1 percent of the incidence; see text.

§Thyroid mortality for males and females. Estimated as 10 percent of incidence.

(UNSCEAR, 1988, 1993) has summarized the committed dose from measurements made in the affected countries from various releases, and these are shown in Table 25-14. Table 25-14 includes environmental releases from most known sources.

Highly radioactive emissions from industrial sources that are "lost," such as the ^{60}Co in Goiania or Thailand, do harm to the few persons involved, often with a few deaths due to very high radiation exposure and dose.

The criticality accident on September 30, 1999, at a fuel reprocessing facility in Tokai-Mura, Japan, resulted in the death of two workers and caused neighbors to receive a small local dose of about 2 mSv (Komura et al 2000).

Local exposures and doses from accidents can only be anticipated to increase, as the use of radioactive materials industrially is widespread.

SUMMARY OF HUMAN CANCER RISKS FROM RADIATION

The details of the five major studies have been given in the preceding sections. The data are summarized in Table 25-15. This table shows the lifetime cancer risks that are significant. The risks are given in units of per gray (or per Sievert where appropriate for alpha emitters).

Within the table, leukemia and cancers of the lung and female breast are the most critical. Osteogenic sarcoma is seen in the radium exposures. There is no clear linear dose response for ^{224,226}Ra. This has been attributed to the existence of an apparent threshold. The cancer risk to individual organs from different study groups is in general agreement regardless of radiation type or whole- or partial-body exposure.

REFERENCES

Adamson HG: A simplified method of x-ray application for the cure of ringworm of the scalp: Kienbock's method, *Lancet* 1:1378–1380, 1909.

Alavanja MCR, Brownson RC, Lubin JH, et al: Residential radon exposure and lung cancer among nonsmoking women. *J Natl Cancer Inst* 86:1829–1837, 1994.

Albert RE, Omran A: A follow-up study of patients treated by x-ray epilation for tinea capitis: I. Population characteristics, posttreatment illnesses, and mortality experience. *Arch Environ Health* 17:899–918, 1968.

Albert RE, Shore RE, Harley NH, Omran A: Follow-up studies of patients treated by x-ray epilation for tinea capitis, in Burns F, Upton AC, Silini G (eds): *Radiation Carcinogenesis and DNA Alterations*. New York: Plenum Press, 1986, pp 1–25.

Andrews HL: *Radiation Biophysics*. Englewood Cliffs, NJ: Prentice-Hall, 1974.

Attix FH, Roesch WC, Tochilin E: *Radiation Dosimetry*. Vol I. New York: Academic Press, 1968.

Aub JC, Evans RD, Hempelmann LH, Martland HS: The late effects of internally deposited radioactive materials in man. *Medicine (Baltimore)* 31:221–329, 1952.

Bethe HA, Ashkin J: Passage of radiations through matter, in Segre E (ed): *Experimental Nuclear Physics*. New York: Wiley, 1953, pp 166–357.

Borak TB, Johnson JA: *Estimating the Risk of Lung Cancer from Inhalation of Radon Daughters Indoors: Review and Evaluation*. Environmental Protection Agency Report EPA 600/6-88/008. Environmental Monitoring Systems Laboratory. Las Vegas, NV: EPA, 1988.

Browne E, Firestone RB, Shirley VS: *Table of Radioactive Isotopes*. New York: Wiley, 1986.

Cember, H. *Introduction to Health Physics*. New York: McGraw-Hill, 1996.

Chemelevsky D, Kellerer AM, Spiess H, Mays CW: A proportional hazards analysis of bone sarcoma rates in German radium-224 patients, in Gossner W, Gerber GB (eds): *The Radiobiology of Radium and Thorotrast*. Munich: Urban & Schwarzenberg, 1986.

Conard RA, Boice JD, Fravwenie JF Jr (eds): Late radiation effects in Marshall Islanders exposed to fallout 28 years ago, in Boice JD, Fraumeni JF Jr (eds): *Radiation Carcinogenesis: Epidemiology and Biological Significance*. New York: Raven Press, 1984, pp 57–71.

Court Brown WM, Doll R: Adult leukemia. Trends in mortality in relation to aetiology. *Br Med J* 1:1063, 1959.

Court Brown WM, Doll R: *Leukemia and Aplastic Anemia in Patients Treated for Ankylosing Spondylitis*. London: Her Majesty's Stationery Office, 1957.

Court Brown WM, Doll R: Mortality from cancer and other causes after radiotherapy for ankylosing spondylitis. *Br Med J* 2: 1327, 1965.

Darby SC, Doll R, Smith PG: Long term mortality after a single treatment course with x-rays in patients treated for ankylosing spondylitis. *Br J Cancer* 55:179–190, 1987.

Darby SC, Nakashima E, Kato H: A parallel analysis of cancer mortality among atomic bomb survivors and patients with ankylosing spondylitis given x-ray therapy. *J Natl Cancer Inst* 72:1, 1985.

Evans RD: *The Atomic Nucleus*. New York: McGraw-Hill, 1955.

Evans RD, Keane AT, Kolenkow RJ, et al: Radiogenic tumors in the radium cases studied at M.I.T., in Mays CW, Jee WSS, Lloyd RD, et al (eds): *Delayed Effects of Bone Seeking Radionuclides*. Salt Lake City: University of Utah Press, 1969, pp 157–194.

George AC, Breslin AJ: The distribution of ambient radon and radon daughters in residential buildings in the New Jersey–New York area, in Gesell TF, Lowder WM (eds): *Natural Radiation Environment III CONF-780422*. Washington, DC: USDOE, 1980, pp 1272–1292.

George AC, Hinchliffe L, Sladowski R: Size distribution of radon daughter particles in uranium mine atmospheres. *Am Ind Hyg Assoc J* 36: 4884, 1975.

Goodhead DT: Initial events in the cellular effects of ionizing radiations: Clustered damage in DNA. *Int J Radiat Biol* 65:7–17, 1994.

Goodhead DT: Track structure considerations in low dose and low dose rate effects of ionizing radiation. *Adv Radiat Biol* 16:7–44, 1992.

Goodhead DT, Nikjoo H: Clustered damage in DNA: Estimates from track structure simulations *Radiat Res* 148:485–486, 1997.

Gossner W: Pathology of radium induced bone tumors. New aspects of histopathology and histogenesis. *Radiat Res* 152 (suppl): S12–S15, 1999.

Harley JH: Dose from residual radioactivity at Hiroshima and Nagasaki, in *New Dosimetry at Hiroshima and Nagasaki and Its Implications for Risk Estimates*. Proc. Number 9. Bethesda, MD: National Council on Radiation Protection, 1987.

Harley NH. Back to background: Natural radioactivity exposed. *Health Physics*. 79:121–128, 2000.

Harley NH: Lung Cancer Risk from Exposure to Environmental Radon. Presented at the 3rd International Conference on Anticarcinogenesis and Radiation Protection, Dubrovnik, 1989.

Harley NH, Albert RE, Shore RE, Pasternack BS: Follow-up study of patients treated by x-ray epilation for tinea capitis: Estimation of the dose to the thyroid and pituitary glands and other structures of the head and neck. *Phys Med Biol* 21:631–642, 1976.

Harley NH, Cohen BS: Updating radon daughter dosimetry, in Hopke

PK (ed): *American Chemical Society Symposium on Radon and Its Decay Products*. Washington, DC: American Chemical Society, 1987, pp 419–429.

Harley NH, Kolber AB, Shore RE, et al: The skin dose and response for the head and neck in patients irradiated with x-ray for tinea capitis: Implications for environmental radioactivity, in *Proceedings in Health Physics Society Mid-Year Symposium*. Albuquerque, NM: Health Physics Society, 1983, pp 125–142.

Holaday DA, Rushing DE, Coleman RD, et al: *Control of Radon and Daughters in Uranium Mines and Calculations on Biologic Effects*. U.S. PHS Report 494. Washington, DC: U.S. Public Health Service, 1957.

Hornung RW, Meinhardt TJ: Quantitative risk assessment of lung cancer in U.S. uranium miners. *Health Phys* 52:417–430, 1987.

Howe GR, Nair RC, Newcombe HB, et al: Lung cancer mortality (1950–80) in relation to radon daughter exposure in a cohort of workers at the Eldorado Beaverlodge Uranium Mine. *J Natl Cancer Inst* 77:357–362, 1986.

Howe GR, Nair RC, Newcombe HB, et al: Lung cancer mortality (1950–80) in relation to radon daughter exposure in a cohort of workers at the Eldorado Port Radium Mine: Possible modification of risk by exposure rate. *J Natl Cancer Inst* 79:1255–1260, 1987.

ICRP: *Recommendations of the International Commission on Radiological Protection.* ICRP Publication 26. New York: Pergamon Press, 1977.

ICRP: *Limits for Intakes of Radionuclides by Workers. International Commission on Radiological Protection.* ICRP Publication 30, Part I. New York: Pergamon Press, 1978.

ICRP: *Limits for Inhalation of Radon Daughters by Workers.* ICRP Publication 32. New York: Pergamon Press, 1981.

ICRP: *Lung Cancer Risk from Indoor Exposures to Radon Daughters.* ICRP Publication 50. Oxford, England: Pergamon Press, 1987.

ICRP: *1990 Recommendations of the International Commission on Radiological Protection.* ICRP Publication 60. New York: Pergamon Press, 1990.

ICRP: *Protection against Radon-222 at Home and at Work.* ICRP Publication 65. New York: Pergamon Press, 1993.

ICRU: *Radiation Quantities and Units in Radiation Protection.* ICRU Report Number 51. Bethesda, MD: International Commission on Radiation Units and Measurements, 1993.

ICRU: *Stopping Powers for Electrons and Positrons.* ICRU Report Number 37. Bethesda MD: International Commission on Radiation Units and Measurements, 1984.

ICRU: *Stopping Powers and Ranges for Protons and Alpha Particles.* ICRU Report Number 49. Bethesda, MD: *International Commission on Radiation Units and Measurements,* 1993.

Kienbock R: Über Radiotherapie und Harrerkrankungen. *Arch Derm Syph Wien* 83:77–111, 1907.

Komura K, Yamamoto M, Muroyama T, et al: The JCO criticality accident at Tokai-Mura, Japan: An overview of the sampling campaign and preliminary results. *J Environ Radioactivity* 50:77–82, 2000.

Kunz E, Sevc J: Radiation risks to underground miners in the light of Czechoslovak epidemiological studies, in Kvasnicka J (ed): Proceedings of the International Workshop on Radiological Protection in Mining, Darwin, Australia, 1988.

Lederer CM, Shirley VS, Browne E, et al: *Table of Isotopes.* New York: Wiley, 1978.

Lewis CA, Smith PG, Stratton M, et al: Estimated radiation doses to different organs among patients treated for ankylosing spondylitis with a single course of x-rays. *Br J Radiol* 61:212–220, 1988.

Lubin JH, Samet JM, Weinberg C: Design issues in studies of indoor exposure to radon and risk of lung cancer. *Health Phys* 59:807–817, 1990.

Marshall JH, Lloyd EL, Rundo J, et al: *Alkaline Earth Metabolism in Adult Man.* ICRP Report Number 20. Elmsford, NY: Pergamon Press, 1972.

Martland HS: The occurrence of malignancy in radioactive persons. *Am J Cancer* 15:2435–2516, 1931.

Mays CW: Alpha particle induced cancer in humans. *Health Phys* 55:637–652, 1988.

Muller J, Kusiak R, Ritchie AC: *Factors Modifying Lung Cancer Risk in Ontario Uranium Miners, 1955–1981.* Ontario Ministry of Labour Report. Toronto: Ministry of Labour, 1989.

NAS: *Health Effects of Exposure to Low Levels of Ionizing Radiation.* National Academy of Sciences Report. BEIR V. Washington, DC: National Academy Press, 1990.

NAS: *Health Effects of Exposure to Radon. National Academy of Sciences Report BEIR VI.* Washington, DC: National Academy Press, 1998.

NAS: *Health Risks of Radon and Other Internally Deposited Alpha Emitters Committee on the Biological Effects of Ionizing Radiation.* National Academy of Sciences Report. BEIR IV. National Research Council Washington, DC: National Academy Press, 1988.

NAS: *The Effects on Populations of Exposure to Low Levels of Ionizing Radiation.* National Academy of Sciences Report. BEIR III. Washington, DC: National Academy Press, 1980.

NAS: *Risk Assessment of Radon in Drinking Water.* National Academy of Sciences. Washington, DC: National Academy Press, 1999.

NCRP: *Evaluation of Occupational and Environmental Exposures to Radon and Radon Daughters in the United States.* National Council on Radiation Protection Report No. 78. Bethesda, MD: NCRP, 1984.

NCRP: *Exposure of the Population in the United States and Canada from Natural Background Radiation.* NCRP Report Number 94, Bethesda, MD: National Council on Radiation Protection and Measurements, 1987b.

NCRP: *Induction of Thyroid Cancer by Ionizing Radiation.* NRCP Report Number 80. Bethesda, MD: National Council on Radiation Protection and Measurements, 1985.

NCRP: *Influence of Dose and Its Distribution in Time of Dose-Response Relationships of Low-LET Radiations.* NCRP Report Number 64. Bethesda, MD: National Council on Radiation Protection and Measurements, 1980.

NCRP: *Limitation of Exposure to Ionizing Radiation.* Report Number 116. National Council on Radiation Protection and Measurements, Bethesda, MD: National Council on Radiation Protection and Measurements, 1993.

NCRP: *Recommendations on Limits for Exposure to Ionizing Radiation.* National Council on Radiation Protection and Measurements, Report Number 91. Bethesda, MD: National Council on Radiation Protection and Measurements, 1987a.

NCRP: *Recommendation on Limits of Exposure to Hot Particles on the Skin.* NRCP Report Number 106. Bethesda, MD: National Council on Radiation Protection and Measurements, 1990.

Nekolla EA, Kellerer AM, Kuse-Isingschulte M, et al: Malignancies in patients treated with high doses of radium-224. *Radiat Res* 152(suppl): S3–S5, 1999.

Neuberger JS: Residential radon exposure and lung cancer. *Health Phys* 63:503–509, 1992.

Neuberger JS: Residential radon exposure and lung cancer (letter). *N Engl J Med* 330:1685, 1994.

Neuberger JS: *Worldwide Studies of Household Radon Exposure and Lung Cancer.* Final Report to the U.S. Department of Energy, Office of Health and Environmental Research. Washington, DC: U.S. Department of Energy, 1989.

NIH: *Radon and Lung Cancer Risk: A Joint Analysis of 11 Underground Miner Studies.* NIH Publication 94-3644. Bethesda, MD: U.S. Department of Health and Human Services, National Institutes of Health, 1994.

Nikjoo H, O'Neill P, Goodhead DT: Computational modeling of low-energy electron-induced DNA damage by early physical and chemical events. *Int J Radiat Biol* 71:467–483, 1997.

Norris WP, Speckman TW, Gustafson PF: Studies of metabolism of radium in man. *AJR* 73:785–802, 1955.

Norris WP, Tyler SA, Brues AM: Retention of radioactive bone seekers. *Science* 128:456, 1958.

NRC: *Comparative Dosimetry of Radon in Mines and Homes*. Washington, DC: National Academy Press, 1991.

Pershagen G, Ackerblow G, Axelson O, et al: IMM Report 2/93—*Radon i bostader och lungcancer* (in Swedish). Stockholm: Institute for Miljomedicin, Karolinska Institute, 1993.

Pershagen G, Ackerblom G, Axelson O, et al: Residential radon exposure and lung cancer in Sweden. *N Engl J Med* 330:159–164, 1994.

Pierce, DA, Preston, DL. Joint analysis of site specific cancer risks for the A-bomb survivors, *Radiat Res* 134:134–142 1993.

Raabe OG, Book SA, Parks NJ: Bone cancer from radium: Canine dose response explains data for mice and humans. *Science* 208:61–64, 1980.

Radford EP, Renard KGS: Lung cancer in Swedish iron miners exposed to low doses of radon daughters. *N Engl J Med* 310:1485–1494, 1984.

RERF: *U.S.–Japan Joint Reassessment of Atomic Bomb Radiation Dosimetry in Hiroshima and Nagasaki*. RERF Final Report DS86. Hiroshima, Japan: Radiation Effect Research Foundation, 1987.

RERF: *U.S.–Japan Joint Reassessment of Atomic Bomb Radiation Dosimetry in Hiroshima and Nagasaki*. Final Report. Radiation Effects Research Foundation. Vol I. Roesch WC (ed). Hiroshima, Japan: Radiation Effects Research Foundation, 1987.

Reuvers AP, Greenstock CL, Borsa J, et al: Studies on the mechanism of chemical protection by dimethyl sulphoxide. *Int J Radiat Biol* 24:533–536, 1973.

Robbins ES, Meyers O: Cycling cells of human and dog tracheobronchial mucosa: Normal and repairing epithelia. *Tech J Franklin Inst* 332A: 35–42, 1995.

Ron E, Modan B: Thyroid and other neoplasms following childhood scalp irradiation, in Boice JD, Fraumeni JF (eds): *Radiation Carcinogenesis: Epidemiology and Biological Significance*. New York: Raven Press, 1984, pp 139–151.

Ron E, Modan B, Preston D: Radiation induced skin carcinomas of the head and neck. *Radiat Res* 125:318–325, 1991.

Rowland RE, Stehney AF, Lucas HF: Dose-response relationships for female radium dial painters. *Radiat Res* 76:368–383, 1978.

Ruzer LS, Nero AV, Harley NH: Assessment of lung deposition and breathing rate of underground miners in Tadjikistan. *Radiat Protect Dosimet*: 58:261–268, 1995.

Saccomanno G, Auerbach O, Kuschner M, et al: A comparison between the localization of lung tumors in uranium miners and in nonminers from 1947 to 1991. *Cancer* 77:1278–1283, 1996.

Samet JM: Radon and lung cancer. *J Natl Cancer Inst* 81:745–757, 1989.

Samet JM, Stolwijk J, Rose SL: Summary: International workshop on residential radon epidemiology. *Health Phys* 60:223–227, 1991.

Schoenberg J, Klotz J: *A Case-Control Study of Radon and Lung Cancer Among New Jersey Women*. NJDH Technical Report, Phase I. Trenton, NJ: New Jersey State Department of Health, 1989.

Schoenberg JB, Klotz JB, Wilcox HB, Szmaciasz SF: A case-control study of radon and lung cancer among New Jersey women, in Cross FT (ed): 29th Hanford Symposium on Health and the Environment: *Indoor Radon and Lung Cancer: Reality or Myth*. Columbus, OH: Battelle Press, 1990, pp 905–922.

Schulz R, Albert RE: Dose to organs of the head from the x-ray treatment of tinea capitis. *Arch Environ Health* 17:935–950, 1963.

Sevc J, Kunz E, Tomasek L, et al: Cancer in man after exposure to Rn daughters. *Health Phys* 54:27–46, 1988.

Shimizu Y, Kato H, Schull WJ, et al: *Life Span Study Report 11, Part 1. Comparison of Risk Coefficients for Site-Specific Cancer Mortality Based on the DS86 and T65DR Shielded Kerma and Organ Doses*. RERF Technical Report TR 12-87. Hiroshima, Japan: Radiation Effects Research Foundation, 1987a.

Shimizu Y, Kato H, Schull WJ: *Life Span Study Report 11, Part 2. Cancer Mortality in the Years 1950–85 Based on the Recently Revised Doses (DS86)*. RERF Report TR-5-88. Hiroshima, Japan: Radiation Effects Research Foundation, 1988.

Shore RE: Issues and epidemiological evidence regarding radiation-induced thyroid cancer. *Radiat Res* 131:98–111, 1992.

Shore RE, Albert RE, Pasternack BS: Follow-up of patients treated by x-ray epilation for tinea capitis. *Arch Environ Health* 31:21–28, 1976.

Shore RE, Albert RE, Reed M, et al: Skin cancer incidence among children irradiated for ringworm of the scalp. *Radiat Res* 100:192–204, 1984.

Shore, RE. Overview of radiation-induced skin cancer in humans. *Int J Radiat Biol* 57:809–827, 1990.

Sinclair WK, Abbatt HE, Farran HE, et al: A quantitative autoradiographic study of radioactive distribution and dosage in human thyroid glands. *Br J Radiol* 29:36–41, 1956.

Smith PG: Late effects x-ray treatment of ankylosing spondylitis, in Boice JD, Fraumeni JF (eds): *Radiation Carcinogenesis: Epidemiology and Biological Significance*. New York: Raven Press, 1984.

Smith PG, Doll R: Mortality among patients with ankylosing spondylitis after a single treatment course with x-rays. *Br Med J* 1:449, 1982.

Smith WM, Doll R: Age- and time-dependent changes in the rates of radiation-induced cancers in patients with ankylosing spondylitis following a single course of x-ray treatment, in *Late Effects of Ionizing Radiation*. Vol 1. Vienna: International Atomic Energy Agency, 1978, p 205.

Spiess FW, Mays CW: Bone cancers induced by Ra-224 (ThX) in children and adults. *Health Phys* 19:713–729, 1970.

Spiess H, Mays CW: Protraction effect on bone sarcoma induction of Ra-224 in children and adults, in Sanders CL, Busch RH, Ballou JE, Mahlum DD (eds): *Radionuclide Carcinogenesis*. Springfield, VA: National Technical Information Service, 1973, pp 437–450.

Sutherland BM, Bennett PV, Sidorkina O, et al: Clustered DNA damages induced in isolated DNA and in human cells by low doses of ionizing radiation. *Proc Natl Acad Sci USA* 97:103–108, 2000.

Tirmarche M, Raphalen A, Allin F, et al: Mortality of a cohort of Rench uranium miners exposure to a relatively low radon exposure. *Br J Cancer* 67:1090–1097, 1993.

Tu KW, Knutson EO: Indoor radon progeny particle size distribution measurements made with two different methods. *Radiat Prot Dosimet* 24:251, 1988.

Turner JE: *Atoms, Radiation and Radiation Protection*. Elmsford, NY: Pergamon Press, 1986.

UNSCEAR: *Sources, Effects and Risks of Ionizing Radiation*. Report of the United Nations Scientific Committee on the Effects of Atomic Radiation. New York: United Nations, 1988.

UNSCEAR: *Sources and Effects of Ionizing Radiation*. Report of the United Nations Scientific Committee on the Effects of Atomic Radiation. New York: United Nations, 1993, pp 125–128.

UNSCEAR: *Sources and Effects of Ionizing Radiation*. Report of the United Nations Scientific Committee on the Effects of Atomic Radiation. New York: United Nations, 1994, pp 60–63.

UNSCEAR: *Sources and Effects of Ionizing Radiation*. Report of the United Nations Scientific Committee on the Effects of Atomic Radiation. New York: United Nations, 2000.

Ward JF: Molecular mechanisms of radiation-induced damage to nucleic acids. *Adv Rad Biol* 5:181–239, 1975.

Ward JF: The complexity of DNA damage: Relevance to biological consequences. *Int J Radiat Biol* 66:427–432, 1994.

Weiss HA, Darby SC, Doll R: Cancer mortality following x-ray treatment for ankylosing spondylitis. *Int J Cancer* 59:327–338, 1994.

Weiss, HA, Darby, SC, Fearn, T: Leukemia mortality following x-ray treatment for ankylosing spondylitis. *Int Radiat Res* 142:1–11, 1995.

Whaling W: The energy loss of charged particles in matter, in Flugge S (ed): *Handbuch der Physik*. Berlin: Springer-Verlag, 1958, pp 193–217.

Wick RR, Chmelevsky D, Gossner W: 224Ra risk to bone and haematopoietic tissue in ankylosing spondylitis patients, in Gossner W, Gerber GB, Hagan U, Luz A (eds): *The Radiobiology of Radium and Thorotrast.* Munich: Urban & Schwarzenberg, 1986, pp 38–44.

Wick RR, Nekolla EA, Gossner W, Kellerer AM: Late effects in ankylosing spondylitis patients treated with ^{224}Ra. *Radiat Res* 152(suppl): S8–S11, 1999.

Woodward A, Roder D, McMichael AJ, et al: Radon daughter exposures at the Radium Hill uranium mine and lung cancer rates among former workers 1952–1987. *Cancer Causes Control* 2:213–220, 1991.

Woodard HQ: *Radiation Carcinogenesis in Man: A Critical Review.* Environmental Measurements Laboratory Report EML-380. New York: U.S. Department of Energy, 1980.

Ziegler JF: *Helium Stopping Powers and Ranges in All Elemental Matter.* New York: Pergamon Press, 1977.

CHAPTER 26

TOXIC EFFECTS OF TERRESTRIAL ANIMAL VENOMS AND POISONS

Findlay E. Russell

Toxinologists generally separates the "venomous" animals from those termed "poisonous." The former are those animals capable of producing a poison in a highly developed secretory gland or group of cells and that can deliver their toxin during a biting or stinging act. Poisonous animals, by contrast, are generally regarded to be those whose tissues, either in part or in their entirety, are toxic. These latter animals have no mechanism or structure for the delivery of their poisons, and poisoning usually takes place through ingestion (Russell, 1965). Venomous or poisonous animals are found in every phylum, even the birds. For the most part, they are widely distributed throughout the animal kingdom, from the unicellular protistan *Alexandrium (Gonyaulax)* to certain of the mammals, including the platypus and the short-tailed shrew. There are at least four hundred species of snakes considered to be of a danger to humans. The number of venomous and poisonous arthropods must be countless, while toxic marine animals number approximately 1500 species and are found in almost every sea and ocean (Halstead, 1965–1970; Russell, 1965, 1984; Russell and Nagabhushanam, 1996).

An animal's venom may have one or several functions. It may play a role in offense, as in the capture and digestion of food, or it may contribute to the animal's defense, as in protection against predators or aggressors. It can also serve both functions. In the snake, the venom provides a food-getting objective. Its secondary function is in its defensive stature. The presence of a toxic venom in the snake is a superior modification to the animal's speed, size, concealment, or strength. In the venomous spiders, the toxin is used to paralyze the prey before it extracts the hemolymph and body fluids. The venom is not primarily designed to kill the prey, only to immobilize the organism for feeding. The same can be said for the scorpions, although they do use their venom in defense. In the fishes, such as the scorpionfishes and stonefishes, and in elasmobranches, such as the stingray, the venom apparatus is generally used in the animal's defense. There does not appear to be any evidence that it is employed in a food-getting capacity, nor would the chemistry or pharmacology so indicate. Venoms used in an offensive posture are generally associated with the oral pole, as in the snakes and spiders, while those used in a defensive function are usually associated with the aboral pole or with spines, as in the stingrays and scorpionfishes. The poisonous animals, on the other hand, usually derive their toxins through the food chain, and as such the poison is often a product of metabolism, sometimes concentrated as it passes through the food chain from one animal to another.

PROPERTIES OF ANIMAL TOXINS

The use to which an animal puts its toxin courses the nature of its chemistry and pharmacology. Whether, in its evolution, the process proceeds by trial and error or by some other means cannot be said. Venoms contain both high- and low-molecular-weight proteins, including polypeptides and enzymes. There may also be amines, lipids, steroids, aminopolysaccharides, quinones, glucosides, and free amino acids as well as 5-hydroxytryptamine (5-HT), histamine, and other substances. Questions then arise as to why and how these substances, most of which are common components of most living tissues, are found in the venom glands, how they came to concentrate there, and why the amounts are sufficient to make them toxic or venomous. It has become apparent that venoms—some snake venoms, for instance—may consist of more than a hundred proteins. Why are there so many? What synergistic and antagonistic mechanisms may be involved, and what autopharmacological phenomena can take place?

One might ask: What is the relationship between the in vitro and in vivo experiment? There is, of course a relationship, but we are finding that putting a single venom component on an isolated tissue preparation (often in far larger amounts than would ever reach that activity site in vivo) does not give us the precise mechanism of action of the full venom; in fact, the data may mislead us, particularly with respect to therapeutics. There is another unfortunate fact in studying the chemistry, pharmacology, and toxicology of venoms in that their structure and function are researched by taking the venoms apart. This has two shortcomings: first, a destructive process is used in attempting to understand what must have been a constructive one; second, the essential quality of the venom may be destroyed before suitable acquaintance of the full toxin has been made. Often, the technology becomes so exacting that the end as to the venom's function is lost sight of in our preoccupation with the means of the examination. Most venoms probably exert their effects on almost every cell and tissue, and their principal pharmacologic properties are usually determined by the amount of a fraction that accumulates at an activity site.

It seems advisable to suggest some general principles on what occurs to a venoms as it passes through the numerous tissues in order to reach an activity site or be metabolized or excreted. The bioavailability of a venom is determined by its composition, molecular size, amount or concentration gradient, solubility, degree of ionization, and the rate of blood flow into that tissue as well as the properties of the engulfing surface itself. The venom can be absorbed by active or passive transport, facilitated diffusion, or even pinocytosis, among other physiologic mechanisms. The role of surface integrins has not been determined for venom components.

In the case of active transport, the cell expends energy and substrates may be accumulated intracellularly against a concentration gradient. In facilitated diffusion, it has been suggested that a "carrier component" combines reversibly with the venom molecule at the membrane's outer surface, and that the carrier-substrate complex can then diffuse more rapidly across the membrane, releasing the molecule (or toxin) to the membrane's inner surface. For some substances it is known that the process of facilitated diffusion is highly selective, accepting only those components that have a relatively specific molecular configuration. There is some evidence to suggest that some fractions of venoms are transported across a membrane by pinocytosis—a process by which a cell engulfs particles or fluids by invaginating and forming a vesicle that later buds off within the interior cell. The venom is then transmitted into the vascular bed, sometimes directly or sometimes through lymphatic channels. This may be determined by the molecular size of its components, by water-oil (or other) partition coefficients, or by some other process causing its movement to the various receptor sites.

The role of the lymphatics and the characteristics in the transport and absorption of snake venom is a much neglected subject in toxicology and toxinology. The lymph circulation not only carries surplus interstitial fluid produced by the venom but also transports the larger molecular components and other particulates back to the bloodstream. Thus, the larger toxins of snake venoms, particularly those of Viperidae, probably enter the lymphatic network preferentially and then transported to the central venous system in the neck. Because lymphatic capillaries (i.e., initial lymphatics), unlike blood capillaries, lack a basement membrane and have fibroelastic "anchoring filaments," they can readily adjust their shape and size, facilitating absorption of excess interstitial fluid along with macromolecules of a venom. Unlike blood flow, which is propelled by a powerful pump, namely the heart, lymph is propelled for the most part by intrinsic segmental contractions of the large and small trunks (lymphangions). With a well-developed intraluminal valve system, the volume of tissue, fluid, and venom components transported is enhanced by both increased rate and greater stroke volume of the lymphangion micropumps (Witte and Witte, 1997).

The receptor sites appear to have highly variable degrees of sensitivity. It is well known that the differences in the rate of metabolism of a venom at a receptor site can vary considerably in mammals. The differences observed in effective amounts of venom between human and laboratory animals does not necessarily reflect any increased sensitivity on the part of the human's target organs but may be directly related to the differences in specific rates of metabolism for the venom as well as the amount of the poison that actually reaches that site. A toxin will produce its pharmacologic effect when the quantity attains a critical minimum concentration at the receptor site. In the case of such complex mixtures as snake venoms, there may be several if not many receptor sites. There is also considerable variability in the sensitivity of those sites for the different components of a venom.

The site of action and metabolism of a venom is dependent on its diffusion and partitioning along the gradient between the plasma and the tissues where the components are deposited. In the case of most snake venoms and fractions so far studied, the distribution is rather unequal, being affected by protein binding, variations in pH, and membrane permeability, among other factors. Once the toxin reaches a particular site, its entry to that site is dependent upon the rate of blood flow into that tissue, the mass of the structure, and the partition characteristics of the toxin between the blood and that particular tissue. Some venom components have a high affinity for certain tissues and exert their most deleterious effects at these sites. This observation has given rise to such terms as *neurotoxin, cardiotoxin, myotoxin,* etc. In such cases the principal effector site may be the nerve, heart, or muscle, but evidence is lacking that these same venoms or fractions do not exert additional deleterious effects, sometimes serious, on other if not most tissues. Then, there is always the problem of how to label a fraction that affects the atrioventricular node. Is this neurologic or cardiovascular? It may seem unwise, in view of our meager knowledge, to claim an understanding of how a venom exerts its exact deleterious effects. One way is to refer to its injurious property, calling it, if we must, neurotoxic, cardiotoxic, or myotoxic, but even those terms circumvent the science of being physiopharmacologically exact.

In addition to the receptor sites, a venom may also be metabolized in several or many different tissues. This is important in considering the pharmacologic activity of a venom or venom fraction, for some components are metabolized distant to the receptor site(s) and may never reach the primary receptor in a quantity sufficient to affect that site. The amount of a toxin that tissues can metabolize without endangering the organisms may also vary. It would be wise, as has been done in some venom studies, to examine tissue slices or homogenates and subcellular fractions of different tissues to determine their metabolic coefficient. In evaluating such data, however, it must be remembered that organs or tissues may contain enzymes that catalyze a host of reactions, including deleterious ones. Enzymes that oxidize venom components by oxygenase mechanisms are for the most part localized in the parenchymal cells of the liver, while other enzymes are found somewhat unevenly distributed throughout many tissues. Again, it should be remembered that these cell types can and do differ between human and other mammals, and particularly the lower animals.

Once a venom component is metabolized or in some way altered, the end substance is excreted, principally through the kidneys. The intestines play a minor role, and what contribution the lungs and biliary system may make has not been determined. Excretion may be complicated by the direct action of the venom on the kidneys themselves, causing an inflammatory reaction that may produce gaps between the endothelial fenestrae, very small pores, so they are more permeable than skeletal muscle capillaries. Intestinal, salivary, and sweat gland capillaries also contain fenestrae. Indeed, the author has been impressed by the damage to the kidneys in humans seen on postmortem examination following crotalid and viperid bites. Although no generalization concerning the damage wrought by a snake venom on the organ systems of humans can be made (as compared with other mammals), the changes in the kidneys would seem only secondary to those occurring in the heart, and of course, the blood vessels (Russell, 1980a, 1980b, 1983). To sum up, applying a venom or venom fraction directly to an isolated tissue preparation of the mouse or other small mammal may provoke a quite different physiopharmacologic response, both qualitatively and quantitatively than the same toxin produces *in vivo* in the human.

ARTHROPODS

There are more than a million species of arthropods, generally divided into 25 orders, of which at least 12 are of importance to humans from an economic standpoint. Medically, however, only about 10 orders are of significant venomous or poisonous importance. These include the arachnids (scorpions, spiders, whipscorpions, solpugids, mites, and ticks); the myriapods (centipedes and millipedes); the insects (water bugs, assassin bugs, and wheel bugs); beetles (blister beetles); Lepidoptera (butterflies, moths, and caterpillars), and Hymenoptera (ants, bees, and wasps). In each of these groups and perhaps in some others, there are additional creatures that have been implicated in poisonings, but in most cases the clinical evidence or chemical nature of the toxin appears to be relatively circumstantial to properly implicate their dangerousness to humans. As noted by many authors, most arthropods do not have fangs or stings long or strong enough to penetrate the human skin.

In treating the subject of venomous arthropods the writer has not included those bites that, because of the trauma of their injury, may be painful. I have also needed to exclude those creatures that are vectors for certain bacterial, viral, or rickettsial disease and those bites or stings that give rise to allergic reactions. There are numerous texts and papers that deal with the general characteristics of venomous and poisonous arthropods. These inlcude those of Minton (1968), Eberling (1975), Maretic and Lebez (1979), Harwood and James (1979), Nutting (1984), and Smith (1997).

The number of deaths from arthropod stings and bites is not known. Most countries do not keep records of the incidence of such deaths or injuries. In Mexico, parts of Central and South America, North Africa, and India, deaths from scorpion stings, for instance, exceed several thousand a year. Spider bites probably do not account for more than 200 deaths a year worldwide. A common problem faced by physicians in suspected spider bites relates to the differential diagnosis. Of approximately 600 suspected spider bites seen in one series of cases, 80 percent were found to be caused by arthropods other than spiders or by other disease states (Russell and Gertsch, 1983). The arthropods most frequently involved in the misdiagnoses were ticks (including their embedded mouthparts), mites, bedbugs, fleas (infected flea bites), Lepidoptera insects, flies, vesicating beetles, water bugs, and various stinging Hymenoptera. Among the disease states that were confused with spider or arthropod bites or stings were erythema chronicum migrans, erythema nodosum, periarteritis nodosum, pyroderma gangrenosum, kerion cell–mediated response to a fungus, Stevens-Johnson syndrome, toxic epidermal necrolysis, herpes simplex, and purpura fulminans.

As with the snake, a spider or any other arthropod may bite or sting and not eject venom. The author has seen many such cases. Finally, some arthropod venom poisonings give rise to the symptoms and signs of an existing undiagnosed subclinical disease. The problem of diverse disease states following bites or stings of various venomous animals has been recognized (Russell, 1979), and when a case of poisoning appears to persist, the patient should be reexamined for the possible presence of some undiagnosed disease. In some cases, stings or bites may induce stress reactions that bring the unrecognized disease to the surface.

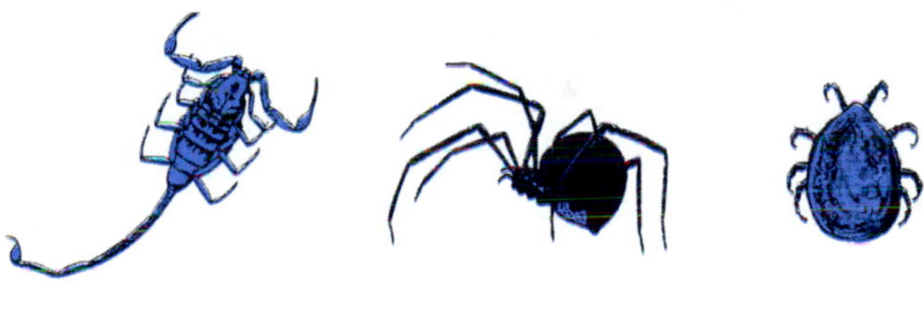

ARACHNIDA

Scorpions

The scorpions are said to be the oldest known terrestrial arthropods. There are at least a thousand species, among which the stings of more than 75 can be considered of sufficient importance to warrant medical attention. Scorpions spend the daylight hours under cover or in burrows. They emerge at night to ambush other arthropods or even small rodents, capture them with their pincers, sting and paralyze them, or tear them apart and digest their body fluids. Because they are carnivorous, the larger ones often feed on the smaller. Scorpions live from 2 to 10 years, although there are reports of a 25-year life span. Some of the more important of these species are noted in Table 26-1. In addition, members of the genera *Pandinus, Hadrurus, Vejovis, Nebo,* and some of the others are capable of inflicting painful and often erythematous lesions. In the United States the sting of *Centruroides exilicauda (sculpturatus)* is dangerous, and in Mexico there were 20,352 deaths over two 9-year periods, chiefly in children less than 3 years of age. It has been said that the total number of scorpion stings per year in Mexico at present may be as high as 250,000, with perhaps 200 deaths. Working in Mexico in 1953, this writer estimated that there were over 40,000 stings that year, of which 10,000 were treated or reported. The total number of deaths appeared to be less than 1500.

The dangerous bark scorpion *Centruroides exilicauda,* so called because of its preference for hiding under the loose bark of trees or in dead trees or logs, often frequents human dwellings. Its general color is straw to yellowish-brown or reddish-brown, and it is often easily distinguishable from other scorpions in the same

Table 26-1
Medically Important Scorpions

GENUS	DISTRIBUTION
Androctonus species	North Africa, Middle East, Turkey
Buthus species	France and Spain to Middle East and north Africa, Mongolia, China
Buthotus species	Africa, Middle East, central Asia
Centruroides species	North, Central, South America
Heterometrus species	Central and southeast Asia
Leiurus species	North Africa, Middle East, Turkey
Mesobuthus species	Turkey, India
Parabuthus species	Southern Africa
Tityus species	Central and South America

habitat by its long, thin telson, or tail, and its thin pedipalps, or pincerlike claws. Adults of this genus show a considerable difference in length. *Centruroides exilicauda* in the southwestern United States and adjacent Mexico reaches a length of approximately 5.5 cm, while *Centruroides vittatus* of the Gulf states and adjacent Mexico is generally slightly larger. *Centruroides suffusus,* a particularly dangerous Mexican species, may attain a length of 9 cm, but *Centruroides noxius,* another important species, seldom exceeds 5 cm in length. Excellent reviews on scorpions have been provided by Keegan (1980) and Polis (1990).

Many scorpion venoms contain low-molecular-weight proteins, peptides, amino acids, nucleotides, and salts, among other components. The neurotoxic fractions are generally classified on the basis of their molecular size, the short-chain toxins being composed of 30 to 40 amino acid residues with three or four disulfide bonds and appear to affect potassium or chloride channels; while the long-chain toxins have 60 to 70 amino acid residues with four disulfide bonds and affect mainly the sodium channels. These particular toxins may have an effect on both voltage-dependent channels. The amino acid content is known for more than 90 species, and there appears to be a high degree of cysteines in most of these venoms. The toxins can selectively bind to a specific channel of excitable cells, thus impairing the initial depolarization of the action potential in the nerve and muscle that results in their neurotoxicity. It appears that the way that some scorpion venoms differently affect mammalian, as opposed to insect tissues is related to the structural basis of the gates in the two organisms. Not all scorpions, however, have fractions that affect neuromuscular transmission. The venoms of most scorpions may be deleterious to other arthropods, but they exert no significant systemic effects on humans. The American scorpion *Vejovis spinigerus* has no effect on mammalian neurotransmission, reflex discharge, or antidromic inhibition, but at high doses it can provoke systemic arterial, venous, and cisternal changes in mammals (Russell, 1968).

The symptoms and signs of scorpion envenomation differ considerably depending on the species. In the United States, the most common offenders are members of the family Vejovidae, generally found in the southwestern and western states as well as in Mexico, Central America, and South America. Their sting gives rise to localized pain, swelling, tenderness, and mild parasthesia. Systemic reactions are rare, although weakness, fever, and muscle fasciculations have been reported. These same findings have been reported for the stings of the giant hairy scorpion, *Hadrurus,* another member of the Vejovidae. Envenomations by some members of the genus *Centruroides* are clinically the most important, particularly in the western United States, where *C. exilicauda* is found. In children, their sting produces initial pain. However, some children do not complain of pain and are unaware of the injury. The area becomes sensitive to touch, and merely pressing lightly over the injury will elicit an immediate retraction. Usually there is little or no local swelling and only mild erythema. The child becomes tense and restless and shows abnormal and random head and neck movements. Often the child will display roving eye movements. In their review of *Centruroides sculpturatus* stings, Rimsza and coworkers (1980) noted visual signs, including nystagmus roving eye and oculogyric movements, in 12 of 24 patients stung by this scorpion. Loud noises, such as banging the examination table behind the child's back, often cause the patient to jump. Tachycardia is usually evident within 45 min as well as some hypertension. Although this is not seen in children as early or as severely as in adults, it is often present within an hour following the sting. Respiratory and heart rates are increased, and by 90 min the child may appear quite ill. Fasciculations may be seen over the face or large muscle masses, and the child may complain of generalized weakness and display some ataxia or motor weakness. Opisthotonos is not uncommon. The respiratory distress may proceed to respiratory paralysis. Excessive salivation is often present and may further impair respiratory function. Slurring of speech may be present, and convulsions may occur. If death does not occur, the child usually becomes asymptomatic within 36 to 48 h.

In adults the clinical picture is somewhat similar, but there are some differences. Almost all adults complain of immediate pain after the sting, regardless of the *Centruroides* species involved. Adults do not show the restlessness seen in children. Instead, they are tense and anxious. They develop tachycardia and hypertension, and respirations are increased. They may complain of difficulties in focusing and swallowing, as may children. In some cases, there is some general weakness and pain on moving the injured extremity. Convulsions are very rare, but ataxia and muscle incoordination may occur. Most adults are asymptomatic within 12 h but may complain of generalized weakness for 24 h or more.

As noted elsewhere (Russell, 1996), a review of the therapy for scorpion stings will provide a fascinating mixture of mythology, folklore, hunches, and a list of all sorts of therapeutic devices from electroshock to mechanical compression. Measures such as bed rest, positive-pressure breathing, mild sedation with diazepam and antihypertensive drugs may be helpful when high blood pressure is a problem. An antivenom produced by Arizona State University for *C. exilicauda* stings is available and approved by the state, but does not have the approval of the U.S. Food and Drug Administration (FDA). An $F(ab)_2$ polyvalent antivenom is produced in Mexico, but the former is preferred for U.S. species. Recently, the continuous infusion of midazolam has been used with considerable success in serious *C. exilicauda* stings in Arizona (Jones et al., 1988).

Spiders

Of the 30,000 or so species, at least 200 have been implicated in significant bites on humans. Some of the more medically important of these spiders are noted in Table 26-2. Spiders are predaceous, polyphagous arachnids that generally feed on insects or other arthropods. A more complete review of spider bites can be found in the excellent work of Kaston (1978), Maretic and Lebez (1979), Gertsch (1979), and the lesser contributions of Southcott (1976) and Russell and Gertsch (1983). It is not possible to describe the chemistry, pharmacology, or immunology of the hundreds (perhaps thousands) of spider venoms that are toxic. Discussed here are only a few that appear to be clinically more important in the United States. There are, however, bites by species of *Pheostica, Pamphobeteus, Bothriocyrtum, Ummidia, Phoneutria, Cupiennius, Lycosa, Heteropoda, Misumenoides, Liocranoides, Neoscona, Araneus, Argiope, Peucetia, Agelenopsis,* and *Tegenaria*. Whether native or imported, all have all been implicated in bites on humans in the United States.

Spider venoms are very complex and have been studied extensively, even as sources for new drugs (Coombs, 1992). From a neuroactive standpoint, the widow and grass spiders, with their neurotranmitter release and channel-affecting properties; the jumping spiders, with their Ca^{2+}–channel blocking activity; and the argiope and orb spinners, with their glutamate and Ca^{2+}–channel blocking activities appear to show much promise as tools in studying neurologic phenomena and perhaps for clinical use.

***Latrodectus* Species (Widow Spiders)** In the United States, these spiders are commonly known as the black widow, brown

Table 26-2
Genera of Spiders for Which Significant Bites on Humans are Known

GENUS	FAMILY	COMMON NAME	DISTRIBUTION
Agelenopsis	Agelenidae	Grass spider	North America
Aganippe species	Idiopidae	Trap-door spider	Australia
Aphonopelma species	Theraphosidiae	Tarantula	North America
Araneus species	Araneidae	Orbweaver	Worldwide
Arbanitis species	Idiopidae	Trap-door spider	Australia, East Indies
Argiope species	Araneidae	Argiope	Worldwide
Atrax species	Hexathelidae	Funnel-web spider	Australia
Bothriocyrtum species	Ctenizidae	Trap-door spider	California
Cheiracanthium species	Miturgidae	Running spider	Europe, north Africa, Orient, North America
Cupiennius species	Ctenidae	Banana spider	Central America
Drassodes species	Gnaphosidae	Running spider	Worldwide
Dyarcyops [=*Misgolas*]	Idiopidae	Trap-door spider	Australia
Dysdera	Dysderidae	Dysderid	Eastern hemisphere, Americas
Elassoctenus [=*Diallomus*]	Zordae	Ctenid	Australia
Filistata species	Filistatidae	Hackled-band spider	Temperate and tropical worldwide
Harpactirella species	Theraphosidae	Trap-door spider	South Africa
Heteropoda species	Sparassidae	Giant crab spider	East Indies, tropical Asia, south Florida
Isopoda species	Sparassidae	Giant crab spider	Australia, East Indies
Ixeuticus [=*Badumna*]	Desidae	Amaurobiid	New Zealand, southern California
Lampona species	Lamponidae	White-tailed spider	Australia, New Zealand
Latrodectus species	Theridiidae	Widow spider	Temperate and tropical regions worldwide
Liocranoides species	Tengellidae	Running spider	Appalachia
Loxosceles species	Loxoscelidae	Brown or violin spider	Americas, Africa, Europe, eastern Asia, Pacific Islands
Lycosa species	Lycosoidae	Wolf spider	Worldwide
Missulena species	Actinopodidae	Trap-door spider	Australia
Misumenoides species	Thomisidae	Crab spider	North and South America
Miturga species	Miturgidae	Running spider	Australia
Mopsus species	Salticidae	Jumping spider	Australia
Neoscona species	Araneidae	Orbweaver	Worldwide
Olios species	Sparassidae	Giant crab spider	North and South America
Pamphobeteus species	Theraphosidae	Tarantula	South America
Peucetia species	Oxyopidae	Green lynx spider	Worldwide
Phidippus species	Salticidae	Jumping spider	North and South America
Phoneutria species	Ctenidae	Hunting spider	Central and South America
Selenocosmia species	Theraphosidae	Tarantula	East Indies, India, Australia, tropical Africa
Steatoda species	Theridiidae	False black widow	Worldwide
Tegenaria	Agelenidae	Funnel-web spider	Worldwide
Ummidia	Ctenizidae	Trap-door spider	North and South America

SOURCE: From Russell, 1996, and revised by NI Planick, American Museum of Natural History, 2000.

widow, or red-legged spider. They, however, have many other common names in English: hourglass, poison lady, deadly spider, red-bottom spider, T-spider, gray lady spider, and shoebutton spider. Widow spiders are found almost circumglobally in all continents with temperate or tropical climates. In the United States, there are at least five species, including the native *L. mactans, L. bishopi, L. variolus, L. hesperus,* and the imported *L. geometricus*. Although both male and female widow spiders are venomous, only the female has fangs large and strong enough to penetrate the human skin. Mature *L. mactans* females range in body length from 10 to 18 mm, whereas males range from 3 to 5 mm. These spiders have a globose abdomen varying in color from gray to brown to black, depending on the species. In the black widow, the abdomen is shiny black with a red hourglass or red spots and sometimes white spots on the venter.

Through the years, one of the difficulties in determining the composition of spider venoms, particularly that of *Latrodectus* spp., has been the procedure of grinding up the venom glands and preparing a homogenate of the glands and then attributing the chemistry or toxicology to that of the actual venom. The manifestations of the poisoning from the glands do not reflect those found in the in vivo state. A family of high-molecular-weight proteins, latrotoxins, have been described in *Latrodectus* venoms. These are proteins of about 1000 amino acid residues (Grishin, 1999). Alpha-latrotoxin is a presynaptic toxin which is said to exert toxic effects on the vertebrate central nervous system in depolarizing neurons by increasing $[Ca^{2+}]i$ and by stimulating uncontrolled proteins described in *Latrodectus* venom. These are proteins of about 1000 amino acid residues (Grishin, 1999). Alpha-latrotoxin is a presynaptic toxin that is said to exert its toxic effects on the vertebrate central nervous system in depolarizing neurons by increasing $[Ca^{2+}]i$, and by exocytosis of neurotransmitters from nerve terminals (Holz and Habener, 1998). Along with the known GTP-binding protein-coupled receptors, five latroinsectotoxins affecting neurotransmitter release from the presynaptic endings of insects and one latrocrustatoxin have been isolated, and a alpha-latrotoxin preparation showed a low-molecular-weight protein structurally related to crustacean hyperglycemic hormones (Greshin, 1998). By thin-layer chromatography (TLC) on silica gel, it was shown that the venom kininase was a thiol endopeptidase (Akhunov et al., 1996).

Clinical Problem Bites by the black widow are described as sharp and pinprick-like, followed by a dull, occasionally numbing pain in the affected extremity and by pain and cramps in one or several of the large muscle masses. Rarely is there any local skin reaction except during the first 60 min following the bite, but piloerection in the bite area is sometimes seen. Muscle fasciculations frequently can be seen within 30 min of the bite. Sweating is common, and the patient may complain of weakness and pain in the regional lymph nodes, which are often tender on palpation and occasionally are enlarged; lymphadenitis is frequently observed. Pain in the low back, thighs, or abdomen is a common complaint, and rigidity of the abdominal muscles is seen in most cases in which envenomation has been severe. Severe paroxysmal muscle cramps may occur, and arthralgia has been reported. Hypertension is a common finding, particularly in the elderly after moderate to severe envenomations. Blood studies are usually normal.

There is no effective first-aid treatment. In most cases, intravenous calcium gluconate will relieve muscle pain, but this may have to be repeated at 4- to 6-h intervals for optimum effect. Muscle relaxants such as methocarbamol 5 to 10 mg can be used. Acute hypertensive crises may require intravenous nitroprusside. The use of antivenom (antivenin, *L. mactans*) should be restricted to more severe cases and when other measures have proved unsuccessful. One ampule administered intravenously is usually sufficient. In patients who are under 16 or over 60 years, have any history of hypertension or hypertensive heart disease, or who show significant symptoms and signs, the use of antivenom seems warranted; it also is appropriate in cases involving pregnancy.

***Loxosceles* Species (Brown or Violin Spiders)** These primitive spiders are variously known in North America as the fiddle-back spider or the brown recluse. There are over 100 species of *Loxosceles*. Twenty of these species range from temperate South Africa northward through the tropics into the Mediterranean region and southern Europe. Another 84 species are known from North, Central, and South America and the West Indies. The most widely distributed is *Loxosceles rufescens,* the so-called cosmopolitan species. It is found in the Mediterranean area, southern Russia, most of north Africa including the Azores, Madagascar, the Near East, Asia from India to southern China and Japan, parts of Malaysia and Australia, some islands of the Pacific, and North America. *Loxosceles laeta* is mostly South American, but it has been introduced into Central America; small areas in Cambridge, Massachusetts; Sierra Madre and Alhambra, California; and the zoology building of the University of Helsinki. The abdomen of these spiders varies in color from grayish through orange and reddish-brown to blackish and is distinct from the pale yellow to reddish-brown background of the cephalothorax. This spider has six eyes grouped in three dyads. Females average 8 to 12 mm in body length, whereas males average 6 to 10 mm. Both males and females are venomous. The most important species in the United States are *Loxosceles reclusa* (brown recluse spider), *Loxosceles deserta* (desert violin spider), and *Loxosceles arizonica* (Arizona violin spider).

The chemistry and toxicology of *Loxosceles* venom were first described by Schenone and Suarez (1978). Early work indicated that the amount of venom protein per spider was about 68 mg. Although the venom is said to contain phospholipase, protease, esterase, collagenase, hyaluronidase, deoxyribonuclease, ribonuclease, dipeptides, dermanecrosis factor 33, dermonecrosis factor 37, the most important factor is sphingomyelinase D. The relationship between these various fractions is not clear, but most recent works treat with the sphingomyelinase D. In *Loxosceles intermedia a* the toxic effects appear to be associated with a 35-kDa protein (1735) which demonstrates a complement-dependent hemolytic activity and a dermonecrotic-inducing factor (Andrade et al., 1998). ^{31}P-Nuclear magnetic resonance assay of the four bands representing proteins, measuring 34 kDa in the venom, produced three proteins with sphingomyelinase D activity (Merchant et al., 1998). An endotoxemic-like shock, showing eosinophilic material in the proximal and distal tubules and tubular necrosis, were the most common histopathologic findings, preceded in mice by prostration, acute cachexia, hypothermia, neurologic changes, and hemoglobinuria (Tambourgi et al., 1998). In Brazil, the sandwich-type enzyme-linked immunosorbent assay (ELISA) for the detection of venom antigens for *L. intermedia* in both animal and human envenomations has been shown to be a useful diagnostic procedure (Chavez-Olortegui et al., 1998). The venom has coagulation and vasoconstriction properties. It causes selective damage to the vascular endothelium. There are adhesions of neutrophils to the capillary wall with sequestration and activation of passing neutrophils by the perturbed endothelial cells (Patel et al., 1994). When the venom is injected into mammals, it produces, in addition to the local tissue reaction, varying degrees of thrombocytopenia, some intravascular hemolysis, and hemolytic anemia.

Clinical Problem The bite of this spider produces about the same degree of pain as does the sting of an ant, but sometimes the patient may be unaware of the bite. In most cases, a local burning sensation, which may last for 30 to 60 min, develops around the injury. Pruritus over the area often occurs, and the area becomes red, with a small blanched area surrounding the reddened bite site. Skin temperature usually is elevated over the lesion area. The reddened area enlarges and becomes purplish during the subsequent 1 to 8 h. It often becomes irregular in shape, and as time passes, hemorrhages may develop throughout the area. A small bleb or vesicle forms at the bite site and increases in size. It subsequently ruptures and a pustule forms. The red hemorrhagic area continues to enlarge, as does the pustule. The whole area may become swollen and painful, and lymphadenopathy is common. During the early stages the lesion often takes on a bull's-eye appearance, with a central white vesicle surrounded by the reddened area and ringed by a whitish or bluish border. The central pustule ruptures, and necrosis to various depths can be visualized. Not all bites, however, take this course, some producing no more than localized pain, slight redness, and minimal swelling (Russell, 1996).

In serious bites, the lesion can measure 8 by 10 cm with severe necrosis invading muscle tissue. On the face, large lesions resulting in extensive tissue destruction and requiring subsequent plastic surgery sometimes are seen after bites by *L. laeta* in South America. Systemic symptoms and signs include fever, malaise, stomach cramps, nausea and vomiting, jaundice, spleen enlargement, hemolysis, hematuria, and thrombocytopenia. Fatal cases, while rare, usually are preceded by intravascular hemolysis, hemolytic anemia, thrombocytopenia, hemoglobinuria, and renal failure. There have been no deaths in the United States from the bites of this spider, contrary to reports in the media.

There are no first-aid measures of value. In fact, all first-aid procedures should be avoided, as the natural appearance of the lesion is most important in determining the diagnosis. A cube of ice may be placed on the wound. At one time, excision of the bite area with ample margins was advised when this could be done within an hour or so of the bite and when *Loxosceles* was definitely implicated. The value of steroids has been questioned. This writer, however, has had seemingly good results with steroids following bites by *L. deserta, L. arizonica, and L. russelli*. The patient should be placed on a corticosteroid such as intramuscular dexamethasone, 4 mg every 6 h during the acute phase. Subsequent doses were determined by clinical judgment, followed by decremental doses over a 4-day period. Antihistamines are of questionable value. The use of dapsone was suggested by King and Rees (1983). The results have been encouraging, but care must be exercised with this drug. If skin grafting becomes necessary, the procedure is best deferred for 4 to 6 weeks after the injury. Systemic manifestations should be treated symptomatically. Antivenom is not commercially available but has been used in Tennessee (King, personal correspondence, 1990).

***Steatoda* Species** The cobweb spiders, *Steatoda* spp., are variously known as the false black widow, combfooted, or cupboard spiders. They are thought to have reached the Americas through trading sources. These spiders are often mistaken for black widow spiders, and indeed the first clinical case of *Steatoda grossa* envenomation directed to the author in 1961 was thought to be caused by *L. mactans*. The female of *S. grossa* differs from *L. mactans* and *L. hesperus* in having a purplish-brown abdomen rather than a black one. It is less shiny, and its abdomen is more oval than round. It may have pale yellow or whitish markings on the dorsum of the abdomen, and no markings on the venter. The abdomen of some species is orange, brown, or chestnut in color and often bears a light band across the anterior dorsum.

Cavalieri et al. (1987) state that the venom of *Steatoda paykulliana* had little effect on guinea pigs and no proteolytic activity was noted, but high concentrations of the venom stimulated release of transmitter substances similar to *Latrodectus* venom. A high-molecular-weight protein was toxic to houseflies. The venom is said to form ionic channels permeable for bi- and monovalent cations. It was found that the living time in the open state depended on the membrane potential (Sokolov et al., 1984). According to Maretić and Lebez (1979), *S. paykulliana* venom gives "strong motor unrest, clonic cramps, exhaustion, ataxia and then paralysis in guinea pigs." Bites by *S. grossa* or *Steatoda fulva* in the United States have been followed by local pain, often severe; induration; pruritus; and the occasional breakdown of tissue at the bite site. Warrell et al. (1991) report a bite by *Steatoda nobilis* with unpleasant local and systemic "symptoms," but whether the envenomation can be termed "neurotoxic" in humans remains questionable. In none of the seven *S. grossa* cases seen by the writer was there any strong evidence of neurotoxicity. Perhaps there is a significant difference in the venoms of the various species. Wounds should be debrided and covered, and signs should be treated symptomatically.

***Cheiracanthium* Species (Running Spiders)** The 160 species of this genus have an almost circumglobal distribution, although only four or five species have been implicated in bites on humans. Maretić and Lebez (1979) named *Cheiracanthium punctorium, Cheiracanthium inclusum, Cheiracanthium mildei,* and *Cheiracanthium diversum* as the spiders most often implicated in envenomations. In Japan, however, *Cheiracanthium japonicum* is a common biting spider. The abdomen is convex and egg-shaped and varies in color from yellow, green, or greenish-white to reddish-brown; the cephalothorax is usually slightly darker than the abdomen. The chelicerae are strong, and the legs are long, hairy, and delicate. The spider ranges in length from 7 to 16 mm. Like *Phidippus* but even more so, *Cheiracanthium* tends to be tenacious and sometimes must be removed from the bite area. For that reason there is a high degree of identification following the bite of these spiders. The most toxic fraction of the venom is said to be a protein of 60 kDa, and the venom is high in norepinephrine and serotonin.

The author's experiences with seven bites by *C. inclusum* have been very similar; the following description is based on those experiences. The patient usually describes the bite as sharp and painful, with the pain increasing during the first 30 to 45 h. The patient complains of dull pain over the injured part. A reddened wheal with a hyperemic border develops. Small petechiae may appear near the center of the wheal. Skin temperature over the lesion is often elevated, but body temperature is usually normal. Lymphadenitis and lymphadenopathy may develop. In Japan, *C. japonicum* produces more severe manifestations than we have seen with the American or European species. These include severe local pain, nausea and vomiting, headache, chest discomfort, severe pruritus, and shock in addition to the local findings.

***Phidippus* Species (Jumping Spiders)** These spiders, variously known as crab spiders and eyebrow spiders, are usually less than 20 mm in length and have a somewhat elevated, rectangular cephalothorax that tends to blunt anteriorly. The abdomen is often oval or elongated. There is a great deal of variation in the color of these spiders. In the female, the cephalothorax may be black, brown, red, orange, or yellowish-orange and the abdomen tends to be slightly lighter in color. In most species there are various white, yellow, orange, or red spots or markings on the dorsum of the abdomen. These spiders are thought to have the sharpest of vision, thus their hunting excellence. They have four large eyes on the face and four smaller eyes on the dorsum of the head. The larger pair of eyes on the face apparently serve for the sharpest vision.

A computer-aided key based on electromorph patterns for five enzyme systems has been developed to determine specific species of *Phidippus*. Digitized, and the gels graphed, the system provides a ready identification of seven species of the spider (Terranova and Roach, 1989). In their comprehensive study of the venom of 26 spider species belonging to 15 families, it was found that the toxic effect of the venom was dramatic with respect to its cytotoxic effect on cultured cells, where there was a dramatic, instantaneous disruption of cell membranes, resulting in the collapse of the neuroblastoma cells (Cohen and Quistad, 1998).

The bite of this spider produces a sharp pinprick of pain, and the area immediately around the wound may become painful and tender. The pain usually lasts 5 to 10 min. An erythematous wheal slowly develops. In cases seen by the author, the wheal measured 2 to 5 cm in diameter. A dull, sometimes throbbing pain may subsequently develop over the injured part, but it rarely requires attention. A small vesicle may form at the bite site. Around this is an irregular, slightly hyperemic area, which in turn may be surrounded by a blanched region that is tender to touch and pressure. Generally, there is only mild lymphadenitis. Swelling of the part may be diffuse and is often accompanied by pruritus. The symptoms and signs usually abate within 48 h. There is no specific treatment for the bite of this spider (Russell, 1970).

Ticks

Tick paralysis is caused by the saliva of certain ticks of the families Ixodidae and Argasidae and perhaps others. An excellent review on the subject has been published by Gregson (1973), while a more recent, shorter review is that of Smith (1997). Tick paralysis is known for both domestic animals and humans, being noted in humans since 1912, although it was known to the American Indians as pajaroella, due to *Ornithodoros corisceus,* long before that time. There are said to be at least 60 species of ticks that have been implicated in paralysis-producing disorders. With respect to tick paralysis rather than tick toxicosis, one must consider the rickettsial, spirochetal, and microbacterial organisms transmitted by ticks (or mites) that cause neurologic disorders similar to those produced by the organism's saliva. Among the diseases due to organisms transmitted by ticks are Lyme disease, Rocky Mountain spotted fever, babesiosis, leptospirosis, Q fever, ehrlichiosis, typhus, tick-borne encephalitis, and others.

The saliva of *Ixodes holocyclus* appears to have been most often studied and has yielded a number of substances that may cause paralysis and, at high doses, death. Peak paralytic activity was found between 60 to 100 kDa, and a lethal nonparalytic fraction was found at 20 kDa. In *Argas* paralysis, the action appears to be directed toward polyneuropathy, with only slight afferent pathways. Respiration is affected and acetylcholine release is reduced, while sensitivity at the neuromuscular junction is affected. Conduction in motor fibers is said to be affected, with a functional deficiency in afferent fibers. It has been suggested that in *Dermacentor andersoni* paralysis, the paralysis represents lower motor neuron injury and irritation of the posterior root of the spinal cord (Amese and Lyday, 1939), while Rose (1954) has provided evidence that the block is at the neuromuscular junction. It must be concluded that the exact mechanism of the paralysis has yet to be determined.

Clinical Problem Except for some species, tick bites are often not felt; the first evidence of envenomation may not appear until several days later, when small macules develop. The macules are 3 to 4 mm in diameter and surrounded by erythema and swelling, often displaying a hyperemic halo. The patient often complains of difficulty with gait, followed by paresis and eventually locomotor paresis and paralysis. Problems in speech and respiration may ensue and lead to respiratory paralysis if the tick is not removed. Since the tick is often in the hair, it may remain unseen, thus confusing the differential diagnosis. Removal of the tick usually results in a rapid and complete recovery, although regression of paralysis may resolve slowly.

It seems probable that the ticks that cause the paralysis in humans and domestic animals may be the same, and that it is the length of the exposure to the feeding tick that determines the degree of poisoning. Obviously, the first signs of poisoning are less likely to be observed in cattle, sheep, dogs, and cats than in humans; as for symptoms (what the patient tells the physician), such reports are not likely to be made. Treatment consists of removal of the tick, using a formamidine derivative or petroleum product, washing with soap and water, and treating specifically for the paralysis or other manifestation. It should be pointed out, again, that these comments are specific only for tick venom poisoning and not for allergic reactions, transmission of disease states, or other complications of tick bites.

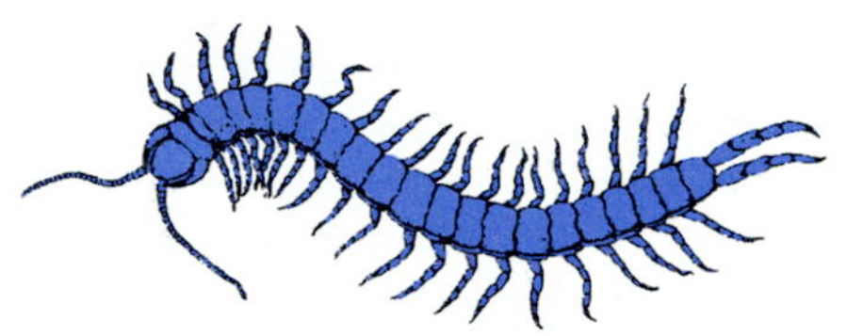

CHILOPODA (CENTIPEDES)

These elongated, many-segmented brownish-yellow arthropods are found worldwide. With a pair of walking legs on most segments, they are fast-moving, secretive, and nocturnal. They feed on other arthropods and even small vertebrates and birds; they are cannibalistic. The first pair of legs behind the head are modified into poison jaws or maxillipeds. Centipedes range in length from 3 to almost 300 mm. In the United States, the prevalent biting genus is a *Scolopendra* species. The venom is concentrated within the intracellular granules, discharged into vacuoles of the cytoplasm of the secretory cells, and moved by exocytosis into the lumen of the gland; from thence ducts carry the venom to the jaws (Ménez et al., 1990).

The venoms of centipedes contain high-molecular-weight proteins, proteinases and esterases, 5-hydroxytrptamine, histamine, lipids, and polysaccharides. In humans, such a venom produces cardiovascular changes and changes associated with acetylcholine release. It produces immediate bleeding, redness, and swelling often lasting 24 h. Localized tissue changes and necrosis have been reported, and severe envenomations may cause nausea and vomiting, changes in heart rate, vertigo, and headache. In the most severe cases, there can be mental disturbances. Treatment is nonspecific, but washing and the application of a cream containing hydrocortisone, diphenhydramine, and tetracaine (Itch Balm Plus, Sawyer) is of value.

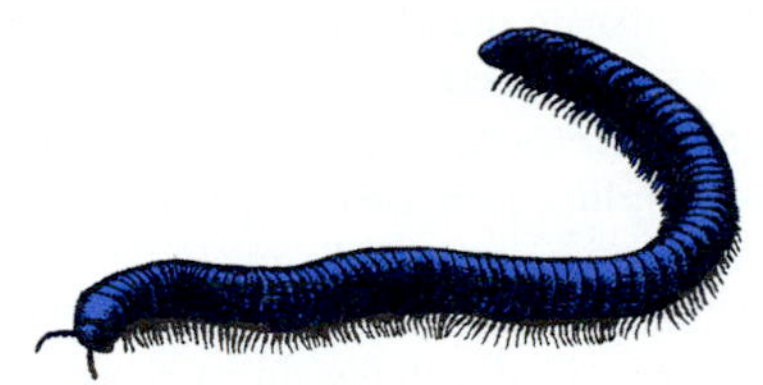

DIPLOPODA (MILLIPEDES)

These arthropods are cylindrical, wormlike creatures, mahogany to dark brown or black in color, bearing two pairs of jointed legs per segment and ranging in length from 20 to 300 mm. In some parts of the world, particularly Australia and New Guinea, the repellent secretions expelled from the sides of their bodies contain a toxin of quinone derivatives and a variety of complex substances such as iodine and hydrocyanic acid, which the animal makes use of to produce hydrogen cyanide. Some species can spray these defensive secretions, and eye injuries, though rare in the United States, are not uncommon.

The lesions produced by millipedes are generally known as "burn" injuries and consist of a burning or prickling sensation and development of a yellowish or brown-purple lesion; subsequently a blister containing serosanguinous fluid forms, which may rupture. Eye contact can cause acute conjunctivitis, periorbital edema, keratosis, and much pain; such an injury must be treated immediately. Skin treatment consists of washing, washing, and washing the area thoroughly with soap and water and applying the cream as previously mentioned.

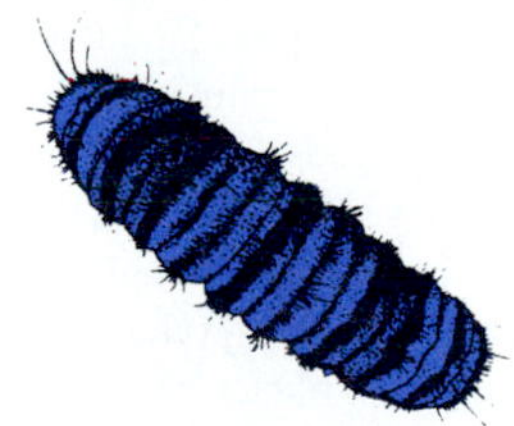

INSECTA

Lepidoptera (Caterpillars, Moths, and Butterflies)

The urticating hairs, or setae, of caterpillars are effective defensive weapons that protect some species from predators. The setae are attached to unicellular poison glands at the base of each hair. Both the larvae and the adults are capable of stinging, either by direct contact with the setae or indirectly when the creature becomes irritated. It appears that contraction of the caterpillar's abdominal muscles is sufficient to release the barbs from their sockets, allowing them to become airborne. Some caterpillars have a disagreeable smell or taste and are avoided by birds and other animals. The toxin found in the venom glands of some caterpillars may be derived from their ingestion of noxious plants, which are then metabolized. Earlier studies showed that the toxic material contained aristolochic acids, cardenolides, and histamine among other substances. In recent studies, fibrinolytic activity has been found at 16 and 18 kDa (isoelectric point of 8.5); coagulation defects such as prolonged prothrombin and partial thromboplastin times have been detected, and decreases in fibrinogen and plasminogen have been noted. It is thought that the hemorrhagic syndrome cannot be classified as being either totally fibrinolytic or a syndrome such as disseminated intravascular coagulopathy; it is also held that the venom has urkinase activity (Kawamoto and Kumada, 1984).

In some parts of the world the stings of several species of Lepidoptera give rise to a bleeding diasthesis, often severe and sometimes fatal. In the United States, envenomation by members of the family Saturniidae, the buck moths, the grapeleaf skeletonizer (family Zygaenidae), the puss moth (family Megalopygie), and the browntailed moth (*Euproctis* species) generally gives rise to little more than immediate localized itching and pain, usually described as burning, followed in some cases by urticaria, edema, and occasionally fever. In the more severe cases abroad—often due to *Megalopygidae, Dioptidae, Automeris, and Hermileucinae* species—there is localized pain as well as papules (sometimes hemorrhagic) and hematomas; on occasion there may also be headache, nausea, vomiting, hematuria, lymphadenitis, and lymphadenopathy. Cerebral edema, hemorrhage (intracranial hypertension), and mental changes have been noted for foreign species.

Treatment consists of placing cellophane tape over the affected area, removing it, and doing this again (to take out the setae); washing the area with warm soap and water and repeating this; and finally applying the cream previously mentioned.

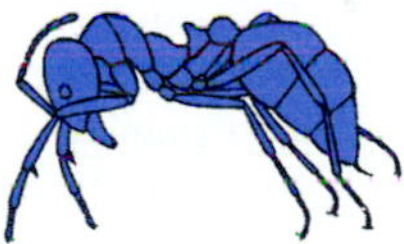

Formicidae (Ants)

The stinging properties of the ants need no introduction. Most species sink their powerful mandibles into the flesh, providing leverage, and then drive their stings into the victim. Most ants have stings, but those that lack them can spray a defensive secretion from the tip of the gaster, which is often placed in the wound of the bite. Ants of the different species vary considerably in length, ranging from less than 1.5 mm to over 35 mm. In the United States, the clinically important stinging ants are the harvesting ants (*Pagonomyrmex*), fire ants (*Solenopsis*), and little fire ants (*Ochetomyrmex*). The harvester ants are large red, dark brown, or black ranging in size from 6 to 10 mm and having fringes of long hairs on the posterior of their heads. They are vicious stingers, and their venom is said to have strong cholinergic properties.

The venoms of the ants vary considerably. The venoms of the Ponerinae and Ecitoninae are proteinaceous in character, as is that of the Pseudomyrmex. The Myrmecinae venoms are a mixture of amines, enzymes and proteinaceous materials, histamine, hyaluronidase, and phospholipase A. Formicinae ant venom contains about 60% formic acid. Fire ants are unique in that while they are poor in polypeptides and proteins, they are rich in alkaloids, some 95%, and these appear to be the cause of pruritic pustules and necrosis (Blum 1989). The sting of the fire ant gives rise to a painful burning sensation, after which a wheal and localized erythema develop, leading in a few hours to a clear vesicle. Within 12 to 24 h, the fluid becomes purulent and the lesion turns into a pustule. It may break down or become a crust or fibrotic nodule. In multiple stingings there may be nausea, vomiting, vertigo, increased perspiration, respiratory difficulties, cyanosis, coma, and even death. Cross exposure to the venom of other species of ants is possible. Treatment of ant stings is dependent upon their number, whether an allergic reaction is involved, and whether there are possible complications.

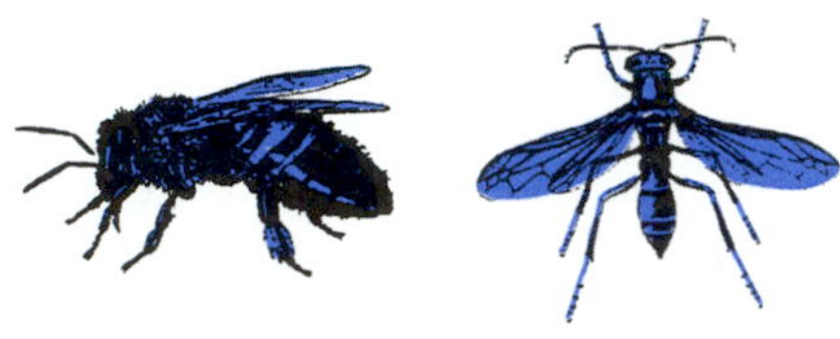

Apidae (Bees)

In this family we include the bumble bees, honey bees, carpenter bees, wasps, hornets, and yellow jackets. The commonest stinging bee is *Apis mellifera,* but with the introduction and rapid spread of the Africanized bee, *Apis mellifer adansonii*, in the United States, the incidence of Hymenoptera poisonings is increasing. In 1996 there were at least 58 deaths and more than 1000 incidents of Africanized bee stings in Mexico and the United States. The venom of the Africanized bee is not remarkably different from that of the European bee, *A. m. mellifer.* The former bee is smaller and gives less venom, but its agressiveness is such that attacks of 50 to 500 bees are not unusual. The overwhelming dose of apamine, which is thought to be lethal factor, results in the serious or even fatal poisoning by this arthropod. In addition to apamine, the venom contains biologically active melittin synergized by phospholipase A_2, hyaluronidase, histamine, dopamine, and a mast cell–degranulating peptide, among other components. It is said that 50 stings can be serious and lead to respiratory dysfunction, intravascular hemolysis, hypertension, myocardial damage, hepatic changes, shock, and renal failure. With 100 or more stings, death can occur. A novel Fab-based antivenom for massive bee attacks has been reported but has not undergone clinical trial at the time of this writing. It could be of value in those cases where the patient survives the initial onslaught of the poisoning and before serious sequelae develop.

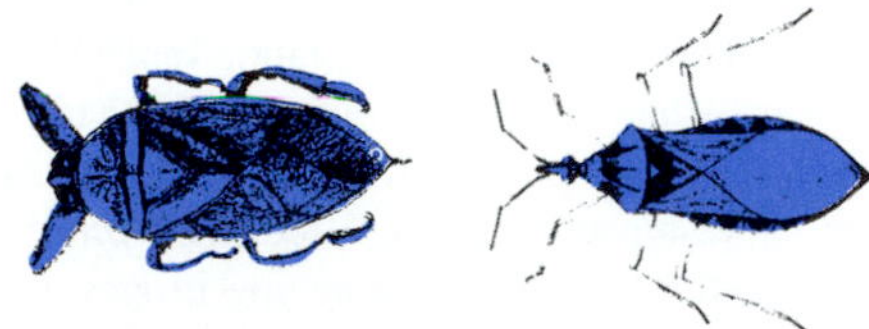

Heteroptera (True Bugs)

The clinically most important of the true bugs are the Reduviidae (the reduviids): the kissing bug, assassin bug, wheel bug, or cone-nose bug of the genus *Triatoma.* Generally, they are parasites of rodents and common in the nests of wood rat or in wood piles. These are elongated bugs with freely movable, cone-shaped heads and straight beaks. The most commonly involved species appear to be *Triatoma protracta, T. rubida, T. magista, Reduvius personatus,* and *Arilus cristatus.* Most are good fliers. During their nocturnal dispersal flights they are attracted to porch or artificial light. Once there, they do not seek to escape until dawn. Indeed, at the author's ranch in Portal, Arizona, more than 100 reduviids have been captured in a single night using bright artificial light. The average length of these bugs was 19 mm.

The venom of these bugs appears to have apyrase activity and to lack 5-nucleotidase, inorganic pyrophosphatase, phosphatase, and adenylate kinase activities, but it is fairly rich in protease properties. It inhibits collagen-induced platelet aggregation. It is said to be a protein of 16 to 19 kDa.

The bites of *Triatoma* species are definitely painful and give rise to erythema, pruritus, increased temperature in the bitten part, localized swelling, and—in those allergic to the saliva—systemic reactions such as nausea and vomiting and angioedema. With some bites the wound area will slough, leaving a depression. Treatment consists of cleansing the area and applying the cream previously described.

The water bugs are water-dwelling true bugs of which there are at least three families: Naucordiae, Belostomatidae, and Notonectidae that are capable of biting and evenomating humans. They are found in lakes, ponds, marshes, quiet fresh water, and swimming pools. The most common biter in the United States is *Lethocerus americanus,* a Belostomatidae, ranging in length from 12 to 70 mm, but some water bugs may reach 150 mm. The dorsal side is usually tan or brown, but it may be brightly colored, while the ventral side is brown. They are very strong insects and can immobilize snails, tadpoles, salamanders, and even small fish and water snakes. They are sometimes known as "toe biters" or "electric light bugs." In some parts of the world they are eaten in stews, but that is not likely to happen in the United States.

The venomousness of the water bugs has been attributed to their saliva, which is said to contain digestive enzymes, neurotoxic components, and hemolytic fractions. ApoLp-III has been isolated from the hemolymph of *Lathocerus medius.* It has a M(r) of 19,000, and an amino acid composition high in methionine. If molested, water bugs will bite, and some species can envenomate in or out of the water. Their bites give rise to immediate pain, some localized swelling, and—in one case seen by the author—induration and the formation of a small papule. Treatment consists of cleansing the areas and applying the cream previously noted.

There are some arthropods that are "poisonous" as opposed to "venomous"; that is, they have no mechanism for delivering their toxin and the poison must come through their being crushed or eaten. These would include, among others, the darkling beetles or stink bugs (*Eleodes*), and the blister beetles (*Epicauta*), for which cantharidin is known.

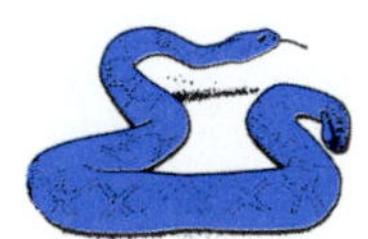

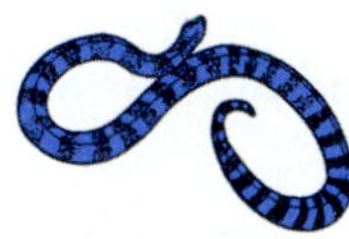

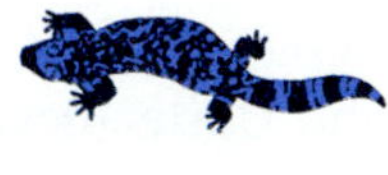

REPTILES

Lizards

The Gila monster (*Heloderma suspectum*) and the beaded lizards (*Heloderma horridum*) are divided into five subspecies. These large, corpulent, relatively slow-moving, and largely nocturnal reptiles have few enemies other than humans. They are far less dangerous than is generally believed. Their venom is transferred from venom glands in the lower jaw through ducts that discharge their contents near the base of the larger teeth of the lower jaw. The venom is then drawn up along grooves in the teeth by capillary action. The venom of this lizard has serotonin, amine oxidase, phospholipase A, and proteolytic as well as hyaluronidase activities but lacks phosphomonoesterase and phosphodiesterase, acetylcholinesterase, nucleotidase, ATP-ase, deoxyribonuclease, ribonuclease, amino acid oxidase, and fibrinogenocoagulase activities. The high hyaluronidase content seems to be consistent with the tissue edema seen in many clinical cases, and the low proteolytic activity is also consistent with the minimal tissue breakdown seen in clinical cases. The injection of large doses of Heloderma venom produces a fall in systemic arterial pressure with a decrease in circulating blood volume, tachycardia, and respiratory distress; in lethal doses, there is a loss of ventricular contractility (Russell and Bogert, 1981). An excellent review on the biology of the Gila monster has been published by Brown and Carmony (1991).

More recently the venom has been shown to contain a 25,376-kDa protein, helothermine, containing 223 amino acids and four pairs of disulfide bonds. Its mode of action appears to involve Ca^{2+} inhibitor from the sarcoplasmic reticulum (Morrissette et al., 1995). Its action on cerebellar granule cells has been described (Nobile et al., 1996). A fraction causing hemorrhage in internal organs and the eye, a glycoprotein of 210 amino acid residues with plasma kallikrein-like properties, has also been described (Dalla and Tu, 1997). According to Horikawa et al. (1998), a 35–amino acid residue, helodermin, that produces hypotension is partially attributed to activation of glibenclamide-sensitive K+ channels. Other definitive works on *Heloderma* venom have been published by Uddman et al. (1999) and Pohl and Wañk (1998). Treatment of Heloderma bites tends to be empiric. An experimental antivenom was once produced at the University of Southern California, but as an IgG product it elicited a large number of sensitivity reactions and its production was halted.

Snakes

From the beginnings of the human record, few subjects have stimulated minds and imaginations more than the study of snakes and snake venoms. No animal has been more worshiped yet more cast out, more loved yet more despised, more collected yet more trampled on than the snake. The essence of the fascination for and fear of snakes lies in their venom. In times past, the consequences of bites by venomous snakes often were attributed to forces beyond nature, sometimes to vengeful deities that were thought to be embodied in the serpents. To early peoples, the effects of snakebite were so surprising and violent that snakes and their poisons were shrouded with myth and superstition.

Among the more than 3500 species of snakes, approximately 400 are considered sufficiently venomous to be dangerous to humans (Dowling et al., 1968; Minton and Minton, 1969; Harding and Welch, 1980; Russell, 1980b, 1983; Junghanss and Budio, 1996). Venomous species can be divided into the Elapidae—the cobras, kraits, mambas, and coral snakes; the Hydrophiidae—the true sea snakes; the Laticaudidae—the sea kraits; the Viperidae—the Old World vipers and adders and the New World Crotalidae (now a subfamily), the rattlesnakes, water moccasins, copperheads, fer-de-lances, and bushmasters and some Asian species; and certain Colubridae, of which clinically the most important are the boomslang and bird snake of Africa and the rednecked keelback of Asia. However, several other colubrids must be viewed with concern (Minton and Minton, 1969; Minton, 1976: Mebs, 1977). There are no poisonous snakes in New Zealand, Hawaii, Ireland, and many other islands. Some medically important venomous snakes and their general distribution are shown in Table 26-3.

Snake Venoms The venoms of snakes are complex mixtures, chiefly proteins, a number of which have enzymatic activities. In some species the most active component of the venom is a peptide or polypeptide. Proteins and peptides make up about 90 to 95 percent of the dry weight of the venom. In addition, snake venoms contain inorganic cations such as sodium, calcium, potassium, magnesium, and small amounts of metals: zinc, iron, cobalt, manganese, and nickel. The importance of the metals in snake venoms is not clear, although in the case of some elapid venoms zinc ions appear to be necessary for anticholinesterase activity, and it has been suggested that calcium may play a role in the activation of phospholipase A and the direct lytic factor. Some proteases appear to be metalloproteins. Some snake venoms also contain carbohydrates (glycoproteins), lipids, and biogenic amines, whereas others contain free amino acid (Russell, 1967, 1980b, 1983; Tu, 1977; Elliott, 1978; Lee, 1979; Habermehl, 1981). A recent contribution on snake toxins, using mass spectrometric immunoassay and bioactive probe techniques, has been published by Tubbs et al. (2000).

Enzymes The venoms of snakes contain at least 25 enzymes, although no single snake venom contains all of them. Enzymes are the proteins responsible for the catalysis of many specific biochemical reactions that occur in living matter. They are the agents on which cellular metabolism depends. Enzymes are universally accepted as proteins, although a few have crucial dependencies on certain nonprotein prosthetic groups, or cofactors. All living cells contain enzymes. Some of the more important snake venom enzymes are shown in Table 26-4.

Proteolytic enzymes catalyze the breakdown of tissue proteins and peptides. They are known as proteolytic enzymes, peptide hydrolases, proteases, endopeptidases, peptidases, and proteinases. There may be several proteolytic enzymes in a single venom. The proteolytic enzymes have molecular weights between 20,000 and 95,000. Some are inactivated by edetic acid (EDTA) and certain reducing agents. The role of metal ions in catalysis was demonstrated many years ago by Wagner and Prescott (1966). Metals appear to be intrinsically involved in the activity of certain venom proteases and phospholipases.

The crotalid venoms examined so far appear to be rich in proteolytic enzyme activity. Viperid venoms have lesser amounts, whereas elapid and sea snake venoms have no proteolytic activity or very little. Venoms that are rich in proteinase activity are associated with marked tissue destruction.

Arginine ester hydrolase is one of a number of noncholinesterases found in snake venoms. The substrate specificities are directed to the hydrolysis of the ester or peptide linkage, to which an argine residue contributes the carboxyl group. This activity is found in many crotalid and viperid venoms and some sea snake venoms but is lacking in elapid venoms with the possible exception of *Ophiophagus hannah.* It was first demonstrated by Deutsch and Diniz (1955) in 15 snake venoms and subsequently has been identified in many others. Some crotalid venoms contain at least three chromatographically separable arginine ester hydrolases. The bradykinin-releasing and perhaps bradykinin-clotting activities of some crotalid venoms may be related to esterase activity.

Thrombin-like enzymes are found in significant amounts in the venoms of the Crotalidae and Viperidae, whereas those of

Table 26-3
Some Medically Important Snakes of the World

SCIENTIFIC AND COMMON NAMES	DISTRIBUTION
Crotalids	
Agkistrodon bilineatus—cantil	Mexico south to Guatemala and Nicaragua
Agkistrodon contortrix—copperhead	New York south to Florida and west to Nebraska and Texas
Agkistrodon halys—mamushi	Caspian Sea to Japan
Agkistrodon piscivorus—eastern cottonmouth	New York to Missouri
Calloselasma (Agkistrodon) rhodostoma—Malayan pit viper	Much of southeast Asia
Bothrops asper and/or *atrox*—fer-de-lance —barba amarillia —terciopelo	Southern Sonora to Peru and northern Brazil
Bothrops jararaca—jararaca	Brazil, Paraguay, and Argentina
Bothrops jararacussu—jararacussu	Brazil, Bolivia, Paraguay, and Argentina
Bothrops neuwiedi—jararaca pintada	Brazil, Bolivia, Paraguay, northern Argentina
Crotalus adamanteus—eastern diamondback rattlesnake	Southeastern United States
Crotalus atrox—western diamondback rattlesnake	Southwestern United States to central Mexico
Crotalus basiliscus—Mexican west-coast rattlesnake	Oaxaca and west coast of Mexico
Crotalus scutulatus—Mojave rattlesnake	Central California to New Mexico
Crotalus viridis helleri—southern Pacific rattlesnake	West Coast, southern California
Trimeresurus flavoviridis—habu	Amami and Okinawa islands
Trimeresurus mucrosquamatus—Chinese habu	Taiwan and southern China west through Vietnam and Loas to India
Viperids	
Bitis arietans—puff adder	Morocco and western Arabia through much of Africa
Bitis caudalis—horned adder	Angola south through Nambia into central and part of south Africa
Causus sp.—night adders	Most of Africa south of the Sahara
Cerastes cerastes—horned viper	Sahara, Arabian peninsula to Lebanon
Cerastes vipera—Sahara sand viper	Central Sahara to Lebanon
Daboi (Vipera) russelli	Indian subcontinent, southeast China to Taiwan and parts of Indonesia
Echis carinatus—saw-scaled viper	Southern India to northern and tropical Africa
Echis coloratus—saw-scaled viper	Eastern Egypt, western Arabian peninsula north to Israel
Vipera ammodytes—long-nosed viper	Italy through southeast Europe, Turkey, Jordan to northwest Iran
Vipera berus—European viper	British Isles through Europe, to northern Asia
Vipera lebetina—Levantine viper	Cyprus through Middle East to Kashmir
Vipera xanthina—Near East viper	European Turkey and Asia Minor
Elapids	
Coral snakes (c.s.)	
Calliophis species—Oriental c.s.	Southeast Asia, Orient
Micrurus alleni—Allen's c.s.	Atlantic Nicaragua to Panama
Micrurus corallinus—c.s.	Southern Brazil to Uruguay, northern Argentina
Micrurus frontalis—southern c.s.	Southwestern Brazil, northern Argentina, Uruguay, Paraguay, and Bolivia
Micrurus fulvius—eastern c.s.	Southeastern, southern United States and north central Mexico
Micrurus mipartitus—black-ringed c.s.	Venezuela and Peru to Nicaragua
Micrurus nigrocinctus—black-banded c.s.	Southern Mexico to northwest Colombia
Cobras	
Hemachatus haemachatus—Ringhals cobra	Southeastern and southern Africa

(*continued*)

Table 26-3 Some Medically Important Snakes of the World *(continued)*

SCIENTIFIC AND COMMON NAMES	DISTRIBUTION
Naja haje—Egyptian or brown cobra	Africa and part of Arabian peninsula
Naja atra—Chinese cobra	Thailand and South China to Taiwan
Naja naja—Indian cobra	Most of Indian subcontinent
Naja nigricollis—spitting cobra	West Africa and southern Egypt to near the Cape
Naja oxiana—Central Asian cobra	Northern Pakistan to Iran, southern Russia
Naja philippinensis—Philippine cobra	Philippines
Naja sputatrix—Malayan cobra	Malayan peninsula and Indonesia
Naja nivea—Cape or yellow cobra	Nambia, Botswana south to the Cape
Ophiophagus hannah—king cobra	Indian subcontinent, China and Philippines
Walterinnesia aegyptia—desert blacksnake or desert cobra	Egypt to Iran
Kraits and mambas	
Bungarus caeruleus—Indian or blue krait	India, Pakistan, Sri Lanka, Bangladesh
Bungarus candidus—Malayan krait	Thailand, Malaysia, Indonesia
Bungarus multicinctus—many-banded krait	Southern China to Hainan, Taiwan
Dendroaspis polylepis—black mamba	Ethiopia and Somalia to Angola, Zambia, Nambia, southwest Africa
Australian elapids	
Acanthophis antarcticus—common death adder	Most of Australia, Moluccas, New Guinea
Notechis scutatus—tiger snake	Southeastern Australia
Oxyuranus scutellatus—Taipan	Northern coastal Australia, parts of New Guinea
Pseudechis australis—mulga	Most of Australia except southeast and southern coast, New Guinea
Pseudonaja nuchalis—western brown snake	Most of Australia except east and southeast coast
Pseudonaja textilis—eastern brown snake	Eastern Australia

NOTE: The common names in this table are those generally employed as literature identifications for the snakes. However, these names may not be the ones used by people in the specific area where the snake abounds.

Elapidae and Hydrophiidae contain little or none. The mechanism of fibrinogen clot formation by snake venom thrombin-like enzymes invokes the preferential release of fibrinopeptide A (or B); thrombin releases fibrinopeptides A and B. Paradoxically, the thrombin-like enzymes have been shown to act as defibrinating anticoagulants in vivo, whereas in vitro they clot plasma, citrated or heparinized plasma, or purified fibrinogen. Because of the obvious clinical potential of these enzymes as defibrinating agents, more attention has been directed toward the characterization and study of the thrombin-like enzymes than toward those of the other venom procoagulant or anticoagulant enzymes. The proteolytic action of thrombin and thrombin-like snake venom enzymes is shown in Table 26-5. This table also shows comparisons of ancrod (from *Calloselasma rhodostoma*), batroxobin (from *Bothrops moojeni*), crotalase (from *Crotalus adamanteus*), gabonase (from *Bitis gabonica*), and venzyme (from *Agkistrodon contortrix*); while Table 26-6 shows the molecular size of some thrombin-like enzymes.

Thrombin-like enzymes have been purified from the venoms of *Crotalus adamanteus* (crotalase) *Crotalus horridus horridus, Calloselasma (Agkistrodon) rhodostoma* (ancrod), *Agkistrodon contortrix contortrix, Deinagkistrodon (Agkistrodon) acutus, Bothrops atrox* (batroxobin), *Bothrops marajoensis, Bothrops moojeni, Trimeresurus gramineus, Trimeresurus okinavensis, and Bitis gabonica.* All these enzymes appear to be glycoproteins; with the exception of two, they appear to have molecular weights in the range of 29,000 to 35,000.

Thrombin-like enzymes have been used clinically and in animals for therapeutic and investigative studies. In experimentally induced venous thrombosis in dogs, treatment with ancrod before the formation of the thrombus prevented thrombosis and ensured vessel patency. However, ancrod had no thrombolytic effect when administered after thrombus formation. Trials of ancrod versus heparin and ancrod versus streptokinase in the treatment of deep venous thromboses of the lower leg have been conducted. Crotalase has been employed to evaluate the role of fibrin deposition in burns in animals (Bajwa and Markland, 1976). The role of fibrin deposition has been evaluated in tumor metastasis, in which fibrinogen is removed by treatment with ancrod or batroxobin. Ancrod also

Table 26-4
Enzymes of Snake Venoms

Proteolytic enzymes	Phosphomonoesterase
Arginine ester hydrolase	Phosphodiesterase
Thrombinlike enzyme	Acetylcholinesterase
Collagenase	RNase
Hyaluronidase	DNase
Phospholipase A_2(A)	5′-Nucleotidase
Phospholipase B	NAD-nucleotidase
Phospholipase C	L-Amino acid oxidase
Lactate dehydrogenase	

SOURCE: Russell, 1983, with permission.

Table 26-5

Proteolytic Action of Thrombin and Thrombin-like Snake Venom Enzymes

	Action on Human Fibrinogen						
ENZYME	FIBRINOPEPTIDES RELEASED	CHAIN DEGRADATION	ACTIVATION OF FACTOR XIII	PROTHROMBIN FRAGMENT CLEAVAGE	PLATELET AGGREGATION AND RELEASE	ACTIVATION OF FACTOR VIII	ACTIVATION OF FACTOR V
Thrombin	A − B	α(A)	Yes	Yes	Yes	Yes	Yes
Thrombinlike enzymes	A*	α(A)† or β(B)‡	No	Yes or no§	No	No	No
Agkistrodon c. contortrix venom	B	n.d.#	Incomplete	n.d.	No	n.d.	n.d.
Bitis gabonica venom	A + B	n.d.	Yes	n.d.	n.d.	n.d.	n.d.

*Includes ancrod, batroxobin, crotalase, and the enzyme from *T. okinavensis*.

†Ancrod [batroxobin degrades α(A) chain of bovine but not human fibrinogen].

‡Crotalase.

§Fragment I released by crotalase and *Agkistrodon contortrix* venom but not by ancrod or batroxobin.

#n.d. = not determined.

SOURCE: Russell, 1983, with permission.

has been used to prevent the deposition of fibrin on prosthetic heart valves implanted in calves (Russell, 1980b, 1983). Ancrod and batroxobin have been used as defibrinogenating agents in clinical conditions of deep venous thrombosis, myocardial infarction, pulmonary embolus, central retinal vein occlusion, peripheral vascular disease, stroke, angina, glomerulonephritis, and renal transplant rejection (Markland, 1998).

Considerable study has been given to the hemostatic properties of venoms (Meier and Stocker, 1991; Ouayang and Huang, 1992; Hutton and Warrell, 1993; Marsh, 1994; Markland, 1998). The hemostatically active components are summarized in Table 26-7.

Collagenase is a specific kind of proteinase that digests collagen. This activity has been demonstrated in the venoms of a number of species of crotalids and viperids. The venom of *Crotalus atrox* digests mesenteric collagen fibers but not other protein. EDTA inhibits the collagenolytic effect but not the argine esterase effect.

Hyaluronidase catalyzes the cleavage of internal glycoside bonds in certain acid mucopolysaccharides. This results in a decrease in the viscosity of connective tissues. The breakdown in the hyaluronic barrier allows other fractions of venom to penetrate the tissues. The enzyme is thought to be related to the extent of edema produced by the whole venom, but the degree to which it contributes to clinical swelling and edema is not known. The enzyme also has been referred to as the "spreading factor."

Phospholipase enzymes are widely distributed throughout the tissues of animals, plants, and bacteria. Some venoms are the richest sources of phospholipase A_2 (PLA_2) enzymes. PLA_2 catalyzes the Ca^{2+}-dependent hydrolysis of the 2-acyl ester bond, producing free fatty acids and lysophospholipid. Many PLA_2s have been sequenced. They have approximately 120 amino acids and 14

Table 26-6

Comparison of Snake Venom Thrombin-like Enzymes

VENOM ENZYME	MOLECULAR WEIGHT	CARBOHYDRATE CONTENT %	NH_2-TERMINAL RESIDUE	ACTIVE SITE SERINE	ACTIVE SITE HISTIDINE
Calloselasma rhodostoma	59,000	36.0	Val	+	+
Crotalus adamantus	32,700	8.3	Val	+	+
Bothrops marajoensis	31,400	High	Val	+	n.d.*
Bothrops moojeni	36,000	5.8	Val	+	n.d.
Crotalus horridus horridus	19,400	Very low	n.d.	n.d.	n.d.
Deinagkistrodon acutus	33,500	13.0	n.d.	+	+
Trimeresurus gramineus	27,000	25.0	n.d.	+	n.d.
Trimeresurus okinavensis	34,000	6.0	n.d.	+	n.d.
Agkistrodon contortrix contortrix	100,000	n.d.	n.d.	+	n.d.
Bitis gabonica	32,500	n.d.	n.d.	n.d.	n.d.

*n.d. = not determined.

SOURCE: Russell, 1983 revised, with permission.

Table 26-7
Snake Venom Proteins Active on the Hemostatic System

GENERAL FUNCTIONAL ACTIVITY	SPECIFIC BIOLOGICAL ACTIVITY
Procoagulant	Factor V activating
	Factor X activating
	Factor IX activating
	Prothrombin activating
	Fibrinogen clotting
	Protein C activating
Anticoagulant	Factor IX/factor X-binding protein
	Thrombin inhibitor
	Phospholipase A
Fibrinolytic	Fibrin(ogen) degradation
	Plasminogen activation
Vessel wall interactive	Hemorrhagic
Platelet active	Platelet aggregation inducers
	Inhibitors of platelet aggregation
Plasma protein inactivators	Inhibitors of SERPINS

SOURCE: From Markland, 1998, with permission.

Cys residues forming seven disulfide bonds. The enzymes are widely distributed in the venoms of elapids, vipers, crotalids, atractaspids, sea snakes, and several colubrids so far studied. Although the sequences of these enzymes are homologous and their enzymatic active sites are identical, they differ widely in their pharmacologic properties. For example, taipoxin, a PLA_2 enzyme from the venom of the Australian elapid *Oxyuranus scutellatus*, has an intravenous LD_{50} in mice of 2 μg/kg, whereas the neutral PLA_2 from *Naja nigricollis* has an LD_{50} of 10,200 μg/kg, even though *N. nigricollis* PLA_2 is enzymatically more active.

Recent studies have shown that PLA_2 enzymes can exert their pharmacologic effects by different mechanisms: hydrolysis of membrane phospholipids, liberation of pharmacologically active products, and effects independent of enzymatic action. Similarly, snake venom PLA_2 enzymes can be separated into three major groupings depending on their pharmacologic activities: low-toxicity enzymes ($LD_{50} > 1$ mg/kg), high-toxicity enzymes (1 mg/kg $> LD_{50} >$ 0.1 mg/kg), and presynaptically acting toxins ($LD_{50} <$ 0.1 mg/kg). Interested readers are referred to reviews by Rosenberg (1978, 1979, 1990).

Phosphomonoesterase (phosphatase) is widely distributed in the venoms of all families of snakes except the colubrids. It has the properties of an orthophosphoric monoester phosphohydrolase. There are two nonspecific phosphomonoesterases, and they have optimal pH at 5.0 and 8.5. Many venoms contain both acid and alkaline phosphatases, whereas others contain one or the other.

Phosphodiesterase has been found in the venoms of all families of poisonous snakes. It is an orthophosphoric diester phosphohydrolase that releases 5-mononucleotide from the polynucleotide chain and thus acts as an exonucleotidase, attacking DNA and RNA. More recently, it has been found that it also attacks derivatives of arabinose.

Acetylcholinesterase was first demonstrated in cobra venom and is widely distributed throughout the elapid venoms. It is also found in sea snake venoms but is totally lacking in viperid and crotalid venoms. It catalyzes the hydrolysis of acetylcholine to choline and acetic acid. The role of the enzyme in snake venoms is not clear.

RNase is present in some snake venoms in small amounts as the endopolynucleotidase RNase. It appears to have specificity toward pyrimidine-containing pyrimidyladenyl bonds in DNA. The optimum pH is 7 to 9 when ribosomal RNA is used as the substrate. This enzyme in *Naja oxiana* venom has a molecular weight of 15,900.

DNase acts on DNA and gives predominantly tri- or higher oligonucleotides that terminate in 3′ monoesterified phosphate. *Crotalus adamanteus* venom contains two DNases, with optimum pH at 5 and 9.

5′-Nucleotidase is a common constituent of all snake venoms; in most instances it is the most active phosphatase in snake venoms. It specifically hydrolyzes phosphate monoesters, which link with a 5′ position of DNA and RNA. It is found in greater amounts in crotalid and viperid venoms than in elapid venoms. The molecular weight as determined from amino acid composition and gel filtration with *Naja naja atra* venom has been estimated at 10,000. The enzyme from *N. naja* venom is enhanced by Mg^{2+}, is inhibited by Zn^{2+}, is inactivated at 75°C at pH 7.0 or 8.4, and has an isoelectric point of about 8.6. That from *Agkistrodon halys blomhoffi* shows a pH optimum of 6.8 to 6.9, with activity being enhanced by Mg^{2+} and Mn^{2+} and inhibited by Zn^{2+}. The enzyme has a low order of lethality, and its pharmacologic role in the venom is not understood (Russell, 1980b, 1983).

Nicotinamide adenine dinucleotide (NAD) nucleotidase has been found in a number of snake venoms. This enzymes catalyzes the hydrolysis of the nicotinamide N-ribosidic linkage of NAD, yielding nicotinamide and adenosine diphosphate riboside. Its optimum pH is 6.5 to 8.5; it is heat-labile, losing activity at 60°C. Its toxicologic contribution to snake venoms is not understood.

L-Amino acid oxidase has been found in all snake venoms examined so far. It gives a yellow color to the venom. This enzyme catalyzes the oxidation of L-α-amino and α-hydroxy acids. This activity results from a group of homologous enzymes with molecular weights ranging from 85,000 to 150,000. It has a high content of acidic amino acids. We found that the mouse intravenous LD_{50} of the enzyme from *Crotalus adamanteus* venom was 9.13 mg/kg body weight, approximately 4 times less than the lethal value of the crude venom, and that this enzyme had no effect on nerve, muscle, or neuromuscular transmission (Russell, 1980b, 1983).

Lactate dehydrogenase catalyzes the equilibrium between lactic acid and pyruvic acid. It is found in almost all animal tissues. It is a tetamer of 140,000 kDa and consists of two subunits of about 35,000 kDa.

Polypeptides Snake venom polypeptides are low-molecular-weight proteins that do not have enzymatic activity. During the past 30 years, a number of peptides of snake venoms have been characterized. In 1965, the first paper on the amino acid composition of a snake venom peptide was published (Yang, 1965), and at the First International Symposium on Animal Toxins in 1966, Tamiya presented a paper on the chromatography, crystallization, electrophoresis, ultracentrifugation, and amino acid composition of the venom of the sea snake *Laticauda semifasciata.* Most of the lethal activity of the poison was recovered as two toxins, erabutoxin a and b, using carboxymethylcellulose chromatography; 30 percent of the proteins were erabutoxins. The homogeneity of the crystalline toxins was demonstrated by rechromatography, disk electrophoresis, and ultracentrifugation (Tamiya et al., 1967). At the same meeting, Su and colleagues (1967) reported the isolation of a cobra "neurotoxin." The toxin was separated by repeated fractionation with ammonium sulfate. Since 1966, more than 80 polypeptides with pharmacologic activity have been isolated from snake venoms. Interested readers will find definitive reviews on these peptides in the works of Tu (1977), Elliott (1978), Rosenberg (1978), Lee (1979), Eaker and Wadstrom (1980), and Gopalakrishnakone and Tan (1992). More recently, erabutoxin a (Ea), a short-chain curamimetic, has been crystallized in monomeric and dimeric forms (Nastopoulos et al., 1998). Erabutoxin b (Eb) is said to be relatively ineffective at the mammalian neuromuscular junction (Vincent et al., 1998). Another curamimetic, a long-chain polypeptide, is alpha-cobratoxin, while a novel "neurotoxin" from *N. naja atra,* having 61 amino acid residues and 8 cystine residues, has been isolated by Chang et al. (1997).

In 1938, Slotta and Fraenkel-Conrat isolated a crystalline protein from the venom of the tropical rattlesnake *Crotalus durissus terrificus.* The protein exhibited most of the toxic properties of the crude venom and was named crotoxin. In addition to the toxic nonenzymatic protein portion, it was found to contain the enzymes hyaluronidase and phospholipase and possibly several others. It did not appear to have proteolytic or coagulant properties or 5′-nucleotidase activity, but it had neurotoxic, indirect hemolytic, and smooth muscle–stimulating properties. After removal of phospholipase A, crotoxin was further separated into a general toxic principle known as crotactin, which was found to have a greater lethal index than that of crotoxin, and a second component that may have been crotamine. The word *crotoxin* has been retained in one form or another in the literature as an identification for 17 different separations of the venom of *C. durissus terrificus* over the past 50 years. This has resulted in considerable confusion and disputes on research techniques, which could be more easily resolved on the basis of a frank statement about the method of isolation. For a thorough review of crotoxin, see Haberman and Breithaupt (1978).

At present, crotoxin is considered a neurotoxic and cytolytic PLA_2 of 30 kDa consisting of two dissimilar subunits: (1) an acidic, nontoxic component (crotapotin) without enzymatic activity and (2) a basic, weakly toxic PLA_2 component. Crotoxin accounts for about 50 percent of the total protein of the venom. The full activity of the complex requires the two components. The principal pharmacologic property appears to be the presynaptic interference with acetycholine release, and secondarily the densensitization of the acelycholine receptor (Haberman and Briethaupt, 1978, Bon et al., 1989, Fortes-Dias et al., 1999). A rabbit-raised antivenom neutralizes the lethal properties of the venom more than an equine preparation (Oshima-Franco et al., 1999). Mojave toxin, from the venom of the rattlesnake *Crotalus scutulatus scutulatus,* is similar to crotoxin. It contains 123 amino acid residues and has an estimated molecular weight of 14 kDa.

Toxicology It is not within the scope of this chapter to discuss all the pharmacologic activities of snake venoms. Interested readers are referred to Russell (1967, 1983), Mebs (1978), to the journal *Toxicon,* and to articles, in the compendia of the *International Society on Toxinology* for a more thorough consideration of the specific toxicologic effects of these poisons and their components. Since these earlier studies, more than 520 papers have been published on the toxinologic and biochemical properties of snake venoms. Some remarks, however, may be made about the venoms of the North American crotalids, particularly the rattlesnakes. The LD_{50}s of some North American snake venoms are shown in Table 26-8.

In general, the venoms of rattlesnakes and other New World crotalids produce alterations in the resistances (and often the integrity) of blood vessels, changes in blood cells and blood coagulation mechanisms, direct or indirect changes in cardiac and pul-

Table 26-8
LD_{50} by Different Routes of Injection

VENOM	INTRAVENOUS	INTRAPERITONEAL	SUBCUTANEOUS
Crotalus viridis helleri	1.29	1.60	3.65
Crotalus adamanteus	1.68	1.90	13.73
Crotalus atrox	2.18	3.71	17.75
Crotalus scutulatus	0.21	0.23	0.31
Agkistrodon piscivorus	4.17	5.10	25.10
Agkistrodon contortrix	10.92	10.50	26.10
Sistrurus miliarius	2.91	6.89	25.10

NOTE: All determinations were made in 20-g female mice of the same group. All mice were injected within a 1-h period and were observed for 48 h.

SOURCE: Russell, 1983, with permission.

monary dynamics, and—with crotalids like *C. durrissus terrificus* and *C. scutulatus*—serious alterations in the nervous system and changes in respiration. In humans, the course of the poisoning is determined by the kind and amount of venom injected; the site where it is deposited; the general health, size, and age of the patient; the kind of treatment; and those pharmacodynamic principles noted earlier in this chapter. Clinical experience indicates that death in humans may occur within less than 1 h or after several days, with most deaths occurring between 18 and 32 h. Hypotension or shock is the major therapeutic problem in North American crotalid bites. In some cases the hypotension is associated with acute blood loss secondary to bleeding and/or hemolysis, but in most patients shock is associated with a decrease in circulating fluid volume, with varying degrees of blood cell loss. It is not surprising, therefore, to find that numerous studies have been directed at determining the mechanisms responsible for snake venom poisoning, hypotension, and shock. These studies have been reviewed elsewhere (Russell, 1983).

Experimentally, it has been found that an intravenous bolus injection of a *Crotalus* venom causes an immediate fall in blood pressure and varying degrees of shock, associated with initial hemoconcentration followed by a decrease in hematocrit values. There is increased blood volume in the lungs, an increase in pulmonary artery pressure with a concomitant decrease in pulmonary artery flow, and a relatively stable heart stroke volume (Russell et al., 1962).

Carlson and colleagues (1975) observed that when *Crotalus* venom is given intravenously and slowly over a 30-min period, there is hypovolemia secondary to an increase in capillary permeability to protein and red blood cells. The laboratory findings showed initial hemoconcentration, lactacidemia, and lipoproteinemia. In cats the same findings are seen, followed by a fall in hematocrit and in some cases hemolysis related to the dose of venom. During this period the cat may be in shock or at a near-shock level, depending on the amount of venom injected or perfused. Respirations become labored, and if the period is prolonged, the animal becomes oliguric, rales develop, and the animal dies.

There appears to be no doubt that the shock or hypotension is caused by a decrease in circulating blood volume secondary to an increase in capillary permeability, which leads to the loss of fluid, protein, and to some extent erythrocytes. The severity of the hypotension is dose-related, and restoration of circulating fluid volume can be achieved with intravenous fluids. In patients with hypovolemic shock due to venom, steroids are of no value, but the use of isoproterenol hydrochloride may be indicated. Antivenom in itself may not reverse a deep shock state, but a combination of parenteral fluids or plasma expanders, isoproterenol hydrochloride, and antivenom is definitely of value. Evidence to the present time indicates that the fraction of the venom that most probably is responsible for the circulatory failure is a peptide. The properties of this peptide have been presented elsewhere (Russell, 1996).

Snakebite Treatment The treatment of bites by venomous snakes is now so highly specialized that almost every envenomation requires specific recommendations. However, three general principles for every bite should be kept in mind: (1) snake venom poisoning is a medical emergency requiring immediate attention and the exercise of considerable judgment; (2) the venom is a complex mixture of substances of which the proteins contribute the major deleterious properties, and the only adequate antidote is the use of specific or polyspecific antivenom; (3) not every bite by a venomous snake ends in an envenomation. Venom may not be injected. In almost 1000 cases of crotalid bites, 24 percent did not end in a poisoning. The incidence with the bites of cobras and perhaps other elapids is probably higher. In the United States, 14 percent of crotalid bites are so trivial that antivenom is not recommended. It would be difficult to detail specific treatments for the almost 400 snakes implicated in snake venom poisoning. Perhaps several recent works will suffice. For the United States, Russell (1980, 1983, 1996, 1998), Dart and Russell (1992), and Heard et al. (1999); for Europe, Persson and Karlson-Stiber (1996) and Sorkine et al. (1996); for Africa, Visser and Chapman (1978) and Chippaux et al. (1996); for Central America, Russell (1997); for Australia, Sutherland (1983) and White (1996); for the carpet viper, Warrell and Arnett (1976); for Russell's viper, Warrell (1989); and in general (worldwide), Dowling et al. (1968), Russell (1983), Warrell (1996), and Junghanss and Bodio (1996).

ANTIVENOM

Because of their protein composition, many toxins produce an antibody response; this response is essential in producing antisera. An antivenom consists of venom-specific antisera or antibodies concentrated from immune serum to the venom. Antisera contain neutralizing antibodies: one antigen (monospecific) or several antigens (polyspecific). Animals immunized with venom develop a variety of antibodies to the many antigens in the venom. The serum is harvested, partially or fully purified, and further processed before being administered to the patient. The antibodies bind to the venom molecules, rendering them ineffective. Antivenoms have been produced against most medically important snake, spider, scorpion, and marine toxins.

Antivenoms are available in several forms: intact IgG antibodies or fragments of IgG such as $F(ab)_2$ and Fab. They are prepared through $(NH_4)_2SO_4$ or Na_2SO_4 precipitation, pepsin or papain digestion, and other procedures, among which the elimination of the Fc, or complement-binding and complement-sensitizing fraction, is one of the most important. The molecular weight of the intact IgG is about 150,000, whereas that of Fab is approximately 50,000.

The molecular size of IgG prevents its renal excretion and produces a volume of distribution much smaller than that of Fab. The elimination half-life of IgG in the blood is approximately 50 h. Its ultimate fate is not known, but most IgG is probably taken up by the reticuloendothelial system and degraded with the antigen attached. Fab fragments have an elimination half-life of about 17 h, and are small enough to permit renal excretion.

Since all antivenom products are produced through the immunization of animals, this increases the possiblity of hypersensitivity. Type I (immediate) hypersensitivity reactions are caused by antigen cross-linking of endogenous IgE bound to mast cells and basophils. Binding of antigen by a mast cell may cause the release of histamine and other mediators, producing an anaphylactic reaction. Once initiated, anaphylaxis may continue despite discontinuation of antivenin administration. An additional concern is an *anaphylactoid* reaction. This is a term for a syndrome resembling an anaphylactic reaction; its etiology is unknown but it appears to be associated with aggregated protein in the antiserum. Protein aggregates may activate the complement cascade, producing an anaphylactic-like syndrome. An important difference between anaphylactic and anaphylactoid reactions is that anaphylactoid reactions are dose-dependent and may be halted by removing the antigen. Type III hypersensitivity (serum sickness) may develop several days after antivenom administration. In these cases, antigen-antibody complexes are deposited in different areas of the body, often producing inflammatory responses in the skin, joints, kidneys, and other tissues. Fortunately, these reactions are rarely serious. The risks of anaphylaxis should always be considered when one is deciding whether to administer antivenom.

It has been said, principally by nonclinical researchers, that antivenoms have little effect on the local tissue changes produced by snake venoms. Perhaps this opinion now needs to be reevaluated on the basis of new knowledge and experience. The supposition is based on the early clinical experience, where antivenom doses were obviously too low to effectively neutralize *all* the deleterious activities of a venom. For instance, in 1950 the dose of Antivenom [Crotalidae] Polyvalent for a minimal crotalid envenomation was 1 to 3 vials, for a moderate envenomation 3 to 5 vials, and for a severe envenomation, 5 to 8 vials. By 1970, these doses had been revised upward (Russell, 1980), and at the present time the average dose of this antivenom in the United States is 11.3 vials, with the average dose at the author's medical center being 17 and as many as 50 vials having been given. Also, hospital time has been reduced from 5 to 8 days to 2 to 3 days, and patients leave the hospital with little or no local tissue destruction.

It has become evident that the ability of an effective antivenom to alleviate or neutralize the deleterious properties of a venom should be dependent on its ability to neutralize the effects of the *whole* venom, and that up until the not too distant past, antivenoms were judged solely on the basis of their ability to neutralize the lethal effect of a venom. I suggest that the best solution at this time is just to use more antivenom. Apparently, the ability of the antigen(s) to produce the antibody(ies) necessary to neutralize the cytolytic effect is either too weak or too small in quantity to stimulate the neutralization necessary to alleviate the cytolytic effects of the venom to the level of other antigen/antibody reactions.

In the United States a new Fab antivenom, CroFab, has been developed by Therapeutic Antibodies (now Protheric). It is an ovine antiserum. One of its advantages over the IgG product is that the former reaches its maximum protein level in the blood in 20 to 25 min, while the IgG product requires 40 to 50 min to reach the same level. Experiences with the efficacy and safety of the CroFab antivenom are found in Dart et al. (1997) and Seifert et al. (1997). It has become obvious that the use of this product may require periodic administration rather than single-bolus doses of the antivenom (Boyer et al., 1999).

ACKNOWLEDGMENT

The author wishes to acknowledge the opinions and assistance of Professors M. Mayersohn, A, Martin, S. Yalkowsky, L. Boyer, M. Witt, C. Witt, R. Smith, and J. McNally of the University of Arizona and Prof F. Markland of the University of Southern California. All errors of commission and omission are those of the author. Drawings are from Smith (1997).

REFERENCES

Akhunov AA, Makevnina L, Golubenko Z, et al: Kininase of the *Latrodectus tredecimguttatus* venom: A study of its enzyme specificity. *Immunopharmacology* 32:190, 1996.

Bajwa SS, Markland FS: Defibrinogenation studies with crotalase: Possible clinical applications. *Proc West Pharmacol Soc* 21:461, 1978.

Bettini S: *Arthropod Venoms*. New York: Springer-Verlag, 1978.

Bettini S, Maroli M: Venoms of Theridiidae, genus *Latrodectus,* in Bettini S (ed): *Arthropod Venoms*. New York: Springer-Verlag, 1978, p 149.

Blum MS: On the chemistry of ant venoms. *J Chem Evol* 15(1):2589, 1989.

Blum MS: Poisonous ants and their venoms, in Tu A (ed) *Insect Poisons, Allergens, and Other Invertebrate Venoms*. Vol 2. New York: Marcel Dekker, 1984, p 225.

Bon C, Bouchier C, Choumet V, et al: Crotoxin, half-century of investigations on a phospholipase A_2 neurotoxin. *Acta Physiol Pharmacol Latinoam* 39(4):439–448, 1989.

Boyer LV, Seifert SA, Clark RF et al: Recurrent and persistent coagulopathy following pit viper envenomation. *Arch Intern Med* 159: 706–710, 1999.

Bonilla CA, Fiero MK: Comparative biochemistry and pharmacology of salivary gland secretions: II. Chromatographic separation of the basic proteins from North American rattlesnake venoms. *J Chromatogr* 56.253, 1971.

Brown DE, Carmony NB: *Gila Monster*. Silver City, N.M. High Lonesome Books, 1991.

Carlson RW, Schaeffer RC, Russell FE, et al: A comparison of corticosteroid and fluid treatment after rattlesnake venom shock in rats. *Physiologist* 18:160, 1975.

Cavaliere M, D'Urso D, Lassa A, et al: Characterization and some properties of the venom gland extract of a theridiid spider (*Steatoda paykulliana*) frequently mistaken for black widow spider (*Latrodectus tredecimguttatus*). *Toxicon* 25(9):965, 1987.

Chang LS, Chou YC, Lin SR, et al: A novel neurotoxin, cobrotoxin b, from *Naja naja atra* venom: Purification, characterization and gene organization. *J Biochem* 122(6):1252–1259, 1997.

Chavez-Olortegui C, Zanetti VC, Ferreira AP: ELISA for the detection of venom antigens in experimental and clinical envenoming by *Loxosceles intermedia* spiders. *Toxicon* 36(4):563, 1998.

Chippaux JP, Amadi-Eddine P, Fagot F, et al: Therapeutic approach to snake bite in tropical Africa, in Bon C, Goyffon M (eds): *Envenomings and Their Treatments:* Paris, Institut Pasteur, 1996, p 247.

Cohen E, Quistad G: Cytotoxic effects of arthropod venoms on various cultured cells. *Toxicon* 36(2):353, 1998.

Dart RC, Russell FE: Animal poisoning, in Hall JB, Schmidt GA, Wood LD (eds): *Principles of Critical Care*. New York: McGraw-Hill, 1992, p 2163.

Dart RC, Seifert SA, Carrol L, et al: Affinity-purified, mixed monospecific crotalid antivenom ovine Fab for the treatment of crotalid venom poisoning. *Ann Emerg Med* 30:33, 1997.

Datta G, Tu AT: Structure and other chemical characterizations of gila toxin, a lethal toxin from lizard venom. *J Peptide Res* 50(6):443, 1997.

Delezenne C: Le zinc, constituant cellullaire de l'organissne animal. Sa presence et son rôle dans le veneendes serpents. *Ann Inst Pasteur* 33:68, 1919.

Deutsch HF, Diniz CR: Some proteolytic activities of snake venoms. *J Biol Chem* 216:17, 1995.

Dowling HG, Minton SA, Russell FE: *Poisonous Snakes of the World*. Washington, DC: U.S. Government Printing Office, 1968.

Dubnoff JW, Russell FE: Isolation of lethal protein and peptide from *Crotalus viridis helleri* venom. *Proc West Pharmacol Soc* 13:98, 1970.

Eaker D, Wadström T (eds): *Natural Toxins*. Elmsford, NY: Pergamon Press, 1980.

Ebeling W: *Urban Entomology*. Los Angeles; University of California Division of Agricultural Sciences, 1975.

Elliott WB: Chemistry and immunology of reptilian venoms, in Gans C (ed): *Biology of the Reptilia*. Vol 8. London: Academic Press, 1978, p 163.

Fortes-Dias CL, Jannotti MLD, Franco FJL et al: Studies on the specificity of CNF, a phospholipase A_2 inhibitor isolated from the blood plasma of the South American rattlesnake (*Crotalus durissus terrificus*): I. Interaction with PLA_2 from *Lachisus muta muta* snake venom. *Toxicon* 37:1747–1759, 1999.

Franca FOS, Benevenuti LA, Fan HW, et al: Severe and fatal mass attacks by "killer" bees (Africanized honey bees—*Apis mellifera scutellata*) in Brazil: Clinicopathological studies with measurement of serum venom concentrations. *Q J Med* 87:269, 1994.

Gertsch WJ: *American Spiders,* 2d ed. New York: Van Nostrand Reinhold, 1979.

Gold BS, Wingert WA: Snake venom poisoning in the United States. *South Med J* 87:579, 1994.

Gopalakrishnakone P, Tan CK (eds): *Recent Advances in Toxinology Research*. Singapore: National University of Singapore, 1992.

Gregson JD: Tick Paralysis an appraisal of natural and experimental data. Monograph 9. *Canada Department of Agriculture,* 1973.

Grishin E: Polypeptide neurotoxins from spider venoms. *Eur J Biochem* 264(2):276, 1999.

Grishin EV: Black widow spider toxins: The present and the future. *Toxicon* 36(11):1693, 1998.

Habermann E, Breithaupt H: The crotoxin complex: An example of biochemical and pharmacological protein complementation. *Toxicon* 16:19, 1978.

Habermehl GG: *Venomous Animals and Their Toxins*. Berlin: Springer-Verlag, 1981.

Harding KA, Welch KRG: *Venomous Snakes of the World: A Checklist.* Elmsford, NY: Pergamon Press, 1980.

Heard K, O'Malley GF, Dart RC: Antivenom therapy in the Americas (review). *Drugs* 58(1)5, 1999.

Holz GG, Habener JF: Alpha-latrotoxin: A presynaptic neurotoxin that shares structural homology with the glucogen-like peptide-1 family of insulin secretagogic hormones. *Comp Biochem Physiol [B]* 121(2):177, 1998.

Horikawa N, Kataha K, Watanabe N, et al: Glibenclamide-sensitive hypotension produced by helodermin assessed in the rat. *Biol Pharm Bull* 21(12):1290, 1998.

Jones RGA, Corteling HP, Bhogal G, et al: A novel Fab-based antivenom for treatment of mass bee attacks. *Am J Trop Med Hyg* 61:361–366, 1999.

Kawamoto F, Kumada N: Biology and venoms of *Ledpidoptera,* in Tu A (ed): *Insect Poisons, Allergens, and Other Invertebrate Venoms*. Vol 2. New York: Marcel Dekker, 1984, p 292.

Kazuni K, McBumey RN, Goldin SM: Venoms and toxins as sources of drug leads, in Coombes, JD (ed): *New Drugs from Natural Sources.* London: IBC Technical Services, 1997, p 143.

Keegan HL: *Scorpions of Medical Importance*. Jackson, MI: University Press of Mississippi, 1980.

King LE, Rees RS: Dapsone treatment of a brown recluse bite. *JAMA* 250:648, 1983.

Lee C-Y (ed): *Snake Venoms*. New York: Springer-Verlag, 1979.

Maeda N, Tamiya N, Pattabhiraman TK, et al: Some chemical properties of the venom of the rattlesnake *Crotalus viridis helleri*. *Toxicon* 16:431, 1978.

Maretić Z: Erfahrungen mit Stichen von Giftfischen. *Acta Trop (Basel)* 14:157, 1957.

Maretić Z, Lebez D: *Araneism*. Belgrade, Yugoslavia: Nolit Belgrade, 1979.

Markland FS: Snake venoms and their hemostatic system. *Toxicon* 36:1749, 1998.

Ménez A, Zimmerman K, Zimmerman S, *et al.*: Venom apparatus and toxicity of the centipede *Ethmostigmus rubripes* (Chilopoda, Scolopendridae). *J Morphol* 206:303, 1990.

Merchant ML, Hinton JF, Geren CR: Sphingomyelinase D activity of brown recluse spider (*Loxosceles reclusa*) venom as studied by ^{31}P-NMR: Effects on the time-course of sphingomyelin hydrolysis. *Toxicon* 36(3):537, 1998.

Mebs D: Bissverletzungen durch "ungiftige" Schlangen. *Dtsch Med Wochenschr* 102:1429, 1977.

Mebs D: Pharmacology of reptilian venoms, in Gans C (ed): *Biology of the Reptilia.* Vol 8. London: Academic Press, 1978, p 437.

Minton SA Jr: A list of colubrid envenomations. *Kentucky Herpetol* 7:4, 1976.

Minton SA Jr, Minton MG: *Venomous Reptiles*. New York: Scribner, 1969.

Morrissette J, Kratezschmar J, Haendler B, et al: Primary structure and properties of helothermine, a peptide toxin that blocks ryanodine receptors. *Biophys J* 68(6):2280, 1995.

Nastopoulis, D. Structure of dimeric and monomeric erabutoxin a refined at I.5A resolution. *Acta Crystallog D* 54(pt 5):964–974, 1998.

Nobile M, Noceti F, Prestipino G, et al: Helothermine, a lizard venom toxin, inhibits calcium current in cerebellar granules. *Exp Brain Res* 110(1):15, 1996.

Oliveira de KC, Andrade de RMG, Giusti AL, et al: Sex-linked variation of *Loxosceles intermedia* spider venoms. *Toxicon* 37:217, 1999.

Oshima-Franco Y, Hyslop S, Prado-Franceschi J et al: Neutralizing capacity of antisera raised in horses and rabbits against *Crotalus durissus terrificus* (South American rattlesnake) venom and its main toxin, crotoxin. *Toxicon* 37:1341, 1999.

Parnas 1, Russell FE: Effects of venoms on nerve muscle and neuromuscular junction, in Russell FE, Saunders PR (eds): *Animal Toxins*. Oxford, England: Pergamon Press, 1967, p 401.

Parrish HM: *Poisonous Snakebites in the United States*. New York: Vantage Press, 1980.

Patel KA, Modur V, Zimmerman GA: The necrotic venom of the brown recluse spider induces dysregulated endothelial cell-dependent neutrophil activation. *Am Soc Clin Invest* 94:631, 1994.

Persson H, Karlson-Stiber C: Clinical features and principles of treatment of envenoming by European vipers, in Bon C, Goyffon M (eds): *Envenomings and Their Treatments*. Paris: Institut Pasteur, 1996, p 281.

Polis, GA (ed) *The Biology of Scorpions*. Stanford, CA: Stanford University Press, 1990, p 482.

Rimsza ME, Zimmerman DR, Bergeson PS: Scorpion envenomation. *Pediatrics* 66:298, 1980.

Rosenberg P: Pharmacology of phospholipase A_2 from snake venoms, in Lee C-Y (ed): *Snake Venoms—Handbook of Experimental Pharmacology.* Vol 52. Berlin: Springer-Verlag, 1979, p 403.

Rosenberg P: Phospholipases, in Shier WT, Mebs D (eds): *Handbook of Toxinology*. New York: Marcel Dekker, 1990, p 67.

Rosenberg P (ed): *Toxins: Animal, Plant, and Microbial*. Elmsford, NY: Pergamon Press, 1978.

Russell FE: Venomous animals and their toxins. *London Times Sci Rev* 49:10, 1963.

Russell FE: Comparative pharmacology of some animal toxins. *Fed Proc* 26:1206, 1967.

Russell FE: Poisons and venoms, in Hoar WS, Randall DJ (eds): *Fish Physiology.* Vol III. New York: Academic Press, 1969, p 401.

Russell FE: Envenomation and diverse disease states (letter). *JAMA* 238:281, 1977.

Russell FE: Pharmacology of venoms, in Eaker D, Wadström T (eds): *Natural Toxins*. Elmsford, NY: Pergamon Press, 1980a, p 13.

Russell FE: Venomous bites and stings, in Berkow R (ed): *The Merck Manual,* 14th ed. Rahway, NJ: Merck Sharp & Dohme, 1982, p 2451.

Russell FE: *Snake Venom Poisoning*. Philadelphia: Lippincott, 1980b; Great Neck, NY: Scholium International, 1983.

Russell FE: Snake venoms, in Ferguson MWJ (ed): *The Structure, Development and Evolution of Reptiles* (Symposia of the Zoological Society of London). London: Academic Press, 1984, p 469.

Russell FE: Snake venom poisoning in the United States of America, in Bon C, Goyffon M (eds): *Envenomings and Their Treatments*. Paris: Institut Pasteur, 1996a, p 235.

Russell FE: Toxic effects of animal venoms, in Klaassen CD (ed): *Casarett and Doull's Toxicology: The Basic Science of Poisons*. 5th ed. New York: McGraw-Hill, 1996b, p 801.

Russell FE: Snakes and snakebite in Central America. *Toxicon* 35(10): 1469–1522, 1997.

Russell FE, Alender CB, Buess FW: Venom of the scorpion *Vejovis spingerus. Science* 159:90, 1968.

Russell FE, Bogert CM: Gila monster, its biology, venom and bite: A review. *Toxicon* 19:341, 1981.

Russell FE, Buess FW. Gel electrophoresis: A tool in systematics studies with *Latrodectus mactans* venom. *Toxicon* 8:81, 1970.

Russell FE, Buess FW, Strassburg J: Cardiovascular response to *Crotalus* venom. *Toxicon* 1:5, 1962.

Russell FE, Carlson RW, Wainschel J, et al: Snake venom poisoning in United States: Experiences with 550 cases. *JAMA* 233 – 341, 1975.

Russell FE, Gertsch WJ: Letter to the editor (arthropod bites). *Toxicon* 21:337, 1983.

Russell FE, Marcus P, Strong JA: Black widow spider envenomation during pregnancy: Report of a case. *Toxicon* 17:188, 1979.

Russell FE, Nagabhushanam, R: *The Venomous and Poisonous Marine Invertebrates of the Indian Ocean*. Enfield, NH: Science Publications, p 271, 1996a, p 271.

Schaeffer RC Jr, Carlson RW, Whigham H, et al: Acute hemodynamic effects of rattlesnake *Crotalus viridis helleri* venom, in Rosenberg P (ed): *Toxins: Animal, Plant, and Microbial*. Oxford, England: Pergamon Press, 1978, p 383.

Schenone H, Suarez G: Venoms of Scytodidae genus *Loxosceles,* in Bettini S (ed): *Arthropod Venoms*. New York: Springer-Verlag, 1978, p 247.

Seifert SA, Boyer LV, Dart RC, et al: Relationship of venom effects to venom antigen and antivenom serum concentration in a patient with *Crotalus atrox* envenomation treated with Fab antivenom. *Ann Emerg Med* 30:49, 1997.

Slotta K, Frankel-Conrat H: Two active proteins from rattlesnake venom. *Nature* 142:213, 1938.

Sokolov IV, Chanturiia AN, Lishko VK: [Channel-forming properties of *Steatoda paykulliana* spider venom] [Russian]. *Biofizika* 29(4):620, 1984.

Sorkine M, Audebert F, Bon C: Clinical and biological evaluation of viper bites in France, in Bon C, Goyffon M (eds): *Envenomings and Their Treatments*. Paris: Institut Pasteur, 1996, p 77.

Southcott RV. Arachnidism and allied syndromes in the Australian region. *Rec Adelaide Child Hosp* 1:97, 1976.

Su C, Chang C, Lee C-Y: Pharmacological properties of the neurotoxin of cobra venom, in Russell FE, Saunders PR (eds): *Animal Toxins*. Oxford, England: Pergamon Press, 1967, p 259.

Sutherland SK: *Australian Animal Toxins*. Melbourne: Oxford University Press, 1983.

Tambourgi DV, Petricevich VL, Magnoli FC, et al: Endotoxemic-like shock induced by *Loxosceles* spider venoms: Pathological changes and putative cytokine mediators. *Toxicon* 36(2):391, 1998.

Tamiya N, Arai H, Sato S: Studies on sea snake venoms: Crystallization of "erabutoxins" a and b from *Laticauda semifasciata* venom and of "laticotoxin"a from *Laticauda laticaudata* venom, in Russell FE, Saunders PR (eds): *Animal Toxins*. Oxford, England: Pergamon Press, 1967, p 249.

Terranova AC, Roach SH: A computer aided key for distinguishing South Carolina (USA) species of the genus *Phidippus* (Aranea: Salticidae). *J Agric Entomol* 6(1):23, 1989.

Tu A: *Chemistry and Molecular Biology*. New York: Wiley, 1977.

Tubbs M: Screening for fibrinolytic activity in 8 viperid venoms. *Comp Biochem Physiol Pharmacol Toxicol Endocrinol* 124(1):91, 1999.

Uddman R, Goadsby PJ, Jansen-Olesen I, et al: Helospectin-like peptides: Immunochemical localization and effects on isolated cerebral arteries and on local cerebral blood flow in the cat. *J Cerebral Blood Flow Metabol* 19(1):61, 1999.

Van Mierop LHS: Poisonous snakebite: A review. *J Fla Med Assoc* 63:191, 1976.

Vick JA, Ciuchta HP, Manthei JH: Pathophysiological studies on ten snake venoms, in Russell FE, Saunders PR (eds): *Animal Toxins*. Oxford, England: Pergamon Press, 1967, p 269.

Vincent A, Jacobson L, Curran L: Alpha-bungarotoxin binding to human muscle acetylcholine receptor. *Neurochem Int* 332(5–6): 427–433, 1998.

Visser J, Chapman DS: *Snakes and Snakebite*. Cape Town: Purnell and Sons, 1978.

Warrell DA: Injuries, envenoming, poisoning, and allergic reactions caused by animals, in Weatherall OK, Leadingham JGG, Warrell, DA (eds): *Oxford Textbook of Medicine*. Oxford, England: Oxford University Press, 1966, pp 1124–1151.

Warrell, DA: Snake venoms in science and clinical medicine: 1. Russell's viper: Biology, venom and treatment of bites. *Trans R Soc Trop Med Hyg* 83:732–740, 1989.

CHAPTER 27

TOXIC EFFECTS OF PLANTS

Stata Norton

INTRODUCTION

In the course of evolution, plants have been attacked by pathogens (viruses, bacteria, and fungi) and eaten by animals from insects to elephants. In response, plants have developed various elegant defenses, including synthesis of chemicals that inhibit the actions of pathogens and rapidly acting chemicals designed to deter attack by inducing negative effects on the gastrointestinal, cardiac, or nervous systems of plant predators. The quickest way for a plant to protect itself from being eaten is to produce chemicals that are irritating on contact. Nausea and gastric irritation occurring in close conjunction with ingestion are also effective deterrents.

Of the many species of plants that contain toxic chemicals, only a few can be described here. Selection has been based on three considerations: frequency with which contact occurs, importance and seriousness of toxic effect, and scientifically interesting nature of the action of the chemical.

It is important to note that toxic effects of the same species of plant may vary with differences in production of the toxic chemical by plants. The reasons for variability in concentration of toxic chemicals are several:

1. Different portions of the plant (root, stem, leaves, seeds) often contain different concentrations of a chemical. For example, paclitaxel (Taxol), an antineoplastic drug from species of *Taxus* (yew), is present in various parts of *Taxus cuspidata.* The needles, bark, wood, and mature cones contain, in that order, decreasing concentrations of paclitaxel (Fett-Netto and DiCosmo, 1992).
2. The age of the plant contributes to variability. Young plants may contain more or less of some constituents than mature plants. For example, in spring pokeweed (*Phytolacca americana*), sprouts and young leaves are safer to eat than mature leaves. The saponin produced in pokeweed as it develops contributes to the toxicity of the mature plant (Blackwell, 1990).
3. Climate and soil influence the synthesis of some chemicals. For example, lichens produce carotenoids in direct relation to the amount of sunlight, with the advantage to the plant that carotenoids protect from excessive ultraviolet light (Czeczuga, 1988).
4. Genetic differences within a species may alter the ability of individual plants to synthesize a chemical. Synthesis of related toxic chemicals often is found in taxonomically related species as a characteristic of a genus and sometimes as a familial characteristic. For example, species of *Ranunculus* (buttercup) produce an acrid juice that releases the irritating chemical anemonin. Some other genera of the same family (Ranunculaceae) also release anemonin.

TOXIC EFFECT BY ORGAN

Skin

Allergic Dermatitis Most people are familiar with dermatitis caused by some plants, such as poison ivy. Equally familiar is the allergenic response of many individuals in the form of "hay fever" or summer rhinitis.

Philodendron (family Araceae, arum family) and *Rhus* (Anacardiaceae, cashew family) are not closely related plants, but species of both genera cause contact dermatitis as an allergic reaction. *Philodendron scandens* is a common houseplant, while *Rhus radicans* (poison ivy) is native to North America. In addition to poison ivy, the toxicodendron group of plants contains *Rhus diversiloba* (poison oak) and *Rhus vernix* (poison sumac). The active ingredients in *P. scandens* are resorcinols, especially 5-*n*-heptadecatrienyl resorcinol (Knight, 1991). In *R. radicans,* the allergenic component is a mixture of catechols called urushiol. The most active compound in urushiol is 3-*n*-pentadecadienyl catechol, representing approximately 60 percent of urushiol (Johnson et al., 1972). As in allergies in general, there is no response to the initial exposure; even with repeated exposure, individuals show marked variation in severity of response. The allergens in urushiol will sensitize about 70 percent of persons exposed, making the response to poison ivy and related plants the most common form of allergic contact dermatitis in the United States. Urushiol is fat-soluble, penetrates the stratum corneum, and binds to Langerhans cells in the epidermis. These haptenated cells then migrate to lymph nodes, where T cells are activated; they then return to the skin, where they are involved in the dermatitis (Kalish and Johnson, 1990). Contact dermatitis also develops with repeated exposures to the sap of mango fruit, because the skin of the fruit contains oleoresins that cross-react with allergens of poison ivy (Tucker and Swan, 1998).

Flower growers and other individuals who handle bulbs and cut flowers of daffodils, hyacinths, and tulips sometimes develop dermatitis from contact with the sap. These conditions occur frequently enough to have achieved common names: "hyacinth itch," "daffodil itch," and "tulip fingers." The rashes are due to irritation from alkaloids (masonin, lycorin, and several related alkaloids) or to needle-like crystals of calcium oxalate in the bulbs (Gude et al., 1998). Most of these alkaloids do not act as allergens, but one, tulipalin-A, which causes "tulip fingers" from sorting and peeling tulip bulbs, has allergenic properties. Tulipalin-A, alpha-methylene-gamma-butyrolactone, is present in some cultivars in a concentration as high as 2 percent. A safe threshold for this allergen is considered to be a concentration of 0.01 percent (Hausen et al., 1983). The advantage to the plant of the tulipalins is not their allergenic properties but that they are strong antifungal agents (Christensen and Kristiansen, 1999).

The allergens of plants tend to be located in the outer cell layers of plant organs. In allergic contact dermatitis to chrysanthemums (*Dendranthema* species), the allergens are sesquiterpene lactones present in small hairs (trichomes) on the stems, undersides of leaves, and in flowering heads (McGovern and Barkley, 1999).

An immunoglobulin-mediated hypersensitivity, called the *latex-fruit syndrome,* results in cross-sensitivity in some individuals to latex in rubber gloves and fruit. The major allergen in natural rubber latex from the rubber tree, *Hevea brasiliensis,* is prohevein, a chitin-binding polypeptide found in several plants. Hevein, a 43–amino acid N-terminal fragment of prohevein, is the major binding component (Alenius et al., 1996). Individuals sensitive to latex rubber may be sensitized to several fruits containing a chitinase with a hevein-like domain, including banana, kiwi, tomato, and avocado (Blanco et al., 1999).

Pollen from several genera in the family Asteraceae (for example, mugwort, *Artemisia vulgaris* in Europe, and ragweed, *Ambrosia artemisiifolia* in North America) contains allergens causing summer rhinitis. Immunoglobulin antibodies produced by sensitized individuals cross-react with mugwort and ragweed pollen. The cross-reactive allergen has been identified as a highly conserved 14-kDa protein, profilin, found as well in birch pollen (Hirschwehr et al., 1998).

Allergy to grass pollen is worldwide in occurrence and causes serious morbidity and economic cost. Individuals with grass pollen allergy react to pollen from a number of species. *Poa* and *Festuca* species are major contributors to the allergic response (Lovborg et al., 1999).

Contact Dermatitis One of the most common exposures to toxic substances in plants reported to poison-control centers in the United States is from the houseplant *Dieffenbachia* (dumb cane, arum family). Children and workers in plant nurseries are the usual patients. *Dieffenbachia* does not cause allergic dermatitis, but when leaves or stems are broken, the juice is immediately irritating to mucous membranes. Children may chew the leaves of the plant and workers in greenhouses cut the plant in the course of their work. Contact of the eye or tongue to the juice results in pain and rapid development of edema and inflammation, which may take days or weeks to subside. The toxicity is due to a combination of factors. The leaves contain irritating calcium oxalate crystals coated with a trypsin-like inflammatory protein. Release of a histamine-like or serotonin-like chemical may be involved in the immediate pain (Pamies et al., 1992). The needle-like crystals of calcium oxalate, called raphides, are located in ampule-shaped ejector cells throughout the surface of the leaf. Slight pressure on these cells causes expulsion of the raphides (McIntire et al., 1990).

Acute dermatitis is caused by contact with the trichomes of species of *Urtica* (nettles). Even gentle contact with the hairs causes pain and erythema from penetration of the skin by the trichomes. In the stinging nettles, *Urtica urens* and *Urtica dioica* (family Urticaceae), the trichomes covering the leaves and stems consist of fine tubes with bulbs at the end that break off in the skin and release fluid containing histamine, acetylcholine, and serotonin, causing the acute response (Oliver et al., 1991). Exposure to *Urtica ferox* (poisonous tree nettle), a plant widespread in New Zealand, has caused death in humans and animals. A defense against ingestion by animals, similar to that of nettles, has been developed by *Mucuna pruriens* (cowhage), a legume, with pods covered with barbed trichomes that cause pain, itching, erythema, and vesication. The trichomes of *M. pruriens* contain mucinain, a proteinase responsible for the pruritus (Southcott and Haegi, 1992).

Several species of *Ranunculus* (buttercup) cause contact dermatitis. These plants contain ranunculin, which releases the toxic principle protoanemonin, also present in *Anemone,* another genus of the buttercup family. Protoanemonin is readily converted to anemonin, which has marked irritant properties. Ingestion of plants containing protoanemonin may result in severe irritation of the gastrointestinal tract (Kelch et al., 1992).

The genus *Euphorbia* (Euphorbiaceae, spurge family) contains hundreds of species dispersed over temperate and tropical regions. Characteristically, the stems and leaves exude milky latex when damaged. The latex contains diterpene esters irritating to the skin. *Euphorbia marginata* (snow-on-the-mountain) is a common plant in the United States, growing wild from Minnesota to Texas and cultivated for its attractive foliage. Individuals using the plant in flower arrangements may come in contact with the latex and develop skin irritation (Urushibata and Kase, 1991). Serious eye irritation has been reported (Frohn et al., 1993). The latex of *Euphorbia pulcherrima,* poinsettia, cultivars of which are common house plants, may cause contact dermatitis (Massmanian, 1998), but the large number of exposures to poinsettia reported to poison-control centers result in minor irritation (Krenzelok et al., 1996). A major ester found in *Euphorbia resinifera* and several other species of *Euphorbia* is resiniferatoxin. It acts at the vanilloid receptor of the primary sensory neurons that mediate pain perception and neurogenic inflammation. Resiniferatoxin is a potent analog of capsaicin but desensitizes with less stimulation of the receptor than capsaicin. This property is being used to desensitize sensory neurons to mitigate neuropathic pain (Appendino and Scallazi, 1997).

Photosensitivity Not all cases of dermatitis from plants are due to skin contact. Poisoning of livestock from *Hypericum perforatum* (St. John's wort) has been reported in the United States, New Zealand, Australia, North Africa, Iraq, and Europe. The toxic principle is hypericin (hexahydroxydimethylnaphthodianthrone), which is present throughout the plant. Sheep are the most commonly affected animals, ingesting the plant in pasturage. The effect in sheep is development of edematous lesions of the skin, especially in areas not well covered with hair, including the ears, nose, and eyes. Hypericin causes photosensitization, and lesions appear after exposure to sunlight (Sako et al., 1993). In human consumption of St. John's wort, photosensitivity is a rare event (Ernst et al., 1998).

Gastrointestinal System

Direct Irritant Effects The most common outcome of ingestion of a toxic plant is gastrointestinal disturbance (nausea, vomiting, and diarrhea) from irritation of the mucous membranes. Many different kinds of chemicals are responsible for this. Some have found a place in medicine as mild purgatives, such as cascara sagrada ("sacred bark"). Cascara is obtained from the bark of *Rhamnus purshiana* (California buckthorn). The active ingredient is emodin.

Tung nut (*Aleurites fordii*) is grown widely in the world, including the southwestern United States, Taiwan, mainland China, Japan, and India. The seeds, from which commercially useful oil is expressed, are the most toxic part. Ingestion of the ripe nuts causes abdominal pain, vomiting, and diarrhea. Outbreaks of poisoning are most common in children (Lin et al., 1996).

Buffalo bean or buffalo pea (*Thermopsis rhombifolia*) is a legume growing wild in the western United States. Loss of life of livestock has been reported from consumption of the mature plant with seeds. Children develop nausea, vomiting, dizziness, and abdominal pain from eating the beans (McGrath-Hill and Vicas, 1997). The active toxic substances are quinolizidine alkaloids.

Aesculus hippocastanum (horse chestnut) and *Aesculus glabra* (Ohio buckeye) are common trees with attractive panicles of flowers in the spring. Nuts of both trees contain a glucoside called esculin. When eaten by humans, the main effect is gastroenteritis, which may be severe if several nuts are consumed. Esculin is poorly absorbed from the gastrointestinal tract of humans, and its systemic effects are limited. In cattle the glucoside may be hydrolyzed in the rumen, releasing the aglycone to cause systemic effects. Cattle develop signs of nervous system stimulation—a stiff-legged gait and, in severe poisoning, tonic seizures with opisthotonus (Casteel et al., 1992). While the most common poisoning of cattle occurs from ingestion of nuts, they may also be poisoned in pasture in spring by eating new leaves and buds.

Antimitotic Effects *Podophyllum peltatum* (May apple) contains the toxic purgative podophyllotoxin, especially in foliage and roots. In low doses, mild purgation predominates. Overdose results in nausea and severe paroxysmal vomiting (Frasca et al., 1997). Podophyllotoxin inhibits mitosis by binding to microtubules, and this property has made the toxin of interest in the treatment of cancer (Schacter, 1996).

Colchicine is best known in western medicine for its antimitotic effect, which is particularly useful in attacks of gout. Colchicine is the major alkaloid in the bulbs of *Colchicum autumnale* (autumn crocus, lily family), native to Asia Minor. Severe gastroenteritis (nausea, vomiting, diarrhea, and dehydration) follows ingestion of the bulbs. Systemic effects may develop, including confusion, delirium, hematuria, neuropathy, and renal failure. Bone marrow aplasia results from block of mitosis in bone marrow. The antimitotic action is caused by block of the formation of microtubules and subsequent failure of the mitotic spindle. Additional toxic effects may be due to lectins in the plant. Several plants, including *Colchicum autumnale,* contain lectins that are potent inducers of a gelatinase by mononuclear white blood cells. It has been suggested that the acute toxicity of many plant lectins may be partially mediated by induction of gelatinase from leukocytes (Dubois et al., 1998). High circulating levels of gelatinase have been shown to be present in circulatory shock.

In southern Europe, hay for cattle may contain the wild autumn crocus and deaths occur if contamination is heavy. In other countries similar poisoning has been found after human ingestion of tubers of *Gloriosa superba* (glory lily), an ornamental lily that contains colchicine. The plant grows wild in Sir Lanka, and poisoning by *Gloriosa* tubers has been reported as the most common plant poisoning in that country. Poisoning has also been reported in India (Mendis, 1989).

Lectin Toxicity *Wisteria floribunda* (family Leguminosae) is a common ornamental climbing vine or small tree with lilac-colored flowers from which pods containing several seeds develop in the fall. The plant is of interest as a research tool because the seeds contain a lectin with affinity for *N*-acetylglucosamine on mammalian neurons. The lectins of legumes are a well-studied family of plant proteins with a wide repertoire of binding to specific cell-surface carbohydrates. Wisteria species also contain saponins (Nohara et al., 1996). The seeds of wisteria cause severe gastroenteritis when ingested. A few seeds can result in headache, nausea, and diarrhea within hours, followed by dizziness, confusion, and hematemesis (Rondeau, 1993).

Ricinus communis (castor bean) is a member of the family Euphorbiaceae, which contains several genera that produce toxic chemicals. The castor bean is an ornamental plant introduced from India and grown in temperate regions as an annual. The seeds are large and attractively mottled. If the seeds are eaten, children and adults experience no marked symptoms of poisoning for several days. In this interval there is some loss of appetite, with nausea, vomiting, and diarrhea developing gradually. After that, gastroenteritis becomes severe, with persistent vomiting, bloody diarrhea, dehydration, and icterus in fatal cases. Death occurs in 6 to 8 days.

The fatal dose for a child can be 5 to 6 seeds; it is about 20 seeds for an adult. Postmortem examination shows foci of necrosis in the liver, spleen, lymph glands, intestine, and stomach. Fatality is low in individuals who eat the seeds—less than 10 percent when a "fatal" dose is consumed—because the toxic protein is largely destroyed in the intestine. Death from castor beans is caused by two lectins in the beans: ricin I and ricin II. The more toxic is ricin II. Ricin II consists of two chains of amino acids. The A chain (molecular weight 30,000) inactivates the 60s ribosomal subunit of cells by catalytic depurination of a single adenosine residue within the 28s rRNA (Bantel et al., 1999) and blocks protein synthesis. The A chain is endocytosed into the cell cytosol after the B chain (molecular weight 33,000) binds to a terminal galactose residue on the cell membrane. The two chains are linked by disulfide bonds. Similar toxic lectins are found in the seeds of *Abrus precatorius* (jequirity bean), attractive scarlet and black beans that are sometimes made into necklaces. Abrin-a, one of four isoabrins from the plant, has the highest inhibitory effect on protein synthesis and consists of an A chain of 250 amino acids and a B chain of 267 amino acids (Tahirov et al., 1994). The LD_{50} of abrin injected in mice is less than 0.1 μg/kg, making abrin one of the most toxic substances known.

Ricin-type lectins with both A and B chains are potentially deadly if they pass, even in small quantities, through the gastrointestinal tract. Plants that produce only A chains offer much less risk when ingested. Young shoots of pokeweed (*Phytolacca americana*) are sometimes used in the spring as a salad green. Mature leaves and berries may cause gastrointestinal irritation with nausea and diarrhea. The plant produces three isozymes of single-chain lectins (PAP, PAPII, and PAP-S; molecular weights about 30,000) that can inhibit protein synthesis in cells by inactivating rRNA. Single-chain, ribosome-inhibiting proteins do not enter intact cells readily, but if the cell membrane has been breached by a virus, they may enter the cell (Monzingo et al., 1993). Lectins that bind strongly to the cells lining the small intestine and are endocytosed by them may be "nutritionally toxic" if they are consumed over a long period. Experimentally, reduction in weight gain has been the major finding from the presence of high quantities of some lectins in the diet. A correlation between strength of binding to the brush border of the jejunum and effectiveness as an antinutrient has been reported (Pusztai et al., 1993).

Lung

In addition to the well-recognized involvement of the lung and airway tissues in allergic asthma in some individuals sensitized to plant allergens, the lung is directly affected by some plant chemicals.

Cough Reflex It has been found that workers who handle two peppers, *Capsicum annum* (cayenne pepper) and *Capsicum frutescens* (chili pepper), have a significantly increased incidence of cough during the day. The major irritant ingredients in *Capsicum* are capsaicin (trans-8-methyl-*N*-vanillyl-6-nonenamide) and dihydrocapsaicin (Surh et al., 1998). Capsaicin-sensitive nerves in the airway are involved in the irritation and cough (Blanc et al., 1991). Sensory endings of C fibers are part of the cough reflex, and the principal neurotransmitter for these fibers, the neuropeptide substance P, is depleted by capsaicin. Capsaicin activates a subtype of the vanilloid receptor found in the airway, spinal cord, dorsal root ganglion, bladder, urethra, and colon. Capsaicin can be irritating to the skin, and individuals handling the peppers may experience irritation and vesication.

Cell Death In the laboratory, rats are highly susceptible to monocrotaline from seeds of *Crotalaria spectabilis* (showy rattlebox, legume family) and develop a condition resembling pulmonary hypertension. In the rat, monocrotaline is converted in the liver into an active pyrrolic metabolite responsible for the cardiopulmonary lesions (Schultze et al., 1991). Apoptosis of arterial endothelial cells may be involved early in the onset of pulmonary hypertension (Thomas et al., 1998). In many other species, hepatitis is the primary toxicity.

Cardiovascular System

Cardioactive Glycosides Several disparate families of plants contain species with cardioactive glycosides, the best known of which is *Digitalis purpurea* (foxglove, Scrophulariaceae family). In the lily family, squill (*Scilla maritima*) contains scillaren, and lily of the valley (*Convallaria majalis*) contains convallatoxin in the bulbs. Both glycosides have actions resembling digitalis. Milkweeds (*Asclepias* species, Asclepiadaceae family) are noted for the glycosides in the plants, which are consumed by monarch butterfly caterpillars during their development. The glycosides are retained into the adult stage and help protect the butterflies from predators. The cardiac glycoside [6′-0-(E-4-hydroxycinnamoyl) desglucouzarin] in *Asclepias asperula,* like digitalis, inhibits Na^+,K^+-ATPase (Abbott et al., 1998). Two plants in the Apocynaceae family contain cardioactive glycosides. *Nereum oleander* (bay laurel) is native to the Mediterranean area but is grown ornamentally in many regions. The major glycosides, oleandrin and nerium, may be present in concentrations as high as 0.5 mg/g plant material. Animals and humans have been poisoned by eating the leaves or seeds. The effect is identical to that of digitalis toxicity: nausea, vomiting, and cardiac arrhythmias (Clark et al., 1991). A related plant, *Thevetia peruviana* (yellow oleander), is a common ornamental in the United States. Human poisoning has also been reported in Australia, Melanesia, Thailand, and India. The seeds are the major source of the cardiac glycosides, the most active of which is thevetin A. The fatal dose to an adult is 8 to 10 seeds (Prabhasankar et al., 1993).

Action on Cardiac Nerves *Veratrum viride* (American hellebore, lily family), native to eastern North America, produces several toxic alkaloids that are distributed in all parts of the plant. European hellebore (*Veratrum album*) and *Veratrum californicum* in western North America have similar alkaloids. *V. album* was part of the "vegetable materia medica" for centuries, employed to "slow and soften the pulse." These species of *Veratrum* contain a mixture of alkaloids, including protoveratrine, veratramine, and jervine. After ingestion, the alkaloids cause nausea, emesis, hypotension, bradycardia, and sometimes muscle spasm. The primary effect of the veratrum alkaloids on the heart is to cause a repetitive response to a single stimulus resulting from prolongation of the sodium current (Jaffe et al., 1990). Several species of *Zigadenus,* including *Zigadenus nuttallii* (death camas), contain *Veratrum*-like alkaloids. The plants grow throughout North America and the white bulbs may be mistaken for wild onions. Cattle are also poisoned in pastures where the plants are common. All parts of the plant are toxic (Heilpern, 1995).

Aconitum species have been used in western and eastern medicine for centuries. The European plant, *Aconitum napellus* (monkshood, Ranunculaceae family), is a perennial grown in gardens for its ornamental blue flowers. The roots of *Aconitum kusnezoffii* (chuanwu) and *Aconitum carmichaeli* (caowu) are in the Chinese materia medica. Poisoning may occur from intentional or accidental ingestion, and the concentration of the alkaloids—aconitine, mesaconitine, and hypoaconitine—varies depending on species, place of origin, time of harvest, and processing procedure (Chan et al., 1994). In addition to cardiac arrhythmias and hypotension, the alkaloids cause gastrointestinal upset and neurologic symptoms, especially numbness of the mouth and paresthesia in the extremities. The alkaloids cause a prolonged sodium current in cardiac muscle with slowed repolarization (Peper and Trautwein, 1967). The neurologic effects are due to a similar action on voltage-sensitive sodium currents in nerve fibers (Murai et al., 1990).

In Greece almost 2500 years ago, Xenophon described a serious condition called "mad honey poisoning" that developed in his soldiers after they had consumed honey. It consists of marked bradycardia, hypotension, oral paresthesias, weakness, and gastrointestinal upset, resembling aconitine poisoning. In severe poisoning there is respiratory depression and loss of consciousness. The condition is caused by eating honey contaminated with grayanotoxins. Some of the action of grayanotoxins is central. Grayanotoxin I (acetylandromedol) slows both the opening and closing of sodium channels in nerves (Narahashi, 1986). Honey poisoning has been reported in Turkey, Japan, Nepal, Brazil, Europe, and some parts of North America. Grayanotoxins are produced exclusively by several genera of Ericaceae (heath family). They have been isolated from *Rhododendron ponticum* (Onat et al., 1991) and *Kalmia angustifolia* (Burke and Doskotch, 1990). The toxin gets into honey from nectar collected by bees from the flowers. The grayanotoxins are present throughout the plants, including leaves, flowers, pollen, and nectar. Livestock have been poisoned by eating leaves of the plants. Toxicity has been reported in goats and sheep eating leaves of *Rhododendron macrophyllum* (Casteel and Wagstaff, 1989).

Vasoactive Chemicals Mistletoe is a parasitic plant on trees and has over the centuries been considered either holy or demonic. The poisonous qualities of mistletoe were recognized by John Gerarde in his herbal in 1597. He described a case of poisoning from mistletoe berries in which the tongue was inflamed and swollen, the mind distraught, and strength of heart and wits enfeebled. The mistletoe that appears in shops at Christmastime in the United States is *Phoradendron tomentosum,* a member of the same family as European mistletoe (*Viscum album,* Loranthaceae family). The American mistletoe contains phoratoxin, a polypeptide with a molecular weight of about 13,000. Experimentally, phoratoxin produces effects in animals that resemble the effects of viscotoxins: hypotension, bradycardia, negative inotropic effects on heart muscle, and vasoconstriction of the vessels of skin and skeletal muscle. Phoratoxin is only one-fifth as active as the viscotoxins (Rosell and Samuelsson, 1988). Viscotoxins are basic polypeptides (molecular weight of about 5000). Serious poisoning from the plants is rare and includes gastrointestinal distress and hypotension.

Vasoconstriction is a primary toxic effect of some plant chemicals. Of the various fungi that produce toxic principles, some are parasitic or symbiotic on grasses used as food by humans and livestock. *Claviceps purpurea* (ergot) is a fungus parasitic on grains of rye. This fungus has caused outbreaks of unusual poisonings in several European countries since the Middle Ages. The condition was called "St. Anthony's fire" from the blackened appearance of the limbs of some sufferers. The main toxic effect of ergot alkaloids is vasoconstriction, primarily in the extremities, followed by gangrene. Abortion in pregnant women is also common after ingestion of contaminated rye flour. Ergot alkaloids are derivatives of lysergic acid. Some of the alkaloids have been used in therapeutics, especially ergotamine and ergonovine.

Another fungus, *Acremonium coenophialum,* grows symbiotically on the forage grass tall fescue (*Festuca arundinacea*) and produces some ergot alkaloids and other lysergic acid derivatives. The fungus causes "fescue toxicosis" in cattle grazing on infected plants (Hill et al., 1994). The condition in cattle includes decreased weight gain, decreased reproductive performance, and peripheral vasoconstriction. In the southwestern United States, *Stirpa robusta* (sleepy grass) also is infected with an *Acremonium* fungus. Horses grazing in areas where the infected perennial grass grows become somnolent, presumably as a result of ingesting lysergic acid amide, ergonovine, and related alkaloids produced by the fungus (Petroski et al., 1992).

Caulophyllum thalictroides (blue cohosh or papoose root, Berberidaceae family) contains a vasoactive glycoside and methylcytisine, causing coronary artery vasoconstriction and uterine stimulation. Toxic effects on the fetal myocardium from maternal ingestion have been reported (Jones and Lawson, 1998).

Liver

Hepatocyte Damage In 1884 cases of "hepatitis" in cattle in Iowa were found to be caused by ingestion of species of *Senecio* (ragwort or groundsel, aster family). *Senecio* is a large genus of plants with worldwide distribution. Species containing significant concentrations of pyrrolizidine alkaloids are responsible for liver damage in the form of hepatic venoocclusive disease. Species of three other genera, *Crotalaria, Heliotropium,* and *Symphytum,* also contain pyrrolizidine alkaloids. *Heliotropium* and *Symphytum* are in the borage family. Different animal species show marked differences in susceptibility to pyrrolizidine alkaloids. Susceptible species are rats, cattle, horses, and chickens; resistant species are guinea pigs, rabbits, gerbils, hamsters, sheep, and Japanese quail. Different susceptibilities are related in general to the rate of hepatic pyrrole formation, although other sources of differences must be present (Huan et al., 1998). Damage to hepatocytes has been proposed to be due to the formation of pyrrole metabolites from the alkaloids by liver microsomes, with cross-linking of DNA strands by the metabolites (Carballo et al., 1992). Human deaths from pyrrolizidine alkaloids have been reported in several countries, including South Africa, Jamaica, and Barbados. In Afghanistan there was an epidemic of hepatic venoocclusive disease from consumption of a wheat crop contaminated with seeds of a species of *Heliotropium* (Tandon et al., 1978). The clinical signs associated with the liver damage resemble those of cirrhosis and some hepatic tumors and may be mistaken for those conditions (McDermott and Ridker, 1990). The clinical condition has been described as a form of the Budd-Chiari syndrome, with portal hypertension and obliteration of small hepatic veins (Ridker et al., 1985). Human consumption also occurs from *Symphytum* and *Senecio* species in some herbal preparations, such as "comfrey tea" or "groundsel tea." Hepatitis in cattle grazing on these plants, most commonly *Senecio,* has been reported in Africa and Asia as well as in the United States. Cows and horses are seriously affected. The condition is progressive, and death occurs after weeks or months of grazing on contaminated pastures. The major toxic alkaloid in *Senecio vulgaris* (common groundsel) is retrorsine; it is jacobine in *Senecio jacobaea* ("stinking willie").

Inhibition of RNA Polymerase Many of the nonedible mushrooms may cause gastrointestinal distress, but most are not life-threatening. Most deaths from mushroom poisoning worldwide are due to liver damage following consumption of *Amanita phalloides,* appropriately called "death cap." *Amanita ocreata* (death angel) is equally dangerous. *A. phalloides* contains two types of toxic chemicals: phalloidin and amatoxins. Phalloidin is a cyclic heptapeptide that may be responsible for some of the diarrhea that develops 10 to 12 h after ingestion of *A. phalloides.* Phalloidin combines with actin in muscle cells to interfere with muscle function but is not readily absorbed from the gastrointestinal tract (Cappell and Hassan, 1992). The amatoxins are bicyclic peptides (molecular weight 900) and are absorbed. The most toxic, alpha-amanitin, has a strong affinity for hepatocytes and binds to RNA polymerase II, thus inhibiting protein synthesis (Jaeger et al., 1993). Serious clinical signs develop slowly, beginning about the third day after ingestion. Treatment in severe cases may require liver transplant; there is no other specific treatment. Administration of silymarin, the active principle of the thistle *Silybum marianum,* in the form of its soluble succinate has been used. Several hypotheses have been proposed for the therapeutic action of silymarin, including free radical scavenging and stimulation of ribosomal RNA polymerase (Flora et al., 1998). Renal lesions are found in cases of severe amanita poisoning, with damage most prominent in proximal tubules. In addition to the amanitas, several species of *Lepiota* (parasol mushrooms) produce amatoxins, notably *Lepiota helveola* and *Lepiota bruneo-incarnata.*

Block of Sphingolipid Biosynthesis Fumonisins are toxins produced by the fungus *Fusarium,* primarily by *Fusarium moniliforme* and *Fusarium proliferatum* growing on corn. Ingestion by horses of corn contaminated with *Fusarium* mold causes "moldy corn poisoning," or equine leukoencephalomalacia. The signs in affected horses are lethargy, ataxia, convulsions, and death (Norred, 1993). There are several target organs, but the liver is a primary target in every species; in horses, it is liver and brain; in pigs, liver and lung; in rats, liver and kidney; in chickens, liver (Riley et al., 1994). In humans, an association with esophageal cancer has been suggested (Yoshizawa et al., 1994). Chemically fumonisins are diesters of propane-1,2,3-tricarboxylic acid and a pentahydroxyicosane containing a primary amino acid (Gurung et al., 1999). The structure of fumonisins is similar to that of sphingosine, and their toxicity has been proposed to be related to the blocking of enzymes in sphingolipid biosynthesis (Norred, 1993).

Lantadene Toxicity *Lantana camara* (Verbenaceae family) has been described as one of the 10 most noxious weeds in the world. It is an attractive flowering shrub, native to Jamaica and commonly cultivated in greenhouses. *L. camara* thrives outdoors in hot, dry climates. An unusual property of the plant is that it inhibits the growth of neighboring plants. In India, livestock poisoning from *L. camara* is a serious problem. Cattle grazing on the plant develop cholestasis and hyperbilirubinemia. The leaves are toxic to some nonruminants, including rabbits and guinea pigs. Several triterpenoids have been isolated from the plant. One that has been shown to induce hepatotoxicity is lantadene A (22-beta-angeloyloxy-3-oxo-olean-12-en-28-oic acid) (Sharma et al., 1991).

Kidney and Bladder

Carcinogenic Chemicals Bracken fern (*Pteridium aquilinum*) grows worldwide and, in the United States, primarily east of the Rocky Mountains. It has been described as one of the five most common plants on the planet and is found locally in heavy concentrations. Bracken fern is the only higher plant known to cause cancer in animals under natural conditions of feeding. The commonest bladder tumors in cattle are epithelial and mesenchymal neoplasms (Kim and Lee, 1998). The major carcinogen is reported to be ptaquiloside, a norsesquiterpene glucoside present in high concentrations in bracken, especially in crosiers and young unfolding fronds. Ptaquiloside alkylates adenines and guanines of DNA (Shakin et al., 1999). It has been proposed that human consumption of bracken fern leads to an increased incidence of esophageal and stomach cancers, based on geographic association of consumption of the fern and cancer incidence.

Kidney Tubular Degeneration Species of *Xanthium* (cocklebur, aster family) are annual plants found in several countries. Toxicosis in livestock is most common in spring and early summer due to ingestion of seedlings and young plants. Pigs, sheep, cattle, horses, and fowl can be affected in pastures where two- and four-leaf seedlings are present. The clinical signs are depression and dyspnea. Pathologic findings include tubular degeneration and necrosis in the kidney and centrilobular necrosis in the liver (del Carmen Mendez et al., 1998).

Most deaths from mushroom poisoning are due to fulminant hepatic failure from *Amanita*-type mushrooms. However, acute renal failure is the cause of death in poisoning from *Cortinarius* species. *Cortinarius* is a large genus of woodland fungi, found especially in northern conifer forests. Species vary widely in habit and in edibility. In one series of poisonings from *Cortinarius orellanus* and related species involving 135 cases in which the mushrooms were eaten, deaths secondary to acute renal failure occurred in almost 15 percent of the cases. Renal biopsy showed acute degenerative tubular lesions with inflammatory interstitial fibrosis (Bouget et al., 1990).

Blood

Anticoagulants Fungal infections in sweet clover (*Melilotus alba*) silage and hay have caused serious toxicity and death in cattle in the northern plains of the United States and Canada and, more recently, in California (Puschner et al., 1998). Deaths are from hemorrhages caused by dicumarol, a fungal metabolite. Dicumarol [3,3′-methylene-bis(4-hydroxycoumarin)] is an effective anticoagulant, causing prothrombin deficiency, and has been used therapeutically for this purpose.

Cyanogenic Chemicals Cyanogens are constituents of several different kinds of plants. One that is present in the kernels of apples, cherries, peaches, and related genera in the rose family is amygdalin, found in the highest amounts in the seeds of the bitter almond *Prunus amygdalus,* var. *amara.* Amygdalin is not present in the seeds of the sweet almond, the nut used for food. The amount of cyanogen in peach (*Prunus persica*) kernels is enough to cause poisoning in small children if several kernels are eaten. The small seeds of apples are unlikely to present a problem. In the stomach, amygdalin releases hydrocyanic acid, which combines with ferric ion in cytochrome oxidase or methemoglobin. The result of ingestion of several bitter almond seeds is classic cyanide poisoning with death as in asphyxia.

Cassava is a staple food starch from *Manihot esculenta* (Euphorbiaceae family), which is grown extensively in some parts of Africa as a major food source. The untreated root contains linamarin, a cyanogenic glucoside. During processing of the root for human consumption, the cyanogen is removed. However, local processing may be inadequate. Chronic ingestion of linamarin in cassava has been proposed as the cause of epidemics of konzo, a form of tropical myelopathy with sudden onset of spastic paralysis (Tylleskar et al., 1992). Degeneration of the corticospinal motor pathway in affected individuals may be caused by production of thiocyanate from linamarin and stimulation of neuronal glutamate receptors by thiocyanate (Spencer, 1999). Another plant containing linamarin is flax, *Linum usitatissumum,* the seed of which is the source of linseed oil. In some European countries, as a domestic remedy, linseeds are soaked overnight and the extract is used as a laxative, exposing these individuals to cyanide from the linamarin (Rosling, 1993).

Central and Autonomic Nervous Systems

Excessive stimulation of neurons results in toxic signs varying with the specific receptors involved. Permanent damage to the nervous system is a serious consequence of excessive neuronal stimulation.

Epileptiform Seizures The parsley family of plants (Apiaceae or Umbelliferae) contains some of the most edible (for example, carrots) and some of the most poisonous plants in the northern hemisphere. The fleshy tubers of *Cicuta maculata* (water hemlock) may be mistaken for other edible wild tubers. A single tuber may cause fatal poisoning, characterized by tonic-clonic convulsions. The toxic principle, cicutoxin (a C_{17}-polyacetylene), has been shown to be a potent blocker of potassium channels of T lymphocytes (Strauss et al., 1996). A similar action on potassium channels of neurons could account for the central nervous system effects.

Several members of the mint family (Labiatae) are noted for their pleasant essential oils, such as pennyroyal (*Hedeoma*), sage (*Salvia*), and hyssop (*Hyssopus*). These oils contain monoterpenes. For example, sage contains thujone, camphor, and cineole. In high doses, taken orally, well above amounts used for flavoring, these monoterpenes can cause tonic-clonic convulsions (Burkhard et al., 1999).

Excitatory Amino Acids Widely divergent species of plants produce amino acids that mimic the action of glutamate on the central nervous system. Most fast excitatory transmission in the mammalian brain is mediated by inotropic receptors for the amino acid glutamate on specialized neurons. Three types of glutamate receptors are named after three different agonists: AMPA (alpha-amino-3-hydroxyl-5-methyl-4-isoxazolepropionate), NMDA (*N*-methyl-D-aspartate), and kainate [kainic acid, 2-carboxy-4-(1-methyleney1)-3-pyrrolidine acetic acid] receptors. The excitatory amino acids (EAAs) from plants act on one or more of these glutamate receptor subtypes. The consequence of ingestion of EAAs is excessive stimulation, which may result in death of neurons. Kainic acid is present in the marine red alga *Digenia simplex.* Under some climatic conditions, the algae reproduce rapidly, causing a "red tide." Filter-feeding mussels eat the algae and humans may be poisoned by eating the mussels. A similar problem exists with the green alga *Chondria aranta,* growing in northern oceans. The alga produces domoic acid, a tricarboxylic amino acid, as does the marine diatom *Nitzschia pungens.* In 1987 there was a serious outbreak of poisoning in Canada in individuals eating mussels containing domoic acid. The acute symptoms were gastrointestinal distress, headache, hemiparesis, confusion, and seizures. Prolonged effects were severe memory deficits and sensorimotor neuronopathy (Teitelbaum et al., 1990). The action of domoic acid is to release glutamate by activating presynaptic kainate- or AMPA-type receptors (Scallet and Ye, 1997).

The fungus *Amanita muscaria* (fly agaric) got its name from its poisonous actions on flies. Poisoning from this woodland mushroom and from *Amanita pantherina* (panther agaric, common in western United States) is due to the content of the EAA, ibotenic acid, and possibly to its derivative, muscimol. The effects are somewhat variable: central nervous system depression, ataxia, hysteria, and hallucinations. Myoclonic twitching and seizures sometimes develop (Benjamin, 1992). The content of ibotenic acid varies with the time of year—more has been reported in spring than in fall.

EAAs are also found in flowering plants. The pea family (Leguminosae) contains several species that produce EAAs in the seeds. Willardiine [1-(2-amino-2-carboxyethyl) pyrimidine-2,4-dione] has been isolated from *Acacia willardiana, Acacia lemmoni, Acacia millefolia,* and *Mimosa asperata* (Gmelin, 1961). Willardiine acts as an agonist on the AMPA and kainate receptors (Jane et al., 1997). Other important EAAs are present in species of *Lathyrus. Lathyrus sylvestris* (flat pea) is a perennial indigenous to Europe and central Asia and naturalized in Canada and the northern United States. The plant is eaten by livestock in these areas. An acute neurologic condition in sheep begins with weakness and progresses to tremors and prostration, sometimes with clonic movements and seizures (Rasmussen et al., 1993). The seeds contain DABA (2,4-diaminobutyric acid) and lower quantities of BOAA (beta-*N*-oxalylamino-L-alanine). Both DABA and BOAA are excitatory neurotoxins acting on the AMPA-type receptor. Seeds of *Lethyrus sativus* (chickling pea) contain more BOAA than DABA, and the seeds of this plant are used as food by humans in parts of Africa. Lathyrism is a condition developing from consumption of large quantities of *L. sativus* seeds over periods of months or longer. Affected individuals have corticospinal motor neuron degeneration with severe spastic muscle weakness and atrophy but little sensory involvement (Spencer et al., 1986).

Mannosidase Inhibitors Swainsonine is an indolizidine alkaloid found in *Swainsonia canescens,* an Australian plant, and in *Astragalus lentiginosus* (spotted locoweed) and *Oxytropis sericea* (locoweed) in the western United States. Cattle consume these weeds in pasture. The common name comes from the most obvious consequence of ingestion of the locoweeds: abberrant behavior with hyperexcitability and locomotor difficulty. In animals dying from locoweed poisoning there is cytoplasmic foamy vacuolation of cerebellar neurons. The toxic ingredient, swainsonine, causes marked inhibition of liver lysosomal and cytosomal alpha-mannosidase and Golgi mannosidase II. Inhibition of the Golgi enzyme results in abnormal brain glycoproteins and accumulation of mannose-rich oligosaccharides (Tulsiani et al., 1988). The pathology is not limited to the nervous system, and the effects of swainsonine poisoning are found in several tissues. A major effect in animals grazing at high altitudes is congestive heart failure. The condition has been called "high mountain disease" (James et al., 1991).

Motor Neuron Demyelination Paralysis develops from some toxins without primary excitation of neurons. *Karwinskia humboldtiana,* family Rhamnaceae, is a shrub of the southwestern United States, Mexico, and Central America. Common names are buckthorn, coyotillo, and tullidora. Anthracenones are found in the seeds, varying with growth; green fruit may be more toxic than ripe fruit (Bermudez et al., 1986). Both human and livestock poisonings occur, occasionally in epidemic proportions. The clinical syndrome that develops after a latency of several days is ascending flaccid paralysis, beginning with demyelination of large motor neurons in the lower legs and, in fatal cases, leading to bulbar paralysis (Martinez et al., 1998). Sensory fibers are largely spared. In addition to neurotoxicity, the anthracenones in *Karwinskia,* especially peroxisomicine A_2 [3,39-dimethyl-3,39,8,89,9,99- hexahydroxy-3,30,4,49-tetrahydro-(7,10-bianthracene)-1,19-2H,29H-dione], cause atelectasis and emphysema in lungs and massive liver necrosis. Inhibition of catalase in peroxisomes has been proposed as a mechanism for the cellular toxicity (Martinez et al., 1997).

Parasympathetic Stimulation Several plant alkaloids affect the autonomic nervous system, mimicking or blocking the transmitter acetylcholine at autonomic ganglia (nicotinic receptors) or the peripheral endings of the parasympathetic system (muscarinic receptors). The postsynaptic receptors at terminations of the parasympathetic nerve fibers are called "muscarinic" after the selective stimulation of these receptors by muscarine, which was first extracted from the mushroom *Amanita muscaria.* However, this mushroom contains only trace amounts of muscarine, and poisoning is due to its content of ibotenic acid. Some mushrooms of the genera *Inocybe, Clitocybe,* and *Omphalatus* contain significant amounts of muscarine, and consumption of toxic species causes diarrhea, sweating, salivation, and lacrimation, all referable to stimulation of parasympathetic receptors (de Haro et al., 1999).

Parasympathetic Block The belladonna alkaloids (l-hyoscyamine, atropine or *d,l*-hyoscyamine, and scopolamine), present in several genera of plants of the family Solanaceae, are best known for their block of muscarinic receptors. The plants are widely distributed and have had a place in the materia medica of many cultures. *Datura stramonium* (jimsonweed) is native to India and contains primarily scopolamine; *Hyoscyamus niger* (henbane) is native to Europe and contains mostly l-hyoscyamine; *Atropa belladonna* (deadly nightshade), also native to Europe, contains atropine; *Duboisia myoporoides* (pituri) in Australia contains l-hyoscyamine. Of the two active alkaloids, l-hyoscyamine and scopolamine, the latter has greater action on the central nervous system, while l-hyoscyamine acts primarily to block muscarinic receptors of the parasympathetic nervous system. The effects of modest doses of l-hyoscyamine or atropine are referable to muscarinic block: tachycardia, dry mouth, dilated pupils, and decreased gastrointestinal motility. Large doses of either or of scopolamine affect the central nervous system: confusion, bizarre behavior, hallucinations, and subsequent amnesia. Deaths are rare, although recovery may take several days. *Datura* (*Brugmansia*) *suaveolens* (angel's trumpet) is used as an ornamental houseplant and contains significant quantities of atropine and scopolamine (Smith et al., 1991). Seeds of the weed *Datura ferox* contain belladonna alkaloids and are contaminants of animal feed in some parts of Europe. In areas where seeds for human consumption are not carefully sorted before milling and where *Datura stramonium* and *Datura metel* are common weeds, millet, wheat, rye, corn and beans sometimes are contaminated with the seeds. The amount needed to poison an adult is about 20 seeds. Symptoms from eating bread made from contaminated flour are typical of poisoning from belladonna alkaloids (van Meurs et al., 1992). An unusual source of belladonna poisoning has been reported from eating wasp honey. Some wasps (*Polistes* species) store enough honey to attract humans to steal their honey. Atropine-like poisoning has been reported from consuming the honey when the wasps have gathered nectar from *Datura inoxia* (Ramirez et al., 1999).

The seeds of *Solanum dulcamara* (woody nightshade, bittersweet) are brilliant orange-red and are gathered for flower arrangements in the fall. The seeds contain solanine, a glycoalkaloid, responsible for the acute toxicity from ingested seeds, including tachycardia, dilated pupils, and hot, dry skin, as in atropine poisoning (Ceha et al., 1997).

Skeletal Muscle and Neuromuscular Junction

Neuromuscular Junction Block Block of the neuromuscular junction of skeletal muscle may result from either block of postsynaptic acetylcholine (nicotinic) receptors by an antagonist or by an agonist causing excessive stimulation of the receptor followed by prolonged depolarization. Nicotine, for which the receptor is named, stimulates autonomic ganglia as well as the neuromuscular junction. An isomer of nicotine, anabasine ($C_{10}H_{14}N_2$), present in *Nicotiana glauca* (tree tobacco), produces prolonged depolarization of the junction. Consumption of the leaves of the plant has caused severe, generalized muscle weakness and respiratory compromise, following flexor muscle spasm and gastrointestinal irritation (Mellick et al., 1999). Curare, the South American arrow poison, is a potent neuromuscular blocking agent for skeletal muscle and kills by stopping respiration. Paralysis is due to block of acetylcholine at the postsynaptic junction. Curare is obtained from tropical species of *Strychnos* and *Chondrodendron.* However, not all plants producing chemicals that block acetylcholine are of tropical origin. In warm weather, blooms of blue-green algae are not uncommon in farm ponds in temperate regions, particularly ponds enriched with fertilizer. Under these conditions, one species of alga, *Anabaena flos-aquae,* produces a neurotoxin, anatoxin A, which depolarizes and blocks acetylcholine receptors, both nicotinic and muscarinic, causing death in animals that drink the pond water. The lethal effects develop rapidly, with death in minutes to hours from respiratory arrest (Short and Edwards, 1990). Anatoxin A is 2-acetyl-9-azabicyclo [4.2.1] non-2-ene (Hyde and Carmichael, 1991).

Methyllycaconitine is a norditerpenoid present in *Delphinium barbeyi* (tall larkspur) and some related species. The plant contaminates western pastures in the United States and causes death of livestock. Poisoned cattle show muscle tremors, ataxia, and prostration and die from respiratory failure. The alkaloid has a high affinity for the acetylcholine receptor and causes death by blocking the action of acetylcholine at the neuromuscular junction, much as curare does (Dobelis et al., 1999). Physostigmine has been used successfully as an antagonist in some cases of methyllycaconitine poisoning (Pfister et al., 1994). Methyllycaconitine is being used experimentally as a selective probe for discriminating different acetylcholine-binding sites in the brain (Davies et al., 1999).

Skeletal Muscle Damage Direct damage to skeletal muscle fibers has been demonstrated in some plant poisonings. Species of *Thermopsis* (family Leguminosae) grow commonly in the foothills of the Rocky Mountains. Mature seeds of these plants form attractive pods, as in many legumes. Seeds of the poisonous species of *Thermopsis* contain quinolizidine alkaloids, principally anagyrine and thermopsine. Human poisoning from eating the seeds is rare, but cases have been reported in young children (Spoerke et al., 1988). The symptoms in children are abdominal cramps, nausea, vomiting, and headache lasting up to 24 h. Serious poisoning has occurred in livestock grazing on *Thermopsis montana* (false lupine). The animals develop locomotor depression with prolonged recumbency. Microscopic areas of necrosis in skeletal muscle are found on autopsy (Keeler and Baker, 1990).

Among the common contaminants of animal feeds are seeds of *Cassia obtusifolia* (sicklepod, family Leguminosae). Consumption of the seeds of *C. obtusifolia* causes illness in cattle, swine, and chickens. The toxic effect is a degenerative myopathy of cardiac and skeletal muscle. It has been shown that extracts of *C. obtusifolia* inhibit NADH-oxidoreductase activity in bovine and porcine heart mitochondria in vitro (Lewis and Shibamoto, 1989), possibly related to the anthraquinone content of the seeds.

Bone

Soft Tissue Calcification In 1967, Worker and Carrillo proposed that a decrease of bone calcification and wasting in cattle grazing along the eastern coastal plains of South America was due to the consumption of *Solanum malacoxylon* (nightshade family, Solanaceae). They recognized the association of the presence of the plant in the fields with the condition. The disease, known in Argentina as *enteque seco,* is characterized by calcification of the entire vascular system, especially the heart and aorta. Lungs, joint cartilage, and kidney are also affected in the worst cases. Sheep and cows are both affected by ingestion of the plant. The general picture resembles vitamin D intoxication. A water-soluble vitamin D–like substance, a glycoside of 1,25-dihydroxycholecalciferol, has been isolated from the plant (Skliar et al., 1992).

Cestrum diurnum (day-blooming jasmine) causes hypercalcemia and extensive soft tissue calcification in grazing animals in Florida, resembling the action of *S. malacoxylon.* A dihydroxyvitamin D_3 glycoside in the leaves is the toxic agent (Durand et al., 1999). *Cestrum laevigatum* causes a similar deposition of calcium in chickens (Mello and Habermehl, 1992). The plant is occasionally a contaminant of hay in Europe. However, ingestion of the dried plant by cattle results primarily in liver damage (van der Lugt et al., 1991).

Reproductive System and Teratogenesis

Embryo loss and teratogenesis in herbivores caused by ingestion of some plants are serious factors in livestock production worldwide. The types of plants and the abortifacient or teratogenic chemicals they contain are diverse.

Teratogens *Veratrum californicum* is native to the mountains of North America where sheep are grazed. An incidence of teratogenesis as high as 25 percent has been reported in pregnant sheep in these areas, along with an incidence of early embryonic death as high as 75 percent (Keeler, 1990). The teratogenic manifestations are dependent on the developmental stage at the time of ingestion, as with many teratogens. Malformations in the offspring involve cyclopia, exencephaly, and microphthalmia. During the fourth and fifth weeks of gestation, limb defects are common; on gestational days 31 to 33, the result of ingestion is stenosis of the trachea (Omnell et al., 1990). The alkaloids in *Veratrum* that are responsible for the defects are jervine, 11-deoxojervine, and 3-*O*-glucosyl-11-deoxojervine. Although there is species difference in sensitivity, birth defects occur in cows and goats grazing on *Veratrum californicum* and can be produced experimentally in chickens, rabbits, rats, and mice (Omnell et al., 1990), hamsters (Gaffield and Keeler, 1993), and rainbow trout embryos (Crawford and Kocan, 1993). The *Veratrum* alkaloids are teratogenic by blocking cholesterol synthesis and thus the response of fetal target tissue to a gene locus (sonic hedgehog locus, Shh). The Shh locus has a role in developmental patterning of head and brain, and block of cholesterol synthesis has been shown experimentally to result in loss of midline facial structures (Cooper et al., 1998).

A cluster of fetal malformations characterized by deformation of limbs and spinal cord is found after ingestion of several related alkaloids from different species of plants during a sensitive gestational period. This syndrome has been found in cattle grazing on *Lupinus caudatus* and *Lupinus formosus* (lupines), *Nicotiana glauca* (tree tobacco), and *Conium maculatum* (poison hemlock), known historically as the plant that Socrates drank when condemned to death by the Athenians. The fatal actions of the poison in that instance are described by Plato in the *Phaedo* dialogue. The active alkaloids in these plants have been identified as anagyrine (*L. caudatus*), ammodendrine (*L. formosus*), anabasine (*N. glauca*), and coniine (*C. maculatum*). It has been proposed that these alkaloids depress fetal movements during susceptible gestational periods and in this way cause malformations (Lopez et al., 1999). Not all species are equally affected by coniine. Notably, rats and hamsters do not show teratogenesis in response to coniine but goat and chick embryos are susceptible (Forsyth et al., 1996).

Abortifacients The active alkaloid in the legumes *Astragalus* and *Oxytropus* is swainsonine. In addition to actions on the nervous system, swainsonine frequently causes abortions when locoweeds are ingested by pregnant livestock (Bunch et al., 1992). Two genera of tropical legumes, *Leucaena* and *Mimosa,* contain a toxic amino acid, mimosine [beta-*N*(3-hydroxy-4-pyridone)-alpha-aminoproprionic acid]. Mimosine is found in large amounts in foliage and seeds of *L. leucocephala, L. glauca* and *M. pudica.* In cattle the amino acid causes incoordinated gait, goiter and reproductive disturbances including infertility and fetal death (Kulp et al., 1996). Mimosine arrests the cell cycle after cells enter S phase (Hughes and Cook, 1996).

Lectins that are ribosome-inactivating proteins may have many biological effects when ingested, including antifertility, abortifacient, and embryotoxic actions. A lectin from bitter melon seeds (*Momordica charantia,* family Cucurbitaceae) has been shown to have such effects. The lectins are alpha- and beta-momorcharins, single-chain glycoproteins with molecular weights of about 29,000.

The momorcharins are known to induce midterm abortion in humans (Wang and Ng, 1998).

SUMMARY

A great number of toxic chemicals have been produced by plants for their own protection from the environment and from predators, including pathogenic organisms. The list of these defensive chemicals is steadily growing in the scientific literature and not all the chemicals are deleterious to humans. Throughout history a select number have been incorporated into therapy against disease and to combat morbidity, often with considerable success. Morphine from the latex of the opium poppy is an ancient historical example. If fungi are included with plants (as they are in this chapter), defensive chemicals of plants are responsible for some of our more recent successful therapies, such as antibiotics of the penicillin type and new treatments for cancer. On balance, in spite of the long list of potentially dangerous agents, it is fair to conclude that toxic chemicals from plants have proved more useful than harmful to humans. Finally, there is simply the pleasure of scientific inquiry into the successful adaptations of plants to their complex and often hostile environments.

REFERENCES

Abbott AJ, Holoubek CG, Martin RA: Inhibition of Na^+,K^+-ATPase by the cardenolide 6′-O-(E-4-hydroxycinnamoyl) desglucouzarin. *Biochim Biophys Res Comm* 251:256–259, 1998.

Alenius H, Kalkkinen N, Reunala T, et al: The main IgE-binding epitope of a major latex allergen, prohevein, is present in its N-terminal 43-amino acid fragment, hevein. *J Immunol* 156:1618–1625, 1996.

Appendino G, Szallasi A: Euphorbium: Modern research on its active principle, resiniferatoxin, revives an ancient medicine. *Life Sci* 60:681–696, 1997.

Bantel H, Engels IH, Voelter W, et al: Mistletoe lectin activates caspase-8/FLICE independently of death receptor signaling and enhances anticancer drug-induced apoptosis. *Cancer Res* 59:2038–2090, 1999.

Benjamin DR: Mushroom poisoning in infants and children. *J Toxicol Clin Toxicol* 30:13–22, 1992.

Bermudez MV, Gonzalez-Spencer D, Guerrero M, et al: Experimental intoxication with fruit and purified toxins of buckthorn (*Karwinskia humboldtiana*). *Toxicon* 24:1091–1097, 1986.

Blackwell WH: *Poisonous and Medicinal Plants.* Englewood Cliffs, NJ: Prentice-Hall, 1990, p 243.

Blanc P, Liu D, Juarez C, et al: Cough in hot pepper workers. *Chest* 99:27–32, 1991.

Blanco C, Diaz-Perales A, Collada C, et al: Class I chitinases as potential panallergens involved in the latex-fruit syndrome. *J Allergy Clin Immunol* 103(pt 1):507–513, 1999.

Bouget J, Bousser J, Pats B, et al: Acute renal failure following collective intoxication by *Cortinarius orellanus. Intens Care Med* 16:506–510, 1990.

Bunch TD, Panter KD, James LK: Ultrasound studies of the effects of certain poisonous plants on uterine function and fetal development in livestock. *J Anim Sci* 70:1639–1643, 1992.

Burke JW, Doskotch RW: High field 1 H- and 13 C-NMR assignments of grayanotoxins I, IV and XIV isolated from *Kalmia angustifolia. J Nat Prod* 53:131–137, 1990.

Burkhard PR, Burkhardt K, Haenggeli C-A, et al: Plant-induced seizures: Reappearance of an old problem. *J Neurol* 246:667–670, 1999.

Cappell MS, Hassan T: Gastrointestinal and hepatic effects of *Amanita phalloides* ingestion. *J Clin Gastroenterol* 15:225–228, 1992.

Carballo M, Mudry MD, Larripa IB, et al: Genotoxic action of an aqueous extract of *Heliotropium curassavicum* var *argentinum. Mutat Res* 279:245–253, 1992.

Casteel SW, Johnson GC, Wagstaff DJ: *Aesculus glabra* intoxication in cattle. *Vet Hum Toxicol* 34:55, 1992.

Casteel SW, Wagstaff DJ: *Rhododendron macrophyllum* poisoning in a group of sheep and goats. *Vet Hum Toxicol* 31:176–177, 1989.

Ceha LJ, Presperin C, Young E, et al: Anticholinergic toxicity from nightshade berry poisoning responsive to physostigmine. *J Emerg Med* 15:65–69, 1997.

Chan TYF, Tomlinson B, Critchley JAJH, et al: Herb-induced aconitine poisoning presenting as tetraplegia. *Vet Hum Toxicol* 36:133–134, 1994.

Christensen LP, Kristiansen K: Isolation and quantification of tuliposides and tulipalins in tulips (*Tulipa*) by high-performance liquid chromatography. *Contact Dermatitis* 40:300–309, 1999.

Clark RF, Selden BS, Curry SC: Digoxin-specific Fab fragments in the treatment of oleander toxicity in a canine model. *Ann Emerg Med* 20:1073–1077, 1991.

Cooper MK, Porter JA, Young RE, et al: Teratogen-mediated inhibition of target tissue response to Shh signalling. *Science* 280:1603–1610, 1998.

Crawford L, Kocan RM: Steroidal alkaloid toxicity to fish embryos. *Toxicol Lett* 66:175–181, 1993.

Czeczuga B: Carotenoids, in Galun M (ed): *Handbook of Lichenology.* Vol III. Boca Raton, FL: CRC Press, 1988, p 25.

Davies ARL, Hardick DJ, Blagbrough JS, et al: Characterization of the binding of [^{3}H]methyllycaconitine: A new radioligand for labelling alpha-7-type neuronal nicotinic acetylcholine receptors. *Neuropharmacology* 38:679–690, 1999.

de Haro L, Prost N, David JM, et al: Syndrome sudorien ou muscarinien. *Presse Med* 28:1069–1070, 1999.

del Carmen Mendez M, dos Santos RS, Riet-Correa F: Intoxication by *Xanthium cavanillesii* in cattle and sheep in southern Brazil. *Vet Hum Toxicol* 40:144–147, 1998.

Dobelis P, Madl JE, Pfister JA, et al: Effects of *Delphinium* alkaloids on neuromuscular transmission. *J Pharmacol Exp Ther* 291:538–546, 1999.

Dubois B, Peumons WJ, vam Damme EJM, et al: Regulation of gelatinase B (MMP-9) in leukocytes by plant lectins. *FEBS Lett* 427:275–278, 1998.

Durand R, Figueredo JM, Mendoza E: Intoxication in cattle from *Cestrum diurnum. Vet Hum Toxicol* 41:26–27, 1999.

Ernst E, Rand JI, Barnes J, et al: Adverse effects profile of the herbal antidepressant St. John's wort. *Eur J Clin Pharmacol* 54:589–594, 1998.

Fett-Netto AG, DiCosmo F: Distribution and amounts of taxol in different shoot parts of *Taxus cuspidata. Planta Med* 58:464–466, 1992.

Flora K, Hahn M, Rosen H, et al: Milk thistle (*Silybum marianum*) for the therapy of liver disease. *Am J Gastroenterol* 93:139–143, 1998.

Forsyth CS, Speth RC, Wecker L, et al: Comparison of nicotinic receptor binding and biotransformation of coniine in the rat and chick. *Toxicol Lett* 89:175–183, 1996.

Frasca T, Brett AS, Yoo SD: Mandrake toxicity. *Arch Intern Med* 157:2007–2009, 1997.

Frohn A, Frohn C, Steuhl KP et al: Wolfsmilchveratzung. *Ophthalmology* 90:58–61, 1993.

Gaffield W, Keeler RF: Implications of C-5, C-6 unsaturation as a key structural factor in steroidal alkaloid-induced mammalian teratogenesis. *Experientia* 49:922–924, 1993.

Gmelin R: Isolierung von Willardiin [3-(1-uracyl)-L-alanin] aus den samen von *Acacia millefolia, Acacia lemmoni* and *Mimosa asperata. Acta Chem Scand* 15:1188–1189, 1961.

Gude M, Hausen MD, Heitsch H, et al: An investigation of the irritant and allergenic properties of daffodils (*Narcissus pseudonarcissus* L., Amaryllidaceae): A review of daffodil dermatitis. *Contact Dermatitis* 19:1–10, 1988.

Gurung NK, Rankens DL, Shelby RA: In vitro ruminal disappearance of fumonisin B_1 and its effects on in vitro dry matter disappearance. *Vet Hum Toxicol* 41:196–199, 1999.

Hausen BM, Prater E, Shubert H: The sensitizing capacity of *Alstroemeria* cultivars in man and guinea pig. *Contact Dermatitis* 9:46–54, 1983.

Heilpern KL: *Zigadenus* poisoning. *Ann Emerg Med* 25:259–262, 1995.

Hill NS, Thompson FN, Dawe DL, et al: Antibody binding by circulating ergot alkaloids in cattle grazing tall fescue. *Am J Vet Res* 55:419–424, 1994.

Hirschwehr R, Heppner C, Spitzauer S, et al: Allergens, IgE, mediators, inflammatory mechanisms. *J Allergy Clin Immunol* 101:196–206, 1998.

Huan J-Y, Mironda CL, Buhler DR, et al: Species differences in the hepatic microsomal enzyme metabolism of the pyrrolizidine alkaloids. *Toxicol Lett* 99:127–137, 1998.

Hughes TA, Cook PR: Mimosine arrests the cell cycle after cells enter S-phase. *Exp Cell Res* 222:275–280, 1996.

Hyde EG, Carmichael WW: Anatoxin-a(s), a naturally occurring organophosphate, is an irreversible active site-directed inhibitor of acetylcholinesterase (E.C.3.1.1.7). *J Biochem Toxicol* 6:195–201, 1991.

Jaeger A, Jehl F, Flesch F, et al: Kinetics of amatoxins in human poisoning: Therapeutic implications. *Clin Toxicol* 31:63–80, 1993.

Jaffe AM, Gephardt D, Courtemanche L: Poisoning due to ingestion of *Veratrum viride* (false hellebore). *J Emerg Med* 8:161–167, 1990.

James LF, Panter KE, Broquist HP, et al: Swainsonine-induced high mountain disease in calves. *Vet Hum Toxicol* 33:217–219, 1991.

Jane DE, Hoo K, Komboj R, et al: Synthesis of willardiine and 6-azawillardiine analogs: Pharmacological characterization on cloned homomeric human AMPA and kainate receptor subtypes. *J Med Chem* 40:3645–3650, 1997.

Johnson RA, Baer H, Kirkpatrick CH, et al: Comparison of the contact allergenicity of the four pentadecylcatechols derived from poison ivy urushiol in human subjects. *J Allergy Clin Dermatol* 49:27–35, 1972.

Jones TK, Lawson BM: Profound neonatal congestive heart failure caused by maternal consumption of blue cohosh herbal medication. *J Pediatr* 132:550–552, 1998.

Kalish RS, Johnson KL: Enrichment and function of urushiol (poison ivy)–specific T lymphocytes in lesions of allergic contact dermatitis to urushiol. *J Immunol* 145:3706–3713, 1990.

Keeler RF: Early embryonic death in lambs induced by *Veratrum californicum. Cornell Vet* 80:203–207, 1990.

Keeler RF, Baker DC: Myopathy in cattle induced by alkaloid extracts from *Thermopsis montana, Laburnum anagyroides* and a *Lupinus* sp. *J Comp Pathol* 103:169–182, 1990.

Keeler RF, Panter KE: Piperidine alkaloid composition and relation to crooked calf disease-inducing potential of *Lupinus formosus. Teratology* 40:423–432, 1989.

Kelch WJ, Kerr LA, Adair HS, et al: Suspected buttercup (*Ranunculus bulbosus*) toxicosis with secondary photosensitization in a Charolais heifer. *Vet Hum Toxicol* 34:238–239, 1992.

Kim D-Y, Lee Y-S: Ovine copper poisoning and *Pteridium aquilinum*–associated bovine urinary bladder tumor in Korea. *J Toxicol Soc* 23(suppl 4):645–646, 1998.

Knight TE: Philodendron-induced dermatitis: Report of cases and review of the literature. *Cutis* 48:375–378, 1991.

Krenzelok EP, Jacobsen TD, Aronis JM: Poinsettia exposures have good outcomes . . . just as we thought. *Am J Emerg Med* 14:671–674, 1996.

Kulp KS, Valliet PR, Richard P: Mimosine blocks cell cycle progression by chelating iron in asynchronous human breast cancer cells. *Toxicol Appl Pharmacol* 139:356–364, 1996.

Lewis DC, Shibamoto T: Effects of *Cassia obtusifolia* (sicklepod) extracts and anthraquinones on muscle mitochondrial function. *Toxicon* 27:519–529, 1989.

Lin T-J, Hsu C-I, Lee K-H, et al: Two outcomes of acute tung nut (*Aleurites fordii*) poisoning. *Clin Toxicol* 34:87–92, 1996.

Lopez TA, Cid MS, Bianchini ML: Biochemistry of hemlock (*Conium maculatum* L) alkaloids and their acute and chronic toxicity in livestock: A review. *Toxicon* 37:841–865, 1999.

Lovborg U, Baker PJ, Taylor DJM, et al: Subtribe-specific monoclonal antibodies to *Lolium perenne. Clin Exp Allergy* 29:973–981, 1999.

Martinez FJ, Duron RR, deTorres NW, et al: Experimental evidence for toxic damage induced by a dimeric anthracenons: Diast T-514 (peroxisomicine A_2). *Toxicol Lett* 90:155–162, 1997.

Martinez HR, Bermudez MV, Rangel-Guerra RA, et al: Clinical diagnosis in *Karwinskia humboldtiana* polyneuropathy. *J Neurol Sci* 154:49–54, 1998.

Massermanian A: Contact dermatitis due to *Euphorbia pulcherrima* Willd, simulating a phototoxic reaction. *Contact Derm* 38:113–114, 1998.

McDermott WV, Ridker PM: The Budd-Chiari syndrome and hepatic veno-occlusive disease. *Arch Surg* 125:525–527, 1990.

McGovern TW, Barkley TM: Botanical briefs: Chrysanthemum—*Dendranthema* spp. *Cutis* 63:319–320, 1999.

McGrath-Hill CA, Vicas JM: Case series of *Thermopsis* exposures. *Clin Toxicol* 35:659–665, 1997.

McIntire MS, Guest JR, Porterfield JF: Philodendron—An infant death. *J Toxicol Clin Toxicol* 28:177–183, 1990.

Mellick LB, Makowski T, Mellick GA, et al: Neuromuscular blockade after ingestion of tree tobacco (*Nicotiana glauca*). *Ann Emerg Med* 34:101–104, 1999.

Mello JR, Habermehl GG: Calcinogenic plants and the incubation effect of rumen fluid. *Dtsch Tierarztl Wochenschr* 99:371–376, 1992.

Mendis S: Colchicine cardiotoxicity following ingestion of *Gloriosa superba* tubers. *Postgrad Med J* 65:752–755, 1989.

Monzingo AF, Collins EJ, Ernst SR, et al: The 2.5A structure of pokeweed antiviral protein. *J Mol Biol* 233:705–715, 1993.

Murai M, Kimura I, Kimura M: Blocking effects of hypaconitine and aconitine on nerve action potentials in phrenic nerve-diaphragm muscles of mice. *Neuropharmacology* 29:567–572, 1990.

Narahashi T: Modulators acting on sodium and calcium channels: Patch-clamp analysis. *Adv Neurol* 44:211–224, 1986.

Nohara T, Yohara S, Kinjo J: Bioactive saponins from solanaceous and leguminous plants. *Adv Exp Med Biol* 404:263–267, 1996.

Norred WP: Fumonisins—Mycotoxins produced by *Fusarium moniliforme. J Toxicol Environ Health* 38:309–328, 1993.

Oliver F, Amon EU, Breathnach A, et al: Contact urticaria due to the common stinging nettle (*Urtica dioica*)—Histological, ultrastructural and pharmacological studies. *Clin Exp Dermatol* 16:1–7, 1991.

Omnell ML, Sun FRP, Keeler RF, et al: Expression of *Veratrum* alkaloid teratogenicity in the mouse. *Teratology* 42:105–119, 1990.

Onat FY, Yegen BC, Lawrence R, et al: Mad honey poisoning in man and rat. *Rev Environ Health* 9:3–9, 1991.

Pamies RJ, Powell R, Herold AH, et al: The *Dieffenbachia* plant: Case history. *J Fla Med Assoc* 79:760–761, 1992.

Peper K, Trautwein W: The effect of aconitine on the membrane current in cardiac muscle. *Pflugers Arch* 296:328–336, 1967.

Petroski RJ, Powell RG, Clay K: Alkaloids of *Stirpa robusta* (sleepygrass) infected with an *Acremonium* endophyte. *Nat Toxins* 1:84–88, 1992.

Pfister JA, Panter KE, Manners GD: Effective dose in cattle of toxic alkaloids from tall larkspur (*Delphinium barbeyi*). *Vet Hum Toxicol* 36:10–11, 1994.

Poyet J-L, Hoeveler A, Jongeneel CV: Analysis of active site residues of the antiviral protein from summer leaves from *Phytolacca americana* by site-directed mutagenesis. *Biochem Biophys Res Commun* 253:582–587, 1998.

Prabhasankar P, Raguputhi G, Sundaravadivel B, et al: Enzyme-linked immunosorbent assay for the phytotoxin thevetin. *J Immunoassay* 14:279–296, 1993.

Puschner B, Galey FD, Holstege DM, et al: Sweet clover poisoning in California. *J Am Vet Med Assoc* 212:857–859, 1998.

Pusztai A, Ewen SWB, Grant G, et al: Antinutritive effects of wheat-germ agglutinin and other *N*-acetylglucosamine–specific lectins. *Br J Nutr* 70:313–321, 1993.

Ramirez M, Rivera E, Ereu C: Fifteen cases of atropine poisoning after honey ingestion. *Vet Hum Toxicol* 41:19–20, 1999.

Rasmussen MA, Allison MJ, Foster JG: Flatpea intoxication in sheep and indications of ruminal adaptation. *Vet Hum Toxicol* 35:123–127, 1993.

Ridker PM, Ohkuma S, McDermott WV, et al: Hepatic venocclusive disease associated with the consumption of pyrrolizidine-containing dietary supplements. *Gastroenterology* 88:1050–1054, 1985.

Riley RT, Hinton DM, Chamberlain WJ, et al: Dietary fumonisin B_1 induces disruption of sphingolipid metabolism in Sprague-Dawley rat: A new mechanism of nephrotoxicity. *J Nutr* 124:594–603, 1994.

Rondeau ES: Wisteria toxicity. *J Toxicol* 31:107–112, 1993.

Rosell S, Samuelsson G: Effect of mistletoe viscotoxin and phoratoxin on blood circulation. *Toxicon* 26:975–987, 1988.

Rosling R: Cyanide exposure from linseed. *Lancet* 341:177, 1993.

Sako MDN, Al-Sultan II, Saleem AN: Studies on sheep experimentally poisoned with *Hypericum perforatum. Vet Hum Toxicol* 35:298–300, 1993.

Scallet AC, Ye X: Excitotoxic mechanisms of neurodegeneration in transmissible spongiform encephalopathies. *Ann NY Acad Sci* 825:194–205, 1997.

Schacter L: Etopside phosphate: What, why, where and how? *Semin Oncol* 23(suppl 13):1–7, 1996.

Schultze AE, Wagner JG, White SM, et al: Early indications of monocrotaline pyrrole–induced lung injury in rats. *Toxicol Appl Pharmacol* 109:41–50, 1991.

Shakin M, Smith BL, Prakash AS: Bracken carcinogens in the human diet. *Mutat Res* 443:69–79, 1999.

Sharma OP, Dawra RK, Pattabhi V: Molecular structure, polymorphism, and toxicity of lantadene A, the pentacyclictriterpenoid from the hepatotoxic plant *Lantana camara. J Biochem Toxicol* 6:57–63, 1991.

Short SO, Edwards WC: Blue green algae toxicosis in Oklahoma. *Vet Hum Toxicol* 32:558–560, 1990.

Skliar MI, Boland RL, Mourino A, et al: Isolation and identification of vitamin D_3, 25-hydroxyvitamin D_3, 1,25-dihydroxyvitamin D_3 and 1,24,25-trihydroxyvitamin D_3 in *Solanum malacoxylon* incubated with ruminal fluid. *J Steroid Biochem Mol Biol* 43:677–682, 1992.

Smith EA, Meloan CE, Pickell JA, et al: Scopolamine poisoning from homemade "moon flower" wine. *J Anal Toxicol* 15:216–219, 1991.

Southcott RV, Haegi LAR: Plant hair dermatitis. *Med J Aust* 156:623–628, 1992.

Spencer PS: Food toxins, AMPA receptors and motor neuron diseases. *Drug Metab Rev* 31:561–587, 1999.

Spencer PS, Roy DN, Ludolph A, et al: Lathyrism: Evidence for the role of the neuroexcitatory amino acid, BOAA. *Lancet* 2:1066–1067, 1986.

Spoerke DG, Murphy MM, Wruck KM, et al: Five cases of *Thermopsis* poisoning. *J Toxicol Clin Toxicol* 26:397–406, 1988.

Strauss U, Wittstock U, Schubert R, et al: Cicutoxin from *Cicuta virosa*—A new and potent potassium channel blocker in T-lymphocytes. *Biochem Biophys Res Commun* 219:332–336, 1996.

Surh Y-J, Lee E, Lee JM: Chemoprotective properties of some pungent ingredients present in red pepper and ginger. *Mutat Res* 402:259–267, 1998.

Tahirov THO, Lu T-H, Liaw Y-C, et al: A new crystal form of arbin-a from the seeds of *Abrus precatorius. J Mol Biol* 235:1152–1153, 1994.

Tandon HD, Tandon BN, Mattocks AR: An epidemic of veno-occlusive disease of the liver in Afghanistan. *Am J Gastroenterol* 70:607–613, 1978.

Teitelbaum JS, Zatorre RJ, Carpenter S, et al: Neurologic sequelae of domoic acid intoxication due to the ingestion of contaminated mussels. *N Engl J Med* 322:1781–1787, 1990.

Thomas HC, Lame MW, Dunston SK, et al: Monocrotaline pyrrole induces apoptosis in pulmonary artery endothelial cells. *Toxicol Appl Pharmacol* 152:236–244, 1998.

Tucker MO, Swan CR: The mango–poison ivy connection. *N Engl J Med* 339:235, 1998.

Tulsiani DR, Broquest HP, James LF, et al: Production of hybrid glycoprotein and accumulation of oligosaccharides in the brain of sheep and pigs administered swainsonine or locoweed. *Arch Biochem Biophys* 264:607–617, 1988.

Tylleskar T, Banca M, Bikongi N, et al: Cassava cyanogens and konzo, an upper motoneuron disease found in Africa. *Lancet* 339:208–211, 1992.

Urushibata O, Kase K: Irritant contact dermatitis from *Euphorbia marginata. Contact Dermatitis* 24:155–157, 1991.

van der Lugt JJ, Nel PW, Kitching JP: The pathology of *Cestrum laevigatum* (Schlechtd) poisoning in cattle. *Onderstepoort J Vet Res* 58:211–221, 1991.

van Meurs A, Cohen A, Edelbroek P: Atropine poisoning after eating chapattis contaminated with *Datura stramonium* (thorn apple). *Trans R Soc Trop Med Hyg* 86:221, 1992.

Wang H, Ng TB: Ribosome inactivating protein and lectin from bitter melon (*Momordica charantia*) seeds: Sequence comparison with related proteins. *Biochem Biophys Res Commun* 253:143–146, 1998.

Worker NA, Carrillo BJ: "Enteque seco," calcification and wasting in grazing animals in the Argentine. *Nature* 215:72–74, 1967.

Yoshizawa T, Yamashita A, Luo Y: Fumonisin occurrence in corn from high- and low-risk areas for human esophageal cancer in China. *Appl Environ Microbiol* 60:1626-1629, 1994.

UNIT 6

ENVIRONMENTAL TOXICOLOGY

CHAPTER 28

AIR POLLUTION*

Daniel L. Costa

AIR POLLUTION IN PERSPECTIVE

The last fifty years have brought remarkable changes in the way we view our environment. In the early 1950s, our industrial prosperity was often depicted as an expanse of factories with smokestacks belching opaque black clouds into the surrounding air. The growing environmental activism in the latter decades of the century—stemming from aesthetic and, more importantly, health concerns—forced regulatory legislation that has now made such scenes rare in most technologically advanced nations. Today, every urban community is in search of "clean industries." Yet ironically, we endure increasingly congested thoroughfares of automobiles commuting to these industries as we fuel a photochemical cauldron of oxidant air pollution—i.e., smog. Moreover, areas once considered "pristine" are today tarnished by the influx of polluted air masses that drift and disperse across hundreds of miles. Clearly, air pollution remains a reality of our twenty-first-century lifestyle, and while great strides have been made to reduce emissions from both stationary and mobile sources, unsatisfactory air quality now plagues much broader geographic areas. As a result, millions of people in the United States live in areas that are not in compliance with current National Ambient Air Quality Standards (NAAQS) (Fig. 28-1).

Most peoples of the western world today face fewer episodes of extreme air pollution; instead, they experience prolonged periods of relatively low-level exposure to complex mixtures of photochemically transformed stationary and mobile emissions. We know most about the health effects of individual pollutants, and we use this knowledge to drive controls where single pollutants dominate the situation. However, much less is understood about the realities of present-day patterns of diurnal and prolonged exposure and how mixtures of pollutants can affect human health. This chapter is intended to inform the reader as to the state of our knowledge of air pollution, with the goal of providing the reader with a fundamental knowledge and appreciation of the nature of the problem, its complexity, and the uncertainties in need of investigation.

*This article has been reviewed by the National Health and Environmental Effects Research Laboratory, U.S. Environmental Protection Agency, and approved for publication. Approval does not signify that the contents necessarily reflect the views and the policies of the Agency.

A Brief History of Air Pollution

For most of history, air pollution has been a problem of microenvironments and domestic congestion. The smoky fires of early cave and hut dwellers choked the air inside their homes. When it was eventually vented outdoors, it combined with that of the neighbors to settle around the village in the damp cold night. With urbanization and the concomitant decrease in forest wood as a source of fuel, the need for heat and energy led to the burning and ambient release of sulfurous, sooty smoke from cheap coal. City dwellers had to endure the bad air, while those with wealth had country homes to which they could escape from time to time. The poor quality of urban air is well documented historically. Seneca, the Roman philosopher, in A.D. 61 wrote: "As soon as I had gotten out of the *heavy air* of Rome, and from the *stink* of the chimneys thereof, which being stirred, poured forth whatever *pestilential vapors and soot* they had enclosed in them, I felt an *alteration to my disposition*" (emphasis added: Miller and Miller, 1993).

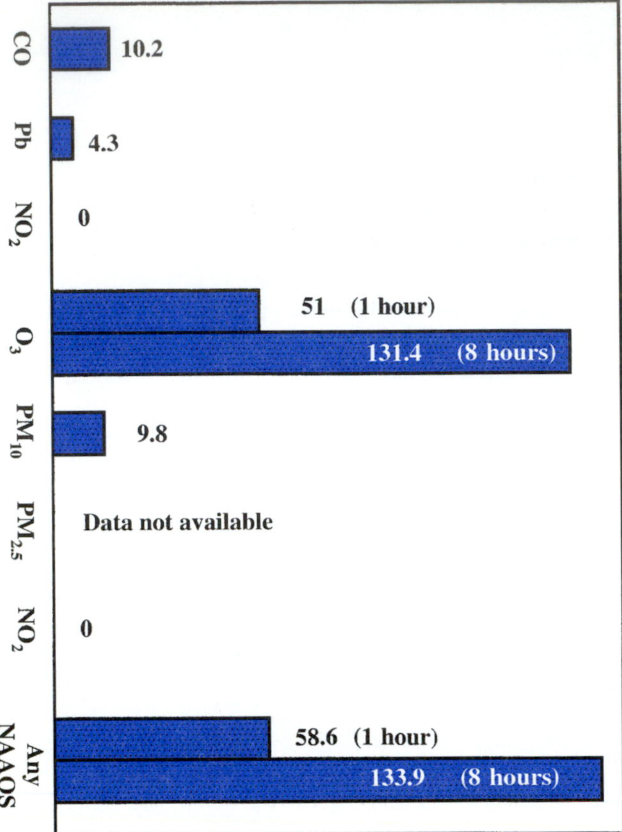

Figure 28-1. Number of people (millions) living in U.S. counties not in compliance with current 1998 NAAQS. (Adapted with permission from National Air Quality & Emission Trends Report, 1998.)

Efforts to regulate air pollution, on the other hand, evolved more slowly. Beginning in the thirteenth century, community-based outcries received some recognition by governing officials, one example being the banning of domestic burning of "sea coal" in London by Edward I. Enforcement, however, was not effective and people largely resigned themselves to polluted air as part of urban life. By the seventeenth century, England, in the middle of several decades some refer to as "the little ice age," experienced further reductions in wood harvests, thus increasing reliance on sea coal for domestic heating. Despite Percival Pott's discovery that soot was related to the occurrence of scrotal cancer in chimney sweeps, the health community offered only a simple recommendation: "Fly the city, shun its turbid air; breathe not the chaos of eternal smoke . . . " (Brimblecombe, 1999)—advice hardly advanced from that of Seneca 1600 years earlier. In the late eighteenth century, the industrial revolution, which was powered by the burning of mined coal, added a second dimension to urban air pollution. These emissions were more acidic and hung in the air longer than the fluffy soot of the cheaper sea coal burned in home heaters. Continued soiling of buildings and damage to nearby crops brought community boards to address sanitary reforms to cut the worse of the pollution peaks and episodes, but any gains were soon offset by growth. By the end of the nineteenth century and into the early twentieth century, power plants were being built to provide energy for factories and eventually to light homes. Steel mills and other industries proliferated along riverbanks and lakeshores, oil refineries rose in port cities and near oilfields, and smelters roasted and refined metals in areas near large mineral deposits.

By 1925, air pollution was common to all industrialized nations, but people became less tolerant of the nuisance of acidic-soot corrosion of all exposed surfaces and the general discomfort that came with smoky air. Public surveys were initiated—as in Salt Lake City in 1926, New York City in 1937, and Leicester, Great Britain, in 1939—to bring political attention to the problem and promote the implementation of controls (Miller and Miller, 1993). However, it was not until the great air pollution disasters in the Meuse Valley, Belgium, in 1930; Donora, Pennsylvania, in 1948; and the great London fog of 1952 that air pollution was indicted primarily as a health issue. In the United States, California was already leading the way with passage of the Air Pollution Control Act of 1947 to regulate the discharge of opaque smokes. Visibility problems in Pittsburgh during the 1940s had also prompted efforts to control smoke from local industries, but it was the initiative of President Truman that provided the federal impetus to deal with air pollution. This early effort culminated in congressional passage of a series of acts starting with the Air Pollution Control Act of 1955.

The prosperity and suburban sprawl of the late 1950s provided the third and perhaps most chemically complex dimension of air pollution. The term *smog,* though originally coined to describe the mixture of smoke and fog that hung over large cities such as London, was curiously adopted for the eye-irritating photochemical reaction products of auto exhaust that blanketed cities such as Los Angeles. Early federal legislation addressing stationary sources was soon expanded to include automobile-derived pollutants (the Clean Air Act of 1963, amended in 1967, and the Motor Vehicle Air Pollution Control Act of 1965). The landmark Clean Air Act (CAA) of 1970 evolved from the early legislation, and despite being only an amendment, it was revolutionary. It recognized the problem of air pollution as a national issue and set forth a plan to control it. The Act established the U.S. Environmental Protection Agency (USEPA) and charged it with the responsibility to protect the public from the hazards of polluted outdoor air. Seven "criteria" air pollutants [ozone (O_3), sulfur dioxide (SO_2), particulate matter (PM), nitrogen dioxide (NO_2), carbon monoxide (CO), lead (Pb), and total hydrocarbons—the last now dropped from the list, leaving six criteria pollutants] were specified as significant health hazards in need of *individual* National Ambient Air Quality Standards (NAAQS). These NAAQS were mandated for review every 5 years as to the adequacy of the existent standard to protect human health (Table 28-1). For each of the criteria pollutants, there was to be developed a Criteria Document, which would provide a detailed summary of the available database on that pollutant and then would be integrated into a staff paper for use by the EPA Administrator to set the NAAQS. With regard to the Primary NAAQS, only health criteria could be used, including a safety factor for the most susceptible groups. Secondary consideration was given to agricultural and structural welfare; economic impacts were not to be involved in standard setting itself—only in the implementation procedures. Other hazardous air pollutants (HAPs), of which there were eight listed at the time, were to undergo health assessments to establish emission controls. The CAA of 1970 was by far the most far-reaching legislation to date.

The accidental release of 30 tons of methyl isocyanate vapor into the air of the shanty village of Bhopal, India, on December 3, 1984, killed an estimated 3000 people within hours of

Table 28-1
U.S. National (Primary) Ambient Air Quality Standards*

POLLUTANT	UNIT	AVERAGING TIME	CONCENTRATION	STATISTIC
Sulfur dioxide	$\mu g/m^3$ (ppm)	Annual	80 (0.03)	Annual mean
		24 h	365 (0.14)	Maximum
Carbon monoxide	$\mu g/m^3$ (ppm)	8 h	10 (9)	Maximum
		1 h	40 (35)	Maximum
Ozone	$\mu g/m^3$ (ppm)	1 h	235 (0.12)	Maximum
		8 h	157 (0.08)	Maximum
Nitrogen dioxide	$\mu g/m^3$ (ppm)	Annual	100 (0.053)	Annual mean
Particulates PM_{10}	$\mu g/m^3$	Annual and 24 h	150 and 50	Annual mean and
		Annual and 24 h	65 and 15	maximum
$PM_{2.5}$				
Lead	$\mu g/m^3$	3 months	1.5	Quarterly average

*For detailed information regarding policy and precise statistical and time-based computations to achieve attainment, contact EPA website: www.epa.gov/airs/criteria.html

the release, with another 200,000 injured and/or permanently impaired. The tragedy shocked the world, and raised the issue of HAPs in the United States to a new level of concern. While such a disaster has never struck the United States, accidental industrial releases or spills of toxic chemicals are surprisingly common, with 4375 cases recorded between 1980 and 1987, inflicting 11,341 injuries and 309 deaths (Waxman, 1994). The HAPs, which had been the stepsister of the criteria pollutants for more than a decade after the passage of the CAA, have since garnered more public and policy attention. There is concern not only for accidental releases of fugitive or secondary chemicals—such as phosgene, benzene, butadiene, and dioxin, into the air of populated industrial centers—but also for potential chronic health effects, with cancer often being the focus of attention. The slow progress of regulatory decisions on HAPs (only eight between 1970 and 1990) led to a mandated acceleration of the process under the CAA amendment of 1990. Section 112(b) currently lists 188 chemicals or classes of chemicals for which special standards and risk assessments are required. The chemicals listed are those of greatest concern on the basis of toxicity (including cancer) and estimated release volumes. These emissions are mandated for control to the maximal achievable control technology (MACT), and any residual health risk after MACT is to be considered in a separate quantitative risk assessment. The database for this process utilizes existing knowledge or, if necessary, mandates further research by the emitter. While many of these chemicals are now better controlled than in the past, most residual risk estimates are yet to be completed.

Emissions from motor vehicles are addressed primarily under the CAA Title II, Emission Standards for Mobile Sources. The reduction of emissions from mobile sources is complex and involves both fuel and engine/vehicle reengineering. Despite continued refinements in combustion engineering through the use of computerized ignition and timing, fuel properties have drawn recent attention for improvement. For example, to reduce wintertime CO, several oxygenates (including ethers and alcohols) have be formulated into fuels both to reduce cold-start emissions and enhance overall combustion. Perhaps the most prominent of the ethers is MTBE (methyl tertiary butyl ether), which became a controversial additive in the early 1990s, arising in part from odor and reports of asthma-like reactions by some individuals during auto refueling at service stations. Today, the controversy has taken an unexpected twist; MTBE has now been removed from fuel, not because health concerns associated with airborne exposure but rather due to leakage from service-station storage tanks into groundwater. Ironically, this prescribed remedy for an air problem has evolved into a new problem: groundwater contamination. This example illustrates the broad complexity of pollution control, measures that transcend engineering. Meanwhile, the introduction of another fuel additive, methylcyclopentadienyl manganese tricarbonyl (MMT)—to boost octane ratings of fuel and improve engine performance and combustion—is being carefully reviewed under Title II because of concerns regarding the potential introduction of manganese into the environment, reminiscent of use lead in fuels from the 1930s to 1970s, when lead fuel additives were banned.

Internationally, the magnitude and control of air pollution sources vary considerably, especially among developing nations, which often forgo concerns for health and welfare because of cost and the desire to achieve prosperity. Fig. 28-2 illustrates the variation among international megacities in regard to three major urban pollutants: total suspended particulate (TSP) matter, sulfur oxides (SO_x), and O_3. The recent political upheaval in eastern Europe has revealed the consequences of decades of uncontrolled industrial air pollution. While vast improvements are now becoming evident in this area, as industries are being modernized and emissions controlled, many Asian, African, and South American cities have virtually unchecked air pollution. Some nations as well as the World Health Organization (WHO) have adopted air quality standards as a rational basis for guiding control measures, but the lack of binding regulations and/or economic fortune has impeded significant controls and improvements (Lipfert, 1994). In addition to local socioeconomic and political concerns, emissions of air pollutants will, in all probability, spawn problems of "international pollution" as we enter the twenty-first century, when the impact of long-range transport of polluted air masses from one country to another fully matures as a global issue (Reuther, 2000). This was the subject of some controversy between Canada and the United States in the late 1980s and into the 1990s as a result of the air mass transport of acid sulfates from industrial centers of the midwestern United States to southern Ontario. However, reduction in SO_2 emissions has somewhat relieved the tension over the last several years (Fig. 28-3).

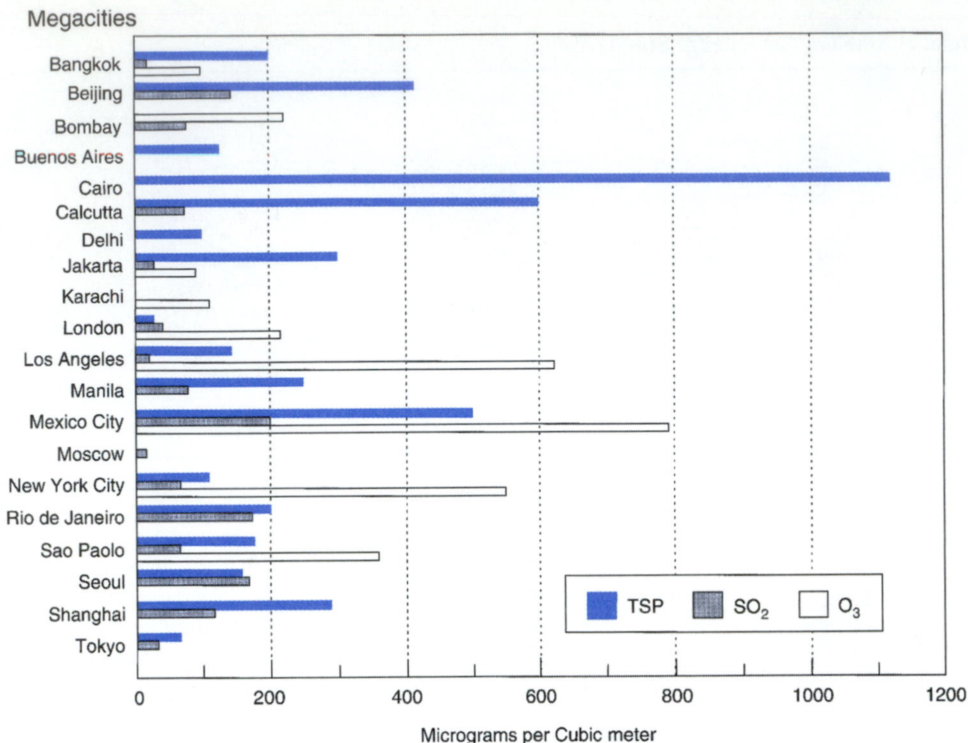

Figure 28-2. Comparison of ambient levels of 1-h maximum ozone, annual average of total suspended particulate matter, and sulfur dioxide in selected cities from around the world to illustrate the variation in these levels from country to country with respect to the United States. (Reproduced with permission from the National Air Quality and Emission Trends Report, 1992.)

ASSESSING RISKS ASSOCIATED WITH AIR POLLUTION

"Risk Assessment" has become a formalized process, originally described in the landmark 1983 National Research Council Report, whereby evidence regarding toxicity, exposure, and dose-dependency are systematically organized to estimate the degree of risk to a population. The health database for any air pollutant comprises data from animal toxicology, controlled human studies, and epidemiology. But, because each of these research approaches has inherent strengths and limitations, an appropriate assessment of an air pollutant requires the careful integration and interpretation of data from all three methodologies. Thus, one should be aware of the attributes of each (Table 28-2).

Epidemiologic studies reveal associations between exposure to a pollutant or pollutants and the health effect or effects in the *community* or *population* of interest. Because data are garnered directly under real exposure conditions and involve large numbers of humans, the data are of direct utility to the regulatory community assessing the impact of that pollution. Moreover, with proper design and analysis, studies can explore either acute or long-term exposures and theoretically can examine trends in mortality and morbidity, accounting irreversible effects as well as responses in population subsets (i.e., sensitive groups). Why, then, is this approach to the study of air pollution not the exclusive choice of regulators in decision making? The problem here is that it is often difficult to control independent and personal variables in the human population because of genetic diversity among individuals and lifestyle differences, their mobility over time, and the lack of adequate exposure data—especially on a personal basis. Also, it is difficult to segregate a single pollutant from copollutants and the influence of meteorologic confounders. Thus, at best, only associations can be drawn between the broad-based exposure data and effects, with these effects typically of a gross nature—mortality, hospitalizations, etc. Rarely is a causal relationship discernible even in the presence of strong statistical significance. However, recent advances in exposure estimation and study design and analysis (e.g., time series) have allowed epidemiologists to examine relationships with greater confidence and specificity. These models limit the impact of covariates and longer time-based influences and thus allow epidemiologists to tease out effects of short-term pollution not accessible formerly (Schwartz, 1991). Similarly, newer approaches that employ field studies—sometimes called *panel studies*—incorporate time-series design and regression analyses of more focused exposure data (ideally personal) and targeted clinical endpoints in the exposed population under study. The endpoints often derive from empiric human and animal studies. These novel approaches are clearly evident in the most recent studies of particulate matter air pollution (see below).

Studies that involve controlled human exposures have been used extensively to evaluate the criteria air pollutants regulated by the USEPA. Because most people are exposed to these pollutants in their daily lives, human volunteers can be ethically exposed to them (with the exception of Pb, which has cumulative and irreversible effects). Exposures are conducted in a controlled environment, are generally of short or limited repeat durations, and all responses must be reversible. Clearly, data of this type are very valuable in assessing potential human risk, since they

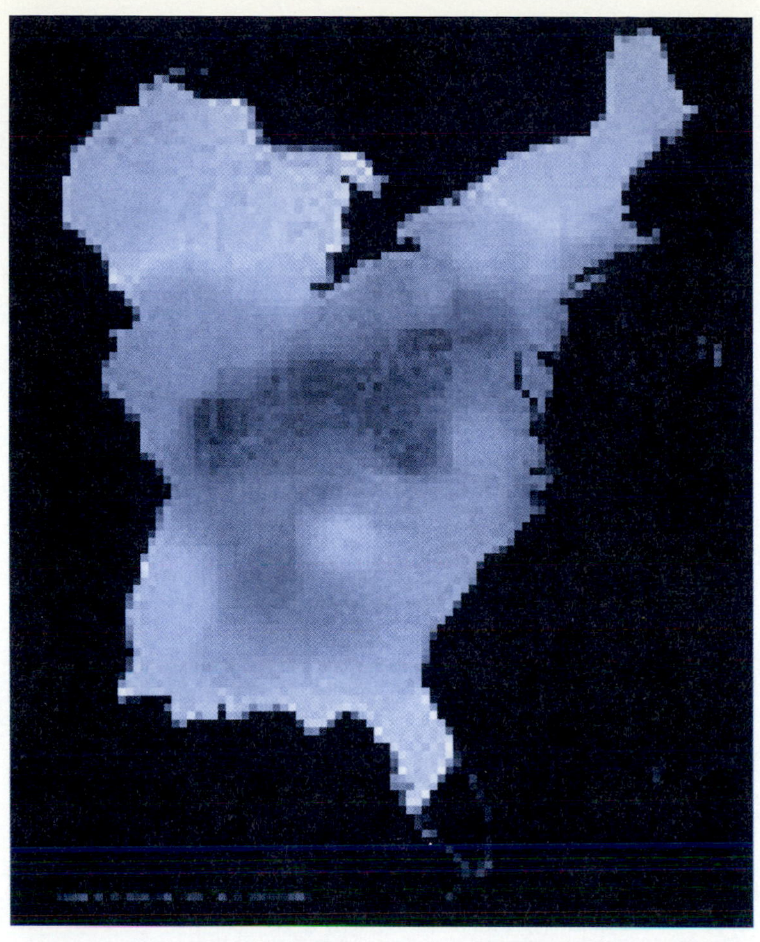

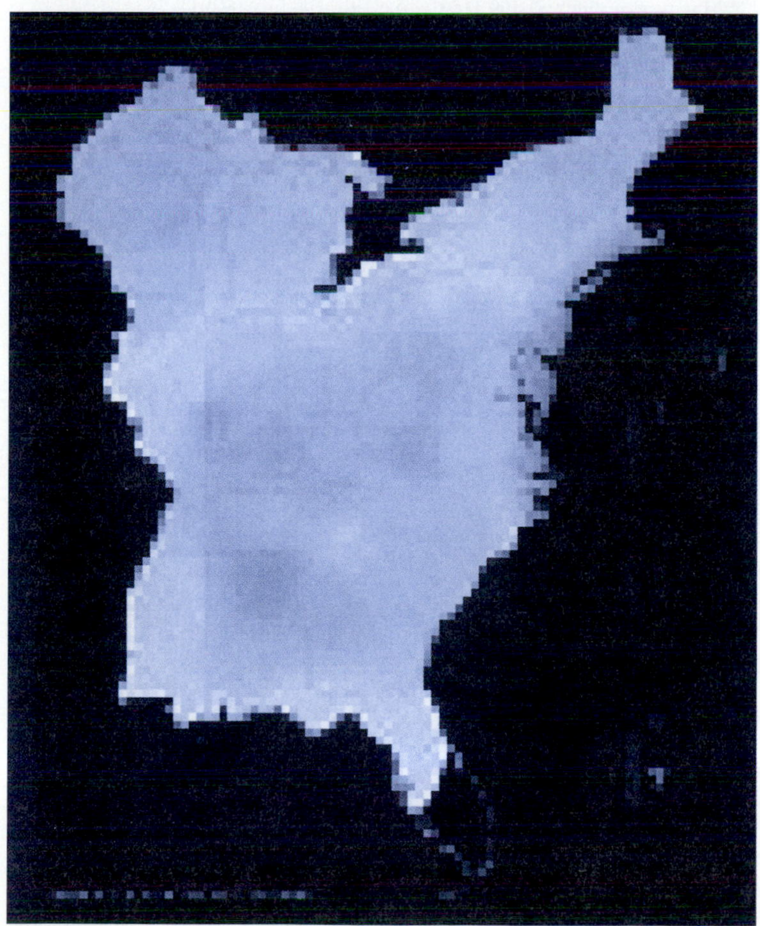

Figure 28-3. Reduction in ambient sulfate concentrations between 1990–1991 and 1997–1998 in the rural U.S. Midwest from CASTNet monitoring data.

The acid sulfates are dispersed by prevailing winds toward the eastern United States and southeastern Canada, contributing to the acid rain deposition (see Fig. 28-9). (Adapted with permission from National Air Quality & Emission Trends Report, 1998.)

Table 28-2
Strengths and Weaknesses of Disciplinary Approaches for Obtaining Health Information

DISCIPLINE	POPULATION	STRENGTHS	WEAKNESSES
Epidemiology	Communities	Natural exposure	Difficult to quantify exposure Many covariates
	Diseased groups	No extrapolation Isolates susceptibility trait Long-term, low-level effects	 Minimal dose–response data Association vs. causation
	Field/Panel groups	Good exposure data Fewer covariates Focus on host traits Utilizes clinical evaluations	Usually short-term Volunteers Expensive
Clinical studies	Experimental Diseased subjects	Controlled exposures Few covariates Isolates susceptibility trait Cause–effect	Artificial exposures Acute effects only Hazards Volunteers
Toxicology	Animals	Maximum control Dose-response data Cause–effect	Human extrapolation Realistic models of human disease?
	In vitro systems	Rapid data acquisition Mechanisms	In vivo extrapolation

SOURCE: Modified from Boubel et al., 1994: with permission.

are derived from the species of concern and are rooted in our well-established clinical knowledge and experience. Additionally, suspected "susceptible or sensitive" individuals representing potential high-risk groups can be studied to better understand the breadth of response in the exposed public. However, clinical studies have practical limitations. Ethical issues are involved in every aspect of a clinical test; potentially irreversible effects and carcinogenicity are also always of concern, along with the definition of an acceptable level of hyperresponsiveness in a so-called sensitive individual who may be subjected to testing. Likewise for any test subject, there are obvious restrictions on the invasiveness of biological procedures, though sophistication in medical technology has made accessible a large array of molecular biomarkers from peripheral blood and nasal, bronchial, and alveolar lavage fluids as well biopsied cells from airway segments (Devlin et al., 1991; Salvi et al., 1999). Finally, the cost, the limited numbers of subjects that usually can be evaluated, and the inability to address chronic exposure issues are also constraints on human testing. Where partnership with animal toxicology studies has been established, studies in laboratory animal species can sometimes open the door for at least limited direct human exposure study. Analogously, in vitro studies in both human and animal cell and tissue systems allow the elucidation of mechanisms of toxicity and identify basic biological responses that serve the extrapolation of animal data to humans as well as supporting the feasibility and ethical limitations of human study even with toxic air pollutants (see below).

Animal toxicology is frequently used to predict or corroborate suspected effects in humans. In the absence of human data, animal toxicology constitutes the essential first step of risk assessment: *hazard identification*. The importance of animal toxicology in elucidating pathogenic mechanisms should not be overlooked, however, as knowledge of the basic in vivo biological processes involved in toxic injury or disease is critical to extrapolating databases across species and to estimating uncertainties. Knowledge of the toxic mechanism(s) provides the underpinnings to the "plausibility" of the findings when extrapolated to humans and, under carefully defined and highly controlled circumstances, may allow *quantitative* estimates of risk. Animal toxicology studies have been used to investigate all of the criteria air pollutants and many of the HAPs as well. The strength of this discipline is that it can involve methods that are not practical in human studies, including a diversity of exposure concentrations and durations, and the inclusion of a wide array of invasive biological procedures. The minimization of uncontrolled variables (e.g., genetic and environmental) may be the greatest strength of the animal bioassay. On the other hand, the clear limitation of this approach lies in the extrapolation of the findings from animals to the day-to-day human life scenario. Ideally, a test animal is selected with knowledge that it responds in a manner similar to that of the human (*homology*). *Qualitative* extrapolation of homologous effects is not unusual with most toxic inhalants, but *quantitative* extrapolation is frequently clouded by uncertainties of the relative *sensitivity* of the animal or specific target tissue compared with that of the human. Uncertainties about the target tissue dose also loom large, as it constitutes the first obstacle to quantitative extrapolation (see below). With respect to the target tissue dose, however, most animal toxicologists make every effort to keep exposure concentrations at 5- to 10-fold that of the anticipated human exposure until appropriate dosimetric data can be ascertained. The higher doses are typically needed to achieve a group response among a limited pool of animals (maybe 6 to 10) to represent a large population effect, where perhaps only a few of hundreds or thousands may be responsive; although it must be appreciated that mechanisms may differ at different dose levels. Despite these limitations, animal studies have provided the largest database on a wide range of air toxicants and have proven utility in predicting human adverse responses to chemicals.

Health scientists must appreciate the strengths and weaknesses of these approaches if an appropriate estimation of toxic risk or potential hazard is to be reached. However, other scientific disciplines also are integral to the full assessment of the impact of air pollution on society. Chemical and engineering methodologies are used together to detect and control pollutants in the atmosphere and develop empiric test systems to gather information used to evaluate individual toxicity and/or physicochemical interactions. Their use in determining local and personal exposure for panel and prospective epidemiologic studies is most important. Other disciplines, such as meteorology and atmospheric chemistry, relate to the real world by yielding information on the dispersion of pollutants from their sources and the conditions leading to the stagnation of air masses and the accumulation of pollutants. Recreating these environments to the extent possible, using surrogate atmospheres, is critical to understanding toxic risks and creating models to estimate human risk. Last, data derived from studies in plants are now being appreciated more than ever. Not only are commercial and native vegetation affected by pollution but plants themselves are being appreciated as sensitive "sentinels," warning us of the impact of pollution. When these elements are considered collectively, the economist can inform regulators and the public at large of the cumulative impact and adversity of pollution on our standard of living (Maddison and Pierce, 1999).

Animal-to-Human Extrapolation: Issues and Mitigating Factors

Extrapolation is the process of relating empiric study findings to real-world scenarios. The utility and value of animal toxicology is most dependent on this process. Thus, the selection of an animal species as a toxicologic model should involve more than considerations of cost and convenience. Whenever possible, effects that are homologous between the study species and humans should guide selection of the test species. For example, if irritant responses to an upper airway irritant (e.g., SO_2 or formaldehyde) are of interest, the guinea pig, with its labile and reactive bronchoconstrictive reflex, should be selected over the rat, which is not particularly responsive to sensory irritants. By contrast, certain strains of rats exhibit a clear neutrophilic response to deep lung irritants, such as O_3, that resembles the human response. Other innate differences in sensitivity among species may relate to differences in lung structure, specific regionally based cell metabolism or polymorphisms, or overall defenses (e.g., antioxidants) (Paige and Plopper, 1999; Slade et al., 1985). When such nuances are unclear or unknown, the replication of responses in multiple species builds confidence in the finding as being the product of conserved mechanisms across species and therefore its relevance to the human. However, new transgenic and knockout strains of mice (and in some cases rats), specially engineered to address hypotheses focused on genetically linked traits, have given toxicologists a new instrument for the study of air pollutants.

An essential part of extrapolating responses from species to species is an accurate assessment of the relative dosimetry of the pollutant along the respiratory tract. Significant advances in studies of the distribution of gaseous and particulate pollutants have been made through the use of empiric and mathematical models, the latter of which incorporate parameters of respirato°ry anatomy and physiology, aerodynamics, and physical chemistry into predictions of deposition and retention. Empiric models combined with theoretical models aid in relating animal toxicity data to humans and help refine the study of injury mechanisms with better estimates of the target dose. Figure 28-4*A* and *B* illustrates the application of such an approach to the reactive gas ozone and insoluble 0.6-μm spherical particles, respectively, as each is distributed along the respiratory tract of humans and rats. Anatomic differences between the species clearly affect the deposition of both gases and particles, but the qualitative and to a large extent quantitative similarities in deposition profiles are noteworthy. This is not surprising if one argues teleologically that the lungs of each species evolved with similar functional demands (i.e., O_2–CO_2 exchange, blood acid/base balance), mechanical impediments, and environmental stresses. One needs only a cursory review of the comparative lung physiology literature to appreciate the allometric consistency of the mammalian respiratory tract to meet the challenge of breathing air. This design coherency has provided the fundamental rationale for the use of animal models for the study of air pollutants.

Susceptible subpopulations that may show exaggerated responsiveness to a pollutant deserve special mention. The existence of hyperresponsive individuals and groups is well accepted among those who study air pollution toxicology, but little is actually known about the host traits that make certain individuals responsive. This appreciation for sensitive populations is specifically noted in the CAA, where their protection is mandated in the promulgation of NAAQS. There are some definable subgroups that are assumed to be susceptible, including children, the elderly, and those with a preexisting disease (e.g., asthma, cardiovascular disease, lung disease). However, the assumption that these groups are indeed susceptible is based more on perceptions than on real data. In some cases susceptibility may reside in some innate responsiveness, while in other cases it may relate more to the loss of functional reserve or compensation, perhaps altering a response threshold. The reasons for paucity of data likely lie in the difficulty in ethically conducting studies in humans who are potentially at higher risk and recruiting such individuals on a volunteer basis. However, inroads into this issue have been made in recent years, in part because of more precise definitions of potential risk factors, allowing researchers to design studies that examine host attributes that need not be at life-threatening stages of impairment and the development of more appropriate animal models of disease or dysfunction. Hence, studies in both animals and human subjects are being devised specifically to investigate the roles of diet (e.g., antioxidant content), exercise (as it relates to dosimetry), and age, gender, and race. In addition, studies in human subjects with mild asthma or heart-lung disease have been conducted to address the degree of sensitivity that these compromised groups exhibit. Analogously, animal models with imposed cardiopulmonary impairments are being used more and more to address the same basic questions.

Recent advances in molecular biology have provided tools to bioengineer mice (and occasionally rats) with virtually any trait that is under the control of identifiable genes. Transgenic strains can express desired traits derived from other animals or even humans, or knockout models can be made devoid of specific traits to isolate the impact of that trait on the animal's responsivity to a toxic challenge. These animal models add to the availability of natural mutants that have been inbred historically to purify a desired genotype to achieve a specific phenotype, ideally one that is analogous to that of the human (Ho, 1994: Glasser et al., 1994). Natural mutant and bioengineered transgenic and knockout rodent models provide unparalleled potential to examine specific genetic factors involved in response (i.e., susceptibility). Current technology can also target genes for specific

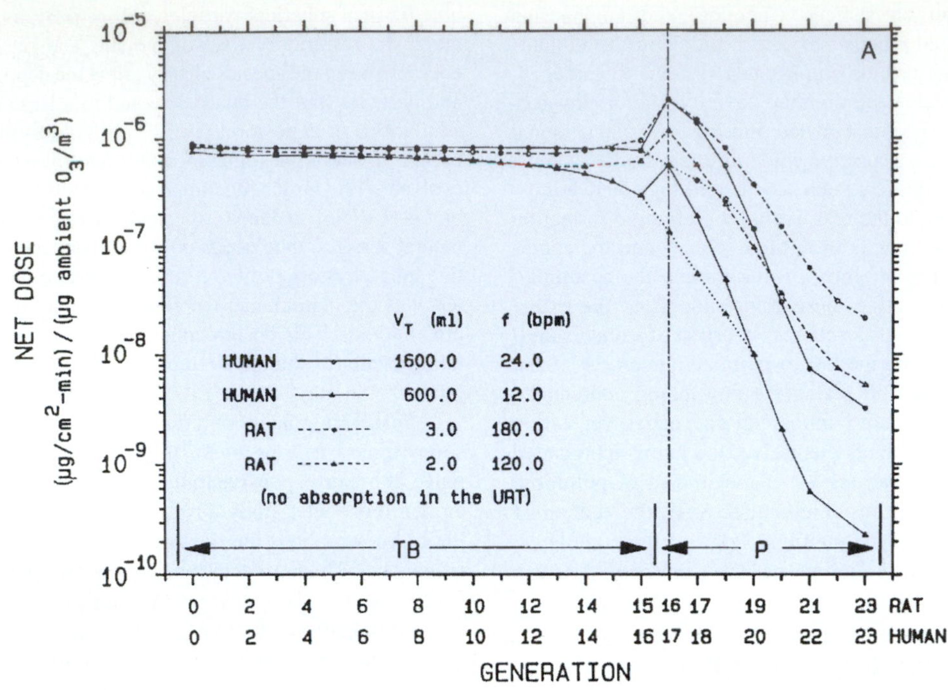

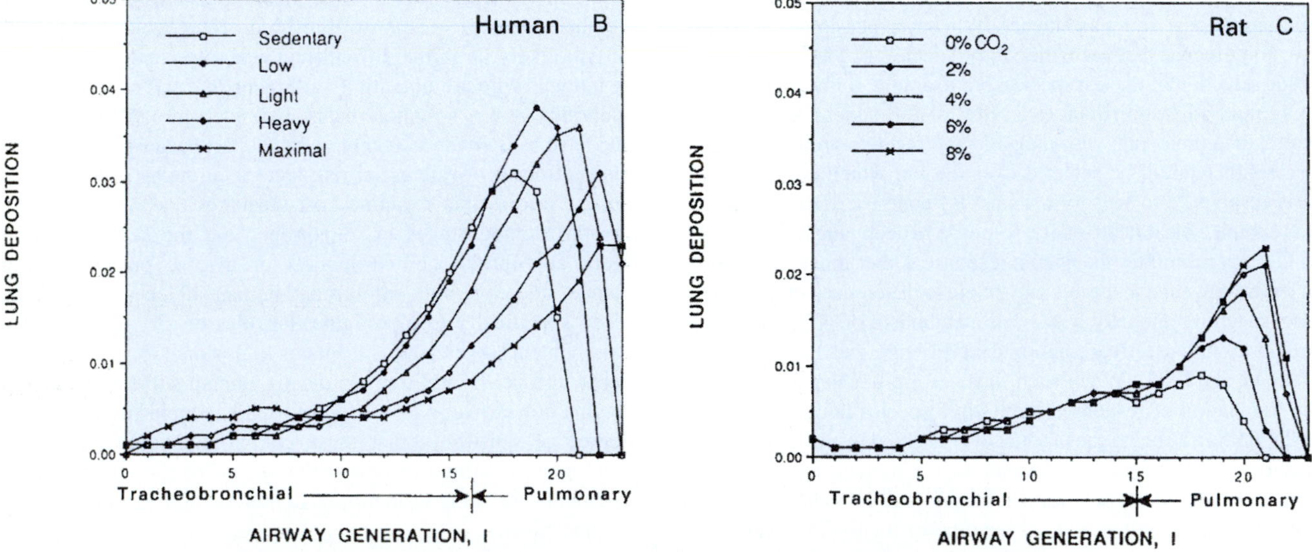

***Figure 28-4.** Theoretical (normalized to the concentration in inspired air) uptake curves for the reactive gas ozone in a resting/exercising human and a rat (**A**). Likewise, the percent deposition in the airways of a 0.6 μm insoluble particle in the respiratory tracts of a resting/exercising human (**B**) and rat (**C**).*

Here 8% inspired CO_2 in the rat augments ventilation up to threefold. Airway generation refers to that airway branch numbered from the trachea (0). [Panel *A* is from Overton and Miller, 1987, and panels *B* and *C* are from Martonen et al., 1992. Reproduced with permission.]

expression in the lung (e.g., linked to surfactant protein C), and in some cases it can even provide a control gene with which an investigator can switch the gene of interest on or off using a pharmacologic or chemical prechallenge. Such advances allow the dissection of underlying mechanisms under very controlled scenarios and avoid the problems of having a gene be inappropriately active or inactive through all life stages (Gossen et al., 1996).

To date the emphasis of studies using these genetically modified animal models have been on mechanisms associated with disease pathogenesis (Recio, 1995; Suga et al., 2000). Among the most popular uses of knockout and transgenic mice has been in the study of inflammatory cytokines and associated products in asthma, as the expression of many of these mediators are thought to be under the control of single genes (e.g., Kakuyama et al., 1999, Kuhn et al., 2000). Clearly these genetically modified mice are ideally suited for the study of mechanism of action where a specific mediator-based hypothesis can be tested as it relates to an impaired function, pathology, or altered inflammatory pattern. When these models are derived to exhibit a desired pathology or disease due to a genetic defect—for example involving lung structure or growth (e.g., emphysema or fibrosis), such that by adulthood the animal exhibits the disease—the model may serve as a surrogate of the human condition (e.g., O'Donnell et al., 1999).

The use or genetically modified animal models in air pollution research has lagged behind that of basic science and toxicology in general. The reasons for this are unclear and may relate to the difficulties in incorporating such data into conventional risk-assessment paradigms. However, with recent interest in potentially susceptible groups, there has been a definitive upswing in the use of pharmacologically or naturally altered as well as bioengineered animals (Kodavanti et al., 1999) and an effort to more closely link mechanistic profiles to basic human biology. Ozone has frequently been the test pollutant in these new studies, since more is known about O_3 and its effects in humans than about any other air pollutant. Frequently, these studies address aspects of inflammation and antioxidant capacity relative to challenge by ozone and other oxidants (Johnston et al., 1999; Kleeberger et al., 2000). But with the current interest in particulate matter (PM) health effects, these and other models are being redirected; for example: strain differences and acid coated PM (Ohtsuka et al., 2000); hypertransferrinemic mice and metal-rich PM (Ghio et al., 2000); and metallothionein-null mice and mercury vapor (Yoshida et al., 1999). The curious are directed to the rapidly evolving literature in this area of research.

Air Pollution: Sources and Personal Exposure

In terms of tons of anthropogenic material emitted annually in the United States (as of 1998), five major air pollutants account for 98 percent of pollution (Fig. 28-5): CO (52 percent), SO_x (14 percent), volatile organic compounds (VOCs; 14 percent), PM (4 percent), and NO_x (14 percent). The remainder consists of Pb, which is down >90 percent since 1983, when it was banned from gasoline, and a myriad of other compounds considered under the category of hazardous air pollutants. On a national basis, since 1996, PM and SO_x increased slightly and NO_x remained the same, while VOCs and CO decreased slightly. Obviously, for any specific locality, this emission picture can vary widely. In the vicinity of a smelter, for example, SO_x, metals, and/or PM dominate the pollutant profile; while a refinery air shed would be dominated by VOCs; and in suburban areas, where the automobile is the main source of pollution, CO, VOCs, and NO_x would prevail along with their primary photochemical product, O_3.

Classically, air pollution has been distinguished on the basis of the chemical redox nature of its primary components. Dickens's eighteenth-century "London's particular," in which SO_2 and smoke from incomplete combustion of coal accumulated as a chilled, acidic fog, was termed "reducing-type" air pollution. This acidic mix would react with surfaces, corroding metal and eroding masonry, as is characteristic of reductive chemistry. Historically, this reducing-type atmosphere has been associated with smelting and related combustion-based industries (as along the Meuse River in 1930 and Donora, Pennsylvania, in 1948) as well as large, coal-based urban centers such as London (1952) and New York (1962). In contrast, Los Angeles has always had a characteristically "oxidant-type" pollution consisting of NO_x and many secondary photochemical oxidants, such as O_3, aldehydes, and electron-hungry hydrocarbon radicals. In photochemical air pollution, atmospheric reaction products of automobile exhaust and sunlight are trapped by regional topography or meteorologic inversion. This condition is today referred to colloquially as "smog" or "haze."

The classic types of air pollution were implicitly seasonal. Reducing air pollution occurred during winter periods of oil and coal combustion and meteorologic inversions, while the oxidant atmospheres occurred during the summertime, when sunlight is most intense and can catalyze reactions among the constituents of auto exhaust. While some regions of the United States may still experience a more reducing-type or oxidant-type atmosphere, today the distinction between these smogs is largely academic. Most modern industrial centers have undergone a considerable reduction in smoky, sulfurous emissions while experiencing a proliferation of automobiles that contribute tons of oxidant precursors into the air. Thus, major metropolitan areas, most notably those in the northeastern United States, have atmospheres with both reducing and oxidant air pollutants. Sulfates may predominate over nitrates in the air, in contrast to the southwestern United States, but no longer is the northeastern smog simply a sulfur-based problem. Nonetheless, Los Angeles (though challenged by Houston for the number-one spot in 1999) remains the prototypical center of photochemical air pollution in the United States. Outside the United States, however, many megacities remain plagued by the classic forms of air pollution. For example, uncontrolled industrial emissions surrounding cities like Beijing and the northern sectors of Mexico City are dominated by oil, coal, and industrial emissions, whereas southern Mexico City, Santiago, and Tokyo have substantially (but not so exclusively) automobile-derived oxidant smogs. The lack of

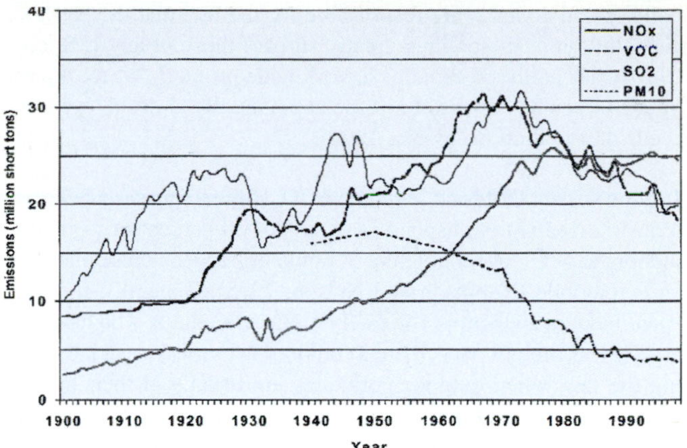

Figure 28-5. Emission trend for volatile organic compounds (VOC), nitrogen oxides (NO_x), sulfur dioxide (SO_2), and particulate matter (PM <10 μm) from 1900 (or when records began) to 1998.

Note that since the passage of the Clean Air Act of 1970, most emissions have decreased or, in the case of nitrogen oxides, have leveled off. (Reproduced with permission from National Air Pollutant Emission Trends Report, 1998.)

policies and controls are responsible for the fact that the levels of air pollution in these cities greatly surpass those of any U.S. city. Clearly, air pollution remains a worldwide problem, where the estimate of people exposed to ozone at potentially harmful levels exceeds 480 million (Schwela, 1996).

Indoor versus Outdoor People in the United States (and in most industrialized nations) spend in excess of 80 percent of their time indoors at work, at school, and at home or between these places in an automobile (Robinson and Nelson, 1995). Generally, the time spent indoors is disproportionately higher for adults, who have relatively less time to participate in outdoor activities, especially during the day, when outdoor pollutants are usually at their highest levels. Children and outdoor workers, by contrast, are much more likely to encounter outdoor air pollution at its worst; in fact, because of the relatively high activity levels of these subgroups compared with inactive office workers, their lungs may incur a considerably larger dose of any given pollutant. Thus, while it is important to characterize and track pollution levels in outdoor air, the most appropriate measure for exposure should involve a paradigm that addresses the total personal exposure of the individual or group of concern, and taken one step further, also dose to the lungs. However, defining typical paradigms of personal exposure can be exceedingly difficult, as personal monitoring is tedious, expensive, and complex given the many potential pollutants one may encounter and can involve a personal dynamic as individual as that person's lifestyle. Frequently, groups of people are monitored in order to develop models for the projection expected exposure values.

The indoor environment has only recently been widely appreciated as a major contributor to total personal exposure. The energy crisis of the 1970s spurred efforts to increase home and building insulation, reduce infiltration of outside air, and minimize energy consumption. At the same time, indoor sources of air contaminants have been on the rise from household products and furnishings, which—when combined with poorly ventilated heating systems and overall reductions in air-exchange rates—give rise to potentially unhealthy indoor air environments. As people began to notice patterns of odors, microbiologic growth, and even ill health, measures of indoor air became a significant part of environmental assessment. Personal exposure has, therefore, come to include the myriad of potential sources, both outdoors and indoors.

It is clear now that indoor air can be even more complex than outdoor air. Indeed, outdoor air permeates the indoor environment in spite of the reduced air exchange in most buildings. However, many variables determine how well components of the outdoor air infiltrate. The current evidence suggests that the average insulated home has about one air change per hour, resulting in indoor concentrations of pollutants that range from 30 to 80% of those outdoors. For nonreactive gases (e.g., CO), there could likely be nearly a 1:1 indoor/outdoor ratio in the absence of a "sink" for that gas; the ratio for fine particulate matter (<2.5 μm) could also be fairly high (~0.4 to 0.7), since these particles can easily penetrate through cracks and open spaces. In contrast, the indoor/outdoor ratio of O_3 would likely be low (<0.3) because of its reactivity. Obviously, household differences in the use of window ventilation and air conditioning would be important variables. Where there are independent sources of contamination indoors, the ratio of an indoor pollutant to that outdoors can even exceed 1 (e.g., NO_2). Unvented space heaters and poorly vented fireplaces and wood stoves or fresh paint and cleaning agents can be significant indoor sources. However, attention now is being directed toward the many and varied insidious sources of indoor contaminants: certain soils and construction masonry (radon), gas cooking appliances (NO_x), sidestream tobacco smoke (PM, CO, and a host of carcinogenic polyaromatics), and carpets, furnishings, dry-cleaned clothes, and household air fresheners (VOCs). Some of these chemicals can even interact with one another as has been found to occur with O_3 diffused indoors reacting with VOCs emitted from household cleaners. The complexity of these multiple sources underscores the importance of appreciating the total exposure scenario if we are to understand the nature of air pollution and its potential effects on humans (Fig. 28-6).

EPIDEMIOLOGIC EVIDENCE OF HEALTH EFFECTS

Outdoor Air Pollution

Acute and Episodic Exposures A number of air pollution incidents have been documented where concentrations of contaminants have risen to levels that are clearly hazardous to human health. When a single chemical has been accidentally released (e.g., methyl isocyanate in Bhopal, India), establishing the relationship between cause and ill effect is typically straightforward. However, most air pollution situations involve complex atmospheres, and establishing a specific cause other than the air pollution incident itself can be difficult. Three acute episodes of community air pollution are considered classic (Meuse Valley, Donora, and London). In each event, community inhabitants were clearly affected adversely; hospitalizations were concomitant with or were followed closely with an elevation in the mortality rate. Although no single contaminant could be fully blamed in any of these, the air pollution was the "reducing-type," in which acrid, coal-derived sulfurous gas and industrial particulate matter (including many metal sulfates) accumulated within a blanket of cool moist air. In each case, a meteorologic inversion (cold air capped above by a blanket of warm air, with little or no vertical air mixing) prevailed for 3 or 5 days, during which time the concentration of pollutants rose well above the normal levels for these already heavily polluted areas. No actual measurements of pollution were made in the Meuse Valley and Donora, but crude measurements of the London fog recorded daily averages of smoke and SO_2. These were estimated at 4.5 mg/m^3 and 1.34 ppm, respectively, on the worst day. Brief (on the order of hours) peak concentrations probably reached even higher levels. During the Meuse Valley episode, 65 people died, while in Donora the number was 20. These deaths were considered "excess" deaths when compared with normal mortality rates for that time of year.

The famous "London smog" of 1952 is estimated to have resulted in 4000 excess deaths. Hospital admissions increased dramatically, mainly among the elderly and those with preexisting cardiac and/or respiratory disease. Even otherwise healthy pedestrians, their visibility limited to as little as 3 ft, covered their noses and mouths in an attempt to minimize their exposure to the "choking" air. Those with preexisting health problems were particularly affected and made up the majority of deaths. It is ironic that 16 years earlier, 3200 deaths had been predicted for London should it experience an episode like that of the Meuse Valley (Firkert, 1936). Although the London 1952 incident brought the issue of air pollution to the public consciousness, many additional episodes oc-

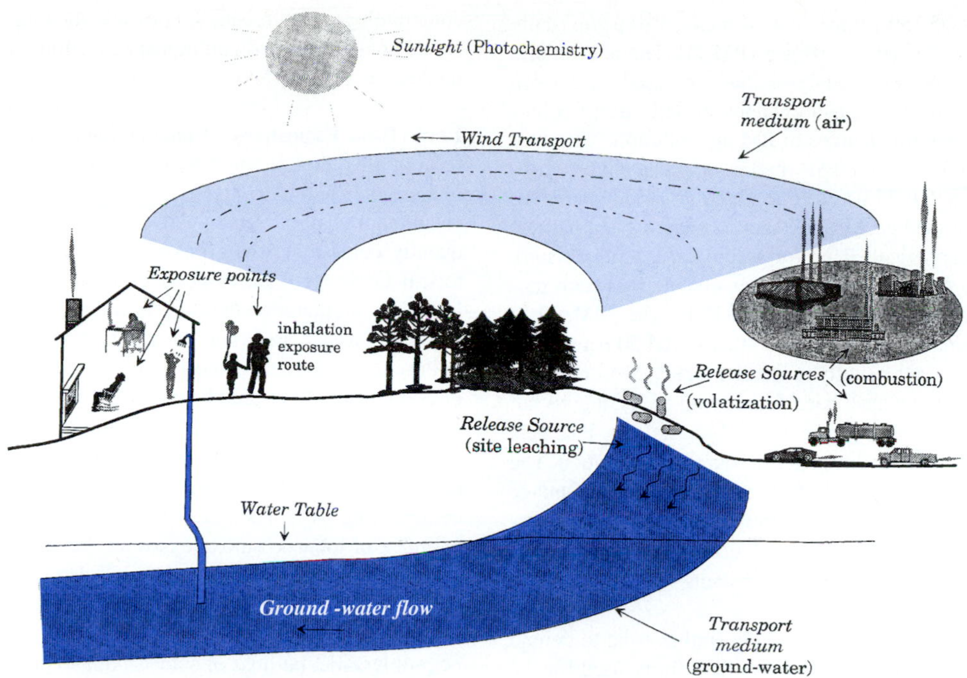

Figure 28-6. Illustration of contributors to the total personal exposure paradigm showing how these indoor and outdoor factors interact.

curred later, with the 1956 and 1962 incidents being among the most notable. As recently as December 1991, London experienced a winter smog alert that exhibited black smoke at 148 $\mu g/m^3$ and SO_2 at 72 ppb (four times and twice the seasonal average, respectively). The difference here was that the polluted atmosphere was far more the result of air contamination by automobile emissions than domestic burning of coal (Anderson, 1999), in keeping with the trends noted above. Mortality and hospital admissions were again affected, and again mostly among the elderly and cardiopulmonary-impaired (mortality: $\uparrow$14 percent cardiovascular and $\uparrow$22 percent respiratory; $\uparrow$43 percent for respiratory admissions). London has not been alone among industrialized cities significantly affected by air pollution episodes in the more recent past. New York; Steubenville, Ohio; Pittsburgh, Pennsylvania; Athens, Greece, and entire regions like those of the Netherlands and the Ruhr Valley of Germany have all had air pollution episodes of note between 1970 and 1990. Air pollution events continue to decrease over time in the modern world, both in their frequency and intensity. What episodes do arise are dwarfed in their impact by the classic smog episodes.

So much has the air improved in recent times that many have thought that the problem of sulfur-based industrial pollution was essentially resolved. However, in the late 1980s, there were revelations regarding acidic pollution of lakes and defoliation of forests (Calvert et al., 1985) as well as new studies showing increased emergency room visits among potentially susceptible populations —asthmatics (Bates and Sizto, 1987). A series of studies showed acute effects of ambient levels of pollution that occur during the summer (summer haze) in areas of central and northeastern North America. These peaks of pollution were typified by increases in O_3 and sulfates, characteristic of the new generation of pollution in most U.S. urban areas. The increase in sulfate consisted of both acidic and atmospherically neutralized forms of sulfuric acid and photochemically derived O_3; such hazes cover large regions and can be widely transported. In one southern Ontario–based study, there was a consistent association in the summer between hospital visits for acute respiratory problems, especially among asthmatic children, and daily levels of both O_3 and sulfate. Interestingly, the apparent combined temporal or sequential patterns of O_3 and sulfate were associated with the health effects, but neither constituent alone. Similar results have been reported for the upstate New York area as well (Thurston et al., 1992), but acidity as $[H^+]$, which is common in summer haze, was thought to play a more dominant role. However, studies of children at summer camps, where they are active and outdoors most of the day, had reported decrements in daily measured pulmonary function on days when both O_3 and acidity levels were elevated but still below those that would be predicted to have a measurable effect (Lippmann, 1989). Animal toxicology and clinical studies in adolescent asthmatics have lent further support to the belief that H^+ can affect airway function, particularly in the presence of O_3. Studies in the South and Southwest similarly have found effects in young asthmatics, but these appear to relate more specifically to O_3, since sulfate is less prominent. This finding is in agreement with earlier data from the Los Angeles area showing a high degree of correlation between diminished performance among high school athletes and increased oxidant levels.

Of the many studies of air pollution over the last 10 to 15 years, none has had more impact on today's perspective of the risks associated with pollution than a series of studies using a relatively new analyses of contemporary or preexistent daily mortality and morbidity trends and regional air monitoring data. These studies showed significant and consistent associations between health impacts of ambient PM at levels thought to be safe. Prior to this period, measurable effects of PM and SO_2 were not easily detected below the 24-h mean for smoke and SO_2 levels of 250 $\mu g/m^3$ and 0.19 ppm, respectively. The new findings showed effects, evidenced by increases in mortality and morbidity rates at or below their contemporaneous NAAQS [50 μg/m^3, annual mean; 150 μg/m^3 daily maximum for PM of diameter <10 μm (PM_{10})]. The new studies made use of novel time-series analyses that are based on Poisson regression modeling to distinguish changes in daily death counts associated with short-term changes in PM air pollution. The studies initially found effects with TSP matter, which includes virtually all particles to about 35 μm in mass median aerodynamic diameter (MMAD—a median particle size normalizing the particle to unit density and spherical shape for aerodynamic comparison). These studies were followed with stronger associations with particles considered almost fully inhalable—PM_{10} (an MMAD at which PM is aerodynamically separated at an initial 50 percent efficiency at 10 μm and increasingly at smaller sizes). Most recently, even stronger associations have been found with an analogous but fully and deeply respirable particle—$PM_{2.5}$. As the PM gets smaller, it represents more anthropogenic sources of pollution. The statistical methodology applied in these studies had an advantage over conventional regression analyses in that it could detect short-term trends and minimized the effects of other pollutants and potential confounders with longer time constants (Schwartz, 1991; reviewed by Pope and Dockery, 1999).

In contrast to the three epidemiologic studies used to defend the 1987 PM_{10} NAAQS, there were more than thirty used for the 1997 revision of the standard and promulgation of a new $PM_{2.5}$ NAAQS [15 μg/m^3, annual mean; 65 μg/m^3 daily maximum for PM of diameter <2.5 μm ($PM_{2.5}$)]. These newer studies have shown a significant health impact of PM, linked to mass and not necessarily sulfate or any other constituent. Although effects are most apparent in individual groups already compromised by cardiopulmonary diseases, there is no one accepted mechanism to account for these findings (Schwartz, 1994; Costa, 2000). That the association is not somehow linked to the composition of the PM has drawn considerable attention from researchers who are trying to establish a "biologically plausible" link to some attribute of PM other than mass alone. The linkage to mass and not composition is somewhat counterintuitive to the toxicology community, especially in light of the fact that all PM is not constitutively identical. Nevertheless, the collective data show that for day-to-day fluctuations in the mass concentration of 10 μg/m^3 airborne PM, there occurs an increase of about 0.6 to 1 percent (excess) mortality. In addition to mortality, morbidity (in terms of hospital visits, inhaler use by asthmatics, and school absenteeism) also is associated with ambient PM levels; other factors such as temperature, humidity, O_3, SO_2, and other pollutants per se do not explain the observed effects. At this point the consistency of the phenomenon from one geographic site to another and over time is remarkable. Even revisiting the mortality data from the 1952 London incident demonstrates that PM was likely the pollutant of most prominence in terms of the adverse health consequences back almost 50 years (Schwartz and Marcus, 1990).

The direction and design of population studies today, frequently referred to as panel or cohort studies, are largely person-based, where groups of people are studied (e.g., nursing home residents, schoolchildren) in their immediate environment using non- or minimally invasive clinical tools (e.g., pulmonary or cardiac function, symptoms, blood screenings, etc.) to correlate effects with ambient and/or personal environmental and air pollutant measures. These studies sacrifice the power of group numbers for more direct and individual data in an attempt to link biomarkers with exposure. These novel approaches have the promise of eventually offering clues as to causality, which is not possible with conventional epidemiology, and recent studies are showing increasingly more subtle changes in cardiopulmonary function with exposure to very modest air pollution.

Long-Term Exposures Epidemiologic studies of the chronic effects of air pollution are difficult to conduct because of the nature of the goal: outcomes associated with long-term exposures. The usual approach of retrospective, cross-sectional studies is frequently confounded with unknown variables and inadequate historical exposure data. A good example of the problem of confounding is cigarette smoking. Without extensive control of both active of passive smoking, the ability to discern the impact of air pollution or a disease outcome such as chronic bronchitis and emphysema would be greatly impaired because of the high background of disease attributable to smoking and the imprecision of most indices of smoking exposure in this type of study. In contrast, prospective studies have the advantage of more precise control of confounding variables, such as the tracking of urinary cotinine as an index of tobacco smoke exposure, but they can be very expensive and require substantial time and dedication on both the part of the investigators as well as the population under study. Depending on the study size and design, exposure aspects can also be problematic, but loss of subjects due to dropout is usually more troublesome.

Despite these deficiencies, there have been several epidemiology studies of both types conducted with the aim of determining long-term air pollution health effects. In general, these studies have suggested a positive association between urban pollution and progressive pulmonary impairment. On the one hand, cross-sectional studies in the Los Angeles Air Basin have found evidence of accelerated "aging-like" loss of lung function in people living for extended periods in regions of high oxidant pollution as compared with areas where sea air circulates and lowers the overall pollutant concentrations (Detels et al., 1991). Similarly, chronic exposure to SO_2 and PM in the Netherlands over a 12-year period was shown prospectively to gradually impair lung function (Van De Lende et al., 1981). And even rural areas in western Pennsylvania, which are swept by reducing-type pollutants transported from midwestern industrial centers, have been shown to have a higher incidence of respiratory symptoms as determined from a questionnaire-based design (Schenker et al., 1983). While the role of any specific pollutant in these studies is difficult to dissect, the message that air pollution contributes to deterioration of lung health seems clear.

Among the most detailed prospective epidemiologic studies of the chronic health effects of current levels of air pollution has been the so-called Harvard Six Cities Study begun in the early 1970s. The cities were chosen to represent a range of air quality (based on SO_2 and PM). Initially, there was great dependence on routine regional air-monitoring data, but over time air analyses of microenvironments by the investigators themselves predominated. The initial design of these studies included the gathering of parental questionnaire data (including some 20,000 people) about the prevalence of respiratory problems in schoolchildren and has been continued over twenty years with tracking of similar data along with periodic assessments of pulmonary function. When compared across cities, [H^+] (measured in four of the six cities) was correlated (Fig. 28-7*A*) better than was sulfate with the prevalence of bronchitis in children age 10 to 12 (Speizer, 1989). However, as the assessment program evolved, more detailed study revealed mortality associations with PM as noted above, and represented in Fig.

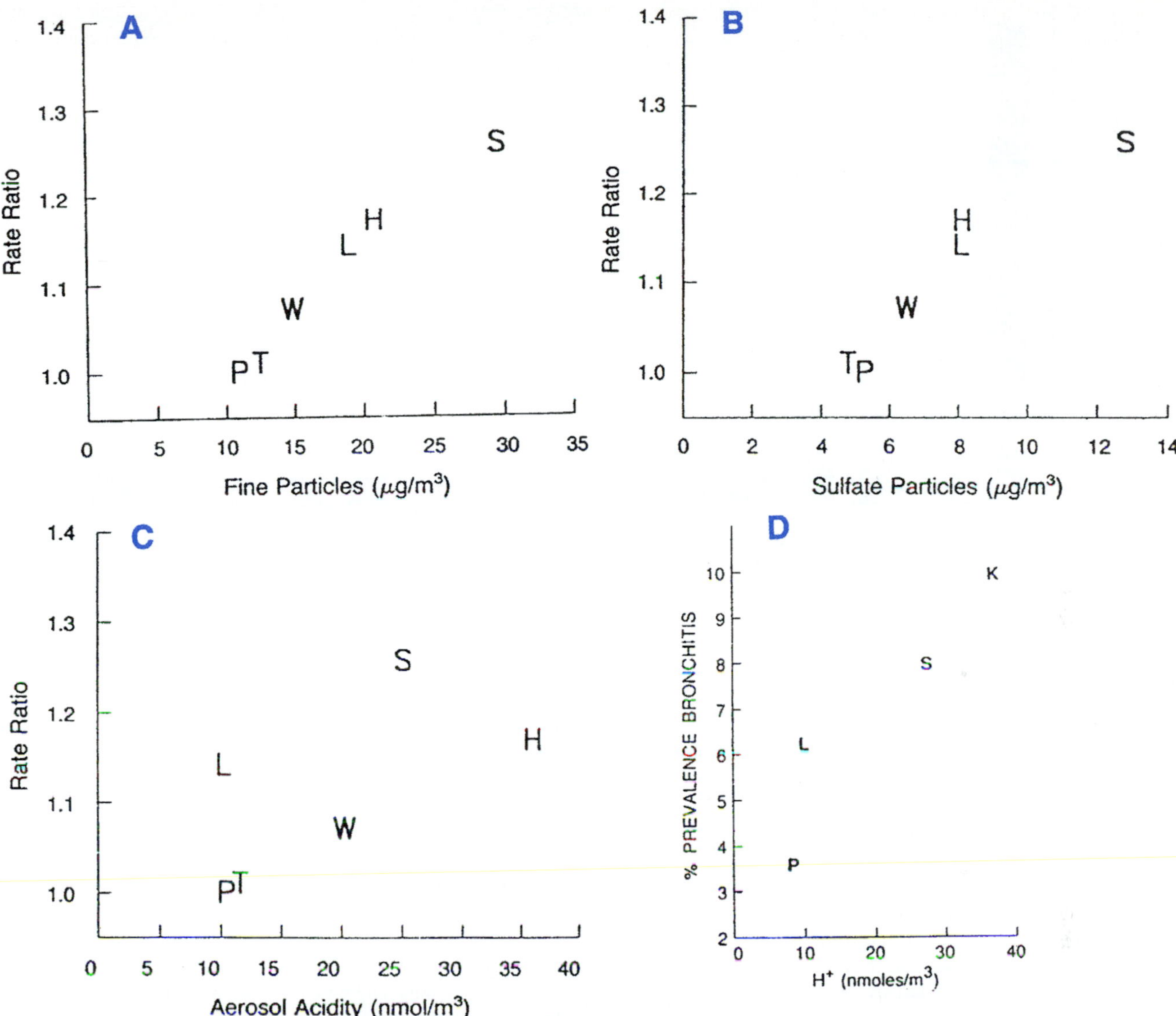

Figure 28-7. Data from the Harvard Six Cities Studies indicating the superior relationship of PM_{10} and sulfate to mortality rates (**A–C**) *in contrast to acidity* (**D**), *which correlates better with the prevalence of bronchitis in children. [Reproduced with permission from Speizer, 1989* (**D**) *and Dockery et al., 1993* (**A–C**).*]*

28-7*B* through *D*, but the role of $[H^+]$ in this relationship with acute mortality was less convincing than that associated with the sulfate or fine ($\leq$2.5 μm) PM (sulfates co-associate with fine PM in the atmosphere) (Dockery et al., 1993). But more importantly with regard to long-term health, this study showed very significant effects of PM on the life spans of people living in Steubenville, Ohio—an area of industrial reducing-type pollution. Over a 15-year period, the average human life span was reduced by about 2 years due to PM exposure. Another cohort-based mortality study of the long-term effects from PM, especially that derived from combustion ($PM_{2.5}$ and sulfate), was conducted using the data from 151 cities (Pope et al., 1995). This study confirmed the impact of PM on mortality, showing a 15 to 17 percent increased risk over 7 years, about equivalent to the risk of smoking over that period. Hence, there is now growing concern for the potential chronic health impacts and heightened risk of premature death from lifelong air pollution exposure.

The role of air pollution in human lung cancer is also difficult to assess because the vast majority of respiratory cancers result from cigarette smoking. However, many compounds that occur as urban air pollutants are known to have carcinogenic potency. Several of these compounds are among the 188 HAPs listed in the CAA Amendment of 1990. However, most of the HAPs and even fewer (about 10 percent) of the more than 2800 compounds that have been identified in the air have been assayed for carcinogenic potency. Figure 28-8 gives estimates of the relative contributions of various chemicals to the lung cancer rate that is *not* associated with cigarette smoking, which, for outdoor air, is estimated to be about 2000 cases per year (Lewtas, 1993). This compares with about 2000 cases per year for passive environmental tobacco smoke and about 100,000 cases per year for smokers. Volatile organic compounds (VOCs) and nitrogen-containing and halogenated organics account for most of the compounds that have been studied with animal and genetic bioassays. Most of these compounds are

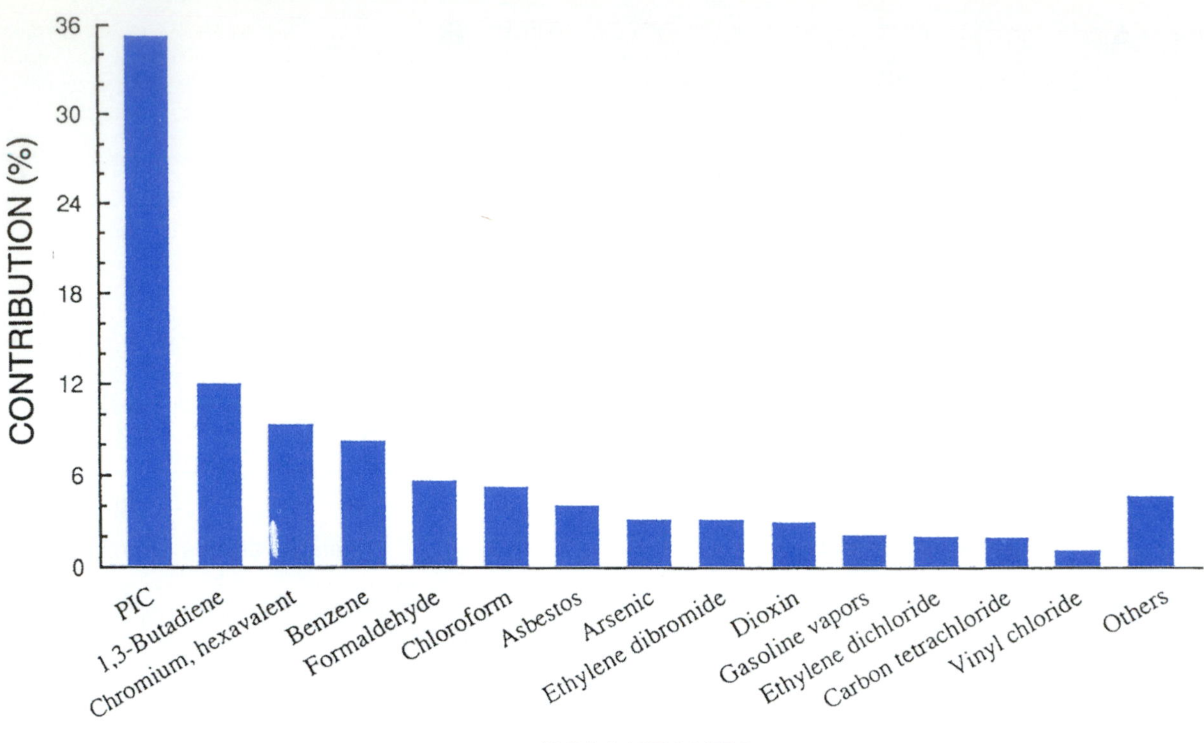

Figure 28-8. Relative contribution of individual airborne hazardous pollutants to lung cancer rates after removal of tobacco smoke cancer.

The total number of cancers from non-tobacco-smoke sources is estimated to be about 2000 per year. (Reproduced with permission from Lewtas, 1993.) PIC = products of incomplete combustion.

derived from combustion sources ranging from tobacco to power plants to incinerators. Other potential carcinogens arise from mobile sources as products of incomplete combustion and their atmospheric transformation products as well as fugitive or accidental chemical releases. This contrasts with indoor air, where the sources are thought to derive largely from environmental tobacco smoke and radon, with some contribution from the off-gassed organics (e.g., adhesives, carpet polymers).

The cancer risk of any individual should be some function of the carcinogenic nature of the substance, the amount of material deposited, which is itself a function of the concentration in the ambient air and the cumulative volume inhaled, and of course the innate susceptibility of the individual (including genotypic traits and environmental factors such as diet, etc.). A significant body of data suggests that the majority of cancer risk from ambient air pollution lies within the particulate fraction. Among the many potent chemicals are the polycyclic organic chemicals, along with a group of less-volatile organics sometimes referred to as "semivolatiles" (including nitroaromatics). These persistent organics associate with the particulate matrix and thus could have a prolonged residence time at deposition sites within the respiratory tract. Genetic bioassays have revealed the potent mutagenicity, and presumably carcinogenicity, of various chemical fractions of ambient aerosols (Lewtas, 1993). Some of these compounds require metabolic transformation to activate their potency while others may be detoxified by their metabolism.

The cells lining the respiratory tract turn over relatively quickly, since they continuously interface with the ambient environment. Conceptually, their DNA would thus be frequently vulnerable to carcinogenic or oxidant-induced replication errors that, when fixed as mutations, could be tumorigenic. Copollutants, such as irritant gases that initiate inflammation, may promote carcinogenic activity by damaging cells and further enhancing their turnover. For example, there is experimental evidence that benzo(a)pyrene inhaled by rats whose respiratory tracts have been chronically irritated by SO_2 inhalation may result in bronchogenic carcinoma. Likewise, epidermoid carcinomas were produced in mice that inhaled ozonized gasoline, containing many reactive organic products, if these mice had been previously infected with influenza virus and had presumably developed inflammation. Many believe that the so-called rural-urban gradient of lung cancer, apparent even when corrected for cigarette smoking, is a product of these complex interactions. Thus, while the phenomenon of environmental lung cancer remains poorly understood, there is general sentiment for the early opinion expressed by Kotin and Falk in 1963: "Chemical, physical and biological data unite to form a constellation that strongly implicates the atmosphere as one dominant factor in the pathogenesis of lung cancer." At the time of this statement, however, the role of tobacco smoke was not widely appreciated.

Indoor Air Pollution

As outdoor air quality has improved over the last 20 to 30 years, there has been a growing awareness of the potential for indoor air pollution to elicit adverse health effects. The concerns about indoor air that at first brought skepticism have gained an element of respectability as various attributes of the indoor environment and its effect on health and well-being are being investigated. However, the issue remains controversial because many of the health problems associated with indoor air pollution generally involve nonspecific symptomatology and appear to involve a wide range of potential toxicants and sources (Molhave et al., 1986). The responses to indoor air pollution also appear to be affected by ambient comfort factors such as temperature and humidity. Two broadly defined illnesses that are largely unique to the indoor environment are discussed below (Brooks and Davis, 1992).

Sick-Building Syndromes This collection of ailments, defined by a set of persistent symptoms enduring at least 2 weeks (Table 28-3), occurs in at least 20 percent of those exposed and is typically of unknown specific etiology but is relieved sometime after an affected individual leaves the offending building (Hayes et al., 1995). Frequently but not always, this syndrome occurs in new, poorly ventilated, or recently refurbished office buildings. The suspected causes include combustion products, household chemicals, biological materials and vapors, and emissions from furnishings; they are exacerbated by the effect of poor ventilation on comfort factors. The perception of irritancy to the eyes, nose, and throat ranks among the predominant symptoms that can become intolerable with repeated exposures. Controlled clinical studies have shown concentration- and duration-dependent worsening of sensory discomfort after exposure to a complex mixture of 22 VOCs commonly found in the indoor environment (Molhave et al., 1986). The many factors contributing to such responses are poorly understood but include various host susceptibility factors such as personal stress and fatigue, diet and alcohol use, and other factors. Current biomarkers of response used in the laboratory include sensory irritancy to the eyes in volunteer test subjects and sometimes in animals as well. Animal studies using standard measures of sensory irritation or other corporal endpoints have had limited success in assessing sick-building syndromes (SBS) and related syndromes. The biggest problem generally lies in the VOC concentrations required to achieve responses in a limited pool of animals that relate to likely human exposures is too high to establish a plausible link to the human condition.

Building-Related Illnesses This group of illnesses, in contrast to the SBS, consists of well-documented conditions with defined diagnostic criteria and generally recognizable causes. These illnesses typically call for a conventional treatment regimen, since simply exiting the building where the illness was contracted does not readily reverse the symptoms. Several of the bicontaminant-related illnesses (e.g., legionnaires' disease, hypersensitivity pneumonitis, humidifier fever) fall into this group, as do allergies to animal dander, dust mites, and cockroaches. Some toxic inhalants might be classified in this group, such as carbon monoxide. In many cases, however, when the concentrations of CO, NO_2, and many VOCs result in less discernible or definable conditions, the responses may be mistaken for or considered to be SBS, thus complicating the assessment of the situation. It should be noted that many inhalants, such as NO_2 and trichloroethylene (a VOC common to the indoor air arising from chlorinated water or dry-cleaned clothes), have been shown in animal toxicology studies to suppress immune defenses and allow opportunistic pathogens to proliferate in the lung. The involvement of immunologic suppression is a particularly controversial yet important attribute of indoor pollution because of its insidious nature and implications for all building-related illnesses. This is further complicated in that complex indoor environments comprising of chemicals and biologicals may also lead to in unexpected interactions that are virtually unstudied and thus are not appreciated in the assessment of indoor pollution.

Table 28-3
Symptoms Commonly Associated with the Sick-Building Syndromes

Eyes, nose, and throat irritation
Headaches
Fatigue
Reduced attention span
Irritability
Nasal congestion
Difficulty breathing
Nosebleeds
Dry skin
Nausea

SOURCE: Modified from Brooks and Davis, 1992, with permission.

POLLUTANTS OF OUTDOOR AMBIENT AIR

Classic Reducing-Type Air Pollution

The acute air pollution episodes of this century have made it clear that high concentrations of the reducing-type air pollution, characterized by SO_2 and smoke, are capable of producing disastrous human health effects. Empiric studies in human subjects and animals have long stressed the irritancy of SO_2 and its role in these incidents, while the full potential for interactions among the copollutants in the smoky, sulfurous mix has not been fully replicated in the laboratory. Nevertheless, the irritancy of most S-oxidation products in the atmosphere is well documented, and there are both empiric and theoretical reasons to suspect that such products act to amplify the irritancy of fossil fuel emission atmospheres via chemical transformations and related interactions.

Sulfur Dioxide ***General toxicology*** Sulfur dioxide is a water-soluble irritant gas. As such, it is absorbed predominantly in the upper airways and, as an irritant, can stimulate bronchoconstriction and mucus secretion in a number of species, including humans. As one of the earliest suspect air pollutants, it has been well studied over the years. Early studies with relatively high exposure concentrations of SO_2 showed airway cellular injury and subsequent proliferation of mucus-secreting goblet cells. This attribute of SO_2 has led to its use ($>$250 ppm) in the production of laboratory animal models of bronchitis and airway injury (Kodavanti et al., 1999). At much lower concentrations ($<$1 ppm), such as might be encountered in the polluted ambient air of industrialized areas, long-term residents experience a higher incidence of bronchitis. In fact, prior to the breakup of the Soviet block, many eastern European cities were renowned for widespread public affliction with bronchitis; now, 20 years later, the prevalence of bronchitis is greatly reduced (von Mutius et al., 1994). While other factors (diet, access to health care, other pollutants) may well have been involved in this reversal, reductions in ambient smoke and SO_2 are generally thought to be most important.

The concentrations of SO_2 likely to be encountered in the United States are lower still—on average, less than 0.1 ppm. Mandated use of cleaner (low-S) fossil fuels, emission control devices, and the use of tall emission stacks have largely been responsible for the reductions. However, on occasional down-drafting of smokestack plumes or meteorological inversions near point-sources result in low ppm levels of SO_2 that may pose a hazard to some individuals. A 2-min exposure to 0.4 to 1.0 ppm can elicit bronchoconstriction in exercising asthmatics within 5 to 10 min (Gong et al., 1995). However, it is the low-level, long-term effects, which erode pulmonary defenses, that continue to worry some regulators. Studies have shown that SO_2 is itself capable of impairing macrophage-dependent bacterial killing in murine models. Exposed mice have a greater frequency and severity of infection, which has been suggested to be linked to diminished ability to generate endogenous oxidants for bacterial killing. Analogously, rats exposed for 70 to 170 h to 0.1, 1.0, and 20 ppm exhibited reduced clearance of inert particles, while dogs exposed to 1 ppm for a year had slowed tracheal mucocilliary transport. The fact that the low-concentration exposures showed marked effects when extended over longer periods is consistent with the epidemiologic associations between SO_2 exposure and bronchitis. The evidence is not clear, however, as some studies show no overt pulmonary pathology. Guinea pigs and monkeys, for example, showed no effect on lung function or pathology after a year of continuous exposure to concentrations of 0.1 to 5 ppm (Alarie et al., 1970, 1972).

The penetration of SO_2 into the lungs is greater during mouth as opposed to nose breathing. An increase in the airflow rate further augments penetration of the gas into the deeper lung. As a result, persons exercising would inhale more SO_2 and, as noted with asthmatics, are likely to experience greater irritation. Once deposited along the airway, SO_2 dissolves into surface lining fluid as sulfite or bisulfite and is readily distributed throughout the body. It is thought that the sulfite interacts with sensory receptors in the airways to initiate local and centrally mediated bronchoconstriction. Labeled $^{35}SO_2$ studies indicate, however, that some residual S (presumably as protein reaction products) persists in the respiratory system for a week or more after exposure, and is slowly excreted in the urine (Yokoyama et al., 1971). In both rabbits and human subjects, sulfite that reaches the plasma has been shown to form *S*-sulfonate products of reaction with the disulfide bonds in plasma proteins (Gunnison and Palmes, 1974). The toxicologic significance of *S*-sulfonate proteins is unknown, but they might serve as markers of exposure.

Pulmonary Function Effects The basic pulmonary response to inhaled SO_2 is mild bronchoconstriction, which is reflected as a measurable increase in airflow resistance due to narrowing of the airways. Concentration-related increases in resistance have been observed in guinea pigs, dogs, and cats as well as humans. Exposure of isolated segments of the nose or airways of dogs and guinea pigs appeared to alter resistance in a manner consistent with receptor-mediated sensory stimulation. Airflow resistance increased more when the gas was introduced through a tracheal cannula than via the nose, since nasal scrubbing of the water-soluble gas was bypassed. Isolated nasal exposures increased nasal airflow resistance through the nose largely as a result of mucosal swelling, but the irritant effect appeared to signal to the more distal airways as well. Direct exposure of the trachea had a more dramatic effect on airflow resistance, but exposure of the intact nose and lungs together gave the most marked responses, consistent with the theory that a neural network involving receptor stimulation is involved in bronchoconstriction (Frank and Speizer, 1965; Nadel et al., 1965). Intravenous injection of atropine (a parasympathetic receptor blocker) or cooling of the cervical vagosympathetic nerves abolishes bronchoconstriction in the cat model; rewarming of the nerve reestablishes the response. The rapidity of the response and its reversal emphasize the parasympathetic tonal change in airway smooth muscle. Studies in human subjects have confirmed the predominance of parasympathetic mediation, but histamine from inflammatory cells may play a secondary role in the bronchoconstrictive responses of asthmatics (Sheppard et al., 1981).

Human subjects exposed to 1, 5, or 13 ppm SO_2 for just 10 min exhibit a rapid bronchoconstrictive response, with 1 to 3 ppm being a threshold for most if exercise is involved. Healthy individuals at rest seem to have a clear response at about 5 ppm, though there is considerable variation among individuals (Frank et al., 1962). Even 0.25 to 1 ppm for a few hours can induce bronchoconstriction in adult and adolescent subjects with clinically defined mild asthma (Sheppard et al., 1981; Koenig et al., 1981). Findings such as these (responses <0.5 ppm) have raised concerns about potential adverse effects in this sensitive subpopulation when it is exposed to peaks of SO_2 that are known to occur near point sources.

Chronic Effects Few long-term studies have been conducted with SO_2 at levels approaching those found in ambient air. Alarie and associates (1970) exposed guinea pigs to 0.13, 1.01, or 5.72 ppm SO_2 continuously for a year without adverse impact on lung mechanics. Similarly, monkeys exhibited no alteration in pulmonary function when exposed continuously for 78 weeks to 0.14, 0.64, and 1.28 ppm SO_2 (Alarie et al., 1972). Even in the presence of 0.1 mg/m^3 sulfuric acid, dogs exposed 16 h a day for 18 months to 0.5 ppm SO_2 showed no impairment in pulmonary function (Vaughan et al., 1969). Only higher levels of SO_2 for protracted periods of time [dogs to 5 ppm for 225 days (Lewis et al., 1969); rats to 350 ppm for 30 days (Reid, 1963)] have been shown to alter airway mucus secretion, goblet cell topography, or lung function, but these results are of little relevance to typical SO_2 levels in ambient air.

Sulfuric Acid and Related Sulfates

The conversion of SO_2 to sulfuric acid is favored in the environment. During oil combustion or the smelting of metal, sulfuric acid condenses downstream of the combustion processes with available metal ions and water vapor to form submicron sulfated fly ash. Sulfur dioxide continues to oxidize to sulfate in dispersing smokestack plumes in the presence of free soluble or partially coordinated transition metals such as iron, manganese, and vanadium within the ash particles. When coal is burned, the acid may adsorb to the surface or solubilize in ultrafine (<0.1 μm) metal oxide particles during emission. These sulfates on the surface of coal ash may constitute as much as 9 percent of the emitted sulfur—the rest is emitted as SO_2 gas. Photochemical environments in the lower troposphere can also promote acid sulfate formation via both metal-dependent and independent mechanisms, but studies have shown that most of the oxidation of SO_2 occurs within diluted plumes drifting in the atmosphere. Stack emissions may undergo long-range transport to areas distant from the emission source, allowing considerable time for sunlight-driven chemical reactions to occur. Although the fine-particle sulfates may exist as fine sulfuric acid (the primary source of free H^+), partially or fully neutralized forms (ammonium bisulfate and ammonium sulfate) predominate due to the abundance of natural atmospheric ammonia. As fine PM sulfates are transported long distances, they may contribute to regional summer haze and pose not only a health hazard to certain groups (e.g., asthmatics)–(Koenig et al., 1989), but may stress the general environment as acid rain (Calvert et al., 1985) (Fig. 28-9).

General Toxicology Sulfuric acid irritates respiratory tissues by virtue of its ability to protonate (H^+) receptor ligands and other biomolecules. This action can either directly damage membranes or activate sensory reflexes that initiate inflammation. Ammonia, which exists in free air at about 25 ppb and in much higher concentrations in the mammalian nasopharynx/oropharynx, is capable of neutralizing most of the irritant potential of acidic sulfates. The efficiency of this process is dependent on temperature, relative humidity, and air mixing and thus is a likely source of variability in biological responses. This is particularly true in animal studies involving standard whole-body exposure-chamber operation, in which excreta and bacteria may interact, giving rise to chamber ammonia concentrations up to 1100 ppb—more than enough to fully neutralize sulfuric acid up to several mg/m^3 (Higuchi and Davies, 1993). Similarly, endogenous ammonia such as that which exists in the mouth has been shown to inhibit responses up to 350 μg/m^3 sulfuric acid in exercising asthmatics (Utell et al., 1989). For this reason, most human test subjects rinse orally with citrus juice before a sulfuric acid study, so as to minimize this phenomenon.

Interestingly, there is considerable species variability in sensitivity to sulfuric acid, with guinea pigs being quite reactive to acid sulfates, in contrast to rats, which are highly resistant. The reasons for this difference are not fully understood but relate to receptor type and density in the airways and probably not on differences in neutralization by ammonia in the airway. The sensitivity of healthy humans appears to fall somewhere in between, with asthmatic humans being perhaps best modeled by the guinea pig. Overall, however, the collective data involving animals and humans are remarkably coherent, as reviewed in an article by Amdur (1989). To illustrate this point, Table 28-4 compares the acute toxicity of SO_2 and sulfuric acid in animals and human subjects, using indices detailed below, airway resistance, and bronchial clearance. To allow direct comparisons, the concentrations are presented as μmol/m^3 of the two compounds.

Pulmonary Function Effects Sulfuric acid produces an increase in flow resistance in guinea pigs due to reflex airway narrowing, or bronchoconstriction, which impedes the flow of air into and out of the lungs. This process can be thought of as a defensive measure to limit the inhalation of air containing noxious gases. The magnitude of the response is related to both acid concentration and particle size (Amdur, 1958; Amdur et al., 1978). Early studies indicated that as particle size was reduced from 7 μm to the submicron range, the concentration of sulfuric acid necessary to induce a response and the time to the onset of the response fell significantly. With large particles, even the sensitive guinea pig was able to withstand an exceedingly high (30 mg/m^3) challenge with little change in pulmonary resistance, in contrast to the <1 mg/m^3 challenge needed with the 0.3 μm particles (Amdur et al., 1978). Human asthmatics exposed to 2 mg/m^3 of acid fog (10 μm) for 1 h, a very high concentration for an asthmatic, experienced variable respiratory symptoms suggesting irritation, but no changes in spirometry were elicited (Hackney et al., 1989). The apparent reason for this PM size–based differential response is probably the scrubbing of large particles in the nose, while the small particles are able to penetrate deep into the lung, reaching receptors that stimulate bronchoconstriction and mucus secretion. The thicker mucus blanket of the nose may blunt (by dilution or neutralization by mucus buffers) much of the irritancy of the deposited acid, thus limiting its effects to mucous cell stimulation and a minor increase in nasal flow resistance. In contrast, the less shielded distal airway tissues, with their higher receptor density, would be expected to be more sensitive to the acid, as reflected by their responsiveness to

4.8
4.7
4.6
4.5
4.4
4.3
4.2
*Shaded areas indicate individual states with emissions of 1,000 kilotonnes of SO_2 and greater.
Contours connect points of equal precipitation pH.

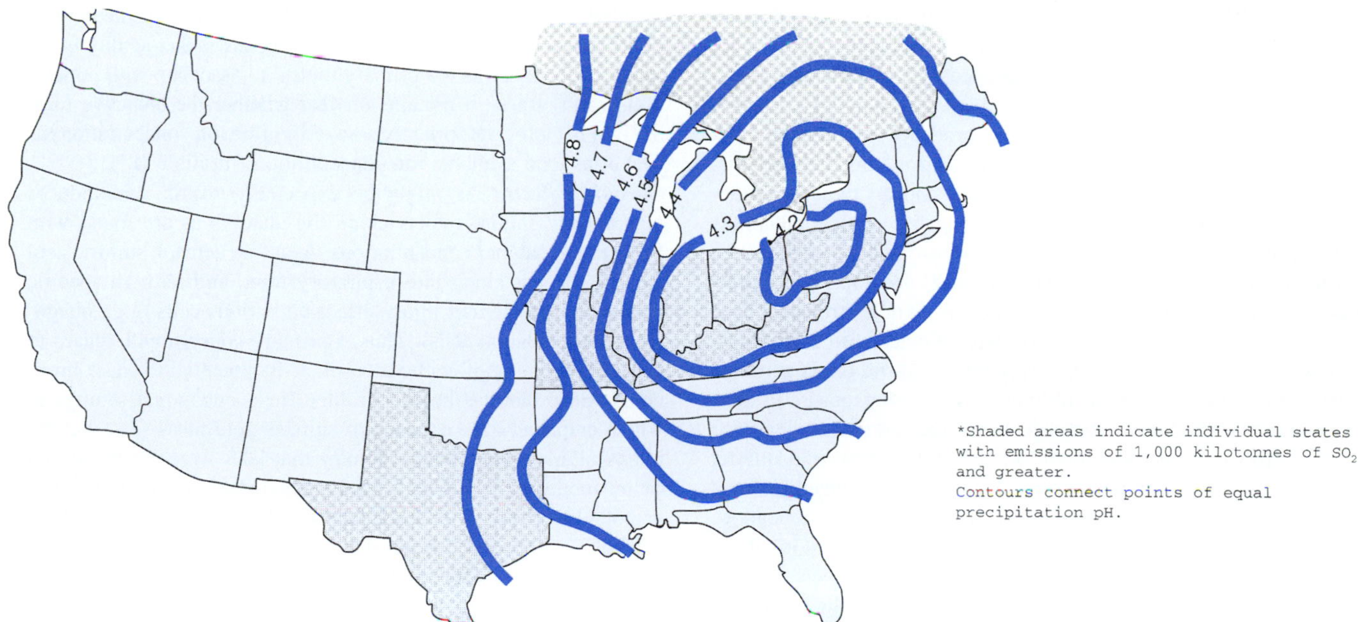

Figure 28-9. Areas in 1988 where precipitation in the East fell below pH 5: acid rain.

The acidity of the air in the east is thought to result from air mass transport of fine sulfated particulate matter from the industrial centers of the Midwest. (Reproduced with permission from National Air Pollutant Emission Trends Report, 1998.)

Table 28-4
Comparative Toxicity of SO_2 and H_2SO_4 in Acute Studies

	μmol		
	SO_2	H_2SO_4	REFERENCE
Guinea pigs: 1 h; 10% ↑ airway resistance	6	1	Amdur, 1974
Donkeys: 30 min; 1-h altered bronchial clearance	8875	2	Spiegelman et al., 1968; Schlesinger et al., 1978
Normal subjects: 7 min; 1-h altered bronchial clearance	520	1	Lippmann and Altshuler, 1976; Leikauf et al., 1981
Normal subjects: 10 min; 5% ↓ tidal volume	29	1.25	Amdur, 1954
Adolescent asthmatics: 40 min; equal ↑ airway resistance	20	1	Koenig et al., 1989

the small particles reaching that area (Costa and Schlegele, 1998). This regional sensitivity and the longer residence time of a deposited particle relative to SO_2 gas probably were reflected in the relatively protracted recovery times observed in acid-exposed guinea pigs compared with animals exposed to SO_2 alone. Alternatively, the particles of ZnO used in this study provided soluble Zn^{+2} when combined with acid.

Asthmatics appear to be somewhat more sensitive to the bronchoconstrictive effects of sulfuric acid than are healthy individuals, but published studies have been inconsistent (Koenig et al., 1989; Utell et al., 1984). Asthma generally is characterized by hyperresponsive airways, so their tendency to constrict at low acid concentrations would be expected, just as asthmatic airways are sensitive to nonspecific airway smooth muscle agonists (e.g., carbachol, histamine, exercise) (Hanley et al., 1992). The variability may well relate to differences in the degree of impairment or underlying inflammation in the subjects, but this hypothesis remains to be confirmed. Airway hyperreactivity has been observed as an acute response in guinea pigs 2 h after a 1-h exposure to 200 μg/m^3 sulfuric acid and appears to be associated with pulmonary inflammation. Likewise in rabbits, increased airway reactivity was associated with arachidonate metabolites, products of epithelial cells as well as inflammatory cells. The general correlation between airway responsiveness and inflammation that appears to be important in grading asthma severity and risk of negative clinical outcomes may also be predictive of responses to environmental stimuli.

Effects on Mucociliary Clearance and Macrophage Function Sulfuric acid alters the clearance of particles from the lung and thus can interfere with a major defense mechanism. Effects on clearance of insoluble, radioactively labeled ferric oxide particles have been observed after as little as a single 1-h exposure in donkeys, rabbits, and human subjects. The impact on mucus clearance appears to vary directly with the acidity ([H^+]) of the acid sulfate, with sulfuric acid having the greatest effect and ammonium sulfate the smallest (Schlesinger, 1984). Curiously, there appears to be a biphasic response to the acid that has been observed in all animal species studies to date as well as in human subjects. In general, brief, single exposures of $<$250 μg/m^3 accelerate clearance, while high concentrations of $>$1000 μg/m^3 clearly depress clearance. Over several days, there also appears to be a cumulative (concentration times duration) dose-related depression of clearance. Longer-term exposure of rabbits to low-level acid ultimately slows clearance in apparent concert with hyperplasia of airway mucosecretory cells (Gearhart and Schlesinger, 1989). Acidification of mucus by H^+ (i.e., a fall in pH), even if localized, is hypothesized to have potential effects on mucus rheology and viscosity (Holma, 1989) as well as on mucus secretion and ciliary function. These effects are not unreasonable in light of the drop in macrophage intracellular pH reported in some acid studies (Qu et al., 1993).

Sulfate effects on bronchial clearance in both rabbits and humans and airway resistance in guinea pigs and in asthmatics (though sensitivities in these subjects can be quite variable) appear coherent relative to the irritant potency of sulfates: sulfuric acid $>$ ammonium bisulfate $>$ ammonium sulfate. Acidity appears to be the primary driving factor on most respiratory effects attributable to the acid sulfates even at the level of pulmonary macrophages. Lavaged rabbit macrophage phagocytosis was affected more after a single exposure to 500 μg/m^3 sulfuric acid than after 2000 μg/m^3 ammonium bisulfate (Schlesinger et al., 1990). However, there is some evidence at the level of cellular activation and arachidonate metabolism suggesting that the anionic component of the aerosol also plays some role. Although the consensus is that acidity is the active toxicant and is the primary metric to associate with population health effects, it remains unclear whether the bioactive form of [H^+] is more appropriately assayed as free ion concentration (as pH) or as total available ion concentration (titratible H^+).

Chronic Effects As might be expected, sulfuric acid induces qualitatively similar effects along the airways as are found with SO_2 at much higher concentrations. As a fine aerosol, sulfuric acid deposits deeper along the respiratory tract, and its high specific acidity imparts greater injury effect on various cells (e.g., phagocytes and epithelial cells). Thus, a primary concern with regard to chronic inhalation of acidic aerosols is its potential to cause bronchitis, since this has been a problem in occupational settings in which employees are exposed to sulfuric acid mists (e.g., battery plants). Early studies in the donkey that later were expanded in a rabbit model have provided fundamental data on this issue. The profound depression of clearance found in donkeys exposed repeatedly (100 μg/m^3 1 h per day for 6 months) promoted the hypothesis that a similar response (i.e., chronic bronchitis) can occur in humans. This argument was strengthened by the similar bronchitogenic responses of the two species when chronically exposed to cigarette smoke.

Many studies conducted with sulfuric acid in the rabbit are in general agreement with the early findings in the donkey (Schlesinger et al., 1979; Schlesinger 1984). These studies have expanded our knowledge of the biological response and its exposure-based relationship. The initial stimulation of clearance with subsequent depression has been shown to occur over 12 months with as little as 2 h per day at 125 $\mu g/m^3$ sulfuric acid (Schlesinger et al., 1992). Related studies also have demonstrated that the airways of exposed animals become progressively more sensitive to challenge with acetylcholine, showed a progressive decrease in diameter, and experienced an increase in the number of secretory cells, especially in the smaller airways (Gearhart and Schlesinger, 1989).

Unlike other irritants, such as O_3 (see below), sulfuric acid does not appear to stimulate a classic neutrophilic inflammation after exposure. Rather, eicosanoid homeostasis appears to be disturbed resulting in macrophage dysfunction and altered host defense, perhaps in part mediated by a decrease in intracellular pH. Long-term disease attributable to connective tissue disturbances induced by sulfuric acid seems to be of lesser concern than is the impact on mucociliary function and the potential effect on ventilation and arterial oxygenation (Alarie et al., 1972, 1975). Therefore, it seems reasonable to postulate that chronic daily exposure of humans to sulfuric acid at levels of about 100 $\mu g/m^3$ may lead to impaired clearance and mild chronic bronchitis. As this is less than an order of magnitude above haze levels of sulfuric acid, the possibility that chronic irritancy may elicit bronchitic-like disease in susceptible individuals (perhaps over a lifetime or in children because of dose differences) appears to be reasonable.

Particulate Matter

Particulate matter in the atmosphere is a mélange of organic, inorganic, and biological materials whose compositional matrix can vary significantly depending on local point sources. The contribution to any regional PM matrix from long-range transport of emissions or transformation products can also be substantial, particularly for fine (<2.5-μm) particles. There is now a large epidemiologic database contending that PM elicits both short- and long-term health effects at current ambient levels (near the NAAQS). According to the epidemiology, these effects appear to be less affected by gross particle composition (e.g., inorganic versus organic) and nominal size (e.g., TSP, PM_{10}, $PM_{2.5}$) than by basic gravimetric measures of ambient exposure. Many have argued that this relationship contradicts the basic tenets of conventional air pollution toxicology, which is rooted in the concept of chemical-specific toxicity. A number of hypotheses that draw upon various physical and chemical attributes of PM have been offered in search of a "biologically plausible" explanation for the reported epidemiologic observations. Prominently included among these hypotheses are PM-associated metals, organics, acidity, size distribution (focusing on the unique bioactivity of ultrafine PM), PM oxidant activity or reactivity, and potentially toxic or allergenic biologicals. However, at present, there is simply not enough basic understanding of the respective roles of PM composition and size to defend one hypothesis overwhelmingly over another, nor is there reason to unseat the PM mass-based correlation with health outcomes. Although the animal and human toxicologic database is growing rapidly with regard to the issue of causation, much remains to learned before new regulatory indices can be adopted.

From research directed initially toward potential occupational hazards, it is known that several metals and silicates that make up at least part of the inorganic phase of PM can be cytotoxic to lung cells, and that organic constituents theoretically can induce toxicity either directly or via metabolism to genotoxic agents. Also, studies focusing on very small, ultrafine (<0.1 μm) particles suggest that though these particles are low in mass, they are high in number and thus provide substantial particle surface to biological surface interaction. Less is known about the role of biologically derived materials such as endotoxin and bioallergen fragments that may elicit rudimentary inflammatory responses, but the involvement of these substances in agricultural and indoor exposures is very real. Finally, in the early days of air pollution toxicology, there was considerable interest in PM–copollutant interactions, but our knowledge in this area beyond the data derived largely from one laboratory (Amdur et al., 1986) is very limited.

Metals There have been many standard acute and subchronic rodent inhalation studies with specific metal compounds, often oxides or sulfates. These relate most appropriately to occupational exposures. The systemic toxicities of metal compounds are presented in detail elsewhere in this text; the effects of many metals delivered by inhalation may differ from their impact when administered systemically. Since virtually any metal can be found at some concentration in ambient PM and many have toxic or prooxidant potential, their role in PM toxicity has garnered considerable interest (Costa and Dreher, 1999). The most common are metals released during oil and coal combustion (e.g., transition and heavy metals), metals derived from the earth's crust as dust (e.g., iron, sodium, and magnesium), and metals used functionally in fuels, such the antiknock gasoline metal lead (much reduced since its ban in 1983) or metals released from engine wear. Metals derived from anthropogenic combustion sources tend to enrich the fine fraction (<2.5 μm) of PM, while coarse (2.5- to 10-μm) PM is made up of metal compounds of crustal origin (e.g., Fe_2O_3, SiO_2).

Metal compounds can be separated physicochemically: those that are essentially water-insoluble (e.g., metal oxides and hydroxides such as those that might be released from high-temperature combustion sources or derived from the geocrustal matrix) and those that are soluble or mostly soluble in water (often chlorides or sulfates such as those that might form under acidic conditions in a smoke plume or leach from acid-hydrated silicate particles in the atmosphere). Solubility appears to play a role in the toxicity of many inhaled metals by enhancing metal bioavailability (e.g., nickel from nickel chloride versus nickel oxide), but insolubility can also be a critical factor in determining toxicity by increasing pulmonary residence time within the lung (e.g., insoluble cadmium oxide versus soluble cadmium chloride). Moreover, some metals, either in their soluble forms or when coordinated on the surface of silicate or bioorganic materials, can promote electron transfer to induce the formation of reactive oxidants (Ghio et al., 1992). Thus, caution is warranted in assessing inhaled metals, as both their chemical and physical attributes and not simply their total mass govern their effects in the lung. It is likely that a number of mechanisms are involved in the action of inhaled PM-associated metals.

Gas-Particle Interactions The coexistence of pollutant gases and particles in the atmosphere raises the concern that these phases may interact chemically or physiologically to yield unpredictable outcomes. Many studies have shown that these generic interactions are feasible as mechanisms for altering the toxicity of either the particle or the gas. The guinea pig bronchoconstriction model used for many years by Amdur and associates has clearly shown that SO_2 can interact with metal salts to potentiate particle irritancy. The mechanism(s) behind this interaction involve the solubility of SO_2 in a liquefied aerosol as well as the ability of the metal to catalyze the oxidation of the dissolved gas to sulfate. In the case of sodium chloride aerosol, potentiation appeared to be governed primarily by the solubility of SO_2 in that salt droplet and its enhanced respiratory penetration, while metal salts such as manganese, iron, and vanadium functioned through the formation of the stronger irritant sulfate (Amdur and Underhill, 1968). The degree of response to the mixture was dictated by the aerosol itself, indicating that it was indeed the proximate irritant. Studies in humans have been less revealing about such interactions, perhaps in part as a result of differences in study design and methodology.

Metal smelting or the combustion of coal can emit sulfuric acid that is physically associated with ultrafine metal oxide particles. Analogous particles can be furnace-generated in the laboratory and diluted in cool clean air to expose animals (Amdur et al., 1986). These ultrafine particles are distributed widely and deeply in the lung and enhance the irritant potency beyond that predicted on the basis of the sulfuric acid concentration alone. Exposure of guinea pigs to 30 to 60 $\mu g/m^3$ sulfuric acid combined with ultrafine zinc oxide produced dose-dependent decreases in DL_{CO}, total lung capacity, and vital capacity and increases in cells, protein, and a variety of enzymes in lavage fluid that were not completely resolved 96 h after exposure (Amdur, 1989). Other studies of combustion products of different coals emphasized again the role of surface associated acidic *S*-compounds. Illinois No. 6 coal, which has a layer of sulfuric acid sorbed on the surface of the ultrafine ash, produced more effects in the guinea pig model than the more alkaline Montana lignite, which has sorbed neutralized sulfate, even though the absolute amount of sulfate was greater in the Montana lignite (Chen et al., 1990). While the exact physicochemical interaction between SO_2 and zinc oxide to bring about enhanced effects is arguably a combination of surface and solubility mechanisms, similar studies using inert carbon black appear consistent with its role as carrier for reactive gases such as ozone and various aldehydes to enhance delivery of toxic materials to the deep lung (Jakab, 1992). The result was enhanced infectivity when the test animals were subsequently exposed to pathologic bacteria. Thus, the combination of the inert or chemically active particles with a toxic gas appears able to enhance the impact of the gas alone, either by altering dose distribution or the formation of a more toxic product.

Another potential interaction may result from the ability of gaseous pollutants to influence the clearance of particles from the lung or alter the metabolism or cellular interactions with lung-deposited particles. The early studies by Laskin at New York University in the 1960s, showing an intriguing interaction of SO_2 and benzo(*a*)pyrene to promote carcinogencity, were noted earlier; however, this result may well have been due to impaired clearance as well as the promoting activity of inflammation. Similarly, rats exposed to an urban 8-h daily profile of ozone for 6 weeks, followed by a 5-h exposure to asbestos, were found to retain three times as many fibers as did the controls 30 days later. In this case, the fibers were deposited in the distal airways and penetrated more deeply into the intercellular areas, where they seemed inaccessible to phagocytic removal (Pinkerton et al., 1989). These studies, together with those focusing on irritancy and infectivity, raise the prospect that realistic exposure scenarios of gaseous and particulate pollutants can interact through either chemical or physiologic mechanisms to enhance either immediate or associated long-term risks of complex polluted atmospheres.

Ultrafine Carbonaceous Matter Carbonaceous material often forms the core of fine PM. The organic materials, which can be of a semivolatile or nonvolatile nature, are more often dispersed within the structure of PM, forming layers or sheaths. Estimates of the carbonaceous content vary considerably but are nominally considered to be about 30 to 60 percent of the total mass of fine PM. The sources of organic carbon are varied and include the combustion products of natural smoke (e.g., forest fires) and engine exhaust as well as stationary sources (fugitive fly ash). Elemental carbon is at the core of most diesel PM, though many complex organics can be associated with its surface. It has been estimated that diesel contributes about 7 percent of the fine urban PM emissions, which, when expressed as an annual U.S. average, are about 2 $\mu g/m^3$ (USEPA, 1993). Because of the higher use of diesel fuel in Europe and along U.S. freeways, the diesel content of ambient PM has been estimated to be as high as 30 percent.

As an air pollutant, the carbonaceous core of PM has been considered largely inert except in experimental "overload" conditions associated with long-term, high-exposure concentrations in rodent bioassays (addressed below). The potential of PM to act as a carrier of certain irritant gases was noted earlier. Recently, however, carbon in the ultrafine mode (<0.1 μm) has been suggested to be more toxic than the same substance in the larger fine-mode range (2.5 μm), perhaps due to differences in surface reactivity or tissue penetration (Oberdorster et al., 1994; Donaldson et al., 1998). Ultrafine PM possesses extremely high surface area while contributing almost negligible mass to $PM_{2.5}$. This is relevant to the diesel issue, since diesel PM is made up of aggregated ultrafine carbon with small amounts of various combustion-derived complex polycyclic and nitroaromatic compounds and only a trace of metals. However, whole diesel exhaust also contains significant amounts of NO_x, CO, and SO_x as well as formaldehyde, acrolein, and other aldehyde compounds, which are known to be irritants. Recent studies of diluted exhaust in humans reveals that the diesel exhaust mix is inflammogenic and to a degree cytotoxic to airway cells (Salvi et al., 1999). Animal and in vitro cell studies with diesel particles themselves, however, have not shown much acute toxicity. But further studies of the same isolated diesel PM reacted in vitro with ozone before testing in a biological system indicate significant enhancement of the inherently low toxicity of diesel PM (Madden et al., 2000). This underscores the potential importance of interactions among air pollutants as the critical factor in air pollution toxicity.

Chronic Effects and Cancer Chronic exposure studies have been conducted with a number of particles ranging from titanium dioxide and carbon to diesel exhaust and coal fly ash aerosol. Of these substances, diesel exhaust has been the most extensively studied (reviewed by Cohen and Nikula, 1999). The diesel particle is of interest because it can constitute a significant portion of an urban particulate load in some cities (especially in Europe). The primary concern with diesel has been the suspicion that it can induce lung cancer and thus is classified as a Class B carcinogen. However, despite evidence from over forty occupational studies (primarily railway yard, truck, and bus workers) implicating diesel exhaust as a mild carcinogen, confounding elements undermine virtually every study. If one looks to empiric studies, potential carcinogenicity is suggested by several chronic exposure studies in animals and in vitro data indicating mutagenicity in *Salmonella* bacteria and enhanced sister chromatid exchange rates in Chinese hamster ovary cells. (These genotoxic effects have been linked to the nitroarenes associated with the diesel PM.) However, animal studies have not resolved the question of carcinogenic health risk from diesel. The in vivo chronic bioassay studies in rats show a pattern of tumorigenesis that appears to be an effect of the bulk loading of particulate material in the lungs. At high concentrations of diesel PM (3.5 and 7 mg/m^3), normal mucociliary clearance in rats is gradually overwhelmed, resulting in a progressive buildup of particles in the lungs. By 12 months (and increasingly upon approaching 18 to 24 months), clearance essentially ceases and there is evidence of ongoing inflammation, oxidant generation, epithelial hyperplasia, and fibrogenic activity around agglomerates of particles and phagocytic cells in the distal areas of the lung. These patchy sites of injury are associated with the eventual development of adenosarcomas and squamous cell carcinomas in the rats involved in these studies. At lower concentrations, where the particle buildup does not occur, tumors do not develop.

The phenomenon of overwhelming mucociliary clearance of inert particles deposited in the rodent lung has been termed "overload" and is a common finding at the highest exposure concentrations of chronic bioassays involving PM exposures. While this phenomenon could not occur in humans exposed to PM in the ambient environment, it is a subject worthy of consideration in a discussion of PM health effects, as it relates to the interpretation of toxicologic data. Several, poorly soluble particles have induced lung tumors in chronic rat bioassays only under the circumstance of overload; tumors have not developed under similar conditions in mice and hamsters. Among these particles are titanium dioxide, carbon black, toner dust, talc, and diesel PM; the potential for tumors is especially marked when the particles are in the ultrafine mode. In the rat, the time course and pattern of accumulation, chronic inflammation, epithelial hyperplasia, and tumorigenesis are essentially the same for all of the particles. In contrast, the degree of active inflammation in the mouse and hamster under similar overload conditions appears much less and thus is thought to be an important distinction among the species that relates to their sensitivities. Classic in vivo genotoxicity seems largely absent. Not surprisingly, the interpretation of cancer data under these conditions remains controversial. The closest analogy in humans would be coal miners who do not appear to have an enhanced risk of lung cancer except when smoking is not involved.

The issue, then, is whether rat bioassay cancer data under conditions of overload are relevant to risk assessment. A recent review by an expert panel (ILSI, 2000) concluded that rats, while apparently unique in this response, may represent a sensitive subgroup, and that tumorigenesis data from the rat bioassay under conditions of overload cannot be summarily dismissed as not relevant to the consideration of cancer risk in humans. However, the data should be interpreted and weighed in the context of lower concentrations and the tumor incidence and pathology found therein.

Photochemical Air Pollution

Photochemical air pollution arises from a series of complex reactions in the troposphere close to the earth's surface and comprises a mixture of ozone, nitric oxides, aldehydes, peroxyacetyl nitrates, and a myriad of reactive hydrocarbon radicals. If SO_2 is present, sulfuric acid PM may also be formed; likewise, the complex chemistry can generate organic PM, nitric acid vapor, and condensate. From the point of view of the toxicology of photochemical air pollutants, the gaseous hydrocarbon component is no longer listed collectively as a Criteria pollutant, although individual compounds may fall into the category of HAPs (most often associated with cancer). In general, the concentrations of the hydrocarbon precursors in ambient air generally do not reach levels high enough to produce acute toxicity. Their importance stems largely from their roles in the chain of photochemical reactions that leads to the formation of oxidant smog or haze.

The oxidant of most toxicologic importance in the so-called photochemical "soup" is O_3. It is important to appreciate that atmospheric O_3 is not summarily undesirable. About 10 km above the earth's surface there is sufficient short-wave ultraviolet (UV) light to directly split molecular O_2 to atomic $O^\bullet$, which can then recombine with O_2 to form O_3. This O_3 accumulates to several hundred ppm within a thin strip of the stratosphere and absorbs incoming short-wavelength UV radiation. The O_3 forms and decomposes and reforms to establish a "permanent" barrier to UV radiation, which lately has become a issue of concern, as this barrier is threatened by various anthropogenic emissions (Cl_2 gas and certain fluorocarbons) that enhance O_3 degradation. The consequence is excess infiltration of UV light to the earth's surface and the potential for excess skin cancer risk and immune suppression.

The issue is different in the troposphere, where accumulation of O_3 serves no known purpose and poses a threat to the respiratory tract. Near the earth's surface, NO_2 from combustion processes efficiently absorbs longer-wavelength UV light, from which a free O atom is cleaved, initiating the following simplified series of reactions:

$$NO_2 + h\nu \text{ (UV light)} \rightarrow O^\bullet + NO^\bullet \quad (1)$$
$$O^\bullet + O_2 \rightarrow O_3 \quad (2)$$
$$O_3 + NO^\bullet \rightarrow NO_2 \quad (3)$$

This process is inherently cyclic, with NO_2 regenerated by the reaction of the $NO^\bullet$ and O_3. In the absence of unsaturated hydrocarbons, this series of reactions would approach a steady state with no excess or buildup of O_3. The hydrocarbons, especially olefins and substituted aromatics, are attacked by the free atomic $O^\bullet$, resulting in oxidized compounds and free radicals that react with $NO^\bullet$ to produce more NO_2. Thus, the balance of the reactions shown in Eqs. (28-1) to (28-3) is upset, leading to buildup of O_3. This reaction is particularly favored when the sun's intensity is greatest at midday, utilizing the NO_2 provided by morning traffic. Aldehydes are also major by-products of these reactions. Formaldehyde and acrolein account for about 50 percent and 5 percent, respectively, of the total aldehyde in urban atmospheres. Peroxyacetyl nitrate (CH_3COONO_2), often referred to as PAN, and its homologs also arise in urban air, most likely from the reaction of the peroxyacyl radicals with NO_2.

Short-Term Exposures to Smog

In the 1950s and 1960s, the complexity of photochemical air pollution challenged toxicologists to ascertain its potential to affect human health adversely. The toxicity of O_3 was shown to be very high even at low ppm concentrations. Concerns that the complex atmosphere was even more hazardous, a number of studies were undertaken with actual (outdoor-derived) or synthetic (photolyzed laboratory-prepared atmospheres) smog in an attempt to assess the potency of a more realistic pollution mix. When human subjects were exposed to actual photochemical air pollution (Los Angeles ambient air pumped into a laboratory exposure chamber), they experienced changes in lung function similar to those described in controlled clinical studies of O_3 alone (i.e., reduction in spirometric lung volumes; see below), thus supporting the view that this is the pollutant of primary concern. Acute animal studies using synthetic atmospheres (usually irradiated auto exhaust) provided evidence indicating deep lung damage, primarily within the small airway and proximal alveolar epithelium. In some of these studies, early evidence of edema appeared in the interstitium, particularly in older animals. Additionally, mice similarly exposed were found to be more susceptible to bacterial challenge and lung pneumonias. With time, after the termination of an acute exposure, end-airway lesions recovered and the susceptibility to infection waned, although some pathology in the distal lung persisted for more than 24 h.

While O_3 appeared to be the prime toxicant in many of these studies, there was some evidence that other copollutants were involved. When guinea pigs were exposed to irradiated auto exhaust, airway resistance increased quickly, in contrast to the pattern of O_3 alone, where less effect is seen on resistance than on breathing rate. This indicated that a more soluble irritant(s) probably was active, presumably reactive aldehydes. Thus, the array of effects of a complex atmosphere may be more diverse than would be predicted if it were assumed that O_3 alone was responsible.

Chronic Exposures to Smog

Studies in animals and human populations have attempted to link degenerative lung disease with chronic exposure to photochemical air pollution. Cross-sectional and prospective field studies have suggested an accelerated loss of lung function in people living in areas of high pollution. However, as with many studies of this type, there are problems with confounding factors (meteorology, imprecise exposure assessment, and population variables). Recently, studies have been conducted in children living in Mexico City, which has oxidant and PM levels far in excess of any city in the United States. These studies have focused on the nasal epithelium as an exposure surrogate for pulmonary tissues, using biopsy and lavage methodologies to assess damage. Dramatic effects were found in exposed children, consisting of severe epithelial damage and metaplasia as well as permanent remodeling of the nasal epithelium. When children migrate into Mexico City from cleaner, nonurban regions were evaluated, even more severe damage was observed, suggesting that the remodeling in the permanent residents imparted some degree of incomplete adaptation. Since the children were of middle-class origin, these observations were not likely confounded by poor diet (Calderon-Garcidueñas et al., 1992). These dramatic nasal effects have raised concerns for the more fragile, deep lung tissues, where substantial deposition of oxidant air pollutants is thought to occur.

An extensive, now classic synthetic smog study in animals was undertaken at the Cincinnati EPA laboratory in the mid-1960s in an attempt to address the potential for long-term lung disease. Beagle dogs were exposed on a daily basis (16 h) for 68 months, followed by a clean-air recovery period of about 3 years (Lewis et al., 1974). A series of physiologic measurements were made on the dogs after the exposure, and after their 3-year recovery. They were then moved to the College of Veterinary Medicine at the University of California at Davis. The lungs of the dogs then underwent extensive morphologic examination to correlate with the physiology. Seven groups of 12 dogs each were studied. These were exposed to nonirradiated auto exhaust (group 1), irradiated auto exhaust (group 2), SO_2 plus sulfuric acid (group 3), the two types of exhaust plus the sulfur mixture (groups 4 and 5), and a high and a low level of NO_x (groups 6 and 7). The irradiated exhaust contained oxidant (measured as O_3) at about 0.2 ppm and NO_2 at about 0.9 ppm. The raw exhaust contained minimal concentrations of these materials and about 1.5 ppm NO. Both forms of exhaust also contained about 100 ppm CO. The controls did not show time-related lung function changes, but all the exposure groups had abnormalities, most of which persisted or worsened over the 3-year recovery period in clean air. Enlargement of airspaces and loss of interalveolar septa in proximal acinar regions were most severe in dogs that were exposed to NO_x and SO_x with irradiated exhaust (Hyde et al., 1978). These studies described a morphologic lesion that was degenerative and progressive in nature, not unlike that of chronic obstructive pulmonary disease (COPD)—a condition most often associated with lifelong tobacco smoking.

More recently, "sentinel" studies have been attempted whereby the animals live in the same highly polluted air to which people are exposed. This approach has had a troubled past, but newer studies appear to have better control for the problems of infection, inappropriate animal care (e.g., heat), and variable exposure atmospheres. One such study, conducted in rats exposed for 6 months to the air of São Paulo, Brazil, found considerable airway damage, lung function alterations, and altered mucus rheology (Saldiva et al., 1992). The concentrations of O_3 and PM in São Paulo frequently exceed daily maximum values (in the summer months of February and March) of 0.3 ppm and 75 $\mu g/m^3$, respectively. This collage of effects is not unlike a composite of injury one might suspect from a mixed atmosphere of oxidants and acid PM on the basis of controlled animal studies in the laboratory. However, the essential conclusion from most sentinel studies is that "pollution is unhealthy," since individual and mixed pollutant effects and interactions cannot be easily addressed.

Ozone *General toxicology* Ozone is the primary oxidant of concern in photochemical smog because of its inherent bioreactivity and concentration. Depending on the meteorologic conditions of a given year, 60 to 80 million Americans live in areas not in absolute compliance with the 1-h NAAQS of 0.12 ppm. (Formal compliance limits use one exceedence per year averaged over 3 years.) Los Angeles frequently attains and occasionally exceeds 1-h levels of 0.2 to 0.3 ppm. Unlike SO_2 and the reducing-type pollution profile discussed above, current mitigation strategies for O_3 have been largely unsuccessful despite significant reductions in individual automobile emissions. These reductions have been offset by population growth, which brings with it additional vehicles. With the spread of suburbia and the downwind transport of air masses from populated areas to more rural environments, the geographic distribution of those exposed has spread, as has the temporal profile of potential exposure. In other words, O_3 exposures are no longer stereotyped as brief 1- to 2-h peaks. Instead, there are prolonged periods of exposure of 6 h or more at or near the NAAQS level and may occur either downtown or in the formerly cleaner suburban or rural areas downwind. This recently noted shift has given rise to concerns that cumulative damage from such prolonged exposures may be more significant than brief pulse-like exposures, and that many more people are at risk than was previously thought. With the recent revision of the O_3 NAAQS in 1997 to include an 8-h maximum average of 0.08 ppm, even more cities and suburban areas find themselves in violation of the standard. The American Lung Association estimates that 132 million Americans live in O_3-noncompliant areas (State of the Air, 2000). Perhaps of greater significance is that of those who might be considered susceptible due to preexistent cardiopulmonary problems, 80 to 90 percent live in these areas that fail to comply with the present O_3 NAAQS.

Ozone has been the subject of considerable toxicologic interest because it induces a variety of effects in humans and experimental animals at concentrations that occur in many urban areas (Lippmann, 1989). These effects include morphologic, functional, immunologic, and biochemical alterations. Because of its low water solubility, a substantial portion of inhaled ozone penetrates deep into the lung, but its reactivity is such that about 17 percent and 40 percent is scrubbed by the nasopharynx of resting rats and humans, respectively (Hatch et al., 1994; Gerrity et al., 1988). The reason for the higher degree of scrubbing in humans is unclear, but the finding is reproducible. Moreover, mouth scrubbing does not differ from nasal scrubbing. However, regardless of species, the region of the lung that is predicted to have the greatest O_3 deposition (dose per surface area) is the acinar region, from the terminal bronchioles to the alveolar ducts, sometimes referred to as the proximal alveolar ductal region (Overton and Miller, 1988). Because O_3 penetration increases with increased tidal volume and flow rate, exercise increases the dose to the target area. Using $^{18}O_3$ (a nonradioactive isotope of oxygen), Hatch and coworkers have shown that the dose to the distal lung and the degree of damage to the lung as determined by extravasated protein into the alveolar space (as collected by bronchoalveolar lavage) in exercising human subjects exposed to 0.4 ppm for 2 h with intermittent periods of 15 min of exercise (threefold normal ventilation on average) are similar to those in resting rats exposed for the same length of time to 2.0 ppm. Thus, it is important to consider the role of exercise in a study of O_3 or any inhalant before making cross-study comparisons, especially if that comparison is across species. With so many years invested in the study of O_3, it is surprising that only now is the nature of species differences with regard to exercise-associated dosimetry being appreciated.

Animal studies indicate that the acute morphologic response to O_3 involves epithelial cell injury along the entire respiratory tract, resulting in cell loss and replacement. The pattern of injury parallels the dosimetry profile, with the majority of damage occurring in the centriacinar region. However, along the airways, ciliated cells appear to be most sensitive to O_3, while Clara cells and mucus-secreting cells are the least sensitive. Studies in the rat nose indicate that O_3 also is an effective mucus secretagogue. In the distal lung, the type 1 epithelium is very sensitive to O_3, in contrast to type 2 cells, which serves as the stem cell for the replacement of type 1 cells. Ultrastructural damage can be observed in rats after a few hours at 0.2 ppm, but sloughing of cells generally requires concentrations above 0.8 ppm. Recovery occurs within a few days, and there appears to be no residual pathology. Hence, from animal studies, it would appear that a single exposure to O_3 at a relatively low concentration is not likely to cause permanent damage. On a gross level, when a bronchoscope is used to peer into the human bronchus after O_3 exposure, the airways appear "sunburned" and, as with mild skin sunburn, recovery is typical. What is uncertain is the impact of repeated "sunburning"of the airways and lung.

The mechanisms by which O_3 causes cellular injury have been studied using cellular as well as cell-free systems. As a powerful oxidant, O_3 seeks to extract electrons from other molecules. The surface fluid lining the respiratory tract and cell membranes that underlie the lining fluid contain a significant quantity of polyunsaturated fatty acids (PUFA), either free or as part of the lipoprotein structures of the cell. The double bonds within these fatty acids have a labile, unpaired electron which is easily attacked by O_3 to form ozonides that progress through a less stable zwitterion or trioxolane (depending on the presence of water); these ultimately recombine or decompose to lipohydroperoxides, aldehydes, and hydrogen peroxide. These pathways are thought to initiate propagation of lipid radicals and autooxidation of cell membranes and macromolecules (Fig. 28-10).

Evidence of free radical–related damage in vivo includes detection of breath pentane and ethane and tissue measurements of diene conjugates. Damage to the air-blood interface disrupts its barrier function and promotes inflammation. Inflammatory cytokines (e.g., interleukins 6, 8 and others) are released from epithelial cells and macrophages that mediate early responses and initiate repair. This inflammatory process is generally transient, but it may also interact with neurogenic irritant responses to affect lung function acutely. This latter response may have implications for those with preexistent inflammation or disease.

Pulmonary Function Effects Exercising human subjects exposed to 0.12 to 0.4 ppm O_3 experience reversible concentration-related decrements in forced exhaled volumes [forced vital capacity (FVC) and forced expiratory volume in 1 s (FEV_1)] after a 2 to 3 h of exposure (McDonnell et al., 1983). With the recent concern that prolonged periods of exposure (6 to 8 h) may lead to cumulative effects, similar protocols with lower exercise levels were extended up to 6.6 h. In these studies, exposures to 0.12, 0.10, and 0.08 ppm induced progressive lung function impairment during the course of the exposure (Horstman et al., 1989). The pattern of response was linearly cumulative as a function of exposure time such that changes not detectable at 1 or 2 h reached significance by 4 to 6 h. Decrements in FEV_1 after 6.6 h at 0.12 ppm averaged 13.6 percent and were comparable to that observed after a 2-h exposure to 0.22 ppm with much heavier exercise. Interestingly, the human lung dysfunction resulting from O_3 does not appear to be vagally mediated, but the response can be abrogated by analgesics such as ibuprofen and opiates, which function to reduce pain and inflammation (see below). Thus pain reflexes involving C-fiber networks are thought to be important in the reductions in forced expiratory volumes. On the other hand, animal studies suggest that cardiac as well as lung function effects of O_3 have a significant parasympathetic component. Other lung function indices, such as nonspecific airway reactivity to various pharmacologic agents, indicate hyperreactivity after acute 2- to 6-h exposures to O_3 to sub-NAAQS levels of 0.08, 0.10, and 0.12 ppm (by 56, 86, and 121 percent, respectively, to methacholine). It is widely thought that

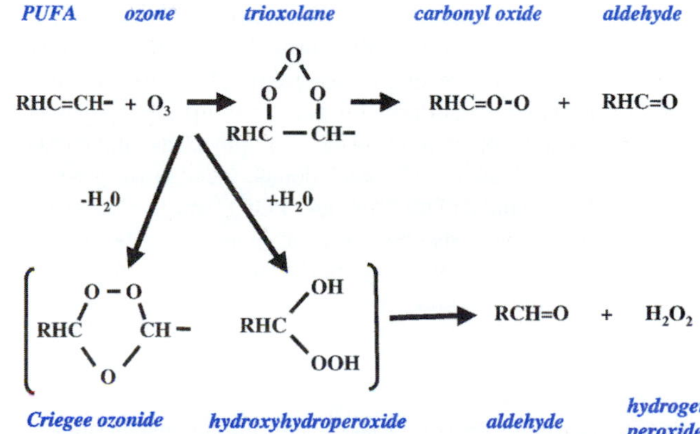

Figure 28-10. Major reactions pathways of O_3 with lipids in lung lining fluid and cell membranes. (Adapted with permission from the Air Quality Criteria Document for Ozone and Photochemical Oxidants. 600/P-93/004cF, NCEA. Research Triangle Park, NC: U.S. EPA, 1996.)

hyperreactive airways may predispose responses to other pollutants such as sulfuric acid or aeroallergens, but such evidence is limited.

When compared with field studies, chamber exposures may underestimate responses for a given exposure to O_3. For a given concentration of O_3, greater decrements in pulmonary function have been reported in children playing outdoors at summer camps than were observed in controlled exposure studies involving exercise (Lippmann, 1989). The reasons for this difference are uncertain but might relate more to cumulative exposure in the children at camp, as they were outside all day, or to the fact that the ambient exposures probably involve other haze copollutants, such as H^+. The responses to the ambient exposures also have slightly altered temporal patterns, whereby responses to O_3 are influenced by previous exposures (Kinney et al., 1988). Animal studies are consistent with the fact that both duration and concentration are important in assessing the response to O_3 exposure (Costa et al., 1989). Pulmonary function decrements increased with $C \times T$ (concentration times time) in rats exposed for 2, 4, or 8 h to ozone at 0.2, 0.4, and 0.8 ppm. Rats exposed for 7 h to 0.5 ppm with 8% CO_2 added to increase the respiratory rate produced functional decrements similar to those observed in human chamber studies of 6.6 h at 0.12 ppm when ventilation-adjusted $C \times T$ products were factored in. This would imply that rats and humans respond with about the same sensitivity and opens the door to the study of various scenarios of exposure to predict human responses under varied conditions. It should be cautioned, however, that it is unknown whether CO_2-stimulated breathing in the rat might alter response thresholds beyond mere incrementing of the dose. On the other hand, in related studies without stimulated breathing, lavage fluid protein content (an index of permeability) 24-h postexposure was also nearly linearly cumulative, with exaggerated responses at the higher concentrations suggestive of an exponential pattern (Highfill et al., 1992) common to other biological functions.

Inflammation of the Lung and Host Defense The mechanism by which O_3 produces decrements in pulmonary function is not fully understood. In contrast to sulfuric acid and SO_2, functional responses to O_3 do not correlate with responsiveness to bronchoconstrictor challenge and are not ostensibly enhanced in asthmatics, as appears to be the general case with the sulfated acids. Because the contribution of vagal mechanisms in the acute human lung functional response to O_3 appears to be minimal, attention has turned to the role of lung inflammation. Koren and colleagues (1989) found an eightfold increase in polymorphonuclear leukocytes (PMNs) in lavage fluid recovered from human subjects 18-h after a 2-h exposure to 0.40 ppm with intermittent exercise. There was also evidence of increased epithelial permeability (a twofold increase in serum proteins and albumin). The inflammatory markers did not correlate well with functional impairment among the individuals tested. Arachidonate metabolism products, including the prostaglandins PGE_2 and PGF_{2a} and the leukotriene thromboxane B_2, have also been seen to increase in human bronchoalveolar lavage fluid after 0.4 ppm ozone for 2-h (Seltzer et al., 1986). Pretreatment with the anti-inflammatory agents indomethacin and ibuprofen (cyclooxygenase inhibitors) decreased the pulmonary function deficit and PGE_2, but other indicators of cell injury and vascular leak in lavage fluid (PMNs, extravasated protein, and lactate dehydrogenase) were not attenuated after exposure to a similar ozone challenge. Because PGE_2 can have either pro- or anti-inflammatory functions under certain conditions as well as bronchodilatory action on constricted airways, it remains to be seen whether there is any causal relationship between arachidonate metabolites and functional responses. Sensitivity to O_3 appears to have a genetic component as well. Studies in inbred stains of mice have shown that O_3-induced pulmonary neutrophilia and permeability are governed by a single gene linked to the Toll4 locus that has been associated with endotoxin sensitivity (Kleeberger et al., 2000). Advances in genetic mapping and molecular biology have yielded significant information on the nature of O_3 susceptibility in mice and may one day explain differences seen among humans.

The potential for O_3 to influence allergic sensitization or challenge-responses has received limited investigation in either humans or animals. In general, animal studies have shown the ability of O_3 to enhance the sensitization process under certain conditions (Osebold et al.,1980), but evidence of this in humans is lacking. Controlled studies of heightened antigen responsiveness in allergic subjects have only been suggestive, with enhancement of allergic rhinitis after 0.5 ppm for 4 h providing the only credible data to date. However, diary studies of asthmatic nurses report worsened allergy symptoms, as well as durations thereof, at concentrations of O_3 near the NAAQS (Schwartz, 1992).

Exposure to O_3 before a challenge with aerosols of infectious agents produces a higher incidence of infection than is seen in control animals (Coffin and Blommer, 1967). Studies have demonstrated that this effect in a mouse model using an aerosol of *Streptococcus* (group C) bacteria is a direct result of altered phagocytosis by macrophages in the O_3-exposed animals (Gilmour et al., 1993), allowing the bacteria to develop a thickened capsule that reduces their attractiveness to phagocytes and enhances their virulence. This host resistance model has shown responsiveness to an exposure as low as 0.08 ppm for 3 h. The susceptibility of mice and hamsters to *Klebsiella pneumoniae* aerosol is also increased by prior exposure to O_3. In the rat, altered microbe-killing ability may relate to membrane damage in macrophages, thus impairing the production of bactericidal superoxide anions. However, the rat appears to have a more vigorous PMN response to bacteria than do mice, which seems to compensate for macrophage impairments and lends the rat less sensitive to bacterial proliferation.

Chronic Effects Morphometric studies of the acinar region of rats exposed for 12 h per day for 6 weeks to 0.12 or 0.25 ppm ozone showed hyperplasia and hypertrophy of type I alveolar cells and major alterations in ciliated and Clara cells in small airways (Barry et al., 1988). When quantitative estimates of type I cell hypertrophy (thickness) from this study and those of another that employed a low-level, urban ambient profile of O_3 through 12 weeks were combined, hypertrophy appeared linearly cumulative to the O_3 $C \times T$(Chang et al., 1991, 1992). This finding suggested that over a season, the impact of O_3 in the distal lung may be cumulative and perhaps more importantly may be without threshold. The biological significance of this change is unclear—it may be part of a compensatory response to "thicken" that part of the distal airway most affected by the oxidant. Although most of the morphologic changes induced by O_3 clearly regress over time when the animals are returned to clean air, there is evidence of interstitial remodeling below the epithelium in this centriacinar region, which may have long-term implications. Examination of autopsied lung specimens from young smokers shows many analogous tissue lesions that come to be described as the "smoldering" precursors of emphysema.

Studies involving episodic exposures of rats and monkeys using a pattern of alternating months of O_3 (0.25 ppm) for 18 months indicate that there may be carry-over effects, notably thickening of interstitial fibrous matrix (Tyler et al., 1988, 1991). These interstitial changes were quantitatively similar regardless of the twofold difference in the cumulative exposure dose (i.e., C × T). This would imply that a pattern of exposure resembling seasonal O_3 patterns might result in more serious lesions than predicted by dose alone—indeed more than would have occurred had the exposure been continuous. Hence, the concept of "more dose . . . more effect" may not hold in chronic scenarios, as it appears to do in acute exposures. The number of episodes experienced may well be more significant to long-term outcomes than total dose—a phenomenon not unlike that of repeated sunburning and deterioration of the skin.

Studies of lung function in animals exposed chronically to O_3 have been conducted but have yielded mixed results. Generally, the dysfunction is reflective of stiffened or fibrotic lungs, particularly at higher concentrations. There have been two prominent chronic O_3 studies—the EPA 18-month chronic study of a realistic urban exposure profile (Chang et al, 1992; Costa et al., 1995) and the National toxicology Program (NTP)—Health Effects Institute (HEI Report, 1994/1995) study of 0.125 to 1 ppm for 20 months (6 h/day; 5days/week). From an environmental relevance perspective, the C × T doses for these studies were similar, but the urban profile study produced evidence for centriacinar interstitial fibrosis suggesting a possible influence of the exposure pattern. There was no general biochemical evidence for fibrosis, however (Last et al., 1994), as observed in monkey and rat studies at higher concentrations. If one attempts to compare these results with the Cincinnati beagle study, one finds that the synthetic smog atmosphere showed degenerative and not fibrotic lung lesions. However, it should be noted that the mixture used in the beagle study was both more complex and involved considerably higher concentrations than most current-day rat and nonhuman primate studies.

One aspect of O_3 that is important in any assessment of potential long-term toxicity is ability of O_3 to induce tolerance to itself. Classic O_3 tolerance takes the form of protection against a lethal dose in animals that received a very low initial challenge 7 days before. The term *tolerance* is sometimes used to describe "adaptation" or acclimatization over time to near ambient levels of O_3. The process begins during and immediately after the initial exposure and progresses to completion in at most 2 to 4 days. This adaptive phenomenon has been reported a number of times for humans with regard to lung function tests and recently has been correlated with inflammatory endpoints (Devlin et al., 1993). Lavage lactate dehydrogenase (LDH; a marker of cell injury) and elastase (enzymatically active against lung matrix), interestingly, did not appear to adapt in humans. An analogous pattern of adaptation of functional and biochemical endpoints (including LDH and elastase) in rodents also takes place with repeated exposures up to a week. But to date, the linkages between acute, adaptive, and long-term process remain unclear, since over longer periods of exposure both morphologic and functional effects do appear to develop. In the short run, however, O_3 adaptation appears in part to be related to the induction of an endogenous acute-phase response (McKinney et al., 1997) as well as lung antioxidants (Wiester et al., 2000) such as ascorbic acid. The significance of this finding in humans is uncertain because ascorbic acid is not endogenously synthesized in humans as it is in the rat. Self-administration of ascorbate has been shown to reduce the lung function decrement to O_3 in humans (Mudway et al., 1999), but the potential role of a regimen of self-administered antioxidants (including ascorbate) to protect from ozone is not confirmed.

Ozone Interactions with Copollutants An approach simplifying the complexity of synthetic smog studies yet addressing the issue of pollutant interactions involves the exposure of animals or humans to binary or tertiary mixtures of pollutants known to occur together in ambient air. Such studies have had a number of permutations, but most have attempted to address the interactions of O_3 and nitrogen dioxide or O_3 and sulfuric acid. Depending on study design, there has been evidence supporting either augmentation or antagonism of lung function impairments, lung pathology, or other indices of injury. This apparent conflict only emphasizes the need to carefully consider the myriad of factors than might affect studies involving multiple determinants.

When O_3 and NO_2 (1 ppm and 14 ppm, respectively) were administered to rats from a premixed retention chamber, the resulting damage evident in bronchoalveolar lavage exceeded that of either toxicant alone, regardless of the temporal sequence of exposure (Gelzleichter et al., 1992). Fibrogenic potential also was increased (Last et al., 1994). Theoretically, the two oxidants formed an intermediate nitrogen radical that was more toxic than either gas alone. At much more realistic concentrations (0.3 ppm O_3 and 3.0 ppm NO_2), where this reaction would not be favored, the impact of these irritants on rabbits was only additive (Schlesinger et al., 1991). This contrast in response serves to illustrate that the tenet of dose-dependency that holds for any single-toxicant response is of equal or more importance when two or more pollutants coexist and have the potential to interact.

Studies of O_3 mixed with acid aerosols also have shown potentiative or antagonistic responses that were time-dependent during the period of exposure. On the one hand, as noted above, field studies of children in camps and asthma admissions in the Northeast and in Canada, have found an apparent interdependence of acid and O_3 underlying responses to summer haze. Yet, over an extended period, there was evidence of enhanced or antagonized secretory cell responses with combined O_3 (0.1 ppm) and sulfuric acid (125 $\mu g/m^3$) at different points in the 1-year exposure of rabbits (Schlesinger et al., 1992). As the number of interacting variables increases, so does the difficulty in interpretation. Studies of complex atmospheres involving acid-coated carbon combined with O_3 at relevant levels show variable strength of evidence of interaction on lung function and macrophage receptor activities (Kleinman et al., 1999). The difficulty with any multicomponent study is the statistical separation of the interacting variables and responses from the individual or combined components. However, it is the complex mixture to which people are exposed that we wish to evaluate for its toxicologic potential. Creative approaches to understanding mixture responses are a likely part of the new agenda that toxicologists will need to address in the next decade (Mauderly, 1999).

Nitrogen Dioxide *General Toxicology* Nitrogen dioxide, like O_3, is a deep lung irritant that can produce pulmonary edema if it is inhaled at high concentrations. It is a much less potent irritant and oxidant than O_3, but NO_2 can pose clear toxicologic problems. Potential life-threatening exposure is a real-world problem for farmers, as sufficient amounts of NO_2 can be liberated from silage. Typically, shortness of breath ensues rapidly with exposures nearing 75 to 100 ppm NO_2, with delayed edema and symptoms of pulmonary damage, collectively characterized as silo-filler's disease. Nitrogen dioxide is also an important indoor pollutant, especially in homes with unventilated gas stoves or kerosene heaters (Spengler and Sexton, 1983). Under such circumstances, very young children and their mothers who spend considerable time indoors may be especially at risk. Sidestream tobacco smoke can also be a source of indoor NO_2. In the outdoor environment, the levels of NO_2 needed to produce clear effects are in general far above those that occur in ambient air. However, more recently, protocols that simulate an urban (rush hour) or household (cooking) pattern of two daily peaks superimposed on a low continuous background concentration have produced effects in experimental animals when continuous exposure to NO_2 did not, suggesting an important dependency on exposure profile.

Although the distal lung lesions produced by acute NO_2 are similar among species, there are considerable differences in species sensitivity. Where a direct comparison is possible, guinea pigs, hamsters, and monkeys are more sensitive than are rats, although comparative dosimetry information might explain some of this difference. As in the case of O_3, theoretical dosimetry studies indicate that NO_2 is deposited along the length of the respiratory tree, with its preferential site of deposition being the distal airways. Not surprisingly, the pattern of damage to the respiratory tract reflects this profile: damage is most apparent in the terminal bronchioles, just a bit more proximal in the airway than is seen with O_3. At high concentrations, the alveolar ducts and alveoli are also affected, with type I cells again showing their sensitivity to oxidant challenge. In the airways of these animals there is also damage to epithelial cells in the bronchioles, notably with loss of ciliated cells, as well as a loss of secretory granules in Clara cells. The pattern of injury of NO_2 is quite similar to that of O_3, but its potency is about an order of magnitude lower.

Pulmonary Function Effects Exposure of normal human subjects to concentrations of $\leq$4 ppm NO_2 for up to 3 h produces no consistent effects on spirometry. However, a study has shown slightly enhanced airway reactivity with 1.5 to 2.0 ppm. Interestingly, ascorbic acid pretreatment of human subjects appeared to protect them from this hyperreactivity (Mohsenin, 1987). Whether asthmatics have a particular sensitivity to NO_2 is a controversial issue. A number of factors appear to be involved (e.g., exercise, inherent sensitivity of the asthmatic subject, exposure method). Some studies have reported effects in some individuals at 0.2 ppm, which is an ambient level in a household with an unvented gas stove. Recent meta-analyses, which have incorporated the findings of many studies to achieve a weight-of-evidence perspective, appear to support an effect of NO_2 on asthmatics. As for an appropriate animal model, only very high concentrations (10 ppm NO_2) invoke an irritancy response in guinea pigs (tachypnea); these levels are well above those a person probably would encounter in everyday life. Recently, NO_2 has been found to be associated with mortality in some time-series studies of air pollution attempting to tease out specific pollutant effects (focusing mainly on PM) (Gold et al., 2000). These studies have found correlates with cardiovascular deaths, which has raised new questions of the mechanisms by which pollutants might affect health in susceptible subgroups.

Inflammation of the Lung and Host Defense Unlike O_3, NO_2 does not induce significant neutrophilic inflammation in humans at exposure concentrations approximating those in the ambient outdoor environment. There is some evidence for bronchial inflammation after 4 to 6 h at 2.0 ppm, which approximates the likely highest transient peak indoor levels of this oxidant. Exposures at 2.0 to 5.0 ppm have been shown to affect T lymphocytes, particularly $CD8^+$ cells and natural killer cells that function in host defenses against viruses. Though these concentrations may be high, epidemiologic studies variably show effects of NO_2 on respiratory infection rates in children, especially in indoor environments. Animal models, by contrast, have for years shown associations between NO_2 and bacterial infection (Gardner, 1984). Susceptibility to infection appears to be governed more by the peak exposure concentration than by exposure duration. The effects are ascribed to suppression of macrophage function and clearance from the lung. Altered function in the form of killing and/or motility was apparent in macrophages from rabbits exposed to 0.3 ppm for 3 days (Schlesinger, 1987) and from humans exposed to 0.10 ppm for 6.6 h (Devlin et al., 1991).

Toxicologic studies of the interaction of NO_2 with viruses are suggestive of enhanced infectivity. Squirrel monkeys infected with nonlethal levels of A/PR-8 influenza virus and then exposed continuously to 5 or 10 ppm NO_2 suffered high mortality rates; 6/6 monkeys exposed to 10 ppm died within 3 days, while only 1/3 exposed to 5 ppm died (Henry et al., 1970). Other experiments suggest that the exposure of squirrel monkeys for 5 months to 5 ppm NO_2 depresses the formation of protective antibodies against the A/PR-8 influenza virus. Controlled human studies, however, have been inconclusive, generally because of low subject numbers. One study showed decreased virus inactivation by alveolar macrophages recovered from 4 of 9 subjects cultured in vitro and exposed to 3.5 h to 0.6 ppm NO_2. These same macrophages also produced interleukin-1, which is a known cytokine modulator of immune cell function (Frampton et al., 1989). Thus, the issue of enhanced viral infection associated with NO_2 exposure remains of concern, especially during seasonal use of unvented gas-heating indoors, but full confirmation of this risk is absent at this time.

Chronic Effects Concern about the chronic effects of NO_2 stem from observations that 30-ppm exposures for 30 days produce emphysema in hamsters. Whether this has a bearing on human exposures at 100-fold lower exposure concentrations is questionable. An 18-month study in rats exposed to an urban pattern of nitrogen dioxide in which a background of 0.5 ppm for 23 h per day peaked at 1.5 ppm for 4 h each day showed little ultrastructural damage to the distal lung (Chang et al., 1988). Other studies utilizing peak-base patterns of exposure have found some effect at near-environmental levels of NO_2 using other biological endpoints. Mice exposed for a year to a base level of 0.2 ppm NO_2 with a 1-h spike of 0.8 ppm twice a day 5 days per week (Miller et al., 1987) yielded effects that differed between base-only and peak-only exposure groups. The base level produced no effects, while the peak-only group experienced slight functional impairment and augmented susceptibility to bacterial infection. Early studies (Ehrlich and Henry, 1968) showed that clearance of bacteria from the lungs is suppressed with 0.5 ppm NO_2 through 12 months of exposure. Interestingly, recent studies with a similar double diurnal peak design for NO_2, with NO used as a negative control, showed more pronounced effects of NO on alveolar septal remodeling than did NO_2 (Mercer et al., 1995). Apparently, NO as an intercellular signal can alter collagen metabolism; the potential for NO_2 to act in this manner is not known. These and similar studies utilizing peak-plus-baseline versus base-only or peak-only exposures indicate that, for NO_2 or its reduction product NO, the exposure profile may be an important determinant of response.

Other Oxidants While a number of reactive oxidants have been identified in photochemical smog, most are short-lived because of their reaction with available volatile organic compounds (VOCs), nitrogen oxides, and other reducing equivalents that have the effect of scrubbing them from the air before they can be breathed.

One reactive, irritating constituent of the oxidant atmosphere is peroxyacetyl nitrate (PAN), which is thought to be responsible for much of the eye-stinging activity of smog. It is more soluble and reactive than ozone and hence rapidly decomposes in mucous membranes before it can get to tissues deep into the lungs. The cornea has many irritant receptors and responds readily, while the PAN absorbed into the thicker mucous fluids of the proximal nose and mouth presumably never reaches its target. A few studies with high levels of PAN have shown that it can cause lung damage and have mutagenic activity in bacteria, but it is not likely that this is relevant to ambient levels of PAN.

Aldehydes Various aldehydes in polluted air are formed as reaction products of the photooxidation of hydrocarbons. The two aldehydes of major interest are formaldehyde (HCHO) and acrolein ($H_2C{=}CHCHO$). These materials contribute to the odor as well as eye and sensory irritations of photochemical smog. Formaldehyde accounts for about 50 percent of the estimated total aldehydes in polluted air, while acrolein, the more irritating of the two, may account for about 5 percent of the total. Acetaldehyde (C_3HCHO) and many other longer-chain aldehydes make up the remainder, but they are not as irritating because of their low concentration and lesser solubility in airway fluids. Formaldehyde and particularly acrolein are found in mainstream tobacco smoke (about 90 and 8 ppm, respectively, per drag) and are likely to be found in sidestream smoke as well. Formaldehyde is also an important indoor air pollutant and can often achieve higher concentrations indoors than outdoors if due to outgassing by new upholstery or other furnishings.

Empiric studies have shown that formaldehyde and acrolein are competitive agonists for similar irritant receptors in the airways. Thus, irritation may be related not to "total aldehyde" concentration but to specific ratios of acrolein and formaldehyde. Their relative difference in solubility, with formaldehyde being somewhat more water-soluble and thus having more nasopharyngeal uptake, may distort this relationship under certain exposure conditions (e.g., exercise). On the other hand, acrolein is very reactive and may interact easily with many tissue macromolecules.

Formaldehyde Formaldehyde is a primary sensory irritant. Because it is very soluble in water, it is absorbed in mucous membranes in the nose, upper respiratory tract, and eyes. The dose–response curve for formaldehyde is steep: 0.5 to 1 ppm yields a detectable odor; 2 to 3 ppm produces mild irritation; and 4 to 5 ppm is intolerable to most people. Formaldehyde is thought to act via sensory nerve fibers that signal through the trigeminal nerve to reflexively induce bronchconstriction through the vagus nerve. In guinea pigs, a 1-h exposure to about 0.3 ppm of formaldehyde induces an increase in airflow resistance accompanied by a lesser decrease in compliance (Amdur, 1960). Respiratory frequency and minute volume also decreased, but these changes do not become statistically significant until >10 ppm. The no observed effect level (NOEL) using these lung function criteria is about 0.05 ppm. The general pattern of the irritant response and its rapid recovery is similar to that produced by higher concentrations of SO_2. And also like SO_2, the introduction of formaldehyde through a tracheal cannula to bypass nasal scrubbing greatly augments the irritant response, indicating that deep lung irritant receptors can also be activated by this vapor.

Formaldehyde, like SO_2, can interact with water-soluble salts during inhalation and produce irritancy beyond that expected for the gas alone. When it was inhaled simultaneously with submicron sodium chloride aerosol, irritancy was augmented in proportion to the aerosol concentration, but this potentiation cannot be accounted for by a simple "carrier" effect of the aerosol (Amdur, 1960). Moreover, reversal of bronchoconstriction was slower than had been observed with SO_2. Thus it appeared that the aerosol itself constituted a new irritant species, the product of a chemical transformation of formaldehyde—perhaps methylene hydroxide (Underhill, 2000). In addition to interactions with water-soluble particles, formaldehyde has been shown to interact with carbon-based particles (Jakab, 1992) to augment bacterial infectivity in a murine model. In this case, the potentiation appears to correlate with the surface carrying capacity of the inhaled particle.

Two aspects of formaldehyde toxicology have brought it from relative obscurity to the forefront of attention in recent years. One is its presence in indoor atmospheres as an off-gassed product of construction materials such as plywood or improperly installed urea-formaldehyde foam insulation. This aspect is discussed at length in a review article (Spengler and Sexton, 1983). Complaints of formaldehyde irritation in industry have been reported at 50 ppb (Horvath et al., 1988). In studies relating household formaldehyde to chronic effects, children were found to have significantly lower peak expiratory flow rates (about 22 percent in homes with 60 ppb) than did unexposed children. Asthmatic children were affected below 50 ppb. Thus, this irritant vapor has the potential to cause respiratory effects at commonly experienced exposure levels (Krzyzanowski et al., 1990), and this may relate to evidence that formaldehyde is a weak allergen.

Nasal cancer has been induced empirically with formaldehyde vapor in rodents. In a 2-year study, rats were exposed to 2, 6, or 14 ppm formaldehyde 6 h per day, 5 days per week. The occurrence of nasal squamous cell carcinomas was zero in the control and 2-ppm groups, 1 percent in the 6-ppm group, and 44 percent in the 14-ppm group. An exposure-related induction of squamous metaplasia occurred in the respiratory epithelium of the anterior nasal passages in all exposed groups. Rats exposed 6 h per day for 5 days to 14 ppm had a greater than 20-fold increase in cell proliferation in the nasal epithelium. Mice were much less sensitive; only one carcinoma was seen at 14 ppm. The detection of DNA adducts in the two species paralleled the difference in the incidence of tumors as well as regional dosimetry. With this collection of data, formaldehyde has been designated as a probable human carcinogen by the IARC. The implications of these findings have been reviewed by Starr and Gibson (1985), but recent epidemiology studies have generally failed to find an increased incidence of nasal cancer in exposed workers.

Acrolein Because acrolein is an unsaturated aldehyde, it is more irritating than formaldehyde. Concentrations below 1 ppm cause irritation of the eyes and the mucous membranes of the respiratory tract. Exposure of guinea pigs to ≥ 0.6 ppm reversibly increased pulmonary flow resistance and tidal volume and decreased respiratory frequency (Murphy et al., 1963). With irritants of this type, flow resistance is increased by concentrations below those that cause a decrease in frequency. This suggests that increases in flow resistance would be produced by far lower concentrations of acrolein than were tested. The mechanism of increased resistance appears to be mediated through a cholinergic reflex. Atropine (muscarinic blocker) and aminophylline, isoproterenol, and epinephrine (sympathetic agonists) partially or completely reversed the changes, while the antihistamines pyrilamine and tripelennamine had no effect.

Exposures of rats to 0.4, 1.4, or 4.0 ppm for 6 h per day 5 days per week for 13 weeks resulted in apparently paradoxical effects on lung function (Costa et al., 1986). The lowest concentration resulted in hyperinflation of the lung with an apparent reduction in small-airway flow resistance, while the highest concentration resulted in airway injury and peribronchial inflammation and fibrosis. The intermediate concentration was functionally not different from the control, but airway pathology was evident. It appears that the high-concentration response reflected the cumulative irritant injury and remodeling as a result of the repeated acrolein, while the low-concentration group had little overt damage and appeared to have slightly stiffened airways, perhaps a result of the protein cross-linking action of acrolein. The pathology in these animals contrasts with that found in formaldehyde studies of similar duration in that there was much more upper airway involvement. Ambient exposure to acrolein probably would be about fivefold to tenfold lower than the low concentration used in the subchronic study discussed above. Thus, as a class the aldehydes can be very irritating and may constitute a significant fraction of the discomfort and sensation experienced during an oxidant episode, especially in mixed atmospheres containing particles.

Carbon Monoxide Carbon monoxide is classed toxicologically as a chemical asphyxiant because its toxic action stems from its formation of carboxyhemoglobin, preventing oxygenation of the blood for systemic transport. The fundamental toxicology of CO and the physiologic factors that determine the level of carboxyhemoglobin attained in the blood at various atmospheric concentrations of carbon monoxide are detailed in Chap. 11.

The normal concentration of carboxyhemoglobin (COHb) in the blood of nonsmokers is about 0.5 percent. This is attributed to endogenous production of CO from heme catabolism. Uptake of exogenous CO increases blood COHb as a function of the concentration in air as well as the length of exposure and the ventilation rate of the individual. Uptake is said to be ventilation-limited, implying that virtually all the CO inspired in a breath is absorbed and bound to the available hemoglobin. Thus, continuous exposure of human subjects to 30 ppm CO leads to an equilibrium value of 5 percent COHb. The Haldane equation is used to compute the COHb equilibrium under a given exposure situation. The equilibrium values generally are reached after 8 h or more of exposure. The time required to reach equilibrium can be shortened by physical activity.

Analysis of data from air-monitoring programs in California indicates that 8 h average values can range from 10 to 40 ppm CO. Depending on the location in a community, CO concentrations can vary widely. Concentrations predicted inside the passenger compartments of motor vehicles in downtown traffic were almost 3 times those for central urban areas and 5 times those expected in residential areas. Occupants of vehicles traveling on expressways had CO exposures somewhere between those in central urban areas and those in downtown traffic. Concentrations above 87 ppm have been measured in underground garages, tunnels, and buildings over highways.

No overt human health effects have been demonstrated for COHb levels below 2 percent, and levels above 40 percent can be fatal due to asphyxia. At COHb levels of 2.5 percent resulting from about 90-min exposure to about 50 ppm CO, there is an impairment of time-interval discrimination; at approximately 5 percent COHb, there is an impairment of other psychomotor faculties. At 5 percent COHb in nonsmokers (the median COHb value for smokers is about 5 percent), however, maximal exercise duration and maximal oxygen consumption are reduced (Aronow, 1981). Cardiovascular changes also may be produced by exposures sufficient to yield COHb in excess of 5 percent. These include increased cardiac output, arteriovenous oxygen difference, and coronary blood flow in patients without coronary disease. Decreased coronary sinus blood PO_2 occurs in patients with coronary heart disease, and this would impair oxidative metabolism of the myocardium. In the early 1990s, a series of studies in subjects with cardiovascular disease were conducted in several laboratories under the sponsorship of the Health Effects Institute (HEI) to determine the potential for angina pectoris when they exercised moderately with COHb levels in the range of 2 to 6 percent (Allred et al., 1989). The results of these studies indicate that premature angina can occur under these conditions but that the potential for the induction of ventricular arrhythmias remains uncertain. Thus, the reduction in ambient CO brought about by newer controls should reduce the risk of myocardial infarct in predisposed persons.

The recent introduction of fuel oxygenates like MTBE and related ether compounds into gasoline was an attempt to enhance fuel combustion and reduce CO emissions. The ensuing problems with MTBE have been discussed earlier, but the goal of achieving lower CO was only partially successful. This finding reinforces the need to carefully consider whether resolution of one problem has the potential for generating others.

Hazardous Air Pollutants Hazardous air pollutants (so-called air toxics or HAPs) represent an inclusive classification for air pollutants that are of anthropogenic origin, are of measurable quantity, and are not covered in the Criteria Pollutant list. Some of the regulatory aspects of the HAPs were discussed above. The inclusive nature of this group of pollutants complicates a discussion of their toxicology because the group includes various classes of organic chemicals (by structure, e.g., acrolein, benzene), minerals (e.g., asbestos), polycyclic hydrocarbon particulate material [e.g., benzo(*a*)pyrene], and various metals and metal compounds (e.g., mercury, beryllium compounds) and pesticides (e.g., carbaryl, parathion).

Most toxic air pollutants are of concern because of their potential carcinogenicity, as shown in chronic bioassays, mutagenicity tests in bacterial systems, structure-activity relationships, or—in a few special cases (e.g., benzene, asbestos)—their known carcinogenicity in humans. These cancers need not be, and generally are not, pulmonary. Noncancer issues frequently relate to direct lung toxicants that, upon accidental release or as fugitive emissions over time, might induce lung damage or lead to chronic lung disease. The assessment of noncancer risk by air toxics to any organ system is based on the computation of long-term risk reference exposure concentrations (RfCs) to which individuals may be exposed over a lifetime without adverse, irreversible injury. This approach to hazardous air pollutant assessment is discussed in detail by Jarabek and Segal (1994). A short-term RfC method for brief or accidental exposures is currently being developed.

Accidental versus "Fence-Line" Exposures The relationship between the effects associated with an accidental release of a large quantity of a volatile chemical into the air from a point source such as a chemical plant and the effects associated with a chronic low-level exposure over many years or a lifetime is not clear. With regard to cancer, which defaults to a linearized model of dose and effect (through some alternative models can be used if there is some data), the issue is fairly straightforward. Any exposure must be minimized if not eliminated if cancer risk is to be kept as close to zero as possible. With noncancer risks, the roles of nonspecific or specific host defenses, thresholds of response, and repair and recovery after exposure complicate the assessment of risk. In large part the issue here relates to C × T. Can we better relate disease or injury to *cumulative dose* or *peak* concentration for protracted exposures? Is there an exposure peak beyond which a cumulative approach fails (i.e., the effect is concentration-driven), or is concentration always the dominant determinant? Many of these questions have yet to be answered, not to mention their specificity with regard to individual compounds and tissues affected.

Methyl isocyanate provides a contrast between the effects of a large accidental release versus those produced by a small release of fugitive vapor such that it is detectable in ambient air, but at very low levels. The reactive nature of methyl isocyanate with aqueous environments is of such magnitude that upon inspiration, almost immediate mucous tissue corrosion can be perceived. The vapor undergoes hydrolysis within the mucous lining of the airways to generate hydrocyanic acid, which destroys the airway epithelium and causes acute bronchoconstriction and edema. The damage is almost immediately life-threatening at concentrations above 50 ppm; at 10 ppm, it is damaging in minutes. These concentrations are in the range of the dense vapor cloud that for several hours enshrouded the village of Bhopal bordering the Union Carbide pesticide plant. Studies in guinea pigs showed the immediate irritancy of this isocyanate, which in just a few minutes also resulted in significant pathology (Alarie et al., 1987). Rats exposed to 10 or 30 ppm for 2 h also showed severe airway and parenchymal damage, which did not resolve in surviving rats; transient effects were seen at 3 ppm. Even 6 months after exposure, the airway and lung damage remained, having evolved into patchy, mostly peribronchial fibrosis with associated functional impairments (Stevens et al., 1987). There was also cardiac involvement secondary to the damage to the pulmonary parenchyma and arterial bed. As a result, there was pulmonary hypertension and right-sided heart hypertrophy. This same spectrum of health effects appeared in the surviving exposed residents of Bhopal and is in large part associated with their above-average death rate.

In the United States, methyl isocyanate has been measured in Katawba Valley, Texas, as a result of small but virtually continual fugitive releases of the vapor into the community air ("fence-line") from an adjoining region with several chemical plants. While these levels of methyl isocyanate are not sufficient to cause the damage seen in Bhopal, there is concern that low-level exposure over many years may have more diffuse, chronic effects. Residents complain of odors and a higher frequency of respiratory disorders, but clear evidence of injury or disease is lacking.

Phosgene is best known for its use as a war gas, but it is also one of the most common intermediate reactants used in the chemical industry, particularly in pesticide formulation. It is also a constituent of photochemical smog. Because of its direct pulmonary reactivity, it lends itself to use as a model pulmonary toxicant for studies addressing C × T relationships. These studies suggest that there may be a threshold below which compensatory and other bodily defenses (e.g., antioxidants) may be able to cope with long-term low-level exposure (tolerance). For phosgene this appears to be at or below the current threshold limit value of 0.1 ppm for 8 h. At higher concentrations, however, concentration appears to be the primary determinant of injury or disease regardless of duration. Thus, even though there is some adaptation with time, there continues to be a concentration-driven response that exceeds that predicted by C × T. This relationship appears to be different from that of ozone at ambient levels, which can be approximated acutely by the C × T paradigm.

WHAT IS AN ADVERSE HEALTH EFFECT?

Any attempt to establish criteria to define an "adverse effect" of air pollution is likely to be questioned. Some effects would pass uncontested, e.g., death, life-threatening dysfunction or disease, irreversible impairment, and pain. Other effects that may reflect minor and temporary dysfunctions or discomfort could be argued by some as not warranting significant or costly concern, especially if effects are minor or transient. The goal of air-quality management is clearly to avoid or, at worse, limit negative impacts of air pollution on public health. However, one must appreciate the distinction between risk to the individual and to a population. Clearly, risk to an individual can be beyond an acceptable limit and can put that person's health in jeopardy, but this response may be lost in a population index. On the other hand, risk to a population is the summation of individual risks such that there is a shift in the normal distribution putting unspecified individuals at risk. These two forms of risk are clearly related, but most often in practice, the population risk is considered most appropriate and most reasonably quantifiable. This population-based risk is that used in the CAA of 1970.

In 1985, the American Thoracic Society issued a position paper that attempted to define an adverse effect related to air pollution. This has recently been revised because of the many advances in clinical medicine and empiric health sciences (ATS, 2000). This statement considers seven broad areas: biomarkers, quality of life, physiologic impacts, symptoms, clinical outcomes, mortality, and population health versus individual risk. The summary conclusion states that caution should be exercised in evaluating the many new biomarkers of effect (especially cell and molecular markers), as there is need for validation that *small* changes in these markers represent a progression along a course to disease or permanent impairment. Admittedly, in the clinical environment many of these markers may appear as salient features of a disease or injury, but the health implications of minor changes in these biomarkers remains uncertain. Significant alterations of standard clinical measures of health due to pollution are clearly adverse. However, a shift from the 1985 ATS statement is that transient pulmonary function deficits (where a 10 percent or more drop in FVC was defined as adverse) may not necessarily be adverse. On the other hand, any irreversible reduction in pulmonary function would be adverse either for an individual or across a population. Any population for which a significant mortality risk can be detected must be considered adverse. Of course, a common thread through all of these subject areas is the influential role of susceptibility, which can take the form of hyper-responsiveness or loss of reserve. What was a minor reversible effect may now be a dysfunction that cannot be reversed or compensated (Fig. 28-11). Obvious examples would be cardiopulmonary compromised individuals who function with little or no reserve. In the end, however, the ATS statement realizes the limits of definitions and the importance of value judgment in the final assessment. Implied in this position is that a loss of quality

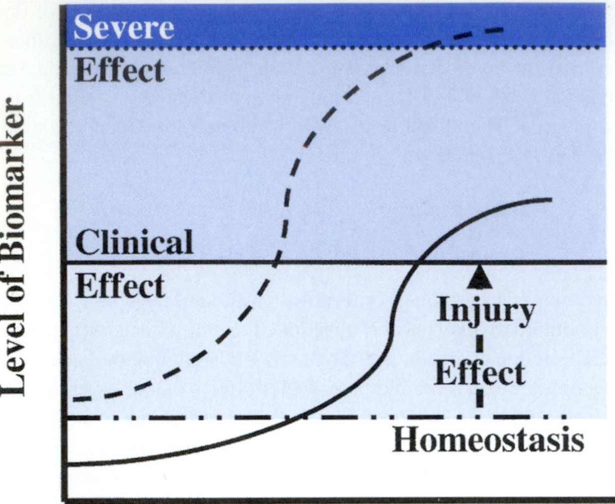

Figure 28-11. Schematic illustration of the elements of a dose response to an air pollutant(s) by a susceptible versus a healthy individual.

The hypothetical susceptible individual has both a *loss of reserve* and an *inability to maintain homeostasis*. The *leftward shift in the slope* of the dose-response curve also suggests an increase in responsiveness. These response elements of the susceptible individual may contribute to apparent sensitivity to challenge and the likelihood of progressing from subtle to severe effects.

of life due to air pollution as well as enduring its associated effects may also be designated as adverse.

CONCLUSIONS

In writing this textbook chapter on air pollution toxicology, the author's goal has been to relate empiric studies in animals to phenomena known to occur in humans through epidemiologic or controlled clinical study. The breadth and complexity of the problem of air pollution—from the development of credible databases to supporting regulatory action and decision making—has been the theme throughout. The classic and still most important air pollutants provide a foundation for understanding and appreciating the nuances of the issues and strategies for air pollution control and protection of public health. The key role of the toxicologist is to develop sensitive methods to assay responses to low pollutant concentrations, apply these methods to relevant exposure scenarios and test species, and develop paradigms to relate empiric toxicologic data to real life through an understanding of mechanism. Last, the toxicologist must continually integrate laboratory data with those of epidemiology and clinical study to ensure their maximum utility.

ACKNOWLEDGMENT

The author would like to thank Mr. James R. Lehmann and Dr. James Samet of the USEPA for their constructive comments on the chapter.

REFERENCES

AlarieY, Ferguson JS, Stock MF, et al: Sensory and pulmonary irritation of methyl isocyanate in mice and pulmonary irritation and possible cyanide-like effects of methyl isocyanate in guinea pigs. *Environ Health Perspect* 72:159–168, 1987.

Alarie YC, Krumm AA, Busey WM, et al: Long-term exposure to sulfur dioxide, sulfuric acid mist, fly ash, and their mixtures: Results of studies in monkeys and guinea pigs. *Arch Environ Health* 30:254–262, 1975.

Alarie YC, Ulrich CE, Busey WM, et al: Long-term continuous exposure of guinea pigs to sulfur dioxide. *Arch Environ Health* 21:769–777, 1970.

Alarie YC, Ulrich CE, Busey WM, et al: Long-term continuous exposure to sulfur dioxide in cynomolgus monkeys. *Arch Environ Health* 24:115–128, 1972.

Allred EN, Bleeker ER, Chaitman BR, et al: Short-term effects of carbon monoxide exposure on individuals with coronary heart disease. *N Engl J Med* 321:1426–1432, 1989.

Altshuler B: Regional deposition of aerosols, in Aharonson FF et al (eds): *Air Pollution and the Lung*. New York: Wiley, 1976.

Amdur MO, Underhill DW: The effect of various aerosols on the response of guinea pigs to sulfur dioxide. *Arch Environ Health* 16:460–468, 1968.

Amdur MO: 1974 Cummings memorial lecture: The long road from Donora. *Am Ind Hyg Assoc J* 35:589–597, 1974.

Amdur MO: Sulfuric acid: The animals tried to tell us: 1989 Herbert E. Stokinger Lecture. *Appl Ind Hyg Assoc J* 4:189–197, 1989.

Amdur MO: The respiratory response of guinea pigs to sulfuric acid mist. *AMA Arch Ind Health* 18:407–414, 1958.

Amdur MO: The response of guinea pigs to inhalation of formaldehyde and formic acid alone and with a sodium chloride aerosol. *Int J Air Pollut* 3:201–220, 1960.

Amdur MO: Toxicological studies of air pollutants. *US Public Health Reports* 69:724–726, 1954.

Amdur MO, Dubriel M, Creasia DA: Respiratory response of guinea pigs to low levels of sulfuric acid. *Environ Res* 15:418–423, 1978.

Amdur MO, Sarofim AF, Neville M, et al: Coal combustion aerosols and SO_2: An interdisciplinary analysis. *Environ Sci Tech* 20:139–145, 1986.

American Thoracic Society: What constitutes an adverse health effect of air pollution? *Am J Respir Crit Care Med* 161:665–673, 2000.

Anderson HR: Health effects of air pollution episodes, in: Holgate ST, Samet JM, Koren H, Maynard RL (eds): *Air Pollution and Health.* London, Academic Press, 1999; pp 461–484.

Aronow WS: Aggravation of angina pectoris by two percent carboxyhemoglobin. *Am Heart J* 101:154–157, 1981.

Barry BE, Mercer RR, Miller FJ, Crapo JD: Effects of inhalation of 0.25 ppm ozone on the terminal bronchioles of juvenile and adult rats. *Exp Lung Res* 14:225–245, 1988.

Bates DV, Sizto R: Air pollution and hospital admissions in southern Ontario: The acid summer haze effect. *Environ Res* 65:172– 194, 1987.

Boubel RW, Fox DL, Turner DB et al: Fundamentals of Air Pollution 3d ed. New York: Academic Press, 1994, p 107.

Brimblecombe P: Air pollution and health history, in: Holgate ST, Samet JM, Koren H, Maynard RL (eds.): *Air Pollution and Health.* London: Academic Press, 1999, p 10.

Brooks BO, Davis WF: *Understanding Indoor Air Quality*. Boca Raton, FL: CRC Press, 1992.

Calderon-Garcidueñas L, Osorno-Velazquez A, Bravo-Alvarez H et al: Histopathological changes of the nasal mucosa in southwest metropolitan Mexico City inhabitants. *Am J Pathol* 140:225–232, 1992.

Calvert JG, Lazrus A, Kok GL, et al: Chemical mechanisms of acid generation in the troposphere. *Nature* 317:27–35, 1985.

Chang L, Huang Y, Stockstill BL, et al: Epithelial injury and interstitial fibrosis in the proximal alveolar regions of rats chronically exposed to a simulated pattern of urban ambient ozone. *Toxicol Appl Pharmacol* 115:241–252, 1992.

Chang L, Miller FJ, Ultman J, et al: Alveolar epithelial cell injuries by subacute exposure to low concentrations of ozone correlate with cumulative exposure. *Toxicol Appl Pharmacol* 109:219–234, 1991.

Chang LY, Mercer RR, Stockstill BL, et al: Effects of low levels of NO_2 on terminal bronchiolar cells and its relative toxicity compared to O_3. *Toxicol Appl Pharmacol* 96:451–464, 1988.

Chen LC, Lam HF, Kim EJ, et al: Pulmonary effects of ultrafine coal fly ash inhaled by guinea pigs. *J Toxicol Environ Health* 29:169–184, 1990.

Coffin DL, Blommer EJ: Acute toxicity of irradiated auto exhaust: Its indication by enhancement of mortality from streptococcal pneumonia. *Arch Environ Health* 15:36–38, 1967.

Costa DL. Particulate matter and cardiopulmonary health: A toxicologic perspective. *Inhal Toxicol* 12(suppl 3):35–44, 2000.

Costa DL, Dreher KL: Bioavailable transition metals in particulate matter mediate cardiopulmonary injury in healthy and compromised animal models. *Environ Health Perspect* 105(suppl. 5):1053–1060, 1997.

Costa DL, Hatch GE, Highfill J, et al: Pulmonary function studies in the rat addressing concentration vs. time relationships for ozone, in Schneider T, Lee SD, Wolters GJR, Grant LD (eds): *Atmospheric Ozone Research and Its Policy Implications*. Amsterdam: Elsevier, 1989, pp 733–743.

Costa DL, Kutzman RS, Lehmann JR, et al: Altered lung function and structure in the rat after subchronic exposure to acrolein. *Am Rev Respir Dis* 133:286–291, 1986.

Costa DL, Schlegele E: Irritant air pollutants, in Swift DL, Foster WM (eds): *Air Pollutants and the Respiratory Tract*. New York: Marcel Dekker, 1998, pp 119–145.

Costa DL, Tepper JS, Stevens MA, et al: Restrictive lung disease in rats chronically exposed to an urban profile of ozone. *Am J Respir Crit Care Med* 151:1512–1518, 1995.

Detels R, Tashkin DP, Sayre JW, et al: The UCLA population studies of CORD: X. A cohort study of changes in respiratory function associated with chronic exposure to SO_x, NO_x, and hydrocarbons. *Am J Public Health* 81:350–359, 1991.

Devlin RB, Folinsbee LJ, Biscardi F, et al: Attenuation of cellular and biochemical changes in the lungs of humans exposed to ozone for five consecutive days. *Am Rev Respir Dis* 147:A71, 1993.

Devlin RB, McDonnell WF, Mann R, et al: Exposure of humans to ambient levels of ozone for 6.6 hours causes cellular and biochemical changes in the lung. *Am J Respir Cell Mol Biol* 4:72–81, 1991.

Dockery DW, Pope CA: Acute respiratory effects of particulate air pollution. *Rev Public Health* 15:107–132, 1994.

Dockery DW, Pope CA, Xu X, et al: An association between air pollution and mortality in six U.S. cities. *N Engl J Med* 329(24):1753–1759, 1993.

Donaldson K, Li XY, MacNee W: Ultrafine (nanometre) particle mediated lung injury, *J Aerosol Sci* 29:553–560, 1998.

Ehrlich R, Henry MC: Chronic toxicity of nitrogen dioxide: I. Effect on resistance to bacterial pneumonia. *Arch Environ Health* 17:860–865, 1968.

Environmental Progress and Challenges: EPA's Update. U.S. EPA, Office of Policy Planning and Evaluation (PM-219), EPA-230-07-88-033. Washington, DC: EPA. 1988, p 29.

Firkert M: Fog along the Meuse Valley. *Trans Faraday Soc* 32:1192–1197, 1936.

Frampton MW, Smeglin AM, Roberts NJJ, et al: Nitrogen dioxide exposure *in vivo* and human macrophage inactivation of influenza virus *in vitro*. *Environ Res* 48:179–192, 1989.

Frank NR, Amdur MO, Worchester J, Whittenberger JL: Effects of acute controlled exposure to SO_2 on respiratory mechanics in healthy male adults. *J Appl Physiol* 17:252–258, 1962.

Frank NR, Speizer FE: SO_2 effects on the respiratory system in dogs: Changes in mechanical behavior at different levels of the respiratory system during acute exposure to the gas. *Arch Environ Health* 11:624–634, 1965.

Gardner DE: Oxidant induced enhanced sensitivity to infection in animal models and their extrapolation to man. *J Toxicol Environ Health* 13:423–439, 1984.

Gearhart JM, Schlesinger RB: Sulfuric acid-induced changes in the physiology and structure of the tracheobronchial airways. *Environ Health Perspect* 79:127–136, 1989.

Gelzleichter TR, Witschi H, Last JA: Synergistic interaction of nitrogen dioxide and ozone on rat lungs: Acute responses. *Toxicol Appl Pharmacol* 116:1–9, 1992.

Gerrity TR, Weaver RA, Bernsten J, et al: Extrathoracic and intrathoracic removal of ozone in tidal breathing humans. *J Appl Physiol* 65:393–400, 1988.

Ghio AJ, Carter JD, Richards JH, et al.: Diminished injury in hypertransferrinemic mice after exposure to a metal-rich particle. *Am J Physiol Lung Cell Mol Physiol* 278(5):L1051–L1061, 2000.

Ghio AJ, Kennedy TP, Whorton AR, et al: Role of surface complexed iron in oxidant generation and lung inflammation induced by silicates. *Am J Physiol Lung Cell Mol Physiol* 263(7):L511–L518, 1992.

Gilmour MI, Park P, Doerfler D, Selgrade MK: Ozone-enhanced pulmonary infection with *Streptococcus zooepidemicus* in mice: The role of alveolar macrophage function and capsular virulence factors. *Am Rev Respir Dis* 147:753–760, 1993.

Glasser SW, Korfhagen TR, Wert S, et al: Transgenic models for study of pulmonary development and disease. *Am J Physiol Lung Cell Mol Physiol* 267(11):L489–L497, 1994.

Gold DR, Litonjua A, Schwartz J et al: Ambient pollution and heart rate variability. *Circulation* 101(11):1267–1273, 2000.

Gong Jr H, Lachenbruch PA, Haber P, et al.: Comparative short term health responses to sulfur dioxide exposure and other common stressors in a panel of asthmatics. *Toxicol Ind Health* 11:467–487, 1995.

Gunnison AF, Palmes ED: S-Sulfonates in human plasma following inhalation of sulfur dioxide. *Am Ind Hyg Assoc J* 35:288–291, 1974.

Hackney JD, Linn WS, Avol EL: Acid fog: Effects on respiratory function and symptoms in healthy asthmatic volunteers. *Environ Health Perspect* 79:159–162, 1989.

Hanley QS, Koenig JQ, Larson TV, et al: Response of young asthmatic patients to inhaled sulfuric acid. *Am Rev Respir Dis* 145:326–331, 1992.

Hatch GE, Boykin E, Graham JA, et al: Inhalable particles and pulmonary host defense: *In vivo* and *in vitro* effects of ambient air and combustion particles. *Environ Res* 36:67–80, 1985.

Hatch GE, Slade R, Harris LP, et al: Ozone dose and effect in humans and rats: A comparison using oxygen-18 labeling and bronchoalveolar lavage. *Am J Respir Crit Care Med* 150:676–683, 1994.

Hayes SM, Gobbell RV, Ganick NR (eds): *Indoor Air Quality: Solutions and Strategies*. New York: McGraw-Hill, 1995.

Hazucha M, Madden M, Pape G, et al: Effect of cycloxygenase inhibition on ozone induced respiratory inflammation and lung function changes. *Environ J Appl Physiol Occup Health.* 73(1–2):17–27, 1996.

Health Effects Report: Consequences of Prolonged Inhalation of Ozone on F344 Rats: Collaborative Studies. Studies I-XIII, Report #65. Boston: Health Effects Institute, 1994–1995.

Henry MC, Findlay J, Spengler J, Ehrlich R: Chronic toxicity of NO_2 in squirrel monkeys: III. Effect on resistance to bacterial and viral infection. *Am Ind Hyg Assoc J* 20:566–570, 1970.

Highfill JH, Hatch GE, Slade R, et al: Concentration time models for the effects of ozone on bronchoalveolar lavage fluid protein in rats and guinea pigs. *Inhal Toxicol* 4:1–16, 1992.

Higuchi MA, Davies DW: An ammonia abatement system for whole-body animal inhalation exposures to acid aerosols. *Inhal Toxicol* 5:323–333, 1993.

Ho YS: Transgenic models for the study of lung biology and disease. *Am J Physiol Lung Cell Mol Physiol* 266(10):L319–L353, 1994.

Holma B: Effects of inhaled acids on airway mucus and its consequences for health. *Environ Health Perspect* 79:109–114, 1989.

Horstman DH, Folinsbee LJ, Ives PJ, et al: Ozone concentration and pulmonary response relationships for 6.6 hours with five hours of moderate exercise to 0.08, 0.10, and 0.12 ppm. *Am Rev Respir Dis* 142:1158–1162, 1989.

Horvath E, Anderson H, Pierce W, et al: Effects of formaldehyde on mucous membranes and lungs: A study of an industrial population. *JAMA* 259:701–707, 1988.

Hyde D, Orthoefer J, Dungworth D, et al: Morphometric and morphologic pulmonary lesions in beagle dogs chronically exposed to high ambient levels of air pollutants. *Lab Invest* 38(4):455–469, 1978.

ILSI Report: The relevance of the rat lung response to particle overload for human risk assessment: A workshop consensus report. ILSI Sponsored Workshop, March, 1998, in S.S. Olin (ed): *Inhal Toxicol* 12:101–117, 2000.

Jakab GJ: Relationship between carbon black particulate-bound formaldehyde, pulmonary antibacterial defenses and alveolar macrophage phagocytosis. *Inhal Toxicol* 4:325–342, 1992.

Jarabek AM, Segal SA: Noncancer toxicity of inhaled toxic air pollutants: Available approaches for risk assessment and risk management, in Patrick DR (ed): *Toxic Air Pollution Handbook.* New York: Van Nostrand Reinhold, 1994, pp 100–132.

Johnston CJ, Finkelstein JN, Oberdorster G, et al.: Clara cell secretory protein-deficient mice differ from wild-type mice in inflammatory chemokine expression to oxygen and ozone, but not to endotoxin. *Exp Lung Res* 25(1):7–21, 1999.

Kakuyama M, Ahluwalia A, Rodrigo J, et al: Cholingergic contraction is altered in nNOS kockouts: Cooperative modulation of neural bronchoconstriction by NOS and COX. *Am J Respir Crit Care Med* 160:2072–2078, 1999.

Kinney PJ, Ware JH, Spengler JD: A critical evaluation of acute epidemiology results. *Arch Environ Health* 43:168–173, 1988.

Kistner A, Gossen M, Zimmermann F, Jerecic J, et al: Doxycycline mediated quantitative and tissue specific control of gene expression in transgenic mice. *Pro. Natl Acad Sci USA* 93:10933–10938, 1996.

Kleeberger SR, Reddy S, Zhang LY, et al: Genetic susceptibility to ozone-induced lung hyperpermeability. Role of toll-like receptor 4. *Am J Respir Cell Mol Biol* 22(5):620–627, 2000.

Kleinman MT, Bailey RM, Whynot JD et al: Controlled exposure to a mixture of SO_2, NO_2, and particulate air pollutants: Effects on human pulmonary function and respiratory symptoms. *Arch Environ Health* 40:197–201, 1985.

Kleinman MT, Mautz WJ, Bjarnason S: Adaptive and non-adaptive responses in rats exposed to ozone, alone and in mixtures, with acidic aerosols. *Inhal Toxicol* 11(3):249–264, 1999.

Kodavanti UP, Costa DL, Bromberg P: Rodent models of cardiopulmonary disease: Their potential applicability in studies of air pollutant susceptibility. *Environ Health Perspect* 106 (suppl 1):111–130, 1998.

Kodavanti UP, Mebane R, Ledbetter A, et al: Variable pulmonary responses from exposure to concentrated ambient air particles in a rat model of bronchitis. *Toxicol Sci.* 54(2):441–451, 2000.

Koenig JQ, Covert DS, Pierson WE: Effects of inhalation of acidic compounds on pulmonary function in allergic adolescent subjects. *Environ Health Perspect* 79:127–137, 173–178, 1989.

Koenig JQ, Pierson WE, Horike M, Frank R: Effects of SO_2 plus NaCl aerosol combined with moderate exercise on pulmonary function in asthmatic adolescents. *Environ Res* 25:340–348, 1981.

Koren HS, Devlin RB, Graham DE, et al: Ozone-induced inflammation in the lower airways of human subjects. *Am Rev Respir Dis* 139:407–415, 1989.

Kotin P, Falk HF: Atmospheric factors in pathogenesis of lung cancer. *Cancer Res* 7:475–514, 1963.

Krzyzanowski M, Quackenboss JJ, Lebowitz MD: Chronic respiratory effects of indoor formaldehyde exposure. *Environ Res* 52:117–125, 1990.

Kuhn III C, Homer RJ, Zhu Z, et al: Airway hyperresponsiveness and air obstruction in transgenic mice: Morphologic correlates in mice overexpressing IL-11 and IL-6 in the lung. *Am J Respir Cell Mol Biol* 22:289–295, 2000.

Last JA, Gelzleichter TR, Harkema J, Hawk S: *Consequences of Prolonged Inhalation of Ozone on Fischer-344/N Rats: Collaborative Studies.* Part I: *Content and Cross-Linking of Lung Collagen*: Res. Report No. 65. Cambridge, MA: Health Effects Institute, April 1994.

Leikauf G. Yeates DB, Wales KA, et al: Effects of sulfuric acid aerosol on respiratory mechanics and mucociliary particle clearance in healthy nonsmoking adults. *Am Ind Hyg Assoc J* 42:273–282, 1981.

Lewis TR, Campbell KI, Vaughan TR Jr: Effects on canine pulmonary function: Via induced NO_2 impairment, particulate interaction, and subsequent SO_x. *Arch Environ Health* 18:596–601, 1969.

Lewis TR, Moorman WJ, Yang YY, Stara JF: Long-term exposure to auto exhaust and other pollutant mixtures. *Arch Environ Health* 21:102–106, 1974.

Lewtas J: Airborne carcinogens. *Pharmacol Toxicol* 72(Suppl 1):S55–S63, 1993.

Lipfert FW: *Air Pollution and Community Health: A Critical Review and Data Sourcebook.* New York: Van Nostrand Reinhold, 1994, pp 10–57.

Lippmann M: Health effects of ozone: A critical review. *J Air Pollut Control Assoc* 39:67–96, 1989.

Madden MC, Richards J, Daily LA, et al: Effect of ozone on diesel exhaust particle toxicity in the rat lung. *Toxicol Appl Pharmacol.* 168: 140–148, 2000.

Maddison D, Pierce D: Costing the health effects of poor air quality, in Holgate ST, Samet JM, Koren H, Maynard RL (eds): *Air Pollution and Health.* London: Academic Press, 1999, pp 917–930.

Martonen TB, Zhang Z, Yang Y: Interspecies modeling of inhaled particle deposition patterns. *J Aerosol Sci* 23(4):389–406, 1992.

Mauderly JL: Toxicological approaches to complex mixtures. *Environ Health Perspect* 101(suppl 4):155–165, 1993.

McDonnell WF, Horstman DH, Hazucha MJ, et al: Pulmonary effects of ozone exposure during exercise: Dose-response characteristics. *J Appl Physiol* 5:1345–1352, 1983.

McKinney WJ, Jaskot RH, Richards JH, et al: Cytokine mediation of ozone-induced pulmonary adaptation. *Am J Respir Cell Mol Biol* 18:696–705, 1998.

Mercer RR, Costa DL, Crapo JD: Effects of prolonged exposure to low doses of nitric oxide on the alveolar septa of the adult rat lung. *Lab Invest* 73(1):1–9, 1995.

Miller FJ, Graham JA, Raub JA, et al: Evaluating the toxicity of urban patterns of oxidant gases: II. Effects in mice from chronic exposure to nitrogen dioxide. *J Toxicol Environ Health* 21:99–112, 1987.

Miller FW, Miller RM: *Environmental Hazards: Air Pollution—A Reference Handbook.* Contemporary World Issues. Santa Barbara, CA: ABC-CLIO, 1993, pp 1–18.

Mohsenin V: Effect of vitamin C on NO_2-induced airway hyperresponsiveness in normal subjects. *Am Rev Respir Dis* 136:1408–1411, 1987.

Molhave LB, Bach B, Pederson O: Human reactions to low concentrations of volatile organic compounds. *Environ Int* 12:165–167, 1986.

Motor vehicle-related air toxics study U.S.EPA. EPA 420-R-93-005. Ann Arbor, MI: Office of Mobile Sources, 1993.

Mudway IS, Krishna MT, Frew AJ et al: Compromised concentrations of ascorbate in fluid lining the respiratory tract in human subjects after exposure to ozone. *Occup Environ Med* 56(7):473–481, 1999.

Murphy SD, Klingshirn DA, Ulrich CE: Respiratory response of guinea pigs during acrolein inhalation and its modification by drugs. *J Pharmacol Exp Ther* 141:79–83, 1963.

Nadel JA, Salem H, Tamplin B, Tokiwa Y: Mechanism of bronchoconstriction during inhalation of sulfur dioxide. *J Appl Physiol* 20:164–167, 1965.

National Air Pollutant Emission Trends, 1988. EPA-230-07-88-033. Research Triangle Park, NC: U.S. EPA, Office of Air Quality Planning and Standards, 1988.

National Air Pollutant Emission Trend Reports, 1998. EPA 454/R-00-002. Research Triangle Park, NC: U.S. EPA: Office of Air Quality Planning and Standards, March 2000, p 21.

National Air Pollutant Emission Trend Reports, 1998. EPA 454/R-00-002. Research Triangle Park, NC: U.S. EPA: Office of Air Quality Planning and Standards, March 2000, p 21.

National Air Quality and Emissions Trends Report, 1992. EPA 454 R-93-031. Research Triangle Park, NC: U.S. EPA: Office of Air Quality Planning and Standards, October 1993.

National Air Quality & Emission Trends Report. EPA 454/R-00-003. Research Triangle Park, NC: U.S. EPA Office of Air Quality Planning and Standards, March 2000, pp 2, 5.

National Research Council (NRC) and Committee on the Institutional Means for Assessment of Risks to Public Health: *Risk Assessment in the Federal Government: Managing the Means*. Washington, DC: National Academy Press, 1983.

Oberdorster G, Ferin J, Lehnert BE: correlation between particle size, *in vivo* particle persistence, and lung injury. *Environ Health Perspect* 102(suppl. 5):173–179, 1994.

O'Donnell MD, O'Conner CM, FitzGerald MX, et al: Ultrastructure of lung elastin and collagen in mouse models of spontaneous emphysema. *Matrix Biol* 18(4):357–360.

Ohtsuka Y, Clarke RW, Mitzner W, et al: Interstrain variation in murine susceptibility to inhaled acid-coated particles. *Am J Physiol Lung Cell Mol Physiol* 278(3): L469-L476, 2000.

Osebold JW, Gershwin LJ, Zee YC: Studies on the enhancement of allergic lung sensitization by inhalation of ozone and sulfuric acid aerosol. *J Environ Pathol Toxicol* 3:221–234, 1980.

Overton JH, Miller FJ: Modeling ozone absorption in the respiratory tract. 80th Annual Meeting of the Air Pollution Control Association, paper no. 87–99.4, 1987.

Paige RC, Plopper CG: Acute and chronic effects of ozone in animal models, in Holgate ST, Samet JM, Koren H, Maynard RL (eds): *Air Pollution and Health,* London: Academic Press, 1999, pp 531–557.

Pinkerton KE, Brody AR, Miller FJ, Crapo JD: Exposure to low levels of ozone results in enhanced pulmonary retention of inhaled asbestos fibers. *Am Rev Respir Dis* 140(4):1075–1081, 1989.

Pope CA, Dockery DW: Epidemiology of particle effects, in Holgate ST, Samet JM, Koren HS, Maynard RL (eds): *Air Pollution and Health.* San Diego, CA: Academic Press, 1999, pp. 673–706.

Qu QS, Chen LC, Gordon T, et al: Alteration of pulmonary macrophage pH regulation by sulfuric acid aerosol exposures. *Toxicol Appl Pharmacol* 121(1):138–143, 1993.

Recio L: Transgeneic animal models and their application in mechanistically based toxicology research. *CIIT Activities* 15(10):1–7, 1995.

Reid L: An experimental study of hypersecretion of mucus in the bronchial tree. *Br J Exp Pathol* 44:437–440, 1963.

Reuther CG: *FOCUS*—Winds of change: Reducing transboundary air pollutants. *Environ Health Perspect* 108(4):A170-A175, 2000.

Robinson J, Nelson WC: *National Human Activity Pattern Survey Data Base.* Research Triangle, Park, NC: U.S. Environmental Protection Agency, 1998.

Saldiva PHN, King M, Delmonte VLC, et al: Respiratory alterations due to urban air pollution: An experimental study in rats. *Environ Res* 57:19–33, 1992.

Salvi S, Blomberg A, Rudell B, et al: Acute inflammatory responses in the airways and peripheral blood after short-term exposure to diesel exhaust in healthy human volunteers. *Am J Respir Crit Care Med* 159:702–709, 1999.

Schenker MB, Samet JM, Speizer FE, et al: Health effects of air pollution due to coal combustion in the Chestnut Ridge region of Pennsylvania: Results of cross-sectional analysis in adults. *Arch Environ Health* 38:325–330, 1983.

Schlesinger RB: Comparative irritant potency of inhaled sulfate aerosol: Effects on bronchial mucociliary clearance. *Environ Res* 34:268–279, 1984.

Schlesinger RB: Intermittent inhalation of nitrogen dioxide: Effects on rabbit alveolar macrophages. *J Toxicol Environ Health* 21:127–139, 1987.

Schlesinger RB, Chen LC, Finkelstein I, Zelikoff JT: Comparative potency of inhaled acidic sulfates: Speciation and the role of hydrogen ion. *Environ Res* 52:210–224, 1990.

Schlesinger RB, Gorczynski JE, Dennison J, et al: Long-term intermittent exposure to sulfuric acid aerosol, ozone, and their combination: Alterations in tracheobronchial mucociliary clearance and epithelial secretory cells. *Exp Lung Res* 18:505–534, 1992.

Schlesinger RB, Halpern M, Albert RE, Lippmann M: Effects of chronic inhalation of sulfuric acid mist upon mucociliary clearance from the lungs of donkeys. *J Environ Pathol Toxicol* 2:1351–1367, 1979.

Schlesinger RB, Lippmann M, Albert RE: Effects of short-term exposures to sulfuric acid and ammonium sulfate aerosols upon bronchial airway function in the donkey. *Am Ind Hyg Assoc J* 39:275–286, 1978.

Schlesinger RB, Weidman PA, Zelikoff JT: Effects of repeated exposures to ozone and nitrogen dioxide on respiratory tract prostanoids. *Inhal Toxicol* 3:27–36, 1991.

Schwartz J: Air pollution and daily mortality: A review and meta analysis. *Environ Res* 64:36–52, 1994.

Schwartz J: Air pollution and the duration of acute respiratory symptoms. *Arch Environ Health* 47(2):116–22, 1992.

Schwartz J. Particulate air pollution and daily mortality in Detroit. *Environ Res* 56:204–213, 1991.

Schwartz J, Marcus A: Mortality and air pollution in London. *Am J Epidemiol* 131:185–194, 1990.

Schwela D: Exposure to environmental chemicals relevant for respiratory hypersensitivity: Global aspects. *Toxicol Lett* 86:131–142, 1996.

Seltzer J, Bigby BG, Stulbarg M, et al: O_3-induced change in bronchial reactivity to methacholine and airway inflammation in humans. *J Appl Physiol* 60:1321–1326, 1986.

Sheppard DA, Saisho A, Nadel JA, Boushey HA: Exercise increases sulfur dioxide induced bronchoconstriction in asthmatic subjects. *Am Rev Respir Dis* 123:486–491, 1981.

Slade R, Stead AG, Graham JA, Hatch GE: Comparison of lung antioxidant levels in humans and laboratory animals. *Am Rev Respir Dis* 131:742–746, 1985.

Speigelman JR, Hanson GD, Lazurus A, et al: Effect of acute sulfur dioxide exposure on bronchial clearance in the donkey. *Arch Environ Health* 17:321, 1968.

Speizer FE: Studies of acid aerosols in six cities and in a new multi-city investigation: Design issues. *Environ Health Perspect* 79:61–68, 1989.

Spengler JD, Sexton K: Indoor air pollution: A public health perspective. *Science* 221:9–17, 1983.

Starr TB, Gibson JE: The mechanistic toxicology of formaldehyde and its implications for quantitative risk assessment. *Annu Rev Pharmacol Toxicol* 25:745–767, 1985.

State of the Air: 2000. American Lung Assoc. www.ala.org, 2000.

Stevens MA, Fitzgerald S, Menache MG, et al: Functional evidence of persistent airway obstruction in rats following a two-hour inhalation exposure to methyl isocyanate. *Environ Health Perspect* 72:89–94, 1987.

Suga T, Kurabayashi M, Sando Y, et al.: Disruption of the klotho gene causes pulmonary emphysema in mice. *Am J Respir Cell Mol Biol* 22:26–33, 2000.

Thurston GD, Ito K, Kinney PL, Lippmann M: A multi-year study of air pollution and respiratory hospital admissions in three New York state metropolitan areas: Results for 1988 and 1989 summers. *J Expos Anal Environ Epidemiol* 2:429–450, 1992.

Tyler WS, Tyler NK, Hinds D, et al: Influence of exposure regimen on effects of experimental ozone studies: Effects of daily and episodic and seasonal cycles of exposure and post-exposure. Presented at the 84th annual meeting of the Air and Waste Management Assoc., Vancouver, BC, Canada. Paper No. 91–141.5, 1991.

Tyler WS, Tyler NK, Last JA, et al: Comparison of daily and seasonal exposures of young monkeys to ozone. *toxicology* 50:131–144, 1988.

Underhill DW. Aerosol synergism and hydrate formation A possible connection. *Inhal Toxicol* 12(suppl 1):189–198, 2000.

Utell MJ, Mariglio JA, Morrow PE, et al: Effects of inhaled acid aerosols on respiratory function: The role of endogenous ammonia. *J Aerosol Med* 2:141–147, 1989.

Utell MJ, Morrow PE, Hyde RW: Airway reactivity to sulfate and sulfuric acid aerosols in normal and asthmatic subjects. *J Air Pollut Control Assoc* 34:931–935, 1984.

Van De Lende R, Kok TJ, Reig RP, et al: Decreases in VC and FEV_1 with time: Indicators for effects of smoking and air pollution. *Bull Eur Physiopathol Respir* 17:775–792, 1981.

Vaughan TR Jr, Jennelle LF, Lewis TR: Long-term exposure to low levels of air pollutants: Effects on pulmonary function in the beagle. *Arch Environ Health* 19:45–50, 1969.

von Mutius E, Martinez FD, Fritzsch C et al.: Prevalence of asthma and atopy in two areas of West and East Germany. *Am J Respir Crit Care Med* 149(2 Pt 1):358–364, 1994.

Waxman HA: Title III of the 1990 Clean Air Act Amendments, in Patrick DR (ed): *Toxic Air Pollution Handbook*. New York: Van Nostrand Reinhold, 1994, pp 25–32.

Wiester MJ, Winsett DW, Richards JE, et al.: Ozone adaptation in mice and its association with ascorbic acid in the lung. *Inhal Toxicol.* 12: 577–590, 2000.

Yokoyama E, Toder RE, Frank NR: Distribution of $^{35}SO_2$ in the blood and its excretion in dogs exposed to $^{35}SO_2$. *Arch Environ Health* 22:389–395, 1971.

Yoshida M, Satoh M, Shimada A, et al: Pulmonary toxicity caused by acute exposure to mercury vapor is enhanced in metallothionein-null mice. *Life Sci* 64(20):1861–1867, 1999.

CHAPTER 29

ECOTOXICOLOGY

Ronald J. Kendall, Todd A. Anderson, Robert J. Baker, Catherine M. Bens, James A. Carr, Louis A. Chiodo, George P. Cobb III, Richard L. Dickerson, Kenneth R. Dixon, Lynn T. Frame, Michael J. Hooper, Clyde F. Martin, Scott T. McMurry, Reynaldo Patino, Ernest E. Smith, and Christopher W. Theodorakis

INTRODUCTION TO ECOTOXICOLOGY

The field of environmental toxicology, particularly as related to the area of ecotoxicology, continues to be a rapidly developing discipline of environmental science (Connell and Miller, 1984; Duffus, 1980; Guthie and Perry, 1980; Hoffman et al., 1995; Moriarity, 1988; Truhaut, 1977). The term *ecotoxicology* was introduced by Truhaut in 1969 (Truhaut, 1977) and this field is a natural extension of toxicology. It is best defined as the study of the fate and effects of toxic substances on an ecosystem and is based on scientific research employing both field and laboratory methods (Kendall, 1982; Kendall, 1992; and Hoffman et al., 1995). Environmental toxicology as it is related to ecotoxicology requires an understanding of ecologic principles and theory as well as a grasp of how chemicals can affect individuals, populations, communities, and ecosystems (Kendall and Lacher, 1994; Hoffman et al., 1995). Measurements of biological impact are accomplished using either species-specific responses to toxicants (Smith, 1987) or impacts on higher levels of organization from individuals to populations, and so on. Ecotoxicology builds on the science of toxicology and the principles of toxicologic testing, though its emphasis is more at the population, community, and ecosystem levels (Moriarty, 1988). The ability to measure chemical transport and fate and exposure of organisms in ecotoxicologic testing is critical to the ultimate development of an ecologic risk assessment (U.S. EPA, 1992 a,b,c; Suter, 1993; Maughan, 1993).

Descriptions of ecotoxicologic methods and procedures have been offered by Cairns (1978) and Cairns et al. (1980) and more recently by Hoffman et al. (1995). Unlike standard toxicologic tests, which seek to define the cause-effect relationship with certain concentrations of toxicant exposure at a sensitive receptor site, ecotoxicologic testing attempts to evaluate cause and effects at higher levels of organization, but particularly on populations (National Academy of Sciences, 1975; Hoffman et al., 1995). To a large extent, the early tests (such as evaluating the effects of pesticides in fish and wildlife populations) generally employed species-specific tests in the laboratory (Smith, 1987). Tests of species included aquatic species such as *Daphnia magna,* fathead minnows (*Pimephales promelas*), the mosquitofish (*Gambusia affinis*); and, among wildlife, the northern bobwhite (*Colinus virginianus*) and mallard duck (*Anas platyrhynchos*) (Lamb and Kenaga, 1981). Arguments have continued over the last decade concerning the relevance of these few organisms to the larger ecosystem at risk. Methods for laboratory bioassays to measure the impact of chemical and nonchemical stressors on aquatic and terrestrial plants and animals continue to evolve. In addition, extrapolation of the results of these assays to field conditions and their utility in an ecologic risk assessment are active areas of research. To an even larger degree, the interrelationship or signals of animal sentinels responding to environmental toxicants as related to human health is an area of increasing interest and under rapid development (Kendall et al., 1998).

A critical component in ecotoxicologic testing is the integration of laboratory and field research (Kendall and Akerman, 1992). Laboratory toxicity bioassays define toxicant impact on individual organisms and on their biochemistry and physiology. Knowledge acquired in the laboratory is integrated with what is occurring under field conditions and is critical to understanding the complex set of parameters with which an organism must deal in order to reproduce or survive under toxicant exposures. Laboratory testing often limits the complexity of stress parameters except perhaps for isolating the toxicant. It is therefore difficult to interpret potential ecotoxicologic effects resulting from laboratory studies without data from pertinent field investigations. For these reasons, integrating laboratory and field research ensures that ecotoxicologic testing methods produce relevant data (Kendall and Lacher, 1994). Demands on ecotoxicologic testing methodologies will continue to increase as concern for environmental protection and chemical impacts increases. Scientific journals continue to publish increasing numbers of manuscripts on ecotoxicologic studies. Furthermore, there is an increasing interest in the relationship of the environment and potential environment toxicant stressors in human health implications. Therefore, this chapter, in addition to outlining some test methodologies for evaluating the effects of toxicants on invertebrates, vertebrates, and plants in aquatic and terrestrial ecosystems, also addresses the relationship of these endpoints to potential human health implications. The complexity and testing strategy in the aquatic versus terrestrial environment can be quite different, and this is one of the challenges currently faced by ecotoxicologic research. For this reason the chapter addresses both aquatic and terrestrial ecotoxicology to reflect the often different parameters involved in evaluating chemical impacts on aquatic versus terrestrial habitats. In recent years, the creation of major new environmental legislation—including the Food Quality Protection Act of 1996 and amendments to the Safe Drinking Water Act—has dictated a renewed evaluation of the relationship between environmental toxicants and potential impacts on the environment as related to human health implications. For this reason, the current chapter addresses some questions and issues related to the integration of environmental signals for toxicant stress and human health implications; in addition, discussion of ecologic risk assessment as related to applications of environmental toxicology data are expanded upon. Those reading this chapter should be aware that the increasing interest on sublethal impacts of contaminants on the environment, including those of biological and nonbiological origin, is being dealt with to a large degree by new environmental laws and by new strategies in risk assessment. These new strategies in risk assessment include probabilistic approaches and increased emphasis on relating environmental information to human health. These issues are addressed in the present chapter.

CHEMICAL MOVEMENT, FATE, AND EXPOSURE

To characterize chemical behavior, it is necessary to measure the chemical in different environmental compartments (e.g., air, soil, water, and biological systems), understand the movement and transport of the chemical within and among these compartments, and follow the chemical as it is metabolized, degraded, stored, or concentrated within each compartment. During the past half-century, intensive effort has been directed toward developing analytic techniques to detect and quantify minute concentrations of chemicals in environmental matrices (Murray, 1993; Blaser et al., 1995). One need only look at the myriad of studies investigating parts per quadrillion (ppq) concentrations of 2,3,7,8-tetrachlorodibenzo-*p*-dioxin (TCDD) to realize that environmental analytic chemistry has progressed substantially to complement the ever-increasing sensitivity of measurable toxicologic endpoints. Consider, for illustrative purposes, the fact that 1 ppq is 1 billion times smaller than a part per million (ppm), equating to approximately 1 g of salt in a billion metric tons of sugar. Nevertheless, it is well documented that environmental concentrations below 1 ppm of certain chemicals can have deleterious effects on different components of the ecosystem.

Chemodynamics

Chemical transport occurs both within environmental compartments (intraphase) and between them (interphase) (Thibodeaux, 1996; Mackay, 1991) and is critical to understanding and interpreting environmental toxicology data. A likely scenario for a chemical released into the environment entails its release into one environmental compartment; it is subsequently partitioned among environmental compartments; it is involved in movement and reactions within each compartment; it is partitioned between each compartment and the biota that reside in that compartment; and it finally reaches an active site in an organism at a high enough concentration for long enough to induce an effect. Chemodynamics is, in essence, the study of chemical release, distribution, degradation, and fate in the environment.

Contaminant transport through the environment is often predicted assuming thermodynamic equilibrium. While this assumption often does not hold, the approach is relatively straightforward and easy to apply. Although intraphase chemical transport is most easily approximated assuming thermodynamic equilibrium, better accuracy is possible using a steady-state model (Mackay, 1991). Abiotic and biotic reactions, which occur within a phase, result in significant changes in the physical and chemical properties of the compound, such as the oxidation state, lipophilicity, and volatility.

Combining these approaches facilitates prediction of the chemical concentration within the immediate vicinity of a particular organism. Chemodynamics can also describe chemical movement or absorption into organisms. Detoxification mechanisms, such as partitioning into adipose tissue, metabolism, and accelerated excretion, can significantly reduce, eliminate, or in some cases increase the toxic action of the chemical. Thus, an appreciation of chemodynamics aids in the prediction of chemical concentrations in compartments and serves as a resource for designing toxicologic experiments using the appropriate concentrations and forms of the chemical in question.

Single-Phase Chemical Behavior

Once a synthetic chemical enters the environment, it is acted upon primarily by natural forces. Models are used to predict the effect of natural forces on the movement of chemicals in the environment. This requires the incorporation of abiotic variables into valid models. These variables include temperature, wind and water-flow directions and velocities, incident solar radiation, atmospheric pressure and humidity, and the concentration of the chemical in one of four matrices: atmosphere (air), hydrosphere (water), lithosphere (soil), and biosphere (living organisms). Intraphase movement consists of mass transfer, diffusion, or dispersion within a single phase (Atkins, 1982). Concentration gradients result in movement within the medium. Contaminant persistence is a function of the stability of that chemical in a phase and its transport within that phase. Stability is a function of the physicochemical properties of a particular chemical and the kinetics of its degradation in the phase; these vary widely in and between classes of chemicals (Howard et al., 1991). Stability issues are difficult to predict and are often better handled by observation rather than modeling. Transport of chemicals in the environment, in contrast, is more predictable and is discussed in detail below.

Air The primary routes of contaminant entry into the atmosphere are through evaporation, stack emissions, and other matrices. Contaminant transport in air generally occurs much more rapidly than in the hydrosphere, as air has lower viscosity. Contaminant transport in air occurs primarily by diffusional processes or advection. Diffusion dominates in the very thin boundary layer between air and the other phases, the thickness of which is less than that of equivalent water-phase interfaces. The diffusion rate for a contaminant in air is approximately 100-fold faster than for the same contaminant in water and is a function of phase viscosity and existing concentration gradients. The contaminant diffusivity in air depends on its molecular weight compared to air, air temperature, the molecular separation at collision, the energy of molecular interaction, and Boltzmann's constant (Atkins, 1982). Wind currents transport airborne contaminants much more rapidly than does diffusion (Wark and Warner, 1981). Atmospheric stability affects the amount of turbulence and thus the degree of vertical mixing in the atmosphere. The stability of the atmosphere is considered neutral when the convective forces—heat transfer from warm ground surfaces and radiative cooling from the top of the cloud layer—are equal. Vertical mixing is at a maximum when heat transfer is greater than radiative cooling and at a minimum during inversion conditions. It is the latter condition that can trap higher concentrations of contaminants near the earth's surface.

Water Contaminants enter the hydrosphere by direct application, spills, wet and dry deposition, and interphase movement. In addition, chemicals enter the hydrosphere by direct dissolution of lighter-than-water spills in the form of slicks or from pools on the bottom of channels, rivers, or other waterways. Chemical movement in the hydrosphere occurs through diffusion, dispersion, and bulk flow of the water. In any flow, a stagnant boundary layer exists at the interface between phases or artificial boundaries. Overlying this layer is a section in which flow is laminar. Finally, above the laminar flow, the fluid is in turbulent flow. Contaminant movement in a mobile phase, in this case, water, is dominated by the turbulence of the mobile phase. If the water is stagnant, (e.g., in close proximity to a stationary phase such as soil or an artificial boundary), the chemical moves by molecular diffusion. As described for the other fluid environmental compartment, air, the diffusion rate depends on fixed characteristics such as the molecular weight of the contaminant (solute), the molecular weight of the water (solvent), water temperature, viscosity, and the association factor for water and dynamic characteristics such as the magnitude of the concentration gradient of the contaminant. These characteristics are referred to as the *diffusivity* of the contaminant-water mixture. Diffusional processes in water are several orders of magnitude faster than in soil.

Away from the boundaries of other media (i.e., air and soil), transport in water is dominated by turbulence. Even in seemingly still water, water is constantly moving in vertical and horizontal eddies. These eddies are small pockets of water that form and subside and, during the process, transport the contaminant. This mode of transport is defined as *eddy diffusion*. In addition, the contaminant can be rapidly transported by bulk flow (also referred to as *advection*) in the cases of streams and rivers. In advection, the rate of transport is proportional to stream velocity.

Soil Chemicals enter the lithosphere by processes similar to those for the hydrosphere. Soils have varying porosities due to their composition (percent sand, silt, clay, organic matter), but pores are invariably filled with either gas or fluids. Chemical movement in the soil occurs by diffusion in these fluids or by the movement of water through the voids between soil particles. Fluid-borne contaminants partition with the solid fraction of soil by processes closely resembling chromatography, in that chemical solubility in pore water, adsorption to soil particles, and pore-water velocity affect the rate of transport (Willard et al., 1988). The direction of diffusion will be from areas of high to areas of low concentration. The chemical diffusion rate in soil depends on molecular weight, soil temperature, the length of the path, and the magnitude of the concentration gradient (Shonnard et al., 1993), among other issues. Contaminants leave the soil by interphase transport or decomposition. Transformation of contaminants (as through microbial degradation) can be significant in soil due to the density and diversity of microorganisms in this compartment compared with water and air.

Chemical Transport between Phases

Once released, a chemical can enter any of the four matrices: the atmosphere by evaporation, the lithosphere by adsorption, the hydrosphere by dissolution, or the biosphere by absorption, inhalation, or ingestion (depending on the species). Once in a matrix, the contaminant can enter another matrix by interphase transport. Absorption by biota is considered under "Chemical Behavior and Bioavailability," below.

Air–Water A chemical can leave the water by volatilization. Conversely, an airborne contaminant can move into an aqueous phase by absorption. At equilibrium, the net rates of volatilization and absorption are equal and the total mass transfer of the contaminant is zero. In nonequilibrium conditions, the rate of net movement of a chemical from one phase to another depends on how far the system is away from equilibrium as well as the magnitude of the overall mass transfer coefficient (Mackay, 1991). In turn, this mass transfer coefficient depends on the physical properties of the solute (such as vapor pressure and solubility) and the magnitude of the bulk flow of both the air and the water. For example, ammonia desorbs most quickly from shallow, rapidly flowing streams with a brisk cross wind. Alternatively, the water–air interface (surface microlayer) can be a concentration point for materials, both natural and anthropogenic (Hardy, 1982; Gever et al., 1996).

Soil–Water A contaminant can leave the soil and enter the water through the process of desorption. Water-borne contaminants can also adsorb on soil particles. Again, the rate of mass transfer depends on the contaminant-specific overall mass transfer coefficient, the bulk flow velocity of the water over the water-soil interface, and physicochemical properties of the soil, such as particle size distribution and organic matter content. Partitioning of contaminants from water to soil or sediment is one of the key processes controlling exposure.

Soil–Air A contaminant may leave the soil and be transported into the overlying air through the process of volatilization. This process is dependent on the vapor pressure of the chemical and its affinity for the soil. Environmental processes that affect the thickness of the soil–air boundary layer (i.e., wind velocity) or contaminant sorption (i.e., soil moisture content), in turn, influence movement from soil to air. For example, more contaminant will be released from contaminated soil at higher wind velocities as well as from wet versus dry soil.

Chemical Behavior and Bioavailability

An appreciation of how physicochemical properties influence contaminant behavior is necessary to anticipate chemical concentrations and speciation in different environmental compartments. Such an appreciation is also valuable in developing an exposure characterization for the contaminant(s) of interest. Ultimately, the goal is to assess the potential bioconcentration (uptake of contaminants from the external environment), bioaccumulation (uptake of contaminants from the external environment and food), and biomagnification (increasing contaminant concentrations at higher trophic levels) in organisms. An investment in careful exposure characterization is worth the expense and effort.

In the environment, only a portion of the total quantity of chemical present is potentially available for uptake by organisms. This concept is referred to as the *biological availability* (or bioavailability) of a chemical. Chemical bioavailability in various environmental compartments ultimately dictates toxicity; therefore it is important to characterize exposure on a site-specific basis. For example, total mercury concentration in aquatic sediments does not necessarily correlate with mercury concentration in midge larvae of the genus *Chironomus*. Important considerations in the case of mercury include the mercury species (e.g., the oxidation state, whether organic or inorganic) as well as physical and chemical characteristics of the sediment matrix (e.g., acid volatile sulfide concentration, pH, pE) (Tinsley, 1979). To complicate matters, in most cases mercury will not exist as a single species but will be distributed among several stable forms. Hence, a simple analytic result of total mercury content does not sufficiently describe the hazard associated with the presence of the metal in sediment. The multiple influences of soil, sediment, and water quality on the bioavailability of environmental chemicals are important research areas.

Chemical bioavailability in the water column has been studied for years, yet many questions are still unanswered. The behavior of dissolved metals, for example, has been studied for over two decades. In the early seventies, much research concerned the influence of pH and water hardness on metal toxicity to algae and other aquatic organisms. This work led to the development of a model to predict metal toxicity based on pH and water hardness [U.S. Environmental Protection Agency (EPA), 1986a].

The behavior and bioavailability of contaminants in the water column have been shown to relate directly to their water solubility. However, the presence of certain constituents in water may affect the apparent water solubility of toxicants. Johnson-Logan and coworkers (1992) demonstrated the apparent solubility of the organochlorine insecticide chlordane (1,2,4,5,6,7,8,8-octachloro-2,3,3a,4,7,7a hexahydro-4,7-methano-1*H*-indene) to be enhanced almost 500 percent in groundwater containing 34 mg/L total organic carbon. This enhanced solubility resulted directly from partitioning of this hydrophobic insecticide into the dissolved organic carbon (DOC) fraction within the water column. The apparent increase in water solubility did not necessarily indicate an increase in pesticide bioavailability. Dissolved organic carbon may increase transport and mobility of organic contaminants in the water column but also reduce their bioavailability.

The behavior and bioavailability of sediment-incorporated xenobiotics is a complex phenomenon studied only recently. The awareness that many aquatic contaminants settle into sediments has prompted studies of metals and organics to characterize their fate and disposition within the complex sediment matrix. Deposition is a combination of physical, chemical, and biological processes that may ultimately change the form of the xenobiotic. Many metals are abiotically or biotically reduced as they are incorporated into sediments. Mercury is methylated through microbial reactions in the sediment. Methylmercury is typically more bioavailable and more toxic than inorganic mercury.

Characterization of processes that control metal bioavailability in sediments would facilitate the development of models to predict toxic threshold concentrations of metals in different sediments. Work with sediment-incorporated metals has emphasized divalent cations in anaerobic environments. Under these conditions, acid volatile sulfides (AVS) preferentially bind divalent cations. Initial work with AVS focused on cadmium (DiToro et al., 1990), which can react with the solid phase AVS to displace iron and form a cadmium sulfide precipitate:

$$Cd^{2+} + FeS(s) \leftrightarrow CdS(s) + Fe^{2+}$$

If the AVS quantity in sediment exceeds the quantity of added cadmium, the cadmium concentration in the interstitial water is not detectable and the cadmium is not bioavailable, hence it is not toxic. This process can be extended to other cations including nickel, zinc, lead, copper, mercury, and perhaps chromium, arsenic, and silver (Ankley et al., 1991). Furthermore, there is thermodynamic evidence that the presence of one divalent cation, copper for example, may displace a previously bound divalent cation with weaker binding strength such as cadmium. This results in a greater concentration of bioavailable cadmium while sulfide-bound copper is less bioavailable. Thus, the bioavailable fraction of metals in sediments can be predicted by measuring AVS and the simultaneously extracted metals (SEM) that result during AVS extraction. If the molar ratio of SEM to AVS is <1, little or no toxicity should be expected; if the molar ratio of SEM to AVS is >1, the mortality of sensitive species can be expected (DiToro et al., 1992). This approach is not without controversy and, while many scientists believe that AVS plays a significant role in the bioavailability of divalent cations in anaerobic sediment, most would agree that AVS alone does not predict metal bioavailability. Other sediment factors including oxide and hydroxide layers undoubtedly play a role in metal bioavailability. In addition, the ability of sediment-dwelling organisms to oxidize their surrounding environment, thus breaking metal-sulfide bonds, should be further studied.

Organic chemicals residing in the sediment matrix undergo a variety of abiotic and biotic transformations. Predicting the intraphase movement of organics in sediments is extremely difficult, and in general, the processes that control such movement are poorly understood. For nonionic, nonmetabolized, nonpolar organics, however; equilibrium partitioning theory has been proposed as the basis for developing sediment quality criteria. This theory suggests that, in the sediment matrix, certain chemicals partition between interstitial water and the organic carbon fraction of the solids. At equilibrium, this partitioning can be predicted using laboratory-generated partitioning coefficients (e.g., K_{oc}). The resulting interstitial water concentration should induce the same exposure as a water-only exposure. Thus, the toxicity of chemicals in interstitial water can be predicted using the results of water column bioassays with the chemical. One assumption of this theory is that, for these chemicals, exposure of sediment-dwelling organisms occurs through interstitial water only and that chemicals partitioned onto solids are not bioavailable. A good review of this theory and supporting data can be found in the 1991 report of DiToro and colleagues.

In soils, sorption also controls the bioavailability of contaminants. An example of the importance of site-specific exposure characterization is highlighted by a series of experiments designed by researchers at the United States Environmental Protection Agency (U.S. EPA) (Weis et al., 1994). The finding that many forms of environmental lead are not well absorbed across the gastrointestinal tract disproved the assumption that all forms of lead in contaminated surface soil are equally hazardous (Table 29-1).

Table 29-1
Studies of Endocrine Disruption in Representative Wildlife Species

SPECIES	COMPOUND	EFFECTS
Invertebrates		
Molluscs	Tributyltin	Imposex
Insects	DDE	Metabolic masculinization
Fish		
White sucker (*Catostomus commersoni*)	Kraft mill effluent	Delayed maturation, induction of vitellogenin in male fish, reduced gonad size and development, altered sex steroid concentrations
Trout (*Salmo gairderi*)	Municipal sewer effluent (containing alkylphenols, and conjugated estrogens	Feminization of male fish, including induction of plasma vitellogenin
Amphibians		
African clawed frog (*Xenopus laevis*)	Estrogens	Sexual imprinting (100% females)
Reptiles		
Red-eared slider (*Trachemys scripta*)	Estrogens, pesticides	Sex reversal, gonadal aberrations, altered sex steroid
American alligator (*Alligator mississippiensis*)	Estrogens, pesticides	Sex reversal, gonadal and phallus malformations, altered sex steroid concentrations
Birds		
Herring gulls (*Larus argentatus*)	PCBs, pesticides	Masculinization, altered gonadal structure
American bald Eagle (*Haliaeetus leucocephalus*)	PCBs, dioxins, pesticides	Eggshell thinning, brain asymmetry
Mammals		
Beluga whale (*Delphinptenus leucas*)	Organochlorines, metals	Tumors, immune suppression, impaired reproduction
Mink (*Mustela vision*)	PCBs, dioxins	Impaired reproduction, fetal mortality

SOURCE: Kendall et al., 1998, with permission.

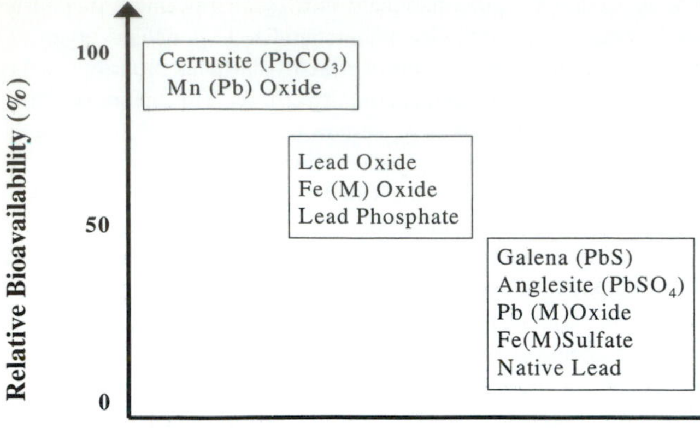

***Figure 29-1.** Gastrointestinal bioavailability of soil lead as a function of the physical and chemical nature of the exposure material (From Weis et al., 1994, with permission.)*

Highly oxidized lead forms found in soils near mining and/or smelting sites is absorbed into blood nearly as well as freely soluble lead, while more reduced forms are only poorly absorbed.

Other lead forms were shown to be nearly as well absorbed as freely soluble lead acetate. Using an immature swine model as a surrogate (Weis and LaVelle, 1991) and a series of highly controlled animal studies, these investigators measured soil lead bioavailability ranging from less than 6 percent to greater than 90 percent relative to a soluble lead acetate reference substance (Fig. 29-1).

Tight sorption or sequestration of contaminants with increasing residence time in soil, often referred to as "aging," has also been documented (Pignatello et al., 1993; Hatzinger and Alexander, 1995), especially for lipophilic organic contaminants. Although the amount of contaminant in soil remains fairly constant, the fraction of the contaminant available to soil organisms is reported to significantly decrease with time. An important issue currently being addressed is the development of methods to assess the magnitude of available contaminant residues in soil (Kelsey and Alexander, 1997), including the use of sampling devices based on passive diffusion (Johnson et al., 1995; Awata et al., 1999).

BIOMARKERS

A fundamental challenge in environmental toxicology is relating the presence of a chemical in the environment with a valid prediction of ensuing hazard to potential biological receptors. Adverse health effects in biological receptors begin with exposure to a contaminant and can progress to damage or alteration in function of an organelle, cell, or tissue. Exposure of wildlife by contact to contaminated environmental media is defined as an *external dose,* whereas internalization of the contaminated media, via inhalation, ingestion, or dermal absorption, results in an *internal dose*. The amount of this internal dose necessary to elicit a response or health effect is referred to as the *biologically effective dose*.

Traditionally, environmental risk was assessed by chemical residue determination in samples of environmental media, combined with comparison to toxicity observed in species in contact with the media. This approach, although it yields useful information, has several limitations. The determination of chemical residues in environmental matrices is not simple and may require extensive sample cleanup leading to high per sample costs (U.S. EPA, 1986b). The availability of the chemicals in the environmental matrix to the biological receptor, or bioavailability, cannot be quantified by this approach. Depending upon the chemical, the environmental matrix, and the species, bioavailability may range from 100 percent to a fraction of a percent. To overcome this problem, chemical residue analysis of tissues containing the biological receptor may be performed [Agency for Toxic Substances and Disease Registry (ATSDR), 1994]. This approach, however, is often more difficult and expensive than the cost of the analysis of environmental matrices and yields no information on toxicologic response. In addition, the toxicokinetics and toxicodynamics of a contaminant in a particular species determines whether an exposure is capable of an adverse response. A biomarker-based approach resolves many of these difficulties by providing a direct measure of toxicant effects in the affected species (Dickerson et al., 1994).

The National Academy of Sciences defines a biomarker or biological marker as a xenobiotically induced alteration in cellular or biochemical components or processes, structures, or functions that is measurable in a biological system or sample (Committee on Biological Markers, 1987). To this list may well be added xenobiotically induced alterations in behavior. Therefore, biomarkers can be broadly categorized as markers of exposure, effects, or susceptibility (ATSDR, 1994). The selection of appropriate biomarkers to be used for hazard evaluation is based on the mechanism of a chemically induced disease state. Moreover, growing awareness of the possibility of using wildlife as sentinels for human environmental disease has created a demand for biomarkers that are nonlethal and correlate with adverse effects in humans.

Dosing with an adequate concentration of a toxicant produces a continuum of responses beginning with exposure and perhaps resulting in the development of a disease. These events begin with external exposure, followed by the establishment of an internal dose leading to delivery of a contaminant to a critical site. This is followed either by reversible or irreversible adverse alterations to the critical site, resulting in the development of recognizable disease states. A clearer understanding of a chemically induced disease state in a species leads to an increase in the number of specific and useful biomarkers that may be extrapolated to other species. It is readily apparent that the earlier these effects can be measured at a critical site, the more sensitive the prediction of hazard or disease. However, in many cases the exact mechanism by which a toxicant induces injury is not well understood and nonspecific indicators of disease must be used.

Biomarkers of Exposure

The presence of a xenobiotic substance or its metabolite(s) or the product of an interaction between a xenobiotic agent and some target molecule or cell that is measured within a compartment of an organism can be classified as a biomarker of exposure (ATSDR, 1994). In general, biomarkers of exposure are used to predict the dose received by an individual, which can then be related to changes resulting in a disease state. In many cases, biomarkers of exposure are among the most convenient to determine because the contaminant or its metabolites can be quantified from nonlethally obtained samples of exhaled air, urine, feces, blood, or breast milk as well as tissues obtained through biopsy or necropsy. The former sources are the most desirable because they can be used for multiple determinations over time, thus making the biomarker more useful by providing more information on the effects of the toxicant with time and by reducing variability.

Some very useful biomarkers of cancer involve detecting the ability of chemical carcinogens to form adducts with cellular macromolecules such as DNA or protein. Most chemical carcinogens are either strong electrophiles or are converted to an electrophilically active substance through metabolic activation (Miller and Miller, 1981). These carcinogens react with nucleophilic biomacromolecules to form adducts. If the biomacromolecule is sufficiently stable, adducts can then be detected by a variety of means and used to determine exposure profiles. Stable biomacromolecules can also provide measurement of the dose of a chemical carcinogen received by animals and humans. Adduct detection can be accomplished by total hydrolysis of the protein to alkylated amino acids (histidine, cysteine adducts), mild hydrolysis to release adducts (adducts that form esters to carboxyl groups or sulfonamides), immunodetection, or modified Edman degradation (adducts to N terminal valines on Hb). These techniques have been used to identify adducts formed by simple alkylating agents and their metabolites, aromatic amines, nitrosamines, and polynuclear aromatic hydrocarbons. One major advantage to this method of cancer risk determination is that blood samples are easily obtained and multiple samples can be obtained to determine patterns of exposure. In addition, the presence of adducts can often be detected by the creation of a point mutation. An example of this is the G-to-T transversion created following the formation of a N7 guanine adduct by benzo[*a*]pyrene 7,8-dihydrodiol-9,10-epoxide (BPDE) (Shibutani et al., 1993). Such point mutations can be detected by restriction fragment length polymorphisms.

Biomarkers of Effect

Biomarkers of effect are defined as measurable biochemical, physiologic, behavioral, or other alterations within an organism that, depending on their magnitude, can be recognized as an established or potential health impairment or disease (ATSDR, 1994). Ideally, a biomarker result must be able to stand alone. As such, it does not need chemical analysis or additional biological tests for confirmation. These tests are highly specific for individual chemicals and thus have a fairly limited application. Examples of such biomarkers include inhibition of brain cholinesterase by organophosphate or carbamate insecticides, induction of delta aminolevulinic acid synthetase and inhibition of aminolevulinic acid dehydratase by lead and certain other metals, and eggshell thinning by 1,1-dichloro-2,2-bis(*p*-chlorophenyl) ethylene (DDE), a metabolite of 1,1,1-trichloro-2,2-bis(*p*-chlorophenyl)ethane (DDT) (Scott, 1977).

Less specific biomarkers are also well validated, but they have wider applications and tend to respond to broader classes of chemicals. Examples of these biomarkers are the induction of mixed-function oxidases, the formation of DNA adducts, other DNA alterations such as sister chromatid exchange and strand breakage, porphyrin profile alterations, induction of vitellogenin in oviparous vertebrates, and immunologic changes such as immunosuppression and hypersensitivity. These assays require either additional biomarker studies or chemical residue analysis in order to link causative agent to adverse effect. For example, the induction of cytochrome P4501Al (CYP1A1) enzymes in fish liver is generally recognized as a useful biomarker of the exposure of fish to anthropogenic contaminants, but these results are not compound-specific, as they may be induced by a variety of polynuclear and halogenated aromatic hydrocarbons as well as by hypoxia (HIF response element; Collier et al., 1995; Chan et al., 1999).

Finally, there is a long list of biomarkers that are under development or have been used with varying degrees of success but require further validation before they can be used in hazard evaluation. Thyroid function, retinol levels, plasma sex steroids, and stress proteins fall into this classification. Challenges exist in interpreting data from measurements of these endpoints because of normal circadian and seasonal variation, multiple known factors involved in the control of these endpoints, and marked interindividual variability.

Biomarkers of Susceptibility

Biomarkers of susceptibility are endpoints that are indicative of an altered physiologic or biochemical state that may predispose the individual to impacts of chemical, physical, or infectious agents. These biomarkers can be useful in predicting human disease states from wildlife sentinels. Low-level exposure to a cytochrome P4501A1 or 1A2 inducer, for example, may result in elevated enzyme activity in wildlife but no observable adverse effects. Such elevations in enzyme activity in humans have been linked to greater risk of a number of cancers due to increased bioactivation of procarcinogens. Similar observations have been made for decreases in conjugation enzymes and their high-energy substrates (Frame et al., 1998). In addition, a number of xenobiotic compounds inhibit the activities of the immune system and thus increase susceptibility to infectious agents, parasites, and cancer. Admittedly, the distinction between biomarkers of effect and susceptibility may be blurred. However, the distinction may be based upon whether the xenobiotic causes a physiologic or biochemical change that is directly indicative of a disease state or whether it reduces resistance to other biological, physical, or chemical agents.

Biomarker Interpretation

Caution must be used in interpreting biomarker results and extrapolating from one species to another. The same chemical may induce different proteins in one species when compared to another and the same enzyme may have different substrate specificities in species as closely related as the mouse and rat. For example, the common environmental contaminant *p,p'*-DDE induces cytochrome P4502B in the laboratory rat (*Rattus rattus*) but induces cytochrome P4501A1 in the deer mouse (*Peromyscus maniculatus*). Moreover, TCDD is a cytochrome P4501A1 inducer in the rat but induces both 1A1 and 2B in the deer mouse as determined by Western blotting, Northern blotting, and enzymatic activities (Nims et al., 1998, Dickerson et al., 1999). Similar differences exist between laboratory rats and birds, fish, and reptiles. Extrapolation of results requires a thorough knowledge of comparative physiology and biochemistry.

Alternatively, an important application of biomarkers is their ability to integrate multiple chemical exposures across an area with a variety of chemical contaminants, the scenario found at most chemical waste sites. CYP1A1 responses to sediments contaminated with dioxin, polychlorinated biphenyls (PCBs), or polynuclear aromatic hydrocarbons (PAHs) can provide insight to the status of the contaminants on site, their bioavailability, and the overall risk that they pose. Similarly, porphyrin profile alterations, metallothionein content, and immune function can provide insight to the combined effects of metals found on mine waste-contaminated sites. It is thus essential in the use of biomarkers to understand both the strengths and the limitations of the techniques and to be cautious in extrapolating between species.

Beyond the current predominance of functionally based biomarkers, new trends in biomarker development appear distinctly molecular. A review of the most recent biomarker literature lists molecular biomarkers for a great many diseases and environmental contaminants ranging from secondhand smoke to suicide. The integration of biomarkers with epidemiology has resulted in a new discipline, molecular epidemiology, which has the potential for creating worldwide databases for environmental and genetic diseases (Albertini, 1999). The integration of biomarkers with molecular biology has revolutionized both medicine and biology by providing new tools by which to determine mechanisms of action (Costa, 1998). Moreover, these techniques can be applied to samples as small as one cell (Rao et al., 1998). Increasing emphasis is being placed upon nonlethal biomarkers such as enzyme-linked immunosorbent assay (ELISA) techniques for measuring fecal steroids in deer mice. A recent study defined four major needs in the development of biomarkers (Ward et al., 1996). New biomarkers are needed to monitor the continuum between exposure and overt disease. An increased knowledge is needed of the relationship between biomarker responses and disease pathology. In addition, better validation and increased sensitivity are required from existing biomarkers in order to better predict disease development. Last, as biomarkers become better tools for predicting environmental and genetic risk, a need to integrate science with policy emerges due to ethics of furnishing risk data to employers and insurance providers.

ENDOCRINE AND DEVELOPMENTAL DISRUPTORS

Endocrine disruption has recently emerged as a major issue, in terms of both science and public policy. A number of compounds, both natural and anthropogenic, cause alterations of the endocrine system (Colborn, 1996). Profound endocrine effects, both in individuals and at the population level, have been documented after exposure to high levels of certain compounds. All available evidence indicates that this issue will continue to evolve because of the controversial nature of the topic and the current insufficiency of data with which to make sound policy decisions (Kendall et al., 1998).

Mechanisms of Endocrine Toxicity and Sensitive Life Stages

It is evident that endocrine-disrupting compounds (EDCs) may interact with multiple targets. There is evidence for EDCs acting at every level of hormone synthesis, secretion, transport, site of action, and metabolism. Some examples of known mechanisms for EDCs include the following.

Receptor-Mediated Effects of EDCs A xenobiotic compound may exert effects at the receptor level through multiple mechanisms beyond the classic ligand-receptor interaction. These include differential effects at multiple receptor types or direct effects on intracellular signaling pathways, thereby directly influencing hormone action at the target tissue. Xenobiotic compounds may act on the endocrine system by affecting transcription and signal transduction and can act through receptor-mediated or nonreceptor-mediated mechanisms. For example, genistein has been shown to be a weak estrogen receptor agonist; however, it also modulates the activity of tyrosine kinases and DNA topoisomerases (Makela et al., 1994; Makela et al., 1995; Okajima et al., 1994; Olsen et al., 1994; Piontek et al., 1993; Whitten et al., 1995).

Effects of EDCs on Hormone Synthesis and Metabolism A compound may adversely alter levels of critical endogenous hormones by inducing or inhibiting biosynthetic or metabolic enzyme activities. Some phytoestrogens can interact with the 17β-dehydrogenase that regulates estradiol and estrone levels, suggesting that they can modulate overall estrogen levels in addition to acting as a ligand for the estrogen receptor. Perchlorate competitively inhibits thyroidal iodine uptake, thereby disrupting thyroid hormone synthesis (Lamm et al., 1999).

Effects on Hormone Secretion and Transport It has been known for many years that Cd^{2+} is a nonselective Ca^{2+} blocker that can disrupt Ca^{2+}-dependent exocytosis in hypothalamic neurosecretory neurons and pituitary endocrine cells, for example. Alternatively, EDCs can affect hormone-binding (sex hormone binding globulin, SHBG; corticosteroid binding globulin, CBG) proteins in blood, thereby disrupting hormone transport by increasing or decreasing the bound-to-free ratio of the hormone in plasma (reviewed in van der Kraak et al., 1998).

Timing of Exposure

There is substantial evidence that the sensitivity of an individual to gonadal steroids is dependent on the life stage of that individual. Specifically, the fetus appears to be the most sensitive life stage for lasting impacts of gonadal steroids or agonists/antagonists (Birnbaum, 1994; Blanchard and Hannigan, 1994; Ojasoo et al., 1992). For example, a compound may have little effect at environmentally relevant concentrations on a postpubescent animal but may prevent normal development if exposure occurs during fetal development or puberty. Research with polychlorinated biphenyls (PCBs) and dioxin has shown that gestational exposure is more critical than lactational exposure in eliciting developmental effects (Bjerke et al., 1994a; Bjerke and Peterson, 1994; Bjerke et al., 1994b). Sensitivity to EDCs is generally higher in fetal and perinatal individuals than in adults. However, in some cases, the presence of fetal serum-binding proteins may result in lower sensitivity to these compounds. For example, the ability of α-fetoprotein to bind 17β-estradiol protects the fetal male rat from maternal estrogen (Herve et al., 1990). Recent U.S. EPA workshops have identified the development of reproductive capability as the highest research priority in consideration of the features discussed above (Ankley et al., 1998).

Hormone Regulation and Feedback Control

There are several important control mechanisms that regulate estrogen biosynthesis during pregnancy. Estrogen levels are not feedback-regulated in a typical homeostatic mechanism; rather, there is a feed-forward mechanism resulting in steadily increasing serum levels of estradiol across most of pregnancy in rodents and humans (Casey et al., 1985). Thus, an exogenous dose of any estrogen agonist will be additive with the endogenous level because feedback will not reduce endogenous production in a compensatory way. Additionally, in rodents and humans, the specific estradiol (E2) serum-binding proteins, α-fetoprotein (AFP), and testosterone-estradiol binding globulin (TEBG), also increase steadily during pregnancy, serving to protect the fetus from the high circulating estrogen level of pregnancy. Xenoestrogens that fail to bind effectively to these proteins have increased bioavailability (Sheehan and Young, 1979). Diethylstilbestrol and ethynylestradiol bind AFP with about 100-fold lower affinity than E2. Hence their bioavailability in newborn rats with high AFP levels is increased to about the same extent as E2, the bioavailability of which is decreased (Sheehan and Barnham, 1987). A fungal estrogen (i.e., Zearalenone) is about 0.066 percent as potent as E2 for adult uterotrophic responses, while equol, a plant estrogen, is about 0.25 percent as potent. In the neonatal rat, these numbers are 5 and 25 percent, respectively (Sheehan et al., 1984).

Species-Dependent Sex Determination

There are major differences in the control of sex determination among vertebrate classes. In mammals, sexual determination is based on the XY/XX system with the female as the homogametic sex. This system requires the synthesis of testosterone and dihydrotestosterone (through modification of testosterone by the action of 5α-reductase) in some target tissues and the presence of functional androgen receptors in the undifferentiated gonad, secondary sexual tissues, and brain (Norris, 1997). In rodents (but not necessarily in primates), the presence of estrogen receptors in the brain is essential for establishing male-type behavior. In order for this to occur, testosterone or a precursor must be aromatized to 17β-estradiol. Failure of any component results in the development of genetic males whose external phenotype or behavioral sex is not concordant with chromosomal sex (Norris, 1997). The sensitivity of this system is so exquisite that effects on reproductive development after in utero exposure may drive the risk assessment for EDCs (EC, 1996). In contrast, birds have a WZ/WW sex chromosomal system with the male as the homogametic sex. In birds, the ability to synthesize and recognize 17β-estradiol is necessary for female central nervous system (CNS) and gonadal sexual development to occur. A number of environmentally relevant chemicals can affect sexual differentiation and behavior in avian species. For example, masculinization of behavior in female birds may be observed following exposure to certain halogenated aromatic hydrocarbons (Fry, 1995; Nisbet et al., 1996; Rattner et al., 1984).

A nonheterogametic chromosome sex determination pathway exists in some reptilian species, predominantly the crocodilians, some turtles, and lizards. In these oviparous species, the temperature of incubation determines the sex of the embryo—a mechanism referred to as *environmental* or *temperature-dependent sex determination* (TSD). The window of sex determination for most animals is fairly narrow, comprising approximately 25 percent of the total incubation period (Norris, 1997). In some species, such as the American alligator (*Alligator mississippiensis*), the relationship between incubation temperature and sex is fairly linear, with lower incubation temperatures producing female offspring and higher incubation temperatures producing male offspring (reviewed in Matter et al., 1998). Moreover, incubation temperatures below 26°C and above 36°C result in embryonic death. For the red-eared slider (*Trachemys scripta*), the relationship is opposite. In other reptilian species, the relationship between sex and incubation temperature is more complex, with intermediate incubation temperatures producing predominantly male offspring and incubation temperatures on either extreme resulting in predominantly female offspring. The molecular mechanism of TSD is not well understood but may be the result of temperature-dependent control of aromatase (Rhen et al., 1999; Chardard and Dournon, 1999; Bergeron et al., 1999; Jeyasuria and Place, 1998). A number of compounds found in the environment can cause a reversal of sex determination in these species. Feminization of alligator and turtle embryos by DDE and hydroxylated PCBs has been reported (Guillette et al., 1999; Bergeron et al., 1994).

Endocrine disruption was initially observed in wildlife species and has received much attention in both the lay and scientific press. Although there are species differences in the response to EDCs, wildlife are sensitive to the effects of EDCs. Studies in wildlife are an important tool in determining the risk posed by EDCs in the environment. Table 29-1 lists a number of studies in various species, the causative agent (if known), and effects observed.

Further Issues on Endocrine and Developmental Toxicants

The Endocrine Disruptor Screening and Testing Advisory Committee (EDSTAC) was formed to develop strategies for evaluating the thousands of products and intermediates currently in use or in development that have the potential of human or environmental exposure. EDSTAC became necessary when the U.S. Congress mandated testing for endocrine-active substances in the Food Quality Protection Act (1996) and the Safe Drinking Water Reauthorization Act and Amendments (1996). These acts required that the U.S. EPA develop a screening program by August 1998, implement the program by August 1999, and report results back to Congress by August 2000. EDSTAC was chartered by the U.S. EPA administrator to provide advice and council to the U.S. EPA on these issues. This legislation increased the number of compounds likely to be tested from a few hundred to most chemicals in production or trials.

Currently, the most widely used tests are the Developmental Toxicology Test and Multigenerational Tests. These have been described previously in this volume. The limitations of the Developmental Toxicology Test are insufficient exposure during sexual differentiation and limited evaluation of reproductive and/or endocrine systems. Limitations of multigenerational tests include not enough diversity in the species tested, insufficient sensitivity of some endpoints, and failure to identify malformations elicited by known endocrine disrupting compounds (e.g., eggshell thinning).

EDSTAC recommended a two-tiered approach, with the first tier concerned with detecting—through the use of a battery of assays in mammalian and nonmammalian organisms—compounds that may be endocrinologically active, affecting the estrogen, androgen, and thyroid hormone systems. The second tier is designed to characterize the dose-response relationship of endocrine-disrupting compounds in wildlife and humans. Compounds are being selected (prioritized) for testing based upon their production volume, potential for exposure, result of high-throughput prescreening, structure, chemical class, and other relevant information. Once selected, the compounds will be evaluated by a series of in vitro and in vivo tests. These in vitro tests include estrogen receptor (ER) binding/transcriptional activation, androgen receptor (AR) binding/transcriptional activation, and steroid hormone synthesis using minced testis. Proposed in vivo tests include uterotrophic assay in adult ovariectomized rat, pubertal female rat assay including thyroid tests, (anti)androgen assay in castrate-T-treated male rat, frog metamorphosis assay for EDCs with thyroid hormone action, and a short-term fish gonadal recrudescence assay.

TERRESTRIAL AND AQUATIC ECOTOXICOLOGY

Many environmental studies include the analysis of contaminant exposure and effects on relatively small scales. However, contaminants can affect ecologic systems over large areas, including ecosystems and landscapes (Holl and Cairns, 1995). Ecosystems are composed of groups of all types of organisms that function together as well as interact with the physical environment, including energy flow and cycling of material between living and nonliving components (Odum, 1983). In turn, ecosystems collectively constitute landscapes with their own functional (nutrient and energy flow) and structural (patches, corridors) attributes. Movement of biotic and abiotic components within these large systems varies depending on several factors, including the species of animal and physical features of the system. Large vertebrates may roam over hundreds of square kilometers, integrating many habitat types within their home range. The area used by small animals may be small on an individual basis; however, dispersal individuals can maintain rather extensive connectivity among otherwise distinct local populations. Cycling and flow of materials maintain varying levels of connectivity within ecologic systems, such that disturbances to one component may be realized at another seemingly distinct component (Holl and Cairns, 1995). In general, ecologic systems are in a constant state of communication, which can potentially facilitate the large-scale effects of pollution.

Ecotoxicology includes all aspects of aquatic and terrestrial systems while attempting to elucidate the effects on biota following contaminant exposure. Exploring exposures to terrestrial systems and the effects of environmental contaminants within them is a recent endeavor relative to work that has been conducted historically in aquatic systems. Studies in aquatic and terrestrial toxicology rely heavily on interdisciplinary scientific exploration. Such research encompasses a variety of topics, including toxicity testing, sublethal responses of individual organisms, effects on populations and communities, and field research (Kendall and Lacher, 1994). A plethora of measurement endpoints exist that can be used to determine exposure and effects in different organisms or ecologic systems (Holl and Cairns, 1995; Melancon, 1995). These biological indicators of pollution may include individual-based measurements of some biochemical, physiologic, or morphologic endpoint (as previously discussed) or higher-order endpoint measurements including perturbations at population or higher levels. Thus, pollution may result in a cascade of events, beginning with effects on homeostasis in individuals and extending through populations, communities, ecosystems, and landscapes. This complexity and potential for large-scale effects extending through ecosystems results in a challenging research environment for environmental toxicologists.

Separation of aquatic and terrestrial environments in ecotoxicology is often impossible, as contaminants can be readily transported between these two systems. For example, contaminants in terrestrial environments may be transported to aquatic systems through surface runoff, resulting in exposure and effects in aquatic organisms located considerable distances from the source of contamination. Conversely, contaminants originating in aquatic environments may move into terrestrial environments following flood events or evaporation. One mechanism of contaminant movement of considerable interest in ecotoxicology is the transfer of contaminants through trophic levels, both within and between aquatic and terrestrial systems. Life-history strategies of many vertebrate and invertebrate organisms routinely integrate aquatic and terrestrial systems, resulting in exposure and effects scenarios that can be quite complex. Thus, although aquatic and terrestrial ecotoxicology are often considered separately, they are often intimately connected through abiotic and biotic mechanisms, examples of which can be found throughout the scientific literature.

Toxicity Tests

Acute and chronic toxicity tests are designed to determine the short- and long-term effects of chemical exposure on a variety of endpoints, including survival, reproduction, and physiologic and biochemical responses. Toxicity testing of terrestrial animal and plant species serves a number of purposes in terrestrial toxicology. Understanding the effects of a single compound provides a foundation for assessing the effects of contaminant mixtures. Because of the complex possibilities under typical field conditions, acute and chronic toxicity testing provides a critical foundation for evaluating the exposures and effects encountered in the field and for linking cause and effect to specific chemicals. For example, brain and plasma cholinesterase (ChE) inhibition has proven to be an excellent tool for monitoring exposure and in some cases for diagnosing the effect in animals exposed to organophosphate and carbamate pesticides (Mineau, 1991). Advances in toxicology have resulted in an expanding search for new sentinel plant and animal species for assessing contaminant exposure and effects. In turn, new sentinel prospects require testing to determine their sensitivity and the precision of their responses. Acute and chronic toxicity testing represents the initial steps toward validating new animal and plant species as useful sentinels of environmental contamination.

Results derived from acute and chronic tests can be used to determine the pathologic effects of contaminants, to provide data necessary to analyze the effects discovered in field tests, identify the potential effects to be aware of under field conditions, and provide dose-response data for comparison to exposure levels in the field. Although they measure effects at the individual level, acute and chronic toxicity tests were designed for the purpose of protecting natural ecosystems from perturbation due to anthropogenic contamination. There are concerns raised by some researchers that laboratory toxicity tests are not realistic predictors of effects in complex field ecosystems. On the other hand, others have argued that short-term toxicity data provide conservative indices by which to judge potential effects of chemicals and effluents on natural populations and ecosystems (Cairns and Mount, 1990). It has even been found that toxicity tests can sometimes be used as indicators of potential effects on community structure (Norberg-King and Mount, 1986; Hartwell, 1997).

Sublethal Effects

Mortality represents a nonreversible endpoint of interest in ecotoxicology. However, documenting die-offs can be challenging, as success is affected by search efficiency and rapid disappearance of carcasses (Rosene and Lay, 1963). Also, many contaminants exist in smaller, nonlethal amounts or in relatively unavailable forms, such that acute mortality is unlikely. Thus, understanding and monitoring the sublethal effects of contaminant exposure in aquatic and terrestrial systems is of great interest. The existence of sublethal effects in exposed organisms has been used as an advantage in monitoring strategies. Biochemical and physiologic measurement endpoints have been developed or adapted from other sources and, in turn, used with various plant and animal sentinels to assess exposure and effect in many different species (Lower and Kendall, 1990; Kendall et al., 1990; Huggett et al., 1992; Adams et al., 1992; Theodorakis et al., 1992). Inhibition of ChEs has proven an excellent marker that is both sensitive and diagnostic for organophosphate and carbamate insecticide exposure (Mineau, 1991). Induction of enzyme systems, such as the mixed-function oxygenases, are also useful as sublethal biomarkers of exposure to many types of environmental pollutants (Elangbarn et al., 1989; Rattner et al., 1989). Other strategies for monitoring sublethal effects include monitoring immune function (McMurry et al., 1995), genotoxicity (McBee et al., 1987), and reproductive endpoints (Kendall et al., 1990). Even though these effects may not result in immediate mortality, they can affect fecundity and reproductive success of aquatic and terrestrial organisms and ultimately have effects on population structure and function. Chemicals may also affect the growth rate of organisms. Because growth rate and body size are related to reproductive maturity in juvenile organisms and its attainment as well as relative fecundity in adults, chemical stressors that inhibit growth rates can also affect the reproductive potential of the population.

Sublethal effects of contaminant exposure reach beyond the intrinsic physiologic and biochemical responses to many behavioral traits of the individual. Decreased predator avoidance capability may expose individuals to increased susceptibility to predation (Bildstein and Forsyth, 1979; Preston et al., 1999). Foraging behavior may be altered by chemicals, such that foraging efficiency or success in prey capture is diminished (Peterle and Bentley, 1989; Smith and Weis 1997). Migration and homing also may be affected, decreasing the general fitness of the individual (Snyder, 1974; Willette, 1996; Vyas et al., 1995). Altered breeding behavior may decrease fecundity through impaired nest-building and courtship behavior, territorial defense, and parental care of the young (McEwen and Brown, 1966; Jones and Reynolds, 1997). In addition, changes in fish behavior patterns or avoidance of contaminated water have been used as indicators of aquatic pollution (Gruber et al., 1994; DeLonay et al., 1996). These may occur at earlier times or at lower doses than overt mortality, providing an early-warning indicator of toxic effects (Gerhardt, 1998).

Determination of sublethal effects is an important component of risk assessments for two reasons. First, these responses may provide information not available from measurements of contaminant tissue concentrations. This is because (1) it may not be possible to measure tissue concentrations of some chemicals because they are rapidly metabolized and (2) the toxic effects of many chemicals, especially when present in complex mixtures (as is usually the case in the environment) may not be predicted from tissue concentrations alone (Lower and Kendall, 1990). Second, alterations of biochemical and molecular physiology have been associated with reductions of fecundity, growth, and bioenergetic status of affected organisms (Adams et al., 1989, Theodorakis et al., 1996, Steinert et al., 1998). Hence, perturbations of subcellular function may affect fitness and health of fish and wildlife, and may ultimately be translated as effects on populations and communities.

Although they are quite similar, sublethal effects in aquatic and terrestrial organisms do differ in some important aspects. For example, there are a number of suborganismal (cellular, molecular, histologic) effects that can be detected in aquatic and terrestrial organisms, and many of these are commonly studied in both types of organisms—e.g., liver mixed function oxidase induction (Goksøyr and Förlin, 1992). However, aquatic and terrestrial organisms may differ in the relative magnitude of these responses. DNA-repair enzyme activity may be lower in fish than in mammals (Wirgin and Walden, 1998). Additionally, some toxicant-responsive genes in terrestrial vertebrates may not have homologs in aquatic organisms, possibly leading to species-specific differences of toxic effect or induction of these genes (Hahn et al., 1992). There are also differences between aquatic and terrestrial biomarkers in relation to the attention given to various endpoints. For example, studies that examine acetylcholinesterase inhibition mainly focus on terrestrial organisms, whereas studies examining DNA damage (Shugart and Theodorakis, 1994) and metallothionein induction (Roesijadi, 1992) are more heavily represented in aquatic studies. Another class of protein that can be induced by contaminant exposure are the stress or "heat-shock" proteins (Sanders, 1993), which participate in the renaturation of damaged proteins. Although they are highly conserved in all organisms from bacteria to mammals and are a major focus of study in the biomedical field, in the field of ecotoxicology, studies on the induction of stress proteins focus almost exclusively on aquatic organisms. Aquatic toxicology studies also differ from those in terrestrial toxicology because aquatic organisms respire through gills. Gills may be constantly exposed to water-borne contaminants and are highly permeable to dissolved substances. As a result, gills may accumulate certain contaminants (Robinson and Avenant-Oldewage, 1997) or their structure and function may be impaired (Karan et al., 1998; Li et al., 1998). Conversely, terrestrial organisms will realize most of their exposure through ingestion of contaminated media.

Population and Community Effects

One of the major objectives of ecotoxicology is the detection and prevention of pollutant effects on population structure and function. These effects may be determined by collection of empiric data or simulated with the use of population models (Albers et al., 2000). In the former case, natural populations are sampled in order to determine the effects of environmental contamination on density, abundance, or biomass of indigenous organisms (Rask, 1992; Welsh and Ollivier, 1998). These values from contaminated populations are then compared with those from reference populations (with no history of contamination) in order to determine pollution effects. Such effects may also be manifest as changes in age structure or sex ratios, which may affect the reproductive potential of the population (DeAngelis et al., 1990). The age structure of populations (relative number of individuals of each age class) may give an indication of pollutant effects, such as reproductive failure or perturbations in recruitment of juveniles into the population (Vuori and Parkko, 1994; Hesthagen et al., 1996). The pattern of population response to pollution may also provide information as to the mechanism of population effect, such as changes in adult mortality, juvenile recruitment, food availability, etc. (Gibbons and Munkittrick, 1994).

Alternatively, effects of pollutants on populations can be predicted or simulated using mathematical models. These models use empiric data such as abundance, age distribution, and age-specific mortality and fecundity in order to predict effects of pollutant exposure on abundance of individuals and rate of population change (growth or decline). The empiric data are gathered from organisms grown in laboratory cultures or from natural populations, and population parameters are calculated using linear or matrix algebra (DeAngelis et al., 1990). Models also exist that use toxicity test data derived from laboratory exposures in combination with population parameters in order to predict effects of pollutants on populations (Barnthouse et al., 1990). Other models use physiologic and behavioral parameters of individuals in order to predict such effects (DeAngelis et al., 1990).

Any effects on populations may ultimately be manifest as effects on communities because, by definition, communities are collections of interacting populations. Environmental contaminants can affect the structure of communities as well as the interactions of species within them. For example, it is well known that exposure to chemicals may cause a reduction of community diversity (relative number of species) and changes in community composition (e.g., LaPoint et al., 1984; Hartwell et al., 1997; Beltman et al., 1999). In addition, the trophic structure of fish and invertebrate communities may also be affected by exposure to anthropogenic chemicals (Camargo, 1992; Paller et al., 1996).

The trophic structure of communities is related to the relative abundance of species that feed on various food items (piscivores, omnivores, detritivores, insectivores, etc.) or have various foraging methods (shredders, scrapers, etc.). These changes in species/trophic composition may come about by direct or indirect mechanisms. The direct effects involve loss of some species due to an increase in pollution-induced mortality or reduced reproductive output. In this case the communities will be dominated by species that are less affected by pollutant exposure. This is the basis of a phenomenon termed *pollution-induced community tolerance,* or PICT (Blanck and Wangberg, 1988), in which algal communities become more pollution-tolerant over time due to the replacement of pollution-sensitive species with more tolerant ones. Some evidence of this phenomenon has also been observed in terrestrial systems where shifts in the composition of rodent communities appears to indicate contaminant-induced reductions of select species in the community in favor of resistant or resilient species (Allen and Otis, 1998).

Alternatively, community structure may change through indirect mechanisms. For example, a species may be absent from a community because the organisms upon which it feeds are exterminated by pollutant exposure. Indirect effects may also be affected by changes in dynamic interactions between species—for example, predator/prey interactions. Analogously, if competing species differ in relative sensitivity to a pollutant, environmental contamination may give one species a competitive edge over the other, resulting in local extinction of the less tolerant species. Finally, it has been suggested that such changes in community structure come about because some species are more genetically adaptable than others and so are better able to adapt to novel stressors such as pollution (Luoma, 1977). Thus, the more sensitive species would not be able to adapt to this stressor and become locally extinct. These types of perturbations in community structure and dynamics may ultimately compromise the stability, sustainability, and productivity of affected ecosystems.

Chemical Interactions and Natural Stressors

As more information becomes available on chemical effects in aquatic and terrestrial organisms, there is increasing interest in understanding the interactive effects of exposure to multiple contaminants as well as the interactions between contaminants and inherent stressors (e.g., nutritional stress, disease, predation, climate, water quality). This area of ecotoxicology is one of the least understood because of the a priori need to understand the more direct exposure and effects scenarios. Nevertheless, it represents an expanding part of ecotoxicology and is generating interest in the research community.

Perhaps the greatest inherent stressors faced by many species of wildlife are nutritional restriction and seasonal shifts in climatic extremes. Daily food restriction of as little as 10 percent below normal intake has been shown to enhance the overall decline in courtship behavior, egg laying and hatching, and number of young fledged by ringed turtle doves (*Streptopelia risoria*) exposed to DDE (Keith and Mitchell, 1993). Antagonistic relationships also exist. Methionine supplementation effectively negated the detrimental effects of selenium toxicity on mortality in mallard ducklings (Hoffman et al., 1992). Similarly, relative magnitude of biomarker responses and tissue distribution of contaminants in fish may be influenced by nutritional status and food deprivation (Joergensen et al., 1999). Effects have also been found for the interaction between temperature and chemical exposure. Cold stress has been shown to augment the effects of pesticide exposure, resulting in increased mortality of several wildlife species (Fleming et al., 1985; Rattner and Franson, 1984; Montz and Kirkpatrick, 1985). However, more subtle interactive effects on energy acquisition and allocation were less conclusive in deer mice exposed to aldicarb—2-methyl-2-(methylthio)propanal *O*-[(methylamino)carbonyl] oxime—and cold stress (French and Porter, 1994). Unlike many wildlife species, fish and aquatic invertebrates are poikilotherms, so their metabolic rate is more dependent on ambient temperature than that of birds or mammals. As a result, toxicity, accumulation, and metabolism of aquatic contaminants may be influenced by water temperature (Odin et al., 1994; Sleiderink et al., 1995; van Wezel and Jonker, 1998). Other environmental variables, such as salinity and pH, may also affect uptake and toxicity of aqueous chemicals (Norrgren et al., 1991; Hall and Anderson, 1995). Conversely, exposure to pollutants may affect an organism's ability to tolerate natural environmental variables such as water oxygen concentrations (Bennett et al., 1995). Other areas of interest include interactions between chemical exposure and social stress (Brown et al., 1986) and interactions between different chemicals (Stanley et al., 1994).

Trophic-Level Transfer of Contaminants

Although contaminant exposure may occur through inhalation, dermal contact, or ingestion from preening or grooming behavior, significant exposure also occurs through food-chain transport. Depending on specific chemical properties, contaminants may accumulate in either soft or hard tissues of prey species. Species not normally in direct contact with contaminated media may become exposed through ingestion of contaminated prey, promoting accumulation or magnification of contaminants into higher trophic levels. Earthworms in soils contaminated with organochlorines and heavy metals can accumulate quantities of contaminants known to be deleterious to sensitive species (Beyer and Gish, 1980; Beyer and Cromartie, 1987). The use of pesticides to control plant pests often coincides with the reproductive periods of many wildlife species, enhancing exposure potential in juveniles that often rely on invertebrates as a primary food source (Korschgen, 1970).

The foraging habits of individual species dictate the potential for contaminant exposure through food-chain transport. In a field study in Canada, Daury and coworkers (1993) found a higher percentage of ring-necked ducks (*Aythya collaris*) with elevated blood lead concentrations compared to American black ducks (*Anas rubripes*). The difference was attributed primarily to foraging habits, as ring-neck ducks are divers and may consume up to 30 percent invertebrates in their diet, compared with American black ducks, which forage on the surface of the water. Even when contaminated prey is ingested, exposure may be minimal in certain species. Adult American kestrels (*Falco sparverious*) fed pine voles (*Microtus pinetorum*) with mean body burdens of 48 μg/g DDE, 1.2 μ/g dieldrin, and 38 μg/g lead accumulated approximately 1 μg/g lead in bone and liver tissue but 232 μg/g DDE and 5.9 μg/g dieldrin in carcasses after 60 days. Mean lead concentration in regurgitated pellets from kestrels was 130 μg/g, demonstrating their lack of lead accumulation from contaminated prey (Stendell et al., 1989). Secondary poisoning from food-chain transfer has also been implicated in the mortality of endangered species. Lead poisoning was apparently responsible for the deaths of several California condors (*Gymnogyps californianus*) found in California. The probable source of the lead was considered to be bullet fragments consumed by condors feeding on hunter-killed deer (Wiemeyer et al., 1988).

The potential exposure of predatory species may be enhanced by the altered behavior of contaminant-exposed prey. Affected prey may be easier to catch, leading predators to concentrate their foraging efforts on contaminated sites and thus increasing their direct exposure and the transfer of contaminants through trophic levels (Bracher and Bider, 1982; Mendelssohn, 1977). As contaminants move through food chains, they may be translocated from their source. Migrating individuals may transport contaminants considerable distances, resulting in potential exposure and effects in organisms that otherwise would not be in contact with contaminated sites (Braestrup et al., 1974).

Genotoxicity

Ecogenotoxicology is a relatively young field that has benefited tremendously from the growth of molecular biology and molecular genetics. It is concerned with the effects of pollutants or chemicals (mutagens, clastogens, aneuogens, and teratogens) on the genetic material of organisms. Such genetic material is usually defined as DNA, RNA, and chromosomes but may also include modifications of proteins. Such effects may be manifest as DNA strand breaks, base modifications, chromosomal rearrangements or fragmentation, and aneuploidy (Shugart and Theodorakis, 1994). While it is possible to damage the genetic material of an organism without any subsequent effect on that individual, it is also possible that mutations in the DNA can result in somatic effects such as cancers. If these effects occur in germinal tissues, this can also result in heritable effects and an increase in the genetic load (i.e., relative frequency of deleterious mutations in the population). Other types of multigenerational effects may not occur by direct interaction of contaminants with the DNA molecule but by selection pressure from chemical contaminants. Because this can change the evolutionary nature of a species, Bickham and Smolen (1994) coined the phrase *evolutionary toxicology* to describe this phenomenon. They proposed that selection resulting from the stress of somatic effects of contaminants could lead to population genetic changes that are not predictable from a knowledge of the mechanisms of toxicology of the contaminants. Also, individuals that have the pollutant-resistant genotypes may be more susceptible to natural stressors (Weis et al., 1982). Furthermore, because changes in the genetic makeup of the population involve alterations in survival and recruitment, such changes may be indicators of adverse chronic effects on population structure and dynamics. Selection for pollutant-resistant genotypes, as well as genetic bottlenecks—a result of reductions in population size or recruitment—may reduce genetic variability in affected populations (Guttman, 1994; Theodorakis and Shugart, 1998). These effects may be indicators of community-level effects, because it has been found that patterns of genetic diversity and community-level pollution effects are correlated in contaminated streams (Krane et al., 1999). These were termed *emergent* effects.

Besides selection and genetic bottlenecks, an elevated mutation rate may also alter population genetic structure. The search for methods to detect mutations easily among millions of base pairs is one of the primary needs of genotoxicology. The mitochondrial DNA has the least effective repair mechanism and should be among the fragments of DNA that permit detection of an elevated mutation rate. However, it is often difficult to detect an increase in the mutation rate because baseline mutation rates are so low that even highly contaminated environments may fail to induce significant changes (reviewed in Cotton, 1997). For example, studies of Chernobyl mice experiencing doses in excess of 15 rads per day (Chesser et al., 2000) failed to detect statistically significant elevation of mutation rates (Baker et al., 1999). In addition, minisatellite and microsatellite mutation frequencies are among the highest documented for the nuclear genome, and this phenomenon appears to have potential in genotoxicology. Makova et al., (1998), however, failed to find an elevated mutation rate in mice at Chernobyl. Dubrova et al. (1996) reported an elevated mutation rate in minisatellite loci in children born to survivors of the Chernobyl disaster.

It is appealing to use native species living in a highly polluted environment to determine multigenerational effects on the genome (McBee and Bickham, 1990). The basic assumption is that living in a polluted environment will result in reduced fitness and deterioration of health of the sentinel species. With an adequate array of biomarkers such as alterations in the DNA (Shugart et al., 1994), mini- and microsatellites (Dubrova et al., 1996; Bickham et al., 1998), micronuclei frequency (Heddle et al., 1991, MacGregor et al., 1995; Rodgers and Baker, 2000), flow-cytometry values (Bickham et al., 1992), enzymatic assays (Jensen et al., 1997; Langlois et al., 1993), and population genetic characteristics (Matson et al., 2000), it should be possible to estimate risk and genotoxicologic damage.

However, the issue is not simple because life is resilient and often highly polluted environments are modified and devoid of other human activities. Some areas with extremely high levels of radioactivity, like Chernobyl, may support population densities and levels of biodiversity reminiscent of conservation parks, suggesting that human activities can be more detrimental to natural ecosystems than the world's worst nuclear power plant disaster. The problem of using native species as sentinel species may be further complicated by adaptation of the local populations to the polluting chemicals (Theodorakis et al., 1998). Undoubtedly, studies that resolve reduced fitness and health issues of wildlife will require excellent experimental design using control populations and multigenerational data.

Terrestrial Ecotoxicology

Terrestrial toxicology is the science of the exposure to and effects of toxic compounds in terrestrial ecosystems. Investigations in terrestrial toxicology are often complex endeavors because of a number of intrinsic and extrinsic factors associated with terrestrial systems. All organisms function at several levels, from the individual level to the level of the ecosystem, interacting with others within the constraints of social ranking, food webs, and niches. Many terrestrial species are very mobile, covering significant areas while defending territories, foraging, migrating, and dispersing. Terrestrial toxicology includes all aspects of the terrestrial system while attempting to elucidate the effects on the biota following contaminant exposure. Exploring exposures to and the effects of environmental contaminants in terrestrial systems is a recent endeavor relative to work that has been conducted historically in aquatic systems. Like aquatic toxicology, however, terrestrial toxicology relies heavily on interdisciplinary scientific exploration.

The early 1900s witnessed the relization that chemicals used in the environment could affect nontarget organisms. Studies were conducted on the exposures to and effects of arsenicals, pyrethrums, mercurials, and others on terrestrial organisms (Reviewed in Peterle, 1991). In later years, synthetic pesticides became increasingly important in controlling pest species in agricultural crops, although little was known about their effects on nontarget organisms. As pesticide development and use continued, however, reports of wildlife mortalities and declining avian populations spawned concern among biologists internationally. Studies were conducted that documented residues of DDT and DDT metabolites, other chlorinated hydrocarbon insecticides, and industrial chemicals, including PCBs, in the tissues of wildlife species. Although reduced nesting success was apparent in some avian species (e.g., osprey, bald eagles, Bermuda petrels, herring gulls, and brown pelicans) (Ames, 1966; Peterle, 1991; Wurster and Wingate, 1968; Keith, 1966; Schreiber and DeLong, 1969), the underlying mechanism was not completely understood until later.

The study of the toxic effects of chemicals on terrestrial organisms witnessed its most dramatic growth in the 1980s (Kendall and Akerman, 1992). Requirements for detailed and accurate information on the effects of pesticides on terrestrial wildlife species played a large part in the development of terrestrial toxicology methodologies. Persistent pesticides such as DDT and mirex [1,1a,2,2,3,3a,4,5,5,5a,5b,6-dodecachlorooctahydro-1,3,4-methano-1*H*-cyclobuta(cd)pentalene] were shown to accumulate in wildlife species. Development of new insecticides, such as organophosphates, lessened the problem of persistence, although toxicity was still a concern. An obvious need existed by which scientifically sound investigations could be conducted to explore the direct and indirect effects of chemicals on terrestrial wildlife populations.

Chemical effects on avian populations were the primary focus for many years. This problem became more apparent as the link was established between DDT contamination and declining bird populations. The classic case of eggshell thinning in raptor eggs was established by Ratcliffe (1967) in studies on declining sparrow hawk (*Accipiter nisus*) and peregrine falcon (*Falco peregrinus*) populations in the United Kingdom. Other studies soon followed and it became apparent that many avian species suffered reduced productivity resulting from eggshell thinning and decreased hatching success. Studies continue to be conducted on the exposure and effects of these persistent pesticides in wildlife species (Bergman et al., 1994; Custer and Custer, 1995; Auman et al., 1997; Allen and Otis, 1998; Elliott and Norstrom, 1998, Creekmore et al., 1999).

Acute and Chronic Toxicity Testing Terrestrial organisms are typically exposed to contaminants through ingestion of some contaminated media, although inhalation and dermal absorption of contaminants do occur. Thus, toxicity tests for terrestrial species are usually designed to test the effects of a chemical dose, administered by oral gavage or injection. Exposure can also be accomplished through consumption of contaminated food or water, resulting in dosages calculated from consumption rates or simply exposure over time to a given concentration of contaminant in the diet. Methods for measuring endpoints in toxicity tests include the LD_{50} and LC_{50}, the ED_{50} and EC_{50}, and reproductive tests (fertility, egg hatchability, neonate survival). These endpoints can be used to assess toxicity in a variety of terrestrial animals, including earthworms (*Eisenia foetida*), honeybees (*Apis mellifera*), northern bobwhite, mallards, mink, and European ferrets (*Mustela purofius furo*) (Menzer et al., 1994). Likewise, specialized tests for determining toxicity in plants are used to assess lethal and nonlethal response to contaminants. Standardized tests for toxicity in plants include germination assays for lettuce seeds (*Latuca sativa*), root elongation in seedlings, and analysis of whole plants such as soybean (*Glycine max*) and barley (*Hordeum vulgare*) (Wang, 1985; Greene et al., 1989; Pfleeger et al., 1991; Ratsch, 1983). Other plant and animal species, including domestic and wild types, can be used in standardized testing systems as dictated by specific site requirements (Lower and Kendall, 1990).

Standardized laboratory toxicity tests performed under U.S. EPA guidelines include acute oral LD_{50}s and dietary LC_{50}s on northern bobwhite quail and mallard ducks. Also, mammalian toxicity tests include acute oral LD_{50}s on rats using estimated environmental concentrations of the chemical in question. Avian and mammalian reproductive toxicity testing may be required under certain circumstances, depending on such factors as food tolerance, indications of repeated or continued exposure, the persistence of chemicals in the environment, and chemical storage or accumulation in plant or animal tissues (U.S. EPA, 1982).

Field Testing Field studies are designed to address exposure to contaminants and resulting effects to organisms outside the highly controlled environment of the laboratory. Field studies may be designed specifically to address concerns suggested by laboratory studies or to test modeled or predicted exposure and effects based on site contaminant levels. As the effects of environmental contaminants on wild populations of animals have become more apparent, the need for more useful field testing methodologies has led to improved assessment strategies. Whether the U.S. EPA requires field testing depends both on laboratory testing results, professional judgment, or the degree of consensus on anticipated exposure and effects. Chemical properties of the compound, intended use patterns (e.g., pesticides), difference between the estimated environmental concentration (EEC) and the lowest observed effect level (LOEL), and dose-response relationships are considered in combination when exploring the need for conducting field studies.

Field studies are conducted in complex ecologic systems where plants and animals are affected by numerous natural stressors (e.g., nutrient restriction, disease, predation) that might possibly confound the measurement of contaminant exposure and effects. In addition, life history characteristics vary dramatically among species. Issues of habitat use, home range size, foraging characteristics, and other factors must be considered in designing a field study. Field study design must be robust to noncontaminant influences, and some important considerations include censusing techniques, sampling units, site replication, scale ecologic similarity among sites, and choice of study organisms. Results from several studies indicate the potential complexity involved with censusing animals exposed to contaminants, as alterations in behavior and observation difficulties may bias results (Grue and Shipley, 1981; Fryday et al., 1996; Hawkes et al., 1996; Madrigal et al., 1996).

Traditional methods used by biologists and wildlife ecologists have been used successfully in terrestrial ecotoxicology field studies, and resources are available that describe the various techniques for trapping, remote sensing, and sampling terrestrial biota (Bookhout, 1994; Menzer et al., 1994). Ligature techniques used for birds have improved the process of collecting food from nestlings raised on contaminated sites, allowing researchers to better determine the composition of the diet and to ascertain the contaminant loads in foodstuffs (Mellott and Woods, 1993). The published results of field studies have provided information on the impacts of contaminants on wildlife abundance and survival (Rowley et al., 1983), acute mortality (Babcock and Flickinger, 1977; Kendall et al., 1992), food-chain relationships (Korschgen, 1970), reproduction (Clark and Lamont, 1976; Hooper et al., 1990), and behavior (Grue et al., 1982). Basic laboratory techniques are often integrated with field methods to determine the ecologic significance and mechanisms of exposure and effects on populations (Hooper et al., 1990).

Techniques for the assessment of wildlife exposure and its effects must incorporate sufficient flexibility to allow their use on sites with a wide variety of physical and chemical characteristics (Fite et al., 1988; Warren-Hicks et al., 1989). To accomplish this goal, three approaches to wildlife assessments are generally used to provide the required breadth. These are the use of (1) endemic species occurring naturally on contaminated sites, (2) enhanced species attracted to the site by creating more favorable breeding habitat, and (3) enclosed species derived from clean laboratory-bred populations (Hooper and La Point, 1994).

Field studies are often designed to study populations of organisms living on contaminated sites, which are then compared with other populations living on noncontaminated reference sites. The primary benefit in these studies is the use of endemic species that receive lifelong exposures to site contaminants of concern. Detracting from the utility of these studies is the lack of control over such factors as exposure history or genetic background of individuals. Although some control is available over other factors such as the test species and habitat type, study design is still subject to the local conditions dictated by the contaminated site. Further, the small sizes of some sites can preclude effective use of some native wildlife species that roam over large areas.

Enhanced species studies generally include assessing the reproductive effects of contaminant exposure on species that inhabit nest boxes, such as the European starling (*Sturnus vulgaris*), which provides a model for assessing other cavity-nesting passerines with similar life history traits (Kendall et al., 1989). Cavity-nesting birds readily occupy artificial nest cavities and will often colonize study sites when provided with nest boxes. Increased numbers of adults and nestlings are thus available, from which information on reproductive success, behavioral response, exposure routes, and physiologic and biochemical perturbations can be obtained during the breeding season. Numerous studies have taken advantage of these traits in other avian species, including eastern bluebirds (*Sialia sialis*), American kestrels, and—more recently—tree swallows (*Tachycineta bicolor*). Tree swallows have been used extensively to assess exposure and effects from a number of contaminants (Shaw, 1984; DeWeese et al., 1985; Custer et al., 1998; Bishop et al., 1999, McCarty and Secord, 1999).

Use of enclosures has greatly enhanced control over many of the environmental factors that can complicate field studies. Enclosure studies incorporate a variety of outdoor, open-air facilities to enclose test organisms during toxicologic testing. The purpose of using enclosures is to simulate natural field conditions while maintaining a level of control over experimental conditions (e.g., exposure period, nutritional condition, test organism, sex ratios, age, genetic similarity, habitat type). In essence, enclosure-based experiments can be used to bridge the gap between laboratory and field investigations. Study organisms are more readily accessible when housed in enclosures, making it easier to take multiple samples from individuals, administer treatments to them, and monitor their behavior and reproduction. The flexibility afforded under these conditions makes it possible to explore a number of questions regarding the potential interactions between the contaminant and natural stressors in the environment. Enclosure studies may be required by the U.S. EPA under the Federal Insecticide, Fungicide and Rodenticide Act (FIFRA) guidelines for pesticide registration if they can potentially yield useful information about pesticide impacts on wildlife.

Enclosure studies have been used successfully with aquatic and terrestrial species to explore the effects of pesticides and chemical contaminants on abundance, reproduction, immune function, and biochemical response (Barrett, 1968; Pomeroy and Barrett, 1975; Barrett, 1988; Dickerson et al., 1994; Gebauer and Weseloh, 1993; Weseloh et al., 1994; Hooper and La Point, 1994; Edge et al., 1996; Caslin and Wolff, 1999). Basic approaches to using enclosures to study the impacts of chemicals on terrestrial organisms vary widely. There is considerable variation in enclosure size; they range from less than 1 m^2 to more than a hectare. Small stainless steel enclosures, approximately 0.5 by 1.5 in, have been used to house laboratory-raised deer mice (*Peromyscus maniculatus*) for the assessment of contaminant uptake and biomarker response in mice on sites contaminated with polynuclear aromatic hydrocarbons (Dickerson et al., 1994). Larger enclosures can be used to monitor population-level responses and community interactions. Barrett (1988) and Pomeroy and Barrett (1975) used large enclosures to assess population and community responses of several rodent species to controlled applications of Sevin (1-naphthyl-*N*-methylcarbamate) insecticide. Studies incorporating pinioned ducks on contaminated waste ponds provide an equivalent method for avian species (Gebauer and Weseloh, 1993; Weseloh, 1994).

Although large enclosures offer the advantage of addressing population- and community-level issues of toxicant effects, they can be restrictive in cost and space. Smaller enclosures are affordable and can be beneficial for site-specific evaluations. They can be easily moved among locations, making them an excellent strategy for short-term testing and determining the efficacy of site remediation. However, the design of enclosures depends on the goals of the study.

Aquatic Ecotoxicology

Aquatic toxicology is the study of effects of anthropogenic chemicals on organisms in the aquatic environment. The aquatic ecosystem is of particular concern because this is where most contaminants released into the environment are eventually deposited, either from direct discharge into bodies of water or from terrestrial runoff and atmospheric deposition (Pritchard, 1993). Furthermore, there are certain features of the aquatic environment that make it unique. First, certain chemicals are not volatile in air but are soluble in water (e.g., metals), so aquatic organisms may be exposed to chemicals via routes that are not present in their terrestrial counterparts. Also, many contaminants are readily degraded in an aerobic environment, but the aquatic environment frequently contains little or no oxygen. Therefore, some contaminants can persist in aquatic ecosystems far longer than in terrestrial systems (Ashok and Saxena, 1995). Finally, aquatic organisms are frequently restricted in their habitat and home range, so they often cannot avoid contaminated areas. These attributes of aquatic systems present unique circumstances and problems that are not applicable to terrestrial systems.

The physiology and anatomy of aquatic organisms can also present problems that are different from those faced in the study of terrestrial organisms. For example, aquatic organisms have highly permeable skin and gills and so are particularly susceptible to the effects of ambient contamination (Pritchard, 1993). Furthermore, aquatic communities are dominated by ectothermic organisms (e.g., invertebrates, fish, amphibians, and, to a lesser extent, aquatic reptiles), whose metabolic rate is determined by ambient water temperature. Thus, the accumulation of contaminants and their toxic effects are influenced by water temperature, which can vary both spatially and temporally. Finally, fish and amphibians are unique among the vertebrates in that they have a highly permeable anamniotic egg (an egg without a shell or amniotic membrane), and the embroyo develops while the egg is completely immersed in water. They are also unique in that they are the only vertebrates that have an aquatic larval life stage that undergoes metamorphosis. For these reasons, the embryo/larval stages are often very sensitive to chemical insult and may be vulnerable to effects experienced by terrestrial vertebrates.

Acute and Chronic Toxicity Testing In aquatic toxicity tests, fish, invertebrates, or algae are exposed to aqueous chemicals in the laboratory. Designs for these tests include static (in which the test water is not renewed for the duration of the test), static renewal (test water is renewed periodically), and flow-through systems (test water is renewed continually). The organisms may be exposed for short (acute toxicity tests) or long periods (chronic toxicity tests). Static designs are usually restricted to acute toxicity tests, and chronic tests frequently have a flow-through design. Acute and chronic tests not only differ in duration but also in the endpoints that are measured. In acute tests, survival is often the only endpoint (ASTM, 1992a). However, in chronic tests, effects on growth and reproduction are also determined. To accomplish this, the duration of the chronic test is designed to span the entire life cycle of the organism (i.e., from zygote to age of first reproduction; U.S. EPA, 1989). However, chronic tests are often difficult to perform because of their long duration (9 to 30 months for fish tests) and are very expensive, which makes their routine use prohibitive. Hence, three alternatives to full life-cycle tests have been developed: partial life-cycle tests, early-life-stage tests, and short-term chronic tests. Partial life-cycle tests are used for fish that require >12 months to reach reproductive maturity. They begin with immature fish prior to gonadal maturation and end after the first reproduction in order to determine the effects of aquatic contaminants on reproductive potential of the fish. Early-life-stage tests determine toxicity in fish exposed from the embryonic through juvenile stages and are typically 1 to 2 months in duration (ASTM, 1992b). The rationale is that the embryo and larvae of fish are thought to be the life-cycle stage that is most sensitive to toxic effects (McKim et al., 1978). Short-term chronic assays are static-renewal tests developed by the EPA that commonly use fathead minnows (*Pimephales promelas*), *Daphnia magna,* or *Ceriodaphnia dubia* (small planktonic crustaceans) and a green algae (*Selenastrum capricornutum*) as test organisms (Birge et al., 1985; U.S. EPA, 1989). These assays examine growth (fathead minnow and algae), survival (minnow and *C. dubia*), and reproduction (*C. dubia*) after a 4- to 7-day exposure. The fathead minnow tests are basically truncated versions of the early-life-stage tests. However, *C. dubia* reach sexual maturity and begin to reproduce within a week of hatching, so the 7-day test for this species essentially encompasses the full life cycle.

Unlike tests on terrestrial organisms, where subjects are dosed with test chemicals via oral or inhalation routes, in aquatic toxicity tests the subjects are immersed in a solution of the contaminant. Therefore, the endpoints of aquatic toxicity tests are not recorded as LD_{50} or ED_{50} but as LC_{50} or EC_{50} (lethal and effective concentration). Results of the chronic tests are sometimes expressed as the maximum allowable toxicant concentration (MATC). This is a range of toxicant concentrations bounded by the *lowest observed effect concentration* (LOEC) at the upper end and the *no observable effect concentration* (NOEC) at the lower end. The LOEC and NOEC are determined by statistical analysis and are defined as the lowest toxicant concentration that elicits an effect that is statistically significantly different from the control and the highest concentration for which the effect is not significantly different from control, respectively (Mount and Stephan, 1967).

Toxicity tests have been used to measure toxic effects of individual chemicals or contaminated water collected from the field. Single-chemical tests are typically used for the purposes of chemical registry, while testing of contaminated water is commonly used for environmental monitoring purposes and to verify compliance with permitting requirements. In the latter case, water can be collected from the source of wastewater discharge ("effluent") or from the body of water receiving the effluent ("receiving water"). In these tests, the water to be tested is collected on site and test organisms are exposed to various concentrations diluted with clean water (ASTM, 1992c). Toxicity tests of undiluted effluent (referred to as *whole-effluent tests* or WETs; U.S. EPA, 1991a) are mandated by the Clean Water Act as part of the requirements for a permit to release effluents—a National Pollutant Discharge and Elimination System (NPDES) permit. Effluents are complex mixtures of multiple chemicals, some of which may contribute to the toxicity and some may not. Identification of toxic components of effluents may be facilitated by a process known as toxicity identification evaluation (TIE; U.S. EPA, 1993). In this process, different samples of the effluent are treated to remove various constituent chemicals (e.g., chelation to remove metals, extraction to remove organic contaminants) and each sample is tested. Reduction of the toxicity in any treated sample indicates that particular constituent has contributed to the toxicity of the whole effluent. TIEs are then followed by a Toxicity Reduction Evaluation (TRE). In this procedure, the source of the toxic constituents in the effluent may be identified and possible methods to remove these toxic components from the effluent or reduce their toxicity are evaluated. This is followed by implementation of methods to control output of the toxic constituents or treat the effluent to reduce its toxicity. Follow-up toxicity testing is used to assess the efficacy of these remedial actions (U.S. EPA, 1991b).

Another type of test used for monitoring purposes is sediment toxicity testing. In this case, sediment is collected from the bottoms of lakes, rivers, bays, etc., and brought into the laboratory. Benthic invertebrates—commonly oligochaet worms, chironomid (midge fly) larvae, amphipod crustaceans, or mollusks—are then subjected to chronic or acute exposures and endpoints such as survival, growth, reproduction, and burrowing or other behaviors are recorded (ASTM, 1995). Important applications of sediment tests include determination of toxicity of sediments that are dredged from one location (e.g., in clearing shipping channels) and need to be disposed of at another location, environmental risk assessments of contaminated areas, and as a part of biomonitoring programs for the purpose of compliance to environmental regulations.

Sublethal Effects In the aquatic environment, concentrations of contaminants in the water or sediment may not be high enough to elicit mortality but may still induce sublethal effects on the health of aquatic organisms. One method by which these health effects can be determined is via histologic evidence of tissue damage or dysfunction (Teh et al., 1997). This type of damage can lead to diseases such as tumors or infectious and parasitic infestations. Tumor prevalence is commonly reported in bottom-dwelling fish and bivalve mollusks from contaminated areas (Van Beneden et al., 1993; Baumann, 1998; Wirgin and Waldman, 1998). Tumors are generally reported more often in feral populations of aquatic than terrestrial organisms. This is perhaps due to the less efficient DNA repair capacity of aquatic organisms (Wirgin and Waldman, 1998). Tumors are commonly reported in organisms that live within or in close proximity to the sediment, which is often highly contaminated with carcinogenic materials such as PAHs. Unlike cancers, infectious and parasitic diseases are not directly induced by contaminant exposure, but such exposure may increase the occurrence and severity of these infections. This is possibly due to suppression of leukocyte function (Chu and Hale, 1994; Couillard et al., 1995). The effects may be physically manifest as deterioration of the fins, skin lesions, or a high load of ecto- and endoparasites (Couillard et al., 1995; Landsberg et al., 1998). These detrimental effects on the health of aquatic organisms do not necessarily result in immediate mortality, but the life expectancy and relative reproductive output of the affected organisms may be compromised. If significant numbers of individuals are affected, this could ultimately have effects at the population level.

Field Studies Aquatic field studies can be classified as either manipulative or observational. In manipulative studies, previously unexposed organisms are used, and the experimenter determines the level of contamination to which they are exposed. In contrast, in observational studies, the level of contamination to which the organisms are exposed is not under the control of the experimenter. The objective of these studies may be collection of data for independent research projects or for monitoring organismal health and environmental quality as mandated by a regulatory authority. In the latter case, these studies are referred to as *biomonitoring*.

Aquatic field experiments in which treatments are applied by the experimenter include microcosms and mesocosms. The difference between microcosms and mesocoms is size. Microcosms are composed of large tanks, aquaria, or artificial pools. Mesocosms are artificially constructed ponds, plastic enclosures in lakes or ponds, or artificial streams. The attributes common to both are that they typically (but not always) contain more than one species of test organism, are located outdoors (although microcosms may also be located indoors), and are more complex than simple aquaria. They frequently contain sediment and/or vegetation or other structures and substrates that provide some degree of complexity and realism. The rationale is to produce a test system that contains some of the realism of the natural environment but is not so complex. Endpoints examined may include comparative acute toxicity (Stay and Jarvinen, 1995), biomarker expression (Eggens et al., 1996), or effects on aquatic populations and communities (Juettner et al., 1995; Barry and Logan, 1998). Although they are useful in providing information in some instances, their utility for regulatory purposes is controversial (Shaw and Kennedy, 1996).

Biomonitoring involves sampling aquatic organisms in the natural environment as an indication of the impact of anthropogenic contamination. Such activities may include confining test organisms in cages or sampling indigenous populations at contaminated sites. The relative advantages of using caged versus field-collected aquatic organisms are basically the same as those expounded in the preceding discussion on terrestrial enclosure studies. One endpoint that is particularly well suited to caging studies is acute and chronic toxicity. These endpoints are assessed by exposing caged organisms to contaminated water, sediment, or both and noting mortality and reproductive impairments. These types of tests are termed *ambient toxicity tests* (Stewart, 1996).

Evidence of overt toxicity is more difficult to determine in indigenous populations except during fish kills or other episodes of massive mortality. Consequently, endpoints other than mortality are more commonly documented in biomonitoring studies. One of the endpoints commonly measured is tissue concentrations of contaminants of concern (van der Oost, 1996a). These data are useful in determining whether chemicals present in the water or sediment are in a form that is bioavailable to aquatic organisms, for determining possible health risks to humans that might consume these organisms, or for modeling accumulation and effects in organisms at higher trophic levels. In addition, biomarkers or other sublethal effects may also be incorporated into aquatic biomonitoring programs (van der Oost et al., 1996b). This provides additional information as to whether the accumulated chemicals may be producing detrimental effects, assessing possible effects of complex mixtures and abiotic variables (e.g., water temperature) on toxic response. Additional endpoints used in biomonitoring may include effects on populations or communities (described above) or calculation of indices of water quality. One such index is known as the *Index of Biotic Integrity* (IBI). The variables used to calculate this index include percent pollution-tolerant species, percent of species from various trophic levels (e.g., herbivores, omnivores, top predators) or with various reproductive strategies, and occurrence of individuals with deformities, diseases, or other lesions (Karr, 1987). Each variable is given a numerical score that reflects its relative similarity to the reference sites. The scores are then summed to give a relative overall score for each sampling site. Analogous indices for benthic invertebrates are Hilsenhoff's biotic index and the Ephemeroptera-Plecoptera-Trichoptera (EPT) index, both of which rely on relative abundances of taxa that are thought to be pollution-tolerant and pollution-sensitive (Hoiland and Rabe, 1992).

A related idea in biomonitoring is the concept of indicator species. These can be species that are particularly tolerant or sensitive to environmental contamination such that their presence or absence is indicative of environmental degradation (Lang and Reymond, 1996). In this regard, indicator species may be used as a basis for biotic indices. For example, insects in the orders Ephemeroptera, Plecoptera, and Trichoptera are indicator species used in the EPT index. Alternatively, indicator species may be those in which biomarker responses to specific chemicals are well characterized, or species that are known to accumulate environmental contaminants. One such application is the Mussel Watch program (Wade et al., 1999) enacted by the United States National Oceanic and Atmospheric Administration (NOAA) in 1985. This program monitors contaminant tissue concentrations of coastal mussel populations as an indication of marine contamination. Indicator organisms such as these are useful in the detection of environmental contamination and its changes over time, and as early-warning indicators of possible ecologic effects.

The most efficacious methods of biomonitoring are those methods that integrate multiple endpoints at various levels of biological organization (e.g., chemical concentrations, biomarkers, community composition). For example, the *sediment quality triad* approach (Chapman, 1989) incorporates analysis of sediment chemical concentrations, acute toxicity, and benthic invertebrate community structure to assess the level of sediment contamination. Concordance between all three endpoints is taken as strong evidence that there are contaminants present in the sediment that could have detrimental effects on the aquatic ecosystem. There are analogous studies in fish that integrate endpoints at multiple levels of organization such as water and tissue chemical concentrations, biomarker expression, and population/community level effects (Adams et al., 1992). Integrated approaches such as these are necessary to evaluate environmental contamination in natural settings accurately, because the aquatic environment is too complex to be accurately assessed by one endpoint alone.

GOOD LABORATORY PRACTICES IN TERRESTRIAL AND AQUATIC ECOTOXICOLOGY

Good scientific practices, which result in high-quality data collection and interpretation, are of paramount importance in the field of toxicology. There is a great public demand for personal and environmental requirements under FIFRA and the Toxic Substances Control Act (TSCA), among other environmental legislation. With regulatory agencies increasingly being held accountable for environmental standards, there is a corresponding strong demand for formal and legal assurance that the toxicologic data generated are accurate and that sufficient documentation exists to support the study conclusions. Requirements are designed to ensure that the studies are conducted under high ethical and scientific standards. It is thus critical in today's regulated environment that toxicologic data are produced and reported in a manner that ensures the study is reconstructible and that there are sufficient assurances of the quality and integrity of the data.

The principles and practices of quality assurance and quality control are perhaps best exemplified by the Good Laboratory Practice Guidelines (GLPs). The GLPs are regulation standards that define conditions under which a toxicology study should be planned, conducted, monitored, reported, and archived. They have been adopted by many national and international governments and agencies. The GLPs outline study management procedures and documentation practices that, if followed, will limit the influence of extraneous factors on study results and interpretations. GLPs include provisions for such factors as personnel management and training, facilities support and operation, equipment design, maintenance and calibration, independent quality assurance monitoring, handling of test systems and materials, documentation of study conduct, written standard operation procedures and study protocols, reporting study results, and retention of records and samples.

The U.S. EPA implemented GLP regulations in 1983 under the mandate of FIFRA (40 CFR Part 160) and TSCA (40 CFR Part 792) for pesticide and toxic chemical registration and use. By 1989, these regulations were amended to cover field studies as well as laboratory studies. Today, significant efforts are under way to provide international harmonization of the regulations/standards in the field of ecotoxicology.

MODELING AND GEOGRAPHIC INFORMATION SYSTEMS

Modeling in ecotoxicology allows the prediction of effects of toxic compounds on the environment, which can be characterized by various ecosystems. Terrestrial ecosystems include forests, grasslands, and agricultural areas, whereas aquatic ecosystems include lakes, rivers, and wetlands. Each of these systems is a collection of interconnected components, or subsystems, that functions as a complete entity. Because the dynamics of real systems are quite complex, an understanding of the impacts of toxicants on a system can be enhanced by modeling that system.

The components, or compartments, of a system are represented by state variables that define the system. Once we have defined the system, it is possible to identify stimuli or disturbances from exogenous toxic substances, called *inputs,* from outside the system. These inputs operate on the system to produce a response called the *output*. The adverse effects of many toxic inputs are directly related to their ability to interfere with the normal functioning of both physiologic and environmental systems. For example, emissions of heavy metals from a lead ore-processing complex caused perturbations to the litter-arthropod food chain in a forest ecosystem (Watson, et al., 1976). Elevated concentrations of lead (Pb), zinc (Zn), copper (Cu), and cadmium (Cd) caused reduced arthropod density and microbial activity, resulting in a lowered rate of decomposition and a disturbance of forest nutrient dynamics.

In applying modeling to ecotoxicology, we are interested in studying a "real world" system and the effects of various toxicants on that system. A model is a necessary abstraction of the real system. The level of abstraction, however, is determined by the objectives of the model. Our objective is to stimulate the behavior of a system perturbed by a toxicant. This requires a mechanistic approach to modeling.

The modeling process involves three steps: (1) identification of system components and boundaries, (2) identification of component interactions, and (3) characterization of those interactions using quantitative abstractions of mechanistic processes. Once the model has been defined, it is implemented on a computer. Measurements obtained from the real system are compared with the model projections in a process of model validation. Improvements are then made to the model by changing parameter values or modifying equations in the model. Several iterations of comparing model behavior to that of the real system are usually required to obtain a satisfactory or "valid" model.

Types of Models

Models can be used to obtain qualitative or quantitative information about a complex system. Qualitative models emphasize the relationship between the variables of interest while minimizing the requirement for tremendous accuracy in the parameters of the model. The disadvantage is that there can be no reliance on the numbers produced from such a model. Quantitative ecotoxicologic models can be classified as (1) individual-based versus aggregated models, (2) stochastic versus deterministic models, and (3) spatially distributed versus lumped models. Such models often have hundreds of thousands of lines of code and are used only at the final stages of a system simulation. The results of such simulations are always regarded with suspicion until they are verified by actual data obtained in real systems. The development of such models usually takes place over a number of years as opposed to hours or days for models that are used for qualitative information.

Individual-Based versus Aggregated Models Models that stimulate all individuals simultaneously are referred to as *individual-based models* (e.g., Huston et al., 1988; DeAngelis and Gross, 1992). Each individual in the simulation has a unique set of characteristics: age, size, condition, social status, and location in the landscape as well as its own history of daily foraging, reproduction, and mortality. The individual-based approach has several advantages. It enables the modeler to include complex behavior and decision making by individual organisms in the model. But importantly, it allows one to model populations in complex landscapes, where different individuals may be exposed to very different levels of toxicant concentration (DeAngelis, 1994).

Models of individuals can be extended to a population as a whole by (1) simulating not just one individual but all individuals that make up the population of interest or (2) aggregating various population members into classes, such as age classes. *Aggregated models,* then, follow not individual organisms but variables representing the numbers of individuals per age class. In simulating a complex environmental system, both individual-based and aggregated models will be needed. Usually individual-based models are used to represent vertebrate species while aggregated models are used to represent organisms at lower classification levels.

Stochastic versus Deterministic Models Model coefficients can be functions not only of other variables but also of random variables; thus they can be random variables themselves. In this way of classifying models, those with random (stochastic) variables are called *stochastic models* and those without are called *deterministic models*. Random variables are used to represent the random variation or "unexplained" variation in the state variables. Stochastic models also can include random variables expressed either as random inputs or as parameters with a random error term.

In a stochastic model, random variables representing state variables, model parameters, or both will take on values according to some statistical distribution. In other words, there will be a probability associated with the value of the parameter or state variable.

Monte Carlo is a numerical technique of finding a solution to a stochastic model. For those random features of the model, values are chosen from a probability distribution. Repeated runs of the model then will result in different outcomes. A probability distribution can be calculated for a state variable in the model along with its mean and variance. Suppose the model has random variables for parameters $p_1, p_2, p_3, \ldots p_n$; the state variable will then be a function of the n parameters. A value for each parameter is calculated by sampling from its individual distribution function. A value for the state variable X then is obtained by running a simulation of the model. We repeat the process until we have N values of the state variable X. Finally we determine the mean (μ) and variance (σ^2) for X.

Spatially Distributed versus Lumped Models Lumped models spatially integrate the entire area being modeled (Moore et al., 1993). Parameters for lumped models are averaged over the same spatial area. Spatially distributed models are based upon identifiable geographic units within the area being modeled. These subunits can represent physiographic areas, such as hydrologic or atmospheric basins, which can be identified using a geographic information systems (GIS). A GIS can be used to further identify homogeneous polygons or grid cells based upon soil and terrain features. Model parameters for each subunit can be geographically referenced and stored in the GIS database. The distributed model can then be used to simulate the response to a spatially distributed toxicant by replicating the model for each geographic subunit. Responses to toxicants are likely to be spatially nonlinear. Therefore, a lumped model using mean parameter values will not yield the expected value of the combined results of a distributed model. Modeling in ecotoxicology usually will involve individual-based, stochastic, spatially distributed models.

Modeling Exposure

Exposure of organisms to toxicants requires contact between organisms and the toxicant of concern. Modeling exposure requires a model that will predict the spatial and temporal distributions of the toxicant and a model that will predict the organism's geographic position relative to the toxicant concentration. Transport and fate models are used to predict the spatial distribution of toxicants. Atmospheric transport models (for example, CALPUFF (U.S. EPA, 1995a) and ISC3 (U.S. EPA, 1995b) predict ground-level concentrations of toxicants from stack emissions. Dixon and Murphy (1979) used an atmospheric transport model to predict exposure concentrations as a series of "plume events" at any point on the ground (Fig. 29-2*A*). Exposure can occur from inhalation, immersion, ingestion, or a combination of these. Some vegetation models CERES (Dixon et al., 1978a,b, Luxmoore et al., 1978) and PLANTX (Trapp et al., 1994) can predict uptake of atmospheric and soil concentrations of toxicants. Surface hydrologic models HSPF (Donigian et al., 1983) and GLEAMS (Leonard et al., 1987) predict the runoff of toxicants from the land surface. Lake and stream models obtain input from surface runoff models and predict the change in toxicant concentration within the water body.

Most vertebrates are mobile enough to move from an area of high toxicant concentration to an area of low toxicant concentration (or vice versa). The actual exposure of an animal will depend upon the concentration levels at the geographic locations visited by the animal at the time of the visit. An integrated time- and space-averaged exposure E_i can be calculated using the model (Ott et al., 1986; Henriques and Dixon, 1996):

$$E_i = \sum_{j=1}^{J} c_j t_{ij} \qquad (1)$$

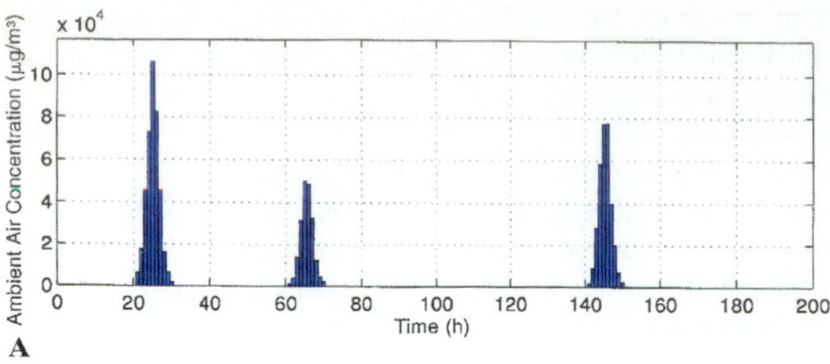

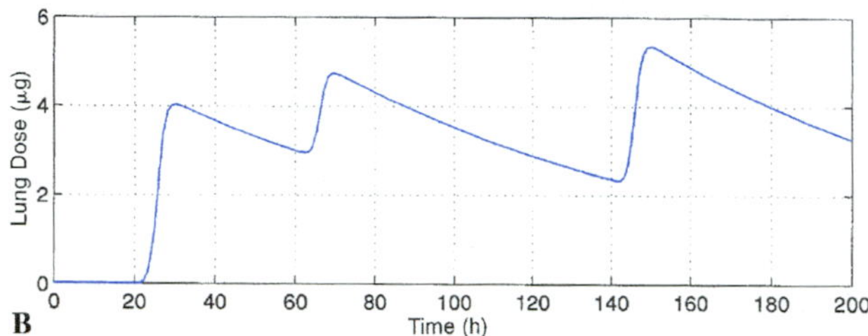

Figure 29-2. **(A).** ***Ambient air concentrations of toxicant predicted by discrete-event gaussian plume model over time. Each pulse represents the ground-level concentration at a given location. The shape of the pulse depends upon wind direction, wind speed, and atmospheric stability.*** **(B).** ***Lung dose of toxicant predicted from the lung model [Eq. (2)] with input from the plume model. The dose increases as plume passes over animal's location. The dose decreases as plume changes direction and concentration in lung decreases by diffusion to the bloodstream.***

where c_j = exposure concentration in microenvironment j
t_{ij} = time spent by animal i in microenvironment j
J = total number of microenvironments occupied by animal i

The prediction of real-time exposure requires linking transport models with behavioral models of animal movement (Sathe, 1997). Models of animal movement can be based upon matching spatial patterns of observed behavior (Siniff and Jessen, 1969), rules based upon mechanisms governing the response of an individual to its environment (Wolff, 1994), or theoretical constructs such as random-walk models (Holgate, 1971; Tyler and Rose, 1994).

Modeling Effects

The effect of a toxicant on an organism depends upon the dose (the concentration reaching the target organ) and the physiologic response to the dose. The dose depends upon the concentration of the chemical at the exposure site and the duration of the exposure. To predict the concentration reaching the target organ, we need to know how much of the chemical is taken up and absorbed by the organism. We also need to know where the chemical is distributed among the organism's tissues and organs, and the rate at which the chemical is excreted from the same tissues and organs.

The dynamics of the disposition of a toxicant in the body of an organism is the subject of toxicokinetics. The dynamics involve the concentration changes over time of a toxicant in various tissues and the rate processes that control the movement from one part of the organism to another. For example, the dynamics of a toxic gas or vapor in the lungs, dC/dt (μg/h), can be simulated with the model:

$$\frac{dC}{dt} = 10^{-6}\, Y \cdot V_T \cdot f - k \cdot C \qquad (2)$$

where Y = exposure concentration (μg/m³)
V_T = tidal volume (milliliters per breath)
f = breathing frequency (breaths per hour)
k = transfer rate from lungs to bloodstream (L/h).

A solution to Eq. (2), with the input from the discrete-event atmospheric exposure model, can be obtained by integrating over a defined time period and initial concentration (Fig. 29-2*B*).

Linking Models to Geographic Information Systems

Geographic information systems (GISs) can be used to map the observed and predicted concentrations of toxic substances as well as the resulting effects of exposure to these concentrations. By linking models with GISs, the ability to explicitly model spatial dynamics of toxicant concentrations is greatly enhanced. There are different levels of integration of models with a GIS. First, a set of utility programs, external to both the model and the GIS, can be used to transfer data between the model and the GIS. Second, routines and macros can be written in the GIS language to run the models and analyze the results. And third, the GIS computer code can be modified to run the models and display the results of the simulations as part of the GIS procedures.

Mapping Exposure and Effects Results from simulation models with spatially referenced output can be mapped as static or dynamic data. Static data are spatially explicit but are expressed as a point (snapshot), an average, or a summed response over time. Dynamic data consider responses of state variables at points in space or a sum of the responses for an area and can be graphed as a function of time, or time series.

In our lung-model example, static exposure can be mapped using the spatial behavior model (Fig. 29-3*A*) and the discrete-event gaussian plume model (Fig. 29-3*B*). The resulting effect (lung dose) also can be mapped spatially (Fig. 29-3*C*). The results from the discrete-event plume model and the lung model can be graphed as a time series (Fig. 29-2*A*,*B*). This response is a result of the animal moving in space and time and the different concentrations of toxicant to which it is exposed at those places and times. A population response can be predicted by repeating the procedure for all the individuals in the exposed population. A spatial map of the steady-state lung concentrations in the population (Fig. 29-4*A*) shows a static response. The population response can also be expressed as a probability distribution (Fig. 29-4*B*) to show the variability in the population that results from the different individual responses.

Displaying both spatial and temporal responses simultaneously is more difficult, although recent developments in the area of computer visualization make this possible. Dynamic shifts in spatial maps of animal behavior (home range) and ambient concentrations can be illustrated in a "movie" sequence of maps. It is also possible to use visualization methods to show "real time" movement of an animal in space and simultaneously display the time-series graph of lung dose. These techniques can enhance our understanding of the effects of toxicants in the environment and provide for more realistic estimates of risk to those toxicants.

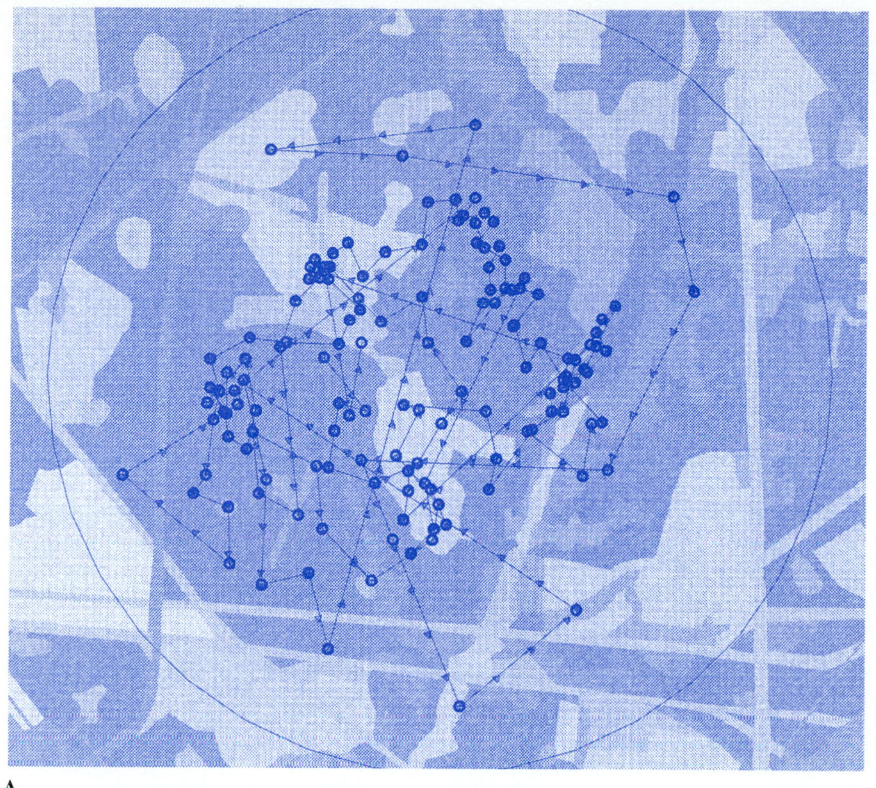

A

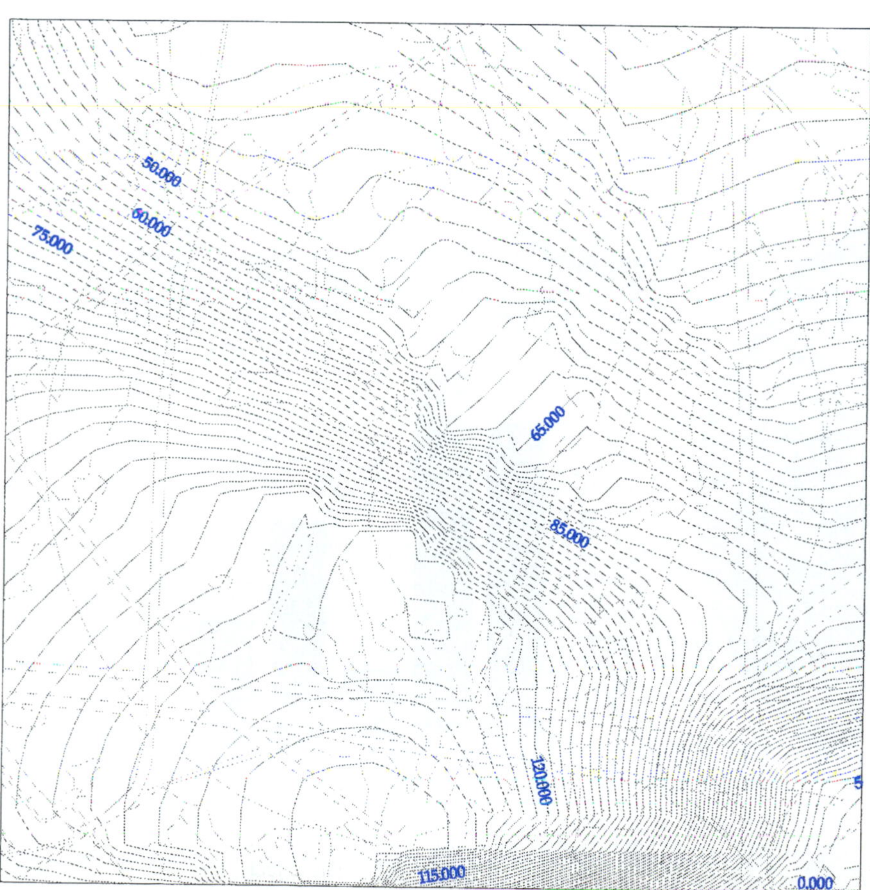

B

***Figure 29-3. Example of an animal's movement predicted by a spatial behavior model* (A). *Example of static ambient ground-level concentrations of a toxicant predicted by Gaussian plume model* (B).**

Isopleths show lines of equal concentration (units are in micrograms per cubic meter.) (From Henriques and Dixon, 1996.) Predicted dose to the lungs from exposure to ambient toxicant concentration as the animal moves according to the pattern in *(A)*. Dose depends upon the exposure concentration *(B)* and the time the animal spends at each location in *(A)*. Isopleths are lines of equal lung dose in units of μg *(C)*. Predicted dose to the lungs from exposure to ambient toxicant concentration as the animal moves according to the pattern in *(A)* depends upon the exposure concentration *(B)* and the time the animal spends at each location in *(A)*. Isopleths are lines of equal lung dose in units of micrograms.

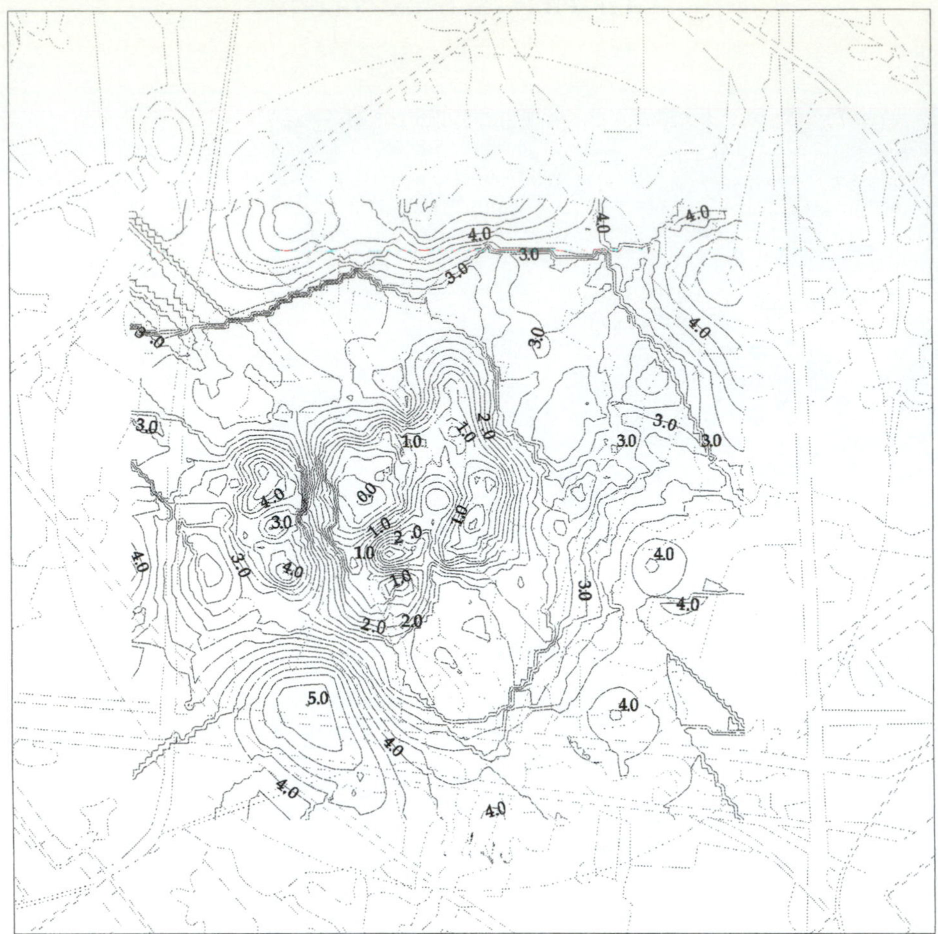

C

Figure 29-3. **(*Continued*)**

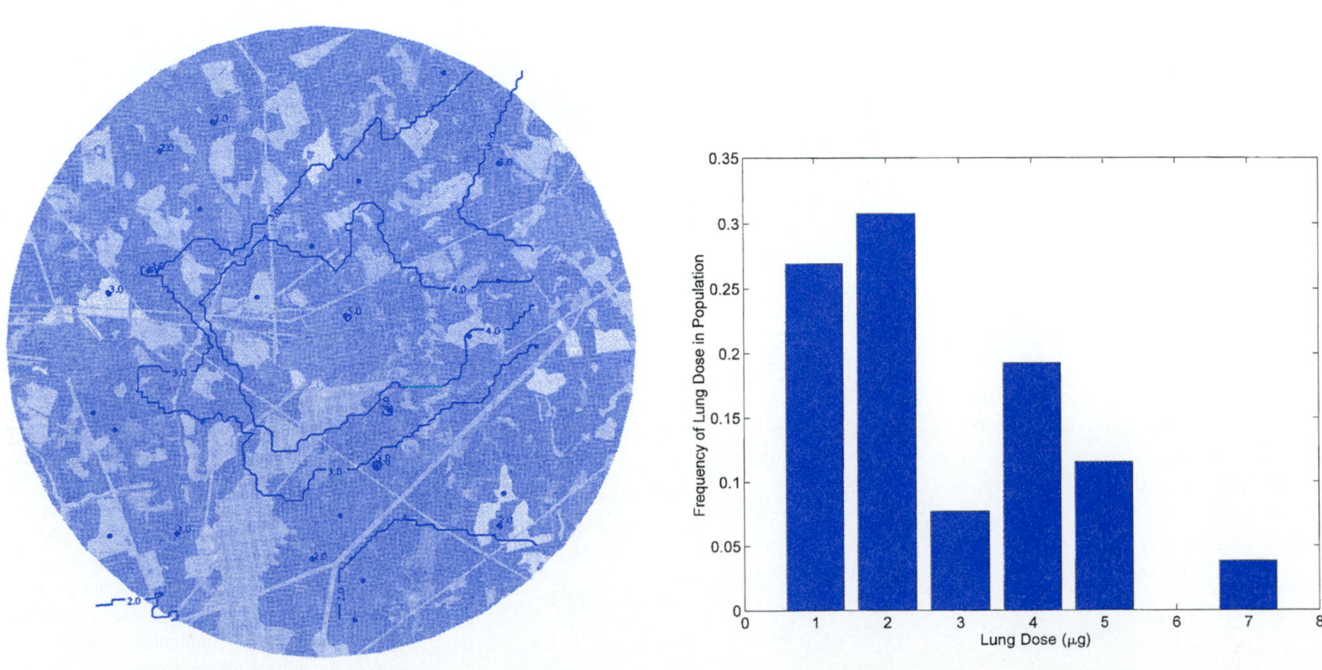

A B

***Figure 29-4.* (A). *Predicted static population lung dose for 26 individual animals. Dose is the maximum for that individual and mapped at the center of the animal's home range. Individual in Fig. 29-2A is found in the northwest quadrant.* (B). *Frequency of occurrence of lung dose in population mapped in* (A).**

ECOLOGIC RISK ASSESSMENT

With the growth of environmental toxicology comes the need to appropriately assess and quantify the impact of toxic chemicals on organisms, their populations, and communities in ecosystems. Earlier techniques to conduct risk assessments utilizing human health approaches were not appropriate for ecologic systems. For this reason, the U.S. EPA issued a framework for conducting ecologic risk assessment (U.S. EPA, 1992a). This framework, which was expanded and modified in 1998 (U.S. EPA, 1998), allows for the assessment of the impact of toxic chemicals as well as other stressors on ecologic systems (Fig. 29-5). In the problem-formulation phase, the potential pathways and species that might be affected by the toxic substance are considered. As part of the problem-formulation phase, a conceptual model is usually developed describing routes of exposure, biota of concern, and anticipated effect endpoints. The actual risk of chemicals to wildlife or other biota is then determined using exposure data and toxic effects of the chemicals of interest (Table 29-2 demonstrates for agriculture chemicals). Toxicity data for species of concern at either the individual or population level are also incorporated (Kendall and Akerman, 1992). In the risk-characterization phase, exposure and effect data accumulated in the analysis phase are combined and the risk potential is characterized. Based on the resulting risk, risk-management steps can be taken, generally involving decreasing the exposure portion of the assessment, in order to decrease the overall risk.

One example involving the assessment of the ecologic risk to wildlife of exposure to the insecticide carbofuran (a carbamate) has been published by the U.S. EPA (Houseknecht, 1993). Ecologic risk assessment revealed widespread and repeated mortality events, particularly in locations where birds ingested carbofuran granules in agricultural ecosystems. According to legislation promulgated by FIFRA and extended to the international sphere by the Migratory Bird Treaty Act, environmental regulations do not permit the killing of migratory songbirds or waterfowl with a pesticide. Under FIFRA, through a special review, the U.S. EPA took regulatory action against a carbamate, carbofuran (2,3-Dihydro-2,2-dimethyl-7-benzofuranol methylcarbamate), used in a large number of agroecosystems in which such use was associated with wildlife mortality.

Under the U.S. EPA's risk-assessment paradigm, risk characterization offers the opportunity to put the ecologic risk in per-

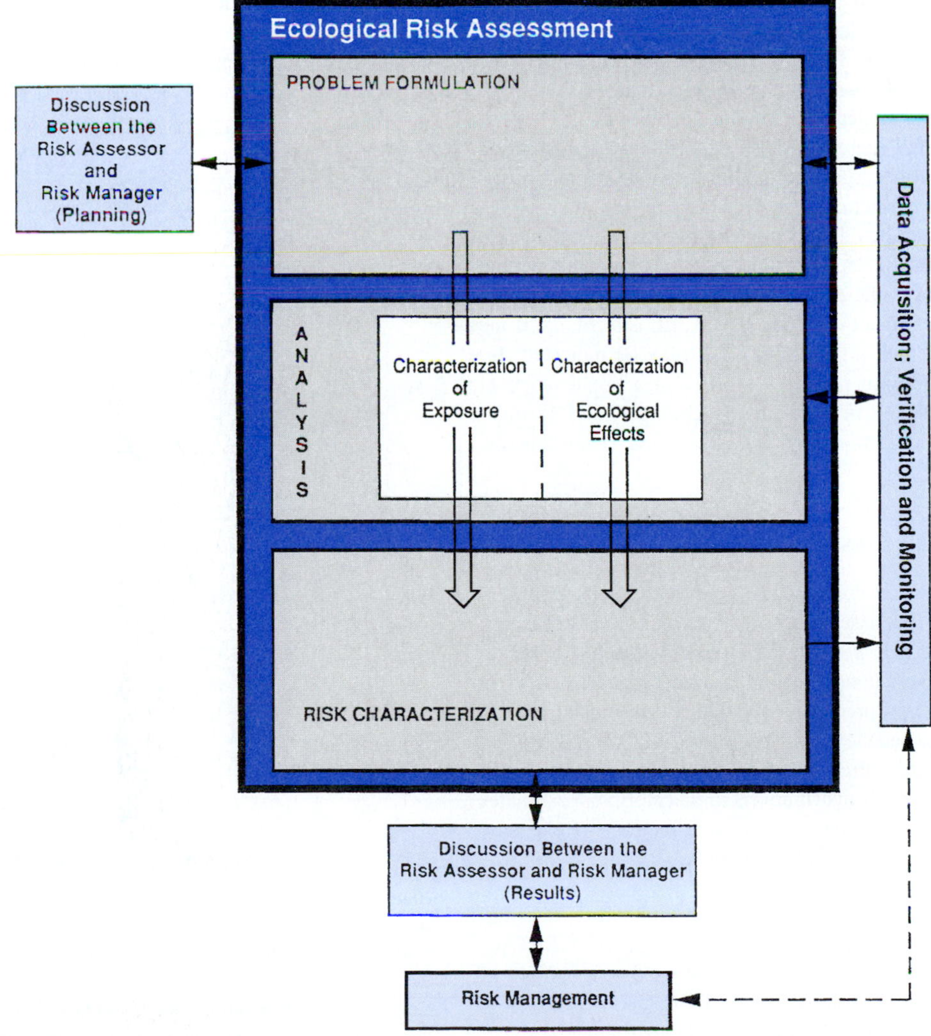

Figure 29-5. Generalized framework for ecologic risk assessment. (From U.S. EPA, 1998.)

Table 29-2
Ecotoxicological Assessment Criteria for Pesticides

PRESUMPTION OF MINIMUM HAZARD	HAZARD THAT MAY BE MITIGATED BY RESTRICTED USE	LEVEL OF CONCERN (LOC)
Mammals and Birds	Granular Formulations	
LD_{50}/sq. ft. $< \frac{1}{5}$ LD_{50}	$\frac{1}{5} \leq LD_{50}$/sq. ft. $< \frac{1}{2}$ LD_{50}	LD_{50}/sq. ft. $> \frac{1}{2}$ LD_{50}
	$LD_{50} \geq 50$mg/kg	
	Acute Toxicity	
EEC* $< \frac{1}{5}$ LC_{50}	$\frac{1}{5}$ $LC_{50} \leq$ EEC $< \frac{1}{2}$ LC_{50}	EEC $\geq \frac{1}{2}$ LC_{50}
mg/kg/day $< \frac{1}{5}$ LD_{50}	$\frac{1}{5}$ $LD_{50} \leq$ mg/kg/day $< \frac{1}{2}$ LD_{50}	mg/kg/day $\geq \frac{1}{2}$ LD_{50}
Aquatic Organisms		
EEC $< \frac{1}{10}$ LC_{50}	$\frac{1}{10}$ $LC_{50} \leq$ EEC $< \frac{1}{2}$ LC_{50}	EEC $\geq \frac{1}{2}$ LC_{50}
Mammals, Birds, and Aquatics	Chronic Toxicity	
EEC < Chronic	N/A	EEC ≥ effect level
No effect level		(including reproductive)

SOURCE: EPA guidelines provided by Edward Fite, Office of Pesticide Programs, Ecological Effects Branch, EPA Headquarters, Washington, DC. From: *Wildlife Toxicology and Population Modeling: Integrated Studies of Agroecosystem.* Boca Raton, FL: CRC/Lewis, 1994, with permission.

*Estimated environmental concentration. This is typically calculated using a series of simple nomographs to complex exposure models.

spective and to identify uncertainty in the development of the risk assessment. Although carbofuran could not be proven to cause significant adverse effects on bird populations, widespread and repeated mortality was evident and regulatory action was taken (Houseknecht, 1993; U.S. EPA, 1989). Evidence of carbofuran killing bald eagles (*Haliaeetus leucocephalus*) added to the overall concern for this chemical. Under the auspices of the Endangered Species Act, endangered species in the United States required special consideration because of their limited numbers and possible susceptibility to extinction.

The quotient method of assessing risk is often utilized in ecologic risk assessment (Bascietto et al., 1990). The quotient method employs the formula of the expected environmental concentration divided by the toxic impact of concern (e.g., LC_{50} or EC_{50}). If the quotient exceeds 1, then a significant risk may be indicated. Indeed, granular carbofuran products utilized in a broad range of agricultural uses resulted in quotients exceeding 1, and, as mentioned earlier, wildlife mortality was identified (Houseknecht, 1993).

Probabilistic Risk Assessment

Ecologic risk assessment continues to evolve as a science (Suter, 1993). Probabilistic risk assessments are used to further refine risk assessments so that they reflect actual risk in the environment. Probabilistic risk assessments have been used for several years in other disciplines such as predicting accidents, systems failure, and weather forecasting, but they have been used in ecologic risk assessments only recently. Probabilistic risk assessments can range from the use of probability distributions in place of point estimates in the Quotient Method to overlapping distributions of exposure and toxicity to stochastic simulation models.

Overlapping Distributions Overlapping probability distributions have been described in detail (Cardwell et al., 1993; SETAC, 1994; Parkhurst et al., 1995) and have been used in a number of ecologic risk assessments (Solomon et al., 1996; Giesy et al., 1999). In this approach, cumulative frequencies of environmental exposure concentrations (EECs, generally in milligrams per kilogram on food items) and toxicity values (LC_{50}, LC_{10}, or LC_5 transformed to a value of milligrams per kilogram per day) are plotted on the same graph. Frequencies are plotted on the *Y* axis using a probability scale and the concentrations plotted on the *X* axis using a logarithmic scale (Fig. 29-6). Toxicity values are ranked in as-

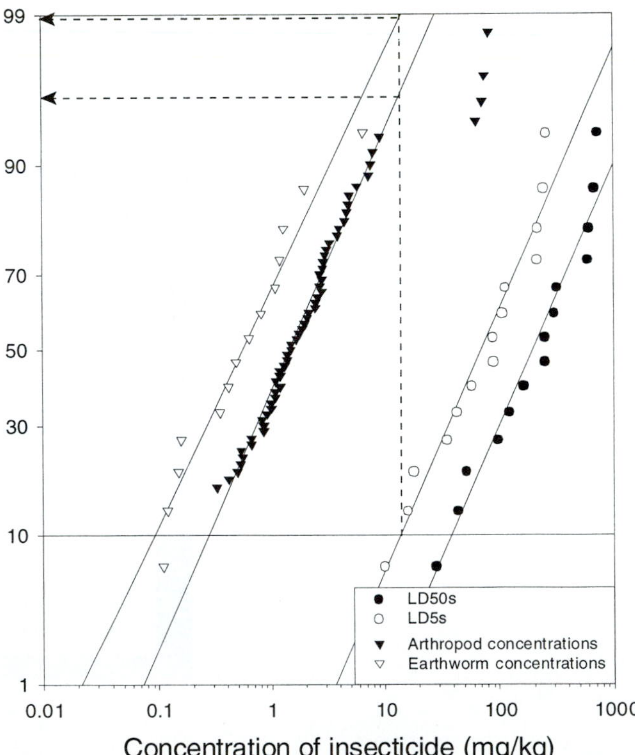

Figure 29-6. Graph showing distributions of insecticide toxicity to birds (expressed as concentration in food items) compared to actual concentrations reported in collected food items.

Comparing the distributions, the 10th centile of avian toxicity (LD_5 values) would be exceeded 1 percent of the time for earthworm consumption and 5 percent of the time for other invertebrates.

cending order and then transformed to cumulative percentages using the transformation:

$$\frac{100 \times i}{n + 1}$$

where i = ith observation of a total of n observations, starting with the lowest toxicity value. The resulting plots show an approximate linear relationship between frequency and the exposure and toxicity data, and linear regression can be used to fit straight lines to the data. The area of overlap between the two lines (if any) then can indicate the level of risk to the organisms exposed to the EECs. In the example shown in Fig. 29-6, exposure concentrations are the residues from the insecticide chlorpyrifos found on arthropods and earthworms. These data were ranked in the same way as the toxicity data. In this example, there is very little overlap of the two distributions. Using the 10th centile as an exceedance level, the LD_5s would exceed this level about 1 percent of the time for consumption of arthropods and about 5 percent of the time for consumption of earthworms (ECOFRAM, 1999).

Stochastic Simulation In probabilistic risk assessments using simulation, probability distributions are measured (or estimated) for parameters to account for natural variation, lack of knowledge, or uncertainty. The actual parameter values used in a simulation are obtained by sampling their distributions in a Monte Carlo process. The resulting model output will contain endpoint values, one value for each set of parameter values in a given simulation (see "Modeling and Geographic Information Systems," above). Several simulations will yield a probability distribution of endpoint values, such as mortality percentage in the simulated population. By altering the mean value of the model parameters and running additional sets of simulations, the percentage of outcomes that exceed a certain level of mortality can be estimated (Fig. 29-7). This curve can be compared with a graph of the "threshold of acceptability" defined by the risk manager to determine whether there is the potential for unacceptable risk.

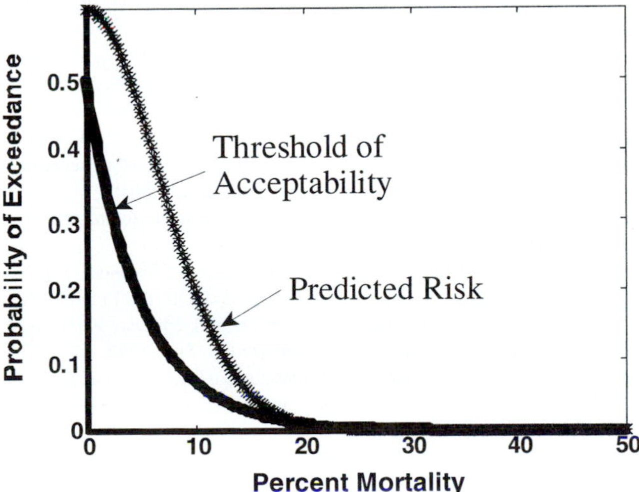

Figure 29-7. Illustration of risk manager's threshold of acceptability (shaded line) and predicted risk from a simulation model (data points).

A comparison of the two curves shows an area where the predicted risk exceeds the acceptability threshold, indicating a potentially unacceptable risk. (Adapted from ECOFRAM, 1999.)

Examples of probabilistic ecologic risk assessments include the effects of the herbicide atrazine [6-chloro-*N*-ethyl-*N*-(1-methylethyl)-1,3,5-triazine-2,4-diamine] on aquatic ecosystems in the midwestern U.S. corn belt (Solomon et al., 1996) and the insecticide chlorpyrifos [*O*,*O*-diethyl *O*-(3,5,6-trichloro-2-pyridinyl) ester] on aquatic ecosystems (Giesy et al., 1999), also in the midwestern United States.

The key to understanding ecologic risk assessment in ecotoxicology is considering more than just chemical toxicity. We must consider ecologic risk assessment in the context of exposure and other issues such as sublethal effects or ecosystem impacts. Indeed, we now know that predator-prey relationships can be affected by chemical exposure in prey (Galindo et al., 1985). In addition, "biomarkers" offer new technologies to assess sublethal impacts of chemicals on fish and wildlife populations (Dickerson et al., 1994).

The availability of data from laboratory and field ecotoxicologic experiments generated under GLPs, as discussed above, will improve the quality and ultimate value of ecologic risk assessments. In probabilistic risk assessments, the amount of data required increases substantially as the point estimates for toxicity and exposure are replaced by distributions and model parameters with error terms. Good Laboratory Practices data may offer new opportunities to integrate validated information into ecologic effect or exposure models for use in risk assessment (Kendall and Lacher, 1994). The contribution of ecologic models in the ecologic risk assessment process is in its infancy and offers significant opportunities for the extrapolation of data from laboratory and field experiments to a broader range of applications for the protection of the environment and its fish, wildlife, and other biotic resources.

ENVIRONMENTAL TOXICOLOGY AND HUMAN HEALTH

Links between wildlife and human health serve as a premise for extrapolation in risk assessment. Humans share many cellular and subcellular mechanisms with wildlife species. Humans and wildlife also overlap in their physical environment and therefore are exposed to many of the same contaminants. There is evidence to suggest that when highly conserved systems are targeted by environmental toxicants, both ecosystem and human health suffer.

There are obvious challenges and concerns in the extrapolation of wildlife data to humans. When there are contaminant-specific alterations in wildlife health, concerns about coordinate adverse effects in humans tend to focus on susceptible developmental periods, including in utero, neonatal, pubertal, lactational, and menopausal stages (Colburn et al., 1993). There is also a real concern about an increased risk of various cancers caused by environmental contaminants (Kavlock et al., 1996) and populations with genetic or environmental susceptibility (Frame et al., 1998). The overall rate of some cancers is increasing, particularly in industrialized countries. Based on animal models, chemical exposure figures in the etiology of many cancers; therefore a link to human cancer incidence seems plausible. Unfortunately, linking known contaminant exposures to an affected human population is difficult, particularly when effects are not identified for many years. By the time human effects are identified, the causative agent may not be present or detectable.

As with wildlife, some human health effects may be reversible while others may involve irreversible changes. In some instances, this may be a matter of dose. A high dose may lead to irreversible direct effects, such as malformations. However, low doses may manifest as subtle or latent functional changes in susceptibility that are not apparent until after the exposure has passed and the individual is "challenged." Particularly because of the longevity of humans, even low-dose exposures may result in a human health risk, predisposing elderly individuals to chronic disease processes. Wildlife may not be affected in the same ways because of their generally shorter life span.

Regardless of species, the process of risk assessment requires four steps: hazard identification, dose-response assessment, exposure assessment, and risk characterization. Often, these processes are difficult in human populations and extrapolations are required, including qualitative interspecies extrapolation from test animal to human and quantitative extrapolation from high to low dose. Uncertainties in these two extrapolations have sometimes resulted in a low confidence in risk estimates for humans. When human data are of low quality or not available, wildlife sentinels can serve a useful role in assessing human risk. For the future, however, much more information is needed to develop the human database regarding exposure, susceptibility, metabolism and disposition, site and mechanisms, tissue repair processes, compensatory responses, and adaptive mechanisms. Obviously, the more human data available for risk assessment, the better, and the more generalized and relevant to real human health effects, the easier it is to define a risk-management strategy (Smith and Wright, 1996).

Thus far, the best wildlife-to-human extrapolations have relied on strong, consistent human data available from high-dose accidental exposures for comparison with wildlife effects from monitoring studies; the Yusho and Yu-Cheng PCB incidents (Masuda et al., 1979; Kuratsune et al., 1976; Hsu, 1985); the TCDD accident in Seveso, Italy (Mocarelli et al., 1991); and human exposure to diethylstilbestrol (DES). The dose-response data collected, the large numbers of affected individuals, and an understanding of biological mechanisms in each of these cases make the comparisons possible. For most low-dose exposures, the ability to show causation is still poor. Future research relating the environmental health problems of wildlife and humans should recognize the scope of environmental disease processes and species-specific endpoints that reflect the divergence as well as the conservation of systems.

The interconnections between ecologic health and human health should not be overlooked. The indirect effects of environmental pollution may, in the end, be more important than the direct effects for human health. The environment is thought to act as a buffer for both toxicants and disease. However, even a buffer has its limits. For instance, the human population is at greater risk for emerging diseases as the natural environment dwindles in relative area. In the future, it is important that researchers focus on closing the artificial gap that views "environmental" or "human" health issues separately.

REFERENCES

Adams, SM, Crumby WD, Greeley MS Jr, et al: Relationships between physiological and fish population responses in a contaminated stream. *Environ Toxicol Chem* 11:1549–1557, 1992.

Adams SM, Shepard KL, Greeley MS, et al: The use of bioindicators for assessing the effects of pollutant stress on fish. Mar Environ Res 28:459–464, 1989.

Agency for Toxic Substances and Disease Registry (ATSDR): *Toxicological Profile for 4,4′-DDT,4,4′-DDE,4,4′-DDD*. TP-93/05. Atlanta: U.S. Department of Health and Human Services, 1994.

Agency for Toxic Substances and Disease Registry (ATSDR): *Toxicology Profile for Pentachlorophenol.* TP 93/13. Atlanta: U.S. Department of Health and Human Services 1994.

Albers PH, Heinz GH, Ohlendorf HM (eds): *Environmental Contaminants and Terrestrial Vertebrates: Effects on Populations, Communities, and Ecosystems*. Pensacola, FL: Society of Environmental Toxicology and Chemistry (SETAC), 2000.

Albertini RJ: Biomarker responses in human populations: Towards a worldwide map. *Mutat Res* 428(1-2):217–226, 1999.

Allen DL, Otis DL: Relationship between deer mouse population parameters and dieldrin contamination in the Rocky Mountain Arsenal National Wildlife Refuge. *Can J Zool* 76:243–250, 1998.

American Society for Testing and Materials (ASTM): *Annual Book of Standards*. Vol 11. Philadelphia: ASTM, 1986.

American Society for Testing and Materials: Standard methods for conducting acute toxicity tests with fishes, macroinvertebrates, and amphibians, in *Annual Book of ASTM Standards*. Vol 11. Designation E 729-88a. Philadelphia: ASTM, 1992a, pp 403–422.

American Society for Testing and Materials: Standard methods for conducting early life-stage tests with fishes, in *Annual Book of ASTM Standards*. Vol 11. Designation E 1241-92. Philadelphia: ASTM, 1992b, pp 885–913.

American Society for Testing and Materials: Standard methods for conducting acute toxicity tests on aqueous effluents with fishes, macroinvertebrates, and amphibians, in *Annual Book of ASTM Standards*. Vol 11. Designation E 1706-95a. Philadelphia: ASTM, 1992c, pp 403–422.

American Society for Testing and Materials: Standard methods for measuring the toxicity of sediment-associated contaminants with freshwater invertebrates, in *Annual Book of ASTM Standards*. Vol 11. Designation E 1706-95a. Philadelphia: ASTM, 1995.

Ames PL: DDT residues in the eggs of the osprey in the northeastern United States and their relation to nesting success. *J Appl Ecol (Suppl)* 3:87–97, 1966.

Ankley G, Mihaich E, Stahl R, et al: Overview of a workshop on screening methods for detecting potential (anti-) estrogenic/androgenic chemicals in wildlife. *Environ Toxicol Chem* 17:68, 1998.

Ankley GT, Phipps GL, Leonard EN, et al: Acid volatile sulfide as a factor mediating cadmium and nickel bioavailability in contaminated sediments. *Environ Toxicol Chem* 10(10):1299–1307, 1991.

Ashok, T, Saxena S: Biodegradation of polycyclic aromatic-hydrocarbons—A review. *J Sci Ind Res* 54:443–451, 1995.

Atkins PW: *Physical Chemistry,* 2d ed. San Francisco: Freeman, 1982.

Auman HJ, Ludwig JP, Summer CL, et al: PCBs, DDE, DDT, and TCDD-EQ in two species of albatross on Sand Island, Midway Atoll, North Pacific Ocean. *Environ Toxicol Chem* 16:498–504, 1997.

Awata H, Johnson KA, Anderson TA: Passive sampling devices as surrogates for evaluating bioavailability of aged chemicals in soil. *Toxicol Environ Chem* 73:25–42, 1999.

Babcock KM, Flickinger EL: Dieldrin mortality of lesser snow geese in Missouri. *J Wildl Mgt* 41:100–103, 1977.

Baker RJ, Chesser RK: The Chernobyl nuclear disaster and subsequent creation of a wildlife preserve. *Environ Toxicol Chem* 19:1231–1232, 2000.

Barnthouse LW, Suter GW III, Rosen AE: Risks of toxic contaminants to exploited fish populations: Influence of life history, data uncertainty, and exploitation intensity. *Environ Toxicol Chem* 9:297–311, 1990.

Barrett GW: Effects of Sevin on small-mammal populations in agricultural and old-field ecosystems. *J Mammal* 69:731–739, 1988.

Barrett GW: The effects of an acute insecticide stress on a semi-enclosed grassland ecosystem. *Ecology* 49:1019–1035, 1968.

Barry MJ, Logan DC: The use of temporary pond microcosms for aquatic toxicity testing: Direct and indirect effects of endosulfan on community structure. *Aqua Toxicol* 41:101–124, 1998.

Bascietto J, Hinckley D, Platkin J, Slimak M: Ecotoxicity and ecological risk assessment. *Environ Sci Technol* 24:10–15, 1990.

Baumann PC: Epizootics of cancer in fish associated with genotoxins in sediment and water. *Mutat Res* 411:227–233, 1998.

Beltman DJ, Clements WH, Lipton J, Cacela D: Benthic invertebrate metals exposure, accumulation, and community-level effects downstream from a hard-rock mine site. *Environ Toxicol Chem* 18:299–307, 1999.

Bennett WA, Sosa A, Beitinger TL: Oxygen tolerance of fathead minnows previously exposed to copper. *Bull Environ Contam Toxicol* 55:517–524, 1995.

Bergeron JM, Crews D, McLacjlan JA: PCBs as environmental estrogens: Turtle sex determination as a biomarker of environmental contamination. *Environ Health Perspect* 102:780–781, 1994.

Bergeron JM, Willingham E, Osborn CT III, et al: Developmental synergism of steroidal estrogens in sex determination. *Environ Health Perspect* 107:93–97, 1999.

Bergman HL, Norstrom RJ, Haraguchi K, et al: PCB and DDE methyl sulfones in mammals from Canada and Sweden. *Environ Toxicol Chem* 13:121–128, 1994.

Beyer AIN, Gish CD: Persistence in earthworms and potential hazards to birds of soil applied DDT, dieldrin and heptachlor. *J Appl Ecol* 17:295–307, 1980.

Beyer WN, Cromartie EJ: A survey of Pb, Cu, Zn, Cd, Cr, As, and Se in earthworms and soil from diverse sites. *Environ Monit Assess* 8:27–36, 1987.

Bickham JW, Rogers WJ, and Theodorakis CW: Transgenerational genetic effects of environmental contamination: Implications for risk assessment. Proceeding of the American Nuclear Society, Topical Meeting on Risk-Based Performance Assessment and Decision Making, Richland/Pasco, WA, 1998, pp 187–194.

Bickham JW, Sawin VL, Burton DW, McBee R: Flow-cytometric analysis of the effects of triethylenemelamine of somatic and testicular tissues of the rat. *Cytometry* 13:368–373, 1992.

Bickham JW, Smolen MJ: Somatic and heritable effects of environmental genotoxins and the emergence of evolutionary toxicology. *Environ Health Perspect Suppl* 12:25–28, 1994.

Bildstein KL, Forsyth DJ: Effects of dietary dieldrin on behavior of white-footed mice (*Peromyscus leucopus*) toward an avian predator. *Bull Environ Contam Toxicol* 21:93–97, 1979.

Birge WJ, Black JA, Westerman AG: Short-term fish and amphibian tests for determining the effects of toxicant stress on early life stages and estimating choric values for single compounds and complex effluents. *Environ Toxicol Chem* 49:807–821, 1985.

Birnbaum LS: Endocrine effects of prenatal exposure to PCBs, dioxins and other xenobiotics: Implications for policy and future research. *Environ Health Perspect* 102:676–679, 1994.

Bishop CA, Mahony NA, Trudeau S, Pettit KE: Reproductive success and biochemical effects in tree swallows (*Tachycineta bicolor*) exposed to chlorinated hydrocarbon contaminants in wetlands of the Great Lakes and St. Lawrence River Basin, USA and Canada. *Environ Toxicol Chem* 18:263–271, 1999.

Bjerke DL, Brown TJ, MacLusky NJ, et al: Partial demasculinization and feminization of sex behavior in male rats by *in utero* and lactational exposure to 2,3,7,8-tetrachlorodibenzo-*p*-dioxin is not associated with alterations in estrogen receptor binding or volumes of sexually differentiated brain nuclei. *Toxicol Appl Pharmacol* 127:258–267, 1994a.

Bjerke DL, Peterson RE: Reproductive toxicity of 2,3,7,8-tetrachlorodibenzo-*p*-dioxin in male rats: Different effects of *in utero* versus lactational exposure. *Toxicol Appl Pharmacol* 127:241–249, 1994.

Bjerke DL, Sommer RJ, Moore RW, Peterson RE: Effects of *in utero* and lactational 2,3,7,8-tetrachlorodibenzo-*p*-dioxin exposure on responsiveness of the male rat reproductive system to testosterone stimulation in adulthood. *Toxicol Appl Pharmacol* 127:250–257, 1994b.

Blanchard BA, Hannigan JH: Prenatal alcohol exposure: Effects on androgen and nonandrogen dependent behaviors and on gonadal development in male rats. *Neurotoxicol Teratol* 16:31–39, 1994.

Blanck H, Wangberg S-A: Induced community tolerance in marine periphyton communities established under arsenate stress. *Can J Fish Aquat Sci* 45:1816–1819, 1988.

Blaser WW, Bredeweg RA, Harner RS, et al: Process analytical chemistry, in *Application Reviews*. Washington, DC: American Chemical Society, 1995, pp 47R–70R.

Bookhout TA: *Research and Management Techniques for Wildlife and Habitats*. Bethesda, MD: The Wildlife Society, 1994.

Bonaventura R, Pedro AM, Coimbra J, Lencastre E: Trout farm effluents: Characterization and impact on the receiving streams. *Environ Pollut* 95:379–387, 1997.

Bracher GA, Bider JR: Changes in terrestrial animal activity of a forest community after an application of aminocarb (Metacil). *Can J Zool* 60:1981–1997, 1982.

Braestrup L, Clausen J, Berg O: DDE, PCB and aldrin levels in arctic birds of Greenland. *Bull Environ Contam Toxicol* 11:326–332, 1974.

Brown C, Gross WB, Ehrich M: Effects of social stress on the toxicity of malathion in young chickens. *Avian Dis* 30:679–682, 1986.

Bulich AA: Use of luminescent bacteria for determining toxicity in aquatic environments, in Marking LL, Kimerle RA (eds): *Aquatic Toxicology: Second Conference*. ATM STP 667. Philadelphia: American Society for Testing and Materials, 1979, pp 98–106.

Cairns J Jr, Dickson KL, Maki AW (eds): *Estimating the Hazard of Chemical Substances to Aquatic Life*. Special Technical Publication 657. Philadelphia: American Society for Testing and Materials, 1978.

Cairns J Jr, Dickson KL, Maki AW: Scenarios on alternative futures for biological monitoring, 1978–1985, in Worf DL (ed): *Biological Monitoring for Environmental Effects*. Lexington, MA: Heath, 1980, pp 11–21.

Cairns J Jr, Mount DI: Aquatic toxicology. *Environ Sci Technol* 24:154–159, 1990.

Camargo JA: Structural and trophic alterations in macrobenthic communities downstream from a fish farm outlet. *Hydrobiologia* 242:41–49, 1992.

Cardwell RD, Parkhurst BR, Warren-Hicks W, Volosin JS: Aquatic ecological risk. *Water Environ Technol* 5:47–51, 1993.

Carpenter SR, Caraco NF, Correll DL, et al: Nonpoint pollution of surface waters with phosphorus and nitrogen. *Ecol Appl* 8:559–568, 1998.

Casey ML, MacDonald PC, Simpson ER: Endocrinological changes of pregnancy, in Wilsom JD, Foster DW (eds): *William's Textbook of Endocrinology*. Philadelphia: Saunders, 1985, pp 422–437.

Caslin TM, Wolff JO: Individual and demographic responses of the gray-tailed vole to Vinclozolin. *Environ Toxicol Chem* 18:1529–1533, 1999.

Chan WK, Yao G, Gu YZ, Bradfield CA: Cross-talk between the aryl hydrocarbon receptor and hypoxia inducible factor signaling pathways. Demonstration of competition and compensation. *J Biol Chem* 274(17):12115–12123, 1999.

Chapman PM: Current approaches to developing sediment quality criteria. *Environ Toxicol Chem* 8:589–599, 1989.

Chardard D, Dournon C: Sex reversal by aromatase inhibitor treatment in the newt *Pleurodeles*. *J Exp Zool* 283:43–50, 1999.

Chesser RK, Sugg DW, Smith MH, et al: Concentrations and dose rate estimates of ^{134,137}cesium and ^{90}strontium in small mammals at Chernobyl. *Environ Toxicol Chem* 19:305–310, 2000.

Chu F-LE, Hale RC: Relationship between pollution and susceptibility to infectious disease in the eastern oyster, *Crassostrea virginica*. *Mar Environ Res* 38:243–256, 1994.

Clark DR, Lamont TG: Organochlorine residues and reproduction in the big brown bat. *J Wildl Mgt* 40:249–254, 1976.

Colborn T: Environmental Estrogens: health implications for humans and wildlife. *Environ Health Perspec* 103(suppl 7):135–136, 1996.

Colborn T, vom Saal FS, Soto AM: Developmental effects of endocrine-disrupting chemicals in wildlife and humans. *Environ Health Perspect* 101(5):378–384, 1993.

Collier TK, Anulacion BF, Stein JE, et al: A field evaluation of cytochrome P4501A as a biomarker of contaminant exposure in three species of flatfish. *Environ Toxicol Chem* 14(1):143–152, 1995.

Committee on Biological Markers of the National Research Council: Biological markers in environmental health research. *Environ Health Perspect* 74:3–9, 1987.

Connell DW, Miller GJ: *Chemistry and Ecotoxicology of Pollution*. New York: Wiley, 1984.

Correll DL: role of phosphorus in the eutrophication of receiving waters: A review. *J Environ Qual* 27:261–266, 1998.

Costa LG: Biochemical and molecular neurotoxicology: relevance to biomarker development, neurotoxicity testing and risk assessment. *Toxicol Lett* 102–103:417–421, 1998.

Cotton RGH: Slowly but surely towards better scanning for mutations. *Trends Genet* 13(2):43–46, 1997.

Couillard CM, Hodson PV, Gagnon P, Dodson JJ: Lesions and parasites in white suckers, *Catostomus commersoni,* in bleached-kraft pulp mill-contaminated and reference rivers. *Environ Toxicol Chem* 14:1051–1060, 1995.

Creekmore TE, Whittaker DG, Roy RR, et al: Health status and relative exposure of mule deer and white-tailed deer to soil contaminants at the Rocky Mountain Arsenal. *Environ Toxicol Chem* 18:272–278, 1999.

Custer CM, Custer TW, Allen PD, et al: Reproduction and environmental contamination in tree swallows nesting in the Fox River drainage and Green Bay, Wisconsin, USA. *Environ Toxicol Chem* 17:1786–1798, 1998.

Custer TW, Custer CM: Transfer and accumulation of organochlorines from black-crowned night-heron eggs to chicks. *Environ Toxicol Chem* 14:533–536, 1995.

Daury RW, Schwab RE, Bateman MC: Blood lead concentrations of waterfowl from unhunted and heavily hunted marshes of Nova Scotia and Prince Edward Island, Canada. *J Wildl Dis* 29:577–581, 1993.

DeAngelis DL: What food web analysis can contribute to wildlife toxicology, in Kendall RJ, Lacher TE Jr (eds): *Wildlife Toxicology and Population Modeling: Integrated Studies of Agroecosystems*. Boca Raton, FL: Lewis/CRC, 1994, pp 365–382.

DeAngelis DL, Barnthouse LW, Van Winkle W, Otto RG: A critical appraisal of population approaches in assessing fish community health. *J Great Lakes Res* 16:576–590, 1990.

DeAngelis DL, Gross LJ (eds): *Individual-Based Models and Approaches in Ecology*. New York: Chapman and Hall, 1992.

DeLonay, AJ, Little EE, Lipton J, et al: Behavioral avoidance as evidence of injury to fishery resources: Applications to natural resource damage assessment. ASTM Spec Tech Publ no. 1262. Conshohocken, PA: ASTM, 1996, pp 268–280.

DeWeese LR, Cohen RR, Stafford CJ: Organochlorine residues and eggshell measurements for tree swallows, *Tachycineta bicolor,* in Colorado. *Bull Environ Contam Toxicol* 35:767–775, 1985.

Dickerson RL, Hooper MJ, Gard NW, et al: Toxicological foundations of ecological risk assessment: Biomarker development and interpretation based on laboratory and wildlife species. *Environ Health Perspect* 102(12):65–69, 1994.

Dickerson RL, McMurry CS, Smith EE, et al: Modulation of endocrine pathways by 4,4'-DDE in the deer mouse *Peromyscus maniculatus. Sci Tot Environ* 233:97–108, 1999.

DiToro DM, Mahony JD, Hansen DJ, et al: Acid volatile sulfide predicts the acute toxicity of cadmium and nickel in sediments. *Environ Sci Technol* 26:96–101, 1992.

DiToro DM, Mahony JD, Hansen DJ, et al: Toxicity of cadmium in sediments: the role of acid volatile sulfides. *Environ Toxicol Chem* 9(12):1487–1502, 1990.

Dixon KR, Luxmoore RJ, Begovich CL: CERES—A model of forest stand biomass dynamics for predicting trace contaminant, nutrient, and water effects. I. Model description. *Ecol Mod* 5:17–38, 1978a.

Dixon KR, Luxmoore RJ, Begovich CL: CERES—A model of forest stand biomass dynamics for predicting trace contaminant, nutrient, and water effects. II. Model application. *Ecol Mod* 5:93–114, 1978b.

Doherty FG, Quershi AA, Razza JB: Comparison of the *Ceriodaphnia dubia* and Microtox inhibition tests for toxicity assessment of industrial and municipal wastewaters. *Environ Toxicol* 14:375–382, 1999.

Donigian AS Jr, Imhoff JC, Bichnell BR: Predicting water quality resulting from agricultural nonpoint source pollution via simulation-HSPF, in Schaller FW, Bailey GW (eds): *Agricultural Management and Water Quality*. Ames, IA: State University Press, 1983, pp 200–249.

Dubrova YE, Nesterov YN, Krouchinsky NG, et al: Human minisatellite mutation rate after the Chernobyl accident. *Nature* 380:683–686, 1996.

Duffus JH: *Environmental Toxicology*. New York: Wiley, 1980.

EC (European Commission): *European Workshop on the Impact of Endocrine Disrupters on Human Health and Wildlife*. Weybridge, UK: EC, 1996.

ECOFRAM (Ecological Committee on FIFRA Risk Assessment Methods): *Terrestrial Draft Report,* Washington, DC: United States Environmental Protection Agency, 1999.

Edge WD, Carey RL, Wolff JO, et al: Effects of Guthion 2S on *Microtus canicaudus:* A risk assessment validation. *J Appl Ecol* 33:269–278, 1996.

Eggens ML, Vethaak AD, Leaver MJ, et al: Differences in CYP1A response between flounder (*Platichthys flesus*) and plaice (*Pleuronectes platessa*) after long-term exposure to harbour dredged spoil in a mesocosm study. *Chemosphere* 32:1357–1380, 1996.

Elangbarn CS, Qualls CW Jr, Lochmiller RL, Novak J: Development of the cotton rat (*Sigmodon hispidus*) as a biomonitor of environmental contamination with emphasis on hepatic cytochrome P-450 induction and population characteristics. *Bull Environ Contam Toxicol* 42:482–488, 1989.

Elliott JE, Norstrom RJ: Chlorinated hydrocarbon contaminants and productivity of bald eagle populations on the Pacific Coast of Canada. *Environ Toxicol Chem* 17:1142–1153, 1998.

Fite EC, Ibmer LW, Cook JJ, et al: *Guidance Document for Conducting Terrestrial Field Studies*. Technical Report 540/09-88-109. Washington, DC: Environmental Protection Agency, 1988.

Fleming WJ, Heinz GH, Franson JC, Rattner BA: Toxicity of ABATE 4E (*Temephos*) in mallard ducklings and the influence of cold. *Environ Toxicol Chem* 4:193–199, 1985.

Frame LT, Ambrosone CB, Kadlubar FF, Lang NP: Host-environment interactions that impact on interindividual variability in susceptibility to human cancer, in *Human Variability in Response to Chemical Exposures: Measures, Modeling and Risk Assessment*. International Life Sciences Institute, 1998, pp 165–204.

Frame LT, Hart RW, Leakey JE: Caloric restriction as a mechanism mediating resistance to environmental disease. *Environ Health Perspect* 106(suppl 1):313–324, 1998.

French JB Jr, Porter WP: Energy acquisition and allocation in *Peromyscus maniculatus* exposed to aldicarb and cool temperatures. *Environ Toxicol Chem* 13:297–933, 1994.

Frey LT, Palmer DA, Kruger HO: LORSBAN insecticide: An evaluation of its effects upon avian and mammalian species on and around corn fields in Iowa. Project 103–366. MVTL Laboratories, New Ulm, MN. Easton, MD: Wildlife International, 1994.

Fry DM: Reproductive effects in birds exposed to pesticides and environmental chemicals. *Environ Health Perspect* 103:(suppl 7):165–171, 1995.

Fryday SL, Hart ADM, Langton SD: Effects of exposure to an organophosphorus pesticide on the behavior and use of cover by captive starlings. *Environ Toxicol Chem* 15:1590–1596, 1996.

Gabric AJ, Bell PRF: Review of the effects of non-point nutrient loading on coastal ecosystems. *Aust J Marine Freshwater Res* 44:261–283, 1993.

Galindo JC, Kendall RJ, Driver CJ, Lacher TE: The effect of methyl parathion on susceptibility of bobwhite quail (*Colinus virginianus*) to domestic cat predation. *Behav Neural Biol* 43:21–36, 1985.

Gallagher SP, Palmer DA, Krueger HO: *Lorsban Insecticide: A Pilot Year Evaluation of Effects upon Avian and Mammalian Species on and Around Citrus Groves in California*. Technical Report ES-2525. MRID# 43730301. Indianapolis, IN: DowElanco, 1994.

Gebauer MB, Weseloh DV: Accumulation of organic contaminants in sentinel mallards utilizing confined disposal facilities at Hamilton Harbour, Lake Ontario, Canada. *Arch Environ Contam Toxicol* 25:234–243, 1993.

Gerhardt A: Whole effluent toxicity testing with *Oncorhynchus mykiss* (Walbaum 1792): Survival and behavioral responses to a dilution series of a mining effluent in South Africa. *Arch Environ Contam Toxicol* 35:309–316, 1998.

Gever GR, Mabury SA, Crosby DG: Rice field surface microlayer: Collection, composition, and pesticide enrichment. *Environ Toxic Chem* 15:1676–1682, 1996.

Gibbons WN, Munkittrick KR: A sentinel monitoring framework for identifying fish population responses to industrial discharges. *J Aquat Ecosyst Health* 3:227–237, 1994.

Giesy JP, Solomon KR, Coates JR, et al: Chlorpyrifos: Ecological risk assessment in North American aquatic environments. *Environ Contam Toxicol* 160:1–129, 1999.

Goksøyr A, Förlin L: The cytochrome P-450 system in fish, aquatic toxicology and environmental monitoring. *Aquat Toxicol* 22:287–312, 1992.

Greene JC, Bartels CL, Warren-Hicks WJ, et al: *Protocols for Short Term Toxicity Screening of Hazardous Waste Sites*. EPA/600/3-881029. Washington, DC: Environmental Protection Agency, 1989.

Gruber D, Frago CH, Rasnake WJ: Automated biomonitors—First line of defense. *J Aquat Ecosyst Health* 3:87–92, 1994.

Grue CE, Powell GVN, McChesney MJ: Care of nestlings by wild female starlings exposed to an organophosphate pesticide. *J Appl Ecol* 19:327–335, 1982.

Grue CE, Shipley BK: Interpreting population estimates of birds following pesticide applications—Behavior of male starlings exposed to an organophosphate pesticide. *Studies Avian Biol* 6:292–296, 1981.

Guillette LJ Jr, Brock JW, Rooney AA, Woodward AR: Serum concentrations of various environmental contaminants and their relationship to sex steroid concentrations and phallus size in juvenile American alligators. *Arch Environ Contam Toxicol* 36:447–455, 1999.

Gupta A: Pollution load of paper mill effluent and its impact on biological environment. *J Ecotoxicol Environ Monit* 7:1010–1112, 1997.

Guthie FE, Perry JJ (eds): *Introduction to Environmental Toxicology*. New York: Elsevier, 1980.

Guttman, SI: Population genetic structure and ecotoxicology. *Environ Health Perse* 102(suppl 12):97–100, 1994.

Guzzella L: Comparison of test procedures for sediment toxicity evaluation with *Vibrio fischeri* bacteria. *Chemosphere* 37:2895–2909, 1998.

Hahn ME, Poland A, Glover E, Stegeman JJ: The Ah receptor in marine animals: Phylogenetic distribution and relationship to cytochrome P4501A inducibility. *Mar Environ Res* 34:87–92, 1992.

Hall LW Jr, Anderson RD: The influence of salinity on the toxicity of various classes of chemicals to aquatic biota. *Crit Rev Toxicol* 25:281–346, 1995.

Hardy JT: The sea-surface microlayer: Biology, chemistry, and anthropogenic enrichment. *Prog Oceanogr* 11:307–328, 1982.

Hartwell, SI: Demonstration of a toxicological risk ranking method to correlate measures of ambient toxicity and fish community diversity. *Environ Toxicol Chem* 16:361–371, 1997.

Hatzinger PB, Alexander M: Effect of aging of chemicals in soil on their biodegradability and extractability. *Environ Sci Technol* 29:537–545, 1995.

Hawkes AW, Brewer LW, Hobson JF, et al: Survival and cover-seeking response of Northern bobwhite and morning doves dosed with Aldicarb. *Environ Toxicol Chem* 15:1538–1543, 1996.

Heddle JA, Cimino MC, Hayashi M, et al: Micronuclei as an index of cytogenetic damage: past, present and future. *Environ Mol Mutagen* 18:277–291, 1991.

Henriques W: A Model of Spatial and Temporal Exposure and Effect of Dieldrin on Badgers at the Rocky Mountain Arsenal. PhD dissertation, Department of Environmental Toxicology. Clemson, SC: Clemson University, 1996.

Henriques WD, Dixon KR: Estimating spatial distribution of exposure by integrating radiotelemetry, computer simulation, and GIS. *Hum Ecol Risk Assess* 2:527–538, 1996.

Herve F, Gentin M, Rajkowski KM, et al: Estrogen binding properties of alpha 1-fetoprotein and its isoforms. *J Steroid Biochem* 36:319–324, 1990.

Hesthagen T, Langeland A, Berger HM: Effects of acidification due to emissions from the Kola Peninsula on fish populations in lakes near the Russian border in northern Norway. *Water, Air, Soil Pollut* 102:17–36, 1998.

Hoffman DJ, Ratter BA, Burton GA Jr, Cairns J Jr: *Handbook of Ecotoxicology*. Boca Raton, FL: Lewis/CRC, 1995.

Hoffman DJ, Sanderson CJ, leCaptain LJ, et al: Interactive effects of selenium, methionine, and dietary protein on survival, growth, and physiology in mallard ducklings, *Arch Environ Contam Toxicol* 23:163–171, 1992.

Hoiland WK, Rabe FW: Effects of increasing zinc levels and habitat degradation on macroinvertebrates communities in three North Idaho streams. *J Freshwat Ecol* 7:373–380, 1992.

Holgate P: Random walk models for animal behavior, in Patil GP, Pielou EC, Waters WC (eds): *Statistical Ecology*. Vol 2. University Park, PA: State University Press, 1971, pp 1–12.

Holl KD, Cairns J Jr: Landscape indicators in ecotoxicology, in Hoffman DJ, Rattner BA, Burton GA Jr, Cairns, J Jr (eds). *Handbook of Ecotoxicology*. Boca Raton, FL: Lewis, 1995, pp 185–197.

Hooper MJ, Brewer LW, Cobb GP Kendall RJ: An integrated laboratory and field approach for assessing hazards of pesticide exposure to wildlife, in Somerville L, Walker CH (eds): *Pesticide Effects on Terrestrial Wildlife*. London: Taylor & Francis, 1990, pp 271–283.

Hooper MJ, La Point TW. Contaminant effects in the environment: their use in waste site assessment. *Ctr Eur J Pub Health* 2(suppl):65–69, 1994.

Houseknecht CR: Ecological risk assessment case study: Special review of the granular formulations of carbofuran based on adverse effects on birds, in *A Review of Ecological Assessment Case Studies from a Risk Assessment Perspective*. Vol 3. Environmental Protection Agency Risk Assessment Forum. EPA/630/R-92-005. Washington, DC: Environmental Protection Agency, 1993, pp 1–25.

Howard PH, Boethling RS, Jarvis WF, et al: *Handbook of Environmental Degradation Rates*. Chelsea, MI: Lewis, 1991.

Hsu St, Ma CI, Hsu SK, et al: Discovery and epidemiology of PCB poisoning in Taiwan: A four-year follow-up. *Environ Health Perspect* 59:5–10, 1985.

Huggett RJ, Kimerle RA, Mehrle PM, Jr, Bergman HL (eds.): *Biomarkers: Biochemical, Physiological, and Histological Markers of Anthropogenic Stress*. Boca Raton, FL: Lewis, 1992.

Huston MA, DeAngelis DL, Post WM: New computer models unify ecological theory. *Bioscience* 38:682–691, 1988.

Jensen RH, Reynolds JC, Robbins J, et al: Glycophorin A as a biological dosimeter for radiation dose to the bone marrow from iodine-131. *Radiat Res* 147:747–752, 1997.

Jeyasuria P, Place AR: Embryonic brain gonadal-axis in temperature dependent sex determination of reptiles: a role for P450 aromatase (CYP19). *J Exp Zool* 281:428–449, 1998.

Joergensen EH, Bye BE, Jobling M: Influence of nutritional status on biomarker responses to PCB in the Arctic charr (*Salvelinus alpinus*). *Aquat Toxicol* 44:233–244, 1999.

Johnson BT: Microtox toxicity test system—new developments and applications, in Wells PG, Lee K, Blaise C (eds): *Microscale Testing in*

Aquatic Toxicology: Advances, Techniques and Practice. Boca Raton, FL: CRC Press, 1998, pp. 201–218.

Johnson KA, Naddy RB, Weisskopf CP: Passive sampling devices for rapid determination of soil contaminant distributions. *Toxicol Environ Chem* 51:31–44, 1995.

Johnson-Logan LR, Broshears RE, Maine SJ: Partitioning behavior and the mobility of chlordane in groundwater. *Environ Sci Technol* 26(11):2234–2239, 1992.

Jones JC, Reynolds JD: Effects of pollution on reproductive behaviour of fishes. *Rev Fish Biol Fish* 7:463–491, 1997.

Juettner I, Peither A, Lay JP, Kettrup A, Ormerod SJ: An outdoor mesocosm study to assess ecotoxicological effects of atrazine on a natural plankton community. *Arch Environ Contam Toxicol* 29:435–441, 1995.

Karan V, Vitorovic S, Tutundzic V, Poleksic V: Functional enzymes activity and gill histology of carp after copper sulfate exposure and recovery. *Ecotoxicol Environ Saf* 40:49–55, 1998.

Karr JR: Biological monitoring and environmental assessment: A conceptual framework. *Environ Mgt* 11:249–256, 1987.

Kavlock RJ, Daston GP, DeRosa C, et al: Research needs for the risk assessment of health and environmental effects of endocrine disruptors: A report of the U.S. EPA-sponsored workshop. *Environ Health Perspect* 104(suppl 4):715–40, 1996.

Keith JA: Reproduction in a population of herring gulls (*Larus argentatus*) contaminated by DDT. *J Appl Ecol* 3(suppl):57–70, 1966.

Keith JO, Mitchell CA: Effects of DDE and food stress on reproduction and body condition of ringed turtle doves. *Arch Environ Contam Toxicol* 25:192–203, 1993.

Kelsey JW, Kottler BD, Alexander M: Selective chemical extractants to predict bioavailability of soil-aged organic chemicals. *Environ Sci Technol* 31:214–217, 1997.

Kendall RJ: Farming with agrochemicals: the response of wildlife. *Environ Sci Technol* 26(2):238–245, 1992.

Kendall RJ: Wildlife toxicology. *Environ Sci Technol* 16(8):448A–453A, 1982.

Kendall RJ, Akerman J: Terrestrial wildlife exposed to agrochemicals: An ecological risk assessment perspective. *Environ Toxicol Chem* 11(12):1727–1749, 1992.

Kendall RJ, Brewer LW, Hitchcock RR, Mayer JR: American wigeon mortality associated with turf application of diazinon AG500. *J Wildl Dis* 28:263–267, 1992.

Kendall RJ, Brewer LW, Lacher TE, et al: *The Use of Starling Nest Boxes for Field Reproductive Studies.* Provisional Guidance Document and Technical Support Document. EPA/600/8-89/056. Washington, DC: Environmental Protection Agency, 1989.

Kendall RJ, Dickerson RL, Giesy JP, Suk WA (eds): *Principles and Processes for Evaluating Endocrine Disruption in Wildlife*. Pensacola, FL: SETAC Press, 1998.

Kendall RJ, Funsch JM, Bens CM: Use of wildlife for on-site evaluation of bioavailability and ecotoxicology of toxic substances in hazardous waste sites, in Sandhu SS, Lower WR, deSerres FJ, et al (eds): *In Situ Evaluations of Biological Hazards of Environmental Pollutants.* New York: Plenum Press, 1990, pp 241–255.

Kendall RJ, Lacher TE Jr (eds): *Wildlife Toxicology and Population Modeling. Integrated Studies of Agroecosystems.* Chelsea, MI: Lewis, 1994.

Kolar CS, Hudson PL, Savino JF: Conditions for the return and simulation of the recovery of burrowing mayflies in western Lake Erie. *Ecol Appl* 7:665–676, 1997.

Korschgen LJ: Soil-food-chain-pesticide wildlife relationships in aldrin-treated sites. *J Wildl Mgt* 34:186–199, 1970.

Krane DE, Sternberg DC, Burton GA: Randomly amplified polymorphic DNA profile-based measures of genetic diversity in crayfish correlated with environmental impacts. *Environ Toxicol Chem* 18:504–508, 1999.

Kuratsune M, Masuda Y, Nagayama J: Some of the recent findings concerning Yusho, in Buckley JL, et al (eds): *National Conference on Polychlorinated Biphenyls.* Washington, DC: Environmental Protection Agency, 1976, pp 14–29.

Kwan KK, Dutka BJ: Evaluation of Toxi-Chromotest direct sediment toxicity testing procedure and Microtox solid-phase testing procedure. *Bull Environ Contam Toxicol* 49:656–662, 1992.

Lamb DW, Kenaga EE (eds): *Avian and Mammalian Wildlife Toxicology: Second Conference.* Philadelphia: American Society for Testing and Materials, 1981.

Lamm SH, Braverman LE, Li FX, et al: Thyroid Health status of ammonium perchlorate workers: A cross-sectional occupational health study. *J Occup Environ Med* 41:248–260, 1999.

Landsberg JH, Blakesley BA, Reese RO, et al: Parasites of fish as indicators of environmental stress. *Environ Monit Assess* 51:211–232, 1998.

Lang C, Reymond OR: Reversal of eutrophication in four Swiss lakes: Evidence from oligochaete communities. *Hydrobiologia* 334:157–162, 1996.

Langlois RG, Akiyama M, Kusunoki Y, et al: Analysis of somatic cell mutations at the glycophorin a locus in atomic bomb survivors: A comparative study of assay methods. *Radiat Res* 136:111–117, 1993.

La Point TW, Melancon SM, Morris MK: Relationships among observed metal concentrations, criteria values, and benthic community structural responses in 15 streams. *J Water Pollut Contr Fed* 56:1030–1038, 1984.

Leonard RA, Knisel WG, Still DA: GLEAMS: Groundwater loading effects of agricultural management systems. *Trans ASAE* 30:1403–1418, 1987.

Li J, Quabius ES, Wendelaar Bonga SE, et al: Effects of water-borne copper on brachial chloride cells and Na^{+}/K^{+}-ATPase activities in Mozambique tilapia (*Oreochromis mossambicus*). *Aquat Toxicol* 43:1–11, 1998.

Lower WR, Kendall RJ: Sentinel species and sentinel bioassay, in McCarthy JF, Shugart LR (eds): *Biomarkers of Environmental Contamination.* Boca Raton, FL: Lewis/CRC, 1990, pp 309–331.

Luoma SN: Detection of trace contaminant effects on aquatic ecosystems. *J Fish Res Board Can* 34:436–439, 1977.

Luxmoore RJ, Begovich CL, Dixon KR: Modelling solute uptake and incorporation into vegetation and litter. *Ecol Mod* 5:137–171, 1978.

MacGregor JT, Tucker JD, Eastmond DA, Wyrobek AJ: Integration of cytogenetic assays with toxicology studies. *Environ Mol Mutagens* 25:328–337, 1995.

Mackay D: *Multimedia Environmental Models. The Fugacity Approach.* Chelsea, MI: Lewis, 1991.

Madrigal JL, Pixton GC, Collings BJ, et al: A comparison of two methods of estimating bird mortalities from field-applied pesticides. *Environ Toxicol Chem* 15:878–885, 1996.

Makela S, Davis VL, Tally WC, et al: Dietary estrogens act through estrogen receptor-mediated processes and show no antiestrogenicity in cultured breast cancer cells. *Environ Health Perspect* 102(6-7):572–578, 1994.

Makela S, Poutanen M, Lehtimaki J, et al: Estrogen specific 17 beta hydroxysteroid oxidoreductase type 1 (E.C. 1.1.1.62) as a possible target for the action of phytoestrogens. *Proc Soc Exp Biol Med* 208:51–59, 1995.

Makova, KD, Patton JC, Krysanov EY, et al: Microsatellite markers in wood mouse and striped field mouse (genus *Apodemus*). *Mol Ecol* 7:247–255, 1998.

Marwood TM, Knoke K, Yau K, et al: Comparison of toxicity detected by five bioassays during bioremediation of diesel fuel-spiked soil. *Environ Toxic Water Qual* 13:117–226, 1998.

Masuda Y, Kagawa R, Kuroki H, et al: Transfer of various polychlorinated biphenyls to the foetuses and offspring of mice. *Food Cosmet Toxicol* 17(6):623–627, 1979.

Matson CW, Rodgers RE, Chesser RK, Baker RJ: Genetic diversity of *Clethrionomys glareolus* populations from highly contaminated sites in the Chernobyl region. *Environ Toxicol Chem* 19:2130–2135, 2000.

Matter JM, Sills C, Anthony AB, Dickerson RL: Development and implementation of endocrine biomarkers of exposure and effects in American alligators (*Alligator mississippiensis*). *Organohalogen Comp* 29:28–32, 1998.

Maughan JT: *Ecological Assessment of Hazardous Waste Sites.* New York: Van Nostrand Reinhold, 1993.

McBee K, Bickham JW: Mammals as bioindicators of environmental toxicology, in Genoways HH (ed): *Current Mammalogy.* Vol 2. New York: Plenum Press, 1990, pp 17–88.

McBee K, Bickham JW, Brown KW, Donnelly KC: Chromosomal aberrations in native small mammals (*Peromyscus leucopus* and *Sigmodon hispidus*) at a petrochemical waste disposal site. 1. Standard karyology. *Arch Environ Contam Toxicol* 16:681–688, 1987.

McCarty JP, Secord AL: Reproductive ecology of tree swallows (*Tachycineta bicolor*) with high levels of polychlorinated biphenyl contamination. *Environ Toxicol Chem* 18:1433–1439, 1999.

McEwen LC, Brown LC: Acute toxicity of dieldrin and malathion to wild sharptailed grouse. *J Wildl Mgt* 30:604–611, 1966.

McKim JM, Eaton JG, Holcombe GW: Metal toxicity to embryos and larvae of eight species of freshwater fish. II: Copper. *Bull Environ Contam Toxicol* 19:608–616, 1978.

McMurry ST, Lochmiller RL, Chandra SAM, Qualls CW Jr: Sensitivity of selected immunological, hematological, and reproductive parameters in the cotton rat (*Sigmodon hispidus*) to subchronic lead exposure. *J Wildl Dis* 31:193–204, 1995.

Melancon MJ: Bioindicators used in aquatic and terrestrial monitoring, in Hoffman DJ, Rattner BA, Burton GA Jr, Cairns J Jr (eds): *Handbook of Ecotoxicology.* Boca Raton, FL: Lewis Publishers, 1995, pp 220–240.

Mellott RS, Woods PE: An improved ligature technique for dietary sampling in nestling birds. *J Field Ornithol* 64:205–210, 1993.

Mendelssohn H: Mass mortality of birds of prey caused by azodrin, an organophosphorus insecticide. *Biol Conservat* 11:163–170, 1977.

Menzer RE, Lewis MA, Fairbrother A: Methods in environmental toxicology, in Hayes AW (ed): *Principles and Methods of Toxicology,* 3d ed. New York: Raven, 1994.

Miller EC, Miller JA: Mechanisms of chemical carcinogenesis. *Cancer* 47:1055–1064, 1981.

Mineau P (ed): *Cholinesterase Inhibiting Insecticides: Their Impact on Wildlife and the Environment.* New York: Elsevier, 1991.

Mocarelli P, Needham LL, Marocchi A, et al: Serum concentrations of 2,3,78-tetrachlorodibenzo-*p*-dioxin and test results from selected residents of Seveso, Italy. *J Toxicol Environ Health* 32(4):357–366, 1991.

Montz WE Jr, Kirkpatrick RL: Effects of cold temperatures on acute mortality of *Peromyscus leucopus* dosed with parathion. *Bull Environ Contam Toxicol* 35:375–379, 1985.

Moore ID, Timer AK, Wilson JP, et al: GIS and land-surface-subsurface process modeling, in Goodchild MR, Parks BO, Steyaert IT (eds): *Environmental Modeling with GIS.* New York: Oxford University Press, 1993, pp 198–230.

Morand P, Briand X: Excessive growth of macroalgae: A symptom of environmental disturbance. *Bot Mar* 39:491–516, 1996.

Moriarty F: *Ecotoxicology: The Study of Pollutants in Ecosystems,* 2d ed. New York: Academic Press, 1988.

Mount DI, Stephen CE: A method for establishing acceptable limits for fish—malathion and the butoxy-ethanol ester of 2,4 D. *Trans Am Fish Soc* 96:185–193, 1967.

Murray RW (ed): Application reviews. *J Anal Chem* 1991 and 1993.

National Academy of Sciences (NAS): *Ecological Knowledge and Environmental Problem Solving. Concepts and Case Studies.* Washington, DC: National Academy Press, 1986.

National Academy of Sciences (NAS): *Principles for Evaluating Chemicals in the Environment.* Washington, DC: National Academy Press, 1975.

National Research Council (NRC): *Testing for Effects of Chemicals on Ecosystems.* Washington, DC: National Academy Press, 1981.

Nims RW, Lubet RA, Fox SD, et al: Comparative pharmacodynamics of CYP2B induction by DDT, DDE, and DDD in male rat liver and cultured rat hepatocytes. *J Toxicol Environ Health* 53:455–477, 1998.

Nisbet IC, Fry DM, Hatch JJ, Lynn B: Feminization of male common tern embryos is not correlated with exposure to specific PCB congeners. *Bull Environ Contam Toxicol* 57:895–901, 1996.

Norberg-King T, Mount DI: *Validity of Effluent and Ambient Toxicity Tests for Predicting Biological Impact, Skeleton Creek, Enid, Oklahoma.* EPA/600/30-85/044. Duluth, MN: Duluth Environmental Research Laboratory, 1986.

Norrgren L, Wicklund GA, Malmborg O: Accumulation and effects of aluminum in the minnow (*Phoxinus phoxinus L.*) at different pH levels. *J Fish Biol* 39:833–847, 1991.

Norris DO: *Vertebrate Endocrinology.* San Diego, CA: Academic Press, 1997.

Odin M, Feurtet-Mazel A, Ribeyre F, Boudou A: Actions and interactions of temperature, pH and photoperiod on mercury bioaccumulation by nymphs of the burrowing mayfly *Hexagenia rigida,* from the sediment contamination source. *Environ Toxicol Chem* 13:1291–1302, 1994.

Odum EP: *Basic Ecology.* New York: Saunders College Publishing, 1983.

Ojasoo T, Vannier B, Pasqualini JR: *Effect of Prenatally Administered Sex Steroids and Their Antagonists on the Hormonal Responses of Offspring in Humans and Animals.* New York: Marcel Dekker, 1992.

Okahima F, Akbar M, Abdul Majid M, et al: Genistein, an inhibitor of protein tyrosine kinase, is also a competitive antagonist for P1-purinergic (adenosine) receptor in FRTL-5 thyroid cells. *Biochem Biophys Res Commun* 203:1488–1495, 1994.

Olsen SC, Atluru D, Erickson HH, Ames TR: Role of the tyrosine kinase inhibitor, genistein, in equine mononuclear cell proliferation and leukotriene B-4 synthesis. *Biochem Arch* 10:11–16, 1994.

Ott W, Wallace L, Mage D, et al: The Environmental Protection Agency's research program on total human exposure. *Environ Int* 12:475–494, 1986.

Paller MH, Reichert MJM, Dean JM: Use of fish communities to assess environmental impacts in South Carolina Coastal Plain streams. *Trans Am Fish Soc* 125:633–644, 1996.

Parkhurst BR, Warren-Hicks W, Etchison T, et al: *Methodology for Aquatic Ecological Risk Assessment.* RP91-AER, Final Report. Alexandria, VA: Water Environment Research Foundation, 1995.

Pelley J: Is coastal eutrophication out of control? *Environ Sci Technol* 32:462A–466, 1998.

Peterle TJ: *Wildlife Toxicology.* New York: Van Nostrand Reinhold, 1991.

Peterle TJ, Bentley R: Effects of a low OP dose on seed/bead discrimination in the kangaroo rat, *Diopodomys. Bull Environ Contain Toxicol* 43:95–100, 1989.

Pfleeger T, McFarlane JC, Sherman R, Volk G: A short-term bioassay for whole plant toxicity, in Gorsuch JW, Lower WR, Lewis MA, Wang W (eds): *Plants for Toxicity Assessment.* Publ. 04-011150-16. Philadelphia: American Society for Testing and Materials, 1991, pp 355–364.

Pignatello JJ, Ferrandino FJ, Huang LQ: Elution of aged and freshly added herbicides from soil. *Environ Sci Technol* 27:1563–1571, 1993.

Piontek M, Hengels KJ, Proschen R, Strohmeyer G: Antiproliferative effect of tyrosine kinase inhibitors in epidermal growth factor-stimulated growth of human gastric cells. *Anticancer Res* 13:2119–2123, 1993.

Pomeroy SE, Barrett GW: Dynamics of enclosed small mammal populations in relation to an experimental pesticide application. *Am Midl Natur* 93:91–106, 1975.

Preston BL, Cecchine G, Snell TW: Effects of pentachlorophenol on predator avoidance behavior of the rotifer *Brachionus calyciflorus. Aquat Toxicol* 44:201–212, 1999.

Pritchard JB: Aquatic toxicology—Past, present, and prospects. *Environ Health Perspect* 100:249–257, 1993.

Rao JY, Apple SK, Hemstreet GP, et al: Single cell multiple biomarker analysis in archival breast fine-needle aspiration specimens: Quantitative fluorescence image analysis of DNA content, p53, and G-actin as breast cancer biomarkers. *Cancer Epidemiol Biomarkers Prev* 7(1):1027–1033, 1998.

Rask M: Changes in the density, population structure, growth and reproduction of perch, *Perca fluviatilis L,* in two acidic forest lakes in southern Finland. *Environ Pollut* 78:121–125, 1992.

Ratcliffe DA: Decrease in eggshell weight in certain birds of prey. *Nature* 215(5097):208–210, 1967.

Ratsch H: *Interlaboratory Root Elongation Testing of Toxic Substances on Selected Plant Species*. NTIS, PB 83-226. Washington, DC: Environmental Protection Agency, 1983.

Rattner BA, Eroschenko VP, Fox GA, et al: Avian endocrine responses to environmental pollution. *J Exp Zool* 232:683–689, 1984.

Rattner BA, Franson JC: Methyl parathion and fenvalerate toxicity in American kestrels: Acute physiological responses and effects of cold. *Can J Physiol Pharmacol* 62:787–792, 1984.

Rattner BA, Hoffman DJ, Marn CM: Use of mixed-function oxygenases to monitor contaminant exposure in wildlife. *Environ Contam Toxicol* 8:1093–1102, 1989.

Rhen T, Willingham E, Sakata JT, Crews D: Incubation temperatures influence sex-steroid levels in juvenile red-eared slider turtles, *Trachemys scripta,* a species with temperature dependent sex determination. *Biol Reprod* 61:1275–1280, 1999.

Robinson J, Avenant-Oldewage A: Chromium, copper, iron and manganese bioaccumulation in some organs and tissues of *Oreochromis mossambicus* from the lower Olifants River, inside the Kruger National Park. *Water, Air, Soil Pollut* 23:387–403, 1997.

Rodgers BE, Baker RJ: Frequencies of micronuclei in bank voles from zones of high radiation at Chernobyl. *Environ Toxicol Chem* 1644–1648, 2000.

Rodgers DW, Schroeder J, Vereecken Sheehan L: Comparison of *Daphnia magna,* rainbow trout and bacterial-based toxicity tests of Ontario Hydro aquatic effluents. *Water Air Soil Pollut* 90:105–112, 1996.

Roesijadi G: Metallothioneins in metal regulation and toxicity in aquatic animals. *Aquat Toxicol* 22:81–114, 1992.

Rosene W Jr, Lay DW. Disappearance and visibility of quail remains. *J Wildl Mgt* 27:139–142, 1963.

Rowley MH, Christian JJ, Basu DK, et al: Use of small mammals (voles) to assess a hazardous waste site at Love Canal, Niagara Falls, New York. *Arch Environ Contam Toxicol* 12:383–397, 1983.

Sanders BM: Stress proteins in aquatic organisms: an environmental perspective. *Crit Rev Toxicol* 23:49–75, 1993.

Sathe SS: A Model to Predict Exposure of Wildlife to Contaminants from an Industrial Point Source. M.S. Thesis, Department of Environmental Toxicology. Clemson, SC: Clemson University, 1997.

Schreiber RW, DeLong RL: Brown pelican status in California. *Audubon Field Notes* 23:57–59, 1969.

Scott, ML: Effects of PCBs, DDT and mercury compounds in chickens and Japanese quail. *Fed Proc* 36:1888–1893, 1977.

Shaw GG: Organochlorine pesticide and PCB residues in eggs and nestlings of tree swallows, *Tachycineta bicolor,* in central Alberta. *Can Field Natur* 98:258–260, 1984.

Shaw JL, Kennedy JH: The use of aquatic field mesocosm studies in risk assessment. *Environ Toxicol Chem* 15:605–607, 1996.

Sheehan DM, Branham WS: Dissociation of estrogen-induced growth and ornithine decarboxylase activity in the postnatal rat. *Teratogenesis Carcinog Mutagen* 7:411–22, 1987.

Sheehan DM, Branham WS, Medlock KL, Shanmugsundaram ER: Estrogenic activity of zearalenone and zearalanol in the neonatal rat uterus. *Teratology* 29:383–392, 1984.

Sheehan DM, Young M: Diethylstilbestrol and estradiol binding to serum albumin and pregnancy plasma of rat and human. *Endocrinology* 104:1442–1446, 1979.

Shibutani S, Margulis LA, Geacintov NE, Grolman AP: Translesional synthesis on a DNA template containing a single stereoisomer of dG-(+) or dG-(−)-anti BPDE (7,8-dihydroxy-anti-9,10-epoxy-7,8,9,10-tetrahydrobenzo[*a*]pyrene. *Biochemistry* 32(29):7531–7541, 1993.

Shonnard DR, Bell RL, Jackman AP: Effects of nonlinear sorption on the diffusion of benzene and dichloromethane from two air-dry soils. *Environ Sci Technol* 27(3):457–465, 1993.

Shugart LR, Theodorakis CW: Environmental genotoxicity: Probing the underlying mechanisms. *Environ Health Perspect* 102(suppl 12):13–17, 1994.

Siniff DB, Jessen CR: A simulation model of animal movement patterns. *Adv Ecol Res* 6:185–219, 1969.

Sleiderink HM, Beyer J, Everaarts JM, Boon J: Influence of temperature on cytochrome P450 1A in dab (*Limanda limanda*) from the southern North Sea: Results from field surveys. *Mar Environ Res* 39:67–71, 1995.

Smith AH, Sciortino S, Goeden H, Wright CC: Consideration of background exposures in the management of hazardous waste sites: A new approach to risk assessment. *Risk Anal* 16(5):619–625, 1996.

Smith GJ: *Pesticide Use and Toxicology in Relation to Wildlife. Organophosphates and Carbamate Compounds*. Resource Publ. 170. Washington, DC: U.S. Dept of the Interior, Fish and Wildlife Service, 1987.

Smith GM, Weis JS: Predator-prey relationships in mummichogs (*Fundulus heteroclitus* L): Effects of living in a polluted environment. *J Exp Mar Biol Ecol* 209:75–87, 1997.

Snyder RL: Effects of dieldrin on homing and orientation in deer mice. *J Wildl Mgt* 38:362–364, 1974.

Society of Environmental Toxicology and Chemistry SETAC Foundation for Education: Report of the aquatic risk assessment and mitigation dialogue group for pesticides. Pensacola, FL: SETAC, 1994.

Solomon KR, Baker DB, Richards RP, et al: Ecological risk assessment of atrazine in North American surface waters. *Environ Toxicol Chem* 15:31–76, 1996.

Stanley TR Jr, Spann JW, Smith GJ, Rosscoe R: Main and interactive effects of arsenic and selenium on mallard reproduction and duckling growth and survival. *Arch Environ Contam Toxicol* 26:444–451, 1994.

Stay FS, Jarvinen AW: Use of microcosm and fish toxicity data to select mesocosm treatment concentrations. *Arch Environ Contam Toxicol* 28:451–458, 1995.

Steinert SA, Streib-Montee R, Leather JM, Chadwick DB: DNA damage in mussels at sites in San Diego Bay. *Mutat Res* 399:65–85, 1998.

Stendell RC, Beyer WN, Stelm RH: Accumulation of lead and organochlorine residues in captive American kestrels fed pine volestrom apple orchards. *J Wildl Dis* 25:388–391, 1989.

Stewart AJ: Ambient bioassays for assessing water-quality conditions in receiving streams. *Ecotoxicology* 5:377–393, 1996.

Suter GW II: *Ecological Risk Assessment*. Chelsea, MI: Lewis, 1993.

Teh SJ, Adams SM, Hinton DE: Histopathologic biomarkers in feral freshwater fish populations exposed to different types of contaminant stress. *Aquat Toxicol* 37:51–70, 1997.

Theodorakis CW, Bickham JW, Elbl T, et al:Genetics of radionuclide-contaminated mosquitofish populations and homology between *Gambusia affinis* and *G. holbrooki. Environ Toxicol Chem* 17(10):1992–1998, 1998.

Theodorakis CW, Blaylock BG, Shugart LR: Genetic ecotoxicology: I. DNA integrity and reproduction in mosquitofish exposed in situ to radionuclides. *Ecotoxicology* 5:1–14, 1996.

Theodorakis CW, D'Surney SJ, Bickham JW, et al: Sequential expression of biomarkers in bluegill sunfish exposed to contaminated sediment. *Ecotoxicology* 1:45–73, 1992.

Thibodeaux LJ: *Environmental Chemodynamics. Movement of Chemicals in Air, Water, and Soil*. New York: Wiley, 1996.

Tinsley IJ: *Chemical Concepts in Pollutant Behavior*. New York: Wiley, 1979.

Trapp S, McFarlane C, Matthies M: Model for uptake of xenobiotics into plants: Validation with bromacil experiments. *Environ Toxicol Chem* 13:413–422, 1994.

Truhaut R: Ecotoxicology: objectives, principles and perspectives. *Ecotoxicol Environ Saf* 1:151–173, 1977.

Tyler JA, Rose KA: Individual variability and spatial heterogeneity in fish population models. *Rev Fish Biol Fish* 4:91–123, 1994.

U.S. EPA: *A User's Guide for the CALPUFF Dispersion Model*. EPA-454/B-95-006. Washington, DC: U.S. EPA, 1995a.

U.S. EPA: *Carbofuran Special Review Technical Support Document*. 540/09-89/027, Washington, DC: U.S. EPA, 1989.

U.S. EPA: *Final Report. Pesticide Assessment Guidelines, Subdivision*

E-Hazard Evaluation: Wildlife and Aquatic Organisms. EPA/540/9-82/024. Washington, DC: U.S. EPA, 1982.

U.S. EPA: *Guidelines for Ecological Risk Assessment*. EPA/630/R-95/002Fa, Washington, DC: U.S. EPA, 1998.

U.S. EPA: *Methods for Aquatic Toxicity Identification Evaluations: Phase II. Toxicity Identification Procedures for Samples Exhibiting Acute and Chronic Toxicity*. EPA-600/r92/081. Washington, DC: U.S. EPA, 1993.

U.S. EPA: *Methods for Estimating the Chronic Toxicity of Effluents and Receiving Waters to Freshwater Organisms*. EPA-600/4-89-001. Cincinnati, OH: Environmental Monitoring Systems Laboratory, 1989.

U.S. EPA: *Methods for Measuring the Acute Toxicity of Effluents to Aquatic Organisms*. EPA-600/4-90-027. Cincinnati, OH: Office of Research and Development, 1991a.

U.S. EPA: *Quality Criteria for Water*. Appendix A. EPA 440/5-86-0001, Washington, DC: U.S. EPA Office of Water Regulation and Standards, 1986a.

U.S. EPA: *Risk Assessment Forum: Framework for Ecological Risk Assessment*. EPA/630/R-92/001. Washington, DC: U.S. EPA, 1992a.

U.S. EPA: *Screening Procedures for Estimating the Air Quality Impact of Stationary Sources*. Revised. EPA-454/R-92-019. Washington, DC: U.S. EPA, 1992b.

U.S. EPA: *Technical Support Document for Water Quality-Based Toxics Control*. EPA-505-2-90-001. Washington, DC: U.S. EPA, 1991b.

U.S. EPA: *Test Methods for Evaluating Solid Waste,* 3d ed. Vol 1C. *Laboratory Manual Physical/Chemical Methods*. SW846. Washington, DC: U.S. EPA, 1986b.

U.S. EPA: *User's Guide for the Industrial Source Complex (ISC2) Dispersion Models: User Instructions*. Vol 1. EPA-450/4-92-008a, Washington, DC: U.S. EPA, 1992c.

U.S. EPA: *User's Guide for the Industrial Source Complex (ISC3) Dispersion Models*. Vols. I-III. EPA-454/B-95-003a-c. Washington, DC: U.S. EPA, 1995b.

Van Beneden RJ, Gardner GR, Blake NJ, Blair DG: Implications for the presence of transforming genes in gonadal tumors in two bivalve mollusk species. *Cancer Res* 53:2976–2979, 1993.

Van Der Kraak GJ, Munkittrick KR, McMaster ME, et al: Exposure to bleached kraft pulp mill effluent disrupts the pituitary gonadal-axis of white sucker at multiple sites. *Toxicol Appl Pharmacol* 115:224–233, 1992.

Van der Oost R, Goksoeyr A, Celander M, et al: Biomonitoring of aquatic pollution with feral eel (*Anguilla anguilla*). 2. Biomarkers: Pollution-induced biochemical responses. *Aquat Toxicol* 36:189–222, 1996b.

Van der Oost R, Opperhuizen A, Satumalay K, et al: Biomonitoring aquatic pollution with feral eel (*Anguilla anguilla*). 1. Bioaccumulation: Biota-sediment ratios of PCBs, OCPs, PCDDs and PCDFs. *Aquat Toxicol* 35:21–46, 1996a.

van Wezel AP, Jonker MTO: Use of the lethal body burden in the risk quantification of field sediments, influence of temperature and salinity. *Aquat Toxicol* 42:287–300, 1998.

Vuori KM, Parkko M: Assessing pollution of the river Kymijoki via hydropsychid caddisflies: Population age structure, microdistribution and gill abnormalities in the *Cheumatopsyche lepida* and *Hydropsyche pellucidula* larvae. *Arch Hydrobiol* 136:171–190, 1996.

Vyas NB, Kuenzel WJ, Hill EF, Sauer JR: Acephate affects migratory orientation of the white-throated sparrow (*Zonotrichia albicollis*). *Environ Toxic Chem* 14(11):1961–1965, 1995.

Wade TL, Sericano JL, Gardinali PR, et al: NOAA's "Mussel Watch" project: Current use organic compounds in bivalves. *Mar Pollut Bull* 37:20–26, 1999.

Wang W: The use of plant seeds in toxicity tests of phenolic compounds. *Environ Int* 11:49–55, 1985.

Ward JB Jr, Ammenheuser MM, Whorton EB Jr, et al: Biological monitoring for mutagenic effects of occupational exposure to butadiene. *Toxicology* 113(1-3):84–90, 1996.

Wark K, Warner C: *Air Pollution: Its Origin and Control*. New York: Harper & Row, 1981, pp 69–73.

Warren-Hicks W, Parkhurst BR, Baker SS: *Ecological Assessments of Hazardous Waste Sites*. A Field and Laboratory Reference Document. EPA/600/3-89/01. Washington, DC: Environmental Protection Agency, 1989.

Watson AP, Van Hook RI, Jackson DR, Reichle DE: Impact of a lead mining-smelting complex on a forest-floor fitter arthropod fauna in the new lead belt region of southeast Missouri. ORNL/NSF/EATC-30. Oak Ridge, TN: Oak Ridge National Laboratory, 1976.

Weis CP, LaVelle JM: Characteristics to consider when choosing an animal model for the study of lead bioavailability. *Sci Technol Lett* 3:113–119, 1991.

Weis CP, Poppenga RH, Thacker BJ, Henningsen GM: Design of pharmacokinetic and bioavailability studies of lead in an immature swine model, in Beard ME, Iske SA (eds): *Lead in Paint, Soil, and Dust: Health Risks, Exposure Studies, Control Measures, Measurement Methods, and Quality Assurance*. ASTM STP 1226. Philadelphia, American Society for Testing and Materials, pp 19103–19187, 1994.

Weis JS, Weis P, Heber M: Variation in response to methylmercury by killifish (*Fundulus heteroclitus*) embryos, in Pearson JG, Foster R, Bishop WE (eds): *Aquatic Toxicology and Risk Assessment: 5th Conference* ASTM S.T.P. 7760. Philadelphia: American Society for Testing and Materials, 1982.

Welsh HH Jr, Ollivier LM: Stream amphibians as indicators of ecosystem stress: A case study from California's redwoods. *Ecol Appl* 8:1118–1132, 1998.

Weseloh DV, Struger J, Hebert C: White Peking ducks (*Anas platyrhynchos*) as monitors of organochlorine and metal contamination in the Great Lakes. *J Great Lakes Res* 20:277–288, 1994.

Whitten Pl, Lewis C, Russell E, Naftolin F: Potential adverse effects of phytoestrogens. *J Nutr* 125:771S–776S, 1995.

Wiemeyer SN, Scott JM, Anderson MP, et al: Environmental contaminants in California condors. *J Wildl Mgt* 52:238–247, 1988.

Willard WW, Merritt LL, Dean JA, Settle FA: *Instrumental Methods of Analysis,* 7th ed. Belmont, CA: Wadsworth, 1988.

Willette M: Impacts of the *Exxon Valdez* oil spill on the migration, growth, and survival of juvenile pink salmon in Prince William Sound. *Am Fish Soc Symp* 18:533–550, 1996.

Wirgin I, Waldman JR: Altered gene expression and genetic damage in North American fish populations. *Mutat Res* 99:193–219, 1998.

Wolff WF: An individual-oriented model of a wading bird nesting colony. *Ecol Mod* 72:75–114, 1994.

Wurster CF, Wingate DB: DDT residues and declining reproduction in the Bermuda petrel. *Science* 159(3818):979–981, 1968.

UNIT 7

APPLICATIONS OF TOXICOLOGY

CHAPTER 30

FOOD TOXICOLOGY

Frank N. Kotsonis, George A. Burdock, and W. Gary Flamm

INTRODUCTION TO FOOD TOXICOLOGY

This chapter describes the general principles of food toxicology and explains how those principles have been shaped by existing food laws and applied to the safety assessment of foods, food ingredients, and food contaminants. Food toxicology is different from other subspecialties in toxicology largely because of the nature and chemical complexity of food. The necessity for practical and workable approaches to the assessment of food safety is addressed throughout the chapter.

The typical western diet contains hundreds of thousands of substances naturally present in food and many more which form in situ when food is cooked or prepared. Many of these substances affect the nutritional and esthetic qualities of food, including appearance and organoleptic properties (i.e., conferring flavor, texture, or aroma) that determine whether or not we will even try the food or take a second bite, respectively. While these or other substances present in food may be nutritional and/or gratifying, they may not necessarily be "safe" in *any* amount or for *any* intended use. The Federal Food, Drug and Cosmetic (FD&C) Act gives the federal government the authority to ensure that all food involved in interstate commerce is safe. Congress, in writing the FD&C Act (and its subsequent amendments), understood that safety cannot be proved absolutely and indicated instead that the safety standard for substances added to food can be no more than a reasonable certainty that no harm will occur. As pointed out in other sections of this chapter, the language of the FD&C Act effectively provides for practical and workable approaches to the assessment of safety for food, food ingredients, and food contaminants. Because food is highly complex, the legal framework provided by Congress for the regulation of food and substances in food was kept simple so that it would work. The basic element of the framework is that food, which is defined as articles or components of articles used for food or drink for humans or animals, bears the presumption of safety [sections 201(f) and 402(a)(1) of the FD&C Act]. This means that a steak or a potato is presumed to be safe unless it contains a poisonous or deleterious substance in an amount shown to make it *ordinarily injurious* to health. In essence, this presumption of safety was born of necessity. If the hundreds of thousands of substances naturally present in food were subject to the same strictures and limitations that apply to added substances, food shortages could easily result. To avoid such crises, Congress developed a safety standard that would not force regulatory authorities to ban common, traditional foods.

In cases where the substance is not naturally present in food but is a contaminant or added ingredient, the safety standard is quite different. This standard decrees a food to be adulterated if it contains any poisonous or deleterious substance that *may render it injurious.* Therefore, the presence of a substance that is not a *natural* component of a food demands a far higher standard of safety. The mere possibility that such a substance *may* render the food injurious to health is sufficient to ban the food containing that substance. Thus, for additives and contaminants, Congress recognized that these substances are not as complex as food and must, therefore, meet a higher standard of safety.

An understanding of the term *safe* is necessary in deciding how many and what types of studies must be conducted to determine that an added substance is safe. Wisely, the act does not give explicit instructions about how safety should be determined and does not explicitly define safety. Because neither the law nor the U.S. Food and Drug Administration (FDA) or the U.S. Department of Agriculture (USDA) regulations explicitly define the term *safety* for substances added to food, scientists and their legal and regulatory counterparts have worked out operational definitions for the safety of food ingredients. The one principle on which there has been nearly unanimous agreement is that safety concerns in regard to an added substance should focus on both the nature of the substance *and* its intended conditions of use. It is recognized that substances are not inherently unsafe, it is only the quantity at which they are presented in the diet that makes them unsafe. The quantity (or "level") present in the diet is determined by the intended conditions of use and limitations of use of the substance.

As with food, practical and workable solutions must be found for the constituents of additives, because all substances contain a myriad of impurities at trace and even undetectable levels. Decisions concerning the safety of impurities and the development of appropriate specifications for food and color additives to assure that they are of suitable purity must similarly constitute a workable approach. In this case, the workable approach involves setting specification limits on contaminants—limits that are intended to exclude the possibility that the level of contaminants present in an additive *may* render the food to which the substance is added unsafe. As a practical matter and because of time and cost considerations, established specifications must be relatively simple and straightforward and must provide reasonable assurance that an ingredient is of suitable purity for its intended conditions of use. However, it generally is not necessary or practical to require extensive analysis and identification of all individual impurities to establish the fact that a substance is of "food-grade purity." It should be emphasized that specifications can serve their purpose of assuring suitable purity only if the manufacturing processes used are adequately controlled to assure consistency in the quality and purity of the product. It should be understood that the philosophy by which specifications are established for substances added to food embodies the belief that not all risks are worthy of regulatory concern and control. Implicit in this philosophy is the concept of *threshold of regulation,* which is an important unifying concept in food safety assessment (Flamm et al., 1994).

To understand the meaning in the FD&C Act of the phrase "safe for intended conditions of use" as applied to a substance added to food, it is important to recognize that such a determination must rest on a general understanding of the risks posed by food itself. The requirement that substances added to food be safe (to a reasonable degree of certainty) demands consideration of the far higher theoretical risk posed by food itself. Food, as stated earlier, contains hundreds of thousands of substances, most of which have not been fully characterized or tested. The presumption that a food is safe is based on a history of common use and on the fact that the consumption of certain foods is deeply rooted in tradition (e.g., "ethnic" foods or those foods traditionally consumed for a holiday celebration). When the uncertainty about the risk of the added substance is small compared with the uncertainties attending food itself, the standard of "reasonable certainty of no harm" for the added substance has been satisfied. Thus, for food-like substances, the presumption is that the substance resembles food, is digested and metabolized as food, and consequently raises fewer toxicologic and safety-related questions than do substances that are not food-like. And such substances are added either directly or indirectly (substances that may migrate into food from packaging or other food contact surfaces) to foods in only very small or trace amounts, the low levels of exposure aid in demonstrating that the intended conditions of use of these substances are safe. These broad generalizations, however, do not suffice to exempt these food ingredients from the requirements of thorough safety testing. The FDA requires that such testing be done but it is tempered by considerations of (1) the basic nature of the substance, (2) the level to which consumers will be exposed as the result of the intended use, and (3) the inherent safety of food and constituents of food.

Over the past several years, there has been increasing interest on the part of consumers in the health-enhancing properties of foods and the components they contain. Substances such as phytosterols from vegetable oils and isoflavones from soy have been isolated and added to other foods at elevated levels to impart cholesterol-lowering abilities. Such products have raised regulatory questions about whether these substances are functioning as drugs and should be regulated as such or whether they should be viewed as new nutrients and allowed in foods, as are vitamin C and iron. At a recent conference, experts in nutritional science concluded that the concept of nutrients should be expanded to include a growing number of desirable food constituents that produce quantifiable health benefits related to disease prevention (Sansalone, 1999). This isolation of new food components and their use in fortifying food products will necessitate a thorough evaluation of safety at the intended level of intake and for the population at large.

Finally, it should be recognized that in most of the world, microbiologic contamination of food represents by far the greatest food-borne risk facing consumers. Thus, while vigilance in assuring the safety of substances added to food under their intended conditions of use is appropriate, we should not lose sight of the major concern of food safety.

Uniqueness of Food Toxicology

The nature of food is responsible for the uniqueness of food toxicology. Food is not only essential to all life but also a major contributor to the quality of life. Food and drink are enjoyed for their appearance, aroma, flavor, and texture. They are significant factors in defining cultures and societies. For example, ethnic foods and gourmet foods have a status that far exceeds their nutritional benefits, but any proposal to ban an ethnic food because new data have raised questions about its safety would be met with strong resistance.

As food occupies a position of central importance in virtually all cultures and because most food cannot be commercially produced in a definable environment under strict quality controls, food generally cannot meet the rigorous standards of chemical identity, purity, and good manufacturing practice met by most consumer products. The fact that food is harvested from the soil, the sea, or inland waters or is derived from land animals, which are subject to the unpredictable forces of nature, makes the constancy of raw food unreliable. Food in general is more complex and variable in composition than are all the other substances to which humans are exposed. However, there is nothing to which humans have greater exposure despite the uncertainty about its chemical identity, consistency, and purity. Experience has supported the safety of commonly consumed foods, and the good agricultural practices under which food is produced mandate the need for quality controls. Nevertheless, it is clear that food is held to a different standard as a practical matter dictated by necessity.

Food also acquires uniqueness from its essential nutrients, which, like vitamin A, may be toxic at levels only 10-fold above those required to prevent deficiencies. The evaluation of food ingredient substances often must rely on reasoning unique to food science in the sense that such substances may be normal constituents of food or modified constituents of food as opposed to the types of substances ordinarily addressed in the fields of occupational, environmental, and medical toxicology. Assessment of the safety of such substances, which are added to food for their technical effects, often focuses on digestion and metabolism occurring in the gastrointestinal (GI) tract. The reason for this focus is that in many cases an ingested substance is not absorbed through the GI tract; only products of its digestion are absorbed, and these products may be identical to those derived from natural food.

Nature and Complexity of Food

Food is an exceedingly complex mixture of nutrient and nonnutrient substances, whether it is consumed in the "natural" (unprocessed) form or as a highly processed ready-to-eat microwaveable meal (Table 30-1). Among the "nutrient" substances, the western diet consists of items of caloric and noncaloric value; that is, carbohydrates supply 47 percent of caloric intake, fats supply 37 percent, and protein supplies 16 percent (all three of which would be considered "macronutrients") (Technical Assessment Systems, Inc., 1992), whereas minerals and vitamins, the "micronutrients," obviously have no caloric value but are no less essential for life.

Nonnutrient substances are often characterized in the popular literature as being contributed by food processing, but nature provides the vast majority of nonnutrient constituents. For instance, in Table 30-2 one can see that even among "natural" (or minimally processed) foods, there are far more nonnutrient than nutrient constituents. Many of these nonnutrient substances are vital for the growth and survival of the plant, including hormones and naturally occurring pesticides (estimated at approximately 10,000 by Gold et al., 1992). Some of these substances may be antinutrient [e.g., goiterogens in *Brassica,* trypsin and/or chymotrypsin inhibitors in soybeans, phytates that may bind minerals (present in soybeans), and antihistamines in fish and plants] or even toxic (e.g., tomatine, cycasin) to humans. An idea of the large number of substances present in food is given in the series edited by Maarse and associates (1993), in which approximately 5500 volatile substances are noted as occurring in one or more of 246 different foods. However, this is only the tip of the iceberg, as the number of unidentified natural chemicals in food vastly exceed the number that have been identified (Miller, 1991).

Nonnutrient substances are also added as a result of processing, and in fact, 21 CFR 170.3(o) lists 32 categories of direct additives, of which there are about 3000 individual substances. Approximately 1800 of the 3000 are flavor ingredients, most of which

Table 30-1
Food as a Complex Mixture

NUTRIENTS	NONNUTRIENTS
Carbohydrates	Naturally occurring substances
Proteins	Food additives
Lipids	Contaminants
Minerals	Products of food processing
Vitamins	

SOURCE: Smith 1991, with permission.

Table 30-2
Nonnutrient Substances in Food

FOOD	NUMBER OF IDENTIFIED NONNUTRIENT CHEMICALS
Cheddar cheese	160
Orange juice	250
Banana	325
Tomato	350
Wine	475
Coffee	625
Beef (cooked)	625

SOURCE: Smith, 1991, with permission.

already occur naturally in food and are nonnutritive. Of the 1800 flavoring ingredients that may be added to food, approximately one-third are used at concentrations below 10 ppm (Hall and Oser, 1968), about the same concentration as is found naturally.

Importance of the Gastrointestinal Tract

It is essential to appreciate the fact that the gut is a large, complex, and dynamic organ with several layers of organization and a vast absorptive surface that has been estimated to be from 200 to 4500 m^2 (Concon, 1988). The GI transit time provides for adequate exposure of ingesta to a variety of environmental conditions (i.e., variable pH), digestive acids and enzymes (trypsin, chymotrypsin, etc., from the pancreas and carbohydrases, lipases, and proteases from the enterocytes), saponification agents (in bile), and a luxuriant bacterial flora providing a repertoire of metabolic capability not shared by the host (e.g., fermentation of "nondigestible" sugars such as xylitol and sorbitol) (Drasar and Hill, 1974). The enterocytes (intestinal epithelium) possess an extensive capacity for the metabolism of xenobiotics that may be second only to that of the liver, with a full complement of phase (type) I and phase (type) II reactions present. The enteric monooxygenase system is analogous to the liver, as both systems are located in the endoplasmic reticulum of cells, require reduced nicotinamide adenine dinucleotide phosphate (NADPH) and O_2 for maximum activity, are inhibited by SKF-525A and carbon monoxide, and are qualitatively similar in their response to enzyme induction (Hassing et al., 1989). Induction of xenobiotic metabolism by the enteric monooxygenase system has been demonstrated in a number of substances, including commonly eaten foods and their constituents (Table 30-3). Dietary factors may also decrease metabolic activity. For example, in one study, iron restriction and selenium deficiency decreased cytochrome P450 values, but a vitamin A rich diet had the same effect (Kaminsky and Fasco, 1991).

The constituents of food and other ingesta (e.g., drugs, contaminants, inhaled pollutants dissolved in saliva and swallowed) are physicochemically heterogeneous, and because the intestine has evolved into a relatively impermeable membrane, mechanisms of absorption have developed that allow substances to gain access to the body from the intestinal lumen. The four primary mechanisms for absorption are passive or simple diffusion, active transport, facilitated diffusion, and pinocytosis. Each of these mechanisms characteristically transfers a defined group of constituents from the lumen into the body (Table 30-4). As noted in the table, xenobiotics and other substances may compete for passage into the body.

Aiding this absorption is the rich vascularization of the intestine, with a normal rate of blood flow in the portal vein of approximately 1.2 L/h/kg. However, after a meal, there is a 30 percent increase in blood flow through the splanchnic area (Concon, 1988). It follows, then, that substances which affect blood flow also tend to affect the absorption of compounds; an example is alcohol, which tends to increase blood flow to the stomach and thus

Table 30-3
Induction of Xenobiotic Metabolism in the Rat Intestine

INDUCER	SUBSTRATE OR ENZYME	REFERENCE
Butylated hydroxyanisole benzo[*a*]pyrene	UDP-glucuronic acid	Goon and Klaassen, 1992
Benzo[*a*]pyrene, cigarette smoke, charcoal-broiled ground beef (vs. ground beef cooked on foil), Purina Rat Chow (vs. semisynthetic diet), chlorpromazine, chlorcyclizine	Phenacetin	Pantuck et al., 1974, 1975
Cabbage or brussels sprouts	Phenacetin, 7-ethoxycoumarin, hexobarbital	Pantuck et al., 1976
Ethanol	Benzo[*a*]pyrene	Van de Wiel et al., 1992
Indole-3-carbinol (present in brussels sprouts)	Pentoxy- and ethoxyresorufin, testosterone	Wortelboer et al., 1992b
Fried meat, dietary fat	7-Ethoxyresorufin *O*-deethylase	Kaminsky and Fasco, 1991
Brussels sprouts	Aryl hydrocarbon hydroxylase, 7-ethoxyresorufin *O*-deethylase	Kaminsky and Fasco, 1991
Brussels sprouts	Ethoxyresorufin deethylation, glutathione *S*-transferase, DT-diaphorase	Wortelboer et al., 1992a

Table 30-4
Systems Transporting Enteric Constituents

SYSTEM	ENTERIC CONSTITUENT
Passive diffusion	Sugars (e.g., fructose, mannose, xylose, which may also be transported by facilitated diffusion), lipid-soluble compounds, water
Facilitated diffusion	D-xylose, 6-deoxy-1,5-anhydro-D-glucitol, glutamic acid, aspartic acid, short-chain fatty acids, xenobiotics with carboxy groups, sulfates, glucuronide esters, lead, cadmium, zinc
Active transport	Cations, anions, sugars, vitamins, nucleosides (pyrimidines, uracil, and thymine, which may be in competition with 5-fluorouracil and 5-bromouracil), cobalt, manganese (which competes for the iron transportation system)
Pinocytosis	Long-chain lipids, vitamin B_{12} complex, azo dyes, maternal antibodies, botulinum toxin, hemagglutinins, phalloidins, *E. coli* endotoxins, virus particles.

enhances its own absorption. Few stimuli tend to decrease flow to this area, with the possible exception of energetic muscular activity and hypovolemic shock.

Lymph circulation is important in the transfer of fats, large molecules (such as botulinum toxin), benzo[*a*]pyrene, 3-methylcholanthrene, and *cis*-dimethylaminostilbene (Chhabra and Eastin, 1984). Lymph has a flow rate of about 1 to 2 mL/h/kg in humans, and few factors—with the exception of tripalmitin, which has been shown to double the flow and therefore double the absorption of *p*-aminosalicylic acid and tetracycline—are known to influence its flow (Chhabra and Eastin, 1984). Another factor that lends importance to lymph is the fact that the lymph empties via the thoracic duct into the point of junction of the left internal jugular and subclavian veins, preventing "first-pass" metabolism by the liver, unlike substances transported by the blood.

Many food ingredients are modified proteins, carbohydrates, fats, or components of such substances. Thus, an understanding of the changes these substances undergo in the GI tract, their possible effect on the GI tract, and whether they are absorbed or affect the absorption of other substances is critical to an understanding of food toxicology and safety assessment. Some of the factors that may affect GI absorption and the rate of absorption are listed in Table 30-5.

SAFETY STANDARDS FOR FOODS, FOOD INGREDIENTS, AND CONTAMINANTS

The Food, Drug and Cosmetics Act Provides for a Practicable Approach

The FD&C Act presumes that traditionally consumed foods are safe if they are free of contaminants. For the FDA to ban such foods, it must have clear evidence that death or illness can be traced to consumption of a particular food. The fact that foods contain many natural substances, some of which are toxic at a high concentration, is in itself an insufficient basis under the act for declaring a food as being unfit for human consumption. Examples of this concept include acceptance of generally recognized as safe status and the implementation of tolerances.

The Application of Experience: Generally Recognized as Safe (GRAS) The FD&C Act permits the addition of substances to food to accomplish a specific technical effect if the substance is determined to be GRAS by experts qualified by scientific training and experience to evaluate food safety. The FD&C Act does not require this determination be made by the FDA, though it does not

Table 30-5
Factors Affecting Intestinal Absorption and Rate of Absorption

FACTOR	EXAMPLE
Gastric emptying rate	Increased fat content
Gastric pH	Antacids, stress, H_2-receptor blockers
Intestinal motility	Diarrhea due to intercurrent disease, laxatives, dietary fiber, disaccharide intolerance, amaranth
Food content	Lectins of *Phaseolus vulgaris* (inhibition of glucose absorption and transport)
Surface area of small intestine	Short-bowel syndrome
Intestinal blood flow	Alcohol
Intestinal lymph flow	Tripalmitin
Enterohepatic circulation	Chlordecanone (prevented by cholestyramine)
Permeability of mucosa	Inflammatory bowel disease, celiac disease
Inhibition of digestive processes	Catechins of tea which inhibit sucrase and therefore glucose absorption
Concomitant drug therapy	Iron salts/tetracycline

SOURCE: Modified from Hoensch and Schwenk, 1984, with permission.

exclude the agency from making such decisions. The act instead requires that scientific experts base a GRAS determination on the adequacy of safety, as shown through scientific procedures or through experience based on common use in food before January 1, 1958, under the intended conditions of use of the substance [FD&C Act, section 201(s)].

In addition to allowing GRAS substances to be added to food, the act provides for a class of substances that are regulated food additives, which are defined as "any substances the intended use of which results in its becoming a component . . . of any food . . . if such substance is not generally recognized . . . to be safe." Hence, a legal distinction is drawn between regulated food additives and GRAS substances. Regulated food additives must be approved and regulated for their intended conditions of use by the FDA under 21 CFR 172–179 before they can be marketed. In section 409 of the act, the requirements for data to support the safe use of a food additive are described in general terms. The requirements or recommended methods for establishing safe conditions of use for an additive are available in the form of a guideline issued by FDA (*Toxicological Principles for the Safety Assessment of Direct Food Additives and Color Additives Used in Food*). These guidelines, referred to as "the Redbook," provide substance and definition to the safety standard applicable to regulated food additives: "reasonable certainty of no harm under conditions of intended use."

Use of Tolerances If a food contains an unavoidable contaminant even with the use of current good manufacturing practices (CGMP), it may be declared unfit as food if the contaminant may render the food injurious to health. Thus, for a food itself to be declared unfit, it must be ordinarily injurious, while an unavoidable contaminant in food need only pose the risk of harm for the food to be found unfit and subject to FDA action. The reason for the dichotomy is practicability. Congress recognized that if authority were granted to ban traditional foods for reasons that go beyond clear evidence of harm to health, the agency would be subject to pressure to ban certain foods.

Foods containing *unavoidable* contaminants are not automatically banned because such foods are subject to the provisions of section 406 of the FD&C Act, which indicates that the quantity of unavoidable contaminants in food may be limited by regulation for the protection of public health and that any quantity of a contaminant exceeding the fixed limit shall be deemed unsafe. This authority has been used by the FDA to set limits on the quantity of unavoidable contaminants in food by regulation (tolerances) or by informal action levels that do not have the force of law. Such action levels have been set for aflatoxin in peanuts, grain, and milk (Table 30-6). Action levels have the advantage of offering greater flexibility than is provided by tolerances established by regulation. Whether tolerances or action levels are applied to unavoidable contaminants of food, the FDA attempts to balance the health risk posed by unavoidable contaminants against the loss of a portion of the food supply. In contrast, contaminants in food that are *avoidable* by CGMP are deemed to be unsafe under section 406 if they are considered poisonous or deleterious. Under such circumstances, the food is typically declared *adulterated* and unfit for human consumption. The extent to which consumers who are already in possession of such food must be alerted depends on the health risk posed by the contaminated food. If there is a reasonable probability that the use of or exposure to such a food will cause serious adverse health consequences or death, the FDA will seek a class I recall which provides the maximum public warning, the greatest depth of recall, and the most follow-up. Classes II and III represent progressively less health risk and require less public warning, less depth of recall, and less follow-up (21 CFR 7.3).

Food and Color Additives

An intentionally added ingredient, not considered GRAS, is either a direct food additive or color additive. As with all ingredients intentionally added to food, there must be a specific and justifiable functionality. While a color additive has only one function, a food additive may have any one of 32 functionalities (Table 30-7).

The term *color additive* refers to a dye, pigment, or other substance made by a process of synthesis or extracted and isolated from a vegetable, animal, or mineral source [FD&C Act 201(t)]. Blacks, whites, and intermediate grays are also included in this definition. When such additives are added or applied to a food, drug, or cosmetic or to the human body, they are capable of imparting color. Color additives are not eligible for GRAS status.

Two distinct types of color additives have been approved for food use: those requiring certification by FDA chemists and those exempt from certification. Certification, which is based on chemical analysis, is required for each batch of most organic synthesized colors because they may contain impurities that may vary from batch to batch. Most certified colors approved for food use bear the prefix FD&C. They include FD&C Blue No. 1, FD&C Blue No. 2, FD&C Green No. 3, FD&C Red No. 3, FD&C Red No. 40, FD&C Yellow No. 5, and FD&C Yellow No. 6. Orange B and Citrus Red No. 2 are the only certified food colors that lack the FD&C designation (21 CFR 74 Subpart A).

The basis for the certification of these color additives is the finding that each batch is of suitable purity and can be safely used

Table 30-6
FDA Action Levels for Aflatoxins (Compliance Policy Guides 7120.26, 7106.10, and 7126.33)

COMMODITY	LEVEL, ng/g
All products, except milk, designated for humans	20
Milk	0.5
Corn for immature animals and dairy cattle	20
Corn for breeding beef cattle, swine, and mature poultry	100
Corn for finishing swine	200
Corn for finishing beef cattle	300
Cottonseed meal (as a feed ingredient)	300
All feedstuffs other than corn	20

Table 30-7
Direct Food Additives by Functionality

NUMBER	DESIGNATION	DESCRIPTION	EXAMPLES
170.3(o) (1)	Anticaking agents and free-flow agents	Substances added to finely powdered or crystalline food products to prevent caking, lumping, or agglomeration	Glucitol, sodium ferrocyanide, silicon dioxide
(2)	Antimicrobial agents	Substances used to preserve food by preventing growth of microorganisms and subsequent spoilage, including fungistats, mold, and rope inhibitors and the effects listed by the NAS/NRC under "preservatives"	Nisin; metyhyl-, ethyl-, propyl-, or butyl-ester of *p*-hydroxybenozoic acid; sodium benzoate; sorbic acid and its salts
(3)	Antioxidants	Substances used to preserve food by retarding deterioration, rancidity, or discoloration due to oxidation	Butylated hydroxyanisole (BHA), butylated hydroxytoluene (BHT), propyl gallate
(4)	Colors and coloring adjuncts	Substances used to impact, preserve, or enhance the color or shading of a food, including color stabilizers, color fixatives, color-retention agents	FD&C Yellow No. 5 (tartrazine), FD&C Red No. 4, β-carotene, annatto, turmeric
(5)	Curing and pickling agents	Substances imparting a unique flavor and/or color to a food, usually producing an increase in shelf life	Calcium chloride, glucitol
(6)	Dough strengtheners	Substances used to modify starch and gluten, producing a more stable dough, including the applicable effects listed by the NAS/NRC under "dough conditioners"	Calcium bromate, baker's yeast extract, calcium carbonate
(7)	Drying agents	Substances with moisture-absorbing ability used to maintain an environment of low moisture	Calcium stearate, cobalt caprylate, cobalt tallate
(8)	Emulsifiers and emulsifier salts	Substances that modify surface tension in the component phase of an emulsion to establish a uniform dispersion or emulsion	Phosphate esters of mono- and diglycerides, acetylated monoglycerides, calcium stearate
(9)	Enzymes	Enzymes used to improve food processing and the quality of the finished food	Papain, rennet, pepsin
(10)	Firming agents	Substances added to precipitate residual pectin, strengthening the supporting tissue and preventing its collapse during processing	Calcium acetate, calcium carbonate
(11)	Flavor enhancers	Substances added to supplement, enhance, or modify the original taste and/or aroma of a food without imparting a characteristic taste or aroma of their own	Monosodium glutamate, inositol
(12)	Flavor agents and adjuvants	Substances added to impart or help impart a taste or aroma in food	Cinnamon, citral, *p*-cresol, thymol, zingerone
(13)	Flour-treating agents	Substances added to milled flour at the mill to improve its color and/or baking qualities, including bleaching and maturing agents	Calcium bromate
(14)	Formulation aids	Substances used to promote or produce a desired physical state or texture in food, including carriers, binders, fillers, plasticizers, film formers, and tableting aids	Palm kernel oil, tallow

(continued)

Table 30-7 *(continued)*

NUMBER	DESIGNATION	DESCRIPTION	EXAMPLES
(15)	Fumigants	Volatile substances used for controlling insects or pests	Aluminum phosphide, potassium bromide
(16)	Humectants	Hygroscopic substances incorporated in food to promote retention of moisture, including moisture-retention agents and antidusting agents	Arabic gum, calcium chloride
(17)	Leavening agents	Substances used to produce or stimulate production of carbon dioxide in baked goods to impart a light texture, including yeast, yeast foods, and calcium salts listed by the NAS/NRC under "dough conditioners"	Carbon dioxide, adipic acid
(18)	Lubricants and release agents	Substances added to food contact surfaces to prevent ingredients and finished products from sticking to them	Mineral oil, acetylated monoglycerides
(19)	Nonnutritive sweeteners	Substances having less than 2 percent of the caloric value of sucrose per equivalent unit of sweetening capacity	Acesulfame, aspartame, saccharin
(20)	Nutrient supplements	Substances that are necessary for the body's nutritional and metabolic processes	Calcium carbonate
(21)	Nutritive sweeteners	Substances that have greater than 2 percent of the caloric value of sucrose per equivalent unit of sweetening capacity	Lactitol, hydrogenated starch hydrolysate
(22)	Oxidizing and reducing agents	Substances that chemically oxidize or reduce another food ingredient, producing a more stable product, including the applicable effects listed by the NAS/NRC under "dough conditioners"	Calcium peroxide, chloride, hydrogen peroxide
(23)	pH control agents	Substances added to change or maintain active acidity or basicity, including buffers, acids, alkalis, and neutralizing agents	Acetic acid, propionic acid, calcium acetate, calcium carbonate, carbon dioxide
(24)	Processing aids	Substances used as manufacturing aids to enhance the appeal or utility of a food or food component, including clarifying agents, clouding agents, catalysts, flocculents, filler aids, and crystallization inhibitors	Carbon dioxide, ammonium carbonate, ammonium sulfate, potassium bromide
(25)	Propellants, aerating agents, and gases	Gases used to supply force to expel a product or reduce the amount of oxygen in contact with the food in packaging	Carbon dioxide, nitrous oxide
(26)	Sequestrants	Substances that combine with polyvalent metal ions to form a soluble metal complex to improve the quality and stability of products	Acetate salts, citrate salts, gluconate salt, metaphosphate, edetic acid, calcium acetate
(27)	Solvents and vehicles	Substances used to extract or dissolve another substance	Acetic acid, acetylated monoglycerides
(28)	Stabilizers and thickeners	Substances used to produce viscous solutions or dispersions, to impart body, improve consistency, or stabilize emulsions, including suspending and bodying agents, setting agents, jellying agents, and bulking agents	Calcium acetate, calcium carbonate

(continued)

Table 30-7 *(continued)*

NUMBER	DESIGNATION	DESCRIPTION	EXAMPLES
(29)	Surface-active agents	Substances used to modify surface properties of liquid food components for a variety of effects other than emulsifiers but including solubilizing agents, dispersants, detergents, wetting agents, rehydration enhancers, whipping agents, foaming agents, and defoaming agents	Sorbitan monostearate, mono- and diglycerides, polysorbate 60, acetostearin
(30)	Surface-finishing agents	Substances used to increase palatability, preserve gloss, and inhibit discoloration of foods, including glazes, polishes, waxes, and protective coatings	Ammonium hydroxide, arabic gum
(31)	Synergists	Substances used to act or react with another food ingredient to produce a total effect different from or greater than the sum of the effects produced by the individual ingredients	Acetic acid, propionic acid
(32)	Texturizers	Substances that affect the appearance or feel of food	Calcium acetate

as prescribed by regulation (FD&C Act, section 721). Certification involves in-depth chemical analysis of major and trace components of each individual batch of color additives by FDA chemists and is required before any batch can be released for commercial use. Such color additives consist of aromatic amines or aromatic azo structures (FD&C Blue No. 1, FD&C Blue No. 2, FD&C Green No. 3, FD&C Red No. 40, FD&C Yellow No. 5, and FD&C Yellow No. 6) that cannot be synthesized without a variety of impurities.

Although aromatic amines are generally considered relatively toxic substances, the FD&C colors are notably nontoxic. Table 30-8, which is adopted from a publication of the National Academy of Sciences (NAS) (Committee on Food Protection, 1971), shows that certified food colors have a low order of acute

Table 30-8
Data on Certified Food Colors Permanently Listed in the United States

COLOR	NO ADVERSE EFFECT DIETARY LEVELS IN ANIMAL STUDIES	SAFE LEVEL FOR HUMANS mg/day	ESTIMATED MAXIMUM INGESTION mg/day PER PERSON
FD&C Blue No.1	5.0% rats 2.0% dogs	363	1.23
FD&C Blue No.2	1.0% rats, dogs	181	0.29
FD&C Green No.3	5.0% rats 1.0% dogs 2.0% mice	181	0.07
Orange B	5.0% rats 1.0% dogs 5.0% mice	181	0.31
Citrus Red No.2	0.1% rats	18	Not applicable
FD&C Red No. 3	0.5% rats 2.0% dogs 2.0% mice	91	1.88
FD&C Yellow No.5	2.0% rats 2.0% dogs	363	16.3
FD&C Yellow No.6	2.0% rats 2.0% dogs 2.0% mice	363	15.5

SOURCE: Committee on Food Protection, 1971.

Table 30-9
Tests for Each Concern Level

CONCERN LEVEL	TESTS REQUIRED
I	Short-term feeding study (at least 28 days in duration) Short-term tests for carcinogenic potential that can be used for determining priority for conduction of lifetime carcinogenicity bioassays and may assist in the evaluation of results from such bioassays, if conducted
II	Subchronic feeding study (at least 90 days in duration) in a rodent species Subchronic feeding study (at least 90 days in duration) in a nonrodent species Multigeneration reproduction study (minimum of two generations with a teratology phase) in a rodent species Short-term tests for carcinogenic potential
III	Carcinogenicity studies in two rodent species A chronic feeding study at least 1 year in duration in a rodent species (may be combined with a carcinogenicity study) Long-term (at least 1 year in duration) feeding study in a nonrodent species Multigenerational reproduction study (minimum of two generations) with a teratology phase in a rodent species Short-term tests for carcinogenic potential

toxicity. The principal reason involves sulfonation of the aromatic amine or azo compound that constitutes a color additive. Such sulfonic acid groups are highly polar, which, combined with their high molecular weight, prevents them from being absorbed by the GI tract or entering cells. All the FD&C food colors have been extensively tested in all Concern Level (CL) tests (Table 30-9) and have been found to be remarkably nontoxic.

Food colors that are exempt from certification typically have not been subjected to such extensive testing requirements. The exempt food colors are derived primarily from natural sources. While synthetic food colors have received the majority of public, scientific, and regulatory attention, natural color agents are also an important class. Currently, 25 color additives have been given exemption from certification in 21 CFR 73. These agents consist of a variety of natural compounds generally obtained by various extraction and treatment technologies. Included in this group of colors are preparations such as dried algae meal, beet powder, grape skin extract, fruit juice, paprika, caramel, carrot oil, cochineal extract, ferrous gluconate, and iron oxide. A problem encountered in attempts to regulate these additives is the lack of a precise chemical definition of many of these preparations. With a few exceptions, such as caramel, which is the most widely used color, the natural colors have not been heavily used. In part, this may be due to economic reasons, but these colors generally do not have the uniformity and intensity characteristic of the synthetic colors, therefore necessitating higher concentrations to obtain a specific color intensity. They also lack the chemical and color stability of the synthetic colors and have a tendency to fade with time.

Intake of color additives varies among individuals. The maximal intake of food colors is estimated to be approximately 53.5 mg/day, whereas the average intake per day is approximately 15 mg (Committee on Food Protection, 1971). Only about 10 percent of the food consumed in the United States contains food colors. The foods that utilize food colors in order of the quantity of color utilized are (1) beverages, (2) candy and confections, (3) dessert powders, (4) bakery goods, (5) sausages (casing only), (6) cereals, (7) ice cream, (8) snack foods, and (9) gravies, jams, jellies, and so forth (Committee on Food Protection, 1971).

Methods Used to Evaluate the Safety of Foods, Ingredients, and Contaminants

Safety Evaluation of Direct Food and Color Additives The philosophy and approach to evaluating the safety of substances added to foods has evolved over the past six decades. The concept that forms the foundation for this evolution is the recognition that the safety of any added substance to food must be established on the basis of specific intended conditions of use or uses in food. Intended conditions of use encompass (1) the foods to which the substance is added, (2) the level of use in such foods, (3) the purpose for which the substance is used, and (4) the population expected to consume the substance.

Exposure: The Estimated Daily Intake Before 1958, the FDA employed the philosophy that additives (and contaminants) should be harmless per se; that is, an additive should not be harmful at *any* level. The impractical nature of this philosophy is illustrated by two examples: A reasonable person would assume that pure, distilled water is harmless, but if enough is ingested to cause electrolyte imbalance, death may result; similarly, sulfuric acid in its concentrated form can dissolve steel, but when used to control pH during the processing of alcoholic beverages or cheeses, it is considered GRAS by the FDA (*Principles,* 1991). Clearly, exposure should be a major criterion for safety evaluation. This philosophy is reflected in the FDA's *Toxicological Principles for the Safety Assessment of Direct Food Additives and Color Additives Used in Food* (U.S. FDA, 1982),[1] in which exposure is a key factor in an algorithm used to determine which types of testing should be carried out on a substance.

Exposure is most often referred to as an estimated daily intake (EDI) and is based on two factors: the daily intake (I) of the food in which the substance will be used and the concentration (C) of the substance in that food:

$$\mathrm{EDI} = C \times I$$

[1]At the time of this writing, *Redbook II* remains in draft form and may undergo significant revision before finalizing. For this reason, the original (1982) version is used in this chapter except where noted.

In most cases, an additive is used in several different food categories, but for the sake of simplicity, we can assume that the additive is used only in baked goods. If the additive is used at a level that does not exceed 10 ppm and the mean daily intake of baked goods is 137 g per person per day, the EDI for this substance is 1370 μg per person per day.

Because most additives are used in more than one food, the total exposure (dose) is the sum of the exposures from each of the food categories. The formula for exposure to substance X is

$$EDI_x = (C_x f \times I_f) + (C_x g \times I_g) + (C_x h \times I_h) + (C \ldots)$$

where $C_x f$ and $C_x g$ are the concentration of X in food category f and the concentration of X in food category g, respectively. I_f and I_g are the daily intake of food category f, food category g, and so on. Therefore, the EDI is the sum of the individual contributions of X in each of the food categories.

Many of the same principles can be applied to an estimation of the consumption of residue from enzyme preparations [total organic solids (TOS)], residue from secondary direct additives (substances not intended to remain in a food after the technical effect has been accomplished; this includes but is not limited to mold release agents, solvents, defoaming agents, or chemicals used in washing fruits), and contaminants.

These principles give rise to two questions: (1) How does one determine how much is added to each of the food categories? and (2) What are the food categories, and how are they determined? First, the agency will use as the basis for its calculations the highest end of the range of use level for the new substance, but what ensures that these food group maximums will not be exceeded by a food manufacturer? This is also covered by a regulation—CGMPs (21 CFR 110)—in which a manufacturer is bound not to add more of an additive than is reasonably required to achieve its specific technical effect. That is, if the desired red color of strawberry ice cream is achieved with the addition of 1 ppm of red dye and additional dye does not increase the color or the intensity of the color, it is in violation of CGMPs to add an amount greater than 1 ppm. (A discussion of CGMPs may be found in the *Food Chemicals Codex,* 1996.)

In regard to the second question on food categories, one set of 43 food categories is listed in 21 CFR 170.3(n), which grew out of a survey of food additives conducted by the National Academy of Sciences/National Research Council and published in 1972. A sample of those categories is shown in Table 30-10. This survey pioneered the use of food categorization, but changing lifestyles of the population and shifts in food preferences have necessitated the generation of additional, more timely data.

The newer food consumption surveys provide more contemporary data on food intake (Table 30-11). All these databases (and others) have characteristics that serve a particular purpose. For example, one database may be only a 3-day "snapshot" of consumption, another may cover average consumption over 14 days, while yet another provides a detailed breakout of particular subpopulations (e.g., teenagers, the elderly, Hispanics). The majority of these databases are available to the public but may not be particularly "user-friendly," and private industry has made some of them available on a fee basis.

In estimates of consumption and/or exposure, one must also consider other sources of consumption for the proposed intended use of the additive if it already is used in food for another purpose, occurs naturally in foods, or is used in nonfood sources (e.g., drugs, toothpaste, lipstick). Thus, to estimate human consumption of a particular food substance, it is necessary to know (1) the levels of the substance in food, (2) the daily intake of each food containing the substance, (3) the distribution of intakes within the population, and (4) the potential consumption of or exposure to the substance from nonfood sources. (A discussion of chemical intake is covered in Rees and Tennant, 1994.)

Before a food additive is approved, regulatory agencies require evidence that it is safe for its intended use(s) and that its EDI is less than its acceptable daily intake (ADI). If such an estimate exceeds the ADI, regulatory agencies may impose restrictions on approvals for certain uses or restrict future approvals for new categories of use. The ADI is generally based on the results from animal toxicology studies, usually lifetime studies in rodents. These studies are used to determine the no-observed-effect level (NOEL) for the additive. The NOEL is usually divided by 100 to determine the ADI for a food additive, thus providing a 100-fold safety factor to account for species differences and the inter-individual variation among humans. This factor provides a reasonable certainty in estimating safe doses in humans from animal studies (Butchko and Kotsonis, 1996).

Assignment of Concern Level (CL) and Required Testing Structure-activity (SA) relationships are now the basis for developing

Table 30-10
Food Categories

NUMBER	DESIGNATION	DESCRIPTION	EXAMPLES
170.3(n)			
(1)	Baked goods and baking mixes	Includes all ready-to-eat and ready-to bake products, flours, and mixes requiring preparation before serving	Doughnuts, bread, croissants, cake mix, cookie dough
(2)	Beverages, alcoholic	Includes malt beverages, wines, distilled liquors, and cocktail mix	Beer, malt liquor, whiskey, liqueurs, wine coolers
(3)	Beverages and beverage bases, nonalcoholic	Includes only special or spiced teas, soft drinks, coffee substitutes, and fruit- and vegetable-flavored gelatin drinks	Herbal tea (non-tea-containing "teas"), soda pop, chicory
(4)	Breakfast cereals	Includes ready-to-eat and instant and regular hot cereals	Oatmeal (both regular and instant) farina, corn flakes, wheat flakes

Table 30-11
Databases for Estimating Food Intake

The Nationwide Food Consumption Survey, USDA, 1987–1988*
Foods Commonly Consumed by Individuals, USDA (Pay et al., 1984)
Continuing Survey of Food Intakes by Individuals, USDA, 1985, 1986, 1989*, 1990, 1991
The 1977 Survey of Industry on the Use of Food Additives by the NRC/NAS, Volume III
Estimates of Daily Intake (NRC/NAS), 1979 (Abrams, 1992)
USDA Economic Research Service Reports
The FDA Total Diet Study (Pennington and Gunderson, 1987)

*Indicates current use by FDA.
SOURCE: Information kindly provided by Technical Assessment Systems, Inc. Washington, D.C.

many therapeutic drugs, pesticides, and food additives. These relationships are put to good use in the *Toxicological Principles for the Safety Assessment of Direct Food Additives and Color Additives Used in Foods* (U.S. FDA, 1982), which describes a qualitative "decision tree" that assigns categories to substances on the basis of the structural and functional groups in the molecule. Additives with functional groups with a high order of toxicity are assigned to category C, those of unknown or intermediate toxicity are assigned to category B, and those with a low potential for toxicity are assigned to category A. For example, a simple saturated hydrocarbon alcohol such as pentanol would be assigned to category A. Similarly, a substance containing an α,β-unsaturated carbonyl function, epoxide, thiazole, or imidazole group would be assigned to category C. Thus, based on structure assignment and calculated exposure, the CLs are assigned (Table 30-12). For example, a substance in structure category B added to food at a level of 0.03 ppm would be assigned to concern level II.

Once the CL is established, a specific test battery is prescribed, as shown in Table 30-9. The tests for CL III are the most demanding and provide the greatest breadth for the determination of adverse biological effects, including effects on reproduction. The tests are comprehensive enough to detect nearly all types of observable toxicity, including malignant and benign tumors, preneoplastic lesions, and other forms of chronic toxicity. The tests for CL II are of intermediate breadth. These tests are designed to detect the most toxic phenomena other than late-developing histopathological changes. The short-term (genotoxicity) tests are intended to identify substances for which chronic testing becomes critical. The CL I test battery is the least broad, as is appropriate for the level of hazard which substances in this category may pose. However, if untoward effects are noted, additional assessment becomes necessary. Studies of the absorption, distribution, metabolism, and elimination characteristics of a test substance are recommended before the initiation of toxicity studies longer than 90 days' duration. Of particular importance for many proposed food ingredients is data on their processing and metabolism in the GI tract.

Unique to food additive carcinogenicity testing is the controversial use of protocols that include an in utero phase. Under such protocols, parents of test animals are exposed to the test substance for 4 weeks before mating and throughout mating, gestation, and lactation. Most countries and international bodies do not subscribe to the combining of an in utero phase with a rat carcinogenicity study, as this presents a series of logistic and operational problems and substantially increases the cost of conducting a rat carcinogenicity study. The FDA began requesting in utero studies of the food industry in the early 1970s, when it was discovered from lifetime feeding studies that the artificial sweetener saccharin produced bladder tumors in male rats when in utero exposure was introduced. Subsequently, the FDA required the food, drug, and cosmetic color industries to conduct lifetime carcinogenicity feeding studies of 18 color additives in rats using an in utero exposure phase. This testing has provided the largest database available to date on the performance of in utero testing.

Special note should also be made of genetic toxicity testing. Genetic toxicity tests are performed for two reasons: (1) to test chemicals for potential carcinogenicity and (2) to assess whether a chemical may induce heritable genetic damage. Currently, genetic toxicity assays can be divided into three major groups: (1) forward and reverse mutation assays (e.g., point mutations, deletions), (2) clastogenicity assays detecting structural and numerical

Table 30-12
Assignment of Concern Level

STRUCTURE CATEGORY A	STRUCTURE CATEGORY B	STRUCTURE CATEGORY C	CONCERN LEVEL
<0.05 ppm in the total diet (<0.0012 mg/kg/day)	<0.025 ppm in the total diet (<0.00063 mg/kg/day)	<0.0125 ppm in the total diet (<0.00031 mg/kg/day)	I
or	or	or	
≥0.05 ppm in the total diet (≥0.0012 mg/kg/day)	≥0.025 ppm in the total diet (≥0.00063 mg/kg/day)	≥0.0125 ppm in the total diet (≥0.00031 mg/kg/day)	II
or	or	or	
≥1 ppm in the total diet (≥0.025 mg/kg/day)	≥0.5 ppm in the total diet (≥0.0125 mg/kg/day)	≥0.25 ppm in the total diet (≥0.0063 mg/kg/day)	III

Table 30-13
Exposure Estimate Calculations (Package Type)

		Food-Type Distribution (f_T)			
PACKAGE CATEGORY	CF*	AQUEOUS	ACIDIC	ALCOHOLIC	FATTY
Glass	0.08	0.08	0.36	0.47	0.09
Metal, polymer-coated	0.17	0.16	0.35	0.40	0.09
Metal, uncoated	0.03	0.54	0.25	0.01†	0.20
Paper, polymer-coated	0.21	0.55	0.04	0.01†	0.40
Paper, uncoated	0.10	0.57	0.01†	0.01†	0.41
Polymer	0.41	0.49	0.16	0.01	0.34

*As discussed in the text, a minimum CF of 0.05 is used initially for all exposure estimates.
†1% or less.

changes in chromosomes (e.g., chromosome aberrations, micronuclei), and (3) assays that identify DNA damage (e.g., DNA strand breaks, unscheduled DNA synthesis).

Because the correlation between carcinogens and mutagens has proved to be less than desirable, as has been demonstrated by false-positive and false-negative findings when carcinogens and noncarcinogens have been examined in genetic toxicity tests, it is recommended that several tests be selected from a battery of tests. It should be kept in mind that as the number of tests employed increases, the possibility of false-negative results increases as well. Consequently, the National Toxicology Program (NTP) has advised that only a single gene mutational assay be used (*Salmonella typhimurium*) to optimize the prediction of carcinogenicity (Tennant and Zeiger, 1993).

Safety Determination of Indirect Food Additives Indirect food additives are substances defined as food additives that are not added directly to food but enter food by migrating from surfaces that contact food. These surfaces may be from packaging material (cans, paper, plastic) or the coating of packaging materials or surfaces used in processing, holding, or transporting food.

Essential to demonstrating the safety of an indirect additive are extraction studies with food-simulating solvents. The FDA recommends the use of three food-simulating solvents—8% ethanol, 50% ethanol, and corn oil or a synthetic triglyceride—for aqueous and acidic, alcoholic, and fatty foods, respectively (FDA, 1988). The conditions of extraction depend in part on the intended conditions of use. If the package material is intended to be retorted, the petitioner must conduct extractions for at least 2 hr at 275°F. For all conditions of use, high-temperature extraction (conducted at 275, 250, or 212°F for 2 h) is followed by a minimum of 238 h at 120°F except for refrigerated foods (in which 70°F is used) and frozen food (in which only 120 h of extraction is required).

Extraction studies are used to assess the level or quantity of a substance which might migrate and become a component of food, leading to consumer exposure. The prescribed extraction tests are believed to overestimate the amount of an indirect additive that is likely to migrate to food and thus are unlikely to underestimate consumer exposure. To convert extraction data from packaging material into anticipated consumer exposure, the FDA has determined the fraction of the U.S. diet which comes into contact with different classes of material: glass, metal-coated, metal-uncoated, paper-uncoated, paper-coated, and polymers. For each class, FDA has assigned a "consumption factor" (CF), which is the fraction of the total diet that comes into contact with an individual class of material (Table 30-13).

The fraction of individual food types (aqueous, acidic, alcoholic, fatty) for which such packaging material is used is referred to as the food-type-distribution factor (f_T). To calculate consumer exposure (EDI), the following equation is used:

$$\text{EDI} = \text{CF} \times [(f_{T\ \text{aqueous}} \times \text{ppm in 8\% ethanol}) + (f_{T\ \text{acidic}} \times \text{ppm in 8\% ethanol}) + (f_{T\ \text{alcohol}} \times \text{ppm in 50\% ethanol}) + (f_{T\ \text{fatty}} \times \text{ppm in corn oil})] \times 3\ \text{kg per person per day} = \text{mg per person per day}^2$$

For additives with virtually no migration (<0.05 ppm), in which the EDIs correspond to 0.15 mg per person per day, acute toxicology data are considered sufficient to provide an assurance of safety for the intended conditions of use of the additive. Migration levels, as determined by extraction studies, that are greater than 0.05 to 1 ppm of exposure generally require subchronic (90-day) feeding studies in rodent and nonrodent (usually the dog) species. Where there is significant migration—that is, more than 1 ppm exposure—carcinogenicity/chronic toxicity testing in rodents, at least a 1 year test in a nonrodent, and multigeneration reproduction testing to a minimum of two generations with a teratology phase in a rodent, are recommended by the FDA. Other studies may be indicated by the data or information available on the substance.

Safety Requirements for GRAS Substances In spite of the fact that the FD&C Act and the relevant regulations (21 CFR 170.3, etc.) scrupulously avoid defining food except in a functional sense—"food means articles used for food or drink for man or other animals . . . [and includes] chewing gum, and . . . articles used for components of any such article"—it regards foods as GRAS when they are added to other food, for example, green beans in vegetable soup (Kokoski et al., 1990). It also regards a number of food ingredients as GRAS, and these ingredients are listed under 21 CFR 182, 184, and 186. However, it is important to note that not all substances regarded as GRAS are listed as such. The language used in 21 CFR 182.1(a) acknowledges that there are substances the FDA considers to be GRAS which are not listed.

[2]The 3 kg is the FDA's value for daily food consumption which, when multiplied by mg/kg (ppm) and the weighting factors, reduces to milligrams of the additive per day.

This accomplishes two things: (1) It leaves the door open for additional nonlisted substances to be affirmed as GRAS by the agency and (2) reinforces the concept that substances can be deemed GRAS whether or not they are listed by the FDA or on a publicly available list. A list of examples of substances regarded as GRAS is given in Table 30-14. It is important to re-emphasize that GRAS substances, though *used* like food additives, are *not* food additives. Although the distinction may seem to be one of semantics, it allows GRAS substances to be exempt from the premarket clearance restrictions enforced by the FDA and exempt from the Delaney clause, because that clause pertains only to food additives.

While the courts have ruled that GRAS substances must be supported by the same quantity and quality of safety data that support food additives, this ruling should not be interpreted to mean that the supporting data must be identical in nature and character to those supporting a food additive. For uses of substances to be eligible for classification as GRAS, there must be common knowledge throughout the scientific community about the safety of substances directly or indirectly added to food (21 CFR 170.30).

The studies relied on for concluding that a given use of a substance is GRAS ordinarily are based on generally available data and information published in the scientific literature. Such data are unlikely to be conducted in accordance with FDA-recommended protocols, as these studies often are conducted for reasons unrelated to FDA approval. GRAS status also can be based on experience with common use in food before January 1, 1958, which further distinguishes GRAS data requirements from those demanded of food additives. Such experience need not be limited to the United States; but if it comes from outside the United States, it must be documented by published or other information that is corroborated by information from an independent source.

Importance of the GRAS Concept

The importance of the GRAS provision is obvious from its many applications. Many substances, for example, that are used in food processing have never received formal FDA approval. The use of these substances in the manufacture of food products is considered appropriate under CGMPs, while the substance itself is considered GRAS for such purposes. Similarly, certain substances are permitted as optional ingredients in standardized foods [foods with standards of identity specified by regulation (21 CFR 130–169)] even though they are not approved food additives and are not on any of the GRAS lists.

The GRAS concept as traditionally applied in the United States also has applicability to certain novel foods which may differ only slightly from traditional foods or which, after careful consideration, can be regarded as raising no issues or questions of safety beyond that raised by the traditional foods they are intended to replace. The GRAS approach may therefore permit the introduction of novel foods that contain less saturated fat and/or cholesterol or more fiber or are in other ways modified.

Transgenic Plant (and New Plant Varieties) Policy Crops have been genetically modified through conventional crop breeding for more than a hundred years to produce new plant varieties. This was usually done by conventional breeding methods. Scientists today can use biotechnology to insert specific genes into a plant to give it new characteristics. For example, approximately 25 percent of the corn crop planted in 1999 in the United States contains a gene from the bacterium *Bacillus thuringiensis* that produces a Bt insecticidal protein (James, 1999). Bt is a protein toxic to certain caterpillar insect pests that destroy corn plants (EPA, 1988; McClintock et al., 1995). By enabling the corn plant to protect itself from this insect pest, the use of this product can reduce the need for and use of conventional insecticides (Gianessi and Carpenter, 1999).

Irrespective of the breeding method used to produce a new plant variety, tests must be done to ensure that the levels of nutrients or toxins in the plants have not changed and that the food is still safe to consume. Clearly, new proteins produced in plant varieties must be nontoxic and not have the characteristics of proteins known to cause allergies. Thus, the proteins produced in genetically modified crops are evaluated for allergenicity (Metcalf et al., 1996). The DNA that is introduced into genetically modified plants to direct the production of such new proteins has been determined to be generally recognized as safe (FDA, 1992). The use of antibiotic resistance marker genes in genetically modified crops has been determined by FDA and other regulatory agencies to be

Table 30-14
Examples of GRAS Substances and Their Functionality

CFR NUMBER	SUBSTANCE	FUNCTIONALITY
	Substances Generally Recognized as Safe 21 CFR 182	
182.2122	Aluminum calcium silicate	Anticaking agent
182.5065	Linoleic acid	Dietary supplement
	Direct Food Substances Affirmed as Generally Recognized as Safe 21 CFR 184	
184.1005	Acetic acid	Several
184.1355	Helium	Processing aid
	Indirect Food Substances Affirmed as Generally Recognized as Safe 21 CFR 186	
186.1025	Caprylic acid	Antimicrobial
186.1374	Iron oxides	Ingredient of paper and paperboard

safe (FDA, 1992). Nonetheless, regulatory agencies have advised researchers to avoid using marker genes in crops that encode resistance to clinically important antibiotics.

The safety of new plant varieties (transgenic plants, genetically modified plants) is regulated primarily under the FDA's postmarket authority [section 402(a)(1) of the FD&C Act]. This section, previously applied to occurrences of unsafe levels of toxicants in food, is now applied to new plant varieties whose composition has been altered by an added substance. The new policy has been applied to plants containing substances that are GRAS [*Federal Register* 57(104):22984–23005]. The *Federal Register* notice (May 29, 1992) indicates that "[i]n most cases, the substances expected to become components of food as a result of genetic modification of a plant will be the same as or substantially similar to substances commonly found in food, such as proteins, fats and oils, and carbohydrates." The notice also indicates the responsibility of the FDA to exercise the premarket review process when the "objective characteristics of the substance raise questions of safety." In regard to substances within the new variety that are not similar to substances commonly found in food, a food additive petition may have to be filed.

The *Federal Register* notice offers points of consideration for the safety assessment of new plant varieties (Table 30-15). Accompanying these points of consideration are a decision flowchart and advice that the FDA be consulted on certain findings, for example, transference of allergens from one plant to another, a change in the concentration or bioavailability of nutrients, and the introduction of a new macroingredient.

In the United States, new plant varieties are regulated not only by FDA but also by the EPA and USDA. FDA is responsible for the safety and labeling of foods and feeds derived from crops, irrespective of the method used to produce the new plant variety. EPA is responsible for assuring the safety of pesticides; thus in the example cited above whereby a pesticide is produced in a new plant variety, this product would also fall under the EPA's jurisdiction. The USDA's Animal and Plant Health Inspection Service has responsibility for the environmental safety of field-testing and commercial planting of new plant varieties.

Methods for Establishing Safe Conditions of Use for Novel Foods Novel foods, including those derived from new plant varieties and macroingredient substitutes, present new challenges and may require new methods of determining safety. For example, with each new additive, it has been traditional (and rooted in a regulation such as 21 CFR 170.22) to establish an ADI, which is usually based on 1/100 of the NOEL established in animal testing. This works well for additives projected to be consumed at a level of 1.5 g/day or less (which is equal to or less than 25 mg/kg), for this extrapolates at a 100-fold safety factor to consumption by a rat at a level of 2500 mg/kg/day (about 5 percent of the rat's diet). The problem arises when a new food or macroingredient substitute becomes a substantive part of the diet (estimated to constitute as much as 15 to 20 percent). For example, a macroingredient substitute or food projected to be consumed at a level of just 5 percent of the diet (150 g/day) would require the test animal (rat) to consume 250 g/kg/day, or slightly more than the rat's body weight. This is an untenable test requirement, for at those levels, the investigator would establish an effect level only for malnutrition, not for the toxicity of the macroingredient. The converse is true for some essential nutrients, such as vitamins A and D and iron, which at doses 100 times the nutritional use level would be toxic (Kokoski et al., 1990). The answer therefore lies in careful interpretation of toxicological data and the conduct, where appropriate, of special studies to assess drug interactions, nutrient interactions, changes in gut flora, changes in gut activity, and the like (Borzelleca, 1992a,b; Munro, 1990). Also, it may be appropriate to consider what effect, if any, macroingredients may have on individuals with compromised digestive tracts, those dependent on laxatives, and those on high-fiber diets.

The regulatory approval of a new food additive is generally based on traditional toxicology studies. The rationale is that data from such studies will adequately predict adverse effects that could occur in humans. However, such studies, especially for novel foods, may not be adequate. Therefore, although human studies are not generally required for food additives, in the case of novel foods, human studies are likely essential in evaluating their safety (Stargel et al., 1996).

Another useful tool in ensuring the safety of a food additive is monitoring it after its approval, or postmarketing surveillance. With widespread use of a food additive, *monitoring for consumption* can determine whether actual consumption exceeds the EDI and *monitoring for anecdotal complaints* may identify adverse health effects that escaped detection in earlier studies. This could be especially important for novel foods when traditional toxicology studies are not done at large multiples of the EDI (Butchko et al., 1994, 1996). Thus, the combination of traditional toxicity studies, special animal and human studies, and possibly postmarketing surveillance will ensure the safety of consumers and provide evidence to justify a safety factor different from 100.

Table 30-15
Points of Consideration in the Safety Assessment of New Plant Varieties

Toxicants known to be characteristic of the host and donor species
The potential that food allergens will be transferred from one food source to another
The concentration and bioavailability of important nutrients for which a food crop is ordinarily consumed
The safety and nutritional value of newly introduced proteins
The identity, composition, and nutritional value of modified carbohydrates or fats and oils

Dietary Supplements Dietary supplements have a special status within the law and the regulations; supplements are regarded as foods or food-type substances but not food additives and not drugs. Although regarded as foods, they cannot be sold as conventional foods. Unique to dietary supplements (or dietary supplement ingredients) is a lesser standard for safety than is required for food ingredients. That is, while a food ingredient must have *demonstrated safety,* a supplement ingredient must have *no history of unsafe use,* a much easier standard to meet. While this distinction is subtle, it permits the use of a substance as a dietary supplement that cannot be used as a food ingredient (e.g., stevioside). In the example of stevioside, because there is no history of unsafe use, the FDA has not objected to its use as a dietary supplement but feels that the safety data are inadequate to support the use of stevioside as an ingredient added to food. Concomitantly, an unapproved health claim cannot be made for the dietary supplement, as it is then regarded as a "drug" and subject to the rigorous drug application process with demonstrations of safety and effectiveness (Burdock, 2000).

Assessment of Carcinogens

Carcinogenicity as a Special Problem As discussed above, Congress provided the FDA with wide latitude in assessing safety and assuring a safe food supply with—one exception. That exception is a provision of the FD&C Act known as the Delaney clause, which prohibits the approval of regulated food additives "found to induce cancer when ingested by man or animals" [section 409(c)(3)(A)]. The Delaney clause is found in two other sections of the act. The three clauses—sections 409(c)(3)(A), 706(b)(5)(B), and 512(d)(1)(H)—constitute the Delaney clause.

It must be emphasized that the Delaney prohibition applies only to the approval of food additives, color additives, and animal drugs; it does not apply to unavoidable contaminants or GRAS substances or ingredients sanctioned by the FDA or USDA before 1958. The clause also does not apply to carcinogenic constituents that are present in food or color additives or animal drugs as nonfunctional contaminants provided that the level of such contaminants can be demonstrated to be safe and the whole additive, including its contaminants (permitted by specification and regulations), is not found to induce cancer in humans or animals. This interpretation of the Delaney clause was set forth by the FDA in its so-called constituent policy published on April 2, 1982, as an Advanced Notice of Proposed Rulemaking (ANPR). The policy mandates the development and use of animal carcinogenicity data and probabilistic risk assessment to establish a safe level for the contaminant in the additive under its intended conditions of use.

The constituent policy and, as discussed further on, the implementation of the so-called DES (diethylstilbestrol) proviso for animal drugs under the Delaney clause, have forced the FDA to develop a means for establishing safe levels for carcinogenic substances. The DES proviso allows the addition of carcinogenic animal drugs to animal feed if they leave no residue in edible tissue as determined by an approved analytic procedure. To do this, the FDA has turned to the use of probabilistic risk assessment in which tumor data in animals are mathematically extrapolated to an upper-bound risk in humans exposed to particular use levels of the additive. The FDA takes the position that, considering the many conservative assumptions inherent in the procedure, an upper-bound lifetime risk of one cancer in a million individuals is the biological equivalent of zero.

Much controversy surrounds the use of risk-assessment procedures, in part because estimates of risk are highly dependent on the many assumptions that must be made. The tendency is to be "risk-averse" and favor assumptions that exaggerate risk. As these exaggerations are multiplicative, the total overestimation of risk can be several orders of magnitude. Table 30-16 provides some rough estimates of potential ranges of uncertainty that might lead to large overestimates (Flamm and Lorentzen, 1988).

The common practice of testing at a maximum tolerated dose (MTD) (Williams and Weisburger, 1991) raises the question of appropriateness to human exposure. Do high test doses cause physiologic changes unlike those from human exposure? The basic assumption in quantitative risk assessment (QRA) that the dose-response curve is linear beneath the lowest observable effect

Table 30-16
Uncertainty Parameters and Their Associated Range of Risk Factors

UNCERTAINTY PARAMETERS	ESTIMATED RANGE, FACTOR
Extrapolation model	1–10,000
Total dose vs. dose rate	30–45
Most sensitive sex/strain vs. average sensitivity	1–100
Sensitivity of human vs. test animal	1–1000
Potential synergism or antagonism with other carcinogens or promoters	1–1000?
Total population vs. target population, potential vs. actual market penetration	1–1000
Absorptive rate (gut, skin, lung) for animals at high dose vs. humans at low dose	1–10
Dose scaling: mg/kg body weight, ppm (diet, water, feed) surface area	1–15
Upper confidence on users or exposed	1–10
Specifics or tolerances	1–10
Limits of detection vs. actual levels	1–1000
Additivity vs. nonadditivity of multiple sites	1–3
Survival or interim sacrifice adjustments	1–2
Knowledge of only high-end plateau dose response	1–10
Error or variation in detection methods	1–10
Adjustments for less than lifetime bioassays	1–100
Adjustments for intermittent and less than lifetime human exposure	1–100
Use vs. nonuse of historical data	1–2
Upper confidence and lower confidence limits vs. expected values in extrapolation level of acceptable risk	1–1000
Level of acceptable risk	1–1000
Adding or not adding theoretical risks from many substances	1–100

SOURCE: Flamm and Lorentzen, 1988.

may result in the calculation of relatively high risks even at doses that are much lower than the lowest dose that produces cancer in experimental animals (Flamm and Lorentzen, 1988). QRA is more a process than a science; many steps in the process are based on assumptions, not proven scientific facts. If only the most conservative assumptions are made throughout the process, many will represent overestimates of human risk by 10- or 100-fold, leading to a combined overestimate of perhaps a millionfold or more.

Risk assessment cannot be used for either food additives or color additives because of the Delaney clause. If these additives are found to induce cancer, they cannot be approved for foods or colors no matter how small the estimated risk. Because of the harsh consequences of finding a food additive to be a carcinogen, the FDA has interpreted this clause as requiring an affirmative finding of a clear and unequivocal demonstration of carcinogenicity upon ingestion. Historically, the FDA has employed a high threshold for establishing that a food or color additive has been found to induce cancer when ingested by humans or animals. Very few substances have been disapproved or banned because of the Delaney clause. Two indirect food additives (Flectol H and mercaptoimidazoline) that migrate from packaging material were banned. Among direct additives, safrole, cinnamyl anthranilate, thiourea, and diethylpyrocarbonate were banned because of the Delaney clause; diethylpyrocarbonate was banned because it forms urethane.

A number of substances [e.g., butylated hydroxyanisole (BHA), xylitol, methylene chloride, sorbitol, trichloroethylene, nitrilotriacetic acid (NTA), diethylhexyl phthalate, melamine, formaldehyde, bentonite] listed in the Code of Federal Regulation as regulated food additives are also listed as carcinogens by National Toxicology Program (NTP), the International Agency for Research on Cancer (IARC), or the state of California (under the Safe Drinking Water and Toxic Enforcement Act of 1986, also known as Proposition 65). How is this possible, and on what basis do these food additive listings continue?

Despite the fact that tests and conditions exist under which each of these substances will produce cancer in animals, the FDA has found it possible to continue listing these substances as food additives. The reasoning applied in almost every case is based on secondary carcinogenesis. The one exception is formaldehyde, which is carcinogenic only on inhalation, and there are compelling reasons to believe that inhalation is not an appropriate test in this case (Flamm and Frankos, 1985). Therefore formaldehyde is not treated as a carcinogen prohibited by the Delaney clause.

For BHA, which induces forestomach cancer, the concept has been advanced that its carcinogenicity is attributable primarily to irritation, restorative hyperplasia, and so on (Clayson et al., 1986). For xylitol, a sugar alcohol, an increase in bladder tumors and adrenal pheochromocytomas is considered secondary to calcium imbalance resulting from the indigestibility of sugar alcohols and their fermentation in the lower GI tract. Sorbitol, another sugar alcohol, behaves in a similar manner. For NTA, the argument is secondary carcinogenesis, and although specific explanations vary, the mechanism involving zinc imbalance has considerable scientific support. The review of diethylhexyl phthalate is ongoing, but the possibility that peroxisome proliferation is involved has been offered, as has the possibility that hepatocellular proliferation is primary to the subsequent development of tumors.

Thus, the FDA has generally interpreted the phrase "found to induce cancer when ingested by man or animals" as excluding cancers that arise through many secondary means. Therefore, to be a carcinogen under the Delaney clause, a food or color additive must be demonstrated to induce cancer by primary means when ingested by humans or animals or to induce cancer by other routes of administration that are found to be appropriate. This is interpreted to mean that the findings of cancer must be clearly reproducible and that the cancers found are not secondary to nutritional, hormonal, or physiologic imbalances. This position allows the agency to argue that changing the level of protein or fat in the diet does not induce cancer but simply modulates tumor incidence (Kritschevsky, 1994). Given the many modulating factors and influences connected with food and diet, the FDA must be careful about what it declares to be a carcinogen under the Delaney clause. Thus, the FDA has always had to look at the mechanistic question and has been doing that for more than 30 years.

Biological versus Statistical Significance Much can be learned about the proper means of assessing carcinogenicity data by studying large databases for substances that have been tested for carcinogenicity many times. The artificial sweetener cyclamate is an example. The existence of more than a dozen studies on cyclamate and the testing of multiple hypotheses at dozens of different organ and tissue sites in all these studies led to the awareness that the overall false-positive error rate (i.e., higher cancer incidence at a specific organ site in treated subjects versus controls as a result of chance) could be inflated if individual findings were viewed out of context (FDA, 1984). Therefore very careful attention must be paid to the totality of the evidence.

The possibility of false-negative error is always of concern because of the need to protect public health. However, it should be recognized that any attempt to prove absolutely that a substance is not carcinogenic is futile. Therefore, an unrelenting effort to minimize false-negative errors can produce an unacceptably high probability of a false positive. Further, demanding certainty (i.e., a zero or implicitly an extremely low probability of false-negative error) has negative consequences for an accurate decision-making process. This is the case because it severely limits the ability to discriminate between carcinogens and noncarcinogens on the basis of bioassays (FDA, 1984).

In addition to the false-positive/false-negative trap, which is a statistical matter, there are many potential biological traps. The appearance of a higher incidence of tumors at a specific organ site in treated animals may not demonstrate by itself a carcinogenic action of the substance employed in the treatment. This is the case because the incidence of tumors at specific organ sites can be influenced and controlled by many biological processes that may affect tumor incidence.

The test substance, typically administered at high MTDs, may affect one or more of the many biological processes known to modulate tumor incidence at a specific organ site without causing an induction of tumors at that or any other site. Nutritional imbalances such as choline deficiency are known to lead to a high incidence of liver cancer in rats and mice. Simple milk sugar (lactose) is known to increase the incidence of Leydig's cell tumors in rats. Caloric intake has been shown to be a significant modifying factor in carcinogenesis. Impairment of immune surveillance by a specific or nonspecific means (stress) affecting immune responsiveness and hormonal imbalance can result in higher incidences of tumors at specific organ sites. Hormonal imbalance, which can be caused by hormonally active agents (e.g., estradiol) or by other substances that act indirectly, such as vitamin D, may result in an increased tumor incidence. Chronic cell injury and restorative hyperplasia resulting from treatment with lemon flavor (*d*-limonene) probably are responsible for renal tumor development in male rats by mechanisms that are of questionable relevance to humans (Flamm and Lehman-McKeeman, 1991).

In these examples, the increases in tumor incidence at specific organ sites probably are secondary to significant changes in normal physiologic balance and homeostasis. Moreover, the increases in tumor incidence, and hence in the risk of cancer, probably would not occur except at toxic doses (Ames and Gold, 1997).

To preserve the ability of a bioassay to discriminate, the possibility of false-positive or false-negative results and of secondary effects must be considered. To be meaningful, evaluations must be based on the weight of evidence, which must be reviewed as carefully as possible. Particular attention must be given to the many factors used in deciding whether tumor incidences are biologically as well as statistically significant. These factors include (1) the historical rate of the tumor in question (is it a rare tumor, or does it occur frequently in the controls?); (2) the survival histories of dosed and test animals (did dosed animals survive long enough to be considered "at risk"? What effect did chemical toxicity and reduced survival have in the interpretation of the data?); (3) the patterns of tumor incidence (was the response dose-related?); (4) the biological meaningfulness of the effect (was it experimentally consistent with the evidence from related studies? Did it occur in a target organ?); (5) the reproducibility of the effect with other doses, sexes, or species; (6) evidence of hyperplasia, metaplasia, or other signs of an ongoing carcinogenic process (is the effect supported by a pattern of related nonneoplastic lesions, particularly at lower doses?); (7) evidence of tumor multiplicity or progression; and (8) the strength of the evidence of an increased tumor incidence (what is the magnitude of the p value? for pairwise comparison? for trend?).

A good discussion of the use of these factors by scientists in deciding whether a substance induces cancer in animals is contained in the notice of a final rule permanently listing FD&C Yellow No. 6 (51 FR 41765–41783, 1988). An elevation of tumor incidence in rats was identified at two organ and/or tissue sites: (1) medullary tumors of the adrenal glands in female rats only and (2) renal cortical tumors in female rats only. Scientists at the FDA concluded that the increase in medullary tumors of the adrenal glands in female rats did not suffice to establish that FD&C Yellow No. 6 is a carcinogen. The basis for the decision was (1) a lack of dose response, (2) the likelihood of false positives, (3) the lack of precancerous lesions, (4) morphologic similarity of adrenal medullary lesions in treated and control rats, (5) an unaffected latency period, (6) a lack of effect in male rats, and (7) a comparison with other studies in which there was no association between exposure to FD&C Yellow No. 6 and the occurrence of adrenal medullary tumors.

A similar judgment was made with respect to the cortical renal lesions in female rats, which were not found to provide a basis for concluding that FD&C Yellow No. 6 can induce cancer of the kidneys. The main reasons leading to this conclusion were (1) the relatively common occurrence of proliferative renal lesions in aged male control rats (28 months or older), (2) the lack of renal tumors in treated males despite their usually greater sensitivity to renal carcinogens, (3) the lack of malignant tumors indicating no progression of adenomas to a malignant state, (4) the lack of a decreased latency period compared with controls, (5) the coincidence of renal proliferative lesions and chronic renal disease, (6) the lack of genotoxicity, and (7) a lack of corroborative evidence from other studies that suggests a treatment-related carcinogenic effect of FD&C Yellow No. 6 on the kidney. Both of these examples emphasize the importance of considering all the evidence in attempting to decide the significance of any subset of data.

As essential elements, vitamins, sugars, and calories per se can increase tumor incidence in test animals; the mechanism by which tumors arise as the result of exposure to food or food ingredients is critically important to assessing the relevance of the finding to the safety of the substance under its intended conditions of use in food. McClain (1994) provides an excellent discussion of mechanistic considerations in the regulation and classification of chemical carcinogens.

Carcinogenic Contaminants The Delaney clause, which prohibits the addition of carcinogens to food, could ban many food additives and color additives if it were strictly interpreted to include carcinogenic contaminants of additives within its definition. Clearly, this was not Congress's intent, and just as clearly, the FDA needed to develop a commonsense policy for addressing the problem that all substances, including food and color additives, may contain carcinogenic contaminants at some trace level.

Toward this end, the agency argued (FDA, 1982) that banning food and color additives simply because they have been found or are known to contain a trace level of a known carcinogen does not make sense because all substances may contain carcinogenic contaminants. The agency asserted in its constituent policy that the mere fact an additive contains a contaminant known to be carcinogenic should not automatically lead the agency to ban that food additive under the Delaney clause but should instead cause the agency to consider the health risks it poses based on its level of contamination and the conditions of its use. The agency stated that by using highly conservative scientific assumptions and a highly conservative methodology for extrapolating cancer risk from high dose to low and from animals to humans, one could estimate such risks in a manner that would assure that the actual risks posed to humans would not be underestimated. This reaffirmed the agency's position taken in the proposal on the addition of carcinogens to the feed of food-producing animals (FDA, 1977).

SAFETY OF FOOD

Adverse Reactions to Food or Food Ingredients

In a survey of Americans, 30 percent indicated that they or someone in their immediate families had a food sensitivity. Although this number is likely too high, as much as 7.5 percent of the population may be allergic to some food or component thereof (Taylor et al., 1989). Lactose intolerance (a deficiency of the disaccharide enzyme lactase) is very high among some groups; for example, there is an incidence of 27 percent in black children age 12 to 24 months, which may increase to 33 percent by age 6 years (Juambeltz et al., 1993). The percentage of young (northern European) children allegedly intolerant to food additives ranges from 0.03 to 0.23 percent (Wuthrich, 1993) to 1 to 2 percent (Fuglsang et al., 1993). Further, there are certain drug-food incompatibilities about which physicians and pharmacists are obligated to warn patients, such as monoamine oxidase (MAO) inhibitors and tyramine in cheese or benzodiazapenes and naringenin in grapefruit juice. People who are prescribed tetracycline also must be alerted not to take milk with this antibiotic. By any standard, there are large numbers of real and perceived adverse reactions to or incompatibilities with food (Thomas and Tschanz, 1994). The first step in understanding these reactions is to define the nomenclature, a task undertaken by the American Academy of Allergy and Immunology (Committee on Adverse Reactions to Foods) and the National Institute of Allergy and Infectious Diseases (Anderson and Sogn, 1984). An adaptation of their attempt at definition and classification is represented in Table 30-17. In the table, the definitions proceed from general to most specific. Obviously, there is little to distinguish the terms *adverse reaction* and *sensitivity* to a food or a food *intolerance* except perhaps in the lexicon of the individual, colored by his or her own experience. That is, an "adverse reaction" may indicate something as simple as an unpleasing esthetic or hedonic quality such as an unpleasant taste, which may in fact have a genetic basis, as in the ability to taste phenylthiocarbamide (Guyton, 1971), or may indicate a fatal outcome resulting from an immune or toxic reaction.

Table 30-17
Adverse Reaction to Food: Definition of Terms

TERM	DEFINITION	CHARACTERISTICS/EXAMPLES
Adverse reaction (sensitivity) to a food	General term that can be applied to a clinically abnormal response attributed to an ingested food or food additive.	Any untoward pathological reaction resulting from ingestion of a food or food additive. May be immune-mediated.
Food hypersensitivity (allergy)	An immunologic reaction resulting from the ingestion of a food or food additive. This reaction occurs only in some patients, may occur after only a small amount of the substance is ingested, and is unrelated to any physiological effect of the food or food additive.	Immune-mediated (cellular or humoral response), requires prior exposure to antigen or cross-reacting antigen. First exposure may have been asymptomatic.
Food anaphylaxis	A classic allergic hypersensitivity reaction to food or food additives.	A humoral immune response most often involving IgE antibody and release of chemical mediators. Mortality may result.
Food intolerance	A general term describing an abnormal physiologic response to an ingested food or food additive; this reaction may be an immunologic, idiosyncratic, metabolic, pharmacologic, or toxic response.	Any untoward pathologic reaction resulting from ingestion of a food or food additive. May be immune-mediated. Celiac disease (intolerance to wheat, rye, barley, oats).
Food toxicity (poisoning)	A term use to imply an adverse effect caused by the direct action of a food or food additive on the host recipient without the involvement of immune mechanisms. This type of reaction may involve nonimmune release of chemical mediators. Toxins may be contained within food or released by microorganisms or parasites contaminating food products.	Not immune-mediated. May be caused by bacterial endo- or exotoxin (e.g., hemorrhagic *E. coli*) fungal toxin (e.g. aflatoxin), tetrodotoxin from pufferfish, domoic acid from mollusks, histamine poisoning from fish (scombroid poisoning), nitrate poisoning (i.e., methemoglobinuria).
Food idiosyncrasy	A quantitatively abnormal response to a food substance or additive; this reaction differs from its physiologic or pharmacologic effect and resembles hypersensitivity but does not involve immune mechanisms. Food idiosyncratic reactions include those which occur in specific groups of individuals who may be genetically predisposed.	Not immune-mediated, Favism (hemolytic anemia related to deficiency of erythrocytic glucose-6-phosphate dehydrogenase), fish odor syndrome, beetanuria, lactose intolerance, fructose intolerance, asparagus urine, red wine intolerance.
Anaphylactoid reaction to a food	An anaphylaxis-like reaction to a food or food additive as a result of nonimmune release of chemical mediators. This reaction mimics the symptoms of food hypersensitivity (allergy).	Not immune-mediated. Scombroid poisoning, sulfite poisoning, red wine sensitivity.
Pharmacological food reaction	An adverse reaction to a food or food additive as a result of a naturally derived or added chemical that produces a drug-like or pharmacologic effect in the host.	Not immune-mediated. Tyramine in patients treated with MAO inhibitors, fermented (alcohol-containing) foods in disulfiram-treated patients.
Metabolic food reaction	Toxic effects of a food when eaten in excess or improperly prepared.	Cycasin, vitamin A toxicity, goitrogens.

SOURCE: Adapted from Anderson and Sogn, 1984.

Clinical descriptions of adverse reactions to food are not new. Hippocrates (460–370 B.C.) first recorded adverse reactions to cow's milk that caused gastric upset and urticaria, and Galen (A.D. 131–210) described allergic symptoms to goat milk. However, the immunologic basis of many adverse reactions to food was not established until the passive transfer of sensitivity to fish was described in the early 1960s (Frankland, 1987; Taylor et al., 1989). This test, which evolved into the (skin) prick test and later the radioallergosorbent (RAST) test, allowed a distinction to be made between immunologically based adverse reactions (true allergies) and adverse reactions with other causation.

Food Allergy ***Description*** Food hypersensitivity (allergy) refers to a reaction involving an immune-mediated response. Such a response is generally IgE-mediated, although IgG_4- and cell-mediated immunity also may play a role in some instances (Fukutomi et al., 1994). What generally distinguishes food allergy from other reactions is the involvement of immunoglobulins, basophils, or mast cells (the latter being a source of mediating substances including histamine and bradykinin for immediate reactions and prostaglandins and leukotrienes for slower-developing reactions) and a need for a prior exposure to the allergen or a cross-reactive allergen. An allergic reaction may be manifest by one or more of the symptoms listed in Table 30-18. The list of foods known to provoke allergies is long and is probably limited only by what people are willing to eat. Although cutaneous reactions and anaphylaxis are the most common symptoms associated with food allergy, the body is replete with a repertoire of responses that are rarely confined to only a few foods.

A curious type of food allergy, the so-called exercise-induced food allergy, is apparently provoked by exercise that has been immediately preceded or followed by the ingestion of certain foods (Kivity et al., 1994), including shellfish, peach, wheat, celery, and "solid" food (Taylor et al., 1989). The exact mechanism is unknown, but it may involve enhanced mast-cell responsiveness to physical stimuli and/or diminished metabolism of histamine similar to red wine allergy (Taylor et al., 1989). On the other hand, food intolerance in patients with chronic fatigue may have less to do with allergic response and has been shown to be a somatization trait of patients with depressive symptoms and anxiety disorders (Manu et al., 1993).

Chemistry of Food Allergens Most allergens (antigens) in food are protein in nature, and although almost all foods contain one or more proteins, a few foods are associated more with allergic reactions than are others. For example, anaphylaxis to peanuts is more common than is anaphylaxis to other legumes (e.g., peas, soybeans). Similarly, although allergies may occur from bony fishes, there is no basis for cross-reactivity to other types of seafood (e.g., mollusks and crustaceans), although dual (and independent) sensitivities may exist (Anderson and Sogn, 1984). Interestingly, patients who are allergic to milk can usually tolerate beef and inhaled cattle dander, and patients allergic to eggs can usually tolerate ingestion of chicken and feather-derived particles (Anderson and Sogn, 1984)—although in the "bird-egg" syndrome, patients can be allergic to bird feathers, egg yolk, egg white, or any combination of the three (DeBlay et al., 1994; Szepfalusi et al., 1994). Some of the allergenic components of common food allergens are listed in Table 30-19.

Table 30-18
Symptoms of IgE-Mediated Food Allergies

Cutaneous	Urticaria (hives), eczema, dermatitis, pruritus, rash
Gastrointestinal	Nausea, vomiting, diarrhea, abdominal cramps
Respiratory	Asthma, wheezing, rhinitis, bronchospasm
Other	Anaphylactic shock, hypotension, palatal itching, swelling including tongue and larynx, methemoglobinemia*

*An unusual manifestation of allergy reported to occur in response to soy or cow milk protein intolerance in infants (Murray and Christie, 1993).

SOURCE: Adapted from Taylor et al., 1989, with permission.

Table 30-19
Known Allergenic Food Proteins

FOOD	ALLERGIC PROTEINS
Cow's milk	Casein (Dorion et al., 1994; Stoger and Wuthrich, 1993)
	β-Lactoglobulin (Piastra et al., 1994; Stoger and Wuthrich, 1993)
	α-Lactalbumin (Bernaola et al., 1994; Stoger and Wuthrich, 1993)
Egg whites	Ovomucoid (Bernhisel-Broadbent et al., 1994)
	Ovalbumin (Fukotomi et al., 1994, Bernhiesel-Broadbent et al., 1994)
Egg yolks	Livetin (de Blay et al., 1994; Szepfalusi et al., 1994)
Peanuts	Ara h II (Dorion et al., 1994)
	Peanut I (Sachs et al., 1981)
Soybeans	β-Conglycinin (7S fraction) (Rumsey et al., 1994)
	Glycinin (11S fraction) (Rumsey et al., 1994)
	Gly mIA (Gonzalez et al., 1992)
	Gly mIB (Gonzalez et al., 1992)
	Kunitz trypsin inhibitor (Brandon et al., 1986)
Codfish	Gad cI (O'Neil et al., 1993)
Shrimp	Antigen II (Taylor et al., 1989)
Green peas	Albumin fraction (Taylor et al., 1989)
Rice	Glutelin fraction (Taylor et al., 1989)
	Globulin fraction (Taylor et al., 1989)
Cottonseed	Glycoprotein fraction (Taylor et al., 1989)
Peach guava, banana, mandarin, strawberry	30-kDa protein (Wadee et al., 1990)
Tomato	Several glycoproteins (Taylor et al., 1989)
Wheat	Gluten (Stewart-Tull and Jones, 1992)
	Gliadin (O'Hallaren, 1992)
	Globulin (O'Hallaren, 1992)
	Albumin (O'Hallaren, 1992)
Okra	Fraction I (Manda et al., 1992)

SOURCE: Modified from Taylor et al., 1989, with permission.

Although food avoidance is usually the best means of protection, it is not always possible because (1) the content of some prepared foods may be unknown (e.g., the presence of eggs or cottonseed oil), (2) there is the possibility of contamination of food from unsuspected sources [e.g., *Penicillium* in cheeses or meat, *Candida albicans* (Dayan, 1993; Dorion et al., 1994), and cow's milk antigens in the breast milk of mothers who have consumed cow's milk (Halken, et al., 1993)], (3) an allergen may be present in a previously unknown place [the insertion of Brazil nut DNA into soybeans and subsequent appearance of the allergic 2S protein in soybean products (Nordlee et al., 1996)], and (4) there is a lack of knowledge about the phylogenetic relationships between food sources (legumes include peas, soybeans, and peanuts; some Americans are not aware that ham is a pork product). While avoidance is not always possible, promising research in the area of probiotics (i.e., promotion of the growth of beneficial intestinal bacteria including lactobacilli or bifidobacteria) may help in management of food allergy (Kirjavainen et al., 1999; Arunachalam, 1999).

Demographics of Food Allergy Although children appear to be the most susceptible to food allergy, with adverse reactions occurring in 4 to 6 percent of infants, the incidence appears to taper off with maturation of the digestive tract, with only 1 to 2 percent of young children (4 to 15 years) susceptible (Fuglsang et al., 1993). The increase in the number of adults exhibiting food allergy may be due in part to an expanded food universe—that is, an increased willingness to try different foods. In one study, allergies among young children were most commonly to milk and eggs, while allergies that developed later in life tended to be to fruit and vegetables (Kivity et al., 1994).

Familial relationships also play a role. Schrander and colleagues (1993) noted that among infants intolerant of cow's milk protein, 65 percent had a positive family history (first- or second-degree relatives) for atopy compared with 35 percent of healthy controls.

Food Toxicity (Poisoning) See "Substances for which Tolerances May Not Be Set" below.

Food Idiosyncrasy Food idiosyncrasies are generally defined as *quantitatively* abnormal responses to a food substance or additive; this reaction differs from the physiologic effect, and although it may resemble hypersensitivity, it does not involve immune mechanisms. Food idiosyncratic reactions include those that occur in specific groups of individuals who may be genetically predisposed. Examples of such reactions and the foods that are probably responsible are given in Table 30-20.

Probably the most common idiosyncratic reaction is lactose intolerance, a deficiency of the lactase enzyme needed for the metabolism of the lactose in cow's milk. A lack of this enzyme re-

Table 30-20
Idiosyncratic Reactions to Foods

FOOD	REACTION	MECHANISM	REFERENCE
Fava beans	Hemolysis, sometimes accompanied by jaundice and hemoglobinuria; also, pallor, fatigue, nausea, dyspnea, fever and chills, abdominal and dorsal pain	Pyramidene aglycones in fava bean cause irreversible oxidation of GSH in G-6-PD-deficient erythrocytes by blocking NADPH supply, resulting in oxidative stress of the erythrocyte and eventual hemolysis	Chevion et al., 1985
Chocolate	Migraine headache	Phenylethylamine-related (?)	Gibb et al., 1991; Settipane, 1987
Beets	Beetanuria: passage of red urine (often mistaken for hematuria)	Excretion of beetanin in urine after consumption of beets	Smith, 1991
Asparagus	Odorous, sulfurous-smelling urine	Autosomal dominant inability to metabolize methanthiol of asparagus and consequent passage of methanthiol in urine	Smith, 1991
Red wine	Sneezing, flush, headache, diarrhea, skin itch, shortness of breath	Diminished histamine degradation: deficiency of diamine oxidase (?) Histamines present in wine	Wantke et al., 1994
Choline- and carnitine-containing foods	Fish odor syndrome: foul odor of body secretions	Choline and carnitine metabolized to trimethylamine in gut by bacteria, followed by absorption but inability to metabolize to odorless trimethylamine *N*-oxide	Ayesh et al., 1993
Lactose intolerance	Abdominal pain, bloating, diarrhea	Lactase deficiency	Mallinson, 1987
Fructose-containing foods	Abdominal pain, vomiting, diarrhea, hypoglycemia	Reduced activity of hepatic aldolase B toward fructose-1-phosphate	Frankland, 1987; Catto-Smith and Adams, 1993

sults in fermentation of lactose to lactic acid and an osmotic effect in the bowel, with resultant symptoms of malabsorption and diarrhea. Lactose intolerance is lowest in northern Europe at 3 to 8 percent of the population; it reaches 70 percent in southern Italy and Turkey and nearly 100 percent in southeast Asia (Gudmand-Hoyer, 1994; Anderson and Sogn, 1984).

Anaphylactoid Reactions Anaphylactoid reactions are historically thought of as reactions mimicking anaphylaxis (and other "allergic-type" responses, including though not limited to itching, chronic urticaria, angioedema, exacerbation of atopic eczema, rhinitis, bronchial obstruction, asthma, diarrhea and other intestinal disturbances, and vasomotor headaches) through direct application of the primary mediator of anaphylactic reactions: histamine. Ingestion of scombroid fish (e.g., tuna, mackerel, bonito) as well as some nonscombroid fish (mahimahi and bluefish) that have been acted upon by microorganisms (most commonly *Proteus morganii, Proteus vulgaris, Clostridium* spp., *Escherichia coli, Salmonella* spp., and *Shigella* spp.) to produce histamine may result in an anaphylactoid reaction also called *scombrotoxicosis* (Table 30-21) (Clark et al., 1999). The condition was reported to be mimicked by the direct ingestion of 90 mg of histamine in unspoiled fish (van Geldern et al., 1992), but according to Taylor (1986), the effect of simply ingesting histamine does not produce the equivalent effect. Instead, Taylor stated that histamine ingested with spoiled fish appears to be much more toxic than is histamine ingested in an aqueous solution, as a result of the presence of histamine potentiators in fish flesh. These potentiators included putrefactive amines (putrescine and cadaverine) and pharmacologic potentiators such as aminoguanidine and isoniazid (histaminase inhibitors). The mechanism of potentiation involves the inhibition of intestinal histamine-metabolizing enzymes (diamine oxidase), which causes increased histamine uptake. Scombrotoxicosis in the absence of high histamine levels (less than the U.S. FDA action level for tuna of 50 mg histamine/100 g fish) was reported by Gessner et al., 1996. Melnik et al., (1997) proposed that anaphylactoid responses may be the sum of several mechanisms: (1) an increased intake of biogenic amines (including histamine) with food, (2) an increased synthesis by the intestinal flora, (3) a diminished catabolism of biogenic amines by the intestinal mucosa, and (4) an increased release of endogenous histamine from mast cells and basophils by histamine-releasing food. Further, improvement was observed in 50 percent of patients with histamine intolerance and atopic eczema who maintained a histamine-depleted diet. Ijomah and coworkers (1991) claimed that dietary histamine is not a major determinant of scombrotoxicosis, since potency is not positively correlated with the dose and volunteers tend to fall into susceptible and nonsusceptible subgroups. Ijomah and coworkers (1991) suggested that endogenous histamine released by mast cells plays a significant role in the etiology of scombrotoxicosis, whereas the role of dietary histamine is minor. An exception to this endogenous histamine theory was described by Morrow and colleagues (1991), who found the expected increase in urinary histamine in scombroid-poisoned individuals but did not find an increase in urinary $9\alpha,11\beta$-dhydroxy-15-oxo-2,3,18,19-tetranorprost-5-ene-1,20-dioic acid, the principal metabolite of prostaglandin D_2, a mast cell secretory product; thus, no mast-cell involvement was indicated. Rittweger et al. (1994) have reported an increase in urinary immunoreaction angiotensin I and angiotensin II following oral provocation tests to patients with a history of anaphylactoid reactions to drugs, foods, and food additives, but unfortunately there are no reports describing urinary angiotensin levels following oral histamine administration.

Smith (1991) described sulfite-induced bronchospasm (sometimes leading to asthma), which was first noticed as an acute sen-

Table 30-21
Anaphylactoid Reactions to Food

FOOD	REACTION	MECHANISM	REFERENCE
Western Australian salmon (*Arripis truttaceus*)	Erythema and urticaria of the skin, facial flushing and sweating, palpitations, hot flushes of the body, headache, nausea, vomiting, and dizziness	Scombroid poisoning; high histamine levels demonstrated in the fish	Smart, 1992
Fish (spiked with histamine)	Facial flushing, headache	Histamine poisoning; histamine concentration in plasma correlated closely with histamine dose ingested	Van Gelderen et al., 1992
Cape yellow tail (fish) (*Seriola lalandii*)	Skin rash, diarrhea, palpitations, headache, nausea and abdominal cramps, paresthesia, unusual taste sensation, and breathing difficulties	Scombroid poisoning, treated with antihistamines	Muller et al., 1992
Sulfite sensitivity	Bronchospasm, asthma	Sulfite oxidase deficiency to metabisulfites in foods and wine	Smith, 1991
Tuna, albacore, mackerel, bonito, mahimahi, and bluefish	Reaction resembling an acute allergic reaction	Scombroid poisoning treated with antihistamines and cimetidine	Lange, 1988
Cheese	Symptoms resembling acute allergic reaction	Responds to antihistamines; histamine poisoning?	Taylor, 1986

sitivity to metabisulfites sprayed on restaurant salads (and salad bars) and in wine. Sulfite is normally detoxicated rapidly to inorganic sulfate by the enzyme sulfite oxidase. In sensitive individuals, there is apparently a deficiency in this enzyme, making them supersensitive to sulfites. (The FDA has taken the position that the addition of sulfite to food is safe only when properly disclosed on the food label.)

Pharmacologic Food Reactions Also referred to as "false food allergies" (Moneret-Vautrin, 1987), these adverse reactions are characterized by exaggerated responses to pharmacologic agents in food (Table 30-22). These reactions are distinguished from other classifications because they are not associated with a specific anomaly of metabolism (e.g., lactose intolerance or favism) but may be a receptor anomaly instead. These, then, are common pharmacologic agents acting in a very predictable manner, but at exceptionally low levels.

Metabolic Food Reactions Metabolic food reactions are distinct from other categories of adverse reactions in that the foods are more or less commonly eaten and demonstrate toxic effects only when eaten to excess or improperly processed (Table 30-23). The susceptible population exists as a result of its own behavior—that is, the "voluntary" consumption of food as a result of a limited food supply or an abnormal craving for a specific food. Such an abnormal craving was reported by Bannister and associates (1977), who noted hypokalemia leading to cardiac arrest in a 58-year-old woman who had been eating about 1.8 kg of licorice per week. In "glycyrrhizism," or licorice intoxication, glycyrrhizic acid is the active component, with an effect resembling that of aldosterone, which suppresses the renin-angiotensin-aldosterone axis, resulting in the loss of potassium. Clinically, hypokalemia with alkalosis, cardiac arrhythmias, and muscular symptoms, together with sodium retention, edema, and severe hypertension are observed. The syndrome may develop at a level of 100 g licorice per day but gradually abates upon withdrawal of the licorice (Tonnesen, 1979).

This category also includes the ingestion of improperly prepared food such as cassava or cycad, which, if prepared properly will result in a toxin-free food. For example, cycad (*Cacaos circinalis*) is a particularly hardy tree in tropical to subtropical habitats around the world. Cycads often survive when other crops have been destroyed (e.g., a natural disaster such as a typhoon or drought) and therefore may serve as an alternative source of food. Among people who have used cycads for food, the method of detoxification is remarkably similar despite the wide range of this plant: the seeds and stems are cut into small pieces and soaked in water for several days; they are then dried and ground into flour. The effectiveness of leaching the toxin (cycasin) from the bits of flesh is most directly dependent on the size of the pieces, the duration of soaking, and the number of water changes. Shortcuts in processing may have grave consequences (Matsumoto, 1985).

Importance of Labeling

Food labeling allows susceptible individuals to avoid foods containing ingredients that may be harmful to them, such as allergens or substances they may be intolerant of, such as lactose. Thus, if a food contained an allergy-causing protein, this would have to be indicated on the label. The FDA has indicated that, at this time, they are not aware of any information that foods developed through genetic engineering differ as a class in any attribute from foods developed through conventional means, and that such foods would therefore not warrant a special label (Thompson, 2000). FDA allows companies to include on the label of a product any statement as long as the statement is truthful and not misleading.

TOLERANCE SETTING FOR SUBSTANCES IN FOODS

Pesticide Residues

A pesticide is defined under the FD&C Act as any substance used as a pesticide, within the meaning of the Federal Insecticide, Fungicide and Rodenticide Act (FIFRA), in the production, storage, or transportation of raw agricultural commodities (food in its raw or natural state) [section 201(q)]. The Pesticide amendments of 1956 to the FD&C Act (section 408) were the first amendments to the FD&C Act requiring premarket clearance evaluations of the safety of chemicals added to food. Currently, the U.S. Environmental Protection Agency (EPA) is responsible for evaluating the safety of pesticides before issuing tolerances.

The regulation of pesticides and their safety is accomplished under both FIFRA and the FD&C Act. FIFRA governs the registration of pesticides. Registration addresses specific uses of a pesticide, and without such registration a pesticide cannot be lawfully sold for such use in the United States. A major part of the registration process involves tolerance setting. Pesticides intended for use on food crops must be granted tolerances or exempted from tolerances under the FD&C Act.

Tolerances for raw agriculture commodities (RAC's) were established under section 408 of the FD&C Act. If the pesticide chemical was found to concentrate in any of the processed fractions from the processing studies on the food crops (usually at least 1.5 or 2.0× of the residue concentration in the RAC), the residues in the

Table 30-22
Pharmacologic Reactions to Food

FOOD	REACTION	MECHANISM	REFERENCE
Cheese, red wine	Severe headache, hypertension	Tyramine from endogenous or ingested tyrosine	Settipane, 1987
Nutmeg	Hallucinations	Myristicin	Anderson and Sogn, 1984
Coffee, tea	Headache, hypertension	Methylxanthine (caffeine) acting as a noradrenergic stimulant	Anderson and Sogn, 1984
Chocolate	Headache, hypertension	Methylxanthine (theophylline) acting as a noradrenergic stimulant	Anderson and Sogn, 1984

Table 30-23
Metabolic Food Reactions

FOOD	REACTION	MECHANISM	REFERENCE
Lima beans, cassava roots, millet (sorghum) sprouts, bitter almonds, apricot and peach pits	Cyanosis	Cyanogenic glycosides releasing hydrogen cyanide on contact with stomach acid	Anderson and Sogn, 1984
Cabbage family, turnips, soybeans, radishes, rapeseed and mustard	Goiter (enlarged thyroid)	Isothiocyanates, goitrin, or *S*-5-vinyl-thiooxazolidone interferes with utilization of iodine	Anderson and Sogn, 1984; vanEtten and Tookey, 1985
Unripe fruit of the tropical tree *Blighia sapida,* common in Caribbean and Nigeria	Severe vomiting, coma, and acute hypoglycemia sometimes resulting in death, especially among the malnourished	Hypoglycin A, isolated from the fruit, may interfere with oxidation of fatty acids, so that glycogen stores have to be metabolized for energy, with depletion of carbohydrates, resulting in hypoglycemia	Evans, 1985
Leguminosae, Cruciferae	Lathyritic symptoms: neurological symptoms of weakness, leg paralysis, and sometimes death	L-2-4-Diaminobutyric acid inhibition of ornithine transcarbamylase of the urea cycle, inducing ammonia toxicity	Evans, 1985
Licorice (glycyrrhizic acid)	Hypertension, cardiac enlargement, sodium retention	Glycyrrhizic acid mimicking mineralocorticoids	Farese et al., 1991
Polar bear and Chicken liver	Irritability, vomiting, increased intracranial pressure, death	Vitamin A toxicity	Bryan, 1984
Cycads (cycad flour)	Amyotrophic lateral sclerosis (humans), hepatocarcinogenicity (rats and nonhuman primates)	Cycasin (methylazoxymethanol); primary action is methylation, resulting in a broad range of effects from membrane destruction to inactivation of enzyme systems	Matsumoto, 1985; Sieber et al., 1980

processed fraction(s) were considered to be intentional food additives and were required to be assigned "Food Additive Tolerances" under Section 409 of the act. If the pesticide chemical in question had been classified by the EPA as a human or animal carcinogen, the Delaney clause would then be invoked, and the section 409 food additive tolerance(s) could be denied on that basis.

Under the new Food Quality Protection Act (FQPA) of 1996, section 201(s) of the FD&C Act excludes pesticides from the definition of *food additive*—even in the case of concentration of residues in processed fractions. Consequently, the Delaney clause is no longer applicable *for pesticides.* The Delaney clause has *not* been repealed from section 409 and continues to apply to intentional food additives *other than pesticides.* In the case of concentration of pesticide residues in a processed fraction above the section 408 tolerances established for the RAC, an additional tolerance for that processed fraction is still established, but now under section 408 rather than section 409.

The FQPA requires that an additional tenfold safety factor "shall be applied for infants and children to take into account potential pre- and post-natal toxicity and completeness of the data with respect to exposure and toxicity to infants and children." Therefore the "default" assumption is that the additional 10× safety factor will be applied to the chemical safety assessment resulting in a total safety factor of 1000×. It further states, however, that "the Administrator may use a different margin of safety for the pesticide chemical residue only if, on the basis of reliable data, such margin will be safe for infants and children." Therefore, the additional 10× safety factor may be reduced depending on such things as adequacy of exposure assessment, adequacy of the toxicologic data-base, and the nature and severity of any adverse effects observed in these studies, the most important being the adequacy of the toxicologic data base.

Drugs Used in Food-Producing Animals

An animal drug "means any drug intended for use for animals other than man" [section 201(w) of the FD&C Act]. Animal drugs, which typically are used for growth promotion and increased food production, present a complex problem in the safety assessment of animal drug residues in human food. Determination of the potential human health hazards associated with animal drug residues is complicated by the metabolism of an animal drug, which results in residues of many potential metabolites. The sensitivity of modern analytic methodologies designed to quantitate small amounts of drugs and their various metabolites has made evaluation more complex.

The primary factors that must be considered in the evaluation of animal drugs are (1) consumption and absorption by the target animal, (2) metabolism of the drug by the target food animal, (3) excretion and tissue distribution of the drug and its metabolites in food animal products and tissues, (4) consumption of food animal products and tissues by humans, (5) potential absorption of the drug and its metabolites by humans, (6) potential metabolism of the drug and its metabolites by humans, and (7) potential excretion and tissue distribution in humans of the drug, its metabolites, and the secondary human metabolites derived from the drug and its metabolites. Thus, the pharmacokinetic and biotransformation characteristics of both the animal and the human must be considered in an assessment of the potential human health hazard of an animal drug.

When an animal drug is considered GRAS, the safety assessment of the drug is handled as described under the section on GRAS, above. With respect to new animal drugs, safety assessment is concerned primarily with residues that occur in animal food products (milk, cheese, etc.) and edible tissues (muscle, liver, etc.). Toxicity studies in the target species (chicken, cow, pig, etc.) should provide data on metabolism and the nature of metabolites along with information on the drug's pharmacokinetics. If this information is not available, these studies must be performed using the animal species that is likely to be exposed to the drug. During this phase, the parent drug and its metabolites are evaluated both qualitatively and quantitatively in the animal products of concern (eggs, milk, meat, etc.). This may involve the development of sophisticated analytic methodologies. Once these data are obtained, it is necessary to undertake an assessment to determine potential human exposure to these compounds from the diet and other sources. If adequate toxicity data are available, it is possible to undertake a safety assessment pursuant to the establishment of a tolerance.

To comply with the congressional intent regarding the use of animal drugs in food-producing animals as required in the "no residue" provision of the Delaney clause, the FDA began to build a system for conducting risk assessment of carcinogens in the early 1970s (FDA, 1977). In the course of developing a policy and/or regulatory definition for "no residue," the FDA was compelled to address the issue of residues of metabolites of animal drugs known to induce cancer in humans or animals. As the number of metabolites may range into the hundreds, it became apparent that, as a practical matter, not every metabolite could be tested with the same thoroughness as the parent animal drug. This forced the FDA to consider threshold assessment for the first time. Threshold assessment combines information on the structure and in vitro biological activity of a metabolite for the purpose of determining whether carcinogenicity testing is necessary (Flamm et al., 1994). If testing is necessary and the substance is found to induce cancer, the FDA's definition states that a lifetime risk of one in a million as determined by a specified methodology is equivalent to the meaning of "no residue" as intended by Congress.

Unavoidable Contaminants

Certain substances—such as polychlorinated biphenyls (PCB's) or heavy metals—are unavoidable in food because their widespread industrial applications or their presence in the earth's crust have resulted in their becoming a persistent and ubiquitous contaminant in the environment. As a result, foods and animal feeds, principally those of animal and marine origin, contain unavoidable contaminants at some level. Tolerances for residues of unavoidable contaminants are established for foods and food ingredients to ensure that they are safe under expected or intended conditions of use.

Heavy Metals There are 92 natural elements; approximately 22 are known to be essential nutrients of the mammalian body and are referred to as *micronutrients* (Concon, 1988). Among the micronutrients are iron, zinc, copper, manganese, molybdenum, selenium, iodine, cobalt, and even aluminum and arsenic. However, among the 92 elements, lead, mercury, and cadmium are familiar as contaminants or at least have more specifications setting their limits in food ingredients (e.g., Food Chemicals Codex, 1996). The prevalence of these elements as contaminants is due to their ubiquity in nature but also to their use by humans.

Lead Although the toxicity of lead is well known, lead may be an essential trace mineral. A lead deficiency induced by feeding rats <50 ppb (versus 1000 ppb in controls) over one or more generations produced effects on the hematopoietic system, decreased iron stores in the liver and spleen, and caused decreased growth (Kirchgessner and Reichmayer-Lais, 1981), but apparently not as a result of an effect on iron absorption (Reichmayer-Lais and Kirchgessner, 1985). Although the toxic effects of lead are discussed elsewhere in this text, it is important to note that the effects are profound (especially in children) and appear to be long-lasting, since mechanisms for excretion appear to be inadequate in comparison to those for uptake (Linder, 1991).

Over the years, recognition of the serious nature of lead poisoning in children has caused the World Health Organization (WHO) and FDA to adjust the recommended tolerable total lead intake from all sources of not more than 100 μg/day for infants up to 6 months of age and not more than 150 μg/day for children from 6 months to 2 years of age to the considerably lower range of 6 to 18 μg/day as a provisional tolerable range for lead intake in a 10-kg child.

Initiatives to reduce the level of lead in foods, such as the move to eliminate lead-soldered seams in soldered food cans that was begun in the 1970s and efforts to eliminate leachable lead from ceramic glazes, have resulted in a steady decline in dietary lead intake. Although food and water still contribute lead to the diet, data from the FDA's Total Diet Study indicated a reduction in mean dietary lead intake for adult males from 95 μg/day in 1978 to 9 μg/day in the period 1986–1988 (Shank and Carson, 1992).

Some lead sources are difficult to curtail, as lead often survives food processing; for example, lead in wheat remains in the finished flour (Linder, 1991). Therefore, reducing the contribution from dietary sources remains a challenge, but elimination of lead-soldered cans, lead-soldered plumbing, and especially the removal of tetraethyl lead as a gasoline additive have produced substantial reductions in lead ingestion. What is needed now is continued vigilance of largely imported lead-based ceramic ware, lead-containing calcium supplements, and lead leaching into groundwater (Shank and Carson, 1992).

Arsenic Arsenic is a ubiquitous element in the environment; it ranks 20th in relative abundance among the elements of the earth's crust and 12th in the human body (Concon, 1988). (Since arsenic is discussed in detail elsewhere in this text, the discussion here is limited to its relationship to foods.) There is some competition for arsenic absorption with selenium, which is known to reduce arsenic toxicity; arsenic is also known to antagonize iodine metabolism and inhibit various metabolic processes, as a result affecting a number of organ systems. There are a number of sources of arsenic, including drinking water, air, and pesticides (Newberne, 1987), but arsenic consumed via food is largely in proportion to the amount of seafood eaten (74 percent of the arsenic in a market basket survey came from the meat-poultry-fish group, of which seafood consistently has the highest concentration) (Johnson et al., 1981). Although arsenic is used as an animal feed additive, this source does not contribute much to the body burden, as 0.1% arsanilic acid or docecylamine-*p*-chlorophenylarsonate fed to turkeys resulted in tissue residues of only 0.31 and 0.24 ppm in fresh muscle (Underwood, 1973).

Acute poisoning with arsenic often results from mistaking arsenic for sugar, baking powder, and soda and adding it to food. The time between exposure and symptoms is 10 min to several days, and the symptoms include burning of the mouth or throat, a metallic taste, vomiting, diarrhea (watery and bloody), borborigmi (rumbling of the bowles caused by movement of gas in the GI tract), painful tenesmus (spasm of the anal or vesical sphincter), hematuria, dehydration, jaundice, oliguria, collapse, and shock. Headache, vertigo, muscle spasm, stupor, and delirium may occur (Bryan, 1984).

Cadmium Cadmium is a relatively rare commodity in nature and is usually associated with shale and sedimentary deposites. It is often found in association with zinc ores and in lesser amounts in fossil fuel. Although rare in nature, it is a nearly ubiquitous element in American society because of its industrial uses in plating, paint pigments, plastics, and textiles. Exposure of humans often occurs through secondary routes as a result of dumping at smelters and refining plants, disintegration of automobile tires (which contain rubber-laden cadmium), subsequent seepage into the soil and groundwater, and inhalation of combustion of cadmium-containing materials. The estimated yearly release of cadmium from automobile tires ranges from 5.2 to 6.0 metric tons (Davis, 1970; Lagerwerff and Specht, 1971).

Although, like mercury, cadmium can form alkyl compounds, unlike mercury, the alkyl derivatives are relatively unstable and consumption almost always involves the inorganic salt. Of two historical incidents of cadmium poisoning, one involved the use of cadmium-plated containers to hold acidic fruit slushes before freezing. Up to 13 to 15 ppm cadmium was found in the frozen confection, 300 ppm in lemonade, and 450 in raspberry gelatin. Several deaths resulted. A more recent incident of a chronic poisoning involved the dumping of mining wastes into rice paddies in Japan. Middle-aged women who were deficient in calcium and had had multiple pregnancies seemed to be the most susceptible. Symptoms included hypercalciuria; extreme bone pain from osteomalacia; lumbago; pain in the back, shoulders, and joints; a waddling gait; frequent fractures; proteinuria; and glycosuria. The disease was called *itai itai* ("ouch-ouch disease") as a result of the pain with walking. The victims had a reported intake of 1000 μg/day, approximately 200 times the normal intake in unexposed populations (Yamagata and Shigematsu, 1970). Cadmium exposure also has been associated with cancer of the breast, lung, large intestine, and urinary bladder (Newberne, 1987).

Chlorinated Organics Chlorinated organics have been with us for some time, and given their stability in water and resistance to oxidation, ultraviolet light, microbial degradation, and other sources of natural destruction, chlorinated organics will continue to reside in the environment for some time to come, albeit in minute amounts. However, with the introduction of chlorinated hydrocarbons as pesticides in the 1930s, diseases associated with an insect vector such as malaria were nearly eliminated. In the industrialized world, chlorinated organics brought the promise of nearly universal solvents, and their extraordinary resistance to degradation made them suitable for use as heat transfer agents, carbonless copy paper, and fire retardants (Table 30-24).

As persistent as these substances are in the environment and despite the degree of toxicity that might be implied, the possible hazard from chlorinated substances is relatively low. Ames et al. (1987) described a method for interpreting the differing potencies of carcinogens and human exposures: the percentage HERP (human exposure dose/rodent potency dose). Using this method, they demonstrated that the hazard from trichloroethylene-contaminated water in Silicon Valley or Woburn, Massachusetts, or the daily dietary intake from DDT (or its product, DDE) at a HERP of 0.0003

Table 30-24
Examples of Levels of Chlorinated Hydrocarbons in British Food

	Chlorinated Hydrocarbons, ug/kg								
FOOD	$CHCl_3$	CCl_4	TCE	TCEY	TTCE	PCE	HCB	HCBD	Per CE
Milk	5.0	0.2		0.3	—	—	1.0	0.08	0.3
Cheese	33.0	5.0		3.0	0.0	0.0	0.0	0.0	2.0
Butter	22.0	14.0		10.0	—	—	—	2.0	13.0
Chicken eggs	1.4	0.5		0.6	0.0	0.0	0.0	0.0	0.0
Beef steak	4.0	7.0	3.0	16.0	0.0	0.0	0.0	0.0	0.9
Beef fat	3.0	8.0	6.0	12.0					1.0
Pork liver	1.0	9.0	4.0	22.0	0.5	0.4			5.0
Margarine	3.0	6.0	—		0.8				7.0
Tomatoes	2.0	4.5	—	1.7	1.0		70.1	0.8	1.2
Bread (fresh)	2.0	5.0	2.0	7.0	—	—	—	—	1.0
Fruit drink (canned)	2.0	0.5	—	5.0		0.8			2.0

KEY: $CHCl_3$ = chloroform; CCl_4 = carbon tetrachloride; TCE = trichloroethane; TCEY = trichloroethylene; TTCE = tetrachloroethane; PCE = pentachloroethane; HCB = hexachlorobenzene; HCBD = hexachlorobutadiene; Per CE = perchloroethylene.

SOURCE: Modified from McConnell et al., 1975, with kind permission from Elsevier Science Ltd, The Boulevard, Langford Lane, Kidlington OX5 1GB, UK.

to 0.004 percent is considerably less than the hazard presented by the consumption of symphytine in a single cup of comfrey herb tea (0.03 percent) or the hazard presented by aflatoxin in a peanut butter sandwich (0.03 percent). The FDA's authority to set tolerances has been used only once in establishing levels for polychlorinated biphenyls (21 CFR 109.15 and 109.30).

Although the possibility always exists, there have been only a few incidents of mass poisonings via food, two of which involved contaminated cooking oil. The first became known as *yusho,* or rice oil disease, from rice oil contamination by polychlorinated biphenyls (PCBs). The most vulnerable individuals were newborn infants of poisoned mothers. The liver and skin were the most severely affected. Symptoms included dark brown pigmentation of nails; acne-like eruptions; increased eye discharge; visual disturbances; pigmentation of the skin, lips, and gingiva; swelling of the upper eyelids; hyperemia of the conjunctiva; enlargement and elevation of hair follicles; itching; increased sweating of the palms; hyperkeratotic plaques on the soles and palms; and generalized malaise. Recovery requires several years (Anderson and Sogn, 1984). The second incident has become known as *Spanish toxic oil syndrome,* and although details are still not fully known, it occurred after aniline-contaminated rapeseed oil was distributed as cooking oil in Spain in 1981. Approximately 20,000 people were affected and there were several deaths. Because symptoms were unique—including respiratory effects, eosinophilia, and muscle wasting—but not typical of aniline poisoning, the exact etiologic agent is still unknown. Because the source of the aniline may have been improperly cleaned tank trucks that had imported industrial chemicals, three hypotheses have been offered: the etiologic agent may have been (1) a contaminant in the aniline, (2) a contaminant introduced during transportation, or (3) a reaction product of normal oil components and the potential contaminants (the fraction of the oil most commonly associated with toxicity contained $C_{18:3}$ anilide, also called oleyl anilide and "fatty acid anilide") (Borda et al., 1998; Posada de la Paz et al., 1996; Wood et al., 1994).

Nitrosamines, Nitrosamides, and *N*-Nitroso Substances Nitrogenous compounds such as amines, amides, guanidines, and ureas can react with oxides of nitrogen (NO_x) to form *N*-nitroso compounds (NOCs) (Hotchkiss et al., 1992). The NOCs may be divided into two classes: the nitrosamines, which are *N*-nitroso derivatives of secondary amines, and nitrosamides, which are *N*-nitroso derivatives of substituted ureas, amides, carbamates, guanidines, and similar compounds (Mirvish, 1975).

Nitrosamines are stable compounds, while many nitrosamides have half-lives on the order of minutes, particularly at pH >6.5. Both classes have members that are potent carcinogens, but by different mechanisms. In general, the biological activity of an NOC is thought to be related to alkylation of genetic macromolecules. *N*-nitrosamines are metabolically activated by hydroxylation at an α-carbon. The resulting hydroxyalkyl moiety is eliminated as an aldehyde, and an unstable primary nitrosamine is formed. The nitrosamine tautomerizes to a diazonium hydroxide and ultimately to a carbonium ion. Nitrosamides spontaneously decompose to a carbonium ion at physiologic pH by a similar mechanism (Hotchkiss et al., 1992). This is consistent with in vitro laboratory findings because nitrosamines require S9 for activity and nitrosamides are mutagenic de novo.

NOCs originate from two sources: environmental formation and endogenous formation (Table 30-25). Environmental sources have declined over the last several years but still include foods (e.g., nitrate-cured meats) and beverages (e.g., malt beverages), cosmetics, occupational exposure, and rubber products (Hotchkiss, 1989). NOCs formed in vivo may actually constitute the greatest exposure and are formed from nitrosation of amines and amides in several areas, including the stomach, where the most favorable conditions exist (pH 2 to 4), although consumption of H_2-receptor blockers or antacids decreases the formation of NOCs.

Table 30-25
Sources of Dietary NOCs

The use of nitrate and/or nitrite as intentional food additives, both of which are added to fix the color of meats, inhibit oxidation, and prevent toxigenesis
Drying processes in which the drying air is heated by an open flame source. NO_x is generated in small amounts through the oxidation of N_2, which nitrosates amines in the foods. This is the mechanism for contamination of malted barley products
NOCs can migrate from food contact materials such as rubber bottle nipples
NOCs can inhabit spices which may be added to food
Cooking over open flames (e.g., natural gas flame) can result in NOC formation in foods by the same mechanism as drying

SOURCE: Hotchkiss et al., 1992, with permission.

Environmentally, nitrite is formed from nitrate or ammonium ions by certain microorganisms in soil, water, and sewage. In vivo, nitrite is formed from nitrate by microorganisms in the mouth and stomach, followed by nitrosation of secondary amines and amides in the diet. Sources of nitrate and nitrite in the diet are given in Table 30-26. Many sources of nitrate are also sources of vitamin C. Another possibly significant source of nitrate is well water; although the levels are generally in the range of 21 μM, average levels of 1600 μM (100 mg/L) have been reported (Hotchkiss et al., 1992). However, on the average, western diets contain 1 to 2 mmol nitrate per person per day (Hotchkiss et al., 1992). Nitrosation reactions can be inhibited by preferential, competitive neutralization of nitrite with naturally occurring and synthetic materials such as vitamin C, vitamin E, sulfamate, and antioxidants such as BHT, BHA, gallic acid, and even amino acids or proteins (Hotchkiss, 1989; Hotchkiss et al., 1992).

N-nitrosoproline is the most common nitrosoamine present in humans and is excreted virtually unchanged in the urine. The basal rate of urinary excretion of nitrosoproline, which is claimed to be noncarcinogenic, is 2 to 7 μg/day in subjects on a low-nitrate diet (Oshima and Bartsch, 1981). Epidemiologic studies have not provided evidence of a causal association between nitrate exposure and human cancer, nor has a causal link been shown between *N*-nitroso compounds preformed in the diet or endogenously synthesized and the incidence of human cancer (Gangolli 1999).

Food-Borne Molds and Mycotoxins Molds have served humans for centuries in the production of foods (e.g., ripening of cheese) and have provided various fungal metabolites with important medicinal uses; they also may produce metabolites with the potential to produce severe adverse health effects. Mycotoxins represent a diverse group of chemicals that can occur in a variety of plant foods. They also can occur in animal products derived from ani-

Table 30-26
Nitrate and Nitrite Content of Food

VEGETABLES	NITRATE, PPM	NITRITE, PPM	MEAT	NITRATE, PPM	NITRITE, PPM
Artichoke	12	0.4	Unsmoked side bacon	134	12
Asparagus	44	0.6	Unsmoked back bacon	160	8
Green beans	340	0.6	Peameal bacon	16	21
Lima beans	54	1.1	Smoked bacon	52	7
Beets	2400	4	Corned beef	141	19
Broccoli	740	1	Cured corned beef	852	9
Brussels sprouts	120	1	Corned beef brisket	90	3
Cabbage	520	0.5	Pickled beef	70	23
Carrots	200	0.8	Canned corn beef	77	24
Cauliflower	480	1.1	Ham	105	17
Celery	2300	0.5	Smoked ham	138	50
Corn	45	2	Cured ham	767	35
Radish	1900	0.2	Belitalia (garlic)	247	5
Rhubarb	2100	NR*	Pepperoni (beef)	149	23
Spinach	1800	2.5	Summer sausage	135	7
Tomatoes	58	NR	Ukranian sausage (Polish)	77	15
Turnip	390	NR	German sausage	71	17
Turnip greens	6600	2.3			

*NR = not reported.
SOURCE: Hotchkiss et al., 1992, with permission

mals that consume contaminated feeds. The current interest in mycotoxicoses was generated by a series of reports in 1960–1963 that associated the death of turkeys in England (so-called turkey X disease) and ducklings in Uganda with the consumption of peanut meal feeds containing mold products produced by *Aspergillus flavus* (Stoloff, 1977). The additional discovery of aflatoxin metabolites (for example, aflatoxin M_1) led to more intensive studies of mycotoxins and to the identification of a variety of these compounds associated with adverse human health effects, both retrospectively and prospectively.

Moldy foods are consumed throughout the world during times of famine, as a matter of taste, and through ignorance of their adverse health effects. Epidemiologic studies designed to ascertain the acute or chronic effects of such consumption are few. Data from animal studies indicate that the consumption of food contaminated with mycotoxins has a high potential to produce a variety of human diseases (Miller, 1991).

With some exceptions, molds can be divided into two main groups: "field fungi" and "storage fungi." The former group contains species that proliferate in and under field conditions and do not multiply once grain is in storage. Field fungi are in fact superseded and overrun by storage fungi if conditions of moisture and oxygen allow. Thus, for instance, *Fusarium* spp., a field fungus commonly found on crops, is seldom found after about 6 weeks of storage, its place being taken by *Aspergillus* and *Penicillium,* both of which represent several species of storage fungi (Harrison, 1971). However, the presence of mold does not guarantee the presence of mycotoxin, which is elaborated only under certain conditions. Further, more than one mold can produce the same mycotoxin (e.g., both *Aspergillus* and *Penicillium* may produce the mycotoxin cyclopiazonic acid) (Truckness et al., 1987; El-Banna et al., 1987). Also, more than one mycotoxin may be present in an intoxication; that is, as in the outbreak of turkey X disease, there is evidence that aflatoxin and cyclopiazonic acid both exerted an effect, but the profound effects of aflatoxin overshadowed those of cyclopiazonic acid (Miller, 1989). Although there are many different mycotoxins and subgroups (Table 30-27), this discussion is confined largely to two of the more toxicologically and economically important ones: the aflatoxins and trichothecenes.

Aflatoxins Among the various mycotoxins, the aflatoxins have been the subject of the most intensive research because of the extremely potent hepatocarcinogenicity and toxicity of aflatoxin B_1 in rats. Epidemiologic studies conducted in Africa and Asia suggest that it is a human hepatocarcinogen, and various other reports have implicated the aflatoxins in incidences of human toxicity (Krishnamachari et al., 1975; Peers et al., 1976).

Generally, aflatoxins occur in susceptible crops as mixtures of aflatoxins B_1, B_2, G_1, and G_2, with only aflatoxins B_1 and G_1 demonstrating carcinogenicity. A carcinogenic hydroxylated metabolite of aflatoxin B_1 (termed aflatoxin M_1) can occur in the milk from dairy cows that consume contaminated feed. Aflatoxins may occur in a number of susceptible commodities and products derived from them, including edible nuts (peanuts, pistachios, almonds, walnuts, pecans, Brazil nuts), oil seeds (cottonseed, copra), and grains (corn, grain sorghum, millet) (Stoloff, 1977). In tropical regions, aflatoxin can be produced in unrefrigerated prepared foods. The two major sources of aflatoxin contamination of commodities are field contamination, especially during times of drought and other stresses, which allow insect damage that opens the plant to mold attack, and inadequate storage conditions. Since the discovery of their potential threat to human health, progress has been made in decreasing the level of aflatoxin in specific commodities. Control measures include ensuring adequate storage conditions and careful monitoring of susceptible commodities for aflatoxin level and the banning of lots that exceed the action level for aflatoxin B_1.

Table 30-27
Selected Mycotoxins Produced by Various Molds

MYCOTOXIN	SOURCE	EFFECT	COMMODITIES CONTAMINATED
Aflatoxins B_1, B_2, G_1, G_2	*Aspergillus flavus, parasiticus*	Acute aflatoxicosis, carcinogenesis	Corn, peanuts, and and others
Aflatoxin M_1	Metabolite of AFB_1	Hepatotoxicity	Milk
Fumonisins B_1, B_2, B_3, B_4, A_1, A_2	*Fusarium moniliforme*	Carcinogenesis	Corn
Trichothecenes	*Fusarium, Myrothecium*	Hematopoietic toxicity, meningeal hemorrhage of brain, "nervous" disorder, necrosis of skin, hemorrhage in mucosal epithelia of stomach and intestine	Cereal grains, corn
T-2 toxin	*Trichoderma*		Corn, barley, sorghum
Trichodermin	*Cephalosporium*		
Zearalenones	*Fusarium*	Estrogenic effect	Corn, grain
Cyclopiazonic acid	*Aspergillus, Penicillium*	Muscle, liver, and splenic toxicity	Cheese, grains, peanuts
Kojic acid	*Aspergillus*	Hepatotoxic?	Grain, animal feed
3-Nitropropionic acid	*Arthrinium sacchari, saccharicola, phaeospermum*	Central nervous system impairment	Sugarcane
Citreoviridin	*Penicillium citreoviride, toxicarium*	Cardiac beriberi	Rice
Cytochalasins E, B, F, H	*Aspergillus and Penicillium*	Cytotoxicity	Corn, cereal grain
Sterigmatocystin	*Aspergillus versiolar*	Carcinogenesis	Corn
Penicillinic acid	*Penicillium cyclopium*	Nephrotoxicity, abortifacient	Corn, dried beans, grains
Rubratoxins A, B	*Penicillium rubrum*	Hepatotoxicity, teratogenic	Corn
Patulin	*Penicillium patulatum*	Carcinogenesis, liver damage	Apple and apple products
Ochratoxin	*A. ochraceus, P. viridicatum*	Balkan nephropathy, carcinogenesis	Grains, peanuts, green coffee
Ergot alkaloids	*Cladosporium purpurea*	Ergotism	Grains

Aflatoxin B_1 is acutely toxic in all species studied, with an LD_{50} ranging from 0.5 mg/kg for the duckling to 60 mg/kg for the mouse (Wogan, 1973). Death typically results from hepatotoxicity. This aflatoxin is also highly mutagenic, hepatocarcinogenic, and possibly teratogenic. A problem in extrapolating animal data to humans is the extremely wide range of species susceptibility to aflatoxin B_1. For instance, whereas aflatoxin B_1 appears to be the most hepatocarcinogenic compound known for the rat, the adult mouse is essentially totally resistant to its hepatocarcinogenicity.

Aflatoxin B_1 is an extremely reactive compound biologically, altering a number of biochemical systems. The hepatocarcinogenicity of aflatoxin B_1 is associated with its biotransformation to a highly reactive electrophilic epoxide that forms covalent adducts with DNA, RNA, and protein. Damage to DNA is thought to be the initial biochemical lesion resulting in the expression of the pathologic tumor growth (Miller, 1978). Species differences in the response to aflatoxin may be due in part to differences in biotransformation and susceptibility to the initial biochemical lesion (Campbell and Hayes, 1976; Monroe and Eaton, 1987).

Although the aflatoxins have received the greatest attention among the various mycotoxins because of their hepatocarcinogenicity in certain species, there is no compelling evidence that they have the greatest potential to produce adverse human health effects.

Trichothecenes Trichothecenes represent a group of toxic substances of which it is likely that several forms may be consumed concomitantly. They represent many different chemical entities all containing the trichothecene nucleus, and are produced by a number of commonly occurring molds, including *Fusarium, Myrothecium, Trichoderma,* and *Cephalosporium.* The trichothecenes were first discovered during attempts to isolate antibiotics, and although some show antibiotic activity, their toxicity has precluded their pharmacologic use. Trichothecenes most often occur in moldy cereal grains. There have been many reported cases of trichothecene toxicity in farm animals and a few in humans. One of the more famous cases of presumed human toxicity associated with the consumption of trichothecenes occurred in Russia during 1944 around Orenburg, Siberia. The disruption of agriculture caused by World War II led to the overwintering of millet, wheat, and barley in the field. Consumption of these grains resulted in vomiting, skin inflammation, diarrhea, and multiple hemorrhages, among other symptoms. This exposure was fatal to over 10 percent of the affected individuals (Ueno, 1977). The extent of toxicity associated with the trichothecenes in humans and farm animals is currently unknown owing to the number of entities in this group and the difficulty of assaying for these compounds. The acute LD_{50}s of the trichothecenes range from 0.5 to 70 mg/kg, and though there have been reports of possible chronic toxicity associated with certain members of this group, more research will be needed before the magnitude of their potential to produce adverse human health effects is understood (Sato and Ueno, 1977).

Fumonisins Fumonisins are recently discovered mycotoxins produced by *Fusarium moniliforme* and several other *Fusarium* species. Corn products contaminated with *Fusarium moniliforme* are responsible for several agriculturally important diseases in horses and swine (Norred, 1993) and are being actively evaluated to determine how great a threat they pose to public health. Initial evidence of the involvement of *F. moniliforme* produced toxins in human disease was reported by Marasas et al. (1988). They found that an increased incidence of esophageal cancer was associated with the consumption of contaminated corn (maize) by humans in a region in South Africa. Corn borer insect pests cause damage to the developing grain, which enables spores of the toxin-producing *Fusarium* fungi to germinate. The fungus then proliferates, which leads to ear and kernel rot and the production of potentially hazardous levels of fumonisins. Corn varieties that express the Bt insecticidal protein have recently been shown to contain significantly reduced levels of fumonisin because the Bt protein significantly reduces corn borer–induced tissue damage in corn products (Munkvold et al., 1997; 1999; Masoero et al., 1999).

Zearalenone Another mycotoxin produced by *Fusarium* is zearalenone. It was first discovered during attempts to isolate an agent from feeds that produced a hyperestrogenic syndrome in swine, characterized by a swollen and edematous vulva and actual vaginal prolapse in severe cases (Stob et al., 1962). Zearalenone can occur in corn, barley, wheat, hay, and oats as well as other agricultural commodities (Mirocha et al., 1977). Zearalenone consumption can decrease the reproductive potential of farm animals, especially swine.

SUBSTANCES FOR WHICH TOLERANCES MAY NOT BE SET

All of the contaminants of food described to this point are those associated with synthesis, growth, production, or storage and are regarded by the FDA as *unavoidable.* Because they are unavoidable, the FDA sets limits rather than banning them, as described earlier. The substances in this section are regarded as (1) *avoidable* or of such hazard that a safe level cannot be set, therefore the FDA has determined that food containing such substances is banned; or (2) beyond the control of the FDA and cannot be regulated (for example, substances produced in the home).

Toxins in Fish, Shellfish, and Turtles

There are a number of seafood toxins (to be distinguished from marine venoms), many of which are not confined to a single species (over 400 species have been incriminated in ciguatera toxicity) and are therefore most likely to be influenced by the environment. However, some seafood toxins are specific to a single species or genus. A complicating factor in the study of seafood toxins is the sporadic frequency and nonpredictability of the presence of the toxin.

Seafood toxins generally can be classified according to the location of the poison. For example: (1) ichthyosarcotoxin is concentrated in the muscles, skin, liver, or intestines or is otherwise not associated with the reproductive system or circulatory system, (2) ichthyootoxin is associated with reproductive tissue, (3) ichthyohemotoxin is confined to the circulatory system, and (4) ichthyohepatotoxin is confined to the liver. In general, seafood toxins under FDA policy have a zero tolerance, with any detectable level considered cause for regulatory action.

Dinoflagellate Poisoning (Paralytic Shellfish Poisoning or PSP; Saxitoxin) The etiologic agent in this type of poisoning is saxitoxin or related compounds and is found in mussels, cockles, clams, soft-shell clams, butter clams, scallops, and shellfish broth. Bivalve mussels are the most common vehicles. Saxitoxin, originally isolated from toxic Alaskan butter clams (*Saxidomus giganticus*) is actually a family of neurotoxins and includes neosaxitin and gonyautoxins 1 through 4. All block neural transmission at the neuromuscular junction by binding to the surface of the sodium channels and interrupting the flow of Na^+ ions; atrioventricular nodal conduction may be suppressed, and there may be direct suppression of the respiratory center and progressive reduction of peripheral nerve excitability. The toxin produces paresthesias and neuromuscular weakness without hypotension and lacks the emetic and hypothermic action of tetrodotoxin. Moderate symptoms are produced by 120 to 180 μg per person and are reversible within hours or days, while 80 μg of purified toxin per 100 g of tissue (0.5 to 2 mg per person) may be lethal, due to asphyxiation, usually within 12 h of ingestion. The toxin is an alkaloid and relatively heat stable. The toxin is produced by several genera of plankton [*Gonyaulax* (now known as *Alexandrium*) *catenella, Gonyaulax acatenella, Gonyaulax tamarensis, Pyrodinium* spp., *Ptychodiscus brevis, Gymnodinium catenaturm,* and others]; and during red tides, blooms of these plankton may reach 20 to 40 million per milliliter. Toxic materials are stored in various parts of the body of shellfish. Digestive organs, liver, gills, and siphons contain the greatest concentrations of poison during the warmer months. Distribution is worldwide (Bryan, 1984; Clark et al., 1999; Liston, 2000).

Amnesic Shellfish Poisoning (Domoic Acid) Consumption of mussels harvested from the area off Prince Edward Island in 1987 resulted in gastroenteritis, and many of the older individuals affected or those with underlying chronic diseases experienced neurologic symptoms including memory loss. Despite treatment, three patients (71 to 84 years old) died within 11 to 24 days. The poisoning was attributed to domoic acid produced by the diatom *Nitzschia pungens* f. *multiseries,* which had been ingested by the mussels during the normal course of feeding. Occurrence of domoic acid has also been reported in California shellfish, produced by *Nitzschia pseudodelicatissima,* and in anchovies (resulting in pelican deaths), produced by *Nitzschia pseudoseriata* (now called *Pseudonitzchia australis*). Domoic acid has been reported in shellfish in other provinces of Canada, Alaska, Washington, and Oregon; it may be as frequent as PSP toxins. Domoic acid has also been reported in seaweed. Domoic acid was reported in Japan in 1958 and was isolated from the red algae *Chondria armata.*

In the Canadian outbreak, mice injected with extracts (as in the PSP assay) died within 3.5 h. The mice exhibited a scratching syndrome uniquely characteristic of domoic acid, followed by increasingly uncoordinated movements and seizures until the mice fell on their sides, rolled over, and died. Levels of domoic acid >40 μg/g wet weight of mussel meat caused the mouse symptoms (Canadian authorities require cessation of harvesting when levels approach 20 μg/g). Mice and rats can generally tolerate 30 to 50 mg/kg (mouse NOEL via intraperitoneal injection is 24 mg/kg). Domoic acid is dose-responsive in humans, with no effect at 0.2 to 0.3 mg/kg, mild (gastrointestinal) symptoms at 0.9 to 1.9 mg/kg, and the most serious symptoms at 1.9 to 4.2 mg/kg. Although rodents may appear to be more tolerant, the fatalities in humans were associated with underlying illness. Domoic acid is an analog of glutamine, a neurotransmitter, and of kainic acid; the toxicity of all three is similar as they are excitatory and act on three types of receptors in the central nervous system, with the hippocampus being the most sensitive. Domoic acid may be a more potent activator of kannic acid receptors than kannic acid itself. The stimulatory action may lead to extensive damage of the hippocampus but less severe injury to the thalamic and forebrain regions (Clark et al., 1999; Todd, 1993).

Ciguatera Poisoning The *cigua* in *ciguatera* is derived from the Spanish name for the sea snail *Turbo pica,* in which the symptoms were first reported. Ciguatera and related toxins (scaritoxin and maitotoxin) are ichthyosarcotoxic neurotoxins (anticholinesterase) and are found in 11 orders, 57 families, and over 400 species of fish as well as in oysters and clams. The penultimate toxin (gambiertoxin) is produced by the dinoflagellate *Gambierdiscus toxicus,* commonly isolated from microalgae growing on or near coral reefs that have ingested the dinoflagellate. The pretoxin appears to pass through the food chain and is biotransformed upon transfer to or by the ingesting fish to the active form, which is consumed by mammals. Other toxins, including palytoxin and okadaic acid, unrelated to gambiertoxin, may be present in ciguarteric fish and may not contribute to toxicity. The asymptomatic period is 3 to 5 h after consumption but may last up to 24 h. The onset of illness is sudden, and symptoms may include abdominal pain, nausea, vomiting, and watery diarrhea; muscular aches; tingling and numbness of the lips, tongue, and throat; a metallic taste; temporary blindness; and paralysis. Deaths have occurred. Recovery usually occurs within 24 h, but tingling may continue for a week or more. The intraperitoneal LD_{50} of maitotoxin in mice is 50 ng/kg (Bryan, 1984; Liston, 2000).

Puffer Fish Poisoning (Tetrodotoxin) Tetrodon or puffer fish poisoning may be caused by the improper preparation and consumption of any of about 90 species of puffer fish (fugu, blowfish, globefish, porcupine fish, molas, burrfish, balloonfish, toadfish, etc.) and has been found in newts, frogs, octopus, starfish, flatworms, various crabs, and gastropods. The toxin (tetrodotoxin) is located in nearly all the tissues, but the ovaries, roe, liver, intestines, and skin are the most toxic. Toxicity is highest during the spawning period, although a species may be toxic in one location but not another. Tetrodotoxin is associated with the presence of several bacteria on and in fish and shellfish and gives the fish an evolutionary advantage in providing protection against predators (i.e., they are *endosymbiotic* bacteria). A total of 21 species can produce tetrodotoxins including *Vibrio, Pseudomonas, E. coli,* and at least two strains of red algae.

Tetrodotoxin is a neurotoxin and causes paralysis of the central nervous system and peripheral nerves by blocking the movement of all monovalent cations. The toxin is water-soluble and is stable to boiling except in an alkaline solution. A fatal dose may be as little as 1 to 4 mg per person. The victim is asymptomatic for 10 to 45 min but may have a reprieve for as long as 3 h or more. Toxicity is manifest as a tingling or prickly sensation of the fingers and toes; malaise; dizziness; pallor; numbness of the lips, tongue, and extremities; ataxia; nausea, vomiting, and diarrhea; epigastric pain; dryness of the skin; subcutaneous hemorrhage and desquamation; respiratory distress; muscular twitching, tremor, incoordination, and muscular paralysis; and intense cyanosis. Fatality rates are high (Bryan, 1984; Liston, 2000).

Moray Eel Poisoning Although the moray eel (*Gymnothorax javanicus*) and other carnivorous fish may accumulate ciguatoxin as the result of eating other contaminated fish, the Indo-Pacific moray eel (*Lycodontis nudivomer*) has been shown to posses a mucous skin secretion with hemolytic, toxic, and hemagglutinating properties. The hemolytic properties can be separated from the hemagglutinating properties. The hemolytic property is lost upon treatment with trypsin and is unstable in the presence of heat or acidic or alkaline media (Randall et al., 1981). The skin mucus of other species of eels, the common European eel (*Anguilla anguilla*) and pike eel (*Muraenesox cinereus*), was found to have proteinaceous toxins immunologically similar to that of the skin mucous toxin from the Japanese eel (*Anguilla japonica*) (Shiomi et al., 1994).

Fish Liver Poisoning This type of poisoning involves an ichthyohepatotoxin and may be related to or cause hypervitaminosis A. It occurs after the consumption of the liver of *sawara* (Japanese mackerel) and *ishingai* (sea bass, sandfish, and porgy). After an asymptomatic period of 30 min to 12 h, the victim experiences nausea, vomiting, fever, headache, mild diarrhea, rash, loss of hair, dermatitis, desquamation, bleeding from the lips, and joint pain (Bryan, 1984).

Fish Roe Poisoning This type of poisoning involves a group of ichthyootoxins found in the roe and ovaries of carp, barbel, pike, sturgeons, gar, catfish, tench, bream, minnows, salmon, whitefish, trout, blenny, cabezon, and other freshwater and saltwater fish. Poisonings have been reported in Europe, Asia, and North America. Within this group of ichthyootoxins are heat-stable toxins and lipoprotein toxins. The asymptomatic period is 1 to 6 h, followed by a bitter taste, dryness of the mouth, intense thirst, headache, fever, vertigo, nausea, vomiting, abdominal cramps, diarrhea, dizziness, cold sweats, chills, and cyanosis. Paralysis, convulsions, and death may occur in severe cases (Bryan, 1984; Furman, 1974).

Abalone Poisoning (Pyropheophorbide) Abalone poisoning is caused by abalone viscera poison (located in the liver and digestive gland) and is unusual in that it causes photosensitization. The toxin, pyropheophorbide a, is stable to boiling, freezing, and salting. It is found in Japanese abalone, *Haliotis discus* and *Haliotis sieboldi.* The development of symptoms is contingent on exposure to sunlight. The symptoms are of sudden onset and include a burning and stinging sensation over the entire body, a prickling sensation, itching, erythema, edema, and skin ulceration on parts of the body exposed to sunlight (Bryan, 1984; Shiomi, 1999). Paralytic shellfish toxin (PST) have been detected in abalone, probably through consumption of the mossworm, a plankton feeder that also clings to seaweed, and some shellfish (Takatani et al., 1997).

Sea Urchin Poisoning The etiologic agent forms during the reproductive season and is confined to the gonads. The sea urchins involved include *Paracentrotus lividus, Tripneustes ventricosus,* and *Centrechinus antillarum.* The symptoms include abdominal pain, nausea, vomiting, diarrhea, and migraine-like attacks (Bryan, 1984). The toxin has been shown to interfere with calcium uptake in nerve preparations (Zhang et al., 1998).

Sea Turtle Poisoning (Chelonitoxin) The etiologic agent here is chelonitoxin, which is found in the liver (greatest concentration) but also in the flesh, fat, viscera, and blood. Toxicity is described as sporadic or even seasonal, indicating that the poison may be derived from toxic marine algae. Most outbreaks occur in the Indo-Pacific region. The turtles involved include the green sea turtle as well as the hawksbill and leatherback turtles. Local custom in Sri Lanka is to first offer the liver to crows, and if the birds eat it, the flesh is regarded as safe. However, because the symptoms appear over a few hours to several days, this bioassay requires patience. Symptoms of intoxication in humans include vomiting; diarrhea; sore lips, tongue, and throat; foul breath; difficulty in swallowing; a white coating on the tongue, which may become covered with pin-sized, pustular papules; tightness of the chest; coma; and death. The toxin has been reported transferred to nursing infants from intoxicated mothers. Postmortem examinations reveal congestion of internal organs, interstitial pulmonary edema, and necrosis of myocardial fibers. Fatality rates of 7 and 25 percent have been reported (Ariyananda and Fernando, 1987; Bryan, 1984; Champetier De Ribes et al., 1997; Chandrasiri et al., 1988).

Haff Disease Haff disease is a syndrome of unknown etiology that occurs following consumption of certain types of fish. The syndrome consists of rhabdomyolysis with a release of muscle cell contents into the blood. Patients are often rigid, sensitive to touch, and unable to move; their urine may have a dark brown color. Symptoms appear 18 h (with a range of 6 to 21 h) after consumption; they resolve within 2 to 3 days, and the fatality rate is approximately 1 percent. "Haff disease" was first reported in the 1920s along the Koenigsberg Haff, a brackish inlet on the Baltic Sea, although outbreaks have been reported in Sweden, the former Soviet Union, and in the United States beginning in 1984. U.S. poisonings have been associated with buffalo fish (*Ictiobus cyprnellus*) caught in California, Missouri (St. Louis), and Louisiana. No etiologic agent has been identified (Anonymous, 1998).

Microbiologic Agents—Preformed Bacterial Toxins

Although the United States likely has the safest and cleanest food supply in the world, most U.S. food-related illness results from microbial contamination. If all the food-borne health concerns could be divided into two large categories—*poisonings* and *infections*—the former would include chemical poisonings (e.g., contaminants such as chlorinated hydrocarbons) and intoxications, which may have a plant, animal, or microbial origin. In the infections category, food acts as a vector for organisms that exhibit their pathogenicity once they have multiplied inside the body. Infections include the two subcategories enterotoxigenic infections (with the release of toxins following colonization of the GI tract) and invasive infections, in which the GI tract is penetrated and the body is invaded by organisms.

Food-borne disease outbreaks are tracked by the Centers for Disease Control and Prevention (CDC), which reports that there are approximately 400 outbreaks of food-borne disease per year, involving 10,000 to 20,000 people. However, the actual frequency may be as much as 10 to 200 times as high because (1) an outbreak is classified as such only when the source can be identified as affecting two or more people and (2) most home poisonings are mild or have a long incubation time; they are therefore not connected to the ingested food and go unreported. Naturally, because of differences in virulence and opportunity, some species are more likely than others to cause outbreaks.

There are a number of food toxins of microbial origin; however, discussion in this chapter is limited to preformed bacterial toxins—that is, those toxins elaborated by bacteria concomitant to their residence and growth in or on the food *prior* to ingestion. There are a number of different types of toxins. An *enterotoxin* is a toxin having action on the *enteric* cells of the intestine and an *endotoxin* is generally a lipopolysaccharide membrane constituent released from a dead or dying gram-negative becteria. These toxins are nonspecific and stimulate inflammatory responses from macrophages, including but not limited to prostaglandins, thromboxans, interleukins, and other mediators of immunity. *Exotoxins* are synthesized and released (usually by gram-positive bacteria) and are not an integral part of the organism; however, they may enhance its virulence. Some bacteria, such as *Shigella, Staphylococcus aureus,* and *E. coli* (which releases the shiga-like Vero toxin), can elaborate both endotoxin and exotoxin.

Clostridium botulinum **and *Clostridium butyricum*** Food botulism, although now relatively rare, still occurs and is important because of its potency. All organisms of the *Clostridium* genus are gram-positive, spore-forming anaerobes. Botulism is due to the toxins A, B, E, and F, which may be produced by one or more strains of *C. botulinum* and *C. butyricum* (type E only); toxins C and D cause botulism in animals. Type G has not caused any human cases. *C. botulinum* organisms are categorized as group I to IV on the basis of toxin produced; additionally, group I is proteolytic in culture (liquefying egg white, gelatin, and other solid proteins). The toxin is elaborated in foods, wounds, and infant gut and is neurotoxic, interfering with acetylcholine at peripheral nerve endings. Although the spores are among the most heat-resistant, the toxins are heat-labile (the toxin may be rendered harmless at 80 to 100°C for 5 to 10 min). Botulinum toxins are large zinc-metalloproteins of ~150,000 Da, composed of two parts: a 50,000-Da piece, the catalytic subunit, and the 100,000-Da piece, containing an N-terminal translocation domain and a C-terminal binding domain. The structural features are similar to those of tetanus toxin. For types B, D, F, and G (and tetanus toxin), the target protein is VAMP/synaptobrevin, a protein associated with the synaptic vesicle. Types A and E cleave a protein associated with the presynaptic memberane, ANAP25. Botulinum toxin C cleaves SNAP25 and syntaxin, another protein involved in exocytosis. Although intracellular mechanisms of botulinum and tetanus toxins are similar, symptoms are different because different populations of neurons are targeted. The symptoms may include respiratory distress and respiratory paralysis that may persist for 6 to 8 months. The case fatality rate is 35 to 65 percent, and the poison is fatal in 3 to 10 days; a lethal dose is approximately 1 ng. Sources and reservoirs include soil, mud, water, and the intestinal tracts of animals. Foods associated with botulinum toxin include improperly canned low-acid foods (green beans, corn, beets, asparagus, chili peppers, mushrooms, spinach, figs, baked potato, cheese sauce, beef stew, olives, and tuna). The toxin also may occur in smoked fish, fermented food (seal flippers, salmon eggs) and improperly home-cured hams. An increasing source of poisonings is from the use of flavored oils or oil infusion, most typically in garlic-in-oil preparations; in 1993, FDA required acidification of such preparations to prevent the growth of *Clostridium.* While a proteolytic strain of *C. botulinum* (group I) may cause the food to appear and smell "spoiled" (by-products include isobutyric acid, isovaleric acid, and phenylpropionic acid), this is not the case with nonproteolytic strains, many of which can flourish and elaborate toxin at temperatures as low as 3°C (Belitz and Grosch, 1999; Bryan, 1984; Crane, 1999; Hobbs, 1976; Loving, 1998; Lund and Peck, 2000).

The successful use of nitrates in meat to prevent spoilage by *C. botulinum* resulted in the petitioning of FDA by the USDA to have sodium and potassium nitrate approved for addition by "prior sanction" (21 CFR 181.33). The mechanism of nitrates is believed to be due to an inactivation by nitric oxide of iron-sulfur proteins such as ferrodoxin and pyruvate oxidoreductase within the germinated cells. The activity is dependent on the pH and is proportional to the level of free HNO_2; 100 mg nitrate/kg of meat is necessary for the antimicrobial effect, although this effect can be enhanced with ascorbates and chelating agents. Other antibacterials that prevent *C. botulinum* include nisin (used in cheese spreads), parabens, phenolic antioxidants, polyphosphates and carbon dioxide (Belitz and Grosch, 1999; Lund and Peck, 2000).

Clostridium perfringens The primary reservoir for *C. perfringens,* unlike *C. botulinum,* is the intestinal tract of warm-blooded animals (including humans). Most incidences of *C. perfringens* food poisoning are associated with the consumption of roasted meat that has been contaminated with intestinal contents at slaughter, followed by roasting and inadequate storage, allowing *C. perfringens* growth and enterotoxin (CPE) to be elaborated (although some CPE may actually be released during a "second sporulation" process in the stomach of the victim). Virtually all food poisoning is produced by type A strain, although a particularly severe form (called "pig-bel") is produced by type C strain and is only seen among natives of the New Guinea highlands. CPE is enterotoxic and follows an ordered series of events, first causing cellular ion permeability, followed by macromolecular (DNA, RNA) synthesis inhibition, morphologic alteration, cell lysis, villus tip desquamation, and severe fluid loss. This is manifest by abdominal cramping diarrhea occurring within 8 to 16 h, although symptoms are of short duration—1 day or less. Foods associated with *C. perfringens* poisoning include cooked meat or poultry, gravy, stew, and meat pies. The curious form called pig-bel follows feasting on pork by New Guinea highlanders, in whom low levels of proteases are inadequate to hydrolyze the toxins, which are subsequently absorbed. *C. perfringens* is also associated with the production of other 11 other toxins, including those associated with gas gangrene (Bryan, 1984; Crane, 1999; Duncan, 1976; Hauschild, 1971; Hobbs, 1979; Hobbs et al., 1953; Labbe, 2000; Walker, 1975).

Bacillus cereus *B. cereus* is also a gram-positive, spore-forming rod, but it is an aerobe. *B. cereus* is a causative agent of emetic or diarrheagenic exo- and enterotoxins elaborated in food. The emetic thermostable toxin (surviving 259°F for 90 min) is called *cerulide* (a small cyclic peptide, of 1.2 kDa that acts on 5-HT_3 receptors, stimulating the vagus afferent nerve) and is produced by serotypes 1, 3, and 8. The diarrheagenic thermolabile toxin (133°F for 20 min) is produced by serotypes 1, 2, 6, 8, 10, and 19 and may also be produced in situ in the lower intestine of the host. The diarrheal form may actually consist of three toxins, one of which is hemolytic. Reservoirs are soil and dust. Foods associated with this organism and its toxic properties include boiled and fried rice (principally the emetic form), while the diarrheal form has a wider occurrence and may be found in meats, stews, pudding, sauces, dairy products, vegetable dishes, soups, and meat loaf (Bryan, 1984; Crane, 1999; Gilbert, 1979; Goepfert et al., 1972; Granum and Lund, 1997).

Evidence is accumulating that other species of *Bacillus* may elaborate food toxins, including *Bacillus thuringiensis, Bacillus subtilis, Bacillus licheniformis,* and *Bacillus pumilis* (Crane, 1999; Granum and Baird-Parker, 2000).

Staphylococcus aureus Staphylococcal intoxication includes staphlyloenterotoxicosis and staphylococcal food poisoning. *S. aureus* produces a wide variety of exoproteins, including toxic shock syndrome toxin-1 (TSST-1), the exfoliative toxins ETA and ETB, leukociden, and the staphylococcal enterotoxins (SEA, SEB, SECn, SED, SEE, SEG, SHE and SEI). TSST-1 and the staphylococcal enterotoxins (SE) are also known as pyrogenic toxin superantigens (PTSAgs) on the basis of their biological characteristics. Although enterotoxemia develops only from the ingestion of large amounts of SE, emesis is produced as the result of stimulation of the putative SE receptors in the abdominal viscera, following which there is a cascade of inflammatory mediator release. All the SE toxins share a number of properties: an ability to cause emesis and gastroenteritis in primates, superantigenicity, intermediate resistance to heat and pepsin digestion, and tertiary structural similarity, including an intramolecular disulfide bond. Sources of *Staphylococcus* include nose and throat discharges, hands and skin, infected cuts, wounds, burns, boils, pimples, acne, and feces. The anterior nares of humans are the primary reservoirs. Other reservoirs include mastitic udders of cows and ewes (responsible for contamination of unpasteurized milk) and arthritic and bruised tissues of poultry. Foods are usually contaminated after cooking by persons cutting, slicing, chopping, or otherwise handling them and then keeping the foods at room temperature for several hours or storing them in large containers. Foods associated with staphylococcal poisoning include cooked ham; meat products, including poultry and dressing; sauces and gravy; cream-filled pastry; potatoes; ham, poultry, and fish salads; milk; cheese; bread pudding; and generally high-protein leftover foods (Bryan, 1976, 1984; Bergdoll, 1979; Cohen, 1972; Crane, 1999; Dinges et al., 2000; Minor and Marth, 1976).

Escherichia coli Although *E. coli* does not produce a preformed toxin, it deserves mention because of the overwhelming publicity the emergent strain O157:H7 has received (H and O refer to flagellar antigens and virulence markers). There are four categories of *E. coli* associated with diarrheal disease: enteropathogenic (EPEC), enterotoxigenic (ETEC), enteroinvasive (EIEC), and Vero cytotoxin–producing *E. coli* (VTEC). The classification VTEC also includes "shiga-like toxin"–producing *E. coli* (or SLTEC) and "shiga toxin"–producing *E. coli* (STEC). *Enterohemorrhagic E. coli* (EHEC) refers to those strains producing bloody diarrhea, which are a subset of VTEC. The reference to shiga toxin is the result of the clinical similarity of the bloody diarrhea caused by EHEC to that caused by *Shigella.* Each of the diseases presented by the four categories is also associated with one or more toxins (Willshaw et al., 2000).

Because cattle are a significant reservoir of *E. coli,* it is logical that most outbreaks in the United States have been associated with hamburgers and other beef products, although raw vegetables (often fertilized with manure) and unpasteurized apple cider and juice have been reported as souces of outbreaks. Outbreaks in Europe are more often associated with contamination of recreational waters (swimming pools, lakes, etc.). Other sources of contamination include person-to-person contact (especially among institutionalized persons and in families) and contact with farm animals, especially following educational farm visits (Karch et al., 1999).

The subject of organic food has increasingly captured the public interest. Within this issue is a debate concerning the use in organic and conventional farming of organic fertilizers (e.g., cow manure) that may contain *E. coli* O157:H7 (Stephenson, 1997). Data reported to the U.S. Centers for Disease Control and Prevention (CDC) in 1996 and tabulated in a CDC document entitled "Clusters/Outbreaks of *E. coli* O157:H7 reported to CDC in 1996" show that approximately 10 percent of all *E. coli* O157:H7 infections reported that year were from organically grown lettuce, although organic foods apparently account for less than 1 percent of the total food supply. This information, although much too preliminary for any meaningful conclusions, nonetheless suggests the need for careful evaluation of the use of manure in conventional and organic farming.

At the basis of the potential problem is the use of inadequately treated manure for fertilizer. Human cases of *E. coli* O157:H7 infection have been reported from consumption of contaminated lettuce, potatoes, radish sprouts, alfalfa sprouts, cantaloupe, and unpasteurized apple cider and juice (Karch et al., 1999). Adequate treating of manure requires composting the manure for a minimum of 3 months, during which the heap must reach a temperature of 60°C; although this may be adequate to kill vegetative pathogens, it will not destroy spore formers such as *Clostridium perfringens* or *Clostridium botulinum*. Survival of viruses and protozoa during composting is not known (Anonymous, 1999).

Bovine Spongiform Encephalopathy

Bovine spongiform encephalopathy (BSE) was first indentified in Great Britain in 1986. BSE is a neurologic disease classified as a transmissible spongiform encephalopathy (TSE) and is similar to TSEs in other species, including scrapie (sheep and goats), transmissible mink encephalopathy (ranch-bred mink), chronic wasting disease (mule deer and elk), exotic ungulate encephalopathy (captive exotic bovoids such as bison, orynx, and kudu), and feline spongiform encephalopathy (domestic cats, zoo Felidae). TSEs among humans include kuru, Creutzfeldt-Jakob disease (CJD) and "new variant" CJD (nvCJD).

Clinically, these diseases all present neurologic deterioration and wasting, with the incubation period and interval from clinical onset to inexorable death determined by the dose of infective agent, its virulence, and the genetic makeup of the victim. The incubation of BSE in cattle is generally 4 to 5 years (range of 20 months to 18 years) and an interval of 1 to 12 months from presentation of clinical signs to death. Characteristic histologic lesions in the brain and spinal cord are vacuolation and "spongiform" changes. BSE fibrils (long strands of host glycoprotein called *prion protein* or PrP) in spinal cord preparations may be seen with electron microscopy following detergent extraction and proteinase K digestion. Scrapie tissues with highest infectivity are brain and spinal cord, followed by spleen, tonsil lymph nodes, distal ileum, and proximal colon. The infective agent can be transferred using preparations of neural tissue from infected animals across species barriers. The most effective method of transfer is direct injection into the brain or spinal cord, but transfer has been reported with intraperitoneal injection and oral dosing. Vertical transfer (mother to offspring) has been reported among domestic cattle, and lateral transfer through biting or injury (especially among mink) has also been reported. It is generally agreed that the infective agent is likely a variant of scrapie (endemic to sheep) and was transferred to cattle from rendered sheep via inadequately processed meat and bone meal protein supplement. Disputes have arisen about other details of BSE, its relationship to other TSEs, and its effects in humans because of an expectation of conformation by BSE to historical principles of disease.

There is mainstream agreement that the infective agents is a prion, a proteinaceous infective particle that does not possess nucleic acid. It is resistant to heat, animicrobials, ultraviolet rays, and ionizing radiation and is not consistently inactivated with alcohol, formaldehyde, glutaraldehyde, or sodium hydroxide. Phenol and sodium hypochlorite disinfection have had variable success.

PrP protein is not the infectious agent, but rather the product of a TSE infection which has switched on the *PrP* gene. While the infectious agent has not been elucidated, investigators have concluded that the agent in nvCJD and BSE is the same strain and that the same agent is also linked to feline spongiform encephalopathy and exotic ungulate encephalopathy. While this information might indicate a simple mode of transmission, workers with the highest potential incidence of exposure to BSE or TSE (sheep farmers, butchers, veterinarians, cooks, and abattoir workers) do not have an unusually high incidence of nvCJD (Collee, 2000; Prusiner, 1991). Likewise, hemophilic patients have not reflected an increased incidence of nvCJD, although CJD transmission has been documented as the result of injections of human growth hormone or gonadotrophin (derived from human pituitary gland), implantation of dura mater and corneas, and even infected EEG electrodes and neurosurgical instruments (Collee, 2000; Lee et al., 1998; Prusiner, 1994).

The final chapter on BSE and other TSEs will not be written for at least 15 to 20 years, the probable conclusion of the incubation period for those exposed to BSE in the late 1980s and early 1990s.

Substances Produced by Cooking

Tolerances cannot be set for contaminants produced as a result of an action taken by the consumer. An example of this type of contaminant is heterocyclic amines, which are generated during cooking. Heterocyclic amines (HCAs) were discovered serendipitously by Japanese investigators who, while examining the mutagenicity of smoke generated by charred foods, found that the extracts of the charred surfaces of the meat and fish were quantitatively more mutagenic than could be accounted for by the presence of polycyclic aromatic hydrocarbons (Sugimura et al., 1989). Collectively, there are more than 20 HCAs. They are formed as a result of high-temperature cooking of proteins (especially those containing high levels of creatinine) and carbohydrates. Normally, as a result of such heating, desirable flavor components are formed, for example, pyrazines, pyridines, and thiazoles. Intermediates in the formation of these substances are dihydropyrizines and dihydropyridines, which in the presence of oxygen form the flavor components; however, in the presence of creatinine, HCAs are formed (Table 30-28) (Chen and Chiu, 1998; Schut and Snyderwine, 1999).

These substances are rapidly absorbed by the GI tract, are distributed to all organs, and decline to undetectable levels within 72 h. HCAs behave as electrophilic carcinogens (Table 30-29). They are activated through *N*-hydroxylation by cytochrome P450 or

Table 30-28
Amounts of Heterocyclic Amines in Cooked Foods

	Amount In Cooked Food, ng/g				
SAMPLE	IQ	MeIQx	4,8-DiMeIQx	Trp-P-1	Trp-P-2
Broiled beef	0.19	2.11		0.21	0.25
Fried ground beef	0.70	0.64	0.12	0.19	0.21
Broiled chicken		2.33	0.81	0.12	0.18
Broiled mutton		1.01	0.67		0.15
Food-grade beef extract		3.10			

SOURCE: Sugimura et al., 1989; Adamson, 1990, with permission.

P448, depending on the specific HCA. The *N*-hydroxy forms require further activation by *O*-acetylation or *O*-sulfonation to react with DNA. DNA adducts are formed with guanosine in various organs, including the liver, heart, kidney, colon, small intestine, forestomach, pancreas, and lung. Unreacted substances are subject to phase II detoxication reactions and are excreted via the urine and feces. In vitro, HCAs require metabolic activation, with some requiring *O*-acetyltransferase and others not requiring it. Although much of the mutagenicity testing has been carried out in TA98 and TA100, these substances are mutagenic in mammalian cells both in vitro and in vivo, *Drosophila,* and other strains of *Salmonella* (Skog et al., 1998; Sugimura and Wakahayashi, 1999)

Miscellaneous Contaminants in Food

Sometimes the items under the "miscellaneous" heading are the most interesting. For example, Rodricks and Pohland (1981) pointed out an interesting historical case of the possible transfer of a toxic botanic chemical from an animal to humans which was first identified by Hall (1979). It is found in the Bible, Book of Numbers, 11:31–33, which describes hungry Israelites inundated with quail blown in from the sea; those who ate the quail quickly died. Hall speculated that the quail had consumed various poisonous berries, including hemlock, while they overwintered in Africa. The hemlock berry contains coniine, a neurotoxic alkaloid to which quail are resistant and that can accumulate in their tissue. Humans are not resistant to coniine, and consumption of large quantities of quail tissue containing the neurotoxin could result in death as described in the biblical text.

Mountain laurel, rhododendron, and azaleas all possess andromedotoxin (now called acetylandromedol) and grayanotoxins (I, II, and II) in their shoots, leaves, twigs, and flowers. Honey made from flowers of these plants is toxic to humans, and after an asymptomatic period of 4 to 6 h, salivation, malaise, vomiting, di-

Table 30-29
Mutagenicity and Carcinogenicity of Heterocyclic Amines

HCA	NUMBER OF REVERTANTS, *u/g* (STRAIN TA98)	*Carcinogenicity* SPECIES	STATISTICALLY SIGNIFICANT TUMORS
MeIQ	47,000,000	Mouse	Liver, forestomach
		Rat	Zymbal gland, oral cavity, colon, skin, mammary gland
IQ	898,000	Mouse	Liver, forestomach, lung
		Rat	Liver, mammary gland, Zymbal gland
		Monkey	Liver, metastasis to lungs
MeIQx	417,000	Mouse	Liver, lung, lymphoma, leukemia
		Rat	Liver, Zymbal gland, clitoral gland, skin
Glu-P-1	183,000	Mouse	Liver, blood vessels
		Rat	Liver, small and large intestine, brain, clitoral gland, Zymbal gland
DiMeIQx	126,000	No data	
Trp-P-2	92,700	Mouse	Liver, lung
		Rat	Liver, clitoral gland
Trp-P-1	8,990	Mouse	Liver
		Rat	Liver, metastasis to lungs
PhIP	1,800	Mouse	Liver, lung, lymphoma
		Rat	Colon, mammary gland
Glu-P-2	930	Mouse	Liver, blood vessels
		Rat	Liver, small and large intestine, Zymbal gland, brain, clitoral gland

SOURCE: Adapted from Sugimura et al., 1989, with permission.

arrhea, tingling of the skin, muscular weakness, headache, visual difficulties, coma, and convulsions occur. Life-threatening bradycardia and arterial hypotension may ensue. Needless to say, beekeepers maintain apiaries well away from these species of plants. A similar poisoning occurs with oleander (*Nerium oleander* and *Nerium indicum*), where honey made from the flowers, meat roasted on oleander sticks, or milk from a cow that eats the foliage can produce prostrating symptoms. The oleander toxin consists of a series of cardiac glycosides: thevetin, convallarin, steroidal, helleborein, ouabain, and digitoxin. Sympathetic nerves are paralyzed; the cardiotoxin stimulates the heart muscles much as digitalis does, and gastric distress ensues (Anderson and Sogn, 1984; VonMalottki and Weichmann, 1996).

Other contaminations include contamination of milk with pyrrolizidine and other alkaloids after a cow has fed on tansy ragwort (*Senecio jacobaea*) and tremetol contamination of milk from white snakeroot (*Eupatorium rugusum*).

CONCLUSIONS

Food toxicology differs in many respects from other subspecialties of toxicology largely because of the nature and chemical complexity of food. Food consists of hundreds of thousands of chemical substances in addition to the macro- and micronutrients that are essential to life. The federal law defining food safety in the United States, the FD&C Act, provides a workable scheme for establishing the safety of foods, food ingredients, and contaminants. While the act does not specify how the safety of food and its components and ingredients is to be demonstrated, it emphasizes the need for reasonable approaches in both the application of tests and their interpretation. The specific examples of reasonable approaches and interpretations of safety data discussed in this chapter illustrate both the means and the necessity for reasonableness. New policies, consistent with the safety provisions of the act, are being developed to provide guidance for determination of the safety-in-use of novel foods and those foods derived from new plant varieties.

Contaminants found in food may be divided into two large classes: those that are unavoidable by current good manufacturing practice and those that are not. The former class is represented by substances such as certain chlorinated organic compounds, heavy metals, and mycotoxins that have been determined to be unavoidable by current food manufacturing practice and for which tolerances or action levels may be established. Additionally, pesticide residues and residues of drugs used in food-producing animals may have tolerances established when necessary to protect public health. For an avoidable class of contaminants, tolerances are not set either because public health concerns dictates that the mere presence of the substance or agent demands immediate regulatory action or because contamination results from food preparation in the home, which is beyond FDA control.

It is important to emphasize that the vast majority of foodborne illnesses in developed countries are attributable to microbiologic contamination of food arising from the pathogenicity and/or toxigenicity of the contaminating organism. Thus, the overwhelming concern for food safety in the United States remains directed toward preserving the microbiologic integrity of food.

REFERENCES

Abrams IJ: Using the menu census survey to estimate dietary intake—Postmarket surveillance of aspartame, in Finley JW, Robinson SF, Armstrong DJ (eds): *Food Safety Assessment.* Washington DC: American Chemical Society, 1992, pp 201–213.

Adamson RH: Mutagens and carcinogens formed during cooking of foods and methods to minimize their formation. *Cancer Prev* 1–7, 1990.

Ames BN, Gold LS: Environmental pollution, pesticides, and the prevention of cancer: Misconceptions. *FASEB J* 11:1041, 1997.

Ames BN, Magaw R, Gold LS: Ranking possible carcinogenic hazards. *Science* 236:271, 1987.

Anderson JA, Sogn DD (eds): *Adverse Reactions to Foods.* Washington, DC: U.S. Department of Health and Human Services, 1984.

Anonymous: Haff disease associated with eating buffalo fish—United States, 1997. *MMWR* 47:1091, 1998.

Anonymous: Organic food. *Food Sci Technol Today* 13:108, 1999.

Ariyananda OL, Fernando SSD: Turtle flesh poisoning. *Ceylon Med* 32:213–215, 1987.

Arunachalam KD: Role of bifidobacteria in nutrition, medicine and technology. *Nutr Res* 19:1559, 1999.

Ayesh R, Mitchell SC, Zhang A, Smith RL: The fish odour syndrome: Biochemical, familial and clinical aspects. *Br Med J* 307:655, 1993.

Bannister B, Gibsburg G, Shneerson T: Cardiac arrest due to licorice induced hypokalemia. *Br Med J* 2:738, 1977.

Belitz HD, Grosch W: *Food Chemistry.* Berlin, Springer-Verlag, 1999.

Bergdoll MS: Staphylococcal intoxication, in Reimann H, Bryan FL (eds): *Foodborne Infections and Intoxications,* 2d ed. New York: Academic Press, 1979, pp 59–73.

Bernaola G, Echechipia S, Urrutia I, et al: Occupational asthma and rhinoconjunctivitis from inhalation of dried cow's milk caused by sensitization to alpha-lactalbumin. *Allergy* 49:189, 1994.

Bernhisel-Broadbent J, Dintzis HM, Dintzis RZ, Sampson HA: Allergenicity and antigenicity of chicken egg ovomucoid (Gal d III) compared with ovalbumin (Gal d I) in children with egg allergy and in mice. *J Allergy Clin Immunol* 93:1047, 1994.

Borzelleca JF: Macronutrient substitutes: Safety evaluation. *Regul Toxicol Pharmacol* 16:253, 1992a.

Borzelleca JF: The safety evaluation of macronutrient substitutes. *Crit Rev Food Sci Nutr* 32:127, 1992b.

Borda IA, Philen RM, Posada de la Paz M, et al: Toxic oil syndrome mortality: The first 13 years. *Int J Epidemiol* 27:1057, 1998.

Brandon DL, Haque S, Friedman M: Antigenicity of native and modified Kunitz soybean trypsin inhibitors. *Adv Exp Med Biol* 199:449, 1986.

Bryan FL: Diseases transmitted by foods—A classification and summary, in Anderson JA, Sogn DN (eds): *Adverse Reactions to Foods.* Washington, DC: U.S. Department of Health and Human Services, 1984, appendix, pp 1–101.

Bryan FL: *Staphylococcus aureus,* in Defigueiredo MP, Splittstoesser DF (eds): *Food Microbiology: Public Health and Spoilage Aspects.* Westport, CT: AVI, 1976.

Burdock GA: Dietary supplements and lessons to be learned from GRAS. *Regul Toxicol Pharmacol* 31:68, 2000.

Butchko H, Kotsonis F: Acceptable daily intake and estimation of consumption, in Tschanz C, Butchko HH, Stargel WW, Kotsonis FN (eds): *The Clinical Evaluation of a Food Additive, Assessment of Aspartame.* Boca Raton, FL: CRC Press, 1996 pp 43–53.

Butchko HH, Tschanz C, Kotsonis FN: Postmarketing surveillance anecdotal medical complaints, in Tschanz C, Butchko HH, Stargel WW, Kotsonis FN (eds): *The Clinical Evaluation of a Food Additive, Assessment of Aspartame.* Boca Raton, FL: CRC Press, 1996 pp 183–194.

Butchko HH, Tschanz C, Kotsonis FN: Postmarketing surveillance of food additives. *Regul Toxicol Pharmacol* 20:105, 1994.

Butzler JP, Skirrow MB: *Campylobacter* enteritis. *Clin Gastroenterol* 8:737, 1979.

Campbell TC, Hayes JR: The role of aflatoxin metabolism in its toxic lesion. *Toxicol Appl Pharmacol* 35:199, 1976.

Catto-Smith AG, Adams A: A possible case of transient hereditary fructose intolerance. *J Inherit Metab Dis* 16:73, 1993.

Champetier De Ribes G, Rasolofonirina RN, Ranaivoson G, et al: [Intoxication by marine animal venoms in Madagascar (ichthyosarcotoxism and chelonitoxism): recent epidemiological data.] *Bull Soc Pathol Exot* 90:286–290, 1997.

Chandrasiri N, Ariyananda PL, Fernando SSD: Autopsy findings in turtle flesh poisoning *Med Sci Law* 28:142–144, 1988.

Chen BH, Chiu CP: Analysis, formation and inhibition of heterocyclic amines in foods: An overview. *J Food Drug Anal* 6:625, 1998.

Chevion M, Mager J, Glaser G: Naturally occurring food toxicants: Favism-producing agents, in Rechcigl M Jr (ed): *CRC Handbook of Naturally Occurring Food Toxicants.* Boca Raton, FL: CRC Press, 1985, pp 63–79.

Chhabra RS, Eastin WC Jr: Intestinal absorption and metabolism of xenobiotics in laboratory animals, in Schiller CM (ed): *Intestinal Toxicology.* New York: Raven Press, 1984, pp 145–160.

Clark RF, Williams SR, Nordt, SP, Manoguerra S: A review of selected seafood poisonings. *Undersea Hyperbaric Med* 26:175, 1999.

Clayson DB, Iverson F, Nera F, et al: Histopathological and radioautographical studies on the forestomach of F344 rats treated with butylated hydroxyanisole and related chemicals. *Food Chem Toxicol* 24:1171, 1986.

Cohen JO (ed): *The Staphylococci.* New York: Wiley-Interscience, 1972.

Collee JG: Transmissible spongiform encephalopathies, in *The Microbiological Safety and Quality of Food,* Gaithersburg, MD: Aspen Publishers, 2000, pp 1589–1624.

Committee on Food Protection: *Food Colors.* Washington, DC: National Academy of Sciences, 1971.

Concon J: *Food Toxicology.* New York: Marcel Dekker, 1988.

Crane JK: Preformed bacterial toxins. *Clin Lab Med* 19:583, 1999.

Davis WE: *National Inventory of Sources and Emissions of Cadmium, Nickel, and Asbestos. Cadmium.* Section 1. Report PB 192250. Springfield, VA: National Technical Information Service, 1970.

Dayan AD: Allergy to antimicrobial residues in food: Assessment of the risk to man. *Vet Microbiol* 35:213, 1993.

DeBlay F, Hoyet C, Candolfi E, et al: Identification of alpha livetin as a cross reacting allergen in bird-egg syndrome. *Allergy Proc* 15:77, 1994.

Dinges MM, Orwin PM, Schlievert PM: Exotoxins of *Staphylococcus aureus. Microbiol Rev* 13:16,2000.

Dorion, BJ, Burks AW, Harbeck R, et al: The production of interferongamma in response to a major peanut allergy, Arh h II, correlates with serum levels of IgE anti-Ara h II. *J Allergy Clin Immunol* 93:93, 1994.

Drasar BS, Hill MJ: *Human Intestinal Flora.* New York: Academic Press, 1974.

Duncan C: *Clostridium perfringens,* in Defigueiredo MP, Splittstoesser DF (eds): *Food Microbiology: Public Health and Spoilage Aspects.* Westport, CT: AVI, 1976.

El-Banna AA, Pitt JI, Leistner L: Production of mycotoxins by *Penicillium* species. *Sys Appl Microbiol* 10(1):42–46, 1987.

EPA: Guidance for the re-registration of pesticide products containing *Bacillus thurigensis* as the active ingredient *Re-registration Standard* 540:RS-89-023, 1988.

Evans CS: Naturally occurring food toxicants: Toxic amino acids, in Rechcigl M Jr (ed): *CRC Handbook of Naturally Occurring Food Toxicants.* Boca Raton, FL: CRC Press, 1985, pp 3–14.

Farese, RV, Biglieri EG, Shackleton CHL, et al: Licorice-induced hypermineralocorticoidism. *N Engl J Med* 325:1223, 1991.

FDA: Food producing animals: Criteria and procedures for evaluating assays for carcinogenic residues. *Fed Reg* 42:15, 636, 1977.

FDA: Policy for regulating carcinogenic chemicals in food and color additives. *Fed Reg* 47:14464, 1982.

FDA: *Recommendations for Chemistry Data for Indirect Food Additive Petitions.* Chemistry Review Branch. Washington, DC: Food and Drug Administration, 1988.

FDA: *Scientific Review of the Long-Term Carcinogen Bioassays Performed on the Artificial Sweetener Cyclamate. Report of the Cancer Assessment Committee for Food Safety and Applied Nutrition.* Washington, DC: Food and Drug Administration, 1984.

FDA: Statement of policy: Foods derived from new plant varieties. *Fed Reg* 57:22984, 1992.

Flamm WG, Frankos V: Nitrates: Laboratory evidence, in Walk NJ, Doll R (eds): *Interpretation of Negative Epidemiological Evidence for Carcinogenicity.* IARC Scientific Publication No 65. Lyons, France: International Agency for Research on Cancer, 1985, pp 85–90.

Flamm WG, Kotsonis FN, Hjelle JJ: Threshold of regulation: A unifying concept in food safety assessment, in Kotsonis F, Mackey M, Hjelle J (eds): *Nutritional Toxicology.* New York: Raven Press, 1994, pp 223–234.

Flamm WG, Lehman-McKeeman LD: The human relevance of the renal tumor-inducing potential of d-limonene in male rats: Implications for risk assessment. *Regul Toxicol Pharmacol* 13:70, 1991.

Flamm WG, Lorentzen RL: Quantitative risk assessment (QRA): A special problem in approval of new products, in Mehlman M (ed): *Risk Assessment and Risk Management.* Princeton, NJ: Princeton Scientific Publishing, 1988, pp 91–108.

Food Chemicals Codex. Washington, DC: National Academy Press, 1996.

Frankland AW: Anaphylaxis in relation to food allergy, in Brostoff J, Challacombe SJ (eds): *Food Allergy and Intolerance.* Philadelphia: Baillière Tindall, 1987, pp 456–466.

Fuglsang G, Madsen C, Saval P, Osterballe O: Prevalence of intolerance to food additives among Danish school children. *Pediatr Allergy Immunol* 4(3):123, 1993.

Fukutomi O, Kondo N, Agata H, et al: Timing of onset of allergic symptoms as a response to a double-blind, placebo-controlled food challenge in patients with food allergy combined with a radioallergosorbent test and the evaluation of proliferative lymphocyte responses. *Int Arch Allergy Immunol* 104(4):352, 1994.

Furman FA: Fish eggs, in Lience IE (ed): *Toxic Constituents of Animal Feedstuffs.* New York: Academic Press, 1974, pp 16–28.

Gangilli SD: Nitrate, nitrite and *N*-nitroso compounds in, Ballantyne B, Marrs T, Turner P: *General and Applied Toxicology.* New York: Stockton Press, 1999, pp 2111–2143.

Gessner BD, Hokama Y Isto S: Scombrotoxicosis-like illness following the ingestion of smoked salmon that demonstrated low histamine levels and high toxicity on mouse bioassay. *Clin Infect Dis* 23:1316, 1996.

Gianessi LP, Carpenter JE: *Agricultural Biotechnology: Insect Control Benefits.* Washington, DC: National Center for Food and Agricultural Policy, 1999.

Gibb CM, Davies PT, Glover V, et al: Chocolate is a migraine-provoking agent. *Cephalalgia* 11(2):93, 1991.

Gilbert R: *Bacillus cereus* gastroenteritis, in Reimann H, Bryan FL (eds): *Food-Borne Infections and Intoxications,* 2d ed. New York: Academic Press, 1979.

Goepfert JM, Spira WM, Kim HU: *Bacillus* cereus: Food poisoning organism: A review. *J Milk Food Technol* 35:213, 1972.

Gold LS, Slone TH, Stern BR, et al: Rodent carcinogens: Setting priorities. *Science* 258: 261, 1992.

Gonzalez R, Polo F, Zapatero L, et al: Purification and characterization of major inhalant allergens from soybean hulls. *Clin Exp Allergy* 22(8):748, 1992.

Goon D, Klaassen CD: Effects of microsomal enzyme inducers upon UDP-glucuronic acid concentration and UDP-glucuronosyltransferase activity in the rat intestine and liver. *Toxicol Appl Pharmacol* 115(2):253, 1992.

Granum PE, Baird-Parker TC: *Bacillus* species, in Lund BM, Baird-Parker TC, Gould GW (eds): *The Microbiological Safety and Quality of* Food. Gaithersburg, MD: Aspen Publishers, 2000, pp 1029–1039.

Granum PE, Lund T: *Bacillus cereus* and its food poisoning toxins. *FEMS Microbiol Lett* 157:223, 1997.

Gudmand-Hoyer E: The clinical significance of disaccharide maldigestion. *Am J Clin Nutr* 59 (suppl 3):735S, 1994.

Guyton AC: The chemical senses—Taste and smell, in *Textbook of Medical Physiology,* 4th ed. Philadelphia: Saunders, 1971, pp 639–646.

Halken S, Host A, Hansen LG, Osterballe O: Preventive effect of feeding high-risk infants a casein hydrolysate formula or an ultrafiltrated whey hydrolysate formula. A prospective, randomized, comparative clinical study. *Pediatr Allergy Immunol* 4(4):173, 1993.

Hall R, Oser B: The safety of flavoring substances. *Residue Rev* 24:1, 1968.

Hall RL: *Proceedings of Marabou Symposium on Foods and Cancer.* Stockholm: Caslan Press, 1979.

Harrison J: Food moulds and their toxicity. *Trop Sci* 13:57, 1971.

Hassing JM, Al-Turk WA, Stohs SJ: Induction of intestinal microsomal enzymes by polycyclic aromatic hydrocarbons. *Gen Pharmacol* 20(5):695, 1989.

Hauschild AHW: *Clostridium perfringens* enterotoxin. *J Milk Food Technol* 34:596, 1971.

Hobbs BC, Smith ME, Oakley CL, Warrack GH: *Clostridium welchii* food poisoning. *J Hyg* 51:75, 1953.

Hobbs G: *Clostridium botulinum* and its importance in fishery products. *Adv Food Res* 22:135, 1976.

Hoensch HP, Schwenk M: Intestinal absorption and metabolism of xenobiotics in humans, in Schiller CM (ed): *Intestinal Toxicology.* New York: Raven Press, 1984, pp 169–192.

Hotchkiss JH: Relative exposure to nitrite, nitrate, and *N*-nitroso compounds from endogenous and exogenous sources, in Taylor SL, Scanlan RA (eds): *Food Taxicology: A Perspective on the Relative Risks.* New York: Marcel Dekker, 1989, pp 57–100.

Hotchkiss JH, Helser MA, Maragos CM, Weng YM: Nitrate, nitrite, and *N*-nitroso compounds: Food safety and biological implications, in Finley JW, Robinson SF, Armstrong DJ (eds): *Food Safety Assessment.* Washington, DC: American Chemical Society, 1992, pp 400–418.

Hubbert WT, McCulloch WF, Schnurrenberger PR (eds): *Disease Transmitted from Animals to Man,* 6th ed. Springfield, IL: Charles C Thomas, 1975.

Ijomah P, Clifford MN, Walker R, et al: The importance of endogenous histamine relative to dietary histamine in the aetiology of scombrotoxicosis. *Food Addit Contam* 8(4):531, 1991.

James C: Preview: Global review of commercialized transgenic crops, in *ISAAA Briefs.* No. 12. Ithaca, NY: International Service for the Acquisition of Agri-Biotech Applications, (ISAAA), 1999.

Johnson RD, Manske DD, New DH, Podrebarac DS: Food and feed pesticides, heavy metal and other chemical residues in infant and toddler total diet samples. *Pest Monit J* 15:39, 1981.

Juambeltz JC, Kula K, Perman, J: Nursing caries and lactose intolerance. *ASDC J Dent Child* 60(4):377, 1993.

Kaminsky LS, Fasco MJ: Small intestinal cytochromes P450. *Crit Rev Toxicol* 21(6):407, 1991.

Karch H, Bielaszewska M, Bitzan M, Schmidt H: Epidemiology and diagonosis of Shiga toxin–producing *Escherichia coli* infections. *Diagn Microbiol Infect Dis* 34:229–243, 1999.

Kirchgessner M, Reichlmayer-Lais AM: *Trace Element Metabolism in Man and Animals (TEMA-4).* Canberra: Australian Academy of Science, 1981.

Kirjavaninen PV, Apostolou E, Salminen SJ, Isolauri E: New aspects of probiotics A novel approach in the management of food allergy. *Allergy* 54:909, 1999.

Kivity S, Sunner K, Marian Y: The pattern of food hypersensitivity in patients with onset after 10 years of age. *Clin Exp Allergy* 24:1, 1994.

Kokoski CJ, Henry SH, Lin CS, Ekelman KB: Methods used in safety evaluation, in Branen AL, Davidson PM, Salminen S (eds): *Food Additives.* New York: Marcel Dekker, 1990.

Krishnamachari KAVR, Bhat RV, Nagarajan V, Tilak TBG: Hepatitis due to aflatoxicosis. *Lancet* 1(7915):1061–1063, 1975.

Kritschevsky D: The role of fat, calories and fiber in disease, in Kotsonis F, Mackey M, Hjelle J (eds): *Nutritional Toxicology.* New York: Raven Press, 1994, pp 67–93.

Labbe RG: *Clostridium perfrungens,* in Lund BM, Baird-Parker TC, Gould GW (eds): *The Microbiological Safety and Quality of Food.* Gaithersburg, MD: Aspen Publishers, 2000, pp 1110–1135.

Lagerwerff JV, Sprecht AW: Occurrence of environmental cadmium and zinc and their uptake by plants, in Hemphill DD (ed): *Proceedings of the University of Missouri 4th Annual Conference on Trace Substances in Environmental Health.* Columbia, MO: University of Missouri, 1971, pp 85–93.

Lange WR: Scombroid poisoning. *Am Fam Physician* 37:163, 1988.

Lee CA, Ironside JW, Bell JE, et al: Retrospective neuropathological review of prion disease in UK haemophilic patients. *Thromb Haemost* 80:909, 1998.

Linder MC: *Nutritional Biochemistry and Metabolism,* 2d ed. Norwalk, CT: Appleton & Lange, 1991.

Liston J: Fish and shellfish poisoning, in Lund BM, Baird-Parker TC, Gould GW (eds): *The Microbiological Safety and Quality* of Food. Gaithersburg, MD: Aspen Publishers, 2000, pp 1518–1544.

Loving AL: Botulism in flavored oils–A review. *Dairy Food Environ Sanit* 18:438, 1998.

Lund BM, Peck MW: Clostridium botulinum, in Lund BM, Baird-Parker TC, Gould GW (eds): *The Microbiological Safety and Quality of Food.* Gaithersburg, MD: Aspen Publishers, 2000, pp 1057–1109.

Maarse H, Visscher CA, Willemsens LC, Boelens MH: *Volatile Compounds in Food: Qualitative and Quantitative Data.* Suppl 4: *TNO Nutrition and Food Research.* Zeist, Netherlands: TNO Nutrition and Food Research, 1993, pp 622.

Mallinson CN: Basic functions of the gut, in Brostoff J, Challacombe SJ (eds): *Food Allergy and Intolerance.* Philadelphia: Baillière Tindall, 1987, pp 27–53.

Manda F, Tadera K, Aoyama K: Skin lesions due to Okra (*Hibiscus esculentus* L.): Proteolytic activity and allergenicity of okra. *Contact Dermatitis* 26(2):95, 1992.

Manu P, Matthews DA, Lane TJ: Food intolerance in patients with chronic fatigue. *Int J East Disord* 13:203, 1993.

Marasas, WFO, Jaskiewicz K, Venter FS, VanSchalkwyk DJ: Fusarium moniliforme contamination of maize in oesophageal cancer areas in the Transkei. *S Afr Med J* 74:110, 1988.

Masoero F, Moschini M, Rossi F, et al: Nutritive value, mycotoxin contamination and *in vitro* rumen fermentation of normal and genetically modified corn [CryIA(B)] grown in northern Italy. *Maydica* 44:205, 1999.

Matsumoto H: Cycasin, in Rechcigl M Jr (ed): *CRC Handbook of Naturally Occurring Food Toxicants.* Boca Raton, FL: CRC Press, 1985, pp 43–61.

McClain RM: Mechanistic considerations in the regulation and classification of chemical carcinogens in, Kotsonis FN, Mackey M, Hjelle JJ (eds): *Nutritional Toxicology.* New York: Raven Press, 1994, pp 273–304.

McClintock JT, Schaffer CR, Sjoblad RD: A comparative review of the mammalian toxicity of *Bacillus thuringiensis*–based pesticides. *Pestic Sci* 45:95, 1995.

McConnell G, Ferguson DM, Pearson CR: Chlorinated hydrocarbons and the environment. *Endeavour* 34:13, 1975.

Melnik B, Szliska C, Noehle M, Schwanitz HJ: Food intolerance: pseudoallergic reactions induced by biogenic amines. *Allergologie* 20:163–167, 1997.

Metcalfe DD, Astwood JD, Townsend R, et al: Assessment of the allergenic potential of foods derived from genetically engineered crop plants. *Crit Rev Food Sci Nutr* 36(S):S165, 1996.

Miller CD: Selected toxicological studies of the mycotoxin cyclopiazonic acid in turkeys (dissertation). Ann Arbor, MI: University of Michigan Dissertation Services, 1989.

Miller EC: Some current perspectives on chemical carcinogenesis in humans and experimental animals: Presidential address. *Cancer Res* 38:1479, 1978.

Miller SA: Food additives and contaminants, in Amdur MO, Doull J, Klaassen CD (eds): *Toxicology: The Basic Science of Poisons*. New York: Raven Press, 1991, pp 819–853.

Minor TE, Marth EH: *Staphylococci and Their Significance in Foods*. Amsterdam: Elsevier, 1976.

Mirocha CJ, Pathre SV, Christensen CM: Zearalenone, in Rodericks JV, Hesseltine CW, Mehlman MA (eds): *Mycotoxins in Human and Animal Health*. Park Forest South, IL: Pathtox, 1977, pp 345–364.

Mirvish SS: Formation of *N*-nitroso compounds: Chemistry kinetics, and *in vivo* occurrence. *Toxicol Appl Pharmacol* 31:325, 1975.

Moneret-Vautrin DA: Food intolerance masquerading as food allergy: False food allergy, in Brostoff J, Challacombe SJ (eds): *Food Allergy and Intolerance*. Philadelphia: Baillière Tindall, 1987, pp 836–849.

Monroe DH, Eaton DL: Comparative effects of butylated hydroxyanisole on hepatic *in vivo* DNA binding and *in vitro* biotransformation of aflatoxin B_1 in the rat and mouse. *Toxicol Appl Pharmacol* 90:401–409, 1987.

Morrow JD, Margiolies GR, Rowland J, Roberts LJ II: Evidence that histamine is the causative toxin of scombroid-fish poisoning. *N Engl J Med* 324(11):716, 1991.

Muller GJ, Lamprecht JH, Barnes JM, et al: Scombroid poisoning: Case series of 10 incidents involving 22 patients. *S Afr Med J* 81(8):427, 1992.

Munkvold GP, Hellmich RL, Rice LR: Comparison of fumonisin concentrations in kernels of transgenic Bt maize hybrids and nontransgenic hybrids. *Plant Dis* 83:130, 1999.

Munkvold GP, Hellmich RL, Showers WB: Reduced fusarium ear rot and symptomless infection in kernels of maize genetically engineered for European corn borer resistance. *Phytopathology* 87:1071, 1997.

Munro IC: Issues to be considered in the safety evaluation of fat substitutes. *Food Chem Toxicol* 28:751, 1990.

Munro IC, Kennepohl E, Erickson RE, et al: Safety assessment of ingested heterocyclic amines: Initial report. *Regul Toxicol Pharmacol* 17:S1, 1993.

Murray KF, Christie DL: Dietary protein intolerance in infants with transient methemoglobinemia and diarrhea. *J Pediatr* 122:90, 1993.

Newberne PM: Mechanisms of interaction and modulation of response, in Vouk VB, Butler GC, Upton AC, et al (eds): *Methods for Assessing the Effects of Mixtures of Chemicals*. New York: Wiley, 1987, pp 555–588.

NRC/NAS (National Research Council/National Academy of Science): *The 1977 Survey of Industry on the Use of Food Additives by the NRC/NAS*. October 1979, U.S. Department of commerce, NTIS PB 80-113418. Vol III: *Estimates of Daily Intake*. Committee on GRAS list survey—Phase III Food and Nutrition Committee. Washington, DC: National Research Council, 1979.

Nordlee JA, Taylor SL, Townsend JA, et al: Transgenic soybeans containing brazil nut 2S storage protein issues regarding allergienicity, in Eisenbrand G et al (eds): *Food Allergies and Intolerances*. New York: VCH Publishers, 1996, pp 196–202.

Norred WP: Fumonisins—Mycotoxins produced. *J Toxicol Environ Health* 38:309, 1993.

O'Hallaren MT: Bakers' asthama and reactions secondary to soybean and grain dust, in Bardana EJ Jr, Montanaro A, O'Hallaren MT (eds): *Occupational Asthma*. Philadelphia: Hanley and Belfus, 1992, pp 107–116.

Ohshima H and Bartsch H: Quantitative estimation of endogenous nitrosation in humans by monitoring *N*-nitrosoproline excreted in the urine. *Cancer Res* 41:3658, 1981.

O'Neil C, Helbling AA, Lehrer SB: Allergic reactions to fish. *Clin Rev Allergy* 11(2):183, 1993.

Pantuck EJ, Hsiao KC, Kuntzman R, Conney AH: Intestinal metabolism of phenacetin in the rat: Effect of charcoal-broiled beef and rat chow. *Science* 187:744, 1975.

Pantuck EJ, Hsiao KC, Maggio A, et al: Effect of cigarette smoking on phenacetin metabolism. *Clin Pharmacol Ther* 15:9, 1974.

Pantuck EJ, Kuntzman R, Conney AH: Intestinal drug metabolism and the bioavailability of drugs, in Mehlman MA, Shapiro RE, Blumenthal H (eds): *New Concepts in Safety Evaluation*. Washington DC: Hemisphere, 1976, pp 345–368.

Pay EM, Fleming KH, Guenther, PM, Mickle SJ: *Foods Commonly Eaten by Individuals: Amount per Day and per Eating Occasion*. Washington, DC: USDA (HERR No. 44), 1984.

Peers FG, Gilman GA, Linsell CA: Dietary aflatoxins and human liver cancer: A study in Swaziland. *Int J Cancer* 17:167, 1976.

Pennington JAP, Gunderson EL: History of the Food Drug Administration total diet study—1961–1987. *J Assoc Off Anal Chem* 70:772, 1987.

Piastra M, Stabile A, Fioravanti G, et al: Cord blood mononuclear cell responsiveness to beta-lactoglobulin: T-cell activity in "atopy-prone" and "non-atopy-prone" newborns. *Int Arch Allergy Immunol* 104:358, 1994.

Posada de la Paz M, Philen RM, Borda IA, et al: Toxic oil syndrome: traceback of the toic oil, and evidence for a point source epidemic. *Food Chem Toxicol* 34:251, 1996.

Principles for Estimating Exposure to Substances Found in or Added to the Diet. Division of food Chemistry and Technology, Regulatory Feed Chemistry Branch. Food and Color Additives Review Section. Washington, DC: U.S. Food and Drug Administration, 1991.

Prusiner SB: *Prion Diseases of Animals and Humans*. Washington, DC: Toxicology Forum, 1991, pp 203–234.

Prusiner SB: Prion diseases of humans and animals. *J R Coll Physicians* 28:1, 1994.

Randall JE, Aida K, Oshima Y, Hori K, Hashimoto Y: Occurrence of a crinotoxin and hemagglutinin in the skin mucus of the moray eel *Lycodontis nudivomer. Mar Biol* 62:179, 1981.

Rees N, Tennant D: Estimation of food chemical intake, in Kotsonis FN, Mackey M, Hjelle J (eds): *Nutritional Toxicology*. New York: Raven Press, 1994 pp 199–221.

Reichlmayer-Lais MM, Kirchgessner M: *Trace Elements in Man and Animals 6*. New York: Plenum Press, 1985.

Rittweger R, Hermann K, Ring J: Increased urinary excretion of angiotensin during anaphylactoid reactions. *Int Arch Allergy Immunol* 104:255–261, 1994.

Rodricks JV, Pohland AE: Food hazards of animal origin, in Roberts HR (ed): *Food Safety*. New York: Wiley, 1981, pp 181–237.

Rumsey GL, Siwicki AK, Anderson DP, Bowser PR: Effect of soybean protein on serological response, nonspecific defense mechanisms, growth, and protein utilization in rainbow trout. *Vet Immunol Immunopathol* 41:323, 1994.

Sachs MI, Jones RT, Yunginger JW: Isolation and partial characterization of a major peanut allergen. *J Allergy Clin Immunol* 67:27, 1981.

Sansalone W (ed): *What Is a Nutrient: Defining the Food-Drug Continuum*. Proceedings, Georgetown University, Center for Food and Nutritional Policy. Washington, DC, 1999, 82 pp.

Sato N, Ueno Y: Comparative toxicities of trichothecenes, in Rodericks JV, Hesseltine CW, Mehlman MA (eds): *Mycotoxins in Human and Animal Health*. Park Forest South, IL: Pathtox, 1977, pp 295–307.

Schrander JJ, van den Bogart JP, Forget PP, et al: Cow's milk protein intolerance in infants under 1 year of age: A prospective epidemiological study. *Eur J Pediatr* 52(8):640, 1993.

Schut HAJ, Snyderwine EG: DNA adducts of heterocyclic amine food mutagens: Implications for mutagenesis and carcinogenesis. *Carcinogenesis* 20:353, 1999.

Settipane GA: The restaurant syndromes. *N Engl Reg Allergy Proc* 8:39, 1987.

Shank FR, Carson KL: What is safe food? in Finely, JW, Robinson SF, Armstrong DJ (eds): *Food Safety Assessment*. Washington, DC: American Chemical Society, 1992, pp 26–35.

Shiomi K: Toxins in marine animals. *J Jpn Assoc Acute Med* 10:4–27, 1999.

Shiomi K, Utsumi K, Tsuchiya S, et al: Comparison of proteinaceous toxins in the skin mucous from three species of eels. Comparative Biochemistry and Physiology B. *Comp Biochem Mol Biol* 107:389, 1994.

Sieber SM, Correa P, Dalgard DW, et al: Carcinogenicity and hepatotoxicity of cycasin and its aglycone methylazoxymethanol acetate in nonhuman primates. *J Natl Cancer Inst* 65:177, 1980.

Skog KI, Johannsson MAE, Jagerstad MI: Carcinogenic heterocyclic amines in model systems and cooked foods: A review on formation, occrurences and intake. *Food Chem Toxicol* 36:879, 1998.

Smart DR: Scombroid poisoning: A report of seven cases involving the Western Australian salmon, *Arripis truttaceus. Med J Aust* 157:748, 1992.

Smibert RM: The genus *Campylobacter. Annu Rev Microbiol* 32:673, 1978.

Smith RL: Does one man's meat become another man's poisons? *Trans Med Soc Lond* Nov. 11, 1991, pp 6–17.

Stargel WW, Sanders PG, Tschanz C, Kotsonis FN: Clinical studies with food additives, in Tschanz C, Butchko HH, Stargel WW, Kotsonis FN (eds): *The Clinical Evaluation of a Food Additive. Assessment of Aspartame.* Boca Raton, FL:CRC Press, 196 pp 11–22.

Stephenson J: Public health experts take aim at a moving target: Foodborne infections. *JAMA* 277:97, 1997.

Stewart-Tull DE, Jones AC: Adjuvanted oral vaccines should not induce allergic responses to dietary antigens. *FEMS Microbiol Lett* 79:489, 1992.

Stob M, Baldwin RS, Tuite J, et al: Isolation of an anabolic, uterotropic compound from corn infected with *Gibberella zeae. Nature* 196:1318, 1962.

Stoger P, Wuthrich B: Type I allergy to cow milk proteins in adults: A retrospective study of 34 adult milk- and cheese-allergic patients. *Int Arch Allergy Immunol* 102:399, 1993.

Stoloff L: Aflatoxins—An overview, in Rodericks JV, Hesseltine CW, Mehlman MA (eds): *Mycotoxins in Human and Animal Health.* Park Forest South, IL: Pathtox, 1977.

Sugimura T, Wakabayashi K: Carcinogens in foods, in Shils ME (ed): *Modern Nutrition in Health and Disease.* Baltimore: Williams & Wilkins, 1999, pp 1255–1261.

Sugimura T, Wakabayashi K, Nagao M, Ohgaki H: Heterocyclic amines in cooked food, in Taylor SL, Scanlan RA (eds): *Food Toxicology: A Perspective on the Relative Risks.* New York: Marcel Dekker, 1989, pp 31–55.

Szepfalusi Z, Ebner C, Pandjaitan R, et al: Egg yolk alpha-livetin (chicken serum albumin) is a cross-reactive allergen in the bird-egg syndrome. *J Allergy Clin Immunol* 93:932, 1994.

Takatani T, Akaeda H, Arakawa O, Noguchi T: Occurrence of paralytic shellfish poison (PSP) in bivalves, along with mossworm adherent to their shells, collected from Fukue Island, Nagasaki, Japan during 1995 and 1996. *J Food Hyg Soc Jpn* 38:430, 1997.

Taylor SL: Histamine food poisoning: Toxicology and clinical aspects. *Crit Rev Toxicol* 17(2):91, 1986.

Taylor SL, Nordlee JA, Rupnow JH: Food allergies and sensitivities, in Taylor SL, Scanlan RA (eds): *Food Toxicology: A Perspective on the Relative Risks.* New York: Marcel Dekker, 1989, pp 255–295.

Technical Assessment Systems: *Evaluation of the Current Dietary Status of the U.S. Population Using the USDA Nationwide Food Consumption Survey Results.* Washington, DC: Technical Assessment Systems, 1992.

Tennant R, Zeiger E: Genetic toxicology: Current status of methods of carcinogen identification. *Environ Health Perspect* 100:307, 1993.

Thomas JA, Tschanz C: Nutrient-Drug Interactions, in Kotsonis FN, Mackey M, HjelleJ J (eds): *Nutritional Toxicology.* New York: Raven Press, 1994, pp 139–148.

Thompsom L: Are Bioengineered Foods Safe? *FDA Consumer* 34:18, 2000.

Todd ECD: Domoic acid and amnesic shellfish poisoning: A review. *J Food Protect* 56:69, 1993.

Tonnesen P: Licorice poisoning. *Ugeskr Laeger* 141:513, 1979.

Truckness MW, Mislivec PB, Young K, et al: Cyclopiazonic acid production by cultures of *Aspergillus* and *Penicillium* species isolated from dried beans, corn meal, macaroni, and pecans. *J Assoc Off Anal Chem* 70:123, 1987.

Ueno Y: Trichothecenes: Overview address, in Rodericks JV, Hesseltine CW, Mehlman MA (eds): *Mycotoxins in Human and Animal Health.* Park Forest South, IL: Pathtox, 1977, pp 189–208.

Underwood JE: Trace elements, in *Taxicants Occurring Naturally in Foods,* 2d ed. Washington, DC: National Academy of Sciences, 1973, pp 178–213.

U.S. FDA: *Toxicological Principles for the Safety Assessment of Direct Food Additives and Color Additives Used in Food.* Washington, DC: U.S. Food and Drug Administration, Bureau of Foods, 1982.

Van de Wiel JA, Meuwissen M, Kooy H, et al: Influence of long-term ethanol treatment on in vitro biotransformation of benzo(*a*)pyrene in microsomes of the liver, lung and small intestine from male and female rats. *Biochem Pharmacol* 44:1977, 1992.

VanEtten CH, Tookey HL: Glucosinolates, in Rechcigl J Jr (ed): *CRC Handbook of Naturally Occurring Food Toxicants.* Boca Raton, FL: CRC Press, 1985, p 15.

Van Gelderen CE, Savelkoul TJ, van Ginkel LA, van Dokkum W: The effects of histamine administered in fish samples to healthy volunteers. *J Toxicol Clin Toxicol* 30(4):585, 1992.

VonMalottki K, Wiechmann HW: Acute life threatening bradycardia: Food poisoning by Turkish wild honey. *Dtsch Med Wochenschr* 121:936, 1996.

Wadee AA, Boting LDA, Rabson AR: Fruit allergy: Demonstration of IgE antibodies to a 302Dkd protein present in several fruits. *J Allergy Clin Immunol* 85:801, 1990.

Walker HW: Foodborne illness from *Clostridium perfringens. CRC Crit Rev Food Sci Nutr* 7:71, 1975.

Wantke F, Gotz M, Jarisch R: The red wine provocation test: Intolerance to histamine as a model for food intolerance. *Allergy Proc* 15(1):27, 1994.

Williams GM, Weisburger JH: Chemical carcinogenesis, in Amdur MO, Doull J, Klaassen CD (eds): *Toxicology: The Basic Science of Poisons.* New York: Raven Press, 1991, pp 127–200.

Willshaw GA, Cheasty T, Smith HR: *Escherichia coli,* in Lund BM, Baird-Parker TC, Gould GW (eds): *The Microbiological Safety and Quality* of Food. Gaithersburg, MD: Aspen Publishers, 2000, pp 1136–1177.

Wogan GN: Aflatoxin carcinogenesis, in Busch H (ed): *Methods in Cancer Research.* New York: Academic Press, 1973, pp 309–344.

Wood GM, Slack PT, Rossell JB, et al: Spanish toxic oil syndrome (1981): Progress in the identification of suspected toxic components in simulated oils. *J Agric Food Chem* 42:2525, 1994. [Correction published in *J Agric Food Chem* 43:854, 1995.]

Wortelboer HM, de Kruif CA, van Iersel AA, et al: Effects of cooked brussels sprouts on cytochrome P450 profile and phase II enzymes in liver and small intestinal mucosa of the rat. *Food Chem Toxicol* 30:17, 1992a.

Wortelboer HM, van der Linden EC, de Kruif CA, et al: Effects of indole-3-carbinol on biotransformation enzymes in the rat: *In vivo* changes in liver and small intestinal mucosa in comparison with primary hepatocyte cultures. *Food Chem Toxicol* 30:589, 1992b.

Wuthrich B: Adverse reactions to food additives. *Ann Allergy* 71(4):379, 1993.

Yamagata N, Shigematsu I: Cadmium pollution in perspective. *Inst Public Health Tokyo Bull* 19:1, 1970.

Zhang YA, Wada T, Ichida S, Nakagawa H: Partially purified sea urchin toxin inhibits $^{45}Ca^{2+}$ uptake in P2 fraction from chick brain under physiological ionic conditions. *Bull Pharm Res Technol Inst* 7:67, 1998.

CHAPTER 31

ANALYTIC/FORENSIC TOXICOLOGY

Alphonse Poklis

It is impossible to consider the topic of forensic toxicology without discussing analytic toxicology in detail. However, analytic toxicology has its roots in forensic applications. Therefore, it is logical to discuss these mutually dependent areas together. Analytic toxicology involves the application of the tools of analytic chemistry to the qualitative and/or quantitative estimation of chemicals that may exert adverse effects on living organisms. Generally, the chemical that is to be measured (the analyte) is a xenobiotic that may have been altered or transformed by metabolic actions of the organism. Frequently, the specimen that is to be analyzed presents a matrix consisting of body fluids or solid tissues from the organism. Both the identity of the analyte and the nature of the matrix present formidable problems to an analytic toxicologist.

Forensic toxicology involves the use of toxicology for the purposes of the law (Cravey and Baselt, 1981). Although this broad definition includes a wide range of applications, such as regulatory toxicology and urine testing to detect drug use, by far the most common application is to identify any chemical that may serve as a causative agent in inflicting death or injury on humans or in causing damage to property. Frequently, as a result of such unfortunate incidents, charges of liability or criminal intent are brought that must be resolved by the judicial system. At times, indirect or circumstantial evidence is presented in an attempt to prove cause and effect. However, there is no substitute for an unequivocal identification of a specific chemical substance that is demonstrated to be present in tissues from the victim at a sufficient concentration to explain the injury with a reasonable degree of scientific probability or certainty. For this reason, forensic toxicology and analytic toxicology have long shared a mutually supportive partnership.

Some forensic toxicologic activities have been deemed so important by society that a great effort is expended to initiate and implement analytic procedures in a forensically credible manner as an aid in deciding whether adverse effects have been produced by certain chemicals. Attempts to control drivers whose driving ability may be impaired by ethanol or certain drugs are evidenced by laws prescribing punishment to individuals who are so impaired. The measurement of ethanol in blood or breath at specific concentrations is generally required to prove impairment by this agent (Fisher et al., 1968). Similarly, the decade of the 1980s saw a growing response by society to the threat of drug abuse. Attempts to identify drug users by testing urine for the presence of drugs or their metabolites, using methods and safeguards developed by forensic toxicologists, have become required by law (Department of Health and Human Services, 1988).

The diagnosis and treatment of health problems induced by chemical substances (Blanke and Decker, 1986) and the closely allied field of therapeutic drug monitoring (Moyer et al., 1986) also rely greatly on analytic toxicology. Although the analytes are present in matrices similar to those seen in forensic toxicology, the results must be reported rapidly to be of use to clinicians in treating patients. This requirement of a rapid turnaround time limits the number of chemicals that can be measured because methods, equipment, and personnel must all be available for an instant response to toxicologic emergencies.

Occupational toxicology (Chap. 33) and regulatory toxicology (Chap. 34) require analytic procedures for their implementation or monitoring. In occupational toxicology, the analytic methods used to monitor threshold limit values (TLVs) and other means of estimating the exposure of workers to toxic hazards may utilize simple, nonspecific, but economical screening devices. However, to determine the actual exposure of a worker, it is necessary to analyze blood, urine, breath, or another specimen by employing methods similar to those used in clinical or forensic toxicology. For regulatory purposes, a variety of matrices (food, water, air, etc.) must be examined for extremely small quantities of analytes. Frequently, this requires the use of sophisticated methodology with extreme sensitivity. Both of these applications of analytic toxicology impinge on forensic toxicology because an injury or occupational disease in a worker can result in a legal proceeding, just as a violation of a regulatory law may.

Other applications of analytic toxicology occur frequently during the course of experimental studies. Confirmation of the concentration of dosing solutions and monitoring of their stability often can be accomplished with the use of simple analytic techniques.

The bioavailability of a dose may vary with the route of administration and the vehicle used. Blood concentrations can be monitored as a means of establishing this important parameter. In addition, an important feature in the study of any toxic substance is the characterization of its metabolites as well as the distribution of the parent drug, together with its metabolites, to various tissues. This requires sensitive, specific, and valid analytic procedures. Similar analytic studies can be conducted within a temporal framework to gain an understanding of the dynamics of the absorption, distribution, metabolism, and excretion of toxic chemicals.

It is evident that analytic toxicology is intimately involved in many aspects of experimental and applied toxicology. Because toxic substances include all chemical types and because the measurement of toxic chemicals may require the examination of biological or nonbiological matrices, the scope of analytic toxicology is broad. Nevertheless, a systematic approach and a reliance on the practical experience of generations of forensic toxicologists can be used in conjunction with the sophisticated tools of analytic chemistry to provide the data needed to understand the hazards of toxic substances more completely. These concepts are described in detail in the rest of this chapter.

ANALYTIC TOXICOLOGY

In light of the statement by Paracelsus five centuries ago, "All substances are poisons: there is none which is not a poison" (Klaassen et al., 1986), analytic toxicology potentially encompasses all chemical substances. Forensic toxicologists learned long ago that when the nature of a suspected poison is unknown, a systematic, standardized approach must be used to identify the presence of most common toxic substances. An approach that has stood the test of time was first suggested by Chapuis in 1873 in *Elements de Toxicologie.* It is based on the origin or nature of the toxic agent (Peterson et al., 1923). Such a system can be characterized as follows:

1. Gases
2. Volatile substances
3. Corrosive agents
4. Metals
5. Anions and nonmetals
6. Nonvolatile organic substances
7. Miscellaneous

Closely related to this descriptive classification is the method for separating a toxic agent from the matrix in which it is embedded. The matrix is generally a biological specimen such as a body fluid or a solid tissue. The agent of interest may exist in the matrix in a simple solution or may be bound to protein and other cellular constituents. The challenge is to separate the toxic agent in sufficient purity and quantity to permit it to be characterized and quantified. At times, the parent compound is no longer present in large enough amounts to be separated. In this case, known metabolites may indirectly provide a measure of the parent substance (Hawks and Chiang, 1986). With other substances, interaction of the poison with tissue components may require the isolation or characterization of a protein adduct (SanGeorge and Hoberman, 1986). Methods for separation have long provided a great challenge to analytic toxicologists. Only recently have methods become available that permit direct measurement of some analytes without prior separation from the matrix.

Gases are most simply measured by means of gas chromatography. Some gases are extremely labile, and the specimen must be collected and preserved at temperatures as low as that of liquid nitrogen. Generally, the gas is carefully liberated by incubating the specimen at a predetermined temperature in a closed container. The gas, freed from the matrix, collects over the specimen's "headspace," where it can be sampled and injected into the gas chromatograph. Other gases, such as carbon monoxide, interact with proteins. These gases can be carefully released from the protein, or the adduct can be measured independently, as in the case of carboxyhemoglobin.

Volatile substances are generally liquids of a variety of chemical types. The temperature at which they boil is sufficiently low that older methods of separation utilized microdistillation or diffusion techniques. Gas-liquid chromatography is the simplest approach for simultaneous separation and quantitation in favorable cases. The simple alcohols can be measured by injecting a diluted body fluid directly onto the column of the chromatograph. A more common approach is to use the headspace technique, as is done for gases, after incubating the specimen at an elevated temperature.

Corrosives include mineral acids and bases. Many corrosives consist of ions that are normal tissue constituents. Clinical chemical techniques can be applied to detect these ions when they are in great excess over normal concentrations. Because these ions are normal constituents, the corrosive effects at the site of contact of the chemical, together with other changes in blood chemistry values, can confirm the ingestion of a corrosive substance.

Metals are encountered frequently as occupational and environmental hazards. Elegant analytic methods are available for most metals even when they are present at extremely low concentrations. Classic separation procedures involve destruction of the organic matrix by chemical or thermal oxidation. This leaves the metal to be identified and quantified in the inorganic residue. Unfortunately, this prevents a determination of the metal in the oxidation state or in combination with other elements, as it existed when the metal compound was absorbed. For example, the toxic effects of metallic mercury, mercurous ion, mercuric ion, and dimethylmercury are all different. Analytic methods must be selected that determine the relative amount of each form present to yield optimal analytic results. The analytic difficulty in doing this has lent support to the unfortunate practice of discussing the toxicity of metals as if each metal existed as a single entity.

Toxic anions and nonmetals are a difficult group for analysis. Some anions can be trapped in combination with a stable cation, after which the organic matrix can be destroyed, as with metals. Others can be separated from the bulk of the matrix by dialysis, after which they are detected by colorimetric or chromatographic procedures. Still others are detected and measured by ion-specific electrodes. There are no standard approaches for this group, and other than phosphorus, they are rarely encountered in an uncombined form.

The *nonvolatile organic substances* constitute the largest group of substances that must be considered by analytic toxicologists. This group includes drugs, both prescribed and illegal, pesticides, natural products, pollutants, and industrial compounds. These substances are solids or liquids with high boiling points. Thus, separation procedures generally rely on differential extractions of tissue specimens (Fig. 31-1). These extractions often are not efficient, and recovery of the toxic substance from the matrix may be poor. When the nature of the toxic substance is known, im-

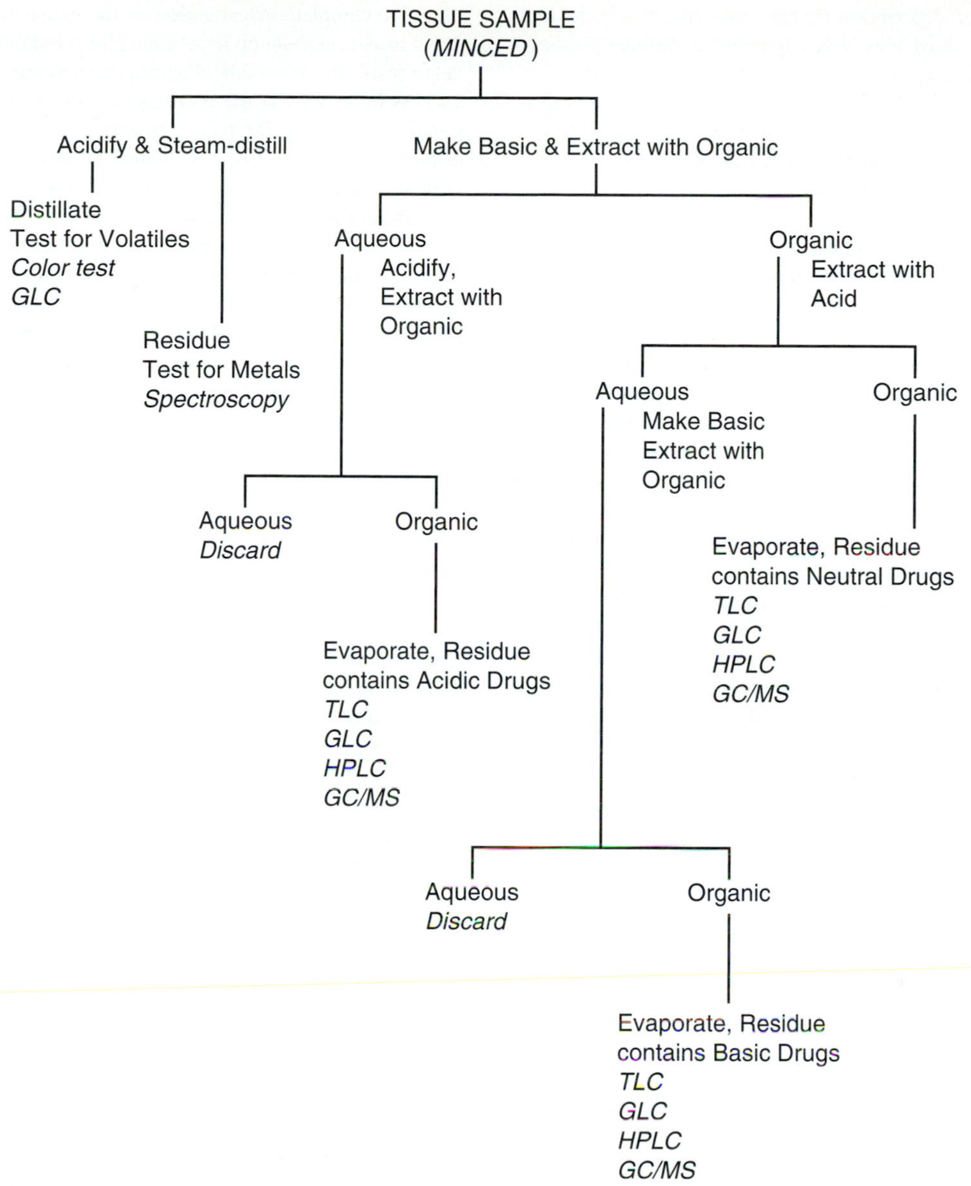

Figure 31-1. ***A scheme of separation for poisons from tissues by steam distillation and differential solvent extraction.***

Abbreviations: GC/MS, gas chromatography/mass spectrometry; GLC, gas-liquid chromatography; HPLC, high-pressure liquid chromatography; TLC, thin-layer chromatography.

munoassay procedures are useful because they allow a toxicologist to avoid using separation procedures. These compounds can be classified as

Organic strong acids
Organic weak acids
Organic bases
Organic neutral compounds
Organic amphoteric compounds

Separation generally is achieved by adjusting the acidity of the aqueous matrix and extracting with a water-immiscible solvent or a solid-phase absorbent material. Finally, a *miscellaneous* category must be included to cover the large number of toxic agents that cannot be detected by the routine application of the methods described above. Venoms and other toxic mixtures of proteins or uncharacterized constituents fall into this class. Frequently, if antibodies can be grown against the active constituent, immunoassay may be the most practical means of detecting and measuring these highly potent and difficult to isolate substances. Unfortunately, unless highly specific monoclonal antibodies are used, the analytic procedure may not be acceptable for forensic purposes. Most frequently, specific analytic procedures must be developed for each analyte of this type. At times, biological endpoints are utilized to semiquantify the concentration of the isolated product.

After this brief description of the scope of analytic toxicology, we shall now show how it is applied to a variety of aspects of toxicology.

ANALYTIC ROLE IN GENERAL TOXICOLOGY

In almost all experimental studies in toxicology, an agent, generally a single chemical substance, is administered in known amounts to an organism. It is universally acknowledged that the chemical under study must be pure or the nature of any contaminants must be known to interpret the experimental results with validity. However, it is common practice to proceed with the experimental study without verifying the purity of the compound. Not only does this practice lead to errors in establishing an accurate dose, but, depending on the nature of the study, other erroneous conclusions may be drawn. For example, the presence of related compounds in the dosage form of a tricyclic antidepressant led to erroneous conclusions about the metabolic products of the drug when it was administered together with the unidentified contaminants (Saady et al., 1981). An even greater error may result when a small amount of a contaminant may be supertoxic. A well-publicized example of this error involved the presence of dioxin in mixtures of the defoliants 2,4-D and 2,4,5-T (Panel on Herbicides, 1971) used during the Vietnam war as Agent Orange. Some of the adverse effects of Agent Orange may have been due to the low concentration of dioxin in those mixtures. Other researchers have reported that the toxicity of mixtures of polybrominated biphenyls may be due to the high toxicity of specific components, while other brominated biphenyls are relatively nontoxic (Mills et al., 1985).

A related application of analytic toxicology is in monitoring dosage forms or solutions for stability throughout the course of an experimental study. Chemicals may degrade in contact with air, by exposure to ultraviolet or other radiation, by interaction with constituents of the vehicle or dosing solution, and by other means. Developing an analytic procedure by which these changes can be recognized and corrected is essential in achieving consistent results throughout a study (Blanke, 1989).

Finally, analytic methods are important in establishing the bioavailability of a compound that is under study. Some substances with low water solubility are difficult to introduce into an animal, and a variety of vehicles may be tried. However, measuring blood concentrations of the compound under study provides a simple means of comparing the effectiveness of vehicles. Introducing a compound to the stomach in an oil vehicle may not be the most effective means of enhancing the absorption of that compound (Granger et al., 1987). Rather than observing dose–effect relationships, it may be more accurate to describe blood (serum) concentration–effect relationships.

ANALYTIC ROLE IN FORENSIC TOXICOLOGY

The duties of a forensic toxicologist in postmortem investigations include the qualitative and quantitative analysis of drugs or poisons in biological specimens collected at autopsy and the interpretation of the analytic findings in regard to the physiologic and behavioral effects of the detected chemicals on the deceased at the time of death.

The complete investigation of the cause or causes of sudden death is an important civic responsibility. Establishing the cause of death rests with the medical examiner, coroner, or pathologist, but success in arriving at the correct conclusion often depends on the combined efforts of the pathologist and the toxicologist. The cause of death in cases of poisoning cannot be proved beyond contention without a toxicologic analysis that establishes the presence of the toxicant in the tissues and body fluids of the deceased.

Many drugs or poisons do not produce characteristic pathologic lesions; their presence in the body can be demonstrated only by chemical methods of isolation and identification. If toxicologic analyses are avoided, deaths resulting from poisoning may be erroneously ascribed to an entirely different cause or poisoning may be designated as the cause of death without definite proof. Such erroneous diagnoses may have significant legal and social consequences.

Additionally, a toxicologist can furnish valuable evidence concerning the circumstances surrounding a death. Such cases commonly involve demonstrating the presence of intoxicating concentrations of ethanol in victims of automotive or industrial accidents or such concentrations of carbon monoxide in fire victims. The degree of carbon monoxide saturation of the blood may indicate whether the deceased died as a result of the fire or was dead before the fire started. Arson is commonly used to conceal homicide. Also, licit or illicit psychoactive drugs often play a significant role in the circumstances associated with sudden or violent death. The behavioral toxicity of many illicit drugs may explain the bizarre or "risk-taking" behavior of the deceased that led to his or her demise. At times, a negative toxicologic finding is of particular importance in assessing the cause of death. For example, toxicology studies may demonstrate that a person with a seizure disorder was not taking the prescribed medication and that this contributed to the fatal event.

Additionally, the results of postmortem toxicologic testing provide valuable epidemiologic and statistical data. Forensic toxicologists are often among the first to alert the medical community to new epidemics of substance abuse (Poklis, 1982) and the dangers of abusing over-the-counter drugs (Garriott et al., 1985). Similarly, they often determine the chemical identity and toxicity of novel analogues of psychoactive agents that are subject to abuse, including "designer drugs" such as "china white" (methylfentanyl) (Henderson, 1988) and "ecstasy" (methylenedioxymethamphetamine) (Dowling et al., 1987).

Today there are numerous specialized areas of study in the field of toxicology; however, it is the forensic toxicologist who is obliged to assist in the determination of the cause of death for a court of law who has been historically recognized by the title "toxicologist."

Until the nineteenth century, physicians, lawyers, and law enforcement officials harbored extremely faulty notions about the signs and symptoms of poisoning (Thorwald, 1965). Unless a poisoner was literally caught in the act, there was no way to establish the fact that the victim died from poison. In the early eighteenth century, a Dutch physician, Hermann Boerhoave, theorized that various poisons in a hot, vaporous condition yield characteristic odors. He placed substances suspected of containing poisons on hot coals and tested their smells. While Boerhoave was not successful in applying his method, he was the first to suggest a chemical method for proving the presence of poison.

White arsenic (arsenic trioxide) has been widely used with murderous intent for over a thousand years. Therefore it is not surprising that the first milestones in the chemical isolation and identification of a poison in body tissues and fluids centered on arsenic. In 1775, Karl Wilhelm Scheele, a Swedish chemist, discovered that white arsenic is converted to arsenous acid by chlorine water. The addition of metallic zinc reduced the arsenous acid to poisonous arsine gas. If gently heated, the evolving gas would deposit metallic arsenic on the surface of a cold vessel. In 1821, Serullas utilized the decomposition of arsine for the detection of small quantities of arsenic in stomach contents and urine in poisoning cases. In 1836, James M. Marsh, a chemist at the Royal British Arsenal in Woolwich, applied Serullas's observations in developing the first reliable method to determine the presence of an absorbed poison in body tissues and fluids such as liver, kidney, and blood. After acid digestion of the tissues, Marsh generated arsine gas, which was drawn through a heated capillary tube. The arsine decomposed, leaving a dark deposit of metallic arsenic. Quantitative measures were performed by comparing the length of the deposit from known concentrations of arsenic with those of the test specimens.

The 1800s witnessed the development of forensic toxicology as a scientific discipline. In 1814, Mathieiv J. B. Orfila (1787–1853), the "father of toxicology," published *Traité des Poisons,* the first systematic approach to the study of the chemical and physiological nature of poisons (Gettler, 1977). Orfila's role as an expert witness in many famous murder trails, particularly his application of the Marsh test for arsenic in the trial of the poisoner Marie Lafarge, aroused both popular and scholarly interest in the new science. As dean of the medical faculty at the University of Paris, Orfila trained numerous students in forensic toxicology.

The first successful isolation of an alkaloidal poison was done in 1850 by Jean Servials Stas, a Belgian chemist, using a solution of acetic acid in warm ethanol to extract nicotine from the tissues of the murdered Gustave Fougnie. As modified by the German chemist Fredrick Otto, the Stas-Otto method was quickly applied to the isolation of numerous alkaloidal poisons, including colchicine, coniine, morphine, narcotine, and strychnine. In the latter half of the nineteenth century, European toxicologists were in the forefront of the development and application of forensic sciences, providing valuable evidence of poisoning. A number of these trials became "causes célèbres" and the testimony of forensic toxicologists captured the imagination of the public and increased awareness of the development and application of toxicology. Murderers could no longer poison with impunity.

In the United States, Rudolph A. Witthaus, professor of chemistry at Cornell University Medical School, made many contributions to toxicology and called attention to the new science by performing analyses for the city of New York in several famous morphine poisoning cases, including the murder of Helen Potts by Carlyle Harris and that of Annie Sutherland by Dr. Robert W. Buchanan. In 1911, Witthaus and Tracy C. Becker edited a four-volume work on medical jurisprudence, forensic medicine, and toxicology, the first standard forensic textbook published in the United States. In 1918, the city of New York established a medical examiner's system, and the appointment of Dr. Alexander O. Gettler as toxicologist marked the beginning of modern forensic toxicology in this country. Although Dr. Gettler made numerous contributions to the science, perhaps his greatest was the training and direction he gave to future leaders in forensic toxicology. Many of his associates went on to direct laboratories within coroners' and medical examiners' systems in major urban centers throughout the country.

In 1949, the American Academy of Forensic Sciences was established to support and further the practice of all phases of legal medicine in the United States. The members of the toxicology section represent the vast majority of forensic toxicologists working in coroners' or medical examiners' offices. Several other international, national, and local forensic science organizations, such as the Society of Forensic Toxicologists and the California Association of Toxicologists, offer a forum for the exchange of scientific data pertaining to analytic techniques and case reports involving new or infrequently used drugs and poisons. The International Association of Forensic Toxicologists, founded in 1963, with over 750 members in 45 countries, permits worldwide cooperation in resolving the technical problems confronting toxicology.

In 1975, the American Board of Forensic Toxicology (ABFT) was created to examine and certify forensic toxicologists. One of the stated objectives of the board is "to make available to the judicial system, and other publics, a practical and equitable system for readily identifying those persons professing to be specialists in forensic toxicology who possess the requisite qualifications and competence." Those certified as diplomats of the board must have a doctor of philosophy or doctor of science degree, have at least 3 years of full-time professional experience, and pass a written examination. In 2000, the board began certifying "forensic toxicology specialists." Specialists must have a master's or bachelor's degree and 3 years of full-time professional experience and must pass a written examination. At present, there are approximately 225 diplomats and 20 specialists certified by the board. In 1998, the board began an accreditation program for forensic toxicology laboratories. ABFT accredited laboratories must meet standards of qualified experienced personnel and forensically sound procedures for the handling of evidence, analysis of specimens, and reporting of results. Laboratories must pass periodic on-site inspections involving a review of laboratory procedures and previous casework since the last inspection in order to maintain their continuous accreditation.

TOXICOLOGIC INVESTIGATION OF A POISON DEATH

The toxicologic investigation of a poison death may be divided into three steps: (1) obtaining the case history and suitable specimens, (2) the toxicologic analyses, and (3) the interpretation of the analytic findings.

Case History and Specimens

Today, thousands of compounds are readily available that are lethal if ingested, injected, or inhaled. Usually a limited amount of specimen is available on which to perform analyses; therefore it is imperative that, before the analyses are initiated, as much information as possible concerning the facts of the case be collected. The age, sex, weight, medical history, and occupation of the decedent as well as any treatment administered before death; the gross autopsy findings; the drugs available to the decedent; and the interval between the onset of symptoms and death should be noted. In a typical year, a postmortem toxicology laboratory will perform analyses for such diverse poisons as prescription drugs (analgesics, antidepressants, hypnotics, tranquilizers), drugs of abuse (hallucinogens, narcotics, stimulants), commercial products (antifreeze, aerosol products, insecticides, rodenticides, rubbing compound, weed killers), and gases (carbon monoxide, cyanide). Obviously, thorough investigation of the death scene including a tentative identification of the administered poison is helpful prior to beginning the analysis (Ernst et al., 1982).

The pathologist at autopsy usually performs the collection of postmortem specimens for analysis. Specimens of many different body fluids and organs are necessary, as drugs and poisons display varying affinities for body tissues (Fig. 31-2). Therefore, detection of a poison is more likely in a tissue in which it accumulates. A large quantity of each specimen is needed for thorough toxicologic analysis because a procedure that extracts and identifies one compound or class of compounds may be ineffective in extracting and identifying others (Table 31-1).

In collecting the specimens, the pathologist labels each container with the date and time of autopsy, the name of the decedent, the identity of the sample, an appropriate case identification number, and his or her signature or initials. It is paramount that the handling of all specimens, their analysis, and the resultant reports be authenticated and documented. A form developed at the collection site that identifies each specimen is submitted to the laboratory with the specimens. The form is signed and dated by the pathologist and subsequently by any individual handling, transferring, or transporting the specimens from one individual or place to another. In legal terms, this form constitutes a "chain of custody" of specimens, documenting by time, date, name, and signature all persons transferring or receiving the specimens. The chain of custody enables a toxicologist to introduce his or her results into legal proceedings, having established that the specimens analyzed came from the decedent.

Specimens should be collected before embalming, as this process may destroy or dilute the poisons present, rendering their detection impossible. Conversely, methyl or ethyl alcohol may be a constituent of embalming fluid, giving a false indication of the decedent's drinking before death.

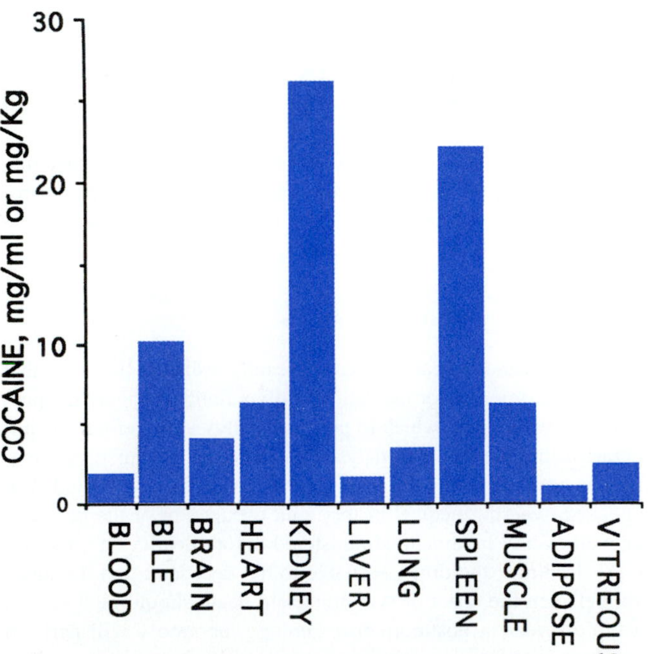

Figure 31-2. Cocaine tissue distribution in a fatal poisoning. (Data drawn from Poklis A, Mackell MA, Graham M: Disposition of cocaine in a fatal poisoning in man. J Anal Toxicol 9:227–229, 1985.)

Table 31-1
Suggested List of Specimens and Amounts to Be Collected at Autopsy

SPECIMEN	QUANTITY
Brain	100 g
Liver	100 g
Kidney	50 g
Heart blood	25 g
Peripheral blood	10 g
Vitreous humor	All available
Bile	All available
Urine	All available
Gastric contents	All available

SOURCE: From Appendix, Report of the Laboratory Guidelines Committee, Society of Forensic Toxicologist and Toxicology Section, American Academy of Forensic Sciences. *J Anal Toxicol* 14:18A, 1990, with permission.

On occasion, toxicologic analysis is requested for cases of burned, exhumed, and skeletal remains. In such instances, it is necessary to analyze unusual specimens such as bone marrow, hair, skeletal muscle, vitreous humor, and even maggots (Inoue, 1992). Numerous drugs have been successfully identified in bone marrow and bone washings from skeletal remains even after decomposition and burial (Benko, 1985). Similarly, the vitreous humor of the eye is isolated and sequestered from putrefaction, charring, and trauma; thus, it is a useful specimen for the detection of most drugs, anions, and even volatile poisons such as alcohols, ketones, and glycols (Coe, 1993). Hair analysis is a rapidly growing technique in forensic toxicology. Recently, numerous therapeutic agents such as antibiotics and antipsychotic drugs as well as drugs subject to abuse (morphine, phencyclidine, and cocaine) have been identified in hair (Tagliro, 1993). Limited data are available to support a direct correlation between hair values and drug doses or between physiologic and behavioral effects; however, qualitative results have been accepted as indicators of drug use. In severely decomposed bodies, the absence of blood and/or the scarcity of solid tissues suitable for analysis have led to the collection and testing of maggots (fly larvae) feeding on the body (Pounder, 1991). The fundamental premise underlying maggot analysis is that if drugs or intoxicants are detected, they could only have originated from the decedents' tissues on which the larvae were feeding. Surprisingly, analysis of maggots is rather straightforward, requiring no special methodology beyond that routinely applied in toxicology laboratories. Case reports have documented the detection of numerous drugs and intoxicants in maggots collected from decomposed bodies. The compounds detected include barbiturates, benzodiazepines, phenothiazines, morphine, and malathion. Controlled studies in which maggots were allowed to feed on tissues to which drugs had been added have demonstrated the accumulation of propoxphene and amitriptyline in the larvae (Goff et al., 1993).

Toxicologic Analysis

Before the analysis begins, several factors must be considered: the amount of specimen available, the nature of the poison sought, and the possible biotransformation of the poison. In cases involving oral administration of the poison, the gastrointestinal (GI) contents are analyzed first, because large amounts of residual unabsorbed poison may be present. The urine may be analyzed next, as the kidney is the major organ of excretion for most poisons and high concentrations of toxicants and/or their metabolites often are present in urine. After absorption from the GI tract, drugs or poisons are carried to the liver before entering the general systemic circulation; therefore, the first analysis of an internal organ is conducted on the liver. If a specific poison is suspected to have caused or contributed to a death, the toxicologist may first analyze the tissues and fluids in which the poison concentrates.

A knowledge of drug biotransformation is often essential before an analysis is performed. The parent compound and any major physiologically active metabolites should be isolated and identified. In some instances, the metabolites provide the only evidence that a drug or poison has been administered. Many screening tests, such as immunoassays, are specifically designed to detect not the parent drug but its major urinary metabolite. An example of the relationship of pharmacokinetic and analytic factors is provided by cocaine. The major metabolites of cocaine biotransformation are benzoylecgonine and ecgonine methylester (Fig. 31-3). The ingestion of alcohol combined with the administration of cocaine results in the hepatic transesterification of cocaine to form cocaethylene (Hime et al., 1991) (Fig. 31-3). The disposition of these compounds in various body fluids and hair is shown in Fig. 31-4. Thus, the initial testing of urine to determine cocaine use is performed with immunoassays specifically designed to detect the presence of benzoylecgonine, the major urinary metabolite. If saliva or hair is tested, parent cocaine is the analyte sought. To determine a cocaine profile of each compound present in a specimen, chromatographic procedures such as gas chromatography/mass spectrometry (GC/MS), that allow the simultaneous separation and quantification of each compound, are used.

The analysis may be complicated by the normal chemical changes that occur during the decomposition of a cadaver. The autopsy and toxicologic analysis should be started as soon after death

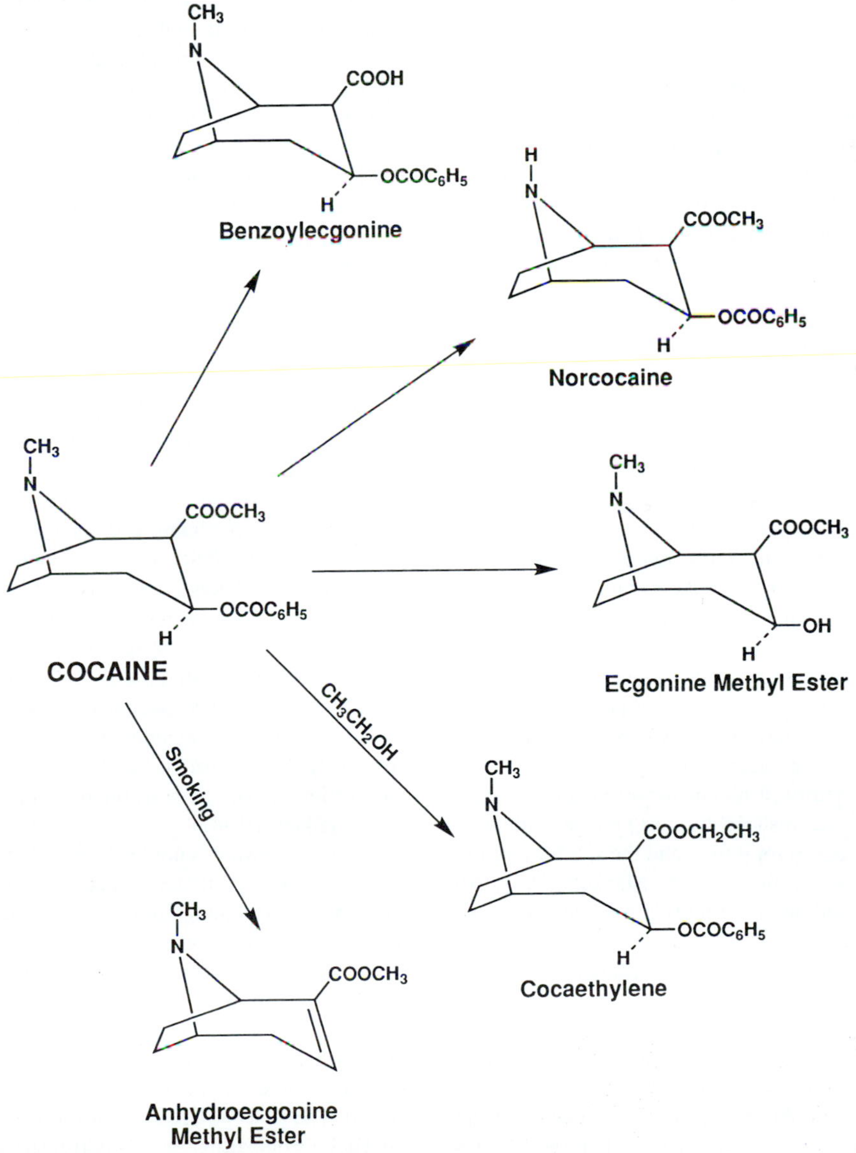

Figure 31-3. Biotransformation and pyrolysis products of cocaine.

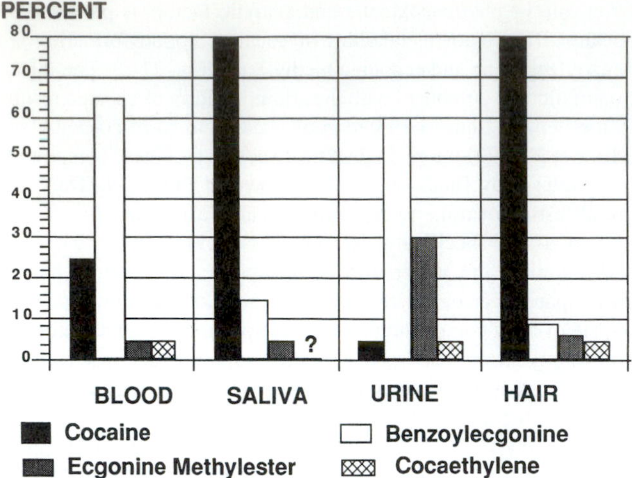

Figure 31-4. Disposition of cocaine and cocaine metabolites in human fluids and hair. (Data redrawn from Spiehler V: Society of Forensic Toxicology Conference on Drug Testing in Hair, Tampa, FL, October 29, 1994.)

as possible. The natural enzymatic and nonenzymatic processes of decomposition and microbial metabolism may destroy a poison that was present at death or produce substances or compounds with chemical and physical properties similar to those of commonly encountered poisons. As early as the 1870s, so-called cadaveric alkaloids isolated from the organs of putrefied bodies were known to produce color test reactions similar to those produced by morphine and other drugs. These cadaveric alkaloids resulted from the bacterial decarboxylation of the amino acids ornithine and lysine, producing putrescine and cadaverine, respectively (Evans, 1963). Similarly, during decomposition, phenylalanine is converted to phenylethylamine, which has chemical and physical properties very similar to those of amphetamine. The hydrolysis, oxidation, or reduction of proteins, nucleic acids, and lipids may generate numerous compounds, such as hydroxylated aliphatic and aromatic carboxylic acids, pyridine and piperidine derivatives, and aromatic heterocyclics such as tryptamine and norharmane (Kaempe, 1969). All these substances may interfere with the isolation and identification of the toxicants being sought. The concentration of cyanide and ethyl alcohol and the carbon monoxide saturation of the blood may be decreased or increased, depending on the degree of putrefaction and microbial activity. However, many poisons—such as arsenic, barbiturates, mercury, and strychnine—are extremely stable and may be detectable many years after death.

Before analysis, the purity of all chemicals should be established. The primary reference material used to prepare calibrators and controls should be checked for purity, and the salt form or degree of hydration should be determined (Blanke, 1989). All reagents and solvents should be of the highest grade possible and should be free of contaminants that may interfere with or distort analytic findings. For example, the chloroform contaminants phosgene and ethyl chloroformate may react with primary or secondary amine drugs to form carbamyl chloride and ethyl carbamate derivatives (Cone et al., 1982). Specimen containers, lids, and stoppers should be free of contaminants such as plasticizers, which often interfere with chromatographic or GC/MS determinations. Care should be exercised to ensure a clean laboratory environment. This is of particular concern in the analysis of metals, as aluminum, arsenic, lead, and mercury are ubiquitous environmental and reagent contaminants.

Forensic toxicology laboratories analyze specimens by using a variety of analytic procedures. Initially, nonspecific tests designed to determine the presence or absence of a class or group of analytes may be performed directly on the specimens. Examples of tests used to rapidly screen urine are the FPN (ferric chloride, perchloric, and nitric acid) color test for phenothiazine drugs and immunoassays for the detection of amphetamines, benzodiazepines, and opiate derivatives. Positive results obtained with these tests must be confirmed by a second analytic procedure that identifies the particular drug. The detection limit of the confirmatory test should be lower than that of the initial nonspecific test. Some analytic procedures identify specific compounds. Even in such instances, a second test should be performed to identify the analyte. The second test should be based on a chemical or physical principle different from that of the first test. Such additional testing is performed to establish an unequivocal identification of the drugs or poisons present. Whenever possible, the most specific test for the compound of interest should be performed. Today, GC/MS or high-performance liquid chromatography (HPLC)/MS is the most widely applied methodology in toxicology and is generally accepted as unequivocal identification for most drugs. Analyte identification is based upon the retention time in the chromatographic system coupled with the ion fragmentation spectrum in the mass spectrometer. The analyte mass spectrum is the pattern of mass to charge ion fragments and their relative abundance. Even drugs such as amitriptyline and cyclobenzaprine that display similar chromatographic behavior and differ in their chemical structure by only a double bond may be readily identified by GC/MS (Fig. 31-5).

The lower limit of detection, the smallest concentration of analyte reliably identified by the assay, and the specificity of all qualitative methods should be well documented. The laboratory must demonstrate that the assay response to blank or negative calibrators does not overlap with the response of the lowest positive calibrator. In certain instances, qualitative identification of a poison or drug is sufficient to resolve forensic toxicology issues. However, most cases require reliable estimates of poison concentrations for forensic interpretation. For quantitative analysis, the linearity, precision, and specificity of the procedure must be established. Linearity should be determined by using at least a drug free and three drug added calibrators whose concentrations bracket the anticipated concentrations in the specimen. Precision, which statistically demonstrates the variance in the value obtained, is determined by replicate analyses of a specimen of a known concentration. For a variety of reasons, a quantitative result occasionally will deviate spuriously from the true value. Therefore, replicate quantitative determinations should be performed on all specimens, at least in duplicate (Blanke, 1987).

When unusual samples such as bone marrow, hair, and maggots are analyzed, the extraction efficiency of a procedure may vary greatly, depending on the nature of the specimens. Therefore, all calibrators and controls should be prepared in the same matrix as the specimens and analyzed concurrently with the specimens. Often the matrix is "unique" or impossible to match, such as decomposed or embalmed tissue. In these instances, the method of "standard additions" may be used. Known amounts of the drug or poison of interest are added to specimen aliquots and these are analyzed. The concentration of poison in the test specimen is determined by comparing the proportional response of the "poison added" specimens to that of the test specimens. When comparable

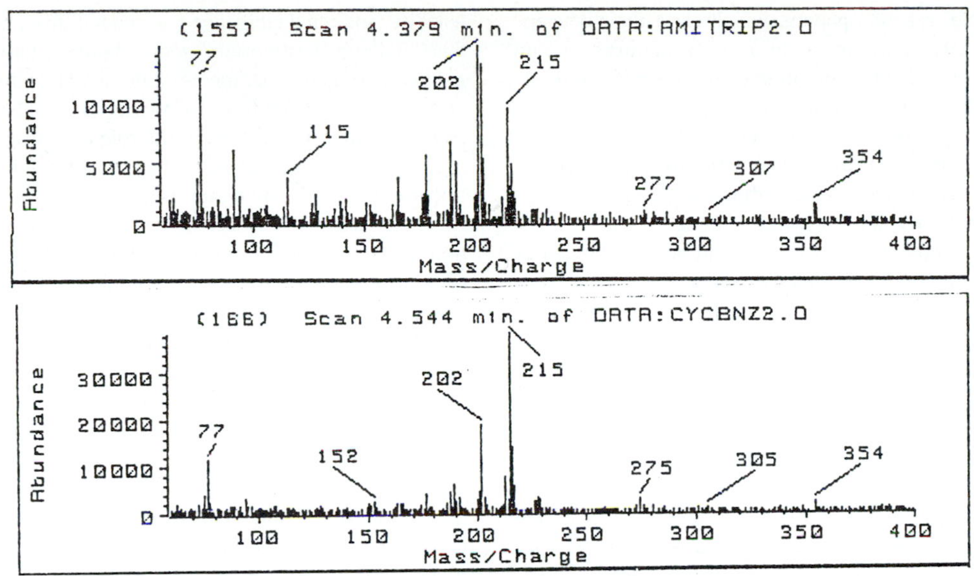

Figure 31-5. Electron impact mass spectra of amitriptyline and cyclobenzaprine, scanning ion mass from 60 to 400 m/e. (From Poklis A: Cyclobenzaprine in emergency toxicology. Clin Chem CC96-3:43–57, 1996. American Society of Clinical Pathologists, with permission.)

results are obtained from analysis of specimens by both direct extraction methods and "standard addition," not only is the efficacy of the extraction method validated, but also the accuracy of the results is assured (Poklis et al. 1998).

Interpretation of Analytic Results

Once the analysis of the specimens is complete, the toxicologist must interpret his or her findings in regard to the physiologic or behavioral effects of the toxicants on the decedent at the concentrations found. Specific questions may be answered, such as the route of administration, the dose administered, and whether the concentration of the toxicant present was sufficient to cause death or alter the decedent's actions enough to cause his or her death. Assessing the physiologic or behavioral meanings of analytic results is often the most difficult problem faced by the forensic toxicologist.

In determining the route of administration, the toxicologist notes the results of the analysis of the various specimens. As a general rule, the highest concentrations of a poison are found at the site of administration. Therefore, the presence of large amounts of drugs and/or poisons in the GI tract and liver indicates oral ingestion, while higher concentrations in the lungs than in other visceral organs can indicate inhalation or intravenous injection. The ratio or relative distribution of drugs in different tissues may also differentiate oral from parenteral administration (Fig. 31-6). Drugs may also be detected in the tissue surrounding an injection site following intramuscular or intravenous injection. Smoking is a popular route of administration for abusers of controlled substances such as cocaine, heroin, and phencyclidine. Pyrolysis of these drugs leads to the inhalation not only of the parent drug but also of characteristic breakdown products of combustion. For example, a major pyrolysis product of "crack" cocaine smoking is anhydroecgonine methylester (Martin et al., 1989) (Fig. 31-3). Thus, identification of relatively high concentrations of this compound along with cocaine or cocaine metabolites in urine or other body fluids or tissues indicates smoking as the route of cocaine administration (Jacob et al., 1990).

The presence of a toxic material in the GI tract, regardless of the quantity, does not provide sufficient evidence to establish that agent as the cause of death. It is necessary to demonstrate that absorption of the toxicant has occurred and that it has been transported by the general circulation to the target organ in order to exert its lethal effect. This is established by blood and tissue analysis. An exception to the rule is provided by strong corrosive chemicals

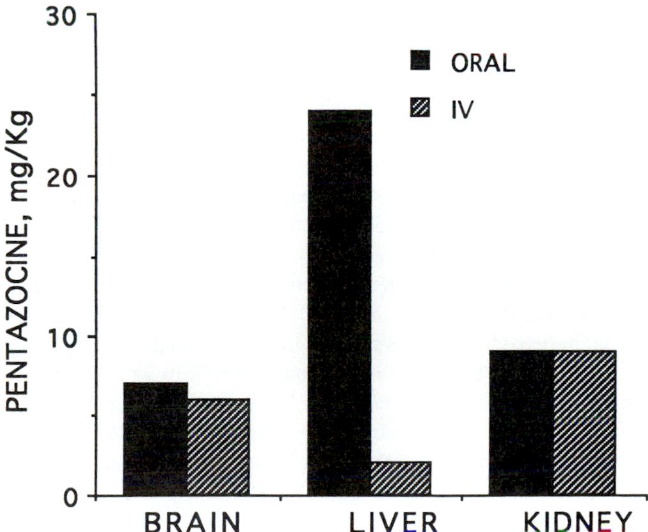

Figure 31-6. Comparison of pentazocine distribution in fatal poisonings due to intravenous injection and oral administration. (Data from Baselt RC: Disposition of Toxic Drugs and Chemicals in Man, 2d ed. Davis, CA: Biomedical Publications, 1982, pp 603–606, and Poklis A, MacKell MA: Toxicological findings in deaths due to pentazocine: A report of two cases. Forensic Sci Int 20:89–95, 1982.)

such as sulfuric acid, lye, and phenol, which exert their deleterious effects by directly digesting tissue, causing hemorrhage and shock. The results of urinalysis are often of little benefit in determining the physiologic effects of a toxic agent. Urine results establish only that the poison was present in the body at some time before death. Correlation of urine values with physiologic effects is poor because of various factors that influence the rate of excretion of specific compounds and the urine volume.

The physiologic effects of most drugs and poisons are correlated with their concentrations in blood or blood fractions such as plasma and serum. Indeed, in living persons, this association is the basis of therapeutic drug monitoring. However, postmortem blood has been described as a fluid resembling blood that is obtained from the vasculature after death. Therefore interpretation of postmortem blood results requires careful consideration of the case history, the site of collection, and postmortem changes. The survival time between the administration of a poison and death may be sufficiently long to permit biotransformation and excretion of the agent. Blood values may appear to be nontoxic or consistent with therapeutic administration. Death from hepatic failure after an acetaminophen overdose usually occurs at least 3 to 4 days after ingestion. Postmortem acetaminophen concentrations in blood may be consistent with the ingestion of therapeutic doses. Therefore, fatal acetaminophen overdose is established by case history, central lobular necrosis of the liver, and, if available, analysis of serum specimens collected from the decedent when he or she was admitted to the emergency department (Price et al., 1991). Emergency medical treatment—such as the administration of fluids, plasma extenders, diuretics, and blood transfusions—may dilute or remove toxic agents. Similarly, prolonged survival on a mechanical respirator, hemodialysis, or hemoperfusion may significantly reduce initially lethal blood concentrations of poisons.

Until recently, it was generally assumed that postmortem blood drug concentrations were more or less uniform throughout the body. However, in the 1970s, several investigators noted that postmortem concentrations of digoxin in heart blood greatly exceeded those in simultaneously collected femoral blood. They also observed that postmortem blood concentrations, particularly in heart blood, exceeded the expected values at the time of death (Vorpahl and Coe, 1978; Aderjan et al., 1979). This postmortem increase in blood digoxin concentrations was apparently due to release of the drug from tissue stores, particularly the myocardium. Recently, other researchers have demonstrated that for many drugs, blood concentrations in the same body vary greatly depending on the site from which the specimen is collected: subclavian vein, thoracic aorta, inferior vena cava, femoral vein, and so forth. For example, in a case of fatal multiple drug ingestion, analysis of postmortem blood collected from 10 different sites demonstrated imipramine concentrations that differed by as much as 760 percent (2.1 to 16.0 mg/L) (Jones and Pounder, 1987). In an extensive investigation, Prouty and Anderson (1990) demonstrated that postmortem blood drug concentrations were not only site-dependent but increased greatly over the interval between death and specimen collection, particularly in heart blood. This increase over the postmortem interval was most pronounced for basic drugs with large apparent volumes of distribution, such as tricyclic antidepressants.

In an overt drug overdose, postmortem blood concentrations are elevated sufficiently to render an unmistakable interpretation of fatal intoxication. However, in many cases, the postmortem redistribution of drugs may significantly affect the interpretation of analytic findings. For drugs whose volume of distribution, plasma half-life, and renal clearance vary widely from person to person or that undergo postmortem redistribution, tissue concentrations readily distinguish therapeutic administration from drug overdose (Apple, 1989). Therefore, to provide a foundation of reasonable medical certainty in regard to the role of a drug in the death of an individual, it is recommended that, in addition to heart blood, a peripheral blood specimen and tissues be analyzed.

The analysis of tissue specimens is important for the estimation of a "minimal administered dose" or body burden of a drug or poison. In order to calculate a minimum body burden, it is necessary to analyze as many different body tissues and fluids as possible to determine the concentrations of the drug present. The concentration of drug in each separate specimen is then multiplied by the total weight or volume of that particular tissue or fluid. In this manner, the total amount of drug in each different tissue or fluid is determined. The amounts of drug in each separate tissue and fluid are then added together to give the total body burden or minimal administered dose. This simple approach has often proven extremely effective in resolving legal medical issues. For example, lidocaine is commonly administered in 50- to 100-mg bolus injections as an antiarrythmic agent for ventricular arrhythmia during resuscitation efforts. Because of poor circulation and tissue perfusion during arrhythmias, lidocaine is not well distributed in the body of the victim of a fatal heart attack. Postmortem bloods often exceed 50 mg/L in such cases, while values for effective antiarrythmic prophylaxis do not exceed 5 mg/L. Therefore, a blood lidocaine value of 50 mg/L may be an artifact of resuscitation efforts or might represent a fatal overdose. Tissue distribution studies have resolved this issue in both accidental and homicidal poisoning with lidocaine (Poklis et al., 1984).

Postmortem toxicology results are often used to corroborate investigative findings. For example, the analysis of sequential sections of hair provides a reliable correlation with the pattern of arsenic exposure. Significant increases in the arsenic content of the root and the first 5 mm of the hair occur within hours after the ingestion of arsenic (Smith, 1964). The germinal cells are in relativity close equilibrium with circulating arsenic; thus, as arsenic concentrations in blood rise or fall, so does arsenic deposition in growing hair. Normal arsenic content in hair varies with nutritional, environmental, and physiologic factors; however, the maximum upper limit of normal with a 99 percent confidence limit in persons not exposed to arsenic is 5 mg/kg (Shapiro, 1967). Hair grows at a rate of approximately 12.5 mm (in.) per month. Therefore, analysis of 1.0-cm segments provides a monthly pattern of exposure (Fig. 31-7). Such analyses are often performed in cases of homicidal poisoning to demonstrate that increases in arsenic deposition in the victim's hair correlate with times when a poisoner had an opportunity to administer the poison. Continuously elevated hair arsenic values indicate chronic rather than acute poisoning as the cause of death.

A new extension of forensic toxicology is the analysis of impurities of illicit drug synthesis in biological specimens. Many drugs of abuse are illicitly manufactured in clandestine laboratories, particularly methamphetamine. There are several popular methods of methamphetamine synthesis; when these are applied in clandestine laboratories, side reactions or incomplete conversion of the reactants yield an impure mixture of methamphetamine and synthetic impurities. These impurities can be characteristic of a particular synthetic method and their detection in biological specimens can indicate use of an illicitly produced drug that is not a legal pharmaceutical product; suggest the synthetic method that

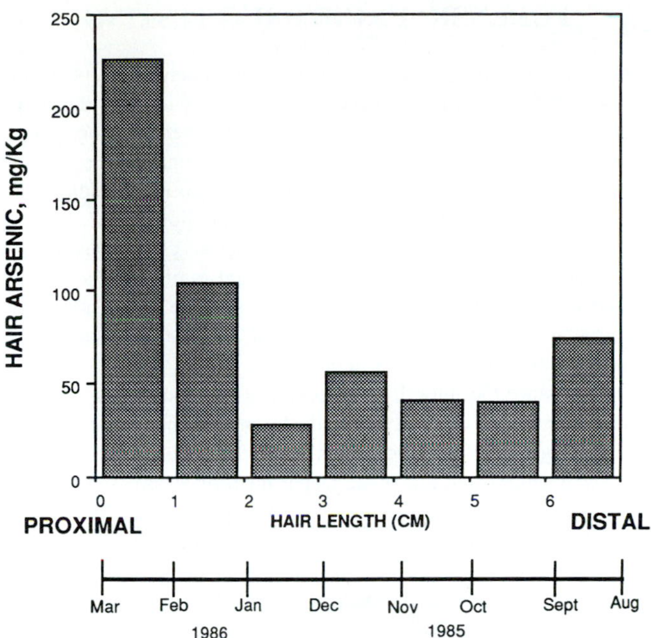

Figure 31-7. Results of neutron activation analysis for arsenic in sequential sections of hair, demonstrating chronic arsenic poisoning. Increased exposure in the first two sections is consistent with fatal events. Lower values in section 3 are consistent with 2 weeks of hospitalization. (Data from Poklis A, Saady JJ: Arsenic poisoning: Acute or chronic? Suicide or murder? Am J Forensic Med Pathol 11:226–232, 1990.)

was used to produce the drug; point to a possible common source of illicit production; and provide a link between manufacturers, dealers, and users. A recent example of impurity analysis was the detection of metabolites of α-benzyl-*N*-methylphenethylamine (BNMPA) in the urine of abusers of methamphetamine (Moore et al., 1996) and in a case of fatal drug overdose involving methamphetamine (Moore et al., 1996). BNMPA is an impurity arising from the synthesis of methamphetamine via the Leukart reaction using phenyl-2-propanone (P2P) synthesized from phenylacetic acid. Clandestine laboratories often must synthesize the P2P starting material, as its sale and distribution is regulated by the federal Drug Enforcement Agency.

CRIMINAL POISONING OF THE LIVING

Over the past few decades, forensic toxicologists have become more and more involved in the analysis of specimens obtained from living victims of criminal poisonings. Generally, this increase in testing has arisen from two types of cases: (1) administration of drugs to incapacitate victims of kidnapping, robbery, or sexual assault and (2) poisoning as a form of child abuse.

For centuries those severely intoxicated from alcohol often became victims of kidnapping, robbery, or sexual assault. In the days of sail, the kidnapping of drunks in seaports was a common way of obtaining sailors for long commercial voyages such as those involved in whaling. Late in the nineteenth century, the mixing of the powerful hypnotic chloral hydrate with alcohol produced the legendary "Mickey Finn." While alcohol is still often a primary factor in cases of alleged sexual assault, common drugs of abuse or other psychoactive drugs are often involved (Table 31-2). Of particular concern are the many potent inductive agents medically administered prior to general anesthesia. Many of these drugs, such as benzodiazepines and phenothiazines, are available today through illicit sources or legal purchase in foreign countries. When administered surreptitiously, they cause sedation and incapacitate the victim while also producing amnesia in the victim as to the events while drugged without causing severe central nervous system depression. These cases often present a difficult analytic challenge to the toxicologist. Usually the victim does not bring forth an allegation of assault until 24 h to several days after the attack. Thus, the intoxicating drug may have been largely eliminated or extensively metabolized such that extremely low concentrations of drug or metabolites are present in the victim's blood, urine, and/or hair specimens. Sophisticated, highly sensitive analytic methods such as GC/MS or HPLC/MS may be required to accurately identify drugs in such specimens. To provide guidance in the choice of analytic approaches to such cases, recommendations for the toxicologic investigation of sexual assaults have recently been formulated by the Toxicology Section of the American Academy of Forensic Sciences (LeBeau et al., 1999).

Poisoning as a form of child abuse involves the deliberate administration of toxic or injurious substances to a child, usually by a parent or other caregiver. The victims of such poisonings range

Table 31-2
Distribution of Drugs of Abuse Encountered Urine Specimens in 578 Cases of Alleged Sexual Assault

RANK	DRUG/DRUG GROUP	INCIDENCE	PERCENT OF CASES*
1.	No drugs found	167	29%
2.	Ethanol	148	26%
3.	Benzodiazepines	70	12%
4.	Marijuana	67	12%
5.	Amphetamines	41	7%
6.	Gamma-hydroxybutyrate	24	4%
7.	Opiate (morphine/codeine)	20	4%
8.	Other drugs	13	3%

*Percentages do not add to 100% due to rounding.

SOURCE: Data from ElSohly MA, et al.: Analysis of flunitrazepam metabolites and other substances in alleged cases of sexual assault. Presentation at the 50th Anniversary Meeting of the American Academy of Forensic Sciences; San Francisco, CA, February 13, 1997.

in age from a few months to the teens. Common agents used to intentionally poison children have included syrup of ipecac, table salt, laxatives, diuretics, antidepressants, sedative-hypnotics, and narcotics (Dine and McGovern, 1982). The motivation for such heinous behavior is in the province of psychiatry, not toxicology. However, toxicologists must have some understanding of the nature of these poisonings to aid in the investigation of such cases. In some instances, it is a form of child battering committed by persons with low tolerance to the child's upsetting behaviors. The poison may be given to an infant to stop its crying or be force-fed to older children as a form of punishment. Such behavior is characteristic of persons with a cultural background where violence toward children is common or who have severe personality disorders or other mental illnesses. "Munchausen syndrome by proxy" is to another form of child poisoning (Murray, 1997). The *term Munchausen syndrome* (MS) is used to describe patients who seek admission to hospitals with apparent illness along with plausible, dramatic, albeit fictitious medical histories. Such people seek medical treatment solely to assume the role of a patient and receive the attention derived from this deception. "MS by proxy" refers to the situation in which an individual, usually a parent, presents not him- or herself but a child with a fictitious illness often induced by physical or chemical means. The purpose of the poisoning is not to kill the child but to induce signs and symptoms of illness that will assure medical attention. Thereby, the parent as caregiver gains the craved attention. Given a fictitious case history and the obvious illness of the child, these cases are almost always and understandably misdiagnosed. Often the child may be chronically poisoned at home and in the hospital for as long as a year before suspicion leads to the collection of specimens for extensive toxicologic testing. Although the parent may not have intended such an outcome, some children have died from fatal poisoning in these situations. As in the case of sexual assault, sophisticated GC/MS testing methods may be required to detect such agents as emetine and cephaeline, the emetic alkaloids in syrup of ipecac. Testing in these cases is best preformed in a laboratory with forensic experience, as positive drug findings will usually result in some form of legal proceeding.

FORENSIC URINE DRUG TESTING

Concerns about the potentially adverse consequences of substance abuse both for the individual and for society have led to widespread urine analysis for the detection of controlled or illicit drugs (Gust and Walsh, 1989). Currently, such testing is conducted routinely by the military services, regulated transportation and nuclear industries, many federal and state agencies, public utilities, federal and state criminal justice systems, and numerous private businesses and industries. Significant ethical and legal ramifications are associated with such testing. Those having positive test results may not receive employment, be dismissed from a job, be court-martialed, or suffer a loss of reputation.

To assure the integrity of workplace urine testing, two certification programs currently accredit forensic urine-testing laboratories. Laboratories conducting testing of federal employees are required to be certified under the Department of Health and Human Services Mandatory Guidelines for Workplace Drug Testing as published in the April 11, 1988, *Federal Register* (Department of Health and Human Services, 1988). The College of American Pathologists (CAP) also conducts a certification program for urine-testing laboratories. The federal program regulates a specific program from specimen collection through testing to the reporting of results, whereas the CAP program allows flexibility in the construction of programs servicing a broad range of clients. Both programs involve periodic on-site inspection of laboratories and proficiency testing.

Forensic urine drug testing (FUDT) differs from other areas of forensic toxicology in that urine is the only specimen analyzed and testing is performed for a limited number of drugs. At present, under the federal certification program, analyses are performed for only five drug classes or drugs of abuse (Table 31-3). While FUDT laboratories typically analyze 100 to 1000 urine specimens daily, only a relatively small number of those specimens are positive for drugs. To handle this large workload, initial testing is performed by immunoassays on high-speed, large-throughput analyzers. A confirmation analysis in FUDT-certified laboratories is performed by GC/MS.

Table 31-3
Forensic Urine Drug-Testing Analytes and Cutoff Concentrations

	Concentration, ng/mL	
	INITIAL TEST	CONFIRMATORY TEST
Marijuana metabolite(s)	50	15†
Cocaine metabolite(s)	300	150‡
Opiate(s)	2000*	—
Morphine	—	300
Codeine	—	300
6-Monoacetylmorphine	—	15
Phencyclidine	25	25
Amphetamines	1000	—
Amphetamine	—	500
Methamphetamine	—	500

*25 ng/mL if immunoassay is specific for free morphine.
†*D*-9-tetrahydrocannabinol-9-carboxylic acid.
‡Benzoylecognine.
SOURCE: Department of Health and Human Services: *Mandatory Guidelines for Federal Workplace Drug Testing Programs, Fed Reg* 53(69), April 11, 1988, p 11983; revised: *Fed Reg* 58(14), January 25, 1993, p 6063.

Proper FUDT is a challenge to good laboratory management. As with all forensic activities, every aspect of the laboratory operation must be thoroughly documented: specimen collection, chain of custody, quality control, procedures, testing, qualifications of personnel, and the reporting of results. The facility must be constructed and operated to assure total security of specimens and documents. Confidentiality of all testing results is paramount; only specifically authorized persons should receive the results. The presence of a controlled or illicit drug in a single random urine specimen is generally accepted as proof of recent or past substance abuse. However, positive urine drug findings are only evidence that, at some time before the collection of the sample, the individual was administered the drug, self-administered it, or was exposed to it. Positive urine tests do not prove impairment from the drug, abuse, or addiction.

FUDT results are reported only as positive or negative for the drugs sought. Cutoff values are established for both the initial and confirmation assays (Table 31-2). The cutoff value is a concentration at or above which the assay is considered positive. Below the cutoff value, the assay is negative. Obviously, drugs may be present below the cutoff concentration. However, the use of cutoff values allows uniformity in the drug testing and reporting of results. All test reports indicate the drug tested and its cutoff value. FUDT laboratories must be thoroughly familiar with all regulatory and analytic issues related to urine testing and devise strategies to resolve uncertainties. Many individuals who are subject to regulated urine testing have devised techniques to mask their drug use either by physiologic means such as the ingestion of diuretics or by attempting to adulterate the specimen directly with bleach, vinegar, or other products that interfere with the initial immunoassay tests (Warren, 1989). Thus, specimens are routinely tested for adulteration by checking urinary pH, creatinine, and specific gravity and noting any unusual color or smell. Recently a mini-industry has developed to sell various products that are alleged to "fool drug testers." These products often have colorful trade names such as UrinAid, Instant Clean ADD-IT-ive, and Klear. They contain chemicals that, when added to a urine specimen, interfere with either the initial or confirmatory drug test. For example, several of these products contain glutaraldehyde, which will react with the nitrogen atoms of the antibody proteins of the immunoassay screening test, thereby cross-linking the antibodies and inactivating the assay. However, this distruction of the test is so complete that the immunoassay analyzer records almost no signal, thus indicating possible adulteration of the specimen. Another adulterant, for the marijuana metabolite urine test, contains sodium nitrite. In acidic urine, the nitrite salt is converted to nitrous acid, which then converts the marijuana metabolites to nitroso derivatives, rendering them undetectable by routine GC/MS analysis (Lewis et al., 1999). Often the pH of the urine is insufficiently acidic for complete nitroso conversion of the tetrahydrocannabinol (THC) metabolite, THC–carboxylic acid. Thus the urine will screen positive by the initial immunoassay. When urine is acidified to extract the THC acid metabolite for MS confirmation testing, the metabolite is completely oxidized and undetectable. However, the deuterated THC–carboxylic acid added to the sample as the internal standard of the confirmation test is also completely destroyed. Failure to detect the internal standard readily alerts the analyst that an oxidant adulterant had been added to the urine. In such cases, a quantitative test for nitrite is performed. Nitrite may be present in urine from numerous internal and external sources such as foods, drugs, pathologic conditions, and infection from nitrate-reducing microorganisms. However, none of these sources produces urinary nitrite concentrations that even begin to approach those obtained by the addition of adulterant amounts of potassium nitrite, >1000 mg/L (Urey et al., 1998). Most chemical adulterants can be detected in urine by specific colorimetric tests that can be readily adapted to high-volume auto-analyzers (Table 31-4). Thus, FUDT laboratories now routinely test not only for drugs of abuse but also for a wide variety of chemical adulterants. In most instances, a positive test result for adulteration has as serious a consequence as a positive drug test.

There may be valid reasons other than substance abuse for positive drug findings, such as therapeutic use of controlled substances, inadvertent intake of drugs via food, and passive inhalation. For example, the seed of *Papaver somniferum,* poppy seed, is a common ingredient in many pastries and breads. Depending on their botanical source, poppy seeds may contain significant amounts of morphine. Several studies have demonstrated that the ingestion of certain poppy-seed foods results in the urinary excretion of readily detectable concentrations of morphine (ElSohly and Jones, 1989). Morphine is a major urinary metabolite of heroin. Therefore, to readily differentiate heroin abuse from poppy seed ingestion, analysis may be performed for 6-monoacetylmorphine, a unique heroin metabolite (Fehn and Megges, 1985).

Even over-the-counter medications may present potential problems for laboratories conducting urine drug testing. Methamphetamine may occur as a racemic mixture of *d* and *l* optical isomers. *d*-Methamphetamine, a Schedule II controlled substance, is a potent central nervous system stimulant subject to illicit drug abuse, while *l*-methamphetamine (*l*-desoxyephedrine) is an alpha-adrenergic stimulant available in over-the-counter Vicks inhalers as a nasal decongestant. Cross-reactivity of *l*-desoxyephedrine with

Table 31-4
Urine Adulterants Detected by Chemical Test

ADULTERANT	DETECTION METHOD
Acids, baking soda	pH
Bleach	Smell, color test (substituted benzene complex)
Detergents, diuretics, salt	Specific gravity
Diuretics	Creatinine
Glutaraldehyde	Altered immunoassay, GC
Nitrite	Color test (azo dye formation)
Pyridium chromate	Color, AAS (chromate), GC (pyridine)

KEY: GC, gas chromatography; AAS, atomic absorption spectrophotometry.

the initial immunoassay screening test may occur after excessive use of the Vicks inhaler (Poklis and Moore, 1995). Additionally, the most popular confirmational GC/MS products for amphetamines are achiral. Therefore, if such analyses are performed, a "false-positive" result for *d*-methamphetamine may be reported. This dilemma is easily resolved if confirmational testing is done with a *chiral* GC/MS procedure, which can readily resolve the stereoisomers of methamphetamine (Fitzgerald et al., 1988).

HUMAN PERFORMANCE TESTING

Forensic toxicology activities also include the determination of the presence of ethanol and other drugs and chemicals in blood, breath, or other specimens and the evaluation of their role in modifying human performance and behavior. The most common application of human performance testing is to determine driving under the influence of ethanol (DUI) or drugs (DUID). While operation of a motor vehicle is a common experience to most people, few appreciate the complexity of mental and physical functioning involved. A driver must simultaneously coordinate fine motor skills in tracking the road course and applying pressure to accelerator or brake—with visual attention immediately in front, to the horizon, and to the periphery of the vehicle—while continuously judging distance, speed, and appropriateness of response to signals, traffic, and unexpected events. The threshold blood ethanol concentration (BAC) for diminished driving performance of these complex functions in many individuals is as low as 0.04 g/dL, the equivalent of ingestion of two beers within an hour's time. The statutory definition of DUI in the United States is a BAC of either 0.08 or 0.10 g/dL, depending on the particular state law. These concentrations are consistent with diminished performance of complex driving skills in the vast majority of individuals. Over the past half century, an enormous amount of data has been developed correlating blood ethanol concentrations with intellectual and physiologic impairment, particularly of the skills associated with the proper operation of motor vehicles. Numerous studies have demonstrated a direct relationship between an increased BAC in drivers and an increased risk of involvement in road accidents (Council on Scientific Affairs, 1986). Alcohol-impaired drivers are responsible for 25 to 35 percent of all crashes causing serious injury in single-vehicle accidents, and 55 to 65 percent of fatally injured drivers have a BAC of 0.10 g/dL or greater.

During the past decade, there has been growing concern about the deleterious effects of drugs other than ethanol on driving performance. Several studies have demonstrated a relatively high occurrence of drugs in impaired or fatally injured drivers (White et al., 1981; Mason and McBay, 1984). These studies tend to report that the highest drug-use accident rates are associated with the use of such illicit or controlled drugs as cocaine, benzodiazepines, marijuana, and phencyclidine. However, most studies test for only a few drugs or drug classes, and the repeated reporting of the same drugs may be a function of limited testing. Before "driving under the influence of drugs" testing is as readily accepted by the courts as ethanol testing, many legal and scientific problems concerning drug concentrations and driving impairment must be resolved (Consensus Report, 1985). The ability of analytic methodology to routinely measure minute concentrations of drug in blood must be established. Also, drug-induced driving impairment at specific blood concentrations in controlled tests and/or actual highway experience must be demonstrated.

COURTROOM TESTIMONY

The forensic toxicologist often is called upon to testify in legal proceedings. As a general rule of evidence, a witness may testify only to facts known to him or her. The witness may offer opinions solely on the basis of what he or she has observed (Moenssens et al., 1973). Such a witness is called a "lay witness." However, the toxicologist is referred to as an "expert witness." A court recognizes a witness as an expert if that witness possesses knowledge or experience in a subject that is beyond the range of ordinary or common knowledge or observation. An expert witness may provide two types of testimony: objective testimony and "opinion." Objective testimony by a toxicologist usually involves a description of his or her analytic methods and findings. When a toxicologist testifies as to the interpretation of his or her analytic results or those of others, that toxicologist is offering an "opinion." Lay witnesses cannot offer such opinion testimony, as it exceeds their ordinary experience.

Before a court permits opinion testimony, the witness must be "qualified" as an expert in his or her particular field. In qualifying someone as an expert witness, the court considers the witness's education, on-the-job training, work experience, teaching or academic appointments, and professional memberships and publications as well as the acceptance of the witness as an expert by other courts. Qualification of a witness takes place in front of the jury members, who consider the expert's qualifications in determining how much weight to give his or her opinions during their deliberations.

Whether a toxicologist appears in criminal or civil court, workers' compensation or parole hearings, the procedure for testifying is the same: direct examination, cross-examination, and redirect examination. The attorney who has summoned the witness to testify conducts direct examination. Testimony is presented in a question-and-answer format. The witness is asked a series of questions that allow him or her to present all facts or opinions relevant to the successful presentation of the attorney's case. During direct examination, an expert witness has the opportunity to explain to the jury the scientific bases of his or her opinions. Regardless of which side has called the toxicologist to court, the toxicologist should testify with scientific objectivity. Bias toward his or her client and prejudgments should be avoided. An expert witness is called to provide informed assistance to the jury. The jury, not the expert witness, determines the guilt or innocence of the defendant.

After direct testimony, the opposing attorney questions the expert. During this cross-examination, the witness is challenged as to his or her findings and/or opinions. The toxicologist will be asked to defend his or her analytic methods, results, and opinions. The opposing attorney may imply that the expert's testimony is biased because of financial compensation, association with an agency involved in the litigation, or personal feelings regarding the case. The best way to prepare for such challenges before testimony is to anticipate the questions the opposing attorney may ask.

After cross-examination, the attorney who called the witness may ask additional questions to clarify any issues raised during cross-examination. This allows the expert to explain apparent discrepancies in his or her testimony raised by the opposing attorney. Often an expert witness is asked to answer a special type of question, the "hypothetical question." A hypothetical question contains only facts that have been presented in evidence. The expert is then asked for his or her conclusion or opinion based solely on this hypothetical situation. This type of question serves as a means by which appropriate facts leading to the expert's opinion are identified. Often these questions are extremely long and convoluted. The witness should be sure he or she understands all the facts and implications in the question. Like all questions, this type should be answered as objectively as possible.

ANALYTIC ROLE IN CLINICAL TOXICOLOGY

Analytic toxicology in a clinical setting plays a role very similar to its role in forensic toxicology. As an aid in the diagnosis and treatment of toxic incidents as well as in monitoring the effectiveness of treatment regimens, it is useful to clearly identify the nature of the toxic exposure and measure the amount of the toxic substance that has been absorbed. Frequently, this information, together with the clinical state of the patient, permits a clinician to relate the signs and symptoms observed to the anticipated effects of the toxic agent. This may permit a clinical judgment as to whether the treatment must be vigorous and aggressive or whether simple observation and symptomatic treatment of the patient are sufficient.

A cardinal rule in the treatment of poisoning cases is to remove any unabsorbed material, limit the absorption of additional poison, and hasten its elimination. The clinical toxicology laboratory serves an additional purpose in this phase of the treatment by monitoring the amount of the toxic agent remaining in circulation or measuring what is excreted. In addition, the laboratory can provide the data needed to permit estimations of the total dosage or the effectiveness of treatment by changes in known pharmacokinetic parameters of the drug or agent ingested.

While the instrumentation and the methodology used in a clinical toxicology laboratory are similar to those utilized by a forensic toxicologist, a major difference between these two applications is responsiveness. In emergency toxicology testing, results must be communicated to the clinician within hours for the results to be meaningful for therapy. A forensic toxicologist may carefully choose the best method for a particular test and conduct replicate procedures to assure maximum accuracy. A clinical laboratory cannot afford this luxury and frequently sacrifices accuracy for a rapid turnaround time. Additionally, because it is impossible to predict when toxicologic emergencies will occur, a clinical laboratory must provide rapid testing 24 h a day every day of the year. The most commonly encountered intoxicants in emergency toxicology testing and the rapid methodologies to detect their presence in serum and/or urine specimens are presented in Table 31-5.

Primary examples of the usefulness of emergency toxicology testing are the rapid quantitative determination of acetaminophen, salicylate, alcohols, and glycol serum concentrations in instances of suspected overdose. Acetaminophen serum values related to the time after ingestion (Chap. 32) not only indicate an overdose, but provide a prognosis for possible delayed hepatotoxicity and the need to continue administration of *n*-acetylcystine antidote. In addition, continuous monitoring of serum values permits an accurate pharmacokinetic calculation of the ingested dose (Melethil et al., 1981). Similarly, salicylate serum values related to the time after ingestion may indicate an overdose, providing a prognosis for possible delayed severe metabolic acidosis and the need for life saving dialysis treatment. Continuous monitoring of serum salicylate values permits an accurate assessment of the efficacy of dialysis.

Ethanol is the most common agent encountered in emergency toxicology. While few fatal intoxications occur with ethanol, serum values are important in the assessment of behavioral and neurologic function, particularly in trauma cases where the patient is unable to communicate and surgery with the administration of anesthetic or analgesic agents is indicated. Intoxications from accidental or deliberate ingestion of other alcohols or glycols—such as methanol from windshield deicer or paint thinner, isopropanol from rubbing alcohol, and ethylene glycol from antifreeze—are often encountered in emergency departments. Following ingestion of methanol or ethylene glycol, patients often present with similar neurologic symptoms and severe metabolic acidosis due to the formation of toxic aldehyde and acid metabolites. A rapid quantitative serum determination for these intoxicants will indicate the severity of intoxication and the possible need for dialysis therapy. Alcohol infusion, in order to saturate the enzyme alcohol dehydrogenase, blocks the conversion of methanol and ethylene glycol to their toxic metabolites. Continuous monitoring of serum values not only permits an assessment of the clear-

Table 31-5
Most Commonly Encountered Drugs and Methods for Analysis in Emergency Toxicology

RANK	DRUG/DRUG GROUP	SPECIMEN	ANALYTICAL METHOD
1.	Drugs of Abuse (amphetamines, cocaine, opiates, phencyclidine)	Urine	Immunoassays
2.	Ethanol	Serum	GC
3.	Benzodiazepines	Urine/Serum	Immunoassay/GC/MS
4.	Acetaminophen, salicylates	Serum	Immunoassay or HPLC
5.	Tricyclic antidepressants	Serum	Immunoassay or HPLC
6.	Ibuprofen	Urine/Serum	TLC/HPLC
7.	Dextropropoxyphene	Urine	Immunoassay
8.	Fluoxetine	Urine/Serum	TLC/HPLC
9.	Barbiturates (50% phenobarbital)	Urine/Serum	Immunoassay/GC
10.	Diphenhydramine	Urine	TLC

KEY: GC, gas chromatography; GC/MS, gas chromatography/mass spectrometry; HPLC, high-pressure liquid chromatography; TLC, thin-layer chromatography.
SOURCE: Data from Year-End 1998 Emergency Department Data from the Drug Abuse Warning Network, Department of Health and Human Services, December 1999.

ance of the intoxicant by dialysis but also assures a proper infusion rate of alcohol for effective antidotal concentrations (Fig. 31-8). To provide effective service to the emergency department, laboratories should have available chromatographic methods for the rapid separation and detection of alcohols and glycols (Edinboro et al., 1993).

The utilization of the analytic capabilities of a clinical toxicology laboratory has increased enormously in recent years. Typically, the laboratory performs not only testing not only for the emergency department but also for a wide variety of other medical departments, as drugs and toxic agents may be a consideration in diagnosis. Urine is analyzed from substance abuse treatment facilities to monitor the administration of methadone or other therapeutic agents and/or to assure that patients do not continue to abuse drugs. Similarly, psychiatrists, neurologists, and physicians treating patients for chronic pain need to know whether patients are self-administering drugs before such patients undergo psychiatric or neurologic examinations. Analysis for drugs of abuse in meconium and urine obtained from neonates is used to corroborate the diagnosis of withdrawal symptoms in newborns and document fetal exposure to controlled substances. Toxic metal determinations, such as blood lead concentration, are often performed to assess possible toxic metal exposure or severity of toxicity (Chap. 23). Analysis of heavy metals in 24-h urine specimens is often used to rule out toxic metal exposure as a cause of symmetrical peripheral neuropathy prior to the diagnosis of neurologic disorders such as Guillian-Barré syndrome. The clinical toxicology laboratory may often perform unique diagnostic tests that require sophisticated analytic capabilities such as GC/MS and HPLC analysis for organic acids and amino acids to detect inborn errors of metabolism in infants and children. Methods for the analysis of abnormal organic acids will also detect acidic drugs and other intoxicants such as salicylates, ethylene glycol, gamma-hydroxybutyric acid, and valproic acid. Another such diagnostic test requiring sensitive chromatography is the timed metabolism of lidocaine to its monoethylglycinexylidide (MEGX) metabolite (O'Neal and Poklis, 1996). The rate of this conversion is a sensitive indicator of hepatic dysfunction and is often used to assess hepatic viability in donor livers prior to transplantation. MEGX formation may also be useful in monitoring the severity of the histologic condition of patients with chronic hepatitis and cirrhosis (Shiffman et al., 1994).

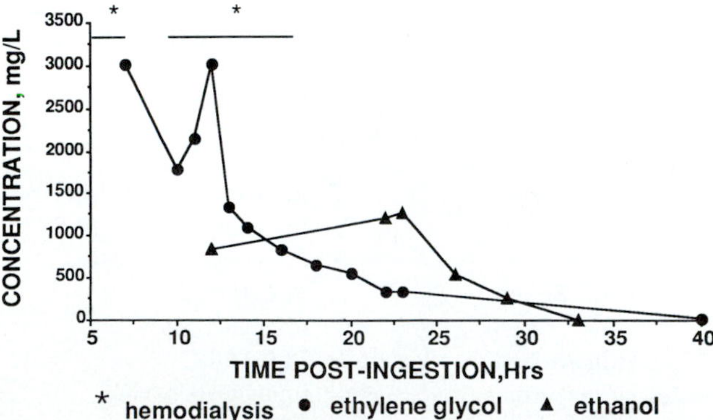

Figure 31-8. Serum ethylene glycol and ethanol concentrations monitored during dialysis and ethanol infusion therapy. (Data from the Toxicology Laboratory, Medical College of Virginia Hospital, Richmond, VA.)

ANALYTIC ROLE IN THERAPEUTIC MONITORING

Historically, the administration of drugs for long-term therapy was based largely on experience. A dosage amount was selected and administered at appropriate intervals based on what the clinician had learned was generally tolerated by most patients. If the drug seemed ineffective, the dose was increased; if toxicity developed, the dose was decreased or the frequency of dosing was altered. At times, a different dosage form might be substituted. Establishing an effective dosage regimen was particularly difficult in children and the elderly.

The factors responsible for individual variability in responses to drug therapy include the rate and extent of drug absorption, distribution and binding in body tissues and fluids, rate of metabolism and excretion, pathologic conditions, and interaction with other drugs (Blaschke et al., 1985). Monitoring of the plasma or serum concentration at regular intervals will detect deviations from the average serum concentration, which, in turn, may suggest that one or more of these variables need to be identified and corrected.

In a given patient, when the various factors are assumed to be constant, the administration of the same dose of a drug at regular intervals eventually produces a steady-state condition (Fig. 31-9) (Moyer et al., 1986). Monitoring of steady-state drug concentra-

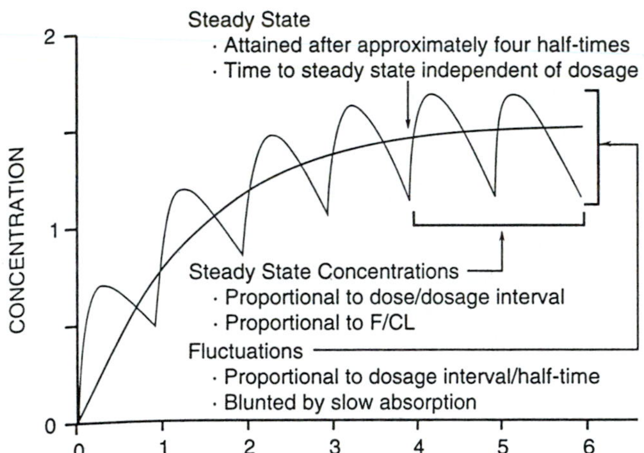

Figure 31-9. Fundamental pharmacokinetic relationships for the repeated administration of drugs.

The blue line is the pattern of drug accumulation during the repeated administration of a drug at intervals equal to its elimination half-time, when drug absorption is ten times as rapid as elimination. As the relative rate of absorption increases, the concentration maxima approach 2 and minima approach 1 during steady-state. The black line depicts the pattern during administration of equivalent dosage by continuous intravenous infusion. Curves are based upon the one-compartment model. Average concentration (Css) when steady state is attained during intermittent drug administration is Css = $F \times$ dose/Cl $\times T$, where F = fractional bioavailability of the dose and T = dosage interval (time). By substitution of infusion rate for $F \times$ dose/T, the formula is equivalent to Eq. (1) and provides the concentration maintained at steady state during continuous intravenous infusion. [From Hardman JG, Limbird LE, Molinoff PB, et al (eds): *Goodman & Gilman's The Pharmacological Basis of Therapeutics,* 9th ed. New York: McGraw-Hill, 1995, p 23.]

Table 31-6
Appropriate Use of Therapeutic Drug Monitoring

USE	EXAMPLES
Optimize efficacy while minimizing toxicity	
Optimal SDC* for clinical effect	
Routine, prophylactic peak serum	aminoglycosides
Poor patient response	antiarrhythmics, antidepressants
Suspected toxicity	
Resolve complicating factors	
Patient characteristics	age, smoking, noncompliance
Disease	renal failure, hepatic disorders
Drug interactions	induction or inhibition of drug metabolism
Sudden change in physiologic state	improved cardiac function on lidocaine therapy increases clearance
Dosage regimen design	
Individualize future dosing (single SDC)	
Pharmacokinetic profiling (multiple SDC)	ideal dosage for aminoglycosides
Follow-up SDC	single steady-state lidocaine
Verify therapy	medicolegal lithium

*SCD, serum drug concentration.

Table 31-7
Drugs Commonly Indicated for Therapeutic Monitoring

THERAPEUTIC USE DRUG	EFFECTIVE SERUM RANGE mg/L	PANIC VALUE = OR > mg/L	ANALYTIC METHODOLOGY
Antiarrythmic			
Digoxin	0.0005–0.002	0.0024	Immunoassay
Procainamide	4–10	12	Immunoassay
NAPA	5–30	40	Immunoassay
Anticonvulsant			
Carbamazepine	4–12	15	Immunoassay
Gabapentin	2–15	20	GC
Lamotrigine	0.5–8	10	HPLC
Phenobarbital	15–30	50	Immunoassay
Phenytoin	10–20	40	Immunoassay
Tropiramate	2–10	Undetermined	GC
Valproic acid	50–100	200	GC
Antidepressants			
Amitriptyline	0.08–0.250	0.5	HPLC
Desipramine	0.125–0.30	0.4	HPLC
Nortriptyline	0.08–0.250	0.5	HPLC
Antimicrobials			
Tobramycin	0.5–1.5 (trough)	2	Immunoassay
	5–10 (peak)	12	
Vancomycin	5–10 (trough)		Immunoassay
	30–40 (peak)	90	
Immunosuppressant			
Cyclosporine	0.1 (trough, whole blood)		HPLC
Neonatal Apnea			
Caffeine	8–20	50	HPLC

KEY: GLC, gas chromatography; HPLC, high-pressure liquid chromatography.

tions assures that an effective concentration is present. For drugs that have a defined correlation between serum values and undesired toxic effects, the lowest serum value immediately prior to dosing (trough) and the highest expected serum concentration (peak) are monitored to assure efficacy and minimize toxicity. Appropriate situations for therapeutic drug monitoring are presented in Table 31-6.

Because the drug being administered is known, qualitative characterization of the analyte generally is not required. Quantitative accuracy is required, however. Frequently, the methodology applied is important, particularly in regard to its selectivity. For example, methods that measure the parent drug and its metabolites are not ideal unless the individual analytes can be quantified separately. Depending on the drug, metabolites may or may not be active to a different degree than the parent drug. The cardiac antiarrythmic drug procainamide is acetylated during metabolism to form *N*-acetylprocainamide (NAPA). This metabolite has antiarrythmic activity of almost equal potency to that of the parent drug, procainamide. There is bimodal genetic variation in the activity of the *N*-acetyltransferase for procainamide, so that, in "fast acetylators," the concentration of NAPA in the serum may exceed that of the parent drug. For optimal patient management, information should be available about the concentrations of both procainamide and NAPA in serum (Bigger and Hoffman, 1985).

Since absolute characterization of the analyte is not necessary for many drugs, immunoassay procedures are commonly used. This is particularly true of drugs with extremely low serum concentrations, such as cardiac glycosides, and drugs that are difficult to extract because of a high degree of polarity, such as the aminoglycoside antibiotics. In these cases, serum can be conveniently assayed directly by using commercially available kits for immunoassays.

The chromatographic methods in which an appropriate internal standard is added are favored when more than one analyte is to be measured or if metabolites with structures similar to those of the parent drugs must be distinguished. Since the nature of drugs is varied, many different analytic techniques may be applied, including atomic absorption spectrophotometry for measuring lithium used to treat manic disorders. Virtually all the tools of the analyst may be used for specific applications of analytic toxicology. Drugs that are commonly monitored during therapy, their usual effective therapeutic serum concentrations, "panic values," and typical analytic methodologies applied to serum measurements are presented in Table 31-7. The term *panic value* denotes a serum drug concentration associated with the development of potentially serious toxicity. In clinical laboratories, the "panic value" alerts the toxicologist that the treating physician must be *immediately* contacted and notified of the test result.

ANALYTIC ROLE IN BIOLOGICAL MONITORING

In the workplace, good industrial hygiene practices require monitoring of the environment to which workers are exposed in order to identify potentially harmful amounts of hazardous chemicals. Despite these precautions, it has become apparent that monitoring a worker directly can be a better indicator of exposure because it can show what has actually been absorbed. This is biological monitoring, and it can take a variety of forms. Often environmental exposures are to a mixture of compounds and/or to compounds that are converted to physiologically important metabolites. Thus, analytic methods must be capable of separating a family of chemical agents and their major metabolites (Fig. 31-10). Additionally, methods must be sufficiently specific and sensitive to measure minute concentrations of the compounds in complex biological matrices.

An example of biological monitoring is presented in Table 31-8, which shows data relating to benzene exposure of chemists engaged in pesticide residue analysis in a state regulatory laboratory. Air-monitoring devices in this laboratory indicated that the ambient benzene concentration never exceeded the time-weighted average (TWA) of 32 mg/m^3 (10 ppm). Monitoring of the breathing zones at different locations around the laboratory where benzene was in use showed other concentrations of this material. When expired air was monitored, one worker showed a significantly greater amount of benzene exposure than did others. Upon questioning, she recalled spilling some of the solvent on a laboratory bench, in the process saturating a portion of her laboratory coat. Presumably, her exposure by inhalation and skin absorption was considerably greater than was indicated by the air monitor.

In addition to the measurement of the chemical or its metabolites in the body fluids, hair, or breath of the worker, other, more indirect methods may be employed. Substances that interact with macromolecules may form adducts that persist for long periods. These adducts can be sampled periodically and potentially can serve as a means of integrating exposure to certain substances over long periods. For example, adducts of ethylene oxide with DNA or hemoglobin have been studied in workers. This technique may

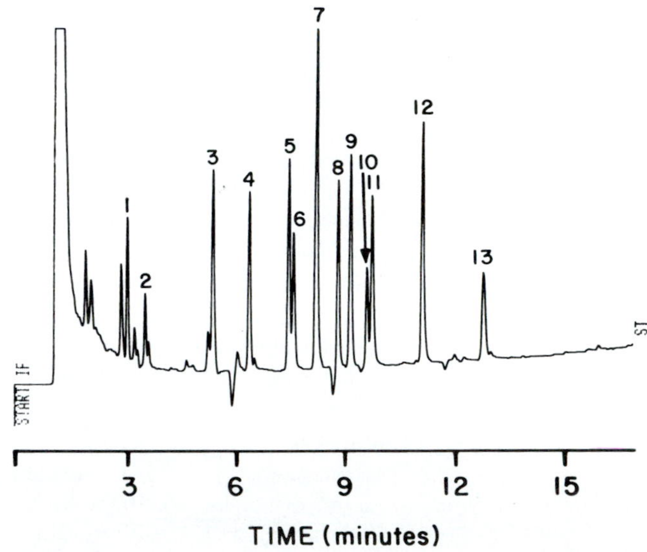

Figure 31-10. Capillary gas chromatographic separation of chlorinated hydrocarbon pesticides added to human serum at concentrations ranging from 1 to 4 ng/mL.

Peak number 1, a-lindane; 2, c-lindane; 3, heptachlor; 4, internal standard; 5, heptachlor epoxide; 6, oxychlordane; 7, c-chlordane; 8, a-chlordane; 9, *trans*-nonachlor; 10, dieldrin; 11, p,p9-DDE; 12, p,p-DDD; 13, p,p9-DDT. (Separation based on the method of Saady JJ, Poklis A: Determination of chlorinated hydrocarbon pesticides by solid phase extraction and capillary GC with electron capture detection. *J Anal Toxicol* 14:301–304, 1990.)

Table 31-8
Benzene Exposure of Chemists Performing Pesticide Residue Analysis

SOURCE	BREATH BENZENE, ppm	AIR BENZENE, ppm
Chemist A	0.45	—
Chemist B	0.13	—
Chemist C	0.41	—
Chemist D	0.48	—
Chemist E	0.34	—
Chemist F	0.37	—
Chemist G	2.50	—
Chemist H	0.56	—
Fume hood breathing zone	—	14.2
Fume hood breathing zone	—	51.2

also be applicable in other situations that are not necessarily related to occupational hazards. Acetaldehyde, a metabolite of ethanol, forms adducts with hemoglobin. This marker may be of use in forensic cases (Stockham and Blanke, 1988).

Another approach that is useful in biological monitoring is to measure changes of normal metabolites induced by xenobiotics. The profile of glucuronic acid metabolites excreted in urine can be altered after exposure to substances that induce monooxygenase activity. Although monitoring the alteration of the urinary excretion of these metabolites may not indicate exposure to specific substances, this technique can be used in a generic fashion to flag a potentially harmful exposure to a hepatotoxic agent (Saady and Blanke, 1990). The early recognition of a toxicologic problem may permit the protection of a worker before irreversible effects occur.

SUMMARY

The analytic techniques initiated by forensic toxicologists have continued to expand in complexity and improve in reliability. Many new analytic tools have been applied to toxicologic problems in almost all areas of the field, and the technology continues to open new areas of research. Forensic toxicologists continue to be concerned about conducting unequivocal identification of toxic substances in such a manner that the results can withstand a legal challenge. The problems of substance abuse, designer drugs, increased potency of therapeutic agents, and widespread concern about pollution and the safety and health of workers present challenges to the analyst's skills. As these challenges are met, analytic toxicologists continue to play a significant role in the expansion of the discipline of toxicology.

REFERENCES

Aderjan R, Bahr H, Schmidt G: Investigation of cardiac glycoside levels in human postmortem blood and tissues determined by a special RIA procedure. *Arch Toxicol* 42:107–114, 1979.

Apple FS: Postmortem tricyclic antidepressant concentrations: Assessing cause of death using parent drug to metabolite ratio. *J Anal Toxicol* 13:197–198, 1989.

Benko A: Toxicological analysis of amobarbital and glutethimide from bone tissue. *J Forensic Sci* 30:708–714, 1985.

Bigger JT Jr, Hoffman BF: Antiarrhythmic drugs, in Gilman AG, Goodman LS, Rall TW, Murad F (eds): *The Pharmacological Basis of Therapeutics,* 7th ed. New York: Macmillan, 1985, p 763.

Blanke RV: Quality assurance in drug-use testing. *Clin Chem* 33: 41B–45B, 1987.

Blanke RV: *Validation of the Purity of Standards.* Irving, TX: Abbott Laboratories, Diagnostic Division, 1989.

Blanke RV, Decker WJ: Analysis of toxic substances, in Tietz NW (ed): *Textbook of Clinical Chemistry.* Philadelphia: Saunders, 1986, pp 1670–1744.

Blaschke TF, Nies AS, Mamelock RD: Principles of therapeutics, in Gilman AG, Goodman LS, Rall TW, Murad F (eds): *The Pharmacological Basis of Therapeutics,* 7th ed. New York: Macmillan, 1985, p 52.

Chapuis E: *Elements de toxicologie,* 1873, cited in Peterson F, Haines WS, Webster RW: *Legal Medicine and Toxicology.* 2d ed. Vol 2. Philadelphia: Saunders, 1923.

Coe JI: Postmortem chemistry update: Emphasis on forensic applications. *Am J Forensic Med Pathol* 14:91–117, 1993.

Cone EJ, Buchwald WF, Darwin WD: Analytical controls in drug metabolism studies: 11. Artifact formation during chloroform extraction of drugs and metabolites with amine substitutes. *Drug Metab Dispos* 10:561–567, 1982.

Consensus report: Drug concentrations and driving impairment. *JAMA* 254:2618–2621, 1985.

Council on Scientific Affairs: Alcohol and the driver. *JAMA* 255: 522–527, 1986.

Cravey RH, Baselt RC: The science of forensic toxicology, in Cravey RH, Baselt RC (eds): *Introduction to Forensic Toxicology.* Davis, CA: Biomedical Publications, 1981, pp 3–6.

Department of Health and Human Services, ADAMHA: Mandatory guidelines for federal workplace drug testing: Final guidelines: Notice. *Fed Reg* 53(69):11970–11989, 1988.

Dowling GP, McDonough ET, Bost RO: "Eve" and "ecstasy": A report of five deaths associated with the use of MDEA and MDMA. *JAMA* 257:1615–1617, 1987.

Edinboro LE, Nanco CR, Soghoian DM, Poklis A: Determination of ethylene glycol in serum utilizing direct injection on a wide bore capillary column. *Ther Drug Monit* 15:220–223, 1993.

ElSohly MA, Jones AB: Morphine and codeine in biological fluids: Approaches to source differentiation. *Forensic Sci Rev* 1:13–22, 1989.

Ernst MF, Poklis A, Gantner, GE: Evaluation of medicolegal investigators' suspicious and positive toxicology findings in 100 drug deaths. *J Forensic Sci* 27:61–65, 1982.

Evans WED: *The Chemistry of Death.* Springfield, IL: Charles C Thomas, 1963.

Fehn J, Megges G: Detection of O6-monoacetylmorphine in urine samples by GC/MS as evidence for heroin use. *J Anal Toxicol* 9:134–138, 1985.

Fisher RS, Hine CH, Stetler CJ (Committee on Medicolegal Problems): *Alcohol and the Impaired Driver: A Manual on the Medicolegal Aspects of Chemical Tests for Intoxication.* Chicago: American Medical Association, 1968.

Fitzgerald RL, Ramos JM, Bogema SC, Poklis A: Resolution of methamphetamine stereoisomers in urine drug testing: Urinary excretion of R(-)-methamphetamine following use of nasal inhalers. *J Anal Toxicol* 12:255–259, 1988.

Garriott JS, Simmons LM, Poklis A, Mackell MS: Five cases of fatal overdose from caffeine-containing "look-alike" drugs. *J Anal Toxicol* 9:141–143, 1985.

Gettler AD: Poisoning and toxicology, forensic aspects: Part 1. Historical aspects. *Inform* 9:3–7, 1977.

Goff ML, Brown WA, Omori AI, LaPointe DA: Preliminary observations of the effects of amitriptyline in decomposing tissue on the development of parasarcophaga ruficornis (Diptera: Sarcophagidae) and implications of this effect to estimation of postmortem interval. *J Forensic Sci* 38:316–322, 1993.

Granger RH, Condie LW, Borzelleca JF: Effect of vehicle on the relative uptake of haloalkanes administered by gavage. *Toxicologist* 40:1, 1987.

Gust SW, Walsh JM: *Drugs in the Workplace: Research and Evaluation Data.* NIDA Research Monograph 91. Washington, DC: U.S. Government Printing Office, 1989.

Hawks RL, Chiang CN: Examples of specific drug assays, in Hawks RL, Chiang CN (eds): *Urine Testing for Drugs of Abuse.* NIDA Research Monograph 73. Rockville, MD: U.S. Department Health and Human Services, PHS, ADAMHA, 1986, p 93.

Henderson GL: Designer drugs: Past history and future prospects. *J Forensic Sci* 33:569–575, 1988.

Hime GW, Hearn WL, Rose S, Cofino J: Analysis of cocaine and cocaethylene in blood and tissues by GC-NPD and GC-Ion Trap mass spectrometry. *J Anal Toxicol* 15:241, 1991.

Inoue T, Seta S: Analysis of drugs in unconventional samples. *Forensic Sci Rev* 4:89–107, 1992.

Jacob P, Lewis ER, Elias-Baker BA, Jones RT: A pyrolysis product, anhydroecgonine methyl ester (methylecgonidine), is in the urine of cocaine smokers. *J Anal Toxicol* 14:353, 1990.

Jones GR, Pounder DJ: Site-dependence of drug concentrations in postmortem blood—A case study. *J Anal Toxicol* 11:186–190, 1987.

Kaempe B: Interfering compounds and artifacts in the identification of drugs in autopsy material, in Stolman A (ed): *Progress in Chemical Toxicology.* Vol 4. New York: Academic Press, 1969, pp 1–57.

Klaassen CD, Amdur MO, Doull J: *Casarett and Doull's Toxicology: The Basic Science of Poisons,* 3d ed. New York: Macmillan, 1986.

LeBeau M, Andollo W, Hearn WL, et al. Recommendations for toxicological investigation of drug-facilitated sexual assaults. *J Forensic Sci* 44:227–230, 1999.

Lewis SA, Lewis LA, Tuinman A:. Potassium nitrite reaction with 11-nor-delta-9-tetrahydrocannabinol-9-carboxylic acid in urine in relation to drug screening analysis. *J Forensic Sci* 44:951–955, 1999.

Martin BR, Lue LP, Boni JP: Pyrolysis and volatization of cocaine. *J Anal Toxicol* 13:158, 1989.

Mason AP, McBay AJ: Ethanol, marijuana, and other drug use in 600 drivers killed in single-vehicle crashes in North Carolina. *J Forensic Sci* 29:987–1026, 1984.

Melethil S, Poklis,A, Schwartz HS: Estimation of the amount of drug absorbed in acetaminophen poisoning: A case report. *Vet Hum Toxicol* 23:421–423, 1981.

Mills RA, Millis CD, Dannan GA, et al: Studies on the structure-activity relationships for the metabolism of polybrominated biphenyls by rat liver microsomes. *Toxicol Appl Pharmacol* 78:96–104, 1985.

Moenssens AA, Moses RE, Inbau FE: *Scientific Evidence in Criminal Cases.* Mineola, NY: Foundation Press, 1973.

Moore KA, Daniel J, Fierro M, et al: Detection of a metabolite of α-benzyl-*N*-methylphenylamine synthesis in a mixed drug fatality involving methamphetamine. *J Forensic Sci* 41:524–526, 1996.

Moore KA, Ismaiel A, Poklis A: α-Benzyl-*N*-methylphenylamine (BNMPA) an impurity of illict methamphetamine synthesis: lII. Detection of BNMPA and metabolites in urine from methamphetamine users. *J Anal Toxicol* 20:89–92, 1996.

Moyer TP, Pippenger CE, Blanke RV: Therapeutic drug monitoring, in Tietz NW (ed): *Textbook of Clinical Chemistry.* Philadelphia: Saunders, 1986, pp 1615–1669.

Murray JB: Munchausen syndrome/Munchausen syndrome by proxy. *J Psychol* 131:343–352,1997.

O'Neal CL, Poklis A: A sensitive HPLC assay for the simultaneous quantitation of lidocaine and its metabolites; monoethylglcinexylididie and glycinexylidide in serum. *Clin Chem* 42:330–331, 1996.

Panel on Herbicides: Report on 2,4,5-T, in *A Report of the Panel on Herbicides of the President's Science Advisory Committee.* Executive Office of the President, Office of Science and Technology, Washington, DC: U.S. Government Printing Office, 1971.

Petersen F, Haines WS, Webster RW: *Legal Medicine and Toxicology,* 2d ed. Vol 2. Philadelphia: Saunders, 1923.

Poklis A: Pentazocine/tripelennamine (T's and blues) abuse: A five year survey of St. Louis, Missouri. *Drug Alcohol Depend* 10:257–267, 1982.

Poklis A, Mackell MA, Tucker E: Tissue distribution of lidocaine after fatal accidental injection. *J Forensic Sci* 29:1229–1236, 1984.

Poklis A, Moore KA: Response of Emit amphetamine immunoassays to urinary desoxyephedrine following Vicks inhaler use. *Ther Drug Monit* 17:89–94, 1995.

Poklis A, Poklis, JL, Trautman D, et al: Disposition of valproic acid in a case of fatal intoxication. *J Anal Toxicol* 22:537–540, 1998.

Pounder DJ: Forensic entomo-toxicology. *J Forensic Sci Soc* 31: 469–472, 1991.

Price LM, Poklis A, Johnson DE: Fatal acetaminophen poisoning with evidence of subendocardial necrosis of the heart. *J Forensic Sci* 36:930–935, 1991.

Prouty BS, Anderson WH: The forensic science implications of site and tempered influences on postmortem blood-drug concentrations. *J Forensic Sci* 35:243–270, 1990.

Saady JJ, Blanke RV: Measurement of glucuronic acid metabolites by high resolution gas chromatography. *J Chromatogr Sci* 28:282–287, 1990.

Saady JJ, Narasimhachari N, Friedel RO: Unsuspected impurities in imipramine and desipramine standards and pharmaceutical formulations. *Clin Chem* 27:343–344, 1981.

SanGeorge RC, Hoberman RD: Reaction of acetaldehyde with hemoglobin. *J Biol Chem* 262:6811–6821, 1986.

Shapiro HA: Arsenic content of human hair and nails: Its interpretation. *J Forensic Med* 14:65–71, 1967.

Shiffman ML, Luketic VA, Sanyal AJ, et al: Hepatic lidocaine metabolism and liver histology in patients with chronic hepatitis and cirrhosis. *Hepatology* 31:933–940, 1994.

Smith H: The interpretation of the arsenic content of human hair. *J Forensic Sci Soc* 4:192–199, 1964.

Stockham TL, Blanke RV: Investigation of an acetaldehyde-hemoglobin adduct in alcoholics: Alcoholism. *Clin Exp Res* 12:748–754, 1988.

Tagliro F (ed): *Hair Analysis as a Diagnostic Tool for Drugs of Abuse Investigation.* Proceeding of the 1st International Meeting, Genoa, Italy, December 10–11, 1992. Special Issue. *Forensic Sci Int* 63: 1–316,1993.

Thorwald J: *The Century of the Detective.* New York: Harcourt, 1965.

Urey FM, Komaromy-Hiller G, Staley B, et al: Nitrite adulteration of workplace urine drug-testing specimens: 1. Sources and associated concentrations of nitrite in urine and distinction between natural sources and adulteration. *J Anal Toxicol* 22:8995, 1998.

Vorpahl TE, Coe JI: Correlation of antemortem and postmortem digoxin levels. *J Forensic Sci* 23:329–334, 1978.

Warren A: Interference of common household chemicals in immunoassay methods for drugs of abuse. *Clin Chem* 35:648–651, 1989.

White JM, Clardy MS, Groves MH, et al: Testing for sedative-hypnotic drugs in the impaired driver: A survey of 72,000 arrests. *Clin Toxicol* 18:945–957, 1981.

CHAPTER 32

CLINICAL TOXICOLOGY

Louis R. Cantilena, Jr.

HISTORY OF CLINICAL TOXICOLOGY

Historical Aspects of the Treatment of Poisoning

The history of poisons and poisoners dates back to ancient times. Homer's *Odyssey* and shastras from approximately 600 B.C. contain references to antidotes. The first documented use of a specific antidote may be found in the *Odyssey,* where it is suggested to Ulysses that he take moli to protect himself from poisoning. Moli may actually be *Galanthus nivalis,* a plant-derived cholinesterase inhibitor that might counteract the effects of the anticholinergic plant *Datura stramonium* (Plaitakis and Duvoisin, 1983).

Galen (A.D. 129 to 200) wrote three books called *De Antidotis I, De Antidotis II,* and *De Theriaca ad Pisonem,* which described the development of a universal antidote known as a alexipharmic or theriac by King Mithridates VI of Pontus, who lived from 132 to 63 B.C. (Wax, 1998). The antidote reportedly contained 36 or more ingredients and was ingested every day, conferring protection against a broad spectrum of poisons such as venomous stings and bites from vipers, spiders, and scorpions (Jarcho, 1972).

The refinement of theriac (antidote) formulations is documented for centuries. Andromachus (first century of the Christian era) was physician to Nero and improved the theriac of Mithridates by modifying the formula to include up to 73 ingredients (Wax, 1998). The use of these ancient antidotes included treatment of acute poisoning and prophylactic treatment to make one "poison-proof." This theriac, with subsequent modifications, remained in use for nearly 2000 years. In 1745, William Heberden wrote *Antitheriaka: An Essay on Mithridatium and Theriaca,* in which he questioned the effectiveness of these products (Jarcho, 1972). However, their use and availability continued until the early twentieth century.

One of the earliest writings on the prevention of the gastrointestinal absorption of poisons was by Nicander (Major, 1934). In this ancient writing, the induction of emesis by ingestion of an emetic agent or mechanical stimulation of the hypopharynx was described as a method to prevent poison absorption. The use of ipecacuanha for induction of emesis was not introduced until the 1600s, when it was recommended by William Piso (Reid, 1970).

The use of charcoal, now a mainstay in the treatment of many human poisonings, can be dated to early Greek and Roman civilization, when wood charcoal was used for the treatment of maladies such as anthrax and epilepsy (Cooney, 1995). The antidotal properties of charcoal were demonstrated in the 1800s by the French, with dramatic demonstrations of a reduction in lethality when charcoal was ingested with potentially lethal doses of arsenic trioxide by Bertrand and strychnine by Touery (Holt and Holz, 1963). One of the earliest reported human studies examining the efficacy of charcoal in poisoning was done in 1948 by the American physician Rand (Holt and Holz, 1963). The use of superheated steam to treat the charcoal so as to enhance its adsorptive capacity was reported by Ostrejko, a Russian scientist, in 1900 (Greensher et al., 1987). By the 1960s, the use of activated charcoal was routinely recommended for the treatment of patients poisoned with substances thought to be adsorbed to charcoal.

Introduction of the Poison Control Center

The evolution in the field of clinical toxicology paralleled the evolution of the poison control centers. In the 1940s, several European communities developed hospital-based treatment facilities for poisoning (Manoguerra and Temple, 1984). A study by the American Academy of Pediatrics completed in 1952 reported that more than half of childhood accidents involved unintentional poisoning in the United States. Possibly in response to this study, Dr. Edward Press started the first poison control center in the United States in Chicago. These centers became valuable resources for providing information about product ingredients and recommendations for treatment of poisoned patients. Poison control centers proliferated over the next two decades. It was estimated that over 650 centers were in operation by 1978. Through regionalization, consolidation, and certification, the number of poison control centers have significantly decreased to less than a hundred since that time.

Staffing of a poison control center usually consists of a medical director (medical toxicologist), administrator or managing director, specialists in poison information, and educators for poison prevention programs. The medical toxicologist, managing director, and specialists in poison information are health care professionals who are credentialed by their respective boards. The American Board of Medical Subspecialties offers a subspecialty certificate to physicians who successfully complete the certifying examination. The American Board of Applied Toxicology (ABAT) offers a certification examination for nonphysicians, and the American Association of Poison Control Centers (AAPCC) provides a certification of the specialists in poison information, who are usually nurses or pharmacists. The managing director is usually either the same person as the medical director or a nonphysician certified by the ABAT.

The public health services provided by poison control centers have been well documented. These services include direct information to patients with recommendations for needed treatment, critical diagnostic and treatment information for health care professionals, education for health care personnel, and poison prevention activities through public education. An example of the cost benefit of poison information centers comes from a 1-year forced closure of the Louisiana State Poison Center. When there was no poison center to call, the community was left with the alternative but a visit to an emergency department (ED) or doctor's office for information on exposures and their possible treatment. It was estimated that the increased costs to the state for emergency medical services was $1.4 million for that year (King, 1991).

CLINICAL STRATEGY FOR TREATMENT OF THE POISONED PATIENT

The initial phases of treatment of the poisoned patient usually occur in the setting of a hospital ED, but initial treatment in other, less ideal settings such as the battlefield, workplace, home. or street setting can be required as well. Most clinical toxicologists agree that a methodically executed, stepwise approach to the treatment of the poisoned patient is required for optimal care (Goldfrank, 1998, Ellenhorn, 1997). This section refers primarily to the treatment of poisoned patients in the ED setting. There, the following general steps represent important components of the initial clinical encounter with a poisoned patient:

1. Stabilization of the patient
2. Clinical evaluation (history, physical, laboratory, radiology)
3. Prevention of further toxin absorption
4. Enhancement of toxin elimination
5. Administration of antidote
6. Supportive care and clinical follow-up

Clinical Stabilization

The first priority in the treatment of the poisoned patient is stabilization. Assessment of the vital signs and the effectiveness of respiration and circulation are the initial concerns. There is a wide range of severity of the clinical toxicity demonstrated by patients poisoned with even lethal doses of toxins early in the course of the poisoning. Some agents, such as a benzodiazepine, can cause pronounced clinical effects, such as sedation, early, but can have a comparatively mild clinical course, while other toxins, such as camphor, show little clinical effect initially but can produce a fatal outcome. Some toxins or drugs can cause seizures early in the course of presentation. Control of toxin-induced seizures can be an important component of the initial stabilization of the poisoned patient. The degree of clinical stabilization required for a poisoned patient therefore is highly variable. The steps and clinical procedures incorporated to stabilize a critically ill poisoned patient are numerous and include assessment—and, if appropriate, support—of ventilation, circulation, and oxygenation. A detailed description of the various clinical methods available to treat abnormalities in these parameters is beyond the scope of this chapter. The reader is referred to textbooks of emergency medicine for further information of this subject. Once the poisoned patient is clinically stabilized, the remaining assessment and treatment steps can proceed.

Clinical History in the Poisoned Patient

The primary goal of taking a medical history in poisoned patients is to determine, if possible, the substance ingested or the substance to which the patient has been exposed as well as extent and time of exposure. Unfortunately, in contrast to most specialties of medicine, the clinical history available during the initial clinical encounter in the treatment of poisoned patients is occasionally unreliable or unobtainable. In the case of intentional self-poisoning, patients may not provide any history or may give incorrect information so as to increase the possibility that they will successfully bring harm to themselves. For these reasons, ancillary sources for the clinical history are often enlisted to determine what substances the patient has been exposed to. Information sources commonly employed in this setting include family members, emergency medical technicians who were at the scene, a pharmacist who can sometimes provide a listing of prescriptions recently filled, or an employer who can disclose what chemicals are available in the work environment.

In estimating the level of exposure to the poison, one should generally maximize one's estimate of the possible dose received. That is, one should assume that the entire prescription bottle contents were ingested, that the entire bottle of liquid was consumed, or that the highest possible concentration of airborne contaminant was present in the case of a patient poisoned by inhalation. Maximizing the potential dose or exposure level reduces the probability of encountering an unexpected clinical outcome in a poisoned patient.

With an estimate of dose, the toxicologist can refer to various information sources to determine what the range of expected clinical effects might be from the exposure. The estimation of expected toxicity greatly assists with the triage of poisoned patients. Poison information specialists working in poison information centers routinely give telephone recommendations regarding the level of medical care required for a given ingestion based on the expected clinical effects from the reported ingestion. The vast majority of in-the-home accidental pediatric exposures are treated with observation or intervention with induction of emesis. In the hospital setting, ED staff use the estimation of expected clinical effects to effectively triage the poisoned patient. For example, a 3-year-old patient who accidentally ingested 25 children's chewable multivitamins without iron would be triaged to a noncritical-care area of the ED, whereas a 42-year-old patient who ingested a hundred 50-mg amitriptyline tablets in an apparent suicide attempt would be triaged to a section of the ED providing intensive care.

Estimating the timing of the exposure to the poison is frequently the most difficult aspect of the clinical history in the setting of treatment of the poisoned patient. Often the toxicologist must turn detective to determine the most likely window of time during which the exposure occurred. For example, if a pediatric patient was being watched by the baby-sitter at all times except for a 20-min period preceding the onset of symptoms and the discovery of an open prescription bottle for a benzodiazepine, one would estimate that the ingestion occurred in that 20-min window. Other situations require estimation of a far broader window for exposure. A person found with a suicide note could have taken the contents of the empty prescription bottle (or anything else available) at any time from when he or she was last seen by someone to a short time before being discovered.

Taking an accurate history in the poisoned patient can be very difficult in some cases. Despite diligent efforts, using both direct and external sources for the medical history information, the clinical toxicologist is sometimes left without a clear indication of the exposure history. In this setting, the treatment proceeds empirically as an "unknown ingestion" poisoning. This type of treatment is discussed further on in this chapter.

Physical Examination One of the most important aspects of the initial clinical encounter in the treatment of the poisoned patient is the physical examination. A thorough examination is required to assess the patient's condition, categorize the patient's mental status, and, if altered, determine possible additional causes such as trauma or central nervous system infection. Because gastric decontamination requires close attention to the patient's ability to protect his or her airway (see below), checking the gag reflex during the physical examination and periodically during the initial treatment phases is important. Whenever possible, the clinical toxicologist categorizes the patient's physical examination parameters into broad classes referred to as *toxic syndromes;* these have also been called *toxidromes* (Mofenson and Greensher, 1970). A toxidrome comprises a constellation of clinical signs and symptoms that, taken together, are likely associated with exposure from certain classes of toxicologic agents. The most important of these are the narcotic, cholinergic, sympathomimetic, and anticholinergic syndromes. Table 32-1 lists the clinical features of the major toxic syndromes.

In some cases, the agent responsible for the poisoning is not known during the critically important phase of initial treatment. Categorization of the patient's presentation into toxic syndromes allows for the initiation of rationale treatment based on the most likely category of toxin responsible. For example, if a patient presents in a coma, with miosis (pinpoint pupils), hypotension, bradycardia, a markedly reduced respiratory rate, and slight hypothermia with an otherwise nonlocalizing neurologic examination, this patient's clinical presentation could be characterized as consistent with the narcotic toxic syndrome. The presence of needle tracks on the skin would support this categorization. The treatment would then be directed at support of respiration and pharmacologic reversal with a mu-receptor opioid antagonist such as naloxone.

Laboratory Evaluation A common misconception concerning the early clinical care of the poisoned patient is that a definitive diagnosis of the specific agent or poison responsible for the patient's clinical presentation is frequently made by the clinical laboratory during the initial evaluation. Unfortunately, the repertoire of specific assays for toxins available in clinical laboratories on a rapid-turnaround basis (e.g., within 1 h) is very limited. Table 32-2 lists drugs, special laboratory tests, or other chemical substances that are typically available for immediate (stat) measurement in a hospital facility of the medical center type. As one can see, the number of agents for which detection, qualitative or quantitative, is possible in the rapid-turnaround clinical setting is extremely limited compared with the number of possible agents that can poison patients. This further emphasizes the importance of recognizing clinical syndromes for poisoning and for the clinical toxicologist to be able to initiate general treatment and supportive care for the patient with poisoning from an unknown substance.

For the relatively few substances that can be measured on a rapid-turnaround basis in an ED setting, the quantitative measurement can often provide both prognostic and therapeutic guidance. In some cases, measurement of an indicator of the biological effect of a poison provides sufficient information to guide the patient's definitive treatment. Measurement of methemoglobin concentration in a patient poisoned by one of many agents that can cause this chemical transformation of the hemoglobin molecule is sufficient to initiate treatment for methemoglobinemia without identification of the specific toxin that caused the condition. Similarly, most hospital laboratories can measure carboxyhemoglobin concentrations rapidly, which permits treatment of carbon monox-

Table 32-1
Clinical Features of Toxic Syndromes

	BLOOD PRESSURE	PULSE	TEMPERATURE	PUPILS	LUNGS	ABDOMEN	NEUROLOGIC
Sympathomimetic	Increased	Increased	Slightly increased	Mydriasis	NC	NC	Hyperalert, increased reflexes
Anticholinergic	Slightly increased or NC	Increased	Increased	Mydriasis	NC	Decreased bowel sounds	Altered mental status
Cholinergic	Slightly decreased or NC	Decreased	NC	Miosis	Increased bronchial sounds	Increased bowel sounds	Altered mental status
Opioid	Decreased	Decreased	Decreased	Miosis	NC or rales (late)	Decreased bowel sounds	Decreased level of consciousness

Table 32-2
Toxins and Special Laboratory Tests Commonly Measured in a Hospital Setting on a Stat Basis

Acetaminophen	Methemoglobin
Acetone	Osmolality
Carbamazepine	Phenobarbital
Carboxyhemoglobin	Phenytoin
Digoxin	Procainamide/NAPA
Ethanol	Quinidine
Ethyl alcohol	Salicylates
Gentamicin	Theophylline
Iron	Tobramycin
Lithium	Valproic acid

ide poisoning based on the laboratory test measuring a surrogate marker for carbon monoxide exposure.

For some commonly ingested drugs, a nomogram has been established to predict the severity of the poisoning; this is important in some cases to guide therapeutic intervention based on the measured plasma concentration of the drug and the time elapsed from the exposure. Proper use of such nomograms is necessary for the clinical management of poisoning cases.

The clinical usefulness of a drug plasma concentration measured by the clinical laboratory was suggested for salicylates approximately 40 years ago. In 1960, Done published a nomogram to predict the clinical outcome from poisoning with salicylates (Done, 1960). The Done nomogram (Fig. 32-1) is still in use today as an aid to interpreting a given salicylate level as long as certain criteria are fulfilled. To use the Done nomogram properly, the blood sample from which the salicylate concentration was measured must be drawn at least 6 h after ingestion. In addition, the nomogram should be applied only to cases with a single, acute ingestion of salicylate. The Done nomogram is not useful in cases of subacute or chronic salicylate intoxication.

In 1975, Rumack and Mathew published the nomogram for acetaminophen poisoning shown in Fig. 32-2. It predicts clinical outcome and is also valuable to guide the clinician in deciding whether or not to administer *N*-acetyl cysteine (NAC), an antidote for significant acetaminophen ingestion. Laboratory evaluation of a patient potentially poisoned with acetaminophen is crucial to assess what hepatic injury may have already occurred and to determine plasma concentrations of acetaminophen. Accurate estimation of acetaminophen in the plasma should be done on samples drawn 4 h after ingestion, when or past the time that peak plasma levels can be expected. Once an accurate plasma concentration of acetaminophen has been obtained and the time of ingestion determined, it should be plotted on the Rumack-Matthew nomogram (Fig. 32-2) to determine whether NAC therapy is indicated. This nomogram is based on a series of patients with and without hepatotoxicity and their corresponding acetaminophen plasma concentrations at presentation.

In the appropriate patient, the decision to treat is based on the plasma concentration of parent acetaminophen plotted on the nomogram. Treatment should be instituted in any patient with an acetaminophen plasma concentration in the "potentially toxic" range. It should be noted, however, that proper use of this nomogram is required: namely, that certain conditions should be met to apply the nomogram to a specific clinical case. The nomogram was validated for a single acetaminophen ingestion; the time of ingestion is critically important to establish the *x*-axis coordinate for the data point and the plasma concentration should have been obtained at least 4 h after ingestion to assure that the peak plasma concentration of parent acetaminophen has occurred.

Similar though perhaps less well established predictive relationships of drug plasma concentration and clinical outcome and/or suggested concentrations that require therapeutic interventions are

Figure 32-1. Done nomogram for salicylate poisoning. (From Done, 1960, with permission. Copyright American Academy of Pediatrics, 1960.)

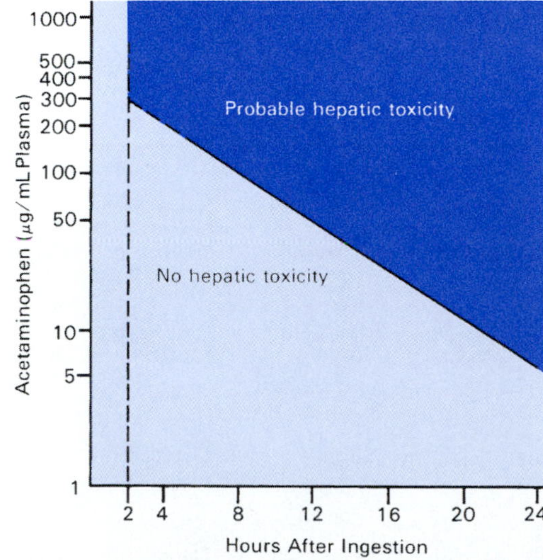

Figure 32-2. Rumack-Mathew nomogram for acetaminophen poisoning. (From Rumack and Mathew, 1975, with permission. Copyright American Academy of Pediatrics, 1975.)

available for several other agents including lithium, digoxin, iron, phenobarbital, and theophylline. Some authors have identified "action levels" or toxic threshold values for the measured plasma concentrations of various drugs or chemicals (Goldfrank, 1998). Generally, these values represent mean concentrations of the respective substance that have been retrospectively shown to produce a significant harmful effect. The pharmaco- (or toxico-) dynamic variability for a given toxin or for a combination of toxins is significant, however. For example, a patient with a "normal" or "nontoxic" digoxin level may display significant toxic effects; conversely, a patient with an elevated or "toxic" plasma concentration of digoxin may not show any sign of harmful effects. The clinical toxicologist must critically evaluate the laboratory data and treat the patient and not just the laboratory value.

Because of the limited clinical availability of "diagnostic" laboratory tests for poisons, toxicologists utilize specific, routinely obtained clinical laboratory data to determine what poisons may have been ingested. There are two laboratory values—the anion gap and the osmol gap—that are routinely obtained in the acute clinical setting and can be helpful to the toxicologist in evaluating certain poisoned patients. An abnormal anion or osmol gap suggests a differential diagnosis for significant exposure. Both calculations are used as diagnostic tools when the clinical history suggests poisoning and the patient's condition is consistent with exposure to agents known to cause elevations of these parameters (i.e., metabolic acidosis, altered mental status, etc.).

The anion gap is calculated as the difference between the serum Na ion concentration and the sum of the serum Cl and HCO_3 ion concentrations.

$$\text{Anion gap} = [\text{Na meq/L} - (\text{Cl meq/L} + \text{HCO}_3 \text{ meq/L})]$$

A normal anion gap is <12. When there is laboratory evidence of metabolic acidosis, the finding of an elevated anion gap would suggest systemic toxicity from a relatively limited number of agents. Table 32-3 lists the agents that include metabolic acidosis with an elevated anion gap as part of the clinical presentation seen when patients have been poisoned by these agents.

The second calculated parameter from clinical chemistry values is the osmol gap. The osmol gap is calculated as the numerical difference between the measured serum osmolality and the serum osmolarity calculated from the clinical chemistry measurements of the serum sodium ion, glucose, and blood urea nitrogen (BUN) concentrations (Smithline and Gardner, 1976).

Table 32-3
Differential Diagnosis of Metabolic Acidosis with Elevated Anion Gap: "AT MUD PILES"

A	Alcohol (ethanol ketoacidosis)
T	Toluene
M	Methanol
U	Uremia
D	Diabetic ketoacidosis
P	Paraldehyde
I	Iron, isoniazid
L	Lactic acid
E	Ethylene glycol
S	Salicylate

$$\text{Osmol gap} = \text{measured serum osmolality (mOsm)} - \text{calculated serum osmolarity}$$

$$\text{where calculated serum osmolarity} = 2 \times \text{Na meq/L} + \text{Glucose mg/dL}/18 + \text{BUN mg/dL}/2.8$$

The normal osmol gap is <10 mOsm. Note that the serum osmolality must be measured by freezing-point depression and not boiling-point elevation, as the latter method can fail to detect the osmolality contribution of volatile, low-molecular-weight substances due to vaporization of the substance during measurement.

An elevated osmol gap in the setting of a poisoned patient suggests the presence of an osmotically active substance in the plasma that is not accounted for by the Na, glucose, or BUN concentrations. Table 32-4 lists several substances that, when ingested, can be associated with an elevated osmole gap in humans.

While calculation of both the anion gap and the osmol gap can provide very useful information from readily available clinical chemistry measurements, these determinations must sometimes be interpreted cautiously in certain clinical settings. For example, even though a patient may have ingested a large, significantly toxic amount of methanol, if measured late in the clinical course of the exposure, the osmol gap may not be significantly elevated, as most of the osmotically active methanol has left the plasma and has been biotransformed or cleared but is still producing serious clinical effects.

Radiographic Examination The use of clinical radiographs to visualize drug overdose or poison ingestions is relatively limited. This is due primarily to the lack of radiopacity of many oral forms of medication. Early radiographic surveys of the radiopacity of oral medications revealed that the vast majority of commercially available tablets and capsules surveyed were essentially undetectable by radiograph (Handy, 1971; O'Brien et al., 1986). These and other studies have shown that relatively few formulations of drugs are radiopaque and would therefore not be likely to be detectable by plain x-ray of the abdomen. Generally, plain radiographs can detect a significant amount of ingested oral medication containing ferrous or potassium salts. However, a study of the in vitro and in vivo visualization of chewable oral formulations of iron supplements showed that once the chewable iron was ingested, it was no longer detectable by plain abdominal radiograph (Everson et al., 1989). In addition, certain formulations that have an enteric coating or certain types of sustained release products are radiopaque as well (Savitt et al., 1987; Nelson et al., 1993).

The most useful radiographs ordered in a case of overdose or poisoning include the chest and abdominal radiographs and the computed tomography (CT) study of the head. The abdominal radiograph has been used to detect recent lead paint ingestion due to pica in children for many years. Although the presence of radiographic evidence of lead-based paint chips probably underrepre-

Table 32-4
Differential Diagnosis of Elevated Osmol Gap

Ethanol
Ethylene glycol
Isopropanol
Methanol

sented the proportion of children with moderate to severe lead poisoning in one study, an abdominal radiograph showing pica was associated with significantly elevated blood lead concentrations (McElvaine et al., 1992). Another situation in which an abdominal radiograph may be helpful is in the setting of a halogenated hydrocarbon such as carbon tetrachloride or chloroform. If a sufficient amount of either liquid is ingested, it is likely that, on the abdominal film, these organic solvents will be visualized as a radiopaque liquid in the gut lumen (Dally et al., 1987). Finally, abdominal plain radiographs have been helpful in the setting where foreign bodies are detected in the gastrointestinal tract. An example of this is in the situation where an international traveler coming to the United States becomes acutely ill with signs of severe sympathomimetic excess and numerous foreign bodies are visualized throughout the gastrointestinal tract. This patient would probably be a "body packer," or one who smuggles illegal substances by swallowing latex or plastic storage vesicles filled with cocaine or some other substance (Beerman et al., 1986; McCarron et al., 1983; Sporer et al., 1997). Occasionally these storage devices rupture and the drug is released into the gastrointestinal tract, with serious and sometimes fatal results. Aside from these relatively uncommon situations, the overall clinical utility for detection and diagnosis of poisons by radiography is limited.

In contrast to the clinical utility of plain radiography to identify a specific poison or diagnose poisoning, plain radiography and other types of diagnostic imaging in clinical toxicology can be extremely valuable for the diagnosis of toxin-induced pathology and to aid the clinical toxicologist in the ongoing treatment and patient management phases of the drug overdose. Detection of drug-induced noncardiac pulmonary edema is associated with serious intoxication with salicylates and opioid agonists (Stern et al., 1968; Heffner, et al., 1990). Plain chest radiography can detect this abnormality, which would likely correlate with the findings observed during physical examination of the lungs. This radiographic finding would increase the severity classification of the poisoning and potentially alter the planned therapeutic strategy for the patient.

Another example of the use of radiologic imaging in clinical toxicology is with CT of the brain. Significant exposure to carbon monoxide (CO) has been associated with CT lesions of the brain consisting of low-density areas in the cerebral white matter and in the basal ganglia, especially the globus pallidus. Although not clinically employed for diagnostic purposes in the acute phases of a CO poisoning, these CT findings of the brain have been useful for estimating the clinical prognosis of a patient who survives the initial phase of such poisoning (Miura et al., 1985; Jones et al., 1994).

The initial clinical evaluation is a critically important phase of the therapeutic process to treat poisoned individuals. The physical, laboratory, and radiologic examination all contribute to the initial diagnostic steps for poison treatment. The physical and laboratory examinations are generally more important from a diagnostic standpoint, while the radiologic examination tends to be more useful for the detection and management of toxin-induced pathology.

Prevention of Further Poison Absorption During the early phases of poison treatment or intervention for a toxic exposure via the oral or the topical route, a significant opportunity exists to prevent further absorption of the poison by minimizing the total amount that reaches the systemic circulation. For toxins presented by the inhalation route, the main intervention to prevent further absorption is removal of the patient from the environment where the toxin is found and providing adequate ventilation and oxygenation for the patient. For topical exposures, clothing containing the toxin must be removed and properly disposed of in airtight wrappings or containers making sure the rescuers and health care providers are adequately protected from secondary exposure. Most topical exposures require gentle washing of the skin with water and mild soap, taking care not to cause cutaneous abrasions of the skin that may enhance dermal absorption.

The optimal time to intervene in order to prevent continued absorption of an oral poison is as soon as possible after the ingestion. The three primary methods currently available for this purpose are: induction of emesis with syrup of ipecac, gastric lavage, and oral administration of activated charcoal. Historically, induction of emesis with a variety of agents was the sole modality employed to treat poisoning by seeking to reduce the gastrointestinal absorption of poisons. "Tartar emetic" was an antimony salt used for induction of emesis and other medicinal purposes. Other emetic agents used later on included mustard mixed in water, concentrated solutions of copper and zinc salts, and various botanical substances. In hospitals, apomorphine injection was given even into the 1980s to cause emesis in patients with a history of potentially toxic ingestion.

Currently syrup of ipecac is the only agent used for induction of emesis in the treatment of a potentially toxic ingestion. Home use of syrup of ipecac upon advice of a poison information center remains the most widely used poison treatment intervention today. Syrup of ipecac has been available in the United States since the early 1960s. Typically, 15 to 20 mL of syrup of ipecac is given orally with water, and vomiting (usually more than a single episode) can be expected within the ensuing 30 min. Controlled studies have demonstrated significant variability in the amount of drug or test markers removed by administration of syrup of ipecac. In addition, a shorter time interval between ingestion and syrup of ipecac administration is more efficacious for gastric emptying (Neuvonen et al., 1983). The accepted contraindications for use of syrup of ipecac are (1) in children less than 6 months of age; (2) in the ingestion of a caustic agent (acid or alkali); (3) in a patient with a depressed level of consciousness or gag reflex or when the toxin ingested is expected to cause either condition within a short period of time; or (4) when there is a significant risk of aspiration of gastric contents, as for ingestion of a liquid hydrocarbon with low viscosity or low surface tension.

The use of gastric lavage—the technique of placing an orogastric tube into the stomach and aspirating fluid, then cyclically instilling fluid and aspirating until the effluent is clear—has diminished significantly in recent years. The reasons for the decline in use of this technique include a growing appreciation of the risk of aspiration during the lavage procedure and growing evidence that the effectiveness of gastric lavage may be more limited than originally thought. Careful attention to the patient's gag reflex prior to initiation of this procedure is important. If the patient does not exhibit a gag reflex, endotracheal intubations must be performed to adequately protect the airway and prevent aspiration. Most clinical toxicologists would agree that the current role of gastric lavage, if there is a role at all, would be in the initial treatment of the overdose patient who had a recent (within 1 h) oral ingestion. It is essential that the orogastric tube be of sufficient size (40 to 44 Fr for an adult) to be useful. Even with a large-bore orogastric tube, some tablets or capsules may not be able to pass through the tube. In the pediatric patient, there are practical limitations to the use of large-bore tubes. In this case, orogastric lavage may be useful only to attempt removal of liquid toxins or possibly dissolved tablets or capsules. Due to recent questioning of the effectiveness of the technique and the availability of data showing that other modalities for prevention of further toxin absorption (e.g., oral activated charcoal) are possibly as or more effective, the use of gastric lavage is decreasing.

As described earlier, the medicinal use of charcoal dates back more than 150 years. The first reported medicinal use of oral charcoal to adsorb an ingested toxin is credited to the American physician Hort, who, in 1834, used large amounts of powdered charcoal to successfully treat a patient poisoned with a chloride salt of mercury. A dramatic demonstration of the adsorptive effect of oral charcoal was that by Tourey, a French pharmacist who reportedly mixed a lethal dose of strychnine with charcoal and consumed the combination before his colleagues at the French Academy in 1930 (Andersen, 1946). Early in vitro investigations of the adsorptive properties of activated charcoal demonstrated the effect of charcoal on various chemical substances in aqueous solutions (Andersen, 1946), the effect of pH on charcoal adsorption properties (Andersen, 1947), and the effect of activated charcoal on the adsorption of strychnine from gastric contents (Andersen, 1948).

During the last 20 to 30 years there has been growing use of oral charcoal as a therapeutic intervention for oral poisoning. For many years, orally administered activated charcoal has been routinely incorporated into the initial treatment of a patient poisoned by the oral route. The term *activated* refers to the substantially increased adsorptive capacity that results from the processing of charcoal obtained from the burning of carbonaceous substances such as wood pulp, sugars, organic material, and industrial wastes. The processing—which involves extensive treatment with steam, carbon dioxide, oxygen, zinc chloride, sulfuric acid, or phosphoric acid at temperatures of 500 to 900° F—"activates" the residue, leading to a significant increase in surface area through the creation of small pores in the material. Many organic molecules are significantly bound to activated charcoal. Generally, low-molecular-weight, polar compounds such as ethanol tend to be less well bound. Substances such as lithium, iron, and certain inorganic salts are not appreciably bound to activated charcoal. In acute oral overdose, activated charcoal is typically administered at a dosage of 1.0 to 2.0 g/kg. When the patient is unable to drink the charcoal slurry safely, it is placed into the stomach via orogastric or nasogastric tube.

Some controversy exists regarding which modality or method of gastric decontamination to employ to prevent further absorption of oral poison. In fact, the data in the majority of published prospective clinical trials show that activated charcoal alone or activated charcoal preceded by gastric lavage is superior to ipecac. By contrast, some studies show that induced emesis results in a greater risk of adverse effects, primarily aspiration pneumonitis resulting from aspiration of gastric contents into the trachea and lung. No published studies show that induced emesis results in fewer adverse effects compared with oral activated charcoal (Kulig et al., 1985; Albertson et al., 1989; Merigian et al., 1990; Rumack, 1985; Vale et al., 1986; Rodgers et al., 1986; Kornberg et al., 1991; Underhill et al., 1990; Saetta et al., 1991; Saetta and Quinton, 1991). Controlled human trials with orally administered radiotracer in capsules have shown that ipecac-induced emesis resulted in removal of more tracer than did gastric lavage (Young et al., 1993). Many treatment centers are beginning to favor use of activated charcoal without gastric decontamination (lavage or ipecac) for treatment of oral poisoning and drug overdose. The use of ipecac syrup is now typically limited to individual patients in whom it is likely to make a difference in outcome, in whom it appears to be the most effective method available in that particular set of circumstances, or in whom it is the only method available to achieve the goal of gastric emptying. Typically, ipecac use is confined to the home at the direction of a poison information center or health care personnel.

Enhancement of Poison Elimination There are several methods available to enhance the elimination of specific poisons or drugs once they have been absorbed into the systemic circulation. The primary methods employed for this use today include alkalinization of the urine, hemodialysis, hemoperfusion, hemofiltration, plasma exchange or exchange transfusion, and serial oral activated charcoal.

The use of urinary alkalinization results in enhancement of the renal clearance of weak acids. The basic principle is to increase the pH of urinary filtrate to a level sufficient to ionize the weak acid and prevent reabsorption of the molecule by the renal tubules. This is also referred to as *ion trapping*. The ion-trapping phenomenon occurs when the pK_a of the agent is such that, after glomerular filtration in the renal tubules, alteration of the pH of the urinary filtrate can ionize and "trap" the agent in the filtrate. Once the toxin is ionized, reabsorption from the renal tubules is impaired; as a result, more of the drug is excreted in the urine.

Clinical use of this alkalinization procedure requires adequate urine flow and close clinical monitoring, including that of the pH of the urine. The procedure is accomplished by adding sterile sodium bicarbonate to sterile water with 5% dextrose for intravenous infusion and titrating the urine pH to 7.5 to 8.5. The drugs for which this procedure has been shown efficacious for are salicylate compounds and phenobarbital, which have pK_as of 3.2 and 7.4, respectively. For example, the increase in total body clearance of salicylate by increasing urinary pH from 5.0 to 8.0 can be substantial.

Although there are potentially similar advantages to be gained from acidification of the urine in order to enhance the clearance of drugs such as amphetamine and phencyclidine (pK_as 9.8 and 8.5, respectively), significant adverse effects are associated with acidification, such as acute renal failure and acid-base and electrolyte disturbances. For this reason, acidification of the urine is no longer recommended as a therapeutic intervention in the treatment of poisoning.

The dialysis technique, either peritoneal dialysis or hemodialysis, relies on passage of the toxic agent through a semipermeable dialysis membrane so that it can equilibrate with the dialysate and subsequently be removed. Hemodialysis incorporates a blood pump to pass blood next to a dialysis membrane, which allows agents permeable to the membrane to pass through and reach equilibrium. In order for this method to be clinically beneficial, the toxin must have a relatively low volume of distribution, low protein binding, a relatively high degree of water solubility as well as a low molecular weight. Treatment with hemodialysis of a toxin with the latter three characteristics but with a relatively high volume of distribution, such as digoxin, would not be clinically beneficial because the vast majority of the drug is not in the physiologic compartment (blood) accessible to the dialysis membrane. Therefore, despite the fact that hemodialysis is able to effectively clear the digoxin in plasma during the dialysis run, most of the body burden of digoxin is located outside the blood compartment and is not appreciably affected by the procedure. Similarly, if a drug is highly protein-bound, only a small percentage (the free fraction) would be available to pass through the dialysis membrane and be cleared from the body. Some drugs, such as phenobarbital, can readily cross these dialysis membranes and go from a high concentration in plasma to a lower concentration in the dialysate. Phenobarbital has a relatively low volume of distribution (0.5 to 0.7 L/kg) and protein binding (30 to 50 percent), so there is a reasonable opportunity for enough drug to be removed from the total body burden to make the technique valuable in serious cases of overdose (Brown et al., 1985; Cutler et al., 1987). Drugs and toxins for which hemodialysis has been shown to be clinically effective in the treatment of poisoning by these agents is shown in Table 32-5.

The technique of hemoperfusion is similar to hemodialysis except there is no dialysis membrane or dialysate involved in the procedure. The patient's blood is pumped through a perfusion cartridge, where it is in direct contact with adsorptive material (usually activated charcoal or Amberlite resin) that has a coating of material such as cellulose or a heparin-containing gel to prevent the adsorptive material from being carried back to the patient's circulation. The principal characteristics for a drug or toxin to be successfully removed by this technique are low volume of distribution and adsorption by activated charcoal. This method can be used successfully with lipid-soluble compounds and with higher-molecular- weight compounds than for hemodialysis. Protein binding does not significantly interfere with removal by hemoperfusion. Because of the more direct contact of the patient's blood with the adsorptive material, the medical risks of this procedure include thrombocytopenia, hypocalcemia, and leukopenia. This technique is primarily used for the treatment of serious theophylline overdose and possibly exposure to *Amanita* as well as paraquat and meprobamate poisoning.

The technique of hemofiltration is relatively new in clinical toxicology applications, and there is much less experience with its use for enhancement of toxin elimination. As in the case of hemodialysis, the patient's blood is delivered through hollow fiber tubes and an ultrafiltrate of plasma is removed by hydrostatic pressure from the blood side of the membrane. Different membrane pore sizes are available, so the size of the filtered molecules can be controlled during the procedure. The perfusion pressure for the technique is generated either by the patient's blood pressure (for arteriovenous hemofiltration) or by a blood pump (for venovenous hemofiltration). Needed fluid and electrolytes removed in the ultrafiltrate are replaced intravenously with sterile solutions. The procedure has the advantage of continuous use compared to the 4- to 6-h limitation for a hemodialysis run. Further studies with this technique for poison treatment are under way. Currently, the most common use of the technique is to aid in the removal of substances such as aminoglycoside antibiotics in the setting of significant renal insufficiency.

Table 32-5
Agents for which Hemodialysis Has Been Shown Effective as a Treatment Modality for Poisoning

Amphetamines	Isoniazid
Antibiotics	Meprobamate
Boric acid	Paraldehyde
Bromide	Phenobarbital
Calcium	Potassium
Chloral hydrate	Salicylates
Fluorides	Strychnine
Iodides	Thiocyanates

The use of either plasma exchange or exchange transfusions has been relatively limited in the field of clinical toxicology. While the techniques afford the potential advantage of being able to remove high-molecular-weight and/or plasma protein–bound toxins, their clinical utility in poison treatment has been limited. Plasma exchange, or pheresis, involves removal of plasma and replacement with frozen donor plasma, albumin, or both with intravenous fluid. The risks and complications of this technique include allergic-type reactions, infectious complications, and hypotension (Mokrzycki et al., 1994). Exchange transfusion involves replacement of a patient's blood volume with donor blood. The use of this technique in poison treatment is relatively uncommon and mostly confined to inadvertent drug overdose in a neonate or premature infant in the setting of a neonatal intensive care unit.

Serial oral administration of activated charcoal, also referred to as multiple-dose activated charcoal (MDAC), has been shown to increase the systemic clearance of various drug substances. The mechanism for the observed augmentation of nonrenal clearance caused by repeated doses of oral charcoal is thought to be transluminal efflux of drug from blood to the charcoal passing through the gastrointestinal tract (Berg et al., 1982). In addition, MDAC is thought to produce its beneficial effect by interrupting the enteroenteric-enterohepatic circulation of drugs. After absorption, a drug may reenter the gut lumen by passive diffusion if the intraluminal drug concentration is lower than the concentration in blood. The rate of this passive diffusion depends on the concentration gradient and the intestinal surface area, permeability, and blood flow. The activated charcoal in the gut lumen serves as a "sink" for toxin. A concentration gradient is maintained and the toxin passes continuously into the gut lumen, where it is adsorbed to charcoal. The characteristics of toxins that favor enhanced elimination by MDAC include (1) significant enteroenteric-enterohepatic circulation, including the formation of active recirculating metabolites; (2) prolonged plasma half-life after an overdose; (3) small ($<$1.0 L/kg) volume of distribution; (4) limited ($<$60 percent) plasma protein binding; (5) a pK_a that maximizes transport of drug across cell membranes; (6) sustained-release/resin-form tablets and/or capsules; and (7) onset of organ failure (e.g., kidney) that results in reduced capacity of the major route of elimination of the toxin so that MDAC may make a considerable contribution to total body clearance.

The technique involves continuing oral administration of activated charcoal beyond the initial dosage (described above) every 2 to 4 h with approximately one-half the initial dose, or 0.5 g/kg. The charcoal is generally mixed as an aqueous slurry and a cathartic substance is not incorporated due to the potential for electrolyte abnormalities with repeated administration of cathartic agents. An alternative technique for MDAC is to give the activated charcoal via an orogastric tube or nasogastric tube a loading dose of 1.0 g/kg of an aqueous slurry of activated charcoal (not the combination product that contains the cathartic sorbitol), followed by a continuous infusion intragastrically of $\geq$12.5 g/h has been recommended for adults. The duration of gastric infusion depends on the clinical status of the patient and repeated monitoring of plasma drug levels where indicated (AACT, EAPCC, 1999; Ilkhanipour et al., 1992; Ohning et al., 1986; Chyka et al., 1993; Goulbourne et al., 1994; Mofenson et al., 1985; Park et al., 1983, 1986; Pollack et al., 1981; Van de Graaff et al., 1982).

Studies in animals and human volunteers have shown that MDAC increases drug elimination significantly, but no prospective randomized, controlled clinical studies in poisoned patients have been published showing a reduction in patient morbidity or mortality when MDAC is employed. The early use of MDAC is an attractive alternative to more complex methods of enhancing toxin elimination, such as hemodialysis and hemoperfusion, although in only a relatively small subset of patients. Generally, patients with certain life-threatening intoxications may benefit the most from MDAC. The decision to use MDAC depends on the clinical situation, including the specific toxin involved, the presence of contraindications (e.g., intestinal obstruction) to the use of MDAC, and the likely effectiveness of alternative methods of therapy. A list of agents for which MDAC has been shown to be an effective means of enhanced body clearance is given in Table 32-6.

Use of Antidotes in Poisoning A relatively small number of specific antidotes are available for clinical use in the treatment of poisoning. This is partially due to a paucity of effort in drug development for antidotes as drugs. There are likely many reasons for this, but they include a small projected market for antidotes and the practical difficulties in performing clinical trials in overdose patients—an important component of an application for drug approval. The U.S. Food and Drug Administration (FDA) has placed incentives for sponsors to develop drugs for rare diseases or conditions through the Orphan Drug Act. Recently, an antidote for a fairly common poisoning was approved using the orphan drug pathway. In December 1997, fomepazole (4-methylpyrazole), a chemical inhibitor of alcohol dehydrogenase, was approved as an antidote for ethylene glycol poisoning. It remains to be seen whether further antidote research and development is stimulated by this regulatory incentive.

The mechanism of action of various antidotes is quite different. For example, a chelating agent or Fab fragments specific to digoxin will work by physically binding the toxin, preventing the toxin from exerting a deleterious effect in vivo, and, in some cases, facilitating body clearance of the toxin. Other antidotes pharmacologically antagonize the effects of the toxin. Atropine, an antimuscarinic, anticholinergic agent is used to pharmacologically antagonize at the receptor level; the effects of organophosphate insecticides which produce cholinergic, muscarinic effects, which if sufficient, can be lethal. Certain agents exert their antidote effects by chemically reacting with biological systems to increase detoxifying capacity for the toxin. For example, sodium nitrite is given to patients poisoned with cyanide to cause formation of methemoglobin, which serves as an alternative binding site for the cyanide ion thereby making it less toxic to the body.

Table 32-6

Agents for which Multiple-Dose Activated Charcoal has been Shown Effective as a Treatment Modality for Poisoning

Carbamazepine
Dapsone
Phenobarbital
Quinine
Theophylline

The time course for the onset of action of currently available antidotes is highly variable. Intravenous naloxone can have a dramatic effect on the level of consciousness of an opiate-poisoned patient within minutes. Chelating agents such as desferoxamine may require multiple dosages over many days before a clinically detectable effect is seen.

Skillful therapeutic use of antidotes is essential to optimize the treatment of the poisoned patient. Many antidotes have a relatively narrow safety margin or low therapeutic index. Excessive dosing with an antidote can in some instances be more harmful than the expected effects of the toxin itself. Some antidotes require an adjustment of their dosage based on a measured blood concentration of the toxin (for example, digoxin Fab fragments) or based on the clinical assessment of the patient, as with sodium bicarbonate usage in a tricyclic antidepressant overdose. A significant part of the clinical training in the field of medical toxicology is devoted to learning the appropriate use of antidotes.

An important area of research in clinical toxicology has been in the study of prognostic indicators of poisoning severity and predictors for the level of treatment required. For practical reasons, much of this work has been retrospective in nature, but it has resulted in significant aids to guide the treatment rendered by clinical toxicologists. Several authors have proposed "action levels" marking the threshold for a certain level of clinical intervention based upon a measured plasma concentration of the toxin or a clinical manifestation of the poisoning. For example, a patient with a measured plasma theophylline concentration of 90 mg/L after a single oral exposure would be expected to exhibit significant toxicity. If the patient's clinical condition correlated with the measured laboratory plasma concentration (i.e., laboratory error was unlikely), the patient would likely require aggressive treatment measures. Similarly, a worker exposed to significant amounts of topical methanol and who demonstrated a metabolic acidosis with an elevated anion gap, an osmol gap, and visual symptoms would likely undergo hemodialysis even in the absence of a confirmatory measurement of the methanol concentration in serum. These relationships, the correlation of serious clinical effects with a theophylline level above 90 mg/L (Weisman, 1998), or visual symptoms in a methanol-poisoned patient (Ellenhorn, 1997) have come from years of observational study by investigators in the field of medical toxicology. Early on, the majority of publications were of the case report type, making it difficult to determine the relative effectiveness of various treatments that were being tried in different parts of the world. The case series or metanalysis type of scientific analysis was an important step to advance the study of clinical outcomes and assess the quality of treatment provided to poisoned patients. An example of the case series study includes the publication that described the relationship of the QRS interval on the patient's 12-lead ECG to the severity of poisoning by tricyclic antidepressant agents (Boehnert et al., 1985). This important observational study helped to stratify patients poisoned with an overdose of first-generation tricyclic antidepressants into risk categories for the development of seizures or cardiac arrhythmias. Later on, the field began to utilize prospective, controlled clinical trials, which have enabled clinicians to validate (or dismiss) new therapeutic modalities and treatment strategies.

Supportive Care of the Poisoned Patient Once the initial treatment phase in the clinical management of the poisoned patient has been completed, those patients who require admission are generally shifted to an inpatient hospital setting. This supportive care phase of poison treatment is very important. Poisoned patients who are unstable or at risk for significant clinical instability are generally admitted to a medical intensive care unit (ICU) for close monitoring. In addition, patients who are excessively sedated from their poisoning or who require mechanical ventilation or invasive hemodynamic monitoring are usually candidates for an ICU stay. Not only are there certain poisonings that have delayed toxicity such as acetaminophen, paraquat, and diphenoxylate, but there are also toxins that exhibit multiple phases of toxicity, including delayed effects (i.e., ethylene glycol, salicylate).

Like other ill, hospitalized patients, those admitted for continued treatment of poisoning are at risk for nosocomial infections, iatrogenic fluid and electrolyte disturbances, and potential harmful effects from the initial therapies they received for treatment of their poisoning. For example, gastric lavage or orogastric infusion of activated charcoal can cause aspiration and lead to pneumonitis. Any drug that severely alters a patient's mental status, causing obtundation, can allow aspiration of gastric contents associated with a loss of the gag reflex. Close clinical monitoring can detect these later-phase poisoning complications and allow for prompt medical intervention to minimize morbidity and mortality. These are but a few of the reasons that close vigilance is a very important component of the support phase of poison treatment.

Another important component of the supportive care phase of poison treatment is the psychiatric assessment. For intentional self-poisonings, a formal psychiatric evaluation of the patient should be performed prior to discharge. In many cases, it is not possible to perform a psychiatric interview of the patient during the early phases of treatment and evaluation. Once the patient has been stabilized and is able to communicate, a psychiatric evaluation should be obtained. Generally a patient who has attempted suicide should be constantly monitored until he or she has been evaluated by the psychiatric consultant and judged to be "safe" (i.e., acceptable risk) to remove from constant surveillance.

Case Examples of Specific Poisonings

Acetaminophen A 36-year-old male patient came to the ED and reported taking "a lot" of acetaminophen approximately 6 h earlier in an attempt to commit suicide. Apparently he was discharged from his job earlier that day and could not face disappointing his family. He now regretted taking the acetaminophen and admitted to taking an entire bottle (500 mg capsules). He reported having some abdominal pain approximately 1 h after the ingestion and vomiting twice approximately 3 to 4 h prior to arrival in the ED. He denied taking any other medications or substances with the acetaminophen. He denied regular or recent use of prescription or over-the-counter medications or dietary supplements as well as regular consumption of alcoholic beverages. The estimate of the maximum amount of acetaminophen consumed was 25 g, well above what is considered a highly toxic dosage.

On physical examination, the vital signs were as follows: blood pressure, 138/88; pulse, 92/min and regular; respiratory rate, 20/min; and temperature 37.2° C. He was awake, alert, and oriented and responded to questions appropriately. The remainder of the physical examination was significant for normal bowel sounds and mild epigastric tenderness without guarding or rebound; the rectal examination was normal and the stool was without detectable occult blood. The neurologic examination was within normal limits.

Routine clinical laboratory studies were ordered stat (electrolytes, creatinine, blood urea nitrogen, glucose, complete blood count with differential, coagulation studies, urine analysis, and urine toxicology screen) and a plasma acetaminophen level. Chest and abdominal radiography were normal.

The patient was given 1.5 g/kg of oral activated charcoal prepackaged with sorbitol cathartic. The patient was closely monitored in the ED while the laboratory tests were being performed. Within 1 h, the laboratory results returned, significant for an acetaminophen concentration of 290 μg/mL. Based on the Rumack-Mathew nomogram (Fig. 32-2), a plasma acetaminophen concentration of 290 μg/kg at approximately 6 h after ingestion is well within the "probable hepatic toxicity" range; therefore treatment with *N*-acetylcysteine (NAC) was required. The patient received his first dosage of oral NAC in the ED and was admitted to the medical ward to complete the treatment course of NAC. Only mild (below four times the upper limit of normal) elevation of hepatic transaminases was measured on follow-up assessments. The patient was seen by the psychiatry consultation service and judged not to be actively suicidal. He was discharged from the hospital 4 days after admission with scheduled psychiatric and medical follow-up appointments.

Acetaminophen has been used as an analgesic and antipyretic since the mid-1950s and has become more prominently recognized as a potential hepatotoxin in the overdose situation since the original British reports in the late 1960s (Proudfoot and Wright, 1970). Work on the mechanisms of the liver toxicity of this drug has provided a theoretical basis for therapy (Mitchell et al., 1973).

The clinical presentation of patients poisoned with acetaminophen is sufficiently confusing, and in some cases it is difficult to estimate the time of ingestion. Due to the paucity of clinical symptoms with acute overdose, waiting for the appearance of symptoms is an inadequate strategy for the clinical decision-making process regarding institution of treatment.

Acetaminophen in normal individuals is inactivated by sulfation (approximately 52 percent) and glucuronide conjugation (42 percent). About 2 percent of the drug is excreted unchanged. The remaining 4 percent is biotransformed by the cytochrome P450 mixed-function oxidase system. The P450 isozyme responsible for acetaminophen biotransformation is CYP2E1. Metabolism by CYP2E1 results in a potentially toxic metabolite that is normally detoxified by conjugation with glutathione and excreted as the mercapturate. Evidence extrapolated from animals estimates that when 70 percent of endogenous hepatic glutathione is consumed, the toxic metabolite becomes available for covalent binding to hepatic cellular components. However, patients who are concurrently using agents that induce CYP2E1, as in the case of chronic ethanol exposure or phenobarbital use, may produce more than 4 percent of the toxic metabolite. In estimating the risk of hepatic necrosis in any given individual, it is therefore important to determine, whenever possible, whether the patient's CYP2E1 system may be induced. When there is evidence (medical history) of concurrent agents that induce CYP2E1, the treatment nomogram for acetaminophen should be modified to a lower threshold for treatment with NAC (Rumack et al., 1981).

Follow-up liver biopsy studies of patients 3 months to a year after their recovery from hepatotoxicity have demonstrated no long-term sequelae or chronic toxicity (Clark et al., 1973). A very small percentage (0.25 percent) of patients in the national multiclinic study conducted in Denver may progress to hepatic encephalopathy with subsequent death. The clinical nature of the overdose is one of a sharp peak of serum glutamic oxaloacetic transaminase (SGOT) by day 3, with recovery to less than 100 IU/L by day 7 or 8. Patients with SGOT levels as high as 20,000 IU/L have shown complete recovery and no sequelae 1 week after ingestion (Arena et al., 1978).

Laboratory evaluation of a potentially poisoned patient is crucial in terms of both hepatic measures of toxicity and plasma levels of acetaminophen. Accurate estimation of acetaminophen in the plasma should be done on samples drawn 4 h after ingestion, when peak plasma levels can be expected.

Once an accurate plasma level has been obtained, it should be plotted on the Rumack-Matthew nomogram to determine whether NAC therapy is indicated (Fig.32-2). This nomogram is based on a series of patients with and without hepatotoxicity and their corresponding blood levels.

Treatment should be instituted in any patient with a plasma level in the potentially toxic range. Standard support with administration of activated charcoal or gastric lavage (for very recent acetaminophen ingestions) should be followed by oral administration of *N*-acetylcysteine (Mucomyst, NAC). The protective effect of NAC in acetaminophen poisoning was demonstrated when NAC-treated patients were contrasted with controls who had not received antidotal therapy (Rumack et al., 1981; Smilkstein et al., 1988). Because NAC is most effective if it is given within 24 h of acetaminophen ingestion, patients in whom blood levels cannot initially be obtained should have NAC treatment instituted and therapy terminated only if their initial blood level is determined to be in the "nontoxic" range. The dosing regimen for NAC is a loading dose of 140 mg/kg orally, followed by 70 mg/kg orally for 17 additional doses (Peterson and Rumack, 1977). An intravenous form of NAC is available in some European countries and under an Investigational New Drug Application (IND) in the United States. Children less than 9 to 12 years of age have a lower incidence of hepatotoxicity after an overdose than do adults (Rumack, 1984) but at present are still treated with NAC according to the same nomogram. Patients with trivial or "nontoxic" acetaminophen ingestions should not be given NAC therapy because the antidote can produce clinical significant adverse events.

Methanol A 27-year-old male was brought to the ED after an apparent suicide attempt. The patient was obtunded but responsive to pain and without obvious signs of trauma. At the scene, emergency medical personnel found no pill containers or chemicals. A suicide note was found but contained no information regarding what might have been taken or used to attempt suicide. No further history was available. Physical exam was significant for a blood pressure of 105/56; pulse, 74/min; respiratory rate, 28/min; and body temperature, 37.0°C. The pupils measured 3 mm and were slowly reactive to light. The lung and heart examinations were normal. Abdominal examination revealed diminished but present bowel sounds, no tenderness, and no organomegaly or masses. The rectal examination was normal and the stool contained no detectable occult blood. The neurologic exam was without focal motor abnormalities with a diminished gag reflex.

The patient was placed on a cardiac monitor, an intravenous line was started, and clinical laboratory specimens were obtained; he was placed on oxygen and given naloxone, thiamine, and dextrose (50%), intravenously. Chest and abdominal radiography was without abnormality. A 12-lead ECG was also normal. Because of the diminished gag reflex, he was endotracheally intubated to protect his airway before an orogastric tube was placed. Activated charcoal (2.0 g/kg) was placed into the stomach along with a cathartic.

Clinical laboratory results returned showing the following:

Serum chemistries: Na, 140 meq/L; K, 3.0 meq/L; Cl, 94 meq/L; HCO_3, 8 meq/L; BUN, 12 mg/dL; glucose, 100 mg/dL

Arterial blood gases (ABG): pH, 7.20; P_{CO_2} 20 mmHg; P_{O_2} 98 mmHg

The complete blood count was normal, the urinalysis was normal, measured serum osmolarity was 330 mOsm/kg, acetaminophen and salicylate levels were below the limits of detection, and the urine toxicology screen was negative.

The laboratory results were interpreted as follows: a metabolic acidosis with elevated anion gap (AG, 38) and an elevated osmole gap (40 mOsm). The primary agents being considered as likely responsible for the poisoning were methanol or ethylene glycol (note cross-referencing Tables 32-3 and 32-4). A blood sample for measurement of methanol and ethylene glycol was sent for analysis. The patient was treated with sodium bicarbonate intravenously and sent for hemodialysis. After 4 h of hemodialysis, his acid-base and electrolyte abnormalities corrected. Approximately 9 h after the blood specimen was sent, the laboratory reported a "toxic" serum methanol concentration of 67 mg/dL. The patient underwent a second 4 h course of hemodialysis 8 h later, when the metabolic acidosis recurred. He regained normal consciousness within 12 h and recovered completely. Subsequently the patient admitted to consuming a methanol-containing gasoline additive to attempt suicide. Psychiatric consultation recommended inpatient psychiatric hospitalization once he was medically stabilized.

This case demonstrates the importance of utilizing the anion and osmole gap calculations in overdose patients. Although not considered diagnostic (Walker et al., 1986), the presence of both a metabolic acidosis with an anion gap and an osmole gap is highly suggestive of either methanol or ethylene glycol, given the patient's presentation and despite a scant history. It is quite possible that if the clinicians had not instituted therapy until the confirmatory laboratory test (i.e., the methanol level) had returned, the patient may have had a fatal or significantly morbid outcome. It is quite common for hospital clinical laboratories to have to "send out" blood specimens for ethylene glycol and methanol analysis, since these are not routinely performed onsite. A turnaround time of 6 to 12 h for this test result to be available is not uncommon.

Methanol exerts is primary toxicity after undergoing biotransformation by alcohol dehydrogenase to formaldehyde and then to formic acid by the action of aldehyde dehydrogenase. The formic acid is thought to be responsible for both the ocular (blindness) and the acid-base toxicity of methanol (Swartz et al., 1981). If untreated or treated too late, methanol poisoning can result in fatal cerebral edema with seizures as a preterminal event. Hemodialysis can remove the unmetabolized methanol, eliminating the substrate for production of the toxic metabolite. If hemodialysis is unavailable, an inhibitor or competing substrate for alcohol dehydrogenase can be administered while the patient is being transported to a health care facility where hemodialysis is available. Ethanol (sterile, for intravenous administration) can be given to effectively inhibit the metabolism of methanol and prevent the potentially devastating effects of the poisoning.

Tricyclic Antidepressants An 18-year-old college freshman came to the ED and told the desk nurse that he had just taken an overdose of a tricyclic antidepressant. The patient was driven to the hospital by friends but walked into the ED. He was immediately taken to the acute or intensive care section of the ED. His friends reported that he took his entire prescription of amitriptyline approximately 90 min prior to arrival at the ED in an apparent suicide attempt. He denied any other ingestion, which was confirmed by his friends. The patient's initial vital signs were blood pressure, 125/70; pulse, 94/min; respiratory rate, 20/min; and temperature, 37.2°C. The unit clerk called his pharmacy to confirm a recent prescription of thirty 50-mg tablets of imipramine. Within 15 min, the patient became unresponsive. His vital signs at that time were blood pressure, 80/55; pulse, 135/min; respiratory rate, 8/min; and temperature, unchanged. Intravenous lines were started, and intravenous fluids were administered as rapidly as possible. The cardiac monitor revealed sinus tachycardia.

The remainder of the physical examination showed the patient to be well dressed without obvious signs of trauma; his skin is warm and dry, without track marks. The pupils measured 7 mm and were poorly reactive to light. Other significant findings included the examination of the abdomen, which showed markedly diminished bowel sounds. The rectal examination was negative for occult blood. The neurologic examination revealed coma without focal motor abnormalities and an absent gag reflex.

Initial laboratory tests showed no significant acid-base disturbance, no elevated anion or osmole gap, and normal glucose, liver function, and renal function tests. The chest and abdominal radiographs were normal. The 12-lead ECG revealed sinus tachycardia, a right-axis deviation, first-degree heart block, and a prolonged QRS interval of 120 ms.

A Foley catheter was inserted and 600 mL of urine obtained. The patient had a generalized seizure lasting approximately 20 s. Endotracheal intubation was performed, followed by gastric lavage; only a few pill fragments were seen in the lavage fluid. Activated charcoal (2.0 g/kg) was administered via the orogastric tube immediately following the lavage procedure. The blood pressure continued to remain low despite intravenous fluid administration. The patient developed intermittent (nonsustained) ventricular tachycardia. Sodium bicarbonate was administered intravenously and an arterial monitor instituted to closely track the arterial pH. The patient then became clinically stabilized, with return of normal blood pressure and cardiac rhythm. He was transferred to the medical ICU and closely monitored. Alkaline intravenous fluid was continued for 8 h to maintain the arterial pH at 7.50. MDAC was employed for approximately 12 h. The patient regained consciousness and was evaluated by the psychiatry service, which recommended close outpatient follow-up after discharge from the hospital.

Tricyclic antidepressants (TCAs) can be very deadly in overdose situations. During the 1980s the TCAs were consistently ranked very high on the list of drugs most frequently involved in cases of fatal drug overdose reported to the AAPCC. No diagnostic laboratory tests are available to acutely aid the clinician treating a patient poisoned with a TCA. Clinically, anticholinergic effects appear early. The TCAs are the most deadly cause of the anticholinergic toxic syndrome. The clinical presentation of the TCA overdose is complex, with central nervous system (CNS), cardiovascular, and respiratory components most prominent. Usually, serious toxicity from TCAs appears within 2 to 3 h of ingestion. The prognostic value of the QRS interval from the 12-lead ECG was discussed above (Boehnert et al., 1985). In this case, the prolonged QRS interval would have predicted the observed systemic toxicity of the reported overdose and specifically an increased likelihood of seizures.

The TCAs are available in a wide variety of brands, including amitriptyline, doxepin, and imipramine, and also in combination with phenothiazine drugs. TCAs have three primary pharmacologic actions: anticholinergic effects, reuptake blockade of catecholamines at the adrenergic neuronal site, and quinidine-like (fast sodium channel) effects on cardiac tissue. The newer TCAs, such as amoxapine, are associated with a significantly higher incidence of seizures and a lower incidence of cardiac arrhythmias than the older TCAs. TCA overdose represents a life-threatening episode (Crome, 1986; Frommer et al., 1987). The initial symptoms seen are CNS depression with manifestations of lethargy, disorientation, ataxia, respiratory depression, hypothermia, and agitation. Severe toxicity may be associated with hallucinations, loss of deep tendon reflexes, muscle twitching, coma, and convulsions. The anticholinergic or atropinic effects of these drugs include dry mouth, hyperpyrexia, dilated pupils, urinary retention, tachycardia, and reduced GI motility, which may result in marked delay of the onset of symptoms. The life-threatening sequelae of the TCAs are the cardiovascular effects, resulting in cardiac arrhythmias such as supraventricular tachycardia, premature ventricular contractions, ventricular tachycardia, ventricular flutter, and ventricular fibrillation frequently associated with hypotension and shock. The ECG characteristically demonstrates a prolonged PR interval, widening of the QRS complex, QT prolongation, T-wave flattening or inversion, ST segment depression, and varying degrees of heart block progressing to asystole. Widening of the QRS complex has been reported to correlate well with the severity of the toxicity after acute overdose ingestions (Bigger, 1977b). Widening of the QRS complex past 100 ms or greater within the first 24 h is an indication of severe toxicity (Boehnert and Lovejoy, 1985).

Lavage as appropriate may be indicated, followed by the administration of activated charcoal. Patients admitted with TCA overdose but without symptoms should be monitored for a minimum of 6 h to detect any possible delayed onset of symptoms. Vital signs and the ECG should be monitored in symptomatic patients, as fatal cardiac arrhythmias have occurred late in the course. Hypotension should be treated with fluids and may respond to sodium bicarbonate as well as vasopressors such as dopamine or norepinephrine. Adjustment of blood pH with bicarbonate to pH greater than 7.45, coupled with appropriate antiarrhythmic drugs (i.e., lidocaine or bretylium), is the primary approach to therapy for cardiac arrhythmias. Seizures may also be responsive to diazepam, phenytoin, or barbiturates.

SUMMARY

Clinical toxicology encompasses the expertise in the specialties of medical toxicology, applied toxicology, and clinical poison information. The clinical science has significantly evolved to the present state of the discipline over the past 50 years or more. The evolution of the poison control center or poison information center has paralleled that of the discipline. The incorporation of evidence-based, outcome-driven practice recommendations has significantly improved the critical evaluation of treatment modalities and methods for poison treatment. Application of a stepwise approach to the poisoned patient as described above is a useful method for the evaluation and treatment of poisoning. A careful diagnostic approach to a poisoned patient is essential, as the important medical history is often absent or unreliable. Skillful use of antidotes is an important component of the practice of medical toxicology. Continued research will increase the repertoire of effective treatments for poisoning and ultimately improve clinical practice.

REFERENCES

Albertson TE, Derlet RW, Foulke GE, et al: Superiority of activated charcoal alone compared with ipecac and activated charcoal in the treatment of acute toxic ingestions. *Ann Emerg Med* 18:56–59, 1989.

American Academy of Clinical Toxicology, European Association of Poison Centres and Clinical Toxicologists, Vale JA, Krenzelok EP, Barceloux DG: Position statement and practice guidelines on the use of multi-dose activated charcoal in the treatment of acute poisoning. *J Toxicol Clin Toxicol*, 37:731–751, 1999.

Anderson AH: Adsorption from gastro-intestinal contents: Experimental studies on the pharmacology of activated charcoal. *Acta Pharmacol* 4:275–284, 1948.

Anderson AH: Adsorption power of charcoal in aqueous solution: Experimental studies on the pharmacology of activated charcoal. *Acta Pharmacol* 2:69–78, 1946.

Anderson AH: The effect of pH on the adsorption by charcoal from aqueous solutions: Experimental studies on the pharmacology of activated charcoal. *Acta Pharmacol* 3:199–218, 1947.

Beerman R, Nunez D, Wetli C: Radiographic evaluation of the cocaine smuggler. *Gastrointest Radiol* 11:351–354, 1986.

Berg MJ, Berlinger WG, Goldberg MJ, et al: Acceleration of the body clearance of phenobarbital by oral activated charcoal. *N Engl J Med* 307:642–644, 1982.

Bigger JT: Tricyclic antidepressant overdose: Incidence of symptoms. *JAMA* 238:135–138, 1977b.

Boehnert MT, Lovejoy FH: Value of the QRS duration versus the serum drug level in predicting seizures and ventricular arrhythmias after an acute overdose of tricyclic antidepressants. *N Engl J Med* 313:474–479, 1985.

Brown TR, Evans JE, Szabo GK, et al: Studies with stable isotopes: II. Phenobarbital pharmacokinetics during monotherapy. *J Clin Pharm* 25:51–58, 1985.

Chyka PA: Mutiple-dose activated charcoal enhancement of systematic drug clearance: Summary of studies in animals and human volunteers. *Clin Toxicol* 33:399–405, 1995.

Clark R, Borirakchanyavat V, Davidson AR, et al: Hepatic damage and death from overdose of paracetamol. *Lancet* 1:66, 1973.

Cooney DO: *Activated Charcoal in Medical Applications.* New York: Marcel Dekker, 1995.

Crome P: Poisoning due to tricyclic antidepressant overdose. *Med Toxicol* 1:261–285, 1986.

Cutler RE, Forland SC, Hammond PGSJ, et al: Extracorporeal removal of drugs and poisons by hemodialysis and hemoperfusion. *Annu Rev Pharm Toxicol* 27:169–191, 1987.

Dally SL, Garneir R, Bismuth C: Diagnosis of chlorinated hydrocarbon poisoning by x-ray examination. *Br J Ind Med* 44:424–425, 1987.

Done AK: Salicylate intoxication: Significance of measurements of salicylate in blood in cases of acute intoxication. *Pediatrics* 26:800–807, 1960.

Ellenhorn MJ: Alcohols and glycols, in Ellenhorn MJ (ed): *Ellenhorn's Medical Toxicology, Diagnosis and Treatment of Poisoning,* 2d ed. Philadelphia: Williams & Wilkins, 1997.

Ellenhorn MJ: *Ellenhorn's Medical Toxicology, Diagnosis and Treatment of Poisoning,* 2d ed. Philadelphia, Williams & Wilkins, 1997.

Everson GW, Oudjhane K, Young LW, et al: Effectiveness of abdominal radiographs in visualizing chewable iron supplements following overdose. *Am J Emerg Med* 7:459–463, 1989.

Frommer DA, Kulig KW, Marx JA, Rumack B: Tricyclic antidepressant overdose: A review. *JAMA* 257:521–526, 1987.

Goldfrank LR: *Principles of managing the poisoned or overdosed patient: An overview,* in Goldfrank NR, Flomenbaum NF, Lewin NA, et al (eds): *Goldfrank's Toxicologic Emergencies,* 6th ed. Stamford, CT: Appleton & Lange, 1998.

Goulbourne KB, Cisek JE: Small-bowel obstruction secondary to activated charcoal and adhesions. *Ann Emerg Med* 24:108–109, 1994.

Greensher J, Mofenson HC, Caraccio TR: Ascendency of the black bottle (activated charcoal). *Pediatrics* 80:949–950, 1987.

Handy CA: Radiopacity of oral non-liquid medications. *Radiology* 98:522–533, 1971.

Heffner JE, Harley RA, Schabel SI: Pulmonary reactions from illicit substance abuse. *Clin Chest Med* 11:151–162, 1990.

Hill JB: Salicylate intoxication. *N Engl J Med* 288:1110–1113, 1973.

Holt LE, Holz PH: The black bottle: A consideration in the role of charcoal in the treatment on poisoning in children. *J Pediatr* 63:306–314, 1963.

Ilkhanipour K, Yealy D, Krenzelok E: The comparative efficacy of various multiple-dose activated charcoal regimens. *Am J Emerg Med* 10:298–300, 1992.

Jarcho S: Medical numismatic notes. VII: Mithridates IV. *Bull NY Acad Med* 48:1059–1064, 1972.

Jones JS, Lagasse J, Zimmerman G: Computed tomographic findings after acute carbon monoxide poisoning. *Am J Emerg Med* 12:448–451, 1994.

King WD, Palmisano PA: Poison control centers: Can their value be measured? *South Med J* 84:722–726, 1991.

Kornberg AE, Dolgin J: Pediatric ingestions: Charcoal alone versus ipecac and charcoal. *Ann Emerg Med* 20:648–651, 1991.

Kulig KW, Bar-Or D, Cantrill SV, et al: Management of acutely poisoned patients without gastric emptying. *Ann Emerg Med* 14:562–567, 1985.

Major RH: History of the stomach tube. *Ann Med Hist* 6:500–509, 1934.

Manoguerra AS, Temple AR: Observations on the current status of poison control centers in the United States. *Emerg Med Clin North Am* 2:185–197, 1984.

McCarron MM, Wood JD: The cocaine "body packer" syndrome. *JAMA* 250:1417–1420, 1983.

McElvaine MD, DeUngria EG, Matte TD, et al: Prevalence of radiographic evidence of paint chip ingestion among children with moderate to severe lead poisoning, St. Louis, Missouri, 1989 through 1990. *Pediatrics* 89:740–742, 1992.

Merigian KS, Woodard M, Hedges JR, et al: Prospective evaluation of gastric emptying in self-poisoned patients. *Am J Emerg Med* 8:479–483, 1990.

Mitchell JR, Jollow DJ, Potter WZ, et al: Acetaminophen-induced hepatic necrosis. *J Pharm Exp Ther* 187:185–194, 1973.

Miura T, Mitomo M, Kawai R, Harada K: CT of the brain in acute carbon monoxide intoxication: Characteristic features and prognosis. *AJNR* 6:739–742, 1985.

Mofenson HC, Caraccio TR, Greensher J, et al: Gastrointestinal dialysis with activated charcoal and cathartic in the treatment of adolescent intoxications. *Clin Pediatr* 24:678–684, 1985.

Mokrzycki MH, Kaplan AA: Therapeutic plasma exhange: Complications and management. *Am J Kidney Dis* 23:817–827, 1994.

Nelson JC, Liu D, Olson KR: Radiopacity of modified release medications. *Vet Hum Toxicol* 35:317, 1993.

Neuvonen P, Vartiainen M, Tokola O: Comparison of activated charcoal and ipecac syrup in prevention of drug absorption. *Eur J Clin Pharm* 24:557–562, 1983.

O'Brien RP, McGeehan PA, Helmeczi, AW, et al: Detectability of drug tablets and capsules by plain radiography. *Am J Emerg Med* 4:302–312, 1986.

Ohning BL, Reed M, Blumer J, et al: Continuous nasogastric administration of activated charcoal for the treatment of theophylline intoxication. *Ped Pharm* 5:241–245, 1986.

Park GD, Radomski L, Goldberg MJ, et al: Effects of size and frequency of oral doses of charcoal on theophylline clearance. *Clin Pharm Ther* 34:663–666, 1983.

Peterson RG, Rumack BH: Treatment of acute acetaminophen poisoning with acetylcysteine. *JAMA* 237:2406–2407, 1977.

Plaitakis A, Duvoisin RC: Homer's moly identified as *Galanthus nivalis:* Physiologic antidote to stramonium poisoning. *Clin Neuropharm;* 6:1–5, 1983.

Pollack MM, Dunbar B, Holbrook P: Aspiration of activated charcoal and gastric contents. *Ann Emerg Med* 10:528–529, 1981.

Proudfoot AT, Wright N: Acute paracetamol poisoning. *Br Med J* 2:557, 1970

Reid DHS: Treatment of the poisoned child. *Arch Dis Child* 45:428–433, 1970.

Rodgers GC, Matyunas, NJ: Gastrointestinal decontamination for acute poisoning. *Pediatr Clin North Am* 33:261–285, 1986.

Rumack BH, Matthew H: Acetaminophen poisoning and toxicity. *Pediatrics* 55:871, 1975.

Rumack BH, Peterson RC, Koch GG, et al: Acetaminophen overdose: 662 cases with evaluation of oral acetylcysteine treatment. *Arch Intern Med* 141:380–385, 1981.

Saetta JP, March S, Gaunt ME, et al: Gastric emptying procedures in self-poisoned patients: Are we forcing gastric contents beyond the pylorus? *J R Soc Med* 84:274–276, 1991.

Saetta JP, Quinton DN: Residual gastric content after gastric lavage and ipecac-induced emesis in self-poisoned patients: An endoscopic study. *J R Soc Med* 84:35–38, 1991.

Savitt DL, Hawkins HH, Roberts JR: The radiopacity of ingested medications. *Ann Emerg Med* 16:331–339, 1987.

Smilkstein MJ, Knapp GL, Kulig KW, et al: Efficacy of oral *N*-acetylcysteine in the treatment of acetaminophen overdose. *N Engl J Med* 319:1557–1562, 1988.

Smithline N, Gardner KD: Gaps: Anionic and osmolal. *JAMA* 236:1594–1597, 1976.

Sporer KA, Firestone J: Clinical Course of crack cocaine body stuffers. *Ann Emerg Med* 29:596–601, 1997.

Stern WZ, Spear PW, Jacobson HG: The roentgen findings in acute heroin intoxication. *AJR* 103:522–532, 1968.

Swartz RD, Millman RP, Billi JE, et al: Epidemic methanol poisoing: Clinical and biochemical analysis of a recent episode. *Medicine* 60:373–382, 1981.

Underhill TJ, Greene MK, Dove AF: A comparison of the efficacy of gastric lavage, ipecacuanha and activated charcoal in the emergency management of paracetamol overdose. *Arch Emerg Med* 7:148–154, 1990.

Vale JA, Meredith TJ, Proudfoot AT, et al: Syrup of ipecacuanha: Is it really useful? *Br Med J* 293:1321, 1986.

Van de Graaff WB, Thompson WL, Sunshine I, et al: Adsorbent and cathartic inhibition of enteral drug absorption. *J Pharmacol Exp Ther* 221:656–663, 1982.

Walker JA, Schwartzbard A, Krauss EA, et al: The missing gap: A pitfall in the diagnosis of alcohol intoxication by osmometry. *Arch Intern Med* 146:1843–1844, 1986.

Wax PM: Analeptic use in clinical toxicology: A historical appraisal. *Clin Toxicol* 35:203–209, 1997.

Weisman, RS: Theophylline, in Goldfrank (ed.): *Goldfrank's Toxicologic Emergencies,* 6th ed. Stanford, CT: Appleton & Lange, 1998.

Young WF, Bivens HG: Evaluation of gastric emptying using radionuclides: Gastric lavage versus ipecac-induced emesis. *Ann Emerg Med* 22:1423–1427, 1993.

CHAPTER 33

OCCUPATIONAL TOXICOLOGY

Peter S. Thorne

INTRODUCTION

For centuries the work environment has contributed significant risk of adverse health effects due to chemical and biological hazards. Early writings by Agricola (1494–1555) and Paracelsus (1492–1541) revealed the toxic nature of exposures in mining, smelting, and metallurgy. A systematic treatise by Ramazzini (1633–1714) described the hazards to miners, chemists, metal workers, tanners, pharmacists, grain sifters, stonecutters, sewage workers, and even corpse bearers. Today we continue to be concerned with occupational health and safety in these and other work environments. Although occupational settings are safer now than in the past, the levels of risk deemed acceptable have decreased and the recognition of the causal link of exposures to chronic diseases or diseases with long latencies has improved.

Occupational toxicology is the application of the principles and methodology of toxicology toward chemical and biological hazards encountered at work. The objective of the occupational toxicologist is to prevent adverse health effects in workers arising from their work environment. Since nonoccupational exposures can act as confounders or can increase the susceptibility of individual workers, occupational toxicologists must evaluate the spectrum of exposures of the work force under their consideration. Occupational toxicology is a discipline that draws on occupational hygiene, epidemiology, occupational medicine, and regulatory toxicology. The occupational toxicologist must have an intimate knowledge of the work environment and be able to recognize and prioritize exposure hazards. Since the work environment often presents exposures to complex mixtures, the occupational toxicologist must also recognize exposure combinations that are particularly hazardous.

It is often difficult to establish a causal link between a worker's illness and job. First, the clinical expressions of occupationally induced diseases are often indistinguishable from those arising from nonoccupational causes. Second, there may be a protracted but biologically predictable latent interval between exposure and the expression of disease. Third, diseases of occupational origin may be multifactorial with personal or other environmental factors contributing to the disease process. Nevertheless, it has been shown repeatedly that the dose of toxicant is a strong predictor of the likelihood, severity, and type of effect.

WORKPLACES, EXPOSURES, AND STANDARDS

The Nature of the Work Force

The demographics and distribution of the work force in industrialized nations has undergone a progressive shift over the past three decades away from jobs in heavy industry and toward jobs in the service sector and high-technology industries. There are currently 134.5 million people in the United States in the civilian, paid work force (seasonally adjusted data). This represents 67.5 percent of all citizens 16 years of age or older and is the highest proportion in history (USDL, 2000b). The 15 countries of the European Union have an estimated 155 million workers (European Union, 1998), and Japan has about 65 million. Table 33-1 shows the breakdown of employment in the United States. This illustrates that there are about 25.4 million workers (18.9 percent) engaged in manufacturing, construction, and agriculture, occupations that have the potential for significant exposure to chemical and biological agents. Furthermore, there are occupations in the service sector, such as automobile repair and employment in botanical gardens, that can also include exposures to hazardous chemicals. Service-producing occupations account for the majority (78.6 percent) of U.S. jobs. On average, weekly hours worked in service-sector jobs are less than in the goods-producing sector. Farm work employs an estimated 3.4 million workers 16 years of age and older and the U.S. Bureau of Labor Statistics has documented an average of 42.2 h

Table 33-1
The U.S. Seasonally Adjusted Civilian Labor Market

SECTOR	NUMBER EMPLOYED	AVERAGE WORK WEEK, HOURS
Nonfarm	131,117,000	
Goods-producing	25,431,000	45.0
Manufacturing	18,372,000	47.0
Construction	6,519,000	39.4
Mining	540,000	45.0
Service-producing	105,686,000	34.2
Retail trade	23,160,000	29.0
Wholesale trade	7,145,000	38.8
Services	40,101,000	32.8
Finance, insurance, real estate	7,696,000	N.A.*
Transportation and utilities	6,937,000	38.6
Government	20,647,000	38.2
Farm	3,369,000	42.2†
Self-employed	2,054,000	43.3†
Wage and salary workers	1,272,000	40.6†
Unpaid family workers	43,000	36.2†
Total	134,486,000	—

*Not available
†Data so marked are for 1998.
SOURCE: U.S. Bureau of Labor Statistics. Data as of April 2000.

worked per week. Work in agriculture is markedly different from most other occupations in four fundamental ways. First, 52 percent of those employed in agriculture are self-employed. Second, the overwhelming majority of farm establishments (91.4 percent) have fewer than 10 employees and these work sites represent 46 percent of the agricultural work force (USDL, 2000a). Third, although the annual average hours worked per week is slightly over 42, many farmers, ranchers, and farm workers have periods when they work as many as 20 h per day, 7 days per week. Fourth, according to the U.S. Bureau of the Census there are in excess of 290,000 children who identify agricultural work as their major employment (GAO/HEHS, 1998). Department of Labor data indicate that, on average, 128,500 hired farm workers between the ages of 14 and 17 were working annually in crop production (GAO/HEHS, 1998). Thus, children make up 7 percent of all hired farm workers working on crops. The presence of children in the work force has important ramifications for body burdens, disease latency, toxicokinetics, and biotransformation of toxicants.

Determinants of Dose

Dose is defined as the amount of toxicant that reaches the target tissue over a defined time span. In occupational environments, exposure is often used as a surrogate for dose. The response to a toxic agent is dependent upon both host factors and dose. Figure 33-1 illustrates the pathway from exposure to subclinical disease or to adverse health effect and suggests that there are important modifying factors: contemporaneous exposures, genetic susceptibility, age, gender, nutritional status, and behavioral factors. These modifying factors can influence whether a worker remains healthy, develops subclinical disease that is repaired, or progresses to illness. Workplace health protection and surveillance programs (shown in blue) can reduce exposures, disrupt the exposure-dose pathway or identify internalized dose and early effects before irreparable disease develops. These programs help to ensure a safe workplace and a healthy workforce.

As illustrated in Fig. 33-1, dose is a function of exposure concentration, exposure duration, and exposure frequency. Individual and environmental characteristics also can affect dose. Table 33-2 indicates determinants of dose for exposure via the inhalation and dermal routes. For inhalation exposure, environmental conditions such as concentration, particle size distribution, and properties of the agent are important. However, respiratory rate and breathing volume as well as other host factors contribute. Protection afforded by personal protective equipment (especially respirators) will reduce but not eliminate exposure. The degree of reduction of exposure for a particular respirator (the workplace protection factor) varies with respirator design, fit, maintenance, and environmental conditions.

Dermal exposures depend upon toxicant concentration; work conditions, including the degree and duration of wetness; and the ambient conditions at the work site (Table 33-2). Some determinants of dermal dosing relate to the physicochemical properties of the chemical as they affect the percutaneous absorption rate. These include solubility, temperature, pH, molecular size, and chemical characteristics of the vehicle. Host factors also influence dermal absorption and distribution. Important factors include the surface area of the skin that is exposed, the integrity of the skin, blood flow, and biotransformation. Since the stratum corneum, the outer layer of the epidermis, is the principal barrier to dermal uptake, the thickness of this layer in the exposed area has great significance. As an example, the absorption of hydrocortisone through the plantar foot arch is 25-fold lower than through the back and 300-fold lower than through scrotal skin (Bason et al., 1991). The

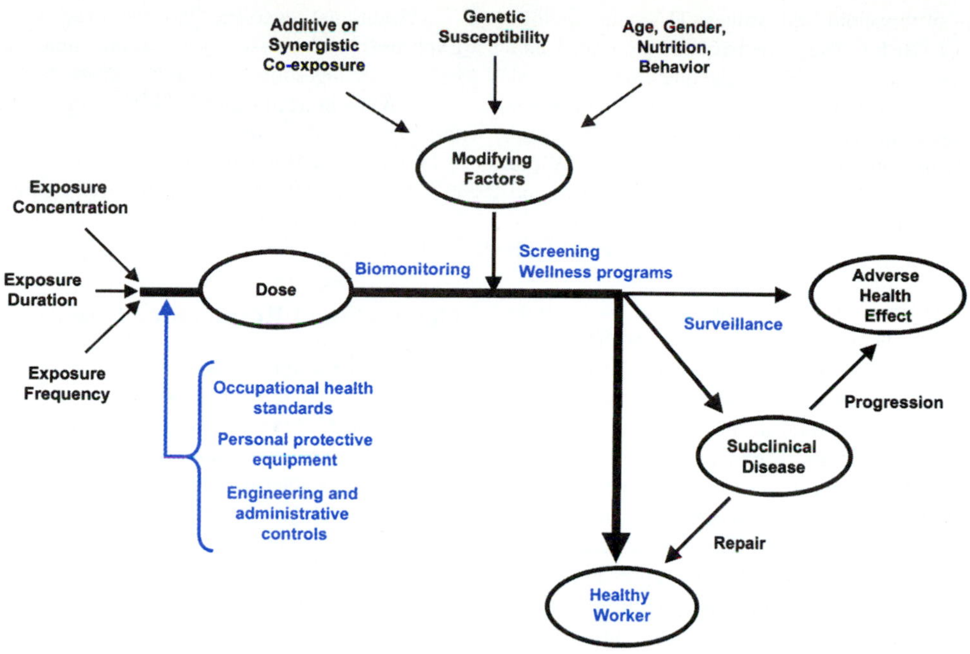

Figure 33-1. Pathway from exposure to disease, showing modifying factors and opportunities for intervention.

use of protective gloves and clothing or aprons and the application of barrier creams can greatly reduce exposure. For maximal protection, it is important that the material of construction of the glove be tailored to the toxicant(s) of concern.

Occupational Exposure Limits

One of the roles of the occupational toxicologist is to contribute data to the process of establishing standards or determining the appropriateness of those standards. Workplace exposure limits exist for chemical, biological, and physical agents and are recommended as guidelines or promulgated as standards in order to promote worker health and safety. For chemical and biological agents, exposure limits are expressed as acceptable ambient concentration levels (occupational exposure limits) or as concentrations of a toxicant, its metabolites, or a specific marker of its effects (biological exposure indices).

Occupational exposure limits (OELs) are established as standards by regulatory agencies or as guidelines by research groups or trade organizations. In the United States, the Occupational Safety and Health Administration (OSHA) under the Department of Labor promulgates legally enforceable standards known as permissible exposure limits (PELs). These are designed to apply the best scientific evidence to assure "to the extent feasible . . . that no employee will suffer material impairment of health or functional capacity" with regular exposure "for the period of his working life." However, there are relatively few PELs compared to the number of compounds to which workers are exposed and some of the existing PELs do not reflect current knowledge. The National Institute for Occupational Safety and Health (NIOSH), under the Centers for Disease Control and Prevention, publishes recommended exposure limits (RELs) that are more frequently updated and are generally more stringent than PELs. NIOSH also performs research and disseminates information on workplace hazards and their prevention. Most developed countries have governmental inspectorate agencies analogous to OSHA that are responsible for establishing and enforcing OELs. In some countries the insurance system also plays a significant role.

The American Conference of Governmental Industrial Hygienists (ACGIH) is a trade organization that annually publishes occupational exposure limits for chemicals and for physical agents.

Table 33-2
Determinants of Toxicant Dose

Inhalation exposure
Airborne concentration
Particle size distribution
Respiratory rate
Tidal volume
Other host factors
Duration of exposure
Chemical, physical, or biological properties of the hazardous agent
Effectiveness of personal protective devices
Dermal exposure
Concentration in air, droplets, or solutions
Degree and duration of wetness
Integrity of skin
Percutaneous absorption rate
Region of skin exposed
Surface area exposed
Preexisting skin disease
Temperature in the workplace
Vehicle for the toxicant
Presence of other chemicals on skin

These take the form of threshold limit values (TLVs) and biological exposure indices (BEIs). They are frequently revisited and generally reflect current knowledge in occupational toxicology and industrial hygiene. They are developed as guidelines and are not enforceable standards; however, many industries adopt TLVs and BEIs as internal occupational exposure limits. As stated by the ACGIH, TLVs "refer to airborne concentrations of substances and represent conditions under which it is believed that nearly all workers may be repeatedly exposed day after day without adverse health effects" (ACGIH, 2000).

Three types of TLVs are suggested, depending on the time scale of adverse effects inducible by the toxicants. The time-weighted average TLV (TLV-TWA) is an occupational exposure limit for exposures averaged over an 8-h day, 5-day week work regimen. These are generally applied to toxicants that exert their effects over long periods. The short-term exposure limit (TLV-STEL) is an occupational exposure limit for a 15-min measurement period. The TLV-STEL should not be exceeded in any 15-min sampling window and there should be 60 min or more between exposures in this range. The ceiling limit (TLV-C) represents a concentration that should never be exceeded. These usually are applied to toxicants that cause acute effects (such as potent sensory irritation) and for which real-time monitoring devices are available. Biological exposure indices are guidelines for biological monitoring and represent levels "most likely to be observed in specimens collected from healthy workers who have been exposed to chemicals to the same extent as workers with inhalation exposure at the Threshold Limit Value" (ACGIH, 2000). BEIs are recommended for analysis of urine, blood, and exhaled air. While hair and fingernails are used in forensic toxicology, there are no BEIs for these specimens. The appendix lists ACGIH TLVs and OSHA PELs for over 800 toxicants.

It is important to recognize that occupational exposure limits do not correspond to exposure conditions devoid of health risk. The concept of acceptable exposure level must be understood as the level of exposure below which the probability of impairing the health of the exposed workers is acceptable. The process of deciding what is an acceptable risk to occupational or environmental hazards blends the scientific disciplines of exposure assessment and toxicology with often vexing policy issues. Historically, acceptable risk in a society is related to the general health of the population and to a host of factors that influence how risks are perceived. To determine that the risks from an occupational hazard are acceptable, it is necessary to characterize the hazard, identify the potential diseases or adverse outcomes, and establish the relationship between exposure intensity or dose and the adverse health effects. If biological markers of exposure or early reversible effects are identified, this can aid in the risk-assessment process.

OCCUPATIONAL DISEASES

Routes of Exposure

Diseases arising in occupational environments involve exposure primarily through inhalation, ingestion, or dermal absorption. In the vast majority of work environments, inhalation of toxicants is a primary concern, with dermal exposure also of importance. Inhalation exposures can occur with gases, vapors, liquid aerosols, particulate aerosols, fumes and mixtures of these. Dermal exposures can arise from airborne materials as well as liquids splashed onto the skin, immersion exposures, or from material handling.

Additional exposure hazards exist for infectious agents. Exposures leading to occupational infections may arise through inhalation or ingestion of microorganisms but can also arise from needlesticks in health care workers or through insect bites among farmers, natural resource workers, and others who work outdoors. Additionally, poisonings from toxic plants or venomous animals can occur through skin inoculation (e.g. zookeepers, horticulturists, or commercial skin divers).

Occupational Respiratory Diseases

Because of the importance of the inhalation route of exposure, many of the major occupational diseases affect the lung and airways. Table 33-3 presents a list of the major occupational diseases and examples of agents that cause them. This is not intended to be all-inclusive. Rather it is meant to highlight what are historically the most important occupational diseases plus those that continue to be prevalent in the workplace. The toxicants listed are those for which there is a strong association with the disease or the most conclusive data to support causality. Examples are shown for cancer and for diseases of the lung and airways, heart, liver, kidney, skin, nervous system, immune system, and reproductive system. Several examples of occupational infectious diseases are also listed to highlight the fact that, in many work settings, infectious agents may constitute the major hazard and may coexist with chemical hazards. Most of the occupational diseases listed in Table 33-3 are associated with industrial chemicals. These are discussed in other chapters throughout this book. Presented below is the prevalence of some very important occupational lung diseases and a discussion of several common diseases in occupational toxicology that are not described elsewhere.

Occupational lung diseases have been studied extensively and are largely responsible for the creation of the occupational regulatory framework. Deaths due to occupational lung diseases such as coal workers' pneumoconiosis, silicosis, asbestosis, byssinosis, and occupational asthma led to important legislation such as the U.S. Occupational Safety and Health Act (1970). These occupational lung diseases continue to have significant morbidity associated with them. Table 33-4 lists the crude U.S. death rate and annual deaths and illustrates that while the death rates are fairly low, there are still about 3600 deaths per year attributable to asbestos, silica, coal dust, and other pneumoconiotic dusts and 343 from hypersensitivity pneumonitis. However, fatalities are just the tip of the iceberg. Hypersensitivity pneumonitis is rarely fatal but is often debilitating. Moreover, there are 11,000 yearly hospital discharges related to cases of asbestosis and 13,500 for coal workers' pneumoconiosis. OSHA has compiled data on inspector-collected samples in a variety of work environments and 3.9 to 24.9 percent of these exceed the PEL for asbestos, coal dust, silica, or cotton dust (Table 33-4).

Many of the diseases listed in Table 33-3 are known by other names that refer to a particular occupation or agent. One example is hypersensitivity pneumonitis, an allergic lung disease marked by interstitial lymphocytic pneumonitis and granulomatous lesions. Hypersensitivity pneumonitis is also known as extrinsic allergic alveolitis, farmer's lung disease, bagassosis (sugar cane), humidifier fever, Japanese summer house fever, pigeon breeder's lung, and maple bark stripper's lung, depending upon the occupational setting in which it arises. Although we often think of these as the same disease, it is important to recognize that the exposures and

Table 33-3
Examples of Occupational Diseases and the Toxicants That Cause Them

ORGAN SYSTEM OR DISEASE GROUP	DISEASE	CAUSATIVE AGENT
Lung and airways	Acute pulmonary edema, bronchiolitis obliterans	Nitrogen oxides, phosgene
	Allergic rhinitis	Pollens, fungal spores
	Asphyxiation	Carbon monoxide, hydrogen cyanide, inert gas dilution
	Asthma	Toluene diisocyanate, α-amylase, animal urine proteins
	Asthma-like syndrome	Swine barn environments, cotton dust, bioaerosols
	Bronchitis, pneumonitis	Arsenic, chlorine
	Chronic bronchitis	Cotton dust, grain dust, welding fumes
	Emphysema	Coal dust, cigarette smoke
	Fibrotic lung disease	Silica, asbestos
	Hypersensitivity pneumonitis	Thermophilic Bacteria, avian proteins, pyrethrum, *Penicillium, Aspergillus*
	Metal fume fever	Zinc, copper, magnesium
	Mucous membrane irritation	Hydrogen chloride, swine barn environments
	Organic dust toxic syndrome	"Moldy" silage, endotoxin
	Upper respiratory tract inflammation	Endotoxin, peptidoglycan, glucans, viruses
Cancer	Acute myelogenous leukemia	Benzene, ethylene oxide
	Bladder cancer	Benzidine, 2-naphthylamine, 4-biphenylamine
	Gastrointestinal cancers	Asbestos
	Hepatic hemangiosarcoma	Vinyl chloride
	Hepatocellular carcinoma	Aflatoxin, hepatitis B virus
	Mesothelioma, lung carcinoma	Asbestos, arsenic, radon, bis-chloro methyl ether
	Skin cancer	Polycyclic aromatic hydrocarbons, ultraviolet irradiation
Skin	Allergic contact dermatitis	Natural rubber latex, isothiazolins, poison ivy, nickel
	Chemical burns	Sodium hydroxide, hydrogen fluoride
	Chloracne	TCDD,† polychlorinated biphenyls
	Irritant dermatitis	Sodium dodecyl sulfate
Nervous system	Cholinesterase inhibition	Organophosphate insecticides
	Neuronopathy	Methyl mercury
	Parkinsonism	Carbon monoxide, carbon disulfide
	Peripheral neuropathy	*N*-hexane, trichloroethylene, acrylamide
Immune system	Autoimmune disease	Vinyl chloride, silica
	Hypersensitivity	See entries for allergic rhinitis, asthma, Hypersensitivity pneumonitis, allergic contact dermatitis
	Immunosuppression	TCDD,† lead, mercury, pesticides
Renal disease	Indirect renal failure	Arsine, phosphine, trinitrophenol
	Nephropathy	Paraquat, 1,4-dichlorobenzene, mercuric chloride
Cardiovascular disease	Arrhythmias	Acetone, toluene, methylene chloride, trichloroethylene
	Atherosclerosis	Dinitrotoluene, carbon monoxide
	Coronary artery disease	Carbon disulfide
	Cor pulmonale	Beryllium
	Systemic hypotension	Nitroglycerine, ethylene glycol dinitrate
Liver disease	Fatty liver (steatosis)	Carbon tetrachloride, toluene
	Cirrhosis	Arsenic, trichloroethylene
	Hepatocellular death	dimethylformamide, TCDD†
Reproductive system	Male	Chlordecone (Kepone), dibromochloropropane, hexane
	Female	Aniline, styrene
	Both sexes	Carbon disulfide, lead, vinyl chloride

(continued)

Table 33-3 *(continued)*

ORGAN SYSTEM OR DISEASE GROUP	DISEASE	CAUSATIVE AGENT
Infectious diseases*	Arboviral encephalidites	Alphavirus, Bunyavirus, Flavivirus
	Aspergillosis	*Aspergillus niger, A. fumigatus, A. flavus*
	Cryptosporidiosis	*Cryptosporidium parvum*
	Hepatitis B	Hepatitis B virus
	Histoplasmosis	*Histoplasma capsulatum*
	Legionellosis	*Legionella pneumophila*
	Lyme disease	*Borrelia burgdorferi*
	Psittacosis	*Chlamydia psittaci*
	Tuberculosis	*Mycobacterium tuberculosis hominis*

*For more on occupational infectious diseases, see Douwes et al., 2001.
†TCDD = 2,3,7,8-tetrachlorodibenzo-*p*-dioxin.

physiologic responses they induce are complex and may differ in the manifestation of the disease.

The U.S. Bureau of Labor Statistics tracks data for respiratory conditions arising from exposure to toxic agents. These conditions include pneumonitis, pharyngitis, rhinitis, and acute lung congestion. Table 33-5 shows data for rates and cases for 1995 by industry division. These data are representative of values over the 1990s and indicate 24,000 cases per year of respiratory conditions attributed to toxic agents. The manufacturing and services industries contributed 72 percent of these cases. Eight specific industries that consistently have case rates exceeding 4.5 per 10,000 workers are listed in the footnote to Table 33-5.

Toxic gas injuries are often characterized by leakage of both fluid and osmotically active proteins from the vascular tissue into the interstitium and airways. Important determinants of the severity and location of injury are the concentration and water solubility of the toxic gas or vapor. Anhydrous ammonia, with its extremely high solubility, primarily damages the eyes, sinuses, and upper airways. The vapors combine with water in the tissue and form ammonium hydroxide, quickly producing liquefaction necrosis. Chemicals with lower solubility, such as nitrogen dioxide, act more on the distal airways and alveoli and take longer to induce tissue damage.

Occupational asthma may be defined as a "disease characterized by a variable air flow limitation and/or airway hyper-responsiveness due to causes and conditions attributable to a particular occupational environment and not to stimuli encountered outside the workplace" (Bernstein et al., 1999). The Third National Health and Nutrition Examination Survey (NHANES III) has provided data on the prevalence of asthma based upon usual industry and smoking status (Table 33-6). These data indicate that asthma prevalence is highest in health services, hospitals, and agriculture and lowest in mining. Interestingly, in some industries current smokers demonstrate the highest prevalence (e.g., rubber, plastics, and leather products), while in other industries the highest prevalence is seen among former smokers (e.g., textile mill products, health services).

There are a variety of industries in which there is increased risk of developing work-related asthma. In chemical-based industries, plastic and rubber polymer precursors, diisocyanates, reactive dyes, and acid anhydrides are recognized low-molecular-weight sensitizing compounds. Biocides and fungicides used in metal fabrication and machining, custodial services, lawn and turf growing, and agriculture are also chemicals associated with occupational asthma. A number of metals can induce sensitization and asthma, including chromium, cobalt, nickel, platinum, and zinc. Many enzymes can pose significant risks for occupational asthma. Examples include α-amylase among bakery workers (Houba et al., 1996) and subtilisin, a protease used in laundry detergents (Flindt, 1969; Sarlo et al., 2000; Thorne et al., 1986). The enzyme pro-

Table 33-4
Crude U.S. Death Rates (1987–1996) and Deaths in 1996 Attributed to Selected Occupational Lung Diseases

DISEASE	DEATH RATE PER MILLION	DEATHS (1996)	INSPECTOR SAMPLES EXCEEDING PEL
Asbestosis	4.83	1,176	3.9%
Coal workers pneumoconiosis	9.16	1,417	7.4%
Silicosis	1.40	212	13.6%
Byssinosis	0.07	9	24.9%
Other pneumoconioses*	1.60	316	
Neoplasms of the pleura	2.62	510	
Hypersensitivity pneumonitis	0.17	343	

*This includes aluminosis, berylliosis, stannosis, siderosis, and fibrosis from bauxite, graphite fibers, wollastonite, cadmium, portland cement, emery, kaolin, antimony, and mica.
SOURCE: U.S. Bureau of Labor Statistics.

Table 33-5
Reported Respiratory Conditions* in Private Industry due to Toxic Agents, 1995 Data

INDUSTRY DIVISION†	RATE PER 10,000	CASES
Manufacturing	5.1	9,400
Services	3.4	7,900
Transportation and public utilities	3.2	1,800
Finance	2.3	1,400
Construction	1.7	800
Mining	1.5	100
Agriculture	1.4	200
Wholesale and retail sales	1.3	2,900
Total	3.0	24,000

*These conditions are pneumonitis, pharyngitis, rhinitis, and acute congestions due to chemicals, dusts, gases, or fumes.

†These occur at rates consistently above 4.5 per 10,000 full-time workers in the following industries: transportation equipment, primary metals industry, electronics fabrication, health services, rubber and plastic products industry, chemical industry, food production, career gardening.

SOURCE: U.S. Bureau of Labor Statistics, *Annual Report of Occupational Injuries and Illnesses.*

duction industry has had to adopt strict environmental and process controls to reduce the risk of occupational asthma in their production facilities.

Those working with animals or animal products are at increased risk of developing occupational asthma. Animal handlers, processors, and laboratory technicians who work with animals can become immunologically sensitized to urine or salivary proteins in many vertebrates; proteins in bat guano and bird droppings; animal dander; serum proteins in blood products; dust from horns, antlers, and tusks; or shells of crustaceans. Very high rates of sensitization can occur in shellfish processors (Glass et al., 1998). Arthropods such as insect larvae, cockroaches, mites, or weevils are recognized inducers of work-related asthma. Plants and plant products (e.g., soy flour, spices, and coffee beans) can also cause asthma among workers. In a variety of occupations, exposure to fungi—especially of the genera *Aspergillus, Penicillium, Rhizopus, Mucor,* and *Paecilomyces* are associated with allergic rhinitis and asthma. These are especially important in sawmills, wood-chip handling, and composting facilities (Duchaine et al., 2000; Eduard et al., 1992; Halpin et al., 1994). Apart from the contaminating microorganisms, certain woods themselves produce chemical sensitizing agents. Examples include western red cedar, redwood, and some tropical hardwoods. Asthma has emerged as a major occupational health concern among health care workers. In order to reduce the risk of hepatitis B and other infectious diseases, health care workers have increasingly adopted the use of natural rubber latex gloves for barrier protection. Proteins from the latex of the rubber tree, *Hevea braziliensis,* are the sensitizing agents. Seven of these high-molecular-weight proteins have now been characterized as allergens. Many other plants of less commercial value produce a similar milky fluid when cut and have similar sensitizing properties.

Studies of asthma prevalence in occupational settings with exposure to low-molecular-weight agents have suggested prevalence rates of 8.3 to 11.0 percent for toluene diisocyanate (Becklake et al., 1999; Pepys et al., 1972a; Weill et al., 1975), 3.2 to 18 percent for anhydrides (Venables et al., 1985; Wernfors et al., 1986), 4 percent for plicatic acid from western red cedar (Chan-Yeung et al., 1984), and 54 percent in a platinum refinery (Pepys et al., 1972b;

Table 33-6
U.S. Asthma Prevalence by Usual Industry and Smoking Status for Selected Industry Codes

INDUSTRY	*Asthma Prevalence, %*		
	NON-SMOKERS	FORMER SMOKERS	CURRENT SMOKERS
Health services	6.3	25.8	14.8
Hospitals	14.4	12.9	8.9
Agriculture services, forestry, and fishing	0.3	11.8	19.8
Trucking service	3.8	8.9	13.6
Paper products, printing	9.7	7.3	8.4
Lumber and wood products	2.8	8.0	12.8
Textile mill products	3.6	15.9	2.8
Repair services	2.0	4.0	15.5
Rubber, plastics, and leather products	1.8	3.5	16.1
Chemicals, petroleum, and coal products	8.4	5.7	4.9
Agriculture production	4.5	9.3	2.6
Metal industries	1.6	5.1	5.9
Mining	1.5	1.3	0

SOURCE: *National Health and Nutrition Examination Survey, NHANES III, 1996* (NIOSH, 2000).

Venables et al., 1989). For high-molecular-weight allergens, prevalence among shellfish processors was estimated at 21 to 26 percent (Cartier et al., 1984; Desjardin et al., 1995; Glass et al., 1998), 11 to 44 percent among lab animal workers (Cullinan et al., 1994; Fuortes et al., 1996, 1997; Hollander et al., 1997), and 26 percent among bakers exposed to wheat and alpha-amylase (Houba et al., 1996). Surveillance through the NIOSH SENSOR program in California, Massachusetts, Michigan, and New Jersey indicates that of 1100 cases reported in 1993–1995, 19 percent were for work-aggravated asthma and 81 percent for new-onset asthma (NIOSH, 2000).

Agricultural workers exposed to grain dust, cotton dust, or atmospheres in swine or poultry confinement barns are at risk for the development of an asthma-like syndrome. This syndrome is an acute nonallergic airway response characterized by self-limited inflammation with neutrophilic infiltrates and increased proinflammatory cytokines (TNF-α, IL-6, and IL-8), but it does not include persistent airway hyperreactivity, as in occupational asthma (Schenker et al., 1998). Asthma-like syndrome includes cough, mild dyspnea, fever, malaise, and cross-shift declines in lung function. Endotoxin in combination with other inflammatory bioaerosols are the likely etiologic agents (Douwes et al., 2001; Schwartz et al., 1994; Schwartz et al., 1995).

Other Occupational Diseases

Occupational toxicants may induce diseases in a variety of sites distant from the lung or skin. These include tumors arising in the liver, bladder, gastrointestinal tract, or hematopoietic system attributable to a variety of chemical classes. For further discussion of other occupational diseases and the toxicants listed in Table 33-3, the reader is referred to the relevant chapters in Units 4 and 5 of this text.

Nervous system damage can be central, peripheral, or both. It may be acute, as with some organophosphate exposures, or chronic, as with organomercury poisoning or acrylamide-induced neuropathy. Injury affecting the immune system may arise from the immunosuppressive effects of chemicals such as dioxins or toxic metals. Many occupational diseases of the immune system occur due to hypersensitivity leading to respiratory or dermal allergy or systemic hypersensitivity reactions. Autoimmune syndromes have been associated with occupational exposures to crystalline silica and vinyl chloride.

Occupational diseases of the cardiovascular system include atherosclerosis, a variety of arrhythmias, problems with coronary blood supply, systemic hypotension, and cor pulmonale (right ventricular hypertrophy usually due to pulmonary hypertension as with chronic obstructive pulmonary disease). Liver diseases such as carbon tetrachloride–induced fatty liver and hepatocellular death due to toxic concentrations of acetaminophen have classically been used to illustrate chemical mechanisms of cellular injury leading to organ failure. These are thoroughly discussed in Chap. 13. Occupational diseases of the reproductive system can be gender- and organ-specific; but several toxicants—including carbon disulfide, lead, and vinyl chloride—may affect both sexes.

Exposures to infectious agents are a part of a variety of occupations. Veterinarians, health care workers, and biomedical researchers studying infectious agents have exposures that are largely known, and infection control strategies can limit their risks. For others, such as farmers and foresters, specific risks may be less obvious. Zoonotic diseases such as Q-fever, rabies, leptospirosis, and brucellosis may affect abattoir workers, zookeepers, animal handlers, and veterinarians. Foresters, field biologists, and natural resource workers who spend time in wooded areas experience tick- and mosquito-borne illnesses with increased frequency over the general population. These illnesses include the arboviral encephalitides, Rocky Mountain spotted fever, Lyme disease, and ehrlichiosis. Occupational infections may arise as a result of work settings bringing people into close proximity with other people or animals, thus facilitating the transmission of microorganisms. Occupational infectious diseases attributable to the clustering of people affect workers in day care centers, schools, health care settings, correctional facilities, dormitories, military barracks, shelters for the homeless, and so on. Industrial settings can place large numbers of workers in a shared space, leading to increased transmission of diseases. This is especially true for diseases with annual outbreaks, such as influenza and Norwalk-like viruses. Exposures to chemicals may increase the susceptibility of workers to infection through irritation of mucosa or the pulmonary epithelium or through immunosuppression leading to impaired host defense.

Both industrial and nonindustrial indoor environments may pose occupational hazards due to the presence of chemical or biological agents. With ineffective ventilation or decreased ventilation rates and increased utilization of synthetic building materials, there has been a rise in complaints associated with occupancy in buildings. In some cases, workers in a problem building develop specific clinical conditions with recognized etiology. This is defined as building-related illness. In other cases, symptoms are nonspecific and disappear when the worker leaves the problem building. When this occurs with sufficient prevalence, it is termed *sick building syndrome*. Volatile and semivolatile chemicals are released from manufacturing process materials, building materials, floor coverings, furniture, cleaning products, biocides, and microorganisms. Office buildings and residences develop a complex ecology consisting of people, molds, mites, volatile organic compounds of microbial and nonmicrobial origin, and sometimes plants, pets, and vermin (Thorne and Heederik, 1999b). An important example of this relationship involves skin cells, fungi, and house dust mites. People slough as much as 1 g of skin cells per person daily. Fungi colonize these skin cells in carpets, bedding, and upholstery, where they then serve as a food source for mites. The mites produce gastric enzymes to aid in the digestion of the fungi and skin cells, and these enzymes are potent human allergens. Excrement from the mites contains these allergenic molecules, which, when inhaled, complete the exposure pathway that can lead to allergy and asthma. Exposure to chemicals and biomolecules such as endotoxin may enhance this process (Michel et al., 1996). In some cases the occupied space of a building may be clean and dry, but local amplification sites for molds may develop. These may arise in ventilation systems, utility closets, subfloors or basements that serve as return air plenums, or in local sites of water damage. Such sites can become sources of microorganisms and aeroallergens of sufficient volume to generate significant bioaerosol exposures throughout the environment. Airborne viruses, bacteria, and fungi are responsible for a variety of building-related illnesses arising from organisms that are pathogenic to humans. Nonpathogenic microorganisms may induce symptoms or diseases through inflammatory processes, by stimulating the immune response, or by releasing noxious odors, allergenic compounds, or bioactive macromolecules. These may combine with industrial chemicals released into the air to create complex exposure environments. There are many challenges to assessing exposures to microorganisms and chemicals in these environments (Thorne and Heederik, 1999a).

TOXICOLOGIC EVALUATION OF OCCUPATIONAL AGENTS

Evaluation of Occupational Risks

In most instances of prolonged exposure to chemicals, there is a continuum between being healthy and being ill. The exposures may impart biochemical or functional changes that are without signs or symptoms, subclinical changes, or more significant toxicity manifest as clinical disease. The health significance of the identified changes resulting from exposure to a particular agent must be assessed in order to determine which are adverse. Following this assessment, one must consider the interindividual variability or susceptibility factors that influence the risks. There is no one single dose-effect relationship but a distribution of responses. Therefore, to recommend an acceptable exposure level to an industrial chemical, one must attempt to define the risk associated with adverse effects in the most sensitive populations exposed. It then remains to decide what proportion of exposed subjects may still develop an adverse effect at the proposed acceptable exposure level. This acceptable risk level will vary according to a value judgment of the severity, permanence, and equality of the potential adverse effects and the characteristics of the most susceptible population. Clearly, inhibition of an enzyme without functional consequences will be viewed as more acceptable than a more serious toxic effect, such as teratogenicity leading to a congenital malformation.

Establishing Causality In complex occupational environments it may be difficult to establish a causal relationship between a toxic substance and a disease. For this reason a number of systematic approaches have been devised to help define causation. In 1890 Robert Koch proposed postulates for "proving" that a specific organism caused a specific disease. T. M. Rivers extended this approach to viruses in 1937. Sir Austin Bradford Hill suggested epidemiologic criteria for assessing causality in 1965. These schema and modern weight-of-evidence determination criteria were later combined to suggest a set of postulates for the evaluation of evidence for disease agents in organic dust (Donham and Thorne, 1994). A matrix was developed and is extended here to evaluate the weight of evidence for a causal association between a toxicant and an occupational disease (Fig. 33-2). Evidence from well-conducted in vitro studies, animal studies, and human challenge studies, case reports, and epidemiologic investigations are evaluated with regard to data quality and clarity of evidence in support of the establishment of causality. This evaluation is guided by seven criteria (shown in blue). If a chemical were thoroughly studied in animals, humans, and in vitro studies and produced clear and convincing evidence of an exposure-response relationship in controlled studies that used appropriate models and relevant endpoints, that would constitute compelling evidence of a causal relationship between that chemical and that disease. Figure 33-2 reminds us that a consortium of study types contributes data used for the evaluation of occupational hazards. These are discussed below.

To evaluate with some degree of confidence the level of exposure at which the risk of health impairment is acceptable, a body of toxicologic information is required. Five sources of data may be available to inform the occupational risk-assessment process.

	Assessment of Exposure to Specific Agents	Consideration or Control of Confounders	Evidence of a Dose-Response Relationship	Consistent Results From Different Studies	Objective Clinical Data	Endpoints Related to Human Pathology	Appropriate Subjects or Models
In Vitro Studies							
Animal Studies							
Human Challenge Studies							
Case Studies							
Epidemiology Studies							

For each type of study listed in the first column weight the quality of data from existing studies based on the criteria listed in the column headings as follows:

0 No evidence or condition is not met
1 Equivocal evidence or condition is partially met
2 Some evidence or condition is mostly met
3 Clear evidence or condition is convincingly met

Figure 33-2. Matrix for assessing the strength of an association between a toxicant and an occupational disease.

- In vitro assays
- Animal toxicology studies
- Human challenge studies
- Case reports
- Epidemiology studies

In Vitro Assays A number of useful in vitro assays have been developed over the past several decades in order to provide screening data and, in some cases, mechanistic insight without the need or expense of exposing animal or human subjects. While at this time there are few validated methods to determine complex toxicologic responses such as immune hypersensitivity or peripheral neuropathy, there are validated and very useful screening assays. Notable examples are the *Salmonella typhimurium* reverse mutation assay, or Ames test, and the Corrositex assay for dermal corrosivity potential of chemicals (NIH-99-4495, 1999). In addition, quantitative structure-activity relationships can help suggest potential toxicologic effects for an unstudied compound if structurally similar compounds have been evaluated.

Animal Toxicology Studies Animal toxicology studies serve an important function in terms of identifying adverse effects, providing mechanistic data, establishing dose-response relationships, and aiding the process of establishing standards. Since animal studies can be conducted before there is any human exposure, these studies play an important role in hazard identification and prevention of human disease. There are numerous animal models for occupational injury and illness; these are described throughout this textbook in the context of the affected organ system and the classes of toxicants. Generation of animal toxicology data to predict health effects in workers is a central function of experimental toxicologists. Toxicologic investigations using animals often serve to establish a tentative acceptable exposure level. Other important information that may also be derived from these investigations concerns the relationships between the metabolic handling of the chemical and its interactions with target molecules (mechanism of action), identification of methods for biological monitoring of exposure and early health effects, and of preexisting pathologic states that may increase susceptibility to the chemical. However, animal testing can provide only an estimate of the toxicity of a chemical for humans. Animals do not always respond to chemical exposure the same way humans do. For instance, there are very significant species and strain differences in responsiveness to aryl hydrocarbon receptor agonists such as polychlorinated dibenzo-*p*-dioxins (Abnet et al., 1999; Whitlock et al., 1996; Wilson and Safe, 1998). In some instances, interspecies differences in metabolism or mechanism of action cause certain chemicals to induce cancer in rodents but not in humans. One such example is kidney cancer, attributable to the accumulation of a rat-specific protein (α_{2u}-globulin) in proximal tubular cells, produced in male rats chronically exposed to unleaded gasoline (Hard et al., 1993). There are a few compounds for which animal models have not been found. As discussed further on, skin and internal cancers caused in humans by excessive oral exposure to inorganic arsenic have not been reproduced during classic carcinogenicity studies in animals (ATSDR, 1993).

Human Challenge Studies Human challenge studies, or clinical exposure studies, are a useful approach for verifying findings from animal toxicology studies in humans and for establishing whether biotransformation pathways in the animal models represent those in exposed humans. Human challenge studies help to establish biomarkers of exposure. For reversible conditions, they can be useful for testing therapeutic options. Extreme caution must be exercised to ensure the safety of subjects. Idiosyncratic responses can cause a subject to be exceptionally sensitive. For inhalation studies, equipment malfunction can result in overexposure. In the past 20 years, there have been several serious injuries and fatalities associated with human challenge studies. These have been attributed to hypersensitivity reactions and generally used mock workplace simulations without rigorous control and monitoring of exposures, as is the current standard of practice.

Case Reports When new toxicants or new combinations of toxicants enter the workplace, a case or outbreak of cases can occur. These may be identified through workplace surveillance systems or through workers associating their disease with workplace exposures. These may end up being reported as case reports or case series. NIOSH has a Health Hazard Evaluation (HHE) program in place in which employees or their authorized representatives or employers at a job site can request an investigation to evaluate a potentially hazardous situation. This program issues HHE Reports to disseminate information regarding the hazard. NIOSH also publishes NIOSH Alerts, Criteria Documents, Special Occupational Hazard Reviews, Occupational Hazard Assessments, and Current Intelligence Bulletins. While useful for hazard identification, case reports and HHE Reports do not establish incidence or prevalence of diseases associated with an occupational hazard.

Epidemiology Studies Epidemiology studies help to unravel the associations between occupational diseases, exposures, and personal risk factors. Several types of epidemiologic studies are used to gather data on the association of workplace exposures with human disease. Cross-sectional studies compare disease prevalence or health status between groups of workers classified according to job title, work site, or exposure status. Cohort studies compare exposed workers versus unexposed workers either prospectively or retrospectively in order to associate the occurrence of disease with exposure. Since many occupational diseases have a long induction period or occur only rarely, prospective cohort studies may require a long time and need a large number of subjects to establish significant findings. Retrospective cohort studies can resolve the latency problem but require that relevant exposure data have been collected over time. Exposure misclassification is frequently a problem in retrospective studies. Case-control studies are useful for investigating rare diseases or diseases with long induction periods. As the name suggests, case-control studies compare workers with disease to workers without disease with regard to their exposure intensity, frequency, and duration, plus other postulated risk factors. In some instances where the exposure-disease relationship is not understood, it may be difficult to identify an appropriate control group

Animal Toxicology Testing for Establishing Acceptable Levels of Exposure

It is evident that certainty as to the complete safety of a chemical can never be obtained whatever the extent of toxicologic investigations performed on animals. Nevertheless, animal studies provide valuable data from which to estimate the level of exposure at which the risk of health impairment is acceptable. Guidelines and protocols for assessing experimentally the toxicologic hazards of chemicals have been formulated by various national and international agencies. These tests include local and systemic acute toxicity tests, tests of toxicity following repeated exposure, investigations of metabolism and mechanism of action, short-term tests for detecting potential mutagens and carcinogens, studies of effect on reproduction and of teratogenic activity, chronic studies to detect carcinogenesis and other long-term effects, interaction studies, tests for immunosuppression, and dermal and pulmonary hypersensitivity tests. The need for performing these testing protocols should be carefully evaluated for any occupational toxicant to which workers will be exposed. In selecting the studies most appropriate for safety evaluation the toxicologist should be guided by an understanding of the following:

- Physicochemical properties of the chemical
- Potential for the generation of toxic derivatives when the chemical is submitted to heat, pH changes, and UV light
- Conditions of use
- Type of exposure (continuous, intermittent, or incidental)
- Degree of exposure

Toxicologic information already available on other chemicals with similar chemical structure and reactive chemical groups can suggest potential hazards and reactivity.

Conclusions drawn from any toxicologic investigation are useful only if the composition and physical state of the tested preparation is known. This would include the nature and concentration of impurities or degradation products, speciation of inorganic compounds, characterization of physical properties for inhaled materials, and characterization of the vehicle (if any). Sensitive and specific methods of analysis of the chemical in solution, air, and biological material also should be available. The assessment of the toxicity of malathion in the 1970s illustrates this point. Malathion is an organophosphate insecticide normally with relatively low human toxicity. This pesticide was responsible for a 1976 episode of mass poisoning among malaria workers in Pakistan because the specific product contained impurities (mainly isomalathion) capable of inhibiting tissue and plasma carboxyesterases (Baker et al., 1978; Aldridge et al., 1979). The toxicity evaluation for malathion had not anticipated isomalathion coexposure.

The duration of tests necessary to establish an acceptable level for occupational exposure is primarily a function of the type of toxic action suspected. It is generally recognized that for systemically acting chemicals, subacute and short-term toxicity studies are usually insufficient for proposing OELs. Subacute and short-term toxicity tests are usually performed to find out whether the compound exhibits immunotoxic properties and cumulative characteristics. They also aid in selection of the doses for long-term-exposure studies and the kind of tests that may be most informative when applied during long-term exposures. A number of studies have drawn attention to the fact that the reproductive system may also be the target organ of industrial chemicals (e.g., glycol ethers, styrene, lead, dibromochloropropane). Thus, studies designed to evaluate reproductive effects and teratogenicity should also be considered during routine toxicologic testing of occupational toxicants.

Information derived from exposure routes similar to those sustained by workers is clearly most relevant. For airborne pollutants, inhalation exposure studies provide the basic data on which provisional OELs are based. Experimental methodology is certainly much more complicated for inhalation studies than for oral administration experiments and requires more specialized equipment and expertise (Thorne, 2000). For example, in the case of exposure to an aerosol, particle size distribution must be evaluated and the degree of retention in the respiratory tract of the animal species under study should be established. Ideally, particle size should be selected according to the deposition pattern of dry or liquid aerosols in the particular animal species used in order to represent human lung deposition with occupational exposures. Particle deposition and retention curves have been published for human, monkey, dog, guinea pig, rat, and mouse (Hsieh et al., 1999; Schlesinger, 1985). It also should be kept in mind that the concentration of the material in the air and the duration of exposure do not give a direct estimate of the dose, since retained dose is also dependent on the minute volume and the proportion of inhaled particles retained. Measurement of pulmonary dust retention following exposure to a radiolabeled or fluorescently tagged test aerosol should be performed prior to conducting acute, subchronic, or chronic studies. This allows one to assess deposition and determine whether the selected levels of exposure may overwhelm pulmonary clearance mechanisms (Lewis et al., 1989; Morrow, 1992).

The choice of what studies to perform using which routes of administration must be evaluated scientifically for each toxicant. Important considerations include its target sites and mechanism of action, metabolism, the nature of its adverse effects, and how workers are exposed to the toxicant. The morphologic, physiologic, and biological parameters that are usually evaluated, either at regular intervals in the course of the exposure period or at its termination, are described in Units 4 and 5 of this text. Knowledge of the absorption, distribution, biotransformation, and excretion of the chemical and its mechanism of action are of major interest. Investigations that can make use of specific physiologic or biochemical tests, based on knowledge of the principal target organ or function, produce highly valuable information and increase confidence in the OEL derived from them.

Worker Health Surveillance

The primary objective of occupational toxicology is to prevent the development of occupational diseases. The monitoring of exposures to toxicants in the workplace may play an important role in detecting excessive exposures before the occurrence of significant biological disturbances and health impairment. A scheme for biological monitoring of exposure and of early biological effects is possible only when sufficient toxicologic information has been gathered from animal studies on the mechanism of action and the metabolism of xenobiotics to which workers are exposed. When a new chemical is being used on a large scale, the careful clinical surveillance of workers and monitoring of workplaces should be instituted in order to address three aims: (1) to identify overexposure or adverse effects on the health of the workers and quickly intervene, (2) to evaluate the validity of a proposed occupational exposure limit derived from animal experiments, and (3) to test the validity of a proposed method for a biological monitoring.

Evaluation of the validity of the proposed OEL derived from animal experiments through workplace surveillance is the major aim, since "studies and observations on [humans] will always be the final basis for deciding whether [an OEL] set originally on the basis of tests on animals is, in fact, truly acceptable as one that will not produce any signs of intoxication" (Barnes, 1963). This means that sensitive clinical, biochemical, physiologic, or behavioral tests for detecting an adverse effect of a toxicant should ideally be performed on the workers concurrent with exposure assessment. It is helpful if human challenge studies or studies on workers can include the same biomarkers as used in prior animal studies. The occupational toxicologist cannot rely solely on the diagnostic tools used in clinical medicine, as they were established primarily to reveal advanced pathologic states and not to detect early adverse effects at a stage when they are still reversible. For example, the measurement of serum creatinine is still a widely used clinical test for assessing renal integrity; yet it is known that the glomerular filtration rate of the kidney must be reduced by more than 50 percent before serum creatinine rises significantly.

The main limitation of current OELs or BEIs is that some are based on limited experimental data or clinical studies in which only late effects have been investigated and correlated with past exposure. Furthermore, several BEIs are derived from the study of external-internal exposure relationships and not from relationships between internal dose and early adverse effects. The validity of an OEL is much stronger if it is based on the study of dose-response relationships in which the dose is expressed in terms of the cumulative target dose and the monitored effect reflects a critical biological event. However, it should be noted that for some chemicals and some adverse effects (e.g., induction of hypersensitivity and possibly genotoxic effects), the frequency of peak exposure may be more important for health risk assessment than the integrated dose. For example, long-term low-level exposures to commercial enzymes rarely induce sensitization. However, a single exposure to a high concentration can produce hypersensitivity and occupational asthma.

Epidemiologic studies designed to assess exposure-response relationships can be carried out by using a variety of variables for assessing the exposure and health changes. Exposure may be characterized using a surrogate measure such as job classification, seniority, or via questionnaire or more directly through ambient or personal exposure monitoring or measurement of the internalized dose. Adverse effects may be expressed in terms of mortality, incidence or prevalence of clinical disease, irreversible or reversible functional changes, or critical biological changes. It is evident that the assessment of the health risk resulting from exposure will have more validity if it results from exposure-response studies in which both the target dose and the critical biological changes are monitored. Of course, the use of such parameters requires knowledge of the fate of the chemical in the organism and its mechanism of action. However, this approach is more expensive than simpler epidemiologic study designs and may result in a trade-off between sophistication and study sample size.

Because early biomarkers of effect are subtle and individual variations exist in the response to a chemical insult, results generally require a statistical comparison between a group of exposed workers and a similar group of workers without the exposure of interest. The group of unexposed workers should be matched on variables such as age, race, gender, socioeconomic status, and smoking habits. The importance of selecting a control group that is well matched with the exposed group and that undergoes the same standardized clinical, biological, or physiologic evaluation at the same time as the exposed group must be emphasized. Comparison with the general population is not valid because an employed population is a highly selected group and may have a higher degree of physical fitness. Since occupational epidemiologic studies often last for several years, all methods of investigation—such as questionnaires, instrumentation, and analytic techniques—must be validated and standardized before the start of the study. The number of subjects under study should be chosen based on a sample size calculation to be able to detect a difference between exposed and unexposed subjects (should there be a difference) and should take into account labor turnover and those declining participation in any aspects of the study. If exposures are high enough to induce an adverse effect, it is expected that these studies may permit establishment of the relationship between integrated exposure (intensity $\times$ time) and frequency of abnormal results and, consequently, a redefinition of the OEL.

In cases where a surveillance program was not instituted before the introduction of a new chemical, it is more difficult to establish the efficacy of the OEL. In this situation, evaluation depends on retrospective cohort studies or case-control studies or on cross-sectional studies on workers who have already sustained exposure. Evaluation of a "no observed adverse effect level" (NOAEL) is difficult because information on past exposures is often incomplete and frank effects are generally the focus of retrospective or case-control studies. Provided that a satisfactory assessment of past exposure is possible, cross-sectional studies that rely on preclinical signs of toxicity may, to a certain extent, overcome these difficulties. Whether or not clinical investigations are planned from the introduction of a new chemical or process, it is essential to keep standardized records of occupational histories and exposure. The need may arise for mortality or case history studies in order to answer an urgent question on a suspected risk.

Case reports of isolated overexposures resulting from specific incidents such as containment breaches, chemical spills, vessel or pipe ruptures can provide useful information. Although such observations are usually not helpful for determining the NOAEL in humans, they may indicate whether human symptomatology is similar to that found in animals and may suggest functional or biological tests that might prove useful for routine monitoring of exposed workers.

Human challenge studies with occupational toxicants are usually designed to answer very specific questions regarding rates of uptake, biotransformation pathways, the time course of metabolite excretion during and after exposure, evaluation of the threshold concentration for sensory responses (odor, irritation of the nasal mucosa, etc.), and acute effects of toxicant exposure on perception, vigilance, and function. For ethical reasons, such studies can be undertaken only when the same results cannot be obtained through other means and under circumstances in which the risk for volunteers can reasonably be estimated as negligible.

In most cases, studies on human subjects encompass the collection of samples from the subjects or data obtained through interaction with the subjects. Since this often includes identifiable private information, subjects are rightfully concerned about issues of confidentiality. The guiding principle is that the value of the study does not outweigh the rights of the subjects. U.S. and international law requires that subjects must always have the right to refuse participation and investigators must have written consent from a duly informed volunteer obtained without coercion.

Linkage of Animal Studies and Epidemiologic Studies

In the field of occupational toxicology, perhaps more than in other areas of toxicology, close cooperation between those conducting animal studies and studies of workers is essential for examining risks associated with overexposure to chemicals and other toxicants. A few examples will serve to illustrate the complementarity of these disciplines.

Several occupational carcinogens have been identified clearly through combined epidemiologic and experimental approaches (IARC, 1987). For example, the carcinogenicity of vinyl chloride was first demonstrated in rats (Viola et al., 1971), and a few years later, epidemiologic studies confirmed the same carcinogenic risk for humans (Creech and Johnson, 1974; Monson et al., 1974). This observation stimulated several investigations on the metabolism of vinyl chloride in animals and on its mutagenic activity in in vitro systems. Identification of vinyl chloride metabolites led to the conclusion that there is microsomal oxidation leading to the formation of an epoxide derivative, which acts as a proximate carcinogen (ATSDR, 1997). This finding triggered further studies on the biotransformation of structurally related halogenated ethylenes, such as vinyl bromide, vinylidene chloride, 1,2-dichloroethene, trichloroethylene, perchloroethylene (Bonse et al., 1975; Uehleke et al., 1977; Dekant et al., 1987). Comparison of their oncogenic activity in relation to their metabolism suggested that an interplay between the stability and reactivity in reaching the DNA target and reacting with it after being formed would determine their genotoxic risk (Bolt, 1984). It is now recognized that vinyl chloride produces DNA adducts by inducing the formation of an additional ring in adenine and cytosine on DNA molecules (Birner et al., 1993; NTP, 2000).

1,3-Butadiene is a known human carcinogen that is used in the manufacture of synthetic rubber products. Experimental studies in rats and mice demonstrated carcinogenicity, with mice being particularly sensitive (NTP, 2000). Subsequent to these findings 1,3-butadiene was shown to follow the same metabolic pathway in humans as in rats and mice forming mutagenic and carcinogenic epoxides. That led to cohort and case-control studies establishing 1,3-butadiene as a human carcinogen (NTP, 2000). Recent studies have considered the relative importance of the metabolic pathway leading to formation of the reactive metabolite 1,2-epoxy-3-butene, which reacts with hemoglobin to form 1- and 2-hydroxy-3-butenyl valine adducts (MHBVal) and with DNA to form guanine adducts. Under the assumption of a genotoxic mechanism and cross-species comparisons of hemoglobin and DNA binding, these data facilitate a more informed cancer risk assessment. This analysis suggests that for exposures to 1,3-butadiene, the cancer risk is lower for humans than rats or mice on an equivalent dose basis (Van Sittert et al., 2000). Furthermore, this work illustrates that the measurement of the MHBVal adducts is a sensitive method for monitoring 1,3-butadiene metabolism via the epoxide-forming pathway in workers.

In 1973, an outbreak of peripheral neuropathy occurred in workers exposed to the solvent methyl butyl ketone (MBK) (McDonough, 1974; Allen et al., 1975). The same lesion was reproduced in animals (Mendell et al., 1974; Spencer et al., 1975). Biotransformation studies were then undertaken in rats and guinea pigs, and some MBK metabolites (2,5-hexanedione, 5-hydroxy-2-hexanone) were also found to possess neurotoxic activity (Spencer and Schaumburg, 1975; DiVincenzo et al., 1976; DiVincenzo et al., 1977). Similar oxidation products are formed from *n*-hexane, the neurotoxicity of which is probably due to the same active metabolite as that produced from MBK. Since methyl isobutyl ketone and methyl ethyl ketone cannot give rise to 2,5-hexanedione, they were suggested as replacement solvents.

These examples demonstrate that studies of the metabolic handling of occupational toxicants in animals are instrumental in the characterization of reactive intermediates and may suggest unsuspected risks or indicate new methods of biological monitoring. Conversely, clinical observations on workers may stimulate studies of the metabolism or the mechanism of toxicity of a toxicant in animals, thereby revealing the health significance of a biological disturbance.

Arsenic is one of the very few compounds for which there are limited data of predictive value from animal studies to human health effects. Arsenic has been used as a medicine since the time of Hippocrates. Initially used to treat ulcers, arsenicals achieved notoriety as medicinals for a wide variety of ailments, and then, in the first half of the twentieth century, for the treatment of syphilis and parasites. Many foods and beverages contaminated with arsenic have been associated with accidental and intentional poisonings. Inorganic pentavalent arsenic (arsenate) is readily absorbed across tissues and converted to the trivalent form (arsenite). This is then methylated to form monomethylarsenic acid and dimethylarsenic acid (NRC, 1999). These are primarily transported in the blood bound to sulfhydryl groups in proteins. The half-life in humans for arsenic compounds is 2 to 4 days and the major excretion is via the urine (Nriagu, 1994). These organic arsenicals have lower toxicity than the inorganic arsenic compounds.

Inorganic arsenic was first noted as a human carcinogen by Hutchinson in 1887 (Hutchinson, 1887). Epidemiologic studies led to classification of arsenic by the International Agency for Research on Cancer (IARC) as a skin and lung carcinogen in 1980 (IARC, 1980). Since then studies among occupationally exposed populations and populations with high arsenic in their drinking water have shown conclusively that arsenic causes human cancers of the skin, lung, bladder, kidney, liver, nasal tissue, and prostate. There is also evidence for arsenic-associated cutaneous effects, cardiovascular and cerebrovascular disease, diabetes mellitus, and adverse reproductive outcomes (EPA, 2000).

A large number of carefully executed cancer bioassays in mice, rats, beagles, and monkeys have been performed using sodium arsenate, sodium arsenite, lead arsenite, arsenic trioxide, and dimethylarsinic acid. These studies have been uniformly negative. A number of subsequent studies that tested for tumor-promotion activity following dosing with recognized tumor initiators also yielded negative results. Negative results in animal studies in the face of unquestionable oncogenic activity in humans suggest that inorganic arsenic may follow a nongenotoxic mode of action (NRC, 1999).

The examples above demonstrate that the occupational toxicologist cannot rely solely on animal or epidemiologic studies. A combined approach is necessary in order to identify, elucidate, and prioritize risks and to develop interventions and techniques for worker health surveillance.

EXPOSURE MONITORING

Two important applications of occupational toxicologic investigations are compared below: environmental monitoring and biological monitoring. As described above under "Occupational Health Standards," both are important in worker health surveillance and are essential elements of toxicology studies with dosing via the inhalation or dermal routes.

Environmental Monitoring for Exposure Assessment

An important objective of experimental and clinical investigations in occupational toxicology is the proposal of safe levels of exposure. It is evident that with the accumulation of new information on the toxicity of industrial chemicals, OELs must be reevaluated at regular intervals. It should also be made clear that these levels may not protect everyone and should not supplant close medical surveillance of workers. Various private and official institutions regularly review the toxicologic information on chemicals in order to propose or update permissible levels of exposure. These include governmental organizations worldwide and trade organizations such as the ACGIH and the European Centre for Ecotoxicity and Toxicology of Chemicals (ECETOC). A critical element of establishing OELs is the accurate and uniform assessment of exposure. Methodology for exposure assessment must be specifically tailored to the agent under study and the environment in which it appears. To assess airborne exposures for compliance purposes, personal samples taken in the breathing zone are generally used. In a few specific environments, area samples form the basis of an exposure standard (e.g. the standard for exposure to raw cotton dust specifies use of the vertical elutriator or an equivalent method). Occupational environmental surveys may use area sampling to determine areas with higher or lower toxicant concentrations. However, concentrations determined from personal samples typically exceed area concentrations, depending on the work practices and environmental controls. For example, geometric mean concentrations of inhalable dust assessed from 159 personal samples in dairy barns were 1.78 mg/m^3, compared with 0.74 mg/m^3 for 252 area samples collected simultaneously in two locations in the same barns (Kullman et al., 1998). Thus, in this environment, area sampling alone would underestimate personal exposures by a factor of 2.4.

Repeated random sampling is theoretically the best approach to developing unbiased measures of exposure. However, this is rarely the approach that is taken. Variability in exposure, especially variability over time, is usually large; therefore a considerable number of repeated measurements are needed to obtain an accurate proxy of the true exposure. When the number of repeats is insufficient, the slope of the exposure-response relationship will be biased, usually leading to considerable underestimation of the relationship (Heederik and Attfield, 2000). Recent studies have demonstrated that group-based approaches are more efficient in terms of measurement effort to obtain a desired level of accuracy. In a group-based approach, workers are grouped by job title or task performed and the group mean is used as the average exposure for each worker (Kromhout et al., 1996). Further statistical modeling of the exposure data can reduce problems of bias and large temporal and spatial variability (Preller et al., 1995; Tielemans et al., 1998). While this approach is gaining acceptance among occupational epidemiologists for evaluating exposure-response data and assessing risks, it is not generally used for compliance monitoring.

Although one cannot assess dose directly through exposure monitoring, it has distinct advantages over biomonitoring. Exposure monitoring allows one to quantify exposure by route through selective air monitoring in the breathing zone of the worker and dermal dosimetry using absorptive material affixed to the workers' skin or clothing. Biomonitoring cannot provide route-specific exposure data. Environmental monitoring techniques are generally less expensive and less invasive than techniques involving the collection and analysis of biological samples such as blood or urine. Thus, a larger population of workers can be studied for the same amount of money. Workers are accustomed to wearing personal samplers for exposure assessment and generally quite willing to do so. However, they are often unwilling to give a blood or urine sample, fearing that the sample will be surreptitiously used for drug testing, DNA testing, or experimentation. Some express fear that they will contract a serious infectious disease during the process of giving a blood sample. Another benefit of air sampling in the workplace is that spatial, temporal, and work practice associations can be established and can suggest better interventions and engineering controls. Finally, analytic interferences and variabilities are generally lower with environmental samples than with biological samples.

A fully validated sampling and analysis method requires specification of the sampling methods, sample duration, sample handling, and storage procedures; the analytic method and measurement technique; the range, precision, accuracy, bias, and limits of detection; quality assurance issues; and known interferences. It is also important to document intralaboratory and interlaboratory variability. Once a standard method is established, it must be followed in every detail in order to assure consistency of results.

The development of accurate and precise analytic methods for environmental assessment is an ongoing effort. NIOSH publishes the extensive *NIOSH Manual of Analytical Methods* (Casinelli and O'Connor, 1994), and these are widely used. The American Society for Testing Materials (ASTM) has also established a rigorous system for the establishment of methods. It generally requires 5 or more years to establish a new ASTM method for exposure assessment. The International Organization for Standardization (ISO) is a global federation of national standards bodies with over 125 member countries. The subcommittee on workplace atmospheres is administered by the American National Standards Institute (ANSI). ISO has completed harmonization on a number of air sampling methods—for example, the determination of the number concentration of airborne inorganic fibers by phase contrast optical microscopy. The American Industrial Hygiene Association (AIHA) and the ACGIH publish compilations with descriptions of analytic devices and methodology (Cohen and Hering, 1995; DiNardi, 1997). Methods have also been developed for bioaerosol exposure assessment, and these have been recently reviewed (Eduard and Heederik, 1998; Heederik et al., 2001; Thorne and Heederik, 1999a; Willeke and Macher, 1999).

Biological Monitoring for Exposure Assessment

Biological monitoring of exposure assesses health risk through the evaluation of the internal dose. Depending on the chemical and the analyzed biological parameter, the term *internal dose* may have different meanings. A biological parameter may reflect the amount of chemical absorbed shortly before sampling, as with the concentration of a solvent in the alveolar air or in the blood during the workshift. It may reflect exposure during the preceding day, as with the measurement of a metabolite in blood or urine collected 16 h after the end of exposure. For toxicants with a long biological half-life, the measured parameter may reflect exposure accumulated over a period of weeks. *Internal dose* may refer to the amount of chemical stored in one or in several body compartments or in the whole body (*the body burden*).

When biological measurements are available to assess the internal dose, the approach offers important advantages over monitoring the air of the workplace. Its greatest advantage is that the biological parameter of exposure is more directly related to the adverse health effects than environmental measurements. Therefore, it may offer a better estimate of the risk than can be determined from ambient monitoring. Biological monitoring accounts for uptake by all exposure routes. Many industrial chemicals can enter the organism by absorption through the skin or the gastrointestinal tract as well as the lung. For example, some solvents (e.g., dimethylformamide) and many pesticide formulations exhibit substantial exposure via the dermal route. In these situations, exposures determined through monitoring airborne concentrations underestimate true exposure.

Several factors can influence uptake. Personal hygiene habits vary from one person to another, and there is some degree of individual variation in the absorption rate of a chemical through the lungs, skin, or gastrointestinal tract. Use of size-selective air sampling to determine the inhalable or respirable fraction can strengthen the exposure estimate. However, biological factors such as ventilatory parameters can affect the strength of such a correlation. For example, increased workload can markedly increase the respiratory uptake of an airborne toxicant. Because of its ability to encompass and evaluate the overall exposure (whatever the route of entry), biological monitoring also can be used to test the overall efficacy of personal protective equipment such as respirators, gloves, or barrier creams. Another consideration with biological monitoring is the fact that the nonoccupational exposures (hobbies, residential exposures, dietary habits, smoking, second jobs) also may be expressed in the biological level. The organism integrates the total external (environmental and occupational) exposure into one internal load. While this is beneficial for worker health and safety, it may be confounding in epidemiologic studies or compliance monitoring.

The value of biological monitoring is heightened when the relationships between external exposure, internal dose, and adverse effects are established. Normally, biological monitoring of exposure cannot be used for assessing exposure to substances that exhibit their toxic effects at the sites of first contact and are poorly absorbed. Examples include dermally corrosive compounds and primary lung irritants. In this situation, the only useful relationship is that between external exposure and the intensity of the local effects.

Relationships between air monitoring and biological monitoring may be modified by factors that influence the fate of an occupational toxicant in vivo. Metabolic interactions can occur when workers are exposed simultaneously to chemicals that are biotransformed through identical pathways. Exposure to chemicals that modify the activity of the biotransformation enzymes (e.g., microsomal enzyme inducers or inhibitors) may also influence the fate of another compound. Furthermore, metabolic interferences may occur between occupational toxicants and alcohol, tobacco, food additives, prescription drugs, natural product remedies, or recreational drugs. Changes in any of several biological variables (weight, body mass, pregnancy, diseases, immune status, etc.) also may modify the metabolism of an occupational chemical. These factors have to be taken into consideration when the results of biological exposure tests are interpreted. Whatever the parameter measured, whether it is the substance itself, its metabolite, or an early biomarker of effect, the test must be sufficiently sensitive and specific to be of practical value.

Some chemicals have a long biological half-life in various body compartments (e.g., blood or urine), and the time of sampling may not be critical. For other chemicals, the time of sampling is critical because, following exposure, the compounds or their metabolites may be rapidly eliminated from the organism. In these cases, the biological sample is usually collected during exposure, at the end of the exposure period, or sometimes just before the next work shift. When biological monitoring consists of the sampling and analysis of urine, it is usually performed in "spot" specimens, because routine collection of 24-h samples from workers is impractical. It is standard practice to correct the results for the dilution of the urine by expressing the results per gram of creatinine. Analyses performed on very dilute urine samples are not reliable. The World Health Organization has specified acceptable limits for urine specimens of between 0.3 and 3.0 g/L creatinine (or 1.010 to 1.030 specific gravity) (ACGIH, 2000). When the large interindividual variability or high "background" level of the biological parameter selected makes the interpretation of a single measurement difficult, it is sometimes useful to analyze biological material collected before and after the exposure period. The change in the biological parameter specifically due to exposure can sometimes be better assessed by this method.

Environmental monitoring plays an important role for evaluating and preventing excessive exposure to toxicants in the workplace. However, the prevention of acute toxic effects on the respi-

Table 33-7
Control Approaches for Occupational Inhalation Hazards

Change the process to use or produce less hazardous compounds.
Automate and enclose the process to isolate the compounds.
Incorporate administrative and work practice controls to reduce duration or intensity of exposure.
Install or upgrade local exhaust systems and dilution exhaust.
Institute a comprehensive program for personal protective equipment use where necessary.

ratory tract, skin, or eye mucosa can only be achieved by keeping the concentration of the irritant substance below a certain level or eliminating exposure. Local acute effects of chemicals do not lend themselves to a biological surveillance program. Likewise, biological monitoring is usually not indicated for detecting peak exposure to dangerous chemicals such as arsine (AsH_3), carbon monoxide, or prussic acid (HCN). Furthermore, identification of emission sources and the evaluation of the efficiency of engineering control measures are usually best performed by ambient air analysis. Table 33-7 lists the approaches most useful for controlling inhalation exposures in the workplace. It should be emphasized that process changes and application of engineering controls are preferable to reliance on personal protective equipment.

In summary, environmental and biological monitoring should not be regarded as opposites but as complementary elements an occupational health and safety program. They should be integrated as much as possible to ensure low levels of contaminants and optimal health for workers.

CONCLUSION

The working environment will always present the risk of overexposure of workers to various toxicants. Recognition of these risks should not wait until epidemiologic studies have defined hazardous levels. A combined experimental, clinical, and epidemiologic approach is the most effective for evaluating the potential risks. One can then promulgate scientifically based occupational health standards, apply effective workplace controls to ensure adherence to those standards, and institute worker health surveillance programs to identify unexpected effects in susceptible individuals.

REFERENCES

Abnet CC, Tanguay RL, Heideman W, Peterson RE: Transactivation activity of human, zebrafish, and rainbow trout aryl hydrocarbon receptors expressed in COS-7 cells: Greater insight into species differences in toxic potency of polychlorinated dibenzo-*p*-dioxin, dibenzofuran, and biphenyl congeners. *Toxicol Appl Pharmacol* 159(1):41–51, 1999.

ACGIH: *2000 TLVs and BEIs: Threshold Limit Values for Chemical Substances and Physical Agents and Biological Exposure Indices.* Cincinnati, OH: American Conference of Governmental Industrial Hygienists, 2000; pp 3–14 and 91–95.

Aldridge WN, Miles JM, Mount DL, Verschoyle RD: The toxicological properties of impurities in malathion. *Arch Toxicol* 42:95–106, 1979.

Allen N, Mendell JR, Billmaier DJ, et al: Toxic polyneuropathy due to methyl n-butylketone. *Arch Neurol* 32:209–218, 1975.

ATSDR (Agency for Toxic Substances and Disease Registry): *Toxicological Profile for Arsenic.* Atlanta: U.S. Department of Health and Human Services, 1993.

ATSDR (Agency for Toxic Substances and Disease Registry): *Toxicological Profile for Vinyl Chloride.* Atlanta: U.S. Department of Health and Human Services, 1997.

Baker EL, Zack M, Miles JV, et al: Epidemic malathion poisoning in Pakistan malaria workers. *Lancet* 1:31–33, 1978.

Barnes JM: The basis for establishing and fixing maximum allowable concentrations. *Trans Assoc Ind Med Off* 13:74–76, 1963.

Bason M, Lammintausta K, Maibach HI: Irritant dermatitis (irritation), in Marzulli FN and Maibach HI (eds): *Dermatotoxicology,* 4th ed. New York: Hemisphere, 1991, pp 223–252.

Becklake MR, Malo J-L, Chan-Yeung M: Epidemiological approaches in occupational asthma, in Bernstein IL et al (eds) *Asthma in the Workplace,* 2d ed. New York:, Marcel Dekker, 1999, pp 27–66.

Bernstein IL, Bernstein DI, Chan-Yeung M, Malo J-L: Definition and classification of asthma, in Bernstein IL et al (eds): *Asthma in the Workplace,* 2d ed. New York: Marcel Dekker, 1999, pp 1–3.

Birner G, Vamvakas S, Dekant W, Henschler D: Nephrotoxic and genotoxic *N*-acetyl-*S*-dichlorovinyl-L-cysteine is a urinary metabolite after occupational 1,1,2-trichloroethylene exposure in humans: Implications for the risk of trichloroethene exposure. *Environ Health Perspect* 99:281–284, 1993.

Bolt HN: Metabolism of genotoxic agents: Halogenated hydrocarbons, in Berlin A, Draper M, Hemminki K, Vainio H (eds): *Monitoring Human Exposure to Carcinogenic and Mutagenic Agents.* No. 59. Lyons, France: International Agency for Research on Cancer, 1984, pp 63–72.

Bonse G, Urban T, Reichert D, Henschler D: Chemical reactivity, metabolic oxirane formation and biological reactivity of chlorinated ethylenes in the isolated perfused rat liver preparation. *Biochem Pharmacol* 24:1829–1834, 1975.

Cartier A, Malo J-L, Forest F, et al: Occupational asthma in snow crab-processing workers. *J Allergy Clin Immunol* 74:261–269, 1984.

Casinelli ME, O'Connor PF (eds): *NIOSH Manual of Analytical Methods* (NMAM), 4th ed. DHHS (NIOSH) Publication 94–113. Washington, DC: National Institute for Occupational Safety and Health, 1994.

Chan-Yeung M, Vedal S, Kus J, et al: Symptoms, pulmonary function and bronchial hyperactivity in western red cedar workers compared with those in office workers. *Am Rev Respir Dis* 130:1038–1041, 1984.

Cohen BS, Hering SV (eds): *Air Sampling Instruments for Evaluation of Atmospheric Contaminants,* 8th ed. Cincinnati, OH: American Conference of Governmental Industrial Hygienists, 1995.

Creech JL, Johnson HM: Angiosarcoma of the liver in the manufacture of polyvinylchloride. *J Occup Med* 16:150–151, 1974.

Cullinan P, Lowson D, Nieuwenhuijsen MJ, et al: Work related symptoms, sensitisation, and estimated exposure in workers not previously exposed to laboratory rats. *Occup Environ Med* 51:589–592, 1994.

Dekant W, Martens G, Vamvakas S, et al: Bioactivation of tetrachloroethylene. *Drug Metab Dispos* 15:702–709, 1987.

Desjardins A, Malo JL, L'Archevêque J, et al: Occupational IgE-mediated sensitization and asthma due to clam and shrimp. *J Allergy Clin Immunol* 96:608–617, 1995.

DiNardi SR (ed.): *The Occupational Environment—Its Evaluation and Control.* Fairfax, VA: American Industrial Hygiene Association, 1997.

DiVincenzo GD, Hamilton ML, Kaplan CJ, Dedinas J: Metabolic fate and disposition of ^{14}C-labeled methyl *n*-butyl ketone in the rat. *Toxicol Appl Pharmacol* 41:547–560, 1977.

DiVincenzo GD, Kaplan CJ, Dedinas J: Characterization of the metabolites of methyl-*n*-butyl ketone, methyl iso-butyl ketone, and methyl ethyl ketone in guinea pig serum and their clearance. *Toxicol Appl Pharmacol* 36:511–522, 1976.

Donham KJ, Thorne PS: Agents in organic dusts: Criteria for a causal relationship. *Am J Ind Med* 25:33–39, 1994.

Douwes J, Thorne PS, Pearce N, Heederik D: Biological agents—recognition, in Perkins JL (ed): *Modern Industrial Hygiene:* Vol III. *Biological Aspects.* Cincinnati, OH: American Conference of Governmental Industrial Hygienists, 2001. In press.

Duchaine C, Meriaux A, Thorne PS, Cormier Y: Assessment of particulates and bioaerosols in Eastern Canadian sawmills. *Am Ind Hyg Assoc J* 61:727–732, 2000.

Eduard W, Heederik D: Methods for quantitative assessment of airborne levels of noninfectious microorganisms in highly contaminated work environments. *Am Ind Hyg Assoc J* 59:113–127, 1998.

Eduard W, Sandven P, Levy F: Relationships between exposure to spores from *Rhizopus microsporus* and *Paecilomyces variotii* and serum IgG antibodies in wood trimmers. *Int Arch Allergy Immunol* 97:274–282, 1992.

EPA. 40 CFR Parts 141 and 142, National primary drinking water regulations; arsenic and clarifications to compliance and new source contaminants monitoring; proposed rule. *Fed Reg* 65(121):38888–38983, 2000.

European Union: Employment rates report 1998 Employment performance in the member states. http://europa.eu.int/comm/employment social/empl&est/empL99/rates en.pd f, pp. 1–31, 1998.

Flindt, MHL: Pulmonary disease due to inhalation of derivatives of *Bacillus subtilis* containing proteolytic enzyme. *Lancet* 1:1177, 1969.

Fuortes LJ, Weih LA, Jones M, et al: Epidemiologic assessment of laboratory animal allergy among university employees. *Am J Ind Med* 29:67–74, 1996.

Fuortes LJ, Weih L, Pomrehn P, et al: Prospective epidemiologic evaluation of laboratory animal allergy among university employees. *Am J Ind Med* 32:665–669, 1997.

GAO/HEHS: Child *Labor in Agriculture—Changes Needed to Better Protect Health and Educational Opportunities*. GAO/HEHS-98-193. Washington, DC: U.S. General Accounting Office, 1998, pp 1–90.

Glass, WI, Power P, Burt R, et al: Work-related respiratory symptoms and lung function in New Zealand mussel openers. *Am J Ind Med* 34:163–168, 1998.

Halpin DMG, Graneek BJ, Lacey J, et al: Respiratory symptoms, immunological responses, and aeroallergen concentrations at sawmills. *Occup Environ Med* 51:165–172, 1994.

Hard GC, Rodgers IS, Baetcke KP, et al: Hazard evaluation of chemicals that cause accumulation of α_{2u}-globulin, hyaline droplet nephropathy, and tubule neoplasia in the kidneys of male rats. *Environ Health Perspect* 99:313–349, 1993.

Heederik D, Attfield M. Characterization of dust exposure for the study of chronic occupational lung disease: A comparison of different exposure assessment strategies. *Am J Epidemiol* 151(10):982–990, 2000.

Heederik D, Thorne PS, Douwes J: Monitoring and evaluation of bioaerosol exposure, in Perkins JL (ed): *Modern Industrial Hygiene:* Vol III. *Biological Aspects.* Cincinnati, OH: American Conference of Governmental Industrial Hygienists, 2001. In press.

Hollander A, Heederik D, Doekes G: Respiratory allergy to rats: exposure—response relationships in laboratory animal workers. *Am J Respir Crit Care Med* 155:562–567, 1997.

Houba R, Heederik DJ, Doekes G, van Run PE: Exposure-sensitization relationship for alpha-amylase in the baking industry. *Am J Respir Crit Care Med* 154:130–136, 1996.

Hsieh TH, Yu CP, Oberdorster G: Deposition and clearance models of Ni compounds in the mouse lung and comparisons with the rat models. *Aerosol Sci Technol* 31:358–372, 1999.

Hutchinson J: Arsenic cancer. *Br Med J* 2:1280–1281, 1887.

IARC (International Agency for Research on Cancer): *IARC Monographs on the Evaluation of Carcinogenic Risks to Humans*. Suppl 7. Lyons, France: IARC, 1987.

IARC: *Metals and metallic compounds*. IARC Monographs on the Evaluation of Carcinogenic Risks to Humans, Vol 23. Lyon, France: International Agency for Research on Cancer, 1980.

Kromhout H, Tielemans E, Preller L, Heederik D: Estimates of individual dose from current measurements of exposure. *Occup Hyg* 3:23–39, 1996.

Kullman GJ, Thorne PS, Waldron PF, et al: Organic dust exposures from work in dairy barns. *Am Ind Hyg Assoc J* 59:403–413, 1998.

Lewis TR, Morrow PE, McClellan RO, et al.: Establishing aerosol exposure concentrations for inhalation toxicity studies. *Toxicol Appl Pharmacol* 99:377–383, 1989.

McDonough JR: Possible neuropathy from methyl-*n*-butyl ketone. *N Engl J Med* 290:695, 1974.

Mendell JR, Saida K, Ganasia MF, et al: Toxic polyneuropathy produced by methyl-*n*-butyl ketone. *Science* 185:787–789, 1974.

Michel O, Kips J, Duchateau J, et al: Severity of asthma is related to endotoxin in house dust. *Am J Respir Crit Care Med* 154:1641–1646, 1996.

Monson RR, Peters JM, Johnson MN: Proportional mortality among vinylchloride workers. *Lancet* 2(7877):397–398, 1974.

Morrow, PE: Contemporary issues in toxicology: Dust overloading of the lungs: Update and appraisal. *Toxicol Appl Pharmacol* 113:1–12, 1992.

NIH-99-4495: *Corrositex: An in Vitro Test Method for Assessing Dermal Corrosivity Potential of Chemicals*. NIH-99-4495. Washington, DC: National Toxicology Program, 1999, pp 1–236.

NIOSH: *Work-Related Lung Disease Surveillance Report*. Number 2000-105. Washington, DC: Department of Health and Human Services (NIOSH), 2000.

NRC (National Research Council): *Arsenic in Drinking Water*. Washington, DC: National Academy Press, 1999, pp 1–200.

Nriagu JO: *Arsenic in the Environment:* Part II: *Human Health Effects and Ecosystem Effects*. New York: Wiley. 1994, pp 1–91.

NTP (National Toxicology Program): *Ninth Report on Carcinogens*. Research Triangle Park, NC: National Toxicology Program, U.S. Department of Health and Human Services, 2000.

Pepys J, Pickering CAC, Breslin ABX, Terry DJ: Asthma due to inhaled chemical agents—Toluene di-isocyanate. *Clin Allergy* 2:225–236, 1972a.

Pepys J, Pickering CAC, Hughes EG: Asthma due to inhaled chemical agents—complex salts of platinum. *Clin Allergy* 2:391–396, 1972b.

Preller L, Kromhout H, Heederik D, Tielen MJM: Modeling long-term average exposure in occupational exposure-response analysis. *Scand J Work Environ Health* 21:504–512, 1995.

Sarlo K, Parris JS, Clark ED, et al: Influence of MHC background on the antibody response to detergent enzymes in the mouse intranasal test. *Toxicol Sci* 58:299–305, 2000.

Schenker MB, Christiani D, Cormier Y, et al: Respiratory health hazards in agriculture. *Am J Respir Crit Care Med* Suppl 158(pt 2):S1–S76, 1998.

Schlesinger RB: Comparative deposition of inhaled aerosols in experimental animals and humans: A review. *J Toxicol Environ Health* 15:197–214, 1985.

Schwartz DA, Thorne PS, Jagielo PJ, et al: Endotoxin responsiveness and grain dust–induced inflammation in the lower respiratory tract. *Am J Physiol* 267:L609–L617, 1994.

Schwartz DA, Thorne PS, Yagla SJ, et al: The role of endotoxin in grain dust–induced lung disease. *Am J Respir Crit Care Med* 152:603–608, 1995.

Spencer PS, Schaumburg HH: Experimental neuropathy produced by 2,5-hexanedione A major metabolite of the neurotoxic industrial solvent methyl-*n*-butyl ketone. *J Neurol Neurosurg Psychiatry* 38:771–775, 1975.

Spencer PS, Schaumburg HH, Raleigh RL, Terhaar CJ: Nervous system degeneration produced by the industrial solvent methyl-*n*-butyl ketone. *Arch Neurol* 32:219–222, 1975.

Thorne PS, Heederik D: Assessment methods for bioaerosols, in Salthammer T (ed): *Organic Indoor Air Pollutants—Occurrence, Measurement, Evaluation*. Weinheim, Germany: Wiley/VCH, 1999a; pp 85–103.

Thorne PS, Heederik D: Indoor bioaerosols—Sources and characteristics, in Salthammer T (ed): *Organic Indoor Air Pollutants—Occurrence, Measurement, Evaluation*. Weinheim, Germany: Wiley/VCH, 1999b; pp 275–288.

Thorne PS: Inhalation toxicology models of endotoxin- and bioaerosol-induced inflammation. *Toxicology* 152:13–23, 2000.

Thorne PS, Hillebrand J, Magreni C, et al: Experimental sensitization to subtilisin: I. Production of immediate and late-onset pulmonary reactions. *Toxicol Appl Pharmacol* 86:112–123, 1986.

Tielemans E, Kupper LL, Kromhout H, et al: Individual-based and group-based occupational exposure assessment: Some equations to evaluate different strategies. *Ann Occup Hyg* 42(2):115–119, 1998.

Uehleke H, Tabarelli-Poplawski S, Bonse G, Henschler D: Spectral evidence for 2,2,3-trichloro-oxirane formation during microsomal trichloroethylene oxidation. *Arch Toxicol* 37:95–105, 1977.

USDL (United States Department of Labor): *Career Guide to Industries: Agricultural Production*. 2000–01 ed. Washington, DC: U.S. Department of Labor, Bureau of Labor Statistics, http://www.bls.gov/oco/cg/cgs001.htm, 2000a.

USDL (United States Department of Labor): *The Employment Situation: April 2000*. USDL 00-126. U.S. Department of Labor, Bureau of Labor Statistics 2000b, pp 1–20.

van Sittert NJ, Megens HJJJ, Watson WP, Boogaard PJ: Biomarkers of exposure to 1,3-butadiene as a basis for cancer risk assessment. *Toxicol Sci* 56:189–202, 2000.

Venables KM, Dally MB, Nunn AJ, et al: Smoking and occupational allergy in workers in a platinum refinery. *Br Med J* 299:939–942, 1989.

Venables KM, Topping MD, Howe W, et al: Interaction of smoking and atopy in producing specific IgE antibody against a hapten protein conjugate. *Br Med J* 290:201–204, 1985.

Viola PL, Bigotti A, Caputo A: Oncogenic response of rat skin, lungs, and bones to vinyl chloride. *Cancer Res* 31:516–522, 1971.

Weill H, Salvaggio JE, Neilson A, et al: Respiratory effects of toluene diisocyanate manufacture: A multidisciplinary approach. *Environ Health Perspect* 11:101–108, 1975.

Wernfors M, Nielsen J, Schültz A, Skerfving S: Phthalic anhydride-induced occupational asthma. *Int Arch Allergy Appl Immunol* 79:77–82, 1986.

Whitlock JP Jr, Okino ST, Dong L, et al: Cytochromes P450 5: induction of cytochrome P4501A1: A model for analyzing mammalian gene transcription. *FASEB J* 10(8):809–818, 1996.

Willeke K, Macher J: Air sampling, in Macher J (ed): *Bioaerosols—Assessment and Control.* Cincinnati, OH: American Conference of Governmental Industrial Hygienists, 1999, pp 11-1–11-25.

Wilson CL, Safe S: Mechanisms of ligand-induced aryl hydrocarbon receptor-mediated biochemical and toxic responses. *Toxicologic Pathol* 26(5):657–671, 1998.

CHAPTER 34

REGULATORY TOXICOLOGY

Richard A. Merrill

THE ROLES OF SCIENCE AND REGULATION

This chapter deals with the use of the results of toxicologic studies by governmental regulatory agencies and with the requirements these agencies impose for the conduct of such studies. It does not attempt to justify government agencies' handling of toxicology-related issues but rather seeks to explore the interaction of scientific and regulatory institutions in this field.

This explanation begins by recognizing a central difference between the goals of science and those of government: Science investigates and attempts to explain natural phenomena; it is cautious, incremental, and truth-seeking. Government, in its capacity as regulator, seeks to affect human behavior and settle human disputes; it is episodic and peremptory and pursues resolution rather than truth. It often happens that a regulator cannot withhold a decision or reserve judgment on a problem even when the facts appear to call for a delay, for even a pause to delay out of respect for "getting all the information" has real-world consequences. Because the field of toxicology continuously generates information about the effects of chemicals (though it less often provides information about the magnitude of their effects or the frequency of exposure associated with these effects), regulators invariably are forced to intervene (i.e., to decide) before knowledge is complete.

Scientists are also often frustrated by another feature of American regulatory institutions. In the United States, government officials are accorded less discretion to make political or social judgments than in any other industrialized society. Government actions affecting private interests are constrained by the demand that they be authorized by the legislature and that they rest on a factual XXX predicate that the legislature has specified for such decisions. Furthermore, our legal system requires regulators to set forth the facts on which they rely, and we allow the opponents of regulatory measures numerous opportunities to contest them. Participants in the regulatory process start from the assumption that the available evidence can be construed in the light most favorable to their position. Regulators, for their part, often overstate the evidence for their decisions, just as those who challenge them do, with the result that both sides frequently appear to distort the facts.

THE RELATIONSHIP BETWEEN THE DISCIPLINE OF TOXICOLOGY AND REGULATORY INSTITUTIONS

The foregoing observations could apply to any scientific discipline whose investigations underpin governmental decision making. But over the past three decades regulation and toxicology have become intertwined in distinctive ways. The most obvious connection is that regulators whose job is to protect health rely heavily on toxicologic principles and experimental data for their evaluation of problems that present the need for a decision. Whether the decision is to assign priorities among a group of compounds or to approve a new substance or restrict the use of an old one, the findings of toxicologic investigations are likely to be influential, and often decisive.

Regulators are not merely consumers of experimental results but also shape toxicologic science in ways that may be unexpected. Regulatory demands have provided a major impetus for improvements in toxicologic methods, and they have stimulated a demand for major toxicologic studies. Some programs, such as the programs of the Food and Drug Administration (FDA) for licensing drugs and food additives and that of the Environmental Protection Agency (EPA) for registering pesticides, explicitly demand toxicologic studies of new, and in some cases marketed, compounds. Such studies constitute a major part of the discipline's research agenda. But even if no government agency were empowered to demand toxicologic studies, concern for public health would lead marketers of new products to turn to toxicology to evaluate their possible health hazards.

Regulatory agencies also have exercised important influence over the design and conduct of toxicologic studies. For example, the EPA is empowered by the Toxic Substances Control Act (TSCA) to promulgate standards for different types of toxicologic (and other scientific) investigations. Likewise, the FDA has long issued guidelines for laboratory studies submitted in support of food additives and drugs. Both agencies have adopted requirements governing laboratory operations and practice. Communication between government officials and laboratory scientists flows in both directions. Government testing standards are influenced strongly by the prevailing consensus among toxicologists, many of whom work in regulatory agencies. The procedures for adopting these standards always permit if not encourage the expression of privately held views by members of the discipline.

The balance of this chapter focuses on two of these prominent linkages between toxicology and regulation. The next section outlines the legal and administrative contexts in which regulators rely on toxicologic data in making critical decisions. In the final section, the focus is on government as a regulator of toxicology—as the source of guidance for and limitations on the design and conduct of laboratory experiments. This chapter does not, however, provide a comprehensive treatment of the legal and regulatory requirements that impinge on toxicology, nor does it discuss every program that relies on toxicologic data. It also omits such topics as the laws and regulations designed to protect laboratory personnel, legal restrictions on the handling of dangerous substances, and local requirements for the operation of laboratories.

REGULATORY PROGRAMS THAT RELY ON TOXICOLOGY

An Overview of Approaches to Toxic Chemical Regulation

This section surveys current federal programs for controlling human exposure to toxic chemicals. The discussion highlights the features of regulatory programs that influence both the quantity and the quality of data needed to support an agency's decisions. One such regulatory feature, sometimes overlooked by nonlawyers, is the law's allocation of the "burden of proof," which is the responsibility for demonstrating whether a substance is safe or hazardous. The range of possible approaches can be observed by comparing laws such as the Food Additives Amendment, which requires users of new substances to prove lack of hazard *before* humans may be exposed, with laws such as the Occupational Safety and Health Act (1970), which requires regulators to show that a substance *is* hazardous *before* exposures can be restricted. The approach chosen by Congress powerfully influences an agency's ability to require comprehensive toxicologic investigation of compounds and thus affects the quality of data on which decisions ultimately are based.

A parallel distinction, observable even in programs that mandate premarket testing of new products, is made between substances not yet on the market and those previously approved on the basis of studies that inevitably appear inadequate as investigatory methods improve.

Typology of Regulatory Approaches

At least two issues must be resolved to justify government action to regulate human exposure to a substance. First, it must be determined that the substance is capable of harming persons who may be exposed. Second, it must be determined that humans are likely to be exposed to the substance in ways that could be harmful. In the absence of affirmative answers to both questions, government intervention to control exposure would be difficult to justify. A few statutes require only these two findings. Most laws under which chemicals are regulated, however, mandate or permit consideration of other criteria as well, such as the *magnitude* of the risk posed by a substance and the *consequences and costs* of regulating it.

Agencies Involved

At the federal level, four agencies are chiefly responsible for regulating human exposure to chemicals: the FDA, the EPA, the Occupational Safety and Health Administration (OSHA), and the Consumer Product Safety Commission (CPSC). Together they administer some two dozen statutes whose primary goal is the protection of health. The statutes administered by these four agencies convey different levels of concern about risks to human health and about the weight to be given economic costs (OTA, 1981). This diversity has several explanations. The statutes were enacted in different eras. They originated with different political constituencies and remain under their influence. Perhaps most significant, statutory standards often reflect differences in the technical capacity to control different types of exposures, and they embody different congressional judgments about the economic implications of limiting exposures.

Summary of Current Approaches

For at least two decades, federal regulatory agencies have distinguished between cancer and all other toxic effects. However, it is in their treatment of carcinogens that existing statutes appear to display the greatest diversity. For other (noncarcinogenic) chemicals, regulators have generally embraced a standard safety assessment formula, built around the concept of *acceptable daily intake* (ADI). (In recent years, the EPA has adopted the term *reference dose* in order to avoid any implication that any exposure to a toxic material is "acceptable.") The ADI for a chemical is derived by applying a safety factor—usually 100, but sometimes a larger number if the toxicologic data are sparse or occasionally a smaller number if the data are complete—to the human equivalent of the lowest "no observed effect level" (NOEL) revealed in animal experiments. When estimated human exposure to a chemical falls below the ADI, it—or the quantity of it that results in that exposure—is adjudged "safe." It is only when exposure is likely to exceed the ADI that the regulator must turn to any other considerations made relevant by the applicable statute.

However, this traditional approach to conventional toxicants has not been considered appropriate for carcinogens. Regulators in the United States and many of their counterparts in other countries have operated on the premise that carcinogens as a class cannot be assumed to have "safe" or threshold doses. Furthermore, they have assumed that any chemical shown convincingly in animal studies to cause cancer should be considered a potential human carcinogen. Accordingly, for this group of compounds, which has grown to exceed 500 as more chemicals have been subjected to long-term testing, U.S. regulators have generally assumed that no finite level of human exposure can be considered risk-free. As research has begun to illuminate the different mechanisms by which chemicals may cause cancer, however, regulatory agencies have cautiously accepted the possibility that "safe" thresholds may be established for particular carcinogens.

No Risk The traditional approach is epitomized, indeed codified, by the famous Delaney clause, enacted in 1958 as part of the Food Additives Amendment. The amendment itself requires that any food additive be found "safe" before the FDA may approve its use (FD&C Act, 1958). The Delaney proviso stipulates that this finding may not be made for a food additive that has been shown to induce cancer in humans or in experimental animals. The Delaney clause has been characterized as a categorical risk-benefit judgment by Congress that no food additive is likely to offer benefits sufficient to outweigh any risk of cancer (Turner, 1971).

Negligible Risk Because the risk posed even by a carcinogenic substance depends on the dose as well as its potency, it may be possible to reduce human exposure to such low levels that any associated risk is small enough to ignore without considering any other criteria. No current health statute explicitly prescribes such a "negligible risk" approach, but the FDA has adopted it administratively for some classes of environmental carcinogens. For example, under a 1962 amendment to the Delaney clause, the FDA may approve a carcinogenic drug for use in food-producing animals if no residue will be found in edible tissues of treated animals (FD&C Act, 1938). The FDA announced that it will calibrate its tests for residues so that they only register toxins with carcinogenic potency (FDA, 1985) and will approve a carcinogenic drug if the sponsor provides an analytic method capable of detecting residues in meat, milk, or eggs large enough to pose a lifetime dietary risk greater than 1 in 1 million, as determined by extrapolation from animal bioassays. In 1996, Congress amended the provisions of the Food, Drug, and Cosmetics (FD&C) Act applicable to pesticide residues on food, adopting a standard that, though not expressed in these words, is understood to permit a tolerance for a carcinogenic pesticide if the estimated cancer risk is extremely small, on the order of 1 in 1 million (Food Quality Protection Act, 1996).

Any "negligible" or "de minimis" risk approach requires data depicting carcinogenic potency. This is not a major problem when an agency can require a product's sponsor to conduct the necessary tests, but programs in which regulation responds to already extant exposures often lack such leverage. The approach also requires a method for quantifying the risk associated with low doses of a carcinogen. As a practical matter, a negligible risk approach will not suffice when exposures to toxic substances cannot be reduced to very low levels without sacrificing other values.

Trade-off Approaches These embrace a variety of verbal formulas that have one common feature: each requires the regulatory agency to weigh factors in addition to the health risks posed by substances targeted for regulation. One version is illustrated by the Occupational Safety and Health Act, which directs OSHA in setting workplace standards for toxic materials, to elect the standard "which most adequately assures, *to the extent feasible* . . . that no employee will suffer material impairment of health or functional capacity" (OSHA, 1970). OSHA has interpreted this language as requiring it to consider, in addition to the risk posed by a substance, the availability of technology for reducing exposure and the financial ability of the responsible industries to pay for the necessary controls. The agency need not, however, balance the health benefits of mandated exposure controls against the costs of achieving them (*American Textile Manufacturers Institute v. Donovan,* 1982).

A more expansive "trade-off" law is the Federal Insecticide, Fungicide, and Rodenticide Act (FIFRA), which requires the EPA to refuse or withdraw registration of a pesticide if its use is likely to result in "unreasonable adverse effects on health or the environment" (FIFRA, 1972). The EPA interprets this language as requiring that it weigh all the effects of a pesticide—its contribution to food production as well as its possible adverse effects on applicators, consumers, and the natural environment—in determining whether, or on what terms, to permit registration. The Toxic Substances Control Act (TSCA, 1976) uses more explicit language to mandate the balancing of risks and benefits. TSCA further dictates that, in seeking the right balance, the EPA must adopt the "least burdensome" controls on the use of or exposure to a chemical (*Corrosion Proof Fittings v. EPA,* 1991).

PROGRAMS FOR REGULATING CHEMICAL HAZARDS

Food and Drug Administration

The oldest of the major health regulation laws, the FD&C Act, was enacted in 1938 and covers food for humans and animals, human and veterinary drugs, medical devices, and cosmetics.

Food The original 1906 Food and Drug Act contained two prohibitions addressed to foods containing hazardous constituents; both remain part of the current law. The first forbids the marketing of any food containing "any *added* poisonous or deleterious *substance which may render it injurious* to health," a provision that the FDA has interpreted as barring foods presenting any significant risk. The second forbids the marketing of foods containing *nonadded* toxicants that make them "*ordinarily injurious* to health," a standard that accords a preferred status to traditional components of the American diet [FD&C Act § 402(a)]. Neither of these original provisions required premarket approval; the FDA had the burden of proving that a food was, in the legal vernacular, "adulterated."

Congress has since amended the act several times to improve the FDA's ability to ensure the safety of foods. Each time, it identified a class of additives for which it prescribed a form of premarket approval, thus giving the FDA the authority not only to evaluate a substance's safety before humans are exposed but also to specify the kinds of studies necessary to obtain approval (FDA, 1994).

The most important of these amendments was the 1958 Food Additives Amendment. For food additives, the law requires safety to be demonstrated prior to marketing. The critical standard for approval is that the substance is "reasonably certain to be safe"; no inquiry into the benefits of an additive is undertaken or authorized (Cooper, 1978). But the amendment does not apply to all food ingredients. Congress excluded substances that are "generally recognized as safe" (GRAS) by qualified scientific experts. In effect, it instructed the FDA to pay less attention to ingredients that had been in use for many years without observable adverse effects. Congress also excepted ingredients sanctioned by either the FDA or the U.S. Department of Agriculture (USDA) prior to 1958. The practical significance of this exception is that a "prior-sanctioned" ingredient is not subject to the Delaney clause because it is not in the technical legal sense a food additive.

Three classes of indirect food constituents—pesticide residues, animal drug residues, and food-contact materials—are subject to distinct regulatory standards. Pesticide residues on raw agricultural commodities for years were regulated by the EPA under a 1954 amendment to the FD&C Act, which allowed residues if they meet a tolerance established by the agency (FD&C Act § 348). In setting tolerances, the EPA could consider both the potential adverse health effects of residues and the value of pesticide uses. If the concentration of a pesticide in a processed food exceeded the established tolerance, however, and the pesticide was a carcinogen, the Delaney clause prohibited its approval for that use (*Les v. Reilly,* 1992). This framework was revised by Congress in 1996 to exempt pesticide residues from the operation of the Delaney clause but also restrict sharply the circumstances in which food production "benefits" could be considered in setting tolerances. The amended law requires that any pesticide tolerance, whether on raw or processed food, whether for a carcinogen or a conventional toxicant, must be "safe," a standard defined as "reasonable assurance of no harm" (Food Quallity Protection Act, 1996).

Any animal drug residue must be shown to be safe for humans under essentially the same standards that apply to food additives, with a notable exception. The FDA has interpreted the 1962 authorization for approval of carcinogenic compounds ("if . . . no residue of the additive will be found") as allowing residues that pose no more than a negligible risk.

A food-contact substance requires approval as a food additive if, when used as intended, it "may reasonably be expected to become a component of food." This vague language presents two issues. First, the Delaney clause appears to preclude approval if the material induces cancer, as some important food-packaging materials, such as acrylonitrile and polyvinyl chloride, clearly do. Second, the scientific principle of diffusion supports the argument that all food-contact substances are properly characterized as food additives. The FDA has attempted to cushion this potential collision between toxicologic findings and advances in analytic chemistry. It has declined to apply the Delaney clause to carcinogenic migrants whose extrapolated risk does not exceed 1 in 1 million, because these migrants present only a minimal risk (FDA, 1984). Before 1997, the law required affirmative FDA approval of all such "indirect food additives," burdening both the agency and producers of food-contact materials with a slow and expensive process for evaluating chemicals that could migrate into food, if at all, only at extremely low levels. In omnibus legislation that addressed most of FDA's regulatory programs, Congress substituted a premarket notification system for food-contact materials that permits the agency to delay introduction if it questions a material's safety but does not require affirmative agency approval (FDA Modernization Act, 1997).

Human Drugs Environmental contaminants constitute the final category of food constituents of concern to regulators. The FDA relies on a provision of the 1938 act authorizing the establishment of tolerances for "added poisonous or deleterious substances" that cannot be avoided through good manufacturing practice. In setting such tolerances, the FDA weighs three factors: (1) the health effects of the contaminant, usually estimated on the basis of animal data; (2) the ability to measure the contaminant; and (3) the effects of various tolerance levels on the price and availability of the food (Merrill and Schewel, 1980).

Preclinical studies in animals play an important role in the FDA's evaluation of human drugs. The current law requires premarket approval, for both safety and efficacy, of all "new" drugs, a category that embraces virtually all prescription drug ingredients introduced since 1938 (Hutt and Merrill, 1991). Investigation of therapeutic agents in humans has long been accepted, and the primary evidence of safety (as well as effectiveness) accordingly comes from clinical and not laboratory studies. However, animal studies are the sole source of information about a substance's biological effects before human trials are begun, and their results influence not only the decision whether to expose human subjects but also the design of clinical protocols (FDA, 1994).

Medical Devices In 1976, Congress overhauled the FD&C Act's requirements for medical devices, according the FDA major new authority to regulate their testing, marketing, and use. The elaborate new scheme contemplates three tiers of control, the most restrictive of which is premarket approval similar to that required for new drugs. To obtain FDA approval of a so-called class III device, the sponsor must demonstrate safety and efficacy. The bulk of the data supporting such applications will be derived from clinical studies but also will include toxicologic studies of any constituents likely to be absorbed by the patient.

Cosmetics The statutory provisions governing cosmetics do not require premarket approval of any ingredient or demand that manufacturers test their products for safety, though most manufacturers routinely do so. The basic safety standard for cosmetics is similar to that for food ingredients: no product may be marketed if it contains "a poisonous or deleterious substance which may render it injurious to health" [FD&C Act § 601(a)]. The case law establishes that this language, too, bars distribution of a product that poses any significant risk of more than transitory harm when used as intended, but it places on the FDA the burden of proving a violation (Hutt and Merrill, 1991). The FDA has brought few cases under this standard, in part because acute toxic reactions to cosmetics are readily detected and immediately result in abandonment of the offending ingredient.

While the law does not require premarket proof of safety for most cosmetic ingredients generally, it does mandate safety testing for color additives. The scheme enacted by Congress in 1960 (FD&C Act § 706) resembles that for food additives except that no colors are exempt; every color additive must be shown, with "reasonable certainty," to be safe. A separate version of the Delaney clause precludes approval of any carcinogenic color additive, no matter how small a risk it presents (*Public Citizen v. Young,* 1987).

Environmental Protection Agency

Created in 1970, the EPA became responsible for administering an expanding portfolio of laws protecting human health and the environment. A comprehensive review of the EPA's numerous programs is not possible here; the following summary focuses on those EPA activities in which toxicologic evidence plays a central role:

pesticide regulation, regulation of industrial chemicals, regulation of drinking water supplies, hazardous waste control, and regulation of toxic pollutants of water and of air.

Pesticides Under the Federal Insecticide, Fungicide, and Rodenticide Act (FIFRA), no pesticide may be marketed unless it has been registered by the EPA. The law specifies that a pesticide shall be registered if it is effective, bears proper labeling, and "when properly used . . . will not generally cause unreasonable adverse effects on the environment" (FIFRA § 136b). Congress defined this last criterion as "any unreasonable risk to man or the environment, taking into account the economic, social and environmental costs and benefits of the use of any pesticide." Most of the data supporting a product's initial registration—mainly toxicologic studies—are provided by the sponsor.

In the early 1970s, the EPA engendered controversy by canceling registrations for a number of pesticides based primarily on studies suggesting that they were carcinogenic in animals. Criticism of its "hair-trigger" approach to regulation, coupled with court rulings that the agency was obligated to initiate the process of cancellation whenever a pesticide's safety came into question, led to important changes in the law. Congress added procedural safeguards for pesticide manufacturers and created a panel of outside scientists to review contemplated actions against pesticides (FIFRA, 1972). The EPA itself established a procedure, now named "special review," for public ventilation of disputes over the risks and benefits of pesticides before the formal cancellation process is undertaken (EPA, 1980). A pesticide will be subjected to close scrutiny if the EPA concludes that it induces cancer in experimental mammalian species or in humans. The agency published guidelines for assessing whether a pesticide or any other substance poses a cancer risk to humans (EPA, 1984), and a decade later issued a proposed revision of these guidelines which remains the subject of fierce debate as this volume goes to press (EPA, 1996). Even if a pesticide is convincingly shown to be a carcinogen, however, the law would allow it to be registered if the EPA concluded that its economic benefits outweighed the risk.

The EPA has for nearly two decades been engaged in a comprehensive review of previously registered pesticides and "reregistration" of those that meet contemporary standards for marketing. Under this program, many older pesticides have been subjected to comprehensive toxicologic testing, including carcinogenicity testing, for the first time, and the results have required modification of the terms of approved use and, in some instances, cancellation for several agents. In 1988, Congress amended the law to require the EPA to accelerate this reregistration effort (FIFRA Amendments, 1988). The agency was specifically requested to increase the stringency of its requirements for neurotoxic and behavioral testing to include tests "related to chronic exposure, prenatal, and neonatal effects." The EPA has since published additional testing data requirements for hundreds of active pesticide ingredients and has issued decisions on reregistration eligibility for over 70, but the project remains a work in progress.

Industrial Chemicals The Toxic Substances Control Act (TSCA, 1976) represents Congress's most ambitious effort to control the hazards of chemicals in commercial production. The TSCA covers all chemical substances manufactured or processed in or imported into the United States, except for substances already regulated under other laws. *A chemical substance* is defined broadly as "any organic or inorganic substance of a particular molecular identity."

The TSCA gives the EPA three main powers. The agency is empowered to restrict or even ban the manufacture, processing, distribution, use, or disposal of a chemical substance when there is a reasonable basis to conclude any such activity poses an "unreasonable risk of injury to health or environment." In determining whether a chemical substance presents an unreasonable risk, the agency is instructed (TSCA § 6) to consider the effects of such substance or mixture on the health and the magnitude of the exposure of human beings to such substance or mixture; the effects of such substance or mixture on the environment and the magnitude of the exposure of the environment to such substance or mixture; the benefits of such substance for various uses and the availability of substitutes; and the reasonably ascertainable economic consequences of the rule, after consideration of the effect on the national economy, small business, technologic innovation, the environment and public health.

The EPA also must consider any rule's positive impact on the development and use of substitutes as well as its negative impact on manufacturers or processors of the chemical and weigh the economic savings to society resulting from reduction of the risk. The TSCA's trade-off approach to regulation has proved a major challenge to the EPA. The agency has not often used its authority often under TSCA § 6. In 1989, it issued a comprehensive rule prohibiting the future manufacture, importation, processing, and distribution of almost all products containing asbestos. Despite the documented hazards of asbestos, a court overturned the rule; the ban failed to satisfy the statutory requirement that the EPA promulgate the "least burdensome" regulation required to protect the environment (*Corrosion Proof Fittings v. Environmental Protection Agency*, 1991). The ban continues to govern products that were not in manufacture as of mid-1989, but even a decade later the EPA has not attempted to issue a new rule regulating existing asbestos-containing products, nor has it attempted to use what was once assumed to be its potent authority under Section 6 to regulate any other chemical substance.

If the EPA suspects that a chemical *may* pose an unreasonable risk but lacks sufficient data to take action, the TSCA empowers it to require testing to develop the necessary data. Similarly, it may order testing if the chemical will be produced in substantial quantities that may result in significant human exposure whose effects cannot be predicted on the basis of existing data. In either case, the EPA must consider the "relative costs of the various test protocols and methodologies" and the "reasonably foreseeable availability of the facilities and personnel" needed to perform the tests (TSCA § 4).

Finally, to enable the EPA to evaluate chemicals before humans are exposed, the TSCA requires the manufacturer of a new chemical substance to notify the agency 90 days prior to production or distribution [TSCA § 5(a)(1)]. The manufacturer's or distributor's notice must include any health effects data it possesses. However, the EPA is not empowered to require that manufacturers routinely conduct testing of all new chemicals to permit an evaluation of their risks; Congress declined to confer the kind of premarket approval authority that the FDA exercises for drugs and food additives and the EPA exercises for pesticides.

The system for regulating new and existing chemical substances in the European Union (E.U.) highlights both the advantages and disadvantages of the U.S. system under the TSCA. Since 1979, the E.U. has required manufacturers of new chemical substances to submit notification to a member state at least 45 days prior to *marketing* the substance. The notification for substances produced in excess of 1 ton per year must include a base set of data that assess acute and subacute toxicity, mutagenicity, and carcinogenic screening. Additional tests may be required if the production level exceeds specified volumes or if the base set of data suggests a possible hazard. In 1992, the E.U. expanded its regulatory scheme by imposing health effects testing requirements on chemicals produced in amounts of less than 1 ton per year and by lengthening the waiting period from 45 to 60 days. In addition, member states that receive notification are now obligated to conduct risk assessments on new substances in accordance with guidelines adopted by the E.U.

The E.U. and U.S. systems for regulating new chemicals thus differ significantly. The E.U. scheme requires manufacturers to generate and submit a base set of data concerning the health risks of most new chemicals; the EPA is authorized to order testing only in limited situations. The TSCA, however, permits regulatory intervention at a much earlier stage than the E.U. by requiring notification prior to manufacturing. Perhaps most importantly, the E.U. system addresses only notification, labeling, and packaging, while member states retain their independent authority over the control of new substances.

In 1993, the E.U. adopted a scheme for regulating approximately 100,000 existing chemicals listed on the European Inventory of Existing Chemical Substances (EINECS). The E.U. system for regulating existing chemicals closely resembles the TSCA approach. Manufacturers of existing chemicals must submit existing data on the chemicals. Based on these data, E.U. regulators select priority chemicals each year and assign the responsibility for assessing these chemicals to member states. Manufacturers of priority chemicals must submit data for the assessments and perform new studies if necessary.

Hazardous Wastes Several statutes administered by the EPA regulate land disposal of hazardous materials. The principal law is the Resource Conservation and Recovery Act (RCRA), enacted in 1976. The RCRA established a comprehensive federal scheme for regulating hazardous waste. Directed to promulgate criteria for identifying hazardous wastes, the EPA specified these as ignitability, corrosivity, reactivity, and toxicity. The agency has identified accepted protocols for determining these characteristics and established a list of substances whose presence will make waste hazardous.

The RCRA directs the EPA to regulate the activities of generators, transporters, and those who treat, store, or dispose of hazardous wastes. Standards applicable to generators, transporters, and handlers of hazardous wastes must "protect human health and the environment." The EPA's regulations applicable to generators and transporters establish a manifest system that is designed to create a paper trail for every shipment of waste, from generator to final destination, to ensure proper handling and accountability. The agency has the broadest authority over persons who own or operate hazardous waste treatment, storage, or disposal facilities. Pursuant to the RCRA, it has issued regulations prescribing methods for treating, storing, and disposing of wastes; governing the location, design, and construction of facilities; mandating contingency plans to minimize negative impacts from such facilities; setting qualifications for ownership, training, and financial responsibility; and requiring permits for all such facilities (EPA, 1993).

Toxic Water Pollutants The EPA has had responsibility for regulating toxic water pollutants since 1972. As originally enacted, Section 307 of the Federal Water Pollution Control Act required the EPA to publish within 90 days and periodically add to a list of toxic pollutants for which effluent standards (discharge limits) would then be established. Section 307(a)(4) of the act originally specified that, in establishing standards for any listed pollutant, the EPA was to provide an "*ample margin of safety*" —a difficult criterion to meet for most toxic pollutants and arguably impossible for any known to be carcinogenic. The law also mandated both a rapid timetable and a complex procedure for standard setting.

The EPA's disturbingly slow implementation of these instructions precipitated a series of lawsuits. The agency eventually reached a court-sanctioned settlement that fundamentally altered the federal approach toward toxic pollutants of the nation's waterways. The settlement allowed the EPA to act under other provisions of the act that focused on economic cost and technologic feasibility in setting limits and thus freed the agency from the rigid demands of Section 307. Congress incorporated the terms of this settlement in 1977 amendments to the statute.

In 1987, Congress again amended the Federal Water Pollution Control Act to toughen standards for toxic pollutants. Under the prior law, the EPA had developed health-based "water quality criteria" for 126 compounds it had identified as toxic. These criteria essentially described *desirable* maximum contamination levels which, because the EPA's discharge limits were technology-based, generally were substantially lower than the levels actually achieved. The 1987 amendments gave what had been advisory criteria real bite by requiring that states incorporate them in their own mandatory standards for water quality and impose additional effluent limits on operations discharging into below-standard waterways (Heineck, 1989).

Drinking Water The 1974 Safe Drinking Water Act (SDWA) was enacted to ensure that public water supply systems "meet minimum national standards for the protection of public health." Under the SDWA, the EPA is required to regulate any contaminants "which may have an adverse effect on human health." The means prescribed was the establishment of national primary drinking water regulations for public water systems. For each contaminant of concern, the agency was to prescribe a maximum contaminant level (MCL) or a treatment technique for its control. The original 1974 act prescribed a two-stage process. The EPA first was required to promulgate *interim* national primary drinking water regulations, uniform minimum standards at levels that would "protect health to the extent feasible . . . (taking costs into consideration)." These interim regulations were later supplanted by regulations formulated on the basis of a series of reports by the National Academy of Sciences (NAS). The charge to the NAS committee was to recommend the MCLs necessary to protect humans from any known or anticipated adverse health effects. In turn, the EPA was to specify enforceable limits as close as feasible to the levels recommended by the NAS. By 1986, the EPA had established MCLs for just 23 contaminants and treatment techniques for none.

In that year Congress amended the Safe Drinking Water Act to cover more contaminants, apply more pressure to states and localities to clean up their drinking water supplies, and strengthen the EPA's enforcement role. The EPA was required to adopt regulations for a total prescribed list of 83 contaminants within 3 years (including all but one of those originally regulated). The 1986 amendments sharpened the distinction between optimal drinking water conditions—renamed maximum contaminant level goals (or MCLGs)—and legally enforceable, technology- and cost-based contaminant levels or treatment requirements, which continued to bear the label "MCL."

Continuing criticism of the EPA SDWA effect through the following decade precipitated yet another legislative attempt at reform. In 1996, Congress once again amended the act to encompass an expanded list of contaminants to be regulated and revise the schedule for standard setting. At the urging of industry, it also included a provision that specifically directs the EPA, in setting MCLGs and MCLs, to use the "best available science."

In March 2000, the latter change in the law led to one of the most significant judicial rulings in the environmental health field. The case was a challenge to the EPA's decision to retain a MCLG for chloroform of zero in the face of evidence, accepted by its own scientists, that the mechanism by which chloroform produces tumors in rodents is threshold-limited. The reviewing court held that given its acceptance of the evidence of a threshold, the EPA was required by the SDWA's "best available" evidence provision to base its decision on that evidence (*Chlorine Chemistry Council v. EPA,* 2000). This ruling marks the first time that a court has directed a federal regulatory agency to recognize a "safe" finite level of exposure for an animal carcinogen.

Toxic Air Pollutants Section 112 of the Clean Air Act (CAA) now provides a list of 189 hazardous air pollutants, which the EPA may modify by adding or deleting items. The EPA must establish national emissions standards for sources that emit any listed pollutant. The original 1970 version of Section 112 required the standards to provide "an ample margin of safety to protect the public health from such hazardous air pollutants." The implication of this language—that standards were to be set without regard to the costs of emissions control—generated intense debate from the beginning and contributed to the EPA's glacial pace of implementation. The EPA finally attempted to escape the strict language of Section 112 when it issued a standard for vinyl chloride in 1986. In this instance the agency claimed it could consider costs and declined to adopt a standard dictated solely by safety. A court ruled that the EPA had improperly considered costs, but it did make clear that in determining what emissions level was safe, even for a carcinogen, the EPA was not obligated to eliminate exposure. The court also said the EPA could consider costs in deciding what, if any, additional margin of protection to prescribe (*Natural Resources Defense Council, Inc., v. United States Environmental Protection Agency*, 1987).

Amendments to the CAA in 1990 responded to the difficulties presented by the strict approach of old Section 112. The amendments replace the health-based standard with a two-tiered system of regulation. The EPA must first issue standards that are technology-based, designed to require the "maximum degree of emission reduction achievable" (MACT) [CAA § 112(d)(2)]. If the MACT controls are insufficient to protect human health with an "ample margin of safety," the EPA must issue residual risk standards [CAA § 112(f)]. The 1990 Amendments essentially define "ample margin of safety" for carcinogens by requiring the EPA to establish added residual risk limits for any pollutant that poses a lifetime excess cancer risk of greater than 1 in 1 million.

Occupational Safety and Health Administration

The 1970 Occupational Safety and Health Act requires employers to provide employees with safe working conditions and empowers OSHA to prescribe mandatory occupational safety and health standards (OSHA, 1970). OSHA's most controversial actions involved its attempts to set exposure limits for toxic chemicals.

While manufacturers of food additives, drugs, and pesticides must demonstrate the safety of their products prior to marketing, no employer need obtain advance approval of processes or materials or conduct tests to ensure that its operations will not jeopardize worker health. OSHA must first discover that a material already in use threatens worker health before it may attempt to control exposure. Standards for toxic chemicals typically set maximum limits on employee exposure and prescribe changes in employer procedures or equipment to achieve this level.

The act specifies that in regulating toxic chemicals, OSHA shall adopt the standard "which most adequately assures, to the extent feasible, on the basis of the best available evidence, that no employee will suffer material impairment of health or physical capacity" [OSH Act § 6 (b)(5)]. The meaning of these contradictory phrases was for many years a source of controversy. Court decisions made clear that the "best available evidence" did not require proof of causation or even positive epidemiologic studies; animal data alone could support regulation of a toxic substance. The debate focused on whether OSHA had an obligation to weigh the economic costs of its standards. The agency acknowledged that it was required to consider technologic achievability and industry viability, but it denied that it was obliged to balance health benefits against economic costs.

Judicial challenges to OSHA standards have clarified OSHA's responsibilities. In a famous case, the U.S. Supreme Court overturned OSHA's benzene standard because the agency had not shown that prevailing worker exposure levels posed a "significant" health risk (*Industrial Union Department, AFL-CIO, v. American Petroleum Institute,* 1980). This prerequisite proved a major obstacle when OSHA attempted to establish standards for 428 air contaminants in a single proceeding in 1989. Although it found that OSHA's generic approach to regulation was permissible in theory, a court vacated the standards because OSHA failed to show that each individual contaminant posed a "significant risk" at current levels (*American Federation of Labor v. OSHA,* 1992). However, the Supreme Court earlier upheld OSHA's cotton dust standard, rejecting arguments that the agency was obligated to weigh the costs of individual standards for concededly hazardous substances (*American Textile Manufacturers Institute v. Donovan,* 1982).

Consumer Product Safety Commission

Of the four agencies discussed here, the CPSC has played the least important role in federal efforts to control toxic chemicals. The commission was created in 1972 by the Consumer Product Safety Act (CPSA) with authority to regulate products that pose an unreasonable risk of injury or illness to consumers. The commission is empowered to promulgate safety standards "to prevent or reduce an unreasonable risk of injury" associated with a consumer product. If no feasible standard "would adequately protect the public from the unreasonable risk of injury" posed by a consumer product, the commission may ban the product (CPSA § 8). In assessing the need for a standard or ban, the agency must balance the likelihood that a product will cause harm, and the severity of harm it will likely cause, against the effects of reducing the risk on the product's utility, cost, and availability to consumers.

The CPSC also administers the older Federal Hazardous Substances Act (FHSA). The FHSA authorizes the CPSC to regulate, primarily through prescribed label warnings, products that are toxic, corrosive, combustible, or radioactive or that generate pressure. The FHSA is unusual among federal health laws because it contains detailed criteria for determining toxicity. It defines "highly toxic" in terms of a substance's acute effects in specified tests in rodents; substances capable of producing chronic effects thus fall within the "toxic" category. The FHSA contains another unique provision [FHSA § 2(h)(2)] specifically addressing the probative weight of animal and human data on acute toxicity: "If the [commission] finds that available data on human experience with any substance indicates results different from those obtained on animals in the above-named dosages or concentrations, the human data shall take precedence."

The CPSC has prescribed labeling for products containing numerous substances that are acutely toxic. It has also acted to ban from consumer products several substances that pose a cancer risk, including asbestos, vinyl chloride as a propellant, benzene, tris(hydroxymethyl)aminomethane (TRIS), and formaldehyde (Merrill, 1981). Its ban of urea formaldehyde foam insulation was set aside by a reviewing court in an opinion that is remarkable for its unsophisticated but critical analysis of the agency's handling of toxicologic data (*Gulf South Insulation v. CPSC,* 1983).

The Labeling of Hazardous Art Materials Act of 1988 (LHAMA) amended the FHSA. The LHAMA authorizes the CPSC to require labeling of art materials that have "the potential for producing chronic adverse health effects with customary or reasonably foreseeable use." The LHAMA also requires a producer or repackager of an art material to submit the material to a toxicologist for review. The toxicologist must determine whether the material presents a chronic health hazard and must recommend appropriate labeling. The CPSC has issued guidelines, applicable to both the LHAMA and the FHSA, for determining whether a material presents a chronic health hazard (CPSC, 1992).

The CPSC's regulation of asbestos under the FHSA illustrates the overlap of regulatory jurisdictions of different agencies. In 1986, the CPSC issued an enforcement policy requiring accurate labeling of the hazards of asbestos for all asbestos-containing household products (CPSC, 1986). It characterized the labeling requirement as an "interim measure" because the EPA had proposed a ban of asbestos in household products under TSCA. However, as discussed earlier, a court later overturned the EPA's asbestos ban (*Corrosion Proof Fittings v. Environmental Protection Agency,* 1991). Neither the EPA nor the CPSC has since attempted to restrict asbestos-containing products.

REGULATORY CONTROLS OVER TOXICOLOGY

Previous sections of this chapter have surveyed legal contexts in which regulators draw on toxicologic data to decide whether and how to control environmental chemicals. Modern toxicology has developed, in substantial part, in response to the information needs of contemporary regulation. But government impinges on the discipline in more direct ways as well. Regulatory agencies often prescribe the specific objectives and design of studies that are conducted to satisfy regulatory requirements. In addition, pressure to protect animals used in research has produced laws and regulations that govern toxicologists themselves.

Different Ways Regulation Impinges on Toxicology

An agency's influence over the conduct of toxicologic studies depends on its regulatory responsibilities. An agency such as the FDA or the EPA, which must confirm the safety of new substances before marketing, can dictate the kinds of tests that manufacturers must conduct to gain approval. By contrast, an agency that has no premarket approval function has less leverage.

Statutory terms often do not reveal an agency's real power. For example, the FD&C Act does not in so many words authorize the FDA to prescribe the kinds of preclinical tests a manufacturer of human drugs must conduct; it merely says that no new drug may be marketed until the manufacturer has satisfied the FDA, "by all methods reasonably applicable," that it is "safe" [FD&C Act § 505(c)]. However, the agency's power to withhold approval when it has doubts about a drug's safety provides it the practical leverage necessary to demand whatever tests its scientific reviewers believe necessary. Some laws, notably the TSCA, explicitly accord power to prescribe testing; but if an agency has the ability to prevent marketing until safety is proved, doubts about its legal authority to prescribe testing requirements are academic. The important issues are the procedures by which its requirements are adopted, their scope and scientific support, and their legal effect.

The last issue is important for laboratory scientists and test sponsors as well as for lawyers. Two significant legal distinctions should be noted. The first is the distinction between the requirements that an agency imposes for testing of specific compounds and generic requirements prescribed for all compounds within a class (e.g., direct food additives). The FDA could impose its views of appropriate toxicologic testing without ever enunciating any general testing standards. When a compound's sponsor seeks approval, it could be told that the tests it had conducted were inadequate. Alternatively, an individual sponsor could solicit the agency's advice about what tests were necessary before it undertook testing. The first approach wastes resources, and the second—unless agency advice is broadly disseminated—fails to guide other potential sponsors and allows inconsistency in the treatment of similar compounds.

For these reasons, the FDA and EPA have moved increasingly toward establishing generic test standards or guidelines. Both agencies have issued guidelines for the design and conduct of studies of the health effects of compounds submitted for agency approval (EPA, 1993; FDA, 1993). In addition, the EPA has established guidelines for several of the tests that it may mandate by rule or consent agreement for individual chemicals under TSCA § 4 (EPA, 1993). Multinational bodies like the Organization for Economic Cooperation and Development have sought to secure multilateral adherence to standardized test guidelines and minimum testing requirements for new chemicals (Page, 1982).

This trend has focused attention on a second legal distinction: that between binding regulations and advisory guidelines. Any time a regulatory agency wants to provide guidance for private behavior, it confronts a choice between establishing standards that have the force of law and merely conveying its current best judgment of what conduct will satisfy the law. A regulation typically specifies what the law mandates; failure to comply (e.g., failure to perform a test or follow a specified protocol) constitutes a violation of law just as if the regulation had been enacted by Congress. A test guideline describes performance that will satisfy legal requirements; but failure to follow the guideline is not forbidden. The agency may accept another approach that employs, for example, a different set of studies or studies conducted using different protocols if it concludes that they meet the law's basic objectives.

Regulations ensure consistency and are more easily enforced than guidelines, but they are more rigid because they restrict the agency, and the procedures for their adoption are cumbersome. The design and conduct of toxicologic studies, it is often argued, should take into account the characteristics of the test compound, the endpoints to be evaluated, the resources available, and perhaps even laboratory capabilities. Accordingly, both the FDA and EPA have preferred to announce their standards as guidelines, permitting sponsors and scientists to consider alternative approaches.

It is increasingly common for U.S. agencies to specify the types of tests they require before they will consider the safety of a compound (e.g., tests for acute toxicity, subchronic effects, and chronic effects). Within each of these categories, an agency might set out more detailed requirements, essentially enumerating its "base set" data demands. As noted above, an agency may also describe methods for executing particular tests, for instance, a bioassay for carcinogenesis. It is these descriptions that in the United States usually take the form of guidelines.

Both the FDA and the EPA have adopted another set of requirements that specify laboratory procedures for conducting tests required or submitted for regulatory consideration. These good laboratory practice (GLP) regulations prescribe essential but often mundane features of sound laboratory science, such as animal husbandry standards and record-keeping practices (EPA, 1999; FDA, 2000). All of these types of requirements are intended to contribute to sound regulatory decision making by ensuring the quality and integrity of toxicologic data submitted to support agency decisions.

FDA and EPA Testing Standards

It would serve little purpose here to detail existing agency requirements for the design and conduct of toxicologic studies; they change frequently enough that any summary would soon be outdated. This chapter thus only attempts to acquaint the reader with the principal federal programs that specify standards for toxicity testing. The discussion focuses on the FDA and the EPA.

Food and Drug Administration The FDA exercises premarketing approval authority over several classes of compounds, of which the most important, for present purposes, are new human drugs and direct additives to food.

Toxicologic Testing Requirements for Human Drugs In 1962, Congress expressly authorized the FDA to exempt investigational drugs from the premarket approval requirement so that they could be shipped for use in clinical testing, subject to conditions the agency believed appropriate to protect human subjects [FD&C Act § 505(i)]. One condition that the FDA established was that an investigational drug first must have been evaluated in preclinical studies. This requirement appears in current regulations that amplify, in the text and in referenced guidelines, the types of tests that are to be performed and the design they should follow (FDA, 1994). Almost invariably, a drug's sponsor will consult agency personnel to get a precise understanding of what sorts of toxicologic studies they expect. Preclinical studies of substances that are candidates for use as human drugs must meet the standards set by the FDA's GLP regulations (FDA, 1994). These regulations apply to all laboratories—university, independent, and manufacturer-owned—in which such studies are conducted. The work of the International Conference on Harmonisation of Technical Requirements for Registration of Pharmaceuticals for Human Use (ICH) highlights the trend toward international agreement on test methods. In 1994 the ICH—comprising the European Union, Japan, and the United States—issued six draft guidelines on various toxicology testing methods for human drugs. The testing requirements applicable in the United States surely will evolve as the international community reaches consensus on the appropriate methodology.

Testing Requirements for Food Additives The Food Additives Amendment and the Color Additive Amendments require premarket approval of new additives to human food. Both laws assume that laboratory studies in animals will provide the principal data for assessing safety. Thus, a petitioner must submit "full reports of investigations made with respect to the safety for use of such additives, including full information as to the methods and control used" [FD&C Act § 409(c)].

The FDA's regulations contain only general statements about the need for and features of toxicologic studies. For many years, the agency maintained an advice-giving system in which it prescribed the type and design of tests to be performed. In 1982, the FDA first codified this "common law" in *Toxicological Principles for the Safety Assessment of Direct Food Additives and Color Additives Used in Food,* known thereafter as the "Red Book." The Red Book describes the types of tests the FDA believes necessary to evaluate an additive's safety. The agency's requirements, which are in the form of guidelines rather than regulations, are calibrated to the purposes for which the additive will be used, to estimated levels of human exposure, and to the results of sequential studies. The FDA later issued a draft revision, "Red Book II," under the same title as the original. Tests of food color and additives must also comply with the FDA's good laboratory practice regulations (FDA, 1993).

Environmental Protection Agency The EPA's premarket approval authority over pesticides places it, like the FDA, in a position to dictate the design and conduct of studies on such compounds. The 1976 Toxic Substances Control Act gave the EPA authority to mandate testing of other chemicals in use or scheduled for introduction and to specify, by regulation, test standards.

Toxicology Requirements for Pesticides The FIFRA clearly contemplates the submission of toxicologic studies, as well as other types of investigations, to support the EPA's evaluation of a pesticide [FIFRA § 136(b)]. The statute also requires the EPA to "publish guidelines specifying the kinds of information which will be required to support the registration of a pesticide and to revise such guidelines from time to time."

The EPA's regulations state broadly that pesticide registration depends on evaluation of "all available, pertinent data," which must satisfy the minimum requirements set forth in registration guidelines (EPA, 1993). The agency has issued regulations outlining the procedures for submission of registration petitions and their basic content (EPA, 1978, 1993). Animal studies of pesticides must also comply with EPA's own good laboratory practice regulations, which were inspired by the same investigations that led the FDA to promulgate its standards for testing laboratories and impose similar requirements.

Testing of Industrial Chemicals The primary means by which the EPA may mandate health effects testing of new or existing industrial chemicals is Section 4(a) of the TSCA. That provision states that the administrator "shall by rule require that testing be conducted to develop data with respect to the health and environmental effects for which there is an insufficiency of data and experience" to permit assessment of whether a substance presents an unreasonable risk. This obligation to order testing is triggered by an administrative finding that a chemical presents a potential risk (based on the suspicion of toxicity) or that humans or the environment will be exposed to substantial quantities. The statute creates an Interagency Testing Committee (ITC) with members from

EPA, OSHA, CEQ, NIOSH, NIEHS, NCI, NSF, and the Department of Commerce to recommend a list of chemicals that should be tested and in what order of priority. Once the ITC has recommended a chemical substance for testing, the EPA must either initiate testing or publish its reasons for not doing so, within 12 months.

This last requirement, coupled with the statute's formal procedures for adopting test rules, led the EPA initially to rely on negotiations with chemical producers to secure voluntary agreements for the conduct of tests it thought appropriate for chemicals identified by the ITC (GAO, 1982). The practice was challenged by public interest organizations, who were excluded from the negotiations, and ultimately it was declared unlawful (*Natural Resources Defense Council, Inc., v. United States Environmental Protection Agency,* 1984). The agency amended its regulations to recognize two forms of mandates for testing: test rules and enforceable testing consent agreements (EPA, 1993).

TSCA test rules are subject to judicial challenge. Manufacturers challenged a 1988 test rule for cumene, arguing that the EPA had failed to support its finding that the substance enters the environment in substantial quantities with the potential for substantial human exposure. Although the court ultimately upheld the rule, it ordered the agency to articulate standards governing the definition of "substantial" (*Chemical Manufacturers Association v. EPA,* 1990). Another court challenge to a test rule requiring neurotoxicity studies of ten widely used and intensively marketed organic solvents resulted in a settlement with the EPA. The settlement required the EPA to enter into consent agreements with reduced testing requirements for seven chemicals, to eliminate testing requirements for two, and to postpone its decision on one. Both test rules and testing consent agreements specify what types of tests are to be done. Their design is governed either by general "test methodology guidelines" that the EPA has issued for several types of tests or by the rule or the agreement itself. All toxicologic studies required by the EPA under the TSCA must comply with its GLP regulations.

Locating Testing Guidelines The EPA usually publishes toxicology testing guidelines that apply to a specific regulatory program in the *Code of Federal Regulations* (*C.F.R.*). For example, the TSCA testing guidelines appear at 40 *C.F.R.* Part 798. The health effects testing guidelines applicable to the FIFRA appear in the *Federal Register* or may be obtained directly from the agency.

The EPA occasionally issues generic guidelines applicable to several of its regulatory programs. In 1996 it released a draft revision of its cancer assessment guidelines (EPA, 1996). The revised guidelines offer a more flexible approach to the assessment of cancer risk. For example, they support the use of several types of data—including biological, pharmacokinetic, and tumor development data—for hazard identification.

Interagency Testing Criteria and Programs

The foregoing summary of regulatory programs that mandate toxicologic tests (see "FDA and EPA Testing Standards," above) suggests the possibility of inconsistencies in testing standards. In the late 1970s, the responsible regulatory agencies (OSHA and the CPSC as well as the FDA and the EPA) combined to form the Interagency Regulatory Liaison Group (IRLG) to secure agreement on the design of standard toxicologic tests. Though the IRLG has long since collapsed, both the FDA and the EPA, along with the White House Office of Science and Technology Policy, have continued to work to achieve internal consistency.

The National Toxicology Program (NTP) was established in 1978 as an administrative umbrella for coordinating the numerous federal efforts to improve test methods and to coordinate toxicologic studies then under way, primarily in the Department of Health and Human Services. NTP assumed responsibility for what had been the bioassay program of the National Cancer Institute (NCI). An NTP committee that includes representatives of all four regulatory agencies is responsible for selecting chemicals to be tested at public expense. Attention continues to be focused on improving health risk assessment research techniques.

Animal Welfare Requirements

Researchers who conduct studies funded by federal agencies must comply with the Animal Welfare Act (AWA), and some may also be subject to restrictions imposed by the Public Health Service (PHS). Recipients of grants from the Department of Education, the Department of Health and Human Services, the Department of Agriculture, or the EPA are subject only to the AWA. Those funded by the Department of Energy or by the PHS must also comply with PHS policies. Restrictions on animal use also appear in the GLP regulations adopted by the FDA and the EPA (Reagan, 1986).

Animal Welfare Act The AWA is administered by the Animal and Plant Health Inspection Service (APHIS), a part of the U.S. Department of Agriculture. The AWA, which protects only warm-blooded animals and excludes birds, rats, and mice, requires all covered research facilities to register with APHIS and agree to comply with applicable AWA standards. Each facility must file an annual report signed by a responsible official that shows that "professionally acceptable standards governing the care, treatment, and use of animals" were followed for the year in question. The report must include the following:

1. Assurances that alternatives to painful procedures were considered in the design of the studies conducted there.
2. A summary and brief explanation of all exceptions to the standards and regulations that were approved by the Institutional Animal Care and Use Committee, including the species and number of animals affected.
3. The common names and the numbers of animals used in three research categories: (a) research involving no pain, distress, or use of pain-relieving drugs; (b) research involving pain and distress and for which pain-relieving drugs were used; and (c) research involving pain or distress in which no pain-relieving drugs were used because of adverse effects on the procedures, results, or interpretation.
4. The common names and the numbers of animals bred, conditioned, or held for research purposes but not yet used.

Pursuant to the AWA, APHIS has established specific requirements for the humane handling, care, and transportation of dogs and cats, guinea pigs and hamsters, rabbits, nonhuman primates, marine mammals, and other warm-blooded animals. The regulations governing facilities address living space, heating, lighting, ventilation, and drainage. The health and husbandry provisions address feeding, watering, sanitation, veterinary care, grouping of animals, and the number and qualifications of caretakers (APHIS, 1994).

The APHIS has strengthened the content and broadened the scope of its regulations, which were amended in an attempt to achieve more consistency with those of the PHS while favoring flexible guidelines rather than strict standards. The 1991 amendments to the specifications for the humane handling, care, and treatment of dogs and nonhuman primates require research facilities to develop plans to ensure appropriate exercise for dogs as well as an environment that promotes the psychological well-being of nonhuman primates (APHIS, 1991). The APHIS also has clarified the question of whether horses and other farm animals are subject to its regulations (APHIS, 1990). Despite these initiatives, several animal welfare groups and individuals have sued the agency in an attempt to further strengthen the regulations. One lawsuit challenged the APHIS's exclusion of rats, mice, and birds from coverage under the AWA (*Animal Legal Defense Fund v. Madigan,* 1992). A second lawsuit challenged the regulations governing the exercise of dogs and the psychological well-being of nonhuman primates on the grounds that the discretionary standard failed to guarantee minimum requirements (*Animal Legal Defense Fund v. Secretary of Agriculture,* 1993). Both suits were dismissed on the ground that the petitioners—including researchers, members of institutional oversight committees, and animal welfare organizations—lacked standing to challenge the regulations. A more recent challenge to USDA regulations to protect nonhuman primates in biomedical research surmounted the government's claim that the plaintiffs lacked standing but proceeded to uphold the regulations on the merits (*Animal Legal Defense Fund, Inc., v. Glickman,* 2000).

The AWA requires each research facility to establish an Institutional Animal Care and Use Committee (IACUC), composed of three or more members, one of whom must be a veterinarian and one of whom must represent community interests and who may not be affiliated with the institution. In 1989, the APHIS expanded the responsibilities of the IACUC. At least one member of the IACUC must now review and approve the animal care and use components of all proposed research activities. Prerequisites to approval include the avoidance or minimization of discomfort, distress and pain; the use of pain-relieving drugs where appropriate; the consideration of pain-free alternatives; and euthanization when an animal would otherwise experience severe or chronic pain or distress that cannot be relieved.

The IACUC is also responsible for conducting semiannual inspections of the facility itself and of the program for humane care and use of animals. Committee reports are filed with the APHIS and with any federal agency funding the research.

Public Health Service Policy The PHS Policy on Humane Care and Use of Laboratory Animals by Awardee Institutions applies to research using all vertebrates, and thus has a broader reach than the AWA. The PHS policy requires each facility to submit an annual report, called an "Assurance," which is evaluated by the National Institutes of Health (NIH) Office for Protection from Research Risks (OPRR) to determine the sufficiency of animal care.

The PHS policy imposes two primary obligations on researchers: each institution must adopt a Program for Animal Care and Use, and it must establish an IACUC. The IACUC must be made up of at least five members, including a veterinarian, an animal research scientist, a nonscientist, and a person who is not affiliated with the facility in any other capacity. The IACUC must review all applications for research funding and review the institution's programs to ensure compliance with NIH standards. The Health Research Extension Act of 1985 requires that PHS-funded institutions provide training on methods to reduce animal suffering similar to that mandated by the AWA for its personnel. It also requires that researchers' grant applications justify any proposed use of animals (NRC, 1988).

Research facilities subject to either the AWA or PHS may wish to consult a National Academy of Sciences report that details suggestions for developing institutional compliance programs (National Research Council, 1991). Scientists working with no federal funding who expect their research to be submitted to the FDA or the EPA are not subject to the AWA or PHS policies, but they must comply with the animal protection provisions of those agencies' GLP regulations. These regulations prescribe adequate living conditions, detail requirements for veterinary treatment, and impose specific record-keeping requirements (EPA, 1999; FDA, 2000).

REFERENCES

Cases

American Federation of Labor v. OSHA, 965 F.2d 962 (11th Cir. 1992).

American Textile Manufacturers Institute v. Donovan, 452 U.S. 490, 495 (1982).

Animal Legal Defense Fund v. Glickman, 204 F.3d 229 (D.C. Cir. 2000).

Animal Legal Defense Fund v. Madigan, 781 F. Supp. 797 (D.D.C. 1992), *vacated and remanded sub nom. Animal Legal Defense Fund v. Espy,* 23 F.3d 496 (D.C. Cir. 1994).

Animal Legal Defense Fund v. Secretary of Agriculture, 813 F. Supp. 882 (D.D.C. 1993), *vacated and remanded sub nom. Animal Legal Defense Fund v. Espy,* 29 F.3d 720 (D.C. Cir. 1994).

Chemical Manufacturers Association v. EPA, 899 F.2d 344 (5th Cir. 1990).

Chlorine Chemistry Council v. EPA, 206 F.3d 1286 (D.C. Cir. 2000).

Corrosion Proof Fittings v. Environmental Protection Agency, 947 F.2d 1201 (5th Cir. 1991).

Environmental Defense Fund, Inc., v. Environmental Protection Agency, 548 F.2d 998 (D.C. Cir. 1976).

Environmental Defense Fund, Inc., v. Ruckelhaus, 439 F.2d 584 (D.C. Cir. 1971).

Environmental Defense Fund, Inc., and National Audubon Society v. Environmental Protection Agency, 510 F.2d 1292 (D.C. Cir. 1975).

Gulf South Insulation v. CPSC, 701 F.2d 1137 (5th Cir. 1983).

Industrial Union Department, AFL-CIO, v. American Petroleum Institute, 448 U.S. 607 (1980).

Industrial Union Department, AFL-CIO, v. Hodgson, 499 F.2d 467 (D.C. Cir. 1974).

Les v. Reilly, 968 F.2d 985 (9th Cir. 1992).

Monsanto v. Kennedy, 613 F.2d 947 (D.C. Cir. 1979).

Natural Resources Defense Council, Inc., v. United States Environmental Protection Agency, 595 F. Supp. 1255 (S.D.N.Y. 1984).

Natural Resources Defense Council, Inc., v. United States Environmental Protection Agency, 824 F.2d 1146 (D.C. Cir. 1987).

NRDC v. Train, 8 E.R.C. 2120 (D.D.C. 1976).

Public Citizen v. Young, 831 F.2d 1108 (D.C. Cir. 1987).

Society of the Plastics Industry, Inc., v. OSHA, 509 F.2d 9301 (2d Cir. 1975).

SECONDARY SOURCES

Berger J, Riskin S: Economic and technological feasibility under the Occupational Safety and Health Act. *Ecology L Q* 7:285, 1978.

Bruser J, Harris R, Page T: Waterborne carcinogens: An economist's view, in *The Scientific Basis of Health and Safety Regulation*. Washington, DC: Brookings Institution, 1981.

Cooper R: The role of regulatory agencies in risk-benefit decision-making. *Food Drug Cosmet L J* 33:755–757, 1978.

Douglas I: Safe Drinking Water Act of 1975—History and critique. *Environ Affairs* 5:501, 1976.

EPA: *Draft Revisions to the Guidelines for Carcinogen Risk Assessment*. Report by the U.S. Environmental Protection Agency. Washington, DC: EPA, 1994.

FDA: *Toxicological Principles for the Safety Assessment of Direct Food Additives and Color Additives Used in Food*. Washington, DC: U.S. Food and Drug Administration, 1982.

FDA: *Toxicological Principles for the Safety Assessment of Direct Food Additives and Color Additives Used in Food*. Draft Report. Washington, DC: U.S. Food and Drug Administration, 1993.

GAO: *EPA Implementation of Selected Aspects of the Toxic Substances Control Act*. Washington, DC: U.S. General Accounting Office, December 1982.

Gray K: The Safe Drinking Water Act Amendments of 1986: Now a tougher act to follow. *Environ L Rep* 16:10338, 1986.

Heineck D: New clean water act toxics control initiatives. *Nat Resources Environ* 1:10, 1989.

HHS: *National Toxicology Program Annual Plan for Fiscal Year 1988*. Washington, DC: U.S. Department of Health and Human Services, January 1988.

Hutt PB, Merrill R: *Food and Drug Law: Cases and Materials*. Mineola, NY: Foundation Press, 1991.

Merrill R: Regulating carcinogens in food: A legislator's guide to the food safety provisions of the federal Food, Drug, and Cosmetics Act. *Mich L Rev* 77:179–184, 1979.

Merrill R: CPSC regulation of cancer risks in consumer products: 1972–81. *Va L Rev* 67:1261, 1981.

Merrill R, Schewel M: FDA regulation of environmental contaminants of food. *Va L Rev* 66:1357, 1980.

National Institute of Health, Department of Health and Human Services: *Guide for the Care and Use of Laboratory Animals,* Publ. No. 23. Guide for Grants and Contracts: Special ed: Laboratory Animal Welfare. Washington, DC: NIH/DHHS, June1985.

National Research Council: *A Guide for Developing Institutional Programs*. Washington, DC: National Academy, 1991.

National Research Council: *Use of Laboratory Animals in Biomedical and Behavioral Research*. Washington, DC: National Academy, 1988.

OTA: *Assessment of Technologies for Determining the Cancer Risks from the Environment*. Report by the Office of Technology Assessment. Washington, DC: US Government Printing Office, June 1981.

Page NP: Testing for health and environmental effects: The OECD guidelines. *Toxic Substances J* 4:135, 1982.

Reagan K: Federal regulation of testing with laboratory animals: Future directions. *Pace Environ L Rev* 3:165, 1986.

Reed PD: The trial of hazardous air pollution regulation. *Environ L Register* 16:10066–10072, 1986.

Turner J: The Delaney anticancer clause: A model environmental protection law. *Vand L Rev* 24:889, 1971.

STATUTES AND REGULATIONS

Animal Welfare, 9 *CFR* Parts 2 & 3 (1994).

Animal Welfare Act (1988), 7 U.S.C. § 2131 et seq.

Animal Welfare; Standards. *Fed Reg* 56(32):6426, 1991.

APHIS: (part of USDA) Intent to Regulate Horses and Other Farm Animals Under the Animal Welfare Act; Technical Amendment and Definition. *Fed Reg* 55(66):12630, 1990.

Applications for FDA Approval to Market a New Drug or an Antibiotic Drug, 21 C.F.R. Part 314 (1994).

Clean Air Act (1976), 42 U.S.C. § 7401 et seq.

Color Additive Amendments of 1960 to the Federal Food, Drug, and Cosmetic Act, 21 U.S.C. § 706.

Color Additive Petitions, 21 C.F.R. Part 71 (1994).

Consumer Product Safety Act (1972), 15 U.S.C. § 2051 et seq.

CPSC: Labeling of Asbestos-Containing Household Products; Enforcement Policy. *Fed Reg* 51(185):33910, 1986.

CPSC: Labeling of Hazardous Art Materials Act (1988), 15 U.S.C. §1277.

CPSC: Labeling Requirements for Art Materials Presenting Chronic Hazards; Guidelines for Determining Chronic Toxicity of Products Subject to the FHSA; Supplementary Definition of "Toxic" Under the Federal Hazardous Substances Act. *Fed Reg* 57(197):46626, 1992.

Data Requirements for Registration, 40 C.F.R. Part 158 (1993).

Drug Amendments of 1962 to the Federal Food, Drug, and Cosmetic Act, 21 U.S.C. § 360(b).

Environmental Effects Testing Guidelines, 40 C.F.R. Part 797 (1993).

EPA: Good Laboratory Practice Standards for Health Effects: Environmental Protection Agency. *Fed Reg* 44(91):27362, 1979.

EPA: Hazardous Waste Management System: General, 40 C.F.R. Part 260 (1993).

EPA: Proposed Guidelines for Carcinogen Risk Assessment; Request for Comments. *Fed Reg* 49(227):46293–46301, 1984.

EPA: Proposed Guidelines for Carcinogen Risk Assessment. *Fed Reg* 61(85):17960–18010, 1996.

FDA: Food Additive Petitions, 21 C.F.R. Part 171 (1994).

FDA: Good Laboratory Practice for Nonclinical Laboratory Studies, 21 C.F.R. Part 58 (2000).

FDA: Indirect Food Additives: Polymers; Acrylonitrile/Styrene Copolymers. *Fed Reg* 49(183):36635–36644, 1984.

FDA Modernization Act, Pub. L. No. 105–115, 1997.

FDA: Policy for Regulating Carcinogenic Chemicals in Food and Color Additives: Advanced Notice of Proposed Rulemaking: Food and Drug Administration. *Fed Reg* 47(64):14464–14469, 1982.

FDA: Sponsored Compounds in Food Producing Animals. *Fed Reg* 50(284): 45530, 1995.

Federal Food, Drug, and Cosmetic Act (1938), 21 U.S.C. § 321 et seq.

Federal Hazardous Substances Act (1976), 15 U.S.C. § 1261 et seq.

Federal Insecticide, Fungicide, and Rodenticide Act (1972), 7 U.S.C. § 135 et seq.

Federal Insecticide, Fungicide, and Rodenticide Act Amendments of 1988, Pub. L. No. 100–532, 102 Stat. 2654.

Federal Water Pollution Control Act Amendments of 1972, 33 U.S.C. § 307.

Food Additive Amendments to the Federal Food, Drug, and Cosmetic Act (1958), 21 U.S.C. § 348 et seq.

Food Quality Protection Act, Pub. L. No. 104–170, 1996.

Good Laboratory Practice Standards, 40 C.F.R. Part 160 (1999).

Good Laboratory Practice Standards, 40 C.F.R. Part 792 (1999).

Health Effects Testing Guidelines, 40 C.F.R. Part 798 (1993).

Identification of Specific Chemical Substance and Mixture Testing Requirements, 40 C.F.R. Part 799 (1993).

New Drugs, 21 C.F.R. Part 310 (1994).

Occupational Safety and Health Act (1970), 29 U.S.C. § 651 et seq.

OSHA: Identification, Classification and Regulation of Potential Occupational Carcinogens: Occupational Safety and Health Act. *Fed Reg* 45(15):5002, 1980.

OSHA: Identification, Classification and Regulation of Potential Occupational Carcinogens: Occupational Safety and Health Act. *Fed Reg* 47(2):187–190, 1982.

Pesticide Residue Amendments to the Federal Food, Drug, and Cosmetic Act (1954), 21 U.S.C. § 348 et seq.

Proposed Guidelines for Registering Pesticides in the United States: Environmental Protection Agency. *Fed Reg* 43(163):37336, 1978.

Proposed Health Effects Test Standards for Toxic Substances Control Act Test Rules: Environmental Protection Agency. *Fed Reg* 44(145):44054, 1979.

Proposed Interim Primary Drinking Water Regulations: Environmental Protection Agency. *Fed Reg* 43(130):29135–29137, 1978 (to be codified at 40 C.F.R. § 141).

Provisional Test Guidelines, 40 C.F.R. Part 795 (1993).

Rebuttable Presumption Against Registration (RPAR) Proceedings and Hearings Under Section 6 of the Federal Insecticide, Fungicide, and Rodenticide Act (FIFRA): Environmental Protection Agency. *Fed Reg* 45(154):52628–52674, 1980.

Resource Conservation and Recovery Act (1976), 42 U.S.C.A. § 6901.

Safe Drinking Water Act (1974), 42 U.S.C. §§ 300f to 300j-9.

Specific Chemical Test Rules, 40 C.F.R. Part 799 (1993).

Sponsored Compounds in Food Producing Animals: Proposed Rule and Notice. *Fed Reg* 50(211):45529–45556, 1985.

Testing Consent Orders, 40 C.F.R. § 799.5000 (1993).

Toxic Substances Control Act (1976), 15 U.S.C. § 2601.

Toxic Substances Control Act, § 4, 15 U.S.C. § 2603(b)(1) (1988).

Toxic Substances Control Act, § 6, 15 U.S.C. § 2605 (1988).

1999–2000 Threshold Limit Values (TLV) and Permissible Exposure Limits (PEL) ***(continued)***

		ACGIH TLV		*OSHA PEL*	
NAME	CAS NO.	TWA	STEL	TWA	STEL
Acrylic acid, methyl ester (methyl acrylate)	000096-33-3	2 ppm Skin Sen A4		10 ppm Skin	
Acrylonitrile (vinyl cyanide)	000107-13-1	2 ppm, A3 Skin		2 ppm Skin	C10 ppm
Adipic acid	000124-04-9	5 m/M			
Adiponitrile	000111-69-3	2 ppm Skin			
Aldrin	000309-00-2	0.25 m/M Skin A3		0.25 m/M Skin	
Allyl alcohol	000107-18-6	0.5 ppm Skin		2 ppm Skin	
Allyl chloride	000107-05-1	1 ppm A3	2 ppm	1 ppm	
Allyl glycidyl ether (AGE)	000106-92-3	1 ppm A4			C10 ppm
Allyl propyl disulfide	002179-59-1	2 ppm	3 ppm	2 ppm	
α-Alumina (aluminum oxide)	001344-28-1	10 m/M		15 m/M	
Aluminum metal dust [7429-90-5]		10 m/M		15 m/M	
Aluminum, alkyls, not otherwise classified as Al		2 m/M			
Aluminum, pyro powders, as Al		5 m/M			
Aluminum, soluble salts, as Al		2 m/M			
Aluminum, welding fumes, as Al		5 m/M			
Aluminum oxide		10 m/M A4		15 m/M	
2-Aminoethanol (ethanolamine)	000141-43-5	3 ppm	6 ppm	3 ppm	
2-Aminopyridine (2-nitro-4-aminophenol)	000504-29-0	0.5 ppm		0.5 ppm	
3-Amino-1,2,4-triazole (amitrole)	000061-82-5	0.2 m/M			
Ammonia	007664-41-7	25 ppm	35 ppm	50 ppm	
Ammonium chloride fume	012125-02-9	10 m/M			
Ammonium perfluoro-octanoate	003825-26-1	0.01 m/M, A3 Skin			
Ammonium sulfamate	007773-06-0	10 m/M		10 m/M	
Amosite (asbestos)	012172-73-5	0.1 f/cc, A1		0.1 f/cc	
n-Amyl acetate	000628-63-7	50 ppm	100 ppm	100 ppm	
sec-Amyl acetate	000626-38-0	50 ppm	100 ppm	125 ppm	
Aniline and homologues	000062-53-3	2 ppm Skin		5 ppm Skin	
Anisidine (*o*-, *p*-isomers)	029191-52-4	0.1 m/M Skin		0.5 m/M Skin	
Antimony [7440-36-0] and compounds, as Sb		0.5 m/M		0.5 m/M	
Antimony trioxide, handling and use, as Sb	001309-64-4	0.5 m/M		0.5 m/M	
ANTU (*α*-naphthylthiourea)	000086-88-4	0.3 m/M		0.3 m/M	
Argon	007440-37-1	Asphyxiant			
Arsenic, elemental [7440-38-2] and inorganic compounds (except arsine), as As		0.01 m/M A1		0.01 m/M	
Arsenous acid, arsenic acid and salts		0.01 m/M A1			
Arsine	007784-42-1	0.05 ppm		0.05 ppm	
Asbestos, all forms		0.1 f/cc A1		0.1 f/cc	1 f/cc
Asphalt (petroleum) fumes	008052-42-4	0.5 m/M A4			
Atrazine	001912-24-9	5 m/M A4			

(continued)

1999–2000 Threshold Limit Values (TLV) and Permissible Exposure Limits (PEL) ***(continued)***

NAME	CAS NO.	*ACGIH TLV* TWA	*ACGIH TLV* STEL	*OSHA PEL* TWA	*OSHA PEL* STEL
Azinphos-methyl (Guthion)	000086-50-0	0.2 m/M Skin		0.2 m/M Skin	
Barium [7440-39-3] soluble compounds, as Ba		0.5 m/M A4		0.5 m/M	
Barium sulfate	007727-43-7	10 m/M		15 m/M	
Beech wood dust		1 m/M SEN A1			
Benomyl	017804-35-2	0.84 ppm		15 m/M	
Benzene	000071-43-2	0.5 ppm Skin A1	2.5 ppm	1 ppm	5 ppm
p-Benzoquinone (quinone)	000106-51-4	0.1 ppm		0.1 ppm	
Benzoyl peroxide	000094-36-0	5 m/M		5 m/M	
Benzo[*a*]pyrene	000050-32-8	A1		0.2 m/M	
Benzylchloride	000100-44-7	1 ppm A3		1 ppm	
Beryllium [7440-41-7] and compounds, as Be		0.002 ppm A1		0.002 m/M	
Biphenyl (diphenyl)	000092-52-4	0.2 ppm		0.2 ppm	
Bismuth telluride, undoped, as Bi_2Te_3	001304-82-1	10 m/M A4		15 m/M	
Bismuth telluride, Se-doped, as Bi_2Te_3	001304-82-1	5 m/M			
Bitumen	008052-42-4	5 m/M A4			
Borates, tetra, sodium salts, anhydrous	001303-96-4	1 m/M			
Borates, tetra, sodium salts, decahydrate	001303-96-4	5 m/M			
Borates, tetra, sodium salts, pentahydrate	001303-96-4	1 m/M			
Boron oxide	001303-86-2	10 m/M		15 m/M	
Boron tribromide	010294-33-4		C1 ppm		
Boron trifluoride	007637-07-2		C1 ppm		C1 ppm
Bromacil	000314-40-9	10 m/M A3			
Bromine	007726-95-6	0.1 ppm	0.2 ppm	0.1 ppm	
Bromine pentafluoride	007789-30-2	0.1 ppm			
Bromochloromethane (chlorobromomethane)	000074-97-5	200 ppm		200 ppm	
Bromoethane (ethyl bromide)	000074-96-4	5 ppm Skin A3		200 ppm	
Bromoform (tribromomethane)	000075-25-2	0.5 ppm Skin A3		0.5 ppm Skin	
1,3-Butadiene	000106-99-0	2 ppm A2		5 ppm	
Butane	000106-97-8	800 ppm			
Butanethiol (butyl mercaptan)	000109-79-5	0.5 ppm		10 ppm	
n-Butanol (*n*-butyl alcohol)	000071-36-3		C50 ppm Skin	100 ppm Skin	
sec-Butanol (*sec*-butyl alcohol)	000078-92-2	100 ppm		150 ppm	
tert-Butanol (*tert*-butyl alcohol)	000075-65-0	100 ppm A4		100 ppm	
2-Butanone (methyl ethyl ketone [MEK])	000078-93-3	200 ppm	300 ppm	200 ppm	
2-Butoxyethanol (ethylene glycol monobutyl ether)	000111-76-2	20 ppm Skin		50 ppm Skin	
n-Butyl acetate	000123-86-4	150 ppm	200 ppm	150 ppm	
sec-Butyl acetate	000105-46-4	200 ppm		200 ppm	
tert-Butyl acetate	000540-88-5	200 ppm		200 ppm	
n-Butyl acrylate (acrylic acid, *n*-butyl ester)	000141-32-2	2 ppm SEN A4			

(continued)

1999–2000 Threshold Limit Values (TLV) and Permissible Exposure Limits (PEL) ***(continued)***

NAME	CAS NO.	ACGIH TLV TWA	ACGIH TLV STEL	OSHA PEL TWA	OSHA PEL STEL
n-Butylamine	000109-73-9		C5 ppm Skin		C5 ppm Skin
tert-Butyl chromate, as CrO_3	001189-85-1		C0.1 m/M Skin		C0.1 m/M Skin
n-Butyl glycidyl ether (BGE)	002426-08-6	25 ppm		50 ppm	
n-Butyl lactate	000138-22-7	5 ppm			
Butyl mercaptan (butanethiol)	000109-79-5	0.5 ppm		10 ppm	
o-sec-Butylphenol	000089-72-5	5 ppm Skin			
p-tert Butyltoluene	000098-51-1	1 ppm		10 ppm	
Cadmium [7440-43-9] and compounds, as Cd		0.01 m/M A2		0.005 m/M	
Calcium carbonate (limestone; marble)	001317-65-3	10 m/M		15 m/M	
Calcium chromate, as Cr	013756-19-0	0.001 m/M A2			
Calcium cyanamide	000156-62-7	0.5 m/M			
Calcium hydroxide	001305-62-0	5 m/M		15 m/M	
Calcium oxide	001305-78-8	2 m/M		5 m/M	
Calcium silicate (synthetic)	001344-95-2	10 m/M A4		15 m/M	
Calcium sulfate (gypsum; plaster of paris)	007778-18-9	10 m/M		15 m/M	
Camphor, synthetic	000076-22-2	2 ppm A4	3 ppm	2 m/M	
Caprolactam dust	000105-60-2	1 m/M A4	3 m/M		
Caprolactam vapor	000105-60-2	5 ppm A4	10 ppm		
Captafol	002425-06-1	0.1 m/M Skin A4			
Captan	000133-06-2	5 m/M A3			
Carbaryl (sevin)	000063-25-2	5 m/M A4			
Carbofuran	001563-66-2	0.1 m/M A4		5 m/M	
Carbon black	001333-86-4	3.5 m/M A4		3.5 m/M	
Carbon dioxide	000124-38-9	5000 ppm	30,000 ppm	5000 ppm	
Carbon disulfide	000075-15-0	10 ppm Skin		20 ppm Skin	
Carbon monoxide	000630-08-0	25 ppm		50 ppm	
Carbon tetrabromide	000558-13-4	0.1 ppm	0.3 ppm		
Carbon tetrachloride (tetrachloromethane)	000056-23-5	5 ppm A2 Skin	10 ppm A3 Skin	10 ppm	C25 ppm
Carbonyl chloride (phosgene)	000075-44-5	0.1 ppm		0.1 ppm	
Carbonyl fluoride	000353-50-4	2 ppm	5 ppm		
Catechol (pyrocatechol)	000120-80-9	5 ppm Skin A3			
Cellulose	009004-34-6	10 m/M		15 m/M	
Cesium hydroxide	021351-79-1	2 m/M			
Chlordane	000057-74-9	0.5 m/M Skin A3		0.3 m/M Skin	
Chlorinated camphene (toxaphene)	008001-35-2	0.5 m/M Skin	1 m/M Skin	0.5 m/M Skin	
Chlorinated diphenyl oxide	031242-93-0	0.5 m/M		0.5 m/M	
Chlorine	007782-50-5	0.5 ppm	1 ppm		C1 ppm
Chlorine dioxide	010049-04-4	0.1 ppm	0.3 ppm	0.1 ppm	
Chlorine trifluoride	007790-91-2		C0.1 ppm		C0.1 ppm
Chloroacetaldehyde	000107-20-0		C1 ppm		C1 ppm
Chloroacetone	000078-95-5		C1 ppm Skin		
α-Chloroacetophenone (phenacyl chloride)	000532-27-4	0.05 ppm A4		0.05 ppm	
Chloroacetyl chloride	000079-04-9	0.05 ppm Skin	0.15 ppm Skin		
Chlorobenzene (monochlorobenzene)	000108-90-7	10 ppm A3		75 ppm	
o-Chlorobenzylidene malononitrile	002698-41-1		C0.05 ppm Skin A4	0.05 ppm	

(continued)

1999–2000 Threshold Limit Values (TLV) and Permissible Exposure Limits (PEL) ***(continued)***

		ACGIH TLV		*OSHA PEL*	
NAME	CAS NO.	TWA	STEL	TWA	STEL
Chlorobromomethane (bromochloromethane)	000074-97-5	200 ppm		200 ppm	
2-Chloro-1,3-butadine (*β*-chloroprene)	000126-99-8	10 ppm Skin		25 ppm Skin	
Chlorodifluoromethane	000075-45-6	1000 ppm A4			
Chlorodiphenyl (42% chlorine)	053469-21-9	1 m/M Skin		1 m/M Skin	
Chlorodiphenyl (54% chlorine)	011097-69-1	0.5 m/M Skin A3		0.5 m/M Skin	
1-Chloro,2,3-epoxypropane (epichlorohydrin)	000106-89-8	0.5 ppm Skin		5 ppm	
Chloroethane (ethyl chloride)	000075-00-3	100 ppm		1000 ppm	
2-Chloroethanol (ethylene chlorohydrin)	000107-07-3		C1 ppm Skin A4	5 ppm	
Chloroethylene (vinyl chloride)	000075-01-4	1 ppm A1	1 ppm	5 ppm	
Chloroform (trichloromethane)	000067-66-3	10 ppm A3			C15 ppm
bis(Chloromethyl) ether	000542-88-1	0.001 ppm A1			
1-Chloro-1-nitropropane	000600-25-9	2 ppm		20 ppm	
Chloropentafluorethane	000076-15-3	1000 ppm			
Chloropicrin (trichloronitromethane)	000076-06-2	0.1 ppm A4		0.1 ppm	
β-Chloroprene	000126-99-8	10 ppm Skin		25 ppm Skin	
2-Chloropropionic acid	000598-78-7	0.1 ppm Skin			
o-Chlorostyrene	002039-87-4	50 ppm	75 ppm		
o-Chlorotoluene	000095-49-8	50 ppm			
2-Chloro-6-(trichloromethyl) pyridine (nitrapyrin)	001929-82-4	10 m/M	20 m/M	15 m/M	
Chlorpyrifos	002921-88-2	0.2 m/M Skin			
Chromates, alkaline, as Cr		0.05 m/M A1			C0.1 m/M
Chromic acid [1066-30-4] and chromates		0.05 m/M A1			C0.1 m/M
Chromite ore processing (chromate), as Cr		0.05 m/M A1			
Chromium (II) compounds, as Cr				0.5 m/M	
Chromium (III) compounds, as Cr		0.5 m/M A4		0.5 m/M	
Chromium (VI) compounds, as Cr, water-soluble		0.05 m/M A1			C0.1 m/M
Chromium (VI) compounds, as Cr, certain water insoluble		0.01 m/M A1			C0.1 m/M
Chromium metal	007440-47-3	0.5 m/M A4		1 m/M	
Chromium trioxide, as Cr	001333-82-0	0.05 m/M A1			C0.1 m/M
Chromyl chloride	014977-61-8	0.025 ppm			
Chrysene	000218-01-9	A3			0.2 m/M
Chrysotile (asbestos, chrysotile)	012001-29-5	0.1 f/cc A1		0.1 f/cc	
Clopidol	002971-90-6	10 m/M		15 m/M	
Coal dust		2 m/M		2 m/M	

(continued)

1999–2000 Threshold Limit Values (TLV) and Permissible Exposure Limits (PEL) *(continued)*

NAME	CAS NO.	ACGIH TLV TWA	ACGIH TLV STEL	OSHA PEL TWA	OSHA PEL STEL
Coal tar pitch volatiles, as benzene solubles	65996-93-20	0.2 m/M A1		0.2 m/M	
Cobalt, elemental [7440-48-4], and inorganic compounds, as Co		0.02 m/M A3		0.01 m/M	
Cobalt carbonyl, as Co	010210-68-1	0.1 m/M			
Cobalt hydrocarbonyl, as Co	016842-03-8	0.1 m/M			
Coke oven emissions				0.15 m/M	
Copper fume	007440-50-8	0.2 m/M		0.1 m/M	
Copper [7440-50-8] dusts and mists, as Cu		1 m/M		1 m/M	
Cotton dust				0.2 m/M	
Cotton dust, raw		0.2 m/M		1 m/M	
Cresol, all isomers	001319-77-3	5 ppm Skin		5 ppm Skin	
Cristobalite (silica-crystalline)	014464-46-1	0.05 m/M			
Crocidolite (asbestos, crocidolite)	012001-28-4	0.1 f/cc A1		0.1 f/cc	
Crotonaldehyde	004170-30-3		C0.3 ppm A3	2 ppm	
Crufomate	000299-86-5	5 m/M A4			
Cumene	000098-82-8	50 ppm Skin		50 ppm Skin	
Cyanamide	000420-04-2	2 m/M			
Cyanide, calcium, as CN	000592-01-8		C5 m/M Skin	5 m/M	
Cyanide, potassium, as CN	000151-50-8		C5 m/M Skin	5 m/M	
Cyanide, sodium, as CN	000143-33-9		C5 m/M Skin	5 m/M	
Cyanogen	000460-19-5	10 ppm			
Cyanogen chloride	000506-77-4		C0.3 ppm		
Cyclohexane	000110-82-7	300 ppm		300 ppm	
Cyclohexanol	000108-93-0	50 ppm Skin		50 ppm Skin	
Cyclohexanone	000108-94-1	25 ppm Skin A4		50 ppm Skin	
Cyclohexene	000110-83-8	300 ppm		300 ppm	
Cyclohexylamine	000108-91-8	10 ppm			
Cyclonite (RDX)	000121-82-4	0.5 m/M Skin A4			
Cyclopentadiene	000542-92-7	75 ppm		75 ppm	
Cyclopentane	000287-92-3	600 ppm			
Cyhexatin (tricyclohexyltin hydroxide)	013121-70-5	5 m/M A4			
2,4-D (2,4-dichlorophenoxyacetic acid)	000094-75-7	10 m/M A4		10 m/M	
DDT (Dichlorodiphenyltrichloroethane)	000050-29-3	1 m/M A3		1 m/M Skin	
Decaborane	017702-41-9	0.05 ppm Skin	0.15 ppm Skin	0.05 ppm Skin	
Demeton-methyl (methyl demeton)	008022-00-2	0.5 m/M Skin			
Demeton (Systox)	008065-48-3	0.01 ppm Skin		0.1 m/M Skin	
Diacetone alcohol (4-hydroxy-4-methyl-2-pentanone)	000123-42-2	50 ppm		50 ppm	
1,2-Diaminoethane (ethylenediamine)	000107-15-3	10 ppm A4		10 ppm	
Diatomaceous earth (silica-amorphous)	061790-53-2	10 m/M		80 m/M	
Diazinon	000333-41-5	0.1 m/M Skin			
Diazomethane	000334-88-3	0.2 ppm		0.2 ppm	

(continued)

1999–2000 Threshold Limit Values (TLV) and Permissible Exposure Limits (PEL) *(continued)*

NAME	CAS NO.	*ACGIH TLV*		*OSHA PEL*	
		TWA	STEL	TWA	STEL
Diborane	019287-45-7	0.1 ppm		0.1 ppm	
Dibrom (naled)	000300-76-5	3 m/M Skin A4		3 m/M	
1,2-Dibromo-3-chloropropane (DBCP)	000096-12-8			0.001 ppm	
1,2-Dibromoethane (ethylene dibromide)	000106-93-4			20 ppm	C30 ppm
2-*N*-Dibutylaminoethanol	000102-81-8	0.5 ppm Skin			
Dibutyl phosphate	000107-66-4	1 ppm	2 ppm	1 ppm	
Dibutyl phenyl phosphate	002528-36-1	0.3 ppm Skin			
Dibutyl phthalate	000084-74-2	5 m/M A3		5 m/M	
Dichloroacetylene	007572-29-4		C0.1 ppm		
o-Dichlorobenzene (1,2-dichlorobenzene)	000095-50-1	25 ppm Skin A4	50 ppm Skin		C50 ppm Skin
p-Dichlorobenzene (1,4-dichlorobenzene)	000106-46-7	10 ppm A3		75 ppm	
1,4-Dichloro-2-butene	000764-41-0	0.005 ppm Skin A2			
Dichlorodifluoromethane	000075-71-8	1000 ppm A4		1000 ppm	
1,3-Dichloro-5,5-dimethyl hydantoin	000118-52-5	0.2 m/M	0.4 m/M	0.2 m/M	
Dichlorodiphenyltrichloro-ethane (DDT)	000050-29-3	1 m/M A3		1 m/M Skin	
1,1-Dichloroethane (ethylidene chloride)	000075-34-3	100 ppm A4		100 ppm	
1,2-Dichloroethane (ethylene dichloride)	000107-06-2	10 ppm		50 ppm	
1,1-Dichloroethylene (vinylidene chloride)	000075-35-4	5 ppm A4			
1,2-Dichloroethylene (acetylene dichloride)	000540-59-0	200 ppm		200 ppm	
Dichloroethyl ether	000111-44-4	5 ppm Skin A4	10 ppm Skin		C15 ppm Skin
Dichlorofluoromethane (dichloromonofluoro-methane)	000075-43-4	10 ppm		1000 ppm	
Dichloromethane (methylene chloride)	000075-09-2	50 ppm A3		25 ppm	
1,1-Dichloro-1-nitroethane	000594-72-9	2 ppm			C10 ppm
2,4-Dichlorophenoxyacetic acid (2,4-D)	000094-75-7	10 m/M A4		10 m/M	
1,2-Dichloropropane (propylene dichloride)	000078-87-5	75 ppm A4	110 ppm	75 ppm	
1,3-Dichloropropene	000542-75-6	1 ppm Skin			
2,2-Dichloropropionic acid	000075-99-0	5 m/M			
Dichlorotetrafluoroethane	000076-14-2	1000 ppm A4		1000 ppm	
Dichlorvos (DDVP)	000062-73-7	0.1 ppm Skin A4		1 m/M Skin	
Dicrotophos	000141-66-2	0.05 m/M Skin A4			
Dicyclopentadiene	000077-73-6	5 ppm			
Dicyclopentadienyl iron (ferrocene)	000102-54-5	10 m/M		15 m/M	
Dieldrin	000060-57-1	0.25 m/M Skin A4		0.25 m/M Skin	
Diethanolamine	000111-42-2	0.46 ppm Skin			
Diethylamine	000109-89-7	5 ppm A4	15 ppm A4	25 ppm	
2-Diethylaminoethanol	000100-37-8	2 ppm Skin		10 ppm Skin	
Diethylene triamine	000111-40-0	1 ppm Skin			
Diethyl ether (ethyl ether)	000060-29-7	400 ppm	500 ppm	400 ppm	

(continued)

1999–2000 Threshold Limit Values (TLV) and Permissible Exposure Limits (PEL) *(continued)*

NAME	CAS NO.	ACGIH TLV		OSHA PEL	
		TWA	STEL	TWA	STEL
Di(2-ethylhexyl)phthalate (DEHP; di-sec-octyl-phthalate)	000117-81-7	5 m/M A3		5 m/M	
Diethyl ketone	000096-22-0	300 ppm			
Diethyl phthalate	000084-66-2	5 m/M A4			
Difluorodibromomethane	000075-61-6	100 ppm		100 ppm	
Diglycidyl ether (DGE)	002238-07-5	0.1 ppm A4			C0.5 ppm
Dihydroxybenzene (hydroquinone)	000123-31-9	2 m/M A3		2 m/M	
Diisobutyl ketone (2,6-dimethyl-4-heptanone)	000108-83-8	25 ppm		50 ppm	
Diisopropylamine	000108-18-9	5 ppm Skin		5 ppm Skin	
Dimethoxymethane (methylal)	000109-87-5	1000 ppm		1000 ppm	
N,N-Dimethyl acetamide	000127-19-5	10 ppm Skin A4		10 ppm Skin	
Dimethylamine	000124-40-3	5 ppm A4	15 ppm	10 ppm	
Dimethylaminobenzene (xylidine)	001300-73-8	0.5 ppm Skin A2		5 ppm Skin	
Dimethylaniline (*N,N*-dimethylaniline)	000121-69-7	5 ppm Skin A4	10 ppm Skin	5 ppm Skin	
Dimethylbenzene (xylene)	001330-20-7	100 ppm A4	150 ppm	100 ppm	
Dimethyl-1,2-dibromo-2,2-dichloroethyl phosphate (dibrom; naled)	000300-76-5	3 m/M Skin A4		3 m/M	
Dimethylethoxysilane	014857-34-2	0.5 ppm	1.5 ppm		
Dimethylformamide	000068-12-2	10 ppm Skin A4		10 ppm Skin	
2,6-Dimethyl-4-heptanone (diisobutyl ketone)	000108-83-8	25 ppm		50 ppm	
1,1-Dimethylhydrazine	000057-14-7	0.01 ppm Skin A3		0.5 ppm Skin	
Dimethylphthalate	000131-11-3	5 m/M		5 m/M	
Dimethyl sulfate	000077-78-1	0.1 ppm Skin A3		1 ppm 1 Skin	
Dinitolmide (3,5-dinitro-*o*-toluamide)	000148-01-6	5 m/M			
Dinitrobenzene	000528-29-0 000099-65-0 000100-25-4 025154-54-5		0.15 ppm Skin		1 m/M Skin
Dinitro-*o*-cresol	000534-52-1	0.2 m/M Skin		0.2 m/M Skin	
3,5-Dinitro-*o*-toluamide (dinitolmide)	000148-01-6	5 m/M			
Dinitrotoluene	025321-14-6	0.2 m/M Skin A3		1.5 m/M Skin	
1,4-Dioxane	000123-91-1	20 ppm Skin A3		100 ppm Skin	
Dioxathion	000078-34-2	0.2 m/M Skin A4			
Diphenyl (biphenyl)	000092-52-4	0.2 ppm		0.2 ppm	
Diphenylamine	000122-39-4	10 m/M			
Diphenylmethane-4,4′-diisocyanate (methylene bisphenyl isocynate; MDI)	000101-68-8	0.005 ppm			C0.02 ppm
Dipropylene glycol methylether	034590-94-8	100 ppm Skin	150 ppm Skin	100 ppm Skin	
Dipropyl ketone	000123-19-3	50 ppm			
Diquat	002764-72-9	0.5 m/M			

(continued)

1999–2000 Threshold Limit Values (TLV) and Permissible Exposure Limits (PEL) ***(continued)***

		ACGIH TLV		*OSHA PEL*	
NAME	CAS NO.	TWA	STEL	TWA	STEL
Di-*sec*-octyl-phthalate [di(2-ethylhexyl) phthalate] (DEHP)	000117-81-7	5 m/M A3		5 m/M	
Disulfiram	000097-77-8	2 m/M			
Disulfoton	000298-04-4	0.1 m/M Skin			
2,6-Di-*tert*-butyl-*p*-cresol	000128-37-0	10 m/M			
Diuron	000330-54-1	10 m/M			
Divinyl benzene	001321-74-0	10 ppm			
Emery	001302-74-5	10 m/M		15 m/M	
Endosulfan	000115-29-7	0.1 m/M Skin A4			
Endrin	000072-20-8	0.1 m/M Skin A4		0.1 m/M Skin	
Enflurane	013838-16-9	75 ppm			
Enzymes, proteolytic (subtilisins)	001395-21-7		C0.00006 m/M		C0.00006 m/M
Epichlorohydrin (1-chloro-2,3-epoxypropane)	000106-89-8	0.5 ppm Skin A3		5 ppm Skin	
EPN	002104-64-5	0.1 m/M Skin A4		0.5 m/M Skin	
1,2-Epoxypropane (propylene oxide)	000075-56-9	20 ppm		100 ppm	
2,3-Epoxy-1-propanol (glycidol)	000556-52-5	2 ppm A3		50 ppm	
Ethanethiol (ethyl mercaptan)	000075-08-1	0.5 ppm			C10 ppm
Ethanol (ethyl alcohol)	000064-17-5	1000 ppm		1000 ppm	
Ethanolamine (2-aminoethanol)	000141-43-5	3 ppm A4	6 ppm	3 ppm	
Ethion	000563-12-2	0.4 m/M Skin			
2-Ethoxyethanol (ethylene glycol, monoethyl ether)	000110-80-5	5 ppm Skin		200 ppm Skin	
2-Ethoxyethyl acetate (ethylene glycol, monoethyl ether acetate	000111-15-9	5 ppm Skin		100 ppm Skin	
Ethyl acetate	000141-78-6	400 ppm		400 ppm	
Ethyl acrylate (acrylic acid, ethyl ester)	000140-88-5	5 ppm A4	15 ppm	25 ppm Skin	
Ethyl alcohol (ethanol)	000064-17-5	1000 ppm A4		1000 ppm	
Ethylamine	000075-04-7	5 ppm Skin	15 ppm Skin	10 ppm	
Ethyl amyl ketone (5-methyl-3-heptanone)	000541-85-5	25 ppm		25 ppm	
Ethyl benzene	000100-41-4	100 ppm	125 ppm	100 ppm	
Ethyl bromide (bromoethane)	000074-96-4	5 ppm A3		200 ppm	
Ethyl butyl ketone (3-heptanone)	000106-35-4	50 ppm	75 ppm	50 ppm	
Ethyl chloride (chloroethane)	000075-00-3	100 ppm A3		1000 ppm	
Ethylene	000074-85-1	Asphyxiant			
Ethylene chlorohydrin (2-chloroethanol)	000107-07-3		C1 ppm Skin A4		5 ppm Skin
Ethylenediamine (1,2-diaminoethane)	000107-15-3	10 ppm A4		10 ppm	
Ethylene dibromide (1,2-dibromoethane)	000106-93-4			20 ppm	
Ethylene dichloride (1,2-dichloroethane)	000107-06-2	10 ppm A3		50 ppm	C100 ppm
Ethylene glycol	000107-21-1		C100 ppm A4		

(continued)

1999–2000 Threshold Limit Values (TLV) and Permissible Exposure Limits (PEL) *(continued)*

NAME	CAS NO.	*ACGIH TLV*		*OSHA PEL*	
		TWA	STEL	TWA	STEL
Ethylene glycol dinitrate	000628-96-6	0.05 ppm Skin			C0.2 ppm Skin
Ethylene glycol methyl ether acetate (2-methoxyethyl acetate)	000110-49-6	5 ppm Skin		25 ppm Skin	
Ethylene glycol monobutyl ether (2-butoxyethanol)	000111-76-2	20 ppm Skin		50 ppm Skin	
Ethylene glycol monoethyl ether (2-ethoxyethanol)	000110-80-5	5 ppm Skin		200 ppm	
Ethylene glycol monoethyl ether acetate (2-ethoxy-ethyl acetate)	000111-15-9	5 ppm Skin		100 ppm Skin	
Ethylene glycol monomethyl ether (2-methoxyethanol)	000109-86-4	5 ppm Skin		25 ppm	
Ethylene glycol monomethyl ether acetate (2-methoxy-ethyl acetate)	000110-49-6	5 ppm Skin		25 ppm	
Ethylene oxide	000075-21-8	1 ppm A2		1 ppm	5 ppm
Ethyleneimine	000151-56-4	0.5 ppm Skin			
Ethyl ether (diethyl ether)	000060-29-7	400 ppm	500 ppm	400 ppm	
Ethyl formate (formic acid, ethyl ester)	000109-94-4	100 ppm		100 ppm	
Ethylidene chloride (1,1-dichloroethane)	000075-34-3	100 ppm A4		100 ppm	
Ethylidene norbornene	016219-75-3		C5 ppm		
N-Ethylmorpholine	000100-74-3	5 ppm Skin		20 ppm Skin	
Ethyl mercaptan (ethanethiol)	000075-08-1	0.5 ppm			C10 ppm
Ethyl silicate (silicic acid, tetraethyl ester)	000078-10-4	10 ppm		100 ppm	
Fenamiphos	022224-92-6	0.1 m/M Skin A4			
Fensulfothion	000115-90-2	0.1 m/M A4			
Fenthion	000055-38-9	0.2 m/M A4			
Ferbam	014484-64-1	10 m/M		15 m/M	
Ferrocene (dicyclopentadienyl iron)	000102-54-5	10 m/M		15 m/M	
Ferrovanadium dust	012604-58-9	1 m/M	3 m/M	1 m/M	
Fluorides as F	None	2.5 m/M A4		2.5 m/M	
Fluorine	007782-41-4	1 ppm	2 ppm	0.1 ppm	
Fluorotrichloromethane (trichlorofluoromethane)	000075-69-4		C1000 ppm A4	1000 ppm	
Fonofos	000944-22-9	0.1 m/M Skin			
Formaldehyde	000050-00-0		C0.3 ppm A2	0.75 ppm	2 ppm
Formamide	000075-12-7	10 ppm Skin			
Formic acid	000064-18-6	5 ppm	10 ppm	5 ppm	
Formic acid, ethyl ester (ethyl formate)	000109-94-4	100 ppm		100 ppm	
Formic acid, methyl ester (methyl formate)	000107-31-3	100 ppm	150 ppm	100 ppm	
Furfural	000098-01-1	2 ppm Skin A3		5 ppm Skin	
Furfuryl alcohol	000098-00-0	10 ppm Skin	15 ppm Skin	50 ppm Skin	
Gasoline	008006-61-9	300 ppm	500 ppm		
Germanium tetrahydride	007782-65-2	0.2 ppm			
Glutaraldehyde	000111-30-8		C0.2 ppm A4		
Glycerin mist	000056-81-5	10 ppm		15 m/M	

(continued)

1999–2000 Threshold Limit Values (TLV) and Permissible Exposure Limits (PEL) ***(continued)***

		ACGIH TLV		*OSHA PEL*	
NAME	CAS NO.	TWA	STEL	TWA	STEL
Glycidol (2,3-epoxy-1-propanol)	000556-52-5	2 ppm		50 ppm	
Glycol monoethyl ether (2-ethoxyethanol)	000110-80-5	5 ppm Skin		200 ppm Skin	
Grain dust (oat, wheat, barley)		4 m/M		10 m/M	
Graphite (natural)	007782-42-5	2 m/M		15 m/M	
Graphite (synthetic)		2 m/M		15 m/M	
Guthion (azinphos-methyl)	000086-50-0	0.2 m/M A4		0.2 m/M	
Gypsum (calcium sulfate)	013397-24-5	10 m/M		15 m/M	
Hafnium	007440-58-6	0.5 m/M		0.5 m/M	
Halothane	000151-67-7	50 ppm A4			
Helium	007440-59-7	Asphyxiant			
Heptachlor and heptachlor epoxide	000076-44-8	0.5 m/M A3		0.5 m/M	
Heptane (*n*-heptane)	000142-82-5	400 ppm	500 ppm	500 ppm	
2-Heptanone (methyl *n*-amyl ketone)	000110-43-0	50 ppm		100 ppm	
3-Heptanone (ethyl butyl ketone)	000106-35-4	50 ppm	75 ppm	50 ppm	
Hexachlorobenzene (HCB)	000118-74-1	0.002 m/M A3 Skin			
Hexachlorobutadiene	000087-68-3	0.02 ppm Skin A3			
γ-Hexachlorocyclohexane (lindane)	000058-89-9	0.5 m/M Skin A3		0.5 m/M Skin	
Hexachlorocyclopentadiene	000077-47-4	0.01 ppm			
Hexachloroethane	000067-72-1	1 ppm Skin A3		1 ppm Skin	
Hexachloronaphthalene	001335-87-1	0.2 m/M Skin		0.2 m/M Skin	
Hexafluoroacetone	000684-16-2	0.1 ppm Skin			
Hexamethylene diisocyanate	000822-06-0	0.005 ppm			
Hexane (*n*-hexane)	000110-54-3	50 ppm		500 ppm	
Hexane, other isomers		500 ppm	1000 ppm		
1,6-Hexanediamine	000124-09-4	0.5 ppm			
2-Hexanone (methyl *n*-butyl ketone)	000591-78-6	5 ppm Skin	10 ppm	100 ppm	
Hexone (methyl isobutyl ketone)	000108-10-1	50 ppm	75 ppm	100 ppm	
sec-Hexyl acetate	000108-84-9	50 ppm		50 ppm	
Hexylene glycol	000107-41-5		C25 ppm		
Hydrazine	000302-01-2	0.01 ppm Skin A2		1 ppm Skin	
Hydrogen	001333-74-0	Asphyxiant			
Hydrogen bromide	010035-10-6		C3 ppm	3 ppm	
Hydrogen chloride	007647-01-0		C5 ppm		C5 ppm
Hydrogen cyanide	000074-90-8		C4.7 ppm Skin	10 ppm Skin	
Hydrogen fluoride, as F	007664-39-3		C3 ppm	3 ppm	
Hydrogen peroxide	007722-84-1	1 ppm A3		1 ppm	
Hydrogen selenide, as Se	007783-07-5	0.05 ppm		0.05 ppm	
Hydrogen sulfide	007783-06-4	10 ppm	15 ppm		C20 ppm
Hydrogenated terphenyls	061788-32-7	0.5 ppm			
Hydroquinone (dihydroxy benzene)	000123-31-9	2m/M A3		2m/M	
4-Hydroxy-4-methyl-2-pentanone (diacetone alcohol)	000123-42-2	50 ppm		50 ppm	
2-Hydroxypropyl acrylate	000999-61-1	0.5 ppm Skin			
Indene	000095-13-6	10 ppm			

(continued)

1999–2000 Threshold Limit Values (TLV) and Permissible Exposure Limits (PEL) ***(continued)***

		ACGIH TLV		*OSHA PEL*	
NAME	CAS NO.	TWA	STEL	TWA	STEL
Indium [7440-74-6] and compounds, as In		0.1 m/M			
Iodine	007553-56-2		C0.1 ppm A4		C0.1 ppm
Iodoform	000075-47-8	0.6 ppm			
Iron oxide dust and fume (Fe_2O_3), as Fe		5 m/M A4		10 m/M	
Iron pentacarbonyl as Fe	013463-40-6	0.1 ppm	0.2 ppm		
Iron salts, soluble, as Fe		1 m/M			
Isoamyl acetate	000123-92-2	50 ppm	100 ppm	100 ppm	
Isoamyl alcohol	000123-51-3	50 ppm	100 ppm	100 ppm	
Isobutyl acetate	000110-19-0	150 ppm		150 ppm	
Isobutyl alcohol	000078-83-1	50 ppm		100 ppm	
Isooctyl alcohol	026952-21-6	50 ppm Skin			
Isophorone	000078-59-1		C5 ppm A3	25 ppm	
Isophorone diisocyanate	004098-71-9	0.005 ppm			
Isopropoxyethanol	000109-59-1	25 ppm Skin			
Isopropyl acetate	000108-21-4	250 ppm	310 ppm	250 ppm	
Isopropyl alcohol	000067-63-0	400 ppm	500 ppm	400 ppm	
Isopropylamine	000075-31-0	5 ppm	10 ppm	5 ppm	
Isopropyl ether	000108-20-3	250 ppm	310 ppm	500 ppm	
Isopropyl glycidyl ether (IGE)	004016-14-2	50 ppm	75 ppm	50 ppm	
N-Isopropylaniline	000768-52-5	2 ppm Skin			
Kaolin	001332-58-7	2 m/M A4		15 m/M	
Ketene	000463-51-4	0.5 ppm	1.5 ppm	0.5 ppm	
Lead elemental [7439-92-1], and inorganic compounds, as Ph		0.05 m/M A3		0.5 m/M	
Lead arsenate, as $Pb(AsO_4)_2$	003687-31-8	0.15 m/M		0.01 m/M	
Lead chromate	007758-97-6	0.05 m/M A2			
Lead phosphate	007446-27-7	0.05 m/M A3		0.05 m/M	
Limestone (calcium carbonate)	001317-65-3	10 m/M		15 m/M	
Lindane (γ-hexachloro-cyclohexane)	000058-89-9	0.5 m/M Skin A3		0.5 m/M Skin	
Lithium hydride	007580-67-8	0.025 m/M		0.025 m/M	
LPG (liquified petroleum gas)	068476-85-7	1000 ppm		1000 ppm	
Magnesite	000546-93-0	10 m/M		15 m/M	
Magnesium oxide fume	001309-48-4	10 m/M		15 m/M	
Malathion	000121-75-5	10 m/M Skin		15 m/M Skin	
Maleic anhydride	000108-31-6	0.1 ppm A4		0.25 ppm	
Manganese, elemental [7439-96-5], and inorganic compounds, as Mn		0.2 m/M			C5 m/M
Manganese fume, as Mn	007439-96-5	0.2 m/M		3 m/M	
Manganese cyclopentadienyl tricarbonyl, as Mn	012079-65-1	0.1 m/M Skin			
Marble (calcium carbonate)	001317-65-3	10 m/M		15 m/M	
Mercury, alkyl compounds, as Hg		0.01 m/M	0.03 m/M	0.01 m/M	C0.04 m/M
Mercury, aryl compounds, as Hg		0.1 m/M Skin			C0.1 m/M Skin
Mercury, inorganic compounds, as Hg		0.025 m/M A4 Skin			C0.1 m/M Skin

(continued)

1999–2000 Threshold Limit Values (TLV) and Permissible Exposure Limits (PEL) ***(continued)***

NAME	CAS NO.	ACGIH TLV		OSHA PEL	
		TWA	STEL	TWA	STEL
Mercury, vapor, as Hg		0.025 A4 Skin		0.05 m/M	
Mesityl oxide	000141-79-7	15 ppm	25 ppm	25 ppm	
Methacrylic acid	000079-41-4	20 ppm			
Methacrylic acid, methyl ester	000080-62-6	50 ppm A4	100 ppm	100 ppm	
Methane	000074-82-8	Asphyxiant			
Methanethiol (methyl mercaptan)	000074-93-1	0.5 ppm			C10 ppm
Methanol (methyl alcohol)	000067-56-1	200 ppm Skin	250 ppm Skin	200 ppm Skin	
Methomyl	016752-77-5	2.5 m/M			
Methoxychlor	000072-43-5	10 m/M		15 m/M	
2-Methoxyethanol (ethylene glycol monomethyl ether)	000109-86-4	5 ppm Skin		25 ppm	
2-Methoxyethyl acetate (ethylene glycol monomethyl ether acetate)	000110-49-6	5 ppm Skin		25 ppm Skin	
4-Methoxyphenol	000150-76-5	5 m/M			
Methyl acetate	000079-20-9	200 ppm	250 ppm	200 ppm	
Methyl acetylene (propyne)	000074-99-7	1000 ppm		1000 ppm	
Methyl acetylene-propadiene mixture (MAPP)		1000 ppm	1250 ppm	1000 ppm	
Methyl acrylate (acrylic acid, methyl ester)	000096-33-3	2 ppm Skin A4		10 ppm Skin	
Methylacrylonitrile	000126-98-7	1 ppm Skin			
Methylal (dimethoxymethane)	000109-87-5	1000 ppm		1000 ppm	
Methyl alcohol (methanol)	000067-56-1	200 ppm Skin	250 ppm Skin	200 ppm Skin	
Methylamine	000074-89-5	5 ppm	15 ppm	10 ppm	
Methyl amyl alcohol (methyl isobutyl carbinol; 4-methyl-2-pentanol)	000108-11-2	25 ppm Skin	40 ppm Skin	25 ppm Skin	
Methyl *n*-amyl ketone (2-hepatone)	000110-43-0	50 ppm		100 ppm	
N-Methyl aniline (monomethyl aniline)	000100-61-8	0.5 ppm Skin		2 ppm Skin	
2-Methylaziridine (propylene imine)	000075-55-8	2 ppm Skin A3		2 ppm Skin	
Methyl bromide	000074-83-9	1 ppm Skin A3			C20 ppm Skin
Methyl-*tert*-butyl ether	001634-04-4	40 ppm A3			
Methyl *n*-butyl ketone (2-hexanone)	000591-78-6	5 ppm Skin	10 ppm	100 ppm	
Methyl cellosolve (2-methoxyethanol)	000109-86-4	5 ppm Skin		25 ppm Skin	
Methyl cellosolve acetate (2-methoxyethyl acetate)	000110-49-6	5 ppm Skin		25 ppm Skin	
Methyl chloride	000074-87-3	50 ppm Skin A4	100 ppm Skin	100 ppm	
Methyl chloroform (1,1,1-trichloroethane)	000071-55-6	350 ppm A4	450 ppm	350 ppm	
Methyl-2-cyanoacrylate	000137-05-3	0.2 ppm			
Methylcyclohexane	000108-87-2	400 ppm		500 ppm	
Methylcyclohexanol	025639-42-3	50 ppm		100 ppm	
o-Methylcyclohexanone	000583-60-8	50 ppm Skin	75 ppm Skin	100 ppm Skin	
2-Methylcyclopentadienyl manganese tricarbonyl, as Mn	012108-13-3	0.2 m/M			

(continued)

1999–2000 Threshold Limit Values (TLV) and Permissible Exposure Limits (PEL) ***(continued)***

		ACGIH TLV		*OSHA PEL*	
NAME	CAS NO.	TWA	STEL	TWA	STEL
Methyl demeton (demeton-methyl)	008022-00-2	0.5 m/M Skin			
Methylene bisphenyl isocyanate (diphenyl-methane-4,4′-diisocyanate; MDI)	000101-68-8	0.005 ppm			
Methylene chloride (dichloromethane)	000075-09-2	50, A2 ppm		25 ppm	
4,4′-Methylene *bis* (2-chloroaniline) (MBOCA)	000101-4-4	0.01 ppm Skin A2			
Methylene *bis*(4-cyclo-hexylisocyanate)	005124-30-1	0.005 ppm			
4,4′-Methylene dianiline	000101-77-9	0.1 ppm Skin A3		0.01 ppm	
Methyl ethyl ketone (MEK; 2-butanone)	000078-93-3	200 ppm	300 ppm	200 ppm	
Methyl ethyl ketone peroxide	001338-23-4		C0.2 ppm		
Methylformate (formic acid, methyl ester)	000107-31-3	100 ppm	150 ppm	100 ppm	
5-Methyl-3-heptanone (ethyl amyl ketone)	000541-85-5	25 ppm		25 ppm	
Methylhydrazine	000060-34-4	0.01 ppm Skin A3			C0.2 ppm Skin
Methyliodide	000074-88-4	2 ppm A2		5 ppm Skin	
Methylisoamyl ketone	000110-12-3	50 ppm		100 ppm	
Methylisobutyl carbinol (methyl amyl alcohol)	000108-11-2	25 ppm Skin	40 ppm Skin	25 ppm Skin	
Methylisobutyl ketone (hexone)	000108-10-1	50 ppm	75 ppm	50 ppm	
Methylisocyanate	000624-83-9	0.02 ppm Skin		0.02 ppm Skin	
Methylisopropyl ketone	000563-80-4	200 ppm			
Methylmercaptan (methanethiol)	000074-93-1	0.5 ppm			C10 ppm
Methylmercury	022967-92-6	0.01 m/M Skin	0.03 m/M Skin	0.01 m/M Skin	C.04 m/M Skin
Methylmethacrylate	000080-62-6	50 ppm A4	100 ppm	100 ppm	
Methylparathion	000298-00-0	0.2 m/M Skin A4			
4-Methyl-2-pentanol (methyl amyl alcohol)	000108-11-2	25 ppm Skin	40 ppm Skin	25 ppm Skin	
Methylpropyl ketone (2-pentanone)	000107-87-9	200 ppm	250 ppm	200 ppm	
Methylsilicate	000681-84-5	1 ppm			
α-Methylstyrene	000098-83-9	50 ppm	100 ppm		C100 ppm
Methyl styrene (all isomers) (vinyl toluene)	025013-15-4	50 ppm	100 ppm	100 ppm	
Metribuzin	021087-64-9	5 m/M			
Mevinphos (Phosdrin)	007786-34-7	0.01 ppm Skin	0.03 ppm Skin	0.01 ppm Skin	
Mica	012001-26-2	3 m/M			
Molybdenum [7439-98-7], soluble compounds, as Mo		5 m/M		5 m/M	
Molybdenum [7439-98-7], insoluble compounds, as Mo		10 m/M			
Monochlorobenzene (chlorobenzene)	000108-90-7	10 ppm A3		75 ppm	

(continued)

1999–2000 Threshold Limit Values (TLV) and Permissible Exposure Limits (PEL) ***(continued)***

NAME	CAS NO.	ACGIH TLV TWA	ACGIH TLV STEL	OSHA PEL TWA	OSHA PEL STEL
Monocrotophos	006923-22-4	0.025 m/M Skin A4			
Morpholine	000110-91-8	20 ppm Skin A4		20 ppm Skin	
Naled (Dibrom)	000300-76-5	3 m/M Skin A4		3 m/M Skin	
Naphtha (coal tar) (rubber solvent)	008030-30-6	400 ppm		100 ppm	
Naphthalene	000091-20-3	10 ppm A4	15 ppm	10 ppm	
α-Naphthylthiourea (ANTU)	000086-88-4	0.3 m/M		0.3 m/M	
Neon	007440-01-9	Asphyxiant			
Nickel, elemental	007440-02-0	1 m/M A1 A5		1 m/M	
Nickel, insoluble compounds, as Ni		0.2 m/M Skin A1		1 m/M	
Nickel, soluble compounds, as Ni		0.1 m/M A4		0.1 m/M	
Nickel, carbonyl, as Ni	013463-39-3	0.05 ppm		0.001 ppm	
Nickel sulfide roasting, fume and dust, as Ni		1 m/M A1			
Nicotine	000054-11-5	0.5 m/M Skin		0.5 m/M Skin	
Nitrapyrin (2-chloro-6-trichloromethyl pyridine)	001929-82-4	10 m/M A4	20 m/M	15 m/M	
Nitric acid	007697-37-2	2 ppm	4 ppm	2 ppm	
Nitric oxide	010102-43-9	25 ppm		25 ppm	
p-Nitroaniline	000100-01-6	3 m/M Skin A4		6 m/M Skin	
Nitrobenzene	000098-95-3	1 ppm Skin A3		1 ppm Skin	
p-Nitrochlorobenzene	000100-00-5	0.1 ppm Skin		1 m/M Skin	
Nitroethane	000079-24-3	100 ppm		100 ppm	
Nitrogen	007727-37-9	Asphyxiant			
Nitrogen dioxide	010102-44-0	3 ppm	5 ppm		
Nitrogen trifluoride	007783-54-2	10 ppm		10 ppm	
Nitroglycerin (NG)	000055-63-0	0.05 ppm Skin			C0.2 ppm Skin
Nitromethane	000075-52-5	20 ppm A3		100 ppm	
1-Nitropropane	000108-03-2	25 ppm A4		25 ppm	
2-Nitropropane	000079-46-9	10 ppm A3		25 ppm	
Nitrotoluene, *o*-isomer	000088-72-2	2 ppm Skin	5 ppm Skin	2 ppm Skin	
Nitrotoluene, *m*-isomer	000099-08-1	2 ppm Skin	5 ppm Skin	2 ppm Skin	
Nitrotoluene, *p*-isomer	000099-99-0	2 ppm Skin	5 ppm Skin	2 ppm Skin	
Nitrotrichloromethane (chloropicrin)	000076-06-2	0.1 ppm A4		0.1 ppm	
Nitrous oxide	010024-97-2	50 ppm A4			
Nonane	000111-84-2	200 ppm			
Nuisance particulates (particulates not otherwise classified [PNOC])		10 m/M		15 m/M	
Octachloronaphthalene	002234-13-1	0.1 m/M Skin	0.3 m/M Skin	0.1 m/M Skin	
Octane	000111-65-9	300 ppm		500 ppm	
Oil mist, mineral, severely refined		5 m/M		5 m/M	
Osmium tetroxide, as Os	020816-12-0	0.0002 ppm	0.0006 ppm	0.0002 ppm	
Oxalic acid	000144-62-7	1 m/M	2 m/M	1 m/M	
Oxygen difluoride	007783-41-7		C0.05 ppm	0.05 ppm	
Ozone	010028-15-6	0.05 ppm		0.1 ppm	
Paraffin wax fume	008002-74-2	2 m/M			
Paraquat	004685-14-7	0.5 m/M		0.5 m/M Skin	
Parathion	000056-38-2	0.1 m/M Skin A4		0.1 m/M Skin	

(continued)

1999–2000 Threshold Limit Values (TLV) and Permissible Exposure Limits (PEL) ***(continued)***

NAME	CAS NO.	ACGIH TLV TWA	ACGIH TLV STEL	OSHA PEL TWA	OSHA PEL STEL
Partic. polycycl. arom. hydrocarb. (PPAH; coal tar pitch volatiles)		0.2 m/M A4		0.2 m/M	
Particulates not otherwise classified (PNOC) (nuisance particulates)		10 m/M		15 m/M	
Pentaborane	019624-22-7	0.005 ppm	0.015 ppm	0.005 ppm	
Pentachloronaphthalene	001321-64-8	0.5 m/M Skin		0.5 m/M Skin	
Pentachloronitrobenzene	000082-68-8	0.5 m/M			
Pentachlorophenol	000087-86-5	0.5 m/M Skin A3		0.5 m/M Skin	
Pentaerythritol	000115-77-5	10 m/M		15 m/M	
Pentane	000109-66-0	600 ppm		1000 ppm	
2-Pentanone (methyl propyl ketone)	000107-87-9	200 ppm	250 ppm	200 ppm	
Perchloroethylene (tetrachloroethylene)	000127-18-4	25 ppm A3	100 ppm	100 ppm	
Perchloromethyl mercaptan	000594-42-3	0.1 ppm		0.1 ppm	
Perchloryl fluoride	007616-94-6	3 ppm	6 ppm	3 ppm	
Perfluoroisobutylene	000382-21-8		C0.01 ppm		
Perlite	093763-70-3	10 m/M		15 m/M	
Petroleum distillates (gasoline; Stoddard solvent; VM&P naphtha)				500 ppm	
Phenacyl chloride (α-Chloroacetophenone)	000532-27-4	0.05 ppm A4		0.05 ppm	
Phenol	000108-95-2	5 ppm Skin A4		5 ppm Skin	
Phenothiazine	000092-84-2	5 m/M Skin			
o-Phenylenediamine	000095-54-5	0.1 m/M A3			
m-Phenylenediamine	000108-45-2	0.1 m/M A4			
p-Phenylenediamine	000106-50-3	0.1 m/M Skin A4		0.1 m/M Skin	
Phenyl ether, vapor	000101-84-8	1 ppm	2 ppm	1 ppm	
Phenyl ether-biphenyl mixture, vapor				1 ppm	
Phenylethylene (Styrene, monomer)	000100-42-5	20 ppm Skin	40 ppm	100 ppm	
Phenyl glycidyl ether (PGE)	000122-60-1	0.1 ppm Skin A3		10 ppm	
Phenylhydrazine	000100-63-0	0.1 ppm Skin A3		5 ppm Skin	
Phenyl mercaptan	000108-98-5	0.5 ppm			
Phenylphosphine	000638-21-1		C0.05 ppm		
Phorate	000298-02-2	0.05 m/M Skin	0.2 m/M		
Phosdrin (mevinphos)	007786-34-7	0.01 ppm Skin	0.03 ppm Skin	0.01 ppm Skin	
Phosgene (carbonyl chloride)	000075-44-5	0.1 ppm		0.1 ppm	
Phosphine	007803-51-2	0.3 ppm	1 ppm	0.3 ppm	
Phosphoric acid	007664-38-2	1 m/M	3 m/M	1 m/M	
Phosphorus (yellow)	007723-14-0	0.02 ppm		0.1 m/M	
Phosphorus oxychloride	010025-87-3	0.1 ppm			
Phosphorus pentachloride	010026-13-8	0.1 ppm		1 m/M	
Phosphorus pentasulfide	001314-80-3	1 m/M	3 m/M	1 m/M	
Phosphorus trichloride	007719-12-2	0.2 ppm	0.5 ppm	0.5 ppm	
Phthalic anhydride	000085-44-9	1 ppm A4		2 ppm	
m-Phthalodinitrile	000626-17-5	5 m/M			
Picloram	001918-02-1	10 m/M A4		15 m/M	
Picric acid (2,4,6-trinitrophenol)	000088-89-1	0.1 m/M		0.1 m/M Skin	

(continued)

1999–2000 Threshold Limit Values (TLV) and Permissible Exposure Limits (PEL) ***(continued)***

		ACGIH TLV		*OSHA PEL*	
NAME	CAS NO.	TWA	STEL	TWA	STEL
Pindone (2-pivalyl-1,3-indandione)	000083-26-1	0.1 m/M		0.1 m/M	
Piperazine dihydrochloride	000142-64-3	5 m/M			
2-Pivalyl-1,3-indandione (pindone)	000083-26-1	0.1 m/M		0.1 m/M	
Plaster of paris (calcium sulfate)	026499-65-0	10 m/M		15 m/M	
Platinum, metal	007440-06-4	1 m/M			
Platinum, soluble salts, as Pt	007440-06-4	0.002 m/M		0.002 m/M	
Portland cement	065997-15-1	10 m/M		15 m/M	
Potassium hydroxide	001310-58-3		C2 m/M		
Precipitated silica (silica—amorphous)	112926-00-8	10 m/M		80 m/M	
Propane	000074-98-6	2500 ppm		1000 ppm	
Propargyl alcohol	000107-19-7	1 ppm Skin			
β-Propiolactone	000057-57-8	0.5 ppm A3			
Propionic acid	000079-09-4	10 ppm			
Propoxur	000114-26-1	0.5 m/M			
n-Propyl acetate	000109-60-4	200 ppm	250 ppm	200 ppm	
n-Propyl alcohol	000071-23-8	200 ppm Skin	250 ppm Skin	200 ppm	
Propylene	000115-07-1	Asphyxiant			
Propylene dichloride (1,2-dichloropropane)	000078-87-5	75 ppm	110 ppm	75 ppm	
Propylene glycol dinitrate	006423-43-4	0.05 ppm Skin			
Propylene glycol monomethyl ether	000107-98-2	100 ppm	150 ppm		
Propylene imine (2-methylaziridine)	000075-55-8	2 ppm Skin A3		2 ppm Skin	
Propylene oxide (1,2-epoxypropane)	000075-56-9	20 ppm A3		100 ppm	
n-Propylnitrate	000627-13-4	25 ppm	40 ppm	25 ppm	
Propyne (methylacetylene)	000074-99-7	1000 ppm		1000 ppm	
Pyrethrum	008003-34-7	5 m/M A4		5 m/M	
Pyridine	000110-86-1	5 ppm		5 ppm	
Pyrocatechol (catechol)	000120-80-9	5 ppm			
Quartz (silica-crystalline)	014808-60-7	0.1 m/M		0.1 m/M	
Quinone	000106-51-4	0.1 ppm		0.1 ppm	
RDX (cyclonite)	000121-82-4	0.5 m/M Skin A4			
Resorcinol	000108-46-3	10 ppm A4	20 ppm		
Rhodium, metal	007440-16-6	1 m/M A4		0.1 m/M	
Rhodium, insoluble compounds, as Rh		1 m/M		0.1 m/M	
Rhodium, soluble compounds, as Rh		0.01 m/M		0.001 m/M	
Ronnel	000299-84-3	10 m/M		15 m/M	
Rotenone (commercial)	000083-79-4	5 m/M A4		5 m/M	
Rouge		10 m/M A4		15 m/M	
Rubber solvent (Naphtha)	008030-30-6	400 ppm		100 ppm	
Selenium [7782-49-2] and compounds, as Se		0.2 m/M		0.2 m/M	
Selenium hexafluoride, as Se	007783-79-1	0.05 ppm		0.05 ppm	
Sesone (sodium-2,4-dichlorophenoxyethyl sulfate)	000136-78-7	10 m/M		15 m/M	

(continued)

1999–2000 Threshold Limit Values (TLV) and Permissible Exposure Limits (PEL) *(continued)*

		ACGIH TLV		*OSHA PEL*	
NAME	CAS NO.	TWA	STEL	TWA	STEL
Silane (silicon tetrahydride)	007803-62-5	5 ppm			
Silica—amorphous diatomaceous earth (uncalcined)	061790-53-2	10 m/M		80 m/M	
Silica—amorphous precipitated silica	112926-00-8	10 m/M			
Silica—amorphous silica fume	069012-64-2	2 m/M			
Silica—amorphous silica, fused	060676-86-0	0.1 m/M			
Silica—amorphous silica gel	112926-00-8	10 m/M			
Silica—crystalline cristobalite	014464-46-1	0.05 m/M			
Silica—crystalline quartz	014808-60-7	0.1 m/M			
Silica—crystalline tridymite	015468-32-3	0.05 m/M			
Silica—crystalline tripoli	001317-95-9	0.1 m/M			
Silica fume (silica—amorphous)	069012-64-2	2 m/M			
Silica, fused (silica—amorphous)	060676-86-0	0.1 m/M			
Silica gel (silica—amorphous)	112926-00-8	10 m/M			
Silica, precipitated (silica—amorphous)	112926-00-8	10 m/M			
Silicic acid, tetraethyl ester (ethyl silicate)	000078-10-4	10 ppm		100 ppm	
Silicon	007440-21-3	10 m/M		15 m/M	
Silicon carbide	000409-21-2	10 m/M A4		15 m/M	
Silicon tetrahydride (silane)	007803-62-5	5 ppm			
Silver, metal	007440-22-4	0.1 m/M		0.01 m/M	
Silver, soluble compounds, as Ag		0.01 m/M		0.01 m/M	
Soapstone		6 m/M			
Sodium azide	026628-22-8		C0.11 ppm		
Sodium bisulfite	007631-90-5	5 m/M A4			
Sodium-2,4-dichlorophenoxyethyl sulfate (sesone)	000136-78-7	10 m/M A4		15 m/M	
Sodium fluoroacetate	000062-74-8	0.05 m/M Skin		0.05 m/M Skin	
Sodium hydroxide	001310-73-2		C2 m/M		
Sodium metabisulfite	007681-57-4	5 m/M			
Starch	009005-25-8	10 m/M		15 m/M	
Stearates		10 m/M			
Stibine	007803-52-3	0.1 ppm		0.1 ppm	
Stoddard solvent	008052-41-3	100 ppm		500 ppm	
Strontium chromate, as Cr	007789-06-2	0.0005 m/M A2			C0.1 m/M
Strychnine	000057-24-9	0.15 m/M		0.15 m/M	
Styrene, monomer (phenylethylene; vinyl benzene)	000100-42-5	20 ppm Skin A4	40 ppm Skin	100 ppm	C200 ppm
Subtilisins (proteolytic enzymes as 100% pure)	001395-21-7		C0.00006 m/M		

(continued)

1999–2000 Threshold Limit Values (TLV) and Permissible Exposure Limits (PEL) ***(continued)***

NAME	CAS NO.	ACGIH TLV		OSHA PEL	
		TWA	STEL	TWA	STEL
Sucrose	000057-50-1	10 m/M A4		15 m/M	
Sulfometuron methy1	074222-97-2	5 m/M A4			
Sulfotep (TEDP)	003689-24-5	0.2 m/M Skin A4		0.2 m/M Skin	
Sulfur dioxide	007446-09-5	2 ppm	5 ppm	5 ppm	
Sulfur hexafluoride	002551-62-4	1000 ppm		1000 ppm	
Sulfuric acid	007664-93-9	1 m/M A2	3 m/M	1 m/M	
Sulfur monochloride	010025-67-9		C1 ppm	1 m/M	
Sulfur pentafluoride	005714-22-7		C0.01 ppm	0.025 ppm	
Sulfur tetrafluoride	007783-60-0		C0.1 ppm		
Sulfuryl fluoride	002699-79-8	5 ppm	10 ppm	5 ppm	
Sulprofos	035400-43-2	1 m/M			
Systox (demeton)	008065-48-3	0.01 ppm Skin		0.1 ppm Skin	
2,4,5-T (2,4,5-Trichloro-phenoxyacetic acid)	000093-76-5	10 m/M A4		10 m/M	
Talc (containing no asbestos fibers)	014807-96-6	2 m/M			
Tantalum metal	007440-25-7	5 m/M		5 m/M	
Tantalum, oxide dusts	001314-61-0	5 m/M		5 m/M	
TEDP (sulfotep)	003689-24-5	0.2 m/M Skin A4		0.2 m/M Skin	
Tellurium (13494-80-9) and compounds, as Te		0.1 m/M		0.1 m/M	
Tellurium hexafluoride, as Te	007783-80-4	0.02 ppm		0.02 ppm	
Temephos	003383-96-8	10 m/M		15 m/M	
TEPP (tetraethyl pyrophosphate)	000107-49-3	0.004 ppm Skin		0.05 m/M Skin	
Terephthalic acid	000100-21-0	10 m/M			
Terphenyls	026140-60-3		C0.53 ppm		C1 ppm
1,1,1,2-Tetrachloro-2,2-difluoroethane	000076-11-9	500 ppm		500 ppm	
1,1,2,2-Tetrachloro-1,2-difluoroethane	000076-12-0	500 ppm		500 ppm	
1,1,2,2-tetrachloroethane	000630-20-6	1 ppm Skin A3		5 ppm Skin	
Tetrachloroethylene (perchloroethylene)	000127-18-4	25 ppm A3	100 ppm A3	100 ppm	
Tetrachloromethane (carbon tetrachloride)	000056-23-5	5 ppm Skin A3	10 ppm Skin	10 ppm Skin	
Tetrachloronaphthalene	001335-88-2	2 m/M		2 m/M Skin	
Tetraethyl lead, as Pb	000078-00-2	0.1 m/M Skin A4		0.075 m/M Skin	
Tetraethyl pyrophosphate (TEPP)	000107-49-3	0.004 ppm Skin		0.05 m/M Skin	
Tetrahydrofuran	000109-99-9	200 ppm	250 ppm	200 ppm	
Tetramethyl lead, as Pb	000075-74-1	0.15 m/M Skin		0.075 m/M Skin	
Tetramethyl succinonitrile	003333-52-6	0.5 ppm Skin		0.5 ppm Skin	
Tetranitromethane	000509-14-8	0.005 ppm A2		1 ppm	
Tetrasodium pyrophosphate	007722-88-5	5 m/M			
Tetryl (2,4,6-Trinitrophen-ylmethylnitramine)	000479-45-8	1.5 m/M		1.5 m/M Skin	
Thallium, soluble compounds, as TI		0.1 m/M Skin		0.1 m/M Skin	
4,4′-Thiobis (6-*tert*-butyl-*m*-cresol)	000096-69-5	10 m/M		15 m/M	
Thioglycolic acid	000068-11-1	1 ppm Skin			
Thionyl chloride	007719-09-7		C1 ppm		
Thiram	000137-26-8	1 m/M		5 m/M	

(continued)

1999–2000 Threshold Limit Values (TLV) and Permissible Exposure Limits (PEL) *(continued)*

		ACGIH TLV		*OSHA PEL*	
NAME	CAS NO.	TWA	STEL	TWA	STEL
Tin, metal	007440-31-5	2 m/M		2 m/M	
Tin, oxide and inorganic compounds, except SnH_4 as Sn		2 m/M		2 m/M	
Tin, organic compounds, as Sn		0.1 m/M Skin A4	0.2 m/M Skin	0.1 m/M Skin	
Tin oxide, as Sn	021651-19-4	2 m/M		2 m/M	
Titanium dioxide	013463-67-7	10 m/M		15 m/M	
Toluene (toluol)	000108-88-3	50 ppm Skin		200 ppm	
Toluene-2,4-diisocyanate (TDI)	000584-84-9	0.005 ppm A4	0.02 ppm	C0.02 ppm	
o-Toluidine	000095-53-4	2 ppm A2 Skin		5 ppm Skin	
m-Toluidine	000108-44-1	2 ppm Skin			
p-Toluidine	000106-49-0	2 ppm Skin A2			
Toluol (toluene)	000108-88-3	50 ppm Skin		200 ppm	
Toxaphene (chlorinated camphene)	008001-35-2	0.5 m/M Skin	1 m/M Skin	0.5 m/M Skin	
Tremolite	001332-21-4	1 f/cc A1		0.1 f/cc	
Tribromomethane (bromoform)	000075-25-2	0.5 ppm Skin A3		0.5 ppm Skin	
Tributyl phosphate	000126-73-8	0.2 ppm		5 ppm	
Trichloroacetic acid	000076-03-9	1 ppm			
1,2,4-Trichlorobenzene	000120-82-1		C5 ppm		
1,1,1-Trichloroethane (methyl chloroform)	000071-55-6	350 ppm	450 ppm	350 ppm	
1,1,2-Trichloroethane	000079-00-5	10 ppm Skin		10 ppm Skin	
Trichloroethylene	000079-01-6	50 ppm A5	100 ppm	100 ppm	
Trichlorofluoromethane (fluorotrichloromethane)	000075-69-4		C1000 ppm	1000 ppm	
Trichloromethane (chloroform)	000067-66-3	10 ppm A3			C50 ppm
Trichloronaphthalene	001321-65-9	5 m/M Skin		5 m/M Skin	
Trichloronitromethane (chloropicrin)	000076-06-2	0.1 ppm		0.1 ppm	
2,4,5-Trichlorophenoxyacetic acid (2,4,5-T)	000093-76-5	10 m/M		10 m/M	
1,2,3-Trichloropropane	000096-18-4	10 ppm Skin		50 ppm	
1,1,2-Trichloro-1,2,2-trifluoroethane	000076-13-1	1000 ppm	1250 ppm	1000 ppm	
Tricyclohexyltin hydroxide (cyhexatin)	013121-70-5	5 m/M			
Tridymite (silica—crystalline)	015468-32-3	0.05 m/M			
Triethanolamine	000102-71-6	5 m/M			
Triethylamine	000121-44-8	1 ppm Skin A4	3 ppm Skin	25 ppm	
Trifluorobromomethane	000075-63-8	1000 ppm		1000 ppm	
Trimellitic anhydride	000552-30-7		C0.04 m/M		
Trimethylamine	000075-50-3	5 ppm	15 ppm		
Trimethyl benzene	025551-13-7	25 ppm			
Trimethyl phosphite	000121-45-9	2 ppm			
2,4,6-Trinitrophenol (picric acid)	000088-89-1	0.1 m/M Skin		0.1 m/M Skin	
2,4,6-Trinitrophenylmethylnitramine (tetryl)	000479-45-8	1.5 m/M		1.5 m/M Skin	
2,4,6-Trinitrotoluene (TNT)	000118-96-7	0.1 m/M Skin		1.5 m/M Skin	

(continued)

1999–2000 Threshold Limit Values (TLV) and Permissible Exposure Limits (PEL) ***(continued)***

		ACGIH TLV		OSHA PEL	
NAME	CAS NO.	TWA	STEL	TWA	STEL
Triorthocresyl phosphate	000078-30-8	0.1 m/M Skin A4		0.1 m/M Skin	
Triphenyl amine	000603-34-9	5 m/M			
Triphenyl phosphate	000115-86-6	3 m/M A4		3 m/M	
Tripoli (silica—crystalline)	001317-95-9	0.1 m/M			
Tungsten [7440-33-7] and insoluble compounds, as W		5 m/M	10 m/M		
Tungsten, soluble compounds, as W		1 m/M	3 m/M		
Turpentine	008006-64-2	100 ppm		100 ppm	
Uranium (natural [7440-61-1], soluble and insoluble compounds), as U		0.2 m/M	0.5 m/M	0.05 m/M	
n-Valeraldehyde	000110-62-3	50 ppm			
Vanadium pentoxide, as V_2O_5, respirable dust or fume	001314-62-1	0.05 m/M			C0.05 m/M
Vegetable oil mists		10 m/M		15 m/M	
Vinyl acetate	000108-05-4	10 ppm A3	15 ppm A3		
Vinyl benzene (styrene, monomer)	000100-42-5	20 ppm Skin A4	40 ppm Skin	100 ppm	
Vinyl bromide	000593-60-2	5 ppm A2			
Vinyl chloride (chloroethylene)	000075-01-4	1 ppm A1		1 ppm	
Vinyl cyanide (acrylonitrile)	000107-13-1	2 ppm Skin A2		2 ppm	
Vinyl cyclohexene	000100-40-3	0.1 ppm A2			
Vinyl cyclohexene dioxide	000106-87-6	0.1 ppm Skin A2			
Vinylidene chloride (1,1-dichloroethylene)	000075-35-4	5 ppm A4			
Vinyl toluene (methyl styrene, all isomers)	025013-15-4	50 ppm	100 ppm	100 ppm	
VM & P Naphtha	008032-32-4	300 ppm			
Warfarin	000081-81-2	0.1 m/M		0.1 m/M	
Welding fumes (NOC)*		5 m/M			
Wood dust (certain hardwoods as beech and oak)		1 m/M			
Wood dust, soft wood		5 m/M			
Wood dust, western red cedar		5 m/M SEN			
Xylene (*o*-, *m*-, *p*-isomers) 1330-20-7; 95-47-6; 108-38-3; 106-42-3		100 ppm	150 ppm	100 ppm	
m-Xylene α, α'-diamine	001477-55-0		C0.1 m/M		
Xylidine (mixed isomers)	001300-73-8	0.5 ppm A2 Skin		2 ppm Skin	
Yttrium [7440-65-5] metal and compounds, as Y		1 m/M		1 m/M	
Zinc beryllium silicate, as Be	039413-47-3	0.0002 m/M A2		0.0002 m/M	
Zinc chloride fume	007646-85-7	1 m/M	2 m/M	1 m/M	
Zinc chromates, as Cr 13530-65-9; 11103-86-9; 37300-23-5		0.01 m/M A1			C0.1 m/M

(continued)

1999–2000 Threshold Limit Values (TLV) and Permissible Exposure Limits (PEL) ***(continued)***

		ACGIH TLV		*OSHA PEL*	
NAME	CAS NO.	TWA	STEL	TWA	STEL
Zinc oxide, dust	001314-13-2	10 m/M		15 m/M	
Zinc oxide, fume	001314-13-2	5 m/M	10 m/M	5 m/M	
Zinc stearate	000557-05-1	10 m/M		15 m/M	
Zirconium (7440-67-7) compounds, as Zr		5 m/M	10 m/M	5 m/M	

INDEX

NOTE: Page numbers in **boldface** refer to major discussions. Page numbers followed by a *t* refer to tables; numbers followed by an *f* indicate figures.

B

D

E

G

O

P

Q

R

S

U

NOTES

NOTES

NOTES

NOTES

NOTES

NOTES

NOTES

NOTES

NOTES

NOTES

NOTES

NOTES

NOTES